M000239819

PRIORITY CONCEPT EXEMPLARS

SENSORY PERCEPTION

SEXUALITY

TISSUE INTEGRITY

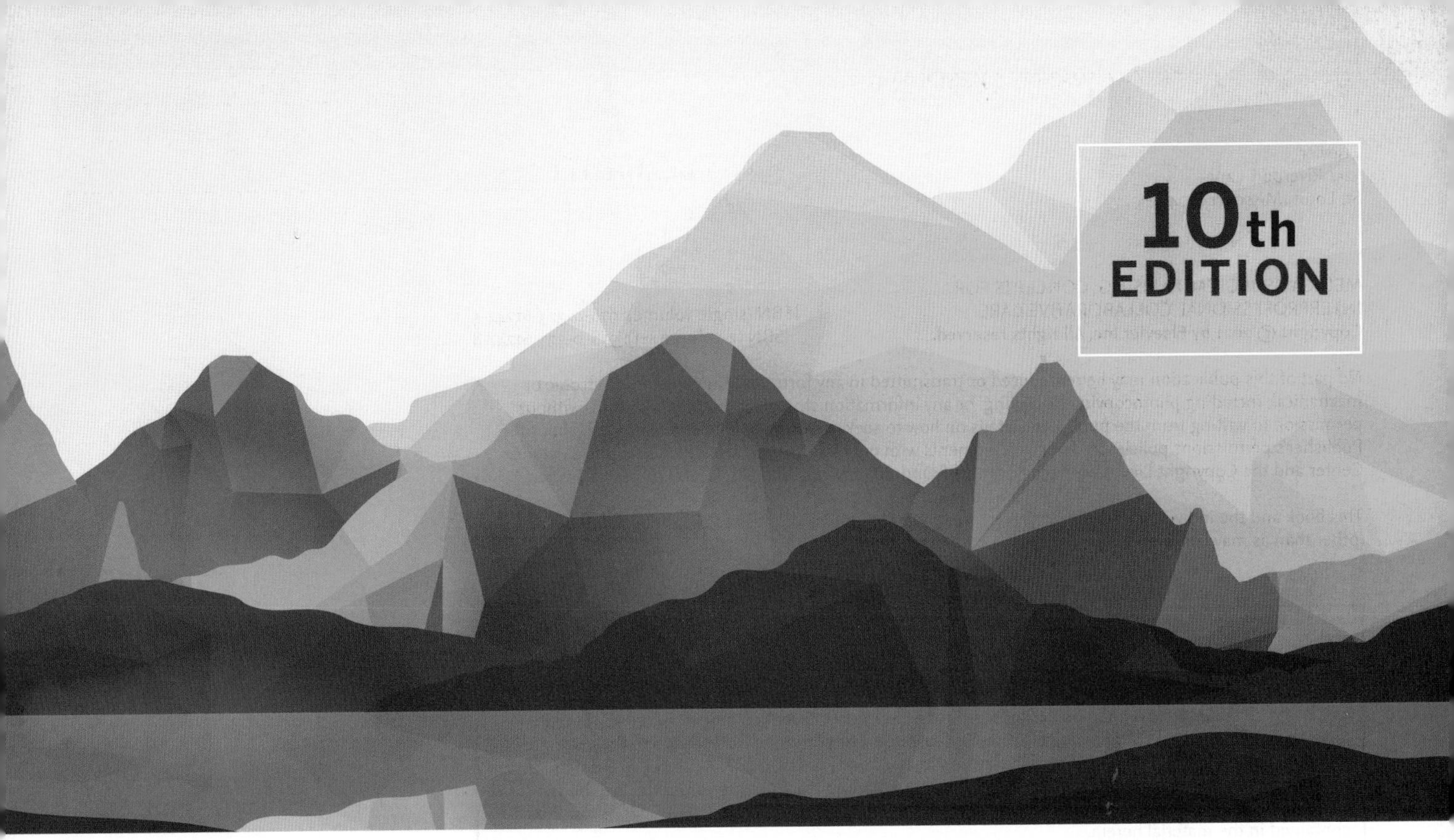

10th EDITION

MEDICAL-SURGICAL NURSING

CONCEPTS FOR INTERPROFESSIONAL COLLABORATIVE CARE

Donna D. Ignatavicius,
MS, RN, CNE, CNEcl, ANEF
Speaker and Nursing Education Consultant;
Founder, Boot Camp for Nurse Educators;
President, DI Associates, Inc.
Littleton, Colorado

M. Linda Workman,
PhD, RN, FAAN
Author and Consultant
Visiting Professor and Former Endowed Professor
Frances Payne Bolton School of Nursing
Case Western Reserve University
Cleveland, Ohio

Cherie R. Rebar,
PhD, MBA, RN, COI
Subject Matter Expert and Nursing Education Consultant
Beavercreek, Ohio;
Professor of Nursing
Wittenberg University
Springfield, Ohio

Nicole M. Heimgartner,
DNP, RN, COI
Subject Matter Expert and Nursing Education Consultant
Louisville, Kentucky;
Adjunct Faculty
American Sentinel University
Aurora, Colorado

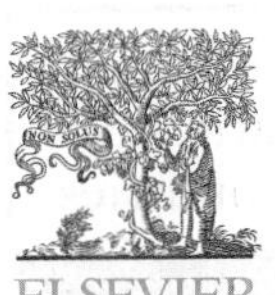

ELSEVIER

Elsevier
3251 Riverport Lane
St. Louis, Missouri 63043

MEDICAL-SURGICAL NURSING: CONCEPTS FOR
INTERPROFESSIONAL COLLABORATIVE CARE

ISBN (single volume): 978-0-323-61242-5
ISBN (2-volume set): 978-0-323-61241-8

Notice

Practitioners and researchers must always rely on their own experience and knowledge in evaluating and using any information, methods, compounds or experiments described herein. Because of rapid advances in the medical sciences, in particular, independent verification of diagnoses and drug dosages should be made. To the fullest extent of the law, no responsibility is assumed by Elsevier, authors, editors or contributors for any injury and/or damage to persons or property as a matter of products liability, negligence or otherwise, or from any use or operation of any methods, products, instructions, or ideas contained in the material herein.

Previous editions copyrighted 2018, 2016, 2013, 2010, 2006, 2002, 1999, 1995, 1991

International Standard Book Number (single volume): 978-0-323-61242-5
International Standard Book Number (2-volume set): 978-0-323-61241-8

Executive Content Strategist: Lee Henderson
Director, Content Development: Laurie Gower
Senior Content Development Specialist: Laura Goodrich
Publishing Services Manager: Julie Eddy
Senior Project Manager: Jodi M. Willard
Design Direction: Brian Salisbury

Printed in India

Last digit is the print number: 9 8 7 6 5 4 3

CONTRIBUTORS

Marie Bashaw, DNP, RN, NEA-BC
Professor and Director of Nursing
Department of Nursing
Wittenberg University
Springfield, Ohio

Cecilia Bidigare, MSN
Professor
Nursing
Sinclair Community College
Dayton, Ohio

Maureen Bishop, MSN, RN, CCRN, CCNS
Clinical Nurse Specialist
Lakeland University
Lakeland Health
St. Joseph, Michigan

Andrea A. Borchers, PhD, RN
Assistant Professor
School of Nursing
Northern Arizona University
Flagstaff, Arizona

Samuel A. Borchers, OD
Optometrist
Vision Clinic
Northern Arizona VA Healthcare System
Prescott, Arizona

Katherine Byar, MSN, ANP, BC, BMTCN
Nurse Practitioner
Hematological Malignancy
Nebraska Medicine
Omaha, Nebraska

Michelle Camicia, PhD, CRRN, CCM, NEA-BC, FAHA
Director of Operations
Kaiser Foundation Rehabilitation Center
Kaiser Permanente
Vallejo, California

Lara Carver, PhD, MSN, RN, CNE
Director
College of Health Professions
Western Governors University
Salt Lake City, Utah

Keelin C. Cromar, MSN, RN
Subject Matter Expert
Nursing Consultant
Wichita County Public Health District
Wichita Falls, Texas

Laura M. Dechant, DNP, CCNS, CCRN
Clinical Nurse Specialist
Heart, Vascular and Interventional Services
Christiana Care Health System
Newark, Pennsylvania

Stephanie M. Fox, PsyD
Clinical Psychologist
Littleton, Colorado

Carolyn J. Gersch, PhD, MSN, RN, CNE
Professor
Wittenberg University
Springfield, Ohio

Darla Green, RN, DNP, FNP-C
Assistant Professor
Del Mar College
Department of Nurse Education
Corpus Christi, Texas

Charity Hacker, RN, MSN-Ed
Assistant Professor
Nursing
Ivy Tech Community College
Madison, Indiana;
Adjunct Faculty
Nursing
Indiana University Purdue University Columbus (IUPUC)
Columbus, Indiana

Linda Laskowski-Jones, MS, APRN, ACNS-BC, CEN, FAWM, FAAN
Vice President
Emergency & Trauma Services
Christiana Care Health System
Newark, Delaware

Cheryl L. Leksan, MSN, MEd, BSN
Formerly, Teaching Professor
School of Nursing
Xavier University
Cincinnati, Ohio

Hannah Lopez, MSN, RN, OCN, CBCN
Clinical Nurse Manager
Hematology/Oncology & Supportive and Palliative Care
Baylor Scott & White Health
Round Rock, Texas

Robyn Mitchell, APRN-CNP, MSN, CCRN, CSC, CMC, AGACNP-AG, AGACNP-BC, ACNP
Critical Care House Officer
Cleveland Clinic
Cleveland, Ohio

Jennifer Dawn Powers, FNP-BC, MSN, BSN
Adjunct Faculty
Department of Nursing
National University
Henderson, Nevada

Harry Rees III, MSN, APRN-CNP
Trauma, Critical Care, and Burn
The Ohio State University Wexner Medical Center
Columbus, Ohio

Jonathon Rospierski, MSN, BS, RN-BC
Nursing Professional Development Specialist/Nurse Residency Program Coordinator
Lakeland University
Lakeland Health
St. Joseph, Michigan

James G. Sampson, DNP, RN
Infectious Disease
Denver Health Medical Center
Denver, Colorado

Karen L. Toulson, DNP, MBA, CEN, NE-BC
Director, Clinical Operations
Emergency Department
Christiana Care Health System
Newark, Delaware

Sharon A. Watts, DNP, MSN, BSN
Endocrinology
Veterans Health Administration
Cleveland, Ohio

CONTRIBUTORS TO TEACHING/LEARNING RESOURCES

PowerPoint Slides

Nicole M. Heimgartner, DNP, RN, COI
Subject Matter Expert and Nursing Education Consultant
Louisville, Kentucky;
Adjunct Faculty
American Sentinel University
Aurora, Colorado

Cherie R. Rebar, PhD, MBA, RN, COI
Subject Matter Expert and Nursing Education Consultant
Beavercreek, Ohio;
Professor of Nursing
Wittenberg University
Springfield, Ohio

Teach® for Nurses Lesson Plans

Nicole M. Heimgartner, DNP, RN, COI
Subject Matter Expert and Nursing Education Consultant
Louisville, Kentucky;
Adjunct Faculty
American Sentinel University
Aurora, Colorado

Cherie R. Rebar, PhD, MBA, RN, COI
Subject Matter Expert and Nursing Education Consultant
Beavercreek, Ohio;
Professor of Nursing
Wittenberg University
Springfield, Ohio

Test Bank

Meg Blair, PhD, MSN, RN, CEN
Professor
Nursing Division
Nebraska Methodist College
Omaha, Nebraska

Donna D. Ignatavicius, MS, RN, CNE, CNEcl, ANEF
Speaker and Nursing Education Consultant;
Founder, Boot Camp for Nurse Educators;
President, DI Associates, Inc.
Littleton, Colorado

Case Studies

Tami Kathleen Little, DNP, RN, CNE
Corporate Director of Nursing
Vista College
Richardson, Texas

Review Questions for the NCLEX® Examination

Donna D. Ignatavicius, MS, RN, CNE, CNEcl, ANEF
Speaker and Nursing Education Consultant;
Founder, Boot Camp for Nurse Educators;
President, DI Associates, Inc.
Littleton, Colorado

M. Linda Workman, PhD, RN, FAAN
Author and Consultant
Visiting Professor and Former Endowed Professor
Frances Payne Bolton School of Nursing
Case Western Reserve University
Cleveland, Ohio

Cherie R. Rebar, PhD, MBA, RN, COI
Subject Matter Expert and Nursing Education Consultant
Beavercreek, Ohio;
Professor of Nursing
Wittenberg University
Springfield, Ohio

Nicole M. Heimgartner, DNP, RN, COI
Subject Matter Expert and Nursing Education Consultant
Louisville, Kentucky;
Adjunct Faculty
American Sentinel University
Aurora, Colorado

REVIEWERS

Rosalinda Alfaro-Lefevre, MSN, RN, ANEF
President
Teaching Smart/Learning Easy
Stuart, Florida

Nell Britton, MSN, RN, CNE
Adjunct Nursing Instructor
Anderson University
Anderson, South Carolina

Mary Dolansky, PhD, RN, FAAN
Associate Professor
Frances Payne Bolton School of Nursing;
Assistant Professor
Department of Population and Quantitative Health Sciences
School of Medicine;
Director, QSEN Institute
Frances Payne Bolton School of Nursing;
Senior Faculty Scholar
VA Quality Scholars Program
Case Western Reserve University
Cleveland, Ohio

Claudia Grobbel, DNP, RN
Associate Professor
Oakland University
Rochester, Michigan

Michael J. Rebar, DO, DPM
Hospitalist
Miami Valley Hospital
Dayton, Ohio

Christy Roberts, MSN, BSN, APRN, FNP-C
Family Nurse Practitioner
One Medical
Mount Washington, Kentucky

Jeffrey Schultz, MS, APRN, ACNP-BC, CCNS, RN-BC, CCRN, CEN, NE-BC, NR-P
Senior APP-CVICU
Cardiothoracic Surgery
North Florida Regional Medical Center
Gainesville, Florida;
Flight Nurse
University of Florida Health
ShandsCair Critical Care Transport Program
Gainesville, Florida

PREFACE

The first edition of this textbook, entitled *Medical-Surgical Nursing: A Nursing Process Approach,* was a groundbreaking work in many ways. The following nine editions built on that achievement and further solidified the book's position as a major trendsetter for the practice of evidence-based adult health nursing. Now in its tenth edition, "Iggy" again charts the cutting-edge approach for the future of adult nursing practice—an approach reflected in its current title: *Medical-Surgical Nursing: Concepts for Interprofessional Collaborative Care.* The focus of this new edition continues to help students learn how to utilize clinical judgment skills to provide safe, quality nursing care that is patient-centered, evidence-based, and interprofessionally collaborative. In addition to print formats as single- and two-volume texts, this edition is available in a variety of electronic formats.

KEY COMPONENTS OF THE TENTH EDITION

Similar to the last edition's conceptual learning approach, the tenth edition organizes the content in each chapter by the most important *professional nursing and/or health concepts* and then presents commonly occurring *exemplars* for each concept. The key components for this edition that strengthen the text's conceptual focus are consistent with the Quality and Safety Education for Nurses' (QSEN) competencies and include *clinical judgment, safety, quality care,* and *patient-centeredness.* Further information about these components are described below.

- **Enhanced Emphasis on Professional Nursing and Health Concepts.** This edition uniquely balances a focus on nursing concepts with a conceptual approach to teaching and learning. Prelicensure programs that embrace the concept-based nursing curriculum, system-focused curriculum, or a hybrid or modified approach will find this edition easy to use. To help students connect previously learned concepts with new information in the text, Chapters 1 and 3 review the main concepts used in this edition, giving a working definition on which the students will reflect and build as they learn new material. These unique features build on basic concepts learned in nursing fundamentals courses, such as gas exchange and safety, to help students make connections between foundational concepts and interprofessional care for patients with medical-surgical conditions. For continuity and reinforcement, a list of specific Priority and Interrelated Nursing Concepts is highlighted at the beginning of each chapter. This placement is specifically designed to help students better understand the priority and associated needs that the nurse will address when providing safe, evidence-based, patient-centered care for individuals with selected health problems.
- **Emphasis on Common Exemplars.** For each priority concept listed in the beginning of the Nursing Care chapters, the authors have identified common or major exemplars. The nursing and interprofessional collaborative care for patients experiencing these exemplar diseases and illnesses is discussed through the lens of the priority and interrelated concepts. In addition, patient problems are presented as a collaborative problem list.
- **Focus on Clinical Judgment.** Stressing the importance of clinical judgment helps to prepare students for professional nursing practice and the current and Next-Generation NCLEX® (NGN) Examination for nursing licensure. A new chapter in this edition (Chapter 2), entitled *Clinical Judgment and Systems Thinking,* focuses on how nurses use clinical judgment in practice. Systems thinking allows the nurse to look beyond an individual action for additional or enhanced methods to promote safety and increase quality of care, which drives more favorable patient outcomes. Inversely, the nurse can look at interventions that have served populations and then navigate ways to bring those to the individual patient level.

  In addition to the new chapter, most chapters in this edition present **Clinical Judgment Challenges** that describe complex clinical situations and require the students to use clinical judgment skills based on the NCSBN's Clinical Judgment Measurement Model (CJMM). This model is the basis for the new test item types on the Next-Generation NCLEX® Examination. Suggested answer guidelines for these Clinical Judgment Challenges are provided on the companion Evolve website (http://evolve.elsevier.com/Iggy/).

  In the tenth edition, the six cognitive skills of the NCSBN's CJMM can be aligned with each nursing process step. The authors use this alignment to help students and faculty transition from the basic foundation of the nursing process to the critical thinking and clinical reasoning required for clinical judgment as follows:
  - Assessment: Recognize Cues
  - Analysis: Analyze Cues and Prioritize Hypotheses
  - Planning and Implementation: Generate Solutions and Take Action
  - Evaluation: Evaluate Outcomes
- **Emphasis on Patient Safety.** Patient safety is emphasized throughout this edition, not only in the narrative but also in **Nursing Safety Priority boxes** that enable students to immediately identify the most important care needed for patients with specific health problems. These highlighted features are further classified as an Action Alert, Drug Alert, or Critical Rescue. We also continue to include our leading-edge **Best Practice for Patient Safety & Quality Care boxes** to emphasize the most important nursing care.
- **Highlight on Quality Care.** The QSEN Institute emphasizes, and clinical practice agencies require, that all nurses have *quality improvement* knowledge, skills, attitudes, and abilities. To help prepare students for that role, this edition includes unique **Systems Thinking and Quality Improvement boxes.** Each box summarizes a quality improvement project published in the literature and discusses the implications of the project's success in improving nursing care.

The inclusion of these boxes disseminates information and research and helps students understand that quality improvement begins at the bedside as the nurse identifies potential evidence-based solutions to practice problems.

- **Enhanced Focus on Patient-Centered Care.** Patient-centered care is enhanced in this tenth edition in several ways. This edition continues to use the term "patient" instead of "client" throughout. Although the use of these terms remains a subject of discussion among nursing educators, we have not defined the patient as a dependent person. Rather, the patient can be an individual, a family, or a group—all of whom have rights that are respected in a mutually trusting nurse-patient relationship. Most health care agencies and professional organizations use "patient" in their practice and publications, and most professional nursing organizations support the term. To help illustrate the importance of Patient-Centered Care, this text incorporates the following special boxes:
    - Patient-Centered Care: Older Adult Considerations
    - Patient-Centered Care: Veterans Health Considerations
    - Patient-Centered Care: Cultural/Spiritual Considerations
    - Patient-Centered Care: Genetic/Genomic Considerations
    - Patient-Centered Care: Gender Health Considerations

  In addition, specific differences in patient values, preferences, and beliefs are addressed in **Chapter 68, Concepts of Care for Transgender Patients.** Along with other individuals in the LGBTQ population, the health needs of transgender patients have gained national attention through their inclusion in *Healthy People 2020* and The Joint Commission's Standards affecting transgender patients. This chapter, first introduced in the eighth edition, continues to provide tools to help prepare students and faculty to provide safe, evidence-based, patient-centered care for transgender patients who are considering, currently undergoing, or have undergone the gender transition process.
- **Emphasis on Evidence-Based Practice.** The tenth edition focuses again on the importance of *using best current evidence in nursing practice* and how to locate and use this information to improve patient care. **Evidence-Based Practice boxes** offer a solid foundation in this essential component of nursing practice. Each box summarizes a useful research article, explains the implications of its findings for nursing practice and further research, and rates the level of evidence based on a well-respected scale.
- **Continued Emphasis on Preparation for the NCLEX® Examination.** An enhanced emphasis on the NCLEX® Examination and consistency with the 2019 NCLEX-RN® test plan has been refined in this edition. The tenth edition emphasizes "readiness"—readiness for the NCLEX® Examination, readiness for disaster and mass casualty events, readiness for safe drug administration, and readiness for the continually evolving world of genetics and genomics. An increased number of new **NCLEX Examination Challenges** are interspersed throughout the text to allow students the opportunity to practice test-taking and decision making. **NCLEX Mastery Questions,** new to the tenth edition, are at the end of each chapter. Answers to these Challenges are provided in the back of the book, and their rationales are provided on the Evolve website (http://evolve.elsevier.com/Iggy). In a world that needs more nurses than ever before, it is critical that students be ready to pass the licensure examination on the first try. To help students and faculty achieve that goal, **Learning Outcomes** at the beginning of each chapter continue to be consistent with the competencies outlined in the 2019 NCLEX-RN® Test Plan. The tenth edition continues to include an innovative end-of-chapter feature called **Get Ready for the Next-Generation NCLEX® Examination!** This unique and effective learning aid consists of a list of **Key Points** *organized by Client Needs Category* as found in the NCLEX-RN® Test Plan. Relevant QSEN and Nurse of the Future competency categories are identified for selected Key Points.
- **Focus on Care Coordination and Transition Management.** Similar to the ninth edition, the tenth edition includes a priority focus on continuity of care via a Care Coordination and Transition Management section in each Nursing Care chapter. Literature continues to emphasize the importance of care coordination and transition management between acute care and community-based care. To help students prepare for this role, this edition of our text provides content focusing on Home Care Management, Self-Management Education, and Health Care Resources.

CLINICAL CURRENCY AND ACCURACY

To ensure currency and accuracy, we listened to students and faculty who have used the previous editions, hearing their impressions of and experiences with the book. A thorough literature search of current best evidence regarding nursing education and clinical practice helped us validate best practices and national health care trends that have shaped the focus of the tenth edition. Further cumulative efforts are reflected in this edition:

- Strong, consistent focus on NCLEX-RN® Examination preparation, clinical judgment, safe patient-centered interprofessional care, pathophysiology, drug therapy, quality improvement, evidence-based clinical practice, and care coordination and transition management
- Foundation of relevant research and best practice guidelines
- Emphasis on critical "need-to-know" information that entry-level nurses must master to provide safe patient care

With the amount of information that continues to evolve in health care practice and education, it is easy for a book to become larger with each new edition. The reality is that today's nursing students have a limited time to absorb and apply essential information to provide safe medical-surgical nursing care. Materials in this edition were carefully scrutinized to determine the essential information that students will actively *use* when providing safe, patient-centered, interprofessional, quality nursing care for adults.

OUTSTANDING READABILITY

Today's students must maximize their study time to read information and quickly understand it. The average reading level of today's learner is 10th to 11th grade. To achieve this level of readability without reducing the quality or depth of material that students need to know, this text uses a direct-address style (where appropriate) that speaks directly to the reader. Sentences are as short as possible without sacrificing essential content. The new edition has continued to improve within consistency among chapters. The result of our efforts is a medical-surgical text of consistently outstanding readability in which content is clear, focused, and accessible.

EASE OF ACCESS

To make this text as easy to use as possible, we have maintained our approach of having smaller chapters of more uniform length. Consistent with our focus on "need-to-know" material, we chose exemplars to illustrate concepts of care versus detailing every health disorder. The focused tenth edition contains 69 chapters. To help decrease the number of chapters and stay focused on essential "need-to-know" content, several changes were made, including:

- Combining the content on skin disorders and burns into one chapter instead of two separate chapters
- Deleting the chapter on Intraoperative Care, a specialized area of expertise that is no longer tested on the NCLEX-RN® Examination
- Combining the preoperative and postoperative content from two chapters into one chapter (Chapter 9: Concepts of Care for Perioperative Patients)
- Deleting the chapter on arthritis and connective tissue disorders but moving essential content into appropriate chapters, including a new chapter in the musculoskeletal section (Chapter 46: Concepts of Care for Patients with Arthritis and Total Joint Arthroplasty)
- Combining the two chapters on disorders of the oral cavity and esophagus into one chapter (Chapter 49) to prevent duplication of content

The overall presentation of the tenth edition has been updated, including more current, high-quality photographs for realism. Design changes have been made to improve accessibility of material. There is appropriate placement of display elements (e.g., figures, tables, and boxes) for a chapter flow that enhances text reading without splintering content or confusing the reader. Instead of including a glossary at the end of the text, each chapter's key terms are now defined at the beginning of the chapters for quick reference. To increase the smoothness of flow and reader concentration, side-turned tables and charts or tables and charts that span multiple pages are infrequently used.

We have maintained the unit structure of previous editions, with larger vital body systems appearing earlier in the book. However, in the tenth edition we expanded complex care content in separate critical care chapters for patients with coronary artery disease, respiratory health problems, and neurologic health problems.

To break up long blocks of text and highlight key information, we continue to include streamlined yet eye-catching headings, bulleted lists, tables, boxes, and in-text highlights. Current references at the end of each chapter include research articles, nationally accepted clinical guidelines, and other sources of evidence when available for each chapter. Classic sources from before 2015 are noted with an asterisk (*).

A PATIENT-CENTERED, INTERPROFESSIONAL COLLABORATIVE CARE APPROACH

As in previous editions, we maintain in this edition a collaborative, interprofessional care approach to patient care. In the real world of health care, nurses, patients, and all other providers who are part of the interprofessional team *share* responsibility for the management of patients and their health problems. Thus we present information in a collaborative framework with an increased emphasis on the interprofessional nature of care. In this framework we make no *artificial* distinctions between medical treatment and nursing care. Instead, under each Interprofessional Collaborative Care heading we discuss how the nurse coordinates care and transition management while interacting with members of the interprofessional team. A new feature for the tenth edition is **Interprofessional Collaboration boxes** that present helpful content on how nurses can collaborate with the interprofessional health care team to help meet optimal patient outcomes. Each box identifies the Interprofessional Education Collaborative (IPEC) Expert Panel's Competency of Roles and Responsibilities that aligns with its content.

Although our approach has a focus on interprofessional care, the text is first and foremost a *nursing* text. We therefore use a nursing process/clinical judgment approach as a tool to organize discussions of patient health problems and their management. Discussions of *major* health problems follow a full nursing process format using this structure:

[Health problem]
Pathophysiology Review
  Etiology (and Genetic Risk when appropriate)
  Incidence and Prevalence
Health Promotion and Maintenance (when appropriate)
Interprofessional Collaborative Care
  Assessment: Recognize Cues
  Analysis: Analyze Cues and Prioritize Hypotheses
  Planning and Implementation: Generate Solutions and Take Action
    [Collaborative Intervention Statement (based on priority patient problems)]
    Planning: Expected Outcomes
    Interventions
  Care Coordination and Transition Management
    Home Care Management
    Self-Management Education
    Health Care Resources
  Evaluation: Evaluate Outcomes

Discussions of less common (but important) or less complex disorders follow a similar yet abbreviated format: a discussion of the problem itself (including pertinent review information on pathophysiology) followed by a section on interprofessional collaborative care of patients with the disorder. To demonstrate our commitment to providing the content foundational to nursing education, and consistent with the recommendations of Benner and colleagues through the Carnegie Foundation for the Future of Nursing Education, we highlight essential pathophysiologic concepts that are key to understanding the basis for collaborative management.

Integral to the interprofessional care approach is a narrative of who on the health care team is involved in the care of the patient. When a responsibility is primarily the nurse's, the text says so. When a decision must be made jointly by various members of the team (e.g., by the patient, nurse, primary health care provider, and physical therapist), this is clearly stated. When health care practitioners in different care settings are involved in the patient's care, this is noted.

ORGANIZATION

The 69 chapters of *Medical-Surgical Nursing: Concepts for Interprofessional Collaborative Care* are grouped into 15 units. Unit I, Concepts for Medical-Surgical Nursing, provides fundamental information for the health care concepts incorporated throughout the text. Unit II consists of three chapters on concepts of emergency care and disaster preparedness.

Unit III consists of three chapters on the management of patients with fluid, electrolyte, and acid-base imbalances. Chapters 13 and 14 review key assessments associated with fluid and electrolyte balance, acid-base balance, and related patient care in a clear, concise discussion. The chapter on infusion therapy (Chapter 15) is supplemented with an online Fluids & Electrolytes Tutorial on the companion Evolve website.

Unit IV provides core content on health problems related to immunity. This material includes information on inflammation and the immune response, altered cell growth and cancer development, and interventions for patients with connective tissue disease, HIV infection, and other immunologic disorders, cancers, and infections.

The remaining 11 units focus on medical-surgical content by body system. Each of these units begins with an Assessment chapter and continues with one or more Nursing Care chapters for patients with selected health problems, highlighted via exemplars, in that body system. This framework is familiar to students who learn the body systems in preclinical foundational science courses such as anatomy and physiology.

MULTINATIONAL, MULTICULTURAL, MULTIGENERATIONAL FOCUS

To reflect the increasing diversity of our society, *Medical-Surgical Nursing: Concepts for Interprofessional Collaborative Care* takes a multinational, multicultural, and multigenerational focus. Addressing the needs of both U.S. and Canadian readers, we have included U.S. and international units for normal values of selected laboratory tests. When appropriate, we identify specific Canadian health care resources, including their websites. In many areas, Canadian health statistics are combined with those of the United States to provide an accurate "North American" picture.

To help nurses provide quality care for patients whose preferences, beliefs, and values may differ from their own, numerous **Patient-Centered Care: Cultural/Spiritual Considerations** and **Patient-Centered Care: Gender Health Considerations boxes** highlight important aspects of culturally competent care. Chapter 68 is dedicated to the special health care needs of transgender patients.

Increases in life expectancy and aging of the baby-boom generation contribute to a steadily increasing older adult population. To help nurses care for this population, the tenth edition continues to provide thorough coverage of the care of older adults. Chapter 4 offers content on the role of the nurse and interprofessional team in promoting health for this population, with coverage of common health problems that older adults may experience, such as falls and inadequate nutrition. **Patient-Centered Care: Considerations for Older Adults boxes** that specify normal physiologic changes to expect in the older population are found in each Assessment chapter. In the Nursing Care chapters, these boxes also present key points for the student to consider when caring for these patients. A new feature for the ninth edition was **Patient-Centered Care: Veterans Health Considerations**. The tenth edition increases emphasis on the special health needs of this population. An increasing number of veterans have multiple physical and mental health concerns that require special attention in today's environment of care.

AN INTEGRATED MULTIMEDIA RESOURCE BASED ON PROVEN STRATEGIES FOR STUDENT ENGAGEMENT AND LEARNING

Medical-Surgical Nursing: Concepts for Interprofessional Collaborative Care, 10th edition, is the centerpiece of a comprehensive package of electronic and print learning resources that break new ground in the application of proven strategies for student engagement, learning, and evidence-based educational practice. This integrated multimedia resource actively engages the student in problem solving and using clinical judgment to make important clinical decisions.

Resources for Instructors

For the convenience of faculty, all Instructor Resources are available on a streamlined, secure instructor area of the Evolve website (http://evolve.elsevier.com/Iggy/). All ancillaries for this edition were developed with direct involvement of the textbook authors. Included among these Instructor Resources are the ***TEACH*® *for Nurses* Lesson Plans.** These Lesson Plans focus on the most important content from each chapter and provide innovative strategies for student engagement and learning. This tenth edition *TEACH for Nurses* product incorporates numerous interprofessional activities that give students an opportunity to practice as an integral part of the health care team. Lesson Plans are provided for each chapter and are categorized into several parts:

Learning Outcomes
Teaching Focus
Key Terms
Nursing Curriculum Standards
- QSEN
- Concepts
- BSN Essentials

Student Chapter Resources
Instructor Chapter Resources
Teaching Strategies

Additional Instructor Resources provided on the Evolve website include:

- A completely revised, updated, high-quality **Test Bank** consisting of more than 1509 items, both traditional multiple-choice and NCLEX-RN® "alternate-item" types. Each question is coded for correct answer, rationale, cognitive level, NCLEX Integrated Process, NCLEX Client Needs Category, and new key words to facilitate question searches. Page references are provided for Remembering (Knowledge)-level and Understanding (Comprehension)-level questions. (Questions at the Applying [Application] and above cognitive level require the student to draw on understanding of multiple or broader concepts not limited to a single textbook page, so page cross references are not provided for these higher-level critical thinking questions.) The Test Bank is provided in the Evolve Assessment Manager and in ExamView and ParTest formats. New to this edition, 75 Next-Generation NCLEX® Examination Review questions are provided within an interactive application for further testing options.
- An electronic **Image Collection** containing all images from the book (approximately 550 images), delivered in a format that makes incorporation into lectures, presentations, and online courses easier than ever.
- A completely revised collection of more than 2000 **PowerPoint slides** corresponding to each chapter in the text and highlighting key materials with integrated images and Unfolding Case Studies. Audience Response System Questions (three discussion-oriented questions per chapter for use with iClicker and other audience response systems) are included in these slide presentations. Answers and rationales to the Audience Response System Questions and Unfolding Case Studies are found in the "Notes" section of each slide.

Also available for adoption and separate purchase:

- Corresponding chapter-by-chapter to the textbook, ***Elsevier Adaptive Quizzing (EAQ)*** integrates seamlessly into your course to help students of all skill levels focus their study time and effectively prepare for class, course exams, and the NCLEX® certification exam. ***EAQ*** is comprised of a bank of high-quality practice questions that allows students to advance at their own pace—based on their performance—through multiple mastery levels for each chapter. A comprehensive dashboard allows students to view their progress and stay motivated. The educator dashboard, grade book, and reporting capabilities enable faculty to monitor the activity of individual students, assess overall class performance, and identify areas of strength and weakness, ultimately helping to achieve improved learning outcomes.
- ***Simulation Learning System (SLS) for Medical-Surgical Nursing*** is an online toolkit designed to help you effectively incorporate simulation into your nursing curriculum, with scenarios that promote and enhance the clinical decision-making skills of students at all levels. It offers detailed instructions for preparation and implementation of the simulation experience, debriefing questions that encourage critical thinking, and learning resources to reinforce student comprehension. Modularized simulation scenarios correspond to Elsevier's leading medical-surgical nursing texts, reinforcing students' classroom knowledge base, synthesizing lecture and clinicals, and offering the remediation content that is critical to debriefing.

Resources for Students

Resources for students include a revised, updated, and retitled Study Guide, a Clinical Companion, Elsevier Adaptive Learning (EAL), Virtual Clinical Excursions (VCE), and Evolve Learning Resources.

The ***Study Guide*** has been completely revised and updated and features a fresh emphasis on clinical decision making, priorities of delegation, management of care, and pharmacology. Unlike earlier editions, the rationales are provided along with the correct responses to allow students the opportunity to enhance their understanding of content and increase their test-taking skills.

The pocket-sized ***Clinical Companion*** is a handy clinical resource that retains its easy-to-use alphabetical organization and streamlined format, with completely revised content for ease of use and on-the-go care. The bulleted format is integrated with key elements of the NCSBN Clinical Judgment Measurement Model. It includes "Critical Rescue," "Drug Alert," and "Action Alert" highlights throughout based on the Nursing Safety Priority features in the textbook. National Patient Safety Goals highlights have been expanded as a QSEN feature, focusing on one of six QSEN core competencies while still underscoring the importance of observing vital patient safety standards. Increased use of illustrations facilitates clinical application of key content. This "pocket-sized Iggy" has been tailored to the special needs of students preparing for clinicals and clinical practice.

Corresponding chapter-by-chapter to the textbook, ***Elsevier Adaptive Learning (EAL)*** combines the power of brain science with sophisticated, patented Cerego algorithms to help students to learn faster and remember longer. It's fun, it's engaging, and it constantly tracks and adapts to student performance to deliver content precisely when it's needed to ensure core information is transformed into lasting knowledge.

Virtual Clinical Excursions, featuring an updated and easy-to-navigate "virtual" clinical setting, is once again available for the tenth edition. This unique learning tool guides students through a virtual clinical environment and helps them "learn by doing" in the safety of a "virtual" hospital.

Also available for students is a dynamic collection of Evolve Student Resources, available at http://evolve.elsevier.com/Iggy/. The Evolve Student Resources include the following:

- Review Questions—NCLEX® Examination
- Review Questions—Next-Generation NCLEX® Examination
- Answer Guidelines for Next-Generation NCLEX® Examination and Clinical Judgment Challenges
- Interactive Case Studies
- Concept Maps

- Concept Map Creator (a handy tool for creating customized Concept Maps)
- Fluid & Electrolyte Tutorial (a complete self-paced tutorial on this perennially difficult content)
- Key Points (downloadable expanded chapter reviews for each chapter)
- Audio Glossary
- Audio Clips and Video Clips

In summary, *Medical-Surgical Nursing: Concepts for Interprofessional Collaborative Care,* tenth edition, together with its fully integrated multimedia ancillary package, provides the tools you will need to equip nursing students to meet the opportunities and challenges of nursing practice both now and in an evolving health care environment. The only elements that remain to be added to this package are those that you uniquely provide—your passion, your commitment, your innovation, *your nursing expertise.*

Donna D. Ignatavicius
M. Linda Workman
Cherie R. Rebar
Nicole M. Heimgartner

We are dedicating this landmark tenth edition to our parents. These wonderful women and men were our first teachers, believed in our dreams, and instilled in us the fortitude to reach high to accomplish our professional and personal goals. It is with love and gratefulness that we honor and remember:

Donna's parents
Mary P. Dennis (1929-1972)
Barney J. Dennis, Jr. (1923-1985)

Linda's parents
M. Eunice R. Workman (1929-2019)
Homer D. Workman (1928-1992)

Cherie's parents
Ruth (Whitt) Carnes (1933-2019)
Charles R. Carnes, Jr. (1930-2008)

Nicole's parents
Edna Surles (1944-2018)
Logan Surles, Jr. (living)

ABOUT THE AUTHORS

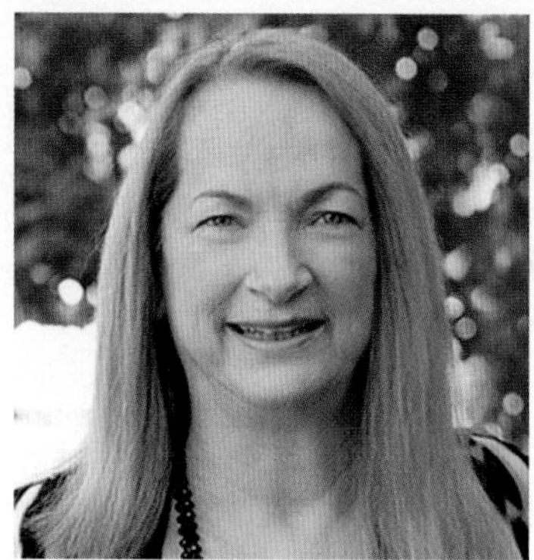

Donna D. Ignatavicius received her diploma in nursing from the Peninsula General School of Nursing in Salisbury, Maryland. After working as a charge nurse in medical-surgical nursing, she became an instructor in staff development at the University of Maryland Medical Center. She then received her BSN from the University of Maryland School of Nursing. For 5 years she taught in several schools of nursing while working toward her MS in Nursing, which she received in 1981. Donna then taught in the BSN program at the University of Maryland, after which she continued to pursue her interest in gerontology and accepted the position of Director of Nursing of a major skilled-nursing facility in her home state of Maryland. Since that time, she has served as an instructor in several associate degree nursing programs. Through her consulting activities, faculty development workshops, and international nursing education conferences (such as Boot Camp for Nurse Educators®), Donna is nationally recognized as an expert in nursing education. She is currently the President of DI Associates, Inc. (http://www.diassociates.com/), a company dedicated to improving health care through education and consultation for faculty. In recognition of her contributions to the field, she was inducted as a charter Fellow of the prestigious Academy of Nursing Education in 2007, received her Certified Nurse Educator credential in 2016, and obtained her Academic Clinical Nurse Educator certification in 2020.

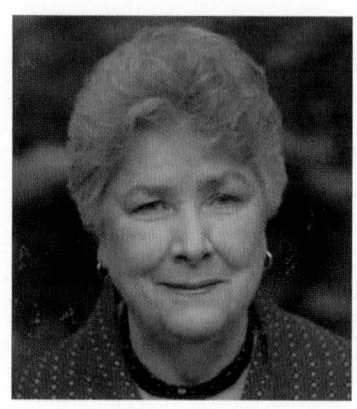

M. Linda Workman, a native of Canada, received her BSN from the University of Cincinnati College of Nursing and Health. After serving in the U.S. Army Nurse Corps and working as an Assistant Head Nurse and Head Nurse in civilian hospitals, Linda earned her MSN from the University of Cincinnati College of Nursing and a PhD in Developmental Biology from the University of Cincinnati College of Arts and Sciences. Linda's 30-plus years of academic experience include teaching at the diploma, associate degree, baccalaureate, master's, and doctoral levels. Her areas of teaching expertise include medical-surgical nursing, physiology, pathophysiology, genetics, oncology, and immunology. Linda has been recognized nationally and internationally for her teaching expertise and was inducted as a Fellow into the American Academy of Nursing in 1992. She received Excellence in Teaching awards at the University of Cincinnati and at Case Western Reserve University. She is a former American Cancer Society Professor of Oncology Nursing and occupied an endowed chair in oncology for 5 years. She has authored several additional textbooks and continues to serve as a consultant for major universities.

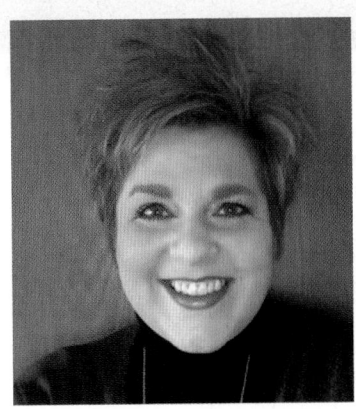

Cherie R. Rebar earned her first degree in education from Morehead State University in Morehead, Kentucky. She returned to school to earn an Associate of Science degree in Nursing from Kettering College, MSN and MBA degrees from the University of Phoenix, a post-masters certificate in Family Nurse Practitioner studies from the University of Massachusetts—Boston, a Psychiatric-Mental Health Nurse Practitioner post-masters certificate from the University of Cincinnati College of Nursing, and a PhD in Psychology (Health Behaviors) from Northcentral University. Combining her loves of nursing and education, Cherie continues to teach students in prelicensure and graduate nursing programs. She has served in numerous leadership positions over the years, including Chair of ASN, BSN Completion, and BSN Prelicensure Nursing Programs, and Director of Nursing. She currently is a Professor of Nursing at Wittenberg University and an Adjunct Faculty Member at Indiana Wesleyan University and Mercy College of Ohio. Her years of clinical practice include medical-surgical, acute care, ear/nose/throat surgery and allergy, community, and psychiatric-mental health nursing. A frequent presenter at national and state nursing conferences, Cherie serves as a consultant to nursing programs and faculty, contributes regularly to professional publications, and holds student success at the heart of all she does.

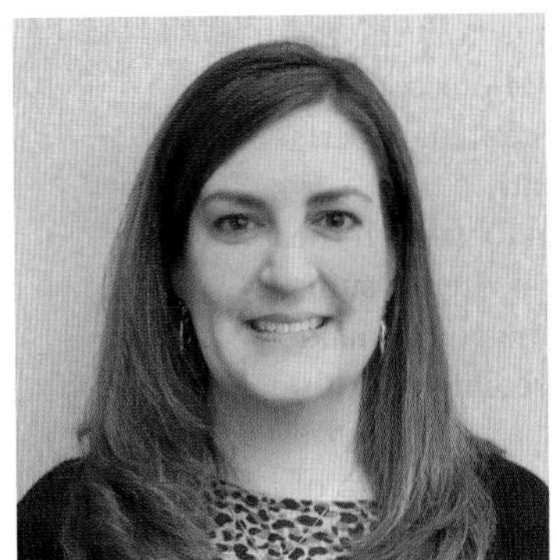

Nicole M. Heimgartner received her BSN from Spalding University in Louisville, Kentucky, her MSN with an emphasis in education from the University of Phoenix, and her Doctorate of Nursing Practice in Educational Leadership from American Sentinel University in Aurora, Colorado. Nicole is also certified in online education.

Nicole has a very diverse clinical background, with extensive practice experience in cardiovascular, medical-surgical, and community nursing. As her love for the nursing profession grew, Nicole started teaching in undergraduate and graduate degree programs. Nicole now has over 17 years of experience as an educator, focusing on innovative educational strategy, nursing leadership, and incorporating online learning into nursing education. Her expertise includes currency in clinical practice as well as teaching and designing curriculum at the undergraduate and graduate levels of nursing education. Nicole also presents at the state and national level on best nursing practice, serves as a consultant with nursing programs and faculty, contributes regularly to professional publications, and is passionate about current practice and engaging the adult learner.

ACKNOWLEDGMENTS

Publishing a textbook and ancillary package of this magnitude would not be possible without the combined efforts of many people. With that in mind, we would like to extend our deepest gratitude to many people who were such an integral part of this journey.

For the tenth edition, we welcomed Nicole M. Heimgartner as a full member of the author and editor team. Nicole has worked with our team previously in contributor, section editor, and ancillary roles over the past editions.

Our contributing authors once again provided excellent manuscripts to underscore the clinical relevancy of this publication. Our reviewers—expert clinicians and instructors from around the United States and Canada—provided invaluable suggestions and encouragement throughout the development of book.

The staff of Elsevier has, as always, provided us with meaningful guidance and support throughout every step of the planning, writing, revision, and production of the tenth edition. Executive Content Strategist Lee Henderson worked closely with us from the early stages of this edition to help us hone and focus our revision plan while coordinating the project from start to finish. Senior Content Development Specialist Laura Goodrich then worked with us to bring the logistics of the tenth edition from vision to publication. Laura also held the reins of our complex ancillary package and worked with the authors and a gifted group of writers and content experts to provide an outstanding library of resources to complement and enhance the text.

Senior Project Manager Jodi Willard was, as always, an absolute joy with whom to work. If the mark of a good editor is that his or her work is invisible to the reader, then Jodi is the consummate editor. Her unwavering attention to detail, flexibility, and conscientiousness helped to make the tenth edition consistently readable, while making the production process incredibly smooth. Also, a special thanks to Publishing Services Manager Julie Eddy.

Designer Brian Salisbury is responsible for the beautiful cover and the new interior design of the tenth edition. Brian's work on this edition has cast important features in exactly the right light, contributing to the readability and colorful beauty of this edition.

Our acknowledgments would not be complete without recognizing our dedicated team of Educational Solutions Consultants and other key members of the Sales and Marketing staff who helped to put this book into your hands.

Donna D. Ignatavicius
M. Linda Workman
Cherie R. Rebar
Nicole M. Heimgartner

CONTENTS

Asterisk (*) denotes a Concept Exemplar.

GUIDE TO SPECIAL FEATURES

PATIENT-CENTERED CARE: CULTURAL/SPIRITUAL CONSIDERATIONS

PATIENT-CENTERED CARE: GENDER HEALTH CONSIDERATIONS

PATIENT-CENTERED CARE: GENETIC/GENOMIC CONSIDERATIONS

PATIENT-CENTERED CARE: OLDER ADULT CONSIDERATIONS

PATIENT-CENTERED CARE: VETERANS HEALTH CONSIDERATIONS

BEST PRACTICE FOR PATIENT SAFETY AND QUALITY CARE

COMMON EXAMPLES OF DRUG THERAPY

EVIDENCE-BASED PRACTICE

FOCUSED ASSESSMENT

HOME CARE CONSIDERATIONS

KEY FEATURES

LABORATORY PROFILE

PATIENT AND FAMILY EDUCATION: PREPARING FOR SELF-MANAGEMENT

SYSTEMS THINKING AND QUALITY IMPROVEMENT

1

Overview of Professional Nursing Concepts for Medical-Surgical Nursing

Donna D. Ignatavicius

http://evolve.elsevier.com/Iggy/

LEARNING OUTCOMES

1. Provide examples of how nurses use the Rapid Response Team (RRT) to ensure patient ***safety.***
2. Identify the six core Quality and Safety Education for Nurses (QSEN) competencies that professional nurses need to provide safe, coordinated ***patient-centered care.***
3. Differentiate the major ***ethics*** principles that help guide professional nursing practice.
4. Communicate patient values, preferences, and expressed needs to other members of the health care team for effective ***teamwork and*** interprofessional ***collaboration.***
5. Describe common methods used to ensure effective hand-off communication in health care agencies.
6. Explain the relationship between ***evidence-based practice*** and ***clinical judgment.***
7. Identify the nurse's role in ***systems thinking*** and the ***quality improvement*** process.
8. State three ways that ***informatics*** is used in health care.
9. Explain why many minority populations and older adults are at risk for ***health care disparities.***
10. Identify the role of the nurse when communicating with members of the LGBTQ community.

KEY TERMS

adverse event A variation in the standard of care.

autonomy An ethical principle in which one is capable of making informed decisions about one's own care; also referred to as *self-determination* or *self-management.*

beneficence An ethical principle in which nurses promote positive actions to help others.

care coordination The deliberate organization of and communication about patient care activities between two or more members of the health care team (including the patient) to facilitate appropriate and continuous health care to meet that patient's needs.

care transition Actions designed to ensure safe, effective coordination and continuity of care as patients experience a change in health status, primary health care provider, or setting; the nurse plays a vital role in patient-centered care transition management.

case management A process to ensure quality and cost-effective services and resources to achieve positive patient outcomes.

clinical judgment The observed outcome of critical thinking and decision making. It is an iterative process that uses nursing knowledge to observe and access presenting situations, identify a prioritized client concern, and generate the best possible evidence-based solutions in order to deliver safe client care (NCSBN, 2019).

culture of safety An environment that provides a blame-free approach to improving care in high-risk, error-prone health care settings using interprofessional collaboration.

delegated responsibility A nursing activity, skill, or procedure that is transferred from a licensed nurse to a delegate, usually an LPN/VN or assistive personnel (AP) in a selected patient care situation.

early warning system (EWS) (also called an early warning scoring system [EWSS]) A guide for the health care team to quickly determine a patient's condition on the basis of a physiologic scoring matrix.

ethics A theoretical and reflective domain of human knowledge that addresses issues and questions about morality in human choices, actions, character, and ends.

Evidence-Based Practice (EBP) A QSEN competency in which the nurse uses the integration of the best current evidence and practices to make decisions about patient care. It considers the patient's preferences and values and one's own clinical expertise for the delivery of optimal health care.

failure to rescue The inability of nurses or other interprofessional health team members to save a patient's life in a timely manner when a health care issue or medical complication occurs.

fidelity An ethical principle that refers to the agreement that nurses will keep their obligations or promises to patients to follow through with care.

health care disparities Differences in patient access to or availability of appropriate health care services.

Informatics A QSEN competency in which the nurse accesses and uses information and electronic technology to communicate, manage knowledge, prevent error, and support decision making.

medication reconciliation A formal evaluative process in which the nurse compares the patient's actual current medications to his or her medications at time of admission, transfer, or discharge to identify and resolve discrepancies.

modified early warning system (MEWS) A screening and scoring tool for medical-surgical nursing assessment to determine a patient's condition based primarily on the patient's level of consciousness and respiratory rate. Most MEWS tools also include measurements of systolic blood pressure, temperature, heart rate, oxygen saturation, and hourly urinary output (previous 2 hours).

nonmaleficence An ethical principle that emphasizes the importance of preventing harm and ensuring the patient's well-being.

Patient-Centered Care A QSEN competency in which the nurse recognizes the patient or designee as the source of control and full partner in providing compassionate and coordinated care based on respect for the patient's preferences, values, and needs.

PICOT A format using a spirit of inquiry to formulate a quality improvement project question.

Plan-Do-Study-Act (PDSA) A commonly used systematic quality improvement model used in health care and other settings.

Quality Improvement (QI) A QSEN competency in which the nurse uses indicators (data) to monitor care outcomes and develop solutions to change and improve care.

Rapid Response Team (RRT) A group of health care professionals who save lives and decrease the risk for harm by providing care before a medical emergency occurs. by intervening rapidly for patients who are beginning to clinically decline. Members of an RRT are critical care experts who are on-site and available at any time.

Safety A QSEN competency in which the nurse keeps the patient and staff free from harm and minimizes errors in care.

SBAR A formal method of communication between two or more members of the health care team or health care agency.

sentinel event A severe variation in the standard of care that is caused by human or system error and results in an avoidable patient death or major harm.

social justice An ethical principle that refers to equality and fairness; that is, all patients should be treated equally and fairly, regardless of age, gender identity, sexual orientation, religion, race, ethnicity, or education.

Systems Thinking The ability to recognize, understand, and synthesize the interactions and interdependencies in a set of components designed for a specific purpose (Dolansky & Moore, 2013).

supervision Guidance or direction, evaluation, and follow-up by the nurse to ensure that a nursing task or activity is performed appropriately and safely.

TeamSTEPPS A systematic communication approach for interprofessional teams designed to improve safety and quality.

Teamwork and Collaboration A QSEN competency in which the nurse functions effectively within nursing and interprofessional teams, fostering open communication, mutual respect, and shared decision making to achieve quality patient care.

telehealth The long-distance use of electronic information and telecommunication technology to support clinical health care by a variety of health care professionals.

telenursing A type or subset of telehealth that allows nurses to provide care through the use of the Internet, telephone, computers, digital assessment tools, and telemonitoring equipment.

veracity An ethical principle related to fidelity in which the nurse is obligated to tell the truth to the best of his or her knowledge.

PRIORITY AND INTERRELATED CONCEPTS

The priority concepts for this chapter are:

- ***Patient-Centered Care***
- ***Safety***
- ***Teamwork and Collaboration***
- ***Evidence-Based Practice***
- ***Quality Improvement***
- ***Informatics***
- ***Clinical Judgment***
- ***Systems Thinking***
- ***Ethics***
- ***Health Care Disparities***

Medical-surgical nursing, sometimes called *adult health nursing,* is a specialty practice area in which nurses promote, restore, or maintain optimal health for patients from 18 to older than 100 years of age (Academy of Medical-Surgical Nurses [AMSN], 2012). A separate chapter on care of older adults is part of this textbook because the majority of medical-surgical patients in most health care settings are older than 65 years (see Chapter 4).

To be consistent with the most recent health care literature, the authors use the term *patient* rather than *client* (except in NCLEX Examination Challenge questions and Clinical Judgment Challenges where *client* is used to reflect that licensure examination). To be patient-centered, be sure to refer to individuals according to the policy of the health care organization and the individual's preference. The *family* refers to the patient's relatives and significant others in the patient's life whom the patient identifies and values as important.

Medical-surgical nursing is practiced in many types of settings, such as acute care hospitals, skilled nursing facilities, ambulatory care settings, and the patient's home, which could be either a single residence or group setting such as an assisted living facility. The role of the nurse in these settings includes care coordinator and transition manager, caregiver, patient educator, leader, and patient and family advocate. To function in these various roles, nurses need to have the knowledge, skills, attitudes, and abilities to keep patients and their families safe.

QUALITY AND SAFETY EDUCATION FOR NURSES' COMPETENCIES

The Institute of Medicine (IOM, now the National Academy of Medicine [NAM]), a highly respected U.S. organization that monitors health care and recommends health policy, published many reports during the past 25 years suggesting ways to improve patient safety and quality care. One of its classic reports, *Health Professions Education: A Bridge to Quality,* identified five broad core competencies for health care professionals to ensure patient safety and quality care (Institute of Medicine [IOM], 2003). All of these competencies are interrelated and include:

- Provide ***patient-centered care.***
- *Collaborate* with the interprofessional health care team.
- Implement ***evidence-based practice.***
- Use ***quality improvement*** in patient care.
- Use ***informatics*** in patient care.

Several years later, the QSEN initiative, now called the *QSEN Institute,* validated the IOM (NAM) competencies for nursing practice and added ***safety*** as a sixth competency to emphasize its importance. More information about the QSEN Institute can be found on www.qsen.org.

In addition to emphasizing the six QSEN competency concepts in this text, the authors integrate these four professional nursing concepts:

- Clinical Judgment
- Systems Thinking
- Ethics
- Health Care Disparities

This chapter briefly reviews each of these professional nursing concepts and includes the concept definition; scope, category, or models of the concept; and attributes (characteristics) of the concept. Each concept analysis review ends with at least one example of how the concept may be used in practice. Many of the concepts in this chapter are interrelated. For instance, ***systems thinking*** is required for ***quality improvement. Clinical judgment*** to make the best patient care decisions promotes ***patient safety.***

PATIENT-CENTERED CARE

Definition of Patient-Centered Care

To be competent in *Patient-Centered Care,* the nurse recognizes "the patient or designee as the source of control and full partner in providing compassionate and coordinated care based on respect for [the] patient's preferences, values, and needs" (Quality and Safety Education for Nurses [QSEN], 2019). Implied in this widely used definition is the need for the nurse to provide safe, culturally competent care for diverse patients and their families. Many patients who are part of minority groups do not have equal access to appropriate and/or culturally sensitive health care. Therefore, the primary interrelated concepts are ***safety*** and ***health care disparities.*** The Joint Commission, a major accrediting organization for health care agencies, uses the term *family-centered care* to emphasize the importance of including the patient's support system as part of interprofessional collaboration.

Scope of Patient-Centered Care

Patient-centered care has been a focus of health professions' education and research for several decades. Before this period of time, patients in inpatient facilities and their families often had little to no input into their health care. Many health care professionals believed that they were better prepared than patients to make care decisions and did not consistently include the patient and family in this process. The Joint Commission and other organizations called for the rights of patients or their designees (e.g., family members, guardians) to make their own informed decisions. The IOM (now NAM) further emphasized the need for all health care agencies to place patients and their families at the center of the interprofessional team to make mutual decisions based on patient preferences and values.

Attributes of Patient-Centered Care

The attributes, or characteristics, of ***patient-centered care*** were identified by researchers as a result of a classic medical study (Frampton et al., 2008). These attributes are listed in Table 1.1 and discussed in this section.

Showing respect and advocating for the patient and family's preferences and needs is essential to ensure a wholistic or "whole person" approach to care. As a patient advocate, the nurse also ensures that the patient's autonomy and self-determination are respected (Gerber, 2018). To help illustrate the importance of Patient-Centered Care, this text incorporates special boxes that include:

- Patient-Centered Care: Older Adult Considerations
- Patient-Centered Care: Gender Health Considerations
- Patient-Centered Care: Veterans Health Considerations
- Patient-Centered Care: Cultural/Spiritual Considerations
- Patient-Centered Care: Genetic/Genomic Considerations

TABLE 1.1 Attributes of the Concept of Patient-Centered Care

- Respect for patients' values, preferences, and expressed needs
- Coordination and integration of care
- Information, communication, and education
- Physical comfort
- Emotional support and alleviation of fear and anxiety
- Involvement of family and friends
- Transition and continuity
- Access to care

Data from Frampton, S., Guastello, S., Brady, C., Hale, M., Horowitz, S., Smith, S. B., et al. (2008). *Patient-centered care improvement guide.* Derby, CT: Planetree.

TABLE 1.2 Examples of Integrative (Complementary and Alternative) Therapies Used in Health Care Organizations

• Pet therapy	• Aromatherapy
• Massage therapy	• Health-focused television
• Guided imagery	• Music therapy
• Biofeedback	• Acupuncture
• Exercise and fitness programs	• Acupressure
• Nutritional supplements	• Disease management programs

Canadian nursing practice includes ***patient-centered care*** and culture from a ***safety*** perspective. Promoting safety requires nursing practice that respects and nurtures the unique and dynamic characteristics of patients and families to meet their needs, preferences, values, and rights (Doane & Varcoe, 2015). *Cultural safety* is part of relational inquiry and practice and is highly valued in Canada as a major competency for professional nursing.

Examples of Context of Patient-Centered Care in Nursing and Health Care

Patient-centered care is a major emphasis in all health care settings. For example, many health care organizations integrate complementary and alternative medicine (CAM) as a supplement to traditional health care to meet the specific preferences of patients and their families. This *integrative care* model is in response to the increasing use of these therapies by consumers to maintain health and help manage chronic health issues, such as joint pain, back pain, and anxiety or depression. Integrative care reflects nursing theories of caring, compassion, and whole person care to *respect the diverse preferences and needs* of patients and their families. Examples of these therapies are listed in Table 1.2. Specific integrative therapies are highlighted throughout this text as appropriate.

All patients have the right to have their *basic physical care and comfort needs* met. For example, patients in a variety of settings often experience acute and/or chronic pain. Nurses continually assess the patient's pain management needs and implement interventions to relieve or reduce pain in a timely manner. Chapter 5 describes pain assessment and interventions in detail.

During a stay in a health care agency, patients have a need for individualized coordinated care. **Care coordination** is the deliberate organization of and communication about patient care activities between two or more members of the health care team (including the patient) to facilitate appropriate and continuous health care to meet that patient's needs (Lamb, 2014). One of the most important members of the health care team who assists with care coordination is the case manager (CM) or discharge planner, who is typically a nurse or social worker in health care agencies.

The purpose of the **case management** process is to ensure quality and cost-effective services and resources to achieve positive patient outcomes. In collaboration with the nurse, the CM coordinates inpatient and community-based care before discharge from a hospital or other facility. Part of that process may involve communicating with other CMs who are employed by third-party health care payers (e.g., Medicare) in the community to keep patients from being readmitted to the hospital.

In addition to care coordination during and after hospital discharge, care transitions are essential to prevent adverse events and hospital readmissions. A **care transition** involves actions designed to ensure safe, effective coordination and continuity of care as patients experience a change in health status, primary health care provider, or setting (Dusek et al., 2015). The medical-surgical nurse plays a vital role in managing patient-centered care transitions, often called *transition management* or *transitional care*. The Joint Commission (2013) recommends these components for effective patient-centered care coordination and transition management:

- Understandable discharge instructions for the patient and family
- Explanation of self-care activities
- Ongoing or emergency care information
- List of community and outpatient (ambulatory care) resources and referrals
- Knowledge of the patient's language, culture, and health literacy
- Medication reconciliation (also a Joint Commission National Patient Safety Goal)

Medication reconciliation is a formal evaluative process in which the patient's actual current medications are compared with his or her medications at time of admission, transfer, or discharge to identify and resolve discrepancies. The types of information that clinicians use to reconcile medications include drug name, dose, frequency, route, and purpose. This comparison addresses duplications, omissions, and interactions and the need to continue current medications. Medication discrepancies can cause negative patient outcomes, including rehospitalizations for medical complications.

Miner et al. (2018) identified six steps for improving the care transition or discharge process as outlined in the Best Practice for Patient Safety & Quality Care: Best Care Transition Practices box.

BEST PRACTICE FOR PATIENT SAFETY & QUALITY CARE QSEN

Best Care Transition Practices

- Educate and coach patients and their caregivers.
- Use transition coaches, if available, to improve care coordination and transition management.
- Follow up with postdischarge visits or phone calls.
- Improve communication handoffs from hospitals to ambulatory care or home care settings.
- Identify high-risk patients for readmission on the basis of age (older than 80), number of comorbidities (≥3), number of prescription drugs (≥5), and difficulty performing at least 1 activity of daily living (ADL).
- Address patient caregiver needs to prevent caregiver role strain.

Data from Miner, M. B., Evans, M. M. & Riley, K. (2018). Using transitional care to improve the discharge process in a medical-surgical setting. *MEDSURG Nursing, 27*(1), 4–6.

In this text the authors use the heading *Care Coordination and Transition Management* to describe the specific activities, including discharge planning, health teaching, and community-based care, that are essential for patients with selected health problems and their families. Nurses play a major role in coordinating this care with the interprofessional team to promote safe, quality care.

SAFETY

Definition of Safety

Safety is the ability to keep the patient and staff free from harm and minimize errors in care. The concept of ***safety*** is interrelated to all of the other professional nursing concepts in this chapter. Health care errors by primary health care providers, nurses, and other professionals have been widely reported for the past 25 years. Many of these errors resulted in patient injuries or deaths, as well as increased health care costs. A number of national and international organizations implemented new programs and standards to combat this growing problem.

Scope of Safety

Safety is essential for patients, staff members, and health care organizations. Although most literature discusses ***safety*** for patients, safety for members of the staff and interprofessional team is equally important. The scope of ***safety*** can be described as *unsafe,* possibly causing harm or even death, or *safe* to help prevent harm or minimize negative outcomes. Nurses have accountability for and play a key role in promoting ***safety*** and preventing errors, including "missed nursing care," the necessary care that should have been provided by one or more nurses.

According to classic research by Benner et al. (2010), patient *harm and errors* caused by nurses generally occur as a result of:

- Lack of clear or adequate communication among patient, family, and members of the interprofessional health care team (discussed later in this chapter)
- Lack of attentiveness and patient monitoring
- Lack of ***clinical judgment*** (discussed later in this chapter and in Chapter 2)
- Inadequate measures to prevent health complications
- Errors in medication administration (discussed later in this section)
- Errors in interpreting authorized provider prescriptions
- Lack of professional accountability and patient advocacy
- Inability to carry out interventions in an appropriate and timely manner (discussed later in this chapter)
- Lack of mandatory reporting

Attributes of Safety

Patient and staff safety is the major priority for professional nurses. Best ***safety*** practices reduce error and harm through established protocols, memory checklists, and systems such as bar-code medication administration (BCMA) (Fig. 1.1). Maintaining ***safety*** requires that nurses and other health care professionals use these systems and practices consistently and as specified to achieve positive outcomes. Working around these systems (often called *work-arounds*) is not acceptable and can increase the risk of error to patients and/or staff.

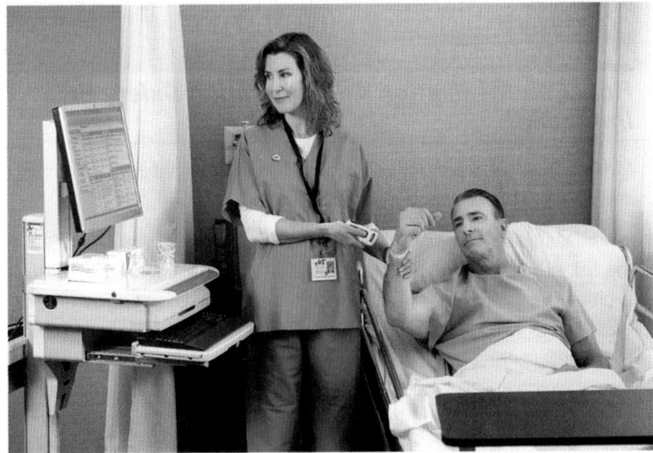

FIG. 1.1 Example of a bar-code medication administration (BCMA) system. (Courtesy Zebra Technologies.)

Three types of *Nursing Safety Priority* boxes are found throughout this text to emphasize its importance in daily practice. These features delineate ***safety*** on the basis of patient and/or staff need. For example, *Nursing Safety Priority: Critical Rescue* emphasizes the need for action for potential or actual life-threatening problems. *Nursing Safety Priority: Action Alert* boxes focus on the need for action but not necessarily for life-threatening situations. As the name implies, *Nursing Safety Priority: Drug Alert* boxes specify actions needed to ensure ***safety*** related to drug administration, monitoring, or related patient and family education.

Examples of Context of Safety in Nursing and Health Care

Medication administration ***safety*** continues to be a major problem in hospitals and other health care agencies. While giving medications, nurses frequently experience work interruptions and distractions, which contribute to medication errors (Cooper et al., 2016). A study by McMahon (2017) found that wearing a medication ***safety*** vest and signage during medication administration can reduce interruptions and minimize these errors (see the Systems Thinking and Quality Improvement box).

In 2002 The Joint Commission (TJC) published its first annual National Patient Safety Goals (NPSGs). These goals require health care organizations to focus on specific priority ***safety*** practices, many of which involve establishing nursing and health system approaches to safe care. Since that time, TJC continues to add new goals each year. NPSGs address high-risk issues such as safe drug administration, prevention of health care–associated infections, and communication effectiveness among the interprofessional team. When appropriate, this textbook includes related NPSGs. A complete list of the latest goals can be found on the TJC website at www.jointcommission.org.

TJC also requires that health care organizations create a culture of safety. A **culture of safety** provides a blame-free approach to improving care in high-risk, error-prone health care settings using interprofessional collaboration. Patients and families are encouraged to become ***safety*** partners in protecting patients from harm. In this environment, nurses and other

SYSTEMS THINKING AND QUALITY IMPROVEMENT QSEN

How Can Medication Administration Safety Be Improved?

McMahon, J. T. (2017). Improving medication administration safety in the clinical environment. *MEDSURG Nursing, 26*(6), 374–377, 409.

Work interruptions and distractions during medication administration increase the risk of medication errors and can cause patient harm. In this quality improvement (QI) project, clinical nurses on a 28-bed medical-surgical unit in a 251-bed regional medical center worked with a project leader to decrease the number of medication errors on their unit. For a period of 4 weeks, nurses wore disposable vests labeled *Do Not Disturb* while they were giving patient medications. As a result of this intervention, medication errors on the unit decreased by 88%.

Commentary: Implications for Practice and Research

The system in this study was the medical-surgical nursing unit. In any clinical setting or system, nurses need to implement interventions to prevent work interruptions and distractions while administering medications. For this QI project, the number of participants was limited to 28 staff nurses, and the study was conducted on only one patient care unit for 4 weeks. The project needs to be repeated using a larger number of nurses working on multiple units and health care organizations. However, this project validated findings from previous studies about the effectiveness of the medication safety vest with signage in reducing errors.

interprofessional health team members should not hesitate to report and document errors or missed care using appropriate internal organizational documents for risk management, ***quality improvement,*** and staff education purposes. A variation in the standard of care is often referred to as an adverse event. The Joint Commission requires that health care organizations report serious adverse events, known as sentinel events. A sentinel event is a *severe* variation in the standard of care that is caused by human or system error and results in an avoidable patient death or major harm.

TEAMWORK AND COLLABORATION

Definition of Teamwork and Collaboration

To provide patient- and family-centered care and be competent in *teamwork and collaboration,* the nurse "functions effectively within nursing and interprofessional teams, fostering open communication, mutual respect, and shared decision making to achieve quality patient care" (QSEN, 2019). Therefore the knowledge and skills needed for this competency are effective communication and team functioning. Communication is an essential process for evaluating patient care together using an interprofessional (IP) plan of care. To help meet this purpose, health care organizations have frequent and regular IP meetings and often conduct IP patient care rounds. The primary interrelated concepts are ***patient-centered care*** and ***ethics.***

Scope of Teamwork and Collaboration

In this textbook the interprofessional health care team includes the patient, family, primary health care providers, nurses, assistive personnel (AP, such as nursing assistants), and other health care professionals and their assistants needed to provide appropriate and safe, evidence-based care. Other older terms used for these members include the *interdisciplinary* or multidisciplinary team, depending on health care organization, context, or setting. Although there are many health care team members, some health care professionals work more closely with nurses than others. For example, the primary health care provider and medical-surgical nurse collaborate frequently in any given day regarding patient care. The occupational therapist may not work as closely with the nurse unless the patient is receiving rehabilitation services. Collaboration with the rehabilitation team is discussed in Chapter 7.

Attributes of Teamwork and Collaboration

In 2016 the Interprofessional Education Collaborative (IPEC) Expert Panel published their latest competencies to guide health professionals in education and practice. The four major IPEC competencies include:

- *Values/Ethics for Interprofessional Practice:* Work with individuals of other professions to maintain a climate of mutual respect and shared values.
- *Role-Responsibilities:* Use the knowledge of one's own role and those of other professions to appropriately assess and address the health care needs of patients and populations served.
- *Interprofessional Communication:* Communicate with patients, families, communities, and other health professionals in a responsive and responsible manner that supports a team approach to the maintenance of health and the treatment of disease.
- *Teams and Teamwork:* Apply relationship-building values and the principles of team dynamics to perform effectively in different team roles to plan and deliver patient-population-centered care that is safe, timely, efficient, effective, and equitable.

Specific competencies for each of these general statements are delineated in the IPEC document. Examples of competencies for *Interprofessional Communication* are listed in Table 1.3. Interprofessional Collaboration boxes that apply some of these competencies are found throughout this textbook.

Examples of Context of Teamwork and Collaboration in Nursing and Health Care

Two examples of nursing ***teamwork and collaboration*** are discussed in this section: communication and delegation/supervision.

Communication. Poor communication between professional caregivers and health care agencies causes many medical errors and patient ***safety*** risks. In 2006 The Joint Commission began to require systematic strategies for improving communication. Two years later, another National Patient Safety Goal mandated that nurses communicate continuing patient care needs such as pain management or respiratory support to postdischarge caregivers for safe transition management.

To improve communication between staff members and health care agencies, procedures for handoff communication were established. An effective procedure used in many agencies today is called SBAR (pronounced S-Bar) (see the Evidence-Based Practice box).

TABLE 1.3 Interprofessional Communication Competencies (CC)

CC1. Choose effective communication tools and techniques, including information systems and communication technologies, to facilitate discussions and interactions that enhance team function.
CC2. Organize and communicate information with patients, families, and health care team members in a form that is understandable, avoiding discipline-specific terminology when possible.
CC3. Express one's knowledge and opinions to team members involved in patient care with confidence, clarity, and respect, working to ensure common understanding of information and treatment and care decisions.
CC4. Listen actively and encourage ideas and opinions of other team members.
CC5. Give timely, sensitive, instructive feedback to others about their performance on the team, responding respectfully as a team member to feedback from others.
CC6. Use respectful language appropriate for a given difficult situation, crucial conversation, or interprofessional conflict.
CC7. Recognize how one's own uniqueness, including experience level, expertise, culture, power, and hierarchy within the health care team, contributes to effective communication, conflict resolution, and positive interprofessional working relationships.
CC8. Communicate consistently the importance of teamwork in patient-centered and community focused care.

Data from the Interprofessional Education Collaborative Expert Panel. (2016). *Core competencies for interprofessional collaborative practice: Report of an expert panel* (2nd ed.). Washington, DC: Interprofessional Education Collaborative.

EVIDENCE-BASED PRACTICE QSEN

How Effective Is SBAR Handoff Communication?

Stewart, K.R. & Hand, K.A. (2017). SBAR, communication, and patient safety: An integrated literature review. *MEDSURG Nursing, 26*(5), 297–305.

The purpose of this systematic review was to analyze studies to determine the effectiveness of using the SBAR handoff communication method in health care. Four themes were identified by researchers from 21 articles included in the review:

- Use of SBAR creates a common language for communication of key patient care information.
- Use of SBAR increases confidence of both the speaker and receiver during the handoff report.
- Use of SBAR improves efficiency, efficacy, and accuracy of the handoff report.
- Use of SBAR improves the perception of effective communication and is well received among health care staff.

Level of Evidence: 1

This study was a systematic review and analysis of multiple research articles.

Commentary: Implications for Practice and Research

The researchers suggest that because communication has been established as a cause of sentinel events, use of SBAR has these two implications for nursing practice: (1) SBAR should be used as a handoff communication method for all interactions, and (2) education regarding the proper use of SBAR should be included in nursing curricula. A limitation of this review was that only one randomized control study was included. This limitation prevents any conclusion about *causation* between SBAR and patient ***safety.***

SBAR is a formal method of communication between two or more members of the health care team or health care agency. The SBAR process includes these four steps:

- **S**ituation: Describe what is happening at the time to require this communication.
- **B**ackground: Explain any relevant background information that relates to the situation.
- **A**ssessment: Provide an analysis of the problem or patient need based on assessment data.
- **R**ecommendation/**R**equest: State what is needed or what the desired outcome is.

Several modifications of SBAR include I-SBAR, I-SBAR-R, and SBARQ. In these methods the "I" reminds the individual to *identify* himself or herself. The last "R" stands for the *response* that the receiver provides based on the information given. "Q" represents any additional questions that need to be answered. Be sure to follow the established documentation and reporting protocols in your health care organization.

TeamSTEPPS is also a systematic communication approach for interprofessional teams that was designed to improve ***safety*** and quality. STEPPS stands for **S**trategies and **T**ools to **E**nhance **P**erformance and **P**atient **S**afety. Adapted from the aviation industry, this model reminds professionals that mistakes can cause negative outcomes, including death. In addition to SBAR or other standardized communication, these common communication tools as part of TeamSTEPPS are effective for promoting communication, patient ***safety,*** and teamwork:

- *CUS words:* State "I'm **c**oncerned; I'm **u**ncomfortable; I don't feel like this is **s**afe."
- *Check backs:* Restate what a person said to verify understanding by all team members.
- *Call outs:* Shout out important information (such as vital signs) for all team members to hear at one time.
- *Two-challenge rule:* State a concern twice as needed; if ignored, follow the chain of command to get the concern addressed.

Many health care agencies have adopted TeamSTEPPS. Gaston et al. (2016) found that initiating this systematic approach was a practical, effective, and low-cost strategy to promote patient ***safety.*** Staff perception of the TeamSTEPPS initiative included improved communication and teamwork.

Delegation and Supervision. As a nursing leader you will delegate certain nursing tasks and activities to assistive personnel (AP) such as patient care technicians (PCTs) or nursing assistants (NAs). A delegated responsibility is a nursing activity, skill, or procedure that is transferred from a licensed nurse to a delegatee, usually an LPN/VN or assistive personnel (AP) in a selected patient care situation (NCSBN-ANA, 2019). These activities, skills, or procedures are not part of the routine care usually performed by the delegatee. This process requires precise and accurate communication. *The nurse is always accountable for what is delegated!*

An important process that is sometimes not consistently performed by busy medical-surgical nurses is supervision of the LPN/VN or AP to whom activities, skills, or procedures have been delegated. Supervision is guidance or direction, evaluation, and follow-up by the nurse to ensure that they are performed appropriately and safely.

Be sure to follow these five rights when you delegate and supervise to a delegatee:

- *Right task:* The task is within the delegatee's scope of practice and competence.
- *Right circumstances:* The patient care setting and resources are appropriate for the delegation.
- *Right person:* The delegatee is competent to perform the delegated activity, skill, or procedure.
- *Right communication:* The nurse provides a clear and concise explanation of the task or activity, including limits and expectations.
- *Right supervision:* The nurse appropriately monitors, evaluates, intervenes, and provides feedback on the delegation process as needed.

Interventions that you can typically delegate or assign in any state are indicated throughout this text. Some of the *NCLEX Examination Challenges* throughout this book will test your understanding of the delegation and supervision process.

NCLEX EXAMINATION CHALLENGE 1.1

Safe, Effective Care Environment

Which nursing activities may be safely delegated to competent assistive personnel (AP)? **Select all that apply.**

A. Discharge teaching
B. Blood pressure monitoring
C. Gastrostomy feeding
D. Oxygen administration
E. Ambulation assistance

EVIDENCE-BASED PRACTICE

Definition of Evidence-Based Practice

Evidence-Based Practice (EBP) is the integration of the best current evidence and practices to make decisions about patient care. It considers the patient's preferences and values and one's own clinical expertise for the delivery of optimal health care (Melnyk & Fineout-Overholt, 2019; QSEN, 2019). The primary interrelated concepts are ***patient-centered care, clinical judgment***, and ***safety.***

Levels of Evidence

The best source of evidence is usually research. Fig. 1.2 shows the level of evidence (LOE) pyramid that is commonly used to rate the quality (strength) or scope of available evidence. The highest levels of evidence are systematic reviews and integrative or meta-analysis studies. In these studies the researcher conducts a thorough literature search for appropriate studies and then analyzes findings of those studies to determine which best practices answer the research question. The types of research in nursing may be limited in some areas and may not reflect the highest or best level of evidence. Some nursing research is designed as small, descriptive studies to explore new concepts. The findings of these studies cannot be generalized, but they provide a basis for future larger and better-designed research.

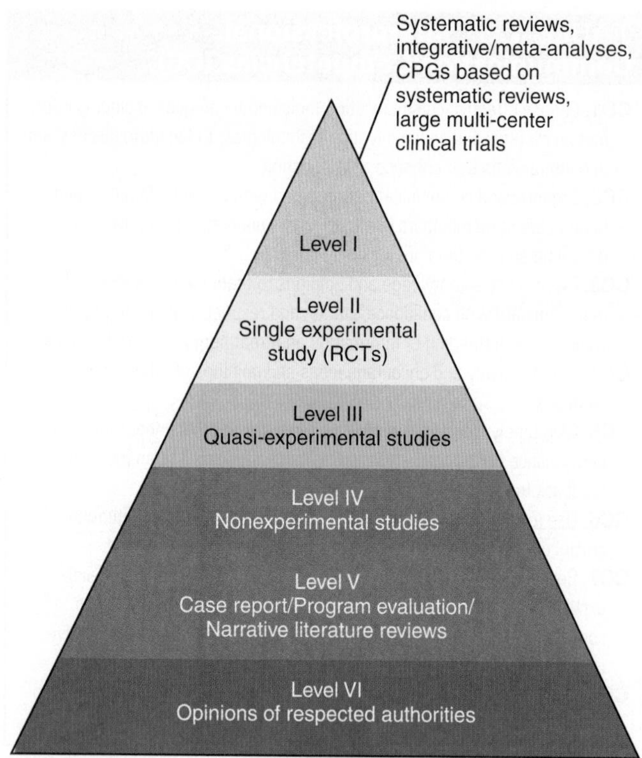

FIG. 1.2 Levels (strength) of evidence. Level 1 is the strongest evidence. (©2010. Rona F. Levin & Jeffrey M. Keefer.)

Evidence-Based Practice boxes are found throughout the text (including this chapter) to provide the most current research that serves as a basis for nursing practice. Each of these features presents a brief summary of the research, identifies the LOE using the scale in Fig. 1.2, and concludes with a "Commentary: Implications for Practice and Research" discussion to help you apply the findings of the study to daily nursing practice.

Attributes of Evidence-Based Practice

EBP promotes ***safety*** for patients, families, staff, and health care systems because it is based on reliable studies, guidelines, consensus, and expert opinion. However, recall that a best practice identified through research or clinical practice guideline may not be consistent with the patient's or family's personal preferences or beliefs. Nurses must be patient centered and respect the values of the patient or designee at all times even if those values differ from their own or those of the interprofessional health care team.

Examples of Context of Evidence-Based Practice in Nursing and Health Care

Health care organizations receiving Medicare and/or Medicaid funding are obligated to follow the evidence-based interprofessional Core Measures to ensure that best practices are followed for selected health problems. Examples of Core Measures are included in this textbook, such as those related to heart failure, stroke, and venous thromboembolism.

In addition to complying with federal mandates and those outlined by The Joint Commission (TJC), many hospitals have achieved or are on the path to achieve the American Nurses

Credentialing Center's Magnet Recognition. This highly desired status requires nurses to demonstrate how best current evidence guides their practice. Many hospitals have nursing research departments with experts to facilitate this process. Using research to guide practice is a way to continuously improve the quality of care, as described as part of the following concept.

QUALITY IMPROVEMENT

Definition of Quality Improvement

Quality Improvement (QI), sometimes referred to as *continuous quality improvement (CQI),* is a process in which nurses and the interprofessional health care team use indicators (data) to monitor care outcomes and develop solutions to change and improve care. This process is also sometimes called the *evidence-based practice improvement (EBPI)* process because the best sources of evidence are used to support the improvement or change in practice. Therefore the primary interrelated concepts are ***evidence-based practice*** and ***safety.***

Models for Quality Improvement

When a patient care or system issue is identified as needing improvement, specific systematic QI models such as the Plan-Do-Study-Act (PDSA) or the *FOCUS-PDCA* are typically used. The steps of the PDSA model include (Connelly, 2018):

1. Identify and analyze the problem (Plan).
2. Develop and test an evidence-based solution (Do).
3. Analyze the effectiveness of the test solution, including possible further improvement (Study).
4. Implement the improved solution to positively impact care (Act).

The steps of the more specific *FOCUS-PDCA* model are:

- **F**ind a process to improve.
- **O**rganize a team.
- **C**larify the current process.
- **U**nderstand variations in current process.
- **S**elect the process to improve.
- **P**lan the improvement.
- **D**o the improvement.
- **C**heck for results.
- **A**ct to hold the gain.

An example of a QI project using the *FOCUS-PDCA* model to prevent hospital-acquired pressure injuries (HAPIs) on a medical-surgical telemetry unit is summarized in the Systems Thinking and Quality Improvement box.

Another QI method called the *DMAIC model* was translated from the business world to health care to more clearly delineate each QI step. This model includes the need to continue the new intervention or change over time. The steps of this model are:

1. **D**efine the issue or problem.
2. **M**easure the key aspects of the current process for the issue (collect data).
3. **A**nalyze the collected data.
4. **I**mprove or optimize the current process by implementing an evidence-based intervention/solution.
5. **C**ontrol the future state of the intervention to ensure continuity of the process.

SYSTEMS THINKING AND QUALITY IMPROVEMENT QSEN

Can a Medical-Surgical Unit Decrease the Incidence of HAPIs?

Amon, B. V., David, A. G., Do, V. H., Ellis, D. M., Portea, D., Tran, P., et al. (2019). Achieving 1,000 days with zero hospital-acquired pressure injuries on a medical-surgical telemetry unit. *MEDSURG Nursing, 28*(1), 17–21.

A nursing team was established on a 32-bed medical-surgical telemetry unit to develop a QI program using a bundled evidence-based practice approach to decrease hospital-acquired pressure injuries (HAPIs). Six strategies were implemented:

- Improved risk assessment
- Individualized pressure injury risk factor reduction
- Specialized skin prevention products and support services
- Early mobility
- Staff education
- Unit skin champions

The result of this QI project was achieving 1000 days (almost 2 years) with no patient developing a HAPI in the unit.

Commentary: Implications for Practice and Research

The system in this study was the medical-surgical nursing telemetry unit. The application of evidence-based practices to decrease HAPI improved system outcomes. The project needs to be repeated using a larger number of nurses working on multiple units and health care organizations.

Attributes of Quality Improvement

As a medical-surgical nurse, you will be expected to participate in the QI process on your unit or in your agency. You will need the knowledge and skills to:

- Employ a spirit of inquiry to formulate PICOT questions. The PICOT format stands for:
  - **P**opulation/**P**atient Problem (such as falls)
  - **I**ntervention (such as bed alarms to help reduce falls)
  - **C**omparison (use of reminder signage for staff instead of or in addition to bed alarms)
  - **O**utcome (fall reduction)
  - **T**ime frame (during night shift, but time may not always be relevant)
- Identify indicators (data) to monitor quality and effectiveness of health care.
- Access and evaluate data to monitor quality and effectiveness of health care.
- Recommend ways to improve care processes.
- Implement activities to improve care processes.

Examples of Context of Quality Improvement in Nursing and Health Care

This textbook features *Systems Thinking and Quality Improvement* boxes that summarize articles on QI projects and end with a "Commentary: Implications for Practice and Research" discussion. These features will help you learn how nurses participate in QI and the benefits to patients, staff, and health care systems or patient care units. Two examples of these boxes are part of this chapter. Additional information about the QI process can be found in nursing leadership and management resources.

INFORMATICS

Definition of Informatics

Although the QSEN competency includes only Informatics, this text recognizes that technology plays an equally important role in patient ***safety.*** *Informatics* is defined as the access and use of information and electronic technology to communicate, manage knowledge, prevent error, and support decision making (QSEN, 2019). Therefore the primary interrelated concepts are ***safety, evidence-based practice,*** and ***quality improvement.***

Categories of Informatics

Many health care organizations have information technology (IT) departments. The most common application of health care ***informatics*** is use of the electronic health record (EHR) (also called electronic patient record [EPR] or electronic medical record [EMR]) for documenting nursing and interprofessional care. Computers may be located at the nurses' workstation, at the patient's bedside (point of care [POC]), or near the nurses' station. Handheld mobile devices or laptops are also popular because of their ease of use and portability.

The most common application of technology is the use of devices and systems to monitor patient care and prevent errors. For example, smart infusion pumps consist of customized software that contains a drug library. The software transforms conventional infusion pumps into computers to alert nurses when medication dosing is not within acceptable parameters. These devices reduce human medication errors caused by incorrect pump settings.

Attributes of Informatics

Although ***safety*** and quality of health care are the major purposes for ***informatics,*** patient and family privacy may be at risk unless precautions are implemented. For example, staff and students may take photos of patients to show their family and friends about the health problems for which they care. In some cases these photos are posted on social media such as Facebook. *This action is a violation of patient privacy and confidentiality.*

Examples of Context of Informatics in Nursing and Health Care

A major purpose of ***informatics*** is for retrieval of data for ***evidence-based practice*** and ***quality improvement.*** the internet and intranets (internal databases) provide ways to search for multiple sources of information efficiently. However, all data sources must be evaluated for their credibility and reliability.

New technologies for patient, staff, and resource (inventory) management are used in health care agencies to promote patient ***safety*** and improve efficiency. For example, radiofrequency identification (RFID) systems allow any person or object to be tracked electronically. BCMA systems ensure that the correct medication is given to the correct patient (see Fig. 1.1).

Another example of health technology is the growing use of telehealth and telenursing. **Telehealth** is the long-distance use of electronic information and telecommunication technology to support clinical health care. **Telenursing** is a type or subset of this technology that allows nurses to provide care through the use of the Internet, telephone, computers, digital assessment tools, and telemonitoring equipment. Most patients who are monitored have chronic diseases such as heart failure and diabetes. The *Healthy People 2030* objectives include the call for a need to increase the use of telehealth to improve access to health services (www.healthypeople.gov).

Regardless of their use, nurses need to be involved in decisions about introducing new or advanced health care technologies into the health care agency or community. They should also be included in designing technology that improves the effectiveness and efficiency of health care while providing for patient and staff privacy.

CLINICAL JUDGMENT

Definition of Clinical Judgment

Clinical judgment, sometimes called nursing judgment, is an iterative process that uses nursing knowledge to observe and access presenting situations, identify a prioritized client concern, and generate the best possible evidence-based solutions in order to deliver safe client care (NCSBN, 2019). Clinical judgment, then, is the observed outcome of critical thinking and decision making (www.ncsbn.org). These solutions may be developed for individual or systems care. Therefore the primary interrelated concepts are ***evidence-based practice, systems thinking,*** and ***safety***. The nursing process, critical thinking, and a variety of reasoning patterns help the medical-surgical nurse make clinical judgments while being respectful of the patient's and family's culture and lifestyle choices. This textbook presents many *Clinical Judgment Challenges* and *NCLEX Examination Challenges* to help you practice how to make clinical judgments on the basis of the best current evidence. Chapter 2 discusses ***clinical judgment*** in more detail.

Scope of Clinical Judgment

Appropriate or "sound" ***clinical judgment*** (also referred to as *sound judgment*) leads to positive patient or staff outcomes. By contrast, inappropriate or "poor" judgment results in negative outcomes that can pose a risk to patient or staff safety. In her classic systematic review, Tanner (2006) concluded that sound ***clinical judgment*** is influenced by how well the nurse knows the patient's typical response pattern and the situational context or culture of the nursing care unit.

The worst result of poor judgment is a growing health care crisis referred to as *failure to rescue.* **Failure to rescue (FTR)** is the inability of nurses or other interprofessional health team members to save a patient's life in a timely manner when a health care issue or medical complication occurs. Patients often have beginning or subtle signs and symptoms 1 to 3 days before cardiopulmonary arrest or multiple organ failure. FTR occurs when those signs and symptoms are not noticed *(failure to recognize)* or accurately interpreted and therefore action to improve the patient's condition is not implemented *(failure to escalate)* (see the Evidence-Based Practice box).

EVIDENCE-BASED PRACTICE (QSEN)

What Is Failure to Rescue?

Musta, J., Rush, L. K., & Andersen, E. (2018). Failure to rescue as a nurse-sensitive indicator. *Nursing Forum, 53*(1), 84–92.

The researchers conducted a systematic review of the literature to analyze the concept of **failure to rescue (FTR).** Four key attributes of this concept were identified:

- Errors of omission
- Failure to recognize changes in patient condition
- Failure to communicate patient changes
- Failures in clinical decision making

The authors also found evidence that strategies which help prevent FTR include early warning system indicators, structured communication, and teamwork.

Level of Evidence: 1

This study was a systematic review and analysis of multiple research articles.

Commentary: Implications for Practice and Research

Medical-surgical nurses can play a pivotal role in preventing FTR through early recognition of and intervention for subtle changes of medical complications. Although this study was a systematic review, more studies are needed to validate best practices for preventing FTR and managing complications to prevent patient death.

Models of Clinical Judgment

According to Tanner, ***clinical judgment*** involves specific reasoning and critical thinking and includes these skills:

- Noticing
- Interpreting
- Responding
- Reflecting

The National Council of State Boards of Nursing (NCSBN) recognizes six cognitive skills or processes of ***clinical judgment*** that can be measured. These skills will serve as the basis for new types of test items on the national nursing licensure examination (NCLEX Examination) in the near future (NCSBN, 2019). In this text, each of these skills is paired with the steps of the nursing process for all exemplar health problems:

- Assessment: Recognize Cues
- Analysis: Analyze Cues and Prioritize Hypotheses
- Planning and Implementation: Generate Solutions and Take Action
- Evaluation: Evaluate Outcomes

The *Clinical Judgment Challenges* in this book will require you to apply these six skills of the NCSBN Clinical Judgment Measurement Model (NCSBN-CJMM). This model is discussed in more detail in Chapter 2.

Examples of Context of Clinical Judgment in Nursing and Health Care

Clinical judgment is needed to improve patient ***safety*** and prevent failure to rescue. Most hospitals have a Rapid Response Team (RRT), also called the *Medical Emergency Team (MET).* **Rapid Response Teams** save lives and decrease the risk for harm by providing care *before* a medical emergency occurs by intervening rapidly when needed for patients who are *beginning* to clinically decline. Members of an RRT are critical care experts who are on-site and available at any time. Although membership varies among agencies, the team may consist of an intensive care unit (ICU) nurse, respiratory therapist, intensivist (physician who specializes in critical care), and/or hospitalist (physician, physician assistant, or nurse practitioner employed by the hospital). The team responds to emergency calls, usually from clinical staff nurses, according to established agency protocols and policies. Patients' families may also activate the RRT.

The Joint Commission's **NPSGs** include the need for early intervention for patients who are clinically deteriorating. They require each health care organization to establish criteria for patients, families, or staff to call for assistance in response to an actual or perceived deterioration in the patient's condition. As a strategy to meet this requirement, many hospitals and other health care agencies use an **early warning system (EWS,** also called an early warning scoring system [EWSS]). An EWSS is a guide for the health care team to quickly determine a patient's condition on the basis of a physiologic scoring matrix.

The most commonly used type of EWS is the **modified early warning system (MEWS).** This guide is a screening and scoring tool for medical-surgical nursing assessment to determine a patient's condition based primarily on the patient's level of consciousness and respiratory rate. Declines in either of these assessments often occur about 6 to 8 hours before a cardiac or respiratory arrest. Most MEWS tools also include measurements of systolic blood pressure, temperature, heart rate, oxygen saturation, and hourly urinary output (previous 2 hours) (Race, 2015). If the patient's condition deteriorates, the MEWS score triggers the need for medical intervention usually initiated by the RRT. More information on this patient safety warning system may be found in Chapter 34 of this text.

Systems Thinking

Definition of Systems Thinking. *Systems thinking* is the ability to recognize, understand, and synthesize the interactions and interdependencies in a set of components designed for a specific purpose. In health care, the nurse must know how the components of a complex health care system influence the care of each patient (Dolansky & Moore, 2013). As part of Systems Thinking, the nurse uses the primary interrelated concepts of ***quality improvement***, ***clinical judgment***, ***evidence-based practice***, and ***patient-centered care*** whether caring for individuals, families, communities, or populations.

Scope of Systems Thinking. ***Systems thinking*** functions on a continuum from individuals to larger environmental components, such as teams, units, and organizations (Dolansky & Moore, 2013). It can transform care provided to an *individual* as a result of patient-centered care or can influence organizational transformation among *teams.* ***Systems thinking*** can also transform the entire health care *organization* as a result of "strengthening organization and clinical reasoning, facilitated decision making, and provision of improved IPP [interprofessional practice] to meet patient outcomes" (Stalter et al., 2017, p. 327).

Attributes of Systems Thinking. In their concept analysis of ***systems thinking,*** Stalter et al. (2017) identified four attributes:

- Is a dynamic system on a continuum
- Has a holistic perspective including multiple aspects
- Seeks to identify patterns within a complex situation
- Is transformative creating change through insight and action

Examples of Context of Systems Thinking in Nursing and Health Care. To promote patient ***safety*** and quality care, nurses identify individual patient or system problems and implement interventions to manage those concerns. For example, the nurse may identify a hospitalized older adult who is at an increased risk for falls. The nurse implements evidence-based interventions to prevent falls for that specific individual patient using ***clinical judgment.*** By expanding to ***systems thinking,*** the nurse may review the fall rate on the nursing unit where the patient is hospitalized and collaboratively plan interventions for all patients at risk for falls using a QI model (see earlier discussion). Further systems thinking may result in updating of policies within the facility that govern fall protocols. Chapter 2 discusses ***systems thinking*** in more detail.

ETHICS

Definition of Ethics

According to the American Nurses Association (ANA), *ethics* is "a theoretical and reflective domain of human knowledge that addresses issues and questions about morality in human choices, actions, character, and ends (ANA, 2015, p. xii). *Applied* professional nursing ***ethics*** is about considering what is right and wrong when using clinical judgment to make clinical decisions. Therefore the primary interrelated concept is ***clinical judgment.***

Categories of Ethics

Clinical decisions are either ethical or unethical and are based on one or more of six principles described under Attributes of Ethics. ***Ethics*** is also described by the type of ethics or setting in which these decisions are made. For example, *organizational* ethics refers to the ethical practices of health care organizations. Applied nursing ***ethics*** is a type of *professional* ethics used in practice by individual nurses.

Attributes of Ethics

Respect for people is the basis for six essential *ethical principles* that nurses and other health care professionals should use as a guide for clinical reasoning and judgment. Respect implies that patients are treated as autonomous individuals capable of making informed decisions about their care. This patient **autonomy** is also referred to as *self-determination* or *self-management.* When the patient is not capable of self-determination, you are ethically obligated to protect him or her as an advocate within the professional scope of practice, according to the American Nurses Association (ANA) Code of Ethics for Nurses (ANA, 2015).

The second ethical principle is **beneficence**, which promotes positive actions to help others. In other words, it encourages the nurse to do good for the patient. **Nonmaleficence** emphasizes the importance of preventing harm and ensuring the patient's well-being. Harm can be avoided only if its causes or possible causes are identified. As described earlier in this chapter, patient ***safety*** is currently a major national focus to prevent deaths and injuries.

Fidelity refers to the agreement that nurses will keep their obligations or promises to patients to follow through with care. **Veracity** is a related principle in which the nurse is obligated to tell the truth to the best of his or her knowledge. If you are not truthful with a patient, his or her respect for you will diminish and your credibility as a health care professional will be damaged.

Social justice, the last principle, refers to equality and fairness; that is, all patients should be treated equally and fairly, regardless of age, gender identity, sexual orientation, religion, race, ethnicity, or education. For example, a patient who cannot afford health care receives the same quality and level of care as one who has extensive insurance coverage. An older patient with dementia is shown the same respect as a younger patient who can communicate. A Hispanic patient who can communicate only in Spanish receives the same level of care as a Euro-American patient whose primary language is English. More information on ethics and ethical principles can be found in your fundamentals textbook.

Examples of Context of Ethics in Nursing and Health Care

Nurses and other members of the interprofessional team are involved in many ethical decisions and dilemmas in daily practice. Examples of these dilemmas include issues surrounding advance directives and aggressive treatment options.

A major resource for nurses and other members of the health care team is the health care organization's *ethics advisory committee.* This diverse group typically consists of clinicians (primary health care providers and nurses), social worker, psychologist, chaplain, attorney, quality improvement manager, and community representatives. The primary goals of the committee are to protect the rights of patients and promote fairness in shared decision making regarding ethical issues through consultation and policy development. Examples of ethical policies include informed consent, organ procurement, and withholding or withdrawing life-sustaining treatments. These issues are discussed as appropriate throughout this textbook.

NCLEX EXAMINATION CHALLENGE 1.2

Physiological Integrity

A nurse assures a client experiencing abdominal surgical pain that comfort measures, including drug therapy, will be provided as the client needs them. Which ethical principles apply in the situation? **Select all that apply.**

A. Beneficence
B. Social justice
C. Autonomy
D. Fidelity
E. Veracity

HEALTH CARE DISPARITIES

Definition of Health Care Disparities

Health care disparities are differences in access to and use of care, quality of care, and health insurance coverage (Ubri & Artiga, 2016). For many groups, they represent gaps in health care experienced by one population when compared with another as a result of numerous factors, including being members of a minority or vulnerable group. Therefore the primary interrelated concepts are ***patient-centered care*** and ***ethics.***

Categories of Health Care Disparities

A major focus of the U.S. *Healthy People 2020* initiative is to decrease ***health care disparities*** caused by poor communication, lack of health care access, inadequate health literacy, and primary health care provider biases and discrimination. The *Healthy People 2030 objectives* call for access to health services for all people (www.healthypeople.gov). Although progress has been made over the past few decades, many minority populations have a high incidence of chronic disease and mortality as a result of Health Care Disparities (Neumayer & Plumper, 2016). The National Center on Minority Health and Health Disparities of the National Institutes of Health leads and coordinates the efforts to reduce these disparities in the United States. Similar organizations in other countries exist for this same purpose.

Attributes of Health Care Disparities

Many factors affect patient access to quality health care services, including geographic location, cultural variables, and resources. For instance, some individuals live in rural areas that do not have quality health care services. In other cases the care is available, but the individual may not have transportation to get to the primary health care provider or value the need for regular preventive health care. Language barriers may also prevent the individual from accessing services. For example, many older individuals in Hispanic communities do not speak English, and most health care professionals do not speak Spanish. This communication barrier and possible mistrust of primary health care providers can prevent access to needed services.

Some individuals remain uninsured or underinsured and cannot afford health care services. "Working poor" patients may have health insurance, but their copayments are too high to seek services. Copayments for a primary health care provider office visit may be $50 or higher. Medication copayments can range from $5 to more than $100 per prescription, depending on which type of insurance the patient has. These expenses are usually not a priority over other personal financial needs such as food and rent.

Examples of Context of Health Care Disparities to Nursing and Health Care

Entire groups of people are vulnerable or likely to experience an inability to access available health care for a variety of reasons. Health care professionals may have biases and beliefs about certain cultures and groups that prevent them from being effective in developing a culturally appropriate individualized plan of care. Examples of these groups include older adults, racial and ethnic minorities, and the lesbian, gay, bisexual, transgender, and questioning/queer (LGBTQ) population.

Special Needs of Older Adults. Older adults are a growing subset of the adult population as "baby boomers" turn 60 to 70. This group of young older adults is different from previous generations as they aged. Many are working well past 65 years of age and have active social lives. Chapter 4 in this text is dedicated to the special health care needs of older adults.

Special Needs of Racial and Ethnic Minorities. Early health care research focused on promoting health or managing health problems among affluent Euro-Americans. More recent research has included implications for or differences in care based on race or ethnicity. ***Health care disparities*** have been identified as they affect various groups and populations. As mentioned earlier in this chapter, many *Patient-Centered Care: Cultural/Spiritual Considerations* features are integrated throughout this textbook to include differences in care needed to meet the special health needs of individuals from a variety of racial and ethnic groups.

Special Needs of the LGBTQ Population. Nurses today have been made aware of cultural variations and learned how to incorporate these differences to individualize patient care. However, one group that is less often addressed in the nursing literature is the LGBTQ population. This terminology is widely accepted by the LGBTQ community and is commonly used, although *LGBT* may be seen more often in health care literature. Questioning and/or queer individuals prefer not having strict labels on their sexualities or genders. Another term that may be used is *LGBTQI* to include intersex individuals. Intersex individuals have sexual or reproductive organs that are not clearly male or female at birth or may have a combination of both male and female organs.

Many studies provide evidence that LGBTQ individuals do not feel comfortable with or trust health care professionals because of previous discrimination. All patients and their families deserve a safe, trusting environment where they can receive health care with dignity (Santori, 2018). Many agencies have signage that assures patients that they are in a Safe Zone (Fig. 1.3).

The *Healthy People 2020* and *Healthy People 2030* initiatives added a category for these individuals because of access to health services in this population and the need to improve LGBTQ health. This textbook includes special health needs of this population as part of its *Patient-Centered Care: Gender Health Considerations* features. A separate chapter in this book on transgender health helps students learn about the special needs of transgender patients.

The health care system, like other facets of society, often overlooks sexualities and genders that are alternative to the mainstream of heterosexuality and clearly delineated maleness or femaleness. *As a health care professional, it is essential to not be restricted by rigid standards of identity.* A good way of rethinking concepts of ***sexuality*** and gender is to think of each as existing along a spectrum rather than categorizing people into heterosexual/homosexual and male/female.

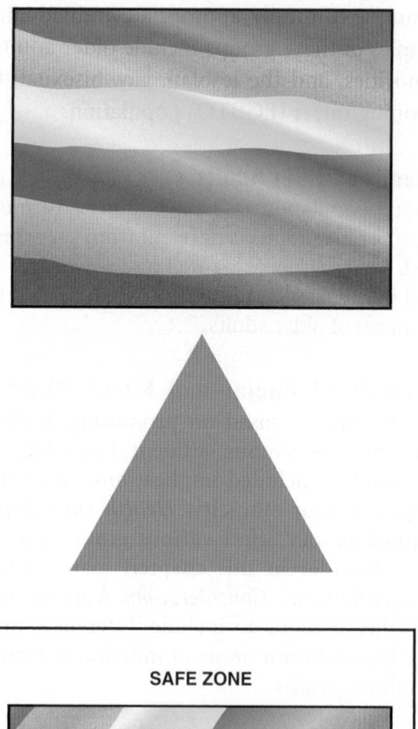

FIG. 1.3 The Safe Zone—Rainbow or Pink Triangles welcome LGBTQ patients in a health care agency.

TABLE 1.4 Recommended Patient Interview Questions About Sexual Orientation, Gender Identity, and Health Care

- Do you have sex with men, women, both, or neither?
- Does anyone live with you in your household?
- Are you in a relationship with someone who does not live with you?
- If you have a sexual partner, have you or your partner been evaluated about the possibility of transmitting infections to each other?
- If you have more than one sexual partner, how are you protecting both of you from infections such as hepatitis B, hepatitis C, or HIV?
- Have you disclosed your gender identity and sexual orientation to your primary health care provider?
- If you have not, may I have your permission to provide that information to members of the health care team who are involved in your care?
- Whom do you consider to be your closest family members?

HIV, Human immune deficiency virus.

To begin to gain trust and show respect for the LGBTQ patient, health care professionals may need to know their patient's sexual orientation and gender identity. Do not assume that every patient is heterosexual or clearly gendered. *Include questions about gender identity and sexual activity as part of your patient's health assessment.* Table 1.4 lists recommended patient interview questions about sexual orientation, gender identity, and health care.

GET READY FOR THE NEXT-GENERATION NCLEX® EXAMINATION!

Key Points

Review these Key Points for each NCLEX Examination Client Needs Category.

Safe and Effective Care Environment

- The Joint Commission requires that health care organizations create a culture of ***safety*** by following the NPSGs. **QSEN: Safety**
- RRTs save lives and decrease the risk for patient harm before a respiratory or cardiac arrest occurs. **QSEN: Safety**
- Remember to always observe for (Notice) changes in patient condition and intervene appropriately using Clinical Judgment. **Clinical Judgment; QSEN: Safety**
- A vital role of the nurse is as an advocate to empower patients and their families to have control over their health care and function as ***safety*** partners. **QSEN: Safety**
- Examples of the provisions of the ANA Code of Ethics for Nurses are listed in Table 1.3. **Ethics**
- Six essential ethical principles to consider when making clinical decisions are autonomy, beneficence, nonmaleficence, fidelity, veracity, and social justice. **Ethics**
- Nurses collaborate by communicating patients' needs and preferences with members of the interprofessional health care team to establish an individualized approach to care. **QSEN: Teamwork and Collaboration**
- The SBAR procedure or similar established method is used for successful hand-off communication between caregivers and between health care agencies. **QSEN: Safety**
- **TeamSTEPPS** A systematic communication approach for interprofessional teams designed to improve safety and quality. **QSEN: Safety, Teamwork and Collaboration**
- When delegating nursing activities, skills, or procedures to LPNs/VNs or assistive personnel (AP), the nurse is always accountable to ensure that they were performed safely and accurately. **QSEN: Safety**
- Evidence-Based Practice (EBP) is the integration of best current evidence to make decisions about patient care. It considers the patient's preferences and values and one's own clinical expertise. **QSEN: Evidence-Based Practice, Patient-Centered Care**
- Nurses are active participants in the systematic Quality Improvement (QI) process in their health care agency and used one of several QI models to improve care and promote patient safety. **QSEN: Quality Improvement**
- Informatics is used for patient documentation, electronic data access, and health care resource tracking. **QSEN: Informatics**
- Systems Thinking is the ability to recognize, understand, and synthesize the interactions and interdependencies in a set of components designed for a specific purpose. **Systems Thinking**

Psychosocial Integrity

- Nurses must show respect and compassion for the uniqueness of every individual to ensure Patient-Centered and family-centered Care. **QSEN: Patient-Centered Care**
- Health Care Disparities are differences in the access or availability of health care; members of minority groups and other vulnerable populations are particularly at risk for health disparities. **Health Care Disparities**
- The lesbian, gay, bisexual, transgender, queer and/or questioning (LGBTQ) population typically does not trust health care professionals; use sensitive questioning about sexual orientation and gender identity as part of your interview with patients in this group (see Table 1.4). **QSEN: Patient-Centered Care**

MASTERY QUESTIONS

1. The nurse provides an SBAR hand-off communication regarding a client whose blood pressure and respiratory rate have decreased. Where will the nurse include these data as part of the SBAR format?
   A. **S**ituation
   B. **B**ackground
   C. **A**ssessment
   D. **R**ecommendation
2. The nurse collaborates with the registered dietitian nutritionist to improve the nutritional status of clients on a hospital unit. Which priority professional nursing concepts apply in this situation? **Select all that apply.**
   A. Quality Improvement
   B. Ethics
   C. Health Care Disparities
   D. Systems Thinking
   E. Teamwork and Collaboration

REFERENCES

Asterisk(*) indicates a classic or definitive work on this subject.

*Academy of Medical-Surgical Nurses (AMSN). (2012). *Scope and standards of medical-surgical nursing practice* (5th ed.). Pitman, NJ: Author.

*American Nurses Association (ANA). (2015). *Code of ethics for nurses with interpretive statements.* Silver Spring, MD: Author.

Amon, B. V., David, A. G., Do, V. H., Ellis, D. M., Portea, D., et al. (2019). Achieving 1,000 days with zero hospital-acquired pressure injuries on a medical-surgical telemetry unit. *Medsurg Nursing, 28*(1), 17–21.

*Benner, P. E., Malloch, K., & Sheets, V. (2010). *Nursing pathways for patient safety.* St. Louis, MO: Elsevier.

Connelly, L. M. (2018). Overview of quality improvement. *Medsurg Nursing, 27*(2), 125–126.

Cooper, C. H., Tupper, R., & Holm, K. (2016). Interruptions during medication administration: A descriptive study. *MEDSURG Nursing, 25*(3), 186–191.

*Doane, G. H., & Varcoe, C. (2015). *How to nurse: Relational inquiry with individuals and families in changing health and health care contexts.* Philadelphia: Wolters Kluwer.

*Dusek, B., Pearce, N., Harripaul, A., & Lloyd, M. (2015). Care transitions: A systematic review of best practices. *Journal of Nursing Care Quality, 30*(3), 233–239.

*Frampton, S., Guastello, S., Brady, C., Hale, M., Horowitz, S., Smith, S. B., et al. (2008). *Patient-centered care improvement guide.* Derby, CT: Planetree.

Gaston, T., Short, N., Ralyea, C., & Casterline, G. (2016). Promoting patient safety: Results of a TeamSTEPPS® initiative. *Journal of Nursing Administration, 46*(4), 201–207.

Gerber, L. (2018). Understanding the nurse's role as a patient advocate. *Nursing, 48*(4), 55–58.

*Institute of Medicine (IOM). (2003). *Health professions education: A bridge to quality.* Washington, DC: National Academies Press.

Interprofessional Education Collaborative Expert Panel. (2016). *Core competencies for interprofessional collaborative practice: Report of an expert panel* (2nd ed.). Washington, DC: Interprofessional Education Collaborative.

*Lamb, G. (2014). *Care coordination: The game changer. Silver Spring.* MD: American Nurses Association.

McMahon, J. T. (2017). Improving medication administration safety in the clinical environment. *Medsurg Nursing, 26*(6), 374–377 409.

Melnyk, B. M., & Fineout-Overholt, E. (2019). *Evidence-based practice in nursing and healthcare* (4th ed.). Philadelphia: Walter Klowers.

Miner, M. B., Evans, M. M., & Riley, K. (2018). Using transitional care to improve the discharge process in a medical-surgical setting. *MEDSURG Nursing, 27*(1), 4–6.

Musta, J., Rush, L. K., & Andersen, E. (2018). Failure to rescue as a nurse-sensitive indicator. *Nursing Forum, 53*(1), 84–92.

National Council of State Boards of Nursing (NCSBN). (2019). The clinical judgment model. *Next Generation NCLEX News. (Winter).* 1–6.

NCSBN-ANA. (2019). *National guidelines for nursing delegation.* https://www.ncsbn.org/NGND-PosPaper_06.pdf.

Neumayer, E., & Plumper, T. (2016). Inequalities of income and inequalities of longevity: a cross-country study. *American Journal of Public Health, 106*(1), 160–165.

Quality and Safety Education for Nurses (QSEN). (2019). Competency KSAs (pre-licensure). www.qsen.org.

*Race, T. K. (2015). Improving patient safety: Modified early warning scoring system. *American Nurse Today, 10*(11).

Santori, C. A. (2018). Ethical nursing practice regarding sexual orientation, gender identification, and caring for intersex, transgender, and transitioning patients. *Medsurg Nursing, 27*(1), 7–9.

Stewart, K. R., & Hand, K. A. (2017). SBAR, communication, and patient safety: An integrated literature review. *Medsurg Nursing, 26*(5), 297–305.

*Tanner, C. A. (2006). Thinking like a nurse: A research-based model of clinical judgment in nursing. *Journal of Nursing Education, 45*(6), 204–211.

*The Joint Commission. (2013). *Transitions of care: The need for a more effective approach to continuing patient care.*

Ubri, P., & Artiga, S. (2016). *Disparities in health care health care: Five key questions and answers.*

2

Clinical Judgment and Systems Thinking

Cherie R. Rebar, Nicole M. Heimgartner

http://evolve.elsevier.com/Iggy/

LEARNING OUTCOMES

1. Discuss elements of critical thinking, clinical reasoning, and ***clinical judgment.***
2. Identify nursing actions within the National Council of State Boards of Nursing (NCSBN) Clinical Judgment Measurement Model.
3. Differentiate environments of care and roles of health care providers within the health care system.
4. Describe the process of incorporating nursing knowledge into ***systems thinking.***
5. Connect the importance of applying appropriate ***clinical judgment*** to ***systems thinking.***

KEY TERMS

clinical judgment The skill of recognizing cues about a clinical situation, generating and weighing hypotheses, taking action, and evaluating outcomes for the purpose of arriving at a satisfactory clinical outcome. Clinical judgment is the observed outcome of two unobserved underlying mental processes, critical thinking and decision making (NCSBN, 2018b).

clinical reasoning The process by which nurses collect cues, process the information, come to an understanding of a patient problem or situation, plan and implement interventions, evaluate outcomes, and reflect on and learn from the process (Levett-Jones, 2013).

critical thinking The skill of using logic and reasoning to identify the strengths and weaknesses of alternative health care solutions, conclusions, or approaches to clinical or practice problems (NCSBN, 2018b).

Evidence-Based Practice A QSEN competency in which the nurse uses the integration of the best current evidence and practices to make decisions about patient care. It considers the patient's preferences and values and the nurse's own clinical expertise for the delivery of optimal health care.

Informatics A QSEN competency in which the nurse uses information and technology to communicate, manage knowledge, mitigate error, and support decision making.

Patient-Centered Care A QSEN competency in which the nurse recognizes the patient or caregiver as the source of control and full partner in providing compassionate and coordinated care based on respect for the patient's preferences, values, and needs.

Quality and Safety Education for Nurses (QSEN) A project addressing the challenge of preparing future nurses with the knowledge, skills, and attitudes (KSAs) necessary to continuously improve the quality and safety of the health care systems in which they work. Competencies include *Patient-Centered Care, Teamwork and Collaboration, Evidence-Based Practice, Quality Improvement, Safety,* and *Informatics.*

Quality Improvement (QI) A QSEN competency in which the nurse uses indicators (data) to monitor care outcomes and develop solutions to change and improve care.

Safety A QSEN competency in which the nurse keeps the patient and staff free from harm and minimizes errors in care.

systems thinking The ability to recognize, understand, and synthesize the interactions and interdependencies in a set of components designed for a specific purpose (Dolansky & Moore, 2013).

Teamwork and Collaboration A QSEN competency in which the nurse functions effectively within nursing and interprofessional teams, fostering open communication, mutual respect, and shared decision-making to achieve quality patient care.

PRIORITY AND INTERRELATED CONCEPTS

The priority concepts for this chapter are:
- ***Clinical Judgment***
- ***Systems Thinking***

The interrelated concepts for this chapter are:
- ***Patient-Centered Care***
- ***Quality Improvement***
- ***Safety***
- ***Teamwork and Collaboration***

OVERVIEW

For over 20 years, nurses have consistently been ranked number 1 in the field of 16 of the most trusted professions, based on their demonstrated honesty and ethics (American Hospital Association, 2018). These are admirable and expected characteristics of nurses, yet just as important as the kind word and gentle touch is the ability to think through decisions that influence care and often make the difference between life and death.

Nurses are present in people's lives when they are the most vulnerable, as well as spend the longest periods of time interfacing with patients in the health care system. Caring holistically requires much more than a kind heart; it requires an elaborate body of knowledge that is used systematically, yet in a patient-centered and personalized manner, each time a nurse cares for a patient.

HEALTH CARE CONCEPTS

At one time in history, knowledge and skills, in addition to a kind heart, were sufficient for a health care provider to meet the needs of an ailing society. Nurses, as well as physicians and other members of the interprofessional health care team, could rely on their appropriate level of education and experience to deliver needed care. As newer treatment options emerged and comorbidities became more common, health care delivery systems expanded. Researchers learned that management of health conditions was no longer well served by only knowledge and experience. Additional factors have been subsequently identified that influence patient outcomes:

- *Behavioral and social determinants of health:* What "health" means to each person within the context of his or her culture, and what actions he or she is willing to take to achieve or maintain it.
- *New approaches to population health management:* Evidence-based methods to reduce health inequities and improve the health of the human population within groups, defined areas, nations, and worldwide using methods of data collection and analysis that allow health care to be proactive rather reactive. A focus on attaining, maintaining, and regaining health, as well as on best practices for improved outcomes, such as those outlined in *Healthy People 2020* and projected in the development of *Healthy People 2030.*
- *Policy and health care reform:* The view that health care is a right rather than a privilege and that individuals should be active participants in health care choices and actions.
- *Available and emerging technologies:* Use of new technologies to assess specific health risks and implement treatment plans based on personal factors rather than on a "one-size-fits-all" traditional approach to prevention and care.
- *Interprofessional practice in the form of* ***teamwork and collaboration****, an emphasis on* ***patient-centered care:*** The involvement, coordination, and respect of all members of the health care team to provide competent, precise, and personalized care to meet the needs of individual patients.
- *Shift toward systems thinking:* The recognition that health maintenance and health care activities and interventions do not occur in isolation and that a systems approach to prevention and care is more likely to have positive health outcomes than actions taken by a single provider.

Nurses and providers who think globally can better work with patients to achieve desired outcomes. Health care finance, interprofessional ***teamwork and collaboration,*** judicial ***clinical judgment*** (Skochelak & Hawkins, 2017), and ***evidence-based practice*** that drives ***quality improvement*** (Billings et al., 2016) affect these outcomes. This idea is reflected in Fig. 2.1, demonstrating that individual patient care is only the tip of an iceberg, with the systemic components under the surface supporting what can be seen immediately above the water.

INDIVIDUAL PATIENT CARE: CRITICAL THINKING, CLINICAL REASONING, AND DECISION MAKING

As nurses, we desire to see maintenance or improvement in our patients' conditions and overall sense of well-being. The evaluation of nursing care can be phrased in relationship to goals of improving health.

To arrive at a place of evaluation, this nurse must first use critical thinking and clinical reasoning to inform decision making about interventions to use with individual patients. Critical thinking "involves the skill of using logic and reasoning to identify the strengths and weaknesses of alternative health care solutions, conclusions, or approaches to clinical or practice problems" (NCSBN, 2018b). Without critical thinking, safety lapses and errors occur that can lead to harm or death (Schuelke & Barnason, 2017). The nurse's willingness to think critically is predicted by caring behaviors, self-reflection, and insight. The desire to truly help each individual patient versus simply being present to cover an assigned shift improves the clinical reasoning (Chen et al., 2018).

Critical thinking in nursing is informed by information that is directed by nursing standards and practice, as well as national competencies. A solid example that contains many of the fundamental elements of critical thinking can be found in the QSEN competencies (QSEN, 2019):

1. *Patient-Centered Care*—recognizing that the patient, with his or her own autonomy, is at the center of all decision making
2. *Safety*—designing all nursing care with the focus on safety at the forefront of planning and execution of care, both at the individual and systems level of care
3. *Evidence-Based Practice*—using the best evidence in conjunction with clinical experience and patient preference to deliver safe care

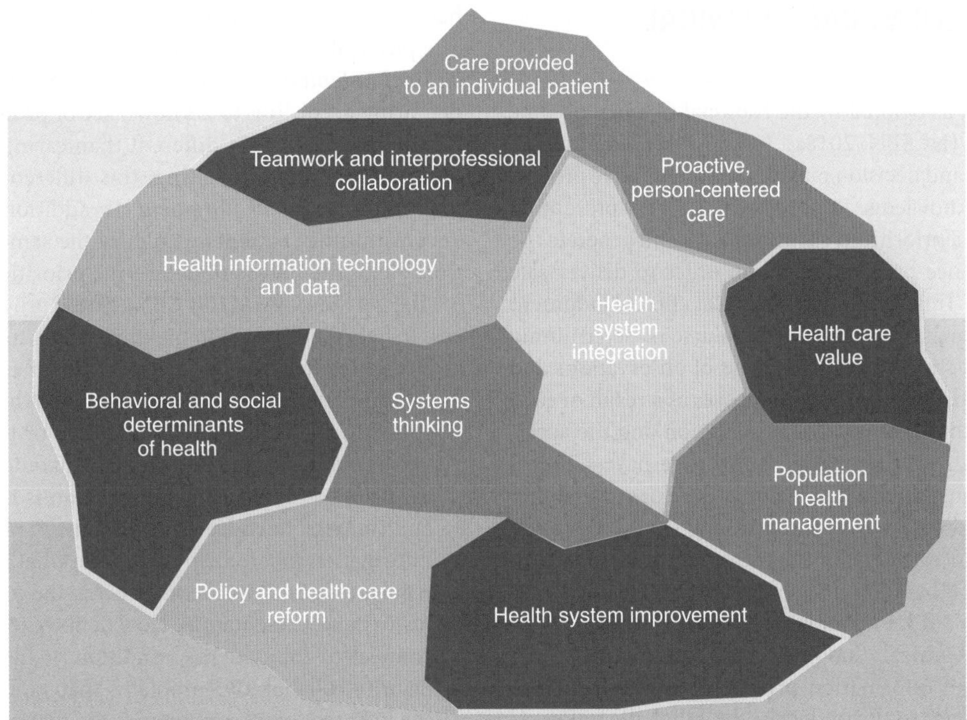

Fig. 2.1 The "Iceberg" of health care concepts impacting health. Numerous factors and concepts are often underappreciated in the provider-patient interaction within a clinic room. Traditionally, these concepts have not been included in the scope of nursing education. (From Skochelak, S., & Hawkins, R. (2017). *Health systems science*. Philadelphia, PA: Elsevier.)

4. *Informatics*—making use of the most up-to-date technology to support decision making, delivery, and documentation of care
5. *Teamwork and Collaboration*—functioning well within the interprofessional team; recognizing that shared decision making contributes to safety and quality
6. *Quality Improvement*—using data to make informed decisions to continually improve health care outcomes

Clinical reasoning is the process by which nurses collect cues, process the information, come to an understanding of a patient problem or situation, plan and implement interventions, evaluate outcomes, and reflect on and learn from the process (Levett-Jones, 2013). It takes place through a process known as ADPIE—Assessing, (Nursing) Diagnosis, Planning, Implementing, and Evaluating (Orlando, 1958, in Toney-Butler and Thayer, 2019; Alfaro-LeFevre, 2020), or AAPIE—Assessing, Analyzing, Planning, Implementing, and Evaluating.

Nursing Process	
• Assessing:	Detecting/**noticing** cues (signs, symptoms, risks)
• Analyzing:	Synthesizing and **interpreting data**; differential diagnosis (creating a list of suspected problems; weighing the probability of one problem against that of another that's closely related)
• Planning:	**Responding**; predicting complications; anticipating consequences; considering actions; setting priorities; decision making
• Implementing:	**Responding**; taking actions; monitoring responses; **reflecting**; making adjustments
• Evaluating:	**Reflecting**; repeating AAPIE as indicated

Adapted from Alfaro-LeFevre, R (2020). *Critical thinking, clinical reasoning, and clinical judgment* (7th ed). St. Louis: Elsevier.

For example, let's assume this nurse is caring for a patient who was admitted to a medical-surgical unit for ongoing dizziness. The patient requests to use the bathroom. When the nurse helps the patient to a sitting position, and then to a standing position, the patient reports feeling light-headed and is noted to seem unstable when standing. The nurse has *assessed* the situation by *noticing* cues: dizziness and instability are noted upon changing positions. At this point, the nurse begins to think through what this could mean and hypothesizes causes associated with this assessment data. The nurse recalls how low blood glucose can cause dizziness and possible instability but then considers that the patient's symptoms began upon changing position. This leads the nurse to think about the pathophysiology associated with orthostatic hypotension. In this process, the nurse has *analyzed* the data collected to *hypothesize* the possible underlying cause. In determining that this is the *most likely* cause of the patient's condition, the nurse then *plans* for management of this concern. Instead of ambulating an unsteady patient, the nurse helps the patient to a urinal or bedpan. Once the patient is safe, the nurse dialogues with the health care provider about obtaining an order for a bedside commode. The nurse *implements* the change via nursing actions by ensuring that the patient is identified as a fall risk. The nurse confirms that a fall risk bracelet is in place, educates other members of the interprofessional team about the patient's status, and *monitors* responses to make sure that these interventions are being consistently put in place. Finally, the nurse *evaluates,* or *reflects* on his or her actions to determine whether the fall risk precautions are working after being put in place. If needed, the nurse can revisit the AAPIE process to make necessary, patient-centered alterations in the plan of care.

INDIVIDUAL PATIENT CARE: CLINICAL JUDGMENT

Clinical judgment, as defined by the National Council of State Boards of Nursing (NCSBN, 2018a), is "the observed outcome of critical thinking and decision making. It is an iterative process that uses nursing knowledge to observe and access presenting situations, identify a prioritized client concern, and generate the best possible evidence-based solutions in order to deliver safe client care" (p. 12). This definition shows that clinical judgment is a continually evolving process for each nurse of determining the best course of action based on analysis of observations and presenting patient data. The process improves as a result of each new encounter with a specific patient condition and the application of the nurse's ever-increasing knowledge base. Clinical judgment is demonstrated when a nurse develops the ability to analyze collected data via critical thinking, apply reasoning to that data (which reflects clinical reasoning), and make an appropriate decision based on the context of the specific situation (Victor-Shmil, 2013, in Sommers, 2018).

The NCSBN Clinical Judgment Measurement Model (CJMM), built as an information-processing framework, was developed in response to the understanding that clinical decision making does not happen in an isolated "bubble." Context surrounding situations influences clinical judgment. Factors such as time constraints, risks, and available resources always impact choices that a nurse makes when determining how to formulate and implement a plan of care (Dickison et al., 2019, p. 12). The CJMM "represents a fundamental shift from the current dichotomous measurement models in which something is either right or wrong" (Dickison et al., 2019, p. 12), allowing for evaluation of comprehensive clinical judgment based on layers of collected information and surrounding context.

Under this model, ***clinical judgment*** can be viewed and evaluated according to four levels of information. Each time the nurse encounters a patient, assessment begins. Whether the setting is in a hospital, a health care provider's office, or in the community, the nurse begins receiving and analyzing cues based on objective and subjective assessment. Nursing analysis is heavily based on formal classroom education coupled with what has been learned in personal clinical experiences. This information becomes the foundation on which the nurse will form hypotheses, prioritize decision making, formulate solutions, and then implement nursing interventions based on the designed plan of care.

The most important part of the CJMM is that another layer—the context of the situation—considers and supports ***clinical judgment.*** The factors within this layer, such as environment, time pressure, availability or content of electronic health records, resources, and individual nursing knowledge, have a direct impact on ***clinical judgment.*** For example, the nurse will respond to a patient with an ankle fracture experienced in a mass casualty or disaster situation differently than to a patient who is in a hospital bed after surgical repair of the ankle. ***Clinical judgment*** may be affected by immediate access to a comprehensive, up-to-date electronic health record versus having to wait to document based on computer availability. The physical environment of care can also have an impact on ***clinical judgment.*** Moving within a familiar environment and operating according to a known set of protocols in a familiar facility may feel vastly different than caring for patients in an international mission setting; this difference in environment may impact ***clinical judgment.*** In addition, previous experience with other patients who have the same or similar conditions helps the nurses to determine priorities of care.

The NCSBN CJMM (NCSBN, 2018a) provides a six-step process to help guide decision making leading to ***clinical judgment.***

1. **Recognize Cues.** Cues are elements of assessment and data that provide important information. What data are *relevant* (directly related to patient outcomes or the priority of care) versus *irrelevant* (unrelated to patient outcomes or priority of care)? What assessment information is the most important and immediate concern to the nurse? Identify the relevant information *first* to help determine what is most important.
2. **Analyze Cues.** Consider the cues in the context of the patient history and presentation. How do the cues (assessment data) connect to the patient's condition or history? Think about priority collaborative problems that support and contradict the information presented in this situation.
3. **Prioritize Hypotheses.** Consider all possibilities and determine their urgency and risk for the patient. What will happen? Which possible outcomes present the greatest concern?
4. **Generate Solutions.** Use the hypothesis to develop expected outcomes. What interventions will lead to the expected outcomes? What interventions should be *avoided* or are *potentially harmful?* Determine the desired outcomes first to help decide which interventions are appropriate.
5. **Take Action.** Use nursing interventions to address the highest priorities of care and indicate how these will be performed. Consider additional assessment, health teaching, documentation, requested health care provider orders or prescriptions, nursing skills, interprofessional collaboration, etc.
6. **Evaluate Outcomes.** Consider patient outcomes in relation to expected outcomes. What signs indicate an improvement, decline, or unchanged patient condition?

The steps within the CJMM reflect multiple models of care including the nursing process and Tanner's Model of Clinical Judgment (Tanner, 2006). The nursing process includes (1) assessment, which corresponds to recognizing and analyzing cues; (2) diagnosis, which corresponds to prioritization of hypotheses; (3) planning, which corresponds to generating solutions; (4) interventions, which correspond to taking action; and (5) evaluation, which corresponds with evaluating outcomes. Tanner's Model (2006) uses patterns of noticing, interpreting, responding, and reflecting, which you will see exhibited in the concept exemplars throughout this book. The NCSBN has also created an action model to help bridge the gap between what is being measured and what is being taught in nursing education. The action model reflects components of behavior that meld textbook knowledge with clinical skills and critical thinking, resulting in the nurse's clinical judgment (NCSBN, 2019). See the Rebar-Heimgartner Model and Theory Comparison graph (Fig. 2.2).

Model/Theory	Components					
NCSBN Clinical Judgment Measurement Model	Recognize Cues	Analyze Cues	Prioritize Hypotheses	Generate Solutions	Take Action	Evaluate Outcomes
Nursing Process (AAPIE)	Assessment	Analysis		Planning	Implementation	Evaluation
Tanner Model	Noticing	Interpreting		Responding		Reflecting

Fig. 2.2 The Rebar-Heimgartner Model and Theory Comparison graph. (Copyright © 2018.)

Throughout the text, the authors have included Clinical Judgment Challenges to help you actively apply the CJMM to clinical scenarios. In the following example, a Clinical Judgment Challenge is presented along with guided answers.

CLINICAL JUDGMENT CHALLENGE 2.1

Patient-Centered Care; Clinical Judgment

A 27-year-old female client with spina bifida with a history of pressure injuries is sent to the hospital by the home health registered nurse who visits once every 2 weeks. The client has a temperature of 101.9°F and multiple stage 2 pressure injuries on her buttocks. The client is allergic to penicillin and has seasonal allergies to mold. During assessment, the client states, "I don't have a life and I can't work, so I don't have any money." The client appears disheveled and is noted to have body odor.

1. **Recognize Cues:** What assessment information in this client situation is the most important and of immediate concern for the nurse? (Hint: Identify the **relevant** information *first* to help you determine what is most important.)
2. **Analyze Cues:** What client conditions are consistent with the **most relevant** information? (Hint: Think about priority collaborative problems that support and contradict the information presented in this situation.)
3. **Prioritize Hypotheses:** Which possibilities or explanations are **most likely** to be present in this client situation? Which possibilities or explanations are the most serious? (Hint: Consider all possibilities and determine their urgency and risk for this client.)
4. **Generate Solutions:** What actions would most likely achieve the desired outcomes for this client? Which actions should be **avoided** or are **potentially harmful?** (Hint: Determine the desired outcomes first to help decide which actions are appropriate and those that should be avoided.)
5. **Take Action:** Which actions are the most appropriate and how should they be implemented? In what **priority order** should they be implemented? (Hint: Consider health teaching, documentation, requested health care provider orders or prescriptions, nursing skills, collaboration with or referral to health team members, etc.)
6. **Evaluate Outcomes:** What client assessment would indicate that actions were **effective**? (Hint: Think about signs that would indicate an improvement, decline, or unchanged client condition.)

THE HEALTH CARE SYSTEM: ENVIRONMENT OF CARE

Primary Health Care

In order to gain a full understanding and appreciation for **systems thinking,** and how the nurse functions within this continuum, you first must understand the components that contribute to the system. Primary care is perhaps the most recognizable form of care provided, as this serves as a point of entry into the health care system for many people (Shi & Singh, 2019). This is the traditional venue in which a patient first encounters a primary care provider who becomes a "gatekeeper" for the patient's care (Shi & Singh, 2019). Although primary care may look different in various parts of the world, the central theme is the same: initial and essential care afforded to everyone. The World Health Organization (WHO, 2019) states that primary care ranges from prevention to management of chronic health conditions and involves three main areas:

- Empowered people and communities
- Multisectoral policy and action
- Primary care and essential public health functions

Inpatient Care

An inpatient stay involves overnight care of 24 hours or greater in a health care facility such as a hospital (Shi & Singh, 2019). This stay may be for observational or monitoring purposes or to actively care for an injury, illness, or other health condition. The largest portion of U.S. national health care spending continues to be directed toward hospitals (Shi & Singh, 2019), despite efforts to shift care to wellness and health promotion and community-based care.

Community Health Care

Community health care has two branches: community-oriented primary care (COPC) and community-based care. COPC exists in some countries outside of the United States and incorporates the model of primary care delivery with a population-based approach. A barrier to implementation in the United States is the lack of clear direction regarding what constitutes a community and how far reaching that definition should be (Shi & Singh, 2019).

Community-based care, a model that is very common in the United States, continues to grow in function and outreach. See Box 2.1 for types of community-based care systems.

Managed Care

The 1990s saw the rise of managed care within the United States. This type of organized delivery of care provides members with needed health services where costs have been determined by the managed care company and health care providers (Shi & Singh, 2019). Even the most recent sweeping health care reform of the Affordable Care Act of 2010 did not do away with the managed care system, which continues to dominate the U.S. health care system (Shi & Singh, 2019).

NCLEX EXAMINATION CHALLENGE 2.1

Safe and Effective Care Environment: Management of Care

Which environments of care will the nurse recognize as components of the health care system? **Select all that apply.**

A. Long-term care
B. Primary care
C. Free-standing emergency department
D. National League of Nursing
E. Patient-centered medical home
F. World Health Organization

BOX 2.1 Types of Community-Based Care in the United States

- Private medical practices
- Hospital-based (outpatient) services such as support groups and health information workshops
- Freestanding points of care, such as small emergency departments, urgent care, or ambulatory surgery facilities
- Retail clinics, such as "minute clinics" located inside drug stores or other retailers
- Mobile medical, diagnostic, and screening services
- Home health care
- Hospice services
- Ambulatory long-term care services
- Public health services
- Community health centers
- Free clinics
- Telehealth access

Medical Home

Medical homes may be visualized as a type of primary care home for Americans (Grumbach & Bodenheimer, 2002). First introduced in 1967, the medical home was developed to meet the needs of ill children whose health care required constant coordination (Shi & Singh, 2019). Today, a medical home serves to decrease fragmentation of care for patients with ongoing health needs. The patient-centered medical home (PCMH) consists of an interprofessional health care team who continually communicate with the patient and family members to ensure that comprehensive care is delivered. Assessment of the medical home is based on The Joint Commission's Primary Care Medical Home Designation Standards and other initiatives (Burton et al., 2012, in Shi & Singh, 2019) and contains these elements:

- Key domains of care including access
- Culturally competent communication
- Care comprehensiveness
- Care continuity
- Patient engagement and self-care
- Coordination of care
- Care planning
- Population management
- Team-based care
- Evidence-based care
- Quality measurement and improvement
- Community resources
- Medical records
- Health information technology
- Congruence between patient and practice

BOX 2.2 Types of Long-Term Care Services (Offered in the United States)

- Private medical practices
- Nursing care
- Rehabilitation care
- Mental health
- Dementia care
- Social support
- Respite care
- End-of-life care

Long-Term Care

Long-term care is a complex system that exists within a larger system of the U.S. health care delivery system (Shi & Singh, 2019). Care received in the long-term setting is highly individualized and well coordinated to help provide partial or total care for a period of time, sometimes indefinitely. Common examples of long-term care services include rehabilitation care and dementia care. Other examples are shown in Box 2.2.

THE HEALTH CARE SYSTEM: ROLE OF THE INTERPROFESSIONAL HEALTH CARE TEAM

The health care system is composed of numerous types of health care professionals who provide services throughout the system. While you are likely familiar with many members of the health care team, it is important to consider each collaborative role in the context of the system as a whole. It is also important to consider each main profession as it fits into the health care system. Nursing is a perfect example to consider. Within the profession, there are licensed practical nurses, registered nurses, nurse practitioners, clinical nurse specialists, nurse anesthetists, and others with various certifications. Think about how these types of nurses contribute to the body of the profession of nursing and then how the profession of nursing contributes to the system in which patients receive care.

Physicians, physician assistants, and nurse practitioners focus their practice on identifying the cause of health care problems and treating them accordingly. This process includes physical examination and may include ordering of diagnostic tests, followed by prescribing methods of treating the condition. Although their roles are similar, the approach of physicians and physician assistants differs from the approach of nurse practitioners. Physicians and physician assistants are educated in, and practice according to, a medical model that applies knowledge of anatomy, biochemistry, histology, and pathology to identify and treat conditions (Fawcett, 2017). Nurse practitioners are educated in, and practice according to, a nursing model. This emphasizes patient-centered care that involves promotion of health and wellness, and quality of life across the lifespan, even when treating conditions that deviate from the expected norm (Fawcett, 2017).

Nurses of various levels of preparation, ranging from licensed practical nurses to those prepared at a doctoral level, are involved in direct care of patients throughout the health care system. Nurse practitioners, certified nurse midwives, clinical nurse specialists, and certified registered nurse anesthetists are all recognized as advanced practice nurses (APRNs) (American Nurses Association [ANA], 2018). APRNs have their own scope of practice that extends beyond the scope of the registered nurse (RN). The scope of practice for the RN, which is determined by each state, includes the who, what, where, when, and why of nursing practice (Table 2.1).

TABLE 2.1 RN Scope of Practice Elements

Who	RNs who are educated and titled and maintain licensure
What	"Nursing is the protection, promotion, and optimization of health and abilities; prevention of illness and injury; facilitation of healing; alleviation of suffering through the diagnosis and treatment of human response; and advocacy in the care of individuals, families, groups, communities, and populations" (ANA, n.d., para. 2).
Where	Wherever there is a patient who is in need of care
When	When there is a need for nursing knowledge, compassion, and the holistic provision of care
Why	Nursing exists to promote positive patient outcomes in keeping with the holistic approach of nursing as an art and a science

American Nurses Association, n.d. Scope of Practice.

There are many other members of the interprofessional health care team that the nurse will work with on a regular basis. It is important to consider these team members and their role within the context of the health care system. While the nursing role is very important, consulting other team members can be equally important in the provision of quality patient care in a complex health care system. See Table 2.2 for "Examples of Interprofessional Health Care Team Members."

NCLEX EXAMINATION CHALLENGE 2.2

Safe and Effective Care Environment: Management of Care

What is the generalist registered nurse's role related to patient care within a system? **Select all that apply.**

1. Caring
2. Teaching
3. Collaborating
4. Advocating
5. Researching
6. Prescribing

TABLE 2.2 Interprofessional Health Care Team Members

Profession	Role
Physician (MD/DO) Physician Assistant (PA)	Examines patients; takes medical histories; prescribes medications; and orders, performs, and interprets diagnostic tests (Bureau of Labor Statistics, U.S. Department of Labor, 2019b). Care is provided according to a medical model of delivery.
Advanced Practice Nurse (APRN)	Diagnoses and treats patients according to a nursing model at an advanced level within the nursing scope of practice. According to the APRN Consensus Model, these roles include certified nurse midwife, clinical nurse specialist, certified registered nurse anesthetist, and certified nurse practitioner (NCSBN, 2018a)
Registered Nurse (RN)	Practices professional nursing as defined by individual state's board of nursing; performs roles of caring, teaching, collaborating, advocating, and researching.
Assistive Personnel (AP)	Umbrella term including paraprofessionals who assist individuals with ADLs and provide care—including basic nursing procedures—all under the supervision of a registered nurse, licensed practical nurse, or other licensed health care professional (American Nurses Association, 2012).
Occupational/Physical Therapist (OT/PT)	OT: Helps patients develop, recover, improve, and maintain ADLs through therapy (Bureau of Labor Statistics, U.S. Department of Labor, 2019c). PT: Uses treatment techniques to promote movement, reduce pain, restore function, and prevent disability (American Physical Therapy Association, 2019).
Speech/Language Pathologist (SLP)	Assesses, diagnoses, treats, and helps to prevent communication and swallowing disorders. (Bureau of Labor Statistics, U.S. Department of Labor, 2019e).
Registered Dietitian Nutritionist (RDN)	A food and nutrition expert who educates individuals about nutrition and healthy eating habits. They may administer medical nutrition therapy and manage food service operations in a system (Academy of Nutrition and Dietetics, n.d.)
Licensed Social Worker (LSW)	Helps people solve and cope with problems in their everyday lives (Bureau of Labor Statistics, U.S. Department of Labor, 2019d).
Pharmacist (PharmD)	Dispenses prescription medications and offer expertise in the safe use of drugs. (Bureau of Labor Statistics, U.S. Department of Labor, 2019a).
Respiratory Therapist (RT)	Treats breathing disorders, manages ventilators and artificial airways, and educates about lung disease (American Association for Respiratory Care, 2019).
Radiography Technologist	Captures images of internal organs, soft tissues, and bones using x-ray equipment (American Registry of Radiologic Technologists, n.d.)

Understanding the role of the nurse and how the nursing profession fits into the overall health care system is an important step in visualizing the system as a whole. Consider the nursing role as an individual piece of a puzzle, which, when combined collaboratively with other puzzle pieces (members of the interprofessional team), produces a well-defined image. This is the goal of interprofessional care and creates a solid foundation for *systems thinking.*

THE NEED FOR SYSTEMS THINKING

Nursing is a profession that values the individual. We place a high degree of importance on personalization of patient care. Nurses recognize that although the same physiological or psychosocial disorder can have similar impacts on patient populations, the uniqueness of each person's physiological or psychosocial makeup affects the ways we design individualized care.

Traditionally, nurses have been taught to focus on the practice of individualized care of the patient (Dolansky & Moore, 2013). This focus was based on the development of critical thinking skills and provides a strong foundation on which nurses could plan individualized care for the patient immediately in front of them. However, as disease comorbidity increases, patients live longer due to innovations in treatment. Points of care continue to grow and change, creating a need for the nurse to continue to think about the individual patient, yet within an evolving system of care.

Stalter and Mota (2018) present the analogy of a single pebble dropping into water and creating widespread ripples on the water surface and below to explain how the nurse's individual actions and awareness can influence and shape the greater context of the health care system. By applying systems thinking to nursing actions for an individual patient issue, nurses can assess for root problems that create or intensify the issue and involve appropriate health care team members to plan and implement evidence-based practices to reduce or prevent the issue system wide. This approach to care reinforces the nurse's role in ***safety*** and ***quality improvement*** while expanding ***clinical judgment*** to include the patient's place within the greater health care system in the context of care decisions.

A good place to start developing ***systems thinking*** is to consider individual nursing actions and relationships within a nursing unit. For example, an individual staff nurse recognizes that effective oral care can dramatically decrease the incidence of ventilator-associated pneumonia (VAP) (Gupta et al., 2016). Because of this knowledge, the nurse follows the protocol closely to provide consistent oral care. ***Systems thinking*** encourages the nurse to look beyond this individual action for additional or enhanced methods to promote ***safety*** and increase ***quality improvement***. To increase compliance with oral care protocols, the nurse places a sign over the patient's bed as a reminder for other nurses to perform oral care. The nurse then decides to bring forward new research related to the prevention of VAP through the use of oral chlorhexidine rinse to the unit staff meeting (Guler & Turk, 2018). The other nurses on the unit may then begin to discuss potential barriers to prevention of VAP, as well as explore methods to decrease incidence within the nursing unit (Atashi et al., 2018). Rates of VAP at the unit level could then be compared with organizational rates of other units within the organization. Analysis of this data may lead to goals and policy changes that could then be enacted to improve patient outcomes.

This progression from clinical judgment used by an individual staff nurse, to systematic change throughout a health care system, reflects ***systems thinking.***

In the process of critical thinking and decision making, with the nurse and patient always at the center, the nurse considers influencers that guide care (Fig. 2.3). These influencers, as noted earlier in the section entitled Health Care Concepts, exist within the system of care and impact clinical judgment. They include:

- Complexity of care
- Interprofessional practice

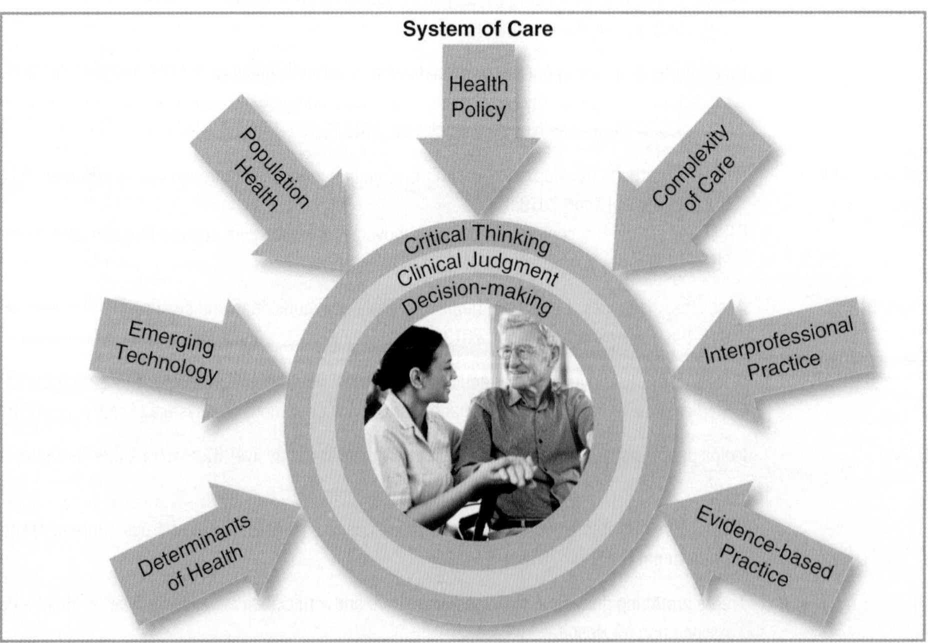

Fig. 2.3 Influencers on clinical judgment within a system of care. (Copyright © Heimgartner and Rebar, 2019.)

- Evidence-based practice
- Determinants of health
- Population health
- Emerging technology
- Health policy

Examples of ways in which these influencers impact the nurse's critical thinking, clinical reasoning, and decision making about a patient cared for in a health system are listed in Table 2.3.

Remember that systems can exist locally, nationally, or globally. Current evidence indicates that continued research is needed to implement ***systems thinking*** across international borders to influence global health (Phillips et al., 2018). Fig. 2.4 demonstrates the Systems-Based Continuum of Care that can begin at any level and influence evaluation of best practices that impact ***safety*** and quality of care within surrounding systems. There are times when ***systems thinking*** will start with care of an individual patient with a specific problem or need. This leads to an awareness of how individual nursing actions within the context of an organization inform practice and policy. Other times, national initiatives, such as Quality and Safety Education for Nurses (QSEN, 2019), inform best practice at multiple levels within the systems-based continuum of care.

Included within Fig. 2.4 are factors that influence outcomes with each of the identified systems of care. For example, at a global level, the trend toward enhancement of population health influences outcomes by placing emphasis on care of many who have similar needs. Similarly, at the national level,

TABLE 2.3 Influences on Critical Thinking and Decision Making

Influencer	Impact on Critical Thinking and Decision Making
Complexity of care	Is the patient's present condition managed or unmanaged? How long has the patient been living with this condition, or is this a new concern? Is there presence of comorbid conditions? If present, are the patient's comorbid conditions managed or unmanaged?
Interprofessional practice	Are members of the interprofessional team available in this environment of care and, if so, which one(s)? What are the schedules of interprofessional team members? (e.g., some environments of care may not have certain specialties staffed on weekends)
Evidence-Based Practice (EBP)	Is there access to evidence-based research available? What level of comfort does the nurse have with seeking and applying evidence?
Determinants of health	What are the physical determinants of health that impact this patient? • Natural environment, such as plants, weather, or climate change • Built environment, such as buildings or transportation • Worksites, schools, and recreational settings • Housing, homes, and neighborhoods • Exposure to toxic substances and other physical hazards • Physical barriers, especially for people with disabilities • Aesthetic elements, such as good lighting, trees, or benches What are the social determinants of health that affect this patient? • Availability of resources to meet daily needs, such as educational and job opportunities, living wages, or healthful foods • Social norms and attitudes, such as discrimination • Exposure to crime, violence, and social disorder, such as the presence of trash • Social support and social interactions • Exposure to mass media and emerging technologies, such as the Internet or cell phones • Socioeconomic conditions, such as concentrated poverty • Quality schools • Transportation options • Public safety • Residential segregation (Determinants of health taken from *Healthy People 2020* https://www.healthypeople.gov/2020/about/foundation-health-measures/Determinants-of-Health)
Population health	How does the shift toward population health impact the care of this patient? What access to care does the patient have within the system? Does the interprofessional health care team embrace involvement of the patient in his or her own care? What lessons can be learned from this patient that could impact the health of a population with similar needs?
Emerging technology	How does the availability of technology in this environment impact the ability to address the patient's needs? What is the comfort level of health care providers and the nurse in using available technology in the care of patients?
Health policy	What local, state, and/or federal health policies affect this patient? (e.g., increasing taxes on tobacco products implemented at the state level may decrease the patient's ability or desire to purchase cigarettes, which could improve respiratory function and elongate life span)

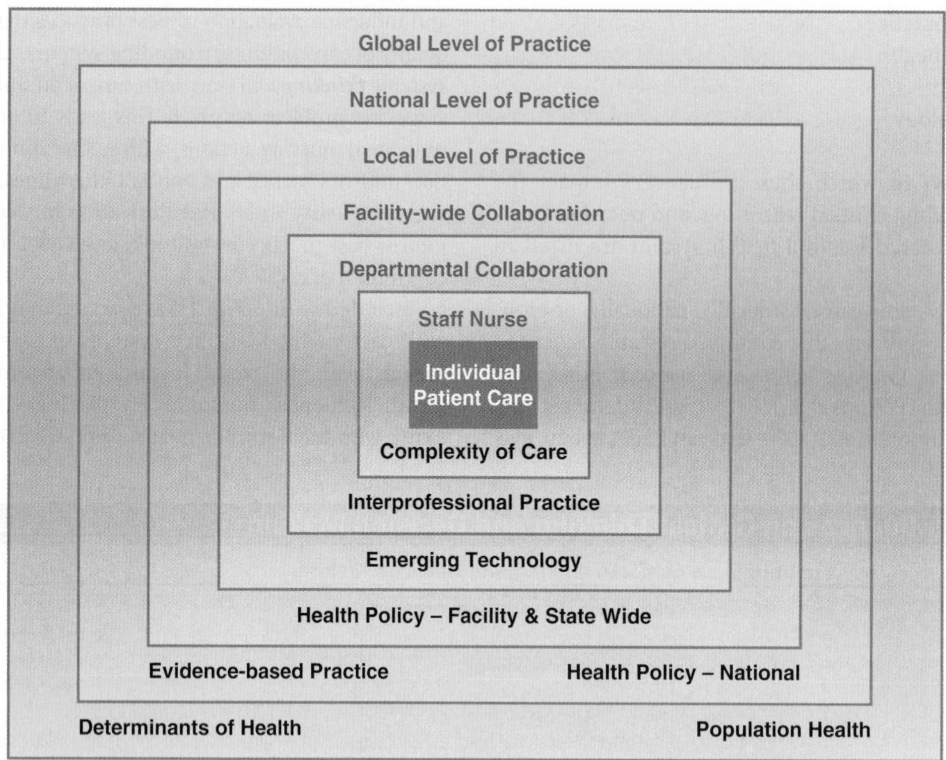

Fig. 2.4 The Heimgartner-Rebar Systems-Based Continuum of Care (Copyright © 2018).

movements toward consistent application of evidence-based practice (like clinical guidelines) influence outcomes by standardizing and delivering best practices, and health policy enacted at a national level (e.g., the Affordable Care Act) influences outcomes by attempting to bring equity to individuals by offering coverage options to all. At the level of departmental collaboration, the amount and quality of interprofessional practice influence outcomes; if health care providers work in silos, care is compartmentalized, whereas if they work in partnership as part of an interprofessional team, patient care is more comprehensive and outcomes are shown to be more favorable.

MOVING FROM CLINICAL JUDGMENT TO SYSTEMS THINKING

While this process of thinking of the patient's place within health care systems may seem complicated, it is actually quite simple. The goal of ***systems thinking*** is to encourage the nurse to develop awareness of the interrelationships that exist between individual care and the overall context of health care ***safety*** and ***quality improvement***. "Nurses must be able to take action to address potential or ongoing ***quality improvement*** and ***safety*** concerns" (Stalter & Mota, 2018, p. 35). Personal effort—the desire to care—and ***clinical judgment*** are crucial elements that lead to the process of ***systems thinking,*** which is essential for today's practicing nurse (Chen et al., 2018; Stalter et al., 2017). In the example regarding prevention of VAP, the nurse needed an awareness that oral care guidelines were developed based on actual evidence that promote quality, as well as an understanding that individual care or lack thereof can affect the overall system. Consider again the image of the iceberg presented in Fig. 2.1. Nursing actions or visible care provided to an individual patient are just the tip of the iceberg. The unseen behaviors and interventions, which are driven by critical thinking, clinical reasoning, and decision making that inform ***clinical judgment,*** help to shape the whole system and its outcomes. ***Quality improvement*** initiatives are examples of behaviors that are often unseen yet lead to changes in visible care for individual patients, which can shape evidence throughout the system.

Understanding the independent yet interdynamic functions of systems helps the nurse to better problem solve, determine priorities of care settings, delegate, act, interact, and collaborate while making important nursing decisions that affect the patient's immediate, as well as long-term, well-being and outcomes (Dolansky & Moore, 2013). The QSEN (2019) initiative has shaped the process of providing effective nursing care while applying the competencies of ***patient centered care,*** *evidence-based practice,* ***safety, quality improvement, informatics,*** and ***teamwork and collaboration*** that are integral to daily nursing practice. At present, these competencies are most often demonstrated in practice at the individual level. The full effect on health outcomes will only be realized through systematic implementation, which requires ***systems thinking*** (Dolansky & Moore, 2013). As a result, the QSEN Institute RN-BSN taskforce has recommended that systems-based practice be added as a practice competency (Stalter et al., 2017). The Massachusetts Nurse of the Future (NOF) Core Nursing Competencies has already identified systems-based practice as a core competency for the registered nurse (Massachusetts Department of Higher Education Nursing Initiative, 2016).

Further, ***systems thinking*** and systems-based practice connect directly to the *Essentials* of baccalaureate nursing education as developed by the American Association of Colleges of Nursing (2008). Nurses are considered the frontrunners within the health care system and, as such, have a responsibility to model the way forward in terms of demonstrating ***clinical judgment*** and ***systems thinking*** to shape today's practice environment (Stalter et al., 2017).

SYSTEMS THINKING AND QUALITY IMPROVEMENT QSEN

Catheter-Associated Urinary Tract Infection (CAUTI) Prevention

Scanlon, K., Wells, C., Woolforde, L., Khameraj, A., & Baumgartner, J. (2017). Saving lives and reducing harm: A CAUTI reductionprogram. *Nursing Economics, 35*(3), 134–141.

The Centers for Medicare and Medicaid Services (CMS), along with the Joint Commission, have identified hospital-acquired infection (HAI) as a priority safety issue. Urinary tract infections, specifically those that are associated with an indwelling urinary catheter (known as catheter-associated urinary tract infections [CAUTIs]), contribute to a significant percentage of HAIs. There are 13,000 CAUTI-related deaths each year, with associated annual costs over $500 million.

Because of the significant impact to patient ***safety***, as well as the extensive and unnecessary financial burden, prevention of CAUTI is imperative. One hospital system developed an interprofessional process that began with the individual patient and then progressed throughout the health care network to reduce the CAUTI rate. Entry points for patients at higher risk for CAUTI were identified with target areas of the emergency department, operating room, postanesthesia unit, and critical care units. Part of the process included educating CAUTI ambassadors or "champions," which were registered nurses who were the clinical army in the consistent use of a proven, effective algorithm for standardized treatment protocols. This action was combined with interprofessional rounds and a monthly "root cause" committee that evaluated every CAUTI incidence to analyze areas for improvement. Over a 12-month period, using this process, this hospital system demonstrated a 46% decrease in the incidence of CAUTI, which resulted in an estimated $62,396 savings. This process also made a significant change in employees by demonstrating their efforts and renewing their passion for transforming front-line care.

Commentary: Implications for Systems Thinking and Quality Improvement

This study shows the impact that nurses can have when system-level thinking is implemented. This study began with nurses who saw an issue (health care–associated infections) in their respective patients. These nurses used bedside data to identify trends within their unit that were then compared with the rest of the hospital and national standards. These data were used to benchmark a change in practice that ultimately created a measurable increase in patient ***safety*** and financial responsibility in the context of quality care.

GET READY FOR THE NEXT-GENERATION NCLEX® EXAMINATION!

Key Points

Review these Key Points for each NCLEX Examination Client Needs Category.

Safe and Effective Care Environment

- Interprofessional care, coordination, and respect for all members of the health care team are essential elements of provision of competent, precise, and personalized care for each individual patient. **QSEN: Teamwork and Collaboration**
- Health interventions do not occur in isolation; a systems approach to care yields better health outcomes. **QSEN: Teamwork and Collaboration**
- Critical thinking, clinical reasoning, and clinical judgment are essential skills that nurses must have to provide safe and effective care. **QSEN: Safety**
- Clinical judgment is informed by recognizing and analyzing cues, prioritizing hypotheses, generating solutions, taking action, and evaluating outcomes. **QSEN: Evidence-Based Practice**
- Care takes place in multiple environments, ranging from the acute care setting, to the community, to the home. **QSEN: Safety**
- The interprofessional team consists of health care providers, nurses, therapists, assistive personnel, speech/language pathologists, registered dietitian nutritionists, social workers, pharmacists, and radiography technologists. **QSEN: Teamwork and Collaboration**
- Systems thinking encourages the nurse to look beyond actions taken to care for individual patients and moving that information into additional or enhanced methods that promote overall safety and increase quality. **QSEN: Safety; Quality Improvement**

Health Promotion and Maintenance

- Behavioral determinants of health influence what "health" means to a person and what actions he or she is willing to take to achieve of maintain it. **QSEN: Patient-Centered Care**
- Population health management is reflected within evidence-based methods to reduce health inequities and improve health of the human population in various locations worldwide **QSEN: Evidence-Based Practice**
- Individuals should be active participants in their own healthcare choices and actions. **QSEN: Patient-Centered Care**

Psychosocial Integrity

- Social determinants of health also influence what "health" means to a person, and what actions he or she is willing to take to achieve of maintain it. **QSEN: Patient-Centered Care**

MASTERY QUESTIONS

1. The nurse is participating in a unit meeting to discuss daily nursing care expectations. Which nursing statement reflects systems level thinking?
   A. "It is important to provide care consistent with the client's expectation."
   B. "I will always consider my client's cultural preferences when delivering care."
   C. "I have been comparing our rates of infection with other units in the hospital."
   D. "I will look for the policy about family visitation to show my client."
2. Which nursing action reflects implementation of systems level thinking?
   A. Conducting a skin assessment on a newly admitted client
   B. Documenting a pressure injury in the electronic health record
   C. Notifying the health care provider of a 2″ × 1″ pressure injury on the coccyx
   D. Participating in a quality improvement project about eliminating pressure injury occurrences
3. How will the experienced nurse explain systems thinking to a new nurse?
   A. Reading a journal article to enhance one's understanding of a specific disorder
   B. Providing patient-centered care to each individual, recognizing his or her uniqueness
   C. Engaging in a professional development activity to earn continuing education credit
   D. Using information from individual client care to improve outcomes at a macro level

REFERENCES

Asterisk (*) indicates a classic or definitive work on this subject.

Academy of Nutrition and Dietetics. (n.d.). *What is a registered dietitian nutritionist?*. https://www.eatrightpro.org/about-us/what-is-an-rdn-and-dtr/what-is-a-registered-dietitian-nutritionist.

Alfaro-LeFevre, R. (2020). *Critical thinking, clinical reasoning, and clinical judgment* (7th ed). St. Louis: Elsevier.

American Association of Colleges of Nursing. (2008). *The essentials of baccalaureate nursing education for professional nursing practice.* http://www.aacnnursing.org/Portals/42/Publications/BaccEssentials08.pdf.

American Association for Respiratory Care. (2019). *What is an RT?*. http://www.aarc.org/careers/what-is-an-rt/.

American Hospital Association. (2018). *Nurse watch: Nurses again top Gallup poll of trusted professions and other nurse news.* https://www.aha.org/news/insights-and-analysis/2018-01-10-nurse-watch-nurses-again-top-gallup-poll-trusted-professions.

American Nurses Association. (2012*). *ANA's principles for delegation by registered nurses to unlicensed assistive personnel (UAP).* https://www.nursingworld.org/~4af4f2/globalassets/docs/ana/ethics/principlesofdelegation.pdf.

American Nurses Association ANA. (2018). *Advanced practice registered nurse. APRN.* https://www.nursingworld.org/practice-policy/workforce/what-is-nursing/aprn/.

American Nurses Association (ANA). (n.d.). *Scope of practice.* https://www.nursingworld.org/practice-policy/scope-of-practice/.

American Physical Therapy Association. (2019). *Who are physical therapists?*. http://www.apta.org/AboutPTs/.

American Registry of Radiologic Technologists. (n.d.). *Radiography.* https://www.arrt.org/about/about-us.

Atashi, V., Yousefi, H., Mahjobipoor, H., & Yazdannik, A. (2018). The barriers to the prevention of ventilator-associated pneumonia from the perspective of critical care nurses: A qualitative descriptive study. *Journal of Clinical Nursing, 27*, e1161–e1170. https://doi.org/10.1111/jocn.14216.

Billings, D., Kowalski, K., & Phillips, J. (2016). Integrating systems thinking into nursing education. *The Journal of Continuing Education in Nursing, 47*(9).

Bureau of Labor Statistics, U.S. Department of Labor. (2019a). *Occupational outlook handbook. Pharmacists.* https://www.bls.gov/ooh/healthcare/pharmacists.htm.

Bureau of Labor Statistics, U.S. Department of Labor. (2019b). *Occupational outlook handbook. Physicians and surgeons.* https://www.bls.gov/ooh/healthcare/physicians-and-surgeons.htm.

Bureau of Labor Statistics, U.S. Department of Labor. (2019c). *Occupational outlook handbook. Occupational therapists.* https://www.bls.gov/ooh/healthcare/occupational-therapists.htm.

Bureau of Labor Statistics, U.S. Department of Labor. (2019d). *Occupational outlook handbook.* Social workers. https://www.bls.gov/ooh/community-and-social-service/social-workers.htm.

Bureau of Labor Statistics, U.S. Department of Labor. (2019e). *Occupational outlook handbook, Speech-language pathologists.* https://www.bls.gov/ooh/healthcare/speech-language-pathologists.htm.

Burton, R., et al. (2012). *Patient-centered medical home recognition tools: A comparison of ten surveys' content and operational detail.* http://web.pdx.edu/~nwallace/CRHSP/PCMHTools.pdf.

Chen, S., Chang, H., & Pai, H. (2018). Caring behaviors directly and indirectly affect nursing students' critical thinking. *Scandinavian Journal of Caring Sciences, 32*(1), 197–203.

Dickison, P., Haerling, K. A., & Lasater, K. (2019). Integrating the national council of state boards of nursing clinical judgment model into nursing educational frameworks. *Journal of Nursing Education, 58*(2), 72–78.

Dolansky, M., & Moore, S. (2013). Quality and Safety Education for Nurses (QSEN): The key is systems thinking. *OJIN: The Online Journal of Issues in Nursing, 18*(3), Manuscript 1.

Fawcett, J. (2017). Thoughts about nursing conceptual models and the "medical model". *Nursing Science Quarterly, 30*(1), 77.

*Grumbach, K., & Bodenheimer, T. A. (2002). A primary care home for Americans: Putting the house in order. *Journal of the American Medical Association, 288*, 889–893.

Guler, E., & Turk, G. (2018). Oral chlorhexidine against ventilator associated pneumonia and microbial colonization in intensive care patients. *Western Journal of Nursing Research*, 1–19. https://doi.org/10.1177/0193945918781531.

Gupta, A., Gupta, A., Singh, T., & Saxsena, A. (2016). Role of oral care to prevent VAP in mechanically ventilated intensive care unit patients. *Saudi Journal of Anaesthesia, 10*(1), 95–97. http://doi.org/10.4103/1658-354X.169484.

Levett-Jones, T. (2013). *Clinical reasoning: learning to think like a nurse.* Frenchs Forest, Australia: Pearson.

Massachusetts Department of Higher Education Nursing Initiative. (2016). *Massachusetts nurse of the future nursing core competencies.* https://www.mass.edu/nahi/documents/NOFRNCompetencies_updated_March2016.pdf.

National Council of State Boards of Nursing. (2019). NGN talks: The clinical judgment model and action model video transcript. https://www.ncsbn.org/Transcript_NGNTalk_Episode07.pdf?fbclid=IwAR0iRkqdh5AoQ_xKDFAIsyfnHcYSoeAobLieNs1dagLfWDuUP3DyhdvFjWw.

National Council of State Boards of Nursing (NCSBN). (2018a). In focus: Measuring the right things. https://www.ncsbn.org/InFocus_Winter_2018.pdf.

National Council of State Boards of Nursing (NCSBN). (2018b). *Next generation NCLEX news.* https://www.ncsbn.org/NCLEX_Next_Winter18_Eng_05.pdf.

Phillips, J., et al. (2018). Systems thinking and incivility in nursing practice: An integrative review. *Nursing Forum, 2018*, 1–13.

QSEN. (2019). *Competencies.* http://qsen.org/competencies/.

Scanlon, K., Wells, C., Woolforde, L., Khameraj, A., & Baumgartner, J. (2017). Saving lives and reducing harm: A CAUTI reduction program. *Nursing Economic, 35*(3), 134–141.

Schuelke, S., & Barnason, S. (2017). Interventions used by nurse preceptors to develop critical thinking of new graduate nurses: A systematic review. *Journal for Nurses in Professional Development, 31*(1), E1–E7.

Shi, L., & Singh, D. (2019). *Delivering health care in America: A systems approach* (7th ed.). Burlington, MA: Jones & Bartlett Learning.

Skochelak, S., & Hawkins, R. (2017). *Health systems science.* Philadelphia: Elsevier.

Sommers, C. L. (2018). Measurement of critical thinking, clinical reasoning, and clinical judgment in culturally diverse nursing students—A literature review. *Nurse Education in Practice, 0*, 91–100.

Stalter, A., & Mota, A. (2018). Using systems thinking to envision quality and safety in healthcare. *Nursing Management*, 32–39.

Stalter, A., Phillips, J., & Dolansky, M. (2017). QSEN Institute RN-BSN Task Force. White paper and recommendation for systems-based practice competency. *Journal of Nursing Care Quality, 32*(4), 354–358.

Tanner, C. (2006). Thinking like a nurse: A research-based model of clinical judgment in nursing. *Journal of Nursing Education, 45*(6), 204–211.

Toney-Butler, T., & Thayer, J. (2019). Nursing process. In *StatPearls* [Internet]. Treasure Island, FL: StatPearls Publishing. https://www.ncbi.nlm.nih.gov/books/NBK499937/.

World Health Organization (WHO). (2019). *Primary health care.* Geneva, Switzerland: WHO. http://www.who.int/primary-health/en/.

3

Overview of Health Concepts for Medical-Surgical Nursing

Donna D. Ignatavicius

http://evolve.elsevier.com/Iggy/

LEARNING OUTCOMES

1. Collaborate with the interprofessional team to help patients meet basic ***nutrition, elimination,*** and ***tissue integrity*** needs.
2. Plan collaborative interventions to manage ***pain*** and promote ***comfort.***
3. Assess risk factors that may result in altered ***sexuality.***
4. Plan nursing interventions to promote ***cognition, mobility***, and ***sensory perception*** and maintain safety.
5. Differentiate the concepts of ***inflammation, immunity,*** and ***infection.***
6. Describe common physiologic consequences when a patient has impaired ***acid-base balance*** and/or impaired ***fluid and electrolyte balance.***
7. Describe how to determine a patient's ***perfusion, gas exchange,*** and ***clotting*** status.
8. Plan patient-centered nursing interventions to help patients meet selected physiologic health needs related to ***cellular regulation*** and ***glucose regulation.***

KEY TERMS

acid-base balance The maintenance of arterial blood pH between 7.35 and 7.45 through control of hydrogen ion production and elimination.

cellular regulation The genetic and physiologic processes that control cellular growth, replication, differentiation, and function to maintain homeostasis.

clotting A complex, multistep process by which blood forms a protein-based structure (clot) in an appropriate area of tissue injury to prevent excessive bleeding while maintaining whole body blood flow.

cognition The complex integration of mental processes and intellectual function for the purposes of reasoning, learning, memory, and personality.

comfort A state of physical well-being, pleasure, and absence of pain or stress. This definition implies that comfort has physical and emotional dimensions.

constipation Hard dry stool that is difficult to pass through the rectum.

delirium Acute fluctuating mental confusion.

dementia Chronic mental confusion.

diarrhea Watery stool without solid form.

elimination The excretion of waste from the body by the GI tract (as feces) and by the renal/urinary system (as urine).

exemplar Selected health problem or issue that represents priority concepts.

fluid and electrolyte balance The regulation of body fluid volume, osmolality, and composition; the regulation of electrolytes by the processes of filtration, diffusion, osmosis, and selective excretion.

gas exchange The process of oxygen transport to the cells and carbon dioxide transport away from the cells through ventilation and diffusion.

glucose regulation The process of maintaining optimal blood glucose levels.

immunity Protection from illness or disease that is maintained by the body's physiologic defense mechanisms.

infection The invasion of pathogens into the body that multiply and cause disease or illness.

inflammation A syndrome of normal responses to cellular injury, allergy, or invasion by pathogens.

mobility The ability of an individual to perform purposeful physical movement of the body.

nutrition The process of ingesting and using food and fluids to grow, repair, and maintain optimal body functions.

pain An unpleasant sensory and emotional experience that may be acute or persistent (chronic).

perfusion Adequate arterial blood flow through the peripheral tissues (peripheral perfusion) and blood that is pumped by the heart to oxygenate major body organs (central perfusion).

sepsis A life-threatening response of the body to infection and widespread inflammation that can cause multiple organ dysfunction syndrome (MODS).

sensory perception The ability to perceive and interpret sensory input into one or more meaningful responses.

sexuality A complex integration of physiologic, emotional, and social aspects of well-being related to intimacy, self-concept, and role relationships.

tissue integrity The intactness of the structure and function of the integument (skin and subcutaneous tissue) and mucous membranes.

PRIORITY AND INTERRELATED CONCEPTS

The priority concepts for this chapter are:

- ***Acid-Base Balance***
- ***Cellular Regulation***
- ***Clotting***
- ***Cognition***
- ***Comfort***
- ***Elimination***
- ***Fluid and Electrolyte Balance***
- ***Gas Exchange***
- ***Glucose Regulation***
- ***Immunity***
- ***Infection***
- ***Inflammation***
- ***Mobility***
- ***Nutrition***
- ***Pain***
- ***Perfusion***
- ***Sensory Perception***
- ***Sexuality***
- ***Tissue Integrity***

Nurses care for adults in a variety of settings to help them meet a multitude of biopsychosocial needs. When these needs are not met, the nurse plans and implements care in collaboration with the interprofessional health team. This chapter reviews the 19 health concepts that are emphasized and built on in this text and are presented alphabetically here for easy access. For more information about these concepts, see your fundamentals of nursing textbook or other concept-based resource. Each chapter in the body systems units applies appropriate health concepts to patient assessment or interventions for selected health problems or issues, identified as **exemplars.**

ACID-BASE BALANCE

Definition of Acid-Base Balance

Acid-base balance is the maintenance of arterial blood pH between 7.35 and 7.45 through control of hydrogen ion production and elimination. Blood pH represents a delicate balance between hydrogen ions (acid) and bicarbonate (base) and is largely controlled by the lungs and kidneys. The primary interrelated concepts are ***elimination, fluid and electrolyte balance,*** and ***nutrition***.

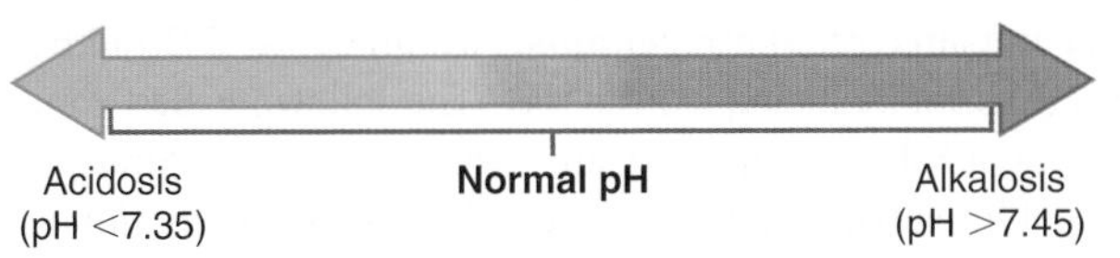

FIG. 3.1 Scope of *acid-base balance.*

Scope of Acid-Base Balance

If the arterial blood pH is either below 7.35 or above 7.45, the patient has a type of acid-base *imbalance* (Fig. 3.1). *Acidosis* occurs if the arterial blood pH level falls below 7.35 and is caused by either too many hydrogen ions in the body or too little bicarbonate. Conversely, *alkalosis* occurs if the pH is greater than 7.45 and is caused by either too few hydrogen ions in the body or too much bicarbonate. Both severe acidosis and alkalosis can lead to death if the patient is not diagnosed accurately and treated quickly.

Common Risk Factors for Acid-Base Imbalance

Any individual is at risk for an acid-base imbalance, but it occurs most commonly as a complication of many acute and chronic health problems. The most common risk factors include:

- Poisoning such as excessive salicylate ingestion
- Medical conditions such as chronic obstructive pulmonary disease (COPD), uncontrolled diabetes mellitus (especially type 1), and chronic kidney disease
- Excessive emesis
- Prolonged diarrhea
- Hyperventilation
- Electrolyte imbalances, especially potassium

A more thorough discussion of acid-base imbalances by specific type may be found in Chapter 14 of this text.

Physiologic Consequences of Acid-Base Imbalance

When the body has an impaired ***acid-base balance,*** several mechanisms are activated in an attempt to correct the imbalance, a process referred to as *compensation*. For example, if the patient is acidotic (pH lower than 7.35), the kidneys typically decrease the amount of bicarbonate ions (base) that is excreted through the urine. The lungs may try to rid the body of carbon dioxide (directly related to hydrogen ions) through increased and deeper respirations. In this case, both compensatory mechanisms aim to restore ***acid-base balance*** by increasing the blood pH to greater than 7.35. These actions can only occur if the individual has healthy lungs and kidneys.

Assessment of Acid-Base Balance

Take a patient health history for chronic illnesses such as diabetes mellitus or COPD and any past experiences of acid-base imbalance. Ask about the presence or recent history of signs and symptoms that could predispose the patient to acidosis or alkalosis such as excessive vomiting or diarrhea. The patient's current or recent use of medications, including over-the-counter drugs (such as acetylsalicylic acid [ASA]) and nutrition supplements (such as calcium), should be reviewed to determine if they could cause acid-base imbalance.

Arterial blood gas monitoring gives the health care team an understanding of the type of acid-base imbalance the patient is experiencing. Assessing the pH determines whether the patient has an imbalance and, if so, how severe it is. The PaO_2 level (normal value is 95 to 100 mm Hg), or partial pressure of oxygen, indicates how well the lungs are functioning. The $PaCO_2$ level (normal value is 35 to 45 mm Hg), or partial pressure of carbon dioxide, indicates how well the lungs are functioning in blowing off or retaining carbon dioxide as needed to help correct the acid-base imbalance. The bicarbonate level, or HCO_3 (normal value is 21 to 28 mEq/L [21 to 28 mmol/L), indicates how well the kidneys are excreting or reabsorbing base as needed.

Health Promotion Strategies to Maintain Acid-Base Balance and Prevent Acid-Base Imbalance

The best way for an individual to maintain ***acid-base balance*** is to practice health promotion measures, including living a healthy lifestyle. For example, most cases of COPD can be prevented by avoiding or quitting smoking. Regular exercise and a healthy diet can decrease the incidence of type 2 diabetes mellitus and help control blood glucose in all types of diabetes.

Teach patients who are at risk for acute or chronic vomiting or diarrhea to be monitored carefully by a primary health care provider to assess for fluid, electrolyte, and acid-base imbalances. (See discussion of ***fluid and electrolyte balance*** later in this chapter and in Chapter 13.)

Interventions for Patients With Acid-Base Imbalances

Managing a patient with an acid-base imbalance depends on which type of imbalance is present. When possible, the health care team aims to diagnose and treat the underlying cause(s) of the imbalance. Chapter 14 describes the pathophysiology and management of common types of acid-base imbalance in detail.

CELLULAR REGULATION

Definition of Cellular Regulation

Cellular regulation is the genetic and physiologic processes that control cellular growth, replication, differentiation, and function to maintain homeostasis. Cellular *growth* refers to division and continued growth of the original cell. Cell *replication* refers to making a copy of a specific cell. Cell *differentiation* refers to the process of the cell becoming specialized to accomplish a specific task. The primary interrelated concepts are ***immunity*** and ***pain.***

Scope of Cellular Regulation

Cellular Regulation may be normal or impaired. When it is impaired with loss of control over cellular reproduction, the result is excessive and abnormal growth of tissue not needed for optimum whole body function. Such abnormal cell growth includes benign or malignant tumors (cancer), fibrosis, and excessive scar tissue formation. Inhibition of cellular regulation can reduce cell production of certain substances (such as insulin or clotting factors) to levels that cannot support homeostasis.

Common Risk Factors for Impaired Cellular Regulation

Risk factors that increase the probability of impaired ***Cellular Regulation*** include:

- Older age (55 years and older, with significant potential for abnormal cell development at ages older than 70)
- Smoking
- Poor ***nutrition***
- Physical inactivity
- Environmental pollutants (such as air, water, soil)
- Radiation
- Selected medications (such as chemotherapy)
- Genetic predisposition or risk

Physiologic Consequences of Impaired Cellular Regulation

Impaired ***cellular regulation*** often results in benign and malignant cell growth. *Benign* cell growth mirrors the original cell, but excessive cells are present. Benign cells do not have the capability to spread to other tissues or organs. However, benign masses can cause health risks because of the ability to obstruct or compress organs in the body, causing significant discomfort or high risk to the individual. For example, a meningioma (benign mass) can compress the brain and lead to increased intracranial pressure (ICP), a potentially fatal complication.

Malignant (cancerous) cells, over time, have no comparison to the original cells from which they are derived. Replication of abnormal cells leads to significant invasion of healthy cells, tissues, and organs through tumor formation and invasion. Chapter 19 discusses the concepts of cancer development in detail.

Assessment of Cellular Regulation

Perform a thorough patient history, extensive family history, and psychosocial history. Completing a thorough and detailed physical examination may identify any visible or palpable masses, pain, or difficulty breathing. Diagnostic tests such as radiographic examination, computed tomography (CT), or magnetic resonance imaging (MRI) may identify the location of any mass. More invasive tests such as a colonoscopy or endoscopy give the primary health care provider an opportunity to directly visualize the mass. Laboratory tests can provide additional information regarding the overall health of the patient and the composition of any mass. For example, tissue biopsies and cell cytology are essential to identify the type of abnormal cell that is present. Grading and staging to identify the extent and severity of the growth are a necessity to diagnose, treat, and offer a prognosis for the patient (see Chapters 19 and 20).

Health Promotion Strategies to Maintain Cellular Regulation and Prevent Impaired Cellular Regulation

Interventions include primary and secondary prevention techniques. *Primary prevention* includes minimizing the risk of developing impaired ***cellular regulation.*** *Healthy People 2030* addresses objectives for reducing cancer risk. The following Best Practice for Patient Safety & Quality Care: Health Promotion Strategies to Prevent Impaired Cellular Regulation box lists key points for health teaching to help prevent impaired ***cellular regulation.*** Additional health promotion strategies are discussed throughout this text.

BEST PRACTICE FOR SAFETY & QUALITY CARE QSEN

Health Promotion Strategies to Prevent Impaired Cellular Regulation

Teach patients to:
- Protect exposed skin with sunscreen of at least 30 SPF.
- Minimize exposure to sunlight or other source of ultraviolet light such as tanning beds (to prevent skin cancers).
- Stop smoking or other tobacco use if applicable (to prevent many cancer types, including lung, oral, and bladder cancers).
- Consume a diet low in saturated fat and high in fiber (to prevent breast and colon cancer).
- Increase physical activity and regular exercise (to prevent all cancer types).
- Avoid exposure to environmental hazards (to prevent all cancer types).

Secondary prevention includes proper and regular screening to identify early any risks or hazards that could be present. Screening also enables the primary health care provider to diagnose cancer early, which often increases the patient's chance for a cure or long-term survival. Objectives for Healthy People 2030 focus on reducing the number of cancer deaths through improved screening and other health promotion practices.

Interventions for Patients With Impaired Cellular Regulation

Collaborative interventions for the patient with impaired ***cellular regulation*** can include surgery, radiation therapy, chemotherapy, hormonal therapy, targeted therapy, biologic therapy, and bone marrow or hematopoietic stem cell transplants. The type and course of interprofessional management depends on the type and severity of cellular regulation impairment. The two chapters on cancer in this textbook discuss the pathogenesis of cancer and its patient-centered management (see Chapters 19 and 20).

CLOTTING

Definition of Clotting

Clotting is a complex, multistep process by which blood forms a protein-based structure (clot) in an appropriate area of tissue injury to prevent excessive bleeding while maintaining whole body blood flow (***perfusion***). A major component of this process involves specialized cells called *platelets* (thrombocytes) that circulate in the blood until they are needed. When injury occurs, platelets are activated to become sticky, causing them to aggregate (clump together) to form a temporary semisolid plug. The platelet aggregation triggers a rapid complex process, known as the *clotting cascade,* in which multiple clotting factors (enzymes and plasma proteins) work together to create a fibrin clot and local blood coagulation (clotting). Another pathway, known as the *fibrinolytic system,* is triggered to cause clot lysis (breakdown) (McCance et al., 2019). The primary interrelated concepts are ***mobility*** and ***perfusion***. Chapter 33 describes ***clotting*** in more detail.

Scope of Clotting

An inability to form adequate clots can result in bleeding and threaten a person's life. In some cases an excess of platelets or excessive platelet stickiness can lead to hypercoagulability (increased clotting ability), which can impair blood flow. Therefore the scope of ***clotting*** can range from increased or excessive clotting to an inability to adequately clot, either locally at the site of an injury or systemically. Fig. 3.2 illustrates the potential scope of ***clotting***.

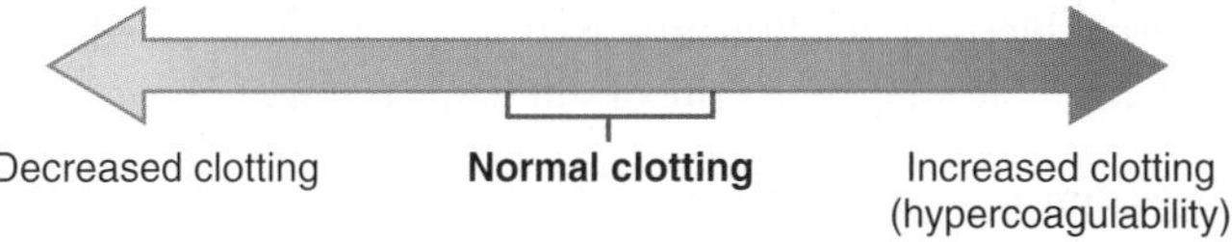

FIG. 3.2 Scope of *clotting.*

Common Risk Factors for Impaired Clotting

When taking a patient and family history, be aware that impaired ***clotting*** may result in either excessive or inadequate clotting. Common risk factors for *increased* clotting include immobility or decreased ***mobility,*** health problems such as polycythemia, and smoking. Immobility slows venous blood flow to the heart and can result in venous stasis and venous thromboembolism (VTE), described later in this text. Certain chronic health problems such as diabetes mellitus are also associated with decreased blood flow, making patients more likely than healthy adults to develop VTE or arterial clots. Polycythemia causes an excessive production of red blood cells, which can lead to multiple clots. Atrial fibrillation causes pooling of blood in the atria (stasis) and often leads to embolic stroke. As people age and smoke, platelets typically become stickier and therefore tend to aggregate more easily. In addition, venous valves that normally prevent the backflow of blood become weak and often inadequate as adults age. The result is venous stasis and an increased risk for VTE.

Decreased clotting most often occurs when there is an inadequate number of circulating platelets (thrombocytopenia). For example, chemotherapeutic drugs and corticosteroids cause bone marrow suppression where platelets and other blood cells are produced. Patients with cirrhosis of the liver also have a decreased production of clotting factors, including prothrombin, causing them to be at an increased risk for bleeding. Some rare genetic diseases such as recessive sex-linked hemophilia A and B are the result of defective clotting factors that also increase the risk for bleeding.

Physiologic Consequences of Impaired Clotting

For patients at risk for *increased* or excessive ***clotting,*** recognize that clots can occur in either venous or arterial blood vessels. Venous thrombosis is a clot formation in either superficial or deep (9most often) veins, usually in the leg. If a thrombus becomes dislodged, it is known as an embolus. Emboli may travel to the brain (causing a stroke) or lung (pulmonary embolus).

For patients with a *decreased* ability to clot, prolonged internal (systemic) or external (localized) bleeding may occur. Internal bleeding may occur in the brain (hemorrhagic stroke), GI tract (frank or occult blood in the stool), and/or urinary tract (hematuria). It may also occur under the skin (purpura).

External bleeding often manifests as epistaxis (nose bleeds) or prolonged bleeding at the site of soft tissue trauma.

Assessment of Clotting

Observe patients for signs and symptoms of *decreased* ***clotting***, especially purpural (hemorrhagic) lesions such as ecchymosis (bruising) and petechiae (pinpoint purpura). Notice if bleeding is prolonged as a result of injury or trauma. Check urine and stool for the presence of occult or frank blood. Observe for frank bleeding from the gums or nose.

For patients with *increased* risk for clotting or excessive ***clotting***, observe for signs and symptoms of *venous* thrombosis such as localized redness, ***pain***, swelling, and warmth.

! NURSING SAFETY PRIORITY (QSEN)

Critical Rescue

An *arterial* thrombosis is not locally observable and is typically manifested by decreased blood flow (***perfusion***) to a distal extremity or internal organ. For example, a femoral arterial clot causes an occlusion (blockage) of blood to the leg. In this case the distal leg becomes pale and cool; distal pulses may be weak or absent; *this is an emergent problem requiring immediate intervention. Do not elevate the affected leg! If these symptoms are present, notify the primary health care provider or Rapid Response Team immediately.* If this condition continues, the leg may become gangrenous and require amputation. A mesenteric artery thrombosis can cause small bowel ileus and gangrene if not treated in a timely manner. A renal artery thrombosis can cause acute kidney injury.

A number of serum laboratory tests are available to measure *clotting* factor levels and bleeding time. The most common tests are prothrombin time (PT) and activated partial thromboplastin time (aPTT). An international normalized ratio (INR) indicating a derived measure of prothrombin is used to monitor the effectiveness of warfarin.

Health Promotion Strategies to Maintain Clotting and Prevent Impaired Clotting

Teach the patient with *decreased* ***clotting*** ability to report unusual bleeding or bruising immediately to the primary health care provider or nurse, depending on where the patient is. Be sure to teach patients at risk for *increased* ***clotting*** to:

- Drink adequate fluids to prevent dehydration.
- Avoid crossing the legs.
- Ambulate frequently and avoid prolonged sitting.
- Explore smoking cessation programs as needed.
- Call your primary health care provider if redness, ***pain,*** swelling, and warmth occur in a lower extremity.

Interventions for Patients With Impaired Clotting

In addition to the previous interventions, for many adults at increased risk for ***clotting,*** *anticoagulants, or antiplatelet drugs* (also called *blood thinners* by many patients) may be prescribed in either community or inpatient settings. Examples of medications that require frequent laboratory testing are sodium heparin and warfarin. *Teach adults the importance of obtaining these tests and monitor results to ensure that they are within the desired range to ensure patient safety.*

Newer anticoagulants called *direct thrombin inhibitors* may be given to decrease the risk of stroke in patients with atrial fibrillation. Monitor patients receiving any of these drugs for signs of bleeding, including bruising and blood in the urine or stool. Continued bleeding can lead to anemia or hemorrhage, depending on the location and severity of the bleeding. Drug therapy to prevent ***clotting*** is discussed in detail in Chapter 33.

NCLEX EXAMINATION CHALLENGE 3.1

Physiological Integrity

Which assessment findings indicate to the nurse that a client taking warfarin may have decreased ***clotting***? **Select all that apply.**

A. Frequent nosebleeds
B. Lower leg swelling
C. Upper extremity bruising
D. Difficulty breathing
E. Intermittent chest pain
F. Dark stools

COGNITION

Definition of Cognition

Cognition is the complex integration of mental processes and intellectual function for the purposes of reasoning, learning, memory, and personality. *Reasoning* is a high-level thinking process that allows an individual to make decisions and judgments. *Memory* is the ability of an individual to retain and recall information for learning or recall of past experiences. *Personality* refers to the way an individual feels and behaves, often based on how he or she thinks. The primary interrelated concepts are ***fluid and electrolyte balance, gas exchange,*** and ***perfusion.***

Scope and Categories of Cognition

An adult may have either intact or adequate cognitive functioning or inadequate cognitive functioning. Examples of inadequate ***cognition*** include **delirium** (acute fluctuating confusion) and **dementia** (chronic confusion). Table 3.1 compares these two major cognitive disorders that are most common in older adults. Chapter 4 describes these health problems in detail. Adults may also have delayed intellectual functioning or amnesia (loss of memory) caused by brain trauma, congenital disorders, or acute health problems such as a stroke. Impaired ***cognition*** may also be classified into two major categories: *global cognitive disorders* (such as dementia or delirium) and *focal cognitive disorders* (such as amnesia [loss of memory]).

Common Risk Factors for Inadequate Cognition

Inadequate ***cognition*** is complex and includes a variety of signs and symptoms. They may be short term and reversible or long term and not reversible. Common risk factors include:

- Advanced age (although dementia is *not* a normal physiologic change of aging)
- Brain trauma at any age, including at birth
- Disease or disorder such as brain tumor, hypoxia, or stroke (infarction)
- Environmental exposure to toxins such as lead

TABLE 3.1 Differences in Characteristics of Delirium and Dementia

Variable	Dementia	Delirium
Description	A chronic, progressive cognitive decline	An acute, fluctuating confusional state
Onset	Slow	Fast
Duration	Months to years	Hours to less than 1 month
Cause	Unknown, possibly familial, chemical	Multiple, such as surgery, infection, drugs
Reversibility	None	May be possible
Management	Treat signs and symptoms	Remove or treat the cause
Nursing interventions	Reorientation is not effective in the late stages; use validation therapy (acknowledge the patient's feelings and do not argue); provide a safe environment; observe for associated behaviors such as delusions and hallucinations	Reorient the patient to reality; provide a safe environment

- Substance use disorder
- Genetic diseases such as Down syndrome
- Depression
- Opioids, steroids, psychoactive drugs, and general anesthesia, especially in older adults
- Fluid and electrolyte imbalances

Physiologic and Psychosocial Consequences of Inadequate Cognition

Common signs and symptoms of inadequate or impaired ***cognition*** include:

- Loss of short- and/or long-term memory
- Disorientation to person, place, and/or time
- Impaired reasoning and decision-making ability
- Impaired language skills
- Uncontrollable or inappropriate emotions such as severe agitation and aggression
- Delusions and hallucinations

These manifestations often result in patient *safety* and communication issues. For example, an adult with impaired short-term memory may forget to turn off a stove burner that could result in a fire. A person who has impaired reasoning and decision-making ability may decide to drive a motor vehicle or operate machinery. Communication with a patient who is disoriented, aggressive, and/or delusional may not be possible.

Assessment of Cognition

Taking a thorough history from either the patient or family is essential to determine potential or actual cognitive impairment. Conduct a mental status assessment using one of several available mental health/behavioral health screening tools such as the Confusion Assessment Method (CAM). Other tools also assess memory, speech and language, judgment, thought processes, calculation, and abstract reasoning. Discussion of assessment tools to screen for specific ***cognition*** problems may be found throughout this text and in mental health textbooks.

Diagnostic testing includes brain imaging procedures such as magnetic resonance imaging (MRI) to determine the presence of brain abnormalities such as trauma, tumors, and infarction. Neuropsychological testing by a licensed clinical psychologist may be performed to diagnose the cause and severity of specific changes associated with cognitive problems.

Health Promotion Strategies to Maintain Cognition and Prevent Inadequate Cognition

Teach adults to avoid risk factors such as substance use and lifestyle behaviors such as motorcycle driving without protective headgear. Teach older adults to stimulate the intellectual part of their brain through new learning activities such as taking music lessons, mastering a new language, or completing crossword puzzles or other "brain teasers."

Interventions for Patients With Inadequate Cognition

Nursing interventions focus on ***safety*** to prevent injury and foster communication. For adults with delirium or *mild* or *early-stage* dementia, provide orientation to person, time, and place. Patients with mild to moderate dementia, especially Alzheimer's disease, may be prescribed cholinesterase inhibitors (e.g., donepezil) to help them maintain function for an undetermined period of time.

Collaborate with the interprofessional health care team to determine the underlying cause of delirium, such as analgesics or hypoxia. Patients with moderate or severe dementia cannot be oriented to reality because they have *chronic* confusion.

! NURSING SAFETY PRIORITY QSEN

Action Alert

Teach families and caregivers to provide a safe environment for the individual with cognitive impairment living in the community! Adults who are confused or cannot follow instructions may be injured by operating machinery or driving a motor vehicle. For those in inpatient facilities, provide a safe environment, depending on the patient's specific cognitive deficit. For example, implement fall precautions for those who need help getting out of bed. Adults with delirium or dementia may wander outside and be injured. Be sure they wear an alarm and identification bracelet.

In some cases the primary health care provider may prescribe psychoactive drug therapy for psychotic behaviors associated with specific cognitive disorders. Some of these drugs are described later in this text but are discussed in more detail in mental health/behavioral health textbooks.

COMFORT

Definition of Comfort

Comfort is a state of physical well-being, pleasure, and absence of pain or stress. This definition implies that ***comfort*** has physical and emotional dimensions. A primary role of the nurse is to promote basic care and ***comfort***. The primary interrelated concepts are ***inflammation*** and ***pain.***

Scope of Comfort

The desired outcome for optimal health and well-being of any individual is to have ***comfort*** or be comfortable. Many health problems can cause decreased ***comfort,*** also called *discomfort*. Most often patients report ***pain*** or other sensation that disrupts their ability to function, either physically or mentally.

Common Risk Factors for Decreased Comfort

Risk factors can be divided into physical causes and emotional, or psychosocial, causes. In some cases patients have risk factors for both physical and emotional discomfort. Decreased ***comfort*** can be acute (short term) or chronic (long term). For example, patients who are having surgery are often anxious and feel stressed about the procedure. They may worry about who will care for them or their family after the surgery. This emotional stress is uncomfortable and can affect the outcomes of surgery. In addition, patients who have surgery typically have *acute* ***pain*** or impaired ***comfort.*** This unpleasant sensation causes more emotional stress and discomfort. Some postoperative patients also have nausea or light-headedness as a result of the anesthesia used during the surgical procedure. All of these symptoms are causes of discomfort.

Patients at the end of life experience various types of discomfort as a result of *persistent* ***pain,*** nausea, vomiting, dyspnea, and GI disturbances. These signs and symptoms decrease patients' quality of life and contribute to a "bad" death (see Chapter 8 for more information about end-of-life care).

Physiologic and Psychosocial Consequences of Decreased Comfort

Physical causes of decreased ***comfort*** (discomfort) such as ***pain,*** nausea, dyspnea, and itching can result in emotional stress and discomfort. The body's "fight or flight" mechanism helps the individual cope with the source and manifestations of the discomfort. If this response is not successful in reducing stress, the individual may develop persistent ***pain*** and anxiety.

Assessment of Comfort

Ask patients if they are comfortable. If ***pain*** is the source of discomfort, assess the patient's pain level and plan interventions to manage it. See Chapter 5 of this text for ***pain*** assessment. If emotional stress is the source of discomfort, be sure to help the patient describe the nature and cause of stress. Once the underlying cause(s) of discomfort is identified, coordinate with the interprofessional health care team to treat or remove it if possible.

Health Promotion Strategies to Maintain Comfort and Prevent Decreased Comfort

Pain and emotional stress are the most common sources of decreased ***comfort.*** To prevent these sensations, anticipate which patient may experience them and provide preplanned interventions. For example, for postoperative ***pain*** control, ensure that the patient receives a basal continuous dose of patient-controlled analgesia. For patients at the end of their lives, palliative care is needed to promote ***comfort*** (see Chapter 8).

Interventions for Patients With Decreased Comfort

Assess patients at risk for discomfort and plan interventions to alleviate it, depending on its source and cause. Collaborate care with members of the interprofessional health care team as needed. For example, refer the patient to a counselor, social worker, or other qualified mental health professional to manage emotional stress. Consult with the primary health care provider and pharmacist to manage acute and persistent ***pain,*** dyspnea, and other sources of impaired ***comfort.***

ELIMINATION

Definition of Elimination

Elimination is the excretion of waste from the body by the GI tract (as feces) and renal/urinary system (as urine). *Bowel* elimination occurs as a result of food and fluid intake and ends with passage of feces (stool) or solid waste products from food into the rectum of the colon. The fecal material remains in the rectum until the urge to defecate occurs. Bowel ***elimination*** control depends on multiple factors, including muscle strength and nerve function.

Urinary ***elimination*** occurs as a result of multiple kidney processes and ends with the passage of urine through the urinary tract. When the urge to void occurs, urine is passed from the bladder through the urinary sphincter, urethra, and meatus. Urine consists of water and waste products (toxins) from many chemical processes in the body. Urinary ***elimination*** control also depends on multiple factors, including muscle strength and nerve function. The primary interrelated concepts are ***fluid and electrolyte balance,*** *tissue integrity,* and ***nutrition.***

Scope of Elimination

Adults desire voluntary control of both bowel and urinary ***elimination,*** a normal condition called *continence.* However, a number of factors can cause *incontinence* (lack of bowel or bladder control) or *retention* (an inability to expel stool or excrete urine).

Bowel ***elimination*** may also be categorized by the consistency of fecal material, which is shown in Fig. 3.3. At one end of the continuum the stool can be watery and without solid form,

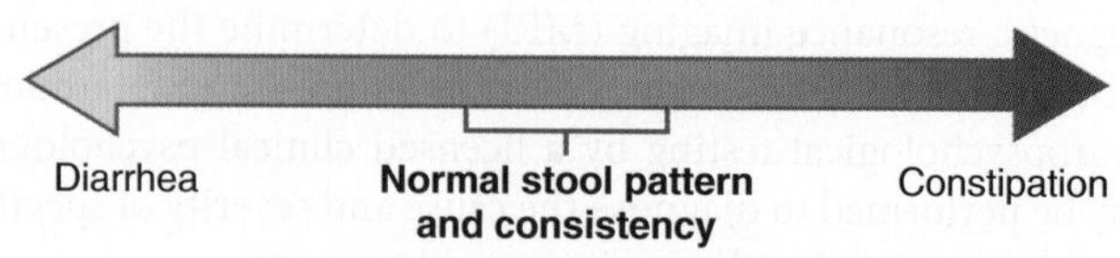

FIG. 3.3 Scope of bowel *elimination.*

a condition called diarrhea. At the other end of the continuum, the stool can be hard, dry, and difficult to pass through the rectum, a condition called constipation.

Common Risk Factors for Changes in Elimination

Incontinence of either the bowel or bladder can occur as a result of aging when pelvic floor muscles become weaker. It may also occur in adults who have neurologic disorders such as stroke, dementia, and multiple sclerosis. Excessive use of laxatives may cause fecal (diarrheal) incontinence. *Diarrhea* also results from acute GI infections such as gastroenteritis and chronic inflammatory bowel diseases such as Crohn's disease. Irritable bowel syndrome causes frequent diarrhea, constipation, or intermittent episodes of diarrhea and constipation.

Urinary retention is often a problem in older men who have benign prostatic hyperplasia (overgrowth). This overgrowth blocks the bladder neck and prevents urination or complete bladder emptying.

Retention of stool, or *obstipation,* is also common in older adults who have decreased peristalsis and/or lack of adequate dietary fiber and fluids to promote fecal passage. Lack of exercise and use of certain medications such as opioids, diuretics, and psychoactive drugs can contribute to constipation in adults of any age. Spinal cord and brain injuries or diseases often cause involuntary control or retention of both bowel and bladder (neurogenic bowel and bladder).

Renal and urinary health problems can alter urinary ***elimination,*** depending on the type of disease or disorder. For example, urinary tract obstructions such as ureteral stones may prevent urine from reaching the bladder. Chronic kidney disease can cause changes in the amount of urinary output, depending on the stage of the disease. In the end stage the patient experiences oliguria (scant urine) or anuria (absence of urine) because the kidneys have lost their ability to make urine.

Physiologic and Psychosocial Consequences of Changes in Elimination

Adults who have urinary or bowel *incontinence* are at risk for damage to ***tissue integrity.*** If not removed promptly from the skin, stool and urine can cause skin irritation, fungal infection, and/or skin breakdown, which are very uncomfortable. Loss of bladder and bowel control can also lead to depression and anxiety. Older adults in both health care and community settings may wear undergarments or briefs to prevent soiling their clothes. Many older adults perceive these protective garments as "diapers" and are embarrassed or feel humiliated when wearing them. Avoid using this term with communicating with patients, family, and staff.

If not treated, patients with prolonged *diarrhea* may develop fluid and electrolyte imbalances, especially dehydration and hypokalemia (decreased serum potassium). These problems are serious and can be life-threatening because hypokalemia often causes cardiac rhythm abnormalities (dysrhythmias).

Urinary or bowel *retention* can result in a buildup of toxins and waste products in the body. Although not common, a large amount of retained urine can cause rupture of the bladder. The most common consequence of urinary retention is a urinary tract infection due to urinary stasis. A large amount of stool can lead to bowel impaction and result in partial or total intestinal obstruction. These conditions can be life threatening.

Assessment of Elimination

Take a patient history to determine risk factors or the underlying cause for impaired or altered ***elimination.*** Ask the patient or designated family member if incontinence or retention is or has been a problem. Assess the perineal area and buttocks for skin breakdown, redness, and fungal infection in patients who have incontinence.

Monitor the frequency, amount, consistency, and characteristics of urine and stool. Listen to bowel sounds in all four quadrants for presence of adequate bowel sounds. Expect overactive bowel sounds in a patient who has diarrhea; anticipate hypoactive bowel sounds in patients who have constipation. Palpate the bladder and bowel for distention.

For some patients, laboratory testing of urine or stool may be useful in determining the cause of ***elimination*** changes. For example, a urinalysis and culture and sensitivity are appropriate for the patient with suspected urinary stones, retention, and infection. Radiologic testing and ultrasonography for stones or other structural abnormalities may also be performed. Bedside bladder scanning is frequently performed by nurses to detect urinary retention that can result in urinary tract infections.

A stool culture and sensitivity may be done for patients suspected of having *Clostridium difficile* ("*C. diff*") infection. This infection often causes severe diarrhea in older adults who have received antibiotic therapy due to decreased ***immunity*** and is easily spread from one patient to another. Be sure to use proper hand hygiene to help prevent ***infection*** transmission!

Health Promotion Strategies to Maintain Elimination and Prevent Changes in Elimination

Maintaining normal ***elimination*** requires adequate ***nutrition*** and hydration. Teach adults to ensure a diet high in fiber, including eating fruits, vegetables, and whole grains, and drinking 8 to 12 glasses of water each day unless medically contraindicated. Remind them to promptly toilet or void when the urge occurs. Patients at risk for *constipation* may need to take bulk-forming agents or stool softeners in addition to a high-fiber diet and fluids. Remind adults who have or are at risk for constipation to exercise frequently to stimulate peristalsis.

Interventions for Patients With Changes in Elimination

Adults with frequent or ongoing *diarrhea* need medical attention to determine the underlying cause of the problem. Monitor the patient for signs and symptoms of fluid and electrolyte imbalances. These problems can be treated to help the patient return to more normal ***elimination*** patterns and restore ***fluid and electrolyte balance.*** The Best Practice for Patient Safety & Quality Care box outlines nursing best practices for care of the patient experiencing diarrhea.

BEST PRACTICE FOR PATIENT SAFETY & QUALITY CARE (QSEN)

Care of the Patient With Diarrhea

- Protect the perineal and buttock area with a topical barrier cream to prevent skin irritation and excoriation, especially for patients who are incontinent.
- Wash and dry skin where stool and urine have made contact, especially for patients who are incontinent.
- Encourage fluid intake and ensure that the patient consumes foods high in potassium such as bananas and potatoes.
- Document food and fluid intake and urinary/stool output.
- Check the patient's weight each day for weight loss.
- Collaborate with the primary health care provider for prescribing an antifungal cream if needed.

Nursing care for patients with *constipation* includes health teaching and collaboration with the interprofessional health care team. In addition to teaching about measures to prevent worsening of constipation as described previously, recommend that the patient take stool softeners, bulk-forming agents, and/or mild laxatives as needed to restore normal elimination patterns. In some cases, enemas may be needed to stimulate peristalsis and empty the rectum.

Adults who experience urinary *incontinence* need frequent toileting every 1 to 2 hours. This routine can prevent incontinence and train the bladder to empty at more regular intervals. A similar toileting schedule, especially after a meal, can help train the bowel to evacuate at about the same time each day.

Patients with short-term urinary *retention* require one or more straight urinary catheterizations to empty the bladder until the usual voiding pattern returns. For those with long-term retention, especially retention caused by lack of nerve stimuli, teach the patient or family/caregiver how to perform catheterizations on a daily routine schedule. Chapter 7 discusses bowel and bladder training in detail.

FLUID AND ELECTROLYTE BALANCE

Definition of Fluid and Electrolyte Balance

Fluid and electrolyte balance is the regulation of body fluid volume, osmolality, and composition and the regulation of electrolytes by the processes of filtration, diffusion, osmosis, and selective excretion. To maintain balance or homeostasis in the body, ***fluid and electrolyte balance*** must be as close to normal as possible. Water makes up 55% to 60% of total body weight. Older adults have less body fluid than younger adults.

Fluid occupies the inside of the cell (intracellular fluid) and the outside of the cell (extracellular fluid). Extracellular fluid is found in the vascular space (plasma) and interstitial space (fluid between cells, often referred to as *third space fluid*). *Electrolytes* are chemicals in the body needed for normal body functioning, especially the heart and brain. Examples of electrolytes are sodium, potassium, calcium, and magnesium. The primary interrelated concepts are ***acid-base balance***, ***elimination***, and ***nutrition***. Chapter 13 discusses ***fluid and electrolyte balance*** in detail.

TABLE 3.2 Common Fluid and Electrolyte Imbalances

Common Fluid Imbalances	Common Electrolyte Imbalances
Fluid volume deficit (dehydration)	Hyponatremia (low serum sodium)
Fluid volume excess (overload)	Hypernatremia (high serum sodium)
	Hypokalemia (low serum potassium)
	Hyperkalemia (high serum potassium)
	Hypocalcemia (low serum calcium)
	Hypercalcemia (high serum calcium)
	Hypomagnesemia (low serum magnesium)
	Hypermagnesemia (high serum magnesium)

Scope of Fluid and Electrolyte Balance

Fluid imbalances range from decreased fluid (deficit), often causing dehydration, to excessive fluid (overload), often causing edema. *Electrolyte imbalances* may also occur as deficits such as hypokalemia (low serum potassium) and excesses such as hyperkalemia (high serum potassium). Table 3.2 lists common fluid and electrolyte imbalances.

Common Risk Factors for Fluid and Electrolyte Imbalance

Examples of risk factors that can alter a person's ***fluid and electrolyte balance*** include:

- Acute illnesses (e.g., vomiting and diarrhea)
- Severe burns
- Serious injury or trauma
- Chronic kidney disease
- Major surgery
- Poor nutritional intake

Older adults are especially at risk for imbalances in fluids and electrolytes because they have less body water, often have inadequate ***nutrition,*** and are most likely to experience acute and chronic illnesses.

Physiologic Consequences of Fluid and Electrolyte Imbalance

Physiologic consequences of *fluid deficit* are the result of lack of poor ***perfusion*** (blood flow) and oxygen delivery to all parts of the body. A decrease in blood volume leads to hypotension (low blood pressure). In an attempt to compensate for hypotension and perfuse major organs, the heart rate increases (tachycardia). Peripheral pulses become weak and thready. For patients with severe dehydration, fever may occur due to inadequate body water. Older adults may also experience delirium due to lack of blood flow to the brain. If fluid deficit is not adequately managed, the kidney function diminishes, as evidenced by a decrease in urinary output. Recall that the minimum urinary output should be at least 30 mL per hour.

Patients with *fluid excess* (overload) usually have an increase in blood pressure due to increased blood volume. Peripheral pulses are often strong and bounding. Many patients experience peripheral edema due to fluid excess. Fluid from the vascular space shifts to the interstitial space (third spacing).

The physiologic consequences of *electrolyte deficit* depend on which electrolyte is decreased. For example, a decrease in serum potassium level (hypokalemia) can result in cardiac dysrhythmias (abnormal heart rhythms) and muscle weakness. A decreased sodium level (hyponatremia) can result in changes in mental status and generalized weakness.

The consequences of *electrolyte excess* also depend on which electrolyte is increased. For example, an increase in serum potassium (hyperkalemia) or calcium (hypercalcemia) can cause cardiac dysrhythmias. In addition, skeletal muscle spasms are likely. An increased calcium level can also result in kidney or urinary tract calculi (stones). Chapter 13 describes specific fluid and electrolyte imbalances in detail.

Assessment of Fluid and Electrolyte Balance

Take a complete health history for past experiences of fluid and electrolyte imbalance and for any risk factors that can lead to an imbalance. Ask about any current episodes of nausea, vomiting, or diarrhea. Inquire about the current use of medications, including prescribed and over-the-counter drugs and herbal supplements.

Monitor vital signs, especially blood pressure and pulse rate and quality, fluid intake and output, and weight. *Changes in weight are the best indicator of fluid volume changes in the body.* Assess skin and mucous membranes for dryness and decreased skin turgor. Monitor and interpret laboratory tests to determine fluid or electrolyte imbalance. Examples of common tests are measurements of serum electrolyte concentration, blood urea nitrogen (BUN), and serum osmolality. Chapter 13 discusses each of these assessments in detail.

Health Promotion Strategies to Maintain Fluid and Electrolyte Balance and Prevent Fluid and Electrolyte Imbalance

Maintaining ***fluid and electrolyte balance*** in the body is essential for normal body functioning. Teach patients to drink adequate fluids to remain hydrated. Eight glasses or more of water a day are often recommended unless medically contraindicated. Older adults may not feel thirsty or want to limit their fluid intake to prevent urinary incontinence. Teach them the importance of drinking adequate fluids to prevent dehydration and potential urinary tract infection.

Remind all adults about the need to eat a well-balanced diet that promotes electrolyte balance. Certain foods contain high concentrations of essential vitamins, minerals, and electrolytes. For instance, milk and other dairy products are a good source of calcium. Bananas and potatoes are good sources of potassium.

Interventions for Fluid and Electrolyte Imbalances

Priority nursing interventions include maintenance of patient ***safety*** and ***comfort*** measures when managing fluid or electrolyte imbalances. For patients with a *fluid deficit,* the primary collaborative intervention is fluid replacement, either orally or parenterally. Depending on the cause of *fluid overload,* patients may require a fluid restriction (e.g., for those with chronic kidney disease). Diuretic therapy is often used for patients with fluid overload caused by chronic heart failure to prevent pulmonary edema, a potentially life-threatening complication. However, diuretics can also cause decreased serum sodium (hyponatremia) and potassium (hypokalemia). If lower extremity edema is present, teach patients the importance of elevating the legs above the heart to promote venous return.

Interprofessional collaborative management of electrolyte imbalance depends on which electrolyte balance is impaired. In general, electrolyte deficits are treated by replacing them, usually parenterally as IV fluids. Electrolyte excesses are managed by restricting additional electrolytes or using a medication or fluids that can help eliminate the excess. For example, sodium polystyrene sulfonate may be used for patients with hyperkalemia to eliminate excess potassium via the GI system.

GAS EXCHANGE

Definition of Gas Exchange

Gas exchange is the process of oxygen transport to the cells and carbon dioxide transport away from the cells through ventilation and diffusion. This process begins with ventilation triggered by neurons in the brain sensing the need for gas exchange. These neurons stimulate contraction of skeletal muscles that expand the chest cavity, causing inhalation of oxygen-containing air into the airways and lungs. From the lung alveoli, oxygen diffuses into blood and red blood cells, and the waste gas carbon dioxide diffuses from the blood into the alveoli. Once in the alveoli, carbon dioxide is exhaled from the body as a result of recoil of lung elastic tissues and contraction of skeletal muscles that constrict the chest cavity. The oxygen in red blood cells bound to hemoglobin is transported through the blood by cardiac effort to tissue cells ***(perfusion),*** where low oxygen concentration allows release of oxygen from hemoglobin and diffusion or cell metabolism. The high concentration of carbon dioxide waste resulting from cellular metabolism allows diffusion of this gas into the blood and red blood cells. The waste gas is then transported back to the lungs to diffuse into the alveoli for removal during exhalation. The primary interrelated concept is ***perfusion***.

Scope of Gas Exchange

Gas exchange is either normal to allow for adequate ***perfusion*** and removal of waste gas (carbon dioxide) or decreased. Decreased ***gas exchange*** can range from minimal to severe.

Common Risk Factors for Decreased Gas Exchange

Adequate ventilation requires normal functioning central (brain and spinal cord) neurons, normal diaphragm function, adequate skeletal muscle contractility (especially the intercostal muscles between the ribs), and an intact chest thorax. Any acute or chronic problems that affect these functions can result in decreased ventilation, which impairs ***gas exchange.*** For example, pneumonia or lung abscess prevents adequate ventilation and gas exchange. A patient who experienced a high cervical spinal cord injury often has decreased ventilation ability due to damage to spinal nerves that control the diaphragm.

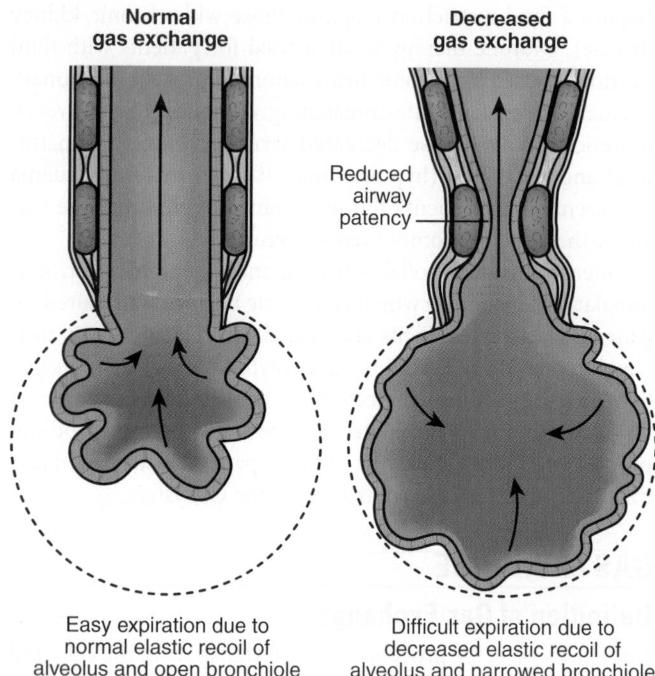

FIG. 3.4 Damaged inelastic alveoli common in patients with chronic obstructive pulmonary disease cause decreases in oxygen and carbon dioxide diffusion.

As adults age, pulmonary alveoli lose some of their elasticity, causing a decrease in ***gas exchange.*** Health problems can also affect lung functioning. Any condition that decreases ventilation such as asthma can impair ***gas exchange.*** Asthma causes bronchospasm and narrowed airways, which diminishes the amount of available oxygen. Other lung diseases such as chronic obstructive pulmonary disease (COPD) directly damage the alveoli, decreasing both oxygen and/or carbon dioxide diffusion (Fig. 3.4). Risk factors for developing these diseases include smoking and environmental pollutants. In addition, prolonged immobility can decrease ***gas exchange*** as a result of inadequate pulmonary ventilation.

Physiologic Consequences of Decreased Gas Exchange

Decreased ***gas exchange*** results in (1) inadequate transportation of oxygen to body cells and organs and/or (2) retention of carbon dioxide. Inadequate oxygen results in cell dysfunction (ischemia) and possible cell death (necrosis or infarction). An excessive buildup of carbon dioxide combines with water to produce carbonic acid. This increase in acid causes respiratory acidosis and lowers the pH of blood. See the previous discussion of ***acid-base balance*** earlier in this chapter and in Chapter 14.

Assessment of Gas Exchange

Take a complete health history and perform a focused respiratory assessment. Ask the patient about current or history of lung disease or trauma. Assess the patient's breathing effort, oxygen saturation, capillary refill, thoracic expansion, and lung sounds anteriorly and posteriorly. Monitor for the presence of a cough; sputum; report of shortness of breath; dizziness; chest pain; presence of cyanosis; or adventitious lung sounds such as wheezing, rhonchi, or crackles. Interpret associated laboratory results, including arterial blood gases (ABGs) and complete blood count (CBC) (Jarvis, 2020). When necessary, a chest x-ray, chest computed tomography (CT), or V/Q scan may be performed to determine the presence and severity of lung disease. Pulmonary function tests can determine the extent of airway disease in the small and large airways of the lungs and their structures. Bronchoscopy can provide direct visualization into the bronchus and its extending structures.

Health Promotion Strategies to Maintain Gas Exchange and Prevent Decreased Gas Exchange

Teach patients the importance of using ***infection*** control measures (primarily proper handwashing), smoking cessation to prevent COPD, and getting immunizations as recommended to prevent influenza and pneumonia. Instruct them to be aware of exposure to specific respiratory conditions, including tuberculosis and influenza.

Interventions for Patients With Decreased Gas Exchange

Managing decreased ***gas exchange*** requires finding the underlying cause and treating it, often with drug therapy. Examples of drugs used to treat respiratory health problems include antihistamines, decongestants, glucocorticoids, bronchodilators, mucolytics, and antimicrobials.

Chest expansion is improved when the patient is sitting or in a semi-Fowlers position. Teach the patient about the need for deep breathing and coughing to further enhance lung expansion and decrease breathing effort. Teach him or her how to correctly use incentive spirometry and inhalers if indicated. Administer oxygen therapy and monitor pulse oximetry to determine its effectiveness.

GLUCOSE REGULATION

Glucose regulation is the process of maintaining optimal blood glucose levels. Although this concept is not a primary concept used throughout this book, it is discussed in connection with multiple interrelated concepts with the ***glucose regulation*** concept exemplar diabetes mellitus in Chapter 59.

IMMUNITY

Definition of Immunity

Immunity is protection from illness or disease that is maintained by the body's physiologic defense mechanisms. *Natural active* immunity occurs when an antigen enters the body and the body creates antibodies to fight off the antigen. *Artificial active* immunity occurs via a vaccination or immunization. *Natural passive* immunity occurs when antibodies are passed from a mother to the fetus through the placenta or using colostrum or the breast milk; *artificial passive* immunity occurs via a specific transfusion such as immunoglobulins.

Multiple organs and cells in the body are involved in the immune response. *Antibody-mediated* ***immunity*** (humoral immunity) includes the antigens and antibodies interacting in an attempt to slow down or destroy the foreign body. B-cells play a major role in this activity, together with the macrophages, T-lymphocytes (T-cells), and spleen. *Cell-mediated* ***immunity*** involves the functions of numerous cells to fight off the antigen, including white blood cells (WBCs), T-cells, natural killer (NK) cells, and multiple cytokines. The thymus and lymph nodes also play a role in this immune process. The primary interrelated concepts are ***cellular regulation, inflammation,*** and ***infection.***

Scope of Immunity

Immunity has the potential to be decreased (suppressed or weakened) or excessive (exaggerated or heightened).

Common Risk Factors for Changes in Immunity

Adult populations at risk for altered ***immunity*** include but are not limited to:

- Older adults (diminished immunity due to normal aging changes)
- Low socioeconomic groups (inability to obtain proper immunizations)
- Nonimmunized adults
- Adults with chronic illnesses that weaken the immune system
- Adults taking chronic drug therapy such as corticosteroids and chemotherapeutic agents
- Adults experiencing substance use disorder
- Adults who do not practice a healthy lifestyle
- Adults who have a genetic risk for decreased or excessive immunity

Physiologic Consequences of Changes in Immunity

An individual with a decreased immune response is susceptible to multiple types of ***infection*** because of the inability to "fight off" particular antigens. An individual with an excessive immune response has allergies or autoimmune reactions or diseases. Reactions are graded types I to IV and have varying degrees of urgency. These types are discussed in detail in Chapter 18.

Assessment of Immunity

A thorough history of the individual and the family is necessary to determine any of the previous risks associated with an immune problem. Identify any patient allergies, current medications, and history of environmental exposures. Ask the patient about an immunization history.

Assess weight, adequate wound healing, ***cognition,*** allergic responses (red, watery eyes; nasal congestion; swelling or rashes), and potential or actual organ dysfunction (cardiovascular, respiratory, renal, or musculoskeletal). Monitor laboratory tests such as complete blood count (CBC) with differential, C-reactive protein (CRP), erythrocyte sedimentation rate (ESR), and allergy testing to identify any susceptibilities that may exist. Specific tests such as the enzyme-linked immunosorbent assay (ELISA) and Western blot tests may be performed to identify the presence of human immune deficiency virus (HIV) antibodies. A complete immune panel, including antinuclear antibody (ANA) and rheumatoid factor (RF) testing, helps to detect autoimmune disease.

Health Promotion Strategies to Maintain Immunity and Prevent Changes in Immunity

Avoiding ***infection,*** frequent handwashing, and having recommended immunizations are essential for promoting healthy immune function (Blevins, 2017). Teach patients to practice a healthy lifestyle, including eating a well-balanced diet to ensure adequate vitamins and minerals, getting at least 7 to 8 hours of sleep each day, and having regular primary health care provider physical examinations. Remind them to avoid environmental hazards such as potential allergens (if sensitive) and people with contagious infections such as influenza.

Interventions for Patients With Changes in Immunity

Patients with a *decreased* immune system for any reason are very prone to infection. Teach them to avoid large crowds or anyone with a transmittable infectious disease or illness. Remind them to wash their hands frequently and use hand sanitizer when water and soap are not available.

Patients with an *excessive* immune function have hypersensitivity reactions. Interprofessional collaborative management of these adults depends on the type and severity of the reaction. The expected outcome of treatment is to decrease symptoms and promote a quality of life. In some cases remission of the health problem can be achieved, but not a cure. Examples of autoimmune diseases that typically have remissions and exacerbations (flare-ups) are rheumatoid arthritis and lupus erythematosus. These disorders are discussed later in this text.

INFECTION

Definition of Infection

Many microorganisms (also called microbes) exist in a person's body and on his or her skin. Some of these microorganisms are normal flora that help protect the body from disease or illness as part of immune function. *Infection* is the invasion of pathogens (harmful microbes) into the body that multiply and cause disease or illness. The primary interrelated concepts are ***pain, immunity, inflammation,*** and ***tissue integrity.***

Categories of Infection

Infections can be classified by type of microorganism, by extent of its spread throughout the body, or by the length of time that the infection exists. The four major classifications of microorganisms that can cause ***infection*** include:

- Bacteria
- Viruses
- Fungi
- Parasites or protozoa

Infections may also be categorized as localized or systemic. *Localized* infections are limited to a specific area of the body. *Systemic* infections affect the entire body and can cause **sepsis,** a life-threatening response of the body to ***infection*** and widespread ***inflammation*** that can cause multiple organ dysfunction syndrome (MODS).

Infections can also be classified as acute or chronic. *Acute* infections resolve in a short period of time, usually a few days

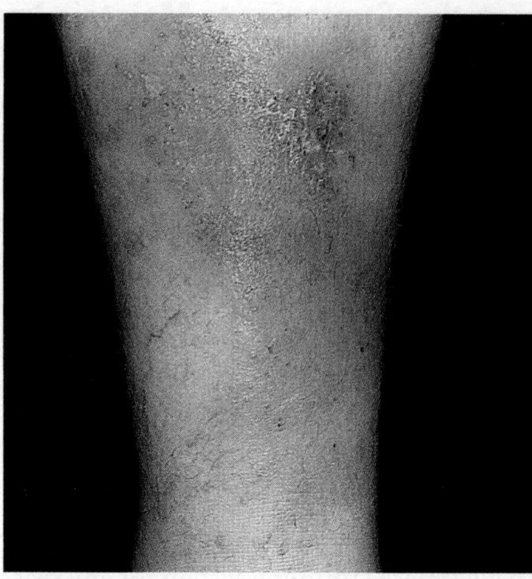

FIG. 3.5 Cellulitis, a localized *infection.* (From Habif, T. P., Dinulos, J. G. H., Capman, M. S., & Zug. K. A. (2018) *Skin disease: Diagnosis and treatment* (4th ed.). Philadelphia: Elsevier.)

or weeks. *Chronic* infections usually last more than 12 weeks and may not be resolved. Chapter 21 discusses ***infection*** in more detail. Sepsis and septic shock are discussed in Chapter 34.

Common Risk Factors for Infection

Populations at risk for ***infection*** include those who:

- Are immunocompromised by disease such as HIV or treatment such as chemotherapy (also called *opportunistic* infections)
- Have chronic illnesses such as chronic obstructive pulmonary disease (COPD) and diabetes mellitus
- Are of advanced age because immune function declines as part of normal aging
- Live in a crowded or unsanitary environment
- Ingest contaminated food or water
- Have impaired ***tissue integrity*** (causing an interruption in the body's first line of defense against infection)
- Are exposed to individuals who have highly contagious infections, such as influenza or tuberculosis
- Experience continuous or frequent stress

Physiologic Consequences of Infection

The physiologic consequences of ***infection*** depend on whether it is localized or systemic. *Localized* infection, such as cellulitis, typically causes ***inflammation*** (Fig. 3.5). Signs and symptoms of ***inflammation*** include redness, warmth, pain, and swelling. If localized infection is not treated or does not respond to treatment, it may spread and affect the entire body, causing a systemic infection (McCance et al, 2019).

Because *systemic* infection affects the entire body, the response of the body is also systemic. Physiologic consequences of systemic infection include fever and an increased white blood cell count (WBC), also known as *leukocytosis*. If the infection is not treated or does not respond to treatment, the patient may become septic and experience decreased ***perfusion*** causing hypotension and eventually organ failure (septic shock). These complications are discussed in detail in Chapter 34.

Assessment of Infection

When performing a nursing assessment, take a thorough history to determine the patient's risk for and exposure to ***infection.*** Observe for signs and symptoms of infection if visible, such as redness, warmth, ***pain***, and swelling. Ask about changes in ***elimination,*** including urinary burning and urgency, diarrhea, and nausea/vomiting. These changes may be indications of urinary or GI system infection.

Monitor laboratory test results including:

- Elevated WBC count with differential (especially lymphocytes and neutrophils)
- Increased erythrocyte sedimentation rate (ESR)
- Increased C-reactive protein
- Positive culture and sensitivity

Additional information about assessment of ***infection*** may be found in Chapter 21.

Health Promotion Strategies to Prevent Infection

Health promotion related to ***infection*** may be categorized as primary and secondary prevention. *Primary* prevention includes measures to prevent ***infection,*** such as immunizations against common illnesses (e.g., pneumococcal 13-valent conjugate vaccine) to prevent pneumonia in older adults). *Secondary* prevention involves screening for existing infection, such as when sexually transmitted infections (STIs) are suspected or the patient is at a high risk for STIs (see Chapter 69). Best health promotion practices to prevent ***infection*** or the transmission of ***infection*** are listed in the Best Practice for Patient Safety & Quality Care box.

Interventions to Manage Patients With Infection

For some adults, infections resolve without medical or collaborative management. For example, viral respiratory infections in adults often respond to self-management with acetaminophen, fluids, and rest. However, nursing and collaborative interventions may be needed to manage some types of ***infection.*** Collaborative interventions include:

- Antimicrobial drug therapy (type depends on type of pathogen)
- Increased fluids and electrolytes

BEST PRACTICE FOR PATIENT SAFETY & QUALITY CARE QSEN

Primary Health Promotion Strategies to Prevent Infection

- Follow accepted recommended immunization guidelines for each adult age group.
- Wash hands for at least 30 seconds or use an alcohol-based hand rub for at least 15 seconds.
- Keep open skin areas covered during the healing process.
- Avoid direct contact with other people's wounds or other infections.
- Do not share personal items such as razors or towels.
- In health care, follow hand hygiene guidelines established by the CDC.
- In health care, use Standard Precautions when caring for all patients
- Employ appropriate Transmission-Based Precautions, depending how the *infection* is transmitted (spread).

- Sufficient rest
- Adequate ***nutrition***

Chapter 21 discusses care of patients with ***infection*** in more detail.

NCLEX EXAMINATION CHALLENGE 3.2

Health Promotion and Maintenance

The nurse is conducting assessments for clients at potential risk for infection. Which client is **most** at risk for acquiring an ***infection?***

A. A client who had an open incision for abdominal surgery
B. A client who has not been immunized for pneumonia or influenza
C. A client who works in a high-stress job for an accounting practice
D. A client who is 85 years old and in good health

INFLAMMATION

Definition of Inflammation

Inflammation is a syndrome of normal responses to cellular injury, allergy, or invasion by pathogens. This reaction may occur anywhere in the body and may not be observable. The primary interrelated concepts are ***immunity, infection, pain,*** and ***tissue integrity.***

Categories of Inflammation

Inflammation may be categorized as either acute or chronic. *Acute* inflammation may be *localized or systemic,* and has a short duration (hours or days). Examples of acute inflammatory health problems include cholecystitis (inflammation of the gallbladder) and appendicitis (inflammation of the appendix). *Chronic* inflammation continues for weeks, months, or possibly years. It is usually *systemic,* affecting a large portion of the body. Examples of chronic ***inflammation*** include chronic inflammatory bowel disease (e.g., ulcerative colitis) and rheumatoid arthritis (RA), which are discussed elsewhere in this textbook.

Common Risk Factors for Inflammation

Anyone is at risk for acute ***inflammation*** because it is a normal reaction to injury. Patients at risk for allergy or chronic inflammatory diseases are most susceptible to chronic ***inflammation.***

Physiologic Consequences of Inflammation

Inflammation is closely related to immune function. The cardinal signs and symptoms of *Inflammation* include:

- Redness
- Warmth
- Swelling
- ***Pain*** or discomfort

For patients with widespread or severe ***inflammation,*** loss of function of the affected part(s) of the body may also be a physiologic consequence. The function of organs or parts of the body that become inflamed also decreases or becomes impaired. For example, synovial joint inflammation as a result of RA causes ***pain,*** stiffness, and decreased ***mobility.*** Chapter 46 discusses RA in detail. Chronic ***inflammation*** may also cause low-grade fever.

Assessment of Inflammation

If localized (e.g., skin or joint inflammation) is suspected, assess for signs and symptoms as listed in the last section. If the ***inflammation*** is not observable because it is confined to inside of the body, monitor for signs and symptoms of organ dysfunction. For example, patients with chronic inflammatory bowel disease have frequent diarrhea. ***Inflammation*** of arterial vessel walls, called arterial *vasculitis,* can cause organ dysfunction due to lack of adequate ***perfusion.*** For example, renal function may be impaired due to lack of adequate blood flow to one or both kidneys.

Serum tests to measure the white blood cell count with differential, C-reactive protein, and erythrocyte sedimentation (ESR) indicate the presence of ***inflammation*** but do not help to determine a specific medical diagnosis. Direct visualization using endoscopy allows the primary health care provider to directly observe signs, symptoms, and extent of ***inflammation.***

Health Promotion Strategies to Prevent Inflammation

Inflammation occurs in response to cellular injury. Therefore avoiding injury is the best way to prevent it.

Interventions to Manage Patients With Inflammation

Manage the signs and symptoms of local ***inflammation*** in one or more extremities by applying RICE:

- <u>R</u>est
- <u>I</u>ce
- <u>C</u>ompression
- <u>E</u>levation

Check for distal circulation in the affected extremity to ensure adequate ***perfusion.*** Swelling can impair circulation and result in ischemia.

Drug therapy is often used for chronic systemic ***inflammation.*** Agents that may be used to manage systemic ***inflammation*** include antipyretics (to reduce fever), nonsteroidal anti-inflammatory drugs (NSAIDs), corticosteroids, and biologic response modifiers. For patients experiencing allergic symptoms, antihistamines and decongestants are often used.

MOBILITY

Definition of Mobility

Mobility is the ability of an individual to perform purposeful physical movement of the body. When a person is able to move, he or she can usually perform activities of daily living (ADLs) such as eating, dressing, and walking. This ability depends primarily on the function of the central and peripheral nervous system and the musculoskeletal system and is sometimes referred to as *functional ability.* The primary interrelated concepts are ***pain*** and ***sensory perception.***

Scope of Mobility

The scope of ***mobility*** can be best understood as continuum of a person's ability to move, with high-level (normal) mobility on one end of the continuum and total immobility on the other end. Many patients have varying degrees of impaired or altered physical ***mobility. Decreased*** physical ***mobility*** is the inability to move purposefully within the environment because of multiple factors, such as severe fatigue, decreased muscle strength, ***pain,*** or advanced dementia.

Common Risk Factors for Decreased Mobility

Patients who have dysfunction of the musculoskeletal or nervous system are most at risk for decreased ***mobility*** or immobility. For example, a patient with a fractured hip is not able to walk because of pain and hip joint instability until the hip is surgically repaired and healed. Patients who have severe brain or spinal cord injuries have decreased ***mobility*** or total immobility caused by lack of neuronal communication or damaged nerve tissues that enable body movement. Any person who is bedridden or on prolonged bedrest is at risk for immobility issues, regardless of health problem or medical diagnosis (Crawford & Harris, 2016).

Physiologic Consequences of Decreased Mobility

Decreases in ***mobility*** or total immobility for even a few days can cause serious and often life-threatening complications (Teodoro et al., 2016). Table 3.3 lists the most common complications seen in adult patients.

Assessment of Mobility

Observe patients within the environment to determine their mobility level. The ***mobility*** level of the patient is adequate if he or she can move purposely to walk with an erect posture and coordinated gait and perform ADLs without assistance. Several functional assessment tools are available to measure the level at which a patient can perform ADLs (see Chapter 7). Assessment of muscle strength and joint range of motion (ROM) can also be measured using a scale of 0 to 5, with 5 being normal and 0 indicating no muscle contractility.

Health Promotion Strategies to Maintain Mobility and Prevent Decreased Mobility

The nurse has a major role in promoting mobility and preventing immobility. First assess the patients who are most at risk for decreased ***mobility.*** In general, to maintain a high level of mobility or prevent decreased mobility in high-risk patients, perform these evidence-based priority interventions for the patient at home or in a health care facility:

- Teach patients to do active ROM exercises every 2 hours. Assess and manage ***pain*** to promote more comfortable movement.
- Teach patients to perform "heel pump" activities and drink adequate fluids to help prevent venous thromboembolism (VTE) such as deep vein thrombosis (DVT).
- In collaboration with the occupational therapist, evaluate the patient's need for assistive devices to promote ADL independence such as a plate guard or splint; encourage self-care.
- Evaluate the patient's need for ambulatory aids such as a cane or walker; encourage ambulation; collaborate with the physical therapist if needed.

TABLE 3.3 Common Complications of Decreased Mobility and Causes

Physiologic Complications (Occur Most Often in Older Adults)

- Pressure injuries (pressure on skin over bony prominences)
- Disuse osteoporosis (increased bone resorption)
- Constipation (decreased GI motility)
- Weight loss or gain (decreased appetite and movement)
- Muscle atrophy (catabolism)
- Atelectasis/hypostatic pneumonia (decreased lung expansion)
- Venous thromboembolism (e.g., deep venous thrombosis and pulmonary embolus [decreased blood circulation])
- Urinary system calculi (stones) (urinary stasis)

Psychosocial Complications

- Depression (isolation, inability to provide self-care)
- Changes in sleep-wake cycle (especially if confined to bed)
- Sensory deprivation (especially if confined to bed)

EVIDENCE-BASED PRACTICE (QSEN)

Is a Nurse-Initiated Ambulation Protocol Effective in Promoting Patient Ambulation?

Teodoro, C. R., Breault, K., Garvey, C., Klick, C., O'Briend, J., Purdue, T., et al. (2016). STEP-UP: Study of the effectiveness of a patient ambulation protocol. *MEDSURG Nursing, 25*(2), 111–116.

Impaired ***mobility*** or immobility in hospitalized patients can cause multiple complications, many of which are life-threatening (e.g., deep vein thrombosis, hospital-acquired pneumonia). The authors assigned 48 patients on a 30-bed medical-surgical unit in a community hospital to one of two randomly assigned matched groups: 22 patients participated in the formal ambulation protocol (STEP-UP group), and 26 patients received usual care. All patients in the study sample were in the hospital for at least 3 days and had orders for ambulation. All patients were alert and oriented and able to be ambulated with the assistance of one or two staff members. Each patient in the sample viewed a short educational video on the importance of ambulation. Each participant wore a pedometer to track the number of steps taken for 2 consecutive study days. The participants in the STEP-UP group had significantly higher numbers of steps when compared with the group who received usual care.

Level of Evidence: 3

The study used a quasi-experimental design.

Commentary: Implications for Practice and Research

This study illustrates the need for staff nurses to ensure that hospitalized patients who are able continue to ambulate using a systematic approach or protocol to prevent impaired mobility and its associated complications. Complications of immobility are often life threatening and costly. In addition, third-party payers such as Medicare do not pay for acquired complications resulting from inadequate care.

More research is needed to follow a larger group of patients for a longer period of time in multiple settings to increase the generalizability of the findings this study. Additional studies are also needed to compare the incidence of complications from impaired mobility in both groups of patients.

A study by Teodoro et al. (2016) found that a practical nurse-led ambulation program designed for hospitalized patients significantly improved ***mobility*** (see the Evidence-Based Practice box).

BEST PRACTICE FOR PATIENT SAFETY & QUALITY CARE QSEN

Nursing Interventions for Patients With Decreased Mobility or Immobility

- Perform passive ROM exercises for patients who are immobile or have severe impaired ***mobility;*** teach passive assist or active ROM exercises to patients and families with the ability to participate in this activity.
- Turn and reposition the patient every 1 to 2 hours as needed; assess for skin redness and intactness.
- Keep the patient's skin clean and dry; use pressure-relieving or pressure-reducing devices as indicated.
- In collaboration with the registered dietitian nutritionist, teach the patient and family the need for adequate ***nutrition,*** including high-fiber and protein-rich foods to promote ***elimination*** and slow muscle loss.
- Teach the patient to eat high-calcium foods to help prevent bone loss; avoid excessive high-calorie foods to prevent obesity.
- Encourage deep-breathing and coughing exercises; teach the patient how and when to use incentive spirometry.
- Teach the patient and family the need for adequate hydration to prevent renal calculi (stones) and constipation.
- Teach the patient and family to report signs and symptoms of complications of immobility such as pressure injuries; swollen, reddened lower leg; and excessive respiratory secretions.
- Collaborate with the physical therapist to ambulate the patient with ***mobility*** aids (e.g., walker, cane) if needed.

Interventions for Patients With Decreased Mobility

For patients who are immobile or have decreased ***mobility,*** perform the evidence-based nursing interventions outlined in the Best Practice for Patient Safety & Quality Care: Nursing Interventions for Patients With Decreased Mobility or Immobility box in collaboration with the interprofessional team at home or in a health care agency.

NUTRITION

Definition of Nutrition

Nutrition is the process of ingesting and using food and fluids to grow, repair, and maintain optimal body functions. Nutrients from food and fluids are used for optimal cellular metabolism and health promotion. Examples of nutrient groups are proteins, carbohydrates, fats, vitamins, and minerals. The primary interrelated concepts are ***elimination*** and ***fluid and electrolyte balance.***

Scope of Nutrition

An optimal nutritional status means that the individual has adequate nutrients for body functioning. However, some adults have decreased or poor nutritional status because of lack of available nutrients or inadequate use of nutrients. *Malnutrition* occurs in adults who are underweight or overweight/obese. Some individuals have *generalized* malnutrition; others have specific nutrient deficiencies such as lack of vitamin D, iron, or protein.

Common Risk Factors for Inadequate or Decreased Nutrition

Older adults are the largest population at risk for malnutrition as a result of acute and chronic diseases, poor oral health, and social isolation. Obesity is a common problem in people who have type 2 diabetes mellitus and metabolic syndrome.

In addition to these high-risk populations, other common risk factors for decreased or inadequate ***nutrition*** in adults include lack of money to purchase healthy food and substance use. Adults with anorexia or bulimia nervosa are also malnourished. These disorders are discussed in textbooks on mental and behavioral health. Table 3.4 summarizes common risk factors for decreased or inadequate ***nutrition.***

Physiologic Consequences of Inadequate or Decreased Nutrition

The physiologic changes that occur as a result of inadequate or decreased ***nutrition*** depend on whether the individual has generalized malnutrition or a lack of specific nutrients such as vitamin D, iron, and protein. For example, an individual who is lactose intolerant may not ingest adequate amounts of vitamin D in the diet. This deficit can cause bone demineralization such as osteoporosis. An adult who does not eat meat or other sources of iron can develop iron-deficiency anemia. Most of these patients have low serum protein, especially albumin and prealbumin, resulting in generalized edema. Serum proteins exert an osmotic pull to keep fluid within the vascular space. When they are decreased, fluid leaves the vascular system and moves into the interstitial space (third spacing).

Assessment of Nutrition

Conduct a complete patient and family history for risk factors that could cause inadequate or decreased ***nutrition.*** Ask about current or recent GI symptoms such as nausea, vomiting, constipation, and diarrhea. Obtain the patient's height and weight and calculate body mass index (BMI). Assess the patient's skin, hair, and nails. Malnutrition often causes very dry skin and brittle hair and nails.

Serum laboratory testing depends on which nutrients are inadequate. For example, older women often have vitamin D and calcium testing to determine risk for bone demineralization risk. Low serum iron levels and anemia indicate an iron deficiency. The most common assessment for generalized malnutrition is

TABLE 3.4 Risk Factors for Inadequate or Decreased Nutrition

- Familial predisposition or genetic risk
- High stress level
- Depression and social isolation, especially among older adults
- Consuming fad diets that do not provide adequate nutrients
- Obesity
- Substance use
- Lack of money to purchase food
- Impaired food intake caused by dysphagia, poor appetite, or poor oral health
- Thyroid disorders
- Chronic diseases such as chronic obstructive pulmonary disease (COPD) and cancer
- GI distress such as excessive diarrhea or vomiting
- Anorexia or bulimia nervosa

prealbumin and albumin measurement. Albumin is a major serum protein that is below normal in patients who have had inadequate nutrition for weeks. Prealbumin assessment is preferred because it decreases more quickly when ***nutrition*** is not adequate. Monitor and interpret these laboratory data to assess the patient's nutritional status. Chapter 48 describes nutritional screening and assessment in more detail.

Health Promotion Strategies to Maintain Nutrition and Prevent Inadequate or Decreased Nutrition

Teach adults to follow a healthy lifestyle that includes regular exercise and adequate nutrients to promote optimal ***nutrition*** and a BMI between 19 and 24.9 kg/m^2 (Jarvis, 2020). Remind them to avoid high-calorie, high-fat foods with no nutritive value. For patients at risk for inadequate or decreased ***nutrition,*** collaborate with the interprofessional team to implement the appropriate interventions discussed in the following section.

Interventions for Patients With Inadequate or Decreased Nutrition

Collaborative interventions to improve ***nutrition*** depend on the cause of inadequate or decreased nutrition. For those with weight loss or low weight, common interventions include high-protein oral supplements, enteral supplements (either oral or by feeding tube), or parenteral nutrition. Collaborate with the registered dietitian nutritionist for specific instructions regarding enteral feedings; consult with the pharmacist to administer parenteral therapy. Drug therapy such as iron or vitamin D to replace selected nutrients may also be given. To determine effectiveness of these interventions, weigh the patient at least once a week or as prescribed, using the same scale at the same time of day and preferably before breakfast.

Patients experiencing obesity may be prescribed drug therapy to help them lose weight. In some cases bariatric surgical procedures are needed to restrict the volume of food that can be ingested and/or decrease the absorptive area for nutrients. These procedures have the potential to cause multiple complications and require an interprofessional team approach for success. Chapter 55 describes these surgeries in detail and their associated nursing and interprofessional collaborative care.

PAIN

Definition of Pain

Pain is generally defined as an unpleasant sensory and emotional experience. Because pain is a subjective symptom, nurses and other health care professionals must respect the patient's description of pain. More detailed information may be found in Chapter 5 of this text. The primary interrelated concepts are ***inflammation*** and ***tissue integrity.***

Categories of Pain

Pain can be categorized by duration as acute or persistent (chronic). *Acute* ***pain*** is short lived, temporary, and typically confined to an injured area of the body (localized). It serves a biologic purpose to activate the sympathetic nervous system and other physiologic responses. *Persistent (chronic)* ***pain*** does not serve this purpose and tends to last more than 3 months. It is often described as diffuse and not confined to one area of the body. The two major types of persistent pain are persistent cancer pain and persistent noncancer pain. Chapter 5 differentiates acute versus persistent ***pain*** in detail.

Pain can also be categorized by its underlying mechanism into nociceptive and neuropathic pain. *Nociceptive* pain results from skin or organ damage or ***inflammation.*** *Neuropathic* pain involves a set of mechanisms related to the nervous system with or without tissue damage. Chapter 5 compares the characteristics of these types of ***pain.***

Common Risk Factors for Pain

Anyone is at risk for ***pain,*** and many adults have experienced one or more types of pain sometime in their lives. Specific risk factors include individuals who experience acute trauma or have chronic diseases, such as osteoarthritis, cancer, or low back pain. These diseases are discussed elsewhere in this text.

Physiologic and Psychosocial Consequences of Pain

Patients experiencing *acute* ***pain*** usually have one or more sympathetic nervous system signs and symptoms including nausea, vomiting, diaphoresis (sweating), increased blood pressure, increased respiratory rate, increased pulse, and dilated pupils (McCance et al., 2019). This "flight or fight" reaction does not occur in patients with *persistent* ***pain***. *Persistent* ***pain*** can cause psychosocial issues including anxiety and depression.

Assessment of Pain

A comprehensive ***pain*** assessment includes these components (Jarvis, 2020):

- Location of pain and whether it radiates or is referred to other areas of the body
- Intensity of pain using one of several valid and reliable pain assessment tools
- Quality of pain (such as burning, stabbing, and sharp in patient's own words)
- Onset and duration of pain
- Aggravating or precipitating factors that cause pain
- Effects of pain on quality of life and daily function
- Psychosocial effects of pain (such as anxiety, fear, and depression)

Chapter 5 describes the nurse's role in ***pain*** assessment in detail.

Health Promotion Strategies to Prevent Pain

Acute pain is often unavoidable. Almost everyone has had a headache, GI discomfort, or acute injury, including small cuts and bruises. Avoiding high-risk activities can help prevent trauma from accidental injury and thus prevent severe acute ***pain***. After surgery, acute pain must be well controlled to prevent *persistent* pain that may last for months or years.

Interventions to Manage Patients With Pain

Nursing and collaborative management of ***pain*** may be categorized by pharmacologic and nonpharmacologic interventions.

Evidence-based *pharmacologic* interventions involve a variety of analgesics and are determined on the basis of severity, type, and source of ***pain.*** Analgesics may be divided into nonopioid drugs and opioid drugs. Nonopioid drugs may be used without concern related to abuse or addiction; however, they have side and adverse effects that require careful monitoring. For example, acetaminophen can cause liver damage if taken in large doses for a prolonged period of time.

Patient education is an important nursing intervention when managing patients who have ***pain.*** For example, teach patients to take drug therapy for *persistent* pain on a continuous regimen basis for the best control. *Persistent* cancer ***pain*** often requires opioids at the end-of-life to provide ***comfort*** and prepare for a "good death."

Nonpharmacologic patient-centered interventions depend on the patient's preferences. Examples of these integrative therapies include imagery, acupressure, acupuncture, and aromatherapy. Chapter 5 discusses interventions for ***pain*** in detail.

PERFUSION

Definition of Perfusion

Perfusion is adequate arterial blood flow through the peripheral tissues (*peripheral* ***perfusion***) and blood that is pumped by the heart to oxygenate major body organs (*central* ***perfusion***). ***Perfusion*** is a normal physiologic process of the body; without adequate ***perfusion,*** cell death can occur. The primary interrelated concepts are ***clotting, gas exchange,*** and ***tissue integrity.***

Scope of Perfusion

The scope of ***perfusion*** can best be understood as a continuum of the heart's ability to adequately supply blood to the body and the patency of arteries to adequately supply blood to peripheral tissues. *Ischemia* refers to impaired ***perfusion***, whereas *infarction* is complete tissue death (Fig. 3.6).

Common Risk Factors for Decreased Perfusion

Risk factors for decreased ***perfusion*** can be either modifiable (can be changed) or nonmodifiable (cannot be changed). *Nonmodifiable* factors include age, gender, and family history (genetics). Older adults are at the most risk for decreased ***perfusion.*** Examples of *modifiable* risk factors are smoking, lack of physical activity, and obesity. Patients with hyperlipidemia, diabetes mellitus, peripheral vascular disease, and arteriosclerosis are at a very high risk for both decreased central and peripheral ***perfusion.***

Physiologic Consequences of Decreased Perfusion

Decreased *peripheral* ***perfusion*** most often occurs in the lower extremities. The distal legs become cool and pale or cyanotic. Pedal pulses may be diminished or absent. If not treated, inadequate ***perfusion*** may result in skin ulcers (see ***tissue integrity*** later in this chapter) or cell death such as gangrene. Decreased *central* ***perfusion*** may result in life-threatening systemic events such as acute myocardial infarction, stroke, and shock as a result of decreased blood flow to major organs discussed elsewhere in this textbook.

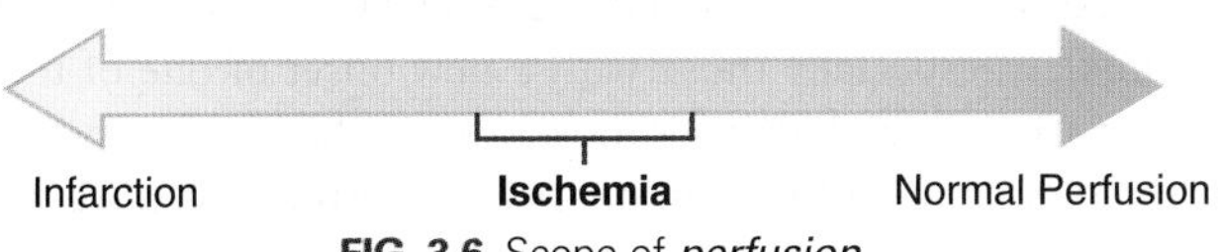

FIG. 3.6 Scope of *perfusion.*

Assessment of Perfusion

Conduct a complete patient and family history for risk factors and existing problems with ***perfusion.*** Assess for signs and symptoms of inadequate *central* ***perfusion,*** including dyspnea, dizziness or syncope, and chest pain. Signs and symptoms of decreased cardiac output include hypotension, tachycardia, diaphoresis, anxiety, decrease in cognitive function, and dysrhythmias. Assess for signs and symptoms of decreased *peripheral* ***perfusion,*** including decreased hair distribution, nonlocalized and diffuse pain or discomfort, coolness, and pallor and/or cyanosis of the extremities (McCance et al., 2019). Document the presence and quality of distal peripheral pulses because severe impaired ***perfusion*** can lead to absent peripheral pulses distal to the arterial occlusion. Notify the Rapid Response Team or primary health care provider if these signs and symptoms occur.

Health Promotion Strategies to Maintain Perfusion and Prevent Decreased Perfusion

The nurse plays a vital role in promoting adequate ***perfusion*** and preventing any impairment. Help the patient identify modifiable risk factors such as inadequate ***nutrition*** and smoking. Teach the importance of a heart-healthy lifestyle that includes a well-balanced diet, regular exercise, and smoking cessation. Encourage the patient to obtain frequent screening and monitoring of blood pressure and relevant laboratory work to detect early signs of decreased ***perfusion.***

Interventions for Patients With Decreased Perfusion

Because decreased ***perfusion*** can cause serious and life-threatening consequences, the primary health care provider may prescribe vasodilating drugs to promote blood flow. However, for many patients, a vascular intervention to open the occluded or narrowed artery is performed. This type of procedure can be done to open coronary arteries (central ***perfusion***) or peripheral arteries such as the femoral or pelvic arteries in the leg.

NCLEX EXAMINATION CHALLENGE 3.3

Safe, Effective Care Environment

A client reports increasing diffuse pain in the entire right leg. What is the nurse's **priority action** at this time?

A. Elevate the right leg on a pillow.
B. Perform a peripheral vascular assessment.
C. Check for swelling in the right leg.
D. Notify the Rapid Response Team immediately.

SENSORY PERCEPTION

Definition of Sensory Perception

Sensory perception is the ability to perceive and interpret sensory input into one or more meaningful responses. Sensory input is usually received through the five major senses of vision, hearing, smell, taste, and touch. The primary interrelated concept is ***mobility.***

Scope and Categories of Sensory Perception

The most likely cause of changes in smell and taste for adults is a dry mouth, which is a common side effect of drug therapy. Examples of drugs that can cause dry mouth include antidepressants, chemotherapeutic agents, antihistamines, and antiepileptic drugs (AEDs). When the causative drug is discontinued, the problem typically subsides. Touch (peripheral sensation loss) is most often affected in patients who have acute and chronic neurologic problems such as stroke, traumatic brain injury, or spinal cord injury. For many patients this sensory deficit is permanent. These health problems are discussed elsewhere in this text.

Problems of ***sensory perception*** that occur in the adult population largely affect vision and hearing. Therefore the following discussion is limited to these two sensory functions.

Vision and hearing abilities (acuity) vary from person to person, depending on a number of factors. Acuity of vision and hearing ranges from optimum through a continuum to complete blindness (vision) and deafness (hearing). Many adults have visual or hearing deficits but are able to function independently.

Common Risk Factors for Changes in Sensory Perception

As adults age, they are at an increased risk for decreased visual and hearing acuity. Older adults typically have *presbyopia* (far-sightedness) and *presbycusis* (sensorineural type) caused by the aging process. Chronic diseases such as diabetes mellitus and hypertension can lead to decreased visual acuity. Although these health problems can occur in any age-group, they most commonly occur in older adults. The older population is also more at risk for glaucoma, cataracts, and macular degeneration, all of which can cause loss of vision.

Other causes for changes in or loss of vision include direct mechanical or chemical trauma, genetic risk, cranial nerve II (optic) damage, and drug therapy such as antihistamines and antihypertensives. Hearing loss may be caused by direct physical trauma, cranial nerve VIII (acoustic, or auditory) damage, occupational factors (e.g., consistent loud noises), genetic risk, and drugs that are ototoxic. Examples of drugs that can cause ototoxicity are salicylates, diuretics, antiepileptic drugs (AEDs), and antibiotics, especially aminoglycosides.

Physiologic Consequences of Changes in Sensory Perception

Adults with visual and hearing acuity loss that cannot be corrected are at risk for physical injury, including falls and other accidents. They may not be able to perform ADLs or ambulate independently and may require assistance. Those with hearing loss may not be able to rely solely on verbal communication. Visually impaired adults may not be able to use written communication.

Assessment of Sensory Perception

Conduct a thorough patient and family history to determine risk factors for vision or hearing loss. Ask the patient about the use of eyeglasses, contacts, or a magnifier to improve vision. Inquire if he or she uses one or more hearing aids or amplifier. If any of these corrective aids are used, determine their effectiveness.

Ask the patient to read from a written text source such as a newspaper. Assess the patient to determine reading ability before requesting this screening. In the community setting a Snellen chart is often used to assess visual acuity. Use a whisper test to determine if the patient can hear. More extensive testing of the eyes and ears, including physical assessment, is performed by the primary health care provider or other qualified health professional.

Health Promotion Strategies to Maintain Sensory Perception and Prevent Changes in Sensory Perception

Primary and secondary preventive interventions are used to promote vision and hearing and prevent sensory deficits. *Primary* measures focus on avoiding risk factors that cause vision and hearing loss or using protective devices to minimize risk. For example, safety goggles help prevent eye injury when working with materials that can get into the eye. Ear plugs or other ear protective devices can minimize the exposure to loud noises such as that caused by machinery. A healthy lifestyle can help prevent the risk for diseases such as diabetes mellitus and hypertension, thus reducing the chance for decreased visual acuity from chronic disease.

The purpose of secondary prevention is to perform screening and diagnostic tests for early detection of beginning sensory loss. Examples of these strategies include regular eye examinations (annually for older adults) and physical examinations to diagnose and manage any chronic diseases early.

Interventions for Patients With Changes in Sensory Perception

For patients who have glaucoma, drug therapy (local or systemic) may decrease intraocular pressure and prevent loss of vision. For some patients, corrective lenses or eye surgery (LASIK) can improve refractory vision problems. Adults with visual changes may have correction with eyeglasses or contact lenses; those with hearing loss may benefit from one or two hearing aids (Fig. 3.7). Adults who are totally blind may use guide dogs and/or braille. Those who are deaf may use closed-caption television, assistive listening devices, and sign language.

Assess patients with vision and hearing loss for self-image and anxiety, especially those with a new onset of one of these deficits. Consult with or refer those who are having psychological distress to a qualified member of the interprofessional health team.

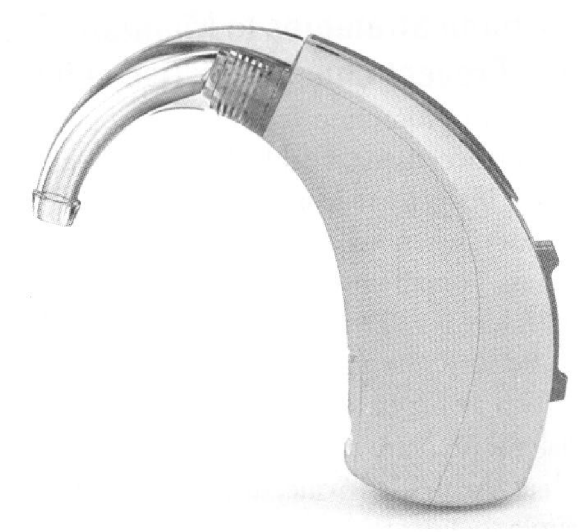

FIG. 3.7 Example of a hearing aid. (Courtesy of Starkey.)

SEXUALITY

Definition of Sexuality

Sexuality is a complex integration of physiologic, emotional, and social aspects of well-being related to intimacy, self-concept, and role relationships. It is not the same as *reproduction,* which is the process of conceiving and having a child. ***Sexuality*** involves sex, sexual acts, and sexual orientation; these terms are *not* the same as gender identity, which is discussed later in Chapter 68. The primary interrelated concept is ***comfort***.

Scope of Sexuality

The concept of ***sexuality*** ranges from positive sexual health and function to negative sexual health, impairment, or dysfunction. Men and women often define sexuality, sex, and sexual health differently. Women usually view sexuality as defined previously; men often associate the term sexuality only with the act of sexual intercourse (Giddens, 2021). Therefore the concept of ***sexuality*** may be perceived differently by different individuals.

Common Risk Factors for Changes in Sexuality

For some adults, changes in ***sexuality*** may be equated with poor sexual health or lack of sexual intercourse. During menopause some women perceive more positive ***sexuality,*** but others feel that changes such as vaginal atrophy and moodiness cause a more negative sexual experience. Men who have problems with penile erection or deal with prostate problems often feel sexually inadequate and have a poor self-concept when they are unable to satisfy their partners. As men get older, the risk of erectile dysfunction (ED) increases. Drug therapy, such as antihypertensive drugs; chronic diseases, such as diabetes mellitus; and decreased testosterone can also contribute to ED.

Physiologic and Psychosocial Consequences of Changes in Sexuality

Depending on the individual, the major consequence of ***sexuality*** changes or sexual dysfunction may not be physiologic. Rather, the adult experiencing changes in ***sexuality*** often has a poor self-image and self-concept. Being able to be intimate with another person is an important human need for most people. Sexual intimacy shows a deep sense of caring for another person.

Assessment of Sexuality

Discussing ***sexuality,*** sexual health, and sexual intercourse is often difficult for both the patient and nurse. Ask patients about their perception of their ***sexuality,*** including both sexual activity and intimacy behaviors. Determine if they have sex and/or intimacy with one or more partners. Ask about protection measures and any history of sexually transmitted infections (STIs) or problems during sexual intercourse.

Health Promotion Strategies to Maintain Sexuality and Prevent Changes in Sexuality

Interventions include STI screening and physical examinations to determine any physical cause of changes in ***sexuality.*** For example, a man may have ED, and a woman may have decreased libido due to menopause. Assess patients for self-concept related to these issues or other intimacy concerns. Encourage patients at risk for STIs to be evaluated for their occurrence.

Interventions for Patients With Changes in Sexuality

Interventions depend on the cause of the sexual impairment. Physical causes such as ED or STIs can be managed by drug therapy and other measures. Refer the patient whose impaired ***sexuality*** is caused by emotional or psychological factors to a qualified primary health care provider.

TISSUE INTEGRITY

Definition of Tissue Integrity

Tissue integrity is the intactness of the structure and function of the integument (skin and subcutaneous tissue) and mucous membranes. The skin is the largest organ of the body and has multiple functions, including protection from infection, fluid preservation, and temperature control. The primary interrelated concepts are ***fluid and electrolyte balance, infection, nutrition,*** and ***perfusion.***

Scope of Tissue Integrity

Tissue integrity can vary from intact (normal) to impaired tissue integrity, often referred to as an injury, wound, or ulcer, depending on its cause. ***Tissue integrity*** changes can occur as a result of infections, burns, local skin reactions, injury/trauma, growths or lesions, and inadequate peripheral ***perfusion*** (decrease in oxygenated blood to a specific area of the body). The degree of tissue damage is referred to as partial- or full-thickness loss. A *partial-thickness* wound extends through the epidermis and dermis. *Full-thickness* wounds extend into the subcutaneous tissue and can expose muscle or bone.

Common Risk Factors for Changes in Tissue Integrity

Changes in ***tissue integrity*** can occur at any age, but older adults are at increased risk. The skin and underlying tissues of older adults become thinner, drier, and more likely to bruise because of increased capillary fragility. Arterial blood flow is often decreased. Certain medical conditions also increase the risk of impaired ***tissue integrity*** and include malnutrition, neurologic disorders, diabetes mellitus, peripheral vascular disease, urinary and bowel incontinence, and immune suppression. Adults who do not protect their skin from sunlight are at high risk for skin cancer. The most common tissue impairment, though, is *pressure injuries,* which account for a significant number of hospital and long-term care admissions (see Chapter 23).

Physiologic Consequences of Changes in Tissue Integrity

Alterations in ***tissue integrity*** can lead to localized (cellulitis) or systemic (sepsis) ***infection.*** Both partial- and full-thickness wounds can be very painful and difficult to heal, especially for patients with diabetes and other diseases in which arterial ***perfusion*** is diminished.

Assessment of Tissue Integrity

Take a thorough health history of previous and current chronic health problems and current medications (prescribed and over-the-counter [OTC]). Assess for change in skin color, moles or lesions, excessive skin dryness, bruising, and hair loss or brittle nails (indicating decreased tissue ***perfusion***). For patients at risk for pressure injury, conduct a risk assessment using the Braden Scale or other evidence-based tool (see Chapter 22).

Document any existing tissue impairment in detail, including wound size, color, depth, and drainage. Monitor serum albumin and prealbumin levels to ensure that the patient has adequate protein for preventing tissue impairment or healing any existing wounds.

Health Promotion Strategies to Maintain Tissue Integrity and Prevent Changes in Tissue Integrity

The primary health promotion focus is on proper hygiene and nutrition to enhance tissue health. Teach patients at risk for changes in ***tissue integrity*** to inspect the skin every day. Keep the skin clean and dry; when needed, moisturize the skin to prevent excessive dryness. For patients who are confined to a bed or chair, ensure that pressure is relieved by changing body position every 1 to 2 hours. Be sure that patients sit or lie on pressure-reducing surfaces such as mattress overlays or chair gel pads. Assess patients at risk for pressure injuries with evidence-based screening tools such as the Braden Scale, discussed in Chapter 22.

Teach people to wear wide brim hats, long sleeves, and long pants when going outside if the environmental temperature is not too warm. Stress the importance of using sunscreen with at least a 30 SPF on all exposed skin areas to prevent skin cancer. Sunglasses are also essential to protect eyes from the harmful effects of the sun.

Interventions for Patients With Changes in Tissue Integrity

Provide preventive interventions as described previously to prevent further skin and tissue breakdown. Ensure that patients eat an adequate diet and receive nutritional supplements as needed for healing. Protein and vitamin C are especially important for preventing skin breakdown and promoting healing of existing wounds. Protein shakes and powders can be added to the daily diet.

Interprofessional collaborative management of any ***tissue integrity*** alteration may include drug therapy (e.g., antibiotics, topical steroids, creams). Chemical and/or surgical wound débridement for necrotic tissue is essential to allow healing. In some cases, the primary health care provider may need to perform an interventional procedure to open arteries that are narrowed or obstructed to increase blood flow and promote wound healing.

GET READY FOR THE NEXT-GENERATION NCLEX® EXAMINATION!

Key Points

Review these Key Points for each NCLEX Examination Client Needs Category.

Safe and Effective Care Environment

- Collaborate with members of the interprofessional health care team as needed to meet the patient's physiologic needs. For example, consult with the registered dietitian nutritionist for patients who have impaired ***nutrition;*** consult with the physical therapist for patients with impaired ***mobility.*** **QSEN: Teamwork and Collaboration**

Health Promotion and Maintenance

- Provide patient education/health teaching to promote physiologic health, including ***nutrition, mobility,*** and ***gas exchange.*** **QSEN: Patient-Centered Care**
- Assess patient lifestyle behaviors and other factors to determine risks for impairments in basic physiologic needs such as ***mobility, gas exchange,*** and ***perfusion*** (see Tables 3.3 and 3.4). **Clinical Judgment**

Psychosocial Integrity

- Differentiate the assessment findings associated with dementia versus delirium (see Table 3.1). **Clinical Judgment**
- Plan interventions to promote ***sensory perception,*** especially in older adults. **QSEN: Patient-Centered Care**
- Risk factors that affect ***sexuality*** include poor sexual health, physiologic changes associated with menopause, and poor self-concept. **Clinical Judgment**

Physiological Integrity

- Recognize that the type, source, and severity of ***pain*** or impaired ***comfort*** determine the priority patient-centered interventions. **QSEN: Patient-Centered Care; Evidence-Based Practice**

- Monitor vital signs and laboratory tests to determine the status of ***gas exchange*** and ***clotting;*** assess the patient's circulation to determine the status of peripheral ***perfusion.*** **QSEN: Safety**
- Provide evidence-based nursing interventions to manage impairments in physiologic needs such as decreased ***nutrition*** and ***mobility*** to maintain patient ***safety.*** **QSEN: Evidence-Based Practice; Safety**

MASTERY QUESTIONS

1. The nurse is assessing an older adult and notes that the client is at risk for constipation. Which statements will the nurse include in health teaching for this client to promote optimum bowel elimination? **Select all that apply.**
A. "Be sure to include plenty of fresh fruits and vegetables in your diet each day."
B. "Eat lots of high fiber foods, including whole grains each day."
C. "Be sure to take a laxative every day to clean out your bowels and prevent toxins."
D. "Exercise several times a week to keep our bowels working for regular elimination."
E. "Drink at least 3 caffeinated beverages every day to keep your bowels stimulated."
F. "Drink plenty of fluids, including water, to prevent having difficulty going to the bathroom."

2. Which of the following factors does the nurse recognize as being a risk for altered sensory perception in the older adult client?
A. Diabetes mellitus
B. Hypotension
C. Osteoarthritis
D. Peptic ulcer disease

REFERENCES

Blevins, S. H. (2017). Immunizations for the adult patient. *Medsurg Nursing, 26*(2), 138–151.

Crawford, A., & Harris, H. (2016). Caring for adults with impaired physical mobility. *Nursing, 46*(12), 36–42.

Giddens, J. F. (2021). *Concepts for nursing practice* (3rd ed.). St. Louis: Elsevier.

Jarvis, C. (2020). *Physical examination and health assessment* (8th ed.). St. Louis: Elsevier.

McCance, K., Huether, S., Brashers, V., & Rote, N. (2019). *Pathophysiology: The biologic basis for disease in adults and children* (8th ed.). St. Louis: Mosby.

Teodoro, C. R., Breault, K., Garvey, C., Klick, C., O'Briend, J., Purdue, T., et al. (2016). STEP-UP: Study of the effectiveness of a patient ambulation protocol. *Medsurg Nursing, 25*(2), 111–116.

4

Common Health Problems of Older Adults

Donna D. Ignatavicius

http://evolve.elsevier.com/Iggy/

LEARNING OUTCOMES

1. Identify common risk factors for decreased ***mobility*** and ***sensory perception*** in older adults who live in the community or are in inpatient facilities.
2. Describe evidence-based falls risk and prevention interventions for older adults in the community or inpatient facilities.
3. Summarize best practices to promote patient safety when using restraints.
4. Plan evidence-based health teaching about lifestyle practices to promote health in older adults.
5. Conduct a medication assessment for potential risks for adverse drug events in older adults.
6. Assess the older patient's risk for and signs of neglect and abuse.
7. Identify ***health care disparities*** within the older-adult population.
8. Identify valid and reliable assessment tools to document inadequate ***cognition*** in the older adult, including depression, delirium, and dementia.
9. Explain factors that contribute to decreased ***nutrition*** and ***elimination*** changes among older adults in the community and inpatient facilities.
10. Prioritize key interventions to prevent ***tissue integrity*** changes in older adults.

KEY TERMS

delirium An acute and fluctuating cognitive disorder that is characterized by the patient's inattentiveness, disorganized thinking, and altered level of consciousness (either hypoalert or hyperalert).

dementia A broad term used for a syndrome that involves a slowly progressive cognitive decline, sometimes referred to as *chronic confusion.* This syndrome represents a global impairment of intellectual function and is generally chronic and progressive.

depression A mood disorder that can have cognitive, affective, and physical manifestations. It can be primary or secondary and can range from mild to severe or major.

fall An unintentional change in body position or descent that results in the person's body coming to rest on the floor or ground.

fallophobia Fear of falling (especially among older adults).

geriatric syndromes Major health issues associated with late adulthood in community and inpatient settings (but that are not normal aging changes).

health literacy The degree to which a person has the ability to obtain, communicate, process, and understand basic health information to make appropriate health decisions.

neglect Failure of a caregiver to provide for an older adult's basic needs such as food, clothing, medications, or assistance with ADLs.

nocturia Urination during the night.

polypharmacy The use of multiple drugs, duplicative drug therapy, high-dosage drugs, and drugs prescribed for too long a period of time.

presbycusis Hearing loss associated with the aging process.

presbyopia Farsightedness that worsens with aging.

relocation stress syndrome The physical and emotional distress that can occur after a person moves from one setting to another.

restraint Any device or drug that prevents the patient from moving freely and must be prescribed by a primary health care provider.

PRIORITY AND INTERRELATED CONCEPTS

The priority concepts for this chapter are:
- ***Mobility***
- ***Nutrition***
- ***Cognition***

The interrelated concepts for this chapter are:
- ***Elimination***
- ***Sensory Perception***
- ***Tissue Integrity***
- ***Health Care Disparities***

About 15% of the people in the United States are currently older than 65 years, but this number is expected to grow dramatically over the next 20 years (www.census.gov). Although Euro-Caucasians are the majority of the current older population, the ethnic and racial makeup of this group is expected to change over the next few decades. In general, women live longer than men, although the exact reason for this difference is not known. Most patients on adult acute care and nursing home units are older than 65 years; many of these patients are discharged for continuing health services. Therefore nurses and other interprofessional team members need to know about the special needs of older adults to care for them in a variety of settings.

This chapter describes the major health issues, sometimes referred to as geriatric syndromes, associated with late adulthood in community and inpatient settings. The care of older adults (sometimes referred to as *elders*) with specific acute and chronic health problems is discussed as appropriate throughout this text. *Older Adult Considerations* boxes highlight the most important information. A brief review of major physiologic changes of aging is listed in the Assessment chapter of each body system unit. A number of gerontologic nursing textbooks and journals are available for additional information about older-adult care.

OVERVIEW

Late adulthood can be divided into four major subgroups:
- 65 to 74 years of age: the young old
- 75 to 84 years of age: the middle old
- 85 to 99 years of age: the old old
- 100 years of age or older: the elite old

The fastest growing subgroup is the old old, sometimes referred to as the advanced older-adult population. Members of this subgroup are sometimes referred to as the *frail elderly,* although a number of 85- to 99-year-olds are very healthy and do not meet the criteria for being frail. *Frailty* is actually a geriatric syndrome in which the older adult has unintentional weight loss; weakness and exhaustion; and slowed physical activity, including walking. Frail older adults are also at high risk for adverse outcomes.

The vast majority of older adults live in the community at home, in assisted-living facilities, or in retirement or independent living complexes. Of all older adults, less than 10% live in long-term care (LTC) facilities (mostly nursing homes), and another 10% to 15% are chronically ill but are cared for at home. Older adults from any setting usually experience one or more hospitalizations in their lifetime. Many older adults will likely be admitted at some time during their life for short-term stays in a skilled unit of an LTC facility, often for rehabilitation or complex medical-surgical follow-up care.

Other institutions also have an increase in aging adults. For example, men older than 50 years are the fastest growing group of prisoners today. Like the rest of the older population, older prisoners have multiple chronic health problems. However, these problems are often complicated by a history of substance use and poor ***nutrition*** that requires specific management strategies. Nurses who work in these settings must have expertise in care of older adults.

The number of homeless people older than 60 years is also growing. The inability to pay for housing and family/partner relationship problems are primary factors that contribute to this trend. Many homeless adults have one or more chronic health problems, including mental health/behavioral health disorders. A growing number are veterans of recent wars.

HEALTH ISSUES FOR OLDER ADULTS IN COMMUNITY-BASED SETTINGS

Many older adults in the community are at risk for poor health due to low health literacy. Health literacy is the degree to which a person has the ability to obtain, communicate, process, and understand basic health information to make appropriate health decisions. A secondary study by Cutilli et al. (2018) found that low health literacy in older adults is associated with having a low income, high school education or less, and fair to poor health. These factors can result in ***health care disparities***. Therefore health literacy is a priority for nurses and other health care professionals.

An older adult's health status can affect his or her ability to perform ADLs and to participate in social activities. A failure to perform these activities may increase dependence on others and may have a negative effect on morale and life satisfaction. If older adults lose the ability to function independently, they often feel empty, bored, and worthless. Loss of autonomy is a painful event related to the physical and mental changes of aging and/or illness.

Older adults may also experience a number of losses that can affect a sense of control over their lives such as the death of a spouse and friends or the loss of social and work roles. Nurses need to support older adults' self-esteem and feelings of independence by encouraging them to maintain as much control as possible over their lives, to participate in decision making, and to perform as many tasks as possible.

Like younger and middle-age adults, older adults need to practice health promotion and illness prevention to maintain or achieve a high level of wellness. Teach them the importance of promoting wellness and practices for meeting this outcome. Examples of these practices are listed in the Patient and Family Education: Preparing for Self-Management: Lifestyles and Practices to Promote Wellness box.

PATIENT AND FAMILY EDUCATION: PREPARING FOR SELF-MANAGEMENT

Lifestyles and Practices to Promote Wellness

Health-Protecting Behaviors

- Have yearly influenza vaccinations (preferably after October 1).
- Obtain pneumococcal vaccinations as recommended.
- Obtain a shingles vaccination; be sure to obtain the most recent available immunization.
- Have a tetanus booster (Tdap) every 10 years.
- Wear seat belts when you are in an automobile.
- Use alcohol in moderation or not at all.
- Avoid smoking; if you do smoke, do not smoke in bed.
- Install grab bars in showers, in tubs, and near toilets.
- Install and maintain working smoke detectors and/or sprinklers.
- Create a hazard-free environment to prevent falls; eliminate hazards such as scatter rugs and waxed floors.
- Use medications, herbs, and nutritional supplements according to your primary health care provider's prescription.
- Avoid over-the-counter medications unless your primary health care provider directs you to use them.

Health-Enhancing Behaviors

- Have a yearly physical examination; see your primary health care provider more often if health problems occur.
- Reduce dietary fat to not more than 30% of calories; saturated fat should provide less than 10% of your calories.
- Increase your daily dietary intake of complex carbohydrate- and fiber-containing food to five or more servings of fruits and vegetables and six or more servings of grain products.
- Increase calcium intake to between 1000 and 1500 mg daily; take a vitamin D supplement as recommended.
- Allow at least 10 to 15 minutes of sun exposure two or three times weekly for vitamin D intake; avoid prolonged sun exposure and use sunscreen.
- Exercise regularly three to five times a week.
- Manage stress through coping mechanisms that have been successful in the past.
- Get together with people in different settings to socialize.
- Reminisce about your life through reflective discussions or journaling.

Common health issues and geriatric syndromes that often affect older adults in the community include:

- Inadequate or decreased ***nutrition*** and hydration
- Decreased ***mobility***
- Stress and coping
- Accidents
- Drug use and misuse
- Inadequate ***cognition***
- Substance use disorder
- Elder neglect and abuse

Inadequate or Decreased Nutrition and Hydration

Chapter 3 includes a concept review of ***nutrition***. The minimum nutritional requirements of the human body remain consistent from youth through old age, with a few exceptions. Older adults need an increased dietary intake of calcium and vitamins D, C, and A because aging changes disrupt the ability to store, use, and absorb these substances. For older adults who have a sedentary lifestyle and decreased metabolic rate, a reduction in total caloric intake to maintain an ideal body weight is needed. Inadequate or decreased ***nutrition***, either underweight or overweight/obesity, can occur in older adults when these needs are not met.

Many physical aging changes influence nutritional status or the ability to consume needed nutrients. For example, diminished senses of taste and smell often result in a loss of desire for food. Older adults often have less ability to taste sweet and salt than to taste bitter and sour. This aging change may result in an overuse of table sugar and salt to compensate. Some older adults consume numerous desserts and other sweet foods, which can cause them to become overweight or obese. Teach older adults how to balance their diets with healthy food selections. Remind them to substitute herbs and spices to season food and vary the textures of food substances to feel satisfied.

Tooth loss and poorly fitting dentures from inadequate dental care or calcium loss can also cause the older adult to avoid important nutritious foods. Unlike today, dental preventive programs were not readily available or stressed as being important when today's older adults were younger. Older people with dentition problems may eat soft, high-calorie foods such as ice cream and mashed potatoes, which lack roughage and fiber. Unless the person carefully chooses more nutritious soft foods, vitamin deficiencies, constipation, and other problems can result. The extensive use of prescribed and over-the-counter (OTC) drugs, including herbal supplements, may decrease appetite, affect food tolerances and absorption, and cause constipation.

Constipation can reduce quality of life for older adults and cause pain, depression, anxiety, and decreased social activities. In some cases it leads to a small or large bowel obstruction, a potentially life-threatening event. Constipation is common among older adults and can be caused by multiple risk factors, including foods, drugs, and diseases.

! NURSING SAFETY PRIORITY QSEN

Action Alert

Teach older adults to increase fiber and fluid intake, exercise regularly, and avoid risk factors that contribute to constipation. Older adults should consume 35 to 50 g of fiber each day and drink at least 2 liters a day unless medically contraindicated. Some people may also add a "colon cocktail" of equal parts of prune juice, applesauce, and psyllium to their daily diet. Remind older adults to take 1 to 2 tablespoons of the mixture daily. If these measures do not prevent constipation, teach them to take a stool softener. For opioid-induced constipation (OIC), drug therapy may be prescribed.

Reduced income, chronic disease, fatigue, and decreased ability to perform ADLs are other factors that contribute to inadequate or decreased ***nutrition*** and constipation among older adults. "Fast food" is often inexpensive and requires no preparation. However, it is generally high in fat, carbohydrates, and calories and lacking in healthy nutrients. Older adults can become overweight or obese when they consume a diet high in fast food.

Other older adults may reduce their intake of food to near-starvation levels, even with the availability of programs such as food stamps (Supplemental Nutrition Assistance

Program [SNAP]), community food banks, and the Older Americans Act (OAA) Nutrition Program. Many senior centers and homeless shelters offer congregate meals and group social activities. The lack of transportation, the necessity of traveling to obtain such services, and the inability to carry large or heavy groceries prevent some older adults from taking advantage of congregate food programs. In this case, the OAA Nutrition Program can provide one meal a day for 5 days a week for home delivery (Mangels, 2018). Some older adults are too proud to accept these free services.

Inadequate or decreased ***nutrition*** may also be related to loneliness. Older adults may respond to loneliness, depression, and boredom by not eating, which can lead to weight loss. Many who live alone lose the incentive to prepare or eat balanced diets, especially if they do not "feel well." Men who live at home alone are especially at risk for poor nutrition (Mangels, 2018).

! NURSING SAFETY PRIORITY QSEN

Action Alert

Perform nutritional screening for older adults in the community who are at risk for inadequate or decreased *nutrition*—either weight loss or obesity. Ask the person about unintentional weight loss or gain, eating habits, appetite, prescribed and OTC drugs, and current health problems. Determine contributing factors for older adults who have or are at risk for poor *nutrition* such as transportation issues or loneliness. Based on these assessment data, develop and implement a plan of care in collaboration with the registered dietitian nutritionist, pharmacist, and/or case manager to manage these problems. Nutritional assessment and management of *nutrition* problems are described in more detail elsewhere in this textbook.

Adults older than 65 years are also at risk for dehydration because they have less body water content than younger adults and tend to have decreased thirst. In severe cases, they require emergency department visits or hospital stays.

! NURSING SAFETY PRIORITY QSEN

Action Alert

Older adults sometimes limit their fluid intake, especially in the evening, because of decreased *mobility*, prescribed diuretics, and urinary incontinence. *Teach older adults that fluid restrictions make them likely to develop dehydration and electrolyte imbalances (especially sodium and potassium) that can cause serious illness or death.*

Incontinence may actually increase because the urine becomes more concentrated and irritating to the bladder and urinary sphincter. Teach older adults the importance of drinking 2 liters of water a day plus other fluids as desired unless medically contraindicated. Remind them to avoid excessive caffeine and alcohol because they can cause dehydration. Chapter 13 discusses fluid and electrolyte imbalances in detail.

Decreased Mobility

Exercise and activity are important for older adults as a means of promoting and maintaining mobility and overall health (Fig. 4.1). A large study of almost 16,000 older adults living in the community found that those with severe limitations in ***mobility*** experienced increased falls that often led to negative health outcomes when compared with those with adequate mobility (Musich, et al., 2018).

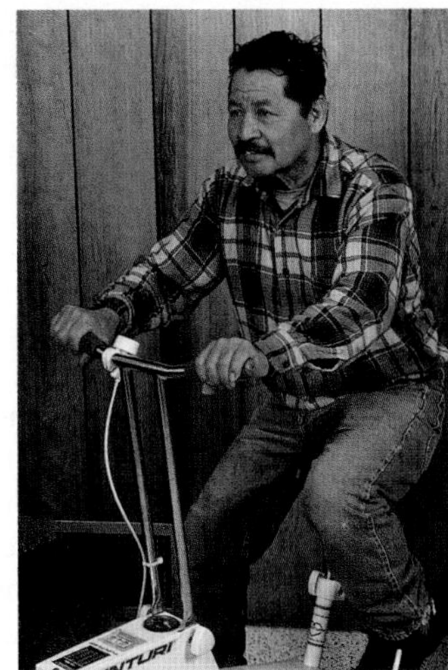

Fig. 4.1 Exercise is important to older adults for health promotion and maintenance.

Physical activity can help keep the body in shape and maintain an optimal level of functioning. Regular exercise has many benefits for older adults in community-based settings. The major advantages of maintaining appropriate levels of physical activity include:

- Decreased risk for falls
- Increased muscle strength and balance
- Increased ***mobility***
- Increased sleep
- Reduced or maintained weight
- Improved sense of well-being and self-esteem
- Decreased risk for constipation
- Improved longevity
- Reduced risks for diabetes, coronary artery disease, and dementia

Assess older adults in any setting regarding their history of exercise and any health concerns they may have. For independent older adults, remind them to check with their primary health care provider to implement a supervised plan for regular physical activity. Teach older adults about the importance and value of physical activity.

For people who are homebound, focus on functional ability such as performing ADLs. For those who are not homebound, teach the importance of exercise. For example, resistance exercise maintains muscle mass. Aerobic exercise such as walking improves strength and endurance. One of the best exercises is walking at least 30 minutes three to five times a week. During the winter, indoor shopping centers and other public places can be used. In addition, many senior centers and community centers offer exercise programs for older adults. For those who have limited ***mobility***, chair exercises may be provided.

Swimming is also a good way to exercise but does not offer the weight-bearing advantage of walking. Weight bearing helps build bone, an especially important advantage for older women to prevent osteoporosis (see Chapter 45). Teach older adults who have been sedentary to start their exercise programs slowly and gradually increase the frequency and duration of activity over time under the direction of their primary health care provider.

Stress and Coping

Stress can speed up the aging process over time, or it can lead to diseases that increase the rate of degeneration. It can also impair the reserve capacity of older adults and lessen their ability to respond and adapt to changes in their environment.

Although no period of the life cycle is free from stress, the later years can be a time of especially high risk. Frequent sources of stress and anxiety for the older population include:

- Rapid environmental changes that require immediate reaction
- Changes in lifestyle resulting from retirement or physical incapacity
- Acute or chronic illness
- Loss of significant others
- Financial hardships
- Relocation

Older-Adult Veterans and Coping. Many older adults experience high stress and anxiety as a result of having served in the U.S. military. Some veterans of war have had to kill their enemies, often resulting in disenfranchised grief, a grief that cannot be openly or socially accepted or mourned. Over 22 million American men and women are veterans, and many of those are older than 60 years. Older veterans can be divided into three groups based on the war in which they served (Smith & Harris, 2017):

- *World War II veterans:* Veterans of World War II are part of a generation of people born before 1946. They tend to be very disciplined and have a high respect for authority. They often do not discuss their war-related issues and do not typically ask for help in managing them.
- *Korean Conflict veterans:* The Korean Conflict (1950–1953) is often referred to as the Forgotten War. Many soldiers who fought in this conflict experienced local injuries and illnesses, including frostbite, blast injuries, and posttraumatic stress disorder (PTSD).
- *Vietnam War veterans:* The Vietnam War (1964–1973) resulted in many deaths and major illnesses and injuries, including those that resulted from chemicals such as Agent Orange. Veterans of this war tend to seek help more often than older veterans as a result of their high risk for suicide, substance use disorder, and PTSD.

Nurses caring for veterans should ask specific questions as part of their health assessment, including (Bartzak, 2017):

- Tell me about your experience in the military.
- Is your military experience affecting you now, and if so, how is it affecting you?
- Were you deployed? If so, for how long?
- Do you have a safe place to live or stay?
- Have you had nightmares or negative thoughts that keep you from sleeping?
- Are you overly anxious and easily startled?
- Do you ever feel detached from other people or your environment?
- Do you have ways that you use to cope with your stress?

How a veteran or any older adult reacts to these stresses may depend on his or her personal coping skills and support networks. A combination of poor physical health and social issues such as homelessness can leave veterans susceptible to stress overload, which can result in illness and premature death.

Adapting to Older Adulthood. The ways in which people adapt to old age depend largely on the personality traits and coping strategies that have characterized them throughout their lives. Establishing and maintaining relationships with others throughout life are especially important to the older person's happiness. Even more important than having friends is the nature of the friendships. People who have close, intimate, stable relationships with others in whom they confide are often more likely to cope with crisis, whether present or past.

Some older adults continue to work well into their 70s and 80s. Those who retired early may choose to return to work on a part-time basis to increase their income and socialize with other people. If a person retires between the ages of 55 and 65 years and lives into his or her 80s or 90s, retirement funds can deplete. As one ages, additional income is needed to meet basic needs, including money for prescription drugs. Although U.S. government Medicare Part A pays for inpatient hospital care and skilled care for a limited time, older adults pay for Medicare Part B to reimburse 80% of the cost of most ambulatory care and diagnostic services. Older adults also pay for Medicare Part D, which covers prescription drugs, and a private Medigap insurance plan or supplement (e.g., United Health or Blue Cross/Blue Shield), to cover the costs not paid for by Medicare B. The premiums for these insurances are very expensive and may still require that older adults pay out-of-pocket copayments for health care services and prescription drugs. If the older adult works after 65 years of age, premiums are higher because they are income adjusted.

In other developed countries, part of or all older-adult care may be provided for publicly by the federal government. For example, in Canada all acute and primary health care provider care is paid for publicly. In Germany all older-adult care, including long-term care, is paid for by the government.

Fortunately most older adults today are relatively healthy and live in and own their own homes. A number of programs have been developed to improve life for older adults such that they can stay in their homes in their communities. One nurse-developed program funded by the National Institutes of Health is CAPABLE (Community Aging in Place—Advancing Better Living for Elders). Other resources include:

- National Aging in Place Council (www.ageinplace.org)
- Village to Village Network (www.vtvnetwork.org)
- AARP Livable Communities (www.aarp.org/livable-communities/about)
- Administration for Community Living (www.acl.gov)

EVIDENCE-BASED PRACTICE QSEN

How Can Nurses Help Prepare Patients and Families for Long-Term Care?

Kokonya, A. & Fitzsimons, V. (2018). Transition to long-term care: preparing older adults and their families. *MEDSURG Nursing, 27*(3), 143–148.

This systematic review of the literature identified evidence-based strategies for assisting patients and their families transition to long-term care. The authors searched major databases for studies published on the topic between 2013 and 2017. Although all types of studies were found, most were qualitative research. Thirteen articles were selected and systematically reviewed and analyzed. All of the studies found that ongoing autonomy and control over care decisions were very important to both the patient and family. Unplanned transitions and poor coping by either the patient or family affected the ability to adapt to the new setting. Other evidence-based strategies to help older adults and families include:

- Early consumer education to prepare patients and families
- Trial of respite care prior to relocation (if possible)
- Establishing a liaison between acute and long-term care staff
- Key consistent nurse for resident until settled in the long-term care facility
- Involving family and friends in care and schedule
- Prolonged stay time for family, especially for first week
- Structured resident introduction to social activities

Level of Evidence: 1

This study was a systematic review and analysis of existing research.

Commentary: Implications for Practice and Research

This study emphasized the role of nurses in acute care and other settings in helping patients and families prepare for the difficult and challenging transition to long-term care. However, many nurses do not have expertise in geriatrics and gerontology. The authors suggested that nursing programs should include these topics as well as transitioning patients to long-term care facilities in their curricula. Future research is needed in this area as "baby boomers" age and eventually need long-term care.

Despite efforts to help older adults stay in their communities, physical and/or mental health/behavioral health problems may force some to relocate to a retirement center, an assisted-living facility, or long-term care, although these facilities can be very expensive. Others move in with family members or to apartment buildings funded and designated for seniors. Older adults usually have more difficulty adjusting to major change when compared with younger and middle-age adults. Being admitted to a hospital or nursing home can be a particularly traumatic experience. Kokonya and Fitzsimons (2018) found that nurses can be very helpful in preparing the patient and family for the transition to long-term care (see the Evidence-Based Practice box).

Older adults often suffer from relocation stress syndrome, also known as *relocation trauma.* **Relocation stress syndrome** is the physical and emotional distress that can occur after a person moves from one setting to another. Examples of physiologic behaviors are sleep disturbance and increased physical symptoms such as GI distress. Examples of emotional manifestations are withdrawal, anxiety, anger, and depression. The Best Practice for Patient Safety & Quality Care: Minimizing the Effects of Relocation Stress in Older Adults box lists nursing interventions that may help decrease the effects of relocation.

BEST PRACTICE FOR PATIENT SAFETY & QUALITY CARE QSEN

Minimizing the Effects of Relocation Stress in Older Adults

- Provide maximum opportunities for the patient to assist in decision making.
- Carefully explain all procedures and routines to the patient before they occur.
- Ask the family or significant other to provide familiar or special keepsakes to keep at the patient's bedside (e.g., family picture, favorite hairbrush).
- Reorient the patient frequently to his or her location.
- If possible, ask the patient about his or her expectations during hospital, assisted-living, or nursing home stay.
- Encourage the patient's family and friends to visit often.
- Establish a trusting relationship with the patient as early as possible.
- Assess the patient's usual lifestyle and daily activities, including food likes and dislikes and preferred time for bathing.
- Avoid unnecessary room changes.
- If possible, have a family member, significant other, staff member, or volunteer accompany the patient when leaving the unit for special procedures or therapies.

Family members and facility staff need to be aware that older adults need personal space in their new surroundings. Older adults need to participate in deciding how the space will be arranged and what they can keep in their new home to help offset potential feelings of powerlessness. Suggest that the patient or family bring in personal items such as pictures of relatives and friends, favorite clothing, and valued knickknacks to help make the new setting seem more familiar and comfortable.

Accidents

Accidents are very common among older adults; falls are the most common. Older women are at the highest risk for falls as a result of taking more opioids and benzodiazepines than men (Haddad et al., 2018). Motor vehicle crashes increase as well because of physiologic changes of aging or chronic diseases such as Alzheimer disease or peripheral neuropathy.

Fall Prevention. Most accidents occur at home. According to the Centers for Disease Control and Prevention (CDC), more than one in four older adults experience at least one fall each year (https://www.cdc.gov/features/falls-older-adults/index.html). Teach older adults about the need to be aware of safety precautions to prevent accidents such as falls. Injury-related accidents are a primary cause of decreased ***mobility*** and chronic pain in old age. Some people develop **fallophobia** (fear of falling) and avoid leaving their homes. This reaction is particularly common for those who have previously fallen and/or have osteoporosis (bone tissue loss). Osteoporosis is especially common in older thin Euro-Caucasian women who typically have a stooped posture (kyphosis), which can cause problems with balance (see Chapter 45).

Home modifications may help prevent falls. Collaborate with the older adult, family, and significant others when recommending useful changes to prevent injury. Safeguards such as handrails, slip-proof pads for rugs, and adequate lighting are essential in the home. Avoiding scatter rugs, slippery floors, and clutter is also important to prevent falls. Installing grab bars and using nonslip bathmats can help prevent falls in the bathroom. Raised toilet seats are also important, especially for those who have hip and knee arthritis. Remind older adults to avoid going out on days when steps are wet or icy and to ask for help when ambulating. To minimize sensory overload, advise the older adult to concentrate on one activity at a time.

Changes in ***sensory perception*** can create challenges for older adults in any environment. For example, **presbyopia** (farsightedness that worsens with aging) may make walking more difficult; the person is less aware of the location of each step. In addition, the older adult may have disorders that affect visual acuity such as macular degeneration, cataracts, glaucoma, or diabetic retinopathy. Teach the person to look down at where he or she is walking and have frequent eye examinations to update glasses or contact lenses to improve vision. Drug therapy or surgery may be needed to correct glaucoma or cataracts (see Chapter 42).

A reduced sense of touch decreases the awareness of body orientation (e.g., whether the foot is squarely on the step). The decreased reaction time that commonly results from age-related changes in the neurologic system may also impair the ability to recognize or move from a dangerous setting. Chronic diseases such as peripheral neuropathy and arthritis can affect ***sensory perception*** in the older adult as well. If needed, encourage the use of visual and/or ambulatory assistive devices. High costs and a fear of appearing old sometimes prevent older adults from obtaining or using these devices.

A major contributing factor to falls in older adults is medication use, discussed in more detail later in this chapter. For example, many older adults, especially women, take psychoactive medications and opioid analgesics that affect the central nervous system, causing drowsiness and acute confusion. Drug therapy for hypertension can cause dizziness and loss of balance as a result of orthostatic hypotension, an adverse drug effect.

In response to the increasing fall rate among older adults as baby boomers age, the CDC recently developed a fall prevention initiative called Stopping Elderly Accidents, Deaths, and Injuries (STEADI) (www.cdc.gov/steadi). The three elements of the STEADI initiative include:

- Screen older adults to determine those at risk for falls
- Assess modifiable risk factors, including medication use
- Intervene by using clinical and community strategies, including health teaching

Evidence-based interventions include referral to vision specialists, medication review and management, and participation in an exercise program (Haddad et al., 2018). For example, for those in the community, tai chi exercise or yoga for seniors is very helpful to improve balance and ***mobility*** and decrease the fear of falling, especially among older women.

NCLEX EXAMINATION CHALLENGE 4.1

Safe and Effective Care Environment

The nurse performs an initial health assessment of an older adult. Which assessment findings indicate that the client may be at risk for falls? **Select all that apply.**

A. Has presbyopia
B. Has peripheral neuropathy
C. Uses a cane
D. Takes multiple medications
E. Has bilateral cataracts
F. Has thin papery skin

Driving Safety. *Motor vehicle crashes are a major cause of accidents and death among the older-adult population.* Increased national concerns about this growing problem have prompted many states to require more frequent testing for older drivers. Several functional abilities decline with normal aging, including reaction time and the ability to multitask. **Presbycusis** (hearing loss associated with the aging process) can prevent older adults from hearing emergency vehicles or vehicle horns. Sleep disturbances, especially insomnia, are also common in older adults but are *not* part of normal aging. Some crashes occur because the person falls asleep while driving.

The older the person, the more likely that he or she will have chronic diseases and the drugs needed to manage them. These health problems and treatments can contribute to motor vehicle crashes (Staplin et al., 2017). For instance, peripheral neuropathy may prevent a driver from feeling whether his or her foot is on the brake or accelerator. Drugs used for hypertension can cause orthostatic hypotension (low blood pressure when changing body position from a supine to sitting or standing position).

Primary health care providers play a major role in identifying driver safety issues. Yet many are reluctant to intervene because older patients think they will lose their independence if they cannot drive. They may also be angry and resistant to the idea of giving up perhaps their only means of transportation. As an alternative, health care professionals can recommend driving refresher courses and suggest that high-risk driving conditions such as wet or icy roads be avoided. Newer vehicles have safety features to help older adults such as large-print digital readouts for speed and rear cameras to see behind the vehicle. The Best Practice for Patient Safety & Quality Care box lists additional ways to address older-adult driver safety.

Drug Use and Misuse

Drug therapy for the older population can be another major health issue. Because of the multiple chronic and acute health problems that occur in this age-group, drugs for older adults account for about one-third of all prescription drug costs. The term *polymedicine* has been used to describe the use of many drugs to treat multiple health problems for older adults. **Polypharmacy** is the use of multiple drugs, duplicative drug

BEST PRACTICE FOR PATIENT SAFETY & QUALITY CARE (QSEN)

Recommendations for Improving Older-Adult Driver Safety

- Discuss driving ability with the older adult to assess his or her perception.
- Assess physical and mental deficits that could affect driving ability, including older adults who:
  - Had a recent medication change
  - Experienced recent falls
  - Present with signs and symptoms of cognitive impairment or decline
  - Have progressive health problems
- Consult with appropriate primary health care providers to manage health problems that could interfere with driving.
- Suggest community-based transportation options, if available, instead of driving.
- Discuss driving concerns with older adults and/or their families.
- Remind the older adult to wear glasses and hearing aids if prescribed.
- Encourage driver-refresher classes, often offered by AARP (formerly the American Association of Retired Persons).
- Refer the older adult to a *certified* driving specialist for an on-road driving assessment.
- Encourage avoiding high-risk driving locations or conditions such as busy urban interstates and wet or icy weather conditions.
- Report unsafe drivers to the state department of motor vehicles if they continue to drive.

therapy, high-dosage drugs, and drugs prescribed for too long a period of time.

Many older adults also take multiple nonprescription or over-the-counter (OTC) drugs such as analgesics, antacids, cold and cough preparations, laxatives, and herbal/nutritional supplements, often without consulting a primary health care provider. Therefore this population is at high risk for adverse drug events (ADEs) directly related to the number of drugs taken and the frequency with which they are taken. Drug-drug, food-drug, drug-herb, and drug-disease interactions are common ADEs that often lead to hospital admission.

Effects of Drugs on Older Adults. Many older adults often do not tolerate the standard dosage of drugs traditionally prescribed for younger adults. The physiologic changes related to aging make drug therapy more complex and challenging. These changes affect the absorption, distribution, metabolism, and excretion of drugs from the body. Even common antibiotics can lead to temporary memory loss or acute confusion. More commonly, long-term antibiotic therapy can cause a *Clostridium difficile* infection or more serious life-threatening complications, as discussed in Chapter 21.

Age-related changes that can potentially affect drug *absorption* from an oral route include an increase in gastric pH, a decrease in gastric blood flow, and a decrease in GI motility. Despite these changes, older adults do not have major absorption difficulties because of age-related changes alone.

TABLE 4.1 Common Adverse Drug Events (ADEs) in Older Adults

• Edema	• Dizziness
• Severe nausea and vomiting	• Syncope
• Anorexia	• Urinary retention
• Dehydration	• Diarrhea
• Dysrhythmias	• Constipation/impaction
• Fatigue	• Acute confusion
• Weakness	• Hypotension

Age-related changes that affect drug *distribution* include smaller amounts of total body water, an increased ratio of adipose tissue to lean body mass, a decreased albumin level, and a decreased cardiac output. Increased adipose tissue in proportion to lean body mass can cause increased storage of lipid-soluble drugs. This leads to a decreased concentration of the drug in plasma but an increased concentration in tissue.

Drug *metabolism* often occurs in the liver. Age-related changes affecting metabolism include a decrease in liver size, a decrease in liver blood flow, and a decrease in serum liver enzyme activity. These changes can result in increased plasma concentrations of a drug. Monitor liver function studies and teach older adults to have regular physical examinations.

Changes in the kidneys can also result in high plasma concentrations of drugs. The *excretion* of drugs usually involves the renal system. Age-related changes in the renal system include decreased renal blood flow and reduced glomerular filtration rate. These changes result in a decreased creatinine clearance (CrCl) and thus a slower excretion time for medications. CrCl values typically decrease with age by 6.5 mL/min per decade of life after age 20 years (Pagana & Pagana, 2018). Consequently serum drug levels can become toxic, and the patient can become extremely ill or die. *Monitor renal studies, especially serum creatinine and creatinine clearance, when giving drugs to older adults!*

When chronic disease is added to the physiologic changes of aging, drug reactions have a more dramatic effect and take longer to correct. Often a lower dose of a drug is necessary to prevent ADEs. The policy of "start low, go slow" is essential when primary health care providers prescribe drugs for older adults (Smith & Kautz, 2018). The physiologic changes of aging are highly individual. Alterations in drug therapy should always be individualized according to the actual physiologic changes present and the occurrence and severity of chronic disease. Common ADEs are listed in Table 4.1.

Opioid Use Among Older Adults. Opioids are increasingly being used by older adults to manage both acute and persistent pain. Persistent pain resulting from health problems such as arthritis and long-term back pain is common among older adults. A study by Musich et al. (2019) showed that high-dose opioid users among the older-adult population were

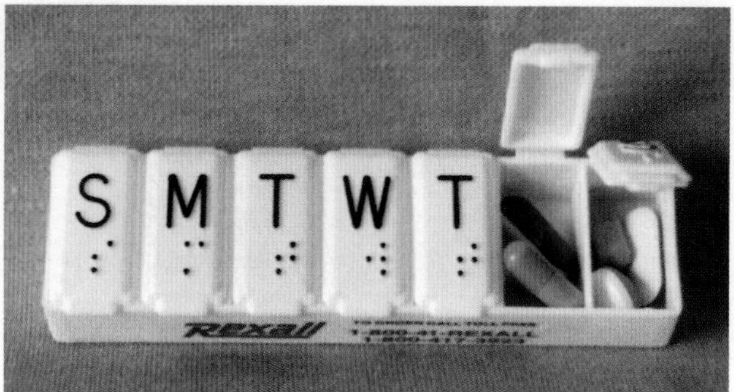

Fig. 4.2 A medication system for safe self-administration.

younger, male, depressed, and in poor health and had back pain. Many of the high-dose users also took benzodiazepines and/or sleep medications and used four or more pharmacies. This study suggests that mental health interventions may be helpful to promote more effective pain management in this population. A proposed objective for *Healthy People 2030* is to reduce the proportion of older adults who use inappropriate medications such as high-dose opioids (https://www.healthypeople.gov).

Self-Administration of Drugs. Most people older than 65 years take their own medications. Because the risk for drug toxicity is considerably increased in the older population, help patients assume this task responsibly. Teach patients and their caregivers, providing clear and concise directions and developing ways to help them overcome difficulties with self-administration.

Older adults may make errors in self-administration or may not adhere to the drug regimen for several reasons. First, they may simply forget. In the rush of daily activities, they may not take their drugs or may take them too often because they cannot remember when or whether they have taken the medications. It is often helpful if they associate pill taking with daily events (e.g., meals) or keep a simple chart or calendar. Pill boxes are available for a daily, weekly, or monthly supply of medicine that can be placed in small compartments (Fig. 4.2). Egg cartons can be very cost-effective pill boxes. Large print on the drug label helps patients who have poor vision. Writing the drug regimen on the top of the bottle with large letters and numbers is helpful for some older adults. Colored labels or dots can also be applied. Easy-open bottle caps help older adults with limited hand mobility or strength.

A second reason for drug errors is poor communication with health care professionals. These problems result from poor explanations that are not understood because of educational limitations, language barriers, or difficulty with hearing and vision. Health care professionals often presume that their patients have learned the information if they have taught them about the drugs. Help older adults plan their drug therapy schedules as needed.

A third reason for errors is the varying ways that older adults take their medications. Many people older than 65 years use a multitude of complementary and integrative therapies. Some add to their drug regimen by taking OTC drugs, which can interact with prescription drugs and cause serious problems. For example, a patient receiving warfarin for anticoagulation may take ibuprofen regularly for arthritis or garlic for hypertension. Because ibuprofen and garlic can inhibit clotting, this combination can cause serious bleeding. When obtaining a drug history, ask patients about all OTC drugs, including herbal and food supplements.

Some older adults avoid taking their prescribed drugs. The fear of dependency or the cost of the drugs may cause many to discontinue their drug therapy too soon or not begin taking the drug. In addition, the actions or side effects of some drugs may not be desirable. For example, diuretics may cause incontinence when patients cannot get to the bathroom quickly enough. Others may think that two pills are twice as effective and therefore it is better to take two rather than just one. Some older adults take drugs that are left over from a previous illness or one that is borrowed from someone else. Teach patients to take their medications exactly as prescribed by their primary health care providers.

BEST PRACTICE FOR PATIENT SAFETY & QUALITY CARE (QSEN)

Recommended Interview Questions for Older-Adult Medication Assessment

- Do you take five or more prescription medications?
- Do you take herbs, vitamins, other dietary supplements, or OTC medications?
- Do you have your prescriptions filled at more than one pharmacy?
- Is more than one health care practitioner prescribing your medications?
- Do you take your medications more than once a day?
- Do you have trouble opening your medication bottles?
- Do you have poor eyesight or hearing?
- Do you live alone?
- Do you have a hard time remembering to take your medications?

Medication Assessment and Health Teaching. The *Healthy People 2020* initiative recommends that older adults be interviewed regarding their medication use, including the questions in the Best Practice for Patient Safety & Quality Care: Recommended Interview Questions for Older-Adult Medication Assessment box.

One of the objectives for the *Healthy People 2030* initiative is to reduce the proportion of older adults who are taking inappropriate medications. The most recent edition of the Beers Criteria for Potentially Inappropriate Medication Use in Older Adults assessment tool, simply known as the *Beers criteria,* is also very useful in screening for medication-related risks in older adults who have chronic health problems (2019 American Geriatric Society Beers Criteria Update Expert Panel, 2019). This tool lists multiple medications and related concerns. Examples of these "at-risk" drugs are listed in Table 4.2.

TABLE 4.2 Examples of Potentially Inappropriate Medication Use in Older Adults

• meperidine	• diazepam
• oxycodone	• promethazine
• cyclobenzaprine	• ketorolac
• digoxin (Should not exceed 0.125 mg daily except for atrial fibrillation)	• short-acting nifedipine
• ticlopidine	• ferrous sulfate (Should not exceed 325 mg daily)
• fluoxetine	• diphenhydramine
• amitriptyline	• chlorpropamide

NURSING SAFETY PRIORITY QSEN

Drug Alert

To reduce drug-related risks in older adults, perform a medication assessment every 6 months or more often if an acute illness or exacerbation of a chronic disease occurs. Be sure to:

- Obtain a list of all medications taken on a regular and as-needed basis; include OTC and prescribed drugs, herbs, and nutritional supplements. If a list is not available, ask the older adult or family to gather all ointments, pills, lotions, eyedrops, inhalers, injectable solutions, vitamins, minerals, herbs, and other OTC medications and place into a bag for review.
- Highlight all medications that are part of the Beers criteria; highlight any medication for which the indication for its use is not clear, any medication that is inappropriate, or any that could be discontinued (e.g., duplicative drug).
- Collaborate with the older adult, family, pharmacist, and primary health care provider if appropriate to determine the need for medication changes. Suggest once-a-day dosing if possible.
- Give older adults verbal and written information (at the appropriate reading level) regarding any change or new medication prescribed.
- Promote adherence to the drug therapy regimen exactly as prescribed; remind older adults to check with their primary health care provider if they want to change their regimen or add an OTC medication or natural product (nutritional or herbal supplement, or probiotic).
- Encourage lifestyle changes and other nonpharmacologic interventions to help manage or prevent health problems.
- Remind older adults not to share or borrow medications.

Inadequate Cognition

Older adults living in the community are usually mentally sound and competent. However, when they are hospitalized or have chronic illness, major changes in ***cognition*** often occur. Some changes have been identified as age related and are linked to specific cognitive functions rather than intellectual capacity. These changes include a decreased reaction time to stimuli and an impaired memory for recent events. *However, severe cognitive impairment and psychosis are not common.*

Two forms of cognitive competence exist: legal competence and clinical competence. A person is *legally competent* if he or she is:

- 18 years of age or older
- Pregnant or a married minor
- A legally emancipated (free) minor who is self-supporting
- Not declared incompetent by a court of law

If a court determines that an older adult is not legally competent, a *guardian* is appointed to make health care decisions. Guardians may be family members or a person who is not related to the patient. When no one is available, a guardian may be appointed from a local Area Agency on Aging, an organization with comprehensive services and resources for older adults.

A person is *clinically competent* if he or she is legally competent and can make appropriate decisions. Decisional capacity is determined by a person's ability to identify problems, recognize options, make decisions, and provide the rationale supporting the decisions. Selected behavioral/mental illnesses often affect both legal and clinical competence.

Nurses are in a unique position to teach older adults about ways to promote ***cognition***. Cognitive training (e.g., learning a new skill), physical and mental activity, social engagement, and proper ***nutrition*** are the most helpful interventions to *prevent* cognitive changes in older adults. In some communities, online cognitive training is playing a role in helping to improve memory in older adults.

As older adults age, they are at increasing risk for cognitive impairments—depression, delirium, and dementia, often referred to as the *3Ds*. The 3Ds are discussed briefly here; more comprehensive discussions can be found in mental health/behavioral health textbooks.

PATIENT-CENTERED CARE: VETERANS HEALTH CONSIDERATIONS QSEN

Many older veterans of the Korean and Vietnam wars also suffer from chronic pain, depression, posttraumatic stress disorder (PTSD), and severe anxiety. Substance use disorder, especially alcoholism, is common among young and older veterans. Alcoholism can contribute to cognitive decline and may be used as a coping mechanism for loss. As a result, many of today's homeless population are veterans of previous and more recent wars.

Depression. *Depression is the most common mental health/behavioral health problem among older adults in the community.* It increases in incidence when older adults are admitted to the hospital or nursing home. **Depression** is broadly defined as a mood disorder that can have cognitive, affective, and physical manifestations. It can be primary or secondary and can range from mild to severe or major. As a *primary* problem, depression is thought to result from a lack of the neurotransmitters *norepinephrine* and *serotonin* in the brain. *Secondary* depression, sometimes called *situational* depression, can result when there is a sudden change in the person's life such as an illness or loss. Common chronic illnesses that can cause secondary depression include stroke, arthritis, and cardiac disease. It is often underdiagnosed by primary health care providers and is therefore undertreated.

Families and nurses are in the best position to suspect depression in an older adult. Several screening tools are available to help determine if the patient has clinical depression. For example, the *Geriatric Depression Scale—Short*

Form (GDS-SF) is a valid and reliable screening tool and is available in multiple languages. The patient selects "yes" or "no" to 15 questions, or a nurse or other health care professional can ask the patient the questions. A score of 10 or higher is consistent with a possible diagnosis of clinical depression (Fig. 4.3). These patients are then evaluated more thoroughly by the primary health care provider for treatment. Without diagnosis and/or adequate treatment, depression can result in:

- Worsening of medical conditions
- Risk for physical illness
- Alcoholism and drug use
- Increased pain and disability
- Delayed recovery from illness
- Suicide (especially in Euro-Caucasian men between 75 and 85 years of age)

Older adults with depression may have early morning insomnia, excessive daytime sleeping, poor appetite, a lack of energy, and an unwillingness to participate in social and recreational activities. The primary treatment for depression usually includes drug therapy and psychotherapy, depending on the severity of the problem. Selective serotonin reuptake inhibitors (SSRIs) are the first choice for drug therapy but take 2 to 3 weeks to work. They act by increasing the amount of serotonin and norepinephrine at nerve synapses in the brain.

! NURSING SAFETY PRIORITY QSEN

Drug Alert

Tricyclic antidepressants should not be used for older adults because they have anticholinergic properties that can cause acute confusion, severe constipation, and urinary retention or incontinence. For older adults who may be prescribed this group of drugs, question the primary health care provider and request an SSRI or other treatment.

Reminiscence and music therapies may also help reduce feelings of depression and despair (see the Evidence-Based Practice box earlier in the chapter). More information about depression, including additional strategies for preventing depression, is available in mental health/behavioral health nursing textbooks.

Geriatric Depression Scale—Short Form

Choose the best answer for how you have felt over the past week:

1. Are you basically satisfied with your life? YES / **NO**
2. Have you dropped many of your activities and interests? **YES** / NO
3. Do you feel that your life is empty? **YES** / NO
4. Do you often get bored? **YES** / NO
5. Are you in good spirits most of the time? YES / **NO**
6. Are you afraid that something bad is going to happen to you? **YES** / NO
7. Do you feel happy most of the time? YES / **NO**
8. Do you often feel helpless? **YES** / NO
9. Do you prefer to stay at home, rather than going out and doing new things? **YES** / NO
10. Do you feel you have more problems with memory than most? **YES** / NO
11. Do you think it is wonderful to be alive now? YES / **NO**
12. Do you feel pretty worthless the way you are now? **YES** / NO
13. Do you feel full of energy? YES / **NO**
14. Do you feel that your situation is hopeless? **YES** / NO
15. Do you think that most people are better off than you are? **YES** / NO

Answers in bold indicate depression. Score 1 point for each bolded answer.

A score > 5 points is suggestive of depression.
A score ≥ 10 points is almost always indicative of depression.
A score > 5 points should warrant a follow-up comprehensive assessment.

FIG. 4.3 The Geriatric Depression Scale—Short Form. (From the Aging Clinical Research Center [ACRC], a joint project of Stanford University and the VA Palo Alto Health Care System, Palo Alto, CA, funded by the National Institute of Aging and the Department of Veterans Affairs.)

NCLEX EXAMINATION CHALLENGE 4.2

Physiological Integrity

A nurse conducts an assessment of an older adult's medications, including both prescription and over-the-counter drugs. Which drug would the nurse identify as being potentially **inappropriate** for older adults?

A. Vitamin D
B. Losartan
C. Nortriptyline
D. Hydrochlorothiazide (HCTZ)

Dementia. Dementia is a broad term used for a syndrome that involves a slowly progressive cognitive decline, sometimes referred to as *chronic confusion*. This syndrome represents a global impairment of intellectual function and is generally chronic and progressive. There are many types of dementia, the most common being Alzheimer's disease. Multi-infarct dementia, the second most common dementia, results from a vascular disorder. Chapter 39 discusses dementias in detail, with a focus on Alzheimer's disease.

Delirium. Whereas dementia is a chronic, progressive disorder, delirium has an *acute* and fluctuating onset. It is often seen among older adults in a setting with which they are unfamiliar, including both acute and long-term care. Delirium is characterized by the patient's inattentiveness, disorganized thinking, and altered level of consciousness (either hypoalert or hyperalert). In addition to cognitive changes, some patients have physical and emotional manifestations and may become psychotic. In hospital settings, older adults commonly have a triad of pain, agitation, and delirium (PAD), sometimes referred to as a syndrome rather than three separate problems (Hartjes et al., 2016).

The major types of delirium are *hyperactive, hypoactive,* and *mixed. Hyperactive* patients may try to climb out of bed or become agitated, restless, and aggressive. *Hypoactive* patients are quiet, apathetic, lethargic, unaware, and withdrawn. They often move very slowly and stare. Patients with hypoactive dementia are often not diagnosed. *Mixed* delirium patients have a combination of hyperactive and hypoactive manifestations.

Identify patients who are at risk for delirium; high-risk patients are usually the old old and those with alcoholism and/or disorders of major body organs. Some health care agencies offer programs to prevent delirium and loss of function in high-risk patients such as the Hospital Elder Life Program (HELP). Marsh and Imgrund (2017) found that a hospital nurse-led quality improvement (QI) project using an established protocol, guidelines, and educational session for clinical staff helped to prevent and manage delirium. Examples of the many factors that can cause delirium are outlined in Table 4.3.

EVIDENCE-BASED PRACTICE QSEN

What Effect Do Music Therapies Have on Older Adults Who Experience Depression?

Quach, J., & Lee, J.A. (2017). Do music therapies reduce depressive symptoms and improve QOL in older adults with chronic disease? *Nursing, 35*(6), 58–62.

Chronic health problems in older adults can increase their risk for depression. The authors conducted a systematic review of the literature to examine the effect of different types of music therapy on depressive symptoms. Although 65 articles were originally located, only 13 randomized controlled trials and quasi-experimental studies were selected for review. All studies used one or more types of music therapy: listening to music, playing an instrument, singing, or a combination of music therapies. In all but one study, the therapies continued for 1 to 3 months. However, sample sizes were often small (less than 55). All of the reviewed studies showed some benefit of music, including reducing anxiety and depressive symptoms, improving quality of life, and improving overall mood.

Level of Evidence: 1

The study was a systematic review and analysis of existing research.

Commentary: Implications for Practice and Research

This study illustrated that music therapies are very beneficial in helping to manage depression and improve overall mood of older adults. Nurses and other health care professionals should consider incorporating these low-cost interventions to help manage older adults with depression as a result of chronic health problems. However, more studies using larger numbers of subjects are needed to enable generalization of the findings to a larger population of older adults.

! NURSING SAFETY PRIORITY QSEN

Action Alert

Delirium is a major predictor of morbidity and mortality. For example, acutely confused patients who are discharged from the hospital are at an increased risk for functional decline, falls, and incontinence at home. Therefore carefully assess older patients in any setting for acute confusion so it can be managed promptly.

A number of tools have been developed for point-of-care screening for delirium, including the Confusion Assessment Method (CAM), Delirium Index (DI), NEECHAM Confusion Scale, and Mini-Cog. The CAM is a short and easy-to-use tool

TABLE 4.3 Common Factors That Can Cause Delirium[a]

- Drug therapy (especially anticholinergics, opioids, and psychoactive drugs)
- Fluid and electrolyte imbalances
- Infections, especially urinary tract infection, pneumonia, and sepsis
- Fecal impaction or severe diarrhea
- Surgery (especially fracture hip repair and posttransplant)
- Metabolic problems such as hypoglycemia
- Neurologic disorders such as tumors
- Circulatory, renal, and pulmonary disorders causing hypoxia
- Nutritional deficiencies
- Hypoxemia (decreased arterial oxygen level)
- Mechanical ventilation
- Insomnia
- Relocation
- Major loss
- Critical care setting

[a]Many patients have more than one of these factors as causes for their delirium.

TABLE 4.4 The Confusion Assessment Method (CAM)

1. Acute onset and fluctuating course (e.g., Is there evidence of an acute change in mental status from the patient's baseline?)
2. Inattention (e.g., Does the patient have difficulty focusing attention or keeping track of what is being said?)
3. Disorganized thinking (e.g., Are the patient's thinking and conversation disorganized or incoherent?)
4. Altered level of consciousness (e.g., Is the patient lethargic, hyperalert, or difficult to arouse?)

The diagnosis of delirium by the CAM is the presence of features 1 and 2 *and* either 3 *or* 4.

Data from Sendelbach, S., & Guthrie, P.F. (2009). Evidence-based guideline—Acute confusion/delirium: Identification, assessment, treatment, and prevention. *Journal of Gerontological Nursing, 35*(11), 11–17.

that consists of nine open-ended questions and a diagnostic algorithm for determining delirium (Table 4.4). This screening tool is easily adaptable for computerized point-of-care charting.

Collaborate with the interprofessional health care team to remove or treat risk or causative factors for acute confusion. For example, if the patient has a low oxygen saturation level, provide supplemental oxygen therapy to increase oxygen to the brain. If the patient has a urinary tract infection (UTI), it is treated. The primary sign of a UTI in older adults is acute confusion.

To help prevent and manage delirium, use a calm voice to frequently reorient the patient. For example, playing tapes of soothing music may have a calming effect. Providing a doll or stuffed animal with which to "fidget" may prevent the patient from removing important medical tubes or equipment. Some nurses believe that providing dolls and stuffed animals is treating the adult like a child, but this intervention can sometimes be very effective when used for therapeutic purposes. If the patient has a favorite item such as a blanket or a picture, ask the family or significant others to provide it for the same purpose.

Table 3.1 in Chapter 3 highlights the major differences between delirium and dementia and lists the major nursing considerations for each. The most difficult challenge is caring for a patient who is experiencing both problems at the same time.

Substance Use Disorder

Excessive substance use (both alcohol and illicit drugs) may increase the risk for falls and other accidents; affects mood and ***cognition***; and may lead to complications of chronic diseases such as diabetes mellitus, hypertension, and heart disease. Isolation, depression, and delirium can also result from substance use. Older adults should decrease or avoid alcohol because they can become more sensitive to its effects. Illicit drugs such as cannabis (marijuana) should be avoided unless they are needed for therapeutic use.

The Short Michigan Alcoholism Screening Test—Geriatric Version (SMAST-G) is often used by nurses and other health care professionals in ambulatory care settings to detect alcohol use or alcoholism. The 10 yes/no question test is available in English and Spanish and can be either self-administered or administered by a clinician. Examples of questions on the tool are:

- Do you drink to take your mind off your problems?
- When you feel lonely, does having a drink help?

A "yes" answer is worth one point. A total score of two or more points indicates that the person has a problem with alcohol.

Other screening tools for alcohol use in older adults include the CAGE questionnaire, the Alcohol-Related Problems Survey (ARPS), and the Short ARPS (shARPS). The acronym *CAGE* comes from four questions:

- Have you ever tried to *c*ut down on your drinking?
- Have people *a*nnoyed you by criticizing your drinking?
- Have you ever felt bad or *g*uilty about your drinking?
- Have you ever had a drink first thing in the morning to settle your nerves or to get rid of a hangover (*e*ye-opener)?

Elder Neglect and Abuse

Another problem for some older adults is neglect and abuse, including verbal, financial, and physical. Some older adults are more vulnerable to these problems than others, especially widows, who may have difficulty being assertive. Elder abuse and neglect is a serious problem that affects many older adults each year. Older people who are neglected or abused are often physically dependent from one or more disabilities. The abuser is often a family member who becomes frustrated or distraught over the burden of caring for the older adult. Unfortunately, only a few cases of elder abuse are reported.

Prolonged caregiving by a family member is a common new role for adult children, usually women. This new role may result in role fatigue, conflict, and strain. As a result, neglect can occur when a caregiver fails to provide for an older adult's basic needs such as food, clothing, medications, or assistance with ADLs. The caregiver refuses to let other people such as nursing assistants or home care nurses into the home. Whether intentional or unintentional, neglect accounts for almost half of all cases of actual elder abuse.

Physical abuse is the use of physical force that results in bodily injury, especially in the "bathing suit" zone (abdomen, buttocks, genital area, upper thighs). Examples of physical abuse are hitting, burning, pushing, and molesting the patient. Sedating the older adult is also abusive. *Financial abuse* occurs when the older adult's property or resources are mismanaged or misused; this is more common than physical abuse. *Emotional abuse* is the intentional use of threats, humiliation, intimidation, and isolation toward older adults.

A number of older adults have been the victims of "scams" in which they are approached via phone or email and asked to send money for specific causes or organizations. These scams are not legitimate and have cost many older adults thousands of dollars. Teach people of all ages, especially older adults, to verify the legitimacy of the caller or email source and the cause or organization to prevent this financial and emotional abuse.

When caring for older adults, assess for indications of physical abuse such as bruises in clusters or regular patterns; burns, commonly to the buttocks or the soles of the feet; unusual hair loss; or multiple injuries, especially fractures. If the older adult is too weak or has no other resources or support systems, he or she may not admit that abuse is occurring. Neglect may be manifested by pressure injuries, contractures, dehydration or

TABLE 4.5 Examples of Elder Abuse Screening Tools

- Elder Abuse Suspicion Index
- Elder Assessment Instrument
- Indicators of Abuse Screen
- Questions to Elicit Elder Abuse
- Hwalek-Sengstock Elder Abuse Screening Tool
- Caregiver Abuse Screen
- Brief Abuse Screen for the Elderly
- Vulnerability to Abuse Screening Scale

malnutrition, urine burns, excessive body odor, and listlessness. Depression and dementia are common in community older adults who are abused or neglected.

Be sure to screen for abuse and neglect of older adults using an appropriate assessment tool. Table 4.5 lists tools that can be used by nurses and other health care professionals to screen for elder abuse and neglect. Refer the older adult to the appropriate service when there is:

- Evidence of mistreatment without sufficient clinical explanation
- A report by an older adult of being abused or neglected
- A belief by the health care professional that there is a high risk for or probable abuse, neglect, abandonment, or exploitation

All states in the United States and other Western countries have laws requiring health care professionals to report suspected elder abuse. In the community, if physical abuse or neglect is suspected, notify the local Adult Protective Services agency or other advocate organization. In a hospital or nursing home, notify the social worker or ombudsman, who then will investigate the case and report the problem to the appropriate agency.

HEALTH ISSUES FOR OLDER ADULTS IN HOSPITALS AND LONG-TERM CARE SETTINGS

Older adults who are admitted to hospitals and long-term care settings such as nursing homes have special needs and potential health problems. Nurses may not be aware that the needs of older adults differ from those of younger adults. Many of these needs are similar to those seen among community older adults as discussed in this chapter.

Since 1996 the Hartford Institute for Nursing has worked to ensure that all hospitalized patients 65 years of age and older be given high-quality care. Some health care systems have designated Acute Care of the Elderly (ACE) units with geriatric resources nurses and geriatric clinical nurse specialists. The patients are cared for by geriatricians who specialize in the care of older adults. Other hospitals have developed interprofessional health programs system-wide to meet the special needs of older patients. The incentive for these new programs is the Nurses Improving Care for Healthsystem Elders (NICHE) project, which continues to generate evidence-based practice guidelines for older-adult care. The purpose of all of these programs and units is to focus on the special health care issues or geriatric syndromes seen in the inpatient older population.

PATIENT-CENTERED CARE: CULTURAL/ SPIRITUAL CONSIDERATIONS (QSEN)

The health of Hispanic older adults continues to lag behind that of non-Hispanic whites due to a number of factors such as language barriers, inadequate health insurance, and lack of health care access. To add to this health disparity, most nurses and other health care professionals are not educated in the language or culture of Hispanic older adults. Some older Hispanic patients may have beliefs and values that conflict with traditional Western health care views. Many have strong religious and spiritual beliefs. For example, traditional Catholicism is practiced among most Hispanic elders in the southwestern United States. Be respectful of these practices and preferences and incorporate them into your patient's plan of care. Become educated about the Hispanic culture and learn to speak basic medical Spanish to foster communication and trust.

PATIENT-CENTERED CARE: GENDER HEALTH CONSIDERATIONS (QSEN)

Significant ***health care disparities*** are also associated with the lesbian, gay, bisexual, transgender, and questioning (LGBTQ) older-adult population. Compared with heterosexual adults, LGBTQ older adults are at an elevated risk for disability from chronic disease, mental distress, and overall poor health. They also tend to engage in risky unhealthy behaviors such as smoking and excessive drinking, which can result in multiple hospitalizations and an earlier need for long-term care when compared with heterosexual older adults (Kraus & Duhamel, 2018). When admitted to the hospital or nursing home, they may hide their gender identity and/or sexual orientation from the nurse and primary health care providers because of fear of rejection or discrimination or lack of adequate health care.

Be culturally competent and do not assume that your older patients or visitors are heterosexual. Establish a safe and trusting relationship with the patient; discuss sexual orientation and gender identity in a private setting to emphasize confidentiality. Do not force patients to answer any questions with which they feel uncomfortable. Teach direct caregivers such as nursing assistants that they may observe patients with sexual organs that conflict with the patient's gender identity. If this situation occurs, remind them not to be offensive or judgmental but, rather, to carry out the task as planned.

Be aware that the Services and Advocacy for Gay, Lesbian, Bisexual and Transgender Elders (SAGE) organization is available to provide services and resources for older LGBTQ adults and their caregivers. Chapter 68 in this text describes care of transgender patients in detail.

The *Fulmer SPICES* framework was developed as part of the NICHE project and identifies six serious "marker conditions" that can lead to longer hospital stays, higher medical costs, and even deaths for older adults. These conditions are:

- *S*leep disorders
- *P*roblems with eating or feeding
- *I*ncontinence
- *C*onfusion
- *E*vidence of falls
- *S*kin breakdown

Each of these problems is described briefly here and also is discussed in more detail in other parts of this chapter and the textbook. Other problems such as depression and constipation are also common in older hospitalized patients. Rather than being fully comprehensive, this classic, well-known SPICES framework is intended to be an easy tool that has been called *geriatric vital signs* (Fulmer, 2007).

Problems of Sleep, Nutrition, and Continence

Sleep disorders are common in hospitalized patients, especially older adults. Adequate rest is important for healing and for physical and mental functioning. Pain, chronic disease, environmental noise and lighting, and staff conversations are a few of the many contributing factors to insomnia in the acute and long-term care setting. Assess the patient and ask how he or she is sleeping. If the patient is not able to answer, observe for restlessness and other behaviors that could indicate lack of adequate rest. Manage the patient's pain by giving appropriate analgesics before bedtime. Attempt to keep patients awake during the day to prevent insomnia. Keep staff conversations as quiet as possible and away from patients' rooms. Dim the lights to make the patient area as dark as possible. Avoid making loud noises such as slamming doors. Postpone treatments until waking hours or early morning if they can be delayed safely. If possible, place a "Do Not Disturb" sign on the patient's door to avoid unnecessary interruptions in sleep.

Problems with eating and feeding prevent the older patient from receiving adequate ***nutrition***. Malnutrition is common among older adults and is associated with poor clinical outcomes, including death. Nurses need to perform nutritional screenings on the first day of patient admission, including a thorough nutritional history and weight, height, and body mass index (BMI) calculation. Chapter 48 describes nutritional assessment in more detail.

Collaborate with the registered dietitian nutritionist (RDN) about the patient's nutritional status as needed to achieve desired health outcomes. Consider cultural preferences and determine which foods the patient likes. Manage symptoms such as pain, nausea, and vomiting. If the patient has difficulty chewing or swallowing, coordinate a plan of care with the speech-language pathologist (SLP) and RDN. If there are no dietary restrictions, encourage family members or friends to bring in food that the patient might enjoy. Additional interventions to prevent or manage nutrition-related problems are discussed in Chapter 55.

Urinary and bowel ***elimination*** *issues* vary in type and severity and may be caused by many factors, including acute or chronic disease, ADL ability, and available staff. Assess the patient to identify causes for incontinence or retention. *These problems are not physiologic changes of aging but are very common in both the hospital and long-term care setting.* Implement a toileting schedule or a bowel or bladder training program, if appropriate. Delegate this activity to assistive personnel and supervise them. Chapter 7 discusses bowel and bladder training in detail; constipation is described earlier in this chapter.

Confusion, Falls, and Skin Breakdown

Acute and chronic confusion affect many older patients in both the hospital and nursing home. Whereas chronic confusion states such as dementia are not reversible, acute confusion, or delirium, may be avoidable and is often reversible when the causes are resolved or removed (see Table 3.1 in Chapter 3). For example, avoiding multiple drugs and promoting adequate sleep can help prevent acute confusion. Help the patient by reorienting him or her to reality as much as needed. Keep the patient as comfortable as possible (e.g., provide interventions to control pain). Delirium is discussed earlier in this chapter. Chapter 39 describes dementia in detail.

NCLEX EXAMINATION CHALLENGE 4.3

Physiological Integrity

An older adult's furosemide dosage was increased 2 days ago to 40 mg daily. This morning the nurse observes that the client has become confused and very weak. What is the nurse's **best** action?

A. Encourage fluid intake.
B. Withhold this morning's dose of furosemide.
C. Review the most recent serum electrolyte levels.
D. Place the patient on strict intake and output.

The most common accident among older patients in a hospital or nursing home setting is falling. A **fall** is an unintentional change in body position or descent that results in the patient's body coming to rest on the floor or ground. Some falls result in serious injuries such as fractures and head trauma. *The Joint Commission's National Patient Safety Goals (NPSGs) require that all inpatient health care settings use admission and daily fall risk assessment tools and a fall reduction program for patients who are at high risk.*

Assess all older patients for risk for falls. Many evidence-based assessment tools such as the Morse Fall Scale and the Hendrich II Fall Risk Model (HIIFRM) have been developed to help the nurse focus on factors that increase an older person's risk for falling. Some of these tools also recommend selected interventions, depending on the patient's fall risk score. The Best Practice for Patient Safety & Quality Care box lists some of the common risk factors that should be assessed and evidence-based, collaborative interventions for preventing falls in high-risk hospitalized patients. *A recent history of falling is the single most important predictor for falls.*

Fall prevention is an interprofessional responsibility and a national nursing quality indicator (Porter, 2018). Both the number of falls and the number of injuries resulting from falls are monitored and tracked in health care agencies. Johnston and Magnan (2019) described a quality improvement project that their nursing unit used to help prevent falls (see the Systems Thinking and Quality Improvement box).

Toileting-related falls are very common, especially at night. Older patients often have *nocturia* (urination during the night) and get out of bed to go to the bathroom. They may forget to ask

BEST PRACTICE FOR PATIENT SAFETY & QUALITY CARE (QSEN)

Assessing Risk Factors and Preventing Falls in Older Adults

Assess for the presence of these risk factors:

- History of falls
- Advanced age (>80 years)
- Multiple illnesses
- Generalized weakness or decreased mobility
- Gait and postural instability
- Disorientation or confusion
- Use of drugs that can cause increased confusion, mobility limitations, or orthostatic hypotension
- Urinary incontinence
- Communication impairments
- Major visual impairment or visual impairment without correction
- Alcohol or other substance use
- Location of patient's room away from the nurses' station (in the hospital or nursing home)
- Change of shift or mealtime (in the hospital or nursing home)

Implement these nursing interventions for all patients, regardless of risk

- Monitor the patient's activities and behavior as often as possible, preferably every 30 to 60 minutes.
- Teach the patient and family about the fall prevention program to become safety partners.
- Remind the patient to call for help before getting out of bed or a chair.
- Help the patient get out of bed or a chair if needed; lock all equipment such as beds and wheelchairs before transferring patients.
- Teach patients to use the grab bars when walking in the hall without assistive devices or when using the bathroom.
- Provide or remind the patient to use a walker or cane for ambulating if needed; teach him or her how to use these devices.
- Remind the patient to wear eyeglasses or a hearing aid if needed.
- Help the incontinent patient to toilet every 1 to 2 hours.
- Clean up spills immediately.
- Arrange the furniture in the patient's room or hallway to eliminate clutter or obstacles that could contribute to a fall.
- Provide adequate lighting at all times, especially at night.
- Observe for side effects and toxic effects of drug therapy.
- Orient the patient to the environment.
- Keep the call light and patient care articles within reach; ensure that the patient can use the call light.
- Place the bed in the lowest position with the brakes locked.
- Place objects that the patient needs within reach.
- Ensure that adequate handrails are present in the patient's room, bathroom, and hall.
- Have the physical therapist assess the patient for mobility and safety.

For patients at a high risk for falls:

- Implement all assessments and interventions listed previously.
- Relocate the patient for best visibility and supervision.
- Encourage family members or significant other to stay with the patient.
- Collaborate with other members of the health care team, especially the rehabilitative services.
- Use technologic devices such as bed and chair alarms to alert staff to patients getting out of bed.
- Use low beds or futon-type beds to prevent injury if the patient is at risk for falling out of bed.

SYSTEMS THINKING AND QUALITY IMPROVEMENT (QSEN)

Can a Checklist Help to Prevent Falls in an Inpatient Unit?

Johnston, M., & Magnan, M.A. (2019). Using a fall prevention checklist to reduce hospital falls: Results of a quality improvement project. *American Journal of Nursing, 119*(3), 43–49.

A group of nurses on an acute hospital unit conducted a quality improvement (QI) project to evaluate the impact of a fall prevention list on the implementation of 14 evidence-based interventions (fall protocol) and the incidence of falls on the study unit. Data were collected for 13 days for 26 shifts, and involved 37 nursing staff members who completed 90 fall prevention checklists. The results showed that the two most commonly missed interventions were setting the bed alarm correctly (should have been on Zone 2 on each bed) and posting signage both inside and outside the patient's room. However, no falls occurred during the 13-day study period. Nurses in the study suggested that additional interventions should be added to the checklist based on patient-specific needs.

Commentary: Implications for Practice and Research

The system in this QI project was the inpatient hospital unit. Monitoring staff use of an established fall prevention protocol is important to assess compliance and the need for additional staff education. More studies conducted on a larger scale may help to standardize fall prevention protocols while allowing for patient-specific concerns.

for assistance and may subsequently fall as a result of disorientation in the darkness in an unfamiliar environment. In some cases they may crawl over the side rail, which can make the fall more serious. Because of this, side rails are used far less often in both hospitals and nursing homes. In both settings side rails are classified as restraints unless the use of rails helps patients increase mobility.

A ***restraint*** is any device or drug that prevents the patient from moving freely and must be prescribed by a primary health care provider. In 1990 the U.S. government passed a law that gives nursing home residents the right to be restraint free. Removing physical restraints from nursing home residents has reduced serious injuries, although falls and minor injuries have increased in some cases. Futon-type beds or "low beds" have helped reduce injury.

Hospitals have also reduced the use of physical restraints. The Joint Commission has specific standards that limit the use of physical restraints in hospitals and nursing homes. Although not appropriate, chemical restraints (psychoactive drugs) such as haloperidol have sometimes been used in place of physical restraints.

Experts, including those at The Joint Commission, agree that older adults should not be placed in a physical restraint or sedated just because they are old. Use alternatives before applying any type of restraint, as outlined in the Best Practice for Patient Safety & Quality Care: Using Restraint Alternatives box.

If all other interventions (e.g., reminding patients to call for assistance when needed; asking a family member to stay with patients) are not effective in fall prevention, a physical restraint may be required for a limited period. Applying a restraint is a serious intervention and should be analyzed for its risk versus

BEST PRACTICE FOR PATIENT SAFETY & QUALITY CARE QSEN

Using Restraint Alternatives

- If the patient is acutely confused, reorient him or her to reality as often as possible.
- If the patient has dementia, use validation to reaffirm his or her feelings and concerns.
- Check the patient often, at least every 30 to 60 minutes.
- If the patient pulls tubes and lines, cover them with roller gauze or another protective device; be sure that IV insertion sites are visible for assessment.
- Keep the patient busy with an activity, pillow or apron, puzzle, or art project.
- Provide soft, calming music.
- Place the patient in an area where he or she can be supervised. (If the patient is agitated, do not place him or her in a noisy area.)
- Turn off the television if the patient is agitated.
- Ask a family member or friend to stay with the patient at night.
- Help the patient to toilet every 1 to 2 hours, including during the night.
- Be sure that the patient's needs for food, fluids, and comfort are met.
- If agency policy allows, provide the patient with a pet visit.
- Provide familiar objects or cherished items that the patient can touch.
- Document the use of all alternative interventions.
- If a restraint is applied, use the least restrictive device (e.g., mitts rather than wrist restraints, a roller belt rather than a vest).

its benefit. Check the patient in a restraint every 30 to 60 minutes and release the restraint at least every 1 to 2 hours for turning, repositioning, and toileting. Physical restraints such as vests have caused serious injury and even death. *If restraint is needed, use the least restrictive device first. Be sure to follow your facility policy and procedure for using restraints.*

Chemical restraints are often overused in hospital settings. Examples include:

- Antipsychotic drugs
- Antianxiety drugs
- Antidepressant drugs
- Sedative-hypnotic drugs

The most potent group of psychoactive drugs is the antipsychotics. These drugs are appropriate only for the control of certain behavioral problems such as delusions, acute psychosis, and schizophrenia. Typical antipsychotic drugs include haloperidol and thiothixene. These drugs should not be used to treat anxiety or induce sedation.

! NURSING SAFETY PRIORITY QSEN

Drug Alert

Closely monitor older adults receiving antipsychotics for adverse drug events (ADEs). Assess patients for:

- Anticholinergic effects, the most common problem, causing constipation, dry mouth, and urinary retention or incontinence
- Orthostatic hypotension, which increases the patient's risk for falls and fractures
- Parkinsonism, including tremors, bradycardia, and a shuffling gait
- Restlessness and the inability to stay still in any one position
- Hyperglycemia and diabetes mellitus, which occur more with drugs such as risperidone and quetiapine

If any of these ADEs occur, notify the primary health care provider immediately.

Skin breakdown, especially pressure injuries, is a major ***tissue integrity*** problem among older adults in hospitals and nursing homes. In some cases these wounds cause death from infection. Therefore prevention is the best approach.

Assess older adults for their risk for pressure injuries, using an assessment tool such as the Braden Scale for Predicting Pressure Injury Risk (see Chapter 23). Implement evidence-based interventions to prevent agency-acquired pressure injuries and maintain ***tissue integrity***. Coordinate these interventions with members of the interprofessional health care team, including the registered dietitian nutritionist and wound care specialist.

! NURSING SAFETY PRIORITY QSEN

Action Alert

Supervise assistive personnel (AP) for frequent turning and repositioning for the patient who is immobile. Assess the skin every 8 hours for reddened areas that do not blanch. Remind UAP to keep the skin clean and dry. Use pressure-relieving mattresses and avoid briefs or absorbent pads that can cause skin irritation and excess moisture. Chapter 23 describes in detail additional interventions for prevention and management of pressure injuries.

Skin tears are also common in older adults, especially the old-old group and those who are on chronic steroid therapy. Teach assistive personnel (AP) to use extreme caution when handling these patients. Use a gentle touch and report any open areas. Avoid bruising because older adults have increased capillary fragility.

CARE COORDINATION AND TRANSITION MANAGEMENT

Some older adults and their families experience a breakdown in communication and coordination of care when transitioning from the hospital or long-term care (LTC) setting (nursing home) to the home setting. If the transition is not optimal, older adults experience high readmission rates and an increase in visits to the emergency department or primary health care provider's office.

Health care professionals, especially nurses, often do not communicate effectively when they prepare for the discharge of older adults. Care is often not coordinated among health care professionals, which leads to confusion for the older adult and family caregivers. To help prevent these problems, establish a system to address patients' communication needs. This system should include follow-up phone calls after discharge to home and having one case manager to coordinate care during and after the transition from the inpatient agency to home. A home care nurse or other health care professional can serve as a "health coach" to ensure understanding of discharge instructions, consistent follow-up appointments, and a designated emergency contact for the patient and family. Discharge instructions should be easy to read, in large print, and accurate. Continuity of care for high-quality transition between settings is essential to achieve positive outcomes for older adults.

GET READY FOR THE NEXT-GENERATION NCLEX® EXAMINATION!

Key Points

Review these Key Points for each NCLEX Examination Client Needs Category.

Safe and Effective Care Environment

- Collaborate with the interprofessional team when providing care to older adults in the community or inpatient setting. For example, consult with the registered dietitian nutritionist for problems with ***nutrition***; consult with the pharmacist to discuss the patient's drug regimen. **QSEN: Teamwork and Collaboration**
- Assess all older adults for risk factors for impaired driving ability such as decreased ***mobility***, ***sensory perception***, and ***cognition***. **QSEN: Safety**
- Assess older adults in the community and inpatient settings for fall risk factors (e.g., cognitive decline and vision impairment) and implement evidence-based prevention measures as delineated in the chapter. **QSEN: Safety; Evidence-Based Practice**
- Do not use physical and chemical restraints for older adults until all other alternatives have been tried. **QSEN: Evidence-Based Practice**
- Follow The Joint Commission's National Patient Safety Goals and federal and state standards to maintain patient safety when using patient restraints. **QSEN: Safety**

Health Promotion and Maintenance

- Teach older adults about the benefits of regular physical exercise to promote ***mobility*** and improve mental health. **QSEN: Evidence-Based Practice**
- Provide information regarding community resources for older adults to help them meet their basic needs. **QSEN: Informatics; Patient-Centered Care**
- Be aware that nonwhite subgroups, such as Hispanics, and elders who identify as LGBTQ often are afraid or unable to obtain adequate health services. **Health Care Disparities**
- Conduct a medication assessment for potential risks in older adults using the Beers criteria. **QSEN: Safety**

Psychosocial Integrity

- Screen older adults for depression, which is the most common yet most underdiagnosed and undertreated mental health/behavioral health disorder among older adults. **Clinical Judgment**
- Delirium is acute confusion that has a sudden onset and fluctuating course; dementia is chronic confusion (see Table 3.1 in Chapter 3). Confusion is not part of the normal aging process. **QSEN: Evidence-Based Practice**
- Screen older adults for alcohol abuse or alcoholism and refer those with identified problems to appropriate resources. **QSEN: Evidence-Based Practice**
- Screen older adults for neglect and abuse, which are serious problems; family caregivers are usually the abusers (see Table 4.5). **QSEN: Safety**
- Assess for relocation stress syndrome, which is the reaction of an older adult when transferred to a different environment, and intervene to prevent or minimize this problem. **QSEN: Evidence-Based Practice**

Physiological Integrity

- Be aware that the four subgroups of the older-adult population are the young old, middle old, old old, and elite old. **QSEN: Patient-Centered Care**
- Be aware that the biggest concern regarding accidents among older adults in both the community and inpatient setting is falls. **QSEN: Safety**
- Recognize that physiologic changes of aging predispose older adults to toxic effects of medication; drugs are absorbed, metabolized, and distributed more slowly than in younger people. They are also excreted more slowly by the kidneys. **QSEN: Safety**
- Be aware that medication use in older adults is often a problem when they commit errors when self-medicating, avoid taking needed medications, or have problems understanding their medication regimen. **QSEN: Safety**
- Promote sleep and rest for older adults to decrease the incidence of delirium and to prevent falls. **QSEN: Evidence-Based Practice**
- Use the SPICES assessment tool for identifying serious health problems that can be prevented or managed early. **QSEN; Evidence-Based Practice**

MASTERY QUESTIONS

1. The nurse is conducting an assessment of an older adult living in the community. Which assessment findings are considered usual physiologic changes of aging? **Select all that apply.**
   A. Dementia
   B. Relocation stress
   C. Urinary incontinence
   D. Presbyopia
   E. Obesity

2. The nurse is caring for an older client who is experiencing acute confusion and agitation following a fractured hip repair this morning. Which risk factors may be contributing to the client's delirium? **Select all that apply.**
   A. Anesthesia used during surgery
   B. Surgical pain
   C. Unfamiliar environment
   D. Noisy hospital unit
   E. Medications used to manage pain

REFERENCES

Asterisk (*) indicates a classic or definitive work on this subject.

American Geriatric Society Beers Criteria Update Expert Panel. *American Geriatric Society 2019 Updated AGS Beers Criteria for potentially inappropriate medication use in older adults.* https://doi.org/10.1111/jgs.15767.

Bartzak, P. J. (2017). The extremes of human experience: Caring for soldiers who have had to take a life in the line of duty. *MEDSURG Nursing, 26*(1), 10–11.

Cutilli, C. C., Simko, L. C., Colbert, A. M., & Bennett, I. M. (2018). Health literacy, health disparities, and sources of health information in U.S. older adults. *Orthopaedic Nursing, 37*(1), 54–65.

*Fulmer, T. (2007). How to try this: Fulmer SPICES. *American Journal of Nursing, 107*(10), 40–48.

Haddad, Y. K., Bergen, G., & Luo, F. (2018). Reducing fall risk on older adults. *The American Journal of Nursing, 118*(7), 21–22.

Hartjes, T. M., Horgas, A. L., & Meece, L. (2016). Assessing and managing pain, agitation, and delirium in hospitalized older adults. *The American Journal of Nursing, 116*(10), 38–46.

Johnston, M., & Magnan, M. A. (2019). Using a fall prevention checklist to reduce hospital falls: Results of a quality improvement project. *American Journal of Nursing, 119*(3), 43–49.

Kokonya, A., & Fitzsimons, V. (2018). Transition to long-term care: Preparing older adults and their families. *MEDSURG Nursing, 27*(3), 143–148.

Kraus, S., & Duhamel, K. V. (2018). Culturally competent care for older LGBTQ patients. *Nursing, 48*(8), 48–52.

Mangels, A. R. (2018). Malnutrition in older adults. *The American Journal of Nursing, 118*(3), 34–41.

Marsh, E., & Imgrund, D. (2017). Implementing a delirium prevention and recognition program. *MEDSURG Nursing, 26*(4), 269–273.

Musich, S., Wang, S. S., Ruiz, J., Hawkins, K., & Wicker, E. (2018). The impact of mobility limitations on health outcomes among older adults. *Geriatric Nursing, 39*(2), 162–169.

Musich, S., Wang, S. S., Slindee, L., Kraemer, S., & Yeh, C. S. (2019). Prevalence and characteristics associated with high-dose opioid users among older adults. *Geriatric Nursing, 40*(1), 31–36.

Pagana, K. D., & Pagana, T. J. (2018). *Mosby's manual of diagnostic and laboratory tests* (6th Ed.). St. Louis, MO: Elsevier.

Porter, R. B. (2018). Exploring clinicians' perceptions about sustaining an evidence-based fall prevention program. *The American Journal of Nursing, 118*(5), 24–34.

Quach, J., & lee, J.-A. (2017). Do music therapies reduce depressive symptoms and improve QOL in older adults with chronic disease? *Nursing, 35*(6), 58–62.

*Sendelbach, S., & Guthrie, P. F. (2009). Evidence-based guideline—Acute confusion/delirium: Identification, assessment, treatment, and prevention. *Journal of Gerontological Nursing, 35*(11), 11–17.

Smith, C. J., & Harris, H. (2017). Caring for our nation's veterans: A shared responsibility. *Nursing, 47*(11), 51–52.

Smith, D. M. R., & Kautz, D. D. (2018). Protect older adults from polypharmacy hazards. *Nursing, 48*(2), 56–59.

Staplin, L., Lococo, K. H., Mastromatto, T., Sifrit, K. J., & Trazzera, K. M. (2017). Can your older patients drive safely? *The American Journal of Nursing, 117*(9), 34–42.

5

Assessment and Concepts of Care for Patients With Pain

Nicole M. Heimgartner

http://evolve.elsevier.com/Iggy/

LEARNING OUTCOMES

1. Identify the role of the nurse as an advocate for patients with acute ***pain*** or persistent (chronic) pain.
2. Collaborate with the interprofessional team to coordinate high-quality care to promote ***comfort*** in patients with ***pain.***
3. Teach the patient and caregiver(s) about drug therapy and complementary and integrative therapies for ***pain*** management.
4. Plan care coordination and transition management for patients with ***pain.***
5. Implement patient- and family-centered nursing interventions to decrease the psychosocial impact caused by ***pain.***
6. Apply knowledge of anatomy and physiology to perform an evidence-based assessment for a patient with ***pain.***
7. Prioritize evidence-based nursing interventions to prevent common side effects of analgesics, including the effects on ***cognition*** and ***sensory perception.***
8. Use clinical judgment to prioritize care for the patient receiving analgesia.
9. Incorporate nonpharmacologic interventions into the patient's plan of care as needed to control ***pain*** and promote ***comfort.***

KEY TERMS

acute pain the unpleasant sensory and emotional experience associated with tissue damage that results from acute injury, disease, or surgery.

breakthrough pain additional pain that "breaks through" the pain being managed by the mainstay analgesic drugs.

half-life the time it takes for the amount of drug in the body to be reduced by 50%.

nociceptive pain the result of actual or potential tissue damage or inflammation and is often categorized as being somatic or visceral.

pain an unpleasant sensory and emotional experience associated with actual or potential tissue damage. The most reliable indication of pain is the patient's self-report.

persistent pain (also called *chronic pain*) pain that persists or recurs for an indefinite period, usually for more than 3 months, often involves deep body structures, is poorly localized, and is difficult to describe.

placebo any medication or procedure, including surgery, which produces an effect in a patient because of its implicit or explicit intent, not because of its specific physical or chemical properties.

PRIORITY AND INTERRSSELATED CONCEPTS

The priority concept for this chapter is:
- ***Pain***

The interrelated concepts for this chapter are:
- ***Comfort***
- ***Cognition***
- ***Sensory Perception***

OVERVIEW OF PAIN

Pain is the most common reason people seek medical care and the number-one reason people take medication. Pain is universal, complex, and a personal experience that everyone has at some point in life. Pain can lead to poor health for many millions of people. Unrelieved pain can alter or diminish quality of life more than any other single health-related problem. Despite more than 30 years of education and dissemination of guideline recommendations, the failure to adequately manage pain remains a major health problem worldwide.

In response to mandates by multiple organizations and The Joint Commission (TJC), many hospitals and other health care agencies have implemented interprofessional pain initiatives to help ensure that patients receive the best possible treatment. Some hospitals address this mandate by establishing pain resource nurse (PRN) programs. As the name implies, one or more nurses per clinical unit are educated to serve as a resource to other members of the health care team in managing pain and promoting ***comfort***. Other hospitals have a formal team or pain service consisting of one or more nurses, pharmacists, case managers, and/or primary health care providers. In larger facilities, pain services may specialize by type of pain (e.g., acute pain service or pain and palliative care team). Although a large part of the interprofessional team's plan may center on drug therapy, these groups also recommend nonpharmacologic measures when appropriate.

Scope of the Problem

Pain is a major economic problem and a leading cause of disability that changes the lives of many people, especially older adults. Persistent noncancer pain such as osteoarthritis, rheumatoid arthritis, and diabetic neuropathy is the most common cause of long-term disability, affecting millions of Americans and others throughout the world.

PATIENT-CENTERED CARE: OLDER ADULT CONSIDERATIONS QSEN

Pain is treated inadequately in almost all health care settings. Populations at the highest risk in medical-surgical nursing are older adults, patients with substance use disorder, and those whose primary language differs from that of the health care professional. Older adults in nursing homes are at especially high risk because many residents are unable to report their pain. In addition, there is often a lack of staff members who have been educated to manage pain in the older adult population.

Inadequate pain management can lead to many adverse consequences affecting the patient and family members (Table 5.1). Therefore nurses have a legal and ethical responsibility to promote ***comfort*** and ensure that patients receive adequate ***pain*** control. Many professional organizations, including the American Society for Pain Management Nursing (ASPMN), the American Pain Society (APS), and TJC state that patients in all health care settings, including home care, have a right to effective pain management.

Patients rely on nurses and other health care professionals to adequately assess and manage their pain. As the coordinator of patient care, be sure to accurately document your assessments and actions, including patient and caregiver teaching. Communication and collaboration among the patient and members of the interprofessional health team about the patient's pain, expectations, and progress toward control are equally important.

Definitions of Pain

Pain is defined as an unpleasant sensory and emotional experience associated with actual or potential tissue damage. McCaffery (1968) offered the more classic and personal definition when she stated that pain is whatever the experiencing person says it is and exists whenever he or she says it exists. This has become the clinical definition of pain worldwide and reflects an understanding that the patient is the authority and the *only* one who can describe the pain experience. *In other words, self-report is always the most reliable indication of pain.* Nurses who approach pain from this perspective can help the patient achieve effective management by advocating for proper control. If the patient cannot provide self-report, a variety of other methods such as observation of behavioral indicators are used for pain assessment (see later in this chapter).

TABLE 5.1 Impact of Unrelieved Pain

Physiologic Impact	Quality-of-Life Impact
• Prolongs stress response • Increases heart rate, blood pressure, and oxygen demand • Decreases GI motility • Causes immobility • Decreases immune response • Delays healing • Poorly managed acute pain increases risk for development of chronic pain	• Interferes with ADLs • Causes anxiety, depression, hopelessness, fear, anger, and sleeplessness • Impairs family, work, and social relationships **Financial Impact** Costs Americans billions of dollars per year Increases length of hospital stay Leads to lost income and productivity

TABLE 5.2 Characteristics of Acute Pain and Persistent Pain

Acute	Persistent (Chronic)
• Has short duration • Usually has a well-defined cause • Decreases with healing • Is usually reversible • Initially serves a biologic purpose (warning sign to withdraw from painful stimuli or seek help) • When prolonged, serves no useful purpose • Ranges from mild-to-severe intensity • May be accompanied by anxiety and restlessness • When unrelieved, can increase morbidity and mortality and prolong length of hospital stay	• Usually lasts longer than 3 months • May or may not have well-defined cause • Usually begins gradually and persists • Serves no useful purpose • Ranges from mild-to-severe intensity • Often accompanied by multiple quality-of-life and functional adverse effects, including depression; fatigue; financial burden; and increased dependence on family, friends, and the health care system • Can impact the quality of life of family members and friends

Categorization of Pain

Pain can be categorized in several ways, and for some patients more than one type of pain may be present. Pain is often described as being acute or persistent (chronic) based on its duration (Table 5.2). *Acute pain* is usually short-lived, whereas *persistent (chronic) pain* can last a person's lifetime. *Acute pain* often results from sudden, accidental trauma (e.g., fractures, burns, lacerations) or from surgery, ischemia, or acute inflammation. *Persistent (chronic) pain* lasts beyond the time that is expected for healing. Persistent (chronic) pain that is not related to cancer is the most common type of pain. Pain is also categorized by cause such as cancer pain, which can be acute or persistent, as well as by type of pain such as nociceptive or neuropathic pain (ANA & ASPMN, 2016).

Acute Pain. Almost everyone experiences acute pain at some time. Brief acute pain serves a biologic purpose in that it acts as a warning signal by activating the sympathetic nervous system and causing various physiologic responses. Although not consistent in all people, when acute pain is severe, you may see responses similar to those found in "fight-or-flight" reactions such as increased vital signs, sweating, and dilated pupils. Most people protect themselves by drawing away from the painful stimulus. Behavioral signs may include restlessness (especially among cognitively impaired older adults who sometimes fidget and pick at clothing), an inability to concentrate, apprehension, and overall distress of varying degrees. These heightened physiologic and behavioral responses are often referred to as the *acute pain model.* It is important to remember that the response to pain is highly individual and that humans quickly adapt physiologically and behaviorally to pain. Be careful not to expect certain responses when assessing any type of pain. *The absence of the physiologic and behavioral responses does not mean the absence of pain.*

Acute ***pain*** is usually temporary, has a sudden onset, and is easily localized. The pain is typically confined to the injured area and may subside with or without treatment. As the injured area heals, the ***sensory perception*** of pain changes and, in most cases, diminishes and resolves. Both the caregiver and the patient can see an end to the pain, which usually makes coping somewhat easier.

Pain that accompanies surgery is one of the most common examples of acute pain, but it is not always well managed. *The response to pain after surgery is highly individual and variable.* There is no evidence that shows that one type of surgery is consistently more or less painful than another. Usually poorly managed postoperative pain is a result of inadequate drug (analgesic) therapy. Poorly managed and prolonged acute pain serves no useful purpose and has many adverse effects, including inability of the patient to participate in the recovery process with subsequent increased disability. The severity of early postoperative pain may be a predictor of long-term pain. Those who experience unrelieved severe postoperative pain are at high risk for the development of chronic persistent postsurgical pain (Czarnecki & Turner, 2018).

Persistent (Chronic) Pain. Persistent pain (also called *chronic pain)* is often defined as pain that lasts or recurs for an indefinite period, usually for more than 3 months. The onset is gradual, and the character and quality of the pain often change over time. *Persistent pain serves no biological purpose.* Because it persists for an extended period, it can interfere with personal relationships and performance of ADLs. Persistent pain can also result in emotional and financial burdens, depression, and hopelessness for patients and their families. It is important to remember that the body adapts to persistent pain; thus vital signs such as pulse and blood pressure may actually be lower than normal in people with persistent pain. *Although many characteristics of persistent pain are similar in different patients, be aware that each patient is unique and requires a highly individualized plan of care.*

Persistent pain that is unrelated to cancer (persistent noncancer pain) is a global health problem, occurring most often in people older than 65 years. There are many sources and types of persistent noncancer pain. Among the most common are neck, shoulder, and low back pain following injury. Chronic conditions such as diabetes, rheumatoid arthritis, Crohn's disease, and interstitial cystitis are often associated with persistent pain. People who have had a stroke or trauma or are paralyzed may report persistent pain as a result of central nervous system (CNS) damage. Sometimes the exact cause of the pain is unclear, as with fibromyalgia.

Categorization of Pain by Etiology

Cancer Pain. Many patients with cancer report ***pain*** at the time of diagnosis, which increases in advanced stages of the disease. Most cancer pain can be managed successfully by giving adequate amounts of oral opioids around the clock, yet patients with cancer are often treated inadequately for what can be persistent, excruciating pain and suffering.

Most cancer pain is persistent and is the result of tumor growth, including nerve compression; invasion of tissue; and/or bone metastasis, an extremely painful condition. Cancer treatments also can cause *acute pain* (e.g., from repetitive blood draws and other procedures, surgery, and toxicities from chemotherapy and radiation therapy).

Procedural Pain. Procedural pain is pain that is associated with medical procedures or surgical interventions. This type of pain is common in the health care setting and is generally acute in nature. Effective control of acute procedural pain is very important as poor pain control can have numerous undesirable consequences including poor patient outcomes, increased chance of readmission, patient dissatisfaction, and increased health care costs (Jungquist et al., 2017). Further, it is suggested that poor control of acute pain can lead to the development of persistent (chronic) pain, a process called the *chronification* of pain (Jungquist et al., 2017).

PATIENT-CENTERED CARE: VETERANS HEALTH CONSIDERATIONS QSEN

American veterans experience pain more often and more severely than nonveterans, with young and middle-aged veterans suffering the most (Nahin, 2017). Over half of the veterans of recent wars report persistent pain, mostly due to musculoskeletal disorders (MSDs) from either trauma or arthritis. Research shows that persistent pain is associated with a much higher incidence of posttraumatic stress disorder (PTSD) (DeCarvalho, 2016). For veterans, persistent pain may exacerbate or cause depression, PTSD, and a decreased sense of well-being. Some of these patients are managed through Veterans Administration Medical Centers in ambulatory care clinics in the United States. Unfortunately, others are jobless and homeless and therefore receive no care to manage their physical or psychological health problems.

Categorization of Pain by Underlying Mechanisms. Pain is also categorized as either nociceptive (normal pain processing) or neuropathic (abnormal pain processing) (Table 5.3). The duration of nociceptive and neuropathic pain can be either acute (short lived) or persistent (chronic), and a person can have both types.

Nociceptive Pain. Nociception is the term that is used to describe how pain becomes a conscious experience. It involves the *normal functioning of physiologic systems* that process noxious stimuli, with the ultimate result being that the stimuli are perceived to be painful. In short, nociception means "normal" pain transmission and is generally discussed in terms of four processes: transduction, transmission,

TABLE 5.3 Physiologic Sources of Nociceptive Pain and Neuropathic Pain

Physiologic Structure	Characteristics of Pain	Sources of Acute Postoperative Pain	Sources of Chronic Pain Syndromes
Nociceptive Pain (Normal Pain Processing)			
Somatic Pain			
Cutaneous or superficial: skin and subcutaneous tissues	Well localized Sharp, throbbing	Incisional pain, pain at insertion sites of tubes and drains, wound complications, orthopedic procedures, skeletal muscle spasms	Bony metastases, osteoarthritis and rheumatoid arthritis, low back pain, peripheral vascular diseases
Deep somatic: bone, muscle, blood vessels, connective tissues	Dull, aching, cramping		
Visceral Pain			
Organs and the linings of the body cavities	Poorly localized Diffuse, deep cramping or pressure, sharp, stabbing	Chest tubes, abdominal tubes and drains, bladder distention or spasms, intestinal distention	Pancreatitis, liver metastases, colitis, appendicitis
Neuropathic Pain (Abnormal Pain Processing)			
Peripheral or central nervous system: nerve fibers, spinal cord, and higher central nervous system	Poorly localized Shooting, burning, fiery, shocklike, tingling, painful numbness	Phantom limb pain, postmastectomy pain, nerve compression	HIV-related pain, diabetic neuropathy, postherpetic neuralgia, chemotherapy-induced neuropathies, cancer-related nerve injury, radiculopathies

HIV, Human immune deficiency virus.

perception, and modulation (Fig. 5.1). Although it is helpful to consider nociception in the context of these four processes, it is important to understand that they do not occur as four separate and distinct entities. They are continuous, and the processes overlap as they flow from one to another.

Transduction is the first process of nociception and refers to the means by which noxious events activate neurons that exist throughout the body (skin, subcutaneous tissue, and visceral [or somatic] structures) and have the ability to respond selectively to specific noxious stimuli. These neurons are called *nociceptors.* When they are stimulated directly, a number of excitatory compounds (e.g., serotonin, bradykinin, histamine, substance P, and prostaglandins) that further activate more nociceptors are released (see Fig. 5.1).

Transmission is the second process involved in nociception. Nociceptors have small-diameter axons—either A-delta or C fibers (see Fig. 5.1). Effective transduction generates an electric signal (action potential) that is transmitted in these nerve fibers from the periphery toward the CNS. *A-delta fibers* are lightly myelinated and conduct faster than unmyelinated C fibers. The endings of A-delta fibers detect thermal and mechanical injury. The ***sensory perception*** accompanying A-delta fiber activation is sharp and well localized and leads to an appropriately rapid protective response such as reflex withdrawal from the painful stimuli. *C fibers* are unmyelinated or poorly myelinated slow conductors and respond to mechanical, thermal, and chemical stimuli. Activation after acute injury yields a poorly localized (more widely distributed), typically aching or burning pain. In contrast to the intermittent nature of A-delta sensations, C fibers usually produce more continuous pain.

Perception is the third broad process involved in nociception. Perception, which may be viewed as the end result of the neural activity associated with transmission of information about noxious events, involves the conscious awareness of pain (see Fig. 5.1). It requires the activation of higher brain structures, including the cortex, and involves both awareness and the occurrence of emotions and drives associated with pain. The physiology of pain perception is very poorly understood but presumably can be targeted by therapies that activate higher cortical functions and ***cognition*** to achieve pain control or coping. Cognitive-behavioral therapy and specific approaches such as distraction and imagery (discussed later in the chapter) have been developed based on evidence that brain processes can strongly influence pain perception.

Modulation of afferent input generated in response to noxious stimuli happens at every level from the periphery to the cortex (see Fig. 5.1). The neurochemistry of modulation is complex and not yet fully understood, but it is known that multiple peripheral and central systems and dozens of neurochemicals are involved. For example, the endogenous opioids (endorphins) are found throughout the peripheral nervous system (PNS) and CNS and, like the exogenous opioids administered therapeutically, they inhibit neuronal activity by binding to opioid receptors. Other central inhibitory neurotransmitters important in the modulation of pain include serotonin and norepinephrine, which are released in the spinal cord and brainstem by the descending fibers of the modulatory system to inhibit pain.

Nociceptive pain is the result of actual or potential tissue damage or inflammation and is often categorized as being somatic or visceral. *Somatic pain* arises from the skin and musculoskeletal structures, and *visceral pain* arises from organs. Examples include pain-associated trauma, surgery, burns, and tumor growth.

Neuropathic Pain. Neuropathic pain is a descriptive term used to refer to pain that is believed to be sustained by a set of mechanisms driven by damage to or dysfunction of the PNS and/or

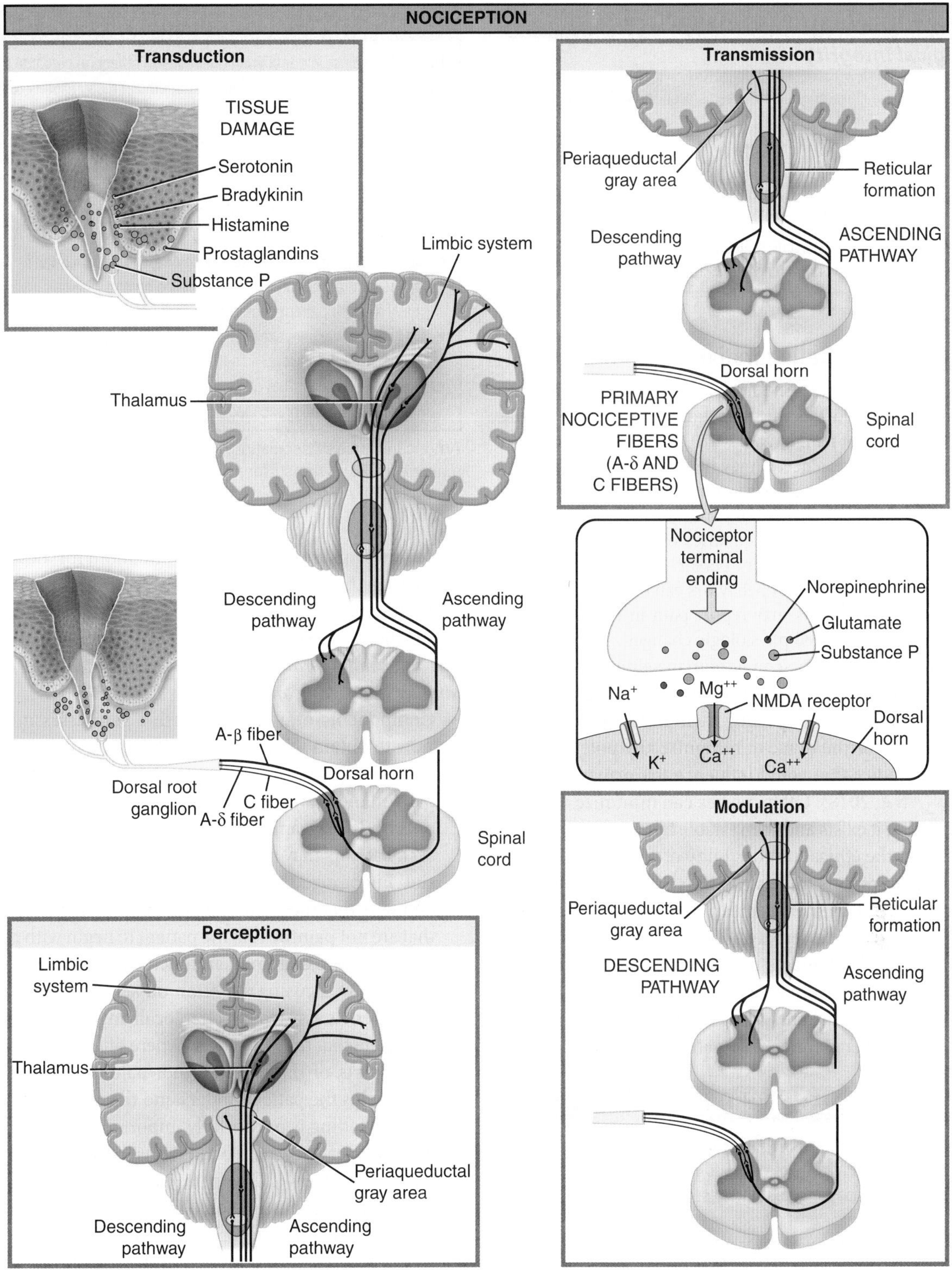

Fig. 5.1 Nociception. (Modified from Pasero, C., & McCaffery, M. (2011). *Pain assessment and pharmacologic management*. St. Louis: Mosby.)

CNS. In contrast to nociceptive pain, which is sustained by ongoing activation of essentially *normal* neural systems, neuropathic pain is sustained by the *abnormal* processing of stimuli. Whereas nociceptive pain involves tissue damage or inflammation, neuropathic pain may occur in the absence of either.

It is not clear why noxious stimuli result in neuropathic pain in some people and not in others and why some treatments work in some and not in others. Neuropathic pain is difficult to treat and often resistant to first-line analgesics. Asking patients to describe it is the best way to identify the presence of neuropathic pain. Common distinctive descriptors include "burning," "shooting," "tingling," and "feeling pins and needles." Much is unknown about what causes and maintains neuropathic pain; it is the subject of intense ongoing research.

NCLEX EXAMINATION CHALLENGE 5.1

Physiological Integrity

The nurse is teaching a class on pain management strategies. Which client statement requires additional teaching?

A. "Persistent pain is a warning in my body that alerts the sympathetic nervous system."
B. "Acute pain has a quick onset and is usually isolated to one area of my body."
C. "My frozen shoulder causes musculoskeletal or somatic pain."
D. "Nociceptive pain follows a normal and predictable pattern."

❖ Interprofessional Collaborative Care

◆ **Assessment: Recognize Cues.** All accepted guidelines identify the patient's self-report as the gold standard for assessing the existence and intensity of pain (ANA, 2018). Because pain is such a private and personal experience, it may be difficult for the person to describe or explain it to others. However, subjective descriptions of the experience and measurement of pain intensity are more reliable and accurate than observable qualities of pain. The amount of pain and responses to it vary from person to person; therefore interpreting it solely on actions or behaviors can be misleading and is not recommended. Patients may report pain in the absence of any observable or documented physiologic changes.

The primary role of the nurse in ***pain*** management is to advocate for patients by *accepting* their reports of pain and acting promptly to relieve it while respecting their preferences and values. It is important for the nurse to recognize any potential personal bias or prejudice that could influence the management of patient's pain (ANA, 2018). Often, nurses can minimize bias just by recognizing that it exists and then establishing a plan to set the bias aside to meet the ethical responsibility of pain management. See Table 5.4 for questions to help the nurse recognize personal bias associated with pain management. To be patient centered, always respect the patient's verbal and nonverbal expressions of pain without making judgments or inferences about its reality. If patients perceive that health care professionals doubt the existence of their pain, mistrust and other negative feelings can arise and interfere with a therapeutic nurse-patient relationship.

ETHICAL/LEGAL CONSIDERATIONS

The American Nurses Association (ANA) has a specific position statement regarding the ethical responsibility of nurses to manage pain (ANA, 2018). Although the opioid crisis has presented obstacles to pain management, effective and unbiased pain management remains an ethical responsibility for the nurse. Interprofessional collaboration is required to develop pain management plans that include thorough assessment, goal setting, and ongoing reassessment to determine the efficacy of pain management. Nurses must recognize personal bias and work to relieve inequities that prevent the relief of pain and suffering (ANA, 2018).

TABLE 5.4 Recognizing Personal Bias

The nurse can use the following questions to reflect on personal experiences and potential bias that could affect the ethical responsibility to manage pain (ANA, 2018, p. 4):

- Do I worry about causing addiction for my patients?
- Do I feel that some patients are trying to work the system to get access to more medication?
- Do I feel anxious when discussing pain management with other team members?
- Do I ever feel guilty about too much or too little pain relief?
- Do I recognize that pain is whatever the person who has it says it is but really feel the patient sometimes is not right?
- Do I impose my own experience with addition, opioid misuse, and drug-seeking behaviors?
- Do I resist the idea that some patients may require more aggressive pain management than prescribed?

American Nurses Association. (2018). The ethical responsibility to manage pain and the suffering it causes. Position Statement. Silver Springs, MD: ANA.

The Comprehensive Pain Assessment. A comprehensive pain assessment should be conducted during the initial interview with the patient, with each new report of pain, and whenever indicated by changes in the patient's condition or treatment plan during the course of care. Pain assessment at these intervals serves as the foundation for developing and evaluating the effectiveness of the treatment plan. Remember that patients' personal preferences and values affect how they report their history. *When culturally appropriate, be sure to make this information-gathering process family centered by including families and significant others.*

Components of a comprehensive pain assessment and tips on how to obtain the information from the patient include:

- *Location(s):* Ask the patient to state or point to the area(s) of pain on the body. Sometimes allowing patients to make marks on a body diagram is helpful in gaining this information (Fig. 5.2). Patients may present with more than one specific painful site. Encourage those who cannot identify the painful areas and state that they "hurt all over" to focus on parts of the body that are not painful. Ask the patient to begin with the hand and fingers of one extremity and identify the presence or absence of pain. By focusing attention on selected areas of the body, the patient is assisted in better localizing painful areas. Patients who state that they hurt everywhere often begin to realize that some parts of the body are not painful. Identifying painful areas helps the patient understand the origin of the pain. This understanding is particularly important for those with cancer because every new pain often raises the suspicion of metastasis (spread of disease). The pain may have other causes such as immobility or constipation. Pain may be described as belonging to one of four categories related to its location:
  - *Localized* pain is confined to the site of origin.
  - *Projected* pain is diffuse around the site of origin and is not well localized.
  - *Referred* pain is felt in an area distant from the site of painful stimuli.
  - *Radiating* pain is felt along a specific nerve or nerves.
- *Intensity:* Ask the patient to rate the severity of the pain using a reliable and valid assessment tool. Various self-report scales have been developed to help patients communicate pain intensity. Once a scale is selected, be sure to use the *same* scale over time for that patient and assess intensity

McGill-Melzack
PAIN QUESTIONNAIRE

Patient's name ______________ Age __________

File No. ______________ Date __________

Clinical category (e.g., cardiac, neurologic)

Diagnosis: __________

____

____

Analgesic (if already administered):

1. Type ______________
2. Dosage ______________
3. Time given in relation to this test ______

Patient's intelligence: circle number that represents best estimate.

1 (low) 2 3 4 5 (high)

****

This questionnaire has been designed to tell us more about your pain. Four major questions we ask are

1. Where is your pain?
2. What does it feel like?
3. How does it change with time?
4. How strong is it?

It is important that you tell us how your pain feels now. Please follow the instructions at the beginning of each part.

Part 1. Where Is Your Pain?

Please mark, on the drawings below, the areas where you feel pain. Put E if external, or I if internal, near the areas you mark. Put EI if both external and internal.

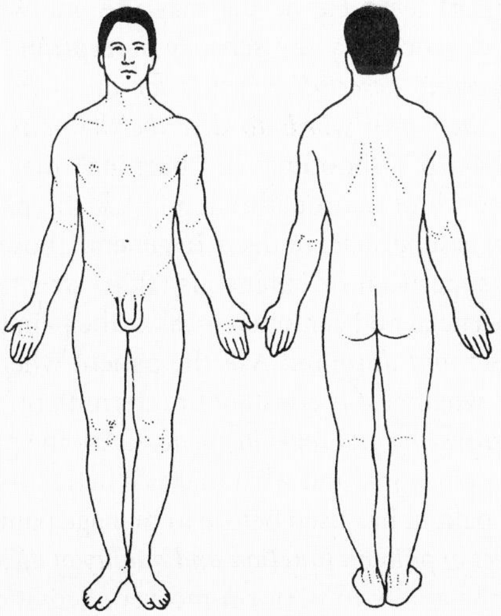

Part 2. What Does Your Pain Feel Like?

Some of the words below describe your *present* pain. Circle *ONLY* those words that best describe it. Leave out any category that is not suitable. Use only a single word in each appropriate category—the one that applies best.

1. Flickering, Quivering, Pulsing, Throbbing, Beating, Pounding
2. Jumping, Flashing, Shooting
3. Pricking, Boring, Drilling, Stabbing, Lancinating
4. Sharp, Cutting, Lacerating
5. Pinching, Pressing, Gnawing, Cramping, Crushing
6. Tugging, Pulling, Wrenching
7. Hot, Burning, Scalding, Searing
8. Tingling, Itchy, Smarting, Stinging
9. Dull, Sore, Hurting, Aching, Heavy
10. Tender, Taut, Rasping, Splitting
11. Tiring, Exhausting
12. Sickening, Suffocating
13. Fearful, Frightful, Terrifying
14. Punishing, Grueling, Cruel, Vicious, Killing
15. Wretched, Blinding
16. Annoying, Troublesome, Miserable, Intense, Unbearable
17. Spreading, Radiating, Penetrating, Piercing
18. Tight, Numb, Drawing, Squeezing, Tearing
19. Cool, Cold, Freezing
20. Nagging, Nauseating, Agonizing, Dreadful, Torturing

Part 3. How Does Your Pain Change With Time?

1. Which word or words would you use to describe the *pattern* of your pain?

1	2	3
Continuous	Rhythmic	Brief
Steady	Periodic	Momentary
Constant	Intermittent	Transient

2. What kind of things *relieve* your pain?
3. What kind of things *increase* your pain?

Part 4. How Strong Is Your Pain?

People agree that the following 5 words represent pain of increasing intensity. They are:

1	2	3	4	5
Mild	Discomforting	Distressing	Horrible	Excruciating

To answer each question below, write the number of the most appropriate word in the space beside the question.

1. Which word describes your pain right now? ____
2. Which word describes it at its worst? ____
3. Which word describes it when it is least? ____
4. Which word describes the worst toothache you ever had? ____
5. Which word describes the worst headache you ever had? ____
6. Which word describes the worst stomachache you ever had? ____

Fig. 5.2 The McGill-Melzack Pain Questionnaire. (From Melzack, R. [1975]. The McGill Pain Questionnaire: Major properties and scoring methods. *Pain, 1*, 272–281.)

TABLE 5.5 Teaching Patients and Their Families How to Use a Pain Rating Scale[a]

Step 1. Show the pain rating scale to the patient and family and explain its primary purpose.

Example: "This is a pain rating scale that many of our patients use to help us understand their pain and set goals for pain relief. We will ask you regularly about pain, but any time you have pain you must let us know so that we can help control it. We don't always know when you hurt."

Step 2. Explain the parts of the pain rating scale. If the patient does not like it or understand it, switch to another scale (e.g., vertical presentation, VDS, or FACES).

Example: "On this pain rating scale 0 means no pain, and 10 means the worst possible pain. The middle of the scale, around 5, means moderate pain. A 2 or 3 would be mild pain, but 7 or higher means severe pain."

Step 3. Discuss pain as a broad concept that is not restricted to a severe and intolerable sensation.

Example: "Pain refers to any kind of discomfort anywhere in your body. Pain also means aching and hurting. Pain can include pulling, tightness, burning, knifelike feelings, and other unpleasant sensations."

Step 4. Verify that the patient understands the broad concept of pain. Ask the patient to mention two examples of pain that he or she has experienced. If the patient is already in pain that requires treatment, use the present situation as the example.

Example: "I want to be sure that I've explained this clearly; so would you give me two examples of pain you've had recently?" If the patient examples include various parts of the body and various pain characteristics, it indicates that he or she understands pain as a fairly broad concept. An example of what a patient might say is "I have a mild, sort of throbbing headache now, and yesterday my back was aching."

Step 5. Ask the patient to practice using the pain rating scale with the present pain or select one of the examples mentioned.

Example: "Using the scale, what is your pain right now? What is it at its worst?" OR "Using the pain rating scale and one of your examples of pain, what is that pain usually? What is it at its worst?"

Step 6. Set goals for comfort and function/recovery/quality of life. Ask patients which pain rating would be acceptable or satisfactory, considering the activities required for recovery or for maintaining a satisfactory quality of life.

Example for a surgical patient: "I have explained the importance of coughing and deep breathing to prevent pneumonia and other complications. Now we need to determine the pain rating that will not interfere with this so that you may recover quickly."

Example for patient with chronic pain or terminal illness: "What do you want to do that pain keeps you from doing? Which pain rating would allow you to do this?"

From Pasero, C., & McCaffery, M. (2011). *Pain assessment and pharmacologic management.* St. Louis: Mosby. Copyright 2011, McCaffery, M., & Pasero, C. Used with permission.

VDS, Verbal descriptor scale.

[a]When a patient is obviously in pain or not focused enough to learn to use a pain rating scale, pain treatment should proceed without pain ratings. Teaching can be undertaken when pain is reduced to a level that facilitates understanding how to use a pain scale.

both with and without activity. See Table 5.5 for strategies that can be used to teach patients and their families how to use a pain rating scale. The most common intensity rating scales are:

- Numeric Rating Scale (NRS): The NRS is usually presented as a horizontal 0-to-10 point scale, with word anchors of "no pain" at one end of the scale, "moderate pain" in the middle of the scale, and "worst possible pain" at the end of the scale. Some patients relate better to a vertical presentation of the scale.
- Wong-Baker FACES Pain Rating Scale: The FACES scale consists of six cartoon faces with word descriptors, ranging from a smiling face on the left for "no pain (or hurt)" to a frowning, tearful face on the right for "worst pain (or hurt)." The faces are most commonly numbered 0 to 10. Patients are asked to choose the face that best describes their pain. It is important to appreciate that faces scales are self-report tools; *clinicians should not attempt to match a face shown on a scale to the patient's facial expression to determine pain intensity.* Fig. 5.3 provides the Wong-Baker FACES scale combined with the NRS.
- Faces Pain Scale—Revised (FPS-R): The FPS-R has six faces to make it consistent with other scales using the 0-to-10 metric. The faces range from a neutral facial expression to one of intense pain. As with the Wong-Baker FACES scale, patients are asked to choose the face that best reflects their pain. Some research shows that the FPS-R is preferred by both cognitively intact and impaired older adults.
- Verbal Descriptor Scale (VDS): A VDS uses different words or phrases to describe the intensity of pain such as "*no pain, mild pain, moderate pain, severe pain, very severe pain,* and *worst possible pain.*" The patient is asked to select the phrase that best describes the pain intensity.
- *Quality:* Ask the patient to describe how the ***pain*** and discomfort feels. He or she may use one word or a group of words to convey the ***sensory perception*** of the pain. *Avoid suggesting descriptive words for the pain; allow patients to use their own words to describe the pain.* Descriptors such as "sharp," "shooting," or "burning" may help identify the presence of neuropathic pain. Ask the patient whether the pain is superficial or deep. In general, those with pain involving superficial or cutaneous (skin) structures describe it as superficial and can often localize the pain to a specific area.
- *Onset and duration:* Ask the patient when the pain started and whether it is constant or intermittent.
- *Aggravating and relieving factors:* Ask the patient what makes the pain worse and what makes it better. Ask about strategies the patient has used before to manage pain.
- *Effect of pain on function and quality of life:* The effect of pain on the ability to perform recovery activities should be evaluated regularly. It is particularly important to ask patients with persistent pain about how it has affected their lives. Is the patient able to sleep? Ask the patient what they could do before the pain began that they can no longer do and what they want to do but cannot do.
- *Comfort-function (pain intensity) outcomes:* For patients with *acute pain,* identify expected short-term functional

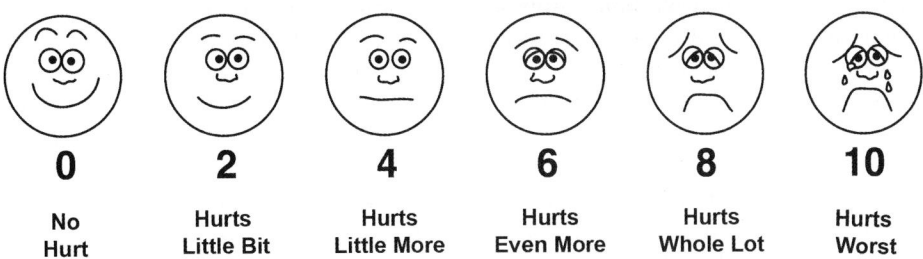

Fig. 5.3 Wong-Baker FACES® pain rating scale. (From Wong-Baker FACES Foundation [2016]. Wong-Baker FACES Pain Rating Scale. Retrieved March 12, 2017, with permission from http://www.WongBakerFACES.org.)

outcomes. Reinforce to the patient that adequate pain control will lead to more successful achievement of those outcomes. For example, tell surgical patients that they will be expected to ambulate or participate in physical therapy after surgery. Ask patients to identify a level of pain that will allow accomplishment of the expected outcomes. A realistic outcome for most patients is 2 or 3 on a scale of 0 to 10. Pain intensity that is consistently above the desired level requires further evaluation and consideration of possible adjustment of the treatment plan.

- *Other information:* Consider the patient's culture, past pain experiences, and pertinent medical history such as comorbidities. Current treatments and diagnostic studies are considered when performing an assessment. For example, patients who are intubated may be awake and alert but unable to speak.

PATIENT-CENTERED CARE: OLDER ADULT CONSIDERATIONS (QSEN)

Pain is not a result of aging; however, the incidence is higher in older adults. Sensitivity to pain does not diminish with age. Many older adults, even those with mild-to-moderate dementia, are able to use a self-report assessment tool if nurses and other caregivers take the time to administer it. Many older adults are reluctant to report pain for a variety of reasons, including the belief that it is normal and that they are bothering the nurse. It is essential that attempts be made to obtain the patient's self-report and that pain be assessed frequently with a focus on functional and quality-of-life indicators in this vulnerable population.

Psychosocial Assessment. **Pain** holds unique meaning for the person experiencing it. Patients having *acute pain* from surgery may interpret it as necessary and expected. It may be viewed with relief as a sign that some greater problem has been resolved or alleviated by the surgery. Knowing that the duration of the pain is limited may be reassuring for a patient. In contrast, acute chest pain associated with angina may mark the beginning of a life of fear and uncertainty.

Various psychosocial factors influence *persistent (chronic)* pain. Some factors are similar to those found in the acute pain experience such as anxiety or fear related to the meaning of the pain. Because chronic pain persists or is perhaps only partially relieved, the patient may feel powerless, angry, hostile, or desperate. He or she is also vulnerable to labels such as "chronic complainer" or "faker." Remember that it is unprofessional and inappropriate to label or stereotype patients. *Remain objective and advocate for proper pain control for all patients.*

Assess the status of family and other close relationships, along with the range of social resources available to the patient with persistent pain. The existence of a pain-specific conflict with a spouse or significant other may affect or limit coping strategies. Other people may react to persistent pain with depression, social withdrawal, and preoccupation with physical symptoms.

PATIENT-CENTERED CARE: CULTURAL/SPIRITUAL CONSIDERATIONS (QSEN)

If persistent pain is associated with a progressive disease such as cancer, rheumatoid arthritis, or peripheral vascular disease, the patient may have worries and concerns about the consequences of the illness. People with cancer-related pain may fear death or body mutilation. Some may think they are being punished for some wrongdoing in life. Others may attach a religious or spiritual significance to lingering pain.

Ask open-ended questions (e.g., "Tell me how your pain has affected your job or your role as a mother.") to allow the patient to describe personal attitudes about pain and its influence on life. This opportunity can help someone whose life has been changed by pain. However, some patients choose not to share their private information or fears. As a patient-centered nurse, always respect patients' preferences and values.

NCLEX EXAMINATION CHALLENGE 5.2

Physiological Integrity

Which documentation will the nurse record for a client who had a total knee replacement 2 days ago and reports sharp pain at the surgical site?

A. Reports acute pain at the surgical site.
B. Persistent pain reported around the surgical site.
C. Experiences neuropathic pain near the surgical site.
D. Discomfort has progressed to chronification of pain.

Assessment Challenges. Patients who are unable to report their pain using the customary self-report assessment tools are at higher risk for undertreated pain than those who can report. These include patients who are cognitively impaired, critically ill (intubated, unresponsive), comatose, or imminently dying. Patients who are receiving neuromuscular blocking agents or are sedated from general anesthetics and other drugs given during surgery are also among this at-risk population.

The *Hierarchy of Pain Measures* is recommended by many professional organizations today as a framework for assessing pain in patients who cannot self-report (Booker & Haedtke, 2016). The key components of the Hierarchy require the nurse to (1) attempt to obtain self-report; (2) consider underlying pathology or conditions and procedures that might be painful (e.g., surgery); (3) observe behaviors; (4) evaluate physiologic indicators; and (5) conduct an analgesic trial. See Table 5.6 for detailed information on each component of the Hierarchy of Pain Measures.

Patients with problems of ***cognition*** are among those at highest risk for undertreated pain because they are unable to report or have difficulty reporting their pain. The Hierarchy of Pain Measures lists several strategies to use when obtaining self-report is a challenge. When these are ineffective, the Hierarchy suggests that a number of behaviors have been shown to be indicators of pain. Behavioral pain assessment tools are often used to systematically evaluate behaviors to help determine the presence of pain. Improvement in the behavioral pain score helps confirm suspicions that pain is present and provides a reference point for assessing the effectiveness of interventions.

It is important for nurses to remember that *a score obtained from the use of a behavioral tool is not the same as a self-reported pain intensity score*. Although it may seem logical to assume that the higher the behavioral score, the more intense the pain, this cannot be proven without the patient's report. Some patients remain nonverbal and lie completely still (which would yield a low behavioral score) despite having severe pain. The reality is that, if a patient cannot report the intensity of pain, the exact intensity is unknown. Two of the most commonly used behavioral assessment tools that are used for patients with problems of ***cognition*** such as delirium (acute confusion) or dementia (chronic confusion) are:

- Pain Assessment Checklist for Seniors with Limited Ability to Communicate–II (PACSLAC-II) has been tested in the acute care setting in patients with varying levels of cognitive impairment (Chan et al., 2014). The tool groups behavioral indicators of pain into six categories. Each category allows a score of 0 if the behavior is not observed and a 1 if the behavior occurred even briefly during activity or rest:
  - Facial expression (e.g., grimacing, crying)
  - Verbalizations or vocalizations (e.g., screaming)

TABLE 5.6 Hierarchy of Pain Measures

1. Attempt to obtain the patient's self-report, the single most reliable indicator of pain. Do not assume that a patient cannot provide a report of pain; many cognitively impaired patients are able to use a self-report tool if simple actions are taken.
   - Try using a standard pain assessment tool (see Fig. 5.3).
   - Ensure that eyeglasses and hearing aids are functioning.
   - Increase the size of the font and other features of the scale.
   - Present the tool in vertical format (rather than the frequently used horizontal).
   - Try using alternative words such as "ache," "hurt," and "sore" when discussing pain.
   - Ask about pain in the present.
   - Repeat instructions and questions more than once.
   - Allow ample time to respond.
   - Remember that head nodding and eye blinking or squeezing the eyes tightly can also be used to signal presence of pain and sometimes to rate intensity.
   - Ask awake and oriented ventilated patients to point to a number on the numeric scale if they are able.
   - Repeat instructions and show the scale each time pain is assessed.
2. Consider the patient's condition or exposure to a procedure that is thought to be painful. If appropriate, *assume pain is present* (APP) and document APP when approved by institution policy and procedure. As an example, pain should be assumed to be present in an unresponsive, mechanically ventilated, critically ill trauma patient. Nurses should assume that certain procedures are painful and premedicate based on that assumption.
3. Observe behavioral signs (e.g., facial expressions, crying, restlessness, and changes in activity). A pain behavior in one patient may not be in another. Try to identify pain behaviors that are unique to the patient ("pain signature"). Many behavioral pain assessment tools are available that will yield a pain behavior score and may help determine if pain is present. However, it is important to remember that a behavioral score is not the same as a pain intensity score. Behavioral tools are used to help identify the presence of pain and whether an intervention is effective, but the pain intensity is unknown if the patient is unable to provide it.
   - A surrogate who knows the patient well (e.g., parent, spouse, or caregiver) may be able to provide information about underlying painful pathology or behaviors that may indicate pain.
   - Although surrogates may be helpful in identifying behaviors that may indicate pain, research has shown that they commonly underestimate or overestimate the intensity of the pain. Therefore they should not be asked to rate the patient's pain intensity.
4. Evaluate physiologic indicators with the understanding that they are the *least* sensitive indicators of pain and may signal the existence of conditions other than pain or a lack of it (e.g., hypovolemia, blood loss). Patients quickly adapt physiologically despite pain and may have normal or below-normal vital signs in the presence of severe pain. The overriding principle is that the absence of an elevated blood pressure or heart rate does not mean the absence of pain.
5. Conduct an analgesic trial to confirm the presence of pain and to establish a basis for developing a treatment plan if pain is thought to be present. An analgesic trial involves administering a low dose of analgesic and observing patient response. The initial low dose may not be enough to illicit a change in behavior and should be increased if the previous dose was tolerated, or another analgesic may be added. If behaviors continue despite optimal analgesic doses, other possible causes should be investigated.
   - In patients who are unresponsive, no change in behavior will be evident, and the optimized analgesic dose should be continued.

From Pasero, C., & McCaffery, M. (2011). *Pain assessment and pharmacologic management.* St. Louis: Mosby.

  - Body movements (e.g., restlessness)
  - Changes in interpersonal interactions
  - Changes in activity patterns or routines
  - Mental status changes (e.g., confusion, increased confusion)
- Pain Assessment in Advanced Dementia (PAINAD) scale has been tested in patients with severe dementia (Herr et al., 2011). The tool groups behavioral indicators into five categories for scoring using a graduated scale of 0 (least intense behaviors) to 2 (most intense behaviors) per category for a maximum behavioral score of 10:
  - Breathing (independent of vocalization)
  - Negative vocalization
  - Facial expression
  - Body language
  - Consolability (ability to calm the patient)

For patients who are mechanically ventilated or may not be able to use other tools for communication, try these interventions:

- Establish a reliable yes-no signal (e.g., thumbs up or down, head nods, or eye blinks) to determine the presence of pain.
- Use communication boards, alphabet boards, computer, or picture boards with word labels for patients with ***cognition*** problems.
- Correctly interpret lip reading by maintaining eye contact, encouraging the patient to speak slowly, and using dentures if required.

◆ **Interventions: Take Action.** ***Pain*** is managed using nonpharmacologic interventions, drug therapy, or both. Although nonpharmacologic interventions are commonly used, they are most often combined with drug therapy as complementary or supplemental therapies. Because drug therapy is the most often used approach to pain management, it is presented first in this chapter.

Drug Therapy. Safe and effective use of analgesics requires the development of an individualized treatment plan based on a comprehensive assessment. This plan includes clarifying the desired outcomes of treatment and discussing options and preferences with the patient and family. Desired outcomes are periodically re-evaluated, and changes made, depending on patient response and in some cases disease progression.

Multimodal Analgesia. Pain is complex, which explains why there is no single, universal treatment for it. Its complexity is also the basis for the widespread recommendation that a multimodal analgesic approach be used to effectively manage pain (Chou et al., 2016; Czarnecki & Turner, 2018). Multimodal treatment involves the use of two or more classes of analgesics or interventions to target different pain mechanisms in the PNS or CNS. It relies on the thoughtful and rational combination of analgesics to maximize relief and prevent analgesic gaps that may lead to worsening pain or unnecessary episodes of uncontrolled pain.

A multimodal approach may allow lower doses of each of the drugs in the treatment plan (Czarnecki & Turner, 2018). Lower doses have the potential to produce fewer side effects. Further, multimodal analgesia can result in comparable or greater relief than can be achieved with any single analgesic. For postoperative pain the use of combination therapy to prevent both inflammatory and neuropathic pain is likely to yield the best immediate results. It also offers the promise of reducing the incidence of prolonged or persistent postsurgical pain.

The multimodal strategy also has a role in the management of persistent pain. The complex nature of the many chronic conditions indicates the need for appropriate combinations of analgesics such as anticonvulsants, antidepressants, and local anesthetics to target differing underlying mechanisms. Multimodal therapy often includes integrative therapies such as biofeedback, medical massage, and physical therapy (ANA & ASPMN, 2016).

Preemptive analgesia involves the administration of local anesthetics, opioids, and other drugs (multimodal analgesia) in anticipation of pain along the continuum of care during the preoperative, intraoperative, and postoperative periods. This continuous approach is designed to decrease pain severity in the postoperative period, reduce analgesic dose requirements, prevent morbidity, shorten hospital stay, and avoid complications after discharge. Continuous multimodal analgesia may inhibit changes in the spinal cord that can lead to changes in the PNS and CNS that initiate and sustain chronic persistent postsurgical pain (see Nociception earlier in the chapter).

Routes of Administration. The oral route is the *preferred* route of analgesic administration. It should be used whenever feasible because it is generally the least expensive, best tolerated, easiest to administer, and replicable at home once the patient is discharged. Other routes of administration are used when the oral route is not possible such as in patients who are NPO, nauseated, or unable to swallow. For example, early postoperative pain and pain that is severe and escalating are managed with the IV route of administration. Then patients are transitioned to oral analgesics when they are able to tolerate oral intake.

Around-the-Clock Dosing. Two basic principles of providing effective interprofessional collaborative care are (1) preventing pain and (2) maintaining a level of pain control that allows the patient to function and have an acceptable quality of life. Accomplishment of these desired outcomes may require the mainstay analgesic to be administered on a scheduled around-the-clock (ATC) basis rather than PRN ("as needed") to maintain stable analgesic levels. *ATC dosing regimens are designed to control pain for patients who report it being present 12 hours or more during a 24-hour period*, such as that associated with most chronic syndromes and pain during the first 24 to 48 hours after surgery or other tissue injury. PRN dosing of analgesics is appropriate for intermittent pain such as before painful procedures and **breakthrough pain** (additional pain that "breaks through" the pain being managed by the mainstay analgesic), for which supplemental doses of analgesic are provided.

Patient-Controlled Analgesia. **Patient-controlled analgesia** (PCA) is an interactive method of management that allows patients to treat their ***pain*** by self-administering doses of analgesics. It is used to manage all types of pain and given by multiple routes of administration, including IV, subcutaneous, epidural, and perineural. A PCA infusion device ("pump") is used when PCA is delivered by invasive routes of administration and is programmed so that the patient can press a button ("pendant") to self-administer a set dose of analgesic ("PCA dose") at a set time interval ("demand" or "lockout") as needed. *Patients who use PCA* *must be able to understand the relationships among pain, pressing the PCA button and taking the analgesic, and pain relief. They must also be cognitively and physically able to use any equipment that is used to administer the therapy.*

PCA may be given with or without a basal rate (continuous infusion). The use of a basal rate is common when patient-controlled epidural analgesia (PCEA) is used. For IV PCA, a basal rate may be added for opioid-tolerant patients to replace their home analgesic regimen. Basal rates are not recommended for opioid-naïve patients receiving IV PCA as evidence shows no improved analgesia when compared with a PCA without basal infusion (Chou et al., 2016). If a basal rate is used, use great caution and remember that the patient has no control over the delivery of a continuous infusion. Essential to the safe use of a basal rate is prompt discontinuation of the basal rate if increased sedation or respiratory depression occurs.

! NURSING SAFETY PRIORITY (QSEN)

Action Alert

Teach patients how to use the PCA device and to report side effects such as dizziness, nausea and vomiting, and excessive sedation. As with all opioids, monitor the patient's sedation level and respiratory status at least every 2 hours. Promptly decrease the opioid dose (i.e., discontinue basal rate) if increased sedation is detected.

The primary benefit of PCA is that it recognizes that only the patient can feel the pain and only the patient knows how much analgesic will relieve the pain. This fact reinforces that *PCA is for patient use only and that unauthorized activation of the PCA button (called "PCA by proxy") can be very dangerous.* Instruct staff, family, and other visitors to contact the nurse if they have concerns about pain control rather than pressing the PCA button for the patient.

The Three Analgesic Groups. Analgesics are categorized into three main groups: (1) nonopioid analgesics, which include acetaminophen and nonsteroidal anti-inflammatory drugs (NSAIDs); (2) opioid analgesics such as morphine, hydrocodone, hydromorphone, fentanyl, and oxycodone; and (3) adjuvant analgesics (sometimes referred to as *co-analgesics*), which make up the largest group and include a variety of agents with unique and widely differing mechanisms of action. Examples are local anesthetics, muscle relaxants, and some anticonvulsants and antidepressants.

Nonopioid Analgesics. Acetaminophen and NSAIDs make up the nonopioid analgesic group. *Acetaminophen* is thought to relieve pain by underlying mechanisms in the CNS. It has analgesic and antipyretic properties but is not effective for treating inflammation. In contrast, *NSAIDs* have analgesic, antipyretic, and anti-inflammatory properties. These drugs produce pain relief by blocking prostaglandins through inhibition of the enzyme *cyclooxygenase (COX)* in the peripheral nervous system (see Nociception and Fig. 5.1 earlier in the chapter).

Nonopioids are available in a variety of formulations and given by multiple routes of administration. They are also flexible analgesics used for a wide range of conditions. Nonopioid drugs are appropriate alone for mild-to-moderate nociceptive pain (e.g., from surgery, trauma, or osteoarthritis) or are added to opioids, local anesthetics, and/or anticonvulsants as part of a multimodal analgesic regimen for more severe nociceptive pain. *However, they have limited benefit for neuropathic pain.*

Acetaminophen and an NSAID may be given together, and there is no need for staggered doses. Unless contraindicated, all surgical patients should routinely be given acetaminophen and an NSAID in scheduled doses as the foundation of the pain treatment plan throughout the postoperative course, preferably initiated before surgery.

The nonopioids are often combined in a single tablet with opioids such as oxycodone or hydrocodone and are very popular for the treatment of mild-to-moderate acute pain. Many people with persistent pain also take a combination nonopioid/opioid analgesic. However, it is important to remember that these combination drugs are not appropriate for severe pain of any type because the maximum daily dose of the nonopioid limits the escalation of the opioid dose.

Oral *acetaminophen* has a long history of safety in recommended doses in all age-groups and most patient populations. It is recommended as first line for musculoskeletal pain (e.g., osteoarthritis) in older adults but has no inflammatory properties. Therefore acetaminophen is less effective than NSAIDs for chronic inflammatory pain (e.g., rheumatoid arthritis). IV acetaminophen is approved for treatment of pain and fever in adults. It can be given alone for mild-to-moderate pain or in combination with opioid analgesics for more severe pain.

The most serious complication of acetaminophen is hepatotoxicity (liver damage) as a result of overdose. A patient's hepatic risk factors must always be considered before administration of acetaminophen. Acetaminophen does not increase bleeding time and has a low incidence of GI adverse effects, making it the analgesic of choice for many people in pain, especially older adults.

! NURSING SAFETY PRIORITY (QSEN)

Drug Alert

Teach patients to tell their primary health care provider about the amounts of acetaminophen and NSAIDs they take each day. Remind patients of the importance of being alert to the adverse effects of the medications they take and to complete any prescribed laboratory tests (e.g., liver enzymes) to identify early indicators of adverse effects.

A benefit of the *NSAID* group is the availability of a wide variety of agents for administration via noninvasive routes. Ibuprofen, naproxen, and celecoxib are the most widely used oral NSAIDs in the United States and Canada. Diclofenac is prescribed in patch and gel form for topical administration. An intranasal patient-controlled formulation of ketorolac has been approved for short-term treatment of acute pain. IV formulations of ketorolac, ibuprofen, and diclofenac are also used to manage acute pain. Each has been shown to produce excellent analgesia alone for mild-to-moderate nociceptive pain and significant opioid dose-sparing effects when administered as part of a multimodal analgesic plan for more severe pain.

NSAIDs have more adverse effects than acetaminophen, with gastric toxicity and ulceration being the most common. Risk factors for NSAID adverse effects include being older than 60 years or having a history of peptic ulcer or cardiovascular (CV) disease. An important principle of NSAID use is to administer the lowest dose for the shortest time necessary.

All NSAIDs carry a risk for CV adverse effects through prostaglandin inhibition. The U.S. Food and Drug Administration (FDA) cautions against the use of any NSAIDs after high-risk open-heart surgery because of an elevated CV risk with NSAIDs in this population. Prostaglandins also affect renal function. Be sure that the patient is adequately hydrated when administering NSAIDs to prevent acute renal failure.

NURSING SAFETY PRIORITY QSEN

Drug Alert

NSAIDs can cause GI disturbances and decrease platelet aggregation (clotting), which can result in bleeding. Therefore observe the patient for gastric discomfort or vomiting and for bleeding or bruising. Tell the patient and family to stop taking these drugs and report these effects to the primary health care provider immediately if any of these problems occur. Celecoxib has no effect on bleeding time and produces less GI toxicity compared with other NSAIDs.

Opioid Analgesics. Opioid analgesics are the mainstay in the management of moderate-to-severe nociceptive types of pain such as postoperative, surgical, trauma, and burn pain. Although it is often used, the term *narcotic* is considered obsolete and inaccurate when discussing the use of opioids for pain management. "Narcotic" is used loosely by law enforcement and the media to refer to a variety of substances of potential abuse. Legally controlled substances classified as narcotics include opioids, cocaine, and others. *The preferred term is "opioid analgesics" when discussing these agents in the context of pain management.* Some patients prefer the term *pain medications* or *pain medicine.*

PATIENT-CENTERED CARE: OLDER ADULT CONSIDERATIONS QSEN

Older adults are at increased risk for NSAID-induced GI toxicity. Acetaminophen should be used for mild pain. If an NSAID is needed for inflammatory pain or additional analgesia, the least ulcer-causing NSAID is recommended. The addition of a proton pump inhibitor (e.g., lansoprazole, omeprazole) to NSAID therapy or use of opioid analgesics rather than an NSAID is recommended for high-risk patients. Topical NSAIDs may be used as needed, especially for musculoskeletal disorder pain. Topical NSAIDs are as effective as oral NSAIDs for localized pain and do not have the risk of systemic side effects (Arnstein et al., 2017).

Opioids produce their effects by interacting with opioid receptor sites located throughout the body, including in the peripheral tissues, the GI system, and the spinal cord and brain. When an opioid binds to the opioid receptor sites, it produces analgesia and unwanted effects such as constipation, nausea, sedation, and respiratory depression. There are three classifications of opioids:

- Pure opioid agonists (or *full opioid agonists*) bind primarily to the mu-type opioid receptors in the CNS, and this results in analgesia (Burchum & Rosenthal, 2019). Pure opioid agonists are often the first-line opioid analgesics for moderate-to-severe nociceptive pain. A major benefit of pure opioid agonists is that they have no ceiling on analgesia. This means that increases in dosage produce increases in pain relief. Dosage can be adjusted based on severity of pain. Pure opioid agonists are subject to abuse as they can produce euphoric effects in conjunction with analgesia (Burchum & Rosenthal, 2019). However, abuse is rare when opioids are used appropriately to treat pain (see Physical Tolerance later in this chapter). Examples are morphine, fentanyl, hydromorphone, oxycodone, oxymorphone, and hydrocodone.
- Agonist-antagonist opioids *(or mixed opioids)* bind to more than one type of opioid receptor. All drugs in this category, with the exception of buprenorphine, bind as agonists to the kappa opioid receptors to produce analgesia and other effects and to the mu opioid receptors as antagonists. This antagonistic property explains why these drugs can trigger severe pain and opioid withdrawal syndrome in patients who have been taking regular daily doses of a pure opioid agonist for several days. Another undesirable effect of these drugs is that they produce a dose-ceiling effect, which means that further increases in dose will not produce further relief. This latter property limits their usefulness in pain management. Occasionally these drugs are used in very low doses to antagonize (in hopes of relieving) opioid-induced side effects such as pruritus. However, this approach risks reversing analgesia; therefore patients must be assessed frequently to ensure that adequate pain control and ***comfort*** are maintained. Examples are butorphanol and nalbuphine.

  Buprenorphine is a *partial agonist opioid* at mu receptors and an antagonist at kappa receptors. Buprenorphine is used to produce analgesia; however, it also has a dose-ceiling effect and is not easily reversed by opioid antagonists such as naloxone (Burchum & Rosenthal, 2019). These properties limit the role of buprenorphine in pain management. While increasing doses of this drug do not increase the level of analgesia, they can block other mu opioid agonist from fully binding to the mu opioid receptors. As such, this drug is approved for use in treating opioid use disorder (OUD) (Broglio & Matzo, 2018).
- Opioid antagonists act as antagonists at mu and kappa receptors, binding to the opioid receptors but producing no analgesia (e.g., naloxone, naltrexone). If an antagonist is present, it competes with opioid molecules for binding sites on the opioid receptors and has the potential to block analgesia and other effects. They are used most often to reverse opioid effects such as excessive sedation and respiratory depression (Burchum & Rosenthal, 2019).

PATIENT-CENTERED CARE: GENETIC/GENOMIC CONSIDERATIONS QSEN

It has long been known that the cytochrome (CY) *P450* enzyme system is important to the metabolism of some opioids. Variations in phenotypes of the *CYP450* enzymes are common, affecting metabolism of selected analgesics in some patients. These variations have clinical implications when the opioid *codeine,* which is metabolized by the *CYP450* enzyme system, is administered. Slow metabolizers may not respond well to codeine, and ultrarapid metabolizers may have an exaggerated response (Czarnecki & Turner, 2018).

Key Principles of Opioid Administration. Many factors are considered when determining the appropriate opioid analgesic for the patient with pain. These include the unique characteristics of the various opioids and patient factors such as type of ***pain,*** pain intensity, age, gender, coexisting disease, current drug regimen and potential drug interactions, prior treatment outcomes, and patient preference.

Titration (dose increases or decreases) of the opioid dose is usually required at the start and throughout the course of treatment when opioids are administered. Whereas patients with cancer pain most often are titrated upward over time for progressive pain, patients with acute pain, particularly postoperative pain, are eventually titrated downward as pain resolves. Although the dose and analgesic effect of pure opioid (mu) agonist have no ceiling, the dose may be limited by side effects. The absolute dose administered is unimportant as long as a balance between pain relief and side effects is favorable. *The desired outcome of titration is to use the smallest dose that provides satisfactory pain relief with the fewest side effects.*

When an increase in the opioid dose is necessary and safe, the increase can be titrated according to patient response and drug effect. The time at which the dose can be increased is determined by the onset and peak effects of the opioid and its formulation. For example, the frequency of IV opioid doses during initial titration may be as often as every 5 to 15 minutes (see later discussion of specific opioids). In contrast, at least 24 hours should elapse before the dose of transdermal fentanyl is increased after the first patch application.

In addition to the concept of titration, nurses must also consider pain medication orders that are prescribed using a *dose range*. Again, because of the wide variability in patient response, many health care providers provide orders for opioids within a dose range. For example, the provider may order morphine 2 to 5 mg IV every 2 hours as needed for pain. This order allows the nurse flexibility to dose the patient based on individual need (Drew et al., 2018). This requires that the nurse use clinical judgment to base decisions on implementation of range orders using thorough pain assessment and accurate pharmacokinetic information of the opioid that is to be administered (Drew et al., 2018). (See Box 5.1.)

PATIENT-CENTERED CARE: OLDER ADULT CONSIDERATIONS QSEN

Although the patient's weight is not a good indicator of analgesic requirement, *age is considered an important factor to consider when selecting an opioid dose.* For older adults the guideline is to "start low and go slow" with all drug dosing. For example, the starting opioid dose may need to be reduced by 25% to 50% in older adults because they are more sensitive to opioid side effects than are younger adults. The subsequent doses are based on patient response, which should be evaluated frequently. Monitor sedation level and respiratory status and promptly reduce the drug dose if sedation occurs or the respiratory rate is markedly decreased, depending on agency policy. Many older adults are admitted to the ED with fractures of the hip, pelvis, and spine, which are very painful and require prompt and adequate ***pain*** management to promote patient ***comfort.*** Best practices for pain assessment and management in the older adult are described in the Patient-Centered Care: Older Adult Considerations box on the next page..

BOX 5.1 Dose Range Orders for Opioid Analgesia

To provide safe administration of range orders for opioid analgesia the nurse will:

- Use clinical judgment, basing decisions on thorough pain assessment
- Consider pain intensity, location, cause of pain, and previous pain relief
- Use the same valid and reliable pain assessment tool
- Consider the pharmacokinetics of the opioid to be administered
- Inform the patient about the drug including the name and dose
- Frequently monitor the patient, evaluating patient response to the dose; monitor for negative side effects including changes in respiratory pattern or breathing difficulty. In turn, be alert to continued pain and treat the patient accordingly, within the range ordered by the health care provider.
- Wait until the peak effect of the first dose has been reached before giving a subsequent dose.

Adapted from: Drew, D., Gordon, D., Morgan, B., & Manworren, R. (2018). "As-needed" range orders for opioid analgesics in the management of pain: A consensus statement of the American Society of Pain Management Nursing and the American Pain Society. Position Statement. *Pain Management Nursing, 19*(3), 207-210.

The Opioid Epidemic. Managing pain is a complex process and when opioids are used appropriately, they can be very effective for acute pain, as well as for palliative care patients. However, administration of opioids for analgesia requires an understanding of the opioid epidemic in the United States, which was declared a national emergency in 2017 (Broglio & Matzo, 2018). In the past decade, prescription opioids were implicated in the growing epidemic. However, in the recent past, the epidemic has been complicated by increased use of the illegal opioid heroin and the development of synthetic opioids such as fentanyl (ANA, 2018). More than 48 million Americans have used illicit drugs or misused prescription drugs (CDC, 2017). On average, 115 Americans die every day from an opioid overdose (CDC, 2017).

While the goal is not to prevent administration of needed opioids, it is to bring about awareness of the problem, as well as an understanding of the patient experiencing opioid use disorder (OUD). "Registered nurses (RNs), who are often the best equipped to assess a patient's pain and need for pharmacologic pain relief, are on the front lines of the opioid epidemic" (ANA, 2018, p. 1). All nurses have an ethical responsibility to manage pain for all patients. However, this ethical responsibility brings a delicate balance between the nurse's duty to manage pain and the duty to avoid harm (ANA, 2018). Prolonged use of opioids is not recommended for persistent (chronic) pain. However, opioids are often needed to control acute pain and prevent the progression of acute pain into chronic pain (Jungquist et al., 2017). In addition, the nurse must be aware of the rise in patients with opioid use disorder, both those patients who are in medication-assisted treatment programs and those patients who are actively using opioids. See Table 5.7 for Pain Management Considerations for the patient with opioid use disorder.

Patients that are actively using opioids may be using prescription opioids or illegal opioids. Fentanyl is similar in effect to morphine and heroin; however, it is 50 to 100 times more potent (PSHSA, 2017). Carfentanil, which is an analog of fentanyl, was originally intended for use in large animals, is 100 times more potent than fentanyl, and is 10,000 times more potent than

PATIENT-CENTERED CARE: OLDER ADULT CONSIDERATIONS (QSEN)

Pain

Prevalence of Pain

- Recognize that older adults are at high risk for undertreated pain and those with cognitive impairment are at even higher risk.
- Common caregiver misconceptions (such as older adults are less sensitive to pain or older adults cannot handle the effects of pain medications) contribute to the undertreatment of pain in older adults.

Beliefs About Pain

- Older adults tend to report pain less often than younger adults, which frequently results in members of the health care team administering suboptimal analgesics and doses.
- Older adults may not report pain due to common beliefs and such as:
  - Pain is an inevitable consequence of aging and little can be done to provide relief.
  - Expressing pain is unacceptable or is a sign of weakness.
  - Reporting pain will result in being labeled as a "bad" patient or a "complainer."
  - Health care providers are too busy to listen to reports of pain.
  - Pain signifies a serious illness or impending death.
- Nurses and other caregivers can overcome their reluctance to administer prescribed analgesics in adequate doses by following the principles of pain management in older people (see Management of Pain section).

Assessment of Pain

- Ask the patient to provide his or her own report of pain.
- Offer various self-report pain tools.
- Always show tools in hard copy with large lettering, adequate space between lines, nonglossy paper, and color for increased visualization.
- Be sure that the patient is wearing glasses and hearing aids if needed and available.
- Provide adequate lighting and privacy to avoid distracting background noise.
- Repeat questions more than once and allow adequate time for response.
- Use verbal descriptions such as "ache," "sore," and "hurt" if the patient seems to have difficulty relating to the word "pain."
- If the patient is able to use a self-report tool, use the same tool and reteach the tool each time pain is assessed.

Considerations for Patients With Cognitive Impairments (also see Table 5.6)

- Remember to "assume that pain is present" in patients with diseases and conditions or procedures commonly associated with pain.
- If the patient is unable to provide self-report, look for behaviors that may indicate the presence of pain.
- Someone who knows the patient well, such as a family member or caregiver, may be helpful in identifying behaviors that might indicate pain. Do not ask others to rate pain intensity and do not attempt to rate it yourself. Only the patient knows how severe the pain is; if he or she cannot rate or describe the intensity, the exact intensity is unknown.
- Assess using a reliable and valid behavioral pain assessment tool.
- Remember that behavioral tools tell us that pain might be present and provide a reference point to help determine the effectiveness of interventions, but the scores on behavioral tools have not been correlated with the ratings on pain intensity scales. A behavioral score is not a pain intensity rating.
- Use the same behavioral assessment tool each time pain is assessed.
- Consider an analgesic trial to help determine the presence of pain and to establish an ongoing treatment plan in patients who are thought to have pain. This involves the administration of a low-dose analgesic; changes or decreases in the intensity of behaviors indicate that pain may be the cause of the behaviors. Doses should be increased, or additional analgesics added as appropriate.

Management of Pain

- Use a multimodal approach that combines analgesics with different underlying mechanisms with the desired outcome of achieving optimal pain relief with lower doses than would be possible with a single analgesic; lower doses result in fewer side effects.
- Consider the type of pain and begin therapy with the first-line analgesics that are recommended for that type of pain.
- Do not give meperidine to older adults because most have decreased renal function and are unable to efficiently eliminate its central nervous system (CNS)-toxic metabolite *normeperidine.*
- Use around-the-clock (ATC) dosing of analgesics for pain that is of a continuous nature (e.g., persistent [chronic] osteoarthritis or cancer pain; persistent [chronic] neuropathic pain, first 24 to 48 hours after surgery).
- Use as-needed (PRN) dosing for intermittent pain and before painful activities, such as before ambulation and physical therapy.
- Be aware of the main side effects of the analgesics that are administered and that they may be more likely to occur or be more severe in older than in younger adults.
- *Start low and go slow* with drug dosing; increase doses to achieve adequate analgesia based on the patient's response to the previous dose.
- Teach the patient and family or other caregiver about the pain management plan (analgesics and nonpharmacologic strategies) and when to notify the primary health care provider for unrelieved pain or unmanageable or intolerable drug side effects.
- To promote adherence to the pain management plan in the home setting, suggest using a pillbox to organize each day's medications and keeping a diary to identify times of the day or activities that increase pain. The diary can be presented to the primary health care provider, who can use it to make necessary adjustments in the treatment plan.

morphine (PSHSA, 2017). With illicit use of synthetic opioids such as fentanyl and carfentanil, the nurse must be aware of the risks associated with secondary exposure. To prevent secondary exposure, nurses should (NIOSH, 2018):

- Review agency specific policy for handling hazardous items like fentanyl.
- In the ED, be aware of decontamination protocol.
- Treat unknown substances as if they are or contain fentanyl (Fentanyl Safety, 2018).
- Do not touch your eyes, nose, or mouth after touching a surface potentially contaminated with illicit fentanyl.
- Wash your hands with soap and water if potential exposure is expected. Do not use alcohol-based hand rubs as this can facilitate cutaneous absorption of the drug.
- Avoid actions that could aerosolize the drug, such as shaking bed linens or tossing linens.
- Never handle any substance that you suspect is illicit without personal protective equipment (PPE).
- Know the symptoms of secondary exposure (drowsiness, difficulty thinking, confusion, pinpoint pupils, trouble breathing, slow breathing, slowed heart rate, decreased blood pressure, cold, clammy skin) (Fentanyl Safety, n.d.).

TABLE 5.7 Pain Management for Patients With Opioid Use Disorder

In 2016, among patients with OUD, 350,000 were treated with methadone, 60,000 were treated with buprenorphine, and more than 10,000 were treated with naltrexone (SAMHSA, 2016). While each of these drugs works on the mu opioid receptors differently, they are all used to block the euphoric effects of opioids and reduce cravings. As such, it is imperative for the nurse to use an evidence-based approach for acute pain management in patients with OUD.

- It is vital to contact the opioid treatment program when a patient with OUD is admitted.
- If medications, such as methadone, are discontinued, the patient may undergo significant withdrawal, complicating the primary reason for admission.
- Be aware that methadone interacts with numerous medications and can prolong the QT interval, thus electrocardiogram (ECG) monitoring should be considered (Broglio & Matzo, 2018).
- Naltrexone must be stopped if a patient requires pain management with opioid therapy as it is an opioid antagonist. When a patient has naltrexone in his or her system, the patient may require 10-20 times the usual opioid dose to control pain (Broglio & Matzo, 2018).
- Do not confuse naltrexone with naloxone (Narcan).
- If buprenorphine is discontinued during hospitalization, the patient may require higher doses of opioids until the medication is out of the patient's system (24 to 72 hours). Nurses must monitor for respiratory depression if higher opioid doses are used to achieve pain control.
- For all patients on medication to treat OUD, nurses should coordinate care between the acute care setting and the providers managing the OUD as this can be a vital measure in the prevention of relapse into active drug use on discharge from the hospital.

Adapted from Broglio & Matzo, 2018.

Physical Dependence, Tolerance, and Addiction. The terms *physical dependence* and *tolerance* often are confused with *addiction;* thus clarification of definitions is important. The most widely accepted definitions of these terms are:

- *Physical dependence is a response* that occurs with repeated administration of an opioid for several days. It is manifested by the occurrence of withdrawal symptoms when the opioid is stopped suddenly or rapidly reduced or an antagonist such as naloxone is given. Withdrawal symptoms may be suppressed by the natural, gradual reduction of the opioid as pain decreases or by gradual, systematic reduction, referred to as *tapering. Physical dependence is not the same as addiction.*
- *Tolerance is also a response* that occurs with regular administration of an opioid and consists of a decrease in one or more effects of the opioid (e.g., decreased analgesia, sedation, or respiratory depression). The body adapts to the drug and, in turn, requires more of the drug to achieve a certain effect (National Institute on Drug Abuse, 2018). Like physical dependence, *tolerance is not the same as addiction.* Tolerance can be beneficial when it occurs to side effects, such as nausea, but problematic if tolerance occurs to analgesia (Gupta & Rosenquist, 2018). Patients do not develop tolerance to opioid-induced constipation. Tolerance to opioids can be treated by adjusting the dose or changing to a different opioid.
- *Opioid addiction is a chronic neurologic and biologic disease.* The development and characteristics of addiction are influenced by genetic, psychosocial, and environmental factors. No single cause of addiction such as taking an opioid for pain relief has been found. It is characterized by one or more of these behaviors: impaired control over drug use, compulsive use, continued use despite risk or actual harm, and craving. *The disease of addiction is a treatable disease; as for any other suspected disease, refer the patient to an expert for diagnosis and treatment.*
- *Pseudoaddiction* is a mistaken diagnosis of addictive disease. When a patient's pain is not well controlled, the patient may begin to manifest symptoms suggestive of addictive disease. For example, in an effort to obtain adequate pain relief, the patient may respond with escalating and frantic requests for more or different medications and repeated requests for opioids on time or before the prescribed interval between doses has elapsed. Pain relief typically eliminates these behaviors and is often accomplished by adjusting opioid doses or decreasing intervals between doses.

Opioid Naïve Versus Opioid Tolerant. Patients are often characterized as being either opioid naïve or opioid tolerant. An *opioid-naïve* person has not recently taken enough opioid on a regular basis to become tolerant to the effects of an opioid. An *opioid-tolerant* person has taken an opioid long enough at doses high enough to develop tolerance to many of the effects, including analgesia and the undesirable effects such as nausea and sedation. There is no set time for the development of tolerance, with wide individual variation among people. Some patients do not develop tolerance at all.

Equianalgesia. The term *equianalgesia* means approximately "equal analgesia." An equianalgesic chart provides a list of analgesic doses, both oral and parenteral (IV, subcutaneous, and IM), that are approximately equal to one another in ability to provide pain relief. Equianalgesic conversion of doses is used to help ensure that patients receive approximately the same pain relief when they are switched from one opioid or route of administration to another. It requires a series of calculations based on the daily dose of the current opioid to determine the equianalgesic dose of the opioid to which the patient is to be switched. Consult and collaborate with the pharmacist whenever equianalgesic conversion is indicated.

Relative potency is the ratio of drug doses required to produce the same effect. For example, a single dose of 1.5 mg of parenteral hydromorphone produces approximately the same analgesia as 10 mg of parenteral morphine. This means that hydromorphone is more po-tent than morphine, but increased potency does not mean that the drug is therapeutically superior or that it provides any advantage. Safe and effective pain management requires nurses to appreciate the differences in the potencies of the various opioids and apply the principles of equianalgesia when administering opioids.

Drug Formulation Terminology. The terms *short acting, fast acting, immediate release (IR),* and *normal release* have been used interchangeably to describe oral opioids that have an onset of action of about 30 minutes and a relatively short duration of 3 to 4 hours. The term *immediate release* is misleading because none of the oral analgesics has an immediate or even a fast onset of analgesia. The term *short acting* is preferred to reflect the short duration of oral opioids. Oral transmucosal and intranasal formulations are appropriately referred to as *ultrafast acting* because they have a peak effect of 5 to 15 minutes, depending on formulation.

The terms *modified release, extended release (ER), sustained release (SR),* and *controlled release (CR)* are used to describe opioids that are formulated to release over a prolonged period of time. For the purposes of this chapter, the term *modified release* will be used when discussing these opioid formulations. *Long acting* is applied to drugs with a long *half-life* such as methadone. The half-life of a drug provides an estimate of how fast the drug leaves the body. By definition, **half-life** is the time it takes for the amount of drug in the body to be reduced by 50%.

! NURSING SAFETY PRIORITY QSEN

Drug Alert

Modified-release opioids should never be crushed, broken, or chewed because doing so alters the formulation of the drug and can result in adverse events, including death from respiratory depression if consumed. Teach the patient to swallow the drug whole and allow the "time-release" function of the drug to take effect.

Selected Opioid Analgesics. *Morphine* is the standard against which all other opioid drugs are compared. It is the most widely used opioid throughout the world, particularly for cancer pain, and its use is established by extensive research and clinical experience. Morphine is a *hydrophilic* drug (readily absorbed in aqueous solution), which accounts for its slow onset and long duration of action when compared with other opioid analgesics. It is available in a wide variety of short-acting and modified-release oral formulations and is given by multiple other routes of administration, including rectal, subcutaneous, and IV.

Fentanyl differs from morphine significantly in characteristics. It is a *lipophilic* (readily absorbed in fatty tissue) opioid and, as such, has a fast onset and short duration of action. These characteristics make it the most commonly used IV opioid when rapid analgesia is desired such as for the treatment of severe, escalating acute pain and for procedural pain when a short duration of action is desirable. Fentanyl is the recommended opioid for patients with end-organ failure because it has no clinically relevant metabolites. It also produces fewer hemodynamic adverse effects than other opioids; therefore it is often preferred in patients who are hemodynamically unstable such as the critically ill.

Fentanyl can be administered by four different routes: parenteral, transdermal, transmucosal, and intranasal. Transmucosal (lozenges, buccal tablets, sublingual tablets, or spray) and intranasal delivery methods are used to manage breakthrough pain in opioid-tolerant patients. Transdermal delivery is used for long-term opioid therapy. After application of the transdermal patch, the drug is slowly released from the patch and absorbed into the skin (Burchum & Rosenthal, 2019). When the first patch is applied, 12 to 18 hours are required for clinically significant analgesia to be obtained. Be aware that the patient may need adequate supplemental analgesia during that time. Change the patch every 48 to 72 hours, depending on patient response.

! NURSING SAFETY PRIORITY QSEN

Drug Alert

Teach patients using transdermal fentanyl not to apply heat (e.g., hot packs, heating pads) directly over the patch because heat increases absorption of the drug and can result in adverse events, including death from fentanyl-induced respiratory depression. Ask patients about the presence of patches on admission and document and communicate this information to other members of the interprofessional health care team.

Hydromorphone is less hydrophilic than morphine but less lipophilic than fentanyl, which contributes to an onset and duration of action that is intermediate between morphine and fentanyl. The drug is often used as an alternative to morphine, especially for acute pain, most likely because the two drugs produce similar analgesia and have comparable side effects. It is a first- or second-choice opioid (after morphine) for postoperative management via IV patient-controlled analgesia (PCA) and is also available in a once-daily modified-release oral formulation for long-term opioid treatment.

Oxycodone is available in the United States for administration by the oral route only and is used to treat all types of pain. In combination with acetaminophen or ibuprofen, it is appropriate for mild-to-some moderate pain. Single-entity, short-acting and modified-release oxycodone formulations are used in patients with moderate-to-severe chronic pain. It has been used successfully as part of a multimodal treatment plan for postoperative pain as well. Like morphine, it is available in liquid form for patients who are unable to swallow tablets.

When used in combination with nonopioids, *hydrocodone* is limited in use to treating mild to moderate pain. It is the most commonly prescribed opioid analgesic in the United States and Canada. However, its use should be evaluated carefully for treatment of persistent pain (except for breakthrough dosing), because it has a ceiling on efficacy and safety due to its nonopioid ingredient. It is also available as a modified-release formulation for persistent (chronic) pain.

Methadone is a unique opioid analgesic that may have advantages over other opioids in carefully selected patients. In addition to being a mu opioid, it is an antagonist at the NMDA (*N*-methyl-D-aspartate) receptor site and thus has the potential to produce analgesic effects as a second- or third-line option for some neuropathic pain states.

Although it has no active metabolites, methadone has a very long and highly variable half-life (5 to 100+ hours; average is 20 hours). Patients must be watched closely for excessive sedation—a sign of drug accumulation during the titration period. Other limitations are its tendency to interact with a large number of medications and prolong corrected QT (QTc) interval. Methadone should be prescribed only by providers who are familiar with its unique properties. While this drug is used to relieve pain in some patients, it is more commonly associated with treatment of opioid use disorder (see Table 5.7).

Dual Mechanism Analgesics. The dual mechanism analgesics *tramadol* and *tapentadol* have been useful additions to the pain management arena. These drugs bind weakly to the mu opioid-receptor site and block the reuptake (resorption) of the inhibitory neurotransmitters *serotonin* and/or *norepinephrine* in the spinal cord and brainstem of the modulatory descending pain pathway (see Nociception earlier in this chapter). This makes these neurotransmitters more available to fight pain. Because they have the opioid receptor-binding property, they are discussed in the Opioid Analgesics section of this chapter. However, they are usually referred to as dual mechanism or mixed analgesics rather than opioid analgesics.

Tramadol is used for both acute and chronic pain and is available in oral short-acting and modified-release formulations, including a short-acting tablet in combination with acetaminophen. It is appropriate for acute pain and has been designated as a second-line analgesic for the treatment of neuropathic pain. Side effects are similar to those of opioids. The drug can lower seizure threshold and interact with other drugs that block the reuptake of serotonin such as the selective serotonin reuptake inhibitor (SSRI) antidepressants. Although rare, this combination can have an additive effect and result in serotonin syndrome, characterized by agitation, diarrhea, heart and blood pressure changes, and loss of coordination.

The newer dual-mechanism analgesic *tapentadol* is also available in short-acting and modified-release formulations and is appropriate for both acute and chronic pain. Major benefits of tapentadol are that it has no active metabolites and a significantly more favorable side effect profile (particularly GI effects) compared with opioid analgesics.

Opioids to Avoid. *Meperidine* was once the most widely used opioid analgesic in the inpatient setting. In recent years it has either been removed from or severely restricted on U.S. hospital formularies for the treatment of pain in an effort to improve patient safety. A major drawback to the use of meperidine is its active metabolite, *normeperidine,* a CNS stimulant that can cause delirium, irritability, tremors, myoclonus, and generalized seizures. It is a particularly poor choice in older adults because they have decreased renal function, which prevents the elimination of the toxic metabolite. Meperidine has no advantages over any other opioid, and it has no place in the treatment of persistent pain or in delivery systems such as PCA.

Codeine in combination with nonopioids has been used for many years for the management of mild-to-moderate pain; however, it has largely been replaced by analgesics that are more efficacious and better tolerated (e.g., hydrocodone combinations). Research has shown that codeine/acetaminophen is less effective and associated with more adverse effects than NSAIDs such as ibuprofen and naproxen for acute pain.

Intraspinal Analgesia. Intraspinal analgesia involves the administration of analgesics via a needle or catheter placed in the epidural space or the intrathecal (subarachnoid) space by an anesthesia provider (see Fig. 5.4). The intraspinal routes of administration are used to manage both acute ***pain*** such as postoperative pain and some persistent (chronic) pain.

Epidural analgesia can be delivered by intermittent bolus technique, continuous infusion, or patient-controlled epidural analgesia (PCEA) with or without continuous infusion. The most commonly administered analgesics by the epidural route are the opioids *morphine, hydromorphone,* and *fentanyl* in combination with a long-acting local anesthetic such as bupivacaine or ropivacaine. This multimodal approach allows lower doses of both the opioid and local anesthetic and produces fewer side effects.

Intrathecal (spinal) analgesia is usually delivered via single bolus technique for patients with acute pain (e.g., hysterectomy) or continuous infusion via an implanted device (pump) for the treatment of persistent (chronic) pain. Because the drug is delivered directly into the aqueous cerebrospinal fluid (CSF), morphine with its hydrophilic nature is used most often for intrathecal analgesia. Extremely small amounts of drug are administered by the intrathecal route because the drug is so close to the spinal action site.

The side effects of intraspinal analgesia depend on the type of drug administered. In other words, if opioids are administered, the same opioid-induced side effects that occur with other routes of administration can occur with intraspinal administration. If local anesthetics are administered, common side effects are urinary retention, hypotension, and numbness and weakness of lower extremities. The latter can occur on a continuum (mild and localized) to a complete block (undesirable and requires prompt anesthesia evaluation). In most cases the side effects that occur during continuous infusion or PCEA can be managed by decreasing the dose.

Complications of intraspinal analgesia are rare but can be life threatening. Complications from the intrathecal pump can be surgical, pump related, or catheter related (Textor, 2016). Perform frequent neurologic assessments and promptly report abnormal findings to the anesthesiologist or nurse anesthetist.

See the Best Practice for Patient Safety & Quality Care box for a summary of best practices needed when caring for a patient who has an intrathecal pump.

! NURSING SAFETY PRIORITY QSEN

Drug Alert

Assess patients receiving epidural local anesthetic for their ability to bend their knees and lift their buttocks off the mattress (if not prohibited by surgical procedure). Ask them to point to any areas of numbness and tingling. Mild, transient lower-extremity motor weakness and orthostatic hypotension may be present, necessitating assistance with ambulation. Most undesirable effects can be managed with a reduction in local anesthetic dose. Promptly report areas of numbness outside of the surgical site, inability to bear weight, and severe hypotension to the anesthesia provider. *Do not delegate assessment of local anesthetic effects to assistive personnel!*

Sensory perception signs and symptoms (e.g., increasing numbness and tingling of extremities), decreasing ability to bear weight, and/or changes in bowel or bladder function can

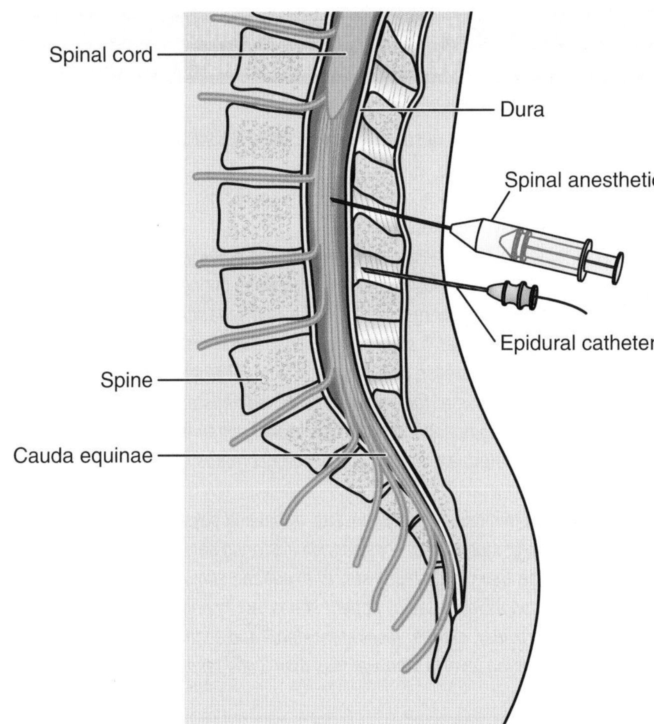

Fig. 5.4 Intraspinal analgesia.

indicate the development of an epidural hematoma or abscess. If not detected, a hematoma or abscess can cause spinal cord compression and paralysis.

Nurses have an extensive role in the management and monitoring of intraspinal techniques, including infusion device operation, replacing empty drug reservoirs, checking and protecting infusion sites and systems, treating side effects, preventing complications, discontinuing therapy, and removing catheters.

Adverse Effects of Opioid Analgesics. The most common side effects of opioid analgesics are constipation, nausea, vomiting, pruritus, and sedation. Respiratory depression is less common but the most feared of the opioid side effects. *Most of the opioid side effects are dose related; therefore simply decreasing the opioid dose is sufficient to eliminate or make the most of the side effects tolerable for most patients.* Table 5.8 lists interventions to prevent and manage opioid-induced side effects.

Most patients experience sedation at the beginning of opioid therapy and whenever the opioid dose is increased significantly. *If undetected or left untreated, excessive sedation can progress to clinically significant respiratory depression.* Like most of the other opioid side effects, sedation and respiratory depression are dose related. Preventing clinically significant opioid-induced respiratory depression begins with administering the lowest effective opioid dose (multimodal analgesia with a nonopioid foundation), careful titration, and closely monitoring sedation and respiratory status throughout therapy. *Unless the patient is at the end of life, promptly reduce opioid dose or stop titration whenever increased sedation is detected to prevent respiratory depression.* In some patients (e.g., those with obstructive sleep apnea, pulmonary dysfunction, multiple comorbidities), mechanical monitoring such as capnography (to measure exhaled carbon dioxide) and pulse oximetry (to measure oxygen saturation) is needed.

BEST PRACTICE FOR PATIENT SAFETY & QUALITY CARE (QSEN)

Care of the Patient Who Has an Intrathecal Pump

Provide postoperative care and health teaching to include:

- Monitor respiratory status, including respiratory rate, oxygen saturation, and level of consciousness every 1 to 2 hours after surgery for at least 12 hours or per agency protocol.
- Apply an abdominal binder in place as prescribed to hold the pump in a flat position.
- Teach the patient that a burning sensation may occur around the pump area. Cold packs and topical lidocaine may provide ***comfort;*** do *not* use heat over the lumbar pump site.
- Teach the patient to avoid lifting more than 5 lb or twisting/bending at the waist for 6 weeks or as instructed by the surgeon.

Monitor for and teach the patient and family to report these potential complications:

- Surgical complications
  - Infection: Observe for fever and localized redness or hematoma at the lumbar site.
  - Cerebrospinal (CSF) fluid leak: Ask about headache; observe for swelling without redness at the lumbar site.
- Catheter-related complications
  - Structural damage, including kinks, occlusion, or disconnection; note change in pain control or signs of opioid withdrawal.
- Pump-related complications (not common)
  - Malfunction or displacement: Observe for opioid overdose or underdosing, causing a change in pain control or opioid withdrawal.

Keep these safety and care precautions in mind when caring for the patient:

- Be sure that the pump is shielded if the patient receives external beam radiation.
- Be sure that the patient does not have an abrupt discontinuation of baclofen (can cause respiratory depression) or clonidine (can cause hypertension and stroke).

Data adapted from Textor, L. (2016). Intrathecal pumps for cancer pain. *AJN, 116*(5), 36–41.

Occasionally drugs that produce significant sedation are used to treat side effects and other conditions that accompany the pain experience. For example, *antianxiety agents* (anxiolytics) such as alprazolam and lorazepam are prescribed to reduce anxiety. Many of the drugs used to treat opioid side effects are sedating, such as the antihistamines (diphenhydramine) for pruritus and the antiemetics *promethazine* and *hydroxyzine* for nausea. It is important to recognize that administration of these drugs together has an additive sedating effect. If administered, closely monitor for sedation and assess respiratory status frequently.

To assess sedation, use a simple, easy-to-understand sedation scale developed for assessment of *unwanted* sedation that includes what should be done at each level of sedation. Table 5.9 presents a widely used sedation scale. The key to assessing sedation is to determine how easy it is to arouse the patient. Assess each person's response to the first dose of an opioid. If opioids are administered by bolus technique, assess sedation level and respiratory status at the opioid's peak time after each bolus.

Respiratory depression is assessed on the basis of what is normal for a particular person and is usually described as

TABLE 5.8 Nursing Interventions to Prevent and Treat Selected Opioid Side Effects

Constipation

- Assess previous bowel habits.
- Keep a record of bowel movements.
- Remind patients that tolerance to this side effect does not develop, so *a preventive approach must be used;* administer a stool softener plus mild stimulant laxative for duration of opioid therapy; do not give bulk laxatives because these can result in obstruction in some patients.
- Provide privacy, encourage adequate fluids and activity, and give foods high in roughage.
- If ineffective, try suppository or Fleet's enema.
- For long-term opioid-induced constipation (OIC) in patients with chronic pain, drug therapy may be used (e.g., lubiprostone, methylnaltrexone).

Nausea and Vomiting (N/V)

- Use a multimodal antiemetic preventive approach (e.g., dexamethasone plus ondansetron in moderate- to high-risk patients).
- Assess cause of nausea and eliminate contributing factors if possible.
- Reduce opioid dose if possible.
- Reassure patients taking long-term opioid therapy that tolerance to this side effect develops with regular daily opioid doses.
- Consider switching to another opioid for unresolved N/V.

Sedation

- Remember that sedation precedes opioid-induced respiratory depression; identify patient and iatrogenic risk factors and monitor sedation level and respiratory status frequently during the first 24 hours of opioid therapy.
- Use a simple sedation scale to monitor for unwanted sedation (see Table 5.9).
- If excessive sedation is detected, reduce opioid dose to prevent respiratory depression.
- Eliminate unnecessary sedating drugs such as antihistamines, anxiolytics, muscle relaxants, and hypnotics. If it is necessary to administer these drugs during opioid therapy, monitor sedation and respiratory status closely.
- Reassure patients taking long-term opioid therapy that tolerance to this side effect develops with regular daily opioid doses.
- Be aware that stimulants such as caffeine may counteract opioid-induced sedation.
- Consider switching to another opioid for unresolved excessive sedation during long-term opioid therapy.

Respiratory Depression

- Be aware that counting respiratory rate alone does not constitute a comprehensive respiratory assessment. Proper assessment of respiratory status includes observing the rise and fall of the patient's chest to determine depth and quality in addition to counting respiratory rate for 60 seconds.
- Recognize that *snoring indicates respiratory obstruction and is an ominous sign requiring prompt intervention.*
- Remember that sedation precedes opioid-induced respiratory depression; identify patient and iatrogenic risk factors and monitor sedation level and respiratory status frequently during the first 24 hours of opioid therapy (see Sedation section).
- Stop opioid administration immediately for clinically significant respiratory depression, stay with patient, continue attempts to arouse patient, support respirations, call for help (consider Rapid Response Team or Code Blue), and consider administration of naloxone.

TABLE 5.9 Pasero Opioid-Induced Sedation Scale (POSS) With Interventions[a]

S = Sleep, easy to arouse
Acceptable; no action necessary; may increase opioid dose if needed.

1 = Awake and alert
Acceptable; no action necessary; may increase opioid dose if needed.

2 = Slightly drowsy, easily aroused
Acceptable; no action necessary; may increase opioid dose if needed.

3 = Frequently drowsy, arousable, drifts off to sleep during conversation
Unacceptable; monitor respiratory status and sedation level closely until sedation level is stable at less than 3 and respiratory status is satisfactory; decrease opioid dose 25% to 50%[b] or notify primary[c] or anesthesia provider for orders; consider administering a nonsedating, opioid-sparing nonopioid such as acetaminophen or a NSAID if not contraindicated; ask patient to take deep breaths every 15 to 30 minutes.

4 = Somnolent; minimal or no response to verbal and physical stimulation
Unacceptable; stop opioid; consider administering naloxone[d,e]; call Rapid Response Team (code blue); stay with patient, stimulate, and support respiration as indicated by patient status; notify primary[c] or anesthesia provider; monitor respiratory status and sedation level closely until sedation level is stable at less than 3 and respiratory status is satisfactory.

Adapted from Pasero, C., & McCaffery, M. (2011). *Pain assessment and pharmacologic management.* St. Louis: Mosby. Copyright 1994. Used with permission.

[a]Appropriate action is given in italics at each level of sedation.

[b]Opioid analgesic prescriptions or a hospital protocol should include the expectation that a nurse will decrease the opioid dose if a patient is excessively sedated.

[c]For example, the physician, nurse practitioner, advanced practice nurse, or physician assistant responsible for the pain management prescription.

[d]For adults experiencing respiratory depression, administer dilute solution of naloxone very slowly while observing the patient's response.

[e]Hospital protocols should include the expectation that a nurse will administer naloxone to any patient suspected of having life-threatening opioid-induced sedation and respiratory depression.

clinically significant when there is a significant decrease in the rate, depth, and regularity of respirations from baseline, rather than just by a specific number of respirations per minute. Risk factors for opioid-induced respiratory depression include age 55 years or older, obesity, obstructive sleep apnea, and preexisting pulmonary dysfunction or other comorbidities.

! NURSING SAFETY PRIORITY QSEN

Critical Rescue

Watch the rise and fall of the patient's chest to determine depth and regularity of respirations in addition to counting the respiratory rate for 60 seconds. For accuracy, respiratory assessment is done before arousing the sleeping patient. *If a patient is difficult to arouse, always stop the opioid, stay with the patient, continue vigorous attempts to arouse, and call for help!*

Listening to the sound of the patient's respiration is critical as well—*snoring indicates airway obstruction and must be attended to promptly* with repositioning, including placing the patient in a sitting position. Depending on severity, collaborate with the respiratory therapist for consultation and further evaluation.

NURSING SAFETY PRIORITY QSEN

Drug Alert

Unless the patient is at the end of life, promptly administer the opioid antagonist naloxone IV to reverse clinically significant opioid-induced respiratory depression, usually when the respiratory rate is less than 8 breaths per minute or according to agency protocol. When giving the opioid antagonist naloxone, administer it slowly until the patient is more arousable and respirations increase to an acceptable rate. The desired outcome is to reverse just the sedative and respiratory depressant effects of the opioid but not the analgesic effects. Giving too much naloxone too fast can not only cause severe ***pain*** but also lead to ventricular dysrhythmias, pulmonary edema, and even death. Continue to closely monitor the patient after giving naloxone because its duration is shorter than that of most opioids and respiratory depression can recur. Sometimes more than one dose of naloxone is needed.

PATIENT-CENTERED CARE: OLDER ADULT CONSIDERATIONS QSEN

The incidence of opioid side effects in the older adult population varies, depending on the side effect. Older adults are sensitive to the sedating effects of opioids, making them higher risk for respiratory depression than in younger adults.

Adjuvant Analgesics. Adjuvant analgesics (sometimes called *co-analgesics*) are drugs that have a primary indication other than pain but are analgesic for some painful conditions. For example, the primary indication for antidepressants is depression, but some antidepressants help relieve some types of pain. The adjuvant analgesics are the largest and most diverse of the three analgesic groups. Drug selection and dosing are based on both experience and evidence-based practice guidelines.

Anticonvulsants and Antidepressants. Some *anticonvulsants* (also called *antiepileptic drugs [AEDs]* when used for seizure management) produce analgesia by blocking sodium and calcium channels in the CNS, thereby diminishing the transmission of pain. The gabapentinoids *gabapentin* and *pregabalin* are used frequently for neuropathic pain. Gabapentin is generally well tolerated, with the primary side effects of sedation and dizziness, which often diminish with continued use (Burchum & Rosenthal, 2019). Pregabalin can produce euphoria and as such is classified as a controlled substance in the United States (Rosenquist, 2018). Side effects of pregabalin, like gabapentin, include sedation and dizziness, as well as weight gain and a risk for hypersensitivity reactions including angioedema.

Antidepressants relieve pain on the descending modulatory pathway by blocking the body's reuptake of the inhibitory neurochemicals *norepinephrine* and *serotonin.* Antidepressant adjuvant analgesics are divided into two major groups: *tricyclic antidepressants* (TCAs) and newer *serotonin and norepinephrine reuptake inhibitors* (SNRIs). Amitriptyline is the most commonly used TCA for persistent pain, although several others (e.g., desipramine, nortriptyline) have been used with success (Rosenquist, 2018). Duloxetine and venlafaxine, SNRIs, are widely studied and used for persistent and neuropathic pain (Rosenquist, 2018).

The most common side effects of the TCAs are dry mouth, sedation, dizziness, mental clouding, weight gain, and constipation. Orthostatic hypotension is a potentially serious TCA side effect. The most serious adverse effect is cardiotoxicity, especially for patients with existing significant heart disease. The SNRIs have a more favorable side effect profile and are better tolerated than the TCAs. The most common SNRI side effects are nausea, headache, sedation, insomnia, weight gain, impaired memory, sweating, and tremors.

PATIENT-CENTERED CARE: OLDER ADULT CONSIDERATIONS QSEN

Older adults are often sensitive to the effects of the adjuvant analgesics that produce sedation and other CNS effects such as anticonvulsants and antidepressants. Therapy should be initiated with low doses, and titration should proceed slowly with systematic assessment of patient response. Caregivers in the home setting must be taught to take preventive measures to reduce the likelihood of falls and other accidents. A home safety assessment is highly recommended and can be arranged by social services before discharge.

Local Anesthetics. Local anesthetics relieve ***pain*** by blocking the generation and conduction of the nerve impulses necessary to transmit pain. The local anesthetic effect is dose related. A high enough dose of local anesthetic can produce complete anesthesia, and a low enough dose (subanesthetic) can produce analgesia.

Local anesthetics have a long history of safe and effective use for the treatment of all types of pain. Allergy to local anesthetics is rare, and side effects are dose related. CNS signs of systemic toxicity include ringing in the ears, metallic taste, irritability, and seizures. Signs of cardiotoxicity include tingling and numbness, bradycardia, cardiac dysrhythmias, and cardiovascular collapse.

The *lidocaine 5% patch* is placed directly over or adjacent to the painful area for absorption into the tissues directly below. A major benefit of the drug is that it produces minimal systemic absorption and side effects. The patch is left in place for 12 hours and then removed for 12 hours (12-hours-on, 12-hours-off regimen). This application process is repeated as needed for continuous analgesia.

Topical local anesthetics are also available for superficial procedures such as IV insertion. In the past, creams such as *EMLA* (eutectic mixture of local anesthetics*) and lidocaine/prilocaine cream* were applied to intact skin for 30 to 60 minutes before the procedure. While still used, especially in the pediatric population, the length of time that it takes these topical anesthetics to provide analgesia limits their use. A newer technique using compressed gas to deliver a liquid form of lidocaine into the skin that produces analgesia within 1 to 3 minutes is becoming more common (Hsu, 2018). Topical local anesthetic side effects are rare and usually transient, with local skin reactions being the most common.

Liposomal bupivacaine for postoperative wound infiltration is a sustained-release formulation injected as a single dose into the surgical site by the surgeon. The sustained-release formulation has been shown to produce prolonged analgesia, which decreases the need for potent opioids.

For many years *regional anesthesia* has been administered by single-injection peripheral nerve blocks using a long-acting local anesthetic such as bupivacaine or ropivacaine to target a specific nerve or nerve plexus. This technique is highly effective in producing pain relief, but the effect is temporary (4 to 12 hours). *Continuous peripheral nerve block* (also called *perineural regional analgesia*) offers an alternative with longer-lasting analgesia. A continuous peripheral nerve block involves establishment by an anesthesia provider of an initial block followed by placement of a catheter through which an infusion of local anesthetic is administered continuously, with or without PCA capability. When PCA capability is added, this is referred to as *patient-controlled regional analgesia* (PCRA). Just as with epidural and intrathecal analgesia, nurses are responsible for monitoring and managing the therapy.

Medical Marijuana (Cannabis). Cannabis is a schedule Icontrolled substance and has been since 1970. However, the use of cannabis and cannabinoids for various medical reasons, including persistent and neuropathic ***pain,*** is increasing. Currently over 31 jurisdictions have legalized the use of medical cannabis, creating a conflict between state and federal law in the United States (NCSBN, 2018). Medical use of cannabis is legal in Canada. Medical marijuana programs (MMPs) that adhere to each jurisdiction's rules and regulations have been established. The health care provider does not prescribe cannabis in any state; however, he or she may assess and determine qualifying conditions in accordance with state law (NCSBN, 2018).

Discovered in 1973, the body contains an endocannabinoid system that is thought to promote homeostasis. Endocannabinoids are naturally occurring substances in the body. Cannabis contains numerous cannabinoids, the most common are: tetrahydrocannabinol (THC), cannabidiol (CBD), and cannabinol (CBN). Because cannabis is a Schedule I controlled substance, the evidence regarding best practice and effectiveness is limited. This is an area of research that is expanding rapidly. Current moderate- to high-quality evidence exists for medical cannabis use for persistent pain from cancer, rheumatoid arthritis, and fibromyalgia, as well as neuropathies that are associated with conditions such as multiple sclerosis (NCSBN, 2018). Medical cannabis is not regulated by the Food and Drug Administration (FDA). As such, there is not standardized dosing. Medical cannabis can be inhaled via smoking, vaporization, and ingestion (Bridgeman & Abazia, 2018). Side effects of medical cannabis include but are not limited to increased heart rate, increased appetite, dizziness, decreased blood pressure, dry mouth, hallucination, paranoia, altered psychomotor function, and impaired attention (NCSBN, 2018).

THC is known to be the psychoactive component of cannabis (Bridgeman & Abazia, 2017). As such, THC is the cause of many of the side effects associated with cannabis use. This component is what creates the potential for abuse with this drug. The use of cannabinoids that do not contain psychoactive components (e.g., CBD and CBN) is increasing, and effects with regard to pain management are promising. Research is ongoing to determine potential use, as well as long-term effects.

It is important that the nurse understand that even if the patient uses medical marijuana, the nurse cannot administer the drug unless specifically authorized by jurisdiction law (NCSBN, 2018). The patient or a designated caregiver must administer the drug. As with all patients, the nurse should provide care without judgement regarding the patient's choice of treatment in managing pain.

Use of Placebos. A placebo is defined as any medication or procedure, including surgery, which produces an effect in a patient because of its implicit or explicit intent, not because of its specific physical or chemical properties. A saline injection is one example of a placebo. Administration of a medication at a known subtherapeutic dose (e.g., 0.05 mg of morphine in an adult) is also considered a placebo.

Placebos are appropriately used as controls in research evaluating the effects of a new medication. Patients or volunteers who participate in placebo-controlled research must be able to give informed consent or have a guardian who can provide informed consent. Unfortunately, occasionally placebos are used clinically in a deceitful manner and without informed consent. This is often done when the clinician does not accept the patient's report of pain. Pain relief resulting from a placebo, should it occur, is mistakenly believed to invalidate a patient's report of pain. This typically results in the patient being deprived of pain-relief measures despite research showing that many patients who have obvious physical stimuli for pain (e.g., abdominal surgery) report pain relief after placebo administration. The use of placebos has both ethical and legal implications, violates the nurse-patient relationship, and deprives patients of more appropriate methods of assessment or treatment.

! NURSING SAFETY PRIORITY

Drug Alert QSEN

Deceitful administration of a placebo violates informed consent law and jeopardizes the nurse-patient therapeutic relationship. Never administer a placebo to a patient. Promptly contact your nursing supervisor if you are given an order to do so.

Nonpharmacologic Management. Most people use self-management and nonpharmacologic strategies to deal with their health issues and promote well-being. Nonpharmacologic methods are appropriate alone for mild- and some moderate-intensity ***pain*** and should be used to complement, not replace, pharmacologic therapies for more severe pain. The effectiveness of nonpharmacologic methods can be unpredictable. Although not all have been shown to relieve pain, they offer many benefits to some patients of all ages. For example, research has shown that nonpharmacologic methods can facilitate relaxation and reduce anxiety, stress, and depression, which often accompany the pain experience (Cornelius et al., 2017; McMillan et al., 2018). Many patients find that the use of nonpharmacologic methods helps them cope better and feel greater control over the pain experience. Nurses play an important role in providing and teaching their patients about nonpharmacologic strategies. Many of the methods are relatively easy for nurses to incorporate into daily clinical practice and may be used individually or in combination with other nonpharmacologic therapies.

Nonpharmacologic interventions are categorized as being body-based (physical) modalities; mind-body (cognitive-behavioral) methods; biologically based therapies; and energy therapies. Biologically based and energy therapies are used most often in the ambulatory care setting and are beyond the scope of this chapter. Body-based and mind-body therapies are often used by patients to self-manage their ***pain*** and enhance ***comfort.***

Physical Modalities. In the acute care setting the physical modalities are used most often because of their ease in implementation and their role in postoperative recovery. In the ambulatory care setting or at home, sustained physical regimens such as regular low-impact exercise, in combination with analgesics and other interventions, improve outcomes for people with persistent (chronic) pain. Many of the physical modalities require a prescription for use and reimbursement. Some require a trained expert to administer the technique (e.g., acupuncture). Among the most effective physical modalities used to manage or prevent pain are:

- Physical therapy
- Occupational therapy
- Aquatherapy
- Functional restoration (also has cognitive-behavioral components)
- Acupuncture
- Low-impact exercise programs such as slow walking and yoga

The physical modalities are often administered using an interprofessional collaborative approach. The assistance of physical and occupational therapists to help design and implement an individualized plan with realistic goal setting promotes effectiveness of these methods. Coordinate with the therapist to implement strategies to decrease pain before therapy sessions with the purpose of increasing function and preventing further deterioration. Teach patients to adhere to their drug regimen to maximize effectiveness of the treatment plan. Expected patient outcomes include an increase in the range of motion, strength, and function of the affected area and an improved quality of life. The occupational therapist may also help decrease pain by making one or more splints to rest severely inflamed joints.

A number of *cutaneous (skin) stimulation* strategies, which apply mild stimulation to the skin and subcutaneous tissues, have been used for many years to relieve pain. Examples of cutaneous stimulation include:

- Application of heat, cold, or pressure
- Therapeutic massage
- Vibration
- Transcutaneous electrical nerve stimulation (TENS)

Cold applications (ice) are especially helpful for inflamed areas such as for patients with rheumatoid arthritis and those who have knee surgery. Heat is appropriate when an increased blood flow is desired such as for patients with osteoarthritis pain. Paraffin dips for the hands can be helpful to increase movement for those patients as well. Warm showers and compresses that can be done at home are useful in reducing stiffness and promoting movement in patients with arthritis, especially after awakening. Local short-acting gels and creams may provide *cryotherapy (cold treatment)* to relieve muscle aches and pains. These products can often be bought over the counter (OTC) (e.g., Bengay, Icy Hot). The effects of this type of application can last up to 2 hours. Discuss this information with the patient before the use of a cutaneous method.

The benefits of cutaneous stimulation are highly unpredictable and may vary from application to application. Despite these potential drawbacks, it can be effective in the management of both acute and persistent pain in selected patients. A major benefit of these methods is that many are easy for patients to self-administer.

TENS is used as an adjunctive treatment for ***pain.*** Although there are several types of **transcutaneous electrical nerve stimulation (TENS)** units, each involves the use of a battery-operated device capable of delivering small electrical currents through electrodes applied to the painful area (Fig. 5.5). The voltage or current is regulated by adjusting a dial to the point at which the patient perceives a prickly "pins-and-needles" ***sensory perception*** rather than the pain. The current is adjusted based on the degree of desired relief. Newer, smaller, and less expensive TENS units are easy for anyone to apply and are often used at home or other community-based setting. The cost for a single unit usually ranges between $100 to $300 per unit, depending on the number of settings and leads.

Spinal cord stimulation is an *invasive* stimulation technique that provides pain control by applying an electrical field over the spinal cord. A trial with a percutaneous epidural stimulator is conducted to determine whether permanent placement of the device is appropriate. If the trial is successful, electrodes are surgically placed in the epidural space and connected to an external or implanted programmable generator. The patient is

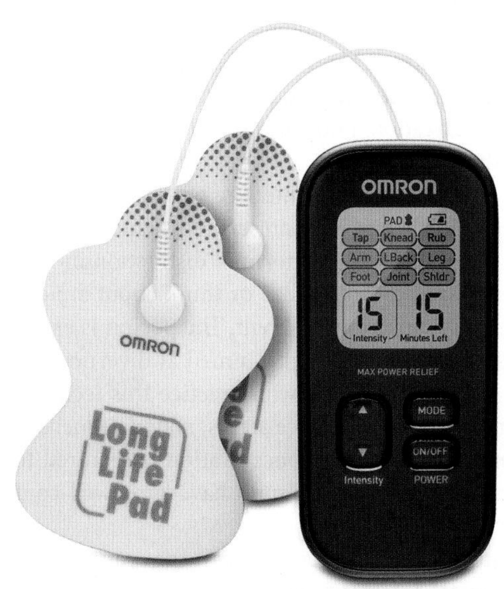

Fig. 5.5 TENS unit used in the home by the patient. (Photo courtesy of OMRON Healthcare, Inc.)

taught to program and adjust the device to maximize ***comfort.*** Spinal cord stimulation can be extremely effective in selected patients but is reserved for intractable neuropathic pain syndromes that have been unresponsive to less invasive methods. Care for the patient with an implanted spinal cord stimulator is the same as that for anyone who has back surgery and epidural anesthesia.

Cognitive-Behavioral Modalities. Cognitive behavioral modalities can be useful in reducing the patient's focus on ***pain*** but do not physiologically block pain transmission. Cognitive-behavioral modalities range from simple (e.g., prayer, relaxation breathing, artwork, reading, and watching television) to more complex (e.g., mindfulness, meditation, guided imagery, hypnosis, biofeedback, and virtual reality). It is important to recognize that many of the methods require patient teaching and subsequent patient participation. Many patients use these methods as part of their self-management and ***comfort*** promotion. Not all patients are receptive to the use of these methods. To respect their wishes, values, and preferences as part of patient-centered care, do not insist that patients use any one particular method. While the use of cognitive behavioral modalities is recommended as part of a multimodal approach to pain management, there is not one specific modality that is superior to another (Chou et al., 2016). Cognitive-behavioral modalities can be provided to patients by a variety of health care providers, including psychologists, psychotherapists, nurses, physicians, and social workers (Chou et al., 2016).

Distraction is probably the most commonly used cognitive-behavioral method. All of us use simple distraction measures in our daily life when we watch television or read a book. Nurses often observe that patients request less pain medication when family members are present and when talking on the phone. After visiting hours it is not unusual for patients to request pain medication because they are no longer distracted.

Visual distracters (e.g., looking at a picture, watching television, playing a video game) can divert the attention to something pleasant or interesting. Auditory distracters (e.g., listening to music or relaxation podcasts) can have a calming effect. Changing the environment involves removing or reducing unpleasant stressors that can interfere with the patient's ability to cope with pain such as loud noise and bright lights.

Imagery is a more complex form of distraction in which the patient is encouraged to visualize or think about a pleasant or desirable feeling, sensation, or event. The person is encouraged to sustain a sequence of thoughts aimed at diverting attention away from the pain. Patients who practice this technique can mentally and vividly experience sights, sounds, smells, events, or other sensations. Intense concentration is required to visualize images; therefore patients must have fairly well-controlled pain to participate.

Before suggesting imagery, assess the patient's level of concentration to determine whether he or she can sustain a particular thought or thoughts for a desired time. The time interval for mental imagery can vary from 5 to 60 minutes. Behaviors that may be helpful in assessing whether a patient is a candidate for teaching guided imagery include that the patient is able to:

- Read and comprehend a newspaper or magazine article
- Tap to a rhythm or sing while listening to music
- Follow the logic and participate in sustained conversation
- Have an interest in environmental surroundings

When the patient has demonstrated ability to concentrate, help him or her identify a pleasant or favorable thought. Encourage the patient to focus on this thought to divert attention away from painful stimuli. CDs or other audio recordings, either commercial or created by the patient and family, may help form and maintain images. Internet-based technology can be used to help patients whose language differs from that of the facilitating practitioner (Morley & Williams, 2015; Wilson et al., 2015; Cornelius et al., 2017).

Mindfulness is similar to imagery except that the patient focuses on his or her actual environment rather than imagining it. For example, in the fall in an area where tree leaves change colors, the patient focuses on the beauty of the colors to appreciate them.

Patients may also use *relaxation techniques* to reduce anxiety, tension, and emotional stress, all of which can exacerbate pain. For example, before and during a painful procedure, patients can be reminded to breathe slowly, deeply, and rhythmically to divert attention and promote relaxation. Relaxation techniques can be both physical and psychological. Physical relaxation techniques include:

- Relaxation breathing
- Receiving a body massage, back rub, or warm bath
- Modifying the environment to reduce distractions
- Moving into a comfortable position

Psychological relaxation techniques include:

- Pleasant conversation
- Laughter and humor
- Music (provide a range of choices)
- Relaxation podcasts or recordings

Care Coordination and Transition Management. Before patients are discharged from any health care setting, collaborate with members of the interprofessional health care team to optimize pain control. Before discharge or transfer ensure that the patient, especially one who will receive opioid analgesia, has appropriate prescriptions and enough doses to last at least until the first follow-up visit with the primary health care provider.

Home Care Management. Fatigue exacerbates ***pain.*** If physical modifications in the home (e.g., installing a downstairs bathroom) are unrealistic, suggest changes in schedules, role responsibilities, and daily routines to help prevent or reduce it.

At home, patients may require a referral for physical therapy, especially to start or continue exercise regimens, treatment with cutaneous stimulation, or heat or cold techniques. Patients may need a social worker to help them develop coping strategies or maintain adequate family dynamics. A hospice or palliative care referral (hospital or community based) can help maintain continuity of care in the management of terminally ill patients and those who require treatment of some chronic conditions.

Home infusion therapy programs provide a wide variety of services to patients who require technology-supported pain management at home. Many of these services depend on approval by the insurance carrier, usually before analgesic options are considered and therapy is started. Case managers can be helpful in answering insurance and other payment questions. Well-defined home agency practices and professional support at home are required if patients leave the hospital with infusion therapy for pain management. Often family members are taught to assume the responsibilities of home infusion therapy.

Self-Management Education. Teach the patient and family about analgesic regimens, including any technical skills needed to administer the analgesic; the purpose and action of various drugs, their side effects, and complications; and the importance of correct dosing and dosing intervals. Explain how to prevent or treat the constipation commonly associated with taking opioid analgesics and other medications. Inform the patient about what to do and whom to contact if the prescribed management regimen is not controlling pain well or when side effects are intolerable or unmanageable.

Help the patient establish an analgesic regimen that does not interfere with sleep, rest, appetite, and level of physical mobility. Ensure that patients are aware of any dangers associated with driving or operating mechanical equipment. Tell patients to ask their primary health care provider when these activities are safe to perform. Older patients and others at risk for falls or accidents in the home setting may benefit from a home safety assessment.

In patients with pain from advanced cancer, all efforts are directed toward maximizing relief and symptom control at home and eliminating unnecessary hospital readmissions. This may mean that the primary health care provider prescribes a flexible analgesic schedule that allows the patient to adjust analgesics according to the amount of pain. Teach the patient and family how to safely treat breakthrough pain and increase drug doses within the prescribed dosing guidelines. If painful ambulatory care treatments or procedures are expected, tell the patient how important it is to talk with his or her primary health care provider to determine available options for preventing procedural pain (e.g., premedicating).

Evaluate family support systems to help the patient adhere to and continue the proposed medical treatment and nursing plan of care. Inform and include family members in activities during and after hospitalization. To achieve a reasonable level of involvement in life activities for the patient, suggest ways to continue participation in household, social, sexual, and work-oriented activities after discharge. Help the patient identify important activities and plan to do them with adequate rest periods.

The patient with persistent (chronic) ***pain*** needs continued support to cope with the anxiety, fear, and powerlessness that often accompany this type of pain. Help the patient and family or significant others identify coping strategies that have worked in the past. Outside support systems are often extremely helpful (e.g., organizations such as the *American Chronic Pain Association* [http://theacpa.org]). This organization has the "10-Step Program from Patient to Person," and it provides numerous educational materials and facilitates the establishment of local support groups for people with chronic pain. Teach patients about the value of nonpharmacologic methods, including mindfulness as part of CBT.

Health Care Resources. Ask the health care provider for a home health care or hospice referral, as appropriate, for patients who require assistance or supervision with the pain management regimen at home. Important information to provide to the home health care nurse includes the patient's condition, level of sedation, weakness or fatigue, possible constipation or nutritional problem, sleep patterns, and functional status. Detailed information about the patient's current pain management regimen and how well it has been tolerated is essential. Use a structured procedure such as SBAR (**s**ituation, **b**ackground, **a**ssessment, **r**ecommendations) to communicate this information.

In addition to explaining the patient's physical status to the home health care nurse, describe his or her level of anxiety and general expectations about pain after discharge. Close relationships and available support networks are important factors in providing ongoing support for effective pain intervention strategies.

Referral to an advanced practice nurse pain specialist, social worker, or psychologist may be necessary for some patients and families to provide continued support, reinforce instructions for complex pharmacologic or nonpharmacologic strategies, or evaluate overall physical and emotional adaptation after discharge. When severe chronic or intractable pain exists, health care professionals should direct the patient and family to appropriate resources such as pain centers or primary health care providers who specialize in long-term pain management.

GET READY FOR THE NEXT-GENERATION NCLEX® EXAMINATION!

Key Points

Review these Key Points for each NCLEX Examination Client Needs Category.

Safe and Effective Care Environment

- The nurse is legally and ethically responsible to act as an advocate for patients experiencing pain.
- Collaborate with the interprofessional team as needed to provide adequate analgesia and nonpharmacologic pain management methods. **QSEN: Teamwork and Collaboration**

Health Promotion and Maintenance

- Provide information to the patient and family about nonpharmacologic physical modalities and cognitive-behavioral strategies for pain management. **QSEN: Evidence-Based Practice**
- Consider the special needs of older adults when assessing and managing pain (See the Patient-Centered Care: Older Adult Considerations: Pain box.) **QSEN: Patient-Centered Care**

- Recognize that many veterans of war have persistent (chronic) pain caused by trauma. **Health Care Disparities**
- Assess and meet the patient's need for pain management promptly to promote relief. **QSEN: Patient-Centered Care**

Psychosocial Integrity

- Be aware that some health care providers may have biases about pain assessment and management; be objective when caring for patients with pain. **Clinical Judgment**
- Assess and document the patient's and family's expectations for management of ***pain*** and promotion of ***comfort.*** Be sensitive to the cultural preferences and values of the patient and family. **QSEN: Patient-Centered Care**

Physiological Integrity

- Remember that pain is what the patient says it is; self-report is always the most reliable indicator of pain. **QSEN: Patient-Centered Care**
- Perform and document a complete pain assessment, including duration, location, intensity, and quality of pain (see Tables 5.5 and 5.6). **QSEN: Informatics**
- Factors that can affect pain and its management include age, gender, genetics, and culture. **QSEN: Patient-Centered Care**
- Pain can be categorized by duration (acute or persistent); etiology (e.g., cancer pain or procedural pain); or underlying mechanism (nociceptive or neuropathic). See Table 5.2.
- Multimodal analgesia combines different drugs with different underlying mechanisms of action with the goal of producing better pain relief at lower analgesic doses than would be possible with any single analgesic alone. **QSEN: Evidence-Based Practice**
- Analgesics are categorized into three main groups: (1) nonopioid analgesics; (2) opioid analgesics; and (3) adjuvant analgesics.
- Registered nurses are on the front lines of the opioid epidemic. All nurses have the ethical responsibility to manage pain, as well as the duty to prevent harm (see Table 5.7).
- Observe for and prevent common side effects of analgesics. **Clinical Judgment**
- Remember that sedation precedes opioid-induced respiratory depression; assess sedation using a sedation scale and decrease the opioid dose if excessive sedation is detected (see Table 5.9). **QSEN: Safety**
- Adjuvant analgesics are drugs that have a primary indication other than pain but are analgesic for some painful conditions.
- Nonpharmacologic therapies may be effective alone for mild pain and are used to complement, not replace, pharmacologic interventions for moderate-to-severe pain. **QSEN: Evidence-Based Practice**

MASTERY QUESTIONS

1. A client taking newly prescribed gabapentin for persistent neuropathic pain reports dizziness. What is the best nursing response?
   A. "This is a common side effect of gabapentin and will decrease with use."
   B. "Stop taking the medication and contact the health care provider."
   C. "The dizziness is caused by the neuropathic pain, not the medication."
   D. "The dizziness is likely from another medication, not the gabapentin."

2. A client has been receiving the same dose of an intravenous opioid for 2 days to manage postsurgical pain. The client reports that the drug is no longer controlling the pain. What does the nurse suspect?
   A. There is likely a history of addiction.
   B. Tolerance to the opioid is developing.
   C. Physical dependence is developing.
   D. The client is opioid naïve.

REFERENCES

Asterisk (*) indicates a classic or definitive work on this subject.

American Nurses Association and American Society for Pain Management Nursing. (2016). *Pain management nursing: scope and standards of practice* (2nd ed). Silver Spring, MD: ANA & ASPMN.

American Nurses Association. (2018). *The ethical responsibility to manage pain and the suffering it causes. [Position Statement].* Silver Spring, MD: ANA.

Arnstein, P., & Herr, K. (2017). Evidence-based practice guideline. Persistent pain management in older adults. *Journal of Gerontological Nursing, 43*(7), 20–31.

Bridgeman, M. B., & Abazia, D. T. (2017). Medicinal Cannabis: History, Pharmacology, And Implications for the Acute Care Setting. *P & T : A Peer-Reviewed Journal for Formulary Management, 42*(3), 180–188.

Booker, S. Q., & Haedtke, C. (2016). Assessing pain in nonverbal older adults. *Nursing, 46*(5), 66–69. https://doi.org/10.1097/01.NURSE.0000480619.08039.50.

Broglio, K., & Portenoy, R. (2019). Commonly used, oral, immediate-release and parenteral pure mu-opioid agonists for chronic pain: Adult dosing and approximate equivalence. *UpToDate.* Retrieved from: https://www.uptodate.com/contents/image

Broglio, K. &Portenoy, R. (2019). Approximate dose conversions for commonly used opioids. [Table]. *UpToDate.* Retrieved from: https://www.uptodate.com/contents/image

Burchum, J., & Rosenthal, L. (2019). *Lehne's pharmacology for nursing care.* St. Louis, MO: Elsevier.

Chan, S., Hadjistavropoulos, T., Williams, J., & Lints-Martindale, A. (2014). Evidence-based development and initial validation of the Pain Assessment Checklist for Seniors with Limited Ability to Communicate-II (PACSLAC-II). *The Clinical Journal of Pain, 30*(9), 816–824.

Chou, r., Gordon, D., de-Leon-Casasola, O., Rosenberg, J., Bickler, S., Brennen, R., et al. (2016). Management of postoperative pain: A clinical practice guideline from the American pain society, the American society of regional anesthesia and pain medicine, and the American society of anesthesiologists' committee on regional anesthesia, executive committee, and administrative council. *Journal of Pain, 17*(2), 131–157.

Centers for Disease Control and Prevention (CDC). (2017). *Understanding the epidemic*. Retrieved from https://www.cdc.gov/drugoverdose/epidemic/index.html.

Cornelius, R., Herr, K., Gordon, D., & Kretzer, K. (2017). Evidence-based practice guideline. Acute pain management in older adults. *Journal of Gerontological Nursing, 43*(2), 18–27.

Czarnecki, M., & Turner, H. (2018). *Core curriculum for pain management nursing* (3rd ed.). St. Louis, MO: Elsevier.

DeCarvalho, L. (2016). *The experience of chronic pain and PTSD: A guide for healthcare providers*. U.S. Department of Veterans Affairs. Retrieved from: https://www.ptsd.va.gov/professional/treat/cooccurring/chronic_pain_guide.asp.

Drew, D., Gordon, D., Morgan, B., & Manworren, R. (2018). "As-needed" range orders for opioid analgesics in the management of pain: A consensus statement of the American Society for pain management nursing and the American pain society. [Position Statement]. *Pain Management Nursing, 19*(3), 207–210.

Fentanyl safety. (n.d.). Handling of suspected drugs. Safety recommendations for first responders. Retrieved from: https://www.fentanylsafety.com/safe-handling/

Gupta, A., & Rosenquist, R. (2018). Use of opioids in the management of chronic non-cancer pain. *UpToDate*. Retrieved from https://www.uptodate.com/contents/use-of-opioids-in-the-management-of-chronic-non-cancer-pain?topicRef=2785&source=-see_link.

*Herr, K., Coyne, P. J., McCaffery, M., Manworren, R., & Merkel, S. (2011). *American Society for Pain Management Nursing position statement with clinical practice recommendations: Pain assessment in the patient unable to self report (revised)*. http://aspmn.org/Documents/PainAssessmentinthePatientUnabletoSelfReport.pdf.

Hsu, D. (2018). *Clinical use of topical anesthetics in children. UpToDate*. Retrieved from https://www.uptodate.com/contents/clinical-use-of-topical-anesthetics-in-children.

Jungquist, C., Vallerand, A., Sicoutris, C., Kwon, K., & Polomano, R. (2017). Assessing and managing acute pain: A call to action. *The American Journal of Nursing, 117*(3), S4–S11.

*McCaffery, M. (1968). *Nursing practice and theories related to cognition, bodily pain, and man-environment interactions*. Los Angeles: University of California at Los Angeles Students' Store.

McMillan, K., Glaser, D., & Radovich, P. (2018). The effect of massage on pain and anxiety in hospitalized patients: An observational study. *MEDSURG Nursing, 27*(1), 14–18.

*Morley, S., & Williams, A. (2015). New developments in the psychological management of chronic pain. *Canadian Journal of Psychiatry, 60*(4), 168–175.

National Council of State Boards of Nursing. (2018). The NCSBN national nursing guidelines for medical marijuana. *Journal of Nursing Regulation, 9*(2). Retrieved from: https://www.ncsbn.org/The_NCSBN_National_Nursing_Guidelines_for_Medical_Marijuana_JNR_July_2018.pdf.

NIDA. (2018, January 17). Principles of Drug Addiction Treatment: A Research-Based Guide (Third Edition). Retrieved from https://www.drugabuse.gov/publications/principles-drug-addiction-treatment-research-based-guide-third-edition on 2018, November 18.

Nahin, R. (2017). Severe pain in veterans: The effect of age and sex, and comparisons with the general population. *Journal of Pain, 18*(3), 247–254.

The National Institute for Occupational Safety and Health (NIOSH). (2018). *Preventing occupational exposure to healthcare personnel in hospital and clinical settings*. Centers for Disease Control and Prevention. Retrieved from: https://www.cdc.gov/niosh/topics/fentanyl/healthcareprevention.html.

*Pasero, C., & McCaffery, M. (2011). *Pain assessment and pharmacologic management*. St. Louis: Mosby.

Public Services Health and Safety Association. (2017). *Fentanyl and carfentanil exposure in health and community care workers*. Retrieved from: https://www.pshsa.ca/wp-content/uploads/2017/11/OOHFCAEN0917-Fentanyl-and-Carfentanil-Exposure-Fast-Fact_Jan-2-2018.pdf.

Rosenquist, E. (2018). *Overview of the treatment of non-cancer pain. UpToDate*. Retrieved from: https://www.uptodate.com/contents/overview-of-the-treatment-of-chronic-non-cancer-pain.

*Textor, L. (2016). Intrathecal pumps for cancer pain. *The American Journal of Nursing, 116*(5), 36–41.

*Wilson, M., Roll, J. M., Corbett, C., & Barbosa-Leiker, C. (2015). Empowering patients with persistent pain using an Internet-based self-management program. *Pain Management Nursing, 16*(4), 503–514.

6

Concepts of Genetics and Genomics

M. Linda Workman

http://evolve.elsevier.com/Iggy/

LEARNING OUTCOMES

1. Collaborate with the interprofessional team to coordinate high-quality ***patient-centered care*** to adults who may have a genetic-based increased risk for a health problem.
2. Apply knowledge of biology, anatomy and physiology, and genetic/genomic principles when performing a genetic assessment and generating a three-generation pedigree to identify adult health problems that have a potential increased genetic risk.
3. Implement patient and family-centered nursing interventions to help people cope with the psychosocial impact caused by genetic assessment, genetic testing, and identification of an increased genetic risk for a specific health problem.
4. Ensure the use of professional ***ethics*** when integrating genomic health into medical-surgical nursing practice, including informed consent procedures.
5. Ensure ***patient-centered care*** by helping the patient and family who undergo genetic testing receive an appropriate level of genetic counseling to interpret the findings.

KEY TERMS

aneuploid A description of cells that have an abnormal number of chromosomes (more or less than the normal number for the species) or broken chromosomes.

carrier An adult who has one mutated allele for a recessive genetic disorder but either does not express the disorder or does not fully express the disorder.

cellular regulation Genetic and physiologic processes that control cellular growth, replication, differentiation, and function to maintain homeostasis.

direct-to-consumer genetic testing (DTC-GT) The marketing of genetic testing by for-profit companies without the involvement of a health care professional.

dominant allele The allele of a single-gene trait that is always expressed whenever it is present, regardless of the nature of the second allele.

epigenetics The changes in gene expression caused by mechanisms that do not involve variation in actual DNA sequences.

euploid A description of cells having the correct number of chromosome pairs for the species.

expressivity The degree of expression a person has when a dominant gene allele or a pair of recessive alleles is present.

gene A segment(s) of DNA that contains the specific code (recipe) for the order of the correct amino acid sequence within a designated protein (see Fig. 6.1) involved in cellular regulation.

gene expression The selective activation (turning on) of a gene to direct the production of its specific protein.

gene therapy An experimental technique that uses genes to treat or prevent disease.

genetics The general mechanisms of heredity and the variation of inherited single-gene traits.

genome The entire set of human nuclear DNA present in nearly all body cells.

genomic health care The use of genetic information and technology to prevent or manage specific health problems.

genomics The function of all of the human DNA, including genes and noncoding DNA regions, and how this affects cellular regulation.

genotype The actual gene alleles a person has for a specific single-gene trait—not just what can be observed.

heritability Characteristic by which the risk for developing the disorder can be transmitted to one's children in a recognizable pattern.

karyotype An organized arrangement of all the chromosomes present in a cell during the metaphase section of mitosis.

microbiome The genomes of all the microorganisms that coexist in and on a person.

mutation DNA base sequence change(s) from the gene wild type that causes a loss of protein function, leading to impaired cellular regulation.

pedigree Graph of a family history for a specific trait or health problem over several generations.

penetrance How often or how well, within a population, a gene is expressed when it is present.

phenotype Gene expression for a person in which a trait or characteristic can actually be observed or, in some cases, determined by a laboratory test.

polymorphism DNA base sequence change(s) from the gene wild type that allows the protein to be made but with differences in how well the protein works.

recessive allele The allele of single-gene trait that is expressed only when the second allele is also recessive and identical.

PRIORITY AND INTERRELATED CONCEPTS

The priority concept for this chapter is:
- ***Cellular Regulation***

The interrelated concepts for this chapter are:
- ***Ethics***
- ***Patient-Centered Care***

OVERVIEW

Differences in DNA and genes are what makes each person unique. Even identical twins, who have identical DNA sequences shortly after conception, have some differences in DNA sequences as adults that can affect their individual health risk. Most of the serious, common adult-onset health disorders have a genetic basis or component. Specific discoveries regarding each adult's genetic/genomic differences are being used to assess disease risk, enhance disease prevention strategies, personalize disease management approaches, and even devise ways to correct a specific genetic problem at its source *(gene therapy)*. Thus genetic and genomic influences are very much part of today's comprehensive ***patient-centered care.***

The use of genetic information and technology to prevent or manage specific health problems is known as **genomic health care** and drives much of today's *precision health.* As a result, all health care professionals, including registered nurses, are expected to have a knowledge of basic genetics sufficient to recognize when a patient or family has a possible genetic risk for a specific health problem (Cheek & Howington, 2017; Montgomery et al., 2017; Paz De Jesus & Mitchel, 2016; Tluczek et al., 2018). Thus nurses are expected to coordinate the attention of interprofessional health team members to ensure adequate care for medical-surgical patients, including the involvement of the appropriate level of genetics professional (Lebet et al., 2019). Table 6.1 lists selected genetic competencies most relevant for medical-surgical nursing practice.

The purpose of genes and genetics is to provide *cellular regulation* in all cells throughout the lifespan. ***Cellular regulation*** is the genetic and physiologic processes that control cellular growth, replication, differentiation, and function to maintain homeostasis. Thus the turning on and off of specific genes determines everything that a cell does, including what it produces, how it functions within a group, when it reproduces, and even when it dies. Chapter 3 provides a summary discussion of cellular regulation.

Although the terms *genetics* and *genomics* often are used interchangeably, there are some differences. **Genetics** is concerned with the general mechanisms of heredity and the variation of inherited single-gene traits. Thus how genetic traits are transmitted from one generation to the next comprises genetics. The definition of **genomics** is both broader and more specific, focusing on the *function* of all of the human DNA, including genes and noncoding DNA regions. Thus how a gene is expressed and its effects on ***cellular regulation*** within a person or family constitute genomics.

Many adult-onset health problems have a genetic basis, meaning that variation of gene sequences and expression contributes to an adult's risk for changes in cellular regulation and disease development. Some of these health problems also demonstrate **heritability**, meaning that the risk for developing the disorder can be transmitted to one's children in a recognizable pattern. Some adult-onset disorders such as Huntington disease are currently unavoidable when a person inherits a specific genetic mutation that causes expression of the disorder. For other health problems, the risk is increased but is not absolute, indicating a *predisposition* or increased *susceptibility* to the problem when a specific genetic mutation is inherited, but the disorder or problem may never occur. For example, inheritance of certain gene variations increases the risk for type 2 diabetes; however, the disease is more likely to develop only when the adult with the genetic variation(s) has a sedentary lifestyle and is overweight. One desired outcome of genomic health care is to identify personal risk for disease development and help the adult reduce the risk by modifying his or her environment. For example, the adult identified as at increased risk for type 2 diabetes can prevent or delay onset of the disorder by maintaining a healthy weight and performing aerobic exercise on a consistent basis. A woman at high risk for breast and ovarian cancer may elect to have these tissues surgically removed before cancer develops.

GENETIC BIOLOGY REVIEW

Genetic Structure and Function

Recall from your biology courses that a **gene** is a segment of DNA that contains the specific code for the order of the correct amino acid sequence within a designated protein (see Fig. 6.1) involved in ***cellular regulation***. For every hormone, enzyme, and other proteins the human body makes, it is the specific genes that tell each cell which protein to make, how to make it, when to make it, and how much to make. Think of each gene as a specific "recipe" for making a protein. Thus proteins are known as *gene products.*

Many proteins are the product of the activation and expression of a single gene. Some proteins require the input and expression of more than one gene for complete production. Much more is known about the inheritance, expression, and

TABLE 6.1 Selected Essential Genetic Competencies for Medical-Surgical Nursing Practice

- Use appropriate genetic terminology.
- Recognize that a person/family with an identified genetic variation is a full member of society deserving of the same quality of health care as that provided to all others.
- Differentiate between genetic predisposition to a health problem and the actual expression or diagnosis of the health problem.
- Recognize the genetic and environmental influences on development of common adult-onset health problems.
- Be aware of genetic-based individual variation in responses to drug therapy.
- Consider genetic transmission patterns when performing a detailed patient and family history assessment with a three-generation pedigree construction using standard symbols.
- Ask appropriate questions during assessment to obtain information relevant to potential genetic risk or predisposition to a specific health problem(s).
- Identify patients/families at increased genetic risk for potential disease development.
- Ensure that patients/families identified to be at increased genetic risk for potential disease development are referred to the appropriate level of genetics professional.
- Individualize patient teaching about genetic issues using terminology and language the patient/family understands.
- Inform patients/families about potential risks and benefits of genetic/genomic testing.
- Advocate for patients with regard to their rights to accurate information, informed consent, competent counseling, refusal of genetic/genomic testing, freedom from coercion, and sharing of testing results.
- Help patients/families find credible resources regarding a specific genetic issue.
- Maintain patient/family confidentiality regarding any issue related to genetic/genomic testing, predisposition, or genetic diagnosis, including whether genetic/genomic testing is even being considered.
- Support the patient's/family's decisions regarding any aspect of genetic/genomic testing or genetic diagnosis.

Data from competencies identified by American Association of Colleges of Nursing. (2008). *The essentials of baccalaureate education for nursing practice*. Washington, DC: Author; and Montgomery, S., Brouwer, W., Everett, P., Hassen, E., Lowe, T., McGreal, S., & Eggert, J. (2017). Genetics in the clinical setting: What nurses need to know to provide the best patient care. *American Nurse Today, 12*(10), 10–15.

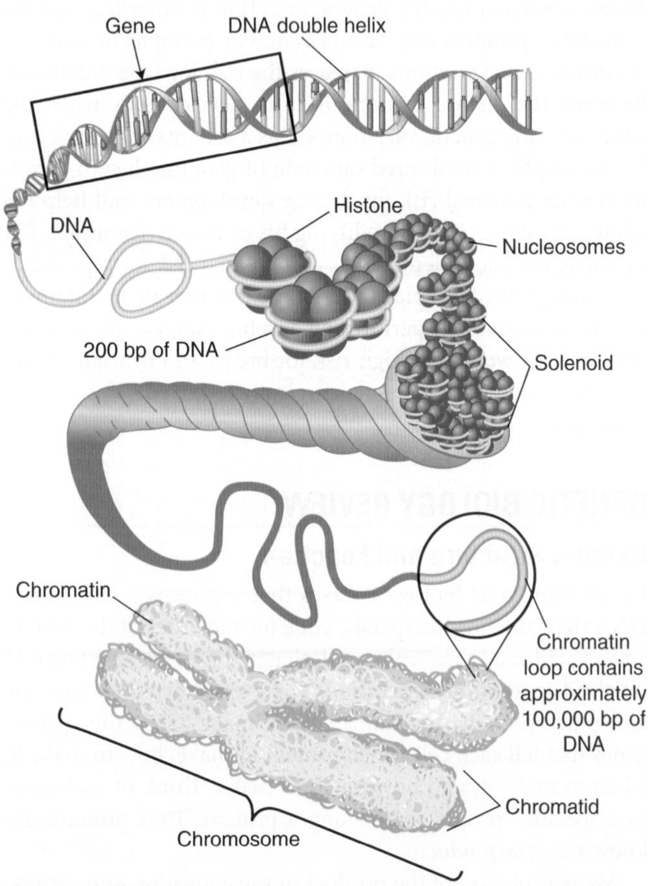

FIG. 6.1 The various forms of DNA from a loose double helix to a form that is coiled tightly into a chromosome. *bp*, Base pair.

suppression of single genes, and these are the current focus of risk assessment, genetic/genomic counseling, and gene therapy.

Every human somatic cell with a nucleus contains the entire set of human nuclear genes, known as the **genome**. The human genome contains between 20,000 and 25,000 genes. **Gene expression** is the selective activation (turning on) of a gene to direct the production of its specific protein. For example, all cells have the gene for insulin. However, expression of the insulin gene to make insulin for ***cellular regulation*** and glucose regulation occurs only in the beta cell of the pancreas. So, although the insulin gene is present in skin cells, heart cells, brain cells, and all other cells, only in the beta cells does selective expression of this gene lead to insulin production when it is needed.

DNA

Genes are composed of DNA, which is present as 46 separate large chunks within the nucleus. During cell division each large chunk of DNA replicates and then organizes into a chromosome form to ensure precise delivery of the genetic information to each of the two new daughter cells. Thus DNA, chromosomes, and genes refer to different structures of the same materials. Genes are the smallest functional unit of the DNA, whereas each chromosome is a large segment of DNA that contains hundreds of genes (Fig. 6.1).

Human DNA is a linear, double-stranded structure composed of multiple units of four different nitrogenous bases. These *bases* are the essential parts of DNA. Many trillions of bases in the DNA are found in the nucleus of just one cell. The four bases in DNA are adenine (A), guanine (G), cytosine (C), and thymine (T). When the two strands of DNA are lined up properly, they twist into a loose helical shape (see Fig. 6.1). In this shape, the DNA is so fine that it can be seen only with electron microscopes. When a cell undergoes mitosis, the DNA super-coils tightly into dense pieces called *chromosomes* (see Fig. 6.1), which can be seen with standard microscopes.

Proteins are made from amino acids. Smaller proteins, such as insulin and glucagon, contain relatively few amino acids (active insulin is 51 amino acids in length; glucagon is 29), whereas a large protein may have hundreds of thousands of amino acids. There are 22 different amino acids. Each amino acid has at least one unique three-base DNA sequence coding for it. Every protein has a specific number of each of the amino acids and a designated order in which they are placed. *If even one amino acid is out of order or completely deleted from the sequence, the protein may be less functional or perhaps nonfunctional and unable to assist with* ***cellular regulation.***

The key for making a functional protein is accurate placement of all the amino acids in the order specified by the gene. When problems exist in the base sequence of a gene, it may not be produced at all or the protein that is produced may have poor function. In addition, the process of protein synthesis involves many steps. A problem at any step could cause failure to produce a functional protein and thus disrupt cellular regulation.

Chromosomes. As shown in Fig. 6.1, a chromosome is a specific large chunk of highly condensed double-stranded DNA that has already replicated (duplicated), with each chunk containing billions of bases and double sets of hundreds (and sometimes thousands) of genes. Each chromosome with replicated DNA forms and moves to the center of the cell that is about to divide. Just before the cell splits into two cells, each chromosome is pulled apart so half of each chromosome with a complete set of genes goes into one new cell and the other half (also with a complete set of genes) goes into the other new cell. Thus chromosomes are temporary structures to ensure the precise delivery of DNA to the two new cells.

Humans have 23 pairs of chromosomes—46 individual chromosomes. The Y chromosome is small and has fewer than 100 genes. Larger chromosomes, such as the number 1 chromosome, contain thousands of genes. There is a specific chromosome location *(locus)* for every gene. For example, the locus of the gene for blood type is on chromosome 9.

Some things about an adult can be known by examining his or her chromosomes, but information obtained by chromosomal analysis is limited because each chromosome is composed of a large chunk of DNA. Only very large deletions, additions, or rearrangements of DNA show up at the level of the chromosome. Losses or gains of even tens of thousands of bases cannot be detected by chromosome analysis. (Remember, in some cases a change in only *one* base can alter the expression of a gene and affect ***cellular regulation.***)

A karyotype is an organized arrangement of all of the chromosomes present in a cell during the metaphase segment of mitosis (Fig. 6.2). A picture of the chromosomes is made and they are paired up and arranged according to size (largest first) and centromere position. This gross organization of DNA can be used to determine missing or extra whole chromosomes and some large structural rearrangements. *A missing gene or a mutated gene would not show up at this level of analysis.* What can be learned about the adult from whom the karyotype in Fig. 6.2 was made is that she is human, female, and euploid (has the correct number of chromosome pairs for the species). She is chromosomally "normal," although she probably has some genes that are different (variant from or mutated) compared with the same genes in other people. If the karyotype is abnormal in any way (has more or fewer than the normal number for the species or has broken chromosomes), the karyotype would be called aneuploid.

Gene Expression

Just like proteins, many human traits are determined by the expression of single genes *(monogenic)* and others require the expression of many genes *(polygenic).* The expression of single genes is related to whether the gene's alleles are dominant or recessive. Recall that for each single-gene trait, there is only one gene. However, genes for many single-gene traits have slight sequence variations within them that are responsible for trait differences. For example, in humans there is only one gene for blood-type group, but there are three different forms of this gene (alleles) that are responsible for the three different blood-type groups (A, B, and O). Under normal circumstances, each of a person's genes has only two alleles, so each person has only *two* alleles of the blood-type group alleles—one inherited from each of his or her parents. Any person's blood-type group is dependent on which two alleles are inherited from his or her parents and how these alleles are expressed. Fig. 6.3 shows all possible inheritance patterns of a single-gene trait for which there are four known alleles.

Expression of the two alleles for any single gene and single-gene trait is related to the nature of the alleles, which depends on the whether an allele is dominant or recessive. A dominant allele of a person's single gene with two alleles is always expressed whenever it is present regardless of the nature of the second allele. A recessive allele of a person's single gene with two alleles is expressed only when the second allele is also recessive and identical.

Phenotype. The phenotype of any gene expression for a person is a genetic trait or characteristic that can actually be observed or, in some cases, determined by a laboratory test. For example, the person who has an A allele and an O allele for blood-type groups (AO) has the phenotype of type A blood (because A is a dominant allele and O is a recessive allele and only the A allele is expressed). A person with curly hair has a curly-hair phenotype, regardless of whether he or she has two alleles for curly hair or one allele for curly hair and one allele for straight hair (because the curly hair allele is dominant and the straight hair allele is recessive and only the curly hair allele is expressed).

Genotype. The genotype for a person's single-gene trait is what the actual alleles are for that trait—not just what can be observed. A person with a phenotype of type A blood could have either an AA allele genotype or an AO allele genotype. (The AA genotype is *homozygous* because both alleles are the same; the AO genotype is *heterozygous* because the two alleles are different.) The person who has type O blood would have an OO genotype (homozygous). When a person has homozygous

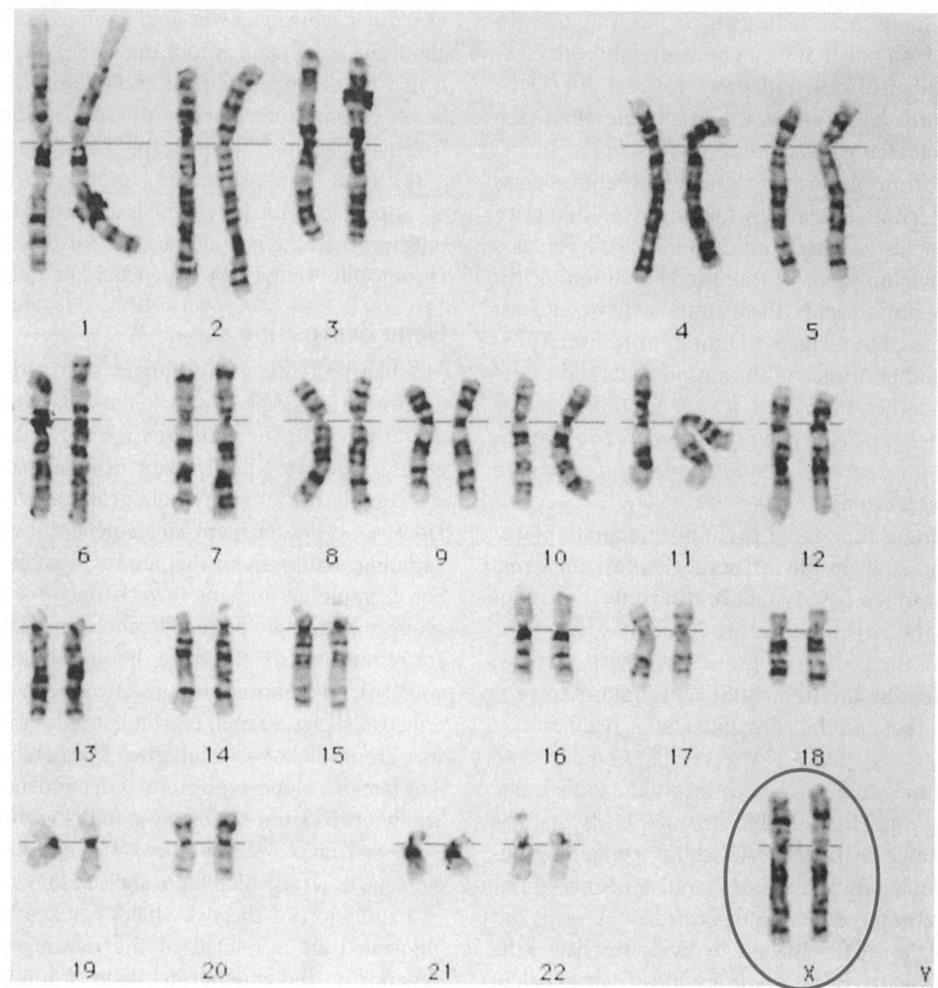

FIG. 6.2 A karyotype of a chromosomally normal female. (The sex chromosomes are *circled in red*.) (Modified from Jorde, L., Carey, J., Bamshad, M., & White, R. [2000]. *Medical genetics* [2nd ed.]. St. Louis: Mosby.)

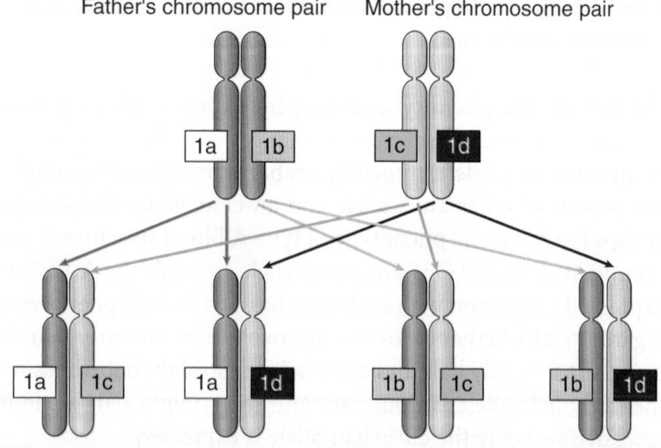

FIG. 6.3 Inheritance of four possible alleles for the single-gene trait 1. (Any one person can have only two alleles for a single-gene trait.)

alleles for a trait, we would expect the genotype and phenotype to be the same. When a person has heterozygous alleles for a trait, the phenotype and the genotype are not always the same. *Recessive traits are expressed only when the person is homozygous for the alleles.* Thus for expressed single-gene recessive traits, phenotype and genotype are the same. Single-gene dominant traits are expressed regardless of whether the person is homozygous for the gene alleles or heterozygous for the gene alleles. Thus for dominant traits phenotype and genotype can be the same but do not have to be the same.

Mutations and Variations

Many human genes have been sequenced, meaning that their base sequence is known and so is the sequence of their amino acids in the expressed proteins. Most people have the same base sequence for a specific gene such as the gene for insulin. When this sequence is the most common one found in a large population of humans, it is referred to as the *wild-type* gene sequence. Think of the term *wild-type* as meaning "normal" or "expected." When a person has a different sequence for a gene compared with the known wild-type sequence, the gene has a variation. Small variations in gene sequences occur more often in very large genes, and the significance of some of these changes is not known. It is these variations in the sequences of some genes from the wild-type that are being examined more closely. Some variations can reduce the function of the protein produced, some can eliminate the function of the protein produced, and a few variations have been found that enhance the function of the produced protein compared with the function of the wild-type protein.

Variations are DNA sequence changes that are passed from one generation to another and thus are inherited. *An inherited variation does not have to mean that it is passed from one human generation to another. It can mean that the variation is passed from one **cell** generation to another and may affect only certain tissues within a person rather than be a problem within a family.* Variations that occur in general body cells (somatic cells) are known as *somatic variations.* Because somatic variations occur in a person's cells after he or she was conceived, the adult cannot pass a somatic variation to his or her children. A possible outcome of somatic variations is a loss of ***cellular regulation*** with increased risk for cancer in cells with such variations.

When variations occur in sex cells, they are known as *germline variations.* A germline variation *can* be passed to a person's children; and each of that child's cells, including his or her somatic cells and sex cells, will contain that DNA variation.

When sequence variations occur in a gene area of the DNA, the change can alter the expression of that gene, and an incorrect gene product (protein) might result. Variations can have a serious impact on cellular regulation, although some may be beneficial. Gene variations that increase the risk for a disorder are known as *susceptibility* genes. Gene variations that decrease the risk for a disorder are known as *protective* or *resistance* genes.

The gene sequences for most proteins are generally the same in all people. Sometimes a base in one person's gene for a specific protein is not the same as that in the wild type. Either this change can be a variation known as a *single nucleotide polymorphism, or SNP* ("snip"), or it can be a mutation. When base changes allow the protein to be made but there are differences in how well the protein works, the change is called a *gene variation* or a **polymorphism**. When a base difference causes a loss of protein function leading to impaired ***cellular regulation***, it is called a **mutation**.

Clinical examples of common SNPs and their influence on health are those that exist within different people in the genes of a large family of enzymes involved in drug metabolism. These enzymes are the cytochrome P-450 family, coded for by at least 10 separate extremely large genes, with as many as 100 subsets of genes. Cytochrome P is abbreviated as CYP (pronounced "sip"). SNPs in these genes can make the resulting enzyme less active than normal or more active than normal. Either way, a change in activity for any of these enzymes can affect a person's response to drug therapy. For example, the drug warfarin is metabolized for elimination primarily by two enzymes from this system, CYP2C9 and CYP2C19. About 17% to 37% of white adults have a SNP variation in the *CYP2CP* gene that slows the metabolism of warfarin. This means that warfarin remains in the patient's system longer, greatly increasing the risk for bleeding and other side effects. For adults who have this gene variation, warfarin doses need to be much lower than those for the general population.

Another example of changes in patient responses to drugs is codeine, an opioid analgesic. When taken orally or given parenterally, codeine is an inactive prodrug that must be metabolized by the CYP2D6 enzyme in the tissues to morphine, which is the active drug. Patients who have nonfunctional or poorly functional CYP2D6 because of a gene variation obtain no pain relief from codeine but do obtain pain relief when given morphine.

PATIENT-CENTERED CARE: CULTURAL/ SPIRITUAL CONSIDERATIONS QSEN

Many adults of Ethiopian heritage have a variation of the *CYP2D6* gene that results in much higher levels of the enzyme produced and are known as "ultrametabolizers." This enzyme deactivates and helps eliminate many drugs, including metoprolol, a beta-blocking agent that is often used to control blood pressure. An adult who ultrametabolizes the drug does not achieve a high enough blood level of the drug for it to be effective because it is eliminated too quickly. Thus any adult of Ethiopian heritage who needs antihypertensive therapy is not likely to respond to metoprolol or any other beta blockers. When patients do not respond to beta-blocker therapy as expected, be sure to ask about their cultural and ethnic heritage.

The most devastating gene mutations are the ones that change the amino acid codes so that a proper protein either is not produced or is produced and nonfunctional. Other changes may impair ***cellular regulation*** by altering how often or how well a group of cells divides. Gene mutations or variations may cause one adult to have a greater-than-normal risk for developing a disease. A different variation in the same gene may cause another adult to have a smaller-than-normal risk for developing the same disease.

Although specific mutations are more common in people of some races and ethnicities, it is important to remember that no health impairment mutation is unique to any one race or ethnicity. For example, although sickle cell disease is more common among African Americans, it also can be found in people of any other race or ethnicity.

PATTERNS OF INHERITANCE

For every single-gene trait, a person inherits one allele for that gene from his or her mother and one allele from his or her father. How these traits are expressed depends on whether one or both alleles are "dominant" or "recessive." Expression also depends on whether the gene for the trait is located on an autosome or on a sex chromosome.

It is possible to determine how the gene for a specific trait is passed from one human generation to the next *(transmitted).* By looking at how that trait is expressed through several generations of a family, patterns emerge that can indicate whether the gene for the trait is dominant or recessive and whether it is located on an autosomal chromosome or on one of the sex chromosomes. This information can be determined through *pedigree analysis.* Determining inheritance patterns for a specific trait makes it possible to predict the relative risk for any one person to have a trait or transmit that trait to his or her children.

Pedigree

A *pedigree* is a graph of a family history for a specific trait or health problem over several generations. Its use by nurses is important for assessing certain ***patient-centered care*** needs. Fig. 6.4 shows common symbols used when creating a pedigree. Fig. 6.5 shows a typical three-generation pedigree. Although the term *pedigree* is the correct genetic term, it can offend patients

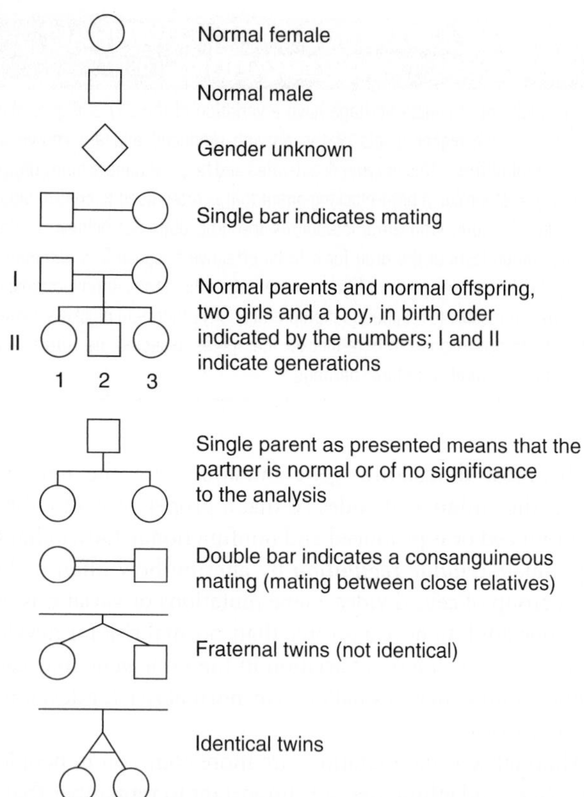

FIG. 6.4 Standard pedigree symbols. (Modified from Jorde, L., Carey, J., & Bamshad, M. [2010]. *Medical genetics* [4th ed.]. St. Louis: Mosby.)

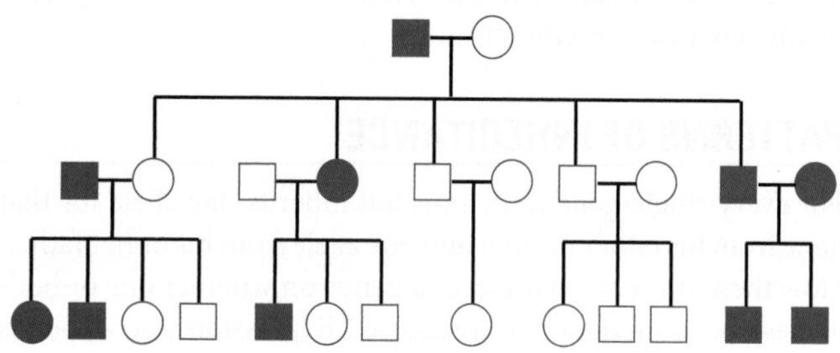

FIG. 6.5 A three-generation pedigree showing an autosomal-dominant pattern of inheritance.

who associate the term with animals. Use the term *family tree* in place of pedigree when talking with patients. Construct a pedigree that includes at least three generations when taking the family history. When analyzing a pedigree, note the answers to these questions:

- Is any pattern of inheritance recognized, or does the trait appear sporadic?
- Is the trait expressed equally among male and female family members or unequally?
- Is the trait present in every generation, or does it skip one or more generations?
- Do only affected adults have children who are affected with the trait, or do unaffected adults also have children who express the trait?

The four types of inheritance patterns associated with single-gene traits are autosomal dominant, autosomal recessive, sex-linked dominant, and sex-linked recessive. Each inheritance pattern has specific defining criteria. Table 6.2 lists the patterns of inheritance for some disorders that occur in adults or may be identified in children who live to adulthood.

TABLE 6.2 Patterns of Inheritance for Genetic Disorders Among Adults

Pattern of Inheritance	Disorder
Autosomal dominant	Breast cancer[a] (mutation of *BRCA1* or *BRCA2* gene)
	Diabetes mellitus type 2[a]
	Familial adenomatous polyposis
	Familial melanoma
	Familial hypercholesterolemia
	Hereditary nonpolyposis colon cancer (HNPCC)
	Huntington disease
	Long QT syndrome and sudden cardiac death
	Malignant hyperthermia (MH)
	Marfan syndrome
	Myotonic dystrophy
	Neurofibromatosis (types 1 and 2)
	Ovarian cancer[a] (mutation of *BRCA1* gene)
	Polycystic kidney disease[b] (types 1 and 2)
	Retinitis pigmentosa[b]
	von Willebrand disease
Autosomal recessive	Alpha$_1$-antitrypsin deficiency
	Beta-thalassemia
	Bloom syndrome
	Cystic fibrosis
	Gaucher disease
	Hereditary hemochromatosis
	Sickle cell disease
	Xeroderma pigmentosum
Sex-linked recessive	Glucose-6-phosphate dehydrogenase deficiency
	Hemophilia
	Red-green color blindness
Complex disorders/familial clustering	Alzheimer's disease
	Autoimmune disorders
	Bipolar disorder
	Parkinson disease
	Hypertension
	Rheumatoid arthritis
	Schizophrenia

[a]Some disorders have both a genetic and a nongenetic form.
[b]Some disorders have more than one genetic form and can also be autosomal recessive.

Autosomal Dominant Pattern of Inheritance

Autosomal dominant (AD) single-gene traits require that the gene alleles controlling the trait be located on an autosomal chromosome. A dominant gene allele is usually expressed, even when only one allele of the pair is dominant. Table 6.2 lists some AD adult disorders and Fig. 6.5 shows a typical pedigree for an AD trait or disorder. Other criteria for AD inheritance include:

- The trait appears in every generation with no skipping.
- The risk for an affected adult to pass the trait to a child is 50% with each pregnancy.

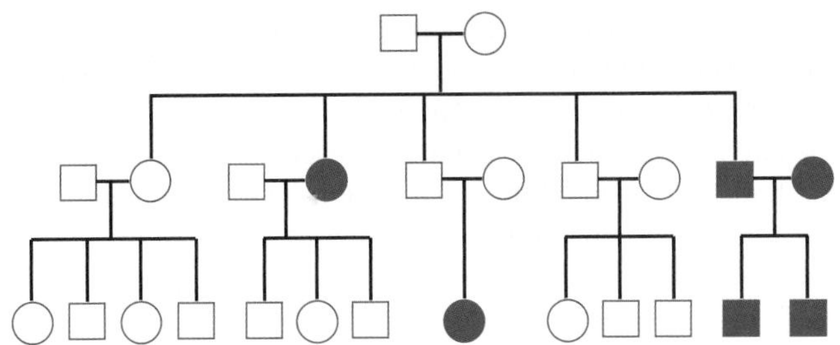

FIG. 6.6 A typical pedigree showing an autosomal-recessive pattern of inheritance.

- Unaffected adults do not have affected children; therefore their risk is essentially 0%.
- The trait is found about equally in males and females.

An example of an AD trait is blood-type A. If a person is homozygous for the blood-type A allele, he or she will express type A blood (with genotype being identical to the phenotype). If a person is heterozygous for the blood-type A allele with the other allele being type O (which is a recessive trait), he or she will also express type A blood. However, in this case the phenotype is *not* identical to the genotype. *When a dominant allele is paired with a recessive allele, only the dominant allele is expressed.* The blood-type B allele is a dominant allele. When a B allele is paired with an O allele, B blood type is expressed. However, when a person has one blood-type A allele and a blood-type B allele, both alleles are expressed because they are equally dominant (co-dominant), and the person has type AB blood.

Some health problems inherited as autosomal-dominant (AD) single-gene traits are not apparent at birth but develop as the person ages (see Table 6.2). Two factors that affect the expression of some AD single-gene traits are penetrance and expressivity.

Autosomal-Recessive Pattern of Inheritance

Autosomal-recessive (AR) single-gene traits require that the gene controlling the trait be located on an autosomal chromosome. Normally the trait can be expressed *only* when both alleles are present. Table 6.2 lists some AR adult disorders. Fig. 6.6 shows a typical pedigree for an AR disorder. Criteria for AR patterns of inheritance include:

- The trait may not appear in all generations of any one branch of a family.
- The trait often first appears only in siblings rather than in parents and children.
- About 25% of a family will be affected and express the trait.
- The children of two affected parents will almost *always* be affected (risk is nearly 100%) but may vary in the intensity of expression of the trait or disorder.
- Unaffected adults who are carriers (heterozygous for the trait) and do not express the trait themselves *can* transmit the trait to their children if their partner either is also a carrier or is affected.
- The trait is found about equally in male and female members of the same family.

An example of an AR trait is type O blood. The blood-type O allele is recessive, and both alleles must be type O (homozygous) for the person to express type O blood. If only one allele is a type O allele and the other allele is either type A or type B, the dominant allele will be expressed and the O allele, although present, is not expressed. For AR single-gene traits, phenotype and genotype are always the same.

An adult who has one mutated allele for a recessive genetic disorder but does not express or does not fully express the disorder is a carrier. A carrier, even though he or she may have one mutated allele, may not have any signs or symptoms of the disorder but can pass this mutated allele to his or her children. For some autosomal-recessive disorders, a carrier may have mild symptoms of the change in ***cellular regulation*** associated with the mutation. One example is sickle cell trait. A patient with two sickle cell alleles has the disease and many associated health problems. A carrier with one sickle cell allele (has "sickle cell trait") may be healthy most of the time and have symptoms only under conditions of severe hypoxia.

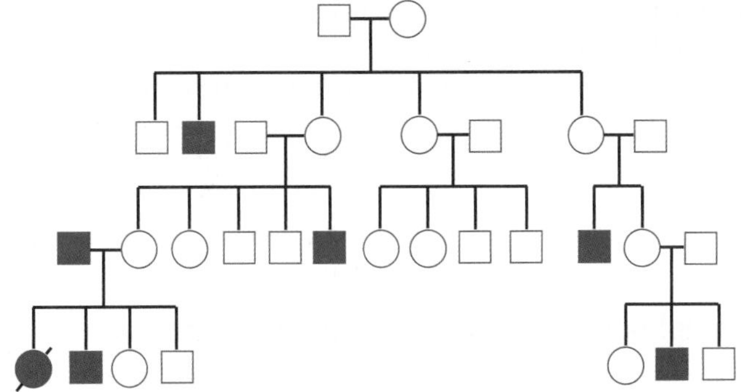

FIG. 6.7 A typical pedigree showing a sex-linked (X-linked) recessive pattern of inheritance.

Sex-Linked Recessive Pattern of Inheritance

Some genes are present only on the sex chromosomes. The Y chromosome has only a few genes that are not also present on the X chromosome. These genes are important for male sexual development. The X chromosome has many unique single genes that are not present on the Y or elsewhere in the genome. Some of these genes are specific for female sexual development, but there are also several hundred genes on the X chromosome that code for other important functions. Few disorders have X-linked dominant expression and are not discussed in this chapter.

Because the number of X chromosomes in males and females is not the same (1:2), the number of X-linked chromosome genes in the two genders is also unequal. Males have only one X chromosome. As a result, X-linked recessive genes have dominant expression in males and recessive expression in females. This difference in expression is because males do not have a second X chromosome to balance the presence of a recessive gene on the first X chromosome.

Sex-linked (X-linked) recessive single-gene traits require that the gene allele be present on both of the X chromosomes for the trait to be expressed in females (homozygous) and on only one X chromosome for the trait to be expressed in males. Fig. 6.7 shows a typical pedigree for a sex-linked recessive disorder. Features of a sex-linked recessive pattern of inheritance are:

- The incidence of the trait is much higher among males in a family than among females.
- The trait cannot be passed down (transmitted) from father to son.
- Transmission of the trait is from father to all daughters (who will be carriers).
- Female carriers have a 50% risk (with each pregnancy) of passing the gene to their children.

Complex Inheritance and Familial Clustering

Some health problems affecting ***cellular regulation*** appear in families at a rate higher than normal and greater than can be accounted for by chance alone; however, no specific pattern occurs within a family. Although clusters suggest a genetic influence, it is likely that additional factors such as gender and the environment also influence disease development or severity. Such disorders include Alzheimer's disease, type 1 diabetes, and many others. These disorders are often called *complex* and *multifactorial,* because although an increased genetic risk may be present, the risk is changed by diet, lifestyle, exposure to toxins, infectious agents, and other factors.

NCLEX EXAMINATION CHALLENGE 6.1

Health Promotion and Maintenance

While a nurse constructs a pedigree during the assessment, the client asks why this is being performed. Which explanation does the nurse provide to the client for this action?

A. "This information will help identify your blood relatives' places within your family and describe their health histories."
B. "I will use this document to find which person in your family is responsible for introducing a possible genetic mutation into the family."
C. "This information will help your primary health care provider decide whether to prescribe genetic/genomic testing for you."
D. "This is a normal way we take information on new clients and is nothing you need to worry about."

Genetic Factors Affecting Single-Gene Expression

Penetrance. *Penetrance* is how often or how well, within a population, a gene is expressed when it is present. Some genes are more penetrant than others. For example, the gene for Huntington disease (HD) has an autosomal-dominant pattern of transmission and is "highly penetrant" (sometimes called *fully penetrant*). This means that if a person has the HD gene allele, his or her risk for expressing the gene and developing the disease is about 99.99%. Therefore a person who has one HD allele is at high risk for developing HD.

Some dominant gene alleles have "reduced" penetrance. A person who has the gene mutation has a lower risk for this gene being expressed and actually developing the disorder.

Penetrance has been calculated by examining a population of people known to have the gene mutation and assessing the percentage that go on to express the gene by developing the disorder. For example, the *BRCA2* gene mutation increases a person's risk for breast cancer. This gene is not fully penetrant; so some women (and men) who have the gene do not develop breast cancer. The penetrance rate for this gene mutation is calculated to be between 60% and 80%, meaning that an adult who has the gene mutation has a 60% to 80% risk for developing breast cancer. Although this risk is far higher than among adults who do not have the mutated gene, the risk is not 100%. Having the gene mutation does not absolutely predict that the adult will develop breast cancer—just that the risk is high. However, the adult with the mutation can pass this genetic mutation to his or her children, who will then also have an increased risk for breast cancer development.

Expressivity. *Expressivity* is the degree of expression a person has when a dominant gene allele or a pair of recessive alleles is present. It is a personal issue, not a population issue. The gene is nearly *always* expressed, but some people have more severe problems than other people. For example, the gene mutation for one form of neurofibromatosis (NF1) is dominant. Some people with this gene mutation have only a few light-brown skin tone areas known as *café au lait spots*. Other people with the same gene mutation develop hundreds of tumors (neurofibromas) that protrude through the skin. Another example is when a person has a pair of gene allele mutations for cystic fibrosis but has only incomplete development of the vas deferens as a physical symptom of the disorder and no pulmonary symptoms. Expressivity accounts for some variation in genetic disease severity and its effects on ***cellular regulation.***

Nongenetic Factors Affecting Single-Gene Expression

Recently some nongenetic factors have been discovered to change how single genes are expressed even when there is no alteration of the actual structure or location of the genes. Two examples of nongenetic factors that can cause unexpected expression and lack of expression for normal genes are epigenetics and the microbiome.

Epigenetics. Epigenetics (also called *epigenomics*) is the changes in gene expression caused by mechanisms that do not involve variation in actual DNA sequences (Jorde et al., 2016). Some of these mechanisms can be inherited when they occur in germline cells; others occur any time after conception. Some changes can be reversed with certain types of therapy. The three known mechanisms that appear to change gene expression without changing the sequence of a gene or genes are the action of DNA methylation, the action of histone modification, and the presence of excessive or inappropriate small pieces of RNA known as microRNAs (miRNAs). Any of these mechanisms can have a profound effect on ***cellular regulation***.

Both DNA methylation and histone modification change the structures that surround segments of cellular DNA and inhibit the transcription of one or more genes, thus "silencing" their expression. The gene or genes are present but do not get expressed. Methylation involves the attachment of chemical methyl group (CH_3) side chains to the DNA. Histone modification involves making the DNA more tightly wound during chromosome formation. The ends of the tightly wound DNA can then be hidden so that genes in this region are not transcribed and thus are not expressed. Both excessive methylation and histone modification can occur as a result of environmental exposures to some chemicals or toxins and dietary intake of oxidating agents, among other possible causes. When the silenced gene is a normal gene important for ***cellular regulation***, the result of silencing can have a detrimental effect on health. For example, if a growth-suppressing gene controlling cell division is silenced, cell growth is less controlled and cancer development is more likely. However, when the silenced gene is a mutation, the resulting disorder may never occur. For example, if the mutated gene allele responsible for development of Huntington disease (HD) is methylated in brain cells, it may not be expressed and the adult with the methylated gene does not develop HD even though he or she has the actual disease-causing mutation. These forms of epigenetic influences help explain why a gene mutation present in two identical twins is not equally expressed. However, it adds a complicating factor for assessment of genetic risk that is not currently part of most genetic/genomic testing.

MicroRNA mechanisms for changing gene expression are slightly different and work at the translation part of protein production rather than at the transcription part. MicroRNAs are small single-stranded pieces of RNA that interfere with translation of RNA into protein. These miRNAs can bind to messenger RNA, making it double-stranded and preventing protein production, which turns off selected gene expression. Just as for methylation and histone modification, the presence of miRNA-induced alteration of gene expression can be positive or negative. Its role in cancer development has been explored to a greater degree than in other health problems. When miRNAs reduce the activity of cancer suppresser genes, the risk for cancer development increases. When miRNAs reduce the activity of oncogenes, the risk for cancer development decreases (see Chapter 19).

At present, the extent of the effect of epigenetics on ***cellular regulation*** and individual risk for disease development or on individual resistance to disease development is unknown, although it is unlikely to be either the primary or only factor. Because epigenetic factors can be reversed and actual gene mutations cannot be reversed at this time, treatment strategies focusing on epigenetics are being explored. Some agents in current use include azacitidine, a chemotherapy drug that suppresses an enzyme that increases DNA methylation. Its use reduces DNA methylation in leukemia and myelodysplastic syndrome and has had some success in the management of these cancers.

Microbiome. The microbiome for an adult is the genomes of all the microorganisms that coexist in and on him or her and can affect ***cellular regulation*** as a type of epigenetic event (**Abbas et al., 2018**). This includes the organisms that live in the mouth, the rest of the GI tract, the nose and sinuses, and the vagina, and on the skin. The number of microbial cell genomes in the body outnumber human cell genomes by about 10 to 1 (**McElroy et al., 2017**). Most of these organisms are part of our "normal flora," which differ somewhat from person to person. These organisms are mostly nonpathogenic (non–disease causing) when they remain confined to the expected area. However, when they manage to escape their normal human habitat and move elsewhere, they may be pathogenic in the new environment. For example, when gut organisms get into the urinary tract or the blood, serious infections can occur.

Adults start acquiring their microbiomes from birth, and their specific microbiome profiles change a little almost daily over time. The interaction between an adult and his or her microbiome is complex and represents all the lifelong experiences of foods eaten, drugs taken, and the touching of other people and animals, along with the specific human genes inherited. To a large extent an adult's microbiome is protective in nature and is important for good health such as helping with food digestion and keeping some pathogenic organisms in check (Abbas et al., 2018). The types of gut organisms an adult has can even change how well he or she responds to immunotherapy for cancer, as well as silence the expression of some genes. As discussed in the epigenetics section, this "silencing" can be helpful or detrimental to overall health.

Changes in the microbiome can influence disease severity and response to therapy. For example, when the gut organisms of obese men with diabetes type 2 and insulin resistance were changed to be more like those of thinner men without diabetes, insulin resistance was reduced and blood glucose levels were more easily controlled (Hartstra et al., 2015). Thus changing the microbiome influenced the expression of the interactions of the multiple genes involved in the risk for type 2 diabetes. Other disorders that appear to be influenced by changes in the microbiome include acne, autism, autoimmune disorders, cancer, and dental cavities. One treatment for some disorders that are made worse by an altered microbiome is the reconstitution of the "healthy" microbiome through fecal transplantation or transfer from one person to another.

NCLEX EXAMINATION CHALLENGE 6.2

Physiological Integrity

How does the presence of microRNA "silence" gene expression?

A. Preventing cytoplasm from coming into contact with the gene
B. Surrounding mRNA and preventing attachment of ribosomes
C. Binding to mRNA and keeping it double-stranded
D. Substituting a thymine for uracil

GENETIC/GENOMIC TESTING

Purpose of Genetic/Genomic Testing

Many adults are eager to have genetic testing but also are fearful of it. The lay public often believe that a single genetic test can "tell everything about you." Although genetic/genomic testing has the potential to be that informative, this is not currently how testing is conducted. *It is important to remember that no single adult is genetically perfect.*

Genetic/genomic testing can be performed with many different techniques. Some tests are specific for a disorder. Others may show a gene variation, but the significance of the variation may not be known. Unexpected information can be found during genetic testing. Some ordinary tests such as blood typing and tissue typing provide genetic information. Tests that measure the amount of an enzyme or protein an adult produces also provide genetic information.

Testing for the purpose of assessing genetic information can be performed at many levels. Cellular or biochemical tests provide information about gene products made by a cell, tissue, or organ, and may determine the cause of altered ***cellular***

TABLE 6.3 Purposes of Genetic/Genomic Testing for Adults

Purpose or Type	Definition
Carrier testing	Determining whether a patient without symptoms has an allele for a recessive disorder that could be transmitted to his or her children. Common disorders for carrier testing include sickle cell disease, hemophilia, hereditary hemochromatosis, cystic fibrosis, beta-thalassemia, and Tay-Sachs disease.
Diagnostic testing	Determining whether a patient has or does not have a mutation that increases the risk for a specific disorder.
Symptomatic	Patient has symptoms; test results confirm a diagnosis.
Presymptomatic	Patient has no symptoms but is at high risk for inheriting a specific genetic disorder for which there is no known prevention or treatment. A disorder for which presymptomatic testing is commonly performed is Huntington disease.
Predisposition	Family history or genetic/genomic testing indicates that risk is high for a known genetic disorder. The patient does not have any symptoms but wants to know whether he or she has the specific mutation and what the chances are that it will be expressed. Common disorders for which predisposition testing is performed include hereditary breast/ovarian cancer and hereditary colorectal cancers. The advantage of predisposition testing is that the patient can then engage in heightened screening activities or medical and surgical interventions that reduce risk.

regulation. Chromosomes and chromosome segments can be assessed for missing, extra, broken, or rearranged chromosomes. The sequence of a gene can be examined to determine variation or mutation. At present not all genes can be analyzed, and the analysis of even one gene may be limited by expense and availability. Specific base pairs can be evaluated for mutations. Many tests are expensive, and the results may not be conclusive. Table 6.3 lists purposes of genetic/genomic testing for adults.

Benefits of Genetic/Genomic Testing

Genetic/genomic testing is different from any other type of testing. Informed consent is required before genetic/genomic testing is performed. The adult tested is the one who gives consent, even though this testing *always* gives information about family members—not just the patient (Jorde et al., 2016). Thus genetic/genomic testing is a unique and personal aspect of ***patient-centered care.***

Benefits of testing include the ability to confirm a diagnosis or to test adults who are at risk for a health problem that can affect ***Cellular regulation*** but do not as yet have any symptoms (presymptomatic testing). The information can help an adult, family, and their primary health care provider develop a specific plan for care and early detection. For example, in the case of a strong genetic predisposition for colon cancer, identifying a patient before symptoms appear allows interventions to prevent the disease or to diagnosis it earlier, when cure is more likely.

Risks and Concerns of Genetic/Genomic Testing

Risks are associated with genetic/genomic testing that are not associated with other types of tests. *These test results do not change.* Thus a positive test result cannot be "taken back." Other risks may include psychological or social risks, as well as a risk for family disruption. Often genetic/genomic tests are expensive and may not be covered by insurance. Some tests have limited value for predicting future risk. Testing may identify a patient at great risk for the future development of a serious health problem that cannot be prevented or managed. Such a disorder is Huntington disease (HD), which currently has no treatment. Knowing positive test results in this case can lead to depression, blame, and guilt.

Another risk of genetic/genomic testing is that positive results may be used to discriminate against an adult or a family. Some protection is in place to prevent health insurance companies from failing to insure a person or dropping the coverage of a person who is at high risk for developing a serious illness (e.g., breast or ovarian cancer). However, there are no protections against rate hikes or exclusions of specific treatments. Patients often fear workplace and personal discrimination if positive test results become known. This problem is less common since the 2008 passage of federal legislation in the Genetic Information and Nondiscrimination Act (GINA), which provides federal protection against employment and insurance discrimination (Lacovara & Bohnenkamp, 2018; Starkweather et al., 2018).

Direct-to-Consumer Genetic/Genomic Testing

An increasing concern of health care and genetics professionals is the risk presented by **direct-to-consumer genetic testing (DTC-GT)**, which is the marketing of genetic/genomic testing by for-profit companies without the involvement of a health care professional. Some companies, such as *AncestryDNA,* focus on providing information about a person's ethnic, racial, and geographic makeup. This type of DTC-GT does **not** pose significant risks. However, other companies offer testing of a person's genetic predisposition and risk for specific disorders, as well as for more general health issues, such as likely response to specific drug categories. The reliability of for-profit DTC-GT for this use has not been proven, and the federal government of the United States through the Food and Drug Administration (FDA) and the Centers for Disease Control and Prevention (CDC) has issued warnings to health care professionals and the general public to discourage their use (U.S. CDC, 2017; U.S. FDA, 2018). Although there may be some perceived benefit to DTC-GT for health risks, many actual and potential issues remain important concerns among health care professionals.

A major concern is the lack of regulation regarding the actual techniques used in the for-profit laboratory-developed tests (LDTs) to assess for mutations that increase the risk for some disorders. The FDA has strict standards for genetic/genomic testing kits as medical devices and laboratory testing used for clinical assessment by medical professionals. These standards provide assurance of quality control in specimen handling, specificity and reliability of complex testing methods, analysis and interpretation of results, and ethical management of personal data. Currently, the only DTC-GT company cleared by the FDA to identify personal risk for development of certain specific genetic-based health problems is *23andMe.* A review of the home DNA test kits provided by other companies showed higher incidences of false positives and false negatives (Starkweather et al., 2017). In 2017 the Centers for Disease Control and Prevention (CDC) identified and warned against the use of 14 for-profit DTC-GT companies that had not received approval or clearance to market their testing kits (U.S. CDC, 2017; U.S. FDA, 2018).

The lack of true and in-depth genetic counseling with DTC-GT is problematic in the interpretation of true risk. For example, some DTC-GT companies offer testing to assess the risk for hereditary breast cancer. The more commonly known genes in which a mutation can increase the risk for breast cancer are the *BRCA1* and *BRCA2* genes. Both are very large genes, and mutations at different sites within them can increase breast cancer risk, whereas other mutations in these genes are not associated with increased risk. Few for-profit laboratories do total sequencing of these genes, instead assessing for only the most common mutations. Thus an adult could be told she or he does not carry the mutation associated with increased breast cancer risk without an accurate explanation of what this result means. The person may believe she or he has no risk for breast cancer and not participate in recommended screening activities. The number of certified genetics professionals qualified to provide such explanations is limited, and most are not associated with for-profit DTC-GT companies. Thus the general public may be relying on incomplete or inaccurate information when making important health decisions (Starkweather et al., 2017; U.S. CDC, 2017).

NCLEX EXAMINATION CHALLENGE 6.3

Health Promotion and Maintenance

A client with a medical problem reports that her brother was diagnosed with schizophrenia last year. She tells the nurse she is considering using a direct-to-consumer genetic/genomic testing service to determine her risk for also developing the disorder. What is the **most relevant** reason for the nurse to discourage this action?

A. Direct-to consumer genetic tests are only performed once the person with a positive diagnosis has first been tested.
B. Such tests are expensive and, when not ordered by a health care provider, they are not covered by insurance.
C. These tests are often misused by employers to support the dismissal of employees at increased genetic risk for a disorder.
D. People using such tests may not receive adequate professional counseling for interpretation of results and accurate risk assessment.

Genetic Counseling

Genetic/genomic testing is not a standard test that any adult should have performed without knowing the benefits and risks. Counseling patients before, during, and after testing is critical and required by the professional ***ethics*** governing genetic/genomic health. Entire families may be a part of the genetic evaluation and follow-up. For example, a 45-year-old woman has breast cancer. In her family, her mother, grandmother, brother, and one sister have all had breast cancer. Genetic testing indicates that she has a *BRCA1* gene mutation. This woman's older daughter wonders whether she has a gene mutation for breast cancer and asks to be tested. When she and her younger sister are tested, the older daughter does not have the mutation, but the younger sister does. Even a negative test result requires ***patient-centered care*** considerations.

Genetic counseling is a process—not a single session or a single recommendation. This process should begin when the patient or family is first identified as potentially having a genetic problem that can affect ***cellular regulation.*** The process continues through actual testing if the decision to test is made, and it continues through interpretation of results and follow-up. The Best Practice for Patient Safety & Quality Care: Steps for Genetic/Genomic Testing and Counseling box lists the steps in the process performed by an appropriately prepared and certified genetics professional.

As a nurse and patient advocate providing ***patient-centered care,*** it is your professional duty to determine whether the patient understands the consequences of testing. Often a patient may request testing even when there is no indication of an increased risk for a genetic disorder. Counseling and evaluation can help patients understand whether any useful information could be obtained from testing.

INTERPROFESSIONAL COLLABORATION

Genetic Counseling

Counseling should be a collaborative effort performed by an interprofessional team with members who have defined expertise in interpretation of genetic testing results. Such professionals include advanced-practice nurses with specialization in genetics, certified genetic counselors, clinical geneticists, and medical geneticists. Each profession has a different level of preparation in genetics and different skills or roles in the counseling process.

Which professional provides genetic counseling depends on the complexity of the issue. For example, an advanced-practice genetic nurse may counsel a patient about the Huntington disease gene mutation because this test is not ambiguous and the gene is highly penetrant. When a genetic/genomic test shows a variation or mutation in an unusual gene region or when penetrance is reduced, the patient may best be served by counseling from a certified genetic counselor or a clinical or medical geneticist.

No matter which professional is involved in genetic counseling, a key feature of this counseling is to be "nondirective" in ensuring ***patient-centered care.*** When using a nondirective approach, the counselor provides as much information as possible about the risks and benefits but does not influence the patient's decision to test or not to test. Once the patient has

BEST PRACTICE FOR PATIENT SAFETY & QUALITY CARE (QSEN)

Steps for Genetic/Genomic Testing and Counseling

Pretesting Assessment and Patient Education (May Take Multiple Sessions)

- Determining patient understanding and why testing or counseling is being sought
- Determining whether testing is reasonable (considering cost of the test, specificity, probable risk, accuracy of testing)
- Establishing a trusting professional relationship
- Ensuring privacy and confidentiality
- Reviewing informed consent procedures
- Assessing the patient's ability to communicate accurately (including language issues, cognitive function, sensory perception)
- Assessing the patient's psychosocial status and availability of social support
- Taking a detailed patient health history (including drugs, diet, exercise, hormonal history, lifestyle issues)
- Obtaining physical assessment data relevant to the at-risk disorder
- Taking a detailed family history and constructing a three-generation pedigree (minimum)
- Obtaining and verifying information obtained from sources such as:
    - Patient and family members
    - Health records
    - Pathology reports
    - Death certificates
- Interpreting the family history
- Discussing the consequences of testing
- Discussing patient rights and obligations regarding disclosure of information
- Discussing testing options
- Assessing to determine whether coercion is occurring
- Obtaining material to be tested (usually blood)

Presentation of Test Results

- Reassessing the patient's wish to know or not know the test results
- Respecting the patient's decision to not know the test results
- Ensuring privacy and confidentiality
- Presenting the test results
- Interpreting the test results
- Assessing the patient's perception of the test results

Follow-Up

- Supporting the patient's decision to disclose or not disclose the information to other family members
- Discussing the potential risks for other family members
- Ensuring privacy and confidentiality
- Addressing the patient's concerns
- Discussing prevention, early detection, and treatment options
- Discussing family concerns
- Addressing psychosocial issues
- Discussing available resources for information, support, and further counseling
- Providing summary of results and consultation to the patient

Adapted from Beery, T., Workman, M.L., & Eggert, J. (2018). *Genetics and genomics in nursing and health care* (2nd ed.). Philadelphia, PA: Davis.

made the decision, the counselor supports the patient and the decision.

Ethical Issues

Ethics and ethical issues are involved at every level of genetic/genomic testing. Some of the most important issues focus on the patient's right to know versus the right to not know his or her gene status, confidentiality, coercion, and sharing of information (Tluczek et al., 2018).

The right to know genetic risk versus the right to not know is the individual patient's choice. Sometimes a patient's right to know has an impact on the right of another family member to not know, especially for disorders that have a severe impact on ***cellular regulation*** and have little or no means to prevent or improve the outcome.

Confidentiality is crucial to the genetic counseling process. *The results of a genetic/genomic test must remain confidential to the patient. The results cannot be given to a family member, other health care provider, or insurance carrier without the patient's permission* (Starkweather et al., 2018). This issue becomes more problematic when patients are asked to give blanket permission for any health care provider to provide information from the patient's electronic health record to a third party, especially an insurance company (Tluczek et al., 2018).

Coercion is possible by other family members and health care professionals. *The final decision to have genetic/genomic testing or to not have it rests with the patient.* Other people may believe it is important for the patient to have the test; however, the patient must make the decision without such pressures. As a patient advocate ensuring ***patient-centered care,*** professional ***ethics*** require you to assess whether the patient is freely making the decision to have testing or whether someone else is urging him or her to be tested. This important issue can be difficult to assess. Ask the patient who in the family wants to know the results of testing.

Sharing test result information, negative or positive, can be stressful. The patient makes the final decision whether to share the information with family members. Some patients choose not to share this information, even when other family members may also be at risk. This can be difficult for the health care provider who knows that the patient has a positive test result for a serious inherited condition and that the patient chooses not to tell other family members who may be at risk. For example, hereditary nonpolyposis colon cancer (HNPCC) has an autosomal-dominant (AD) inheritance pattern, and each child of the patient has a 50% risk for having the gene. If the patient chooses not to tell his or her grown children, they then do not have the opportunity for increased screening to find the cancer at an early stage when cure is possible. Ethical dilemmas arise when the primary health care provider or specialist wants to inform the children of their risk.

THE ROLE OF THE MEDICAL-SURGICAL NURSE IN GENETIC COUNSELING

Medical-surgical nurses providing ***patient-centered care*** help patients during the assessing, testing, and counseling processes, although they do not provide in-depth genetic counseling. Patients often feel most comfortable sharing information with nurses and asking nurses to clarify information.

Nurses may be the first health care professionals to identify a patient at specific genetic risk. Some of the "red flags" that a patient may have a genetic risk for a disease or disorder are:

- The disease or disorder occurs at a higher incidence within the family compared with the general population.
- The patient or close family members have another identified genetic problem.
- The incidence of a specific disease or disorder occurs in the patient or in family members at an unusually early age.
- A rare disease is present in two or more family members.
- More than one type of cancer is present in any one adult.
- The specific physical characteristic is associated with one or more genetic disorders (e.g., unusual freckling or skin pigmentation, bicuspid aortic valve, deafness).

The nurse may be the health care professional who first verifies information to bring a genetic problem to light. For example, during an assessment a patient reveals that her mother died of bone cancer when she was 40 years old. Bone cancer is rare among adults; thus the nurse might then ask, "Did your mother ever have any other type of cancer?" Often the patient may then reveal that her mother had breast cancer some years before ("bone cancer" was actually breast cancer that had spread to the bones). Breast cancer occurring before menopause can indicate a genetic predisposition.

Patients may ask questions that indicate they have an interest in genetic testing. These are examples of questions that may be cues that the patient has genetic concerns:

- Will my children get this disease?
- Because my sister has this problem, what are the chances I might also develop it?
- Is there a way to test and see whether my chances of getting this disease or problem are high or low?

There are many areas of responsibility for any medical-surgical nurse providing ***patient-centered care*** when working with a patient who is considering or having genetic testing. These areas include communication, privacy and confidentiality, information accuracy, patient advocacy, and support.

Communication

Using professional ***ethics,*** act as a patient advocate by ensuring that communication between the patient and whoever is providing the genetic information is clear. First assess the patient's ability to receive and process information. Can he or she see and hear clearly, or are assistive devices needed? Does the patient understand English, or will an interpreter be needed? Does the patient have adequate cognition at the time of meeting with the genetics professional, or is it impaired by medication, disease, anxiety, or fear?

If the patient appears not to understand terms or jargon during a discussion between him or her and a genetics professional, ask the professional to use common terms and examples for the patient. Verify with the patient that he or she understands or does not understand.

After any discussion about genetic risk or genetic/genomic testing, assess the patient's understanding of what was said. Ask the patient to explain, in his or her own words, what the issue means and what his or her expectations are.

Privacy and Confidentiality

Professional ***ethics*** require that all conversations regarding potential diagnoses or genetic/genomic testing need to occur in a private environment. The patient has the right to determine who may be a part of the discussion and can decide to exclude the primary health care provider and any family member from the discussion with a genetics professional. It is important that health care professionals who may be present during such discussion do not disclose information, formally or informally, without the patient's permission. It is the nurse's ethical duty and responsibility in providing ***patient-centered care*** to protect this information from improper disclosure to family members, other health care professionals, other patients, insurance providers, or anyone not specified by the patient.

Information Accuracy

Correct myths about genetic disorders and teach patients about the nature of genetic/genomic testing. Medical-surgical nurses are not genetics experts and would not be expected to be the final source of definitive information; however, with interprofessional collaboration they can help ensure that the patient is referred to the correct level of genetic counseling. If you are present during the patient's discussions with a genetics professional, assess whether he or she understands the issues regarding the health problem. Help patients find accurate and helpful resource materials or websites. Encourage them to avoid relying on unapproved for-profit genetic/genomic testing companies for health care advice.

Patient Advocacy and Support

Professional ***ethics*** require you to ensure that the patient's rights are not neglected or ignored. Ask the patient privately what his or her wishes are regarding genetic/genomic testing. Ask whether another adult or agency is insisting on the testing. Remind the patient that he or she does not have to agree to be tested. Verify that he or she has signed an informed consent statement for the test.

Considering or having genetic/genomic testing is a stressful experience. The patient and family require support and may need help with coping. Ethically, testing should be performed only *after* genetic counseling has occurred and should be followed with more counseling.

Patients may feel anger, depression, guilt, or hopelessness. Patients who have positive results (results indicating that a specific mutation is present) from genetic testing may have issues of risk for early death or disability and the possibility of having passed the risk for a health problem on to children. Patients who have a test result of unknown significance may feel that they have agonized over a decision, spent money, and still have no clear answer. Even patients who have negative genetic/genomic test results (result indicating that a specific mutation is not present) need counseling and support as part of ***patient-centered care.*** Some patients may have an unrealistic view of what a negative result means for their general health. Others may feel guilty they were "spared" when other family members were not.

Assess the patient's response to genetic/genomic testing results. Determine which coping methods were used successfully in the past. If the patient has disclosed information to family members, assess whether they can help provide support or need support themselves. Assess whether the information about positive test results has strained family relationships. Refer the patient to appropriate support groups and interprofessional counseling services.

For some positive genetic test results such as having a *BRCA1* gene mutation, the risk for developing breast cancer is high but is not a certainty. With high risk the patient needs a plan for prevention and risk reduction. One form of prevention is early detection. Thus a patient who tests positive for a *BRCA1* mutation should have at least annual mammograms and ovarian ultrasounds to detect cancer at an early stage when it is more easily cured. Provide ***patient-centered care*** by teaching the patient who has positive test results that indicate an increased risk for a specific health problem about the types of screening procedures that are available and how often screening should occur. For example, some patients at known high genetic risk for breast cancer and ovarian cancer choose the primary prevention methods of bilateral prophylactic mastectomies (surgical removal of the breasts) and oophorectomies (surgical removal of the ovaries). Although these strategies are severe, they are effective, and the patient must be informed about their availability.

Teach patients at known high risk for a specific disorder how to modify the environment to reduce risk. For example, a patient who has a specific mutation in the *a1AT* (alpha$_1$-antitrypsin) gene is at increased risk for early-onset emphysema. The onset of emphysema is even earlier when the patient smokes or has chronic particulate matter exposure to inhalation irritants. By modifying such exposures, the disease can be delayed, or the symptoms reduced.

NCLEX EXAMINATION CHALLENGE 6.4

Psychosocial Integrity

A client whose father has Huntington disease (HD) has been told that by his father's neurologist that genetic/genomic testing for this disorder is possible. He is frightened of knowing for certain he may develop a disabling disease for which there is no cure. He asks a nurse what she would do if one of her parents had the disease. Which responses are the **most ethical** for the nurse to provide to this client? **Select all that apply.**

A. "I would have the test so I could decide whether to have biological children."
B. "Although I can tell you the benefits and the risks of testing, you must make this decision yourself."
C. "Because there is no cure for this disease and testing would not be beneficial, I would not have the test."
D. "I would only have testing if my parent had an early onset of the disease and experienced rapid deterioration."
E. "You need to check with your primary health care provider to determine whether testing for this disease would be appropriate for you."
F. "You sound conflicted. Would you like me to put you in contact with a genetics counselor who can provide you with the most up-to-date information?"

GENE THERAPY

For decades, geneticists and other scientists have considered the ultimate treatment for an inherited genetic disorder to be one in which a defective gene is replaced with a healthy one that will ensure proper gene expression and permanent function. At this time, no therapy does exactly that. The U.S. National Institutes of Health (NIH) defines *gene therapy* as an experimental technique that uses genes to treat or prevent disease (U.S. NIH, 2018). It is envisioned that gene therapy would have the greatest effect on genetic disorders when these actions are available:

- Replacing a mutated gene that causes disease with a healthy copy of the gene
- Inactivating, or "knocking out," a mutated gene that is functioning improperly
- Introducing a new gene into the body to help fight a disease

Although no current specific therapy has been found to cause a permanent cure for an inherited single-gene disorder, this hope for the future is getting closer. In late 2017 the U.S. FDA approved a type of gene therapy to correct a specific genetic defect causing a rare form of retinal dystrophy and blindness. This therapy, known as voretigene neparvovec-rzyl (Luxturna), neither replaces nor removes the defective *RPE65* gene allele but rather causes the insertion of an additional healthy allele into retinal cell DNA. This third allele, when expressed, can result in the person having a significant level of visual improvement, some cases of which have lasted as long as 4 years. The drug as a liquid suspension is injected under the retina in a surgical setting by an ophthalmic surgeon. The long-term effects and outcomes of the therapy are not yet known. The cost of the therapy, which is $850,000.00 for a one-time injection given at separate times to each eye, is a limiting factor for its use.

By definition, gene therapy is still an experimental treatment modality, although many other types of treatments can modify, and sometimes correct, a single-gene disorder. For example, when a hematopoietic stem cell transplant (HSCT) is successfully performed for a variety of single-gene disorders such as sickle cell disease or Gaucher disease, the transplanted cells permanently produce the correct gene product and result in a disease cure. Therefore HSCT is a form of gene therapy. Other drugs and techniques that take advantage of genetic differences in some cancer cells have been effective in controlling cancer. Similar techniques have been used to manage some autoimmune diseases with "biologic" agents. These techniques could be considered a combination of immunotherapy and gene therapy.

In research laboratories, scientists have been able to remove or "splice out" defective genes and replace or "splice in" healthy ones. Often these early techniques used viruses as carriers (vectors) to move the genes into an organism's DNA. Problems with this type of gene replacement therapy are many, and include efficiency of the technique (low), controlling where in a genome the replacement genes were spliced in (not a lot of control), time and expense of the procedures (huge), and duration of expression for the inserted gene (relatively short).

In recent years some technical breakthroughs in "gene editing" have occurred that may speed up the process of true gene therapy for single-gene disorders. The CRISPR/Cascade 9 system has been able to overcome the barriers of efficiency and placement control. CRISPR is short for *c*lustered *r*egularly *i*nterspersed *p*alindromic *r*epeats, which are a type of RNA-guided protection for bacteria against invading viruses. When the RNA sequences are used with the special enzyme system Cascade 9 (Cas9), laboratory-generated gene sequences can be placed in the correct areas of an organism's genome at high efficiency and relatively low costs (Roy et al., 2018; U.S. NIH, 2018). Many other issues with the technique remain, and it may take years or even decades before this gene-editing type of gene therapy becomes a reality. However, just as putting humans on the moon first required development of a rocket capable of reaching the moon, the CRISPR/Cascade 9 system represents a huge first step for the dream of gene therapy.

GET READY FOR THE NEXT-GENERATION NCLEX® EXAMINATION!

Key Points

Review these Key Points for each NCLEX Examination Client Needs Category.

Safe and Effective Care Environment

- Ensure that an adult or family with indications of an increased genetic risk for a disease or disorder is referred to an appropriate genetics professional. **QSEN: Teamwork and Collaboration**
- Advocate for the patient with regard to whether or not to have genetic/genomic testing, informed consent before testing, and sharing of test results. **QSEN: Patient-Centered Care**
- Ensure that confidentiality of genetic/genomic test results is maintained by all health care team members. **QSEN: Safety**

Health Promotion and Maintenance

- Identify patients and families at increased genetic risk for disease or disorder. **QSEN: Patient-Centered Care**
- Teach patients and families at known increased genetic risk for disease or disorder about screening procedures and any appropriate environmental modifications that can reduce risk, delay disease onset, or reduce symptom severity (check specific disorder chapters for the appropriate screening guidelines). **QSEN: Evidence-Based Practice**

Psychosocial Integrity

- Assess patients who have received results of genetic/genomic testing for responses such as anger, guilt, or depression. **QSEN: Patient-Centered Care**
- Ensure that the patient who undergoes genetic/genomic testing is appropriately counseled before testing, while waiting for test results, and after test results are obtained. **QSEN: Teamwork and Collaboration**
- Support the decision of the patient and family to have or not to have genetic counseling or testing. **QSEN: Patient-Centered Care**

Physiological Integrity

- Be aware that mutations or variations in gene sequences can change the activity of a protein and have adverse effects on health.
- Keep in mind that many common adult diseases or disorders have a genetic basis (hypertension, diabetes, cancer), although some of these diseases also may occur among adults with no genetic risk.
- Remind the patient that having a gene variation that increases the risk for a disorder does not necessarily mean the disorder will ever develop.
- Construct a three-generation pedigree from data obtained during the family history section of patient assessment.
- Be prepared to assume the accepted roles of the medical-surgical nurse in genetic counseling, which include examining assessment data for indications of genetic risk, acting as a patient advocate, correcting myths about genetic disorders and genetic/genomic testing, protecting the patient's privacy and rights, and helping to ensure that the patient and family at increased genetic risk are referred to a genetics professional.

MASTERY QUESTIONS

1. Which activity would a medical-surgical nurse be expected perform as part of client-focused genomic care?
   A. Calculating recurrence risk for a woman who was recently diagnosed with unilateral breast cancer
   B. Informing a client that his or her genetic/genomic testing results are positive for a genetic disorder
   C. Obtaining an accurate family history and physical assessment data
   D. Requesting a consultation visit from a clinical geneticist

2. Which observations made by the nurse constructing a client pedigree indicate a probable autosomal-recessive (AR) trait transmission of a health problem? **Select all that apply.**
   A. Siblings are affected when parents are unaffected.
   B. The trait appears to "skip" generations.
   C. Males are affected eight times more often than females.
   D. One affected parent does not have affected children.
   E. The problem is expressed in both siblings in identical (monozygotic) twins.
   F. Males and females are equally affected.
   G. Over five generations, 8 out of 32 family members are affected.

3. What response does the nurse expect for a client who has a normal gene allele and an abnormal gene allele for insulin and the area around the abnormal gene allele is heavily methylated?
   A. Normal insulin is produced in lower-than-normal amounts.
   B. Normal insulin is produced in normal amounts.
   C. Abnormal insulin is produced in high amounts.
   D. No insulin is produced.

4. A client who has been found to have a mutation in a gene allele that greatly increases the risk for future development of polycystic kidney disease that may eventually require kidney transplantation as therapy has received counseling from a genetics professional. The client now asks the nurse who was present during the counseling to be present during disclosure of this information to the family. What is/are the nurse's role(s) in this situation? **Select all that apply.**
   A. Interpreter of the findings
   B. Assurer of the client's correct understanding
   C. Genetic counselor
   D. Client support
   E. Client advocate
   F. Family advocate
   G. Assessor of who might be a kidney donor

REFERENCES

Abbas, A., Lichtman, A., & Pillai, S. (2018). *Cellular and molecular immunology* (9th ed.). Philadelphia: Elsevier.

Cheek, D., & Howington, J. (2017). Patient care in the dawn of the genomic age. *American Nurse Today, 12*(3), 16–21.

Hartstra, A., Bouter, K., Backhed, F., & Nieuwdorp, M. (2015). Insights into the role of the microbiome in obesity and type 2 diabetes. *Diabetes Care, 38*(1), 159–165.

Jorde, L., Carey, J., & Bamshad, M. (2016). *Medical genetics* (5th ed.). Philadelphia: Elsevier.

Lacovara, J., & Bohnenkamp, S. (2018). Genetic testing in oncology for the medical-surgical nurse. *MEDSURG Nursing, 27*(2), 117–120

Lebet, R., Joseph, P., & Aroke, E. (2019). Knowledge of precision medicine and health care: An essential nursing competency. *American Journal of Nursing, 119*(10), 34-42.

McElroy, K., Chung, S.-Y., & Regan, M. (2017). Health and the human microbiome: A primer for nurses. *American Journal of Nursing, 117*(7), 24–30.

Montgomery, S., Brouwer, W., Everett, P., Hassen, E., Lowe, T., McGreal, S., et al. (2017). Genetics in the clinical setting: What nurses need to know to provide the best patient care. *American Nurse Today, 12*(10), 10–15.

Paz De Jesus, M., & Mitchel, M. (2016). Today's nurses need genetics education. *Nursing2016, 46*(10), 68.

Roy, B., Zhao, J., Yang, C., Luo, W., Xiong, T., Fang, X., et al. (2018). CRISPR/Cascade9-mediated genome editing: Challenges and opportunities. *Frontiers in Genetics, 9*(article 240), 1–12. https://www.frontiersin.org/articles/10.3389/fgene.2018.00240.

Starkweather, A., Coleman, B., Barcelona de Mendoza, V., Fu, M., Menzies, V., O'Keefe, M., et al. (2017). Strengthen federal regulation of laboratory-developed and direct-to-consumer genetic testing. *Nursing Outlook, 66*(1), 101–104.

Starkweather, A., Coleman, B., Barcelona de Mendoza, Hickey, K., Menzies, V., Fu, M., et al., The Genomics Nursing & Health Care Expert Panel, & The Informatics & Technology Expert Panel. (2018). Strengthen federal and local policies to advance precision health implementation and nurses' impact on healthcare quality and safety. *Nursing Outlook, 66*(4), 401–406.

Tluczek, A., Twal, M., Beamer, L., Burton, C., Darmofal, L., Kracun, M., et al. (2018). How American Nurses Association code of ethics informs genetic/genomic nursing. *Nursing Ethics, 25*, 1–13.

U.S. Centers for Disease Control and Prevention (2017). Genomics and health impact blog: Direct to consumer genetic testing: Think before you spit, 2017 ed. https://blogs.cdc.gov/genomics/2017/04/18/direct-to-consumer.2/

U.S. Food and Drug Administration. (2018). *Safety communications: The FDA warns against the use of many genetic tests with approved claims to predict patient response to specific medications.* https//www.fda.gov/MedicalDevices/Safety/AlertsandNotices/ucm6247.htm.

U.S. National Institutes of Health (NIH). Department of Health and Human Services (2018). *Genetics Home Reference: What is gene therapy.* https://ghr.nlm.nih.gov/primer/therapy/genetherapy.

7

Concepts of Rehabilitation for Chronic and Disabling Health Problems

Michelle Camicia, Nicole M. Heimgartner

http://evolve.elsevier.com/Iggy/

LEARNING OUTCOMES

1. Identify the roles of each member of the interprofessional rehabilitation team.
2. Identify care organizations within the health system where rehabilitation care is provided.
3. Explain how to use safe patient-handling practices based on current evidence to prevent self-injury.
4. Plan care coordination and transition management for patients with chronic and disabling health problems.
5. Teach patients with chronic and disabling health problems how to prevent complications associated with decreased ***mobility,*** including impaired ***tissue integrity.***
6. Implement patient and family-centered nursing interventions to decrease the psychosocial impact of living with a chronic and disabling health problem.
7. Interpret health assessment findings associated with conditions that require acute or long-term rehabilitation.
8. Create an evidence-based plan of care for the patient who must use assistive-adaptive devices to promote ***mobility*** and ***sensory perception.***
9. Use clinical judgment to plan nursing care to promote health and function in patients in rehabilitative settings.

KEY TERMS

activities of daily living (ADLs) Activities performed in the course of a normal day, such as bathing, feeding, dressing, and ambulating.

activity limitation Difficulty executing an action or task.

aphasia Inability to use or comprehend spoken or written language due to brain injury or disease.

areflexic bladder Urinary retention and overflow (dribbling) caused by injuries or neurologic conditions affecting the lower motor neuron. Also called *flaccid bladder.*

assistive-adaptive device Any item that enables the patient to perform all or part of an activity independently and safely.

assistive technology Electronic equipment that increases the ability of patients who are disabled to care for themselves.

bowel retraining A program for patients with neurologic problems that is designed to include a combination of suppository use and a consistent toileting schedule.

chronic health condition A medical condition that has existed for at least 1 year and requires ongoing medical attention and/or limits activities of daily living (CDC, 2018a).

Credé maneuver Technique used to assist in urination.

disabling health condition Any physical or mental health/behavioral health problem that can cause disability.

disability A broad term that encompasses physical and cognitive impairments, limitations, and restrictions (WHO, 2018).

dysphasia Slurred speech.

impairment An issue with body function or structure.

instrumental activities of daily living (IADLs) Activities necessary for living in the community, such as using the telephone, shopping, preparing food, and housekeeping.

nocturia The need to urinate excessively at night.

orthostatic hypotension A decrease in blood pressure (20 mm Hg in systolic pressure and/or 10 mm Hg in diastolic pressure) that occurs during the first few seconds to minutes after changing from a sitting or lying position to a standing position.

paralysis Absence of movement.

paresis Weakness.

physiatrist A physician who specializes in rehabilitative medicine.

postvoid residual (PVR) The amount of urine remaining in the bladder after voiding.

rehabilitation assistants Assistants to rehabilitation therapists.

rehabilitation therapists The collective group of physical therapists (PRs), occupational therapist (OTs), and speech-language pathologists (SLPs).

resident A person who lives in an inpatient facility and has all the rights of anyone living in his or her home.

robotic technology Technology that provides mechanical parts for extremities when they are not functional or have been amputated.

spastic bladder Incontinence characterized by sudden, gushing voids, usually without complete emptying of the bladder; caused by neurologic problems affecting the upper motor neuron.

work-related musculoskeletal disorders (MSDs) Disorders of the muscles, nerves, tendons, joints, cartilage, and spinal disks that were caused or worsened by working conditions (CDC, 2018b).

PRIORITY AND INTERRELATED CONCEPTS

The priority concepts for this chapter are:

- ***Mobility***
- ***Elimination***
- ***Cognition***

The interrelated concepts for this chapter are:

- ***Tissue Integrity***
- ***Nutrition***
- ***Sensory Perception***
- ***Systems Thinking***

The philosophy of practice and an attitude toward caring for people with disabilities and chronic health conditions is known as rehabilitation (Larsen, 2018). The practice of rehabilitation nursing is recognized as the specialty of managing care of people with disabilities and chronic health conditions across the lifespan. This text focuses primarily on physical health problems; psychosocial health problems are integrated throughout the text as needed to describe whole-person care. They are discussed in more detail in textbooks on mental health/behavioral health nursing.

Patients with chronic and disabling health conditions need the integration of rehabilitation nursing concepts into their care, regardless of setting (e.g., acute care hospital, inpatient rehabilitation, home health), to prevent further disability, maintain function, and restore them to optimal functioning and participation in their community. This desired outcome requires care coordination and collaboration with the patient, the family, and the interprofessional health care team.

OVERVIEW

Chronic and Disabling Health Conditions

Chronic diseases and conditions are among the most common, costly, and preventable of all health problems in the United States. Eighty-six percent of all health care spending in 2010 was for people with one or more chronic health conditions (Gerteis et al., 2014). The rate of chronic and disabling conditions is expected to increase as more "baby boomers" approach late adulthood.

Stroke, coronary artery disease, cancer, chronic obstructive pulmonary disease (COPD), diabetes, asthma, and arthritis are common chronic diseases that can result in varying degrees of disability. Most occur in people older than 65 years. However, younger adults are living longer with potentially disabling genetic disorders that in the past would have shortened life expectancy. Some of these more common disorders are discussed throughout this text.

COVID-19, the most recent global pandemic, has created a new population with intense rehabilitation needs. Some patients with severe COVID-19 symptoms experience debilitating physical changes. New strategies are being developed to begin rehabilitation while patients are still in the hospital with COVID-19, requiring innovative approaches such as virtual therapy and telemedicine (Johns Hopkins, 2020).

Chronic and disabling conditions are not always illnesses (e.g., heart disease); they may also result from accidents. Accidents (e.g., motor vehicle, falls, suicide) are a leading cause of trauma and death among young and middle-age adults. Increasing numbers of people survive accidents with severe injuries because of advances in medical technology and safety equipment such as motor vehicle airbags. As a result, they are often faced with chronic, disabling neurologic conditions such as traumatic brain injury (TBI) and spinal cord injury (SCI). Because people are living longer with chronic and disabling health problems, the need for rehabilitation is increasing.

PATIENT-CENTERED CARE: VETERANS HEALTH CONSIDERATIONS QSEN

Combat in war is another major source of major disability. Many military men and women who served in recent wars such as those in Iraq and Afghanistan have one or more physical or mental health/behavioral health disabilities, most commonly TBI, single or multiple limb amputations, and posttraumatic stress disorder (PTSD). There is also a large population of veterans living with disabilities from wars of the past. These disabilities require months to years of follow-up rehabilitation after return to the community. *Physical* veteran disabilities are described in this text; PTSD is discussed in your mental health/behavioral health book.

Rehabilitation Settings

Many people with chronic and disabling conditions live independently or with assistance in the community. For example, a new-onset condition such as a stroke may require postacute care (PAC) following the initial hospitalization for rehabilitation. This continuing care can be in an acute inpatient rehabilitation facility (IRF), skilled nursing facility (SNF), long-term care hospital (LTCH), or home health agency (HHA). Rehabilitation in each of these health care organizations seeks to minimize activity limitations as a result of an impairment, and to maximize participation in meaningful activities. Each of these care settings varies in the amount and type of rehabilitation and the nursing, health care provider, and other services offered.

People requiring rehabilitation are referred to as *clients, patients,* or *residents,* depending on the setting. For the purpose of consistency within this text, the term *patient* is used throughout this chapter. *However, be sure to refer to people in rehabilitation programs by the term that is consistent with the setting and according to patient preference.*

The determination of the right level of PAC must be based on the patient's biopsychosocial and ecologic assessment (Camicia et al., 2014). Factors that are considered include biologic, social, financial, environmental, and systems factors. Biologic factors include the patient's medical needs, preinjury or preillness level

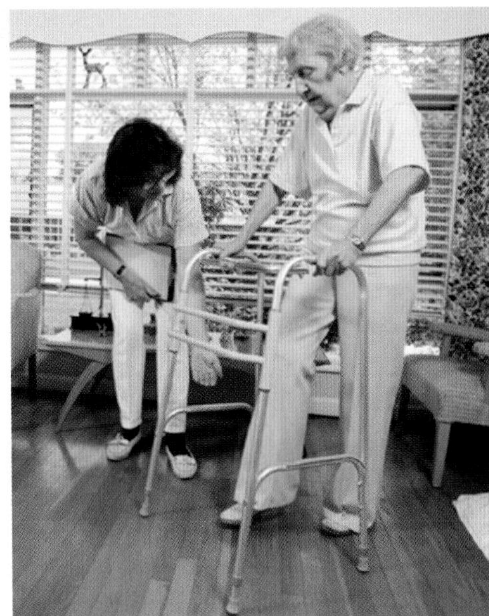

FIG. 7.1 Patient (resident) in a skilled nursing facility rehabilitation unit. (From Potter, P., Perry, A., Stockert, P., Hall, A., & Ostendorf W. [2017]. *Fundamentals of Nursing* [9th ed.]. St. Louis: Mosby.)

of function, and tolerance of rehabilitation. Social factors include psychological, informal, and formal community supports. Other important considerations are financial resources and stressors and the physical environment of the community living setting. Systems factors include the components of care and services, the intensity of service provision (e.g., number of hours of nursing care or therapy), and the structure and process of the program. The PAC setting must be matched to the patients' needs. The nurse coordinates care from acute through community-based care to ensure the person's optimal function and participation in the community.

Rehabilitation care occurs on a continuum. The intensity of services decreases across the continuum from the inpatient rehabilitation facility (IRF) or skilled nursing facility (SNF) to home health to comprehensive ambulatory care (outpatient) programs. The most resource-intensive level of PAC is the IRF. These health care organizations are freestanding rehabilitation hospitals or rehabilitation units within hospitals. Skilled nursing facilities (SNFs)are part of either a hospital or a long-term care (nursing home) setting (Fig. 7.1). For older adults in the United States, rehabilitation services for the first 100 days of inpatient care are paid for by Medicare A.

People in skilled nursing facilities, custodial nursing homes, and assisted-living facilities are called *residents*. The term **resident** implies that the person lives in the facility and has all the rights of anyone living in his or her home. Residents wear street clothes rather than hospital gowns and have choices in what they eat and how they plan each day.

Ambulatory care rehabilitation departments and home rehabilitation programs may be needed for continuing less intensive services. Some agencies have specialized clinics focused on rehabilitation of patients with specific health problems such as those that care for people with strokes; amputations; and large, chronic, and/or nonhealing wounds.

People who are able to rehabilitate to independence or who have a caregiver and an accessible home are able to return home following a disabling medical event. Some people may not be able to return home due to environmental barriers or the absence of a willing and capable caregiver. Alternative living environments include the home of a friend or family, senior citizens' housing units, transitional living apartment, or assisted-living facilities. Part-time rehabilitation services may be provided in any of these home settings by a variety of health care professionals. The cost of these services may be reimbursed by Medicare B or other private health insurance.

Group homes are facilities in which people live independently together with others with disabilities. Each patient or group of patients has a care provider such as a personal care aide to assist with ADLs. The patients may or may not be actively employed. In some cases the care home offers employment opportunities to the residents. The purpose of these homes is to provide independent living arrangements outside an institution, especially for younger people with TBI or SCI.

The desired outcome of rehabilitation is that the patient will return to the best possible physical, mental, social, vocational, and economic capacity and participate fully in society. Rehabilitation is not limited to the return of function in posttraumatic situations. It also includes education and therapy for any chronic conditions characterized by a change in a body system function or body structure. Rehabilitation programs related to neurologic, respiratory, cardiac, and musculoskeletal health problems are common examples that do not involve trauma.

The Rehabilitation Interprofessional Team

Successful rehabilitation depends on the coordinated team effort of the patient, family, and health care professionals in planning, implementing, and evaluating care. The focus of the interprofessional rehabilitation team is to minimize activity limitations and restore and maintain the patient's function to the greatest extent possible.

In addition to the patient, family, and/or significant others, members of the interprofessional health care team in the rehabilitation setting may include:

- Nurses and nursing assistants
- Rehabilitation nurse case managers
- Physicians and physicians assistants
- Advanced practice nurses (APNs) such as nurse practitioners and clinical nurse specialists
- Physical therapists and assistants
- Occupational therapists and assistants
- Speech-language pathologists and assistants
- Rehabilitation assistants/restorative aides
- Recreational or activity therapists
- Cognitive therapists or neuropsychologists
- Social workers
- Clinical psychologists
- Vocational counselors
- Spiritual care counselors
- Registered dietitian nutritionists (RDNs)
- Pharmacists

Not all settings that offer rehabilitation services have all of these members on their team. Not all patients require the services of all health care team members. The team should be

TABLE 7.1 Nurse's Role in the Rehabilitation Team

- Advocates for the patient and family
- Creates a therapeutic rehabilitation milieu
- Provides and coordinates whole-person patient care in a variety of health care settings, including the home
- Collaborates with the rehabilitation team to establish expected patient outcomes to develop a plan of care
- Coordinates rehabilitation team activities to ensure implementation of the plan of care
- Acts as a resource to the rehabilitation team who has specialized knowledge and clinical skills needed to care for patient with chronic and disabling health problems
- Communicates effectively with all members of the rehabilitation team, including the patient and family
- Plans continuity of care when the patient is discharged from the health care facility
- Evaluates the effectiveness of the interprofessional plan of care for the patient and family

Adapted from Association of Rehabilitation Nurses. (2014). *Standards and scope of rehabilitation nursing practice* (6th ed.). Glenview, IL: Author.

TABLE 7.2 Utilizing Systems Thinking to Improve Quality Care

Quality Improvement	The staff have concern that pressure injury quality data are now publicly reported and that facility scores are unfavorable. The staff initiate a quality improvement project with the support of nurse leaders, utilizing the Plan-Do-Study-Act (PDSA) process.
Evidence-Based Practice	The first step in planning is to identify the evidence for providing high-quality care for the prevention of pressure injury. A study was conducted and it was identified that using a reliable and valid risk assessment scale and then developing a plan of care to identify the areas of risk resulted in the absence of pressure injuries.
Clinical Judgment	In studying the problem with the facility skin management team, it was identified that there were many variations in the assessment of skin using the facility pressure injury prevention scale (e.g., Braden Scale). The plan to maintain tissue integrity is dependent on accurate nursing assessment and revision of the plan of care as needed. The variations and inaccuracies of scoring were identified as a root cause for the high incidence of pressure injuries on the unit as the scores provided resulted in a treatment plan that did not adequately address the patient's risk. The staff were provided education to ensure inter-rater reliability and accurate use of the Braden Scale within the facility.
Patient-Centered Care	The staff identified that there is an ethical imperative to implement the evidence-based practices they identified to maintain skin integrity. Proper assessment using a facility-based scale combined with collaboration between the patient, family system, and other health care team members is essential to patient-centered care.

Data from Stalter, A., & Mota, A. (2018). Using systems thinking to envision quality and safety in healthcare. *Nursing Management,* February, 32–39; and Stalter, A., Phillips, J., & Dolansky, M. (2017). QSEN Institute RN-BSN Task Force. White Paper and Recommendation for Systems-Based Practice Competency. *Journal of Nursing Care Quality, 32*(4), 354–358.

composed of providers who are clinically indicated for each patient.

- *Rehabilitation nurses* create a rehabilitation milieu in the care setting, which includes:
- Allowing time for patients to practice self-management skills
- Encouraging patients and providing emotional support
- Promoting self-esteem (e.g., providing emotional support during bowel training for a person with a spinal cord injury [SCI])
- Making the inpatient unit a more homelike environment

Because of an increase in the need for older-adult rehabilitation, some nurses specialize in gerontologic rehabilitation. Nurses and other health care professionals may be designated as *rehabilitation case managers.* Table 7.1 summarizes the nurse's role as part of the rehabilitation team. Nurses caring for people with a disability must know how the components of a complex health care system influence the care of each patient (Dolansky & Moore, 2013). As part of ***systems thinking,*** the nurse uses the primary interrelated concepts of quality improvement, clinical judgment, evidence-based practice, and patient-centered care whether caring for individuals, families, communities, or populations. Table 7.2 provides an example of Systems Thinking in relation to quality care.

A physician who specializes in rehabilitative medicine is called a **physiatrist**. Physiatrists oversee the rehabilitation medical plan of care from the emergency department, intensive care unit, telemetry unit, and medical surgical unit into the community. The physiatrist is the attending physician at the IRF with consultation from other health care providers. They may also provide consultation in the SNF and LTCH.

Physical therapists (PTs), also called *physiotherapists,* intervene to help the patient achieve self-management by focusing on *gross* ***mobility*** skills (e.g., by facilitating ambulation and teaching the patient to use an assistive device such as a walker) (Fig. 7.2). They may also teach techniques for performing activities such as transferring (e.g., moving into and out of bed), ambulating, and toileting. In some settings PTs play a major role in providing wound care. Physical therapy assistants (PTAs) may be employed to help the PT.

Occupational therapists (OTs) work to develop the patient's *fine* motor skills used for ADL self-management such as those required for eating, bathing, grooming, and dressing. They also teach patients how to perform independent living skills such as cooking and shopping. To accomplish these outcomes, OTs teach skills related to coordination (e.g., hand movements) and cognitive retraining (Fig. 7.3). Occupational therapy assistants (OTAs) may be available to help the OT.

Speech-language pathologists (SLPs) evaluate and retrain patients with speech, language, or swallowing problems. *Speech* is the ability to say words, and *language* is the ability

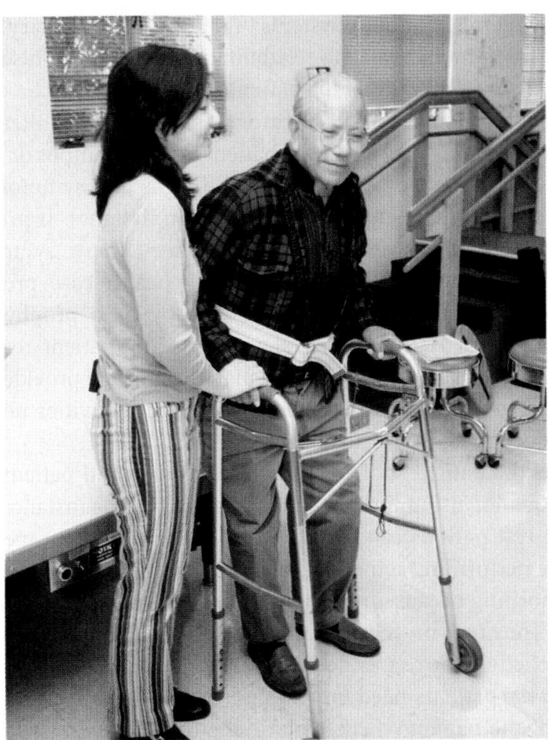

FIG. 7.2 A physical therapist helping a patient ambulate with a walker.

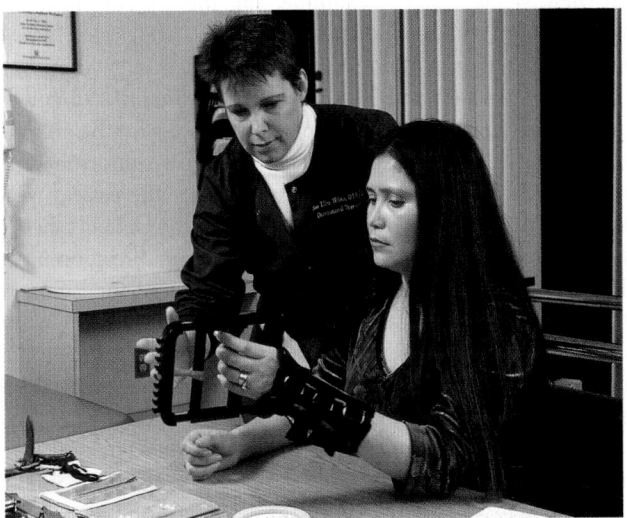

FIG. 7.3 A registered occupational therapist working with a patient on improving hand strength.

to understand and put words together in a meaningful way. Some patients, especially those who have experienced a head injury or stroke, have difficulty with both speech and language. Those who have had a stroke also may have dysphagia (difficulty with swallowing). SLPs provide screening and testing for dysphagia. If the patient has this problem, the SLP recommends appropriate foods and eating techniques. Speech-language pathology assistants (SLPAs) may be employed to help the SLP.

PTs, OTs, and SLPs are collectively referred to as **rehabilitation therapists**. Assistants to PTs, OTs, and SLPs are called **rehabilitation assistants**. In long-term care settings, *restorative aides* may enhance the therapy team to continue the rehabilitation therapy plan of care when therapists are not available.

Recreational or *activity therapists* work to help patients continue or develop recreation or leisure interests to bring meaning to the person's life. These activities may also contribute to strengthening fine motor skills.

Cognitive therapists, usually neuropsychologists, work primarily with patients who have experienced a stroke, brain injury, brain tumor, or other conditions resulting in cognitive impairment. Computer programs are often used to assist with cognitive retraining.

Various professionals promote community reintegration of the patient and acceptance of the disability or chronic conditions. For example, *social workers* help patients identify support services and resources, including financial assistance. *Clinical psychologists* assess and diagnose mental health/behavioral health or ***cognition*** issues resulting from the disability or chronic condition and help both the patient and family identify strategies to foster coping. *Spiritual counselors* specialize in spiritual assessments and care and are able to address the needs of a wide array of patient preferences and beliefs.

Vocational counselors help with job placement, training, or further education. Work-related skills are taught if the patient needs to change careers because of the disability. If the patient has not yet completed high school, tutors may help with completion of the requirements for graduation.

Registered dietitian nutritionist (RDNs) help ensure that patients meet their needs for ***nutrition***. For example, for patients who need weight reduction, a restricted-calorie diet can be planned. For patients who need additional calories or other nutrients, including vitamins, dietitians can plan a patient-specific diet.

Pharmacists collaborate with the other members of the health care team to ensure that the patient receives the most appropriate drug therapy, if required. They oversee the prescription and preparation of medications and provide the interprofessional team with essential information regarding drug safety, interactions, and side effects.

Depending on the patient's health care needs, additional team members may be included in the rehabilitation program such as the geriatrician, respiratory therapist, and prosthetist. Interprofessional team conferences for planning care and evaluating the patient's progress are held regularly with the patient, the family and significant others, and the health care team.

NCLEX EXAMINATION CHALLENGE 7.1

Psychosocial Integrity

The nurse is caring for a 25-year old client with a new spinal cord injury resulting in tetraplegia. The client states, "I won't be able to do any activities that I enjoy now." What is the **priority** nursing intervention?

A. Encourage the client to explore new activities that they can do.
B. Teach the client about reasonable goals for activities.
C. Allow the client time to discuss feelings of loss related to the injury.
D. Consult pastoral care to provide encouragement to the client.

Interprofessional Collaborative Care

Assessment: Recognize Cues

History. Collect the history of the patient's present condition, any current medications (prescribed and over the counter [OTC]), and any treatment programs in progress. Begin by obtaining general background data about the patient and family. This information includes cultural and spiritual practices and the patient's home environment and support system. In collaboration with the occupational therapist, the nurse or case manager assesses the physical layout of the home and determines whether the layout, including stairs or the width of doorways, will present architectural barriers for the patient after discharge.

Assess the patient's usual daily schedule and habits of everyday living. These data include hygiene practices, ***nutrition, elimination,*** sexual activity, and sleep. Ask about the patient's preferred method and time for bathing and hygiene. In assessing dietary patterns, note food likes and dislikes. Also obtain information about the patient's bowel and bladder function and the usual pattern of elimination.

In assessing sexuality patterns, ask about changes in sexual function since the onset of the disability. The patient's current and previous sleep habits, patterns, usual number of hours of sleep, and use of hypnotics are also determined. Question whether the patient feels well rested after sleep. Sleep patterns have a significant impact on activity patterns. The assessment of activity patterns focuses on work, exercise, and recreational activities.

Many people with a disabling health condition require the assistance of a caregiver. Assess the caregiver's commitment and capacity to perform the caregiving role. This includes the caregiver's physical and mental health, financial resources, other roles and responsibilities, and the strength of the relationship (Camicia et al., 2019).

> **PATIENT-CENTERED CARE: OLDER ADULT CONSIDERATIONS** QSEN
>
> Older adults who need rehabilitation often have other chronic diseases that need to be managed, including diabetes mellitus, coronary artery disease, osteoporosis, and arthritis. These health problems, added to the normal physiologic changes associated with aging, predispose older adults to secondary complications such as falls, pressure injuries, and pneumonia. When discharged from the acute care setting, some older patients are undernourished, which causes weakness and fatigue. The longer the hospital stay, the more debilitated the older adult can become. For some patients severe undernutrition results in decreased serum albumin and prealbumin, causing third spacing. Assess the older adult for generalized edema, especially in the lower extremities. Be sure to collaborate with the RDN to improve the patient's nutritional status, with a focus on increasing protein intake that is needed for healing and decreasing edema.
>
> Health teaching may be challenging because some older patients may have beginning changes in ***cognition,*** including short-term memory loss. Sensory loss, like vision and hearing, may also affect their ability to understand new information.

Physical Assessment/Signs and Symptoms. On admission for baseline and at least daily (depending on agency policy and type of setting), collect physical assessment data systematically according to major body systems (Table 7.3). The primary focus of the assessment related to rehabilitation and chronic disease is the *functional* abilities of the patient.

Cardiovascular and Respiratory Assessment. An alteration in cardiac status may affect the patient's cardiac output or cause activity intolerance. Assess associated signs and symptoms of decreased cardiac output (e.g., chest pain, fatigue). If present, determine when the patient experiences these symptoms and what relieves them. The primary health care provider may prescribe a change in drug therapy or a prophylactic dose of nitroglycerin to be taken before the patient resumes activities. Collaborate with the primary health care provider and appropriate therapists to determine whether activities need to be modified.

For the patient showing fatigue, the nurse and patient plan methods for using limited energy resources. For instance, frequent rest periods can be taken throughout the day, especially before performing activities. Major tasks might be performed in the morning because most people have the most energy at that time. The nurse must communicate needs for breaks in the therapy schedule for rest as needed. Schedule nursing care according to the patient's need for rest.

Ask the patient whether he or she has shortness of breath, chest pain, or severe weakness and fatigue during or after activity. *Determine the level of activity that can be accomplished without these symptoms.* For example, can the patient climb one flight of stairs without shortness of breath, or does shortness of breath occur after climbing only two steps?

Gastrointestinal and Nutritional Assessment. Monitor the patient's oral intake and pattern of eating. Assess for the presence of anorexia, dysphagia, nausea, vomiting, or discomfort that may interfere with oral intake. Determine whether the patient wears dentures and, if so, assess the fit. Review the patient's height, weight, hemoglobin and hematocrit levels, serum prealbumin and albumin, and blood glucose levels. (See Chapter 55 for discussion of how to perform a screening for ***nutrition*** status and Chapter 3 for a description of basic nutritional assessments.) Weight loss or weight gain is particularly significant and may be related to an associated disease or to the conditions that caused the disability.

Bowel ***elimination*** habits vary from person to person. They are often related to daily job or activity schedules, dietary patterns, age, and family or cultural background. Ask about usual bowel patterns before the injury or the illness. Note any changes in the patient's bowel routine or stool consistency. The most common problem for rehabilitation patients is constipation.

If the patient reports any alteration in ***elimination*** patterns, try to determine whether it is caused by a change in diet, activity pattern, or medication use. Always assess bowel habits according to what is normal for that person.

Ask whether the patient can manage bowel function independently. Independence in bowel elimination requires adequate cognition, manual dexterity, sensation, muscle control, and mobility. If the patient requires help, provide education to the caregiver on the bowel regimen. Also assess the patient's and family's ability to cope with any dependency in bowel elimination. Assessment of ***elimination*** is summarized in Chapter 3.

TABLE 7.3 Assessment of Patients in Rehabilitation Settings

Body System	Relevant Data
Cardiovascular system	Chest pain Fatigue Fear of heart failure
Respiratory system	Shortness of breath or dyspnea Activity tolerance Fear of inability to breathe
Gastrointestinal system and nutrition	Oral intake, eating pattern Anorexia, nausea, and vomiting Dysphagia Laboratory data (e.g., serum prealbumin level) Weight loss or gain Bowel elimination pattern or habits Change in stool (constipation or diarrhea) Ability to get to toilet
Renal-urinary system	Urinary pattern Fluid intake Urinary incontinence or retention Urine culture and urinalysis
Neurologic system	Motor function Sensation Perceptual ability Cognitive abilities
Musculoskeletal system	Functional ability Range of motion Endurance Muscle strength
Integumentary system	Risk for skin breakdown Presence of skin lesions

Renal and Urinary Assessment. Ask about the patient's baseline urinary ***elimination*** patterns, including the number of voidings. Determine whether he or she routinely awakens during the night to empty the bladder (**nocturia**) or sleeps through the night. Record fluid intake patterns and volume, including the type of fluids ingested and the time they were consumed.

Question whether the patient has ever had any problems with urinary incontinence or retention. Monitor laboratory reports, especially the results of the urinalysis and culture and sensitivity, if needed. *Urinary tract infections (UTIs) among older adults are often missed because acute confusion may be the only indicator of the infection.* Unfortunately, some health care professionals expect older patients to be confused and may not detect this problem. If untreated, UTIs can lead to kidney infection and possible failure.

Neurologic and Musculoskeletal Assessment. The neurologic assessment includes motor function (***mobility***), ***sensory perception***, and ***cognition***. Chapter 3 reviews general assessment of these concepts. Assess the patient's pre-existing problems, general physical condition, and communication abilities. Patients may have dysphasia (slurred speech) or aphasia (inability to express thoughts verbally or comprehend) because of damage to the language centers of the brain commonly occurring in those with a stroke or traumatic brain injury (TBI). These communication problems are discussed in detail in the chapters on problems of the nervous system.

Determine if the patient has paresis (weakness) or paralysis (absence of movement). Observe the patient's gait. Identify changes in ***sensory perception*** such as visual acuity that could contribute to risk for injury. Assess his or her response to light touch, hot or cold temperature, and position change in each extremity and on the trunk. For a perceptual assessment, evaluate the patient's ability to receive and understand what is heard and seen and the ability to express appropriate motor and verbal responses. During this part of the assessment, begin to assess short-term and long-term memory.

Assess the patient's cognitive abilities, especially if there is a brain injury or stroke. The Confusion Assessment Method (CAM) is used to determine if the patient has delirium, an acute confusional state. (See Chapter 4 for description of the CAM tool.)

As with other body systems, nursing assessment of the musculoskeletal system focuses on function. Assess the patient's musculoskeletal status; response to the impairment; and demands of the home, work, or school environment. Determine his or her endurance level and measure active and passive joint range of motion (ROM). Review the results of manual muscle testing by physical therapy, which identifies the patient's ROM and resistance against gravity. In this procedure the therapist determines the degree of muscle strength present in each body segment.

Skin and Tissue Integrity Assessment. Persons with mobility impairments are at high risk for alteration in skin and ***tissue integrity***. This may be magnified by other conditions, such as urinary or fecal incontinence, or poor nutrition. Identify actual or potential interruptions in skin and ***tissue integrity***. Chapter 3 reviews the general assessment of this concept. To maintain healthy skin, the body must have adequate food, water, and oxygen intake; intact waste-removal mechanisms; sensation; and functional ***mobility***. Changes in any of these variables can lead to rapid and extensive skin breakdown.

If a pressure injury or other change in ***tissue integrity*** develops, accurately assess the problem and its possible causes. In the inpatient setting inspect the skin every 8 to 12 hours. Teach the patient or caregiver to inspect the skin daily at home. Measure the depth and diameter of any open skin areas in inches or centimeters, depending on the policy of the facility or country. Assess the area around the open lesion to determine the presence of cellulitis or other tissue damage. Chapter 23 includes several widely used classification systems for assessing skin breakdown. Determine the patient's knowledge about the cause and treatment of skin conditions and his or her ability to inspect the skin and participate in maintaining ***tissue integrity***.

In most health care agencies, the skin assessment is documented on a special form or part of the electronic health record to keep track of each area of skin breakdown. A baseline assessment is conducted on admission and updated periodically, depending on organization policy, and more frequently as indicated. In most long-term care, acute care, and rehabilitation settings and with the patient's (or family's if the patient cannot communicate) permission, photographs of the skin are taken on admission and at various intervals to pictorially document the appearance of the wound.

NCLEX EXAMINATION CHALLENGE 7.2

Physiological Integrity

The rehabilitation nurse is teaching a client with multiple sclerosis who is wheelchair bound strategies to protect skin integrity. Which teaching will the nurse include? **Select all that apply.**

A. Dry the skin carefully after bathing.
B. Do not use pillows to support the body.
C. Apply a moisture barrier on the perineum.
D. Rub reddened areas of skin to help improve circulation.
E. Perform pressure-relief strategies at least once an hour.
F. Use an air mattress to decrease the need for repositioning.

Assessment of Functional Ability. *Functional ability* refers to the ability to perform activities of daily living (ADLs) such as bathing, dressing, eating, using the toilet, and ambulating. Instrumental activities of daily living (IADLs) refer to activities necessary for living in the community such as using the telephone, shopping, preparing food, and housekeeping. Functional assessment tools are used to assess a patient's abilities. Rehabilitation nurses, physiatrists, or rehabilitation therapists complete assessment tools to document functional levels. The Centers for Medicare and Medicaid Services (CMS) requires cross-setting assessment measures to evaluate a patient's function, regardless of the postacute care (PAC) setting where they receive rehabilitation. These tools include functional assessment items for self-care and mobility (Table 7.4) on the Inpatient Rehabilitation Facility Patient Assessment Instrument (IRF-PAI) used in the IRF, the Minimum Data Set (MDS) used in the SNF, and the Outcome and Assessment Information Set (OASIS) used in home health agencies. These assessments are also used for reimbursement from the CMS in the United States.

Another commonly used classic assessment tool is the Functional Independence Measure (FIM) developed by Granger and Gresham (1984). This tool is intended to measure the burden of care for a patient, not what a person should do or how the person would perform under different circumstances. Categories for assessment are self-care, sphincter control, ***mobility*** and locomotion, communication, and ***cognition***. Scoring is on a 1-to-7 scale in which 1 is dependent and 7 is independent. Each score has a definition for every item. The patient is evaluated when he or she is admitted to and discharged from a rehabilitation provider and at other specified times to determine progress toward desired outcomes (also referred to as *goals*). The FIM system has also been adapted for use in across-care settings, including acute care and home care, and is available in multiple languages.

Psychosocial Assessment. In addition to determining ***cognition***, assess the patient's body image and self-esteem through verbal indicators and descriptions of self-care. Encourage the family to allow the patient to independently perform as many functions as possible to build feelings of self-worth.

Assess the patient's use of defense mechanisms and manifestations of anxiety. If indicated, ask him or her to describe feelings concerning the loss of a body part or function. Assess for the presence of any stress-related physical problem. Some patients have symptoms such as fatigue, a change in appetite, or feelings of powerlessness. This may be the result of adjusting to a new disability or signs of depression. See Chapter 8 for a thorough discussion of loss and grieving and Chapter 4 for a brief discussion of depression in the older-adult population.

PATIENT-CENTERED CARE: CULTURAL/SPIRITUAL CONSIDERATIONS QSEN

Determine the availability of support systems for the patient. The major support system is typically the family or significant others; those who do not have these support systems are more likely to develop depression. Ask patients what is important to them and gives meaning to their lives. Identify the patient's cultural, spiritual, and/or religious needs and refer to an appropriate health care team member as needed. Assess sexuality and intimacy needs. Reinforce that many people with disabilities report having a good quality of life.

Vocational Assessment. Patients in the United States should be informed about the Americans With Disabilities Act, which was passed by Congress in 1991 to prevent employer discrimination against people with disabilities. The employer must offer *reasonable* assistance to an employee with a disability to allow him or her to perform the job. For example, if an employee with limited upper extremity mobility caused by a spinal cord injury needs dictation software and an adapted keyboard to perform essential job functions, these should be provided.

The rehabilitation team assesses the cognitive and physical demands of the patient's job to determine whether he or she can return to the position or if retraining in another field is necessary. The physical demands of jobs range from light in sedentary occupations (0 to 10 lb [4.54 kg] often lifted) to heavy (more than 100 lb [45.45 kg] often lifted). The nurse must also consider other required aspects of the job such as ***mobility*** or ***sensory perception*** (e.g., hearing).

Job analysis also involves assessing the work environment of the patient's former or current job. Collaborate with the vocational counselor to determine whether the environment is conducive to the patient's return to work because job modifications may be needed. If an injured worker requires vocational rehabilitation, refer him or her to vocational rehabilitation personnel to evaluate skills and necessary skill development. In many states, Workers' Compensation insurance helps support vocational rehabilitation.

◆ **Analysis: Analyze Cues and Prioritize Hypotheses.** Regardless of age or specific disability, these priority patient problems are common. Additional problems depend on the patient's specific chronic condition or disability. The priority collaborative problems for patients with chronic and disabling health conditions typically include:

1. Decreased ***mobility*** due to neuromuscular impairment, sensory-perceptual impairment, and/or chronic pain
2. Decreased functional ability due to neuromuscular impairment and/or impairment in perception or cognition
3. Risk for pressure injury due to altered sensation and/or altered nutritional state

TABLE 7.4 Cross-Setting Functional Assessment Measures

Functional Domain Examples	Activities Assessed	Measurement Scale and Score
Self-Care	Eating Oral hygiene Toileting hygiene Shower/bathe self Upper body dressing Lower body dressing Putting on/taking off footwear	**Independent:** Patient completes the activity by himself/herself with no assistance from a helper. **Score: 6** **Setup or clean-up assistance:** Helper sets up or cleans up; patient completes activity. Helper assists only prior to or following the activity. **Score: 5** **Supervision or touching assistance:** Helper provides verbal cues and/or touching/steadying and/or contact guard assistance as patient completes activity. Assistance may be provided throughout the activity or intermittently. **Score: 4** **Partial/moderate assistance:** Helper does LESS THAN HALF the effort. Helper lifts, holds, or supports trunk or limbs, but provides less than half the effort. **Score 3** **Substantial/maximal assistance:** Helper does MORE THAN HALF the effort. Helper lifts or holds trunk or limbs and provides more than half the effort. **Score 2** **Dependent:** Helper does ALL of the effort. Patient does none of the effort to complete the activity. Or, the assistance of 2 or more helpers is required for the patient to complete the activity. **Score: 1** **Patients are evaluated on admission, and discharge goals are developed.**
Mobility	Roll left and right Sit to lying Lying to sitting on side of bed Sit to stand Chair/bed to chair transfer Toilet transfer Car transfer Walk 10 feet Walk 50 feet with two turns Walk 150 feet Walking 10 feet on uneven surfaces 1 step up with curb 4 steps up or down 12 steps Picking up objects If in wheelchair, ability to wheel 50 feet with two turns; 150 feet in a corridor	

Data from Centers for Medicare and Medicaid Services (CMS). (2018). Inpatient rehabilitation facility: Patient assessment instrument (IRF-PAI). Retrieved from https://www.cms.gov/Medicare/Quality-Initiatives-Patient-Assessment-Instruments/IRF-Quality-Reporting/Downloads/Final-IRF-PAI-Version-20-Effective-October-1-2018.pdf

TABLE 7.5 Resources for Safe Patient Handling

Organization	Website
American Nurses Association	https://www.nursingworld.org/practice-policy/work-environment/health-safety/handle-with-care
Association of Rehabilitation Nurses	https://rehabnurse.org/resources/position-statements/safe-patient-handling
Centers for Disease Control and Prevention (CDC) National Institute for Occupational Safety and Health (NIOSH)	www.cdc.gov/niosh/topics/safepatient/
U.S. Department of Veterans Affairs (mobile safe patient handling app)	https://mobile.va.gov/app/safe-patient-handling

4. Urinary incontinence or urinary retention due to neurologic dysfunction and/or trauma or disease affecting spinal cord nerves
5. Changes in bowel function due to neurologic impairment, inadequate ***nutrition,*** or decreased mobility

◆ Planning and Implementation: Generate Solutions and Take Action

Increasing Mobility

Planning: Expected Outcomes. The patient with a disabling chronic condition is expected to reach the highest level of physical ***mobility*** that can be obtained with or without assistive devices and be free of complications of immobility.

Interventions. Patients with neurologic disease or injury (e.g., stroke, brain injury, spinal cord injury, tumor), amputations, or other condition resulting in disability usually experience some degree of decreased or impaired physical ***mobility.*** Coordinate care with physical and occupational therapists as the key rehabilitation team members in helping patients meet their mobility outcomes. Complications of decreased ***mobility*** or immobility and how to help prevent them are described in Chapter 3.

Safe Patient Handling and Mobility Practices. Before learning to become independent, patients with decreased ***mobility*** in any health care setting or at home often need assistance with positioning in bed and transfers such as from a bed to a chair, commode, or wheelchair. Patients may not be able to bear full weight due to paralysis or poor strength and/or may have inadequate balance. For many years nurses relied on "body mechanics" to prevent staff injury when assisting patients with mobility. This traditional, but outdated, approach was based on the belief that correct body positioning by staff members would protect them from the force of lifting and moving.

The person with a mobility limitation must be assessed for the level of assistance needed for the specific mobility activity (e.g., bed to chair). The necessary safe patient-handling equipment (e.g., stand-assist device, total lift assistance, friction-reducing surface) must be used to prevent **work-related musculoskeletal disorders (MSDs)**, most often back and shoulder injuries, which can often be prevented. Many online educational resources are available and are listed in Table 7.5.

There is strong evidence that implementation of safe patient-handling practices by nurses reduces occupational-related patient-handling injuries (Teeple et al., 2017; Black et al., 2018). Because each patient has unique needs and characteristics, assess his or her mobility level with a standardized tool to plan interventions for safe patient handling and mobility (SPHM). An example of an appropriate assessment tool for this purpose is shown in Fig. 7.4. Before moving the patient, assess the environment for potential hazards that could cause injury, such as a slippery or uneven floor.

Use these general SPHM practices and teach staff members to:

- Maintain a wide, stable base with your feet.
- Place the bed at the correct height—waist level while providing direct care and hip level when moving patients.
- Keep the patient or work directly in front of you to prevent your spine from rotating.
- Keep the patient as close to your body as possible to prevent reaching.
- Use the appropriate safe patient-handling equipment.

The Veterans Health Administration and many other health care systems follow a no-lift or limited-lift policy for all of their facilities. This means that nurses and therapists either rely on the patient to independently move and transfer or use a powered, mechanical full-body lift that is either ceiling- or wall-mounted or portable (mobile) (Fig. 7.5). Most lifts use slings that are comfortable, safe, and easy to apply. Electric-powered, portable sit-to-stand devices are also available.

For patients who are learning to become independent in transfer or bed ***mobility*** skills, the physical or occupational therapist usually consults with the nurse on the procedure for these maneuvers. For example, a patient with quadriplegia may use a sliding board for transfer, whereas a patient with paraplegia may be able to transfer when the wheelchair arms are removed. A patient may be taught to turn independently using the side rails. In any case, for safety always plan or teach the patient to plan the transfer technique before initiating it. The desired outcome is that the patient will eventually be able to transfer safely, providing his or her maximum effort while assistance is provided by equipment and caregivers as needed.

It is important to include the family or caregiver when teaching the patient mobility and transfer skills. Caregivers commonly report physical strain from efforts to assist older family members. Although many organizations have adopted a no-lift policy, often the equipment that is available in the hospitals is either not available or very different from the equipment that is provided in the home (Powell-Cope et al., 2017). When a caregiver is more confident, the patient experiences more functional independence. See Box 7.1 for specific teaching points and safety reminders for the caregiver.

SYSTEMS THINKING AND QUALITY IMPROVEMENT QSEN

Monitoring Agitation for Improved Care

Wilson, H. J., Dasgupta, K., & Michael, K. (2018). Implementation of the Agitated Behavior Scale in the electronic health record. *Rehabilitation Nursing Journal, 43*(1), 21–25.

Staff at a brain injury unit in an inpatient rehabilitation facility identified that they did not have an objective assessment tool to evaluate agitation in patients as a routine component of clinical practice. This was a barrier to optimal participation in the therapeutic rehabilitation program. An interprofessional team was formed to develop an improvement process to integrate the Agitated Behavior Scale (ABS) into the electronic health record (EHR).

During this three-phase project the nurses were trained regarding the importance of assessing for agitation as well as the potential risk of agitation to overall safety of the patient and the nurse. Use of the ABS was demonstrated using case studies, and nurses were provided positive reinforcement for consistent assessment, response, and documentation of agitation using the ABS. The ABS was integrated into the EHR in addition to a note that included antecedents to the behavior, the ABS score, interventions implemented, and the resulting ABS score.

Medical records were audited, and staff were surveyed regarding the new process. The EHR review revealed an effective management of patients with agitation. Twenty-three nurses participated in the survey. The results indicated 92.2% adherence with the established process in the EHR. The usability of the ABS with the nurses was evaluated using a standardized survey. The nurses indicated an acceptable level of usability.

Commentary: Implications for Research and Practice

This quality improvement change project represents the value of a standardized assessment scale for patients with agitation. Furthermore, this study shows the seamless integration of this assessment into an existing EHR, allowing for consistent assessment and improved recognition of potential agitation triggers for patients with agitation from brain injury. Improved recognition enabled prompt intervention to decrease agitation and foster rehabilitation outcomes. Additional research with a larger sample size using this model for assessment in conjunction with the EHR is suggested to advance safety and thorough assessment in specialty patient populations.

Cognitive impairment can also present unique safety and mobility concerns in the rehabilitation setting. Cognitive impairment can manifest as agitated behavior that may be unpredictable. This behavior can occur as a result of traumatic brain injury but can also be present with other injury to the brain as a result of cancer or stroke. When caring for a patient with cognitive impairment, nurses must implement strategies to prevent injury of the patient and workplace injuries of the nurse. Patients with cognitive impairment may not move as directed or may respond with agitated behavior such as striking, biting, or kicking. Successful nursing care of agitated patients involves assessing patterns of agitation and identifying what is causing the agitation (referred to as the *trigger*). Once the trigger has been identified, the nurse should attempt to decrease exposure to it. For example, if bladder fullness causes agitation, a scheduled bladder management program may be implemented. Monitoring agitation and preventing triggers can decrease safety risks for the patient and the nurse. Identification of triggers and the interventions that decrease agitation are incorporated into a plan of care that is shared with the patient and the family.

! NURSING SAFETY PRIORITY QSEN

Action Alert

Assess the patient and the situation before any transfer. Orthostatic, or postural, hypotension is a common problem and may contribute to falls. If the patient moves from a lying to a sitting or standing position too quickly, his or her blood pressure may drop; as a result, he or she can become dizzy or faint. This problem is worsened by antihypertensive drugs, especially in older adults. To prevent this situation, help the patient change positions slowly, with frequent pauses to allow the blood pressure to stabilize. If needed, measure blood pressure with the patient in the lying, sitting, and standing positions to examine the differences. **Orthostatic hypotension** is indicated by a drop of more than 20 mm Hg in systolic pressure or 10 mm Hg in diastolic pressure between positions. Notify the health care provider and the therapists about this change.

If the patient has problems maintaining blood pressure while out of bed, the physical therapist may start him or her on a tilt table to gradually increase tolerance. Low blood pressure is a particularly common problem for patients with quadriplegia because they have a delayed blood flow to the brain and upper part of the body.

Weight gain as a result of a decreased metabolic rate is another potential problem for patients with decreased ***mobility***. Excessive weight hinders transfers both for the health care professional or caregiver who is assisting with mobility and for the patient who is learning to transfer independently. Weight is usually checked every week to monitor gains or losses. If needed, collaborate with the dietitian to develop a weight-reduction plan.

Gait Training. The physical therapist works with patients for gait training if ambulation is a realistic goal. While regaining the ability to ambulate, patients may need to use assistive devices such as a variety of canes or walkers (Fig. 7.6). The specific device selected for each patient depends on the amount of weight bearing that is allowed or tolerated. For example, a stroke patient who has problems with maintaining balance or a steady gait when walking might need a cane that provides greater steadying. Some patients use walkers with rollers (e.g., tennis-ball material); others who tire easily may need a walker with a built-in seat to rest at intervals (sometimes referred to as a *rollator*). A patient who had a total hip replacement 6 weeks ago may be able to use a straight (also called *single-point*) cane.

When working with patients who are using these devices, also known as ambulatory aids, the physical therapist ensures that there is a level surface on which to walk. The therapist or nurse may use a gait belt to guide him or her during ambulation to help prevent falls.

Reinforce the physical therapist's instructions and encourage practice, with the outcome being optimal mobility for the person. See the Best Practice for Patient Safety & Quality Care: Gait Training With Selected Ambulatory Aids box about teaching patients how to use ambulatory aids.

Some patients never regain the ability to walk because of their impairment such as advanced multiple sclerosis or complete spinal cord injury. They may require the use of a wheelchair and need to learn wheelchair or motorized-scooter mobility skills. With the help of physical and occupational therapy, most patients can learn to move anywhere in a wheelchair or electric scooter. For example, patients with high cervical injuries resulting in quadriplegia may require a motorized wheelchair that can be directed and propelled by moving their head or blowing into a device. A patient with severe, advanced multiple sclerosis may use a scooter because of fatigue or mobility impairment.

BEST PRACTICE FOR PATIENT SAFETY & QUALITY CARE QSEN

Gait Training With Selected Ambulatory Aids

Walker-Assisted Procedure

- Apply a transfer belt around the patient's waist.
- Guide the patient to a standing position.
- Remind the patient to place both hands on the walker.
- Ensure that the patient's body is well balanced.
- Teach the patient repeatedly to perform this sequence:
  - Lift the walker.
  - Move the walker about 2 feet forward and set it down on all legs.
  - While resting on the walker, take small steps.
  - Check balance.
  - Repeat the sequence.

Cane-Assisted Procedure

- Apply a transfer belt around the patient's waist.
- Guide the patient to a standing position.
- Be sure the cane is at the height of the patient's wrist when the arm is placed at his or her side. (Many canes can be adjusted to the required height.)
- Remind the patient to place his or her strong hand on the cane.
- Ensure that the patient's body is well balanced.
- Teach the patient to perform this sequence repeatedly:
  - Move the cane and weaker leg forward at the same time.
  - Move the stronger leg one step forward.
  - Check balance and repeat the sequence.

One way to increase ***mobility*** is through range of motion (ROM) exercises. ROM techniques are beneficial for any patient with decreased mobility. Specific ROM techniques are presented in your basic foundations nursing textbook.

Increasing Functional Ability

Planning: Expected Outcomes. The patient with chronic conditions or disability is expected to increase functional ability in self-care and other self-management skills with or without assistive-adaptive devices.

Interventions. ADLs, or self-care activities, include eating, bathing, dressing, grooming, and toileting. Encourage the patient to perform as much self-care as possible. Allow time to complete the task as independently as possible. Collaborate with the occupational therapist (OT) to identify ways in which self-care activities can be modified so the patient can perform them as independently as possible and with minimal frustration. For example, teach a patient with hemiplegia to put on a shirt by first placing the affected arm in the sleeve, followed by the unaffected arm. Slip-on shoes or shoes with Velcro straps may be recommended for some patients. Encourage patients to practice and allow them time to try to be independent in ADLs.

In SNF settings federal regulations require that the health care providers have a plan to prevent residents from losing their

Assessment Tool and Care Plan for Safe Patient Handling and Movement

I. Patient's Level of Assistance

____Independent—Patient performs task safely, with or without staff assistance, with or without assistive devices.
____Partial Assist—Patient requires no more help than standby, cueing, or coaxing, or caregiver is required to lift no more than 35 lb of a patient's weight.
____Dependent—Patient requires nurse to lift more than 35 lb of the patient's weight, or patient is unpredictable in the amount of assistance offered. In this case, assistive devices should be used.

An assessment should be made before each task if the patient has a varying level of ability to assist because of medical reasons, fatigue, medications, etc. When in doubt, assume the patient cannot assist with the transfer/repositioning.

II. Weight-Bearing Capability

____Full
____Partial
____None

III. Bilateral Upper-Extremity Strength

____Yes
____No

IV. Patient's Level of Cooperation and Comprehension

____Cooperative—May need prompting; able to follow simple commands.
____Unpredictable or variable (patient whose behavior changes frequently should be considered unpredictable)—Not cooperative or unable to follow simple commands.

V. Weight________ **Height** ________

Body Mass Index (BMI) (needed if patient's weight is over 300 lb)*
If BMI exceeds 50, institute Bariatric Algorithms.

The presence of the following conditions is likely to affect the transfer/repositioning process and should be considered when identifying equipment and techniques needed to move the patient.

VI. Check Applicable Conditions Likely to Affect Transfer/Repositioning Techniques

____Hip/knee/shoulder replacements
____History of falls
____Paralysis/paresis
____Unstable spine
____Severe edema
____Very fragile skin
____Respiratory/cardiac compromise
____Wounds affecting transfer/positioning
____Amputation
____Urinary/fecal stoma
____Contractures/spasms
____Tubes (IV, chest, etc.)
____Fractures
____Splints/traction
____Severe osteoporosis
____Severe pain/discomfort
____Postural hypotension

Comments:____
____
____
____
____

VII. Appropriate Lift/Transfer Devices Needed

Vertical Lift:
Horizontal Lift:
Other Patient-Handling Devices Needed:

Sling Type

____Seated
____Supine
____Seated (Amputee)
____Ambulation
____Standing
____Limb Support

Sling Size ________

Signature ______________________________ **Date** ____________

*If patient weighs more than 300 lb, the BMI is needed. For online BMI table and calculator, see http://www.nhlbi.nih.gov/guidelines/obesity/bmi_tbl.htm.

FIG. 7.4 Example of a tool to assess physical mobility.

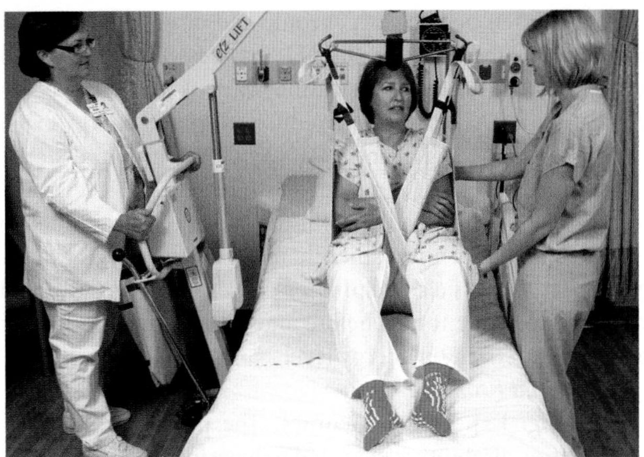

FIG. 7.5 Example of powered, mechanical full-body lift. (From Potter, P., Perry, A., Stockert, P., Hall, A., & Ostendorf, W. [2017]. *Fundamentals of nursing* [9th ed.]. St. Louis: Mosby.)

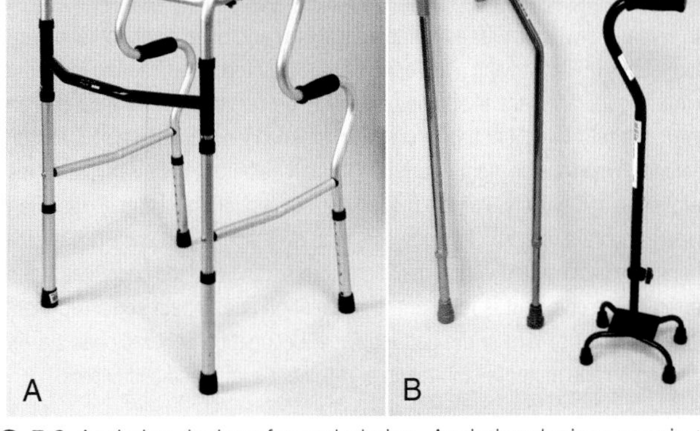

FIG. 7.6 Assistive devices for ambulation. Assistive devices vary in the amount of support they provide. A straight (single-point) cane **(B)** provides less support than a walker (A) or quadripod cane (B).

BOX 7.1 Caregiver Safety

Transfer From a Chair to Standing
- Chose a sturdy chair with arms.
- Remind the care recipient to scoot forward in the chair.
- Encourage the use of both hands to push down on the chair when rising. Do not place both hands on a walker or grab bar to pull up.
- Lean forward to stand (nose over toes).

Transfer From Lying to Sitting up in Bed
- Encourage the care recipient to push up, using the forearms while sliding the legs off the side of the bed.

Car Transfer
- Remind the care recipient to push off the seat. Do not use the car door to pull upward.
- Have the care recipient turn in the seat so that both feet are firmly on the ground before attempting to stand.
- If transferring to a wheelchair, make sure the wheelchair is in a locked position.

Shower and Bathtub Transfers
- Never use the towel bars for support. These are not anchored and are not designed to bear supportive weight.
- Remind the care recipient about the edge of the tub or shower, assisting to navigate if necessary. A shower bench or a transfer bench can be used to help the patient scoot across; both are common mobility aides used in the home.

General Reminders
- When lifting, remember to reduce the load whenever possible. If using a wheelchair, the weight can be reduced by removing the seat and the leg rests allowing for easier lifting.
- It is instinctive to grab the patient's arm to assist. Avoid grabbing the arm or pulling the arm to assist. Rather, provide support with your hand on the low back.

Adapted from Powell-Cope, G., Pippins, K., & Young, H. (2017). Teaching family caregivers to assist safely with mobility. *American Journal of Nursing, 117*(12).

functional skills while they are in the facility. Most facilities have developed *restorative nursing* programs and have coordinated these programs with rehabilitation therapy and activities therapy. The focus of this coordinated effort includes:
- Bed mobility
- Walking
- Transfers
- Dressing
- Grooming
- Active range of motion
- Communication

A variety of devices are available for patients with chronic conditions and disability for *assisting with self-care*. An **assistive-adaptive device** is any item that enables the patient to perform all or part of an activity independently and safely. Examples include long-handled shoehorns and "reachers" to prevent bending and losing one's balance. Table 7.6 identifies common devices and describes their use.

Many medical equipment stores and large pharmacies carry clothing and assistive-adaptive devices designed for patients with disabilities. The occupational therapist determines the specific needs for this equipment. Collaborate with the occupational therapist to look for creative and inexpensive alternatives to meeting these needs. For example, barbecue tongs may be used as "reachers" for pulling up pants or obtaining items on high shelves. A foam curler with the plastic insert removed may be placed over a pencil or eating utensil to make a built-up device. The patient might use an extended shoehorn to operate light switches from wheelchair height. Hook-and-loop fasteners (Velcro) sewn on clothes can prevent the frustrations caused by buttons and zippers.

Assistive technology has further increased the ability of people with disabilities to care for themselves. For example, room lights, door locks, mobile devices, telephones, and computer keyboards can be operated by voice-activation devices. **Robotic technology** provides mechanical parts for the extremities when they are not functional or have been amputated. However, the cost of these aids has prevented their widespread use.

CLINICAL JUDGMENT CHALLENGE 7.1

Teamwork and Collaboration; Safety

A 76-year-old woman was admitted from acute care to the inpatient rehabilitation facility (IRF) following a fall at home that resulted in hip fracture, requiring a total hip replacement. In addition, the client broke her left wrist and index finger in the fall. The client has a functional independence measure of 3. History includes hypertension, poorly controlled type II diabetes mellitus, hypercholesterolemia, and anxiety. Prior to the fall and subsequent hip surgery, the client lived at home alone; she has one son, who lives across the country. Physical therapy was consulted within the acute care setting and the client has transferred to the chair but is resistant to ambulation due to pain and anxiety and does not want to turn in the bed regularly. Occupational therapy has started working on fine motor rehabilitation of the client's left hand and fingers.

1. **Recognize Cues:** What assessment information in this client situation is the most important and immediate concern for the nurse? (Hint: Identify the **relevant** information first to determine what is most important.)
2. **Analyze Cues:** What client conditions are consistent with the **most relevant** information? (Hint: Think about priority collaborative problems that support and contradict the information presented in this situation.)
3. **Prioritize Hypotheses:** Which possibilities or explanations are **most likely** to be present in this client situation? Which possibilities or explanations are the most serious? (Hint: Consider all possibilities and determine their urgency and risk for this client.)
4. **Generate Solutions:** What actions would most likely achieve the desired outcomes for this client? Which actions should be **avoided** or are **potentially harmful?** (Hint: Determine the desired outcomes first to decide which interventions are appropriate and those that should be avoided.)
5. **Take Action:** Which actions are the most appropriate and how should they be implemented? In what **priority order** should they be implemented? (Hint: Consider health teaching, documentation, requested health care provider orders or prescriptions, nursing skills, collaboration with or referral to health team members, etc.)
6. **Evaluate Outcomes:** What client assessment would indicate that the nurse's actions were **effective**? (Hint: Think about signs that would indicate an improvement, decline, or unchanged client condition.)

Fatigue often occurs with chronic and disabling conditions. Therefore collaborate with the OT to assess the patient's self-care abilities and determine possible ways of *conserving energy*. Preparation for ADLs can help reduce effort and energy expenditure (e.g., gathering all necessary equipment before starting grooming routines). If a patient has high energy levels in the morning, he or she can be taught to schedule energy-intensive activities in the morning rather than later in the day or evening. Spacing activities is also helpful for conserving energy. In addition, allowing time to rest before and after eating and toileting decreases the strain on energy level.

Preventing Pressure Injury

Planning: Expected Outcomes. The patient with chronic conditions or disability is expected to have intact skin and ***tissue integrity***.

Interventions. *The best intervention to prevent pressure injury and maintain* ***tissue integrity*** *is frequent position changes in combination with adequate skin care and sufficient nutritional intake. Teach staff to assist with turning and repositioning at least every 2 hours* if patients are unable to perform this activity independently. This time frame may not be sufficient for people who are frail and have thin skin, especially older adults. To determine the best turning schedule, assess the patient's skin condition during each turning and repositioning. For example, if the patient has been sleeping and the nursing assistant decides to postpone turning and repositioning, reddened areas over the bony prominences may be present. If reddened areas do not fade within 30 minutes after pressure relief or do not blanch, they may be classified as pre–pressure injury areas, or stage I pressure areas (see Chapter 23).

Patients who sit for prolonged periods in a wheelchair need to be repositioned at least every 1 to 2 hours. Each patient is evaluated by the physical or occupational therapist for the best seating pad or cushion that is comfortable yet reduces pressure on bony prominences. Patients who are able are taught to perform pressure relief by using their arms to lift their buttocks off the wheelchair seat for 20 seconds or longer every hour or

TABLE 7.6 Examples and Uses of Common Assistive-Adaptive Devices

Device	Use
Buttonhook	Threaded through the buttonhole to enable patients with weak finger mobility to button shirts Alternative uses include serving as pencil holder
Extended shoehorn	Assists in the application of shoes for patients with decreased mobility or ability to reach Alternative uses include turning light switches off or on while patient is in a wheelchair
Plate guard and spork (spoon and fork in one utensil)	Applied to a plate to assist patients with weak hand and arm mobility to feed themselves; spork allows one utensil to serve two purposes
Gel pad	Placed under a plate or glass to prevent dishes from slipping and moving Alternative uses include placement under bathing and grooming items to prevent them from moving
Foam buildups	Applied to eating utensils to help patients with weak hand grip Alternative uses include application to pens and pencils to assist with writing or over a buttonhook to assist with grasping the device
Hook and loop fastener (Velcro) straps	Applied to utensils, a buttonhook, or a pencil to slip over the hand and provide a method of stabilizing the device when the patient's hand grasp is weak
Long-handled reacher	Assists in obtaining items located on high shelves or at ground level for patients who are unable to change positions easily
Elastic shoelaces or Velcro shoe closure	Eliminates the need for tying shoes

more often if needed (sometimes referred to as *wheelchair push-ups*). The PT or OT helps them strengthen their arm muscles in preparation for performing pressure relief.

Many patients with neurologic problems have decreased or absent sensation and may not be able to feel the discomfort of increased pressure. Check any areas where there may be pressure, including places such as the lower legs where the leg of the wheelchair could rub against the skin.

Adequate skin care is an essential component of prevention. Perform or help patients complete skin care each time they are turned, repositioned, or bathed. Delegate and supervise skin care to assistive personnel (AP), including cleaning soiled areas, drying carefully, and applying a moisturizer. If a patient is incontinent, use topical barrier creams or ointments to help protect the skin from moisture, which can contribute to skin breakdown. To prevent damage to the already fragile capillary system, teach AP to avoid rubbing reddened areas. Instead, carefully observe the areas for further breakdown and relieve pressure on the areas as much as possible. Bed pillows are often good pressure-relieving devices. (See Chapter 23 for a complete discussion of skin care interventions.)

Sufficient ***nutrition*** is needed both to repair wounds and to prevent pressure injuries. Collaborate with the dietitian to assess the patient's food selection and ensure that it contains adequate protein and carbohydrates. Both the nurse and the dietitian closely monitor the patient's weight and serum prealbumin levels. If either of these indices decreases significantly, he or she may need high-protein, high-carbohydrate food supplements (e.g., milkshakes) or commercial preparations. Chapter 55 describes nutritional supplementation in detail.

Pressure-relieving or pressure-reducing devices include air mattresses, low–air loss overlays or beds, and air-fluidized beds. Mattress overlays such as air and replacement mattresses are often effective in reducing pressure. *The use of any mechanical device (except air-fluidized beds) does not eliminate the need for turning and repositioning.* Chapter 23 describes skin care in detail.

Establishing Urinary Continence

Planning: Expected Outcomes. Most patients with chronic conditions or disability are expected to have normal patterns of urinary ***elimination*** without retention, infection, or incontinence.

Interventions. Neurologic disabilities often interfere with successful bladder control. These disabilities result in two basic functional types of neurogenic bladder: overactive (e.g., reflex or spastic bladder) and underactive (e.g., hypotonic or flaccid bladder).

An overactive **spastic** (upper motor neuron) **bladder** causes incontinence with sudden voiding. The bladder does not usually empty completely, and the patient is at risk for urinary tract infection. Neurologic problems affecting the upper motor neuron typically occur in patients with strokes or with high-level spinal cord injuries (cervical) or those above the mid-thoracic region. These injuries result in a failure of impulse transmission from the lower spinal cord areas to the cortex of the brain. When the bladder fills and transmits impulses to the spinal cord, the patient cannot perceive the sensation. Because there is no injury to the *lower* spinal cord and the voiding reflex arc is intact, the efferent (motor) impulse from a distended bladder is relayed, and the bladder contracts.

Nonpharmacologic Management. An underactive flaccidor **areflexic** (lower motor neuron) **bladder** results in urinary retention and overflow (dribbling). Injuries that damage the lower motor neuron at the spinal cord level of S2-4 (e.g., multiple sclerosis, spinal cord injury or tumor below T12) may directly interfere with the reflex arc or may result in inaccurate interpretation of impulses to the brain. The bladder fills, and afferent (sensory) impulses conduct the message via the spinal cord to the brain cortex. Because of the injury, the impulse is not interpreted correctly by the bladder center of the brain, and there is a failure to respond with a message for the bladder to contract.

Patients who cannot completely empty their bladder are at risk for postvoid residual urine and subsequent possible urinary tract infection. **Postvoid residual (PVR)** is the amount of urine remaining in the bladder after voiding. PVR assessments using a noninvasive ultrasound device called the *BladderScan* are performed by nurses at the bedside. The residual amount measured is accurate if the device is used correctly. Obesity may interfere with accuracy. The outcome of bladder ultrasonography is to prevent the unnecessary use of an indwelling urinary catheter. Long-term urinary catheters cause urinary tract infections that are often chronic. A picture of the BladderScan device is in Chapter 60.

The nurse can teach a variety of techniques to assist the patient in bladder management, including (Table 7.7):

- Facilitating, or triggering, techniques
- Intermittent catheterization
- Consistent scheduling of toileting routines ("timed void")

TABLE 7.7 Management of Neurogenic Bladder

Functional Type	Neurologic Disability	Dysfunction	Re-establishing Voiding Patterns
Reflex (spastic)	Upper motor neuron spinal cord injury above T12	Urinary frequency, incontinence but may not empty completely	Triggering or facilitating techniques Drug therapy, as appropriate Bedside bladder ultrasound Intermittent catheterization Consistent toileting schedule Indwelling urinary catheter (as last resort) Increased fluids
Flaccid	Lower motor neuron spinal cord injury below T12 (affects S2-4 reflex arc)	Urinary retention, overflow	Valsalva and Credé maneuvers Increased fluids Intermittent or indwelling urinary catheterization

These techniques may not be as effective in patients with physiologic changes associated with aging, including stress incontinence in women with weak pelvic floor muscles and overflow incontinence in men with enlarged prostate glands.

Facilitating (triggering) techniques are used to stimulate voiding. If there is an upper motor neuron problem but the reflex arc is intact (reflex bladder pattern), the voiding response can be initiated by any stimulus that sends the message to the spinal cord level S2-4 that the bladder might be full. Such techniques include stroking the medial aspect of the thigh, pinching the area above the groin, massaging the peno-scrotal area, pinching the posterior aspect of the glans penis, and providing digital anal stimulation.

When the patient has a lower motor neuron problem, the voiding reflex arc is not intact (flaccid bladder pattern), and additional stimulation may be needed to initiate voiding. Two techniques used to facilitate voiding are the Valsalva maneuver and the Credé maneuver. For the Valsalva maneuver, teach the patient to hold his or her breath and bear down as if trying to defecate. This technique should not be used by a spinal cord–injured patient who is at risk for bradycardia as a result of loss of vagus nerve control. Help the patient perform the Credé maneuver by placing his or her hand in a cupped position directly over the bladder area. Then instruct him or her to push inward and downward gently as if massaging the bladder to empty.

Intermittent catheterization may be needed for a flaccid or spastic bladder. Initially a urinary catheter is inserted to drain urine every few hours—after the patient has attempted voiding and has used the Valsalva and Credé maneuvers. If less than 100 to 150 mL of postvoid residual is obtained, the nurse typically increases the interval between catheterizations. *The patient should not go beyond 8 hours between catheterizations.* If intermittent self-catheterization is needed at home after discharge from the rehabilitation facility, the patient may use a specialized appliance to help perform the procedure, especially if he or she has problems with manual dexterity. For those who cannot catheterize themselves, a family member or significant other may need to be taught how to perform the procedure.

Most patients who need intermittent catheterization have chronic bacteriuria (bacteria in the urine with a positive culture), especially those with spinal cord injury (SCI). Unless the patient has symptoms of a urinary tract infection (UTI) such as fever or burning when voiding, the infection is not treated. *Older adults may become acutely confused as the only indication of a UTI.*

Consistent toileting routines may be the best way to re-establish voiding continence when the patient has an overactive bladder. Assess the patient's previous voiding pattern and determine his or her daily routine. At a minimum the nurse or nursing staff helps the patient void after awakening in the morning, before and after meals, before and after physical activity, and at bedtime. *Remind the staff to toilet the patient every 2 hours during the day and every 3 to 4 hours at night.*

Consider the patient's bladder capacity, which may range from 100 to 500 mL; ***mobility*** limitations; and restrictive clothing. Bladder capacity is determined by measuring urine output. Ensure that the patient is aware of nearby bathrooms at all times or has a call system to contact the nurse or assistive personnel for assistance. Chapter 61 also describes methods of achieving bladder control.

PATIENT-CENTERED CARE: OLDER ADULT CONSIDERATIONS QSEN

When urinary antispasmodic drugs are used in older adults, observe for, document, and report hallucinations, delirium, or other acute cognitive changes caused by the anticholinergic effects of the drugs.

Drug Therapy. Drugs are not commonly used for urinary ***elimination*** problems. Mild overactive bladder problems may be treated with antispasmodics such as oxybutynin, solifenacin, or tolterodine to prevent incontinence on a short-term basis.

Patients with symptomatic UTIs are managed with short-term antibiotics such as trimethoprim or trimethoprim/sulfamethoxazole. Patients who have frequent UTIs may be placed on pulse antibiotic therapy in which they alternate 1 week of antibiotic therapy with 3 weeks without antibiotics. Report progress in bladder training to the rehabilitation team so the best decision regarding drug therapy can be made.

Establishing Bowel Continence

Planning: Expected Outcomes. The patient with chronic conditions or disability is expected to have regular evacuation of stool without constipation. If possible, patients control their bowel ***elimination*** schedule.

Interventions. Neurologic problems often affect the patient's bowel pattern by causing a reflex (spastic) bowel, a flaccid bowel, or an uninhibited bowel. Bowel retraining programs are designed for each patient to best meet the expected outcomes (Table 7.8). Pires et al. (2018) found that the management of bowel dysfunction with an effective program can enhance the quality of life for patients who have a spinal cord injury (SCI).

Upper motor neuron diseases and injuries such as a cervical or mid-level spinal cord injury (e.g., quadriplegia) may result in a reflex (spastic) bowel pattern, with defecation occurring suddenly and without warning. With this intact reflex pattern, any facilitating or triggering mechanism may lead to defecation if the lower colon contains stool. An example of facilitating or triggering techniques is digital stimulation. For this technique, use a lubricated glove or finger cot and massage the anus in a circular motion for no less than 1 full minute.

NURSING SAFETY PRIORITY QSEN

Action Alert

Do not use digital stimulation for patients with cardiac disease because of the risk for inducing a vagal nerve response. This response causes a rapid decrease in heart rate (bradycardia).

Lower motor neuron diseases and injuries (e.g., paraplegia) interfere with transmission of the nervous impulse across the reflex arc and may result in a flaccid bowel pattern, with defecation occurring infrequently and in small amounts. The use of manual disimpaction may get the best results. Some patients also need oral laxatives and/or stool softeners. Digital stimulation or suppositories are usually unsuccessful because of loss of the reflex for elimination.

TABLE 7.8 Management of Neurogenic Bowel

Functional Type	Neurologic Disability	Dysfunction	Re-establishing Defecation Patterns
Reflex (spastic)	Upper motor neuron spinal cord injury above T12	Defecation without warning, but may not empty completely	Triggering mechanisms Facilitation techniques High-fiber diet Increased fluids Laxative use (for some patients) Consistent toileting schedule Manual disimpaction
Flaccid	Lower motor neuron spinal cord injury below T12 (affects S2-4 reflex arc)	Usually absent stools for patients with complete lesions	Triggering or facilitating techniques Increased fluids High-fiber diet Suppository use Consistent toileting schedule Manual disimpaction

Neurologic injuries that affect the brain may cause an uninhibited bowel pattern, with frequent defecation, urgency, and reports of hard stool. Patients may manage uninhibited bowel patterns through a consistent toileting schedule, a high-fiber diet, and the use of stool softeners.

In some cases patients are not able to regain their previous level of control over their bowel function. The rehabilitation team assists in designing a bowel ***elimination*** program that accommodates the disability.

Collaborate with patients to schedule bowel ***elimination*** as close as possible to their previous routine. For example, a patient who had stools at noon every other day before the illness or injury should have the bowel program scheduled in the same way. An exception is the patient who prefers another time that best fits into his or her daily routine. If he or she is employed during the day, a time-consuming bowel elimination program in the morning may not work. The bowel protocol can then be changed to the evening when there is more time.

Bowel retraining programs for patients with neurologic problems are often designed to include a combination of methods. Although drug therapy should not be a first choice when formulating a bowel training program, consider the need for a suppository if the patient cannot re-establish defecation habits through a consistent toileting schedule, dietary modification, or digital stimulation.

Bisacodyl, a commonly used laxative, may be prescribed either rectally or orally as part of a bowel training program. Suppositories must be placed against the bowel wall to stimulate the sacral reflex arc (if intact) and promote rectal emptying.

PATIENT-CENTERED CARE: OLDER ADULT CONSIDERATIONS QSEN

Many rehabilitation patients are at high risk for constipation, especially older adults. Encourage fluids (at least eight glasses a day) and 20 to 35 g of fiber in the diet. Teach patients to eat two to three daily servings of whole grains, legumes, and bran cereals and five daily servings of fruits and vegetables. Do not offer a bedpan for toileting. Instead, be sure that the patient sits upright on a bedside commode or bathroom toilet to facilitate defecation. Additional information regarding managing constipation can be found in Chapter 3.

Results occur in 15 to 30 minutes. Administer the suppository when the patient expects to defecate (e.g., after a meal) to coincide with the gastrocolic reflex. Using the suppository every second or third day is usually effective in re-establishing defecation patterns for patients with upper motor neuron problems where the reflex arc is not damaged.

NCLEX EXAMINATION CHALLENGE 7.3

Physiological Integrity

The nurse is caring for a client with a complete spinal cord injury resulting in paraplegia. Which client statement indicates understanding of a bowel retraining program?

A. "I'll use a suppository to help empty my rectum."
B. "I will avoid stool softeners so I don't experience diarrhea."
C. "I'll eat high-fiber foods each day to help prevent constipation."
D. "Digital stimulation for 1 full minute may be needed in order to produce stool."

Care Coordination and Transition Management. Care coordination and transition management begin at the time of the patient's admission. If the patient is transferred from a hospital to an inpatient rehabilitation facility (IRF) or skilled nursing facility (SNF), orient him or her to the change in routine and emphasize the goal of optimal independence in performing self-care activities. When the patient is admitted, a case manager and/or occupational therapist (OT)/physical therapist (PT) assess his or her current living situation at home. Together with the patient and family or significant others, they determine the adequacy of the current situation and the potential needs after discharge to home. The patient with chronic conditions and disability may require home care, assistance with ADLs, nursing care, or physical or occupational therapy after discharge.

Other health care professionals may be necessary to meet the patient's needs. For example, patients with traumatic brain injury (TBI) may benefit from life planning—a process that examines and plans to meet lifelong needs. External case managers specializing in life planning may be part of the interprofessional rehabilitation team.

Home Care Preparation. Before the patient returns home, the nurse assesses his or her readiness for discharge from the institutional setting. The home may be assessed in multiple ways and points in time.

Predischarge Assessment. Before discharge the home must be assessed to ensure accessibility for the patient, given a new mobility impairment. This may be completed by having the family videotape or photograph the home and provide measurements to the PT or OT. Some facilities use a live stream service such as Skype or FaceTime to "walk through" the home with the patient's family. Other programs provide a PT or OT visit to the home to assess its layout, accessibility, and potential barriers or environmental risks. For example, a patient with a fractured hip who is ambulating well with a walker may neglect to explain to the nurse that the bathroom in the home is accessible by stairway only. The patient may not consider that it is important to mention that throw rugs, which can cause falls, are scattered throughout the apartment. Fall prevention strategies in the home environment for older adults are discussed in Chapter 4.

The accessibility of bathrooms, bedrooms, and kitchen is assessed. If the patient will use a wheelchair after discharge from the facility, home modifications such as ramps to replace steps may be needed. Doorways should be checked for adequate width. A doorway width of 36 to 38 inches (slightly less than 1 meter [m]) is usually sufficient for a standard-size wheelchair. Obese patients require bariatric wheelchairs and furniture and therefore need a wider door opening. Any room that the patient needs to use is assessed. The bedroom should have sufficient space for the patient to maneuver transfers to and from the wheelchair and the bed, if needed. The bathroom may need a toilet seat raised to at least 17 inches (43 cm).

Space requirements depend on the patient's need to use a wheelchair, walker, or cane. In the bathroom, grab bars may need to be installed before the patient comes home. Bathtub benches can provide support for the person who has difficulty with mobility and, when used in combination with a handheld showerhead, can provide easily accessible bathing facilities. Assessment of the kitchen may or may not be critical, depending on whether the patient has help with cooking and preparing meals. If the patient will be cooking after discharge, the kitchen may need to be assessed for wheelchair or walker accessibility, appliance accessibility, and the need for adaptive equipment.

Therapeutic Leave-of-Absence Visit. A second method of assessing the patient's home, if the insurance company allows, is through a brief home visit, also called a *leave-of-absence (LOA) visit,* before discharge. Explain the need for the trial home visit and assess the patient's comfort level with this idea. The patient who has been hospitalized for a lengthy period may feel intense anxiety about returning home. The nurse may allay such anxieties with careful preparation. Before the visit the rehabilitation nurse meets with the patient and family members or significant others to set goals for the visit and identify specific tasks to be attempted while at home. After the home visit, interview the patient to determine the success of the visit and to assess additional education or training needs before final discharge and transition of care.

Going home may not be an option for everyone. Some patients may not have a support network of family members or significant others. For example, many older adults have no spouse or close friends living nearby. Children may live far away, which can make home care difficult. If no caregiver is available, the family must decide whether care can be provided in the home by an outside resource. The patient may need to be admitted to a 24-hour supervised health care setting such as a transitional living apartment, board and care facility, assisted-living facility, or nursing home. The least restrictive, least institutional discharge environment is the desired outcome for all patients.

Self-Management Education. The OT and PT teach the pat ient to perform ADLs and IADLs independently. This education is reinforced by the nurse. The patient's learning potential and cognitive capacity are assessed. He or she is asked to perform or direct each skill or technique independently to verify understanding. Written material explaining the steps in the procedure is provided to the patient and family members to reinforce learning and provide support with the technique after discharge. Before distributing written material, the rehabilitation team assesses the reading level of the material and determines whether it is appropriate for the patient's reading ability and language skills.

Any chronic conditions or disability necessitates changes in lifestyle and body image. Help the patient deal with such changes by encouraging verbalization of feelings and emotions. A focus on existing capabilities instead of disabilities is emphasized.

The patient may fail to relate psychologically to the disability during hospitalization. For example, he or she may display anger or frustration in attempting to perform self-care routines before discharge from the rehabilitation facility. Encourage the patient to be open about such feelings and to talk about ways to prevent worries from becoming realities after discharge. If needed, refer the patient to a mental health/behavioral health care professional to help with adjustment and coping strategies.

The LOA home visit assists the patient and family members or significant others in psychosocial preparation for discharge. It allows the experience of the home situation while the patient is able to return to the hospital environment after a few hours. Often he or she finds new problems in the home that must be addressed before discharge. Review this information in preparation for transition to the home.

Health Care Resources. After discharge to the home, various health care resources (e.g., physical therapy, home care nursing, vocational counseling) are available to the patient with chronic conditions and disabilities. Assess the need for additional care and support throughout the hospitalization and coordinate with the case manager and health care provider in arranging for home services. A newer process using technology called *telehealth* or *telerehabilitation* allows for care coordination in the home setting. Through the use of various electronic devices, a phone, or computer software, a health care team member can monitor the patient's vital signs, weight, and other assessment data. Other programs allow patients to perform therapeutic exercises at home using Wii, a webcam, and a computer.

◆ **Evaluation: Evaluate Outcomes.** The patient and rehabilitation team evaluate the effectiveness of interdisciplinary interventions based on the common patient problems. Expected outcomes may include that the patient will:

- Reach a level of ***mobility*** that allows him or her to function independently with or without assistive devices
- Prevent complications of decreased ***mobility***
- Perform self-care and other self-management skills independently or with minimal assistance, possibly using assistive-adaptive devices
- Have intact skin and underlying tissues
- Establish urinary ***elimination*** without infection, incontinence, or retention
- Have regular evacuation of stool without constipation or incontinence

GET READY FOR THE NEXT-GENERATION NCLEX® EXAMINATION!

Key Points

Review these Key Points for each NCLEX Examination Client Needs Category.

Safe and Effective Care Environment

- Rehabilitation is the process of learning to live with chronic and disabling conditions; the role of the rehabilitation nurse is outlined in Table 7.1.
- Collaborate with members of the interprofessional rehabilitation team, including physicians, nurse practitioners, staff nurses, physiotherapists, occupational therapists, dietitians, and speech-language pathologists; the patient and family are the center of and members of the team. **QSEN: Teamwork and Collaboration**
- Know that acute (short-term) rehabilitation care occurs in a variety of settings, including inpatient rehabilitation facilities (IRFs) and skilled nursing facilities (SNFs) in either a nursing home or hospital. **Health Care Organizations**
- After assessing the home environment, the case manager, OT, and/or rehabilitation nurse makes recommendations to the patient and family about home modifications. **QSEN: Teamwork and Collaboration**
- Use evidence-based safe patient-handling practices such as using mechanical lifts and working with other team members when assessing and moving patients to prevent injury and improve mobility. **QSEN: Evidence-Based Practice; Safety**
- Encourage the patient to be as independent as possible when performing ADLs and mobilization.

Health Promotion and Maintenance

- In coordination with the PT and OT, assess the patient's ability to perform ADLs, IADLs, and ***mobility*** skills using a functional assessment instrument. **QSEN: Teamwork and Collaboration**
- Prevent complications of immobility (pressure injuries, contractures, urinary calculi, constipation, and venous thromboembolism) for clients, and teach caregivers how to prevent complications by using interventions discussed in Chapter 3. **QSEN: Evidence-Based Practice**

Psychosocial Integrity

- Assess the patient's self-esteem and changes in body image caused by chronic or disabling health problems.
- Assess the patient's ***cognition*** to screen for depression, delirium, and dementia using tools such as the Confusion Assessment Method (CAM), especially for older adults. **QSEN: Safety**
- Assist patients in coping with their loss and assess the availability of support systems, especially for older adults. **QSEN: Patient-Centered Care**

Physiological Integrity

- Assess rehabilitation patients as outlined in Table 7.3 to help plan appropriate collaborative care.
- Assess patients in rehabilitation for risk factors that make them likely to develop skin breakdown; interventions to prevent skin problems include repositioning and adequate ***nutrition***. **QSEN: Quality Improvement**
- Patients with neurogenic bladder and bowel ***elimination*** problems are treated with training programs; overactive (spastic or reflex) and underactive (hypotonic or flaccid) elimination problems are managed differently (see Tables 7.7 and 7.8).
- In collaboration with the rehabilitation therapists, evaluate the ability of clients to use assistive-adaptive devices to promote independence. **QSEN: Teamwork and Collaboration**
- Determine patient and family needs regarding discharge to home or other community-based setting.

MASTERY QUESTIONS

1. While assessing functional ability, which activities will the nurse document as instrumental activities of daily living (IADLs)? **Select all that apply.**
   A. Cooking a meal
   B. Walking down the hallway
   C. Getting dressed for the day
   D. Answering the telephone
   E. Taking a shower before bed
   F. Shopping at the local market

2. The assistive personnel (AP) is preparing to transfer a client with limited weight bearing from the bed to the chair. Which action by the AP would require intervention from the nurse?
   A. Places the bed at hip level
   B. Applies a gait belt to the client
   C. Extends arms to reach out to client
   D. Creates a wide base with the feet

REFERENCES

Asterisk (*) indicates a classic or definitive work on this subject.

*Association of Rehabilitation Nurses. (2014). *Standards and scope of rehabilitation nursing practice*. Glenview, IL: Author.

Black, J. M., Salsbury, S., & Vollman, K. M. (2018). Changing the perceptions of a culture of safety for the patient and the caregiver integrating improvement initiatives to create sustainable change. *Critical Care Nursing Quarterly*, *41*(3), 226–239. https://doi.org/10.1097/CNQ.0000000000000203.

Camicia, M., Lutz, B., Kim, K., Harvath, T., Drake, C., & Joseph, J. (2019). Development of an instrument to assess stroke caregivers' readiness for the transition home. *Rehabilitation Nursing*. https://doi.org/10.1097/rnj.0000000000000204.

*Camicia, M., Black, T., Farrell, J., Waites, K., Wirt, S., & Lutz, B. (2014). The essential role of the rehabilitation nurse in facilitating care transitions: A white paper by the association of rehabilitation nurses. *Rehabilitation Nursing*, *39*(1), 3–15. https://doi.org/10.1002/rnj.135.

Centers for Disease Control and Prevention (CDC). (2018a). *About chronic diseases*. Retrieved from https://www.cdc.gov/chronicdisease/.

Centers for Disease Control and Prevention (CDC). (2018b). *Work-related musculoskeletal disorders and ergonomics*. Retrieved from: https:///www.cdc.gov/workplacehealthpromotionstrategies/musculoskeletal-disorders/index/htm.

Centers for Medicare and Medicaid Services (CMS). (2018). *Inpatient rehabilitation facility- Patient assessment instrument (IRF-PAI)*. Retrieved from: https://www.cms.gov/Medicare/Quality-Initiatives-Patient-Assessment-Instruments/IRF-Quality-Reporting/Downloads/Final-IRF-PAI-Version-20-Effective-October-1-2018.pdf.

Dolansky, M., & Moore, S. (2013). Quality and Safety Education for Nurses (QSEN): The key is systems thinking. *OJIN: The Online Journal of Issues in Nursing*, *18*(3), Manuscript 1.

Gerteis, J. I. D., Deitz, D., LeRoy, L., Ricciardi, R., Miller, T., & Basu, J. (2014). *Multiple chronic conditions chartbook*. http://www.ahrq.gov/sites/default/files/wysiwyg/professionals/prevention-chronic-care/decision/mcc/mccchartbook.pdf.

Johns Hopkins. (2020). *Innovative approaches to patient rehabilitation maximize COVID-19 recovery at Johns Hopkins*. https://www.hopkinsmedicine.org/coronavirus/articles/innovative-rehabilitation.html.

Larsen, P. (Ed.). (2018). *Chronic illness: Impact and interventions* (10th ed.). Burlington, MA: Jones and Bartlett.

Pires, J. M., Ferreira, A. M., Rocha, F., Andrade, L. G., Campos, I., Margalho, P., & et al (2018). Assessment of neurogenic bowel dysfunction impact after spinal cord injury using the international classification of functioning, disability and health. *European Journal of Physical and Rehabilitation Medicine*. https://doi.org/10.23736/s1973-9087.18.04991-2.

Powell-Cope, G., Pippins, K., & Young, H. (2017). Teaching family caregivers to assist safely with mobility. *American Journal of Nursing*, *117*(12).

Stalter, A., Phillips, J., & Dolansky, M. (2017). QSEN Institute RN-BSN Task Force. White paper and recommendation for systems-based practice competency. *Journal of Nursing Care Quality*, *32*(4), 354–358.

Stalter, A., & Mota, A. (2018). Using systems thinking to envision quality and safety in healthcare. *Nursing Management*, *February*, 32–39.

Teeple, E., Collins, J. E., Shrestha, S., Dennerlein, J. T., Losina, E., & Katz, J. N. (2017). Outcomes of safe patient handling and mobilization programs: A meta-analysis. *Work*, *58*(2), 173–184. https://doi.org/10.3233/wor-172608.

Wilson, H. J., Dasgupta, K., & Michael, K. (2018). Implementation of the agitated behavior scale in the electronic health record. *Rehabilitation Nursing Journal*, *43*(1), 21–25. https://doi.org/10.1002/rnj.297.

World Health Organization (WHO). (2018). *Health topics: Disabilities*. Retrieved from www.who.int/topics/disabilities/en/.

8

Concepts of Care for Patients at End of Life

Darla Green, Nicole M. Heimgartner

http://evolve.elsevier.com/Iggy/

LEARNING OUTCOMES

1. Collaborate within the interprofessional health care team to promote high-quality care for the patient at the end of life, including family or other caregivers.
2. Discuss the ethical and legal obligations of the nurse with regard to end-of-life (EOL) care.
3. Explain to patients and their families the purpose of and procedure for advance directives.
4. Assess the patient's and family's ability to cope with the dying process.
5. Assess and plan interventions to meet the dying patient's spiritual needs.
6. Incorporate the patient's cultural practices and beliefs when promoting ***comfort*** and providing care during the dying process and death.
7. Assess patients for signs and symptoms related to the end of life.
8. Provide evidence-based end-of-life nursing care to the dying patient, including managing symptoms that may result from impaired ***cognition*** and ***perfusion.***

KEY TERMS

advance care planning A process by which patients and families discuss end-of-life care, clarifying values and goals and then expressing those goals in an advance directive.

advance directive (AD) A written document prepared by a competent person to specify what, if any, extraordinary actions he or she would want when no longer able to make decisions about personal health care.

bereavement Grief and mourning experienced by survivors before and after a death.

Cheyne-Stokes respirations Common sign of nearing death in which apnea alternates with periods of rapid breathing.

death When illness or trauma overwhelms the compensatory mechanisms of the body and the lungs and heart cease to function.

death rattle Loud, wet respirations caused by secretions in the respiratory tract and oral cavity of a patient who is near death.

do-not-resuscitate (DNR) Order from physician or other authorized primary health care provider, which instructs that CPR not be attempted in the event of cardiac or respiratory arrest.

durable power of attorney for health care (DPOAHC) A legal document in which a person appoints someone else to make health care decisions in the event he or she becomes incapable of making decisions.

euthanasia Term used to describe the process of ending life. Active euthanasia implies that primary health care providers take action (e.g., give medication or treatment) that purposefully and directly causes the patient's death.

grief The emotional feeling related to the perception of the loss.

hospice An interprofessional approach to facilitate quality of life and a "good" death for patients near the end of their lives, with care provided in a variety of settings.

life review A structured process of reflecting on one's life that is often facilitated by an interviewer.

living will A legal document that instructs health care providers and family members about what life-sustaining treatment is wanted (or not wanted) if the patient becomes unable to make decisions.

mourning The outward social expression of loss.

palliative care A compassionate and supportive approach to patients and families who are living with life-threatening illnesses; involves a holistic approach that provides relief of symptoms experienced by the dying patient.

palliative sedation A care management approach involving the administration of drugs such as benzodiazepines for the purpose of decreasing suffering by lowering patient consciousness.

peaceful death A death that is free from avoidable distress and suffering for patients and families, in agreement with patients' and families' wishes, and consistent with clinical practice standards.

presence A type of communication that consists of listening and acknowledging the legitimacy of the patient's and/or family's impending loss and pain.

religions Formal belief systems that provide a framework for making sense of life, death, and suffering and responding to universal spiritual questions.

reminiscence The process of randomly reflecting on memories of events in one's life.

PRIORITY AND INTERRELATED CONCEPTS

The priority concept for this chapter is:

- ***Comfort***

The ***Comfort*** concept exemplar for this chapter is End of Life.

The interrelated concepts for this chapter are:

- ***Cognition***
- ***Perfusion***
- ***Ethics***

OVERVIEW OF DEATH, DYING, AND END OF LIFE

Dying is often feared as a time of pain and suffering; however, it is part of the normal life cycle. For the family, death of a member is a life-altering loss that can cause significant and prolonged suffering. As sad and difficult as the death may be, the experience of dying need not be physically painful for the patient or emotionally agonizing for the family. The dying process can be an opportunity to change a difficult situation into one that is tolerable, peaceful, comfortable, and meaningful for the patient and the family left behind.

Because nurses spend more time with patients than any other members of the interprofessional health care team, it is the nurse who often has the greatest impact on an adult's experience with death. A nurse can provide a positive impact on the dying process, to prevent death without dignity (sometimes referred to as a *bad death*) from occurring while striving to promote a peaceful and meaningful death (sometimes referred to as a *good death*). A peaceful death is one that is free from avoidable distress and suffering for patients and families, in agreement with patients' and families' wishes, and consistent with clinical practice standards.

Table 8.1 lists the most common causes of death in the United States. Of all people who die, only a small percentage of them die suddenly and unexpectedly. Most people die after a long period of chronic illness (e.g., cardiac, renal, respiratory disease), with gradual deterioration until a significant decline preceding death. Most who die are older than 65 years, and most qualify for Medicare. In many countries family and other lay caregivers provide the majority of long-term home care. In some countries such as Canada, the local or provincial government may compensate these caregivers for the health care they provide.

The U.S. health care system continues to be based on the acute care model, which is focused on prevention, early detection, and cure of disease. This focus and advances in survival rates for diseases that were once considered deadly have made it difficult for patients and providers to accept death as an outcome. Many health care providers view death as a failure. These views have led to a major deficiency in the quality of care provided to many at the end of life, and multiple barriers remain, often related to the reluctance of the patient, family, or health care provider to stop treatment when the end of life is near.

Pathophysiology of Dying

Death is defined as the cessation of integrated tissue and organ function, manifesting with lack of heartbeat, absence of spontaneous respirations, or irreversible brain dysfunction. It generally occurs as a result of an illness or trauma that overwhelms the compensatory mechanisms of the body, eventually leading to cardiopulmonary failure or arrest. Direct causes of death include:

- Heart failure (HF) secondary to cardiac dysrhythmias, myocardial infarction, or cardiogenic shock
- Respiratory failure secondary to pulmonary embolism, HF, pneumonia, lung disease, or respiratory arrest caused by increased intracranial pressure
- Shock secondary to infection, blood loss, or organ dysfunction, which leads to lack of blood flow (i.e., ***perfusion***) to vital organs

Inadequate ***perfusion*** to body tissues deprives cells of their source of oxygen, which leads to anaerobic metabolism with acidosis, hyperkalemia, and tissue ischemia. Dramatic changes in vital organs lead to the release of toxic metabolites and destructive enzymes, referred to as *multiple organ dysfunction syndrome (MODS).* As illness or organ damage progresses, the syndrome occurs with renal and liver failure. Renal or liver failure can also *start* the dying process.

When the body is hypoxic and acidotic, a lethal dysrhythmia such as ventricular fibrillation or asystole can occur, which ultimately leads to lack of cardiac output and ***perfusion.*** Shortly after cardiac arrest, respiratory arrest occurs. When respiratory arrest occurs first, cardiac arrest follows within minutes.

TABLE 8.1 Leading Causes of Death in the United States

- Heart disease
- Cancer (malignant neoplasms)
- Accidents (unintentional injuries)
- Chronic lower respiratory diseases
- Cerebrovascular diseases
- Alzheimer's disease
- Diabetes mellitus
- Influenza and pneumonia
- Kidney disease (nephritis, nephrotic syndrome, and nephrosis)
- Suicide (intentional self-harm)

Data from Centers for Disease Control and Prevention. (2017). *Leading causes of death.* https://www.cdc.gov/nchs/data/hus/2017/019.pdf

COMFORT CONCEPT EXEMPLAR: END OF LIFE

In 1991 the U.S. Congress passed the Patient Self-Determination Act (PSDA), which granted Americans the right to determine the medical care they wanted if they became incapacitated. Documentation of self-determination is accomplished by completing an advance directive (AD), which is part of the process of advance care planning. The PSDA requires that a representative in every health care agency ask patients when admitted if they have written advance directives. Patients who do not have ADs should be provided with information on the value of having an AD in place and be given the opportunity to complete the state-required forms. Ideally, advance directives should be completed long before a medical crisis occurs.

The American Nurses Association and the Hospice and Palliative Nurses Association (HPNA) support the nurse's role in advance care planning as a patient advocate to facilitate informed decisions about future health care. Nurses are often in a position to help patients process advance care planning and discuss how those decisions align with the patient's values, beliefs, and goals (HPNA, 2018). It is important to note that advance care planning does not stop with just asking about advance directives. Rather, **advance care planning** is a process whereby patients and families discuss end-of-life (EOL) care, clarifying values and goals and then expressing those goals in an advance directive (HPNA, 2018).

Advance directives vary from state to state but are readily available through CaringInfo, an online program of the National Hospice and Palliative Care Organization (www.caringinfo.org). Anyone can complete the forms without legal consultation. Titles for ADs vary from state to state. Generally speaking, most have a section in which one names a **durable power of attorney for health care (DPOAHC)** (Fig. 8.1). The DPOAHC is not the same as durable power of attorney for one's finances. It may or may not be the same person, depending on who the patient designates.

The DPOAHC, often referred to as a *health care proxy, health care agent,* or *surrogate decision maker,* does not make health care decisions until the health care provider states that the person lacks capacity to make his or her own health care decisions. This is usually the result of impairment in ***cognition.***

To have decision-making ability, a person must be able to perform three tasks:

- Receive information (but not necessarily be totally oriented)
- Evaluate, deliberate, and mentally manipulate information
- Communicate a treatment preference

By definition, the comatose patient does not have decisional ability.

The second part of the advance directive is a **living will** (LW), which identifies what one would (or would not) want if he or she were near death. Treatments that are discussed include cardiopulmonary resuscitation (CPR), artificial ventilation, and artificial nutrition or hydration. The third type of advance directive is a do-not-resuscitate (DNR) or do-not-attempt-to-resuscitate (DNAR) order, signed by a physician or other authorized primary health care provider, which instructs that CPR not be attempted in the event of cardiac or respiratory arrest. DNRs/DNARs are intended for people with life-limiting conditions, for whom resuscitation is not prudent. Depending on the state of residence, people who have made the decision not to be resuscitated may have portable DNR documents and or bracelets to identify themselves as having directions not to resuscitate. Some states also have directives referred to as *POLST* (physician orders for life-sustaining treatment), which document additional instructions in case of cardiac or pulmonary arrest. Like portable DNRs/DNARs, POLST directives follow the patient across health care settings.

By law, all primary health care providers in the United States must initiate CPR for a person who is not breathing or is pulseless unless that person has a DNR order. The problem with performing CPR is that it can be a violent and likely painful intervention that prevents a peaceful death. CPR may also be unsuccessful or result in the patient being more compromised than they were before the event, perhaps for life. Many patients and families do not understand the limitations of CPR and do not realize that it was never intended to be performed on patients with end-stage disease.

Hospice and Palliative Care

The concept of hospice in the United States and other countries came about from a grassroots effort in response to the unmet needs of people who were terminally ill. As both a philosophy and a system of care, **hospice** is considered to be the model for high-quality, compassionate care for people facing a life-limiting illness or injury. Hospice uses a team-oriented approach, providing expert medical care, pain management, and emotional and spiritual support expressly tailored to the person's needs and wishes. Support is also provided to the person's loved ones. Hospice systems of care are provided in a variety of settings, including the client's home, nursing homes, and inpatient hospice facilities. They are often affiliated with home care agencies, and many clients may transition from home health services into hospice services as health declines. Some communities in larger urban cities have hospice houses, which provide care to patients in the terminal phase of their lives. Hospice services may also be provided in specialty areas such as prisons and in facilities designed for veterans and the homeless (see the Evidence-Based Practice box).

EVIDENCE-BASED PRACTICE (QSEN)

Palliative Care for Veterans

Carpenter, J., McDarby, M., Smith, D., Johnson, M., Thorpe, J., & Ersek, M. (2017). Associations between timing of palliative care consults and family evaluation of care for veterans who die in a hospice/palliative care unit. *Journal of Palliative Medicine, 20*(7), 745–751.

Palliative care has been proven to improve quality of life during the end-of-life stage for the terminally ill, yet often comes too late in the course of the illness to be most beneficial for both the patient and family. A retrospective study of 5592 terminally ill veterans was conducted using records of veterans who died while receiving palliative care or hospice services. Surveys completed by families of veterans who had been receiving these services longer rated the care as excellent more often than the veterans who had been receiving care services for less time. In this sample, the family members of veterans held higher perceptions of end-of-life care when palliative care consultations (PCCs) occurred more than 1 week before death. This association was even higher when the PCC occurred 6 months before death. In addition, mean scores in survey categories of respectful care and communication and emotional and spiritual support were significantly higher in the group that had been in palliative care for 91 to 180 days.

The conclusion of this study demonstrated that positive outcomes are seen for patients introduced to palliative care in the earlier stage of end of life, and strategies aimed at earlier palliative transition to care are needed. Health care providers in the past have perceived the PCC as a failure, often continuing various treatments and hoping for a better outcome, with palliative care mentioned only when all other treatment options have failed. This can create distress for the patient, with considerable physical, emotional, and financial burden for both patients and families. By initiating PCCs earlier, health care providers have more time to develop a relationship with the patient and the family. This also allows for more time to develop end-of-life care goals and allows the connection between health care providers, patients, and families to deepen, which fosters trust throughout the end-of-life stage.

Commentary: Implications for Practice and Research

The research shows the value of palliative care for veterans, emphasizing that earlier consultations with palliative care providers lead to more positive outcomes and higher satisfaction with end-of-life care. Nurses can advocate for palliative care earlier, recognizing that this is not a failure of care, but rather a measure to provide valuable options that can promote death with dignity. Further research regarding the timing of PCCs as well as the identification of more specific criteria for PCC is warranted.

INSTRUCTIONS	
PRINT YOUR NAME PRINT THE NAME AND ADDRESS OF YOUR AGENT INSTRUCTION STATEMENTS CIRCLE AND INITIAL THE RESPONSES THAT REFLECT YOUR WISHES TERMINAL ILLNESS PERMANENTLY UNCONSCIOUS ARTIFICIAL NUTRITION AND HYDRATION ADD PERSONAL INSTRUCTIONS (IF ANY) ALTERNATE AGENT PRINT THE NAME AND ADDRESS OF YOUR ALTERNATE AGENT LOCATION OF THE ORIGINAL AND COPIES DATE AND SIGN THE DOCUMENT HERE WITNESSING PROCEDURE WITNESSES MUST SIGN AND PRINT THEIR ADDRESSES AND A NOTARY PUBLIC OR JUSTICE OF THE PEACE MUST COMPLETE THIS SECTION ©2005 National Hospice and Palliative Care Organization 2014 Revised	

NEW HAMPSHIRE ADVANCE DIRECTIVE
PART I: NEW HAMPSHIRE DURABLE POWER OF ATTORNEY FOR HEALTH CARE

I,__________________________, hereby appoint __________________________
(name) (name of agent)
of ______________________________________
(address)

as my agent to make any and all health care decisions for me, except to the extent I state otherwise in this directive or as prohibited by law. This durable power of attorney for health care shall take effect in the event I lack the capacity to make my own health care decisions.

In the event the person I appoint above is unable, unwilling or unavailable, or ineligible to act as my health care agent, I hereby appoint __________________________ of __________________________
(name of an alternate agent) (address)
as alternate agent.

When making health care decisions for me, my agent should think about what action would be consistent with past conversations we have had, my treatment preferences as expressed in this advance directive, my religious and other beliefs and values, and how I have handled medical and other important issues in the past. If what I would decide is still unclear, then my health care agent should make decisions for me that my health care agent believes are in my best interest, considering the benefits, burdens, and risks of my current circumstances and treatment option.

STATEMENT OF DESIRES, SPECIAL PROVISIONS, AND LIMITATIONS REGARDING HEALTH CARE DECISIONS.

For your convenience in expressing your wishes, some general statements concerning the withholding or removal of life-sustaining treatment are set forth below. (Life-sustaining treatment is defined as procedures without which a person would die, such as but not limited to the following: mechanical respiration, kidney dialysis or the use of other external mechanical and technological devices, drugs to maintain blood pressure, blood transfusions, and antibiotics.) There is also a section which allows you to set forth specific directions for these or other matters. If you wish, you may indicate your agreement or disagreement with any of the following statements and give your agent power to act in those specific circumstances.

A. LIFE-SUSTAINING TREATMENT.

1. If I am near death and lack the capacity to make health care decisions, I authorize my agent to direct that:
(Initial beside your choice of (a) or (b).)
____(a) life-sustaining treatment not be started, or if started, be discontinued.
OR ____(b) life-sustaining treatment continue to be given to me.
2. Whether near death or not, if I become permanently unconscious I authorize my agent to direct that:
(Initial beside your choice of (a) or (b).)
____(a) life-sustaining treatment not be started, or if started, be discontinued.
OR ____(b) life-sustaining treatment continue to be given to me.

B. MEDICALLY ADMINISTERED NUTRITION AND HYDRATION.

1. I realize that situations could arise in which the only way to allow me to die would be to not start or to discontinue medically administered nutrition and hydration. In carrying out any instructions I have given in this document, I authorize my agent to direct that: (Initial beside your choice of (a) or (b).)
____(a) medically administered nutrition and hydration not be started or, if started, be discontinued.
OR ____(b) even if all other forms of life-sustaining treatment have been withdrawn, medically administered nutrition and hydration continue to be given to me.

INITIAL THE RESPONSES THAT REFLECT YOUR WISHES

C. ADDITIONAL INSTRUCTIONS. Here you may include any specific desires or limitations you deem appropriate, such as when or what life-sustaining treatment you would want used or withheld, or instructions about refusing any specific types of treatment that are inconsistent with your religious beliefs or are unacceptable to you for any other reason. You may leave this question blank if you desire.

____
____
____
(attach additional pages as necessary)

I hereby acknowledge that I have been provided with a disclosure statement explaining the effect of this directive. I have read and understand the information contained in the disclosure statement. The original of this document will be kept at: __________________, and the following persons and institutions will have signed copies:
____________________ Name ____________________ Name
____________________ Address ____________________ Address

ADD OTHER INSTRUCTIONS, IF ANY, REGARDING YOUR ADVANCE CARE PLANS
THESE INSTRUCTIONS CAN FURTHER ADDRESS YOUR HEALTH CARE PLANS, SUCH AS YOUR WISHES REGARDING HOSPICE TREATMENT, BUT CAN ALSO ADDRESS OTHER ADVANCE PLANNING ISSUES, SUCH AS YOUR BURIAL WISHES

PART II. NEW HAMPSHIRE DECLARATION

Declaration made this __________ day of ________________. (day) (month, year)
I, ______________________________, (name) being of sound mind, willfully and voluntarily make known my desire that my dying shall not be artificially prolonged under the circumstances set forth below, do hereby declare:

If at any time I should have an incurable injury, disease or illness and I am certified to be near death or in a permanently unconscious condition by 2 physicians or a physician and an ARNP, and two physicians or a physician and an ARNP have determined that my death is imminent whether or not life-sustaining treatment is utilized and where the application of life-sustaining treatment would serve only to artificially prolong the dying process, or that I will remain in a permanently unconscious condition, I direct that such procedures be withheld or withdrawn, and that I be permitted to die naturally with only the administration of medication, the natural ingestion of food or fluids by eating or drinking, or the performance of any medical procedure deemed necessary to provide me with comfort care. I realize that situations could arise in which the only way to allow me to die would be to discontinue medically administered nutrition and hydration.

In carrying out any instruction I have given under this section, I authorize that:
(Initial beside your choice of (a) or (b).)
____(a) medically administered nutrition and hydration not be started or, if started, be discontinued,
OR
____(b) even if other forms of life-sustaining treatment have been withdrawn, medically administered nutrition and hydration continue to be given to me.

Other directions:
____

Fig. 8.1 An example of a durable power of attorney for health care (DPOAHC). (©2005. National Hospice and Palliative Care Organization, 2007 Revised. All rights reserved. Reproduction and distribution by an organization or organized group without the written permission of the National Hospice and Palliative Care Organization is expressly forbidden. Visit caringinfo.org for more information.)

The *Medicare hospice benefit* serves as a guide for hospice care in the United States. This benefit pays for hospice services for Medicare recipients who have a prognosis of 6 months or less to live and who agree to forego curative treatment for their terminal illness. Historically those with terminal cancer made up the majority of patients receiving hospice care. However, the proportion of patients with terminal cancer has decreased, with increases in numbers of patients with other terminal illnesses (e.g., dementia, end-stage chronic obstructive pulmonary disease [COPD], cardiac disease, or neurologic disease).

Guidelines are available to help primary health care providers and families identify who is entitled to hospice care under Medicare. Patients who do not qualify for Medicare may have benefits through private insurance or government medical assistance programs (e.g., Medicaid).

PATIENT-CENTERED CARE: OLDER ADULT CONSIDERATIONS QSEN

In the last 15 years, twice as many older adults died in hospice care as in a hospital or nursing home compared with the previous decade. Despite increase in use, hospice is often a last resort after aggressive critical care. Earlier referrals to hospice care would be of benefit to older adults and their families.

Palliative care is a philosophy of care for people with life-threatening disease that helps patients and families identify their outcomes for care, assists them with informed decision making, and facilitates high-quality symptom management. The goal of palliative care is to improve the quality of life for the patient and the family. An interprofessional team of health care providers (doctor, nurse, social worker, and chaplain) work together to address the unique needs that are associated with serious and chronic illness (Meier & Bowman, 2017). Palliative care consultations (PCCs) are provided in a large number of hospitals and on an ambulatory care basis in some communities. Table 8.2 compares palliative care and hospice care. Classic research as well as current evidence demonstrates the benefits of early initiation of PCCs (Campbell et al., 2012; Carpenter et al., 2017). (See the Evidence-Based Practice Box.) Despite these benefits, palliative care is often not implemented until late in the patient's illness (Institute of Medicine [IOM], 2014). Because of their proximity to patients, nurses are in an excellent position to identify people who would benefit from palliative consultation. To accomplish this desired outcome, nurses need to have knowledge of end-of-life (EOL) care, compassion, advocacy, and therapeutic communication skills. Knowing how to initiate a conversation regarding palliative care is a critical step in achieving earlier access to high-quality end-of-life care (Croson et al., 2018).

TABLE 8.2 Comparison of Hospice and Palliative Care

Hospice Care	Palliative Care
Patients have a prognosis of 6 months or less to live.	Patients can be in any stage of serious illness.
Care is provided when curative treatment such as chemotherapy has been stopped.	A consultation is provided that is concurrent with curative therapies or therapies that prolong life.
Care is provided in 60- and 90-day periods with an opportunity to continue if eligibility criteria are met.	Care is not limited by specific time periods.
Ongoing care is provided by registered nurses, social workers, chaplains, and volunteers.	Care is in the form of a consultation visit by a primary health care provider who makes recommendations; follow-up visits may be provided.

❖ Interprofessional Collaborative Care

◆ **Assessment: Recognize Cues.** Obtain information about the patient's diagnosis, past medical history, and recent state of health to identify the risks for symptoms of distress at the end of life. People with lung cancer, heart failure (HF), or chronic respiratory disease are at high risk for respiratory distress and dyspnea as they decline. Those with brain tumors are at risk for seizure activity. Patients with tumors near major arteries (e.g., head and neck cancer) are at risk for hemorrhage. Those who have been experiencing pain often continue to have pain at the end of life, which may increase, decrease, or remain at the same level of intensity.

Physical Assessment/Signs and Symptoms. As death nears, patients often have signs and symptoms of decline in physical function, manifesting as weakness; increased sleep; anorexia; and changes in cardiovascular function, breathing patterns, and genitourinary function. Level of consciousness often declines to lethargy, unresponsiveness, or coma. Cardiovascular dysfunction leads to decreases in peripheral circulation and poor tissue ***perfusion*** manifesting as cold, mottled, and cyanotic extremities. Blood pressure decreases and often is only palpable. The dying person's heart rate may increase, become irregular, and gradually decrease before stopping. Changes in breathing pattern are common, with breaths becoming very shallow and rapid. Periods of apnea and Cheyne-Stokes respirations (apnea alternating with periods of rapid breathing) are also common. Death occurs when respirations and heartbeat stop.

As the patient's level of consciousness decreases, he or she may lose the ability to speak. When caring for those who are unable to communicate their distress or needs, identify alternative ways to assess symptoms of distress. Teach family caregivers to watch closely for objective signs of impaired ***comfort*** (e.g., restlessness, grimacing, moaning) and identify when these symptoms occur in relation to positioning, movement, medication, or other

PATIENT AND FAMILY EDUCATION: PREPARING FOR SELF-MANAGEMENT

Common Physical Signs and Symptoms of Approaching Death With Recommended Comfort Measures

Coolness of Extremities
Circulation to the extremities is decreased; the skin may become mottled or discolored.
- Cover the patient with a blanket.
- Do not use an electric blanket, hot water bottle, or electric heating pad to warm the patient.

Increased Sleeping
Metabolism is decreased.
- Spend time sitting quietly with the patient.
- Do not force the patient to stay awake.
- Talk to the patient as you normally would, even if he or she does not respond.

Fluid and Food Decrease
Metabolic needs have decreased.
- Do not force the patient to eat or drink.
- Offer small sips of liquids or ice chips at frequent intervals if the patient is alert and able to swallow.
- Use moist swabs to keep the mouth and lips moist and comfortable.
- Coat the lips with lip balm.

Incontinence
The perineal muscles relax.
- Keep the perineal area clean and dry. Use disposable underpads and disposable undergarments.
- Offer a Foley catheter for comfort.

Congestion and Gurgling
The person is unable to cough up secretions effectively.
- Position the patient on his or her side. Use toothette to gently clean mouth of secretions.
- Administer medications to decrease the production of secretions.

Breathing Pattern Change
Slowed circulation to the brain may cause the breathing pattern to become irregular, with brief periods of no breathing or shallow breathing.
- Elevate the patient's head.
- Position the patient on his or her side.

Disorientation
Decreased metabolism and slowed circulation to the brain.
- Identify yourself whenever you communicate with the person.
- Reorient the patient as needed.
- Speak softly, clearly, and truthfully.

Restlessness
Decreased metabolism and slowed circulation to the brain.
- Play soothing music and use aromatherapy.
- Do not restrain the patient.
- Talk quietly.
- Keep the room dimly lit.
- Keep the noise level to a minimum.
- Consider sedation if other methods do not work.

Adapted from the Hospice of North Central Florida.

external stimuli. Teach them how to perform interventions that can help relieve discomfort and stress as described in the Patient and Family Education: Preparing for Self-Management: Common Physical Signs and Symptoms of Approaching Death With Recommended Comfort Measures box.

Although the patient's point of view is the most valid indicator of comfort or distress, the family's perception of symptoms and ***comfort*** level is also important. Family caregivers, health care providers, and dying patients may differ in their perceptions of symptoms in terms of intensity, significance, and meaning. Whereas primary health care providers are often able to identify symptoms of distress, families are often more knowledgeable about the patient's habits and preferences. Incorporate all pertinent information into the plan for symptom management, and work with patients and families toward a common outcome.

Assess any symptom of distress in terms of intensity, frequency, duration, quality, exacerbating (worsening) and relieving factors, and effect on the patient's comfort when awake or asleep. A method for rating the intensity of symptoms should be used to facilitate ongoing assessments and evaluate treatment response. A rating scale of 0 to 10 is commonly used, with 0 indicating no distress and 10 indicating the worst possible distress. The intensity of the symptom before and after an intervention (e.g., medication) is documented by the nurse or the family caregiver and is used daily to evaluate the patient's overall ***comfort.***

Psychosocial Assessment. People facing death may have fear and/or anxiety about their impending death with difficulty coping. Assess cultural considerations, values, and religious beliefs of the patient and family for their influence on the dying experience, control of symptoms, and family bereavement.

PATIENT-CENTERED CARE: CULTURAL/ SPIRITUAL CONSIDERATIONS QSEN

Be aware that patients differ in their needs at the end of life, depending on their cultural and spiritual beliefs. If possible, ask the patient what to tell the family about the patient's condition. In some cultures, families may not want to know about the terminal conditions of their loved ones. This decision may be based on respect for older family members. Ask the family what they want to know and if they desire the assistance of a language interpreter.

At the end of life, adults may feel challenged about their spirituality or want spirituality to become a bigger part of their lives (Finocchiaro, 2016). Many patients reaffirm their faith and/or spirituality with hope that they will have a peaceful death and eternal hope and life. Other patients who do not believe in an afterlife may still experience hope for a cure and a comfortable death.

When assessing a patient's spirituality at the end of life, use this classic *HOPE* mnemonic as a guide. Determine the patient's:

- *H:* Sources of hope and strength
- *O:* Organized religion (if any) and role that it plays in the patient's life
- *P:* Personal spirituality, rituals, and practices
- *E:* Effects of religion and spirituality on care and end-of-life decisions (Finocchiaro, 2016)

Families of people near death often manifest fear, anxiety, and knowledge deficits regarding the process of death and their role in providing care. Assess the patient and family for fear and anxiety

PATIENT AND FAMILY EDUCATION: PREPARING FOR SELF-MANAGEMENT

Common Emotional Signs of Approaching Death

Withdrawal
The person is preparing to "let go" of surroundings and relationships.

Vision-Like Experiences
The person may talk to people you cannot see or hear and see objects and places not visible to you. These are not hallucinations or drug reactions.
- Do not deny or argue about what the person claims.
- Affirm the experience.

Letting Go
The person may become agitated or continue to perform repetitive tasks. Often this indicates that something is unresolved or is preventing the person from letting go. As difficult as it may be to do or say, the dying person takes on a more peaceful demeanor when loved ones are able to say things such as "It's okay to go. We'll be alright."

Saying Goodbye
When the person is ready to die and the family is ready to let go, saying "goodbye" is important for both the patient and the family. Touching, hugging, crying, and saying "I love you," "Thank you," "I'm sorry," or "I'll miss you so much" are all natural expressions of sadness and loss. Verbalizing these sentiments can bring comfort both to the dying person and to those left behind.

Adapted from the Hospice of North Central Florida.

and their expectations of the death experience. Provide them with information about the process itself, emphasizing that symptoms of distress do not always occur and, if they do occur, can be treated and controlled. Ask them if they want to talk to a bereavement (grief) counselor or want guidance from clergy. Explain the common emotional signs of approaching death as described in the Patient and Family Education: Preparing for Self-Management box.

◆ **Analysis: Analyze Cues and Prioritize Hypotheses.** The priority collaborative problem for a patient near the end of life is:
- Potential for symptoms of distress that would prevent a peaceful death

◆ **Planning and Implementation: Generate Solutions and Take Action.** The desired outcomes for a patient near the end of life (EOL) are that the patient will have:
- Needs and preferences acknowledged and met
- Control or management of symptoms of distress
- Meaningful interactions with family and other loved ones
- A peaceful death

Interventions are planned to meet the physical, psychological, social, and spiritual needs of patients by using a coordinated interprofessional health team approach to end-of-life care. *Although the perception of hospice is that it provides care for the dying, the major focus of hospice care is on quality of life.*

When developing a plan of care for people nearing the end of their lives, consideration should be given for where the person wants to die. A large percentage of Americans would like to die at home. If this is the patient's preference, work with the patient, family, and health care provider to determine if this desired outcome is possible. Arrange for patients and families to meet with hospice representatives who are educated in end-of-life care in a variety of settings. In some situations, the patient may wish to die at home but the family members are reluctant to see this happen. Making certain the patients and families understand what to expect, including assistance such as respite care, can often ease this decision making.

Managing Symptoms of Distress. The most common end-of-life symptoms that can cause the patient distress are:
- Pain
- Weakness
- Breathlessness or dyspnea
- Nausea and vomiting
- Agitation and delirium
- Seizures

Interventions to relieve symptoms of distress include positioning, administration of medications, and a variety of complementary and integrative therapies. When medications are used, they are often scheduled around the clock to maintain ***comfort*** and prevent recurrence of the symptom.

Managing Pain. *Pain is the symptom that dying patients fear the most.* Diseases such as cancer often cause tumor pain as a result of the infiltration of cancer cells into organs, nerves, and bones. Other causes of impaired ***comfort*** in dying patients include osteoarthritis, muscle spasms, and stiff joints secondary to immobility.

Both nonopioid and opioid analgesics play a role in pain management near the end of life. Patients who have had their pain controlled with either short- or long-acting opioids should continue their scheduled doses to prevent recurrence of the pain. However, as patients get closer to death, they often lose the ability to swallow. Long-acting oral opioids generally cannot be crushed, and rotation to rectal, transdermal, intravenous, or a subcutaneous route may be necessary. Short-acting nonopioids such as acetaminophen or opioids such as morphine sulfate, oxycodone, or hydromorphone elixir can be given sublingually. They may also be given rectally if the patient and family are receptive to this route. Short-acting analgesics are quick acting; effective; and safe to administer, even to comatose patients.

PATIENT-CENTERED CARE: OLDER ADULT CONSIDERATIONS QSEN

Pain in older adults is often underreported and undertreated. Do not withhold opioid drugs from older adults at the end of their lives. Instead administer low doses of opioids initially as prescribed, with slow increases, monitoring for changes in mental status or excessive sedation.

Some experts in symptom management at the end of life (EOL) recommend discontinuing routine doses of opioids such as morphine when patients become oliguric or anuric. The rationale for this decision is to decrease the risk for delirium that may occur as the result of the inability of a failing kidney to excrete morphine metabolites from the body. If delirium is causing distress for the patient, the health care provider may consider changing the opioid to fentanyl, which does not have active metabolites. The delirium may improve. For patients with known renal failure, fentanyl should ideally be used from the start of opioid administration. When it cannot be easily obtained (i.e., when not available by sublingual or IV route), oxycodone may be a better choice than morphine. Chapter 5 describes in detail the management of persistent (chronic) pain.

Medical Marijuana (Cannabis). The use of medical marijuana, or cannabinoid-based medicines (CBMs), is increasing in palliative and end-of-life care. CBM has been shown to reduce pain, especially pain associated with cancer. However, CBM is recommended only for refractory cancer pain as an adjunct to other prescribed analgesics (Cyr et al., 2018). Although the majority of patients who use CBM do so in an attempt to relieve pain, other common symptoms associated with end-of-life care have also been positively affected. These symptoms include fatigue, anorexia, sleep problems, anxiety, and nausea and vomiting. Research in this area is rapidly expanding, and nurses should be aware of the respective state laws regarding the use of medical marijuana. See Chapter 5 for more detail on medical marijuana.

Complementary and Integrative Health. Nonpharmacologic interventions are often integrated into the pain management plan. Some common approaches are presented here and in Chapter 5.

Massage involves manipulating the patient's muscles and soft tissue, which can improve circulation and promote relaxation. Research indicates that massage, when used effectively, reduces pain and anxiety (McMillan et al., 2018). Massage is one of the most popular complementary interventions used for patients at the end of life. Patients who are severely weak, arthritic, or of advanced age may not tolerate extensive massage but may benefit from a short treatment to sites of their choice. In working with patients with cancer, use light pressure and avoid deep or intense pressure. Massage should not be performed over the site of tissue damage (e.g., open wounds, tissue undergoing radiation therapy), in patients with bleeding disorders, and in those who are uncomfortable with touch (Westman & Blaisdell, 2016).

Music therapy is another complementary therapy used by people near the end of life that has been shown to decrease pain by promoting relaxation. Allow the patient to select music that he or she enjoys, as this has been shown to increase the potential benefit (Hamlin & Robertson, 2017). *Therapeutic Touch* involves moving one's hands through the patient's energy field to relieve pain. *Guided imagery* is the use of mental images through guided imagination or memory to reach a therapeutic goal. Research indicates that use of guided imagery, specifically in palliative care, can decrease pain (Coelho et al., 2018) *Aromatherapy* and *essential oils* can be used in conjunction with other treatments to relieve pain near the end of life. Aromatherapy is thought to decrease pain by promoting relaxation and reducing anxiety. The most researched essential oil is lavender, with associated analgesic effects. Other essential oils that have been used effectively in pain management include chamomile, sweet marjoram, dwarf pine, rosemary, and ginger (Hamlin & Robertson, 2017).

NCLEX EXAMINATION CHALLENGE 8.1

Physiological Integrity

A client receiving palliative care who has advanced dementia is nonverbal and restless and moans when the family attempts to touch or comfort the client. Which nursing intervention is appropriate for this client?

A. Administer acetaminophen rectally for pain.
B. Instruct the family to avoid touching the client to prevent pain.
C. Provide passive range of motion to increase mobility once a shift.
D. Obtain a prescription for transdermal fentanyl for pain.

Managing Weakness. Patients commonly experience weakness and fatigue as death nears. At this point they are generally advised to remain in bed to avoid falls and injuries. Mechanical or electric beds are often obtained to elevate the patient's head to promote air exchange and facilitate administration of medications, food, or fluids. Insertion of a long-term urinary (e.g., Foley) catheter to avoid the need for exertion with voiding should be offered as a ***comfort*** measure. Risk for infection should not be a consideration when a person is near death.

Weakness combined with decreased neurologic function may impair the ability to swallow (dysphagia). Once the patient has difficulty swallowing, oral intake should be limited to soft foods and sips of liquids, offered but not forced. Teach families about the risk for aspiration and reassure them that anorexia is normal at this stage. Families often have difficulty accepting that their loved ones are not being fed and may request that IV fluids be started. With great sensitivity, reinforce that having no appetite or desire for food or fluids is expected. Inform families that giving fluids can actually increase discomfort in a person with multisystem slowdown. Impaired ***comfort*** from fluid replacement could lead to respiratory secretions (and distress), increased GI secretions, nausea, vomiting, edema, and ascites. Most experts believe that dehydration in the last hours of life (i.e., terminal dehydration) does not cause distress and may stimulate endorphin release that promotes the patient's sense of well-being. To avoid a dry mouth and lips, moisten them with soft applicators and apply an emollient to lips.

! NURSING SAFETY PRIORITY QSEN

Drug Alert

Dysphagia near death presents a problem for oral drug therapy. Although some tablets may be crushed, drugs such as sustained-release capsules should not be taken apart. Reassess the need for each medication. Collaborate with the health care provider about discontinuing drugs that are not needed to control pain, dyspnea, agitation, nausea, vomiting, cardiac workload, or seizures. In collaboration with a pharmacist experienced in palliation, identify alternative routes and/or alternative drugs to promote *comfort* and maintain control of symptoms. Choose the least invasive route such as oral, buccal mucosa (inside cheek), transdermal (via the skin), or rectal. Some oral drugs can be given rectally. Depending on patient needs, the subcutaneous or IV route may be used if access is available. The intramuscular (IM) route is almost never used at the end of life because it is considered painful and drug distribution varies among patients.

Managing Breathlessness or Dyspnea. Dyspnea is a subjective experience in which the patient has an uncomfortable feeling of breathlessness, often described as terrifying. It is a common symptom of distress near the end of life, especially among older adults because of decreased oxygen reserves associated with aging. Patients, families, and health care providers often consider it the major cause of suffering at the end of life. Dyspnea can be:

- Directly related to the primary diagnosis (e.g., lung cancer, breast cancer, coronary artery disease, chronic obstructive pulmonary disease [COPD])
- Secondary to the primary diagnosis (e.g., pleural effusion)

- Related to treatment of the primary disease (e.g., heart failure [HF] caused by chemotherapy, pneumonitis or constrictive pericarditis caused by radiation therapy, anemia related to chemotherapy)
- Unrelated to the primary disease (e.g., pneumonia or HF).

Perform a thorough assessment of the patient's dyspnea. Include onset, severity (e.g., 0-to-10 scale), and precipitating factors. Precipitating factors may include time of day, position, anxiety, pain, cough, or emotional distress. *Pharmacologic interventions should begin early in the course of dyspnea.* Nonpharmacologic interventions are used in conjunction with but not in place of drug therapy.

Opioids such as morphine sulfate are the standard treatment for dyspnea near death. They work by (1) altering the perception of air hunger, reducing anxiety and associated oxygen consumption, and (2) reducing pulmonary congestion. Patients who have not been receiving opioids will likely be started on lower doses of oral morphine administered every 4 hours (Dudgeon, 2019). Those who are taking morphine or other opioids for pain may need higher doses for breathlessness.

If a patient is having severe respiratory distress and poor oxygenation, morphine by mouth may need to be repeated as often as every 30 minutes, and an IV or subcutaneous route may need to be established.

Oxygen therapy for dyspnea near death has not been established as a standard of care for all patients. However, those who do not respond promptly to morphine or other drugs should be placed on oxygen to assess its effect. Patients often feel more comfortable when the oxygen saturation is greater than 90%. If possible, provide oxygen by nasal cannula because masks can be frightening. If oxygen is not effective, discontinue it.

! NURSING SAFETY PRIORITY QSEN

Action Alert

Offer oxygen to any patient with dyspnea near death, regardless of his or her oxygen saturation, because *comfort* is the desired outcome. If the patient is feeling dyspneic even though the oxygen saturation is above 90%, be sure that he or she receives oxygen to relieve respiratory distress. In addition, offer an electric fan directed toward the patient's face. Some patients find the circulating air more helpful than oxygen therapy.

Bronchodilators such as albuterol or ipratropium bromide via a metered dose inhaler (MDI) or nebulizer may be given for symptoms of bronchospasm (heard as wheezes). *Corticosteroids* such as prednisone may also be given for bronchospasm and inflammatory problems within and outside the lung. Superior vena cava syndrome and cancer-related lymphangitis causing dyspnea may also respond to corticosteroids (also see Chapter 20).

Patients who have fluid overload with dyspnea, crackles on auscultation, peripheral edema, and other signs of chronic heart failure (HF) may be given a *diuretic* such as furosemide to decrease blood volume, reduce vascular congestion, and reduce the workload of the heart. Furosemide can be administered by mouth, IV, or subcutaneously. IV push administration, which is effective within minutes, may be preferred for HF and pulmonary edema.

Antibiotics may be indicated for dyspnea related to a respiratory infection. A trial of an appropriate antibiotic may be considered to make the patient comfortable.

Secretions in the respiratory tract and oral cavity may also contribute to dyspnea near death. Loud, wet respirations (referred to as **death rattle**) are disturbing to family and caregivers even when they do not seem to cause dyspnea or respiratory distress. Reposition the patient onto one side to reduce gurgling and place a small towel under his or her mouth to collect secretions. *Anticholinergics* such as atropine ophthalmic solution or hyoscyamine are commonly administered sublingually to dry up secretions. Scopolamine may also be given transdermally to reduce secretion production. Oropharyngeal suctioning is not recommended for loud secretions in the bronchi or oropharynx because it is often not effective and may only agitate the patient.

Fear and anxiety may be components of respiratory distress at the end of life. For this reason benzodiazepines are commonly given when morphine does not fully control the person's dyspnea. Low-dose lorazepam is administered orally, sublingually, or IV every 4 hours as needed or around the clock.

Other nonpharmacologic interventions include:

- Limiting exertion to avoid exertional dyspnea
- Inserting a long-term urinary (Foley) catheter to avoid dyspnea on exertion
- Positioning the patient with the head of the bed up either in a hospital bed or a reclining chair to increase chest expansion
- Applying wet cloths to the patient's face
- Encouraging imagery and deep breathing

NCLEX EXAMINATION CHALLENGE 8.2

Physiological Integrity

The family of a client who is near death is concerned about a loud rattling that occurs with the client's breathing. What nursing intervention is appropriate? **Select all that apply.**

A. Administer hyoscyamine as prescribed to dry up secretions.
B. Turn the client onto one side to help decrease the gurgling with respirations.
C. Suction the client regularly to remove secretions in the bronchi and oropharynx.
D. Assess the client for signs of dyspnea or respiratory distress.
E. Administer diuretics as prescribed to help decrease the wet respirations.
F. Teach the family about the buildup of secretions that occurs when a client is near death.

Managing Nausea and Vomiting. Although not as common as pain or dyspnea, nausea and vomiting occur frequently among terminally ill patients during the last week of life. It is particularly common in patients with HIV Stage III (acquired immune deficiency syndrome [AIDS]) and with breast, stomach, or gynecologic cancers.

Other causes of nausea and vomiting at the end of life include:

- Uremia (increased serum urea nitrogen)
- Hypercalcemia
- Increased intracranial pressure
- Constipation or impaction
- Bowel obstruction

If constipation is identified as the cause of nausea and vomiting, give the patient a biphosphate enema (e.g., Fleet) to remove stool quickly. If stool in the rectum cannot be evacuated, a mineral oil enema followed by gentle disimpaction may relieve the patient's distress. Nausea and vomiting related to other causes can be controlled with one or more antiemetic agents such as prochlorperazine, ondansetron, dexamethasone, or metoclopramide. In addition to providing medications, be sure to remove sources of odors and keep the room temperature at a level that the patient desires.

Complementary and Integrative Health. Aromatherapy using chamomile, camphor, fennel, lavender, peppermint, and rose may reduce or relieve vomiting. A study of aromatherapy using peppermint oil for nausea and vomiting showed positive results in the majority of participants (Lyons, 2018). However, aromas may worsen nausea for some patients. Ask the patient and family about their preferences and respect culturally established practices.

Managing Agitation and Delirium. Agitation at the end of life first requires assessing for pain or urinary retention, constipation, or another reversible cause. If pain, urinary retention, and constipation are ruled out as causes, delirium (acute confusion) is suspected. Delirium is an acute and fluctuating change in mental status and is accompanied by inattention, disorganized thinking, and/or an altered level of consciousness. It can be hyperactive, hypoactive, or mixed (both). *Hypoactive (quiet)* delirium is probably not uncomfortable for patients. *Agitated (noisy)* delirium with psychotic and behavioral symptoms (e.g., yelling, hallucinations) can be uncomfortable, especially for family. Chapter 4 discusses delirium in more detail.

When delirium occurs in the week or two before death, it is referred to as *terminal delirium.* Possible causes include the adverse effects of opioids, benzodiazepines, anticholinergics, or steroids. If medications are suspected causes, they may be decreased or discontinued. Ideally, antipsychotic drugs are given only to control psychotic symptoms such as hallucinations and delusions. However, if they are needed to facilitate ***comfort,*** they should be available.

! NURSING SAFETY PRIORITY QSEN

Drug Alert

Do not give the patient more than one antipsychotic drug at a time because of the risk for adverse drug events (ADEs). A neuroleptic drug such as a low dose of haloperidol orally, IV, subcutaneously, or rectally is commonly used at the end of life. Although haloperidol has the potential to cause extrapyramidal symptoms or adverse cardiovascular events and death in older adults with dementia, the benefits of treating psychosis associated with delirium usually outweigh the risks.

Benzodiazepines generally are not used as a first choice for older adults with agitation because of their risk for causing delirium. Development of increased agitation after receiving a benzodiazepine could represent a paradoxical reaction—the opposite of what is expected.

Complementary and Integrative Health. Music therapy may produce relaxation by quieting the mind and promoting a restful state. Some patients, whether in the home setting or in inpatient hospice units, benefit from pet therapy. Aromatherapy with chamomile or lavender may also help decrease anxiety, tension, stress, and insomnia in dying patients (Lyons, 2018).

Managing Seizures. Seizures are not common at the end of life but may occur in patients with brain tumors, advanced AIDS, and pre-existing seizure disorders. Around-the-clock drug therapy is needed to maintain a high seizure threshold for patients who can no longer swallow antiepileptic drugs (AEDs). Benzodiazepines such as diazepam and lorazepam are the drugs of choice. For home use, rectal diazepam gel or sublingual lorazepam oral solution may be preferred.

Managing Refractory Symptoms of Distress. Patients receiving opioids for pain or dyspnea and other drugs such as antiemetics or antianxiety agents may experience mild sedation as a side effect of therapy. Depending on the patient and how soon death is expected, sedation may decrease with time. What is important to understand is that drug therapy for symptoms of distress at the end of life is guided by protocols, using medications believed to be safe, with the intent of alleviating suffering. *There is no evidence that administering medications for symptoms of distress using established protocols hastens death.* The ethical responsibility of the nurse in caring for patients near death is to follow guidelines for drug use to manage symptoms and to facilitate prompt and effective symptom management until death.

A small percentage of patients have refractory symptoms of distress that do not respond to treatment near the end of life. These patients may be candidates for **palliative sedation**—a care management approach involving the administration of drugs such as benzodiazepines (e.g., midazolam), barbiturates, or short-acting anesthetic agents (e.g., propofol) for the purpose of decreasing suffering by lowering patient consciousness (Cherny, 2017). *The intent of palliative sedation to promote comfort and not hasten death distinguishes it from euthanasia (discussed later in this chapter).*

Meeting Psychosocial Needs. The personal experience of dying or of losing a loved one through death is life altering. Unexpected deaths, particularly in young people, tend to be most traumatic. When a person has a chronic life-threatening disease, he or she and the family may have some knowledge of the expected outcome. However, others may have never considered their illness to be potentially terminal. It is important to first assess what patients and family understand about the illness and then help them identify the desired outcomes for care in its context.

Whereas death is the termination of life, dying is a process. People facing death may demonstrate emotional signs and symptoms of their response to the dying process through behaviors that equate to saying goodbye or through actual withdrawal. Some patients attempt to make families feel better by reassuring them that everything will be fine. Teach families that such behaviors are normal. See the Patient and Family Education: Preparing for Self-Management: Common Emotional Signs of Approaching Death box earlier in this chapter.

Assisting Patients During the Grieving Process. **Grief** is the emotional feeling related to the perception of the loss. Patients who are dying suffer not only from the anticipated death but also from the loss of the ability to engage with others and in the world. **Mourning** is the outward social expression of the loss. Interventions to help patients and families grieve and mourn are based on cultural beliefs, values, and practices. Some patients and their families express their grief openly and loudly, whereas others are quiet and reserved. Table 8.3 lists basic beliefs regarding death, dying, and afterlife for some of the major religions.

Nursing interventions are aimed at providing appropriate emotional support to allow patients and their families to verbalize their fears and concerns. Support includes keeping the patient and family involved in health care decisions and emphasizing that the goal is to keep the patient as comfortable as possible until death.

Intervene with those grieving an impending death by "being with" as opposed to "being there." "Being with" implies that you are physically and psychologically with the grieving patient, empathizing to provide emotional support. Listening and acknowledging the legitimacy of the patient's and/or family's impending loss are often more therapeutic than speaking; this concept is often referred to as **presence.** Being present with a patient and family fosters trust, which helps to build a therapeutic relationship (Croson et al., 2018). This relationship can help to facilitate the expression of grief by giving the person who is mourning permission to express himself or herself. Your manner and words show that these expressions of grief are acceptable and expected. An example of therapeutic communication might be "This must be very difficult for you" or "I'm sorry this is happening."

Do not minimize a patient's or family member's reaction to an impending loss or death. Avoid trite assurances such as "Things will be fine. Don't cry," "Don't be upset. She wouldn't want it that way," or "In a year you will have forgotten." Such comments can be barriers to demonstrating care and concern. Accept whatever the grieving person says about the situation. Remain present, be ready to listen attentively, and guide gently. In this way you can help the bereaved family and significant others prepare for the necessary reminiscence and integration of the loss.

Storytelling through reminiscence and life review can be an important activity for patients who are dying. **Life review** is a structured process of reflecting on what one has done through his or her life. This is often facilitated by a trained interviewer. **Reminiscence** is the process of randomly reflecting on memories of events in one's life. The benefits of storytelling through either method provide the ability to attain perspective and enhance meaning. Suggest that the patient and family record autobiographic stories (print or video), write memories in a journal, or develop a scrapbook. Young dying parents often write letters or record videos for their children when they are older.

Perform a spiritual assessment to identify the patient's spiritual needs and facilitate open expression of his or her beliefs and needs. A spiritual assessment could start with questions such as "What is important to you?" or "What gives you meaning or purpose in your life?"

When assessing the spiritual needs of the dying patient, consider end-of-life preferences based on cultural beliefs and practices. For example, the medicine wheel represents the spiritual

TABLE 8.3 Basic Beliefs Regarding Care at End of Life and Death Rituals for Selected Religions

Christianity

- There are many Christian denominations, which have variations in beliefs regarding medical care near the end of life.
- Roman Catholic tradition encourages people to receive Sacrament of the Sick, administered by a priest at any point during an illness. This sacrament may be administered more than once. Not receiving this sacrament will *not* prohibit them from entering heaven after death.
- People may be baptized as Roman Catholics in an emergency situation (e.g., person is dying) by a layperson. Otherwise they are baptized by a priest.
- Christians believe in an afterlife of heaven or hell once the soul has left the body after death.

Judaism

- The dying person is encouraged to recite the confessional or the affirmation of faith, called the *Shema*.
- According to Jewish law, a person who is extremely ill and dying should not be left alone.
- The body, which was the vessel and vehicle of the soul, deserves reverence and respect.
- The body should not be left unattended until the funeral, which should take place as soon as possible (preferably within 24 hours).
- Autopsies are not allowed by Orthodox Jews, except under special circumstances.
- The body should not be embalmed, displayed, or cremated.

Islam

- Based on belief in one God, Allah, and his prophet Muhammad. Qur'an is the scripture of Islam, composed of Muhammad's revelations of the Word of God (Allah).
- Death is seen as the beginning of a new and better life.
- God has prescribed an appointed time of death for everyone.
- Qur'an encourages humans to seek treatment and not to refuse treatment. Belief is that only Allah cures but that Allah cures through the work of humans.
- At death the eyelids are to be closed, and the body should be covered. Before moving and handling the body, contact someone from the person's mosque to perform rituals of bathing and wrapping body in cloth.

Data from Giger, J. N. (2013). *Transcultural nursing: Assessment and intervention* (6th ed.). St. Louis: Mosby.

PATIENT-CENTERED CARE: CULTURAL/ SPIRITUAL CONSIDERATIONS QSEN

Spirituality is whatever or whoever gives ultimate meaning and purpose in one's life that invites particular ways of being in the world in relation to others, oneself, and the universe. A person's spirituality may or may not include belief in God. **Religions** are formal belief systems that provide a framework for making sense of life, death, and suffering and responding to universal spiritual questions. Religions often have beliefs, rituals, texts, and other practices that are shared by a community. Spirituality and religion can help some patients cope with the thought of death, contributing to quality of life during the dying process.

journey to find one's own path for indigenous people in many countries, including American Indians (e.g., Cherokee, Navajo, Lakota) and Aboriginal people (e.g., Inuit, First Nations) in Canada and Alaska (also known as *Canada or Alaska Natives*). The medicine wheel helps people in these groups maintain balance and harmony within four life dimensions (Fig. 8.2). Depending on specific tribal practices and beliefs, the dimensions may be represented by colors, seasons, or directions.

As part of the dying process, certain tribal ceremonies must take place for patients to have a peaceful transition into the spirit world and experience a "good death." One special ceremony involves smudging: selected tribal medicines are burned, and the smoke is passed over the patient's body to cleanse it.

Regardless of whether a person has had an affiliation with a religion or a belief in God or other Supreme Being, he or she can experience what is referred to as *spiritual* or *existential distress.* Existential distress is brought about by the actual or perceived threat to one's continued existence. Terminal illness and facing death can pose a profound threat to one's personhood. The main task for a person at the end of life is coming to terms with one's losses, which may include loss of meaning, loss of relationships, and facing the unknown. Acknowledge the patient's spiritual pain and encourage verbalization. If the patient or family prefers, arrange for counseling with chaplains, spiritual leaders, or others trained in end-of-life care. *Do not try to explain the loss in philosophic or religious terms.* Statements such as "Everything happens for the best" or "God sends us only as much as we can bear" are not helpful when the person has yet to express feelings of anguish or anger. Provide quiet spaces or environments that allow the family members to support one another and the patient. Quiet spaces can offer a place to reflect or pray while processing the intense emotions that accompany terminal illness (Croson et al., 2018).

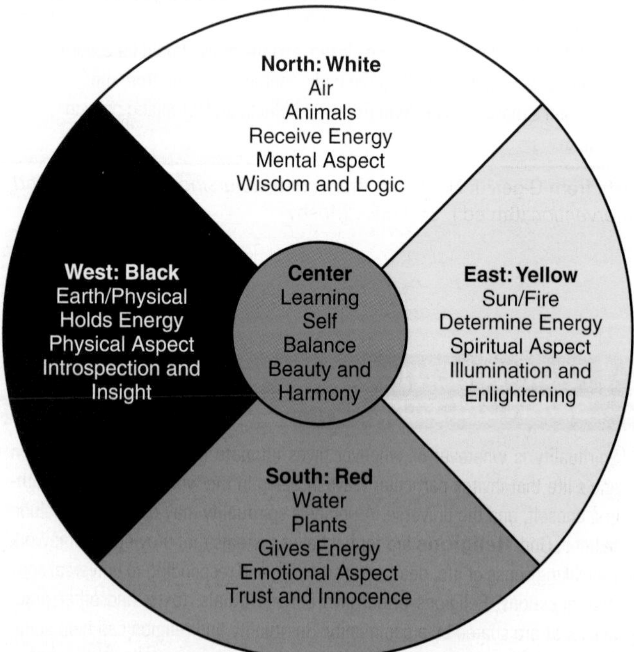

Fig. 8.2 An example of a medicine wheel used by indigenous people to provide harmony and balance in life and transition into the spirit world after death.

Although emotionally challenging, witnessing the death of a loved one may help facilitate the family's acceptance of death. Witnessing how ill a person is makes the event real and enhances an understanding of how disease affects bodily function and decline. Describe the physical signs in detail—realistic enough to be unmistakable, yet not so graphic as to alarm the listeners (see the Patient and Family Education: Preparing for Self-Management boxes). Booklets with this information should be provided to families to help them see what is expected and "normal" to the dying process.

Families witnessing the dying process often have difficulty distinguishing what is a normal finding of decline from signs and symptoms of distress. Instructing families about signs and symptoms of pain (e.g., grimacing, moaning, guarding behaviors) or dyspnea is essential. Emphasize that in the absence of dyspnea or pain, patients often die very peacefully with cessation of breathing. Nurses and family members know that a person has died when he or she stops breathing (see the Patient and Family Education: Preparing for Self-Management: Physical Signs Indicating That Death Has Occurred box).

Nurses, patients, and families may benefit from written information about the dying process and what is known about the patient experience and needs. *Fast Facts and Concepts* are a group of evidence-based summaries on key palliative care topics available on the Palliative Care Network of Wisconsin (2018) website (http://www.mypcnow.org). They provide concise, practical, peer-reviewed information on topics common to patients facing serious illness.

In Canada, the Canadian Hospice Palliative Care Association provides information for patients, families, lay caregivers and volunteers, and members of the interprofessional health care team. A number of documents on palliative care and hospice services are available on the website (www.chpca.net).

Postmortem Care. If the death was in the home and expected, emergency assistance (911) should *not* be called. If the person was a patient in a hospice program, the family calls the hospice service. If a death is unexpected or suspicious, the medical examiner is notified. Otherwise the nurse or primary health care provider performs the pronouncement and completes a death certificate. Most states allow nurses to pronounce death in nursing homes and other long-term care facilities, but only a few states permit nurses to pronounce in acute care facilities such as hospitals. Be sure to check your health care agency policies

PATIENT AND FAMILY EDUCATION: PREPARING FOR SELF-MANAGEMENT

Physical Signs Indicating That Death Has Occurred

- Breathing stops.
- Heart stops beating.
- Pupils become fixed and dilated.
- Body color becomes pale and waxen.
- Body temperature drops.
- Muscles and sphincters relax.
- Urine and stool may be released.
- Eyes may remain open, and there is no blinking.
- The jaw may fall open.

BEST PRACTICE FOR PATIENT SAFETY & QUALITY CARE QSEN

Pronouncement of Death

- Note time of death—the time at which the family or staff reported the cessation of respirations.
- Identify the patient by identification (ID) tag if in facility. Note the general appearance of the body.
- Ascertain that the patient does not rouse to verbal or tactile stimuli. Avoid overtly painful stimuli, especially if family members are present.
- Auscultate for the absence of heart sounds; palpate for the absence of carotid pulse.
- Look and listen for the absence of spontaneous respirations.
- Document the time of pronouncement and all notifications in the medical record (i.e., to attending physician). Document if the medical examiner needs to be notified (may be required for unexpected or suspicious death). Document if an autopsy is planned per the attending primary health care provider and family.
- If your state and agency policy allows an RN to pronounce death, document as indicated on the death certificate.

for who can pronounce death and the specific procedure to follow. See the Best Practice for Patient Safety & Quality Care: Pronouncement of Death box.

After the patient has died, ask the family or other caregivers if they would like to spend time with the patient to help them cope with what has happened and to say their goodbyes. Even if the death has been anticipated, no one knows how he or she will feel until it occurs. It may take hours to days to weeks or months for each person to realize the full effect of the event. Some family members may find it therapeutic to bathe and prepare the person's body for transfer to the funeral home or the hospital morgue. Offer families this opportunity if it is culturally acceptable.

Before preparing the body for transfer, ask the primary health care provider whether an autopsy will be required. When the death is expected, an autopsy is not likely. An autopsy is generally performed only when the cause of death is not known. Some religions such as Orthodox Judaism do not allow autopsies.

After the family or significant others view the body, follow agency procedure for preparing the patient for transfer to either the morgue or a funeral home. In the hospital a postmortem kit is generally used with a shroud and identification tags. See the Best Practice for Patient Safety & Quality Care: Postmortem Care box.

◆ **Evaluation: Evaluate Outcomes.** Evaluate the care of the patient based on the identified priority patient problem. In end-of-life care, evaluation is not related to improvements in overall condition; rather, it is specific to promoting a peaceful death. The expected outcomes are that the patient with end-of-life care will:

- Have needs and preferences acknowledged and met
- Have control or management of symptoms of distress
- Experience meaningful interactions with family and other loved ones
- Experience a peaceful death

ETHICS AND DYING

Euthanasia is a term that has been used to describe the process of ending one's life. *Active euthanasia* implies that

BEST PRACTICE FOR PATIENT SAFETY & QUALITY CARE QSEN

Postmortem Care

- Provide all care with respect to communicate that the person was important and valued.
- Ask the family or significant others if they wish to help wash the patient or comb his or her hair; respect and follow their cultural practices for body preparation.
- If no autopsy is planned, remove or cut all tubes and lines according to agency policy.
- Close the patient's eyes unless the cultural or religious practice is for a family member or other person to close the eyes.
- Insert dentures if the patient wore them.
- Straighten the patient and lower the bed to a flat position.
- Place a pillow under the patient's head.
- Wash the patient as needed and comb and arrange the patient's hair unless the family desires to perform bathing and body preparation.
- Place waterproof pads under the patient's hips and around the perineum to absorb any excrement.
- Clean the patient's room or unit.
- Allow the family or significant others to see the patient in private and to perform any religious or cultural customs they wish (e.g., prayer).
- Assess that all who need to see the patient have done so before transferring to the funeral home or morgue.
- Notify the hospital chaplain or appropriate religious leader if requested by the family or significant others.
- Ensure that the nurse or physician has completed and signed the death certificate.
- Prepare the patient for transfer to either a morgue or a funeral home; wrap the patient in a shroud (unless the family has a special shroud to use), and attach identification tags per agency policy.

primary health care providers take action (e.g., give medication or treatment) that purposefully and directly causes the patient's death. *Active euthanasia, even with the patient's permission, is not supported by most health professional organizations in the United States, including the American Nurses Association.*

Physician-assisted death (PAD), sometimes referred to as assisted dying or physician-assisted suicide, is gaining worldwide public support. A few European countries, including Belgium, Switzerland, Luxembourg, and the Netherlands, have had legalized physician-assisted death for terminally ill patients for a number of years. In 2016 physician-assisted death became legal in Canada. In the United States PAD is now legally approved in Oregon, Washington, Vermont, Montana, California, Colorado, and the District of Columbia (Quill & Battin, 2018). Many other states are considering legislation on end-of-life options. At this time nurses are generally not involved in physician-assisted death but need to be knowledgeable about the legislation in the state where they practice. Nurses are often in the position to educate patients and therefore must be aware of factual information related to aid in dying. Patients and families that are struggling with this issue need a safe place to ask questions and seek clarity, and it is important that the nurse provide open discussion without judgment (Hamric et al., 2018).

Withdrawing or withholding life-sustaining therapy, formerly called *passive euthanasia,* involves discontinuing one or more therapies that might prolong the life of a person who cannot be cured by the therapy. Another phrase sometimes used is "letting the person die naturally" or "allowing natural death." *In this situation, the withdrawal of the intervention does not directly cause the patient's death.* The progression of the patient's disease or poor health status is the cause of death. Professional health care organizations and some religious communities support the right of patients and their surrogate decision makers to refuse or stop treatment when patients are close to death and interventions are considered medically futile or capable of causing harm. The U.S. court system also supports withdrawal of aggressive treatment and the rights of surrogate decision makers to refuse or stop treatment.

An alternative method for hastening death is called *voluntary stopping of eating and drinking (VSED).* For some patients, VSED is viewed as the only legal or moral alternative to relieve intolerable suffering (Hamric et al., 2018). With VSED, competent patients with a terminal or incurable disease or illness refuse to eat or drink to hasten their death. Many patients want control over their lives and wish to die rather than continue experiencing severe pain and suffering. In addition, patients often want to end the caregiver burden that is often assumed by the family or significant other for their care. VSED leads to terminal dehydration (as described earlier in this chapter), which can be managed to promote comfort with palliative measures.

Nurses are usually in the best and most immediate position to discuss these issues. To do this, they must be knowledgeable about terminology and ethical issues related to death and dying. In all cases the principles of informed consent must be met: the patient is competent, the death is voluntary, and the patient understands the benefit, burden, and consequences of the death.

GET READY FOR THE NEXT-GENERATION NCLEX® EXAMINATION!

Key Points

Review these Key Points for each NCLEX Examination Client Needs Category.

Safe and Effective Care Environment

- Hospice care uses an interprofessional approach to medical care, pain management, and emotional and spiritual support expressly tailored to each patient's needs and wishes, including family and loved ones. **QSEN: Teamwork and Collaboration**
- The decision by the person with a durable power of attorney for health care (DPOAHC) to withdraw or withhold life-sustaining therapy is supported by the U.S. Supreme Court and other professional/religious organizations.
- Be aware that physician-assisted death is legal in several countries and multiple states in the United States. **Ethics**
- Nurses have an ethical obligation to provide timely information about expected care outcomes so patients and families can make the best end-of-life decisions. **Ethics**

Health Promotion and Maintenance

- Assess the patient and family for written advance directives such as a DPOAHC, a living will, or portable DNR/DNAR.
- Teach the importance of having a DPOAHC to inform health care providers of your wishes if you lack capacity.
- Teach the patient and family that an advance directive is a written document that specifies what, if any, extraordinary actions the patient would want if he or she could no longer make decisions about care.

Psychosocial Integrity

- Assess the patient's emotional signs of impending death; assess coping ability of the patient and family or other caregiver.
- Incorporate the patient's personal cultural practices and spiritual beliefs regarding death and dying (see Table 8.3). **QSEN: Patient-Centered Care**
- Be aware that people facing death may experience fear and anxiety about their impending death and have difficulty coping.
- Provide psychosocial interventions to support the patient and family during the dying process.

Physiological Integrity

- Death is defined as the cessation of integrated tissue and organ function, manifested by cessation of heartbeat, absence of spontaneous respirations, or irreversible brain dysfunction.
- Hospice and palliative care are different, as described in Table 8.2.
- Assess the patient for pain, dyspnea, agitation, nausea, and vomiting, which are common problems at the end of life. **QSEN: Evidence-Based Practice**
- Recognize that older adults are often undertreated for pain or other symptoms at the end of life.
- Assess for the common physical signs of approaching death, as listed in the Patient and Family Education: Preparing for Self-Management: Physical Signs Indicating That Death Has Occurred box.
- Medications are frequently given to control dyspnea, pain, nausea, vomiting, delirium, and seizures in patients near death.
- Because of the risk for delirium, particularly in older adults, providers may avoid use of benzodiazepines for treatment of anxiety, even at the end of life. Development of increased agitation after receiving benzodiazepine could represent a paradoxical reaction. **QSEN: Safety**
- Terminal delirium may occur in a week or two before death. Haloperidol given orally or IV is the drug of choice to manage psychosis associated with delirium.

- Assessment of oxygen saturation for patients at the end of life is not necessary. Oxygen should be provided based on comfort. **QSEN: Evidence-Based Practice**
- Common complementary and integrative therapies used for symptom management at the end of life include aromatherapy, music therapy, and energy therapies such as Therapeutic Touch.
- Follow best-practice guidelines for performing postmortem care; incorporate the patient's cultural and religious beliefs in body preparation and burial (see Table 8.3). **QSEN: Patient-Centered Care**

MASTERY QUESTIONS

1. A client receiving palliative care for a terminal cancer diagnosis asks the nurse, "Why is this happening to me?" What is the best nursing response?
   A. "I don't know. God knows when your time is up on this earth."
   B. "I'm sorry. I know that this is a very difficult time for you."
   C. "It's going to be OK; at least you aren't leaving any family behind."
   D. "We'll make sure that all of your needs are met, so don't worry."

2. The family of a client experiencing terminal dehydration requests that intravenous fluids be started. What is the best response?
   A. "We can start fluids to help ease the dehydration."
   B. "Intravenous fluids can increase discomfort for the client."
   C. "Intravenous fluids will likely prolong life."
   D. "Terminal dehydration can be managed better with pain medication."

REFERENCES

Asterisk (*) indicates a classic or definitive work on this subject.

*Campbell, M. L., Weissman, D. E., & Nelson, J. E. (2012). Palliative care consultation in the ICU. *Journal of Palliative Medicine, 15*(6), 715–716.

Carpenter, J., McDarby, M., Smith, D., Johnson, M., Thorpe, J., & Ersek, M. (2017). Associations between timing of palliative care consults and family evaluation of care for veterans who die in a hospice/palliative care unit. *Journal of Palliative Medicine, 20*(7), 745–751.

Centers for Disease Control and Prevention. (2017). Leading cause of death and numbers of deaths. Retrieved from https://www.cdc.gov/nchs/data/hus/2017/019.pdf.

Cherny, N. (2017). Palliative sedation. *UpToDate*. Retrieved from https://www.uptodate.com/contents/palliative-sedation.

Coelho, A., Parola, V., Sandgren, A., Fernanded, O., Kolcaba, K., & Apostolo, J. (2018). The effects of guided imagery on comfort in palliative care. *Journal of Hospice & Palliative Nursing, 20*(4), 392–399. https://doi.org/10.1097/NJH.0000000000000460.

Croson, E., Keim-Malpass, J., Bohnenkamp, S., & LeBaron, V. (2018). The medical-surgical nurses' guide to understanding palliative care and hospice. *Medsurg Nursing, 27*(4), 215–222.

Cyr, C., Arboleda, M., Aggarwal, S., Balneaves, L., Daeninck, P., Neron, A., Prosk, E., & Vigano, A. (2018). Cannabis in palliative care: Current challenges and practical recommendations. *Annals of Palliative Medicine, 7*(4), 463–477.

Dudgeon, D. (2019). Assessment and management of dyspnea in palliative care. *UpToDate*. Retrieved from https://www.uptodate.com/contents/assessment-and-management-of-dyspnea-in-palliative-care.

*Finocchiaro, D. N. (2016). Supporting the patient's spiritual needs at the end of life. *Nursing, 46*(5), 57–59.

*Giger, J. N. (2013). *Transcultural Nursing: Assessment and Intervention* (6th ed.). St. Louis: Mosby.

Hamlin, A., & Robertson, M. (2017). Pain and complementary therapies. *Critical Care Nursing Clinics of North America, 29*(4), 449–460.

Hamric, A., Schwarz, J., Cohen, L., & Mahon, M. (2018). Assisted suicide/Aid in dying: What is the nurse's role? *American Journal of Nursing, 118*(5), 50–59.

Hospice and Palliative Nurses Association. (2018). HPNA position statement advance care planning. *Journal of Hospice and Palliative Nursing, 20*(5), E1–E3.

*Institute of Medicine. (2014). Dying in America: Improving quality and honoring individual preferences near the end of life. http://www.nationalacademies.org/hmd/~/media/Files/Report%20Files/2014/EOL/Report%20Brief.pdf.

Lyons, M. (2018). The use of aromatherapy for symptom management. *Pain Management Nursing, 19*(2), 111.

McMillan, K., Glaser, D., & Radovich, P. (2018). The effect of massage on pain and anxiety in hospitalized patients: An observational study. *Medsurg Nursing, 27*(1), 14–18.

Meier, D., & Bowman, B. (2017). The changing landscape of palliative care. *Journal of the American Society on Aging, 41*(1), 74–80.

Quill, T., & Battin, M. (2018). Physician assisted dying: Understanding, evaluating, and responding to requests for medical aid in dying. *UpToDate*. Retrieved from https://www.uptodate.com/contents/physician-assisted-dying-understanding-evaluating-and-responding-to-requests-for-medical-aid-in-dying.

Westman, K. F., & Blaisdell, C. (2016). Many benefits, little risk: The use of massage in nursing practice. *AJN, 116*(1), 34–41.

9

Concepts of Care for Perioperative Patients

Cherie Rebar, Marie Bashaw

http://evolve.elsevier.com/Iggy/

LEARNING OUTCOMES

1. Collaborate with the interprofessional team to coordinate high-quality care for patients in the perioperative setting.
2. Ensure safety by protecting patients from injury, ***infection,*** and complications of surgery during the postoperative phase.
3. Teach the patient and family or caregiver about preoperative preparations and postsurgical interventions to prevent ***infection*** and minimize ***pain.***
4. Teach the postoperative patient and family or caregiver about self-management resources within the community.
5. Implement nursing interventions to decrease the psychosocial impact of the perioperative phase.
6. Apply knowledge of anatomy, physiology, and pathophysiology to perform perioperative assessments.
7. Use clinical judgment to analyze diagnostic findings within the perioperative phase.
8. Plan care coordination and transition management for patients who are discharged after surgery.
9. Use clinical judgment to plan evidence-based care to promote ***tissue integrity*** and prevent complications in patients who have had surgery.

KEY TERMS

ambulatory patient See *outpatient.*

ASA Physical Status Classification system From the American Society of Anesthesiologists (ASA), a system that assesses the fitness of patients for surgery.

atelectasis Collapse of lung tissue; can occur postoperatively if the patient does not change positions and breathe deeply.

autologous donation Blood donation given by the patient before surgery for the purpose of reinfusing for self; reinfusing the patient's own blood during surgery.

carboxyhemoglobin Carbon monoxide on oxygen-binding sites of the hemoglobin molecule.

dehiscence Partial or complete separation of the outer wound layers.

dysuria Painful urination.

evisceration Total separation of all wound layers and protrusion of internal organs through the open wound.

hyperkalemia Increased serum potassium level.

hypokalemia Decreased serum potassium level.

inpatient A patient who is admitted to a hospital.

intraoperative phase During surgery.

malignant hyperthermia (MH) Inherited muscle disorder; an acute, life-threatening complication of certain drugs used for general anesthesia.

morbidity Illness or an abnormal condition or quality; number of serious diseases.

mortality Death.

myoglobinuria Muscle proteins in the urine due to rhabdomyolysis.

nocturia The need to urinate excessively at night.

NPO No eating, drinking (including water), smoking, or oral medications.

oliguria Scant urine output; usually less than 400 mL per day.

outpatient A patient who goes to the surgical area the day of surgery and returns home the same day.

perioperative Operative experience consisting of the preoperative, intraoperative, and postoperative time phases.

postoperative phase After surgery.

preoperative phase Before surgery.

pulse deficit Difference between the apical and peripheral pulses.

sanguineous Bloody (as in drainage).

serosanguineous Yellowish mixed with light red or pale pink (as in drainage).

serous Serum-like, or yellow (as in drainage).

PRIORITY AND INTERRELATED CONCEPTS

The priority concepts for this chapter are:
- ***Gas Exchange***
- ***Pain***

The interrelated concepts for this chapter are:
- ***Infection***
- ***Tissue Integrity***

History shows that rudimentary surgical procedures were done as early as 10,000 BCE, when trepanation, the process of boring or cutting parts of bone out from the skull, was performed (Ellis & Abdalla, 2018). Modern surgery is performed under strict conditions, designed to enhance patient safety, for a multitude of purposes ranging from diagnosis to cure (Table 9.1). Nurses provide critical patient care in periods of time before (preoperative phase), during (intraoperative phase), and after (postoperative phase) all of these types of surgeries. Together, these times are known as the perioperative experience. The generalist nurse will not attend the actual surgical procedure within the intraoperative phase; therefore this chapter focuses on the preoperative and postoperative phases of time.

SURGERY OVERVIEW

Surgical procedures are categorized by the purpose, body location, extent, and degree of urgency. Table 9.2 explains select categories by urgency and approach. Surgery takes place in hospitals and outpatient ambulatory surgical centers (ASCs) that are part of a hospital or may be freestanding. Very minor surgeries can be accomplished in an outpatient office. Inpatient refers to a patient who is admitted to a hospital. The patient may be admitted on the day of surgery (often termed *same-day admission* [SDA]) or may already be an inpatient when surgery is needed. An outpatient or ambulatory patient goes to the surgical area the day of the surgery and returns home on the same day (i.e., same-day surgery [SDS]).

Advantages of outpatient surgery centers include cost-effective care, service-oriented processes, and a high degree of patient satisfaction. The complexity of procedures being performed in outpatient surgery centers (e.g., laparoscopic cholecystectomy) places more responsibility on the patient and family or caregiver, especially for care after surgery. Often a case manager is used to coordinate postdischarge care for the patient to ensure follow-up treatments and avoid postoperative hospital admission.

Regardless of the surgical setting, patient safety, teamwork and interprofessional collaboration, and use of professional ethics are priorities. The Association of periOperative Registered Nurses (AORN) is the specialty organization that provides guidelines for ethical and safe care for patients undergoing operative and other invasive procedures.

Safety During the Surgical Experience

Nurses and other members of the interprofessional health care team consistently anticipate safety needs prior to, during, and after the surgical experience, and carry out initiatives to enhance patient well-being. Because surgery is invasive and involves exposure to various anesthetic agents and drugs, positioning, and other environmental hazards, interventions can be taken to prevent problems that are anticipated. Some complications are considered preventable or "never events." Numerous initiatives that are focused on standardization of care and communication are in place to enhance patient safety and prevent all types of complications.

National Patient Safety Goals. The Joint Commission's National Patient Safety Goals (NPSGs) have long been focused on communication with and between the surgical team so that correct actions are taken to achieve desired outcomes. These NPSGs continue into 2020. See the National Patient Safety Goals box.

! NATIONAL PATIENT SAFETY GOALS: SURGERY

For 2020, National Patient Safety Goals for Surgery focus on (1) having the correct procedure done on the correct patient at the correct body location; (2) marking the correct site of surgery on the patient's body where surgery will take place; and (3) pausing before surgery to make sure that mistakes are not being made (The Joint Commission, 2020).

SBAR. As noted in Chapter 1, SBAR is an effective system of communication used in many agencies for hand-off purposes. Following this format ensures that *s*ituation, *b*ackground, *a*ssessment, and *r*ecommendation/*r*equest information is consistently conveyed between two or more members of the health care team or agency. See Chapter 1 for more information.

Surgical Care Improvement Project. The Surgical Care Improvement Project (SCIP), a set of core compliance measures, was initiated in 2006 to reduce surgical complications. Examples of focus included administration of prophylactic antibiotics, correct hair removal processes, the timing of discontinuation of urinary catheterization after surgery, and venous thromboembolism (VTE) prophylaxis. These practices are now standard in surgical care.

Surgical Safety Checklist. Fig. 9.1 shows a surgical safety checklist as recommended by the World Health Organization (WHO), The Joint Commission, and the Association of periOperative Registered Nurses (AORN). Quality measures such as wrong-site surgery, patient falls, hospital-acquired pressure injuries, and vascular catheter-associated infections must be reported to the Centers for Medicare and Medicaid Services (CMS). These data are used for tracking patient outcomes and ensuring patient-centered care and accountability on the part of health care agencies.

TeamSTEPPS®. TeamSTEPPS® is a system designed to facilitate communication between health care providers to enhance patient safety and quality of care. Designed by the Department of Defense (DOD) and the Agency for Healthcare Research and Quality (AHRQ), TeamSTEPPS has been shown to be effective when used in the surgical environment (AHRQ, 2017). This system

TABLE 9.1 Reasons for Surgical Procedures

Purpose	Definition	Example
Cosmetic[a]	Performed to reshape normal body structures to improve the patient's appearance or self-image Usually is elective in nature	Body contouring (e.g., abdominoplasty—"tummy tuck") Facelift Rhinoplasty
Curative[b]	Performed to resolve a health problem by repairing or removing the cause	Removal of cancerous tumor Removal of gallbladder
Diagnostic[b]	Performed to determine the origin and cause of a disorder by taking a tissue sample with the intention of diagnosing (and staging, if applicable) a condition	Breast biopsy after an abnormal finding on a mammogram Joint arthroscopy
Palliative[b]	Performed to increase the quality of life (often to reduce ***pain***) while reducing stressors on the body; noncurative in nature	Ileostomy creation Stent placement to alleviate obstruction Thoracentesis to drain fluid to reduce ***pain***
Preventative[b]	Performed with the intention that a condition will not develop	Prophylactic bilateral mastectomy in women who carry the *BRCA1* or *BRCA2* gene
Reconstructive[a]	Performed on abnormal or damaged body structures to improve functional ability	Total hip replacement Total knee replacement
Transplantation	Performed to replace a malfunctioning structure	Heart transplant Kidney transplant

[a]Adapted from the American Board of Cosmetic Surgery. https://www.americanboardcosmeticsurgery.org/patient-resources/cosmetic-surgery-vs-plastic-surgery/
[b]Adapted from National Cancer Institute. https://training.seer.cancer.gov/treatment/surgery/types/

TABLE 9.2 Selected Categories of Surgical Procedures by Urgency and Approach

Urgency of Surgery		
Elective	Planned for correction of a nonacute problem	Cataract removal Hernia repair Hemorrhoidectomy Total joint replacement
Urgent	Requires prompt intervention; may be life threatening if treatment is delayed more than 24-48 hr	Intestinal obstruction Bladder obstruction Kidney or ureteral stones Bone fracture Eye injury Acute cholecystitis
Emergent	Requires immediate intervention because of life-threatening consequences	Gunshot or stab wound Severe bleeding Abdominal aortic aneurysm Compound fracture Appendectomy
Surgical Approach		
Simple	Only the most overtly affected areas involved in the surgery	Simple or partial mastectomy
Minimally invasive surgery (MIS)	Surgery performed in a body cavity or body area through one or more endoscopes; can correct problems, remove organs, take tissue for biopsy, reroute blood vessels and drainage systems; is a fast-growing and ever-changing type of surgery	Arthroscopy Tubal ligation Hysterectomy Lung lobectomy Coronary artery bypass Cholecystectomy
Radical	Extensive surgery beyond the area obviously involved; is directed at finding a root cause	Radical prostatectomy Radical hysterectomy

promotes communication, safety, and interprofessional teamwork and collaboration, which has been shown by evidence to result in better patient outcomes and quality of care. See Chapter 1 for more information.

PREOPERATIVE PHASE

The preoperative phase begins when the patient is scheduled for surgery and ends at the time of transfer to the surgical suite. The patient's readiness for surgery is critical to the outcome.

COMPREHENSIVE SURGICAL CHECKLIST

Blue = World Health Organization (WHO) Green = The Joint Commission - Universal Protocol 2016 National Patient Safety Goals Teal = Joint Commission and WHO

PREPROCEDURE CHECK-IN	SIGN-IN	TIME-OUT	SIGN-OUT
In Preoperative Ready Area	**Before Induction of Anesthesia**	**Before Skin Incision**	**Before the Patient Leaves the Operating Room**
Patient or patient representative actively confirms with registered nurse (RN):	**RN and anesthesia professional confirm:**	**Initiated by designated team member:** All other activities to be suspended (except in case of life-threatening emergency)	**RN confirms:**
Identity ☐ Yes Procedure and procedure site ☐ Yes Consent(s) ☐ Yes Site marked ☐ Yes ☐ N/A by the person performing the procedure **RN confirms presence of:** History and physical ☐ Yes Preanesthesia assessment ☐ Yes Nursing assessment ☐ Yes Diagnostic and radiologic test results ☐ Yes ☐ N/A Blood products ☐ Yes ☐ N/A Any special equipment, devices, implants ☐ Yes ☐ N/A Include in Preprocedure check-in as per institutional custom: Beta blocker medication given ☐ Yes ☐ N/A Venous thromboembolism prophylaxis ordered ☐ Yes ☐ N/A Normothermia measures ☐ Yes ☐ N/A	Confirmation of the following: identity, procedure, procedure site, and consent(s) ☐ Yes Site marked ☐ Yes ☐ N/A by person performing the procedure Patient allergies ☐ Yes ☐ N/A Pulse oximeter on patient ☐ Yes Difficult airway or aspiration risk ☐ No ☐ Yes (preparation confirmed) Risk of blood loss (> 500 mL) ☐ Yes ☐ N/A # of units available ________ Anesthesia safety check completed ☐ Yes **Briefing:** All members of the team have discussed care plan and addressed concerns ☐ Yes	Introduction of team members ☐ Yes **All:** Confirmation of the following: identity, procedure, incision site, consent(s) ☐ Yes Site is marked and visible ☐ Yes ☐ N/A Fire Risk Assessment and Discussion ☐ Yes (prevention methods implemented) ☐ N/A Relevant images properly labeled and displayed ☐ Yes ☐ N/A Any equipment concerns ☐ Yes ☐ N/A **Anticipated Critical Events** **Surgeon:** States the following: ☐ Critical or nonroutine steps ☐ Case duration ☐ Anticipated blood loss **Anesthesia professional:** Antibiotic prophylaxis within 1 hour before incision ☐ Yes ☐ N/A Additional concerns ☐ Yes ☐ N/A **Scrub person and RN circulator:** Sterilization indicators confirmed ☐ Yes Additional concerns ☐ Yes ☐ N/A **RN:** Documented completion of time out ☐ Yes	Name of operative procedure: ________ Completion of sponge, sharp, and instrument counts ☐ Yes ☐ N/A Specimens identified and labeled ☐ Yes ☐ N/A Equipment problems to be addressed ☐ Yes ☐ N/A Discussion of Wound Classification ☐ Yes **To all team members:** What are the key concerns for recovery and management of this patient? ________ ________ ________ ________ **Debriefing with all team members:** Opportunity for discussion of - team performance - key events - any permanent changes in the preference card January 2019

The Joint Commission does not stipulate which team member initiates any section of the checklist except for site marking. The Joint Commission also does not stipulate where these activities occur. See the Universal Protocol for details on the Joint Commission requirements.

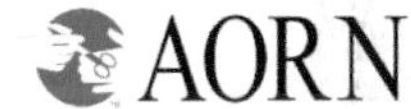

FIG. 9.1 Comprehensive surgical checklist. (Created in collaboration with AORN Perioperative Nursing Specialist Robin Chard, PhD, RN, CNOR, AORN; President Charlotte Guglielmi, RN, BSN, MA, CNOR; contributors to the WHO Surgical Safety Checklist, including Atul Gawande, MD, MPH; and representatives from The Joint Commission.)

Preoperative care focuses on preparing the patient for the surgery and ensuring safety. This care includes assessing patient knowledge and educational needs. Implement interventions needed before surgery to reduce anxiety and complications and to promote patient adherence to the treatment plan after surgery. During the nursing assessment before surgery, validate, clarify, and reinforce information the patient has received from the surgical team. Problems identified may warrant further patient assessment or intervention before the procedure.

❖ Interprofessional Collaborative Care

◆ **Assessment: Recognize Cues.** The surgical patient assessment begins in the preoperative phase and continues throughout the perioperative experience. Using a patient-centered approach focuses the assessment on the patient's physical, psychosocial, cultural, and spiritual needs. The assessment process is key to identifying potential patient problems, planning care, and anticipating potential outcomes.

History. Nurses communicate information about the patient's surgery in multiple capacities. This can take place during a face-to-face meeting in the surgeon's office, in the preadmission or admission office of a hospital, or on an inpatient unit on a floor. It may also take place over the telephone or in a conference call via the Internet. Completing an assessment and gathering data should take place in a private setting to ensure that the patient's confidentiality is protected, regardless of the setting. Privacy increases the patient's comfort with the interview process and may help reduce the stress associated with surgery.

The preoperative assessment will be conducted in various ways at different agencies. The time provided for assessment depends on agency policy, patient condition, and type of surgery that will be performed. In some agencies, the preoperative assessment takes place weeks in advance of a scheduled surgery, where the patient receives a full preoperative physical and diagnostic testing all at once. In other agencies, the nurse who has cared for the patient as an inpatient may perform the preoperative assessment. Another model of care involves a preoperative nurse who conducts a quick assessment before the patient meets with the anesthesia provider and surgeon immediately before surgery. The following information reflects a comprehensive preoperative assessment.

! NURSING SAFETY PRIORITY (QSEN)

Action Alert

Ask about a history of joint replacement, and document the exact location of any prostheses. Communicate this information to operative personnel to ensure that electrocautery pads, which could cause an electrical burn, are not placed on or near the area of the prosthesis. Other areas to avoid when placing electrocautery pads include on or near bony prominences, pacemakers, scar tissue, hair, tattoos, weight-bearing surfaces, pressure points, and metal piercings.

When taking a history as in Box 9.1, be especially alert for problems that may increase the risk for complications during and after surgery, particularly as this relates to anesthesia. Some of these problems are listed in Table 9.3. The American Society of Anesthesiologists (ASA) created the **ASA Physical Status Classification System** (Table 9.4) to assess the preanesthesia status of patients before surgery and to determine existing comorbidities (ASA, 2019). The ASA Classification System facilitates the assessment of a patient's risks before surgery and provides a baseline for intraoperative care. Each surgical patient is assigned a classification by the anesthesia provider to indicate overall physical health or sickness before surgery.

Begin collecting the history by confirming the patient's *age* and *general status of health.* A *review of systems* involves the collection of information about body symptoms in an effort to understand what signs or symptoms the patient has experienced or may be currently experiencing (CMS, 2018). Box 9.2 contains the elements included in a review of systems, with specific examples of items to ask about. Conduct a thorough inquiry about each system, noting specific information that may need further assessment or notification to the health care provider or surgeon.

Medical history is important to obtain because many chronic illnesses increase surgical risks and must be considered when planning care. For example, a patient with systemic lupus erythematosus may need additional drugs to offset the stress of the surgery. A patient with immunity issues such as rheumatoid arthritis may need special considerations during the positioning process because of decreased movement and mobility. Any ***infection*** present requires intervention before surgery, which may involve cancellation of the procedure.

Ask the patient specifically about any cardiac problems because complications from anesthesia occur more often in patients with a cardiac history. Be aware that:

- Coronary artery disease, angina, myocardial infarction (MI) within 6 months before surgery, heart failure, hypertension, and dysrhythmias increase risk.
- These problems impair the patient's ability to withstand hemodynamic changes and alter the response to anesthesia.
- The risk for an MI during surgery is higher in patients who have existing heart problems.
- Patients with cardiac disease who are prescribed beta-blocking drugs should continue the therapy before surgery and in the immediate postoperative phase (Devereaux et al., 2020).

BOX 9.1 Taking a Preoperative History

- Age
- General status of health
- Review of systems
- Medical history
  - Current medical problems and their treatment
  - Allergies, including sensitivity to latex products
  - History of any type of prostheses
- Surgical history
  - Prior surgical procedures and how these were tolerated
  - Prior experience with anesthesia (e.g., difficulty being aroused after surgery, ongoing nausea and vomiting)
  - Prior experience with postsurgical ***pain*** control
- Social history
  - Use of tobacco, alcohol, or illicit substances, including marijuana (which may be legalized in certain states)
  - Current drugs taken (prescribed and over-the-counter)
  - Use of complementary or alternative therapies or practices such as vitamins, minerals, herbal preparations, folk remedies, or acupuncture
- Family history
  - Relevant information about similar familial surgeries and outcomes
  - History of malignant hyperthermia (MH), cancer, or a bleeding disorder
  - History of reactions or complications associated with anesthesia
- Psychosocial status
  - Knowledge about and understanding of events during the perioperative phase
  - Comfort level with understanding the type of surgery planned and the anticipated outcomes
  - Adequacy of the patient's support system
- Cultural or spiritual needs
  - Desire for (or against) autologous or directed blood (or blood product) donations
  - Requests for postsurgical cultural needs, or spiritual support

Determine if the patient has a history of pulmonary problems. Pulmonary complications during or after surgery are more likely to occur in older adults, those with chronic respiratory problems, and smokers because of smoking- or age-related lung changes. Increased chest rigidity and loss of lung elasticity reduce anesthetic excretion. Smoking increases the blood level of **carboxyhemoglobin** (carbon monoxide on oxygen-binding sites of the hemoglobin molecule), which decreases oxygen delivery to organs. Action of cilia in pulmonary mucous membranes decreases, which leads to retained secretions and predisposes the patient to ***infection*** (pneumonia) and **atelectasis** (collapse of alveoli). Atelectasis reduces ***gas exchange*** and causes intolerance of anesthesia. It is also a common problem after general anesthesia.

Chronic lung problems such as asthma, emphysema, and chronic bronchitis also reduce the elasticity of the lungs, which reduces ***gas exchange.*** As a result, patients with these problems have reduced tissue oxygenation.

Previous surgical procedures and anesthesia affect the patient's readiness for surgery. Previous experiences, especially with complications, may increase anxiety about the scheduled surgery. Assess the patient's past experiences with anesthesia and all allergies. These data provide information about tolerance of and possible fears about the use of anesthesia. The family medical history and problems with anesthetics may indicate possible reactions to anesthesia such as

TABLE 9.3 Selected Factors That Increase the Risk for Surgical Complications

Age
- Older than 65 years

Medications
- Antihypertensives
- Tricyclic antidepressants
- Anticoagulants
- NSAIDs
- Immunosuppressive drugs

Medical History
- Decreased immunity
- Diabetes
- Pulmonary disease
- Cardiac disease
- Hemodynamic instability
- Multisystem disease
- Coagulation defect or disorder
- Anemia
- Dehydration
- Infection
- Hypertension
- Hypotension
- Any chronic disease

Prior Surgical Experiences
- Less-than-optimal emotional reaction
- Anesthesia reactions or complications
- Postoperative complications

Health History
- Malnutrition or obesity
- Drug, tobacco, alcohol, or illicit substance use or misuse
- Altered coping ability
- Use of herbal preparations

Family History
- Malignant hyperthermia
- Cancer
- Bleeding disorder
- Anesthesia reactions or complications

Type of Surgical Procedure Planned
- Neck, oral, or facial procedures (airway complications)
- Chest or high abdominal procedures (pulmonary complications)
- Abdominal surgery (risk for paralytic ileus, venous thromboembolism)

TABLE 9.4 American Society of Anesthesiologists (ASA) Physical Status Classification System

Class	Definition	Examples, Including but Not Limited to:
ASA I	Normal healthy patient	Healthy, nonsmoking, no or minimal alcohol use
ASA II	Patient with mild systemic disease	Mild diseases only, without substantive functional limitations; examples include (but not limited to): current smoker, social alcohol drinker, pregnancy, obesity (30 < BMI < 40), well-controlled diabetes mellitus or hypertension, mild lung disease
ASA III	Patient with severe systemic disease	Substantive functional limitations; one or more moderate-to-severe diseases; examples include (but not limited to): poorly controlled diabetes mellitus or hypertension; chronic obstructive pulmonary disease; morbid obesity (BMI ≥40); active hepatitis; alcohol dependence or abuse; implanted pacemaker; moderate reduction of ejection fraction; end-stage renal disease, undergoing regularly scheduled dialysis; premature infant, postconceptual age <60 wk; history (>3 mo) of myocardial infarction, cerebrovascular accident, transient ischemic attack, or coronary artery disease or stents
ASA IV	Patient with severe systemic disease that is a constant threat to life	Examples include (but not limited to): recent (<3 mo) myocardial infarction, cerebrovascular accident, transient ischemic attack, or coronary artery disease or stents; ongoing cardiac ischemia or severe valve dysfunction; severe reduction of ejection fraction; sepsis; disseminated intravascular coagulopathy; acute renal dysfunction or end-stage renal disease not undergoing regularly scheduled dialysis
ASA V	Moribund patient who is not expected to survive without the operation	Examples include (but not limited to): ruptured abdominal or thoracic aneurysm, massive trauma, intracranial bleeding with mass effect, ischemic bowel in the face of significant cardiac pathology or multiple organ or system dysfunction
ASA VI	Declared brain-dead patient whose organs are being removed for donor purposes	

The addition of "E" denotes emergency surgery. (An emergency is defined as existing when delay in treatment of the patient would lead to a significant increase in the threat to life or body part.) Originally approved in 2014; last amended in 2019 by the American Society of Anesthesiologists (ASA). Retrieved from https://www.asahq.org/standards-and-guidelines/asa-physical-status-classification-system.
BMI, Body mass index.

malignant hyperthermia. This information will be critical to the anesthesia team's plan of care.

Ask if there is a history of **malignant hyperthermia (MH)**, an inherited muscle disorder, which is an acute, life-threatening complication of certain drugs used for general anesthesia. It is characterized by many problems, including inadequate thermoregulation. The reaction begins in skeletal muscles exposed to the drugs, causing increased calcium levels in muscle cells and increased muscle metabolism. Serum calcium and potassium levels are increased, as is the metabolic rate, leading to acidosis, cardiac dysrhythmias, and a high body temperature.

BOX 9.2 Review of Systems

General (Constitutional)
- Fevers and/or chills
- Generalized weakness

Eyes
- Dryness or infection of conjunctiva and/or lids
- Blurring or changes in vision

Ears, Nose, Mouth, Throat
- Ear drainage or pain
- Difficulty or changes in hearing or breathing through nose
- Sinus tenderness
- Oral lesions
- Changes in dentition (e.g., cavities, dentures)
- Difficulty in swallowing

Cardiovascular
- Edema
- Exercise intolerance
- Pain
- Palpitations
- Venous thromboembolism
- History of ischemic heart disease

Respiratory
- Cough with sputum or blood
- Pain or shortness of breath when breathing
- Obstructive sleep apnea

Gastrointestinal
- New or unusual masses or tenderness
- Bowel changes or difficulty

Genitourinary
- Pain or burning on urination
- Frequency, urgency, or incontinence
- Bladder changes or difficulty

Musculoskeletal
- Clubbing or cyanosis in digits or nails
- Pain in joints
- Symmetry of extremities
- Loss of or change in range of motion

Integumentary (Includes Skin and Breast)
- Dryness, rashes, lesions, or ulcerations

Neurologic
- Changes in memory or usual state of orientation
- One-sided weakness
- Numbness or tingling
- Loss of balance
- History of cerebrovascular disease

Psychiatric
- General mood
- Depression over diagnosis, or anxiety about surgery

Endocrine
- Increased thirst or urination
- Unexplained weight loss or gain

Hematologic and Lymphatic
- Swollen nodes
- New or unusual bleeding
- Nonhealing wounds

Allergic and Immunologic
- Seasonal, food, chemical allergies
- Changes in immune system

! NURSING SAFETY PRIORITY QSEN

Critical Rescue

Recognize that you must monitor surgical patients at all times for the cluster of elevated end-tidal carbon dioxide level, decreased oxygen saturation, and tachycardia to identify symptoms of malignant hyperthermia (MH). If these changes begin, respond by alerting the surgeon and anesthesia provider immediately.

MH may start immediately after anesthesia induction, several hours into the procedure, or after anesthesia is completed. Symptoms include tachycardia, dysrhythmias, muscle rigidity of the jaw and upper chest, hypotension, tachypnea, skin mottling, cyanosis, and myoglobinuria (muscle proteins in the urine due to rhabdomyolysis). The most sensitive indication is an unexpected rise in the end-tidal carbon dioxide level with a decrease in oxygen saturation and tachycardia. Extremely elevated temperature, as high as 111.2°F (44°C), is a late sign of MH. Survival depends on early diagnosis and the immediate actions of the entire surgical team. Dantrolene sodium, a skeletal muscle relaxant, is the only drug specifically approved for treatment of MH (Malignant Hyperthermia Association of the United States, 2020a).

PATIENT-CENTERED CARE: GENETIC/GENOMIC AND GENDER HEALTH CONSIDERATIONS QSEN

Always ask the patient about previous experiences with anesthesia, especially young adult males (Litman, 2019). The patient with a genetic predisposition for malignant hyperthermia (MH) is at risk when exposed to halothane, enflurane, isoflurane, desflurane, sevoflurane, and succinylcholine. The muscle biopsy tested with the caffeine halothane contracture test (CHCT) is the most commonly used MH test (Malignant Hyperthermia Association of the United States, 2020b). There is also a genetic test that is performed on blood to assess whether a mutation in the *RYR1* gene is present (U.S. National Library of Medicine, 2020). Remind the patient that cost of the genetic test may not be covered by insurance.

Older patients are at increased risk for complications from anesthesia and surgery. The normal aging process decreases immune system functioning and delays wound healing. The frequency of chronic illness increases in older patients. ***Gas exchange*** is more profoundly affected by general anesthetic agents and opioid analgesics. Age-related changes in kidney and liver function may delay the elimination of anesthetic and analgesic agents, increasing the risk for adverse reactions. See Table 9.5 for other changes in older adults that may alter the operative response or risk.

Drugs and substance use may affect patient responses to surgery. Tobacco use increases the risk for pulmonary complications because of changes to the lungs, blood vessels, and chest cavity. Alcohol and illicit substance use can alter the patient's responses to anesthesia and ***pain*** medication. Withdrawal of alcohol before surgery may result in delirium tremens. Prescription and over-the-counter drugs, as well as herbal supplements, may also affect how the patient reacts to the operative experience. Thoroughly assess and document past and current use of herbs or botanicals.

The presence of allergies to certain substances alerts you to a possible reaction to anesthetic agents or to substances that are used before or during surgery. Although historically some patients may have received misinformation about a connection between shellfish allergy and iodine, the shellfish allergy is actually an allergy to tropomyosin, not to iodine, which is a naturally occurring element in the body. Evidence shows no cross-reactivity between shellfish allergy and topical povidone-iodine solutions or iodinated contrast (Long et al., 2019; Sicherer, 2019; Davenport & Newhouse, 2018). The patient with an allergy to avocados, bananas, strawberries, and other fruits may also have a latex sensitivity or allergy. Patients who have an egg, peanut, or soy allergy may be at risk for a reaction to propofol. Carefully assess all patients for food allergies during the preoperative phase, and document this in the electronic health

TABLE 9.5 Age-Related Changes as Surgical Risk Factors

Physiologic Change	Nursing Intervention(s)	Rationale(s)
Cardiovascular System		
Decreased cardiac output Increased blood pressure	Determine normal activity levels and note when the patient tires.	Knowing limits helps prevent fatigue.
Decreased peripheral circulation	Monitor vital signs, peripheral pulses, and capillary refill.	Having baseline data helps detect deviations.
Respiratory System		
Reduced vital capacity Loss of lung elasticity	Teach coughing and deep-breathing exercises.	Pulmonary exercises help prevent pulmonary complications.
Decreased oxygenation of blood	Monitor respirations and breathing effort.	Having baseline data helps detect deviations.
Renal/Urinary System		
Decreased blood flow to kidneys Reduced ability to excrete waste Decline in glomerular filtration rate	Monitor intake and output. Assess overall hydration. Monitor electrolyte status.	Ongoing assessment helps detect fluid and electrolyte imbalances and decreased renal function.
Nocturia	Assist frequently with toileting needs, especially at night.	Frequent toileting helps prevent incontinence and falls.
Neurologic System		
Sensory deficits Slower reaction time Cognitive impairment	Orient the patient to the surroundings. Allow extra time for teaching the patient. Keep patient informed of activities before implementation.	An individualized preoperative teaching plan is developed based on the patient's orientation and any neurologic deficits.
Decreased ability to adjust to changes in the surroundings	Provide for the patient's safety.	Safety measures help prevent falls and injury.
Musculoskeletal System		
Increased incidence of deformities related to osteoporosis or arthritis	Assess the patient's mobility. Teach turning and positioning. Encourage ambulation.	Interventions help prevent complications of immobility.
	Place on falls precautions, if indicated.	Safety measures help prevent injury.
Skin		
Dry with less subcutaneous fat places the skin at greater risk for damage; slower skin healing increases risk for ***infection***	Assess the patient's skin before surgery for lesions, bruises, and areas of decreased circulation.	Having baseline data helps detect changes and evaluate interventions.
	Pad bony prominences.	Padding can protect at-risk areas.
	Use pressure-avoiding or pressure-reducing overlays.	Overlays can prevent pressure injury formation by redistributing body weight.
	Avoid applying tape to skin.	Tape removal damages thin skin.
	Teach the patient to change position at least every 2 hours. Use safe patient-handling devices to avoid shearing during patient movement.	Changing position frequently helps prevent reduced blood flow to an area and changes external pressure patterns.

record. Promptly communicate any allergies to all members of the perioperative team.

In some cases, *blood donation* for surgery can be made by the patient (**autologous donations**) a few weeks before the scheduled surgery date. See the agency policy, as specific criteria, which may vary by surgical type and the patient's health status, must be met to qualify for autologous transfusion. If the patient meets criteria and provides an autologous donation, and blood is needed during or after surgery, the autologous transfusion can be given. This practice eliminates transfusion reactions and reduces the risk for acquiring bloodborne disease.

A special tag is placed on the blood bag when an autologous blood donation has been made to ensure that patients receive only their own donated blood. The blood donor center gives the patient a matching tag that he or she wears or brings to the surgical area before surgery as required by the American Association of Blood Banks (AABB) (AABB, 2019).

Patients may wish to have family and friends donate blood exclusively for their use, if needed. This practice, a *directed blood donation,* is possible only if the blood types are compatible and the donor's blood is acceptable. Directed donation is not practiced in all blood donation centers. When directed blood donations are used, a special tag is attached to the blood bag. This tag notes the names of the patient and the donor and bears the patient's signature.

Ask whether autologous or directed blood donations have been made and document this information in the electronic health record. It is important to know the specific blood collection center where the donation was made and whether the blood has arrived before the patient goes into surgery. The hospital receives and stores the blood units until they are used or are no longer needed. Unused blood is returned to the collection center.

Increased use of "bloodless surgery" and minimally invasive surgery (MIS) provides alternatives for patients with religious or medical restrictions to blood transfusions. Professional ethics require that you, and the interprofessional team members, honor patient requests based on religious views. These programs reduce the need for transfusion during and after surgery. Some techniques used are limiting blood samples (the number of samples and the volume of blood drawn per sample) before surgery and stimulating the patient's own red blood cell production with epoetin alfa. Supplemental iron, folic acid, vitamin B_{12}, and vitamin C may be prescribed to help red blood cell formation.

Current equipment and surgical techniques cause less blood loss. Such advances include intraoperative cell salvage machines commonly known as *cell savers,* which suction, wash, and filter blood so it can be given back to the patient's body instead of being discarded. One advantage to this is that the patient receives his or her own blood instead of donor blood, so there is no risk of contracting outside diseases. Because the blood is recirculated, there is no limit to the amount of blood that can be given back to the patient. The cell salvage is a cost-effective and safe option for autologous transfusion. Cell salvage is also a viable alternative for patients with religious objections to receiving blood transfusions (Campbell et al., 2016). As you do for all individuals, assess, monitor, teach, and advocate for the patient during the bloodless surgery process.

Discharge planning is started before surgery. Assess the patient's home environment, self-care capabilities, and support systems, and anticipate postoperative needs before surgery. *All patients, regardless of how minor the procedure or how often they have had surgery, should have discharge planning.* Do not assume that health care professionals who are having surgery know about their own procedure or discharge instructions. Treat them as if they were laypersons, and provide full assessment and teaching. Older patients and dependent adults may need transportation referrals to and from the health care provider's office or the surgical setting. A home care nurse may be needed to monitor recovery and provide instructions. Patients with few support systems may need follow-up care at home. Some patients need a planned direct admission to a rehabilitation agency or center for physical therapy after surgery, especially joint-replacement surgery. Shortened hospital stays require thorough discharge planning to achieve the desired outcomes after surgery.

NCLEX EXAMINATION CHALLENGE 9.1

Physiological Integrity

The surgery for a client scheduled for an 8:00 a.m. procedure is delayed until 11:00 a.m. What is the appropriate nursing action regarding administration of preoperative prophylactic antibiotic?

A. Administer at 8:00 a.m. as originally prescribed.
B. Adjust the administration time to be given at 10:00 a.m.
C. Do not administer, as preoperative prophylactic antibiotics are optional.
D. Hold the antibiotic until immediately following surgery, and then administer.

Physical Assessment/Signs and Symptoms. Depending on where you work as a medical-surgical nurse, you may perform a physical assessment well in advance of surgery, or immediately before sending an inpatient to surgery. The same principles for conducting a thorough assessment apply, regardless of setting or timing, as this information is used for baseline comparison purposes. Compare your assessment findings with the history and review of systems that were collected to identify any new or immediate health problems, information that indicates potential anesthesia complications, and/or risk for concerns that may occur after surgery.

Begin the assessment by obtaining a complete set of vital signs. You may need to obtain vital signs several times at different time intervals for accurate baseline values. Previous vital signs from another admission (if available) are helpful for purposes of comparison. Abnormal vital signs may indicate a health problem that warrants postponement of surgery until the problem is treated. Recognize that anxiety can increase blood pressure, pulse, and respiratory rate.

The older adult (see also Chapter 4) or patient with a chronic health condition is at increased risk for complications during and after surgery. The numbers of serious diseases (**morbidity**) and deaths (**mortality**) during or after surgery are higher in patients who are older and chronically ill. See the Patient-Centered Care: Older Adult Considerations box.

! NATIONAL PATIENT SAFETY GOALS

Report any abnormal assessment findings to the surgeon and to anesthesia personnel right away, as required by The Joint Commission's National Patient Safety Goals.

PATIENT-CENTERED CARE: OLDER ADULT CONSIDERATIONS QSEN

When planning care for preoperative older adults, recognize that these patients may have:

- Greater incidence of chronic illness (e.g., hypertension, diabetes)
- Greater incidence of malnutrition and dehydration
- More allergies
- An increased number of abnormal laboratory values (anemia, low albumin level)
- Increased incidence of impaired self-care abilities
- Inadequate or absent support systems
- Decreased ability to withstand the stress of surgery and anesthesia
- Increased risk for cardiopulmonary complications after surgery
- Risk for a change in mental status when admitted (e.g., related to unfamiliar surroundings, change in routine, drugs)
- Increased risk for falls and resultant injury
- Mobility changes that affect recovery efforts

Assess *cardiovascular status,* as cardiac problems are associated with many surgery-related deaths. Check the patient for hypertension, which is common, is often undiagnosed, and can affect the response to surgery. Document rate, regularity, and abnormalities of heart sounds. Ask whether the patient has ever had a venous thromboembolism (VTE). Assess hands and feet for temperature, color, peripheral pulses, capillary refill, and edema. Report absent peripheral pulses, pitting edema, cardiac symptoms, chest pain, shortness of breath, and/or dyspnea to the surgeon for further assessment and evaluation. (Cardiac assessment is discussed in Chapter 30.) Determine functionality of any implantable cardiovascular devices such as a pacemaker or implantable cardioverter defibrillator (ICD); report the presence of these to the perioperative team.

Respiratory status is established by age, smoking history (including exposure to secondhand smoke), and any chronic illness. Patients with obesity may have undiagnosed respiratory problems such as obstructive sleep apnea (OSA), which can lead to complications from anesthesia (Olson et al., 2018). Observe the patient's posture and respiratory effort, rate, rhythm, and depth, and auscultate lung sounds. Document clubbing of the fingertips (swelling at the base of the nail beds caused by a chronic lack of oxygen) or cyanosis. (More information on respiratory assessment can be found in Chapter 24.)

Kidney function affects the excretion of drugs and waste products. If the glomerular filtration rate is reduced, excretion of drugs and anesthetic agents is decreased. Opioids, benzodiazepines, and barbiturates can cause confusion, apprehension, and/or restlessness in patients with decreased kidney function. Fluid and electrolyte balance can also be altered, especially in older adults. Review whether the patient has problems such as urinary frequency, **dysuria** (painful urination), **nocturia** (awakening during nighttime sleep because of a need to void), difficulty starting urine flow, and **oliguria** (scant amount of urine). Ask the patient about the appearance and odor of the urine. Assess the patient's usual fluid intake and degree of continence. If the patient has kidney or urinary problems, consult with the surgeon about further workup. (Kidney and urinary assessment is discussed further in Chapter 60.)

Neurologic status includes mental status, level of consciousness, orientation, and ability to follow commands. A problem in any of these areas affects the type of care needed during the surgical experience. Determine if the patient's current neurologic status is in keeping with the baseline findings, and assess for motor or sensory deficits. (See Chapter 38 for complete nervous system assessment.) Evaluate mental status, muscle strength, steadiness of gait, and sense of independence to determine the patient's risk. Document the patient's ability to ambulate and the steadiness of gait as baseline data.

! NATIONAL PATIENT SAFETY GOALS

The Joint Commission's National Patient Safety Goals require that you ensure safety by assessing the patient's risk for falling.

It may be challenging to address the baseline status of a patient who is mentally impaired. Recognize that assessment of coping skills, a mental health history, and notation of any recent behavioral changes is the minimum standard of care for patients at risk or patients with previously diagnosed mental illness. The patient who has been independent and oriented at the place of residence may become disoriented in the hospital setting. Family or caregivers can often provide information about what the patient was like under normal living conditions.

Musculoskeletal status problems may interfere with positioning during and after surgery. For example, patients with arthritis may have discomfort after surgery from prolonged joint immobilization. Document any anatomic features, such as the shape and length of the neck and the shape of the chest cavity, that may interfere with respiratory or cardiac function, or that may require special positioning during surgery. Remember to note the presence of any prostheses, and report these to operative personnel.

Nutrition status, especially undernutrition or obesity, can increase surgical risk. Surgery increases metabolic rate and depletes potassium and vitamins C and B, which are needed for wound healing and blood clotting. Decreased serum protein levels may slow recovery. Negative nitrogen balance may result from depleted protein stores. This problem increases the risk for skin breakdown, delayed wound healing, possible dehiscence or evisceration, dehydration, and sepsis.

Some older patients may have poor nutrition because of chronic illness, diuretic or laxative use, poor dietary planning or habits, anorexia, disinterest in food, or financial limitations (Touhy & Jett, 2020). Indications of poor fluid intake or nutrition status include:

- Brittle nails
- Muscle wasting
- Dry or flaky skin, decreased skin turgor, and hair changes (e.g., dull, sparse, dry)
- Orthostatic (postural) hypotension
- Decreased serum protein levels and abnormal serum electrolyte values

The patient with obesity may be malnourished because of an imbalanced diet. Obesity increases the risk for poor wound healing because of excessive *adipose* (fatty) tissue. Fatty tissue has few blood vessels, little collagen, and decreased nutrients, all of which are needed for wound healing. Obesity places additional stress on the heart and reduces the lung volumes, which can affect surgery and recovery. Recognize that patients with obesity may need larger drug doses and may retain them longer after surgery.

Skin assessment is critical; many insurers no longer reimburse hospitals for care provided to patients who develop skin breakdown or pressure injuries. A thorough assessment includes notation of skin color, turgor, and temperature; signs of breakdown; open lesions; and areas that may be exposed to excessive pressure during the surgical procedure. Be attentive to body piercings, body modifications, and tattoos. Document these findings and communicate pertinent information to members of the interprofessional perioperative team so precautions can be taken to prevent injury during surgery.

Psychosocial Assessment. Most patients have some degree of anxiety or fear before surgery. The extent of these reactions varies according to the type of surgery, the perceived effects of the surgery and its potential outcome, and the patient's personality. Surgery may be seen as a threat to life, body image, self-esteem, self-concept, or lifestyle. Patients may fear death, ***pain,*** helplessness, a change in role or work status, a diagnosis of life-threatening conditions, possible disabling or crippling effects, or the unknown.

Anxiety or fear can affect the patient's ability to learn, cope, and cooperate with teaching and operative procedures. Perform a psychosocial assessment to determine the patient's level of anxiety, coping ability, and support systems. Indications of anxiety include anger, crying, restlessness, profuse sweating, increased pulse rate, palpitations, sleeplessness, diarrhea, and urinary frequency. Ask open-ended questions about the patient's feelings about the entire surgical experience. Provide information and support to the patient and family or caregivers as needed. Identify coping mechanisms used by the patient under similar situations or in the past when confronted with a stressful situation. If performing this assessment well in advance of surgery, refer to appropriate support systems as indicated.

Laboratory Assessment. Presurgical laboratory tests provide baseline data about the patient's health and can help predict potential complications. The patient scheduled for surgery in an ambulatory surgical center (ASC) or admitted to the hospital on the morning of or day before surgery may have preadmission testing (PAT) performed from 24 hours to 28 days before the scheduled surgery. These test results are usually valid unless there has been a change in the patient's condition that warrants repeated testing or the patient is taking drugs that can alter laboratory values (e.g., warfarin, aspirin, diuretics). Some agencies have time limits for tests, especially pregnancy testing or any other test results that would require altering the surgical plan. Follow agency policy accordingly.

The choice of laboratory testing before surgery varies and depends on the patient's age, medical history, and type of anesthesia planned (Rothrock, 2019). The most common tests include:

- Urinalysis
- Blood type and screen
- Complete blood count (or hemoglobin and hematocrit)
- Clotting studies (prothrombin time [PT], international normalized ratio [INR], activated partial thromboplastin time [aPTT], platelet count)
- Metabolic panel (including serum glucose, serum electrolytes, kidney function, liver function, and serum proteins)
- Pregnancy test for the female patient

Urinalysis is performed to assess for abnormal substances in the urine such as protein, glucose, blood, and bacteria. If kidney disease is suspected or if the patient is older, the health care provider may request other tests. For example, baseline arterial blood gas (ABG) values may be assessed for patients with chronic pulmonary problems.

Report electrolyte imbalances or other abnormal laboratory results to the anesthesia team and the surgeon before surgery begins. **Hypokalemia** (decreased serum potassium level) increases the risk for toxicity if the patient is taking digoxin, slows recovery from anesthesia, and increases cardiac irritability. **Hyperkalemia** (increased serum potassium level) increases the risk for dysrhythmias, especially with the use of anesthesia.

SYSTEMS THINKING AND QUALITY IMPROVEMENT QSEN

Preventing Surgical Cancellations and Decreasing Unnecessary Testing

Leite, K.A., Hobgood, T., Hill, B., & Muckler, V.C. (2019). Reducing preventable surgical cancellations: Improving the preoperative anesthesia interview process. *Journal of PeriAnesthesia Nursing 34*(5), 929–937.

An important purpose of the preoperative assessment is to identify health conditions that require further investigation prior to surgery. These types of assessments should be personalized in order to provide patient-centered care, to avoid unnecessary testing, and to capture individualized information that could affect the patient before, during, or after surgery. Missed information can lead to surgical cancellations. This affects not only the patient in terms of scheduling and of finances; it also affects the entire interprofessional team that has been identified to provide care and treatment for the patient, as well as the agency. The nurse must be astute in capturing personalized information during the full assessment process in order to ensure that critical findings that could have an impact on the operative plan are not missed.

One way to bring consistency to the preoperative assessment is through training of nurses who work with preoperative patients. Leite et al. (2019) found that use of online educational modules, as well as implementation of standardized anesthesia interview guidelines, was effective in reducing cancellation rates from 34.3% to 20% in a 3-month period, which resulted in $30,000 savings for the agency. It was also noted that nursing documentation compliance increased, and unnecessary laboratory testing decreased, during this intervention.

Commentary: Implications for Practice and Research

Nurses contribute to patient-centered care by integrating and reconciling data from diverse sources. Accuracy on the part of the nurse can contribute to better patient satisfaction, more favorable outcomes, and lessened financial burden for the patient and agency. Implementation of educational modules and a standardized preoperative anesthesia interview developed specifically for registered nurses has the ability to bring unity to the preoperative assessment process. Following a standardized approach helps the nurse to better identify concerns on a consistent basis. This decreases the chance that pertinent findings are missed in the preoperative phase, which could lead to unnecessary testing or surgical cancellation. These findings are transferrable to the larger system of care, recognizing that standardization of processes decreases the likelihood for missed information that affects patient care.

! NURSING SAFETY PRIORITY QSEN

Critical Rescue

Recognize potassium imbalance when reviewing laboratory reports. If hypokalemia or hyperkalemia is present, respond by communicating this information to the surgeon and perioperative team so the imbalance can be corrected before surgery.

Imaging Assessment. A chest x-ray may be ordered before surgery for patients with a history of respiratory problems.

In addition to providing baseline data, it can show presence of pneumonia or tuberculosis. Abnormal x-ray findings alert the surgeon to conditions such as heart failure, cardiomyopathy, pneumonia, or infiltrates that may cause cancellation or delay of surgery. For emergency surgery, x-ray results help the anesthesia provider select the anesthesia type.

Other imaging studies may be ordered depending on patient history and the nature of surgery. For example, a patient with back pain may have CT scans or MRI done before spinal surgery to identify the exact location of the problem.

Other Diagnostic Assessment. An electrocardiogram (ECG) may be required for patients with a history of, or risk for, cardiac disease who are to have general anesthesia. Some agencies have an age threshold, such as 40 or 45 years old, beyond which all patients must have an ECG. This provides baseline information on new or existing cardiac problems such as an old myocardial infarction (MI). For a patient with a known cardiac problem, a cardiology consultation may be required before surgery.

Drugs for problem prevention, such as nitroglycerin, beta blockers, and antibiotics, may be needed throughout the perioperative phase to reduce or prevent stress on the heart. Abnormal or potentially life-threatening ECG results may cause the cancellation of surgery until the patient's cardiac status is stable.

See the Focused Assessment: The Preoperative Patient box for a summary of findings during the presurgical assessment that must be reported to the surgeon and perioperative team.

FOCUSED ASSESSMENT

The Preoperative Patient

Report pertinent cardiovascular and respiratory findings:

- Chest pain
- Irregular heart rate
- Hypotension or hypertension
- Heart rate <60 or >100 beats/min
- Shortness of breath, dyspnea, tachypnea
- Pulse oximetry reading of less than 94%
- Presence of implantable cardiovascular devices such as a pacemaker or implantable cardioverter defibrillator (ICD)

Report any signs or symptoms of ***infection,*** including:

- Fever
- Purulent sputum
- Increased white blood cell count
- Dysuria or cloudy, foul-smelling urine
- Any red, swollen, draining IV or wound site

Report laboratory data that could contraindicate surgery, including:

- Hypokalemia or hyperkalemia
- Positive pregnancy test result (or patient report of actual or possible pregnancy)
- Increased prothrombin time (PT), international normalized ratio (INR), or activated partial thromboplastin time (aPTT)

Report other clinical conditions that may need further evaluation before proceeding with the surgical plans, including:

- Rash
- Vomiting
- Change in mental status
- Recent administration of an anticoagulant drug

NCLEX EXAMINATION CHALLENGE 9.2

Physiological Integrity: Reduction of Risk Potential

The nurse is caring for a client who is to undergo surgery at 6:00 a.m. today. Which assessment data will the nurse communicate immediately to the surgeon and anesthesia provider? **Select all that apply.**

A. Blood pressure 130/72 mm Hg
B. Serum potassium 3.5 mEq/L
C. Diffuse rash on upper torso
D. Took 650 mg of aspirin yesterday
E. Has not had food or water since 9:00 p.m. last night

◆ **Analysis: Analyze Cues and Prioritize Hypotheses.** The priority collaborative problems for preoperative patients are:

1. Need for health teaching due to unfamiliarity with surgical procedures and preparation
2. Anxiety due to fear of a new or unknown experience, ***pain,*** and/or surgical outcomes

◆ **Planning and Implementation: Generate Solutions and Take Action.** The role of the nurse is to serve as the patient's advocate and coordinate all aspects of care before surgery. The nurse who cares for the patient in the preoperative phase participates in the assessment of risk and collaborates with the perioperative team to safely transition the patient to the intraoperative phase of care.

Need for Health Teaching: Providing Information

Planning: Expected Outcomes. The patient needs to know what to expect during and after surgery, as well as how to participate in his or her recovery.

Interventions. Because the surgical experience is new to many people, focus on teaching the patient and family or caregivers before surgery. Assess the amount of current knowledge. Determine the preferred learning method(s), and provide pamphlets, written instructions, approved websites, and video recordings or DVDs that help to support understanding. Some agencies hold classes or show videos before surgery for groups of patients having the same procedure. Depending on the agency, a tour of the surgical suite and the postanesthesia care unit (PACU) may be included.

If the patient is receiving sedation or general anesthesia in an ambulatory surgical setting, stress the importance of having another adult drive the patient home after the procedure. Document information in the electronic health record about who was involved in teaching, what specifically was taught, and which education materials were given.

! NATIONAL PATIENT SAFETY GOALS

The Joint Commission's National Patient Safety Goals require that you provide information about informed consent, dietary restrictions, specific preparation for surgery (bowel and skin preparations), exercises after surgery, and plans for pain management to promote the patient's participation and to help achieve the expected outcome.

A sample educational checklist is shown in Table 9.6.

Ensuring Informed Consent. Surgery of any type involves invasion of the body and therefore requires informed consent from the patient or legal guardian (Fig. 9.2).

Consent implies that the patient has sufficient information to understand:

- The nature of and reason for surgery
- Who will be performing the surgery and whether others will be present during the procedure (e.g., students, vendors)
- All available treatment options, and the benefits and risks associated with each option
- The risks associated with the surgical procedure and its potential outcomes
- The risks associated with the use of anesthesia
- The risks, benefits, and alternatives to the use of blood or blood products during the procedure

Informed consent is one way to help ensure patient safety. This process reflects professional ethics. It helps protect the patient from any unwanted procedures and protects the surgeon and the agency from lawsuit claims related to unauthorized surgery or uninformed patients. Written record of informed consent is documented on a specific form, and can also be documented in the surgeon's notes. The consent form documents the patient's consent and signature for the procedure(s) listed.

It is the surgeon's responsibility to provide a complete explanation of the planned surgical procedure and to have the consent form signed before sedation is given and before surgery is performed. The perioperative nurse *is not* responsible for providing detailed information about the surgical procedure. The nurse's role is to *clarify* facts that have been presented by the surgeon and dispel myths that the patient, family, or caregiver may have about the surgical experience. The nurse must verify that the consent form is signed, dated, and timed, and he or she may serve as a witness to the signature, not to the adequacy of the patient's understanding, which is the surgeon's responsibility (The Joint Commission, 2016).

! NATIONAL PATIENT SAFETY GOALS

The Joint Commission's National Patient Safety Goals state that patients must be informed and involved in decisions affecting their health care.

As a competent adult, it is the patient's right to refuse treatment for any reason, even when refusal might lead to compromise in the patient's health condition, or death.

! NURSING SAFETY PRIORITY (QSEN)

Action Alert

If you believe that the patient has not been adequately informed, that he or she has questions about his or her procedure, or there is a discrepancy related to the surgical site, it is your professional and ethical duty to contact the surgeon and request that he or she see the patient for further clarification. Document this action in the electronic health record.

Patients who cannot write may sign with an X, which must be witnessed by two people, one of whom can be the nurse. If the patient is not capable of giving consent and has no designated medical power of attorney, the court can appoint a legal guardian to represent the patient's best interests. For a life-threatening situation in which the patient cannot give consent, and every effort has been made to contact the person with medical power of attorney (without success), written consultation with at least two health care providers not associated with the case may be requested by the surgeon. This formal consultation legally supports the decision for surgery until the appropriate person can sign a consent form.

TABLE 9.6 Preoperative Teaching Checklist

Consider these items when planning individualized preoperative teaching for patients and families:

- Addressing fears and anxieties
- Outlining the surgical procedure
- Explaining preoperative routines (e.g., NPO, blood samples, showering)
- Informing about invasive mechanisms (e.g., lines, catheters) to expect
- Teaching about methods of pain control in the postoperative and recovery time frames
- Teaching about coughing, turning, deep breathing, and use of incentive spirometry
- Teaching about lower extremity exercises; stockings; and pneumatic compression devices
- Teaching about splinting and its importance in pain management
- Reinforcing the importance of early ambulation

A blind patient may sign his or her own consent form, which usually needs to be witnessed by two people. Patients who do not speak the general language of the agency or who are hearing impaired require a qualified translator and a second witness. Many agencies have consent forms written in more than one language and also have health care professionals who are proficient with American Sign Language. Qualified translators may be health care professionals or other people employed or contracted by the hospital. Translators are part of the interprofessional care team and are required to keep patient information confidential. Family members should not serve as translators because the health care team cannot validate that the medical information is being translated accurately.

Some surgical procedures such as sterilization and experimental procedures, or administration of anesthesia or blood products, may require a special permit in addition to the standard consent. National and local governing bodies and the individual agency determine which procedures require separate consent.

Surgical procedures that are site specific, such as left, right, or bilateral, require identification before surgery. Marking the surgical site is the role and responsibility of the surgeon (with the patient, when the patient is able); all operative team members are accountable to confirm this site marking during the "time-out" process before surgery commences. This marking should take place outside of the surgical suite and before the patient has been given any sedation. Using a single-use surgical marker to draw a marking that will remain visible after skin preparation, the surgeon is to verify the site with the patient, and place the marking (often the surgeon's initials) as close as anatomically possible to the incision site (AORN, 2020). Document this in the electronic health record. Once inside the surgical suite, further verification of the marking, and the "time-out" process, will take place.

GENERAL REQUEST AND CONSENT

FOR OFFICE USE ONLY:
Patient Name: ______
Date of Birth: ______
Date of Procedure: ______

I ______ request and give consent to ______
(Type or print patient name) (Type or print Doctor or Practitioner Name(s))

to perform the following procedure(s) ______
(Please list site and side if appropriate)

______

______

The benefits, risks, complications, and alternatives to the above procedure(s) have been explained to me.

I understand that the procedure(s) will be performed at Christiana Care by and under supervision of my doctor or practitioner. My doctor or practitioner may use the services of other doctors or practitioners, or members of the resident staff as he or she deems necessary or advisable.

I authorize my doctor or practitioner and his or her associates and assistants to perform such additional procedures, which in their judgment are necessary and appropriate to carry out my diagnosis or treatment.

I authorize the hospital to retain, preserve and use for scientific, teaching or transplant purposes, or to make other dispositions of, at their convenience, any specimens, tissues, or parts taken from my body during the course of this operation.

I consent to observers in the operating room in accordance with hospital policy. I consent to photography or video taping of my surgical procedure for educational purposes, provided my identity remains anonymous and confidential.

I agree to being given blood or blood products as deemed advisable during the course of my procedure. The risks, benefits, and alternatives to receiving blood or blood products have been explained to me.

I consent to the administration of sedation or analgesia during my procedure. The risks, benefits, and alternatives to receiving sedation or analgesia have been explained to me.

If anesthesia is required, I consent to the administration of anesthesia by members of the Department of Anesthesiology. I also consent to the use of non-invasive and invasive monitoring techniques as deemed necessary. I understand that anesthesia involves risks that are in addition to those resulting from the operation itself including, but not limited to, dental injury, hoarseness, vocal cord injury, infection, nerve injury, corneal abrasion, seizures, heart attack, stroke and even death.

Please initial one of the following statements (females only):

______ To the best of my knowledge I am not pregnant. ______ I believe I am pregnant.

I certify that I have read and understand the above consent statements. In addition, I have been offered the opportunity to ask my doctor or practitioner any questions I have regarding the procedure(s) to be performed and they have been answered to my satisfaction. I acknowledge that I have been given no guarantee or assurance as to the results that may be obtained from the procedure(s).

Signature of Patient or Decision Maker	Date and Time	Doctor or Practitioner Signature	Date and Time
Relationship to Patient if Decision Maker		Doctor ID # or Print Name	
Witness Signature	Date and Time	Practitioner Print Name/Title	
Witness Print Name			

Telephone Consent: ______
Name of person obtained from/Relationship to Patient

Witness's (es') Signature(s)	Date and Time	Witness's (es') Signature(s)	Date and Time
Witness's (es') Print Name(s)		Witness's (es') Print Name(s)	

FIG. 9.2 Surgical informed consent form. (Courtesy Christiana Care Health Services, Newark, DE.)

! NATIONAL PATIENT SAFETY GOALS

As required by The Joint Commission's National Patient Safety Goals, to ensure that the correct site is selected and the wrong site is avoided, the site is marked by a licensed independent practitioner and, whenever possible, the marking involves the patient's participation.

! NURSING SAFETY PRIORITY (QSEN)

Action Alert

The surgeon is accountable to mark the surgical site. This is to take place in a setting prior to the patient being moved to the surgical suite. If this is done in your setting (e.g., on a medical-surgical unit before transport to surgery), document this in the electronic health record.

Patient Self-Determination. Patients receiving medical care have the right to have or to initiate advance directives such as a living will or durable power of attorney, as mandated by the Patient Self-Determination Act. Advance directives provide legal instructions to the primary health care providers about the patient's wishes and are to be followed. *Surgery does not provide an exception to a patient's advance directives or living will* (AORN, 2020). Chapter 8 discusses advance directives in more detail.

Implementing Dietary Restrictions. Regardless of the type of surgery and anesthesia planned, the patient is restricted to NPO status before surgery. NPO means no eating, drinking (including water), smoking (nicotine stimulates gastric secretions), or intake of oral medication (unless directed by the surgeon). NPO status ensures that the stomach contains a limited volume of gastric secretions, which decreases the risk for aspiration. Outpatients and patients who are scheduled for admission to the hospital on the same day that surgery is performed must receive written and oral instructions about when to begin NPO status.

The exact amount of time a patient must be NPO before surgery depends on the timing of the planned procedure. Patients, especially older adults, who fast for 8 or more hours may have imbalances of fluids, electrolytes, and blood glucose levels. Current recommendations include having no fried or fatty food, or meat, within 8 hours of surgery; no other food within 6 hours of surgery; and no clear liquids within 2 hours of surgery, although some surgeons will recommend a more stringent timeline (Crowley, 2020). For patients with diabetes, check with the primary health care provider or surgeon for specific guidance on eating before surgery.

! NURSING SAFETY PRIORITY (QSEN)

Action Alert

Emphasize the importance of adhering to the prescribed NPO restriction. Failure to adhere can result in postponing or canceling surgery and an increased risk for aspiration during or after surgery.

Regularly Scheduled Drugs. On the day of surgery, the patient's usual drug schedule may need to be altered. Consult the surgeon and the anesthesia provider for instructions about drugs such as those taken for diabetes, cardiac disease, or glaucoma and regularly scheduled anticonvulsants, antihypertensives, anticoagulants, antidepressants, and corticosteroids. The surgeon may determine that some drugs and supplements, including over-the-counter drugs such as aspirin, other NSAIDs, and herbal preparations, must be stopped at a certain time until after surgery. Other drugs may be given IV to maintain the drug level in the blood. *Drugs for cardiac disease, respiratory disease, seizures, and hypertension are commonly allowed with a sip of water before surgery.* Some antihypertensive or antidepressant drugs are withheld on the day of surgery to reduce adverse effects on blood pressure during surgery. Even when beta blockers are not part of a patient's usual medications, they may be prescribed for those at risk for cardiac problems. Check with the primary health care provider, surgeon, or anesthesia provider to determine whether a specific patient requires perioperative therapy with beta-blocking drugs.

There are different approaches in how patients with diabetes are managed in the preoperative phase. In general, those who take oral hypoglycemic agents or noninsulin injectable medications are told to continue their normal routine until the morning of surgery. At that time, they are to hold the oral hypoglycemia agent(s) and noninsulin injectable (Khan et al., 2018). People with type 1 diabetes or insulin-treated type 2 diabetes who are to have morning surgery that is short (under 2 hours) and noncomplex may continue their subcutaneous insulin (Khan et al., 2018). For patients who are undergoing morning surgery where breakfast and lunch are anticipated to be missed, undergoing long and complex procedures, or undergoing surgery later in the day, check with the primary health care provider or surgeon for specific instructions (Khan et al., 2018). (See Chapter 59 for more information about diabetes.)

Intestinal Preparation. Bowel or intestinal preparations are performed to prevent injury to the colon and reduce the number of intestinal bacteria. Bowel evacuation is needed for major abdominal, pelvic, perineal, or perianal surgery. The surgeon's preference and the type of procedure to be performed determine the type of bowel preparation. Recognize that enemas given until clear, or potent laxatives, can be stressful to a patient. Electrolyte imbalance, fluid volume imbalances, vagal stimulation, and postural (orthostatic) hypotension can occur. Enemas also cause severe anal discomfort in patients with hemorrhoids. When teaching about, or performing, bowel preparation, include safety precautions that should be undertaken to prevent falls.

Skin Preparation. The skin is the body's first line of defense against infection. A break in this barrier increases the risk for infection, especially for older patients. Skin preparation before surgery is the first step to reduce the risk for *surgical site infection* (SSI) (AORN, 2019).

The surgeon may ask the patient to shower 1 or 2 days before the scheduled surgery using an antiseptic solution, often chlorhexidine gluconate (Bashaw & Keister, 2019). This cleaning reduces contamination of the surgical field and the number of organisms at the site. Instruct the patient to be especially careful to clean well around the proposed surgical site. If the patient is hospitalized before surgery, showering and cleaning are repeated the night before surgery or in the morning before transfer to the surgical suite. Remove any soil or debris from the surgical site and surrounding areas.

Factors that increase risk for wound contamination and SSI include bacteria found in hair follicles, disruption of the normal protective mechanisms of the skin, and nicks in the skin. Shaving of hair creates the potential for ***infection.*** Hair removal is to be accomplished, per The Joint Commission's NPSGs, by a method that is evidence based or endorsed by professional organizations

> **! NATIONAL PATIENT SAFETY GOALS**
>
> Hair removal before surgery must be done according to an evidence-based resource or by using a method that is endorsed by professional organizations.

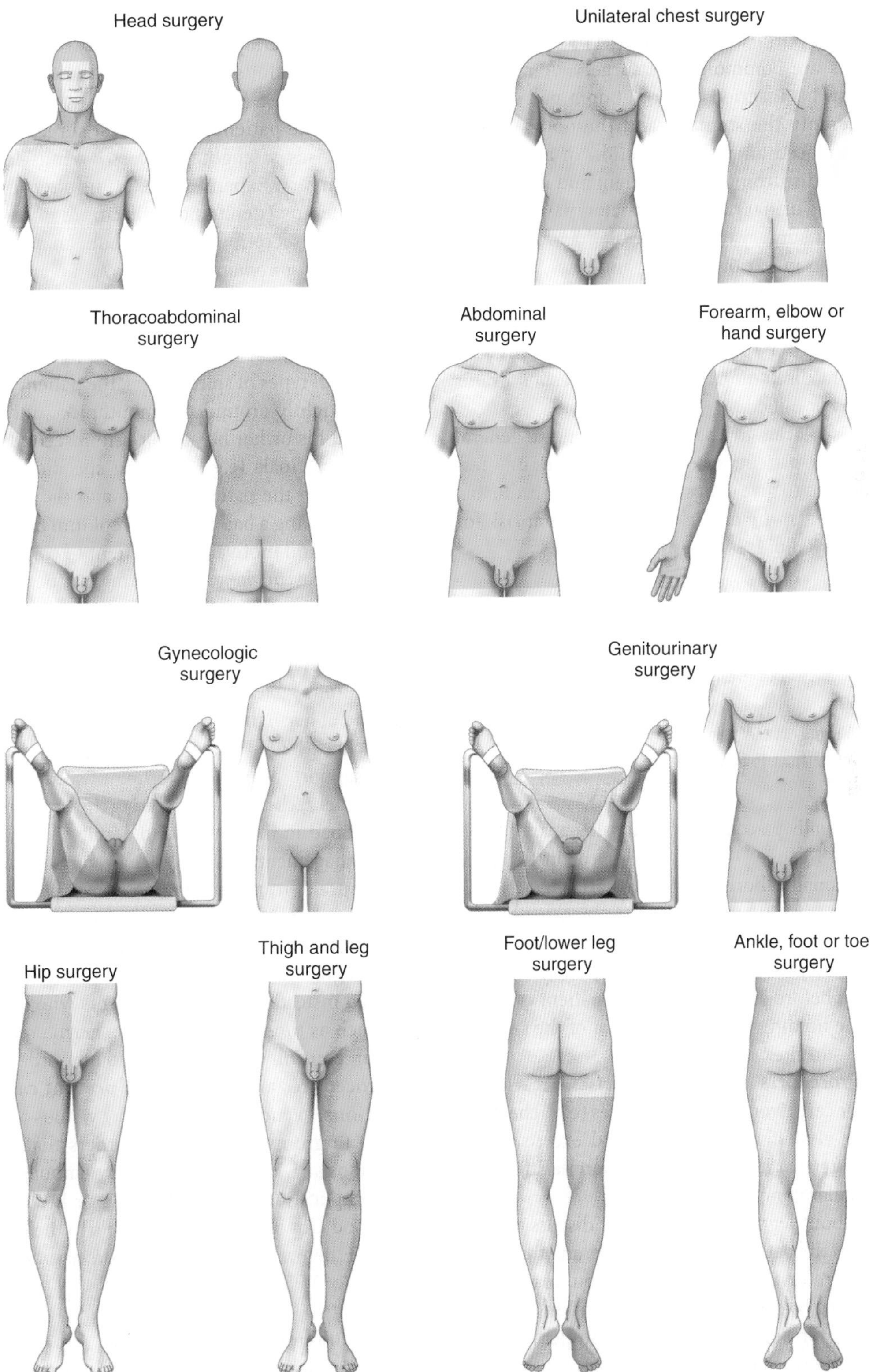

FIG. 9.3 Skin preparation of common surgical sites. Shaded areas indicate preparation sites.

(The Joint Commission, 2019); the recommended way to do this is by using aseptic principles immediately before the start of surgery with electrical clippers or a depilatory agent prior to surgery (Centers for Disease Control and Prevention, n.d.). Fig. 9.3 shows areas of skin preparation for various surgical procedures.

Preparation for Tubes, Drains, and Vascular Access. Prepare the patient for possible placement of tubes, drains, and vascular access devices that may be present after surgery. Teaching about these devices, and their purpose, reduces anxiety.

Tubes of all sorts are common after surgery. A nasogastric (NG) tube may be inserted before abdominal surgery to decompress or empty the stomach and the upper bowel. Usually the tube is placed after the induction of anesthesia, when insertion is less disturbing to the patient and is easier to perform. An indwelling urinary (Foley) catheter may be placed before, during, or after surgery to keep the bladder empty.

Drains, which come in various shapes and sizes, are often placed during surgery to help remove fluid from the surgical site. Some drains are under the dressing; others are visible and require emptying. Teach that these are generally not painful but may cause some mild discomfort. Discuss the reasons drains should not be kinked or pulled.

Vascular access is placed for patients receiving a general anesthetic and for most patients receiving other types of anesthetics. Access is needed to give drugs and fluids before, during, and after surgery. Patients who are dehydrated or are at risk for dehydration may receive fluids before surgery.

PATIENT-CENTERED CARE: OLDER ADULT CONSIDERATIONS QSEN

Older-adult patients are at greater risk for dehydration because their fluid reserves are lower than those of young or middle-age adults. Hemodynamic monitoring of older-adult patients and patients with cardiac disease receiving IV fluids is essential. (See Chapter 15 for more information on IV therapy.)

The IV access is usually placed in the arm using a large-bore, short catheter (e.g., 18-gauge, 1-inch catheter) or in the back of the hand using a smaller-bore (20-gauge) catheter. A larger vein provides the least resistance to fluid or blood infusion, especially in an emergency when rapid infusion may be needed. Depending on the patient's needs and agency policies, the IV access can be placed before surgery when the patient is in the hospital room, in the holding or admission area of the surgical suite, or in the surgical suite.

Postoperative Procedures and Leg Exercises. Teach the patient and family or caregiver about procedures (e.g., checking dressings, obtaining vital signs frequently) and exercises that will be performed after surgery. Teach that exercises decrease respiratory and vascular complications.

When teaching about leg exercises, provide discussion and demonstration. Allow the patient time to practice, and then have the patient provide a return demonstration to you. Instruction should include any leg exercises (see the Patient and Family Education: Preparing for Self-Management: Postoperative Leg Exercises box) to be performed after surgery. Stress the need to begin exercises early in the recovery phase with 5 to 10 repetitions each, every 1 to 2 hours after surgery, and to continue them for at least the first 48 hours. Explain that the patient may need to be awakened for these exercises.

Procedures and exercises to prevent respiratory complications. *Breathing exercises* include deep, or diaphragmatic, breathing to enlarge the chest cavity and expand the lungs. After demonstrating and explaining the technique, urge the patient to practice deep breathing. See the Patient and Family Education: Preparing for Self-Management: Perioperative Respiratory Care box.

For older adults and the patients with chronic lung disease or limited chest expansion, teach expansion breathing exercises. For the patient having chest surgery, expansion breathing exercises strengthen accessory muscles and are started before surgery. Expansion breathing after surgery during chest physiotherapy (percussion, vibration, postural drainage) may help loosen secretions and maintain an adequate air exchange.

Incentive spirometry promotes complete lung expansion and helps to prevent pulmonary problems. Various types of incentive spirometers are available; Fig. 9.4 shows a patient using one type.

With all types of spirometers, the patient must be able to seal the lips tightly around the mouthpiece, inhale spontaneously, and hold his or her breath for 3 to 5 seconds for effective lung expansion. Goals (e.g., attaining specific volumes) can be set according to the patient's ability and the type of incentive spirometer. Seeing a ball move up a column or a bellows expanding reinforces and motivates the patient to continue performance.

Teach that *coughing* and *splinting* may be performed along with deep breathing every 1 to 2 hours after surgery. The purposes of coughing are to expel secretions, keep the lungs clear, allow full aeration, and prevent pneumonia and atelectasis. Coughing may be uncomfortable for the patient but when performed correctly should not harm the incision. Splinting (i.e., holding) the incision area with a folded bath blanket or pillow while coughing provides support, promotes a feeling of security, and reduces ***pain.*** The proper technique for splinting the incision site and coughing is described in the Patient and Family Education: Preparing for Self-Management: Perioperative Respiratory Care box. .

The use of routine coughing exercises after surgery will vary depending on the surgeon's preference and the type of surgery performed. If coughing may harm the surgical wound, deep-breathing and incentive spirometer exercises will be ordered instead. For specific patients who should avoid coughing, such as those who have had a hernia repair or craniotomy, the surgeon will write a "do not cough" order.

Procedures and exercises to prevent cardiovascular complications. Venous stasis and venous thromboembolism (VTE) (a group of vascular disorders that includes deep vein thrombosis [DVT] and pulmonary embolism [PE]) are potential complications of surgery. VTE or DVT can lead to a PE if the blood clot breaks off and travels to the lungs. Always assess for VTE before surgery. Risk factors associated with the development of VTE include:

- Obesity
- Age 40 years or older
- Cancer; spinal cord injury; hip fracture; total hip or total knee replacement surgery

PATIENT AND FAMILY EDUCATION: PREPARING FOR SELF-MANAGEMENT

Postoperative Leg Exercises

Exercise No. 1

1. Lie in bed with the head of your bed elevated to about 45 degrees.
2. Beginning with your right leg, bend your knee, raise your foot off the bed, and hold this position for a few seconds.
3. Extend your leg by straightening your knee, and lower the leg to the bed.
4. Repeat this sequence four more times with your right leg; then perform this same exercise five times with your left leg.

Exercise No. 2

1. Beginning with your right leg, point your toes toward the bottom of the bed.
2. With the same leg, point your toes up toward your face.
3. Repeat this exercise several times with your right leg; then perform this same exercise with your left leg.

Exercise No. 3

1. Beginning with your right leg, make circles with your ankle, first to the left and then to the right.
2. Repeat this exercise several times with your right leg; then perform this same exercise with your left leg.

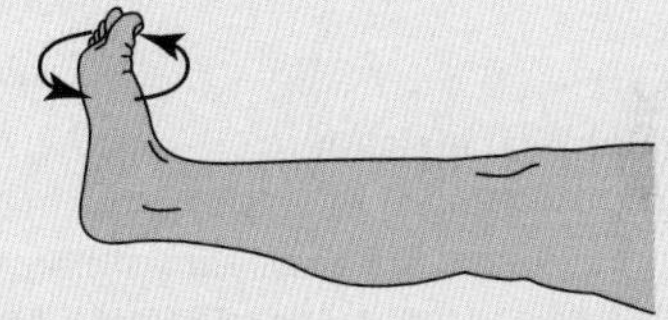

Exercise No. 4

1. Beginning with your right leg, bend your knee and *push* the ball of your foot into the bed or floor until you feel your calf and thigh muscles contracting.
2. Repeat this exercise several times with your right leg; then perform this same exercise with your left leg.

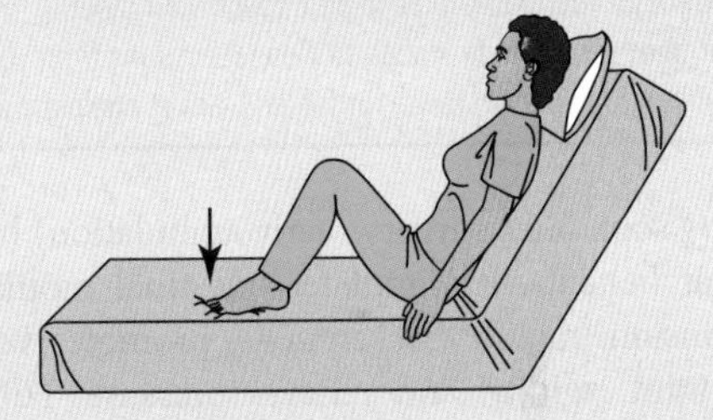

- Decreased mobility or immobility
- History of VTE, DVT, PE, varicose veins, or edema
- Oral contraceptives use
- Smoking
- Decreased cardiac output

Sudden swelling in one leg accompanied by a dull ache in the calf (that becomes worse with ambulation) is a classic assessment finding of VTE caused by DVT. Report this finding immediately to the surgeon. Careful assessment is necessary to prevent the potentially fatal complication of pulmonary embolism. Communicate with the surgeon to determine if an anticoagulant drug will be prescribed prior to surgery, and teach the patient about how to take this if it is ordered. Teach the patient that compression stockings and/or pneumatic compression devices may also be used after surgery.

Remind the patient about leg exercises outlined in the Patient and Family Education: Preparing for Self-Management: Preparing for Self-Management: Postoperative Leg Exercises box, and urge the patient to practice them before surgery. Teach that these help to promote venous return.

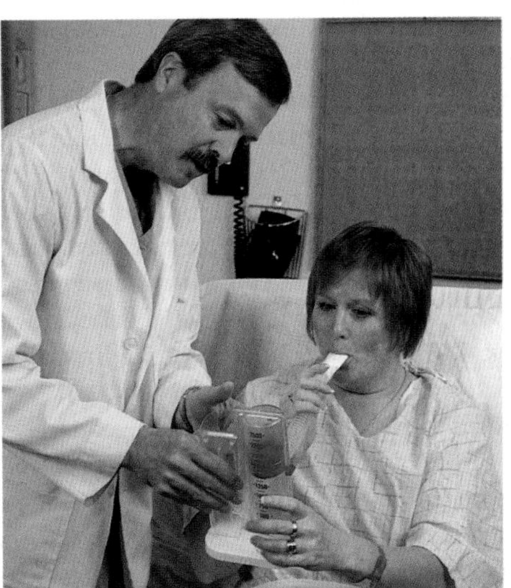

FIG. 9.4 Patient using an incentive spirometer. (From deWit, S.C., & O'Neill, P. [2014]. *Fundamental concepts and skills for nursing* [4th ed.]. St. Louis: Saunders.)

PATIENT AND FAMILY EDUCATION: PREPARING FOR SELF-MANAGEMENT

Perioperative Respiratory Care

Deep (Diaphragmatic) Breathing

1. Sit upright on the edge of the bed or in a chair, being sure that your feet are placed firmly on the floor or a stool. (After surgery, deep breathing is done with the patient in Fowler position or in semi-Fowler position.)
2. Take a gentle breath through your mouth.
3. Breathe out gently and completely.
4. Take a deep breath through your nose and mouth, and hold this breath to the count of five.
5. Exhale through your nose and mouth.

Expansion Breathing

1. Find a comfortable upright position, with your knees slightly bent. (Bending the knees decreases tension on the abdominal muscles and decreases respiratory resistance and discomfort.)
2. Place your hands on each side of your lower rib cage, just above your waist.
3. Take a deep breath through your nose, using your shoulder muscles to expand your lower rib cage outward during inhalation.
4. Exhale, concentrating first on moving your chest, then on moving your lower ribs inward, while gently squeezing the rib cage and forcing air out of the base of your lungs.

Splinting of the Surgical Incision

1. Unless coughing is contraindicated, place a pillow, towel, or folded blanket over your surgical incision and hold the item firmly in place.
2. Take three slow, deep breaths to stimulate your cough reflex.
3. Inhale through your nose and exhale through your mouth.
4. On your third deep breath, cough to clear secretions from your lungs while firmly holding the pillow, towel, or folded blanket against your incision.

Mobility soon after surgery (early ambulation) has many cardiovascular benefits. It stimulates intestinal motility, enhances lung expansion, mobilizes secretions, promotes venous return, prevents joint rigidity, and relieves pressure. For most types of surgery, teach the patient that he or she will need to turn at least every 2 hours after surgery while confined to bed; reassure the patient that nursing staff will turn them initially if they are unable to turn themselves. Teach patients how to use the bedside rails safely for turning and how to protect the surgical wound by splinting when moving. Assure patients that assistance and pain medication will be given as needed to reduce ***pain*** they may have with this activity.

For certain surgical procedures, such as some brain, spinal, and orthopedic procedures, the surgeon may prescribe turning restrictions. Ask the surgeon about other interventions to prevent complications of immobility in patients with turning restrictions. During preoperative teaching, inform the patient of any anticipated turning restrictions.

Most patients are allowed and encouraged to get out of bed the day of or the day after surgery. Teach the patient that he or she will be helped to a dangling position at the side of the bed, then into a chair or with ambulation after the surgery; the next day, or when the surgeon specifies.

Minimizing Anxiety

Planning: Expected Outcomes. An important goal of providing preoperative information is to minimize or eliminate anxiety. The informed, educated patient is better able to anticipate events and maintain self-control and is therefore less anxious.

NCLEX EXAMINATION CHALLENGE 9.3

Physiological Integrity: Reduction of Risk Potential

The nurse is teaching a client about postoperative leg exercises. What teaching will the nurse include? **Select all that apply.**

A. Begin practicing leg exercises prior to surgery.
B. Repeat leg exercises several times daily for each leg.
C. Push the ball of the foot into the bed until the calf and thigh muscles contract.
D. If pain or warmth in the calf is present, discontinue exercises and contact the surgeon.
E. Point toes of one foot toward bed bottom; then point toes of same leg toward face. Switch.

Interventions. Anxiety can cause restlessness and sleeplessness. Assess his or her level of anxiety as discussed in the Psychosocial Assessment section. Provide factual information to promote the patient's understanding. Allow ample time for questions. Respond to the questions accurately and refer unanswered questions to the proper professional.

Encourage communication by allowing the patient to express feelings, fears, and concerns. Use an honest and open approach so the patient can express feelings freely without fear of ridicule or judgment.

Promote rest because the stress and anxiety of impending surgery often interfere with the patient's ability to sleep and rest during the nights before surgery. To help the patient relax, determine what he or she usually does to relax and fall asleep. If these are in keeping with healthy sleep hygiene, urge him or her to continue these methods of relaxation. The surgeon may also prescribe a sedative or hypnotic drug to help the patient rest for surgery.

Distraction may be used as an intervention for anxiety, especially in the 24 hours immediately before surgery. Recommend listening to music, watching television, reading, or visiting with family members or friends.

Teaching the family or caregiver helps reduce anxiety by increasing the likelihood of support and involvement in the patient's care. Be sure to obtain the patient's consent to involve the family or caregiver in teaching. If the patient gives consent for their involvement, assess their readiness and desire to take an active part in the patient's care. A positive sign of interest is the family or caregiver asking questions about the surgical experience.

Inform the patient and family or caregiver of the time for surgery, if known, and of any schedule changes. If the patient is an outpatient, provide clear directions regarding any specific night-before procedures, what time and where to report, and what to bring. Encourage the family or caregiver to stay with the patient before surgery for support.

Most family members and caregivers are anxious about the surgery planned for their loved one. To reduce their anxiety, explain the routines expected before, during, and after surgery. Explain that after the patient leaves the hospital room or admission area, there is usually a 30- to 60-minute preparation period in the operating area (holding room, treatment area) before the surgery actually begins. After surgery, the patient is taken to the postanesthesia care unit (PACU) usually for 1 to 2 hours before returning to the hospital room or discharge area. The length of stay in the PACU depends on the type of surgery, the type of anesthesia, any complications, and the patient's responses. Tell them the best place to wait for the patient or surgeon according to the agency policy. Many hospitals and surgical centers have surgical waiting areas so family and caregivers can wait in comfortable surroundings and be easily located when the procedure is completed. They are often provided with a beeper to let them know when to report to a specific area to receive updates about the patient's status, meet with the surgeon, or see the patient.

Preoperative Electronic Health Record Review. Review the patient's electronic health record to ensure that all documentation, preoperative procedures, and orders are completed. Check the surgical informed consent form (and any other special consent forms) to see that they are signed and dated and that they contain the witnesses' signatures. Confirm that the scheduled procedure is in agreement with what is listed on the consent form. Ensure that the site for surgery has been marked before the procedure begins. Document allergies according to agency policy. Accurate measuring and recording of height and weight are important for proper dosage of the anesthetic agents. Ensure that the results of all laboratory, radiographic, and diagnostic tests are included in the electronic health record. Document any abnormal results, and report them to the surgeon and the anesthesia provider. If the patient is an autologous blood donor or has had directed blood donations made, those special slips must be included in the electronic health record. Record a current set of vital signs (within 1 to 2 hours of the scheduled surgery time), and document any significant physical or psychosocial observations.

Review special needs, concerns, and instructions (including advance directives) and be sure these are all communicated to the surgical team.

Preoperative Patient Preparation. Agencies usually require the patient to remove most clothing and wear a hospital gown into the surgical suite; however, underpants may be worn in above-the-waist surgery; and socks may be worn, except in foot or leg surgery. If prescribed by the surgeon, apply antiembolism stockings or pneumatic compression devices before surgery. In some ambulatory settings, such as for cataract surgery, no or minimal clothing is removed.

Patients who have preplanned surgery are advised to leave all valuables at home. If valuables are present, including jewelry, money, or clothes, they are given to a family member or caregiver, or locked in a safe place, according to the agency policy. If rings cannot be removed, assess the risk for swelling. If swelling makes it necessary, rings may need to be cut off to avoid further injury. It is preferable that all pierced jewelry be removed before surgery. Care must be provided to avoid loss or theft of the patient's items. If desired, religious emblems may be pinned or fastened securely to the patient's gown. Some agencies have paper emblems from religious organizations.

Check the patient's identification band to be sure that the first and last name, hospital number, surgeon, and birthdate are correct. An additional bracelet, usually red, identifies any allergies. A bracelet indicating that a blood sample for type and screen has been drawn may be worn, depending on the agency policy.

Denture removal or lack of removal before anesthesia will be at the anesthesia provider's discretion. Although the denture plate may come loose and obstruct the airway, the anesthesia provider may request that dentures be left in place to ensure a snug fit of the bag-mask. If dentures are to be removed, including partial dental plates, place them in a labeled denture cup. If a patient has any capped teeth, document this finding.

In some agencies, patients may wear eyeglasses and hearing aids until after anesthesia induction. Follow agency policy for collection and storage if they cannot be taken or worn to the surgical suite.

Prosthetic devices, such as artificial eyes and limbs, are removed and given to a family member or caregiver, or safely stored, as are contact lenses, wigs, and toupees. Check and remove hairpins and clips, which can conduct electrical current used during surgery and cause scalp burns.

Most agencies have a policy about fingernail polish or artificial nails worn by the patient. Evidence is mixed regarding whether pulse oximetry is affected by the presence of nail polish (Gillespie et al., 2019). Follow policy, recognizing that some agencies still require that at least one artificial nail or the polish from one nail be removed.

After the patient is prepared for surgery and just before transport into the surgical suite, ask the patient to empty the bladder, or assist with this process. This action prevents incontinence or overdistention and is a starting point for intake and output measurement.

Preoperative Drugs for Hospitalized Patients. Administration of preoperative drugs to hospitalized patients is usually done in the preoperative area right before surgery. This practice permits the surgical team and anesthesia personnel to make more accurate assessments and have last-minute discussions with the patient. Follow agency policy regarding how and when preoperative drugs are administered, including prophylactic antibiotics, which are usually given 1 hour prior to surgery.

Patient Transfer to the Surgical Suite. Right before transfer, review and update the electronic health record, reinforce teaching, ensure that the patient is correctly dressed for surgery, and administer any prescribed preoperative drugs. Use a preoperative checklist for a smooth, efficient transfer to the surgical suite (Fig. 9.5). The patient, along with the signed consent form, the completed preoperative checklist, and the patient identification card, is then ready to be transported to the surgical suite.

Most patients in the hospital setting are transferred to the surgical suite on a stretcher with the side rails up. In special circumstances (e.g., patients requiring traction, those having some types of orthopedic surgery, those who should be moved as little as possible), are transferred in the hospital bed. Other factors that influence the decision to transfer in a bed are the patient's age, size, and physical condition. In ambulatory settings, patients may walk, ride in a wheelchair, or be transferred to the surgical suite on a stretcher.

Prepare for Surgery Checklist

Nearly everyone has concerns heading into surgery. We pride ourselves on helping you feel prepared so that things go smoothly.

72 Hours Before Surgery

- ☐ Wash with special soap from your surgeon's office 2–3 days before surgery. This soap is very important for decreasing your risk of infection.

Day Before Surgery

- ☐ Do not eat after 11 p.m. the night before surgery, regardless of your surgery time.
- ☐ You may drink black coffee (no milk or cream), water, or 7UP® until five hours before your surgery.
- ☐ Bathe and use clean sheets and clean pajamas the night before surgery.
- ☐ Do not smoke, chew tobacco or drink alcohol for at least 24 hours prior to surgery.
- ☐ Do not shave from the neck down.
- ☐ Do not use any lotions, body spray or perfumes deodorant.

Day of Surgery

- ☐ Take medication with a sip of water as directed by your surgeon. If you are having same day surgery, consult with your surgeon for specific directions.
- ☐ Bring a responsible adult (parent or guardian if patient is under 18) to drive you and take care of you for at least 24 hours after surgery.
- ☐ Bring a photo ID, insurance card, advance directives (Living Will), and any payment required prior to surgery
- ☐ Wear loose, comfortable clothing and walking shoes so these can be easily stored or taken home by family members.
- ☐ If you use eyeglasses or dentures, please wear these and they will be returned to you after surgery.

FIG. 9.5 Preoperative checklist.

NCLEX EXAMINATION CHALLENGE 9.4

Physiological Integrity: Reduction of Risk Potential

The nurse has prepared a client for transport from the medical-surgical unit to surgery. Which client statement will the nurse respond to as the **priority**?

A. "When I eat shrimp, my tongue swells and I have trouble breathing."
B. "I'm feeling more anxious about my surgery than I thought I would be."
C. "I'm not sure what I will do if insurance doesn't cover this expensive hip replacement."
D. "My sister had anesthesia a few months ago and she said she didn't like the way she felt."

◆ Evaluation: Evaluate Outcomes

Evaluate the care of the preoperative patient based on the identified patient problems. The expected outcomes include that the patient:

- States understanding of the informed consent and preoperative procedures
- Demonstrates postoperative exercises and techniques for prevention of complications
- Verbalizes reduced anxiety

POSTOPERATIVE PHASE

The **postoperative phase** starts with completion of the surgical procedure and transfer of the patient to a specialized area for monitoring such as the PACU or an ICU. This phase may extend beyond discharge from the hospital until activity restrictions have been lifted. The period of postanesthesia care is divided into three phases that are based on the level of care needed, not the physical place of care (American Society of PeriAnesthesia Nurses, 2019). Not every patient needs to transition through all three phases.

Phase I care occurs immediately after surgery, most often in a PACU. For patients who have very complicated procedures or many serious health problems, phase I care may occur in an ICU. The length of time the patient remains at a phase I level of care depends on health status, the surgical procedure, anesthesia type, and rate of progression to regain alertness and hemodynamic stability. It can range from less than 1 hour to days. This level requires ongoing monitoring of the airway, vital signs, and evidence of recovery that varies from every 5 to 15 minutes initially. The time between assessments gradually increases as the patient progresses toward recovery.

Phase II care focuses on preparing the patient for care in an extended-care environment such as a medical-surgical unit, step-down unit, skilled nursing agency, or home. This phase can occur in a PACU, on a medical-surgical unit, or in the same-day surgery (SDS) unit (ambulatory care unit) and may last only 15 to 30 minutes, although 1 to 2 hours is more typical. Patients are discharged from this phase when the presurgical level of consciousness has returned, oxygen saturation is at baseline, and vital signs are stable. Some patients achieve this level of recovery in phase I and can be discharged directly to home. Others may require further observation.

Phase III care, known as the *extended-care environment,* most often occurs on a hospital unit or in the home. For patients who have continuing care needs that cannot be met at home, discharge may be from the hospital unit to an extended-care agency. Although vital signs continue to be monitored in this type of environment, the frequency ranges from several times daily to just once daily.

Ambulatory surgery units provide same-day procedural care. Patients recover in a PACU environment that advances them quickly from a phase I to a phase III level, preparing them for discharge to home. Discharge criteria must be met before the patient is discharged from the agency. If the patient experiences ongoing issues related to unstable vital signs, poor ***gas exchange,*** excessive nausea and vomiting, or unmanageable ***pain,*** admission to an acute care setting or extended-care agency may be necessary.

For patients who were hospitalized before surgery and/or are anticipated to be hospitalized after surgery, the circulating nurse and the anesthesia provider accompany the patient to the PACU. For patients in critical condition, transfer may be directly from the operating room (OR) to the ICU. On arrival, the anesthesia provider and the circulating nurse give the PACU nurse a verbal "hand-off" report to communicate the patient's condition and care needs.

! NATIONAL PATIENT SAFETY GOALS

A hand-off report that meets The Joint Commission's National Patient Safety Goals requires effective communication between the anesthesia provider, circulating nurse, and PACU (or ICU) nurse.

This report involves communication reflective of a process like TeamSTEPPS®, a systematic communication approach for interprofessional teams to improve quality and safety (see Chapter 1). See the Best Practice for Patient Safety & Quality Care: Postoperative Hand-off Report box for an example of critical information to include in a standard hand-off report.

The PACU nurse is skilled in the care of patients with multiple medical and surgical problems immediately after a surgical procedure. This area requires in-depth knowledge of anatomy and physiology, anesthetic agents, pharmacology, ***pain*** management, airway management, surgical procedures, and Advanced Cardiac Life Support (ACLS). The PACU nurse is skilled in assessment and can make knowledgeable, critical decisions if emergencies or complications occur. The patient is monitored continuously, and the anesthesia provider and surgeon are consulted as needed.

BEST PRACTICE FOR PATIENT SAFETY & QUALITY CARE (QSEN)

Postoperative Hand-off Report

- Type and extent of the surgical procedure
- Type of anesthesia used, and length of time the patient was under anesthesia
- Allergies (especially to latex or drugs)
- Primary language, any sensory impairments, any communication difficulties
- Special requests that were verbalized by the patient before surgery, including communications with the family or caregiver
- Preoperative and intraoperative respiratory function and dysfunction
- Any health problems or pathophysiologic conditions
- Any relevant events or complications during anesthesia or surgery such as a traumatic intubation
- If intraoperative complications occurred, how they were managed and the patient's responses (e.g., laboratory values, excessive blood loss, injuries)
- Intake and output, including current IV fluid administration and estimated blood loss
- Type and amount of IV fluids or blood products administered
- Medications administered and when last dose of pain medication was given
- When the next dose of antibiotics, cardiac drugs, and other medications are due
- Location and type of incisions, dressings, catheters, tubes, drains, or packing
- Prosthetic devices (existing or applied)
- Joint or limb immobility while in the operating room, especially in the older patient
- Other intraoperative positioning that may be relevant in the postoperative phase
- Status of current vital signs, including temperature and oxygen saturation

The nurse generalist will receive the patient from the PACU nurse after the patient has been determined stable for transfer. A hand-off report similar to that shown in the Best Practice for Patient Safety & Quality Care: Postoperative Hand-off Report should be received at that time.

❖ Interprofessional Collaborative Care

◆ Assessment: Recognize Cues

History. Using the surgical team's records and the PACU nurse's hand-off report, the generalist nurse receiving a patient from PACU to discharge, or to receive back to the medical-surgical floor, creates an individualized plan of care. Review the preoperative assessment and the electronic health record for information about the patient's history, physical condition, and emotional status. Table 9.7 identifies potential complications of surgery to consider when designing the plan of care and planning for discharge teaching.

Physical Assessment/Signs and Symptoms. Criteria for discharge to home for patients in an ambulatory surgical setting will be agency specific. These may include stable vital signs; normal body temperature; no overt bleeding; return of gag, cough, and swallow reflexes; the ability to take liquids; and adequate urine output.

! NURSING SAFETY PRIORITY (QSEN)

Action Alert

Perform an initial assessment and continue to monitor respiratory assessment for any patient who has undergone general anesthesia or moderate sedation or has received sedative or opioid drugs.

FOCUSED ASSESSMENT

The Patient on Arrival at the Medical-Surgical Unit After Discharge From the Postanesthesia Care Unit (PACU)

Airway
- Is it patent?
- Is the neck in proper alignment?

Breathing
- What are the quality and pattern of the breathing?
- What are the respiratory rate and depth?
- Are accessory muscles used to breathe?
- Is the patient receiving oxygen? At which setting and method of delivery?
- What is the pulse oximetry reading?

Cardiovascular Status
- Are blood pressure and pulse within the patient's baseline range?
- Are peripheral pulses palpable?
- What are the rate and rhythm of the heartbeat?
- Are these values significantly different from when the patient was in the PACU?

Mental Status
- Is the patient awake, able to be aroused, oriented, and aware?
- Does the patient respond to verbal stimuli?

Surgical Incision Site
- How is it dressed?
- Review the amount of drainage on the dressing immediately.
- Is there any bleeding or drainage underneath the patient?
- Are drains present? If so, what kind? Quantify amount present, and describe drainage characteristics.
- Are the drains set properly (e.g., compressed if they should be compressed, not kinked, patient not lying on them)?

Temperature
- Is the value significantly different from baseline and when the patient was in the PACU?

Intravenous Fluids
- Which type of solution is infusing and with which additives?
- How much solution was remaining on arrival?
- How much solution was infused in the transport time from the PACU?
- At what rate is the infusion supposed to be set?

Other Tubes
- Is there a nasogastric or intestinal tube?
- What is the color, consistency, and amount of drainage?
- Is suction applied to the tube if ordered? Is the suction setting correct?
- Is there a Foley catheter? If so, is it draining properly?
- What is the color, clarity, and volume of urine output?

NCLEX EXAMINATION CHALLENGE 9.5

Physiological Integrity: Reduction of Risk Potential

The nurse is caring for a client who has been readmitted to the medical-surgical unit following surgery for a hernia repair completed under general anesthesia. What is the **priority** nursing assessment?

A. Perform thorough auscultation of the lungs
B. Assess response to pinprick stimulation from feet to mid-chest level
C. Determine level of consciousness and response to environmental stimuli
D. Compare blood pressure findings from preoperative assessment to the present

! NURSING SAFETY PRIORITY (QSEN)

Critical Rescue

During the postoperative phase, recognize that all patients remain at risk for pneumonia, shock, cardiac arrest, respiratory arrest, venous thromboembolism (VTE), and GI bleeding. These serious complications can be prevented, or consequences reduced, by using prudent clinical judgment. If any signs or symptoms of these conditions are noted, respond by immediately notifying the surgeon.

If receiving the patient back to a medical-surgical unit, perform a full assessment once the patient has been transferred to your care. See the Focused Assessment: The Patient on Arrival at the Medical-Surgical Unit After Discharge From the Postanesthesia Care Unit (PACU) box. Fully evaluate and continue to monitor level of consciousness, oxygen saturation, the surgical area for bleeding, and vital signs per agency policy or surgeon's orders. Monitor more frequently if the patient's condition warrants.

Respiratory System. When the patient is admitted to the medical-surgical floor following surgery, immediately assess for a patent airway. *Although some patients may be awake and able to speak, talking is not a reliable indicator of adequate* ***gas exchange.*** An artificial airway such as an endotracheal tube (ET), a nasal trumpet, or an oral airway may be in place. If the patient is receiving oxygen, document the type of delivery device and the concentration or liter flow of the oxygen. Continuously monitor pulse oximetry for oxygen saturation (Spo_2). The Spo_2 should be above 95% (or at the patient's presurgical baseline). Check the lungs at least every 4 hours during the first 24 hours following surgery and then every 8 hours, or per agency policy. Older patients, those who smoke, and patients with a history of lung disease or obesity are at greater risk for respiratory complications after surgery and should be assessed more frequently.

! NURSING SAFETY PRIORITY (QSEN)

Critical Rescue

If you recognize that your patient's oxygen saturation drops below 95% (or below his or her presurgical baseline), immediately respond by notifying the surgeon or anesthesia provider. If the patient's condition continues to deteriorate or other symptoms arise, an emergency response is imperative.

Assess the rate, pattern, and depth of breathing to determine adequacy of ***gas exchange.*** A respiratory rate of less than 10 breaths/min may indicate anesthetic- or opioid analgesic–induced

TABLE 9.7 Potential System Complications of Surgery

Respiratory Complications	Neuromuscular Complications
• Atelectasis • Laryngeal edema • Pneumonia • Pulmonary edema • Pulmonary embolism (PE) • Ventilator dependence	• Hyperthermia • Hypothermia • Joint contractures • Nerve damage and paralysis
Cardiovascular Complications	**GI Complications**
• Anaphylaxis • Anemia • Disseminated intravascular coagulation (DIC) • Dysrhythmias • Heart failure • Hypertension • Hypotension • Hypovolemic shock • Sepsis • Venous thromboembolism (VTE), especially deep vein thrombosis (DVT)	• GI ulcers and bleeding • Paralytic ileus **Kidney/Urinary Complications** • Acute kidney injury (AKI) • Acute urinary retention • Electrolyte imbalances • Stone formation • Urinary tract infection **Skin Complications** • Pressure injuries • Skin rashes or contact allergies • Wound infection • Wound dehiscence • Wound evisceration
Neurologic Complications	
• Cerebral infarction • Cognitive decline • Visual loss	

respiratory depression. Rapid, shallow respirations may signal shock, cardiac problems, increased metabolic rate, or ***pain.***

Auscultate all lung fields to fully assess breath sounds. Check symmetry of breath sounds and chest wall movement. Continue to inspect the chest wall for accessory muscle use, sternal retraction, and diaphragmatic breathing. These symptoms may indicate an excessive anesthetic effect, airway obstruction, or paralysis, which could result in hypoxia. Listen for snoring and ***stridor*** (a high-pitched crowing sound). These occur with airway obstruction resulting from tracheal or laryngeal spasm or edema, mucus in the airway, or blockage of the airway from edema or tongue relaxation. When neuromuscular blocking agents are retained, muscle weakness could affect the diaphragm and impair ***gas exchange.*** Symptoms include the inability to maintain a head lift, weak hand grasps, and an abdominal breathing pattern.

Cardiovascular System. Assess vital signs after surgery for trends and compare them with those taken before surgery. Report blood pressure changes that are 25% higher or lower than values obtained before surgery (or a 15- to 20-point difference, systolic or diastolic) to the surgeon or anesthesia provider. Decreased blood pressure, pulse pressure, and abnormal heart sounds can be indicative of possible cardiac depression, fluid volume deficit, shock, hemorrhage, or the effects of drugs (see Chapters 13 and 34).

Bradycardia could indicate an anesthesia effect or hypothermia. Older patients are at risk for hypothermia because of age-related changes in the hypothalamus (the temperature regulation center), low levels of body fat, or prolonged exposure to the cool environment of the surgical suite (Touhy & Jett, 2020). An increased pulse rate could indicate hemorrhage, shock, or ***pain.***

Cardiac monitoring may be ordered on return to the medical-surgical unit. In assessing the vital signs of a patient who is not being monitored continuously, compare the rate, rhythm, and quality of the apical pulse with that of a peripheral pulse such as the radial pulse. A **pulse deficit** (a difference between the apical and peripheral pulses) could indicate a dysrhythmia.

Peripheral vascular assessment needs to be performed daily because anesthesia and surgical positioning may impair peripheral circulation and contribute to clotting and venous thromboembolism (VTE), especially deep vein thrombosis (DVT). Compare distal pulses on both feet for pulse quality, observe the color and temperature of extremities, evaluate sensation and motion, and determine the speed of capillary refill. Palpable pedal pulses indicate adequate circulation and perfusion of the legs.

Because surgery-related VTE can be prevented and because pulmonary embolism is the leading cause of preventable in-hospital death, prophylaxis is the most important patient safety strategy (*British Medical Journal,* 2020). The patient may be prescribed antiembolism (compression) stockings, pneumatic compression devices (sequential compression devices), and/or a drug for prophylaxis such as enoxaparin following surgery.

! NURSING SAFETY PRIORITY (QSEN)

Action Alert

Evaluate all patients for VTE risk, and ensure that prophylactic measures are in place. These may include antiembolism stockings, pneumatic compression devices, leg exercises, early mobility, and/or drug therapy.

Antiembolism stockings (thromboembolism-deterrent [TED] or compression stockings) provide graduated compression of the legs, starting at the end of the foot and ankle. Measure the patient's leg length and circumference before ordering the stocking size. Elastic wraps can be used when the legs are too large or too small for stockings. Help the patient apply the stockings or wraps and ensure that

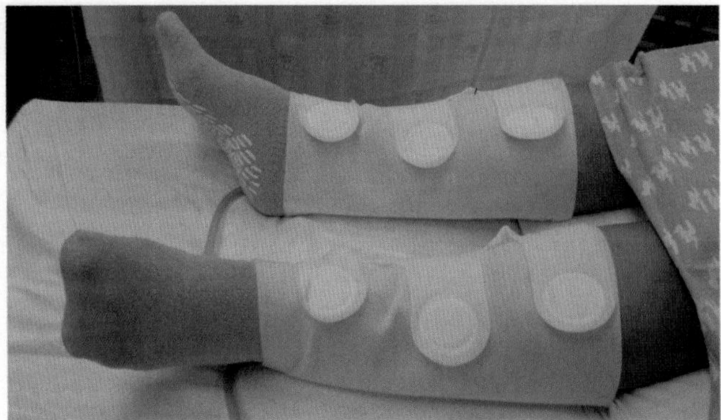

FIG. 9.6 External pneumatic compression device used to promote venous return and prevent venous thromboembolism (VTE). (From Angelo, R., Ryu, R., & Esch, J. [2010]. *AANA advanced arthroscopy: The shoulder*. Philadelphia: Saunders.)

they are neither too loose (are ineffective) nor too tight (inhibit blood flow). They need to be worn properly and should be removed two to three times per day for 30 minutes for skin inspection and skin care.

Pneumatic compression devices (Fig. 9.6) enhance venous blood flow by providing intermittent periods of compression on the legs. Measure the patient's legs and order the correct size. Place the boots on the patient's legs, then set and check the compression pressures (usually 35 to 55 mm Hg).

Neurologic System. *Cerebral functioning* and the level of consciousness or awareness must be assessed in *all* patients who have received general anesthesia (Table 9.8) or any type of sedation. Observe for lethargy, restlessness, or irritability and test coherence and orientation. Determine awareness by observing responses to calling the patient's name, touching the patient, and giving simple commands such as "Open your eyes" and "Take a deep breath." Eye opening in response to a command indicates wakefulness or arousability, but not awareness. Assess the degree of orientation to person, place, and time by asking the conscious patient to answer questions such as, "What is your name?" (person), "Where are you?" (place), and "What day is it?" (time).

PATIENT-CENTERED CARE: OLDER ADULT CONSIDERATIONS QSEN

An older adult may take longer than a younger adult to return to his or her level of presurgical orientation. Preoperative drugs and anesthetics can slow the process. Prevention of delirium involves being mindful of sensory needs (glasses, hearing aids), early ambulation (if possible), bedside presence of a family member or caregiver (if possible), effective pain management, mindfulness of sleep and nutrition status, maintenance of a calm environment, and cognitive stimulation (Touhy & Jett, 2020).

Compare the patient's presurgical neurologic status with the findings after surgery, and monitor level of consciousness every 4 to 8 hours (or per agency policy). Patients who had altered cerebral functioning before surgery because of another condition usually continue to have the same alteration after surgery.

Motor and sensory function after general anesthesia, particularly after spinal or epidural procedures, will be altered, as general anesthesia depresses all voluntary motor function. Regional anesthesia alters the motor and sensory function of only a part of the body.

CLINICAL JUDGMENT CHALLENGE 9.1

Patient-Centered Care

A 60-year old client with a history of opioid misuse fell a week ago and did not seek care until 2 days ago, when a grandchild found him lying in the kitchen of his residence. He was then brought and admitted to the hospital with the diagnosis of a hip fracture. Having just had hip replacement surgery, he is now readmitted to the medical-surgical unit from the PACU. He is responsive when asked his name, yet is mildly confused about where he is. He is pulling at his oxygen cannula but does allow it to be replaced into his nostrils. Initial vital signs on return to the medical-surgical unit included BP 140/90 mm Hg, pulse 100 beats/min, respirations 22 breaths/min. Vital signs taken 15 minutes later show BP 142/92 mm Hg, pulse 100 beats/min, respirations 22 breaths/min. He says he hurts "really badly" and wants to know when he will receive pain medication.

1. **Recognize Cues:** What assessment information in this client situation is the most important and immediate concern for the nurse? (Hint: Identify the **relevant** information *first* to determine what is most important.)
2. **Analyze Cues:** What client conditions are consistent with the **most relevant** information? (Hint: Think about priority collaborative problems that support and contradict the information presented in this situation.)
3. **Prioritize Hypotheses:** Which possibilities or explanations are **most likely** to be present in this client situation? Which possibilities or explanations are the most serious? (Hint: Consider all possibilities and determine their urgency and risk for this client.)
4. **Generate Solutions:** What actions would most likely achieve the desired outcomes for this client? Which actions should be **avoided** or are **potentially harmful**? (Hint: Determine the desired outcomes first to decide which interventions are appropriate and those that should be avoided.)
5. **Take Action:** Which actions are the most appropriate and how should they be implemented? In what **priority order** should they be implemented? (Hint: Consider health teaching, documentation, requested health care provider orders or prescriptions, nursing skills, collaboration with or referral to health team members, etc.)
6. **Evaluate Outcomes:** What client assessment would indicate that the nurse's actions were **effective**? (Hint: Think about signs that would indicate an improvement, decline, or unchanged client condition.)

Assess the level of sensation loss remaining by lightly pricking the patient's skin with a monofilament and having the patient indicate when the sensation feels sharp rather than dull (just pressure).

Evaluate motor function by asking the patient to move each extremity. Assess the strength of each limb and compare the results on both sides. Test for the return of sympathetic nervous system tone by gradually elevating the patient's head and monitoring for hypotension. Begin this evaluation after the patient's sensation has returned to at least the spinal dermatome level of T10 (see Chapter 38).

Specific assessment findings for complications of spinal and epidural anesthesia are listed in the Best Practice for Patient Safety & Quality Care: Recognizing Serious Complications of Spinal and Epidural Anesthesia box.

Fluid, Electrolyte, and Acid-Base Balance. NPO status before surgery, the loss of fluid during surgery, and the type and amount of blood or fluid given affect postsurgical fluid and electrolyte balance. Fluid volume deficit or fluid volume overload may occur. Sodium, potassium, chloride, and calcium imbalances may also result, as may changes in other electrolyte levels. Fluid and electrolyte imbalances occur more often in older patients and in those with chronic health problems such as diabetes mellitus or heart failure.

BEST PRACTICE FOR PATIENT SAFETY & QUALITY CARE QSEN

Recognizing Serious Complications of Spinal and Epidural Anesthesia

Respiratory Depression (Can Occur if the Anesthetic Agent Moves Higher in the Epidural or Subarachnoid Space)

- What is the quality and pattern of the breathing?
- What are the respiratory rate and depth?
- Is the patient receiving oxygen? At which setting and method of delivery? What is the pulse oximetry result?
- Notify the anesthesia provider if pulse oximetry drops below 95% or if the patient is unable to increase the depth of respiration.

Hypotension (Can Occur When Regional Anesthesia Causes Widespread Vasodilation)

- What is the patient's blood pressure?
- Is the blood pressure now lower than in the preoperative or operative phase?
- Has the pulse pressure widened?
- Notify the anesthesia provider if systolic blood pressure remains more than 10 mm Hg below the patient's baseline or if other symptoms of shock are present.
- Notify the anesthesia provider if hypotension is accompanied by other symptoms of autonomic nervous system blockade (bradycardia, nausea, vomiting).

Epidural Hematoma

- Assess for delayed or regressing return of sensory and motor function; if delayed or taking longer than usual, alert the anesthesia provider immediately.
- Determine whether sensory or motor deficits are improving, remaining the same, or worsening; if worsening or decreasing after brief improvement, notify the anesthesia provider immediately.
- Assess for return of deep tendon reflexes of extremities on both sides, and compare from one side of the body with the other; if reflexes regress, notify the anesthesia provider immediately.
- Assess pain level in the back; if the patient feels pressure or increasing back ***pain*** while coughing or straining, notify the anesthesia provider immediately.

Infection (Meningitis)

- Assess for mental status changes.
- Assess for increasing temperature.
- Assess for ability to turn the neck.
- Notify the anesthesia provider immediately for temperature elevations above 101°F (38.3°C), inability to move the neck, or acute confusion.

Postdural Puncture Headache

- Assess for report of headache in the occipital region, especially when the patient is permitted to sit upright.

Intake and output measurement should be continued in the postoperative phase. Document IV fluid intake, vomitus, urine, wound drainage, and nasogastric (NG) tube drainage.

Hydration status can be assessed by inspecting the color and moisture of mucous membranes; the turgor, texture, and "tenting" of the skin (test over the sternum or forehead of an older patient); the amount of drainage on dressings; and the presence (or absence) of axillary sweat. Measure and compare total output (e.g., NG tube drainage, urine output, wound drainage) with total intake to identify a possible fluid imbalance. Consider insensible fluid loss such as sweat when reviewing total output.

IV fluids are closely monitored to promote fluid and electrolyte balance. Isotonic solutions such as lactated Ringer's (LR), 0.9% sodium chloride (normal saline), and 5% dextrose with lactated Ringer's (D5/LR) may have been used as IV fluid replacement in the PACU. After the patient returns to the medical-surgical unit, the type and rate of IV infusions are based on need.

Acid-base balance is affected by the patient's respiratory status; metabolic changes during surgery; and losses of acids or bases in drainage. For example, NG tube drainage or vomitus causes a loss of hydrochloric acid and leads to metabolic alkalosis. Monitor arterial blood gas (ABG) values and other laboratory values to identify potential consequences of an acid-base imbalance. (See Chapter 14 for more detailed information on acid-base imbalances.)

Kidney/Urinary System. Urinary control may return immediately after surgery or may not return for hours after general or regional anesthesia. The effects of preoperative drugs (especially atropine), anesthetic agents, or manipulation during surgery can cause urine retention. Assess for this by inspection, palpation, and percussion of the lower abdomen for bladder distention or use a bladder scanner (see Chapter 60). Urine retention or incontinence may occur early after surgery and requires

NCLEX EXAMINATION CHALLENGE 9.6

Physiological Integrity: Reduction of Risk Potential

In the early postoperative phase, which assessment finding in a client who had an epidural during surgery requires **immediate** nursing intervention?

A. Blood pressure of 142/90 mm Hg
B. Headache of 4 on a 1-10 scale
C. Gradual return of motor function
D. Increase in back pain when coughing

TABLE 9.8 Immediate Postoperative Neurologic Assessment: Return to Preoperative Level

Order of Return to Consciousness After General Anesthesia

1. Muscular irritability
2. Restlessness and delirium
3. Recognition of pain
4. Ability to reason and control behavior

Order of Return of Motor and Sensory Functioning After Local or Regional Anesthesia

1. Sense of touch
2. Sense of pain
3. Sense of warmth
4. Sense of cold
5. Ability to move

intervention such as intermittent (straight) catheterization or an indwelling catheter to empty the bladder.

If the patient has an indwelling urinary (Foley) catheter, assess the urine for color, clarity, and amount. If the patient is voiding, assess the frequency, amount per void, and any symptoms, and remind the patient that you need to have this information communicated to you for documentation purposes. Place a urine hat-type specimen collector on the toilet as a reminder.

Urine output should be close to the total intake for a 24-hour period. Consider sweat, vomitus, or diarrhea stools as sources of fluid output. Report a urine output of less than 30 mL/hr (240 mL per 8-hour nursing shift) to the surgeon, as this may indicate hypovolemia or renal complications. (See Chapter 60 for kidney and urinary assessment.)

Gastrointestinal System. *Postoperative nausea and vomiting (PONV)* is the most common reaction after surgery. Many patients who receive general anesthesia have some form of GI upset within the first 24 hours after surgery. Patients with a history of motion sickness are at high risk for developing PONV, as are patients with obesity because many anesthetics are retained by fat cells and remain in the body longer. Abdominal surgery and the use of opioid analgesics reduce intestinal peristalsis, which also increases the risk.

Preventive drug therapy, often started in the preoperative phase, is effective in reducing the incidence. Drugs often used include ondansetron and dexamethasone. Be aware that dexamethasone may slightly increase glucose levels in patients *without* diabetes in the first 12 hours postoperatively (Blanchard & van Wissen, 2019).

Assess the patient continuously for PONV, which can stress and irritate abdominal and GI wounds, increase intracranial pressure in those who had head and neck surgery, elevate intraocular pressure in those who had eye surgery, and increase the risk for aspiration. Patients may experience nausea if the head of the bed is raised early after surgery. Help reduce this distressing symptom by having the patient assume a side-lying position before raising the head slowly.

Intestinal peristalsis return may be delayed because of prolonged anesthesia time, the amount of bowel handling during surgery, and treatment with opioid analgesics. Assess for the return of peristalsis. Patients who are recovering from pelvic or abdominal surgery often have decreased or no peristalsis for at least 24 hours; this may persist for several days for those who have GI surgery (Rothrock, 2019).

Listen for bowel sounds in all four abdominal quadrants and at the umbilicus. If NG suction is being used, turn off the suction before listening to prevent mistaking the sound of the suction for bowel sounds. *The presence of active bowel sounds usually indicates return of peristalsis; however, the absence of bowel sounds does not confirm a lack of peristalsis. The true indicator of intestinal activity is the passage of flatus or stool* (Rothrock, 2019). Abdominal cramping along with distention denotes trapped, nonmoving gas—not peristalsis.

Decreased peristalsis occurs in patients with a paralytic ileus. The abdominal wall is distended with no visible intestinal movement. Assess for signs and symptoms of paralytic ileus (distended abdomen, abdominal discomfort, vomiting, no passage of flatus or stool). In some patients, bowel sounds can be heard even when a true paralytic ileus is present. The passage of flatus or stool is the only indicator of resolution of a paralytic ileus (Rothrock, 2019).

A nasogastric (NG) tube may be inserted during surgery to decompress and drain the stomach, promote GI rest, and allow the lower GI tract to heal. It may also be used to monitor any gastric bleeding and prevent intestinal obstruction. Usually, low suction is applied to promote drainage. Suction is either continuous or intermittent.

Record the color, consistency, and amount of the NG drainage every 8 hours or per agency policy. An occult blood test (Gastroccult) may be performed. Normal NG drainage fluid is greenish yellow. Red or pink drainage fluid indicates active bleeding, and brown liquid or drainage with a coffee-ground appearance indicates old bleeding. The NG tube should be secured to prevent any chance of displacement.

Assess the patient for complications related to NG tube use such as fluid and electrolyte imbalances, aspiration, and nares discomfort. To prevent aspiration, check the tube placement every 4 to 8 hours and before instilling any liquid, including drugs, into the tube. (See Chapter 50 for information on tube placement and care.) Electrolyte imbalances, such as fluid volume deficit, hypokalemia, hyponatremia (Chapter 13), hypochloremia, and metabolic alkalosis (Chapter 14) can result from NG drainage and tube irrigation with water instead of saline.

! NURSING SAFETY PRIORITY (QSEN)

Action Alert

After gastric surgery do not move or irrigate the NG tube unless ordered.

Constipation may occur after surgery as a result of anesthesia, opioid analgesia, decreased activity, and decreased oral intake. Assess the abdomen by inspection, auscultation, and palpation (the health care provider can provide percussion), and document the elimination pattern to determine whether intervention is needed. *Auscultate before palpation because these two maneuvers can affect peristalsis.* Increased dietary fiber intake, mild laxatives or bulk-forming agents, or enemas may be prescribed. Encourage ambulation as early as possible after surgery to promote peristalsis.

Integumentary System. The clean surgical wound regains ***tissue integrity*** at skin level in about 2 weeks in the absence of trauma, ***infection***, connective tissue disease, malnutrition, or the use of certain drugs such as steroids. Complete tissue integrity (healing) of all layers within the surgical wound may take 6 months to 2 years. Those at risk for delayed wound healing include older adults, patients with obesity, those who are immunocompromised or have diabetes; and people who smoke. The physical health and age of the patient, size and location of the wound, and stress on the wound all affect healing time. Head and facial wounds heal more quickly than abdominal and leg wounds because there is less stress on these locations and better blood flow to the head and neck area.

Normal Wound Healing. During the first few days of normal wound healing, the incised tissue regains blood supply and begins to bind together. Fibrin and a thin layer of epithelial cells seal the incision. After 1 to 4 days, epithelial cells continue growing in the fibrin, and strands of collagen begin to fill in the wound gaps. This process continues for 2 to 3 weeks. At that time ***tissue integrity*** appears regained; however, healing is not complete for up to 2 years, until the scar is strengthened. (See Chapters 22 and 23 for discussion of wound healing and wound infection.)

If the patient has stayed in the hospital following surgery, the surgeon usually removes the original dressing on the first or second day after surgery. Assess the ***tissue integrity*** of the incision on a regular basis, at least every 8 hours, for redness, increased warmth, swelling, tenderness or ***pain,*** and the type and amount of drainage. Some drainage change from **sanguineous** (bloody) to **serosanguineous** (yellowish mixed with light red or pale pink) to **serous** (serum-like, or yellow) is normal during the first few days. Serosanguineous drainage continuing beyond the fifth day after surgery, or in an increasing amount, is a sign of possible dehiscence, and the surgeon should be notified. Crusting on the incision line is normal, as is a pink color to the line itself, which is caused by inflammation from the surgical procedure. Slight swelling under the sutures or staples is also normal. Redness or swelling of or around the incision line, excessive tenderness or ***pain*** on palpation, and/or purulent or odorous drainage indicates surgical site infection (SSI) and must be reported to the surgeon.

Impaired Wound Healing. Impaired healing and a breakdown of the surgical wound with loss of ***tissue integrity*** may be caused by ***infection,*** distention, stress at the surgical site, and other health problems that cause delayed wound healing (e.g., diabetes, renal disease, immune deficiency). Wound **dehiscence** is a partial or complete separation of the outer wound layers, sometimes described as a *splitting open of the wound.* **Evisceration** is the total separation of all wound layers and protrusion of internal organs through the open wound (Fig. 9.7). *Evisceration is a surgical emergency; the surgeon is contacted immediately, and the patient returned to the surgical suite.* Dehiscence or evisceration may follow forceful coughing, vomiting, straining, or not properly splinting the surgical site during movement. The patient may report, "I feel like something popped" or "I feel as if I just split open."

Both dehiscence and evisceration occur most often between the fifth and tenth days after surgery. Dehiscence occurs more often in patients with diabetes, obesity, immune deficiency, or malnutrition, or in those who use steroids. Care for these conditions is covered later in this chapter.

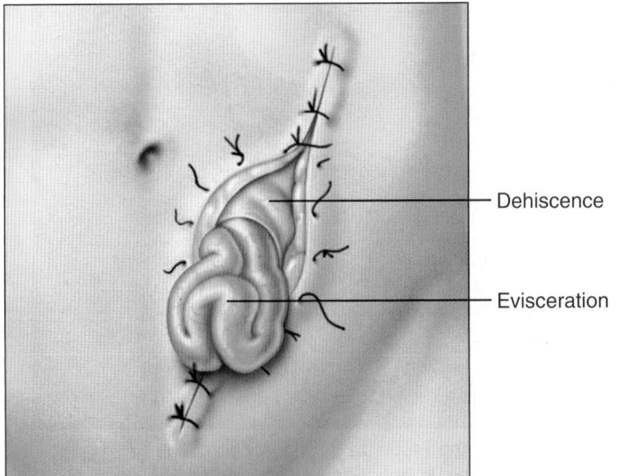

FIG. 9.7 Complications of surgical wound healing. (From Harkreader, H., Hogan, M.A., & Thobaben, M. [2007]. *Fundamentals of nursing: Caring and clinical judgment.* [3rd ed.]. Philadelphia: Saunders.)

Dressings and Drains. Assess all dressings, including casts and elastic bandages, for bleeding or other drainage on admission to the medical-surgical unit and routinely thereafter, at least every 8 hours. Check for drainage and record its amount, color, consistency, and odor. If drainage is present on a dressing or cast, monitor its progression by outlining it with a pencil and indicating the date and time. Large amounts of sanguineous drainage may indicate poor clotting and possible internal bleeding. Check the area underneath the patient also, because drainage or blood may leak from the side of the dressing and not appear on the dressing itself.

Ensure that the dressing does not restrict circulation or sensation. This problem is most likely to occur when dressings are tight or completely encircle an arm or a leg. Chest dressings that are too tight or that encircle the chest can restrict breathing.

The surgeon inserts a drain into or close to the wound if more than a minimal amount of drainage is expected. A Penrose drain (a single-lumen, soft, open, latex tube) is a gravity-type drain under the dressing. Drainage on the dressing is expected with open-tube drains. Closed-suction drains such as Hemovac and Jackson-Pratt drains include a reservoir that collects drainage. Drainage on the dressing around the drain is not usually present. Assess closed drainage systems for maintenance of suction. Specialty drains such as a T-tube may be placed for specific drainage purposes. For example, a T-tube drains bile after a cholecystectomy. Chronic wounds or wounds that heal by delayed primary intention are typically drained with a negative-pressure wound device. Negative-pressure wound therapy (NPWT) has been shown to improve healing of closed surgical incisions and reduce SSIs (Gestring, 2020). Fig. 9.8 shows commonly used drains.

Pain Assessment. ***Pain*** assessment is continuous during recovery. Most patients experience some degree of discomfort after surgery. Pain is a subjective experience and must be assessed based on individual conditions. Pain after surgery can be related to the surgical wound, tissue manipulation during surgery, drains or tube placement, surgical posturing, and/or the patient's experience with pain, among other factors.

Assess the patient's discomfort by checking physical and behavioral signs of acute pain, such as increased pulse and blood pressure, increased respiratory rate, profuse sweating, restlessness, confusion (in the older adult), wincing, moaning, and crying. When possible, ask the patient to rate the ***pain*** before and after drugs are given (e.g., on a scale of 0 to 10, with 0 being no pain and 10 being extreme pain). Plan the patient's activities around the timing of analgesia to improve mobility. Reassess within 20

PATIENT-CENTERED CARE: OLDER ADULT CONSIDERATIONS QSEN

Pain remains poorly assessed in the older adult, and specific care should be taken to determine the level of pain in this population, especially in those who have cognitive impairment. Challenges in assessing pain in the older patient include communication difficulty (in the presence of cognitive deficits), comorbidities, stoic character, and a reluctance to report pain. Drug dosages may need to be adjusted for the older patient to account for age-related changes that affect metabolism and excretion of medication.

to 30 minutes after pain medication has been given to determine its efficacy, and document results in the electronic health record. (See Chapter 5 for further discussion of ***pain*** assessment.)

Psychosocial Assessment. Consider the psychological, social, cultural, and spiritual issues of the patient as postoperative care is provided. The patient's age and health history; surgical procedure; and impact of surgery on recovery, body image, roles, and lifestyle are all considerations to take into account.

Assess for signs of anxiety such as restlessness; increased pulse, blood pressure, and respiratory rate; and crying. The patient may be anxious and ask questions about the results or findings of the surgical procedure. Reassure the patient that he or she is safe and that the surgeon will speak with him or her soon. If the surgeon has already spoken with the patient, reinforce what was said. Assess the family or caregiver for any psychosocial discomfort or need for additional support related to the patient's condition and postoperative plan of care. Be prepared to refer to social services or external support systems as appropriate.

Laboratory Assessment. Laboratory tests ordered after surgery are based on the surgical procedure, the patient's health history, and clinical signs and symptoms after surgery. Common tests include electrolytes, a complete blood count, urinalysis, and kidney function tests.

Changes in electrolyte, hematocrit, and hemoglobin levels often occur during the first 24 to 48 hours after surgery because of blood and fluid loss and the body's reaction to the surgical process. Fluid loss with minimal blood loss may cause elevated laboratory values. Such test results appear increased but actually are concentrated normal values.

An increase in the band cells (immature neutrophils) in the white blood cell differential count, known as a "left-shift" or

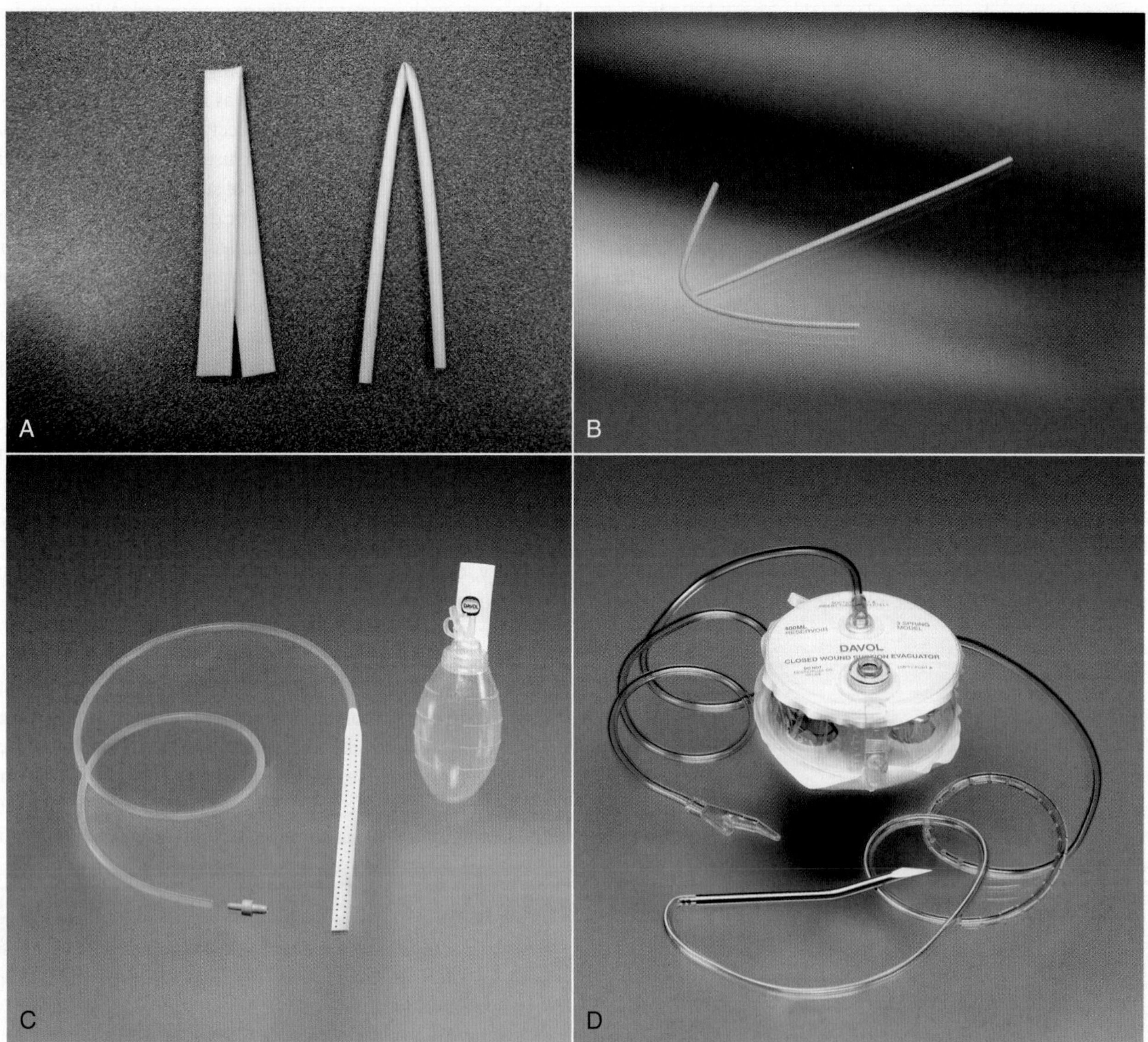

FIG. 9.8 Types of surgical drains. Gravity drains such as the Penrose (A) and the T-tube (B) drain directly through a tube from the surgical area. In closed-wound drainage systems such as the Jackson-Pratt (C) and Hemovac (D), drainage collects in a collecting vessel by means of compression and re-expansion of the system. (A from Sirois, M. [2011]. *Principles and Practice of Veterinary Technology* [3rd ed.]. St. Louis: Mosby; B courtesy 2014 C.R. Bard, Inc. Covington, GA. Used with permission; C and D courtesy C.R. Bard, Inc., Covington, GA.)

"bandemia," is an indication of ***infection***. The source of infection may be the respiratory system, urinary tract, surgical wound, or IV site. Obtain specimens for culture and sensitivity testing as ordered, and review the culture reports at 24, 48, and 72 hours. Notify the surgeon of positive culture results. (See Chapters 16 and 21 for information on infection.)

Arterial blood gas (ABG) tests may be needed for patients who have respiratory or cardiac disease, those undergoing mechanical ventilation after surgery, and those who had chest surgery. Review ABG results and notify the surgeon of any acid-base imbalance or hypoxemia that indicates poor ***gas exchange.*** (For more discussion on arterial blood gases and acidosis, see Chapter 14.)

◆ **Analysis: Analyze Cues and Prioritize Hypotheses.** The priority collaborative problems for patients in the immediate postoperative phase are:

1. Potential for decreased ***gas exchange*** due to the effects of anesthesia, ***pain,*** opioid analgesics, and immobility
2. Potential for ***infection*** and delayed healing due to wound location, decreased mobility, drains and drainage, and tubes
3. Acute ***pain*** due to the surgical incision and procedure, and surgical positioning
4. Potential for decreased peristalsis due to surgical manipulation, opioid use, and fluid and electrolyte imbalances

◆ **Planning and Implementation: Generate Solutions and Take Action**

Improving Gas Exchange

Planning: Expected Outcomes. The patient is expected to attain and maintain optimal lung expansion and breathing patterns after surgery.

Interventions

Monitoring. Monitor the patient's oxygen saturation (Spo_2) for adequacy of ***gas exchange*** with pulse oximetry with each set of vital signs or at least hourly, according to the patient's condition. The highest incidence of impaired ***gas exchange*** after surgery occurs on the second postoperative day.

Patients who normally have a low Pao_2 such as those with lung disease or older adults are at higher risk for hypoxemia. An older adult is often prescribed low-dose oxygen therapy for the first 12 to 24 hours after surgery to reduce confusion from anesthesia and sedation. Patients who received moderate sedation with a benzodiazepine such as midazolam or lorazepam may be overly sedated or have respiratory depression sufficient to need reversal with flumazenil (see the Best Practice for Patient Safety & Quality Care: Emergency Care of the Patient Experiencing a Benzodiazepine Overdose box).

Hypothermia after surgery causes shivering, which increases oxygen demand and can induce hypoxemia. Many rewarming methods can be used, although prevention is more important.

For patients whose only airway is a tracheostomy or laryngectomy stoma, alert other staff members by posting signs in the room and notes on the chart.

Positioning. The patient can be placed in semi-Fowler position unless contraindicated. If the patient has difficulty tolerating the head of the bed in a raised position, place him or her in a side-lying position or turn the head to the side to prevent aspiration.

BEST PRACTICE FOR PATIENT SAFETY & QUALITY CARE (QSEN)

Emergency Care of the Patient Experiencing a Benzodiazepine Overdose

- Secure the airway and IV access before starting benzodiazepine antagonist therapy.
- Administer oxygen as prescribed, if hypoxia is present or if respirations are below 10 breaths/min.
- Prepare to administer flumazenil as prescribed.
- Repeat drug every 2 to 3 minutes up to 3 mg, as prescribed, depending on the patient's response.
- Have suction equipment available because flumazenil can trigger vomiting, which increases the risk for aspiration.
- Continuously monitor vital signs and level of consciousness for reversal of overdose.
- Do not leave the patient until fully responsive.
- Continue to monitor vital signs and level of consciousness every 10 to 15 minutes for the first 2 hours because flumazenil is eliminated from the body more quickly than is the benzodiazepine.
- Be aware that additional flumazenil therapy may be prescribed 1 to 2 hours after the patient initially becomes fully responsive.
- Observe for tremors or convulsions because flumazenil can lower the seizure threshold in those with seizure disorders.
- Assess the IV site every shift because flumazenil can cause thrombophlebitis at the injection site.
- Observe for side effects of flumazenil, including skin rash, hot flushes, dizziness, headache, sweating, dry mouth, and blurred vision. The incidence of these side effects increases with higher total doses of flumazenil.

Oxygen Therapy. Apply oxygen by face tent, nasal cannula, or mask as prescribed to eliminate inhaled anesthetic agents, increase oxygen levels, raise the level of consciousness, and reduce confusion. After the patient is fully reactive and stable, raise the head of the bed to support respiratory function.

Oxygen therapy may continue through the second day after surgery. When hypoxemia occurs despite preventive care, respiratory treatments and mechanical ventilation may be used to manage the cause of hypoxemia.

Breathing Exercises. As soon as the patient is awake enough to follow commands, urge routine coughing, using the incentive spirometer, and hourly coughing and breathing while awake throughout the postoperative phase to promote ***gas exchange.*** Teach the patient splint the incision while coughing and deep breathing. See the Patient and Family Education: Preparing for Self-Management: Perioperative Breathing Exercises box.

The patient who is unable to remove mucus or sputum requires oral or nasal suctioning. Perform mouth care after removing secretions.

Movement. Early ambulation reduces the risk for pulmonary complications, especially after abdominal, pelvic, or spinal surgery. It increases circulation to extremities and reduces the risk for clotting and venous thromboembolism (VTE), especially deep vein thrombosis (DVT). Assist the patient in getting out of bed to ambulate as soon as possible to help remove secretions and promote ventilation. Even when the patient has had extensive surgery, the expectation may be to get out of bed the day of or the first day after surgery. If this is not possible, help him or her turn at least every 2 hours (side to side) and ensure that breathing exercises and leg exercises are performed (see both Patient and Family Education: Preparing for Self-Management boxes).

The patient may resist getting up, but you must stress the importance of activity to prevent complications. When indicated, offer the patient pain medication in advance of scheduled activities to allow for maximum effect of the analgesic agent.

Preventing Wound Infection and Delayed Healing

Planning: Expected Outcomes. The patient is expected to have incision healing without wound complications.

Interventions. Although most wound complications do not require additional surgical intervention, emergency surgical procedures may be needed.

Nonsurgical Management. Wound care includes reinforcing the dressing, changing the dressing, and assessing the wound for healing and ***infection***; caring for drains, including emptying drainage containers and reservoirs; measuring drainage; and documenting findings. Urge the patient to bend the hips when in the supine position to reduce tension on a chest or abdominal wound. Remind him or her to always splint the chest or abdominal incision when coughing. Promote wound healing and protection of the skin, especially for the older patient. See the Patient-Centered Care: Older Adult Considerations: Best Practice in Postoperative Skin Care box for best practices for skin care of the older patient after surgery.

PATIENT-CENTERED CARE: OLDER ADULT CONSIDERATIONS

Best Practice in Postoperative Skin Care

To promote wound healing and protection of the older adult's skin:

- Maintain adequate hydration to facilitate cardiac output.
- Keep the airway patent and provide adequate oxygenation.
- Monitor pulse oximetry for values at or above 95%.
- Use strict aseptic technique (e.g., IV or other catheters, indwelling urethral catheter, wound).
- Promote adequate sleep and rest periods throughout the day.
- If necessary, administer drugs to address ***pain*** and sleeplessness.
- Control room temperature for comfort.
- Institute fall protocols to enhance safety.
- Maintain psychosocial health.
- Assist with personal hygiene as needed.
- Protect fragile skin.
- Minimize the use of tape on the skin; use hypoallergenic tape or Montgomery straps if necessary.
- Change dressings as soon as they become wet.
- With assistive personnel (AP), lift the patient during transfer or repositioning.

Dressings. Dressings vary with the surgical procedure and the surgeon's preference. Common dressings for large incisions consist of gauze or nonadherent pads covered with a larger absorbent pad held in place by tape, a tubular stretchy net, or Montgomery straps (Fig. 9.9). Some incisions may be covered with a transparent plastic surgical dressing (e.g., OpSite) or a spray in the surgical suite. This type of dressing stays intact for 3 to 6 days, allows direct observation of the wound, prevents contamination, and eliminates the need for dressing changes.

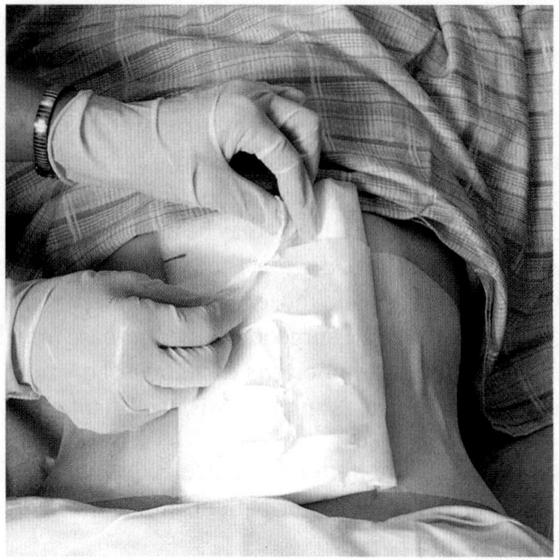

FIG. 9.9 Patient with a dressing held in place with Montgomery straps. (From Harkreader, H., Hogan, M.A., & Thobaben, M. [2007]. *Fundamentals of nursing: Caring and clinical judgment.* [3rd ed.]. Philadelphia: Saunders.)

The surgeon usually performs the first dressing change after surgery to assess the wound, remove any packing, and advance (pull partially out) or remove drains. Follow agency policy regarding timing of the first dressing change; you may need to institute the first change even before the surgeon, or be required to reinforce the dressing (add more dressing material to the existing dressing) if it becomes wet from drainage. If reinforced, document the added material and the color, type, amount, and odor of drainage fluid and time of observation. Assess the surgical site at least every 8 hours and report any unexpected findings to the surgeon.

After removal of the dressing, the surgeon may leave the suture or staple line open to the air, which allows easy assessment of the wound and early detection of poor wound edge approximation, drainage, swelling, or redness. Even if open to air, a healing wound is always covered with a dressing.

Frequency of wound care and dressing changes are usually prescribed by the surgeon; however, the agency or unit may have standards or policies that dictate specific protocols to avoid ***infection.*** Use aseptic technique until sutures or staples are removed. For large dressing changes or drain removal, offer the patient a prescribed analgesic before the procedure. Always assess the skin for redness, rash, or blisters in areas where tape has been used. Tape can cause a skin reaction after surgery even among patients who are not known to be tape sensitive.

Wound or suture line care consists of changing gauze dressings at least once during a nursing shift or per agency policy, and may include cleaning the area with sterile saline or another prescribed solution. Some suture lines are left open to air without any dressing to cover the incision.

Skin sutures or staples are usually removed by the surgeon or nurse (depending on agency policy) 5 to 10 days after surgery. This may vary up to 30 days, depending on the type of surgery and the recovery process. Clean the incision with the prescribed solution before removing sutures or staples, and examine the condition and healing stage of the wound. First, remove every other suture or staple and reassess the wound for integrity. If wound healing is progressing normally, the rest of the sutures or staples may then be removed. If the wound does not appear to be healing well or if any signs or symptoms of ***infection*** are present, notify the surgeon before removing any sutures. After sutures or staples are removed, the incision may then be secured with wound closure tape, which stays in place until it falls off on its own.

Drains. Drains (see Fig. 9.8) may be placed in the wound or through a separate small incision (known as a *stab* wound) close to the incision during surgery. Drains provide an exit route for air, blood, and bile. Drains also help prevent deep infection and abscess formation during healing.

The Penrose drain is placed into the external aspect of the incision and drains directly onto the dressing and skin around the incision. Change a damp or soiled dressing and carefully clean under and around the Penrose drain. Then place absorbent pads under and around the exposed drain to prevent skin irritation, wound contamination, and infection. Whether sutured in place or not, the drain can be dislodged or pulled out accidentally during a dressing change. It is also possible for the drain to slip back through the wound into the patient. Usually this complication is prevented when the drain is first placed in the surgical suite. The surgeon pins a sterile safety pin through the drain at an angle perpendicular to the drain and the wound, which prevents the drain from slipping. As the wound heals, the surgeon or nurse shortens (advances) the drain by pulling it out a short distance and trimming off the excess external part so only 2 to 3 inches of drain protrudes through the incision. The safety pin must be repositioned each time the drain is advanced. The drain remains in place until drainage stops.

Assess that Jackson-Pratt and Hemovac drains are sutured in place with a suture that seals the area when the drain is removed. Use sterile technique to empty the reservoir. Record the amount and color of drainage during every nursing shift or more often if necessary or prescribed. After emptying and compressing the reservoir to restore suction, secure the drain to the patient's gown (never to the sheet or mattress) to prevent pulling and stress on the surgical wound.

Drug therapy. Wound ***infection*** is a major complication after surgery. It usually results from contamination during surgery, preoperative infection, debilitation, or immunosuppression. A patient at risk for wound infection may have received antibiotic therapy with drugs that are effective against organisms common to the specific surgical site both before and during surgery. The need for these antibiotics is re-evaluated at 24 hours after surgery. If signs or symptoms of infection are not present, the antibiotic is discontinued at that time. If signs or symptoms of wound ***infection*** are present, they are documented to justify continuation of antibiotic therapy.

Wounds that become infected and open are treated with dressing changes and systemic antibiotic therapy. Follow the surgeon's prescription for irrigation, packing, and covering the wound. A negative-pressure wound device may be prescribed to help close the wound. Chapter 23 discusses these systems.

Surgical Management. Poorly healing, infected, or complicated wounds may require surgical intervention.

Management of dehiscence. If dehiscence (wound opening) occurs, apply a sterile nonadherent (e.g., Telfa) or saline dressing to the wound and notify the surgeon. Instruct the patient to bend the knees and avoid coughing. A wound that becomes infected dehisces by itself, or it may be opened by the surgeon through an incision and drainage (I&D) procedure. In either case, the wound is left open and is treated as described previously.

Management of evisceration. Remember that *an evisceration is a surgical emergency.* See the Best Practice for Patient Safety & Quality Care: Emergency Care of the Patient With Surgical Wound Evisceration box for emergency care. Provide support by explaining what happened and reassuring the patient that the emergency will be handled quickly and with expertise.

Special Considerations. The best treatment is prevention. If a postoperative patient is at risk for poor healing, encourage adequate supplies of protein, vitamins, and calories. Monitor dietary intake, identify deficiencies, and discuss with the surgeon and the registered dietitian nutritionist (RDN).

The surgeon may prescribe a nasogastric (NG) tube to decompress the stomach and relieve internal pressure, or to remove the stomach's contents if the patient has been eating and general anesthesia is needed. Prepare the patient for surgery to close the wound. Regional or local anesthesia may be used, depending on the location and type of wound, in an effort to

BEST PRACTICE FOR PATIENT SAFETY & QUALITY CARE (QSEN)

Emergency Care of the Patient With Surgical Wound Evisceration

1. Call for another nurse to notify the surgeon and/or Rapid Response Team (RRT) immediately and to bring any needed supplies.
2. Provide reassurance and support to ease the patient's anxiety. Stay with the patient and instruct him or her to remain in bed.
3. Place the patient in a supine position with the hips and knees bent.
4. Raise the head of the bed 15 to 20 degrees.
5. Using sterile technique, unfold a sterile towel to create a sterile field.
6. Open an irrigation set and place the basin and syringe on the sterile field.
7. Open several large abdominal dressings and place them on the sterile field.
8. Don sterile gloves and place one or two of the large abdominal dressings into the basin to saturate them with warm saline solution.
9. Place the moistened dressings over the exposed viscera. Then, place a sterile, waterproof drape over the dressings to prevent the sheets from getting wet.
10. If saline is not immediately available, cover the wound with gauze and moisten with sterile saline when available.
11. Do not attempt to reinsert the protruding organ or viscera.
12. Assess for symptoms of shock, and document vital signs.
13. Continue assessing the patient, including vital signs assessment every 5 to 10 minutes until the surgeon or RRT arrives.
14. Keep dressings continuously moist by adding warmed sterile saline to the dressing as often as necessary. Do not let the dressing become dry.
15. When the surgeon or RRT arrives, report finding and interventions.
16. Document the incident, the activity in which the patient was engaged at the time of the incident, your assessment, and interventions taken.
17. If necessary, prepare the patient for emergency surgery; start an IV infusion as ordered.
18. Don't allow the patient to have anything by mouth, to decrease the risk of aspiration if surgery is necessary.

NURSING SAFETY PRIORITY QSEN

Critical Rescue

Monitor surgical incisions at least every 8 hours to recognize an impending evisceration. If a surgical wound evisceration occurs, respond by staying with the patient while calling for another nurse to immediately notify the surgeon and/or Rapid Response Team.

reduce the chance for nausea and vomiting. To increase the incision's integrity, stay or retention sutures of wire or nylon may be used along with standard sutures or staples.

Managing Pain

Planning: Expected Outcomes. The postoperative patient is expected to attain and maintain optimal levels of comfort.

Interventions. ***Pain*** management after surgery includes drug therapy and other methods of management such as positioning, relaxation techniques, and diversion. Often the patient has better pain relief from a combination of approaches. Assess the patient's pain and the effectiveness of the therapies. See Chapter 5 for discussion of pain assessment and management. The patient who has optimal pain control is better able to cooperate with the therapies and exercises to prevent complications and promote rehabilitation.

Drug Therapy. The use of opioids or other analgesics for ***pain*** management may mask or increase the severity of symptoms of an anesthesia reaction. Administer these drugs with caution.

In some cases, epidural analgesia is given intermittently by the anesthesia provider or by continuous infusion through an epidural catheter left in place after epidural anesthesia. Common drugs given by epidural catheter include the opioids fentanyl, preservative-free morphine, and bupivacaine.

Opioid analgesics given during the first 24 to 48 hours after surgery help manage acute ***pain***. Around-the-clock scheduling or the use of patient-controlled analgesia (PCA) systems is more effective and allows more consistent blood levels than "on-demand" scheduling. In PCA the patient adjusts the dose of the analgesic based on the pain level and response to the drug. This method allows more consistent pain relief and more control by the patient. The maximum dose per hour is "locked in" to the pump so the patient cannot accidentally overdose. Drugs are changed from injectable or PCA to oral as soon as the patient can tolerate oral agents.

Common drugs used for pain management include morphine, hydromorphone, ketorolac, codeine, butorphanol, and oxycodone with aspirin or oxycodone with acetaminophen. Antianxiety drugs may be given with an opioid analgesic to decrease pain-related anxiety, reduce muscle tension, and control nausea.

NURSING SAFETY PRIORITY QSEN

Drug Alert

The usual dosage for hydromorphone is **much smaller** that of morphine. Check dosages carefully.

Assess the type, location, and intensity of the ***pain*** before and after giving pain medication, using a 0-to-10 scale. Monitor the patient's vital signs for hypotension and hypoventilation after giving opioid drugs. See the Common Examples of Drug Therapy: Management of Postoperative Pain box for information about analgesics used after surgery.

Take care not to overmedicate or undermedicate, especially when caring for older patients. In assessing for overmedication, monitor vital signs, especially blood pressure and respiratory rate, and level of consciousness. Complications from the use of opioid analgesics include respiratory depression, hypotension, nausea, vomiting, and constipation. An opioid antagonist such as naloxone may be needed to reverse the acute effects of opioid depression.

PATIENT-CENTERED CARE: OLDER ADULT CONSIDERATIONS QSEN

Special care is needed when using PCA with older adults to prevent undertreating ***pain.*** Assess the patient's level of understanding of the delivery system and his or her comfort with the self-medication process. Reassure the patient that the system prevents accidental overdose.

COMMON EXAMPLES OF DRUG THERAPY QSEN

Management of Postoperative Pain

Drug Category	Selected Nursing Implications
Opioids	
Morphine sulfate and hydromorphone hydrochloride	Monitor respiratory rate and blood pressure; *respiratory depression can be severe and require immediate intervention.*
	Monitor GI motility and urine output; *constipation and urinary retention can occur.*
Codeine sulfate	Monitor respiratory status; *respiratory depression can occur.*
	Monitor GI motility; *constipation can occur.*
Butorphanol tartrate	Monitor neurologic status and for changes in level of consciousness; *increased intracranial pressure can occur.*
	Monitor respiratory status; *respiratory depression can occur.*
Oxycodone and aspirin	Monitor for GI tolerance and function; *the aspirin component of this drug can irritate the stomach, and constipation and GI bleeding can occur.*
	Monitor coagulation studies (PT, aPTT); *the aspirin component of this drug may influence bleeding times and other coagulation study results.*
Oxycodone and acetaminophen	Monitor blood pressure and respiratory status; *hypotension and respiratory depression can occur.*
	Monitor GI motility; *constipation can occur.*
NSAIDs	
Ketorolac tromethamine	Monitor for GI tolerance; *GI bleeding, ulceration, and perforation can occur.*
	Monitor kidney function, especially in older adults; *decreased urine output, increased serum creatinine, hematuria, and proteinuria can occur.*
Ibuprofen	Monitor for GI tolerance; *GI bleeding, ulceration, and perforation can occur.*

[a]*PTT*, Activated partial thromboplastin time; *PT*, prothrombin time.

BEST PRACTICE FOR PATIENT SAFETY & QUALITY CARE QSEN

Emergency Care of the Patient Experiencing an Opioid Overdose

- Naloxone may be administered IV, IM, subcutaneously, or via intranasal spray. The IV route has the most rapid onset and is recommended in emergency situations.
- Maintain an open airway.
- Prepare to administer naloxone hydrochloride as prescribed via IV.
- If the desired degree of improvement in respiratory function is not obtained, it may be repeated at 2- to 3-minute intervals if needed and as prescribed, depending on the patient's response.
- Administer oxygen if hypoxia is present or if respirations are below 10 breaths/min.
- Have suction equipment available because naloxone can trigger vomiting, and a drowsy patient is at risk for aspiration.
- Continuously monitor vital signs and level of consciousness for opioid reversal every 10 to 15 minutes for the first hour. Naloxone is eliminated from the body more quickly than is the opioid; and it may induce side effects, including blood pressure changes, tachycardia, and dysrhythmias.
- Do not leave the patient until he or she is fully responsive.
- Assess the patient for ***pain*** because reversal of the opioid also reverses the analgesic effects.
- The health care provider will determine the need for additional antagonist therapy 1 hour after the patient initially becomes fully responsive.

Adapted from Stolbach, A., & Hoffman, R. (2019). *Acute opioid intoxication in adults*. In *UpToDate*, Traub, S., (Ed.). Waltham, MA. https://www.uptodate.com/contents/acute-opioid-intoxication-in-adults

Because of the short effect of the opioid antagonist, monitor the patient's blood pressure and respirations every 15 to 30 minutes until the full effect of the opioid analgesic has passed. More doses of the antagonist may need to be given during this time because it is eliminated from the body more quickly than is the opioid. (See the Best Practice for Patient Safety & Quality Care: Emergency Care of the Patient Experiencing an Opioid Overdose box for more information on using opioid antagonists to reverse opioid overdose.) In addition, the patient may experience breakthrough ***pain*** after the opioid antagonist is given; therefore other interventions to control pain may be needed.

Assess for undermedication by asking the patient about degree of pain relief and observing for nonverbal cues of discomfort (e.g., restlessness, increased confusion, "picking" at bed linens). Offer prescribed drug(s) after checking for hypotension and respiratory depression.

As recovery progresses, reduce the doses and frequency of drugs for ***pain*** control as prescribed. Nonopioid analgesics such as acetaminophen and NSAIDs such as ibuprofen and ketorolac may be used alone or with an opioid analgesic.

! NURSING SAFETY PRIORITY QSEN

Action Alert

Unless pillow support is ordered, do not place pillows under the knees and do not raise the knee gatch because this position could restrict circulation and increase the risk for venous thromboembolism.

BEST PRACTICE FOR PATIENT SAFETY & QUALITY CARE QSEN

Nonpharmacologic Interventions to Reduce Postoperative Pain and Promote Comfort

- Find a general position of comfort for the patient.
- Use ice to reduce and prevent swelling as indicated.
- Cushion and elevate painful areas; avoid placing tension or pressure on these areas. (Do not place pillows under the knees; do not raise the knee gatch.)
- Control or remove noxious stimuli.
- Provide adequate rest to increase pain tolerance.
- Encourage the patient's participation in diversional activities.
- Teach relaxation techniques; use music and breathing exercises.
- Provide opportunities for meditation.

Nonpharmacologic Interventions. Use gentle massage on stiff joints or a sore back to decrease discomfort, as long as these were not the site of surgery. Assist the patient to a side-lying position and apply lotion with smooth, gentle strokes to increase blood flow to the area and promote relaxation. *Do not massage the calves because of the risk for loosening a clot and causing a life-threatening pulmonary embolus.*

Relaxation and diversion (such as listening to music) may also be used to manage acute episodes of ***pain*** during dressing changes and injections. (See Chapter 5 for how to instruct and guide the patient through these pain control methods.) See the Best Practice for Patient Safety & Quality Care: Nonpharmacologic Interventions to Reduce Postoperative Pain and Promote Comfort box for other nonpharmacologic interventions that can help the patient.

Promoting Peristalsis. Decreased intestinal peristalsis with the possible development of a postoperative ileus (POI) can occur as a result of drug therapy; anesthesia or analgesia; operative manipulation; and increased sympathetic nervous system excitation from stress after any surgery but is most common after open abdominal procedures. All postoperative patients are at some risk for POI, which can lead to other avoidable complications such as wound dehiscence, nausea, vomiting, and deconditioning.

Planning: Expected Outcomes. The patient is expected to have return of intestinal peristalsis after surgery.

Interventions. Nursing interventions to promote peristalsis include monitoring, ensuring adequate hydration, promoting mobility, managing ***pain*** with nonopioid interventions, and when appropriate, performing pharmacologic management.

Monitoring the abdomen is key to determining recovery of intestinal peristalsis and recognizing possible POI early. As described earlier in this chapter, assess for the presence and quality of bowel sounds, degree of distention, and firmness whenever vital signs are taken. Observe for distention and document whether this has increased or decreased since the last observation. Auscultate for bowel sounds in all four abdominal quadrants for up to 1 minute in each quadrant. Gently palpate the abdomen to determine degree of softness or whether any rigidity is present. Although the presence of bowel sounds, especially lower in the tract, does not indicate full peristalsis, the absence of sound does correlate with hypomotility. Ask the patient whether he or she has passed flatus or stool. Although passage of either indicates some intestinal motility, it does not rule out POI.

Ensuring adequate hydration helps promote peristalsis because dehydration, fluid loss, and crystalloid excess can potentially decrease intestinal motility, leading to POI. Monitor IV fluid volume compared with urine output. Fluid volumes infused should be sufficient (for the adult without known kidney or cardiac problems) to maintain adequate urine output that is dilute in appearance.

Increased mobility, especially early ambulation, assists in return of peristalsis. Help the patient ambulate at least once per shift and increase the distance and time spent ambulating with each opportunity. Document the time and distance of each ambulation so progression can be continued by other health care professionals.

*Nonopioid **pain** management* strategies can help reduce the amount of opioids needed to manage pain adequately. Opioids bind to GI receptors and contribute to decreased peristalsis and POI development. Collaborate with the interprofessional team to use alternative pain control measures in addition to opioids in the postoperative phase. See Chapter 5 for more discussion of nonopioid and nonpharmacologic pain management strategies.

Drug therapy can be helpful. One drug, alvimopan, has been approved to accelerate the time to GI recovery following certain gastrointestinal surgeries. Metoclopramide promotes peristalsis by directly stimulating GI motility.

Care Coordination and Transition Management. Except in the cases of emergent surgery, discharge planning, teaching, and referrals begin before the procedure and continue after surgery is completed.

NCLEX EXAMINATION CHALLENGE 9.7

Psychosocial Integrity

The nurse is caring for a client who reports being fearful of becoming dependent on opioid pain medication after surgery. What is the appropriate nursing response? **Select all that apply.**

A. "Why do you think you're going to get hooked?"
B. "Don't worry, I won't give you any opioid medications."
C. "Have you had concerns with drug dependence in the past?"
D. "Tell me what makes you most fearful about taking opioid medication."
E. "There are proper ways of taking opioids so you will not become dependent."

Home Care Management. If the patient is discharged directly to home, assess information about the home environment for safety and the availability of family or caregivers. Use the data obtained before surgery to determine the patient's needs. For example, if the patient is unable or not allowed to climb stairs and lives in a two-story house with only one bathroom upstairs, inform about ways to rent a bedside commode. Other assistive devices may be needed such as a shower chair, walker, or recliner, based on assessment of the patient's living arrangements. Collaborate with the social worker or discharge planner to identify individualized needs related to care after surgery, meal preparation, dressing changes, drain management, drug administration, physical therapy, personal hygiene, and financial needs. A referral to a home care nursing or physical therapy agency may be indicated.

Some patients may need long-term acute care following surgery, in order to recover more fully. When discharging to another agency, follow best practices for SBAR and hand-off (see Chapter 1).

Self-Management Education. The teaching plan for the patient and family or caregiver after surgery includes:

- ***Pain*** management
- Drug therapy with reconciliation of postoperative drugs
- Safety (e.g., who to contact in case of complications, how to progressively increase activity, which assistive devices are needed)
- Prevention of infection with assessment and care of the surgical wound
- Management of drains or catheters
- Nutrition therapy
- Follow-up with the surgeon

If dressing changes and drain or catheter care are needed, teach the importance of proper handwashing to prevent infection. Explain and demonstrate wound care, and then require a return demonstration. During teaching sessions, evaluate learning, as this promotes adherence after discharge. At the same time, teach about the symptoms of complications such as wound ***infection*** and when to contact the health care provider.

Perform a drug reconciliation with the patient before discharge. Ensure that drugs for other health problems are resumed, as needed. Also ensure that drugs specific for the surgical procedure (and its complications) are available to the patient and that he or she understands how they are to be used, any associated side effects, and when they are to be discontinued. Teach the patient about drugs for ***pain,*** especially the proper dosage and frequency. Instruct the patient to notify the surgeon if pain is not controlled or if it suddenly increases. If antibiotics are prescribed, stress the importance of completing the entire prescription, even if the patient feels better.

A diet high in protein, calories, and vitamins promotes wound healing. Supplemental vitamin C, iron, zinc, and other vitamins are often prescribed after surgery to aid in wound healing and red blood cell formation. Instruct the patient who needs dietary restrictions about the importance of following the prescribed diet while recovering from surgery.

Surgery stresses the body, and time and rest are needed for healing. Teach the patient to increase activity level slowly, rest often, and avoid straining the wound or the surrounding area. Reinforce the surgeon's instructions about when the patient may lift (and how much), climb stairs, return to work, drive, and resume other usual ADLs. Instruct the patient in the use of proper lifting techniques and remind him or her about weights of frequently used items such as grocery bags, handbags, and

NURSING SAFETY PRIORITY QSEN

Action Alert

Provide written discharge instructions (including medication education sheets) to follow at home. Request that the patient and family or caregiver explain the regimen in their own words back to you to assess understanding.

common household items. Stress the importance of adherence to the plan of care to prevent complications or disability.

Health Care Resources. In addition to a referral for a home care nurse (if needed), other referrals may include Meals on Wheels, support groups, housekeeping services, and grocery delivery by third-party shoppers.

◆ **Evaluation: Evaluate Outcomes.** Evaluate the care of the patient after surgery based on the identified priority patient problems. The expected outcomes include that the patient:

- Attains and maintains adequate lung expansion and respiratory function
- Has appropriate wound healing without complications
- Has acceptable ***pain*** management
- Has return of peristalsis

GET READY FOR THE NEXT-GENERATION NCLEX® EXAMINATION!

Key Points

Review these Key Points for each NCLEX Examination Client Needs Category.

Safe and Effective Care Environment

- Use at least two appropriate identifiers when providing instruction, administering drugs, marking surgical sites, and performing any procedure. **QSEN: Safety**
- Confirm that the presurgical checklist is complete and accurate. **QSEN: Safety**
- Communicate to the perioperative team any physical or laboratory change(s) that may alter the patient's response to drugs, anesthesia, or surgery. **QSEN: Teamwork and Collaboration**
- Ask the patient to explain in his or her own words which surgical procedure is being done and why. **QSEN: Safety**
- If the patient's understanding of the scheduled surgery is not consistent with the documentation, notify the surgeon to speak to the patient. **QSEN: Safety**
- Confirm that informed consent and any other legal documents are signed before preoperative drug administration. **Ethics**
- If preoperative drugs are administered on the unit before going the surgical suite, keep the side rails up and the bed in the low position. **QSEN: Safety**
- Communicate with the interprofessional team regarding all care that has been provided and what care may still be needed. **QSEN: Teamwork and Collaboration**
- Examine potential risks for surgical site ***infection,*** hypoventilation, hypotension, venous thromboembolism, or injury following surgery. **QSEN: Safety**
- Use aseptic technique during all dressing changes. **QSEN: Safety**
- Keep suction equipment, oxygen, and artificial breathing equipment near each patient bedside. **QSEN: Safety**

Health Promotion and Maintenance

- Teach preoperative preparations **QSEN: Patient-Centered Care**
- Teach postoperative interventions that prevent complications (e.g., hand hygiene, incision splinting, deep-breathing exercises, range-of-motion exercises). **QSEN: Evidence-Based Practice**
- Encourage and assist with early ambulation. **QSEN: Safety**
- Stress the importance of following activity restrictions prescribed by the surgeon. **QSEN: Safety**
- Teach about drugs to be continued after discharge from the agency. **QSEN: Safety**
- Teach signs and symptoms of complications and when to contact the health care provider. **QSEN: Safety**

Psychosocial Integrity

- Assess the patient's and family's or caregivers' knowledge about the scheduled surgical procedure to identify learning needs. **QSEN: Patient-Centered Care**
- Encourage expression of feelings regarding the surgical procedure or its possible outcome(s). **QSEN: Patient-Centered Care**
- Explain and provide written information regarding all diagnostic procedures, restrictions, and follow-up care. **Ethics**
- Communicate patient concerns, fears, or preferences to the perioperative team. **Ethics**
- Implement appropriate interventions to reduce patient anxiety. **QSEN: Patient-Centered Care**
- Reassure the patient that taking ***pain*** medication for the short term as prescribed is highly unlikely to lead to drug abuse. **QSEN: Patient-Centered Care**

Physiological Integrity

- Collect a full preoperative history, and perform a complete and accurate preoperative assessment. **QSEN: Patient-Centered Care**
- Ensure that dentures and any other personal items are removed from the patient before he or she is transferred to the surgical suite. **QSEN: Patient-Centered Care**
- Begin every assessment of the patient after surgery by checking the airway and breathing effectiveness. **QSEN: Safety**
- Assess the incision site each shift for signs of healing or ***infection.*** **Clinical Judgment**

- Offer alternative therapies for relaxation, ***pain*** reduction, and distraction. **QSEN: Patient-Centered Care**
- Apply prescribed antiembolic stockings and sequential compression devices to reduce or prevent vascular complications. **QSEN: Evidence-Based Practice**
- Have the patient with evisceration or dehiscence lie flat (supine) with knees bent to reduce intra-abdominal pressure; apply sterile, nonadherent dressing materials to the wound and notify the surgeon immediately. **QSEN: Safety**

MASTERY QUESTIONS

1. The nurse is completing a preoperative physical assessment for a client who will have surgery this afternoon. Which assessment finding will the nurse report to the operative team? **Select all that apply.**
   A. Left arm prosthesis
   B. Skin turgor <3 seconds
   C. Blood pressure 160/100 mm Hg
   D. Presence of chest rigidity
   E. Has been NPO since midnight
   F. Expressed concern about surgery payment
2. The nurse is caring for a postoperative patient who has asked for pain medicine an hour before it is due. What is the **priority** nursing response?
   A. "You cannot have more pain medicine until an hour from now."
   B. "Can you describe the pain you are having, and rate it on a 1-to-10 scale?"
   C. "I can help you begin a pain diary so we can see trends when your pain worsens."
   D. "Let's try some relaxation exercises to help address the discomfort you are feeling."

REFERENCES

Agency for Healthcare Research and Quality. (2017). *Improving Communication and Teamwork in the Surgical Environment*. Retrieved from https://www.ahrq.gov/hai/tools/ambulatory-surgery/sections/implementation/training-tools/improving-slides.html.

American Association of Blood Banks. (2019). *Standards for perioperative autologous blood collection and administration* (8th ed.). Bethesda, MD: Author.

American Society of Anesthesiologists. (2019). *ASA physical status classification system*. Retrieved from https://www.asahq.org/resources/clinical-information/asa-physical-status-classification-system.

American Society of PeriAnesthesia Nurses. (2019). *2019-2020 perianesthesia nursing standards, practice recommendations and interpretive statements*. Cherry Hill, NJ.

Association of periOperative Registered Nurses (AORN). (2020). Sentinel events: Prevention and reduction of wrong-patient, wrong-site, wrong-procedure events. Retrieved from https://www.aorn.org/education/staff-development/prevention-of-sentinel-events/wrong-site-surgery.

Association of periOperative Registered Nurses (AORN). (2020). *Guidelines for perioperative practice*. Denver: Author.

Association of periOperative Registered Nurses (AORN). (2019). *Preoperative patient skin antisepsis*. Denver: Author.

Bashaw, M., & Keister, K. (2019). Perioperative strategies for surgical site infection prevention. *AORN Journal, 109*(1), 68–78.

Blanchard, D., & van Wissen, K. (2019). Adverse effects of dexamethasone in surgical patients. *American Journal of Nursing, 119*(12), 19.

British Medical Journal - BMJ Best Practice. (2020). *VTE prophylaxis*. Retrieved from https://bestpractice.bmj.com/topics/en-us/1087.

Campbell, Y., Machan, M., & Fisher, M. (2016). The Jehovah's Witness population: Considerations for preoperative optimization of hemoglobin. *American Association of Nurse Anesthetists (AANA) Journal, 84*(3), 173–178.

Centers for Disease Control and Prevention. (n.d.). Top CDC recommendations to prevent healthcare-associated infections. Retrieved from https://www.cdc.gov/HAI/pdfs/hai/top-cdc-recs-factsheet.pdf.

Centers for Medicare and Medicaid Services (CMS). (2018). *2017-2018 Evaluation and Management*. Retrieved from https://www.cms.gov/Outreach-and-Education/Medicare-Learning-Network-MLN/MLNProducts/MLN-Publications-Items/CMS1243514.

Crowley, M. (2020). Preoperative fasting guidelines. In *UpToDate*, Holt, N. (Ed.). Waltham, MA.

Davenport, M., & Newhouse, J. (2018). Patient evaluation prior to oral or iodinated intravenous contrast for computed tomography. In *UpToDate*, Kressel, H. (Ed.). Waltham, MA.

Devereaux, P. et al. (2020). Management of cardiac risk for noncardiac surgery. In *UpToDate*, Pellika, P., & Jaffe, S. (Eds.). Waltham, MA.

Ellis, H., & Abdalla, S. (2020). *A history of surgery*. CRC Press.

Gestring, M. (2020). Negative pressure wound therapy. In *UpToDate*, R. Berman, & A. Cochran (Eds.), *Negative pressure wound therapy* Waltham, MA.

Gillespie, B. M., Walker, R. M., McInnes, E., Moore, Z., Eskes, A. M., O'Connor, T. ,., & Chaboyer, W. (2019). Preoperative and postoperative recommendations to surgical wound care interventions: A systematic meta-review of Cochrane reviews. *International Journal of Nursing Studies*, 103486.

Khan, N., et al. (2018). Perioperative management of blood glucose in adults with diabetes mellitus. In *UpToDate*, Nathan, D., & Jones, S. (Eds.). Waltham, MA.

Leite, K. A., Hobgood, T., Hill, B., & Muckler, V. C. (2019). Reducing preventable surgical cancellations: Improving the preoperative anesthesia interview process. *Journal of PeriAnesthesia Nursing, 34*(5), 929–937.

Litman, R. (2019). Malignant hyperthermia: Diagnosis and management of acute crisis. In *UpToDate*, Jones, S. (Ed.). Waltham, MA.

Long, B., Chassee, T., & Jones, J. (2019). BET 2: Is there an association between iodine, shellfish, and contrast agent allergies? *Emergency Medicine Journal*, 36(11), 698-699.

Malignant Hyperthermia Association of the United States. (2020a). *How does the antidote dantrolene work?* Retrieved from https://www.mhaus.org/faqs/how-does-the-antidote-dantrolene-work/.

Malignant Hyperthermia Association of the United States. (2020b). *Muscle Biopsy CHCT*. Retrieved from https://www.mhaus.org/testing/muscle-biopsy-chct/.

Olson, E., Chung. F., & Ping, E. (2018). Intraoperative management of adults with obstructive sleep apnea. In *UpToDate,* Jones, S., & Collop, N. (Eds.). Waltham, MA.

Rothrock, J. (2019). *Alexander's care of the patient in surgery* (16th ed.). St. Louis: Elsevier.

Sicherer, S. (2019). Seafood allergies: Fish and shellfish. In *UpToDate,* Wood, R. (Ed.). Waltham, MA.

The Joint Commission. (2020). *Hospital National Patient Safety Goals.* Retrieved from https://www.jointcommission.org/assets/1/6/2020_HAP_NPSG_goals_final.pdf.

The Joint Commission. (2019). *National Patient Safety Goals Effective January 2019.* Retrieved From https://www.jointcommission.org/-/media/tjc/documents/standards/national-patient-safety-goals/npsg_chapter_hap_jan2019.pdf?db=web&hash=3060F486CA146BD9071F7C2DBF7796A4.

The Joint Commission. (2016). *Informed consent: More than getting a signature.* Retrieved from https://www.jointcommission.org/-/media/deprecated-unorganized/imported-assets/tjc/system-folders/joint-commission-online/quick_safety_issue_twenty-one_february_2016pdf.pdf?db=web&hash=5944307ED39088503A008A70D2C768AA.

Touhy, T., & Jett, K. (2020). *Ebersole & Hess' toward healthy aging* (10th ed.). St. Louis: Elsevier.

U.S. National Library of Medicine. (2020). RYR1 gene. Retrieved from https://ghr.nlm.nih.gov/gene/RYR1.

10

Concepts of Emergency and Trauma Nursing

Linda Laskowski-Jones, Karen L. Toulson

http://evolve.elsevier.com/Iggy/

LEARNING OUTCOMES

1. Describe the emergency department (ED) environment, including vulnerable populations served.
2. Engage in ***teamwork and collaboration*** with interprofessional team members to maintain staff and patient ***safety.***
3. Explain selected core competencies required of ED nurses.
4. Prioritize order of ED care delivery via triage and based on assessment of the injured patient.
5. Implement nursing interventions to support survivors after the death of a loved one.
6. Describe the expected sequence of events from admission through disposition of a patient treated in the ED.

KEY TERMS

acceleration-deceleration Types of forces that involve rapid or sudden movement forward then backward.

blast effect The damage sustained from the force of an explosion.

blunt trauma A type of trauma resulting from impact forces such as a motor vehicle accident, fall, or assault.

Canadian Triage Acuity Scale (CTAS) A standardized model for triage in which lists of descriptors are used to establish the triage level.

critical access hospital A small rural facility of 25 or fewer inpatient beds that provides around-the-clock emergency care services 7 days per week. Considered a necessary provider of health care to community residents who are not close to other hospitals in a given region.

emergency medical technician (EMT) Prehospital care provider who supplies basic life-support interventions such as oxygen, basic wound care, splinting, spinal motion restriction, and monitoring of vital signs.

emergency medicine physician A member of the emergency health care team with education and training in the specialty of emergency patient management.

Emergency Severity Index (ESI) A standardized model for triage that categorizes both patient acuity and resource utilization into five levels, from most urgent to least urgent.

emergent triage In a three-tiered triage scheme, the category that includes any condition or injury that poses an immediate threat to life or limb, such as crushing chest pain or active hemorrhage.

forensic nurse examiner (RN-FNE) Specialist nurse who is trained to recognize evidence of abuse and to intervene on the patient's behalf. This specialist obtains patient histories, collects forensic evidence, and offers counseling and follow-up care for victims of rape, abuse, and domestic violence.

Glasgow Coma Scale (GCS) An assessment that scores eye opening, verbal response, and motor response.

mechanism of injury (MOI) The method by which a traumatic event occurred.

nonurgent triage In a three-tiered triage scheme, the category that includes patients who can generally tolerate waiting several hours for health care services without a significant risk of clinical deterioration, such as those with sprains, strains, or simple fractures.

paramedic A trained first responder who provides care for patients who require care that exceeds basic life support resources. Advanced life support (ALS) may include cardiac monitoring, advanced airway management and intubation, establishing IV access, and administering drugs, often en route to the emergency department.

penetrating trauma Injuries caused by piercing; classified by the velocity of the vehicle (e.g., knife or bullet) causing the injury.

prehospital care provider Typically, any of the first caregivers encountered by the patient if he or she is transported to the emergency department by an ambulance or helicopter.

primary survey Priorities of care addressed in order of immediate threats to life as part of the initial assessment in the emergency department. Survey is based on the *ABC* mnemonic with *D* and *E* added for trauma patients.

psychiatric crisis nurse team An emergency department specialty team whose nurses interact with patients and families in crisis.

secondary survey In the emergency department, a more comprehensive head-to-toe assessment performed to identify other injuries or medical issues that need to be managed or that might affect the course of treatment.

trauma Bodily injury.

trauma center Specialty care facility that provides competent and timely trauma services to patients depending on its designated level of capability.

trauma-informed care (TIC) An approach to patient care that provides ways for health care providers to view and understand the negative effects of trauma on patient symptoms and behaviors.

trauma system An organized and integrated approach to trauma care designed to ensure that all critical elements of trauma care delivery are aligned to meet the injured patient's needs.

triage In the emergency department, sorting or classifying patients into priority levels depending on illness or injury severity, with the highest-acuity needs receiving the quickest evaluation and treatment.

urgent triage In a three-tiered triage scheme, the category that indicates that the patient should be treated quickly but that an immediate threat to life does not exist at the moment.

PRIORITY AND INTERRELATED CONCEPTS

The priority concepts for this chapter are:

- ***Safety***
- ***Teamwork and Collaboration***
- ***Communication***

Functioning as a safety net for communities of all sizes, emergency departments (EDs) provide services to insured and uninsured patients seeking care. They are also responsible for ***safety*** through public health surveillance and emergency disaster preparedness. Some hospital-based EDs also offer observation, procedural care, and employee or occupational health services. Larger hospital-based EDs often have interprofessional specialty teams that take part in ***teamwork and collaboration*** to provide first-line care for patients with stroke and cardiac disorders. The role of the ED is so vital that the Centers for Medicare and Medicaid Services has a process for designating small rural facilities of 25 acute care inpatient beds or fewer as **critical access hospitals** as long as they provide around-the-clock emergency care services 7 days a week (RHIhub, 2019). Critical access hospitals are considered *necessary providers of health care* to community residents who live in areas more than 35 miles from another hospital.

Emergency departments play a unique role within the U.S. health care system because of the multispecialty nature of the environment. More than 136.9 million people visit the ED each year, or 43.4 visits per 100 people (Centers for Disease Control and Prevention [CDC], 2017). Although the demand for emergency care has greatly increased over the past two decades and the health care consumer has higher expectations, the capacity to provide necessary resources has not kept pace in many systems. Emergency department crowding occurs when the demand for care exceeds available resources in the department, hospital, or both. Poor patient outcomes and inability of staff to provide care according to treatment guidelines are well-documented concerns associated with overcrowding (Morley et al., 2018).

In 2010, the Affordable Care Act became the impetus for health care initiatives that affected emergency services; the full spectrum of that impact has continued to evolve and may change again if this Act is ever repealed. Cost and continued or changed availability of health insurance will continue to influence how patients use emergency departments, primary care networks, disease management programs, home care services, and community resources. The widespread availability of health insurance could produce an increase in the number of patients who use the ED once they have greater access to financial resources. Emergency department use may actually decrease for some types of patients as hospitals and providers partner in Accountable Care Organization models. This change may better control costs by managing patient outcomes through primary care networks and disease management programs. Emergency departments may continue to experience the shift from admitting the majority of acutely ill patients to the hospital to employing ***teamwork and collaboration*** with home care and community resources that enable patients to be safely discharged home from the ED when possible.

THE EMERGENCY DEPARTMENT ENVIRONMENT OF CARE

In the emergency care environment rapid change is expected. The typical ED is fast paced and, at the height of activity, might even appear chaotic. Patients seek treatment for a number of physical, psychological, spiritual, and social reasons. Many nurses work in this environment because they thrive in challenging, stimulating work settings. Although most EDs have treatment areas that are designated for certain populations such as patients with trauma or cardiac, psychiatric, or gynecologic problems, care can actually take place almost anywhere. In a crowded ED patients may receive initial treatment outside of the usual treatment rooms, including the waiting room and hallways.

The ED is typically alive with activity and noise, although the pace decreases at times because arrivals are random. Emergency nurses can expect background sounds that include ringing telephones, monitor alarms, vocal patients, crying children, and radio transmissions between staff and incoming ambulance or helicopter personnel. Interruptions and distractions are the norm, and the nurse must ensure that these events do not impact patient ***safety***.

During any given shift the emergency nurse may function as a cardiac nurse, a geriatric nurse, a psychiatric nurse, a pediatric nurse, and a trauma nurse. Patient acuity typically ranges from life-threatening emergencies to minor symptoms that could be addressed in a primary care office or community clinic. Some of the most common reasons that people seek ED care are:

- Abdominal pain
- Breathing difficulties
- Chest pain
- Fever
- Headache
- Injuries (especially falls in older adults)
- Pain (the most common symptom)

Demographic Data and Vulnerable Populations

Emergency department staff members provide care for people across the life span with a broad spectrum of needs, illnesses, and injuries, as well as varying cultural, spiritual, and religious beliefs and practices. Vulnerable populations who visit the ED include the homeless, the poor, patients with mental health needs, those with substance use concerns, and older adults.

The Impact of Homelessness. Homelessness affected 568,000 people in the United States on a single night in 2019 (U.S. Department of Housing and Urban Development, 2020). The homeless population is made up of both adults and children; an increasing number are young, single mothers, as well as lesbian, gay, bisexual, and transgender youths (Stevenson & Purpuro, 2018). Factors that contribute to being homeless include economic hardship, the need to escape domestic abuse, behavioral health issues, and substance abuse (Stevenson & Purpuro, 2018). People who are homeless have a high incidence of acute and chronic health conditions such as physical disabilities, alcoholism, diabetes, hypertension, and pulmonary disease (Stevenson & Purpuro, 2018). They are vulnerable to physical trauma, weather exposure, sexually transmitted diseases, infestation, and infectious diseases such as tuberculosis and influenza.

Patients who are homeless often seek ED care for a variety of reasons. Because the ED is open 24 hours per day and is mandated by federal law to perform an emergency medical screening examination on all of its patients, those who are homeless may know that they will gain entry despite an inability to pay for services. The ED represents a safe place to go for shelter in poor weather and to obtain food, medical care, pain relief, and human interaction. Some patients who are homeless simply seek a temporary respite from their current living conditions, which may be a park, shelter, car, abandoned building, or cardboard box. People who have been persistently homeless may assimilate into the homeless culture, learn to take great pride in their survival skills, and fiercely protect their few belongings and their living space. They may develop a distrust of outsiders, including members of the health care profession, and are especially sensitive to any perceived bias or stereotyping.

Patients who are homeless bring special challenges to their ED evaluation, treatment, and disposition. Some visit the ED frequently and do not adhere to treatment recommendations or follow up with community referrals.

The key nursing action is to demonstrate nonjudgmental behaviors that promote trust. These include making eye contact (if culturally appropriate), speaking calmly, avoiding any prejudicial or stereotypical remarks, being patient, showing genuine care and concern by listening, following through on promises, and exercising caution when there is a need to enter into the patient's personal space. Nurses must always maintain their situational awareness and attend to their own needs for personal safety. These include anticipating the potential for violent behavior, which can pose a ***safety*** risk to self, staff, and patients. Clear professional boundaries must be communicated if the patient becomes disruptive, profane, or sexually inappropriate.

You will always use Standard Precautions and assess the need to isolate the patient in a negative-pressure room if airborne disease such as tuberculosis is a concern. While collaborating with the emergency care provider to ensure that the patient's health needs are identified and treated, consult a social worker or case manager to work with the patient to identify safety needs, referral options, and community resources. When possible, place emphasis on prevention efforts. Social services can assist by recommending resources for healthier food pantries, employment opportunities, health coverage, and housing (McEnroe-Petitte, 2020). It is also important to develop an individual care plan with the interprofessional health care team if the patient uses the ED frequently. This type of care plan is extremely beneficial in establishing a consistent approach to patient management, especially when the patient has complex conditions or exhibits drug-seeking and disruptive behavior.

PATIENT-CENTERED CARE: OLDER ADULT CONSIDERATIONS QSEN

Older adults often visit the ED because of worsening of an existing chronic condition or because the condition affects their ability to perform ADLs. Older adults are also sometimes admitted from nursing homes or assisted-living facilities for procedures (e.g., insertion of a percutaneous endoscopic gastrostomy [PEG] tube or peripherally inserted central catheter [PICC]) or treatments (e.g., blood transfusions). Some hospitals plan direct admission of the patient to same-day surgery or hold a bed for the procedure or treatment to bypass the ED. This arrangement decreases the patient's wait time and therefore decreases the risks for adverse events such as pressure injury development or hospital-acquired infection (HAI). Incorporating caregivers of older adults into the process of care can aid in overall patient evaluation, decision making, and satisfaction with the ED experience.

Special Nursing Teams—Members of the Interprofessional Team

Many EDs have specialized nursing teams that work with high-risk populations of patients. **Forensic nurse examiners (RN-FNEs)** are educated to obtain patient histories, collect forensic evidence, and offer counseling and follow-up care for victims of rape, abuse, and domestic violence—also known as *intimate partner violence (IPV)* (International Association of Forensic Nurses, 2019). They intervene on the patient's behalf. Forensic nurses who specialize in helping victims of sexual assault are called *sexual assault nurse examiners (SANEs)* or *sexual assault forensic examiners (SAFEs)*.

Interventions performed by forensic nurses may include providing information about developing a ***safety*** plan or how to escape a violent relationship. Forensic nurse examiners document injuries and collect physical and photographic evidence. They may also provide testimony in court as to what was observed during the examination and information about the type of care provided.

Some patients who visit the ED for acute problems also have chronic mental health needs. Patients who are experiencing an acute psychiatric crisis situation as their primary problem such as a suicide attempt secondary to severe depression, or a new onset of psychosis, may also arrive in the ED. The availability of mental health/behavioral health nurses can improve the quality of care delivered to these patients who require specialized interventions in the ED and can offer valuable expertise to the emergency health care staff. The psychiatric crisis nurse team evaluates patients with emotional behaviors or mental illness and facilitates the follow-up treatment plan, including possible admission to an appropriate facility. These nurses interact with patients and families when sudden illness, serious injury, or death of a loved one may have precipitated a crisis.

Some EDs have a specialized area to treat patients with psychiatric disorders that is designed to promote optimal safety. Features may include closed-circuit video monitoring, access-control door locks, solid ceilings (to prevent patients from climbing into the ceiling), a secured area to retain patient belongings, metal detectors, panic alarms, and elimination of any items or room features that could pose a safety risk to self, other patients, or staff.

Interprofessional Team Collaboration

The emergency nurse is one member of the large interprofessional team that provides care for patients in the ED. A team approach to emergency care using ***teamwork and collaboration*** is considered a standard of practice (Fig. 10.1). In this setting the nurse coordinates care with all levels of health care team providers, from prehospital emergency medical services (EMS) personnel to physicians and other providers, hospital technicians, and other professional and essential support staff.

Prehospital care providers are typically the first caregivers that patients see before transport to the ED by an ambulance or helicopter (Fig. 10.2). Local protocols define the skill level of the EMS responders dispatched to provide assistance. Emergency medical technicians (EMTs) offer basic life support (BLS) interventions such as oxygen, basic wound care, splinting, spinal motion restriction, and monitoring of vital signs. Some units carry automatic external defibrillators (AEDs) and may be authorized to administer selected drugs such as an epinephrine autoinjector, intranasal naloxone (Narcan), or nitroglycerin based on training and established protocols. For patients who require care that exceeds BLS resources, paramedics may be dispatched. Paramedics are advanced life support (ALS) providers who can perform advanced techniques, which may include cardiac monitoring, advanced airway management and intubation, needle chest decompression, establishing IV or intraosseous access, and administering drugs en route to the ED (Fig. 10.3).

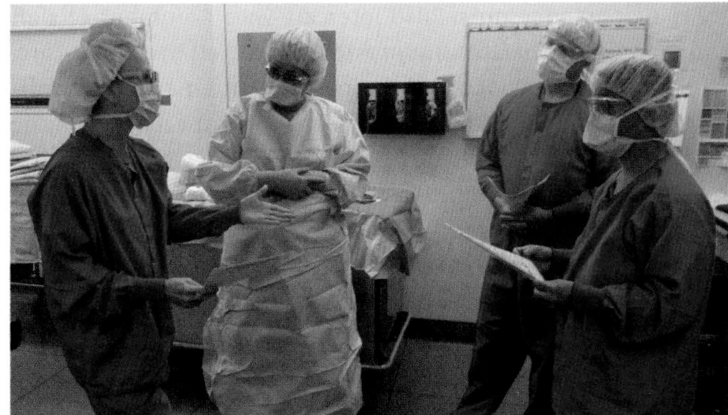

Fig. 10.1 The ability to work as part of an interprofessional team is crucial to positive outcomes for emergency department (ED) patients. (From Rothrock, J. C. [2015]. *Alexander's care of the patient in surgery.* [15th ed.]. St. Louis: Mosby.)

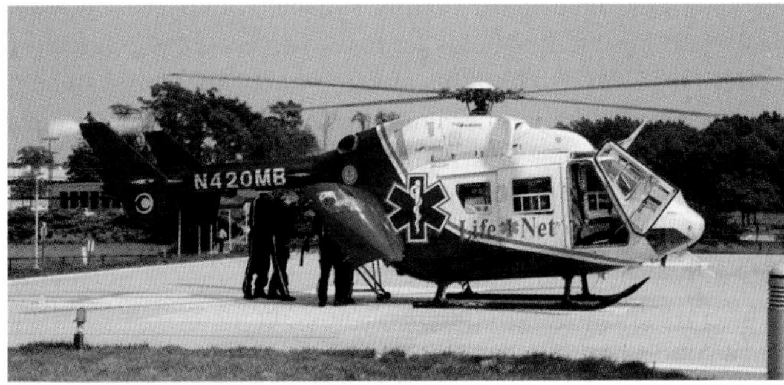

Fig. 10.2 Advanced life support helicopter arriving at emergency department landing zone. Helicopters are used to rapidly transport critically ill and injured patients to the hospital for emergent care.

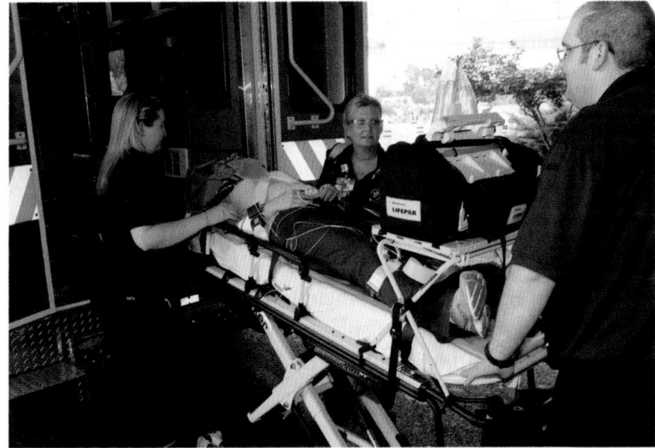

Fig. 10.3 Prehospital providers take a patient from the ambulance to be brought into the emergency department.

The prehospital provider is a key source for valuable patient data. Emergency nurses rely on these providers to be the "eyes and ears" of the health care team in the prehospital setting and to ensure ***communication*** of this information to other staff members for continuity of care.

Another integral member of the emergency health care team is the emergency medicine physician. These medical professionals receive specialized education and training in emergency patient management. Emergency medicine is a recognized physician specialty practice.

The emergency nurse also interacts with a number of staff and community health care providers involved in patient care, yet is involved in closest collaboration with emergency medicine physicians. Even though other physician specialists may be involved in ED patient treatment, the emergency medicine physician typically directs the overall care in the department. Many EDs also employ nurse practitioners (NPs) and physician assistants (PAs) to assume designated roles in patient assessment and treatment. Teaching hospitals have resident physicians who train in the ED. They act in collaboration with or under the supervision of the emergency medicine physician to assist with emergency care delivery.

The emergency nurse interacts and regularly takes part in ***teamwork and collaboration*** with *professional and essential support staff.* These personnel include radiology and ultrasound technicians, respiratory therapists, laboratory technicians, social workers, case managers, nursing assistants, and clerical staff. Each support staff member is key to the success of the emergency health care team. For example, the respiratory therapist can help the nurse troubleshoot mechanical ventilator issues. Laboratory technicians can offer information regarding best practice techniques for specimen collection. During the discharge planning process, social workers or case managers can be tremendous patient advocates in locating community resources, including temporary housing, durable medical equipment (DME), drug and alcohol counseling, health insurance information, follow-up care, and prescription services. The ED nurse is accountable for ***communication*** of pertinent staff considerations, patient needs, and restrictions to support staff (e.g., physical limitations, safety concerns, Transmission-Based Precautions) to ensure that ongoing patient and staff safety issues are addressed.

The emergency nurse's interactions extend beyond the walls of the ED. ***Communication*** with nurses from the inpatient units is necessary to ensure continuity of patient care. Providing a concise but comprehensive report of the patient's ED experience is essential for the *hand-off communication* process and patient ***safety***. Information should include the patient's:

- Situation (reason for being in the ED) and admitting diagnosis
- Pertinent medical history, including implantable devices and any history of organ transplant
- Assessment and diagnostic findings, particularly critical results
- Transmission-Based Precautions and safety concerns (e.g., fall risk, allergies) as indicated
- Interventions provided in the ED and response to those interventions

Many agencies use the SBAR method (situation, background, assessment, response) or some variation of that method to ensure complete and clearly understood ***communication***. Chapter 1 discusses the SBAR technique in more detail.

! NATIONAL PATIENT SAFETY GOALS

The Joint Commission (TJC) (2017) advocates that hospitals and other health care agencies use a standardized approach to hand-off communications to prevent errors caused by poor or inadequate communication.

Emergency nurses and nurses on inpatient units need to understand the unique aspects of their two practice environments to prevent conflicts. For example, nurses on inpatient units may be critical of the push to move patients out of the ED setting quickly, particularly when their unit activity is high. Similarly the emergency nurse may be critical of the inpatient unit's lack of understanding or enthusiasm for accepting admissions rapidly. Effective interpersonal ***communication*** skills and respectful negotiation can optimize ***teamwork and collaboration*** between the emergency nurse and the inpatient unit nurse.

STAFF AND PATIENT SAFETY CONSIDERATIONS

In the emergency department (ED) setting, staff and patient ***safety*** are major concerns. Interventions to minimize risk are noted in the Best Practice for Patient Safety & Quality Care: Maintaining Patient and Staff Safety in the Emergency Department box.

BEST PRACTICE FOR PATIENT SAFETY & QUALITY CARE (QSEN)

Maintaining Patient and Staff Safety in the Emergency Department

Safety Consideration	Interventions to Minimize Risk
Patient identification	Provide an identification (ID) bracelet for each patient. Use two unique identifiers (e.g., name, date of birth). If patient identity is unknown, use a special identification system.
Injury prevention for patients	Keep rails up on stretcher. Keep stretcher in lowest position. Remind the patient to use call light for assistance. Reorient the confused patient frequently. If patient is confused, ask a family member or significant other to remain with him or her. Implement measures to protect skin integrity for patients at risk for skin breakdown.
Risk for errors and adverse events	Obtain a thorough patient and family history. Check the patient for a medical alert bracelet or necklace. Search the patient's belongings for weapons or other harmful items such as drugs and drug paraphernalia when he or she has an altered mental status or presents with behavioral health concerns.
Injury prevention for staff	Use Standard Precautions at all times. Anticipate hostile, violent patient, family, and/or visitor behavior. Plan and practice options if violence occurs, including assistance from the security department.

Staff Safety

Staff safety concerns center on the potential for transmission of disease and on personal safety when working with patients or visitors who are aggressive, agitated, or violent. The emergency nurse uses Standard Precautions at all times when a potential for contamination by blood or other body fluids exists. Patients with tuberculosis or other airborne pathogens are preferentially placed in a negative-pressure room if available. The nurse wears a powered air-purifying respirator (PAPR) or a specially fitted facemask before engaging in any close interaction with these patients (see Chapter 21).

! NURSING SAFETY PRIORITY QSEN

Action Alert

Patients or visitors who display hostile behaviors also pose injury risks to staff members. Be alert for volatile situations or people who demonstrate aggressive or violent tendencies through verbal or nonverbal behaviors. Follow the hospital security plan, including identifying the nearest escape route, attempting de-escalation strategies before harm can occur, and notifying security and supervisory staff of the situation. Emergency visits resulting from gang or domestic violence can produce particularly hazardous conditions. Report all episodes of assaultive or violent behaviors through the hospital event documentation process so leaders and risk managers are aware of the scope of the problem and can plan safety strategies, including staff education, accordingly.

Emergency departments use several methods of ensuring ***safety***. Many EDs have at least one security guard present at all times for immediate assistance with these situations. Metal detectors may be used as a screening device. Strategically located panic buttons and remote door access controls allow staff to get help and secure major entrances. The triage reception area—a particularly vulnerable access point into the ED—is often designed to serve as a security barrier with bulletproof glass and staff-controlled door entry into the treatment area. Hospitals may employ canine units made up of specially trained officers and dogs to patrol high-risk areas and to respond threatening situations.

Patient Safety

Hospital emergency departments have unique factors that can affect patient ***safety***. These factors include the provision of complex emergency care, constant interruptions, and the need to interact with the many providers involved in caring for one patient.

Some of the most common *patient* ***safety*** issues noted in the ED are:

- Fall risk
- Medical errors or adverse events
- Patient misidentification
- Skin breakdown

Correct *patient identification* is critical in all health care settings. All patients are issued an identification bracelet at their point of entry in the ED—generally at the triage registration desk or at the bedside if emergent needs exist. For patients with an unknown identity and those with emergent conditions that prevent the standard identification process (e.g., unconscious patient without identification, emergent trauma patient), hospitals commonly use a "Jane/John Doe" or other system of identification.

! NATIONAL PATIENT SAFETY GOALS

Always verify the patient's identity using two unique identifiers before each intervention and before medication administration per The Joint Commission's (TJC) 2020 National Patient Safety Goals (TJC, 2020). Examples of appropriate identifiers include the patient's name, birth date, agency identification number, home telephone number or address, and Social Security number.

Fall prevention starts with identifying patients at risk for falls and then implementing appropriate fall precautions and ***safety*** measures like application of a fall risk bracelet (Fig. 10.4). Patients can enter the ED without apparent fall risk factors, but because of interventions such as pain medication, sedation, or lower extremity cast application, they can develop a risk for falls. Falls can also occur in patients with medical conditions or drugs that cause syncope ("blackouts"). Some older adults experience orthostatic (postural) hypotension as a side effect of cardiovascular drugs. In this case patients become dizzy when changing from a lying or sitting position (see Chapter 4).

! NURSING SAFETY PRIORITY QSEN

Action Alert

Help patients move slowly from a supine to an upright position. Assist when ambulating. When the patient is on a stretcher, confirm that side rails are up and locked, that the call light is within reach, and that a patient's fall risk is communicated clearly to staff members who may assume responsibility for care, as well as caregivers.

Older adults who are on beds or stretchers should *always* have side rails up and the bed or stretcher in the lowest position. Access to a call light is especially important; instruct the patient to call for the nurse if assistance is needed rather than attempting independent ambulation. Some older adults have difficulty adjusting to the noise and pace of the ED and/or have illnesses or injuries that cause delirium, an acute state of confusion. Reorient the patient frequently and reassess mental status. Undiagnosed delirium increases the risk for mortality for older adults who are admitted to the hospital. Assess the need for a caregiver or safety companion to stay with the patient to prevent falls and help with reorientation. Additional safety strategies are listed in the Best Practice for Patient Safety & Quality Care: Maintaining Patient and Staff Safety in the Emergency Department box.

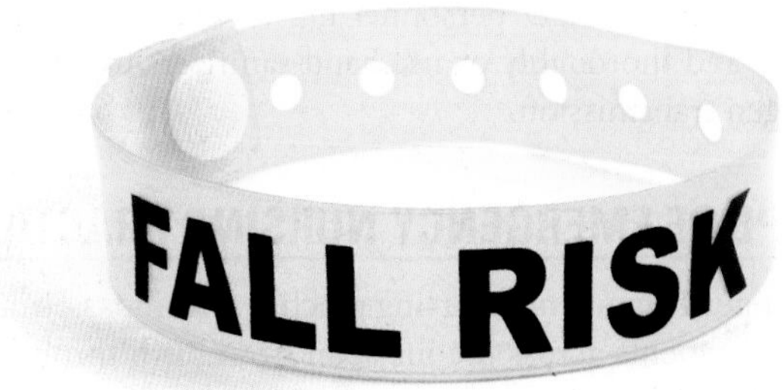

Fig. 10.4 Fall risk bracelet. (©Thinkstock.com/iStock/Image Pixel.)

Some patients spend a lengthy time on stretchers while awaiting unit bed availability. During that time, basic health needs require attention, including providing nutrition, hygiene, ***safety***, and privacy. Waiting in the ED can cause increased pain in patients with back pain or arthritis.

Protecting skin integrity also begins in the ED. Emergency nurses need to assess the skin frequently and implement preventive interventions as part of the ED plan of care, especially when caring for older adults or people who are immobilized. Interventions that promote clean, dry skin for incontinent patients, pressure-relieving skin care products placed over pressure points, mobility techniques that decrease shearing forces when moving the immobile patient, and routine turning help prevent skin breakdown. Chapter 23 describes additional nursing interventions for preventing skin breakdown.

A significant ***safety*** risk for all patients who enter the emergency care environment is the *potential for medical errors or adverse events,* especially those associated with medication administration. The episodic and often chaotic nature of emergency management in an environment with frequent interruptions can easily lead to errors.

To reduce error potential, the emergency nurse makes every attempt to obtain essential and accurate medical history information from the patient and caregivers. When working with patients who arrive with an altered mental status, a quick survey to determine whether the person is wearing a medical alert bracelet or necklace is important. A two-person search of patient belongings may yield medication containers or a medication list; or the name of a health care provider, pharmacy, or caregiver contact. Some EDs employee pharmacists or pharmacy technicians to help gather medication history to improve timeliness and accuracy of the information recorded. Through these processes the nurse may find information that promotes ***safety*** and influences the overall emergency treatment plan.

Automated electronic tracking systems are also available in some EDs to help staff identify the location of patients at any given time and monitor the progress of care delivery during the visit. These valuable safety measures are especially important in large or busy EDs with a high population of older adults (Laskowski-Jones, 2008).

In addition to falls and pressure injury development, another adverse event that can result from a prolonged stay in the ED is a *hospital-acquired infection* (HAI). Older adults in particular are at risk for urinary tract or respiratory infections. Patients who are immunocompromised, especially those on chronic steroid therapy or immunomodulators, are also at a high risk. Nurses and other ED personnel must wash their hands frequently and thoroughly or use hand sanitizers to help prevent pathogen transmission.

SCOPE OF EMERGENCY NURSING PRACTICE

The scope of emergency nursing practice encompasses management of patients across the life span from birth through death and all health conditions that prompt a person of any age to seek emergency care.

CLINICAL JUDGMENT CHALLENGE 10.1

Safety

An 84-year old female client with advanced dementia is brought to the emergency department after an unwitnessed fall at a long-term care facility. The paramedic reports that the nurse at the facility stated that the client had been found lying in the hallway approximately 1 hour earlier. She has been unable to ambulate since then, and one leg is noted to be shorter than the other. The client is crying, yet cannot give any history. The emergency department nurse assesses the client's vital signs: T 98.8°F, 160/98 BP, 90 P, 22 R.

1. **Recognize Cues:** What assessment information in this client situation is the most important and immediate concern for the nurse? (Hint: Identify the **relevant** information *first* to determine what is most important.)
2. **Analyze Cues:** What client conditions are consistent with the **most relevant** information? (Hint: Think about priority collaborative problems that support and contradict the information presented in this situation.)
3. **Prioritize Hypotheses:** Which possibilities or explanations are **most likely** to be present in this client situation? Which possibilities or explanations are the most serious? (Hint: Consider all possibilities and determine their urgency and risk for this client.)
4. **Generate Solutions:** What actions would most likely achieve the desired outcomes for this client? Which actions should be **avoided** or are **potentially harmful**? (Hint: Determine the desired outcomes first to decide which interventions are appropriate and those that should be avoided.)
5. **Take Action:** Which actions are the most appropriate and how should they be implemented? In what **priority order** should they be implemented? (Hint: Consider health teaching, documentation, requested health care provider orders or prescriptions, nursing skills, collaboration with or referral to health team members, etc.)
6. **Evaluate Outcomes:** What client assessment would indicate that the nurse's actions were **effective**? (Hint: Think about signs that would indicate an improvement, decline, or unchanged client condition.)

Core Competencies

Emergency nursing practice is highly dynamic and requires core skills and competencies in patient assessment, priority setting, clinical decision making, documentation, and ***communication***, along with a sound cognitive knowledge base (Sweet, 2018). Flexibility and adaptability are vital traits because situations within the ED and individual patients can change rapidly.

Like that of any practicing nurse, the foundation of the emergency nurse's skill base is *assessment.* The ED nurse must be able to rapidly and accurately interpret assessment findings according to acuity and age. For example, mottling of the extremities may be a normal finding in a newborn, but it may indicate poor peripheral perfusion and a shock state in an adult.

PATIENT-CENTERED CARE: OLDER ADULT CONSIDERATIONS QSEN

Some older adults may not be able to provide an accurate history because of memory loss or acute delirium. If possible, review their prior hospitalization records to obtain past histories or ask a caregiver for pertinent information. Older adults may have pre-existing conditions (comorbidities) that must be considered as part of the assessment. *Knowing the history is important because these conditions might adversely affect or complicate the cause for the ED visit.* For example, a patient who has rib fractures but has a history of severe chronic obstructive pulmonary disease (COPD) may not be able to maintain adequate gas exchange without endotracheal intubation and mechanical ventilatory support in the ED.

Another consideration for assessment of older adults is that their presenting signs and symptoms may be different or less specific than those of younger adults. For example, increasing weakness, fatigue, and confusion may be the only admission concerns. These vague symptoms can be caused by serious illnesses such as an acute myocardial infarction (MI), urinary tract infection, or pneumonia.

Another skill for the emergency nurse is *priority setting*, which is essential in the triage process. Priority setting depends on accurate assessment and appropriate clinical judgment. These skills are gained through hands-on clinical experience in the ED. Discussion of case studies and the use of human patient simulation and simulation software and aids can also help nurses to acquire this skill base in a safe environment and then apply it in the actual clinical situation (Lavoie & Clark, 2017).

The knowledge base for emergency nurses is broad and ranges from critical care emergencies to less common problems such as snakebites and hazardous materials contamination (see Chapters 11 and 12). ED nurses also learn to recognize signs of societal problems such as domestic violence, child or adult abuse, and sexual assault.

Although most EDs have providers available around the clock who are physically located within the ED, the nurse often initiates collaborative interprofessional protocols for lifesaving interventions such as cardiac monitoring, oxygen therapy, insertion of IV catheters, and infusion of appropriate parenteral solutions. In many EDs nurses function under clearly defined medical protocols that allow them to initiate drug therapy for emergent conditions such as anaphylactic shock and cardiac arrest. Emergency care principles extend to knowing which essential laboratory and diagnostic tests may be needed and, when necessary, obtaining them.

The emergency nurse must be proficient in performing a variety of technical skills, sometimes in a stressful, high-pressure environment. He or she may also need to be proficient with critical care equipment such as invasive pressure-monitoring devices and mechanical ventilators. This type of equipment is commonly found in EDs that are part of Level I and Level II trauma centers.

The nurse also collaborates with and assists the ED provider of care with procedures. Knowledge and skills related to procedural setup, patient preparation, teaching, and postprocedure care are key aspects of emergency nursing practice. Common ED procedures include:

- Central line insertion
- Chest tube insertion
- Endotracheal intubation and initiation of mechanical ventilation
- Fracture management
- Foreign body removal
- Lumbar puncture
- Paracentesis
- Pelvic examination
- Wound closure by suturing

More than one nurse may be necessary to assist with some procedures. For example, if deep or moderate procedural sedation is used to produce amnesia and relaxation during fracture reduction, one nurse assists the provider with the actual procedure while the other nurse monitors the patient before, during, and after administration of the moderate procedural sedation medications.

Perhaps the most essential component of the emergency nurse's skill base is ***communication***. The ED environment is complex; multiple barriers to effective communication are likely. It is important to respect each patient's belief system and practice, even if these differ significantly from those of the health care team. Assess each patient as an individual and do not stereotype based on culture, socioeconomic status, gender identity, spirituality, or religious beliefs.

PATIENT-CENTERED CARE: CULTURAL/SPIRITUAL CONSIDERATIONS (QSEN)

Be aware of the various cultural and spiritual values of patients that may influence the care you provide. People often have distinct beliefs that are of importance to them, and these should be respected in the health care setting. Examples of beliefs include the importance of modesty, the interpretation of eye contact (or the lack thereof), specific dietary needs, preferences for health care providers of a certain gender, and decisions about receiving or declining methods of treatment (e.g., blood or animal products).

The population of people who do not speak English, or speak English as a second language, continues to rapidly increase in the United States. Access available resources such as telephone language lines and dedicated interpreters contracted by the hospital to ensure an understanding of all aspects of care. Similarly, deaf interpreters are essential when providing care for patients who are hearing impaired.

PATIENT-CENTERED CARE: GENDER HEALTH CONSIDERATIONS (QSEN)

Be aware that not all patients identify as male or female. Some patients may be in the process of gender transition from male to female or female to male (transgender people), whereas others identify as gender neutral or gender fluid. Demonstrate professional behaviors that promote trust. Ask the patient which name and pronouns (he, she, they, or other term) the person prefers, and use them appropriately. Chapter 68 discusses the special care for the transgender population in more detail.

ED crowding and insufficient nursing personnel to meet the demand for services also create difficulties with ***communication*** of pertinent patient information and quality of written documentation. The high-stress ED environment can strain effective interpersonal behaviors, particularly when nurses are confronted with angry, violent, or challenging patients.

Training and Certification

Two general types of certification are referred to in emergency nursing practice: the "certification" that marks successful completion of a particular course of study, and emergency nursing specialty certification (Table 10.1). As part of the orientation and employment requirements for staff nurses in most US EDs, successful completion of the Basic Life Support (BLS) for Healthcare Providers, Advanced Cardiac Life Support (ACLS), and Pediatric Advanced Life Support (PALS) provider courses through the American Heart Association is necessary. These courses provide instruction in fundamental, evidence-based management

TABLE 10.1 Descriptions of Training and Certifications for Emergency Nursing

Certification	Description
Basic Life Support (BLS) (required)	Noninvasive assessment and management skills for airway maintenance and cardiopulmonary resuscitation (CPR)
Advanced Cardiac Life Support (ACLS) (usually required)	Invasive airway-management skills, pharmacology, and electrical therapies; special resuscitation situations
Pediatric Advanced Life Support (PALS) (may be required)	Neonatal and pediatric resuscitation
Trauma Nursing Core Course (may be required)	Trauma nursing priorities, interventions, diagnostic studies, injury management
Certified Emergency Nurse (CEN) (optional)	Validates core emergency nursing knowledge base

theory and techniques for cardiopulmonary resuscitation (CPR). Course participants include physicians, physician assistants, nurse practitioners, nurses, and prehospital personnel. The ACLS course builds on the BLS content to include:

- Advanced concepts in cardiac monitoring
- Invasive airway-management skills
- Pharmacologic and electrical therapies
- Intravascular access techniques
- Special resuscitation situations
- Postresuscitation management considerations

Additional certification may be required through successful completion of trauma continuing education courses, particularly the Trauma Nursing Core Course through the Emergency Nurses Association.

EMERGENCY NURSING PRINCIPLES

Triage

The organization of emergency care and the ED is structured through triage principles. **Triage** is an organized system for sorting or classifying patients into priority levels, depending on illness or injury severity. The key concept is that patients in the ED with the highest-acuity needs receive the quickest evaluation; treatment; and prioritized resource utilization such as x-rays, laboratory work, and computed tomography (CT) scans. These patients also have priority for hospital service areas such as the operating room or cardiac catheterization laboratory. A person with a lower-acuity problem may wait longer in the ED because a high-acuity patient is moved to the "head of the line." The staff needs to communicate information about this system to the patient and family who may not understand why other patients are treated first, despite having arrived later.

The triage nurse is pivotal in ensuring that patients with the highest-acuity health care needs are prioritized in the emergency care system. When patients come to the ED, regulatory standards dictate that a registered nurse (RN), physician, physician assistant (PA), or nurse practitioner (NP) perform a rapid assessment to determine the triage priority. The RN is typically assigned to perform the triage function in most hospitals. The triage nurse requires appropriate training and experience in both emergency nursing and triage decision-making concepts to develop an expert knowledge base and provide ongoing mentoring and quality improvement feedback (Dippenaar & Bruijns, 2016). The triage nurse may seek the input of an emergency physician, an advanced practice nurse (e.g., nurse practitioner [NP]), or a PA to help establish the acuity level if the patient's presentation is highly unusual.

TABLE 10.2 Three-Tiered Triage System and Examples of Patients Triaged in Each Tier

Tier Level	Examples of Patients Triaged in Each Tier
Emergent (life threatening)	Chest pain with diaphoresis Hemorrhage Respiratory distress Stroke Vital sign instability
Urgent (needs quick treatment, but not immediately life threatening)	Abdominal pain (severe) Fractures (displaced or multiple) Renal colic Respiratory infection (especially pneumonia in older adults) Soft-tissue injuries (complex or multiple)
Nonurgent (could wait several hours if needed without fear of deterioration)	Fracture (simple) Rashes Strains and sprains Urinary tract infection

Based on the triage priority, patients may be rushed into a treatment room, directed to a lower-acuity area within the ED, or asked to sit in the waiting room. Variations include:

- Triage nurse–initiated protocols for laboratory work or diagnostic studies that may be performed before the patient is actually evaluated by an ED provider of care
- Initiation of care while the patient is on a stretcher in the hallway of a crowded ED

These protocols are especially beneficial for certain populations that require rapid diagnosis and collaborative treatment within a defined time frame from ED arrival to meet established standards of care. Examples are patients with chest pain or those with a clinical presentation indicative of stroke, sepsis, or pneumonia.

Emergent, Urgent, and Nonurgent Categories. Various triage systems can be used by a hospital ED. Whatever system is selected must be applied consistently by triage nursing staff and endorsed by the emergency medicine provider staff. Based on the severity of the patient's condition, a well-known triage scheme used in the United States is the three-tiered model of "emergent, urgent, and nonurgent" (Table 10.2). With this system, a patient experiencing crushing substernal chest pain, shortness of breath, and diaphoresis would be classified as emergent and triaged immediately to a treatment room within the ED. Similarly, a critically injured trauma patient or a person with an active hemorrhage would also be prioritized as emergent. The **emergent triage** category implies that a condition exists that poses an immediate threat to life or limb.

The **urgent triage** category indicates that the patient should be treated quickly but that an immediate threat to life does not exist at the moment. Reassessment is needed if a health care provider cannot evaluate the patient in a timely manner. In case of clinical deterioration, triage priority may be upgraded from urgent to emergent. Examples of patients who typically fall into the urgent category are those with a new onset of pneumonia (as long as respiratory failure does not appear imminent), renal colic, complex lacerations not associated with major hemorrhage, displaced fractures or dislocations, and temperature higher than 101°F (38.3°C). Those placed in the **nonurgent triage** category can generally tolerate waiting several hours for health care services without a significant risk for clinical deterioration. Conditions within this classification include patients with sprains and strains, simple fractures, general skin rashes, and uncomplicated urinary tract infections.

Other Multitiered Models. To further sort patient conditions within an acuity classification or triage priority system, four- and five-tier triage models also exist. Such models are based either on comprehensive lists of conditions that indicate the particular triage priority to which a patient should be assigned or on the nature of resources that a patient will use in the ED setting. A patient situation may generate various triage classifications in different hospitals, depending on the triage priority system used at that particular institution. Some schemes may even take into account the presence of pre-existing conditions such as a history of anticoagulant use, diabetes, heart disease, and organ transplantation.

It is surprising that there is no universally accepted triage system recognized in the United States. Thus there is no standardization of triage data to compare patient acuity among hospitals. Health care providers, health insurance companies, and patients often disagree on the definition of an emergent versus a nonurgent ED visit, making it essential to use a practical triage system to maintain department efficiency and allocation of resources. Years ago, the Emergency Nurses Association in collaboration with the American College of Emergency Physicians studied the available research literature on acuity scales and concluded that two standardized five-level systems, the **Emergency Severity Index (ESI)**and the **Canadian Triage Acuity Scale (CTAS)**, were the most reliable (Shelton, 2010). The ESI model uses an algorithm that fosters rapid, reliable, and clinically pertinent categorization of patients into five groups, from Level 1 (emergent) to Level 5 (nonurgent). The CTAS model differs from ESI in that lists of descriptors are used to establish the triage level.

Whatever triage model is used, triage nurses must use a systematic approach, apply solid clinical decision-making skills, and maintain a caring ethic. Compassion fatigue, or burnout, can hinder objectivity in working with patients in the ED. A biased approach threatens the ED nurse's ability to triage patients accurately. Mistriage is a patient ***safety*** risk that can be the "root cause" of delayed or inadequate treatment, with potentially deadly consequences.

Disposition

At the conclusion of the assessment, the provider must make a decision regarding patient disposition (i.e., where the patient should go after being discharged from the ED). Should he or she be admitted to the hospital, transferred to a specialty care center, or discharged to home with instructions for continued care and follow-up? Usually the answer is straightforward. For example, a patient who has an evolving myocardial infarction, sepsis, stroke, or acute surgical need is admitted.

Sometimes, however, the ED disposition decision is less clear. The ED provider of care may discuss this decision in collaboration with other consulted providers and the emergency nurse. The nurse may have a greater sense of how well a patient will manage in a home setting, depending on whether caregivers are reliable and available to assist. For example, in the event that a patient with a minor head injury has sustained a loss of consciousness, someone is typically expected to remain with that person for the first 12 to 24 hours to be sure that he or she does not show any evidence of neurologic deterioration. If the patient does not have a reliable caregiver to perform ongoing neurologic checks in that 12- to 24-hour window, the patient may need admission for observation. Another common scenario involves the potential risk to the patient in cases of actual or suspected domestic violence. If discharge to home is not deemed safe, the patient may be admitted to the hospital in an observation status until resources can be organized to provide for a safe environment. Coordinate the discharge plan and continuing care with the social worker or case manager.

NCLEX EXAMINATION CHALLENGE 10.1

Safe and Effective Care Environment

Which client does the oncoming ED nurse see **first** when assigned to care for four clients?

A. 21-year-old with a skin rash who has been waiting 2 hours to see a provider
B. 30-year-old with influenza who has infusing IV fluids and is resting quietly
C. 47-year-old who fell off of a curb, resulting in a sprained ankle
D. 56-year-old reporting chest pain and diaphoresis that started 30 minutes prior

PATIENT-CENTERED CARE: OLDER ADULT CONSIDERATIONS (QSEN)

If discharge from the emergency department (ED) to home is possible, ensure that safety issues are considered. For example, collaborate with the ED provider to evaluate the patient's current prescriptions and over-the-counter medications to determine if the drug regimen should be continued. Involve the ED-based pharmacist if one is available for consultation when necessary. If the drug regimen needs to be changed, be sure that the patient and caregiver have the new information in writing and that it is explained verbally. If needed, assess whether the patient has someone who can pre-sort and place drugs into a medication dispenser to ensure accuracy and prevent adverse drug events. Consider a social services or case-management referral for patients in need of financial resources to obtain prescribed drugs.

To prevent future ED visits, screen older adults per agency policy for functional assessment, cognitive assessment, and risk for falls. Depression screening is also critical because suicide rates are two times higher among older adults compared with younger adults. Older adult males who are white are at the highest risk (Touhy & Jett, 2019).

Older adults are often admitted to the hospital directly from the ED. If hospitalization is needed, determine if the patient has advance directives or is able to make decisions about advance directives before admission. If the patient was admitted from a nursing home, contact the facility to let them know the patient's status. If the patient was receiving home health services, notify the agency about the hospital admission. Contact the patient's primary health care provider and designated caregiver if he or she is not present with the patient.

Case Management. Some EDs employ registered nurse case managers who screen ED patients and intervene when necessary to arrange appropriate referral and follow-up. This is an evolving role in the ED setting that can be beneficial in providing comprehensive care and as a strategy to avoid inappropriate use of resources.

ED case managers, supported by electronic information systems, can review the ED census on both a "real-time" and a retrospective basis to determine which patients have visited the ED frequently in a given period. The case manager can then determine the reasons they sought emergency services, which may include lack of a primary health care provider, exacerbation ("flare-up") of a chronic condition, lack of health education, or lack of the financial resources necessary to manage the health condition. Collaborative case-management interventions include facilitating referrals to primary health care providers or to subsidized community-based health clinics for patients or families in need of routine services.

For those with needs related to chronic conditions, the case manager can arrange referral into appropriate disease management programs in the community, if available. Disease management programs are specific to a particular condition such as asthma, COPD, diabetes, hypertension, heart failure, and renal failure. They help patients learn how to manage their condition on a day-to-day basis to prevent exacerbations or clinical deterioration. The desired outcome is to keep the person healthier and out of the hospital for as long as possible. Health teaching is a key component of these programs. For other health teaching needs, the ED case manager directs the patient to the appropriate educational resources such as a health educator, registered dietitian, or community organization (e.g., the American Diabetes Association, the American Heart Association).

Other functions of the ED case manager might include working in collaboration with staff to plan disposition for people who are homeless or veterans, locating a safe environment for victims of domestic violence or elder abuse, or providing information on resources for low-cost or free prescriptions. Adults who are homeless often have multiple chronic medical illnesses for which they visit EDs frequently. A study demonstrated a decrease in ED visits of homeless people as a result of use of a case manager, who helped patients become more familiar with resources in the health care system beyond the ED (Bodenmann et al., 2017). (See the Evidence-Based Practice box.)

Patient and Family Education. A key role of the emergency nurse is health teaching. At the most basic level, nurses review discharge instructions with the patient and family before signing them out of the department.

In addition to discharge instructions, the ED environment and community-at-large present many opportunities for health education. Emergency nurses are in an ideal position to educate the public about wellness and injury prevention strategies. If the patient is seen after a minor motor vehicle crash, for instance, the nurse can reinforce the need to wear seat belts or use child safety seats correctly. ED visits that result from mishaps in the home provide an excellent opportunity to discuss home ***safety*** issues (e.g., the need for smoke detectors and carbon monoxide detectors) and fall prevention tips (e.g., the need for proper lighting, removal of throw rugs). A new onset or an exacerbation of a medical condition also allows for education, such as how to measure blood glucose and ways to control blood pressure or reduce the risk for heart disease.

EVIDENCE-BASED PRACTICE (QSEN)

Case Management May Reduce Frequent Use of the Emergency Department in a Universal Health Coverage System: A Randomized Controlled Trial

Bodenmann, P., Velonaki, V. S., Griffin, J. L., Baggio, S., Iglesias, K., Moschetti, K., ... & Schupbach, J. (2017). Case management may reduce emergency department frequent use in a universal health coverage system: a randomized controlled trial. *Journal of General Internal Medicine,* 32(5), 508-515.

This study sought to determine whether a case management (CM) intervention, compared with standard emergency care, reduced emergency department (ED) visits for frequent users.

The sample included 250 patients who frequently used a specific public urban ED, which was defined as have or more visits in the prior 12-month period. Half of the patients were placed into a control group and the other half were placed in the intervention group for a 12-month period.

The individualized CM intervention consisted of tangible assistance in obtaining income entitlements, referrals to primary or secondary providers of care, facilitation of access to mental health care or substance abuse treatment if needed, and counseling on at-risk behaviors and utilization of health care (Bodenmann et al., 2017). These interventions took place at baseline and in months 1, 3, and 5.

A generalized linear model was used for negative binomial distribution to compare the number of ED visits during the 12-month follow-up period between the patients who received the CM intervention versus those who had standard emergency care. Data demonstrated that the patients who received the CM intervention visited the ED 2.71 times in the follow-up period, versus patients in the control group, who visited 3.35 times in the subsequent 12 months following the study. Poor social determinants of health were identified as a significant predictor of use of the ED.

Level of Evidence: 2

This was a randomized controlled trial (RCT).

Commentary: Implications for Practice and Research

Nurses must recognize that patients seek emergency care for a variety of reasons. Although those reasons are indeed often emergent in nature, lack of education about the health care system (a social determinant of health) may influence a patient's choice to use emergency care instead of primary care. Case management interventions may help patients become better acquainted with the resources of the health care system outside of the emergency department, and thus decrease nonemergent use of ED resources.

PATIENT AND FAMILY EDUCATION: PREPARING FOR SELF-MANAGEMENT

Providing Discharge Instructions

Most discharge instructions are either preprinted or computer generated and can be customized to address the patient's needs. Consider reading level, primary language, and visual acuity. For those with visual deficits, large-print materials may be helpful. Educational materials and instructions should be available at no higher than the sixth-grade reading level. For patients who do not speak English or who speak English as a second language, many hospitals have educational materials available in Spanish and other regional languages. Interpreters may be necessary to help the interprofessional health care team customize the information appropriately.

Death in the Emergency Department. Not all critically ill or injured patients who come to the ED can be saved. Sometimes a patient's death is expected by family members, typically when they have dealt with a loved one's terminal condition or age-related decline. In other instances, a death in the ED is a sudden and unexpected event that produces a state of crisis and chaos for family and significant others. Emergency department staff members need to address the needs of the family members during this overwhelming time.

If resuscitation efforts are still under way when the family arrives, one or two family members may be given the opportunity to be present during lifesaving procedures. Family presence during resuscitation has gained wider acceptance in the health care community; however, a significant number of hospitals still have not devised clear policies or guidelines to facilitate family-witnessed resuscitation (Powers & Candela, 2017).

If the patient dies before family members arrive, ED staff members will usually prepare the body and the room for viewing by the family. However, certain types of ED deaths may require forensic investigation or become medical examiner's cases. Therefore, ED staff may not be able to remove IV lines and indwelling tubes or clean the patient's skin if these actions could potentially damage evidence. Trauma deaths, suspected homicide, or cases of abuse always fall into this category. In these situations, cover the body with a sheet or blanket while leaving the patient's face exposed and dim the lights before family viewing.

When dealing with family members in crisis, simple and concrete ***communication*** is best. Words such as *death* or *died,* although seemingly harsh, create less confusion than terms such as *expired* or *passed away.* Demonstrate caring, compassion, and empathy during all interactions, even in periods of heightened emotions. Intense grief can provoke a range of family reactions from silence to violence. If available, coordinate with crisis staff (security, social workers, or psychiatric nurses) to assist families and maintain ***safety*** during this time. Offer the family the option of speaking with clergy or calling someone of their choice for additional support. A family member may even need to be admitted to the ED to be treated for anxiety or physical signs and symptoms of stress such as chest pain, difficulty breathing, or severe headache.

Dealing with death is often difficult for ED personnel, especially during busy periods when the ability to console family members may be limited. In response, some EDs have developed bereavement committees that focus on meeting the needs of grieving families. Actions such as sending sympathy cards, attending funerals, making follow-up phone calls, and creating memory boxes are common. These actions facilitate ***communication*** of caring and compassion after the moment of crisis.

TRAUMA NURSING PRINCIPLES

The general public tends to use the term *trauma* to mean any type of crisis, ranging from a heart attack to psychological stress. Among health care professionals, **trauma** refers to bodily injury. In 2018 240,583 people in the United States died as a result of injuries and over 2 million were hospitalized, often with permanent and disabling consequences (Centers for Disease Control and Prevention [CDC] & National Center for Injury Prevention and Control [NCIPC], 2020). Injuries can be categorized as either intentional (i.e., assault, homicide, suicide) or unintentional (i.e., accidents). *Unintentional injury* such as poisoning or a motor vehicle crash is the leading cause of death for Americans younger than 35 years and is one of today's most significant public health problems (CDC & NCIPC, 2020).

Trauma nursing is a field that encompasses the continuum of care from injury prevention and prehospital services to acute care, rehabilitation, and ultimately community reintegration. Injury management is a key component of ED services. Approximately 22 million people in the United States visit the ED each year to receive treatment for nonfatal injuries (CDC & NCIPC, 2020). Therefore a core competency in general trauma care is an important part of emergency nursing practice. For emergency nurses who work in accredited trauma centers, opportunities typically exist to further develop expertise in trauma nursing through ongoing clinical practice, specialty training programs, and continuing education. One special skill practiced by trauma nurses that benefits survivors of trauma is that of **trauma-informed care (TIC)**. TIC is a model of care that ensures patient safety through four key practices: "realizing the widespread effect of trauma, recognizing the signs and symptoms of trauma, responding by fully integrating trauma knowledge into practices and procedures, and seeking to actively resist retraumatization" (National Center for Trauma-Informed Care and Alternatives to Seclusion and Restraint [NCTIC], 2018, in Li et al., 2019, p. 93). Practicing according to the model of trauma-informed care allows the nurse to better understand the patient's symptoms and behaviors based on what the patient experienced during and as a result of the trauma event (Li et al., 2019).

Trauma Centers and Trauma Systems

Trauma centers have their roots in military medicine. Injured soldiers who received rapid transport from the battlefield and treatment from skilled health care personnel had a survival advantage in the mobile army surgical hospital (MASH) units first deployed in the Korean and Vietnam wars. Consequently the MASH unit became the original model for the development of civilian trauma centers. In modern society the **trauma center** in the United States is a specialty care facility that provides competent and timely trauma services to patients, depending on its designated level of capability.

Trauma Centers. Not all EDs that offer around-the-clock emergency services are trauma centers. The American College of Surgeons Committee on Trauma (2020) has set forth national standards for trauma center accreditation and categorizes the resource requirements necessary for the highest-capability trauma center (Level I) to the lowest (Level IV) (Table 10.3).

A *Level I trauma center* is a regional resource facility that is capable of providing leadership and total collaborative care for every aspect of injury, from prevention through rehabilitation. These centers also have a responsibility to offer professional and community education programs, conduct research, and participate in system planning. Because a significant resource and

TABLE 10.3 Levels and Functions of Trauma Centers

Levels of Trauma Center	Functions of Trauma Center
Level I	Usually located in large teaching hospitals in densely populated areas Provides a full continuum of trauma services for adult and/or pediatric patients Conducting research is a requirement for trauma center verification
Level II and Level III	Both typically located in community hospitals **Level II** • Provides care to most injured patients • Transfers patient if needs exceed resource capabilities **Level III** • Stabilizes patients with major injuries • Transfers patient if needs exceed resource capabilities
Level IV	Usually located in rural and remote areas Provides basic trauma patient stabilization and advanced life support within resource capabilities Arranges transfer to higher trauma center levels as necessary

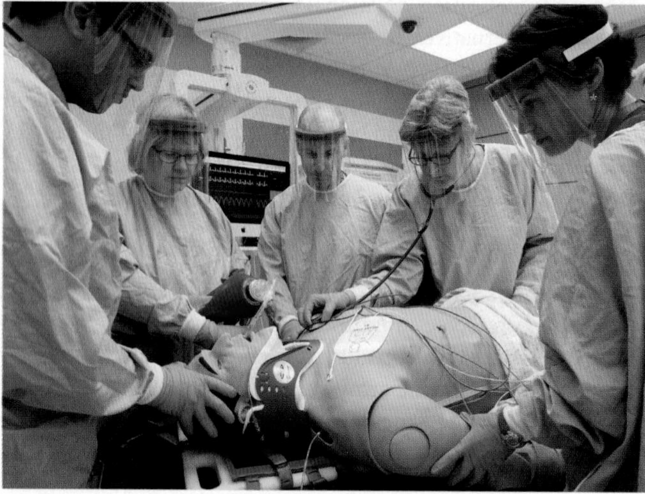

Fig. 10.5 A trauma team participates in a realistic trauma resuscitation simulation. This type of training ensures that staff remain proficient in skills and able to care for any situation that might occur in the emergency department.

experience commitment is required to maintain strict accreditation standards, Level I trauma centers are usually located in large teaching hospitals and serve dense population areas (Fig. 10.5).

Level II trauma centers are usually located in community hospitals and are capable of providing care to the vast majority of injured patients. However, a Level II trauma center may not be able to meet the resource needs of patients who require very complex or multisystem injury management. These people are generally transferred to a Level I trauma center for specialty care. In communities without a Level I trauma center, Level II centers play a significant leadership role in injury management, education, prevention, and emergency preparedness planning.

A *Level III trauma center* is a critical link to higher-capability trauma centers in communities that do not have ready access to Level I or II centers. The primary focus is initial injury stabilization and emergent patient transfer if necessary. Level III trauma centers are often found in smaller, rural hospitals and serve areas with lower population density. Because Level III trauma centers have general surgeons and orthopedic surgeons immediately available, patients with some major injuries may be admitted for care. However, if the injuries are severe or critical, transfer to a Level I or II trauma center occurs after ED assessment, resuscitation, and stabilization—sometimes after emergent, lifesaving surgery. Patients are typically transported out in either an advanced life support ambulance or a helicopter, with critical care transport personnel in attendance.

The function of a *Level IV trauma center* is to offer advanced life support care in rural or remote settings that do not have ready access to a higher-level trauma center such as a ski area. Patients are stabilized to the best degree possible before transfer, using available personnel such as advanced practice nurses, physician assistants, nurses, and paramedics. Resources, including the consistent availability of a physician, may be extremely limited. Transport time to the final care center can be prolonged because of both distance and weather conditions that may prevent transfer by air.

Level III and Level IV trauma centers establish close collaborative relationships with Level I and Level II trauma centers. Based on accreditation standards, care providers at Levels I and II trauma centers have a responsibility to readily accept injured patients in transfer. They provide timely feedback to trauma personnel at referring hospitals and share expertise by offering educational opportunities to advance trauma care delivery in the region. In addition, personnel from all levels of trauma centers participate in focused system improvement and patient safety initiatives that enhance quality of care and solve identified problems.

Trauma Systems. Trauma centers save lives, but a trauma center is only as good as the overall trauma system that supports it. A **trauma system** is an organized and integrated approach to trauma care designed to ensure that all critical elements of trauma care delivery are aligned to meet the injured patient's needs. These elements include (Cooper & Laskowski-Jones, 2006):

- Access to care through ***communication*** technology (e.g., an enhanced 911 service)
- Timely availability of prehospital emergency medical care
- Rapid transport to a qualified trauma center
- Early provision of rehabilitation services
- System-wide injury prevention, research, and education initiatives

The overall desired outcome of an organized trauma system is to enable an injured patient not only to recover from trauma but also to return to a productive role in society.

A well-functioning trauma system is also essential to general public health and ***safety***. It provides the structure necessary for disaster readiness and community emergency preparedness (see Chapter 12). Although most states in the United States now have at least some basic elements of a trauma system in place, gaps still exist in some regions.

Mechanism of Injury

The **mechanism of injury (MOI)** describes how the patient's traumatic event occurred, such as a high-speed motor vehicle crash, a fall from a standing height, or a gunshot wound to the torso. Knowing key details about the MOI can provide insight into the energy forces involved and may help trauma care providers predict injury types and, in some cases, patient outcomes. Prehospital care providers report the MOI as a ***communication*** standard when handing off care to ED and trauma personnel. Similarly, patients who come to the ED for medical care will often relate the MOI by describing the particular chain of events that caused their injuries.

Two of the most common injury-producing mechanisms are blunt trauma and penetrating trauma. **Blunt trauma** results from impact forces such as those sustained in a motor vehicle crash; a fall; or an assault with fists, kicks, or a baseball bat. **Blast effect** from an exploding bomb also causes blunt trauma. The energy transmitted from a blunt-trauma mechanism, particularly the rapid **acceleration-deceleration** forces involved in high-speed crashes or falls from a great height, produces injury by tearing, shearing, and compressing anatomic structures. Trauma to bones, blood vessels, and soft tissues occurs.

Penetrating trauma is caused by injury from sharp objects and projectiles. Examples are wounds from knives, ice picks, other comparable implements, and bullets (gunshot wounds [GSWs]) or pellets. Fragments of metal, glass, or other materials that become airborne in an explosion (shrapnel) can also produce penetrating trauma. Each mechanism has the risk for specific injury patterns and severity that the trauma team considers when planning diagnostic evaluation and management strategies. Certain injury mechanisms such as a gunshot wound to the chest or abdomen or a stab wound to the neck are so highly associated with life-threatening consequences that they automatically require trauma team intervention for a rapid and coordinated resuscitation response.

NCLEX EXAMINATION CHALLENGE 10.2

Safe and Effective Care Environment

What mechanism of injury will the nurse document for a client in a motor vehicle accident whose airbag deployed when the car struck a tree at 40 miles per hour? **Select all that apply.**

A. Blast
B. Blunt
C. Laceration
D. Penetration
E. Acceleration-deceleration

Primary Survey and Resuscitation Interventions

A basic tenet of emergency care in any environment is scene ***safety***. In the prehospital setting, emergency care providers must ensure that they are aware of any hazards that might pose a threat to rescuers and take actions to decrease or eliminate the risk. This same concept applies to the hospital ED setting. Before engaging in trauma resuscitation as a nurse member of the trauma team, keep in mind that there is a high risk for contamination with blood and body fluids. For this reason use Standard Precautions in *all* resuscitation situations and at other times when exposure to blood and body fluids is likely. Proper attire consists of an impervious cover gown, gloves, eye protection, a facemask, surgical cap, and shoe covers (if *significant* blood loss is anticipated such as during an ED thoracotomy).

The initial assessment of the trauma patient is called the **primary survey**, which is an organized framework used to rapidly identify and effectively manage immediate threats to life. The primary survey is typically based on a standard *ABC* mnemonic plus a *D* and an *E* for trauma patients: airway/cervical spine *(A)*; breathing *(B)*; circulation *(C)*; disability *(D)*; and exposure *(E)*. Resuscitation efforts occur simultaneously with each element of the primary survey (Emergency Nurses Association, 2020). Even though the resuscitation team may encounter multiple clinical problems or injuries, issues identified in the primary survey are managed before the team engages in interventions of lower priority such as splinting fractures and dressing wounds.

There is one notable exception to the standard *ABCDE* trauma resuscitation approach. Lessons learned from the military and continued research have made it clear that in the presence of massive, uncontrolled external bleeding, hemorrhage control techniques are the highest-priority intervention (Ferrada et al, 2018; Emergency Nurses Association, 2020). In this situation, the sequence of priorities shifts to *CAB* (circulation, airway, breathing), whereby the initial focus of resuscitation is to effectively stop the active bleeding (Emergency Nurses Association, 2020).

A: Airway/Cervical Spine. Even minutes without an adequate oxygen supply can lead to brain injury that can progress to anoxic brain death. Establishing a patent airway is the highest-priority intervention when managing a trauma patient unless massive, life-threatening external hemorrhage as described previously is present.

! NURSING SAFETY PRIORITY (QSEN)

Critical Rescue

Recognize that you must clear the airway of any secretions or debris with a suction catheter or manually if necessary. Respond by protecting the trauma patient's cervical spine by manually aligning the neck in a neutral, in-line position and using a jaw-thrust maneuver when establishing an airway. Provide supplemental oxygen as ordered for patients who require resuscitation.

A nonrebreather mask is generally best for the spontaneously breathing patient. Bag-valve-mask (BVM) ventilation with the appropriate airway adjunct and a 100% oxygen source is indicated for the person who needs ventilatory assistance during resuscitation. A patient with significantly impaired consciousness (Glasgow Coma Scale [GCS] score of 3 to 8, which is indicative of severe head injury) requires an endotracheal tube and mechanical ventilation (Emergency Nurses Association, 2020).

B: Breathing. After the airway has been successfully secured, breathing becomes the next priority in the primary survey. *This assessment determines whether or not ventilatory efforts are effective—not only whether or not the patient is breathing.* Listen to breath sounds and evaluate chest expansion, respiratory effort, and any evidence of chest wall trauma or physical abnormalities. Both apneic patients and those with poor ventilatory effort need BVM ventilation for support until endotracheal intubation is performed and a mechanical ventilator is used. If cardiopulmonary resuscitation (CPR) becomes necessary, the mechanical ventilator is disconnected, and the patient is manually ventilated with a BVM device. Lung compliance can be assessed through sensing the degree of difficulty in ventilating the patient with the BVM.

C: Circulation. When effective ventilation is ensured, the priority shifts to circulation. The adequacy of heart rate, blood pressure, and overall perfusion becomes the focus of the assessment. Common threats to circulation include cardiac arrest, myocardial dysfunction, and hemorrhage leading to a shock state. Interventions are targeted at restoring effective circulation through cardiopulmonary resuscitation, hemorrhage control, IV vascular access with fluid and blood administration as necessary, and drug therapy. *External* hemorrhage is usually quite obvious and best controlled with firm, direct pressure on the bleeding site with thick, dry dressing material. This method is effective in decreasing blood flow for most wounds. *Tourniquets that occlude arterial blood flow distal to the injury should be used to manage severe, compressible bleeding from extremity trauma when direct pressure fails to achieve hemorrhage control; wound packing and the use of hemostatic dressings (e.g., dressings impregnated with substances that speed the formation of a blood clot) are other essential methods to manage life-threatening hemorrhage. Internal* hemorrhage is a less obvious complication that must be suspected in injured patients or in those in a shock state.

In a resuscitation situation systolic blood pressure (BP) can be quickly and easily estimated before a manual cuff pressure can be obtained by palpating for the presence or absence of peripheral and central pulses:

- Presence of a radial pulse: BP at least 80 mm Hg systolic
- Presence of a femoral pulse: BP at least 70 mm Hg systolic
- Presence of a carotid pulse: BP at least 60 mm Hg systolic

By the time hypotension occurs, compensatory mechanisms used by the body in an attempt to maintain vital signs in a shock state have been exhausted. Timely, effective intervention is critical to preserve life and vital organ function.

IV access is best achieved initially with insertion of large-bore (16-gauge) peripheral IV lines in the antecubital area (inside bend of the elbow). Additional access can be obtained via central veins in the femoral, subclavian, or jugular sites using large-bore (8.5 Fr) central venous catheters. Intraosseous access is an excellent initial approach for critically ill patients when veins cannot be rapidly accessed by the resuscitation team (see Chapter 15 for discussion of intraosseous infusion therapy). Ringer's lactate and 0.9% normal saline (NS) are the crystalloid solutions of choice for resuscitation; hypertonic saline may also be prescribed in some situations, particularly in the case of head trauma. Fluids and blood products should be warmed before administration, to prevent hypothermia. Anticipate the need for rapid blood component administration in a hemorrhagic shock state using packed red blood cells, fresh frozen plasma, and platelets to both replace blood loss and prevent coagulopathy. However, the priority intervention is always to stop the bleeding.

D: Disability. The disability examination provides a rapid baseline assessment of neurologic status. A simple method to evaluate level of consciousness is the *AVPU* mnemonic:

- *A:* **A**lert
- *V:* Responsive to **v**oice
- *P:* Responsive to **p**ain
- *U:* **U**nresponsive

Another common way of determining and documenting level of consciousness is the **Glasgow Coma Scale (GCS)**, an assessment that scores eye opening, verbal response, and motor response. The lowest score is 3, which indicates a totally unresponsive patient; a normal GCS score is 15. Metabolic abnormalities (e.g., severe hypoglycemia), hypoxia, neurologic injury, and illicit drugs or alcohol can impair level of consciousness. Frequent reassessment is needed for rapid intervention in the event of neurologic compromise or deterioration.

E: Exposure. The final component of the primary survey is exposure. If evidence preservation is needed, handle items per institutional policy. Evidence may include articles of clothing, impaled objects, weapons, drugs, and bullets. Emergency nurses are often called on to provide testimony in court regarding their recall of the presentation and treatment of patients in the ED. Examples of types of cases in which evidence collection is vital are rape, abuse of a child or older adult, domestic violence, homicide, suicide, drug overdose, and assault.

! NURSING SAFETY PRIORITY (QSEN)

Action Alert

Remove all clothing to allow for thorough assessment. Always carefully cut away clothing with scissors:

- During resuscitation when rapid access to the patient's body is critical
- When manipulating a patient's limbs to remove clothing could cause further injury
- When thermal or chemical burns have caused fabrics to melt into the patient's skin

Once clothing has been removed, hypothermia (body temperature less than or equal to 96.8°F [36°C]) poses a risk to injured patients (Saqe-Rockoff et al., 2018), especially those with burns and traumatic shock states. Hypothermia is discussed in detail in Chapter 11.

Table 10.4 highlights the primary survey and associated resuscitation interventions.

NCLEX EXAMINATION CHALLENGE 10.3

Safe and Effective Care Environment

On entry to the ED of a client who fell from a roof, what is the nurse's **priority** action?

A. Place nasal cannula to administer oxygen.
B. Apply pressure to small bleeding wounds.
C. Assess airway and stabilize cervical spine.
D. Initiate large-bore IV to infuse normal saline.

TABLE 10.4 The Primary Survey and Resuscitation Interventions

Priorities of the Primary Survey	Examples of Specific Interventions
A: Airway/cervical spine	Establish a patent airway by positioning, suctioning, and administering oxygen as needed. Protect the cervical spine by maintaining alignment; use a jaw-thrust maneuver if there is a risk for spinal injury. If the Glasgow Coma Scale (GCS) score is 8 or lower or the patient is at risk for airway compromise, prepare for endotracheal intubation and mechanical ventilation.
B: Breathing	Assess breath sounds and respiratory effort. Observe for chest wall trauma or other physical abnormality. Prepare for chest decompression if needed. Prepare to assist ventilations if needed.
C: Circulation	Monitor vital signs, especially blood pressure and pulse. Maintain vascular access with a large-bore catheter. Use direct pressure for external bleeding; anticipate need for a tourniquet for severe, uncontrollable extremity hemorrhage, wound packing, and/or use of a hemostatic dressing.
D: Disability	Evaluate the patient's level of consciousness (LOC) using the GCS. Re-evaluate the patient's LOC frequently.
E: Exposure	Remove all clothing for a complete physical assessment. Prevent hypothermia (e.g., cover the patient with blankets, use heating devices, infuse warm solutions).

The Secondary Survey and Resuscitation Interventions

After the ED resuscitation team has addressed the immediate life threats, other activities that the emergency nurse can anticipate include insertion of a gastric tube for decompression of the GI tract to prevent vomiting and aspiration, insertion of a urinary catheter to allow careful measure of urine output, and preparation for diagnostic studies. The resuscitation team also performs a more comprehensive head-to-toe assessment, known as the secondary survey, to identify other injuries or medical issues that need to be managed or that might affect the course of treatment. Splints will be applied to fractured extremities, and temporary dressings will be placed over wounds while the patient undergoes diagnostic testing or preparation for more definitive management.

Disposition

The patient may be transported immediately to the operating room or interventional radiology suite directly from the ED, depending on the nature of the injury. When no immediate procedural intervention is indicated, patients are admitted to inpatient units for management and nursing care based on the nature and severity of their injuries and any other pre-existing medical conditions that could complicate trauma care. However, if the facility does not have the resource capabilities to manage the injured patient, the provider arranges for transfer to a higher level of care at a trauma center.

After the immediate health need has been addressed, and before the patient's disposition is determined, you should also thoroughly assess psychosocial needs. Work in collaboration with the interprofessional team to address the trauma patient's complex care needs, including early consultation with social services and the rehabilitation team. Coordinate with other support services as necessary such as pastoral care, nutrition support, psychiatry, mental health/behavioral health specialists, and substance abuse counselors.

Be alert for any signs of human trafficking, which affects more than 20 million people globally, with up to 80% of the victims being seen by a health care provider while under the trafficker's control (Byrne et al., 2017). This practice of sexual exploitation is a type of modern-day slavery in which the victim is forced or coerced to provide sex to others in exchange for money or valuables that are given to the trafficker. Nurses must be aware that patients seen for recurrent sexually transmitted infections (STIs), pregnancy tests, and abortions may be victims of human trafficking. Physical signs of trafficking include headaches, dizziness, back pain, missing patches of hair (where it has been pulled out), burns, bruises, vaginal or rectal trauma, jaw problems, and head injuries. The victim may also have unusual tattooing or "branding" marks, which are a sign of trafficker ownership. Psychosocial symptoms experienced by victims include stress, paranoia, fear, suicidal ideation, depression, anxiety, shame, and self-loathing (Scannell et al., 2018). The patient may be unable to verify a home address, deny having finances, and defer to the controlling presence of an individual who has accompanied them to the ED (Murray & Smith, 2019). You can assess the patient by asking questions such as, "Do you feel free to come and go anywhere as you please?", "Does anyone you work for make you feel unsafe?", and "Have you ever felt like you cannot leave your employer?" (Office on Trafficking in Persons, 2017). If you suspect that a patient is a trafficking victim, follow agency policy, contact local authorities, and report to the National Human Trafficking Resource Center.

Trauma centers are required to incorporate systems to identify patients with high-risk alcohol use (American College of Surgeons Committee on Trauma, 2020). An effective strategy is to implement an SBIRT (*s*creening, *b*rief *i*ntervention, and *r*eferral to *t*reatment) program in which interprofessional trauma team members, including emergency and trauma nurses, are educated to assess patients for problem drinking. The typical interaction involves a brief, respectful conversation that offers feedback, counsel, and motivation to reduce alcohol consumption.

Consider the needs of caregivers and loved ones in crisis and address them when planning nursing care. A trauma advanced practice nurse, if available, can help coordinate trauma care by offering clinical expertise; facilitating ***communication*** among caregivers; and serving as an educator for the patient, staff, and family. He or she can organize family meetings with the interprofessional team and arrange for necessary resources. If this resource is not available, a case manager or specially educated direct-care nurse may perform these functions.

GET READY FOR THE NEXT-GENERATION NCLEX® EXAMINATION!

Key Points

Review these Key Points for each NCLEX Examination Client Needs Category.

Safe and Effective Care Environment

- Emergency departments (EDs) are fast-paced, often crowded environments where the interprofessional team cares for patients with a variety of health problems across the life span. **QSEN: Teamwork and Collaboration**
- Vulnerable populations who seek ED care include older adults and patients who are uninsured or underinsured, economically disadvantaged, or homeless. **Health Care Disparities**
- Patients commonly seek ED care for chest or abdominal pain, difficulty breathing, injury, headache, fever, and generalized pain. **QSEN: Safety**
- Members of the interprofessional team collaborate at all points of emergency care. **QSEN: Teamwork and Collaboration**
- ED nurses are accountable for preventing or reducing risks such as falls, medication errors, pressure injuries, and hospital-acquired infections. **QSEN: Safety**
- Core competencies for ED nurses include patient assessment, priority setting, clinical decision making, documentation, communication, and a sound cognitive knowledge base. **QSEN: Safety**
- The three-level triage model categorizes patients as emergent, urgent, and nonurgent (see Table 10.2). **QSEN: Safety**
- Trauma centers are categorized as Levels I through IV, based on their resource capabilities as listed in Table 10.3. **QSEN: Safety**
- Two common injury-producing mechanisms are blunt trauma and penetrating trauma. **QSEN: Safety**
- Prioritize resuscitation interventions based on the primary survey of the injured patient as outlined in Table 10.4. **QSEN: Safety**

Psychosocial Integrity

- Collaborate with the behavioral health crisis team as needed. **QSEN: Teamwork and Collaboration**

Physiological Integrity

- The expected sequence of events in the ED includes (1) treatment, (2) stabilization, and (3) discharge or admission. **QSEN: Safety**
- Older adults who visit the ED are frequently admitted to the hospital. **QSEN: Patient-Centered Care**
- ***Communication*** with the older adult may be challenging if the patient has memory loss or acute delirium while in the ED. **QSEN: Patient-Centered Care**

MASTERY QUESTIONS

1. What is the nurse's **priority** action for the unconscious patient who is breathing who has been brought to the ED?
   A. Assess breath sounds and respiratory efforts
   B. Establish vascular access with a large-bore catheter
   C. Remove clothing to perform a complete physical assessment
   D. Evaluate level of consciousness (LOC) using the Glasgow Coma Sale (GCS)
2. After assessing four clients, which will the triage nurse identify to be seen first in the ED?
   A. Client with fever of 101.2°F
   B. Client who reports slurred speech
   C. Client who reports bilateral ear pain
   D. Client with urinary burning and frequency

REFERENCES

Asterisk (*) indicates a classic or definitive work on this subject.

American College of Surgeons Committee on Trauma. (2020). *Clarification document: Resources for optimal care of the injured patient, Version 21*. Chicago: Author. Retrieved from https://www.facs.org/~/media/files/quality%20programs/trauma/vrc%20resources/clarification_document.ashx.

Bodenmann, P., Velonaki, V. S., Griffin, J. L., Baggio, S., Iglesias, K., Moschetti, K., … & Schupbach, J. (2017). Case management may reduce emergency department frequent use in a universal health coverage system: a randomized controlled trial. *Journal of General Internal Medicine, 32*(5), 508–515.

Byrne, M., Parsh, B., & Ghilain, C. (2017). Victims of human trafficking: Hiding in plain sight. *Nursing, 47*(3), 49–52.

Centers for Disease Control and Prevention (CDC). (2017). *FastStats: Emergency department visits*. https://www.cdc.gov/nchs/fastats/emergency-department.htm.

Centers for Disease Control and Prevention (CDC) and National Center for Injury Prevention and Control. (NCIPC). (2020). *Injury prevention and control: Data & statistics (WISQARS)*. Retrieved from https://www.cdc.gov/injury/wisqars/index.html.

*Cooper, G., & Laskowski-Jones, L. (2006). Development of trauma care systems. *Prehospital Emergency Care, 10*(3), 328–331.

Dippenaar, E., & Bruijns, S. (2016). Triage is easy, said no triage nurse ever. *International Emergency Nursing, 29*, 1–2.

Emergency Nurses Association. (2020). *Trauma nursing core course* (8th ed.). Burlington, MA: Jones & Bartlett Learning.

Ferrada, P., et al. (2018). Circulation first – The time has come to question the sequencing of care in the ABCs of trauma; An American Association for the Surgery of Trauma multicenter trial. *World*

Journal of Emergency Surgery, 23(8). https://doi.org/10.1186/s13017-018-0168-3.

International Association of Forensic Nurses. (2019). Retrieved from https://www.forensicnurses.org.

*Laskowski-Jones, L. (2008). Change management at the hospital front door: Integrating automatic patient tracking in a high volume emergency department and Level I trauma center. *Nurse Leader, 6*(2), 52–57.

Lavoie, P., & Clark, S. P. (2017). Simulation in nursing education. *Nursing, 47*(7), 18–20. https://doi.org/10.1016/j.ienj.2016.09.005.

Li, Y., et al. (2019). Current state of trauma-informed education in the health sciences: Lessons for nursing. *Journal of Nursing Education, 58*(2), 93–101.

McEnroe-Petitte, D., (2020). *Caring for patients who are homeless. Nursing 2020, 50*(3), 24–29.

Morley, C., Unwin, M., Peterson, G. M., Stankovich, J., & Kinsman, L. (2018). Emergency department crowding: A systematic review of causes, consequences and solutions. *PLoS ONE, 13*(8), e0203316. https://doi.org/10.1371/journal.pone.0203316.

Murray, A., & Smith, L., (2019). Implementing evidence-based care for women who have experienced human trafficking. *Nursing for Women's Health, 23*(2), 98–104.

National Center for Trauma-Informed Care and Alternatives to Seclusion and Restraint. (2018). *Trauma-informed approach and trauma-specific interventions.* Retrieved from https://www.samhsa.gov/nctic/trauma-interventions.

Office on Trafficking in Persons. (2017). *Human trafficking webinar for health care providers: SOAR to Health and Wellness.* Retrieved from https://www.acf.hhs.gov/archive/otip/resource/soarhealthcare.

Powers, K. A., & Candela, L. (2017). Nursing practice and policies related to family presence during resuscitation. *Dimensions of Critical Care Nursing, 36*(1), 53–59. https://doi.org/10.1097/DDC.0000000000000218.

RHIhub. (2019). *Critical access hospitals (CAHs).* Retrieved from https://www.ruralhealthinfo.org/topics/critical-access-hospitals.

Saqe-Rockoff, A., Schubert, F. D., Ciardiello, A., & Douglas, E. (2018). Improving thermoregulation for trauma patients in the emergency department: An evidence-based practice project. *Journal of Trauma Nursing, 25*(1), 14–20. https://doi.org/10.1097/JTN.0000000000000336.

Scannell, M., MacDonald, A. E., Berger, A., & Boyer, N. (2018). Human trafficking: How nurses can make a difference. *Journal of Forensic Nursing, 14*, 117–121. https://doi.org/10.1097/JFN.0000000000000203.

*Shelton, R. (2010). ESI: A better triage system? *Nursing Critical Care, 5*(6), 34–37.

Stevenson, E., & Purpuro, T. (2018). Homeless people: Nursing care with dignity. *Nursing, 48*(6), 58–62.

Sweet, V. (Ed.). (2018). *Emergency nursing core curriculum* (7th ed.). Emergency Nurses Association. St. Louis: Elsevier.

The Joint Commission (TJC). (2020). *National Patient Safety Goals.* Retrieved from https://www.jointcommission.org/-/media/tjc/documents/standards/national-patient-safety-goals/2020/simplified_2020-hap-npsgs-eff-july-final.pdf.

The Joint Commission (TJC). (2017). *Sentinel event alert: Inadequate handoff communication.* Retrieved from https://www.jointcommission.org/assets/1/18/SEA_58_Hand_off_Comms_9_6_17_FINAL_(1).pdf.

Touhy, T. A., & Jett, K. (2019). *Ebersole & Hess' toward healthy aging: Human needs and nursing response* (10th ed.). St. Louis: Mosby.

U.S. Department of Housing and Urban Development. (2020). *The 2019 annual homeless assessment report (AHAR) to Congress.* Retrieved from https://www.hudexchange.info/resources/documents/2018-AHAR-Part-1.pdf.

11

Concepts of Care for Patients With Common Environmental Emergencies

Linda Laskowski-Jones

http://evolve.elsevier.com/Iggy/

LEARNING OUTCOMES

1. Collaborate with the interprofessional health care team when providing care for patients with environmental emergencies.
2. Teach people at risk how to prevent environmental emergencies.
3. Prioritize first aid/prehospital interventions for patients who have thermoregulation problems, arthropod bites or stings, or venomous snake bites affecting ***tissue integrity*** and ***pain.***
4. Apply knowledge of pathophysiology to identify best practices for care of patients with environmental emergencies.
5. Create an evidence-based plan of care for patients who have experienced an environmental emergency.

KEY TERMS

acclimatization The process of adapting to a high altitude; involves physiologic changes that help the body compensate for less available oxygen in the atmosphere.

acute mountain sickness (AMS) A condition that affects individuals at high altitudes due to lower air pressure and lower oxygen levels.

classic heat stroke A form of heat stroke in which the body's ability to dissipate heat is significantly impaired; occurs over time as a result of long-term exposure to a hot, humid environment such as a home without air-conditioning in the high heat of the summer.

climate action Taking active measures to mitigate (lessen the effect of) and adapt to circumstances, and foster resilience in persons who are affected by actions that are a result of climate change.

climate change Global phenomena resulting from weather pattern alterations and burning of fossil fuels that result in weather extremes.

exertional heat stroke A form of heat stroke with a sudden onset, typically due to strenuous physical activity in hot, humid conditions. Lack of acclimatization to hot weather and wearing clothing too heavy for the environment are common contributing factors.

frostbite A cold injury characterized by the degree of tissue freezing and the resultant damage it produces. Frostbite injuries can be superficial, partial, or full thickness.

frostnip A form of superficial frostbite (typically on the face, fingers, or toes) that produces pain, numbness, and pallor but is easily remedied with the application of warmth and does not induce tissue injury.

heat exhaustion A syndrome primarily caused by dehydration from heavy perspiration and inadequate fluid and electrolyte consumption during heat exposure over hours to days; if left untreated, can be a precursor to heat stroke.

heat stroke A true medical emergency in which the victim's heat regulatory mechanisms fail and are unable to compensate for a critical elevation in body temperature; if uncorrected, organ dysfunction and death will ensue.

high-altitude cerebral edema (HACE) A form of acute mountain sickness, often seen with high-altitude pulmonary edema (HAPE), in which fluid accumulates on the brain. Signs and symptoms include confusion, clumsiness, stumbling, excessive emotion or violence, and drowsiness and loss of consciousness before death.

high-altitude disease (HAD) See *high-altitude illnesses.*

high-altitude illnesses Pathophysiologic responses in the body caused by exposure to low partial pressure of oxygen at high elevations.

high-altitude pulmonary edema (HAPE) A form of acute mountain sickness often seen with high-altitude cerebral edema (HACE). Signs and symptoms include persistent dry cough, cyanosis of the lips and nail beds, tachycardia and tachypnea at rest, and fever. Pink, frothy sputum is a late sign.

hyperemia Increased blood flow to an area.

hypocapnia Decreased arterial carbon dioxide levels.

hypothermia A core body temperature less than 95° F (35° C).

Lichtenberg figures Branching or feathering marks that appear on the skin as a result of a lightning strike. Also called *keraunographic markings* or *erythematous arborization.*

rhabdomyolysis The breakdown or disintegration of muscle tissue; associated with excretion of myoglobin in the urine.

PRIORITY AND INTERRELATED CONCEPTS

The priority concepts for this chapter are:
- ***Tissue Integrity***
- ***Pain***

Health conditions, and thus life span and social determinants of health, are influenced by environmental issues such as food and water insecurities or contamination, air quality, and vector-borne diseases (Leffers et al, 2017). Nurses must recognize those vulnerable to these factors when considering the influence of the environment on health. Vulnerable populations include people of color, those who have low income, immigrants, children, pregnant women, older adults, those with disabilities or chronic health conditions, and those who work in certain occupations (McDermott-Levy et al, 2019).

Climate norms and changes also can affect the health of individuals and populations. For example, temperature extremes affect health, particularly for those who do not have access to proper heat or air-conditioning. If travel is affected, nutrition can be compromised. Displacement due to floods and wildfires that have resulted from **climate change**—global phenomena resulting from weather pattern alterations and the burning of fossil fuels that result in weather extremes—affects physical and mental health (McDermott-Levy et al).

When nurses are aware of the effect of climate change on health, they can be part of **climate action**, which involves taking active measures to mitigate (lessen the effect of) and adapt to circumstances. The nurse can also help to foster resilience in patients who are affected by circumstances that are a result of climate change.

Climate also influences the recreational activities that bring enjoyment to the lives of people who leave their homes. There are activities that, although seemingly harmless, can have environmental risks, especially for older adults. Some bites, stings, and environmental conditions also pose concerns when people are indoors. This chapter provides an overview of selected environmental emergencies, their initial emergency management (first aid), and acute care interventions.

HEAT-RELATED ILLNESSES

The most common environmental factors causing heat-related illnesses are high environmental temperature (above 95°F [35°C]) and high humidity (above 80%). Conditions related to this problem with thermoregulation include heat exhaustion and heat stroke. Some of the most vulnerable, at-risk populations for these problems are older adults (who have less body fluid volume and can easily become dehydrated), people with mental health/behavioral health conditions, those who work outside, homeless individuals, those who use substances, athletes who engage in outdoor sports, and military members stationed in hot climates.

Conditions such as obesity, heart disease, fever, infection, strenuous exercise, seizures, mental health disorders, and all degrees of burns (even sunburn) can increase the risk for heat-related illness. The use of prescribed drugs such as lithium, neuroleptics, beta-adrenergic blockers, anticholinergics, angiotensin-converting enzyme (ACE) inhibitors, and diuretics have also been shown to increase the risk.

Health Promotion and Maintenance

Teach adults how to take steps to eliminate or minimize risks before participating in any hot weather activity. Ask them to have a family member, friend, or neighbor check on them several times each day to ensure that there are no signs of heat-related illness. The Patient-Centered Care: Older Adult Considerations: Heat-Related Illness Prevention box lists other essential heat-related illness prevention strategies for older adults, many of which apply to adults of any age.

PATIENT-CENTERED CARE: OLDER ADULT CONSIDERATIONS

Heat-Related Illness Prevention

- Avoid alcohol and caffeine.
- Prevent overexposure to the sun; use a sunscreen with an SPF of at least 30 with UVA and UVB protection.
- Rest frequently and take breaks from being in a hot environment. Plan to limit activity at the hottest time of day.
- Wear clothing suited to the environment. Lightweight, light-colored, and loose-fitting clothing is best.
- Pay attention to personal physical limitations; modify activities accordingly and take the time necessary to properly acclimate to a hot environment (typically 2 weeks).
- Take cool baths or showers to help reduce body temperature.
- Stay indoors in air-conditioned buildings if possible.
- Ask a neighbor, friend, or family member to check on the older adult at least twice a day during a heat wave.

SPF, Sun protection factor; *UVA*, ultraviolet A; *UVB*, ultraviolet B.

HEAT EXHAUSTION

Pathophysiology Review

Heat exhaustion is a syndrome resulting primarily from dehydration. It is caused by heavy perspiration and inadequate fluid and electrolyte intake during heat exposure over hours to days. Profuse diaphoresis can lead to profound, even fatal, dehydration and hyponatremia caused by excessive sodium lost in perspiration. *If untreated, heat exhaustion can lead to heat stroke, which is a true medical emergency that has a very high mortality rate.*

❖ Interprofessional Collaborative Care

Patients with heat exhaustion usually have flulike symptoms with headache, weakness, nausea, and/or vomiting. Body temperature may not be significantly elevated in this condition. The patient may continue to perspire despite dehydration.

! NURSING SAFETY PRIORITY (QSEN)

Action Alert

Patients should be assessed for orthostatic hypotension and tachycardia, especially the older adult who can dehydrate quickly. Older adults with dehydration often experience acute confusion and are at risk for falls.

Instruct the patient to immediately stop physical activity and move to a cool place. Use cooling measures such as placing cold packs on the neck, chest, abdomen, and groin. Soak the individual in cool water or fan while spraying water on the skin. Remove constrictive clothing. Sports drinks or an oral rehydration-therapy solution can be provided. Mistakenly drinking plain water can worsen the sodium deficit. *Do not give salt tablets,* which can cause stomach irritation, nausea, and vomiting. If signs and symptoms persist, call an ambulance to transport the patient to the hospital.

In the clinical setting, monitor vital signs. Rehydrate the patient with intravenous solution as prescribed if nausea or vomiting persists. Draw blood for serum electrolyte analysis. Hospital admission is indicated only for patients who have other health problems that are worsened by the heat-related illness or for those with severe dehydration and evidence of physiologic compromise. The management of hypovolemic dehydration is discussed in more detail in Chapter 13.

HEAT STROKE

Pathophysiology Review

Heat stroke is a *medical emergency* in which body temperature may exceed 104°F (40°C). It has a high mortality rate if not treated in a timely manner. The victim's thermoregulation mechanisms fail and cannot adjust for a critical elevation in body temperature. If the condition is not treated or the patient does not respond to treatment, organ dysfunction and death can result.

Exertional heat stroke has a sudden onset and is often the result of strenuous physical activity (especially when wearing too heavy clothing) in hot, humid conditions. **Classic heat stroke**, also referred to as *nonexertional heat stroke,* occurs over a period of time as a result of chronic exposure to a hot, humid environment such as living in a home without air conditioning in the high heat of summer.

❖ Interprofessional Collaborative Care

◆ **Assessment: Recognize Cues.** Victims of heat stroke have a profoundly elevated body temperature (above 104°F [40°C]). Although the patient's skin is hot and dry, the presence of sweating does not rule out heat stroke—people with heat stroke may continue to perspire.

Mental status changes occur as a result of thermal injury to the brain and are the hallmark findings in heat stroke. *Key Features: Heat Stroke* demonstrates common signs and symptoms of this condition. Cardiac troponin I (cTnI) is frequently elevated during nonexertional heat-related illnesses; research indicates that this test can be used to cost effectively predict severity and organ damage at the beginning of heat stroke, even in a remote setting (Knoll et al., 2019; Ramirez et al., 2018).

◆ **Interventions: Take Action.** Coordinate with the interprofessional health care team to recognize and treat immediately and aggressively to achieve optimal patient outcomes. The Best Practice for Patient Safety & Quality Care: Emergency Care of the Patient With Heat Stroke: Restoring Thermoregulation box lists evidence-based emergency care of patients with heat stroke.

KEY FEATURES
Heat Stroke

- Body temperature more than 104°F (40°C)
- Hot and dry skin; may or may not perspire
- Mental status changes such as:
  - Acute confusion
  - Bizarre behavior
  - Anxiety
  - Loss of coordination
  - Hallucinations
  - Agitation
  - Seizures
  - Coma
- Vital sign changes, including:
  - Hypotension
  - Tachycardia
  - Tachypnea (increased respiratory rate)
- Electrolyte imbalances, especially sodium and potassium
- Decreased renal function (oliguria)
- Coagulopathy (abnormal clotting)
- Pulmonary edema (crackles)

BEST PRACTICE FOR PATIENT SAFETY & QUALITY CARE (QSEN)
Emergency Care of the Patient With Heat Stroke: Restoring Thermoregulation

At the Scene

- Ensure a patent airway.
- Remove the patient from the hot environment (into air-conditioning or into the shade).
- Contact emergency medical services to transport the patient to the emergency department.
- Remove the patient's clothing.
- Pour or spray cold water on the patient's body and scalp.
- Fan the patient (not only the person providing care, but all surrounding people should fan the patient with newspapers or whatever is available).
- If available, place ice in cloth or bags and position the packs on the patient's scalp, in the groin area, behind the neck, and in the armpits.
- If immediate immersion in cold water is possible, support the patient in the water for rapid cooling and protect the patient's airway. (Note: this is the best method to treat heat stroke.)

At the Hospital

- Give oxygen by mask or nasal cannula; be prepared for endotracheal intubation.
- Start at least one IV with a large-bore needle or cannula.
- Administer fluids as prescribed, using cooled solutions if available.
- Use a cooling blanket.
- Obtain baseline laboratory tests as quickly as possible: urinalysis, serum electrolytes, cardiac enzymes, liver enzymes, and complete blood count (CBC).
- Do not administer aspirin or any other antipyretics.
- Insert a rectal probe to measure core body temperature continuously or use a rectal thermometer and assess temperature every 15 minutes.
- Insert an indwelling urinary drainage catheter.
- Monitor vital signs frequently as clinically indicated.
- Assess arterial blood gases.
- Administer muscle relaxants or benzodiazepines as prescribed if the patient begins to shiver.
- Measure and monitor urine output and specific gravity to determine fluid needs.
- Stop cooling interventions when core body temperature is reduced to 102°F (39°C).

EVIDENCE-BASED PRACTICE QSEN

What Does Evidence Say About Cold Injuries of Veterans?

Young, C., Conard, P. L., Armstrong, M. L., & Lacy, D. (2018). Older military veteran care: Many still believe they are forgotten. *Journal of Holistic Nursing, 36*(3), 291–300.

Since the advent of professional nursing that began with Florence Nightingale, nurses have cared for holistic needs of patients by addressing physiologic, psychosocial, developmental, sociocultural, and spiritual needs. Veterans have unique needs based on the conditions they experienced under which they served their country; some served in regions of extreme hot or cold that have left physiologic and psychologic scars. This study investigated specific types of injuries encountered by certain populations of veterans and also explored the perception that veterans reported of being forgotten by the health care system. Nurses must recognize the impact of these physiologic conditions, and these psychologic perceptions, and be prepared to respond with evidence-based care and compassion to needs that these veterans experience today.

Those who served in the Korean War are much more prone to cold-related injuries and disabilities than veterans who served in other conflicts. In one major assault during the first year of the Korean War from 1950 into 1951, temperatures plummeted to −50° F, with a wind chill factor of −100° F (U.S. Department of Veterans Affairs, 2020). Without adequate protection from the environment, some troops died before treatment could be sought (Wright, 2013). This event accounted for 16% of the U.S. Army's injuries sustained outside of the actual battle field, requiring evacuation from Korea of over 5,000 U.S. troops who experienced cold injuries (U.S. Department of Veterans Affairs, 2015) such as frostbite, hypothermia, and immersion foot—an injury experienced when the foot is wet for prolonged period of time.

Additional References

U.S. Department of Veterans Affairs. (2015). Public health: Cold injuries. Retrieved from https://www.publichealth.va.gov/PUBLICHEALTH/exposures/cold-injuries/index.asp

Wright, J. (2013, July 23). What we learned from the Korean War. Atlantic. Retrieved from https://www.theatlantic.com/international/archive/2013/07/what-we-learnedfrom-the-korean-war/278016/

Level of Evidence: 3

This article reflects evidence from numerous descriptive and qualitative studies.

Commentary: Implications for Practice and Research

As these veterans have grown older and developed other conditions such as diabetes and peripheral vascular disease, they are likely to experience extremity stiffness, pain and/or numbness, and skin cancer in areas of frostbite scars. They are also at higher risk for amputations due to these comorbid conditions. Strengths of this review of the literature include the numerous resources reviewed in the creation of this article. A weakness could be the level of evidence, but this is outweighed by the importance of veterans' health issues that are continuing to arise as the population ages. The key nursing implication from this evidence is that nurses must recognize conditions that have arisen based on the patient's military service and address these as part of holistic care.

! NURSING SAFETY PRIORITY QSEN

Critical Rescue

After ensuring that the patient has a patent airway, effective breathing, and adequate circulation, recognize that you must use rapid cooling as the first priority of care. Respond by implementing methods for rapid cooling, which include removing clothing; placing ice packs on the neck, axillae, chest, and groin; immersing the patient or wetting the patient's body with cold water; and fanning rapidly to aid in evaporative cooling.

First Aid/Prehospital Care. Do not give food or liquid by mouth because vomiting and aspiration are risks in patients with neurologic impairment. Immediate medical care using advanced life support is essential.

Hospital Care. The first priority for interprofessional collaborative care is to monitor and support the patient's airway, breathing, and circulatory status. Follow other interventions as listed in the Best Practice for Patient Safety & Quality Care: Emergency Care of the Patient With Heat Stroke: Restoring Thermoregulation box.

If shivering occurs during the cooling process, midazolam or propofol may be prescribed (Jain et al., 2018). Be aware that midazolam places the patient at high risk for delirium, and propofol carries a risk of hypotension (Jain et al., 2018). Seizure activity can further elevate body temperature and is also treated with an IV benzodiazepine. Once the patient is stabilized, admission to a critical care unit may be warranted to monitor for complications such as multisystem organ dysfunction syndrome and severe electrolyte imbalances, both of which increase mortality risk.

NCLEX EXAMINATION CHALLENGE 11.1

Health Promotion and Maintenance

What teaching will the nurse provide to an older adult who has a history of heat exhaustion? **Select all that apply.**

A. Take frequent rest breaks when doing activities
B. Drink caffeinated beverages before going in the sun
C. Wear dark clothing to protect the skin from burning
D. Stay indoors in an air-conditioned room when possible
E. Take warm baths or showers to regulate the body temperature

SNAKEBITES AND ARTHROPOD BITES AND STINGS

Most snakes fear humans and attempt to avoid contact with them. Sudden, unexpected confrontations at close range often lead to defensive strikes. Awareness is the key to snakebite prevention. Although most snake species are nonvenomous (nonpoisonous) and harmless, there are two families of poisonous snakes in North America: pit vipers *(Crotalidae)* and coral snakes *(Elapidae)*. See the Patient and Family Education: Preparing for Self-Management: Snakebite Prevention box for common-sense actions to avoid being bitten by a poisonous snake.

PATIENT AND FAMILY EDUCATION: PREPARING FOR SELF-MANAGEMENT

Snakebite Prevention

- Do not keep venomous snakes or constricting snakes as pets.
- Be extremely careful in locations where snakes may hide, such as tall grass, rock piles, ledges and crevices, woodpiles, brush, boxes, and cabinets. Snakes are most active on warm nights.
- Wear protective attire such as boots, heavy pants, and leather gloves.
- When walking or hiking, use a walking stick or trekking poles.
- Inspect suspicious areas before placing hands and feet in them.
- Do not harass any snakes you may encounter. Striking distance can be up to two thirds the length of the snake. Even young snakes pose a threat; they are capable of envenomation from birth.
- Be aware that newly dead or decapitated snakes can inflict a bite for up to an hour after death because of persistence of the bite reflex.
- Do not transport the snake with the victim to the medical facility for identification purposes; instead, take a digital photo of the snake at a safe distance if possible.

! NURSING SAFETY PRIORITY (QSEN)

Critical Rescue

Recognize that the first priority is to move the person to a safe area away from the snake and encourage rest to decrease venom circulation. Respond (when in the safe area) by removing jewelry and constricting clothing before swelling worsens. Call for immediate emergency assistance. Do not attempt to capture or kill the snake, but do take digital photographs at a safe distance if possible to aid in snake identification.

Pit vipers are named for the characteristic depression or pit between each eye and nostril that serves as a heat-sensitive organ for locating warm-blooded prey. They include various species of rattlesnakes, copperheads, and cottonmouths and account for the majority of the poisonous snakebites in the United States (Figs. 11.1 and 11.2). Management of a patient who has a snakebite from a pit viper depends on the severity of envenomation (venom injection), as noted in Table 11.1.

Coral snakes (Fig. 11.3) are found from North Carolina to Florida and in the Gulf states through Texas and the southwestern United States. They have broad bands of red and black rings separated by yellow or cream rings. Several harmless snake species closely resemble the coral snake. If a black band lies between the red and yellow bands, the snake is usually nonvenomous. If the red band touches the yellow band, the snake is venomous. A helpful memory aid for identifying coral snakes is "red on yellow, kill a fellow" and "red on black, venom lack." *Be aware that this saying applies only to coral snakes found in the United States!* These nonaggressive snakes have short, fixed fangs and inject highly neurotoxic venom into prey. The World Health Organization maintains a database of venomous snakes and available antivenom at https://apps.who.int/bloodproducts/snakeantivenoms/database/.

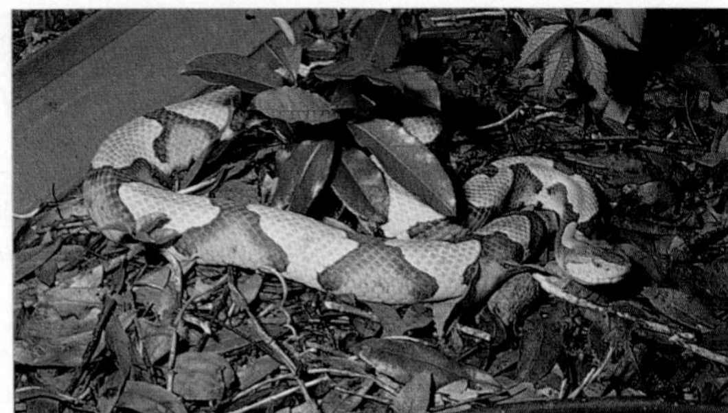

Fig. 11.1 Southern copperhead *(Agkistrodon contortrix)* has markings that make it almost invisible when lying in leaf litter. (From Auerbach, P. S. [2017]. *Wilderness medicine* [7th ed.]. Philadelphia: Mosby; courtesy Michael Cardwell & Carl Barden Venom Laboratory.)

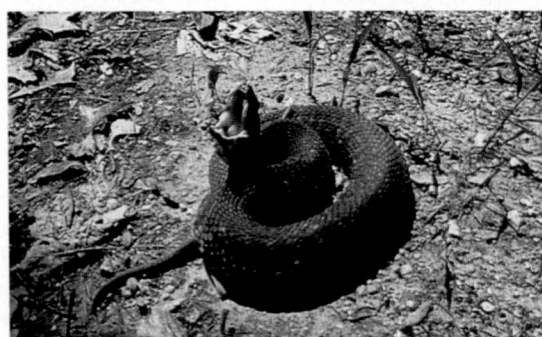

Fig. 11.2 Cottonmouth water moccasin *(Agkistrodon piscivorus)*. The open-mouthed threat gesture is characteristic of this semiaquatic pit viper. (From Auerbach, P. S. [2017]. *Wilderness medicine* [7th ed.]. Philadelphia: Mosby; courtesy Sherman Minton, MD.)

TABLE 11.1 Grades of Pit Viper Envenomation

Envenomation	Characteristics
None	Fang marks, but no local or systemic reactions
Minimal	Fang marks, local swelling and ***pain,*** but no systemic reactions
Moderate	Fang marks and swelling progressing beyond the site of the bite; systemic signs and symptoms such as nausea, vomiting, paresthesias, or hypotension
Severe	Fang marks present with marked swelling of the extremity; subcutaneous ecchymosis; severe symptoms including coagulopathy

From Auerbach, P. S., Donner, H. J., & Weiss, E. A. (2019). *Field guide to wilderness medicine* (5th ed.). St. Louis: Mosby.

! NURSING SAFETY PRIORITY (QSEN)

Critical Rescue

Recognize that the most significant risk to the victim of a snakebite is airway compromise and respiratory failure. Respond by ensuring that the patient's IV lines are patent and that resuscitation equipment is immediately available. Contact Poison Control in collaboration with the health care provider to receive guidance for possible antivenin (also known as antivenom) administration and patient management.

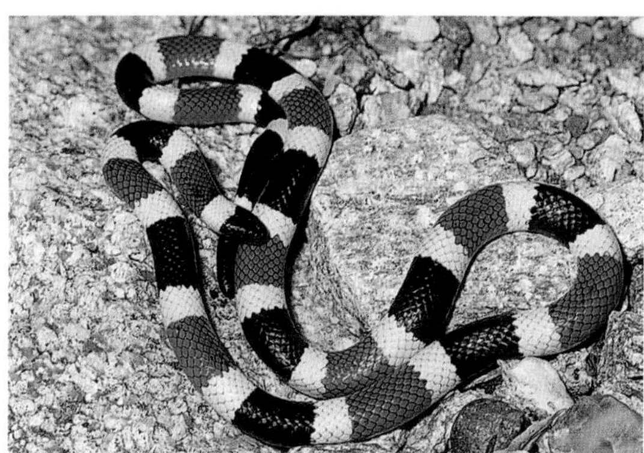

Fig. 11.3 Sonoran coral snake *(Micruroides euryxanthus)* is also known as the *Arizona coral snake.* No documented fatality has followed a bite by this species. (From Auerbach, P. S. [2017]. *Wilderness medicine* [7th ed.]. Philadelphia: Mosby; courtesy Michael Cardwell & Jude McNally.)

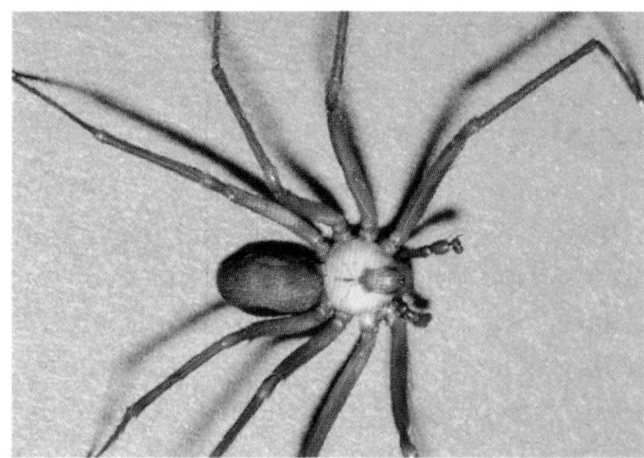

Fig. 11.4 Brown recluse spider *(Loxosceles reclusa).* (From Auerbach, P. S. [2017]. *Wilderness medicine* [7th ed.]. Philadelphia: Mosby; courtesy Indiana University Medical Center.)

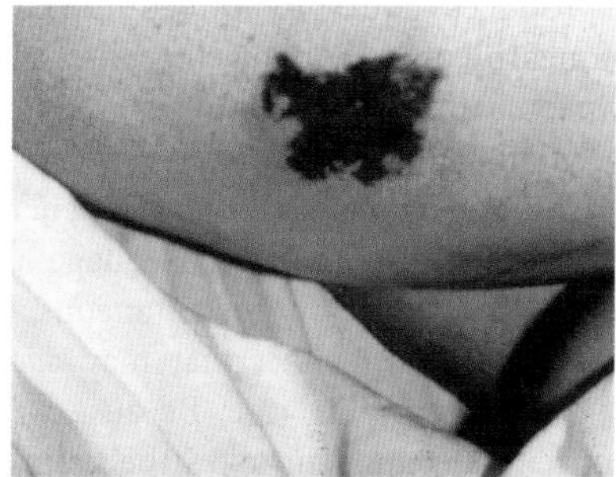

Fig. 11.5 Brown recluse spider bite after 24 hours, with central ischemia and rapidly advancing cellulitis. (From Auerbach, P. S. [2017]. *Wilderness medicine* [7th ed.]. Philadelphia: Mosby; courtesy Paul S. Auerbach, MD.)

Arthropods include spiders, scorpions, bees, and wasps. Unlike snakes, almost all species of spiders are venomous to some degree—most are not harmful to humans, however, because their mouth is too small to pierce human skin or the quantity or quality of their venom is inadequate to produce major health problems. Brown recluse (Figs. 11.4 and 11.5) and black widow spiders, scorpions (Fig. 11.6), bees, and wasps are examples of venomous arthropods that can cause toxic reactions in humans. The Patient and Family Education: Preparing for Self-Management: Arthropod Bite/Sting Prevention box lists actions that help prevent arthropod bites and stings.

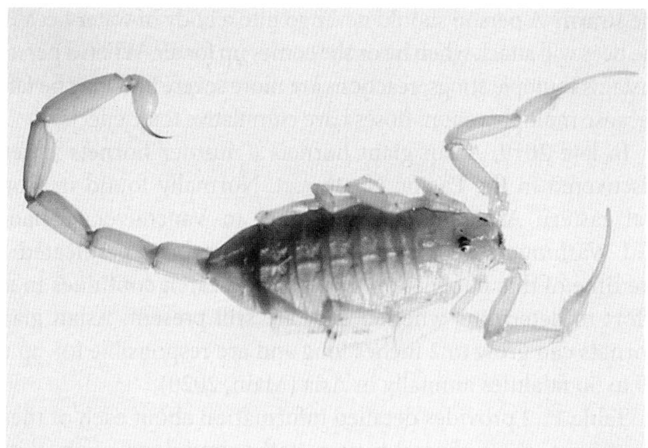

Fig. 11.6 The bark scorpion of Arizona *(Centruroides sculpturatus).* (From Auerbach, P. S. [2012]. *Wilderness medicine* [6th ed.]. Philadelphia: Mosby.)

PATIENT AND FAMILY EDUCATION: PREPARING FOR SELF-MANAGEMENT

Arthropod Bite/Sting Prevention

- Wear protective clothing, including gloves and shoes, when working in areas known to harbor venomous arthropods such as spiders, scorpions, bees, and wasps.
- Cover garbage cans. Bees and wasps are attracted to uncovered garbage.
- Use screens in windows and doors to prevent flying insects from entering buildings.
- Inspect clothing, shoes, and gear for insects before putting on these items.
- Shake out clothing and gear that have been on the ground to prevent arthropod "stowaways" and inadvertent bites and stings.
- Consult an exterminator to control arthropod populations in and around the home. Eliminating insects that are part of the arthropod's food source may also limit their presence.
- Identify nesting areas such as yard debris and rock piles; remove them whenever possible.
- Do not place unprotected hands where the eyes cannot see.
- Avoid handling insects and arthropods or keeping them as "pets."
- Do not swat insects, wasps, and Africanized bees because they can send chemical signals that alert others to attack.
- Carry a prescription epinephrine autoinjector and antihistamines if known to be allergic to bee and wasp stings. Ensure that at least one significant other person is also able to use the autoinjector.

Bee and wasp stings can produce a wide range of reactions from mild discomfort at the sting site to severe ***pain,*** multisystem problems, and life-threatening anaphylaxis in people who are allergic. Bumblebees, hornets, and wasps are capable of stinging repeatedly when disturbed. They have a smooth stinger that may or may not become lodged in the victim. Honeybees can sting just once. When a honeybee stings a person, the stinger and venom sac pull away from the bee. The bee dies, but venom injection continues because the stinger and sac remain in the victim.

"Africanized" bees, also called "killer bees," are a very aggressive species that are found primarily from mid-California across the southern border into Florida. They are known to attack in groups and can remain agitated for several hours. People under attack should attempt to outrun the bees and seek immediate shelter in a building, if possible, and keep the mouth and eyes protected from the swarm. A person should never go into a body of water because the bees will attack when he or she comes up for air. When a person sustains multiple stings, reactions are more severe and may be fatal because multiple venom doses have cumulative toxic effects.

In late 2019, Asian giant hornets ("murder hornets") were discovered in the Pacific Northwest. Normally found in tropical eastern Asia, the hornets found in Vancouver, Canada, and Washington state are thought to have been eradicated at the time of this publication. However, research continues in an effort to determine whether they are still present. Asian giant hornets can grow to 2 inches long and are responsible for up to 30 to 50 fatalities annually in Asia (Main, 2020).

Table 11.2 provides detailed information about each of these organisms, their characteristics, pathophysiology of the bite/sting, first aid and prehospital care, and interprofessional collaborative care that takes place in an acute care setting. The Patient and Family Education: Preparing for Self-Management: Arthropod Bite/Sting Prevention box lists actions that may help prevent arthropod bites and stings.

CLINICAL JUDGMENT CHALLENGE 11.1

Safety

A client arrives at the emergency department with a friend, reporting being bitten on the left foot by a snake 15 minutes prior to arrival. Fishing while barefoot in a marshy area of nearby water, the client describes a sensation of being bitten and then seeing the snake appear to swim away. The client cannot describe characteristics of the snake except that it was estimated to be 18 to 24 inches long and brown or black in color. Nursing assessment reveals two puncture wounds over the left fifth metatarsal with surrounding swelling and mild redness. The client reports mild pain of 3 on a scale of 0–10 at the puncture sites and the sensation of muscle twitching in the lower extremities. There has been no vomiting, but the client reports an onset of nausea and weakness soon after being bitten. Vital signs include BP 98/60, T 99.9° F, P 100 beats per minute, and R 20 breaths per minute. The client reports no prehospital care was given other than to be transported by the friend to the ED.

1. **Recognize Cues**: What assessment information in this client situation is the most important and immediate concern for the nurse? (Hint: Identify the **relevant** information first to determine what is most important.)
2. **Analyze Cues:** What client conditions are consistent with the **most relevant** information? (Hint: Think about priority collaborative problems that support and contradict the information presented in this situation.)
3. **Prioritize Hypotheses:** Which possibilities or explanations are **most likely** to be present in this client situation? Which possibilities or explanations are the most serious? (Hint: Consider all possibilities and determine their urgency and risk for this client.)
4. **Generate Solutions:** What actions would most likely achieve the desired outcomes for this client? Which actions should be **avoided** or are **potentially harmful?** (Hint: Determine the desired outcomes first to decide which interventions are appropriate and those that should be avoided.)
5. **Take Action:** Which actions are the most appropriate and how should they be implemented? In what **priority order** should they be implemented? (Hint: Consider health teaching, documentation, requested health care provider orders or prescriptions, nursing skills, collaboration with or referral to health team members, etc.)
6. **Evaluate Outcomes:** What client assessment would indicate that the nurse's actions were **effective**? (Hint: Think about signs that would indicate an improvement, decline, or unchanged client condition.)

! NURSING SAFETY PRIORITY QSEN

Action Alert

Teach anyone who develops an allergic reaction to bee or wasp stings to always carry a prescription epinephrine autoinjector and wear a medical alert tag or bracelet.

! NURSING SAFETY PRIORITY QSEN

Action Alert

All patients who have sustained multiple stings (particularly more than 50) are observed in an emergency care setting for several hours to monitor for the development of toxic venom effects. Be prepared for the possibility that the patient may need admission to critical care.

LIGHTNING INJURIES

Pathophysiology Review

Lightning is responsible for multiple injuries and deaths each year. It is caused by an electric charge generated within thunderclouds that may become cloud-to-ground lightning—the most dangerous form to people and structures. Most lightning-related injuries occur in the summer months during the afternoon and early evening because of increased thunderstorm activity and greater numbers of people spending time outside. Anyone without adequate shelter, including golfers, hikers, campers, beach-goers, and swimmers, is at risk.

Lightning produces injury by directly striking a victim, splashing off a nearby object, or traveling through the ground. Although few people die after a lightning strike, many survivors are left with permanent disabilities.

Lightning has an enormous magnitude of energy and a different current flow than a typical high-voltage electric shock. The duration of contact is nearly instantaneous, resulting in a flashover phenomenon—an effect that may account for the relatively low overall mortality rate. Because water is a conductor of electricity and current takes the path of least resistance to the ground, any wetness on the body increases the flashover effect of a lightning strike. Lightning flashover produces an explosive force that can injure victims directly and cause them to fall or to be thrown. The clothing and shoes of victims may be damaged or blown off in the process.

Health Promotion and Maintenance

Injuries caused by lightning strike are highly preventable. Teach people to stay indoors during an electrical storm. The Patient and Family Education: Preparing for Self-Management: Lightning Strike Prevention box lists common prevention strategies.

❖ Interprofessional Collaborative Care

◆ **Assessment: Recognize Cues.** Lightning injuries are classified as mild, moderate, or severe (Andrews, 2018). Those with a

TABLE 11.2 Quick Reference for Bites and Stings

Organism and Characteristics	Pathophysiology	First Aid/ Prehospital Care	Assessment: Recognize Cues	Interventions: Take Action: Hospital Care
Pit viper (rattlesnakes, cotton-mouths, copperheads) Triangular head Two retractable curved fangs Single row of ventral subcaudal scales Rattlesnakes have vibrating horny rings in their tails	Venom immobilizes and aids in digestion of prey; may be lethal Has local and systemic effects Enzymes break down human tissue proteins, alter tissue integrity	Move to safety, away from snake Call for immediate emergency assistance Encourage rest to decrease venom circulation Remove jewelry and constrictive clothing Take photos of snake from a safe distance to aid in identification Immobilize affected extremity in position of function—maintain at level of heart Keep patient warm, provide calm environment Do ***not*** incise or suck wound, apply ice, or use a tourniquet	Assess for: • Puncture wounds • ***Pain,*** swelling, redness, and/or bruising around bite(s) • Vesicles or hemorrhagic bullae (may form later) • Report of minty, rubbery, or metallic taste • Tingling or paresthesias on scalp, face, and lips. • Muscle twitching, weakness • Nausea and vomiting • Hypotension, seizures • Clotting abnormalities or DIC	Obtain complete history of event (snake appearance, time of bite, prehospital interventions, and any past snakebites or antivenin therapy) Give supplemental oxygen Insert two large-bore IV lines Infuse fluids as prescribed Monitor heart function and blood pressure Administer opioids to decrease ***pain*** Obtain coagulation panel, CBC, CK, type and crossmatch, urinalysis Obtain ECG Mark, measure, and record circumference of bitten extremity q15-30 minutes See Table 11.1 for envenomation severity Contact regional poison control for specific advice on antivenin dosing and further management Administer crotalidae polyvalent immune fab (if prescribed)
Coral snakes Bands of black, red, and yellow that encircle the snake's body Small maxillary fangs	Venom contains nerve and muscle toxins Blocks neurotransmission Toxic effects may be delayed up to 10-12 hours and then produce rapid clinical deterioration (Norris, 2019)	Move to safety, away from snake Call for immediate emergency assistance Encourage rest to decrease venom circulation Remove jewelry and constrictive clothing Take photos of snake from a safe distance to aid in identification Identify snake as a coral snake, if possible Encircle affected extremity with an elastic bandage or roller gauze dressing (do not wrap so tightly that arterial flow is impeded); then splint. Leave on until the patient is treated at an acute care facility.	Assess for: • Weakness, cranial nerve deficits (ptosis, diplopia, swallowing difficulty), altered level of consciousness, and respiratory paralysis (Norris, 2019) • ***Pain*** at the site, which may be mild and transient • Fang marks that are difficult to locate	Identify snake as a coral snake if possible. If unidentifiable, treat as if venom were injected. Monitor for toxic effects that may be delayed. Monitor for CK level elevation from muscle breakdown and myoglobinuria. Monitor cardiac function, blood pressure, and pulse oximetry. Anticipate admission to a critical care unit. Be prepared to provide aggressive airway management if respiratory insufficiency or severe neurologic impairment occurs. Initiate interventions to decrease risk for aspiration. Coral snake antivenin is not currently manufactured in the United States (although some existing stock may remain). Supportive care is recommended (Norris, 2019). Teach that effects of a severe bite can persist for many days (Norris, 2019). Contact regional poison control for specific advice on management.
Brown recluse spiders Medium-size, light brown, fiddle-shaped mark from eyes down their back Live in boxes, closets, basements, sheds, garages	Venom causes cellular damage and impaired tissue integrity	Move to safety, away from snake Call for immediate emergency assistance Encourage rest to decrease venom circulation Remove jewelry and constrictive clothing Take photos of snake from a safe distance to aid in identification Apply cold compresses over site of bite. Do not apply heat because it increases enzyme activity and potentially worsens wound. Elevate affected extremity, provide local wound care, and rest.	Assess for: • Center of bite to become bluish-purple or necrotic over the following 1-3 days (Fig. 11.5) in some patients. This is the classic *red, white, and blue sign* associated with severe bites. • Objective description of bite as painless, stinging, or sharp • Systematic toxicity, although rare, which includes rash, fever, chills, nausea, vomiting, malaise, joint ***pain*** • Rare, severe systemic complications (loxoscelism), which may include hemolytic anemia, thrombocytopenia, DIC, and death	Hospitalization is rarely indicated unless complications are present. Topical antiseptic and sterile dressings can be applied to wound. Administer tetanus prophylaxis as needed. Teach supportive care measures. Teach to take full course of antibiotics, if prescribed. Teach that débridement and skin grafting may be needed for extensive wounds.

Continued

TABLE 11.2 Quick Reference for Bites and Stings—cont'd

Organism and Characteristics	Pathophysiology	First Aid/ Prehospital Care	Assessment: Recognize Cues	Interventions: Take Action: Hospital Care
Black widow spiders Female: shiny black with a red hourglass pattern on abdomen (hourglass pattern is faint in males) Inhabit cool, damp environments such as log piles, vegetation, and rocks; also live in barns, sheds, and garages	Venom is neurotoxic; produces a syndrome known as latrodectism in which the venom causes neurotransmitter release from nerve terminals	Apply ice pack to decrease action of neurotoxin. Monitor for systemic toxicity; support airway, breathing, and circulation as needed. Transport to acute care facility as soon as possible.	Assess for: • Description of bite as nearly painless to sharply painful • Tiny papule or small, red punctate mark • Systemic muscular complications, which usually develop within an hour of bite • Severe abdominal ***pain***, muscle rigidity and spasm, hypertension, nausea, and vomiting. • Very rare complications may include ileus, priapism, cardiomyopathy, or pulmonary edema	Monitor older adults, especially those with cardiovascular disease, for hypertensive complications. Monitor vital signs; these are normal in most patients although hypertension, tachycardia, and tachypnea may arise from anxiety, pain, or venom effects (Swanson et al., 2020). Administer opioid pain medication and muscle relaxants as prescribed. Administer tetanus prophylaxis as needed. Contact regional poison control for specific advice on antivenin dosing and further management. Administer antivenin as prescribed. Monitor for signs of anaphylaxis and serum sickness.
Scorpions Found within the United States, although not typically in the Midwest or New England Bark scorpion lives in southwestern United States; its sting can be potentially fatal (Fig. 11.6)	Venom injected via stinging apparatus on tail; effects are neurotoxic	Transport to acute care facility as soon as possible.	Assess for: • Symptoms that arise immediately after the sting, reaching crisis level within 5 hours. • Gentle tapping at the site of sting, which usually causes increased ***pain.*** • A sting site that may not be reddened. • Grade I envenomation: Localized pain and paresthesias at the sting site • Grade II envenomation: Local and systemic pain and paresthesias • Grade III envenomation: Cranial nerve dysfunction (dysphagia, drooling, abnormal eye movements, slurred speech) ***or*** somatic skeletal neuromuscular dysfunction (restlessness, abnormal movements, back arching) • Grade IV envenomation: Cranial nerve ***and*** somatic skeletal neuromuscular dysfunction	Monitor vital signs, especially heart rate and respiratory function. Patients with Grade III or IV symptoms require admission for intensive supportive care. Provide basic wound care with antiseptic agent and apply ice pack to sting site. Administer tetanus prophylaxis as needed. Use caution if administering sedative agents, opioids, benzodiazepines, and barbiturates, as these increase risk for respiratory failure. Contact regional poison control for specific information on pharmacologic agents for scorpion stings.
Bees and wasps Found all over United States; "Africanized" or "killer" bees found in southern United States	Venom injected through stings; most can sting repeatedly when disturbed; only honeybees can sting just once	Quickly remove stinger with tweezers or by gently scraping or brushing it off with the edge of a knife blade, credit card, or needles (if present) (Auerbach, 2016) and apply ice pack. Ensure that airway, breathing, and circulation are maintained. If patient has history of allergic reactions to stings or has wheezing, facial swelling, and respiratory distress, epinephrine must be given immediately. Allergic adult patients typically carry an epinephrine autoinjector. (See Chapter 18 for further discussion of epinephrine administration for anaphylaxis management.) Follow with antihistamines (H1 and H2 blockers) and albuterol if carried by the patient and available.	Assess for: • Wheal-and-flare skin reactions; swelling can be extensive and involve an entire limb or body area. • Urticaria (hives), pruritus (itching), and lip/tongue edema in patients with venom allergy. • Signs of anaphylaxis such as bronchospasm, laryngeal edema, hypotension, decreased mental status, and cardiac dysrhythmias. • Systemic effects that develop based on venom load and patient sensitivity, including generalized edema, nausea, vomiting, diarrhea, acute kidney injury, renal failure, liver injury, cardiac complications, and multisystem organ failure.	Administer oxygen. Monitor cardiac function and blood pressure. Administer epinephrine, antihistamines (both H1 and H2 blockers), albuterol, and corticosteroids as prescribed. Ensure that advanced life support drugs and resuscitation equipment are readily available. Observe anyone with multiple stings for several hours. Anticipate admission to critical care if toxic venom effects are noted.

CBC, Complete blood count; *CK*, creatine kinase; *DIC*, disseminated intravascular coagulation; *ECG*, electrocardiogram.

PATIENT AND FAMILY EDUCATION: PREPARING FOR SELF-MANAGEMENT

Lightning Strike Prevention

- Observe weather forecasts when planning to be outside.
- A lightning strike is imminent if your hair stands on end, you see a blue halo around objects, and you hear high-pitched or crackling noises. If you cannot move away from the area immediately, crouch on the balls of your feet and tuck your head down to minimize the target size; do not lie on the ground or make contact with your hands to the ground.
- Seek shelter when you hear thunder. Go inside the nearest building or an enclosed vehicle. Avoid isolated sheds and cave entrances. Do not stand under an isolated tall tree or structure (e.g., ski lift, flagpole, boat mast, power line) in an open area such as a field, ridge, or hilltop; lightning tends to strike high points. Instead, seek a low area under a thick growth of saplings or small trees.
- Leave water immediately (including an indoor shower or bathtub) and move away from any open bodies of water.
- Avoid metal objects such as chairs or bleachers; put down tools, fishing rods, garden equipment, golf clubs, and umbrellas; stand clear of fences, exposed pipes, motorcycles, bicycles, tractors, and golf carts.
- If inside a car with a solid hood, close the windows and stay inside. If in a convertible, leave the car at least 49 yards (45 meters) away and huddle on the ground.
- If inside a tent, stay away from the metal tent poles and wet fabric of the tent walls.
- If you are caught out in the open and cannot seek shelter, attempt to move to lower ground such as a ravine or valley; stay away from any tall trees or objects that could result in a lightning strike splashing over to you; place insulating material between you and the ground (e.g., sleeping pad, rain parka, life jacket).
- If inside a building, stay away from open doors, windows, fireplaces, metal fixtures, and plumbing.
- Turn off electrical equipment, including computers, televisions, and stereos to avoid damage.
- Stay off land-line telephones. Lightning can enter through the telephone line and produce head and neck trauma, including cataracts and tympanic membrane disruption. Death can result. Avoid use of cellular phones, which can transmit loud static that can cause acoustic damage.

Data from Auerbach, P. S., Donner, H. J., & Weiss, E. A. (2019). *Field guide to wilderness medicine* (5th ed.). St. Louis: Mosby.

mild injury may only be stunned or confused. Those with moderate injury may have confusion or be comatose, and experience temporary paralysis (Andrews, 2018). Severely injured patients often experience cardiac arrest, as the cardiopulmonary and the central nervous systems are profoundly affected by lightning injuries. *The most lethal initial effect of massive electrical current discharge on the cardiopulmonary system is cardiac arrest.* Because cardiac cells are autorhythmic, an effective cardiac rhythm may return spontaneously. However, prolonged respiratory arrest from impairment of the medullary respiratory center can produce hypoxia and subsequently a second cardiac arrest. Therefore when attempting to manage multiple victims of a lightning strike, provide care to those who are in cardiopulmonary arrest first. Initiate resuscitation measures with immediate airway and ventilatory management, chest compressions, and other appropriate life support interventions.

People with mild or moderate injury may be treated in a less emergent fashion. However, these victims can have serious myocardial complications, which may be indicated by electrocardiogram (ECG) and myocardial perfusion abnormalities such as angina and dysrhythmias. The initial appearance of mottled skin and decreased-to-absent peripheral pulses usually arises from arterial vasospasm and typically resolves spontaneously in several hours.

Central nervous system (CNS) injury is common in lightning strike victims. Temporary paralysis, known as *keraunoparalysis,* affects the lower limbs to a greater extent than the upper limbs. This condition usually resolves within hours, but the patient must be evaluated for spinal injury. Other signs, symptoms, and complications resulting from lightning strikes include cataracts, tympanic membrane rupture, cerebral hemorrhage, depression, and posttraumatic stress disorder. Lightning strikes also cause skin burns, most of which are superficial and heal without incident. Patients may have full-thickness burns, charring, and contact burns from overlying metal objects. Tree-like branching or ferning marks on the skin called **Lichtenberg figures** or *keraunographic markings* are characteristic skin findings on those struck by lightning. These are not considered burns and are thought to be caused by the coagulation of blood cells in the capillaries.

◆ Interventions: Take Action

First Aid/Prehospital Care. Because of lightning's powerful impact to the body, patients are at great risk for multisystem trauma. The full extent of injury may not be known until thorough monitoring and diagnostic evaluation can be performed in the hospital. Initial care includes spinal stabilization with priority attention to maintenance of an adequate airway, effective breathing, and circulation through standard basic and advanced life support measures. Cardiopulmonary resuscitation (CPR) is performed immediately when a patient is in cardiac arrest. If cardiopulmonary or CNS injury is present, skin burns are *not* the initial priority. However, if time and resources permit, a sterile dressing may be applied to cover the sites.

Victims of lightning strike are not electrically charged; the rescuer is in no danger from physical contact. Nonetheless, the storm can present a continued threat to everyone in the vicinity who lacks adequate shelter. Contrary to popular belief, lightning can and does strike in the same place more than once.

Hospital Care. Once in the acute care hospital setting, the focus of care is advanced life support management, including cardiac monitoring to detect cardiac dysrhythmias and a 12-lead ECG. The patient may require mechanical ventilation until spontaneous breathing returns. Collaborate with the interprofessional health care team to perform a thorough evaluation to identify obvious and occult (hidden) traumatic injuries because the patient may have suffered a fall or blast effect during the strike. A computed tomography (CT) scan of the head may be performed to identify intracranial hemorrhage. A creatine kinase (CK) measurement may be requested to detect skeletal muscle damage resulting from the lightning strike.

In severe cases, rhabdomyolysis (circulation of by-products of skeletal muscle destruction) can lead to renal failure. Burn wounds are assessed and treated according to standard burn care protocols. Tetanus prophylaxis is necessary if the patient has experienced burns or any break in skin integrity. Some agencies transfer these victims to a burn center for follow-up management.

COLD-RELATED INJURIES

Two common cold-related injuries are hypothermia and frostbite. Both types of injury can be prevented by implementing protection from the cold. Teach patients ways to prevent these injuries through methods to maintain thermoregulation, which can range from minor ***pain*** to major systemic complications.

Health Promotion and Maintenance

When participating in cold-weather activities, clothing choices are critical to the prevention of hypothermia and frostbite. Teach the importance of wearing synthetic clothing because it moves moisture away from the body and dries fast. Cotton clothing, especially worn as an undergarment, holds moisture, becomes wet, and contributes to the development of hypothermia. It should be strictly avoided in a cold outdoor environment; this rule applies to gloves and socks as well because wet gloves and socks promote frostbite in the fingers and toes. Wearing too many pairs of socks can decrease circulation and lead to frostbite.

Clothing should be layered so that it can be easily added or removed as the temperature changes. The inner layers, such as polyester fleece, provide warmth and insulation. The outer layer blocks wind and provides moisture protection. This layer is best made of a windproof, waterproof, breathable fabric. Body heat is lost through the head, so a hat should always be worn. A facemask should be used on particularly cold days when wind chill poses a risk. Sunscreen (minimum sun protection factor [SPF] 30) and sunglasses are also important to protect skin and eyes from the sun's harmful rays.

Teach people to keep water, extra clothing, blankets, food, and essential personal medications in their car when driving in cold climates and in winter in case the vehicle becomes stranded. Maintaining personal fitness and conditioning is an important consideration to prevent hypothermia and frostbite. People should not diet or restrict food or fluid intake when participating in winter outdoor activities. Undernutrition and dehydration contribute to cold-related illnesses and injuries. Finally, it is important for people to know their physical limits and to come in out of the cold before those limits have been reached.

HYPOTHERMIA

Pathophysiology Review

Hypothermia is a core body temperature below 95°F (35°C). Common predisposing conditions that promote hypothermia include:

- Cold-water immersion
- Acute illness (e.g., sepsis)
- Traumatic injury
- Shock states
- Immobilization
- Cold weather (especially for people who are homeless or work outdoors)
- Older age
- Use of medications (e.g., phenothiazines, barbiturates)
- Inappropriate alcohol and substance use
- Undernutrition
- Hypothyroidism
- Inadequate clothing or shelter (e.g., the homeless population)

An environmental temperature below 82°F (28°C) can produce impaired thermoregulation and hypothermia in any susceptible person. *Therefore people, especially older adults, are actually at risk on a year-round basis in most areas of the world.* Wind chill is a significant factor: heat loss increases as wind speed rises. Wet conditions further increase heat loss through evaporation. Weather is a common cause of hypothermia.

❖ Interprofessional Collaborative Care

◆ **Assessment: Recognize Cues.** Hypothermia is commonly divided into three categories by severity: *mild* (90° to 95°F [32° to 35°C]); *moderate* (82.4° to 90°F [28° to 32°C]); and *severe* (below 82.4°F [28°C]). Treatment decisions are based on the severity of hypothermia. *Key Features: Hypothermia* summarizes the common key features by category for the patient who is hypothermic.

◆ Interventions: Take Action

First Aid/Prehospital Care. The patient with *mild hypothermia* needs to be sheltered from the cold environment, have all wet clothing removed, and undergo passive or active external rewarming. Passive methods involve applying warm clothing or blankets. Active methods incorporate use of heating blankets,

KEY FEATURES
Hypothermia

Mild
- Shivering
- Dysarthria (slurred speech)
- Decreased muscle coordination
- Impaired cognition ("mental slowness")
- Diuresis (caused by shunting of blood to major organs)

Moderate
- Muscle weakness
- Increased loss of coordination
- Acute confusion
- Apathy
- Incoherence
- Possible stupor
- Decreased clotting (caused by impaired platelet aggregation and thrombocytopenia)

Severe
- Bradycardia
- Severe hypotension
- Decreased respiratory rate
- Cardiac dysrhythmias, including possible ventricular fibrillation or asystole
- Decreased neurologic reflexes to coma
- Decreased ***pain*** responsiveness
- Acid-base imbalance

warm packs, and convective air heaters or warmers. If a heating blanket is used, monitor the patient's skin at least every 15 to 30 minutes to reduce the risk for burn injury.

In the case of mild, uncomplicated hypothermia as the only health problem, having the victim drink warm high-carbohydrate liquids that do not contain alcohol or caffeine can aid in rewarming. Alcohol is a peripheral vasodilator; both alcohol and caffeine are diuretics. These effects can potentially worsen dehydration and hypothermia.

Hospital Care. General management principles apply to both *moderate* and *severe* hypothermia. Protect patients from further heat loss and handle them gently to prevent ventricular fibrillation. Positioning the patient in the supine position prevents orthostatic changes in blood pressure from cardiovascular instability. Follow standard resuscitation efforts with special attention to maintenance of airway, breathing, and circulation as recommended by the American Heart Association (2015):

- Administer drugs with caution and/or spaced at longer intervals because metabolism is unpredictable in hypothermic conditions.
- Remember that drugs can accumulate without obvious therapeutic effect while the patient is cold but may become active and potentially lead to drug toxicity as effective rewarming is under way.
- Collaborate with the health care provider to consider withholding IV drugs, except vasopressors, until the core temperature is above 86° F (30° C).
- Initiate CPR for patients without spontaneous circulation.
- For a hypothermic patient in ventricular fibrillation or pulseless ventricular tachycardia, one defibrillation attempt is appropriate. Be aware that defibrillation attempts may be ineffective until the core temperature is above 86° F (30° C).

Treatment of *moderate* hypothermia may involve both active external and core (internal) rewarming methods. Applying external heat with heating blankets can promote core temperature "after-drop" by producing peripheral vasodilation. **After-drop** is the continued decrease in core body temperature after the victim is removed from the cold environment; it is caused by the return of cold blood from the periphery to the central circulation. Therefore the patient's trunk should be actively rewarmed before the extremities. Core rewarming methods for moderate hypothermia include administration of warm IV fluids; heated oxygen or inspired gas to prevent further heat loss via the respiratory tract; and heated peritoneal, pleural, gastric, or bladder lavage.

! NURSING SAFETY PRIORITY (QSEN)

Critical Rescue

Recognize that patients who are *severely* hypothermic are at high risk for cardiac arrest. Respond by avoiding active *external* rewarming with heating devices because it is dangerous and contraindicated in this population due to rapid vasodilation.

The treatment of choice for *severe* hypothermia is to use *extracorporeal* rewarming methods such as cardiopulmonary bypass or hemodialysis. Cardiopulmonary bypass, which requires specialized personnel and resources, is the fastest core rewarming technique. However, this device is not available in all hospitals. Monitor for early signs of complications that can occur after rewarming such as fluid, electrolyte, and metabolic abnormalities; acute respiratory distress syndrome (ARDS); acute renal failure; and pneumonia.

A long-standing principle in the treatment of patients with hypothermic cardiac arrest is that "no one is dead until he or she is warm and dead." There is a factual basis to this statement when considering the number of survivors who have suffered a prolonged hypothermic cardiac arrest. Prolonged resuscitation efforts may not be reasonable in cases in which survival appears highly unlikely such as in an anoxic event followed by a hypothermic cardiac arrest.

FROSTBITE

Pathophysiology Review

Another significant cold-related injury that may or may not be associated with hypothermia is frostbite. The main risk factor is inadequate insulation against cold weather (i.e., the skin is exposed to the cold, or the person's clothing offers insufficient protection, which leads to injury). Wet clothing is a poor insulator and facilitates the development of frostbite. Fatigue, dehydration, and poor nutrition are other contributing factors. People who smoke, consume alcohol, or have impaired peripheral circulation have a higher incidence of frostbite. Any previous history of frostbite further increases a person's susceptibility.

NCLEX EXAMINATION CHALLENGE 11.2

Physiological Integrity

When caring for four clients, which does the nurse identify as at the **highest** risk for frostbite?

A. 19-year old who takes antihistamines
B. 28-year old who is a vegetarian
C. 41-year old who is being treated for hypothyroidism
D. 57-year old who drinks 4-5 beers per day

❖ Interprofessional Collaborative Care

◆ **Assessment: Recognize Cues.** **Frostbite** occurs when body tissue freezes and causes damage to ***tissue integrity***. Like burns, frostbite injuries can be superficial, partial, or full thickness. By contrast, **frostnip** is a type of superficial cold injury that may produce ***pain,*** numbness, and pallor or a waxy appearance of the affected area but is easily relieved by applying warmth. It does not cause impaired ***tissue integrity***. Frostnip typically develops on areas such as the face, nose, finger, or toes. Untreated, it is a precursor to more severe forms of frostbite.

Grade 1 frostbite, the least severe type of frostbite, involves **hyperemia** (increased blood flow) of the involved area and edema formation. In *Grade 2 frostbite,* large, clear-to-milky, fluid-filled blisters develop with partial-thickness skin necrosis (Fig. 11.7). *Grade 3 frostbite* appears as small blisters that contain dark fluid and an affected body part that is cool, numb, blue, or red and does not blanch. Full-thickness and subcutaneous tissue necrosis occurs and requires débridement. In *Grade 4 frostbite,* the most severe

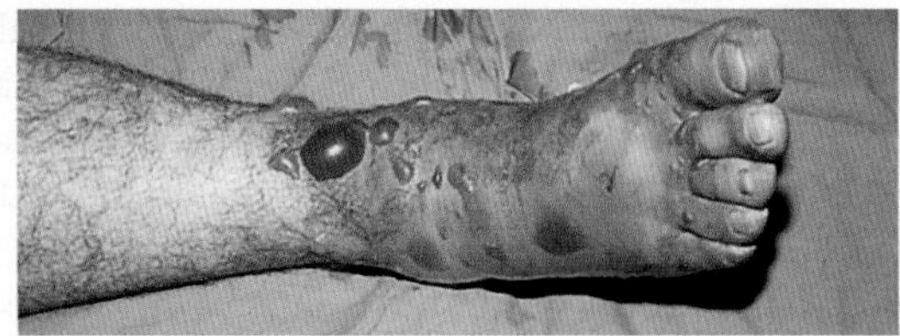

Fig. 11.7 Edema and blister formation 24 hours after frostbite injury occurring in an area covered by a tightly fitted boot. (From Auerbach, P. S. [2008]. *Wilderness medicine* [5th ed.]. Philadelphia: Mosby; courtesy Cameron Bangs, MD)

form, there are blisters over the carpal or tarsal (instead of just the digit) (Zafren & Mechem, 2020); the part is numb, cold, and bloodless. The full-thickness necrosis extends into the muscle and bone. At this stage, gangrene develops, which may require amputation of the affected part. Of note, except for frostnip, other degrees of frostbite may all have the same general appearance while the body part is frozen; the differentiating features of each degree of frostbite only become apparent after the part is thawed. Gangrene may evolve over days to weeks after injury.

◆ Interventions: Take Action

First Aid/Prehospital Care. *Recognition of frostbite is essential to early, effective intervention and prevention of further damage to* ***tissue integrity***. Asking a significant other to frequently observe for early signs of frostbite such as a white, waxy appearance to exposed skin, especially on the nose, cheeks, and ears, is an effective strategy to identify the problem before it worsens. In people with dark skin, skin becomes paler, waxy, and somewhat gray. In this case the best remedy is to have the person seek shelter from the wind and cold and attend to the affected body part. Superficial frostbite is easily managed using body heat to warm the affected area. Teach patients to place their warm hands over the affected areas on their face or to place cold hands under the arms.

Hospital Care. Patients with more severe and deeper forms of frostbite need aggressive management. For all degrees of partial-thickness–to–full-thickness frostbite, rapid rewarming in a water bath at a temperature range of 99° to 102° F (37° to 39° C) is indicated to thaw the frozen part (Freer et al., 2017). The part should be swirled in the water and not allowed to touch the sides of the container to prevent tissue damage. Because patients experience severe ***pain*** during the rewarming process, this intervention is best accomplished in a health care facility; however, it may be done in another setting if no other options exist for prompt transport or rescue. Administer analgesics, IV opiates, and IV rehydration as prescribed. Ibuprofen should also be administered as prescribed, as it decreases thromboxane production in the inflammatory cascade and may reduce secondary tissue injury in frostbite (Auerbach, 2016).

> **! NURSING SAFETY PRIORITY (QSEN)**
>
> ***Critical Rescue***
>
> Recognize that dry heat or massage should not be used as part of the warming process for frostbitten areas because these actions can produce further damage to ***tissue integrity.*** Respond by using other interventions such as a rapid rewarming water bath of 99° to 102° F (37° to 39° C), to preserve tissue.

When the rewarming process is complete, handle the injured areas gently and elevate them above heart level if possible to decrease tissue edema. Sometimes splints are used to immobilize extremities during the healing process. Assess the person at least hourly for the development of compartment syndrome—a limb-threatening complication caused by severe neurovascular impairment. Observe for early signs and symptoms, which include increasing ***pain*** (even after analgesics are given) and paresthesias (painful tingling and numbness). Compare the affected extremity with the unaffected one to assess for pallor. Assess for pulses and muscle weakness. Management of compartment syndrome is discussed in detail in Chapter 47.

Frostbite destroys tissue and produces a deep tetanus-prone wound; so the patient should be immunized to prevent tetanus. Apply only loose, nonadherent sterile dressings to the damaged areas. Avoid compression of the injured tissues. Both topical and systemic antibiotics may be used. Once a patient's frozen part has thawed, do not allow it to refreeze, which worsens the injury. Anticipate diagnostic studies such as arteriography to evaluate perfusion to the injured part.

In cases of severe, deep frostbite, débridement of necrotic tissue may be needed to evaluate tissue viability and provide wound management. Amputation may be indicated for patients with severe injuries or those who develop gangrene or severe compartment syndrome.

ALTITUDE-RELATED ILLNESSES

Pathophysiology Review

High-altitude illness, also known as **high-altitude disease (HAD)** or *altitude sickness,* causes pathophysiologic responses in the body as a result of exposure to low partial pressure of oxygen at high elevations. Although most consider high altitude to be an elevation over 5000 meters, millions of people worldwide who ascend to or live at altitudes above 2500 meters are at risk for acute and chronic high-altitude illness. For purposes of consistency in definition, high-altitude environments are considered to be at an elevation of 1500 meters or higher (Prince & Hubner, 2019).

As altitude increases, atmospheric (barometric) pressure decreases. Oxygen makes up 21% of the pressure. Therefore as this pressure falls, the partial pressure of oxygen in the air decreases, resulting in less available oxygen to breathe. The pathophysiologic consequence is hypoxia, which is more pronounced as elevation increases. Elevations higher than 18,000 feet are considered extreme altitudes. Supplemental oxygen is necessary at these levels in nonacclimatized people to prevent altitude-related illnesses, including death, from occurring during abrupt ascent. Of note, unrecognized or untreated HAD can cause death in susceptible individuals even at lower altitudes.

The cause of HAD is an interaction of environmental and genetic factors. Those with obesity or chronic illnesses, especially cardiovascular problems, are at higher risk than those who are healthier. Dehydration and use of CNS depressants such as alcohol also increase the risk. The age of the person does not seem to be a factor in altitude-related illnesses.

PATIENT-CENTERED CARE: GENETIC/GENOMIC CONSIDERATIONS QSEN

Genetic differences among certain ethnic groups who live in high-altitude areas have been studied. For example, chronic mountain sickness (a type of HAD) is uncommon in Tibetans, even those who have lived in lower altitudes and then reascend to higher altitudes (Bjertness et al., 2017).

The pathogenesis of mountain sickness is associated with unidentified variations in hypoxia-related genes and the genes responsible for the human leukocyte antigen (HLA) system.

At this time, no clinical genetic testing to determine a person's risk for altitude sickness is available; however, research has identified genes that are implicated in susceptibility (Ashmore et al., 2018).

The process of adapting to high altitude is called *acclimatization.* **Acclimatization** involves physiologic changes that help the body adapt to less available oxygen in the atmosphere. As the carotid bodies sense a decline in PaO_2 at about 5000 feet, they increase the respiratory rate to improve oxygen delivery. This mechanism is called the *hypoxic-ventilatory response*. Increased respiratory rate causes **hypocapnia** (decreased carbon dioxide) and respiratory alkalosis, which limit further increases in respiratory rate. Rapid eye movement (REM) sleep is impaired. Hypoxia can occur from periods of apnea. Within 24 to 48 hours of being at high altitude, the kidneys excrete the excess bicarbonate, which helps the pH to return to normal and ventilatory rate to again increase.

Increased sympathetic nervous system activity increases heart rate, blood pressure, and cardiac output. Pulmonary artery pressure rises as an effect of generalized hypoxia-induced pulmonary vasoconstriction. Cerebral blood flow increases to maintain cerebral oxygen delivery. Hypoxia also induces red blood cell production by stimulating the release of erythropoietin. The result is an increase in red blood cells and hemoglobin concentration. Over time polycythemia can develop in people who remain in a high-altitude environment.

People who plan to climb to high altitudes are advised to ascend slowly, over the course of days or even weeks, depending on the degree of elevation. Ascending too rapidly is the primary cause of altitude-related illnesses (and less commonly, death), particularly for those who sleep at elevations above 8000 feet.

The three most common clinical conditions that are considered high-altitude illnesses are **acute mountain sickness (AMS)**, **high-altitude cerebral edema (HACE)**, and **high-altitude pulmonary edema (HAPE)**. AMS may occur with HACE and/or HAPE; the underlying pathophysiology is hypoxia. Chronic mountain sickness can occur in people who live at high elevations. Although each syndrome has several unique signs and symptoms, the basic assessment and management approach are the same.

Health Promotion and Maintenance

Acetazolamide, a carbonic anhydrase inhibitor, is commonly prescribed to prevent or treat AMS. It acts by causing a bicarbonate diuresis, which rids the body of excess fluid and induces metabolic acidosis. The acidotic state increases respiratory rate and decreases the occurrence of periodic respiration during sleep at night. In this way it helps patients acclimate faster to a high altitude. For best results, the drug should be taken 24 hours before ascent and be continued for the first 2 days of the trip.

! NURSING SAFETY PRIORITY QSEN

Drug Alert

Acetazolamide is a sulfa drug. Ask about sulfa allergy before the patient takes the drug because it may cause hypersensitivity reactions in those who are sulfa sensitive.

❖ Interprofessional Collaborative Care

◆ **Assessment: Recognize Cues.** Assessment findings for the typical patient with AMS include throbbing headache, anorexia, nausea, vomiting, chills, irritability, and apathy. The syndrome produces effects similar to an alcohol-induced hangover, and the patient may report a feeling of extreme illness. Vital signs are variable: the patient can be tachycardic or bradycardic, have normal blood pressure, or have postural hypotension. He or she may experience dyspnea both on exertion and at rest. Exertional dyspnea is expected as a person adjusts to high altitude. However, dyspnea at rest is abnormal and may signal the onset of HAPE.

If AMS progresses to high-altitude cerebral edema (HACE), the extreme form of this disorder, the patient cannot perform ADLs and has extreme apathy. A key sign of HACE is the development of ataxia (defective muscular coordination). The patient also experiences a change in mental status with confusion and impaired judgment. Cranial nerve dysfunction and seizures may occur. If untreated, a further decline in the patient's level of consciousness can occur. Stupor, coma, and death can result from brain swelling and the subsequent damage caused by increased intracranial pressure over the course of 1 to 3 days.

High-altitude pulmonary edema (HAPE) often appears in conjunction with HACE but may occur during the progression of AMS within the first 2 to 4 days of a rapid ascent to high altitude, commonly on the second night. It is the most common cause of death associated with high altitude. Patients notice poor exercise tolerance and a prolonged recovery time after exertion. Fatigue, weakness, and other signs and symptoms of AMS are present. Important signs and symptoms of HAPE include a persistent dry cough and cyanosis of the lips and nail beds. Tachycardia and tachypnea occur at rest. Crackles may be auscultated in one or both lungs. Pink, frothy sputum is a late sign of HAPE. A chest x-ray will show pulmonary infiltrates and pulmonary edema. Pneumonia may also be present. Arterial blood gas analysis shows respiratory alkalosis and hypoxemia (decreased oxygen). Pulmonary artery pressure is usually very elevated because of pulmonary edema.

◆ **Interventions: Take Action**

First Aid/Prehospital Care/Hospital Care. *The most important intervention to manage serious altitude-related illnesses is descent to a lower altitude.* Patients must be monitored carefully for evidence of symptom progression. The patient with mild AMS should be allowed to rest and acclimate at the current altitude. The person is instructed not to ascend to a higher altitude, especially for sleep, until symptoms lessen. If symptoms persist or worsen, he or she should be moved to a lower altitude as soon as possible. Even a descent of about 1600 feet may improve the patient's condition and reverse altitude-related pathologic effects. If available, oxygen should be administered to effectively treat symptoms of AMS.

One drug that is indicated in the treatment of moderate-to-severe AMS is dexamethasone. The mechanism of action of this drug is unclear for AMS treatment, but it appears to reduce cerebral edema by acting as an anti-inflammatory in the CNS. It does not speed acclimatization like acetazolamide does, but it does relieve the symptoms of AMS. If the drug is stopped before acclimatization takes place, symptoms of AMS may recur (Centers for Disease Control and Prevention, 2017).

For the treatment of HACE, early recognition of ataxia or a change in level of consciousness should prompt a rapid descent by rescuers or companions to a lower altitude. While undergoing descent, the patient can be given supplemental oxygen and dexamethasone. If mental status is severely impaired and the patient's airway is at risk, all drugs should be given parenterally. Ultimately the patient with HACE must be admitted to the hospital. Critical care management may be necessary.

Like HACE, early recognition of HAPE is essential to improve the patient's chance for survival. Phosphodiesterase inhibitors such as tadalafil and sildenafil have been shown in small studies to prevent development of HAPE because of their pulmonary vasodilatory effects; agreed-upon doses and regimens are not established (Gallagher & Hackett, 2018). The calcium channel blocker *nifedipine* can also be used to decrease pulmonary vascular resistance.

When it occurs, HAPE is a serious condition that requires quick evacuation to a lower altitude, oxygen administration, and bedrest to save the patient's life. If descent must be delayed because of weather conditions or other factors, oxygen administration as soon as possible is essential. Keep the patient warm at all times. Drugs are not substitutes for descent and oxygen. Hospital admission is required. In uncomplicated cases of HAPE, recovery occurs quickly, but effects such as weakness and fatigue may persist for weeks.

The Best Practice for Patient Safety & Quality Care: Preventing, Recognizing, and Treating Altitude-Related Illnesses box summarizes interventions for preventing, recognizing, and treating altitude-related illnesses.

BEST PRACTICE FOR PATIENT SAFETY & QUALITY CARE (QSEN)

Preventing, Recognizing, and Treating Altitude-Related Illnesses

- Plan a slow ascent to allow for acclimatization.
- Learn to recognize signs and symptoms of altitude-related illnesses.
- Avoid overexertion and overexposure to cold; rest at present altitude before ascending further.
- Ensure adequate hydration and nutrition.
- Avoid alcohol and sleeping pills when at high altitude.
- For progressive or advanced acute mountain sickness (AMS), recognize symptoms and implement an immediate descent; provide oxygen at high concentration.
- To prevent the occurrence of AMS, discuss the use of acetazolamide or dexamethsone as indicated with your health care provider.
- Protect skin and eyes from the harmful ultraviolet rays of the sun at high altitude. Wear sunscreen (at least SPF 30) and high-quality wraparound sunglasses or goggles.

SPF, Sun protection factor.

NCLEX EXAMINATION CHALLENGE 11.3

Physiological Integrity

When caring for a client who become ill while mountain climbing, which assessment finding requires **immediate** nursing intervention? **Select all that apply.**

A. Blue nail beds
B. Lung crackles
C. Tachypnea at rest
D. Pink, frothy sputum
E. Persistent dry cough
F. Pulmonary infiltrates per x-ray
G. Increased pulmonary artery pressure

DROWNING

Pathophysiology Review

Drowning is a leading cause of accidental death in the United States. It occurs when a person suffers primary respiratory impairment from submersion or immersion in a liquid medium (usually water). The drowning process is considered a continuum with outcomes that range from survival to death.

Health Promotion and Maintenance

Prevention is the key to avoiding drowning incidents. When providing health teaching, include these points:

- Constantly observe people who cannot swim and are in or around water.
- Do not swim alone.
- Test the water depth before diving in head first; never dive into shallow water.
- Avoid alcoholic beverages and substance use when swimming and boating and while in proximity to water.
- Ensure that water rescue equipment such as life jackets, flotation devices, and rope is immediately available when around water.

❖ Interprofessional Collaborative Care

◆ **Assessment: Recognize Cues.** When water is aspirated into the lungs, the quantity and makeup of the water are key factors in the pathophysiology of the drowning event. Aspiration of both fresh water and salt water causes surfactant to wash out of the lungs. Surfactant reduces surface tension within the alveoli, increases lung compliance and alveolar radius, and decreases the work of breathing. Loss of surfactant destabilizes the alveoli and leads to increased airway resistance. Salt water—a hypertonic fluid—also creates an osmotic gradient that draws protein-rich fluid from the vascular space into the alveoli. In both cases, pulmonary edema results. Salt water and fresh water aspiration cause similar degrees of lung injury. Another concern is water quality; the victim's outcome may be negatively affected by contaminants in the water such as chemicals, algae, microbes, sand, and mud. These substances can worsen lung injury and cause infection.

The duration and severity of hypoxia are the two most important factors that determine outcomes for victims of drowning. Very cold water seems to have a protective effect.

Successful resuscitations have been reported even after prolonged arrest intervals. Hypothermia might offer some protection to the hypoxic brain by reducing the cerebral metabolic rate. The diving reflex is a physiologic response to asphyxia, which produces bradycardia; a reduction in cardiac output; and vasoconstriction of vessels in the intestine, skeletal muscles, and kidneys. These physiologic effects are thought to reduce myocardial oxygen use and enhance blood flow to the heart and cerebral tissues. Survival is thought to be linked to some combination of the effects of hypothermia and the diving reflex.

The cause of the drowning should also be determined if possible. The patient may have experienced an event that caused the drowning event such as a seizure, myocardial infarction, brain attack, or spinal cord injury while in the water. Injuries sustained from diving into shallow water or body surfing, such as cervical spine trauma, can also increase the difficulty of rescue and resuscitation efforts.

◆ Interventions: Take Action

First Aid/Emergency Care. Potential rescuers must consider their own swimming abilities and limitations and any natural or human-made hazards before attempting to save the victim; failure to do so could place additional lives in jeopardy. *Once rescuers gain access to the victim, the priority is safe removal from the water.* Spine stabilization with a board or flotation device should be considered only for victims who are at high risk for spine trauma (e.g., history of diving, use of a water slide, signs of injury or alcohol intoxication), as opposed to all drowning victims. Time is critical; efforts directed toward a rapid rescue have the most potential benefit. Initiate airway clearance and ventilatory support measures, including delivering rescue breaths, as soon as possible while the patient is still in the water. If hypothermia is a concern, handle the victim gently to prevent ventricular fibrillation.

! NURSING SAFETY PRIORITY (QSEN)

Critical Rescue

Recognize that you must not attempt to get the water out of the victim's lungs; respond by delivering abdominal or chest thrusts *only* if airway obstruction is suspected.

Hospital Care. Once the person is safely removed from the water, airway and cardiopulmonary support interventions begin, including oxygen administration, endotracheal intubation, CPR, and defibrillation, if necessary. In the clinical setting, gastric decompression with a nasogastric or orogastric tube is needed to prevent aspiration of gastric contents and improve ventilatory function. After a period of artificial ventilation by mask, the patient typically has a distended abdomen, which impairs movement of the diaphragm and decreases lung ventilation. Patients who experience drowning require complex care. The full spectrum of critical care technology may be needed to manage the pathophysiologic complications of drowning, including pulmonary edema, infection, acute respiratory distress syndrome (ARDS), and CNS impairment.

GET READY FOR THE NEXT-GENERATION NCLEX® EXAMINATION!

Key Points

Review these Key Points for each NCLEX Examination Client Needs Category.

Safe and Effective Care Environment

- Collaborate with the interprofessional health care team to provide the most comprehensive care for patients with environmental emergencies. **QSEN: Teamwork and Collaboration**

Health Promotion and Maintenance

- Teach people methods of preventing all types of environmental emergencies. **QSEN: Safety**

Physiological Integrity

- Assess ***tissue integrity*** for patients with bites, stings, lightning injury, and cold injury. **QSEN: Safety**
- Establish the airway and cool the patient with heat stroke as quickly as possible. **QSEN: Safety**
- Management of a patient who has a snakebite depends on the severity of envenomation (venom injection) (see Table 11.1). **QSEN: Safety**
- Administer antivenin drugs as prescribed for the patient with a poisonous snakebite. **QSEN: Safety**
- Recommend cold applications, such as ice, to be used as first aid/prehospital care for the patient with a poisonous spider bite. **QSEN: Safety**
- Be prepared to administer epinephrine as prescribed for bee and wasp sting allergic reactions, followed by antihistamine drugs. **QSEN: Safety**
- Assess the patient with lightning injury for central nervous system and cardiovascular complications, and skin burns. **Clinical Judgment**
- Assess for signs and symptoms of coagulopathy (abnormal clotting) or cardiac failure in the patient with moderate-to-severe hypothermia. **Clinical Judgment**
- Avoid alcohol as a means of warming for the patient with a cold injury. **QSEN: Safety**
- Prepare to administer cardiopulmonary support, including CPR, for a drowning victim.
- Assess the drowning victim for pulmonary edema, infection, ARDS, and central nervous system impairment. **Clinical Judgment**

MASTERY QUESTIONS

1. What is the priority nursing action when a nurse observes an adult drowning in a lake?
   A. Stabilize the spine with a board
   B. Consider personal swimming abilities
   C. Safely remove person from the water
   D. Initiate airway clearance and deliver rescue breaths

2. In addition to calling 911, what is the appropriate nursing response when a client calls the telehealth nurse to report being bitten on the arm by an unknown type of snake?
   A. Apply ice to the site of the wound
   B. Extract venom by sucking the wound
   C. Apply a tourniquet to the affected arm
   D. Immobilize the extremity at the level of the heart

REFERENCES

Asterisk (*) indicates a classic or definitive work on this subject.

*American Heart Association. (2015). *Advanced cardiovascular life support provider manual.* Dallas: Author.

Andrews, C. J. (2018). Treatment of lightning injury. In *Lightning injuries* (pp. 115–139). CRC Press.

Ashmore, T., Inman, J., Cross, E., & Baugher, P. (2018). Association between NOS3 and EPAS1 gene polymorphisms and susceptibility to acute mountain sickness. *International Journal of Exercise Science: Conference Proceedings, 8*(6), 17.

Auerbach, P. S. (2016). *Medicine for the outdoors: The essential guide to first aid and medical emergencies* (6th ed.). Philadelphia: Elsevier.

Auerbach, P. S., Donner, H. J., & Weiss, E. A. (2019). *Field guide to wilderness medicine* (5th ed.). St. Louis: Elsevier.

Baillie, K., et al. (2020). *Altitude sickness.* Retrieved from https://www.altitude.org/altitude-sickness.

Bjertness, E., Wu, T., Stigum, H., & Nafstad, P. (2017). Acute mountain sickness, arterial oxygen saturation and heart rate among Tibetan students who reascend to Lhasa after 7 years at low altitude: A prospective cohort study. *BMJ Open, 7*(7), e016460.

Centers for Disease Control and Prevention. (2017). *CDC Yellow Book 2018: Health Information for International Travel.* New York: Oxford University Press.

Freer, L., Handford, C., & Imray, C. H. E. (2017). Frostbite. In P. S. Auerbach (Ed.), *Auerbach's wilderness medicine* (7th ed.) (pp. 197–221). Philadelphia: Mosby Elsevier.

Gallagher, S., & Hackett, P. (2018). *High altitude pulmonary edema.* In: *UpToDate,* Danzl, D., & Grayzel, J. (Eds.), Waltham, MA.

Jain, A., Gray, M., Slisz, S., Haymore, J., Badjatia, N., & Kulstad, E. (2018). Shivering treatments for targeted temperature management: A review. *The Journal of Neuroscience Nursing, 50*(2), 63.

Knoll, J. M., Knight, L. R., Quiroz, D., Popat, S. M., Pederson, T. G., & Morton-Gonzaba, N. (2019). Variation in clinical presentations and outcomes of heat stroke victims in the mass-casualty setting. *The Journal of Emergency Medicine, 57*(6), 866–870.

Laskowski-Jones, L., & Jones, L. J. (2018a). Chapter 13: Cold injuries. In S. C. Hawkins (Ed.), *Wilderness EMS* (pp. 241–254). Philadelphia: Wolters Kluwer.

Laskowski-Jones, L., & Jones, L. J. (2018b). Frostbite: Don't be left out in the cold. *Nursing, 48*(2), 26–34.

Leffers, J., Levy, R. M., Nicholas, P. K., & Sweeney, C. F. (2017). Mandate for the nursing profession to address climate change through nursing education. *Journal of Nursing Scholarship, 49*(6), 679–687.

LoVecchio, F. (2020). Scorpion envenomation causing neuromuscular toxicity. In *UpToDate,* Danzl, D., Traub, S., & Burns, M. (Eds.). Waltham, MA.

Main, D. (2020). *"Murder hornets" have arrived in the U.S.* Retrieved from https://www.nationalgeographic.com/animals/2020/05/asian-giant-hornets-arrive-united-states/.

McDermott-Levy, R., Jackman-Murphy, K. P., Leffers, J. M., & Jordan, L. (2019). Integrating climate change into nursing curricula. *Nurse Educator, 44*(1), 43–47.

Norris, R. L. (2019). *Coral snake envenomation.* Retrieved from http://emedicine.medscape.com/article/771701-overview.

Prince, T., & Huebner, K. (2019). Acute mountain sickness. In *StatPearls.* Treasure Island, FL: StatPearls Publishing.

Ramirez, O., Malyshev, Y., & Sahni, S. (2018). It's getting hot in here: A rare case of heat stroke in a young male. *Cureus, 10*(12):e3724.

Swanson, D., et al. (2020). Clinical manifestations and diagnosis of widow spider bites. In *UpToDate,* Traub, S., & Danzl, D. (Eds.). Waltham, MA.

Zafren, K. & Mechem, C. (2020). Frostbite: Emergency care and prevention. In *UpToDate,* Danzl, D. (Eds.). Waltham, MA.

U.S. Department of Veterans Affairs. (2020). *Military exposures: Cold injuries.* Retrieved from https://www.publichealth.va.gov/exposures/cold-injuries/index.asp.

12

Concepts of Disaster Preparedness

Linda Laskowski-Jones

http://evolve.elsevier.com/Iggy/

LEARNING OUTCOMES

1. Apply triage principles to prioritize safe delivery of care in a disaster or mass casualty situation.
2. Identify the roles of the nurse and interprofessional team in emergency preparedness and response.
3. Describe components of facility and personal emergency preparedness and response plans.
4. Describe the role of the nurse in supporting people coping with life changes after disaster.

KEY TERMS

command center See *emergency operations center.*

containment The act of limiting the expansion or spread of a contagion.

debriefing After a mass casualty incident or disaster, (1) the provision of sessions for small groups of staff in which teams are brought in to discuss effective coping strategies (critical incident stress debriefing), and (2) the administrative review of staff and system performance during the event to determine opportunities for improvement in the emergency management plan.

disaster A mass casualty incident in which the number of casualties exceeds the resource capabilities of a particular community or hospital facility.

disaster triage tag system A system that categorizes triage priority by colored and numbered tags.

emergency operations center (EOC) A designated location in the Hospital Incident Command System (HICS) with accessible communication technology. Also called the *command center.*

emergency preparedness A goal or plan to meet an extraordinary need for hospital beds, staff, drugs, personal protective equipment, supplies, and medical devices such as mechanical ventilators.

go bag See *personal readiness supplies.*

Hospital Incident Command System (HICS) An organizational model for disaster management in which roles are formally structured under the hospital or long-term care facility incident commander, with clear lines of authority and accountability for specific resources.

hospital incident commander As defined in a hospital's emergency response plan, the person (either an emergency physician or administrator) who assumes overall leadership for implementing the institutional plan at the onset of a mass casualty incident. This person has a global view of the entire situation, facilitates patient movement through the system, and brings in resources to meet patient needs.

isolation Complete separation from others of a patient with an infectious condition.

mass casualty event A situation affecting public health that is defined based on the resource availability of a particular community or hospital facility. When the number of casualties exceeds the resource capabilities, a disaster situation is recognized to exist.

medical command physician As defined in a hospital's emergency response plan, the person responsible for determining the number, acuity, and medical resource needs of victims arriving from the incident scene and for organizing the emergency health care team response to injured or ill patients.

multicasualty event A disaster event in which a limited number of victims or casualties are involved and can be managed by a hospital using local resources.

pandemic A general epidemic spread over a wide geographic area and affecting a large proportion of the population.

personal emergency preparedness plan An individual plan that outlines specific arrangements in the event of disaster, such as child care, pet care, and older adult care.

personal readiness supplies A preassembled disaster supply kit for the home and/or automobile that contains clothing and basic survival supplies. Also called a *go bag.*

quarantine Isolation for a period of time of people or animals that have been exposed to a contagion or have been in an area in which contagion is present.

triage The process of sorting or classifying patients into priority levels depending on illness or injury severity, with the highest acuity needs receiving the quickest evaluation and treatment.

triage officer In a hospital's emergency response plan, the person who rapidly evaluates each patient who arrives at the hospital. In a large hospital, this person is generally a physician who is assisted by triage nurses; however, a nurse may assume this role when physician resources are limited.

PRIORITY AND INTERRELATED CONCEPTS

The priority concepts for this chapter are:
- *Safety*
- *Teamwork and Collaboration*
- *Communication*

A **disaster** is defined as an event in which illness or injuries exceed resource capabilities of a health care facility or community because of destruction and devastation. This kind of event can be either *internal* to a health care facility or *external* from situations that create casualties in the community. Both internal and external disasters can occur simultaneously, such as when Hurricane Michael incapacitated health care facilities in the Florida Panhandle and in Texas during the 2018 Atlantic hurricane season (Fig. 12.1).

TYPES OF DISASTERS

An event occurring inside a health care facility or campus that could endanger the ***safety*** of patients or staff is considered an *internal* disaster. The event creates a need for evacuation or relocation. It often requires extra personnel and the activation of the facility's emergency preparedness and response plan (also called an *emergency management plan*). Examples of internal disasters include fire, explosion, loss of critical utilities (e.g., electricity, water, computer systems, and ***communication*** capabilities), and violence (e.g., an active-shooter situation). Each health care organization develops policies and procedures for preventing these events through organized facility and security management plans. The most important outcome for any internal disaster is to maintain patient, staff, and visitor safety.

An event outside the health care facility or campus, somewhere in the community, that requires the activation of the facility's emergency management plan is considered an *external* disaster. The number of facility staff and resources may not be adequate for the incoming emergency department (ED) patients. External disasters, like a hurricane, earthquake, or tornado, can be natural, or they can be technologic such as an act of terrorism with explosive devices or a malfunction of a nuclear reactor with radiation exposure. Examples of external disasters include the Coronavirus Disease 2019, also known as COVID-19, pandemic; the mass shootings at the Pulse nightclub in Orlando, Florida in 2016 and at the Las Vegas Harvest Music Festival in 2017; and Hurricane Harvey, which incapacitated parts of Texas in 2017 (Fig. 12.2).

Internal and external disasters can result in many casualties, including death. Multicasualty and mass casualty (disaster) events are not the same. The main difference is based on the scope and scale of the incident, considering the number of victims or casualties involved and the severity of the effects. Both types of disasters require specific response plans to activate necessary resources. In general, a **multicasualty event** can be managed by a hospital using local resources; a **mass casualty event** overwhelms local medical capabilities and may require the collaboration of numerous agencies and health care facilities to handle the crisis. State, regional, and/or national resources may be needed to support the areas affected by the event. Trauma centers have a special role in all emergency preparedness activities because they provide a critical level of expertise and specialized resources for complex injury management.

To maintain ongoing disaster preparedness, hospital personnel participate in emergency training and drills regularly. In the United States, The Joint Commission (2020) mandates that hospitals have an emergency preparedness plan that is tested through drills or actual participation in a real event at least twice a year. One of the drills or events must involve community-wide resources and an influx of actual or simulated patients to assess the ability of collaborative efforts and command structures. Accredited health care organizations are required to take an "all-hazards approach" to disaster planning. Using this approach, preparedness activities must address *all credible threats* to the ***safety*** of the community that could result in a disaster situation. Disaster drills are ideally planned based on a risk assessment or vulnerability analysis that identifies the events most likely to occur in a particular community. For example, a flood is more likely in the Gulf of Mexico, and an avalanche is more likely in ski areas of the Rocky Mountains. Because the threat of gun violence is now a risk in all communities, active-shooter drills are commonplace in health care settings. It is essential that staff actively and seriously participate in these drills to increase their

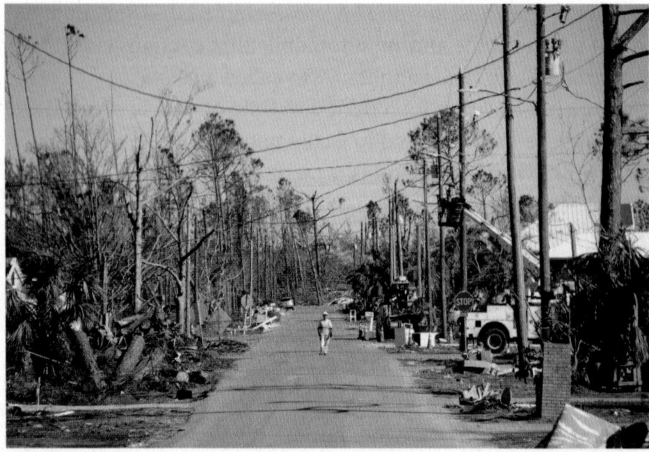

Fig. 12.1 The destruction after Superstorm Sandy ravaged the East Coast in 2012. (Copyright © iStock/Jason Whitman.)

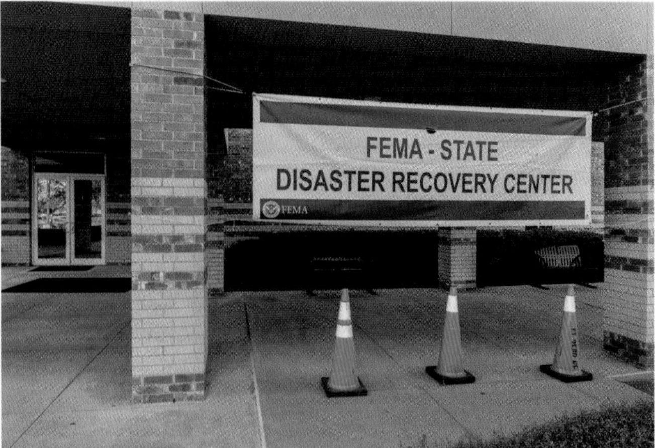

Fig. 12.2 Temporary shelter set up for homeless victims of Hurricane Harvey in Houston, Texas. (Copyright © iStock/michelmond.)

ability to act rapidly and maintain their ongoing competency. The importance of training has been emphasized in the wake of many disaster responses and has been credited with saving lives. Furthermore, literature shows that nurse leaders bring caring and resiliency to disaster response (Barker et al., 2018), so it is critical to stay prepared. After the Pulse nightclub shooting of 2016, Orlando Regional Medical Center (ORMC) treated 44 victims, of whom 35 survived; although there is grief for those lost, effective disaster planning and team preparedness accomplished well before this tragedy helped to save lives on the night of this event (Glasofer & Laskowski-Jones, 2018).

Nursing homes and other long-term care (LTC) facilities are also mandated to have annual drills to prepare for mass casualty events. For these agencies, as well as home care agencies and group homes, part of the response plan must include a method for evacuation of residents from the facility in a timely and safe manner in the event of a disaster.

An evacuation plan is part of fire prevention and preparedness plans for health care facilities. The Life Safety Code published by the National Fire Protection Association (2018) provides guidelines for building construction, design, maintenance, and evacuation. The Centers for Medicare and Medicaid Services (CMS) (2019) requires every health care facility to practice at least one fire drill or actual fire response once a year. Patient evacuation is not required if the event is a drill. All facility personnel are mandated to have training in fire prevention and responsiveness each year. The Best Practice for Patient Safety & Quality Care: Nurse's Role in Responding to Health Care Facility Fires box lists general guidelines for fire responsiveness and building evacuation to ensure ***safety***.

IMPACT OF EXTERNAL DISASTERS

The events of September 11, 2001, substantially changed hospital and community disaster planning efforts. With the shocking terrorist attacks on the Twin Towers of the World Trade Center and on the Pentagon, the loss of life in a field in Pennsylvania, and the actual and perceived threat of domestic terrorism, including the anthrax exposure that followed, hospital emergency preparedness concepts became integrated into the daily operations of emergency departments (EDs) by necessity. Weapons of mass destruction (WMDs) became a focus of public health risk.

The term "NBC" was coined to describe *n*uclear, *b*iologic, and *c*hemical threats. In response, emergency medical services (EMS) agencies and hospitals improved ***safety*** by upgrading their decontamination facilities, equipment, and all levels of personal protective equipment to better protect staff. ED physicians, providers, and nursing staff now routinely undergo hazardous materials (HAZMAT) training and learn how to recognize patterns of illness in patients who present for treatment that potentially indicate biologic terrorism agents such as anthrax or smallpox (Fig. 12.3). Protocols for the pharmacologic treatment of infectious disease agents and stockpiles of antibiotics and nerve agent antidotes are generally more readily available than in the past.

The most significant outcome of improving emergency preparedness after September 11, 2001, was that the ability to competently handle the more typical multicasualty or mass casualty event such as a bus crash, tornado, chemical plant incident, or building collapse was greatly improved in many communities. However, disaster situations even today can still exceed the scope of usual day-to-day crisis operations, pointing to the necessity of well-defined personal, facility, regional, and national emergency preparedness plans, as well as ongoing drills.

From another historical perspective, Hurricane Katrina made landfall in 2005 in Louisiana and other Gulf states as a category 4 storm that caused more than 1000 deaths and devastating environmental and property damage. Volunteers from all over the United States and local, regional, and federal agencies took part in the large-scale disaster evacuation, rescue, and relief effort, which severely challenged available resources and established disaster plans. However, offices that provide and maintain licensure requirements were damaged or inoperable immediately following Katrina, which greatly affect the speed of allowing nurses into the state to provide needed care (Benton,

BEST PRACTICE FOR PATIENT SAFETY & QUALITY CARE (QSEN)

Nurse's Role in Responding to Health Care Facility Fires

- Remove any patient or staff from immediate danger of the fire or smoke.
- Discontinue oxygen for all patients who can breathe without it.
- For patients on life support, maintain their respiratory status manually until removed from the fire area.
- Direct ambulatory patients to walk to a safe location.
- If possible, ask ambulatory patients to help push wheelchair patients out of danger.
- Move bedridden patients from the fire area in bed, by stretcher, or in a wheelchair; if needed, have one or two staff members move patients on blankets or carry them.
- After everyone is out of danger, seek to contain the fire by closing doors and windows and using an ABC extinguisher (which can put out any type of fire) if possible.
- Do not risk injury to yourself or staff members while moving patients or attempting to extinguish the fire.

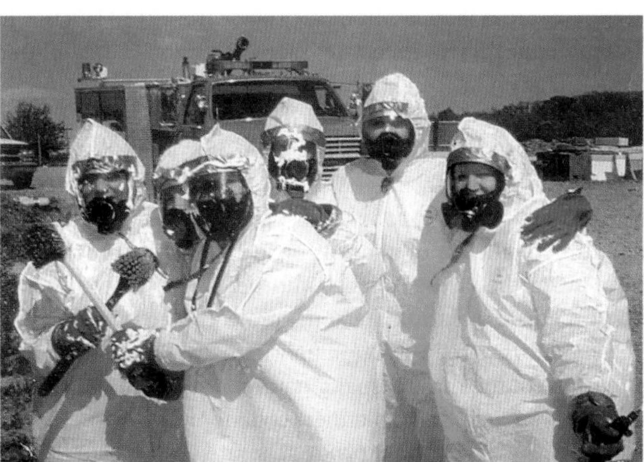

Fig. 12.3 Hazardous materials (HAZMAT) training to decontaminate people exposed to toxic agents in an outdoor decontamination area. (Courtesy Meg Blair, PhD, RN.)

2018). Critical systems failed and were eventually re-established through ***teamwork and collaboration*** among multiple agencies to ensure that the most basic human needs were met. Hurricane Katrina overwhelmed the existing emergency care system and caused the mobilization of a national mutual aid response on a level that had not been experienced in previous U.S. history.

Superstorm Sandy, the historic event that made landfall in New York City in October 2012, was downgraded from a category 1 hurricane. However, the flooding that occurred destroyed critical hospital equipment, including emergency power generators, in the lower levels of several health care facilities, causing the loss of utilities and crippling operations. Hospitals that were severely affected had to evacuate patients to other facilities, many of which were already overwhelmed by an influx of patients from the storm's damage in the community. Staff worked for several days in harsh conditions, carrying glow sticks and flashlights and wearing headlamps while evacuating critically ill and injured patients via stairwells because elevators were nonfunctional.

Lessons learned from September 11, Hurricane Katrina, Superstorm Sandy, earthquakes in Japan and Haiti, tsunamis, and terrorist attacks prompt improved facility design, staff preparation, and coordination of efforts that are beneficial for future disasters. Health care facilities must proactively address structural changes to provide ***safety*** and protection from flooding and utilities failures. These insights also can be applied to health care facility and community agency plans for pandemic infections, including influenza.

A **pandemic** (an infection or disease that occurs throughout the population of a country or the world) leads a vast number of people to seek medical care, even the "worried well." Although not yet ill, the "worried well" want evaluation, preventive treatment, or reassurance from a health care provider. A recent global biologic threat was the Ebola virus disease crisis that devastated West Africa from 2014 to 2016 (World Health Organization, 2020). This outbreak, although better managed, still continues (Fig. 12.4). The most recent global pandemic, the novel Coronavirus Disease 2019 (known as COVID-19, caused by the virus severe acute respiratory syndrome coronavirus 2 [SARS-CoV-2]), arose at the end of 2019 as the causative agent of pneumonia (McIntosh, 2020). It quickly spread worldwide. In a response larger than has been seen since the 1918 H1N1 influenza epidemic, global industries closed or relocated employees to work from home. Retail establishments, restaurants, flights, and cruises were closed and canceled for months. Schools serving K-12 students, colleges, and universities shifted to remote online learning to discourage large assemblies of people in classrooms. Many general populations were sequestered at home under different levels of **quarantine** in an effort to provide **containment** of the virus. Patients who were exposed were placed into immediate **isolation**. Personal protective equipment (PPE) and ventilators were in scarce supply in many parts of the world.

Because of the mass casualty nature of pandemic influenza, emergency preparedness planners collaborated during the outbreak of COVID-19 to incorporate strategies for handling an influx of ill patients into the system. Quarantine of selected nursing units or the entire hospital became necessary in some demographics. At the time of publication, the global response to COVID-19 is still emerging as countries, nations, and states within the United States attempt to reopen safely and possibly prepare for another wave of infection. See Chapters 21 and 28 for more information on COVID-19.

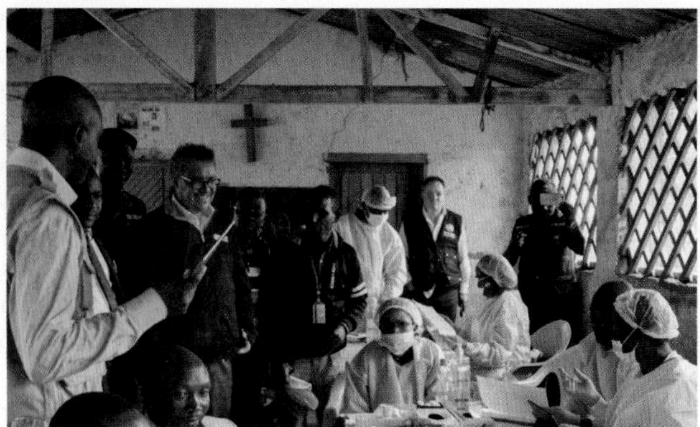

Fig. 12.4 WHO Director-General Dr. Tedros Adhanom Ghebreyesus visiting Ebola-affected areas in the Democratic Republic of the Congo (DRC) to review the response to date.

Common to all mass casualty events, the goal of **emergency preparedness** is to effectively meet the extraordinary need for resources such as hospital beds, staff, drugs, PPE, supplies, and medical devices. The U.S. government stockpiles critical equipment and supplies in case they are needed for a pandemic influenza outbreak and organizes large-scale vaccination programs. Each state has its own specific emergency preparedness plan. In the case of COVID-19, the United States has learned that these methods of preparedness need modification and enhancement to better meet the needs that arose as part of this pandemic influenza outbreak. Future needs after a vaccine for COVID-19 is developed includes planning for how mass inoculations will actually occur in a timely and efficient manner in a way that will reach the at-risk population, including those who are homebound.

EMERGENCY PREPAREDNESS AND RESPONSE

Emergency management includes actions or steps taken to decrease the potential loss during a disaster, and it involves mitigation, preparedness, response, and recovery (Federal Emergency Management Agency [FEMA], 2020b; Nielson, 2017). *Mitigation* involves preplanning for a disaster, analyzing potential risk and loss, and putting processes in place to minimize the impact (Nielson, 2017). *Preparedness* involves active steps taken to prepare to handle an emergency; *response* involves the actions taken to rescue and care for those affected by a disaster, and *recovery* involves steps taken to return to normal after the event (Ohio Emergency Management Agency, 2017).

Mass Casualty Triage

Bystanders will always be first on the scene of a disaster. Resources such as the Department of Homeland Security's (2020) "Stop the Bleed" campaign (Fig. 12.5) can be helpful teaching tools so people know what to do before professional emergency services arrive. A key process in any multicasualty or mass casualty response is effective **triage** to rapidly sort ill or injured patients into priority categories based on their acuity and survival potential.

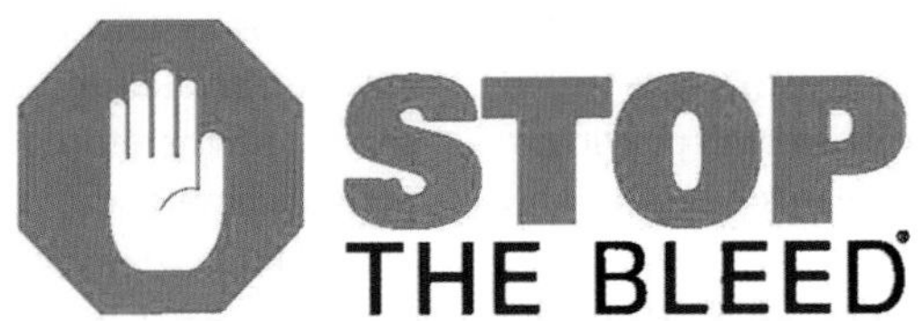

No matter how rapid the arrival of professional emergency responders, bystanders will always be first on the scene. A person who is bleeding can die from blood loss within five minutes, so it's important to quickly stop the blood loss.

Remember to be aware of your surroundings and move yourself and the injured person to safety, if necessary.

Call 911.

Bystanders can take simple steps to keep the injured alive until appropriate medical care is available. Here are three actions that you can take to help save a life:

1. Apply Pressure with Hands

EXPOSE to find where the bleeding is coming from and apply **FIRM, STEADY PRESSURE** to the bleeding site with both hands if possible.

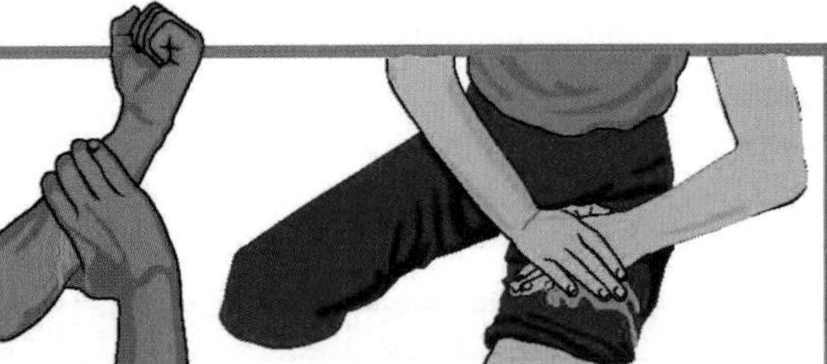

2. Apply Dressing and Press

EXPOSE to find where the bleeding is coming from and apply **FIRM, STEADY PRESSURE** to the bleeding site with bandages or clothing.

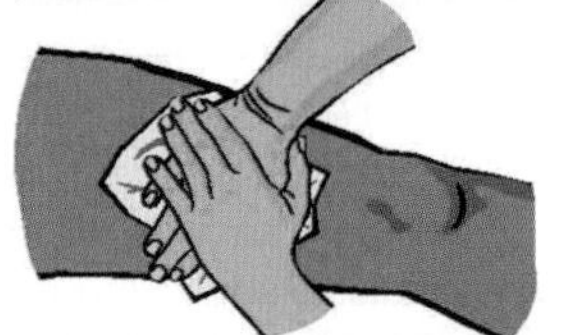

3. Apply Tourniquet(s)

If the bleeding doesn't stop, place a tourniquet as high on the extremity as possibe above the wound. The tourniquet may be applied and secured over clothing.

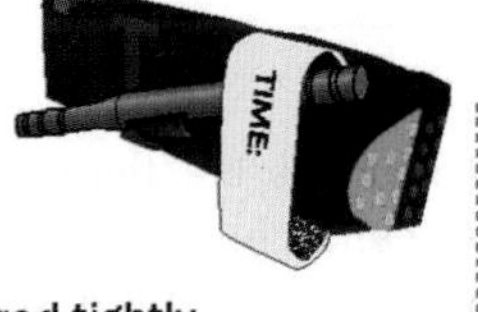

If the bleeding still doesn't stop, place a second tourniquet next to the first tourniquet.

PULL the strap through the buckle, **TWIST** the rod tightly, **CLIP** and **SECURE** the rod with the clasp or the Velcro strap.

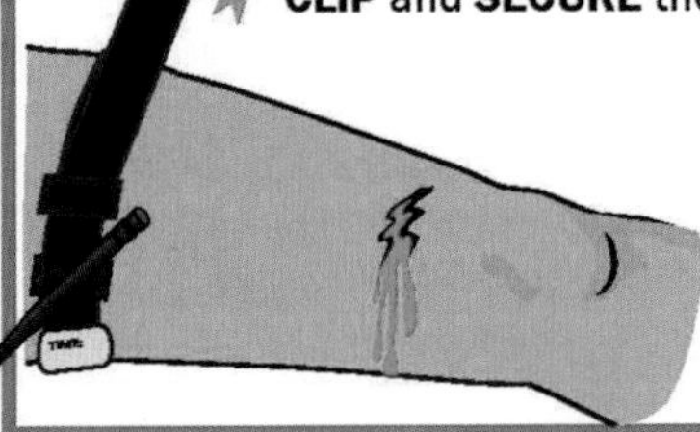

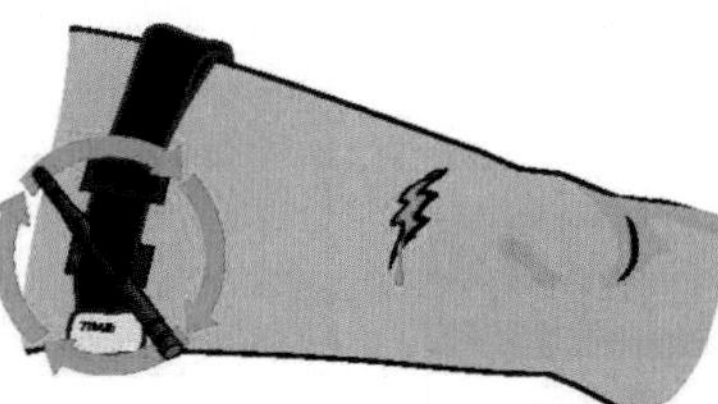

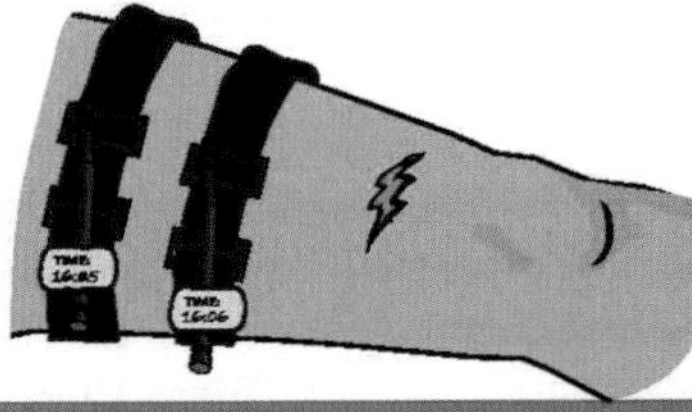

The 'Stop the Bleed' campaign was initiated by a federal interagency workgroup convened by the National Security Council Staff, The White House. The purpose of the campaign is to build national resilience by better preparing the public to save lives by raising awareness of basic actions to stop life threatening bleeding following everyday emergencies and man-made and natural disasters. Advances made by military medicine and research in hemorrhage control during the wars in Afghanistan and Iraq have informed the work of this initiative which exemplifies translation of knowledge back to the homeland to the benefit of the general public. The Department of the Defense owns the 'Stop the Bleed' logo and phrase.

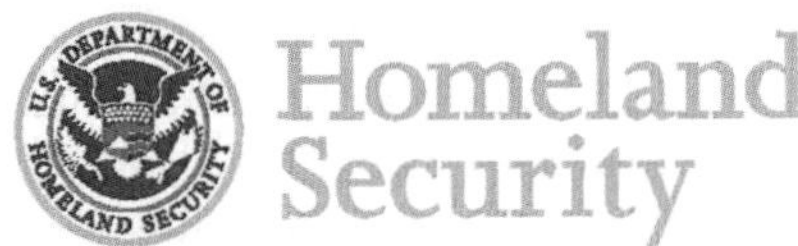

Fig. 12.5 Department of Homeland Security "Stop the Bleed" program. (From U.S. Department of Homeland Security. *Stop the Bleed.* [2020]. https://www.dhs.gov/stopthebleed.)

Triage functions may be performed by EMS providers in the field such as:

- Emergency medical technicians (EMTs) and paramedics
- Nurse, provider, and physician field teams that are called from the hospital to a disaster scene to assist EMS providers
- Nurse, provider, and physician hospital teams to assess and reassess incoming patients

Triage concepts in a mass casualty incident differ from the "civilian triage" methods discussed in Chapter 10 that are practiced during usual emergency operations (Table 12.1). Although disaster triage practices can vary widely based on local EMS protocols, some concepts are fairly universal. Most mass casualty response teams in the field (at the disaster site) and in the hospital setting use a **disaster triage tag system** that categorizes triage priority by color and number:

- Emergent (class I) patients are identified with a red tag.
- Patients who can wait a short time for care (class II) are marked with a yellow tag.
- Nonurgent or "walking wounded" (class III) patients are given a green tag.
- Patients who are expected (and allowed) to die or are dead are issued a black tag (class IV).

! NURSING SAFETY PRIORITY QSEN

Action Alert

In mass casualty or large-scale disaster situations, implement a military form of triage with the overall desired outcome of doing the greatest good for the greatest number of people. If resources are severely limited, this means that patients who are critically ill or injured and might otherwise receive attempted resuscitation during usual operations may be triaged into an "expectant" or "black-tagged" category and allowed to die or not be treated until others have received care.

Typical examples of *black-tagged* patients are those with massive head trauma, extensive full-thickness body burns, and high cervical spinal cord injury necessitating mechanical ventilation. The rationale for this very difficult decision is that limited resources must be dedicated to saving the most lives rather than expending valuable resources to save one life at the possible expense of many others.

TABLE 12.1 Comparison of Triage Under Usual Versus Mass Casualty Conditions

Triage Under Usual Conditions	Triage Under Mass Casualty Conditions
Emergent (immediate threat to life)	Emergent or class I (red tag) (immediate threat to life)
Urgent (major injuries that require immediate treatment)	Urgent or class II (yellow tag) (major injuries that require treatment)
Nonurgent (minor injuries that do not require immediate treatment)	Nonurgent or class III (green tag) (minor injuries that do not require immediate treatment)
Does not apply	Expectant or class IV (black tag) (expected and allowed to die)

In this system of triage, *red-tagged* patients have immediate life-threatening conditions such as airway obstruction or shock and therefore require immediate attention. *Yellow-tagged* patients have major injuries such as open fractures with a distal pulse and large wounds that need treatment within 30 minutes to 2 hours. *Green-tagged* patients have minor injuries that can be managed after a delay, generally more than 2 hours. Examples of green-tagged injuries include closed fractures, sprains, strains, abrasions, and contusions.

Green-tagged patients are often referred to as the "walking wounded" because they may actually evacuate themselves from the mass casualty scene and go to the hospital in a private vehicle. Green-tagged patients usually make up the greatest number in most large-scale multicasualty situations. Therefore they can overwhelm the system if provisions are not made to handle them as part of the disaster plan. A related concern is that green-tagged patients who self-transport may unknowingly carry contaminants from a nuclear, biologic, or chemical incident into the hospital environment, with potentially disastrous consequences. ED staff must anticipate these issues and collaborate to devise emergency response plans accordingly, including appropriate decontamination measures.

PATIENT-CENTERED CARE: CULTURAL/SPIRITUAL CONSIDERATIONS QSEN

As a component of culturally competent care, disaster triage processes should also incorporate strategies to accommodate vulnerable patient populations such as very young infants and children, older adults, people with disabilities, those who have psychological concerns, and those who require devices such as a mechanical ventilator or home oxygen.

NCLEX Examination Challenge 12.1

Safe and Effective Care Environment

After a mass casualty event, which client will the nurse triage with a yellow tag?

A. 29-year old with third-degree burns over 80% of the body
B. 36-year old with closed fractures of both legs
C. 48-year old with wheezing and difficulty breathing
D. 52-year old with multiple abrasions and contusions

Once patients are in the triage area of the hospital, they typically receive a special bracelet with a disaster number. Preprinted labels with this number can be applied to chart forms and personal belongings. Digital photos may be used as part of the identification process in some systems. The standard hospital registration process and identification band can be applied after the patient's identity has been confirmed.

Automated tracking systems using infrared, radiofrequency, or ultrasound technology are available in some EDs to track a patient's triage priority on arrival, location, and process of care. The interactions the patient has with caregivers can also be tracked. This is an important ***safety*** strategy if the patient is later found to have contaminants or a disease that could pose a risk to staff members who had close contact and require decontamination or prophylaxis (Laskowski-Jones, 2008). These systems are valuable components of the hospital's emergency preparedness infrastructure because they can rapidly portray the overall census and acuity of patients. They also enable ED leaders to determine how many casualties of a particular acuity level a hospital can safely accept from the incident scene.

Notification and Activation of Emergency Preparedness/Management Plans

When the number of casualties exceeds the usual resource capabilities, a disaster situation exists. What may be considered a routine day in the ED of a large urban trauma center could be defined as a disaster for a small rural community hospital if the same numbers of patients arrive. Therefore each facility decides when criteria to declare a disaster have been met. Flexibility is needed because resources may change by time of day and by day of the week. For example, hospitals typically have the fewest staff available after midnight on the weekend. An incident that occurs in this time frame may require activation of the emergency preparedness plan to bring extra resources into the hospital. The same incident during weekday business hours might be handled with on-site personnel alone without the need for activation of the plan.

Notification that a multicasualty or mass casualty situation exists usually occurs by radio, cellular, or electronic ***communication*** between the ED and EMS providers at the scene. A state or regional emergency management agency may also notify the ED of the event. Each hospital has its own policy that specifies *who* has the authority to activate and *how* to activate the disaster or emergency preparedness plan. Group texting or paging systems, telephone trees, and instant computer-based automated alert messages are the most common means of notifying essential personnel of a mass casualty incident or disaster.

A catastrophic event such as a major earthquake or tornado, or a terrorist incident involving weapons of mass destruction (WMDs), also requires the ***teamwork and collaboration*** of volunteers from all members of the health care team in the region. The media may be contacted to facilitate ***communication*** by broadcasting messages to the health care community-at-large via television, radio, or social media. Social media continue to be used more frequently in times of disaster for citizen reporting, community organizing, problem solving, and volunteer recruitment (Kim & Hastak, 2018; Palen & Hughes, 2018). For such incidents, the National Guard, the American Red Cross, the public health department, various military units, a Medical Reserve Corps (MRC), or a Disaster Medical Assistance Team (DMAT) can be activated by state and federal government authorities.

- An MRC is made up of a group of volunteer medical and public health care professionals, including physicians, providers, and nurses. They offer their services to health care facilities or to the community in a supportive or supplemental capacity during times of need such as a disaster or pandemic disease outbreak. This group may help staff hospitals or community health settings that face personnel shortages and establish first aid stations or special-needs shelters. As a means to alleviate ED and hospital overcrowding, the MRC may also set up an acute care center (ACC) in the community for patients who need acute care (but not intensive care) for days to weeks.
- A DMAT is a medical relief team made up of civilian medical, paraprofessional, and support personnel that is deployed to a disaster area with enough medical equipment and supplies to sustain operations for 72 hours (U.S. Department of Health and Human Services, 2019). DMATs are part of the National Disaster Medical System (NDMS) in the United States. They provide relief services ranging from primary health care and triage to evacuation and staffing to assist health care facilities that have become overwhelmed with casualties. *Because licensed health care providers such as nurses act as federal employees when they are deployed, their professional licenses are recognized and valid in all states.* Additional examples of services provided by the NDMS include:
  - Disaster Mortuary Operational Response Teams (DMORTs) to manage mass fatalities
  - National Veterinary Response Teams (NVRTs) for emergency animal care
  - International Medical Surgical Response Teams (IMSURTs) to establish fully functional field surgical facilities wherever they are needed in the world

Nurses can join these teams, complete the required training, and offer their expertise as part of a coordinated federal response team in times of critical need (U.S. Department of Health and Human Services, 2017).

Before going to the incident in the field, all members of the interprofessional team must have adequate training to prepare them to recognize the risks in an unstable environment (Laskowski-Jones, 2010; Clutter, 2016). Such risks can include the potential for structural collapse, becoming the secondary target of a terrorist attack, interpersonal violence in unsecured locales, and working in an environment in which contagious diseases and natural hazards are possible (e.g., poisonous snake bites and mosquito-borne illnesses). Disaster workers must take measures such as obtaining prophylactic medications and vaccinations, having a personal evacuation plan, and ensuring access to necessary supplies and protective equipment so they do not become victims as well.

The National Disaster Life Support Foundation (2020) offers Core, Basic, and Advanced Disaster Life Support training courses that include all essential aspects of disaster response and management. They include the core competencies of disaster management to all levels of health care professionals. In addition, the Federal Emergency Management Agency (FEMA) (2020a) provides numerous online resources, including Community Emergency Response Team (CERT) training so people are better prepared for disasters and are able to respond more self-sufficiently to incidents and hazard situations in their own communities. These courses include mass casualty triage education.

Hospital Emergency Preparedness: Personnel Roles and Responsibilities

Nurses play a major role in the emergency preparedness or emergency management plan. Because multiple health system resources are necessary to effectively manage the disaster, the Hospital Incident Command System is typically established for organization and structure.

Hospital Incident Command System. The facility-level organizational model for disaster management is the **Hospital Incident Command System (HICS)**, which is a part of the National Incident Management System (NIMS) implemented by the Department of Homeland Security and FEMA to standardize disaster operations. In this system, roles are formally structured under the hospital or long-term care facility incident commander with clear lines of authority and accountability for specific resources (FEMA, 2020a). Officers are named to oversee essential emergency preparedness functions such as public information, ***safety*** and security, and medical command. Chiefs are appointed to manage logistics, planning, finance, and operations as appropriate to the type and scale of the event. In turn, chiefs delegate specific duties to other departmental officers and unit leaders. The idea is to achieve a manageable span of control over the personnel or resources allocated to achieve efficiency. FEMA offers free courses on the NIMS model and HICS structure through its website at www.training.fema.gov/IS/.

Because mass casualty events typically involve large numbers of people and can create a chaotic work environment, many EMS agencies and health care facilities use brightly colored vests with large lettering to help identify key leadership positions. Specific job action sheets are distributed to all personnel with leadership roles in HICS that predefine reporting relationships and list prioritized tasks and responsibilities. The HICS personnel also establish an **emergency operations center (EOC)** or **command center** in a designated location with accessible communication technology. They then use their collective expertise to manage the overall incident. All internal requests for additional personnel and resources and ***communication*** with field teams and external agencies should be coordinated through the EOC to maintain unity of command.

The roles and responsibilities of health care personnel in a mass casualty event or disaster are defined within the institution's emergency response or preparedness plan (Table 12.2). Each plan is as individualized as the particular facility's operations, yet virtually all plans identify certain key functions. One of the primary roles to be established at the onset of an incident is that of a **hospital incident commander** who assumes overall leadership for implementing the institutional plan. This person is usually either a physician in the ED or a hospital administrator who has the authority to activate resources. This role can also be fulfilled by a nursing supervisor functioning as the on-site hospital administrator after usual business hours until hospital leadership personnel arrive. The hospital incident commander's role is to take a global view of the entire situation and facilitate patient movement through the system, while bringing in personnel and supply resources to meet patient needs. For example, a hospital incident commander might dictate that all patients due to be discharged from an inpatient unit be moved to a lounge area immediately to free up hospital beds for mass casualty victims. He or she could also direct departments such as physical therapy or a surgical clinic to cancel their usual operations to convert the space into a minor treatment area. The incident commander assists in the organization of hospital-wide services to rapidly expand hospital capacity, recruit paid or volunteer staff, and ensure the availability of medical supplies.

TABLE 12.2 Summary of Key Personnel Roles and Functions for Emergency Preparedness and Response Plan

Personnel Role	Personnel Function
Hospital incident commander	Physician or administrator who assumes overall leadership for implementing the emergency plan
Medical command physician	Physician who decides the number, acuity, and resource needs of patients
Triage officer	Physician or nurse who rapidly evaluates each patient to determine priorities for treatment
Community relations or public information officer	Person who serves as a liaison between the health care facility and the media

Another typical role defined in hospital or other health care emergency preparedness plans is that of the **medical command physician**. He or she focuses on determining the number, acuity, and medical resource needs of victims arriving from the incident scene to the hospital and organizing the emergency health care team response to the injured or ill patients. Responsibilities include identifying the need for and calling in specialty-trained providers such as:

- Surgeons (trauma, neuro, orthopedic, plastic, and/or burn)
- Anesthesiologists
- Radiologists
- Pulmonologists
- Infectious disease physicians
- Industrial hygienists
- Radiation safety personnel

In smaller hospitals with limited specialty resources, the medical command physician might also help determine which patients should be transported out of the facility to a higher level of care or to a specialty hospital (e.g., burn center).

Closely affiliated with the medical command physician is the **triage officer**. This person is generally a physician in a large hospital who is assisted by triage nurses. When physician resources are limited, an experienced nurse may assume this role. The triage officer rapidly evaluates each person who presents to the hospital, even those who come in with triage tags in place. Patient acuity is re-evaluated for appropriate disposition to the area within the ED or hospital best suited to meet the patient's needs.

Many other roles and responsibilities can be defined within the institutional emergency response plan and may include the supply officer, the ***communication*** officer, the infection control officer, and the community relations or public information officer, to name a few. The community relations or public information officer is an especially important role to delineate in advance. Mass casualty incidents tend to attract a large amount of media attention. This staff member can draw media away from the clinical areas so essential hospital operations are not hindered. He or she can also serve as the liaison between hospital administration and the media to release only appropriate and accurate information.

Role of Nursing in Health Care Facility Emergency Preparedness and Response. Nurses function in key roles before, during, and after a disaster. The core components of the nursing process apply in the overall assessment of the emergency situation; the identification of needs, capabilities, and priorities (assessment and determination of need); and planning, implementing, and evaluating the disaster response. Before an event, nurses contribute to developing internal and external emergency response plans, including defining specific nursing roles. Nurses take into account the security needs; ***communication*** methods; training; alternative treatment areas; staffing for high-demand or surge situations; and requirements for resources, equipment, and supplies. They then test the plans by actively participating in disaster drills and evaluating the outcomes. If outcomes are not as desired, nurses help to modify the plan of action.

During an actual disaster, the ED charge nurse, trauma program manager, and other ED and hospital nursing leadership personnel act in collaboration with the medical command physician and triage officer to organize nursing and ancillary services to meet patient needs. Telephone trees or automated group notification systems may be activated to call in ED nurses who are not working or are not scheduled to work. ED areas are identified and prepared to stage, triage, resuscitate, and treat the disaster victims. Efforts are made to quickly discharge or admit other ED patients as appropriate to make room for the new arrivals. ED nurses apply principles of triage to prioritize care delivery as disaster victims enter the system and direct patients to the designated areas best suited to meet their needs.

Nursing roles in a disaster extend to all areas within a health care facility. The level of involvement is determined by the scope and scale of the disaster. In any mass casualty event, nurses from critical care and medical-surgical nursing units may be asked, in collaboration with the health care provider, to recommend patients for transfer or discharge to free up inpatient beds for disaster victims. Patients who are the most medically stable may be discharged early, including those who:

- Were admitted for observation and are not bedridden
- Are having diagnostic evaluations and are not bedridden
- Are soon scheduled to be discharged or could be cared for at home with support from family or home health care services
- Have had no critical change in condition for the past 3 days
- Could be cared for in another health care facility such as rehabilitation or long-term care

NCLEX Examination Challenge 12.2

Safe and Effective Care Environment

Which assignment will the ED charge nurse make when nurses from within the hospital are floated to the ED to care for clients affected by an earthquake? **Select all that apply.**

A. GI laboratory nurse assigned to clients needing sedation
B. Psychiatric nurse assigned to care for clients with lacerations
C. Orthopedic nurse assigned to accompany clients to radiology
D. Nurse administrator assigned to sit with loved ones in the waiting room
E. Medical-surgical nurse assigned to health care worker who is feeling overwhelmed

General staff nurses also may be recruited to collaborate in providing care for stable ED patients, thus allowing ED nurses to focus their efforts on caring for the mass casualty victims. Critical care unit nurses need to identify patients who can be transferred out of the unit to rapidly expand bed capacity. They can supplement ED nurses in the resuscitation setting or assist in monitored care and transport to critical care units. Hospital and ED nurse leaders also typically direct the ancillary departments to deliver supplies, instrument trays, medications, food, and personnel to meet service demands.

Hospital staff of all levels may be required to alter their routine operations to accommodate a high volume of patients, including those with special needs such as decontamination, burn management, or quarantine. Inpatient unit nurses may be assigned a higher number of patients than usual. They may also be asked to provide care in nontraditional locations such as hallways or waiting rooms to help rapidly decompress the ED so new arrivals can be readily managed.

Emergency plans dictate specific actions by all members of the interprofessional team such as who should be called when the plan is activated, who should report, where to report, which supplies or equipment carts should be brought to a predesignated location, and which type of paperwork or system should be implemented for patient identification in a large-scale event. Some staff may even have their roles changed completely. For example, administrative nurses may be reassigned to fulfill a clinical responsibility for a nursing unit. The key concept is that staff members are expected to remain flexible in a mass casualty situation and perform at their highest level and scope of practice to address the needs of the health care system and the patients. The greatest good for the greatest number of people is still the organizing principle when considering roles and responsibilities in mass casualty events—not necessarily individual staff preferences. However, the ***safety*** of all patients is vital.

EVENT RESOLUTION AND DEBRIEFING

When the last major casualties have been treated and no more are expected to arrive in numbers that could overwhelm the

ETHICAL/LEGAL CONSIDERATIONS

Creativity and flexibility of nursing leaders and nursing staff are essential to provide the staffing coverage necessary for a large-scale or extended incident. The willingness of staff to come to work is directly affected by personal concerns. When called to respond to work during a disaster, mass casualty event, or pandemic infectious disease outbreak, nurses may experience ethical and moral conflict among their own personal preparedness for disaster response, family obligations, and professional responsibilities (Lam et al., 2018). The American Nurses Association (ANA) Code of Ethics for Nurses With Interpretive Statements (2015) offers general guidance that can be helpful to nurses. Each nurse has to make a personal choice about whether to be involved in helping during the emergency or when to become involved.

A **personal emergency preparedness plan** developed in advance of a disaster by each individual nurse can help in such situations (Casey, 2017). It should outline the preplanned specific arrangements that are to be made for child care, pet care, and older adult care if the need arises, especially if the event prevents returning home for an extended period.

NCLEX Examination Challenge 12.3

Safe and Effective Care Environment

When creating a personal emergency preparedness plan, which does the nurse include? **Select all that apply.**

A. Assembling a go bag
B. Arranging for child care
C. Determining who will care for pets
D. Noting who will be called when the plan is activated
E. Identifying how long the emergency is expected to last
F. Noting where a nurse is expected to report if the emergency plan is activated
G. Collecting names, addresses, and telephone numbers to be used if a crisis occurs

! NURSING SAFETY PRIORITY (QSEN)

Action Alert

Include emergency contact names, addresses, and telephone numbers to use in a crisis as part of a personal emergency preparedness plan. In addition, preassemble **personal readiness supplies** or a **go bag** (disaster supply kit) for the home and automobile with clothing and basic survival supplies (Fig. 12.6), which allows for a rapid response for disaster staffing coverage (Box 12.1). Go bags are needed for all members of the family, including pets, in the event the disaster requires evacuation of the community or people to take shelter in their own homes.

health care system, the incident commander considers "standing down" or deactivating the emergency response plan. Although the casualties may have left the ED, other areas in the hospital may still be under stress and need the support of the supplemental resources provided by emergency plan activation. Before terminating the response, it is essential to ensure that the needs of the other hospital departments have been met and all are in agreement to resume normal operations.

A vital consideration in event resolution is staff and supply availability to meet ongoing operational needs. If nursing staff and other personnel were called in from home during their

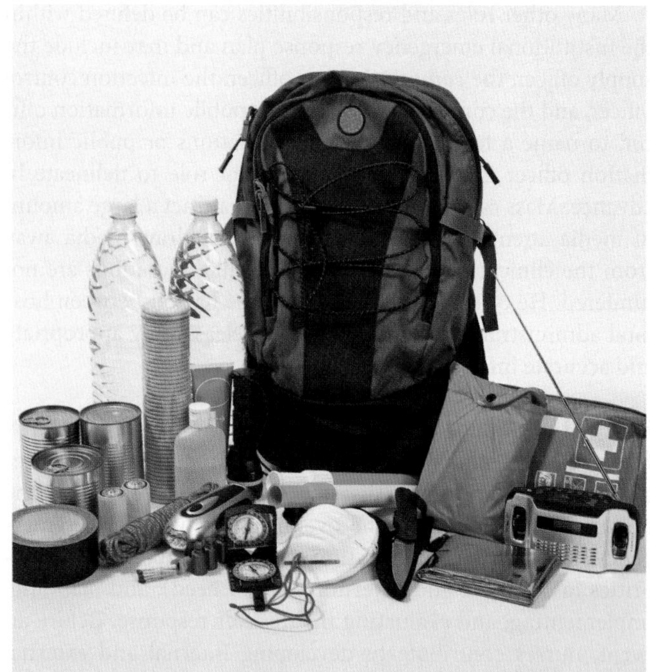

Fig. 12.6 Example of a personal readiness supplies, also known as a "Go Bag." (Copyright © istockphoto.com/schfer.)

off hours or if they worked well beyond their scheduled shifts to meet patient and departmental needs, provision for adequate rest periods should be made. Exhaustion poses a risk to patient ***safety*** and to the nurse when he or she must drive home. Sleeping quarters at the hospital might be necessary in this case, especially if the disaster event contributed to treacherous travel conditions.

Severe shortages of supplies pose a threat to usual operations. Taking inventory and restocking the ED are high-priority assignments following a disaster or mass casualty event. ***Teamwork and collaboration*** between the ED and the central supply department are essential to resolving stock availability problems. Instrument trays must be washed, packaged, and resterilized. Contracts with key external vendors outlining emergency resupply expectations and arrangements should be a part of the hospital's overall emergency preparedness plan so that service can be undertaken quickly after an event.

Two general types of **debriefing**, or formal systematic review and analysis, occur after a mass casualty incident or disaster. The first type entails bringing in crisis support teams to provide sessions for small groups of staff, to promote effective coping strategies. The second type of debriefing involves an administrative review of staff and system performance during the event to determine whether opportunities for improvement in the emergency management plan exist.

Crisis Support

Crisis workers with special education and training in psychological first aid and behavioral health address pre-crisis through postcrisis interventions for small-to-large groups, including communities. After working through the turmoil and the emotional impact of the incident and

BOX 12.1 Basic Supplies for Personal Preparedness (3-Day Supply)

- Backpack
- Clean, durable weather-appropriate clothing; sturdy footwear
- Potable water—at least 1 gallon per person per day for at least 3 days
- Food–nonperishable, no cooking required
- Headlamp or flashlight—battery powered; extra batteries and/or chemical light sticks (**Note:** a headlamp is superior because it allows hands-free operation)
- Pocket knife or multitool
- Personal identification (ID) with emergency contacts and phone numbers, allergies, and medical information; lists of credit card numbers and bank accounts (keep in watertight container)
- Towel and washcloth; towelettes, soap, hand sanitizer
- Paper, pens, and pencils; regional maps
- Cell phone and charger
- Sunglasses; protective and/or corrective eyewear
- Emergency blanket and/or sleeping bag and pillow
- Work gloves
- Personal first aid kit with over-the-counter (OTC) and prescription medications
- Rain gear
- Roll of duct tape and plastic sheeting
- Radio—battery powered or hand-crank generator
- Toiletries (toothbrush and toothpaste, comb, brush, razor, shaving cream, mirror, menstrual supplies, deodorant, shampoo, soap, lip balm, sunscreen, insect repellent, toilet paper)
- Plastic garbage bags and ties, resealable plastic bags
- Matches in a waterproof container
- Whistle
- Household liquid bleach for disinfection

the aftermath, the staff may find it difficult to "get back to normal." Without intervention during *and* after the emergency, they are at risk to develop acute stress disorder (ASD) or posttraumatic stress disorder (PTSD). ASD, although similar to PTSD, focuses on dissociative symptoms such as numbing, reduced awareness, depersonalization, derealization, or amnesia, experienced within the first month after a traumatic event. PTSD can lead to multiple characteristic psychological and physical effects, including flashbacks, avoidance, less interest in previously enjoyable events, detachment, rapid heart rate, and insomnia. People with PTSD can have great difficulty relating in their usual way to family and friends. Ultimately, professional "burnout" can stem from the inability to cope with the stress effectively. A resource is the International Critical Incident Stress Foundation (2019); their mission is "to provide leadership, education, training, consultation, and support services in comprehensive crisis intervention and disaster behavioral health services to the emergency response professions, other organizations, and communities worldwide." Research indicates that education and training in disaster management before an incident occurs is associated with improved confidence and better coping after the incident (Brooks, et al., 2018).

BEST PRACTICE FOR PATIENT SAFETY & QUALITY CARE (QSEN)

Preventing Staff Acute Stress Disorder and Posttraumatic Stress Disorder Following a Mass Casualty Event

- Use available counseling.
- Encourage and support co-workers.
- Monitor each other's stress level and performance.
- Take breaks when needed.
- Talk about feelings with staff and managers.
- Drink plenty of water and eat healthy snacks for energy.
- Keep in touch with family, friends, and significant others.
- Do not work more than 12 hours per day.

Adapted from Papp, E. (2005). Preparing for disasters: Helping yourself as you help others. *The American Journal of Nursing, 105*(5), 112.

The Best Practice for Patient Safety & Quality Care: Preventing Acute Stress Disorder and Posttraumatic Stress Disorder Following a Mass Casualty Event box lists recommendations proposed by several national organizations to help prevent staff ASD and PTSD following an emergency situation.

Administrative Review

The second type of debriefing is an administrative evaluation, also known as a "hot wash," directed at analyzing the hospital or agency response to an event while it is still in the forefront of the minds of everyone who participated in it. The goal of this debriefing is to discern what went right and what could be improved during activation and implementation of the emergency preparedness plan so that needed changes can be made. Typically, representatives from all groups who were involved in the incident come together soon after plan activation has been discontinued. They each are given an opportunity to hear and express positive and negative comments related to their experiences with the event. In the days after the plan activation, written critique forms are also solicited to gain additional information after participants have had time to consider their overall impressions of the response and the impact it had on their respective departments or clinical areas.

Although drills are important, implementing the emergency preparedness plan during an actual mass casualty event is the most effective means of "reality testing" the plan's utility. Feedback provided by participants can be used to modify or revise the plan and create new processes in preparation for future events.

ROLE OF NURSING IN COMMUNITY EMERGENCY PREPAREDNESS AND RESPONSE

During a community disaster, nurses and other emergency personnel may be needed for triage, first aid or emergency care, and shelter assistance. The initial action of first responders in a disaster is to remove people from danger, both the injured and uninjured. Firefighters and other disaster-trained emergency personnel typically manage this job; unless they have had specific prehospital search-and-rescue training, nurses are not usually involved in this process. In all cases, developing and maintaining accurate *situational awareness* are critical for appropriate priority setting and ***safety*** in a rapidly changing environment.

After removal from danger, victims are triaged by health care personnel as described earlier in this chapter. After triage, nurses often provide on-site first aid and emergency care. They may also be involved in teaching and supervising volunteers.

The American Red Cross sets up shelters for people who have lost their homes or have been evacuated from their homes. Nurses may need to teach those living temporarily in shelters about procedures that will be needed for ***safety*** when they return home. For example, clean drinking water may not be available for several days or longer, so community residents may need to boil their water before drinking. If electricity and gas are not available, an outdoor grill or camp stove can be used for this purpose. As alternative procedures, commercial water purification filters, sterilizing ultraviolet pens, or 10 to 20 drops of chlorine bleach added to a gallon of water will make the water safe to drink.

Human waste management creates another challenge if toilets do not flush. If not managed safely, enteric pathogens spread disease. A toilet bowl or bucket lined with a plastic bag can be used for human waste. To sanitize it and provide odor control, chlorine bleach can be added, and the bag tied and sealed. Portable toilet chemicals or chlorinated lime may be used as an alternative. To prevent a toxic gas reaction, remind residents not to mix any chemicals. Treated human waste bags can be buried in the ground. In an austere environment, a pit can be dug in the ground as an improvised toilet. In all cases, emphasize the importance of handwashing with soap and water or using a hand sanitizer to prevent disease transmission.

PSYCHOSOCIAL RESPONSE OF SURVIVORS TO MASS CASUALTY EVENTS

One of the most important roles of the nurse during and after a community disaster is health assessment (also known as *recognizing cues*) including psychosocial health. Experiencing a disaster can produce both immediate and long-lasting psychological and psychosocial effects in people personally affected by the event. Depending on the nature and magnitude of the incident, survivors experience the tragic loss of loved ones, pets, property, and valued possessions. They and their loved ones may have experienced injuries or illnesses brought about by the catastrophe. Lifestyles, roles, and routines are drastically altered, preventing people from achieving any sense of normalcy in the hours, days, and perhaps even weeks and months that follow a disaster. Coping abilities in survivors are severely stressed, leading to many individual responses, which can range from functional and adaptive behaviors to maladaptive coping.

Survivors have to confront feelings of vulnerability resulting from the devastating event, knowing that it could occur again. This may be a particularly relevant issue for people who live in areas prone to acts of terrorism or natural disasters. The decision, be it voluntary or involuntary, to abandon a family home or geographic region and then relocate to a "safe" area either temporarily or permanently can result in a sense of loss, grief, and disorientation. Some people may feel guilty about living through an event that caused others to die. The range of intense emotions can manifest as physical illness, as well as psychological and social dysfunction.

When helping people in crisis after a mass casualty event, be calm and reassuring. Establish rapport through active listening and honest ***communication***. Survivors benefit from talking about their experiences and putting them in chronological order, which provides clarity and helps them begin to problem solve. Offer resources whenever possible to help survivors gain a sense of personal control. Help survivors adapt to their new surroundings and routines through simple, concrete explanations. Convey caring behaviors, and provide a sense of ***safety*** and security to the best extent possible. If available, request that crisis counselors respond and assist in providing compassionate support to victims and their families.

Survivors also are at risk for development of acute stress disorder (ASD) or posttraumatic stress disorder (PTSD), as noted earlier.

Nurses caring for survivors with symptoms of ASD or PTSD should perform further assessment by using a tool such as the Impact of Event Scale—Revised (IES-R) (Weiss, 2007). The IES-R is a 22-item self-administered questionnaire that includes several subscales such as avoidance. Before giving the tool, determine the patient's reading level because it is written at a 10th-grade reading level. The tool should not be used for patients with short-term memory loss. For this reason, many older survivors often are not adequately assessed for postdisaster PTSD. Depending on the patient's presentation and the results of your assessment, remember that behavioral health evaluation and referral to counseling may be appropriate.

! NURSING SAFETY PRIORITY (QSEN)

Action Alert

A total score of 33 or higher (out of a possible 88) on the Impact of Event Scale—Revised (IES-R) is indicative of probable PTSD. Refer the patient to a psychiatrist, psychiatric mental health nurse practitioner, or qualified mental health counselor. A high score on any IES-R subscale indicates a need for further evaluation and counseling; again, make the appropriate referral to a mental health specialist to evaluate the possibility of current or past trauma, such as abuse or neglect.

CLINICAL JUDGMENT CHALLENGE 12.1

Patient-Centered Care

You are a nurse on a DMAT team that has been dispatched to help a community after a category 4 hurricane came ashore in a rural, underserved area. You have been notified that so far, 10 people have been declared dead on the scene and over 200 have been identified as injured. The first person you encounter is a 21-year old woman whom you quickly triage with a green tag, as she has experienced only a few abrasions from brushing her legs against a downed tree. Her blood pressure is 150/90 and her pulse rate is 94 beats/min. She breathlessly tells you that she cannot find her 69-year-old grandmother, and she is quickly becoming panicked.

1. **Recognize Cues:** What assessment information in this client situation is the most important and immediate concern for the nurse? (Hint: Identify the **relevant** information *first* to determine what is most important.)
2. **Analyze Cues:** What client conditions are consistent with the **most relevant** information? (Hint: Think about priority collaborative problems that support and contradict the information presented in this situation.)
3. **Prioritize Hypotheses:** Which possibilities or explanations are **most likely** to be present in this client situation? Which possibilities or explanations are the most serious? (Hint: Consider all possibilities and determine their urgency and risk for this client.)
4. **Generate Solutions:** What actions would most likely achieve the desired outcomes for this client? Which actions should be **avoided** or are **potentially harmful?** (Hint: Determine the desired outcomes first to decide which interventions are appropriate and those that should be avoided.)
5. **Take Action:** Which actions are the most appropriate and how should they be implemented? In what **priority order** should they be implemented? (Hint: Consider health teaching, documentation, requested health care provider orders or prescriptions, nursing skills, collaboration with or referral to health team members, etc.)
6. **Evaluate Outcomes:** What client assessment would indicate that the nurse's actions were **effective?** (Hint: Think about signs that would indicate an improvement, decline, or unchanged client condition.)

GET READY FOR THE NEXT-GENERATION NCLEX® EXAMINATION!

Key Points

Review these Key Points for each NCLEX Examination Client Needs Category.

Safe and Effective Care Environment

- Understand that nurses play a major role in triage, first aid and emergency care, and shelter assistance after disasters or mass casualty events. **QSEN: Safety**
- Recognize that all hospitals are required to have a hospital emergency preparedness and response team in place in case of mass casualty (disaster). **QSEN: Safety**
- Use a triage system that is implemented in a mass casualty situation (see Table 12.1). **Ethics**
- Recognize roles of interprofessional team members in a mass casualty incident as identified in Table 12.2. **QSEN: Teamwork and Collaboration**
- Maintain a personal emergency preparedness plan (see Box 12.1). **QSEN: Safety**

Psychosocial Integrity

- Assess survivors and families for their ability to adapt to the effects of disaster changes or traumatic events. **QSEN: Patient-Centered Care**
- Recognize that people and/or families will experience life changes resulting from a disaster; support them through active listening and make appropriate referrals. **QSEN: Patient-Centered Care**
- Be honest with victims and their families; offer orienting information and help them adapt to their changed or new situation. **Ethics**
- Take precautions to prevent staff from developing ASD or PTSD. **QSEN: Safety**
- Properly assess victims of disaster for ASD or PTSD. **Health Care Disparities**

Physiological Integrity

- Know your own limitations and develop situational awareness when responding to disaster or mass casualty events. **QSEN: Safety**

MASTERY QUESTIONS

1. What is the appropriate nursing action when assessing that a client scored 40 on the IES-R?
A. Triage with a black tag
B. Prepare for discharge to home
C. Administer oxygen and assess saturation
D. Refer to a psychiatrist or mental health counselor

2. What is the appropriate nursing response when asked to report to work to assist with a mass casualty event?
A. Report to work when asked by a supervisor
B. Refrain from working to care for family members
C. Refer to the ANA Code of Ethics for Nurses for direction
D. Agree to work for several hours until other nurses arrive to assist

REFERENCES

Asterisk (*) indicates a classic or definitive work on this subject.

American Nurses Association. (2015). Code of Ethics for Nurses With Interpretive Statements. Retrieved from http://www.nursingworld.org/MainMenuCategories/EthicsStandards/CodeofEthicsforNurses/Code-of-Ethics-For-Nurses.html.

Barker, C., Bell, E., Zhao, M., & Dyess, S. (2018). Caring & resiliency: Nurse educator leaders respond to hurricane harvey. *Nurse Leader, 16*(3), 177–180.

Benton, D. (2018). Disasters, regulation, and proactive response. *American Nurse Today, 13*(1), 32–33.

Brooks, S. K., Dunn, R., Amlot, R., Greenberg, N., & Rubin, G. J. (2018). Training and post-disaster interventions for the psychological impacts on disaster-exposed employees: A systematic review. *Journal of Mental Health.* https://www.ncbi.nlm.nih.gov/pubmed/29447058.

Casey, D. (2017). Ethical considerations during disaster. *MedSurg Nursing, 26*(6), 411–413.

Centers for Medicare and Medicaid Services (CMS). (2019). *Emergency Preparedness Rule.* https://www.cms.gov/Medicare/Provider-Enrollment-and-Certification/SurveyCertEmergPrep/Emergency-Prep-Rule.html.

Clutter, P. L. (2016). Unique roles of the emergency nurse. In J. Solheim (Ed.), *Emergency nursing: The profession, the pathway, the practice* (pp. 41–58). Indianapolis: Sigma Theta Tau International Honor Society of Nursing.

Department of Homeland Security. (2020). *Stop the bleed.* https://www.dhs.gov/stopthebleed.

Federal Emergency Management Agency (FEMA). (2020a). *Training.* https://training.fema.gov/is/.

Federal Emergency Management Agency (FEMA). (2020b). *What is mitigation?* https://www.fema.gov/what-mitigation.

Glasofer, A., & Laskowski-Jones, L. (2018). Mass shootings: A call for nursing awareness and action. *Nursing, 48*(12), 51–55.

International Critical Incident Stress Foundation, Inc. (2019). Mission statement. http://www.icisf.org/about-us/mission-statement/.

Kim, J., & Hastak, M. (2018). Social network analysis: Characteristics of online social networks after a disaster. *International Journal of Information Management, 38*(1), 86–96.

Lam, S. K. K., Kwong, E. W. Y., Hung, M. S. Y., Pang, S. M. C., & Chiang, V. C. L. (2018). Nurses' preparedness for infectious disease outbreaks: A literature review and narrative synthesis of qualitative evidence. *Journal of Clinical Nursing, 27*(7-8), e1244–e1255.

*Laskowski-Jones, L. (2008). Change management at the hospital front door: Integrating automatic patient tracking in a high-volume emergency department and level I trauma center. *Nurse Leader, 6*(2), 52–57.

*Laskowski-Jones, L. (2010). When disaster strikes: Ready, or not? (Editorial). *Nursing, 40*(4), 6.

McIntosh, K. (2020). Coronavirus disease 2019 (COVID-19): Epidemiology, virology, clinical features, diagnosis, and prevention. In *UpToDate*, Hirsch, M. (Ed.). Waltham, MA.

National Disaster Life Support Foundation. (2020). Retrieved from https://www.ndlsf.org

National Fire Protection Association. (2018). *The Life Safety Code.* Retrieved from https://catalog.nfpa.org/NFPA-101-Life-Safety-Code-P1220.aspx?icid=A292.

Nielson, M. (2017). When disaster strikes, will you be ready? *Nursing, 47*(12), 52–56.

Ohio Emergency Management Agency. (2017). The four phases of emergency management. https://ema.ohio.gov/Documents/COP/The%20Four%20Phases%20of%20Emergency%20Management.pdf.

*Papp, E. (2005). Preparing for disasters: Helping yourself as you help others. *American Journal of Nursing, 105*(5), 112.

Palen, L., & Hughes, A. L. (2018). Social media in disaster communication. In *Handbook of disaster research* (pp. 497–518). Cham: Springer.

The Joint Commission. (2020). *Emergency management resources.* http://www.jointcommission.org/emergency_management.aspx.

U.S. Department of Health and Human Services. (2017). *Disaster Medical Assistance Team (DMAT).* Retrieved from https://www.phe.gov/Preparedness/responders/ndms/ndms-teams/Pages/dmat.aspx.

U.S. Department of Health and Human Services. (2019). *National disaster medical system.* http://www.phe.gov/Preparedness/responders/ndms/Pages/default.aspx.

*Weiss, D. S. (2007). The impact of event scale: Revised. In J. P. Wilson, & C. S. Tang (Eds.), *Cross-cultural assessment of psychological trauma and PTSD* (pp. 219–238). New York: Springer.

World Health Organization. (2020). *Ebola virus disease.* Retrieved from https://www.who.int/news-room/fact-sheets/detail/ebola-virus-disease.

13

Concepts of Fluid and Electrolyte Balance

M. Linda Workman

http://evolve.elsevier.com/Iggy/

LEARNING OUTCOMES

1. Collaborate with the interprofessional team to perform a complete assessment of ***fluid and electrolyte balance***.
2. Explain how physiologic aging changes the effectiveness of mechanisms to maintain ***fluid and electrolyte balance*** and increases the risk for imbalance.
3. Apply knowledge of anatomy, physiology, and pathophysiology to perform an evidence-based assessment for the patient with a disturbance of ***fluid and electrolyte balance***.
4. Interpret assessment findings for the patient experiencing a disturbance of ***fluid and electrolyte balance***.
5. Protect the patient with a problem of ***fluid and electrolyte balance*** from injury and complications, especially those related to ***perfusion***.
6. Teach the patient and caregiver(s) how home safety is affected by problems of ***fluid and electrolyte balance***.

KEY TERMS

anions Negatively charged electrolytes.

calcium (Ca^{2+}) An important body electrolyte ion having two positive charges (divalent cation).

cations Positively charged electrolytes.

dehydration Body fluid volume (especially plasma volume) deficit caused by fluid intake or retention below what is needed to meet the body's daily fluid needs.

diffusion Movement of particles (solute) across a permeable membrane from an area of higher particle concentration to an area of lower particle concentration (down a concentration gradient).

electrolytes (ions) Solute particles that express and overall electrical charge (positive or negative). Also known as *ions*.

extracellular fluid (ECF) The compartment composing fluids outside of the cells (interstitial fluid and plasma volumes).

facilitated diffusion Movement across a cell membrane that requires a membrane-altering system.

filtration Movement of fluid through a cell or blood vessel membrane because of hydrostatic pressure (water pressure) differences.

fluid and electrolyte balance Regulation of body fluid volume, osmolarity, and composition; the regulation of electrolytes by the processes of filtration, diffusion, osmosis, and selective excretion.

hydrostatic pressure Pressure exerted by water molecules against the surfaces (membranes or walls) of a confining space. Also known as *water pressure.*

hypercalcemia Total serum calcium level above 10.5 mg/dL or 2.62 mmol/L.

hyperkalemia Serum potassium level higher than 5.0 mEq/L (mmol/L).

hypermagnesemia Serum magnesium level above 2.6 mEq/L or 1.07 mmol/L.

hypernatremia Serum sodium level over 145 mEq/L (mmol/L).

hyperosmotic/hypertonic Fluid with an osmolarity greater than 300 mOsm/L.

hypervolemia Fluid overload.

hypocalcemia Total serum calcium (Ca^{2+}) level below 9.0 mg/dL or 2.25 mmol/L.

hypokalemia Serum potassium level below 3.5 mEq/L (mmol/L).

hypomagnesemia Serum magnesium (Mg^{2+}) level below 1.8 mEq/L or 0.74 mmol/L.

hyponatremia Serum sodium (Na^{+}) level below 136 mEq/L (mmol/L).

hypo-osmotic/hypotonic Fluid with an osmolarity less than 270 mOsm/L.

hypovolemia Lower than normal circulating blood volume.

insensible water loss Body water loss that has no mechanisms for control, including losses through the skin, the lungs, GI tract, salivation, drainage from fistulas and drains.

interstitial fluid The part of extracellular fluids present between cells, also called the *third space,* that includes blood, lymph, water in the bones and connective tissue water, and the transcellular fluids.

intracellular fluid (ICF) The compartment composing fluids inside of the cells (cellular fluid).

isosmotic/isotonic Fluid that has the solute (particle) concentration (osmolarity) within the normal range for human body fluids, 270 to 300 mOsm/L.

magnesium (Mg^{2+}) A divalent cation that is stored mostly in bones and cartilage.

obligatory urine output Minimum amount of urine output per day needed to excrete toxic waste products (400 to 600 mL).

osmolality The number of milliosmoles in a kilogram of solution.

osmolarity The number of milliosmoles in a liter of solution.

osmosis Movement of water only through a selectively permeable (semipermeable) membrane to achieve an equilibrium of osmolarity.

potassium (K^+) The major cation of the intracellular fluid (ICF).

sodium (Na^+) The major cation (positively charged particle) in the extracellular fluid (ECF).

solute Particles dissolved in the solvent of body fluids.

solvent The water portion of body fluids.

PRIORITY AND INTERRELATED CONCEPTS

The priority concept for this chapter is:
- ***Fluid and Electrolyte Balance***

The ***Fluid and Electrolyte Balance*** concept exemplar for this chapter is Dehydration.

The interrelated concept for this chapter is:
- ***Perfusion***

ANATOMY AND PHYSIOLOGY REVIEW

The composition of the human body is more than 50% fluid (by weight). However, this fluid is more than pure water, much like the composition of the ocean, with particles dissolved or suspended in water. Thus water is the **solvent** portion of body fluids and **solute** is the particles dissolved or suspended in the water. When dissolved solute particles express an overall electrical charge (positive or negative), they are known as **electrolytes** or **ions**.

Body fluids deliver dissolved nutrients and electrolytes to all organs, tissues, and cells. Thus maintaining the volume of fluid and the electrolyte composition of the major fluid spaces *(compartments)* within the normal range is critical to optimal body function. Changes in either the amount of water or the amount of electrolytes in various body fluid compartments can reduce the function of all cells, tissues, and organs. To prevent changes, the body has many homeostatic mechanisms for maintaining the critical balance of body fluids and electrolytes. ***Fluid and electrolyte balance*** is the regulation of body fluid volume, osmolarity, and composition, as well as the regulation of electrolytes by the processes of filtration, diffusion, osmosis, and selective excretion. Although it is easier to understand how body water and each individual electrolyte are regulated separately, remember that these substances and their regulation are interrelated and control actions usually occur simultaneously. Thus the processes involved in fluid and electrolyte balance are never truly separate.

Total body water (fluid) in adults varies by age and gender. Water makes up about 55% to 60% of total weight for younger adults and 50% to 55% of total weight for older adults. Women of all ages usually have a lower percentage of body water than do men of the same ages. This is because men generally have greater muscle mass than women and muscle cells contain a lot of water. Women usually have a greater percentage of body fat than men and fat cells contain practically no water.

Body fluid is divided into two main compartments (spaces)—the fluid outside the cells (**extracellular fluid [ECF]**) and the fluid inside the cells (**intracellular fluid [ICF]**). The ECF space is about one third (about 15 L) of the total body water. The ECF includes **interstitial fluid** (fluid between cells, "third space"); blood, lymph, bone, and connective tissue water; and transcellular fluids. Transcellular fluids include cerebrospinal fluid, synovial fluid, peritoneal fluid, and pleural fluid. ICF is about two thirds (about 25 L) of total body water. Fig. 13.1 shows normal total body fluid distribution. Solute particles vary in type and amount from one fluid space to another.

Three processes control ***fluid and electrolyte balance*** to prevent dangerous changes regardless of differences in fluid ingestion and fluid excretion (McCance et al., 2019). For example, on one day you may drink less than a liter of fluid and on another day you may drink 4 L of different types of beverages. Even with this variation of fluid intake from day to day, overall body fluid volumes and compositions remain within the normal ranges because of effective homeostatic mechanisms for ***fluid and electrolyte balance***. These mechanisms involve the actions of the processes of filtration, diffusion, and osmosis that determine whether water and particles move across cell membranes and in which direction.

Filtration

Actions. **Filtration** is the movement of fluid (water) through a cell or blood vessel membrane because of hydrostatic pressure *(water pressure)* differences on both sides of the membrane. **Hydrostatic pressure** is the pressure exerted by water molecules against the surfaces (membranes or walls) of a confining space. Water molecules in a confined space constantly press outward against the membranes, creating hydrostatic pressure. This is a "water-pushing" pressure because it forces water outward from a confined space through a membrane (Fig. 13.2).

The amount (volume) of water in any body fluid space determines the hydrostatic pressure of that space. Blood, which is "thicker" than water (more *viscous*), is confined within the blood vessels. Blood has hydrostatic pressure because of its weight and volume and also from the pressure in arteries generated by the pumping action of the heart.

The hydrostatic pressures of two fluid spaces can be compared whenever a porous *(permeable)* membrane separates the two spaces. If the hydrostatic pressure is the same in both fluid spaces, there is no pressure difference between the two spaces, and the hydrostatic pressure is at *equilibrium*. If the hydrostatic pressure is not the same in both spaces, *disequilibrium* exists. This means that the two spaces have a graded difference *(gradient)* for hydrostatic pressure: one space has a higher hydrostatic pressure than the other. *The human body constantly seeks equilibrium.* When a gradient exists, water movement through membranes (filtration) occurs until the hydrostatic pressure is the same in both spaces (see Fig. 13.2).

Water moves through the porous membrane *(filters)* from the space with higher hydrostatic pressure to the space with lower pressure. Filtration continues only as long as a hydrostatic pressure gradient exists. Equilibrium is reached when enough fluid leaves one space and enters the other space to make the hydrostatic pressure in both spaces equal. Then water molecules are evenly exchanged between the spaces, and neither space gains or loses water molecules. Thus the hydrostatic pressure in both spaces is the same.

Clinical Examples. Blood pressure is an example of a hydrostatic filtering force. It moves blood from the heart to capillaries where capillary walls are thin enough for filtration to exchange water, nutrients, and waste products between the blood and the tissue spaces. The hydrostatic pressure difference between the capillary blood and the interstitial fluid (fluid in the tissue spaces between cells) determines whether water leaves the blood vessels and enters the tissue spaces.

Capillary membranes are only one cell layer thick, making a thin "wall" to hold blood in the capillaries. Large spaces *(pores)* in the capillary membrane help water filter freely in either direction when a hydrostatic pressure gradient is present (Fig. 13.3). Thus depending on which compartment has the higher hydrostatic pressure, capillaries can allow fluid to move from the blood into the interstitial space or from the interstitial space back into the blood.

Excess tissue fluid *(edema)* forms with changes in hydrostatic pressure differences between the blood and the interstitial fluid, such as in right-sided heart failure (McCance et al., 2019). In this condition the volume of blood in the right side of the heart increases because the right ventricle is too weak to pump blood well into lung blood vessels. As blood backs up into the venous and capillary systems, the capillary hydrostatic pressure rises until it is higher than the pressure in the interstitial space. Excess filtration from the capillaries into the interstitial tissue space then forms visible edema.

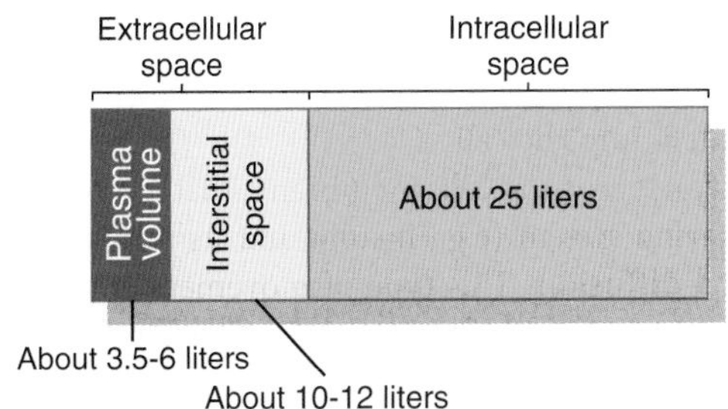

Fig. 13.1 Normal distribution of total body water in adults.

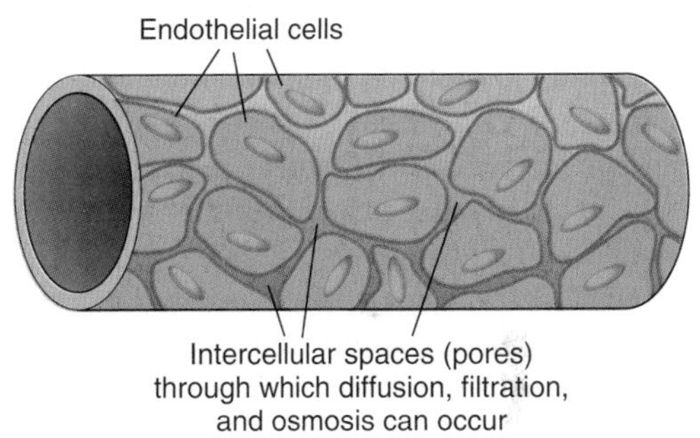

Fig. 13.3 Basic structure of a capillary.

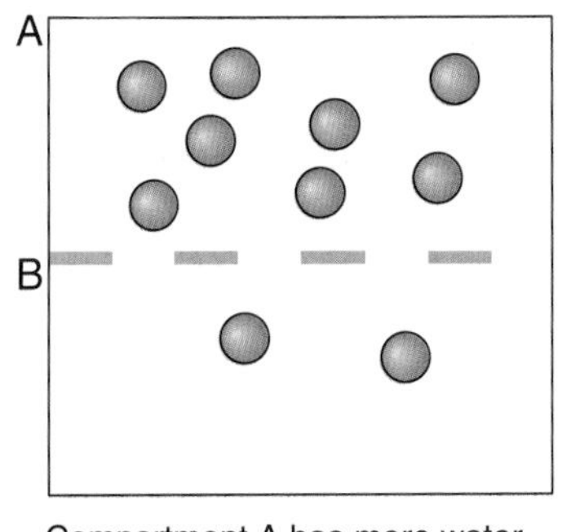

Compartment A has more water molecules and greater hydrostatic pressure than does compartment B.

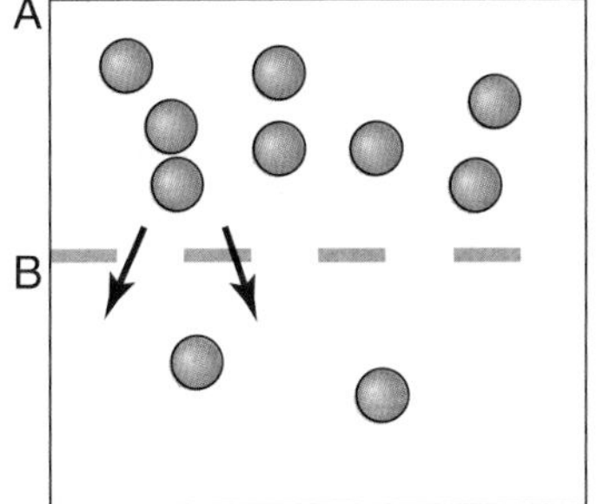

Water molecules move down the hydrostatic pressure gradient from compartment A through the permeable membrane into compartment B, which has a lower hydrostatic pressure.

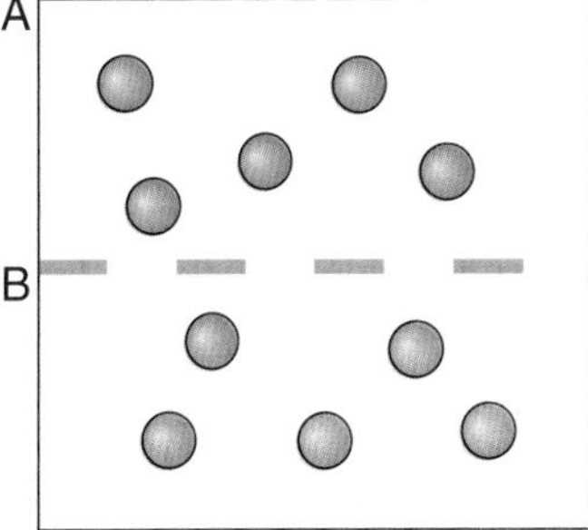

Enough water molecules have moved down the hydrostatic pressure gradient from compartment A into compartment B that both sides now have the same amount of water and the same amount of hydrostatic pressure. An equilibrium of hydrostatic pressure now exists between the two compartments, and no further *net* movement of water will occur.

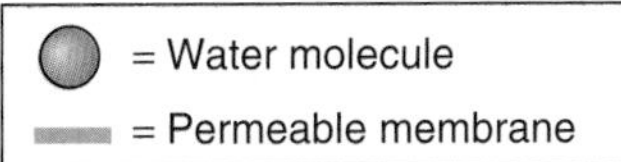

Fig. 13.2 Process of filtration.

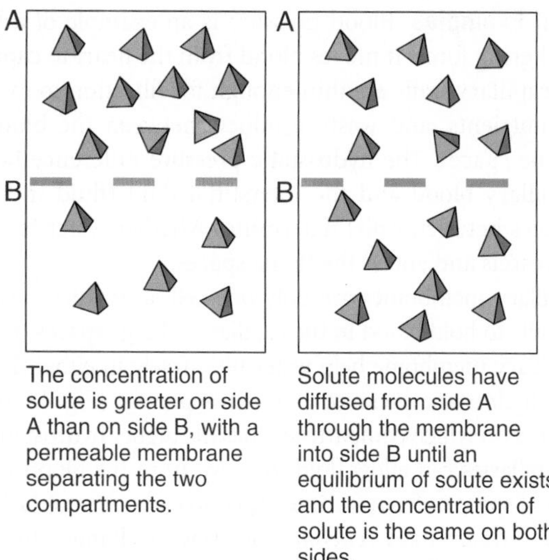

A
B
A
B
The concentration of solute is greater on side A than on side B, with a permeable membrane separating the two compartments.
Solute molecules have diffused from side A through the membrane into side B until an equilibrium of solute exists and the concentration of solute is the same on both sides.

Fig. 13.4 Diffusion of solute particles through a permeable membrane from an area of higher solute concentration to an area of lower solute concentration until an equilibrium is reached.

Diffusion

Actions. Diffusion is the movement of particles (solute) across a permeable membrane from an area of higher particle concentration to an area of lower particle concentration (*down a concentration difference or "gradient"*). Particles in a fluid have random movement from the vibration of atoms in their nuclei. Random movement allows molecules to bump into each other in a confined fluid space. Each collision increases the speed of particle movement. The more particles (higher concentration) present in the confined fluid space, the greater the number of collisions.

As a result of the collisions, particles in a solution spread out evenly through the available space. They move from an area of higher particle concentrations to an area of lower concentrations until an equal concentration (amount) is present in all areas. Spaces with many particles have more collisions and faster particle movement than spaces with fewer particles.

A *concentration gradient* exists when two fluid spaces have different concentrations of the same type of particles. Particle collisions cause them to move down the concentration gradient. Any membrane that separates two spaces is struck repeatedly by particles. When the particle strikes a pore in the membrane that is large enough for it to pass through, diffusion occurs (Fig. 13.4). The chance of any single particle hitting the membrane and going through a pore is much greater on the side of the membrane with a higher solute particle concentration.

The speed of diffusion is related to the difference in amount of particles (concentration gradient) between the two sides of the membrane. The degree of difference is the *steepness* of the gradient: the larger the concentration difference between the two sides, the steeper the gradient. Diffusion is more rapid when the gradient is steeper (just as a ball rolls downhill faster when the hill is steep than when the hill is nearly flat). Particles move from the fluid space with a higher concentration of solute particles to the fluid space with a lower concentration of solute particles.

Particle diffusion continues as long as a concentration gradient exists between the two sides of the membrane. When the concentration of particles is the same on both sides of the membrane, the particles are in equilibrium, and only an equal exchange of particles continues.

Clinical Examples. Diffusion transports most electrolytes and other particles through cell membranes. Cell membranes, unlike capillary membranes, are *selective* for which particles can diffuse. They permit diffusion of some particles but not others. Some particles cannot move across a cell membrane, even when a steep "downhill" gradient exists, because the membrane is *impermeable* (closed) to that particle type. For these particles the concentration gradient is maintained across the membrane.

Impermeability and special transport systems cause differences in the amounts of specific particles from one fluid space to another. For example, usually the fluid outside the cell (the *extracellular fluid [ECF]*) has 10 times more sodium ions than the fluid inside the cell (the *intracellular fluid [ICF]*). This extreme difference is caused by cell membrane impermeability to sodium and by special "sodium pumps" that move any extra sodium present inside the cell out of the cell "uphill" against its concentration gradient and back into the ECF.

For some particles diffusion cannot occur without help, even down steep concentration gradients, because of selective membrane permeability. One example is glucose. Even though the amount of glucose may be much higher in the ECF than in the ICF (creating a steep gradient for glucose), glucose cannot cross some cell membranes without the help of insulin. Insulin binds to insulin receptors on cell membranes, which then makes the membranes much more permeable to glucose. Then glucose can cross the cell membrane down its concentration gradient into the cell.

Diffusion across a cell membrane that requires a membrane-altering system (e.g., insulin and its receptors) is called facilitated diffusion. This type of movement is still a form of diffusion because it does not require extra energy.

Osmosis

Actions. Osmosis is the movement of *water only* through a selectively permeable (*semipermeable*) membrane to achieve an equilibrium of osmolarity. For osmosis to occur, a membrane must separate two fluid spaces and one space must have particles that cannot move through the membrane. (The membrane is *impermeable* to this particle.) A concentration gradient of this particle must also exist between the two spaces. Because the membrane is impermeable to these particles, they cannot cross the membrane to establish an equilibrium, but water molecules can.

For the fluid spaces to have equal concentrations of all the particles, the water molecules move down their concentration gradient from the side with the higher concentration of water molecules (and a lower concentration of particles along with a greater hydrostatic pressure) to the side with the lower concentration of water molecules (and a higher concentration of particles along with a lower hydrostatic pressure). This movement continues until both spaces contain the same proportions of particles to water and thus have an equilibrium of osmolarity. At this point the *concentrations* of particles in the fluid spaces on both sides of the membrane are equal even though the total amounts of particles and volumes of water are different. *The*

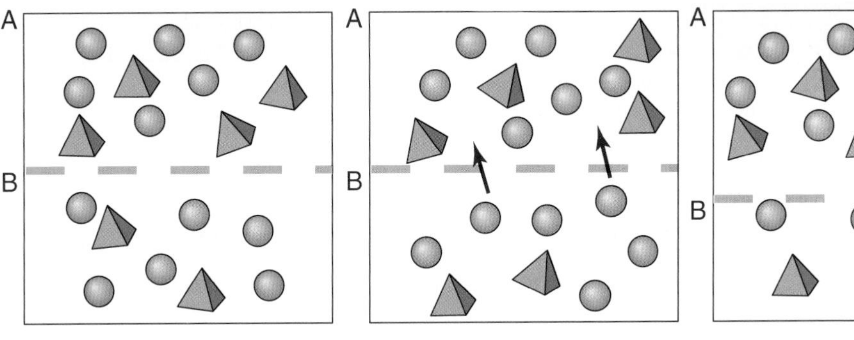

Side A has more solute molecules than does side B, even though the number of water molecules is the same on both sides. Thus side A has a greater osmotic (water pulling) pressure than does side B.

DISEQUILIBRIUM
Side A 1.5:1 ratio of water to solute
Side B 3:1 ratio of water to solute

Movement of water occurs by osmosis toward side A because it has greater osmotic pressure. The membrane is *not* permeable to the solute molecules, so the actual number of solute molecules on side A and side B does not change. *Only the water molecules move, because the membrane is not permeable to the solute molecules.*

Enough water molecules have moved from side B into side A that the actual concentration of solute is now the same on both sides, with a ratio of water to solute of 2:1. An equilibrium of osmotic pressure now exists between the two compartments, and no further *net* movement of water molecules or solute molecules will occur.

EQUILIBRIUM
Side A 2:1 ratio of water to solute
Side B 2:1 ratio of water to solute

= Water molecule
= Permeable membrane
= Solute molecule

Fig. 13.5 The process of osmosis to generate a concentration equilibrium (but not a volume equilibrium) for a solute particle that cannot move through a cell membrane.

concentration equilibrium occurs by the movement of water molecules rather than the movement of solute particles.

Dilute fluid is less concentrated and has fewer particles and more water molecules than more concentrated fluid. Thus water moves by osmosis down its hydrostatic pressure gradient from the dilute fluid to the more concentrated fluid until a fluid concentration of solute (osmolarity) equilibrium occurs (Fig. 13.5).

Particle concentration in body fluid is the major factor that determines whether and how fast osmosis and diffusion occur (McCance et al., 2019). This concentration is expressed in milliequivalents per liter (mEq/L), millimoles per liter (mmol/L), and milliosmoles per liter (mOsm/L). **Osmolarity** is the number of milliosmoles in a *liter* of solution; **osmolality** is the number of milliosmoles in a *kilogram* of solution. Because 1 L of water weighs 1 kg, in human physiology osmolarity and osmolality are considered the same, although osmolarity is the actual concentration measured most often. The normal osmolarity value for plasma and other body fluids ranges from 270 to about 300 mOsm/L. The body functions best when the osmolarity of all body fluid spaces is close to 300 mOsm/L. When all fluids have this solute (particle) concentration, the fluids are **isosmotic** or **isotonic** (also called *normotonic*) to each other.

Fluids with osmolarities greater than 300 mOsm/L are **hyperosmotic**, or **hypertonic**, compared with isosmotic fluids. These fluids have a *greater* osmotic pressure than do isosmotic fluids and tend to pull water from the isosmotic fluid space into the hyperosmotic fluid space until an osmotic balance occurs.

Clinical Examples. If a hyperosmotic (hypertonic) IV solution (e.g., 3% or 5% saline) were infused into a patient with normal extracellular fluid (ECF) osmolarity, the infusing fluid would make the patient's blood hyperosmotic. To balance this situation, the interstitial fluid would be pulled into the circulation in an attempt to dilute the blood osmolarity back to normal. In addition, fluid would also be drawn from the intracellular fluid (ICF) compartment. As a result, the interstitial and ICF volumes would shrink, and the plasma volume would expand.

Fluids with osmolarities of less than 270 mOsm/L are **hypo-osmotic**, or **hypotonic**, compared with isosmotic fluids. Hypo-osmolar fluids have a *lower* osmotic pressure than isosmotic fluids, and water is pulled from the hypo-osmotic fluid space into the isosmotic fluid spaces of the interstitial and ICF fluids. As a result, the interstitial and ICF fluid volumes would expand, and the plasma volume would shrink. An example of a hypotonic IV fluid is 0.45% saline.

Osmosis and filtration act together at the capillary membrane to maintain both extracellular fluid (ECF) and intracellular fluid (ICF) volumes within their normal ranges. The thirst mechanism is an example of how osmosis helps maintain homeostasis. The feeling of thirst is caused by the activation of cells in the brain that respond to changes in ECF osmolarity. These cells, so very sensitive to changes in ECF osmolarity, are called *osmoreceptors*. When an adult loses body water but most of the particles remain, such as through excessive sweating, ECF volume is decreased and its osmolarity is increased (is hypertonic). The cells in the thirst center shrink as water moves from the cells into the hypertonic ECF. The shrinking of these cells triggers awareness of thirst and increases the urge to drink. Drinking replaces the amount of water lost through sweating and dilutes the ECF osmolarity, restoring it to normal.

Plasma volume	Interstitial fluid	Intracellular fluid
Volume 3.5-5.5 L Osmolarity 270-300 mOsm Sodium 136-145 mEq/L Potassium 3.5-5.0 mEq/L Chloride 96-109 mEq/L Calcium 9.0-10.5 mg/dL Magnesium 1.3-2.1 mEq/L Protein 7-8 g/L	Volume ~10 L Osmolarity 270-300 mOsm Sodium 135-145 mEq/L Potassium 3.5-5.0 mEq/L Chloride ~118 mEq/L Calcium 7.0-9.0 mg/dL Magnesium ~1.3 mEq/L Protein ~2 g/L	Volume 25-30 L Osmolarity 270-300 mOsm Sodium 14 mEq/L Potassium 140 mEq/L Chloride ~4-6 mEq/L Calcium 1.0-8.0 mg/dL Magnesium 6-30 mEq/L Protein 16 g/L

Fig. 13.6 Electrolyte composition of various body fluids.

NCLEX EXAMINATION CHALLENGE 13.1

Physiological Integrity

What responses does the nurse expect as a result of infusing 500 mL liter of a 3% saline intravenous solution into a client over a 1-hour time period?

A. Plasma volume osmolarity increases; blood pressure increases
B. Plasma volume osmolarity decreases; blood pressure increases
C. Plasma volume osmolarity increases; blood pressure decreases
D. Plasma volume osmolarity decreases; blood pressure decreases

FLUID AND ELECTROLYTE BALANCE

As indicated earlier, fluid balance is linked to and affected by electrolyte balance. **Electrolytes (ions)** are dissolved substances (solute) that express an electrical charge. Most of the common blood electrolytes are mineral elements. **Cations** are positively charged electrolytes; **anions** are negatively charged electrolytes. Body fluids are electrically neutral, which means that the number of positive ions is balanced by an equal number of negative ions. Most ions have different concentrations in the extracellular fluid (ECF) and the intracellular fluid (ICF) (Fig. 13.6). This concentration difference helps maintain membrane excitability and allows nerve impulse transmission. The normal ranges of blood electrolytes are narrow, so even small changes in these levels can cause major problems.

Electrolyte imbalances can occur in healthy people as a result of changes in fluid intake and output. These imbalances are usually mild and are easily corrected. Severe electrolyte imbalances with actual losses or retention of electrolytes are life threatening and can occur in any setting. Adults at greatest risk for severe imbalances are older patients, patients with chronic kidney or endocrine disorders, and those who are taking drugs that alter fluid and electrolyte balance. *All ill adults are at some risk for electrolyte imbalances.*

The Laboratory Profile: Fluid and Electrolyte Assessment box lists the normal ranges of the major serum electrolytes. Most electrolytes enter the body in ingested food. Electrolyte balance occurs when dietary intake of electrolytes matches kidney electrolyte excretion or reabsorption. For example, serum potassium level is maintained between 3.5 and 5.0 mEq/L (mmol/L). The high potassium level in foods such as meat and citrus fruit could increase the ECF potassium level and lead to major problems. In health, kidney excretion of potassium keeps pace with potassium intake and prevents major changes in the blood potassium level.

PATIENT-CENTERED CARE: OLDER ADULT CONSIDERATIONS QSEN

Older adults are at risk for fluid and electrolyte imbalances as a result of age-related organ changes. Always ask the older adult which drug(s) he or she takes because older adults are more likely to be taking drugs that affect *fluid and electrolyte balance.*

LABORATORY PROFILE

Fluid and Electrolyte Assessment

Electrolyte	Normal Ranges	Significance of Abnormal Values
Sodium (Na+)	136-145 mEq/L (mmol/L)	*Elevated:* Hypernatremia; dehydration; kidney disease; hypercortisolism *Low:* Hyponatremia; fluid overload; liver disease; adrenal insufficiency
Potassium (K+)	3.5-5.0 mEq/L (mmol/L)	*Elevated:* Hyperkalemia; dehydration; kidney disease; acidosis; adrenal insufficiency; crush injuries *Low:* Hypokalemia; fluid overload; diuretic therapy; alkalosis; insulin administration; hyperaldosteronism
Calcium (Ca^{2+})	9.0-10.5 mg/dL (2.25-2.75 mmol/L)	*Elevated:* Hypercalcemia; hyperthyroidism; hyperparathyroidism *Low:* Hypocalcemia; vitamin D deficiency; hypothyroidism; hypoparathyroidism; kidney disease; excessive intake of phosphorus-containing foods and drinks
Chloride (Cl^-)	98-106 mEq/L (mmol/L)	*Elevated:* Hyperchloremia; metabolic acidosis; respiratory alkalosis; hypercortisolism *Low:* Hypochloremia; fluid overload; excessive vomiting or diarrhea; adrenal insufficiency; diuretic therapy
Magnesium (Mg^{2+})	1.8-2.6 mEq/L (0.74-1.07 mmol/L)	*Elevated:* Hypermagnesemia; kidney disease; hypothyroidism; adrenal insufficiency *Low:* Hypomagnesemia; malnutrition; alcoholism; ketoacidosis
Osmolarity	270-300 mOsm/L	*High:* Dehydration; hypernatremia; hyperglycemia *Low:* Fluid overload; hyponatremia; hypoproteinemia; malnutrition

Data from Pagana, K., & Pagana, T. (2018). *Mosby's manual of diagnostic and laboratory tests* (6th ed.). St. Louis: Mosby.

Fluid Balance

Age, gender, and amount of fat affect the amount and distribution of body fluids. An older adult has less total body water than a younger adult. An obese adult has less total water than a lean adult of the same weight because fat cells contain almost no water. See the Patient-Centered Care: Older Adult Considerations box for expected age-related changes in fluid balance and the Patient-Centered Care: Gender Health Considerations box for gender differences in fluid balance.

PATIENT-CENTERED CARE: OLDER ADULT CONSIDERATIONS QSEN

System/Organ	Change	Result
Skin	Loss of elasticity Decreased turgor	Skin becomes an unreliable indicator of fluid status
	Decreased oil production	Dry, easily damaged skin
Kidney	Decreased glomerular filtration	Poor excretion of waste products
	Decreased concentrating capacity	Increased water loss, increasing the risk for dehydration
Muscular	Decreased muscle mass	Decreased total body water Greater risk for dehydration
Neurologic	Reduced thirst reflex	Decreased fluid intake, increasing the risk for dehydration
Endocrine	Adrenal atrophy	Poor regulation of sodium and potassium balance, increasing the risk for hyponatremia and hyperkalemia

Data from Touhy, T., & Jett, K. (2020). *Ebersole and Hess' toward health aging* (10th ed.). St. Louis: Mosby.

PATIENT-CENTERED CARE: GENDER HEALTH CONSIDERATIONS QSEN

Women of any age have less total body water and a higher risk for dehydration than men of similar sizes and ages. This difference is because men tend to have more muscle mass than women and because women have more body fat. (Muscle cells contain mostly water, and fat cells have little water.)

Body fluids are constantly filtered and replaced as fluid balance is maintained through intake and output. The total amount of water in each fluid space is stable, but water in all spaces is exchanged continually while maintaining a constant fluid volume.

Fluid intake is regulated through the thirst drive. Fluid enters the body as liquids and as solid foods, which contain up to 85% water (Table 13.1). A rising blood osmolarity or a decreasing blood volume triggers the sensation of thirst (McCance et al., 2019). An adult takes in about 2300 mL of fluid daily from food and liquids.

Fluid loss occurs through several routes (see Table 13.1). The kidney is the most important and the most sensitive water loss route because it is regulated and adjustable. The volume lost through urine elimination daily varies, depending on the amount of fluid taken in and the body's need to conserve fluids.

TABLE 13.1 Routes of Fluid Ingestion and Excretion

Intake	Output
Measurable	
Oral fluids	Urine
Parenteral fluids	Emesis
Enemas[a]	Feces
Irrigation fluids[a]	Drainage from body cavities
Not Measurable	
Solid foods	Perspiration
Metabolism	Vaporization through the lungs

[a]Measured by subtracting the amount returned from the amount instilled.

The minimum amount of urine output per day needed to excrete toxic waste products is 400 to 600 mL. This minimum volume is called the **obligatory urine output**. If the 24-hour urine output falls below the obligatory output amount, wastes are retained and can cause lethal electrolyte imbalances, acidosis, and a toxic buildup of nitrogen.

The ability of the kidneys to make either concentrated or very dilute urine helps maintain fluid balance. The kidney works with various hormones to maintain fluid balance when extracellular fluid (ECF) concentrations, volumes, or pressures change (Ellison & Farrar, 2018).

Other normal water loss occurs through the skin, lungs, and intestinal tract. Water losses also can result from salivation, drainage from fistulas and drains, and GI suction. This loss is called **insensible water loss** because no mechanisms control it. In a healthy adult insensible water loss is about 500 to 1000 mL/day. This loss increases greatly during thyroid crisis, trauma, burns, states of extreme stress, and fever. Patients at risk for excess insensible water loss include those being mechanically ventilated, those with rapid respirations, and those undergoing continuous GI suctioning. Water loss through stool increases greatly with severe diarrhea or excessive fistula drainage. If not balanced by intake, insensible loss can lead to severe dehydration and electrolyte imbalances.

Regulation of Fluid Balance

Hormones. Three hormones help control ***fluid and electrolyte balance***. These are aldosterone, antidiuretic hormone (ADH), and natriuretic peptide (NP).

Aldosterone is secreted by the adrenal cortex whenever sodium levels in the extracellular fluid (ECF) are low. Aldosterone prevents both water and sodium loss. When aldosterone is secreted, it acts on the kidney nephrons, triggering them to reabsorb sodium and water from the urine back into the blood. This action increases blood osmolarity and blood volume. Aldosterone also promotes kidney potassium excretion.

Antidiuretic hormone (ADH), or vasopressin, is released from the posterior pituitary gland in response to changes in blood osmolarity. The hypothalamus contains osmoreceptors, which are sensitive to changes in blood osmolarity. Increased blood osmolarity, especially an increase in the level of plasma sodium, results in

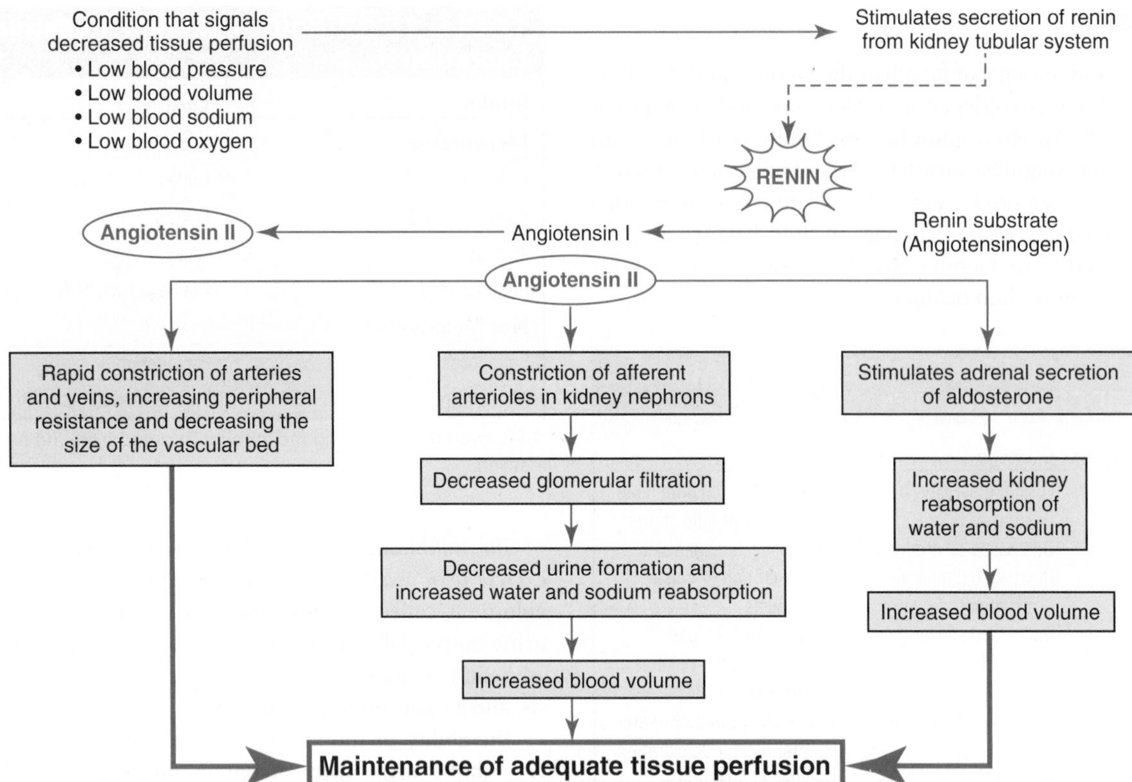

Fig. 13.7 The renin-angiotensin-aldosterone system (RAAS) in fluid and electrolyte balance and blood pressure regulation.

a slight shrinkage of these cells and triggers ADH release from the posterior pituitary gland. Because the action of ADH retains just water, it only indirectly regulates electrolyte retention or excretion.

ADH acts on kidney nephrons, making them more permeable to water. As a result, more water is *reabsorbed* by these tubules and returned to the blood, decreasing blood osmolarity by making it more dilute. When blood osmolarity decreases with low plasma sodium levels, the osmoreceptors swell slightly and inhibit ADH release. Less water is then reabsorbed, and more is excreted in the urine, bringing extracellular fluid (ECF) osmolarity up to normal.

Natriuretic peptides (*NPs*) are hormones secreted by special cells that line the atria of the heart (atrial natriuretic peptide [ANP]) and ventricles of the heart. (The peptide secreted by the heart ventricular cells is known as *brain natriuretic peptide* [BNP]). These peptides are secreted in response to increased blood volume and blood pressure, which stretch the heart tissue. NP binds to receptors in the nephrons, creating effects that are opposite of aldosterone. Kidney reabsorption of sodium is inhibited at the same time that urine output is increased. The outcome is decreased circulating blood volume and decreased blood osmolarity.

Renin-Angiotensin-Aldosterone System (RAAS)

Actions. The most important body fluids to keep in balance for optimal function are the blood volume (plasma volume) and fluid inside the cells (intracellular fluid). Changes in these volumes, especially decreases, can lead to poor organ perfusion and cellular dysfunction. Maintaining blood volume at a sufficient level for blood pressure to remain high enough to ensure adequate ***perfusion*** is critical for life. Cellular volumes must be maintained for continued individual cellular work. Thus neither compartment tolerates large changes in volume. The interstitial compartment, however, can tolerate significant changes in volume. Fluid in this compartment is often changed to help maintain the volumes of the other two compartments. A major regulator of fluid balance is the *renin-angiotensin-aldosterone system (RAAS)*, also known as the *renin-angiotensin II pathway.*

Because low blood volume and low blood pressure can rapidly lead to death, the body has many compensatory mechanisms that guard against low plasma volume. These involve specific responses to change how water and sodium are handled to maintain blood pressure.

Because the kidney is a major regulator of water and sodium balance to maintain blood pressure and perfusion to all tissues and organs, the kidneys monitor blood pressure, blood volume, blood oxygen levels, and blood osmolarity (related to sodium concentration). When the kidneys sense that any one of these parameters is getting low, they begin to secrete a substance called *renin* that sets into motion a group of hormonal and blood vessel responses to ensure that blood pressure is raised back up to normal (Ellison & Farrar, 2018). Fig. 13.7 summarizes these responses.

So the triggering event for renin secretion is any change in the blood indicating that ***perfusion*** is at risk. Low blood pressure is a triggering event because it reduces perfusion to tissues and organs. Anything that reduces blood volume (e.g., dehydration, hemorrhage) below a critical level *always* lowers blood pressure. Low blood oxygen levels also are triggering events because with too little oxygen in the blood, it cannot supply the needed oxygen and the tissues and organs could die. A low blood sodium level also is a triggering event because sodium and water are closely linked. Where sodium goes, water follows. So anything that causes the blood to have too little sodium prevents water from staying in the blood. The result is low blood volume with low blood pressure and poor tissue perfusion (Bertschi, 2020).

Once the kidneys sense that ***perfusion*** is at risk, special cells in the kidney tubule start the RAAS by secreting renin into the blood. Renin then activates *angiotensinogen*. Activated angiotensinogen is *angiotensin I*, which is activated by the enzyme *angiotensin-converting enzyme (ACE)* to its most active form, angiotensin II (McCance et al., 2019).

Angiotensin II starts several actions to increase blood volume and blood pressure. First it constricts arteries and veins throughout the body. This action increases peripheral resistance and reduces the size of the vascular bed, which raises blood pressure as a compensatory mechanism without adding more blood volume. Angiotensin II also constricts the size of the arterioles that feed the kidney nephrons. This action results in a lower glomerular filtration rate and a huge reduction of urine output. Decreasing urine output prevents further water loss, so more is retained in the blood to help raise blood pressure. Angiotensin II also causes the adrenal glands to secrete the hormone aldosterone. Aldosterone is nicknamed the "water-and-sodium-saving hormone" because it causes the kidneys to reabsorb water and sodium, preventing them from being excreted into the urine. This response allows more water and sodium to be returned to the blood, increasing blood pressure, blood volume, and ***perfusion***.

Clinical Examples. The renin-angiotensin-aldosterone system (RAAS) is stimulated whenever the patient is in shock. This is why urine output is used as an indicator of ***perfusion*** adequacy after surgery or any time the patient has undergone an invasive procedure and is at risk for hemorrhage.

RAAS is also related to management of *hypertension* (high blood pressure). Patients who have hypertension are often asked to limit their intake of sodium. The reason for this is that a high sodium intake raises the blood level of sodium, causing more water to be retained in the blood volume and raising blood pressure. Drug therapy for hypertension management may include diuretic drugs that increase the excretion of sodium so that less is present in the blood, resulting in a lower blood volume. Another class of drugs often used to manage blood pressure is the "ACE inhibitors" (ACEIs). These drugs disrupt the RAAS pathway by reducing the amount of angiotensin-converting enzyme (ACE) made, so less angiotensin II is present. With less angiotensin II, there is less vasoconstriction and reduced peripheral resistance, less aldosterone production, and greater excretion of water and sodium in the urine. All of these responses lead to decreased blood volume and blood pressure. Another class of drugs used to manage hypertension is the angiotensin receptor blockers (ARBs). These drugs disrupt the renin-angiotensin II pathway by blocking the receptors that bind with angiotensin II so that the tissues cannot respond to it and blood pressure is lowered. The most recent class of drugs to manage hypertension by changing the RAAS is the direct renin inhibitors. These drugs act early in the pathway and prevent the enzyme renin from changing angiotensinogen into angiotensin I. They may be combined with an ARB to block the pathway in more than one place, leading to greater reduction in blood pressure. See Chapter 33 for more information about antihypertensive drugs.

Electrolyte Balance

Although all electrolytes play a role in homeostasis, the more critical ones are sodium, potassium, calcium, and magnesium. Many of the same control mechanisms that regulate fluid balance are also critical for regulating the balance of these important electrolytes.

Sodium. Sodium (Na^+) is the major *cation* (positively charged particle) in the extracellular fluid (ECF) and maintains ECF osmolarity. Sodium levels of the ECF are high (136 to 145 mEq/L [mmol/L]), and the intracellular fluid (ICF) sodium levels are low (about 14 mEq/L [mmol/L]). Keeping this difference in sodium levels between the two compartments is vital for muscle contraction, cardiac contraction, and nerve impulse transmission. Sodium levels and movement influence water balance because "where sodium goes, water follows." The ECF sodium level determines whether water is retained, excreted, or moved from one fluid space to another. Changes in plasma sodium levels seriously change fluid volume and the distribution of other electrolytes.

Sodium enters the body through the ingestion of many foods and fluids. Foods with the highest sodium levels are those that are processed or preserved, such as smoked or pickled foods, snack foods, and many condiments. Foods lowest in sodium include fresh fish and poultry and most fresh vegetables and fruit.

Despite variation in daily sodium intake, blood sodium levels usually remain within the normal range. Serum sodium balance is regulated by the kidney under the influences of aldosterone, antidiuretic hormone (ADH), and natriuretic peptide (NP) (see the Hormones section of the Regulation of Fluid Balance section).

Low serum sodium levels inhibit the secretion of ADH and NP and trigger renin-angiotensin-aldosterone system (RAAS). Together these compensatory actions increase serum sodium levels by increasing kidney reabsorption of sodium and enhancing kidney loss of water.

High serum sodium levels inhibit aldosterone secretion and stimulate secretion of ADH and NP. Together these hormones increase kidney sodium excretion and water reabsorption.

Potassium. Potassium (K^+) is the major cation of the intracellular fluid (ICF). The normal plasma potassium level ranges from 3.5 to 5.0 mEq/L (mmol/L) (see the Laboratory Profile: Fluid and Electrolyte Assessment box). The normal ICF potassium level is about 140 mEq/L (mmol/L). Keeping this large difference in potassium concentration between the ICF and the extracellular fluid (ECF) is critical for excitable tissues to be able to depolarize and generate action potentials.

Because potassium levels in the blood and interstitial fluid are so low, any change seriously affects physiologic activities (Pagana & Pagana, 2018). For example, a decrease in blood potassium of only 1 mEq/L (from 4 mEq/L [mmol/L] to 3 mEq/L) [mmol/L] is a 25% difference in total ECF potassium concentration.

Almost all foods contain potassium. It is highest in meat, fish, and many (but not all) vegetables and fruits. It is lowest in eggs, bread, and cereal grains. Typical potassium intake is about 2 to 20 g/day. Despite heavy potassium intake, the healthy adult keeps plasma potassium levels within the narrow range of normal values.

The main controller of ECF potassium level is the sodium-potassium pump within the membranes of all body cells. This pump moves extra sodium ions from the ICF and moves extra potassium ions from the ECF back into the cell. In this way, the serum potassium level remains low and the intracellular potassium remains high. At the same time, this action also helps the serum sodium level remain high and the cellular sodium level remain low. Another influencing factor for potassium balance is adequate magnesium levels. Low magnesium levels often result in a corresponding low potassium level.

About 80% of potassium is removed from the body by the kidney. Kidney excretion of potassium is enhanced by aldosterone.

Calcium. Calcium (Ca^{2+}) is an ion having two positive charges *(divalent cation)* that exists in the body in a bound form and an ionized (unbound or free) form. Bound calcium is usually attached to serum proteins, especially albumin. Ionized calcium is present in the blood and other extracellular fluid (ECF) as free calcium. Free calcium is the active form and must be kept within a narrow range in the ECF (see the Laboratory Profile: Fluid and Electrolyte Assessment box). Calcium has a steep gradient between ECF and intracellular fluid (ICF) because the amount of calcium in the ICF is very low. This mineral is important for maintaining bone strength and density, activating enzymes, allowing skeletal and cardiac muscle contraction, controlling nerve impulse transmission, and enhancing blood clotting.

Calcium enters the body by dietary intake and absorption through the intestinal tract. Absorption of dietary calcium requires the active form of vitamin D. Most body calcium is stored in the bone matrix rather than in any fluid compartment. When more calcium is needed, parathyroid hormone (PTH) is released from the parathyroid glands. PTH increases serum calcium levels by:

- Releasing free calcium from bone storage sites (bone *resorption* of calcium)
- Stimulating vitamin D activation to help increase intestinal *absorption* of dietary calcium
- Inhibiting kidney calcium excretion
- Stimulating kidney calcium *reabsorption* into the blood

When excess calcium is present in plasma, PTH secretion is inhibited and the secretion of *thyrocalcitonin (TCT)*, a hormone secreted by the thyroid gland, is increased. TCT causes the plasma calcium level to decrease by inhibiting bone resorption of calcium, inhibiting vitamin D–associated intestinal uptake of calcium, and increasing kidney excretion of calcium in the urine.

Magnesium. Magnesium (Mg^{2+}) is an ion that is stored mostly in bones and cartilage. Little magnesium is present in the blood (see Table 13.1). Just like for potassium and calcium, the intracellular fluid (ICF) has more magnesium, and this mineral has more functions inside the cells than in the blood. It is important for skeletal muscle contraction, carbohydrate metabolism, generation of energy stores, vitamin activation, blood coagulation, and cell growth. Adequate amounts of intracellular magnesium are particularly essential for the health and maintenance of cardiac muscle. Within cells and the blood, magnesium levels are related to the levels of potassium and calcium and help maintain proper balance of these two electrolytes (Pagana & Pagana, 2018).

FLUID AND ELECTROLYTE BALANCE CONCEPT EXEMPLAR: DEHYDRATION

Pathophysiology Review

In **dehydration** fluid intake or retention is less than what is needed to meet the body's fluid needs, resulting in a deficit of fluid volume, especially plasma volume. It is a condition rather than a disease and can be caused by many factors (Table 13.2).

TABLE 13.2 Common Causes of Fluid Imbalances

Dehydration	Fluid Overload
• Hemorrhage • Vomiting • Diarrhea • Profuse salivation • Fistulas • Ileostomy • Profuse diaphoresis • Burns • Severe wounds • Long-term NPO status • Diuretic therapy • GI suction • Hyperventilation • Diabetes insipidus • Difficulty swallowing • Impaired thirst • Unconsciousness • Fever • Impaired motor function	• Excessive fluid replacement • Kidney failure (late phase) • Heart failure • Long-term corticosteroid therapy • Syndrome of inappropriate antidiuretic hormone (SIADH) • Psychiatric disorders with polydipsia • Water intoxication

Dehydration may be an *actual* decrease in total body water caused by either too little intake of fluid or too great a loss of fluid. It can also occur without an actual loss of total body water, such as when water shifts from the plasma into the interstitial space. This condition is called *vascular* dehydration.

PATIENT-CENTERED CARE: OLDER ADULT CONSIDERATIONS QSEN

Older adults are at high risk for dehydration because they have less total body water than younger adults resulting from age-related muscle mass loss. Many older adults have decreased thirst sensation and may have difficulty with walking or other motor skills needed for obtaining fluids. They also may take diuretics, antihypertensives, and laxatives that increase fluid excretion. Assess the *fluid and electrolyte balance* status of older adults in any setting, especially among those in long-term care (Namasivayan-MacDonald et al., 2017).

Dehydration may occur with just water loss or with water and electrolyte loss (isotonic dehydration). *Isotonic dehydration is the most common type of fluid loss problem.* Fluid is lost only from the extracellular fluid (ECF) space, including both the plasma and the interstitial spaces. There is no shift of fluids between spaces, so the intracellular fluid (ICF) volume remains normal (Fig. 13.8). Circulating blood volume is decreased (**hypovolemia**) and leads to reduced perfusion. The body's defenses compensate during dehydration to maintain ***perfusion*** to vital organs in spite of hypovolemia. The main defense is increasing vasoconstriction and peripheral resistance to maintain blood pressure and circulation.

Health Promotion and Maintenance

Mild dehydration is very common among healthy adults and is corrected or prevented easily by matching fluid intake with fluid output. Teach adults to drink more fluids, especially water, whenever they engage in heavy or prolonged physical activity or live in dry climates or at higher altitudes. Beverages with

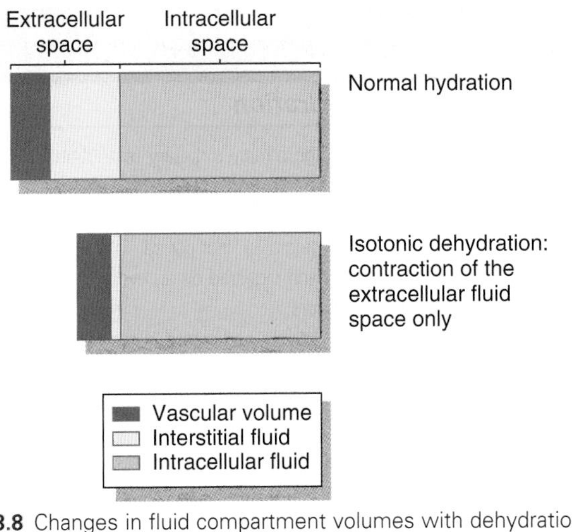

Fig. 13.8 Changes in fluid compartment volumes with dehydration. (© 1992 by M. Linda Workman. All rights reserved.)

caffeine can increase fluid loss, as can drinks containing alcohol; thus these beverages should not be used to prevent or treat dehydration.

❖ Interprofessional Collaborative Care

Dehydration can occur in any setting. Mild dehydration can be managed in the home or other residential setting. Severe dehydration may require temporary hospitalization, depending on the cause and the effects on ***perfusion***.

◆ Assessment: Recognize Cues

History. Ask about food and liquid intake, including the types of fluids and foods ingested to determine amount and osmolarity. Foods such as ice cream, gelatin, and ices are liquids at body temperature and are included when calculating fluid intake.

Ask about exact intake and output volumes, and obtain serial daily weight measurements. If possible, weigh the patient directly rather than asking what he or she weighs. Weight loss is an indication of dehydration. *Because 1 L of water weighs 2.2 lb (1 kg), changes in daily weights are the best indicators of fluid losses or gains. A weight change of 1 lb corresponds to a fluid volume change of about 500 mL.*

Ask specific questions about prescribed and over-the-counter drugs and check the dosage, the length of time taken, and the patient's adherence to the drug regimen. Older adults may use diuretics or laxatives that can lead to impaired ***fluid and electrolyte balance***.

Ask about the presence of kidney or endocrine diseases. Assess the patient's level of consciousness and mental status, which is often changed with fluid imbalance. Ask the patient about changes in ring or shoe tightness. A sudden decrease in tightness may indicate dehydration.

Physical Assessment/Signs and Symptoms. Nearly all body systems are affected by dehydration to some degree. The most obvious changes occur in the cardiovascular and integumentary systems (Sheills & Morrell-Scott, 2018).

Cardiovascular changes are good indicators of hydration status because of the relationship between plasma fluid volume, blood pressure, and ***perfusion***. Heart rate increases to help maintain blood pressure with less blood volume. Peripheral pulses are weak, difficult to find, and easily blocked. Blood pressure also decreases, as does pulse pressure, with a greater decrease in systolic blood pressure. Hypotension is more severe with the patient in the standing position than in the sitting or lying position *(orthostatic* or *postural hypotension)*. Measure blood pressure first with the patient lying down, then sitting, and finally standing. As the blood pressure decreases when changing position, perfusion to the brain decreases, causing light-headedness and dizziness. This problem increases the risk for falling, especially among older adults.

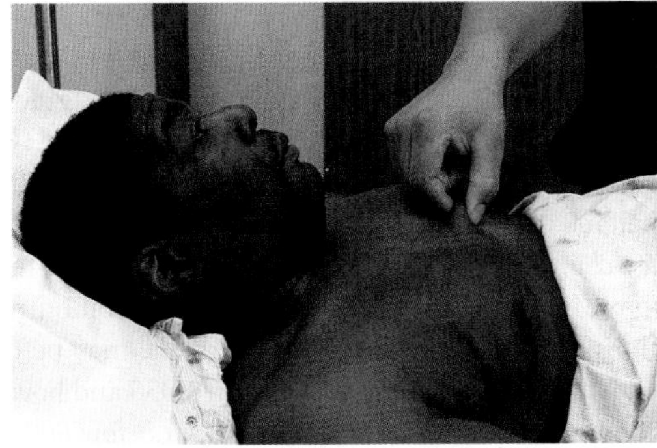

Fig. 13.9 Examining the skin turgor of an older patient.

Neck veins are normally distended when a patient is in the supine position, and hand veins are distended when lower than the level of the heart. Neck veins normally flatten when the patient moves to a sitting position. With dehydration, neck and hand veins are flat, even when lying down and when the hands are not raised above the level of the heart.

Respiratory changes include an increased rate because the decreased blood volume reduces ***perfusion*** and gas exchange. The increased respiratory rate is a compensatory mechanism that attempts to maintain oxygen delivery when perfusion is decreased.

Skin changes can indicate dehydration. Assess the skin and mucous membranes for color, moisture, and turgor. Assess skin turgor by checking:

- How easily the skin over the back of the hand and arm can be gently pinched between the thumb and forefinger to form a "tent"
- How soon the pinched skin resumes its normal position after release

In dehydration, skin turgor is poor, with the tent remaining for minutes after pinching the skin. The skin is dry and scaly.

> **PATIENT-CENTERED CARE: OLDER ADULT CONSIDERATIONS** QSEN
>
> Assess skin turgor in an older adult by pinching the skin over the sternum or on the forehead, rather than on the back of the hand (Fig. 13.9). With aging the skin loses elasticity and tents on hands and arms even when the adult is well hydrated.

In dehydration oral mucous membranes may be dry and covered with a thick, sticky coating and may have cracks and fissures. The tongue surface may have deep furrows.

Neurologic changes with dehydration include changes in mental status and temperature with reduced ***perfusion*** to and within the brain. Changes in cognition are more common among older adults and may be the first indication of a fluid imbalance (Sheills & Morrell-Scott, 2018).

The patient with dehydration often has a low-grade fever, and fever can also cause dehydration. For every degree (Celsius) increase in body temperature above normal, a minimum of an additional 500 mL of body fluid is lost.

Kidney changes in dehydration affect urine volume and concentration. Monitor urine output, comparing total output with total fluid intake and daily weights. The urine may be concentrated, with a specific gravity greater than 1.030 and have a dark amber color and a strong odor. *Urine output below 500 mL/day for a patient without kidney disease is cause for concern* (Ellison & Farrar, 2018). Use daily weights to assess fluid loss. Weight loss over a half pound per day is fluid loss.

Laboratory Assessment. No single laboratory test result confirms or rules out dehydration. Instead, dehydration is determined by laboratory findings along with signs and symptoms (see the Laboratory Profile: Fluid and Electrolyte Assessment box). Usually laboratory findings with dehydration show elevated levels of hemoglobin, hematocrit, serum osmolarity, glucose, protein, blood urea nitrogen, and electrolytes because more water is lost and other substances remain, increasing blood concentration *(hemoconcentration). Hemoconcentration is not present when dehydration is caused by hemorrhage because loss of all blood cells and plasma products occurs together.*

Imaging Assessment. In intensive care settings ultrasono graphy together with basic echocardiography can be used to evaluate fluid status. These techniques are most useful in identifying hypovolemia caused by fluid shifts to other body areas such as the abdomen. This type of volume assessment of the heart, lungs, pleura, and vasculature can help detect causes of fluid imbalance and guide management (Bailey et al., 2017).

BEST PRACTICE FOR PATIENT SAFETY & QUALITY CARE (QSEN)

The Patient With Dehydration

- Provide oral fluids that meet the patient's dietary restrictions (e.g., sugar-free, low-sodium, thickened).
- Collaborate with other members of the interprofessional team to determine the amount of fluids needed during a 24-hour period.
- Ensure that fluids are offered and ingested on an even schedule at least every 2 hours throughout 24 hours.
- Teach assistive personnel to actively participate in the hydration therapy and not to withhold fluids to prevent incontinence.
- Infuse prescribed IV fluids at a rate consistent with hydration needs and any known cardiac, pulmonary, or kidney problems.
- Monitor the patient's response to fluid therapy at least every 2 hours for indicators of adequate rehydration or the need for continuing therapy, especially:
  - Pulse quality and pulse pressure
  - Urine output
  - Weight (every 8 hours)
- Monitor for and report indicators of fluid overload, including:
  - Bounding pulse
  - Difficulty breathing
  - Neck vein distention in the upright position
  - Presence of dependent edema
- Assess IV infusion site hourly for indications of infiltration or phlebitis (e.g., swelling around the site, pain, cordlike veins, reduced drip rate).
- Give drugs prescribed to correct the underlying cause of the dehydration (e.g., antiemetics, antidiarrheals, antibiotics, antipyretics).

◆ **Analysis: Analyze Cues and Prioritize Hypotheses.** The priority problems for the patient who has dehydration are:

1. Poor ***perfusion*** due to excess fluid loss or inadequate fluid intake
2. Potential for injury due to blood pressure changes and muscle weakness

◆ **Planning and Implementation: Generate Solutions and Take Action.** The focus of management for the patient with dehydration is to prevent further fluid loss, to increase fluid volumes to normal, and to prevent injury. Nursing priorities include fluid replacement, drug therapy, and patient safety.

Restoring Fluid Balance

Planning: Expected Outcomes. The patient with dehydration is expected to have sufficient fluid volume for adequate ***perfusion***.

Interventions. Interventions for restoring fluid balance include fluid replacement and drug therapy.

Fluid Replacement. Replacement of fluids is key to correcting dehydration and preventing death from reduced ***perfusion***. Use the interventions listed in the Best Practice for Patient Safety & Quality Care box for nursing care of the patient with dehydration.

Mild to moderate dehydration is corrected with oral fluid replacement if the patient is alert enough to swallow and can tolerate oral fluids. Encourage fluid intake and measure the amount ingested. For patients who lack the strength or coordination to lift a glass and drink unassisted, a bedside water device can be useful in preventing dehydration (Sheills & Morrell-Scott, 2018). These devices are water bottles with long strawlike tubes that have a mouthpiece for the patient to use at will to ingest fluids by sucking. The device can rest on a table near the patient and also can be attached to a wheelchair.

Provide fluid the patient enjoys and time the intake schedule. Dividing the total amount of fluids needed by nursing shifts helps meet fluid needs more evenly over 24 hours with less danger of overload. Offer the conscious patient small volumes of fluids hourly.

Coordinate with assistive personnel (AP) to meet patients' specific fluid needs. Teach AP to offer 60 to 120 mL of fluid every hour to patients who are dehydrated or who are at risk for dehydration. If incontinence is a concern, ensure that AP understand that withholding fluids is not appropriate to prevent the problem. Instruct them to take the time to stay with patients while they drink the fluid and to note the exact amount ingested.

Use of oral rehydration solutions (ORSs) for rehydration therapy is an effective way to replace fluids. Specially formulated solutions containing glucose and electrolytes are absorbed even when the patient is vomiting or has diarrhea. These solutions are more often used in the home setting; in long-term care; and for patients who have poor veins, making IV therapy difficult. A variety of commercial ORSs are available over the counter.

TABLE 13.3 Osmolarity of Common Intravenous Therapy Solutions

Solution	Osmolarity (mOsm/L)
0.9% saline	308 Isotonic
0.45% saline	154 Hypotonic
5% dextrose in water (D_5W)	272 Isotonic[a]
10% dextrose in water ($D_{10}W$)	500 Hypertonic[a]
5% dextrose in 0.9% saline	560 Hypertonic[a]
5% dextrose in 0.45% saline	406 Hypertonic[a]
5% dextrose in 0.225% saline	321 Isotonic[a]
Ringer's lactate	273 Isotonic
5% dextrose in Ringer's lactate	525 Hypertonic[a]

[a]Solution tonicity at the time of administration. Within a short time after administration, the dextrose is metabolized and the tonicity of the infused solution decreases in proportion to the osmolarity or tonicity of the nondextrose components (electrolytes) within the water.

When dehydration is severe or the patient cannot tolerate oral fluids, IV fluid replacement is needed. Calculation of how much fluid to replace is based on the patient's weight loss and symptoms. The rate of fluid replacement depends on the degree of dehydration and the patient's cardiac, pulmonary, and kidney status.

The type of fluid prescribed varies with the patient's cardiac status and blood osmolarity (Gross et al., 2017; Pierce et al., 2016). Crystalloids are IV fluids that contain water, minerals (electrolytes), and sometimes other water-soluble substances such as glucose. These fluids rapidly disperse to all body fluid compartments and are most useful when dehydration includes both the intracellular and extracellular compartments. Colloids are IV fluids that contain larger non–water-soluble molecules that increase the osmotic pressure in the plasma volume. These fluids can help maintain or expand plasma volume with a lower infused volume (Gross et al., 2017; Pierce et al., 2016). Table 13.3 lists types of common IV fluids. *The two most important areas to monitor during rehydration are pulse rate and quality and urine output.*

Drug Therapy. Drug therapy may correct some causes of the dehydration. Antidiarrheal drugs are prescribed when diarrhea causes dehydration. Antimicrobial therapy may be used in patients with bacterial diarrhea. Antiemetics may be used when vomiting causes dehydration. Antipyretics to reduce fever are helpful when fever makes dehydration worse. Desmopressin is used to control fluid loss in diabetes insipidus (Goad & Levesque, 2020).

Preventing Injury

Planning: Expected Outcomes. The patient with dehydration is expected to avoid injury.

Interventions. Patient safety issues and strategies are priorities of care before and during other therapies for dehydration. Monitor vital signs, especially heart rate quality and blood pressure. The patient with dehydration is at risk for falls because of orthostatic hypotension, dysrhythmia, muscle weakness, and possible confusion. Assess his or her muscle strength, gait stability, and level of alertness. Instruct the patient to get up slowly from a lying or sitting position and to immediately sit down if he or she feels light-headed. Stress the importance of asking for assistance to ambulate. Implement other falls precautions as described in Chapter 4.

Care Coordination and Transition Management. Because dehydration is a symptom or complication of another health problem or drug therapy, dehydration is often resolved before patients return home or to residential care. Education is the most important management strategy to prevent recurrence among adults who remain at some risk for recurrence such as patients who have diabetes insipidus or diabetes mellitus (Hutto & French, 2017). See Chapter 57 for a detailed discussion of the care coordination needed for diabetes insipidus and Chapter 59 for care coordination for diabetes mellitus.

◆ **Evaluation: Evaluate Outcomes.** Most patients return to an acceptable fluid balance with proper management. Indications that the patient's underlying cause of dehydration is well managed and that the imbalance is corrected include that the patient:

- Maintains a daily fluid intake of at least 1500 mL (or drinks at least 500 mL more than his or her daily urine output)
- Maintains blood pressure at or near his or her normal range
- Has moist mucous membranes and normal skin turgor
- Asks for assistance when ambulating
- Does not fall
- Can state the indications of dehydration
- Starts fluid replacement at the first indication of dehydration
- Correctly follows treatment plans for ongoing health problems that increase the risk for dehydration

NCLEX EXAMINATION CHALLENGE 13.2

Safe and Effective Care Environment

Which clinical indicators are **most relevant** for the nurse to monitor during IV fluid replacement for a client with dehydration? **Select all that apply.**

A. Blood pressure
B. Deep tendon reflexes
C. Hand-grip strength
D. Pulse rate and quality
E. Skin turgor
F. Urine output

FLUID OVERLOAD

Pathophysiology Review

Fluid overload, also called *overhydration,* is an excess of body fluid. It is a clinical indication of a problem in which fluid intake or retention is *greater* than the body's fluid needs. The most common type of fluid overload is **hypervolemia** (Fig. 13.10) because the problems result from excessive fluid in the extracellular fluid (ECF) space. Most problems caused by fluid overload are related to excessive fluid in the vascular space or to dilution of specific electrolytes and blood components. The conditions leading to fluid overload are

KEY FEATURES

Fluid Overload

Cardiovascular Changes
- Increased pulse rate
- Bounding pulse quality
- Elevated blood pressure
- Decreased pulse pressure
- Elevated central venous pressure
- Distended neck and hand veins
- Engorged varicose veins
- Weight gain

Respiratory Changes
- Increased respiratory rate
- Shallow respirations
- Shortness of breath
- Moist crackles present on auscultation

Skin and Mucous Membrane Changes
- Pitting edema in dependent areas
- Skin pale and cool to touch

Neuromuscular Changes
- Altered level of consciousness
- Headache
- Visual disturbances
- Skeletal muscle weakness
- Paresthesias

GI Changes
- Increased motility (in acute fluid overload; decreased in conditions causing chronic overload)
- Enlarged liver

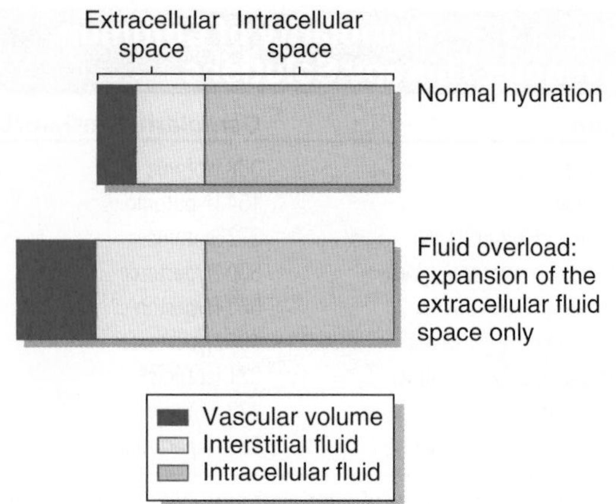

Fig. 13.10 Changes in fluid compartment volumes with fluid overload. (© 1992 by M. Linda Workman. All rights reserved.)

related to excessive intake or inadequate excretion of fluids. See Table 13.2 for causes of fluid overload. Fig. 13.11 outlines the adaptive changes the body makes in response to mild or moderate fluid overload, especially increased urine output and edema formation. When overload is severe or occurs in an adult with poor cardiac or kidney function it can lead to heart failure and pulmonary edema. Dilution of sodium and potassium can lead to seizures, coma, and death (Reynolds, 2016).

Interprofessional Collaborative Care

Assessment: Recognize Cues. Patients with fluid overload often have pitting edema in dependent areas, which vary with patient position (Fig. 13.12). Other symptoms, listed in the Key Features: Fluid Overload box, are usually seen in the cardiovascular, respiratory, neuromuscular, integumentary, and GI systems.

Fluid overload is diagnosed based on assessment findings and the results of laboratory tests. Usually serum electrolyte values are normal in isotonic fluid overload, but decreased hemoglobin, hematocrit, and serum protein levels may result from excessive water in the vascular space *(hemodilution).*

Interventions: Take Action. The focus of priority nursing interventions is to ensure patient safety, restore normal fluid balance, provide supportive care until the imbalance is resolved, and prevent future fluid overload. Drug therapy, nutrition therapy, and monitoring are the basis of intervention.

Patient safety is the first priority. Interventions are implemented to prevent fluid overload from becoming worse, leading to pulmonary edema, heart failure, and complications of electrolyte dilution. Any patient with fluid overload, regardless of age, is at risk for these complications, especially when the onset is acute. Older adults or those with cardiac problems, kidney problems, pulmonary problems, or liver problems are at greater risk.

NURSING SAFETY PRIORITY: CRITICAL RESCUE (QSEN)

Assess the patient with fluid overload at least every 2 hours to recognize pulmonary edema, which can occur very quickly and can lead to death. If signs of worsening overload are present (bounding pulse, increasing neck vein distention, lung crackles, increasing peripheral edema, reduced urine output), respond by notifying the primary health care provider.

The patient with fluid overload and edema is at risk for skin breakdown. Use a pressure-reducing or pressure-relieving overlay on the mattress. Assess skin pressure areas daily for signs of redness or open area, especially the coccyx, elbows, hips, and heels. Help the patient change positions every 2 hours or ensure that assistive personnel (AP) perform this action.

Drug therapy focuses on removing excess fluid. Diuretics are used for fluid overload if kidney function is normal. Drugs may include high-ceiling (loop) diuretics such as furosemide. If there is concern that too much sodium and other electrolytes would be lost using loop diuretics or if the patient has syndrome of inappropriate antidiuretic hormone (SIADH), conivaptan or tolvaptan may be prescribed (Hutto & French, 2017).

Monitor the patient for response to drug therapy, especially weight loss and increased urine output. Observe for indications of electrolyte imbalance, especially changes in electrocardiogram (ECG) patterns. Assess sodium and potassium values whenever they are drawn.

Nutrition therapy for the patient with chronic fluid overload may involve restrictions of both fluid and sodium intake. Often sodium restriction involves only "no added salt" to ordinary table foods when fluid overload is mild. For more severe fluid overload, the patient may be restricted to 2 g/day to 4 g/day of sodium. Teach the patient and family how to check food labels for sodium content and how to keep a daily record of sodium ingested.

Monitoring intake and output and weight provides information on therapy effectiveness. Teach UAP that these measurements need to be accurate, not just estimated, because treatment decisions are based on these findings. Schedule fluid offerings throughout the 24 hours. Teach UAP to check urine for color and character and to report these findings.

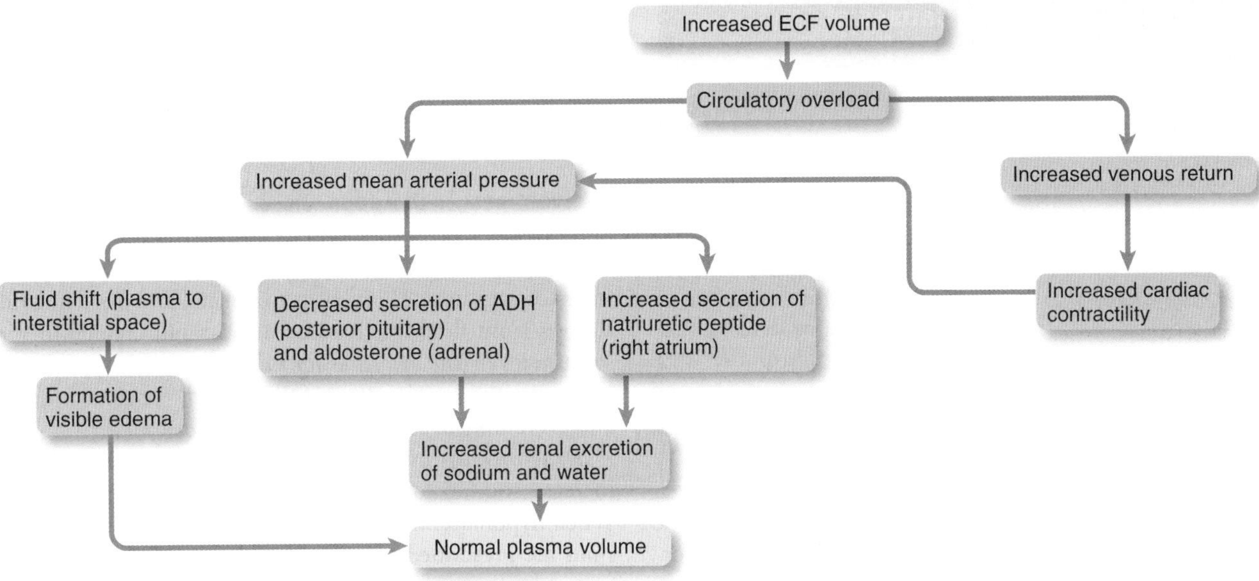

Fig. 13.11 Adaptive actions and mechanisms to prevent cardiac and pulmonary complications during fluid overload. (*ADH,* Antidiuretic hormone; *ECF,* extracellular fluid.)

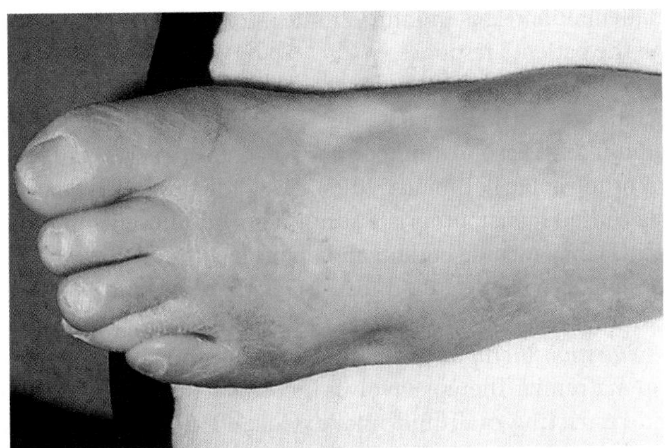

Fig. 13.12 Pitting edema of the left foot and ankle.

Fluid retention may not be visible. Rapid weight gain is the best indicator of fluid retention and overload. Metabolism can account for only a half pound (250 g) of weight gain in 1 day. Each pound (0.5 kg) of weight gained (after the first half pound) equates to about 500 mL of retained fluid. Weigh the patient at the same time every day (before breakfast), using the same scale. Have the patient wear the same type of clothing for each weigh-in. When in-bed weights are taken, lift tubing and equipment off the bed. Record the number of blankets and pillows on the bed at the initial weigh-in and ensure that ongoing weights always include the same number.

If the patient is discharged to home before the fluid overload has completely resolved or has continuing risk for fluid overload, teach him or her and the family to monitor weight at home. Teach them to keep a record of daily weights to show the health care provider at checkups. Patients may choose to use mobile "apps" to record and trend this information. Instruct the patient to call the primary health care provider for more than a 3-lb (1.5-kg) gain in a week or more than a 2-lb (1-kg) gain in 24 hours.

NCLEX EXAMINATION CHALLENGE 13.3

Safe and Effective Care Environment

The client who is confined to bed in the recumbent position has gained 5 lb (2.3 kg) in the past 24 hours. In which area does the nurse assess skin turgor for accurate determination of dependent edema?

A. Foot and ankle
B. Forehead
C. Sacrum
D. Chest

SODIUM IMBALANCE: HYPONATREMIA

Pathophysiology Review

Hyponatremia is an electrolyte imbalance in which the serum sodium (Na^+) level is below 136 mEq/L (mmol/L). Sodium imbalances often occur along with a fluid imbalance because the same hormones regulate both sodium and water balance. The problems caused by hyponatremia occur from two changes—reduced excitable membrane depolarization and cellular swelling.

Excitable cell membrane depolarization depends on high extracellular fluid (ECF) levels of sodium being available to cross cell membranes and move into cells in response to a stimulus. Hyponatremia makes depolarization slower, so excitable membranes are less excitable.

With hyponatremia the osmolarity of the ECF is lower than that of the intracellular fluid (ICF). As a result, water moves into the cell, causing swelling (Bertschi, 2020). Even a small amount of swelling can reduce cell function. Larger amounts of swelling can make the cell burst *(lysis)* and die.

Many conditions and drugs can lead to hyponatremia (Table 13.4). A common cause of low sodium levels is the prolonged use and overuse of diuretics, especially in older adults. When these drugs are used to manage fluid overload, sodium is lost along with water. Hyponatremia can result from the loss of total body sodium,

TABLE 13.4 Common Causes of Hyponatremia

Actual Sodium Deficits	Relative Sodium Deficits (Dilution)
• Excessive diaphoresis • Diuretics (high-ceiling diuretics) • Wound drainage (especially GI) • Decreased secretion of aldosterone • Hyperlipidemia • Kidney disease (scarred distal convoluted tubule) • Nothing by mouth • Low-salt diet • Cerebral salt-wasting syndrome • Hyperglycemia	• Excessive ingestion of hypotonic fluids • Psychogenic polydipsia • Freshwater submersion accident • Kidney failure (nephrotic syndrome) • Irrigation with hypotonic fluids • Syndrome of inappropriate antidiuretic hormone secretion • Heart failure

the movement of sodium from the blood to other fluid spaces, or the dilution of serum sodium from excessive water in the plasma.

❖ Interprofessional Collaborative Care

◆ **Assessment: Recognize Cues.** The signs and symptoms of hyponatremia are caused by its effects on excitable cellular activity. The cells especially affected are those involved in cerebral, neuromuscular, and intestinal smooth muscle, and cardiovascular functions.

Cerebral changes are the most obvious problems of hyponatremia. Behavioral changes result from cerebral edema and increased intracranial pressure. Closely observe and document the patient's behavior, level of consciousness, and cognition. A sudden onset of acute confusion or increased confusion is often seen in older adults who have low serum sodium levels (Touhy & Jett, 2020). When sodium levels become very low, seizures, coma, and death may occur (Pagana & Pagana, 2018).

Neuromuscular changes are seen as general muscle weakness. Assess the patient's neuromuscular status during each nursing shift for changes from baseline. Deep tendon reflexes diminish, and muscle weakness is worse in the legs and arms. Assess muscle strength and deep tendon reflex responses as described in Chapter 38.

! NURSING SAFETY PRIORITY (QSEN)

Action Alert

If muscle weakness is present, immediately check respiratory effectiveness because ventilation depends on adequate strength of respiratory muscles.

Intestinal changes include increased motility, causing nausea, diarrhea, and abdominal cramping. Assess the GI system by listening to bowel sounds and observing stools. Bowel sounds are hyperactive, and bowel movements are frequent and watery.

Cardiovascular changes are seen as changes in cardiac output. The cardiac responses to hyponatremia with hypovolemia include a rapid, weak, thready pulse. Peripheral pulses are difficult to palpate and are easily blocked. Blood pressure is decreased, and the patient may have severe orthostatic hypotension, leading to light-headedness or dizziness. The central venous pressure is low.

When hyponatremia occurs with hypervolemia (fluid overload), cardiac changes include a full or bounding pulse with normal or high blood pressure. Peripheral pulses are full and difficult to block; however, they may not be palpable if edema is present.

◆ **Interventions: Take Action.** The cause of the low sodium level must first be determined to plan appropriate management. Interventions with drug therapy and nutrition therapy are used to restore serum sodium levels to normal and prevent complications from fluid overload or a too-rapid change in serum sodium level. *The priorities for nursing care of the patient with hyponatremia are monitoring the patient's response to therapy and preventing hypernatremia and fluid overload.*

Drug therapy involves reducing the doses of any drugs that increase sodium loss such as most diuretics (Thomas, 2017). When hyponatremia occurs with a fluid deficit, IV saline infusions are prescribed to restore both sodium and fluid volume. Severe hyponatremia may be treated with small-volume infusions of hypertonic saline, most often 3% saline (Jones et al., 2017), although 5% saline can be used for extreme hyponatremia. These infusions are delivered using a controller to prevent accidental increases in infusion rate. Monitor the infusion rate and the patient's response.

When hyponatremia occurs with fluid excess, drug therapy includes drugs that promote the excretion of water rather than sodium (e.g., vasopressin receptor antagonists such as conivaptan or tolvaptan) (Thomas, 2017). Drug therapy for hyponatremia caused by inappropriate secretion of antidiuretic hormone (ADH) may include lithium and demeclocycline. Assess hourly for signs of excessive fluid loss, potassium loss, and increased sodium levels.

Nutrition therapy can help restore sodium balance in mild hyponatremia. Therapy involves increasing oral sodium intake and restricting oral fluid intake. Collaborate with the registered dietitian nutritionist (RDN) to teach the patient about which chronic foods to increase in the diet. Fluid restriction may be needed long term when chronic fluid overload is the cause of the hyponatremia or when kidney fluid excretion is impaired. Nursing actions for patient safety, skin protection, monitoring, and patient and family teaching are the same as those for fluid overload.

SODIUM IMBALANCE: HYPERNATREMIA

Pathophysiology Review

Hypernatremia is a serum sodium level over 145 mEq/L (mmol/L). It can be caused by or can cause changes in fluid volume. Table 13.5 lists causes of hypernatremia.

As serum sodium level rises, a larger difference in sodium levels occurs between the extracellular fluid (ECF) and intracellular fluid (ICF). More sodium is present to move rapidly across cell membranes during depolarization, making excitable tissues more easily excited. This condition is called *irritability*, and excitable tissues overrespond to stimuli. In addition, water moves from the cells into the ECF to dilute the hyperosmolar ECF (Bertschi, 2020). Thus when serum sodium levels are high, severe cellular

TABLE 13.5 Common Causes of Hypernatremia

Actual Sodium Excesses	Relative Sodium Excesses
• Hyperaldosteronism	• Nothing by mouth
• Kidney failure	• Increased rate of metabolism
• Corticosteroids	• Fever
• Cushing syndrome or disease	• Hyperventilation
• Excessive oral sodium ingestion	• Infection
• Excessive administration of sodium-containing IV fluids	• Excessive diaphoresis
	• Watery diarrhea
	• Dehydration

dehydration with cellular shrinkage occurs. Eventually the dehydrated excitable tissues may no longer be able to respond to stimuli.

Interprofessional Collaborative Care

Assessment: Recognize Cues. Symptoms of hypernatremia vary with the severity of sodium imbalance and whether a fluid imbalance is also present. Changes are first seen in excitable membrane activity, especially nerve, skeletal muscle, and cardiac function.

Nervous system changes start with altered cerebral function. Assess the patient's mental status for attention span and cognitive function. In hypernatremia with normal or decreased fluid volumes, the patient may have a short attention span and be agitated or confused. When hypernatremia occurs with fluid overload, the patient may be lethargic, stuporous, or comatose.

Skeletal muscle changes vary with the degree and stage of sodium increases. Mild rises in early stages cause muscle twitching and irregular muscle contractions. As hypernatremia continues to worsen, the muscles and nerves are less able to respond to a stimulus and muscles become progressively weaker. In later stages, the deep tendon reflexes are reduced or absent. Muscle weakness occurs bilaterally and has no specific pattern. Observe for twitching in muscle groups. Assess muscle strength by having the patient perform handgrip and arm flexion against resistance as described in Chapters 38 and 44. Assess deep tendon reflexes by lightly tapping the patellar (knee) and Achilles (heel) tendons with a reflex hammer and measuring the movement.

Cardiovascular changes include decreased contractility because high sodium levels slow the movement of calcium into the heart cells, which is needed for effective cardiac contraction. Measure blood pressure and the rate and quality of the apical and peripheral pulses. Pulse rate is increased in patients with hypernatremia and hypovolemia. Peripheral pulses are difficult to palpate and are easily blocked. Hypotension and severe orthostatic (postural) hypotension are present, and pulse pressure is reduced. Patients with hypernatremia and hypervolemia have slow to normal bounding pulses. Peripheral pulses are full and difficult to block. Neck veins are distended, even with the patient in the upright position. Blood pressure, especially diastolic blood pressure, is increased.

Interventions: Take Action. Drug and nutrition therapies are used to prevent further sodium increases and to decrease high serum sodium levels. Nursing care priorities for the patient with hypernatremia include monitoring his or her response to therapy and ensuring patient safety by preventing hyponatremia and dehydration.

Drug therapy is used to restore fluid balance when hypernatremia is caused by fluid loss. Isotonic saline (0.9%) and dextrose 5% in 0.45% sodium chloride are most often prescribed. Although the dextrose 5% in 0.45% sodium chloride is hypertonic in the IV bag, once it is infused, the glucose is rapidly metabolized making the infused fluid hypotonic. Hypernatremia caused by reduced kidney sodium excretion requires drug therapy with diuretics that promote sodium loss such as furosemide or bumetanide. Assess the patient hourly for indications of excessive losses of fluid, sodium, or potassium.

Nutrition therapy to prevent or correct mild hypernatremia involves ensuring adequate water intake, especially among older adults. Dietary sodium restriction may be needed to prevent sodium excess when kidney problems are present. Collaborate with the registered dietitian nutritionist to teach the patient how to determine the sodium content of foods, beverages, and drugs. Nursing actions for patient safety, skin protection, monitoring, and patient and family teaching are similar to those for fluid overload.

POTASSIUM IMBALANCE: HYPOKALEMIA

Pathophysiology Review

Hypokalemia is a serum potassium level below 3.5 mEq/L (mmol/L). As discussed earlier in the Electrolyte Balance section, most potassium (K^+) is inside cells and minor changes in extracellular potassium levels cause major changes in cell membrane excitability. *This imbalance can be life threatening because every body system is affected.*

Low serum potassium levels reduce the excitability of cells. As a result, the cell membranes of all excitable tissues such as nerve and muscle are less responsive to normal stimuli. Gradual potassium loss may have no symptoms until the loss is extreme. Rapid reduction of serum potassium levels causes dramatic changes in function. Table 13.6 lists causes of hypokalemia.

Actual potassium depletion occurs when potassium loss is excessive or when potassium intake is not adequate to match normal potassium loss. Relative hypokalemia occurs when total body potassium levels are normal but the potassium distribution between fluid spaces is abnormal or diluted by excess water. This can also occur during rapid infusions of insulin because this drug increases the activity of the sodium-potassium pump, forcing more blood potassium into the cells. In the ICF and ECF potassium levels are linked to that of magnesium; low blood levels of magnesium are often accompanied by hypokalemia.

Interprofessional Collaborative Care

Assessment: Recognize Cues. *Age* is important because urine concentrating ability decreases with aging, which increases potassium loss. Older adults are more likely to use drugs that lead to potassium loss.

Drugs, especially diuretics, corticosteroids, and beta-adrenergic agonists or antagonists, can increase kidney potassium loss. Ask about prescription and over-the-counter drug use. Ask whether the patient takes a potassium supplement such as potassium chloride (KCl) or eats foods that have high concentrations of potassium, such as bananas, citrus juices, raisins,

TABLE 13.6 Common Causes of Hypokalemia

Actual Potassium Deficits	Relative Potassium Deficits

• Inappropriate or excessive use of drugs:
  • Diuretics
  • Corticosteroids
• Increased secretion of aldosterone
• Cushing syndrome
• Diarrhea
• Vomiting
• Wound drainage (especially GI)
• Prolonged nasogastric suction
• Heat-induced excessive diaphoresis
• Kidney disease impairing reabsorption of potassium
• Nothing by mouth
	• Alkalosis
	• Hyperinsulinism
	• Hyperalimentation
	• Total parenteral nutrition
	• Water intoxication
	• IV therapy with potassium-poor solutions

and meat. The patient may not be taking the supplement as prescribed because of its unpleasant taste.

Disease can lead to potassium loss. Ask about chronic disorders, recent illnesses, and medical or surgical interventions. A thorough nutrition history, including a typical day's food and beverage intake, helps identify patients at risk for hypokalemia.

Respiratory changes occur because of respiratory muscle weakness, resulting in shallow respirations. Assess the patient's breath sounds, ease of respiratory effort, color of nail beds and mucous membranes, and rate and depth of respiration.

! NURSING SAFETY PRIORITY (QSEN)

Action Alert

Assess respiratory status of a patient with hypokalemia at least every 2 hours because respiratory insufficiency is a major cause of death from hypokalemia.

Musculoskeletal changes include skeletal muscle weakness. A stronger stimulus is needed to begin muscle contraction. Patients may be too weak to stand. Hand grasps are weak, and deep tendon reflexes are reduced *(hyporeflexia)*. Severe hypokalemia causes flaccid paralysis. Assess for muscle weakness and the patient's ability to perform ADLs.

Cardiovascular changes are assessed by palpating the peripheral pulses. In hypokalemia the pulse is usually thready and weak. Palpation is difficult, and the pulse is easily blocked. Pulse rate ranges from very slow to very rapid, and an irregular heartbeat (dysrhythmia) may be present. Measure blood pressure with the patient in the lying, sitting, and standing positions because orthostatic (postural) hypotension occurs with hypokalemia.

Neurologic changes from hypokalemia include altered mental status. The patient may have short-term irritability and anxiety followed by lethargy that progresses to acute confusion and coma as hypokalemia worsens.

Intestinal changes occur with hypokalemia because GI smooth muscle contractions are decreased, which leads to decreased peristalsis. Bowel sounds are hypoactive, and nausea, vomiting, constipation, and abdominal distention are common. Observe for abdominal distension and auscultate for bowel sounds in all four abdominal quadrants. *Severe hypokalemia can cause the absence of peristalsis (paralytic ileus).*

Laboratory data confirm hypokalemia (serum potassium value below 3.5 mEq/L [mmol/L]). Hypokalemia causes ECG changes in the heart, including ST-segment depression, flat or inverted T waves, and increased U waves. *Dysrhythmias can lead to death, particularly in older adults who are taking digoxin.*

NCLEX EXAMINATION CHALLENGE 13.4

Safe and Effective Care Environment

With which client does the nurse remain alert for and assess most frequently for signs and symptoms of hypokalemia to **prevent harm**?

A. 72-year-old taking the diuretic spironolactone for control of hypertension
B. 62-year-old receiving an IV solution of Ringer's lactate at a rate of 200 mL/hr
C. 42-year-old trauma victim receiving a third infusion of packed red blood cells in 12 hours
D. 22-year-old receiving an IV infusion of regular insulin to manage an episode of ketoacidosis

◆ **Interventions: Take Action.** Interventions for hypokalemia focus on preventing potassium loss, increasing serum potassium levels, and ensuring patient safety. Drug and nutrition therapies help restore normal serum potassium levels. *The priorities for nursing care of the patient with hypokalemia are ensuring adequate gas exchange, patient safety for falls prevention, prevention of injury from potassium administration, and monitoring the patient's response to therapy.* Review the nursing care activities listed in the Best Practice for Patient Safety & Quality Care: The Patient With Dehydration box.

Drug therapy for management and prevention of hypokalemia includes additional potassium and drugs to prevent potassium loss. Most potassium supplements are potassium chloride, potassium gluconate, or potassium citrate. The amount and route of potassium replacement depend on the degree of loss.

Potassium is given IV for severe hypokalemia. The drug is available in different concentrations, and this drug carries a high alert warning as a concentrated electrolyte solution.

Before infusing any IV solution containing potassium chloride (KCl), check and recheck the dilution of the drug in the IV solution container.

! NATIONAL PATIENT SAFETY GOALS (NPSG)

The Joint Commission's National Patient Safety Goals mandate that concentrated potassium be diluted and added to IV solutions only in the pharmacy by a registered pharmacist and that vials of concentrated potassium not be available in patient care areas.

! NURSING SAFETY PRIORITY (QSEN)

Drug Alert

A dilution no greater than 1 mEq (mmol/L) of potassium to 10 mL of solution is recommended for IV administration. The maximum recommended infusion rate is 5 to 10 mEq/hr (mmol/hr); **this rate is never to exceed 20 mEq/hr (mmol/hr) under any circumstances.** In accordance with National Patient Safety Goals (NPSGs), potassium is **not** given by IV push to avoid causing cardiac arrest.

Potassium is a severe tissue irritant and is never given by IM or subcutaneous injection. Tissues damaged by potassium can become necrotic, causing loss of function and requiring surgery. IV potassium solutions irritate veins and cause phlebitis. Check the prescription carefully to ensure that the patient receives the correct amount of potassium. Assess the IV site hourly and ask the patient whether he or she feels burning or pain at the site.

! NURSING SAFETY PRIORITY (QSEN)

Action Alert

If infiltration of a solution containing potassium occurs, stop the IV solution immediately, remove the venous access, and notify the health care provider or Rapid Response Team. Document these actions and provide a complete description and photograph of the IV site.

Oral potassium preparations may be taken as liquids or solids. Potassium has a strong, unpleasant taste that is difficult to mask, although it can be mixed with many liquids. Because potassium chloride can cause nausea and vomiting, give the drug during or after a meal and advise patients using the drug at home not to take it on an empty stomach.

Diuretics that increase the kidney excretion of potassium can cause hypokalemia, especially high-ceiling (loop) diuretics (e.g., furosemide and bumetanide) and thiazide diuretics. These drugs are avoided in patients with hypokalemia. A potassium-sparing diuretic such as spironolactone, triamterene, or amiloride may be prescribed to increase urine output without increasing potassium loss.

Nutrition therapy involves collaboration with an RDN to teach the patient how to increase dietary potassium intake. Eating foods rich in potassium helps prevent further loss, but supplementation is needed to restore normal potassium levels.

Implement safety measures with a patient who has muscle weakness from hypokalemia, including the falls precautions listed in Chapter 4. Be sure to have the patient wear a gait belt when ambulating with assistance.

Respiratory monitoring is performed at least hourly for severe hypokalemia. Also check oxygen saturation by pulse oximetry to determine breathing effectiveness. Assess respiratory muscle effectiveness by checking the patient's ability to cough. Examine the face, oral mucosa, and nail beds for pallor or cyanosis. Evaluate arterial blood gas values (when available) for decreased blood oxygen levels *(hypoxemia)* and increased arterial carbon dioxide levels *(hypercapnia)*, which indicate inadequate gas exchange.

POTASSIUM IMBALANCE: HYPERKALEMIA

Pathophysiology Review

Hyperkalemia is a serum potassium level higher than 5.0 mEq/L (mmol/L). Even small increases above normal values can affect excitable tissues, especially the heart.

A high serum potassium increases cell excitability, causing excitable tissues to respond to less intense stimuli. The heart is very sensitive to serum potassium increases; and hyperkalemia interferes with electrical conduction, leading to heart block and ventricular fibrillation.

The problems that occur with hyperkalemia are related to how rapidly ECF potassium levels increase. Sudden potassium rises cause severe problems at serum levels between 6 and 7 mEq/L (mmol/L). When serum potassium rises slowly, problems may not occur until potassium levels reach 8 mEq/L (mmol/L) or higher.

TABLE 13.7 Common Causes of Hyperkalemia

Actual Potassium Excesses	Relative Potassium Excesses

• Overingestion of potassium-containing foods or medications:
  • Salt substitutes
  • Potassium chloride
• Rapid infusion of potassium-containing IV solutions
• Bolus IV potassium injections
• Transfusions of whole blood or packed cells
• Adrenal insufficiency
• Kidney failure
• Potassium-sparing diuretics
• Angiotensin-converting enzyme inhibitors (ACEIs)
	• Tissue damage
	• Acidosis
	• Hyperuricemia
	• Uncontrolled diabetes mellitus

Hyperkalemia is rare in people with normal kidney function (Ellison & Farrar, 2018; McCance et al., 2019). Most cases of hyperkalemia occur in hospitalized patients and in those undergoing medical treatment (Adis Medical Writers, 2015). Those at greatest risk are chronically ill patients, debilitated patients, older adults, and those taking potassium-sparing diuretics (Table 13.7).

Interprofessional Collaborative Care

Assessment: Recognize Cues. Age is important because kidney function decreases with aging. Ask about kidney disease, diabetes mellitus, recent medical or surgical treatment, and urine output, including frequency and amount of voidings. Ask about drug use, particularly potassium-sparing diuretics, angiotensin-converting enzyme inhibitors (ACEIs), and angiotensin receptor blockers (ARBs). Obtain a nutrition history to determine the intake of potassium-rich foods and the use of salt substitutes (which contain potassium).

Ask whether the patient has had palpitations, skipped heartbeats, or other cardiac irregularities; muscle twitching; leg weakness; or unusual tingling or numbness in the hands, feet, or face. Ask about recent changes in bowel habits, especially diarrhea.

Cardiovascular changes are the most severe problems from hyperkalemia and are the most common cause of death in patients with hyperkalemia. Cardiac symptoms include bradycardia, hypotension, and ECG changes of tall, peaked T waves, prolonged PR intervals, flat or absent P waves, and wide QRS complexes. Ectopic beats may appear. Complete heart block, asystole, and ventricular fibrillation are life-threatening complications of severe hyperkalemia.

Neuromuscular changes with hyperkalemia have two phases. Skeletal muscles twitch in the early stages of hyperkalemia, and the patient may be aware of tingling and burning sensations, followed by numbness in the hands and feet and around the mouth *(paresthesia)*. As hyperkalemia worsens, muscle weakness occurs, followed by flaccid paralysis. The weakness moves up from the hands and feet and first affects the muscles of the arms and legs. Respiratory muscles are not affected until serum potassium levels reach lethal levels.

Intestinal changes include increased motility with diarrhea and hyperactive bowel sounds. Bowel movements are frequent and watery.

Laboratory data confirm hyperkalemia (potassium level over 5.0 mEq/L [mmol/L]). If it is caused by dehydration, levels of other electrolytes, hematocrit, and hemoglobin are also elevated. Hyperkalemia caused by kidney failure occurs with elevated serum creatinine and blood urea nitrogen, decreased blood pH, and normal or low hematocrit and hemoglobin levels.

◆ **Interventions: Take Action.** Interventions for hyperkalemia focus on reducing the serum potassium level, preventing recurrences, and ensuring patient safety. Drug therapy is key. *The priorities for nursing care of the patient with hyperkalemia are assessing for cardiac complications, patient safety for falls prevention, monitoring the patient's response to therapy, and health teaching.*

Drug therapy can restore potassium balance by enhancing potassium excretion and promoting the movement of potassium from the extracellular fluid (ECF) into the cells. The oral drug patiromer binds with potassium in the GI tract and decreases its absorption.

Stop potassium-containing infusions and keep the IV access open. Withhold oral potassium supplements and collaborate with an RDN to help the client select foods low in potassium.

Increasing potassium excretion helps reduce hyperkalemia if kidney function is normal. Potassium-excreting diuretics are prescribed. When kidney problems exist, more invasive interventions may be needed (see Chapter 63).

Movement of potassium from the extracellular fluid (ECF) to the intracellular fluid (ICF) can help reduce serum potassium levels temporarily. Potassium movement into the cells is enhanced by insulin. Insulin increases the activity of the sodium-potassium pumps, which move potassium from the ECF into the cell. IV fluids containing glucose and insulin may be prescribed to help decrease serum potassium levels. These IV solutions are hypertonic and are infused through a central line or in a vein with a high blood flow to avoid local vein inflammation. Observe the patient for indications of hypokalemia and hypoglycemia during this therapy.

Cardiac monitoring allows for the early recognition of dysrhythmias and other symptoms of hyperkalemia on cardiac muscle. Compare recent ECG tracings with the tracings obtained when the patient's serum potassium level was close to normal.

! NURSING SAFETY PRIORITY QSEN

Critical Rescue

Assess anyone who has or is at risk for hyperkalemia to recognize cardiac changes. If the patient's heart rate falls below 60 beats/min or if the T waves become spiked, both of which accompany hyperkalemia, respond by notifying the Rapid Response Team.

Health teaching is key to the prevention of hyperkalemia and the early detection of complications. The teaching plan includes diet, drugs, and recognition of the indicators of hyperkalemia. Collaborate with the registered dietitian nutritionist (RDN) to teach the patient and family about which foods to avoid (those high in potassium). Instruct the patient and family to read the labels on drug and food packages to determine the potassium content. Warn them to avoid salt substitutes, which contain potassium.

NCLEX EXAMINATION CHALLENGE 13.5

Safe and Effective Care Environment

In reviewing the electrolytes of a client, the nurse notes the serum potassium level has increased from 4.6 mEq/L (mmol/L) to 6.1 mEq/L (mmol/L). Which assessment does the nurse perform first to **prevent harm**?

A. Deep tendon reflexes
B. Oxygen saturation
C. Pulse rate and rhythm
D. Respiratory rate and depth

CALCIUM IMBALANCE: HYPOCALCEMIA

Pathophysiology Review

Hypocalcemia is a total serum calcium (Ca^{2+}) level below 9.0 mg/dL or 2.25 mmol/L. Because the normal blood level of calcium is so low, any change in calcium levels has major effects on function.

Calcium is an excitable membrane stabilizer, regulating depolarization and the generation of action potentials. It decreases sodium movement across excitable membranes, slowing the rate of depolarization. Low serum calcium levels increase sodium movement across excitable membranes, allowing depolarization to occur more easily and at inappropriate times.

Hypocalcemia is caused by many chronic and acute conditions, as well as medical or surgical treatments. Table 13.8 lists causes of hypocalcemia. Acute hypocalcemia results in the rapid onset of life-threatening symptoms. Chronic hypocalcemia occurs slowly over time, and excitable membrane symptoms may not be severe because the body has adjusted to the gradual reduction of serum calcium levels.

PATIENT-CENTERED CARE: GENDER HEALTH CONSIDERATIONS QSEN

Postmenopausal women are at risk for chronic calcium loss. This problem is related to reduced weight-bearing activities and a decrease in estrogen levels. As they age, many women decrease weight-bearing activities such as running and walking, which allows osteoporosis to occur at a more rapid rate. In addition, the estrogen secretion that protects against osteoporosis diminishes. Teach older women to continue walking and other weight-bearing activities.

❖ Interprofessional Collaborative Care

◆ **Assessment: Recognize Cues.** Assess the nutrition history for the risk for hypocalcemia. Ask the patient about his or her intake of dairy products and whether he or she takes a calcium supplement regularly.

One indicator of hypocalcemia is a report of frequent, painful muscle spasms ("charley horses") usually in the thigh, calf, or foot during rest or sleep. Ask about a history of recent orthopedic surgery or bone healing. Thyroid surgery, therapeutic irradiation of the upper middle chest and neck area, or a recent anterior neck injury increases the risk for hypocalcemia. Most symptoms of acute hypocalcemia are caused by overstimulation of the nerves and muscles.

TABLE 13.8 Common Causes of Hypocalcemia

Actual Calcium Deficits	Relative Calcium Deficits

• Inadequate oral intake of calcium
• Lactose intolerance
• Malabsorption syndromes:
  • Celiac disease, sprue
  • Crohn's disease
• Inadequate intake of vitamin D
• End-stage kidney disease
• Diarrhea
• Steatorrhea
• Wound drainage (especially GI)
	• Hyperproteinemia
	• Alkalosis
	• Calcium chelators or binders
	• Citrate
	• Mithramycin
	• Penicillamine
	• Sodium cellulose phosphate (Calcibind)
	• Aredia
	• Acute pancreatitis
	• Hyperphosphatemia
	• Immobility
	• Removal or destruction of parathyroid glands

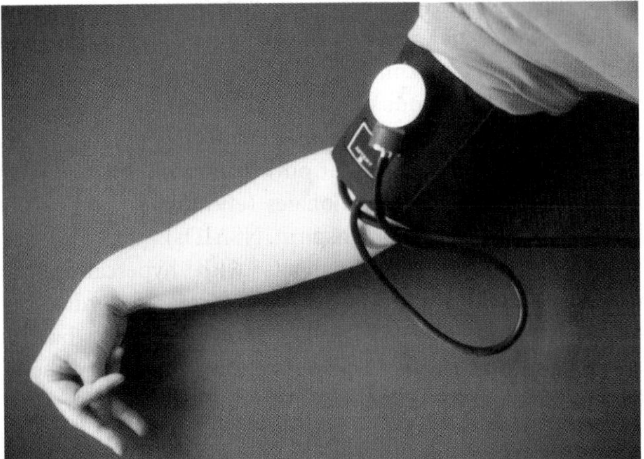

Fig. 13.13 Palmar flexion indicating a positive Trousseau sign in hypocalcemia.

Neuromuscular changes often occur first in the hands and feet. Paresthesias occur at first, with sensations of tingling and numbness. If hypocalcemia continues or worsens, muscle twitching or painful cramps and spasms occur. Tingling may also affect the lips, nose, and ears. These problems may signal the onset of neuromuscular overstimulation and tetany.

Assess for hypocalcemia by testing for Trousseau's and Chvostek's signs. To test for Trousseau's sign, place a blood pressure cuff around the arm, inflate the cuff to greater than the patient's systolic pressure, and keep the cuff inflated for 1 to 4 minutes. Under these hypoxic conditions, a positive Trousseau's sign occurs when the hand and fingers go into spasm in palmar flexion (Fig. 13.13). To test for Chvostek's sign, tap the face just below and in front of the ear to trigger facial twitching of one side of the mouth, nose, and cheek (Fig. 13.14).

Cardiovascular changes involve heart rate and ECG changes. The heart rate may be slower or slightly faster than normal, with a weak, thready pulse. Severe hypocalcemia causes severe hypotension and ECG changes of a prolonged ST interval and a prolonged QT interval.

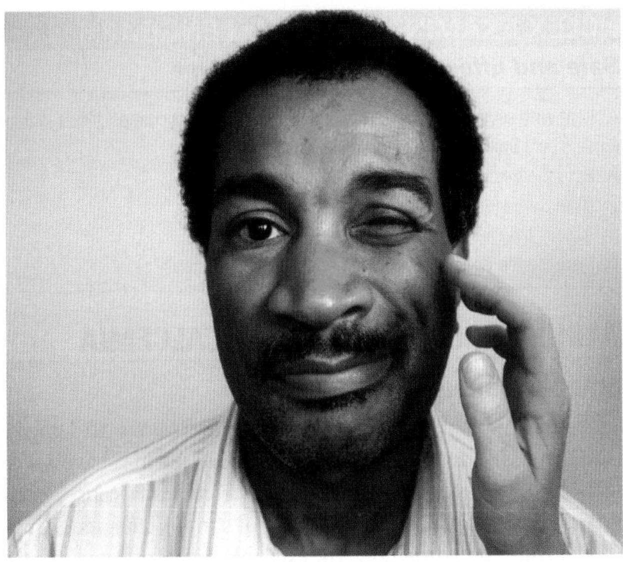

Fig. 13.14 Facial muscle response indicating a positive Chvostek sign in hypocalcemia.

Intestinal changes include increased peristaltic activity. Assess the abdomen for hyperactive bowel sounds. The patient may report painful abdominal cramping and diarrhea.

Skeletal changes are common with chronic hypocalcemia. Calcium leaves bone storage sites, causing a loss of bone density (osteoporosis). The bones are less dense, more brittle, and fragile and may break easily with slight trauma. Vertebrae become more compact and the spine may bend forward, leading to an overall loss of height. See Chapter 45 for discussion of osteoporosis.

Ask about changes in height and any unexplained bone pain. Observe for spinal curvatures and any unusual bumps or protrusions in bones that may indicate old fractures.

◆ **Interventions: Take Action.** Interventions focus on restoring normal calcium levels and preventing complications. These include drug therapy, nutrition therapy, reducing environmental stimuli, and preventing injury. Patient safety during restoration of serum calcium levels is a nursing care priority.

Drug therapy includes direct calcium replacement (oral and IV) and drugs that enhance the absorption of calcium, such as vitamin D. When neuromuscular symptoms are troublesome, drugs that decrease nerve and muscle responses may also be used.

Nutrition therapy involves a calcium rich diet for patients with mild hypocalcemia and for those who are at continuing risk for hypocalcemia. Collaborate with the registered dietitian nutritionist (RDN) to help the patient select calcium-rich foods.

Environmental management for safety is needed because the excitable membranes of the nervous system and the skeletal system are overstimulated in hypocalcemia. Reduce stimulation by keeping the room quiet, limiting visitors, adjusting the lighting, and using a soft voice.

Injury prevention strategies are needed because the patient with long-standing calcium loss may have brittle, fragile bones that fracture easily despite causing little pain. When lifting or moving a patient with fragile bones, use a lift sheet rather than pulling the patient. Observe for normal range of joint motion and for any unusual surface bumps or depressions over bony areas that may indicate bone fracture.

NCLEX EXAMINATION CHALLENGE 13.6

Safe and Effective Care Environment

A client with severe diarrhea reports tingling lips and foot cramps. What is the nurse's best first action to **prevent harm**?

A. Hold the next dose of the prescribed antidiarrheal drug
B. Assess bowel sounds in all four abdominal quadrants
C. Assess the client's response to the Chvostek test
D. Increase the IV flow rate of the normal saline infusion

CALCIUM IMBALANCE: HYPERCALCEMIA

Pathophysiology Review

Hypercalcemia is a total serum calcium level above 10.5 mg/dL or 2.62 mmol/L. Even small increases above normal have severe effects, and all systems are affected. Hypercalcemia causes excitable tissues to be less sensitive to normal stimuli, thus requiring a stronger stimulus to function. The excitable tissues affected most by hypercalcemia are the heart, skeletal muscles, nerves, and intestinal smooth muscles. Causes of hypercalcemia are listed in Table 13.9.

TABLE 13.9 Common Causes of Hypercalcemia

Actual Calcium Excesses	Relative Calcium Excesses
• Excessive oral intake of calcium	• Hyperparathyroidism
• Excessive oral intake of vitamin D	• Malignancy
• Kidney failure	• Hyperthyroidism
• Use of thiazide diuretics	• Immobility
	• Use of glucocorticoids
	• Dehydration

❖ Interprofessional Collaborative Care

◆ **Assessment: Recognize Cues.** The signs and symptoms of hypercalcemia are related to its severity and how quickly the imbalance occurred. The patient with a mild but rapidly occurring calcium excess often has more severe problems than the patient whose imbalance is severe but has developed slowly.

Cardiovascular changes are the most serious and life-threatening problems of hypercalcemia. Mild hypercalcemia at first causes increased heart rate and blood pressure. Severe or prolonged calcium imbalance depresses electrical conduction, slowing the heart rate.

Measure pulse rate and blood pressure, and observe for indications of poor ***perfusion*** such as cyanosis and pallor. Examine ECG tracings for dysrhythmias, especially a shortened QT interval.

Hypercalcemia allows blood clots to form more easily whenever blood flow is slow or impaired. Blood clotting is more likely in the lower legs, the pelvic region, areas where blood flow is blocked by internal or external constrictions, and areas where venous obstruction occurs.

Assess for slowed or impaired ***perfusion***. Measure and record calf circumferences with a soft tape measure. Assess the feet for temperature, color, and capillary refill to determine perfusion to and from the area.

Neuromuscular changes include severe muscle weakness and decreased deep tendon reflexes without paresthesia. The patient may be confused and lethargic.

Intestinal changes are first reflected as decreased peristalsis. Constipation, anorexia, nausea, vomiting, abdominal distention, and pain are common. Bowel sounds are hypoactive or absent. Assess abdominal size by measuring abdominal girth with a soft tape measure in a line circling the abdomen at the umbilicus.

◆ **Interventions: Take Action.** Interventions for hypercalcemia focus on reducing serum calcium levels through drug therapy; rehydration; and, depending on the cause and severity, dialysis. Cardiac monitoring is also important.

Drug therapy involves preventing increases in calcium and drugs to lower calcium levels. IV solutions containing calcium (e.g., Ringer's lactate) are stopped. Oral drugs containing calcium or vitamin D (e.g., calcium-based antacids) are discontinued.

Fluid volume replacement can help restore normal serum calcium levels. IV normal saline (0.9% sodium chloride) is usually given because sodium increases kidney excretion of calcium.

Thiazide diuretics are discontinued and replaced with diuretics that enhance the excretion of calcium, such as furosemide. Calcium chelators (calcium binders) help lower serum calcium levels. Such drugs include plicamycin and penicillamine.

Drugs to prevent hypercalcemia include agents that inhibit calcium resorption (movement out) from bone such as phosphorus, calcitonin, bisphosphonates (etidronate), and prostaglandin synthesis inhibitors (aspirin, NSAIDs).

Cardiac monitoring of patients with hypercalcemia is needed to identify dysrhythmias and decreased cardiac output. Compare recent ECG tracings with the patient's baseline tracings. Especially look for changes in the T waves and the QT interval and changes in rate and rhythm.

MAGNESIUM IMBALANCE: HYPOMAGNESEMIA

Pathophysiology Review

Hypomagnesemia is a serum magnesium (Mg^{2+}) level below 1.8 mEq/L or 0.74 mmol/L. It is most often caused by decreased absorption of dietary magnesium or increased kidney magnesium excretion. Two major causes of hypomagnesemia are inadequate intake and the use of loop or thiazide diuretics. Table 13.10 lists additional causes of hypomagnesemia.

The effects of hypomagnesemia are caused by increased membrane excitability and the accompanying serum calcium and potassium imbalances. Excitable membranes, especially nerve cell membranes, may depolarize spontaneously.

Cardiovascular changes associated with hypomagnesemia are serious. Low magnesium levels increase the risk for hypertension, atherosclerosis, hypertrophic left ventricle, and a variety of dysrhythmias (McCance et al., 2019). The dysrhythmias include premature contractions, atrial fibrillation, ventricular fibrillation, and long QT intervals. One aspect of the conduction problems is that, when serum magnesium levels are low, intracellular potassium levels are also low. These changes alter the resting membrane potential in cardiac muscle cells, shortening the ST segment, prolonging the PR and QRS intervals, and triggering ectopic beats. Low magnesium levels also are associated with greater cardiac muscle cell damage after myocardial infarction.

TABLE 13.10 Common Causes of Magnesium Imbalance

Hypomagnesemia	Hypermagnesemia
• Malnutrition • Starvation • Diarrhea • Steatorrhea • Celiac disease • Crohn's disease • Drugs (diuretics, aminoglycoside antibiotics, cisplatin, amphotericin B, cyclosporine) • Citrate (blood products) • Ethanol ingestion	• Increased magnesium intake: • Magnesium-containing antacids and laxatives • IV magnesium replacement • Decreased kidney excretion of magnesium resulting from kidney disease

Neuromuscular changes are caused by increased nerve impulse transmission. Normally magnesium inhibits nerve impulse transmission at synapse areas. Decreased levels increase impulse transmission from nerve to nerve or from nerve to skeletal muscle. The patient has hyperactive deep tendon reflexes, numbness and tingling, and painful muscle contractions. Positive Chvostek and Trousseau signs may be present because hypomagnesemia may occur with hypocalcemia (see the earlier discussion of these assessment signs of neuromuscular changes in the Hypocalcemia section). The patient may have tetany and seizures as hypomagnesemia worsens.

Intestinal changes are from decreased intestinal smooth muscle contraction. Reduced motility, anorexia, nausea, constipation, and abdominal distention are common. A paralytic ileus may occur when hypomagnesemia is severe.

Interprofessional Collaborative Care

Interventions for hypomagnesemia aim to correct the imbalance and manage the specific problem that caused it. In addition, because hypocalcemia often occurs with hypomagnesemia, interventions also aim to restore normal serum calcium levels.

Drugs that promote magnesium loss such as high-ceiling (loop) diuretics, osmotic diuretics, aminoglycoside antibiotics, and drugs containing phosphorus are discontinued. Magnesium is replaced intravenously with magnesium sulfate ($MgSO_4$) when hypomagnesemia is severe. Assess deep tendon reflexes at least hourly in the patient receiving IV magnesium to monitor effectiveness and prevent hypermagnesemia. If hypocalcemia is also present, drug therapy to increase serum calcium levels is prescribed.

MAGNESIUM IMBALANCE: HYPERMAGNESEMIA

Hypermagnesemia is a serum magnesium level above 2.6 mEq/L or 1.07 mmol/L. Table 13.10 lists the specific causes of hypermagnesemia.

Magnesium is a membrane stabilizer. Most symptoms of hypermagnesemia occur as a result of reduced membrane excitability. They usually are not apparent until serum magnesium levels exceed 4 mEq/L (1.6 mmol/L).

Cardiac changes include bradycardia, peripheral vasodilation, and hypotension. These problems become more severe as serum magnesium levels increase. ECG changes show a prolonged PR interval with a widened QRS complex. Bradycardia can be severe, and cardiac arrest is possible. Hypotension is also severe, with a diastolic pressure lower than normal. *Patients with severe hypermagnesemia are in grave danger of cardiac arrest.*

Central nervous system changes result from depressed nerve impulse transmission. Patients may be drowsy or lethargic. Coma may occur if the imbalance is prolonged or severe.

Neuromuscular changes include reduced or absent deep tendon reflexes. Voluntary skeletal muscle contractions become progressively weaker and finally stop.

Hypermagnesemia has no direct effect on the lungs; however, when the respiratory muscles are weak, respiratory insufficiency can lead to respiratory failure and death.

Interventions for hypermagnesemia focus on reducing the serum level and correcting the underlying problem that caused the imbalance. All oral and parenteral magnesium is discontinued. When kidney failure is not present, giving magnesium-free IV fluids can reduce serum magnesium levels. High-ceiling (loop) diuretics such as furosemide can further reduce serum magnesium levels. When cardiac problems are severe, giving calcium may reverse the cardiac effects of hypermagnesemia.

GET READY FOR THE NEXT-GENERATION NCLEX® EXAMINATION!

Key Points

Review these Key Points for each NCLEX Examination Client Needs Category.

Safe and Effective Care Environment

- Use a pump or controller to deliver IV fluids to patients with fluid overload. **QSEN: Safety**
- Do not give IV potassium at a rate greater than 20 mEq/hr (mmol/hr). **QSEN: Safety**
- Never give potassium supplements by the IM, subcutaneous, or IV push routes. **QSEN: Safety**
- Use a pump or controller when giving IV potassium-containing solutions. **QSEN: Safety**
- Assess the IV site hourly of an adult receiving IV solutions containing potassium, and document its condition. **QSEN: Safety**
- Use a lift sheet to move or reposition a patient with chronic hypocalcemia. **QSEN: Safety**

Health Promotion and Maintenance

- Teach all adults to increase fluid intake when exercising, when in hot or dry environments, or during conditions that increase metabolism (e.g., fever). **QSEN: Patient-Centered Care**
- Ensure access to adequate fluids for patients who cannot talk or who have limited mobility. **QSEN: Patient-Centered Care**
- Instruct caregivers of older adults who have cognitive impairments or mobility problems to schedule offerings of fluids at regular intervals throughout the day. **QSEN: Evidence-Based Practice**
- Teach patients how to determine electrolyte content of processed foods by reading labels. **QSEN: Patient-Centered Care**

Psychosocial Integrity

- Assess patients who have a sudden change in cognition for a change in ***fluid and electrolyte balance***. **QSEN: Patient-Centered Care**

Physiological Integrity

- Assess skin turgor on the forehead or the sternum of older patients. **QSEN: Evidence-Based Practice**
- Use daily weights to determine fluid gains or losses. **QSEN: Evidence-Based Practice**
- Ask patients about the use of drugs such as diuretics, laxatives, salt substitutes, and antihypertensives that may alter ***fluid and electrolyte balance***. **QSEN: Patient-Centered Care**
- Monitor the cardiac and pulmonary status at least every hour when patients with dehydration are receiving IV fluid replacement therapy. **QSEN: Patient-Centered Care**
- Collaborate with the registered dietitian-nutritionist (RDN) to teach patients about diets that are restricted in potassium, sodium, or calcium. **QSEN: Teamwork and Collaboration**
- Immediately stop the infusion of potassium-containing solutions if infiltration is suspected. **QSEN: Evidence-Based Practice**
- Assess all patients with hyperkalemia for cardiac dysrhythmias and ECG abnormalities, especially tall T waves, conduction delays, and heart block. **QSEN: Evidence-Based Practice**
- Assess the respiratory status of all patients with hypokalemia. **QSEN: Evidence-Based Practice**
- Assess the bowel sounds; heart rate, rhythm and quality; and muscle strength to evaluate the patient's responses to therapy for an electrolyte imbalance. **QSEN: Evidence-Based Practice**

MASTERY QUESTIONS

1. Which electrolytes are most detrimentally affected by low magnesium levels? Select all that apply.
   A. Calcium
   B. Chloride
   C. Hydrogen
   D. Potassium
   E. Sodium
   F. Sulfate
2. Which condition or manifestation in the client with a serum sodium level of 149 mEq/L indicates to the nurse that this electrolyte imbalance may be caused by excessive fluid loss?
   A. The client has calf muscle cramping.
   B. The serum chloride level is low.
   C. The urine specific gravity is high.
   D. The hematocrit is 52%.
3. A client is receiving an intravenous infusion of 100 mEq (mmol) of potassium chloride in 1000 mL of normal saline. How many mEq (mmol) of potassium per hour does the nurse calculate the client will receive if the IV is infused at a rate of 150 mL/hour?
   A. 12 mEq (mmol)
   B. 15 mEq (mmol)
   C. 18 mEq (mmol)
   D. 20 mEq (mmol)
4. Which assessment data is most **relevant** for the nurse to obtain from a client who has a serum potassium level of 2.9 mEq/L?
   A. Asking about the use of sugar substitutes
   B. Determining what drugs are taken daily
   C. Measuring the client's response to Chvostek testing
   D. Asking about a history of kidney disease

REFERENCES

Asterisk(*) indicates a classic or definitive work on this subject.

*Adis Medical Writers. (2015). Minimize drug-induced hyperkalemia by increasing awareness and using preventative strategies. *Drugs & Therapy Perspectives*, *31*(1), 28–33.

Bailey, B., Davis, S., & Witherspoon, B. (2017). Assessment of volume status using ultrasonography. *Nursing Clinics of North America*, *52*(2), 269–279.

Bertschi, L. (2020). Concentration and volume: Understanding sodium and water in the body. *American Journal of Nursing*, *120*(1), 51-56.

Ellison, D., & Farrar, F. (2018). Kidney influence on fluid and electrolyte balance. *Nursing Clinics of North America*, *53*, 469–480.

Goad, N., & Levesque, M. (2020). Role of desmopressin in the critical care setting. *AACN Advanced Critical Care*, *31*(1), 5-11.

Gross, W., Samarin, M., & Kimmons, L. (2017). Choice of fluids for resuscitation of the critically ill: What nurses need to know. *Critical Care Nursing Quarterly*, *40*(4), 309–322.

Hutto, C., & French, M. (2017). Neurologic intensive care unit electrolyte management. *Nursing Clinics of North America*, *52*(2), 321–329.

Jones, G. M., Bode, L., Riha, H., & Erdman, M. (2017). Safety of continuous peripheral infusion of 3% sodium chloride solution in neurocritical care patients. *American Journal of Critical Care*, *26*(1), 37–42.

McCance, K., Huether, S., Brashers, V., & Rote, N. (2019). *Pathophysiology: The biologic basis for disease in adults and children* (8th ed.). St. Louis: Mosby.

Namasivayan-MacDonald, A., Slaughter, S., Steele, C., Carrier, N., Langyel, C., & Keller, H. (2017). Inadequate fluid intake in long term care residence: Prevalence and determinants. *Geriatric Nursing*, *39*(3), 330–335.

Pagana, K., & Pagana, T. (2018). *Mosby's manual of diagnostic and laboratory tests* (6th ed.). St. Louis: Mosby.

Pierce, J., Shen, Q., & Thimmesch, A. (2016). The ongoing controversy: Crystalloids versus colloids. *Journal of Infusion Nursing*, *39*(1), 40–44.

Reynolds, G. (2016). Recognizing acute hyponatremia. *American Nurse Today*, *10*(7), 26.

Sheills, R., & Morrell-Scott (2018). Prevention of dehydration in hospital patients. *British Journal of Nursing*, *27*(10), 565–569.

Thomas, S. (2017). Acute hypervolemic hypernatremia: A case report. *Nursing*, *47*(10), 53–57.

Touhy, T., & Jett, K. (2020). *Ebersole and Hess' toward health aging* (10th ed.). St. Louis: Mosby.

14

Concepts of Acid-Base Balance

M. Linda Workman

http://evolve.elsevier.com/Iggy/

LEARNING OUTCOMES

1. Collaborate with the interprofessional team to perform a complete assessment of ***acid-base balance***.
2. Explain how physiologic aging changes the effectiveness of mechanisms to maintain ***acid-base balance*** and increases the risk for imbalance.
3. Apply knowledge of anatomy, physiology, and pathophysiology to perform an evidence-based assessment for the patient with a disturbance of ***acid-base balance***.
4. Interpret assessment findings for the patient with a disturbance of ***acid-base balance***.

KEY TERMS

acid-base balance The maintenance of arterial blood pH between 7.35 and 7.45 through control of hydrogen ion production and elimination.

acidosis Arterial blood pH level below 7.35.

acids Substances that release hydrogen ions when dissolved in water (H_2O) or body fluids, increasing the amount of free hydrogen ions in that solution.

alkalosis Arterial blood pH level above 7.45.

bases Substances that bind free hydrogen ions in solution and lower the amount of free hydrogen ions in solution.

buffers Substances that when dissolved in fluid can react as either an acid (releasing a hydrogen ion) or a base (binding a hydrogen ion) depending on the pH of that fluid.

hyperventilation Rate and depth of breathing increased above normal.

hypoventilation Rate and depth of breathing decreased below normal.

Kussmaul respiration A pattern of breathing associated with acidosis in which breaths are deep and rapid.

PRIORITY AND INTERRELATED CONCEPTS

The priority concept for this chapter is:

- ***Acid-Base Balance***

The ***Acid-Base Balance*** concept exemplar for this chapter is Acidosis.

Acid-base balance is the maintenance of arterial blood pH between 7.35 and 7.45 through regulation of hydrogen ion (H^+) production and elimination. Arterial pH is a measure of the free hydrogen ion level in the blood and other body fluids. Maintaining the pH within the normal range is part of homeostasis and is critical for optimal body function. Free hydrogen ions are the most tightly controlled substances in the human body and have the narrowest range of normal. This rigid regulation is needed because free hydrogen ions are constantly formed as a result of normal metabolism. Even small increases in the free hydrogen ion level (lower pH) of body fluids can reduce body function and lead to death.

The normal blood level of free hydrogen ions is quite low (less than 0.0001 mEq/L [mmol/L]), and its concentration is calculated in negative logarithm units. This calculation makes the value of pH *inversely* related (negatively related) to the concentration of free hydrogen ions. Thus the *lower* the pH value of a fluid, the *higher* the level of free hydrogen ions in that fluid. A pH of 1 is as acidic as possible, and a pH of 14 is as alkaline as possible. A pH of 7.0 is neutral. *A change of 1 pH unit actually represents a 10-fold change in free hydrogen ion level* (McCance et al., 2019). Thus any pH unit increase (e.g., a change from 7.4 to 7.3) represents a huge increase in the free hydrogen ion level.

When ***acid-base balance*** is disrupted, the following actions can result:

- Reduced function of hormones, enzymes, and many drugs
- Fluid and electrolyte imbalances
- Changed excitable membrane activity, making the heart, nerves, muscles, and GI tract either less or more active than normal

NCLEX EXAMINATION CHALLENGE 14.1

Physiological Integrity

Which normal physiologic process contributes most to the need for ***acid-base balance?***

A. Continuous organ production of bicarbonate from carbonic acid
B. Continuous alveolar exchange of oxygen and carbon dioxide
C. Continuous metabolic production of free hydrogen ions
D. Continuous kidney formation of urine from blood

MAINTAINING ACID-BASE BALANCE

Arterial blood normally has a slightly alkaline pH between 7.35 and 7.45 even though it contains acids and bases. With ***acid-base balance*** the pH remains at this near-neutral value when the rate of continuous free hydrogen ion production is matched with its loss.

ACID-BASE CHEMISTRY

Acids

Acids are substances that release hydrogen ions when dissolved in water (H_2O) or body fluids, *increasing* the amount of free hydrogen ions in that solution. The strength of an acid is measured by how easily it releases a hydrogen ion in solution. A strong acid such as hydrochloric acid (HCl) separates completely in water and releases *all* of its hydrogen ions, as shown in Fig. 14.1.

$$HCl + H_2O \leftrightarrow H^+ + Cl^- + H_2O$$

Hydrochloric acid | Water | Hydrogen ion | Chloride ion | Water

Fig. 14.1 Release of hydrogen ions by a strong acid (hydrochloric acid) in which the strong acid completely dissociates in water.

On the other hand, a weak acid usually has more free hydrogen ions per molecule but releases only *some,* not all, of its hydrogen ions. For example, each molecule of acetic acid (CH_3COOH), a weak acid, contains a total of four hydrogen molecules. When acetic acid combines with water, it releases only *one* of its four hydrogen molecules, keeping the other three hydrogen molecules bound to the molecule (CH_3COO^-).

Bases

Bases bind free hydrogen ions in solution and *lower* the amount of free hydrogen ions in solution. The most common base in human physiology is bicarbonate (HCO_3^-). Although it is a weak base, the many bicarbonate ions in the body are critical in preventing major changes in body fluid pH without harming body tissues.

Buffers

Buffers are substances that, when dissolved in fluid, can react as either an acid (releasing a hydrogen ion) or a base (binding a free hydrogen ion) depending on the pH of that fluid. Buffers always try to keep body fluid pH as close as possible to the pH of 7.35 to 7.45. If a body fluid is basic (with few free hydrogen ions), the buffer *releases hydrogen ions* into the fluid (Fig. 14.2). If a body fluid is acidic (with many free hydrogen ions), the buffer *binds some of the excess hydrogen ions.* In this way buffers act like hydrogen ion "sponges," soaking up hydrogen ions when too many are present and squeezing out hydrogen ions when too few are present. This flexibility allows buffers to help keep body fluid pH in the normal range.

Arterial blood with a pH of 7.35 to 7.45 is considered balanced for free hydrogen ion level with the concentration of acids and bases being nearly equal. Fig. 14.3 shows the concept of normal pH in which the concentrations of all acids are equal to the concentrations of all bases within a given solution. With physiologic ***acid-base balance***, the concentrations of acids and bases are nearly equal and remain so because normal hydrogen ion production is balanced with hydrogen ion loss so that the overall free hydrogen ion levels remain constant.

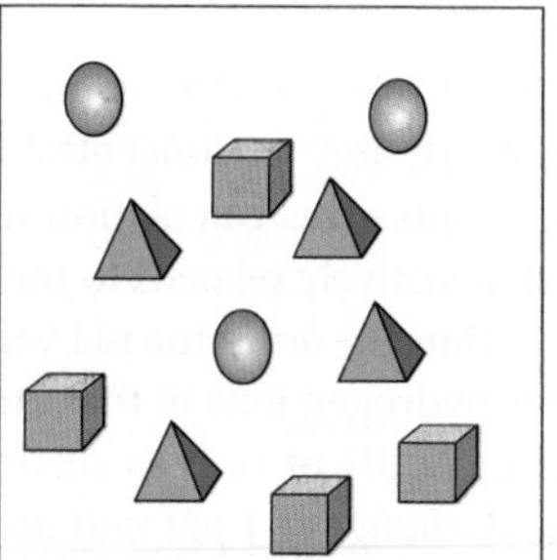

Fluid pH 7.38 (normal). The number and strength of acid components are equal to the number and strength of base components. Hydrogen ion concentration is limited and constant.

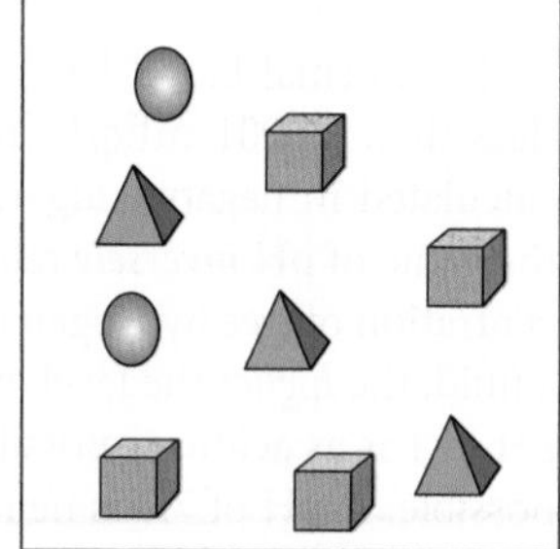

Fluid pH 7.51 (alkaline). The number and strength of base components are greater than the number and strength of acid components. Hydrogen ion concentration is below normal.

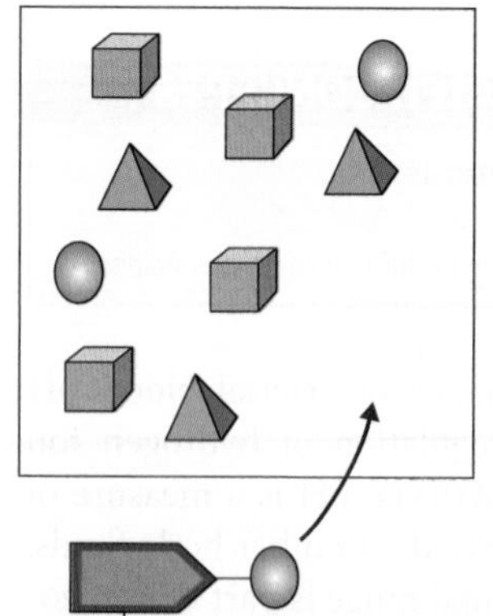

Buffer is added to the alkaline fluid.

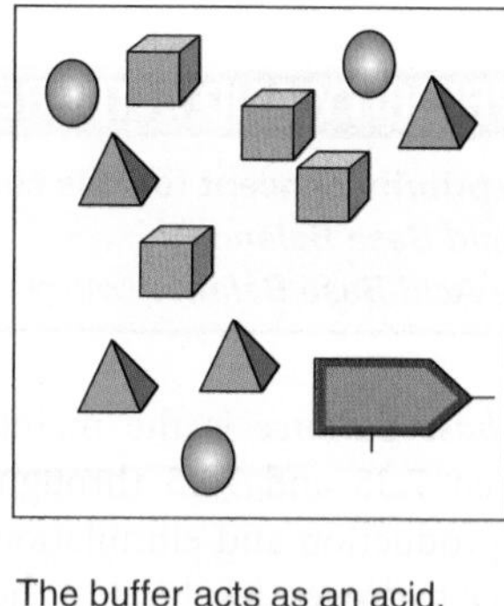

The buffer acts as an acid, releasing a hydrogen ion.

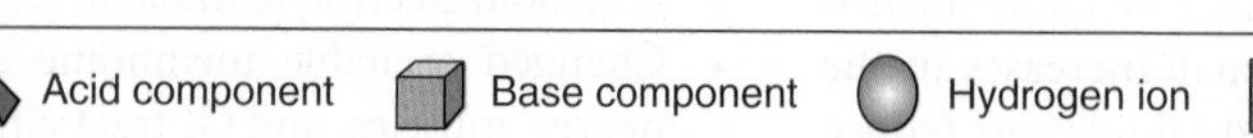

Fig. 14.2 Action of buffer in solution. (© 1992 by M. Linda Workman. All rights reserved.)

Body fluids with a pH less than 7.35 have a higher concentration of acids compared with bases. These fluids are *acidic* (see Fig. 14.3), with more free hydrogen ions released than bound, increasing the amount of free hydrogen ions in the fluid.

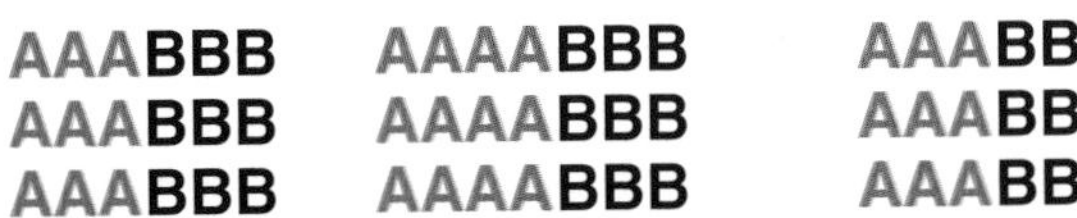
AAABBB AAAABBB AAABB
AAABBB AAAABBB AAABB
AAABBB AAAABBB AAABB
Neutral or acid-base balance
Acidic (acid excess) (actual acidosis)
Acidic (base deficit) (relative acidosis)

Fig. 14.3 Concept of acidic versus normal pH. (A = acid; B = base.)

Body fluids with a pH higher than 7.45 have a higher concentration of bases compared with acids. These fluids are *basic,* in which more hydrogen ions are being bound than released, decreasing the amount of free hydrogen ions (Fig. 14.4).

AAABBB	AAABBBB	AABBB
AAABBB	AAABBBB	AABBB
AAABBB	AAABBBB	AABBB
Neutral	Alkaline (base excess)	Alkaline (acid deficit)

Fig. 14.4 Concepts of alkaline versus normal pH and relative versus actual alkalosis. (A = acid; B = base.)

BODY FLUID CHEMISTRY

Bicarbonate Ions

Body fluids contain different types of acids and bases. The most common base in human body fluid is bicarbonate (HCO_3^-); the most common acid is carbonic acid (H_2CO_3). In health the body keeps these substances at a constant ratio of 1 molecule of carbonic acid to 20 free bicarbonate ions (1:20) (Fig. 14.5). To maintain this ratio, both carbonic acid and bicarbonate must be carefully controlled. This constant ratio is related to balancing the production and elimination of carbon dioxide (CO_2) and hydrogen ions (H^+).

Relationship Between Carbon Dioxide and Hydrogen Ions

A key process in understanding ***acid-base balance*** is the carbonic anhydrase equation. This equation, driven by the enzyme carbonic anhydrase, shows how free hydrogen ion levels and carbon dioxide levels are *directly* related to one another, so an increase in one causes an equal increase in the other (Fig. 14.6).

$$CO_2 + H_2O \leftrightarrow H_2CO_3 \leftrightarrow HCO_3^- + H^+$$

Fig. 14.6 The carbonic anhydrase equation showing that the concentration of carbon dioxide is directly related to the concentration of hydrogen ions.

Carbon dioxide (CO_2) is a gas that forms carbonic acid when combined with water, making carbon dioxide a part of carbonic acid. Carbonic acid is not stable, and the body needs to keep a

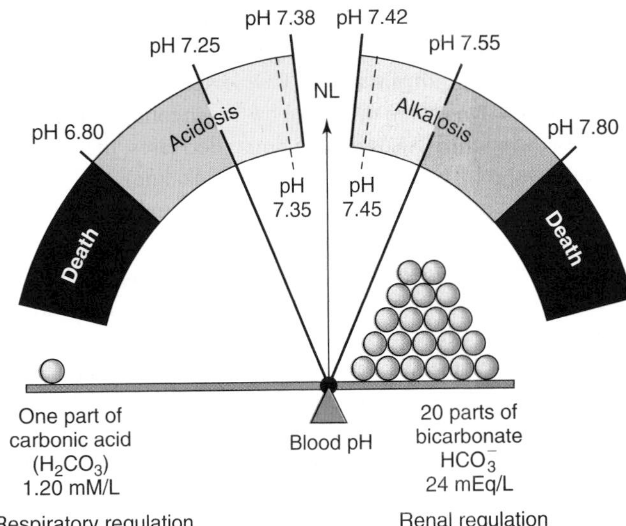

Fig. 14.5 Normal ratio of carbonic acid to bicarbonate is 1:20. (From McCance, K., Huether, S., Brashers, V., & Rote, N. [2019]. *Pathophysiology: The biologic basis for disease in adults and children* [8th ed.]. St. Louis: Mosby.)

1:20 ratio of carbonic acid to bicarbonate. When carbonic acid is formed from water and carbon dioxide, it begins to separate into free hydrogen ions and bicarbonate ions. *Therefore the carbon dioxide content of a fluid is directly related to the amount of free hydrogen ions in that fluid. Whenever conditions cause carbon dioxide to increase, more free hydrogen ions are created. Likewise, whenever free hydrogen ion production increases, more carbon dioxide is produced.*

When excess carbon dioxide is produced, the equation shifts to the *right,* causing an *increase* in hydrogen ions (and a *decrease* in pH), as shown in Fig. 14.7. When very little carbon dioxide is produced, no free hydrogen ions are created by this equation.

$$CO_2 + H_2O \rightarrow H_2CO_3 \rightarrow HCO_3^- + H^+$$

Fig. 14.7 Increased carbon dioxide levels force the equation to the right and increase the concentration of hydrogen ions proportionately.

When excess hydrogen ions are present, the carbonic anhydrase equation shifts to the *left,* causing the creation of more carbon dioxide, as shown in Fig. 14.8. When the amount of free hydrogen ions in body fluids is low, no extra carbon dioxide is produced.

$$CO_2 + H_2O \leftarrow H_2CO_3 \leftarrow HCO_3^- + H^+$$

Fig. 14.8 Increased hydrogen ion levels force the equation to the left and increase the concentration of carbon dioxide levels proportionately.

How is the relationship between free hydrogen ions and carbon dioxide helpful? Carbon dioxide is a gas that can be eliminated during exhalation, and this action is important for ***acid-base balance.*** When any condition causes the blood free hydrogen ion concentration to increase, extra CO_2 is produced in the same proportion. This extra CO_2 is eliminated during exhalation, helping to bring the hydrogen ion concentration down to normal. Whenever the CO_2 level changes, the pH changes to the same degree, in the opposite direction. Thus when the CO_2 level of a liquid increases, the pH drops, indicating more free hydrogen ions (more acidic). Likewise, when the CO_2 level of a liquid decreases, the pH rises, indicating fewer free hydrogen ions (more alkaline).

An increase in bicarbonate causes the amount of free hydrogen ions to decrease and the pH to increase, becoming more alkaline *(basic)*. Likewise, a decrease in bicarbonate causes the free hydrogen ion level to increase and the pH to decrease, becoming more *acidic*.

Because the kidneys control bicarbonate levels and the lungs control CO_2 levels, ***acid-base balance*** and pH are also the result of how well the kidneys are functioning to retain or eliminate bicarbonate divided by how well the lungs are functioning to eliminate carbon dioxide (Fig. 14.9). A problem in either organ system can lead to an acid-base imbalance, most often acidosis.

$$\text{pH} = \frac{\overset{\text{(Slow but powerful response)}}{\textbf{Kidney function = Bicarbonate levels}}}{\underset{\text{(Rapid but limited response)}}{\textbf{Lung function = Carbon dioxide levels}}}$$

Fig. 14.9 Contribution of pH balance by kidney and lung function.

Sources of Acids and Bicarbonate

When acids are present in body fluids, free hydrogen ions are released and must be controlled for ***acid-base balance***. Acids and hydrogen ions are produced continuously through normal body physiologic work and metabolism.

Normal metabolism of carbohydrate, protein, and fat creates natural waste products. Carbohydrate metabolism forms carbon dioxide (CO_2), which is exhaled by the lungs during breathing. One factor that determines blood pH is how much CO_2 is produced by body cells during metabolism versus how rapidly that CO_2 is removed by breathing. Protein breakdown forms sulfuric acid. Fat breakdown forms fatty acids and ketoacids.

Lactic acid production occurs when cells metabolize under *anaerobic* (no oxygen) conditions, such as hypoxia, sepsis, and shock. Excessive fat breakdown forms ketoacids.

Cell destruction allows cell contents to be released, including the structures that contain acids. These released acids in the extracellular fluid (ECF) increase free hydrogen ion levels.

Bicarbonate is produced from carbonic acid primarily in the pancreas, kidneys, and inside red blood cells. It also can be reabsorbed from urine in the kidney and returned to the blood. Unlike free hydrogen ion production, no natural pathologic conditions lead to excessive production of bicarbonate.

ACID-BASE REGULATORY ACTIONS AND MECHANISMS

As long as body cells are healthy, they continuously produce acids, carbon dioxide, and free hydrogen ions. Despite this production, hydrogen ion, bicarbonate, oxygen, and carbon dioxide levels are kept within normal limits when ***acid-base balance*** controlling actions are normal. This homeostasis depends on:

TABLE 14.1 Acid-Base Regulatory Mechanisms

Mechanism Type	Key Characteristics
Chemical	
Protein buffers (albumin, globulins, hemoglobin) Chemical buffers (bicarbonate, phosphate)	Very rapid response Provide immediate response to changing conditions Can handle relatively small fluctuations in hydrogen ion production during normal metabolic and health conditions
Respiratory	
Increased hydrogen ions or increased carbon dioxide: Triggers the brain to increase the rate and depth of breathing, causing more carbon dioxide to be lost and decreasing the hydrogen ion concentration Decreased hydrogen ions or decreased carbon dioxide: Inhibits brain stimulation, leading to decreased rate and depth of breathing, causing carbon dioxide to be retained and increasing the hydrogen ion concentration	Primarily assist buffering systems when the fluctuation of hydrogen ion concentration is acute Response occurs quickly, within seconds to minutes
Kidney	
Actions to decrease pH: Increased kidney excretion of bicarbonate Increased kidney reabsorption of hydrogen ions Actions to increase pH: Decreased kidney excretion of bicarbonate Decreased kidney reabsorption of hydrogen ions	The most powerful regulator of acid-base balance Respond to large or chronic fluctuations in hydrogen ion production or elimination Slowest response (hours to days) Longest duration

- Hydrogen ion production being consistent and not excessive
- CO_2 loss from the body through breathing, keeping pace with all forms of hydrogen ion production

To keep the free hydrogen ion level (pH) of the ECF within the narrow normal range, the body has chemical, respiratory, and kidney actions (mechanisms) for acid-base balance (Table 14.1). The laboratory profile lists the normal values for arterial blood gases (ABGs) and other substances important for assessing acid-base balance.

Chemical Acid-Base Control Actions

Buffers are the first line of defense against changes in free hydrogen ion levels. These buffers are always present in body fluids and act fast to reduce or raise the amount of free hydrogen ions to normal. By acting as hydrogen ion "sponges," buffers can bind free hydrogen ions when too many are present or release them when not enough are present. Bicarbonate, a weak base, is the main buffer of the ECF. It comes from the GI absorption

LABORATORY PROFILE

Acid-Base Assessment: Normal Ranges/ Significance of Changes

Test	Normal Range	Significance of Changes From Normal
pH	7.35-7.45	*Increased:* Metabolic alkalosis, loss of gastric fluids, decreased potassium intake, diuretic therapy, fever, salicylate toxicity, respiratory alkalosis, hyperventilation *Decreased:* Metabolic or respiratory acidosis, ketosis, renal failure, starvation, diarrhea, hyperthyroidism
Pao_2	80-100 mm Hg	*Increased:* Increased ventilation, oxygen therapy *Decreased:* Respiratory depression, high altitude, carbon monoxide poisoning, decreased cardiac output
$Paco_2$	35-45 mm Hg	*Increased:* Respiratory acidosis, emphysema, pneumonia, cardiac failure, respiratory depression *Decreased:* Respiratory alkalosis, hyperventilation, diarrhea
Bicarbonate	21-28 mEq/L (21-28 mmol/L)	*Increased:* Metabolic alkalosis, bicarbonate therapy, metabolic compensation for chronic respiratory acidosis *Decreased:* Metabolic acidosis, diarrhea, pancreatitis
Lactate	Arterial 3-7 mg/dL (0.3-0.8 mmol/L) Venous 5-20 mg/dL (0.6-2.2 mmol/L)	*Increased:* Hypoxia, exercise, insulin infusion, alcoholism, pregnancy, dehydration sepsis *Decreased:* Fluid overload

$Paco_2$, Partial pressure of arterial carbon dioxide; *Pao_2*, partial pressure of arterial oxygen.
Data from Pagana, K., & Pagana, T. (2018). *Mosby's manual of diagnostic and laboratory tests* (6th ed.). St. Louis: Elsevier.

of ingested bicarbonate, pancreatic production of bicarbonate, movement of cellular bicarbonate into the ECF, kidney reabsorption of filtered bicarbonate, and the breakdown of carbonic acid.

Other common buffers are phosphate (which is active in the ICF) and proteins. Blood protein buffers are albumin and globulins. A major intracellular protein buffer is hemoglobin (McCance et al., 2019). When the amount of free hydrogen ions in the blood increases, some of the excess hydrogen ions cross the membranes of red blood cells and bind to the large numbers of hemoglobin molecules in each red blood cell. Binding of free hydrogen ions to hemoglobin results in fewer hydrogen ions remaining in the blood, bringing blood pH back up toward normal.

Respiratory Acid-Base Control Actions

When chemical buffers alone cannot prevent changes in blood pH, the respiratory system is the second line of defense against changes. Breathing controls the amount of free hydrogen ions by controlling the amount of carbon dioxide (CO_2) in arterial blood. Because CO_2 is converted into free hydrogen ions with the carbonic anhydrase reaction and vice versa, the CO_2 level is *directly* related to the hydrogen ion level. Breathing rids the body of any excess CO_2, which results in fewer free hydrogen ions.

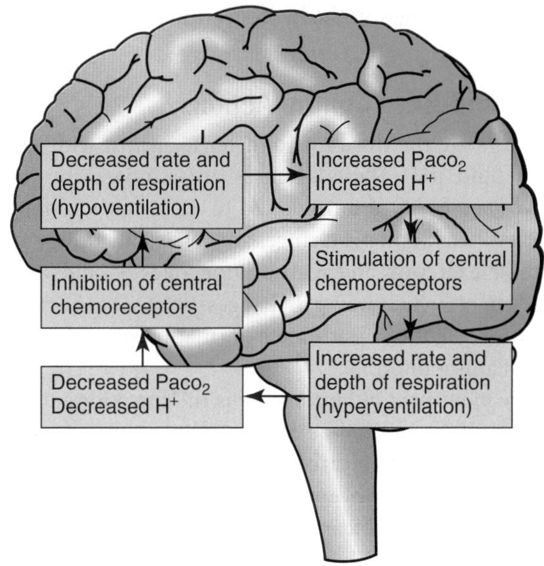

Fig. 14.10 Neural regulation of respiration and hydrogen ion concentration. (*H^+*, Hydrogen ion; *$Paco_2$*, partial pressure of arterial carbon dioxide.)

The CO_2 level in venous blood increases with metabolism. This CO_2 moves into lung capillary blood. Because the amount (pressure) of CO_2 is far higher in lung capillary blood than it is in the air in the alveoli, CO_2 diffuses freely from the blood into the alveolar air. Once in the alveoli, CO_2 is exhaled during breathing and is lost from the body. Because the amount of CO_2 in room air is nearly zero, CO_2 can continue to be exhaled even when breathing is somewhat impaired.

Respiratory regulation of ***acid-base balance*** is under the control of the central nervous system (Fig. 14.10). Special receptors in the respiratory areas of the brain are sensitive to changes in the amount of CO_2 in brain tissues. As the amount of CO_2 begins to rise above normal in brain blood and tissues, these central receptors trigger the neurons to increase the rate and depth of breathing (**hyperventilation**). As a result, more CO_2 is exhaled ("blown off") from the lungs and the CO_2 level in the ECF decreases. When the arterial CO_2 level returns back down to normal, the rate and depth of breathing return to levels that are normal for the patient.

If the amount of ECF free hydrogen ions is too low, the CO_2 level is also too low. Central receptors sense these low CO_2 levels and stop or slow the neuron activity in the respiratory centers of the brain, decreasing the rate and depth of breathing (**hypoventilation**). As a result, less CO_2 is lost through the lungs and more CO_2 is retained in arterial blood. This retention of already-formed CO_2, together with the normal production of CO_2 from metabolism, results in a rapid return of the arterial CO_2 levels (and free hydrogen ion levels) back up to normal. When these levels are normal, the rate and depth of breathing also return to normal levels.

The respiratory system's response in acid-base balance is rapid. Changes in the rate and depth of breathing occur within minutes after changes in the hydrogen ion level or CO_2 level of the ECF occur.

Kidney Acid-Base Control Actions

The kidneys are the third line of defense against wide changes in body fluid pH. These defenses are stronger for regulating ***acid-base balance*** but take 24 to 48 hours to completely respond. When blood pH changes are persistent, kidney actions to increase excretion and reabsorption rates of acids or bases (depending on which way pH changes) start. These actions are kidney movement of bicarbonate, formation of acids, and formation of ammonium.

Kidney movement of bicarbonate is the first kidney pH control action. It occurs in the kidney tubules in two ways: (1) kidney movement of bicarbonate produced elsewhere in the body, and (2) kidney movement of bicarbonate produced in the kidneys. Much of the bicarbonate made in other body areas is excreted in the urine. When blood hydrogen ion levels are high, this bicarbonate is reabsorbed from the kidneys back into circulation, where it can help buffer excess hydrogen ions. The kidney tubules can also make additional bicarbonate and reabsorb it to increase the buffer effect. When blood hydrogen ion levels are low, the bicarbonate stays in the urine and is excreted.

Formation of acids occurs through the phosphate-buffering system inside the cells of the kidney tubules. When the newly created bicarbonate made in kidney cells is reabsorbed into the blood, the urine has an excess of anions, including phosphate (HPO_4^{2-}). This negatively charged fluid draws free hydrogen ions (which have a positive charge) into the urine. Once in the urine, the hydrogen ions bind to phosphate ions, forming an acid (H_2PO_4) that is then excreted in the urine.

Formation of ammonium converts the ammonia (NH_3) normally formed during protein breakdown, into ammonium (NH_4^+) in the urine. The ammonium "traps" the hydrogen ions by binding them tightly, which then allows them to be excreted in the urine. The result is a loss of hydrogen ions and an increase in blood pH.

Compensation

In the process of *compensation,* the body adapts to attempt to correct changes in blood pH and maintain ***acid-base balance*** (Pompey & Abraham-Settles, 2019). A pH below 6.9 or above 7.8 is usually fatal. Both the kidneys and the lungs can compensate for acid-base imbalances, but they are not equal in their final responses. The respiratory system is much more sensitive to acid-base changes and can begin compensation efforts within seconds to minutes after a change in pH. However, these efforts are limited and can be overwhelmed easily. The kidney compensatory actions are much more powerful and result in rapid changes in ECF composition. However, these more powerful actions are not fully triggered unless the acid-base imbalance continues for several hours to several days.

Respiratory compensation occurs through the lungs, usually to correct for acid-base imbalances from metabolic problems. For example, when prolonged running causes buildup of lactic acid, hydrogen ion levels in the ECF increase, causing the pH to drop. To bring the pH back to normal, breathing is triggered in response to increased carbon dioxide levels. Both the rate and depth of respiration increase. These respiratory efforts cause the blood to lose carbon dioxide with each exhalation, so ECF levels of carbon dioxide and free hydrogen ions gradually decrease. When the lungs can *fully compensate,* the pH returns to normal.

Kidney compensation results when a healthy kidney works to correct for changes in blood pH that occur when the respiratory system either is overwhelmed or is not healthy. For example, in an adult with chronic obstructive pulmonary disease (COPD), the respiratory system cannot exchange gases adequately. Carbon dioxide is retained continuously, hydrogen ion levels increase, and the blood pH falls (becomes more acidic). The kidneys oppose this by excreting more hydrogen ions and increasing the movement of bicarbonate back into the blood. Then blood pH remains either within or closer to the normal range. When adaptive actions are completely effective, acid-base problems are *fully compensated* and the pH of the blood returns to normal even though the levels of oxygen and bicarbonate may be abnormal.

However, sometimes the respiratory problem causing the acid-base imbalance is so severe that kidney actions can only *partially compensate* and the pH is not quite normal. Partial compensation prevents the acid-base imbalance from becoming even more severe.

NCLEX EXAMINATION CHALLENGE 14.2

Physiological Integrity

Which set of client arterial blood gas (ABG) values indicates to the nurse that some mechanisms are working to partially compensate for an acid-base imbalance?

A. pH 7.42; Pao_2 92 mm Hg; CO_2 41 mm Hg; HCO_3^- 28 mEq/L (mmol/L)
B. pH 7.46; Pao_2 98 mm Hg; CO_2 38 mm Hg; HCO_3^- 30 mEq/L (mmol/L)
C. pH 7.22; Pao_2 60 mm Hg; CO_2 80 mm Hg; HCO_3^- 22 mEq/L (mmol/L)
D. pH 7.29; Pao_2 78 mm Hg; CO_2 82 mm Hg; HCO_3^- 36 mEq/L (mmol/L)

ACID-BASE IMBALANCES

Acid-base imbalances are problems of ***acid-base balance*** resulting from changes in the blood free hydrogen ion level or pH. These changes are caused by problems with the acid-base regulatory actions or exposure to dangerous conditions. Imbalances in which blood pH is below normal reflect **acidosis**, and imbalances in which blood pH is above normal reflect **alkalosis**. Acid-base imbalances impair the function of many organs and can be life threatening. It is important to remember that neither acidosis nor alkalosis is an actual disease or disorder. Both are conditions resulting from other acute or chronic health problems that disrupt or overwhelm the balancing mechanisms. Thus the origin of acidosis and alkalosis can be respiratory, metabolic, or both. Therefore interventions to restore acid-base balance must be focused on correcting the health problem causing the imbalance. *Health problems are more likely to cause acidosis rather than alkalosis because there are no specific disorders that cause the overproduction of bicarbonate, whereas many conditions can lead to excess free hydrogen ion production or retention.*

ACID-BASE BALANCE CONCEPT EXEMPLAR: ACIDOSIS

Pathophysiology Review

In acidosis the acid-base balance of arterial is upset by an excess of free hydrogen ions (H^+). This is seen as an arterial blood pH below 7.35. The amount of acids present is greater than normal compared with the amount of bases.

Acidosis is not a disease; it is a condition caused by a disorder or pathologic process. It can be caused by metabolic problems, respiratory problems, or both. Patients at greatest risk for acute acidosis are those with problems that impair breathing. Older adults with chronic health problems are at greater risk for developing acidosis (McCance et al., 2019). The Patient-Centered Care: Older Adult Considerations box lists areas to specifically assess in the older adult to determine risk for an acid-base imbalance.

PATIENT-CENTERED CARE: OLDER ADULT CONSIDERATIONS QSEN

Acid-Base Balance

When Obtaining a Patient's History

- Assess risk factors for acid-base imbalance, including drugs, chronic health problems (especially kidney disease, pulmonary disease), and acute health problems.
- Ask the patient to list all prescribed and over-the-counter drugs and herbal supplements (especially diuretics and antacids). If the patient is unable to provide this information, ask the family to bring the drugs in from home.
- Ask the patient to recall which liquids were taken in the past 24 hours and whether urination amounts have changed.

Assessment Points

- Compare the patient's mental status with what the family, significant other, or health record states is the patient's baseline.
- Check the rate and depth of respiration.
- Determine whether the patient can complete a sentence without stopping for breath.
- Examine the color of nail beds and mucous membranes.
- Examine skin turgor for dehydration. Attempt to pinch the skin to form a tent over the sternum and on the forehead. If a tent forms, record how long it remains.
- Measure the rate and quality of the pulse.
- Monitor clinical responses and laboratory values while the acid-base imbalance is being corrected.

Modified from Touhy, T., & Jett, K. (2020). *Ebersole & Hess' toward healthy aging* (10th ed). St. Louis: Elsevier.

Acidosis can result from an actual or relative increase in the amount or strength of acids. An *actual acid excess* results in acidosis by either overproducing acids (and release of free hydrogen ions) or undereliminating normally produced acids (retention of free hydrogen ions). Either way, more free hydrogen ions are present than should be. Problems that increase acid production include diabetic ketoacidosis and seizures. Problems that decrease acid elimination include respiratory impairment and kidney impairment.

In *relative* acidosis, the amount of acids does not increase. Instead, the amount or strength of the bases decreases (to create a *base deficit*), which makes the fluid relatively more acidic than basic. A relative acidosis *(base deficit)* is caused by either over eliminating or underproducing bicarbonate ions (HCO_3^-) (see Fig. 14.3). Problems that underproduce bases include pancreatitis and dehydration. A condition that overeliminates bases is diarrhea.

Regardless of its cause, acidosis causes major changes in body function. The main problems occur because free hydrogen ions are positively charged ions. An increase in hydrogen ions creates imbalances of other positively charged electrolytes, especially potassium. The changes in potassium levels because of excess hydrogen ions are described in the Laboratory Assessment section for acidosis. These electrolyte imbalances then disrupt the functions all excitable tissues, especially nerves, cardiac muscle, and skeletal muscle. Symptoms of acidosis first appear in the musculoskeletal, cardiac, respiratory, and central nervous systems. Even slight increases in blood free hydrogen ion levels reduce the activity of many hormones and enzymes, leading to death.

Acidosis can be caused by metabolic problems, respiratory problems, or combined metabolic and respiratory problems. Specific causes of acidosis are listed in Table 14.2.

Metabolic Acidosis. Four processes can result in metabolic acidosis: overproduction of hydrogen ions, underelimination of hydrogen ions, underproduction of bicarbonate ions, and overelimination of bicarbonate ions.

TABLE 14.2 Common Causes of Acidosis

Pathology	Condition
Metabolic Acidosis	
Overproduction of hydrogen ions	Excessive oxidation of fatty acids: Diabetic ketoacidosis Starvation Hypermetabolism: Heavy exercise Seizure activity Fever Hypoxia, ischemia Excessive ingestion of acids: Ethanol or methanol intoxication Salicylate intoxication
Underelimination of hydrogen ions	Kidney failure
Underproduction of bicarbonate	Kidney failure Pancreatitis Liver failure Dehydration
Overelimination of bicarbonate	Diarrhea
Respiratory Acidosis	
Underelimination of hydrogen ions	Respiratory depression: Anesthetics Drugs (especially opioids) Electrolyte imbalance Inadequate chest expansion: Muscle weakness Airway obstruction Alveolar-capillary block

Overproduction of hydrogen ions can occur with excessive breakdown of fatty acids, anaerobic glucose breakdown *(lactic acidosis)*, and excessive intake of acids. Excessive breakdown of fatty acids occurs with diabetic ketoacidosis or starvation. Lactic acidosis occurs when cells use glucose without adequate oxygen *(anaerobic metabolism)*; glucose is then incompletely broken down and forms lactic acid. Lactic acidosis occurs whenever the body has too little oxygen to meet metabolic oxygen demands (e.g., heavy exercise, seizure activity, reduced oxygen). Excessive intake of acids floods the body with hydrogen ions. Agents that cause acidosis when ingested in excess include ethyl alcohol, methyl alcohol, and acetylsalicylic acid (aspirin).

Underelimination of hydrogen ions leads to acidosis when free hydrogen ions are produced at the normal rate but are not removed at the same rate they are produced. The most common causes are severe lung impairment (with retention of CO_2) and kidney failure (with retention of hydrogen ions).

Underproduction of bicarbonate ions (base deficit) leads to acidosis when free hydrogen ion production and removal are normal but too few bicarbonate ions are present to balance the hydrogen ions. Because bicarbonate is made in the kidneys and pancreas, kidney failure and impaired liver or pancreatic function can cause a base-deficit acidosis.

Overelimination of bicarbonate ions (base deficit) leads to acidosis when hydrogen ion production and removal are normal but too many bicarbonate ions have been lost. A common cause of base deficit acidosis is diarrhea.

Respiratory Acidosis. Respiratory acidosis results when respiratory function is impaired and the exchange of oxygen (O_2) and carbon dioxide (CO_2) is reduced. This problem causes CO_2 retention, which leads to the same increase in free hydrogen ion levels and acidosis (McCance et al., 2019). (See the carbonic anhydrase equation in Fig. 14.6.)

Unlike metabolic acidosis, respiratory acidosis results from only one cause—retention of CO_2, causing increased production of free hydrogen ions. Table 14.2 lists common causes of respiratory acidosis.

Respiratory depression results from depressed function of the brainstem neurons that trigger breathing movements. This lowered rate and depth of breathing leads to poor gas exchange and retention of carbon dioxide. Respiratory depression also occurs when respiratory neurons are damaged or destroyed by trauma or when problems in the brain increase the intracranial pressure.

Inadequate chest expansion reduces gas exchange and leads to acidosis. Chest expansion can be restricted internally by skeletal trauma or skeletal deformities, as well as by respiratory muscle weakness. External constriction such as casts, tight scar tissue around the chest, or obesity can also restrict chest movement.

Airway obstruction prevents air movement into and out of the lungs *(ventilation)* and leads to poor gas exchange, CO_2 retention, and acidosis.

Reduced alveolar-capillary diffusion causes poor gas exchange and leads to CO_2 retention and acidosis. Disorders that reduce diffusion include pneumonia, pneumonitis, tuberculosis, emphysema, acute respiratory distress syndrome, chest trauma, pulmonary emboli, pulmonary edema, and drowning.

In addition to pathologic conditions, improper mechanical ventilation can cause respiratory acidosis. If either the tidal volume or the number of ventilations per minute is set too low, the patient can develop respiratory acidosis because the ventilations are not sufficient to rid the body of excess CO_2.

Combined Metabolic and Respiratory Acidosis. Metabolic and respiratory acidosis can occur at the same time (McCance et al., 2019; Pompey & Abraham-Settles, 2019). For example, an adult who has diabetic ketoacidosis and chronic obstructive pulmonary disease has a combined metabolic and respiratory acidosis. Combined acidosis is more severe than either metabolic acidosis or respiratory acidosis alone.

❖ Interprofessional Collaborative Care

Episodes of acidosis that are severe enough to require intervention are usually managed in an acute care setting. Patients are discharged from the hospital when ***acid-base balance*** is restored. For patients who are at continuing risk for acidosis, especially respiratory acidosis, management interventions that focus on the chronic health problem leading to acidosis must be continued in the home or other residential setting.

◆ Assessment: Recognize Cues

History. Collect data about risk factors related to the development of acidosis. Information about age, nutrition, and current symptoms is especially important.

Older adults are more at risk for problems leading to acid-base imbalance, including cardiac, kidney, or pulmonary impairment (Touhy & Jett, 2020). They may also be taking drugs that disrupt ***acid-base balance***, especially diuretics and aspirin. Ask about specific risk factors such as any type of breathing problem, kidney failure, diabetes mellitus, diarrhea, pancreatitis, and fever.

Ask about headaches, behavior changes, increased drowsiness, reduced alertness, reduced attention span, lethargy, anorexia, abdominal distention, nausea or vomiting, muscle weakness, or increased fatigue. Ask the patient to relate activities of the previous 24 hours to identify activity intolerance, behavior changes, and fatigue. If the central nervous system is depressed or the patient is confused, obtain this information from the patient's family.

Physical Assessment/Signs and Symptoms. Symptoms of acidosis are similar whether the cause is metabolic or respiratory and are listed in the Key Features: Acidosis box. Acidosis reduces the ability of excitable membranes to respond appropriately, especially in cardiovascular tissue, neurons, skeletal muscle, and GI smooth muscle.

Cardiovascular changes are first seen with mild acidosis and become more severe as the condition worsens. Early changes include increased heart rate and cardiac output. With worsening acidosis or with acidosis and *hyperkalemia* (elevated blood potassium levels), heart rate decreases, T waves become tall and peaked, and QRS complexes are widened. Peripheral pulses may be hard to find and are easily blocked. Hypotension occurs with vasodilation.

KEY FEATURES

Acidosis

Cardiovascular Signs and Symptoms
- Ranges from bradycardia to heart block
- Tall T waves
- Widened QRS complex
- Prolonged PR interval
- Hypotension
- Thready peripheral pulses

Central Nervous System Signs and Symptoms
- Depressed activity (lethargy, confusion, stupor, coma)

Neuromuscular Signs and Symptoms
- Hyporeflexia
- Skeletal muscle weakness
- Flaccid paralysis

Respiratory Signs and Symptoms
- Kussmaul respirations (in metabolic acidosis with respiratory compensation)
- Variable respirations (generally ineffective in respiratory acidosis)

Integumentary Signs and Symptoms
- Warm, flushed, dry skin in metabolic acidosis
- Pale-to-cyanotic and dry skin in respiratory acidosis

NURSING SAFETY PRIORITY QSEN

Critical Rescue

Assess the cardiovascular system **first** in any patient at risk for acidosis because acidosis can lead to cardiac arrest from the accompanying hyperkalemia. If cardiac changes are present, respond by reporting these changes immediately to the health care provider.

Central nervous system (CNS) changes include depression of CNS function. Problems may range from lethargy to confusion, especially in older patients. As acidosis worsens, the patient may become unresponsive.

Neuromuscular changes include reduced muscle tone and deep tendon reflexes as a result of the accompanying hyperkalemia. Assess arm muscle strength by having the patient squeeze your hand. Assess leg muscle strength by having the patient push both feet against a flat surface (such as a box or a board) while you apply resistance to the opposite side of the surface. Muscle weakness is bilateral and can progress to paralysis.

Respiratory changes may cause the acidosis and can be caused by the acidosis. Assess the patient's rate, depth, and ease of breathing. Use pulse oximetry to determine how well oxygen is delivered to the peripheral tissues.

If acidosis is metabolic in origin, the rate and depth of breathing increase as the hydrogen ion level rises. Breaths are deep and rapid and not under voluntary control, a pattern called **Kussmaul respiration**. The high levels of arterial CO_2 in the brain caused by the elevated free hydrogen ion concentration excessively excite the respiratory neurons, leading to this breathing pattern to increase the rate at which CO_2 is exhaled by the lungs to help correct the acidosis.

If acidosis is caused by respiratory problems, breathing efforts are reduced. Respirations are usually shallow and rapid. Muscle weakness makes this problem worse.

Skin changes occur with metabolic or respiratory acidosis. With metabolic acidosis breathing is unimpaired and the excessive free hydrogen ions cause vasodilation and make the skin and mucous membranes warm and dry with reddish undertones. With respiratory acidosis, breathing is ineffective and skin and mucous membranes are pale to cyanotic.

Psychosocial Assessment. *Cognitive changes may be the first signs of acidosis.* Assess the patient's mental status for awareness of time, place, and person (see Chapter 38). Check the patient's cognitive abilities by asking him or her to count backward by threes. Ask family members whether the patient's behavior is typical for him or her and establish a baseline for comparison with later assessment findings.

Laboratory Assessment. Arterial blood pH is the laboratory value used to confirm acidosis. Acidosis is present when arterial blood pH is less than 7.35. However, this test alone does not indicate what is causing the acidosis. Symptoms of metabolic acidosis and respiratory acidosis are similar, but their treatments are different. *Therefore it is critical to obtain and interpret other laboratory data such as arterial blood gas (ABG) values and blood levels of electrolytes* (Gooch, 2015).

Metabolic acidosis is reflected by several changes in ABG values shown in the Key Features box. The pH is low (<7.35) because buffering and respiratory compensation are not adequate to keep the amount of free hydrogen ions at a normal level. The bicarbonate level is usually low (<21 mEq/L [mmol/L]) because bicarbonate has been lost or its production is inadequate as causes of the acidosis. The classic ABG values that distinguish metabolic acidosis from respiratory acidosis when pH is below 7.35 are a normal partial pressure of arterial oxygen (Pao_2) together with a normal or even slightly low partial pressure of arterial carbon dioxide ($Paco_2$).

KEY FEATURES

Metabolic Acidosis: Expected Arterial Blood Gas Values

Test	Expected Value	Significance
pH	Below 7.35	Represents an increase in the free hydrogen ion concentration of arterial blood.
Pao_2	80-100 mm Hg	Represents the patient's normal value because oxygen intake is unimpaired
$Paco_2$	35-40 mm Hg	Retention of carbon dioxide is not a feature of metabolic acidosis because ventilation is not impaired. The value may be *low* because of respiratory compensation from a metabolic origin acidosis.
Bicarbonate	15-20 mEq/L (15-20 mmol/L) or lower	Loss of bicarbonate or inadequate production of bicarbonate is often the cause of metabolic acidosis, except for diabetic ketoacidosis.

$Paco_2$, Partial pressure of arterial carbon dioxide; *Pao_2*, partial pressure of arterial oxygen.

The serum potassium level is often high in acidosis as the body attempts to maintain electroneutrality during buffering. Fig. 14.11 shows the movement of potassium ions as serum pH changes. As the blood hydrogen ion level rises, some of the excess hydrogen ions enter red blood cells for intracellular buffering. The movement of hydrogen ions into the cells creates an excess of positive ions inside the cells. To balance these extra positive charges, an equal number of potassium ions (that also have a positive charge) moves from the cells into the blood. This increases the blood potassium level, causing hyperkalemia.

Respiratory acidosis is reflected by several changes in ABG values in addition to the low pH, as shown in the Key Features box. Buffering and kidney compensation are not adequate to keep the amount of free hydrogen ions at a normal level. If the kidneys partially compensate for this acidosis, pH is low but not as abnormal as could be expected with the degree of CO_2 retention.

The partial pressure of arterial oxygen (Pao_2) is low, and the partial pressure of arterial carbon dioxide ($Paco_2$) is high because the pulmonary problem impairs gas exchange, causing poor oxygenation and CO_2 retention. (*The hallmarks of respiratory acidosis are a decreasing* Pao_2 *coupled with a rising* $Paco_2$*.*) Because carbon dioxide diffuses more easily across the alveolar membrane than oxygen, a decreased Pao_2 usually occurs before an increased $Paco_2$.

The serum bicarbonate level is variable. A patient with rapid onset of respiratory acidosis often has a normal bicarbonate level because kidney compensation has not started. When acidosis persists for 24 hours or longer, kidney compensation increases the levels of bicarbonate. Chronic respiratory acidosis is indicated by an elevated bicarbonate level and increased $Paco_2$.

Serum potassium levels are elevated in acute respiratory acidosis. They are normal or low in chronic respiratory acidosis when kidney compensation is present.

◆ **Analysis: Analyze Cues and Prioritize Hypotheses.** Patients with acidosis have problems associated with decreased excitable tissues, including hypotension and decreased perfusion, impaired memory and cognition, and increased risk for falls. For patients who have respiratory acidosis in addition to the general problems, life-threatening problems are related to the cause of the respiratory impairment. The priority patient problem for the patient experiencing respiratory acidosis is:

1. Reduced gas exchange resulting from underlying pulmonary disease

KEY FEATURES

Respiratory Acidosis: Expected Arterial Blood Gas Values

Test	Expected Value	Significance
pH	Below 7.35	Represents an increase in the free hydrogen ion concentration of arterial blood.
Pao_2	<90 mm Hg	Represents greatly reduced gas exchange and inadequate oxygenation from the patient's underlying acute or chronic respiratory problems.
$Paco_2$	>50 mm Hg and can even be >100 mm Hg	Represents greatly reduced gas exchange and retention of CO_2 from the patient's underlying acute or chronic respiratory problems.
Bicarbonate	21-28 mEq/L (21-28 mmol/L) or higher	Bicarbonate is not lost in pure respiratory acidosis and the level is usually normal in acute respiratory acidosis. The level is elevated in chronic respiratory acidosis because of kidney compensation.

$Paco_2$, Partial pressure of arterial carbon dioxide; *Pao_2*, partial pressure of arterial oxygen.

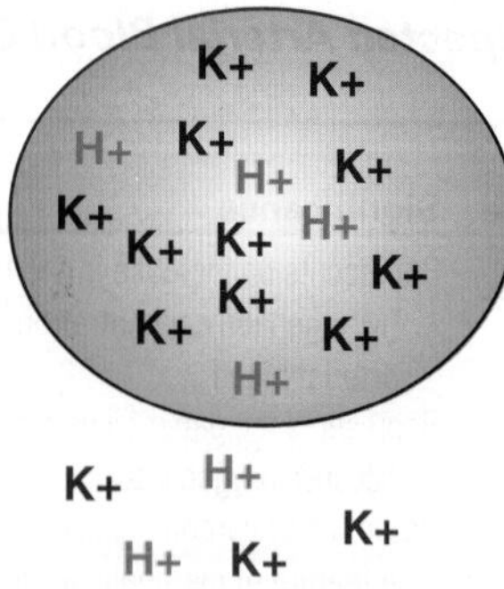

Under normal conditions, the intracellular potassium content is much greater than that of the extracellular fluid. The concentration of hydrogen ions is low in both compartments.

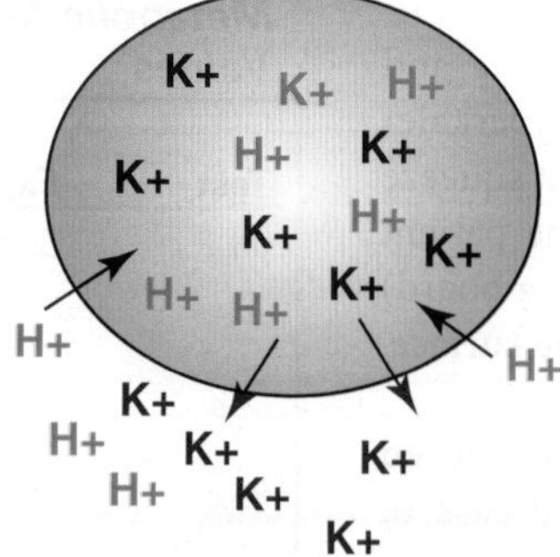

In acidosis, the extracellular hydrogen ion content increases and the hydrogen ions move into the intracellular fluid. To keep the intracellular fluid electrically neutral, an equal number of potassium ions leave the cell, creating a relative hyperkalemia.

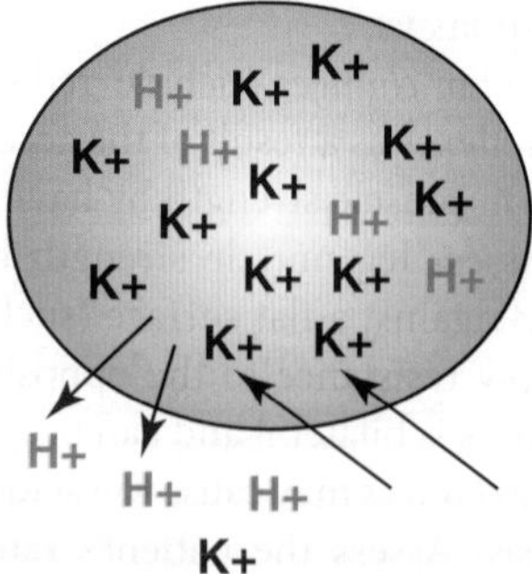

In alkalosis, more hydrogen ions are present in the intracellular fluid than in the extracellular fluid. Hydrogen ions move from the intracellular fluid into the extracellular fluid. To keep the intracellular fluid electrically neutral, potassium ions move from the extracellular fluid into the intracellular fluid, creating a relative hypokalemia.

Fig. 14.11 Movement of potassium (K^+) in response to changes in the extracellular fluid hydrogen ion (H^+) concentration.

◆ **Planning and Implementation: Generate Solutions and Take Action.** Interventions for acidosis focus on correcting the underlying problem and monitoring for changes. Remember that acidosis is not a disease. It is a symptom of another health problem. To ensure appropriate interventions, first identify the specific type of acidosis present.

Metabolic Acidosis. Interventions for metabolic acidosis include hydration and drugs or treatments to control the problem causing the acidosis. For example, if the acidosis is a result of diabetic ketoacidosis, insulin is given to correct the hyperglycemia and halt the production of ketone bodies. Rehydration and antidiarrheal drugs are given if the acidosis is a result of prolonged diarrhea. *Bicarbonate is given only if serum bicarbonate levels are low and the pH is less than 7.2.*

Nursing priorities include continuously monitoring the patient for indications that he or she is either responding to the treatment or the acidosis is becoming worse. The cardiovascular and skeletal muscle systems are sensitive to acidosis and are the most important systems to monitor. Interpreting ongoing ABG results is an important part of monitoring.

Respiratory Acidosis

Improving Gas Exchange

Planning: Expected Outcomes. The patient being managed for respiratory acidosis is expected to have a reduction in acidosis signs and symptoms.

Interventions. Interventions for the patient who has a condition that causes him or her to remain at continued risk include drug therapy, oxygen therapy, pulmonary hygiene (positioning and breathing techniques), and ventilatory support. These interventions are the same as those used for a patient who has chronic obstructive pulmonary disease (COPD), which is the most common health problem associated with continuing risk for respiratory acidosis. A brief overview of these interventions is provided here. For in-depth discussion of these interventions, see Chapter 27 under the Gas Exchange Exemplar: Chronic Obstructive Pulmonary Disease.

Drug therapy is focused on improving ventilation and gas exchange rather than directly on altering pH. Drug categories useful for respiratory acidosis include bronchodilators, anti-inflammatories, and mucolytics.

Oxygen therapy helps promote gas exchange for patients with respiratory acidosis. Carefully monitor oxygen saturation levels to ensure that the lowest flow of oxygen that prevents hypoxemia is used to avoid oxygen-induced tissue damage.

Ventilation support with mechanical ventilation may be needed for patients who cannot keep their oxygen saturation at 90% or who have respiratory muscle fatigue. Chapter 29 discusses the nursing care needs of patients who are being mechanically ventilated.

Preventing complications is a nursing priority when caring for a patient with respiratory acidosis. Monitoring breathing status hourly and intervening when changes occur are critical in preventing complications. Listen to breath sounds and assess how easily air moves into and out of the lungs. Check for any muscle retractions, the use of accessory muscles (especially the neck muscles [sternocleidomastoids]), and whether breathing produces a grunt or wheeze that can be heard without a stethoscope. Assess nail beds and oral membranes for cyanosis (a late finding).

Care Coordination and Transition Management. Because respiratory acidosis is a symptom or complication of another health problem, most often COPD, care during the acute phase occurs in a hospital setting. Ongoing management for continuing risk is the same as for COPD. See Chapter 27 for a detailed discussion of the care coordination needed for this problem.

◆ **Evaluation: Evaluate Outcomes.** Depending on the cause of the respiratory acidosis and the patient's continuing risk, some patients may not return to full ***acid-base balance***, even with meticulous care. Indications that the patient's underlying disease process is well managed and that the imbalance is reduced include the expected outcomes that he or she:

- Maintains adequate gas exchange
- Has an arterial pH above 7.2 and closer to 7.35
- Has a Pao_2 level above 90 mm Hg or at least 10 mm Hg higher than admission level
- Has a $Paco_2$ levels below 45 mm Hg or at least 15 mm Hg below admission level

ALKALOSIS

Pathophysiology Review

In patients with alkalosis the ***acid-base balance*** of the blood is disturbed and has an excess of bases, especially bicarbonate (HCO_3^-). The amount of bases is greater than normal compared with the amount of the acids. Alkalosis is a *decrease* in the free hydrogen ion level of the blood and is reflected by an arterial blood pH *above* 7.45. Like acidosis, alkalosis is not a disease but rather an indication of a problem. It can be caused by metabolic problems, respiratory problems, or both (Table 14.3).

Alkalosis can result from an actual or relative increase in the amount of bases. In an actual base excess, alkalosis occurs when base (usually bicarbonate) is either overproduced or undereliminated.

In *relative* alkalosis, the actual amount bases does not increase, but the amount of the acids decreases, creating an *acid deficit*. A relative base-excess alkalosis (actual acid deficit) results from an overelimination or underproduction of acids (see Fig. 14.4).

The problems of alkalosis are serious and can be life threatening. Management focuses on correcting the cause after identifying whether the alkalosis origin is respiratory or metabolic.

Whether metabolic, respiratory, or both, alkalosis affects specific functions. The pathologic effects are caused by the electrolyte imbalances that occur in response to decreased blood cation (positively charged particles) levels. Most problems of alkalosis are related to increased stimulation of the nervous, neuromuscular, and cardiac systems.

Metabolic alkalosis is an acid-base imbalance caused by either an increase of bases (base excess) or a decrease of acids (acid deficit). Base excesses are caused by excessive intake of bicarbonates, carbonates, acetates, and citrates. Excessive use of

TABLE 14.3 Common Causes of Alkalosis

Pathology	Condition
Metabolic Alkalosis	
Increase of base components	Oral ingestion of bases: Antacids Parenteral base administration: Blood transfusion Sodium bicarbonate Total parenteral nutrition
Decrease of acid components	Prolonged vomiting Nasogastric suctioning Hypercortisolism Hyperaldosteronism High ceiling (loop) and thiazide diuretics (in higher dosages)
Respiratory Alkalosis	
Excessive loss of carbon dioxide	Hyperventilation, fear, anxiety Mechanical ventilation Salicylate toxicity High altitudes Early-stage acute pulmonary problems

bicarbonate-containing antacids can cause a metabolic alkalosis. Other base excesses can occur during medical treatments such as citrate excesses during massive blood transfusions and IV sodium bicarbonate given to correct acidosis. The hallmark of a base excess alkalosis is an ABG result with an elevated pH and an elevated bicarbonate level, along with normal oxygen and carbon dioxide levels.

Acid deficits can be caused by disease processes or medical treatment. Disorders causing acid deficits include prolonged vomiting, excess cortisol, and hyperaldosteronism. Treatments that promote acid loss causing metabolic alkalosis include thiazide diuretics and prolonged gastric suctioning.

Respiratory alkalosis is usually caused by an excessive loss of CO_2 through hyperventilation (rapid respirations). Patients may hyperventilate in response to anxiety, fear, or improper settings on mechanical ventilators. Hyperventilation can also result from direct stimulation of central respiratory centers because of fever, central nervous system lesions, and salicylates. The hallmark of respiratory alkalosis is an ABG result with an elevated pH coupled with a low carbon dioxide level. Usually the oxygen and bicarbonate levels are normal.

Interprofessional Collaborative Care

Assessment: Recognize Cues. Symptoms of problems with ***acid-base balance*** regulation are the same for metabolic and respiratory alkalosis. Many symptoms are the result of the low calcium levels *(hypocalcemia)* and low potassium levels *(hypokalemia)* that usually occur with alkalosis (see Fig. 14.11). These problems change the function of the nervous, neuromuscular, cardiac, and respiratory systems as shown in the Key Features: Alkalosis box.

Central nervous system (CNS) changes are caused by overexcitement of the nervous systems. Patients have dizziness, agitation, confusion, and hyperreflexia, which may progress to seizures. Tingling or numbness may occur around the mouth and in the toes. Other indicators of alkalosis with hypocalcemia are positive Chvostek and Trousseau signs (see Chapter 13).

KEY FEATURES

Alkalosis

Central Nervous System Signs and Symptoms
- Increased activity
- Anxiety, irritability, tetany, seizures
- Positive Chvostek sign
- Positive Trousseau sign
- Paresthesias

Neuromuscular Signs and Symptoms
- Hyperreflexia
- Muscle cramping and twitching
- Skeletal muscle weakness

Cardiovascular Signs and Symptoms
- Increased heart rate
- Normal or low blood pressure
- Increased digoxin toxicity

Respiratory Signs and Symptoms
- Hyperventilation in respiratory alkalosis (often the cause of the acidosis)
- Decreased respiratory effort associated with skeletal muscle weakness in metabolic alkalosis

Neuromuscular changes are related to the hypocalcemia and hypokalemia that occur with alkalosis. Nervous system activity increases, causing muscle cramps, twitches, and "charley horses." Deep tendon reflexes are hyperactive. **Tetany** (continuous contractions) of muscle groups may also be present. Tetany is painful and indicates a rapidly worsening condition.

Skeletal muscles may contract as a result of nerve stimulation, but they become weaker because of the hypokalemia. Handgrip strength decreases, and the patient may be unable to stand or walk. Respiratory efforts become less effective as the respiratory muscles weaken.

Cardiovascular changes occur because alkalosis increases myocardial irritability, especially when accompanied by hypokalemia. Heart rate increases, and the pulse is thready. When decreased blood volume is also present, the patient may have severe hypotension. The hypokalemia increases heart sensitivity to digoxin, which increases the risk for digoxin toxicity.

Respiratory changes, especially increases in the rate of breathing, are the main causes of respiratory alkalosis. Although the volume of air inhaled and exhaled with each breath is nearly normal, the total volume of air inhaled and exhaled each minute rises with the increased respiratory rate. The increased minute volume may be caused by anxiety or physiologic changes.

Arterial blood pH greater than 7.45 confirms alkalosis, but this test alone does not identify its cause. Because the symptoms of metabolic alkalosis and respiratory alkalosis are similar, it is critical to obtain additional laboratory data, especially arterial blood gas (ABG) values and specific serum electrolyte levels.

◆ **Interventions: Take Action.** Interventions are planned to prevent further losses of hydrogen, potassium, calcium, and chloride ions; to restore fluid balance; to monitor changes; and to provide for *patient safety*. Treatments that may have caused alkalosis (e.g., prolonged gastric suctioning, excessive infusion of certain IV solutions, drugs that promote hydrogen ion excretion) are modified or stopped. Drug therapy is prescribed to resolve the causes of alkalosis and to restore normal fluid, electrolyte, and acid-base balance. For example, the patient with metabolic alkalosis caused by diuretic therapy receives fluid and electrolyte replacement, and the diuretic therapy is adjusted or stopped. Antiemetic drugs are prescribed for vomiting. Monitor the patient's progress and adjust fluid and electrolyte therapy. Monitor electrolytes daily until they return to near normal.

During correction of alkalosis, a nursing care priority is prevention of injury from falls. The patient with alkalosis has hypotension and muscle weakness, which increase the risk for falls, especially among older adults. Implement the falls prevention nursing interventions presented in Chapter 4.

NCLEX EXAMINATION CHALLENGE 14.3

Safe and Effective Care Environment

With which clients does the nurse remain alert for the possibility of metabolic alkalosis? Select all that apply.

A. Client who has been NPO for 36 hours without fluid replacement
B. Client receiving a rapid infusion of normal saline
C. Client who has been self-managing indigestion with chronic ingestion of bicarbonate
D. Client who has had continuous gastric suction for 48 hours
E. Client having a sudden and severe asthma attack
F. Client with uncontrolled diabetes mellitus

GET READY FOR THE NEXT-GENERATION NCLEX® EXAMINATION!

Key Points

Review these Key Points for each NCLEX Examination Client Needs Category.

Safe and Effective Care Environment

- Assess the cardiovascular system first in any patient at risk for acidosis because acidosis can lead to cardiac arrest from the accompanying hyperkalemia. **QSEN: Safety**
- Assess the airway of any patient who has acute respiratory acidosis. **QSEN: Safety**
- Monitor the neurologic status at least every 2 hours in patients being treated for a problem with ***acid-base balance.*** **QSEN: Safety**
- Use fall precautions for any patient with a problem in ***acid-base balance.*** **QSEN: Safety**

Health Promotion and Maintenance

- Teach patients to take drugs as prescribed, especially diuretics, antihypertensives, and cardiac drugs to prevent an acid-base imbalance. **QSEN: Patient-Centered Care**

Psychosocial Integrity

- Perform a mental status assessment in any patient with or at risk for problems of ***acid-base balance.*** **QSEN: Patient-Centered Care**

Physiological Intxegrity

- Be aware of how the following principles, processes, and mechanisms influence the regulation of ***acid-base balance:***
  - The normal pH of the body's extracellular fluids (including blood) is 7.35 to 7.45.
  - The more hydrogen ions present, the more acidic the fluid; the fewer hydrogen ions present, the more alkaline the fluid.
  - pH values below 7.35 indicate acidosis; pH values above 7.45 indicate alkalosis.
  - Anything that increases the CO_2 level in the blood increases the hydrogen ion content and lowers the pH.
  - Acids are normally formed in the body as a result of metabolism.
  - Chemical blood buffers are the immediate way that acid-base imbalances are corrected.
  - The lungs control the amount of CO_2 that is retained or exhaled.
  - The kidneys regulate the amount of hydrogen and bicarbonate ions that are retained or excreted by the body.
  - If a lung problem causes retention of carbon dioxide, the healthy kidney compensates by increasing the amount of bicarbonate that is produced and retained.
  - Acidosis reduces the excitability of cardiovascular muscle, neurons, skeletal muscle, and GI smooth muscle.
  - Alkalosis increases the sensitivity of excitable tissues, allowing them to overrespond to normal stimuli and respond even without stimulation.
- Check the serum potassium level for any patient who has acidosis. **QSEN: Evidence-Based Practice**
- Monitor arterial blood gas (ABG) values to evaluate the effectiveness of therapy for acid-base imbalances. **QSEN: Patient-Centered Care**

MASTERY QUESTIONS

1. How does the corresponding increase in carbon dioxide levels that occurs when arterial pH drops assist in maintaining acid-base balance?
   A. Carbon dioxide loss through exhalation can raise arterial pH levels.
   B. Carbon dioxide retention during exhalation can lower arterial pH levels.
   C. Carbon dioxide is a base that can convert free hydrogen ions into a neutral substance.
   D. Carbon dioxide is a buffer that can bind free hydrogen ions and form a neutral substance.

2. The handgrasp strength of a client with metabolic acidosis has diminished since the previous assessment 1 hour ago. What is the nurse's best first action?
   A. Measure the client's pulse and blood pressure
   B. Apply humidified oxygen by nasal cannula
   C. Assess the client's oxygen saturation
   D. Notify the Rapid Response Team

REFERENCES

Asterisk (*) indicates a classic or definitive work on this subject.

*Gooch, M. (2015). Identifying acid-base and electrolyte imbalances. *The Nurse Practitioner*, *40*(8), 37–42.

McCance, K., Huether, S., Brashers, V., & Rote, N. (2019). *Pathophysiology: The biologic basis for disease in adults and children* (8th ed.). St. Louis: Elsevier.

Pagana, K., & Pagana, T. (2018). *Mosby's manual of diagnostic and laboratory tests* (6th ed.). St. Louis: Elsevier.

Pompey, J., & Abraham-Settles, B. (2019). Clarifying the confusion of arterial blood gas analysis: Is it compensation or combination? *American Journal of Nursing*, *119*(3), 52–56.

Touhy, T., & Jett, K. (2020). *Ebersole & Hess' Toward healthy aging* (10th ed.). St. Louis: Elsevier.

15

Concepts of Infusion Therapy

Cheryl L. Leksan, Nicole M. Heimgartner

http://evolve.elsevier.com/Iggy/

LEARNING OUTCOMES

1. Use evidence-based practice to prevent infusion administration errors.
2. Describe the benefits and limitations of selected safety-enhancing technologies used for infusion therapy.
3. Identify the evidence-based guidelines for prevention of intravenous (IV) catheter-related bloodstream infection (CRBSI).
4. Describe the population-specific care for older adults receiving infusion therapy, including careful monitoring of ***fluid and electrolyte balance.***
5. Teach the patient and family about the patient's type of infusion therapy and associated care.
6. Explain the process of determining infusion and drug order accuracy to promote patient safety.
7. Explain the evidence-based process of peripheral and central IV therapy, including site selection, insertion, and maintenance.
8. Explain nursing interventions with associated rationale that prevent impaired tissue integrity at the infusion site.
9. Prioritize nursing interventions for maintaining an infusion system.
10. Use clinical judgment to prevent, assess, manage, and document complications related to infusion therapy and vascular access devices (VADs).
11. Describe nursing care associated with intra-arterial, intraperitoneal, subcutaneous, intraosseous, and intraspinal infusion therapy.

KEY TERMS

adverse drug events (ADEs) An unintended harmful reaction to an administered drug.

ambulatory pumps Infusion therapy pump generally used with a home care patient to allow a return to his or her usual activities while receiving infusion therapy.

catheter-related bloodstream infection (CRBSI) Health care–acquired bloodstream infections caused by the presence of any type of intravenous catheter.

catheter-related bloodstream infection (CRBSI) prevention bundle A nationally recognized set of evidence-based practices to prevent CRBSIs.

central line–associated bloodstream infection (CLABSI) Health care–acquired bloodstream infections caused by the presence of a central intravenous line.

compartment syndrome A condition in which increased tissue pressure in a confined anatomic space causes decreased blood flow to the area, leading to hypoxia and pain.

extravasation Escape of fluids or drugs into the subcutaneous tissue; a complication of intravenous infusion therapy.

implanted port A surgically implanted vascular access device (VAD) where the port is placed in a subcutaneous pocket; used for long-term or frequent infusion therapy.

infiltration Leakage of IV solution into the tissues around the vein.

infusate Solution that is infused into the body.

infusion therapy Delivery of parenteral medications and fluids through a variety of catheter types and locations using multiple techniques and procedures, such as intravenous therapy to deliver solutions into the vascular system.

midline catheters A VAD that is 3 to 8 inches long and inserted through the veins of the antecubital fossa.

nontunneled central venous catheter (CVC) A multilumen VAD inserted through the subclavian or jugular vein using sterile technique.

peripheral IV therapy IV therapy in which a vascular access device (VAD) is placed in a peripheral vein, usually in the arm.

peripherally inserted central catheter (PICC) A long VAD inserted through a vein at the antecubital fossa.

phlebitis Inflammation of a vein that can predispose patients to thrombosis.

short peripheral catheter (SPC) A VAD composed of a plastic cannula, built around a sharp stylet for venipuncture, which extends slightly beyond the cannula and is advanced into the vein.

secondary (piggyback) administration set A short tubing set that is attached to the primary administration set and used to deliver intermittent medications.

smart pumps Infusion pumps with dosage calculation software.

syringe pumps Pump for infusion therapy that uses a battery-powered piston to push the plunger continuously at a selected rate; limited to small-volume or intermittent infusions.

thrombophlebitis Presence of a thrombus associated with inflammation.

thrombosis Formation of a blood clot within a blood vessel.

tunneled central venous catheter A surgically implanted VAD used for long-term infusion therapy in which the catheter lies in a subcutaneous tunnel, separating the points where the catheter enters the vein from where it enters the skin.

vascular access device (VAD) An infusion catheter placed in a blood vessel to deliver fluids and medications.

vesicant medications Drugs that cause severe tissue damage if they escape into the subcutaneous tissue; also referred to as *vesicants.*

PRIORITY AND INTERRELATED CONCEPTS

The priority concept for this chapter is:
- ***Fluid and Electrolyte Balance***

The interrelated concept for this chapter is:
- ***Tissue Integrity***

Infusion therapy is the delivery of medications in solution or fluids by a parenteral route, which requires piercing of the skin with a needle or catheter. There are many catheter types and access locations. IV therapy is the most common route for infusion therapy, delivering solutions directly into the veins of the vascular system. This chapter focuses on access for and administration of all types of infusion therapy.

OVERVIEW

Infusion therapy is delivered in all health care settings, including hospitals, home care, ambulatory care clinics, primary health care providers' offices, and long-term care facilities. The most common reasons for using infusion therapy are to:
- Maintain ***fluid balance*** or correct fluid imbalance
- Maintain *electrolyte* or acid-base ***balance*** or correct electrolyte or acid-base imbalance
- Administer medications
- Replace blood or blood products

Infusion therapy is the most common invasive therapy administered to hospitalized patients. Many patients depend on long-term infusion therapies for health maintenance and management of disease progression. Advances in medicine and technology have made it possible for people with chronic diseases such as diabetes mellitus, chronic kidney disease, and malabsorption syndromes to live long and productive lives. Patients with chronic conditions who require long-term infusion therapy often have poor vascular integrity. This can make intravenous access difficult and requires a high level of skill.

A specialized team of infusion nurses to initiate and maintain infusion therapy is recommended as best practice by the Centers for Disease Control and Prevention (CDC) to reduce complications of infusion therapy. These teams have demonstrated value in cost savings, patient satisfaction, and patient outcomes.

Infusion nurses may perform any or all of these activities:
- Develop evidence-based policies and procedures.
- Insert and maintain various types of peripheral, midline, and central venous catheters and subcutaneous and intraosseous accesses.
- Monitor patient outcomes of infusion therapy.
- Educate staff, patients, and families regarding infusion therapy.
- Consult on product selection and purchasing decisions.
- Provide therapies such as blood withdrawal, therapeutic phlebotomy, hypodermoclysis, intraosseous infusions, and administration of medications.

The registered nurse (RN) generalist is taught to insert peripheral IV lines; most institutions have a process for demonstrating competency for this skill. Depending on each state's nurse practice act, licensed practical/vocational nurses (LPNs/LVNs) and technicians may be trained and verified competent to perform the skill of peripheral IV insertion and assist with infusions.

The RN is ultimately accountable for all aspects of infusion therapy and delegation of associated tasks (Infusion Nurses Society, 2016).

The Infusion Nurses Society (INS) publishes guidelines and standards of practice for policy and procedure development in all health care settings. These standards establish the criteria for all nurses delivering infusion therapy. The Infusion Nurses Certification Corporation (INCC) offers a written certification examination. Nurses who successfully complete this examination have mastered an advanced body of knowledge in this specialty and may use the initials *CRNI,* which stand for *certified registered nurse infusion* (Vizcarra, 2016).

Types of Infusion Therapy Fluids

Many types of parenteral fluids are used for infusion therapy. These fluids are IV solutions, including parenteral nutrition, blood and blood components, biologics, and pharmacologic therapy.

Intravenous Solutions. More than 200 IV fluids (solutions) that meet the requirements established by the U.S. Pharmacopeia (USP) are available. Each solution is classified by its tonicity (concentration) and pH. Tonicity is typically categorized by comparison with normal blood plasma as osmolarity (mOsm/L). As discussed in Chapter 13, normal serum osmolarity for adults is between 270 and 300 mOsm/L. Parenteral solutions within that normal range are **isotonic,** fluids greater than 300 mOsm/L are **hypertonic,** and fluids less than 270 mOsm/L are **hypotonic.**

When an *isotonic* **infusate** (solution that is infused into the body) is used, water does not move into or out of the body's cells and remains in the extracellular compartments. Therefore patients, especially older adults, receiving isotonic solutions are at risk for fluid overload (see Chapter 13) (Coulter, 2016). *Hypertonic* solutions are used to correct altered ***fluid and electrolyte balance*** and acid-base imbalances by moving water out of the body's cells and into the interstitial spaces and bloodstream. Electrolytes and other particles also move across cell membranes across a concentration gradient (from higher concentration to lower concentration). Parenteral nutrition solutions are hypertonic (see Chapter 55). Instead of moving water out of cells, *hypotonic* infusates move water into cells to expand them. Patients receiving either hypertonic or hypotonic fluids are at risk for phlebitis and infiltration. **Phlebitis** is the inflammation of a vein caused by mechanical, chemical, or bacterial irritation. **Infiltration** occurs when IV solution leaks into the tissues around the vein.

The pH of IV solutions is a measure of acidity or alkalinity and usually ranges from 3.5 to 6.2. Extremes of both osmolarity and pH can cause vein damage, leading to phlebitis and **thrombosis** (blood clot in the vein). Thus fluids and medications with a pH value less than 5.0 and more than 9.0 and with an osmolarity more than 600 mOsm/L are best infused in the central circulation where greater blood flow provides adequate hemodilution (Kear, 2017).

For example, total parenteral nutrition (TPN) solutions have an osmolarity greater than 1400 mOsm/L. TPN should never be infused in peripheral circulation because it can damage blood cells and the endothelial lining of the veins and decrease perfusion.

! NURSING SAFETY PRIORITY (QSEN)

Drug Alert

Drugs such as amiodarone, vancomycin, and ciprofloxacin are venous irritants that have a pH less than 5.0. Phlebitis can occur when patients require long-term infusion of these drugs in peripheral circulation. Drugs with vasoconstrictive action (e.g., dopamine or chemotherapeutic agents) are **vesicants** (chemicals that damage body tissue on direct contact) that can cause extravasation. **Extravasation** results in severe ***tissue integrity*** impairment as manifested by blistering, tissue sloughing, or necrosis from infiltration into the surrounding tissues. (See the Complications of Intravenous Therapy section for further explanation and Chapter 20 for more detail.) The IV insertion site should be assessed carefully for early signs of infiltration, including swelling, coolness, tingling, or redness. If any of these symptoms are present, discontinue the drug immediately and notify the infusion therapy team, if available. If an infusion specialist is not available, remove the IV catheter and notify the primary health care provider.

Blood and Blood Components. Blood transfusion is given by using packed red blood cells, created by removing a large part of the plasma from whole blood. Other available blood components include platelets, fresh frozen plasma, albumin, and several specific clotting factors. Each component has specific detailed requirements for blood-type compatibility and infusion techniques.

! NATIONAL PATIENT SAFETY GOALS

For patient safety, The Joint Commission's (TJC) 2020 National Patient Safety Goals (NPSGs) require agencies to have processes in place to help eliminate transfusion errors related to patient misidentification. Positive patient identification using two patient identifiers and requiring two qualified health care professionals is essential before any blood or blood component is administered. Automated bar coding can be used for positive patient identification in ambulatory care, acute care, and critical access hospitals and office-based surgery-accredited programs.

Most organizations use the International Society of Blood Transfusion (ISBT) universal bar-coding system to ensure the right blood for the right patient (Fig. 15.1). The ISBT system includes four components that must be present on the blood label both in bar code and in eye-readable format. These four components are (1) a unique facility identifier, (2) the lot number relating to the donor, (3) the product code, and (4) the ABO group and Rh type of the donor. Chapter 37 describes blood and blood product administration in more detail.

Drug Therapy. IV drugs provide a rapid therapeutic effect but can lead to immediate serious reactions, called **adverse drug events (ADEs)**. Hundreds of drugs are available for infusion by a variety of techniques. As with all drug administration, nurses must be knowledgeable about drug indications, proper dosage, contraindications, and precautions. IV administration also requires knowledge of appropriate dilution, rate of infusion, pH and osmolarity, compatibility with other IV medications, appropriate infusion site (peripheral versus central circulation), potential for vesicant/irritant effects, and specific aspects of patient monitoring because of its immediate effect. *Regardless of familiarity with the drug, never assume that IV administration is the same as giving that drug by other routes.* Because new drugs are being created and trade names and doses of medications change, it is the professional responsibility of the nurse to be familiar with a medication before administration.

Medication safety is extremely important in all health care settings today.

! NATIONAL PATIENT SAFETY GOALS

The Joint Commission's 2020 NPSGs include as a major goal improving the safety of using medications. This safety goals includes labeling drugs appropriately, using special precautions with the use of anticoagulants, and medication reconciliation. Electronic medication administration records (MARs) and multiple checks by nurses and pharmacists, as required by The Joint Commission's NPSGs, help reduce errors.

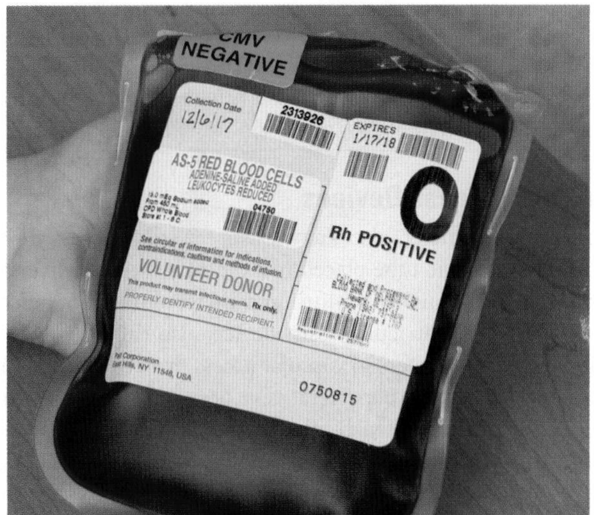

Fig. 15.1 Unit of blood showing the International Society of Blood Transfusion (ISBT) universal bar code for blood transfusions. (From Perry, A., Potter, P., & Ostendorf, W. [2017]. *Clinical nursing skills & techniques* [9th ed.]. St. Louis: Mosby.)

Strategies to reduce errors include awareness of high-alert drugs including look-alike, sound-alike drugs; limiting available concentrations of drugs; and dispensing all drugs, including catheter flush solutions, in single-dose, single-use containers. Smart pumps with drug libraries (see Infusion Systems section), in combination with computer provider (physician, nurse practitioner, physician assistant) order entry (CPOE) and bar-code medication administration (BCMA) systems, use recent technology to help reduce adverse drug events (ADEs).

Prescribing Infusion Therapy

A prescription for infusion therapy written by an authorized primary health care provider (physician, nurse practitioner, or physician assistant) is necessary before IV therapy begins. To be complete, the prescription for infusion fluids should include:

- Specific type of fluid to be infused
- Rate of administration written in milliliters per hour (mL/hr) or the total amount of fluid and the total number of hours for infusion (e.g., 125 mL/hr or 1000 mL/8 hr)
- Specific drugs and dose to be added to the solution such as electrolytes or vitamins

A drug prescription should include:

- Drug name, preferably by generic name
- Specific dose and route
- Frequency of administration
- Time(s) of administration
- Length of time for infusion (number of doses/days)
- Purpose (required in some health care agencies, especially nursing homes)

Some continuously infused drugs such as those for pain management are prescribed as milligrams per hour. The type and volume of dilution for infusion medications may be included in the prescription or calculated by the infusion pharmacist.

! NURSING SAFETY PRIORITY (QSEN)

Action Alert

Determine that the IV prescription is appropriate for the patient and clarify any questions with the primary health care provider before administration. Be sure to check for the accuracy and completeness of the treatment prescription. For example: "5% dextrose in water to keep the vein open" (TKO or KVO) does not specify the rate of infusion and is an incomplete prescription.

Vascular Access Devices

An infusion catheter, also known as a **vascular access device (VAD)**, is a plastic tube placed in a blood vessel to deliver fluids and medications. This infusion catheter should not be confused with the ventricular assist device, also called a VAD. In this chapter VAD refers to vascular access devices. The location of the VAD, either a peripheral vein or a large central vein in the chest, is determined by the specific type and purpose of the therapy. Advances in catheter materials and insertion techniques have radically expanded the types of VADs currently used. This discussion includes the description of each type of catheter used for peripheral and central IV therapy including:

- Short peripheral catheters (SPC)
- Midline catheters

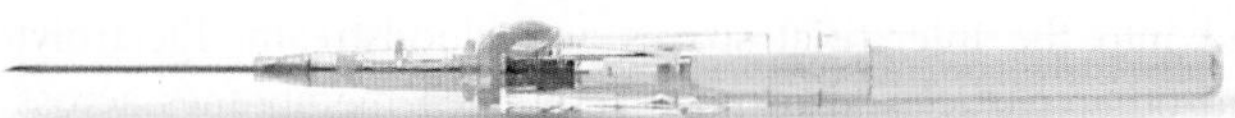

Fig. 15.2 BD Insyte Autoguard IV catheter. With the push of a button, the needle instantly retracts, reducing the risk for accidental needlestick injuries. (Courtesy and © Becton, Dickinson and Company.)

- Peripherally inserted central catheters (PICCs)
- Nontunneled percutaneous central venous catheters (CVCs)
- Tunneled catheters
- Implanted ports
- Hemodialysis catheters

Assess the patient's needs for vascular access and choose the device that has the best chance of infusing the prescribed therapy for the required length of time. Depending on the patient and type of VAD needed, a topical anesthetic agent or intradermal lidocaine HCl 1% may be helpful to decrease patient discomfort. Obtain a primary health care provider's prescription and always check for patient allergies before administering any anesthetic.

NCLEX EXAMINATION CHALLENGE 15.1

Safe and Effective Care Environment

A client had a 20-gauge short peripheral catheter (SPC) inserted for antibiotic administration 48 hours ago. Which nursing intervention is appropriate?

A. Discontinue the SPC.
B. Relocate the SPC for infection control.
C. Assess the SPC for redness, swelling, or pain.
D. Change the occlusive dressing covering the SPC.

PERIPHERAL INTRAVENOUS THERAPY

Short infusion catheters are the most commonly used vascular access devices (VADs) for **peripheral IV therapy**. They are usually placed in the veins of the arm. Another catheter used for peripheral IV therapy is a midline catheter.

Short Peripheral Catheters

Short peripheral catheters are composed of a plastic cannula built around a sharp stylet extending slightly beyond the cannula (Fig 15.2). The stylet allows for the venipuncture, and the cannula is advanced into the vein. Once the cannula is advanced into the vein, the stylet is withdrawn. A federal law enacted in 2000 amended the Bloodborne Pathogen Standards from the Occupational Safety and Health Administration (OSHA) requiring the use of catheters with an engineered safety mechanism to prevent needlesticks. Therefore these catheters are designed with a safety mechanism to cover the sharp end of the stylet after it is removed from the patient to decrease the risk of accidental injury. The stylet is a hollow-bore, blood-filled needle that carries a high risk for exposure to bloodborne pathogens if needlestick injury occurs.

Insertion and Placement Methods. Short peripheral catheters are most often inserted into superficial veins of the forearm. In emergent situations, these catheters can also be used in the external jugular vein of the neck. *Avoid the use of veins in the* *lower extremities of adults, if possible, because of an increased risk for deep vein thrombosis and infiltration.*

Short catheters range in length from ¾ inch to 1¼ inch, with gauge sizes from 26-gauge (the smallest) to 14-gauge (large bore). Choose the smallest-gauge catheter capable of delivering the prescribed therapy with consideration of all the contributing factors, including expected duration, vascular characteristics, and comorbidities (INS, 2016). Current design improves the fluid flow through the catheter while using a smaller gauge and thereby decreases the possibility of vein irritation from a large catheter. For example, a thin-walled 24-gauge catheter has about the same flow-rate ability as a 22-gauge non–thin-walled catheter. Larger-gauge sizes allow for faster flow rates but also cause phlebitis more often. Table 15.1 lists each gauge size and its common uses.

There is no specific timeframe that short peripheral catheters may stay in (dwell). The recommendations from both the Centers for Disease Control and Prevention (CDC) and the INS are that the catheter should be removed and/or rotated to a different site based on clinical indications (e.g., signs of phlebitis [warmth, tenderness, erythema, or palpable venous cord], infection, or malfunction) (INS, 2016). This process requires conscientious and frequent assessment of the site. INS (2016) recommends assessment at least every 4 hours—every 1 to 2 hours for vulnerable patients and every 4 hours for continuous infusions for outpatient and home care patients; otherwise, site assessment should be done once a day. When selecting the site for insertion of a peripheral catheter, consider the patient's age, history, and diagnosis; the type and duration of the prescribed therapy; and, whenever possible, the patient's preference. See the Best Practice for Patient Safety & Quality Care: Placement of Short Peripheral Venous Catheters box for the major criteria for the placement of short peripheral venous catheters.

Vascular visualization technology (e.g., near infrared and ultrasound devices) are now available as tools to assist in IV line placement. Several different types of portable *vein transilluminators* are available such as VeinViewer, Veinlite LED, and AccuVein AV 300 (Fig. 15.3). Although they may have different mechanisms of action (some use infrared light and some use laser), these devices penetrate only up to about 10 mm and are limited to finding *superficial* veins.

Ultrasound-guided peripheral IV insertion can allow insertion into *deeper* veins (Fabiani et al., 2017). This technology has been shown to be valuable in assisting with cannulation of peripheral veins that the nurse cannot access with sight and touch. However, there are risks the nurse must be aware of when using ultrasound guidance. This technology should be used only by nurses who have been trained and whose competencies are maintained. Arteries and nerves often lie parallel to deep veins, and training is essential to learn to identify these structures and avoid damaging them. In addition, when deeper veins are used, infiltration may go undetected until a significant amount of fluid has collected in the tissues. This complication can be particularly devastating if the solution is an irritant or vesicant.

For patients who need IV access but are at risk for fluid overload or do not need additional IV fluids, the peripheral vascular access device (VAD) can be converted into an intermittent IV lock, also called a *saline lock*. This device allows administration of specific drugs given IV push (e.g., furosemide) or on an intermittent basis using a medication administration set. IV antibiotics are frequently administered using a saline lock. For

BEST PRACTICE FOR PATIENT SAFETY & QUALITY CARE (QSEN)

Placement of Short Peripheral Venous Catheters

- Verify that the prescription for infusion therapy is complete and appropriate for infusion through a short peripheral catheter.
- For adults, choose a site for placement in the upper extremity. DO NOT USE THE WRIST.
- Choose the patient's nondominant arm when possible.
- Choose a distal site and make all subsequent venipunctures proximal to previous sites.
- Do not use the arm on the side of a mastectomy, lymph node dissection, arteriovenous shunt or fistula, or paralysis.
- Avoid choosing a site in an area of joint flexion.
- Avoid choosing a site in a vein that feels hard or cordlike.
- Avoid choosing a site close to areas of cellulitis, dermatitis, or complications from previous catheter sites.
- Choose a vein of appropriate length and width to fit the size of the catheter required for infusion.
- Limit unsuccessful attempts to two per clinician and no more than four total (INS, 2016).

TABLE 15.1 Choosing the Gauge Size for Peripheral Catheters

Catheter Gauge	Indications	Approximate Flow Rates
24-26 gauge Smallest, shortest (¾-inch length)	Not ideal for viscous infusions Expect blood transfusion to take longer Preferred for infants and small children	24 mL/min (1440 mL/hr)
22 gauge	Adequate for most therapies; blood can infuse without damage	38 mL/min (2280 mL/hr)
20 gauge (1- to 1¼-inch length)	Adequate for all therapies Most providers of anesthesia prefer not to use a smaller size than this for surgery cases	65 mL/min (3900 mL/hr)
18 gauge	Preferred size for surgery Vein needs to be large enough to accommodate the catheter	110 mL/min (6600 mL/hr)
14-16 gauge	For trauma and surgical patients requiring rapid fluid resuscitation Needs to be in a vein that can accommodate	Over 200 mL/min (12,000 mL/hr)

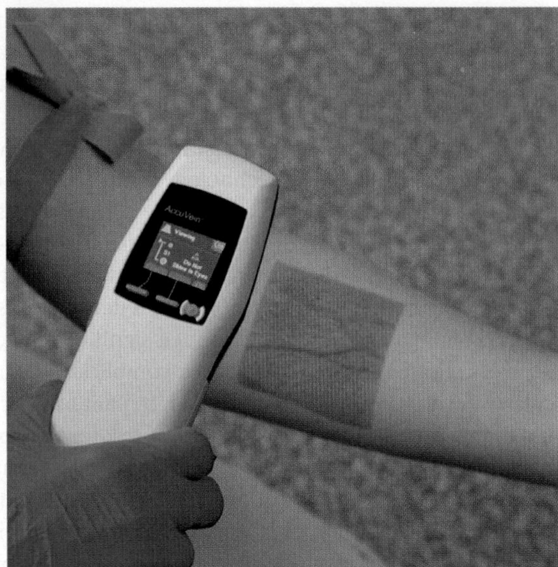

Fig. 15.3 The AccuVein AV300 is a vein illumination device that helps health care professionals locate veins for blood draw, IV infusion, and blood donation by projecting a pattern of light on the patient's skin to reveal the position of underlying veins on the skin's surface. The device uses red and infrared light, which the hemoglobin in blood absorbs to detect the position of the vein. (Courtesy AccuVein, LLC.)

many patients, the saline lock is placed in case there is a need for emergency drug administration via IV push. The intermittent device is flushed with saline before and after drug administration to ensure patency and prevent occlusion with a blood clot. These VADs are not recommended for obtaining routine blood samples due to the risk of hemolysis.

Site Selection and Skin Preparation. The most appropriate veins for peripheral catheter placement include the dorsal venous network (i.e., basilic, cephalic, and median veins and their branches) (Fig. 15.4). *However, cannulation of veins on the hand is not appropriate for older patients with a loss of skin turgor and poor vein condition or for active patients receiving infusion therapy in an ambulatory care clinic or home care. Use of veins on the dorsal surface of the hands should be reserved as a last resort for short-term infusion of nonvesicant and nonirritant solutions in young patients.*

Mastectomy, axillary lymph node dissection, lymphedema, paralysis of the upper extremity, and the presence of dialysis grafts or fistulas alter the normal pattern of blood flow through the arm. Using veins in the extremity affected by one of these conditions requires a primary health care provider's order.

! NURSING SAFETY PRIORITY QSEN

Critical Rescue

Avoid veins on the palmar side of the wrist because the median nerve is located close to veins in this area, making the venipuncture more painful and difficult to stabilize. The cephalic vein begins above the thumb and extends up the entire length of the arm. This vein is usually large and prominent, appearing as a prime site for catheter insertion. Reports of tingling, feeling "pins and needles" in the extremity, or numbness during the venipuncture procedure can indicate nerve puncture. If any of these symptoms occur, stop the IV insertion procedure immediately, remove the catheter, and choose a new site.

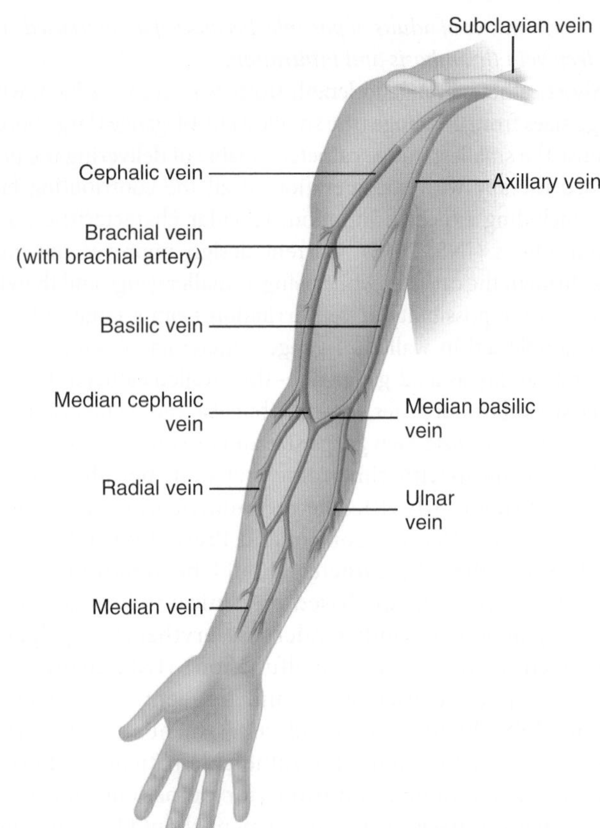

Fig. 15.4 Common IV sites in the inner arm.

Winged needles ("butterfly needles") are easy to insert but are associated with a high frequency of infiltration. They are most commonly used for injecting single-dose drugs or drawing blood samples. Like a short peripheral catheter, winged needles should also have an engineered safety mechanism to house the needle when removed.

Aseptic skin preparation and technique before IV insertion are crucial. **Catheter-related bloodstream infection (CRBSI)** can occur from a peripheral IV site. Both the CDC and the INS have best practice guidelines developed to prevent infection. Bundling best practice into sequential steps to prevent complications reflects evidence-based practice (Crowell, O'Neil, & Drager, 2017). The HANDS mnemonic (Box 15.1) has been used to effectively demonstrate bundling of best practice (Caguioa et al. as cited in Crowell, O'Neil, & Drager, 2017).

Midline Catheters

Midline catheters can be anywhere from 3 to 8 inches long, 3 to 5 Fr, and double or single lumen. They are inserted into a vein of the upper arm. The median antecubital vein is used most often if insertion is done without the aid of ultrasound guidance. With ultrasound guidance, deeper veins can be accessed and the insertion site can be farther above the antecubital fossa. The basilic vein is preferred over the cephalic vein because of its larger diameter and straighter path. It also allows greater hemodilution of the fluids and medications being infused, resulting in less potential irritation from the IV solution. The catheter tip is located in the upper arm, with the tip residing no farther into the venous network than the axillary vein (Fig. 15.5).

BOX 15.1 HANDS Mnemonic

H: Hygiene—Wash your hands and use gloves before inserting a peripheral catheter or drawing blood. Ensure that skin is clean. If visibly soiled, cleanse with soap and water.
A: Antisepsis—Prepare clean skin with a skin antiseptic (chlorhexidine 2% with 70% alcohol, 70% isopropyl alcohol, or povidone-iodine) with a back-and-forth motion for 30 seconds and allow the solution to dry before peripheral venous catheter insertion.
N: No-Touch Technique—Once the area has been prepped, do not touch the site.
D: Documentation—Document assessment of the site, dressing, and tubing. Ensure that the date is clear for all infusion sites.
S: Scrub the Hub—Scrub the hub of the catheter site with an alcohol pad for at least 15 seconds each time you access an infusion site.

From Crowell, J., O'Neil, K., & Drager, L. (2017). Project HANDS. A bundled approach to increase short peripheral catheter dwell time. *Journal of Infusion Nursing, 40*(5), 274–280. doi: 10.1097/NAN.0000000000000237.

Midline catheters reduce the number of repeated IV cannulations, which reduces patient discomfort, increases patient satisfaction, and contributes to organizational efficiency (Xu et al., 2016). A midline catheter can be used when skin integrity or limited peripheral veins make it difficult to maintain a short peripheral catheter. Indications for midline catheters include fluids for hydration and drug therapy that are given longer than 6 days and up to 14 days (Moureau & Chopra, 2016; Chopra, 2018). Because of the extended dwell time, strict sterile technique is used for insertion and dressing changes for a midline catheter. Additional education and skill assessment are required for the nurse to be qualified to insert midline catheters.

Midline catheters are considered to dwell in the peripheral circulation; the recommendations for infusates (fluids or drugs) are the same as for short peripheral IV lines. Fluids and medications infused through a midline catheter should have a pH between 5 and 9 and a final osmolarity of less than 600 mOsm/L (Kear, 2017). The pH and osmolarity outside these parameters increase the risk for complications such as phlebitis and thrombosis. Midline catheters should not be used for infusion of **vesicant medications**—drugs that cause severe tissue damage if they escape into the subcutaneous tissue (**extravasation**). There is concern that at a midline tip location, larger amounts of the drug may extravasate before the problem is detected.

All parenteral nutrition formulas, including those with low concentrations of dextrose and solutions that have an osmolarity greater than 600 mOsm/L, should not be infused through a midline. Do not draw blood from these catheters routinely. Midline catheters should not be placed in extremities affected by mastectomy with lymphedema, paralysis, or dialysis grafts and fistulas. When using a double-lumen midline catheter, do not administer incompatible drugs simultaneously through both lumens because the blood flow rate in the axillary vein is not high enough to ensure adequate hemodilution and prevention of drug interaction in the vein. Currently new midlines with power-injectable technology are available for use with computed tomography.

NCLEX EXAMINATION CHALLENGE 15.2

Physiological Integrity

The primary health care provider has prescribed 1 L of D_5NS to infuse at a rate of 125 mL/hr. The nurse begins the infusion at 0700 (7 a.m.). When will the nurse anticipate completion of the infusion?

A. 1300 hours (1 p.m.)
B. 1500 hours (3 p.m.)
C. 1900 hours (7 p.m.)
D. 2100 hours (9 p.m.)

CENTRAL INTRAVENOUS THERAPY

In **central IV therapy** the vascular access device (VAD) is placed in the central circulation, specifically within the superior vena cava (SVC) near its junction with the right atrium, also called the *caval-atrial junction (CAJ)*. Blood flow in the SVC is about 2 L/min compared with about 200 mL/min in the axillary vein. Most central vascular access devices require confirmation of tip location at the CAJ by chest x-ray before solutions are infused. However, newer technologies use either a magnet tip locator or identification of the CAJ by electrocardiogram rather than by x-ray. Both the Sherlock 3CG by Bard and the VasoNova/Teleflex systems have received Food and Drug Administration (FDA) approval as alternatives to chest x-ray or fluoroscopy to verify PICC tip location.

A number of types of central vascular access devices (CVADs) are available, depending on the purpose, duration, and insertion site availability. Several recent improvements in catheter materials allow antimicrobial and heparin coatings to reduce infection risk and improve the longevity of the catheter. Not all central-line catheters are approved for power injection used in radiologic tests. The catheter can rupture if it is not designed to handle the injection pressure necessary for some tests such as pulmonary CT angiography or CT angiography of the aorta. Be sure to confirm if the PICC is designed as power injectable to ensure safe patient care.

Peripherally Inserted Central Catheters

A **peripherally inserted central catheter (PICC)** is a long catheter inserted through a vein of the antecubital fossa (inner aspect of the bend of the arm) or the middle of the upper arm. Nurses who insert these CVADs require special training and competency confirmation.

In adults the PICC length ranges from 18 to 29 inches (45 to 74 cm), with the tip residing in the superior vena cava (SVC) ideally at the caval-atrial junction (CAJ) (Fig. 15.6). Placement of the catheter tip in veins distal to the SVC is avoided. This inappropriate tip location, often called a *midclavicular catheter*, is associated with much higher rates of thrombosis than when the tip is located in the SVC at the CAJ. Midclavicular tip locations are used only when anatomic or pathophysiologic changes prohibit placing the catheter into the SVC.

PICCs should be inserted early in the course of therapy before veins of the extremity have been damaged from multiple venipunctures and infusions. Insertion methods using guidewires and ultrasound systems greatly improve insertion success.

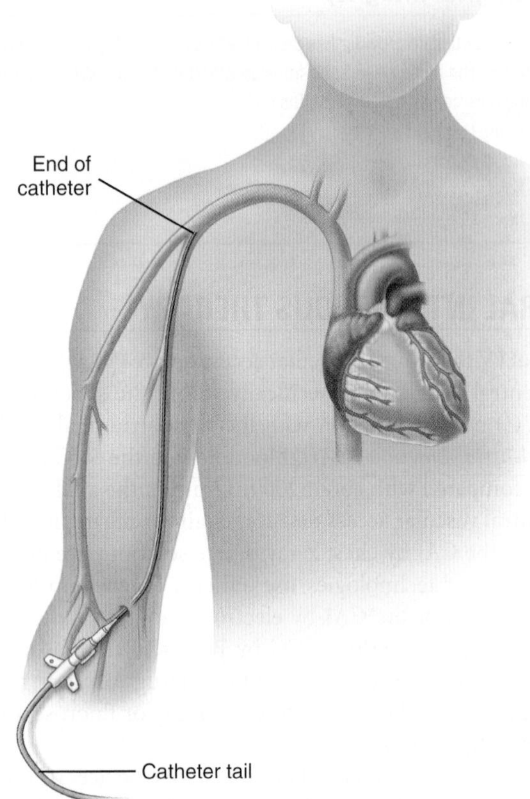

Fig. 15.5 Midline catheter; the tip of this catheter resides in a peripheral vein.

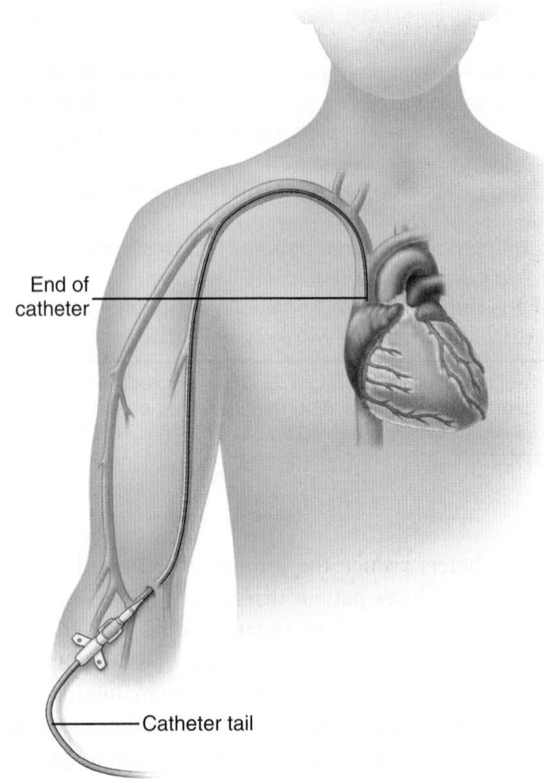

Fig. 15.6 Peripherally inserted central catheter (PICC) is placed peripherally in a vein of the upper arm with the tip resting in the superior vena cava.

The basilic vein is the preferred site for insertion; the cephalic vein can be used if necessary. Two brachial veins are not recommended because they are more difficult to access; they are deeper in the arm and run close to the brachial artery. *Sterile technique is used for insertion to reduce the risk for CRBSI. Before the catheter can be used for infusion, a chest x-ray indicating that the tip resides in the lower SVC is required when the catheter is not placed under fluoroscopy or with the use of the electrocardiogram tip-locator technique.*

PICCs are available in single-, dual-, or triple-lumen configurations and with both the Groshong valve and the pressure-activated safety valve (PASV). PICCs are also available as "Power PICCs" and can be used for contrast injection at a maximum of 5 mL/sec and a maximum pressure of 300 psi. They can also be connected to transducers and used to monitor central venous pressure.

The most common complications from PICCs include phlebitis, thrombophlebitis, deep vein thrombosis (DVT), and CRBSIs. When infections occur from a central line, they are also referred to as **central line–associated bloodstream infection, or CLABSI**. Thrombophlebitis and DVT can be very serious, threaten the integrity of the vein, and decrease perfusion. The smallest possible French size should be used to decrease the rate of upper-extremity DVT, a potentially life-threatening event.

CRBSI has been noted to be less common in PICCs than in other central venous catheters (CVCs) because of the insertion site in the upper extremity. The cooler, drier skin of the upper arm has fewer types and numbers of microorganisms, leading to lower rates of infection. Accidental arterial puncture or excessive bleeding can occur on insertion and is controlled by direct pressure. Infiltration and extravasation are rare. Insertion complications such as pneumothorax associated with other CVCs do not occur with PICCs.

PICCs can accommodate infusion of all types of therapy because the tip resides in the SVC where the rapid blood flow quickly dilutes the fluids being infused. Therefore there are no limitations on the pH or osmolality of fluids that can be infused through a PICC. For example, patients requiring lengthy courses (more than 14 days) of antibiotics, chemotherapy agents, parenteral nutrition formulas, and vasopressor agents can benefit from this type of catheter (Chopra, 2018). PICCs have been reported to dwell successfully for several months; however, the optimal dwell time is not known (Chopra, 2018).

PICCs can be used for blood sampling; however, lumen sizes of 4 Fr or larger are recommended. Using lumens with small diameters may not yield a sample capable of producing the needed test results. In addition, frequent entry into any central line should be minimized and treated with strict aseptic technique to prevent CRBSI. Transfusion of blood through a PICC usually requires the use of an infusion pump. Packed red blood cells are cold and viscous. The length of the catheter adds resistance and may prevent the blood from infusing within the 4-hour limit.

Teach patients with a PICC to perform usual ADLs; however, the patient should avoid excessive physical activity. Muscle contractions in the arm from physical activity such as heavy lifting can lead to catheter dislodgment and possible lumen occlusion. PICCs may be contraindicated in paraplegic patients who rely on their arms for mobility and in patients using crutches that provide support in the axilla.

PICC insertion is commonly performed in the patient's hospital room, an ambulatory care treatment facility, or the imaging department. Regardless of the environment of care where they are inserted, the same precautions must be taken as with any other central line insertion using the **catheter-related bloodstream infection (CRBSI) prevention bundle**. Major components of this prevention bundle include:

- Proper aseptic hand hygiene
- Measuring upper arm circumference as a baseline before insertion (INS, 2016)
- Maximal barrier precautions on insertion
- Chlorhexidine skin antisepsis
- Optimal catheter site selection and postplacement care with avoidance of the femoral vein for central venous access in adult patients
- Daily review of line necessity with prompt removal of unnecessary lines

Other helpful interventions include use of a checklist for sterility during the procedure, a line cart with all equipment, and a stop sign on the door of the room to stop unnecessary traffic through the room during the procedure. The checklist should be completed by another professional health care member who can stop the inserter when any breaks in technique are observed (INS, 2016).

! NURSING SAFETY PRIORITY (QSEN)

Action Alert

The INS recommends that PICC lines not actively in use be flushed with heparin at least daily when using a nonvalved catheter and at least weekly with a valved catheter. Be sure to refer to agency policy and give extra attention to heparin concentration. Use 10 mL of sterile saline to flush before and after medication administration; 20 mL of sterile saline flush after drawing blood. *Always use 10-mL barrel syringes to flush any central line because the pressure exerted by a smaller barrel poses a risk for rupturing the catheter.*

Nontunneled Percutaneous Central Venous Catheters

Nontunneled central venous catheters (CVCs) are inserted percutaneously with the catheter exiting the skin near the cannulation site. These catheters can be inserted by a physician, physician assistant, nurse practitioner, or qualified RN through the subclavian vein in the upper chest or the internal jugular veins in the neck using sterile technique (Plohal et al., 2017). Occasionally the patient's condition may require insertion of the CVC in a femoral vein, but the rate of infection is very high. If the femoral site must be used, it is removed as soon as possible.

CVCs are usually 7 to 10 inches (18 to 25 cm) long and have one to as many as five lumens (Fig. 15.7). These catheters are also available with antimicrobial coatings such as chlorhexidine and silver sulfadiazine. The tip resides in the superior vena cava unless the CVC was inserted using the femoral vein. CVCs inserted using the femoral vein terminate in the inferior vena cava (Androes & Heffner, 2020). Placement is confirmed by chest x-ray. Nontunneled CVCs are most commonly used for emergent or trauma situations, critical care, and surgery. There is no recommendation for optimal dwell time. However, these catheters are commonly used for short-term situations and are *not* the catheter of choice for home care or ambulatory clinic settings.

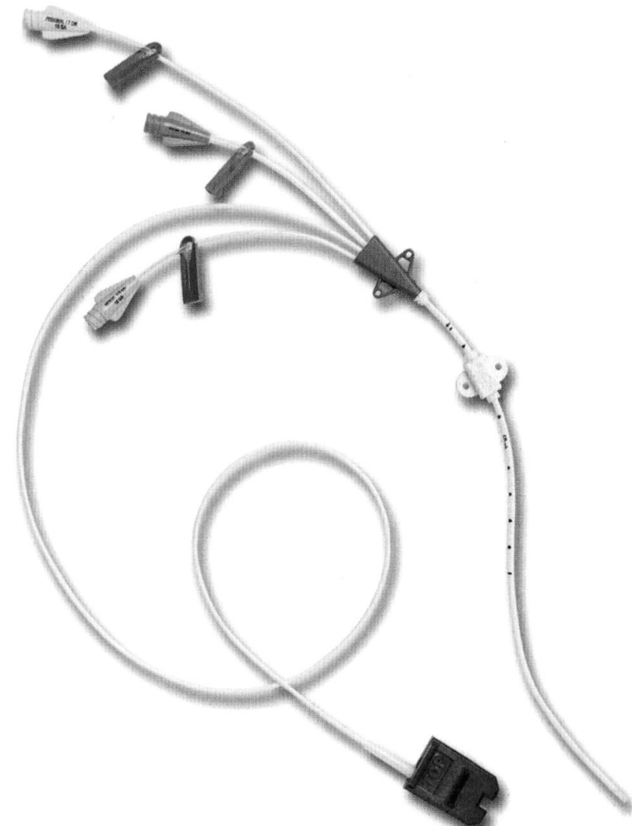

Fig. 15.7 Edwards Lifesciences PreSep central venous catheter (CVC); often placed in the subclavian or internal jugular vein with the tip of the catheter resting in the superior vena cava. (Courtesy Edwards Lifesciences, Irvine, CA.)

Insertion of these central catheters requires the patient to be placed in the Trendelenburg position, usually with a rolled towel between the shoulder blades. This position may be difficult or contraindicated for patients with respiratory conditions, spinal curvatures, and increased intracranial pressure, especially for older adults (Coulter, 2016). Trauma, surgery, or radiation in the neck or chest prohibits the use of these devices as well. Insertion with ultrasound guidance has been demonstrated to improve the safety of insertion in the internal jugular site. The presence of a tracheotomy increases the risk for cross-contamination of the insertion site. The warmer, moister skin of the neck and upper chest has more types and higher numbers of microorganisms, resulting in more CRBSIs with this type of catheter.

Tunneled Central Venous Catheters

Tunneled central venous catheters are VADs that have part of the catheter lying in a subcutaneous tunnel, separating the

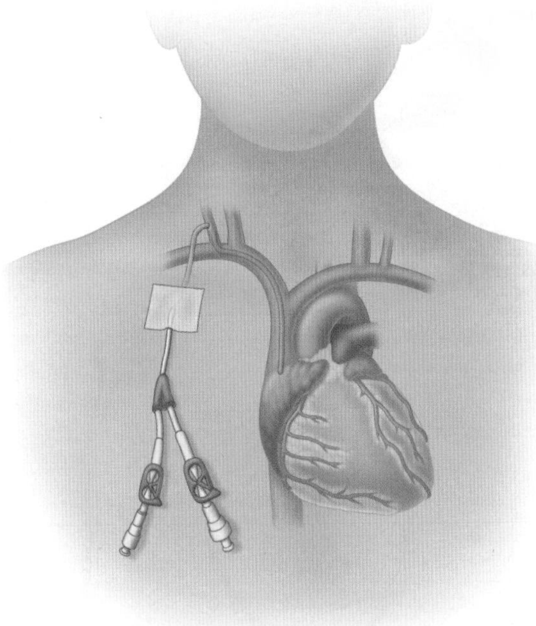

Fig. 15.8 Tunneled catheter. Part of this catheter lies in a subcutaneous tunnel, separating the point where the catheter enters the vein from where it exits the skin.

points where the catheter enters the vein from where it exits the skin. This separation is intended to prevent the organisms on the skin from reaching the bloodstream (Fig. 15.8). These catheters are usually inserted by physicians in the radiology suite rather than placed surgically. The catheter has a cuff made of a rough material that is positioned inside the subcutaneous tunnel. These cuffs commonly contain antibiotics, which also reduce the risk for infection. The tissue granulates into the cuff, providing a mechanical barrier to microorganisms and anchoring the catheter in place.

The design of tunneled CVCs requires surgical techniques for insertion and removal. Single, dual, and triple lumens are available. These catheters were originally named for the physicians who designed them, including Broviac, Hickman, and Leonard catheters.

Tunneled catheters are used primarily when the need for infusion therapy is frequent and long term. Tunneled catheters are chosen when several weeks or months of infusion therapy are needed and a PICC is not a good choice. For example, paraplegic patients needing 6 to 8 weeks of antibiotics are not good candidates for a PICC because of the excessive use of the upper extremities for mobility. Some oncology patients may prefer a tunneled catheter instead of an implanted port because they cannot tolerate the needlesticks required for accessing those devices.

Implanted Ports

Totally implanted ports are very different from other central vascular access devices (CVADs). This type of device is chosen for patients who are expected to require IV therapy for more than a year (Conley et al., 2017). Implanted ports typically are inserted by a physician in the radiology department or a surgeon in the operating suite. Implanted ports consist of a portal body, a dense septum over a reservoir, and a catheter. They can be single or double lumen and come in various sizes. A subcutaneous pocket is surgically created to house the port body. The catheter is inserted into the vein and attached to the portal body. The septum is made of self-sealing silicone and is located in the center of the port body over the reservoir; the catheter extends from the side of the port body. The incision is closed, and no part of the catheter is visible externally; therefore this device has the least impact on body image (Fig. 15.9).

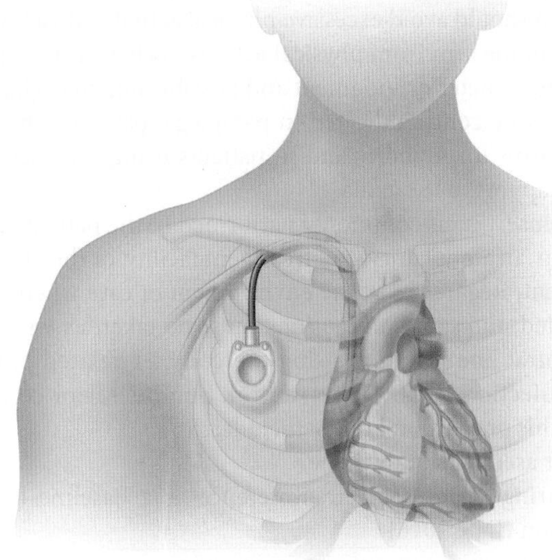

Fig. 15.9 Positioning of an implanted port.

Some implanted ports are power injectable and can be used for obtaining contrast-enhanced computed tomography (CECT). These devices can withstand 5 mL/sec at up to 300 psi pressure. The BARD PowerPort can be identified by palpation of three bumps on the top of the septum and a triangular-shaped port. Be careful not to press firmly on the bumps because it can be painful to the patient. Be sure to use a power-injection–rated noncoring needle with this type of port when used for this purpose. These needles come with labeling identifying that they are power-injection rated (Fig. 15.10).

Venous ports may be placed on the upper chest or the upper extremity and may enter either the subclavian or internal jugular vein. Although an implanted port is most commonly used in the venous system, the catheter may be placed in arteries, the epidural space, or the peritoneal cavity, with the port pocket located over a bony prominence.

Implanted ports are accessed by using a noncoring needle (a common brand name is *Huber*) that is specially designed with a deflected tip. This design slices through the dense septum without coring out a small piece of it, thus preserving the integrity of the septum. Port bodies placed in the chest have a larger septum and usually tolerate about 2000 punctures. Port bodies placed in the upper extremity are smaller and are rated to tolerate about 750 punctures.

Port access should be done only by formally trained health care professionals using a mask and aseptic technique.

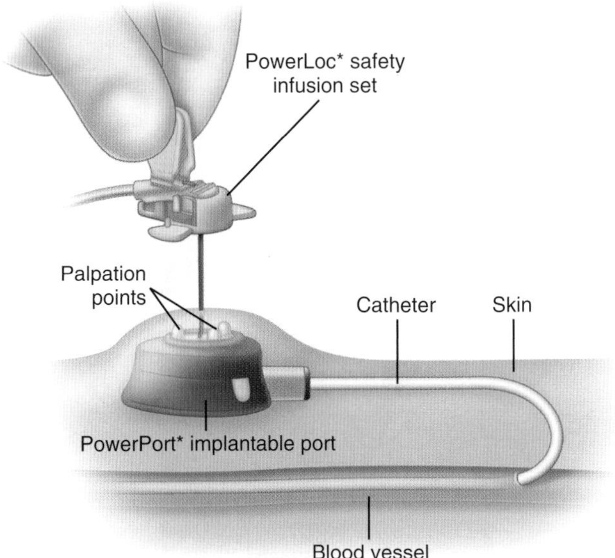

Fig. 15.10 A noncoring needle for accessing an implanted power port.

Implanted ports are used most often for patients receiving chemotherapy. These patients are immune compromised, making them highly susceptible to infection. Before puncture, palpate the port to locate the septum. Carefully palpate to feel the shape and depth of the port body to ensure puncture of the septum, not the attached catheter. Some have attached extension sets and wings to stabilize the needle. One important feature is an engineered safety mechanism to contain the needle when it is removed from the septum. Because the dense septum holds tightly to the needle, there can be a rebound when it is pulled from the septum, which can result in needlestick injury to the nurse.

Implanted ports need to be flushed after each use and at least once a month between courses of therapy. This procedure is done to prevent clot formation in the internal chamber of the port and is often referred to as "locking" or "de-accessing." The INS recommendation for locking or de-accessing a port is the use of a 10-mL syringe with either heparin 10 units per milliliter or preservative-free 0.9% normal saline (INS, 2016). When the port is not accessed, there is no external catheter requiring a dressing. Puncture of the skin over the port is required to gain access to the port body, causing pain for some patients. Topical anesthetic creams can be used to make the access procedure more tolerable.

! NURSING SAFETY PRIORITY QSEN

Drug Alert

Before giving a drug through an implanted port, always check for blood return. INS (2016) defines blood return "as the color and consistency of whole blood upon aspiration" (p. S147). If there is no blood return, withhold the drug until patency and adequate noncoring needle placement of the port are established. Serious extravasations of vesicant drugs can occur because a fibrin sheath (flap or tail) may occur at the tip of the catheter, clot it, and cause retrograde subcutaneous leakage.

Hemodialysis Catheters

Hemodialysis catheters have very large lumens to accommodate the hemodialysis procedure or a pheresis procedure that harvests specific blood cells. They may be tunneled for long-term needs or nontunneled for short-term needs. A hemodialysis catheter is critical to the management of renal failure and must function well. CRBSIs and vein thrombosis are common complications; therefore this catheter should not be used for administration of other fluids or drugs except in an emergency. Because these catheters have very large lumens, heparin is injected and dwells within the lumen to maintain patency. To prevent systemic anticoagulation and subsequent bleeding, the heparin must be aspirated from the lumens before use. The generalist RN generally does not access hemodialysis catheters. These are maintained by specially trained hemodialysis nurses.

INFUSION SYSTEMS

Nurses administering infusion therapies need to understand how infusion systems work. This knowledge ensures that the patient can benefit from a particular system's advantages while minimizing any potential complications.

Containers

Infusion containers are made of glass or plastic. *Glass* bottles were the original fluid container to be mass produced. They are easily sterilized, and it is easy to read the amount of fluid remaining in the bottle. Also, glass is inert and cannot interact with some drugs like plastic can. However, glass bottles are heavy and cannot be used easily in many situations such as patient transport during emergencies. These containers require an air vent for fluids to flow freely from them. The most common method is to use an administration set with a special filtered vent.

Plastic containers are considered *closed systems* because they do not rely on outside air to allow the fluid to infuse. Instead, atmospheric pressure pushes against the flexible sides of the container, allowing the fluid to flow by gravity. For this reason plastic containers do not require vented administration sets. These containers are lightweight, resistant to breaking, easier to store, and easy to use in emergency conditions. Therefore they are used more frequently than glass containers.

All plastic containers were commonly made of polyvinyl chloride (PVC). To increase flexibility and strength, PVC required the addition of a plasticizer such as di-2-ethylhexyl-phthalate or DEHP. Concern has been growing in the past few years over the exposure of patients to this chemical because it can leach from the plastic fluid container or tubing and infuse into the patient with the IV fluid or medication. However, the FDA has determined that there is little to no risk posed to most patients by the limited exposure to the amount of DEHP released from IV bags with infusion of crystalloids or drugs. However, there is concern about the buildup of chemical exposure from many sources over a lifetime of patients who frequently undergo infusion therapy and specifically the potential effects of DEHP on the development of the male reproductive system (Rowdhwal et al., 2018). Therefore many hospitals are using PVC-free and DEHP-free IV bags, especially for high-risk groups.

One disadvantage of removing DEHP from the plastic bags is that the bags are less pliable and more prone to rupture. Some institutions do not allow these bags to be sent through a pneumatic tube system because the pressure exerted has caused the bags to rupture during transport.

A problem with some plastic containers is that they are not compatible with insulin, nitroglycerin, lorazepam, fat emulsions, and lipid-based drugs. Nitroglycerin and insulin adhere to the walls of the PVC container, making it impossible to know exactly how much medication the patient is receiving. Another concern with plastic bags is the accuracy of reading the amount of fluid remaining in the container and the residual volume in some sets.

! NURSING SAFETY PRIORITY (QSEN)

Action Alert

Regardless of the type of fluid container used, it is necessary to check it for cracks, damage, or pinholes before use. Always observe the fluid for turbidity (cloudiness), particulate matter, or any unusual color that could indicate contamination.

Administration Sets

The administration set is the connection between the catheter and the fluid container. Numerous sets are available in many different configurations. The type and purpose of the infusion determine the type of administration set needed. Some sets are *generic,* meaning that they are appropriate for most infusions. Other sets are used for specific types of infusions such as blood transfusion. Still others are *dedicated,* meaning that they must be used with a specific manufacturer's infusion controlling device. Information that describes their proper use is provided on the packaging of administration sets.

Secondary Administration Sets. A primary continuous administration set is used to infuse the primary IV fluid by either a gravity infusion or an electronic infusion pump. A short **secondary administration set,** also known as a **piggyback set,** is attached to the primary set at a Y–injection site and is used to deliver intermittent medications (Fig. 15.11). Directions and diagrams for use are typically on the packaging. Once attached, these sets should remain connected as an infusion system. Primary and secondary continuous infusion administration sets used to infuse fluids other than parenteral nutrition and lipids can be used for up to 96 hours unless the closed system has been compromised (INS, 2016).

Intermittent Administration Sets. When no primary continuous fluid is being infused, use an intermittent administration set to infuse multiple doses of medications through a catheter that has been capped with a needleless connection device. Remove the medication bag from the previous dose and attach the new one. Remove the sterile cap covering the distal end of the set and attach the set to the catheter. Because both ends of the set are being manipulated with each dose, the INS standards of practice state that this set should be changed every 24 hours. When the administration set is used for infusion of parenteral nutrition or lipid solution, change it every 24 hours. Change blood tubing within 4 hours.

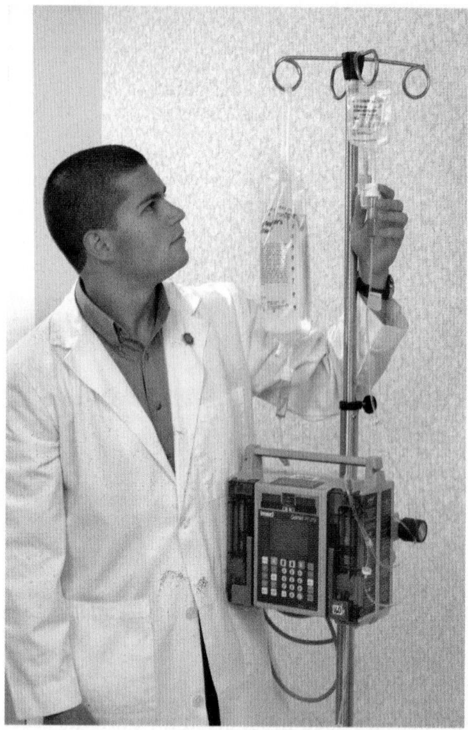

Fig. 15.11 Secondary IV administration set attached to the primary set at a Y-injection site. (Courtesy Rick Brady, Riva, Maryland. In Lilley, L., Collins, S., & Snyder, J. [2014]. *Pharmacology and the nursing process* [7th ed.]. St. Louis: Mosby.)

Administration sets are sterile in the fluid pathway and under the sterile caps on each end of the set. The set is not packaged as a completely sterile product and cannot be added to a sterile field. Careful attention is required to maintain the sterility of the spike and the connection end of the tubing to prevent introduction of microorganisms into the catheter and bloodstream.

Add-on Devices. Several other types of add-on devices include short extension sets, injection caps, and filters. Extension sets may be packaged as a sterile product for adding to a sterile field; however, always check the product label for this information.

Administration sets have two ways to connect to the catheter hub: a slip lock or a Luer-Lok. The *slip lock* is a male end that slips into the female catheter hub. A *Luer-Lok* connection has the same male end with a threaded collar that requires twisting onto the corresponding threads of the catheter hub. All connections, including *extension sets,* should have a Luer-Lok design to ensure that the set remains firmly connected. Loose connections lead to fluid leakage and increase the risk for contamination and subsequent bloodstream infection. When using a central venous catheter, a Luer-Lok connection is critical to reduce the risk for air embolism. Tape is not considered an adequate mechanism for securing set connections.

Luer-Lok devices may be purposefully or accidentally disconnected. Patients or visitors may disconnect the system to allow the patient to get out of bed or the chair, or the device may become accidentally disconnected when the patient turns or moves. In either case be sure to reconnect the device by following the proper sequence to reassemble the IV system components.

Fatalities have resulted when nurses have accidently reconnected IV tubing to a tracheostomy or other inappropriate port.

Filters may be part of the administration set or separate add-on pieces. Their purpose is to remove particulate matter, microorganisms, and air from the infusion system. Filter sizes depend on the pore size, with common sizes being 1.2 microns used to filter lipid-containing parenteral nutrition and 0.2 microns intended to remove all particles and bacteria. Filters should be placed as close to the catheter hub as possible.

Particulate matter in the IV fluid, a primary reason to use filters, comprises undissolved, unintended substances and may include rubber pieces, glass particles, cotton fibers, drug particles, paper, and metal fibers. These particles become trapped in the small circulation of the lungs. A red blood cell is about 5 microns in diameter and is the largest size that can pass through the pulmonary capillary bed; IV fluids may contain particles larger than 5 microns. For patients receiving infusion therapy for long periods, a significant number of particles could block the blood flow through the pulmonary circulation. Microcirculation in the spleen, kidneys, and liver could also be affected. Particulate matter has also been implicated in the development of phlebitis in peripheral veins.

Other concerns with using filters include the possibility for their rupture, their use with certain drugs that bind to the filter surface, using the incorrect size of filter for drugs with large molecules, and choosing a filter that will not tolerate the pressure exerted by infusion pumps. Rupture is most commonly associated with the exertion of high pressure exceeding the limit tolerated by the specific filter. Some drugs cannot be filtered because they are retained inside the filter because of their chemical nature or molecule size. For these reasons medication filtration during the process of admixing is commonly used today as an alternative to final filtration at the bedside. Drugs of a very small quantity should be administered below the filter.

Filters used on blood administration sets have much larger pore size and are not interchangeable with filters used for fluids and medications. A standard blood filter ranges from 170 to 260 microns and removes microclots and other debris caused by blood collection and storage. Microaggregate filters have a pore size of 20, 40, or 80 microns and are used to remove degenerating platelets, white blood cells, and fibrin strands. Leukocyte-removal filters are used to remove white blood cells that cause febrile and allergic blood transfusion reactions.

Needleless Connection Devices. In July 1992, the Occupational Safety and Health Administration (OSHA) published guidelines entitled *Occupational Exposure to Bloodborne Pathogens, Final Rule.* This document requires health care organizations to initiate engineering controls "that isolate or remove the bloodborne pathogen hazard from the workplace." This standard was amended in 2001 with the passage of the Needlestick Safety and Prevention Act. This regulation requires the use of devices engineered with safety mechanisms and mandates that staff who perform these tasks be directly involved with selecting products. It also requires each employer to maintain a sharps injury log with details of each incident. Many products are designed to minimize health care workers' exposure to contaminated needles. Luer-lock–activated devices are the most common design for needleless systems today.

Although these devices have reduced the incidence of accidental needlesticks for health care professionals, it is imperative that the connector be disinfected with alcohol or chlorhexidine/alcohol before and after each use with a *vigorous scrub* for 5 to 60 seconds (INS, 2016). This method is often referred to as "scrub the hub" (The Joint Commission, 2013). Blood and bacteria can be trapped in the crevices, and meticulous disinfecting is required with each use.

Various designs are available for connectors that provide positive or negative displacement of fluid when the needleless syringe is removed. Needleless positive-pressure valve (PPV) connectors were developed to prevent backflow of blood into the IV catheter, thereby decreasing chances of thrombus formation and CRBSI. Several newer connectors are silver impregnated to reduce bacterial growth (Fig. 15.12). Be sure to check which type of connector valve is used in your facility because the flushing technique differs depending on type.

To reduce infection risk in all needleless systems, implement these interventions:

- Clean all needleless system connections vigorously with an antimicrobial (usually 70% alcohol or alcohol and 2% chlorhexidine swabs) for 10 to 15 seconds before connecting infusion sets or syringes, paying special attention to the small ridges in the Luer-Lok device. The "scrub the hub" technique suggests generating friction by scrubbing the connection hubs in a twisting motion as if you were juicing an orange (The Joint Commission, 2013). Newer caps that are impregnated with alcohol or chlorhexidine may be used to keep the port aseptic; however, these will increase costs, and research is needed to demonstrate the benefit.
- Do not tape connections between tubing sets.
- Use evidence-based hand hygiene guidelines from the CDC and OSHA.

Rate-Controlling Infusion Devices

The ability to regulate the rate and volume of infusions is critical to the safe and accurate administration of medications and fluids to patients. Nurses have a choice of numerous devices that can be electronically or mechanically regulated, adapted to a variety of situations, and handle multiple medication infusions simultaneously.

Electronic infusion devices (IV pumps) are used universally in acute care institutions. They are also used in long-term care

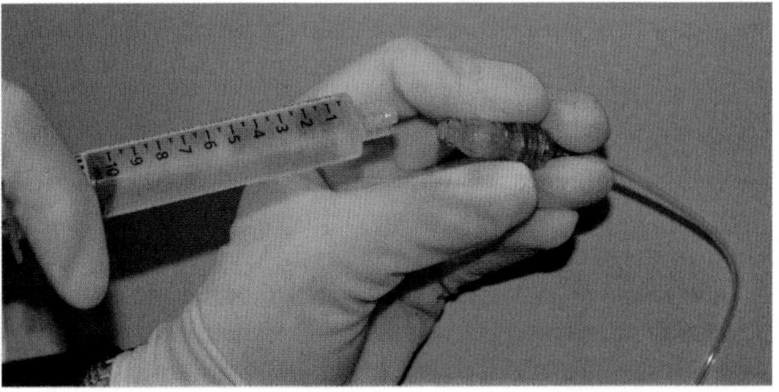

Fig. 15.12 Example of a needleless connector.

settings and in the home. In addition, "smart pumps" provide the latest infusion computer technology to promote patient safety and save nursing time. *Remember that the use of pumps does not decrease the nurse's responsibility to carefully monitor the patient's infusion site and the infusion rate.*

In inpatient settings IV pumps are mobile as they are generally mounted on a pole that has wheels. As their name implies, these electronic devices with battery backup pump drugs or fluids under pressure. These pumps accurately measure the volume of fluid being infused by using one of three mechanisms:

- A syringe-type mechanism that fills and empties
- A wavelike, peristaltic action that pushes fluid along the tubing
- A series of microchambers that fill and empty

Regardless of the pumping mechanism, these devices require dedicated cassette tubing designed to match the pump.

Syringe pumps use an electronic or battery-powered piston to push the plunger of a large syringe inserted into the pump mechanism continuously at a selected milliliter-per-hour rate. The use of syringe pumps is limited to small-volume continuous or intermittent infusions and depends on the syringe size. Antibiotics and patient-controlled analgesia are frequently delivered with syringe pumps. Patients requiring fluid restrictions can also benefit from using a syringe pump because smaller yet accurate volumes can be used to dilute medications.

Ambulatory pumps are generally used for home care patients and allow them to return to their usual activities while receiving infusion therapy. These pumps have a wide range of sizes, with some requiring a backpack, but they usually weigh less than 6 lb. They are typically used to accurately deliver continuous infusions such as parenteral nutrition, pain medication, and many programmable drug schedules. Frequent battery recharging or replacement is usually necessary.

Electronic infusion devices can be programmed in many different ways and require a thorough knowledge of the specific brand being used. Infusion rate and the volume to be infused are usually entered in single milliliter increments, but some can be programmed as fractions of a milliliter. Some pumps allow the rate to be programmed to taper or ramp up and down at the beginning and ending of the infusion. Secondary syringe infusion, secondary infusion rate, remote site programming, adjustable infusion pressure, and integration into the nurse call system are also possible.

Electronic infusion devices have a variety of alarms such as air-in-line, upstream and downstream occlusion, infusion complete, and low-battery or power warnings. All devices must have some mechanism to prevent free flow of the infusing fluid or medication. When the cassette or tubing is removed from the pump, this mechanism automatically stops fluid flow until it is properly replaced in the pump. This safety measure prevents accidental rapid infusion of large amounts of fluid or medication, which could lead to serious clinical problems.

In the past few years, **smart pumps** (infusion pumps with dosage calculation software) have been promoted to reduce adverse drug events (ADEs). Incorrect programming of pumps without this feature is one of the most common types of drug errors, especially in hospitals. Multiple libraries of drug information are stored in the pump manufacturer's medical management system. This software allows the facility to preprogram dosing limits, especially for high-alert drugs. Examples of smart pumps are the B. Braun Outlook 400ES and the Baxter Sigma Spectrum infusion system.

A more recent development in smart pumps is a wireless network connection. Drug libraries can be updated via a wireless connection, thus eliminating the necessity of manually updating each pump. In addition to preventing drug errors, smart-pump systems record potential errors that would have occurred without these safety mechanisms.

Dose-track technology is intended to transmit the infusion data to the institution's pharmacy so that the correct patient receives the correct medication. Dose-guard technology alerts the nurse if institution-defined dose limits are exceeded. These newer technologies provide safeguards for patients to keep them safe. However, the "smarter" the pump, the more extensive the programming steps and the more alarms to which the nurse must respond. In addition, technology and wireless connections can fail. The challenge for nurses is to maintain the skill of manual dose calculation and rate control, acknowledge and validate all alarms, and guard against becoming desensitized to alarms.

> **! NATIONAL PATIENT SAFETY GOALS**
>
> Recognizing and responding to clinical alarms continues to be a top national patient safety goal (The Joint Commission, 2020). The Joint Commission 2020 NPSGs require that hospitals establish alarm safety as a priority. These measures include educating staff of the importance of alarms and the risks that can occur when alarms are dismissed or ignored.

Mechanically regulated devices can be used to deliver intermittent medications such as antibiotics or continuous pain medications in community-based health or home care settings. In acute care settings, devices called "infusers" may be found in surgical services. They are powered by positive pressure from the collapsing balloon or roller returning to its coiled position.

The systems include elastomeric balloons, spring-coiled syringes and containers, and a multichambered fluid container placed in a mechanical roller (Accufuser or ON-Q PainBuster) (Fig. 15.13). These small portable devices do not require power sources such as batteries or electricity. They deliver a preset infusion rate, and fluid volume is determined by the size of the fluid container; however, most hold only 50 to 100 mL, which limits usability.

NURSING CARE FOR PATIENTS RECEIVING INTRAVENOUS THERAPY

Educating the Patient

The current trend in health care requires health care professionals to partner with patients in the provision of patient-centered, evidence-based care.

> **! NATIONAL PATIENT SAFETY GOALS**
>
> The Joint Commission NPSGs require that all patients who have central venous catheters placed must have education on prevention of catheter-related bloodstream infection (CRBSI) (TJC, 2020).

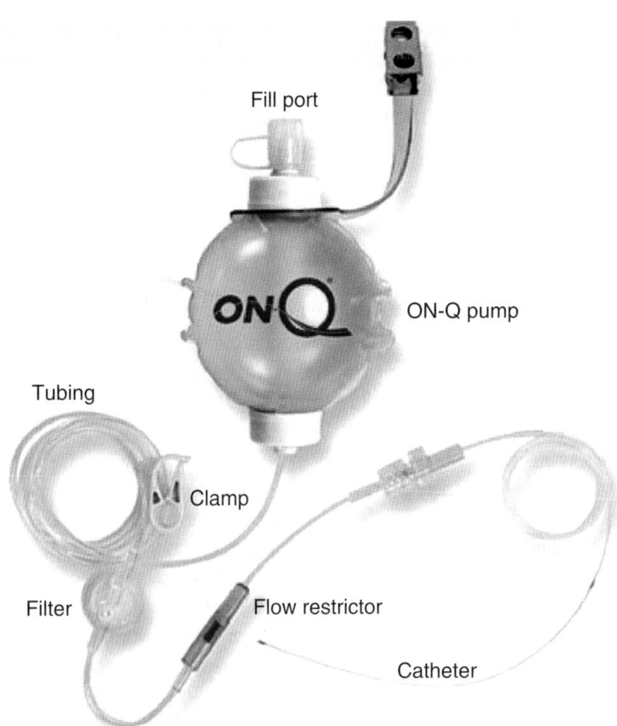

Fig. 15.13 ON-Q PainBuster pump (mechanical infuser). (Courtesy Kimberly-Clark Corporation.)

Before catheter insertion, educate the patient and family about:

- The type of catheter to be used
- Hand hygiene and aseptic technique for care of the catheter
- The therapy required
- Alternatives to the catheter and therapy
- Activity limitations
- Any signs or symptoms of complications that should be reported to a health care professional

Provide written information before placement of a long-term catheter and continue to assess the patient's knowledge level and provide more information or answers as needed. Most manufacturers of PICCs, tunneled catheters, and implanted ports provide patient information booklets. However, specific information about the chosen procedures and supplies may be required. Conversation and pictures are helpful for patients who are literacy challenged (have a low reading level ability). Patients who do not speak or read English will need an appropriate translator.

Performing the Nursing Assessment

All central VADs require documentation of tip location at the caval-atrial junction (CAJ) by electrocardiogram technology, fluoroscopy, or chest x-ray. The initial verbal and subsequent written report should contain specific information about the catheter tip location in relation to anatomic structures. The nurse's knowledge of accurate tip location is required before beginning infusion through the catheter. Repeating the x-ray during catheter use may be necessary if the patient reports unusual pain or sensation.

Nursing assessment for all infusion systems should be systematic beginning at the insertion site, working upward following the tubing to the infusion bag. Know the type of catheter your patient has in place. Be sure to find out the length of catheter, the insertion site, and tip location to perform a complete assessment. Assess the insertion site by looking for redness, swelling, hardness, or drainage. Also assess the skin underneath the dressing, especially for signs of medical adhesive–related skin injury (MARSI) (INS, 2016). When a midline catheter or PICC is used, assess the entire extremity and upper chest for signs of phlebitis and thrombosis. When a tunneled catheter is used, assess the exit site, the entire length of the tunnel, and the point where the catheter enters the vein. For a well-healed catheter, it may not be possible to detect the vein entrance site. On newly inserted catheter sites, there could be a small puncture with a suture or other securement device. For implanted ports, assess the incision and surgically created subcutaneous pocket.

Assess the integrity of the dressing, making sure that it is clean, dry, and adherent to the skin on all sides. Check all connections on the administration set and ensure that they are secure. Be sure that they are not taped. Check the rate of infusion for all fluids by either counting drops or checking the infusion pump. Assess that the amount of fluid that has infused from the container is correct. Is it accurate, or is it infusing too fast or too slow? Adjust the rate to the prescribed flow rate. Check all labels on containers for the patient's name and fluid or medication. *Be sure that the correct solution is being infused!*

! NURSING SAFETY PRIORITY (QSEN)

Action Alert

Remind assistive personnel (AP) to avoid taking blood pressures in an extremity with any type of catheter in place. If a short peripheral catheter is being used for continuous infusion, the compression while taking the blood pressure can increase venous pressure, causing fluid to overflow from the puncture site and infiltration. When a midline catheter or PICC is being used, compression from the blood pressure cuff could increase vein irritation and lead to phlebitis.

Draw blood samples in the extremity opposite from all catheters. Blood should not be drawn from a venipuncture site proximal to (above) an infusing peripheral catheter because the infusing fluid could alter the results of the test to be performed. Venipuncture at or near the insertion site of a midline catheter or PICC could damage the catheter, add to areas of venous inflammation, and decrease perfusion.

Securing and Dressing the Catheter

Securing the catheter is an important step in the prevention of complications. Tape, sutures, and specially designed securement devices can be used for this purpose. For a short peripheral catheter, tape strips are most common; however, the tape should be *clean* and tape strips from a peripheral IV start kit are preferred. Strips of tape should not be taken from rolls of tape moved between patient's rooms, from other procedures, or from uniform pockets. Precutting tape and placing it on the patient's bedrails, your uniform or scrubs, or other object should also be avoided to prevent transmission of microorganisms.

Newer *securement devices* are designed for all catheter types and provide an evidence-based method to prevent VAD movement (INS, 2016). Recent studies have shown that these devices such as the StatLock IV stabilization device prevent peripheral and central catheters from becoming dislodged (Fig. 15.14) (see the Evidence-Based Practice box). In addition, they prevent complications such as phlebitis and infiltration. To prevent skin tears, remove the adhesive on a StatLock with 70% alcohol.

PICCs and nontunneled central catheters may be sutured in place; however, this creates additional breaks in the skin that could become infected. If these sutures are loose or broken, notify the primary health care provider to replace them. IV catheter sutures are being replaced with securement devices and Dermabond glue in some facilities, which can decrease infection and avoid the need to remove sutures after infusion therapy is discontinued.

Tunneled catheters usually have sutures placed near the skin exit site, which are removed after the tunnel has healed. The incision over an implanted port pocket will have sutures until it has healed. After it is healed and when it is not accessed, no dressing is required. When an implanted port is accessed, the sterile occlusive dressing should cover the entire needle and insertion site.

Sterile dressings used over the insertion site protect the skin and puncture site. For a short *peripheral* catheter, the transparent membrane dressings do not require routine changes. Short peripheral lines do not usually dwell longer than a few days, and as long as the dressing is dry, clean, and intact, it does not have to be changed. Any VAD dressing should be changed when it is loose or soiled.

For central lines and midline catheters, tape and sterile gauze or a transparent membrane dressing may be used. Change tape and gauze dressings every 48 hours; change transparent membrane dressings, such as Tegaderm, every 5 to 7 days (INS, 2016). The initial dressing on a midline catheter or PICC is usually tape and gauze, changed within 24 hours after insertion because some bleeding is likely. Transparent membrane dressings can be used for subsequent dressing. For patients who develop erythema (redness) from Tegaderm, the IV3000 dressing from Smith and Nephew may be used. Document when you change the sterile dressing and your IV site assessments in the appropriate electronic health record according to agency policy.

When changing the dressing, remove it by pulling laterally from side to side. It can also be removed by holding the external catheter and pulling it off toward the insertion site. *Never pull it off by pulling away from the insertion site because this could dislodge the catheter!*

After removing the dressing from a midline catheter or any central venous catheter, note the external catheter length. Compare this length with the original length at insertion. If the length has changed, the catheter tip location has also changed and may no longer be in a vein appropriate for infusion. Follow agency policy or notify the primary health care provider about the length change. A chest x-ray may be needed, and careful assessment of the type of therapy and remaining length of therapy will likely be required.

Protect the external catheter, dressing, and all attached tubing from water because it is a source of contamination. *Remind assistive personnel (AP) to cover the extremity where the IV line is located when giving the patient a bath.* A plastic bag or wrap can be taped over the extremity to keep the dressing and site dry.

EVIDENCE-BASED PRACTICE QSEN

What Is the Best Method for Securing a Patient's Peripheral Venous Catheter?

Marsh, N., Webster, J., Mihala, G., & Rickard, C. M. (2017). Devices and dressings to secure peripheral venous catheters: A Cochrane systematic review and meta-analysis. *International Journal of Nursing Studies, 67,* 12–19. https://doi.org/10.1016/J.IJNURSTU.2016.11.007

Venous catheterizations are the most frequent invasive procedures performed in hospitalized patients, and peripheral venous lines are the most common type of VAD (venous access device). It is of significant concern that over 30% of peripheral venous catheters fail before infusion therapy concludes, frequently due to catheter dislodgement or accidental removal. Peripheral venous catheters require stabilization to ensure extended use. Dislodgment is one of the major complications associated with failure of the access device. This study included a systematic review and meta-analysis methodology to explore the fundamental principles of securement and dressing products to prevent peripheral venous access device failure. Comparisons within the study included a variety of dressing and securement devices including transparent dressings versus gauze; bordered transparent dressings versus a securement device; bordered transparent dressings versus tape; and transparent dressings versus adhesive plaster.

Results concluded that there was no one best option in terms of dressing or securement device when compared with the others studied. The researchers concluded that while there was no one best option in terms of reducing accidental dislodgement, there was limited evidence that transparent dressings were more effective than gauze dressings. Future studies are needed to determine the most effective securement that is cost-effective for all populations.

Level of Evidence: 1

This study used a systematic review and meta-analysis to examine current research findings from six randomized control studies (1539 participants) comparing a variety of dressings and securement devices.

Commentary: Implications for Practice and Research

This research study examined the current methods and effectiveness of peripheral VAD securement devices. The results concluded that based on the studies reviewed, there was no one dressing or securement device that was more effective than any other in terms of reducing the frequency of dislodgement. Health care providers need to recognize the priority of securing a peripheral IV and dressing the site appropriately. Agencies are encouraged to collect data and identify procedures and processes to recognize the long-term savings of using securement and dressings to prevent catheter failure for improved patient outcomes. Future clinical research is needed.

Changing Administration Sets and Needleless Connectors

Plan the change of administration sets and fluid containers to occur at the same time, if possible, to minimize the number of times the system is opened. For short peripheral catheters, the administration set and catheter should also be changed at the same time to avoid excessive manipulation of the catheter. Document these changes per agency policy.

Needleless connector devices can be changed when the administration set is changed. If it is being used for intermittent infusions, the device should be changed at least once per

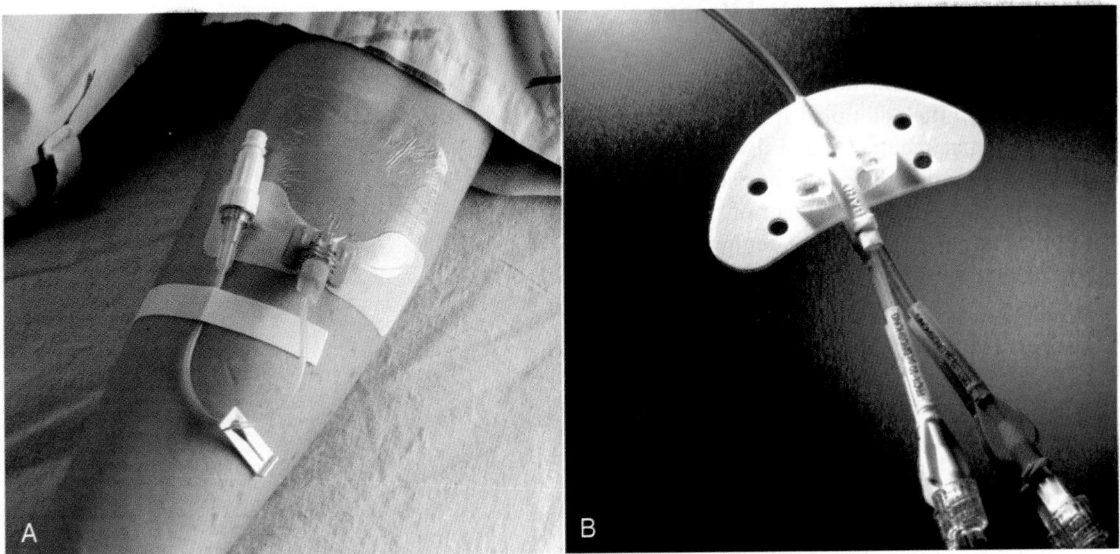

Fig. 15.14 (A and B) The StatLock provides a standardized method to prevent catheter movement. (Courtesy Venetec International, San Diego, CA.)

week. Fluid leakage from the device or tubing indicates that the integrity has been compromised and should be changed immediately. Be sure to date the tubing and document IV site/tubing changes per agency policy.

Precautions to prevent *air emboli* are required when changing the set or connectors attached to any catheter; however, central venous catheters require special attention. Most catheters have a pinch clamp that should be closed during this procedure. Techniques used to increase the intrathoracic pressure and prevent air embolism during IV set change include:

- Placing the patient in a flat or Trendelenburg position to ensure that the catheter exit site is at or below the level of the heart
- Asking the patient to perform a Valsalva maneuver by holding his or her breath and bearing down
- Timing the IV set change to the expiratory cycle when the patient is spontaneously breathing
- Timing the IV set change to the inspiratory cycle when the patient is receiving positive-pressure mechanical ventilation

Controlling Infusion Pressure

In order for fluid to flow through the system, the pressure on the external side must be greater than the pressure at the catheter tip. Fluid flow can be slowed or obstructed from the catheter tip impinging on the vein wall, a thrombus distal to the catheter, or a venous spasm. Inside the catheter lumen, resistance is created by the catheter length and diameter or deposits of fibrin, thrombus, or drug precipitate.

All catheter manufacturers have warnings about the use of excessive pressure. Gravity and infusion pumps do not exert pressure too high for the catheter to handle; however, excessive pressure from syringes can lead to catheter damage. For this reason, use 10-mL syringes when performing an IV push through a central venous catheter. Although these larger syringes generate less pressure, it is still possible to reach excessive pressure levels if great force is applied to a syringe attached to a catheter that is partially occluded.

Flushing the Catheter

Catheter flushing prevents contact between incompatible drugs and maintains patency of the lumens. Normal saline alone or normal saline followed by heparinized saline may be used, depending on the device recommendations. When using valved catheters and certain positive fluid-displacement needleless devices, normal saline alone is acceptable because these devices have mechanisms that prevent backflow of blood into the catheter lumen.

! NURSING SAFETY PRIORITY QSEN

Critical Rescue

Assess catheter patency carefully before each use. Flush the catheter with normal saline while applying slow, gentle pressure to the syringe plunger. If you feel any resistance, stop the procedure immediately! If you continue to exert pressure on the syringe, catheter rupture or forcing a blood clot into circulation could result. During the flushing procedure always aspirate for a brisk blood return from the catheter lumen. If the catheter does not yield a blood return, further diagnostic studies may be needed to determine the cause of the problems.

For short peripheral catheters, usually 3 mL of normal saline is adequate to flush the catheter. For all other catheters 5 to 10 mL of preservative-free normal saline is needed. Bacteriostatic normal saline is limited to no more than 30 mL in a 24-hour period in adults. By using 10 mL before and after each dose of medication, it is easy to exceed this limitation. The specific flushing amounts will vary depending on the device used and individual agency policies. Many facilities are now using prefilled flush syringes or single-dose containers. This approach decreases the risk of contamination, as well as the potential for error (Lenz et al., 2017). Flush catheters immediately after each use. Any delay in disconnecting the intermittent administration set and flushing the catheter could cause lumen occlusion from blood that backflows into the lumen when the infusion pressure is lower than venous pressure.

Obtaining Blood Samples From Central Venous Catheters

Short peripheral catheters should not be used routinely for obtaining blood samples. The additional manipulation could lead to vein irritation that requires removal of the catheter. Central venous catheters and midlines can be used for obtaining blood samples after a careful assessment of the risks versus benefits. If a patient has no peripheral venipuncture sites, requires frequent blood draws, or is fearful of needles, using the central venous catheter may be appropriate. The risks associated with obtaining blood samples from a central venous catheter are numerous. This procedure requires additional hub manipulation, which is a major cause of CRBSI. Consider the laboratory tests needed and the types of fluids that have recently been infused. For example, heparin interferes with coagulation studies, and electrolytes in the IV fluid may alter the results of serum electrolytes. Drawing blood from catheters for blood culture should not be done within an hour of completion of antimicrobial infusions.

If blood sampling from a central venous catheter is the best alternative, vigorous cleaning of the connections with 70% alcohol is necessary. Vacuum tubes attached via a "vacutainer" to the catheter hub eliminate the need to transfer the blood from a syringe into the tubes and therefore do not require exposed needles. For small-diameter catheters, the vacuum in the tube may cause the catheter to temporarily collapse, preventing backflow of blood into the tube. In this situation small syringes should be used because they create less pressure on aspiration, the opposite of what small syringes do on injection. Transfer of the blood from the syringe to the vacuum tube requires the use of a "vacutainer needle holder." This device keeps the needle housed in a plastic case and covered, preventing accidental needlestick injuries (Fig. 15.15). After blood draw from any catheter, a flush of 10 to 20 mL sterile normal saline is necessary to ensure a patent line. Be sure to clear the line and cap of blood to prevent a breeding ground for infection.

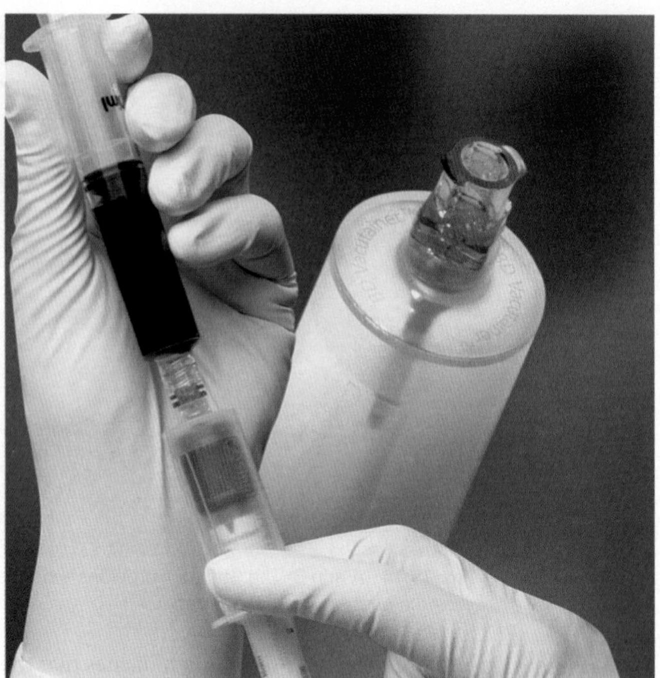

Fig. 15.15 Vacutainer needle holder prevents needlestick injuries when drawing blood. (Courtesy and © Becton, Dickinson and Company.)

Removing the Vascular Access Device

To remove a short peripheral IV line, after explaining the procedure to the patient, lift opposite sides of the transparent dressing and pull laterally to remove the dressing from the site while stabilizing the catheter. Slowly withdraw the catheter from the skin and immediately cover the puncture site with dry gauze. Hold pressure on the site until hemostasis is achieved. Assess the catheter tip to make sure that it is intact and completely removed. Document the time of catheter removal and appearance of the IV site.

Removal of midline catheters and PICCs must be performed with the same slow, gentle techniques used to insert the catheter. Veins can develop venospasms when rapid or forceful techniques are used. After explaining to the patient that this procedure will not be painful, remove the dressing and withdraw the catheter in short segments by pulling from the insertion site. *If you feel resistance, always stop and never apply force to the catheter. Extreme traction or force could cause the catheter to break and embolize (travel) to the heart or pulmonary circulation.*

Simple distraction techniques and deep breathing may be sufficient to relax the patient and facilitate the removal of the catheter. If these fail, replace the dressing and apply heat; allow time for the vein wall to relax. Keeping the extremity warm and dry and asking the patient to drink warm liquids could facilitate removal. Use of medications to relax the vein wall may be required if the catheter cannot be removed after several hours. Imaging studies may also be needed to determine whether the cause is a thrombosis instead of venospasm.

Nontunneled percutaneous central catheters are removed by removing the dressing as noted above, clipping any sutures, and gently withdrawing the catheter in short segments. Venospasm does not commonly occur when removing these catheters because the vein diameter is large and less reactive.

To prevent venous air embolism when removing any central venous catheter (including PICCs), position the patient in a flat supine or Trendelenburg position according to agency policy. To ensure that the intrathoracic pressure is higher than atmospheric pressure, have the patient hold his or her breath or perform a Valsalva maneuver during removal. If the patient is mechanically ventilated, time the removal to the delivery of an inhalation breath by the ventilator. Be sure to keep the catheter clamped during this procedure. When a central venous catheter is removed, a tract between the skin and vein may create a conduit that could allow air to be pulled into the vein, causing a venous air embolism.

After removal, measure the catheter length and compare it with the length documented on insertion. If the entire catheter length was not removed, contact the primary health care provider immediately as this constitutes a medical emergency! Removal of tunneled catheters and implanted ports is usually performed by physicians or nurse practitioners.

TABLE 15.2 Catheter-Related Bloodstream Infection (CRBSI) Prevention Bundle

- Use a checklist during insertion to make sure that everything is done correctly. Tell anyone who violates the correct steps to stop the procedure immediately.
- Hand hygiene before inserting a central line must be thorough (i.e., no quick scrub). Anyone who touches the central line must also perform thorough hand hygiene.
- Maximal barrier precautions during line insertion require that the patient be draped from head to toe with a sterile barrier.
- The primary health care provider who inserts the VAD wears sterile gloves, a gown, and a mask. Anyone in the room during the procedure must also wear a mask.
- Traffic in and out of the room must be minimized. Many institutions use a "stop" sign on the door of the room to prevent people from coming in and going out during the procedure. A special "central line cart" is often used to ensure that all needed equipment is readily available.
- Chlorhexidine is used for skin disinfection because it has the best outcomes for preventing infection.
- Use preferred sites. The upper arm and subclavian veins are the first choice for PICC placement. The next preference is the internal jugular vein, and the least preferred is the femoral vein.
- Postplacement care requires meticulous dressing changes and care of all parts of the IV system, such as keeping ports and stopcocks clean, hanging bags using sterile technique, and vigorously scrubbing catheter hub with alcohol when used.
- Review daily the need for the patient's VAD. The incidence of CRBSI increases each day the device is in place. As soon as it is determined that the patient no longer needs the IV line, it should be removed.

PICC, Peripherally inserted central catheter; *VAD,* vascular access device.

Documenting Intravenous Therapy

Intravenous therapy is risk prone; however, nurses are in a unique position to assess, prevent, and provide early intervention if a problem occurs. Nurses can protect themselves from negligence and malpractice claims with conscientious assessment, intervention, and documentation. Be sure to document after insertion of a vascular access device (VAD) and throughout the course of the therapy. When inserting a venous catheter, remember to document the following:

- Date and time of the VAD insertion
- Name of the nurse (you) who inserted the VAD
- Vein/location that was used for insertion
- Type of VAD used including gauge and length of catheter
- Number of insertion attempts and locations of attempts before successful insertion
- Response of the patient to the VAD insertion process
- Type of dressing applied
- Type of securement device, if used
- Special barrier precautions used, if any
- Patient and family education provided related to IV therapy

During the course of the patient's infusion therapy, be sure to continue documenting in the electronic health record your assessments and any interventions needed as a result of complications. Follow your agency's policies and procedures for additional requirements.

COMPLICATIONS OF INTRAVENOUS THERAPY

Complications from IV therapy can be minor and limited or life threatening. Serious life-altering or life-threatening complications are dramatically increasing in frequency and severity, and present a tremendous financial burden to the U.S. health care system. Catheter-related bloodstream infection (CRBSI) is one of the most serious problems, often resulting in patient death. These infections are more common in patients with central VADs but can also occur with peripheral catheters.

Catheter-Related Bloodstream Infection

The Institute for Healthcare Improvement identified CRBSI as one of several preventable hospital-acquired infections (HAIs). As part of their previous *100,000 Lives Campaign*, a number of evidence-based interventions were combined into the CRBSI prevention bundle. Nurses are accountable for ensuring that these interventions are followed correctly (Table 15.2).

Other Complications of Intravenous Therapy

Local complications of IV therapy occur at or near the catheter. A priority of care for patients with IV therapy is to prevent, assess, and detect these complications. In some cases nurses also manage these problems. Definitions, causes, signs and symptoms, treatment, and prevention of local complications are summarized in Table 15.3. *Systemic complications* of IV therapy involve the entire vascular system or multiple systems. Information on common systemic complications can be found in Table 15.4. For central venous catheters (CVCs), complications can occur during the insertion procedure or during the dwell time (Table 15.5). Tables 15.6 and 15.7 are the INS criteria for grading phlebitis and infiltrations. Document all assessments and complications in the patient's electronic health record. Notify the infusion therapy team and/or primary health care provider per agency policy when complications occur.

INTRAVENOUS THERAPY AND CARE OF THE OLDER ADULT

The aging process causes numerous changes in all body functions, and yet aging occurs differently in each person. Nutrition, environment, genetics, social factors, and education are just a few of the factors that influence the older adult's needs. Because all body functions are affected, IV therapy can be affected by these changes.

Skin Care

Aging skin becomes thinner and loses subcutaneous fat, decreasing the skin's ability for thermal regulation. Fewer nerve endings may alter the way an individual experiences pain and other sensations. Older patients may not perceive acute pain from traumatic venipuncture and may tolerate probing or multiple attempts (Coulter, 2016). However, this action increases

TABLE 15.3 Local Complications of Intravenous Therapy

Complication	Common Causes	Signs and Symptoms	Interventions	Prevention
Infiltration				
Leakage of a nonvesicant IV solution or medication into the extravascular tissue	Peripheral catheter has punctured opposite vein wall Inflammatory process causing fluid leakage at the capillary level Retrograde flow and leakage from venipuncture site Dislodged port access needle	IV rate slows Increasing edema around site Skin tightness; coolness of skin; burning, tenderness, or general discomfort at the insertion site; fluid leaking from puncture site; absence of a blood return (although this may not be reliable with a short peripheral catheter)	Stop infusion and remove short peripheral catheter immediately after identification of problem Apply sterile dressing if weeping from tissue occurs Elevate extremity Warm or cold compresses may be used according to organizational policy. Warm compresses increase circulation to the area and speed healing Cool compresses may be used to relieve discomfort and reduce swelling Insert a new catheter in the opposite extremity Rate the infiltration using the INS Infiltration Scale and document (Table 15.7)	Catheter stabilization—use smallest catheter appropriate; avoid area of flexion or use armboard Avoid placing restraints at IV site Make successive venipunctures proximal to the previous site Assess site frequently; educate patient about activities and signs and symptoms of infiltration Central venous catheters—obtain a brisk blood return before using the catheter for infusion Frequently assess proper positioning of port access needle
Extravasation				
Leakage of a vesicant IV solution or medication into the extravascular tissue Can occur with both peripheral and central catheters	Same as for infiltration	Same as for infiltration Blistering and tissue sloughing may not appear for a few days and resolves over 1-4 wks with infiltration of some chemotherapeutic agents	Stop infusion and disconnect administration set If possible, aspirate drug from SPC, CVC, or port access needle Leave SPC, CVC, or port access needle in place to deliver antidote, if indicated by established policy Apply cold compresses for all drugs EXCEPT vinca alkaloids and epipodophyllotoxins Photograph site Assess at 24 hr, 1 wk, 2 wk, and as needed Surgical interventions may be required Provide written instructions to patient and family	Same as for infiltration Recognize the vesicant potential before administering any IV medication **Prevention is key**
Phlebitis				
Inflammation of the vein Postinfusion phlebitis presents within 48-96 hrs after the catheter has been removed	Mechanical cause: insertion technique, catheter size, or lack of catheter securement Chemical cause: extremes of pH and/or osmolarity of the fluid or medication Bacterial/pathogenic cause: a break in aseptic technique, extended dwell time	pain at the IV site; vein may appears red and inflamed; vein may become hard and cordlike (Table 15.6)	Remove SPC at the first sign of phlebitis; use warm compresses to relieve pain Assess frequently Document using Phlebitis Scale Insert a new catheter using the opposite extremity Phlebitis occurring in the first week after PICC insertion: may be treated without catheter removal. Apply continuous heat; rest and elevate the extremity. Significant improvement is seen in 24 hrs, and complete resolution is seen within 72 hrs. Remove catheter if treatment is unsuccessful	Choose the smallest-gauge catheter for the required therapy Avoid sites of joint flexion or stabilize with an armboard Avoid infusing fluids or medications with a pH below 5.0 or above 9.0 through a peripheral vein Avoid infusing fluids or medications with a final osmolarity above 500 mOsm/L through a peripheral vein Adequately secure the catheter Use aseptic technique For PICCs, teach patient to avoid excessive physical activity with the extremity

TABLE 15.3 Local Complications of Intravenous Therapy—cont'd

Complication	Common Causes	Signs and Symptoms	Interventions	Prevention
Thrombosis				
Blood clot inside the vein	Anything that damages the endothelial lining of the intima can initiate clot formation Traumatic venipuncture Multiple venipuncture attempts Use of catheters too large for the chosen vein Hypercoagulable state and venous stasis	Slowed or stopped infusion rate Swollen extremity Tenderness and redness For CVCs, engorged peripheral veins of the ipsilateral chest and extremity	Stop infusion and remove SPC immediately Apply cold compresses to decrease blood flow and stabilize the clot Elevate extremity Surgical intervention may be required For CVCs, notify the health care provider for a diagnostic study. Low-dose thrombolytic agents may be used to lyse the clot	Use evidence-based venipuncture technique Make only two attempts to perform venipuncture Choose the smallest-gauge catheter in the largest vein possible Secure catheter adequately Use armboards if SPCs are placed in areas of joint flexion
Thrombophlebitis				
Presence of a blood clot and vein inflammation	Same as for phlebitis and thrombosis	Same as for phlebitis and thrombosis	Same as for phlebitis and thrombosis Apply cold pack initially, followed by warm compress	Same as for phlebitis and thrombosis
Ecchymosis and Hematoma				
Ecchymosis results from infiltration of blood into the surrounding tissue Hematoma results from uncontrolled bleeding	Unskilled or multiple IV insertion attempts Patients with coagulopathy or fragile skin and veins (e.g., older adults and patients on steroids Accidental laceration of a large vein or artery	Swelling Bruising Pain or tenderness	When removing device, apply light pressure; excessive pressure could cause other fragile veins in the area to rupture For hematoma, apply direct pressure until bleeding has stopped. Elevate extremity, apply ice pack for first 24 hr and then warm compress for comfort	Avoid veins that cannot be easily seen and/or palpated Use extra caution in patients with coagulopathies Use evidence-based venipuncture technique
Site Infection				
Invasion of microorganisms at the insertion site in the absence of simultaneous bloodstream infection Infection localized at the insertion site, the port pocket, or subcutaneous tunnel	Break in aseptic technique during insertion or the handling of sterile equipment Lack of proper hand hygiene and skin antisepsis	Site appears red, swollen, and warm; tenderness at site; may observe purulent or malodorous exudates	Clean exit site with alcohol, expressing drainage if present For SPC, midline catheter, or PICC, remove using sterile technique and avoid contact between skin and catheter Send catheter tip for culture, if requested Clean site with alcohol and cover with dry, sterile dressing; health care provider to evaluate for septic phlebitis; possible need for antimicrobial therapy or surgical intervention	Use strict aseptic technique when inserting, maintaining, or removing catheters Practice evidence-based hand hygiene Ensure that dressing remains clean, dry, and adherent to skin at all times
Venous Spasm				
Sudden contraction of the vein	Normal response to irritation or injury of the vein wall	Cramping or pain at or above the insertion site Numbness in the area Slowing of the infusion rate Inability to withdraw midline catheter or PICC	Temporarily slow infusion rate Apply warm compress Do not immediately remove SPC If occurring during midline catheter or PICC removal, do not apply tension or attempt forceful removal Reapply a dressing, apply heat, encourage patient to drink warm liquids, and keep extremity covered and dry; 12-24 hr may be required before catheter can be removed	Allow time for vein diameter to return to normal after tourniquet removal and before advancing catheter Infuse fluids at room temperature if possible For a midline catheter or PICC, gently withdraw the catheter in short segments

Continued

TABLE 15.3 Local Complications of Intravenous Therapy—cont'd

Complication	Common Causes	Signs and Symptoms	Interventions	Prevention
Nerve Damage				
Inadvertent piercing or complete transection of a nerve	Venipuncture near known nerve locations Unanticipated nerve locations	Reports of pain, tingling, or feeling "pins and needles" at or below the insertion site Numbness at or near the insertion site	Immediately stop the insertion procedure if the patient reports extreme pain Remove the catheter if reports of discomfort do not improve when the catheter is secured	Avoid using the cephalic vein near the wrist Avoid using veins on the palm side of the wrist Adequately secure the catheter, but avoid tape that is too tight Support areas of joint flexion with an armboard

CVC, Central venous catheter; *INS,* Infusion Nurses Society; *PICC,* peripherally inserted central catheter; *SPC,* short peripheral catheter.

TABLE 15.4 Systemic Complications of Intravenous Therapy

Complication	Cause	Signs and Symptoms	Interventions	Prevention
Circulatory Overload				
Disruption of fluid homeostasis with excess fluid in the circulatory system	Infusion of fluids at a rate greater than the patient's system can accommodate	Patient may report shortness of breath and cough; patient's blood pressure is elevated, and there is puffiness around the eyes and edema in dependent areas; patient's neck veins may be engorged, and nurse may hear moist breath sounds May exhibit DOE, decreased SaO_2	Slow the IV rate and notify physician; raise patient to an upright position; monitor vital signs and administer oxygen as prescribed; administer diuretics as prescribed	Monitor intake and output carefully and notify physician as soon as an imbalance is noticed between the patient's intake and output
Speed Shock				
Systemic reaction to the rapid infusion of a substance unfamiliar to the patient's circulatory system	Rapid infusion of drugs or bolus infusion, which causes the drug to reach toxic levels quickly	Patient may report light-headedness or dizziness and chest tightness; nurse may note that patient has a flushed face and an irregular pulse; without intervention, patient may lose consciousness and go into shock and cardiac arrest	Immediately discontinue the drug infusion and hang isotonic solution to keep the vein open; monitor vital signs carefully and notify physician for further treatments	Be aware of the appropriate infusion rate of medications and adhere to them; use of infusion control devices helps to prevent speed shock
Catheter Embolism				
A shaving or piece of catheter breaks off and floats freely in the vessel	Anything that damages the catheter—during insertion, dressing change, excessive force with flushing, or medication administration	Depending on where the catheter embolizes, this could be life threatening Cardiopulmonary arrest could occur	Emergently notify the physician. Remove the catheter and apply a tourniquet high on the limb of the catheter site; inspect catheter to determine how much may have embolized; an x-ray is taken to determine the presence of any catheter piece; surgical intervention may be necessary	When inserting over-the-needle catheters, never reinsert the needle into the catheter; avoid pulling a through-the-needle catheter back through the needle during insertion Avoid scissors near the catheter with dressing changes

the risk for fluid leakage and subsequent infiltration or extravasation injury. Inserting and removing a catheter and dressing could tear the skin layers.

Skin antisepsis is extremely important because of the decreased immunity seen as part of the aging process. Lipids are normally found in skin as a protective agent, and alcohol easily dissolves lipids. Although greater numbers of organisms may be killed, the skin can also become excessively dry and cracked. Current recommendations call for using friction when cleaning the skin to penetrate the layers of the epidermis. However, excessive friction may damage fragile skin and cause impaired ***tissue integrity***. Chlorhexidine is the preferred agent, and the product currently available contains alcohol. Check for allergies to iodine before using iodine or iodophors. Iodophors such as povidone-iodine require contact with the skin for a minimum of 2 minutes to be effective. All antiseptic solutions must be thoroughly dry before applying the dressing or tape to ensure adequate adherence to the skin.

TABLE 15.5 Complications During the Dwell of Central Venous Catheters

Complication	Possible Causes	Signs and Symptoms	Treatment	Prevention
Catheter Migration				
Movement of a properly placed catheter tip to another vein No change in the external catheter length	Changes in intrathoracic pressure caused by coughing, vomiting, sneezing, heavy lifting, and congestive heart failure	For migration to the jugular vein—reports of hearing a running stream or gurgling sound on the side of catheter insertion For migration to the azygos vein—back pain between the shoulder blades Neurologic complications if medications are infused	Stop all infusions and flush catheter Notify health care provider Obtain a chest x-ray, if required, to assess tip location Spontaneous repositioning back to the SVC is possible Repositioning by radiology may be required	Place catheter tip properly in the lower third of the SVC near the junction with the right atrium Instruct patient to perform usual ADLs but to avoid excessive physical activity
Catheter Dislodgment				
Movement of catheter into or out of the insertion site	Inadequate catheter securement Excessive physical activity with a PICC	External catheter length has changed, also changing the internal tip location No other signs or symptoms may be noticed immediately	Stop all infusions and flush catheter NEVER readvance the catheter into the insertion site Determine the amount of external catheter length and compare with the length documented on insertion Notify the health care provider inserting the catheter for further assessment May require an x-ray	Use proper catheter securement device Instruct patient to perform normal ADLs but to avoid excessive physical activity
Catheter Rupture				
Catheter is broken, damaged, or separated from hub or port body	Forcefully flushing a catheter with any size syringe against resistance Using scissors to remove a dressing Catheter compression of a subclavian-inserted catheter between the clavicle and first rib (also known as *pinch-off syndrome*)	Fluid leaking from insertion site Pain or swelling during infusion Reflux of blood into the catheter extension Inability to aspirate blood from catheter	Repair the damaged segment; depends on the availability of a repair kit designed for the specific brand of catheter being used; repair may be considered a temporary measure instead of a permanent treatment Remove catheter	NEVER use excessive force when flushing a catheter, regardless of syringe size On injection, small syringes generate more pressure than larger syringes. Use of a 10-mL syringe is generally recommended for flushing procedures Insert catheter through jugular or upper-extremity sites instead of subclavian site
Lumen Occlusion				
Catheter lumen is partially or totally blocked	Drug or mineral precipitate (calcium, diazepam, and phenytoin are common) Lipid sludge from long-term infusion of fat emulsion Blood clots and fibrin sheath caused by blood reflux into lumen Allowing administration sets to remain connected for extended periods after medication has infused	Infusion stops or pump alarm sounds Inability or difficulty administering fluids Inability or difficulty drawing blood Increased resistance to flushing of the catheter	Assess history of catheter use. A suddenly developing problem may indicate contact between incompatible medications. A problem that develops over an extended period may indicate a gradual clot formation For drug precipitate, determine the pH of the precipitated drug. Use hydrochloric acid for acidic drug. Use sodium bicarbonate for alkaline drugs For blood clot, use thrombolytic enzymes such as alteplase	Always flush with normal saline between, before, and after each medication given through the catheter Use positive-pressure flushing techniques when a negative fluid-displacement needleless connector is being used Use a positive fluid-displacement needleless connector Flush catheters immediately when medication infusion is complete

Continued

TABLE 15.5 Complications During the Dwell of Central Venous Catheters—cont'd

Complication	Possible Causes	Signs and Symptoms	Treatment	Prevention
Catheter-Related Bloodstream Infection (CRBSI)				
Pathogenic organisms invade the patient's circulation The CDC has specific criteria to classify these infections	Lack of sterile field during insertion Inadequate skin antiseptic agents and application techniques Manipulation of the catheter hub leading to intraluminal contamination Inadequate hand hygiene Long dwell time	Early symptoms include fever, chills, headache, and general malaise Later symptoms include tachycardia, hypotension, decreased urinary output	Change the entire infusion system from solution to IV device; notify health care provider, obtain cultures, and administer antibiotics as prescribed If the infusate is the suspected cause, send a specimen to the laboratory for evaluation If the catheter is the suspected cause, send catheter tip to the laboratory for evaluation	Maintain sterile technique Use the recommended CRBSI prevention bundle

CDC, Centers for Disease Control and Prevention; *PICC,* peripherally inserted central catheter; *SVC,* superior vena cava.

TABLE 15.6 Phlebitis Scale From INS Standards of Practice

Grade	Clinical Criteria
0	No symptoms
1	Erythema with or without pain
2	Pain at access site with erythema and/or edema
3	Pain at access site with erythema and/or edema Streak formation Palpable cord
4	Pain at access site with erythema and/or edema Streak formation Palpable venous cord more than 1 inch long Purulent drainage

Data from Infusion Nurses Society (INS). (2016). Infusion therapy standards of practice. *Journal of Infusion Nursing, 39*(1S), S96.

TABLE 15.7 Infiltration Scale From INS Standards of Practice

Grade	Clinical Criteria
0	No symptoms
1	Skin blanched Edema <1 inch in any direction Cool to touch With or without pain
2	Skin blanched Edema 1-6 inches in any direction Cool to touch With or without pain
3	Skin blanched, translucent Gross edema >6 inches in any direction Cool to touch Mild-to-moderate pain Possible numbness
4	Skin blanched, translucent Skin tight, leaking Skin discolored, bruised, swollen Gross edema >6 inches in any direction Deep pitting tissue edema Circulatory impairment Moderate-to-severe pain Infiltration of any amount of blood product, irritant, or vesicant

Data from Infusion Nurses Society (INS). (2016). Infusion therapy standards of practice. *Journal of Infusion Nursing, 39*(1S), S96.

Skin should never be shaved before venipuncture as shaving causes microabrasions that can lead to infection. Shaving can also more easily nick the thin, delicate skin of an older adult. If necessary, excessive amounts of hair should be clipped to ensure the bandage adheres to the skin.

Skin and ***tissue integrity*** can easily be compromised by the application of tape or dressings. The use of skin protectant solutions puts a protective barrier between the skin and dressing and improves the adherence of the dressing to the skin. Removal of tape and dressings may require adhesive remover solutions, or an alcohol pad may accomplish the same purpose. Securement devices such as the StatLock require the use of a skin protectant (e.g., Skin-Prep) before applying the device. The protectant prevents skin tearing when the device is removed.

Vein and Catheter Selection

Vein and catheter selection are of highest importance in older adults. Choose insertion sites carefully after considering the patient's skin integrity, vein condition, and functional ability. The general principle of starting with the most distal sites usually indicates use of hand veins. *However, avoid fragile skin and small, tortuous veins on the back of the hand (dorsum); select the initial IV site higher on the arm.*

Venous distention must be accomplished with a flat tourniquet; however, the veins may require longer to adequately distend. Allowing a tourniquet to remain in place for extended periods causes an overfilling of the vein and can result in a hematoma when the vein is punctured. On extremely fragile skin the tourniquet application can lead to ecchymotic areas or skin tears. Protect the skin by placing a washcloth or the patient's gown between the skin and tourniquet. A tourniquet may not be required in veins that are already distended; however, carefully palpate these veins to determine their condition. Avoid hard, cordlike veins. Blood pressure cuffs can also be used for venous distention. Inflate the cuff and release until the pressure is slightly less than diastolic pressure. Other methods to distend veins include:

- Tapping the vein lightly, but avoiding forceful slapping
- Asking the patient to open and close the fist so the muscles can force blood into the veins, making sure that the hand is relaxed when the venipuncture is attempted
- Placing the extremity lower than the heart
- Applying warm compresses or a heating pad (be careful not to make it too hot) to the entire extremity for 10 to 20 minutes and removing just before making the venipuncture

As with all patients, venipuncture technique requires adequate skin and vein stabilization during the puncture and complete catheter advancement. Veins of an older adult are more likely to roll away from the needle as veins become firmer and more difficult to puncture with aging (Coulter, 2016; Kear, 2017). Low angles of 10 to 15 degrees between the skin and catheter will improve success with venipuncture.

As soon as the catheter enters the vein, it may be necessary to release the tourniquet. Release of venous pressure from the puncture can lead to ecchymosis. Allowing the tourniquet to remain in place during the complete catheter advancement could increase this problem.

! NURSING SAFETY PRIORITY (QSEN)

Action Alert

Catheter securement may be a challenge when a patient is confused. The nurse may need to move the IV equipment out of easy reach of the patient and provide other means to protect the VAD. A device such as the IV House UltraDressing shown in Fig. 15.16 can protect the site while keeping it visible for easy assessment. Another alternative is a flexible netting material that covers both the insertion site and the tubing. Regardless of the method used, it is essential that the site be visible for assessing the insertion site for signs of complications.

Choosing a midline catheter or PICC may be best in older patients with poor skin turgor; limited venous sites; or veins that are fragile, tortuous, or hard. These catheters are placed in the upper extremity where venous distention techniques can be used. Inserting nontunneled percutaneous central catheters in older adults can be much more challenging. Venous distention for insertion requires the Trendelenburg position and a well-hydrated patient to ensure that the veins are adequately distended. Fluid volume deficit prevents adequate distention of the subclavian or jugular veins. Patients with conditions such as chronic obstructive pulmonary disease and kyphosis cannot tolerate the Trendelenburg position. Tunneled catheters and implanted ports may be appropriate after considering the surgical techniques required to insert these catheters.

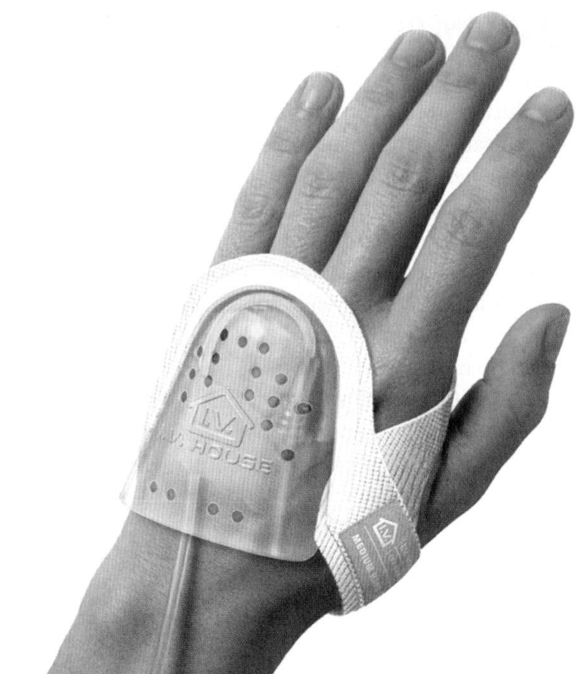

Fig. 15.16 I.V. House UltraDressing IV site protector, a safety device used for IV site protection, guards the integrity of the older adult's skin while helping secure the site. (Courtesy I.V. House, Hazelwood, MO.)

Cardiac and Renal Changes

Because of changes in cardiac and renal status in older adults, the accuracy of infusion volume and flow rate measurements is very important in the older adult. Older adults are more prone to fluid overload with resulting heart failure or dehydration with subsequent poor perfusion (Coulter, 2016). The primary health care provider's prescription for infusion therapy should be assessed for appropriateness for the patient's condition. Electronic controlling devices may be required to ensure the necessary accuracy. Signs and symptoms of fluid overload are described in Chapter 13.

When fluid restrictions are required, medications could be diluted in small quantities and delivered using a syringe pump or a manual IV push. Consult with a pharmacist to determine the smallest amount of diluent required. This alternative may allow the patient to have more fluid to drink. Serum sodium levels should be considered when normal saline is routinely used for dilution in patients with hypertension or cardiac problems.

An increasing number of patients with chronic illness require repeated and frequent IV therapies. Many of these patients are vein depleted and need vein preservation. Subcutaneous and intraosseous routes have demonstrated effectiveness in emergency resuscitation. These procedures may also be beneficial for routine infusion of isotonic, nonirritant, nonvesicant solutions in patients with chronic illness and vein depletion (Coulter, 2016; Johnson et al., 2016).

Specific therapies requiring infusion into arteries and peritoneal, epidural, and intrathecal space are also available. These therapies are most commonly used to administer chemotherapy, lytic therapy, or pain medication.

SUBCUTANEOUS INFUSION THERAPY

Subcutaneous infusion therapy has been used for a variety of drug infusions. Most commonly it is used for administration of pain medications and insulin therapy. It is beneficial for palliative care patients who cannot tolerate oral medications, when IM injections are too painful, or when vascular access is not available or is too difficult to obtain.

Hypodermoclysis or "clysis" involves the slow infusion of isotonic fluids into the patient's subcutaneous tissue for the purpose of slow, steady rehydration. Although common in the early twentieth to mid-twentieth century, this method was not widely used again until the 1990s. The growth of geriatric and palliative health care has helped spur the use of this method of infusion therapy for selected patients and the emergent biologics.

Hypodermoclysis can be used for short-term fluid volume replacement. The patient must have sufficient sites of intact skin without infection, inflammation, bruising, scarring, or edema. The most common sites are the front and sides of the thighs and hips, the upper abdomen, and the area under the clavicle. Unlike IV therapy, the upper extremities should not be used because fluid is absorbed more readily from sites with larger stores of adipose tissue. Hypodermoclysis is not appropriate for emergency resuscitations and should not be used for high quantity or emergent fluid replacement needs (Jan, 2017). Hyaluronidase, an enzyme that improves the absorption of the infusion, may be prescribed by the primary health care provider and is mixed with each liter of infusion fluid.

A small-gauge (25 to 27) winged infusion or "butterfly" needle, a small-gauge short peripheral catheter, or an infusion set specially designed for subcutaneous infusion can be chosen. The subcutaneous infusion sets have a small needle extending at a right angle from a flat disk that helps stabilize the needle.

When choosing the infusion site, consider the patient's level of activity. The area under the clavicle or the abdomen prevents difficulty with ambulation. Clip excess hair in the area and clean the chosen site with the antiseptic solution, preferably 2% chlorhexidine gluconate in 70% isopropyl alcohol to prevent infection. Prime the infusion tubing and the attached subcutaneous infusion set or winged needle. Gently pinch an area of about 2 inches (5 cm) and insert the needle using sterile technique. After securing the needle, cover the site with a transparent dressing. Flow rates for hydration fluids begin at 30 mL/hr. After 1 hour the rate can be increased if the patient has experienced no discomfort. The maximum rate is usually 2 mL/min or 120 mL/hr. Assess the site every 4 hours while in a hospital setting and at least twice daily while at home. Redness, warmth, leakage, bruising, swelling, and reports of pain indicate tissue irritation and possible impaired tissue integrity. If these symptoms occur, remove the infusion needle. Rotate the site at least once a week. More frequent rotation may be needed, depending on ***tissue integrity*** (INS, 2016).

Other complications include pooling of the fluid at the insertion site and an uneven fluid drip rate. Both of these problems may be resolved by restarting the infusion in another location. An infusion pump may also be used. Small ambulatory infusion pumps can be used to allow for greater mobility.

INTRAOSSEOUS INFUSION THERAPY

Intraosseous (IO) therapy allows access to the rich vascular network in the red marrow of bones. Although IO has previously been regarded as a pediatric procedure, it is now considered acceptable for use in adults. Victims of trauma, burns, cardiac arrest, diabetic ketoacidosis, and other life-threatening conditions benefit from this therapy because health care providers often cannot access these patients' vascular systems for traditional IV therapy. IO catheters may be established in the prehospital setting when IV access cannot be readily obtained in an emergency (Johnson et al., 2016).

Absorption rates of large-volume parenteral (LVP) infusions and drugs administered via the IO route are similar to those achieved with peripheral or central venous administration. The IO route is for short-term therapy and should be used only during the immediate period of resuscitation and should not be used longer than 24 hours (Johnson et al., 2016). After establishing access, efforts should continue to obtain IV access as well.

There are few contraindications for IO infusion. The only absolute contraindication is fracture in the bone to be used as a site. Conditions such as severe osteoporosis, osteogenesis imperfecta, or other conditions that increase the risk for fracture with insertion of the IO needle and skin infection over the site may also be contraindications for some patients. Repeated attempts to access the same site should be avoided.

Any needle can be used to provide IO therapy and access the medullary space (marrow). However, 15- or 16-gauge needles specifically designed for IO therapy are preferred. New technology using a battery-powered drill has improved the ease of IO insertion. A number of sites can be used, including the proximal tibia (tibial tuberosity), distal femur, medial malleolus (inner ankle), proximal humerus, and iliac crest. The proximal tibia is the most common site accessed for IO therapy (Fig. 15.17). During insertion, the leg is restrained, and the site cleaned with an antiseptic agent such as chlorhexidine.

After successful insertion the needle must be secured to prevent movement out of the bone. The same doses of fluids and medications can be infused by IO therapy as IV, and an infusion pump should be used for rapid flow rates.

During the procedure most patients rate the pain as a 2 or 3 on a scale of 0 to 10. Lidocaine 1% is used to anesthetize the skin, subcutaneous tissue, and periosteum to promote comfort. Pain is also reported during the initial infusion. This may be reduced by injecting 0.5 mg/kg of preservative-free lidocaine through the IO port before initiating the infusion. However, this may be omitted if the decision to use an IO device is based on an emergent or trauma situation.

Improper needle placement with infiltration into the surrounding tissue is the most common complication of IO therapy. Accumulation of fluid under the skin at either the insertion site or on the other side of the limb indicates that the needle either is not far enough in to penetrate the bone marrow or is too far into the limb and has protruded through the other side of the shaft. Needle obstruction occurs when the puncture has been accomplished but flushing has been delayed. This delay may cause the needle to become blocked with bone marrow.

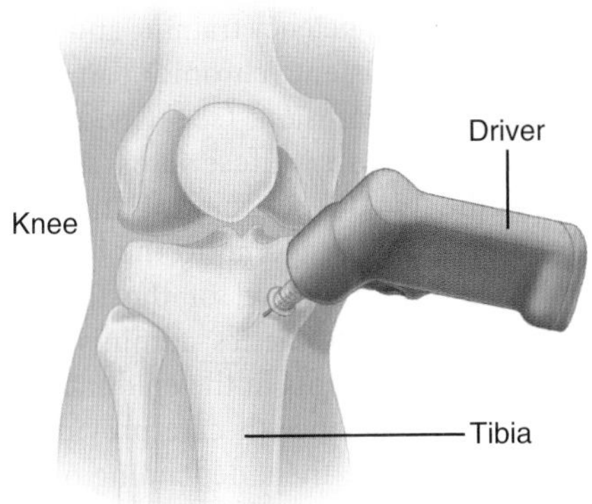

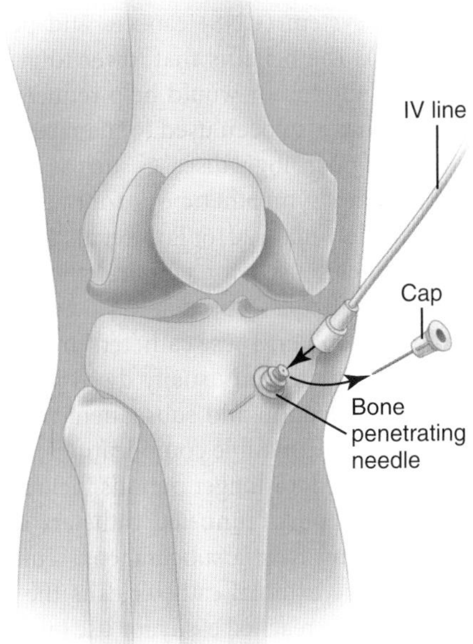

Fig. 15.17 Proximal tibial intraosseous (IO) access.

Osteomyelitis is an unusual but serious complication of IO therapy. You can help prevent this with meticulous aseptic technique, proper hand hygiene, and removal of the catheter as soon as it is no longer needed.

Compartment syndrome is a condition in which increased tissue pressure in a confined anatomic space causes decreased perfusion (peripheral blood flow to the area). The decreased circulation to the area leads to hypoxia and pain in the area. Although the complication is rare in IO therapy, the nurse should monitor the site carefully and alert the primary health care provider promptly if the patient exhibits any signs of decreased circulation to the limb such as coolness, swelling, mottling, or discoloration. Without improvement in perfusion to the limb, the patient could ultimately require amputation of the limb. Nursing assessment and interventions for compartment syndrome are discussed in detail in Chapter 47.

INTRA-ARTERIAL INFUSION THERAPY

Catheters are placed into arteries to obtain repeated arterial blood samples, monitor various hemodynamic pressures continuously, and infuse chemotherapy agents or fibrinolytics (**intra-arterial infusion therapy**). Catheters placed in the radial, brachial, or femoral arteries are used for obtaining blood samples and arterial pressure monitoring. Arterial waveforms and pressures are converted to digital values displayed on attached monitors. Between the catheter and the monitor is a special administration set capable of handling high infusion pressure, a pressurized fluid container, a continuous flush attachment, a three-way stopcock, and a transducer. The transducer is positioned at the level of the patient's atrium and secured to an IV pole to enable correct arterial pressure measurements.

The pulmonary artery is used to monitor pressures in the heart and lungs. This artery is cannulated via the large central venous system and through the right side of the heart. Hemodynamic monitoring and how to interpret these values are described in Chapter 35.

Use of an intra-arterial catheter for infusion therapy is not common and is generally used for direct treatment of tumor sites. Chemotherapy agents administered arterially allow infusion of a high concentration of drug directly to the tumor site before it is diluted in blood or metabolized by the liver or kidneys. Drug infusion through the same blood supply feeding the tumor optimizes cell destruction at the tumor site while minimizing systemic side effects. The most common arterial sites include the hepatic and celiac arteries for liver tumors, although the carotid artery for tumors of the head, neck, or brain and pelvic arteries for cervical tumors have been used. Arterial catheter insertion can be performed through the skin via a surgical procedure or by an interventional radiologist. Implanted ports are commonly used for extended therapies. For short-term therapy, an external catheter may be used for 3 to 7 days, although the risks for complications increase during dwell time.

! NURSING SAFETY PRIORITY QSEN

Critical Rescue

All arterial lines must be carefully and appropriately secured with Luer-Lok devices. These devices use a male and female adaptor that are twisted together to prevent accidental detachment. Life-threatening hemorrhage can occur if an accidental disconnection occurs! When an infusion pump is used, be sure that it has a pressure high enough to overcome arterial pressure. Closely monitor the arterial insertion site and affected extremity. Assess the extremity for warmth, sensation, capillary refill, and pulse to ensure adequate perfusion distal to the insertion site.

When the carotid artery is used for intra-arterial infusion, perform neurologic and cognitive assessments to determine adequate blood flow to the brain. When a femoral catheter is used, the patient will have very limited movement, so apply antiembolic stockings or other measures to prevent deep vein thrombosis. Complications from arterial catheters are similar to those from venous catheters, including infection, bleeding from the insertion site, hemorrhage from a catheter disconnection, catheter migration, infiltration, and catheter lumen or arterial occlusion. However, it is important to remember that any occlusion or hemorrhage from an arterial site is likely to result in more serious consequences than those in a vein. Specialized training is required to manage care of patients with arterial catheters.

INTRAPERITONEAL INFUSION THERAPY

Intraperitoneal (IP) infusion therapy is the administration of chemotherapy agents into the peritoneal cavity. IP therapy is used to treat intra-abdominal malignancies such as ovarian and GI tumors that have moved into the peritoneum after surgery.

Catheters used for IP therapy may be an implanted port for long-term treatment or an external catheter for temporary use. These catheters, including those attached to an implanted port, have large internal lumens with multiple side holes along the catheter length to allow for delivery of large quantities of fluid. Administration of IP therapy includes three phases: the instillation phase; the dwell phase, usually 1 to 4 hours; and the drain phase. Because this treatment involves the delivery of biohazardous agents, additional competency is required to handle the infusion properly.

The patient should be placed in the semi-Fowler position for the infusion. He or she may experience nausea and vomiting caused by increasing pressure on the internal organs from the infusing fluid. Pressure on the diaphragm may cause respiratory distress. Reducing the flow rate and treatment with antiemetic drugs can reduce these symptoms. Severe pain may indicate that the catheter has migrated, and an abdominal x-ray is needed to determine its location.

During the dwell and drainage phases, the patient may need assistance in frequently moving from side to side to distribute the fluid evenly around the abdominal cavity. After the fluid has drained, the catheter is flushed with normal saline, although heparinized saline may be used in implanted ports. Catheter lumen occlusion can result from the formation of fibrous sheaths or fibrin clots or plugs inside the catheter or around the tip.

Exit site infection, indicated by redness, tenderness, and warmth of the tissue around the catheter, can occur. Microbial peritonitis and inflammation of the peritoneal membranes from the invasion of microorganisms are other complications. If peritonitis occurs, the patient may experience a fever, abdominal rigidity, paralytic ileus, and rebound tenderness and report abdominal pain. This condition is preventable by using strict aseptic technique in the handling of all equipment and infusion supplies. Management of peritonitis includes antimicrobial therapy administered either IV or intraperitoneally and may require removal and replacement of the IP catheter.

INTRASPINAL INFUSION THERAPY

The spinal column is covered by three layers: the dura mater, or outermost covering; the arachnoid, or middle layer; and the pia mater, which is closest to the spinal cord. Two spaces used for infusion are the **epidural** space between the dura mater and vertebrae and the **subarachnoid** space. The epidural space consists of fat, connective tissue, and blood vessels that protect the spinal cord. Medications infused into the epidural space must diffuse through the dura mater, and there is the possibility that some drug will be absorbed systemically. **Intrathecal** medications are infused into the subarachnoid space and directly into the cerebral spinal fluid, allowing reduced doses (Pope et al., 2016). Care of patients with these therapies requires competency training and validation.

Postoperative and persistent (chronic) pain is the primary indication for epidural infusion (see Chapter 5). Opioids administered epidurally slowly diffuse across the dura mater to the dorsal horn of the spinal cord. They lock onto receptors and block pain impulses from ascending to the brain. The patient receives pain relief from the level of the injection caudally (toward the toes). Local anesthetics administered epidurally work on the sensory nerve roots in the epidural space to block pain impulses. The primary health care provider administers the first dose of medication; then, depending on state law, the type of medication, and facility policies, nurses trained in epidural therapy may administer subsequent doses.

Intrathecal infusion of chemotherapy is used for treating central nervous system (CNS) cancers and postoperative pain (Yi et al., 2017). The belief is that lower total body doses delivered directly to the tumor would help reduce side effects. Intrathecal infusion has also been used to manage chronic pain and treat spasticity of neurologic diseases such as cerebral palsy, multiple sclerosis, reflex sympathetic dystrophy, and traumatic brain injuries (Lumsden et al., 2016; Pope et al., 2016).

A temporary catheter used for epidural therapy can be a percutaneous catheter that is secured at the site and extends up the back toward the shoulder. These catheters are used for postoperative pain management and usually dwell for only several hours or a few days. Infection and subsequent meningitis and catheter migration are the possible complications.

Epidural catheters used for longer periods include a tunneled catheter and implanted port. Tunneled catheters are tunneled toward the abdomen and have a subcutaneous cuff to act as a barrier to infection. The external catheter exits the skin on the abdomen so that it can be reached easily for use by the patient or caregiver. An epidural implanted port is the same design as an IV implanted port and is accessed with the same noncoring needle. The catheter extends from the lumbar puncture site to the port pocket and is located over a bony prominence on the abdomen through a subcutaneous tunnel. Surgically implanted pumps can also be used to deliver epidural and intrathecal infusion.

Using sterile technique, an intraspinal catheter is usually inserted in the lumbar region. The external part of a temporary epidural catheter is laid along the back toward the head and usually extends over the shoulder. The entire catheter length is taped for added security. Dressings are usually not routinely changed because they are used only for short periods. If bleeding or fluid leakage requires dressing removal, use extreme care to prevent dislodging the catheter.

For a tunneled catheter or implanted port, the entire subcutaneous tunnel and port pocket should be assessed frequently. Measurement of an external catheter segment could help identify catheter migration.

An in-line filter is used on all intraspinal infusions to block the infusion of particulate matter. Medications commonly contain preservatives such as alcohol, phenols, or sulfites; however, these are toxic to the CNS. All medications used for intraspinal infusion must be free of preservatives. Alcohol and products containing alcohol should not be applied to the insertion site because the solution could track along the catheter and cause nerve damage. Povidone-iodine solutions are preferred for skin antisepsis before insertion and during catheter dwell, including tunneled catheter exit sites and implanted port pockets.

Complications from epidural and intrathecal infusion can be caused by the type of medication being infused or can be related to the catheter. It is important to know the specific location of the intraspinal catheter because the doses of medications are quite different. When used for pain management, doses are usually 10 times greater for epidural than for intrathecal infusion. Assess the patient for response to the drugs being given, level of alertness, respiratory status, and itching.

Catheter-related complications include infection, bleeding, leakage of cerebrospinal fluid (CSF), occlusion of the catheter lumen, and catheter migration. It is important to be aware of coagulopathy and timing of anticoagulant therapy when epidural catheters are inserted. An epidural hematoma can cause neurologic damage if not corrected promptly. Infection in the patient receiving either epidural or intrathecal therapy could be the result of a lack of asepsis when handling the medication or during the administration. Evidence of local infection such as redness or swelling at the catheter exit site may be present. The patient may also exhibit neurologic and systemic signs of infection (e.g., meningitis) such as headache, stiff neck, or temperature higher than 101° F (38.3° C). Report any neurologic change to the primary health care provider immediately!

GET READY FOR THE NEXT-GENERATION NCLEX® EXAMINATION!

Key Points

Review these Key Points for each NCLEX Examination Client Needs Category.

Safe and Effective Care Environment

- Use smart pumps and other technology-based safety systems and always check infusion administration prescriptions for accuracy and completeness before implementing them. **QSEN: Safety & Informatics**
- Devices engineered with safety mechanisms are required by OSHA to reduce the risk of staff injuries from needles, thus preventing bloodborne pathogen hazards. **QSEN: Safety**
- Use the evidence-based catheter-related bloodstream infection (CRBSI) prevention bundle during insertion and care of patients who have central lines (see Table 15.2). **QSEN: Evidence-Based Practice**

Health Promotion and Maintenance

- Older adults present special challenges when infusion therapy is used; physiologic changes of ***tissue integrity*** and cardiac/renal systems must be considered.
- Use small IV catheters for older adults and insert using a 10- to 15-degree angle to prevent rolling of the vein. **QSEN: Patient-Centered Care**
- Teach patients and their families about the patient's infusion therapy, including purpose, type, potential complications, and safety precautions. **QSEN: Patient-Centered Care**

Physiological Integrity

- Infusion therapy is the delivery of parenteral medications and fluids through a wide variety of catheters and locations.
- Infusion therapy is used for establishing ***fluid and electrolyte balance,*** achieving optimum nutrition, maintaining hemostasis, and treating or preventing illnesses with medications.
- Vascular access devices (VADs) are catheters that are used to deliver fluids and electrolytes and medications into the intravascular space; the type used depends on the reason for infusion therapy, patient condition, and plan of care. **Clinical Judgment**
- Use best practice for placement of short peripheral VADs, including avoiding the small veins of the hands. **QSEN: Evidence-Based Practice**
- Document care for the patient receiving IV therapy, including the type of VAD inserted. **QSEN: Informatics**
- Use normal saline to flush IV catheters on a periodic basis per agency policy.
- Assess, prevent, and manage systemic complications related to peripheral and central IV therapies as outlined in Tables 15.4 and 15.5. **Clinical Judgment**
- Assess, prevent, and manage complications during the course of central IV therapy as listed in Table 13-5. **Clinical Judgment**
- Other methods of infusion therapy include subcutaneous therapy of fluids (hypodermoclysis), intraosseous therapy, arterial therapy, intraperitoneal therapy, and epidural and intrathecal administration.

MASTERY QUESTIONS

1. A client receiving gentamycin intravenously reports that the peripheral IV insertion site has become painful and reddened. What is the priority nursing action?
   A. Contact the primary health care provider
   B. Document findings in the electronic health record
   C. Change the IV site to a new location
   D. Stop the infusion of the drug
2. An older adult client receiving an infusion of 5% dextrose in 0.9% normal saline at 150 mL/hour has developed shortness of breath with a decrease in oxygen saturation to 86%. What is the priority nursing intervention?
   A. Notify the health care provider
   B. Place the client on oxygen
   C. Sit the client upright in bed
   D. Assess the client's lung sounds

REFERENCES

Asterisk (*) indicates a classic or definitive work on this subject.

Androes, M., & Heffner, A. (2020). Placement of femoral venous catheters. *UpToDate*. Retrieved: https://www.uptodate.com/contents/placement-of-femoral-venous-catheters.

Chopra, V. (2018). *Central venous access devices and approach to selection in adults*. UpToDate. Retrieved from https://www.uptodate.com/contents/central-venous-access-devices-and-approach-to-selection-in-adults.

Conley, S., Buckley, P., Magarace, L., Hsieh, C., Pedulla, & Vitale, L. (2017). Standardizing best nursing practice for implanted ports: Applying evidence-based professional guidelines to prevent central line-associated bloodstream infections. *Journal of Infusion Nursing, 40*(3), 165–174.

Coulter, K. (2016). Successful infusion therapy in older adults. *Journal of Infusion Nursing, 39*(6), 352–358. https://doi.org/10.1097/NAN.0000000000000196.

Crowell, J., O'Neil, K., & Drager, L. (2017). Project HANDS. A bundled approach to increase short peripheral catheter dwell time. *Journal of Infusion Nursing, 40*(5), 274–280. https://doi.org/10.1097/NAN.0000000000000237.

Fabiani, A., Dreas, L., & Sanson, G. (2017). Ultrasound-guided deep-arm veins insertion of long peripheral catheters in patients with difficult venous access after cardiac surgery. *Heart & Lung, 46*, 46–53.

Infusion Nurses Society. (2016). Infusion therapy standards of practice. *Journal of Infusion Nursing, 39*(1S), S96.

Jan, L. (2017). The hypodermoclysis – comfortable way to rehydration in patients with end-stage dementia. *Journal of Psychiatry, 20*, 397. https://doi.org/10.4172/2378-5756.1000397.

Johnson, M., Inaba, K., Byerly, S., Falsgraf, E., Lydia, L., Benjamin, E., et al. (2016). Intraosseous infusion as a bridge to definitive access. *American Surgeon, 82*(10), 876–880.

Kear, T. M. (2017). Fluid and electrolyte management across the age continuum. *Nephrology Nursing Journal, 44*(6), 491–497.

Lenz, J., Degnan, D., Hertig, J., & Stevenson, J. (2017). A review of best practices for intravenous push medication administration. *Journal of Infusion Nursing, 40*(6), 354–358.

Lumsden, D., Ashmore, J., Ball, G., Charles-Edwards, G., Selway, R., Ashkan, K., et al. (2016). Fractional anisotropy in children with dystonia or spasticity correlates with the selection for DBS or ITB movement disorder surgery. *Neuroradiology, 58*(4), 401–408. https://doi.org/10.1007/s00234-015-1639-9.

Marsh, N., Webster, J., Mihala, G., & Rickard, C. M. (2017). Devices and dressings to secure peripheral venous catheters: A cochrane systematic review and meta-analysis. *International Journal of Nursing Studies, 67*, 12–19. https://doi.org/10.1016/J.IJNURSTU.2016.11.007.

Moureau, N., & Chopra, V. (2016). Indications for peripheral, midline and central catheters: summary of the MAGIC recommendations. *British Journal of Nursing, 25*(8), S15–S24.

Plohal, A., Dumont, C., Perry, C., Biddix, V., Bird, D. B., Darst, T., et al. (2017). The role of the registered nurse in the insertion of nontunneled central vascular access devices. *Journal of Infusion Nursing, 40*(6), 339–345. https://doi.org/10.1097/NAN.0000000000000255.

Pope, J. E., Deer, T. R., Bruel, B. M., & Falowski, S. (2016). Clinical uses of intrathecal therapy and its placement in the pain care algorithm. *Pain Practice, 16*(8), 1092–1106. https://doi.org/10.1111/papr.12438.

Rowdhwal, S., & Chen, J. (2018). Toxic effects of Di-2-ethylhexyl phthalate: An overview. *BioMed Research International, 18*. https://doi.org/10.1155/2018/1750368.

*The Joint Commission. (2013). *Preventing central line–associated bloodstream infections: Useful tools, an international perspective.* Nov 20, 2013. Accessed November 2, 2018. http://www.jointcommission.org/CLABSIToolkit.

The Joint Commission. (2020). *2020 National patient safety goals*. Retrieved from https://www.jointcommission.org/-/media/tjc/documents/standards/national-patient-safety-goals/2020-hap-npsg-goals-final.pdf..

Vizcarra, C. (2016). The Role of unlicensed assistive personnel in the provision of infusion therapy. *Journal of Infusion Nursing, 39*(4), 196–200. https://doi.org/10.1097/NAN.0000000000000172.

Xu, T., Kingsley, L., DiNucci, S., Messer, G., Jeong, J., Morgan, B., et al. (2016). Safety and utilization of peripherally inserted central catheters versus midline catheters at a large academic medical center. *American Journal of Infection Control, 44*(12), 1458–1461. https://doi.org/10.1016/J.AJIC.2016.09.010.

Yi, T., Xu, T., Qinghua, W., & Hui, Z. (2017). Intrathecal morphine versus femoral nerve block for pain control after total knee arthroplasty: A meta-analysis. *Journal of Orthopaedic Surgery & Research, 12*(1), 1–8. https://doi.org/10.1186/s13018-017-0621-0.

16

Concepts of Inflammation and Immunity

M. Linda Workman

http://evolve.elsevier.com/Iggy/

LEARNING OUTCOMES

1. Explain how physiologic aging affects ***immunity*** and ***inflammation*** and the associated care of older adults.
2. Distinguish between innate-native ***immunity*** and adaptive ***immunity*** with regard to initiating triggers, cell types, responses, and duration of protection.
3. Interpret laboratory findings to assess the patient's risk for an ***immunity*** problem or an increased risk for ***infection.***

KEY TERMS

absolute neutrophil count (ANC) Actual number of mature circulating neutrophils.

agglutination An antibody-antigen action in which a clumping action occurs when antibodies link antigens together, forming large and small immune complexes.

antibody Immunoglobulin produced by sensitized B-lymphocytes (plasma cells or memory cells) that bind to a specific antigen.

antibody-mediated immunity (AMI) The type of adaptive immunity that uses antibodies produced by sensitized B-lymphocytes to stimulate antigen-antibody interactions that neutralize, eliminate, or destroy foreign proteins.

antigens Proteins (usually) considered as non-self by a person's immune system that will stimulate the immune system to have an immunity response and make antibodies directed against the antigen.

cell-mediated immunity (CMI) The type of adaptive immunity that is provided by T-lymphocytes.

complement activation and fixation An antibody-antigen action by the IgG and IgM classes of antibodies to activate the 20 different inactive complement proteins that then form membrane attack complexes on the surface of antigens to enhance phagocytosis and antigen destruction.

cytokines Small hormone-like proteins produced by the many leukocytes (and some other tissues) that help modify inflammation and immunity.

erythrocytes Red blood cells (RBCs).

five cardinal symptoms of inflammation Warmth, redness, swelling, pain, and decreased function.

human leukocyte antigens (HLAs) Unique surface proteins that present on all of a person's cells that are specific to him or her. Also known as a person's "tissue type."

immunity Protection from illness or disease that is maintained by the body's physiologic defense mechanisms.

immunocompetent Having maximum protection against infection.

inactivation (neutralization) An antibody-antigen action in which antibody binding covers the antigen's active site, making it harmless without destroying it.

infection Invasion of pathogens into the body that multiply and cause disease or illness.

inflammation A syndrome of normal tissue responses to cellular injury, allergy, or invasion by pathogens.

left shift A condition in which the most prevalent type of neutrophil in circulation is not the mature, segmented neutrophil but is the less mature "band" neutrophil. Also called "bandemia."

leukocytes White blood cells (WBCs).

lysis An antibody-antigen binding action in which the antibody causes the antigen's cell membrane to be destroyed.

memory cell A sensitized B-lymphocyte that produces specific antibodies on all subsequent exposures to the initial sensitizing antigen.

microbiome All the microorganisms of normal flora that coexist in and on a person.
neutrophilia Increased number of circulating neutrophils.
phagocytosis Cellular engulfment and destruction of invading microorganisms and debris.
plasma cell A sensitized B-lymphocyte that immediately starts to produce antibodies against the sensitizing antigen.
precipitation An antibody-antigen action in which large antigen-antibody complexes are formed that precipitate in the blood, allowing other cells to destroy them through phagocytosis.
self-tolerance The special ability of immune system cells to recognize self versus non-self and avoid actions that would harm self cells.
stem cells Immature undifferentiated cells produced in the bone marrow that are pluripotent with the potential to mature into any blood cell type.

PRIORITY AND INTERRELATED CONCEPTS

The priority concepts for this chapter are:
- *Immunity*
- *Inflammation*

The interrelated concept for this chapter is:
- *Infection*

OVERVIEW

Immunity is protection from illness or disease that is maintained by the body's physiologic defense mechanisms. Complete protection requires the interaction of immunity and inflammation working together and includes both adaptive responses, as well as general or nonspecific responses and protections. *Inflammation* is a syndrome of normal tissue responses to cellular injury, allergy, or invasion by pathogens. This syndrome is nonspecific. The cellular components of immunity involve many different white blood cells (WBCs) and their products. In addition to certain WBCs, other nonspecific immunity protections are intact skin and mucous membranes, along with the person's microbiome. An adult's **microbiome** is all the microorganisms of normal flora that coexist in and on him or her. These includes the organisms that live in the mouth, the rest of the GI tract, the nose and sinuses, the vagina, and on the skin. The microbiome differs somewhat from person to person, and the organisms are *nonpathogenic* (non–disease causing) when they remain confined to the expected area. Organisms of the microbiome help promote the effectiveness of immunity and cellular regulation.

Most adults are healthy more often than they are ill even though communicable diseases and infectious agents are constantly present in the environment. ***Immunity*** and ***inflammation*** working together are critical to maintaining health, preventing disease, and repairing tissue damage. When all the different parts and functions of immunity are working well, the adult is **immunocompetent** and has maximum protection against infection.

Immunity is reduced by many diseases, injuries, and medical therapies. *Whether immunity is reduced temporarily or permanently, this reduction always endangers the patient's health.* Chapter 17 discusses reduced and inadequate immunity. Other problems occur when immunity is excessive or it occurs at inappropriate times. Chapter 18 discusses issues related to excess or inappropriate immunity responses, such as hypersensitivity and autoimmune disorders.

Adults interact with many other large and small living organisms (bacteria, viruses, molds, spores, pollens, protozoa, and cells from other people or animals). As long as organisms do not enter the body, they pose no health threat. Nonspecific body defenses to prevent organisms from entering include intact skin and mucous membranes, the microbiome, and natural chemicals that inhibit bacterial growth. These defenses are not perfect, and invasion can occur. However, most invasions do not result in disease or illness because of proper immunity.

Immunity and the immune system stimulate processes that neutralize, eliminate, or destroy invading organisms. To protect without causing harm, immune system cells exert actions only against non-self proteins and cells. Immune system cells have the special ability to distinguish between the body's own healthy self cells and non-self proteins and cells, a feature known as **self-tolerance**.

Self Versus Non-Self

Non-self proteins and cells include infected body cells, cancer cells, cells from other people, and invading organisms. Self-tolerance prevents the different immune system cells and products from harming healthy body cells. Self-tolerance is possible because of the different proteins present on cell membranes and the actions of T-lymphocytes known as *T-regulator cells* or *Tregs*.

Cells are surrounded by plasma membranes with different proteins on or through the surface (Fig. 16.1). For example, many different protein types are present on the liver cell membranes. Each of these protein types differs from that of all other protein types. Some protein types are specific markers for human tissues and are found only on human cells. In addition, each person's cells have unique surface proteins that are specific to that person, known as **human leukocyte antigens (HLAs)**. These genetically determined HLAs serve as a "universal product code" for that person and are identical only to the HLAs of an identical sibling. One adult's HLAs are recognized as "foreign," or non-self, by the immune system of another adult. Because the cell-surface proteins are non-self to another adult's immune system, they are **antigens**, which are proteins capable of triggering an ***immunity*** response.

HLAs are on the surfaces of most body cells—not just leukocytes. They are a normal part of the individual person and determine the *tissue type* of that person, which is coded for by the specific genes he or she inherits from both parents. Other names for these HLAs are *human histocompatibility antigens* and *class I antigens*.

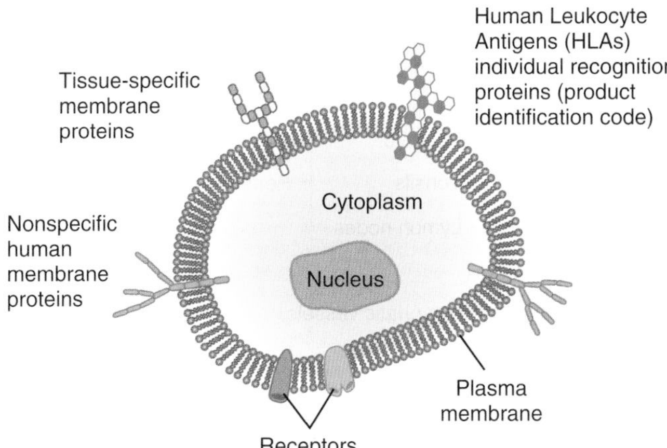

Fig. 16.1 Proteins on human cell plasma membranes.

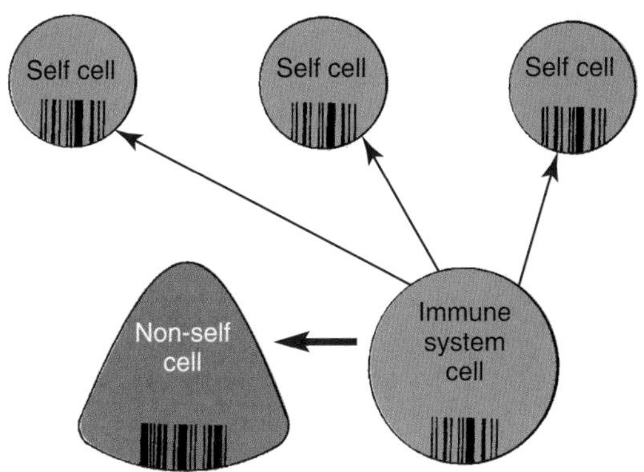

Fig. 16.2 Determination by immune system cell of self versus non-self cells.

The HLAs are key for recognition and self-tolerance. The immune system cells constantly come into contact with other body cells and with any invader that enters the body. At each encounter the immune system cells compare the surface protein HLAs to determine whether the encountered cell belongs in the body (Fig. 16.2). If the encountered cell's HLAs match the HLAs of the immune system cell, the encountered cell is "self" and is not attacked. If the encountered cell's HLAs do not perfectly match the HLAs of the immune system cell, the encountered cell is non-self, or foreign. The immune system cell then takes action to neutralize, destroy, or eliminate this foreign invader.

A key element for recognition of non-self by cells involved in general immunity and those involved in adaptive immunity is the presence of *toll-like receptors (TLRs)* on these cells. Toll receptors were first discovered in fruit flies as a way that this insect recognizes and rids itself of *pathogenic* (disease-causing) microorganisms. TLRs, which closely resemble the toll receptors, also are present on immune system cells of humans and other animals, as well as on defensive cells of insects and plants (Abbas et al., 2018). Their protective purpose is to interact with the surface of any invading organism and allow recognition of non-self, especially microorganisms, so that appropriate actions are taken to rid the body of this invader. TLRs also help immune system cells recognize injured, stressed, or unhealthy self cells.

Organization of the Immune System

The immune system is present throughout the body (Fig. 16.3) and is not confined to any single tissue or organ. The bone marrow is the source of all blood cells and many immune system cells. The bone marrow produces immature, undifferentiated cells called **stem cells**. Stem cells are *pluripotent,* meaning that each cell has more than one potential outcome for mature blood cells and immune system cells. When the stem cell is first generated in the bone marrow, it is undifferentiated, not yet committed to maturing into a specific blood cell type. This flexible or pluripotent stem cell could become any one of many mature blood or immune cell types. Fig. 16.4 shows the possible outcomes for maturation of stem cells. The type of mature cell that the stem cell becomes depends on which pathway it follows. Some cells mature in the bone marrow; others leave the bone marrow and mature in different body sites. When mature, many immune system cells are released into the blood, where they circulate to most body areas and have specific effects.

The maturational pathway of any stem cell depends on body needs and the presence of specific growth factors that direct the cell to a pathway. For example, erythropoietin is a growth factor for **erythrocytes** (red blood cells [RBCs]). When immature stem cells are exposed to erythropoietin, they commit to the erythrocyte pathway and eventually become mature RBCs.

Leukocytes (white blood cells [WBCs]) are the immune system cells that use a variety of actions to provide ***immunity.*** Table 16.1 lists the functions of different immune system cells. Some WBCs are classified as granulocytes because they have large granules in the cytoplasm. These include the neutrophils, basophils, and eosinophils, along with tissue mast cells. The monocytes, macrophages, and lymphocytes are classified as *agranulocytes,* although they do have fine granules in the cytoplasm. The leukocytes provide protection through these defensive actions:

- Recognition of self versus non-self for the initiation of defensive ***inflammation*** and ***immunity*** actions for protection
- Destruction of foreign invaders, cellular debris, and unhealthy or abnormal self cells
- Production of antibodies directed against invaders
- Complement activation forming membrane attack complexes to enhance phagocytosis
- Maintenance of self-tolerance
- Production of cytokines that stimulate increased formation of leukocytes in bone marrow and increase specific leukocyte activity

The three processes needed for human protection through ***immunity*** are the innate-native actions of (1) ***inflammation*** and the specific adaptive responses of (2) antibody-mediated immunity (AMI), and (3) cell-mediated immunity (CMI). Each process uses different defensive actions, and each influences or requires assistance from the other two processes (Fig. 16.5). *Full immunity (immunocompetence) requires the function and interaction of all three processes.*

Age-Related Changes in Immunity

Immunity changes during an adult's life as a result of nutrition status, environmental conditions, drugs, disease, and age.

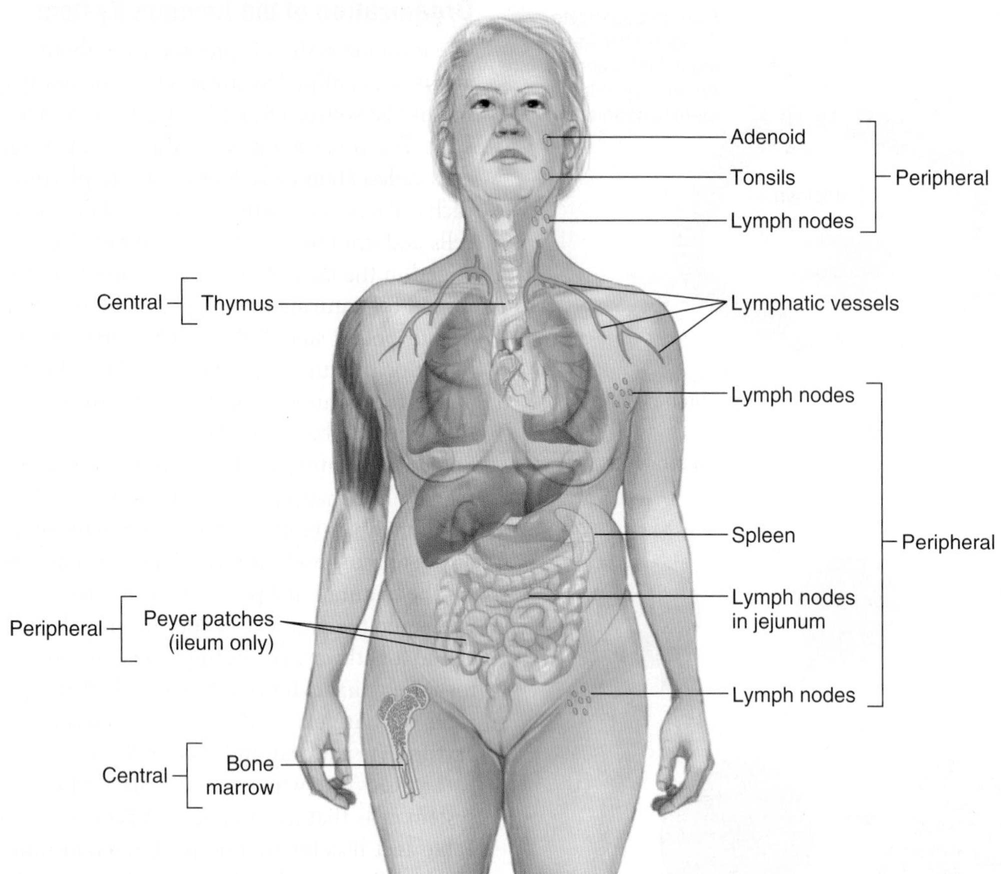

Fig. 16.3 The immune system and major sites of B-cell and T-cell maturation. (From McCance, K., Huether, S., Brashers, V., & Rote, N. [2019]. *Pathophysiology: The biologic basis for disease in adults and children* [8th ed.]. St. Louis: Mosby.)

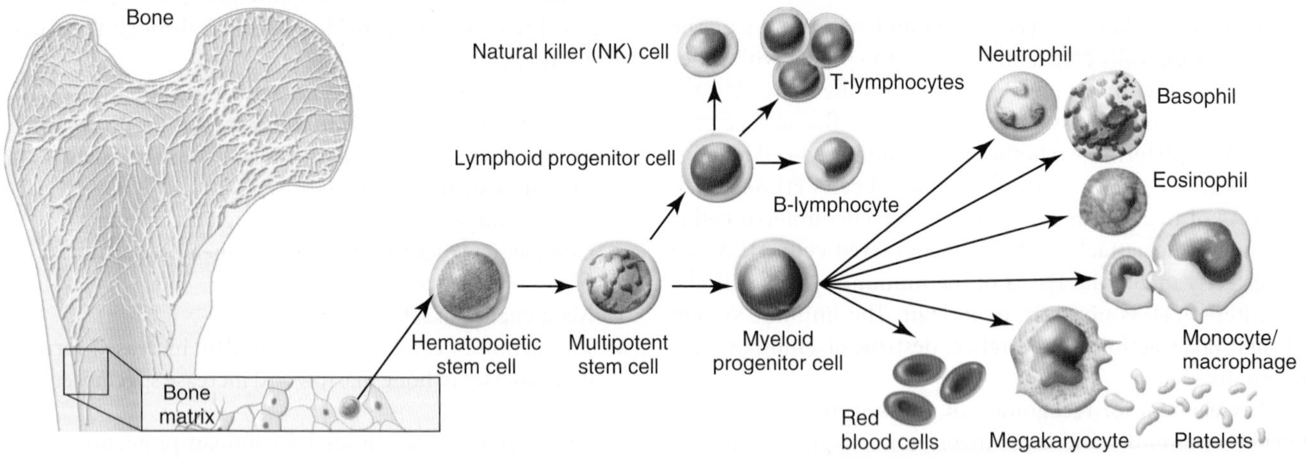

Fig. 16.4 Stem cell differentiation and maturation. (Modified from Goldman, L., & Schafer, A. [Eds.], [2012]. *Goldman's Cecil medicine* [24th ed.]. Philadelphia: Saunders.)

Immunity is most efficient in healthy adults who are in their 20s and 30s and slowly declines with increasing age (Touhy & Jett, 2020). Older adults have decreased function of both nonspecific general immunity and specific adaptive immunity. This decreased function increases the risk for infection and development of autoimmune diseases. The Patient-Centered Care: Older Adult Considerations box lists nursing implications of age-related changes in immune function.

The normal flora (microbiome) of skin, mucous membranes, and the GI tract changes, and overgrowth of more pathogenic organisms occurs (Touhy & Jett, 2020). The numbers of neutrophils and macrophages are reduced, as are their functions. As a result, some of the normal responses to infection and injury are reduced. The older adult may not have a fever or any temperature elevation even with severe infection. The usual response of an increased white blood cell count is

TABLE 16.1 Immune Functions of Specific Leukocytes

Variable	Leukocyte	Function
Inflammation	Neutrophil	Nonspecific ingestion and phagocytosis of microorganisms and foreign proteins
	Macrophage	Nonspecific recognition of foreign proteins and microorganisms; ingestion and phagocytosis Assists with antibody-mediated immunity and cell-mediated immunity
	Monocyte	Destruction of bacteria and cellular debris; matures into macrophage
	Eosinophil	Releases vasoactive amines during allergic reactions and in response to parasite infestations
	Basophil	Releases histamines, kinins, and heparin in areas of tissue damage
Antibody-mediated immunity	B-lymphocyte	Becomes sensitized to foreign cells and proteins with the assistance of macrophages and helper T-cells
	Plasma cell	Secretes immunoglobulins in response to the presence of a specific antigen
	Memory cell	Remains sensitized to a specific antigen and can secrete increased amounts of immunoglobulins specific to the antigen on re-exposure
Cell-mediated immunity	Helper T-cell	Enhances immune activity of all parts of general and specific immunity through secretion of various factors, cytokines, and lymphokines
	Cytotoxic T-cell	Selectively attacks and destroys non-self cells, including virally infected cells, grafts, and transplanted organs
	Regulator T-cell	Regulates a balance between offensive and defensive inflammation and immunity actions, and maintains self-tolerance
	Natural killer cell	Nonselectively attacks non-self cells, especially body cells that have undergone mutation and become malignant; also attacks grafts and transplanted organs

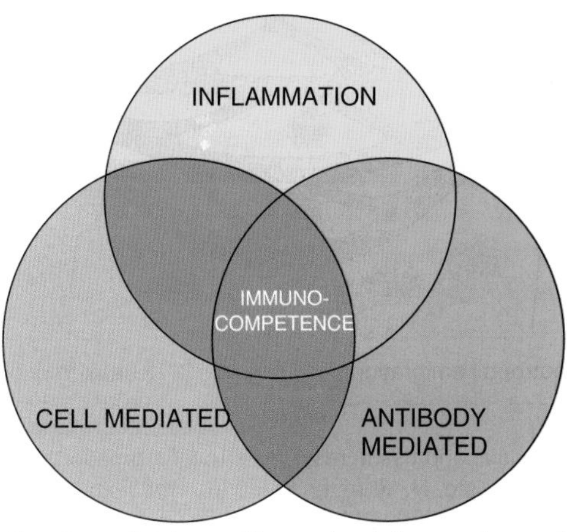

Fig. 16.5 The three divisions of immunity: inflammation, antibody-mediated immunity, and cell-mediated immunity. Optimal function of all three divisions is necessary for complete immunity.

delayed or absent. The number of toll-like receptors (TLRs) decreases (McCance et al., 2019). These changes result in less recognition of pathogens and an increased risk for infections of all types. In addition, because some of the usual responses are absent, identification and management of infection may be delayed until sepsis is present.

Changes in adaptive ***immunity*** include lower T-cell function (although lymphocyte numbers do not decrease). B-lymphocytes take longer to become sensitized and begin to make antibodies to new antigen exposures. Memory cells are much slower to respond to re-exposure of antigens. For these reasons, repeat vaccinations to boost adaptive immunities developed in childhood are needed for older adults (Rittle & Francis, 2016). With the loss of recognition of self, the amount of circulating autoantibodies increases, increasing the risk for autoimmune diseases in older adults (McCance et al., 2019).

PATIENT-CENTERED CARE: OLDER ADULT CONSIDERATIONS QSEN

Age-Related Changes in Immunity

Change	Nursing Implications
Inflammation	
Reduced neutrophil function.	Neutrophil counts may be normal, but activity is reduced, increasing the risk for infection.
Leukocytosis does not occur during acute infection.	Patients may have an infection but not show expected changes in white blood cell counts.
Older adults may not have a fever during inflammatory or infectious episodes.	Not only is there potential loss of protection through inflammation, but also minor infections may be overlooked until the patient becomes severely infected or septic.
Antibody-Mediated Immunity	
The total number of B-lymphocytes and their ability to mature into antibody-secreting cells are diminished.	Older adults are less able to make new antibodies in response to the presence of new antigens. Thus they should receive immunizations such as "flu shots," the pneumococcal vaccination, and the shingles vaccination.
The natural antibody response to antigens declines and the amount of time formed antibodies remain present is reduced.	Older adults may not have sufficient antibodies to provide protection when they are re-exposed to microorganisms against which they have already generated antibodies. Thus older patients need to receive "booster" shots for old vaccinations and immunizations, especially tetanus and pertussis (whooping cough).
Cell-Mediated Immunity	
The number of circulating T-lymphocytes decreases.	Skin tests for tuberculosis may have falsely negative results. Older patients are more at risk for bacterial and fungal infections, especially on the skin and mucous membranes, in the respiratory tract, and in the genitourinary tract.

GENERAL IMMUNITY: INFLAMMATION

Inflammation is part of the general ***immunity***, also called *innate-native immunity* or *natural immunity*, which is the first line of protection. It is nonspecific, is present in health, is not an adaptive response, and cannot be transferred from one adult to another. As part of general immunity, inflammation helps provide immediate protection against the effects of tissue injury and invading foreign proteins. Innate-native immunity is any natural protective feature of a human. It is a barrier to prevent organisms from entering the body and can attack organisms that have already entered the body.

General immunity comprises ***inflammation*** responses, the skin, mucosa, antimicrobial chemicals on the skin, complement, and natural killer cells. Inflammation is critical for health. General immunity and inflammation differ from specific adaptive immunity in two ways:

- Protection by inflammation is immediate but short-term and does not provide true ***immunity*** on repeated exposure to the same organisms.
- Inflammation is a *nonspecific* body defense to invasion or injury and can be started quickly by almost any event, regardless of where it occurs or what causes it.

So inflammation responses triggered by a scald burn to the hand are the same as inflammation responses triggered by bacteria in the middle ear. How widespread the symptoms of inflammation are depend on the intensity, severity, and duration of exposure to the initiating event. For example, a splinter in the finger triggers inflammation only at the splinter site, whereas a 50% burn injury leads to an inflammatory response involving the entire body.

Inflammation starts vascular and tissue actions causing visible and uncomfortable symptoms that are important in ridding the body of harmful organisms. However, if the inflammation responses are excessive, tissue damage may result. Inflammation also helps start the adaptive immunity responses of both antibody-mediated and cell-mediated actions to activate full ***immunity.*** Fig. 16.6 shows the vascular and tissue responses that occur with acute inflammation.

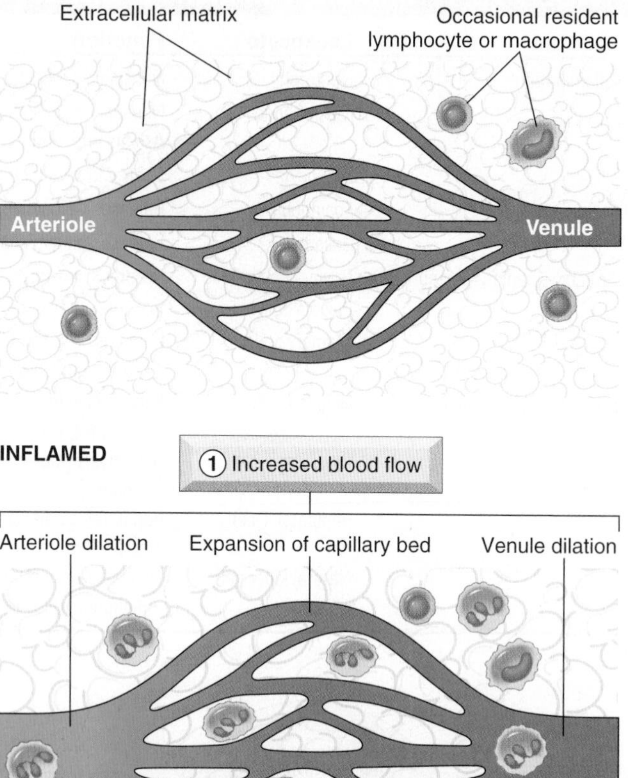

Fig. 16.6 Vascular and tissue responses to inflammation. (From Kumar, V., Abbas, A., Fausto, N., & Aster, J. [2010]. *Robbins and Cotran pathologic basis of disease* [8th ed.]. Philadelphia: Saunders.)

Infection

Infection is the invasion of pathogens into the body that multiply and cause disease or illness. Infection usually triggers ***inflammation*** and most often is accompanied by it. Examples of inflammation from infection include otitis media, appendicitis, and viral hepatitis, among many others. However, inflammation can occur without infection when the triggering event is tissue injury or a noninfectious invasion. Examples of ***inflammation*** without infection include joint sprains, myocardial infarction, and blister formation. Examples of inflammation caused by noninfectious invasion include allergic rhinitis, contact dermatitis, and other allergic reactions. *Thus inflammation does not always mean that an infection is present.*

Cell Types Involved in Inflammation

The leukocytes (white blood cells [WBCs]) involved in ***inflammation*** are neutrophils, macrophages, eosinophils, and basophils. An additional cell type important in inflammation is the tissue mast cell. Neutrophils and macrophages destroy and eliminate foreign invaders. Basophils, eosinophils, and mast cells release chemicals, such as histamine and kinins, that act on blood vessels to cause tissue-level responses that help neutrophil and macrophage actions.

Neutrophils. *Mature neutrophils* make up between 55% and 70% of the normal total WBC count. Neutrophils come from the stem cells and complete the maturation process in the bone marrow (Fig. 16.7). They are also called *granulocytes* because of the large number of granules present inside each cell. Other names for neutrophils are based on their appearance and maturity. Mature neutrophils are also called *segmented neutrophils* ("segs") or *polymorphonuclear cells* ("polys," PMNs) because of their segmented nucleus. Less mature neutrophils are called *band neutrophils* ("bands" or "stabs") and have a more U-shaped nucleus.

Usually growth of a stem cell into a mature neutrophil requires 12 to 14 days. This time can be shortened by the presence of

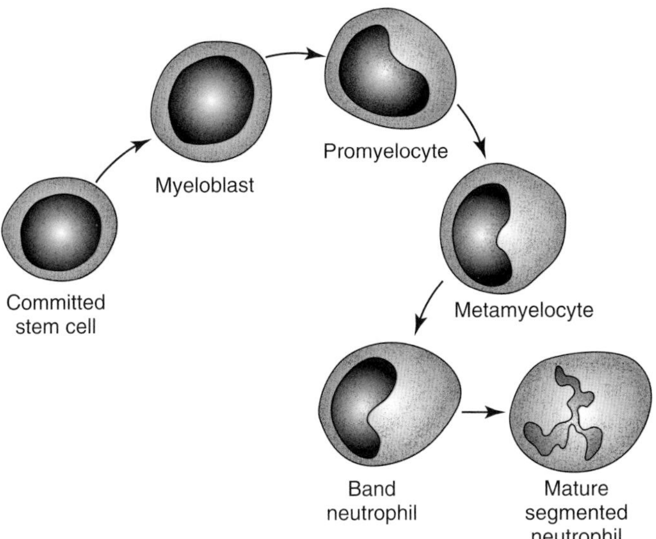

Fig. 16.7 Stem cell maturation into fully functional segmented neutrophils.

specific growth factors (cytokines) such as granulocyte-macrophage colony-stimulating factor (GM-CSF) and granulocyte colony-stimulating factor (G-CSF). The purpose and action of cytokines are described in the Cytokines section. In the healthy adult with full ***immunity***, more than 100 billion fresh, mature neutrophils are released from the bone marrow into the circulation daily. This huge production is needed because the life span of each neutrophil is short—about 12 to 18 hours.

Neutrophil function provides protection after invaders, especially bacteria, enter the body. This powerful army of small cells destroys invaders by phagocytosis and enzymatic digestion, although each cell is small and can take part in only one episode of phagocytosis.

Mature neutrophils are the only stage of this cell capable of phagocytosis. Because this cell type causes continuous, instant, nonspecific protection against organisms, the percentage and actual number of mature circulating neutrophils are used to measure a patient's risk for infection: the higher the numbers, the greater the resistance to ***infection***. This measurement is the **absolute neutrophil count (ANC)**.

The differential of a normal WBC cell count shows the number and percent of the different types of circulating leukocytes, as shown in the Laboratory Profile box. Most circulating neutrophils are segmented neutrophils; only a small percentage are band neutrophils or less mature forms. Problems such as sepsis cause the circulating neutrophils to change from being mostly segmented neutrophils to being less mature forms. This situation is a **left shift** or *bandemia* (sometimes called a "shift to the left") because the segmented neutrophil (at the far right of the neutrophil pathway in Fig. 16.7) is no longer the most numerous type in circulation. Instead, more of the circulating cells are bands—the less mature cell type found farther left on the neutrophil maturational pathway.

A left shift indicates that the patient's bone marrow cannot produce enough mature neutrophils to keep pace with the continuing infection and is releasing immature neutrophils into the blood. Most of these immature cells are of minimal benefit because they are not capable of phagocytosis.

LABORATORY PROFILE

Normal White Blood Cell (WBC) Count With Differential

WBC Type	%	/mm^3	× 10^9/L
Total	100	5000-10,000	5-10
Segs	55-70	2500-7000	3.0-5.8
Bands	5	250-500	0.25-0.5
Monos	2-8	100-800	0.3-0.5
Lymphs	20-40	1000-4000	1.5-3.0
Eosins	1-4	50-400	0.0-0.25
Basos	0.5-1.0	25-100	0.01-0.04

Data from Pagana, K., & Pagana, T. (2018). *Mosby's manual of diagnostic and laboratory tests* (6th ed.). St. Louis: Elsevier.

Macrophages. *Macrophages* come from the committed myeloid stem cells in the bone marrow and form the mononuclear-phagocyte system. The stem cells first form monocytes, which are released into the blood at this stage. Until they mature, monocytes have limited activity. Most monocytes move from the blood into body tissues, where they mature into macrophages. Some macrophages become "fixed" in position within the tissues, whereas others can move within and between tissues. Macrophages in various tissues have slightly different appearances and names. The liver, spleen, and intestinal tract contain large numbers of these cells.

Macrophage function helps stimulate immediate responses of ***inflammation*** and also stimulates the longer-lasting immune responses of antibody-mediated ***immunity*** (AMI) and cell-mediated immunity (CMI). Macrophage functions include phagocytosis, repair, antigen presenting/processing, and secretion of cytokines for immune system control.

The inflammatory function of macrophages is phagocytosis. Macrophages can easily distinguish between self and non-self, and their large size makes them very effective at trapping invading cells. They have long life spans, and each cell can take part in many phagocytic events.

Basophils. *Basophils* come from myeloid stem cells and make up only about 1% of the total circulating WBC count. These cells cause the signs and symptoms of ***inflammation*** shown in Fig. 16.6.

Basophil function acts on blood vessels with basophil chemicals (vasoactive amines), which include heparin, histamine, serotonin, kinins, and leukotrienes. Basophils have sites that bind the stem part of immunoglobulin E (IgE) molecules, which binds to and is activated by allergens. When allergens bind to the IgE on the basophil, the basophil membrane opens and releases the vasoactive amines into the blood, where most of them act on smooth muscle and blood vessel walls. Heparin inhibits blood and protein clotting. Histamine dilates arterioles and constricts small veins, slowing blood flow and decreasing venous return. This effect causes blood to collect in capillaries and arterioles. Kinins dilate arterioles and increase capillary permeability, causing blood plasma to leak into the interstitial space *(vascular leak syndrome)*. Basophils stimulate both general inflammation and the inflammation of allergic reactions.

Eosinophils. *Eosinophils* come from the myeloid line and contain many vasoactive chemicals. Only 1% to 4% of the total WBC count normally is composed of eosinophils.

Eosinophil function is most active against infestations of parasitic larvae and also works in the later reactions of ***inflammation*** to prolong the response. For many people with allergic asthma, eosinophils are the cell type in the respiratory tract that triggers mediators of inflammation and asthma attacks. The number of circulating eosinophils increases during an allergic response; when the numbers are very high *(eosinophilia)*, they can cause allergic responses or make them worse (Abbas et al., 2018).

Tissue Mast Cells. *Tissue mast cells* look like and have functions very similar to basophils and eosinophils. Although mast cells do originate in the bone marrow, they come from a different parent cell than leukocytes and do not circulate as mature cells (Abbas et al., 2018). Instead they differentiate and mature in tissues, especially those near blood vessels, lung tissue, skin, and mucous membranes. Mast cells have binding sites for the stems of IgE molecules and, when activated, are involved in allergic reactions. They also respond to the inflammatory products released by T-lymphocytes. Thus tissue mast cells maintain and prolong ***inflammation*** and allergic reactions.

Complement. The complement system is a part of innate ***immunity***. It is composed of a system of 20 different types of inactive plasma proteins that, when activated, act as enzymes and attracting agents to enhance (or "complement") cell actions of innate immunity. When stimulated, each type of complement protein is activated, joins other activated complement proteins, surrounds an antigen, and "fixes" or sticks to the antigen, quickly forming a membrane attack complex (MAC) on the antigen surface. This action makes immune cell attachment to antigens and phagocytosis more efficient.

NCLEX EXAMINATION CHALLENGE 16.1

Physiological Integrity

Which change would the nurse expect to see in the white blood cell differential of a client who has a prolonged, severe intestinal helminth infestation?

A. Band neutrophils outnumber segmented neutrophils.
B. Macrophage count is low.
C. Monocyte count is high.
D. Eosinophil count is high.

Phagocytosis

A key process of ***inflammation*** is phagocytosis, the engulfing and destruction of invaders, which also rids the body of debris after tissue injury. Neutrophils and macrophages are most efficient at phagocytosis. Phagocytosis involves the seven steps shown in Fig. 16.8.

Exposure and invasion occur as the first step in response to injury or invasion. Leukocytes that engage in phagocytosis and trigger inflammation are present in the blood and extracellular fluids. Phagocytosis starts with invasion by organisms or foreign proteins.

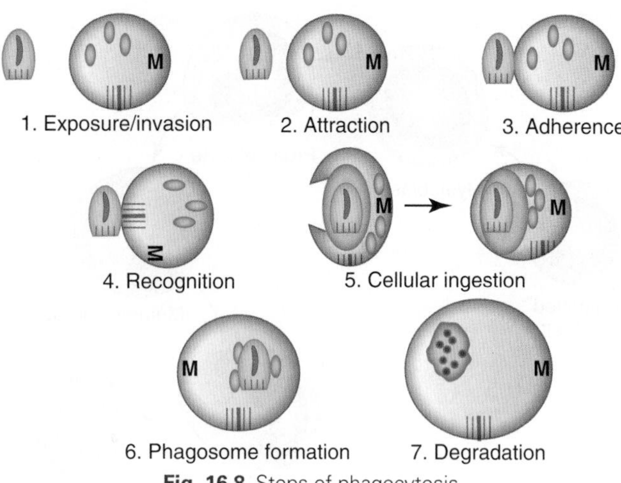

Fig. 16.8 Steps of phagocytosis.

Attraction is the second step and brings the WBC into direct contact with the target (antigen, invader, or foreign protein). Damaged tissues secrete *chemotaxins* that attract neutrophils and macrophages and release debris that binds to the surface of invading proteins.

Adherence binds the phagocytic cell to the surface of the target. *Opsonins* are substances that increase contact of the cell with its target by coating the target cell (antigen or organism). During ***inflammation***, coating the target makes it easier for phagocytic cells, especially macrophages, to stick to it. Substances that are opsonins include dead neutrophils, antibodies, and the membrane attack complexes formed by activated (fixated) complement components.

Recognition occurs when the phagocytic cell sticks to the target cell and "recognizes" it as non-self. The phagocytic cells examine the universal product codes (human leukocyte antigens [HLAs]) of whatever they encounter. Recognition of non-self is made easier by opsonins on the target cell surface. Phagocytic cells start phagocytosis only when the target cell is recognized as non-self or debris.

Cellular ingestion occurs when the target cell is brought inside the phagocytic cell by phagocytosis (engulfment).

Phagosome formation occurs when the phagocyte's granules break and release enzymes that attack the ingested target.

Degradation is the final step. The enzymes in the phagosome digest the engulfed target.

Sequence of Inflammation

Inflammation (inflammatory responses) occurs in a predictable three-stage sequence. The sequence is the same regardless of the triggering event. Responses at the tissue level cause the five cardinal symptoms of inflammation: warmth, redness, swelling, pain, and decreased function (see Fig. 16.6). The timing of the stages may overlap.

Stage I is a vascular response that starts changes in blood vessels. Injured tissues and the leukocytes and tissue mast cells in this area secrete histamine, serotonin, and kinins (especially bradykinin) that constrict small veins and dilate arterioles. These changes cause redness and warmth of the tissues. This increased blood flow increases delivery of nutrients to injured tissues.

Blood flow to the area increases *(hyperemia),* and edema forms at the site of injury or invasion. Capillary leak also occurs, allowing blood plasma to leak into the tissues. This response causes swelling and pain. Edema protects the area from further injury by creating a cushion of fluid. The duration of these responses depends on the severity of the initiating event, but usually they subside within 24 to 72 hours.

The macrophage is the major cell involved in stage I of ***inflammation***. The action is rapid because macrophages are already in place at the site of injury or invasion and also is limited because the number of macrophages is so small. To enhance the response, tissue macrophages secrete many proinflammatory cytokines. One is colony-stimulating factor (CSF), which triggers the bone marrow to shorten the time needed to produce some mature WBCs from 14 days to just hours. Some cytokines cause neutrophils from the bone marrow to move to the site of injury or invasion, which leads to the next stage of inflammation.

Stage II is the cellular exudate part of the response. In this stage **neutrophilia** (an increased number of circulating neutrophils) occurs. Exudate in the form of pus forms, containing dead WBCs, necrotic tissue, and fluids that escape from damaged cells.

Neutrophils, basophils, eosinophils, and tissue mast cells are active in this stage, with continuing activation triggered by the release of cytokines from macrophages in the area. The eosinophils and mast cells promote a continued inflammatory response. Under the influence of cytokines, the neutrophil count can increase hugely within 12 hours after inflammation starts. Neutrophils attack and destroy organisms and remove dead tissue through phagocytosis. Basophils and tissue mast cells continue or sustain the initial responses

In acute ***inflammation***, the healthy adult produces enough mature segmented neutrophils to keep pace with invasion and prevent the organisms from growing. At the same time the WBCs and inflamed tissues secrete cytokines, which allow tissue macrophages to increase and trigger bone marrow production of monocytes.

During this phase the arachidonic acid cascade starts to increase inflammation. This action begins by the conversion of fatty acids in plasma membranes of injured or infected cells into arachidonic acid (AA). The enzyme *cyclooxygenase* (COX) converts AA into chemicals that are further processed into the substances *(mediators)* that promote continued inflammation. Mediators of inflammation include histamine, leukotrienes, prostaglandins, serotonin, and kinins. Many anti-inflammatory drugs stop this cascade by preventing cyclooxygenase from converting AA into inflammatory mediators.

When an infection stimulating ***inflammation*** lasts longer than just a few days, the bone marrow begins to release immature neutrophils, reducing the number of circulating mature neutrophils. This problem limits helpful effects of inflammation and increases the risk for sepsis.

Stage III features tissue repair and replacement. Although this stage is completed last, it begins at the time of injury and is critical to the final function of the inflamed area.

WBCs involved in ***inflammation*** start the replacement of lost tissues or repair of damaged tissues by inducing the remaining healthy cells to divide. In tissues that cannot divide, WBCs trigger new blood vessel growth and scar tissue formation. Because scar tissue does not act like the tissue it replaces, function is lost wherever scar tissue forms as replacement for normal tissue. For example, when heart muscles are destroyed by a myocardial infarction (heart attack), scar tissue forms in the area to prevent a hole from forming in the muscle wall as the ischemic cells die. The scar tissue serves only as a patch; it does not contract or act in any way like heart muscle. So if 20% of the left ventricle is replaced with scar tissue, the effectiveness of left ventricular contraction is reduced by at least 20%.

Inflammation alone cannot provide long-lasting ***immunity***. Lymphocytes are the cells needed for long-lasting antibody-mediated immunity (AMI) and cell-mediated immunity (CMI).

NCLEX EXAMINATION CHALLENGE 16.2

Physiological Integrity

How do macrophages contribute to the neutrophilia that occurs in response to an acute bacterial infection?

A. When invasion occurs, macrophages mature into neutrophils, increasing their circulating numbers.
B. Macrophages have only an indirect role in neutrophilia by secreting substances that reduce bone marrow production of erythrocytes and platelets.
C. At the onset of invasion, macrophages secrete a colony-stimulating factor to induce the bone marrow to increase production and release of neutrophils.
D. Inflammatory damage to macrophages allows release of proteolytic enzymes that enhance liver production of all white blood cell types, including mature segmented neutrophils.

ADAPTIVE IMMUNITY

Adaptive ***immunity*** is a protective response that is specific and results in long-term resistance to the effects of invading microorganisms. This means that the responses are not automatic, which is why adaptive immunity is also known as *acquired immunity.* The body has to learn or acquire the ability to generate specific immune responses when it is infected by or exposed to specific organisms. Lymphocytes develop actions and products that provide true, long-lasting immunity. These cells develop specific actions in response to specific invasion (Fig. 16.9). The two divisions of adaptive immunity are antibody-mediated immunity and cell-mediated immunity. As indicated by Fig. 16.5, activation of both types of specific immunity requires interactions with actions and cells of innate-native immunity (Munro, 2019).

Antibody-Mediated Immunity

Antibody-mediated immunity (AMI), also known as *humoral immunity,* is a type of adaptive immunity that uses antigen-antibody interactions to neutralize, eliminate, or destroy foreign proteins. **Antibodies** are proteins known as immunoglobulins produced by sensitized B-lymphocytes (B-cells) that bind to specific antigens.

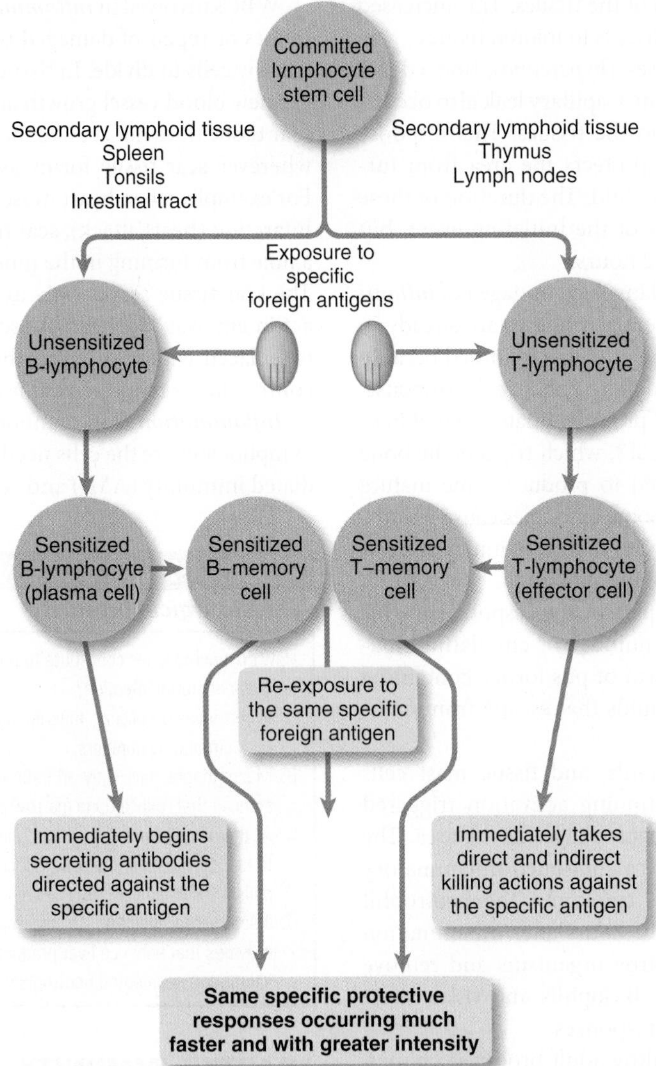

Fig. 16.9 B-lymphocyte and T-lymphocyte differentiation, maturation, and function.

B-cells become sensitized to a specific foreign protein (antigen) and produce antibodies directed specifically against that protein. The antibody, rather than the B-cell, then causes actions to neutralize, eliminate, or destroy that antigen. B-cells have the most direct role in AMI.

Macrophages and T-lymphocytes (discussed the Cell-Mediated Immunity section) work with B-cells to generate antigen-antibody interactions. *For optimal AMI the entire immune system must function adequately.*

B-cells start as stem cells in the bone marrow, the primary lymphoid tissue, that commit to the lymphocyte pathway (see Fig. 16.4) and are then restricted in development. The lymphocyte stem cells released into the blood then migrate into many secondary lymphoid tissues to mature. As shown in Fig. 16.3, the secondary lymphoid tissues for B-cells are the spleen, parts of lymph nodes, tonsils, and the mucosa of the intestinal tract (McCance et al., 2019).

Antigen-Antibody Interactions. The body adapts and learns to make enough of any specific antibody to provide long-lasting ***immunity*** against specific organisms or toxins. The seven steps for specific antibody production against a specific antigen are shown in Fig. 16.10 and described in the following paragraphs.

Exposure or invasion is needed for the antigen to enter the adult to generate an antibody, although not all exposures result in antibody production. Invasion by the antigen must occur in such large numbers that some of the antigen evades detection by the body's innate-native general defenses or overwhelms the ability of ***inflammation*** to get rid of the invader.

For example, an adult who has never been exposed to the viral disease *influenza A* now baby-sits three children who develop influenza symptoms within the next 10 hours. These children, in the presymptomatic stage, shed many millions of live influenza A virus particles by droplets from the upper respiratory tract. They expose the baby-sitter by drinking out of the baby-sitter's cup, kissing her on the lips, and sneezing and coughing into her face. During the 5 hours spent with the children, the baby-sitter is heavily invaded by the influenza A virus and will become sick with this disease within 2 to 4 days. While the virus is growing and the disease is developing, the baby-sitter's sensitized B-lymphocytes

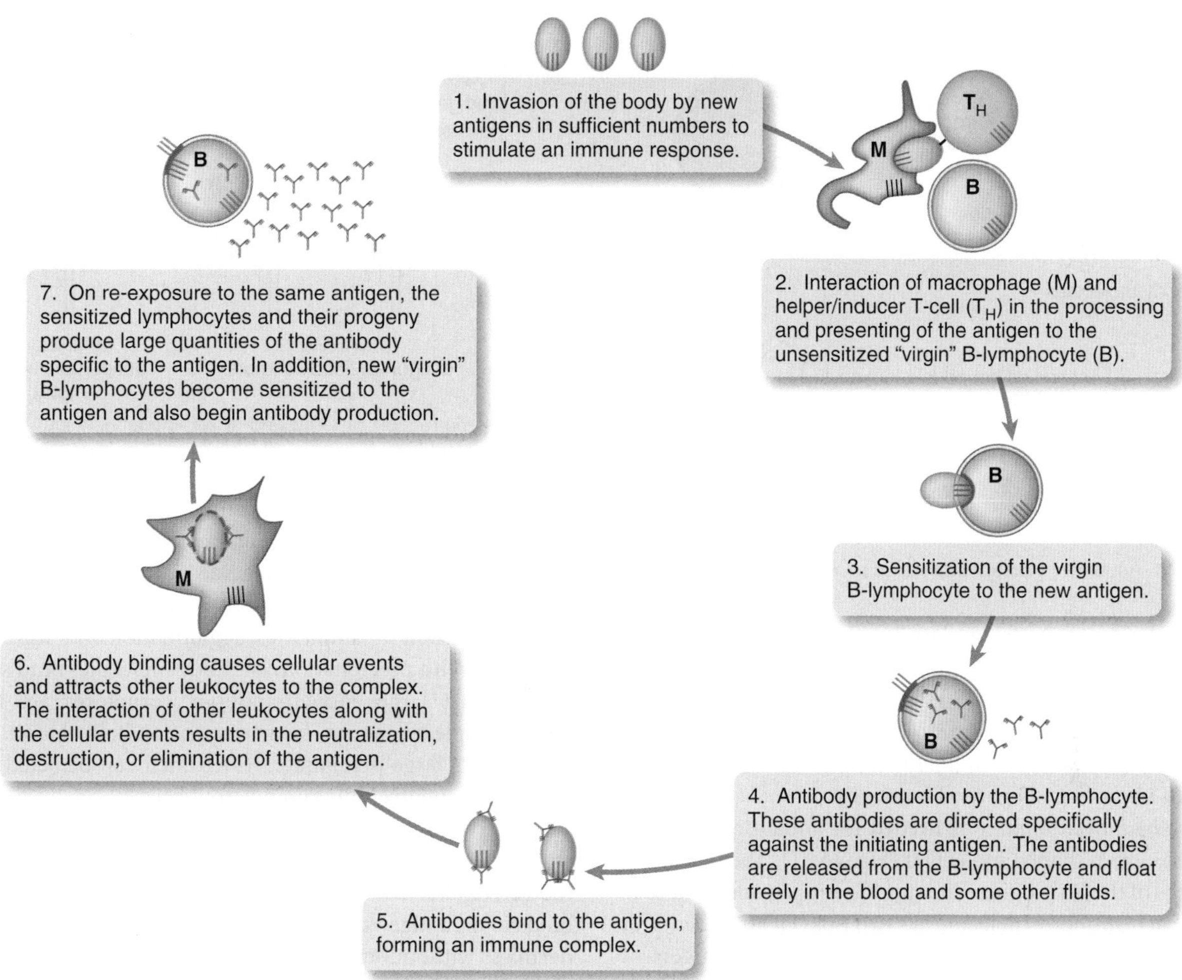

1. Invasion of the body by new antigens in sufficient numbers to stimulate an immune response.
M
T_H
B
2. Interaction of macrophage (M) and helper/inducer T-cell (T_H) in the processing and presenting of the antigen to the unsensitized "virgin" B-lymphocyte (B).
B
3. Sensitization of the virgin B-lymphocyte to the new antigen.
B
4. Antibody production by the B-lymphocyte. These antibodies are directed specifically against the initiating antigen. The antibodies are released from the B-lymphocyte and float freely in the blood and some other fluids.
5. Antibodies bind to the antigen, forming an immune complex.
6. Antibody binding causes cellular events and attracts other leukocytes to the complex. The interaction of other leukocytes along with the cellular events results in the neutralization, destruction, or elimination of the antigen.
M
7. On re-exposure to the same antigen, the sensitized lymphocytes and their progeny produce large quantities of the antibody specific to the antigen. In addition, new "virgin" B-lymphocytes become sensitized to the antigen and also begin antibody production.
B

Fig. 16.10 Sequence of the seven steps required to stimulate antibody-mediated immunity.

(B-cells) are taking part in antibody-antigen actions to prevent her from having influenza A more than once.

Antigen recognition is the recognition of the antigen by unsensitized B-cells. This action requires the help of macrophages and helper/inducer T-cells.

Recognition is started by the macrophages of innate immunity. After the antigen surface has been altered by opsonization (see discussion of adherence in the Phagocytosis section), macrophages recognize the invading antigen as non-self and attach to the antigen. This attachment allows macrophages to "present" the attached antigen to the helper/inducer T-cell. Then the helper/inducer T-cell and the macrophages together process the antigen to expose the antigen's recognition sites (universal product code). After processing the antigen, the helper/inducer T-cells bring the antigen into contact with the B-cell so that the B-cell can recognize the antigen as non-self.

Sensitization occurs when the B-cell recognizes the antigen as non-self and is now "sensitized" to this antigen. A single unsensitized B-cell can become sensitized only once. *So each B-cell can be sensitized to only one type of antigen.*

Sensitizing allows this B-cell to respond to any substance that carries the same antigens (codes) as the original antigen. The sensitized B-cell always remains sensitized to that specific antigen. In addition, all cells produced by that sensitized B-cell also are already presensitized to that same specific antigen.

Immediately after it is sensitized, the B-cell divides and forms two types of B-lymphocytes, each one remaining sensitized to that specific antigen (see Fig. 16.9). One new cell becomes a **plasma cell**, which starts immediately to produce antibodies against the sensitizing antigen. The other new cell becomes a memory cell. The **memory cell** is a sensitized B-cell but does not produce antibodies until the next exposure to the same antigen (see discussion of sustained immunity [memory] later in the Antigen-Antibody Interactions section).

Antibody production and release allow the antibodies to search out specific antigens. Antibodies are produced by plasma cells; each plasma cell can make as many as 300 molecules of antibody per second. A plasma cell produces antibodies specific only to the antigen that originally sensitized the parent B-cell. For example, in the case of the baby-sitter who was invaded by the influenza A virus, the plasma cells from those B-cells sensitized to the influenza A virus can make only anti–influenza A antibodies. The antibody class (e.g., immunoglobulin G [IgG] or immunoglobulin M [IgM]) that the plasma cell produces may vary, but the antibody can be forever directed against only the influenza A virus.

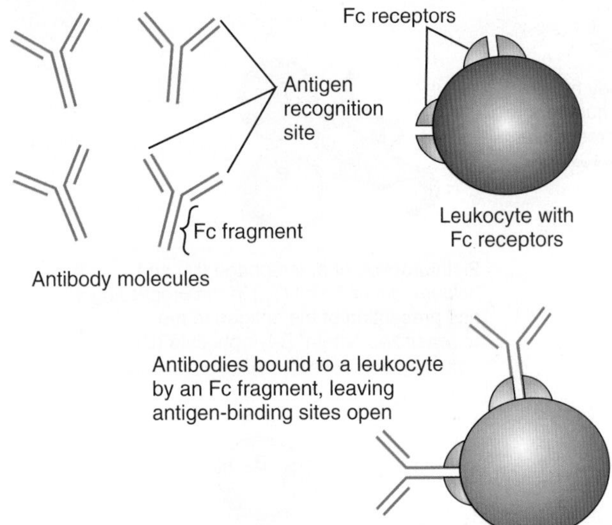

Fig. 16.11 Antibody structure and the Fc receptors on leukocytes.

Antibody molecules from plasma cells are released into the blood and body fluids (body "humors") as free antibodies that are separate from the B-cells. So this type of adaptive ***immunity*** may be called *humoral* immunity. *Circulating antibodies can be transferred from one adult to another and provide the receiving adult with immediate short-term immunity.*

Antibody-antigen binding is needed for antiantigen actions. Antibodies are Y-shaped molecules (Fig. 16.11). The tips of the short arms of the Y recognize the specific antigen and bind to it. Because each antibody molecule has two tips (Fab fragments, or arms), each antibody can bind either to two separate antigens or to two areas of the same antigen.

The stem of the Y is the "Fc fragment." This area can bind to Fc receptor sites on some WBCs. The WBC then not only has its own means of attacking antigens but also has the added power of having surface antibodies that can stick to antigens (see Fig. 16.11).

The binding of antibody to antigen may not be lethal to the antigen. Instead antibody-antigen binding starts other actions that neutralize, eliminate, or destroy the antigen.

Antibody-binding actions are triggered when an antibody binds to an antigen. The resulting actions of agglutination, lysis, complement fixation, precipitation, and inactivation can then neutralize, eliminate, or destroy the bound antigen.

Agglutination is a clumping action occurring when the antibodies link antigens together, forming large and small immune complexes (Fig. 16.12). The irregular shape of the antigen-antibody complex (see Fig. 16.12) increases the actions of macrophages and neutrophils.

Lysis is cell membrane destruction, and it occurs when antibodies bind to membrane-bound antigens of some invaders. Antibody binding makes holes in the invader's membrane, weakening the invader, especially bacteria and viruses. This response usually requires that complement be activated and "fixed" to the immune complex.

Complement activation and fixation is the activation by the IgG and IgM classes of antibodies of the 20 different inactive complement proteins that then form membrane attack complexes on the surface of antigens to enhance phagocytosis and

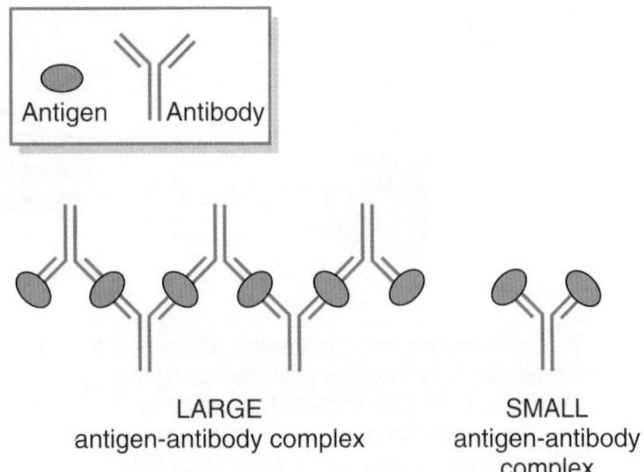

Fig. 16.12 Formation of large and small antigen-antibody complexes (immune complexes).

antigen destruction. Binding of either IgG or IgM to an antigen provides a binding site for the first component of complement. Once the first complement molecule is activated, other proteins of the complement system are activated in a cascade.

Precipitation is similar to agglutination but has a larger response. With precipitation, antibody molecules bind so much antigen that large antigen-antibody complexes are formed. These complexes cannot stay in suspension in the blood. Instead they form a large precipitate, which then can be acted on and removed by neutrophils and macrophages.

Inactivation (neutralization) makes an antigen harmless without destroying it. Usually only a small area of the antigen, the active site, causes the harmful effects. When an antibody binds to an antigen's active site, covering it, the antigen is made harmless without being destroyed.

Sustained immunity (memory) provides us with long-lasting, true adaptive ***immunity*** to a specific antigen. This immunity results from memory B-cells made during lymphocyte sensitization. These memory cells remain sensitized to the specific antigen to which they were originally exposed. On re-exposure to the same antigen, the memory cells rapidly respond by dividing and forming new sensitized blast cells and plasma cells. The blast cells continue to divide, producing many more sensitized plasma cells. These new sensitized plasma cells rapidly make large amounts of the antibody specific for the sensitizing antigen.

Having memory cells respond on re-exposure to the same antigen that originally sensitized the B-cell allows a rapid and large immune response *(anamnestic response)* to the antigen. When so much antibody is made, the invading organisms may be removed completely, and illness does not result. This process prevents adults from becoming ill with any infectious disease more than once, even though they are exposed many times to the same causative organism. Without immunologic memory, adults would be susceptible to the same diseases at every exposure to the causative organisms, and no long-term ***immunity*** would be generated (Abbas et al., 2018).

Antibody Classification. All antibodies are immunoglobulins, also called *gamma globulins.* A globulin is a protein that is globular rather than straight. Because antibodies are globular proteins, they are "globulins." The term *immunoglobulin* is used because they are globular proteins that provide ***immunity.***

TABLE 16.2 **Antibody Classification**

Antibody	Function
IgA	"Secretory" antibody that is present in high concentrations in the secretions of mucous membranes and the intestinal mucosa to provide mucosal immunity Most responsible for preventing infection in the upper and lower respiratory tracts, the GI tract, and the genitourinary tract
IgD	Acts as a B-cell antigen receptor
IgE	Associated with antibody-mediated immediate hypersensitivity reactions Provides protection against parasite infestations, especially helminths
IgG	Accounts for the largest amount of circulating antibodies Is heavily expressed on second and subsequent exposures to antigens to provide sustained, long-term immunity against invading microorganisms Activates classic complement pathway and enhances neutrophil and macrophage actions
IgM	First antibody formed by a newly sensitized B-lymphocyte plasma cell Effective at the antibody actions of agglutination and precipitation because of having 10 binding sites per molecule Activates complement pathway

Antibodies also are called *gamma globulins* because all free antibodies in the plasma separate out in the gamma fraction of plasma proteins during electrophoresis. The five antibody types are classified by differences in size, location, amount, and function (Table 16.2).

On first exposure to an antigen, the newly sensitized B-cell produces the IgM antibody type against the antigen. IgM is special because it is large and forms itself into a five-member group with 10 antigen binding sites. So even though antibody production is slow on first exposure, IgM is very efficient at antigen binding (Munro, 2019). This process ensures that the initial illness (e.g., influenza A) lasts only 5 to 10 days (instead of weeks to months). On re-exposure to the same antigen, the already sensitized B-cell makes large amounts of the IgG type of antibody against that antigen. Although IgG does not form groups of five, the enormous amounts produced make IgG antibodies efficient at clearing the antigen and protecting the patient from becoming ill with the disease again.

Acquiring Antibody-Mediated Immunity. Antibody-mediated ***immunity*** (AMI) is adaptive immunity in which a person's body learns to make an adaptive response to invasion by organisms or foreign proteins. Antibody-mediated immunity therefore is an *acquired immunity.* Adaptive immunity occurs either naturally or artificially through lymphocyte responses and can be either active or passive. Fig. 16.13 shows differences in how active and passive antibody-mediated immunity are acquired and their long-range effects.

Active immunity occurs when antigens enter a human and he or she responds by making specific antibodies against the antigen. This type of adaptive ***immunity*** is *active* because the body takes an active part in making antibodies.

Natural active ***immunity*** occurs when an antigen enters your body naturally without human assistance and your body responds by actively making antibodies against that antigen (e.g., influenza A virus). Usually the invasion that triggers antibody production also causes the disease. However, processes occurring in your body at the same time as infection create immunity to that antigen so illness does not occur again after a second exposure to the same antigen. *Natural active immunity is the most effective type of adaptive immunity and is the longest lasting.*

Artificial active ***immunity*** is the protection developed by vaccination or immunization (Hogue & Meador, 2016). This type of protective immunity is used to prevent serious and potentially deadly illnesses (e.g., tetanus, diphtheria, polio). Small amounts of specific antigens are placed as an oral or injected vaccination into your body. Your immune system then responds by actively making antibodies against the antigen. Because antigens used for this procedure have been specially processed to make them less likely to grow in the body *(attenuated),* this exposure usually does not cause the disease. Artificial active immunity lasts many years, although repeated but smaller doses of the original antigen are required as a "booster" to retain the protection.

Passive immunity occurs when the antibodies against an antigen are transferred to a human after first being made in the body of another human or animal. Although the antibodies were generated because of adaptation, the person receiving the antibodies did not make the adaptations. Because these antibodies are foreign to the receiving human, they are recognized as non-self and eliminated quickly. For this reason passive immunity provides only immediate, short-term protection against a specific antigen. It is used when an adult is exposed to a serious disease for which he or she has little or no actively acquired immunity. Instead the injected antibodies are expected to inactivate the antigen. For example, an immigrant patient who has never received a vaccination or an immunization has a deep puncture wound that is probably contaminated with the tetanus bacterium. He has no adaptive immunity to tetanus and could develop this deadly disease. This patient should first receive an injection that contains a large concentration of antitetanus antibodies to provide immediate protection as passive immunity from the bacteria in the contaminated wound. A few weeks later, he should then receive the usual tetanus toxoid vaccination to start developing his own antitetanus antibodies, generating artificial active immunity against this disease. A recent example of artificial passive immunity is the current use of "convalescent serum" of patients who have recovered from COVID-19 coronavirus influenza. This serum has a high concentration of anti–COVID-19 antibodies that can help prevent a person who is exposed to the virus from becoming ill with the influenza and,

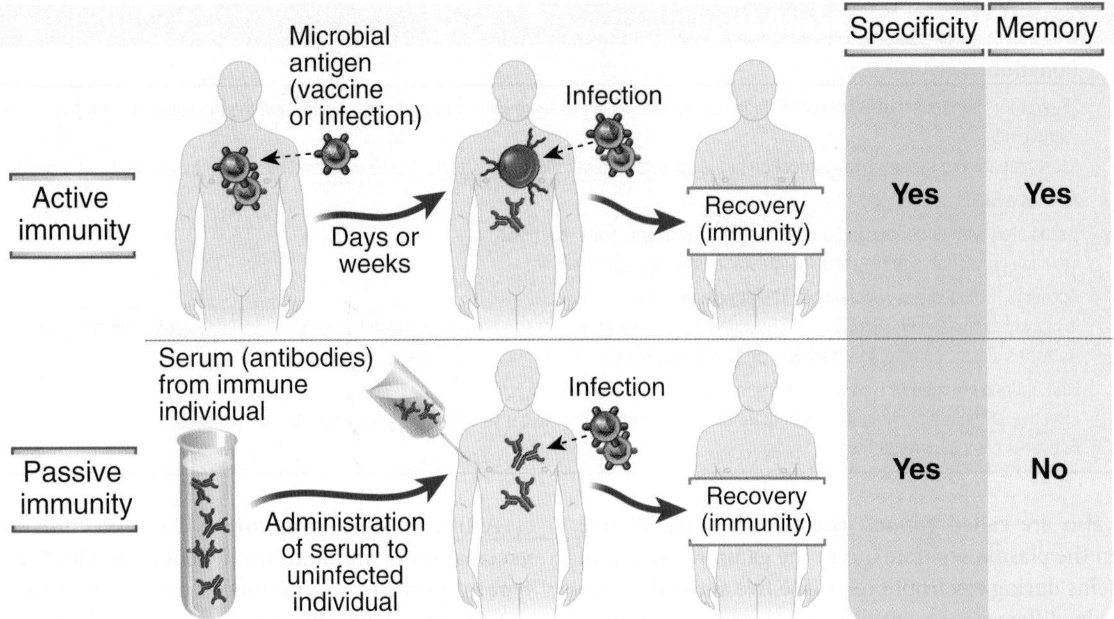

Fig. 16.13 Comparison of active and passive antibody-mediated immunity. (From Abbas, A., Lichtman, A., & Pillai, S. [2018]. *Cellular and molecular immunology* [8th ed.]. Philadelphia: Saunders.)

when given to a person who is already ill with the disease, can reduce its severity and duration.

Artificial passive immunity is most commonly used to prevent disease or death in a patient exposed to rabies, tetanus, poisonous snake bites, or any other serious infectious diseases to which he or she has little or no active immunity. Fig. 16.13 compares active and passive immunity.

Natural passive immunity occurs when antibodies are passed from the mother to the fetus via the placenta or to the infant through colostrum and breast milk.

AMI works with inflammation to protect against infection. It provides effective long-lasting immunity only when its actions are combined with those of cell-mediated immunity.

NCLEX EXAMINATION CHALLENGE 16.3

Physiological Integrity

Which cells, products, or actions are involved in long-lasting immunity resulting from exposure to a specific antigen? **Select all that apply.**

A. Antibody attenuation
B. Interleukin 10 (IL-10)
C. Memory B-cells
D. Monocyte maturation
E. Neutrophilia
F. Phagocytosis

Cell-Mediated Immunity

Cell-mediated immunity (CMI), or cellular immunity, involves many white blood cell (WBC) actions and interactions. CMI also is adaptive, long-lasting ***immunity*** that is provided by lymphocyte stem cells that mature in the secondary lymphoid tissues of the thymus and pericortical areas of lymph nodes (see Fig. 16.3). Certain CMI responses influence and regulate the activities of antibody-mediated immunity (AMI) and innate immunity (***inflammation***) by producing and releasing cytokines. For total or full immunity, CMI must function optimally.

Cell Types Involved in Cell-Mediated Immunity. The WBCs with the most important known roles in CMI include several specific T-lymphocytes (T-cells) along with a special population of cells known as *natural killer (NK) cells.* T-cells have a variety of subsets, each of which has a specific function.

Different T-cell subsets can be identified by the presence of "marker proteins" (antigens) on the cell membrane's surface. More than 200 different T-cell proteins have been identified on cell membrane surfaces, and some of these are commonly used clinically to identify specific cells (Abbas et al., 2018). Most T-cells have more than one antigen on their cell membrane. For example, all mature T-cells contain T1, T3, T10, and T11 proteins. An interesting feature of most T-lymphocytes is that very early in development these cells form groups or colonies called *clones.* The cells in a clone all develop receptors on the cell surface against one specific environmental antigen, most commonly a microorganism. Healthy adults have millions of T-lymphocyte clones that are able to recognize millions of environmental antigens. Thus the T-cell population is excellent at recognizing non-self antigens quickly.

The names that identify specific T-cell subsets include the specific membrane antigen and the overall actions of the cells in a subset. The three T-lymphocyte subsets that appear most important for the development and continuation of CMI are helper T-cells, regulator T-cells, and cytotoxic T-cells. The natural killer cell (NK cell) also contributes to CMI.

Helper T-cells have the T4 protein on their membranes. These cells are usually called *T4+ cells* or T_H *cells*. The most correct name for helper/inducer T-cells is *CD4+* (cluster of differentiation 4). They are called "helper" T-cells because they are responsible for enhancing all aspects of ***immunity.***

Helper T-cells easily recognize self cells versus non-self cells. When they recognize non-self (antigen), helper T-cells secrete cytokines that can enhance the activity of other WBCs and increase overall immune function. These cytokines increase bone marrow production of stem cells and speed up their maturation. Thus helper T-cells act as organizers in "calling to arms" various squads of WBCs involved in ***inflammation,*** as well as in adaptive antibody-mediated immunity, and cellular protective actions.

Regulator T-cells, known as *Tregs,* start out as a type of T4 cells and become sensitized for self-recognition in the thymus. They have CD25 receptors on the cell surface and are activated by interleukin-2 (IL-2) and the transcription factor FoxP3. At one time they were known as suppressor T-cells but have been found to have a larger role in regulation of ***immunity.***

Tregs prevent hypersensitivity and ***immunity*** *overreactions* on exposure to non-self cells or proteins. This action prevents the formation of antibodies directed against normal, healthy self cells, which is the basis for many autoimmune diseases. Tregs secrete cytokines, especially interleukin-10 (IL-10), that have an overall *inhibitory* action on most cells of the immune system. When Tregs are less active or nonfunctional, immunity is unchecked resulting in systemic inflammatory disease and continuous WBC activation. Both innate-native immunity and adaptive immunity actions are greatly increased as is the risk for development of autoimmune disorders (Abbas et al., 2018).

Cytotoxic T-cells are also called CTLs and T_C*-cells.* Cytotoxic T-cells destroy cells that contain a processed antigen's human leukocyte antigens (HLAs) while maintaining self-tolerance through the secretion of cytotoxic T-lymphocyte–associated protein 4 (CTLA-4). This activity is most effective against self cells infected by parasites, such as viruses or protozoa. The CTLA-4 prevents other immune system cells from attacking self cells.

Parasite-infected self cells have both self HLA proteins (universal product code) and the parasite's antigens on the cell surface. This allows immune system cells to recognize the infected self cell as abnormal, and the CTLs can bind to it, punch a hole, and deliver a "lethal hit" of enzymes to the infected cell, causing it to lyse and die.

Natural killer (NK) cells are also known as *CD16+ cells* and are very important in providing CMI. These cells have direct cytotoxic effects on some non-self cells without first being sensitized. They conduct "seek and destroy" missions in the body to eliminate non-self cells. The NK cells are most effective in destroying unhealthy or abnormal self cells such as cancer cells and virally infected body cells (Abbas et al., 2018).

Cytokines. Cell-mediated immunity (CMI) regulates the immune system by producing cytokines. **Cytokines** are small hormone-like proteins produced by many WBCs (and some other tissues) that help modify ***inflammation*** and ***immunity***. Cytokines made by the macrophages, neutrophils, eosinophils, and monocytes are called *monokines.* Those produced by T-cells are called *lymphokines.* In addition, many other body cell types can produce and respond to cytokines.

Cytokines work like hormones: one cell produces a cytokine, which in turn exerts its effects on other cells of the immune system and on other body cells. The cells responding to the cytokine may be located close to or remote from the cytokine-secreting cell. Thus cytokines act like "messengers" that tell specific cells how and when to respond. The cells that change their activity when a cytokine is present are "responder" cells. For a responder cell to respond to the presence of a cytokine, the responder cell must have a specific receptor to which the cytokine can bind. Once the cytokine binds to its receptor, the responder cell changes its activity.

Cytokines control many inflammatory and immune responses and are controlled by interactions with other systems. Cytokines include the interleukins (ILs), interferons (IFNs), colony-stimulating factors (CSFs), tumor necrosis factors (TNFs), and transforming growth factors (TGFs). The interleukins are the largest group of cytokines. Some cytokines have families and other classifications. Some cytokines are "proinflammatory" and increase the actions of ***inflammation***. These currently include TNF-α, IL-1, IL-10, IL-12, IL-17, IL-23, and interferons (α [alpha], β [beta], and γ [gamma]). In particular, IL-17 is an important mediator of neutrophil-rich inflammatory responses. IL-17 also increases production of antimicrobial substances such as defensins from both immune system cells and nonimmune system cells. Other cytokines have a major influence on AMI and CMI activities. These include IL-2, IL-4, IL-5, IL-10, TGF-β, and IFN-γ. Although there are many cytokines (at least 40), not all functions are known or clinically useful at this time. Table 16.3 lists the cytokines that have current clinical importance. Chapters discussing specific diseases (e.g., lymphoma, rheumatoid arthritis) caused by or treated with certain cytokines have more information about the role of specific cytokines in the disease and its management.

Protection Provided by Cell-Mediated Immunity. Cell-mediated immunity (CMI) helps protect the body through the ability to differentiate self from non-self. The non-self cells most easily recognized by CMI are cancer cells and self cells infected by organisms that live within host cells, especially viruses. CMI watches for and rids the body of self cells that might potentially harm the body. *CMI is important in preventing the development of cancer and metastasis after exposure to carcinogens.*

TABLE 16.3 Activity of Selected Cytokines

Cytokine	Actions
Proinflammatory Cytokines	
Interleukin-1 (IL-1)	Induces fever Triggers inflammation and coagulation
Interleukin-2 (IL-2)	Increases growth, differentiation, and activation of all T-lymphocytes and B-lymphocytes Enhances natural killer cell activity against cancer cells
Interleukin-5 (IL-5)	Secreted by T-helper cells and targets eosinophils Increases activity of eosinophils triggering local inflammation Increases reproduction of eosinophils
Interleukin-6 (IL-6)	Stimulates liver to produce fibrinogen and protein C Increases rate of bone marrow production of stem cells Increases numbers and activity of sensitized B-lymphocytes
Interleukin-17 (IL-17)	Increases proinflammatory cytokine production, especially GM-CSF and G-CSF
Interleukin-23 (IL-23)	Increases differentiation and expansion of Th17 cells, which direct bacterium-specific killing actions in the intestinal tract
Inhibitory-Suppressive Cytokines	
Interleukin-10	Secreted by macrophages and regulator T-cells Suppresses release of proinflammatory cytokines Helps maintain self-tolerance
Tumor necrosis factor (TNF) (many subtypes)	Induces fever Major cytokine involved in rheumatoid arthritis damage Major cytokine involved in the acute inflammatory response to infectious bacteria and starts many of the systemic complications of severe infection or sepsis Participates in graft rejection Induces cell death Stimulates delayed hypersensitivity reactions and allergy
Growth Factors	
Granulocyte colony-stimulating factor (G-CSF)	Increases numbers and maturity of neutrophils
Granulocyte-macrophage colony-stimulating factor (GM-CSF)	Increases growth and maturation of myeloid stem cells
Erythropoietin	Increases growth and differentiation of erythrocytes
Thrombopoietin	Increases growth and differentiation of platelets

GET READY FOR THE NEXT-GENERATION NCLEX® EXAMINATION!

Key Points

Review these Key Points for each NCLEX Examination Client Needs Category.

Health Promotion and Maintenance

- Remind adults, especially older adults, that vaccinations providing artificial active adaptive ***immunity*** require periodic "boosting" for best long-term effects. **QSEN: Evidence-Based Practice**
- Remember that older adults may not have typical symptoms of ***infection*** and ***inflammation*** or responses to tests as a result of reduced ***immunity***.

Physiological Integrity

- The five cardinal symptoms of ***inflammation*** are warmth, redness, swelling, pain, and decreased function.
- The presence of ***inflammation*** does not always indicate an ***infection*** is present.
- Innate-native ***immunity*** provides only immediate protection of short duration.
- The differential of the WBC count can help determine the patient's risk for ***infection***, the presence or absence of infection, the presence or absence of an allergic reaction, and whether an infection is bacterial or viral.
- Adaptive ***immunity*** requires that the body adapt to learn to generate responses to invasion and provides longer-lasting protection.
- Antibody-mediated ***immunity*** can be transferred from one person to another for short-term specific protection.

MASTERY QUESTIONS

1. A nursing assistant in a nursing home reports to the nurse that an 87-year-old nursing home client has a 6-inch reddened wound with pus draining from it on his shin where he scratched it open yesterday. After directly assessing the client's wound, what are the **most relevant priority actions** for the nurse to take? **Select all that apply.**
   A. Take a photo of the wound to show the primary health care provider when rounds are made 2 days from now.
   B. Assess the client for signs and symptoms of systemic infection, including temperature elevation.
   C. Notify the primary health care provider now and request a prescription for antibiotic therapy.
   D. Ask the primary health care provider to prescribe a tetanus booster vaccination.
   E. Immediately obtain a specimen for culture and sensitivity testing.
   F. Cleanse the wound and apply a dry dressing to it.
2. The white blood cell count with differential of a client undergoing preadmission testing before surgery indicates a total count of 5000 cells per cubic millimeter (mm^3) of blood. Which of the follow differential counts or percentages does the nurse report to the surgeon to **prevent harm**?
   A. Eosinophils 300/mm^3
   B. Monocytes 600/mm^3
   C. Segmented neutrophils 2000/mm^3
   D. Lymphocytes 2100/mm^3
3. How do plasma cells provide immune protection?
   A. They actively secrete immunoglobulins against specific antigens.
   B. They interact with virgin B lymphocytes at first exposure to an antigen, enhancing B-lymphocyte sensitization.
   C. They regulate the function of natural killer cells, preventing unnecessary damage or death to normal healthy body cells.
   D. They are responsible for balancing helper cell activity with regulator T-cell activity, ensuring that an immunologic response can be mounted whenever the body is invaded by pathologic microorganisms but limiting the response when the body receives antigens as drugs or food.

REFERENCES

Abbas, A., Lichtman, A., & Pillai, S. (2018). *Cellular and molecular immunology* (8th ed.). Philadelphia: Saunders.

Hogue, M., & Meador, A. (2016). Vaccines and immunization practice. *Nursing Clinics of North America, 51*(1), 121–136.

McCance, K., Huether, S., Brashers, V., & Rote, N. (2019). *Pathophysiology: The biologic basis for disease in adults and children* (7th ed.). St. Louis: Mosby.

Munro, N. (2019). Immunology and immunotherapy in critical care: An overview. *AACN Advanced Critical Care, 30*(2), 113–125.

Pagana, K., & Pagana, T. (2018). *Mosby's manual of diagnostic and laboratory tests* (6th ed.). St. Louis: Elsevier.

Rittle, C., & Francis, R. (2016). The critical role of nurses in promoting immunization for adults. *American Nurse Today, 11*(9), 42.

Touhy, T., & Jett, K. (2020). *Ebersole and Hess' toward health aging* (10th ed.). St. Louis: Mosby.

17

Concepts of Care for Patients With HIV Disease

James G. Sampson, M. Linda Workman

http://evolve.elsevier.com/Iggy/

LEARNING OUTCOMES

1. Collaborate with the interprofessional team to coordinate high-quality care and promote ***immunity*** in patients who have human immune deficiency virus (HIV) disease or acquired immune deficiency syndrome (AIDS, also known as *stage HIV-III*).
2. Use clinical judgment to plan care for patients during periods of extremely reduced ***immunity***.
3. Teach the patient and caregiver(s) about common drugs used for reduced ***immunity***, HIV prevention, or HIV disease and its complications.
4. Teach the patient and family with reduced ***immunity*** from advanced HIV disease about self-care management in the community.
5. Apply knowledge of anatomy, physiology, and pathophysiology to assess all adults for high-risk behaviors and complications related to any stage of HIV disease.
6. Implement patient- and family-centered nursing interventions to help people cope with the psychosocial impact caused by changes related to HIV disease.
7. Analyze signs, symptoms, and laboratory data to assess for reduced ***immunity*** and its complications.
8. Plan care coordination and transition management for patients experiencing reduced ***immunity*** from advanced HIV disease (AIDS).

KEY TERMS

anergy Inability to mount an immune response to an antigen.

immunity Protection from illness or disease that is maintained by the body's physiologic defense mechanisms.

infection Invasion of pathogens into the body that multiply and cause disease or illness.

leukopenia Decreased numbers of all circulating white blood cells (WBCs).

lymphocytopenia Decreased numbers of circulating lymphocytes.

opportunistic infections Infections caused by organisms that are present as part of the body's microbiome and usually kept in check by normal immunity.

pre-exposure prophylaxis (PrEP) Use of HIV antiretroviral drugs by an HIV-uninfected adult to prevent HIV infection.

retrovirus Family of viruses that use RNA as their genetic material instead of DNA and can insert their RNA into a human cell's DNA with the enzyme reverse transcriptase to exert control over the human cell's actions.

viremia Presence of detectable virus in the blood.

PRIORITY AND INTERRELATED CONCEPTS

The priority concept for this chapter is:

- ***Immunity***

The ***Immunity*** concept exemplar for this chapter is HIV Infection and AIDS (HIV-III).

The interrelated concepts for this chapter are:

- ***Gas Exchange***
- ***Tissue Integrity***
- ***Infection***
- ***Nutrition***
- ***Pain***

Immunity is the resistance to infection usually associated with the presence of antibodies or cells that act on specific microorganisms. This protection from illness or disease is started and maintained with the defensive actions provided by the cells, products, and actions of the immune system (Chapter 16). Immunity prevents the reproduction and growth of invading infectious organisms and disease development. It is also detects body cells that are no longer normal. With reduced or disrupted immunity, the patient is at risk for life-threatening ***infection*** and cancer.

IMMUNITY CONCEPT EXEMPLAR: HIV INFECTION AND AIDS (HIV-III)

Pathophysiology Review

The human immune deficiency virus (HIV) causes ***infection*** and disease that can progress along a continuum known as *HIV disease*. This serious and common chronic ***infection*** causing impaired ***immunity*** is a worldwide problem (World Health Organization [WHO], 2019).

The continuum of HIV disease has three identified stages. Stage HIV-I begins with the onset of acute infection responses after an initial invasion by the virus causes overt symptoms. This stage is relatively short and in most infected adults can progress over time to the HIV disease chronic stage of HIV-II. With current drug therapy, stage HIV-II can last for years and even decades before progressing to the final and most serious disease stage of HIV-III, known as AIDS (acquired immune deficiency syndrome). This stage is characterized by a profound reduction of ***immunity*** with poor protection against infection and increased risk for cancer development. However, with adequate care and drug therapy, patients in this stage of HIV disease may live for years before succumbing to the complications of the disease.

Etiology and Genetic Risk. The cause of HIV ***infection*** is a virus—the human immune deficiency virus (McCance et al., 2019). This virus, just like all other viruses, must use the infected cell's metabolic resources to reproduce. HIV can infect a cell and take over its control to force the cell to make more copies of the virus (viral particles). These newly formed viral particles bud off from the host cell to infect more cells, repeating the cycle as long as there are new host cells to infect. Unlike most viruses, HIV is a type of retrovirus, which is a family of viruses that use RNA as their genetic material instead of DNA. These viruses can insert their RNA into a human cell's DNA with the enzyme reverse transcriptase to exert control over the human cell's actions. Thus the HIV retrovirus is very efficient at infecting host cells.

The HIV Infectious Process. *HIV viral particles* have an outer coat with special "docking proteins," known as *gp41* and *gp120*, which assist in finding a host (Fig. 17.1). Inside, HIV has RNA genetic material along with the enzymes *reverse transcriptase (RT), HIV protease,* and *HIV integrase*. To infect, HIV must first enter the host's bloodstream and then "hijack" certain cells, especially the *CD4+ T-cell*, also known as the *CD4+ cell, helper T-cell,* or *T4-cell* (see Chapter 16). This cell directs ***immunity*** and increases the activity of most immune system cells. When HIV enters a CD4+ T-cell, this host cell stops being an active immune system cell and becomes a virus factory, creating more virus particles.

Virus-host interactions are needed after ***infection*** for HIV disease development. When an adult is infected with HIV, the virus randomly "bumps" into many cells. The docking proteins on the outside of the virus must bump into and bind to special receptors on a host cell and then enter the cell. The CD4+ T-cell has surface receptors known as *CD4, CCR5,* and *CXCR4* (Fig. 17.2). The gp120 and gp41 proteins on the HIV particle surface recognize these receptors on the CD4+ T-cell. For the virus to

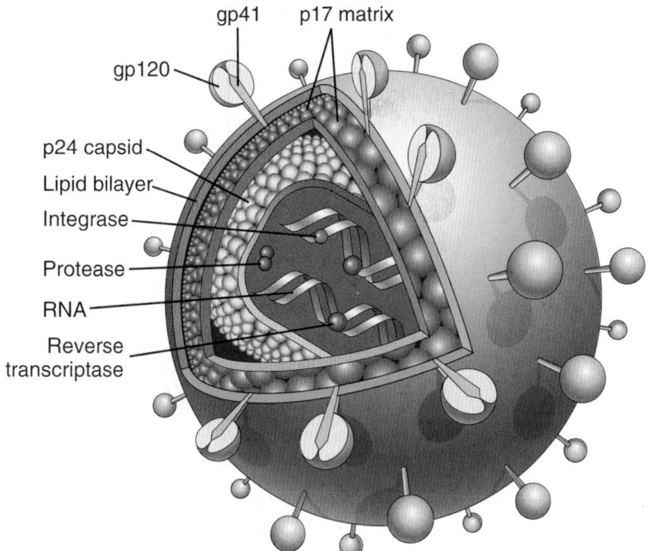

Fig. 17.1 The human immune deficiency virus (HIV). (From Kumar, V., Abbas, A., & Fausto, N. [2010]. *Robbins & Cotran pathologic basis of disease* [8th ed.]. Philadelphia: Saunders.)

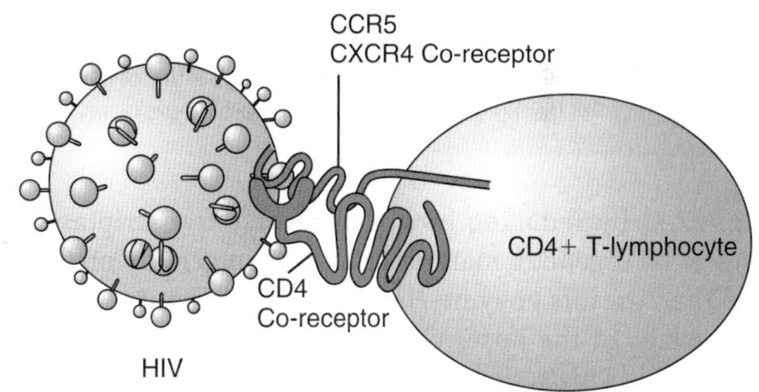

Fig. 17.2 The HIV "docking" proteins and the successful interaction of these proteins with the CD4+ T-lymphocyte receptors.

enter this cell, *both* the gp120 and gp41 must bind to the receptors. The gp120 first binds to the CD4 receptor, which changes its shape and allows the gp120 to bind to either the CCR5 co-receptor or the CXCR4 co-receptor. Once co-receptor binding occurs, gp41 reels the virus and T-cell into physical contact, allowing HIV to insert a fusion peptide into the T-cell membrane, boring a hole to allow insertion of viral genetic material and enzymes into the host cell. This attachment allows the virus to then enter the CD4+ T-cell (see Fig. 17.2). *Viral binding to the CD4 receptor and to either of the co-receptors is needed to enter the cell.* (The drug class known as *fusion inhibitors* works here to prevent the interaction needed for entry of HIV into the CD4+ T-cell. Another class of drugs known as *CCR5 antagonists* work by disrupting the gp120-CCR5 interaction to *prevent* infection.)

Once inside a host cell, HIV must insert its genetic material into the host cell's DNA. Because HIV is a retrovirus, it is able to insert its single-stranded ribonucleic acid (ss-RNA) genetic material into the host's DNA. The HIV enzyme *reverse transcriptase (RT)* converts HIV's RNA into DNA, which makes the viral genetic material compatible with the host cell DNA. (The drug classes known as *nucleoside reverse transcriptase inhibitors [NRTIs]* and *non-nucleoside reverse transcriptase inhibitors [NNRTIs]* work here to prevent viral replication

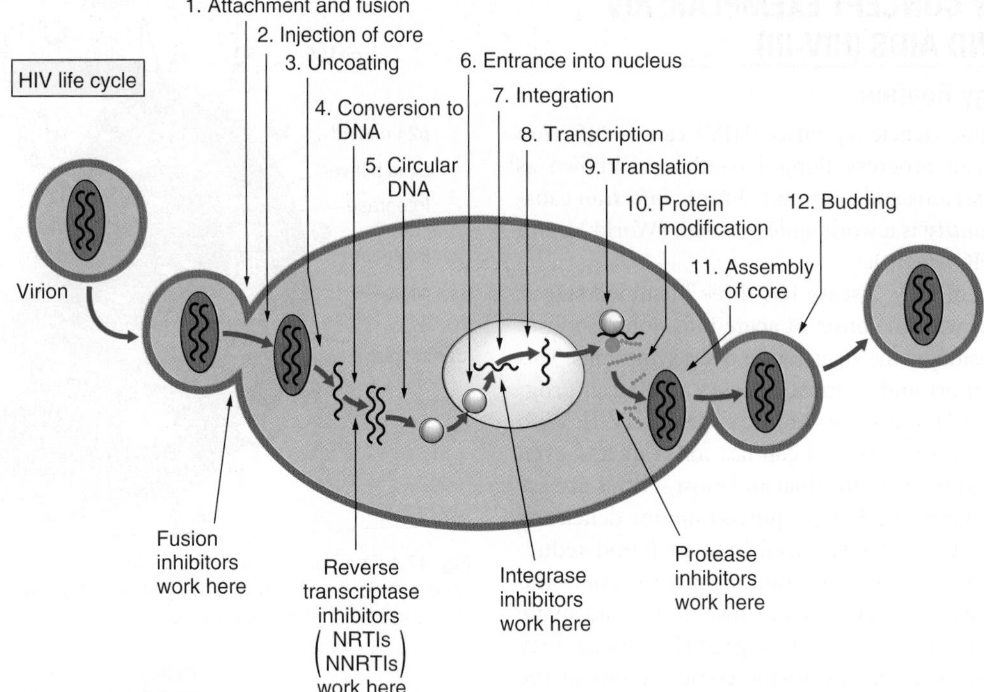

Fig. 17.3 Life cycle of HIV and sites of action for anti-HIV therapy. (From McCance, K. L., & Huether, S.E. [2002]. Pathophysiology: *The biologic basis for disease in adults and children* [4th ed.]. St. Louis: Mosby.)

[Fig. 17.3] by reducing how well reverse transcriptase can convert HIV genetic material into human genetic material.) HIV then uses its enzyme *HIV-integrase* to get its DNA into the nucleus of the host's CD4+ T-cell and insert it into the host's DNA. This action completes the ***infection*** of the CD4+ T-cell. (The drug class known as *integrase inhibitors* works here to prevent viral DNA from integrating into the host's DNA.)

HIV particles are made within the infected CD4+ T-cell, using the host cell's protein synthesis processes. The new virus particle is made as one long inactive protein strand. The strand is clipped by the enzyme *HIV protease* into smaller active pieces. These pieces are formed into a new finished viral particle. (The drug class known as *protease inhibitors* works here to inhibit HIV protease.) Once the new virus particle is finished, it fuses with the infected cell's membrane and then buds off in search of another CD4+ T-cell to infect (see Fig. 17.3).

Effects of HIV ***infection*** are related to the new genetic instructions that now direct CD4+ T-cells to become an "HIV factory," making billions of new viral particles daily. The immune system is made weaker by changing the action of some T-cells from monitoring for infection to being an HIV factory. In early HIV infection before HIV disease is evident, the immune system can still attack and destroy most of the newly created virus particles. However, with time the number of HIV particles overwhelms the immune system's capacity to make more T-cells. Gradually CD4+ T-cell counts fall, viral numbers *(viral load)* rise, and without treatment, the patient eventually dies of opportunistic infection or cancer.

NCLEX EXAMINATION CHALLENGE 17.1

Physiological Integrity

Which part of the HIV infection process is disrupted by the antiretroviral drug class of protease inhibitors?

A. Activating the viral enzyme "integrase" within the infected host's cells
B. Binding of the virus to the CD4+ receptor and either of the two co-receptors
C. Clipping the newly generated viral proteins into smaller functional pieces
D. Fusing of the newly created viral particle with the infected cell's membrane

Everyone who has AIDS (disease stage HIV-III) has HIV infection; however, not everyone who has HIV infection has AIDS (Centers for Disease Control and Prevention [CDC], 2017c). The distinction is the number of CD4+ T-cells and whether any opportunistic infections have occurred. A healthy adult usually has at least 800 to 1000 CD4+ T-cells per cubic millimeter (mm^3) (0.8 to 1.0 x 10^9/L) of blood. This number is reduced in HIV disease.

Most adults develop an acute ***infection*** reaction within 4 weeks of first being infected. Symptoms of acute HIV infection (stage HIV-I) can be fever, sore throat, rash, night sweats, chills, headache, and muscle aches, similar to those of *any* viral infection—not just HIV. The infected adult may not even consider the possibility of HIV infection at this time because the response is so general. With time these symptoms cease and the patient feels well again, although a "war is going on" between HIV and the immune system. Especially in this early acute phase of the disease, the viral numbers in the bloodstream and genital tract are high, and sexual transmission is possible (Grimes et al., 2016; McCance et al., 2019).

TABLE 17.1 Centers for Disease Control and Prevention Laboratory Classification of HIV Disease

Class	Defining Features (all stages require a positive HIV test result)	Stage
0	Patient develops a first positive HIV test result within 6 months after a negative HIV test result. CD4+ T-cell counts are usually in the normal range, and no AIDS-defining condition is present.	HIV-II
1	Patient has a CD4+ T-cell count of greater than 500 cells/mm^3 (0.5 × 10^9/L) or a percentage of 29% or greater. No AIDS-defining illnesses are present.	
2	Patient has a CD4+ T-cell count between 200 and 499 cells/mm^3 (0.2 to 0.499 × 10^9/L) or a percentage between 14% and 28%. No AIDS-defining illnesses are present.	
3	Patient has a CD4+ T-cell count of less than 200 cells/mm^3 (0.2 × 10^9/L) or a percentage of less than 14%. Any patient, regardless of CD4+ T-cell counts or percentages who has an AIDS-defining illness. AIDS diagnosis.	HIV-III
Unknown	Patient has a confirmed HIV infection but no information regarding CD4+ T-cell counts, CD4+ T-cell percentages, and AIDS-defining illnesses is available.	HIV-?

Progression with transition to stage HIV-II is when infected adults are most often diagnosed with HIV disease and management with drug therapy is started. Appropriate drug therapy in stage HIV-II suppresses viral reproduction, allowing the patient to maintain a relatively level of ***immunity*** for protection. However, because drug therapy only suppresses viral reproduction and does not actually kill the organisms, eventually many patients progress to stage HIV-III. During stage HIV-II some patients respond so well to drug therapy that they have undetectable levels of active virus. Controversy exists as to whether this response may actually represent a "cure" or could be considered life-time control until the patient dies from an unrelated health problem.

For most patients, more and more CD4+ T-cells are infected over time and taken out of immune system service, marking the progression on the continuum to stage HIV-III (AIDS). The count decreases, and those that remain function poorly. Poor CD4+ T-cell function leads to these ***immunity*** abnormalities:

- Leukopenia (decreased numbers of all circulating white blood cells [WBCs]
- Lymphocytopenia (decreased numbers of lymphocytes)
- Production of incomplete and nonfunctional antibodies
- Abnormally functioning macrophages

As the CD4+ T-cell level drops, the patient is at risk for bacterial, fungal, and viral infections, as well as opportunistic cancers. Opportunistic infections are caused by the nonpathogenic organisms present as part of the body's microbiome that usually are kept in check by normal ***immunity*** (see Chapter 6 for an explanation of the microbiome). For example *Candida albicans* is a normal part of oral and vaginal flora. When the immune system is working well, the organism is present in controlled areas and amounts and does not cause infection symptoms. The profoundly reduced immunity in the adult with AIDS allows usually harmless organisms to over grow and cause symptomatic ***infection***.

A diagnosis of AIDS (HIV-III) requires that the adult be HIV positive and have either a CD4+ T-cell count of less than 200 cells/mm^3 (0.2 × 10^9/L) or less than 14% (even if the total CD4+ count is above 200 cells/mm^3 [0.2 × 10^9/L]) or an opportunistic infection.

NCLEX EXAMINATION CHALLENGE 17.2

Health Promotion and Maintenance

Which statement made by the client with stage HIV-III disease (AIDS) whose CD4+ T-cell count has increased from 125 cells/mm^3 (0.2 × 10^9/L) to 400 cells/mm^3 (0.2 × 10^9/L) indicates to the nurse that more teaching is needed?

A. "Now my viral load is also probably lower."
B. "I am so relieved that my drug therapy is working."
C. "Although I am still HIV positive, at least I no longer have AIDS."
D. "This change means I am less likely to develop an opportunistic infection."

Once HIV-III (AIDS) is diagnosed, even if the patient's T-cell count improves or if the percentage rises above 14%, or the infection is successfully treated, the AIDS diagnosis remains.

HIV Classification. The Centers for Disease Control and Prevention (CDC) defines five subclasses of HIV disease after initial infection (Table 17.1) based on laboratory confirmation of HIV ***infection*** plus CD4+ T- lymphocyte count or percentage and the presence or absence of the 27 AIDS-defining conditions (Table 17.2) (CDC, 2019). *The adult with HIV infection can transmit the virus to others at all stages of disease, but the recently infected adult with a high viral load and those at end-stage without drug therapy are particularly infectious.* The results of large cohort studies presented in July 2018 at the International AIDS Conference strongly suggest that if the viral load is suppressed to undetectable levels (<20 copies/mL) consistently for greater than 6 months, the virus cannot be passed sexually. This is referred to as *U = U*, in which *undetectable equals untransmittable;* however, it is not known whether or for how long this situation may be sustained (Betancourt, 2018).

HIV Progression. The time from the beginning of HIV-I ***infection*** to progression to stage HIV-III (AIDS) ranges from months to years, depending on how HIV is acquired, other health problems, personal factors, and interventions. When HIV results from a single sexual encounter, progression takes longer. Personal factors influencing time to progression include frequency of re-exposure to HIV, presence of other sexually transmitted infections (STIs), ***nutrition*** status, and stress.

TABLE 17.2 Centers for Disease Control and Prevention Classification of AIDS-Defining Conditions in Adults

- Bacterial infections, multiple or recurrent
- Candidiasis of bronchi, trachea, or lungs
- Candidiasis of esophagus
- Cervical cancer, invasive
- Coccidioidomycosis, disseminated or extrapulmonary
- Cryptococcosis, extrapulmonary
- Cryptosporidiosis, chronic intestinal (>1-month duration)
- Cytomegalovirus disease (other than liver, spleen, or nodes)
- Cytomegalovirus retinitis (with loss of vision)
- Encephalopathy, HIV-related
- Herpes simplex: chronic ulcers (>1-month duration) or bronchitis, pneumonitis, or esophagitis
- Histoplasmosis, disseminated or extrapulmonary
- Isosporiasis, chronic intestinal (>1-month duration)
- Kaposi sarcoma
- Lymphoid interstitial pneumonia or pulmonary lymphoid hyperplasia complex
- Lymphoma, Burkitt (or equivalent term)
- Lymphoma, immunoblastic (or equivalent term)
- Lymphoma, primary, of brain
- *Mycobacterium avium* complex or *Mycobacterium kansasii*, disseminated or extrapulmonary
- *Mycobacterium tuberculosis* of any site, pulmonary, disseminated, or extrapulmonary
- *Mycobacterium*, other species or unidentified species, disseminated or extrapulmonary
- *Pneumocystis jiroveci* pneumonia
- Pneumonia, recurrent (two instances within 12 months)
- Progressive multifocal leukoencephalopathy
- Salmonella septicemia, recurrent
- Toxoplasmosis of brain
- Wasting syndrome attributed to HIV

From Schneider, E., Whitmore, S., Glynn, K. M., Dominguez, K., Mitsch, A., McKenna, M.T.: Centers for Disease Control and Prevention. (2008). Revised surveillance case definitions for HIV infection among adults, adolescents, and children aged <18 months and for HIV infection and AIDS among children aged 18 months to <13 years—United States, 2008. *Morbidity and Mortality Weekly Report: Recommendations and Reports, 57*(RR-10), 9; www.cdc.gov/mmwr/preview/mmwrhtml/rr5710a2.htm.

PATIENT-CENTERED CARE: GENETIC/GENOMIC CONSIDERATIONS QSEN

About 1% of adults with HIV infection are *long-term nonprogressors (LTNPs)* who have been infected with HIV for at least 10 years and have remained asymptomatic, with normal CD4+ T-cell counts and a low or undetectable viral load.

A genetic difference for this group is that their CCR5/CXCR4 co-receptors on the CD4+ T-cells are nonfunctional as a result of gene mutations for these co-receptors. The defective co-receptors cannot bind to the HIV docking proteins, allowing cells to resist HIV entrance. Adults who have only one mutated co-receptor gene allele have lower levels of normal co-receptors and can be infected with HIV, but progression is slow. Remind patients that as long as viral levels are detectable, they can still transmit the disease to others.

Incidence and Prevalence. Since the beginning of the epidemic in the United States, more than 692,789 people have died of stage HIV-III (AIDS). Currently about 40,000 people are diagnosed annually and more than 1,122,900 people in the United States are living with HIV disease (CDC, 2019). Worldwide about 1.8 million people per year are newly infected with HIV, at least 35 million deaths from AIDS have occurred since the start of the epidemic, and about 37.9 million people are currently living with HIV (WHO, 2019) and are known as people living with HIV (PLWH).

Most stage HIV-III (AIDS) cases in North America occur among men who have sex with men (MSM) or adults of either gender who have used injection drugs (16%) (CDC, 2019). *However, the perception that HIV disease is only a problem for homosexual white men is false. The highest rates of new infections occur among adults of color.*

PATIENT-CENTERED CARE: CULTURAL/SPIRITUAL CONSIDERATIONS QSEN

Most new HIV infections reported in the United States and Canada occur among racial and ethnic minorities, particularly among blacks/African Americans and Hispanics (CDC, 2019). An additional group with an increasing incidence of HIV infection is the transgender community, especially transgender women (Kwong, 2019). More culturally sensitive efforts targeted to these groups for prevention and treatment are needed.

PATIENT-CENTERED CARE: GENDER HEALTH CONSIDERATIONS QSEN

About 25% of newly diagnosed cases of PLWH are women. In less affluent countries 50% of cases occur in women (WHO, 2019). The largest risk factor is sexual exposure. Women with HIV disease have a poorer outcome with shorter mean survival time than that of men. This outcome may be the result of late diagnosis and social or economic factors that reduce access to medical care. Encourage all sexually active women to monitor their HIV status.

Often the gynecologic problems of persistent or recurrent vaginal candidiasis are the first signs of HIV disease in women. Other problems include pelvic inflammatory disease, genital herpes, other STIs, and cervical dysplasia, or cancer.

Effects of HIV on pregnancy outcomes include higher incidence of premature delivery, low-birth-weight infants, and transmission of the disease to the infant. Antiretroviral drug therapy during pregnancy reduces the risk for transmitting the infection to the infant. (See the discussion in the "Perinatal Transmission" section.)

PATIENT-CENTERED CARE: OLDER ADULT CONSIDERATIONS QSEN

Infection with HIV can occur at any age (Gray, 2019). Assess the older patient for risk behaviors, including a sexual and drug use history. Age-related reduced ***immunity*** increases the likelihood that the older adult will develop the infection after an HIV exposure.

Health Promotion and Maintenance

HIV-III (AIDS) has a high morbidity and rapid mortality rate when untreated. Although HIV disease and AIDS cannot yet be cured, the continued correct use of antiretroviral therapy allows HIV patients to live longer, healthier lives. The increasing number of adults who, during stage HIV-II, have had viral loads reduced to undetectable levels provide hope that induction of a "cure" may be possible in the near future. Prevention of HIV infection and antiretroviral treatment for all who are HIV positive remain major foci for world health (WHO, 2019).

HIV is found in the blood, semen, vaginal secretions, breast milk, amniotic fluid, urine, feces, saliva, tears, cerebrospinal fluid, lymph nodes, cervical cells, corneal tissue, and brain tissue of infected patients. Contact with tears, saliva, and sweat is low risk for transmission unless obvious blood is present. Infected body fluids with highest HIV concentrations are semen, blood, breast milk, and vaginal secretions. HIV is transmitted most often in these three ways:

- Sexual: genital, anal, or oral sexual contact with exposure of mucous membranes to infected semen or vaginal secretions
- Parenteral: sharing of needles ("sharps") or equipment contaminated with infected blood or receiving contaminated blood products
- Perinatal: from the placenta, from contact with maternal blood and body fluids during birth, or from breast milk from an infected mother to child

Teach all adults about the transmission routes and ways to reduce their exposure (discussed next). Also stress that HIV is not transmitted by casual contact in the home, school, or workplace. Sharing household utensils, towels and linens, and toilet facilities does not transmit HIV. HIV is not spread by mosquitos or other insects.

NURSING SAFETY PRIORITY (QSEN)

Action Alert

Teach all adults, regardless of age, gender, ethnicity, or sexual orientation, that they are susceptible to HIV ***infection*** (Gray, 2019).

PATIENT AND FAMILY EDUCATION: PREPARING FOR SELF-MANAGEMENT

CDC Recommendations for Annual HIV Testing and One-Time Screening

You should be tested annually for HIV if you:

- Have a sexually transmitted infection
- Use injection drugs
- Consider yourself at risk
- Are a woman of childbearing age with identifiable risks, including:
  - Used injection drugs
  - Engaged in sex work
  - Had sexual partners who were infected or at risk
  - Had sexual contact with men from countries with high HIV prevalence
- Received a blood products transfusion between 1978 and 1985
- Plan to get married
- Are undergoing medical evaluation or treatment for symptoms that may be HIV related
- Have been or are in a correctional institution such as jail and prison
- Are a sex worker or have had sex with a sex worker

In the absence of any of the above conditions, you should be tested (screened) once:

- If you are between the ages of 18 and 65 years
- As part of routine prenatal screening when you are pregnant

Modified from Centers for Disease Control and Prevention, 2018a.

PATIENT-CENTERED CARE: VETERANS HEALTH CONSIDERATIONS (QSEN)

The Veterans Health Administration (VHA) is a major health care provider in the United States and has eliminated the need for written consent for including HIV screening as part of routine testing. However, many veterans still do not know their HIV status. Most believe they are HIV negative because they believe that the VHA would have notified them of positive results. This lack of knowledge is a problem because of the high prevalence of behaviors such as substance use and unsafe sexual practices among the VHA patient population. When interacting with veterans and discussing the issue of being aware of their HIV status as part of disease prevention, be sure to inform them that HIV screening is available to them through the VHA.

HIV Status. Currently there are about 1.2 million PLWH in the United States and about another 63,000 PLWH live in Canada (CDC, 2019; Government of Canada, 2018). In both countries about one in seven infected people are unaware of their HIV infection. Many new transmission events come from those who are unaware of their HIV-positive status. Early diagnosis allows for early treatment and prevention, a concept known as *Treatment As Prevention (TAP)*. When an HIV-positive adult starts combination antiretroviral therapy (cART) and the viral load is undetectable for greater than 6 consecutive months, the risk for sexual transmission of HIV is reduced to zero.

Recommendations for HIV screening is a one-time screen for all adults between the ages of 15 and 65, an annual screening of those who are at greater risk for HIV infection, prenatal screening, and frequent testing in adults with repeated high-risk exposures (CDC, 2018a).

HIV testing requires interpretation, counseling, and confidentiality. Testing helps prevention because tests can diagnose HIV ***infection*** before ***immunity*** changes or disease symptoms develop. This allows HIV-positive adults to modify their behaviors to prevent transmission to others. *All sexually active adults should know their HIV status.* The Patient and Family Education: Preparing for Self-Management box lists the recommendations for HIV testing.

Pretest and post-test counseling is performed by professionals trained in HIV issues. These counselors include nurses, physicians, social workers, health educators, or lay educators who have specialized training. Counseling helps the patient make an informed decision about testing and provides an opportunity to teach risk-reduction behaviors. Post-test counseling is needed to interpret the results, discuss risk reduction, and provide psychological support and provide health promotion information for anyone with a positive test result. Care for the newly diagnosed adult appears most effective when it is provided by infectious disease health care providers. Patients are counseled on how to inform sexual partners and those with whom they have shared needles. Testing methods are listed in the Laboratory Assessment section.

Sexual Transmission. Abstinence or mutually monogamous sex with a noninfected partner is the *only* absolute method of preventing ***infection*** by sexual contact. Many forms of sexual expression can spread HIV infection if one partner is infected. *The risk for becoming infected from a partner who is HIV positive and has a detectable viral load is always present. Some sexual practices are riskier than others.* Because the virus concentrates in blood, seminal fluid, and vaginal secretions, risk differs by gender, sexual act, and the viral load of the infected partner.

PATIENT-CENTERED CARE: GENDER HEALTH CONSIDERATIONS (QSEN)

Gender affects HIV transmission, and the infection is more easily transmitted from infected male to uninfected female. This is because HIV is most easily transmitted when infected body fluids come into contact with mucous membranes or nonintact skin. A vagina has more mucous membrane surface area than does the penile urethra. Teach women the importance of always using a vaginal or dental dam or a female condom or having male partners use a condom.

Sexual acts or practices in which infected seminal fluid comes into contact with mucous membranes or nonintact skin are the most risky for sexual transmission of HIV. Anal intercourse with the penis and seminal fluid of an infected adult *(inserting or active or top partner)* coming into contact with the mucous membranes of the uninfected partner's rectum *(receiving or bottom partner)* has the highest risk for transmission regardless of whether the receiving partner is male or female. Anal intercourse allows seminal fluid to make contact with the rectal mucous membranes and also tears the mucous membranes, making ***infection*** more likely. Teach patients who engage in anal intercourse that the top partner needs to wear a condom during this act.

PATIENT-CENTERED CARE: CULTURAL/ SPIRITUAL CONSIDERATIONS (QSEN)

In some cultures male-to-female anal-receptive intercourse is a contraceptive practice. Instruct couples to use condoms, regardless of whether intercourse is vaginal or anal.

Viral load, the amount of virus present in blood and other body fluids, affects transmission. The higher the blood level of detectable HIV (**viremia**), the greater the risk for sexual and perinatal transmission. Current combination antiretroviral therapy (cART) can reduce the viral load of some patients to below detectable levels. *Although there is less virus in seminal or vaginal fluids of patients receiving cART, the risk for transmission still exists if the viral load is detectable.*

Safer sex practices are those that reduce nonintact skin or mucous membranes coming in contact with infected body fluids and blood. Teach all adults the importance of consistently using these safer sex practices:

- A latex or polyurethane condom for genital and anal intercourse
- A water-based lubricant with a latex condom
- A condom or latex barrier (dental dam) over the genitals or anus during oral-genital or oral-anal sexual contact
- Latex gloves for finger or hand contact with the vagina or rectum

Pre-exposure Prophylaxis. Pre-exposure prophylaxis (PrEP) is the use of HIV antiretroviral drugs by an HIV-uninfected adult to prevent HIV ***infection*** (CDC, 2018b; Wilmont, 2018). The currently approved drug combinations for PrEP are Truvada (tenofovir/emtricitabine) and Discovy (emtricitabine/tenofovir). These drugs are taken only once daily for protection. Both drugs have FDA Black Box warnings to avoid in patients who are infected with hepatitis B virus (HBV) because severe acute exacerbations of hepatitis B have occurred when patients have stopped using PrEP.

PrEP is for people who are at high risk for acquiring HIV infection, such as men who have sex with men, nonmonogamous heterosexually active men and women, injection drug users, and relationships in which one partner is HIV positive and one partner is HIV negative (Kerns & Sheridan, 2018). After an adult is identified as at risk, blood and urine testing is done to ensure that it is safe to use PrEP. First, it is important to ensure the adult is HIV negative using a fourth-generation HIV antigen/antibody test. Other necessary tests include kidney function tests; tests for other STIs; liver function tests; and hepatitis A, B, and C. If the adult has active hepatitis B, PrEP is not started and the patient is referred to an infectious disease specialist or hepatologist.

After starting PrEP, ongoing testing of kidney function and HIV infection is performed usually every 3 months because both drugs can be toxic to the kidney and liver. The person using PrEP is not protected until 7 days of consistent dosing allows a steady-state blood drug level to be achieved. Once the initial protection period is completed, one dose can be missed and protection is still adequate. However, two consecutively missed doses greatly reduce protection and the patient needs to start over with another 7-day lead-in period until a new steady state is achieved before being sexually active. When PreEP is used consistently and correctly, it is very effective in HIV infection prevention but does not protect against other STIs or pregnancy.

NURSING SAFETY PRIORITY (QSEN)

Drug Alert

PrEP does **not** replace the standard safer sex practices to prevent HIV transmission. If this drug therapy is used in patients who become infected with HIV-1, the risk for developing drug resistance greatly increases. Therefore remind adults prescribed PrEP to use the safer sex practices described previously and to adhere to an every-3-month HIV testing schedule along with monitoring for side effects of either of these drugs.

Postexposure Prophylaxis. Postexposure prophylaxis (PEP) with cART is used for adults who have had an occupational exposure (e.g., a sharps injury), those who have had a nonoccupational exposure (e.g., consensual sexual exposure with a person of unknown HIV status), and those who have suffered a sexual assault. Starting cART as soon as possible (within the first 36 hours) is critical to preventing HIV ***infection***. Current recommendations indicate that significant exposures be treated with the same three-drug regimen of cART for 28 days or until the HIV status of the source has been determined to be negative (Fig. 17.4A) (New York State Department of Health AIDS Institute, 2018).

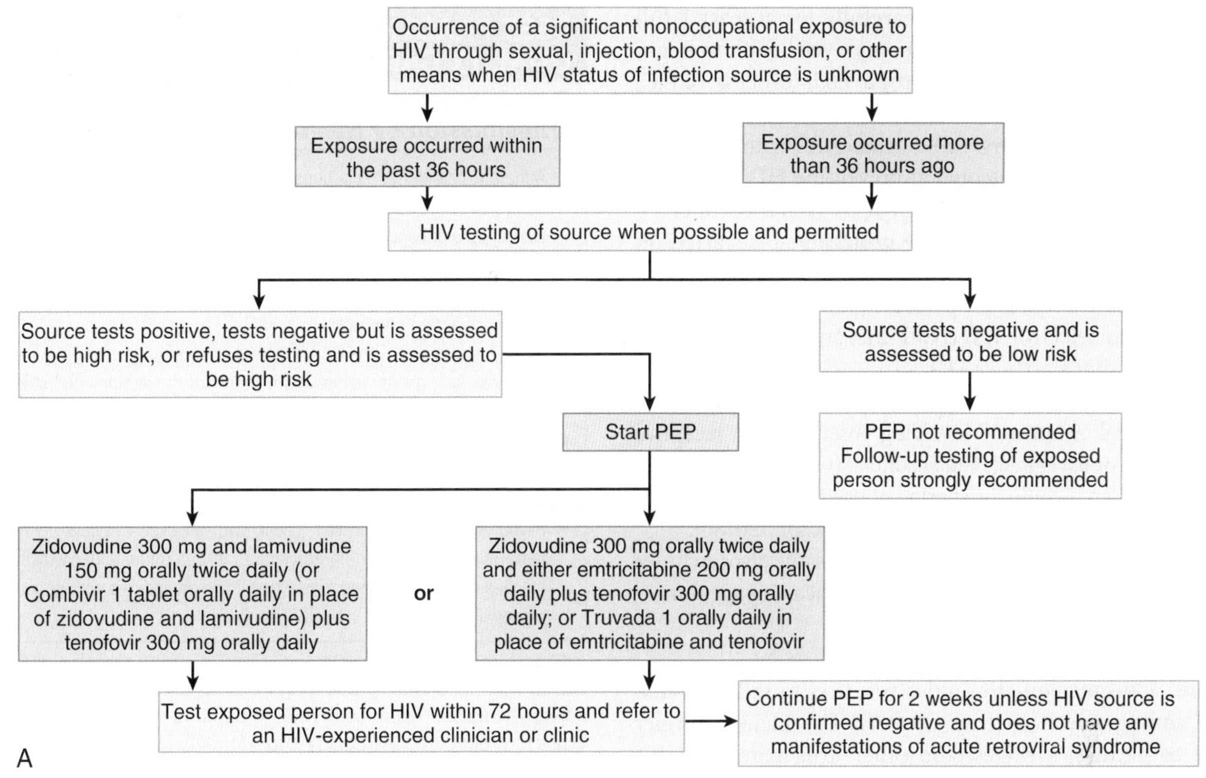

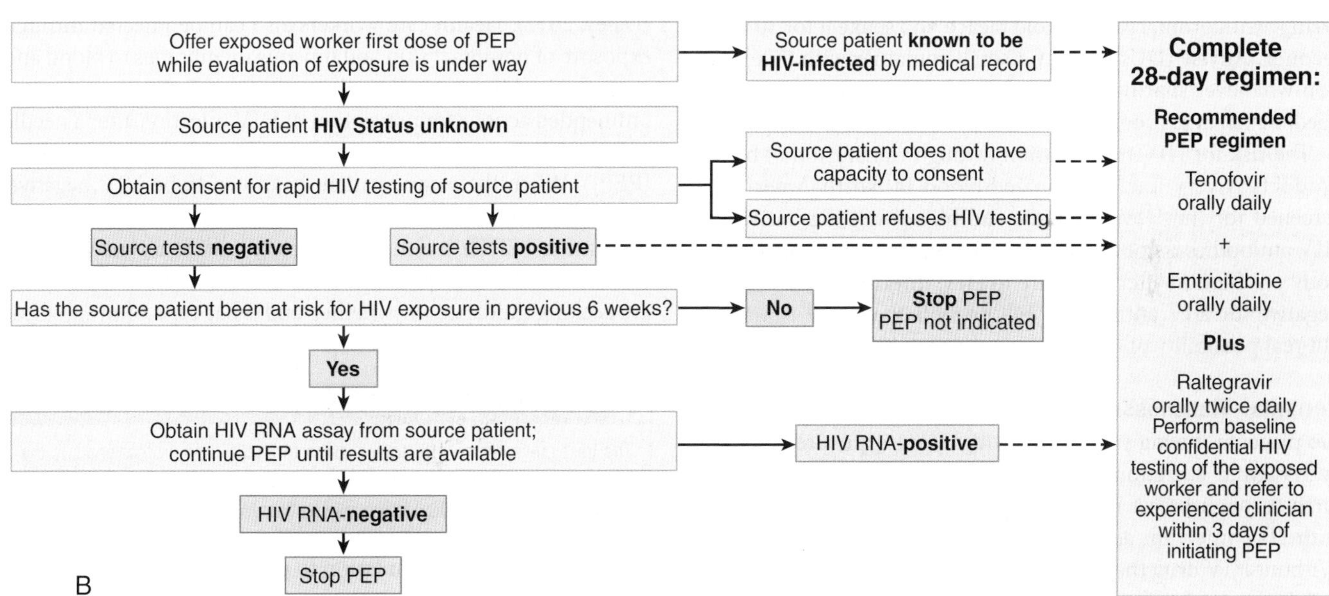

Fig. 17.4 New York State Health Department HIV guidelines. PEP, postexposure prophylaxis. A, Recommendations for nonoccupational postexposure prophylaxis for HIV infection. B, Recommendations for occupational postexposure prophylaxis for HIV infection. (Adapted from New York State Department of Health AIDS Institute. [2018]. *Clinical Guidelines Program*. Free compilation of current guidelines for clinical practice. From: www.hivguidelines.org.)

Occupational exposure is contact between blood, tissue, or selected body fluids (e.g., blood, cerebrospinal fluid, pleural fluid, synovial fluid, peritoneal fluid, pericardial fluid, breast milk, amniotic fluid, semen, and vaginal secretions) from a patient who is positive for HIV *(source patient)* and the blood, broken skin, or mucous membranes of a health care professional. Substances not considered infectious for HIV unless obviously bloody (e.g., feces, nasal secretions, sputum, saliva, sweat, tears, urine, vomit) do not require prophylaxis.

Most cases of occupational exposure requiring PEP involve a percutaneous needle stick with a needle (Daley, 2017; Kerns & Sheridan, 2019). Another common exposure is fluid contact with mucous membranes (e.g., eyes, nose, mouth) (Mitchell & Powel, 2018). For sharps injuries, initial steps include washing the wound carefully for at least 1 full minute and immediately contacting employee health to begin the documentation, testing, and prophylaxis process (CDC, 2013).

Once the exposure occurs, three-drug cART within 2 hours of exposure has the best outcome in preventing HIV ***infection***. Best outcomes decrease when prophylaxis is started after 36 hours. Thus the exposed health care professional is started on cART *before* all test results are known. The professional receiving prophylaxis must return for periodic HIV testing at 1, 3, and 6 months and for electrolytes, creatinine, and complete blood counts 2 weeks after starting cART.

Common nonoccupational exposures are consensual and nonconsensual sexual exposures, involving insertive and receptive types of sex with oral, vaginal, or anal contact (CDC, 2017b). Other types of contact can include the sharing of needles and inadvertent percutaneous or mucosal contact in the home (CDC, 2018c).

Exposure to HIV as a result of sexual assault also includes testing for other STIs. For women of child-bearing age, emergency contraception is offered.

Parenteral Transmission. Preventive practices to reduce transmission among injection drug users (IDUs) include proper cleaning of needles, syringes, and other drug paraphernalia. Instruct IDUs to clean a used needle and syringe by first filling and flushing them with clear water. Teach them to then fill the syringe with ordinary household bleach and shake it for 30 to 60 seconds. Advise IDUs to carry a small container with this solution whenever sharing needles or to participate in community needle-exchange programs, if they are available.

The risk for HIV transmission through transfusion of blood products is very low. All donated blood in North America is screened for the HIV antibody, and blood that is positive for HIV antibodies is not transfused. Because of the time lag in antibody production after exposure to HIV, infected blood can test negative for HIV antibodies. Tell patients that there is a small but real possibility of transmission through blood products.

Perinatal Transmission. HIV transmission can occur across the placenta during pregnancy, with infant exposure to blood and vaginal secretions during birth, or with exposure after birth through breast milk. Inform women of childbearing age with HIV infection about the risks for perinatal transmission. Without HIV drug therapy during pregnancy, the risk for transmission to infants from pregnant HIV-positive women is about 25%. This risk drops to less than 8% for women who are using HIV drug therapy (CDC, 2017c). Encourage HIV-positive women who are pregnant to continue the therapy or, if they are not on antiviral therapy, to start the therapy as soon as possible.

Transmission and Health Care Workers. Needlestick and "sharps" injuries are the main means of occupation-related HIV ***infection*** for health care workers (Mitchell & Parker, 2018; Mitchell, 2020). The incidence dropped after implementation of the use of sharps with engineered sharps injury protection (SESIPs), but preventable sharps injuries continue when health care workers fail to use SESIP features, especially during disposal (Daley, 2017). Health care workers also can be infected through exposure of nonintact skin and mucous membranes to blood and body fluids (Mitchell & Powell, 2018). Fig. 17.4B shows the recommended actions for prevention of HIV infection after a needle stick or other occupational exposure (postexposure prophylaxis [PEP]). When the source patient is known to be HIV negative, PEP is not recommended. The Centers for Disease Control and Prevention (CDC) maintains a special hotline to answer questions for health care professionals who have been exposed and are seeking guidance on whether and what type of prophylaxis would be appropriate for them (1-888-448-4911).

BEST PRACTICE FOR PATIENT SAFETY & QUALITY CARE

Recommendations for Preventing HIV Transmission by Health Care Workers

- Adhere to Standard Precautions.
- If you have exudative lesions or weeping dermatitis, do not perform direct patient care or handle patient care equipment and devices used in invasive procedures.
- Follow guidelines for disinfection and sterilization of reusable equipment used in invasive procedures.
- If you are infected with HIV, you may perform non–exposure-prone procedures, as long as you comply with Standard Precautions and sterilization and disinfection recommendations.
- Identify exposure-prone procedures by institutions where they are performed.
- If you perform exposure-prone procedures, know your HIV antibody status.
- If you are infected with HIV, check with an expert review panel before performing exposure-prone procedures to determine under which circumstances you may continue to practice these procedures with notification of prospective patients of your HIV positivity.

Adapted from Centers for Disease Control and Prevention. (1991). Recommendations for preventing transmission of human immunodeficiency virus and hepatitis B virus to patients during exposure-prone invasive procedures. *Morbidity and Mortality Weekly Report: Recommendations and Reports, 40*(RR-8), 1–9.

! NATIONAL PATIENT SAFETY GOALS

The best prevention of HIV transmission to health care professionals is the consistent use of Standard Precautions (see Chapter 21) for all patients as recommended by the CDC and required by The Joint Commission.

To prevent HIV transmission to patients, health care workers must wear gloves when in contact with patients' mucous membranes or nonintact skin. Infected workers with weeping dermatitis or open lesions must wear gloves or not perform direct patient care. The CDC guidelines for preventing HIV transmission by health care workers during exposure-prone procedures in which the health care the worker's blood is likely to make contact with the patient's body cavity, subcutaneous tissues, or mucous membranes are listed in the Best Practice for Patient Safety & Quality Care box.

Interprofessional Collaborative Care

With treatment, HIV disease at stage HIV-II is a chronic ***infection*** and PLWH may live for decades. The disease course may have

KEY FEATURES

AIDS (HIV-III)

Immunologic Indications
- Low white blood cell counts
  - CD4+/CD8+ ratio <2
  - CD4+ count <200/mm^3 (0.2 × 10^9/L)
- High blood immunoglobulin levels
- Opportunistic infections
- Lymphadenopathy

Integumentary Indications
- Dry skin, skin lesions
- Poor wound healing
- Night sweats

Respiratory Indications
- Cough, shortness of breath

GI Indications
- Diarrhea
- Weight loss
- Nausea and vomiting

Central Nervous System Indications
- Confusion, dementia, memory loss
- Headache
- Fever
- Visual changes
- Personality changes
- Seizures

Opportunistic Infections

Protozoal-like Infections
- Toxoplasmosis
- Cryptosporidiosis
- Isosporiasis, microsporidiosis
- Strongyloidiasis
- Giardiasis

Fungal Infections
- Candidiasis
- *Pneumocystis jiroveci* pneumonia
- Cryptococcosis
- Histoplasmosis
- Coccidioidomycosis

Bacterial Infections
- *Mycobacterium avium* complex
- Tuberculosis
- Nocardiosis

Viral Infections
- Cytomegalovirus
- Herpes simplex virus
- Varicella-zoster virus

Malignancies
- Kaposi's sarcoma
- Non-Hodgkin's lymphoma
- Hodgkin's lymphoma
- Invasive cervical carcinoma

intermittent acute infections and periods of relative wellness. This period is often followed by chronic, progressive debilitation. The cyclic nature of HIV disease and AIDS (HIV-III) results in the patient practicing self-care most of the time in the community between hospital admissions. New techniques and strategies, including mHealth, to promote self-care include the use of mobile devices for reminders and information. Newer combination drugs with once-daily dosing lessen the burden of drug management for PLWH.

In an acute care setting, the disease is best managed using an interprofessional team approach. Team members include physicians, nurses, registered dietician nutritionists (RDNs), infectious disease specialists, social workers, and wound care specialists among others.

◆ Assessment: Recognize Clues. The adult who has HIV disease at stages HIV-II or HIV-III is monitored regularly for changes in ***immunity*** or health status that indicate disease progression and the need for intervention. Monitoring schedules vary from every 2 to 6 months based on disease progression and responses to treatment. Monitoring of patient responses and changes is needed to assess for treatment-related issues and problems caused by disease in many organ systems and to ensure drug therapy effectiveness. Assess for subtle changes so that problems can be found early and managed.

History. Ask about age, gender, occupation, and home environment. Assess the current illness, including when it started, the severity of symptoms, associated problems, and any interventions to date. Ask the patient about when the HIV ***infection*** was diagnosed and which symptoms led to that diagnosis. Ask him or her to give a chronologic history of infections and problems since the diagnosis. Ask the immigrant patient about his or her history of transfusion therapy before coming to North America. All of this information is critical to obtain for patients who are newly diagnosed with HIV disease. For patients who have been under treatment for years at the same practice setting, this information is usually part of the patient's record and a complete history may be not only unnecessary but also annoying to the patient.

Ask the patient about sex practices, STIs, and infectious diseases, including TB and hepatitis. If the patient has hemophilia, ask about treatment with clotting factors. Ask whether he or she has engaged in past or present injection drug usage. Assess the patient's cognitive function and knowledge level of the diagnosis, symptom management, diagnostic tests, treatments, community resources, and modes of HIV transmission. Also assess his or her understanding and use of safer sex practices, and provide appropriate patient teaching.

Physical Assessment/Signs and Symptoms. The patient with HIV disease may have few symptoms, but as the disease progresses, more severe health problems occur. Assess for clusters of symptoms that may indicate disease progression as described in the Key Features: AIDS (HIV-III) box.

Opportunistic Infections. The patient with HIV disease at stage HIV-III (AIDS) often develops pathogenic infections and opportunistic infections. *Pathogenic infections* are caused by virulent organisms and occur even among adults with normal ***immunity***. *Opportunistic infections* are those caused by overgrowth of the patient's microbiome (normal flora). Only when immunity is depressed are such organisms capable of causing ***infection***.

Opportunistic ***infection*** occurs because of the profoundly reduced ***immunity*** with HIV disease. It may result from new infection or reactivation of a previous infection, usually protozoan, fungal, bacterial, or viral. More than one infection may be present at the same time. Opportunistic infections usually indicate disease progression or a temporary further reduction of immunity and *can result in death if treatment is not started quickly*. Priority nursing actions when caring for a patient who is HIV positive are continually assessing for and documenting the presence of an opportunistic infection and monitoring the patient's response to therapy. Report any changes that may indicate an infection to the immunity health care professional.

An opportunistic ***infection*** rarely poses a threat to the health care worker who has normal ***immunity*** when caring for a patient with HIV disease at any stage. However, when the patient has a pathogenic infection, health care personnel must use precautions appropriate to the specific disease to prevent disease spread. For example, when the patient with HIV disease also has tuberculosis at a transmissible stage, Airborne Precautions are needed in addition to Standard Precautions (Chapter 21).

Protozoal and fungal infections are common among patients with AIDS (HIV-III), especially *Pneumocystis jiroveci* pneumonia (PCP). Assess for shortness of breath, tachypnea, persistent dry cough, and persistent low-grade fever. The patient may report fatigue and weight loss. Assess breath sounds for crackles.

Toxoplasmosis encephalitis, caused by *Toxoplasma gondii,* is acquired through contact with contaminated cat feces or by ingesting infected undercooked meat. Assess the patient for subtle changes in mental status, neurologic deficits, headaches, and fever. Other changes may include difficulties with speech, gait, and vision; seizures; lethargy; and confusion. Perform a comprehensive mental status examination and monitor the patient to detect subtle changes.

Cryptosporidiosis is an intestinal ***infection*** caused by *Cryptosporidium* organisms. In AIDS this illness ranges from mild diarrhea to severe wasting with electrolyte imbalance. Diarrhea may result in significant fluid loss. Ask the patient about diarrhea and whether he or she has had an unplanned weight loss of 5 lb (2.3 kg) or more.

Fungal ***infection*** is most often an overgrowth of normal body flora. *Candida albicans* is part of the intestinal tract's natural flora. In stage HIV-III (AIDS), overgrowth of the *Candida* fungus occurs because the reduced ***immunity*** can no longer control fungal growth. *Candida* stomatitis or esophagitis occurs often. Patients may report food tasting "funny," mouth pain, difficulty swallowing, and pain behind the sternum. When examining the mouth and throat, you may see cottage cheese–like, yellowish white plaques and inflammation (Fig. 17.5). Women with HIV disease may have persistent vaginal candidiasis with severe pruritus (itching), perineal irritation, and a thick, white vaginal discharge.

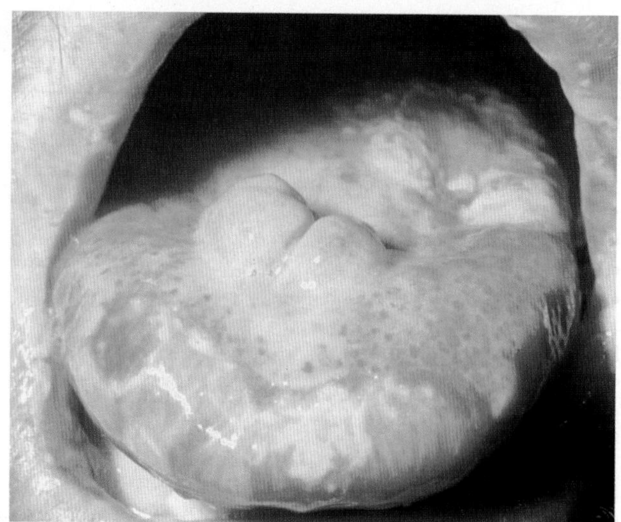

Fig. 17.5 Oral candidiasis (thrush). (From Marks, J., & Miller, J. [2006]. *Lookingbill & Marks' principles of dermatology* [4th ed.]. Philadelphia: Saunders.)

Cryptococcosis, caused by *Cryptococcus neoformans,* is a debilitating meningitis and can be a widely spread infection in HIV-III (AIDS). Ask about fever, headache, blurred vision, nausea and vomiting, neck stiffness, confusion, and other mental status changes. Patients may have seizures and other neurologic problems, or they may have mild malaise, fever, and headaches.

Histoplasmosis, caused by *Histoplasma capsulatum,* begins as a respiratory ***infection*** and progresses to widespread infection in HIV-III (AIDS). Assess for dyspnea, fever, cough, and weight loss. Check for enlargement of lymph nodes, the spleen, or the liver.

Bacterial infections are acquired from other people or sources and as overgrowth of skin flora. *Mycobacterium avium* complex (MAC) is a common bacterial ***infection*** with later-stage HIV disease and is caused by *M. intracellulare* or *M. avium,* which infects the respiratory or GI tract of patients with advanced HIV disease. MAC is a systemic infection. Assess for fever, physical weakness, weight loss, malaise, and sometimes swollen lymph glands or organ disease.

Tuberculosis (TB), an ***infection*** caused by *Mycobacterium tuberculosis,* occurs in 2% to 10% of adults with AIDS (CDC, 2016; CDC, 2017a). More than 50% of all patients at the HIV-III (AIDS) stage who also have TB have *extrapulmonary* (beyond the lungs) disease sites. Ask about cough, dyspnea, chest pain, fever, chills, night sweats, weight loss, and anorexia. Symptoms of extrapulmonary infection vary with the site. *The adult with TB and a CD4+ T-cell count below 200/mm^3 (0.2 x 10^9) may not have a positive TB skin test (purified protein derivative [PPD]) because of an inability to mount an immune response to the antigen, a condition known as anergy*. Blood analysis by the fully automated nucleic acid amplification test (NAAT) for TB with results available in less than 2 hours is the most sensitive and rapid test. It is useful in the acute care setting to determine whether a symptomatic patient actually has TB. Other diagnostic tests include a chest x-ray, acid-fast sputum smear, and sputum culture.

NURSING SAFETY PRIORITY (QSEN)

Action Alert

Maintain Airborne Precautions along with Standard Precautions for a patient with HIV-III (AIDS) who also has TB symptoms until parameters other than a skin test come back negative for TB.

TB is spread by airborne routes (see Chapter 28). When particles from an infected patient's respiratory tract are aerosolized, anyone near him or her is at risk for inhaling the particles and the bacillus. In some settings the interprofessional team member who gives cough-inducing aerosol treatments such as pentamidine isethionate is screened every 6 months to determine whether he or she has been infected with TB.

Pneumonia from bacterial ***infection*** recurs often in patients at stage HIV-III (AIDS), and two or more episodes of any type of bacterial pneumonia in a 12-month period are an AIDS case definition. Assess for chest pain, productive cough, fever, and dyspnea.

Viral infection from a virus other than HIV is common among adults with HIV disease that has progressed to stage HIV-III (AIDS). Cytomegalovirus (CMV) can infect many sites, including the eye (CMV retinitis), respiratory and GI tracts, and the central nervous system. CMV ***infection*** causes many nonspecific problems such as fever, malaise, weight loss, fatigue, and swollen lymph nodes. CMV retinitis impairs vision, ranging from slight impairment to total blindness. The infection can also cause diarrhea, abdominal bloating and discomfort, and weight loss. Ask the patient whether he or she has any of these symptoms. Other problems caused by CMV include encephalitis, pneumonitis, adrenalitis, hepatitis, and disseminated infection.

Herpes simplex virus (HSV) ***infection*** in HIV disease or AIDS occurs in the perirectal, oral, and genital areas. The symptoms are more widespread and of longer duration than among adults who have full ***immunity***. Numbness or tingling at the site of infection occurs up to 24 hours before blisters form. Lesions are painful, with chronic open areas after blisters rupture. Assess for fever, headache, pain and enlarged lymph nodes in the affected area, and malaise.

Varicella-zoster virus (VZV) ***infection*** *(shingles)* is not a new infection for adults with AIDS. This virus causes chickenpox with rash and fever. Once these symptoms have resolved, the virus remains hidden in the nerve ganglia. When adults who have had chickenpox previously have reduced ***immunity***, VZV leaves sensory nerve ganglia and enters other tissue areas, causing shingles. Ask whether the patient has pain and burning along sensory nerve tracts (see Chapter 38 for sensory nerve dermatomes), headache, and low-grade fever. Assess the skin for fluid-filled blisters with or without crusts.

Malignancies. Weakened ***immunity*** increases the risk for cancer, especially Kaposi sarcoma, lymphomas, invasive cervical cancer, lung cancer, GI cancer, and anal cancer.

Kaposi sarcoma (KS) is the most common AIDS-related malignancy. The risk for KS is related to co-infection of HIV and human herpesvirus 8.

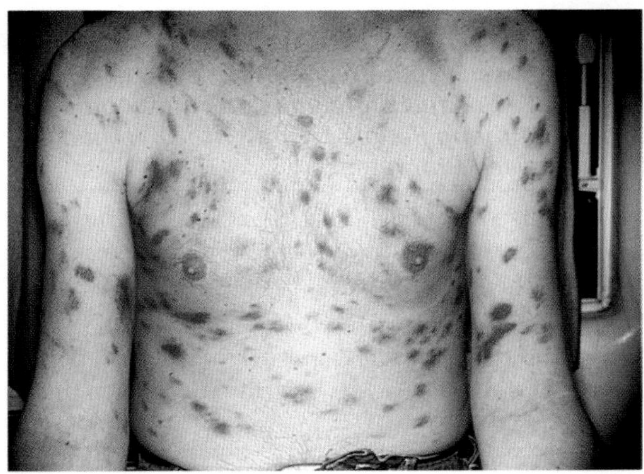

Fig. 17.6 Kaposi sarcoma lesions. (From Leonard, P. C. [2012]. Building a medical vocabulary [8th ed.]. St. Louis: Saunders.)

KS develops as small, purplish-brown, raised lesions on skin and mucous membranes that are usually not painful or itchy (Fig. 17.6). In some patients lesions develop in the lymph nodes, mouth and throat, intestinal tract, or lungs. Assess KS lesions for number, size, location, and whether they are intact, and monitor their progression.

Malignant lymphomas occurring at stage HIV-III are Hodgkin lymphoma, non-Hodgkin lymphomas, and primary brain lymphoma. Symptoms include swollen lymph nodes, weight loss, fever, and night sweats.

Human papilloma virus (HPV) ***infection*** results in many malignancies, including head and neck cancer, but the most common in HIV infection are cervical and anal dysplasia that can advance to cancer. Cervical Papanicolaou (Pap) testing every 6 months is recommended for HIV-positive patients. In PLWH having anal intercourse, an anal Pap test is used for the early detection and treatment of anal dysplasia.

Endocrine Complications. Patients with HIV disease may have disease-related and treatment-related endocrine problems, such as gonadal dysfunction, body shape changes, adrenal insufficiency, diabetes, and elevated triglycerides and cholesterol (which increase the risk for cardiovascular problems) (Kwong, 2019).

Many HIV-positive men have low testosterone levels, and HIV-positive women often have irregular menstrual cycles. Changes in gonadal function decreases muscle mass for both genders, along with weight loss, decreased libido, decreased energy, and increased fatigue.

Body shape changes from fat redistribution or fat deposition *(lipodystrophy)* are common with older antiretroviral drug therapies, especially protease inhibitors and nucleoside reverse transcriptase inhibitors. (Newer cART drugs are less associated with lipoatrophy and lipodystrophy.) Symptoms include "buffalo humps" or neck fat development and large belly fat accumulation. Other areas such as the face, arms, and legs appear wasted and show prominent vein patterns or sunken facial cheeks from *loss* of subcutaneous fat *(lipoatrophy)*.

Decreased adrenal function can result when the glands are infected by opportunistic organisms, causing adrenal insufficiency. This life-threatening problem causes fatigue, weight loss,

EVIDENCE-BASED PRACTICE QSEN

Do Supervised Programs of Physical Activity Have More Positive Outcomes on Functional Capacity Among People Living With HIV Than Do Unsupervised Programs?

Voigt, N., Cho, H., & Schnall, R. (2018). Supervised physical activity and improved functional capacity among adults living with HIV: A systematic review. *Journal of the Association of Nurses in AIDS Care, 29*(5), 667–680.

Previous studies indicate that people living with HIV benefit from regular physical activity consisting of 20 to 40 minutes of combined aerobic and resistance exercise at least 3 times weekly. The objective of this systematic review was to determine whether supervised physical activity was more effective in maintaining or improving functional capacity compared with self-reports of similar activity that was not supervised. The review incorporated the results of 15 studies of 537 adult participants living with HIV. Supervised physical activity was defined as physical activity interventions actually supervised by a health care or allied health professional. Actual functional capacity measurements for muscle strength, cardiovascular fitness, and flexibility were obtained and compared with self-reported measures of physical activity. The programs of physical activity ranged in duration from 6 weeks to 24 weeks. The results of the systematic review were consistent with the results of previous reviews and showed that consistent implementation of aerobic and/or progressive resistance exercise interventions improved overall functional capacity, including cardiovascular parameters, with greater improvement seen when participation continued over longer periods. Results of supervised interventions showed consistent improvement in all areas of functional capacity, whereas self-report of exercise performance regularity and intensity did not consistently show improvement in measurements of functional capacity.

Level of Evidence: 1

The analysis was performed as a systematic review of 15 randomized controlled trials (RCT) with documentation of functional capacity measurements.

Commentary: Implications for Practice and Research

This review confirmed previous findings that supervised physical activity programs have a reduced "drop-out" rate and greater efficacy for improved functional capacity among PLWH than exercise programs that are not supervised. Nurses are health care professionals with sufficient education and skill to supervise physical activity programs and can serve as leaders in this intervention. With nurse-supervised physical activity programs, especially those with consistent involvement of the same nurses, the likely development of interpersonal trusting relationships with participants can help motivate participants to remain in such programs and try harder to reach long-term goals. In view of the fact that nurses comprise the largest available group of health care professionals, future studies could compare the efficacy, adherence, and satisfaction of nurse-supervised physical activity programs for PLWH with those led by other health care or allied health professionals. Additional studies that examine functional capacity changes when programs are continued over longer periods of time are also needed to determine the durability of improvements.

nausea, vomiting, low blood pressure, and electrolyte disturbances (see Chapter 57).

Patients taking older protease inhibitors have a higher-than-expected incidence of type 2 diabetes and hyperlipidemia. These problems are seen even among patients who have no other risks for the disorders.

Cardiovascular Complications. As PLWH lead longer lives now that HIV disease can be managed more as a chronic health problem, cardiovascular complications are reducing life expectancy (Kwong, 2019). These complications result from both the disease and its associated drug therapy. Fat metabolism is disordered and the common problem of diabetes mellitus adds to the risk for hypertension and atherosclerosis. Cardiovascular complications are now a leading cause of death for PLWH (Farahani et al., 2017). Just as for all other populations, a sedentary lifestyle can further increase the risk, whereas participation in regular physical activity of at least 150 minutes per week can lower the risk (see the Evidence-Based Practice box).

Other Symptoms. All body systems are affected in stage HIV-III (AIDS). HIV-associated neurocognitive disorder (HAND) and *HIV-associated dementia complex* (HADC) are symptoms of central nervous system (CNS) involvement. HADC occurs in many patients as a result of ***infection*** within the CNS by HIV. HAND and HADC cause cognitive and motor impairments and behavioral changes. Symptoms range from being just noticeable to confusion and severe dementia.

Some neurologic problems may be a result of HIV infection or drug side effects, including peripheral neuropathy and myopathy. Assess for peripheral neuropathy symptoms, which include paresthesias and burning sensations, reduced sensory perception, pain, and gait changes. Myopathies are accompanied by leg weakness, ataxia, and muscle pain.

Assess the patient with neurologic symptoms for increased intracranial pressure (ICP). If not recognized and managed early, ICP can lead to permanent brain damage and death.

! NURSING SAFETY PRIORITY QSEN

Critical Rescue

Assess patients frequently to recognize any changes in level of consciousness (an early sign of increased ICP), vital signs, pupil size or reactivity, or limb strength. If any of these are present, respond by reporting them immediately to the immunity health care provider.

AIDS wasting syndrome in HIV-III is not caused by any single factor. Diarrhea, malabsorption, anorexia, and oral and esophageal lesions can all contribute to persistent weight loss, and the patient may appear emaciated.

Skin changes include dry, itchy, irritated skin and many types of rashes. Folliculitis, eczema, or psoriasis may occur. Ask the patient about skin sensation changes and examine any rash or irritation. When the platelet count is low, petechiae or bleeding gums may be present.

Kidney problems including HIV-associated nephropathy (HIVAN) are common. These problems range from minor glomerular injury to acute and chronic kidney diseases. Patients with HIV have a far higher risk for requiring a renal replacement intervention.

Psychosocial Assessment. Patients with HIV-III (AIDS) suffer from enormous loss and psychological stress. Assess baseline neurologic and mental status by using neurologic assessment tools (see Chapter 38) to compare any changes. Evaluate the patient for subtle changes in memory, ability to concentrate, affect, and behavior. Ask about the social support system, including family, significant others, and friends. To protect confidentiality, learn who in this support system is aware of the diagnosis so that it is not mentioned inadvertently. Health care professionals must respect the patient's choices as much as possible without compromising care. Offer resources to help with disclosure to sexual partners or significant others.

The patient may be closest to a partner or friend who is not legally recognized as next of kin. Obtain the name and telephone number of that person and determine whether a health care proxy or durable power-of-attorney document has been signed. Encourage all patients to have advanced directive documents (living will and durable power of attorney) included in their medical records.

Ask about the patient's ADLs and any changes that may have occurred since the diagnosis. Assess his or her employment status and occupation, immigration status, social activities and hobbies, living arrangements, and financial resources, including health insurance. Ask whether he or she uses tobacco, alcohol, supplements, opioids, or other drugs.

To plan care and monitor changes, assess the patient's feelings, thoughts, and behaviors, which include anxiety level, mood, cognition, energy, and activity level. Work with him or her to identify strengths and coping strategies. Ask about any feelings of depression; suicidal ideation, intent, or plan, as well as other psychosocial concerns. Also ask about the use of support groups or other community resources.

The patient with HIV disease at stage HIV-III has less energy as the disease progresses. Pace interviews, assessments, and interventions to match his or her energy level. Document the psychosocial assessment and the patient's use of interventions using his or her own words. Communicate this information to all members of the interprofessional team.

Laboratory Assessment

Lymphocyte Counts. Lymphocyte counts are performed as part of a complete blood count (CBC) with differential (see Chapter 16). The normal white blood cell (WBC) count is between 5000 and 10,000 cells/mm^3 (5 and 10 × 10^9/L), with a differential of about 30% to 40% lymphocytes (an absolute number of 1500 to 4500 [1.5 to 4.5 10 × 10^9/L]). Patients with AIDS are often *leukopenic,* with a WBC count of less than 3500 cells/mm^3 (3.5 10 × 10^9/L), and *lymphopenic* (<1500 lymphocytes/mm^3 [<1.5 × 10^9/L]) (Pagana & Pagana, 2018).

CD4+ T-cell and CD8+ T-cell counts and percentages are part of an ***immunity*** profile. Adults with HIV disease and AIDS usually have a lower-than-normal number of CD4+ T-cells and a normal number of CD8+ T-cells. The normal ratio of CD4+ to CD8+ T-cells is 2:1. In HIV disease and AIDS, because of the low number of CD4+ T-cells, this ratio is low. Low CD4+ T-cell counts and a low ratio are associated with more disease symptoms.

Antibody-Antigen Tests. Antibody tests measure the patient's response to the virus (the antigen) and are indirect tests for HIV. When the body is first infected with HIV, it makes an antibody to the virus within 3 weeks to 3 months after ***infection***, although some adults do not make detectable antibodies for up to 36 months. *If an adult has a positive test result for HIV antibodies, it does not indicate severity or disease progression—only that he or she has been infected with the virus.*

HIV antibodies can be measured by enzyme-linked immunosorbent assay (ELISA) and Western blot analysis, which is an older testing algorithm. This algorithm was the gold standard for many years and, while highly accurate, is more time consuming and expensive than more recently developed tests. A third-generation test looks specifically for HIV IgG antibodies. When a positive test result is found, a confirmatory Western blot test is done, which is more sensitive and specific for HIV (co-infection with influenza A can cross-react with the third-generation test, leading to a false-positive result). HIV antibodies are not detected for at least 14 to 21 days after exposure, and the confirmatory Western blot requires an additional 7 days before results can confirm ***infection***. This time frame is known as the "window period" in which an adult is first infected with the virus and when viral replication is occurring but the immune system has not yet started making antibodies. Using this older algorithm, the period from the point of suspected infection to confirmation can take up to 28 days. *Therefore if the patient has unprotected sex with an HIV-positive adult one night and comes in for testing a week later, the ELISA will be negative, even though the patient may have active HIV. Thus testing during the window does not provide useful information* (Grimes et al., 2016).

New technology allows for faster and more accurate initial diagnosis of HIV ***infection***. The CDC recommends the use of a fourth-generation HIV assay that detects HIV-IgM and IgG antibodies (positive in 21 days) and detects the presence of the p24 antigen (an HIV capsid protein) in serum (positive in 14 days). This type of testing reduces the window period in which false negatives are often reported. If the sample is negative, no further testing is required. If the sample is positive, step 2 follows to differentiate between HIV-1 and HIV-2. If this step result is indeterminate, HIV-1 NAT (nucleic acid test) testing is done to detect HIV RNA, not only antibodies and antigens specific for HIV. An HIV-1 NAT+ result indicates acute HIV-1 infection. An HIV-1 NAT- result indicates the sample is negative for HIV infection.

Viral Load Testing. *Viral load testing* directly measures the actual amount of HIV viral RNA particles present in 1 mL of blood and is used to measure therapy effectiveness. An uninfected adult has no viral load for HIV. A positive viral load test can measure as few as 20 particles/mL, but the viral load can be greater than 1 million HIV particles/mL. *The higher the viral load, the greater the risk for transmission.* Current tests are not sensitive enough to measure viral loads less than 20/mL.

In a newly infected adult a viral load is present about 10 days after ***infection***. HIV viral loads can be processed in as little as 24 hours. If positive, this is a clear diagnosis of HIV infection. One caution is that some immune systems can be strong enough to control the viral replication to result in an undetectable viral load. So in addition to running an HIV RNA, the fourth-generation testing should also be done and the results reported together. If the viral load is negative and the fourth-generation testing is negative, the specimen is truly negative.

HIV home screening tests can use blood or oral transmucosal exudate (not saliva). Some tests with specimens collected at home can be performed at home. Other tests involve sending specimens to a laboratory. Patient privacy is maintained when specimens have code numbers for test results. A positive result indicates the need for additional testing.

Other Laboratory Assessment. Other tests monitor the patient's overall health and detect any ***infection*** or problem related to HIV disease (e.g., blood chemistries; urinalysis; CBC with differential; toxoplasmosis antibody titer; liver function tests; tests for STIs, hepatitis viruses A, B, and C; lipid profile; QuantiFERON TB testing or PPD; and cervical and anal Pap testing). Other tests may be performed to monitor toxicities from antiretroviral drugs.

PATIENT-CENTERED CARE: GENETIC/GENOMIC CONSIDERATIONS QSEN

The HIV genotype test is used before starting antiretroviral drugs to determine whether any mutations causing drug resistance exist in the strain of HIV the patient has. It helps determine which antiretroviral drugs are most likely to be effective. It is also useful in PLWH who first show successful viral control and then have rapid disease progression. Ensure that newly diagnosed patients have a genotype test performed.

The human leukocyte antigen (HLA) B5701 allele test is a genetic test to determine whether a patient will have a hypersensitivity reaction to abacavir that ranges from mild fever, rash, nausea, and vomiting to fatal anaphylaxis. Testing is done *before* abacavir therapy; if the patient is positive for the hypersensitivity mutation, abacavir is never used.

The Trofile test determines the degree of expression of the CCR5 receptor on CD4+ cells. This test is needed before starting drug therapy with maraviroc, which is a CCR5 antagonist drug in the entry inhibitor class. If no CCR5 receptors are present, the drug is ineffective.

Other Diagnostic Assessments. Other diagnostic tests are performed on the basis of the patient's symptoms. These may include testing stool for ova and parasites; biopsies of the skin, lymph nodes, lungs, liver, GI tract, or brain; chest x-ray; gallium scans; bronchoscopy, endoscopy, or colonoscopy; liver and spleen scans; CT scans; pulmonary function tests; and arterial blood gas analysis.

◆ **Analysis: Analyze Cues and Prioritize Hypotheses.** The priority problems for patients at stage HIV-III disease (AIDS) include:

1. Potential for infection due to reduced ***immunity***
2. Inadequate ***gas exchange*** due to anemia, respiratory infection, pulmonary Kaposi sarcoma, or anemia
3. ***Pain*** due to neuropathy, myelopathy, cancer, or infection
4. Inadequate ***nutrition*** due to increased metabolic need, nausea, vomiting, diarrhea, difficulty chewing or swallowing, or anorexia
5. Diarrhea due to ***infection,*** food intolerance, or drugs
6. Potential for reduced ***tissue integrity*** due to KS, ***infection***, reduced ***nutrition***, incontinence, immobility, hyperthermia, or cancer

◆ **Planning and Implementation: Generate Solutions and Take Action**

Preventing Infection. The patient with HIV-III (AIDS) is susceptible to opportunistic ***infection*** because of reduced ***immunity***. Initial management focuses on supporting the patient's immunity by controlling the HIV infection with antiretroviral therapy. When the patient's immunity declines, management includes prevention and treatment of opportunistic infections.

Planning: Expected Outcomes. The patient is expected to remain free of opportunistic diseases and other infection.

Interventions. Adults who have HIV disease with reduced ***immunity*** are at greater risk for any type of ***infection***. Teach them to avoid exposure to infectious agents as listed in the Patient and Family Education: Preparing for Self-Management box for prevention of infections. Use the actions in the Best Practices for Patient Safety & Quality Care box for prevention of infection in a hospitalized patient with reduced immunity.

PATIENT AND FAMILY EDUCATION: PREPARING FOR SELF-MANAGEMENT

Prevention of Infection

- During the times when your white blood cell counts are low:
  - Avoid crowds and other large gatherings of people.
  - Do not share personal articles such as toothbrushes, toothpaste, washcloths, or deodorant sticks.
  - If possible, bathe daily, using an antimicrobial soap. If total bathing is not possible, wash the armpits, groin, genitals, and anal area twice a day with an antimicrobial soap.
  - Clean your toothbrush at least weekly by either running it through the dishwasher or rinsing it in liquid laundry bleach (and then rinsing out the bleach with hot running water).
  - Wash your hands thoroughly with an antimicrobial soap before you eat or drink, after touching a pet, after shaking hands with anyone, as soon as you come home from any outing, and after using the toilet.
  - Avoid eating undercooked meat, fish, and eggs.
  - Wash dishes between use with hot, sudsy water or use a dishwasher.
  - Do not change pet litter boxes. If unavoidable, use gloves and wash hands immediately.
  - Avoid turtles and reptiles as pets.
  - Do not feed pets raw or undercooked meat.
  - Take your temperature at least once a day and whenever you do not feel well.
- Report any of these indications of infection to your primary health care provider immediately:
  - Temperature greater than 100° F (37.8° C)
  - Persistent cough (with or without sputum)
  - Pus or foul-smelling drainage from any open skin area or normal body opening
  - Presence of a boil or abscess
  - Urine that is cloudy or foul smelling or that burns on urination
- Take all prescribed drugs.
- Do not dig in the garden or work with houseplants.
- Avoid travel to areas with poor sanitation or primitive health care facilities.

Identifying an infection early reduces the risk for development of sepsis. Continually assess the patient for the presence of infection. This task is difficult because symptoms are not obvious in the patient who is leukopenic. He or she may have a severe infection without pus and with only a low-grade fever.

Monitor the patient's daily complete blood count (CBC) with differential WBC count and absolute neutrophil count (ANC). Inspect the mouth every shift for lesions and mucosa breakdown. Assess the lungs every 8 hours for crackles, wheezes, and reduced breath sounds that indicate impaired ***gas exchange***. Assess urine for odor and cloudiness. Ask about any urgency, burning, or pain on urination. Assess any areas for loss of ***tissue integrity*** and open sores for indications of ***infection,*** especially in the perirectal region. Take vital signs every 4 hours and assess for fever.

Drug Therapy. Approved antiretroviral drugs have excellent activity against HIV replication. However, *it is important to*

BEST PRACTICE FOR PATIENT SAFETY & QUALITY CARE

Care of the Patient With Reduced Immunity

- Place the patient in a private room whenever possible.
- Use good handwashing technique or alcohol-based hand rubs before touching the patient or any of his or her belongings.
- Ensure that the patient's room and bathroom are cleaned at least once each day.
- Do not use supplies from common areas. For example, keep a dedicated box of disposable gloves in his or her room and do not share this box with other patients. Provide single-use food products, individually wrapped gauze, and other individually wrapped items.
- Limit the number of personnel entering the patient's room.
- Monitor vital signs, including temperature, every 4 hours.
- Inspect the patient's mouth and skin and mucous membranes (including the anal area) for the presence of fissures and abscesses at least every 8 hours.
- Inspect open areas such as IV sites every 4 hours for signs of infection.
- Change gauze-containing wound dressings daily.
- Obtain specimens of all suspicious areas for culture (as specified by the agency) and promptly notify the primary health care provider.
- Help the patient perform coughing and deep-breathing exercises.
- Keep frequently used equipment in the room for use with this patient only (e.g., blood pressure cuff, stethoscope, thermometer).
- Limit visitors to healthy adults.
- Use strict aseptic technique for all invasive procedures.

remember that this therapy does not kill the virus; it only controls viral replication. Treatment with multiple drugs from different classes are used together in combinations known as *combination antiretroviral therapy (cART).* This approach reduces viral load, improves CD4+ T-cell counts, and slows disease progression. Teach PLWH that they must take the drugs correctly 90% of the time, making sure that, out of 10 doses, 9 are taken on time and correctly.

An important issue with cART is the development of drug-resistant mutations in the HIV organism. When resistance develops, viral replication is no longer suppressed by the drugs. Testing is now possible to determine whether a strain of HIV has developed resistance to specific drugs (see the Patient-Centered Care: Genetic/Genomic Considerations box on the previous page). The most important factor leading to development of drug resistance to cART is missed drug doses (Penkalski et al., 2017). When doses are missed, the blood drug levels become lower than that needed for inhibition of viral replication. HIV then can replicate and produce new viral particles that are resistant to the drugs being used.

Once a patient has HIV with resistant mutations, the resistant virus is stored in the body indefinitely *(archiving)* and the drugs to which the virus is resistant are no longer used for him or her. Even years later, if the drug to which the HIV demonstrated resistance is tried again, the resistant viruses come out of archival storage and do not respond to the drug. A patient who has resistant virus and is not currently on cART (or not taking it consistently) risks passing on that resistant virus to another person via sexual transmission or sharing needles. This person could then become infected with the resistant virus and now has the same drug limitations, and not all of the current cART drugs will work to suppress the virus.

The cART drug classes and actions are listed in the Common Examples of Drug Therapy: HIV Infection box and include

! NURSING SAFETY PRIORITY (QSEN)

Drug Alert

Ensure that cART drugs are not missed, delayed, or given in lower-than-prescribed doses. Teach patients the importance of taking the cART drugs exactly as prescribed to maintain their effectiveness (Penkalski et al., 2017). Even a few missed doses per month promote drug resistance (remember the 90% rule).

nucleoside reverse transcriptase inhibitors (NRTIs), nonnucleoside reverse transcriptase inhibitors (NNRTIs), protease inhibitors (PIs), integrase inhibitors, and fusion inhibitors. Drawbacks to cART include the expense of the drugs, food and timing requirements, and the number of daily drugs. New combination drugs have reduced the number of tablets and capsules that need to be taken daily (in some cases to just one tablet or capsule daily); however, the daily regimen is lifelong and can be burdensome (Hussar, 2019).

Most antiretroviral drugs have significant side effects and many drug interactions. Protease inhibitors require combining with a pharmacoenhancer for best antiviral effect (Cluck & Underwood, 2018). Be sure to consult a drug reference book for usual dosages, side effects, and nursing interventions (Burcham & Rosenthal, 2019).

NCLEX EXAMINATION CHALLENGE 17.3

Health Promotion and Maintenance

The client on combination antiretroviral therapy calls the nurse to report that he is on vacation and the bag with his drugs was accidentally left on the airplane, so he missed all of yesterday's dosages. What action does the nurse recommend?

A. "Take today's dosages as normally prescribed and continue to follow your therapy program."
B. "Don't worry. Unless you miss your drugs for 4 days consecutively, there is not a problem."
C. "Take double doses of the drugs for the next 2 days and do not have sex for at least 4 days."
D. "Go to the nearest emergency department and have an immediate blood test for assessment of viral load."

A complication of effective cART in some patients whose CD4+ T-cell counts rise and ***immunity*** returns to normal is the development of *immune reconstitution inflammatory syndrome (IRIS)* (Kwong, 2020). As the drugs suppress HIV replication and the T-cells increase, the T4 cells "recognize" opportunistic infections (e.g., tuberculosis, cryptococcosis, *Mycobacterium avium* complex, pneumocystis pneumonia, cytomegalovirus, hepatitis) that were present before but not recognized because of severely reduced immunity. With the increased T-cell numbers and activity, they begin to sound the alarm about the presence of these infections. The T4-cells start an inflammatory reaction with high fever, chills, and, depending on which ***infection*** the immune system is reacting against, worsening disease. For example, IRIS is common with those co-infected with HIV and TB. TB symptoms initially become much worse after starting cART. Because some symptoms are similar to those of drug therapy side effects and

COMMON EXAMPLES OF DRUG THERAPY

HIV Infection

Drug Class	Nursing Implications
Nucleoside Reverse Transcriptase Inhibitors (NRTIs)	
These drugs have a similar structure to the four bases of DNA, making them "counterfeit" bases. They fool the HIV enzyme *reverse transcriptase* into using these counterfeit bases so that viral DNA synthesis and replication are suppressed.	
Abacavir Didanosine Emtricitabine Lamivudine Tenofovir Zidovudine	Remind patients to avoid fatty and fried foods with these drugs *because they cause digestive upsets and may lead to pancreatitis when combined with NRTIs.* Teach patients to use precautions to prevent injury *because these drugs induce peripheral neuropathy.* Teach patients taking abacavir to report flulike symptoms to the health care provider immediately *because these symptoms may indicate a hypersensitivity reaction that requires discontinuing the drug.* Instruct patients to avoid or severely limit alcoholic beverages *to reduce the risk for liver damage while on these drugs (which are also toxic to the liver).*
Non-Nucleoside Reverse Transcriptase Inhibitors (NNRTIs)	
These drugs work by binding directly to the HIV-1 enzyme reverse transcriptase, preventing viral cell DNA replication, RNA replication, and protein synthesis, which suppresses viral replication of the HIV-1 virus.	
Doraverine Efavirenz Etravirine Nevirapine Rilpivirine	Check for increased liver enzymes and decreased red blood cells *because common side effects are anemia and liver toxicity.* Teach patients to take these drugs at least 1 hour before or 2 hours after taking an antacid *to avoid inhibiting drug absorption* (except doraverine). Instruct patients to notify the prescriber if a sore throat, fever, different types of rashes, blisters, or multiple bruises develop *because these are indications of a serious adverse drug effect.* Do not give delavirdine or efavirenz to pregnant women *because these two drugs may cause birth defects and developmental problems.*
Protease Inhibitors (PIs)	
These drugs block the HIV protease enzyme, preventing viral replication and release of viral particles. The HIV initially produces all of its proteins in one long strand, which must be broken down into separate smaller proteins by HIV protease to be active. Thus when inhibited, viral proteins are not functional and viral particles do not leave the cell to infect other cells.	
Atazanavir Darunavir Fosamprenavir Lopinavir/ritonavir Nelfinavir Saquinavir Tipranavir	Instruct patients to not chew or crush these drugs *because this causes rapid absorption and increases the risk for side effects.* Teach patients to report jaundice, nausea and vomiting, or severe abdominal pain *because these drugs can induce liver toxicity.* Remind patients to avoid St. John's wort while taking these drugs *because the supplement reduces the effectiveness of all PIs.* Teach patients taking atazanavir and ritonavir to check their pulse daily and report low heart rate to the prescriber *because these two drugs can impair electrical conduction and lead to heart block.* Do not give darunavir or fosamprenavir to patients who have a known sulfa allergy *because these two drugs contain sulfa.*
Integrase Inhibitors	
These drugs inhibit the HIV enzyme integrase, which the virus uses to insert the viral DNA into human DNA. Thus viral proteins are not made and viral replication is inhibited.	
Bictegravir Dolutegravir Elvitegravir Raltegravir	Suggest that patients take the drug with food *to reduce the expected GI side effects of diarrhea, nausea, and abdominal pain.* Instruct patients to not chew or crush these drugs *because this causes rapid absorption and increases the risk for side effects.* Instruct patients to report new-onset muscle pain or weakness *because these drugs can cause muscle breakdown (rhabdomyolysis), especially in adults taking a "statin" type of lipid-lowering drug.* Teach patients with diabetes to closely monitor blood glucose levels *because these drugs increase hyperglycemia.* For patients with diabetes taking metformin and dolutegravir, the maximum daily dose of metformin is 1000 mg. Do not give raltegravir or dolutegravir to pregnant women *because it is associated with an increased risk for birth defects.*
Fusion Inhibitors/CCR5 Antagonists	
These drugs halt cellular infection with HIV by blocking the gp41 to prevent fusion of virus to host cells or blocks the CCR5 receptors on CD4+ T-cells, which prevents the virus's gp120 from binding to the CCR5 receptor and entering the host cells.	
Enfuvirtide Maraviroc	Instruct patients to not chew or crush maraviroc *because this action may cause the drug to be absorbed too rapidly and increase the risk for side effects.* Teach patients to change positions slowly *because hypotension is common.* Teach patients to report jaundice, nausea and vomiting, or severe abdominal pain *because these drugs can induce liver toxicity.* Instruct patients to report pain or numbness in the hands or feet *because this drug can induce peripheral neuropathy.* Maraviroc therapy first requires a positive Trophile test indicating the presence of the CCR5 receptor. Teach patients how to prepare and inject enfuvirtide subcutaneously *to ensure correct dosage and effectiveness.* Assess injection sites for warmth, swelling, redness, skin hardening, or bumps *because these are indications of injection site reactions.*
Combination Products	
Atripla (emtricitabine, tenofovir, efavirenz) [a]Biktarvy (bictegravir, emtricitabine, tenofovir) Combivir (lamivudine, zidovudine) Complera (emtricitabine, rilpivirine, tenofovir) Descovy (emtricitabine, tenofovir) [a]Dovato (dolutegravir, lamivudine) Epzicom (lamivudine, abacavir)	[a]Genvoya (elvitegravir, cobicistat, emtricitabine, tenofovir) [a]Juluca (dolutegravir, rilpivirine) Odefsey (emtricitabine, rilpivirine, tenofovir) Prezcobix (darunavir, cobisistat) Stribild (elvitegravir, cobicistat, emtricitabine, tenofovir) Truvada (emtricitabine, tenofovir) [a]Triumeq (dolutegravir, abacavir, lamivudine)

[a]Denotes single-dose daily tablet regimen.

other problems, IRIS may go undiagnosed and untreated, increasing the risk for death. When IRIS is recognized, short-term therapy with corticosteroids can reduce the inflammatory responses.

NCLEX EXAMINATION CHALLENGE 17.4

Physiological Integrity

What is the **most important** question for the nurse to ask before giving the first dose of fosamprenavir to a client newly prescribed this drug?

A. "Do you have glaucoma or any other problem with your eyes?"
B. "Do you take medications for a seizure disorder?"
C. "Are you allergic to sulfa drugs?"
D. "Are you a diabetic?"

Complementary and Alternative Therapies. Complementary therapies are often used by PLWH, although their effectiveness has not been established. Some products alter the effects of cART drugs. Ask the patient which botanical or homeopathic agents he or she is using, and check with the pharmacist to determine known drug interactions.

Enhancing Gas Exchange

Planning: Expected Outcomes. The patient is expected to maintain ***gas exchange*** with oxygenation and perfusion and to have minimal dyspnea.

Interventions. The nurse or respiratory therapist uses drug therapy, respiratory support and maintenance, comfort, and rest to enhance gas exchange.

Drug therapy is a mainstay for ***gas exchange*** problems resulting from ***infection***. It is started after an infectious cause is identified. A common respiratory infection in adults with HIV disease is *P. jiroveci* pneumonia (PCP). The treatment of choice for PCP is trimethoprim with sulfamethoxazole. Many patients have adverse reactions to this drug, including nausea, vomiting, hyponatremia, rashes, fever, leukopenia, thrombocytopenia, and hepatitis.

Pentamidine isethionate, usually given IV or IM, is also used to treat PCP. Aerosolized pentamidine isethionate is used as prophylaxis for patients with CD4+ T-cell counts below 200 ($0.2 \times 10^9/L$) or 14% and for those who have already had PCP.

Other therapies to improve ***gas exchange*** include bronchodilators to improve airflow and dapsone and atovaquone as alternative therapies to trimethoprim-sulfamethoxazole for existing PCP or as prophylaxis. For moderate to severe PCP, glucocorticoids can reduce the inflammation.

Respiratory support helps maintain ***gas exchange*** and avoids complications. Assess the respiratory rate, rhythm, and depth, breath sounds, and vital signs and monitor for cyanosis at least every 8 hours. Apply oxygen and humidify the room as prescribed. Monitor mechanical ventilation, perform suctioning and pulmonary hygiene, and evaluate blood gas results.

Comfort can help improve ***gas exchange***. Assess the patient's comfort. The patient with difficulty breathing is often more comfortable with the head of the bed elevated. Pace activities to reduce shortness of breath and fatigue.

Rest and activity changes are needed when gas exchange is impaired. Most patients with HIV infection have fatigue, especially when respiratory problems are also present. Work with the patient to pace activities to conserve energy. Schedule activities such as bathing so that he or she is not fatigued at mealtime. Eliminate or reschedule activities that do not have a direct and immediate positive outcome for the patient.

NCLEX EXAMINATION CHALLENGE 17.5

Psychosocial Integrity

Which activities can the nurse postpone or eliminate for the client who has extreme fatigue today? **Select all that apply.**

A. Administering prescribed drug therapy
B. Ambulating in the hall
C. Culturing suspected infectious drainage
D. Performing pulmonary hygiene
E. Performing oral care
F. Providing a complete bed bath
G. Teaching about nutrition therapy

Managing Pain. The patient with severe advanced HIV disease (stage HIV-III [AIDS]) often has pain from many causes. ***Pain*** can result from enlarged organs stretching the viscera or compressing nerves. Tumor invasion of bone and other tissues can cause pain, as can compression of nerves from swollen lymph nodes. Many patients have peripheral neuropathy-induced pain from the disease or drug therapies. Many have generalized joint and muscle pain.

Planning: Expected Outcomes. The patient is expected to achieve an acceptable level of comfort and ***pain*** reduction.

Interventions. Drug therapy and other approaches are used together to manage pain associated with HIV disease, depending on the cause of the pain.

Comfort measures include the use of pressure-relieving mattress pads, warm baths or other forms of hydrotherapy, massage, and applying heat or cold to painful areas to reduce pain levels, with or without drug therapy. Take care when moving or assisting the patient. Use lift sheets to avoid pulling or grasping the patient with joint pain. The patient may be thin and have poor circulation, contributing to ***pain.*** Help him or her change positions often.

Drug therapy with different drug classes is used to manage different types of pain, although opioids are no longer recommended as first-line therapy (Bruce et al., 2017). For arthralgia and myalgia, NSAIDs may reduce inflammation and increase comfort. Acetaminophen also can help reduce pain. Pregabalin may provide some relief from muscle and joint pain. Neuropathic pain may respond to tricyclic antidepressants such as amitriptyline or to anticonvulsant drugs such as gabapentin, phenytoin, or carbamazepine, or antidepressant drugs such as venlafaxine or duloxetine, although these drugs may interact with antiretroviral drugs and often take days to weeks before effective and opioids may be needed to control pain.

When opioids are used, assess the patient for pain intensity and quality. Mild to moderate acute ***pain*** is managed with weaker opioids such as hydrocodone or codeine. More intense pain requires stronger opioids such as oxycodone, morphine, hydromorphone, or fentanyl. Combining opioids along with nonopioid drugs may provide sustained pain relief and allow the patient to participate in activities to the extent that he or she wishes.

Enhancing Nutrition. Many patients at stage HIV-III (AIDS) have inadequate ***nutrition,*** and a registered dietitian nutritionist (RDN) is part of the interprofessional health care team. Fatigue, anorexia, nausea, difficulty swallowing, diarrhea, poor GI absorption, or wasting syndrome all reduce nutrition (Clark & Cress, 2018).

Planning: Expected Outcomes. The patient is expected to maintain optimal weight through adequate ***nutrition*** and hydration.

Interventions. Because of the many factors for poor ***nutrition*** in HIV-III (AIDS), diagnostic procedures are needed to determine the cause. Once the cause is determined, appropriate therapy is initiated. For example, in candidal esophagitis, nutrition is affected by swallowing difficulties. A soft or liquid diet with cooler foods can help reduce discomfort and increase oral intake.

Drug therapy can include ketoconazole or fluconazole orally, or IV amphotericin B. Give the drug as prescribed, and monitor for side effects such as nausea and vomiting, which also affect ***nutrition***. Provide mouth care and ice chips, and keep unpleasant odors out of the patient's environment. Antiemetics are used as needed.

Nutrition therapy includes monitoring weight, intake and output, and calorie count. Assess food preferences and dietary cultural or religious practices. Collaborate with the RDN to teach the patient about the need for a high-calorie, high-protein diet. Encourage him or her to avoid dietary fat, because fat intolerance often occurs as a result of the disease and as a side effect of HIV drug therapy. Often small, frequent meals are better tolerated than large meals. Supplemental vitamins and fluids are indicated in some cases. For the patient who cannot achieve adequate ***nutrition*** through food, enteral or parenteral nutrition may be needed.

Mouth care can improve appetite. When delegating this nursing action to assistive personnel (AP), instruct them to offer the patient rinses of sodium bicarbonate with sterile water or normal saline several times a day. Explain to AP why the patient needs to use a soft toothbrush and the need to drink plenty of fluids. For oral ***pain,*** general analgesics or oral anesthetic gels and solutions may be needed. Avoid the use of alcohol-based mouthwashes.

NCLEX EXAMINATION CHALLENGE 17.6

Health Promotion and Maintenance

Which dietary change does the nurse suggest for the client who has esophageal candidiasis?

A. "Avoid drinking alcoholic beverages."
B. "Eat soft, cool food such as pudding and smoothies."
C. "Limit your intake of fluid to no more than 1 L daily."
D. "Increase your intake of cooked leafy green vegetables."

Managing Diarrhea. Patients with stage HIV-III (AIDS) often have diarrhea. Sometimes an infectious cause (e.g., *Giardia, Cryptosporidium,* or amoeba) can be determined and treated; or the cause is determined, but no effective therapy is available. Many patients are lactose intolerant, and HIV disease worsens this problem. Diarrhea may be a side effect of drug therapy. At times no cause can be identified.

Planning: Expected Outcomes. The patient is expected to have decreased diarrhea; to maintain fluid, electrolyte, and ***nutrition*** status; and to reduce incontinence.

Interventions. For most patients with HIV-III (AIDS) and diarrhea, symptom management is all that is available. Antidiarrheals such as diphenoxylate hydrochloride or loperamide, given on a regular schedule, provide some relief. Consult with the registered dietitian nutritionist (RDN), and teach about appropriate foods. Recommended dietary changes include less roughage; less fatty, spicy, and sweet food; and no alcohol or caffeine. Some patients obtain relief when they eliminate dairy products or eat smaller amounts of food more often. If dehydration also occurs, IV fluids may be needed.

Assess the perineal skin every 8 to 12 hours for a change in ***tissue integrity*** or indication of ***infection,*** such as an open sore or pimple. Provide a bedside commode or a bedpan if the patient cannot reach the bathroom in time. Teach AP to provide the patient with privacy, support, and understanding. Explain the need to keep the perineal area clean and dry and to wear gloves during this care. Instruct AP to report any skin changes in the perineal area, including redness, rashes, blisters, or open areas. Collaborate with a wound care specialist for interventions to manage anal excoriation and discomfort.

Restoring Skin Integrity. Impaired ***tissue integrity*** may be related to Kaposi sarcoma (KS) of the skin, mucous membranes, and internal organs. Lesions may be localized or widespread. Large lesions can cause pain, restrict movement, and impede circulation, causing open, weeping, painful lesions. Another cause of impaired tissue integrity may be skin ***infection*** with herpes simplex virus (HSV) or varicella zoster virus (VZV) (shingles).

Planning: Expected Outcomes. The patient is expected to have healing of existing lesions and avoid increased skin breakdown or secondary infection.

Interventions. KS responds well to antiretroviral drug therapy, and many lesions disappear over time. For lesions that do not respond to cART, KS can be treated with local radiation, local or systemic chemotherapy, interferon, cryotherapy, or topical retinoids to restore ***tissue integrity***.

Management of painful KS lesions includes analgesics and comfort measures. Keep open, weeping KS lesions clean and dressed to prevent infection. Many patients with KS are concerned about their appearance and the risk for being identified as HIV positive. Makeup (if lesions are closed), long-sleeved shirts, and hats may help maintain a normal appearance.

For the patient with a herpes simplex virus (HSV) outbreak, provide good skin care directly or delegate this care to AP. Stress the importance of keeping the area clean and dry. Teach AP to clean abscesses at least once per shift with normal saline and allow them to air-dry. This ***infection*** is painful and requires analgesics, assistance with position, and other comfort measures. Modified Burow solution soaks promote healing for some patients. Drug therapy for HSV infection includes acyclovir or valacyclovir.

Care Coordination and Transition Management. The management of HIV disease as a chronic progressive disease occurs in many settings, most often at home. Hospitalizations occur during periods of severe ***infection*** or acute exacerbations of symptoms, especially at stage HIV-III (AIDS). As the illness progresses, the patient may need referral to a long-term care facility, home care agency, or hospice. In collaboration with the social worker, RDN, and others, work with patients to plan what will be needed and how they will manage at home with self-care and ADLs.

Home Care Management. Before the patient is discharged to home, assess his or her status, ability to perform self-care activities, and plans to maintain communication with primary health care

FOCUSED ASSESSMENT

Patient at Stage HIV-III (AIDS)

Cardiovascular and Respiratory Status
- Vital signs
- Presence of acute chest pain or dyspnea
- Presence of cough
- Presence of fever
- Activity tolerance

Assess Nutrition Status
- Food intake
- Weight loss or gain
- General condition of skin

Neurologic Status
- Cognitive changes
- Motor changes
- Sensory disturbances

GI Status
- Mouth and oropharynx
- Presence of dysphagia
- Presence of abdominal pain
- Presence of nausea, vomiting, diarrhea, constipation

Psychological Status
- Feelings, thoughts, and behaviors
- Presence of anxiety, fear, or depression
- Suicide ideation, intent, or plan
- Support systems within the family and community
- Patient's and caregiver's coping skills

Activity and Rest
- ADLs
- Mobility and ambulation
- Fatigue
- Sleep pattern
- Presence of pain

Home Environment
- Safety hazards
- Structural barriers affecting functional ability

Assess Patient's and Caregiver's Adherence and Understanding of Illness and Treatment
- Symptoms to report to nurse
- Medication schedule and side or toxic effects

PATIENT AND FAMILY EDUCATION: PREPARING FOR SELF-MANAGEMENT

Infection Control for Home Care of the Patient at Stage HIV-III (AIDS)

Direct Care
- Follow Standard Precautions and good handwashing techniques.
- Do not share razors or toothbrushes.

Housekeeping
- Wipe up feces, vomit, sputum, urine, or blood or other body fluids and the area with soap and water. Dispose of solid wastes and solutions used for cleaning by flushing them down the toilet. Disinfect the area by wiping with a 1:10 solution of household bleach (1 part bleach to 10 parts water). Wear gloves during cleaning.
- Soak rags, mops, and sponges used for cleaning in a 1:10 bleach solution for 5 minutes to disinfect them.
- Wash dishes and eating utensils in hot water and dishwashing soap or detergent.
- Clean bathroom surfaces with regular household cleaners and then disinfect them with a 1:10 solution of household bleach.

Laundry
- Rinse clothes, towels, and bedclothes if they become soiled with feces, vomit, sputum, urine, or blood. Dispose of the soiled water by flushing it down the toilet. Launder these clothes with hot water and detergent with 1 cup of bleach added per load of laundry.
- Keep soiled clothes in a plastic bag.

Waste Disposal
- Dispose of needles and other "sharps" in a labeled puncture-proof container such as a coffee can with a lid or empty liquid bleach bottle, using Standard Precautions, to avoid needlestick injuries. Decontaminate full containers by adding a 1:10 bleach solution. Then seal the container with tape and place it in a paper bag. Dispose of the container in the regular trash.
- Remove solid waste from contaminated trash (e.g., paper towels or tissues, dressings, disposable incontinence pads, disposable gloves); then flush the solid waste down the toilet. Place the contaminated trash items in tied plastic bags and dispose of them in the regular trash.

providers. Home care can range from help with ADLs for those with weakness, or limited function to around-the-clock nursing care, drugs, and ***nutrition*** support for severely ill patients. Assess available resources, including family members and significant others willing and able to be caregivers. Help the family make arrangements for outside caregivers or respite care, if needed. Patients may need referrals or help in planning housing, finances, insurance, legal services, and spiritual counseling. Coordinate with the case manager to ensure that these issues are addressed.

Usually a home care nurse makes an initial visit to the patient at stage HIV-III (AIDS) for assessment purposes, and care is followed up by home care aides. Reassessment is needed if the patient becomes more debilitated. Assessment areas for the patient at home are listed in the Focused Assessment: Patient at Stage HIV-III (AIDS) box.

Self-Management Education. *Teaching the patient, family, and friends is a high priority when preparing for discharge.* Instruct about modes of transmission and preventive behaviors (e.g., guidelines for safer sex; not sharing toothbrushes, razors, and other potentially blood-contaminated articles). Caregivers also need instruction about best practices to prevent transmission while caring for the patient in the home (as listed in the Patient and Family Education: Preparing for Self-Management: Infection Control for Home Care of the Patient at Stage HIV-III (AIDS) box), nursing techniques to use in the home, and coping or support strategies.

Teach the patient, family, and friends how to protect the patient from ***infection***, how to identify the presence of infections, and what to do if these appear. Teach about the use of self-care strategies such as good hygiene, balanced rest and exercise, skin care, mouth care, and safe administration and potential side effects of all prescribed drugs. During diet teaching stress good ***nutrition;*** the need to avoid raw or rare fish, fowl, or meat; thorough washing of fruits and vegetables; and proper food refrigeration.

Teach the patient to avoid large crowds, especially in enclosed areas, not to travel to areas with poor sanitation, and to avoid cleaning pet litter boxes. The Patient and Family Education: Preparing for Self-Management box on prevention of infection lists more strategies to teach the patient and family how to avoid ***infection***.

Psychosocial Preparation. Patients advanced HIV disease often fear social stigma and rejection, even from health care professionals. Help patients identify strengths and coping strategies for difficult situations. Support family members and friends in efforts to help the patient and provide protection from discrimination.

Encourage patients to continue as many usual activities as possible. Except when too ill or too weak, they can continue to work and participate in most social activities. Support them in their selection of friends and relatives with whom to discuss the diagnosis. Stress that sexual partners and care providers should be informed; beyond that, it is up to the patient. Some patients have depression or anxiety about the future. Almost all feel the burden of having a complicated disease widely considered unacceptable and feel compelled to maintain some secrecy about the illness. Referrals to community resources, mental health professionals, and support groups can help the patient verbalize fears and frustrations and cope with the illness.

Health Care Resources. Community groups and volunteers often assist adults at stage HIV-III (AIDS). The types of services vary but may include HIV testing and counseling, clinic services, buddy systems, support groups, respite care, education and outreach, referral services, and housing. Patients may need referrals to other local resources such as home care agencies, companies that provide home IV therapy, community mental health/behavioral health agencies, Meals on Wheels, transportation services, and others. Educational materials and support groups are available through the Internet.

◆ **Evaluation: Evaluate Outcomes.** The overall outcomes for care of PLWH are to maintain the highest possible level of function for as long as possible, reduce ***infection***, and maintain quality of life and dignity during the course of progressive illness. Evaluate the care of the patient with HIV-III (AIDS) on the basis of the identified priority problems. Expected outcomes include that he or she will:

- Adhere to the prescribed drug therapy regimen at least 90% of the time
- Practice safer sex techniques all of the time
- Remain free from opportunistic and other ***infections***
- Have adequate ***gas exchange***
- Achieve an acceptable level of ***pain*** relief and physical comfort
- Attain adequate weight and ***nutrition*** and fluid status
- Maintain ***tissue integrity***
- Have enough energy to participate in ADLs and other activities as desired
- Maintain a support system and involvement with others

CLINICAL JUDGMENT CHALLENGE 17.1

Patient-Centered Care; Evidence-Based Practice; Safety

The client is a 31-year-old female certified emergency medical technician (EMT) who passed out on the job and was brought to the emergency department with shortness of breath and a pulse oximetry reading of 88%. She is found to have pneumonia by auscultation and chest x-ray. Her vital signs are temperature 101° F (38.3° C), pulse 126, respiratory rate of 32, and blood pressure of 102/60. She is now alert and able to answer questions. On being told that she has pneumonia, she sighs and say that this is the third time in the past year she has had pneumonia.

The admitting nurse documents the following history and physical assessment data:

- Most recent episode of pneumonia (community acquired, 10 weeks ago) was treated with amoxicillin
- Has a productive cough that kept her awake last night
- Was once homeless and an injection drug user who also misused alcohol
- Is not on speaking terms with her parents
- Was admitted 5 years ago with an opioid overdose
- Has worked as an EMT for 3 years
- Is married with no children
- Uses oral contraceptives as her preferred method of birth control
- Was admitted to an inpatient rehabilitation center after the overdose and has been clean and sober ever since
- Other hospitalizations include surgery for appendicitis 15 years ago and emergency treatment for a fractured wrist 2 years ago
- Married the EMT who transported her during the overdose episode
- Other current daily drugs include a multiple vitamin and NSAIDs for perceived job-related muscle pain
- Admitting white blood cell count = 3400/mm^3

1. **Recognize Cues:** What assessment information in this client situation is the most important and immediate concern for the nurse? (Hint: Identify the **relevant** information *first* to help the nurse determine what is most important.)
2. **Analyze Cues:** What client conditions are consistent with the **most relevant** information? (Hint: Think about priority collaborative problems that support and contradict the information presented in this situation.)
3. **Prioritize Hypotheses:** Which possibilities or explanations are **most likely** to be present in this client situation? Which possibilities or explanations are the most serious? (Hint: Consider all possibilities and determine their urgency and risk for this client.)
4. **Generate Solutions:** What interventions would most likely achieve the desired outcomes for this client? Which interventions should be **avoided** or are **potentially harmful**? (Hint: Determine the desired outcomes first to help the nurse decide which interventions are appropriate and those that should be avoided.)
5. **Take Action:** Which interventions are the most appropriate, and how should they be implemented? In what **priority order** should they be implemented? (Hint: Consider health teaching, documentation, requested health care provider orders or prescriptions, nursing skills, collaboration with or referral to health team members, etc.)
6. **Evaluate Outcomes:** What client assessment would indicate that the nurse's interventions were **effective**? (Hint: Think about signs that would indicate an improvement, decline, or unchanged client condition.)

GET READY FOR THE NEXT-GENERATION NCLEX® EXAMINATION!

Key Points

Review these Key Points for each NCLEX Examination Client Needs Category.

Safe and Effective Care Environment

- Use Standard Precautions for all patients, regardless of age, gender, race or ethnicity, sexual orientation, education level, and profession. **QSEN: Safety**
- Protect the hospitalized immunosuppressed patient from ***infection.*** **QSEN: Safety**
- Teach assistive personnel (AP) to use Standard Precautions. **QSEN: Safety, Teamwork and Collaboration**
- Collaborate with immunity health care providers, registered dietitian nutritionist (RDN), respiratory therapist, pharmacist, social worker, and case manager to individualize patient care for the adult with HIV disease at any stage in any care setting. **QSEN: Teamwork and Collaboration**
- Teach the patient and family about the indications of ***infection*** and when to seek medical advice. **QSEN: Safety**

Health Promotion and Maintenance

- Urge all patients who are HIV positive to use condoms and other precautions during sexual intimacy even if the partner is also HIV positive. **QSEN: Evidence-Based Practice**
- Urge patients to adhere to their antiviral drug regimen. **QSEN: Evidence-Based Practice**
- Refer patients newly diagnosed with HIV ***infection*** to local resources and support groups. **QSEN: Patient-Centered Care**

Psychosocial Integrity

- Urge all patients who are HIV positive to inform their sexual partners of their HIV status. **QSEN: Patient-Centered Care**
- Respect the patient's right to inform or not to inform family members about his or her HIV status. **Ethics**
- Ensure the confidentiality of the patient's HIV status. **Ethics**

Physiological Integrity

- Use prescribed oxygen therapy, drug therapy, and respiratory support to improve ***gas exchange*** for the patient with respiratory problems related to reduced ***immunity.*** **QSEN: Evidence-Based Practice**
- Use pharmacologic and nonpharmacologic therapies to reduce ***Pain*** for the patient with advanced HIV disease. **QSEN: Patient-Centered Care**
- Teach the patient and caregivers the schedule, side effects, and possible drug interactions of combination antiretroviral therapy (cART). **QSEN: Patient-Centered Care**
- Assess the patient with impaired ***immunity*** every shift for signs of ***infection.*** Document the assessment findings, and report any indication of infection immediately to the immunity health care provider. **QSEN: Safety**
- Assess the ***tissue integrity*** of the perianal region of a patient with AIDS-related diarrhea after every bowel movement. **QSEN: Evidence-Based Practice**

MASTERY QUESTIONS

1. Which part of the HIV infection process is disrupted by the antiretroviral drug class of entry inhibitors?
   A. Activating the viral enzyme "integrase" within the infected host's cells
   B. Binding of the virus to the CD4+ receptor and either of the two co-receptors
   C. Clipping the newly generated viral proteins into smaller functional pieces
   D. Fusing of the newly created viral particle with the infected cell's membrane
2. Which food, drink, or herbal supplement does the nurse teach the client taking tipranavir to avoid?
   A. Caffeinated beverages
   B. Grapefruit juice
   C. Dairy products
   D. St. John's wort
3. A client who is HIV positive and receiving combination antiretroviral therapy tells the nurse she is now pregnant. Which drug does the nurse expect to be suspended during this patient's pregnancy?
   A. Abacavir
   B. Darunivir
   C. Tripanavir
   D. Raltegravir

REFERENCES

Asterisk (*) indicates a classic or definitive work on this subject.

Betancourt, J. (2018). Learning from the past while looking to the future: Nurses' continuing roles as advocates in the era of U=U. *Journal of the Association of Nurses in AIDS Care, 29*(5), 628–634.

Bruce, R. D., Merlin, J., Lum, P. J., Ahmed, E., Alexander, C., Corbett, A., Foley, K., Leonard, K., Treisman, G. J., & Selwyn, P. (2017). 2017 HIVMA of IDSA clinical practice guideline for the management of chronic pain in patients living with HIV. *Clinical Infectious Diseases, 65*(10), e1–e37.

Burcham, J. R., & Rosenthal, L. D. (2019). *Lehne's pharmacology for nursing care* (10th ed.). St. Louis: Elsevier.

*Centers for Disease Control and Prevention (CDC). (1991). Recommendations for preventing transmission of human immunodeficiency virus and hepatitis B virus to patients during exposure-prone invasive procedures. *Morbidity and Mortality Weekly Report, 40*(RR-8), 1–9.

Centers for Disease Control and Prevention (CDC). (2013). *Updated Public Health Service guidelines for the management of occupational exposures to HIV and recommendations for postexposure prophylaxis.* https://stacks.cdc.gov/view/cdc/20711.

Centers for Disease Control and Prevention (CDC). (2016). *TB elimination: Special considerations for the treatment of TB disease in persons infected with HIV.* https://www.cdc.gov/tb/publications/factsheets/treatment/treatmenthivpositive.pdf.

Centers for Disease Control and Prevention (CDC). (2017a). *HIV and Tuberculosis.* https://www.cdc.gov/hiv/pdf/library/factsheets/hiv-tb.pdf.

Centers for Disease Control and Prevention (CDC). (2017b). *CDC's HIV Basics: PEP 101.* https://www.cdc.gov/hiv/pdf/library/factsheets/cdc-hiv-pep101.pdf.

Centers for Disease Control and Prevention (CDC). (2017c). *CDC's HIV Basics: Preventing mother-to-child transmission of HIV.* https://www.hiv.gov/authors/cdc-s-hiv-basics//hiv-prevention/reducing-mother-to-child-risk/preventing-mother-to-child-transmission-of-hiv.

Centers for Disease Control and Prevention (CDC). (2018a). *CDC's HIV Basics: HIV testing 101.* https://www.cdc.gov/hiv/pdf/library/factsheets/hiv-testing.

Centers for Disease Control and Prevention (CDC). (2018b). *CDC's HIV basics: PrEP.* From https://www.cdc.gov/hiv/basics/prep.html-101-info-sheet.pdf.

Centers for Disease Control and Prevention (CDC). (2018c). *Updated Guidelines for Antiretroviral Postexposure Prophylaxis After Sexual, Injection Drug Use, or other Nonoccupational Exposure to HIV-United States*, 2016. https://stacks.cdc.gov/view/cdc/38856.

Centers for Disease Control and Prevention (CDC). (2019). *Diagnosis of HIV infection in the United States and dependent areas, 2018* (vol. 28). From: http://www.cdc.gov/hiv/library/reports/hiv-surveillance.html.

Clark, W., & Cress, E. (2018). Nutritional issues and positive living in human immunodeficiency virus/AIDS. *Nursing Clinics of North America, 53*(1), 13–24.

Cluck, D., & Underwood, R. (2018). A therapeutic perspective of living with human immunodeficiency virus/AIDS in 2017. *Nursing Clinics of North America, 53*(1), 97–110.

Daley, K. (2017). Sharps injuries: Where we stand today. *American Nurse Today, 12*(2), 23–24.

Farahani, M., Mulinder, H., Farahani, A., & Marlink, R. (2017). Prevalence and distribution of non-AIDS causes of death among HIV-infected individuals receiving antiretroviral therapy: A systematic review and meta-analysis. *International Journal of STD and AIDS, 28*(7), 636–650.

Government of Canada. (2018). *HIV in Canada-Surveillance Report, 2017.* From: https://www.canada.ca/content/dam/phac-aspc/documents/services/reports-publications/canada-communicable-disease-report-ccdr/monthly-issue/2018-44/issue-12-december-6-2018/ccdrv44i12a03-eng.pdf.

Gray, T. (2019). Burdened by a secret: Caring for older adults with HIV in critical care. *AACN Advances in Critical Care, 30*(1), 79–84.

Grimes, R., Hardwicke, R., Grimes, D., & DeGarmo, S. (2016). When to consider acute HIV infection in the differential diagnosis. *The Nurse Practitioner, 41*(1), 1–5.

Hussar, D. (2019). New drugs 2019: Part 2. *Nursing 2019, 49*(5), 32–41.

Kerns, R., & Sheridan, D. (2019). HIV postexposure prophylaxis for healthcare professionals. *Nursing 2019, 49*(1), 67–68.

Kerns, R., & Sheridan, D. (2018). Should your patient be PrEPared? *Nursing 2018, 48*(3), 69.

Kwong, J. (2019). HIV update: An epidemic transformed. *American Journal of Nursing, 119*(9), 30–39.

Kwong, J. (2020). New drug treatment options for HIV. *The Nurse Practitioner, 45*(3), 28–39.

McCance, K., Huether, S., Brashers, V., & Rote, N. (2019). *Pathophysiology: The biologic basis for disease in adults and children* (8th ed.). St. Louis: Elsevier.

Mitchell, A. (2020). Sharps injury prevention. *American Nurse Today, 15*(4), 38.

Mitchell, A., & Parker, G. (2018). Building programs to reduce sharps injuries from insulin injection. *American Nurse Today, 13*(2), 13–14.

Mitchell, A., & Powell, L. (2018). Splash safety-Protecting your eyes. *American Nurse Today, 13*(3), 22–23.

New York State Department of Health AIDS Institute. (2018). *Clinical Guidelines Program. Free compilation of current guidelines for clinical practice.* From www.hivguidelines.org.

Pagana, K., & Pagana, T. (2018a). *Mosby's manual of diagnostic and laboratory tests* (6th ed.). St. Louis: Mosby.

Penkalski, M., Felicilda-Reynaldo, R., & Patterson, K. (2017). Antiviral medications, Part 2: HIV antiretroviral therapy. *MEDSURG Nursing, 26*(5), 327–331.

Voigt, N., Cho, H., & Schnall, R. (2018). Supervised physical activity and improved functional capacity among adults living with HIV: A systematic review. *Journal of the Association of Nurses in AIDS Care, 29*(5), 667–680.

World Health Organization (WHO). (2019). *HIV/AIDS.* Fact Sheet. From: http://www.who.int/news-room/fact-sheets/detail/hiv-aids.

Wilmont, S. (2018). A missed opportunity in HIV prevention? *American Journal of Nursing, 118*(1), 18–19.

18

Concepts of Care for Patients With Hypersensitivity (Allergy) and Autoimmunity

M. Linda Workman

http://evolve.elsevier.com/Iggy/

LEARNING OUTCOMES

1. Collaborate with the interprofessional team to coordinate high-quality care and protect the patient experiencing problems of excessive ***inflammation*** or overactive ***immunity***, including allergic reactions and autoimmunity.
2. Apply knowledge of anatomy, physiology, pathophysiology, and genetics to assess patients who have health problems related to excessive ***inflammation*** or overactive ***immunity***.
3. Teach patients with allergies how to protect themselves against harm from a hypersensitivity reaction and from therapies used to treat excessive ***inflammation*** or overactive ***immunity***.
4. Use clinical judgment to plan care for patients during periods of ***inflammation*** or overactive ***immunity***.
5. Implement nursing interventions to help the patient and family cope with the psychosocial impact caused by hypersensitivity or autoimmunity.
6. Teach the patient and caregiver(s) about common drugs used for control of systemic lupus erythematosus and other forms of excessive ***inflammation*** or overactive ***immunity***.

KEY TERMS

allergen An antigen that triggers excessive inflammation or immunity overreactions only in susceptible individuals.

allergy See ***hypersensitivity***.

anaphylaxis A condition in which a type I hypersensitivity reaction involves all blood vessels and bronchiolar smooth muscle, causing widespread blood vessel dilation, decreased cardiac output, and bronchoconstriction.

angioedema A severe type I hypersensitivity reaction that involves the blood vessels and all layers of the skin, mucous membranes, and subcutaneous tissues in the affected area.

antigens Proteins (usually) considered as non-self by a person's immune system that will stimulate the person's immune system to have an ***immunity*** response and make antibodies directed against the antigen.

autoantigens Antibodies directed against self tissues and cells.

autoimmunity A process whereby an inappropriate ***immunity*** develops to an adult's own tissues.

five cardinal symptoms of inflammation Warmth, redness, swelling, pain, and decreased function.

human leukocyte antigens (HLAs) Unique surface proteins present on all of a person's cells that are specific to him or her. Also known as a person's *tissue type*.

hypersensitivity Overactive ***immunity*** with excessive ***inflammation*** occurring in response to the presence of an antigen to which the patient usually has been previously exposed (also known as *allergy*).

immunity Protection from illness or disease that is maintained by the body's physiologic defense mechanisms.

inflammation A syndrome of normal tissue responses to cellular injury, allergy, or the invasion of pathogens.

Lyme disease A reportable systemic infectious disease caused by the spirochete *Borrelia burgdorferi*.

self-tolerance The special ability of immune system cells to recognize self versus non-self and avoid actions that would harm self cells.

systemic lupus erythematosus (SLE) A chronic and progressive autoimmune disorder in which inflammatory and immune attacks occur against multiple self tissues and organs.

Inflammation, which is a syndrome of normal tissue responses to cellular injury, allergy, or the invasion of pathogens, is an important protective mechanism and also starts the critical processes needed for wound healing. **Immunity**, which is protection from illness or disease that is maintained by the body's physiologic defense mechanisms, is provided by antibodies and other special secretions or cells that result in sustained, long-term protective actions. Both inflammation and immunity are necessary and helpful protective responses when their reactions are directed against only appropriate targets and the duration of

PRIORITY AND INTERRELATED CONCEPTS

The priority concepts for this chapter are:
- ***Immunity***
- ***Inflammation***

The ***Immunity*** concept exemplar for this chapter is Systemic Lupus Erythematosus.

The interrelated concepts for this chapter are:
- ***Gas Exchange***
- ***Tissue Integrity***

any increased response is limited. However, when the responses are excessive, widespread, or directed against normal body tissues, damage can result (Abbas et al., 2018; McCance et al., 2019). These excessive responses are responsible for the problems associated with hypersensitivity and autoimmunity.

HYPERSENSITIVITIES/ALLERGIES

Hypersensitivity (also known as **allergy**) is overactive ***immunity*** with excessive ***inflammation*** occurring in response to the presence of an antigen to which the patient usually has been previously exposed. (Recall from Chapter 16 that an **antigen** is a protein considered as non-self by a person's immune system that will stimulate the immune system to have an immunity response and make antibodies directed against the antigen.) It can cause problems that range from being uncomfortable (e.g., itchy, watery eyes, or sneezing) to life threatening (e.g., allergic asthma, angioedema, anaphylaxis, bronchoconstriction, or circulatory collapse). The terms *hypersensitivity* and *allergy* are interchangeable. These reactions are classified into four basic types, determined by differences in timing, pathophysiology, and symptoms (Table 18.1). Each type may occur alone or along with one or more of the other types (McCance et al., 2019).

Although the predisposition to have allergies is genetic, specific allergies are *not* inherited. For example, a woman who has an allergy to penicillin but not to peanuts may have a child with an allergy to peanuts but not to penicillin.

TYPES OF HYPERSENSITIVITY REACTIONS

Type I hypersensitivity, or rapid hypersensitivity, also called *atopic allergy,* is the most common type of hypersensitivity from excessive ***inflammation*** caused by overactive ***immunity***. Usually the target of the actions is appropriate but the responses are excessive. Type I reactions result from the increased production of the immunoglobulin E (IgE) antibody class. Acute inflammation occurs when IgE responds to an antigen such as pollen and causes the release of histamine, bradykinin, and other vasoactive amines from basophils, eosinophils, and mast cells. Examples of type I reactions include angioedema, anaphylaxis, and allergic asthma; atopic allergies such as hay fever and allergic rhinosinusitis; and allergies to substances such as latex, bee venom, peanuts, iodine, shellfish, drugs, and many other antigens that act as allergens. An **allergen** is an antigen that triggers excessive inflammation or

TABLE 18.1 Mechanisms and Examples of Types of Hypersensitivities

Mechanism	Clinical Examples
Type I: Rapid or Immediate	
Reaction of IgE antibody on mast cells with antigen, which results in release of mediators, especially histamine	Hay fever (rhinosinusitis) Allergic asthma Anaphylaxis Angioedema
Type II: Cytotoxic	
Reaction of IgG with host cell membrane or antigen adsorbed by host cell membrane	Autoimmune hemolytic anemia Goodpasture syndrome Myasthenia gravis
Type III: Immune Complex–Mediated	
Formation of immune complex of antigen and antibody, which deposits in walls of blood vessels and results in complement release and inflammation	Serum sickness Vasculitis Systemic lupus erythematosus Rheumatoid arthritis
Type IV: Delayed	
Reaction of sensitized T-cells with antigen and release of lymphokines, which activates macrophages and induces inflammation	Poison ivy Graft rejection Positive TB skin tests Sarcoidosis

IgE, Immunoglobulin E; *IgG,* immunoglobulin G; *TB,* tuberculosis.

immunity overreactions only in susceptible individuals. Allergens can be contacted in these ways:
- Inhaled (plant pollens, fungal spores, animal dander, house dust, grass, ragweed)
- Ingested (foods, food additives, drugs)
- Injected (insect or other venom, drugs, biologic substances such as contrast dyes)
- Skin or mucous membrane contacted (latex, pollens, foods, environmental proteins)

Some reactions occur just in the areas exposed to the antigen such as the mucous membranes of the nose and eyes, causing symptoms of rhinorrhea, sneezing, and itchy, red, watery eyes. Other reactions may lead to the condition of anaphylaxis with involvement of all blood vessels and bronchiolar smooth muscle, causing widespread blood vessel dilation, decreased cardiac output, and bronchoconstriction. This condition is a medical emergency and must be treated immediately (see the Anaphylaxis section).

The mechanism for type I reactions is the same regardless of whether they are widespread and severe, or localized and annoying. On first exposure to an allergen, the patient initially responds by making antigen-specific IgE. This IgE binds to the surface of basophils and mast cells (Fig. 18.1). These cells have many granules containing vasoactive amines (including histamine) that are released when stimulated. Once the antigen-specific IgE is formed, the patient is sensitized to that allergen.

When the sensitized patient is re-exposed to the allergen, the resulting response has a primary phase and a secondary phase. In the primary phase, the allergen binds to two adjacent

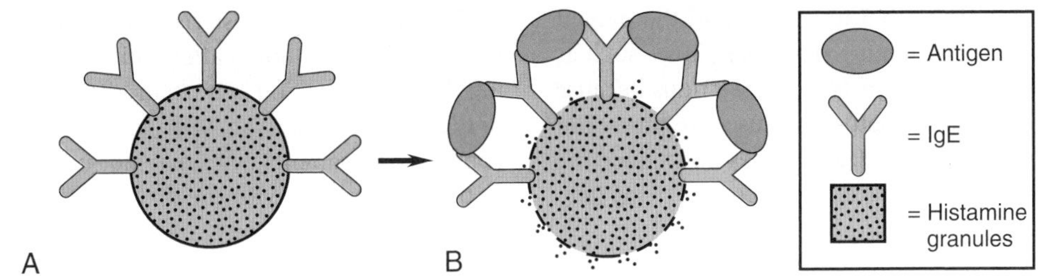

Fig. 18.1 Degranulation and histamine release. (A) Mast cell with IgE. (B) Mast cell degranulation and histamine release when allergen binds to IgE.

IgE molecules on the surface of a basophil or mast cell, which alters the cell's membrane. The membrane opens and releases the vasoactive amines into tissue fluids (see Fig. 18.1).

The most common vasoactive amine is *histamine,* a short-acting biochemical. Histamine results in the **five cardinal symptoms of inflammation** (warmth, redness, swelling, pain, and decreased function) caused by capillary leak, nasal and conjunctival mucus secretion, and pruritus (itching), often occurring with redness (erythema). These symptoms last for about 10 minutes after histamine is first released. When the allergen is continuously present, mast cells continuously release histamine and other inflammatory proteins, prolonging the response.

The secondary phase results from the release of other cellular proteins. These proteins draw more white blood cells to the area and stimulate a more general inflammatory reaction through actions of leukotriene, bradykinin, and prostaglandins (other mediators of ***inflammation***; see Chapter 16). This reaction occurs in addition to the allergic reaction stimulated in the primary phase. The resulting inflammation increases the symptoms and continues the response.

The production of high IgE levels in response to antigen exposure is genetically based on the inheritance of many genes. However, as stated earlier, specific allergies are not inherited.

Type II cytotoxic reactions occur when the body makes autoantibodies directed against self cells that have some form of foreign protein attached to them. The autoantibody binds to the self cell and forms an immune complex (see Fig. 16.12 in Chapter 16). The self cell is then destroyed along with the attached protein. Examples of type II reactions include immune hemolytic anemias, immune thrombocytopenic purpura, hemolytic transfusion reactions (when a patient receives the wrong blood type during a transfusion), and drug-induced hemolytic anemia.

Management of type II reactions begins with discontinuing the offending drug or blood product. *Plasmapheresis* (filtration of the plasma to remove specific substances) to remove autoantibodies may be beneficial. Otherwise treatment is symptomatic. Complications such as hemolytic crisis and kidney failure can be life threatening.

Type III immune complex reactions result from excess antigens causing immune complexes to form in the blood (Fig. 18.2). These circulating complexes then lodge in small blood vessels of the kidneys, skin, and joints. The complexes trigger inflammation, and tissue or vessel damage results.

Most immune complex disorders (autoimmune disorders) are caused by type III reactions. For example, the symptoms of rheumatoid arthritis are caused by immune complexes that

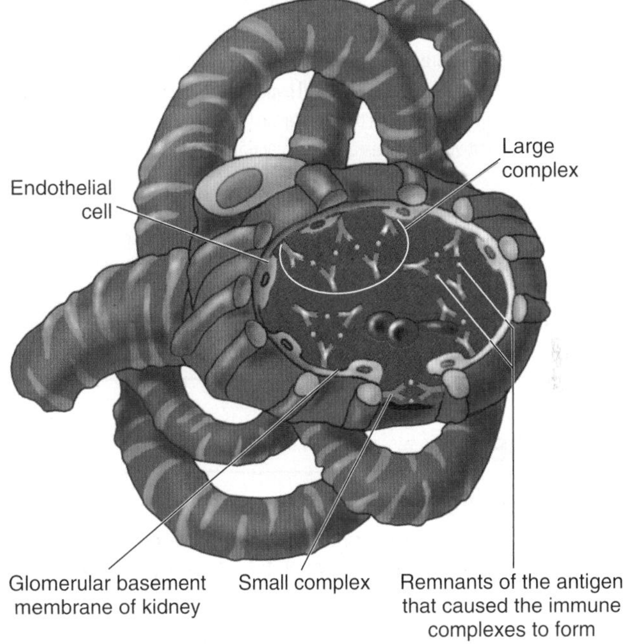

Fig. 18.2 An immune complex in a type III hypersensitivity reaction.

lodge in joint spaces followed by tissue destruction, scarring, and fibrotic changes. Systemic lupus erythematosus (SLE) has immune complexes lodged in blood vessels (causing vasculitis), the glomeruli (causing glomerulonephritis), the joints (causing arthralgia, arthritis), and other organs and tissues, leading to loss of ***tissue integrity*** and permanent damage.

Type IV delayed hypersensitivity reactions have T-lymphocytes (T-cells) as the activated immune system component triggering the excessive responses. Antibodies and complement are not involved (Abbas et al., 2018). Sensitized T-cells (from a previous exposure) respond to an antigen by releasing chemical mediators and triggering macrophages to destroy the antigen. A type IV response typically occurs hours to days after exposure. It consists of edema, induration, ischemia, and tissue damage at the site of the exposure.

Common examples of type IV reactions include contact dermatitis such as poison ivy skin rashes or metal-induced skin irritations from jewelry, local response to insect stings, and sarcoidosis. A classic example of a small type IV reaction is a positive purified protein derivative (PPD) test for tuberculosis (TB). In a patient previously exposed to TB, an intradermal injection of this agent causes sensitized T-cells to clump at the injection site, release lymphokines, and activate macrophages. Induration and erythema at the injection site appear after about 24 to 72 hours.

The reaction is self-limiting in 5 to 7 days, and the patient is treated symptomatically. Histamine (H_1) antagonists such as diphenhydramine are not useful for type IV reactions because histamine is not the main mediator. Because IgE does not cause this type of reaction, desensitization does not reduce the response. Corticosteroids can reduce the discomfort and help resolve the reaction more quickly.

NCLEX EXAMINATION CHALLENGE 18.1

Physiological Integrity

Which statement(s) regarding type III hypersensitivity reactions is/are true? **Select all that apply.**

A. Type III responses are usually directed against self cells and tissues.
B. Susceptibility for developing a type III hypersensitivity response follows an autosomal dominant pattern of inheritance.
C. The hypersensitivity starts as a type II reaction that progresses to a type III reaction.
D. The major mechanism of the reaction is the release of mediators from sensitized T-cells that trigger antigen destruction by macrophages.
E. Rheumatoid arthritis is an example of a health problem caused by this type of hypersensitivity.
F. The second phase of the reaction with accumulation of excess bradykinin is responsible for development of angioedema.

ANGIOEDEMA

Pathophysiology Review

Angioedema is a severe type I hypersensitivity reaction that involves the blood vessels and all layers of the skin, mucous membranes, and subcutaneous tissues in the affected area (Abbas et al., 2018). Unlike the superficial responses of allergic rhinosinusitis, the angioedema response is a deep-tissue problem of IgE-mediated release of inflammatory proteins, especially bradykinin.

Although angioedema can occur in any part of the body, it is most often seen in the lips, face, tongue, larynx, and neck (Fig. 18.3). Intestinal angioedema can also occur, with problems of severe abdominal pain, cramping, nausea, and vomiting. It can be difficult to differentiate this problem from any other acute abdominal problem.

Exposure to any ingested drug or chemical can cause the problem. The most common drugs associated with angioedema are angiotensin-converting enzyme inhibitors (ACEIs) used for hypertension (Banerji et al., 2017; Hirschy et al., 2018) and NSAIDs. Bradykinin is the inflammatory mediator most responsible for ACEI-induced angioedema. This mediator is a strong vasodilator and promoter of deep-tissue ***inflammation***. It is rapidly deactivated by angiotensin-converting enzyme (ACE). Drugs that inhibit ACE lead to increasing tissue accumulation of bradykinin over time, which is responsible the delayed onset of ACEI-induced angioedema even though it is a type I hypersensitivity reaction (Hirschy et al., 2018).

About 0.7% of adults taking ACEIs develop angioedema from the drug. These reactions are responsible for at least 40,000 emergency department visits in the United States annually (Banerji et al., 2017). This high incidence reflects how commonly these drugs are prescribed.

Although the greatest risk for angioedema from ACEIs is within the first 24 hours after taking the first dose of an offending drug, the reaction can occur after days, weeks, and months of therapy (Banerji et al., 2017). Any new onset of symptoms is confusing to patients, who may not understand the association of the angioedema with the drug or drugs they have been taking, often for months or years.

PATIENT-CENTERED CARE: CULTURAL/SPIRITUAL CONSIDERATIONS QSEN

Black adults, especially African Americans, have a higher incidence of angioedema and laryngeal edema from ACEIs, about five times higher than in whites (Hirschy et al., 2018; Nguyen, 2018). Any ACEI should be used cautiously in black patients. Be sure to observe the patient carefully for any signs and symptoms of angioedema and laryngeal edema after the first dose. Teach black patients taking an ACEI about the indications of angioedema and the need to go to an emergency department or to call 911 immediately if symptoms appear.

Interprofessional Collaborative Care

Angioedema from a drug exposure can occur in any setting but is more likely to happen in the home or community. Management requires at least a brief hospitalization.

Assessment: Recognize Cues. An accurate and detailed history helps identify the possible cause of angioedema. Ask the patient to list all drugs taken on a regular basis, especially drugs for blood pressure control. Although more information can be helpful, intervention is critically important because laryngeal edema can cause the patient to lose his or her airway. Defer further history taking until interventions have been implemented.

Often a patient may have only lip swelling or a slight itching in the back of the throat from time to time before a fully developed case of angioedema occurs. Ask the patient specifically about whether he or she has had such a problem, when it occurred, how long it lasted, and whether any drugs were taken to reduce the symptoms. Also ask about any other allergies the patient may have.

The patient with ACEI-induced angioedema (with or without laryngeal edema) has deep, firm swelling of the face, lips, tongue, and neck. He or she may have difficulty speaking or drinking because the lips are so stiff from swelling. The face can be so distorted that friends and relatives may not recognize the patient. Often, nasal swelling interferes with breathing through the nose. Problems that indicate a need for immediate intervention are the inability to swallow, the feeling of a lump in the throat, or stridor, indicating the edema has spread to the larynx. Usually the patient with ACEI-induced angioedema is diagnosed based on the signs and symptoms. No specific test can diagnose angioedema, and valuable time should not be wasted in laboratory testing during an acute episode.

Interventions: Take Action. Interventions focus on stopping the reaction and ensuring an adequate airway. Prompt intervention can reverse angioedema before laryngeal edema forms and

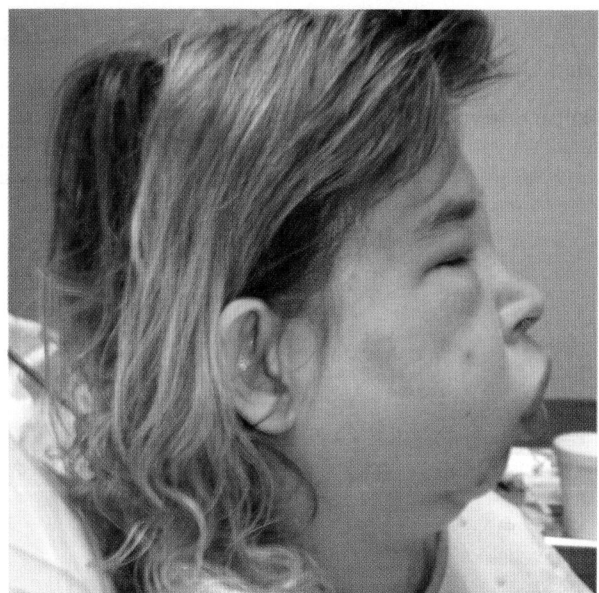

Fig. 18.3 Angioedema of the face, lips, and mouth. (From Auerbach, P. [2008]. *Wilderness medicine* [5th ed.]. Philadelphia: Mosby; courtesy Sheryl Olson.)

intubation is needed. Oxygen by nasal cannula is applied to help maintain ***gas exchange***. Because the reaction is mediated through antibodies and release of vasoactive amines (especially bradykinin), the most useful drugs are corticosteroids and epinephrine. Indications for intubation are the presence of stridor and the inability of the patient to swallow.

Drug therapy may need to continue for several hours after angioedema has initially resolved. Usually the agent that caused the angioedema has a longer half-life than the drugs used to treat it. Thus initial drug therapy can successfully shrink the facial, oral, and airway edema to the extent that symptoms are no longer felt or observed. However, if drug therapy is completely stopped at this point, the agent remaining in the blood can cause angioedema to redevelop. Once drug therapy has stopped, the IV access remains, and the patient is closely monitored for 2 to 6 hours. If the angioedema does not recur, the patient is usually discharged to home.

In some patients ACEI-induced angioedema may not be responsive to standard drug therapy and edema progresses despite corticosteroids and epinephrine. Experimental therapy with the use of fresh-frozen plasma replacement or the drug icatibant (used for management of hereditary angioedema) have been tried but do not show a clear benefit. The cost of a single dose of icatibant is more than $11,000, and it is not a commonly available agent (Riha et al., 2017).

If laryngeal edema forms and intubation is not possible, an emergency tracheostomy is needed. Location of the tracheotomy (incision into the trachea) must be below the level of the edema to ensure adequate airflow to the site of ***gas exchange***. Mechanical ventilation is usually not needed. The tracheostomy tube is discontinued when the patient can easily breathe around the tube. (See Chapter 25 for detailed information about tracheostomy.)

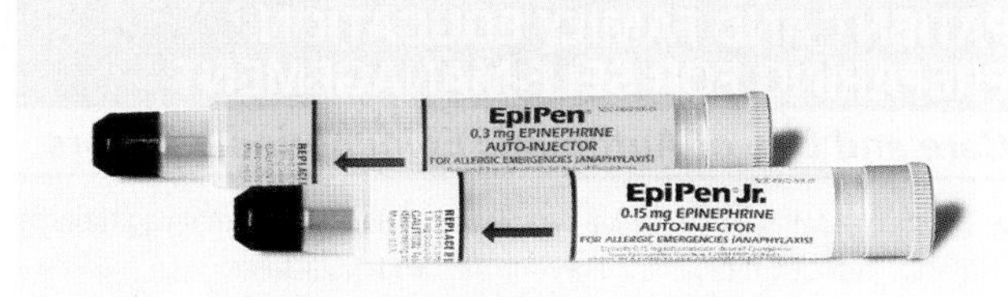

Fig. 18.4 EpiPen and EpiPen Jr. self-injectors for epinephrine. (Courtesy Dey, Napa, CA.)

Severe angioedema of the face or mouth is an acute emergency. With successful management the patient is discharged to resume his or her usual activities. The most important aspects of care coordination are to determine the cause of the angioedema, teach the patient to avoid the offending agent, and ensure that he or she knows to seek emergency care as soon as any signs or symptoms of the problem occur.

ANAPHYLAXIS

Pathophysiology Review

Anaphylaxis is a condition in which a type I hypersensitivity reaction involves of all blood vessels and bronchiolar smooth muscle, causing widespread blood vessel dilation, decreased cardiac output, and bronchoconstriction within seconds to minutes after allergen exposure. It is the most life-threatening example of a type I hypersensitivity reaction and occurs rapidly and systemically. Anaphylaxis episodes can vary in severity and can be fatal. *The major factor in fatal outcomes for anaphylaxis is a delay in the administration of epinephrine (Hayden, 2019).* Such a failure to rescue is an important negative nursing quality indicator (NQI). Almost any substance can trigger anaphylaxis in a susceptible adult. Drugs and injectable imaging contrast media ("dyes") are some causes of anaphylaxis in acute care settings; food and insect stings or bites are common causes in community settings.

Health Promotion and Maintenance

Anaphylaxis has a rapid onset and a potentially fatal outcome (even with appropriate intervention); thus prevention and early intervention are critical. *Teach the patient with a history of allergic reactions to avoid known allergens whenever possible, to wear a medical alert bracelet, and to alert health care personnel about specific allergies.* Some patients must carry an emergency anaphylaxis kit (e.g., a kit with injectable epinephrine, sometimes called a *bee sting kit*) or an epinephrine autoinjector (EAI). Recently the U.S. Food and Drug Administration approved generic EAIs with a much lower cost per dose than the original EpiPen product (Palmer, 2018). Spring-loaded epinephrine auto-injectors that deliver a specific dose are available for subcutaneous or intramuscular injection (Fig. 18.4). Teach patients how to care for and use the device as described in the Patient and Family Education: Preparing for Self-Management: Care and Use of Automatic Epinephrine Injectors box.

PATIENT AND FAMILY EDUCATION: PREPARING FOR SELF-MANAGEMENT

Care and Use of Automatic Epinephrine Injectors

- Practice assembly of injection device with a non–drug-containing training device provided through the injection device manufacturer.
- Keep the device with you at all times.
- When needed, inject the drug into the top of your thigh, slightly to the outside, holding the device so the needle enters straight down.
- You can inject the drug right through your pants; just avoid seams and pockets where the fabric is thicker.
- Use the device when any symptom of anaphylaxis is present and before you call 911 (Hayden, 2019). **It is better to use the drug when it is not needed than to not use it when it is needed!!!**
- Whenever you need to use the device, get to the nearest hospital for monitoring for at least the next 4 to 6 hours.
- Have at least two drug-filled devices on hand in case more than one dose is needed.
- Protect the device from light and avoid temperature extremes.
- Carry the device in the case provided by the manufacturer.
- Keep safety cap in place until you are ready to use the device.
- Check the device for:
  Expiration date—If the date is close to expiring or has expired, obtain a replacement device.
  Drug clarity—If the drug is discolored, obtain a replacement device.
  Security of cap—If the cap is loose or comes off accidently, obtain a replacement device.

NURSING SAFETY PRIORITY (QSEN)

Action Alert

The medical records (paper and electronic) of patients with a history of anaphylaxis should prominently display the list of specific allergens. Ask the patient about drug allergies before giving any drug or agent. If he or she has a known allergy, be sure to document the allergen and the specific type of response the patient experienced and communicate the allergy and its response to other members of the interprofessional care team. Be aware of common cross-reacting agents. For example, a patient who is allergic to penicillin is also likely to react to cephalosporins because both have a similar chemical structure.

Take precautionary measures if a drug or agent must be used despite a history of allergic reactions. Start an IV, and place intubation equipment and a tracheostomy set at the bedside. The patient is often premedicated with diphenhydramine or a corticosteroid.

KEY FEATURES

Anaphylaxis

Clinical Criteria 1

Onset within minutes to hours of skin or mucous membrane problems involving swollen lips, tongue, soft palate, uvula; widespread hives; pruritus; or flushing along with any one of these new-onset symptoms:

- Respiratory distress or ineffectiveness:
- Dyspnea
- Bronchospasms
- Wheezes
- Stridor
- Hypoxia
- Cyanosis
- Peak expiratory rate flow lower than the patient's usual rate
- Hypotension or any indication of reduced perfusion resulting in organ dysfunction:
  - Loss of consciousness
  - Incontinence
  - Hypotonia
  - Absent deep tendon reflexes

Clinical Criteria 2

Onset within minutes to hours of two or more of these symptoms after a patient has been exposed to a potential allergen:

- Skin or mucous membrane problems involving swollen lips, tongue, soft palate, uvula; widespread hives; pruritus; or flushing
- Respiratory distress or ineffectiveness as evidenced by any dyspnea, bronchospasms, wheezes, stridor, hypoxia, cyanosis, or peak expiratory rate flow lower than the patient's usual
- Hypotension or any indication of reduced perfusion resulting in organ dysfunction such as loss of consciousness, incontinence, hypotonia, or absent deep tendon reflexes
- Persistent GI problems such as nausea or vomiting, cramping, abdominal pain

Clinical Criteria 3

Onset within minutes to hours of hypotension with systolic blood pressure lower than 90 mm Hg or 30% lower than the patient's baseline systolic pressure

Adapted from Simons, E., Ardusso, L., Bilo, M.B., El-Gamal, Y., Ledford, D., Ring, J., et al. (2011). World Allergy Organization guidelines for the assessment and management of anaphylaxis. *WAO Journal, 4*(2), 13–37.

❖ Interprofessional Collaborative Care

◆ **Assessment: Recognize Cues.** A major problem with anaphylaxis management is that initial symptoms may be subtle, such as sudden severe abdominal cramping and diarrhea. A set of three criteria, listed in the Key Features: Anaphylaxis box, is used for diagnosis of anaphylaxis. A patient is considered to have anaphylaxis whenever any *one* of these three criteria is met, and interventions are started immediately.

Patients often have feelings of apprehension, weakness, and impending doom early in the reaction and are anxious and frightened. These feelings are followed quickly by generalized itching and urticaria (hives). Erythema and angioedema of the eyes, lips, or tongue may occur next. Intensely itchy hives may appear and may merge to form large, red blotches.

Histamine and other mediators cause inflammation, bronchoconstriction, mucosal edema, and excess mucus production. Respiratory symptoms include congestion, rhinorrhea, dyspnea, and increasing respiratory distress as audible wheezing with reduced ***gas exchange***.

On auscultation, crackles, wheezing, and reduced breath sounds are heard. Patients may have laryngeal edema as a "lump in the throat," hoarseness, and *stridor* (a crowing sound). Distress increases as the tongue and larynx swell and more mucus is produced. Stridor increases as the airway begins to close. Increasing bronchoconstriction can lead to reduced chest movement and impaired airflow. Respiratory failure may follow from laryngeal edema, suffocation, or lower airway constriction causing *hypoxemia* (poor blood oxygenation).

BEST PRACTICE FOR PATIENT SAFETY & QUALITY CARE (QSEN)

Emergency Care of the Patient With Anaphylaxis

- Immediately assess the respiratory status, airway, and oxygen saturation of patients who show any symptom of an allergic reaction.
- Call the Rapid Response Team.
- Ensure that intubation and tracheotomy equipment is ready.
- Apply oxygen using a high-flow, nonrebreather mask at 90% to 100%.
- Immediately discontinue the IV drug or infusing solution of a patient having an anaphylactic reaction to that drug or solution. Do not discontinue the IV, but change the IV tubing and hang normal saline.
- If the patient does not have an IV, start one immediately and infuse normal saline.
- Be prepared to administer epinephrine IM. Repeat drug as needed every 5 to 15 minutes until the patient responds.
- Keep the head of the bed elevated about 10 degrees if hypotension is present; if blood pressure is normal, elevate the head of the bed to 45 degrees or higher to improve ventilation.
- Raise the feet and legs.
- Stay with the patient.
- Reassure the patient that the appropriate interventions are being instituted.

! NURSING SAFETY PRIORITY (QSEN)

Critical Rescue

Closely monitor any patient receiving a drug that is associated with anaphylaxis to recognize symptoms early. If you suspect anaphylaxis, respond by immediately notifying the Rapid Response Team because most anaphylaxis deaths occur from dysrhythmias, shock, and cardiopulmonary arrest that are related to treatment delay.

The patient is hypotensive and has a rapid, weak, irregular pulse from extensive capillary leak and vasodilation. He or she is faint and anxiety and confusion.

◆ **Interventions: Take Action.** Assess ***gas exchange*** first. Emergency respiratory management is critical during an anaphylactic reaction because the severity of the reaction increases with time. The upper and lower airways become constricted, which impairs airflow and leads to arrest. Establish or stabilize the airway. If an IV drug is suspected to be causing the anaphylaxis, stop the drug immediately but do not remove the venous access because restarting an IV is difficult when the patient is hypotensive. Change the IV tubing and hang normal saline. Other emergency interventions for patients with anaphylaxis are listed in the Best Practice for Patient Safety & Quality Care: Emergency Care of the Patient with Anaphylaxis box.

The patient with anaphylaxis is usually anxious or frightened and often expresses a sense of impending doom. Stay with the patient and reassure him or her that the appropriate interventions are being instituted.

Epinephrine is the first-line drug for anaphylaxis. (Dosage is dependent on patient size.) It is most often given IM when symptoms appear. This drug constricts blood vessels, improves cardiac contraction, and dilates the bronchioles. The same dose may be repeated every 5 to 15 minutes if needed.

! NURSING SAFETY PRIORITY (QSEN)

Critical Rescue

Monitor susceptible patients for signs and symptoms of anaphylaxis. When you recognize anaphylaxis, respond by administering epinephrine as quickly as possible. *Most deaths from anaphylaxis are related to delay in epinephrine administration.*

Antihistamines such as diphenhydramine are second-line drugs and are given IV or IM for angioedema and urticaria. Other drugs used to support cardiovascular function during anaphylaxis are the same as those used in hypovolemic shock (see Chapter 34). If needed, an endotracheal tube may be inserted or an emergency tracheostomy may be performed.

If the patient can breathe independently, give oxygen to reduce hypoxemia and promote ***gas exchange.*** Start oxygen therapy via a high-flow nonrebreather facemask at 90% to 100% *before* arterial blood gas results are obtained. Monitor pulse oximetry to determine gas exchange adequacy. Arterial blood gases may be drawn to determine therapy effectiveness. Use suction to remove excess mucus and other secretions, if indicated. Continually assess the respiratory rate and depth, and assess breath sounds continually for bronchospasm, wheezing, crackles, and stridor. Elevate the bed to 45 degrees unless severe hypotension is present.

For bronchospasms the patient may be given an inhaled beta-adrenergic agonist such as metaproterenol or albuterol via high-flow nebulizer every 2 to 4 hours. Corticosteroids are added to emergency interventions, but they are not effective immediately. Oral steroids are continued (at lower doses) after the anaphylaxis is under control to prevent the late recurrence of symptoms.

Continually assess for changes in any system or for effects of drug therapy. For severe anaphylaxis the patient is admitted to an ICU for cardiac, pulmonary arterial, and capillary wedge pressure monitoring. The patient is discharged from the hospital when respiratory and cardiovascular functions have returned to normal.

GENERAL AUTOIMMUNITY

Autoimmunity is a process whereby an inappropriate ***immunity*** develops to an adult's own tissues. In this response the body's antibodies or lymphocytes are directed against the body's own healthy normal cells and tissues, not just against invaders. The immune system loses some ability to tolerate self cells and tissues. (Chapter 16 discusses the principles of immunity self-tolerance.) Some disorders with an autoimmune cause are listed in Table 18.2. Some, such as type 1 diabetes mellitus, may have multiple causes, one of which is autoimmune. Autoimmune disorders are common, chronic, progressive, self-perpetuating, and at this time cannot be cured, although spontaneous remissions have occurred (rarely). The incidence of autoimmunity within the general population is about 5% (Abbas et al., 2018; Jorde et al., 2016). However, the incidence is far higher in some families than in others. Gender and racial differences in incidence are obvious and also support a genetic basis for susceptibility.

CLINICAL JUDGMENT CHALLENGE 18.1

Safety; Evidence-Based Practice

A 45-year-old client is an inpatient with type I diabetes who has just started receiving the antibiotic ceftriaxone intravenously for a facial abscess that is close to her right eye. Her other health problems include moderate hypertension, well controlled with lisinopril, and osteoarthritis of the left knee for which she takes meloxicam daily. She has documented allergies to peanuts, other tree nuts, and penicillin. She is married, has two children, and is a full-time third-grade teacher. She puts on her call light to report that she feels dizzy and is having shortness of breath. When the nurse reaches the bedside, the following observations are noted:

- Oxygen saturation by pulse oximetry is 86%.
- All the food on the lunch tray has been eaten.
- There is normal saline hanging and 125 mL of the 250 mL total of the ceftriaxone remains in the piggyback bag.
- She received her premeal insulin dose 45 minutes ago.
- Vital sign assessment reveals a respiratory rate of 34, heart rate of 110, and BP of 94/50.
- She can talk but is having a hard time finding words.

1. **Recognize Cues:** What assessment information in this client situation is the most important and immediate concern for the nurse? (Hint: Identify the **relevant** information *first* to determine what is most important.)
2. **Analyze Cues:** What client conditions are consistent with the **most relevant** information? (Hint: Think about priority collaborative problems that support and contradict the information presented in this situation.)
3. **Prioritize Hypotheses:** Which possibilities or explanations are **most likely** to be present in this client situation? Which possibilities or explanations are the most serious? (Hint: Consider all possibilities and determine their urgency and risk for this client.)
4. **Generate Solutions:** What actions would most likely achieve the desired outcomes for this client? Which actions should be **avoided** or are **potentially harmful**? (Hint: Determine the desired outcomes first to decide which interventions are appropriate and those that should be avoided.)
5. **Take Action:** Which actions are the most appropriate and how should they be implemented? In what **priority order** should they be implemented? (Hint: Consider health teaching, documentation, requested health care provider orders or prescriptions, nursing skills, collaboration with or referral to health team members, etc.)
6. **Evaluate Outcomes:** What client assessment would indicate that the nurse's actions were **effective**? (Hint: Think about signs that would indicate an improvement, decline, or unchanged client condition.)

TABLE 18.2 Disorders With an Autoimmune Basis

- Ankylosing spondylitis (AS)
- Autoimmune hemolytic anemia
- Autoimmune thrombocytopenic purpura
- Celiac disease (CeD)
- Crohn's disease (CD)
- Diabetes (type 1)
- Dermatomyositis
- Erythema nodosum leprosum (ENL)
- Glomerulonephritis
- Goodpasture syndrome
- Graves disease
- Hashimoto thyroiditis
- Hepatitis
- Idiopathic Addison disease
- Irritable bowel disease (IBD)
- Multiple sclerosis (MS)
- Myasthenia gravis
- Pernicious anemia
- Psoriasis (PS)
- Psoriatic arthritis (PSA)
- Rheumatoid arthritis (RA)
- Reiter syndrome
- Scleroderma
- Sjögren syndrome (SS)
- Systemic lupus erythematosus (SLE)
- Ulcerative colitis (UC)
- Uveitis
- Vasculitis

PATIENT-CENTERED CARE: GENDER HEALTH CONSIDERATIONS QSEN

All autoimmune disorders occur much more commonly among women than men (McCance et al., 2019). The risk for autoimmune disease among women compared with men ranges from 5:1 to 20:1 (Abbas et al., 2018).

Development of autoimmune disorders is complex, involving genetic susceptibility and environmental interactions. The two major problems thought to lead to development of autoimmune disorders are reduced self-tolerance combined with changes in normal body cells, tissues, or organs that result in false recognition as non-self. These changes then make normal cells and tissues targets for attack and destruction by many components of normal ***immunity***. Some of the factors considered to help make normal cells become inappropriate targets of autoimmune attacks include infection, injury, drugs, hormones, and exposure to environmental substances. However, these factors must work in concert with an immune system that is more susceptible to loss of self-tolerance.

PATIENT-CENTERED CARE: GENETIC/GENOMIC CONSIDERATIONS QSEN

Twin studies have confirmed the strong link between genetic inheritance and autoimmunity. For dizygotic twins (fraternal twins), when one twin is diagnosed with an autoimmune disease, the incidence of autoimmune disease development in the other twin is about 6%, nearly the same as in the general population. For monozygotic twins (identical twins), when one twin is diagnosed with an autoimmune disease, development of an autoimmune disorder (but not necessarily the same disorder) in the other twin is about 50% (Abbas et al., 2018; Jorde et al., 2016).

Specific inherited tissue types are much more associated with autoimmunity. Susceptible tissue types, known as *human leukocyte antigens (HLAs)*, include DR2, DR3, DRB, DQA, DQB, and Cw6. Ask any patient diagnosed with autoimmune disease whether other family members have an autoimmune disease.

During development most immune system cells learn to recognize and tolerate the body's own cell surface antigens without initiating any immunologic response. As described in Chapter 16, self-tolerance is possible because of the different proteins present on cell membranes and the actions of T-lymphocytes known as T-regulator cells or *Tregs*. Tregs secrete cytokines, especially interleukin-10 (IL-10), that have an overall *inhibitory* action on most cells of the immune system. Usually those immune system cells that do not tolerate self cells and become self-reacting are either eliminated early from the immune system or are held in check by suppressive elements. Genetically susceptible adults have reduced numbers of Tregs or nonfunctional Tregs. Then immunity is unchecked, resulting in failure to recognize certain tissues as self, and both antibody- and cell-mediated responses and products are directed against normal body cells (McCance et al., 2019). (Antibodies directed against self tissues or cells are known as autoantibodies.) Through the actions of intracellular enzymes known as Janus kinases (JAKs), regulation of immune system cells and products is reduced and the production of proinflammatory cytokines, especially interleukins 12, 17, and 23 (IL-12, IL-17, IL-23); gamma interferon; and different subtypes of tumor necrosis factor (TNF) is greatly increased. These actions are the basis for the ***inflammation*** that is characteristic of all autoimmune disorders and lead to reactions that can result in tissue damage and loss of ***tissue integrity***. In addition to damaging tissues, these cytokines also increase the growth rate for white blood cells (especially macrophages), which then continue the attack on self tissues.

Self-reactions can form against one type of cell and cause problems only for a specific tissue, organ, or system. An example of a selective autoimmune disorder is myasthenia gravis, in which the person makes antibodies against acetylcholine or the acetylcholine receptor on muscle cells, and transmission of nerve impulses to the skeletal muscles for contraction does not occur.

Self-reactions can also be directed against a specific tissue component or multiple components that are present in many organs or tissues, resulting in widespread problems or symptoms such as in systemic lupus erythematosus (SLE). Another common autoimmune disorder is rheumatoid arthritis (RA). See Chapter 46 for a full discussion of this disorder.

IMMUNITY CONCEPT EXEMPLAR: SYSTEMIC LUPUS ERYTHEMATOSUS

Systemic lupus erythematosus (SLE) is a chronic and progressive autoimmune disorder in which inflammatory and immune attacks occur against multiple self tissues and organs. Over time the progressive loss of ***tissue integrity*** through excessive ***inflammation*** and overactive ***immunity*** leads to organ failure and death. A less common form of lupus is *cutaneous lupus erythematosus (CLE)* (formerly called discoid lupus erythematosus) in which only the skin is affected by autoimmune attack. However, about 70% to 80% of patients initially diagnosed with CLE eventually develop SLE (McCance et al., 2019), suggesting that CLE may not be a distinct disorder from SLE.

Pathophysiology Review

Etiology and Genetic Risk. SLE is not a new disorder and was described as a chronic health problem even in ancient times (Norman, 2016). As with other types of autoimmune disorders, its development in adults represents a failure of self-tolerance and results from gene-environment interactions. Although the genetic connection is strong, the relationship is complex and appears to reflect a multiple gene *(polygenic)* origin for susceptibility that has not yet been clearly elucidated. Exactly how specific immune components lose self-tolerance and develop antiself responses remains unclear, but the physical consequences of these actions are well known. Triggers for expression of SLE in a genetically susceptible adult include infection, injury, drugs, hormones, and exposure to environmental substances, especially ultraviolet (UV) light.

Both innate and specific immune reactions are involved in the symptoms and tissue damage caused by SLE. Autoantibodies are largely directed against many different proteins in the nucleus of cells, particularly of cells making up connective tissue rather than glandular tissue.

Circulating autoantibodies attack tissues, causing a type III hypersensitivity reaction with formation of immune complexes that precipitate and deposit in various tissues, resulting in some degree of impaired ***tissue integrity***. These actions cause systemic ***inflammation*** and attract other immune cells and products to the sites, which then stimulate chronic tissue injury and destruction. Compounding this general problem, blood vessels are major targets, leading to chronic inflammation in the vessels *(vasculitis)*, which reduces perfusion to organs and increases the risk for injury and permanent damage. Although any and all organs and tissues may be affected, the most common causes of death are chronic kidney disease and cardiovascular impairment. Arthritis and joint pain occur in about 90% of patients with SLE. The percentage of major tissue and organ SLE involvement includes vasculitis and rash, 70% to 80%; kidney damage to the glomeruli and tubular basement membranes, 40% to 50%; hematologic problems, 50%; and cardiovascular problems, 30% to 50% (McCance et al., 2019).

Although progressive in nature and chronic, symptoms may be present at a constant level, at a reduced level *(remission)*, or as an acute episode of increased symptoms known as a "flare" or exacerbation. (The degree of presentation in which symptoms are continually present at a constant level or during a flare is known as *SLE activity*.) Variation in presentation and severity contribute to difficulty in diagnosis. As a result, SLE has been called "the great imitator" and "the disease with a thousand faces." Although SLE symptoms and laboratory changes can arise temporarily from chronic use of certain drugs (e.g., hydralazine, isoniazid, penicillamine D, procainamide), these problems resolve when the offending drug is discontinued.

Incidence and Prevalence. SLE is not a reportable disorder. Current estimates are that about 18,000 new cases are diagnosed annually in the United States and Canada (Lupus Canada, 2017; Lupus Foundation of America, 2019a). With proper management adults with SLE are living 20 years or longer. About 1.6 million adults are currently living with SLE in North America, and the worldwide prevalence is estimated at 5 million.

Interprofessional Collaborative Care

The onset of SLE is usually slow and the symptoms may be so mild, general, and vague that diagnosis often is difficult and delayed (Chaplin, 2018; Richard-Eaglin & Smallheer, 2018). The average time from initial mild symptoms to actual diagnosis is 6 years (Lupus Foundation of America, 2019a). However, progression of the disorder can be delayed when it is diagnosed and

PATIENT-CENTERED CARE: GENDER HEALTH CONSIDERATIONS QSEN

Systemic lupus erythematosus (SLE) is present in women about 10 times more frequently than in men, with great variation across different races (Yen & Singh, 2018). The incidence in African Americans compared with whites is 8:1 (although the disorder is rare in Africa), and is also higher in most populations of nonwhites (McCance et al., 2019). SLE is most commonly diagnosed in women 30 to 44 years old. The overwhelming prevalence of the disorder in women during childbearing years strongly suggests estrogen as a potential trigger for expression of the disorder. When caring for any woman who has a history of chronic fatigue, recurring fevers of unknown origin, and persistent joint and muscle pain, report these findings to the primary health care provider for consideration of SLE.

managed earlier in its course. Exacerbations *(flares)* accelerate organ damage.

Patients usually live in the community and require acute care only during periods of exacerbation, which can be so life threatening that intensive care may be required. When mobility or function compromises ADLs, the patient may require assisted living or long-term care. With most patients living 20 years or longer with SLE, they also may be hospitalized for non-SLE problems, during which time the drug treatment plan continues.

A primary health care provider is often the first medical professional to suspect SLE. After diagnosis, a rheumatology specialist is the health care provider who is most responsible for day-to-day management of the disorder. When other organ involvement is present, other specialty health care providers are included in the management team.

◆ Assessment: Recognize Cues.

History. Ask the patient to tell you about any physical difference(s) she or he has noticed about herself or himself over the past 5 years because any tissue can be affected and initial symptoms are often vague. Ask specifically whether pain without injury is present continually or intermittently because generalized pain is common and is the health problem that drives most patients to seek medical help (Lupus Foundation of America, 2019a). Also determine whether the patient or any close relatives either have SLE or have been diagnosed with another autoimmune disorder, because of the gene-environment interaction. Ask whether any specific infection or environmental exposure occurred before the onset of a new symptom or symptoms. Many patients experience unexplained intermittent fevers. Ask whether he or she has noticed any pattern of fever with increased fatigue when no other family members have been ill.

Certain drugs can cause an SLE-like reaction. Drug-induced SLE can be caused by hydralazine, isoniazid, penicillamine D, and procainamide. Determine whether these or any other drugs were taken on a long-term basis within the year before symptoms were first noticed.

Physical Assessment/Signs and Symptoms. As stated earlier, any tissue or organ can be affected, and each patient's pattern of signs and symptoms is unique, making diagnosis difficult. Presenting physical changes and laboratory analyses are used together to determine the presence of

KEY FEATURES
Systemic Lupus Erythematosus (SLE)

- Red, macular, facial rash over the cheeks and nose in the shape of a butterfly
- Coin-shaped lesions (discoid rash) on the face, scalp, and sun-exposed areas
- Sensitivity to sunlight (photosensitivity) with rash development after exposure
- Chronic lesions on the mucous membranes of the mouth and throat
- Nonerosive arthritis of two or more peripheral joints with pain and swelling
- Inflammation of serosal membranes, especially pericarditis and pleurisy
- Kidney changes with persistent casts and protein in the urine
- Neurologic problems such as seizures or psychosis without previous history
- Hematologic problems with hemolytic anemia (most common), decreased white blood cells (leukopenia), decreased lymphocytes (lymphopenia), decreased platelets (thrombocytopenia)
- Immunity problems such as autoantibodies to cell nuclear structures and false-positive results of serologic tests for syphilis
- Presence of antinuclear antibodies (ANAs)

Adapted from McCance, K., Huether, S., Brashers, V., & Rote, N. (2019). *Pathophysiology: The biologic basis for disease in adults and children* (8th ed.). St. Louis: Mosby.

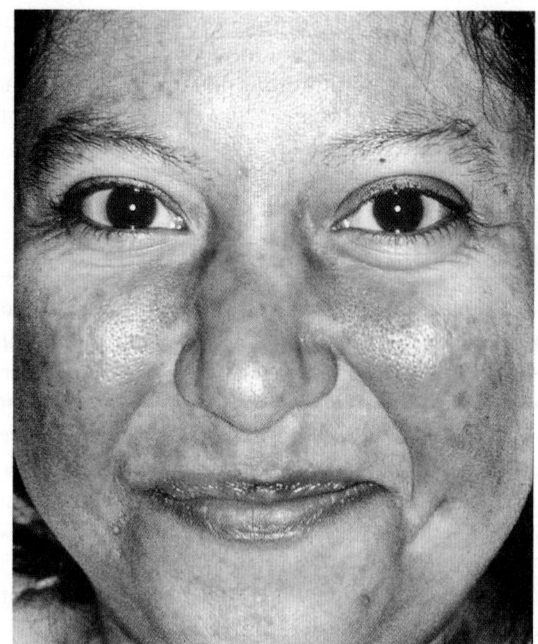

Fig. 18.5 The characteristic "butterfly" rash of systemic lupus erythematosus.

SLE. The Key Features: Systemic Lupus Erythematosus box lists the 11 most common changes associated with SLE. Few patients have all of these, and the presence of any four of them is considered diagnostic for SLE when it is supported by specific laboratory indicators. Most often, patients come to a primary health care professional's office with the three symptoms of fever, rash, and painful swollen joints (Richard-Eaglin & Smallheer, 2018).

Skin changes in SLE may be the first observable symptom and include a dry, scaly, raised rash on the face ("butterfly" rash) that may also appear on other sun-exposed areas (Fig. 18.5). Skin involvement indicates that the ***inflammation*** of SLE is systemic

(Pullen, 2018). Rashes are initially nonscarring and may increase in a lupus flare and become less apparent or disappear when the disorder is in remission. Individual round discoid (coinlike) lesions are the scarring lesions of cutaneous lupus. The lesions are especially evident when the patient is exposed to sunlight or UV light.

For some patients with SLE, the skin of the face (cheeks, nose, and chin) can darken significantly and cheek volume decreases as the fatty tissue beneath the skin is destroyed by vasculitis. This rare condition is known as *lupus profundus* and can drastically change an adult's facial appearance. Alopecia is also common in lupus. Observe and document all skin changes and monitor them daily while the patient is in an acute care setting or during an ambulatory care or home visit. Also assess for the presence of ulcers in the mouth and throat.

Intermittent fever is a common finding and caused by chronic systemic ***inflammation***. Most often, fever is associated with an exacerbation or flare.

Chronic fatigue is a physical problem reported by more than 80% of patients with SLE (Lupus Foundation of America, 2019a). The fatigue can interfere with all aspects of life and can be debilitating during periods of increased SLE activity and flare. Although the precise cause of fatigue is unknown, major factors intensifying it include persistent systemic inflammation with an increased metabolic rate generated by greatly increased activity of cells involved in the response. Fatigue is worsened when fever also is present.

Musculoskeletal changes with SLE are common and include arthritis, muscle aches *(arthralgias)*, and muscle inflammation *(myositis)* because of the systemic inflammation and the hypoxia caused by blood vessel changes *(vasculitis)*. The joints most commonly involved are in the feet, ankles, knees, wrists, and fingers. The synovial lining is inflamed, causing painful swelling. However, because the bone and cartilage are not eroded, joint deformities, like those seen in rheumatoid arthritis, are not present. Usually joint involvement occurs bilaterally. *Osteonecrosis* (bone necrosis from lack of oxygen) is often seen in patients who have been treated for at least 5 years with steroids like prednisone that can restrict blood flow to the joint.

Some patients with SLE have generalized muscle pain similar to fibromyalgia with symptoms of pain and sensitivity at 18 "tender points." These points occur bilaterally, especially in the neck, shoulders, chest, hips, knees, and elbows.

Assess for painful, red, and swollen joints. Determine the patient's range of motion with involved joints and to what extent the arthritis interferes with ADLs.

Kidney changes occur as a result of the autoantibody attack on the connective tissues of glomerular capillaries and the basement membranes of the kidney tubules with loss of ***tissue integrity*** in these structures. As the glomerular capillaries are damaged, proteins filter through the glomerulus and remain in the urine. Persistent proteinuria is an indicator of reduced kidney function regardless of the cause and in SLE is known as *lupus nephritis*. Examine urine for cloudiness, the presence of obvious blood in the urine, and whether the urine appears foamy (caused by protein in the urine). Changes in nonglomerular kidney blood vessels lead to hypoxic injury, all of which can cause chronic kidney disease, which is a common cause of death for adults with SLE.

Cardiac changes with SLE occur as a result of immune complexes being deposited in any layer of the heart and its functional structures, such as valves and cords. Chronic ***inflammation*** in cardiac tissues develops with these deposits, leading to pericarditis and valve thickening. Any cardiac change can affect gas exchange and perfusion. Assess heart rate and pulse quality. Also assess blood pressure. Auscultate for abnormal heart sounds, especially murmurs. Assess for jugular-venous distention, peripheral edema, capillary refill, and oxygen saturation with pulse oximetry.

Psychosocial Assessment. The psychosocial responses to SLE as a chronic, progressive disorder that can have disfiguring changes and the potential for significant organ damage can be extensive. Chronic fatigue and generalized weakness may prevent the patient from being as active as in the past. He or she may avoid social gatherings and may withdraw from family activities. The unpredictability and chronicity of SLE can cause fear and anxiety. Fear may increase if the patient knows another person with the disease, particularly if the other person has more advanced and severe changes.

Unfortunately the myth that lupus is fatal is still common. Inform the patient and family that control of SLE is generally possible with regular medical monitoring, drugs, and healthy practices such as limiting sun exposure to prevent exacerbation of the disease.

Assess the patient's and family's feelings about the disorder to identify areas requiring intervention. Determine their usual coping mechanisms and support systems before developing a plan of care.

Laboratory Assessment. Classic laboratory assessment for diagnosis of SLE is based on the presence of circulating autoantibodies to components of cellular nuclei, as well as general indicators of ***inflammation***, such as the erythrocyte sedimentation rate and serum complement levels for C3 and C4. Autoantibody tests include antinuclear antibodies (ANAs); antibodies to double-stranded DNA (anti-dsDNA), single-stranded DNA (anti-ssDNA), Smith antibodies (anti-SM), and extractable nuclear proteins (anti-ENA); and antibodies to nuclear membrane phospholipids. Nearly all (97%) patients with SLE have ANAs, making the test very sensitive but not specific because the test result often is positive in patients with other autoimmune disorders (Cadet, 2018). Thus the lack of circulating ANAs can exclude an SLE diagnosis but does not confirm it. No single laboratory test is used to definitively diagnose the disorder.

A newer technique available in some areas is the use of microarray technology to generate an immune profile of autoantibodies, which allows each patient suspected of having SLE to have all serum autoantibodies evaluated in one test. Currently the assay is used to definitively rule out the disorder (Cohen, 2016). However, because this method also establishes the strength of autoantibody responses, it not only has the potential to indicate the presence of a specific autoantibody, but may link individual responsiveness to the assay with the degree of target organ involvement. Although not yet a standard laboratory test for SLE, it is hoped microarray technology will make diagnosis less complex and more timely, and will indicate which organs may be at higher risk for ongoing injury in any individual patient.

Other Diagnostic Assessments. During periods of greater SLE activity, the disorder causes progressive injury in many tissues and organs as a result of primary attack by autoantibodies on specific tissues within an organ or secondary to poor perfusion caused by widespread vasculitis within any organ. As a result, blood and urine tests for assessing bone marrow, cardiac, kidney, and liver function are usually performed at initial diagnosis to determine whether and which additional organs may be affected by the disorder. When blood or urine tests indicate reduced or unusual function of any major organ, more in-depth laboratory and imaging studies are performed. (See the body system assessment chapters for diagnostic assessment techniques to determine specific organ involvement.)

◆ Analysis: Analyze Cues and Prioritize Hypotheses.

The priority collaborative problems for patients with systemic lupus erythematosus (SLE) are:

1. Persistent pain due to chronic ***inflammation*** and hypoxia from vasculitis-related reduced perfusion in many tissues and organs
2. Fatigue due to chronic ***inflammation*** and hypoxia from vasculitis-related reduced perfusion in many tissues and organs, especially during flares
3. Potential for loss of ***tissue integrity*** and organ failure with progression of the disorder and increased ***inflammation*** and/or vasculitis
4. Potential for decreased self-esteem due to changes in body image from disorder progression or drug therapy

◆ Planning and Implementation: Generate Solutions and Take Action.

Managing Persistent Pain

Expected Outcomes. With intervention the patient with SLE is expected to have pain reduced to a level acceptable to him or her between and during periods of increased SLE activity.

Interventions. Pain management involves the use of drug therapy to control the disorder, as described in the section Preventing Organ Failure and Reducing SLE Activity Periods. In addition to drug therapy for disorder management, drug therapy with acetaminophen and NSAIDs can help moderate daily joint and muscle pain. (Acetaminophen can alter pain perception but does not reduce the ***inflammation*** associated with or causing the pain.) Patients vary in their responses to different NSAIDs, and a trial period may be needed to determine which one is best. During periods of increased SLE activity and more intense pain, corticosteroids are used. If corticosteroids are already part of the patient's SLE drug management routine, the dosage is increased and then tapered to her or his usual dosage when the flare is over. Remind the patient taking an increased dose of prescribed corticosteroids to follow the tapering schedule exactly and not suddenly return to her or his base dose, to prevent adrenal crisis.

Many patients find moist heat helps relieve muscle and joint pain. Warm baths and showers or the use of spa tubs can be especially helpful. The temporary use of ice and cold applications is recommended only when muscles and joints have been strained or sprained (Lupus Foundation of America, 2019a).

Currently SLE is not a disorder approved for pain therapy with medical marijuana, although studies with patients who have other autoimmune disorders have reported positive results with the experimental synthetic cannabinoid JBT-101 (lenabasum). This drug does not produce the "high" associated with other marijuana products and is currently in clinical trials for its effectiveness in reducing pain in adults with SLE.

Managing Fatigue

Expected Outcomes. The patient with SLE is expected to understand the nature of chronic fatigue and take steps to avoid worsening the duration or intensity of the problem.

Interventions. Fatigue associated with SLE is chronic and often occurs at the point in life (ages 20 to 50 years) when adults are expected to be most active and productive in their career and family roles. Management focuses on helping patients recognize that their health must come first and learning to make lifestyle choices to improve endurance and prevent excessive fatigue.

Ask the patient to list all work-, family-, and leisure-related activities that she or he is required to perform or has always performed. Work with her or him to determine which are "must" activities versus are less essential based on the patient's desires and expectations. For example, is making a home-cooked meal for the family more important to the patient than routine household cleaning? If this is the case, perhaps housekeeping chores could be delegated to a family member or, if finances permit, outside services. Help the patient plan for completion of daily must or essential activities first. Then, depending on energy level, some less essential activities can be performed that day or delayed for another time.

Determine the nature of the patient's work activity. Is it indoors or out? Is heavy labor involved? What adjustments can be made to perform well and not incur excessive fatigue? In some cases the patient may plan for potential future changes in activity tolerance by taking courses or learning a different trade to reduce excess physical demands. For example, a nurse who has always worked in areas requiring much standing, lifting, running, and other physical demands might change positions to less physical areas such as preadmission testing or nurse navigator or, with an advanced degree, might become an instructor or advanced practice nurse.

Some adults with SLE believe that any physical exercise should be avoided. In fact, aerobic exercise is known to be effective in improving endurance in lupus fatigue. Although high-impact exercises should be performed only on the advice of the rheumatology specialist, daily performance of lower-impact activities and strength-building exercises are helpful. For adults whose fitness level is low, walking and stretching exercises are appropriate for initial activity. Duration and intensity can gradually be increased.

No matter at what level the patients starts his or her exercise routine, these activities should be followed by a short period of rest. Some patients benefit from dividing the exercises into two shorter sessions (15 to 30 minutes) daily. Other energy-saving, fatigue-managing tips recommended by the Lupus Foundation of America are listed in the Patient and Family Education: Preparing for Self-Management: Systemic Lupus Erythematosus (SLE) box.

PATIENT AND FAMILY EDUCATION: PREPARING FOR SELF-MANAGEMENT

Systemic Lupus Erythematosus (SLE)

- Accept fatigue as a continuing but manageable condition of SLE.
- Avoid self-blame for the need to alter activity. It is not your fault that you have lupus.
- Keep in mind that your health comes first.
- Establish good sleep patterns and a healthy diet for more energy.
- Make rest time a priority, and make sure your family knows why. If you rest now, you can participate later. However, be aware that sleeping during the day may make sleeping at night more difficult.
- If you smoke, stop and avoid nicotine in any form. Nicotine use reduces your available energy by restricting blood flow to your heart and lungs.
- Plan ahead and prioritize your activities, keeping in mind that you do not have to be a "super" person involved in everything. It is okay to say "no."
- Group your errands when driving, starting with those farther from home and heading toward home.
- When possible, shop online and have items delivered directly to you, especially heavy items such as groceries.
- Prepare meals in advance on less busy days; engage other family members in prepping items to cook.
- When possible, prepare items while sitting (e.g., cutting vegetables).
- Carefully select which activities and events you can attend or participate in and which ones you must regretfully decline. For example, you might not want to volunteer to take and chaperone first graders on a trip to the zoo but may be able to organize volunteers or type meeting minutes.
- Work on asking for what you need. Asking for help will become easier with time and practice. (You may be able to help those who help you by performing tasks for them that are less physically challenging).
- Accept help offered by others. This practice often results in stronger bonds between you and those who care about you.
- Make adjustments in your life that will help you live better, such as joining a support group or carving out some "me" time (perhaps for a relaxing massage).

Adapted from Lupus Foundation of America. (2019c). *Strategies for managing fatigue.* https://www.lupus.org/resources/strategies-for-managing-fatigue

Preventing Organ Failure and Reducing SLE Activity Periods

Expected Outcomes. The patient being managed for SLE is expected to have positive treatment outcomes and avoid or delay organ dysfunction.

Interventions. Drug therapy and lifestyle changes are the mainstays of treatment for inducing and prolonging remissions and preventing or delaying major organ damage.

Drug Therapy. Drug therapy for SLE often involves a combination of general immunosuppressant agents and selective immunosuppressive agents. Patient responses to therapy drive the types and combinations of drugs used.

Corticosteroids such as prednisone remain a common cornerstone of therapy for SLE. This systemic drug is a general anti-inflammatory immunosuppressant that enters and affects every type of body cell and produces many side effects. Common side effects that appear within a week of corticosteroid therapy include acne, sodium and fluid retention, hypertension, sensation of "nervousness," difficulty sleeping, and emotional changes such as crying easily. Side effects with long-term therapy include weight gain, fat redistribution (moon face; buffalo hump between the shoulders), increased risk for GI ulcers and bleeding, fragile skin that bruises easily, reduced muscle mass and strength, thinning scalp hair, increased facial and body hair, increased susceptibility to colds and other infections, and stretch marks.

! NURSING SAFETY PRIORITY QSEN

Drug Alert

The most important precaution to teach patients taking long-term corticosteroids is to never stop taking the drug abruptly because adrenal crisis can result and may be life threatening. If the patient becomes ill and cannot tolerate the prescribed oral corticosteroid, instruct her or him to immediately contact the rheumatology health care provider to receive the drug parenterally.

Antimalarial drugs, such as hydroxychloroquine and chloroquine, were once a standard drug therapy for SLE. Use of these drugs has recently increased especially for those whose symptoms have not responded to other therapies. In particular, hydroxychloroquine has both immunomodulating and anticlotting effects (which may be needed in patients with vasculitis to prevent thrombotic events). This drug decreases the absorption of ultraviolet (UV) light by the melanin-containing skin cells and therefore decreases the risk for skin lesions. A major complication of this drug is its toxicity to retinal cells, causing retinitis that can lead to an irreversible loss of central vision. *Teach patients prescribed hydroxychloroquine to have frequent eye examinations with visual field testing (before starting the drug and every 6 months thereafter).*

Immune modulators, also known as disease-modifying antirheumatic drugs (DMARDs) and cytotoxic agents, are used to control inflammation and suppress the overactive immune system when either corticosteroids are not effective or the patient cannot tolerate the dose needed (Lupus Foundation of America, 2019b). They work by destroying some immune system cells and preventing their reproduction. The three most commonly used drugs in this category are cyclophosphamide, methotrexate, and azathioprine. These drugs may be used individually on a continuing basis or only during flares.

Monoclonal antibodies have been used successfully to help control many other autoimmune disorders. These drugs, usually given intravenously or subcutaneously, block specific proinflammatory cytokines that stimulate immune attacks on self tissues. One drug, belimumab, is specific for management of SLE. It binds to stimulatory receptors on B-lymphocytes, reducing their ability to reproduce and secrete autoantibodies. It is used parenterally in combination with standard therapies, especially during flares, to reduce the duration of flares and prevent tissue damage. Infusion-related reactions, including severe hypersensitivity reactions, are possible, and the drug must be given by a health care professional in a setting prepared to manage anaphylaxis. Patient monitoring during infusion and for up to 2 hours after infusion is required.

Janus kinase inhibitors have been used to manage rheumatoid arthritis. Drugs in this class block the Janus kinase enzyme pathway, which stimulates the production of many proinflammatory cytokines. Although none of these drugs are approved at this time for management of SLE, one oral drug, baricitinib, has

NCLEX EXAMINATION CHALLENGE 18.2

Physiological Integrity

Which new-onset condition or symptom in a client who has systemic lupus erythematosus (SLE) now taking hydroxychloroquine does the nurse deem to have the **highest** priority for immediate reporting to **prevent harm**?

A. Increased bruising
B. Increased daily output of slightly foamy urine
C. Failure to see letters in the middle of a word
D. Sensation of nausea within an hour of taking the drug

! NURSING SAFETY PRIORITY QSEN

Drug Alert

All immunosuppressants reduce protective *immunity* to some degree and increase the patient's risk for new infections and reactivation of dormant infections such as tuberculosis (TB). Lower doses of general immunosuppressants do not require TB testing before drug therapy initiation but should not be started in any patient with a current infection. Tuberculosis testing is usually performed before starting any selective immunosuppressant. Teach patients taking these drugs to practice social distancing. Also teach them to contact their rheumatology specialist at the first sign of an infection.

been fast-tracked for phase III clinical trials for patients with high-activity SLE.

Lifestyle Changes. Some lifestyle changes are needed to manage SLE and prevent more frequent flares. Changes that focus on managing fatigue were described earlier. An extremely important intervention for patients with SLE is to avoid exposure to UV light, especially sunlight. UV light exacerbates all aspects of the disorder, not just the skin symptoms.

! NURSING SAFETY PRIORITY QSEN

Action Alert

Instruct patients to avoid prolonged exposure to sunlight and other forms of ultraviolet lighting, including certain types of fluorescent light. Remind them to wear long sleeves and a large-brimmed hat when outdoors. Patients should use sun-blocking agents with a sun protection factor (SPF) of 30 or higher on exposed skin surfaces.

Instruct patients to avoid sun exposures during times of most direct sunlight. In addition to wearing exposure protective clothing, discuss engaging in outdoor activities, such as gardening or golfing, in the early morning or later evening when sunlight is less direct. When possible at outdoor events such as sports or picnics, stay in the shade or use an umbrella.

Enhancing Self-Esteem

Expected Outcomes. The expected outcome is that the patient will be able to express a positive perception of herself or himself as a result of interprofessional interventions.

Interventions. Self-esteem changes resulting from a diagnosis of SLE may be complicated by many factors, including the patient's perception of self before the disorder was diagnosed, as well as by the types and degree of support that surround her or him. Nursing interventions for supporting positive coping mechanisms and listening to patient concerns are important. However, depending on the patient's self-perception, collaboration with mental health professionals may also be needed by the patient and family.

Many patients are frustrated that family members, friends, and co-workers may not understand the remission and flare nature of the disorder. She or he may be able to participate in activities at a near prediagnosis level during remissions or whenever the disorder is less active, and may be close to incapacitated during severe flares. Educate the patient and family about this issue and help them consider providing accurate information to their co-workers (when confidentiality is not an issue) to explain how and when participation levels must change or be modified. Managing fatigue has been shown to decrease depression in patients with SLE and improve self-esteem (see the Patient and Family Education: Preparing for Self-Management: Systemic Lupus Erythematosus [SLE] box in the section Managing Fatigue). Encouraging the patient to be an active partner in management of the disorder can help improve self-esteem by helping the patient feel she or he has some control over the situation.

Self-esteem also may be negatively affected by changes in work ability and role within the family. The obvious skin-associated changes can be devastating, especially because facial skin is often involved. Women who never had a blemish are confronted with a rash that may not be completely covered with makeup. If chronic steroid therapy is used, side effects such as acne, striae, fat pads, and weight gain intensify the problem of an already altered body image.

Care for the skin can help improve appearance and self-esteem. Teach patients to clean the skin with mild soap (e.g., Ivory, Dove) and to avoid harsh, perfumed substances that may irritate the skin further. The skin should be rinsed and dried well and lotion applied. Excess powder and other drying substances should be avoided. Cosmetics must be selected carefully and should include moisturizers and sun protectors. If desired, refer the patient to a medical cosmetologist who specializes in applying makeup for skin lesions of all types. Some patients have achieved good results in covering lesions with theatrical-grade cosmetics. Newer skin rejuvenating techniques, such as laser resurfacing and injection of "plumping" agents, are available, but no studies have determined whether these relatively costly procedures improve appearance to an acceptable degree or whether positive results are long-lasting.

Care Coordination and Transition Management

Home Care Management. Most patients with SLE are managed for years in the ambulatory care setting and self-manage at home. When a severe exacerbation develops, the patient often returns home after hospitalization. During flares with increased joint pain and swelling, accommodations for one-floor living in the home may be needed temporarily. For those with advanced disease, 24-hour care may be needed for ADLs and for monitoring. If home care is not possible, placement in a long-term care setting may be needed.

Self-Management Education. Patients with SLE and their families need to know as much about the disease as possible so they can better manage it and themselves. They should be able to discuss drug therapy, correct timing of drug doses, indications of adverse drug reactions, signs of infection, and when to seek medical help.

Instruct them to identify and avoid stressors that can worsen the disease. Reinforce the strategies that promote reduced pain and longer periods of reduced SLE activity, such as regular exercise, not smoking or using nicotine in any form, pacing themselves, and using all the other strategies listed in the Patient and Family Education: Preparing for Self-Management: Systemic Lupus Erythematosus (SLE) box in the Managing Fatigue section.

Stress the importance of protecting themselves from sun exposure. Remind patients that this exposure can trigger systemic flares, not just increased skin symptoms. Also reinforce that their health needs to come first to enable them to maintain their involvement in desired activities for as long as possible. Because the two most common causes of death among adults with SLE result from chronic kidney disease and cardiovascular damage, urge them to continue to be monitored with tests for kidney and cardiovascular function at least annually to identify changes early when management is most effective at preventing complications.

Health Care Resources. The Lupus Foundation of America (www.lupus.org) and Lupus Canada (www.lupuscanada.org) are comprehensive resources specific for patients with lupus. These national organizations have chapters nationwide to provide information and assistance for patients with lupus and their families. Some of the resources offered include blogs, videos with experts explaining different aspects of SLE management, and directories of local support groups and services.

◆ **Evaluation: Evaluate Outcomes.** Evaluate the care of the patient with SLE based on the identified priority patient problems. The expected outcomes of care are that the patient will:

- Understand the basis of the disorder and its management
- Accept the lifestyle changes needed to protect herself or himself to prevent complications
- Be an active partner in the prescribed long-term SLE management plan
- Have pain levels reduced to the extent that she or he can participate in job-related, family, and social activities to a degree acceptable to her or him
- Have reduced number and severity of flares and longer periods of remission with low SLE activity
- Remain free from infection
- Express a positive perception of herself or himself

LYME DISEASE

Pathophysiology Review

Lyme disease is a reportable systemic infectious disease caused by the spirochete *Borrelia burgdorferi*. The organism is common in rodents and is spread to humans through the bite of an infected deer tick *(Ixodes),* also known as the "black-legged tick." It is the most common vector-borne disease in North America and Europe. Most cases of the disease in North America are seen in New England; the mid-Atlantic states, including Maryland and Virginia; the upper Midwest, including Wisconsin and Minnesota; northern California; southern Ontario, southern Quebec; and New Brunswick, especially during the summer months. Although about 40,000 cases of Lyme disease are reported in North America annually, it is a vastly underreported problem with estimates of incidence between 200,000 and 300,000 (Saccomano & Hrelic, 2018).

The disease is not a true autoimmune disorder because the antibodies generated in response to the infection are directed against the organism, not to self tissues. However, the continuing attack on the organism causes chronic ***inflammation*** with release of cytokines that intensify the tissue injury initiated by the spirochete. Thus the disease is presented in this chapter because of the tissue results of the chronic nature of the continuing ***immunity*** that attempts to eliminate the invading organism.

B. burgdorferi has some unique features that allow it to escape immune capture and destruction in some adults. Just like every other organism, the spirochete has unique proteins on its cell surface that can be recognized as non-self by immune system cells and products in order for general secretion of proinflammatory cytokines, especially tumor necrosis factor, and adaptive ***immunity*** actions to eliminate it or destroy it. After infection with this organism the immune system responds in the usual way and generates antibodies specifically against *B. burgdorferi's* surface proteins. However, this spirochete can switch out parts of its unique surface proteins with a process known as "antigenic variation" (Verhey et al., 2018). This switching changes the ability of sensitized immune system cells and antibodies to recognize the existing infecting organism, allowing it to "hide." Eventually the immune system catches up with the new parts of the surface proteins, treats them like a new infection, and develops new antibodies and inflammatory responses to them. Then the infecting spirochetes switch again, keeping all general and specific immunity actions in continual but ineffective attack mode. The switching continues through all stages of the disease process, allowing the organism to penetrate and continually reproduce in many cells, including the skin, lymphoid tissues, meninges, neurons, pericardium, myocardium, and joint tissues. As the immune system continues to recognize "switched" spirochetes as newly infecting organisms, inflammatory responses in affected tissues continue and enhance the damage inflicted by the organism.

❖ Interprofessional Collaborative Care

In the early and localized stage I, the patient appears with flu-like symptoms, erythema migrans (round or oval, flat or slightly raised rash often in a bull's eye pattern), and pain and stiffness in the muscles and joints. Symptoms begin within 3 to 30 days of the tick bite, but most present in 7 to 14 days. Antibiotic therapy such as doxycycline or amoxicillin is prescribed during this uncomplicated stage for 14 to 21 days. Erythromycin can be used for patients who are allergic to penicillin. With treatment, the disease process can be halted at this stage. Even without treatment these symptoms may disappear in about 4 to 5 weeks, but the organism disseminates beyond the initial bite area.

If not treated or if treatment is not successful, the patient may progress to the more serious complications of Lyme disease. Stage II (early disseminated stage) occurs 2 to 12 weeks after the tick bite. The patient may develop carditis with dysrhythmias, dyspnea, dizziness, or palpitations and central nervous system disorders such as meningitis, facial paralysis (often misdiagnosed as Bell palsy), and peripheral neuritis. For severe disease, IV antibiotics (e.g., ceftriaxone or cefotaxime) are given for at least 30 days.

If Lyme disease is not diagnosed and treated in the two earlier stages, later chronic complications (e.g., arthritis, chronic fatigue, memory and thinking problems) can result. This late stage III (chronic persistent stage) occurs months to years after the tick bite (Patton & Phillips, 2018). For some patients the first and only sign of Lyme disease is arthritis. In some cases the disease may not respond to antibiotics in any stage, and the patient develops permanent damage to joints and the nervous system. Prevention is the best strategy for Lyme disease. Teach patients to follow the measures outlined in the Patient and Family Education: Preparing for Self-Management box to prevent Lyme and other tick-borne diseases. Tell them about community resources, such as the Lyme Disease Foundation (www.lyme.org) and the Centers for Disease Control and Prevention website (www.cdc.gov/lyme/index.html), for more information.

PATIENT AND FAMILY EDUCATION: PREPARING FOR SELF-MANAGEMENT

Prevention and Early Detection of Lyme Disease

- Avoid heavily wooded areas or areas with thick underbrush, especially in the spring and summer months.
- Walk in the center of the trail.
- Avoid dark clothing. Lighter-colored clothing makes spotting ticks easier.
- Use an insect repellent (DEET) on your skin and clothes when in an area where ticks are likely to be found.
- Wear long-sleeved tops and long pants; tuck your shirt into your pants and your pants into your socks or boots.
- Wear closed shoes or boots and a hat or cap.
- Bathe immediately after being in an infested area and inspect your body for ticks (about the size of a pinhead); pay special attention to your arms, legs, and scalp.
- Check your pets for ticks.
- Gently remove with tweezers or fingers covered with tissue or gloves any tick that you find (do not squeeze). Dispose of the tick by flushing it down the toilet (burning a tick could spread infection).
- After removal, clean the tick area with an antiseptic such as rubbing alcohol.
- Wait 4 to 6 weeks after being bitten by a tick before being tested for Lyme disease (testing before this time is not reliable).
- Report symptoms such as a rash or influenza-like illness to your primary health care provider immediately.

GET READY FOR THE NEXT-GENERATION NCLEX® EXAMINATION!

Key Points

Review these Key Points for each NCLEX Examination Client Needs Category

Safe and Effective Care Environment

- Verify that all allergies are documented in a prominent place in the patient's medical record or electronic health record. **QSEN: Safety**
- Keep emergency equipment and drugs (epinephrine, diphenhydramine, cortisol) in or near the room of a patient with known severe allergies or a history of anaphylaxis. **QSEN: Safety**
- Teach patients to remove common allergens from the home or avoid direct contact with them. **QSEN: Safety**
- Ensure that patients with systemic lupus erythematosus (SLE) who are hospitalized for any reason continue with prescribed drug therapy for the disorder to prevent increased SLE activity. **QSEN: Safety**

Health Promotion and Maintenance

- Urge all patients with severe allergies or those who have a history of anaphylaxis to wear a medical alert bracelet. **QSEN: Patient-Centered Care**
- Teach the patient and family about the symptoms of allergic reactions and when to seek medical help. **QSEN: Patient-Centered Care**
- Teach the patient who carries an automatic epinephrine injector how to care for, assemble, and use the device. Obtain a return demonstration. **QSEN: Patient-Centered Care**
- Provide information to patients and families experiencing SLE for community resources such as the Lupus Foundation of America and Lupus Canada. **QSEN: Patient-Centered Care**
- Teach patients with SLE to protect themselves from direct sunlight to prevent more rapid progression of the disorder. **QSEN: Evidence-Based Practice**
- Because the two most common causes of death in patients with SLE are chronic kidney disease and cardiac complications, urge them to participate with annual monitoring of these systems to identify changes early when management is more effective. **QSEN: Evidence-Based Practice**
- Teach patients with SLE to use the strategies listed in the Patient and Family Education: Preparing for Self-Management of SLE guide to reduce the severity and negative effects of chronic fatigue. **QSEN: Patient-Centered Care**
- Teach patients taking immunosuppressive drugs for management of autoimmune disorders to protect themselves from infection by avoiding crowds and people who are ill, as well as keeping up-to-date with recommended vaccinations. **QSEN: Evidence-Based Practice**
- Educate adults about how to avoid tick bites in Lyme disease–associated geographic areas. **QSEN: Evidence-Based Practice**

Psychosocial Integrity

- Stay with the patient in anaphylaxis. **QSEN: Patient-Centered Care**
- Reassure patients who are in anaphylaxis that the appropriate interventions are being instituted. **QSEN: Patient-Centered Care**

- Help patients with SLE understand that the disorder does not result from anything they did and could not have been prevented. **QSEN: Patient-Centered Care**
- Recognize that patients with SLE are often frustrated that family members, friends, and co-workers may not understand the activity changes and physical symptoms that vary with the remission and flare nature of the disorder. **QSEN: Patient-Centered Care**
- Allow patients with SLE who have changes in facial appearance and physical abilities time to mourn these changes. **QSEN: Patient-Centered Care**

Physiological Integrity

- Identify patients at risk for hypersensitivity reactions, especially anaphylaxis. **QSEN: Safety**
- $ Communicate a patient's allergies, especially drug allergies, to all members of the interprofessional health care team. **QSEN: Safety**
- Immediately assess the respiratory status and airway of patients who show any symptoms of an allergic reaction. **QSEN: Evidence-Based Practice**
- Immediately discontinue the IV drug or solution of a patient having an anaphylactic reaction to that drug or solution. **Do not** discontinue the IV, but change the IV tubing and hang normal saline. **QSEN: Evidence-Based Practice**
- Hold the dose of any prescribed drug when a patient develops angioedema or has indications of anaphylaxis. **QSEN: Safety**
- Recall that the symptoms for SLE can be varied and vague, contributing to delay in diagnosis and treatment. **QSEN: Physiological Integrity**
- Suggest moist heat to reduce the joint and muscle pain associated with SLE. **QSEN: Evidence-Based Practice**

MASTERY QUESTIONS

1. Which statement(s) regarding type I hypersensitivity reactions is/are true? **Select all that apply.**
   A. Antihistamines are of minimal benefit because the reactions are mediated by IgE rather than histamine.
   B. The response is characterized by the five cardinal symptoms of inflammation.
   C. Type I responses are usually directed against non-self but the response is excessive.
   D. Susceptibility for developing a type I hypersensitivity response follows an X-linked recessive pattern of inheritance.
   E. This type of hypersensitivity reaction is most strongly associated with systemic lupus erythematosus.
   F. Responses always occur within minutes of exposure to the allergen.
   G. The second phase of the reaction with accumulation of excess bradykinin is responsible for development of angioedema.
2. Which action will the nurse perform **first** for a client in anaphylaxis to **prevent harm**?
   A. Applying oxygen by nonrebreather mask
   B. Administering IV diphenhydramine
   C. Injecting epinephrine
   D. Initiating IV access
3. Which specific information will the nurse teach to the client with systemic lupus erythematosus newly prescribed belimumab therapy?
   A. Avoid injecting it in a site near a cutaneous lesion.
   B. The drug can only be given by a health care professional.
   C. Do not chew, crush, or split the tablet containing this drug.
   D. The drug must be taken at bedtime because it causes extreme drowsiness.

REFERENCES

Abbas, A., Lichtman, A., & Pillai, S. (2018). *Cellular and molecular immunology* (9th ed.). Philadelphia: Elsevier.

Banerji, A., Blumenthal, K., Lai, K., & Zhou, L. (2017). Epidemiology of ACE inhibitor angioedema using a large electronic health record. *Journal of Allergy and Clinical Immunology in Practice*, *5*(3), 744–749.

Cadet, M. (2018). Identification and management of lupus nephritis: An overview. *Journal for Nurse Practitioners*, *14*(1), 1–6.

Chaplin, S. (2018). Management of systemic lupus erythematosus in adults. *Prescriber*, *29*(9), 31–34.

Cohen, I. (2016). Antigen-microarray profiling of antibodies in SLE: A personal view of translation from basic science to the clinic. *Lupus Open Access*, *1*(118), 1–6.

Hayden, M. L. (2019). Review of controversial areas in anaphylaxis for the nurse practitioner. *The Journal for Nurse Practitioners*, *14*(7), 531–537.

Hirschy, R., Shah, T., Davis, T., & Rech, M. (2018). Treatment of life-threatening ACE-Inhibitor-Induced angioedema. *Advanced Emergency Nursing Journal*, *40*(4), 267–277.

Jorde, L., Carey, J., & Bamshad, M. (2016). *Medical genetics* (5th ed.). St. Louis: Elsevier.

Lupus Canada. (2017). *Lupus Canada: Questions and answers.* https://www.lupuscanada.org/lupus-questions/.

Lupus Foundation of America. (2019a). *Lupus facts and statistics.* https://www.lupus.org/resources/lupus-facts-and-statistics.

Lupus Foundation of America. (2019b). *Medications used to treat lupus.* https://www.lupus.org/resources/medications-used-to-treat-lupus.

Lupus Foundation of America. (2019c). *Strategies for managing fatigue.* https://www.lupus.org/resources/strategies-for-managing-fatigue.

McCance, K., Huether, S., Brashers, V., & Rote, N. (2019). *Pathophysiology: The biologic basis for disease in adults and children* (8th ed.). St. Louis: Mosby.

Norman, R. (2016). The history of lupus erythematosus and discoid lupus: From Hippocrates to the present. *Lupus: Open Access*, *1*(1), 1–10.

Nguyen, T. (2018). Angioedema related to angiotensin-converting enzyme inhibitors and angiotensin receptor blockers. *Journal for Nurse Practitioners*, *14*(9), 690–691.

Palmer, C. (2018). FDA approves first EpiPen and EpiPen Jr. generic. *Chest Physician*, *13*(9), 8.

Patton, S., & Phillips, B. (2018). Lyme disease: Diagnosis, treatment, and prevention. *American Journal of Nursing*, *118*(4), 38–45.

Pullen, R. (2018). Cutaneous manifestations in lupus: A clinical case study. *MEDSURG Nursing*, *27*(2), 92–102.

Richard-Eaglin, A., & Smallheer, B. (2018). Immunosuppressive/autoimmune disorders. *Nursing Clinics of North America*, *53*(3), 319–334.

Riha, H., Summers, B., Rivera, J., & Van Berkel, M. (2017). Novel drug therapies for angiotenin-converting enzyme inhibitor-induced angioedema: A systematic review of current evidence. *Journal of Emergency Medicine*, *53*(5), 662–679.

Saccomano, S., & Hrelic, D. (2018). Recognizing and treating Lyme disease. *The Nurse Practitioner*, *43*(8), 13–21.

Verhey, T., Castellanos, M., & Chaconas, G. (2018). Antigenic variation in the Lyme spirochete: Insights into recombinational switching with a suggested role for error-prone repair. *Cell Reports*, *23*, 2595–2605.

Yen, E., & Singh, R. (2018). Lupus-An unrecognized cause of death in young females: A population-based study using nationwide death certificates, 2005-2015. *Arthritis & Rheumatology*, *70*(8), 1251–1255.

Concepts of Cancer Development

M. Linda Workman

http://evolve.elsevier.com/Iggy/

LEARNING OUTCOMES

1. Help adults identify behaviors that reduce the risk for cancer development.
2. Teach adults the recommended screening practices and schedules for specific cancer types.
3. Apply knowledge of basic biology to understand the factors that allow or cause normal cells to lose ***cellular regulation,*** overgrow and become malignant, including the roles of oncogenes and suppressor genes.
4. Distinguish the features of normal cells from those of benign tumors and cancer cells.
5. Interpret laboratory results for cancer grading, ploidy, and staging reports.

KEY TERMS

aneuploidy A condition in which cells have abnormal structures or numbers.

benign tumor cells A type of abnormal cell growth in which normal cells grow in the wrong place or at the wrong time as a result of a problem with ***cellular regulation***.

cancer (malignancy) A type of abnormal cell growth in which ***cellular regulation*** is lost, resulting in new tissues that serve no useful function, are harmful to the function of normal cells and organs, and can lead to death if left untreated.

carcinogenesis (oncogenesis, malignant transformation) Cancer development with changing of a normal cell into a cancer cell.

carcinogens Substances that change the activity of a cell's genes so the cell becomes a cancer cell.

cellular regulation Genetic and physiologic processes that control cellular growth, replication, differentiation, and function to maintain homeostasis.

malignancy See ***cancer***.

malignant transformation See ***carcinogenesis***.

metastasis The ability of cancer cells to invade and spread into other tissues and organs.

metastatic tumors (secondary tumors) Cancerous tumor cells that move from the primary location by breaking off from the original group and establishing remote colonies.

mitosis Cell division.

neoplasia Any new or continued cell growth not needed for normal development or replacement of dead and damaged tissues.

oncogenes Proto-oncogenes promoting cell growth that no longer respond to signals from suppressor genes for ***cellular regulation***.

oncogenesis See ***carcinogenesis***.

oncoviruses Viruses that are known to cause cancer.

primary cancer prevention The use of strategies to prevent the actual occurrence of cancer.

primary tumor The original cancer cells and tumor resulting from carcinogenesis.

secondary cancer prevention The use of screening strategies to detect cancer early, at a time when cure or control is more likely.

secondary tumors See ***metastatic tumors.***

PRIORITY AND INTERRELATED CONCEPTS

The priority concept for this chapter is:
- ***Cellular Regulation***

The interrelated concept for this chapter is:
- ***Immunity***

Cancer, also called **malignancy**, is a type of abnormal cell growth in which cellular regulation is lost, resulting in new tissues that serve no useful function, are harmful to the function of normal cells and organs, and can lead to death if left untreated. It is a common disease worldwide, although the types of cancer vary with a country's affluence. In the United States and Canada about 1.8 million people are newly diagnosed with cancer each year (American Cancer Society [ACS], 2020; Canadian Cancer Society, 2019). The risk for cancer differs for each adult depending on genetic, immunologic, and environmental factors. Some types of cancer can be prevented and many others have better cure rates if diagnosed early. With more extensive use of cancer prevention strategies, the cancer incidence and death rate in the United States and Canada have decreased during the past 5 years. As a nurse you can have a vital impact in educating the public about cancer prevention and early detection methods.

PATHOPHYSIOLOGY REVIEW

During childhood continued orderly growth of cells and tissues must occur for body development and maturation. In adults well-controlled continued growth of some cell types after maturation is needed to replace dead or damaged cells for normal cellular regulation. ***Cellular regulation*** is the genetic and physiologic processes that control cellular growth, replication, differentiation, and function to maintain homeostasis. All steps in the processes of cellular regulation are the result of gene interactions. Tissues that continue to grow by undergoing mitosis in adulthood include cells of the skin, hair, mucous membranes, bone marrow, and linings of organs such as the lungs, stomach, intestines, bladder, breast ducts, and uterus. These tissues are located in areas in which constant damage or wear is likely and continued cell growth is needed to replace dead tissues. This continued growth is controlled by cellular regulation to ensure that the right number of healthy cells is always present in any tissue or organ.

For fully developed tissues and organs that stop growing by mitosis after maturation is complete, such as heart muscle, skeletal muscle, and neurons, damaged cells are replaced with scar tissue. Cardiac muscle cells in the heart therefore do not undergo mitosis in adults, but fibroblastic scar tissue does to help "patch" damaged tissue. The scar tissue does not resemble normal cardiac tissue and does not perform the differentiated function of rhythmic cardiac muscle contraction.

Any new or continued cell growth not needed for normal development or replacement of dead and damaged tissues is called neoplasia. This cell growth is abnormal even if it causes no harm (is *benign*). Whether the new cells are benign or cancerous, neoplastic cells develop from normal cells *(parent cells)*. Thus cancer cells all were once normal cells but underwent genetic mutations to no longer look, grow, or function normally. The strict processes of ***cellular regulation*** controlling normal growth and function have been lost (McCance et al., 2019). To understand how cancer cells grow, it is helpful to understand the growth regulation and function of normal cells.

Biology of Normal Cells

Many different normal cells work together to make the whole body function at an optimal level. For optimal body function, each cell must perform in a predictable manner.

Specific morphology is the feature in which each normal cell type has a distinct and recognizable appearance, size, and shape, as shown in Fig. 19.1.

A smaller nuclear-to-cytoplasmic ratio means that the nucleus of a normal cell occupies a relatively small amount of space inside the cell. As shown in Fig. 19.1, the size of the normal cell nucleus is small compared with the size of the rest of the cell, including the cytoplasm.

Differentiated function means that every normal cell has at least one function it performs to contribute to whole-body function. For example, skin cells make keratin, liver cells make bile, cardiac muscle cells contract, and red blood cells make hemoglobin.

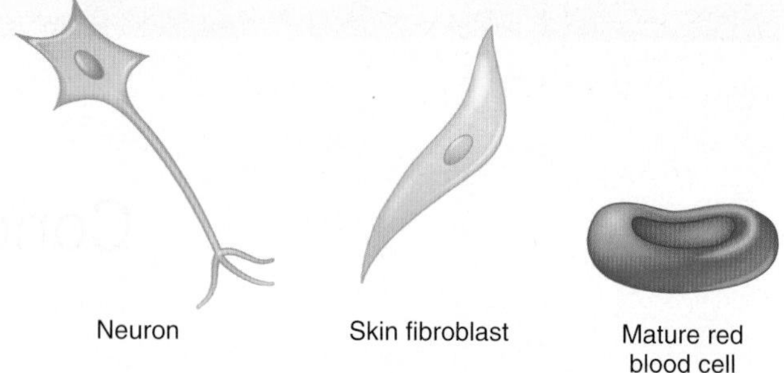

Fig. 19.1 Distinctive morphology of some normal cells.

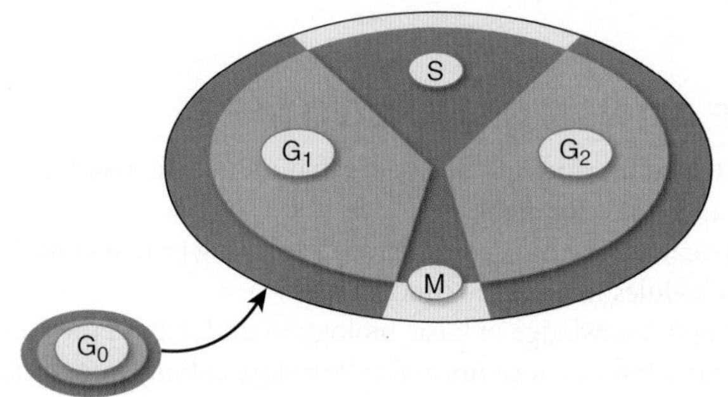

Fig. 19.2 The cell cycle.

Tight adherence occurs because normal cells make sticky cell adhesion molecules (CAMs) that protrude from the membranes, allowing cells to bind closely and tightly together. Exceptions are blood cells that circulate freely as individual cells. Red blood cells and white blood cells produce no CAMs and do not usually adhere together.

Nonmigratory means that normal cells do not wander throughout the body (except for blood cells). Normal cells are nonmigratory because they are tightly bound together with CAMs, which prevents cells from wandering from one tissue into the next. Thus the normal liver does not overgrow and crowd out the space the right kidney should occupy.

Orderly and well-regulated growth by ***cellular regulation*** is a very important feature of normal cells. They divide (undergo mitosis) for only two reasons: (1) to develop normal tissue or (2) to replace lost, damaged, or aged normal tissue. Even when they are capable of mitosis, normal cells divide only when body conditions are just right. Cell division (mitosis), occurring in a well-recognized pattern, is described by the cell cycle. Fig. 19.2 shows the phases of the cell cycle. Living cells not actively reproducing are in a reproductive resting state termed G_0. During the G_0 period, cells actively carry out their functions but do not divide. Normal cells spend most of their lives in the G_0 state rather than in a reproductive state.

Mitosis makes one cell divide into two new cells that are identical to each other and to the cell that began mitosis. The steps of entering and completing the cell cycle are tightly controlled. Whether a cell enters and completes the cell cycle to form two new cells depends on the presence and absence of specific ***cellular regulation*** proteins. Proteins that promote cells to enter and complete cell division are produced by proto-oncogenes and are known as *cyclins*. When cyclins are activated by external or internal signaling, they allow a cell to leave G_0 and enter the cycle. These activated cyclins then drive the cell to progress through the different phases of the cell cycle and undergo

TABLE 19.1 Characteristics of Normal and Abnormal Cells

Characteristic	Normal Cell	Benign Tumor Cell	Malignant Cell
Cell division	None or slow	Continuous or inappropriate	Rapid or continuous
Appearance	Specific morphologic features	Specific morphologic features	Anaplastic
Nuclear-to-cytoplasmic ratio	Smaller	Smaller	Larger
Differentiated functions	Many	Many	Some or none
Adherence	Tight	Tight	Loose
Migratory	No	No	Yes
Growth	Well regulated	Expansion	Invasion
Chromosomes	Diploid (euploid)	Diploid (euploid)	Aneuploid[a]
Mitotic index	Low	Low	High[a]

[a]Depends on the degree of malignant transformation.

cell division. Proteins produced by suppressor genes control the amount of cyclins present and ensure that cell division occurs only when it is needed. *Thus cellular regulation of division is a balance between the proto-oncogene protein products that promote cell division (cyclins) and the proteins that limit cell division (suppressor gene products).*

Contact inhibition is the part of ***cellular regulation*** that stops further rounds of cell division when the dividing cell is completely surrounded and touched (contacted) by other cells. Of the normal cells that can divide, each cell divides only when some of its surface is not in direct contact with another cell. Once a normal cell is in direct contact on all surface areas with other cells, it no longer undergoes mitosis. Thus normal cell division is contact inhibited.

Apoptosis is programmed cell death. Not only do normal cells have to divide only when needed and have to perform their specific differentiated functions, some cells also have to die at the appropriate time to ensure optimum body function. Thus normal cells have a finite life span. With each cell division, the telomeric DNA at the ends of the cell's chromosomes shortens (see Chapter 6). When this DNA is gone, the cell responds to ***cellular regulation*** signals for apoptosis. This ensures that each organ has an adequate number of cells at their functional peak.

Euploidy, having a complete set of chromosomes, is a feature of most normal human cells. These cells have 23 pairs of chromosomes, the correct number for humans.

Biology of Abnormal Cells

Body cells are exposed to a variety of conditions that can alter how cells grow or function. When either cell growth or cell function is changed, the cells are considered abnormal. Table 19.1 compares features of normal, benign tumor, and cancer (malignant) cells.

Features of Benign Tumor Cells. Benign tumor cells are normal cells growing in the wrong place or at the wrong time as a result of a problem with ***cellular regulation***. Examples include moles, uterine fibroid tumors, skin tags, endometriosis, and nasal polyps. Benign tumor cells have these characteristics:

- *Specific morphology* occurs with benign tumors. They look like the tissues they come from, retaining the specific morphology of parent cells.
- *A smaller nuclear-to-cytoplasmic ratio* is a feature of benign tumors just like completely normal cells.
- *Specific differentiated functions* continue to be performed by benign tumors. For example, in endometriosis, a type of benign tumor, the normal lining of the uterus (endometrium) grows in an abnormal place (e.g., on an ovary or elsewhere in the abdominal or even the chest cavity). This displaced endometrium acts just like normal endometrium by changing each month under the influence of estrogen. When the hormone level drops and the normal endometrium sheds from the uterus, the displaced endometrium, wherever it is, also sheds.
- *Tight adherence* of benign tumor cells to one another occurs because they continue to make cell adhesion molecules.
- *No migration* or wandering of benign tissues occurs because they remain tightly bound and do not invade other body tissues.
- *Orderly growth* with normal growth patterns occurs in benign tumor cells even though their growth is not needed. The fact that growth continues beyond an appropriate time or occurs in the wrong place indicates some problem with ***cellular regulation***, but the rate of growth is normal. The benign tumor grows by expansion. *It does not invade.*
- *Euploidy* (normal chromosomes) are usually found in benign tumor cells, with a few exceptions. Most of these cells have 23 pairs of chromosomes, the correct number for humans.

Features of Cancer Cells. Cancer (malignant) cells are abnormal, serve no useful function, and are harmful to normal body tissues. Cancers commonly have these features:

- *Anaplasia* is the cancer cells' loss of the specific appearance of their parent cells. As a cancer cell becomes more malignant, it becomes smaller and rounded. Thus many different types of cancer cells look alike under the microscope, rather than looking like their parent cells.
- *A larger nuclear-cytoplasmic ratio* occurs because the cancer cell nucleus is larger than that of a normal cell and the cancer cell is smaller than a normal cell. The nucleus occupies much of the space within the cancer cell, especially during mitosis, creating a large nuclear-to-cytoplasmic ratio.
- *Specific functions are lost* partially or completely in cancer cells. *Cancer cells serve no useful purpose.*
- *Loose adherence* is typical for cancer cells because they do not make cell adhesion molecules. As a result, cancer cells easily break off from the main tumor.
- *Migration* occurs because cancer cells do not bind tightly together and have many enzymes on their cell surfaces. These features allow the cells to slip through blood vessel walls and between tissues, spreading from the main tumor site to many other body sites. The ability to spread by undergoing metastasis is unique to cancer cells and is

a major cause of death. Cancer cells invade other tissues, both close by and more remote from the original tumor. Invasion and persistent growth make untreated cancer deadly.

- *Contact inhibition* does not occur in cancer cells because of lost ***cellular regulation***, even when all sides of these cells are in continuous contact with the surfaces of other cells. This persistence of cell division makes the disease difficult to manage.
- *Rapid or continuous cell division* occurs in many types of cancer cells because they do not respond to checkpoint control of cell division because of gene changes that reduce the effectiveness of ***cellular regulation***, and they re-enter the cell cycle for mitosis almost continuously. In addition, these cells also do not respond to signals for apoptosis. Most cancer cells have a lot of the enzyme *telomerase,* which maintains telomeric DNA. As a result, cancer cells do not respond to apoptotic signals and have an unlimited life span (are "immortal").
- *Abnormal chromosomes* in which the chromosome number and/or structure is not normal (**aneuploidy**) are common in cancer cells as they become more malignant. Chromosomes are lost, gained, or broken; thus cancer cells can have more than 23 pairs or fewer than 23 pairs. Cancer cells also may have broken and rearranged chromosomes with mutated genes.

CANCER DEVELOPMENT

Carcinogenesis, Oncogenesis, and Malignant Transformation

Carcinogenesis, **oncogenesis**, and **malignant transformation** are different terms for cancer development, which is the process of changing a normal cell into a cancer cell. This process occurs through loss of ***cellular regulation*** leading to the steps of initiation, promotion, progression, and metastasis.

Initiation is the first step in carcinogenesis. Normal cells can become cancer cells if they lose ***cellular regulation*** by having their genes promoting cell division (proto-oncogenes) turn on excessively (are overexpressed), becoming **oncogenes**, and produce more cyclins. Initiation is a change in gene expression caused by anything that can damage cellular DNA, leading to loss of cellular regulation. Such changes can activate proto-oncogenes that should have only limited expression to oncogene status and can damage suppressor genes, which normally limit proto-oncogene activity. Thus initiation leads to excessive cell division through DNA damage that results in loss of cellular regulation by either loss of suppressor gene function or enhancement of proto-oncogene function.

Initiation is an irreversible event that can lead to cancer development. After initiation a cell can become a cancer cell if the cellular regulation loss that occurred during initiation continues. *If growth conditions are right, widespread metastatic disease can develop from just one cancer cell.*

Substances that change the activity of a cell's genes so the cell becomes a cancer cell are **carcinogens**. Carcinogens may be chemicals, physical agents, or viruses. More than 62 agents, substances, mixtures, and exposures are known to cause cancer in humans, and about another 186 are suspected to be carcinogens (U.S. Department of Health and Human Services [USDHHS] National Toxicology Program [NTP], 2016). The NTP's website (http://ntp.niehs.nih.gov/pubhealth/roc/index.html) lists these substances. Chapters presenting the care of patients with specific cancers discuss specific known carcinogens for these cancers in the Etiology sections.

Promotion is the enhanced growth of an initiated cell by substances known as promoters. Once a normal cell has been initiated by a carcinogen and is a cancer cell, it can become a tumor if its growth is enhanced. Many normal hormones and body proteins, such as insulin and estrogen, can act as promoters and make cells divide more frequently. The time between a cell's initiation and the development of an overt tumor is called the *latency period,* which can range from months to years. Exposure to promoters can shorten the latency period.

Progression is the continued change of a cancer, making it more malignant over time. After cancer cells have grown to the point that a detectable tumor is formed (a 1-cm tumor has at least 1 billion cells in it), other events must occur for this tumor to become a health problem. First the tumor must develop its own blood supply. The tumor makes vascular endothelial growth factor (VEGF) that triggers nearby capillaries to grow new branches into the tumor, ensuring the tumor's continued nourishment and growth.

As tumor cells continue to divide, some of the new cells undergo genetic mutations that change features from the original, initiated cancer cell and form different groups. Some of the mutations, known as *driver mutations,* provide these cell groups with advantages *(selection advantages)* that allow them to live and divide no matter how the conditions around them change (Abbas et al., 2018; Beery et al., 2018). These tumor changes may allow it to become more malignant. Over time the tumor cells have fewer and fewer normal cell features. Other mutations, known as *passenger mutations,* also occur but do not appear to induce significant changes, although they can be used as unique cancer identifiers and serve as specific "targets" for newer cancer therapies. For this reason, genetic testing of all cancers is recommended to allow more precise and effective treatment.

The original group of cancer cells or tumor caused by carcinogenesis is called the **primary tumor**. It is usually identified by the tissue from which it arose *(parent tissue)* such as in breast cancer or lung cancer. When primary tumors are located in vital organs such as the brain or lungs, they can grow and either lethally damage the vital organ or interfere with that organ's ability to perform its vital function. At other times the primary tumor is located in soft tissue that can expand without damage as the tumor grows. One such site is the breast. The breast is not a vital organ, and even with a large tumor the primary tumor alone would not cause the patient's death. When the tumor spreads from the original site into vital areas *(metastasizes),* life functions can be disrupted and death may follow.

Metastasis occurs when cancer cells move from the primary location by breaking off from the original group and establishing remote colonies. These additional tumors are called **metastatic tumors** or **secondary tumors**. *Even though the tumor is* *now in another organ, it is still a cancer from the original altered tissue. For example, when breast cancer spreads to the lung and the bone, it is still breast cancer in the lung and bone—not lung cancer and not bone cancer.* Metastasis occurs through many steps, as shown in Fig. 19.3.

Tumors first extend into surrounding tissues by secreting enzymes that open up areas of surrounding tissue. Pressure, created as the tumor increases in size, forces tumor cells to invade new territory.

Spread to distant organs and tissues requires cancer cells to penetrate blood vessels. *Bloodborne metastasis* (tumor cell release into the blood) is a common cause of cancer spread. Enzymes secreted by tumor cells also make large pores in the patient's blood vessels, allowing tumor cells to enter the blood and circulate. Because tumor cells are loosely held together, clumps of cells break off from the primary tumor into blood vessels for transport.

Tumor cells circulate through the blood and enter tissues at remote sites. Clumps of cancer cells can become trapped in capillaries. These clumps damage the capillary wall and allow cancer cells to leave the capillary and enter the surrounding tissue.

When conditions in the remote site can support tumor cell growth, the cells stop circulating (arrest) and invade the surrounding tissues, creating secondary tumors. Table 19.2 lists the common sites of metastasis for specific tumor types.

Another way cancers metastasize is by *lymphatic spread.* Lymphatic spread is related to the number, structure, and location of lymph nodes and vessels. Primary sites that are rich in lymphatics have earlier metastatic spread than areas with few lymphatics.

NCLEX EXAMINATION CHALLENGE 19.1

Psychosocial Integrity

A client asks the nurse why his colorectal cancer is being tested for genetic mutations even though no one else in the family has ever had cancer. What is the nurse's **best** response?

A. "Colorectal cancer is rare and most cases are caused by a genetic mutation."
B. "The results of this testing will indicate what caused your cancer so you can avoid further exposure."
C. "Many tumors have one or more genetic differences that can help determine the most effective treatment options."
D. "Genetic testing of tumor cells can help determine the stage of your cancer and whether it has spread to other organs."

Cancer Classification

Cancers are classified according to the type of tissue from which they arise (e.g., glandular, connective) (McCance et al., 2019), as described in Table 19.3. Other ways to classify cancer include biologic behavior, anatomic site, and degree of differentiation.

About 100 different types of cancer arise from various tissues or organs. Fig. 19.4 compares cancer distribution by site and gender. Cancers are either solid or hematologic. Solid tumors develop from specific tissues (e.g., breast cancer and lung cancer). Hematologic cancers arise from blood cell–forming tissues (e.g., leukemias and lymphomas).

Cancer Grading, Ploidy, and Staging

Systems of grading and staging have been developed to help standardize cancer diagnosis, prognosis, and treatment. *Grading* of a tumor classifies cellular aspects of the cancer. *Ploidy* classifies the number and structure of tumor chromosomes as normal or abnormal. *Staging* classifies clinical aspects of the cancer.

Grading is needed because some cancer cells are "more malignant" than others, varying in their aggressiveness and sensitivity to treatment. Some cancer cells barely resemble the mature tissue from which they arose (are "poorly differentiated"), are aggressive, and spread rapidly. These cells are a "high-grade" cancer. Less malignant cancer cells that are "well differentiated" and more closely resemble the tissue from which they arose are less aggressive. Grading compares the appearance and activity of the cancer cell with the normal parent tissue from which it arose. It is a means of evaluating the patient with cancer for prognosis and appropriate therapy. Grading also allows health care professionals to evaluate the results of management.

Clinical groups have established specific grading systems for different types of cancer cells, but overall they resemble the standard system listed in Table 19.4. This system rates cancer cells, with the lowest rating given to those cells that closely resemble normal cells and the highest rating given to cancer cells that barely resemble normal cells. Grading systems for different cancers are presented in the clinical chapters in which care is discussed.

Ploidy is the description of cancer cells by chromosome number and appearance. Normal human cells have 46 chromosomes (23 pairs), the normal diploid number *(euploidy).* When malignant transformation occurs, changes in the genes and chromosomes also occur. Some cancer cells gain or lose whole chromosomes and may have structural abnormalities of the remaining chromosomes, a condition called *aneuploidy.* The degree of aneuploidy increases with the degree of malignancy. Some chromosome changes are associated with specific cancers, and their presence is used for diagnosis and prognosis. One example is the *Philadelphia chromosome* abnormality often present in chronic myelogenous leukemia cells (see Chapter 37). Other gene changes in cancerous tumors alter the tumor's susceptibility to specific treatment. Some changes form the basis of "targeted therapy" for cancer (see Chapter 20).

Staging determines the exact location of the cancer and whether metastasis has occurred. Cancer stage influences selection of therapy. Staging is done by clinical staging, surgical staging, and pathologic staging. *Clinical staging* assesses the patient's symptoms and evaluates tumor size and possible spread. *Surgical staging* assesses the tumor size, number, sites, and spread by inspection at surgery. *Pathologic staging* is the most definitive type, determining the tumor size, number, sites, and spread by pathologic examination of tissues obtained at surgery.

The *tumor, node, metastasis (TNM)* system is used to describe the anatomic extent of cancers. The TNM staging systems have specific prognostic value for each solid tumor type. Table 19.5 shows a basic TNM staging system. TNM staging is not useful for leukemia or lymphomas (see Chapter 37). Additional specific staging systems include the Dukes staging system for colon and rectal cancer and the Clark levels method for staging skin cancer.

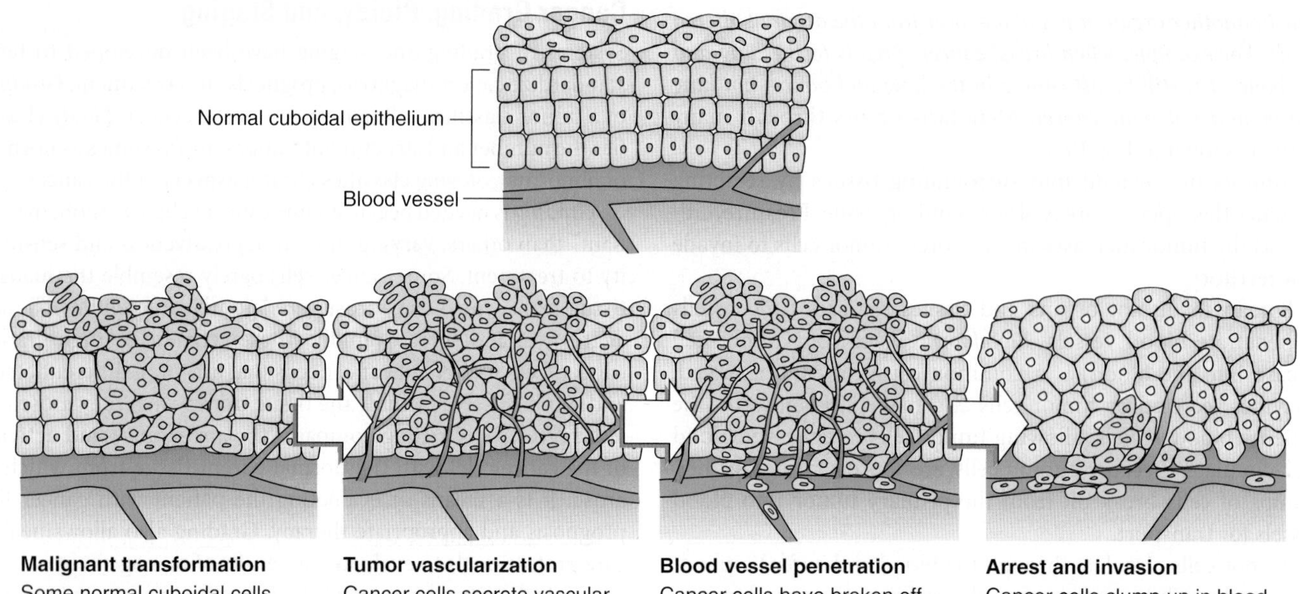

Normal cuboidal epithelium
Blood vessel
Malignant transformation
Some normal cuboidal cells have undergone malignant transformation and have divided enough times to form a tumorous area within the cuboidal epithelium.
Tumor vascularization
Cancer cells secrete vascular endothelial growth factor (VEGF), stimulating the blood vessels to bud and form new channels that grow into the tumor.
Blood vessel penetration
Cancer cells have broken off from the main tumor. Enzymes on the surface of the tumor cells make holes in the blood vessels, allowing cancer cells to enter blood vessels and travel around the body.
Arrest and invasion
Cancer cells clump up in blood vessel walls and invade new tissue areas. If the new tissue areas have the right conditions to support continued growth of cancer cells, new tumors (metastatic tumors) will form at this site.

Fig. 19.3 The steps of metastasis.

TABLE 19.2 Common Sites of Metastasis for Different Cancer Types

Breast Cancer • Bone[a] • Lung[a] • Liver • Brain **Lung Cancer** • Brain[a] • Bone • Liver • Lymph nodes • Pancreas **Colorectal Cancer** • Liver[a] • Lymph nodes • Adjacent structures	**Prostate Cancer** • Bone (especially spine and legs)[a] • Pelvic nodes **Melanoma** • GI tract • Lymph nodes • Lung • Brain **Primary Brain Cancer** • Central nervous system

[a]Most common site of metastasis for the specific cancer.

Tumor growth is assessed in terms of *doubling time* (the amount of time it takes for a tumor to double in size) and *mitotic index* (the percentage of actively dividing cells within a tumor). The smallest detectable tumor is about 1 cm in diameter and contains 1 billion cells. A tumor with a mitotic index of less than 10% is a slower-growing tumor; a tumor with an index of 85% is faster growing. Different tumor types have a wide range of growth rates.

Cancer Etiology and Genetic Risk

Carcinogenesis usually takes years and depends on several tumor and patient factors (Jorde et al., 2016; McCance et al., 2019). Three interacting factors influence cancer development: exposure to carcinogens, genetic predisposition, and ***immunity***. These factors account for variation in cancer development from one adult to another, even when each adult is exposed to the same hazards.

Proto-oncogene activation to oncogene status is the main mechanism of carcinogenesis regardless of the specific cause. These proto-oncogenes are turned on (expressed) under controlled conditions for ***cellular regulation*** when cells divide for normal growth and replacement of dead or damaged tissues. At other times they are turned off, controlled, or suppressed by products of "suppressor genes."

When a normal cell is exposed to any carcinogen (initiator), the normal cell's DNA can be damaged and mutated. The mutations damage suppressor genes, preventing them from producing proteins that control ***cellular regulation*** for the expression of proto-oncogenes. As a result, the proto-oncogenes are overexpressed (overexpressed proto-oncogenes are called *oncogenes*) and can cause the cells to change from normal cells to cancer cells. When oncogenes are overexpressed in a cell, excessive amounts of cyclins are produced and upset the balance between cell growth enhancement and cell growth limitation. The effect of the presence of these excessive cyclins is greater than the normal effect of the suppressor gene products; thus cell regulation is lost, allowing uncontrolled cell division.

Oncogenes are not abnormal genes but are part of every cell's normal makeup and start out as proto-oncogenes. Oncogenes are problematic when they are overexpressed as a result of exposure to carcinogenic agents or events with loss of ***cellular regulation***. External and personal factors can activate proto-oncogenes to oncogenes.

TABLE 19.3 Classification of Tumors by Tissue of Origin

Prefix	Tissue of Origin	Benign Tumor	Malignant Tumor[a]
Adeno	Epithelial glands	Adenoma	Adenocarcinoma
Chondro	Cartilage	Chondroma	Chondrosarcoma
Fibro	Fibrous connective	Fibroma	Fibrosarcoma
Glio	Glial cells (brain)	Glioma	Glioblastoma
Hemangio	Blood vessel	Hemangioma	Hemangiosarcoma
Hepato	Liver	Hepatoma	Hepatocarcinoma
Leiomyo	Smooth muscle	Leiomyoma	Leiomyosarcoma
Lipo	Fat/adipose	Lipoma	Liposarcoma
Lympho	Lymphoid tissues		Malignant lymphomas Hodgkin lymphoma Non-Hodgkin lymphoma Burkitt lymphoma Cutaneous T-cell
Melano	Pigment-producing skin		Melanoma
Meningioma	Meninges	Meningioma	Malignant meningioma
Neuro	Nerve tissue	Neuroma Neurofibroma	Neurosarcoma
Osteo	Bone	Osteoma	Osteosarcoma
Renal	Kidney		Renal cell carcinoma
Rhabdo	Skeletal muscle	Rhabdomyoma	Rhabdomyosarcoma
Squamous	Epithelial layer of skin, mucous membranes, and organ linings	Papilloma	Squamous cell carcinoma of skin, bladder, lungs, cervix

[a]Carcinomas are tumors of glandular tissue; sarcomas are tumors of connective tissue; blastomas are tumors of less differentiated, embryonal tissues.

External Factors Causing Cancer. External factors, including environmental exposure, are responsible for about 80% of cancer in North America, although personal and genetic factors may determine how a specific adult's body responds to the exposures (ACS, 2020; Beery et al., 2018). Environmental carcinogens are chemical, physical, or viral agents that cause cancer (USDHHS, 2016).

Chemical carcinogenesis can occur from exposures to many known chemicals, drugs, and other products used in everyday life. Chemicals vary in how carcinogenic they are. For example, tobacco and alcohol appear to be only mildly carcinogenic. For these substances, chronic, long-term exposure to large amounts is required before ***cellular regulation*** is lost and cancer develops. However, these two substances can act as *co-carcinogens,* meaning that when they are taken together, they enhance each other's carcinogenic activity.

Not all cells are susceptible to carcinogenesis to the same degree. Normal cells that have the ability to divide are at greater risk for cancer development than are normal cells that are not capable of cell division. For example, cancers commonly arise in bone marrow, skin, lining of the GI tract, ductal cells of the breast, and lining of the lungs. All of these cells normally undergo cell division. Cancers of nerve tissue, cardiac muscle, and skeletal muscle are rare. These cells do not normally undergo cell division.

At least 30% of cancers diagnosed in North America are related to tobacco use (ACS, 2020; Canadian Cancer Society, 2019). Tobacco is the single most preventable source of carcinogenesis. It contains many carcinogens and co-carcinogens. The risk for cancer development from tobacco use depends on an adult's ***immunity***, genetic susceptibility, and amount and types of tobacco exposure. Chapter 24 discusses the types of tobacco and tobacco smoke exposure.

Tissues at greatest risk for tobacco-induced cancer are those that have direct contact with tobacco or tobacco smoke such as the lungs and airways. Cigarette smoking and tobacco use also promote the development of pancreatic, oral and laryngeal, bladder, and cervical cancers.

PATIENT-CENTERED CARE: VETERANS HEALTH CONSIDERATIONS QSEN

The incidence of tobacco-related cancers is high among military veterans, as is the incidence of smoking (Centers for Disease Control and Prevention [CDC], 2018). One reason is that at one time cigarette smoking was considered "manly" among military personnel. The cost of cigarettes was low in stores on military installations (no state taxes were applied). In addition, military field meals such as "C-rations" or "K-rations" at one time included free cigarettes. Ask patients about military service and whether cigarette smoking started, continued, or increased during that time.

Physical carcinogenesis from physical agents or events also causes cancer by DNA damage. Two physical agents that are known to cause cancer are radiation and chronic irritation.

Even small doses of radiation affect cells. Some effects are temporary and are self-repaired. Other effects cannot be repaired and may induce cancer in the damaged cells. Both ionizing and ultraviolet (UV) radiation can cause cancer. Some ionizing radiation is found naturally in radon, uranium, and radium found in rocks and soil. Other sources of ionizing radiation include x-rays for diagnosis and treatment of disease, as well as cosmic radiation. UV radiation is a type of solar radiation, coming from the sun. Other sources of UV radiation include tanning beds and germicidal lights. UV rays do not penetrate deeply, and the most common cancer type caused by UV exposure is skin cancer. Both ionizing and UV radiation exposure mutates genes.

Chronic irritation and tissue trauma are suspected to cause cancer. The incidence of skin cancer is higher in the scars of adults with burn scars or other types of severe skin injury. Chronically irritated tissues undergo frequent cell division and thus are at an increased risk for DNA mutation.

Viral carcinogenesis occurs when viruses infect body cells and break DNA strands. Viruses then insert their own genetic material into the human DNA. Breaking the DNA, along with viral gene insertion, mutates the cell's DNA and can either activate an oncogene or damage suppressor genes. Viruses that cause cancer are **oncoviruses**. Table 19.6 lists cancers of known viral origin.

Dietary factors related to cancer are poorly understood but are suspected to increase cancer risk. Suspected dietary factors include low fiber intake and a high intake of red meat or animal fat. Preservatives, preparation methods, and additives (dyes, flavorings, sweeteners) may have cancer-promoting effects. The

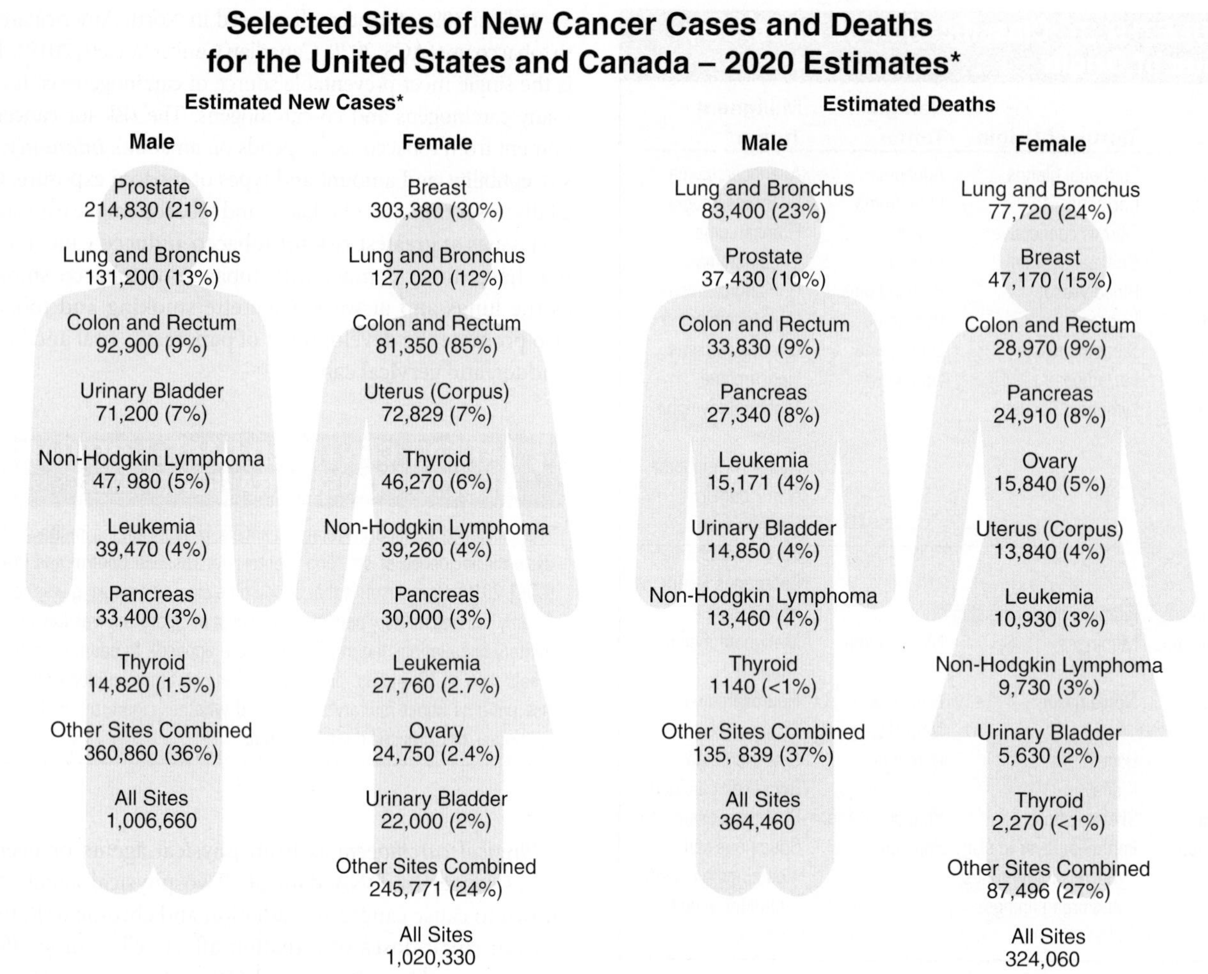

Selected Sites of New Cancer Cases and Deaths for the United States and Canada – 2020 Estimates*

Estimated New Cases*		Estimated Deaths	
Male	**Female**	**Male**	**Female**
Prostate 214,830 (21%)	Breast 303,380 (30%)	Lung and Bronchus 83,400 (23%)	Lung and Bronchus 77,720 (24%)
Lung and Bronchus 131,200 (13%)	Lung and Bronchus 127,020 (12%)	Prostate 37,430 (10%)	Breast 47,170 (15%)
Colon and Rectum 92,900 (9%)	Colon and Rectum 81,350 (85%)	Colon and Rectum 33,830 (9%)	Colon and Rectum 28,970 (9%)
Urinary Bladder 71,200 (7%)	Uterus (Corpus) 72,829 (7%)	Pancreas 27,340 (8%)	Pancreas 24,910 (8%)
Non-Hodgkin Lymphoma 47, 980 (5%)	Thyroid 46,270 (6%)	Leukemia 15,171 (4%)	Ovary 15,840 (5%)
Leukemia 39,470 (4%)	Non-Hodgkin Lymphoma 39,260 (4%)	Urinary Bladder 14,850 (4%)	Uterus (Corpus) 13,840 (4%)
Pancreas 33,400 (3%)	Pancreas 30,000 (3%)	Non-Hodgkin Lymphoma 13,460 (4%)	Leukemia 10,930 (3%)
Thyroid 14,820 (1.5%)	Leukemia 27,760 (2.7%)	Thyroid 1140 (<1%)	Non-Hodgkin Lymphoma 9,730 (3%)
Other Sites Combined 360,860 (36%)	Ovary 24,750 (2.4%)	Other Sites Combined 135, 839 (37%)	Urinary Bladder 5,630 (2%)
All Sites 1,006,660	Urinary Bladder 22,000 (2%)	All Sites 364,460	Thyroid 2,270 (<1%)
	Other Sites Combined 245,771 (24%)		Other Sites Combined 87,496 (27%)
	All Sites 1,020,330		All Sites 324,060

*Excludes basal and squamous cell skin cancers and in situ carcinoma except urinary bladder.

Fig. 19.4 Cancer incidence and death by site and sex. (Data from American Cancer Society, 2020, and Canadian Cancer Society, 2019.)

TABLE 19.4 Grading of Malignant Tumors

Grade	Cellular Characteristics
G_x	Grade cannot be determined.
G_1	Tumor cells are well differentiated and closely resemble the normal cells from which they arose. This grade is considered a low grade of malignant change. These tumors are malignant but are relatively slow growing.
G_2	Tumor cells are moderately differentiated; they still retain some of the characteristics of normal cells but also have more malignant characteristics than do G_1 tumor cells.
G_3	Tumor cells are poorly differentiated, but the tissue of origin can usually be established. The cells have few normal cell characteristics.
G_4	Tumor cells are poorly differentiated and retain no normal cell characteristics. Determination of the tissue of origin is difficult and perhaps impossible.

TABLE 19.5 Staging of Cancer—TNM Classification

Primary Tumor (T)	
T_x	Primary tumor cannot be assessed
T_0	No evidence of primary tumor
T_{is}	Carcinoma in situ
T_1, T_2, T_3, T_4	Increasing size and/or local extent of the primary tumor
Regional Lymph Nodes (N)	
N_x	Regional lymph nodes cannot be assessed
N_0	No regional lymph node metastasis
N_1, N_2, N_3	Increasing involvement of regional lymph nodes
Distant Metastasis (M)	
M_x	Presence of distant metastasis cannot be assessed
M_0	No distant metastasis
M_1	Distant metastasis

PATIENT AND FAMILY EDUCATION: PREPARING FOR SELF-MANAGEMENT

Dietary Habits to Reduce Cancer Risk

- Avoid excessive intake of animal fat.
- Avoid nitrites (prepared lunch meats, sausage, bacon).
- Minimize your intake of red meat.
- Keep your alcohol consumption to no more than one or two drinks per day.
- Eat more bran.
- Eat more cruciferous vegetables such as broccoli, cauliflower, Brussels sprouts, and cabbage.
- Eat foods high in vitamin A (e.g., apricots, carrots, leafy green and yellow vegetables) and vitamin C (e.g., fresh fruits and vegetables, especially citrus fruits).

TABLE 19.6 Cancers Associated With a Known Viral Origin

Virus	Malignancies
Epstein-Barr virus	Burkitt lymphoma, B-cell lymphoma, nasopharyngeal carcinoma
Hepatitis B virus	Primary liver carcinoma
Hepatitis C virus	Primary liver carcinoma, possibly B-cell lymphomas
Human papillomavirus	Cervical carcinoma, vulvar carcinoma, penile carcinoma, other anogenital carcinomas, and head and neck carcinoma
Human lymphotropic virus type I	Adult T-cell leukemia
Human lymphotropic virus type II	Hairy cell leukemia

Data from U.S. Department of Health and Human Services National Toxicology Program. (2016). *Report on carcinogens* (14th ed.). http://ntp.niehs.nih.gov/go.roc13

Patient and Family Education: Preparing for Self-Management: Dietary Habits to Reduce Cancer Risk box lists dietary habits that may help reduce cancer risk.

Personal Factors and Cancer Development. Personal factors, including ***immunity***, age, and genetic risk, also affect whether an adult is likely to develop cancer.

Immunity protects the body from foreign invaders and non-self cells (see Chapter 16). Non-self cells include cells that are not normal such as cancer cells. Cell-mediated immunity, especially natural killer (NK) cells and helper T-cells, provides immune surveillance (Abbas et al., 2018).

Cancer incidence increases among patients with reduced ***immunity***. Adults older than 60 years have reduced immunity and a higher incidence of cancer compared with that of the general population. Organ transplant recipients taking immunosuppressive drugs to prevent organ rejection also have a higher incidence of cancer. In patients with stage HIV-III disease (acquired immune deficiency syndrome [AIDS]), cancer incidence is very high (ACS, 2020).

Advancing age is the single most important risk factor for cancer (ACS, 2020; Canadian Cancer Society, 2019). As an adult ages, immunity decreases and external exposures to carcinogens accumulate. Teach older adults to be aware of and report symptoms such as the seven warning signs of cancer (Table 19.7) to health care providers. Primary health care providers should investigate all symptoms suggestive of disease. Refer to the Patient Centered Care: Older Adult Considerations box on the next page for assessment areas for the most common cancers that occur among older adults.

TABLE 19.7 The Seven Warning Signs of Cancer

C	*C*hanges in bowel or bladder habits
A	*A* sore that does not heal
U	*U*nusual bleeding or discharge
T	*T*hickening or lump in the breast or elsewhere
I	*I*ndigestion or difficulty swallowing
O	*O*bvious change in a wart or mole
N	*N*agging cough or hoarseness

PATIENT-CENTERED CARE: GENETIC/ GENOMIC CONSIDERATIONS QSEN

A hereditary genetic risk for cancer occurs only in a small percent of the population; however, adults who have a genetic predisposition are at very high risk for cancer development (Beery et al., 2018; Jorde et al., 2016). Mutations in suppressor genes or oncogenes can be inherited when they occur in sperm and ova and are then passed on to one's children, in whom all body cells will contain the inherited mutations. Thus for some adults tight ***cellular regulation*** is lost as a result of a mutation in a suppressor gene, which reduces or halts its function and allows proto-oncogene overexpression as oncogenes. In other adults, the suppressor genes are normal and the proto-oncogene is mutated and does not respond to suppressor gene signals, thus reducing cellular regulation and increasing the risk for cancer development. Table 19.8 lists conditions associated with an increased genetic risk for cancer development. Be sure to include questions about these conditions when obtaining a family history, and develop at least a three-generation pedigree (Mahon, 2016).

NCLEX EXAMINATION CHALLENGE 19.2

Physiological Integrity

An older client reports all of the following changes since his last checkup. Which changes alert the nurse to the possibility of prostate cancer? **Select all that apply.**

A. Bloody urine
B. Constipation intermittent with diarrhea
C. Erectile dysfunction
D. Night sweats and fever
E. Persistent pain in the lower back and legs
F. Reduced urine stream

Genetic testing for cancer predisposition is available to confirm or rule out an adult's genetic risk for some specific cancer types. (See Chapter 6 for explanation of genetic terminology.) These tests usually are performed on blood and are expensive. Genetic testing should not be performed unless a family history clearly indicates the possibility of increased genetic risk and the patient wants to have the test results. *These tests do not*

PATIENT-CENTERED CARE: OLDER ADULT CONSIDERATIONS QSEN

Cancer Type	Assessment Consideration
Colorectal cancer	Ask the patient whether bowel habits have changed over the past year (e.g., in consistency, frequency, color). Ask whether the patient has noticed any obvious blood in the stool. Test at least one stool specimen for occult blood during the patient's hospitalization. Urge the patient to have a baseline colonoscopy. Encourage the patient to reduce dietary intake of animal fats, red meat, and smoked meats. Encourage the patient to increase dietary intake of bran, vegetables, and fruit.
Lung cancer	Observe the skin and mucous membranes for color. How many words can the patient say between breaths? Ask the patient about: • Cough • Hoarseness • Smoking history (including use of electronic cigarettes or "vaping") • Particulate matter exposure to inhalation irritants • Exposure to asbestos • Shortness of breath • Activity tolerance • Frothy or bloody sputum • Pain in the arms, shoulders, or chest • Difficulty swallowing
Prostate cancer	Ask the patient about: • Hesitancy • Change in the size of the urine stream • New onset pain in the lower back or legs • History of persistent urinary tract infections
Skin cancer	Examine skin areas for moles or warts. Ask the patient about changes in moles (e.g., color, edges, sensation). Recommend use of sunscreen and protective clothing when outdoors.
Leukemia	Observe the skin for color, petechiae, or ecchymosis. Ask the patient about: • Fatigue • Bruising • Bleeding tendency • History of infections and illnesses • Night sweats and/or fevers
Bladder cancer	Ask the patient about the presence of: • Pain on urination • Blood in the urine • Cloudy urine • Increased frequency or urgency

diagnose the presence of cancer; they only provide risk information. Personal and family history facts that are considered "red flags" suggesting a genetic predisposition for cancer include:

- Cancer of any type appears in multiple members of every generation of a family, especially if an autosomal dominant pattern of inheritance emerges.
- Similar cancers appear in multiple first-degree relatives.
- Multiple instances of rare cancer types occur within a family.
- Cancer occurs at ages several decades younger than the national average.
- Cancer develops in both of paired organs (e.g., bilateral breast cancer).
- Breast cancer is present in a genetic male adult, regardless of gender identity.

A variety of issues and potential problems exist with genetic testing for cancer risk. Correct interpretation of the results is critical. Ideally a genetic counselor is involved in giving the patient information *before*, as well as after, testing is performed. *When a patient tests positive for a known cancer-causing gene mutation, his or her risk for cancer development is greatly increased; however, the cancer still may never develop.* A negative result means that the particular gene mutation tested for is not present. In addition, testing might not find the particular mutation but may indicate a different mutation with an unknown significance. This result is particularly frustrating for patients and health care providers.

Other issues regarding genetic testing include who will have access to the information and whether to share the test results with family members. Genetic testing has implications for the entire family, not just the patient being tested. For more information on genetic testing, see Chapter 6.

When risks for cancer development are assessed, behavior and socioeconomic factors are assessed along with ethnicity and

PATIENT-CENTERED CARE: CULTURAL/SPIRITUAL CONSIDERATIONS QSEN

The incidence of cancer varies among races. American Cancer Society (ACS) data (2020, 2019a, 2019b) show that African Americans have a higher incidence of cancer than whites, and the death rate is higher for African Americans. Since 1960 the overall incidence among African Americans has increased 27%, whereas for whites it has increased only 12%. Cancer sites and cancer-related mortality also vary by race. A possible reason for the difference is that more African Americans have less access to health care. They are more often diagnosed with later-stage cancer that is more difficult to cure or control. However, this disparity in access does not explain all differences.

The rates for cancer types among Hispanic/Latino adults living in the United States vary from the non-Hispanic white population. Hispanic/Latino adults have a lower rate of lung cancer, breast cancer, colorectal cancer, and prostate cancer than do non-Hispanic whites; however, the rates for the infection-related cancers such as liver, gallbladder, and stomach cancers is higher (ACS, 2018). In addition, Hispanic/Latino adults are often diagnosed at later stages, especially for breast cancer and melanoma (ACS, 2018).

NCLEX EXAMINATION CHALLENGE 19.3

Physiological Integrity

Which specific cancer types have a higher rate of occurrence among the Hispanic/Latino population of the United States compared with the non-Hispanic white population? **Select all that apply.**

A. Breast
B. Colorectal
C. Gall bladder
D. Liver
E. Lung
F. Prostate
G. Stomach

TABLE 19.8 Conditions Associated With a Genetic Predisposition for Cancer

Condition	Specific Cancer Type
Inherited cancers[a]	Breast cancer
	Prostate cancer
	Ovarian cancer
Familial clustering	Breast cancer
	Melanoma
Bloom syndrome	Leukemia
Familial polyposis	Colorectal cancer
Chromosomal aberrations	
Down syndrome (47 chromosomes)	Leukemia
Klinefelter syndrome (47,XXY)	Breast cancer
Turner syndrome (45,X)	Leukemia
	Gonadal carcinoma
	Meningioma
	Colorectal cancer

[a]Not all breast, prostate, or ovarian cancers are inherited.

genetic predisposition. The American Cancer Society (2018) has reported that cancer incidence and survival are often related to socioeconomic factors. These factors include the availability of health care services or the belief that seeking early health care has a positive effect on the outcome of cancer diagnosis.

HEALTH PROMOTION: CANCER PREVENTION

Cancer prevention activities focus on primary prevention and secondary prevention. **Primary cancer prevention** is the use of strategies to prevent the actual occurrence of cancer. This type of cancer prevention is most effective when there is a known cause for a cancer type. **Secondary cancer prevention** is the use of screening strategies to detect cancer early, at a time when cure or control is more likely.

Primary Prevention

Avoidance of known or potential carcinogens is an effective prevention strategy when a cause of cancer is known and avoidance is easily accomplished. For example, teach adults to use skin protection during sun exposure to avoid skin cancer. Most lung cancer can be avoided by not using tobacco and eliminating exposure to loose asbestos particles (ACS, 2019b). Teach all adults about the dangers of cigarette smoking and other forms of tobacco use (see the Health Promotion and Maintenance box in Chapter 24). Teach adults who are exposed to carcinogens in the workplace to use personal protective equipment that reduces direct contact with this substance. As more cancer causes are identified, avoidance may become even more effective.

Modifying associated factors appears to help reduce cancer risk. Absolute causes are not known for many cancers, but some conditions appear to increase risk. Examples are the increased incidence of cancer among adults who consume alcohol; the association of a diet high in fat and low in fiber with colon cancer, breast cancer, and ovarian cancer; and a greater incidence of cervical cancer among women who have multiple sexual partners (ACS, 2020). Modifying behavior to reduce the associated factor may decrease the risk for cancer development. Therefore teach all adults to limit their intake of alcohol to no more than 1 ounce per day and to include more fruits, vegetables, and whole grains in their diets. Instruct women about the importance of limiting the number of sexual partners and to use safer sex practices to avoid exposure to viruses that can increase the risk for cervical cancer (ACS, 2019b) (see Table 19.6 for a listing of cancer-causing viruses).

Removal of "at-risk" tissues reduces cancer risk for an adult who has a known high risk for developing a specific type of cancer. Examples include removing moles to prevent conversion to skin cancer, removing colon polyps to prevent colon cancer, and removing breasts to prevent breast cancer. Not all "at-risk" tissues can be removed (e.g., those that are part of essential organs).

Chemoprevention is a strategy that uses drugs, chemicals, natural nutrients, or other substances to disrupt one or more steps important to cancer development. These agents may be able to reverse existing gene damage or halt the progression of the transformation process. Only a few agents have been found effective for chemoprevention. These include the use of aspirin and celecoxib to reduce the risk for colon cancer, the use of vitamin D and tamoxifen to reduce the risk for breast cancer, and the use of lycopene to reduce the risk for prostate cancer (ACS, 2020).

Vaccination is a newer method of primary cancer prevention (ACS, 2019b). Currently the only vaccines approved for cancer prevention are related to prevention of infection from several forms of human papillomavirus (HPV). These vaccines are Gardasil and Cervarix. As more cancer-causing organisms are identified, it is hoped that vaccines will be developed to prevent those infections.

Secondary Prevention

Regular screening for cancer does not reduce cancer incidence but can greatly reduce some types of cancer deaths. Teach all adults the benefits of participating in specific routine screening techniques annually as part of health maintenance. General screening recommendations are listed in chapters discussing cancers by organ system. The age and type of participation in specific screening tests are different for adults who have an identified increased risk for a specific cancer type. In addition, there is some controversy about the age at which and frequency with which screening has the greatest benefit. Examples of recommended screenings include (ACS, 2020):

- The choice of annual mammography for women 40 to 44 years of age, annual mammography for women 45 to 54 years of age, and annual or biennial mammography for women older than 55 years
- Annual clinical breast examination for women older than 40 years, and every 3 years for women age 20 to 39 years
- Annual fecal occult blood text for adults of all ages
- Digital rectal examination (DRE) for men older than 50 years

Because cancer development clearly involves gene changes (either inherited gene mutations or acquired damage-induced gene mutations), adults can be screened for some gene mutations that increase the risk for cancer (Lacovara & Bohnenkamp, 2018). A few examples of known gene mutations that increase cancer risk are found in the *BRCA1* gene, the *BRCA2* gene, and the *CHEK2* gene (which increase the risk for breast cancer) and mutations in the *APC*, *MLH1*, and *MSH2* genes (which increase the risk for colon cancer).

When a patient has a strong family history of either breast or colon cancer, create a three-generation pedigree to more fully explore the possibility of genetic risk (Mahon, 2016). If a pattern of risk emerges, inform the person about the possible benefits of genetic screening and advise him or her to talk with an oncology health practitioner or genetics professional for more information. Genetic screening can help an adult at increased genetic risk for cancer to alter lifestyle factors, participate in early detection methods, initiate chemoprevention, or even have at-risk tissue removed. Genetic screening has some personal risks as well as potential benefits (see Chapter 6).

GET READY FOR THE NEXT-GENERATION NCLEX® EXAMINATION!

Key Points

Review these Key Points for each NCLEX Examination Client Needs Category.

Health Promotion and Maintenance

- Teach adults to avoid tanning beds and to use sunscreen and wear protective clothing during sun exposure. **QSEN: Patient-Centered Care**
- Encourage patients to participate in the recommended cancer-screening activities for their age-group and cancer risk category. **QSEN: Patient-Centered Care**
- Assist adults interested in smoking cessation to find an appropriate smoking cessation program (see Chapter 24). **QSEN: Patient-Centered Care**
- Assess the patient's knowledge about causes of cancer and his or her screening and prevention practices. **QSEN: Patient-Centered Care**
- Ask all patients about their exposures to environmental agents that are known or suspected to impair ***cellular regulation*** and increase the risk for cancer. **QSEN: Evidence-Based Practice**
- Obtain a detailed family history (at least three generations) and use this information to create a pedigree to assess the patient's risk for familial or inherited cancer. **QSEN: Patient-Centered Care**
- Teach anyone, especially older adults, the "seven warning signs of cancer" (see Table 19.7). **QSEN: Evidence-Based Practice**

Physiological Integrity

- Be aware of these facts regarding cancer risk and cancer development:
  - Cancer cells originate from normal body cells.
  - Transformation of a normal cell into a cancer cell involves mutation of the genes (DNA) of the normal cell and results in the loss of ***cellular regulation.***
  - Oncogenes that are overexpressed can cause a cell to develop into a tumor.
  - Most tumors arise from cells that are capable of cell division.
  - A key feature of cancer cells is the loss of ***cellular regulation*** and apoptosis. These cells have an "infinite" life span.
  - Tobacco use is a causative factor in 30% of all cancers.
  - Adults with reduced ***immunity*** have a higher risk for cancer development.
  - Tumors that metastasize from the primary site into another organ are still designated as tumors of the originating tissue.
  - Cancer cells that are less differentiated and have a higher mitotic index are "more malignant" and harder to cure.

MASTERY QUESTIONS

1. How does a mutation in a suppressor gene, such as *BRCA1*, increase the risk for cancer development?
   A. Converting a proto-oncogene into an oncogene
   B. Removing the control over proto-oncogene expression
   C. Reducing the amount of cyclins produced by the oncogenes
   D. Inhibiting the recognition of abnormal cells through immunosurveillance
2. A client's cancer is staged as T1, N2, M1 according to the TNM classification system. How does the nurse interpret this report?
   A. The client has two tumors that are nonresponsive to treatment.
   B. The client has leukemia confined to the bone marrow.
   C. The client has a 2-cm tumor with one regional lymph node involved and no distant metastasis.
   D. The client has a small primary tumor extension into two lymph nodes and one site of distant metastasis.
3. Which statements made by a 62-year-old client alert the nurse to the possibility that he may be at increased genetic risk for cancer development? **Select all that apply.**
   A. An older aunt died from a brain tumor while she had breast cancer.
   B. He had two benign colon polyps removed during his most recent routine colonoscopy.
   C. His sister died from cancer of the appendix.
   D. His brother is being treated for breast cancer.
   E. His 32-year-old daughter has been recently diagnosed with cervical cancer.
   F. One person in each of the previous three generations of his family died from lung cancer.

REFERENCES

Abbas, A., Lichtman, A., & Pillai, S. (2018). *Cellular and molecular immunology* (9th ed.). Philadelphia: Elsevier.

American Cancer Society (ACS). (2020). *Cancer facts and figures-2020*. Atlanta: Author Report No. 00-300M-No. 500820.

American Cancer Society (ACS). (2019a). *Cancer facts and figures for African Americans-2019-2021*. Atlanta: Author. Report No. 861419.

American Cancer Society (ACS). (2019b). *Cancer prevention and early detection: Facts & figures-2019-2020*. Atlanta: Author. Report No. 860019.

American Cancer Society (ACS). (2018). *Cancer facts and figures for Hispanics/Latinos-2018-2020*. Atlanta: Author. Report No. 862318.

Beery, T. A., Workman, M. L., & Eggert, J. A. (2018). *Genetics and genomics in nursing and health care* (2nd ed.). Philadelphia: F.A. Davis.

Canadian Cancer Society, Statistics Canada. (2019). *Canadian Cancer Statistics, 2019*. Toronto, ON: Canadian Cancer Society.

Centers for Disease Control and Prevention (CDC). (2018). *About three in ten US veterans use tobacco products: Veterans use tobacco at much higher rates than most non-veterans*. https://www.cdc.gov/media/releases/2018/p0111-tobacco-use-veterans.html.

Jorde, L., Carey, J., & Bamshad, M. (2016). *Medical genetics* (5th ed.). Philadelphia: Elsevier.

Lacovara, J., & Bohnenkamp, S. (2018). Genetic testing in oncology for the medical-surgical nurse. *MEDSURG Nursing, 27*(2), 117–120.

Mahon, S. (2016). The three-generation pedigree: A critical tool in cancer genetics care. *Oncology Nursing Forum, 43*(5), 655–660.

McCance, K., Huether, S., Brashers, V., & Rote, N. (2019). *Pathophysiology: The biologic basis for disease in adults and children* (8th ed.). St. Louis: Mosby.

U.S. Department of Health and Human Services National Toxicology Program (NTP). (2016). *Report on carcinogens* (14th ed.). http://ntp.niehs.nih.gov/pubhealth/roc/index.html.

20

Concepts of Care for Patients With Cancer

Hannah M. Lopez

http://evolve.elsevier.com/Iggy/

LEARNING OUTCOMES

1. Collaborate with the interprofessional team to coordinate high-quality care to patients receiving cancer treatment.
2. Protect yourself and others from cytotoxic agents and radiation.
3. Teach the patient and caregiver(s) how impaired ***immunity***, impaired ***clotting***, and other changes caused by cancer or cancer treatment affect safety.
4. Identify community resources for patients with cancer.
5. Implement nursing interventions to help the patient and family cope with the psychosocial impact caused by cancer and cancer treatment.
6. Apply knowledge of pathophysiology to assess patients with common side effects and complications caused by cancer and cancer treatment, including oncologic emergencies.
7. Teach the patient and caregiver(s) about common drugs used for cancer therapy and the side effects, including impaired ***immunity*** and impaired ***clotting.***
8. Use clinical judgment to assess laboratory data and signs and symptoms to prioritize nursing care for patients with cancer.
9. Prioritize interprofessional collaborative care for patients who experience an oncologic emergency.

KEY TERMS

alopecia Loss of hair.

cachexia Extreme tissue and muscle wasting due to malnourishment.

chemotherapy Cytotoxic drugs aimed to reduce tumor burden and destroy cancer cells.

chemotherapy-induced peripheral neuropathy (CIPN) The loss of sensory perception or motor function of peripheral nerves associated with exposure to certain anticancer drugs.

dose-dense chemotherapy A chemotherapy regimen that is more frequently administered for aggressive cancer treatment.

emetogenic A substance that can induce nausea and vomiting.

exposure The amount of radiation that is delivered to a tissue.

extravasation Leakage or infiltration of a vesicant into the surrounding tissue.

gray Unit of measurement for an absorbed radiation dose.

immune-related adverse events (irAEs) Adverse events related to immunotherapy.

immunotherapy Drugs designed to activate the body's immune system to attack cancer cells, causing cell death.

metastatic Cancer spreading into vital organs (e.g., brain, liver, bone marrow) from the primary location.

mucositis Inflammatory response leading to sores or ulcers of the mucus membranes.

nadir The period in which the bone marrow suppression is the greatest and the patient is at highest risk for complications.

neutropenia Decreased numbers of neutrophil white blood cells leading to immunosuppression.

radiation dose The amount of radiation absorbed by the tissue.

thrombocytopenia Decreased numbers of platelets leading to impaired clotting and bleeding.

vesicants Drugs, such as cytotoxic agents, that can cause severe tissue damage to surrounding tissue if they escape into subcutaneous tissue.

PRIORITY AND INTERRELATED CONCEPTS

The priority concept for this chapter is:
- ***Immunity***

The interrelated concepts for this chapter are:
- ***Cellular Regulation***
- ***Clotting***
- ***Gas Exchange***
- ***Sensory Perception***

It is estimated that 1.7 million new cases of cancer were diagnosed in 2019. Early detection and treatment have had an impact on overall survival, and many patients are cured or live long term (5 years or longer) with cancer. However, cancer-related conditions are the second leading cause of death in the United States and the leading cause of death in Canada (American Cancer Society [ACS], 2019; Canadian Cancer Society [CCS], 2019). Survivors may have exacerbations and remissions of the disease over their lifetime. *Regardless of the treatment received,*

TABLE 20.1 Text Location of Specific Cancer Content

Cancer Type	Chapter
Bladder (urothelial)	61
Brain	41
Breast	65
Cervical	66
Colorectal	51
Esophageal	49
Head and neck	26
Leukemia	37
Lung	27
Lymphoma	37
Ovarian	66
Prostate	67
Renal cell carcinoma	62
Skin	23
Stomach (gastric)	50

cancer has a negative impact on the adult's physical and psychological functioning and quality of life.

Providing care to patients experiencing cancer and their families is complex, challenging, and best accomplished with an interprofessional team approach. This chapter describes the general interventions for cancer and the problems associated with cancer treatment. For treatments and patient problems that occur with specific cancer types, consult the chapters in which the cancer is described. Table 20.1 lists common cancer types and the specific locations within this text where the interventions are presented.

IMPACT OF CANCER ON PHYSICAL FUNCTION

Cancer can develop in any organ or tissue. Cancer can be localized (near site of origin) or metastatic (spread to distant sites in the body—e.g., brain, liver, or bone). Metastatic cancers are considered incurable, but people are living longer with advanced disease. Treatment strategies and goals of care are different for the patient with curable intent versus a metastatic diagnosis.

Cancer and treatments will often have an impact on:

- ***Immunity*** and clotting
- GI function
- Peripheral nerve sensory perception
- Central motor and sensory function
- Respiratory and cardiac function
- Comfort and quality of life

IMPAIRED IMMUNITY AND CLOTTING

Impaired ***immunity*** and decreased production of healthy bone marrow can occur when cancer starts in *or* invades the bone marrow, where blood cells are formed. Tumor cells can metastasize into the bone marrow and reduce the production and function of healthy white blood cells (WBCs) that are needed for normal immunity. Some cancer treatments, especially chemotherapy, reduce neutrophil WBC numbers, making the patient more prone to infection.

Bone marrow dysfunction causes anemia and thrombocytopenia by decreasing the number of red blood cells and platelets, respectively. The patient with anemia can have fatigue, shortness of breath, and tachycardia. The patient with thrombocytopenia will have impaired ***clotting*** and increased risk of bleeding. These changes may be caused by the disease or by cancer treatment, especially chemotherapy.

ALTERED GI FUNCTION

Tumors of the GI tract or advanced cancers increase the metabolic rate and the need for nutrients; however, many patients develop disease-related and treatment-related appetite loss, and alterations in taste that have a negative impact on nutrition, leading to weight loss. Cachexia (extreme body wasting and malnutrition) may occur during treatment or with advanced cancer. Nutritional support for the cancer patient is complex. Maintaining weight and nutritional intake during treatment is critical. A registered dietitian nutritionist (RDN) is an integral part of the interprofessional team and can provide different nutritional approaches such as smaller, frequent meals, general healthy eating recommendations, or help to facilitate enteral tube or parenteral nutrition if warranted.

Abdominal tumors may obstruct or compress structures anywhere in the GI tract, reducing the ability to absorb nutrients and eliminate wastes. This problem needs to be addressed promptly to avoid complications such as a bowel obstruction.

Tumors that invade the liver have profound effects on this organ, which has many important metabolic functions. This can lead to liver failure and death.

ALTERED PERIPHERAL NERVE FUNCTION

Although tumors in the spine can change peripheral nerve function, the more common cause is chemotherapy. Physical assessment of the degree of sensory perception loss can be performed by using monofilaments as described in Chapter 59. Neurotoxic chemotherapy agents injure peripheral nerves, leading to peripheral neuropathy with reduced ***sensory perception.*** Patients with chemotherapy-induced peripheral neuropathy (CIPN) report loss of sensation, especially in the lower extremities. Symptoms include numbness, tingling, neuropathic pain, and changes in gait and balance.

MOTOR AND SENSORY DEFICITS

Motor and ***sensory perception*** deficits occur when cancers invade bone or the brain or compress nerves. In patients with bone metastasis, the primary cancer started in another organ (e.g., lung, prostate, breast). Bones become thinner, with an increased risk for fractures that can occur with minimal trauma. Bone metastasis causes pain, fractures, spinal cord compression (SCC), and hypercalcemia, each of which reduces mobility. SCC and hypercalcemia are oncologic emergencies and require immediate attention (see section Oncologic Emergencies).

ALTERED RESPIRATORY AND CARDIAC FUNCTION

Cancer can disrupt respiratory function, capacity, and ***gas exchange*** and may result in death. Tumors that grow in the airways cause obstruction. If lung tissue is involved, lung capacity is decreased, leading to dyspnea and hypoxemia. Patients are at risk for hypoxemia and hypoxia with either primary or metastatic lung tumors or if pleural effusion develops.

Tumors can also press on blood and lymph system in the chest, which results in airway compression and dyspnea. Superior vena cava (SVC) syndrome is an oncologic emergency that results from compression of this vessel.

Both radiation therapy and certain chemotherapy agents can affect cardiac function. Following radiation to the chest, even with appropriate shielding, cardiac events may occur at a younger age in cancer patients compared with the general population. Cardiac conditions from radiation include pericarditis, coronary artery disease, myocardial dysfunction, and valvular heart disease. Higher risk for heart disease has been noted in patients with classic risk factors for cardiac problems such as hypertension, smoking, and hypercholesterolemia. Chemotherapy agents can also contribute to cardiac dysfunction through loss of myocardial muscle mass, leading to heart failure. These late effects of therapy are sometimes reversible but may be permanent.

CANCER PAIN AND QUALITY OF LIFE

The patient with cancer may have pain and is at risk for chronic pain. Pain does not always accompany cancer, but it can be a major problem. An interprofessional team that includes an oncologist, advanced oncology nurse practitioner, oncology nurse, interventional radiologist, radiation oncologist, and pain management or palliative care specialists can work together to help control pain and improve quality of life during and after treatment. Patient education is needed to manage side effects of pain drugs, including constipation. Chapter 5 discusses the causes and management of pain.

CANCER MANAGEMENT

The purpose of cancer management is to cure or control the disease while minimizing the side effects of therapy. For certain cancer types such as acute leukemia, failure to treat the disease would result in death within weeks to months. Cancer treatment can include surgery, radiation, chemotherapy, immunotherapy, targeted therapy, and hormonal therapy. These therapies may be used separately or in combination to kill cancer cells. The types of therapy used depend on the specific type of cancer, whether the cancer has spread, and the overall health and functional status of the patient. Treatment regimens *(protocols)* have been established for most types of cancer. The National Comprehensive Cancer Network (NCCN) provides evidence-based guidelines and standardized treatment plans based on the diagnosis and stage of cancer and monitoring of treatment response.

SURGERY

Overview

Surgery often plays a part in the diagnosis and/or management of cancer. Surgery is only one part of a comprehensive treatment approach for cancer therapy. Surgery is used for prophylaxis, diagnosis, cure, control, palliation, and tissue reconstruction.

Prophylactic surgery removes potentially cancerous tissue as a means of preventing cancer development. It is performed when a patient has either an existing premalignant condition or a strong predisposition for development of a specific cancer. For example, removing the opposite breast in a patient who has a genetic mutation (e.g., *BRCA1, BRCA2*) to prevent cancer in the unaffected breast is considered prophylactic surgery.

Diagnostic surgery (e.g. excisional biopsy) is the removal of all or part of a suspected lesion for examination and testing to confirm or rule out a cancer diagnosis. Cancer treatment is not initiated without tissue confirmation of a cancer diagnosis.

Curative surgery removes all cancer tissue. Surgery alone can result in a cure when all visible and microscopic tumor is removed. It is most effective for small localized tumors or non-invasive skin cancers such as basal cell lesions.

Debulking surgery removes part of the tumor if removal of the entire mass is not possible. It decreases the size of the tumor and the number of cancer cells, which may help alleviate symptoms, enhance the success of other types of cancer treatment, and increase survival time.

Palliative surgery focuses on providing symptom relief and improving the quality of life but is not curative. Examples include removal of tumor tissue that is causing pain, obstruction, or difficulty swallowing.

Reconstructive or restorative *surgery* increases function, enhances appearance, or both. Examples include breast reconstruction after mastectomy, bowel reconstruction, revision of scars, and cosmetic reconstruction in head and neck cancer.

Side Effects of Surgical Treatment

Cancer surgery often involves the loss of a body part or its function to ensure removal of all cancerous tissue. Surgery can remove all or part of the affected body part. *Any organ loss reduces function.* Some cancer surgeries result in scarring or disfigurement. For example, the tongue and part of the mandible or larynx may be removed in patients with head and neck cancers (see Chapter 26). Following some cancer surgeries, the removal of the affected area can cause significant changes in appearance or activity level. Patients may need supportive care and help in adapting to their new normal.

❖ Interprofessional Collaborative Care

The overall care needs following surgery for cancer are similar to the care required for patients who undergo surgery for other reasons (see Chapter 9). Additional priority care needs are psychosocial support and helping the patient achieve maximum functioning after surgery.

Cancer treatment often begins shortly after the diagnosis, before the patient and family have time to adjust to a cancer diagnosis. The stress of the diagnosis can have a significant impact on the patient's and family's ability to understand any teaching provided. The nurse should continually assess the patient's understanding of the disease process and treatment plan. Assessment of the patient's and family's ability to cope with the cancer diagnosis, the planned treatment, and the potential changes in body image and role is crucial. For example, surgery involving the reproductive organs, urinary tract, colon, or rectum may permanently damage these organs, resulting in changes or losses that have an impact on sexual expression or control of elimination.

Coordinate with the interprofessional team to provide support and assistance to the patient and his or her family. Encourage the patient and family to ask questions and express their concerns. Help the patient accept changes in appearance or function by allowing them to participate in their care. Provide information about support groups such as those sponsored by the ACS (www.cancer.org) and the Canadian Cancer Society (www.cancer.ca). Some organizations also have support groups for patients' spouses, caregivers, and children and may provide peer support from cancer survivors who have coped with the same cancer or concerns. Such visits can help show the patient that many aspects of life can be the same after cancer treatment. For patients who have anxiety or depression as a result of the cancer experience, initiation of drug therapy and/or inclusion of a mental health professional as part of the interprofessional team may be warranted. Nurses are uniquely positioned to assess and intervene on behalf of the patient.

Physical rehabilitation to improve physical functioning may be indicated before or after cancer surgery. For example, a modified radical mastectomy for breast cancer can lead to shoulder muscle weakness and reduced arm function on the affected side. Performing specific exercises can reduce functional loss. Teaching patients about the importance of performing the exercises to regain as much function as possible and prevent complications is an important nursing function. Even though therapy can be painful and challenging, the patient needs encouragement to perform the expected activities. Head and neck cancer surgery often requires speech therapy to improve swallowing and speech. The physical therapist, occupational therapist, and speech-language pathologist coordinate with other members of the interprofessional team to plan strategies individualized to each patient to regain or maintain optimal function. Research indicates that patients have improved quality of life when exercises and support are provided before surgery (Chou et al., 2018).

The role of surgery in cancer care continues to change. Laparoscopic and robotic-assisted surgeries can decrease incision and healing time. Regardless of the surgical approach, nurses have a critical role in the patient's recovery after surgery, such as reinforcing the importance of early mobility, pain management, and prevention of infection.

The use of surgery in combination with other treatments has increased and can include intraoperative radiation therapy, the placement of a radioactive source, or the administration of chemotherapy into a body cavity. Other surgical procedures include placement of central lines for long-term IV access or electronic pumps for pain control or administration of chemotherapy.

RADIATION THERAPY

Overview

Radiation therapy uses high-energy radiation to kill cancer cells, with the intent to cure or relieve symptoms (palliative). The goal of radiation is to kill the cancer cells while having minimal damaging effects on the surrounding normal tissue.

The effects of radiation are seen only in tissues within the radiation field or path, and radiation is considered a *local* treatment. For example, radiation to the chest for lung cancer causes skin changes and hair loss only on the chest area that is treated. Occasionally, systemic radiation therapy uses an intravenous radioactive substance that travels throughout the body to target cancerous cells. Radiation therapy has both short- and long-term effects, depending on the area(s) radiated. For example, a short-term effect is redness or desquamation of the skin, whereas a long-term effect can be pulmonary fibrosis from radiation of the chest.

When cancer cells are exposed to radiation, the cell's DNA is damaged directly, resulting in a change in ***cellular regulation.*** These damaged cells usually can no longer reproduce or function, leading to cell death. Normal cells in the field of radiation are also affected by radiation. Careful planning of the radiation field by a radiation physicist, dosimetrist, and radiation oncologist is necessary to minimize damage to normal tissues and organs.

The amount of radiation delivered to a tissue is the **exposure**; the amount of radiation absorbed by the tissue is the **radiation dose**. The dose is always less than the exposure because some energy is lost as it travels to the destination. The three factors determining the absorbed dose are the *intensity* of exposure, the *duration* of exposure, and the *closeness* (distance) of the radiation source to the cells. Absorbed radiation doses are described in units called **grays** (Gy). The total dose of radiation used depends on tumor size and location and on the sensitivity of the tumor and nearby tissues.

Radiation therapy usually is given as a series of divided doses (fractionation) over a set time. This allows greater destruction of cancer cells while reducing the damage to normal tissues.

The intensity of the radiation decreases with the increasing distance from the radiation source.

! NURSING SAFETY PRIORITY QSEN

Action Alert

When a nurse is caring for a patient undergoing radiation treatment, there are precautions that the nurse needs to take. Using the general guidelines below, the nurse reduces exposure to ionizing radiation.

- *Time* is length of exposure to the radiation field. Try to coordinate care to limit time directly at the radiation source.
- *Distance* is how far from the radiation source you remain. The farther away from the radiation source, the less exposure.
- *Shielding* is using a material (such as a lead apron) to avoid exposure.

From Center for Nuclear Science and Technology Information. (2018). *Protecting against exposure*. http://nuclearconnect.org/know-nuclear/science/protecting

Radiation may be used as a stand-alone treatment or may be combined with other cancer treatments. Combining treatments requires careful planning of sequencing, timing, and dose of each treatment to maximize tumor kill and limit damage to normal cells. Combining radiation with chemotherapy involves giving chemotherapy agents that radiosensitize the tumor to enhance the radiation damage. This will result in a greater cell kill than either therapy used alone. Side effects of combined therapy can be more severe and may require more frequent interventions.

Radiation Delivery Methods and Devices

Radiation cancer treatment can be delivered by external beam or internal devices (brachytherapy). The treatment plan depends on the patient's general health and on the shape, size, and location of the tumor.

External beam is radiation delivered from a source outside of the patient. Since the radioactive source is external, the patient is not radioactive, and there is no hazard to others around the patient once the treatment is complete. The technique called *intensity-modulated radiation therapy* (IMRT) reduces the amount of normal tissue exposed to radiation by breaking up the single beam into thousands of smaller beams, allowing differing intensities to be delivered to specific areas of the tumor. Stereotactic body radiation therapy (SBRT) uses three-dimensional tumor imaging to identify the exact tumor location, which allows precise delivery of higher radiation doses and spares more of the surrounding tissue. Usually the total dosage is delivered in one to five separate treatment sessions. Other specialized radiation application techniques used in combination with surgery are known as *radiosurgery.* This type of treatment uses ionizing radiation as the surgical instrument instead of a cutting blade. Examples are the Gamma Knife and the CyberKnife, which are used for the treatment of brain tumors by carefully aiming the radiation target point within the brain, sparing normal brain tissue.

Regardless of the delivery method, the exact tumor location is first determined, and the skin is marked for therapy precision. The markings may be small "tattoos" that are ink outlines on the skin; if the tumor is in the head or extremities, a mesh mask will be made to hold the patient in the exact same position for every treatment (Fig. 20.1). Radiation oncology therapists ensure the patient's ability to get into and maintain this position during the radiation treatment.

Brachytherapy is also known as internal radiation therapy. The radiation source (seeds, ribbons, or capsules) comes into direct, continuous contact with the tumor for a specific time period. This method provides a higher dose of radiation in the tumor over a specified time period, while limiting the dose in surrounding normal tissues.

NURSING SAFETY PRIORITY (QSEN)

Action Alert

Ingested isotopes enter body fluids and eventually are eliminated in waste products. These wastes are radioactive, and you must ensure that they are not directly touched by anyone. Handle the wastes according to guidelines established by the institution. During hospitalization for radiation, pregnant women and children are not allowed to visit the patient. After the isotope has been completely eliminated from the body, neither the patient nor the body wastes are radioactive.

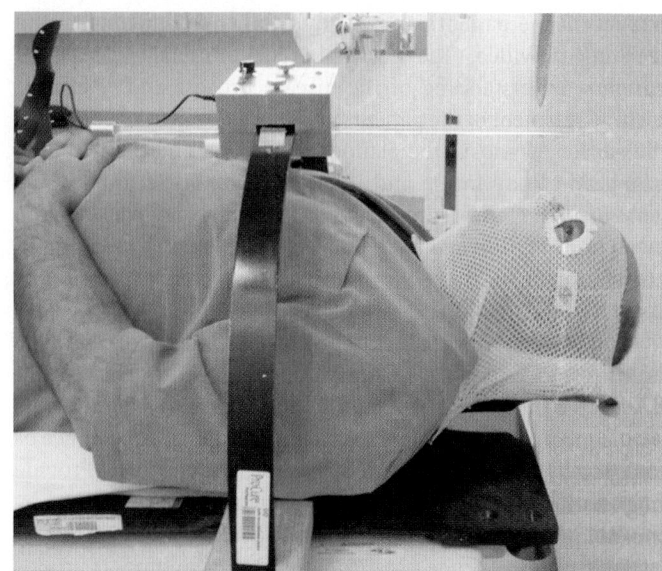

Fig. 20.1 Radiation mask. (From Hartsell, W.F., Kapur, R., Hartsell, S.O., Sweeney, P., Lopes, C., Duggal, A., et al. [2016]. Feasibility of proton beam therapy for ocular melanoma using a novel 3D Treatment planning technique. *International Journal of Radiation Oncology*Biology*Physics, 95*[1], 353–359.)

Brachytherapy uses radioactive isotopes either in solid form or within body fluids. This may include placement of an external catheter in the tumor bed where the radiation is placed or it may involve ingestion of a radioactive source. An example of ingestion is the use of iodine-131 (^{131}I) used to treat some thyroid cancers. The external radiation source is placed in a catheter and then removed after the correct length of treatment. The patient emits radiation for a period of time while being irradiated and is a potential hazard to others during that time. Once the source is removed, the patient is no longer considered radioactive.

Solid radiation sources are implanted within or near the tumor. These sources can be temporary or permanent and emit continuous, low-energy radiation. Some implants (e.g., seeds) can be placed into the tumor and stay in place by themselves. Seeds are so small and the half-life of the isotope is so short that this device is permanently left in place (often for prostate cancer) and over time completely loses its radioactivity. Some sources must be held in place with special applicators during therapy. While the solid implants are in place, the patient emits radiation, but excreta are not radioactive. The patient poses a hazard to others, but the excreta do not.

Traditional implants deliver low-dose-rate (LDR) radiation continuously, and patients may be hospitalized for several days. High-dose-rate (HDR) implant radiation is another delivery type. The patient comes into the radiation therapy department several times a week, and a stronger radiation implant is placed within a catheter near the cancer bed for short duration. The patient is radioactive only when the implant is in place. Refer to the Best Practice for Patient Safety & Quality Care: Care of the Patient With Sealed Implants of Radioactive Sources box for the care of the patient with a sealed radiation implant.

BEST PRACTICE FOR PATIENT SAFETY & QUALITY CARE QSEN

Care of the Patient With Sealed Implants of Radioactive Sources

- Assign the patient to a private room with a private bath.
- Place a "Caution: Radioactive Material" sign on the door of the patient's room.
- If portable lead shields are used, place them between the patient and the door.
- Keep the door to the patient's room closed as much as possible.
- Wear a dosimeter film badge at all times while caring for patients with radioactive implants. The badge offers no protection but measures a person's exposure to radiation. Each person caring for the patient should have a separate dosimeter to calculate his or her specific radiation exposure.
- Wear a lead apron while providing care. Always keep the front of the apron facing the source of radiation (do not turn your back toward the patient).
- If you are attempting to conceive, do not perform direct patient care, regardless of whether you are male or female.
- Nurses who are pregnant should not care for these patients; do not allow women who are pregnant or children younger than 16 years to visit.
- Limit each visitor to 1 half-hour per day. Be sure visitors stay at least 6 feet from the source.
- Never touch the radioactive source with bare hands. In the rare instance that it is dislodged, use long-handled forceps to retrieve it. Deposit the radioactive source in the lead container kept in the patient's room.
- After the source is removed, dispose of dressings and linens in the usual manner. Other equipment can be removed from the room at any time without special precautions and does not pose a hazard to other people.

NCLEX EXAMINATION CHALLENGE 20.1

Safe and Effective Care Environment

A client with prostate cancer is receiving external beam radiation for treatment. What teaching will the nurse provide following the radiation treatment?

A. "After the treatment, there is no radiation hazard to others."
B. "Do not share a bathroom with your spouse for 2 days."
C. "Visitors should be limited to 30 minutes to avoid prolonged radiation exposure."
D. "Report a temperature of 99.1°F to the primary health care provider."

Side Effects of Radiation Therapy

Radiation therapy can result in both acute and long-term side effects (Table 20.2). These side effects vary according to the radiation site and largely are limited to the areas exposed to radiation. Changes to the skin, known as *radiation dermatitis*, are the most common side effect of radiotherapy and can range from redness and rash to skin desquamation (Lucas et al., 2018). Multiple factors, including total radiation dose, duration of radiation, and whether concurrent chemotherapy is prescribed, can affect skin response to radiation. Radiation to the head may result in permanent hair loss.

Some systemic side effects such as altered taste, fatigue, and bone marrow suppression may also occur. Fatigue may be related to the increased energy demands needed to repair damaged cells. Radiation-induced fatigue can be debilitating and may last for months. Some degree of bone marrow suppression and reduced ***immunity*** occurs, regardless of the treatment site. The intensity of marrow suppression is related to the dose, site, and size of the area irradiated.

TABLE 20.2 Acute and Late Site-Specific Effects of Radiation Therapy

Acute Effects	Late Effects
Brain	**Subcutaneous and Soft Tissue**
• Alopecia and dermatitis of the scalp	• Radiation-induced fibrosis
• Ear and external auditory canal irritation	**Central Nervous System**
• Cerebral edema and increased intracranial pressure	• Brain necrosis
• Nausea and vomiting	• Leukoencephalopathy
• Blurry vision	• Cognitive and emotional dysfunction
Head and Neck	• Pituitary and hypothalamic dysfunction
• Oral mucositis	• Spinal cord myelopathies
• Taste changes	**Head and Neck**
• Oral candidiasis, herpes, or other infections	• Xerostomia and dental caries
• Acute xerostomia	• Trismus
• Dental caries	• Osteoradionecrosis
• Esophagitis and pharyngitis	• Hypothyroidism
Breast and Chest Wall	**Lung**
• Skin reactions	• Pulmonary fibrosis
• Esophagitis	**Heart**
Chest and Lung	• Pericarditis
• Esophagitis and pharyngitis	• Cardiomyopathy
• Taste changes	• Coronary artery disease
• Pneumonia	**Breast/Chest Wall**
• Cough	• Atrophy, fibrosis of breast tissue
Abdomen and Pelvis	• Lymphedema
• Anorexia	**Abdomen and Pelvis**
• Nausea and vomiting	• Small and large bowel injury
• Diarrhea	• Diarrhea
• Cystitis or proctitis	
• Vaginal dryness/vaginitis	
• Sexual and fertility problems	
Eye	
• Conjunctival edema and tearing	

Radiation damage to normal tissues during therapy can start inflammatory responses that lead to tissue fibrosis and scarring. These effects may appear years after radiation treatment. Because radiation can damage and mutate normal cell DNA, which disrupts ***cellular regulation,*** radiation therapy increases the risk for development of second malignancies.

Not all patients experience the same degree of side effects to normal tissues, even when receiving the same dose of radiation therapy.

❖ Interprofessional Collaborative Care

Patients and family members are anxious about radiation and look to the nurse and radiation technician to explain the treatment specifics and side effects of radiation therapy. Accurate information about radiation therapy helps patients cope with the treatment.

Skin in the radiation path becomes dry and itchy and may break down. Teaching patients about skin care needs during radiation therapy is a priority intervention. Instruct the patient not to remove temporary ink markings when cleaning the skin until radiation therapy is completed. There are no universal evidence-based interventions for skin care during radiation therapy. It is important to teach patients to avoid skin irritation and friction from clothing. Avoiding deodorant and lotions on the day of treatments may be warranted depending on the location being treated.

Good skin hygiene involves washing the irradiated area with mild soap and water and avoiding skin scrubbing. Limited evidence supports the use of any lotion or ointment to decrease radiation dermatitis (Bauer, 2016). The Patient and Family Education: Preparing for Self-Management: Skin Protection During Radiation Therapy box provides an example of an established skin-care protocol during external radiation therapy.

! NURSING SAFETY PRIORITY QSEN

Action Alert

Skin in the radiation path becomes *photosensitive,* increasing the risk for sunburn and sun damage. Advise against direct skin exposure to the sun during treatment and for at least 1 year after completion of radiation therapy.

The normal tissues most sensitive to radiation are bone marrow cells, skin, mucous membranes, hair follicles, and germ cells (ova and sperm). When possible, these tissues are shielded from radiation during therapy. The long-term problems of radiation vary with the location and dose received (see Table 20.2). For example, radiation to the throat and upper chest can cause difficulty in swallowing and can lead to reduced oral intake and weight loss. Head and neck radiation may damage the salivary glands and cause dry mouth (xerostomia), which has a negative impact on speaking, chewing, and swallowing, and increases the patient's lifelong risk for tooth decay.

PATIENT AND FAMILY EDUCATION: PREPARING FOR SELF-MANAGEMENT

Skin Protection During Radiation Therapy

- Wash the irradiated area gently each day with either water or a mild soap and water as prescribed by your radiation therapy team. Rinse soap thoroughly from your skin.
- Avoid friction to the area being treated. Use your hand rather than a washcloth.
- If ink or dye markings are present to identify exactly where the beam of radiation is to be focused, take care not to remove them.
- Dry the treatment area with patting rather than rubbing motions; use a clean, soft towel or cloth.
- Use only powders, ointments, lotions, or creams that are prescribed by the radiation oncology department on your skin at the radiation site.
- Wear soft clothing over the skin at the radiation site.
- Avoid wearing belts, buckles, straps, or any type of clothing that binds or rubs the skin at the radiation site.
- Avoid exposure of the irradiated area to the sun:
- Protect this area by wearing clothing over it.
- Try to go outdoors in the early morning or evening to avoid the more intense sun rays.
- When outdoors, stay under awnings, umbrellas, and other forms of shade during the times when the sun's rays are most intense (10 a.m. to 4 p.m.).
- Avoid heat exposure.

Interventions such as saliva-substitute sprays, lozenges, and mouth rinses may be helpful. Teach patients that regular dental visits are essential. Bone exposed to radiation therapy is less dense and breaks more easily. Fatigue remains a common and often persistent problem during and for some time after radiation therapy. Exercise and sleep interventions have shown some benefit in reducing fatigue. Teach about the symptoms that might be expected based on the specific location and dose of radiation (see Table 20.1 for the location of information within this text for different cancer types).

NCLEX EXAMINATION CHALLENGE 20.2

Safe and Effective Care Environment

A client receiving radiation for head and neck cancer reports that the skin in the radiation field is itching and painful. What teaching will the nurse provide? **Select all that apply.**

A. "This is likely from medication, not the radiation treatment."
B. "Cover the area with soft clothing."
C. "Be sure to wash your hands well before touching the area."
D. "Sunlight to the radiated area can help the skin heal."
E. "Use a washcloth to thoroughly clean the area with soap and water."
F. "Do not remove the ink markings on the skin."

CYTOTOXIC SYSTEMIC THERAPY

Cytotoxic systemic therapy refers to the use of antineoplastic (**chemotherapy**) drugs that are used to kill cancer cells and disrupt their ***cellular regulation.*** Chemotherapy may be used as the only cancer treatment received, before or after other treatments, or in combination with other cancer treatments. Unlike surgery or radiation, cytotoxic chemotherapy kills cancer cells (and normal cells) throughout the body. Some areas of the body, such as the blood-brain barrier, are difficult for chemotherapy agents to penetrate.

Depending on the plan of care, chemotherapy agents may be used to shrink a tumor before surgery or radiation. This is called *neoadjuvant chemotherapy.* When chemotherapy is used to kill remaining cancer cells following surgery or radiation, it is known as *adjuvant chemotherapy.*

PATIENT-CENTERED CARE: GENETIC/GENOMIC CONSIDERATIONS QSEN

Precision medicine is revolutionizing cancer care, and great potential exists to cure more types of cancer, increase survival, and improve overall patient care (Brant & Mayer, 2017). Genomic profiling allows a more individualized approach to treatment selection and side effect management. In addition, checking the genetic profile of the tumor can determine its sensitivity to various chemotherapy and targeted therapy agents. This practice individualizes cancer treatment and improves outcomes. Treatment can now be based on the specific genetic makeup for a given patient rather than on a tumor type or stage of disease. Pharmacogenomics allows the health care team to look at genetic mutations that may influence the way one responds to pharmacologic agents and prescribe medications tailored to a specific patient's genes.

Selection of specific agents is based on tumor type, tumor markers, growth rate of cells (found on pathology report), and patient's performance status. Most of the cytotoxic agents are not cancer cell specific and thus affect all cells in the body. This effect is especially seen on rapidly dividing cells such as those in the bone marrow, GI tract, hair, and oral mucosa. The time when bone marrow activity and white blood cell counts are at their lowest levels after cytotoxic therapy is the **nadir**. It occurs at different times for different drugs, usually 7 to 10 days. To prevent greatly reduced ***immunity*** and immunosuppression, avoid using cytotoxic combinations with nadirs that occur at or near the same time. Patients undergoing chemotherapy are at high risk for infection, immunosuppression, and complications of treatment. Care of a neutropenic patient will be discussed in the side effects section of this chapter.

Chemotherapy

Overview. Chemotherapy, the treatment of cancer with chemical agents, is used to cure and to increase survival. This killing effect on cancer cells is related to the ability of chemotherapy to damage DNA and interfere with cell division and ***cellular regulation.*** Tumors with rapid growth are often more sensitive to chemotherapy.

As described in Chapter 19, cancer cells can separate from the original tumor and spread to surrounding areas and to distant sites within the body (metastasize). Treatment of patients with metastatic cancer is not considered to be of curative intent, but with newer treatment options, patients are living longer. Chemotherapy is useful in treating cancer because its effects are systemic, providing the opportunity to kill cancer cells, and it may provide protection from cells that have started to metastasize. Drugs used for chemotherapy also exert their cell-damaging (cytotoxic) effects on healthy cells. The normal cells most affected by chemotherapy are those that divide rapidly, including skin, hair, intestinal tissues, reproductive cells, and blood-forming cells.

Chemotherapy Drug Categories. Chemotherapy has many different categories and mechanisms of action specific to the way the drug kills the cell. Chemotherapy drugs can prevent cellular division, break DNA strands to prevent replication, impede cellular and enzyme reactions, and prevent mitosis. This prevents the cell from dividing, or limits division. See Table 20.3 for specific chemotherapy drug categories.

Combination Chemotherapy. *Combination chemotherapy* is using more than one drug for treatment of a specific cancer. Combination therapy is more effective in killing cancer cells than using just one drug because different mechanisms of action work together to affect cell division. However, the side effects and damage caused to normal tissues also increase with combination chemotherapy.

Treatment Issues. Drugs selected for use with a given patient are based on the sensitivity of cancer cells to the drug and the stage or extent of disease. Selected treatment protocols have been developed for many cancers through use of well-established clinical guidelines for initial treatment and relapsed

TABLE 20.3 Categories of Chemotherapeutic Drugs

Drug Categories	Nursing Implications
Antimetabolites Closely resemble normal metabolites and act as "counterfeit" metabolites that fool cancer cells into using the antimetabolites in cellular reactions.	
Some examples are: • Azacitidine • Capecitabine (oral) • Cytarabine • Decitabine • 5-Fluorouracil • Gemcitabine	• Used for some bone marrow and GI cancers. • Risk of neutropenia is high. • Patient education and assessment are crucial. • Patient will be prone to diarrhea.
Antitumor Antibiotics Damage the cell's DNA and interrupt DNA or RNA synthesis. The exact mechanism of interruption varies with each agent.	
Some examples are: • Bleomycin • Daunorubicin • Doxorubicin • Doxorubicin liposomal • Epirubicin	• Lifetime maximum dosage for these agents. • Cardiac and pulmonary toxicity can occur. • Additional monitoring of ejection fraction or pulmonary function tests are required. • These agents are vesicants and can cause severe tissue damage with extravasation.
Antimitotics/Mitosis Inhibitors Interfere with the formation and actions of microtubules so cells cannot complete mitosis during cell division.	
Some examples are: • Docetaxel • Paclitaxel • Vinblastine • Vincristine • Vinorelbine	• May cause peripheral neuropathy. • Patients may experience extreme constipation, and an aggressive bowel regimen may be required.
Alkylating Agents Cross-link DNA, making the DNA strands bind tightly together. This action prevents proper DNA and ribonucleic acid (RNA) synthesis, which inhibits cell division.	
Some examples are: • Carboplatin • Cisplatin • Cyclophosphamide • Dacarbazine • Ifosfamide • Temozolomide (oral)	• May cause peripheral neuropathy. • May cause renal failure if not adequately hydrated. • May cause severe nausea and vomiting.
Topoisomerase Inhibitors Disrupt an enzyme (topoisomerase) essential for DNA synthesis and cell division. When drugs disrupt the enzyme, proper DNA maintenance is prevented, resulting in increased DNA breakage and eventual cell death.	
• Irinotecan • Topotecan	• May cause significant diarrhea.
Miscellaneous Agents Have mechanisms of action that either are unknown or do not fit those of other drug categories.	
• Arsenic trioxide • Hydroxyurea (oral)	• Side effects are based on specific drug profile. • Usually used for blood, bone marrow, and lymph system cancers.

Data from the U.S. Food and Drug Administration website at www.fda.gov/cder/index.html.

disease (National Comprehensive Cancer Network [NCCN] guidelines). Dosages for most chemotherapy drugs are calculated according to the patient's size, based on milligrams per square meter (mg/m^2) of body surface area (BSA). This is a calculation of the patient's height and weight at the time of chemotherapy administration. Dosages may change if the patient experiences significant weight loss between cycles.

Chemotherapy drugs are given on a regularly scheduled basis timed to maximize cancer cell kill and minimize damage to normal cells. Regimens vary in frequency between days, weeks, and number of cycles depending on which protocol is selected. The intent is to allow normal cells time to recover from any injury but prevent cancer cell recovery. **Dose-dense chemotherapy** protocols involve giving chemotherapy rounds closer together, supplemented with bone marrow growth factors to prevent neutropenia. Dose-dense therapy also results in more intense side effects. *Maintaining the intended dosage and timing schedule to ensure that the patient receives the maximum recommended doses is a critical factor in the successful response to chemotherapy and overall survival.*

Patient and family education is critical in helping patients adhere to the prescribed schedule for best outcomes, managing side effects, and preventing therapy complications. Side effects of chemotherapy are generally managed in the home. Nurses are uniquely positioned to educate, reinforce self-care measures, and evaluate interventions to help patients maintain the best quality of life during treatment.

Many chemotherapy drugs are given IV, although other routes may be used. For specific cancer types, the chemotherapy may be infused or instilled into a body cavity. The *intrathecal* route delivers drugs into the cerebrospinal fluid (CSF). *Intraperitoneal* instillations place the drugs within the abdominal cavity, most often for ovarian cancer. Drugs for bladder cancer can be instilled directly into the bladder (*intravesicular* route). In some instances drugs may be applied as a *topical* preparation for skin lesions. *Intra-arterial* infusions may be used to deliver a higher dose locally. For example, with liver tumors an interventional radiologist places a catheter into the artery supplying the liver tumor. The concentrated chemotherapy drug, delivered in sponge-like beads, is infused, and the beads become trapped in the small arteries feeding the tumor. Regardless of the route, chemotherapy agents are designated hazardous drugs (HDs) and must be handled as such.

The standard of care designated by the Oncology Nursing Society (ONS) and supported by the American Society of Clinical Oncology (ASCO) for safe administration of IV chemotherapy is that giving these drugs requires special education and handling (Neuss et al., 2017; Oncology Nursing Society, 2017). *Chemotherapy is to be given only by registered nurses who have completed an approved chemotherapy program and have demonstrated competence in administering these agents. However, responsibility for monitoring the patient during chemotherapy administration rests with all nurses providing patient care.*

Chemotherapy drugs can absorbed through the skin and mucous membranes. As a result the nurses and pharmacists who prepare or give these drugs are at risk for absorbing them. Anyone preparing, giving, or disposing of chemotherapy drugs or handling excreta from patients within 48 hours of receiving IV chemotherapy must wear approved personal protective equipment (PPE) (Neuss et al., 2017). Such equipment includes eye protection, masks, double gloves or "chemo" gloves, and nonpermeable gown. The Occupational Safety and Health Administration (OSHA) and the Oncology Nursing Society (ONS) have established practice guidelines and protective standards (OSHA, n.d.; ONS, 2018).

A serious complication of IV infusion is **extravasation**, which occurs when drug leaks into the surrounding tissues (also called *infiltration*). When the drugs given are **vesicants** (chemicals that damage tissue on direct contact), the results of extravasation can include pain, infection, and tissue loss (Fig. 20.2). Reconstructive surgery is sometimes warranted for severe tissue damage.

Monitoring of blood return at the access site during the infusion at regular intervals is critical during chemotherapy administration to prevent extravasation. Institutions have established evidence-based policies and procedures that are drug specific to guide extravasation management. With some drugs, cold compresses to the area are prescribed; for other agents warm compresses are used. Antidotes may be injected into the site of extravasation. Coordinate with the oncologist and pharmacist to determine the specific antidote needed for the extravasated drug. When vesicants are part of therapy, the use of an implanted port or central line to decrease extravasation risk is highly recommended. Even with these devices, the nurse must observe closely for any indication of leakage, pain, or swelling and initiate management guidelines immediately.

Many anticancer drugs are available currently as oral agents, and more are in development. Oral drugs are more convenient for the patient and can be taken at home. However, oral

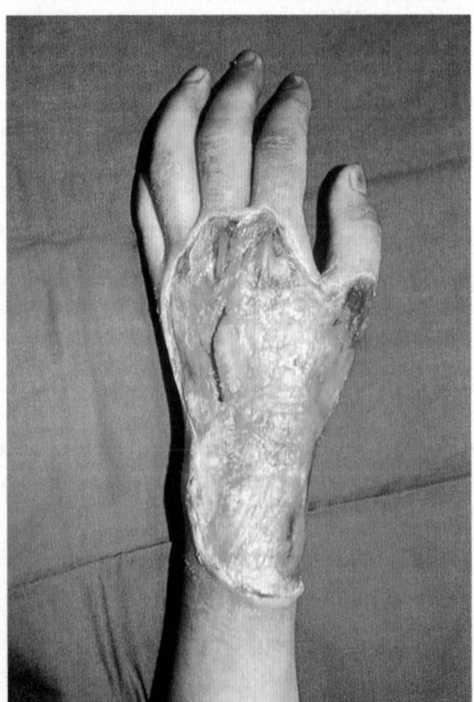

Fig. 20.2 Appearance of tissue damage and loss after chemotherapy extravasation. (From Weinzweig, J., & Weinzweig, N. [2005]. *The mutilated hand.* St. Louis: Mosby.)

regimens are not without challenges. A big misperception by patients and nononcology nurses is that oral anticancer drugs are less toxic than IV chemotherapy. This is *not* true. *Oral anticancer drugs are just as toxic to the patient taking the drug and to the person handling the drug as are IV chemotherapy agents.* The responsibility for administering these drugs often shifts from the oncology clinic to the home or to nononcology acute care settings, and issues of home storage, accurate administration, adherence to prescribed schedule, and recognition and management of side effects are major concerns. There is a critical need for patient and family education and support to self-manage this therapy, as patients are responsible for administration, rather than coming to the clinic for an infusion.

Because these oral agents can be absorbed through skin and mucous membranes and exert toxic effects, the person who handles and administers them needs to use PPE in the same way as during IV chemotherapy administration. *Oral agents must not be crushed, split, broken, or chewed.* These drugs are biohazardous and must be discarded in accordance with agency policy.

This becomes a more critical issue when nononcology nurses are administering the drugs. The Oncology Nursing Society (ONS) stresses nursing education for competence in the administration of chemotherapy drugs (ONS, 2017). All nurses administering these drugs must know the indications for drug use, dosage ranges, side effects and adverse effects, schedules, and specific precautions.

In the home environment, it is important that the patient and family understand the importance of avoiding direct skin contact with oral chemotherapy agents and how to dispose of the medication properly. Teach patients or whoever prepares the dosages how to avoid touching the drugs. Tablets and capsules in blister packs are pressed into a small paper cup. Those in traditional medication bottles are "poured" first into the bottle cap and then into a paper cup. The patient then "drinks" the tablet/capsule from the cup into his or her mouth. These drugs are to be stored separately from all other drugs. Consult a drug handbook or a pharmacist for timing of the drug in relation to meals and what to do if a dose is missed. For many of these oral drugs, missed doses are *not* taken when remembered. The patient just takes the next scheduled drug dose.

Disposal of expired or discontinued oral chemotherapy agents can be a challenge. Do not flush oral chemotherapy drugs in the toilet. These drugs should not be directly touched. Taking them to a community drug disposal event or the police station can be hazardous to others. Instruct the patient to take the expired or discontinued oral chemotherapy agents back to the dispensing pharmacy for disposal when possible.

Adherence to defined oral chemotherapy schedules and dosages is up to the patient or caregiver. Even some highly motivated patients with cancer can have difficulty remembering the dosing schedule. Many reasons such as lack of understanding, cost of medication, side effects, or simply forgetting can affect adherence to the prescribed regimen. Any disruption of the schedule or reduction of dosage can have a negative impact on therapy outcomes and lead to drug resistance among cancer cells, disease progression, and reduced survival. The Systems Thinking and Quality Improvement box describes the effectiveness of an electronic intervention in promoting adherence (Wu et al., 2018).

SYSTEMS THINKING AND QUALITY IMPROVEMENT QSEN

Use of a Smartphone to Improve Adherence to Oral Anticancer Agents

Wu, Y.P., Linder, L.A., Kanokvimankul, P., Fowler, B., Parsons, B.G., Macpherson, C.F., et al. (2018). Use of a smartphone application for prompting oral medication adherence among adolescents and young adults with cancer. *Oncology Nursing Forum, 45*(1), 69–76.

During the past 30 years, adolescents and young adults (AYAs) with cancer have experienced less improvement in survival than children or older adults with cancer. Suboptimal adherence to oral cancer therapy medications has been cited as a key contributor to adverse cancer outcomes, such as disease relapse. Reasons for nonadherence to oral medications include factors related to medications themselves (e.g., side effects, frequent or complex dosing), as well as factors particularly relevant to AYAs, such as forgetting, having lifestyle disruptions, and lacking physical and social support for taking medication. With frequent direct patient contact, nurses are well positioned to intervene with strategies that promote adherence to treatment.

The development of interventions to promote oral medication adherence among AYAs with cancer is an urgent priority because this type of resource is scarce and data to support clinical use are limited. The goal of the current study was to explore use of a smartphone medication reminder application to promote adherence to oral medication regimens among AYAs with cancer.

Eligible persons were able to participate in the 12-week study if they were aged 15 to 29 years, were receiving treatment for any type of cancer, and were receiving at least one outpatient scheduled oral chemotherapy or supportive care medication related to their cancer.

The mobile application provided visual and audible reminder notifications on the participant's phone based on individual medication dosing schedules entered by the participant. When participants received a medication reminder, they were offered the option of selecting "take dose now," "postpone," or "skip," and the reminder was adjusted accordingly. If participants chose to postpone the dose, they were prompted to enter the number of minutes until the medication reminder, and response options were provided again. More than half of the participants took the medication immediately when receiving the reminder notification.

A majority of the participants reported that the application was easy to use and helpful for improving adherence to their regimen.

Commentary: Implications for Research and Practice

As health care technologies such as alerts (i.e., automated emails and telephone calls) become standard practice and continue to evolve, such resources also could be leveraged and integrated into e-health interventions. E-health interventions provide a promising avenue for patient support. This includes improving medication adherence as well as follow-up care.

With further research, specific to improved overall outcomes, health care providers could introduce the use of such an application to patients as part of routine clinical care.

Side Effects of Chemotherapy. Temporary and permanent damage can occur to normal tissues from chemotherapy. Chemotherapy is systemic and exerts its effects on all cells within the body. Common Terminology for Cancer Adverse Events (CTCAE) has a standardized grading scale to evaluate and document common side effects (National Cancer Institute [NCI], 2018). Some problems include bladder toxicity (hemorrhagic cystitis), cardiac muscle damage, and loss of bone density. For some cancer drugs, agents that protect specific healthy cells (cytoprotectants or chemoprotectants) are given ahead of or with chemotherapy drugs to decrease the impact of these

PATIENT-CENTERED CARE: GENDER HEALTH CONSIDERATIONS QSEN

One significant issue that patients can experience with cancer treatment is the risk of infertility or sterility. For some cancers, surgical removal of the reproductive organs (testicles, uterus or ovaries), is required and will permanently eliminate the possibility of reproduction.

Chemotherapy and radiation can also cause fertility or family planning issues. Patients of childbearing age must abstain from conceiving or fathering children and must use reliable methods of birth control while in treatment. Female patients undergoing chemotherapy may not have a menstrual cycle but can still ovulate, so contraception is needed to prevent pregnancy. Chemotherapy can cause premature ovarian failure and early menopause, which can lead to fertility issues and long-term effects.

Young adults may need to place family planning on hold, which can have an impact on hopes and dreams. Nurses should discuss this topic with patients and evaluate their desire for a biologic family. It is important to inform patients of this risk and make appropriate referrals for sperm banking or fertility specialists, if time allows. Distress related to fertility may affect other areas of psychosocial functioning.

drugs on normal tissues. For example, mesna binds toxic metabolites to decrease bladder toxicity and prevent hemorrhagic cystitis from ifosfamide and high-dose cyclophosphamide use. Agents such as the anthracycline drug doxorubicin can result in cardiotoxicity, leading to heart failure and decreased ejection fraction (EF). Dexrazoxane can be prescribed to protect the heart. Loss of bone density is associated with the use of oral aromatase inhibitors for breast cancer treatment. These patients will require a vitamin D supplement or bisphosphonate therapy in an attempt to offset the known risk.

Serious short-term side effects occur with cytotoxic chemotherapy. The side effects on the hematopoietic (blood-producing) system can be life threatening and are the most common reason for changing the dosage or the treatment plan. The suppressive effects on the bone marrow blood-forming cells cause anemia (decreased numbers of red blood cells and hemoglobin); reduced ***immunity*** with **neutropenia** (decreased numbers of neutrophil white blood cells, leading to immunosuppression); and **thrombocytopenia** (decreased numbers of platelets), which leads to impaired ***clotting*** and bleeding. Common distressing side effects include nausea and vomiting, alopecia (hair loss), mucositis (open sores or ulcers on mucous membranes), skin changes, anxiety, sleep disturbance, altered bowel elimination, and changes in cognitive function. The impact of side effects can create distress, which can vary from patient to patient. Cancer symptom distress is measured using the National Comprehensive Cancer Network (NCCN) Distress Thermometer (Fig. 20.3). Assessing for distress is important to

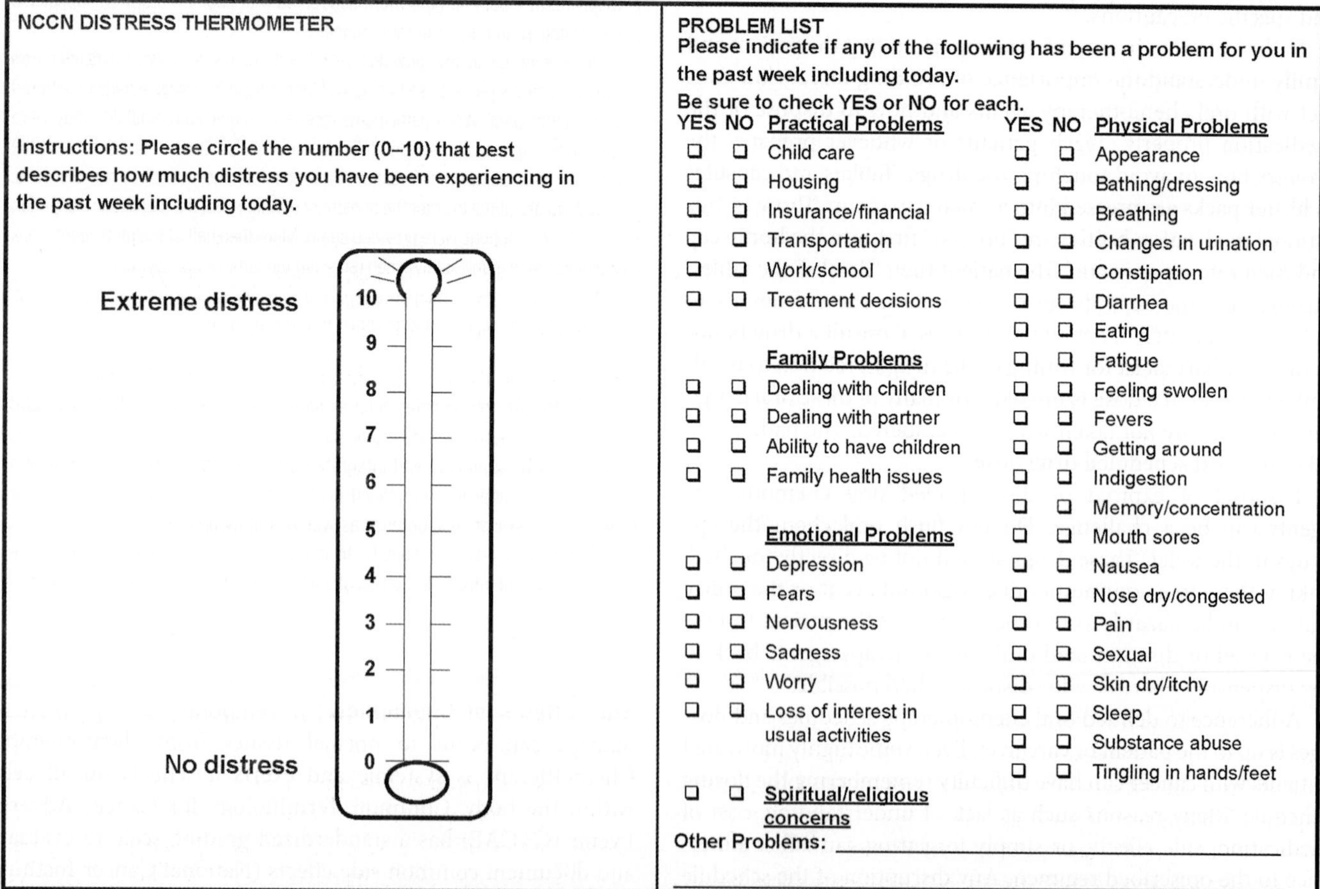

NCCN DISTRESS THERMOMETER

Instructions: Please circle the number (0–10) that best describes how much distress you have been experiencing in the past week including today.

PROBLEM LIST
Please indicate if any of the following has been a problem for you in the past week including today.
Be sure to check YES or NO for each.

YES	NO	Practical Problems
☐	☐	Child care
☐	☐	Housing
☐	☐	Insurance/financial
☐	☐	Transportation
☐	☐	Work/school
☐	☐	Treatment decisions
		Family Problems
☐	☐	Dealing with children
☐	☐	Dealing with partner
☐	☐	Ability to have children
☐	☐	Family health issues
		Emotional Problems
☐	☐	Depression
☐	☐	Fears
☐	☐	Nervousness
☐	☐	Sadness
☐	☐	Worry
☐	☐	Loss of interest in usual activities
☐	☐	**Spiritual/religious concerns**

YES	NO	Physical Problems
☐	☐	Appearance
☐	☐	Bathing/dressing
☐	☐	Breathing
☐	☐	Changes in urination
☐	☐	Constipation
☐	☐	Diarrhea
☐	☐	Eating
☐	☐	Fatigue
☐	☐	Feeling swollen
☐	☐	Fevers
☐	☐	Getting around
☐	☐	Indigestion
☐	☐	Memory/concentration
☐	☐	Mouth sores
☐	☐	Nausea
☐	☐	Nose dry/congested
☐	☐	Pain
☐	☐	Sexual
☐	☐	Skin dry/itchy
☐	☐	Sleep
☐	☐	Substance abuse
☐	☐	Tingling in hands/feet

Other Problems: ______________________

Fig. 20.3 The NCCN Distress Thermometer for patients.

allow for prompt symptom management and overall improvement in quality of life (NCCN, 2018).

Drug therapy is used to reduce symptom distress from some of these side effects. For other problems such as alopecia, no evidence-based prevention strategies exist, but patients can use techniques to be more comfortable with its presence. Nonpharmacologic interventions for symptom distress include distraction, massage, guided imagery, and complementary therapies, such as yoga.

Psychosocial issues can occur during chemotherapy. For many chemotherapy regimens, drugs are given over a period ranging from 30 minutes to 8 hours or longer. During this time the patient may be confined to a treatment area, which is a constant reminder of the disease and its treatment. Distraction methods such as virtual reality, guided imagery, reading, watching television, and talking with visitors may help reduce the sense of unpleasantness.

❖ Interprofessional Collaborative Care

The priority care issues during chemotherapy are protecting the patient from the life-threatening side effects and managing the associated distressing symptoms. For some patients the symptoms are so unpleasant that they choose to stop treatment. Nursing education and intervention are key to supporting the patient and helping manage side effects.

Bone Marrow Suppression. In addition to killing cancer cells, chemotherapy also destroys circulating blood cells and further reduces ***immunity*** by decreasing bone marrow activity. All circulating white and red blood cells and platelets are decreased. Reduced white blood cell numbers, especially neutrophils, greatly increase the risk for infection. Decreased red blood cells cause anemia, hypoxia, and fatigue, and decreased platelets impair ***clotting,*** leading to increased risk of bleeding.

Infection risk results from reduced ***immunity*** with neutropenia, placing the patient at risk for sepsis. *Reduced immunity is the greatest dose-limiting side effect of chemotherapy and can lead to death if sepsis is not managed appropriately and in a timely manner.* Many chemotherapy drugs cause myelosuppression to some degree and decrease the patient's natural responses to infection. Neutropenia is temporary, and immunity usually recovers within weeks after chemotherapy completion. The risk of potential infection is a serious concern of treatment. *Most infections during neutropenia result from overgrowth of the patient's own normal flora (microbiome) and entrance of these organisms into the bloodstream.* Common infections can be fungal, bacterial, and viral in nature. Reactivation of dormant viruses in the body such as *varicella* can occur. Diagnosed infections are managed with anti-infective drugs such as antibiotic, antifungal, and antiviral drugs. Just as for any other infection, anti-infective therapy is specific for the organism(s) causing the infection.

Impaired ***immunity*** with increased infection risk can be managed, and prevented, with the use of growth factors to stimulate bone marrow production of granulocytes. Although not appropriate for all types of cancer, this supportive treatment can reduce the risk for infection during chemotherapy.

PATIENT-CENTERED CARE: OLDER ADULT CONSIDERATIONS QSEN

Older adults are at even greater risk for treatment-related complications and exacerbations of pre-existing comorbidities.

Caring for the older adult receiving cancer treatment is challenging because physiologic changes with aging and comorbidities may affect the ability to tolerate treatment and recover following treatment. Goals of care can include medication management, maintaining functional status, and managing cardiac, pulmonary, and diabetes processes (Goldberg et al., 2018).

NURSING SAFETY PRIORITY QSEN

Action Alert

The priority interventions for the patient with neutropenia are protecting him or her from infection within the health care system and teaching the patient and family how to reduce infection risk in the home. Total patient assessment, including a review of common symptoms associated with infection (e.g., fever, sore throat, urinary frequency or discomfort, purulent drainage), skin and mucous membrane inspection, lung sounds, and inspection of venous access device insertion sites, must be performed routinely or as often as agency policy and the patient's condition warrant by a registered nurse for hospitalized patients. Review the patient's laboratory work, monitoring for decreased neutrophil count. Notify the primary health care provider if the neutrophil count decreases; additional precautions, growth factors, or antibiotics may be required. Additional education is required for the patient taking oral chemotherapy at home because the patient needs to understand the signs of infection and when to contact the primary health care provider.

Explain to the patient the importance of reporting fever, signs and symptoms of infection, any change in skin and mucous membranes, including rash, or other changes in health status. Also teach him or her to report a cough, burning on urination, pain around the venous access site, or new drainage from a wound or any area of the body. Monitoring for indicators of infection is critical for the patient with neutropenia. The reduced numbers of neutrophils can limit the presence of common infection symptoms. Often the patient with neutropenia does not develop a high fever or have purulent drainage even when a severe infection is present. A patient with neutropenia is at risk for sepsis, which is an oncologic emergency, and can be life threatening.

Good handwashing before contact with the patient is essential for infection prevention. Use aseptic technique with any invasive procedure. Review the Best Practice for Patient Safety & Quality Care: Care of the Patient With Myelosuppression and Neutropenia.

Hospital units specializing in care of patients with impaired ***immunity*** and neutropenia often have standard protocols that nurses initiate as soon as infection is suspected, because treatment delay can result in sepsis and death. These protocols specify which types of cultures to obtain (e.g., blood, urine, sputum, central line, wound), which diagnostic tests to obtain (e.g., chest x-ray), and which antibiotics to start immediately. It is crucial to draw blood cultures *before* starting antibiotics.

BEST PRACTICE FOR PATIENT SAFETY & QUALITY CARE QSEN

Care of the Patient With Myelosuppression and Neutropenia

- Place the patient in a private room whenever possible.
- Use good handwashing technique or alcohol-based hand rubs before touching the patient or any of the patient's belongings.
- Ensure that the patient's room and bathroom are cleaned at least once each day.
- Limit the number of health care personnel entering the patient's room.
- Monitor vital signs every 4 hours, including temperature.
- Inspect the patient's skin and mucous membranes for the presence of fissures and abscesses per facility policy.
- Inspect IV sites for indications of infection.
- Change wound dressings daily or as ordered.
- Use strict aseptic technique for all invasive procedures.
- Promptly notify the primary health care provider if any area appears infected and obtain order for culture, per protocol.
- Encourage activity at a level appropriate for the patient's current health status.
- Keep frequently used equipment in the room for use with this patient only (e.g., blood pressure cuff, stethoscope, thermometer).
- Visitors with signs or symptoms of illness should be restricted.
- Monitor the white blood cell count daily.
- Avoid the use of indwelling urinary catheters if possible. Provide perineal hygiene per protocol and at least daily.
- Follow agency policy for restriction of fresh flowers and potted plants in the patient's room.

When delegating any nursing care activity to assistive personnel (AP), teach the importance of protecting the neutropenic patient from infection. Stress the ways that cross-contamination can occur and how to avoid this source of infection. Also, ensure that AP understand that even when the neutropenic patient is very tired and does not feel well, certain aspects of personal hygiene cannot be deferred.

NCLEX EXAMINATION CHALLENGE 20.3

Safe and Effective Care Environment

The nurse is observing the assistive personnel (AP) provide care to a client who is neutropenic. Which action by the AP requires the nurse to intervene?

A. Performing a bed bath because the client is too tired to get in the shower
B. Using the unit mobile blood pressure machine to assess the client's vitals
C. Using alcohol-based hand foam before touching the client
D. Cleaning the client's bathroom with disinfectant

! NURSING SAFETY PRIORITY QSEN

Critical Rescue

Monitor patients with reduced *immunity* to recognize signs of infection. When any temperature elevation (above 100.4°F or 38°C) is present, respond by reporting this to the primary health care provider immediately and implement standard infection protocols. When IV anti-infective drugs are started, the neutropenic patient is admitted to the hospital. The patient with neutropenia does *not* pose an infection risk to other people; however, other people can be an infection risk to the patient.

Many patients remain at home during periods of neutropenia and are at continuing risk for infection. The focus remains on keeping the patient's own normal flora under control and preventing transmission of organisms from others. Teach patients and families self-care actions to reduce the risk for infection, especially handwashing. See the Patient and Family Education: Preparing for Self-Management: Prevention of Infection box.

NCLEX EXAMINATION CHALLENGE 20.4

Safe and Effective Care Environment

The nurse is teaching about infection prevention to a client with cancer who is neutropenic. Which client statement indicates a need for additional teaching?

A. "I will call the primary health care provider if I get a temperature of 100.4 or greater.
B. "I will wash my hands after attending church."
C. "I will wear a condom when having intercourse."
D. "I will not drink anything that has been at room temperature for more than an hour."

Anemia and *thrombocytopenia* also result from the bone marrow suppression caused by some chemotherapy drugs. Anemia causes patients to feel fatigued from a lack of adequate red blood cells to transport oxygen throughout the body. Thrombocytopenia increases the risk for bleeding from impaired ***clotting.*** When the platelet count is less than 50,000/mm^3 (50 × 10^9/L), small trauma or injury can lead to prolonged bleeding. With a count lower than 20,000/mm^3 (20 × 10^9/L), spontaneous and uncontrollable bleeding may occur. Both anemia and thrombocytopenia may require transfusion support.

PATIENT AND FAMILY EDUCATION: PREPARING FOR SELF-MANAGEMENT

Prevention of Infection

During the times your white blood cell counts are low:

- Avoid crowds and other large gatherings of people who might be ill.
- Do not share personal toiletries.
- If possible, bathe daily. If total bathing is not possible, wash the armpits and entire perineal area twice a day with an antimicrobial soap.
- Wash your hands thoroughly with an antimicrobial soap before you eat and drink, after touching a pet, after shaking hands with anyone, as soon as you come home from any outing, and after using the toilet.
- Do not drink perishable liquids that have been standing at room temperature for longer than an hour.
- Use food safety when preparing meals.
- Wash fresh fruits and vegetables prior to eating.
- Do not change pet litter boxes or clean up after pets. Wear gloves if necessary.
- Take your temperature at least once a day and whenever you do not feel well.
- Report any of these indicators of infection to your oncologist immediately:
  - Temperature greater than 100.4°F (38°C)
  - Persistent cough (with or without sputum)
  - Pus or foul-smelling drainage from any open skin area or normal body opening
  - Presence of a boil or abscess
  - Urine that is cloudy or foul smelling or that causes burning on urination
- Take all drugs as prescribed.
- Wear gardening gloves when working in the garden or with houseplants.
- Wear a condom when having sex. If you are a woman having sex with a male partner, ensure that he wears a condom.

BEST PRACTICE FOR PATIENT SAFETY & QUALITY CARE (QSEN)

Prevention of Injury for the Patient With Thrombocytopenia

- Use caution when repositioning or assisting the patient.
- Use and teach assistive personnel (AP) to use a lift sheet when moving and positioning the patient in bed.
- Avoid IM injections and venipunctures. If platelets are <50,000/mm^3 (50 × 109/L), invasive procedures may be postponed.
- When injections or venipunctures are necessary, use the smallest-gauge needle for the task.
- Apply firm pressure to the needlestick site until the site no longer oozes blood.
- Apply ice to areas of trauma.
- Test urine and stool for the presence of occult blood as ordered.
- Observe IV sites every 4 hours for bleeding.
- Instruct patients to notify nursing personnel immediately if any trauma occurs and if bleeding or bruising is noticed.
- Avoid trauma to rectal tissues:
  - Do not administer enemas.
  - If suppositories are prescribed, lubricate liberally and administer with caution.
- Instruct the patient and AP that the patient should use an electric shaver rather than a razor.
- When providing mouth care or supervising others in providing mouth care:
  - Use a soft-bristled toothbrush or tooth sponges.
  - Do not use water-pressure gum cleaners.
  - Make certain that dentures and other dental devices fit and do not irritate the gums.
- Instruct the patient not to forcefully blow the nose or insert objects into the nose.
- Instruct AP and the patient that the patient should wear shoes with firm soles whenever ambulating.
- Practice fall prevention strategies according to the agency's policies.
- Keep pathways and walkways clear and uncluttered.

PATIENT AND FAMILY EDUCATION: PREPARING FOR SELF-MANAGEMENT

Preventing Injury or Bleeding

During the time your platelet count is low:

- Use an electric shaver.
- Use a soft-bristled toothbrush.
- Do not have dental work performed without consulting your cancer health care provider.
- Do not take aspirin or any aspirin-containing products unless prescribed. Read the label to be sure that the product does not contain aspirin or salicylates.
- Do not participate in contact sports or any activity likely to result in your being bumped, scratched, or scraped.
- Avoid hard foods that would scrape the inside of your mouth.
- Eat only warm, cool, or cold foods to avoid burning your mouth.
- Check your skin and mouth daily for bruises; swelling; or areas with small, reddish-purple marks (petechiae) that may indicate bleeding.
- Notify your cancer health care provider if you:
  - Are injured and persistent bleeding results
  - Have menstrual bleeding that is excessive for you
  - See blood in your vomit, urine, or bowel movement
- Avoid trauma with intercourse.
- Avoid anal intercourse.
- Take a stool softener to prevent straining during a bowel movement.
- Do not use enemas or rectal suppositories.
- Do not wear clothing or shoes that are tight or that rub.
- Avoid blowing your nose or placing objects in your nose. If you must blow your nose, do so gently without blocking either nasal passage.
- Avoid activities that increase the pressure in your brain.

The use of growth factors to stimulate production of red blood cells has been shown to increase the patient's risk for hypertension, blood clots, strokes, and heart attacks, especially among older adults. In addition, certain types of cancer cells grow faster in the presence of these growth factors; and their use may be restricted.

The priority for nursing care for the patient with thrombocytopenia is to provide a safe environment. The Best Practice for Patient Safety & Quality Care box includes best practices for injury prevention for the patient with thrombocytopenia. Teach AP the importance of using Bleeding Precautions and the need to report any evidence of bleeding immediately. Caregivers at home also need to know these practices.

Teach patients with thrombocytopenia and their families to avoid injury and when to report bleeding. The Patient and Family Education: Preparing for Self-Management box reviews precautions to teach patients to prevent bleeding and what to do if bleeding occurs.

Chemotherapy-Induced Nausea and Vomiting. Chemotherapy-induced nausea and vomiting (CINV) arises from various pathways in the GI tract or brain. It may manifest as *anticipatory* (before receiving the chemotherapy, often triggered by thoughts, sights, and sounds related to the anticipated chemotherapy), *acute* (within the first 24 hours after chemotherapy), *delayed* (occurring after the first 24 hours), *breakthrough* (occurring intermittently), or any combination of these. Many cancer drugs are **emetogenic** (vomiting inducing); some agents cause more nausea and vomiting than others. Although there are advances in prevention and control of CINV, it remains a common and distressing issue. Nausea often persists, even when vomiting is controlled.

Acute CINV is the most common type. It may start immediately after chemotherapy is given. A few drugs, such as dacarbazine, may trigger CINV almost as soon as the drug is started. Other drugs, such as cisplatin, induce delayed nausea and vomiting that can continue as long as 5 to 7 days after receiving it. Considered the single most distressing side effect of chemotherapy, CINV often can be well controlled with appropriate evidence-based antiemetic therapy, especially with serotonin (5-HT3) antagonist drugs. For moderately and highly emetogenic regimens, adding a neurokinin-1 (NK1) receptor antagonist drug to the regimen has greatly improved control of CINV. The development of standardized protocols for CINV prevention and management are widely used.

Drug Therapy. Many antiemetics are available to relieve nausea and vomiting. These drugs vary in the side effects they produce and how well they control CINV. Antiemetics are usually given before chemotherapy in IV form and after chemotherapy as a prescription for home use. Drugs commonly used on a short-term basis to control CINV are listed in the Common Examples of Drug Therapy: Chemotherapy-Induced Nausea and Vomiting box.

Regardless of which drugs are prescribed to prevent or reduce CINV, they are most effective when used with an evidence-based approach on a scheduled basis for prevention and management. Drug therapy for CINV works best when given

Common Examples of Drug Therapy

Chemotherapy-Induced Nausea and Vomiting

Drug Categories	Nursing Implications
Serotonin Antagonists	
Prevent CINV by blocking the 5-HT3 receptors of the chemotrigger zones in the brain and intestines. This action prevents serotonin from binding to the receptors and activating the nausea and vomiting centers.	
Ondansetron *Oral or IV* Granisetron *IV* Granisetron transdermal *patch* Palonosetron *IV or Oral*	Teach patient to change positions slowly to avoid falls *because these drugs may induce bradycardia, hypotension, and vertigo.* Assess the patient for headache, which is *a common side effect of drugs from this class.* *Constipation may occur. Assess patients for bowel habits and ensure stool softeners or laxatives are ordered if needed.*
Neurokinin 1 Receptor Antagonists	
Reduce CINV by blocking the substance P neurokinin receptor. When used together with a serotonin antagonist and a corticosteroid, both acute and delayed nausea and vomiting are controlled.	
Aprepitant *Oral* Fosaprepitant *IV*	Teach patients who are also taking warfarin to have their INR checked before and after the 3 days of this therapy *because this drug interferes with warfarin effectiveness.* Teach women who are using oral contraceptives to use an additional form of birth control while taking this drug *because it reduces the effectiveness of oral contraceptives, increasing the risk for an unplanned pregnancy.*
Corticosteroids	
Reduce CINV by decreasing swelling in the brain's chemotrigger zone.	
Dexamethasone *Oral or IV*	*These drugs cause sodium retention and hypertension. Dietary sodium restriction may be necessary.* *Can affect quality of sleep if taken late in the day.* Monitor patient's blood sugar if diabetic. *These drugs cause hyperglycemia.*
Prokinetic Agents	
Reduce CINV by blocking dopamine receptors in the brain's chemotrigger zone.	
Metoclopramide *IM or IV*	Teach the patient to avoid driving or operating heavy machinery *because these drugs induce drowsiness.*
Benzodiazepines	
Reduce CINV by enhancing cholinergic effects and decreasing the patient's awareness.	
Lorazepam *Oral or IV*	Teach the patient and family that the patient should avoid driving, operating heavy machinery, making legal decisions, and going up and down staircases unassisted *because drugs from this class induce amnesia and profound drowsiness.*

CINV, Chemotherapy-induced nausea and vomiting; *INR*, international normalized ratio.
Data from Burchum, J., & Rosenthal, L. (2019). Lehne's pharmacology for nursing care. St. Louis: Elsevier; Food and Drug Administration, (2019). Drugs@FDA: FDA-approved drugs. Retrieved from: https://www.accessdata.fda.gov/scripts/cder/daf/.

NURSING SAFETY PRIORITY (QSEN)

Drug Alert

5-HT3 antagonists, such as ondansetron, can prolong the QT interval within the cardiac conduction cycle. ECG monitoring is recommended in patients with electrolyte abnormalities (e.g., hypokalemia or hypomagnesemia), heart failure, or bradyarrhythmias or patients taking other medications that can cause QT prolongation (Burchum & Rosenthal, 2019).

PATIENT-CENTERED CARE: OLDER ADULT CONSIDERATIONS (QSEN)

The older adult can become dehydrated more quickly than a younger adult if CINV is not controlled. Teach older adults to be proactive with taking their prescribed antiemetics and to contact their health care provider if the CINV either does not resolve within 12 hours or becomes worse.

before the nausea and vomiting begin. Ensure that antiemetics are given before chemotherapy and are repeated based on the response and duration of CINV. When patients receive dose-dense chemotherapy, the intensity of CINV also increases, and more aggressive antiemetic therapy is needed. Teach patients to continue the therapy even when CINV appears controlled. *The nursing priority is to coordinate with the patient and cancer health care provider to ensure adequate control of CINV. Patients should take an antiemetic at the first sign of nausea to prevent it from becoming uncontrollable.*

Mucositis. Mucositis (inflammatory process that affects the mucous membranes of the oral mucosa and GI tract) is a dose-limiting side effect of cancer therapy, and severe cases may stop or delay treatment (Nawi, et al., 2018). Mucositis is a complex, multiphase process at the cellular level started in response to cytotoxic chemotherapy. Mouth sores cause pain and interfere with hydration, nutrition, and quality of life (Oral Cancer Foundation, 2019). The Patient and Family Education: Preparing for Self-Management: Mouth Care for Patients With Mucositis box lists patient education for self-management of mucositis.

Oral cryotherapy with ice water or ice chips can be used for the prevention of mucositis. Instruct patients to suck on ice chips before, during, and after rapid infusions of specific mucositis-causing agents, such as fluorouracil (5-FU). It is believed that vasoconstriction caused by the cold temperature decreases exposure of the oral mucous membranes to the mucositis-causing agents. Interventions are mostly focused on prevention, and management is based on supportive therapies (Nawi, et al., 2018). For multiple mouth lesions, patients may require systemic pain medications.

Frequent mouth assessment and oral hygiene are key in managing mucositis. The nurse must stress the importance of thorough and frequent oral hygiene.

PATIENT AND FAMILY EDUCATION: PREPARING FOR SELF-MANAGEMENT

Mouth Care for Patients With Mucositis

- Examine your mouth (including the roof, under the tongue, and between the teeth and cheek) regularly.
- If sores or drainage is present, contact your cancer health care provider.
- Brush the teeth and tongue with a soft-bristled brush or sponges at least every 8 hours and after meals.
- Avoid the use of mouthwashes that contain alcohol.
- "Swish and spit" room-temperature tap water, normal saline, or salt and soda water on a regular basis (at least four times a day) and as needed according to changes in the oral cavity.
- Drink 2 or more liters of water per day if another health problem does not require limiting fluid intake.
- Take all drugs, including antibiotics and drugs for nausea and vomiting, as prescribed.
- Use topical analgesic drugs as prescribed.
- Take pain medications on schedule as needed.
- Apply a water-based moisturizer to your lips as needed.
- Use prescribed "artificial saliva" or mouth moisturizers as needed.
- Avoid using tobacco or drinking alcoholic beverages.
- Avoid spicy, salty, acidic, dry, rough, or hard food.
- Use caution when drinking and eating hot foods to prevent burns.
- If you wear dentures, keep them clean and make sure they fit well.

Recommendations include *gentle* flossing, salt and baking soda rinse, or a non–alcohol-based mouth rinse at frequent intervals during the day and night when awake. Frequency is guided by the intensity of the mucositis. Teach patients to avoid mouthwashes that contain alcohol or other drying agents that may further irritate the mucosa. Because most patients with mucositis also have bone marrow suppression, the risk for impaired ***clotting*** with bleeding exists. Extra caution must be used to avoid injuring the oral mucosa. Instruct patients to use a soft-bristled toothbrush or disposable mouth sponges.

Alopecia. Alopecia, hair loss, can be a very distressing side effects of cancer treatment, especially for women (Katz, 2017). Hair loss may occur as whole-body hair loss or may be as mild as only a thinning of the scalp hair. When body hair loss includes pubic hair, patients may struggle with their body image and sexuality. Reassure patients that hair loss is temporary. Regrowth usually begins about 1 month after completion of chemotherapy; however, the new hair may differ from the original hair in color, texture, and thickness. No known evidence-based treatment fully prevents alopecia; however, scalp cooling is a newer treatment option to decrease hair loss with chemotherapy. Reports of 50% of hair retained or the lack of need for a wig or head covering can be satisfying to patients (Mikel Ross & Fischer-Cartlidge, 2018). Patients wear cooling caps on the head while receiving chemotherapy to help decrease rates of alopecia. However, cost may be prohibitive for some patients to receive this treatment, which may not be covered by insurance.

The hairless scalp is at risk for injury from friction or environmental factors. Teach the patient to avoid direct sunlight on the scalp by wearing a hat or other head covering. Sunscreen use is essential to prevent sunburn because many drugs increase sun sensitivity, regardless of skin tone. Head coverings are needed during cold weather and in cool environments to reduce body heat loss and prevent hypothermia. Help patients select a type of head covering that suits their income and lifestyle.

Suggest that patients obtain a wig before treatment begins and have their hairdresser shape it to mimic their usual hairstyle to reduce appearance changes. High-quality wigs are expensive but can look very much like the patient's own hair. Patients also can disguise hair loss with caps, scarves, and head wraps. The Look Good Feel Better program is available free to patients (Look Good Feel Better, 2019). Licensed cosmetologists teach how to apply makeup and how to use accessories to improve appearance and how patients feel about themselves. The priority nursing actions are to teach patients how to avoid scalp injury and to help them cope with this body image change.

Changes in Cognitive Function. Some patients receiving chemotherapy report changes in cognitive function. It can be reported as a reduced ability to concentrate, memory loss, and difficulty learning new information. This problem, termed *chemo brain,* is often reported during treatment and can last for years after completion of treatment. Cognitive impairment has been reported in up to 75% of patients with breast cancer (Bender et al., 2018). Although the etiology of cognitive impairment is not clear, genetic and aging considerations are being researched. Cognitive training and rehabilitation; physical activity; and pharmaceuticals may help improve quality of life.

The priorities for nursing care are supporting the patient who reports this side effect and providing resources for cognitive training. Listen to the patient's concerns and tell him or her that other patients have also reported such problems. Warn patients against participating in other behaviors that could alter cognitive functioning, such as excessive alcohol intake, recreational drug use, and activities that increase the risk for head injury.

Chemotherapy-Induced Peripheral Neuropathy. Chemotherapy-induced peripheral neuropathy (CIPN) is the loss of ***sensory perception*** or motor function of peripheral nerves associated with exposure to certain anticancer drugs. Some patients undergoing chemotherapy with nerve-damaging drugs (e.g., vincristine and cisplatin) can have onset of severe CIPN. The degree of CIPN is related to the dosage of the nerve-damaging drugs; higher doses or longer duration lead to greater neuropathy. CIPN is a dose-limiting chemotherapy treatment. The development or increased severity of CIPN may result in a reduction of chemotherapy, potentially changing the outcome of cancer treatment. The results of CIPN on function are widespread, with the most common problems including loss of sensation in the hands and feet, impaired gait and balance, orthostatic hypotension, erectile dysfunction, neuropathic pain, loss of taste discrimination, and constipation. Patients may also lose the ability to perform functional or fine motor abilities such as holding a pen, buttoning a shirt, playing an instrument, or feeling the ground while walking. These symptoms can last for months to years after treatment and may decrease quality of life. CIPN may be permanent in some adults. No known evidence-based interventions are available to prevent CIPN; however, some patients have reduced pain and improved function and quality of life when taking duloxetine.

PATIENT AND FAMILY EDUCATION: PREPARING FOR SELF-MANAGEMENT

Chemotherapy-Induced Peripheral Neuropathy

- Protect feet and other body areas where sensation is reduced; always wear shoes with a protective sole.
- Be sure that shoes are well fitting to prevent creating sores or blisters from friction.
- Inspect your feet daily (with a mirror, if needed) for open areas or redness.
- Avoid extremes of temperature; wear warm clothing in the winter, especially over hands, feet, and ears.
- Test water temperature with a thermometer when washing dishes or bathing. Use warm water rather than hot water (less than 105°F or 40.6°C).
- Use gloves when washing dishes or gardening.
- Do not eat foods that are too hot; allow them to cool before placing them in your mouth.
- Eat foods that are high in fiber (e.g., fruit, whole-grain cereals, vegetables).
- Drink 2 to 3 liters of fluid (nonalcoholic) daily unless your primary health care provider orders a fluid-restricted diet.
- Get up slowly from a lying or sitting position. If you feel dizzy, sit back down until the dizziness fades before standing; then stand in place for a few seconds before walking or using the stairs.
- To prevent tripping or falling, look at your feet and the floor or ground where you are walking to assess how the ground, floor, or step changes.
- Avoid using area rugs, especially those that slide easily.
- Keep floors free of clutter that could lead to a fall.
- Use handrails when going up or down steps.

The priority for nursing care of patients experiencing CIPN is teaching them to prevent injury. Loss of ***sensory perception*** increases the patient's risk for injury because he or she may not be aware of excessive heat, cold, or pressure. Falls are more likely because of changes in gait and balance, decreased sensation in the feet, and orthostatic hypotension. Coordinate with an occupational therapist to help the patient adjust for ***sensory perception*** deficits in performing activities. The Patient and Family Education: Preparing for Self-Management: Chemotherapy-Induced Peripheral Neuropathy box lists teaching priorities for the patient with CIPN.

Erectile dysfunction may be helped with drug therapy (see Chapter 67) for options for erectile dysfunction). Other issues may not be correctable and affect quality of life. Assess the patient's ability to cope with these changes and seek referrals as needed for supportive care.

Immunotherapy, Monoclonal Antibodies, and Targeted Therapies

As cancer research continues regarding cellular pathways, new drugs are being developed for the treatment of cancer. These drugs work directly within the cell or they can use the body's own immune system to attack the cancer. Targeted therapies used in cancer treatment are drugs that act on specific components needed for cellular function and reproduction. These therapies include monoclonal antibodies and small molecule drugs. **Immunotherapy**, a new classification in cancer treatment, is use of the body's own defense system to attack the foreign cells. Although this treatment has less cytotoxic side effects and is generally well tolerated, it still can have some significant and life-threatening complications.

Immunotherapy. The immune system has internal regulatory mechanisms that provide alerts when abnormal cells are detected and require attack (Bayer at al., 2017). Tumor cells can evade these mechanisms, which enables them to survive and multiply. Immunotherapy drugs prevent tumor cells from hiding from the immune system. The immune system is then able to recognize tumor cells and flag them for destruction (Warren, 2018).

Immunotherapy offers a treatment regimen for patients who may not be able to tolerate cytotoxic therapy. The patient who receives immunotherapy for cancer treatment does not experience the typical cytotoxic effects. Immunotherapy works to activate the immune system rather than destroy all cells. Fatigue, rash, and risk of infection are common immunotherapy side effects.

Immune-related adverse events (irAEs) occur when the stimulation of the immune system affects healthy cells as well. When healthy cells are targeted instead of cancerous cells, a patient experiences an exacerbation of an inflammatory response caused by the immune system activation (Bayer et al., 2017). Patients may develop symptoms such as colitis, hepatitis, pneumonitis, thyroiditis, endocrinopathies, and dermatologic toxicities, including pruritus and rash. These symptoms should be assessed and reported to the cancer health care provider. Most toxicities are mild, but some can be severe, leading to hospitalization, termination of treatment, or death. Monitoring of laboratory values can also alert the provider of changes. Careful monitoring of laboratory tests at regular intervals, including thyroid panel, pituitary function test, liver function test, and pancreatic enzymes, is needed for early detection of potential gland and organ toxicity (Bayer et al., 2017). Side effects are treated differently than in traditional chemotherapy, and management almost always includes some level of immunosuppression with corticosteroids. Prompt assessment and management of symptoms are key to improving patient outcomes.

Patient education is extremely important in the care of the patient receiving immunotherapy because the patient may not realize that a minor change, such as increasing fatigue or change in sleeping habits, is worth reporting (Bayer et al., 2017).

Monoclonal Antibodies. Monoclonal antibody therapy combines actions from immunotherapy and targeted therapy to help treat specific cancers. The body normally responds to foreign substances by producing antibodies. These proteins are able to target the antigen when present in the body, attacking and destroying the foreign antigen (non-self cells). In cancer therapy human and/or mouse proteins are used to form antibodies against given targets known to be present in or on certain types of cancer cells.

Monoclonal antibodies bind to their target antigens, which are often specific cell surface membrane proteins (Abramson, 2018). Binding prevents the protein from performing its functions; monoclonal antibodies therefore change ***cellular regulation*** and prevent cancer cell division. Some monoclonal antibodies make tumor cells more sensitive to therapy and increase the effectiveness of immune system attacks on the cancer cells. A commonly used monoclonal antibody for targeted therapy is rituximab. It binds to the protein CD20, which is often overexpressed on the surface of non-Hodgkin lymphoma cell membranes.

Infusion-related reactions, or hypersensitivity reactions (HSRs), may occur in patients receiving monoclonal antibodies. Many newer monoclonal antibodies have been "humanized," reducing the risk for infusion-related reactions. Nursing assessment is key for early recognition of a potentially life-threatening infusion-related reaction. Infusion reactions usually occur during the infusion and typically develop within 30 minutes to 2 hours of initiation of the drug (LaCasceet al., 2019). Monoclonal antibody infusion-related reactions include fever, chills, rigors, rash, headache, hypotension, shortness of breath, bronchospasm, nausea, vomiting, and abdominal pain. Side effects can vary from mild to life threatening (Laudati et al., 2018). Premedications, such as diphenhydramine and acetaminophen, can decrease the incidence of infusion-related reactions. Because this is an infusion reaction due to a cytokine response to the antigen, it may be possible to resume the infusion according to patient response and agency protocol or drug manufacturer's recommendation (Laudati et al., 2018).

Targeted Therapy. Targeted therapies block the growth and spread of cancer by interfering with the specific cellular growth pathways or molecules involved in the ***cellular regulation*** of growth and progression of cancer cells. Certain cancers, such as non–small cell lung cancer and pancreatic cancer, may have a known cellular pathway, which is known as the epidermal growth factor receptor (EGFR). Targeted therapies work by acting directly on the cancerous cell, and they have less of an impact on normal cells that do not have this pathway. With increased understanding of the biology of cancer cells, targeted therapies are an effective treatment option that provides patients with a new sense of hope against a challenging disease. Patients need to understand that this is a cancer treatment and there are side effects and required safety precautions. Oral therapy is primarily home-based treatment, rather than received in the clinic. Nurses need to provide detailed education for the patient who has been prescribed oral therapy to help increase adherence and side effect reporting. Teaching should include the need to report side effects in a timely manner, because this may prevent complications of treatment.

As discussed in Chapter 19, normal cells have tightly controlled regulation over when and to what extent a cell divides; cancer cells have altered features that evade this normal control.

Drugs for targeted therapy are classified based on the mechanism of action, and some have more than one action (Table 20.4). *It is important to remember that these drugs will not work unless the cancer cell overexpresses a certain protein or mutation. Therefore not all patients with the same cancer type would benefit from the use of targeted therapy.* Each patient's cancer cells are evaluated to determine whether the cells have a specific pathway to be affected by targeted therapy. Side effects and management of the patient vary from drug to drug, and these targeted agents usually do not have systemic side effects like chemotherapy. However, they have unique side effect profiles including dermatologic, endocrine, vascular, immunologic, and pulmonary toxicities (NCI, 2019). Because of the varying mechanisms of action, a priority nursing action is careful assessment for adverse reactions to treatment.

! NURSING SAFETY PRIORITY QSEN

Drug Alert

Many new cancer treatments come in oral form. This presents challenges for the provider, patient, and family. Adherence can be an issue, because patients take the oral drugs at home versus coming into the cancer health care provider for scheduled dosing. Emphasize with patients and their family members and caregivers the importance of taking the drugs as prescribed and using safe handling techniques. Education should include that only the patient should handle the oral chemotherapy agent and that if the patient is unable, the family member or caregiver needs to wear gloves when handling the chemotherapy drug. Oral anticancer medications should not be stored in the same container as other medications.

Targeted therapy agents are classified based on their action. Discussion in this section focuses on the tyrosine kinase inhibitors (TKIs), epidermal growth factor receptor inhibitors (EGFRIs), vascular endothelial growth factor receptor inhibitors (VEGFRIs), multikinase inhibitors (MKIs), proteasome inhibitors, and angiogenesis inhibitors.

Tyrosine Kinase Inhibitors. Drugs with the main action of inhibiting activation of tyrosine kinases (TKs) are tyrosine kinase inhibitors (TKIs). Some are unique to the cell type; others may be present only in cancer cells that express a specific gene mutation. As a result, the different TKI drugs are effective in disrupting the ***cellular regulation*** and growth of some cancer cell types and not others. An example of a TKI is imatinib mesylate. This drug binds to the energy site of the enzyme TK and prevents its activation. The drug is useful in cancers such as chronic myeloid leukemia (Ph+ CML) and metastatic GI stromal tumors (GISTs).

Side effects common to most TKIs include nausea, vomiting, fluid retention, electrolyte imbalances, and bone marrow suppression that reduces ***immunity*** with neutropenia, anemia, and thrombocytopenia. The problems associated with bone marrow suppression are further increased when the patient also receives traditional chemotherapy with drugs that suppress bone marrow.

Epidermal Growth Factor Receptor Inhibitors. The epidermal growth factor receptor inhibitors (EGFRIs) block epidermal growth factor from binding to its cell surface receptor. When this receptor is blocked, it cannot activate tyrosine kinase. As a result, the signal transduction pathway for promotion of cell division is inhibited.

An example of an EGFRI drug is cetuximab, which binds the excessive amounts of EGFR produced by some colon and head and neck cancers. Binding to this receptor inhibits cancer cell division and increases cellular apoptosis and reduces growth factor production.

The most common side effects of EGFRIs include hypersensitivity reactions and a variety of skin reactions because skin cells also have EGFRs. These side effects may be as mild as a rash or result in excessive skin peeling and fissures (Wallner et al., 2016). A good skin regimen needs to be started at the time of the infusion and maintained during treatment. Patient education is crucial to maintain skin integrity. EGFR treatments cause

TABLE 20.4 Common Targeted Therapy Agents

Drug Classification	Nursing Implications
Tyrosine Kinase Inhibitors (TKIs)	
Some examples are: • Dasatinib (oral) • Erlotinib (oral) • Imatinib (oral) • Lapatinib (oral)	Side effects common to most TKIs include nausea, vomiting, fluid retention, electrolyte imbalances, and bone marrow suppression.
Epidermal Growth Factor Receptor Inhibitors (EGFRIs)	
Some examples are: • Cetuximab • Panitumumab • Trastuzumab	Used for some lung and colon cancers. Common side effects include hypersensitivity reactions and a variety of skin reactions; as mild as a rash or progressing to excessive skin peeling and fissures. A good skin regimen needs to be started at the time of the infusion and maintained during treatment. Patient education is crucial to maintain skin integrity. EGFRI treatments cause significant skin rashes, and although these may look like acne, they are not treated like acne. Using a moisturizing lotion and avoiding sun exposure are key elements.
Vascular Endothelial Growth Factor Receptor Inhibitor (VEGFRI)	
• Bevacizumab	This drug inhibits formation of new blood vessels within a tumor. As a result, tumor cells are poorly nourished and growth is inhibited. The most common side effects are hypertension and impaired wound healing. Patients must not have surgery within 28 days of receiving bevacizumab. Serious and life-threatening complications include gastrointestinal perforation and hemorrhage.
Multikinase Inhibitors	
• Crizotinib (oral) • Sorafenib (oral) • Sunitinib (oral)	A common side effect of this class of drugs is hypertension. Other side effects include nausea and vomiting, diarrhea, constipation, mucositis, erythematous rash on the hands and feet (palmar-plantar erythrodysesthesia), and mild neutropenia and thrombocytopenia.
Proteasome Inhibitors	
• Bortezomib	Common side effects are nausea, vomiting, anorexia, abdominal pain, bowel changes, hypotension, and peripheral neuropathy. Other side effects include headache, rash, back and bone pain, muscle aches, and tumor lysis syndrome.
Angiogenesis/mTOR Kinase Inhibitors	
• Everolimus (oral) • Lenalidomide (oral) • Pomalidomide (oral) • Temsirolimus	Hyperglycemia, hyperlipidemia, and hypersensitivity reactions to these drugs are common. Bone marrow suppression is moderate to severe. Other general side effects include headache, nausea and vomiting, back pain, muscle and joint pain, mucositis, diarrhea, hepatic impairment and skin problems. Lenalidomide is highly regulated, and prescribers must be enrolled in the Risk Evaluation and Mitigation Strategy (REMS) program.
Monoclonal Antibodies	
• Daratumumab • ^{90}Y ibritumomab tiuxetan • Pertuzumab • Rituximab • Trastuzumab	Infusion-related reactions, or hypersensitivity reactions (HSRs), may occur in patients receiving monoclonal antibodies. Nursing assessment is key for early recognition of a potentially life-threatening infusion-related reaction. Infusion reactions usually occur during the infusion. Premedications, such as diphenhydramine and acetaminophen, can decrease the incidence of infusion-related reactions.
Checkpoint Inhibitors: PD1, PD-L1, and CTLA-4 Inhibitors	
• Avelumab • Atezolizumab • Durvalumab • Ipilimumab • Nivolumab • Pembrolizumab	Fatigue, rash, and risk of infection are common immunotherapy side effects.

significant skin rashes, and although it may look like acne, it is not treated like acne. Using a moisturizing lotion and avoiding sun exposure are key elements. Help patients understand that the rash may show a positive outcome to treatment, and teach coping strategies for physical changes that can occur with EGFR treatment.

Vascular Endothelial Growth Factor Receptor Inhibitors. An example of a vascular endothelial growth factor receptor inhibitor drug is bevacizumab. It binds to vascular endothelial growth factor (VEGF) and prevents the binding of VEGF with its receptors on the surfaces of endothelial cells present in blood vessels. This inhibits formation of new blood vessels within a tumor. As a result, tumor cells are poorly nourished and growth is inhibited. This drug is used with standard chemotherapy for many cancers that overexpress the VEGF receptor, such as colorectal, lung, and renal cell cancers.

The most common side effects are hypertension and impaired wound healing. Serious life-threatening complications including gastrointestinal perforation or hemorrhage may also occur. Bone marrow suppression with reduced ***immunity*** and neutropenia and thrombocytopenia also occur, especially when the drug is used in combination with chemotherapy drugs that cause bone marrow suppression.

Multikinase Inhibitors. The multikinase inhibitors (MKIs) inhibit the activity of specific kinases in cancer cells and tumor blood vessels. An example of an MKI is sunitinib. These drugs are most effective in preventing the activation of tyrosine kinases that have a specific gene mutation found most often in some renal cell carcinomas, GI stromal tumors (GISTs), and pancreatic neuroendocrine (pNET) cancers.

A common side effect of this class of drugs is hypertension. Other side effects include nausea and vomiting, diarrhea, constipation, mucositis, erythematous rash on the hands and feet (palmar-plantar erythrodysesthesia), and mild neutropenia and thrombocytopenia.

Proteasome Inhibitors. Proteasome inhibitors prevent the formation of a large complex of proteins (proteasome) in cells. This affects multiple signaling cascades within the cell, impairing the tumor's ***cellular regulation***, promoting cell death. The proteasome inhibitor bortezomib is used in the treatment of multiple myeloma and mantle cell lymphoma.

The most common side effects of bortezomib are nausea, vomiting, anorexia, abdominal pain, bowel changes, hypotension, and peripheral neuropathy. Other side effects include headache, rash, back and bone pain, muscle aches, and tumor lysis syndrome (TLS).

Angiogenesis Inhibitors. Angiogenesis inhibitors target a specific protein kinase known as the *mammalian target of rapamycin (mTOR)*. An example of an angiogenesis inhibitor is temsirolimus, used for renal cell cancer. When the drug binds to an intracellular protein, a protein-drug complex forms that inhibits the activity of mTOR. When mTOR is inhibited, the concentrations of vascular endothelial growth factor (VEGF) are greatly reduced, and many pro–cell division signal transduction pathways are disrupted.

Hyperglycemia, hyperlipidemia, and hypersensitivity reactions to these drugs are common. Bone marrow suppression is moderate to severe, with anemia, neutropenia, and thrombocytopenia. Other general side effects include headache, nausea and vomiting, back pain, muscle and joint pain, mucositis, diarrhea, hepatic impairment, and skin problems.

Endocrine Therapy

Some hormones cause hormone-sensitive tumors to grow more rapidly. By decreasing the amount of these hormones that reach hormone-sensitive tumors, it can slow cancer growth. Breast cancer is one example of a cancer that can be hormonally driven. Pathology reveals if it is estrogen or progesterone positive or negative.

Endocrine therapy may include the use of aromatase inhibitors, gonadotropin-releasing hormone analogs, antiandrogens, and antiestrogens. Many of these agents are used to block receptors and thus affect ***cellular regulation*** by preventing the cancer cells from receiving growth stimulation. As a result, tumor growth is slowed or stopped and the risk of cancer progression decreases (NCI, 2018).

For women with hormone-positive breast cancer, selection of treatment will depending on menopausal status. For men who have prostate cancer, androgen deprivation therapy may be warranted. Table 20.5 lists drugs used in endocrine therapy for cancer treatment.

Side effects of endocrine therapy are different from chemotherapy. Adherence can be a challenge for some patients owing to side effects. Side effects include fatigue, arthralgias, joint stiffness and/or bone pain, hot flashes, and sexual dysfunction. Long-term side effects include osteoporosis, increased cardiovascular risks, and risk of thrombotic events.

Teach patients and families about expected side effects. Encouraging an exercise regimen will help to prevent

CLINICAL JUDGMENT CHALLENGE 20.1

Patient-Centered Care; Safety

The nurse is caring for a 68-year-old female client with stage II diffuse large B-cell lymphoma. The current treatment plan consists of six cycles of chemotherapy. The client received the first dose of chemotherapy without complications at the infusion center in the oncologist's office. The client also received a pegfilgrastim injection 24 hours after chemotherapy to help prevent severe neutropenia.

Three days after the first chemotherapy infusion, the client presented to the emergency department (ED) with reports of fever and fatigue. The client reported a fever of 100.5°F the previous night and 100.8°F 1 hour before she arrived at the ED. Initial nursing assessment revealed:

Temperature: 101°F
Heart rate: 118

Laboratory report revealed the following:

White blood cell count: 2900/mm
Absolute neutrophil count: 400/mm^3
Hematocrit: 37.2%
Hemoglobin: 11.9 g/dL
Platelet count: 230,000/mm^3

1. **Recognize Cues:** What assessment information in this client situation is the most important and immediate concern for the nurse? (Hint: Identify the **relevant** information *first* to determine what is most important.)
2. **Analyze Cues:** What client conditions are consistent with the **most relevant** information? (Hint: Think about priority collaborative problems that support and contradict the information presented in this situation.)
3. **Prioritize Hypotheses:** Which possibilities or explanations are **most likely** to be present in this client situation? Which possibilities or explanations are the most serious? (Hint: Consider all possibilities and determine their urgency and risk for this client.)
4. **Generate Solutions:** What actions would most likely achieve the desired outcomes for this client? Which actions should be **avoided** or are **potentially harmful**? (Hint: Determine the desired outcomes first to decide which interventions are appropriate and those that should be avoided.)
5. **Take Action:** Which actions are the most appropriate and how should they be implemented? In what **priority order** should they be implemented? (Hint: Consider health teaching, documentation, requested health care provider orders or prescriptions, nursing skills, collaboration with or referral to health team members, etc.)
6. **Evaluate Outcomes:** What client assessment would indicate that the nurse's actions were **effective**? (Hint: Think about signs that would indicate an improvement, decline, or unchanged client condition.)

TABLE 20.5 Common Agents Used for Endocrine Therapy for Cancer

Drug Classification	Nursing Implications
Hormone Agonists	
• Luteinizing hormone–releasing hormone (LHRH) • Leuprolide • Goserelin	Injections are given to induce menopause or reduce testosterone levels in patients with prostate cancer. Educate patients on hot flashes, vaginal dryness, and sexual dysfunction.
Hormone Antagonists	
• Antiandrogens • Abiraterone (oral) • Bicalutamide (oral) • Enzalutamide (oral)	Used for prostate cancer. Side effects include infertility, osteoporosis, hot flashes, sexual dysfunction (including loss of libido and erectile dysfunction).
• Antiestrogens • Fulvestrant (oral) • Raloxifene (oral) • Tamoxifen (oral)	Side effects include bone pain, hot flashes, increased cardiovascular risks, risk of thrombotic events (deep vein thrombosis, pulmonary embolism), and increased risk of uterine cancer.
Aromatase Inhibitors	
• Anastrozole (oral) • Exemestane (oral) • Letrozole (oral)	Used in postmenopausal women who have hormone-positive breast cancer. Side effects include fatigue, arthralgias, joint stiffness, and/or bone pain, hot flashes, and sexual dysfunction.

skeletal-related events as well as improve associated musculoskeletal symptoms. Patient who have hormone-positive cancer will need to avoid hormonal replacement that is sometimes used to help alleviate symptoms. For example, estrogen may be prescribed to treat vaginal dryness that can occur with menopause. Bisphosphonates are prescribed to help improve skeletal strength and decrease the risk for osteoporosis and pathologic bone fractures.

Colony-Stimulating Factors as Supportive Therapy

Colony-stimulating factors (CSFs) are used as supportive therapy during chemotherapy by enhancing recovery of bone marrow function after treatment-induced myelosuppression. These are also referred to as *growth factors* (Table 20.6). These factors affect ***cellular regulation*** and stimulate rapid recovery of bone marrow cells after suppression by chemotherapy. This effect has two benefits. First, when impaired ***immunity*** is shortened or less severe, patients have a decreased risk for life-threatening infections. Second, because the growth factors allow more rapid bone marrow recovery, patients can receive their chemotherapy regimen as scheduled, avoid dose reductions, and potentially increase the likelihood of remission or cure.

Side Effects of Colony-Stimulating Factors. Bone pain is a common side effect in patients receiving colony-stimulating factors. Usually acetaminophen or ibuprofen will control the pain, but occasionally an opioid prescription is required. It is important to educate patients about this side effect because it is distressing and can affect overall quality of life. This side effect is usually short-lived. Other side effects include headache, injection site soreness, nausea, vomiting, dizziness, fatigue, dyspnea, and swelling in the face or ankles.

TABLE 20.6 Common Supportive Therapy Agents for Cancer

Drug Classification	Nursing Implications
Colony-Stimulating Factors (CSFs)	
• Filgrastim • Pegfilgrastim • Sargramostim	Used for chemotherapy-induced neutropenia or leukopenia. Pegfilgrastim is a long-acting dose given the day after chemotherapy to help reduce incidence of neutropenia in regimens known to have at least 20% risk of febrile neutropenia. Bone pain is a troublesome side effect. Educate patients on management of this unpleasant side effect.
Erythropoietin-Stimulating Agents (ESAs)	
• Epoetin alfa • Darbepoetin	Used for chemotherapy-induced anemia. Used for anemia induced by renal failure. Use caution for patients receiving curative cancer treatment as these agents may shorten survival or increase tumor progression.

Data from Burchum, J., & Rosenthal, L. (2019). Lehne's pharmacology for nursing care. St. Louis: Elsevier.

ONCOLOGIC EMERGENCIES

With improvements in cancer treatments, many cancers have become chronic diseases. However, acute complications from the cancer or its treatment can occur at any time. This chapter presents select acute complications of cancer or cancer treatment, including sepsis and disseminated intravascular coagulation (DIC), syndrome of inappropriate antidiuretic hormone (ADH), spinal cord compression (SCC), hypercalcemia, superior vena cava (SVC) syndrome, and tumor lysis syndrome (TLS) as oncologic emergencies. Early diagnosis and immediate intervention for these emergency conditions are essential to avoid life-threatening situations. The role of the nurse is to implement interventions to prevent and detect these complications early for immediate treatment.

SEPSIS AND DISSEMINATED INTRAVASCULAR COAGULATION

Sepsis, or septicemia, is a condition in which organisms enter the bloodstream through any site of skin breakdown and cause a severe infection. Severe sepsis can result in septic shock, a life-threatening condition. Adults with cancer who have low white blood cell (WBC) counts (neutropenia) and impaired ***immunity*** from cancer treatment are at risk for infection and sepsis. Chapter 34 describes the pathophysiology of sepsis and septic shock. Patients with neutropenia do not have enough WBCs to produce the typical signs and symptoms of infection (i.e., erythema, swelling, warmth, high fever). Often a low-grade fever (100.4°F or 38°C) is the only sign of infection. Infection and sepsis have a high mortality rate in adults with neutropenia (McCance et al., 2019). Teach patients the importance of notifying the primary health care provider at the first sign of infection or fever.

Disseminated intravascular coagulation (DIC) is a problem with the blood-***clotting*** process. DIC is triggered by many severe illnesses, including cancer. In patients with cancer DIC often is caused by sepsis from a variety of organisms (bacterial, fungal, viral, or parasitic).

Extensive, abnormal ***clotting*** occurs throughout the blood vessels of patients with DIC. This widespread clotting depletes circulating clotting factors and platelets. As this happens, extensive bleeding occurs. Bleeding from many sites is the most common problem and ranges from oozing to fatal hemorrhage. Clots block blood vessels and decrease blood flow to major body organs and result in pain, ischemia, strokelike symptoms, dyspnea, tachycardia, reduced kidney function, and bowel necrosis.

! NURSING SAFETY PRIORITY (QSEN)

Critical Rescue

DIC is a life-threatening problem with a high mortality rate, even when proper treatment is initiated. Identify patients at greatest risk for sepsis and DIC. Prevention of sepsis and DIC is a priority nursing intervention. Practice strict adherence to aseptic technique during invasive procedures and during contact with nonintact skin and mucous membranes. Teach patients and families the early indicators of infection and to seek prompt assistance.

When sepsis is present and DIC is likely, management focuses on reducing the infection and halting the DIC process. IV antibiotic therapy is initiated. During the early phase of DIC, anticoagulants (especially heparin) are given to limit ***clotting*** and prevent the rapid consumption of circulating clotting factors. When DIC has progressed and hemorrhage is the primary problem, clotting factors are given. See Chapter 34 for a detailed discussion of DIC.

SYNDROME OF INAPPROPRIATE ANTIDIURETIC HORMONE

In healthy adults, antidiuretic hormone (ADH) is secreted by the posterior pituitary gland only when more fluid (water) is needed in the body, such as when plasma volume is decreased. Certain conditions induce ADH secretion when not needed by the body, which leads to syndrome of inappropriate antidiuretic hormone (SIADH). SIADH is a disorder of impaired water retention (McCance et al., 2019).

Cancer is a common cause of SIADH, especially small cell lung cancer. SIADH also may occur with other cancers or when metastatic tumors are present in the brain. Some cancers make and secrete ADH, whereas others stimulate the posterior pituitary to secrete ADH. Drugs used for cancer treatment or supportive therapy also can cause SIADH. Older adults are at risk for SIADH due to medications (McCance et al., 2019).

In SIADH, water is reabsorbed in excess by the kidneys and put into systemic circulation. The retained water dilutes blood sodium levels, causing hyponatremia. Normal range for sodium is 136 to 145 mEq/L (mmol/L) (Pagana & Pagana, 2018). Mild symptoms include weakness, muscle cramps, loss of appetite, and fatigue. With greater fluid retention and decreased sodium levels, weight gain, nervous system changes, personality changes, confusion, and extreme muscle weakness occur. As the sodium level drops toward 110 mEq/L (mmol/L), seizures, coma, and death may follow depending on how rapidly hyponatremia occurs.

SIADH is managed by treating the condition and the cause. Nursing priorities focus on patient safety, restoring normal fluid balance, and providing supportive care. Management includes fluid restriction, increased sodium intake, and drug therapy. Immediate cancer treatment with radiation or chemotherapy may cause enough tumor regression that ADH production returns to normal. See Chapter 57 for a detailed discussion of SIADH management.

! NURSING SAFETY PRIORITY (QSEN)

Critical Rescue

Monitor patients at least every 2 hours to recognize signs and symptoms of increasing fluid overload (bounding pulse, increasing neck vein distention [jugular venous distention (JVD)], presence of crackles in lungs, increasing peripheral edema, or reduced urine output) because pulmonary edema can occur very quickly and lead to death. When symptoms indicate that the fluid overload from SIADH either is not responding to therapy or is becoming worse, respond by notifying the primary health care provider immediately.

SPINAL CORD COMPRESSION

Spinal cord compression (SCC) is an oncologic emergency that requires immediate intervention to relieve pain and prevent permanent neurologic damage. Damage from SCC occurs either when a tumor directly enters the spinal cord or spinal column or when the vertebrae collapse from tumor degradation of the bone. The most frequent area for SCC is the thoracic spine.

The symptoms of SCC can vary depending on the severity and location of the compression. Back pain is a common first symptom and occurs before other problems or nerve deficits. Other symptoms include weakness, loss of sensation, urinary retention, and constipation. Loss of or reduced deep tendon reflexes along with reduced pinprick and vibratory sensations are other findings that may be present at physical assessment. Neurologic problems are specific to the level of spinal compression and can lead to paralysis, which is usually permanent if the compression is not alleviated promptly.

Early recognition and treatment of SCC are key to a positive outcome. Assess for back pain that worsens over time; neurologic changes; muscle weakness or a sensation of heaviness in the arms or legs; numbness or tingling in the hands or feet; inability to distinguish pinprick, touch, or hot and cold sensation; and an unsteady gait. Depending on how low the compression occurs, constipation, incontinence, and difficulty starting or stopping urination also may be present. Teach patients and families to recognize and report the symptoms of early SCC, and instruct them to seek help immediately.

If SCC is suspected on the basis of clinical symptoms, treatment should begin immediately to preserve function. MRI is the preferred imaging test that can be used to confirm the diagnosis (Brigle et al., 2017). Treatment is often palliative, with high-dose corticosteroids given first as an IV bolus to reduce swelling around the spinal cord and relieve symptoms, followed by a tapered dose over time. High-dose radiation may be used to reduce the size of the tumor in the area and relieve compression. Surgery may be performed to remove the tumor and trim the bony tissue so less pressure is placed on the spinal cord or to repair the spine if the spinal column is unstable. External back or neck braces may be used to reduce the weight carried by the spinal column and to reduce pressure on the spinal cord or spinal nerves.

NCLEX EXAMINATION CHALLENGE 20.5

Safe and Effective Care Environment

The nurse is assessing a client who has advanced bone cancer. Which client assessment finding causes the nurse to suspect spinal cord compression? **Select all that apply.**

A. Reports of a headache for the past 7 hours
B. Decreased breath sounds in the left lung
C. Worsening mid-thoracic back pain
D. Tingling in the right lower extremity
E. Unsteady gait when ambulating to the bathroom
F. Reports of difficulty sleeping

HYPERCALCEMIA

Hypercalcemia (increased serum calcium level) occurs frequently in patients with cancer. It is a metabolic emergency and can lead to death. Multiple myeloma and metastatic cancer to the bone is a risk for hypercalcemia (Brigle et al., 2017). Bone metastasis can stimulate bone breakdown (osteoclast activity) and bone resorption, which releases more calcium from bone and leads to hypercalcemia. In addition, systemic secretion of vitamin D analogs by the tumor can also cause elevated calcium levels in the bloodstream. Dehydration worsens hypercalcemia.

Early symptoms of hypercalcemia are nonspecific. Common symptoms include fatigue, loss of appetite, nausea, vomiting, constipation, and increased urine output. Additional symptoms include skeletal pain, kidney stones, abdominal discomfort, and altered cognition that can range from lethargy to coma. More serious problems include severe muscle weakness, loss of deep tendon reflexes, paralytic ileus, dehydration, and ECG changes (Shane & Bereson, 2017). Symptom severity depends on how high the calcium level is and how quickly it increased (see Chapter 13).

Cancer-induced hypercalcemia often develops slowly for many patients, which allows the body time to adapt to this electrolyte change. As a result, symptoms of hypercalcemia may not be evident until the serum calcium level is greatly elevated.

For patients who have elevated serum calcium levels and symptoms of hypercalcemia, aggressive IV hydration with normal saline is prescribed. Correcting the dehydration that often accompanies hypercalcemia restores urine output. Assess the patient for volume overload and notify the primary health care provider if this occurs. Loop diuretics can promote calcium loss in urine. Thiazide diuretics are avoided because they can increase calcium reabsorption from urine. Many drugs such as bisphosphonates (which block bone resorption of calcium) and calcitonin (combined with corticosteroids) can temporarily lower serum calcium levels. Treatment of the cancer is needed for long-term control of calcium blood levels. When cancer-induced hypercalcemia is life threatening or occurs with kidney disease, dialysis can temporarily reduce serum calcium levels.

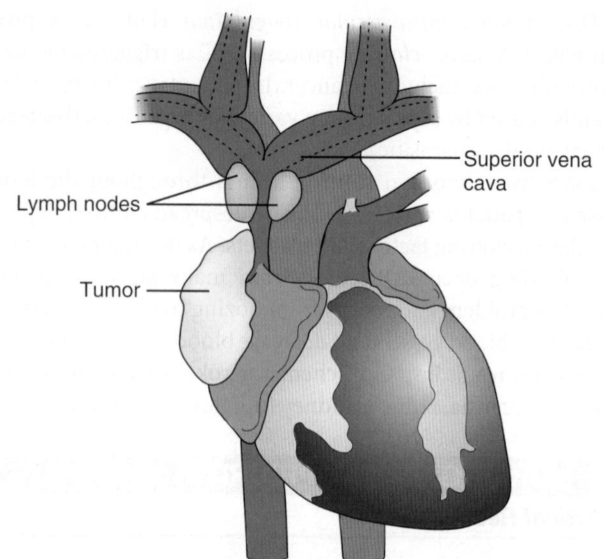

Fig. 20.4 Compression of the superior vena cava by lymph nodes and tumors in superior vena cava syndrome.

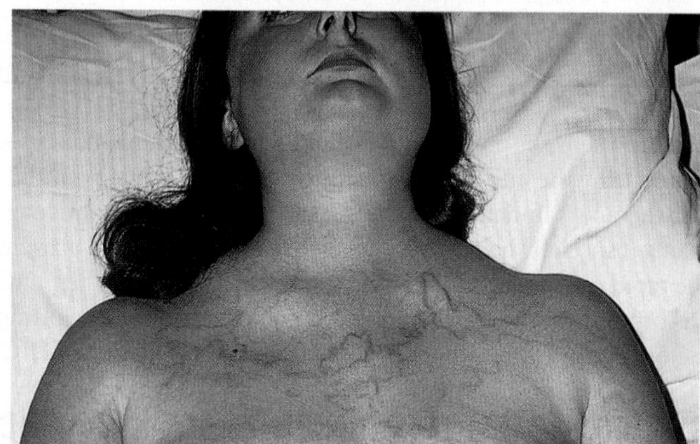

Fig. 20.5 Appearance of the face, neck, upper arms, and chest in a patient with superior vena cava syndrome. (From Forbes, C.D., & Jackson, W.F. [2003]. *Colour atlas and text of clinical medicine* [3rd ed.]. London: Mosby.)

SUPERIOR VENA CAVA SYNDROME

The superior vena cava (SVC) returns all blood from the head, neck, and upper extremities to the heart. Compression or obstruction by tumor growth or by clots in this vessel leads to congestion of blood returning to the body (Fig. 20.4). This is known as SVC syndrome and can occur quickly or develop gradually over time. SVC syndrome occurs most often in patients with mediastinal tumors, or tumors near the chest wall or indwelling catheters.

Compression of the SVC is painful and can be life threatening. Symptoms result from the blockage of venous return from the head, neck, and upper trunk. Early signs and symptoms include edema of the face, especially around the eyes (periorbital edema) on arising in the morning, and reports of head fullness. As the compression worsens, the patient develops engorged blood vessels and erythema of the upper body (Fig. 20.5), edema in the arms and hands, and dyspnea. The development of stridor (a high-pitched crowing sound) indicates narrowing of the pharynx or larynx and is an alarming sign of rapid progression. Symptoms are more apparent when the patient is in the supine position. Late symptoms include hemorrhage, cyanosis, mental status changes, decreased cardiac output, and hypotension. Imaging with CT or MRI is essential for diagnosis and treatment planning. Death results if compression is not relieved.

SVC syndrome is often associated with late-stage disease when the tumor is widespread. SVC syndrome occasionally occurs from an indwelling vascular device as a result of a blood clot. This type of obstruction can be treated successfully with systemic anticoagulation as well as the removal of the catheter.

High-dose radiation therapy to the upper chest area may be used to provide temporary relief of airway obstruction. Chemotherapy may be the only option for long-term control of the cancer causing the compression. Surgery is rarely performed for this condition. A metal stent can be placed in the vena cava in an interventional radiology department to relieve swelling. Follow-up angioplasty may keep this stent open for a longer period.

TUMOR LYSIS SYNDROME

In tumor lysis syndrome (TLS) large numbers of tumor cells are destroyed rapidly. The intracellular contents and subsequent cellular by-products of damaged cancer cells are released into the bloodstream faster than the body can eliminate them (Fig. 20.6).

Severe or untreated TLS can cause acute kidney injury (AKI) and death. Serum potassium levels increase, causing hyperkalemia, which can lead to cardiac dysfunction (see Chapter 13). The large amounts of cellular by-products form uric acid, causing hyperuricemia. These uric acid crystals precipitate in the kidney, blocking kidney tubules and leading to AKI. Sudden development of hyperkalemia, hyperuricemia, and hyperphosphatemia has life-threatening effects on the heart muscle, kidneys, and central nervous system.

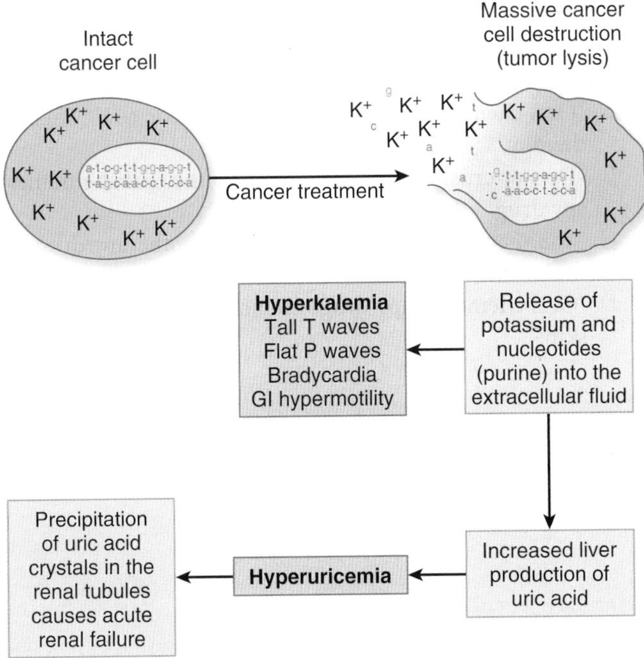

Fig. 20.6 Pathway of tumor lysis syndrome.

TLS is usually seen in patients with high-grade cancers or those with bulky tumor burden, such as diffuse non-Hodgkin lymphoma. Adults receiving radiation or chemotherapy for high-grade cancers are at risk for TLS. Early symptoms of TLS stem from electrolyte imbalances and can include lethargy, nausea, vomiting, anorexia, flank pain, muscle weakness, cramps, seizures, and altered mental status.

Hydration prevents and manages TLS by increasing the kidney flow rates, preventing uric acid buildup in the kidneys, and diluting the serum potassium levels.

With tumors known to be very sensitive to cancer treatment, instruct patients to drink at least 3000 mL (3 L) a day leading up to and during treatment to help prevent TLS. Stress the importance of keeping fluid intake consistent throughout the 24-hour day, and help patients draw up a schedule of fluid intake.

Because some patients have nausea and vomiting after chemotherapy and may not feel like drinking fluids, stress the importance of following the antiemetic regimen. Instruct patients to contact the oncologist immediately if nausea prevents adequate fluid intake so parenteral fluids can be started.

If cancer treatment is expected to rapidly decrease tumor burden, prophylaxis is necessary. Monitor daily weights and serum electrolyte values. Management becomes more aggressive for patients who develop hyperkalemia or hyperuricemia. In addition to fluids, diuretics are given to increase urine flow through the kidney. These agents are used cautiously to avoid dehydration. Drugs that promote uric acid excretion, such as allopurinol, rasburicase, or febuxostat, are given. To reduce serum potassium levels for mild-to-moderate hyperkalemia, sodium polystyrene sulfonate can be given orally or as a retention enema. For more severe hyperkalemia, IV infusions containing glucose and insulin may be given. Patients who have severe hyperkalemia and hyperuricemia may need dialysis and intensive care.

SURVIVORSHIP

As the landscape of cancer care is changing, patients are living longer with the disease. What used to be a death sentence is now being considered a chronic disease. Survivors have unique physical and psychosocial needs, including long-term effects from treatment. NCCN (2018) specifically outlines follow-up care and considerations for survivors. Routine imaging, blood work, and follow-up care with the primary health care provider are of utmost priority. Patients need to be educated on the importance of routine follow-ups and adherence to the recommended schedule. Chemotherapy can lead to cardiac and pulmonary toxicity, infertility, menopause, and peripheral neuropathy as well as an increased risk of secondary malignancies. If lymph nodes were removed during surgery, the risk of lymphedema is lifelong. Radiation can cause fibrosis and permanent skin changes in the radiation path. Nurses are uniquely positioned to provide acute cancer care and also support the patient through the survivorship journey.

GET READY FOR THE NEXT-GENERATION NCLEX® EXAMINATION!

Key Points

Review these Key Points for each NCLEX Examination Client Needs Category.

Safe and Effective Care Environment

- Use aseptic technique during care for open skin areas or any invasive procedure to prevent infection. **QSEN: Safety**
- During chemotherapy administration, assess venous access device to verify blood return per facility protocol. **QSEN: Safety**
- Use appropriate PPE when handling the excreta of a patient receiving chemotherapy and for 48 hours afterward. **QSEN: Safety**
- Inspect the oral mucosa of patients with neutropenia regularly. **QSEN: Safety**
- Teach the patient and family about symptoms of infection and when to contact their oncologist. **QSEN: Safety**
- Report any temperature higher than 100.4°F (38°C) in a patient with neutropenia. **QSEN: Evidence-Based Practice**
- Monitor the patient at risk for bleeding and use bleeding precautions if thrombocytopenia is present. **QSEN: Safety**
- Ensure proper shielding and waste disposal when patients in inpatient settings are receiving brachytherapy. **QSEN: Safety**
- Teach patients receiving radiation therapy how to care for the skin in the radiation path. **QSEN: Safety**
- Instruct patients to contact the pharmacy to determine the proper disposal of expired or discontinued oral chemotherapy agents. **QSEN: Safety**

Health Promotion and Maintenance

- Assist patients and families to find appropriate community resources for support, supplies, care, and other assistance. **QSEN: Patient-Centered Care**

Psychosocial Integrity

- Allow the patient and family the opportunity to express concerns regarding the diagnosis of cancer or the treatment regimen. **QSEN: Patient-Centered Care**
- Encourage the patient to verbalize feelings about changes in appearance resulting from cancer treatment. **QSEN: Patient-Centered Care**

Physiological Integrity

- Perform a total assessment of the patient with cancer. Notify provider of abnormal assessment findings. **QSEN: Patient-Centered Care**
- Assess the patient's pain level on a regular basis. Use pharmacologic and nonpharmacologic therapies to reduce pain. **QSEN: Patient-Centered Care**
- Instruct patients to use prescribed antiemetic drugs on a schedule for control of nausea and vomiting. **QSEN: Evidence-Based Practice**
- Closely monitor patients receiving any type of targeted therapy for severe side effects or adverse drug reactions. **QSEN: Patient-Centered Care**
- Stress the importance of adhering to the prescribed schedule for oral chemotherapy agents. **QSEN: Evidence-Based Practice**
- Demonstrate to the patient and whomever prepares oral chemotherapy agents at home how to do so without touching the tablets or capsules. **QSEN: Patient-Centered Care**
- Teach patients and families the symptoms of oncologic emergencies and when to notify the health care provider. **QSEN: Patient-Centered Care**

MASTERY QUESTIONS

1. A client with chemotherapy-induced neutropenia is prescribed filgrastim. The client states, "The bones in my legs are aching so bad." What is the appropriate nursing response?

A. "The pain in your legs is likely from the cancer."
B. "Bone pain is a side effect of filgrastim that improves with time."
C. "Increasing activity will help with the bone pain."
D. "Have you had any fever or nausea?"

2. The nurse is caring for a client with a sealed radiation implant for the treatment of cancer. Which nursing intervention is appropriate? **Select all that apply.**

A. Place a caution sign on the door of the client's room.
B. Wear a dosimeter badge for protection when providing care.
C. Allow the client's spouse to stay with the client at least 6 feet away for 4 hours.
D. Do not allow children to visit the client for any length of time.
E. Keep the door to the client's room closed.

3. The nurse is teaching a client who has been prescribed an oral chemotherapy agent. What teaching will the nurse include?

A. "Oral chemotherapy drugs are not as toxic as IV chemotherapy."
B. "Do not crush, split, break, or chew the oral chemotherapy drug."
C. "You may dispose of unused oral chemotherapy drugs in the trash."
D. "Oral chemotherapy drugs are not absorbed through the skin."

REFERENCES

Abramson, R. (2018). *Overview of targeted therapies for cancer*. My Cancer Genome (Updated May 25). https://www.mycancergenome.org/content/molecular-medicine/overview-of-targeted-therapies-for-cancer/.

American Cancer Society. (2019). *Cancer facts and figures*. Retrieved from: https://www.cancer.org/research/cancer-facts-statistics/all-cancer-facts-figures/cancer-facts-figures-2019.html.

Bauer, C. (2016). Understanding radiation dermatitis. *American Nurse Today*, *11*(1), 13–15.

Bayer, V., Amaya, B., Baniewicz, D., Callahan, C., Marsh, L., & McCoy, A. S. (2017). Cancer immunotherapy: An evidence-based overview and implications for practice. *Clinical Journal of Oncology Nursing*, *21*(Suppl.), 13–21. https://doi.org/10.1188/17.CJON.S2.13-21.

Bender, C. M., Merriman, J. D., Sereika, S. M., Gentry, A. L., Casillo, F. E., Koleck, T. A., et al. (2018). Trajectories of cognitive function and associated phenotypic and genotypic factors in breast cancer. *Oncology Nursing Forum*, *45*(3), 308–326. https://doi.org/10.1188/18.ONF.308-326.

Brant, J. M., & Mayer, D. K. (2017). Precision medicine: Accelerating the science to revolutionize cancer care. *Clinical Journal of Oncology Nursing*, *21*(6), 722–729. https://doi.org/10.1188/17.CJON.722-729.

Brigle, K., Pierre, A., Finley-Oliver, E., Faiman, B., Tariman, J. D., Miceli, T., & The International Myeloma Foundation Nurse Leadership Board (2017). Myelosuppression, bone disease, and acute renal failure: evidence-based recommendations for oncologic emergencies. *Clinical Journal of Oncology Nursing*, *21*(5), 60–76. https://doi.org/10.1188/17.CJON.S5.60-76.

Burchum, J., & Rosenthal, L. (2019). *Lehne's pharmacology for nursing care*. St. Louis: Elsevier.

Canadian Cancer Society. (2019). *Canadian Cancer Statistics*. Retrieved from: https://www.cancer.ca/~/media/cancer.ca/CW/cancer%20information/cancer%20101/Canadian%20cancer%20statistics/Canadian-Cancer-Statistics-2019-EN.pdf?la=en.

Center for Nuclear Science and Technology Information. (2018). *Protecting against exposure*. Retrieved from: http://nuclearconnect.org/know-nuclear/science/protecting.

Chou, Y.-J., Kuo, H.-J., & Shun, S.-C. (2018). Cancer rehabilitation programs and their effects on quality of life. *Oncology Nursing Forum*, *45*(6), 726–736. https://doi.org/10.1188/18.ONF.726-736.2018.

Goldberg, J. I., Burhenn, P. S., & Ginex, P. K. (2018). Nursing education: Review of assessment, clinical care, and implications for practice regarding older adult patients with cancer. *Clinical Journal of Oncology Nursing*, *22*(6), 19–25. https://doi.org/10.1188/18.CJON.S2.19-25.

Katz, A. (2017). Scalp cooling: The prevention of chemotherapy-induced alopecia. *Clinical Journal of Oncology Nursing*, *21*(4), 413–415. https://doi.org/10.1188/17.CJON.413-415.

LaCasce, A., Castells, M., Burstein, H., & Meyerhardt, J. (2019). *Infusion-related reactions to therapeutic monocolonal antibodies used for cancer therapy. UpToDate*. Retrieved from: https://www.uptodate.com/contents/infusion-related-reactions-to-therapeutic-monoclonal-antibodies-used-for-cancer-therapy1.

Laudati, C., Clark, C., Knezevic, A., Zhang, Z., & Barton-Burke, M. (2018). Hypersensitivity reactions: Priming practice change to reduce incidence in first-dose rituximab treatment. *Clinical Journal of Oncology Nursing*, *22*(4), 407–414. https://doi.org/10.1188/18.CJON.407-414.

Look Good Feel Better. (2019). *About the program*. Retrieved from: http://lookgoodfeelbetter.org/about/about-the-program/.

Lucas, A. S., Lacouture, M. E., Thompson, J. A., & Schneider, S. M. (2018). Radiation dermatitis: A prevention protocol for patients with breast cancer. *Clinical Journal of Oncology Nursing*, *22*(4), 429–437. https://doi.org/10.1188/18.CJON.429-437.

McCance, K., Huether, S., Brashers, V., & Rote, N. (2019). *Pathophysiology: The biologic basis for disease in adults and children* (8th ed.). St. Louis: Mosby.

Mikel Ross, M., & Fischer-Cartlidge, E. (2018). Scalp cooling: A literature review of efficacy, safety, and tolerability for chemotherapy-induced alopecia. *Clinical Journal of Oncology Nursing*, *21*(2), 226–233. https://doi.org/10.1188/17.CJON.226-233.

National Comprehensive Cancer Network. (2018). *NCCN clinical practice guidelines in oncology (NCCN Guidelines®)*. Survivorship [v.3.2017]. Retrieved from https://www.nccn.org/professionals/physician_gls/pdf/survivorship.pdf.

National Cancer Institute. (2018). *Common terminology criteria for adverse events* (2018). Retrieved from https://ctep.cancer.gov/protocolDevelopment/electronic_applications/docs/CTCAE_v5_Quick_Reference_8.5x11.pdf.

National Cancer Institute. (2019). *Target cancer therapies*. Retrieved from https://www.cancer.gov/about-cancer/treatment/types/targeted-therapies/targeted-therapies-fact-sheet#q7.

Nawi, R. I., Chui, P. L., Ishak, W. Z. W., & Chan, C. M. H. (2018). Oral cryotherapy: Prevention of oral mucositis and pain among patients with colorectal cancer undergoing chemotherapy. *Clinical Journal of Oncology Nursing*, *22*(5), 555–560. https://doi.org/10.1188/18.CJON.555-560.

Neuss, M., Gilmore, T., Belderson, K., Billett, A., Conti-Kalchik, T., Harvey, B., et al. (2017). 2016 Updated american society of clinical oncology/oncology nursing society chemotherapy administration safety standards, including standards for pediatric oncology. *Oncology Nursing Forum*, *44*(1), 31–43.

Oncology Nursing Society. (2017). [Position statement]. *Education of the nurse who administers and cares for the individual receiving chemotherapy, targeted therapy, and immunotherapy*. Retrieved from: https://www.ons.org/make-difference/ons-center-advocacy-and-health-policy/position-statements/education-nurse-who.

Oncology Nursing Society. (2018). *Toolkit for safe handling of hazardous drugs for nurses in oncology*. Retrieved from https://www.ons.org/sites/default/files/2018-06/ONS_Safe_Handling_Toolkit_0.pdf.

Oral Cancer Foundation. (2019). *Mucositis*. Retrieved from https://oralcancerfoundation.org/complications/mucositis/.

Occupational Safety and Health Administration. (n.d.). Health Care Facilities. Hazardous Drugs. https://www.osha.gov/SLTC/healthcarefacilities/otherhazards.html

Pagana, K., & Pagana, T. (2018). *Mosby's manual of diagnostic and laboratory tests* (6th ed.). St. Louis: Elsevier.

Shane, E., & Bereson, J. R. (2017). *Treatment of hypercalcemia. UptoDate.*

Wallner, M., Kock-Hodi, S., Booze, S., White, K., & Mayer, H. (2016). Nursing management of cutaneous toxicities from epidermal growth factor receptor inhibitors. *Clinical Journal of Oncology Nursing, 20*(5), 529–536.

Warren, C. B. (2018). Immunotherapy in pediatric oncology: An overview of therapy types and nursing implications. *Clinical Journal of Oncology Nursing, 22*(6), 649–655. https://doi.org/10.1188/18.CJON.649-655.

Wu, Y. P., Linder, L. A., Kanokvimankul, P., Fowler, B., Parsons, B. G., Macpherson, C. F., et al. (2018). Use of a smartphone application for prompting oral medication adherence among adolescents and young adults with cancer. *Oncology Nursing Forum, 45*(1), 69–76.

21

Concepts of Care for Patients With Infection

Donna D. Ignatavicius

http://evolve.elsevier.com/Iggy/

LEARNING OUTCOMES

1. Use clinical judgment to determine ***infection*** control measures based on infection transmission method.
2. Describe evidence-based infection control measures used in hospitals and other inpatient health care facilities.
3. Identify common risk factors for infection, including impaired ***tissue integrity*** and decreased ***immunity.***
4. Identify common assessment findings associated with local and systemic infection, including signs and symptoms of ***inflammation.***
5. Interpret laboratory test findings for patients with infections.
6. Describe collaborative infection control interventions to prevent an increase in antimicrobial resistance.
7. Plan actions to manage fever in the patient with systemic infection.

KEY TERMS

bacteremia The presence of bacteria in the bloodstream.

carrier A person who harbors an infectious agent without signs and symptoms of active disease.

catheter-associated urinary tract infection (CAUTI) A urinary tract infection that occurs as a result of having an indwelling urinary catheter.

Clostridium difficile **infection (CDI)** An infection that destroys normal bowel flora and causes moderate-to-severe diarrhea.

cohorting The practice of grouping patients who are colonized or infected with the same pathogen.

colonization The presence of microorganisms (often pathogenic) in the tissues of the host that do not cause symptomatic disease because of normal flora.

communicable Infection that can be transmitted from person to person.

culture Isolation of a pathogen by cultivation in tissue cultures or artificial media.

disinfection A cleaning process that does not kill spores and only ensures a reduction in the level of disease-causing organisms. High-level disinfection is adequate when an item is going inside the body where the patient has resident bacteria or normal flora (e.g., GI and respiratory tracts).

fecal microbiota transplantation (FMT) A treatment to manage *C. difficile* infection in which healthy normal flora is placed into the lower GI system of the infected patient who does not respond to antibiotic therapy or has recurrent disease.

hand hygiene Handwashing and alcohol-based hand rubs (ABHRs) ("hand sanitizers").

hantaviruses Infections that are caused by exposure to rodent-infected areas such as old sheds or cabins.

health care–associated infection (HAI) Infection acquired in the inpatient health care setting (not present or incubating on admission).

immunity The protection from illness or disease that is maintained by the body's physiologic defenses.

infection The invasion of pathogens (harmful microorganisms) into the body that multiply and cause disease or illness.

particulate matter exposure (PME) A person's exposure to harmful environmental factors (e.g., mold, smoke, metals, toxic organic compounds) that can cause respiratory infections and other health problems, including death.

pathogens Harmful microorganisms in the body that multiply and cause disease or illness.

personal protective equipment (PPE) Items that protect transmission of infection; includes gloves, isolation gowns, face protection (masks, goggles, face shields), and powered air-purifying respirators (PAPRs) or N95 respirators.

powered air-purifying respirator (PAPR) A device that has a high-efficiency particulate air (HEPA) filter and battery to promote positive-pressure airflow and is more effective than N95 respirators in preventing airborne infection transmission.

sterilization A cleaning process that destroys all living microorganisms and bacterial spores. All items or devices that invade human tissue where bacteria are not commonly found should be sterilized.

toxins Protein molecules released by bacteria to affect host cells at a distant site.

PRIORITY AND INTERRELATED CONCEPTS

The primary concept for this chapter is:
- ***Infection***

The interrelated concepts for this chapter are:
- ***Immunity***
- ***Inflammation***
- ***Tissue Integrity***

INFECTION

As defined in Chapter 3, *infection* is the invasion of **pathogens** (harmful microorganisms) into the body that multiply and cause disease or illness. Microorganisms with differing levels of pathogenicity, also referred to as *virulence* (ability to cause disease) surround everyone. However, virulence is related more to the frequency with which a pathogen causes disease (degree of communicability) and its ability to invade and damage a host. It can also indicate the severity of the disease.

PATIENT-CENTERED CARE: GENETIC/GENOMIC CONSIDERATIONS QSEN

A current related issue in genomics is the microbiome. As described in Chapter 6, the microbiome for an adult consists of genomes of all the microorganisms that coexist in and on him or her. Many microorganisms live in or on the human host without causing disease and may be beneficial. These include the organisms that live in the mouth, the rest of the GI tract, the nose and sinuses, and the vagina and on the skin. Most of these organisms are part of our normal flora, which differ somewhat from person to person. Normal flora are mostly nonpathogenic (non–disease causing) when they remain confined to the expected area. However, when they manage to escape their normal human habitat and move elsewhere, they may be pathogenic in the new environment. For example, when GI organisms get into the urinary tract or the blood, serious infections can result. In some instances microorganisms that are often pathogenic may be present in the tissues of the host and yet not cause symptomatic disease because of normal flora; this process is called **colonization**.

In the United States, the Centers for Disease Control and Prevention (CDC) collect information about the occurrence and nature of infections and infectious diseases. It then recommends guidelines to health care agencies for infection control and prevention. Certain diseases such as tuberculosis (TB) must be reported to health departments and the CDC. In Canada the Public Health Agency of Canada also provides guidelines for infection control and for prevention of common infections. The infection control practitioner (ICP) for each health care organization is responsible for tracking infections (surveillance) and ensuring compliance with federal, provincial, and local requirements and accreditation standards.

Transmission of Infectious Agents

Infections can be **communicable** (transmitted from person to person [e.g., influenza]) or not communicable (e.g., peritonitis). Transmission of ***infection*** requires three factors:

- Reservoir (or source) of infectious agents
- Susceptible host with a portal of entry
- Route and method of transmission

TABLE 21.1 Host Factors That Influence the Development of Infection

Host Factor	Increased Risk for Infection
Natural immunity	Congenital or acquired immune deficiencies
Normal flora	Alteration of normal flora by antibiotic therapy
Age	Infants and older adults
Hormonal factors	Diabetes mellitus, corticosteroid therapy, and adrenal insufficiency
Phagocytosis	Defective phagocytic function, circulatory disturbances, and neutropenia
Skin, mucous membranes, normal excretory secretions	Break in skin or mucous membrane integrity; interference with flow of urine, tears, or saliva; interference with cough reflex or ciliary action; changes in gastric secretions
Nutrition	Malnutrition or dehydration
Environmental factors	Tobacco and alcohol consumption and inhalation of toxic chemicals
Medical interventions	Invasive therapy such as endoscopy, urinary catheters, IVs; chemotherapy, radiation therapy, and steroid therapy (suppress immune system); surgery

Reservoirs (sources of infectious agents) are numerous. Animate reservoirs include people, animals, and insects. Inanimate reservoirs include soil, water, handheld mobile devices (especially cell phones), and medical equipment (e.g., IV tubing, urine collection devices). Stethoscopes used for auscultation by many health care professionals carry *Staphylococcus aureus* from the skin of one patient to another. These devices should be cleaned with an antibacterial solution between patients. The host's body can be a reservoir; pathogens colonize skin and body substances (e.g., feces, sputum, saliva, wound drainage). A person with an active infection or an asymptomatic **carrier** (a person who harbors an infectious agent without signs and symptoms of active disease) is a reservoir.

One group of inanimate reservoirs are environmental factors that have recently been categorized as particulate matter, including mold, smoke, dust, metals, and toxic organic compounds. **Particulate matter exposure (PME)** can increase respiratory infections, especially in people who have chronic respiratory diseases such as asthma. PME has also been linked to increased mortality among older adults and other health problems such as ischemic stroke, dementia, and hypertension (Castner & Polivka, 2018).

Continued multiplication of a pathogen is sometimes accompanied by toxin production. **Toxins** are protein molecules released by bacteria to affect host cells at a distant site. *Exotoxins* are produced and released by certain bacteria into the surrounding environment. Botulism, tetanus, diphtheria, and *Escherichia coli* O157:H7–related systemic diseases are attributed to exotoxins. *Endotoxins* are produced in the cell walls of certain bacteria and released only with cell lysis. For example, typhoid and meningococcal diseases are caused by endotoxins.

Host factors influence the development of ***infection*** (Table 21.1). Host defenses provide the body with an efficient system for immunity against pathogens. As defined in Chapter 3, **immunity** is the protection from illness or disease that is maintained by the body's physiologic defenses. Breakdown of these defense mechanisms may increase the susceptibility (risk) of the host for infection.

The patient's immune status plays a large role in determining risk for infection. Congenital abnormalities and acquired health problems (e.g., chronic kidney disease, steroid dependence, cancer) can result in numerous immunologic deficiencies. Decreased ***immunity*** may make the host more susceptible to infection or impair the ability to combat organisms that have gained entry. Chapter 16 discusses the immune system and immunity in detail.

Environmental factors can also influence patients' immune status and thus their susceptibility to or ability to fight ***infection.*** Examples include alcohol consumption, nicotine use, and certain vitamin deficiencies. Malnutrition, especially protein-calorie malnutrition and obesity, places patients at increased risk for infection. Diseases such as diabetes mellitus also predispose a patient to infection. Older adults have decreased ***immunity*** and other physiologic changes that make them very susceptible to infection as outlined in the Patient-Centered Care: Older Adult Considerations box.

PATIENT-CENTERED CARE: OLDER ADULT CONSIDERATIONS QSEN

Factors That May Increase Risk for Infection in the Older Patient

Factor	Aging-Associated Changes or Conditions
Immune system	Decreased antibody production, lymphocytes, and fever response
Integumentary system	Thinning skin, decreased subcutaneous tissue, decreased vascularity, slower wound healing
Respiratory system	Decreased cough and gag reflexes
GI system	Decreased gastric acid and intestinal motility
Chronic illness	Diabetes mellitus, chronic obstructive pulmonary disease, neurologic impairments
Functional and cognitive impairments	Immobility, incontinence, dementia
Invasive devices	Urinary catheters, feeding tubes, IV devices, tracheostomy tubes
Institutionalization	Increased person-to-person contact and transmission

Medical and surgical interventions may impair normal immune responses. Steroid therapy, chemotherapy, and antirejection drugs increase the risk for ***infection.*** Medical devices (e.g., intravascular or urinary catheters, endotracheal tubes, synthetic implants) may also interfere with normal host defense mechanisms. Surgery, trauma, radiation therapy, and burns result in impaired ***tissue integrity.*** *The body's skin is one of the best barriers or defenses against infection.* When this barrier is broken, infection often results. Microorganisms may also enter the body in other ways, including the respiratory tract, GI tract, genitourinary tract, skin and mucous membranes, and bloodstream.

Routes of Transmission. Pathogens may enter the body through the *respiratory tract.* Microbes in droplets are sprayed into the air when people with infected oral or nasal tissues talk, cough, or sneeze. A susceptible host then inhales droplets, and pathogens localize in the lungs or are distributed via the lymphatic system or bloodstream to other areas of the body. Microorganisms that enter the body by the respiratory tract and produce distant infection include influenza virus, coronavirus, *Mycobacterium tuberculosis,* and *Streptococcus pneumoniae.*

Other pathogens enter the body through the *GI tract.* Some stay there and produce disease (e.g., *Shigella* causing self-limited disease). Others invade the GI tract to produce local and distant infection (e.g., *Salmonella enteritidis*). Some produce limited GI symptoms, causing systemic infection (e.g., *Salmonella typhi*) or profound involvement of other organs (e.g., hepatitis A virus). Millions of foodborne illness cases occur each year in the United States. This type of illness results in many hospitalizations and deaths.

Microorganisms also enter through the *genitourinary tract. Urinary tract infection (UTI) is one of the most common health care–associated infections (HAIs).* Indwelling urinary catheters are the primary cause of **catheter-associated urinary tract infections (CAUTIs),** especially in older adults. CAUTIs can increase hospital costs by prolonging the patient's length of stay and complicating his or her recovery. In many settings nurse-driven protocols have helped decrease the use of urinary catheters and associated infections (Scanlon et al., 2017).

Although intact skin is the best barrier to prevent most infections, some pathogens such as *Treponema pallidum* can enter the body through intact *skin* or *mucous membranes.* However, most pathogens enter through breaks in these normally effective surface barriers. Sometimes a medical procedure causes impaired ***tissue integrity*** or a break in mucous membranes, as in catheter-acquired **bacteremia** (bacteria in the bloodstream) and surgical-site infections (SSIs). *Fragile skin of older patients and of those receiving prolonged steroid therapy increases infection risk.*

Microorganisms can gain direct access to the *bloodstream,* especially when invasive devices or tubes are used. The incidence of bloodstream infections (BSIs) continues to increase in hospitals throughout the United States. Central venous catheters (CVCs) are a primary cause of these infections (see Chapter 15 for further discussion of CVC-related BSIs). In the community setting biting insects such as mosquitos can inject organisms into the bloodstream, causing infection (e.g., West Nile viral encephalitis).

Methods of Transmission. For infection to be transmitted from an infected source to a susceptible host, a transport mechanism is required. According to the CDC's classic 2007 infection control guidelines and its 2017 update, microorganisms are transmitted by several routes (www.cdc.gov/infectioncontrol/guidelines/isolation/index.html):

- Contact transmission (indirect and direct)
- Droplet transmission
- Airborne transmission

Contact transmission is the usual mode of transmission of most infections. Many infections are spread by direct or indirect contact. With *direct contact* the source and host have physical contact. Microorganisms are transferred directly from skin to skin or from mucous membrane to mucous membrane. Often called *person-to-person transmission,* direct contact is best illustrated by the spread of the "common cold."

Indirect contact transmission involves the transfer of microorganisms from a source to a host by passive transfer from a contaminated object. Contaminated articles or hands may be sources of infection. For example, patient care devices such as glucometers and electronic thermometers may transmit pathogens if they are contaminated with blood or body fluids. Uniforms, laboratory coats, and isolation gowns used as part of personal protective equipment (PPE) may also be contaminated.

Indirect transmission may involve contact with infected secretions or *droplets*. Droplets are produced when a person talks or sneezes; the droplets travel short distances. Susceptible hosts may acquire ***infection*** through contact with droplets deposited on the nasal, oral, or conjunctival membranes. Therefore the CDC recommends that staff stay 3 or more feet (1 or more m) away from a patient with droplet infection depending on the pathogen. An example of droplet-spread infection is influenza. Another infection spread by droplets and close contact is coronavirus (COVID-19). The recommended distance to stay away from patients who are positive for COVID-19 is at least 6 feet (2 m). This distance is referred to as social distancing.

Airborne transmission occurs when small airborne particles containing pathogens leave the infected source and enter a susceptible host. These pathogens can be suspended in the air for a prolonged time. The particles carrying pathogens are usually contained in droplet nuclei or dust; they are usually propelled from the respiratory tract by coughing or sneezing. A susceptible person then inhales the particles directly into the respiratory tract. For example, tuberculosis (TB) is spread via airborne transmission.

Preventing the spread of microbes that are transmitted by the airborne route requires the use of special air-handling and ventilation systems in an airborne infection isolation room (AIIR). *M. tuberculosis* and the varicella-zoster virus (chickenpox) are examples of airborne agents that require one of these systems. In addition to the AIIR, respiratory protection using a certified **powered air-purifying respirator (PAPR)** is recommended for health care personnel entering the patient's room. This device has a high-efficiency particulate air (HEPA) filter and battery to promote positive-pressure airflow and is more effective than N95 respirators.

Other sources of infectious agents are found in the environment, such as contaminated food, water, or vectors. *Vectors* are insects that carry pathogens between two or more hosts, such as the deer tick that causes Lyme disease and, a more current concern, the mosquito that carries the Zika virus.

The *portal of exit* completes the chain of infection. Exit of the microbe from the host often occurs through the portal of entry. An organism such as *M. tuberculosis* enters the respiratory tract and then exits the same tract as the infected host coughs. Some organisms can exit from the infected host by several routes. For example, varicella-zoster virus can spread through direct contact with infective fluid in vesicles and by airborne transmission.

Physiologic Defenses for Infection

Strong and intact host defenses can prevent microbes from entering the body or can destroy a pathogen that has entered. Impaired host defenses may be unable to defend against microbial invasion, allowing entry of organisms that can destroy cells and cause infection. Common defense mechanisms include (Table 21.2):

- Body tissues
- Phagocytosis
- Inflammation
- Immune systems

TABLE 21.2 Common Physiologic Defenses to Infection

Defense Mechanism	Physiologic Purpose
Body tissues	Intact skin (most important barrier to infection) Mucous membranes (contains lysozymes) Respiratory tract (through filtration, humidification, mucociliary transport, coughing) GI tract (gastric acid, peristalsis, digestive enzymes) Urinary tract (low urinary pH)
Phagocytosis	Neutrophils engulf, ingest, and destroy invading organisms
Inflammation	Inflammatory enzymes, histamine, and fibrinogen "wall off" damaged tissue area
Immune systems	Antibody-mediated and cell-mediated immune processes

Health Promotion and Maintenance

Infections occur most often in high-risk patients such as older adults and those who have inadequate or impaired ***immunity*** (immunocompromised). Because older adults are susceptible to infection, a number of immunizations are recommended for that population as listed in the Patient-Centered Care: Older Adult Considerations box.

Additional interventions to prevent ***infection*** are described in Chapter 3.

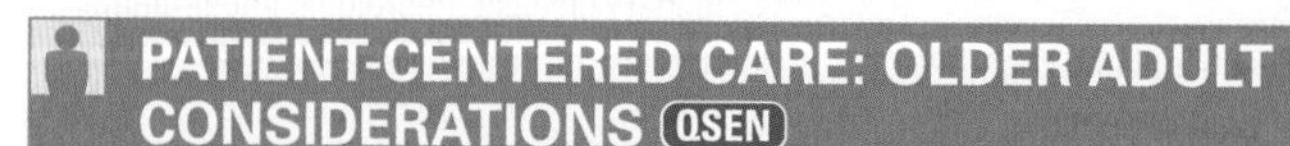

Recommended Immunizations for Older Adults

- Pneumococcal 13-valent conjugate vaccine to prevent pneumonia
- Pneumococcal vaccine polyvalent vaccine to prevent pneumonia
- Yearly influenza vaccine (trivalent or quadrivalent) to prevent influenza (flu)
- Zoster vaccine recombinant to prevent shingles (herpes zoster)
- Adult Tdap vaccine to prevent tetanus, diphtheria, and pertussis (whooping cough) (and Tdap booster every 10 years)

Infection Control in Health Care Settings

Infection acquired in the inpatient health care setting (not present or incubating on admission) is termed a **health care–associated infection (HAI)**. When occurring in a hospital setting, it is sometimes referred to as a *hospital-acquired infection*, but the former term is more accurate. HAIs can be *endogenous* (from a patient's flora) or *exogenous* (from outside the patient, often from the hands of health care workers (HCWs), tubes, or implants). HAIs, including surgical site infections (SSIs), cause increased health care costs and many deaths (see discussion in

Chapter 9). These infections tend to occur most often because HCWs do not follow basic infection control principles.

Infection control within a health care facility is designed to reduce the risk for HAIs and thus reduce morbidity and mortality, as recommended in The Joint Commission's National Patient Safety Goals (NPSGs). This expected outcome is consistent with the desire for health care facilities to create a *culture of safety* within their environments (see Chapter 1). Infection control and prevention are interprofessional efforts and include (Soule & Arias, 2018):

- Health organization–specific and department-specific infection control policies and procedures
- Surveillance and analysis
- Patient and staff education
- Community and interprofessional collaboration
- Product evaluation with an emphasis on quality and cost savings
- Bioengineering for designing health care facilities that help control the spread of infections

The ***infection*** control program of a hospital is coordinated and implemented by a health care professional certified in infection control (CIC) who has clinical and administrative experience. The Centers for Disease Control and Prevention (CDC) recommends one person with CIC credentials for every 100 occupied acute care beds. Long-term care facilities may not have a practitioner who specializes in infection control. However, every facility must designate a health care professional to be responsible for coordinating and implementing an infection prevention and control program.

Long-term care facilities are unique in that they have a large group of older adults who are together in one setting for weeks to years. Nursing homes in particular are required to provide a homelike environment in which residents can move and interact freely. Therefore infection control in these settings can be challenging. As a result, many infectious outbreaks may occur, such as pneumonia, *Clostridium difficile,* and multidrug-resistant organisms (MDROs; discussed in the section Multidrug-Resistant Organism Infections and Colonizations).

Ambulatory and home health care are the fastest-growing segments of the health care system. ***Infection*** remains a common cause of death for dialysis patients. Little information is available about acquired infections in home health settings because data are not systematically collected, surveillance programs are not established, and best practices for infection prevention and control are not widespread.

Methods of Infection Control and Prevention

All health care workers (HCWs) who come in contact with patients or care areas are involved in some aspect of the infection control program of the agency. According to the CDC, infection can be prevented or controlled in several ways:

- Hand hygiene
- Disinfection and sterilization
- Standard Precautions
- Transmission-Based Precautions
- Staff and patient placement and cohorting

BEST PRACTICE FOR PATIENT SAFETY & QUALITY CARE (QSEN)

Hand Hygiene

- When hands are visibly soiled or contaminated with proteinaceous material or visibly soiled with blood or other body fluids, wash hands with soap and water.
- If hands are not visibly soiled, use an alcohol-based hand rub (ABHR) for decontaminating hands or wash hands with soap and water.
- Use either ABHR or wash with soap and water (decontaminate hands) before having direct contact with patients.
- Decontaminate hands before donning (putting on) sterile gloves to perform a procedure such as inserting an invasive device (e.g., indwelling urinary catheter).
- Decontaminate hands after contact with a patient's intact skin (e.g., taking a pulse) or with body fluids or excretions or secretions.
- Decontaminate hands after removing gloves.
- Decontaminate hands after contact with inanimate objects (including medical equipment) in the immediate vicinity of the patient.

Hand Hygiene. HCWs' hands are the primary way in which infection is transmitted from patient to patient or staff to patient. **Hand hygiene** refers to both handwashing and alcohol-based hand rubs (ABHRs) ("hand sanitizers").

In 2002 the U.S. CDC released the classic document "CDC Hand Hygiene Recommendations." These recommendations are summarized in the Best Practice for Patient Safety & Quality Care: Hand Hygiene box.

Handwashing is still an important part of hand hygiene, but it is recognized that in some health care settings, sinks may not be readily available. Despite years of education, HCWs do not wash their hands or perform hand hygiene on a consistent basis.

Effective handwashing includes wetting, soaping, lathering, applying friction under running water for at least 15 seconds, rinsing, and adequate drying. Friction is essential to remove skin oils and disperse transient bacteria and soil from hand surfaces. Performing adequate handwashing takes time that HCWs may not think they have. Handwashing can also cause dry skin; therefore hand moisturizers are essential to maintain good hand health and hygiene.

Alcohol-based hand rubs (ABHRs) allow HCWs to spend less time seeking sinks and more time delivering care. However, these hand rubs have their limitations.

Sterilization and Disinfection. Sterilization and disinfection have helped invasive procedures become much more common and safe. **Sterilization** is a cleaning process that destroys all living microorganisms and bacterial spores. All items or devices that invade human tissue where bacteria are not commonly found should be sterilized. **Disinfection** does not kill spores and only ensures a reduction in the level of disease-causing organisms. High-level disinfection is adequate when an item is going inside the body where the patient has resident bacteria or normal flora (e.g., GI and respiratory tracts). As with sterilization, no high-level disinfection can occur without first cleaning the item. This can be especially difficult with items that have narrow lumens in which organic debris can become

! NURSING SAFETY PRIORITY (QSEN)

Action Alert

If your hands are visibly dirty or soiled or feel sticky or if you have just toileted, *wash your hands instead of using ABHRs.* Keep in mind that ABHRs are also ineffective against spore-forming organisms such as *C. difficile,* a common cause of health care–associated diarrhea, especially in older adults. Do not use an ABHR before inserting eyedrops, ointments, or contact lenses because alcohol can irritate the patient's eyes, causing burning and redness. The Joint Commission's National Patient Safety Goals (NPSGs) require that health care agencies monitor handwashing practices and the use of ABHRs to make sure that HCWs are performing hand hygiene on a regular basis.

The CDC recommends using antiseptic solutions such as chlorhexidine for handwashing in caring for patients who are at high risk for *infection* (e.g., those with decreased *immunity*).

The classic CDC guidelines (CDC, 2002) also address the issue of artificial fingernails, which have been linked to a number of outbreaks because of poor fingernail health and hygiene. The guidelines recommend that artificial fingernails and extenders not be worn while caring for patients at high risk for infections, such as those in critical care units or operating suites. Health care agencies have banned artificial nails for all HCWs providing direct patient care and require that natural nails be short. Some agencies also ban the use of nail polish or gel.

trapped and is not easily visible. For example, endoscopes have been especially challenging to clean and have been linked to a number of infectious outbreaks.

Standard Precautions. The classic 2007 guidelines from the CDC focus on transmission mechanisms and the precautions needed to prevent the spread of infection. Included in these guidelines are Standard Precautions and Transmission-Based Precautions, including Airborne, Droplet, and Contact Precautions (Tables 21.3 and 21.4).

Standard Precautions are based on the belief that all body excretions, secretions, and moist membranes and tissues, excluding perspiration, are potentially infectious. As barriers to potential or actual infections, **personal protective equipment (PPE)** is used. PPE refers to gloves, isolation gowns, face protection (masks, goggles, face shields), and powered air-purifying respirators (PAPRs) or N95 respirators (Fig. 21.1).

! NURSING SAFETY PRIORITY (QSEN)

Action Alert

Remember that gloves are an essential part of infection control and should always be worn as part of Standard Precautions. Either handwashing or use of alcohol-based hand rubs (ABHRs) should be done before donning (putting on) and after removing gloves. The combination of hand hygiene and wearing gloves is the most effective strategy for preventing infection transmission!

The respiratory hygiene/cough etiquette (RH/CE) requirement is directed at patients and visitors with signs of respiratory illness such as sinus or chest congestion, cough, or rhinorrhea ("runny nose"). The elements for RH/CE include:

- Patient, staff, and visitor education
- Posted signs
- Hand hygiene
- Covering the nose and mouth with a tissue and prompt tissue disposal or using surgical masks (or sneezing or coughing into a shirt sleeve rather than the hand)
- Separation from the person with respiratory infection by more than 3 to 6 feet (1 to 2 m)

Transmission-Based Precautions. Transmission-Based Precautions may also be referred to as *Isolation Precautions.* The word *isolation,* however, implies that the patient is physically separated from everyone, which is not always the case.

Airborne Precautions are used for patients known or suspected to have infections transmitted by the airborne transmission route. These infections are caused by organisms that can be suspended in air for prolonged periods. Negative-airflow rooms are required to prevent airborne spread of microbes. Enclosed booths with high-efficiency particulate air (HEPA) filtration or ultraviolet light may be used for sputum induction procedures. Tuberculosis (TB), measles (rubeola), and chickenpox (varicella) are examples of airborne diseases.

Droplet Precautions are used for patients known or suspected to have infections transmitted by the droplet transmission route. Such infections are caused by organisms in droplets that may travel 3 to 6 feet and can be suspended for long periods. Examples of infectious conditions requiring Droplet Precautions include influenza, COVID-19, pertussis, and meningitis caused by either *Neisseria meningitidis* or *Haemophilus influenzae* type B.

Contact Precautions are used for patients known or suspected to have infections transmitted by direct contact or contact with items in the environment. Patients with significant multidrug-resistant organism (MDRO) infection or colonization, such as methicillin-resistant *Staphylococcus aureus* (MRSA) or vancomycin-resistant *Enterococcus* (VRE), are placed on Contact Precautions. Other infections requiring Contact Precautions include pediculosis (lice), scabies, respiratory syncytial virus (RSV), and *C. difficile. C. difficile* infection causes moderate-to-severe diarrhea and is discussed later in this chapter in the section Emerging Infectious Diseases and Bioterrorism.

Staff and Patient Placement and Cohorting. *Adequate staffing* of nurses is an essential method for preventing infection. In addition to a ratio of one infection control practitioner to 100 occupied acute care beds, nurse staffing is critical. When possible, bedside nurse staffing should consist of full-time nurses assigned regularly to the unit to ensure consistent practices.

Patient placement has been used as a way to reduce the spread of infection. The CDC does not mandate that all patients with infections have a private room. It does recommend that private rooms always be used for patients on Airborne Precautions and those in a protective environment (PE). A PE is architecturally designed and structured to prevent infection from occurring in patients who are at extremely high risk, such as those undergoing stem cell therapy. The CDC also prefers private rooms for patients who are on Contact and Droplet Precautions. If private rooms are not available, keep these patients at least 3 to 6 feet apart. Many hospitals are becoming totally private-room facilities. Large health care systems have biomedical engineers to assist in designing the best environment to reduce the spread of infection, including ventilation systems and physical layout.

TABLE 21.3 Recommendations for Application of Standard Precautions for the Care of All Patients in All Health Care Settings

Component	Recommendations
Hand hygiene	Perform hand hygiene after touching blood, body fluids, secretions, excretions, contaminated items; immediately after removing gloves; between patient contacts
Personal protective equipment (PPE)	Use appropriate PPE, including:
• Gloves	• For touching blood, body fluids, secretions, excretions, contaminated items; for touching mucous membranes and nonintact skin
• Gown	• During procedures and patient care activities when contact of clothing/exposed skin with blood/body fluids, secretions, and excretions is anticipated
• Mask, eye protection (goggles), face shield[a]	• During procedures and patient care activities likely to generate splashes or sprays of blood, body fluids, secretions, especially suctioning, endotracheal intubation
Soiled patient care equipment	Handle in a manner that prevents transfer of microorganisms to others and to the environment; wear gloves if visibly contaminated; perform hand hygiene
Environmental control	Develop procedures for routine care, cleaning, and disinfection of environmental surfaces, especially frequently touched surfaces in patient care areas
Textiles and laundry	Handle in a manner that prevents transfer of microorganisms to others and to the environment
Needles and other sharps	Do not recap, bend, break, or hand manipulate used needles; use safety features such as needleless systems when available; place used sharps in puncture-resistant container
Patient resuscitation	Use mouthpiece, resuscitation bag, other ventilation devices to prevent contact with mouth and oral secretions
Patient placement	Prioritize for single-patient room if patient is at increased risk for transmission, is likely to contaminate the environment, does not maintain appropriate hygiene, or is at increased risk for acquiring infection or developing adverse outcome following infection
Respiratory hygiene/cough etiquette (RH/CE) (source containment of infectious respiratory secretions in symptomatic patients, beginning at initial point of encounter [e.g., triage and reception areas in emergency departments and physician offices])	Instruct symptomatic people to cover mouth/nose when sneezing/coughing; use tissues and dispose in no-touch receptacle; observe hand hygiene after soiling of hands with respiratory secretions; wear surgical mask if tolerated or maintain spatial separation greater than 3 to 6 feet if possible

[a]During aerosol-generating procedures on patients with suspected or proven infections transmitted by respiratory aerosols, wear a powered air-purifying respirator (PAPR) (most effective) or N95 mask in addition to gloves, gown, and face and eye protection.

Cohorting is another method of patient placement. **Cohorting** is the practice of grouping patients who are colonized or infected with the same pathogen. This method has been used the most with patients who have an outbreak of an MDRO such as methicillin-resistant *Staphylococcus aureus* (MRSA). It is particularly effective in long-term care settings.

Infection control principles for *patient transport* include limiting movement to other areas of the facility, using appropriate barriers such as covering infected wounds, and notifying other departments or agencies who are receiving the patient about the necessary precautions. *Accurate hand-off communication between agencies is also very important to prevent the spread of infection, according to The Joint Commission's National Patient Safety Goals (NPSGs).*

Protection of Visitors of Patients on Transmission-Based Precautions. Many agencies have policies regarding visitors of patients who are on Transmission-Based Precautions. However, visitors are seldom monitored to ensure that they are following these policies. Munoz-Price et al. (2015) made the following classic recommendations for visitors:

- Use proper hand hygiene before and after the patient visit. (Health care organizations should provide conveniently located alcohol-based rub stations.)
- Wear gowns and gloves (Contact Precautions) to prevent the spread of enteric pathogens or drug-resistant organisms.
- Wear a surgical mask if visiting a patient on Droplet or Airborne Precautions.
- Do not visit patients if you have an active cough or fever.

NCLEX EXAMINATION CHALLENGE 21.1

Safe and Effective Care Environment

Which statements by assistive personnel indicate **understanding** regarding infection control measures needed to care for a client who has possible *Clostridium difficile* infection? **Select all that apply.**

A. "I'll wear an isolation gown when providing direct care."
B. "I'll wear gloves when providing direct care."
C. "I'll wear a mask each time I enter the client's room."
D. "I'll use a hand sanitizer when I can't wash my hands."
E. "I'll wear goggles to protect my eyes."

ANTIMICROBIAL RESISTANCE

Antibiotics have been available for many years. Unfortunately these drugs were commonly prescribed for conditions that did not need them or were given at higher doses and for longer periods of time than were necessary. As a result, a number

TABLE 21.4 Transmission-Based Infection Control Precautions

Precautions (in Addition to Standard Precautions)	Examples of Diseases in Category
Airborne Precautions	
1. Private room required with monitored negative airflow (with appropriate number of air exchanges and air discharge to outside or through HEPA filter); keep door(s) closed 2. Special respiratory protection: • Wear PAPR for known or suspected TB • Susceptible people not to enter room of patient with known or suspected measles or varicella unless immune caregivers are not available • Susceptible people who must enter room must wear PAPR or N95 HEPA filter[a] 3. Transport: patient to leave room only for essential clinical reasons, wearing surgical mask	Diseases that are known or suspected to be transmitted by air: • Measles (rubeola) • *Mycobacterium tuberculosis,* including multidrug-resistant TB (MDRTB) • Varicella (chickenpox)[b]; disseminated zoster (shingles)[b] • COVID-19 (likely spread as airborne)
Droplet Precautions	
1. Private room preferred: if not available, may cohort with patient with same active infection with same microorganisms if no other infection present; maintain distance of at least 3 feet from other patients if private room not available 2. Mask: required when working within 3 to 6 feet of patient 3. Transport: as for Airborne Precautions	Diseases that are known or suspected to be transmitted by droplets: • Diphtheria (pharyngeal) • Streptococcal pharyngitis • Pneumonia • Influenza • Rubella • Invasive disease (meningitis, pneumonia, sepsis) caused by *Haemophilus influenzae* type B or *Neisseria meningitidis* • Mumps • Pertussis • COVID-19 (coronavirus)
Contact Precautions	
1. Private room preferred: if not available, may cohort with patient with same active infection with same microorganisms if no other infection present 2. Wear gloves when entering room 3. Wash hands with antimicrobial soap before leaving patient's room 4. Wear gown to prevent contact with patient or contaminated items or if patient has uncontrolled body fluids; remove gown before leaving room 5. Transport: patient to leave room only for essential clinical reasons; during transport, use needed precautions to prevent disease transmission 6. Dedicated equipment for this patient only (or disinfect after use before taking from room)	Diseases that are known or suspected to be transmitted by direct contact: • Clostridium difficile • Colonization or infection caused by multidrug-resistant organisms (e.g., MRSA, VRE) • Pediculosis • Respiratory syncytial virus • Scabies

[a]Before use: training and fit testing required for personnel.
[b]Add Contact Precautions for draining lesions.
HEPA, High-efficiency particulate air; *MRSA,* methicillin-resistant *Staphylococcus aureus; PAPR,* powered air-purifying respirator; *TB,* tuberculosis; *VRE,* vancomycin-resistant *Enterococcus.*

of microorganisms have become resistant to certain antibiotics—that is, drugs that were once useful no longer control these infectious agents (multidrug-resistant organisms [MDROs]). New antibiotics are not keeping up with preventing antimicrobial resistance (AMR); therefore patients are at risk for increased morbidity and mortality because of health care–associated infections (HCAIs) (Plavskin, 2016). *For this reason, a culture of safety related to infection control has been mandated by the CDC, the Institute for Healthcare Improvement (IHI), and The Joint Commission. Standard Precautions must be strictly followed in all health care settings to prevent more of these difficult and deadly infections.*

One of the newest discoveries to explain the increase in HCAIs, especially the rise in drug-resistant infections, is the formation of biofilms. A *biofilm,* also called *glycocalyx,* is a complex group of microorganisms that functions within a "slimy" gel coating on medical devices such as urinary catheters, orthopedic implants, and enteral feeding tubes; on parts of the body such as the teeth (plaque) and tonsils; and in chronic wounds. These reservoirs become sources of infection for which antibiotics and disinfection are not effective. Antibiotic therapy may increase the growth of microbes within biofilms.

Biofilms are extremely difficult to treat, and mechanical disruption strategies are the mainstay of management and research. Studies on biofilms that cause the most common HCAIs, such as catheter-associated urinary tract infections (CAUTIs) and wound infections, continue to be conducted. Many specific biofilms have been identified, and methods to remove or disrupt them are being researched.

Examples of the most common MDROs are methicillin-resistant *S. aureus,* vancomycin-resistant *Enterococcus,* and carbapenem-resistant *Enterococcus.* Infections caused by these organisms have a high mortality rate when compared with other types of infection. The *Shigella sonnei* bacterium has shown signs of becoming more resistant to ciprofloxacin and other

PATIENT-CENTERED CARE: GENETIC/GENOMIC CONSIDERATIONS (QSEN)

Evidence-Based Practice

A new area of research is the study of genetics and genomics of pathogens to help reduce antimicrobial resistance. For example, genomic bacterial analysis can provide information about sources of infection and how they can be controlled. Population genetic studies can track pathogen transmission and identify infection prevalence and incidence. Transmission mapping can help identify the characteristics of infectious agents, how they are spread, and where carriers of infections are likely to occur within an institution (Plavskin, 2016).

New emerging therapies are being researched that will have major implications for nursing practice in the near future. Examples of these therapies include bacteriophage, more commonly called *phage therapy,* and the development of new vaccines. Phages are bacteria-specific viruses that inject their DNA or RNA to kill bacterial cells. Clinical trials of IV phage therapy were approved in 2019 by the U.S. Food and Drug Administration (Voelker, 2019). While a number of vaccines are currently used, newer ones that are more effective are being developed. For example, current influenza vaccines are changed every year to match circulating viral influenza strains. A universal influenza vaccine developed from a region in the viral genome that is common to all influenza strains is currently being tested to provide long-term immunity (Plavskin, 2019).

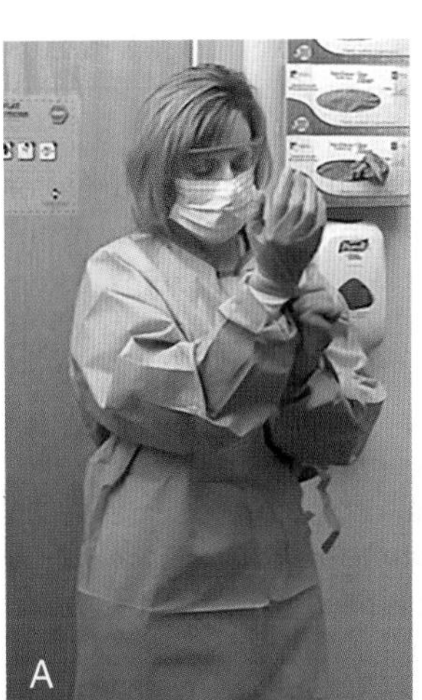
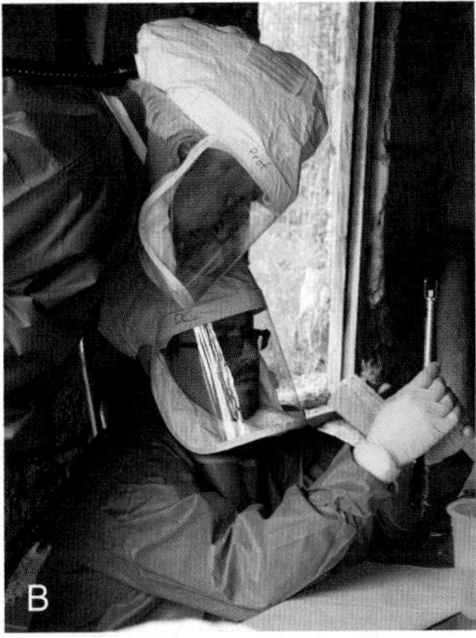

Fig. 21.1 (A) Nurse in personal protective equipment (PPE) caring for a patient in a private room. (B) Powered air-purifying respirator (PAPR). (A copyright © Mosby's Clinical Skills: Essentials Collection. B courtesy of the CDC.)

antibiotics. As a result, shigellosis has become another public health concern in the United States.

Methicillin-Resistant *Staphylococcus aureus* (MRSA)

S. aureus is a common bacterium found *on* the skin and perineum and in the nose of many people. It is usually not infectious when in these areas because the number of bacteria is controlled by good hygiene measures. However, when skin or mucous membranes are not intact, localized infection such as boils or conjunctivitis may occur. If the organism enters into deep wounds, surgical incisions, the lungs, or the bloodstream, more serious or systemic infections occur that require strong antibiotics such as methicillin.

Within the past 40 years, more and more *S. aureus* infections have not responded to methicillin or other penicillin-based drugs. Known as *MRSA,* these infections are one of the fastest growing and most common in health care today. This type of infection is called *health care–associated MRSA,* or *HA-MRSA.* Patients who have HA-MRSA have increased hospital stays at a very high cost. To add to this problem, some patients may be colonized with the organism. Health care staff members may also colonize. Patients who develop HA-MRSA pneumonia, skin infections, or bacteremia (bloodstream infection [BSI]) can quickly progress to bacteremia (Plavskin, 2019).

MRSA is spread by direct contact and invades hospitalized patients, most often older adults, through indwelling urinary catheters, vascular access devices, open wounds, and endotracheal tubes. It is susceptible to only a few antibiotics, such as IV vancomycin and oral linezolid. IV ceftaroline fosamil is the first cephalosporin antibiotic approved to treat MRSA (Burchum & Rosenthal, 2019).

NURSING SAFETY PRIORITY (QSEN)

Drug Alert

Delafloxacin is the first fluoroquinolone demonstrated to be effective against MRSA infections. Delafloxacin is available as an oral and IV drug and tends to bind to other drugs containing metal cations, making it less effective. If prescribed orally, therefore, be sure to administer the drug at least 2 hours before or 6 hours after antacids and vitamin or mineral supplements. When giving the drug as an IV preparation, avoid administering it with any solution containing metal cations, such as magnesium.

Most health care agencies have specific policies regarding MRSA transmission preventive measures. For example, some health care facilities have a MRSA-surveillance program in which each patient's nose is swabbed and cultured for MRSA. Staff may also be cultured. All patients with HA-MRSA infection or colonization should be placed on Contact Precautions.

Nursing research has contributed to these policies by identifying interventions to decrease microbes in their patients. Examples include bathing patients with chlorhexidine wipes and administering nasal mupirocin ointment (Donskey & Deshpande, 2016).

Community-associated MRSA, or CA-MRSA, causes infections in healthy, nonhospitalized people, especially those living in college housing and prisons. It is easily transmitted among family members and can cause serious skin and soft-tissue infections, including abscesses, boils, and blisters. The best way to decrease the incidence of this growing problem is health teaching, including:

- Performing frequent hand hygiene, including using hand sanitizers
- Avoiding close contact with people who have infectious wounds
- Avoiding large crowds
- Avoiding contaminated surfaces
- Using good overall hygiene

Minocycline and doxycycline are usually effective in treating CA-MRSA (Burchum & Rosenthal, 2019).

Vancomycin-Resistant *Enterococcus* (VRE)

Enterococci are bacteria that live in the intestinal tract and are important for digestion. When they move to another area of the body, such as during surgery, they can cause an infection, which is usually treatable with vancomycin. However, in recent years many of these infections have become resistant to the drug, and VRE results. Risk factors for this infection include prolonged hospital stays, severe illness, abdominal surgery, enteral nutrition, and immunosuppression. Common infections caused by VRE include urinary tract infection, endocarditis, pelvic infection, and bacteremia. Place patients with VRE infections on Contact Precautions to prevent contamination from body fluids.

Unfortunately VRE can live on almost any surface for days or weeks and still be able to cause an infection. Contamination of toilet seats, door handles, and other objects is very likely for a lengthy period. Therefore the most current recommendation is to discontinue Contact Precautions after at least one negative stool or rectal swab culture after antimicrobial therapy is discontinued. Some facilities require up to three consecutive negative cultures at least 1 week apart before Contact Precautions are discontinued (Banach et al., 2018).

Carbapenem-Resistant Enterobacteriaceae (CRE)

Carbapenem antibiotics, most often given for peritonitis and bacterial meningitis, have been used extensively for the past 20 years. Examples of this class of antibiotics include imipenem and meropenem.

Klebsiella and *E. coli* are types of Enterobacteriaceae that are located within the intestinal tract. Carbapenem-resistant Enterobacteriaceae (CRE) are a family of pathogens that are difficult to treat because they have a high level of resistance to carbapenems caused by enzymes that break down the antibiotics. *Klebsiella pneumoniae* carbapenemase (KPC) and New Delhi metallo-beta-lactamase are examples of these enzymes. Examples of infections caused by CRE include urinary tract infection, pneumonia, and bacteremia (Plavskin, 2019).

! NURSING SAFETY PRIORITY (QSEN)

Action Alert

Patients who are high risk for CRE include those in critical care units or nursing homes and patients who are immunosuppressed, including older adults. To prevent the transmission of this infection, place patients who are at high risk on Contact Precautions. The CDC recommends chlorhexidine (2% dilution) bathing to prevent CRE or decrease colonization and other types of infections from MDROs.

OCCUPATIONAL AND ENVIRONMENTAL EXPOSURE TO SOURCES OF INFECTION

The U.S. Occupational Safety and Health Administration (OSHA) is a federal agency that protects workers from injury or illness at their place of employment. Unlike the voluntary guidelines developed by the CDC, OSHA regulations are law. Employers can be fined or disciplined for noncompliance with OSHA regulations. The regulation for prevention of exposure to bloodborne pathogens, such as hepatitis B, hepatitis C, or human immune deficiency virus (HIV), is one example of an OSHA regulation.

Reduction of skin and soft-tissue injuries (e.g., needlesticks) is essential to reduce bloodborne pathogen transmission to health care personnel. *OSHA mandates that sharp objects ("sharps") and needles be handled with care.* Many contaminated sharp-object exposures involve nurses. Needleless devices have helped decrease these exposures, especially when caring for patients receiving infusion therapy (see Chapter 15).

Other infection control concerns that nurses and other HCWs have are the possibilities of pandemic influenza or biologic agent exposure. A large outbreak of one of the MDROs is also worrisome, especially if no drug is sensitive enough for successful management. Nurses may fear that they will accidentally bring the infectious agent to their homes and families.

! NURSING SAFETY PRIORITY (QSEN)

Action Alert

To help prevent the transmission of an MDRO, wear scrubs and change clothes before leaving work. Keep work clothes separate from personal clothes. Take a shower when you get home, if possible, to rid your body of any unwanted pathogens. Be careful not to contaminate equipment that is commonly used such as your stethoscope.

Another environmental source for infection is animals or insects. For example, **hantavirus** infections are caused by exposure to rodent-infested areas such as old sheds or cabins. Saliva and excrement from mice and rats living in the southwestern part of the United States are the primary sources of hantaviruses. Although hantavirus is not a common infection, patients can die from complications such as *hantavirus pulmonary syndrome,* a severe and potentially lethal respiratory disease. Teach patients to avoid potential exposure to hantaviruses by avoiding rodent-infested areas. If infested areas need to be cleaned, teach patients to wear rubber or nonlatex gloves and either a tight-seal negative-pressure respirator or a positive-pressure powered air-purifying respirator (PAPR) equipped with an N100 or P100 filter.

EMERGING INFECTIOUS DISEASES AND BIOTERRORISM

Additional current concerns related to infection and infection control are the risk for emerging infectious diseases and global bioterrorism. Many of these diseases are transmitted via global travel (Chapman & Delahanty, 2018). As with any pathogen, strict infection control measures can prevent transmission of these microbes to you and your patients. Some of the most serious infections are briefly described here.

Pandemic infections such as influenza are another threat to the population. Health care workers (HCWs) are encouraged to have annual influenza vaccines to prevent infection with common strains of the virus. The federal government and health care agencies around the United States include the risk for pandemic disease in their disaster planning.

Contaminated food is another source of ***infection.*** The incidence of foodborne infections has risen in the United States as contaminated fresh spinach, ground beef, and other foods were found to contain *E. coli* O157:H7 and other pathogens. Major restaurant chains such as Chipotle have been the source of GI infections for many of their customers. Multiple illnesses and deaths in the United States have been caused by these infections. Safer food preparation practices and increased monitoring by federal agencies have resulted from demand for public safety, but more oversight is needed to prevent large outbreaks.

Another pathogen, *C. difficile,* can overgrow in the intestine most often as a result of antibiotic therapy. Some patients are colonized with the pathogen and have no infection. Other patients have **Clostridium difficile infection (CDI)**, which destroys normal bowel flora and causes moderate-to-severe diarrhea. CDI can be fatal, especially among older adults (Wilson, 2018). A new, more virulent strain of this pathogen has developed in the past decade as a result of the use of fluoroquinolone antibiotics such as ciprofloxacin.

C. difficile is spread by direct contact among people and indirect contact with inanimate objects such as medical equipment and commodes. CDI toxins cause colon dysfunction and cell death from sepsis. CDI is best diagnosed by means of clinical symptoms and a positive laboratory test confirmation. Patients who have three or more liquid stools within 24 hours with no laxative use are suspected of having the ***infection.*** Although several laboratory tests are available, a fecal gastrointestinal pathogen panel–polymerase chain reaction (GIP-PCR) is one of the most specific to confirm a diagnosis. This test requires a stool specimen and is most reliable when the specimen is unformed or liquid (Chapman & Foley, 2018).

The patient should be placed on Contact Precautions to prevent infection transmission, and the patient's room should be disinfected with a sporicidal cleaning product (Houghton, 2019). Fever and abdominal pain and cramping commonly occur with diarrheal stools. Oral metronidazole and vancomycin have been the drugs of choice to treat CDI. However, some patients experience recurrence of infection after treatment with these drugs. Two new oral antibacterial drugs available for specifically managing *C. difficile* are fidaxomicin and teicoplanin (Wilson, 2018). A recent publication by the Society for Healthcare Epidemiology of America (SHEA) recommends that Contact Precautions for *C. difficile* be continued for at least 48 hours after diarrhea has stopped (Banach et al., 2018).

A recently approved treatment for CDI is **fecal microbiota transplantation (FMT)** to place healthy normal flora into the lower GI system of the infected patient who does not respond to antibiotic therapy or has recurrent disease. Potential donors of fecal material should not have impaired ***immunity,*** history of drug abuse, chronic GI disorders, or recent exposure to potential pathogens such as those that could be present from tattooing or travel to endemic areas. Before the FMT, the donor is screened with a variety of blood and stool tests to rule out active or chronic infections such as hepatitis A, B, or C.

Fecal transplantation is most commonly performed by colonoscopy. Therefore the pre-procedure and follow-up care are the same as for any patient having a colonoscopy (see Chapter 48). FMT has been very successful for many patients with *C. difficile.* It is being investigated for use in patients who have other lower GI diseases such as inflammatory bowel disease and irritable bowel syndrome (Kelly et al., 2015). However, the U.S. Food and Drug Administration (FDA) published a MedWatch regarding the presence of multidrug-resistant organisms, such as enteropathogenic *Escherichia coli,* in donor stool (FDA, 2019). Primary health care providers are encouraged to inform patients eligible for FMT about this risk, which can be fatal.

In addition to concerns about emerging infections, preparation for and education about *bioterrorism* have been a major focus of the U.S. government since September 11, 2001. In some cases vaccines are no longer given for biologic agents such as smallpox. Many people in the United States have never been vaccinated, and those who had vaccinations many years ago are not guaranteed to have lifelong immunity. Anthrax, usually seen in animals, may be spread to the skin or inhaled. These infections have a high fatality rate in humans. Plague, once seen centuries ago, is one of the biggest threats because the survival rate is low. Vaccines are being researched and stockpiled by the U.S. government for some of the common biologic agents.

PROBLEMS RESULTING FROM INADEQUATE ANTIMICROBIAL THERAPY

Inadequate antimicrobial therapy may range from an incorrect choice of drug to inadequate drug dosing. Drug regimen nonadherence (accidental failure to take the drug) also contributes to resistant-organism development.

Some diseases such as tuberculosis (TB) have legal sanctions that require that a patient complete treatment. Patients who are at risk for noncompliance or nonadherence with an anti-TB drug regimen may be placed on *directly observed therapy (DOT).* This means that an HCW must observe and validate patient compliance with the drug regimen. DOT has been very effective at reducing the spread of multidrug-resistant TB.

Serious complications of ***infection*** may also result from incomplete or inadequate antibiotic therapy. Local infections that could be cured without complications such as cellulitis and pneumonia may progress to abscess formation or systemic infection if appropriate drug therapy is not continued. Although drug therapy does not always prevent abscess, early therapy may prevent or limit the size of an abscess.

In addition to abscess formation, inadequate therapy or a missed diagnosis may lead to systemic spread, or sepsis. *Sepsis is the number-one cause of hospitalized patient deaths* (Plavskin, 2016). If the infection is not resolved or if it is treated with drugs that are ineffective for the offending microorganism, the pathogen may enter the bloodstream (referred to as *bacteremia, septicemia,* or *bloodstream infection [BSI]*). Inadequately treated local infections may also lead to widespread *sepsis* with leukocytosis (increased white blood cell count) and inflammation. In severe or advanced cases, leukopenia (decreased white blood cell count) and life-threatening disseminated intravascular coagulation (DIC) may occur. After pathogens invade the bloodstream, no site is protected from invasion.

BSI may progress to *septic shock,* more accurately called *sepsis-induced distributive shock.* In septic shock, insufficient cardiac output is compounded by hypovolemia. Inadequate blood supply to vital organs leads to hypoxia (lack of oxygen) and multiple organ failure. Chapter 34 describes sepsis, septic shock, and patient management in detail.

❖ Interprofessional Collaborative Care

◆ Assessment: Recognize Cues

History. The patient's age, history of tobacco or alcohol use, current illness or disease (e.g., diabetes), past and current drug use (e.g., steroids), and poor nutritional status may place him or her at increased risk for infection. Patients with impaired ***immunity*** as a result of disease or therapies such as chemotherapy and radiation are also at a high risk for infection. Ask the patient about previous vaccinations or immunizations, including the dates of administration.

Ask the patient if he or she has recently been in a hospital or nursing home as a patient or visitor. Inquire about any invasive testing, such as a colonoscopy, or recent surgery. Ask if the patient had an indwelling urinary catheter or IV line. These invasive treatments often are the source of ***infection.***

Determine whether the patient has been exposed to infectious agents. A history of recent exposure to someone with similar clinical symptoms or to contaminated food or water, as well as the time of exposure, helps to identify a possible source of infection. This information helps determine the incubation period for the disease and thus provides a clue to its cause.

! NURSING SAFETY PRIORITY (QSEN)

Action Alert

Ask the patient about particulate matter exposure (PME) factors. Using the I-PREPARE environmental exposure history will help prompt you to investigate these factors (Castner & Polivka, 2018). Ask the patient about:

- **P**resent work
- **R**esidence
- **E**nvironmental concerns
- **P**ast work
- **A**ctivities

Once environmental or particular matter exposure has been identified using *P-R-E-P:* provide **R**eferrals (and resources as needed) and **E**ducate the patient on ways to lessen or prevent exposure.

Contact with animals, including pets, may also increase exposure to ***infection.*** Question the patient about recent animal contact at home or work or in leisure activities (e.g., hiking). Insect bites should be documented.

Obtain a travel history. Travel to areas both within and outside the patient's home country may expose a susceptible person to infectious organisms not encountered in the local community.

A thorough sexual history may reveal behavior associated with an increased risk for sexually transmitted infections (STIs). Obtain a history of IV drug use and a transfusion history to assess the patient's risk for hepatitis B, hepatitis C, and HIV infections.

Identifying the type and location of symptoms may point to affected organ systems. The onset order of symptoms gives clues to the specific problem. Gathering a history of past ***infection*** or colonization with MDROs will help determine which type of Transmission-Based Precautions is needed.

Physical Assessment/Signs and Symptoms. Disorders caused by pathogens vary depending on the infection cause and site. Common signs and symptoms are associated with specific sites of infection. Wounds can easily become infected when ***tissue integrity*** is impaired (also see Chapter 3). Carefully inspect the skin for symptoms of *local* infection at any site (pain, swelling, heat, redness, pus). Extended wound redness and/or phlebitis (venous inflammation) indicates that the infection has become *systemic.*

Fever (generally a temperature above 101° F [38.3°C]), possible chills, and malaise are primary indicators of a *systemic* infection. The patient may also have tachycardia due to dehydration that can result from a fever. Fever may accompany other noninfectious health problems; and infection can be present without fever, especially in patients who have decreased ***immunity.***

PATIENT-CENTERED CARE: OLDER ADULT CONSIDERATIONS (QSEN)

The older adult, whose normal temperature may be 1° to 2° lower than the normal temperature in younger adults, may have a fever at 99°F (37.2°C). In most patients with an *infection,* fever (hyperthermia) is a normal immune response that can help destroy the pathogen. Assess the patient for these signs and symptoms and carefully ask about their history and pattern. Assess for signs and symptoms of dehydration, such as tachycardia, acute confusion, and restlessness.

Lymphadenopathy (enlarged lymph nodes), pharyngitis, and GI disturbance (usually diarrhea or vomiting) are often associated with infection. To detect enlargement, palpate the cervical, axillary, and other lymph nodes; examine the throat for redness. Ask about changes in stool and if the patient has had any nausea or vomiting.

NCLEX EXAMINATION CHALLENGE 21.2

Safe and Effective Care Environment

The nurse takes a history for a client admitted to the hospital. Which factors in the nursing history indicate that the client is at risk for infection? **Select all that apply.**

A. Diabetes mellitus type 2 for 20 years
B. 52-pack year history of cigarette smoking
C. Admitted from a long-term care facility
D. Has a history of multiple urinary tract infections
E. Is 84 years of age

Psychosocial Assessment. The patient with an ***infection*** or infectious disease often has psychosocial concerns. Delay in diagnosis because of the need to await clinical test results produces anxiety. Assess the patient's and family's level of understanding about various diagnostic procedures and the time required to obtain test results. Plan education on infection risk reduction at a time when they are ready to learn.

Feelings of malaise and fatigue often accompany ***infection.*** Assess the patient's current level of activity and the impact of these symptoms on family, occupational, and recreational activities.

The potential spread of infection to others is an additional stress associated with the diagnosis. The patient may curtail family and social interactions for fear of spreading the illness. Determine the patient's and family's understanding of the ***infection,*** the mode of transmission, and mechanisms that may limit or prevent transmission. Special precautions, although sometimes necessary for preventing transmission of the organism, can be emotionally difficult for the patient and family.

A number of transmissible infectious diseases, especially those identified with social stigma (e.g., IV drug abuse), are associated with labeling. The patient may feel socially isolated or have guilt related to behavior that increased the risk for ***infection.*** Observe carefully for the patient's reaction to labels and how these feelings further affect socialization.

Laboratory Assessment. The definitive diagnosis of an ***infection*** or infectious disease requires identification of a microorganism in the tissues of an infected patient. Direct examination of blood, body fluids (such as urine), and tissues under a microscope may not yield a definitive identification. However, laboratory assessment usually provides helpful information about organisms, such as amount, shape, motility, and reaction to staining agents. Even when direct microscopy does not provide a conclusive specific diagnosis, often enough information is obtained for starting appropriate antimicrobial therapy.

The best procedure for identifying a microorganism is a culture, or isolation of the pathogen by cultivation in tissue cultures or artificial media. Specimens for culture can be obtained from almost any body fluid or tissue. The primary health care provider usually decides when and where the specimen for culture is taken.

Proper collection and handling of specimens for culture, using Standard Precautions, are essential for obtaining accurate results. Specimens collected must be appropriate for the suspected infection. Be sure that the specimen is of adequate quantity and is freshly obtained and placed in a sterile container to preserve the specimen and microorganism. Label the specimen properly, including the date and time it was collected. Follow your health care organization's policy if you have any questions about how to perform a culture.

After isolation of a microorganism in culture, antimicrobial *sensitivity* testing is performed to determine the effects of various drugs on that particular microorganism. For example, an agent that is killed by acceptable levels of an antibiotic is considered sensitive to that drug. An organism that is not killed by tolerable levels of an antibiotic is considered resistant to that drug. Preliminary results are usually available in 24 to 48 hours, but the final results generally take 72 hours. *Antimicrobial therapy should not begin until after the culture specimen has been obtained.*

Rapid cultures or assays are used in ambulatory care settings to provide quicker assessments of infections. The most popular is the rapid antigen detection test for group A streptococci to rule out "strep throat" in patients with pharyngitis (sore, inflamed throat). Other examples of rapid testing are those for tuberculosis (TB) and influenza ("flu").

A *white blood cell (WBC) count with differential* is often done for the patient with a suspected infection. The normal range for WBCs is 5000/mm^3 (5.0 × 10^9/L) to 10,000/mm^3 (10.0 × 10^9/L). Five types of leukocytes (WBCs) are measured as part of the results:

- Neutrophils
- Lymphocytes
- Monocytes
- Eosinophils
- Basophils

In most active infections, especially those caused by bacteria, the total leukocyte count is elevated. Various infections are characterized by changes in the percentages of the different types of leukocytes. The differential count usually shows an increased number of immature neutrophils, or a *shift to the left* ("left shift"). However, a few infectious diseases such as malaria and infectious mononucleosis are associated with neutropenia (decreased neutrophils). Chapter 36 describes hematologic testing in more detail.

The *erythrocyte sedimentation rate (ESR)* measures the rate at which red blood cells fall through plasma. This rate is most significantly affected by an increased number of acute-phase reactants, which occurs with inflammation. Thus an elevated ESR (>20 mm/hr) indicates ***inflammation*** or infection somewhere in the body. Chronic ***infection,*** especially osteomyelitis and chronic abscesses, is commonly associated with an elevated ESR. The ESR is chronically elevated with inflammatory arthritis, such as rheumatoid arthritis (see Chapter 46). The effectiveness of therapy is often determined by a decrease in this value.

Serologic testing is performed to identify pathogens by detecting antibodies to the organism. The antibody titer tends to *increase* during the acute phase of infectious diseases such as hepatitis B. The titer *decreases* as the patient's condition improves. Other examples of testing for viruses include the enzyme-linked immunosorbent assay (ELISA) and the reverse transcriptase–polymerase chain reaction (RT-PCR).

Imaging Assessment. X-ray films may be obtained to determine activity of or destruction by an infectious microorganism. Radiologic studies (e.g., chest films, sinus films, joint films, GI studies) are available for diagnosis of infection in a specific body site.

More sophisticated techniques for ***infection*** diagnosis include computed tomography (CT) scans and magnetic resonance imaging (MRI). CT and ultrasonography are helpful in assessing for abscesses. CT scans help identify suspected osteomyelitis and fluid collections that point to possible infection. MRI scans provide a cross-sectional assessment for infection.

Another diagnostic tool for the evaluation of a patient with a possible ***infection*** or infectious disease is ultrasonography. This noninvasive procedure is particularly helpful in detecting infection involving the heart valves.

Scanning techniques using radioactive substances such as gallium can determine the presence of inflammation caused by infection. Inflammatory tissue is identified by its increased uptake of the injected radioactive material.

◆ **Analysis: Analyze Cues and Prioritize Hypotheses.** The priority collaborative problem for patients with a systemic infection is *fever due to the immune response triggered by the pathogen.* In addition, the patient has a potential for developing sepsis and septic shock, which are discussed in detail in Chapter 34.

◆ Planning and Implementation: Generate Solutions and Take Action

Managing Fever

Planning: Expected Outcomes. Patients with an infection are expected to have a body temperature within normal limits as a result of effective interprofessional collaborative care.

Interventions. The primary concern is to provide measures to eliminate the underlying cause of fever and to destroy the causative microorganism. In collaboration with the interprofessional health care team, nurses use a variety of methods to manage fever.

Drug therapy plays a major role in interprofessional collaborative care of patients with infection. *Antimicrobials,* also called *anti-infective agents,* are the cornerstone of drug therapy. Antipyretics are used to decrease patient discomfort and reduce fever.

Antibiotics, antiviral agents, and antifungals are common types of antimicrobial drugs that are given for infection, depending on its type. Effective antibiotics are available to treat nearly all bacterial infections, but misuse of antibiotics has contributed to the development of antibiotic resistance and multidrug-resistant organisms (MDROs) discussed earlier in this chapter.

Effective antimicrobial therapy requires delivery of an appropriate drug, sufficient dosage, proper administration route, and sufficient therapy duration. These four requirements ensure delivery of a concentration of drug sufficient to inhibit or kill infecting microorganisms. To ensure effectiveness of antibiotic therapy such as vancomycin, primary health care providers may require serum trough and peak levels to be drawn. A specimen for a *trough level* (lowest serum drug concentration) is drawn about 30 minutes before the next scheduled vancomycin dose. A specimen for a *peak level* (highest serum drug concentration) is drawn 30 to 60 minutes after medication administration (Burchum & Rosenthal, 2019).

Primary health care providers collaborate on selecting drugs and dosing. Antimicrobials act on susceptible pathogens by:

- Inhibiting cell wall synthesis (e.g., penicillins and cephalosporins)
- Injuring the cytoplasmic membrane (e.g., antifungal agents)
- Inhibiting biosynthesis, or reproduction (e.g., erythromycin and gentamicin)
- Inhibiting nucleic acid synthesis (e.g., actinomycin)

! NURSING SAFETY PRIORITY QSEN

Drug Alert

Before administering an antimicrobial drug, check to see that the patient is not allergic to it. Be sure to take an accurate allergy history before drug therapy begins to prevent possible life-threatening reactions, such as anaphylaxis!

Teach the drug's actions, side effects, and toxic effects to patients and their families. Observe and report side effects and adverse events. These reactions vary according to the specific classification of the drug. Most antibiotics can cause nausea, vomiting, diarrhea, and rashes. Stress the importance of completing the entire course of drug therapy, even if symptoms have improved or disappeared.

PATIENT-CENTERED CARE: OLDER ADULT CONSIDERATIONS QSEN

For older adults, be sure to teach the need to drink additional fluids if diarrhea occurs as result of antibiotic therapy. Observe older adults in inpatient facilities carefully for signs and symptoms of dehydration as described in Chapter 13. Acute confusion, hypotension, and tachycardia are common indicators of dehydration and require interventions such as IV fluids. Serum electrolyte levels may increase, causing additional risks to the older adult.

Antipyretic drugs such as acetaminophen are often given to reduce fever. Because these drugs mask fever, monitoring the course of the disease may be difficult. Therefore unless the patient is very uncomfortable or if fever presents a significant risk (e.g., in the patient with heart failure, febrile seizures, or head injury), antipyretics are not always prescribed.

Teach patients that they may have waves of sweating after each dose. Sweating may be acconmpanied by a fall in blood pressure followed by return of fever. These unpleasant side effects of antipyretic therapy can often be alleviated by increasing fluid intake and regular scheduling of drug administration.

Other interventions to reduce fever may include external cooling and fluid administration. Perform a thorough assessment before and after interventions are implemented.

External cooling with hypothermia blankets or ice bags or packs can be an effective mechanism for reducing a high fever. Alternative cooling methods may be used. Sponging the patient's body with tepid water or applying cool compresses to the skin and pulse points to reduce body temperature is sometimes helpful. Ice packs and cooling blankets may be used for patients with extremely high temperatures. *Teach assistive personnel (AP) to observe for and report shivering during any form of external cooling. Shivering may indicate that the patient is being cooled too quickly.*

The use of fans is discouraged because they can disperse airborne- or droplet-transmitted pathogens. Fans can also disturb air balance in negative-pressure rooms, making them positive-pressure rooms and allowing possible transmission of the agent to those outside the room.

In patients with fever, fluid volume loss is increased from rapid evaporation of body fluids and increased perspiration. As body temperature increases, fluid volume loss increases.

CLINICAL JUDGMENT CHALLENGE 21.1

Physiological Integrity

A 75-year old woman fell in her yard and injured her leg on a leaf rake 2 days ago. The prongs of the rake caused a large laceration on her right calf. Her husband took her to the local Urgent Care Center, where her wound was cleaned and dressed. She was placed on an oral antibiotic and told to follow up with her primary health care provider (PHCP). This morning she noticed increased redness, swelling, and a "red streak" above her wound. Her husband called her PHCP, who arranged for a direct admission to the local hospital. On admission to the hospital, the nurse collects this information based on admission assessment:

Client History

- Has had diabetes mellitus type 2 and hypertension for over 10 years
- Takes amlodipine 5 mg orally each morning
- Takes metformin 500 mg twice a day
- Lives at home with her husband
- Is able to perform ADLs independently
- Does not drive
- Has two daughters who live several hours away

Current Assessment

- Reports affected leg pain is 8/10
- Oral temperature = 102.6°F (39.2°C)
- Apical pulse = 100 beats/min; respiratory rate = 22 breaths/minute
- Blood pressure = 88/54 mm Hg
- Laboratory findings:
  - Hemoglobin (Hgb) = 13 g/dL (130 g/L)
  - Hematocrit (Hct) = 40% (0.40 volume fraction)
  - WBC = 14,000/mm^3 (14.0 × 10^9/L)
  - Erythrocyte sedimentation rate (ESR) = 46 mm/hr
  - Fasting blood glucose = 289 mg/dL (12.4 mmol/L)

1. **Recognize Cues:** What assessment information in this client situation is the most important and immediate concern for the nurse? (Hint: Identify the **relevant** information first to determine what is most important.)
2. **Analyze Cues:** What client conditions are consistent with the **most relevant** information? (Hint: Think about priority collaborative problems that support and contradict the information presented in this situation.)
3. **Prioritize Hypotheses:** Which possibilities or explanations are **most likely** to be present in this client situation? Which possibilities or explanations are the most serious? (Hint: Consider all possibilities and determine their urgency and risk for this client.)
4. **Generate Solutions:** What actions would most likely achieve the desired outcomes for this client? Which actions should be **avoided** or are **potentially harmful?** (Hint: Determine the desired outcomes first to decide which interventions are appropriate and those that should be avoided.)
5. **Take Action:** Which actions are the most appropriate and how should they be implemented? In what **priority order** should they be implemented? (Hint: Consider health teaching, documentation, requested health care provider orders or prescriptions, nursing skills, collaboration with or referral to health team members, etc.)
6. **Evaluate Outcomes:** What client assessment would indicate that the nurse's actions were **effective?** (Hint: Think about signs that would indicate an improvement, decline, or unchanged client condition.)

Care Coordination and Transition Management. Patients with infections may be cared for in the home (group or individual), hospital, nursing home, or ambulatory care setting, depending on the type and severity of the infection. Infections among older adults in nursing homes and assisted-living facilities are common. Residents often have meals together in a communal dining room and participate in group activities. Confused residents may not wash their hands or may enter other resident rooms. Immunizing them against common infections is highly recommended because these illnesses can cause severe complications or death in older adults.

Home Care Management. The patient with an infectious disease such as osteomyelitis may require continued, long-term antibiotic therapy at home or in a long-term care facility. Emphasize the importance of a clean home environment, especially for the patient who continues to have compromised ***immunity*** or who is uniquely susceptible to superinfection (i.e., reinfection or a second infection of the same kind) to reduce the chance of infection. Drugs often need to be refrigerated. Ensure that the patient has access to proper storage facilities, and teach him or her to check for signs of improper storage, such as discoloration of the drug.

Ask about the availability of handwashing facilities in the home and check that supplies and instructions are provided as needed. Most people do not know how to wash hands correctly. Demonstrate the procedure with the patient and family and request a repeat demonstration.

Self-Management Education. Explaining the disease and making certain that the patient understands what is causing the illness are the primary purposes of health teaching. Discuss whether the pathogen causing the infection can be spread to others and the modes of transmission.

If the patient has an infection that is potentially transmissible, teach the patient, family, and other home caregivers about precautions. Explain whether any special household cleaning is necessary and, if so, what those special steps include. If syringes with needles are used to administer drug therapy, explain how to dispose of needles safely and legally in the community. Clothing soiled with blood or other body fluids can be washed with bleach or disinfectant. Recommended cleaning measures should be based on actual available equipment and facilities.

For the patient who is discharged to the home setting to complete a course of antimicrobial therapy, the importance of adherence to the planned drug regimen needs to be stressed. Explain the importance of both the timing of doses and the completion of the planned number of days of therapy. Teach the patient (and family as appropriate) how the agents need to be taken (e.g., before meals, with meals, without other agents) and the possible side effects. Side effects include those that are expected (e.g., gastric distress) and adverse reactions that are more severe (e.g., rash, fever, other systemic signs and symptoms). Teach the patient about allergic manifestations and the need to notify a primary health care provider if an adverse reaction occurs. Also discuss what to do if a drug dose is missed (e.g., doubling the dosage, waiting until the next dose time).

Many patients are discharged with an infusion device to continue drug therapy at home or in other inpatient facilities. The patient, family member, or home care nurse administers the drugs. Home care services are often used to teach appropriate administration of drug therapy in the patient's home. Health teaching and wound care may also be needed. These services have proven to be efficient, effective, psychologically supportive,

! NATIONAL PATIENT SAFETY GOALS

Hand-off communication such as the SBAR between the two facilities is required to facilitate a smooth transition from the hospital to the intermediate care setting, according to The Joint Commission's National Patient Safety Goals.

and less expensive than hospitalization or skilled nursing facilities (SNFs).

The patient is often anxious and fearful that the infection will be transmitted to family members or friends. Teaching the patient and the family ways of preventing the spread of disease allays these fears. Pay careful attention to the patient's and family's concerns. Making concrete suggestions (e.g., "Your partner can wear gloves when changing your dressing") to address specific concerns may reduce these fears.

The patient with an infection associated with lifestyle behaviors such as sexual activity or IV drug abuse may have guilt related to the disease. Encourage discussion of feelings associated with the illness, and assist in locating support systems that may help alleviate these feelings, such as clergy or other spiritual or cultural leaders.

Health Care Resources. At times a patient who has been hospitalized for an infection may not be able to return to the home setting because of lack of caregiver support. In such cases temporary placement in an SNF may be needed. Document care requirements, patient history of infection or colonization with MDROs, medication schedules, and personal needs and preferences on transfer forms.

◆ Evaluation: Evaluate Outcomes. Evaluating the care of the patient with an infection on the basis of the identified priority problems is important. The expected outcomes include that the patient:

- Has body temperature and other vital signs within baseline
- Does not experience complications such as dehydration and sepsis
- Adheres to drug therapy regimen

GET READY FOR THE NEXT-GENERATION NCLEX® EXAMINATION!

Key Points

Review these Key Points for each NCLEX Examination Client Needs Category.

Safe and Effective Care Environment

- Handwashing and alcohol-based hand rubs (ABHRs) are two methods of hand hygiene to prevent infection. **QSEN: Safety; Quality Improvement**
- The Centers for Disease Control and Prevention (CDC) recommends a ban on artificial fingernails for health care professionals when they are caring for patients at high risk for infection. **QSEN: Evidence-Based Practice**
- Use clinical judgment to prevent or control infection through hand hygiene, disinfection and sterilization, personal protective equipment (PPE), patient placement, and adequate staffing. Proper hand hygiene and gloves are the most important interventions because the hands of health care workers (HCWs) are the primary way in which disease is transmitted from patient to patient. **Clinical Judgment; QSEN: Evidence-Based Practice**
- Standard Precautions are used with all patients in health care settings, assuming that all body excretions and secretions are potentially infectious (see Table 21.2). **QSEN: Safety**
- Airborne Precautions are used for patients who have infections transmitted through the air such as tuberculosis (TB). **QSEN: Evidence-Based Practice**
- Droplet Precautions are used for patients who have infections transmitted by droplets such as influenza and certain types of meningitis. **QSEN: Evidence-Based Practice**
- Contact Precautions are used for patients who have infections transmitted by direct contact or contact with items in the patient's environment. **QSEN: Evidence-Based Practice**

Health Promotion and Maintenance

- Health teaching about signs and symptoms of infection and drug therapy is important for the patient with an infection being managed at home; some patients may need health care nursing services for IV antimicrobial therapy. **Clinical Judgment**
- Teach patients about antimicrobial therapy and protective measures to prevent infection transmission. **QSEN: Safety**
- Teach patients how to avoid community-acquired MRSA by performing frequent hand hygiene and by avoiding crowds and direct contact with others who have infections. **QSEN: Safety**
- Teach patients about how to prevent transmission of ***infection*** (e.g., using insect repellent to prevent tick and mosquito bites). **QSEN: Safety**

Psychosocial Integrity

- Help patients cope with feelings about having an infection through verbalization and collaboration with the health care team. **QSEN: Teamwork and Collaboration**

Physiological Integrity

- Patients at the highest risk for infection include older adults, health care professionals at risk for needlesticks, and patients who have chronic disease (e.g., diabetes) or impaired ***immunity***. Patients who take long-term steroid therapy or have had invasive procedures or impaired ***tissue integrity*** are also at a high risk for infection. **QSEN: Safety**
- Multidrug-resistant organisms (MDROs), which are the result of the overuse of antibiotic therapy, include methicillin-resistant *Staphylococcus aureus* (MRSA), vancomycin-resistant *Enterococcus* (VRE), and carbapenem-resistant Enterobacteriaceae (CRE). Follow agency policies to prevent these infections and their transmission. **QSEN: Evidence-Based Practice**

- A biofilm, also called *glycocalyx,* is a complex group of microorganisms that function within a "slimy" gel coating on medical devices such as urinary catheters, orthopedic implants, and enteral feeding tubes; on parts of the body such as the teeth (plaque) and tonsils; and in chronic wounds. **QSEN: Evidence-Based Practice**
- Common signs and symptoms of ***infection*** include fever and lymphadenopathy. If infections are not treated or are inadequately treated by the interprofessional health care team, systemic sepsis (septicemia), septic shock, and disseminated intravascular coagulation (DIC) may result. **QSEN: Safety**
- A culture is the most definitive way to confirm and identify microorganisms; sensitivity testing determines which antibiotics will destroy the identified microbes. **QSEN: Evidence-Based Practice**
- Antimicrobials and antipyretics are the most common types of drugs used when infection is accompanied by fever. **QSEN: Evidence-Based Practice**
- Antipyretics are used only when the fever presents a significant risk or the patient is very uncomfortable because antipyretics may mask the disease. **QSEN: Evidence-Based Practice**
- Critical issues for the next decade include bioterrorism, emerging infectious diseases (such as Ebola), and multidrug-resistant organisms (MDROs). **QSEN: Safety**
- Foodborne infections are becoming increasingly common as a result of contaminated food consumed by restaurant customers. **QSEN: Safety**
- Fecal microbiota transplantation (FMT) is a recent therapy for managing chronic *Clostridium difficile*–associated infection. Fecal transplantation restores normal flora to the infected patient. **QSEN: Evidence-Based Practice**

MASTERY QUESTIONS

1. A client who was bitten by a spider develops cellulitis of the left lower arm. What assessment findings will the nurse expect when caring for this client? **Select all that apply.**
   A. Fever
   B. Pain
   C. Redness around the spider bite
   D. Warmth in the affected arm
   E. Swelling of the affected arm

2. A client is diagnosed with *C. difficile* infection. What nursing action is the priority for the client?
   A. Provide meticulous skin care.
   B. Place the client on Contact Precautions.
   C. Give the client an antipyretic medication.
   D. Encourage the client to drink extra fluids.

REFERENCES

Asterisk (*) indicates a classic or definitive work on this subject.

Banach, D. B., Bearman, G., Barnden, M., & Hanrahan, J. A. (2018). Duration of contact precautions for acute-care settings. *Infection Control and Hospital Epidemiology, 39*(2), 127–144.

Burchum, J., & Rosenthal, L. (2019). *Lehne's pharmacology for nursing* (10th ed.). St. Louis: Elsevier.

Castner, J., & Polivka, B. J. (2018). Nursing practice and particulate matter exposure. *The American Journal of Nursing, 118*(8), 52–56.

*Centers for Disease Control and Prevention (CDC). (2002). Guideline for hand hygiene in health-care settings: Recommendations of the healthcare infection control practices advisory committee and the HICPAC/SHEA/APIC/IDSA hand hygiene task force. *MMWR. Morbidity and Mortality Weekly Report, 51*(RR–16), 1–44.

Chapman, C., & Delahanty, K. (2018). Global convergence of emerging infectious diseases: Only a plane ride away. *Nursing, 48*(2), 14–16.

Chapman, C., & Foley, C. (2018). The *C. difficile* puzzle: Putting it all together. *Nursing, 48*(11), 34–40.

Donskey, C. J., & Deshpande, A. (2016). Effect of chlorhexidine bathing in preventing infections and reducing skin burden and environmental contamination: A review of the literature. *American Journal of Infection Control, 44*(5), Supplement, 17–21.

Houghton, D. (2019). Infection in acute care: Evidence for practice. *The American Journal of Nursing, 119*(10), 24–32.

*Kelly, C. R., Kahn, S., Kashyap, P., Laine, L., Rubin, D., Atreja, A., et al. (2015). Update on fecal microbiota transplantation 2015: Indications, methodologies, mechanisms, and outlook. *Gastroenterology, 149*(1), 223–237.

*Munoz-Price, L. S., Banach, D. B., Bearman, G., Gould, J. M., Leekha, S., Morgan, D. J., et al. (2015). Isolation precautions for visitors. *Infection Control and Hospital Epidemiology*. Available on CJO 2015 https://doi.org/10.1017/ice.2015.67.

Plavskin, A. (2019). Fighting antimicrobial resistance with genetics and genomics. *MEDSURG Nursing, 28*(5), 297–302.

Plavskin, A. (2016). Genetics and genomics of pathogens: Fighting infections with genome-sequencing technology. *Medsurg Nursing, 25*(2), 91–96.

Scanlon, K., Wells, C., Woolforde, L., Khameraj, A., & Baumgartner, J. (2017). Saving lives and reducing harm: A CAUTI reduction program. *Nursing Economic$, 35*(3), 134–141.

Soule, B. M., & Arias, K. M. (2018). *The APIC/JCR infection prevention and control workbook* (3rd ed.). Oak Brook, IL: Joint Commission.

U.S. Food and Drug Administration (FDA). (2019). *Fecal microbiota for transplantation: Safety communication: Role of serious adverse reactions due to transmission of multi-drug resistant organisms.* https://www.fda.gov/safety/medical-product-safety-information/fecal-microbiota-transplantation-safety-communication-risk-of-serious-adverse-reactions-due-to-transmission-of-multi-drug-resistant-organisms.

Voelker, R. (2019). FDA approves bacteriophage trial. *Journal of the American Medical Association, 321*(7), 638.

Wilson, A. (2018). Antibiotic treatment for *clostridium difficile* infection in adults. *The American Journal of Nursing, 118*(7), 63.

22

Assessment of the Skin, Hair, and Nails

Cherie R. Rebar

http://evolve.elsevier.com/Iggy/

LEARNING OUTCOMES

1. Collaborate with the interprofessional team to perform a complete skin assessment.
2. Prioritize evidence-based care for patients having invasive integumentary diagnostic testing affecting ***tissue integrity.***
3. Teach evidence-based ways for adults to protect their skin and decrease their risk for cancer development.
4. Explain how physiologic aging changes of the integumentary system affect ***tissue integrity.***
5. Implement nursing interventions to decrease the psychosocial impact for the patient undergoing assessment testing of the skin.
6. Apply knowledge of anatomy and physiology, genetic risk, and principles of aging to perform a focused assessment of the skin, hair, and nails.
7. Use clinical judgment to document the integumentary assessment in the electronic health record.
8. Interpret assessment findings for patients with a suspected or actual integumentary problem.

KEY TERMS

acute paronychia Inflammation of the skin around the nail, which usually occurs with a torn cuticle or an ingrown toenail.

bioburden Number of microorganisms living on a surface.

chronic paronychia Inflammation of the skin around the nail that persists for months.

dandruff An accumulation of patchy or diffuse white or gray scales on the surface of the scalp.

dermal papillae Fingerlike projections of dermal tissue that anchor the epidermis to the dermis.

dystrophic Abnormal in appearance.

ecchymoses Large purple, blue, or yellow bruises of the skin resulting from small hemorrhages; these bruises are larger than petechiae.

ground substance A lubricant composed of protein and sugar groups that surrounds the dermal cells and fibers and contributes to the skin's normal suppleness and turgor.

hirsutism Abnormal growth of body hair, especially on the face, chest, and the linea alba of the abdomen of women.

keratin The protein produced by keratinocytes; makes the outermost skin layer waterproof.

keratinocytes Basal skin cells attached to the basement membrane of the epidermis that undergo cell division and differentiation to continuously renew skin tissue integrity and maintain optimal barrier function. As basal cells divide, keratinocytes are pushed upward and flattened to form the stratified layers of the epithelium (malpighian layers).

lichenified An abnormal thickening of the skin to a leathery appearance; can occur in patients with chronic dermatitis because of their continual rubbing of the area to relieve itching.

lunula The white, crescent-shaped part of the nail at the lower end of the nail plate.

macular Referring to a macula, a discolored spot on the skin that is not raised above the surface.

nits Lice eggs.

papular Referring to a papule, a small, solid elevation of the skin.

petechiae Pinpoint red spots on the mucous membranes, palate, conjunctivae, or skin.

primary lesions In describing skin disease, the initial reaction to a problem that alters one of the structural components of the skin.

pruritus An unpleasant itching sensation.

purpura Purple patches on the skin that may be caused by blood disorders, vascular abnormalities, or trauma.

rete pegs The fingers of epidermal tissue that project into the dermis.

sebum A mildly bacteriostatic, fat-containing substance produced by the sebaceous glands. Sebum lubricates the skin and reduces water loss from the skin surface.

secondary lesions Description of skin disease in terms of changes in the appearance of the primary lesion. These changes occur with progression of an underlying disease or in response to a topical or systemic therapeutic intervention.

stratum corneum The outermost horny skin layer.

taut Tightly stretched.

turgor The amount of skin elasticity.

PRIORITY AND INTERRELATED CONCEPTS

The priority concepts for this chapter are:

- ***Tissue Integrity***
- ***Infection***

Skin, hair, and nails make up the integumentary system. The largest organ of the body is intact skin; it has barrier, alarm, and combat functions. Skin ***tissue integrity*** plays a major role in protection by protecting the body against invasion of pathogenic organisms by providing first, second, and third lines of defense. The normal flora on the surfaces of skin and mucous membranes repels some of the more harmful microorganisms. Specialized cells in the skin engulf foreign substances (antigens) that invade the body when ***tissue integrity*** is lost and then alert the immune system to the presence of the invader. Localized tissue inflammation and swelling work to contain the invading pathogen until white blood cells can respond and remove this threat.

Intact skin helps regulate body temperature and maintains fluid and electrolyte balance. Emotional stress, systemic disease, certain drugs, and skin injury or disease can alter skin function, appearance, and texture. The skin's sensory function allows the use of touch as an intervention to provide comfort, relieve pain, and communicate caring.

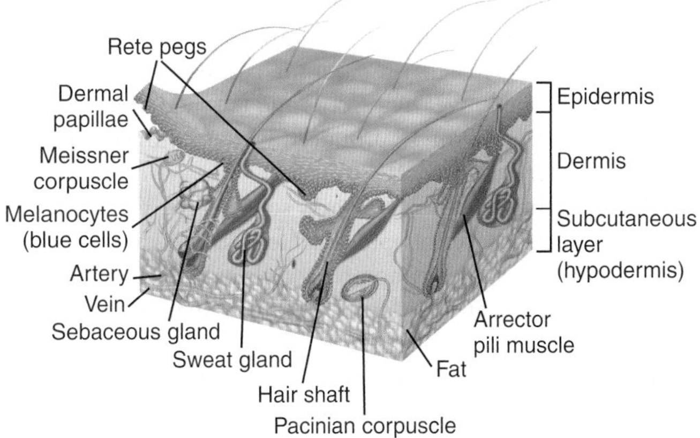

Fig. 22.1 Anatomy of the skin. (From Kumar, V., Aster, J., Robbins, S.L., Abbas, A.K., & Fausto N. [2009]. *Robbins & Cotran pathologic basis of disease* [8th ed.]. St. Louis: Saunders.)

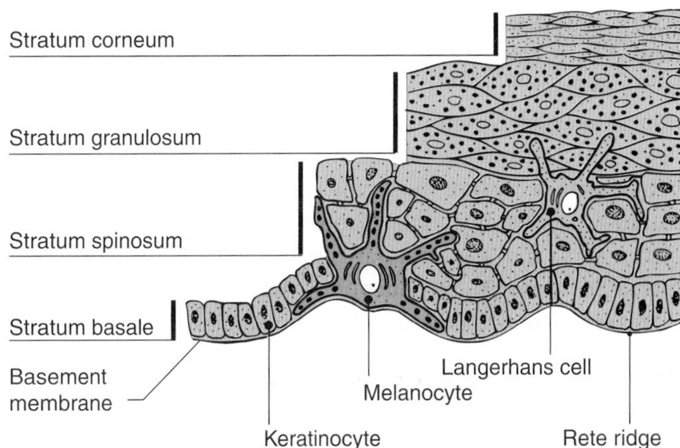

Fig. 22.2 Anatomy of the epidermis. (From Gawkrodger, D., & Ardern-Jones, M.R. [2012]. *Dermatology* [5th ed.]. Philadelphia: Churchill Livingstone.)

ANATOMY AND PHYSIOLOGY REVIEW

Structure of the Skin

There are three skin layers: subcutaneous tissue (fat), dermis, and epidermis (Fig. 22.1). Each layer has unique properties that help the skin perform its complex functions.

Subcutaneous fat (adipose tissue [fat]) is the innermost layer of the skin, lying over muscle and bone. Fat distribution varies with body area, age, and gender. Fat cells insulate the body and absorb shock, padding internal structures. Blood vessels go through the fatty layer and extend into the dermis, forming capillary networks that supply nutrients and remove wastes.

The dermis (corium) is the layer above the fat layer and contains no skin cells but does contain some protective mast cells and macrophages (see Chapter 16). The dermis is composed of interwoven collagen and elastic fibers that give the skin flexibility and strength.

Collagen, the main component of dermal tissue, is a protein produced by fibroblast cells. Its production increases in areas of tissue injury and helps form scar tissue. Fibroblasts also produce **ground substance,** a gel-like substance the fills the spaces between cells and contributes to skin suppleness and turgor. Skin elasticity depends on the amount and quality of the dermal elastic fibers, which are primarily composed of elastin.

The dermis has capillaries and lymph vessels for the exchange of oxygen and heat. Sensory nerves transmit the sensations of touch, pressure, temperature, pain, and itch.

The epidermis is the outermost skin layer. It is anchored to the dermis by fingerlike projections (**rete pegs**) that interlock with dermal structures called **dermal papillae.** Less than 1 mm thick, the epidermal layer is the first line of defense between the body and the environment.

The epidermis (Fig. 22.2) does not have its own blood supply. Instead it receives nutrients by diffusion from the blood vessels in the dermal layer. Attached to the basement membrane of the epidermis are the basal **keratinocytes**—skin cells that undergo cell division and differentiation to continuously renew skin and maintain optimal barrier function. As basal cells divide, keratinocytes are pushed upward and form the *spinous layer (stratum spinosum).* Together the basal layer and the spinous layer are referred to as the *germinative layer (stratum germinativum)* because these layers are responsible for new skin growth (McCance & Huether, 2019). The keratinocytes continue to enlarge and flatten as they move upward to form the outermost horny skin layer (**stratum corneum**). When these cells reach the stratum corneum (in 28 to 45 days), they are no longer living cells and are shed from the skin surface. **Keratin**, a protein produced by keratinocytes, makes the horny layer waterproof.

On the palms of the hands and soles of the feet an additional thick, clear layer of epidermis forms, known as the *stratum lucidum.* This layer of nonliving cells pads and protects the underlying dermal and epidermal structures in these vulnerable areas.

Vitamin D is activated in the epidermis by ultraviolet (UV) light, such as sunlight. Once activated, it is distributed by the blood to the GI tract to promote uptake of dietary calcium.

Melanocytes are pigment-producing cells found at the basement membrane. These cells give color to the skin and account for the ethnic differences in skin tone. Darker skin tones are not caused by increased numbers of melanocytes; rather, the size of the pigment granules *(melanin)* contained in each cell determines the color. Melanin protects the skin from damage by UV light, which stimulates melanin production. For this reason, people with dark skin (and thus more melanin) are less likely to experience sunburn than people with lighter skin. Freckles, birthmarks, and age spots are lesions caused by patches of increased melanin production. Melanin production also increases in areas that have endocrine changes or inflammation.

Structure of the Skin Appendages

Hair differs in type and function in various body areas. Hair growth varies with race, gender, age, and genetic predisposition. Individual hairs can differ in both structure and rate of growth, depending on body location.

Hair follicles are located in the dermal layer of the skin but are actually extensions of the epidermal layer (see Fig. 22.1). Within each hair follicle, a round column of keratin forms the hair shaft. Hair color is genetically determined by a person's rate of melanin production.

Hair growth occurs in cycles of a growth phase followed by a resting phase. Growth is dependent on a good blood supply and adequate nutrition. Stressors can alter the growth cycle and result in temporary hair loss. Permanent baldness, such as male pattern baldness, is inherited.

Nails protect and enhance sensation of the fingertips and toe tips, have cosmetic value, and are useful for grasping and scraping. Like hair follicles, the nails are extensions of the keratin-producing epidermal layers of the skin.

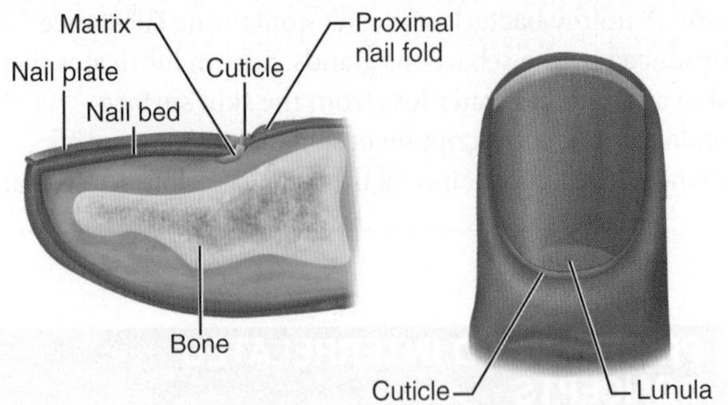

Fig. 22.3 Anatomy of the nail.

The **lunula**—the white, crescent-shaped part of the nail at the lower end of the nail plate—is where nail keratin is formed and nail growth begins (Fig. 22.3). Nail growth is a continuous, slow process. Fingernail replacement takes 3 to 4 months. Toenail replacement may take up to 12 months.

The cuticle attaches the nail plate to the soft tissue of the nail fold. The nail body is translucent, and the pinkish hue reflects a rich blood supply beneath the nail surface. Nail growth and appearance are often altered during systemic disease or serious illness.

Sebaceous glands are distributed over the entire skin surface except for the palms of the hands and soles of the feet. Most of these glands are connected directly to the hair follicles (see Fig. 22.1).

Sebaceous glands produce **sebum**, a mildly bacteriostatic, fat-containing substance. Sebum lubricates the skin and reduces water loss from the skin surface.

Sweat glands of the skin are of two types: eccrine and apocrine. Eccrine sweat glands arise from the epithelial cells. They are found over the entire skin surface and are not associated with the hair follicle. The odorless, colorless secretions of these glands are important in body temperature regulation. This sweat and the resultant water evaporation can cause the body to lose up to 10 to 12 liters of fluid in a single day.

Apocrine sweat glands are in direct contact with the hair follicle and are found mostly in the axillae, nipple, umbilical, and perineal body areas. The interaction of skin bacteria with the secretions of these glands causes body odor.

Functions of the Skin

The skin is a complex organ responsible for the regulation of many body functions throughout the life span (Table 22.1) (McCance & Huether, 2019). In addition to the skin's protective and regulatory functions, its exterior location makes it an important way to visually communicate a patient's state of health.

Skin Changes Associated With Aging

The process of aging begins at birth. As changes in physiology progress with aging, the skin also undergoes age-related changes in structure and function. Figs. 22.4 to 22.6 show age-related skin changes.

TABLE 22.1 **Functions of the Skin**

Epidermis	Dermis	Subcutaneous Tissue
Protection		
Provides protection from injury by corrosive materials via keratin Inhibits proliferation of microorganisms because of dry external surface Provides mechanical strength through intercellular bonds	Provides cells for wound healing Provides mechanical strength: Collagen fibers Elastic fibers Ground substance Houses sensory nerve receptors that signal skin injury and inflammation	Absorbs mechanical shock Insulates energy reserve
Homeostasis (Water Balance)		
Prevents systemic dehydration and electrolyte loss due to low permeability to water and electrolytes	Responds to inflammation, injury, and ***infection*** via lymphatic and vascular tissues	No function
Temperature Regulation		
Eccrine sweat glands allow dissipation of heat through evaporation of sweat secreted onto the skin surface	Cutaneous vasculature promotes or inhibits heat loss from the skin surface	Fat cells insulate and assist in retention of body heat
Sensory Organ		
Transmits a variety of sensations through the neuroreceptor system	Relays sensations to the brain via nerve receptors	Contains large pressure receptors
Vitamin Synthesis		
Allows photo conversion of 7-dehydrocholesterol to active vitamin D	No function	No function
Psychosocial		
Body image alterations occur with many epidermal diseases	Body image alterations occur with many dermal diseases	Body image alterations may result from changes in body fat stores

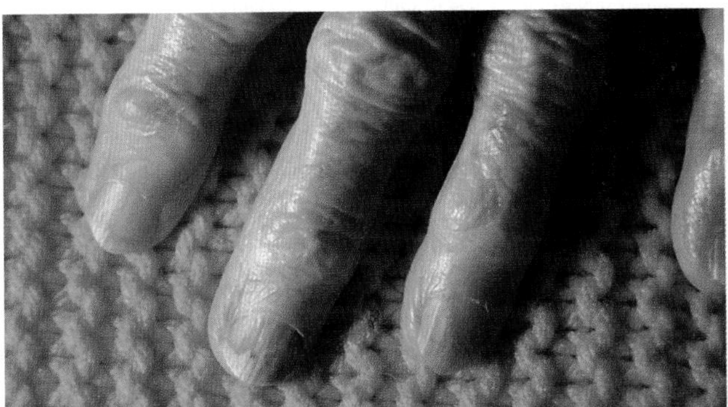

Fig. 22.4 Nail changes, longitudinal ridges, and thickening.

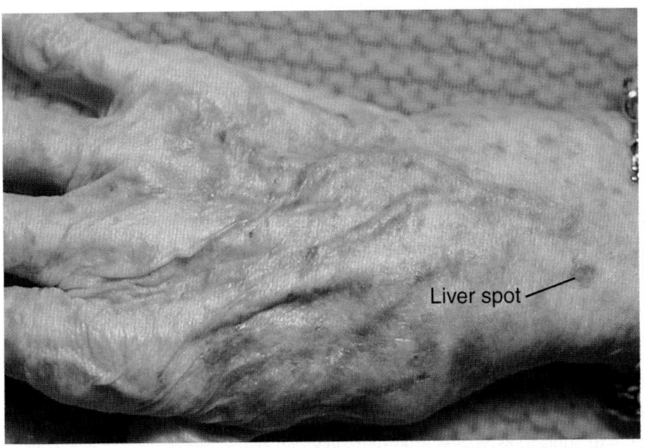

Fig. 22.5 Paper thin, transparent skin with actinic lentigo (liver spots).

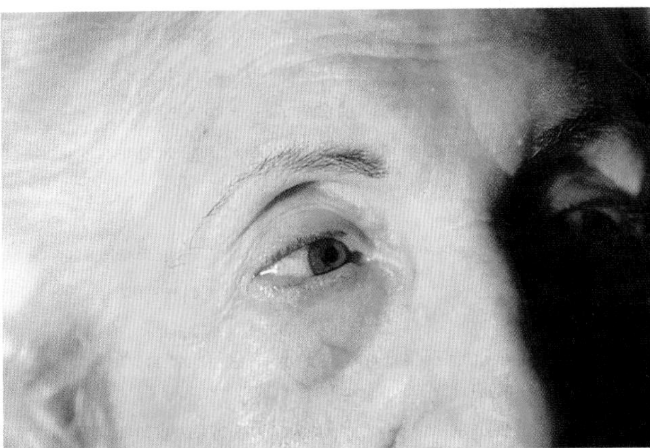

Fig. 22.6 Eyelid eversion, deepening of the eye orbit, and "bags" under the eye.

Individual differences exist in how quickly and to what degree the skin ages, although there are commonalities seen in all aging skin (Touhy & Jett, 2020). (See the Patient-Centered Care: Older Adult Considerations: Changes in the Integumentary System Related to Aging box). Although genetic factors, hormonal changes, and disease may change skin appearance over time, chronic sun exposure is the highest risk factor that leads to degeneration of the skin components.

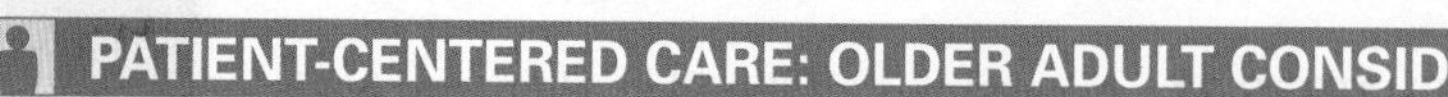

PATIENT-CENTERED CARE: OLDER ADULT CONSIDERATIONS QSEN

Changes in the Integumentary System Related to Aging

Physical Changes	Clinical Findings	Nursing Actions
Epidermis		
Decreased epidermal thickness	Skin transparency and fragility	Handle patients carefully to reduce skin friction and shear. Assess for excessive dryness or moisture. Teach those with excessive dryness to limit warm baths to 3 times weekly and to use skin emollient (Kirkland-Kyhn, 2018). Avoid taping the skin.
Decreased cell division	Delayed wound healing	Avoid skin trauma and protect open areas.
Decreased epidermal mitotic homeostasis	Skin hyperplasia and skin cancers (especially in sun-exposed areas)	Assess non–sun-exposed areas for baseline skin features. Assess exposed skin areas for sun-induced changes.
Increased epidermal permeability	Increased risk for irritation	Teach patients how to avoid exposure to skin irritants.
Decreased immune system cells	Decreased skin inflammatory response	Do not rely on degree of redness and swelling to correlate with the severity of skin injury or localized **infection.**
Decreased melanocyte activity	Increased risk for sunburn	Teach patients to wear hats, sunscreen (minimum of SPF30), and protective clothing. Teach patients to avoid sun exposure from 10 a.m. to 4 p.m.
Hyperplasia of melanocyte activity (especially in sun-exposed areas)	Changes in pigmentation (e.g., liver spots, age spots)	Teach patients to keep track of pigmented lesions. Teach which changes should be evaluated for malignancy.
Decreased vitamin D production	Increased risk for osteomalacia	Urge patients to take a multiple vitamin or a calcium supplement with vitamin D.
Flattening of the dermal-epidermal junction	Increased risk for shearing forces, resulting in blisters, purpura, skin tears, and pressure-related injuries	Never pull or drag patients. Help patients confined to bed or chairs change positions at least every 2 hours. Avoid using adhesives unless necessary (Kirkland-Kyhn, 2018) and use care when removing adhesive wound dressings. Encourage a well-balanced diet with protein and adequate hydration (Kirkland-Kyhn, 2018).
Dermis		
Decreased dermal blood flow	Increased susceptibility to dry skin	Teach patients to apply moisturizers when the skin is still moist and to avoid agents that promote skin dryness.
Decreased vasomotor responsiveness	Increased risk for heat stroke and hypothermia	Teach patients to dress for the environmental temperatures.
Decreased dermal thickness	Paper-thin, transparent skin with an increased susceptibility to trauma	Handle patients gently and avoid the use of tape or tight dressings. Use lift sheets when positioning patients.
Degeneration of elastic fibers	Decreased tone and elasticity	Check skin turgor on the forehead or chest.
Benign proliferation of capillaries	Cherry hemangiomas	Teach patients that these are benign.
Reduced number and function of nerve endings	Reduced sensory perception	Tell patients to use a bath thermometer and lower the water heater temperature to prevent scalds.
Subcutaneous Layer		
Thinning subcutaneous layer	Increased risk for hypothermia	Teach patients to dress warmly in cold weather.
	Increased risk for pressure injury	Help patients confined to bed or chairs change positions at least every 2 hours.
Hair		
Decreased number of hair follicles and rate of growth	Increased hair thinning	Suggest wearing hats to prevent heat loss in cold weather and to prevent sunburn.
Decreased number of active melanocytes in follicle	Gradual loss of hair color (graying)	Inform patients that hair color loss can occur at any age.
Nails		
Decreased rate of growth	Increased risk for fungal ***infection***	Inspect the nails of all older adults. Teach patients to keep feet clean and dry.
Decreased nail bed blood flow	Longitudinal nail ridges	Assess oral mucosa for cyanosis.
Thickening of the nail	Toenails thicken and may overhang the toes	Use fingernails to assess capillary refill. Cut toenails straight across. Do not use nail appearance alone to assess for a fungal ***infection.*** Assess skin next to the nail to determine whether the thick nail is irritating it.
Glands		
Decreased sebum production	Increased size of nasal pores; large comedones	Teach patients not to squeeze the pores or comedones to prevent skin trauma.
Decreased eccrine and apocrine gland activity	Increased susceptibility to dry skin	Urge patients to use soaps with a high fat content. Teach patients to avoid frequent bathing with hot water. Teach patients to apply moisturizers after bathing while skin is moist.
	Decreased perspiration with decreased cooling effect	Do not use sweat production as an indicator of hyperthermia.

BEST PRACTICE FOR PATIENT SAFETY & QUALITY CARE QSEN

Obtaining an Accurate History of the Patient With a Skin Problem

Medical-Surgical History
- Do you have any current or previous medical problems?
- Have you undergone any previous or recent surgical procedures?

Family History
- Is there a family history of skin problems?
- Do any members of your immediate family have skin problems?

Medication History
- Are you allergic to any drugs? If so, describe the reaction.
- What prescription drugs and/or supplements have you taken recently? When was the drug and/or supplement started? What is the dose or frequency of administration? When was the last dose taken?
- What over-the-counter (OTC) drugs have you taken recently? When was the drug started? What is the dose or frequency of administration? When was the last dose taken?

Social History
- What is your occupation?
- What recreational activities do you take part in?
- Have you traveled recently? If so, where?
- What is your nutrition status?
- Do you use tobacco, drugs, or alcohol? If so, what type and how much do you use? How frequently do you use? When did you last take or use?

Current Health Problem
- When did you first notice the skin problem?
- Where on the body did the problem begin?
- Has the problem gotten better or worse?
- Has a similar skin condition ever occurred before? If so, describe it, and how was it treated?
- Is the problem associated with any itching, burning, stinging, numbness, pain, fever, nausea and vomiting, diarrhea, sore throat, cold, stiff neck, new foods, new soaps or cosmetics, new clothing or bed linens, or stressful situations?
- What makes the problem worse?
- What makes the problem better?

ASSESSMENT: RECOGNIZE CUES

Patient History

Take an accurate history from the patient so skin problems can be readily identified. The Best Practice for Patient Safety & Quality Care: Obtaining an Accurate History of the Patient With a Skin Problem box highlights specific questions to ask during a skin assessment.

Collect *demographic data* including age, race, occupation, and hobbies or recreational activities. This information can help identify causative or aggravating factors. Knowing the patient's age is important because certain changes in the skin, hair, and nails are normal as part of the aging process.

Ethnicity is also important. Some variations in skin appearance are normal for patients of some ethnicities but are abnormal for those of other races or ethnicities.

Information about occupation and hobbies can provide clues to chronic skin exposure to chemicals, irritants, and other substances that can contribute to skin problems.

Socioeconomic status data can help identify environmental factors that might contribute to skin disease. Unhealthy or crowded living conditions promote the spread of contagious skin pathogens. Recent or frequent travel to tropical climates may be a source of unusual skin ***infection*** or infestation.

Regardless of skin color or ethnicity, always ask patients about the amount of time spent in the sun and tanning booths to identify skin problems caused by sun overexposure. Teach the patient about the harmful aspects of sun exposure and how to reduce risk by avoiding time in the sun and wearing sunscreen. Because one in five Americans is expected to develop skin cancer in their lifetime (American Academy of Dermatology, 2020), simple preventive actions are important. Also determine whether he or she regularly assesses the skin for lesion development or changes.

Skin problems caused by poor hygiene are common. Ask about living conditions and bathing practices. Teach patients that keeping the skin and hair clean by bathing and shampooing regularly helps maintain the skin's health.

Collect information about drug and substance use. Prescribed drugs, over-the-counter (OTC) drugs, herbal preparations or remedies, and tobacco use can cause skin reactions or affect skin appearance or function. Determine when each drug was started, the dose and frequency of the drug, and the time the last dose was taken. Ask the patient whether skin changes began after starting a new drug. A drug history also helps identify skin changes that result from management of other health problems, such as the changes that occur with long-term steroid or anticoagulant therapy.

Allergies to environmental substances often have skin implications. Ask about the use of any new personal care product (e.g., shaving products, perfume, soap, shampoo, lotion, makeup, hair gel), laundry detergents and softeners, and home cleaning products. Ask whether the patient wears gloves to avoid direct contact with cleaning solutions. New clothing may contain chemicals that irritate the skin.

Nutrition Status

Document the patient's weight, height, body build and fat distribution, and food preferences. Protein and vitamin deficiencies and obesity can increase the risk for skin lesions and delay wound healing. Fat-free diets and chronic alcoholism can lead to vitamin deficiencies and related skin changes. Skin problems such as chronic urticaria and acne may be worsened by certain foods or food additives.

Hydration influences overall skin health, and the skin reflects hydration status. Reduced fluid intake can lead to dry skin. Loose skin that tents when pinched together can be indicative of severe fluid loss. Fluid overload with edema can stretch the skin, masking wrinkles and allowing the formation of skin "pits" (i.e., pitting edema) when pressure is applied to it.

Family History and Genetic Risk

Some skin problems (e.g., psoriasis, keloid formation, eczema) have a familial predisposition. Ask about immediate family members' current health to identify a transmittable disorder (e.g., ringworm, scabies).

Current Health Problems

Begin by gathering information about skin changes and skin care practices (see the Best Practice for Patient Safety & Quality Care: Obtaining an Accurate History of the Patient With a Skin Problem box).

If a skin problem is identified, obtain more information about the specific problem, such as when the patient first noticed the rash or skin change, where the rash began, and whether the problem has improved or become worse. Ask if there is pain associated with problem and if there are any factors that relieve the pain (Brennan, 2019). For lower extremity conditions, determine if the patient has experienced decreased sensation (Brennan, 2019).

If the problem has occurred before, ask the patient to describe the course of the skin lesion and how it was treated. Try to link the problem with other symptoms, such as itching, burning, numbness, pain, fever, sore throat, stiff neck, or nausea and vomiting. Ask the patient to identify anything that seems to make the problem better or worse.

Skin Assessment

Inspection. A thorough assessment of the skin is best performed with the patient undressed. (Always provide privacy to maintain the patient's dignity.) Inspect the patient's skin surfaces in a well-lighted room; natural or bright fluorescent lighting makes subtle skin changes more visible. Use a penlight to closely inspect lesions and to illuminate the mouth.

Incorporate skin examination as a routine part of daily care during the bath or when assisting with hygiene. Check the cleanliness of the various body areas to determine whether the patient's self-care activities need to be evaluated.

Assess each skin surface systematically, including the scalp, hair, nails, and mucous membranes. Give particular attention to the skinfold areas, because these moist, warm environments can harbor organisms such as yeast or bacteria. Observe and document changes in color and vascularity, moisture presence or absence, edema, skin lesions, and skin integrity.

Skin color is affected by blood flow, gas exchange, body temperature, and pigmentation. The wide variation in skin tones requires different techniques for patients who have darker skin. (See the Patient-Centered Care: Cultural/Spiritual Considerations box for methods of assessing patients with darker skin.)

PATIENT-CENTERED CARE: CULTURAL/SPIRITUAL CONSIDERATIONS QSEN

Pallor, erythema, cyanosis, and other skin color changes are less visible in patients with naturally dark skin tones. Although physiologic processes are the same for both light-skinned and dark-skinned patients, the amount of skin pigmentation alters how the skin appears in response to physiologic alterations. Careful assessment skills are needed to detect subtle color changes. Become familiar with the normal appearance of mucous membranes, nail beds, and skin tone of a patient with darker skin, so variations from baseline can be identified. The Best Practice for Patient Safety & Quality Care: Assessing Changes in Patients With Dark Skin box later in this chapter lists evidence-based techniques for this assessment.

Describe and document changes in skin color by their appearance (Table 22.2). Include whether the changes are general or confined to one body region. Color changes are more visible in the areas of least pigmentation, such as the oral mucosa, sclera, nail beds, and palms and soles. Inspect these areas to help confirm more subtle color changes of general body areas.

Lesions are clinically described in terms of being primary or secondary (Fig. 22.7). **Primary lesions** develop as a direct result of a disease process. **Secondary lesions** evolve from primary lesions or develop as a consequence of the patient's activities. These changes occur with progression of an underlying disease or in response to a topical or systemic therapeutic intervention. For example, acute dermatitis often occurs as primary vesicles with associated **pruritus** (itching). Secondary lesions in the form of crusts occur as the patient scratches, the vesicles are opened, and the exudate dries. With chronic dermatitis, the skin often becomes **lichenified** (thickened) because of the patient's continual rubbing or scratching of the area to relieve itching.

Describe lesions or breaks in skin integrity by color, size, location, shape, and presence (or absence) of odor. Note whether they are isolated or are grouped and form a distinct pattern. Table 22.3 defines terms used to describe lesions. Use of a tool such as the WoundVision Scout, an imaging device, can be helpful in photographing and measuring wounds, as well as quantifying and visualizing characteristics below the skin's surface (Sabour, 2017). Follow agency policy for measuring size, because all staff must follow the same protocol to ensure that measurements are recorded and trended accurately (Brennan, 2019). Be sure to remeasure if debridement is done (Brennan, 2019). Document characteristics of the outer edge of the wound, known as the *periwound*, because this can be helpful in determining how long a wound has been present (Cox, 2019).

The evaluation of partial- and full-thickness wounds, including objective criteria that describe progress toward healing, is discussed in Chapter 23. A model such as the Skin Safety Model (SSM) (Campbell et al., 2016) can help you thoroughly evaluate the potential for skin injury and associated outcomes, especially for older adults. Implementation of a protocol such as the Champions for Skin Integrity model can lead to improved skin outcomes in older adults when nurses consistently use evidence-based wound prevention strategies (Edwards et al., 2017). The most current clinical guideline for caring for older adult skin is found in the International Skin Tear Advisory Panel's (2018) Best Practice Recommendations for Prevention and Management of Skin Tears in Aged Skin.

Assess each lesion for these ABCDE features that are associated with skin cancer (The Skin Cancer Foundation, 2020):

- *A*symmetry of shape
- *B*order irregularity
- *C*olor variation within one lesion
- *D*iameter greater than ¼ inch or 6 mm
- *E*volving or changing in any feature (shape, size, color, elevation, itching, bleeding, or crusting)

Because of the continued incidence of melanoma (U.S. Cancer Statistics Working Group, 2019), routinely teach patients signs of skin cancer and encourage them to perform skin self-examination on a monthly basis. High-risk patients may benefit from taking the Melanoma Risk Assessment Tool quiz to self-assess their relative risk for developing melanoma (National Cancer Institute,

TABLE 22.2 **Common Alterations in Skin Color**

Alteration	Underlying Cause	Location	Significance
White (pallor)	Decreased hemoglobin level	Conjunctivae	Anemia
	Decreased blood flow to the skin (vasoconstriction)	Mucous membranes Nail beds Palms and soles Lips	Shock or blood loss Chronic vascular compromise Sudden emotional upset Edema
	Genetically determined defect of the melanocyte (decreased pigmentation)	Generalized	Albinism
	Acquired patchy loss of pigmentation	Localized	Vitiligo, tinea versicolor
Yellow-orange	Increased total serum bilirubin level (jaundice)	Generalized Mucous membranes Sclera	Hemolysis of red blood cells Liver disorders
	Increased serum carotene level (carotenemia)	Perioral Palms and soles Ears and nose Absent in sclera and mucous membranes	Increased ingestion of carotene-containing foods (carrots) Pregnancy Thyroid deficiency Diabetes
	Increased urochrome level	Generalized Absent in sclera and mucous membranes	Chronic kidney disease (uremia)
Red (erythema)	Increased blood flow to the skin (vasodilation)	Generalized	Generalized inflammation (e.g., erythroderma)
		Localized (to area of involvement)	Localized inflammation (e.g., sunburn, cellulitis, trauma, rashes)
		Face, cheeks, nose, upper chest	Fever, increased alcohol intake
		Area of exposure	Exposure to cold
Blue	Increase in deoxygenated blood (cyanosis)	Nail beds Mucous membranes Generalized	Cardiopulmonary disease Methemoglobinemia
	Bleeding from vessels into tissue:		
	Petechiae (1-3 mm)	Localized	Thrombocytopenia
	Ecchymosis (>3 mm)	Localized	Increased blood vessel fragility
Reddish blue	Increased overall amount of hemoglobin	Generalized	Polycythemia vera
	Decreased peripheral circulation	Distal extremities, nose	Inadequate tissue perfusion
Brown	Increased melanin production	Localized (to area of involvement) Pressure points, areolae, palmar creases, and genitalia	Chronic inflammation Exposure to sunlight Addison disease
		Face, areolae, vulva, linea nigra	Pregnancy; oral contraceptives (melasma)
	Café au lait spots (tan-brown patches):		
	Fewer than six spots	Localized	Nonpathogenic
	More than six spots	Generalized	Possible neurofibromatosis
	Melanin and hemosiderin deposits (bronze or grayish-tan color)	Distal lower extremities	Chronic venous stasis
		Exposed areas or generalized	Hemochromatosis

n.d.). *A patient who has a lesion with one or more of the ABCDE features should be evaluated by a dermatologist or surgeon.*

In describing location, determine whether lesions are generalized or localized. If localized, identify the specific body areas involved. This information is important because some diseases have a specific pattern of skin lesions. For example, involvement of only the sun-exposed areas of the body is important when considering possible causes. Rashes limited to the skinfold areas (e.g., on the axillae, beneath the breasts, in the groin) may reflect problems related to friction, heat, and excessive moisture.

Edema causes the skin to appear shiny, **taut** (tightly stretched), and paler than uninvolved surrounding skin. During skin inspection, document the location, distribution, and color of areas of edema.

Skin elasticity is affected by edema. Using moderate pressure, place the tip of a finger against edematous tissue to determine the degree of indentation, or pitting (see Chapter 13).

Primary lesions

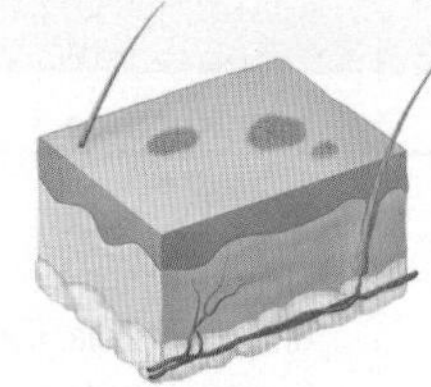

Macules
(such as *freckles, flat moles* or *rubella*) are flat lesions of less than 1 cm in diameter. Their color is different from that of the surrounding skin—most often white, red or brown.

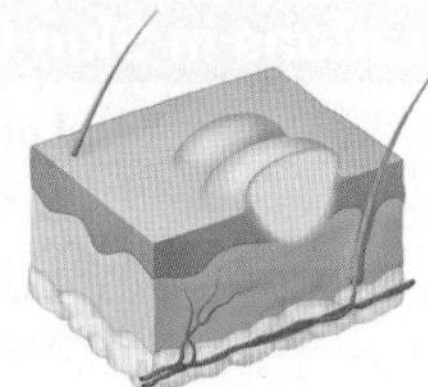

Nodules
(such as *lipomas*) are elevated marble-like lesions more than 1 cm wide and deep.

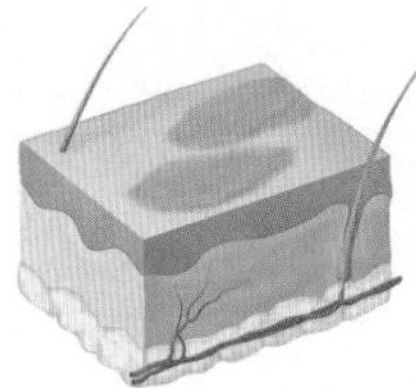

Patches
(such as *vitiligo* or *café au lait spots*) are macules that are larger than 1 cm in diameter. They may or may not have some surface changes—either slight scale or fine wrinkles.

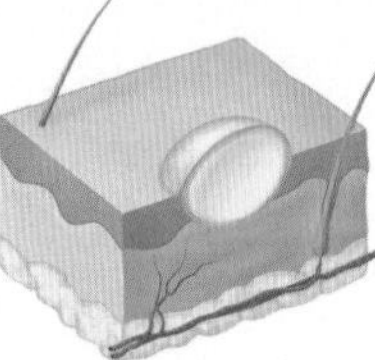

Cysts
(such as *sebaceous cysts*) are nodules filled with either liquid or semisolid material that can be expressed.

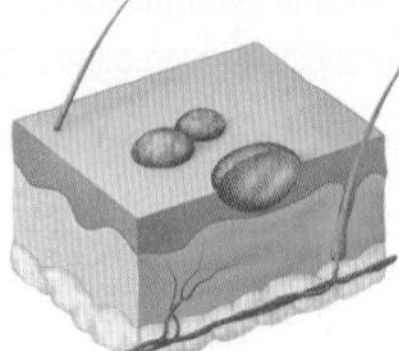

Papules
(such as *warts* or *elevated moles*) are small, firm, elevated lesions less than 1 cm in diameter.

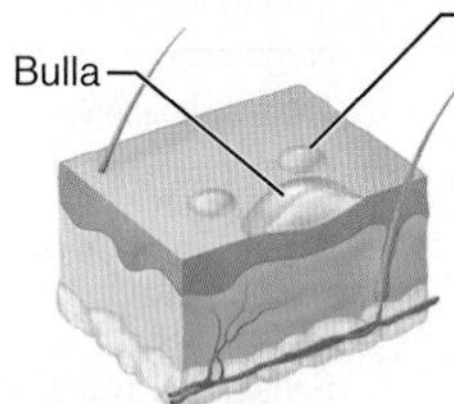

Vesicles
(such as in *acute dermatitis*) and **Bullae** (such as *second-degree burns*) are blisters filled with clear fluid. Vesicles are less than 1 cm in diameter, and bullae are more than 1 cm in diameter.

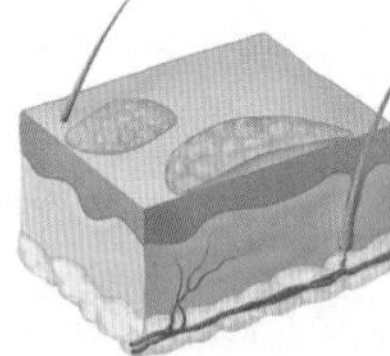

Plaques
(such as in *psoriasis* or *seborrheic keratosis*) are elevated, plateau-like patches more than 1 cm in diameter that do not extend into the lower skin layers.

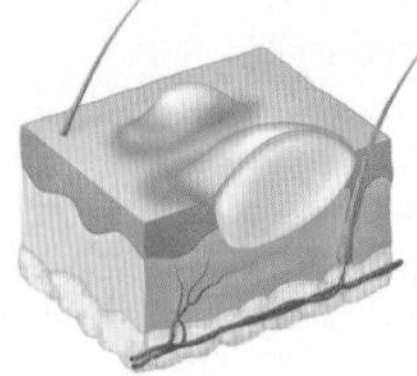

Pustules
(such as in *acne* and *acute impetigo*) are vesicles filled with cloudy or purulent fluid.

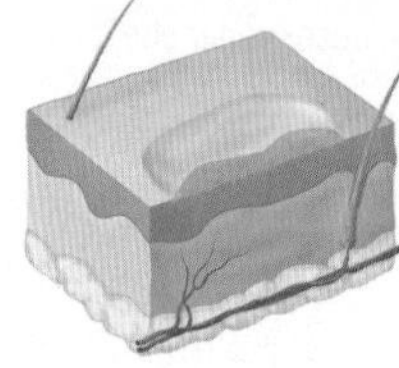

Wheals
(such as *urticaria* and *insect bites*) are elevated, irregularly shaped, transient areas of dermal edema.

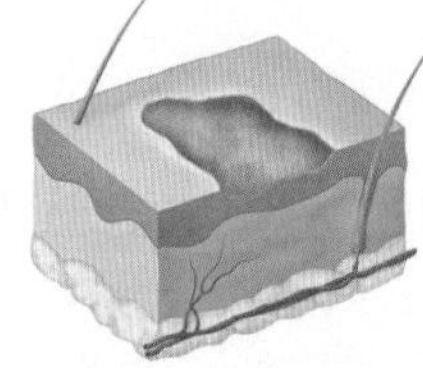

Erosions
(such as in *varicella*) are wider than fissures but involve only the epidermis. They are often associated with vesicles, bullae, or pustules.

Secondary lesions

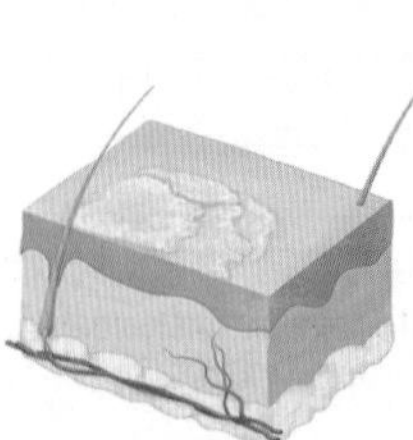

Scales
(such as in *exfoliative dermatitis* and *psoriasis*) are visibly thickened stratum corneum. They appear dry and are usually whitish. They are seen most often with papules and plaques.

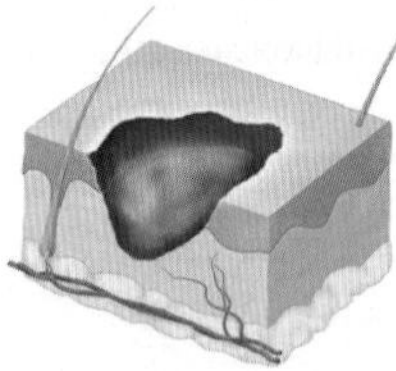

Ulcers
(such as *stage 3 pressure injuries*) are deep erosions that extend beneath the epidermis and involve the dermis and sometimes the subcutaneous fat.

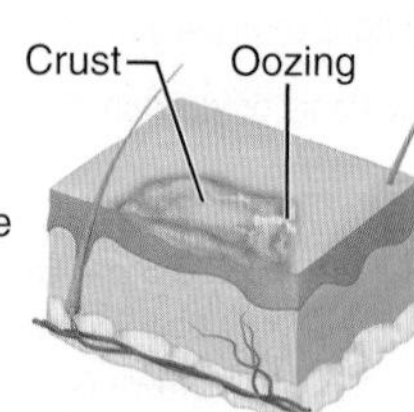

Crusts and oozing
(such as in *eczema* and *late-stage impetigo*) are composed of dried serum or pus on the surface of the skin, beneath which liquid debris may accumulate. Crusts frequently result from broken vesicles, bullae, or pustules.

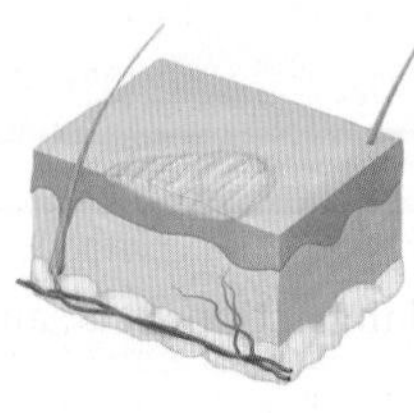

Lichenifications
(such as in *chronic dermatitis*) are palpably thickened areas of epidermis with accentuated skin markings. They are caused by chronic rubbing and scratching.

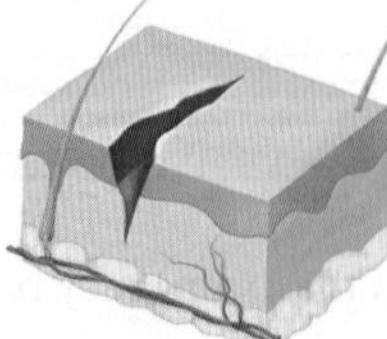

Fissures
(such as in *athlete's foot*) are linear cracks in the epidermis that often extend into the dermis.

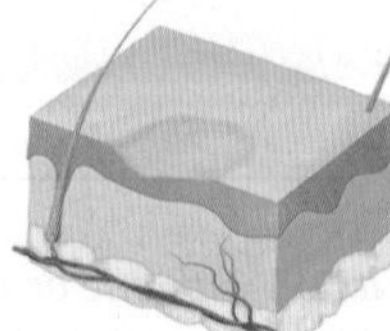

Atrophy
(such as *striae* [stretch marks] and *aged skin*) is characterized by thinning of the skin surface with loss of skin markings. The skin is translucent and paper-like. Atrophy involving the dermal layer results in skin depression.

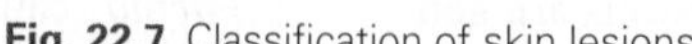

Fig. 22.7 Classification of skin lesions.

TABLE 22.3 Terms Commonly Used to Describe Skin Lesion Configurations

annular Ringlike with raised borders around flat, clear centers of normal skin
circinate Circular
circumscribed Well defined with sharp borders
clustered Several lesions grouped together
coalesced Lesions that merge with one another and appear confluent
diffuse Widespread, involving most of the body with intervening areas of normal skin; generalized
linear Occurring in a straight line
serpiginous With wavy borders, resembling a snake
universal All areas of the body involved, with no areas of normal-appearing skin

Moisture content is assessed by noting the thickness and consistency of secretions. Normally, increased moisture, in the form of sweat, occurs with increased activity or elevated environmental temperatures. When air circulation to skinfold areas is impaired, dampness occurs. Excess moisture can cause impaired ***tissue integrity*** with skin breakdown.

Overly dry skin is caused by a dry environment, poor skin lubrication, inadequate fluid intake, and the normal aging process. Dry skin is marked by scaling and flaking and may be especially marked in areas of lesser circulation such as the feet and lower legs. It is a common problem during the winter months when the air contains less moisture, for those living in geographic areas with little humidity, and in a hospital environment where humidity is often low.

Vascular changes or markings may be normal or abnormal, depending on the cause. Normal vascular markings include birthmarks, cherry angiomas (Fig. 22.8), spider angiomas, and venous stars. Bleeding into the skin is abnormal and results in **purpura** (bleeding under the skin that may progress from red to purple to brownish-yellow), petechiae, and ecchymosis.

Petechiae are small, reddish-purple lesions (<0.5 mm in diameter) that do not fade or blanch when pressure is applied (Fig. 22.9). They often indicate increased capillary fragility. Petechiae of the lower extremities often occur with stasis dermatitis, a condition usually seen with chronic venous insufficiency.

! NURSING SAFETY PRIORITY (QSEN)

Action Alert

Carefully assess the skin for petechiae. If found below the nipple line, petechiae can be indicative of a serious underlying problem such as disseminated intravascular coagulation (DIC).

NCLEX EXAMINATION CHALLENGE 22.1

Physiological Integrity

Which assessment data regarding a lesion found on a 39-year-old client who uses a tanning bed requires nursing intervention? **Select all that apply.**

A. Symmetrical and light pink
B. Brownish-purple with irregular borders
C. Changed in shape since last appointment
D. 8 mm wide and described as itching often
E. Regular border with fixed size and elevation

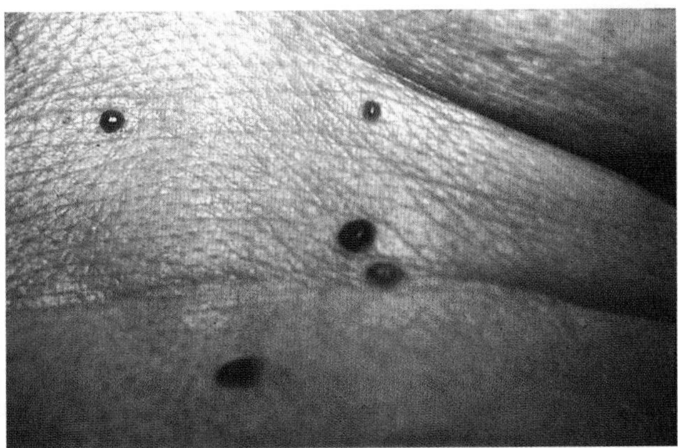

Fig. 22.8 Senile (cherry) angiomas.

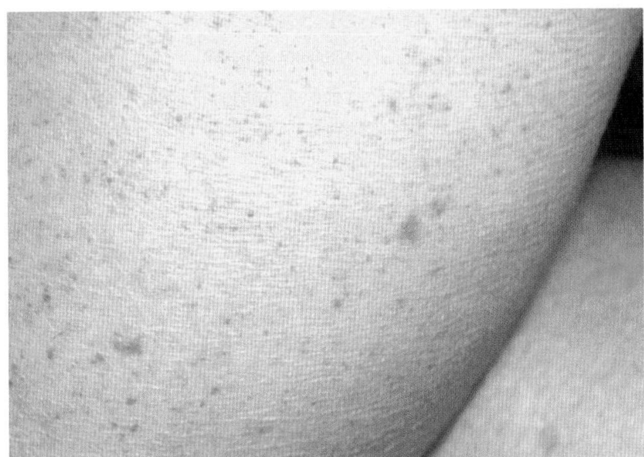

Fig. 22.9 Petechiae. (Modified from Marks, J., & Miller, J. [2013]. *Lookingbill and Marks' principles of dermatology* [5th ed.]. Philadelphia: Saunders.)

Ecchymoses (bruises) are larger areas of hemorrhage. In older adults, bruising is common after minor trauma to the skin. Certain drugs (e.g., aspirin, warfarin, corticosteroids) and low platelet counts lead to easy or excessive bruising. Anticoagulants and decreased numbers of platelets disrupt clotting action, resulting in ecchymosis.

Tissue integrity is assessed by first examining areas with actual breaks or open areas. For example, skin tears are a common finding in older adults. The thin, fragile skin is easily damaged by friction or shearing forces, especially if bruising is already present. Look for skin tears where clothing rubs against the skin, on upper extremities where skin may be grasped to assist with ambulation, and where adhesive tapes or dressings have been applied and removed. Check for the presence of multiple abrasions or early pressure-related skin changes.

Document the presence and characteristics of any wound drainage or ***infection.*** Drainage should be documented as serous, serosanguinous, sanguineous, or purulent, and the amount should also be noted (Brennan, 2019). Note whether there is odor and whether it decreases after cleaning the wound (Brennan). If odors remains, a **bioburden** (number of microorganisms living on a surface) may be present, and this needs to be reported to the primary health care provider (Brennan, 2019).

Cleanliness of the skin is evaluated to learn about self-care needs. Inspect the hair, nails, and skin closely for excessive soiling and offensive odor. Depending on a patient's degree of ability to perform ADLs, hard-to-reach areas (e.g., perirectal and inguinal skinfolds, axillae, feet) may be less clean than other skin surface areas.

Patients who have cognitive problems may not observe hygiene measures. Assess the cognition of any patient whose hygiene of the skin, hair, or nails appears inadequate.

Tattoos, piercings, and henna staining can contribute to or cover skin problems and must be examined carefully. Bruises and rashes may be difficult to see in tattooed areas. Examine newly pierced areas for inflammation or ***infection.*** Scars may be present in old tattoos or pierced areas and should be documented. Closely examine any areas where tattoos have been removed, because skin cancer is more likely to occur in these areas.

Palpation. Skin inspection can be misleading in areas of color changes, tattoos, and piercings. Use gentle palpation to gather additional information about skin lesions, moisture,

TABLE 22.4 Common Clinical Findings in Skin Palpation

Clinical Findings	Cause	Location	Examples of Predisposing Conditions
Edema			
Localized	Inflammatory response	Area of involvement	Trauma
Dependent or pitting	Fluid and electrolyte imbalance Venous and cardiac insufficiency	Ambulatory: dorsum of foot and medial ankle Bedridden: buttocks, sacrum, and lower back	Heart failure Kidney disease Liver cirrhosis Venous thrombosis or stasis
Nonpitting	Endocrine imbalance	Generalized, but more easily seen over the tibia	Hypothyroidism (myxedema)
Moisture			
Increased	Autonomic nervous system stimulation	Face, axillae, skinfolds, palms, and soles	Fever Anxiety Activity Hyperthyroidism
Decreased	Dehydration Endocrine imbalance	Buccal mucous membranes with progressive involvement of other skin surfaces	Fluid loss Postmenopausal status Hypothyroidism Normal aging
Temperature			
Increased	Increased blood flow to the skin	Generalized	Fever Hypermetabolic states Neurotrauma
		Localized	Inflammation
Decreased	Decreased blood flow to the skin	Generalized	Impending shock Sepsis Anxiety Hypothyroidism
		Localized	Interference with vascular flow
Turgor			
Decreased	Decreased elasticity of the dermis (tenting when pinched)	Abdomen, forehead, or radial aspect of the wrist	Severe dehydration Sudden severe weight loss Normal aging
Texture			
Roughness or thickness	Irritation, friction	Pressure points (e.g., soles, palms, elbows) Localized areas of pruritus	Calluses Chronic eczema Atopic skin diseases
	Sun damage	Areas of sun exposure	Normal aging
	Excessive collagen production	Localized or generalized	Scleroderma Scars and keloids
Softness or smoothness	Endocrine disturbances	Generalized	Hyperthyroidism

temperature, texture, and turgor (Table 22.4). Wash hands thoroughly before and after palpating a patient's skin. Use gloves to examine skin, and use Standard Precautions when skin areas are draining.

Palpation confirms lesion size and whether the lesions are flat or slightly raised. Consistency of larger lesions can vary from soft and pliable to firm and solid. Subtle changes, such as the difference between a fine **macular** (flat) rash and a **papular** (raised) rash, are best determined by palpating with your eyes closed. Ask the patient if skin palpation causes pain or tenderness.

In areas of excess dryness, rub your finger against the skin surface to determine the degree of flaking or scaling. Changes in skin temperature are detected by placing the back of your gloved hand on the skin surface, as long as your hands are warm. Cold hands interfere with accurate assessment.

Palpate skin surfaces to assess texture, which differs according to body area and exposure to irritants. For example, areas of long-term sun exposure have a rougher texture than protected skin surfaces. The patient who has repeated exposure to harsh soaps or chemicals may show skin changes related to this exposure. Increased skin thickness from scarring, lichenification, or edema usually decreases elasticity.

Turgor indicates the amount of skin elasticity. Skin turgor can be altered by water content and aging. Gently pinch the patient's skin between your thumb and forefinger and then release. If skin turgor is normal, the skin immediately returns to its original state when released. Poor skin turgor is seen as "tenting" of the skin, with a slower and more gradual return to the original state (see Chapter 13). Although usually checked on the back of the hand, you may also check for turgor on the abdomen, forehead, or radial aspect of the wrist.

! NURSING SAFETY PRIORITY (QSEN)

Action Alert

To avoid mistaking dehydration for dry skin in an older adult, assess skin turgor on the forehead or chest.

Hair Assessment

During the skin assessment, inspect and palpate the hair for general appearance, cleanliness, distribution, quantity, and quality. Hair is normally found in an even distribution over most of the body surfaces. The hair on the scalp, in the pubic region, and in the axillary folds is thicker and coarser than hair on the trunk, arms, and legs. Although color and growth patterns vary, sudden changes in hair characteristics may reflect an underlying disorder. Assess abnormal findings and obtain a detailed history of the change.

How well the hair is cleaned and groomed can provide information about a patient's health care needs. If the patient has intense itching or scratches continually, examine the scalp and pubis for lice and **nits** (lice eggs), scaling, redness, open areas, crusting, and tenderness.

Dandruff, a collection of patchy or diffuse white or gray scales on the surface of the scalp, is a common assessment finding. The flaking that occurs with dandruff causes many adults to mistakenly think the scalp is too dry; however, it is actually a problem of excessive oil production. Dandruff by itself is a cosmetic problem, but a very oily scalp can induce inflammatory changes with redness and itching. Severe inflammatory dandruff can extend to the eyebrows and the skin of the face and neck. *If severe dandruff is not treated, alopecia (hair loss) can occur.* Teach the patient that dandruff is not caused by dryness and should be treated to prevent hair loss.

Although gradual hair loss expectedly occurs with aging, sudden asymmetric or patchy hair loss at any age is of concern. Assess the scalp for hair distribution and thickness, and document variations. Body hair loss, especially on the feet or lower legs, may occur with decreased blood flow to the area and also is a part of aging.

Hirsutism is excessive growth of body hair or hair growth in abnormal body areas. Increased hair growth across the face and chest in women is a sign of hirsutism. It may occur on the face of a woman as part of aging, as a sign of hormonal imbalance, or as a side effect of drug therapy. If hirsutism is present, look for changes in fat distribution and capillary fragility, which can occur in Cushing disease, and ask about clitoral enlargement and deepening of the voice, which may indicate ovarian dysfunction.

Nail Assessment

Dystrophic (abnormal-appearing) nails may occur with a serious systemic illness or local skin disease involving the epidermal keratinocytes. Assess the fingernails and toenails for color, shape, thickness, texture, and the presence of lesions.

Many variations in color, texture, and grooming of the nails are influenced by factors unrelated to disease, such as occupation. When assessing the older adult, observe for minor variations associated with the aging process, such as a gradual thickening of the nail plate, the presence of longitudinal ridges, or a yellowish-gray discoloration.

Color of the nail plate depends on nail thickness and transparency, amount of red blood cells, arterial blood flow, and pigment deposits (Table 22.5). Fig. 22.10 shows normal variations in nail pigmentation. Changes in color can be caused by chemical damage that occurs with some occupations, with the long-term use of nail polish, or with the use of cosmetic nail enhancements. Regardless of skin color, the healthy nail blanches (lightens) with pressure.

During examination, the patient's fingers and toes should be free of any surface pressure that interferes with local blood flow or alters the appearance of the digits. To differentiate between color changes from the underlying blood supply and those from pigment deposits, blanch the nail bed to see whether the color changes with pressure. Gently squeeze the end of the finger or toe, exerting downward pressure on the nail bed, and then release the pressure. Color caused by blood flow changes as pressure is applied and returns to the original state when pressure is released. Color caused by pigment deposits remains unchanged.

Nail shape changes may be related to systemic disease. For example, fingernail clubbing occurs with impaired gas exchange (see Table 22.6 for examples of early and late clubbing.)

Assess nail shape by examining the curve of the nail plate and surrounding tissue from all angles. Palpate the fingertips to

TABLE 22.5 Common Alterations in Nail Color

Alteration	Clinical Findings	Significance
White	Horizontal white banding or areas of opacity	Chronic liver or kidney disease (hypoalbuminemia)
	Generalized pallor of nail beds	Shock Anemia Early arteriosclerotic changes (toenails) Myocardial infarction
Yellow-brown	Diffuse yellow-to-brown discoloration	Jaundice Peripheral lymphedema Bacterial or fungal ***infection*** of the nail Psoriasis Diabetes Cardiac failure Staining from tobacco, nail polish, or dyes Long-term tetracycline therapy Normal aging (yellow-gray color)
	Vertical brown banding extending from the proximal nail fold distally	Normal finding in dark-skinned patients Nevus or melanoma of nail matrix in light-skinned patients
Red	Thin, dark red vertical lines 1-3 mm long (splinter hemorrhages)	Bacterial endocarditis Trichinosis Trauma to the nail bed Normal finding in some patients
	Red discoloration of the lunula	Cardiac insufficiency
	Dark red nail beds	Polycythemia vera
Blue	Diffuse blue discoloration that blanches with pressure	Respiratory failure Methemoglobinuria Venous stasis disease (toenails)

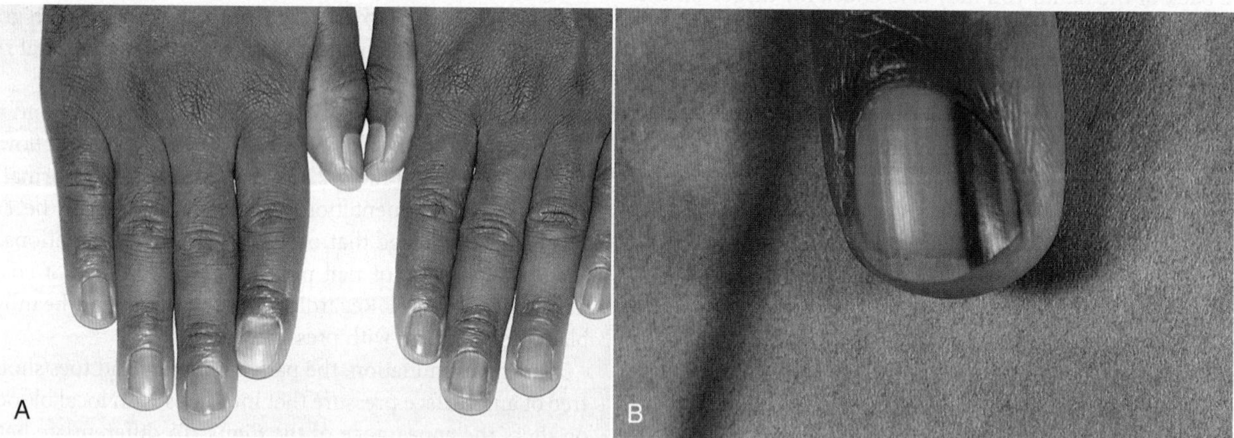

Fig. 22.10 (A) Diffuse nail pigmentation. (B) Linear nail pigmentation.

assess for sponginess, tenderness, or edema. Table 22.6 describes common variations in nail shape.

Thickness of the nail plate varies with age, trauma, dermatologic disease, or decreased arterial blood flow. Nails that have undergone frequent cosmetic enhancement may be very thin and peel easily. In older patients, look for a layered appearance of the toenails, which occurs with fungal ***infection*** *(onychomycosis).*

Consistency of the nail is described as hard, soft, or brittle. Nail plates become hard, with thickening. A warm-water soak is required to soften the nail plates before they can be trimmed. Soft nail plates, which are thin and bend easily with pressure, are associated with malnutrition, chronic arthritis, myxedema, peripheral neuritis, and the use of cosmetic enhancement.

Brittle nails can split, as with onychomycosis or advanced psoriasis involving the fingers or toes. Splitting of the nail plate is caused by repeated exposure to water and detergents, which damage the plate over time.

Lesions can occur around, on, within, or under the nail. Separation of the nail plate from the nail bed *(onycholysis)* creates an air pocket beneath the plate. The pocket first appears as a grayish-white opacity. The color changes as dirt and keratin

TABLE 22.6 Common Variations in Nail Shape

Nail Shape	Clinical Findings	Significance
Normal	Angle of 160 degrees between the nail plate and the proximal nail fold Nail surface slightly convex Nail base firm when palpated	Normal finding
Clubbing		
Early clubbing	Straightening of angle between the nail plate and the proximal nail fold to 180 degrees Nail base spongy when palpated	Hypoxia Lung cancer
Late clubbing	Angle between the nail plate and the proximal nail fold exceeds 180 degrees Nail base visibly edematous and spongy when palpated Enlargement of the soft tissue of the fingertips gives a "drumstick" appearance when viewed from above	Prolonged hypoxia Emphysema Chronic obstructive pulmonary disease Advanced lung cancer Cystic fibrosis Chronic heart disease
Spoon nails (koilonychia)		
Early koilonychias	Flattening of the nail plate with an increased smoothness of the nail surface	Iron deficiency (with or without anemia) Poorly controlled diabetes >15 yr in duration Local injury
Late koilonychias	Concave curvature of the nail plate	Psoriasis Chemical irritants Developmental abnormality
Beau's lines (grooves)	1-mm–wide horizontal depressions in the nail plates caused by growth arrest (involves all nails)	Acute, severe illness Prolonged febrile state Isolated periods of severe malnutrition
Pitting	Small, multiple pits in the nail plate May be associated with plate thickening and onycholysis Most often involves the fingernails (several or all)	Psoriasis Alopecia areata

collect in the pocket, and the area begins to have a bad odor. This problem occurs with a fungal ***infection*** and after trauma. Separation of the nail plate may also occur with psoriasis or with prolonged chemical contact.

Inspect the tissue folds around the nail plate for redness, heat, swelling, and tenderness. Acute paronychia (inflammation of the skin around the nail) often occurs with a torn cuticle or an ingrown toenail.

Chronic paronychia is common and is an inflammation that persists for months. Adults at risk for this condition are those with frequent exposure to water, such as homemakers, bartenders, laundry workers, and health care workers.

Skin Assessment Techniques for Patients With Darker Skin

Pallor can be detected in people with dark skin by first inspecting the mucous membranes for an ash-gray color (Jarvis, 2020). If the lips and the nail beds are not heavily pigmented, they appear paler than normal for that patient. Use good lighting to assess for the absence of the underlying red tones that normally give heavily pigmented skin a healthy glow. With decreased blood flow to the skin, brown skin appears yellow-brown, and very dark brown skin appears ash gray.

Cyanosis can be present when gas exchange is impaired. Examine the lips, tongue, nail beds, conjunctivae, and palms and soles for subtle color changes (Jarvis, 2020). In a patient with cyanosis, the lips and tongue are gray; and the palms, soles, conjunctivae, and nail beds have a bluish tinge. To support these findings, assess for other indicators of hypoxia, including tachycardia, hypotension, changes in respiratory rate, decreased breath sounds, and changes in cognition.

Inflammation in patients with dark skin appears as excessive warmth and changes in skin consistency or texture (Jarvis, 2020). Use the back of your hand to palpate areas of suspected inflammation for increased warmth. With the fingertips, palpate for hardened areas deep in the tissue. Inflamed skin is often tender and edematous. If edema is extensive, the skin is taut and shiny.

Skin areas where inflammation has recently resolved appear *darker* than the patient's normal skin tone. This change is caused by stimulation of the melanocytes during the inflammatory process and the increased pigment production that continues after inflammation subsides. Deep skin injury with destruction of melanocytes (e.g., deep injury, full-thickness burn) may heal with color changes that are *lighter* than the normal skin tone. Chronic inflammatory changes are not tender. Scarred skin feels less supple, especially over the joints. If chronic inflammatory changes are suspected, ask the patient about a history of skin problems in that area.

Jaundice in a patient with dark skin is best assessed by inspecting the oral mucosa, especially the hard palate, for yellow discoloration. Yellowness of the conjunctivae and adjacent sclera may be misleading because normal deposits of fat produce a yellowish hue that is visible in contrast to the dark skin around the eyes (Jarvis, 2020). Examine the sclera closest to the cornea for a more accurate determination of jaundice. The palms and soles of patients with dark skin may appear yellow if they are calloused, even when jaundice is not present.

Skin bleeding with purpuric lesions may not be visible with deep pigmentation. Areas of ecchymoses appear darker than normal skin; they may be tender and easily palpable, depending on whether hematoma is present. Often the patient relates a history of trauma to the area that confirms the assessment. Petechiae are rarely visible in dark skin and may be seen only in the oral mucosa and conjunctiva.

BEST PRACTICE FOR PATIENT SAFETY & QUALITY CARE (QSEN)

Assessing Changes in Patients With Dark Skin

Cyanosis

- Examine lips and tongue for gray color.
- Examine nail beds, palms, and soles for blue tinge.
- Examine conjunctiva for pallor.

Inflammation

- Compare affected area with nonaffected area for increased warmth.
- Examine the skin of the affected area to determine whether it is shiny or taut or pits with pressure.
- Compare the skin color of affected area with the same area on the opposite side of the body.
- Palpate the affected area and compare it with unaffected area to determine whether texture is different (affected area may feel hard).

Jaundice

- Check for yellow tinge to oral mucous membranes, especially the hard palate.
- Examine the sclera nearest to the iris rather than the corners of the eye.

Bleeding

- Compare the affected area with the same area on the unaffected body side for swelling or skin darkening.
- If the patient has thrombocytopenia, petechiae may be present on the oral mucosa or conjunctiva.

Psychosocial Assessment

Skin changes, especially of the face, hair, and hands, can affect body image. Encourage the patient to express feelings about a change in appearance. Assess body language for clues indicating a disturbance in self-concept. Avoidance of eye contact or the use of clothing to cover the affected areas may suggest concern about appearance. Patients with chronic skin diseases can become socially isolated related to a fear of rejection by others or a belief that the skin problem is contagious.

Skin changes linked to poor hygiene are common among people who are homeless and those who have reduced cognitive functioning. Assess the patient's overall appearance for excessive soiling, matted hair, body odor, or other self-care deficits. Confirm unsanitary living conditions by obtaining a social history. Patients may relate similar skin problems among family members, friends, and sexual contacts.

If skin problems related to poor hygiene are identified in older patients, also evaluate any physical limitations that might interfere with grooming. For example, visual or mobility problems can make it difficult for them to see or reach skin surfaces to clean them.

Diagnostic Assessment

Laboratory Tests. When a fungal, bacterial, or viral ***infection*** of the skin is suspected, confirmation by microscopic examination is necessary. *Always wear gloves (use Standard Precautions) when examining skin.*

CLINICAL JUDGMENT CHALLENGE 22.1

Patient-Centered Care

The home health care nurse is assessing a 59-year-old African-American client who has a history of chronic obstructive pulmonary disease. Assessment reveals moist, pink, and pale oral mucous membranes without petechiae; pink and pale nail beds, hand palms, and feet soles; and symmetrical warmth in all extremities. Vital signs include BP 130/80 mm Hg, P 80 beats/min, R 20 breaths/min, and T 98.0°F. The client reports having cut the lawn earlier in the day and feeling "a bit tired but otherwise fine."

1. **Recognize Cues:** What assessment information in this client situation is the most important and immediate concern for the nurse? (Hint: Identify the **relevant** information *first* to determine what is most important.)
2. **Analyze Cues:** What client conditions are consistent with the **most relevant** information? (Hint: Think about priority collaborative problems that support and contradict the information presented in this situation.)

Cultures for fungal ***infection*** are obtained by using a tongue blade and gently scraping scales from skin lesions into a clean container. Fingernail clippings and hair can also be placed into individual clean containers. Waiting for culture results can delay treatment of a superficial fungal infection. For this reason, the specimen is also treated with a potassium hydroxide (KOH) solution and examined microscopically. A positive fungal infection shows branched hyphae when viewed under a microscope after treatment with KOH and may eliminate the need for a culture.

For deeper fungal infections, a piece of tissue is obtained for culture. The primary health care provider obtains the specimen by punch biopsy (see Skin Biopsy section). Check with the laboratory for any specific instructions related to specimen handling.

Cultures for bacterial ***infection*** are obtained from intact primary lesions (abscess, bullae, vesicles, or pustules), if possible. Express material from the lesion, collect it with a cotton-tipped applicator, and place it in a bacterial culture medium specified by the laboratory. For intact lesions, *unroofing* (lifting or puncturing of the outer surface) may be needed using a sterile small-gauge needle before the material can be easily expressed. If crusts are present, the nurse or other health care professional may remove them with normal saline and then swab the underlying exudate to obtain a specimen for culture.

A biopsy of deep bacterial infections may be needed to obtain a specimen for culture. If bacterial cellulitis is suspected, the primary health care provider can inject nonbacteriostatic saline deep into the tissue and then aspirate it back; the aspirant is sent for culture.

Cultures for viral ***infection*** are indicated if a herpes virus infection is suspected. A cotton-tipped applicator is used to obtain vesicle fluid from intact lesions. Viral culture specimen tubes must be refrigerated at 2° to 8°C or placed on ice immediately after specimens have been obtained, and they must be transported to the laboratory as soon as possible (Quest Diagnostics, 2019).

The presence of a viral infection can be confirmed by *Tzanck smear,* although the exact virus is not identified. A smear is obtained from the base of the lesion and examined under a microscope. The presence of multinucleated giant cells confirms a viral infection.

Other Diagnostic Tests. Other tests for diagnosis of skin problems include biopsy, special noninvasive examination techniques, and skin testing for allergy (discussed in Chapter 18).

Skin Biopsy. A small piece of skin tissue may be obtained for diagnosis or to assess the effectiveness of an intervention. Check with the primary health care provider to determine the number, location, and type of skin biopsies to be performed. Depending on the size, depth, and location of the skin changes, the provider may perform a punch biopsy, shave biopsy, or scalpel excision (excisional biopsy).

Punch biopsy is the most common technique. A small circular cutting instrument, or "punch," ranging in diameter from 2 to 6 mm, is used. After the site is injected with a local anesthetic, a small plug of tissue is cut and removed. The site may be closed with sutures or may be allowed to heal without suturing.

Shave biopsies remove only the part of the skin that rises above the surrounding tissue when injected with a local anesthetic. A scalpel or razor blade is moved parallel to the skin surface to remove the tissue specimen. Shave biopsies are usually indicated for superficial or raised lesions. Suturing is not needed.

Excisional biopsy is accomplished by deep excision with a scalpel followed by closure with sutures. Excisional biopsies are more uncomfortable than punch or shave biopsies while healing.

Patient Preparation. Explain to the patient what to expect and that a biopsy is a minor procedure with few anticipated complications. Ensure that informed consent has been obtained. If a punch or shave biopsy is planned, reassure the patient that only a small amount of skin is removed and scarring is minimal. For an excisional biopsy, teach that a scar similar to that of a healed surgical incision will result.

NCLEX EXAMINATION CHALLENGE 22.2

Safe and Effective Care Environment

How will the nurse describe a shave biopsy to a client?

A. "A scalpel will be used to remove a deep sample of skin."
B. "A small plug of tissue will be removed with a circular cutting instrument."
C. "A deep specimen of skin will be taken, and the area will be sutured closed."
D. "A razor blade will be gently moved across the skin's surface to obtain a sample."

Procedure. Establish a sterile field and assemble all needed supplies and instruments. Local anesthesia is administered using a small-gauge (25-gauge) needle to reduce discomfort during injection. Preparation of the biopsy site differs by health care provider preference.

The injection of a local anesthetic agent, which produces a burning or stinging sensation, may be uncomfortable. Reassure the patient that the discomfort will subside as the anesthetic takes effect. Talking the patient through the procedure with a quiet voice along with a gentle touch may have a calming effect.

After removal, tissue specimens for pathologic study are placed in 10% formalin for fixation. Specimens for culture are placed in sterile saline solution. Bleeding of the site may be controlled by applying localized pressure, applying a topical hemostatic agent, or suturing.

Follow-up Care. After bleeding is controlled and any sutures are placed, the site is covered with an adhesive bandage or a dry gauze dressing. Teach the patient to keep the dressing dry and in place for at least 8 hours, and to clean the site daily after the dressing is removed. Tap water or saline is used to remove any dried blood or crusts. An antibiotic ointment may be prescribed to reduce the risk for ***infection.*** The site may be left open or covered for cosmetic reasons or because the site is an area often soiled. Teach the patient to report any redness or excessive drainage, and to return for suture removal (if sutures were placed) 7 to 10 days after biopsy.

Wood Lamp Examination. A handheld, long-wavelength ultraviolet (black) light or Wood lamp may be used during examination. Exposure of certain skin infections with this light produces a specific color, such as blue-green or red, that can be used to identify the ***infection.*** Hypopigmented skin is more prominent when it is viewed under black light, making evaluation of pigment changes in lighter skin easier. This examination is carried out in a darkened room and does not cause discomfort.

Diascopy. Diascopy is a painless technique to eliminate erythema caused by increased blood flow to the skin, thereby easing the inspection of skin lesions. A glass slide or lens is pressed down over the area to be examined, blanching the skin and revealing the shape of the lesions.

GET READY FOR THE NEXT-GENERATION NCLEX® EXAMINATION!

Key Points

Review these Key Points for each NCLEX Examination Client Needs Category.

Safe and Effective Care Environment

- Assist patients to change positions at least every 2 hours, noting areas of compromised ***tissue integrity.*** **QSEN: Safety**
- Wash hands and use Standard Precautions when providing care to a patient with impaired ***tissue integrity.*** **QSEN: Safety**
- Use lift sheets when moving patients to avoid shearing. **QSEN: Safety**
- Position patients to promote air circulation to skinfolds and minimize pressure over bony prominences. **QSEN: Safety**

Health Promotion and Maintenance

- Teach adults to use sunscreen and reduce exposure to sun and ultraviolet (UV) light. **QSEN: Safety**
- Teach adults to examine all skin on a monthly basis for new lesions and changes to existing lesions using the ABCDE method. **QSEN: Evidence-Based Practice**
- Encourage patients to bathe, shampoo hair, and keep fingernails clean and trimmed. **QSEN: Patient-Centered Care**

Psychosocial Integrity

- Use effective communication when teaching patients and caregivers what to expect during tests and procedures associated with skin assessment. **QSEN: Patient-Centered Care**

Physiological Integrity

- Assess the cognitive function of any patient whose hygiene appears inadequate. **QSEN: Patient-Centered Care**
- Assess skin changes according to normal pigmentation of each patient's skin. **Clinical Judgment**
- Be aware of specific allergies that impact skin. **QSEN: Patient-Centered Care**
- Assess if skin changes have occurred since a patient has started taking a new drug. **QSEN: Patient-Centered Care**
- Distinguish between normal variations and abnormalities regarding skin color, texture, warmth, elastic turgor, and moisture. **Clinical Judgment**

MASTERY QUESTIONS

1. Which intervention will the nurse delegate to assistive personnel (AP) for a client who has poor personal hygiene? **Select all that apply.**
   A. Obtain a social history.
   B. Assist the client with bathing.
   C. Help the client with brushing of teeth.
   D. Tell the client that he or she smells bad.
   E. Consult social services to assess the client's living conditions.
   F. Teach client and family members how to help with personal hygiene.
   G. Notify the health care provider of suspected drug or alcohol addiction.
   H. Assess for cognitive function or physical limitations that can interfere with grooming.
2. Which teaching will the nurse provide to the client who just underwent a skin biopsy and had sutures placed to close the wound? **Select all that apply.**
   A. Use antibiotic ointment as prescribed.
   B. Return for suture removal in 2 to 3 days.
   C. Report redness to the health care provider.
   D. Keep dressing moist so skin does not dry out.
   E. Use tap water or saline to remove any crusting.

REFERENCES

American Academy of Dermatology. (2020). *Skin cancer*. Retrieved from https://www.aad.org/media/stats/conditions/skin-cancer.

Brennan, M. (2019). Wound assessment: A step-by-step process. *Nursing, 49*(8), 62–64.

Campbell, J., Coyer, F., & Osborne, S. (2016). The Skin Safety Model: Reconceptualizing skin vulnerability in older patients. *Journal of Nursing Scholarship, 48*(1), 14–22.

Cox, J. (2019). Wound care 101. *Nursing, 49*(10), 33–39.

Edwards, H., Change, A., Gibb, M., Finlayson, K., Parker, C., O'Reilly, M., McDowell, J., & Shuter, P. (2017). Reduced prevalence and severity of wounds following implementation of the Champions for Skin Integrity model to facilitate uptake of evidence–based practice in aged care. *Journal of Clinical Nursing, 26*(23-24), 4276–4285.

International Skin Tear Advisory Panel. (2018). *Best practice recommendations for prevention and management of skin tears in aged skin*. Retrieved from https://www.woundsinternational.com/uploads/resources/57c1a5cc8a4771a696b4c17b9e2ae6f1.pdf.

Jarvis, C. (2020). *Physical examination & health assessment* (8th ed.). St. Louis: Elsevier.

Kirkland-Kyhn, H., et al. (2018). Caring for aging skin. *American Journal of Nursing, 118*(2), 60–63.

McCance, K., & Huether, S. (2019). *Pathophysiology: The biologic basis for disease in adults and children* (8th ed.). St. Louis: Elsevier.

National Cancer Institute. (n.d.). Melanoma Risk Assessment Tool. Retrieved from https://mrisktool.cancer.gov/calculator.html

Quest Diagnostics. (2019). *Herpes simplex/Varicella zoster virus rapid culture*. Retrieved from https://www.questdiagnostics.com/testcenter/BUOrderInfo.action?tc=16829&labCode=AMD.

Sabour, S. (2017). The scout device's reliability: methodological issues. *Advances in skin & wound care, 30*(8), 344.

The Skin Cancer Foundation. (2020). *Melanoma warning signs and images: Do you know your ABCDEs?* Retrieved from https://www.skincancer.org/skin-cancer-information/melanoma/melanoma-warning-signs-and-images/do-you-know-your-abcdes.

Touhy, T., & Jett, K. (2020). *Ebersole & Hess' toward healthy aging* (10th ed.). St. Louis: Elsevier.

U.S. Cancer Statistics Working Group. (2019). *U.S. Cancer Statistics Data Visualizations Tool, based on November 2018 submission data (1999-2016)*. U.S. Department of Health and Human Services, Centers for Disease Control and Prevention and National Cancer Institute. Retrieved from www.cdc.gov/cancer/dataviz.

23

Concepts of Care for Patients With Skin Problems

Cherie R. Rebar, Cecilia Bidigare

http://evolve.elsevier.com/Iggy/

LEARNING OUTCOMES

1. Collaborate with the interprofessional team to coordinate high-quality care for patients with a skin problem.
2. Describe factors that place a patient at high risk for a skin problem, and teach ways to minimize risk.
3. Implement patient-centered nursing interventions to decrease the psychosocial impact of living with a skin problem.
4. Apply knowledge of anatomy, physiology, and pathophysiology to assess patients with a skin problem.
5. Use clinical judgment to analyze assessment findings and diagnostic data in the care of patients with a skin problem.
6. Prioritize evidence-based care for patients with a skin problem affecting ***tissue integrity, fluid and electrolyte balance,*** or ***gas exchange,*** or that induces ***pain.***
7. Plan care coordination and transition management for patients with a skin problem.

KEY TERMS

acute (healing) phase The second phase of a burn injury, beginning at about 36 to 48 hours after the injury and continuing until the wound closure is complete.

approximated In a clean laceration or a surgical incision to be closed with sutures or staples, the act of bringing together the wound edges with the skin layers lined up in correct anatomic position so they can be held in place until healing is complete.

contraction The closure of a wound as new collagen replaces damaged tissue, pulling the wound edges inward along the path of least resistance.

debris Dead cells and tissues in a wound.

emergent (resuscitation) phase The first phase of a burn injury, beginning at the onset of injury and continuing for about 48 hours.

first intention Healing in which the wound can be easily closed and dead space eliminated without granulation, which thus shortens the phases of tissue repair; inflammation resolves quickly, and connective tissue repair is minimal, resulting in a thin scar.

granulation The formation of scar tissue for wound healing to occur.

mechanical débridement Mechanical entrapment and detachment of dead tissue.

natural chemical débridement Promotion of self-digestion of dead tissues by naturally occurring bacterial enzymes *(autolysis).*

nevus Mole.

pediculosis Infestation by lice.

pressure injury (PI) A loss of tissue integrity caused when the skin and underlying soft tissue are compromised between a bony prominence and an external surface.

pruritus Itching.

re-epithelialization In partial-thickness (superficial) wounds involving damage to the epidermis and upper layers of the dermis, a form of healing by means of the production of new skin cells by undamaged epidermal cells in the basal layer of the dermis.

rehabilitative (restorative) phase The third phase of a burn injury, beginning with wound closure and ending when the patient achieves his or her highest level of functioning.

resurfacing Regrowth across the open area of a wound.

second intention Healing of deep tissue injuries or wounds with tissue loss in which a cavity-like defect requires gradual filling of the dead space with connective tissue, which prolongs the repair process.

sharp débridement (also known as *surgical débridement*) A process performed by a health care provider on a draining, necrotic injury before dressing débridement is begun or continued; it facilitates removal of excessive exudate and loose debris without damaging healthy epithelial cells or new granulation tissue.

skin care bundle A tool used to provide consistency in the assessment and planning of care for patients who are at risk for pressure injuries.

surgical débridement See *sharp débridement.*

third intention Delayed primary closure of a wound with a high risk for infection. The wound is intentionally left open for several days until inflammation has subsided and is then closed by first intention.

topical chemical débridement Topical enzyme preparations to loosen necrotic tissue.

tunneling "Hidden" wounds that extend from the primary wound into surrounding tissues.

PRIORITY AND INTERRELATED CONCEPTS

The priority concepts for this chapter are:
- ***Tissue Integrity***
- ***Pain***

The ***Tissue Integrity*** concept exemplar for this chapter is Pressure Injury.

The interrelated concepts for this chapter are:
- ***Fluid and Electrolyte Balance***
- ***Gas Exchange***

As the largest organ, the skin protects the body by providing a strong barrier to harmful microorganisms and other foreign proteins (antigens). Changes in ***tissue integrity*** of the skin can indicate underlying health problems and interfere with management of others.

Age-related changes increase the older patient's risk for skin damage and loss of ***tissue integrity.*** Pressure injuries reflect one of the most concerning skin conditions for which nurses provide care. Nurses are on the forefront of preventing pressure injuries from developing while a patient is hospitalized.

TISSUE INTEGRITY CONCEPT EXEMPLAR: PRESSURE INJURY

Pathophysiology Review

A **pressure injury** (PI) is a loss of ***tissue integrity.*** It is caused when the skin and underlying soft tissue are compressed between a bony prominence and an external surface. This results in *reduced tissue perfusion and* ***gas exchange,*** *which eventually leads to cell death.* Most frequently found on the sacrum, hips, and heels, *pressure injuries can occur on any body surface.* For example, unrelieved pressure from a nasal cannula or endotracheal tube can result in a pressure injury (Kayser et al., 2018; McCance et al., 2019).

Risk factors for development of a pressure injury include lack of mobility, exposure of skin to excessive moisture (e.g., urinary or fecal incontinence), undernourishment, and aging skin. Patients with cognitive decline or impairment are at even higher risk, as they may not be able to fully participate in care. People with peripheral vascular disease and/or diabetes mellitus are at risk, as they may experience impaired sensory perception as well as delayed wound healing. Once formed, these chronic wounds are slow to heal, resulting in increased morbidity and health care costs. Complications include sepsis, kidney failure, infectious arthritis, and osteomyelitis.

Etiology and Genetic Risk. The degree of injury is dependent on mechanism and timing. Friction and shear are mechanical forces that move parallel to skin, causing injury (McCance et al., 2019). *Friction* occurs when surfaces rub the skin and irritate or tear fragile epithelial tissue. Such forces are generated when the patient is dragged or pulled across bed linen. *Shearing forces* are generated when the skin itself is stationary and the tissues below the skin (e.g., fat, muscle) shift or move (Fig. 23.1). The movement of the deeper tissue layers reduces the blood supply to the skin, leading to skin hypoxia, anoxia, ischemia, inflammation, and necrosis.

Although mechanical factors are the causative agent for pressure injuries, research continues regarding exploration of the role that gene expression may have in pressure injury formation (Wang et al., 2016).

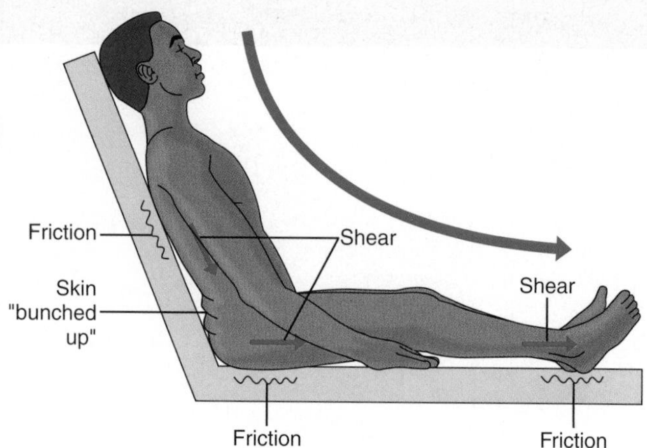

Fig. 23.1 Shearing forces pulling skin layers away from deeper tissue. The skin is "bunched up" against the back of the mattress while the rest of the bone and muscle in the area presses downward on the lower part of the mattress. Blood vessels become kinked, obstructing circulation and leading to tissue death.

Incidence and Prevalence. Prevalence of pressure injuries has not changed significantly over the last 20 years, with 3 million adults affected annually in the United States (Mervis & Phillips, 2019). A retrospective analysis of the 2016 International Pressure Ulcer Prevalence Survey data found the prevalence of medical device–related pressure injuries to be 0.6%, with the ears (due to oxygen tubing) and feet most commonly affected (Kayser et al., 2018).

Health Promotion and Maintenance. Pressure injuries can be prevented if the risk is recognized, interventions to prevent the injury are undertaken before ***tissue integrity*** is compromised, and intervention for any existing injury begins early (see the Best Practice for Patient Safety & Quality Care: Preventing Pressure Injuries box). Deliberate and consistent interventions based on an evidence-based **skin care bundle**, as described in the Systems Thinking and Quality Improvement: Using a Skin Integrity Care Bundle to Prevent Pressure Injuries box, are needed to prevent pressure injuries across the health care continuum, particularly for patients who are older adults and/or critically ill. Key health care team members for pressure injury prevention and management are the nurse, the certified wound care specialist, and the registered dietitian nutritionist (RDN). Involving assistive personnel (AP) in pressure injury prevention under appropriate supervision enhances prevention program effectiveness.

Interprofessional Collaborative Care

Care of the patient with a pressure injury, depending on stage and associated health issues, takes place in all settings, including the home. Members of the interprofessional team who collaborate most closely to care for the patient with pressure injury include the primary health care provider, who continually assesses the wound condition and prescribes treatment; the nurse; and the registered dietitian nutritionist (RDN), who assesses nutrition status and recommends dietary modification to speed wound healing.

BEST PRACTICE FOR PATIENT SAFETY & QUALITY CARE QSEN

Preventing Pressure Injuries

1. Determine risk level.
   a. Use a reliable scale (e.g., Braden Scale) to assess risk, and assess entire skin daily.
   b. Use a proven **skin care bundle** so that all health care professionals are following consistent interventions.
   c. Ensure that a nutrition consultation with the RDN takes place.
   d. Ensure that fluid intake is 2000 to 3000 mL/day.
   e. Help the patient consume the determined amount of protein and calories.
   f. Monitor changes in weight, skin turgor, urine output, renal function, serum sodium, and calculated serum osmolality.
   g. Document interventions thoroughly, and communicate with the interprofessional team regularly to promote continuity of care.
2. Reduce pressure.
   a. Do not keep the head of the bed elevated above 30 degrees to prevent shearing.
   b. When positioning a patient on his or her side, position at a 30-degree tilt (avoiding 90-degree positions).
   c. Examine the source of pressure, and determine how to reduce it.
   d. Help patients in chairs or wheelchairs to stand and march in place, five steps per hour (if they are able).
   e. Use pressure-offloading devices or foam dressings for bony prominences (e.g., float the heels off of a sturdy pillow.
   f. Use devices such as air-fluidized beds or surfaces and powered mattress overlays to manage the microclimate (the area between the patient's skin and the support surface).
   g. Refrain from using donut-shaped pillows; these can damage capillary beds and increase tissue necrosis.
   h. For patients who cannot stand or turn themselves, turn and reposition a minimum of every 2 hours or as needs are assessed.
3. Improve pressure tolerance.
   a. Place pillows or foam wedges between two bony surfaces or between bony surfaces and the bed.
   b. Preserve skin integrity.
      i. Clean the skin as soon as possible after soiling occurs and at routine intervals.
      ii. Moisturize the skin with dimethazone, zinc oxide, lanolin, or petrolatum.
      iii. Change incontinence products regularly.
      iv. Inspect skin, especially under incontinence products, at least every 2 hours.
      v. Wash skin with clean, warm water, and mild soap. Take care not to scrub; use only the amount of pressure needed to provide cleansing; pat skin dry (instead of rubbing).
      vi. Do not massage reddened areas; this increases risk for skin breakdown.
      vii. Perform perineal care every 2 hours; use a disposable cleaning cloth with skin-barrier agents.
      viii. Refrain from putting skin directly on any type of plastic device.
      ix. Keep skin-to-skin areas dry (e.g., under breasts that touch torso, etc.)

Data from Black, J. (2018). Take three steps forward to prevent pressure injury in the medical-surgical patient: Pressure injuries...Prevention across the acute care continuum. *American Nurse Today*, Supplement to May 2018, 10-11, 39; European Pressure Ulcer Advisory Panel, National Pressure Injury Advisory Panel, and Pan Pacific Pressure Injury Alliance. (2019). *Prevention and treatment of pressure ulcers/injuries: Quick Reference Guide 2019* (3rd ed.); Kalowes, P. (2018). Preventing pressure injuries in critically ill patients. *American Nurse Today*, Supplement to May 2018, 8-9, 39; Long, D. (2018). Best practices for pressure injury prevention in the ED: Pressure injuries...Prevention across the acute care continuum. *American Nurse Today*, Supplement to May 2018, 8-9, 39; and Sidor, D., & Sieggreen, M. (2018). Take three steps forward to prevent pressure injury in the medical-surgical patient: Pressure injuries...Prevention across the acute care continuum. *American Nurse Today*, Supplement to May 2018, 35-37.

SYSTEMS THINKING AND QUALITY IMPROVEMENT QSEN

Using a Skin Integrity Care Bundle to Prevent Pressure Injuries

Gallagher-Ford, L., et al. (2019). The STAND skin bundle. *American Journal of Nursing, 119*(10), 45-48.

This initiative sought to determine whether introducing a bundle of prevention interventions would reduce the incidence of hospital-acquired pressure injuries (HAPIs). The Ohio State University Wexner Medical Center noted a rise in HAPIs, a similar and concerning trend seen in many institutions. An interprofessional team was assembled in January 2017, composed of nursing quality experts, information technologists, nutrition services professionals, and wound-ostomy nurses. The team reviewed literature for best practices and created an evidence-based bundle of interventions to prevent HAPIs.

The STAND bundle was developed to describe the interventions to:

- Score (using the Braden Scale for Predicting Pressure Injury Risk)
- Turn (repositioning tubes and devices, turning the patient)
- Apply (bordered foam dressing or barrier cream)
- Nutrition (attention given to nutrition status)
- Discuss (involvement of specialists)

Once the bundle was created, stakeholders were involved to discuss the initiative and offer feedback and input. Staff were notified 4 to 6 weeks prior to implementation, giving them time to learn the protocol and plan ahead (as opposed to learning about implementation only days before the process began). At assessment, if a score of less than 18 on the Braden Scale was found, the other interventions were implemented. Over an 18-month period, a 22.5% overall decrease in HAPIs was noted.

Commentary: Implications for Practice and Research

The Centers for Medicare and Medicaid Services identifies HAPIs as preventable events. Use of a bundle, with an easy-to-remember mnemonic, can make a significant difference when implemented across an agency. Involving key stakeholders, especially nursing staff, well before implementation can increase success of evidence-based initiatives. Using a specific and unified process across a system increases the chances of improving patient outcomes.

NATIONAL PATIENT SAFETY GOALS

Per The Joint Commission's (TJC's) National Patient Safety Goals (NPSGs) (TJC, 2018), all patients admitted to a health care facility or home care agency are to be assessed for pressure injury risk, particularly in skin areas where medical devices are used. The use of a risk assessment tool increases the chances of identifying patients at greater risk for skin breakdown. The Braden Scale (Fig. 23.2) is a commonly used valid skin risk assessment tool. Using it helps the nurse assess and document risk categories for pressure injury formation (e.g., mental status, activity and mobility, nutritional status, incontinence).

NURSING SAFETY PRIORITY QSEN

Action Alert

Teach all nursing care personnel and caregivers to refrain from massaging reddened skin areas directly and from using donut-shaped pillows for pressure relief. These can damage capillary beds and increase tissue necrosis.

◆ Assessment: Recognize Cues

History. If the patient has no pressure injuries, obtain a history with risk factors in mind. See the Focused Assessment: The Patient at Risk for Pressure Injuries box.

For the patient who already has a pressure injury, identify the cause of ***tissue integrity*** loss and factors that may impair healing. Ask about the circumstances of the skin loss. Patients with chronic pressure injuries may have a history of delayed healing or recurrence of the injury after healing has occurred. Assess for any of these contributing factors:

- Prolonged bedrest and/or immobility
- Incontinence
- Diabetes mellitus and/or peripheral vascular disease
- Undernutrition
- Decreased sensory perception or cognitive problems

Physical Assessment/Signs and Symptoms. Inspect the entire body, including the back of the head, for areas of ***tissue integrity*** loss or pressure. Give special attention to bony prominences (e.g., heels, sacrum, elbows, knees, trochanters, and iliac spines), areas with excessive moisture, and areas in which medical devices are present. Assess the patient's general appearance for issues related to skin health, such as the proportion of weight to height, remembering that individuals who are inadequately nourished are at increased risk. Note cleanliness of the skin, hair, and nails. Determine whether any loss of mobility or range of joint motion has occurred. *Do not delegate this assessment to AP because it is beyond their scope of practice.*

Wound Assessment. The appearance of pressure injuries changes with the depth of the ulcer. The Key Features: Pressure Injuries box lists the features of the stages of pressure ulceration, and Fig. 23.3 shows examples.

Document location, size, color, extent of tissue involvement, cell types in the wound base and margins, exudate, condition of surrounding tissue, and presence of foreign bodies for each wound. Assess based on the frequency of the agency policy and as needed. *At each dressing change, compare the existing wound features with those documented previously to determine the current state of healing or deterioration.*

FOCUSED ASSESSMENT

The Patient at Risk for Pressure Injuries

Assess cardiovascular status:
- Presence or absence of peripheral edema
- Hand-vein filling in the dependent position
- Neck-vein filling in the recumbent and sitting positions
- Weight gain or loss

Assess cognition and mental status:
- Level of consciousness
- Orientation to time, place, and person

Assess nutrition status:
- Change in muscle mass
- Lackluster nails, sparse hair
- Recent weight loss of more than 5% of usual weight
- Impaired oral intake
- Difficulty swallowing
- Generalized edema

KEY FEATURES

Pressure Injuries

Stage 1—nonblanchable erythema of intact skin
- Intact skin with localized area of nonblanchable erythema (may appear differently in skin with darker pigmentation).
- May be preceded by changes in sensation, temperature, or firmness.
- Color changes are not purple or maroon.

Stage 2—partial-thickness loss with exposed dermis
- Partial-thickness loss of skin with exposed dermis.
- Wound bed is viable, pink or red, and moist.
- May look like intact or ruptured serum-filled blister.

Stage 3—full-thickness skin loss
- Full-thickness skin loss with adipose (fat) visible in the ulcer.
- Granulation tissue and rolled wound edges are often present.
- Slough and/or eschar may be present.
- Undermining and tunneling may be present.
- Subcutaneous tissues may be damaged or necrotic.

Stage 4—full-thickness loss of skin and tissue
- Full-thickness skin loss with exposed or palpable fascia, muscle, tendon, ligament, cartilage, or bone.
- May have slough or eschar.
- Rolled edges, undermining, or tunneling may be present.

Unstageable—obscured full-thickness skin and tissue loss
- Full-thickness skin and tissue loss.
- The extent of damage cannot be confirmed because it is obscured by eschar or slough.

Suspected deep-tissue injury—persistent nonblanchable deep red, maroon, or purple discoloration
- Intact or nonintact skin.
- Localized area of persistent nonblanchable deep red, maroon, or purple discoloration (may appear differently in skin with darker pigmentation).
- Epidermal separation reveals dark wound bed or blood-filled blister.

Mucosal membrane pressure injury
- Found on mucous membranes where a medical device is in use.
- These are unstageable ulcers.

Data from National Pressure Ulcer Advisory Panel. (2016). *NPUAP pressure injury stages.* https://npiap.com/page/PressureInjuryStages.

Patient's name ______	Evaluator's name ______			Date of assessment		
Sensory perception Ability to respond meaningfully to pressure-related discomfort	**1. Completely limited** Unresponsive to painful stimuli (does not moan, flinch, or grasp) because of diminished level of consciousness or sedation OR limited ability to feel pain over most of body surface	**2. Very limited** Responds only to painful stimuli; cannot communicate discomfort except by moaning or restlessness OR has a sensory impairment that limits the ability to feel pain or discomfort over half of the body	**3. Slightly limited** Responds to verbal commands but cannot always communicate discomfort or need to be turned OR has some sensory impairment that limits ability to feel pain or discomfort in one or two extremities	**4. No impairment** Responds to verbal commands; has no sensory deficit that would limit ability to feel or voice pain or discomfort		
Moisture Degree to which skin is exposed to moisture	**1. Constantly moist** Skin is kept moist almost constantly by perspiration, urine; dampness is detected every time the client is moved or turned	**2. Very Moist** Skin is often but not always moist; linen must be changed at least once a shift	**3. Occasionally moist** Skin is occasionally moist, requiring an extra linen change approximately once a day	**4. Rarely moist** Skin is usually dry; linen requires changing only at routine intervals		
Activity Degree of physical activity	**1. Bedfast** Confined to bed	**2. Chairfast** Ability to walk severely limited or nonexistent; cannot bear own weight and must be assisted into chair or wheelchair	**3. Walks occasionally** Walks occasionally during the day but for very short distances, with or without assistance; spends the majority of each shift in bed or chair	**4. Walks frequently** Walks outside the room at least twice a day and inside the room at least once every 2 hours during waking hours		
Mobility Ability to change or control body position	**1. Completely immobile** Does not make even slight changes in body or extremity position without assistance	**2. Very limited** Makes occasional slight changes in body or extremity position but unable to make frequent or significant changes independently	**3. Slightly limited** Makes frequent though slight changes in body or extremity position independently	**4. No limitations** Makes major and frequent changes in position without assistance		
Nutrition Usual food intake pattern	**1. Very poor** Never eats a complete meal; rarely eats more than a third of any food offered; eats two servings or less of protein (meat or dairy products) per day; takes fluids poorly; does not take a liquid dietary supplement OR is NPO or maintained on clear liquids or IV for more than 5 days	**2. Probably inadequate** Rarely eats a complete meal and generally eats only about half of any food offered; protein intake includes only three servings of meat or dairy products per day; occasionally will take a dietary supplement OR receives less than optimal amount of liquid diet or tube feeding	**3. Adequate** Eats over half of most meals; eats a total of four servings of protein (meat, dairy products) each day; occasionally will refuse a meal, but will usually take a supplement if offered OR is receiving tube feeding or total parenteral nutrition, which probably meets most nutritional needs	**4. Excellent** Eats most of every meal; never refuses a meal; usually eats a total of four or more servings of meat and dairy products; occasionally eats between meals; does not require supplementation		
Friction and shear	**1. Problem** Requires moderate to maximum assistance in moving; complete lifting without sliding against sheets is impossible; frequently slides down in bed or chair, requiring frequent repositioning with maximum assistance; spasticity, contractures, or agitation leads to almost constant friction	**2. Potential problem** Moves feebly or requires minimum assistance during a move; skin probably slides to some extent against sheets, chair, restraints, or other devices; maintains relatively good position in chair or bed most of the time but occasionally slides down	**3. No apparent problem** Moves in bed and in chair independently and has sufficient muscle strength to lift up completely during move; maintains good position in bed or chair at all times			
Scoring system: 15-16 = mild risk, 12-14 = moderate risk, <11 = severe risk				Total score		

Fig. 23.2 The Braden Scale for predicting pressure sore risk. (From Barbara Braden and Nancy Bergstrom. ©1988. Reprinted with permission.)

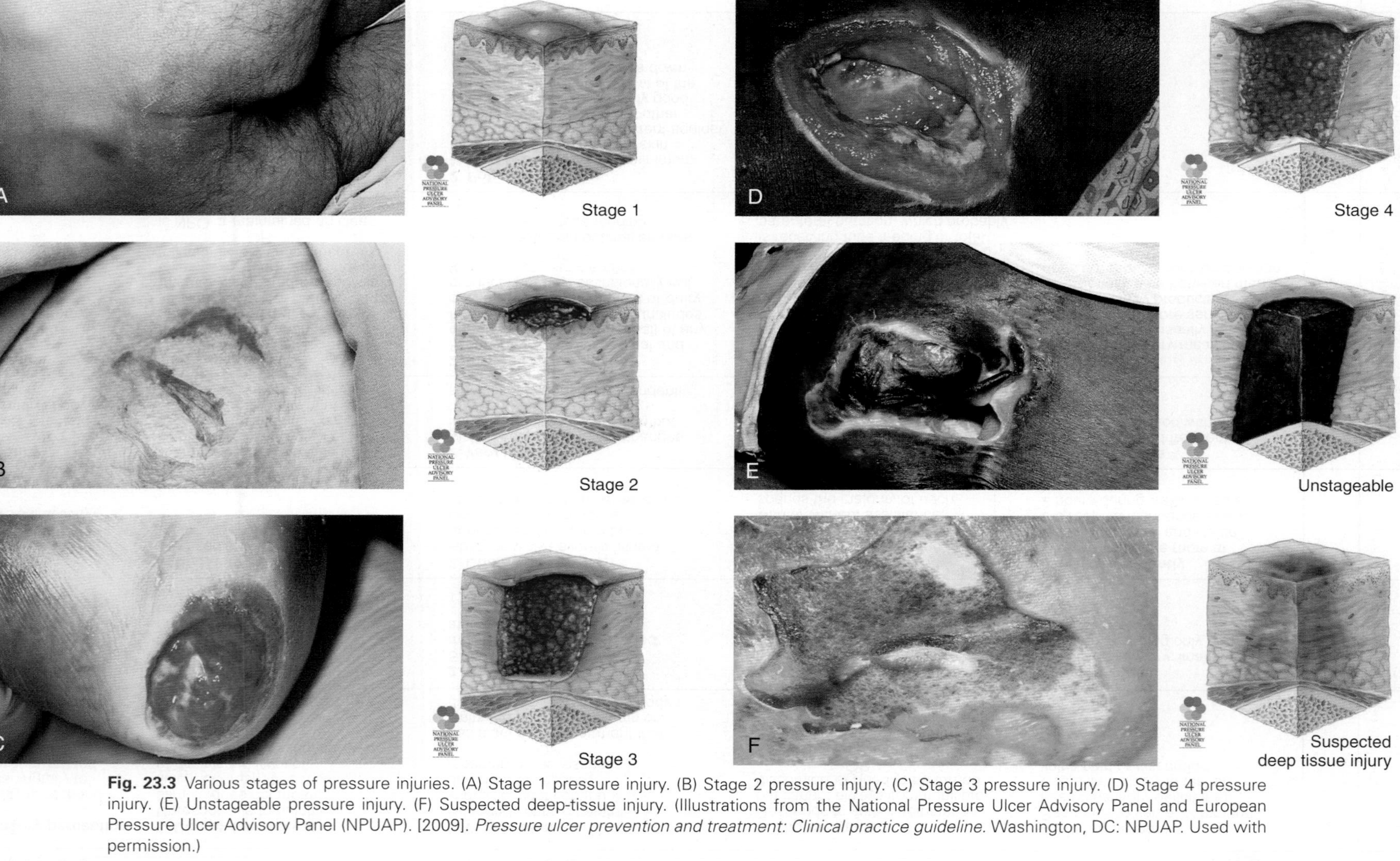

Fig. 23.3 Various stages of pressure injuries. (A) Stage 1 pressure injury. (B) Stage 2 pressure injury. (C) Stage 3 pressure injury. (D) Stage 4 pressure injury. (E) Unstageable pressure injury. (F) Suspected deep-tissue injury. (Illustrations from the National Pressure Ulcer Advisory Panel and European Pressure Ulcer Advisory Panel (NPUAP). [2009]. *Pressure ulcer prevention and treatment: Clinical practice guideline.* Washington, DC: NPUAP. Used with permission.)

Measurement, recorded by length, width, and depth (using millimeters or centimeters), is a key way to determine progression or healing of a wound. To document wound depth, touch the bottom of the wound with a cotton-tipped applicator or swab and mark the place on the swab that is level with the skin surface. Then measure the area of the swab between the tip and the mark. If **tunneling** is present ("hidden" wounds that extend from the primary wound into surrounding tissues), use a cotton-tipped applicator to probe gently for a much larger tunnel or pocket of necrotic tissue beneath the opening. Estimate the size and location of any tunneled areas, and document accordingly. Many agencies use the "clock concept" for documenting tunneling, where the patient's head is considered to be at the 12 o'clock position, and the feet are at the 6 o'clock position.

Blanchable erythema of intact skin over a bony prominence is an early sign of pressure-related complications. For patients with light skin, press the reddened area firmly with a gloved finger and release the pressure. An area that blanches (lightens) when pressure is briefly applied and reddens again when pressure is released suggests adequate tissue perfusion. A reddened area that does not blanch indicates impaired capillary blood flow and early tissue damage. For patients with darker skin, assess for blanching, and also assess skin temperature, edema presence (or absence), ***pain,*** and induration (Black, 2018b). Techniques to better assess darker skin include (Black, 2018b):

- Moisten the skin, which can highlight skin color changes.
- Use long-wave infrared thermography. Compare gradations of the color scale on image results between injured and adjacent skin, recognizing that warm skin is perfused and cool skin is not.

In addition to blanching and tunneling, assess for presence of other wound characteristics:

- Cellulitis—inflammation of the skin and subcutaneous tissue extending beyond the area of injury.
- Eschar—necrotic tissue that appears like a layer of black, gray, or brown collagen; may be dry and leathery (in early stages), or full of exudate and yellow or tan in appearance (Table 23.1).
- Granulation tissue—may be pale pink (early **granulation** [the formation of scar tissue for wound healing to occur]) to beefy red; healthy tissue is moist and slightly spongy.
- Undermining—separation of the skin layers at the wound margins from the underlying granulation tissue.

Serial photographs of the wound are very helpful in documenting changes in wound appearance and progress toward healing. Policies on photographic documentation vary between agencies and require informed consent from the patient or durable power of attorney. Remote visualization and monitoring via telehealth, and use of technology such as augmented reality glasses (ARGs), can also be very effective in prevention and management of patients with pressure injuries (Kaylor et al., 2019; Mazboori et al., 2019).

Psychosocial Assessment. Pressure injuries are often costly to treat and may affect a patient's body image. Assess the patient's and caregiver's desired treatment outcomes, knowledge of how to provide care at home, and ability to adhere to the prescribed treatment regimen. Refer to social services or a case worker if financial barriers are noted, and/or to a home care nurse if the patient or caregiver is unable to safely carry out the plan of care.

TABLE 23.1 Types of Wound Exudate

Characteristics	Significance
Serosanguineous Exudate	
Blood-tinged amber fluid consisting of serum and red blood cells	Normal for first 48 hr after injury Sudden increase in amount precedes wound dehiscence in wounds closed by first intention
Purulent Exudate	
Creamy yellow pus	Colonization with *Staphylococcus*
Greenish-blue pus causing staining of dressings and accompanied by a "fruity" odor	Colonization with *Pseudomonas*
Beige pus with a "fishy" odor	Colonization with *Proteus*
Brownish pus with a "fecal" odor	Colonization with aerobic coliform and *Bacteroides* (usually occurs after intestinal surgery)

Laboratory Assessment. Wound culturing is not routinely performed unless there is lack of healing and signs of persistent infection are present (Boyko et al., 2018). Rather, clinical indicators of infection (e.g., cellulitis, exudate changes, increase in injury size or depth) and systemic signs of bacteremia (e.g., fever, elevated white blood cell [WBC] count) are used to diagnose an infection. If wound culturing is to be performed, a tissue culture is done, not simply a wound swab (Boyko et al., 2018).

Other Diagnostic Assessments. Noninvasive and invasive arterial blood flow studies may be considered if arterial occlusion is suspected in delayed healing of a pressure injury on the heel or ankle. Duplex ultrasound imaging may be performed to assess for venous disease and venous thromboembolism (DeMarco, 2020). Blood tests to determine nutritional deficiencies (e.g., prealbumin, albumin, total protein) are helpful in managing the patient with undernourishment who has a pressure injury.

◆ **Analysis: Analyze Cues and Prioritize Hypotheses.** The priority collaborative problems for patients with pressure injuries include:

1. Compromised ***tissue integrity*** due to vascular insufficiency and trauma
2. Potential for infection due to insufficient wound management

◆ Planning and Implementation: Generate Solutions and Take Action

Improving Tissue Integrity

Planning: Expected Outcomes. The patient with a pressure injury is expected to progress to regain ***tissue integrity*** while not developing new pressure injuries.

Interventions. Wound care for pressure injuries varies significantly. Dressings, topical solutions, débridement, and/or surgery may be indicated.

Nonsurgical Management. General interventions for wound management of pressure injuries are listed in the Best Practice for

CLINICAL JUDGMENT CHALLENGE 23.1

Safety

A 79-year-old client with osteoporosis and urinary incontinence has been admitted to a long-term care facility after having an ischemic stroke. The client's partner reports that before the stroke, the client still needed help with ADLs. Assessment shows a slender, frail older adult with significant left-sided weakness who requires assistance dressing, eating, and transferring between the wheelchair and the bed. While assisting the client with changing clothes, the nurse notes a large reddened area on the left hip that doesn't change color when it is pressed.

1. **Recognize Cues:** What assessment information in this client situation is the most important and immediate concern for the nurse? (Hint: Identify the **relevant** information *first* to determine what is most important.)
2. **Analyze Cues:** What client conditions are consistent with the **most relevant** information? (Hint: Think about priority collaborative problems that support and contradict the information presented in this situation.)
3. **Prioritize Hypotheses:** Which possibilities or explanations are **most likely** to be present in this client situation? Which possibilities or explanations are the most serious? (Hint: Consider all possibilities and determine their urgency and risk for this client.)
4. **Generate Solutions:** What actions would most likely achieve the desired outcomes for this client? Which actions should be **avoided** or are **potentially harmful**? (Hint: Determine the desired outcomes first to decide which interventions are appropriate and those that should be avoided.)
5. **Take Action:** Which actions are the most appropriate and how should they be implemented? In what **priority order** should they be implemented? (Hint: Consider health teaching, documentation, requested health care provider orders or prescriptions, nursing skills, collaboration with or referral to health team members, etc.)
6. **Evaluate Outcomes:** What client assessment would indicate that the nurse's actions were **effective**? (Hint: Think about signs that would indicate an improvement, decline, or unchanged client condition.)

Patient Safety & Quality Care: Wound Management of Pressure Injuries box. Nonsurgical intervention of pressure injuries is often left to the discretion of the nurse, who coordinates with the primary health care provider and certified wound care specialist (if available) to select an appropriate method of wound dressing and management. Many agencies have guidelines for wound dressings based on wound size and depth and presence of drainage.

Dressings. A well-designed dressing helps healing by removing surface debris, protecting exposed healthy tissues, and creating a barrier until the wound is closed. Different dressing materials help remove debris by **mechanical débridement** (mechanical entrapment and detachment of dead tissue), **topical chemical débridement** (topical enzyme preparations to loosen necrotic tissue), or **natural chemical débridement** (promoting self-digestion of dead tissues by naturally occurring bacterial enzymes *[autolysis]*) (Table 23.2). **Sharp débridement** (also known as surgical débridement) may be performed by a health care provider on a draining, necrotic injury before dressing débridement is begun or continued. This process facilitates removal of excessive exudate and loose debris without damaging healthy epithelial cells or new granulation tissue.

Specific dressings, because there are so many and recommendations are so specialized based on the individual patient's needs, are often recommended by the wound nurse. Collaborate closely with this member of the interprofessional team to

BEST PRACTICE FOR PATIENT SAFETY & QUALITY CARE (QSEN)

Wound Management of Pressure Injuries

- Conduct comprehensive ongoing assessments of the patient, including notation of pain.
- Use a standardized form of measurement so that all health care professionals use the same approach.
- Use nonpharmacologic pain management interventions as first-line strategy for discomfort associated with pressure injuries.
- Use cleansing agents with antimicrobials to clean pressure injuries with actual or anticipated infection.
- Cleanse the skin gently around the pressure injury with normal saline.
- Assess the injury for presence of necrotic tissue and amount of exudate; report findings to the primary health care provider.
- Avoid disturbance of stable, hard, dry eschar (in heels and limbs) unless infection is anticipated.
- Evaluate for signs of infection and/or biofilm; obtain tissue biopsy order if needed.
- Evaluate for signs of osteomyelitis if bone is exposed or feels soft, or if injury fails to heal with treatment; report findings to the primary health care provider.
- Optimize nutrition by consulting with the RDN.
- Select dressings (with certified wound care nurse) based on wound assessment, goals, and ability of patient or caregiver to carry out self-care.
- Reposition the patient frequently to avoid injury extension or generation of new injuries.

Data from European Pressure Ulcer Advisory Panel, National Pressure Injury Advisory Panel, and Pan Pacific Pressure Injury Alliance. (2019). *Prevention and treatment of pressure ulcers/injuries: Quick Reference Guide 2019* (3rd ed.).

TABLE 23.2 Common Dressing Techniques for Wound Débridement

Technique	Mechanism of Action
Wet-to-damp saline-moistened gauze	As with the wet-to-dry technique, necrotic debris is mechanically removed but with less trauma to healing tissue.
Continuous wet gauze	The wound surface is continually bathed with a wetting agent of choice, promoting dilution of viscous exudate and softening of dry eschar.
Topical enzyme preparations	Proteolytic action on thick, adherent eschar causes breakdown of denatured protein and more rapid separation of necrotic tissue.
Moisture-retentive dressing	Spontaneous separation of necrotic tissue is promoted by autolysis.

determine the most appropriate dressing. See Table 23.3 for various types of wound dressings.

Wounds should be gently cleansed at each dressing change (and more frequently if needed). See the Best Practice for Patient Safety & Quality Care: Wound Management of Pressure Injuries box.

Physical therapy. Physical therapists are important members of the interprofessional team who can help plan and implement therapeutic strategies to redistribute and offload pressure, maximize overall function, and improve quality of life for patients with chronic wounds. They can also provide electrical stimulation therapy and ultrasound, which have been shown to be an effective adjuvant to traditional pressure injury treatment (Karsli et al., 2017).

Drug therapy. Clean, healthy granulation tissue has a blood supply and is capable of providing white blood cells and antibodies to the wound to combat infection. If extensive necrosis is present or if local tissue defenses are impaired, topical antibacterial agents or dressing materials are often needed to control bacterial growth (see Table 23.3). As in other clinical situations, antibiotic use is avoided in the absence of infection to reduce the development of resistant bacterial strains.

Nutrition therapy. Successful healing of pressure injuries depends on adequate intake of calories, protein, vitamins, minerals, and water. Nutrition deficiencies are common among patients who are chronically ill; this state of undernutrition increases the risk for skin breakdown and delayed wound healing. Severe protein deficiency inhibits healing and impairs host infection defenses.

Coordinate with the registered dietitian nutritionist (RDN) to help the patient eat a well-balanced diet, especially emphasizing protein. Fats also are needed to ensure formation of cell membranes. (See Chapter 55 for interventions to ensure adequate nutrition.) If the patient cannot eat sufficient amounts of food, other types of feedings may be needed to increase protein and caloric intake, and supplementation may be indicated (see Chapter 55).

Adjuvant therapies. Therapies such as electrical stimulation, negative-pressure wound therapy (NPWT), therapeutic ultrasound, hyperbaric oxygen, and topical growth factors may be prescribed (Berlowitz, 2020). There are varying degrees of evidence for each of these therapies, which is why they may be used adjuvantly, but not as the primary means for treatment of pressure injuries.

Electrical stimulation is the application of a low-voltage current to a wound area to increase blood vessel growth and promote granulation. This treatment is usually delivered twice daily through a wound overlay and is usually performed by a physical therapist or certified wound care specialist. The voltage is delivered in "pulses" that may cause a tingling sensation in the skin. It is not used with patients who have a pacemaker, a wound over the heart, or a skin cancer involving the wound or periwound skin.

Negative-pressure wound therapy (NPWT) increases wound healing by increasing blood flow, minimizing edema, and enhancing formation of granulation tissue. Often called vacuum-assisted wound closure, these systems continuously or

TABLE 23.3 Wound Dressings

Dressing Type	Description	Indication
Alginate	Highly absorbent fabrics or yarns that are derived from natural polysaccharide fibers or seaweed; may be combined with collagen. Alginate forms a gel when it comes in contact with the pressure injury.	Stage 3 and 4 pressure injuries with moderate exudate
Antimicrobial	Impregnated with antimicrobial agents, such as medical-grade honey, chlorhexidine, or silver ions.	For pressure injuries with infection
Collagens	Gels, pads, particles, pastes, powders, sheets, or solutions. Made from bovine, equine, porcine, or avian sources. Used with secondary dressings.	Stage 3 or 4 pressure injuries
Foam (including hydropolymers)	Sheets or other shapes of foamed, polymer solutions (usually polyurethane) that have open cells that can hold fluid. May be impregnated or layered.	Stage 2 and greater pressure injuries with moderate or heavy exudate
Gauze (moist)	Dry, woven or nonwoven sponges and wraps made of cotton, polyester, or rayon.	Pressure injuries that cannot be dressed with an advanced wound dressing, yet need a moist environment
Hydrocolloid (e.g., 3M Tegaderm hydrocolloid dressing)	Wafers, powders, or pastes (powder and pastes need a secondary dressing). Used in areas that require contouring (e.g., heels).	Noninfected stage 2 pressure injuries
Hydrogel	Amorphous, impregnated, or in sheet form. Designed to maintain a moist environment.	Noninfected stage 2 pressure injuries Noninfected stage 3 and 4 pressure injuries with minimal exudate
Superabsorbent (e.g., 3M Tegaderm superabsorbent dressing)	Highly absorptive fiber layers (e.g., cellulose, cotton, rayon). Minimizes adherence to the wound while collecting exudate.	Heavily exuding pressure injuries
Transparent films (e.g., 3M Tegaderm)	Polymer membranes that are impermeable to liquid, water, and bacteria. Can see through the dressing. (Also used to cover IV sites, lacerations, second-degree burns.)	Noninfected stage 2 pressure injuries; also for pressure injuries as a secondary dressing when advanced wound dressings are not an option

Data from Kestrel Health Information. (2020). Dressings. Available at woundsource.com/product-category/dressings; and Westby, M., et al. (2017). Dressings and topical agents for treating pressure ulcers. *Cochrane Database of Systematic Reviews.* Available at https://www.cochranelibrary.com/cdsr/doi/10.1002/14651858.CD011947.pub2/full#.

intermittently apply subatmospheric pressure to a wound's surface (Gestring, 2019). In this therapy (Gestring, 2019):

- A foam sponge is trimmed to fit and placed into the wound; it is then secured beneath an adhesive sheet.
- A hole is cut in the adhesive sheet, and one or more suction ports are introduced with placement of tubing, which empties into a disposable container.
- The portable pump is connected to the suction tubing, and continuous or intermittent suction is applied. This reduces the foam size by up to 80%.

The dressing and tubing are changed every 24 to 36 hours, and the foam is changed a minimum of three times weekly (usually every 48 to 72 hours).

NURSING SAFETY PRIORITY QSEN

Action Alert

Recognize that continuous negative-pressure wound therapy is used with caution with patients on anticoagulant therapy. Respond by consulting with members of the interprofessional team, such as the primary health care provider and wound nurse, to ascertain that anticoagulant status is appropriately monitored (Boxall et al., 2017).

Hyperbaric oxygen therapy (HBOT) is the administration of oxygen under high pressure, raising the tissue oxygen concentration. Evidence is not conclusive regarding sustained benefit in the treatment of pressure injuries (Gestring, 2019). This type of therapy is usually reserved for life- or limb-threatening wounds such as burns, necrotizing infections, brown recluse spider bites, osteomyelitis, and diabetic ulcers. The patient is enclosed in a large chamber and exposed to 100% oxygen at pressures greater than normal atmospheric pressure (Fig. 23.4). Systemic oxygen enhances the ability of white blood cells to kill bacteria and reduce swelling. Treatment usually lasts from 60 to 90 minutes per session.

Topical growth factors are normal body substances that stimulate cell movement and growth. These factors are deficient in chronic wounds, and topical application is used to stimulate wound healing. Although evidence is mixed regarding many of these agents, research shows that becaplermin gel (a platelet-derived growth factor) is a cost-effective means for treating pressure injuries (Gilligan et al., 2018).

Skin substitutes are engineered products that aid in the closure of different types of wounds. These products vary widely in design and application and are being studied with more emphasis to determine their efficacy.

Ultrasound-assisted wound therapy (USWT) uses energy produced by low-frequency (40 kHz) sound waves to cleanse and débride necrotic tissue over time, thus reducing microbial bioburden. Again, evidence is mixed regarding usefulness.

Surgical Management. Surgical management of a pressure injury includes removal of necrotic tissue and skin grafting or use of muscle flaps to close wounds that do not heal by re-epithelialization and contraction. Not all wounds are candidates for grafting. Those with poor blood flow are unlikely to have successful graft take and healing. The procedures are very similar to the surgical management of burn wounds.

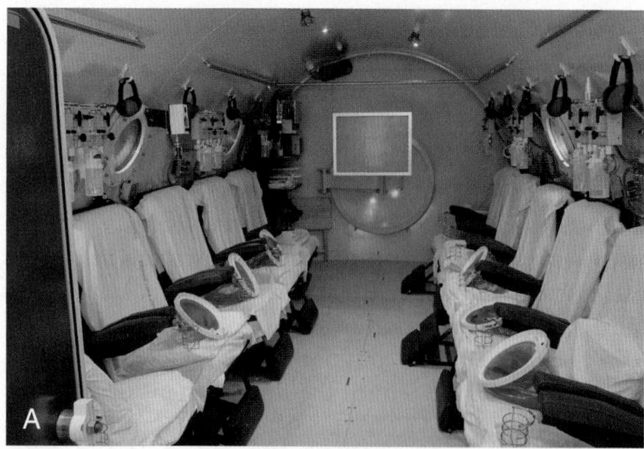

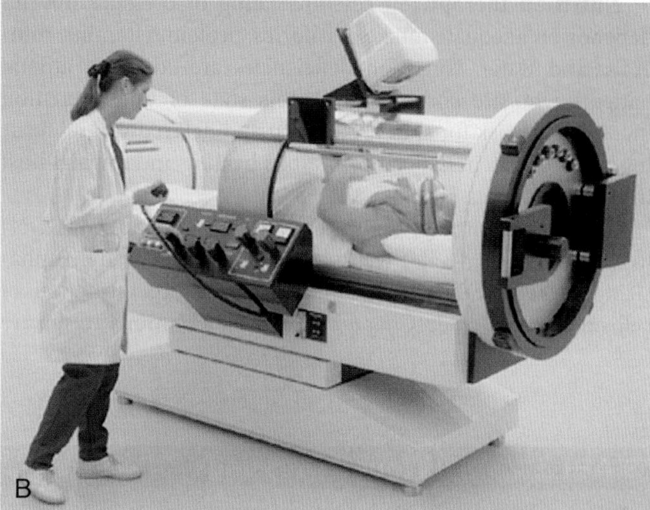

Fig. 23.4 (A and B) Hyperbaric oxygen chambers. (A from Coughlin, M.J., Mann, R.A., & Saltzman, C.L. [2017]. *Surgery of the foot and ankle* [8th ed.]. Philadelphia: Elsevier. B from Auerbach, P.S., Cushing, T.A., & Harris, S. [2017]. *Auerbach's wilderness medicine* [7th ed.]. Philadelphia: Elsevier.)

Preventing Infection

Planning: Expected Outcomes. The patient with a pressure injury is expected to remain free of localized or systemic wound infection.

Interventions. Priority nursing interventions focus on preventing wound infection and identifying it early to prevent complications. *Preventing infection* and its complications starts with monitoring the wound's progress. Routinely check for signs and symptoms of wound infection: increased ***pain,*** tenderness, and redness at the wound margins, edema, and purulent and malodorous drainage. The Best Practice for Patient Safety & Quality Care: Monitoring the Wound box outlines objectives of monitoring wounds with and without tissue loss. Report these changes to the primary health care provider, which may occur with or without signs and symptoms of bacteremia, such as fever, an elevated WBC count, and positive blood cultures:

- Sudden deterioration of the wound, with an increase in the size or depth of the lesion
- Changes in the color or texture of the granulation tissue
- Changes in the quantity, color, or odor of exudate

Use the previously described interventions to prevent the formation of new pressure injuries and to prevent early-stage injuries from progressing to deeper wounds (see the Best Practice for Patient Safety & Quality Care: Preventing Pressure Injuries box).

Maintaining a safe environment can help prevent wound infection. Because of the variety of organisms in the environment, keeping an injury totally free of bacteria is impossible. Optimal management is based on maintaining acceptably low levels of organisms through meticulous wound care and reducing contamination with pathogenic organisms that could lead to sepsis and death. *Teach all personnel to use Standard Precautions and to properly dispose of soiled dressings and linens.*

BEST PRACTICE FOR PATIENT SAFETY & QUALITY CARE (QSEN)

Monitoring the Wound

Variable	Frequency of Assessment	Rationale
Wounds Without Tissue Loss		
Examples		
Surgical incisions and clean lacerations closed primarily by sutures or staples		
Observations (Using First Postoperative Dressing Change as Baseline)		
Check for the presence or absence of increased: • Localized tenderness • Swelling of the incision line • Erythema of the incision line >1 cm on each side of wound • Localized heat	At least every 24 hr until sutures or staples are removed	To detect cellulitis (bacterial infections)[a]
Check for the presence or absence of: • Purulent drainage from any portion of the incision site • Localized fluctuance (from fluid accumulation) and tenderness beneath a *portion* of the wound when palpated	At least every 24 hr until sutures or staples are removed	To detect abscess formation related to presence of foreign body (suture material) or deeper wound infection[a]
Check for the presence or absence of: • Approximation (sealing) of wound edges with or without serosanguineous drainage • Necrosis of skin edges	At least every 24 hr until sutures or staples are removed	To detect potential for wound dehiscence
Wounds With Tissue Loss		
Examples		
Partial- or full-thickness skin loss caused by pressure necrosis, vascular disease, trauma, etc., and allowed to heal by secondary intention		
Observations		
Wound Size		
Measure wound size at greatest length and width using a disposable paper tape measure or, for asymmetric wounds by tracing the wound onto a piece of plastic film or sheeting (plastic template) Measure depth of full-thickness wounds using cotton-tipped applicator Compare all subsequent measurements against the initial measurement	Once per week	To detect increase in wound size and depth secondary to infectious process (Expect an increase in wound size after débridement of necrotic tissue in deep wounds.)
Wound Base		
Check for the presence or absence of: • Necrotic tissue (loose or adherent) • Foul odor from wound when dressing is changedNote the frequency of dressing changes or dressing reinforcements owing to drainage	At least every 24 hr	To detect the need for débridement or the response to treatment (necrotic tissue) and to detect local wound infection (frequent dressing changes and foul odor)
Wound Margins		
Check for the presence or absence of: • Erythema and swelling extending outward >1 cm from wound margins • Increased tenderness at wound margins	At least every 24 hr or at each dressing change	To detect wound infection[a]
Systemic Response		
Check for the presence or absence of elevated body temperature or WBCs or positive blood culture	Check temperature daily; if elevated, check WBCs and blood culture	To detect bacteremia

[a]The wounds of patients who are severely immunosuppressed or wounds with compromised blood supply may not exhibit a typical inflammatory response to local wound infection.

WBCs, White blood cells.

Care Coordination and Transition Management. Even if hospitalized for the pressure injury or another condition, most patients are discharged before complete wound closure is achieved. Discharge may be to the home setting or to another setting, depending on the degree of debilitation and other factors. Coordinate carefully with nurses at other agencies to promote continuity of care if the patient is discharged to a long-term care or subacute setting.

Home Care Management. Care of pressure injuries in the patient's home is similar to care in the hospital. Coordinate with the case manager for ways to obtain dressing supplies and pressure-relief devices. If the patient or caregiver cannot change dressings, arrange for home health nursing services. For the patient who is immobile, home health providers may be able to assist with around-the-clock repositioning to prevent further breakdown.

Self-Management Education. Before discharge, have the patient or caregiver demonstrate competence in removing the dressing, cleaning the wound, and applying the dressing. Coordinate with the wound care professional to determine which dressings will work in the home environment and are affordable to the patient. Explain the signs and symptoms of wound infection and remind the patient and caregiver to report these to the primary health care provider or wound care clinic.

Encourage a balanced diet, including high-protein snacks. Discuss diet preferences with the patient and consult with the registered dietitian nutritionist (RDN) as needed to design a food and supplement plan to promote wound healing.

If the patient is incontinent, emphasize the need to keep the skin clean and dry. If bowel and bladder training are not possible, discuss the use of absorbent underpads, briefs, and topical moisture barrier creams and ointments as methods to reduce skin exposure to urine and feces.

Health Care Resources. Home health services may be needed to follow wound progress after discharge. Provide a thorough hand-off report to the home health nurse, who can then use clinical judgment to determine changes in wound appearance. Collaborate with the case manager if a physical therapist or occupational therapist may benefit the patient's rehabilitation in the home setting.

◆ **Evaluation: Evaluate Outcomes.** Evaluate the care of the patient with a pressure injury on the basis of the identified priority patient problems. The expected outcomes include that the patient will:

- Experience progress toward wound healing by second intention as evidenced by granulation, epithelialization, contraction, and reduction or resolution of wound size
- Re-establish skin ***tissue integrity*** and restore skin barrier function
- Remain free from local or systemic infections

IRRITATION SKIN DISORDERS

PRURITUS

Pathophysiology Review

Skin irritation is often associated with **pruritus** (itching), a distressing and often debilitating condition caused by stimulation of itch-specific nerve fibers. Physical or chemical agents either activate nerve fibers directly or stimulate the release of chemical mediators (i.e., histamine), which then act on itch receptors. An example of a physical agent that invokes itching is scabies; an example of a chemical agent is a detergent. Other conditions that make itching worse include dry skin, perspiration, decreased or increased blood flow to an area (e.g., feet, legs), and emotional stress.

Pruritus can be localized or generalized and can occur with or without a skin rash. It is a subjective condition similar to pain, in which severity varies. Regardless of the cause, patients often report that itching is worse at night when there are fewer distractions.

❖ Interprofessional Collaborative Care

Priority nursing interventions focus on increasing patient comfort and preventing skin injury with loss of ***tissue integrity.*** Patients usually try to relieve itching by scratching or rubbing the skin. This can cause a cycle—an *"itch-scratch-itch" cycle.* Itching with skin lesions can often be relieved by treating the underlying skin disorder with topical or systemic drugs. If prescribed an antihistamine, teach the patient about possible side effects like drowsiness. Remind him or her to avoid driving, use of machinery, concurrent use of alcohol or other drugs, and making decisions that require clarity of thought.

Plan care to promote comfort and prevent disruption of skin tissue integrity from vigorous scratching. Because dry skin worsens itching, teach interventions to prevent it (see the Patient and Family Education: Preparing for Self-Management: Prevention of Dry Skin box). Encourage patients to keep the fingernails trimmed short, with rough edges filed to reduce damage from scratching and secondary infection. Wearing mittens or gloves at night can help prevent scratching during sleep. If self-care cannot be performed, teach the caregiver (for home care) and assistive personnel (AP) to trim the patient's fingernails and apply mittens or gloves. Stress the importance of not breaking the skin

PATIENT AND FAMILY EDUCATION: PREPARING FOR SELF-MANAGEMENT

Prevention of Dry Skin

- Use a room humidifier during the winter months or whenever the furnace is in use.
- Take a complete bath or shower only every other day (wash face, axillae, perineum, and any soiled areas with soap daily), using tepid water.
- Use a superfatted, nonalkaline soap instead of deodorant soap, and rinse soap thoroughly from skin.
- Colloidal oatmeal baths can be very soothing.
- If desired, add oil to the water at the end of the bath. Take care to avoid falls; oil makes the tub slippery.
- Pat skin surfaces dry; do not rub the skin.
- Avoid clothing that continuously rubs the skin, such as tight belts and pantyhose.
- Maintain a daily fluid intake of 3000 mL unless contraindicated for another medical reason.
- Do not apply rubbing alcohol, astringents, or other drying agents to the skin.
- Avoid caffeine and alcohol ingestion.
- Maintain a cool sleeping environment.

or digging into fingernail corners of patients with diabetes, and remind them never to cut the toenails. This should be done by a podiatrist.

URTICARIA

Pathophysiology Review

Urticaria (hives) is a rash of white or red edematous papules or plaques of various sizes. This problem is usually caused by exposure to allergens, which releases histamine into the skin. Blood vessel dilation and plasma protein leakage lead to formation of lesions or wheals. Common causes of urticaria include drugs, temperature extremes, foods, infection, diseases, cancer, and insect bites.

Interprofessional Collaborative Care

Management focuses on removal of the triggering substance and symptom relief. Because the skin reaction is caused by histamine release, antihistamines such as diphenhydramine are often recommended; provide safety teaching as noted in the Pruritus section. Teach the patient to avoid overexertion, alcohol consumption, and warm environments, which further dilate blood vessels and make urticaria worse.

INFLAMMATORY SKIN DISORDERS

GENERAL INFLAMMATORY DISORDERS

Pathophysiology Review

Most skin inflammations are related to allergic immune responses. The responses may be triggered by external skin exposure to allergens or internal exposure to allergens and irritants. The result is tissue destruction or skin changes induced by the immune system (see Chapter 16).

The specific cause of skin inflammation is not always known. When this is the case, the catch-all diagnosis of *nonspecific eczematous dermatitis,* or *eczema,* is usually used. See the Key Features: Common Inflammatory Skin Conditions box for symptoms of many types of inflammatory skin conditions.

Interprofessional Collaborative Care

Because all skin eruptions from inflammation appear similar, personal data are needed to identify the cause. Inflammatory skin problems differ from eczematous dermatitis in chronicity, lesion distribution, and associated signs and symptoms.

If the cause of the rash is identified, avoidance therapy is used to reverse the reaction and clear the rash. For example, if a new soap causes contact dermatitis of the hands, teach the patient to avoid that substance. Even when the cause is unclear, certain irritants may worsen the rash and increase discomfort. Additional interventions promote comfort through suppression of inflammation.

Steroid therapy with topical, intralesional, or systemic steroids may be prescribed to suppress inflammation. They are not curative agents. Because a side effect of oral corticosteroids (e.g., prednisone) is adrenal suppression, patients receiving long-term systemic therapy must taper their drug dosages rather than stop them abruptly.

Antihistamines provide some relief of itching but may not keep the patient totally comfortable. The sedative effects of these drugs may be better tolerated if most of the daily dose is taken near bedtime. Provide safety teaching as noted in the Pruritus section.

KEY FEATURES

Common Inflammatory Skin Conditions

Signs and Symptoms	Distribution
Nonspecific Eczematous Dermatitis (Eczema)	
Evolution of lesions from vesicles to weeping papules and plaques. Lichenification occurs in chronic disease. Oozing, crusting, fissuring, excoriation, or scaling may be present. Itching is common.	Anywhere on the body; localized eczema commonly involves the hands or feet
Contact Dermatitis	
Localized eczematous eruption with well-defined, geometric margins that are consistent with contact with an irritant or allergen. Usually seen in the acute form but may become chronic if exposure is repeated. Allergy to plants (e.g., poison ivy or oak) classically occurs as linear streaks of vesicles or papules.	Cosmetic/perfume allergy: head and neck Hair product allergy: scalp Shoe/rubber allergy: dorsum of feet Nickel allergy: earlobes Mouthwash/toothpaste allergy: perioral region Airborne contact allergy (e.g., paint, ragweed): generalized
Atopic Dermatitis	
Hallmark in adults is lichenification with scaling and excoriation. Extremely itchy. Face involvement is seen as dry skin with mild-to-moderate erythema, perioral pallor, and skinfolds beneath the eyes (Dennie-Morgan lines). Associated with linear markings on the palms.	Face, neck, upper chest, and antecubital and popliteal fossae
Drug Eruption	
Bright red erythematous macules and papules are found. Skin blisters in extreme cases. Lesions tend to be confluent in large areas. Moderately itchy. Fever is rare. Dehydration and hypothermia can occur with extensive involvement. Condition clears only after offending drug has been discontinued.	Generalized Involvement begins on trunk, proceeds distally (legs are the last to be involved)

NURSING SAFETY PRIORITY QSEN

Drug Alert

Polypharmacy combined with the sedating effects of H_1-antihistamines (e.g., diphenhydramine) puts older adults at increased risk for falls. Institute fall precautions, and teach patients how to remain safe in the home environment as well.

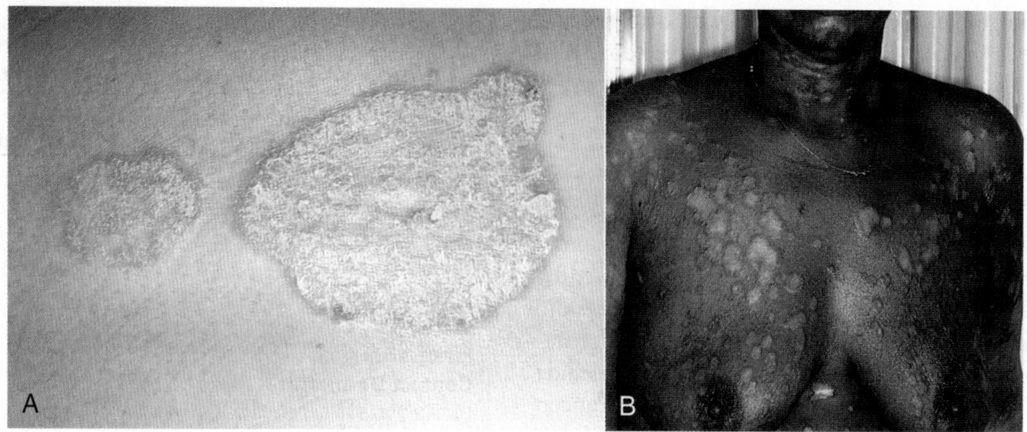

Fig. 23.5 (A) Psoriasis in a patient with white skin. (B) Psoriasis in a patient with dark skin.

Comfort measures such as cool, moist compresses and lukewarm baths with bath additives such as colloidal oatmeal have a soothing effect, decrease inflammation, and help débride crusts and scales.

PSORIASIS

Pathophysiology Review

Psoriasis is a chronic autoimmune disorder marked by exacerbations and remissions in which T-lymphocytes, dendritic cells, and cytokines are involved. In the hyperproliferative state, plaques form on the skin (Fig. 23.5). Psoriasis lesions are scaled with underlying dermal inflammation from an abnormality in the growth of epidermal cells. Normally, basal cells take about 28 days to reach the outermost layer, where they are shed. In a person with psoriasis the rate of cell division is speeded up so that cells are shed every 4 days (Feldman, 2019). Even though psoriasis cannot be cured, patients can often achieve control of symptoms with proper management.

Environmental factors can trigger outbreaks, yet these are very subjective to the individual person. Stress, skin injuries, certain medications (lithium, propranolol, indomethacin, quinidine, and antimalarials), and infection are known triggers (National Psoriasis Foundation, 2020b). Smoking, alcohol use, and obesity have been shown to exacerbate symptoms (Feldman, 2019).

Some patients with psoriasis also develop debilitating *psoriatic arthritis.* This inflammatory musculoskeletal disorder may lead to severe joint changes similar to those seen in rheumatoid arthritis.

❖ Interprofessional Collaborative Care

Care of the patient with psoriasis most often takes place in an outpatient setting. When a patient with psoriasis is hospitalized for another health problem, psoriasis therapy may continue in this setting. Members of the interprofessional team who collaborate most closely to care for the patient with psoriasis include the primary health care provider and the nurse.

◆ Assessment: Recognize Cues

History. Ask the patient about any family history of psoriasis, as there is a strong genetic connection to development of this disorder. Ask the age at onset, a description of the disease progression, and the pattern of recurrences (for the patient, as well as any affected family members). Have the patient describe the current flare-up of psoriasis, including whether the onset was gradual or sudden, where the lesions first appeared, whether there have been any changes in severity over time, and whether fever and itching are present. Explore possible precipitating factors and ask about the effectiveness of any previous interventions.

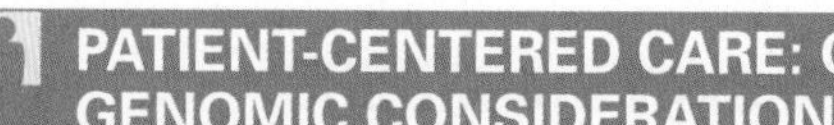

PATIENT-CENTERED CARE: GENETIC/ GENOMIC CONSIDERATIONS QSEN

Always ask about a family history when assessing the patient with psoriasis, as there is a strong genetic predisposition for this disorder (Online Mendelian Inheritance in Man [OMIM], 2018).

Physical Assessment/Signs and Symptoms. The appearance of psoriasis and its course vary among patients. During flare-ups, lesions may thicken and extend into new body areas. As psoriasis responds to treatment, lesions become thinner with less scaling.

There are five types of psoriasis:

1. Plaque psoriasis
2. Guttate psoriasis
3. Inverse psoriasis
4. Pustular psoriasis
5. Erythrodermic psoriasis

See Table 23.4 for characteristics of the various types of psoriasis (National Psoriasis Foundation, 2020a).

◆ Interventions: Take Action.

Treatment, whether topical or systemic, is chosen based on severity, comorbid conditions, efficacy of treatment, the patient's response to treatment, and whether treatment is affordable (Feldman, 2019). Because these treatments are helpful to manage, but not cure, the disorder, *nursing strategies include teaching about the disease and its treatment, and providing emotional support due to changes in body image.*

Topical Therapy. Emollients work to keep the skin soft while minimizing itching or ***pain.*** Corticosteroids provide anti-inflammatory action. These are the two most commonly used topical therapies.

TABLE 23.4 Type of Psoriasis

Type	Description
Plaque psoriasis (most common type)	Raised, red patches covered with silvery white scales (Fig. 23.5) Usually found on scalp, knees, elbows, lower back May be itchy, painful, or bleeding
Guttate psoriasis	Small, dotlike lesions Usually starts after a strep infection
Inverse psoriasis	Very red lesions in folds of the body (e.g., groin, behind knees, under arms) Smooth and shiny Most people have another type of psoriasis in addition to inverse psoriasis
Pustular psoriasis	White pustules surrounded by reddened skin Not infectious nor contagious; the pustules contain white blood cells Usually occurs on hands and feet
Erythrodermic psoriasis	Severe form of psoriasis with widespread, fiery redness over most of the body Causes severe itching and pain Skin may come off in sheets Rare; usually seen in people who also have unstable plaque psoriasis

Anthralin, a hydrocarbon similar in action to tar, can help to relieve chronic psoriasis. Teach the patient to apply this drug, which is suspended in a stiff paste, to each lesion for short periods of time as directed by the primary health care provider. It is a strong irritant and can cause chemical burns if left on lesions too long or not washed off completely after each treatment. Remind the patient to check for local tissue reaction and to avoid allowing it to come into contact with uninvolved skin.

Tar preparations applied to the skin suppress cell division and reduce inflammation. These drugs have been used historically as a primary form of treatment but are messy, cause staining on clothing, and have an unpleasant odor. Although other forms of treatment are available, some still prefer tar preparations that are available as solutions, ointments, lotions, gels, and shampoos.

Tazarotene, a topical retinoid, can be combined with topical corticosteroid therapy. As this is a teratogenic substance, teach women who are pregnant, or who plan to become pregnant, to avoid use of this drug. Teach women to use effective contraception even if pregnancy is not desired.

Other topical therapies may include calcipotriene, a synthetic form of vitamin D that regulates skin cell division. This drug can mildly irritate the skin. Calcitriol has been shown to work as well as calcipotriene, although both of these drugs are more expensive than other corticosteroids.

! NURSING SAFETY PRIORITY (QSEN)

Drug Alert

Tazarotene and other vitamin A derivatives are *teratogenic* (can cause birth defects) even when used topically. Teach sexually active women of childbearing age who are using any of these drugs to adhere to strict contraceptive measures.

Light Therapy. Ultraviolet (UV) irradiation has been shown to be beneficial in controlling psoriatic lesions. Mode of phototherapy is chosen based on availability of modality and supervision of a dermatologist. Office-based treatment with ultraviolent B (UVB) phototherapy involves therapeutic doses of UV light three times weekly; home-based units are available by prescription (Feldman, 2019).

Photochemotherapy (PUVA) can be given by administration of psoralen, a photosensitizer, taken either orally or within a bath, followed by ultraviolent A (UVA) radiation. Because of the variability of UV output from tanning beds, this modality is not often recommended for patients with psoriasis. This type of therapy is not used for patients who have a history of melanoma or other skin cancer.

Excimer lasers emit UVB light and can be used for localized lesion treatment. Whether administered in a continuous or pulsed exposure, this modality allows for better focus on the lesions and reduces exposure to the surrounding normal skin.

Teach patients to inspect the skin carefully each day for signs of overexposure. If tenderness on palpation occurs and severe erythema or blister formation develops, notify the primary health care provider before therapy is resumed.

Systemic Therapy. Oral systemic agents are often prescribed for patients with more than 5% body surface area affected by psoriasis (Feldman, 2019). Methotrexate, folic acid, and systemic retinoids (vitamin A derivatives) are examples of systemic therapy. Teach patients taking a vitamin A derivative to use strict contraceptive measures, as these drugs are teratogenic.

A number of biologic agents are also used for psoriasis, including etanercept, a tumor necrosis factor (TNF)-alpha inhibitor. Teach patients who have been prescribed etanercept to report any signs of tuberculosis or viral, fungal, or bacterial infections. Evidence shows that some latent infections have been activated by use of certain biologics, especially in patients with immune compromise associated with conditions such as diabetes, human immune deficiency virus (HIV) infection, or rheumatoid arthritis. Biologics currently approved for the treatment of psoriasis are listed in the Common Examples of Drug Therapy: Plaque Psoriasis box.

! NURSING SAFETY PRIORITY (QSEN)

Drug Alert

Instruct patients to discontinue the biologic agent and notify the primary health care provider immediately if signs and symptoms of an active infection occur.

Emotional Support. Often patients' self-esteem suffers because of the presence of skin lesions. Encourage the patient to express feelings about having an incurable skin problem that can alter appearance. Support groups for individuals with psoriasis are available in many communities. Urge patients and families to consider participating.

The use of therapeutic touch takes on an added significance for patients with psoriasis. If patients are open to physical contact, shake their hands during introductions or pat them on the shoulder gently as they leave, while you thank them for trusting you with their health care. *Do not wear gloves during these social interactions. Touch, more than any other gesture, communicates acceptance of the person and the skin problem.*

COMMON EXAMPLES OF DRUG THERAPY

Plaque Psoriasis

Drug	Nursing Implications
Adalimumab	Given by pen injection After loading dose is given as two injections, the maintenance dose is given every other week starting on day 8 after the loading dose Black box warning: serious infection risk (especially for TB, *Legionella, Listeria*); risk for malignancy (lymphoma and other malignancies)
Etanercept	Given by SureClick auto-injector Given twice weekly for 3 months Black box warning: serious infection risk (especially for TB, *Legionella, Listeria*); risk for malignancy (lymphoma and other malignancies)
Infliximab	Given IV on Weeks 0, 2, and 6 Black box warning: serious infection risk (especially for TB, *Legionella, Listeria*); risk for malignancy (lymphoma and other malignancies)
Secukinumab	Given by pen injection weekly for 4 or 5 weeks Although no black box warning, monitor for signs of infection
Ustekinumab	Given by pen injection Initial dose given, followed by a dose 4 weeks later and then every 12 weeks Although no black box warning, monitor for signs of infection

TB, Tuberculosis.

NCLEX EXAMINATION CHALLENGE 23.1

Physiological Integrity

The nurse is caring for a client who has been on biologic therapy for plaque psoriasis. Which assessment finding requires **immediate** nursing intervention?

A. Increased itching
B. Temperature of 100°F
C. Presence of new plaques on leg
D. Expression of impaired self-image

SKIN INFECTIONS

Pathophysiology Review

Skin infections can be bacterial, viral, or fungal in origin. The Key Features: Common Skin Infections box lists key characteristics of each type (McCance et al., 2019), with associated nursing implications.

Health Promotion and Maintenance. Preventing skin infection, especially bacterial and fungal infections, involves avoiding the offending organism and practicing good hygiene to remove the organism before infection can occur. *Handwashing and not sharing personal items with others are the best ways to avoid contact with these organisms, including MRSA.* The Patient and Family Education: Preparing for Self-Mangement: Preventing the Spread of MRSA box lists strategies to teach patients and family members to prevent infection spread to other body areas and to others.

NURSING SAFETY PRIORITY (QSEN)

Action Alert

Consider the possibility of bioterrorism whenever lesions consistent with cutaneous anthrax appear in patients who do not have a history of exposure to infected animals.

PATIENT AND FAMILY EDUCATION: PREPARING FOR SELF-MANAGEMENT

Preventing the Spread of MRSA

- Avoid close contact with others, including participation in contact sports, until the infection has cleared.
- Take all prescribed antibiotics exactly as prescribed for the entire time prescribed.
- Keep the infected skin area covered with clean, dry bandages.
- Change the bandage whenever drainage seeps through it.
- Place soiled bandages in a plastic bag and seal it closed before placing it in the regular trash.
- Wash your hands with soap and warm water before and after touching the infected area or handling the bandages.
- Shower (rather than bathe) daily, using an antibacterial soap.
- Wash all uninfected skin areas before washing the infected area or use a fresh washcloth to wash the uninfected areas.
- Use each washcloth only once before laundering and avoid using bath sponges or puffs.
- Sleep in a separate bed from others until the infection is cleared.
- Avoid sitting on or using upholstered furniture.
- Do not share clothing, washcloths, towels, athletic equipment, shavers or razors, or any other personal items.
- Clean surfaces that may have come into contact with your infected skin, drainage, or used bandages (e.g., bathroom counters, shower and bath stalls, toilet seats) with household disinfectant or bleach water mixed daily (1 tablespoon of liquid bleach to 1 quart of water).
- Wash all soiled clothing and linens with hot water and laundry detergent. Dry clothing either in a hot dryer or outside on a clothesline in the sun.
- Urge family members and close friends to shower daily with an antibacterial soap.
- If another person helps you change the bandages, make certain that he or she uses disposable gloves, pulls them off inside out when finished, places them with the soiled bandages in a sealed bag, and washes his or her hands thoroughly.

NURSING SAFETY PRIORITY (QSEN)

Drug Alert

Shingrix (recombinant zoster vaccine) and Zostavax (zoster vaccine live) are "shingles vaccines." Shingrix should not be given to anyone with a history of having already had this vaccine delivered in a previous dose. Zostavax should not be given to patients with severe immunosuppression, those who are taking drugs that affect the immune system, persons who are undergoing radiation or chemotherapy, or those with cancer affecting the bone marrow or lymphatic system (Centers for Disease Control and Prevention [CDC], 2018). Always collaborate with the primary health care provider before giving any vaccines to ensure that the correct one has been prescribed.

KEY FEATURES

Common Skin Infections

Signs and Symptoms	Distribution	Nursing Implications
Bacterial Infections		
Cutaneous Anthrax		
Caused by Bacillus anthracis Usually caused by contact with an infected animal (e.g., by a farm worker, veterinarian, etc.). Often resembles an insect bite, and itches, but is painless. May have only one lesion, or multiple ones. In days, the vesicle center sinks inward and begins necrosing. Surrounding tissues has significant edema. Eschar forms (Fig. 23.6B) regardless of treatment. Systemic symptoms are flulike (e.g., fever, chills, lymphadenopathy).	May be localized or systemic (Fig. 23.6A).	Oral or IV antibiotics are prescribed based on whether infection is localized or systemic. Cutaneous anthrax has been used in bioterrorism; ask questions to determine if the patient has been exposed to animals. If not, report to the appropriate authorities per agency policy.
Folliculitis		
Inflammation of the hair follicles. Can be caused by bacteria, viruses, or fungi, or can be noninfectious (e.g., trauma, or plugging of the follicle). Lesions appear as pustules and papules, with surrounding erythema. Can be caused by poor hygiene, prolonged skin moisture, occlusive clothing.	Most commonly scalp and extremities, although can occur anyplace on the body where there is hair.	Teach proper hygiene methods. Remind patient to keep skin (especially folds) clean and dry. Topical antibiotics may be prescribed.
Furuncles and Carbuncles		
Furuncles (Fig. 23.7)		
Often called "boils" Inflammation of the hair follicles. Usually associated with *Staphylococcus aureus.* Initial nodule is deep, firm, red, and painful (1-5 cm in diameter). Lesion changes in a few days of cystic nodule (cellulitis may be present).	Areas of hair-bearing skin, especially buttocks, thighs, abdomen, posterior neck regions, and axillae.	Warm compresses can be used. If abscess forms, it will need incision and drainage. Systemic antibiotics may be prescribed.
Carbuncles		
Collection of infected hair follicles. Lesion is a firm mass that is red, painful, and swollen; it drains through multiple openings. Abscess may develop. May have systemic flulike symptoms (fever, chills, malaise).	Back of neck, upper back, lateral thighs.	As above for furuncles.
Cellulitis		
Dermal and subcutaneous tissue infection. Often extends from another skin wound (e.g., ulcer, furuncle, carbuncles). Usually caused by *Staphylococcus*, community-acquired methicillin-resistant *Staphylococcus aureus* (CA-MRSA), or group B streptococci. Infected area is red, warm, swollen, and painful. Can extend to lymph nodes and blood.	Can occur anywhere, but more common on lower legs, areas of persistent lymphedema, and areas of other skin wound.	Systemic treatment with antibiotics is needed.
Methicillin-resistant* Staphylococcus aureus *(MRSA)		
Can range from mild folliculitis to extensive furuncles. Can be life threatening if a wound infection erupts or MRSA enters the bloodstream.		See the Patient and Family Education: Preparing for Self-Management: Preventing the Spread of MRSA box and Chapter 21 for more information. If this patient is hospitalized, Transmission-Based Precautions must be instituted and IV antibiotics such as vancomycin or daptomycin may be given.
Viral Infections		
Herpes Simplex		
Grouped vesicles are present on an erythematous base. Vesicles, which may evolve to pustules, rupture, weep, and crust. Lesions last 2-6 wk. Older lesions may appear as punched-out, shallow erosions with well-defined borders. Lesions are associated with itching, stinging, or ***pain.*** Secondary bacterial infection with necrosis is possible in immunocompromised patients.	Type 1 classically on the face and type 2 on the genitalia, but either may develop in any area where inoculation has occurred; recurrent infections occur repeatedly in the same skin area.	This infection is very transmissible; teach to have others avoid contact with lesions. Topical and/or oral antiviral drugs may be prescribed. Teach that ultraviolet light, skin irritations, fever, fatigue, menses, or stress may increase chance of reactivation.

KEY FEATURES—CONT'D

Signs and Symptoms	Distribution	Nursing Implications
Herpes Zoster (Varicella Zoster)		
Lesions are similar in appearance to herpes simplex and also progress with weeping and crusting (Fig. 23.8). Grouped lesions present unilaterally along a segment of skin following the pathway of a spinal or cranial nerve (dermatomal distribution). Eruption is preceded by deep ***pain*** and paresthesia. Postherpetic neuralgia is common in older adults. Secondary infection with necrosis is possible in immunocompromised patients.	Anterior or posterior trunk following involved dermatome; face, sometimes involving trigeminal nerve and eye In complicated cases, full-thickness skin necrosis has been noted.	Teach that antiviral drugs such as acyclovir, valacyclovir, or famciclovir, if prescribed, are most helpful in the first 72 hours following eruption. Vaccination is available, and is recommended for those older than 60. Teach about possible complications including Bell palsy, or eye infection if the virus is introduced to the eyes. Compresses, calamine lotion, or baking soda can be soothing.
Fungal Infections ***Tinea (Mycosis Disorders Caused by Dermatophytes)***		
Annular or serpiginous patches are present with elevated borders, scaling, and central clearing. Itching is common. Lesions may be single or multiple.	Anywhere on the body; in adults, usually seen on the foot (tinea pedis, also known as "athlete's foot").	Teach patients to keep feet clean and dry, and to avoid public showers, locker rooms, and pools where fungi live. Advise patients to avoid sharing footwear and clothing. Topical antifungal therapy may be prescribed.
Candidiasis		
Erythematous macular eruption occurs with isolated pustules or papules at the border (satellite lesions). Candidiasis is associated with burning and itching. Oral lesions (thrush) appear as creamy white plaques on an inflamed mucous membrane. Cracks or fissures at the corners of the mouth may be present. In the body, infected skin appears moist, red, and irritated; it usually burns and/or itches.	Skinfold areas: perineal and perianal region, axillae, beneath breasts, and between the fingers; under wet or occlusive dressings. Lesions possibly present on the oral or vaginal mucous membranes.	Antifungal medications may be prescribed; route is dependent on where the infection is located. Teach the patient to keep skin clean and dry. If the patient is unable to self-turn, reposition frequently to enhance airflow to the skin.

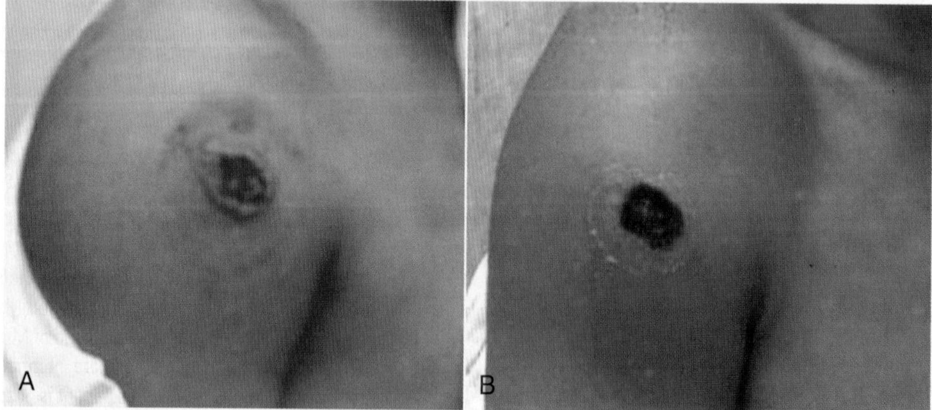

Fig. 23.6 Cutaneous anthrax. Note ulcer with vesicular ring, induration, and erythema (A). As eschar forms, induration lessens and surrounding desquamation occurs, but erythema persists (B). (From Centers for Disease Control and Prevention, Atlanta, GA. [https://www.cdc.gov/anthrax].)

❖ Interprofessional Collaborative Care

Depending on the type of infection and associated health issues, patients with minor skin infections are generally treated on an outpatient basis. For more severe infections, hospitalization for IV antibiotics may be recommended. Members of the interprofessional team who collaborate most closely to care for this patient include the primary health care provider and the nurse.

◆ Assessment: Recognize Cues

History. Concentrate on risk factors for each type of infection. If the location and appearance of lesions suggest a bacterial infection, ask about a recent history of skin trauma or recent staphylococcal or streptococcal infections. Assess living conditions, home sanitation, personal hygiene habits, and leisure or sport activities. Ask whether fever and malaise are also present.

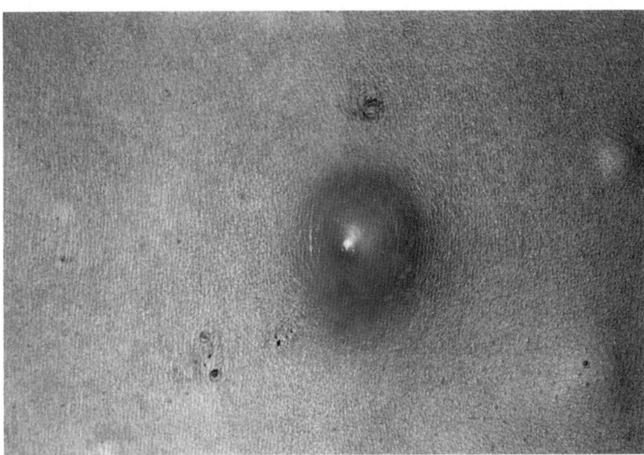

Fig. 23.7 A furuncle.

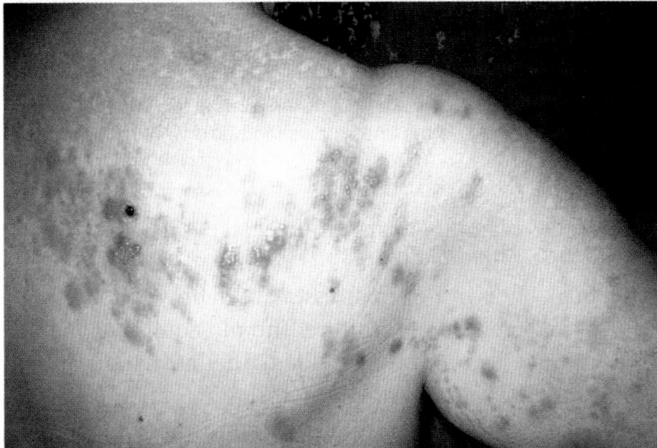

Fig. 23.8 Herpes zoster (shingles).

Lesions appearing on the lips, in the mouth, or in the genital region are more likely to be a possible viral infection. Ask about:

- A history of similar lesions in the same location
- Presence of burning, tingling, or ***pain***
- Recent stress factors that preceded the outbreak
- Recent contact with an infected person

Determine if the patient has had similar lesions before. This information often helps to differentiate viral from bacterial lesions. Ask whether the patient has had chickenpox in the past, if he or she has a history of shingles, and if the patient has received a shingles vaccination.

Physical Assessment/Signs and Symptoms. Because many skin infections are contagious, take precautions to prevent the spread of infection when performing a physical assessment. The Key Features: Common Skin Infections box lists the signs and symptoms of common skin infections.

Laboratory Assessment. When pustules are present in bacterial infections, the infecting organism may be confirmed by swab culture of the purulent material. Blood cultures may be ordered if fever and malaise are present. Various cultures and other techniques are used to identify viral and fungal infections (see Chapter 21).

◆ **Interventions: Take Action.** Most skin infections heal well with nonsurgical management and appropriate drug therapy. Priority nursing interventions focus on patient and family education to prevent infection spread to other body areas or to other people (see the Patient and Family Education: Preparing for Self-Management: Preventing the Spread of MRSA box). Meticulous skin care is needed for prevention of infection spread.

Teach all patients with skin infections to shower daily and to keep the skin clean and dry. Advise avoidance of extreme moisture, and teach ways of promoting air flow to skin through positioning and wearing nonconstrictive clothing. See the Key Features: Common Skin Infections box for specific teaching related to the type of skin infection.

PARASITIC DISORDERS

Parasitic skin disorders occur most often in patients with poor hygiene. Examine any patient who shows obvious signs of a self-care deficit for contagious parasitic infections, remembering that some parasites may carry disease (e.g., typhus).

Pediculosis

Pediculosis is a lice infestation: *pediculosis capitis* (head lice), *pediculosis corporis* (body lice), and *pediculosis pubis* (pubic, or crab, lice). Human lice are oval and 2 to 4 mm long. The female louse lays many eggs *(nits)* at the hair shaft base in hair-bearing areas.

The most common symptom of pediculosis is itching (pruritus). Excoriation from scratching also may be present. Examine the scalp for visible white flecks of the nits attached to the hair shaft near the scalp. Matting and crusting of the scalp and a foul odor indicate a probable secondary infection. Assess the body for excoriation on the trunk, abdomen, or extremities.

Pediculosis pubis causes intense itching of the vulvar or perirectal region. Pubic lice are more compact and crablike in appearance than body lice and can be contracted from infested bed linens or during sexual intercourse with an infected individual. Although these lice are usually found in the genital region, they can also infest the axillae, the eyelashes, and the chest.

The treatment of pediculosis involves chemical killing of the parasites with topical sprays, creams, and shampoos. Topical agents include permethrin cream or malathion lotion. Oral agents such as ivermectin may also be used. Areas where the patient has slept or sat (e.g., pillows, bed, chairs, sofa) will also need to be treated. Clothing and bed linens should be washed in hot water with detergent or dry cleaned. The use of a fine-tooth comb helps remove nits from hair but does not cure the infection. For any louse infestation, social contacts should be treated when possible.

! NURSING SAFETY PRIORITY QSEN

Drug Alert

Over-the-counter lindane, a topical drug, has been used in the past as a pediculocide. It is no longer recommended as the first line of treatment for pediculosis because of rare occurrences of neurologic adverse effects (including seizures and death) and widespread resistance (Goldstein & Goldstein, 2019a). As of publication, this product is currently banned in California and in certain countries (Goldstein & Goldstein, 2019a).

NCLEX EXAMINATION CHALLENGE 23.2

Physiological Integrity

When preparing to discharge a client who has a history of pediculosis, what teaching will the nurse provide? **Select all that apply.**

A. Nits can be removed with a fine-tooth comb.
B. Parasites eventually die off without treatment.
C. Wash bed linens in hot water to remove lice and eggs.
D. Lice can live on clothing items and any surface that is covered by fabric.
E. Lice can infest any place on the body with hair, including eyelashes and axillae.

Scabies

Scabies is a contagious skin infection caused by mite infestations. It is transmitted by close contact with a person or bedding that has been infested. Infestation is common among patients with poor hygiene or crowded living conditions such as in long-term care facilities.

Curved or linear ridges in the skin are characteristic of scabies (Fig. 23.9). The itching is very intense, and patients often report that it becomes unbearable at night. Scabies can present all over the body, although the back and head are usually not affected (Goldstein & Goldstein, 2019b).

The visible, horizontal white skin ridges are formed by burrowing of the mite into the outer skin layers. In classic scabies, the patient usually has 10 to 15 mites present in an initial episode; in crusted scabies, millions of mites can infest the body (Goldstein & Goldstein, 2019b).

Examine the skin on the sides and in the webs of the fingers, and on the inner aspects of the wrists, where these ridges are most common. A hypersensitivity reaction to the mite results in excoriated erythematous papules; pustules; and crusted lesions on the elbows, nipples, lower abdomen, buttocks, and thighs and in the axillary folds. Males can have lesions on the penis.

Infestation is confirmed by taking a scraping of a lesion and examining it under the microscope for mites and eggs. Close contacts also should be examined for possible infestation. Use strict Contact Precautions while caring for the patient with scabies.

Treatment involves the use of scabicides, such as topical permethrin, or oral or topical ivermectin (Goldstein & Goldstein, 2018). Patients with crusted scabies may receive topical and oral treatment together. Laundering clothes and personal items with hot water and detergent will eliminate the mites in these items.

Bedbugs

A common parasite is the bedbug, *Cimex lectularius* and *Cimex hemipterus*. Infestations are increasingly common as a result of travel and resistance to pesticides. Teach patients preventative measures such as to (Elston & Kells, 2017):

- Examine hotel rooms and sleeping quarters, especially in crevices of box springs
- Place luggage on a rack away from the bed when traveling
- Place used or worn clothing into a sealed plastic bag when traveling

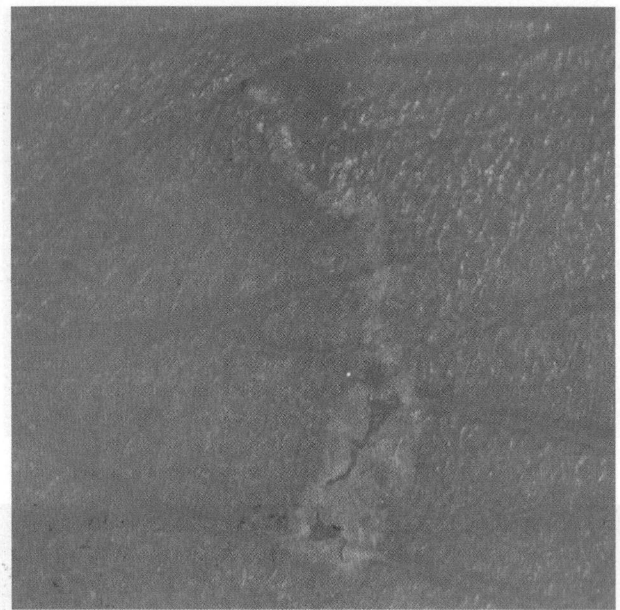

Fig. 23.9 Scabies. Note the lines indicating burrowing of the organism under the skin.

- Carefully examine items from garage sales and resalers before bringing them home

Bedbugs often live in mattresses and fabric upholstery and in cracks and crevices of furniture. They do not live on humans; however, they feed on human blood. The bite causes an itchy discomfort. The most common mode of infestation is carrying the bug home from an infested environment such as a hotel room. This problem is not related to socioeconomic level or to a lack of cleanliness.

The adult bedbug is about the size, shape, and color of an apple seed. After feeding, it may double in size and have a red or black color. The insect bites a human host (often at night) and feeds for 5 to 10 minutes, although the host usually does not notice this process. The bite area resembles a mosquito or flea bite of about 2 to 5 mm, with a reddened, raised bite mark surrounded by a wheal that often itches. Secondary infections such as cellulitis can occur.

Usually, bedbug bites spontaneously resolve. Topical corticosteroids and/or oral antihistamines may be recommended to manage pruritus. If present, secondary infections are treated with antibiotics.

Eradicating the infestation and preventing re-infestations require considerable effort and can be frustrating. Often the home environment needs the extensive eradication efforts of a licensed professional pest-control company with experience in the management of bedbugs (Elston & Kells, 2017).

SKIN TRAUMA

Pathophysiology Review

Skin trauma can vary from an aseptic surgical incision to a grossly infected, draining pressure injury with deep-tissue destruction. Injury to the skin starts a series of actions to repair the skin and restore ***tissue integrity*** to a protective barrier.

TABLE 23.5 Normal Wound Healing

Inflammatory Phase
- Begins at the time of injury or cell death and lasts 3 to 5 days.
- Immediate responses are vasoconstriction and clot formation.
- After 10 minutes, vasodilation occurs with increased capillary permeability and leakage of plasma (and plasma proteins) into the surrounding tissue.
- White blood cells (especially macrophages) migrate into the wound.
- Signs and symptoms of local edema, ***pain***, erythema, and warmth are present.

Proliferative Phase
- Begins about the fourth day after injury and lasts 2 to 4 weeks.
- Fibrin strands form a scaffold or framework.
- Mitotic fibroblast cells migrate into the wound, attach to the framework, divide, and stimulate the secretion of collagen.
- Collagen, together with ground substance, builds tough and inflexible scar tissue.
- Capillaries in areas surrounding the wound form "buds" that grow into new blood vessels.
- Capillary buds and collagen deposits form the "granulation" tissue in the wound, and the wound contracts.
- Epithelial cells grow over the granulation tissue bed.

Maturation Phase
- Begins as early as 3 weeks after injury and may continue for a year or longer.
- Collagen is reorganized to provide greater tensile strength.
- Scar tissue gradually becomes thinner and paler in color.
- The mature scar is firm and inelastic when palpated.

Phases of Wound Healing. Wound healing occurs in three phases: inflammatory phase, proliferative phase, and maturation phase. Table 23.5 lists the key events for each stage of normal wound healing. The length of each phase depends on the type of injury and degree of loss of ***tissue integrity,*** the patient's overall health, and whether the wound is healing by first, second, or third intention (Fig. 23.10).

A wound without tissue loss, such as a clean laceration or a surgical incision, can be closed with sutures, staples, or adhesives. The wound edges are brought together with the skin layers lined up in correct anatomic position (**approximated**) and held in place until healing is complete. This type of wound represents healing by **first intention**, in which the closed wound eliminates dead space and shortens the phases of tissue repair. Inflammation resolves quickly, and connective tissue repair is minimal, resulting in less remodeling and a thin scar. Fig. 23.11 shows the appearance of a normally healing surgical wound over time.

Deeper-tissue injuries with greater loss of ***tissue integrity,*** such as a chronic pressure injury or venous ulcer, result in a cavity that requires gradual filling in of the dead space with connective tissue. This represents healing by **second intention** and prolongs the repair process.

Wounds at high risk for infection, such as surgical incisions into a nonsterile body cavity or contaminated traumatic wounds, may be intentionally left open for several days. After **debris** (dead tissues) and exudate have been removed by débridement, and inflammation has subsided, the wound is closed by first intention. This type of healing represents delayed primary closure (**third intention**) and results in a scar similar to that found in wounds that heal by first intention. Healing can be impaired by many factors (Table 23.6).

PATIENT-CENTERED CARE: OLDER ADULT CONSIDERATIONS QSEN

Any wound in any patient—especially an older adult—with undernutrition, incontinence, or immobility has the potential to become a chronic wound. Although prevention strategies provide the best outcome, aggressive intervention to preserve ***tissue integrity*** should be started as soon as a problem is discovered in an older adult (Touhy & Jett, 2020).

Mechanisms of Wound Healing. When skin injury occurs, the body restores ***tissue integrity*** through three processes: re-epithelialization, granulation, and wound contraction. The depth of injury and extent of tissue integrity loss determine to what degree each process contributes to wound healing.

Partial-Thickness Wounds. Partial-thickness wounds are superficial with minimal loss of ***tissue integrity*** from damage to the epidermis and upper dermal layers. These wounds heal by **re-epithelialization**, the production of new skin cells by undamaged epidermal cells in the basal layer of the dermis, which also lines the hair follicles and sweat glands (Fig. 23.12). Injury is followed immediately by local inflammation that causes the formation of a fibrin clot and releases growth factors that stimulate epidermal cell division (mitosis). New skin cells move into open spaces on the wound surface where the fibrin clot acts as a frame to guide cell movement. Regrowth across the open area (**resurfacing**) is only one cell layer thick at first. As healing continues, the cell layer thickens, stratifies (forms layers), and produces keratin to resemble normal skin.

In a healthy adult, healing of a partial-thickness wound takes about 5 to 7 days. This process is more rapid in skin that is hydrated, is well oxygenated, and has few microorganisms.

Full-Thickness Wounds. In deep partial-thickness wounds and full-thickness wounds, loss of tissue integrity and damage extend into the lower layers of the dermis and subcutaneous tissue. As a result, most of the epithelial cells at the base of the wound are destroyed, and the wound cannot heal by re-epithelialization alone. Removal of the damaged tissue results in a defect that must be filled with scar tissue (**granulation**) for healing to occur. During the second phase of healing, new blood vessels form at the base of the wound, and fibroblast cells begin moving into the wound space. These cells deposit new collagen to replace the lost tissue.

Fibroblasts also begin to pull the wound edges inward along the path of least resistance (**contraction**) (see Fig. 23.12). This causes the wound to decrease in size at a uniform rate. Complete wound closure by contraction depends on the mobility of the surrounding skin as tension is applied to it. If tension in the surrounding skin exceeds the force of wound contraction,

The process of wound healing

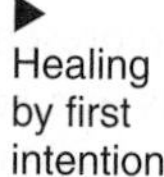

Healing by first intention

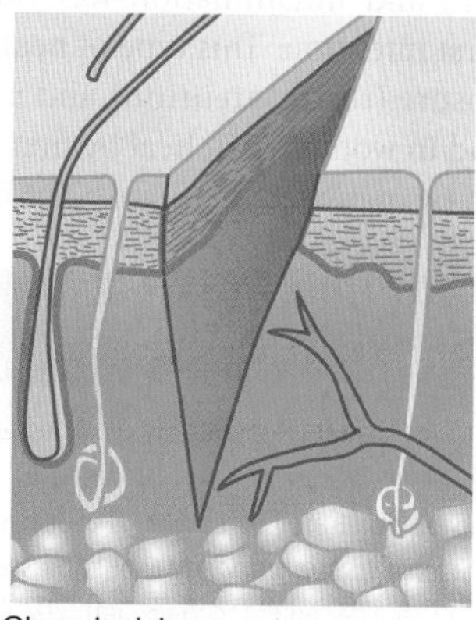

Clean incision

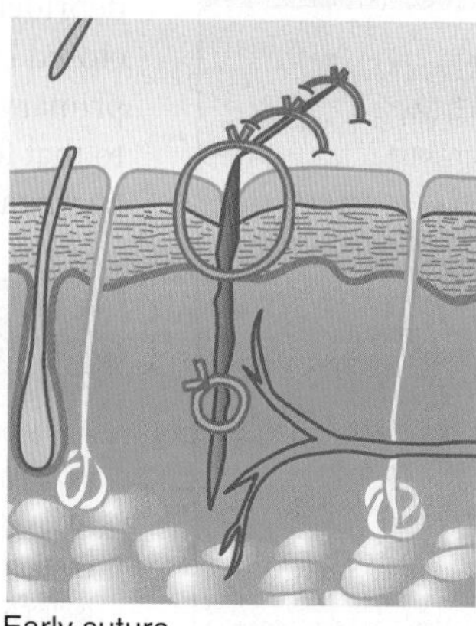

Early suture

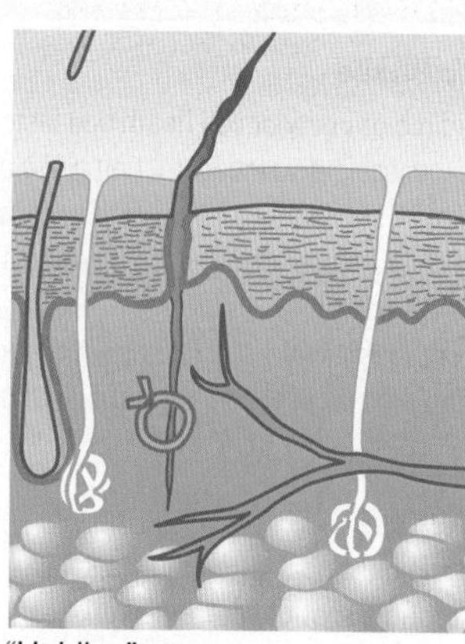

"Hairline" scar

An aseptically made wound with minimal tissue destruction and minimal tissue reaction begins to heal as the edges are approximated by close sutures or staples. No open areas or dead spaces are left to serve as potential sites of infection.

Healing by second intention (granulation) and contraction

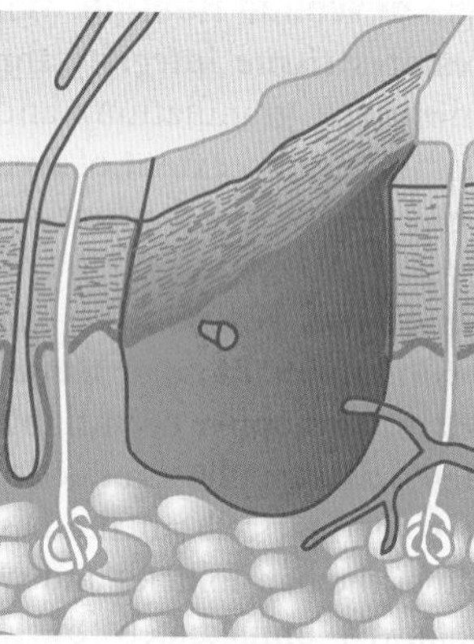

Gaping, irregular wound

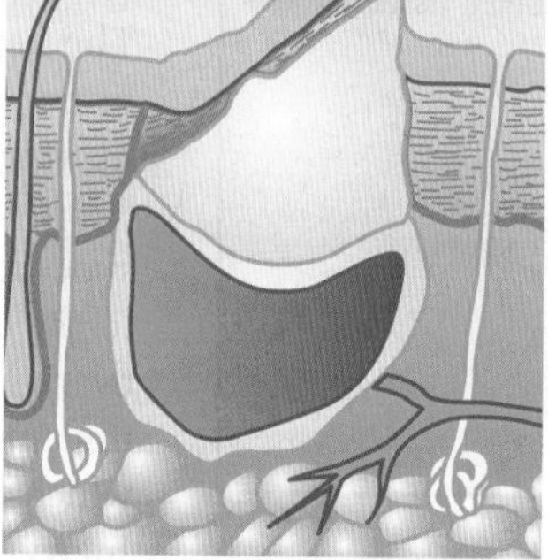

Granulation and contraction

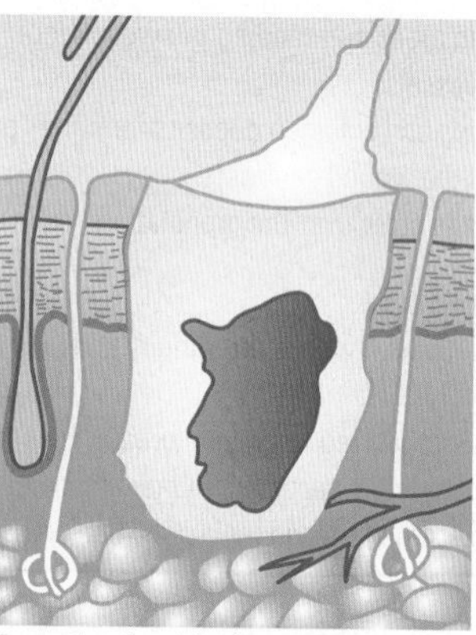

Growth of epithelium over scar

An infected or chronic wound or one with tissue damage so extensive that the edges cannot be smoothly approximated is usually left open and allowed to heal from the inside out. The nurse periodically cleans and assesses the wound for healthy tissue production. Scar tissue is extensive, and healing is prolonged.

Healing by third intention (delayed closure)

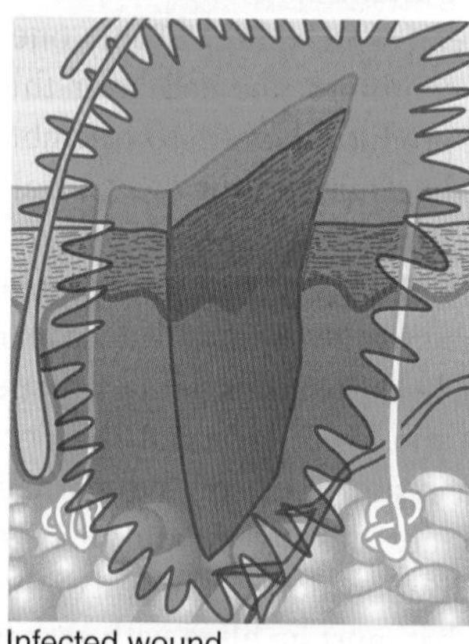

Infected wound

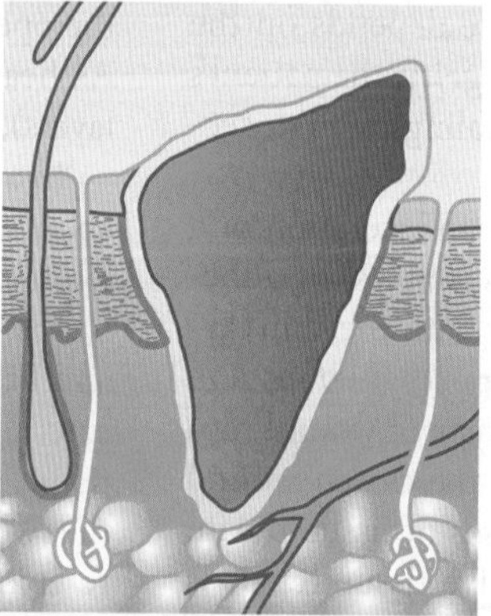

Granulation

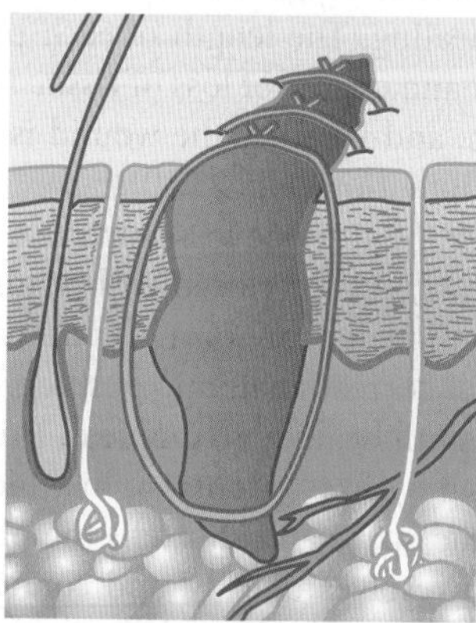

Closure with wide scar

A potentially infected surgical wound may be left open for several days. If no clinical signs of infection occur, the wound is then closed surgically.

Fig. 23.10 The process of wound healing.

healing will be delayed until undamaged epidermal cells at the wound edges can bridge the defect. The bridging of epithelial cells across a large area of granulation tissue results in an unstable barrier rather than near-normal skin. A venous leg ulcer is one example of a skin defect that heals poorly by contraction. Re-epithelialization of these chronic wounds often results in a thin epidermal barrier that is easily reinjured.

The natural healing processes of re-epithelialization, granulation, and contraction can slow and even stop in the presence of chronic infection, unrelieved pressure, or mechanical obstacles.

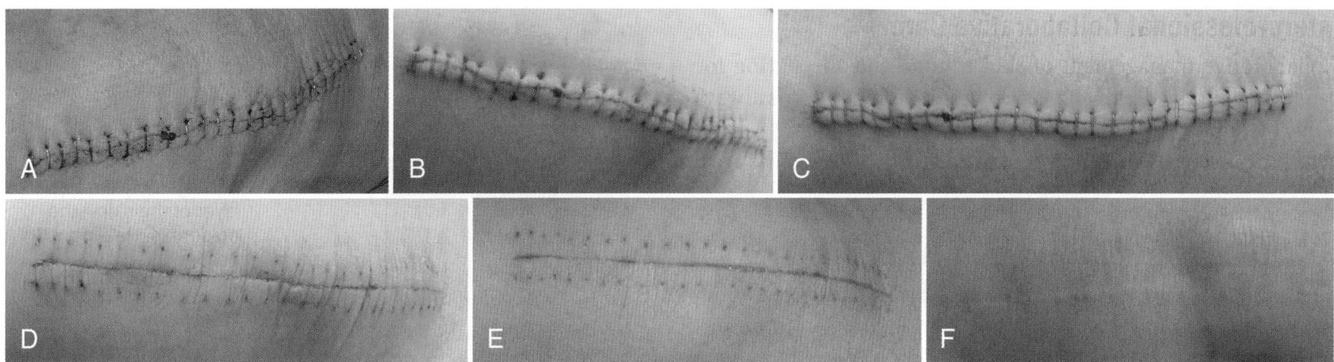

Fig. 23.11 Appearance of a normally healing surgical wound over time.

TABLE 23.6 Causes of Impaired Wound Healing

Cause	Mechanism
Altered Inflammatory Response	
Local	
Arteriosclerosis Crush injuries Diabetes Irradiated tissue Lymphedema Primary closure under tension Thrombosis Vasculitis Venous insufficiency Vasoconstriction (pharmacologic)	Reduced local tissue circulation, resulting in ischemia, impaired leukocytic response to wounding, and increased probability of wound infection
Systemic	
Leukemia Prolonged administration of high-dose corticosteroids or aspirin	Systemic inhibition of leukocytic response, resulting in impaired host resistance to infection
Impaired Cellular Proliferation	
Local	
Biofilm formation Foreign body Necrotic tissue Repeated injury or irritation Wound desiccation or maceration Wound infection Wound movement (e.g., across a joint)	Prolonged inflammatory response, which can result in low tissue oxygen tension and further tissue destruction
Systemic	
Aging Chronic stress Cirrhosis Coagulation disorders Cytotoxic drugs Hypothermia (prolonged) Nutrition deficiencies Oxygenation impairment Uremia	Impaired cellular proliferation and collagen synthesis Decreased wound contraction

For example, dead tissue not only supports bacterial growth but also obstructs collagen deposition and wound contraction. Once dead tissue is removed, the larger majority of chronic wounds remain colonized with communities of bacteria that grow together in an extracellular matrix on the wound surface in the form of a biofilm. Stress-response mediators and other factors alter the cutaneous microbiome, leading to chronic inflammation and allowing biofilm bacteria to become more virulent and resistant to antimicrobials (Holmes et al., 2015). Thus, thorough wound cleansing and débridement are essential for healing. In the case of chronic wounds, healing may stop spontaneously without an obvious cause. In addition, infection in chronic wounds may not show the expected signs or symptoms. Often the only sign is an increase in wound size or failure of the wound to decrease in size. Nonhealing chronic wounds that remain open for extended periods are of particular concern. Although rare, these wounds are at higher risk for evolving into an aggressive malignancy (Marjolin ulcer) (Shah & Crane, 2020).

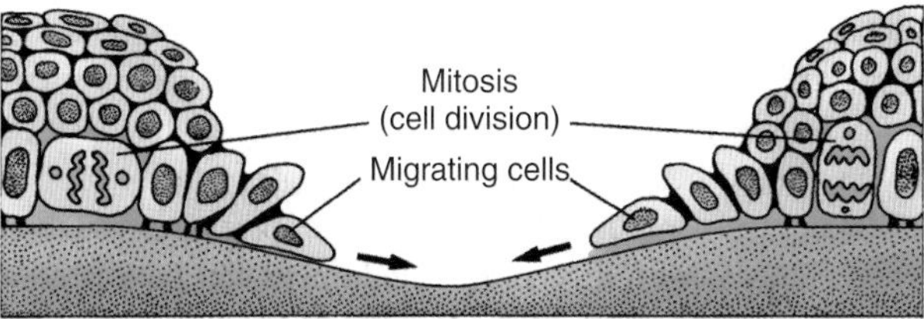

Skin cells at the edge of the wound begin multiplying and migrate toward the center of the wound.

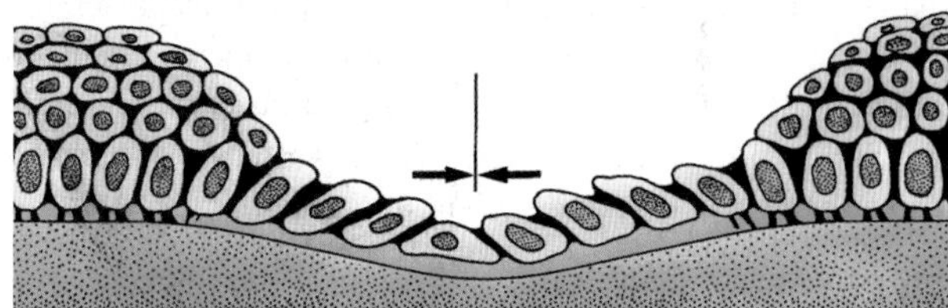

Once advancing epidermal cells from the opposite sides of the wound meet, migration halts.

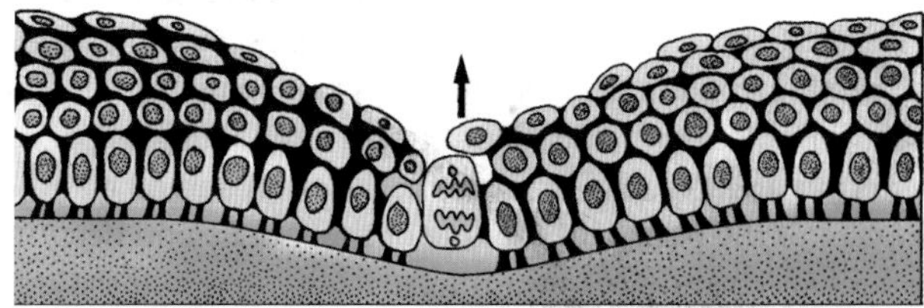

Epithelial cells continue to divide until the thickness of the new skin layer approaches normal.

Fig. 23.12 Re-epithelialization and wound contraction. (Modified from Swaim, S.F. [1980]. *Surgery of traumatized skin.* Philadelphia: Saunders.)

❖ Interprofessional Collaborative Care

Collaborative management of skin trauma and the setting for care vary with the depth and type of injury. Interventions always focus on supporting a healing environment, enhancing wound healing, preventing infection, and restoring function to the area.

BURNS

Burns range in severity from minor sunburns to life-threatening trauma. ***Tissue integrity*** is lost, and the function of numerous body systems can be changed when the skin is injured.

The extent of injury is related to age, general health, size and depth of burn, and the specific body area injured. Even after healing, the burn injury may cause late complications such as contracture formation and scarring. Priorities of care are the prevention of infection and closure of the burn wound. A lack of or delay in wound healing is a key factor for all systemic problems and a major cause of disability and death among patients who are burned. Patients with less complicated burns can be treated and released, whereas individuals with severe burns may need comprehensive care for weeks to months just in order to survive.

Nurses function as vital members of the interprofessional team composed of health care providers, nurses, registered dietitian nutritionists, social workers, counselors, therapists, and religious and spiritual leaders (if requested by the patient) to provide the best care and patient outcomes.

Skin Changes

Anatomic Changes. The skin is the largest organ of the body (see Chapter 22). The epidermis does not have blood vessels. However, it can regrow after a burn injury because the epidermal cells surrounding sweat and oil glands and hair follicles extend into dermal tissue. Skin can regrow as long as parts of the dermis are present. For example, the sweat and oil glands in the palm of the hand and the sole of the foot extend deep into the dermis. This allows for healing of deep burns in these areas. When the entire dermal layer is burned, all cells and dermal appendages are destroyed, and the skin can no longer restore itself. The subcutaneous tissue lies below the dermis and is separated from the dermis by the basement membrane, a thin, noncellular protein surface. Bone, tendon, and muscles maybe exposed if burns are deep. See Fig. 23.13 for tissues involved in burns of various depths.

Functional Changes. The skin has many functions when ***tissue integrity*** is intact. It is a protective barrier against injury and microbial invasion. It helps to maintain normal body temperature, and activates vitamin D when exposed to sun. It maintains the delicate ***fluid and electrolyte balance*** essential for life. Sensory perception allows the individual to feel pain, pressure, and touch; when burned, nerve endings can be exposed or destroyed. Burns break this protective layer barrier, greatly increasing the risk for infection and dysfunction.

Psychosocial Changes. Self-concept—how people think about, evaluate, or perceive themselves—is partly determined by body image. A patient who sustains a major burn often develops reduced self-concept and other psychosocial concerns related to changes in appearance.

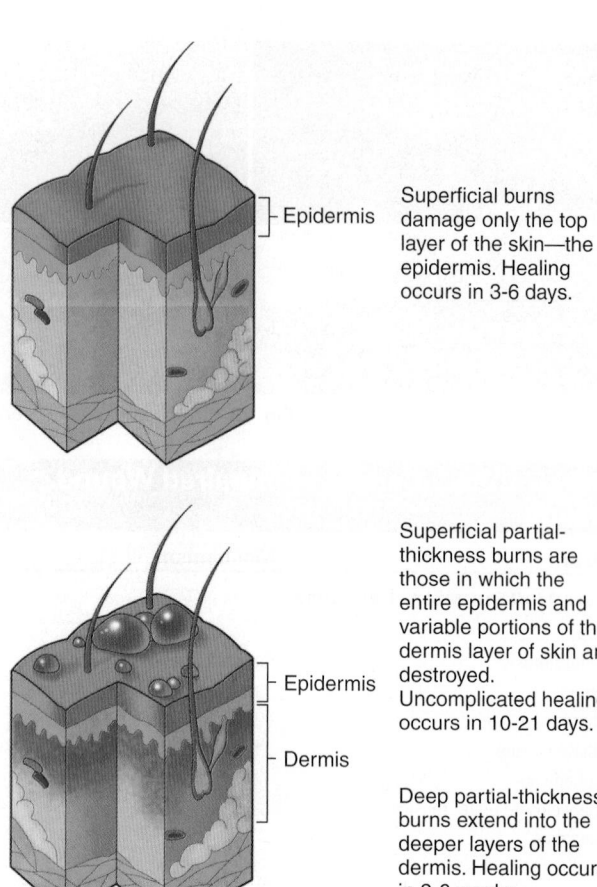

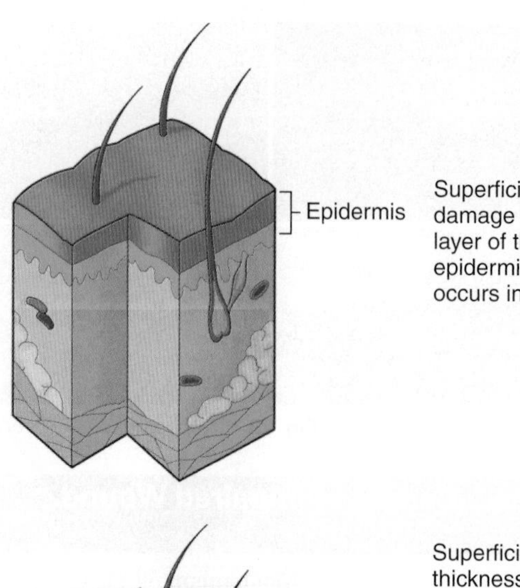

Superficial burns damage only the top layer of the skin—the epidermis. Healing occurs in 3-6 days.

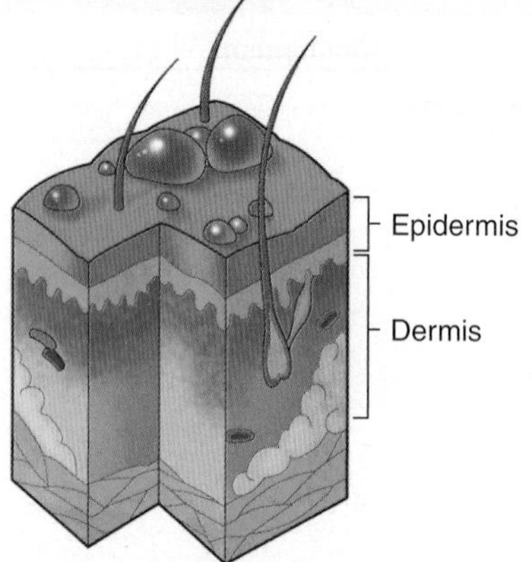

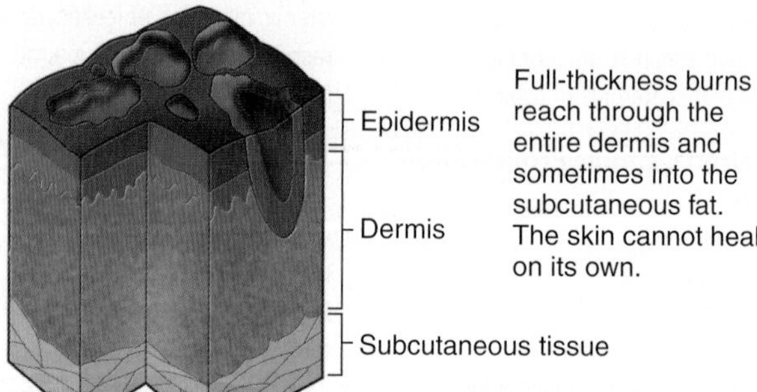

Fig. 23.13 Tissues involved in burns of various depths.

Extent of Burn Injury

The severity of a burn is determined by how much of the body surface area is involved. The quickest method for calculating the size of a burn injury in adult patients whose weights are in normal proportion to their heights is the *rule of nines* (Fig. 23.14). With this method, the body is divided into areas that are multiples of 9%. It is useful at the site of injury. More accurate evaluations using other methods are made in a burn unit.

Burn Classification

Burns can be classified by depth of destruction. The amount of ***tissue integrity*** loss is related to the agent causing the burn, the temperature of the heat source, and how long the skin is exposed to it. Two primary systems of classification exist: (1) degree of burn (first, second, third, and fourth degree), and (2) degree of thickness (superficial or deep, with thickness designations). Table 23.7 demonstrates various types of burns. See Figs. 23.15, 23.16, and 23.17 for appearances of various burn injuries classified by degree of thickness.

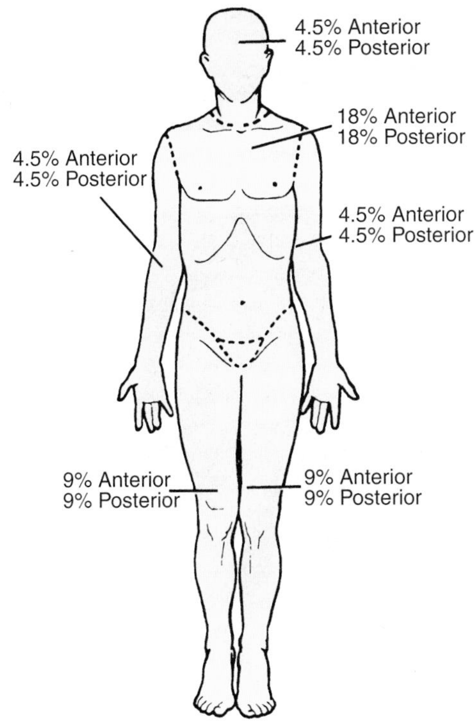

Fig. 23.14 Rule of nines for estimating burn percentage.

Differences in skin thickness in various parts of the body also affect burn depth. In areas where the skin is thin (e.g., eyelids, ears, nose, genitalia, tops of the hands and feet, fingers, and toes), a short exposure to high temperatures causes a deep burn injury. Older adults have thinner skin, which increases their risk for greater injury, even at lower temperatures and with exposure of a shorter duration.

Burns can be also classified as minor, moderate, or major, depending on the depth, extent, and location of injury (Table 23.8). Criteria for referral to a burn center are included in Table 23.8.

Patients with major third-degree or fourth-degree (full-thickness) burns experience tissue destruction that leads to local and systemic problems affecting ***fluid and electrolyte balance*** and changes in metabolic, endocrine, respiratory, cardiac, hematologic, and immune functioning.

These patients need very specialized care, often in an intensive care or a burn center setting, due to the extreme changes in body systems. Care for significant and/or severe burns is found in critical care textbooks. This textbook focuses on care for patients with *uncomplicated* burns that can usually be treated on an ambulatory basis.

Pathophysiology Review

Etiology. Burn injuries are chemical, electrical, radiation, smoke-related, or thermal (heat-related) in nature. The cause of the injury affects both the prognosis and the treatment. *Chemical burns* can occur in homes, in manufacturing industries, or as the result of assault. The severity of the injury depends on the duration of contact, the concentration of the chemical, the amount of tissue exposed, and the chemical's action.

True *electrical injury* occurs when an electrical current enters the body (Fig. 23.18). Tissue injury occurs when electrical energy

TABLE 23.7 Classification of Burn Depth

	Damage	Appearance	Edema	Blistering	Pain	Eschar	Method of Healing	Healing Time
Superficial								
Superficial first-degree burns	Above basal layer of epidermis	Dry Pink to red	No	No	Yes	No	Injured epidermis peels away; reveals new epidermis	About 1 wk
Superficial second-degree burns (superficial partial-thickness)	Into dermis	Moist Red Blanching Blistering	Mild to moderate	Yes	Yes (much)	No	Re-epithelialization from skin adnexa	About 2 wk
Deep								
Deep second-degree burns (deep partial-thickness)	Deeper into dermis	Less moist Less blanching Less painful	Moderate	Rare	Some	Yes, soft and dry	Scar deposition, contraction, limited re-epithelialization; may need grafting	2-6 wk
Third-degree burns (full-thickness)	Entire thickness of skin destroyed, into fat	Any color (black, red, yellow, brown, white) Dry	Severe	No	No	Yes, hard and inelastic	Contraction and scar deposition; requires grafting	Weeks to months
Fourth-degree burns	Damage extends into muscle, tendon, bone	Black	Severe	No	No	Yes	Need specialized care; grafting does not work	Weeks to months, if at all

Data from Rice, P., & Orgill, D. (2019). Assessment and classification of burn injury. In Jeschke, M. (Ed.). Available at www.uptodate.com; and U.S. Department of Health and Human Services. (2019). Burn triage and treatment. Available at https://chemm.nlm.nih.gov/burns.htm.

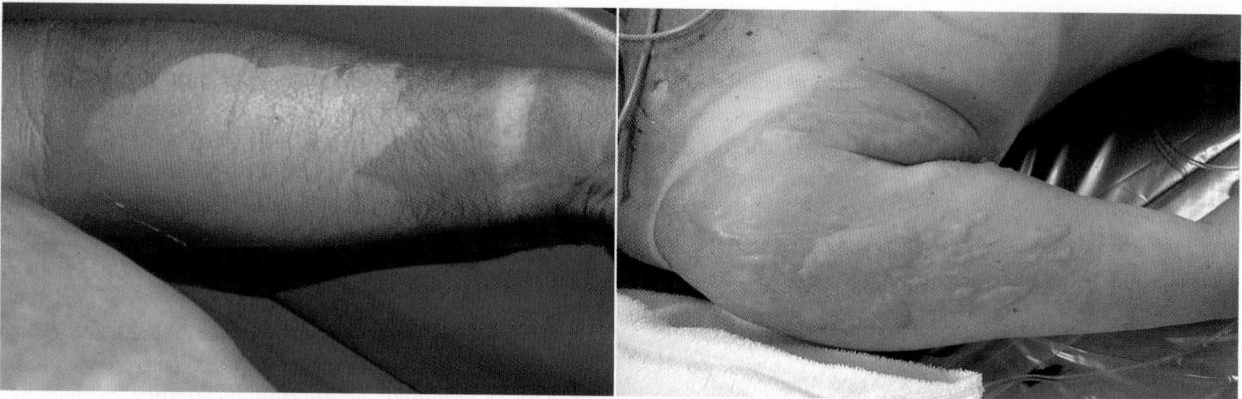

Fig. 23.15 Typical appearance of a superficial partial-thickness burn injury.

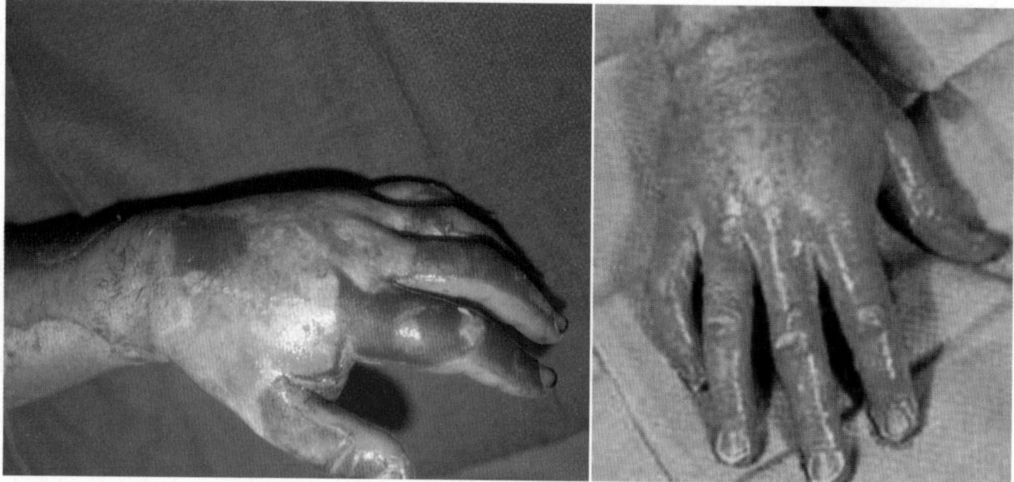

Fig. 23.16 Typical appearance of a deep partial-thickness burn injury.

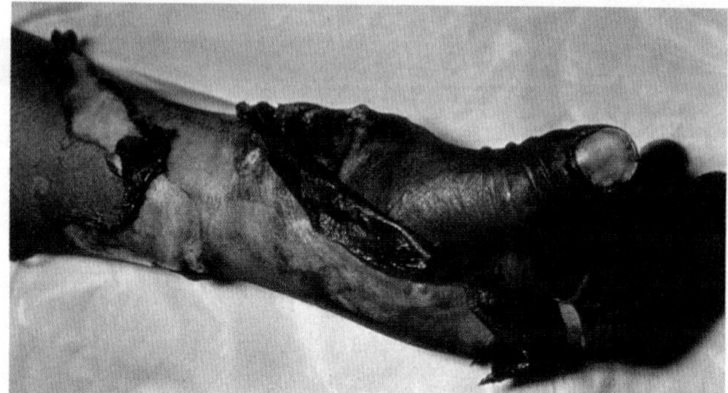

Fig. 23.17 Typical appearance of a full-thickness burn injury.

converts to heat energy as it travels through the body. These injuries are described as having an "iceberg effect" because the surface injuries may look small, but the associated internal injuries can be significant. Once the current penetrates the skin, causing the entry wound, it flows through the body and damages tissues until it leaves the body at the exit wound (Fig. 23.19). The extent of injury depends on the type of current, the pathway of flow, the local tissue resistance, and the duration of contact. The longer the electricity is in contact with the body, the greater the damage. The duration of contact is increased by tetanic contractions of the strong flexor muscles in the forearm, which can prevent the person from releasing the electrical source.

Radiation burns occur with prolonged exposure to the sun or to sources of such as x-rays or therapeutic radiation treatment. Individuals who work in the nuclear industry are also at risk for radiation burns associated with cancer due to exposure to ionizing radiation (Rice & Orgill, 2019).

Smoke-related burn injuries can occur on inhalation. Orofacial burns can cause edema that impairs breathing. *Even if you believe the patient has experienced only a minor burn, it is critical to assess the mouth, throat, and nose for signs of soot.* Listen for coughing, shortness of breath, or hoarseness of the voice, which may indicate smoke inhalation.

Thermal burns are caused by contact with flames (dry heat burns), hot liquids (moist heat [scald] burns), or hot objects or substances (contact burns). *Dry heat injuries* are caused by open flame and explosions. Explosions usually result in flash burns because they produce a brief exposure to very high temperatures. *Moist heat (scald) injuries* are caused by contact with hot liquids or steam and are common among older adults. Hot liquid spills usually burn the chest or arms. Immersion scald injuries usually involve the legs. Thermal burns to the respiratory tract are usually limited to the upper airway above the glottis (nasopharynx, oropharynx, and larynx).

Contact burns occur from hot metal, tar, or grease, often leading to a full-thickness injury. Hot metal injuries occur when a body part contacts a hot surface, such as a space heater or

TABLE 23.8 Mild, Moderate, and Major Burn Injuries and Burn Center Referral Criteria

Characteristics	Comments
Minor Burns	
Partial-thickness burns less than 10% TBSA Full-thickness burns less than 2% TBSA No burns of eyes, ears, face, hands, feet, or perineum No electrical burns No inhalation injury No complicated additional injury Patient is younger than 60 years and has no chronic cardiac, pulmonary, or endocrine disorder	Patients in this category should receive emergency care at the scene and be taken to a clinic or emergency department for evaluation. These patients are treated with outpatient management.
Moderate Burns	
Partial-thickness burns less than 10% TBSA Full-thickness burns 2%-10% TBSA No burns of eyes, ears, face, hands, feet, or perineum No electrical burns No inhalation injury No complicated additional injury Patient is younger than 60 years and has no chronic cardiac, pulmonary, or endocrine disorder	Patients should receive emergency care at the scene and be transferred to either a hospital or a designated burn center.
Major Burns	
Partial thickness burns greater than 10% TBSA Burns that involve the face, hands, feet, genitalia, perineum, or major joints Third-degree burns in any age-group Electrical burns, including lightning injury Chemical burns Inhalation injury Burn injury in patients with preexisting medical disorders that could complicate management, prolong recovery, or affect mortality Any patient with burns and concomitant trauma (such as fractures) in which the burn injury poses the greatest risk of morbidity or mortality; in such cases, if the trauma poses the greater immediate risk, the patient may be initially stabilized in a trauma center before being transferred to a burn unit; physician judgment will be necessary in such situations and should be in concert with the regional medical control plan and triage protocols Burned children in hospitals without qualified personnel or equipment for the care of children Burn injury in patients who will require special social, emotional, or rehabilitative intervention	Patients who meet *any one* of the criteria within this list should receive emergency care at the nearest emergency department and then be transferred to a designated burn center once stable.

TBSA, Total body surface area.
Data from American Burn Association. (2006). *Burn Center Referral Criteria.* Available at http://ameriburn.org/wp-content/uploads/2017/05/burncenterreferralcriteria.pdf.

iron. They also occur in industrial settings from molten metals. Tar and asphalt temperatures usually are greater than 400°F (204.4°C), and deep injuries occur within seconds. Hot grease injuries from cooking are usually deep because of the high temperatures.

Acids and alkalines are the most common chemical substances that can inflict burns. Acids are found in bathroom cleaners, rust removers, pool chemicals, and industrial drain cleaners. Damaged ***tissue integrity*** is caused by coagulating cells and skin proteins, which can limit the depth of tissue damage. Injury is related to the acid's concentration. Alkalines found in oven cleaners, fertilizers, drain cleaners, and heavy industrial cleaners damage the tissues by causing the skin and its proteins to liquefy. This allows for deeper injury below the skin including damage to tissue and muscle. Some chemicals cause a systemic effect that can damage internal organs. Decontamination is the focus for prehospital emergency responders. Contaminated clothing is removed and chemicals in powder form are brushed off. Then the burn is cautiously irrigated with large amounts of water.

Incidence and Prevalence. Burns continue to be a leading cause of unintentional death and injury worldwide. Lifetime odds of dying from exposure to fire, flames, or smoke are 1 in 1498 (National Safety Council, 2017). Males are affected more than females, and most injuries treated have occurred in the home or workplace (National Center for Injury Prevention and Control, 2017).

Health Promotion and Maintenance. Nurses play an important role in teaching strategies to prevent burn injuries. Instruct people to assess water temperature before bathing or showering. Hot water heaters should be set below 120°F (49°C). Stress the importance of never adding a flammable substance (e.g., gasoline, kerosene, alcohol, lighter fluid, charcoal starter) to an open flame. Suggest the use of sunscreen agents and protective clothing to avoid sunburn.

Teach people to reduce the risk for house fires by never smoking in bed and avoiding smoking when drinking alcohol or taking drugs that induce sleep. Keep matches and lighters out of the reach of children or people who are cognitively impaired.

When space heaters are used, stress the importance of keeping clothing, bedding, and other flammable objects away from them. Remind people to keep the screens and doors closed on the fronts of fireplaces and to have chimneys swept each year. Also remind patients using home oxygen not to smoke or have open flames in a room where oxygen is in use.

NCLEX EXAMINATION CHALLENGE 23.3

Health Promotion and Maintenance

When teaching a community group about burn prevention, which education will the nurse include?

A. "Have a smoke detector in one central spot in the home."
B. "If you use home oxygen, turn it down when you are smoking."
C. "Set your water heater temperature below 160°F (71°C.)."
D. "Plan several ways of escape from the home in case the primary exit is blocked."

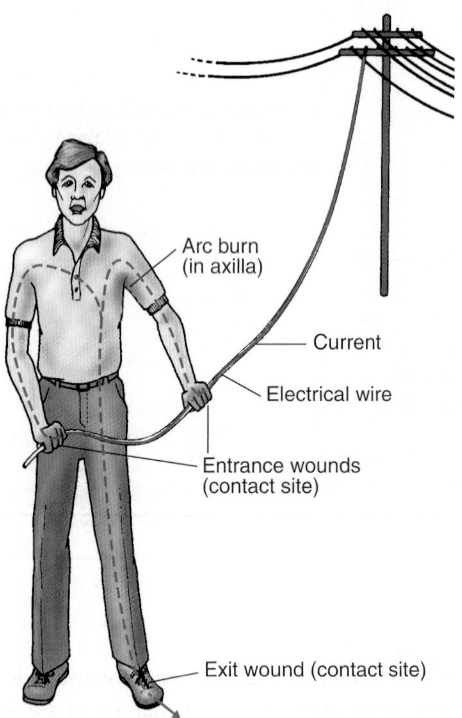

Fig. 23.18 Mechanism of electrical injury: currents passing through the body follow the path of least resistance to the ground.

Teach people to use home smoke and carbon monoxide detectors and to ensure that these are in good working order. The number of detectors needed depends on the size of the home. It is recommended that each bedroom have a separate smoke detector. There should be at least one detector in the hallway of each story and at least one detector for the kitchen, each stairwell, and each home entrance. Teach adults to develop a planned escape route with alternatives for when a main route is blocked by fire. Reinforce that no one should ever re-enter a burning building to retrieve belongings.

Remember to take extra time to speak with older adults about ways in which to minimize their risk for burns. Teach how to avoid common injuries as noted in the Patient-Centered Care: Older Adult Considerations box.

PATIENT-CENTERED CARE: OLDER ADULT CONSIDERATIONS (QSEN)

Adults over 60 are at increased risk for burns. Focus on kitchen and bathroom safety. Teach how to check the temperature of water before entering a bath or shower. Remind to keep loosely fitted clothes away from the stove and how to safely distribute hot food onto a plate without experiencing steam burns.

❖ Interprofessional Collaborative Care

Burn care takes place in three phases: emergent (resuscitation), acute (healing), and rehabilitative (restorative). The **emergent (resuscitation) phase** of a burn injury begins at the onset of injury and continues for about 24 to 48 hours. During this phase, the injury is evaluated and priorities of care are determined based on extent and severity of the burn. The priorities of care during the emergent phase include (1) securing the airway, (2) supporting circulation and perfusion, (3) maintaining body temperature, (4) keeping the patient comfortable with analgesics, and (5) providing emotional support.

The **acute (healing) phase** of burn injury begins about 36 to 48 hours after injury, when the fluid shift resolves, and lasts until wound closure is complete. During this phase, the nurse coordinates interprofessional care that is directed toward continued assessment and maintenance of the cardiovascular and respiratory systems, as well as toward nutrition status, burn wound care to preserve ***tissue integrity, pain*** control, and psychosocial interventions.

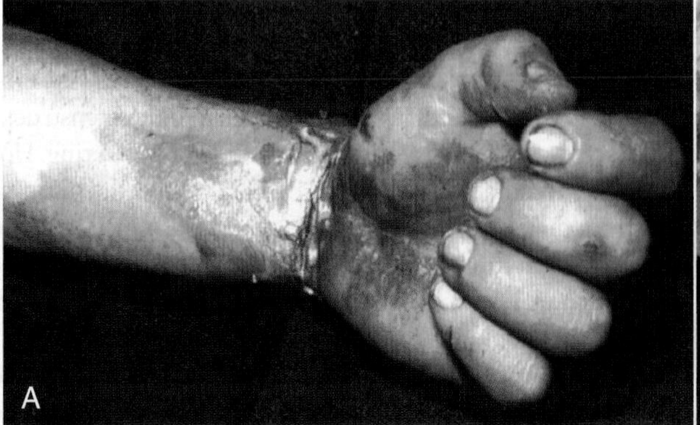

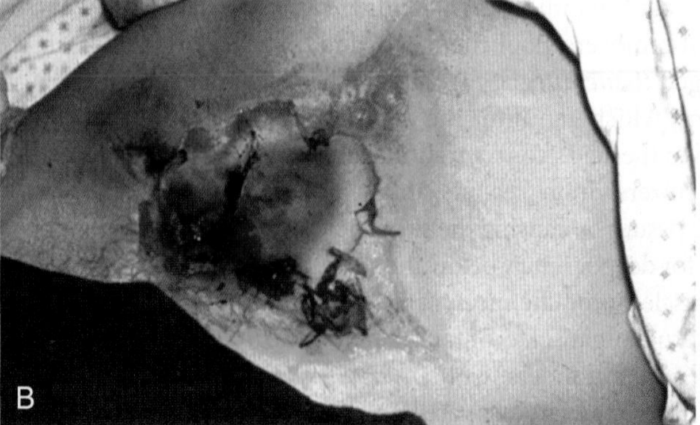

Fig. 23.19 Electrical entrance and exit wounds. (A) Possible entrance site. (B) Possible exit site.

Although rehabilitation efforts are started at the time of admission, the technical **rehabilitative (restorative) phase** begins with wound closure and ends when the patient achieves his or her highest level of functioning. The emphasis is on the psychosocial adjustment of the patient, the prevention of scars and contractures, and the resumption of preburn activity, including resuming work, family, and social roles. This phase may take years or even last a lifetime, depending on the degree and impact of burn(s).

Care of the patient with superficial first- or second-degree burns may take place in various locations depending on the severity of injury. Patients with localized burns may be treated in an outpatient setting such as an urgent care center or an emergency department.

◆ Assessment: Recognize Cues

History. Knowledge of circumstances surrounding the burn injury is valuable in planning the management of a patient who has experienced a burn. Obtain information directly from the patient and/or ask those who witnessed the event to provide context. Ask about the what the patient was doing when the burn occurred, the time and place where it happened, and the source and cause of injury. Asked detailed questions about how the burn occurred and the events that took place from the time of injury until help arrived. Obtain age, weight, and height, and a full health history (including pre-existing medical history, alcohol or drug use, and any history of any other injuries). Obtain a list of allergies, current medications, and immunizations. Ask if other events took place at the time of the burn, such as a fall, which could indicate that other injuries may be present.

Remember that the rate of complications from burn injuries is increased among older adults who are experiencing age-related physiologic changes. See the Patient-Centered Care: Older Adult Considerations: Age-Related Changes That Increase Complications From Burn Injury box.

PATIENT-CENTERED CARE: OLDER ADULT CONSIDERATIONS (QSEN)

Age-Related Changes That Increase Complications From Burn Injury

Age-Related Changes	Complications and Nursing Considerations
Thinner skin, sensory impairment, decreased mobility	Sensory impairment and decreased mobility increase the risk for burn injury. Thinner skin increases the depth of injury even when the exposure to the cause of injury is of shorter duration.
Slower healing time	Longer time with open areas results in a greater risk for infection, metabolic derangements, and loss of function from contracture formation and scar tissue.
Reduced inflammatory and immune responses	Increases the risk for infection and sepsis. Patient may not have a fever when infection is present.
More likely to have pre-existing medical conditions such as diabetes mellitus	Can interfere with wound healing.

Physical Assessment/Signs and Symptoms. Physical assessment findings in the resuscitation phase differ greatly from findings later in the course of the injury.

Respiratory Assessment. Assessment of the respiratory system is most critical to prevent life-threatening complications for those with inhalation injuries. *Even if you think a burn to the skin is minor, inspect the mouth, nose, and pharynx. Continuous airway assessment is a nursing priority.* The degree of inhalation damage depends on the fire source, temperature, environment, and types of toxic gases generated (Box 23.1). Facial burns and singed hair, eyebrows, and /or eyelashes are strong indicators that an inhalation injury is present. Black carbon particles in the nose, mouth, and sputum and edema of the nasal septum indicate smoke inhalation, as does a "smoky" smell to the patient's breath.

A change in respiratory pattern, drooling, or difficulty swallowing may indicate a pulmonary injury and impairment of ***gas exchange.*** Listen for hoarseness, cough, wheezes, and stridor. Place the patient upright, apply oxygen, and report any of these signs immediately to the health care provider.

! NURSING SAFETY PRIORITY (QSEN)

Critical Rescue

Monitor the patient's respiratory efforts closely to recognize possible airway involvement, even if you think a burn injury is minor. For a burn patient in the resuscitation phase who is hoarse, has a brassy cough, drools, has difficulty swallowing, or produces an audible breath sound on exhalation, respond by immediately positioning the patient upright, applying oxygen, and notifying the Rapid Response Team.

Upper airway edema and inhalation injury are most common in the trachea and mainstem bronchi, even in the presence of what may appear to be a minor skin burn injury. Auscultation of these areas may reveal wheezes, which indicate partial obstruction impairing ***gas exchange.*** *Patients with severe inhalation injuries may have such rapid obstruction that within a short time they cannot force air through the narrowed airways. As a result, the wheezing sounds disappear. This finding indicates airway obstruction and demands immediate intubation.* Many patients are intubated when an inhalation injury is first suspected. Waiting for signs of hypoxia may make intubation difficult or impossible.

! NURSING SAFETY PRIORITY (QSEN)

Action Alert

Heat damage of the pharynx is often severe enough to produce edema and upper airway obstruction, especially the epiglottitis, impairing ***gas exchange.*** The problem can occur at any time during the resuscitation phase. If the airway was exposed to heat, early intubation may be performed before obstruction occurs. If intubation is not performed in a patient whose upper airways were mildly exposed to heat or toxic gases, continually assess the upper airway for edema and obstruction.

! NURSING SAFETY PRIORITY QSEN

Critical Rescue

Monitor patients' respiratory efforts closely to recognize possible development of pulmonary edema. When signs and symptoms of pulmonary edema are present, respond by elevating the head of the bed to at least 45 degrees, applying oxygen, and notifying the burn team or the Rapid Response Team.

Skin Assessment. Assess the skin to determine the extent and depth of burn injury. The size of the injury is first estimated in comparison with the *total body surface area (TBSA).* For example, a burn that involves 40% of the TBSA is a 40% burn. The size of the injury is important not only for diagnosis and prognosis but also for calculating drug doses, fluid replacement volumes, and caloric needs.

Inspect the skin ***tissue integrity*** to identify injured areas and changes in color and appearance. Except with electrical burns, this initial size assessment usually can be made accurately with specific assessment tools and charts.

Because specific treatments are related to the depth of the burn injury, initial assessment of the skin includes estimations of burn depth. Criteria for depth of injury are based on appearance and associated characteristics (see Table 23.7).

Laboratory Assessment. For the patient with a burn that can be treated on an ambulatory basis, laboratory assessment is unlikely unless drug or alcohol intoxication is suspected, in which case those screens may be ordered.

Other Diagnostic Assessment. If a burn injury involves the eye, an ophthalmic evaluation is performed to detect corneal damage (see Chapter 42 for specific eye and vision evaluation procedures).

BOX 23.1 Carbon Monoxide Poisoning

Carbon monoxide (CO) is one of the leading causes of death from a fire. It is a colorless, odorless, tasteless gas released in the process of combustion. Inhalation injury is a risk for carbon monoxide poisoning (Woodson et al., 2018).

CO is rapidly transported across the lung membrane and binds tightly to hemoglobin in place of oxygen to form carboxyhemoglobin (COHb), which impairs oxygen unloading at the tissue level. Even though the oxygen-carrying capacity of the hemoglobin is reduced, the blood gas value of partial pressure of arterial oxygen (Pao_2) is normal (Rose et al., 2017). The vasodilating action of carbon monoxide causes the "cherry red" color in these patients. Symptoms vary with the concentration of COHb (Table 23.9). Administer high-flow oxygen for at least 6 hours to patients with suspected or confirmed carbon monoxide poisoning (International Society for Burn Injury, 2016).

TABLE 23.9 Physiologic Effects of Carbon Monoxide Poisoning

Carbon Monoxide Level	Physiologic Effects
1%-10% (normal)	Increased threshold to visual stimuli Increased blood flow to vital organs
11%-20% (mild poisoning)	Headache Decreased cerebral function Decreased visual acuity Slight breathlessness
21%-40% (moderate poisoning)	Headache Tinnitus Nausea Drowsiness Vertigo Altered mental state Confusion Stupor Irritability Decreased blood pressure, increased and irregular heart rate Depressed ST segment on ECG and dysrhythmias Pale to reddish-purple skin
41%-60% (severe poisoning)	Coma Convulsions Cardiopulmonary instability
61%-80% (fatal poisoning)	Death

◆ Interventions: Take Action

Nonsurgical Management. Interventions for the patient receiving burn care on an ambulatory basis are designed to facilitate airway maintenance, ***pain*** control, infection control, and wound healing. Although most patients treated on an ambulatory basis will not have airway compromise, tailor interventions to your respiratory assessment findings. For any patient suspected of an inhalation injury, be prepared to administer oxygen and keep emergency airway equipment near the bedside. This equipment includes oxygen, masks, cannulas, manual resuscitation bags, laryngoscope, endotracheal tubes, and equipment for tracheostomy in case of emergency.

Pain management is tailored to the patient's tolerance level, expectation of pain control, coping mechanisms, and physical status. Because dressing changes can be uncomfortable, medicating at least 30 minutes ahead of time can make the patient more comfortable. The patient with burns that are managed on an ambulatory basis may be able to use ibuprofen or acetaminophen for adequate pain control. If the patient is prescribed an opioid, teach about possible side effects like constipation, and emphasize using the drug for the shortest amount of time necessary.

To reduce risk for infection and to enhance wound healing, teach the proper dressing technique, and to take any prescribed oral antibiotics for the full course, even if the burn begins to look or feel better. For uncomplicated burns, a topical antimicrobial drug may be prescribed, to be covered with a gauze dressing. Remind about the importance of engaging in strict handwashing before and after wound care. Teach the patient to contact the primary health care provider if signs or symptoms of infection arise, such as increasing redness, warmth to the touch, purulent drainage, or fever. A tetanus vaccination may be administered if the patient has not had one in the past 10 years or does not recall when the last vaccine was obtained (Hibberd, 2020).

Depending on the burn type, severity and location, a compression garment may be applied to prevent contractures and tight hypertrophic scars. These garments also inhibit venous stasis

TABLE 23.10 Common Premalignant Lesions and Skin Cancers

Signs and Symptoms	Distribution	Course
Actinic (Solar) Keratosis (Premalignant)		
Small (1-10 mm) macule or papule with dry, rough, adherent yellow or brown scale Base may be erythematous Associated with yellow, wrinkled, weather-beaten skin Thick, indurated keratoses more likely to be malignant	Cheeks, temples, forehead, ears, neck, backs of hands, and forearms	May disappear spontaneously or reappear after treatment Slow progression to squamous cell carcinoma possible
Squamous Cell Carcinoma		
Firm, nodular lesion topped with a crust or a central area of ulceration Indurated margins Fixation to underlying tissue with deep invasion	Sun-exposed areas, especially head, neck, and lower lip Sites of chronic irritation or injury (e.g., scars, irradiated skin, burns, leg ulcers)	Rapid invasion with metastasis via the lymphatics in 10% of cases Larger tumors more prone to metastasis
Basal Cell Carcinoma		
Pearly papule with a central crater and rolled, waxy borders Telangiectasias and pigment flecks visible on close inspection	Sun-exposed areas, especially head, neck, and central portion of face	Metastasis rare May cause local tissue destruction; 50% recurrence rate related to inadequate treatment
Melanoma		
Irregularly shaped, pigmented papule or plaque Variegated colors, with red, white, and blue tones	Can occur anywhere on the body, especially where nevi (moles) or birthmarks are evident Commonly found on upper back and lower legs Soles of feet and palms in dark-skinned people	Horizontal growth phase followed by vertical growth phase Rapid invasion and metastasis with high morbidity and mortality

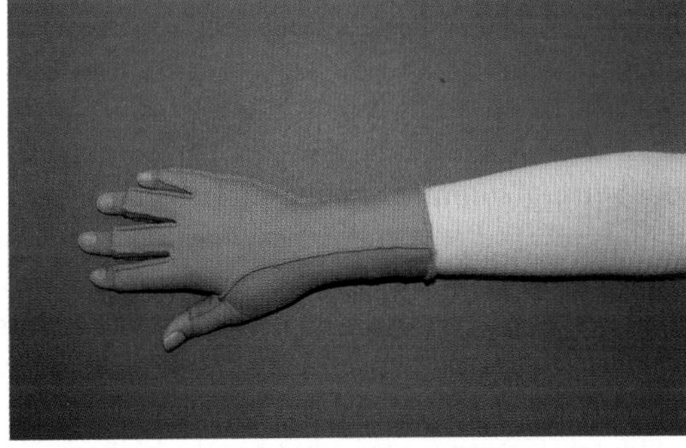

Fig. 23.20 Compression dressing. (From Williams, T., & Berenz, T. [2017]. Postburn upper extremity occupational therapy. *Hand Clinics, 33*(2), 293–304. https://doi.org/10.1016/j.hcl.2016.12.015.)

and edema in areas with decreased lymph flow. Compression dressings may be elastic wraps or specially designed, custom-fitted, elasticized clothing (Fig. 23.20) that provides continuous pressure.

SKIN CANCER

Pathophysiology Review

Overexposure to sunlight is the major cause of skin cancer, although other factors also are associated. Because sun damage is an age-related skin finding, screening for suspicious lesions is an important part of physical assessment of the older adult. The most common precancerous lesions are actinic (solar) keratosis, and the most common skin cancers are squamous cell carcinoma (SCC), basal cell carcinoma, and melanoma, as described in Table 23.10. A biopsy of suspicious lesions is necessary to determine whether a skin lesion is malignant.

Etiology and Genetic Risk. *Actinic (solar) keratoses* are premalignant lesions of the cells of the epidermis. These lesions are common in adults with chronically sun-damaged skin. Progression to squamous cell carcinoma may occur if lesions are untreated. These appear as pink, reddish, or reddish-brown scaly macules or papules (McCance et al., 2019).

Squamous cell carcinoma (SCC) is a cancer of the epidermis. These cancers can invade locally and are potentially metastatic (Fig. 23.21). SCC is the most common cause of lip cancer, often seen in older Caucasian men (McCance et al., 2019). Chronic skin damage from repeated injury or irritation increases risk for this malignancy. Chronic wounds that remain open for long periods are also at increased risk for malignant transformation to cancer.

Basal cell carcinoma arises from the basal cell layer of the epidermis (Fig. 23.22) and is the most common skin cancer worldwide (McCance et al., 2019). Early lesions often go unnoticed, and although metastasis is rare, underlying tissue destruction can occur. Genetic predisposition and chronic irritation are risk factors; however, UV exposure is the most common cause.

Melanomas are pigmented cancers arising in the melanin-producing epidermal cells (Fig. 23.23). Most often they start as the benign growth of a **nevus** (mole) (Skin Cancer Foundation, 2020). Normal nevi have regular, well-defined borders and are uniform in color, ranging from light colors to dark brown. The lesion's surface may be rough or smooth; those

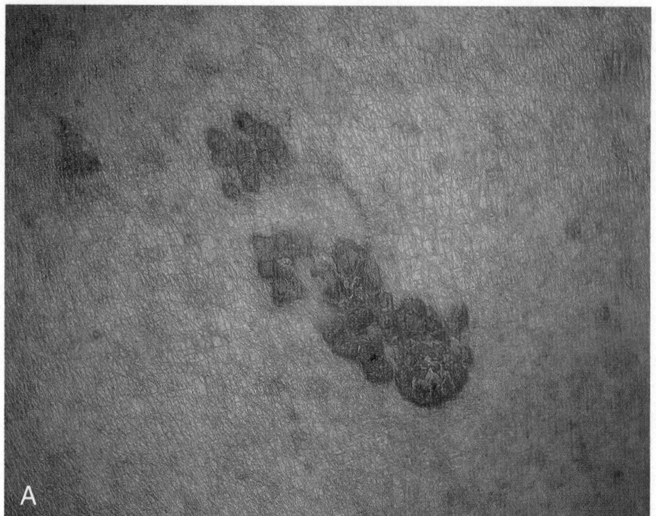

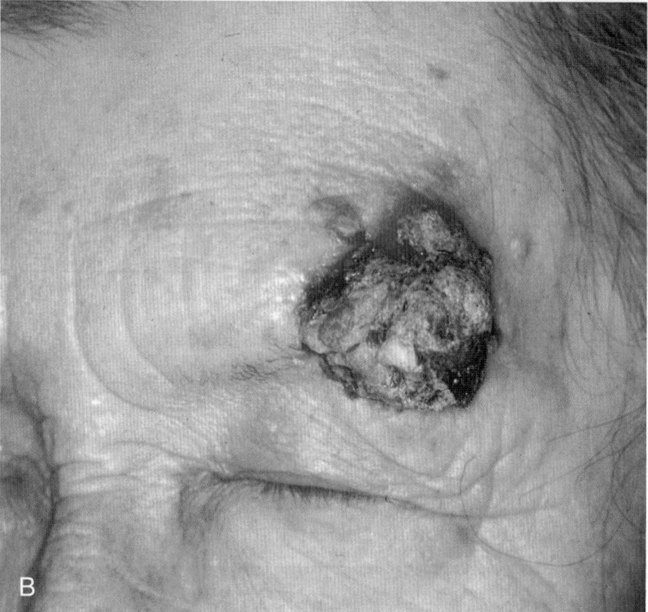

Fig. 23.21 Varying presentations of squamous cell carcinoma. (From Bolognia, J.L., Jorizzo, J.L., & Schaffer, J.V. [2012]. *Dermatology* [3rd ed.]. St. Louis: Saunders.)

with irregular or spreading borders, and/or multiple colors, are abnormal. Other suspicious features include sudden changes in lesion size and reports of itching or bleeding.

Risk factors include genetic predisposition, excessive exposure to UV light or certain occupational chemical carcinogens, and the presence of one or more precursor lesions that resemble unusual moles. *Melanoma is highly metastatic, and survival depends on early diagnosis and treatment.*

PATIENT-CENTERED CARE: GENETIC/ GENOMIC CONSIDERATIONS QSEN

Genetic mutations in the *CDKN2A* and *CDK4* genes have been identified for some cases of familial melanoma (OMIM, 2019), so ask about family history. Other genetic considerations for melanoma are that some specific mutations in the genes of the actual tumor cells increase the response of these cells to targeted therapy.

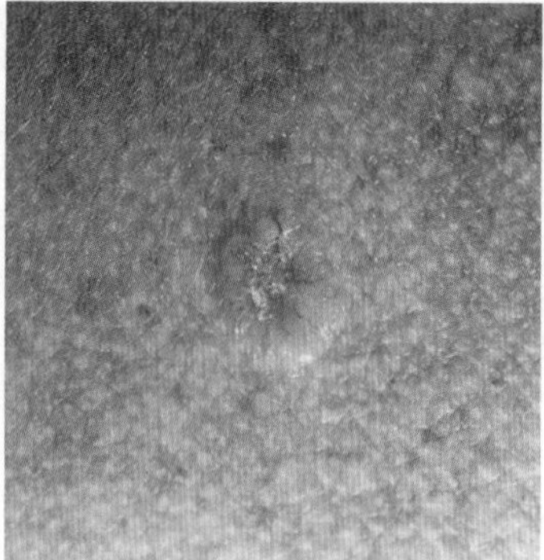

Fig. 23.22 Basal cell carcinoma.

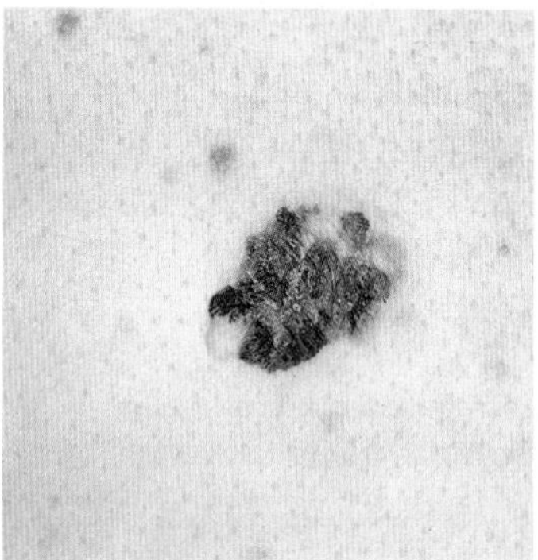

Fig. 23.23 Melanoma.

Incidence and Prevalence. The incidence of basal cell and squamous cell (nonmelanoma) skin cancer is difficult to determine because cases are not required to be reported to cancer registries (American Cancer Society [ACS], 2020). Incidence of melanoma is most common among non-Hispanic white individuals (ACS, 2020). Rates are higher for women than men in those under 50 years of age; by age 65, men's rates double, and by age 80, men's rates triple (ACS, 2020). Skin cancer occurs more often among people who spend extensive time outside exposed to the sun or who use tanning beds. Invasive melanoma reflects only 1% of total skin cancer cases but has the highest associated mortality rates (ACS, 2020).

Health Promotion and Maintenance. The most effective prevention strategy for skin cancer is avoiding or reducing skin exposure to sunlight (or tanning beds). Teach common prevention practices as listed in the Patient and Family Education: Preparing for Self-Management: Prevention of Skin Cancer box.

Teach everyone to evaluate all skin lesions using the ABCDE guide for melanoma (see Chapter 22) and to consult his or her health care provider to examine any lesion having unusual features. When lesions such as moles are present, they should be monitored annually by a dermatologist or other health care professional.

❖ Interprofessional Collaborative Care

Care of the patient with skin cancer, depending on the degree of cancer and associated health concerns, may be treated in the hospital, ambulatory surgical, or outpatient setting. Members of the interprofessional team who most often care for patients with

PATIENT AND FAMILY EDUCATION: PREPARING FOR SELF-MANAGEMENT

Prevention of Skin Cancer

- Avoid sun exposure between 11 a.m. and 3 p.m.
- Avoid all tanning beds.
- Use sunscreens with the appropriate skin protection factor for your skin type.
- Wear a hat, opaque clothing, and sunglasses when you are in the sun.
- Examine your body monthly for possibly cancerous or precancerous lesions.
- Taking pictures of lesions and comparing them month by month can demonstrate changes.
- Keep a "body map" of your skin spots, scars, and lesions to detect when changes have occurred.
- Contact your primary health care provider if you note any of these:
  - A change in the color of a lesion, especially if it darkens or shows evidence of spreading
  - A change in the size of a lesion, especially rapid growth
  - A change in the shape of a lesion, such as a sharp border becoming irregular or a flat lesion becoming raised
  - Redness or swelling of the skin around a lesion
  - A change in sensation, especially itching or increased tenderness of a lesion
  - A change in the character of a lesion, such as oozing, crusting, bleeding, or scaling

skin cancer include the primary health care provider, the nurse, the surgeon or dermatologist who removes cancerous lesions, the oncologist to manage radiation and/or chemotherapy, the pharmacist to dispense medication, the social worker to assist with care coordination and payer sources, and the spiritual leader of the patient's choice (if desired) to provide comfort.

◆ **Assessment: Recognize Cues.** In addition to age and race, ask the patient about any family history of skin cancer and any past surgery for removal of skin growths. Recent changes in the size, color, or sensation of any mole, birthmark, wart, or scar are also significant. Ask in which geographic regions the patient has lived and where he or she currently resides. Obtain information about occupational and recreational activities in relation to sun exposure and any occupational history of exposure to chemical carcinogens (e.g., arsenic, coal tar, pitch, radioactive waste, radium). Ask whether any skin lesions are repeatedly irritated by the rubbing of clothing.

Skin that has been injured previously is at greater risk for cancer development. Ask if the patient has ever experienced a severe skin injury that resulted in a scar. Examine all scarred skin areas for the presence of potentially cancerous lesions. A biopsy may be required to rule out cancer in a chronic open wound that fails to close with proper treatment.

Although most skin cancers appear in sun-exposed areas of the body, inspect the entire skin surface and any unusual lesions, particularly moles, warts, birthmarks, and scars. Also examine hair-bearing areas of the body, such as the scalp and genitalia. Palpate lesions with gloves to determine surface texture. Document the location, size, color, and features of all lesions and any reports of tenderness or itching. Use the ABCDE method of evaluating all lesions for possible melanoma (see Chapter 22).

◆ **Interventions: Take Action.** Surgical and nonsurgical interventions are combined for the effective management of skin cancer. Treatment is determined by the size and severity of the malignancy, the location of the lesion, and the age and general health of the patient.

Surgical intervention can range from local removal of small lesions to a massive excision of large areas of the skin and underlying tissue. Surgical types for skin cancer include:

- Cryosurgery—Cell destruction by the local application of liquid nitrogen (−200°C) to isolated lesions, causing cell death and tissue destruction
- Curettage and electrodesiccation—Removal of cancerous cells with the use of a dermal curette to scrape away cancerous tissue, followed by the application of an electric probe to destroy remaining tumor tissue
- Excision—Surgical removal of small lesions, often done as first-line treatment for squamous cell carcinomas
- Mohs surgery—A specialized form of excision usually for basal and squamous cell carcinomas
- Wide excision—Deep skin resection often involving removal of full-thickness skin in the area of the lesion. Depending on tumor depth, subcutaneous tissues and lymph nodes may also be removed

Actinic keratoses can be treated by excision, cryotherapy, dermabrasion, photodynamic therapy, topical medications, or field ablations (e.g., chemical peels, laser treatment) (Jorizzo, 2019). Determination of best treatment is influenced by number and distribution of lesions, the characteristics of the lesions, potential side effects, and availability and cost of methods (Jorizzo, 2019). Often cryosurgery or excision is chosen owing to their ease and low cost. Topical therapies such as imiquimod and fluorouracil are effective as long as the patient is adherent to the treatment regimen. These medications can cause skin irritation, so some patients prefer to avoid drug therapy.

Squamous cell carcinoma and basal cell carcinoma are usually treated by surgical excision in an outpatient setting with local anesthesia. Curettage and electrodessication, in which a dermal curette is used to scrape away cancerous tissue, followed by the application of an electric probe to destroy remaining tumor tissue, is also effective. Mohs micrographic surgery, in which tissue is sectioned horizontally in layers and examined histologically, layer by layer, to assess for cancer cells, can also be performed. *Radiation therapy* can be used for older patients with low-risk basal cell carcinoma or squamous cell carcinoma who are not candidates for surgery (Aasi et al., 2020). It can also be used for very large tumors or in areas where surgical excision is challenging (ACS, 2019a). Targeted therapy is often used for advanced basal cell cancers, and immunotherapy is often used for squamous cell carcinomas.

Melanoma is usually treated by excision or Mohs micrographic surgery. Lymph node dissection may be necessary, if lesions are found to be abnormally hard or large, or if melanoma is found in a node (ACS, 2019b). Immunotherapy and targeted therapy (e.g., BRAF and MEK inhibitors) are often used early in treatment of melanoma. Chemotherapy can be used if other treatments have not worked, but it is not as effective in treating melanoma as immunotherapy and targeted therapy agents. Radiation is not usually used to treat melanoma unless surgery cannot be done; it is given following lymph node removal or is offered as palliative therapy.

NCLEX EXAMINATION CHALLENGE 23.4

Physiological Integrity

A client with a large, irregularly shaped mole on the upper chest expresses concern about the cosmetic appearance of the lesion. What is the **priority** nursing intervention?

A. Refer to a dermatologic health care provider.
B. Ask if there are any other lesions that are bothersome.
C. Perform a head-to-toe skin assessment and document the findings.
D. Teach about the importance of avoiding excessive sun exposure and tanning beds.

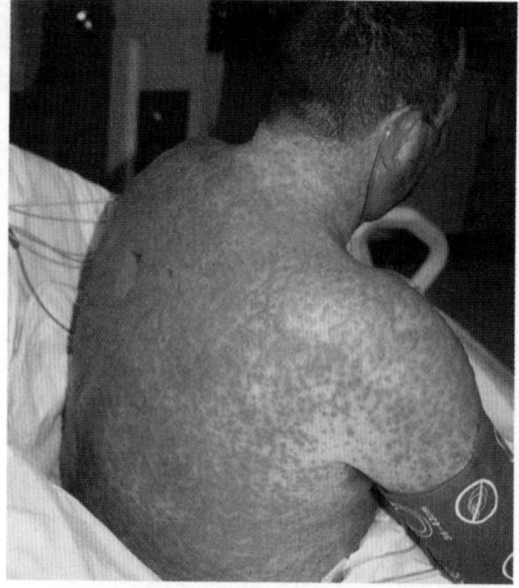

Fig. 23.24 Stevens-Johnson syndrome. (Courtesy Stevens Johnson Syndrome Foundation, Littleton, CO.)

LIFE-THREATENING SKIN DISORDERS

STEVENS-JOHNSON SYNDROME AND TOXIC EPIDERMAL NECROLYSIS

Stevens-Johnson syndrome (SJS) (Fig. 23.24) and toxic epidermal necrolysis (TEN) are life-threatening cutaneous reactions most commonly triggered by a drug. The disorder is characterized by fever, extensive necrosis, epidermal detachment, and mucous membrane involvement in most cases (High, 2019). The disorders are classified by percentage of body surface affected (High, 2019):

- SJS involves skin detachment of less than 10% of the body surface.
- SJS/TEN overlap describes patients in whom more than 10% but less than 30% of the body surface is detached.
- TEN involves detachment of more than 30% of the body surface.

Drugs most commonly associated with SJS/TEN include allopurinol, carbamazepine, lamotrigine, phenobarbital, phenytoin, and sulfasalazine. Immediate treatment involves withdrawal of the suspected drug. Supportive care following drug discontinuation includes skin care, nutrition balance, correction of ***fluid and electrolyte balance*** (if needed), and prevention of infection (High, 2019). Patients with TEN are often cared for in intensive care or burn units, once the disorder is diagnosed, so that sterile handling and reverse-isolation procedures can be followed.

GET READY FOR THE NEXT-GENERATION NCLEX® EXAMINATION!

Key Points

Review these Key Points for each NCLEX Examination Client Needs Category.

Safe and Effective Care Environment

- Wash hands before and after touching any skin lesions, and always use gloves when inspecting the skin. **QSEN: Safety**
- Ensure that the skin of all patients, especially those with incontinence, is kept clean and dry. **QSEN: Evidence-Based Practice**
- Assist patients with limited mobility to change positions regularly, at a minimum of every 2 hours, while using interventions to eliminate friction and shearing. **QSEN: Evidence-Based Practice**
- Use an evidence-based tool (e.g., Braden Scale) to evaluate the pressure injury risk for all patients at admission and regularly thereafter. **QSEN: Evidence-Based Practice**
- Use an evidence-based skin bundle to prevent compromise in skin integrity for all patients. **QSEN: Evidence-Based Practice**
- Use pressure-redistribution devices for patients at risk for, or who have, pressure injuries. **QSEN: Safety**
- Encourage adults to have and maintain home smoke and carbon monoxide detectors. **QSEN: Safety**
- Use strict aseptic technique when caring for patients who have open burn wounds to prevent infection. **QSEN: Safety**

Health Promotion and Maintenance

- Teach the patient and caregivers how to redistribute skin pressure in the home environment. **QSEN: Patient-Centered Care**
- Encourage adults to reduce exposure to the sun and to ultraviolet (UV) light. **QSEN: Safety**
- Teach adults how to keep a record or "body map" and to examine all skin areas monthly for new and changing lesions. **QSEN: Evidence-Based Practice**
- Urge patients to engage in proper hygiene and to keep all skinfolds clean and dry. **QSEN: Patient-Centered Care**
- Teach patients with infected skin lesions or infestations how to limit transmission. **QSEN: Safety**
- Teach patients to not smoke in bed or where home oxygen is in use and to refrain from smoking when taking sedative-inducing substances (drugs or alcohol). **QSEN: Safety**

- Instruct adults to set hot water tank temperatures to manufacturer recommendations and to check water temperature before bathing or showering. **QSEN: Safety**
- Teach patients to avoid exposing burned skin to the sun or to temperature extremes. **QSEN: Safety**
- Teach patients the ABCDE method of evaluating a lesion for melanoma. **QSEN: Patient-Centered Care**

Psychosocial Integrity

- Assess the patient's and family's feelings about how a condition of the skin, hair, or nails has affected body image. **QSEN: Patient-Centered Care**
- Support the patient and family in coping with changes in skin integrity and body image. **QSEN: Patient-Centered Care**
- Encourage the patient with a skin problem to participate in wound care. **QSEN: Patient-Centered Care**
- Professionally demonstrate acceptance of the patient with skin changes. **Ethics**
- Refer patients with chronic skin problems, especially those that alter appearance, to community support groups. **QSEN: Patient-Centered Care**

Physiological Integrity

- Keep skin well hydrated to promote ***tissue integrity*.** **QSEN: Evidence-Based Practice**
- Use appropriate assessment tools to determine risk for pressure injury development. **Clinical Judgment**
- Ask the patient if skin changes have occurred since starting a newly prescribed drug. **QSEN: Patient-Centered Care**
- Evaluate skin lesions daily for size, depth, exudate, presence of infection, and indicators of healing. **Clinical Judgment**
- Differentiate the signs and symptoms for all pressure injury stages. **Clinical Judgment**

MASTERY QUESTIONS

1. Which client statement regarding treatment of a skin infection requires intervention by the nurse?
   A. "I am not going to share my clothes with anyone else."
   B. "Because I am over 60, I am going to get the shingles vaccine."
   C. "It is important to keep my skin very moist, so I will use lotion."
   D. "If I get a fever or chills, I will contact my primary health care provider."
2. What teaching will the nurse provide when educating about carbon monoxide prevention?
   A. "Carbon monoxide is only dangerous if accompanied by fire."
   B. "Black smoke can be seen when carbon monoxide is in the air."
   C. "Your skin will turn a blue color if you have carbon monoxide poisoning."
   D. "Put carbon monoxide detectors in your home, because this is an odorless gas."
3. A client shows the nurse two pictures of the same lesion, taken 1 month apart. Which assessment finding requires nursing intervention?
   A. The light pink color of the lesion is the same in both photographs.
   B. The lesion has almost disappeared by the time of the second photograph.
   C. The lesion borders have expanded and are shaped differently in the second picture.
   D. The lesion's well-approximated margins and size look no different in either photograph.

REFERENCES

Aasi, S., et al. (2020). *Treatment and prognosis of low-risk cutaneous squamous cell carcinoma*. In *UpToDate*, Stern, R., & Robinson, J. (Eds.) Waltham, MA.

American Cancer Society (ACS). (2019a). *Radiation Therapy for Basal and Squamous Cell Skin Cancers*. Retrieved from https://www.cancer.org/cancer/basal-and-squamous-cell-skin-cancer/treating/radiation-therapy.html.

American Cancer Society (ACS). (2019b). *Surgery for Melanoma Skin Cancer*. Retrieved from https://www.cancer.org/cancer/melanoma-skin-cancer/treating/surgery.html.

American Cancer Society (ACS). (2020). *Cancer Facts and Figures 2020*. Retrieved from http://www.cancer.org/content/dam/cancer-org/research/cancer-facts-and-statistics/annual-cancer-facts-and-figures/2020/cancer-facts-and-figures-2020.pdf.

Berlowitz, D. (2020). *Clinical staging and management of pressure-induced skin and soft tissue injury*. In *UpToDate*, Berman, R., & Schmader, K. (Eds.) Waltham, MA.

Black, J. (2018a). Take three steps forward to prevent pressure injury in the medical-surgical patient: Pressure injuries...Prevention across the acute care continuum. *American Nurse Today, 39*, 10–11 Supplement to May 2018.

Black, J. (2018b). Using thermography to assess pressure injuries in patients with dark skin. *Nursing, 48*(9), 60–61.

Boxall, S., et al. (2017). Treatment of anticoagulated patients with negative pressure wound therapy. *International Wound Journal, 14*(6), 950–954.

Boyko, T., Longaker, M., & Yang, G. (2018). Review of the current management of pressure ulcers. *Advances in Wound Care, 7*(2), 57–67.

Centers for Disease Control and Prevention (CDC). (2018). *What Everyone Should Know About Zostavax*. Retrieved from https://www.cdc.gov/vaccines/vpd/shingles/public/zostavax/index.html.

DeMarco, S. (2020). *Wound and Pressure Ulcer Management*. Johns Hopkins Medicine Lecture Series. Retrieved from https://www.hopkinsmedicine.org/gec/series/wound_care.html.

Elston, D., & Kells, S. (2020). *Bedbugs*. In *UpToDate,* Dellavalle, R., & Rosen, T. (Eds.) Waltham, MA.

European Pressure Ulcer Advisory Panel, National Pressure Injury Advisory Panel, and Pan Pacific Pressure Injury Alliance. (2019). *Prevention and Treatment of Pressure Ulcers/Injuries: Quick Reference Guide 2019* (3rd ed.) .

Feldman, S. (2019). *Psoriasis: Epidemiology, clinical manifestations, and diagnosis*. In *UpToDate,* Dellavalle, R., & Duffin, K. (Eds.) Waltham, MA.

Gestring, M. (2020). *Negative pressure wound therapy. UpToDate,* Berman, R., & Cochran, A. (Eds.) Waltham, MA.

Gilligan, A., et al. (2018). Cost effectiveness of becaplermin gel on wound closure for the treatment of pressure injuries. *Wounds, 30*(6), 197.

Goldstein, A., & Goldstein, B. (2018). *Scabies: Management*. In *UpToDate,* Dellavalle, R., Levy, M., & Rosen, T. (Eds.) Waltham, MA.

Goldstein, A., & Goldstein, B. (2019a). *Pediculosis capitis*. In *UpToDate,* Dellavalle, R., Levy, M., & Rosen, T. (Eds.) Waltham, MA.

Goldstein, A., & Goldstein, B. (2019b). *Scabies: Epidemiology, clinical features, and diagnosis*. In *UpToDate*, Dellavalle, R., Levy, M., & Rosen, T. (Eds.) Waltham, MA.

Hibberd, P. (2020). *Tetanus-diphtheria toxoic vaccination in adults*. In *UpToDate*, Weller, P. (Ed.) Waltham, MA.

High, W. (2019). *Stevens-Johnson syndrome and toxic epidermal necrolysis: Management, prognosis, and long-term sequelae*. In UpToDate, N. Adkinson, & M. Levy (Eds.). MA: Waltham.

Holmes, C. J., Plichta, J. K., Gamelli, R. L., & Radek, K. A. (2015). Dynamic role of host stress responses in modulating the cutaneous microbiome: Implications for wound healing and infection. *Advances in Wound Care, 4*(1), 24–37.

International Society for Burn Injury. (2016). Practice guidelines for burn care. *Burns, 42*, 953–1021.

Jorizzo, J. (2019). *Treatment of actinic keratosis*. In *UpToDate*, Dellavalle, R., & Robinson, J. (Eds.) Waltham, MA.

Karsli, P., et al. (2017). High-voltage electrical stimulation versus ultrasound in the treatment of pressure ulcers. *Advances in Skin & Wound Care, 30*(12), 565–570.

Kaylor, J., Hooper, V., Wilson, A., Burkert, R., Lyda, M., Fletcher, K., et al. (2019). Reliability testing of augmented reality glasses technology: Establishing the evidence base for telewound care. *The Journal of Wound, Ostomy and Continence Nursing, 46*(6), 485–490.

Kayser, S., et al. (2018). Prevalence and analysis of medical device-related pressure injuries: Results from the international pressure ulcer prevalence survey. *Advances in Skin & Wound Care, 31*(6), 276–286.

Long, D. (2018). Best practices for pressure injury prevention in the ed: pressure injuries…prevention across the acute care continuum. *American Nurse Today, 39*, 8–9. Supplement to May 2018.

Mazboori, N., Javidan, A. N., & Bahmani, P. (2019). The effect of remote patient monitoring on patients with spinal cord injury: A mini-review. *Archives of Neuroscience*, (in press).

McCance, K., & Huether, S. (2019). *Pathophysiology: The biologic basis for disease in adults and children* (8th ed.). St. Louis: Elsevier.

Mervis, J., & Phillips, T. (2019). Pressure ulcers: pathophysiology, epidemiology, risk factors, and presentation. *Journal of the American Academy of Dermatology, 81*(4), 881–890.

National Center for Injury Prevention and Control, CDC. (2017). *WISQARS Data Source, National Center for Health Statistics (NCHS), National Vital Statistics System.*

National Psoriasis Foundation. (2020a). *About Psoriasis*. Retrieved from https://www.psoriasis.org/about-psoriasis.

National Psoriasis Foundation. (2020b). *Causes and Triggers*. Retrieved from https://www.psoriasis.org/about-psoriasis/causes.

National Safety Council. (2017). *Injury facts, "lifetime odds of death for selected causes, united states." 2017 Edition*. Itsaca, IL: Author.

Online Mendelian Inheritance in Man (OMIM). (2018). *Susceptibility to Psoriasis*. www.omim.org/entry/177900.

Online Mendelian Inheritance in Man (OMIM). (2019). *Melanoma, Cutaneous Malignant*. susceptibility to www.omim.org/entry/155600.

Rice, P., & Orgill, D. (2019). *Assessment and classification of burn injury*. In *UpToDate*, In Jeschke, M. (Ed.) Waltham, MA.

Rose, J. J., et al. (2017). Carbon monoxide poisoning: pathogenesis, management, and future directions of therapy. *American Journal of Respiratory and Critical Care Medicine, 195*(5), 596–606.

Shah, M., & Crane, J. (2020). Marjolin ulcer. In *StatPearls [Internet]*. Treasure Island (FL): StatPearls Publishing; 2019 Jan-. Available from: https://www.ncbi.nlm.nih.gov/books/NBK532861/.

Sidor, D., & Sieggreen, M. (2018). Take three steps forward to prevent pressure injury in the medical-surgical patient: Pressure injuries…Prevention across the acute care continuum. *American Nurse Today*, 35–37, Supplement to May 2018.

Skin Cancer Foundation. (2020). *Melanoma Overview*. Retrieved from www.skincancer.org/skin-cancer-information/melanoma.

The Joint Commission. (2018). *Quick Safety 43: Managing Medical Device-Related Pressure Injuries*. Retrieved from https://www.jointcommission.org/resources/news-and-multimedia/newsletters/newsletters/quick-safety/quick-safety-43-managing-medical-devicerelated-pressure-injuries/.

Touhy, T., & Jett, K. (2020). *Ebersole and Hess' towards healthy aging* (10th ed.). St. Louis: Mosby.

Wang, Y., et al. (2016). Hypoxia-inducible factor-1α gene expression and apoptosis in ischemia–reperfusion injury: A rat model of early-stage pressure ulcer. *Nursing Research, 65*(1), 34–46.

Woodson, L., et al. (2018). Diagnosis and treatment of inhalation injury. In D. N. Herndon (Ed.), *Total burn care*. Edinburgh: Elsevier. 2018.

24

Assessment of the Respiratory System

Harry Rees

http://evolve.elsevier.com/Iggy/

LEARNING OUTCOMES

1. Collaborate with the interprofessional team to perform a complete respiratory assessment, including indicators of ***gas exchange*** and ***perfusion,*** applying knowledge of anatomy, physiology, pathophysiology, and genetics.
2. Explain how age-related physiologic changes of the respiratory system affect ***gas exchange, perfusion,*** and the associated care of older adults.
3. Teach all adults measures to take to protect the respiratory system, including the avoidance of tobacco use.
4. Implement patient-centered nursing interventions to help patients and families cope with the psychosocial impact caused by a respiratory system problem.
5. Use clinical judgment to interpret assessment findings for the patient with a respiratory health problem affecting ***gas exchange***.
6. Teach the patient and caregivers about diagnostic procedures used to assess for respiratory health problems.

KEY TERMS

atelectasis Alveolar collapse.

bronchoscopy The insertion of a tube in the airways as far as the secondary bronchi to view airway structures and obtain tissue samples to diagnose and manage pulmonary diseases.

crepitus Air trapped in and under the skin (subcutaneous emphysema) felt as a crackling sensation beneath the fingertips.

fremitus Vibration of the chest wall felt on the surface by palpation when the patient speaks (tactile or vocal fremitus).

gas exchange Oxygen transport to the cells and carbon dioxide transport away from cells through ventilation and diffusion.

hemoptysis Blood in the sputum.

mediastinal shift A shift of central (midline) thoracic structures toward one side.

methemoglobinemia The conversion of normal hemoglobin to methemoglobin, which is an altered iron state that does not carry oxygen, resulting in tissue hypoxia.

orthopnea Shortness of breath that occurs when lying down and is relieved by sitting up.

oxyhemoglobin dissociation The process in which oxyhemoglobin in arterial blood unloads its oxygen molecules for diffusion into the tissues to allow cellular ***gas exchange*** to occur.

pack-years The number of packs per day multiplied by the number of years the patient has smoked.

perfusion Arterial blood flow through the tissues (peripheral perfusion) and blood that is pumped by the heart (central perfusion).

respiratory diffusion The movement of gases down their concentration gradients across the alveolar and capillary membranes.

surfactant A fatty protein that lines alveoli and reduces alveolar surface tension.

thoracentesis The needle aspiration of pleural fluid or air from the pleural space for diagnostic or management purposes.

ventilation Movement of atmospheric air higher in oxygen into the lungs and removal of the carbon dioxide produced during metabolism.

PRIORITY AND INTERRELATED CONCEPTS

The priority concept for this chapter is:

- ***Gas Exchange***

The interrelated concept for this chapter is:

- ***Perfusion***

ANATOMY AND PHYSIOLOGY REVIEW

The respiratory system includes the upper airways, lungs, lower airways, and alveolar air sacs. It starts the all-important gas exchange process to ensure adequate oxygenation to all cells, tissues, and organs. *Gas exchange* is the oxygen transport to the cells and carbon dioxide transport away from cells through ventilation and diffusion. **Ventilation**, movement of atmospheric air higher in oxygen into the lungs and removal of the carbon dioxide produced during metabolism, is the major function of the respiratory system. **Respiratory diffusion** is the movement of gases down their concentration gradients across the alveolar and capillary membranes. Oxygen diffuses from inhaled atmospheric air into the blood, and carbon dioxide diffuses from the blood into alveolar air, which is then exhaled. Once ventilation and diffusion exchange these gases in the lungs, blood oxygen is then available to cells by perfusion with a second diffusion into the cells. *Perfusion* is the arterial blood flow through the tissues (peripheral perfusion) and blood that is pumped by the heart (central perfusion). All systems depend on adequate ***gas exchange*** for tissue ***perfusion***. Any respiratory problem can affect total body health and well-being. See Chapter 3 for overviews of the concepts of gas exchange and perfusion.

Upper Respiratory Tract

The upper airways include the nose, the sinuses, the pharynx, and the larynx (Fig. 24.1). In addition to inhaling and exhaling, this part of the respiratory system influences speech and the sense of smell.

Nose and Sinuses. The nose is the organ of smell, with receptors from cranial nerve I *(olfactory)* located in the upper areas. The nose is rigid with a bony upper portion and a cartilaginous moveable lower portion. The septum divides the nose into two cavities that are lined with mucous membranes and have a rich blood supply. The *anterior nares* are the external openings into the nasal cavities. The posterior nares are openings from the nasal cavity into the throat.

The *turbinates* are the bones that protrude into the nasal cavities from the internal portion of the nose and are covered with mucous membranes (see Fig. 24.1). They increase the nasal surface area for filtering, warming, and humidifying inspired air before it passes into the nasopharynx.

The *paranasal sinuses* are air-filled cavities within the bones that surround the nasal passages (Fig. 24.2). Lined with ciliated mucous membrane, the sinuses give resonance to speech, decrease the weight of the skull, and act as shock absorbers in the event of facial trauma.

Pharynx. The *pharynx* (throat) is a passageway for both the respiratory and digestive tracts. It is located behind the oral and nasal cavities and is divided into the nasopharynx, the oropharynx, and the laryngopharynx (see Fig. 24.1).

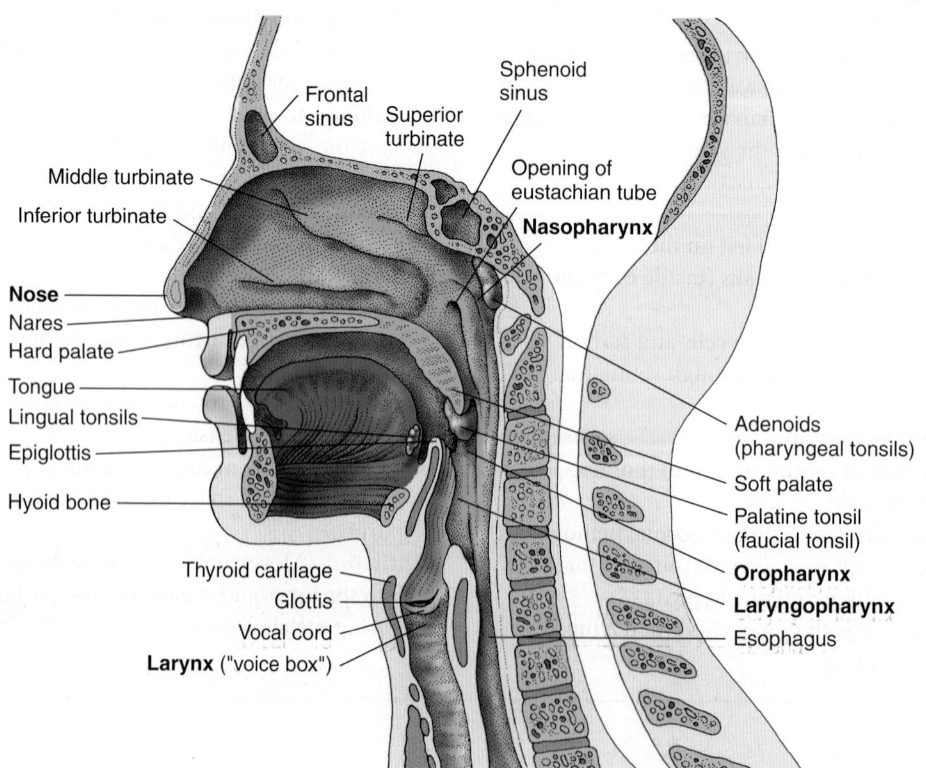

FIG. 24.1 Structures of the upper respiratory tract.

The *nasopharynx* is located behind the nose, above the soft palate. It contains the adenoids and the opening of the eustachian tubes. The adenoids trap organisms that enter the nose or mouth. The *eustachian tubes* connect the nasopharynx with the middle ears and help equalize pressure within the middle ear.

The *oropharynx* is located behind the mouth, below the nasopharynx. It extends from the soft palate to the base of the tongue and is used for breathing and swallowing. The *palatine tonsils,* which are part of the immune system, are located on the sides of the oropharynx and protect against invading organisms that enter through the mouth or nose.

The *laryngopharynx* is the area located behind the larynx from the base of the tongue to the esophagus. It is the dividing point between the larynx and the esophagus.

Larynx. The *larynx* ("voice box") is located above the trachea, just below the throat at the base of the tongue. It is composed of several cartilages (Fig. 24.3). The *thyroid cartilage* is the largest and is commonly called the *Adam's apple.* The *cricoid cartilage,* which contains the vocal cords, lies below the thyroid cartilage. The *cricothyroid membrane* is located below the level of the vocal cords and joins the thyroid and cricoid cartilages. This site is used in an emergency for access to the lower airways through a *cricothyroidotomy,* which is an opening made between the thyroid and cricoid cartilage and results in a tracheostomy.

Inside the larynx are two pairs of vocal cords: the false vocal cords and the true vocal cords. The *glottis* is the opening between the true vocal cords (Fig. 24.4). The *epiglottis* is a small, elastic flap attached to the top of the larynx. It opens during breathing and prevents food from entering the trachea (aspiration) by closing over the glottis during swallowing.

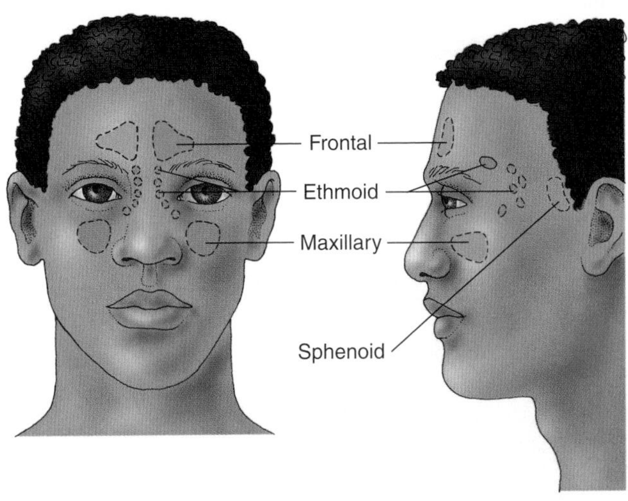

FIG. 24.2 Paranasal sinuses.

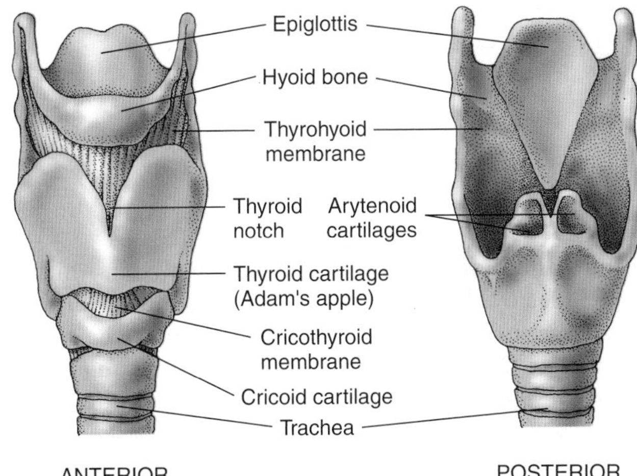

FIG. 24.3 Structures of the larynx.

Lower Respiratory Tract

Airways. The lower airways are the trachea; two mainstem bronchi; lobar, segmental, and subsegmental bronchi; bronchioles; alveolar ducts; and alveoli (Fig. 24.5). The lower respiratory tract *(tracheobronchial tree)* is the branching tubes formed by muscle, cartilage, and elastic tissues. These tubes decrease in size from the trachea to the respiratory bronchioles and allow gases to move to and from the lungs. ***Gas exchange*** takes place in the lung tissue, with diffusion occurring between the alveoli and the lung capillaries, not in the airways, which are too thick to allow diffusion.

The trachea is in front of the esophagus. It branches into the right and left mainstem bronchi at the *carina* junction. The trachea contains 6 to 10 C-shaped rings of cartilage. The open portion of the C is the back of the trachea and shares a muscular wall with the esophagus.

The mainstem bronchi, or primary bronchi, begin at the carina and contain the same tissues as the trachea. The right bronchus is slightly wider, shorter, and more vertical than the left bronchus and can be accidentally intubated when an endotracheal tube is passed. When a foreign object is aspirated from the throat, it usually enters the right bronchus.

The mainstem bronchi branch into the secondary (lobar) bronchi that enter each of the five lobes of the two lungs. Each lobar bronchus branches into progressively smaller divisions. The cartilage rings of the bronchi are complete and resist collapse. The bronchi are lined with a ciliated, mucus-secreting membrane that moves particles away from the lower airways.

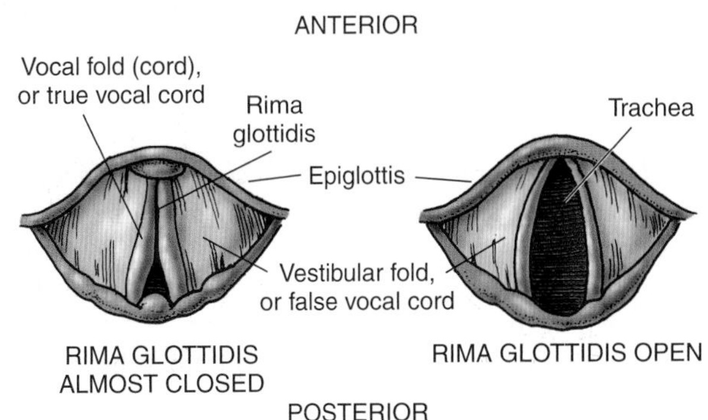

FIG. 24.4 Detail of the glottis (two vocal folds and the intervening space, the rima glottidis).

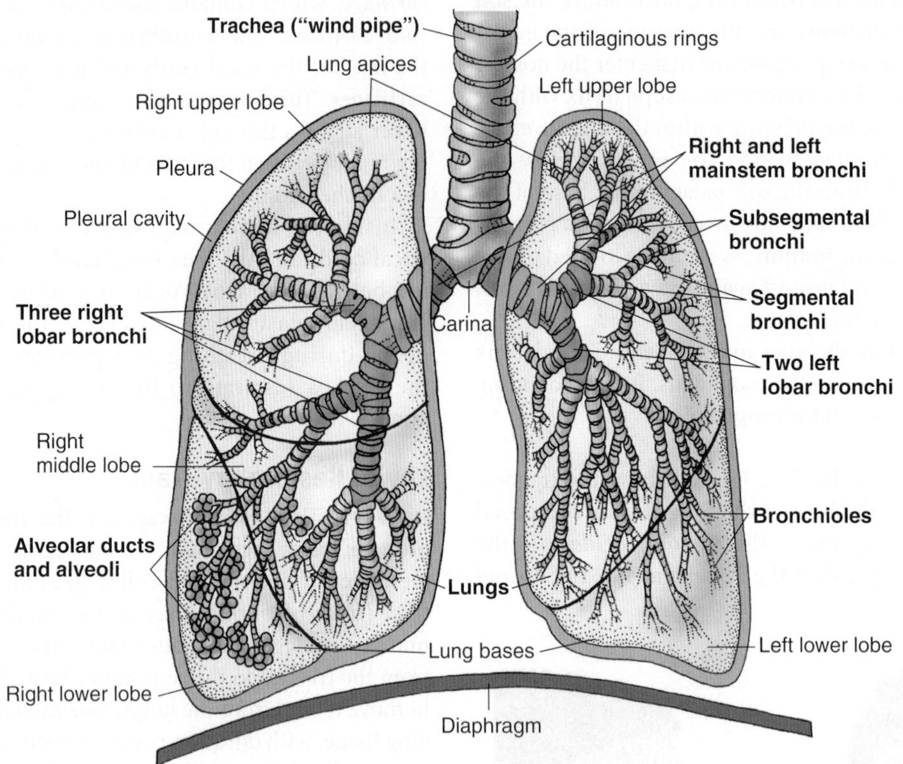

FIG. 24.5 Structures of the lower respiratory tract.

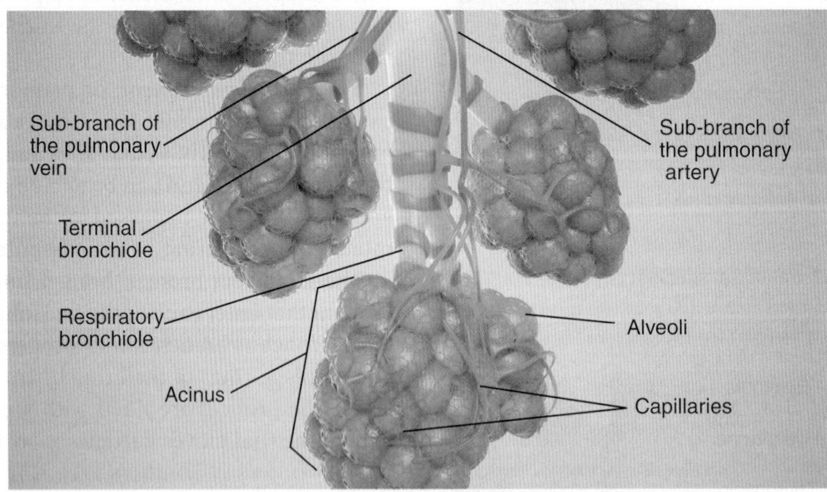

FIG. 24.6 The terminal bronchioles and the acinus. (© Elsevier Animation Collection.)

The bronchioles branch from the secondary bronchi and divide into smaller and smaller tubes, which are the terminal and respiratory bronchioles (Fig. 24.6). These tubes have a small diameter, have no cartilage, and depend entirely on the elastic recoil of the lung to remain open.

Alveolar ducts branch from the respiratory bronchioles and resemble a bunch of grapes. Alveolar sacs arise from these ducts and contain groups of alveoli, which is where respiratory ***gas exchange*** occurs (see Fig. 24.6). A pair of healthy adult lungs has about 290 million alveoli, which are surrounded by lung capillaries. These numerous small alveoli are a large surface area for gas exchange (about the size of a tennis court). *Acinus* is a term for the structural unit consisting of a respiratory bronchiole, an alveolar duct, and alveolar sacs.

The alveolar walls have cells called *type II pneumocytes* that secrete **surfactant**, a fatty protein that lines alveoli and reduces alveolar surface tension. Without surfactant, **atelectasis** (alveolar collapse) occurs, which inhibits ***gas exchange*** because the alveolar surface area is reduced.

Lungs. The lungs are two elastic, elongated cone-shaped organs located in the pleural cavity in the chest. The apex (top) of each lung extends above the clavicle; the base (bottom) of each lung lies just above the diaphragm. The lungs are composed of millions of alveoli and their related ducts, bronchioles, and bronchi. However, the two lungs are not equal in size or gas exchange. The right lung, which is larger and wider than the left, is divided into three lobes: upper, middle, and lower. The left lung is divided into only two lobes. About 55% to 60% of lung function occurs in the right lung. Any problem with the right lung interferes with ***gas exchange*** and ***perfusion*** to a greater degree than a problem in the left lung.

The *pleura* is a continuous smooth membrane with two surfaces that totally enclose the lungs. The parietal pleura lines the inside of the chest cavity and the upper surface of the diaphragm. The visceral pleura covers the lung surfaces. These surfaces are lubricated by a thin fluid that allows the surfaces to glide across each other smoothly during breathing.

Blood flow in the lungs occurs through two separate systems: bronchial and pulmonary. The bronchial system carries the blood needed to oxygenate lung tissues. These vessels are part of systemic circulation and do not participate in gas exchange.

The pulmonary circulation is a highly vascular capillary network. Oxygen-poor blood travels from the right ventricle of the heart into the pulmonary artery. This artery eventually branches into arterioles to form capillary networks that are meshed around and through the alveoli—the actual site of respiratory ***gas exchange*** (see Fig. 24.6). Oxygenated blood travels from the capillaries to the pulmonary veins and then to the left atrium. From the left atrium, oxygenated blood flows into the left ventricle, where it is pumped throughout the systemic circulation.

Accessory Muscles of Respiration. Breathing occurs through changes in the size of and pressure within the chest cavity. Contraction and relaxation of chest muscles (and the diaphragm) cause changes in the size and pressure of the chest cavity. At times, back and abdominal muscles are used in addition to chest muscles when the work of breathing is increased.

NCLEX EXAMINATION CHALLENGE 24.1

Physiological Integrity

Why are the terminal bronchioles more prone to collapse than are the other airways? **Select all that apply.**

A. The cartilage is an incomplete C shape rather than a true ring.
B. The mucous membrane lining contains minimal active cilia.
C. Lung elastic recoil is the only force that keeps them patent.
D. Their walls are too thick to permit gas exchange.
E. They are surrounded by capillaries.
F. The lumens have a small diameter.
G. Their walls contain no cartilage.

Oxygen Delivery and the Oxygen-Hemoglobin Dissociation Curve

Oxygen delivery to the tissues requires the binding of oxygen to hemoglobin in red blood cells (RBCs). Each molecule of hemoglobin can bind four oxygen molecules, which fills *(saturates)* all of its binding sites. Each RBC normally has millions of hemoglobin molecules. When blood passes through the lung alveoli, where oxygen concentration is the greatest, oxygen diffuses from the alveoli into RBCs and binds to all those hemoglobin molecules. This oxygen-rich blood then goes to the left side of the heart and is pumped out into systemic circulation (***perfusion***). In tissues away from the source of oxygen, **oxyhemoglobin dissociation**, in which arterial hemoglobin unloads its oxygen molecules for diffusion into the tissues, allows cellular ***gas exchange*** to occur. Fig. 24.7 shows the oxygen-hemoglobin dissociation curve and its shifts as oxygen needs change.

Tissue oxygen delivery through dissociation or "unloading" from hemoglobin is based on tissues' need for oxygen. The curve in Fig. 24.7 shows that the rate of this unloading changes depending on how much oxygen is already in the tissues. When blood perfuses tissues in which the oxygen levels are high, as indicated in the upper right corner of the figure, hemoglobin binding of oxygen remains very tight, and little oxygen is unloaded or dissociated from the hemoglobin into the tissues. This prevents oxygen delivery from being wasted by unloading it where it is not needed. When blood perfuses tissues in which oxygen levels are very low, as indicated in the lower left corner of Fig. 24.7, hemoglobin binds oxygen less tightly, and rapidly and easily unloads its remaining oxygen to provide these tissues with needed oxygen. So how rapidly and easily hemoglobin dissociates oxygen to the tissues changes depending on tissue oxygen need. The S-shaped curve indicates that it is harder for oxygen to dissociate from hemoglobin in tissues that are well oxygenated and much easier in tissues that are "starving" for oxygen.

The curve in Fig. 24.7 indicates that, on average, 50% of hemoglobin molecules have completely dissociated their

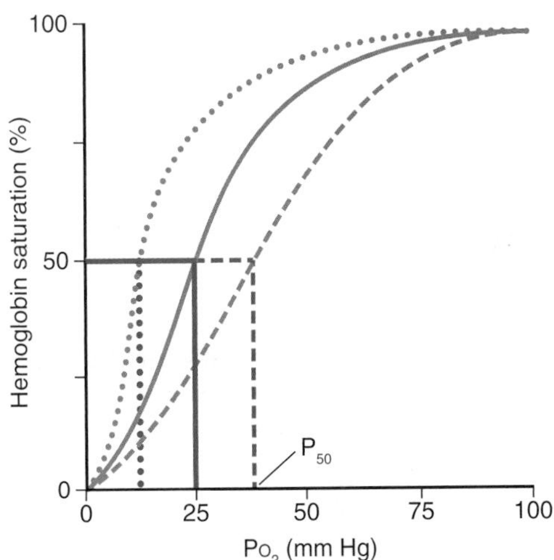

FIG. 24.7 The oxygen-hemoglobin dissociation curve and its shifts as tissue oxygen needs change. P_{50}, The partial pressure of O_2 at which hemoglobin is 50% saturated; Po_2, oxygen partial pressure.

oxygen molecules when blood perfuses tissues that have an oxygen tension (concentration) of 26 mm Hg. This is considered a "normal" point at which 50% of hemoglobin molecules are no longer saturated with oxygen (McCance et al., 2019).

When the need for oxygen is greater in tissues, this curve shifts to the *right,* which means the hemoglobin will dissociate oxygen faster even when the tissue oxygen tension levels are greater than 26 mm Hg. Conditions that shift the curve to the right include increased tissue temperature, increased tissue carbon dioxide concentration, decreased tissue pH (acidosis), chronic hypoxia, and increased levels of a by-product of glucose metabolism, diphosphoglycerate (DPG). (All of these conditions occur during periods of increased tissue metabolism.) This means that it is easier for hemoglobin to unload oxygen to these tissues because they need it to support the higher metabolism. The "right shift" is a tissue protection that increases oxygen delivery to the tissues that need it the most.

When tissues need less oxygen because they are metabolizing more slowly than usual, the oxygen-hemoglobin dissociation curve shifts to the *left,* which means that the tissue oxygen tension level has to be even *lower* for hemoglobin to unload oxygen. Tissue conditions that cause a shift to the left include decreased tissue temperature, decreased carbon dioxide levels, decreased glucose breakdown products (including DPG), and a higher tissue pH (alkalosis). This shift to the left prevents wasting oxygen delivery to tissues that are not using the oxygen they already have. Aging blood cells, including banked blood, have lower levels of DPG. Thus massive blood transfusions may shift the curve to the left, even when tissues could use more oxygen (Hooley, 2015).

A clinical example of how these actions are helpful is one in which a person is having a myocardial infarction (heart attack). Blood flow to the area is reduced; and the heart muscle is metabolizing under hypoxic conditions, which creates more carbon dioxide in the tissue and acidosis. As a result, the hemoglobin that reaches this hypoxic tissue unloads more oxygen at a faster rate to prevent ischemia and cardiac muscle cell death. What if this person believes that he or she is having indigestion, which can have similar symptoms, and tries to correct the problem by taking in large amounts of bicarbonate-based antacids? The antacids increase the pH in the blood and all tissues, shifting the oxygen-hemoglobin dissociation curve to the left. As a result, the hypoxic cardiac muscle cells receive even less oxygen, and more of them die.

Respiratory Changes Associated With Aging

The respiratory changes that occur with aging are described in the Patient-Centered Care: Older Adult Considerations: Age-Related Changes in the Respiratory System box. Other respiratory changes in older adults result from heredity and a lifetime of exposure to environmental pollutants (e.g., cigarette smoke, bacteria, industrial irritants).

Respiratory disease is a major cause of illness and chronic disability in older patients. Respiratory function declines slowly with age, but there is usually no problem keeping pace with the demands of ordinary activity. However, the sedentary older adult often feels breathless during exercise (Touhy & Jett, 2020).

It is difficult to determine which respiratory changes in older adults are related to normal aging and which changes are caused by respiratory disease. Age-related changes in the muscles and the cardiovascular system also may cause abnormal breathing, even if the lungs are normal.

NCLEX EXAMINATION CHALLENGE 24.2

Physiological Integrity

The nurse assessing an 88-year-old client notices a severe kyphosis that curves the client's spine to the right and bends her forward. Which change in respiratory function does the nurse expect as a result of this age-related change?

A. Decreased gas exchange as a result of reduced airway elasticity
B. Decreased gas exchange as a result of ineffective chest movement
C. Reduced pulmonary perfusion as a result of decreased alveolar diffusion capacity
D. Reduced pulmonary perfusion as a result of decreased blood return to the right atrium

HEALTH PROMOTION AND MAINTENANCE

Lung and breathing problems are common causes of death in North America (McCance et al., 2019). Some respiratory problems are chronic, and the patient has physical and lifestyle limitations. Many acute health problems, medical therapies, and surgeries adversely affect respiratory function temporarily or permanently. Exposure to inhalation irritants, especially to cigarette smoke, is the most common cause of chronic respiratory problems and physical limitations. Smoking is a modifiable factor that also greatly increases the risk for cardiovascular disease, stroke, and many types of cancer. Three compounds in cigarette smoke that have been implicated in the development of these serious diseases are tar, nicotine, and carbon monoxide. In the years after a patient has stopped smoking, his or her risk for respiratory-related disorders decreases significantly. Therefore assessing smoking habits, actively promoting smoking cessation, determining exposure to other inhalation irritants, and teaching adults to protect the respiratory system are important nursing functions. Although cigarette smoking has declined in both the United States and Canada, about 15% to 16% of the populations of both countries continue to smoke cigarettes (Centers for Disease Control and Protection [CDC], 2018b).

Assessing Smoking Habits

Begin assessing smoking habits by asking whether the patient is a current smoker or has ever smoked. The smoking history includes the number of cigarettes smoked daily, the duration of the smoking habit, and the age of the patient when smoking started, even for patients who are not current smokers. Record the smoking history in **pack-years,** which is the number of packs smoked per day multiplied by the number of years the patient has smoked.

Ask those who do not currently smoke whether and to what extent they are exposed to the smoke of others. Passive

PATIENT-CENTERED CARE: OLDER ADULT CONSIDERATIONS QSEN

Age-Related Changes in the Respiratory System

Change	Nursing Implications
Alveolar surface area decreases. Diffusion capacity decreases. Elastic recoil decreases. Bronchioles and alveolar ducts dilate. Ability to cough decreases. Airways close early.	Encourage vigorous pulmonary hygiene (i.e., encourage patient to turn, cough, and deep breathe) and use of incentive spirometry, especially if he or she is confined to bed or has had surgery to reduce the risk for infectious respiratory or mechanical complications. Encourage upright position to minimize ventilation-perfusion mismatching.
Residual volume increases. Vital capacity decreases. Efficiency of oxygen and carbon dioxide exchange decreases. Elasticity decreases.	Include inspection, palpation, percussion, and auscultation in lung assessments to detect normal age-related changes. Help patient actively maintain health and fitness to keep losses in respiratory functioning to a minimum. Assess patient's respirations for abnormal breathing patterns, such as Cheyne-Stokes, which can occur in older adults without pathology . Encourage frequent oral hygiene to aid in the removal of secretions.
Muscles atrophy. Vocal cords become slack. Laryngeal muscles lose elasticity, and airways lose cartilage.	Have face-to-face conversations with patient when possible because the patient's voice may be soft and difficult to understand.
Vascular resistance to blood flow through pulmonary vascular system increases. Pulmonary capillary blood volume decreases. Risk for hypoxia increases.	Assess patient's level of consciousness and cognition because hypoxia from acute respiratory conditions can cause the patient to become confused.
Body's response to hypoxia and hypercarbia decreases.	Assess for subtle manifestations of hypoxia to prevent complications.
Respiratory muscle strength, especially the diaphragm and the intercostals, decreases.	Encourage pulmonary hygiene and help patient actively maintain health and fitness to promote maximal functioning of the respiratory system and prevent respiratory illnesses.
Effectiveness of the cilia decreases. Immunoglobulin A decreases. Alveolar macrophages are altered.	Encourage pulmonary hygiene and help patient actively maintain health and fitness to promote maximal functioning of the respiratory system and prevent respiratory illnesses.
Anteroposterior diameter increases. Thorax becomes shorter. Progressive kyphoscoliosis occurs. Chest wall compliance (elasticity) decreases. Mobility of chest wall may decrease.	Discuss the normal changes of aging to help reduce anxiety about changes that occur. Discuss the need for increased rest periods during exercise because exercise tolerance decreases with age.
Osteoporosis is possible, leading to chest wall abnormalities.	Encourage adequate calcium intake (especially during a woman's premenopause phase) to help prevent or reduce later osteoporosis.

smoking has two origins: direct exposure to smoke by being in the same environment with an adult(s) who is actively smoking (*secondhand smoke [SHS]*); and indirect exposure from smoke that clings to hair and clothing (*thirdhand smoke*). Passive smoking contributes to health problems, especially when chronic exposure occurs in small, confined spaces (Middleton & Bruns, 2019).

Social smokers are adults who smoke cigarettes only in the presence of others, borrow rather than purchase cigarettes, prefer the company of nonsmokers, and do not smoke for stress relief. Often the social smoker does not consider himself or herself to be a smoker and must be asked specifically, "Do you ever smoke in social situations?" Even intermittent smoking has adverse effects on respiratory and cardiovascular health and may lead to nicotine addiction.

Hookah or water-pipe smoking is increasing in North America, especially among young adults. Many smokers have the false belief that hookah smoking is safer than cigarette smoking. The exposure to inhaled toxins during hookah smoking is as great or greater than with cigarette smoking.

Electronic nicotine delivery systems (ENDSs) with either battery-powered electronic cigarettes or a vape pen, also known as *vaping,* are alternatives to traditional cigarettes and sometimes are used as a method of quitting smoking (American Lung Association, 2018; Zborovskaya, 2017). A vape pen is a larger device with a greater volume of liquid and is often worn as a pendant or necklace around the neck. The lithium batteries contained in e-cigarettes have been the cause of burns and traumatic injuries incurred from battery fire and explosions (U.S. Fire Administration [USFA], 2017). The liquids and the vapors produced contain nicotine; and new evidence indicates that other lung toxins are present in the flavorings, especially diacetyl (Hua & Talbot, 2016). These toxins appear responsible for new-onset bronchiolitis obliterans ("popcorn lung") and for worsening of other existing lung injury conditions. In addition, heating of the metal coil in the devices to create the vapors contaminates the liquids with toxic metals (e.g., cadmium, nickel, chromium, and manganese), which are then inhaled by the smoker (Olmedo et al., 2018). These issues are especially problematic for adults using vape pens because the devices allow almost continuous use and exposure to the liquids.

In 2019 the CDC and the Food and Drug administration (FDA) began a joint investigation into a national outbreak of e-cigarette, or vaping, product use-associated lung injury (CDC, 2019). As of December 2019, 2506 cases of hospitalized e-cigarette, or vaping, product use-associated lung injury (EVALI) have been reported in the United States with 54 deaths. About 78% of the deaths occurred in adults under 35 years of age. Some adults with serious lung injuries have been using these products for fewer than 2 years. These data suggest that use of e-cigarettes and vaping have more detrimental health effects occurring more rapidly than the use of any other form of nicotine. Many states have now limited the sale of these products to individuals over 21 years of age.

PATIENT CENTERED CARE: CULTURAL/ SPIRITUAL CONSIDERATIONS (QSEN)

The prevalence of smoking is highest among Native Americans and Canadian First Nations peoples, adults with a General Educational Development (GED) certificate, and people living below the poverty level (CDC, 2018b). In addition, many Native Americans and Canadian First Nations peoples use smoking as part of ceremonies and rituals. Development of culturally appropriate smoking-cessation programs and research examining barriers to cessation in these populations may help reduce this disparity.

Promoting Smoking Cessation

Smoking cessation is a sensitive and sometimes uncomfortable issue for nurses and other health care professionals to approach with patients who smoke. However, this opportunity for a "teachable moment" may be the beginning support a patient needs to be successful in this healthful pursuit, especially if the patient is hospitalized for a smoking-related illness (Keating, 2016) or in an emergency department facing a stressful situation (Simerson & Hackbarth, 2018). Acute care settings have automatic smoking-cessation protocols that attach to the patient's electronic health record when an active smoking history is recorded. A simple, straightforward set of questions, known as *the 5 As,* was developed by the U.S. Public Health Service as part of their 2008 Clinical Practice Guideline on treating tobacco dependence. It is designed as a brief intervention lasting less than 3 minutes (U.S. Department of Health and Human Services, 2008). For health promotion and maintenance, nurses can follow the 5 *As* model to promote smoking cessation after assessing the patient's nicotine dependence (Wetter, 2017) (see the Best Practice for Patient Safety & Quality Care: Promotion of Smoking Cessation box).

BEST PRACTICE FOR PATIENT SAFETY & QUALITY CARE (QSEN)

Promotion of Smoking Cessation

The 5 *As* Model for Treating Tobacco Use and Dependence by Nurses

"A" Category	Action
*A*sk about tobacco use	Identify and document tobacco use and status for every patient at every visit.
*A*dvise to quit	In a clear, strong, and personalized manner, urge every tobacco user to quit.
*A*ssess willingness to make a quit attempt	Determine whether the tobacco user is willing to make a quit attempt at this time.
*A*ssist in quit attempt	For the patient willing to make a quit attempt, offer to request a prescription from the primary health care provider for drug therapy or assist the patient to obtain over-the-counter nicotine replacement therapy (NRT) drugs. Also refer the patient to counseling and local support groups. For the patient unwilling to make a quit attempt at this time, provide information about the harmful effects of tobacco and the benefits of quitting. Assess for patient indications that he or she may be interested in quitting in the future, such as statements of desire to reduce use or not use tobacco in the home. Reinforce the patient's tobacco reduction word choices.
*A*rrange follow-up	For the patient willing to make a quit attempt, arrange for follow-up contacts, beginning within the first week after the quit date. For the patient unwilling to make a quit attempt at the time, address tobacco dependence and willingness to quit at next clinic visit.

Adapted from U.S. Department of Health and Human Services, Public Health Service. (2008). *Treating tobacco use and dependence: 2008 update.* https://www.ahrq.gov/professionals/clinicians-providers/guidelines-recommendations/tobacco/index.html

! NATIONAL PATIENT SAFETY GOALS

As part of its quality measures, The Joint Commission requires documentation of screening for tobacco use and that a tobacco treatment program be offered or provided.

Ask about the patient's desire to quit, past attempts to quit, and the methods used. A "yes" response to any of the following questions indicates nicotine dependence. The more "yes" responses, the greater the nicotine dependence. Ask the smoker these questions:

- How soon after you wake up in the morning do you smoke?
- Do you wake up in the middle of your sleep time to smoke?
- Do you find it difficult not to smoke in places where smoking is prohibited?
- Do you smoke when you are ill?

PATIENT AND FAMILY EDUCATION: PREPARING FOR SELF-MANAGEMENT

Smoking Cessation

- Make a list of the reasons you want to stop smoking (e.g., your health and the health of those around you, saving money, social reasons).
- Set a date to stop smoking and keep it. Decide whether you are going to begin to cut down on the amount you smoke or are going to stop "cold turkey." Whichever way you decide to do it, keep this important date!
- Ask for help from those around you. Find someone who wants to quit smoking and "buddy up" for support. Look for assistance in your community, such as formal smoking-cessation programs, counselors, and certified acupuncture specialists or hypnotists.
- Consult your primary health care provider about nicotine replacement therapy (NRT; e.g., patch, gum) or other pharmacologic therapy to assist in smoking cessation.
- Remove ashtrays and lighters from your view.
- Talk to yourself! Remind yourself of all the reasons you want to quit.
- Reward yourself with the money you save from not smoking for a year.
- Avoid places that might tempt you to smoke. If you are used to having a cigarette after meals, get up from the table as soon as you are finished eating. Think of new things to do at times when you used to smoke (e.g., taking a walk, exercising, calling a friend).
- Find activities that keep your hands busy: needlework, painting, gardening, even holding a pencil.
- Take five deep breaths of clean, fresh air through your nose and out your mouth if you feel the urge to smoke.
- Keep plenty of healthy, low-calorie snacks, such as fruits and vegetables, on hand to nibble on. Try sugarless gum or mints as a substitute for tobacco.
- Drink at least eight glasses of water each day.
- Begin an exercise program with the approval of your primary health care provider. Be aware of the positive, healthy changes in your body since you stopped smoking.
- List the many reasons why you are glad that you quit. Keep the list handy as a reminder of the positive things you are doing for yourself.
- If you have a cigarette, think about the conditions that caused you to light it. Try and think of a strategy to avoid that (or those) conditions.
- Don't beat yourself up for backsliding; just face the next day as a new day.
- Think of each day without tobacco as a major accomplishment. It is!

Drug therapies are available over the counter and by prescription to help those addicted to nicotine to modify their behavior and stop smoking. Over-the-counter nicotine replacement therapies (NRTs) include nicotine transdermal patches, gums, and lozenges. Prescribed NRT products include nasal sprays and inhalers. NRT products have a good success rate for smoking cessation, especially when used along with a smoking-cessation program. The Patient and Family Education: Preparing for Self-Management: Smoking Cessation box lists suggestions for providing support to the person interested smoking cessation.

! NURSING SAFETY PRIORITY (QSEN)

Drug Alert

Teach adults using drugs for nicotine replacement therapy (NRT) that smoking while taking these drugs greatly increases circulating nicotine levels and the risk for stroke or heart attack.

Additional drug therapy for smoking cessation includes the oral drugs bupropion and varenicline. Bupropion decreases cravings and withdrawal symptoms, as well as reducing the depression associated with nicotine-withdrawal symptoms. Varenicline interferes with the nicotine receptors. This promotes smoking cessation by reducing the pleasure derived from nicotine and the symptoms of nicotine withdrawal.

! NURSING SAFETY PRIORITY (QSEN)

Drug Alert

Both bupropion and varenicline carry a black box warning that use of these drugs can cause manic behavior and hallucinations. These drugs also may unmask serious mental health issues. Teach the patient prescribed either of these drugs and their families to report any change in behavior or thought processes to the prescriber immediately.

PATIENT-CENTERED CARE: VETERANS HEALTH CONSIDERATIONS (QSEN)

Cigarette smoking among military veterans remains higher (about 33%) than among the general nonveteran population (CDC, 2018a). The slower decline appears to be related to a remaining high smoking prevalence among veterans who have psychiatric and substance use disorders and among female veterans. Be sure to assess the smoking status of all veterans and inform them of Veterans Health Administration smoking-cessation assistance.

Assessing Particulate Matter Exposure

Particulate matter exposure (PME) to inhalation irritants is a common cause of chronic lung disease and can make acute problems worse. Assessing PME exposure must be part of any health history assessment. A commonly used tool is the I PREPARE model shown in the Best Practice for Patient Safety & Quality Care: Assessment of Particulate Matter Exposure Using the I PREPARE Model box.

Protecting the respiratory system starts with making adults aware of the sources of PME and inhalation irritants. Teach adults who live in areas with high levels of air pollution to remain indoors with windows closed on days when air quality is poor and not to engage in heavy physical activity. Teach adults who have workplace or home exposure to inhalation irritants to wear protective masks during these exposures and ensure that the area is well ventilated.

ASSESSMENT: RECOGNIZE CUES

Patient History

Accurate patient information is important for identifying the type and severity of breathing problems that may interfere with ***gas exchange***. Age, gender, and race can affect the physical and diagnostic findings related to breathing (Jarvis, 2020). Many diagnostic studies for respiratory disorders (e.g., pulmonary function tests [PFTs]) use these data for determining predicted normal values. As described in the Health Promotion and Maintenance section, explore the home, community, and workplace for environmental factors that could cause or worsen lung disease. Use this opportunity to teach patients about measures to protect the respiratory system.

BEST PRACTICE FOR PATIENT SAFETY & QUALITY CARE QSEN

Assessment of Particulate Matter Exposure Using the I PREPARE Model

Investigate

Ask the patient specific questions to assess for all possible current and past particulate matter exposures to inhalation irritants including issues regarding current and past geographic living area, home conditions, occupation, and hobbies.

Present Work

Ask about exposure to industrial dusts, fumes, or chemical that may cause breathing disorders. Occupations with higher risk for exposures include bakers, coalminers, stone masons, cotton handlers, woodworkers, welders, potters, plastic and rubber manufacturers, printers, farm workers, those working in grain elevators or flour mills, and steel foundry workers. Ask whether breathing difficulties are less severe when away from the work environment.

Residence

Ask about the type of heat used at home (e.g., gas heater, wood-burning stove, fireplace, kerosene heater). Determine whether other people in the same residence have similar breathing problems. Ask whether any construction, especially in an older home, has recently been performed. Ask about the presence of mold or chronic dampness in the residence.

Environment

Determine the geographic location of the residence and whether it is in an area with higher levels of air pollution. Ask whether heavy industries, factories, farms, airports, or landfills are nearby. How close to an interstate or busy highway does the patient live?

Past Work

Because chronic particulate matter exposure may take years to affect respiratory function, ask the patient about all previous types of work and work environments.

Activities

Ask about hobbies in which the patient or other members of the household may engage, such as painting, ceramics, model airplanes, refinishing furniture, or woodworking, for possible exposure to harmful chemical fumes.

Resources and Referrals

Provide the patient with informative pamphlets and websites that can help him or her understand risk for particulate matter exposure and what types of protection can be used.

Educate

Determine the patient's literacy level and how he or she best acquires new information. Provide information and encourage the use of credible resources. A few examples include the National Center for Environmental Health (NCEH); Centers for Disease Control and Prevention (CDC) resource General Information on Air Pollution and Human Health; Environmental Protection Agency (EPA); Occupational Safety and Health Administration (OSHA); and National Institute for Occupational Safety and Health (NIOSH).

Adapted from Paranzino, G.K., Butterfield, P., Nastoff, T., & Ranger C. (2005). I PREPARE: development and clinical utility of an environmental exposure history mnemonic. *American Association of Occupation Health Nurses Journal, 53*(1), 37–42.

PATIENT-CENTERED CARE: GENDER HEALTH CONSIDERATIONS QSEN

Women, especially smokers, have greater bronchial responsiveness (i.e., bronchial hyperreactivity) and larger airways than men. This factor increases the risk for a more rapid decline in lung function as a woman ages, especially in women who were or are smokers. Be sure to measure ***gas exchange*** adequacy with pulse oximetry when assessing women.

PATIENT-CENTERED CARE: CULTURAL/SPIRITUAL CONSIDERATIONS QSEN

Pulse oximetry results may be lower in adults with dark skin. This is due to deeper coloration of the nail bed and does not reflect true oxygenation status. Use additional respiratory assessment techniques to assess ***gas exchange*** in adults with dark skin, such as examination of the color within the oral cavity and arterial blood gas results.

Ask patients about their respiratory history (Table 24.1), including smoking history, drug use, travel, and area of residence. Document the smoking history in pack-years.

Drug use, both prescribed drugs and illicit drugs, can affect lung function, even when taken systemically. Ask about drugs taken for breathing problems and those taken for other conditions. For example, a cough can be a side effect of some antihypertensive drugs (angiotensin-converting enzyme inhibitors [ACEIs] and angiotensin receptor blockers [ARBs]). Determine which over-the-counter drugs (e.g., cough syrups, antihistamines, decongestants, inhalants) the patient uses. Assess use of complementary and integrative therapies. Ask about past drug use. Some drugs for other conditions can cause permanent changes in lung function. For example, patients may have pulmonary fibrosis if they received bleomycin as chemotherapy for cancer or amiodarone for cardiac problems. Marijuana and illicit drugs, such as cocaine, are often inhaled and can reduce lung function.

Allergies to foods, dust, molds, pollen, bee stings, trees, grass, animal dander and saliva, or drugs can affect breathing. Ask the patient to describe specific allergic responses. For example, does he or she wheeze, have trouble breathing, cough, sneeze, or have rhinitis after exposure to the allergen? Has he or she ever been treated for an allergic response? If the patient has allergies, ask about the specific cause, treatment, and response to treatment.

NURSING SAFETY PRIORITY QSEN

Action Alert

Document any known allergies, especially to drugs, and the specific type of allergic response experienced in a prominent place in the patient's medical record.

TABLE 24.1 Important Respiratory Assessment Issues

• Smoking history
• Childhood illnesses:
  • Asthma
  • Pneumonia
  • Communicable diseases
  • Hay fever
  • Allergies
  • Eczema
  • Frequent colds
  • Croup
  • Cystic fibrosis
• Adult illnesses:
  • Pneumonia
  • Sinusitis
  • Tuberculosis
  • HIV and AIDS (HIV-III)
  • Lung disease such as emphysema and sarcoidosis
  • Diabetes
  • Hypertension
  • Heart disease
  • Influenza, pneumococcal (Pneumovax), and BCG vaccinations
	• Surgeries of the upper or lower respiratory system
	• Injuries to the upper or lower respiratory system
	• Hospitalizations
	• Date of last chest x-ray, pulmonary function test, tuberculin test, or other diagnostic tests and results
	• Recent weight loss
	• Night sweats
	• Sleep disturbances
	• Lung disease and condition of family members
	• Geographic areas of recent travel
	• Occupation and leisure activities

AIDS, Acquired immune deficiency syndrome; *BCG,* bacille Calmette-Guérin; *HIV,* human immune deficiency virus.

Travel and geographic area of residence may reveal exposure to certain diseases. For example, *histoplasmosis,* a fungal disease caused by inhalation of contaminated dust, is found in the central parts of the United States and Canada. *Coccidioidomycosis* is found in the western and southwestern parts of the United States, in Mexico, and in parts of Central America, as is *hantavirus.* With veterans, ask about location of deployments within the past year.

Family History and Genetic Risk. Obtain a family history to assess for respiratory disorders that have a genetic component, such as cystic fibrosis and emphysema. Patients with asthma often have a family history of allergy. Ask about a history of infectious disease, such as tuberculosis, because family members may have similar environmental exposures.

Current Health Problems. Whether the breathing problem is acute or chronic, the current health problem usually includes cough, sputum production, chest pain, and shortness of breath at rest or on exertion. Explore the current illness in chronological order. Ask about the onset of the problem, how long it lasts, the location of the problem, how often it occurs, whether the problem has become worse over time, which symptoms occur with it, which actions or interventions provide relief and which ones make it worse, and which treatments have been used.

Cough is a sign of lung disease. Ask the patient how long the cough has been present and whether it occurs at a specific time of day (e.g., on awakening in the morning) or in relation to any physical activity. Ask whether the cough produces sputum or is dry, tickling, or hacking.

Sputum production is an important symptom associated with coughing. Check the color, consistency, odor, and amount of sputum.

Describe the consistency of sputum as thin, thick, watery, or frothy. Smokers with chronic bronchitis have mucoid sputum. Excessive pink, frothy sputum is common with pulmonary edema. Bacterial pneumonia often produces rust-colored sputum, and a lung abscess may cause foul-smelling sputum. **Hemoptysis** (blood in the sputum) may be seen in patients with chronic bronchitis or lung cancer. Grossly bloody sputum may occur with tuberculosis, pulmonary infarction, lung cancer, or lung abscess.

Ask the patient to quantify sputum by describing its volume in terms such as teaspoon, tablespoon, and cup. Normally the lungs produce up to 90 mL of sputum per day.

Chest pain can occur with other health problems in addition to pulmonary problems. A detailed description of chest pain helps distinguish its cause. Ask whether the pain is continuous or made worse by coughing, deep breathing, or swallowing. Cardiac pain is usually intense and "crushing" and may radiate to the arm, shoulder, or neck. Pulmonary pain varies, depending on the cause, and most often feels like something is "rubbing" inside. Pain may appear only on deep inhalation or be present at the end of inhalation and the end of exhalation. Pulmonary pain is not made worse by touching or pressing over the area.

Dyspnea (difficulty in breathing or breathlessness) is a subjective perception and varies among patients (Campbell, 2017). Some patients with chronic lung disease can reliably report dyspnea levels that accurately correspond to the severity of their disease. However, others have difficulty describing their symptoms or responding to the question "Are you short of breath?" Therefore asking about breathlessness and using a visual analog scale (Fig. 24.8) to assess its severity may provide more accurate information about changes from a patient's baseline ease of breathing. Ask about the onset (slow or abrupt), the duration, relieving factors (position changes, drug use, activity cessation), and whether wheezing or stridor occurs with dyspnea.

Try to quantify dyspnea by asking whether this symptom interferes with ADLs and, if so, how severely. For example, does dyspnea occur after walking one block or climbing one flight of stairs? Table 24.2 classifies dyspnea with changes in ADL performance. Because dyspnea can be a predictor of life-threatening illness, early assessment helps optimize care, improve symptom management, and ensure the appropriate level of intervention and care.

Ask about **orthopnea**—shortness of breath that occurs when lying down and is relieved by sitting up. Assess for paroxysmal nocturnal dyspnea (PND), which awakens the patient from sleep with the feeling of an inability to breathe. PND also occurs while lying flat and is relieved by sitting up. It often occurs with chronic lung disease and left-sided heart failure.

Physical Assessment

Assessment of the Nose and Sinuses. Inspect the patient's external nose for deformities and the nares for symmetry of size and shape. To observe the interior nose, ask the patient to tilt the head back for a penlight examination. The experienced nurse may use a nasal speculum and nasopharyngeal mirror for a more thorough inspection of the nasal cavity.

Inspect for color, swelling, drainage, bleeding, and polyps. Nasal mucous membranes normally appear redder than the oral mucosa but are pale, engorged, and bluish-gray in patients with allergic rhinitis. Check the nasal septum for bleeding, perforation, or deviation. Septal deviation is common and appears as an S shape, tilting toward one side or the other. A perforated septum is present if the light shines through the perforation into the opposite side; this condition is often found in cocaine users. Nasal polyps are pale, shiny, gelatinous lumps or "bags" on the turbinates. Block one naris at a time to check how well air moves through the unblocked side.

Assessment of the Pharynx, Trachea, and Larynx. Assessment of the pharynx begins with inspection of the mouth. To examine the posterior pharynx, use a tongue depressor to press down one side of the tongue at a time (to avoid stimulating the gag reflex). As the patient says "ah," observe the rise and fall of the soft palate and inspect for color and symmetry, drainage, edema or ulceration, and enlarged tonsils.

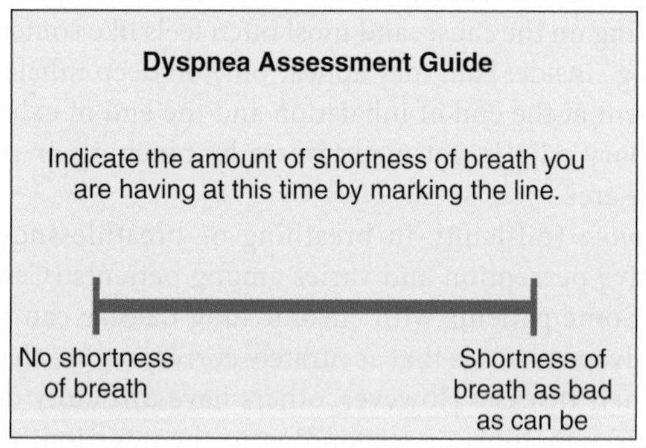

Dyspnea Assessment Guide
Indicate the amount of shortness of breath you are having at this time by marking the line.
No shortness of breath
Shortness of breath as bad as can be

FIG. 24.8 A visual analog scale (VAS) for dyspnea assessment.

Inspect the neck for symmetry, alignment, masses, swelling, bruises, and the use of accessory neck muscles in breathing. Palpate lymph nodes for size, shape, mobility with palpation, consistency, and tenderness.

Gently palpate the trachea for position, mobility, tenderness, and masses. The trachea should be in the midline. Lung disorders that cause the trachea to move *away* from the affected area include tension pneumothorax, large pleural effusion, mediastinal mass, and neck tumor. Pneumonectomy, fibrosis, and atelectasis pull it *toward* the affected area.

The larynx is usually examined by a specialist with a laryngoscope. An abnormal voice, especially hoarseness, may be heard when there are problems of the larynx.

Assessment of the Lungs and Thorax

Inspection. Inspect the front and back of the thorax with the patient sitting up. Normal landmarks of the chest front (anterior) and back (posterior) are shown in Fig. 24.9. The patient should be undressed to the waist. Observe the chest and compare one side with the other. Work from the top (apex) and move downward toward the base, going from side to side, while inspecting for discoloration, scars, lesions, masses, and spinal curvatures. Assessing from side to side allows you to compare the findings for each lung at the same level (Jarvis, 2020).

Observe the rate, rhythm, and depth of inspirations and the symmetry of chest movement. Impaired movement or unequal expansion may indicate disease. Observe the type of breathing (e.g., pursed-lip or diaphragmatic breathing) and the use of accessory muscles.

Examine the shape of the patient's chest, and compare the anteroposterior (AP or front-to-back) diameter with the lateral (side-to-side) diameter. This ratio normally is about 1:1.5,

TABLE 24.2 Correlation of Dyspnea Classification With Performance of ADLs

Classification	ADLs Key
Class I: No significant restrictions in normal activity. Employable. Dyspnea occurs only on more-than-normal or strenuous exertion.	*4:* No breathlessness, normal.
Class II: Independent in essential ADLs but restricted in some other activities. Dyspneic on climbing stairs or on walking on an incline but not on level walking. Employable only for sedentary job or under special circumstances.	*3:* Satisfactory, mild breathlessness. Complete performance is possible without pause or assistance but not entirely normal.
Class III: Dyspnea commonly occurs during usual activities such as showering or dressing, but the patient can manage without assistance from others. Not dyspneic at rest; can walk for more than a city block at own pace but cannot keep up with others of own age. May stop to catch breath partway up a flight of stairs. Is not likely to be employed.	*2:* Fair, moderate breathlessness. Must stop during activity. Complete performance is possible without assistance, but performance may be too debilitating or time consuming.
Class IV: Dyspnea produces dependence on help in some essential ADLs such as dressing and bathing. Not usually dyspneic at rest. Dyspneic on minimal exertion; must pause on climbing one flight, walking more than 100 yards, or dressing. Often restricted to home if lives alone. Has minimal or no activities outside of home.	*1:* Poor, marked breathlessness. Incomplete performance; assistance is necessary.
Class V: Entirely restricted to home and often limited to bed or chair. Dyspneic at rest. Dependent on help for most needs.	*0:* Performance not indicated or recommended; too difficult.

depending on body build. It increases to 1:1 in patients with emphysema, which results in the typical barrel-chest appearance.

Normally the ribs slope downward. Patients with air trapping in the lungs caused by emphysema have ribs that are more horizontal. Observe or palpate the distance between the ribs *(intercostal space)*. This distance is usually one finger-breadth (2 cm). It increases in disorders that cause air trapping, such as emphysema. Observe for retraction of muscle between the ribs and at the sternal notch. Retractions are areas that get sucked inward when the patient inhales. This does not occur in healthy adults during normal respiratory effort. Retractions may occur when the patient is working hard to inhale around an obstruction.

Palpation. Palpate the chest after inspection to assess respiratory movement symmetry and observable abnormalities. Palpation also can help identify areas of tenderness and check for tactile fremitus.

Assess chest expansion by placing your thumbs on the patient's spine at the level of the ninth ribs and extending the fingers sideways around the rib cage. As the patient inhales, both sides of the chest should move upward and outward together in one symmetric movement, moving your thumbs apart. On exhalation, the thumbs should come back together as they return to the midline. Unequal expansion may be a result of pain, trauma, or air in the pleural cavity. Respiratory lag or slowed movement on one side indicates a pulmonary problem (Jarvis, 2020).

Palpate any abnormalities found on inspection (e.g., masses, lesions, swelling). Also palpate for tenderness, especially if the patient reports pain. **Crepitus** (air trapped in and under the skin, also known as *subcutaneous emphysema*) is felt as a crackling sensation beneath the fingertips. Document this finding and report it to the primary health care provider when it occurs around a wound site or a tracheostomy site or if a pneumothorax is suspected.

Fremitus is felt as a vibration of the chest wall produced when the patient speaks. Fremitus is decreased if sound wave transmission from the larynx to the chest wall is slowed, such as when the pleural space is filled with air *(pneumothorax)* or fluid *(pleural effusion)* or when the bronchus is obstructed. Fremitus is increased with pneumonia and lung abscesses because the increased density of the chest enhances vibration transmission.

Percussion. Use percussion to assess for pulmonary resonance, the boundaries of organs, and diaphragmatic excursion. Percussion involves tapping the chest wall, which sets the underlying tissues into motion and produces audible sounds (Fig. 24.10). This action produces five different sounds that help determine whether the lung tissue contains air or fluid or is solid (Table 24.3).

Auscultation. Lung auscultation is listening with a stethoscope for normal breath sounds, abnormal *(adventitious)* sounds, and voice sounds. It provides information about the flow of air through the trachea and lungs and helps identify fluid, mucus, or obstruction in the respiratory system.

Begin auscultation with the patient sitting in an upright position. With the stethoscope pressed firmly against the chest wall (clothing can muffle sounds), instruct the patient to breathe slowly and deeply through an open mouth. (Breathing through the nose sets up turbulent sounds that are transmitted to the lungs.) Use a systematic approach, beginning at the lung apices and moving from side to side down through the intercostal spaces to the lung bases (Fig. 24.11). Avoid listening over bony

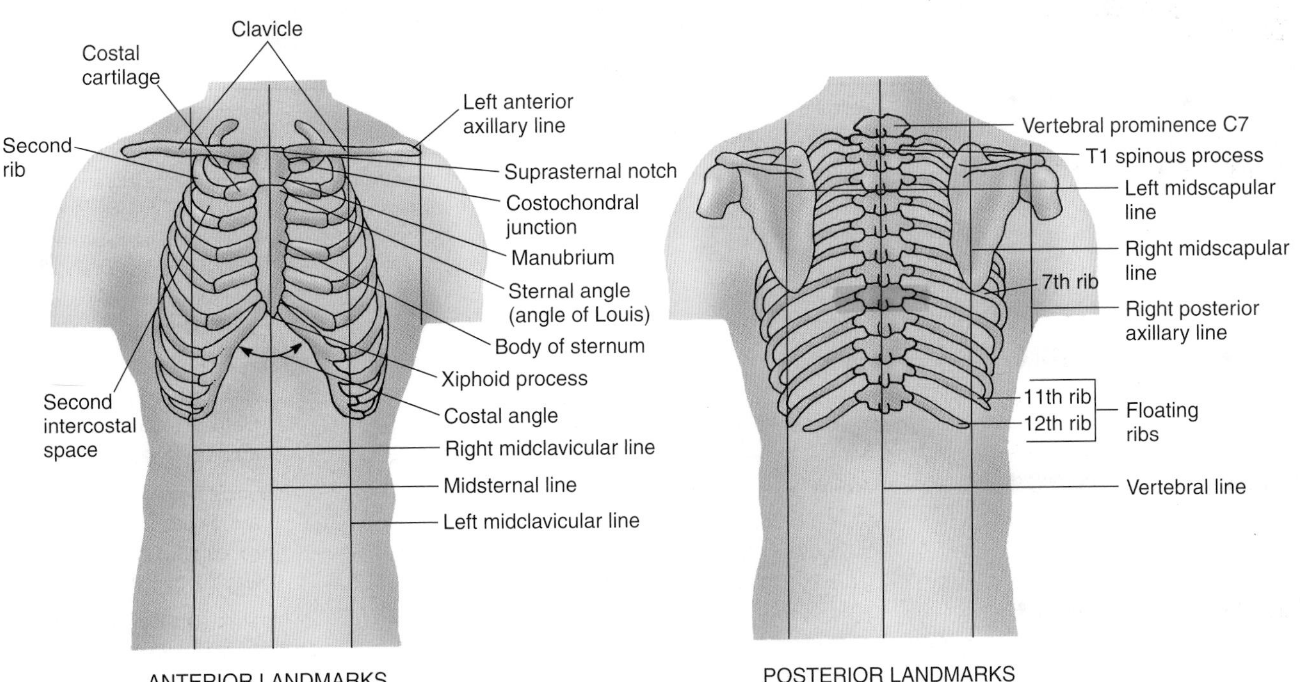

FIG. 24.9 Anterior and posterior chest landmarks.

structures. Listen to a full respiratory cycle, noting the quality and intensity of the breath sounds.

Normal breath sounds are produced as air vibrates while moving through the passages from the larynx to the alveoli. Breath sounds are identified by their location, intensity, pitch, and duration within the respiratory cycle (e.g., early or late inspiration and expiration). Normal breath sounds are known as "bronchial" or "tubular" (harsh hollow sounds heard over the trachea and mainstem bronchi), "bronchovesicular" (heard over the branching bronchi), and "vesicular" (soft rustling sounds heard in lung tissue over small bronchioles) (Table 24.4). Describe these sounds as *normal, increased, diminished,* or *absent.*

Bronchial breath sounds heard at the lung edges are abnormal and occur when the bronchial sounds are transmitted to an area of increased density, such as with atelectasis, tumor, or pneumonia. When heard in an abnormal location, bronchovesicular breath sounds may indicate normal aging or an abnormality such as consolidation and chronic airway disease.

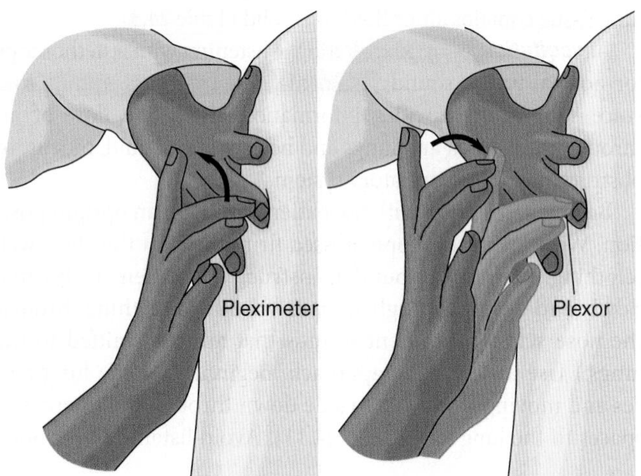

FIG. 24.10 Percussion technique.

Adventitious sounds are additional breath sounds along with normal sounds, and indicate pathologic changes in the lung. Table 24.5 describes adventitious sounds: crackle, wheeze, rhonchus, and pleural friction rub. These sounds vary in pitch, intensity, and duration, and can occur in any phase of the respiratory cycle. Document exactly what you hear on auscultation.

Voice sounds (vocal resonance) through the normally air-filled lung are muffled and unclear because sound vibrations travel poorly through air. These sounds become louder and more distinct when the sound travels through a solid tissue or liquid. The presence of pneumonia, atelectasis, pleural effusion, tumor, or abscess causes increased vocal resonance.

Other Indicators of Respiratory Adequacy. Assess other indicators of respiratory adequacy, because ***gas exchange*** affects all body systems. Some indicators (e.g., cyanosis) reflect immediate gas exchange and ***perfusion*** problems. Other changes (e.g., finger clubbing, weight loss) reflect long-term oxygenation problems.

Skin and mucous membrane changes (e.g., pallor, cyanosis) indicate inadequate ***gas exchange*** and ***perfusion***. Assess the nail beds and the mucous membranes of the oral cavity. Examine the fingers for clubbing (see Fig. 27.10), which indicates long-term hypoxia.

General appearance includes muscle development and general body build. Long-term respiratory problems lead to weight

TABLE 24.3 Characteristics of the Five Percussion Notes

Note	Pitch	Intensity	Quality	Duration	Findings
Resonance	Low	Moderate to loud	Hollow	Long	Resonance is characteristic of normal lung tissue.
Hyperresonance	Higher than resonance	Very loud	Booming	Longer than resonance	Hyperresonance indicates the presence of trapped air, so it is commonly heard over an emphysematous or asthmatic lung and occasionally over a pneumothorax.
Flatness	High	Soft	Extreme dullness	Short	An example location is the sternum. Flatness percussed over the lung fields may indicate a massive pleural effusion.
Dullness	Medium	Medium	Thudlike	Medium	Example locations are over the liver and the kidneys. Dullness can be percussed over an atelectatic lung or a consolidated lung.
Tympany	High	Loud	Musical, drumlike	Short	Examples are the cheek filled with air and the abdomen distended with air. Over the lung, a tympanic note usually indicates a large pneumothorax.

loss and a loss of general muscle mass. Arms and legs may appear thin or poorly muscled. Neck and chest muscles may be hypertrophied, especially in the patient with chronic obstructive pulmonary disease (COPD) (McCance et al., 2019).

Endurance decreases when breathing is inadequate for ***gas exchange***. Observe how easily the patient moves and whether he or she is short of breath while resting or becomes short of breath when walking 10 to 20 steps. Note how often the patient stops for breath between words while speaking.

Psychosocial Assessment

Breathing difficulty often induces anxiety either because of cerebral hypoxia or because the sensation of not getting enough air is

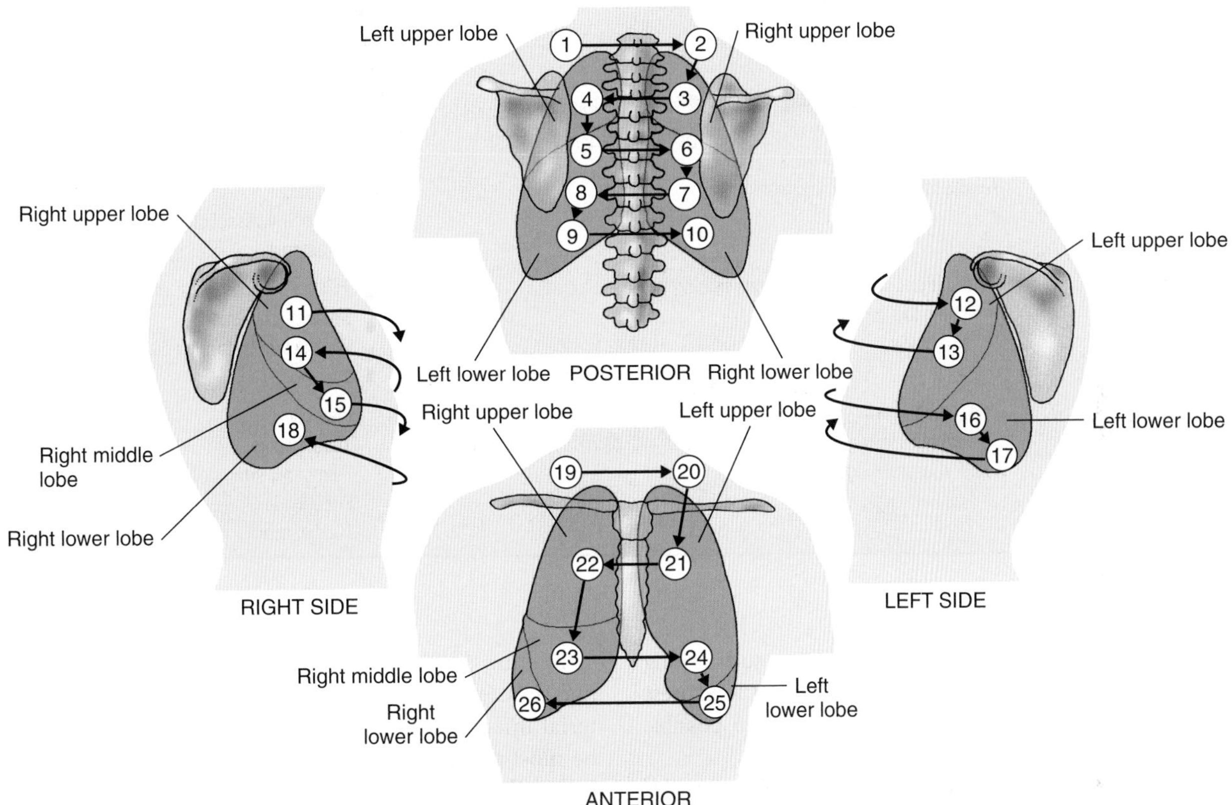

FIG. 24.11 Sequence for percussion and auscultation.

TABLE 24.4 Characteristics of Normal Breath Sounds

	Pitch	Amplitude	Duration	Quality	Normal Location
Bronchial (tubular, tracheal)	High	Loud	Inspiration < expiration	Harsh, hollow, tubular, blowing	Trachea and larynx
Bronchovesicular	Moderate	Moderate	Inspiration = expiration	Mixed	Over major bronchi where fewer alveoli are located; posterior, between scapulae (especially on right); anterior, around upper sternum in first and second intercostal spaces
Vesicular	Low	Soft	Inspiration > expiration	Rustling, like the sound of the wind in the trees	Over peripheral lung fields where air flows through smaller bronchioles and alveoli

From Jarvis, C. (2020). *Physical examination and health assessment* (8th ed.). St. Louis: Saunders.

TABLE 24.5 **Characteristics of Adventitious Breath Sounds**

Adventitious Sound	Character	Association
Fine crackles Fine rales High-pitched rales	Popping, discontinuous sounds caused by air moving into previously deflated airways; sounds like hair being rolled between fingers near the ear "Velcro" sounds late in inspiration usually associated with restrictive disorders	Asbestosis Atelectasis Interstitial fibrosis Bronchitis Pneumonia Chronic pulmonary diseases
Coarse crackles Low-pitched crackles	Lower-pitched, coarse, rattling sounds caused by fluid or secretions in large airways; likely to change with coughing or suctioning	Bronchitis Pneumonia Tumors Pulmonary edema
Wheeze	Squeaky, musical, continuous sounds associated with air rushing through narrowed airways; may be heard without a stethoscope Arise from the small airways Usually do not clear with coughing	Inflammation Bronchospasm (bronchial asthma) Edema Secretions Pulmonary vessel engorgement (as in cardiac "asthma")
Rhonchus (rhonchi)	Lower-pitched, coarse, continuous snoring sounds Arise from the large airways	Thick, tenacious secretions Sputum production Obstruction by foreign body Tumors
Pleural friction rub	Loud, rough, grating, scratching sounds caused by the inflamed surfaces of the pleura rubbing together; often associated with pain on deep inspirations Heard in lateral lung fields	Pleurisy Tuberculosis Pulmonary infarction Pneumonia Lung cancer

frightening. The thought of having a serious problem, such as lung cancer, can also induce anxiety. Encourage the patient to express his or her feelings and fears about symptoms and their possible meaning.

Chronic respiratory disease may cause changes in family roles or relationships, social isolation, financial problems, and unemployment or disability. Discuss coping mechanisms to assess the patient's reaction to these stressors and identify strengths. For example, the patient may react to stress with dependence on family members, withdrawal, or failure to adhere to interventions. Help the patient identify available support systems.

Diagnostic Assessment

Laboratory Assessment. The Laboratory Profile: Respiratory Assessment box lists common tests that are useful in assessing respiratory problems. A red blood cell (RBC) count provides data about oxygen transport. Hemoglobin, found in RBCs, transports oxygen to the tissues. A deficiency of hemoglobin could cause hypoxemia.

Arterial blood gas (ABG) analysis assesses ***gas exchange*** and ***perfusion*** as oxygenation (partial pressure of arterial oxygen [PaO_2]), alveolar ventilation (partial pressure of arterial carbon dioxide [$PaCO_2$]), and acid-base balance. Blood gas studies provide information for monitoring treatment results, adjusting oxygen therapy, and evaluating the patient's responses. See Chapter 14 for more details on blood gas analysis.

Sputum specimens can help identify organisms or abnormal cells. Sputum culture and sensitivity analyses identify bacterial infection and determine which specific antibiotics will be most effective. Cytologic examination can identify cancer cells. Allergic conditions may be identified by cytologic testing.

Imaging Assessment. *Chest x-rays* with digital images are used for patients with pulmonary problems to evaluate chest status and provide a baseline for comparison with future changes. These chest x-rays are performed from *posteroanterior* (PA; back-to-front) and left lateral (LL) positions.

Chest x-rays are used to assess lung pathology such as with pneumonia, atelectasis, pneumothorax, and tumor. They also can detect pleural fluid and the placement of an endotracheal tube or other invasive catheters. A computer-enhanced image can be adjusted to emphasize a specific area. However, these images have limitations and may appear normal, even when severe chronic bronchitis, asthma, or emphysema is present.

Sinus and facial x-rays are used to assess fluid levels in the sinus cavities to assist in the diagnosis of acute or chronic sinusitis.

Computed tomography (CT) assesses soft tissues with consecutive cross-sectional views of the entire chest. This type of imaging can verify the identity of a suspicious lesion or clot. CT scans may require a contrast agent injected IV to enhance the visibility of tumors, blood vessels, and heart chambers. Your role is to provide information to the patient and determine

LABORATORY PROFILE

Respiratory Assessment

Test	Normal Ranges (SI Units)	Significance of Changes From Normal
Blood Studies		
Complete Blood Count		
Red blood cells	*Females:* $4.2\text{-}5.4 \times 10^6$/mcL ($4.2\text{-}5.4 \times 10^{12}$ cells/L) *Males:* $4.7\text{-}6.1 \times 10^6$/mcL ($4.7\text{-}6.1 \times 10^{12}$ cells/L)	*Elevated levels* (polycythemia) are often related to the excessive production of erythropoietin in response to a chronic hypoxic state, as in COPD, and from living at a high altitude. *Decreased levels* indicate possible anemia, hemorrhage, or hemolysis.
Hemoglobin, total	*Females:* 12-16 g/dL (7.4 -9.9 mmol/L) *Males:* 14-18 g/dL (8,7-11.2 mmol/L)	Same as for red blood cells.
Hematocrit	*Females:* 37%-47% (0.37-0.47 volume fraction) *Males:* 42%-52%, or 0.42-0.52 volume fraction	Same as for red blood cells.
WBC count (leukocyte count, WBC count)	Total: 5,000-10,000/mm³, or $5\text{-}10 \times 10^9$/L	*Elevations* indicate possible acute infections or inflammations. *Decreased levels* may indicate an overwhelming infection, an autoimmune disorder, or immunosuppressant therapy.
Differential White Blood Cell (Leukocyte) Count		
Neutrophils	2500-8000/mm³, or 55%-70% of total, or $5\text{-}6.2 \times 10^9$/L	*Elevations* indicate possible acute bacterial infection (pneumonia), COPD, or inflammatory conditions (smoking). *Decreased levels* indicate possible viral disease (influenza).
Eosinophils	50-500/mm³, or 1%-4% of total, or $0.0\text{-}0.3 \times 10^9$/L	*Elevations* indicate possible COPD, asthma, or allergies. *Decreased levels* indicate pyogenic infections.
Basophils	15-50/mm³, or 0.5%-1% of total, or $0.02\text{-}0.05 \times 10^9$/L	*Elevations* indicate possible inflammation; seen in chronic sinusitis, hypersensitivity reactions. *Decreased levels* may be seen in an acute infection.
Lymphocytes	1000-4000/mm³, or 20%-40% of total, or $1.0\text{-}4.0 \times 10^9$/L	*Elevations* indicate possible viral infection, pertussis, and infectious mononucleosis. *Decreased levels* may be seen during corticosteroid therapy.
Monocytes	100-700/mm³, or 2%-8% of total, or $0.1\text{-}0.7 \times 10^9$/L	*Elevations:* see Lymphocytes; also may indicate active tuberculosis. *Decreased levels:* see Lymphocytes.
Arterial Blood Gases		
PaO_2	80-100 mm Hg *Older adults:* values may be lower	*Elevations* indicate possible excessive oxygen administration. *Decreased levels* indicate possible COPD, asthma, chronic bronchitis, cancer of the bronchi and lungs, cystic fibrosis, respiratory distress syndrome, anemias, atelectasis, or any other cause of hypoxia.
$Paco_2$	35-45 mm Hg	*Elevations* indicate possible COPD, asthma, pneumonia, anesthesia effects, or use of opioids (respiratory acidosis). *Decreased levels* indicate hyperventilation/respiratory alkalosis.
pH	*Up to 60 yr:* 7.35-7.45 *60-90 yr:* 7.31-7.42 *>90 yr:* 7.26-7.43	*Elevations* indicate metabolic or respiratory alkalosis. *Decreased levels* indicate metabolic or respiratory acidosis.
HCO_3^-	21-28 mEq/L (21-28 mmol/L)	*Elevations* indicate possible respiratory acidosis as compensation for a primary metabolic alkalosis. *Decreased levels* indicate possible respiratory alkalosis as compensation for a primary metabolic acidosis.
SpO_2	95%-100% *Older adults:* values may be slightly lower	*Decreased levels* indicate possible impaired ability of hemoglobin to release oxygen to tissues.

COPD, Chronic obstructive pulmonary disease; HCO_3^-, bicarbonate ion; *$Paco_2$,* partial pressure of arterial carbon dioxide; *Pao_2,* partial pressure of arterial oxygen; *Spo_2,* peripheral oxygen saturation; *WBC,* white blood cell.

Data from Pagana, K., & Pagana, T. (2018). *Mosby's manual of diagnostic and laboratory tests* (6th ed.). St. Louis: Elsevier.

whether he or she has any sensitivity to the contrast material. Ask the patient whether he or she has a known allergy to iodine or shellfish. In addition, IV contrast medium can be nephrotoxic. Ask about his or her kidney function and whether he or she takes drugs for type 2 diabetes. If the patient usually takes metformin, the drug is stopped at least 24 hours before contrast medium is used and is not restarted until adequate kidney function is confirmed (see Chapter 59).

Other Noninvasive Diagnostic Assessment

Pulse Oximetry. Pulse oximetry identifies hemoglobin saturation with oxygen. Usually hemoglobin is almost 100% saturated with oxygen in superficial tissues. The pulse oximeter uses a wave of infrared light and a sensor placed on the patient's finger, toe, nose, earlobe, or forehead (Fig. 24.12). Ideal normal pulse oximetry values are 95% to 100%. Normal values are a little lower in older patients and in those with dark skin. To avoid confusion with the Pao_2 values from arterial blood gases (ABGs), pulse oximetry readings are recorded as the Spo_2 (peripheral arterial oxygen saturation) or Sao_2.

Pulse oximetry can detect desaturation before symptoms (e.g., dusky skin, pale mucosa, pale or blue nail beds) occur. Causes for low readings include patient movement, hypothermia, decreased peripheral blood flow, ambient light (sunlight, infrared lamps), decreased hemoglobin, edema, and fingernail polish. When patients have any degree of impaired peripheral blood flow, the most accurate place to test oxygen saturation is on the forehead. Some brands of inexpensive portable oximeters have been shown to produce unreliable results in acutely ill patients compared with arterial blood sampling for Sao_2 and should not be used in patients who have known abnormal oxygen saturation values.

Results lower than 91% in an adult who does not have a chronic respiratory problem (and certainly below 86%) are an emergency and require immediate assessment and treatment. When the Spo_2 is below 85%, body tissues have a difficult time becoming oxygenated. An Spo_2 lower than 70% is usually life threatening, but in some cases values below 80% may be life threatening. Pulse oximetry is less accurate at lower values.

Capnometry and Capnography. Capnometry and capnography are methods that measure the amount of carbon dioxide present in exhaled air, which is an indirect measurement of arterial carbon dioxide levels. These noninvasive tests measure the partial pressure of end-tidal carbon dioxide ($PETco_2$, also known as $ETco_2$) levels in both intubated patients and those breathing spontaneously. With capnometry, the exhaled air sample is tested with a sensor that changes the CO_2 level into a color or number for analysis. With capnography, the CO_2 level is graphed as a specific waveform along with a number. These methods provide information about CO_2 production, pulmonary perfusion, alveolar ventilation, respiratory patterns, ventilator effectiveness, and possible rebreathing of exhaled air. Because capnography is a more sensitive indicator of ***gas exchange*** adequacy than pulse oximetry, it can be especially useful in early detection of respiratory depression. Fig. 24.12 shows the use of capnography equipment in a nonventilated patient.

The normal value of the partial-pressure of end-tidal carbon dioxide ($PETco_2$) ranges between 20 and 40 mm Hg. Changes in $PETco_2$ reflect changes in breathing effectiveness and ***gas exchange***. These changes occur before hypoxia can be detected using pulse oximetry because even in the presence of diseased lungs, carbon dioxide moves out of the body more easily than oxygen moves into it. The use of both pulse oximetry and $PETco_2$ for patients at risk for respiratory problems can provide information to direct early intervention.

Conditions that increase $PETco_2$ above normal levels are those that reflect inadequate ***gas exchange*** or an increase in cellular metabolism, both of which increase production of carbon dioxide (CO_2). Conditions of inadequate gas exchange include hypoventilation, partial airway obstruction, and rebreathing

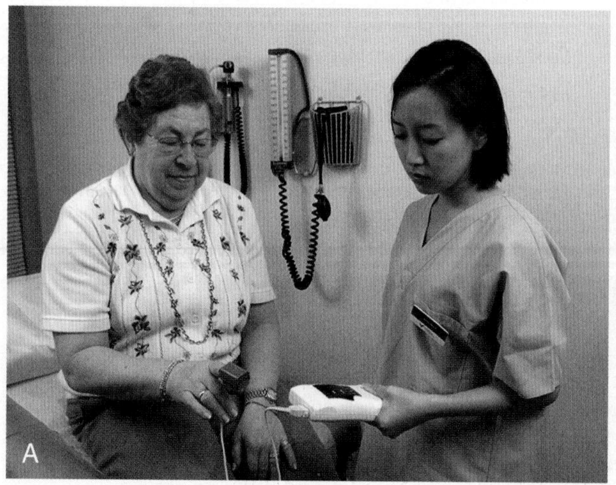

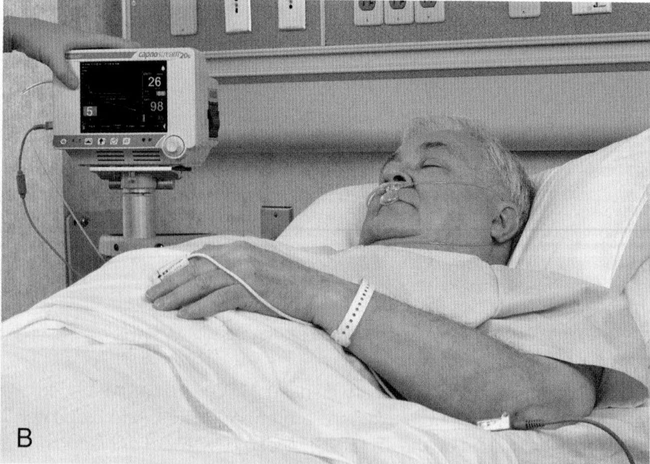

FIG. 24.12 (A) A typical pulse oximeter. (B) Typical capnography equipment without the use of an endotracheal tube. (A from Young, A. P., & Proctor, D. [2008]. *Kinn's the medical assistant: An applied learning approach* [10th ed.]. St. Louis: Saunders. B copyright ©2016 Medtronic. All rights reserved. Used with the permission of Medtronic.)

exhaled air. Conditions that increase cellular metabolism include fever, acidosis, and heavy exercise.

Conditions that decrease $PETco_2$ below normal levels are those that reflect poor pulmonary ventilation, such as pulmonary embolism, apnea, total airway obstruction, and malposition of an endotracheal tube. Other causes of low $PETco_2$ include hyperventilation not based on oxygen need, in which CO_2 is blown off faster than it is generated in the tissues. Cardiopulmonary arrest decreases $PETco_2$, and $PETco_2$ may be used to determine the effectiveness of cardiopulmonary resuscitation (CPR) and whether there is a spontaneous return of circulation.

Pulmonary Function Tests. Pulmonary function tests (PFTs) assess lung function and breathing problems. These tests measure lung volumes and capacities, flow rates, diffusion capacity, ***gas exchange***, airway resistance, and distribution of ventilation. The results are interpreted by comparing the patient's data with expected findings for age, gender, race, height, weight, and smoking status.

PFTs are useful in screening patients for lung disease even before the onset of symptoms. Repeated testing over time provides data that may be used to guide management (e.g., changes in lung function can support a decision to continue, change, or discontinue a specific therapy). Testing before surgery may identify patients at risk for lung complications after surgery. The most common reason for performing PFTs is to determine the cause of dyspnea. When performed while the patient exercises, PFTs help determine whether dyspnea is caused by lung problems or cardiac problems or by muscle weakness (Pagana & Pagana, 2018).

Patient Preparation. Explain the purpose of the tests and advise the patient not to smoke for 6 to 8 hours before testing. Depending on the reasons for testing, bronchodilator drugs may be withheld for 4 to 6 hours before the test. The patient with breathing problems often fears further breathlessness and is anxious before these "breathing" tests. Help reduce anxiety by describing what will happen during and after the testing.

Procedure. PFTs can be performed at the bedside or in the respiratory laboratory by a respiratory therapist or respiratory technician. The patient is asked to breathe through the mouth only. A nose clip is used to prevent air from escaping. The patient performs different breathing maneuvers while measurements are obtained. Table 24.6 describes the most commonly used PFTs and their uses.

Follow-up Care. Because many breathing maneuvers are performed during PFTs, assess the patient for increased dyspnea or bronchospasm after these studies. Document any drugs given during testing.

Exercise Testing. Exercise increases metabolism and increases gas transport because energy is used. Exercise testing assesses the patient's ability to work and perform ADLs, differentiates reasons for exercise limitation, evaluates disease influence on exercise capacity, and determines whether supplemental oxygen is needed during exercise. These tests are performed on a treadmill or bicycle or by a self-paced 12-minute walking test. Exercise in the patient with normal pulmonary function is limited by circulatory factors, whereas exercise in the pulmonary patient is limited by breathing capacity, ***gas exchange*** compromise, or both. Explain exercise testing, and assure the patient that he or she will be closely monitored by trained professionals throughout the test.

TABLE 24.6 Characteristics and Purposes of Pulmonary Function Tests

Test	Purpose
FVC (forced vital capacity) records the maximum amount of air that can be exhaled as quickly as possible after maximum inspiration.	Indicates respiratory muscle strength and ventilatory reserve. Reduced in obstructive and restrictive diseases.
FEV_1 (forced expiratory volume in 1 sec) records the maximum amount of air that can be exhaled in the first second of expiration.	Is effort dependent and declines normally with age. It is reduced in certain obstructive and restrictive disorders.
FEV_1/FVC is the ratio of expiratory volume in 1 sec to FVC.	Indicates obstruction to airflow. This ratio is the hallmark of obstructive pulmonary disease. It is normal or increased in restrictive disease.
$FEF_{25\%-75\%}$ records the forced expiratory flow over the 25%-75% volume (middle half) of the FVC.	This measure provides a more sensitive index of obstruction in the smaller airways.
FRC (functional residual capacity) is the amount of air remaining in the lungs after normal expiration. FRC test requires use of the helium dilution, nitrogen washout, or body plethysmography technique.	Increased FRC indicates hyperinflation or air trapping, often from obstructive pulmonary disease. FRC is normal or decreased in restrictive pulmonary diseases.
TLC (total lung capacity) is the amount of air in the lungs at the end of maximum inhalation.	Increased TLC indicates air trapping from obstructive pulmonary disease. Decreased TLC indicates restrictive disease.
RV (residual volume) is the amount of air remaining in the lungs at the end of a full, forced exhalation.	RV is increased in obstructive pulmonary disease such as emphysema.
DLCO (diffusion capacity of the lung for carbon monoxide) reflects the surface area of the alveolocapillary membrane. The patient inhales a small amount of CO, holds for 10 sec, and then exhales. The amount inhaled is compared with the amount exhaled.	Is reduced whenever the alveolocapillary membrane is diminished (emphysema, pulmonary hypertension, and pulmonary fibrosis). It is increased with exercise and in conditions such as polycythemia and heart disease.

Other Invasive Diagnostic Assessment

Endoscopic Examinations. Endoscopic studies to assess breathing problems include bronchoscopy, laryngoscopy, and mediastinoscopy. With *laryngoscopy*, a tube for visualization is inserted into the larynx to assess the function of the vocal cords, remove foreign bodies caught in the larynx, or obtain tissue samples for biopsy or culture. A *mediastinoscopy* is the insertion of a flexible tube through the chest wall just above the sternum into the area between the lungs. It is performed in the operating room with the patient under general anesthesia to examine for the presence of tumors and obtain tissue samples for biopsy or culture. Most complications are related to the anesthetic agents and bleeding. The most common procedure is bronchoscopy.

Bronchoscopy is the insertion of a tube in the airways as far as the secondary bronchi to view airway structures and obtain tissue samples. It is used to diagnose and manage pulmonary diseases. Rigid bronchoscopy usually requires general anesthesia in the operating room. Flexible bronchoscopy can be performed in the ICU or a special endoscopy suite with low-dose sedation. It is used to evaluate the airway and to help with placing or changing an endotracheal tube, collecting specimens, and diagnosing infections. It is often used for lung cancer staging and removal of secretions that are not cleared with normal suctioning. Stents can be placed during bronchoscopy to open up strictures in the trachea and bronchus.

Patient Preparation. Explain the procedure to the patient and verify that consent for the procedure was obtained. Expected outcomes, risks, and benefits of the procedure must be discussed with the patient by the primary health care provider performing the procedure. Document patient allergies. Other tests before the procedure may include a complete blood count, platelet count, prothrombin time, electrolytes, and chest x-ray. The patient is NPO for 4 to 8 hours before the procedure to reduce the risk for aspiration. Premedication with one of the benzodiazepines may be used to provide both sedation and amnesia. Opioids may also be used.

> **! NATIONAL PATIENT SAFETY GOALS**
>
> In accordance with The Joint Commission's National Patient Safety Goals, verify the patient's identity with *two* types of identifiers (name and at least one person-specific number such as birth date, medical record number, or social security number) before a bronchoscopy.

Benzocaine spray as a topical anesthetic to numb the oropharynx is used cautiously, if at all. This agent may induce a condition called **methemoglobinemia**, which is the conversion of normal hemoglobin to methemoglobin. Methemoglobin is an altered iron state that does not carry oxygen, resulting in tissue hypoxia. Other topical anesthetic sprays, such as lidocaine, are less likely to induce this problem.

The normal blood level of methemoglobin is less than 1%. When this level increases, tissue ***gas exchange*** is reduced. Cyanosis occurs with methemoglobin levels between 10% and 20%, and death can occur when levels reach 50% to 70%. Suspect methemoglobinemia if a patient becomes cyanotic after receiving a topical anesthetic, if he or she does not respond to supplemental oxygen, and if blood is a characteristic chocolate-brown in color. It can be reversed with oxygen and IV injection of 1% methylene blue (1 to 2 mg/kg).

> **! NURSING SAFETY PRIORITY (QSEN)**
>
> ***Critical Rescue***
>
> Assess patients who receive a benzocaine topical anesthetic to the oropharynx to recognize indications of methemoglobinemia. These include cyanosis that is unresponsive to oxygen therapy and chocolate-brown–colored blood. If either of these symptoms is present, respond by initiating the Rapid Response Team.

Procedure. The procedure can be done in a bronchoscopy suite or at the ICU bedside. The bronchoscope is inserted through either the naris or the oropharynx. Maintain IV access and continuously monitor the patient's pulse, blood pressure, respiratory rate, and oxygen saturation. Apply supplemental oxygen.

Follow-up Care. Monitor the patient until the effects of the sedation have resolved and a gag reflex has returned. Continue to monitor vital signs, including oxygen saturation, and assess breath sounds every 15 minutes for the first 2 hours. Also assess for potential complications, including bleeding, infection, or hypoxemia.

Thoracentesis. **Thoracentesis** is the needle aspiration of pleural fluid or air from the pleural space for diagnostic or management purposes. Microscopic examination of the pleural fluid helps in making a diagnosis. Pleural fluid may be drained to relieve blood vessel or lung compression and the respiratory distress caused by cancer, empyema, pleurisy, or tuberculosis. Drugs can also be instilled into the pleural space during thoracentesis.

Patient Preparation. Patient preparation is essential before thoracentesis to ensure cooperation during the procedure and prevent complications. Tell the patient to expect a stinging sensation from the local anesthetic agent and a feeling of pressure when the needle is pushed through the posterior chest. Stress the importance of not moving, coughing, or deep breathing during the procedure to avoid puncture of the pleura or lung.

Ask the patient about any allergy to local anesthetic agents. Verify that he or she has signed an informed consent. The entire chest or back is exposed, and the hair on the skin over the aspiration site is clipped if necessary. The site depends on the volume and location of the fluid.

Fig. 24.13 shows the best position for thoracentesis, which widens the spaces between the ribs and permits easy access to the pleural fluid. Properly position and physically support the patient during the procedure. Use pillows to make the patient comfortable and to provide physical support. When the sitting position is used for the procedure, stand in front of the patient to prevent the table from moving and the patient from falling.

Procedure. Thoracentesis is often performed at the bedside by a nurse practitioner or a physician, although CT or ultrasound

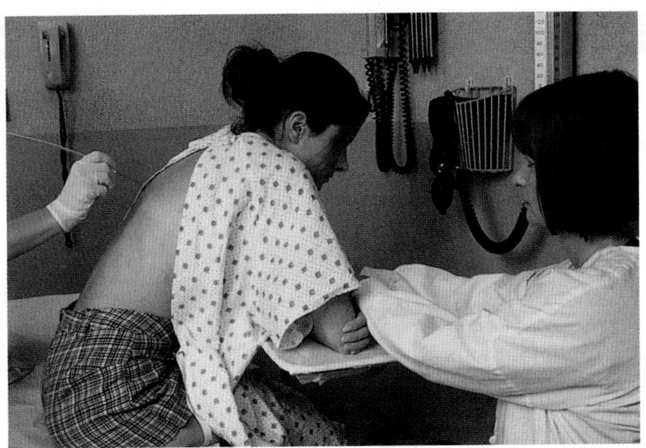

FIG. 24.13 Position for thoracentesis. (From Harkreader, H., Hogan, M. A., & Thobaben, M. [2007]. *Fundamentals of nursing: Caring and clinical judgment* [3rd ed.]. Philadelphia: Saunders.)

may be used to guide it. The person performing the procedure and any assistants wear goggles and masks to prevent accidental eye or oral splash exposure to the pleural fluid. After the skin is prepped, a local anesthetic is injected into the selected site. Keep the patient informed of the procedure while observing for shock, pain, nausea, pallor, diaphoresis, cyanosis, tachypnea, and dyspnea.

The short 18- to 25-gauge thoracentesis needle (with an attached syringe) is advanced into the pleural space. Fluid in the pleural space is slowly aspirated with gentle suction. A vacuum collection bottle may be needed to remove larger volumes of fluid. To prevent re-expansion pulmonary edema, usually no more than 1000 mL of fluid is removed at one time. If a biopsy is performed, a second, larger needle with a cutting edge and collection chamber is used. After the needle is withdrawn, pressure is applied to the puncture site, and a sterile dressing is applied. In some cases, a drainage catheter may be left in place to a water-seal drainage system, rather than doing a thoracentesis aspiration on a recurring basis.

Follow-up Care. After thoracentesis, a chest x-ray is performed to rule out possible pneumothorax and **mediastinal shift** (shift of central thoracic structures toward one side). Monitor vital signs, and listen to the lungs for absent or reduced sounds on the affected side. Check the puncture site and dressing for leakage or bleeding. Assess for complications, such as reaccumulation of fluid in the pleural space, subcutaneous emphysema, infection, and tension pneumothorax. Urge the patient to breathe deeply to promote lung expansion. Document the procedure, including the patient's response; the volume and character of the fluid removed; any specimens sent to the laboratory; the location of the puncture site; and respiratory assessment findings before, during, and after the procedure.

Subcutaneous emphysema is the presence of air in the tissue layers of the skin and usually is seen as skin swelling around the puncture site. Air in these tissues makes a crackling sound when pressure is applied to it. The presence of subcutaneous emphysema may indicate a persistent air leak caused by a puncture that tears the pleura. When confined to a small area, the leak may not require treatment. However, when the affected area increases to include the neck tissues, the patient's airway could be affected.

Teach the patient about the symptoms of a *pneumothorax* (partial or complete collapse of the lung), which can occur within the first 24 hours after a thoracentesis. Symptoms include:

- Pain on the affected side that is worse at the end of inhalation and the end of exhalation
- Rapid heart rate
- Rapid, shallow respirations
- A feeling of air hunger
- Prominence of the affected side that does not move in and out with respiratory effort
- Trachea slanted more to the unaffected side instead of being in the center of the neck
- New onset of "nagging" cough
- Cyanosis

Instruct the patient to go to the nearest emergency department immediately if these symptoms occur.

Lung Biopsy. A lung biopsy is performed to obtain tissue for histologic analysis, culture, or cytologic examination. The samples are used to make a definitive diagnosis of inflammation, cancer, infection, or lung disease. There are several types of lung biopsies. The site and extent of the lesion determine which one is used. Transbronchial biopsy (TBB) and transbronchial needle aspiration (TBNA) are performed during bronchoscopy. Transthoracic needle aspiration is performed through the skin (percutaneous) for areas that cannot be reached by bronchoscopy.

Patient Preparation. The patient may worry about the outcome of the biopsy and may associate the term *biopsy* with *cancer*. Explain what to expect before and after the procedure, and explore the patient's feelings. An analgesic or sedative may be prescribed before the procedure. Inform the patient undergoing percutaneous biopsy that discomfort is reduced with a local anesthetic agent but that pressure may be felt during needle insertion and tissue aspiration. Open lung biopsy is performed in the operating room with the patient under general anesthesia, and the usual preparations before surgery apply (see Chapter 9).

Procedure. Percutaneous lung biopsy is usually performed in the radiology department after an informed consent has been obtained. Fluoroscopy or CT is used to visualize the

NCLEX EXAMINATION CHALLENGE 24.3

Safe and Effective Care Environment

When assessing the client 2 hours after a thoracentesis, the nurse notes the skin around the puncture site is swollen and a crackling is felt and heard when pressure is applied to the area. What is the nurse's **best** action?

A. Assess the client's SpO_2 levels at two separate sites.
B. Obtain a prescription to culture the site.
C. Document the finding as the only action.
D. Notify the respiratory health care provider.

CLINICAL JUDGMENT CHALLENGE 24.1

Patient-Centered Care; Safety

The client is a 37-year-old man with a diagnosis of pneumonia. He reports that he has felt more tired than usual for several days but only noticed a breathless sensation this morning. He has had a chronic cough for years and noted that it is worse today. During the nurse's admission assessment, he reports that he is a two-pack per day smoker but recently converted to an e-cigarette in an effort to quit smoking because he believes it is a healthier alternative. He lives with his wife, a former smoker. Other client information the nurse collects is below.

Client History

- Has high a high blood cholesterol level and hypertension
- Takes lisinopril 20 mg orally each morning
- Takes atorvastatin 20 mg orally each evening
- Lives with his wife, a former smoker, in an affluent suburban neighborhood
- Is an attorney in a large law firm
- Plays golf twice weekly
- Has two school-aged children
- Last "flu shot" was 10 years ago

Current Assessment

- Oral temperature = 102.6°F (39.2°C)
- Apical pulse = 120 beats/min; respiratory rate = 28 breaths/min
- Blood pressure = 138/84
- Oxygen saturation by pulse oximetry = 90%
- Productive cough

Laboratory Findings

- Hemoglobin (Hgb) = 18 g/dL
- Hematocrit (Hct) = 45%
- WBCs = 13,000/mm^3
- Total cholesterol = 198 mg/dL
- Low-density lipoprotein = 102 mg/dL

1. **Recognize Cues:** What assessment information in this client situation is the most important and immediate concern for the nurse? (Hint: Identify the **relevant** information *first* to determine what is most important.)
2. **Analyze Cues:** What client conditions are consistent with the **most relevant** information? (Hint: Think about priority collaborative problems that support and contradict the information presented in this situation.)

area and guide the procedure. The patient is usually placed in the side-lying position, depending on the location of the lesion. The skin is cleansed with an antiseptic agent, and a local anesthetic is given. Under sterile conditions, a spinal-type needle is inserted through the skin into the desired area, and tissue is obtained for microscopic examination. A dressing is applied after the procedure. A CT scan or chest x-ray must follow the biopsy to confirm that there is no pneumothorax.

An open-lung biopsy is performed in the operating room. The patient undergoes a thoracotomy in which lung tissue is exposed and appropriate tissue specimens are taken. A chest tube is placed to remove air and fluid so the lung can reinflate, and then the chest is closed.

Follow-up Care. Monitor the patient's vital signs and breath sounds at least every 4 hours for 24 hours and assess for signs of respiratory distress (e.g., dyspnea, pallor, diaphoresis, tachypnea). Pneumothorax is a serious complication of needle biopsy and open-lung biopsy. Report reduced or absent breath sounds immediately. Monitor for hemoptysis (which may be scant and transient) or, in rare cases, for frank bleeding from vascular or lung trauma.

GET READY FOR THE NEXT-GENERATION NCLEX® EXAMINATION!

Key Points

Review these Key Points for each NCLEX Examination Client Needs Category.

Safe and Effective Care Environment

- Assess any patient's geographic, home, occupational, and recreational exposure to inhalation irritants. **QSEN: Safety**
- Document any known specific allergies that have respiratory symptoms. **QSEN: Safety**
- Assess the patient's respiratory status every 15 minutes for at least the first 2 hours after he or she undergoes an endoscopic test for respiratory disorders. **QSEN: Safety**

Health Promotion and Maintenance

- Teach the older adult about the effects of aging on the respiratory system. **QSEN: Patient-Centered Care**
- Encourage all adults to use protective masks and adequate ventilation to reduce or prevent particulate matter exposure in the presence of inhalation irritants. **QSEN: Evidence-Based Practice**
- Promote smoking cessation for adults who smoke. **QSEN: Patient-Centered Care**

Psychosocial Integrity

- Allow the patient the opportunity to express fear or anxiety about tests of respiratory function or about a potential change in respiratory function. **QSEN: Patient-Centered Care**

Physiological Integrity

- Ask the patient about respiratory problems in any other members of the family because some problems have a genetic component. **QSEN: Patient-Centered Care**
- Ask the patient about current and past drug use (prescribed, over-the-counter, and illicit), and evaluate drug use for potential lung damage. **QSEN: Patient-Centered Care**

- Ask about current and past nicotine use in any form and calculate the pack-year smoking history for the patient who smokes or who has ever smoked cigarettes. **QSEN: *Patient-Centered Care***
- Distinguish between normal and abnormal (adventitious) breath sounds. **QSEN: Patient-Centered Care**
- Interpret arterial blood gas (ABG) values to assess the patient's respiratory status. **QSEN: Patient-Centered Care**
- Assess the degree to which breathing problems interfere with the patient's ability to perform ADLs. **QSEN: Patient-Centered Care**
- Assess the airway and breathing effectiveness for any patient who has shortness of breath or any change in mental status. **QSEN: Evidence-Based Practice**
- Teach patients and caregivers about what to expect during tests and procedures to assess respiratory function and respiratory disease. **QSEN: Patient-Centered Care**
- Explain nursing care needs for the patient after bronchoscopy or open lung biopsy. **QSEN: Patient-Centered Care**

MASTERY QUESTIONS

1. Which respiratory side effect does the nurse teach the client who is now prescribed an angiotensin-converting enzyme (ACE) inhibitor to expect?
   A. Wheezing on exertion
   B. Increased secretions
   C. Persistent dry cough
   D. Orthopnea

2. While responding to questions in a health history, the client reports that he usually expectorates about 2 ounces of thin, clear, colorless sputum daily, usually on getting up in the morning. What is the nurse's best action related to this finding?
   A. Document the report as the only action.
   B. Arrange for the client to have tuberculosis testing.
   C. Collect a sputum specimen for laboratory analysis.
   D. Alert the primary health care provider about this funding.

REFERENCES

Asterisk (*) indicates a classic or definitive work on this subject.

American Lung Association. (2018). *E-cigarettes and lung health.* www.lung.org/stop-smoking/smoking-facts/e-cigarettes-and-lung-health.html?referrer=https://www.google.com.

Campbell, M. (2017). Dyspnea. *Critical Care Nursing Clinics of North America, 29*(4), 461–470.

Centers for Disease Control and Prevention (CDC). (2018a). *About three in ten US veterans use tobacco products: Veterans use tobacco at much higher rates than most non-veterans.* https://www.cdc.gov/media/releases/2018/p0111-tobacco-use-veterans.html.

Centers for Disease Control and Prevention (CDC). (2018b). *Fact Sheet: Current cigarette smoking among adults in the United States.* www.cdc.gov/tobacco/data_statistics/fact_sheets/adult_data/cig_smoking/index.htm.

Centers for Disease Control and Prevention (CDC). (2019). *Outbreak of lung injury associated with the use of e-cigarette, or vaping, products.* https://www.cdc.gov/tobacco/basic_information/e-cigarettes/severe-lung-disease.html.

*Hooley, J. (2015). Decoding the oxyhemoglobin dissociation curve. *American Nurse Today, 10*(1), 18–23.

Hua, M., & Talbot, P. (2016). Potential health effects of electronic cigarettes: A systematic review of case reports. *Preventive Medicine Reports, 4,* 169–178.

Jarvis, C. (2020). *Physical examination & health assessment* (8th ed.). St. Louis: Elsevier.

Keating, S. (2016). Presurgical tobacco cessation counseling. *American Journal of Nursing, 116*(3), 11.

McCance, K., Huether, S., Brashers, V., & Rote, N. (2019). *Pathophysiology: The biologic basis for disease in adults and children* (8th ed.). St. Louis: Mosby.

Middleton, C., & Bruns, D. (2019). Improving screening and education for secondhand smoke exposure in primary care settings. *American Journal of Nursing, 119*(8), 51–57.

Olmedo, P., Goessler, W., Tanda, S., Grau-Perez, M., Jarmul, S., Aherrera, A., Chen, R., Hilpert, M., Cohen, J., Navas-Acien, A., & Rule, A. (2018). Metal concentrations in e-cigarette liquid and aerosol samples: The contribution of metallic coils. *Environmental Health Perspectives, 126*(2). 027010-1–027010-11 Https://doi.org/10.1289/EHP2175.

Pagana, K., & Pagana, T. J. (2018). *Mosby's manual of diagnostic and laboratory tests* (6th ed.). St. Louis: Elsevier.

*Paranzino, G. K., Butterfield, P., Nastoff, T., & Ranger, C. (2005). I Prepare Development and clinical utility of an environmental exposure history mnemonic. *American Association of Occupation Health Nurses Journal, 53*(1), 37–42.

Simerson, D., & Hackbarth, D. (2018). Emergency nurse implementation of the brief smoking-cessation intervention: Ask, advise, and refer. *Journal of Emergency Nursing, 44*(3), 242–248.

Touhy, T., & Jett, K. (2020). *Ebersole and Hess' toward healthy aging: Human needs & nursing response* (9th ed.). St. Louis: Mosby.

*U.S. Department of Health and Human Services, Public Health Service. (2008). *Treating tobacco use and dependence: 2008 update.* https://www.ahrq.gov/professionals/clinicians-providers/guidelines-recommendations/tobacco/index.html.

U.S. Fire Administration. (2017). *Electronic cigarette fires and explosions in the united states 2009 - 2016.* https://www.usfa.fema.gov/downloads/pdf/publications/electronic_cigarettes.pdf.

Wetter, V. (2017). Educating patients on smoking cessation success. *Medsurg Nursing, 26*(6), 417–418.

Zborovskaya, Y. (2017). E-cigarettes and smoking cessation: A primer for oncology clinicians. *Clinical Journal of Oncology Nursing, 21*(1), 54–63.

25

Concepts of Care for Patients Requiring Oxygen Therapy or Tracheostomy

Harry Rees

http://evolve.elsevier.com/Iggy/

LEARNING OUTCOMES

1. Collaborate with the interprofessional team to coordinate high-quality, evidence-based care and promote ***gas exchange*** in patients requiring oxygen therapy or tracheostomy.
2. Teach the patient and caregiver(s) about how oxygen therapy or tracheostomy affects home safety.
3. Identify community resources for patients requiring oxygen therapy or tracheostomy to maintain ***gas exchange***.
4. Implement patient- and family-centered nursing interventions to help people cope with the psychosocial impact caused by the need for oxygen therapy or tracheostomy.
5. Apply knowledge of anatomy, physiology, and pathophysiology to assess patients with respiratory problems affecting ***gas exchange*** who require oxygen therapy or tracheostomy.
6. Use clinical judgment and appropriate techniques to administer prescribed oxygen therapy and provide tracheostomy care to promote ***gas exchange*** and prevent ***infection***.

KEY TERMS

anatomic dead space Places in the airways where air flows but the structures are too thick for ***gas exchange***.

hypercarbia Increased partial pressure of arterial carbon dioxide ($Paco_2$) levels.

hypoxemia Low levels of oxygen in the blood.

hypoxia Decreased tissue oxygenation.

oxygen concentrator (oxygen extractor) A machine that removes nitrogen from room air, increasing oxygen levels to more than 90%.

tracheostomy The tracheal *stoma* (opening) in the neck that results from the tracheotomy.

tracheotomy The surgical incision into the trachea to create an airway to help maintain ***gas exchange***.

PRIORITY AND INTERRELATED CONCEPTS

The priority concept for this chapter is:
- ***Gas Exchange***

The interrelated concepts for this chapter are:
- ***Tissue Integrity***
- ***Infection***

Many respiratory and cardiac problems can reduce ***gas exchange*** as an acute or chronic issue. For these problems, respiratory support with oxygen therapy with or without tracheostomy can promote adequate ***gas exchange*** and tissue perfusion.

OXYGEN THERAPY

Overview

Oxygen (O_2) is both an atmospheric gas and a drug. It is prescribed whenever health problems cause **hypoxemia** (low levels of oxygen in the blood) and **hypoxia** (decreased tissue oxygenation) in a patient who is breathing atmospheric air with an oxygen concentration of 21%. In addition to respiratory and cardiac problems, conditions that can increase the need for oxygen therapy include fever, sepsis, and anemia, which either increase oxygen demand or reduce the oxygen-carrying capacity of the blood.

Ideally, oxygen therapy uses the lowest *fraction of inspired oxygen (Fio_2)* to have an acceptable blood oxygen level without causing harmful side effects. *Although oxygen improves the Pao_2 level, it does not cure the cause of the problem.* Most patients with hypoxia require an oxygen flow of 2 to 4 L/min via nasal cannula or up to 40% via Venturi mask to achieve an oxygen saturation of at least 95%. For a patient who is hypoxemic and has chronic **hypercarbia** (increased partial pressure of arterial carbon dioxide [$Paco_2$] levels), the Fio_2 delivered is adjusted to correct the hypoxemia and achieve generally acceptable oxygen saturations in the range of 88% to 92% (Siela & Kidd, 2017).

Interprofessional Collaborative Care

Oxygen therapy is used in any setting. Most patients are prescribed oxygen therapy through their primary health care provider without first having been hospitalized.

Assessment: Recognize Cues

Arterial blood gas (ABG) analysis is the best measure to determine the need for oxygen therapy and to evaluate its effects. Oxygen need is also determined through noninvasive monitoring, such as pulse oximetry and capnography.

Interventions: Take Action

You must be knowledgeable about oxygen hazards before starting oxygen therapy and while caring for a patient receiving oxygen therapy. Always know the rationale and the expected outcome of oxygen therapy for each patient prescribed to receive oxygen. Follow the guidelines listed in the Best Practice for Patient Safety & Quality Care: Oxygen Therapy box.

Hazards and Complications of Oxygen Therapy

Combustion. Oxygen enhances combustion so fire burns better in its presence, but it does not burn or explode. For example, when the oxygen content of the air around a lighted cigarette is nearly 50%, the entire cigarette flames up, and nearby items can catch fire. Open fires, even small ones such as candles or cigarettes, are not to be in the same room during oxygen therapy. Post an "oxygen in use" sign on the door of the patient's room. Smoking is prohibited in the patient's room, including at home, when oxygen is in use.

BEST PRACTICE FOR PATIENT SAFETY & QUALITY CARE (QSEN)

Oxygen Therapy

- Check the prescription for the type of delivery system and liter flow or percentage of oxygen to be applied.
- Use humidification if oxygen is being delivered at 4 L/min or higher.
- Be sure the equipment is functioning properly.
- Check the skin around the patient's ears, back of the neck, and face every 4 to 8 hours for pressure points and signs of irritation and impaired ***tissue integrity***.
- Provide mouth care every 8 hours and as needed; assess nasal and oral membranes for cracks or other signs of dryness or impaired ***tissue integrity***.
- Pad the elastic band and change its position often to prevent skin breakdown.
- Clean the cannula or mask by rinsing with clear, warm water every 4 to 8 hours or as needed. Clean skin under the tubing, straps, and mask every 4 to 8 hours or as needed.
- Lubricate the patient's nostrils, face, and lips with nonpetroleum cream to relieve the drying effects of oxygen.
- Position the tubing so it does not pull on the patient's face, nose, or artificial airway.
- Ensure that there is no smoking and that no other sources of sparks or flames (e.g., candles or matches) are used in the immediate area.
- Assess and document the patient's response to oxygen therapy.
- Avoid hypoxia or hyperoxia.
- Ensure that the patient has an adequate oxygen source during any periods of transport.
- Collaborate with the respiratory therapist for optimum management.

Ensure that all electrical equipment in rooms where oxygen is in use are grounded (have three prongs) and are plugged into grounded outlets to prevent fires from electrical arcing sparks. Frayed cords are not used because they can spark and ignite a flame. Flammable solutions (containing high concentrations of alcohol or oil) are not used in rooms in which oxygen is in use. (This restriction does not include alcohol-based hand rubs.) Surgical fires in the operating room, although rare, occur when an ignition source (e.g., cautery or lasers) are used in the presence of a fuel source and an oxidizer (oxygen or nitrous oxide). Improvements have been made by limiting the oxygen-rich atmosphere (without causing hypoxia) and minimizing the exposure to flammable pharmaceutical agents such as large volumes of alcohol-based skin preparation liquids.

Oxygen Toxicity. Oxygen toxicity is related to the concentration of oxygen delivered, duration of oxygen therapy, and degree of lung disease present. A continuous oxygen level greater than 50% for more than 24 to 48 hours may injure the lung and reduce ***tissue integrity***. Excess tissue oxygen levels increase the concentration of damaging substances known as reactive oxygen species (ROS), which are oxygen free radicals that can combine with most cellular elements and induce oxidative stress (McCance et al., 2019; Siela & Kidd, 2017). Such stress can cause cell damage and cell death.

The causes and indications of lung injury from oxygen toxicity are the same as those for acute respiratory distress syndrome (ARDS) (see Chapter 29). Symptoms start with dyspnea, nonproductive cough, chest pain beneath the sternum, GI upset, and crackles on auscultation. As exposure to high levels of oxygen continues, problems become more severe, with decreased vital capacity, decreased compliance, and hypoxemia. Continued prolonged exposure to high oxygen levels leads to atelectasis, pulmonary edema, hemorrhage, and hyaline membrane formation. Surviving oxygen toxicity depends on correcting the underlying disease process and decreasing the oxygen amount delivered.

The toxic effects of oxygen are difficult to manage, and prevention is a priority. The lowest level of oxygen needed to maintain ***gas exchange*** and prevent oxygen toxicity is prescribed. Monitor prescribed arterial blood gases (ABGs) during oxygen therapy and notify the respiratory health care provider when Pa_{O_2} levels become greater than 90 mm Hg. Also monitor the prescribed oxygen level and length of therapy to identify patients at risk. The use of noninvasive positive airway pressure techniques with oxygen or the use of mechanical ventilation (see Chapter 29) may reduce the amount of oxygen needed. As soon as the patient's condition allows, the prescribed amount of oxygen is decreased.

Absorptive Atelectasis. Normally nitrogen in the air maintains patent airways and alveoli. Making up 79% of room air, nitrogen prevents alveolar collapse. When high oxygen levels are delivered, nitrogen is diluted, oxygen diffuses from the alveoli into the blood, and the alveoli collapse. Collapsed alveoli

! NURSING SAFETY PRIORITY (QSEN)

Action Alert

Monitor the patient receiving high levels of oxygen closely to recognize indications of absorptive atelectasis (new onset of crackles and decreased breath sounds) every 1 to 2 hours when oxygen therapy is started and as often as needed thereafter.

cause *absorptive atelectasis,* which is detected as crackles and decreased breath sounds on auscultation.

Drying of the Mucous Membranes. When the prescribed oxygen flow rate is higher than 4 L/min, humidify the delivery system to prevent tissue injury and loss of ***tissue integrity*** (Fig. 25.1). Ensure that oxygen bubbles through the water in the humidifier.

Oxygen can also be humidified via a large-volume jet nebulizer in mist form *(aerosol).* A heated nebulizer raises the humidity even more and is used for oxygen delivery through an artificial airway. Usually the upper airway passages warm and humidify the air during breathing, but these passages are bypassed with an artificial airway, such as an endotracheal tube.

For the patient to receive humidified oxygen, the humidifier or nebulizer must have a sufficient amount of sterile water, and the flow rate must be adequate. Condensation often forms in the tubing and can be a source of ***infection***. Remove condensation as it collects by disconnecting the tubing and emptying the water. Minimize the time the tubing is disconnected because the patient does not receive oxygen during this period. Some humidifiers and nebulizers have a water trap that hangs from the tubing so condensation can be drained without disconnecting. Check the water level and change the humidifier as needed, especially when the water is cloudy or contains particles.

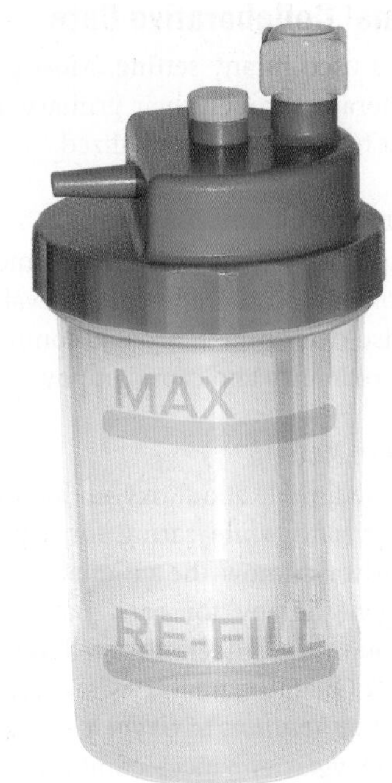

FIG. 25.1 A bubble humidifier bottle used with oxygen therapy.

! NURSING SAFETY PRIORITY QSEN

Action Alert

Assess the tubing system used for oxygen delivery to recognize buildup of condensation. Respond by draining condensation. To prevent bacterial contamination of the oxygen delivery system and prevent ***infection,*** never drain the fluid from the tubing or water trap back into the humidifier or nebulizer.

Infection. The humidifier or nebulizer may be a source of bacteria and fungus, increasing the risk for ***infection***. Oxygen delivery equipment such as cannulas and masks can also harbor organisms. Change equipment per agency policy, which ranges from every 24 hours for humidification systems to every 7 days or whenever necessary for cannulas and masks.

NCLEX EXAMINATION CHALLENGE 25.1

Physiological Integrity

Which statements about oxygen and oxygen therapy are true? **Select all that apply.**

A. An oxygen concentrator reduces the amount of carbon dioxide in atmospheric air.
B. Clients must provide informed consent to receive oxygen therapy.
C. Excessive oxygen use is a contributing cause of chronic obstructive pulmonary disease.
D. In nonemergency situations, a health care provider's prescription is needed for oxygen therapy.
E. Oxygen can explode when handled improperly.
F. Oxygen is a beneficial element but can harm lung tissue.
G. The liquid form of oxygen is a drug to manage hypoxia, whereas the gaseous form is only an atmospheric element.
H. Unless humidity is added, therapy with oxygen dries the upper and lower mucous membranes.

Oxygen Delivery Systems. Oxygen can be delivered by many systems with different indications, advantages, and disadvantages. Use the equipment properly and ensure appropriate equipment maintenance. Consult with a respiratory therapist whenever there is a question or concern about an oxygen delivery system. The type of delivery system used depends on:

- Required oxygen concentration
- Oxygen concentration that can be achieved by a specific delivery system
- Importance of accuracy and control of the oxygen concentration
- Patient comfort
- Use of humidity
- Patient mobility

Oxygen delivery systems are classified by the rate of oxygen delivery as either low-flow or high-flow systems. Low-flow systems deliver a lower fraction of inspired oxygen (FiO_2). These devices do not supply the total oxygen volume because the oxygen is diluted as the patient breathes room air. The total level of oxygen inspired depends on respiratory rate and breathing pattern. High-flow systems have a flow rate designed to supply the total oxygen volume by adjusting the amount of room air that is entrained within the delivery system. These systems are used for critically ill patients and when delivery of precise levels of oxygen is needed.

If the patient needs a mask but is able to eat, request an order for a nasal cannula to be used at mealtimes only. Reapply the mask after the meal is completed. To increase mobility, up to 50 feet of connecting tubing can be used with connecting pieces, although long tubing can be a safety issue for patients who are unsteady while ambulating.

Low-Flow Oxygen Delivery Systems. Low-flow systems include the ordinary nasal cannula, simple facemask, partial

TABLE 25.1 Comparison of Low-Flow Oxygen Delivery Systems

FiO_2 Delivered	Nursing Considerations
24%-40% FiO_2 at 1-6 L/min ≈ 24% at 1 L/min ≈ 28% at 2 L/min ≈ 32% at 3 L/min ≈ 36% at 4 L/min ≈ 40% at 5 L/min ≈ 44% at 6 L/min	Ensure that prongs are in the nares properly to prevent hypoxemia and skin breakdown with loss of ***tissue integrity***. Apply water-soluble jelly to nares PRN to reduce mucosal irritation from the drying effect of oxygen therapy. Assess the patency of the nostrils to detect conditions that prevent effective oxygen delivery such as congestion or a deviated septum. Assess the patient for changes in respiratory rate and depth because these changes reflect how well oxygen is being delivered.
40%-60% FiO_2 at 5-8 L/min; flow rate must be set at least at 5 L/min to flush mask of carbon dioxide ≈ 40% at 5 L/min ≈ 45%-50% at 6 L/min ≈ 55%-60% at 8 L/min	Be sure that mask fits securely over nose and mouth because a poorly fitting mask reduces the FiO_2 delivered. Assess skin and provide skin care to the area covered by the mask because pressure and moisture under it can cause loss of ***tissue integrity***. Monitor the patient closely for risk for aspiration because the mask limits the patient's ability to clear the mouth, especially if vomiting occurs. Provide emotional support to the patient who feels claustrophobic *to decrease anxiety and increase acceptance of the device.* Suggest to the respiratory health care provider to switch the patient from a mask to the nasal cannula during eating *to promote **gas exchange** while eating.*
60%-75% at 6-11 L/min, a liter flow rate high enough to maintain reservoir bag two-thirds full during inspiration and expiration	Make sure that the reservoir does not twist or kink, which results in a deflated bag that can decrease the amount of oxygen delivered and increases rebreathing of exhaled air. Adjust the flow rate to keep the reservoir bag inflated *to meet the patient's oxygen needs.*
80%-95% FiO_2 at a liter flow high enough to maintain reservoir bag two-thirds full	Interventions as for partial rebreather mask; this patient requires close monitoring *to ensure proper functioning of the device.* Make sure that valves and rubber flaps are patent, functional, and not stuck. Valves must open during exhalation and close during inhalation to prevent dramatic decrease in FiO_2, which could lead to suffocation. Closely assess the patient on increased FiO_2 via nonrebreather mask to determine whether the patient's oxygen needs are adequately met or if intubation is needed.

FiO_2, Fraction of inspired oxygen.

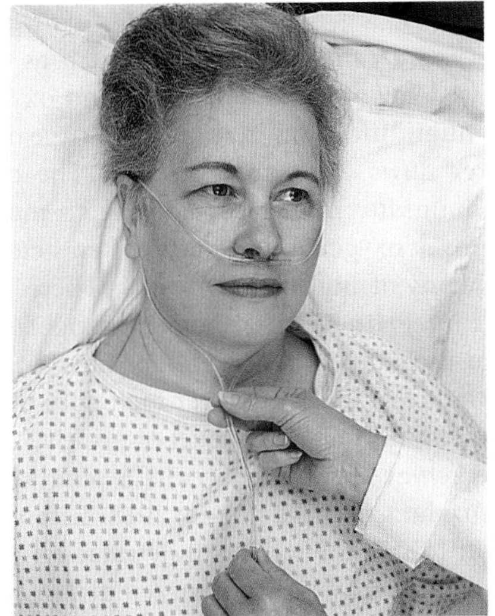

FIG. 25.2 An ordinary (low-flow) nasal cannula (prongs).

rebreather mask, and nonrebreather mask (Table 25.1). These systems are easy to use and fairly comfortable, but the amount of oxygen delivered varies and depends on the patient's breathing pattern. The oxygen is diluted with room air, which lowers the amount actually inspired.

Nasal Cannula. The nasal cannula (prongs) (Fig. 25.2) is used at flow rates of 1 to 6 L/min. Oxygen concentrations of 24% (at 1 L/min) to 44% (at 6 L/min) can be achieved. Flow rates greater than 6 L/min do not increase ***gas exchange*** because the **anatomic dead space** (places in the airways where air flows but the structures are too thick for gas exchange) is full. High flow rates also increase mucosal irritation and injury to ***tissue integrity***.

The nasal cannula is often used for chronic lung disease and for any patient needing long-term oxygen therapy. Place the nasal prongs in the nostrils, with the openings facing the patient, following the natural anatomic curve of the nares.

Facemasks. Facemasks can deliver a wide range of oxygen flow rates and concentrations.

Simple facemasks are used to deliver oxygen concentrations of 40% to 60% for short-term oxygen therapy or in an emergency (Fig. 25.3). A minimum flow rate of 5 L/min is needed to prevent rebreathing of exhaled air. Ensure that the mask fits well to maintain inspired oxygen levels. Care for the skin under the mask and strap to prevent breakdown.

Partial rebreather masks provide oxygen concentrations of 60% to 75% with flow rates of 6 to 11 L/min. These masks have a reservoir bag but no flaps (Fig. 25.4). With each breath, the patient rebreathes one-third of the exhaled tidal volume, which is still high in oxygen and increases the fraction of inspired

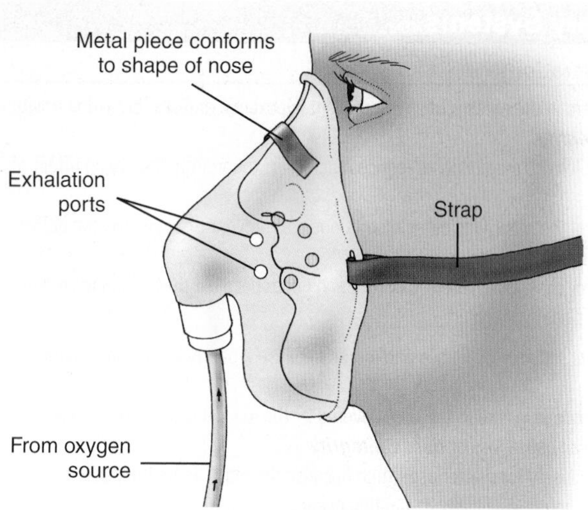

FIG. 25.3 A simple facemask used to deliver oxygen.

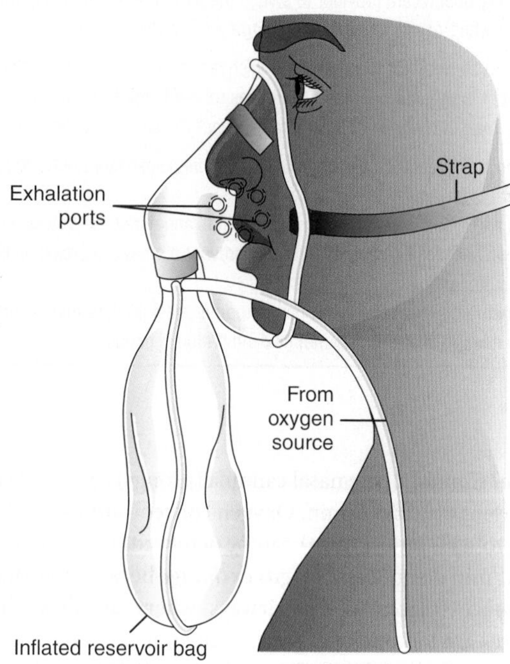

FIG. 25.4 A partial rebreather mask.

oxygen (FiO_2). For best oxygen delivery, be sure that the bag remains slightly inflated at the end of inspiration. If needed, call the respiratory therapist for assistance.

Nonrebreather masks provide the highest oxygen level of the low-flow systems and can deliver an FiO_2 greater than 90%, depending on the patient's breathing pattern. This mask is often used with patients whose respiratory status is unstable and who may require intubation.

The nonrebreather mask has a one-way valve between the mask and the reservoir and usually has two flaps over the exhalation ports (Fig. 25.5). The valve allows the patient to draw all needed oxygen from the reservoir bag, and the flaps prevent room air from entering through the exhalation ports (which would dilute the oxygen concentration). During exhalation, air leaves through these exhalation ports while the one-way valve prevents exhaled air from re-entering the reservoir bag. The flow rate is kept high (10 to 15 L/min) to keep the bag inflated during inhalation. Assess for this safety feature at least hourly.

! NURSING SAFETY PRIORITY (QSEN)

Critical Rescue

Check to ensure that the valve and flaps on a nonrebreather mask are intact and functional during each breath. If the flaps or valve should fail, the patient would inhale room air and exhaled CO_2 with each breath, which decreases oxygen delivery. Ensure that the reservoir does not fully deflate so that the full volume of gas is available with each breath.

NCLEX EXAMINATION CHALLENGE 25.2

Safe and Effective Care Environment

The SpO_2 of a client receiving oxygen therapy by nasal cannula at 6 L/min has dropped from 94% an hour ago to 90%. Which action does the nurse perform **first** to improve gas exchange before reporting the change to the primary health care provider?

A. Tighten the straps on the nasal cannula
B. Increase the oxygen flow rate to 8 L/min
C. Check the tubing for kinks, leaks, or obstructions
D. Check to determine whether the oxygen delivery system is adequately humidified

High-Flow Oxygen Delivery Systems. High-flow systems (Table 25.2) include the Venturi mask, aerosol mask, face tent, high-flow nasal cannula (HFNC), tracheostomy collar, and T-piece. These devices deliver an accurate oxygen level when properly fitted, with oxygen concentrations from 24% to 100% at 8 to 15 L/min.

High-flow nasal cannulas (HFNCs), such as Vapotherm, are widely used for better temperature and oxygen control along with humidification. A precise FiO_2 can be maintained at liter flows of 30 to 60 L/min. The combination of heat and humidity minimizes damage to mucous membranes, improves oxygenation, and is often better tolerated than other forms of high-flow systems. There may be less loss of ***tissue integrity*** because there is no tight-fitting mask to cause skin breakdown. Some studies have suggested that better secretion clearance and lower incidence of respiratory infections occur and that a low level of positive airway pressure may be achieved, which recruits alveoli and increases end-expiratory lung volume (Dries, 2018; Lamb et al., 2018; Nishimura, 2015). The FiO_2 and flow rates can be adjusted independently and may achieve an actual FiO_2 close to the predicted FiO_2 (see the Evidence-Based Practice box). Use pulse oximetry to adjust the HFNC to patient response. Fig. 25.6 shows the workings of HFNCs.

Venturi masks (Ventimasks) deliver the most accurate oxygen concentration without intubation. They work by pulling in a proportional amount of room air for each liter flow of oxygen. An adapter is located between the bottom of the mask and the

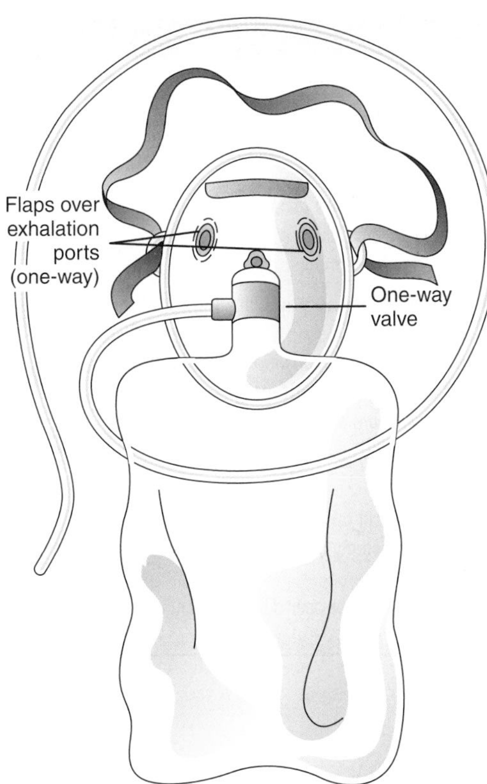

FIG. 25.5 A nonrebreather mask.

oxygen source (Fig. 25.7). Adapters with holes of different sizes allow specific amounts of air to mix with the oxygen, resulting in more precise delivery of oxygen. Each adapter requires a different flow rate. For example, to deliver 24% of oxygen, the flow rate must be 4 L/min. Another type of Venturi mask has one adapter with a dial that is used to select the amount of oxygen desired.

Other high-flow systems are used to provide high humidity with oxygen delivery. A dial on the humidity source regulates the delivered oxygen level. A face tent fits over the chin, with the top extending halfway across the face. Although the oxygen level delivered varies, the face tent is useful for patients who have facial trauma or burns. An aerosol mask is used when high humidity is needed. The tracheostomy collar is used to deliver high humidity and the desired oxygen to the patient with a tracheostomy. A special adapter (the *T-piece*) is used to deliver any desired FiO_2 to the patient with a tracheostomy, laryngectomy, or endotracheal tube (Fig. 25.8). Adjust the flow rate so the aerosol appears on the exhalation side of the T-piece.

Noninvasive Positive-Pressure Ventilation. Noninvasive positive-pressure ventilation (NPPV) is a type of noninvasive ventilation (NIV). This technique uses positive pressure to keep alveoli open and improve ***gas exchange*** without the dangers of intubation. It is used to manage dyspnea, hypercarbia, and acute exacerbations of chronic obstructive pulmonary disease (COPD), cardiogenic pulmonary edema, and acute asthma attacks. Although NPPV prevents the complications associated with intubation, including ventilator-associated pneumonia (VAP) and other ventilator-associated events (VAEs), it still has risks and complications. Masks must fit tightly to form a proper seal, which can lead to loss of ***tissue integrity*** with skin breakdown over the nose or face. Full face masks cause fewer skin problems than do nasal-oral masks. Leaks can cause uncomfortable pressure around the eyes, and gastric insufflation can lead to vomiting and the potential for aspiration. Thus NPPV is recommended only for use in alert patients who have the ability to protect their airway, although a nasogastric (NG) tube may still be required for safety.

EVIDENCE-BASED PRACTICE

Is High-Flow Nasal Cannula Equal to Noninvasive Ventilation for Preventing Postextubation Respiratory Failure?

Hernandez, G., Vaquero, C., Colina, L., Cuena, R., Gonzalez, P., Canabal, A., et al. (2016). Effect of postextubation high-flow nasal cannula vs noninvasive ventilation on reintubation and postextubation respiratory failure in high risk patients: A randomized clinical trial. *JAMA: The Journal of the American Medical Association, 316*(15), 1565–1574.

Respiratory failure after extubation, especially in high-risk patients, places those patients at increased risk for complications and prolonged ICU and hospital stays. Noninvasive ventilation (NIV) can reduce the need for reintubation in high-risk patients with postextubation respiratory failure. However, high-flow nasal cannula (HFNC) oxygen has some advantages, including comfort, lower cost, ability to clear secretions, and ability to communicate compared with other forms of NIV. This study sought to determine if HFNC oxygen delivery was equal to NIV for high-risk patients with postextubation respiratory failure. Some of the high-risk factors for reintubation include age above 65 years, Acute Physiology and Chronic Health Evaluation (APACHE) score greater than 12 points, a body mass index (BMI) greater than 30, moderate-to-severe chronic obstructive pulmonary disease (COPD), mechanical ventilation for longer than 7 days, and heart failure as the primary indication for mechanical ventilation. Patients also had to have more than one comorbidity. The primary outcome was reintubation within 72 hours. HFNC was equal to NIV in this study but some limitations were noted. There is no validated model to predict extubation failure. No other studies were available that reported the reintubation rates of high-risk patients who were treated with HFNC oxygen therapy. The study could not be blinded, so bias could not be completely excluded.

Level of Evidence: 1

This was a multicenter randomized controlled trial (RCT).

Commentary: Implications for Practice and Research

HFNC oxygen therapy can be used to effectively manage postextubation respiratory failure in high-risk patients. Those patients treated with HFNC tolerated the therapy better, ***tissue integrity*** was maintained, and patients retained the ability to communicate effectively. Although NIV can be effective in preventing reintubation, it is important to consider the least invasive methods and the ones with the fewest disadvantages that still produce the desired outcomes. In general, HFNC oxygen delivery appears better tolerated than continuous positive airway pressure (CPAP) or bi-level positive airway pressure (BiPAP), but more research into patient comfort and satisfaction with HFNC are needed. As part of the interprofessional health team, nurses may be able to identify potential candidates, such as those who are very anxious or who have some degree of claustrophobia, who would benefit from this form of oxygen therapy.

TABLE 25.2 Comparison of High-Flow Oxygen Delivery Systems

Fio_2 Delivered	Nursing Considerations
24%-50% Fio_2 with flow rates as recommended by the manufacturer, usually 4-10 L/min; provides high humidity	Perform constant surveillance *to ensure an accurate flow rate for the specific Fio_2.* Keep the orifice for the Venturi adapter open and uncovered *because the adapter does not function when the orifice is covered and oxygen delivery varies.* Provide a mask that fits snugly and tubing that is free of kinks *because these conditions can reduce Fio_2.* Assess the patient for dry mucous membranes *to ensure patient comfort.* Change to a nasal cannula during mealtime *to ensure continued oxygen therapy while eating.*
24%-100% Fio_2 with flow rates of at least 10 L/min; provides high humidity	Assess that aerosol mist escapes from the vents of the delivery system during inspiration and expiration *to ensure humidification is adequate.* Empty condensation from the tubing *because preventing condensation buildup promotes an adequate flow rate, ensures a continued prescribed Fio_2, and helps prevent* ***infection****.* Change the aerosol water container as needed *to ensure adequate humidification.*
24%-100% Fio_2 with flow rates of at least 10 L/min; provides high humidity	Empty condensation from the tubing *to prevent it from interfering with flow rate delivery of Fio2 or draining into the tracheostomy.* Keep the exhalation port open and uncovered *to prevent patient suffocation.* Position the T-piece so it does not pull on the tracheostomy or endotracheal tube, *which can cause pain and loss of* ***tissue integrity****.* Make sure the humidifier creates enough mist. A mist should be seen during inspiration and expiration *to demonstrate an adequate flow rate.*

Fio_2, Fraction of inspired oxygen.

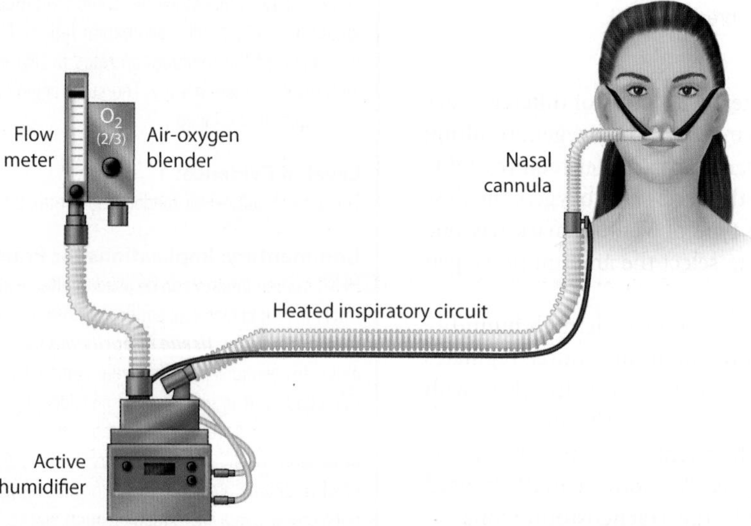

FIG. 25.6 An example of a high-flow nasal cannula oxygen delivery system.

NPPV can deliver oxygen or may use just room air. A nasal mask, nasal pillows, or full-face mask delivery system allows mechanical delivery. The three most common modes of delivery for NPPV are (1) continuous positive airway pressure (CPAP), which delivers a set positive airway pressure throughout each cycle of inhalation and exhalation; (2) volume-limited or flow-limited, which delivers a set tidal volume with the patient's inspiratory effort; and (3) pressure-limited, which includes pressure support, pressure control, and bi-level positive airway pressure (BiPAP), which cycles different pressures at inspiration and at expiration.

For BiPAP, a cycling machine delivers a set inspiratory positive airway pressure each time the patient begins to inspire. As he or she begins to exhale, the machine delivers a lower set end-expiratory pressure. Together, these two pressures improve tidal volume, can reduce respiratory rate, and may relieve dyspnea.

For CPAP, the effect is to open collapsed alveoli. Patients who may benefit from this form of oxygen or air delivery include those with atelectasis after surgery, those with cardiac-induced pulmonary edema, and those with COPD. It is not helpful for patients with respiratory failure following extubation. CPAP and BiPAP are both commonly used after extubation to prevent respiratory failure and the need for reintubation. However, the use of a high-flow nasal cannula (HFNC) has shown promise as an alternative without some of the limitations of NPPV. HFNC

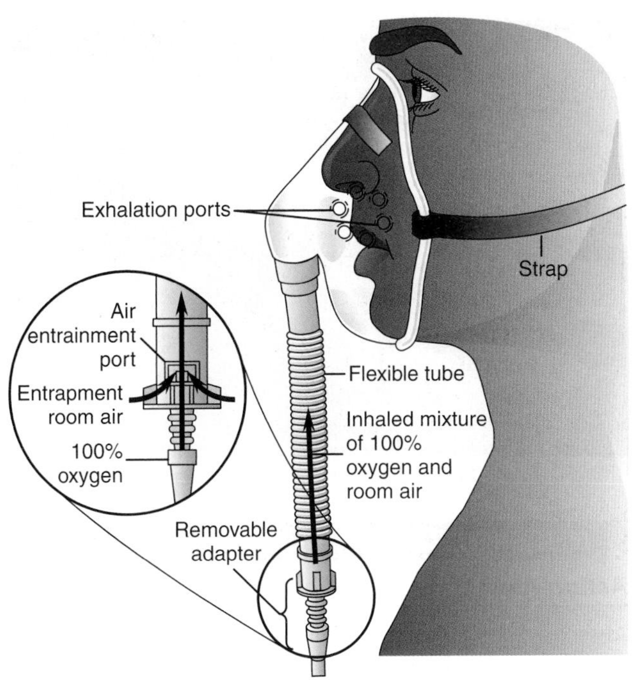

FIG. 25.7 A Venturi mask for precise oxygen delivery.

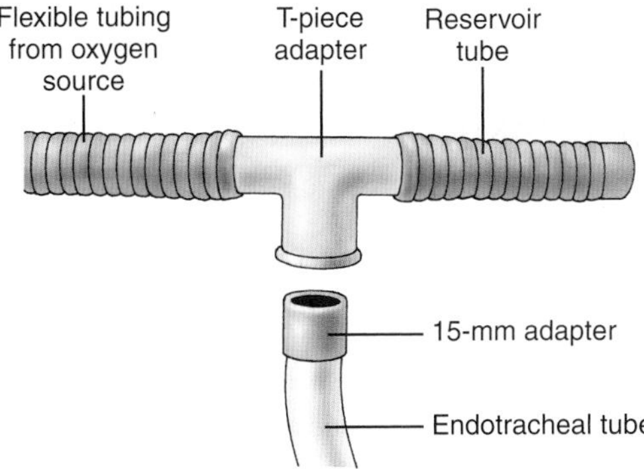

FIG. 25.8 A T-piece apparatus for attachment to an endotracheal or tracheostomy tube.

improves the patient's ability to effectively clear secretions and communicate with the health care team. NPPV is used in palliative care to relieve dyspnea, including for those patients with "do-not-intubate" requests. However, this practice is controversial. The Society of Critical Care Medicine recommends discussing goals and expected outcomes with the patient and family before initiating therapy.

NPPV is used commonly for sleep apnea. The effect is to hold open the upper airways (Fig. 25.9). Patients using CPAP or BiPAP at home for sleep apnea often bring their home equipment to the hospital. They feel more comfortable using their own equipment. The reasons for using NPPV remain when the patient enters the hospital, and the need continues while hospitalized.

The number of patients using NPPV therapy is increasing in every setting. Nurses caring for the patient with NPPV must be knowledgeable about the equipment, technique, and potential complications. Respiratory therapy support can help safely manage a patient receiving NPPV.

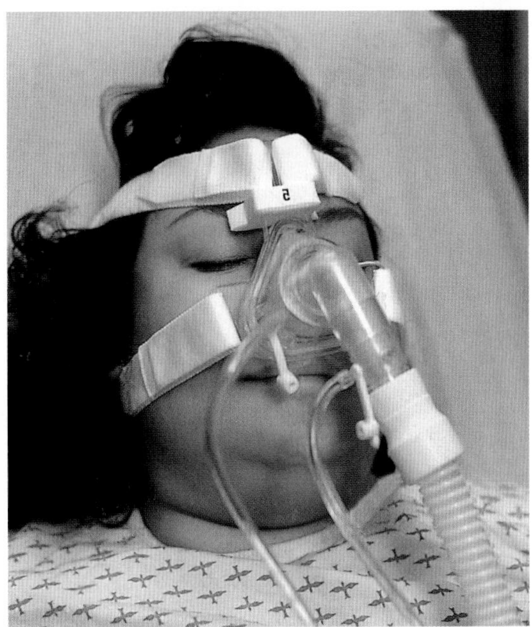

FIG. 25.9 Nasal continuous positive airway pressure (CPAP).

Transtracheal Oxygen Therapy. Transtracheal oxygen (TTO) is a long-term method of delivering oxygen directly into the lungs. A small, flexible catheter is passed into the trachea through a small incision with the patient under local anesthesia. TTO reduces loss of ***tissue integrity*** from nasal prongs and is less visible. A TTO team provides patient education, including the purpose of TTO and care of the catheter. Different flow rates are prescribed for rest and for activity. A flow rate also is prescribed for the nasal cannula, which is used when the TTO catheter is being cleaned.

Care Coordination and Transition Management

Home Care Management. The patient must be stable before home oxygen is considered. For Medicare to cover the cost of home oxygen therapy, the patient must have severe hypoxemia defined as a partial pressure of arterial oxygen (Pao_2) level of less than 55 mm Hg or arterial oxygen saturation (Spo_2) of less than 88% on room air and at rest. The criteria vary when hypoxemia is caused by nonpulmonary problems or when oxygen is needed only at night or with exercise.

Self-Management Education. When home oxygen therapy is prescribed, begin a teaching plan about it. In collaboration with the respiratory therapist teach the patient and family about the equipment needed for home oxygen therapy and the safety aspects of using and maintaining the equipment. Equipment may include oxygen source, delivery devices, and humidity sources. Work with the discharge planner to help the patient select a durable medical equipment (DME) company to deliver oxygen equipment and select a community health nursing agency for follow-up care in the home. Re-evaluation of the need for oxygen therapy occurs on a periodic basis.

While providing discharge planning and teaching, be sensitive to the patient's emotional adjustment to oxygen therapy. Encourage the patient to share feelings and concerns. He or

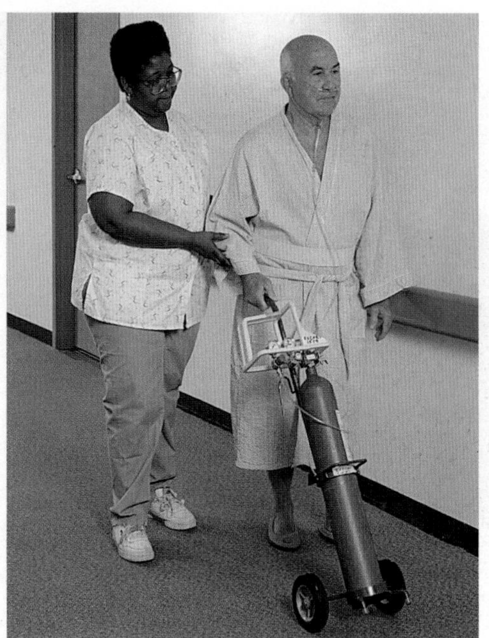

FIG. 25.10 Small E size oxygen tank (cylinder) for portability.

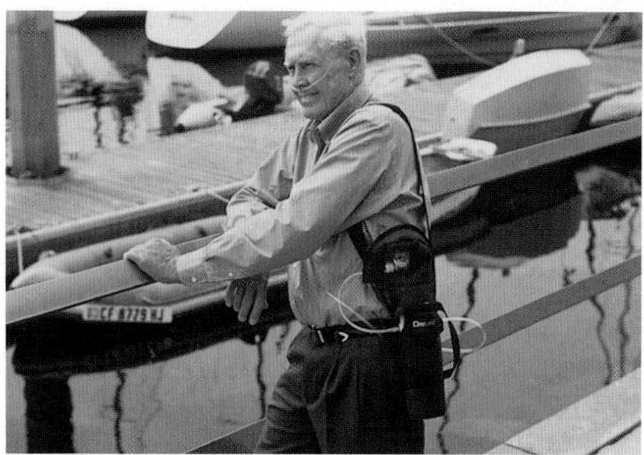

FIG. 25.11 Portable liquid oxygen.

she may be concerned about social acceptance. Help him or her realize that adherence to oxygen therapy is important for being able to participate in ADLs and other events that bring enjoyment.

Home Care Preparation. Home oxygen therapy is provided in one of three ways: compressed gas in a tank or a cylinder, liquid oxygen in a reservoir, or an oxygen concentrator. Compressed gas in an oxygen tank (green) is the most often used oxygen source. The large H cylinder may be used as a stationary source, and the smaller E tank is available for transporting the patient (Fig. 25.10). Even smaller cylinders are available for the patient to carry. Teach the patient and family to check the gauge daily to assess the amount of oxygen left in the tank. As a safety precaution, the tanks must always be in a stand or rack. A tank that is accidentally knocked over could suddenly decompress and move around in an uncontrolled manner.

Liquid oxygen for home use is oxygen gas that has been liquefied. A concentrated amount of oxygen is available in a lightweight and easy-to-carry container similar to a Thermos bottle (Fig. 25.11). This portable tank is filled from a large stationary liquid vessel. Liquid oxygen lasts longer than gaseous oxygen but is more expensive. Patient satisfaction with these units is high, and mobility is less affected (Mussa et al., 2018).

The **oxygen concentrator** or *oxygen extractor* is a machine that removes nitrogen from room air, increasing oxygen levels to more than 90%. This stationary device is the least expensive system and does not need to be filled. Portable units, similar in size and weight to small portable liquid oxygen bottles, are now available and are very convenient (Fig. 25.12). The high cost of these portable units (beginning at $2000) limits their acceptance and use.

Regardless of the type of oxygen delivery system used, review safety issues with the patient and all family members.

! NURSING SAFETY PRIORITY QSEN

Action Alert

Assess the patient's and caregivers' knowledge of oxygen therapy to recognize any deficiencies. Respond by providing safety information and stressing the importance of not smoking where oxygen is in use. *Teach the patient and all family members that smoking materials, candles, gas burners, and fireplaces (and other open flames) are not to be used in the same room in which oxygen is being used.*

TRACHEOSTOMY

Overview

Tracheotomy is the surgical incision into the trachea to create an airway to help maintain ***gas exchange***. **Tracheostomy** is the tracheal *stoma* (opening) in the neck that results from the tracheotomy. A tracheotomy can be an emergency procedure or a scheduled surgery. Tracheostomies can be temporary or permanent. Indications for tracheostomy include acute airway obstruction, the need for airway protection, laryngeal or facial trauma or burns, and airway involvement during head or neck surgery. They also are used for prolonged unconsciousness, paralysis, or the inability to be weaned from mechanical ventilation. With temporary tracheostomies, the nurse is key in evaluating patient readiness for progression toward decannulation (removal of the tracheostomy tube).

❖ Interprofessional Collaborative Care

The initial tracheotomy to form a tracheostomy is usually performed in an acute care setting. When the tracheostomy is permanent, care of the patient often occurs in the home, long-term care, and community settings.

INTERPROFESSIONAL COLLABORATION

The Patient With a Tracheostomy

Care for the patient requiring long-term tracheostomy is best when a team approach is used. In addition to the nurse, interprofessional team members often include the primary health care provider, respiratory therapist, registered dietitian nutritionist, discharge planner, and social worker.

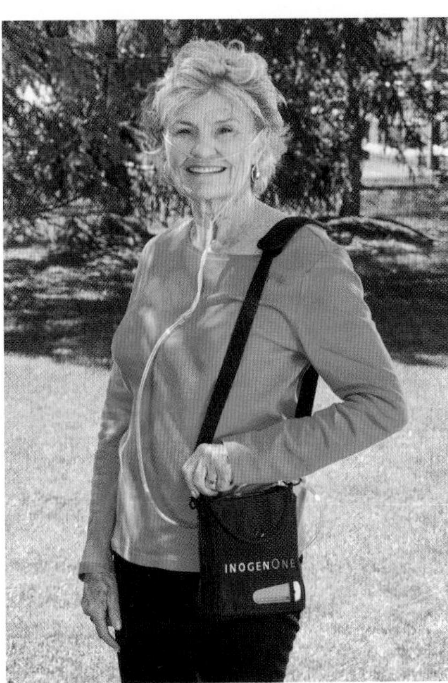

FIG. 25.12 Portable oxygen concentrator.

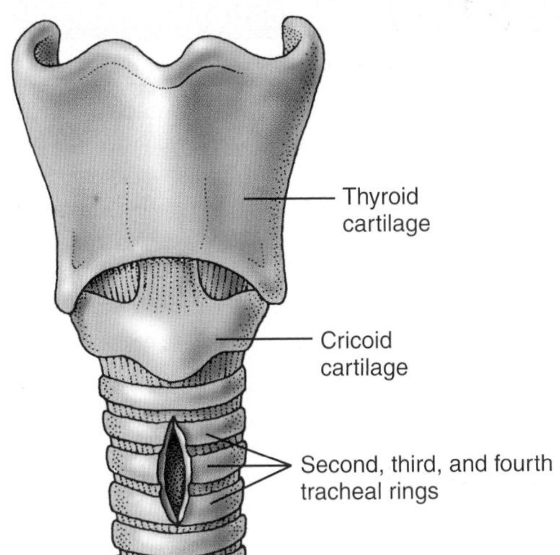

FIG. 25.13 A vertical tracheal incision for a tracheostomy.

◆ Interventions: Take Action

Preoperative Care. The care for the patient having a tracheotomy is similar to that for a laryngectomy (see Chapter 26). Focus on his or her knowledge deficits through teaching and discuss tracheostomy care, communication, and speech.

Operative Procedures. Initially the neck is extended, and an endotracheal (ET) tube is placed by the anesthesia provider to maintain the airway. Incisions are made through the neck and the tracheal rings to enter the trachea (Fig. 25.13).

After the trachea is entered, the ET tube is removed while the tracheostomy tube is inserted. The tracheostomy tube is secured in place with sutures and tracheostomy ties or Velcro tube holders. A chest x-ray determines proper placement of the tube.

Postoperative Care. Immediately after surgery, focus care on ensuring a patent airway. Confirm the presence of bilateral breath sounds. Perform a respiratory assessment at least hourly. Assess the patient for complications from the procedure.

Complications. Major complications can arise after surgery. Table 25.3 lists symptoms, management, and prevention of complications of tracheostomy.

Tube obstruction can occur as a result of secretions or by cuff displacement. Indicators are difficulty breathing; noisy respirations; difficulty inserting a suction catheter; thick, dry secretions; and high peak pressures (if a mechanical ventilator is used). Assess the patient at least hourly for tube patency. Prevent obstruction by helping the patient cough and deep breathe, providing inner cannula care, humidifying oxygen, and suctioning. If tube obstruction results from cuff prolapse over the end of the tube, the respiratory health care provider repositions or replaces the tube.

Tube dislodgment and accidental decannulation can occur when the tube is not secure. Prevent this problem by securing the tube in place to reduce movement and traction or accidental pulling by the patient. *Tube dislodgment in the first 72 hours after surgery is an emergency because the tracheostomy tract has not matured and replacement is difficult. The tube may end up in the subcutaneous tissue instead of in the trachea (also referred to as "false passage"). The patient will not be able to be ventilated.* Obese patients or those with short, large necks may be particularly difficult to recannulate if the tracheostomy tube is dislodged.

! NURSING SAFETY PRIORITY (QSEN)

Critical Rescue

For safety, ensure that a tracheostomy tube of the same type (including an obturator) and size (or one size smaller) is at the bedside at all times, along with a tracheostomy insertion tray. Monitor the patient for tube placement. When you recognize that the tube is dislodged on an immature tracheostomy, respond by ventilating the patient using a manual resuscitation bag and facemask while another nurse calls the Rapid Response Team, as well as the surgical service that placed the tracheostomy. If a stay suture technique was used during the tracheostomy procedure, gentle tension on the sutures can reopen the trachea.

If decannulation occurs after 72 hours, extend the patient's neck and open the tissues of the stoma with a curved Kelly clamp to secure the airway. With the obturator inserted into the tracheostomy tube, quickly and gently replace the tube and remove the obturator. Check for airflow through the tube and for bilateral breath sounds. *If you cannot secure the airway, notify a more experienced nurse, respiratory therapist, or respiratory health care provider for assistance. Ventilate with a bag-valve-mask (Vo et al., 2017). If the patient is in distress, call the Rapid Response Team for help.* To reduce tube dislodgment problems, many institutions have a "difficult airway" cart for high-risk patients.

Pneumothorax (air in the chest cavity) can develop during the tracheotomy procedure if the chest cavity is entered. Chest x-rays after placement are used to assess for pneumothorax.

Subcutaneous emphysema occurs when there is an opening or tear in the trachea and air escapes into the fresh tissue planes of the neck. Air can progress throughout the chest and other tissues into the face. Inspect and palpate for air under the skin around the new tracheostomy.

TABLE 25.3 Complications of Tracheostomy

Complications and Description	Indications	Management	Prevention
Tracheomalacia: Constant pressure exerted by the cuff causes tracheal dilation and erosion of cartilage, leading to loss of ***tissue integrity***.	An increased amount of air is required in the cuff to maintain the seal. A larger tracheostomy tube is required to prevent an air leak at the stoma. Food particles are seen in tracheal secretions. The patient does not receive the set tidal volume on the ventilator.	No special management is needed unless bleeding occurs.	Use an uncuffed tube as soon as possible. Monitor cuff pressure and air volumes closely and detect changes.
Tracheal stenosis: Narrowed tracheal lumen is caused by scar formation from irritation of tracheal mucosa and impaired ***tissue integrity*** by the cuff.	Stenosis is usually seen after the cuff is deflated or the tracheostomy tube is removed. The patient has increased coughing, inability to expectorate secretions, or difficulty breathing or talking.	Tracheal dilation or surgical intervention is used.	Prevent pulling of and traction on the tracheostomy tube. Properly secure the tube in the midline position. Maintain proper cuff pressure. Minimize oronasal intubation time.
Tracheoesophageal fistula (TEF): Excessive cuff pressure causes erosion of the posterior wall of the trachea and loss of ***tissue integrity***. A hole is created between the trachea and the anterior esophagus. The patient at highest risk also has a nasogastric tube present.	Similar to tracheomalacia: Food particles are seen in tracheal secretions. Increased air in cuff is needed to achieve a seal. The patient has increased coughing and choking while eating. The patient does not receive the set tidal volume on the ventilator.	Manually administer oxygen by mask to prevent hypoxemia. Use a small, soft feeding tube instead of a nasogastric tube for tube feedings. A gastrostomy or jejunostomy may be performed by a physician. Monitor the patient with a nasogastric tube closely; assess for TEF and aspiration.	Maintain cuff pressure. Monitor the amount of air needed for inflation and detect changes. Progress to a deflated cuff or cuffless tube as soon as possible.
Trachea—innominate artery fistula: A poorly positioned tube causes its distal tip to push against the lateral wall of the tracheostomy. Continued pressure causes necrosis and erosion of the innominate artery. ***This is a medical emergency!***	The tracheostomy tube pulsates in synchrony with the heartbeat. There is heavy bleeding from the stoma. This is a life-threatening complication.	Remove the tracheostomy tube immediately. Apply direct pressure to the innominate artery at the stoma site. Prepare the patient for immediate surgical repair.	Correct the tube size, length, and midline position. Prevent pulling or tugging on the tracheostomy tube. Immediately notify the surgeon of the pulsating tube.

! NURSING SAFETY PRIORITY QSEN

Critical Rescue

Assess the skin around a new tracheostomy to recognize subcutaneous emphysema. If it is puffy and you can feel a crackling sensation when pressing on this skin, respond by notifying the surgeon immediately.

Bleeding in small amounts from the tracheotomy incision is expected for the first few days, but constant oozing is abnormal. Wrap gauze around the tube and pack gauze gently into the wound to apply pressure to the bleeding sites. Ensure that the tracheostomy cuff is properly inflated. Bleeding can occur in the trachea itself or in the tissues surrounding the incision. If hemorrhage occurs, the site may need surgical exploration or ligation of blood vessels.

Infection can occur at any time. In the hospital, use sterile technique to prevent ***infection*** during suctioning and tracheostomy care. Assess the stoma site at least once every 8 hours for purulent drainage, redness, pain, swelling, or changes in ***tissue integrity***. Tracheostomy dressings may be used to keep the stoma clean and dry. These dressings resemble a 4 × 4 gauze pad with an area removed to fit around the tube. If tracheostomy dressings are not available, fold standard sterile 4 × 4s to fit around the tube. *Do not cut the dressing because small bits of gauze could then be aspirated through the tube.* Change these dressings often because moist dressings provide a medium for bacterial growth. Careful wound care prevents local ***infection***.

Tracheostomy Tubes. Many types of tracheostomy tubes are available (Fig. 25.14). Selection is based on patient needs. Tubes are available in many sizes and are made of plastic or metal. Most tubes are disposable. A tracheostomy tube may have a cuff and may have an inner cannula. A cuffed tube is used for patients receiving mechanical ventilation. The cuff is a small balloon surrounding the outside of the tracheostomy tube (see Fig. 25.14). When inflated to the proper size and pressure, the cuff comes into contact with the trachea and seals it off so that all air movement occurs within the tracheostomy tube, not around it. Usually, the cuff is inflated through the use of a pilot balloon, which remains on the outside of the body where it can be accessed. As shown in Fig. 25.14, the pilot balloon is a small balloon with a valve on one end and a thin long tube on the other end. The thin tube is connected to the cuff. To inflate the cuff, an air-filled syringe is attached

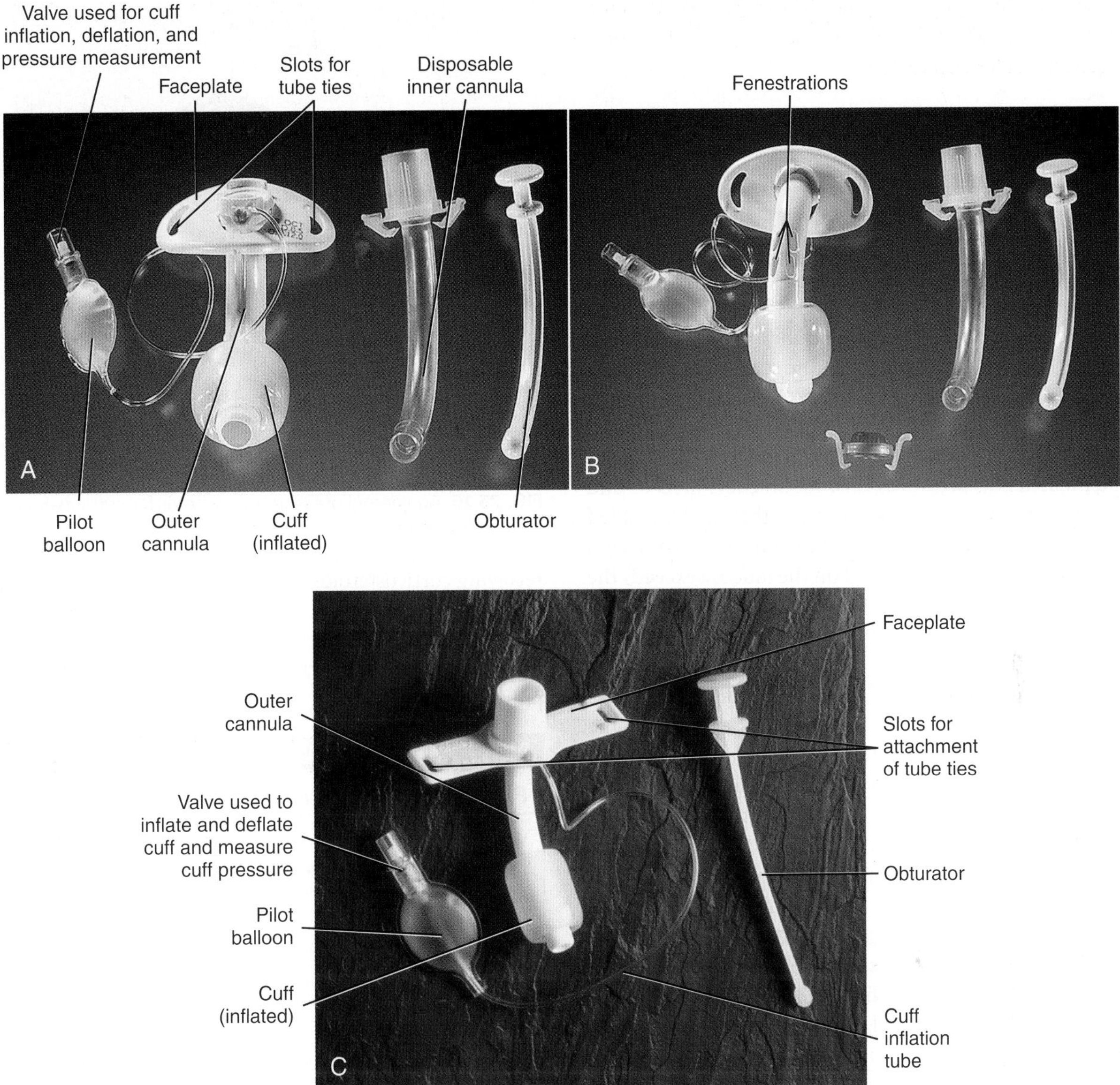

FIG. 25.14 Tracheostomy tubes. (A) Dual-lumen cuffed tracheostomy tube with disposable inner cannula. (B) Dual-lumen cuffed fenestrated tracheostomy tube. (C) Single-lumen cannula cuffed tracheostomy tube.

to the pilot balloon valve. As the syringe is pressed, air first enters the pilot balloon and then moves through the thin tube to inflate the cuff. In addition to the function of inflating the cuff, the pilot balloon can determine whether any air is in the cuff because the pilot balloon remains inflated when the cuff is inflated. It does not indicate air volume or pressure in the cuff.

For tubes with a reusable inner cannula, inspect, suction, and clean the inner cannula. During the first 24 hours after surgery, perform cannula care as often as needed, perhaps hourly. Thereafter care is determined by the patient's needs and agency policy. In planning for self-care, teach the patient to remove the inner cannula and check for cleanliness. Instruct him or her about suctioning and tracheostomy cleaning to prevent ***infection***.

Because breathing and swallowing move the tube, even a cuffed tube does not protect against aspiration. Having a cuffed tube inflated may give a false sense of security that aspiration cannot occur during feeding or mouth care. In addition, the pilot balloon does not reflect whether the correct amount of air is present in the cuff.

A fenestrated tube functions in many different ways. When the inner cannula is in place, the fenestration is closed, and this tube works like a double-lumen tube. With the inner cannula removed and the plug or stopper locked in place, air can pass through the fenestration, around the tube, and up through the natural airway so the patient can cough and speak. If the patient has trouble with these actions, he or she should be evaluated for proper tube placement, patency, size, and fenestration. *Do not cap the tube until the problem is identified and corrected.*

A fenestrated tube may or may not have a cuff. With a cuff, some air flows through the natural airway when the patient is not being mechanically ventilated.

! NURSING SAFETY PRIORITY (QSEN)

Action Alert

Always deflate the cuff before capping the tube with the decannulation cap; otherwise the patient has no airway.

Patients with metal tracheostomy tubes scheduled for MRI need to change to a plastic tube. Metal tubes may be dislodged or heat up in the magnetic field during the scan.

Care Issues for the Patient With a Tracheostomy

Preventing Tissue Injury. Loss of ***tissue integrity*** can occur where the inflated cuff presses against the tracheal mucosa and is considered a "never event" pressure injury that can be avoided with proper care (Dixon et al., 2018). Mucosal ischemia occurs when the pressure exerted by the cuff on the mucosa exceeds the capillary perfusion pressure. To reduce tracheal damage, keep the cuff pressure between 14 and 20 mm Hg or 20 and 30 cm H_2O (ideally, 25 cm H_2O or less).

Most cuffs use a high volume of air while keeping low pressure on the tracheal mucosa. Inflate the cuff to form a seal between the trachea and the cuff using the least amount of pressure. If the cuff cannot be inflated to seal well enough, a larger-diameter tube may be needed. A pressure cuff inflator can be used to inflate the cuff to a specified pressure or to check the cuff pressure (Fig. 25.15).

Check the cuff pressure at least once during each shift using either a pressure cuff inflator or the minimal leak technique. When using an inflator, keep the pressure at 14 to 20 mm Hg or 20 to 30 cm H_2O. In rare situations, the cuff pressure is increased to maintain ventilator volumes when peak pressures are greater than 50 mm Hg (65 cm H_2O) and positive end-expiratory pressure (PEEP) is greater than 10 mm Hg (14 cm H_2O). High PEEP values can deflate the cuff over time, and more air may need to be added to maintain a proper seal. Manufacturers have guidelines for the specific volumes for each cuff size. Most cuffs are adequately inflated with less than 10 mL of air.

When using the minimal leak technique to ensure adequate cuff pressure and reduce the risk for pressure injury, a pressure cuff inflator is not used. Instead, after completing tracheostomy care and suctioning the airway above the cuff, attach a 10-mL Luer-Lok syringe to the valve in the pilot balloon. Place a stethoscope on the side of the patient's neck near the tracheostomy tube and slowly deflate the cuff with the syringe while listening for a loud, gurgling air rush as the seal is broken and air bypasses the tracheostomy tube on inhalation. Then, while reinjecting the air in the syringe, continue to listen for air passing the cuff. When air is no longer heard passing the cuff, the airway is sealed. At this point, remove 1 mL of air from the cuff. This ensures that the airway is sealed sufficiently to allow adequate ventilation and that the tube fit is kept just loose enough to prevent tracheal injury.

Although a high cuff pressure alone can injure tracheal ***tissue integrity***, other factors contribute to the risk for damage. The patient who is malnourished, dehydrated, hypoxic, older, or receiving corticosteroids is at risk for greater tissue damage. Tube friction and movement damage the mucosa and lead to tracheal stenosis. Reduce local airway damage by maintaining proper cuff pressures, stabilizing the tube, suctioning only when needed, and preventing malnutrition, dehydration, and hypoxia.

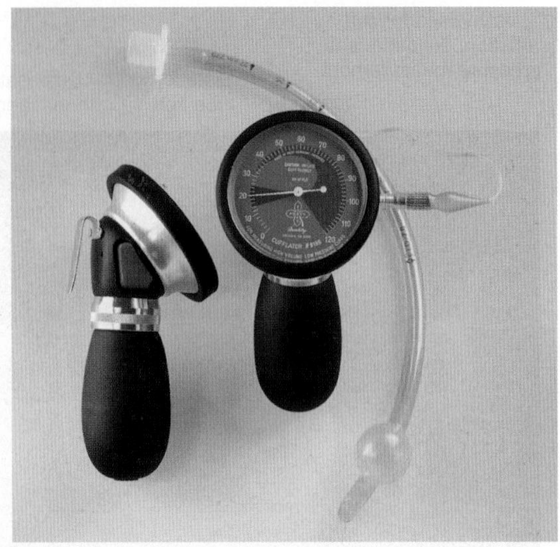

FIG. 25.15 An aneroid pressure manometer for cuff inflation and measuring cuff pressures.

NCLEX EXAMINATION CHALLENGE 25.3

Physiological Integrity

Which action does the nurse use to **prevent harm** by loss of tracheal tissue integrity in a client with a tracheostomy?

A. Providing meticulous oral care every 8 hours
B. Deflating the cuff for 15 minutes every 2 hours
C. Feeding the client liquids rather than solid foods
D. Maintaining cuff inflation pressure less than 25 cm H_2O

Ensuring Air Warming and Humidification. The tracheostomy tube bypasses the nose and mouth, which normally humidify and warm the inspired air. If humidification and warming are not adequate, tracheal damage can occur. Inadequate humidity promotes thick, dried secretions that can occlude the airways and increase the risk for ***infection***.

To prevent these complications, humidify the air as ordered. Continually assess for a fine mist emerging from the tracheostomy collar or T-piece during ventilation. To increase the amount of humidity delivered, a warming device can be attached to the water source with a temperature probe in the tubing circuit. Monitor the circuit temperature hourly by feeling the tubing and by checking the reading on the probe. Ensure adequate hydration, which also helps liquefy secretions. Increasing the flow rate at the flowmeter increases the amount of delivered humidity.

! NURSING SAFETY PRIORITY (QSEN)

Action Alert

Keep the temperature of the air entering a tracheostomy between 98.6°F and 100.4°F (37°C and 38°C) and never exceed 104°F (40°C).

BEST PRACTICE FOR PATIENT SAFETY & QUALITY CARE (QSEN)

Suctioning the Artificial Airway

- Assess the need for suctioning.
- Wash hands. Don protective eyewear. Maintain Standard Precautions.
- Explain to the patient that sensations such as shortness of breath and coughing are to be expected but that any discomfort will be very brief.
- Check the suction source. Occlude the suction source, and adjust the pressure dial to between 80 and 120 mm Hg to prevent hypoxemia and trauma to the mucosa.
- Set up a sterile field.
- Preoxygenate the patient with 100% oxygen for 30 seconds to 3 minutes (at least three hyperinflations) to prevent hypoxemia. Synchronize hyperinflations with inhalation.
- Quickly insert the suction catheter until resistance is met. *Do not apply suction during insertion.*
- Routine instillation of normal saline is ***not*** supported. ***Gas exchange*** is impaired due to hypoxia and there is an increased risk for ***infection***.
- Withdraw the catheter 0.4 to 0.8 inch (1 to 2 cm), and begin to apply suction. Apply continuous suction and use a twirling motion of the catheter during withdrawal to avoid impairing tissue integrity. *Never suction for longer than a total of 10 to 15 seconds.*
- Hyperoxygenate for 1 to 5 minutes or until the patient's baseline heart rate and oxygen saturation are within normal limits.
- Repeat as needed for up to *three* total suction passes.
- Document secretion characteristics and patient responses.

Suctioning. Suctioning maintains a patent airway and promotes ***gas exchange*** by removing secretions when the patient cannot cough adequately. Use the techniques listed in the Best Practice for Patient Safety & Quality Care: Suctioning the Artificial Airway box for suctioning when there is a need for it (e.g., audible or noisy secretions; crackles or wheezes heard on auscultation; restlessness, increased pulse or respiratory rates; or mucus present in the artificial airway). Other indications include patient requests for suctioning or an increase in the peak airway pressure on the ventilator. Routine unnecessary suctioning is not performed without indications to prevent mucosal damage, bleeding, or bronchospasm.

! NURSING SAFETY PRIORITY (QSEN)

Action Alert

It is important to note that airway suction, unlike nasogastric suction, is performed only on an intermittent basis and not continuously. However, during an actual suctioning episode, suction is applied continuously during catheter withdrawal to prevent dropping of secretions from the catheter back into the airway.

Deep endotracheal suctioning is painful. Unconscious patients may still feel pain, and this should be kept in mind during the suctioning procedure. At the very least, acknowledge the discomfort and reassure him or her of when the procedure will end.

Suctioning is often performed through an artificial airway, but the nose or mouth also can be used. Suctioning of both routes is routine for the patient with retained secretions.

Suctioning through the nose has complications and can be painful. Selecting a small suction catheter and coating it with a water-soluble sterile lubricant helps minimize trauma and increase comfort. Slow, careful placement of the catheter following the nasopharyngeal anatomy reduces pain and prevents injury and changes in ***tissue integrity***. Placing a nasopharyngeal airway and suctioning through it can prevent trauma to the nasal mucosa. Advance the catheter through the nasopharynx and into the laryngopharynx while the patient receives oxygen by mask or nasal cannula. Once the catheter enters the larynx, the patient may cough. On inhalation, insert the catheter into the trachea.

Suctioning can cause hypoxia, injury to mucosal ***tissue integrity***, trauma, ***infection***, vagal stimulation, bronchospasm, and cardiac dysrhythmias.

Hypoxia can be caused by these factors in the patient with a tracheostomy:

- Ineffective oxygenation before, during, and after suctioning
- Use of a catheter that is too large for the artificial airway
- Prolonged suctioning time
- Excessive suction pressure
- Too frequent suctioning
- Use of normal saline instillation with suctioning

Prevent hypoxia by hyperoxygenating the patient with 100% oxygen using a manual bag-valve-mask attached to an oxygen source (Vo et al., 2017). Instruct the patient to take deep breaths three or four times with the existing oxygen delivery system before suctioning. Monitor the heart rate or use a pulse oximeter while suctioning to assess tolerance of the procedure. Assess for hypoxia (e.g., increased heart rate and blood pressure, oxygen desaturation, cyanosis, restlessness, anxiety, dysrhythmias). Oxygen saturation below 90% by pulse oximetry indicates hypoxemia. If hypoxia occurs, stop the suctioning procedure. Using the 100% oxygen delivery system, reoxygenate the patient until his or her baseline oxygen saturation level returns.

Use a correct-size catheter to reduce the risk for hypoxia and still remove secretions effectively. The size should not exceed half of the size of the tracheal lumen. The standard catheter size for an adult is 12 or 14 Fr.

*Loss of **tissue integrity*** by trauma results from frequent suctioning, prolonged suctioning, excessive suction pressure, and nonrotation of the catheter. Prevent trauma to the mucosa by suctioning only when needed and lubricating the catheter with sterile water or saline before insertion. *Apply only continuous suction during catheter withdrawal because the practice of intermittent suction during catheter withdrawal does **not** protect the mucosa and can lead to "dropping" of secretions in the airway.* Use a twirling motion during withdrawal to prevent grabbing of the mucosa.

Apply suction for only 10 to 15 seconds because longer can lead to alveolar collapse. Estimate this time frame by holding your own breath and counting to 10 or 15 while suctioning.

Infection is possible because each catheter pass introduces bacteria into the trachea. In the hospital, use sterile technique for suctioning and for all equipment (e.g., suction catheters, gloves, saline or water) to prevent ***infection***. Suction the mouth or nose *after* suctioning the artificial airway. Clean technique can be used at home.

! NURSING SAFETY PRIORITY (QSEN)

Action Alert

Never use oral suction equipment for suctioning an artificial airway because this can introduce oral bacteria into the lungs and increase the risk for ***infection***.

Vagal stimulation and bronchospasm are possible during suctioning. Vagal stimulation results in bradycardia, hypotension, heart block, ventricular tachycardia, or other dysrhythmias. *If vagal stimulation occurs, stop suctioning immediately and oxygenate the patient manually with 100% oxygen.* Bronchospasm may occur when the catheter passes into the airway. The patient may need a bronchodilator to relieve bronchospasm and respiratory distress. The hypoxia caused by suctioning can stimulate a variety of cardiac dysrhythmias. If the patient has cardiac monitoring in place, check the monitor during suctioning.

NCLEX EXAMINATION CHALLENGE 25.4

Safe and Effective Care Environment

Which conditions or changes indicate to the nurse that a client with a tracheostomy requires suctioning? **Select all that apply.**

A. The client has a fever.
B. Crackles and wheezes are heard on auscultation.
C. The client requests that suctioning be performed.
D. Suctioning was last performed more than 3 hours ago.
E. The tracheostomy dressing has a moderate amount of serosanguineous drainage.
F. The skin around the tracheostomy is puffy and makes a crunching sound when touched.

Providing Tracheostomy Care. Tracheostomy care keeps the tube free of secretions, maintains a patent airway, and provides wound care. It is performed whether or not the patient can clear secretions. Before tracheostomy care, assess the patient as described in the Focused Assessment: The Patient With a Tracheostomy box. Perform tracheostomy care according to agency policy, usually every 8 hours and as needed using the techniques listed in the Best Practice for Patient Safety & Quality Care: Tracheostomy Care box (Schreiber, 2015).

The need for suctioning and tracheostomy care is determined by the secretions, the specific disorder, the ability of the patient to cough, the need for mechanical ventilation, and wound care. Using a penlight, inspect the inner lumen of the tube to assess for secretions.

Secure tracheostomy tubes in place using either twill tape ties or commercial tube holders (Smith & Pietrantonio, 2016). These devices require changing when soiled or at least daily to keep them clean, to prevent ***infection***, and to assess ***tissue integrity*** under the ties. Whenever possible, use the assistance of a coworker to stabilize the tube and prevent decannulation when changing the ties or tube holders. Because of the emergent nature of a decannulation in the postoperative period, some health care facilities have policies requiring a second licensed person be present during suctioning or moving a patient within the first 72 hours after tracheostomy. A properly secured tie or holder allows space for only one finger to be placed between the tie or holder and the neck. Tube movement causes irritation and coughing and may lead to decannulation, reducing ***gas exchange***. Include the patient in tracheostomy care as a step toward self-care. Fig. 25.16 shows correct placement of a tracheostomy dressing.

FOCUSED ASSESSMENT

The Patient With a Tracheostomy

- Note the quality, pattern, and rate of breathing and compare with the patient's baseline. Tachypnea can indicate hypoxia, and dyspnea can indicate secretions in the airway.
- Assess for cyanosis, especially around the lips, which could indicate hypoxia.
- Check the patient's oxygen saturation with pulse oximetry.
- If oxygen is prescribed, ensure that the patient is receiving the correct amount, with the correct equipment and humidification.
- Assess the tracheostomy site for color, consistency, and amount of secretions in the tube or externally.
- If the tracheostomy is sutured in place, assess for redness, swelling, or drainage from suture sites.
- If the tracheostomy is secured with ties, assess the condition and security of the ties. Change if they are moist or dirty.
- Assess the skin around the tracheostomy and neck for impaired ***tissue integrity,*** including behind the neck, from the ties or from excess secretions.
- Assess behind the faceplate for the size of the space between the outer cannula and the patient's tissue and whether any secretions have collected in this area.
- If the tube is cuffed, check cuff pressure or collaborate with the respiratory therapist to confirm cuff pressure.
- Auscultate the lungs.
- Ensure that a second (emergency) tracheostomy tube and obturator of the correct size are available.

BEST PRACTICE FOR PATIENT SAFETY & QUALITY CARE (QSEN)

Tracheostomy Care

- Assemble the necessary equipment and maintain Standard Precautions.
- Suction the tracheostomy tube if necessary.
- Remove old dressings and excess secretions.
- Set up a sterile field.
- Remove and clean the inner cannula. Use half-strength hydrogen peroxide (if ordered) to clean the cannula and sterile saline to rinse it. If the inner cannula is disposable, remove the cannula and replace it with a new one.
- Clean the stoma site and then the tracheostomy plate with half-strength hydrogen peroxide followed by sterile saline. Ensure that none of the solutions enters the tracheostomy.
- Change tracheostomy ties if they are soiled. Secure new ties in place before removing soiled ones to prevent accidental decannulation. If a knot is needed, tie a square knot that is visible on the side of the neck. Only one finger should be able to be placed between the tie tape and the neck.
- Document the type and amount of secretions and the general condition of the stoma and surrounding skin tissue integrity. Document the patient's response to the procedure.

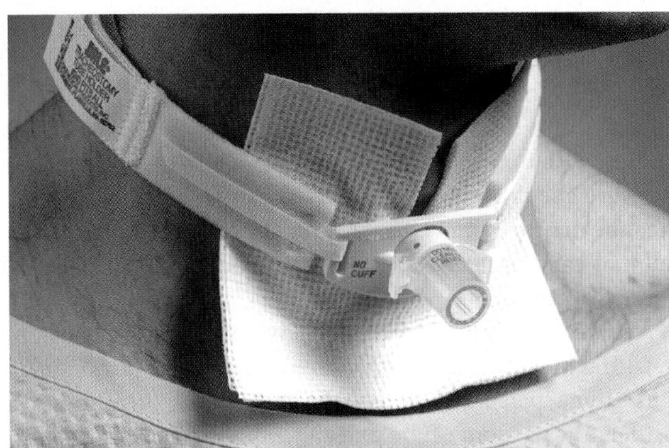

FIG. 25.16 Placement of tracheostomy gauze dressing and Velcro tracheostomy tube holder.

NURSING SAFETY PRIORITY (QSEN)

Action Alert

Prevent decannulation during tracheostomy care by keeping the old ties or holder on the tube while applying new ties or holder or by keeping a hand on the tube until it is securely stable. (This is best performed with the assistance of a coworker. Some hospitals require a second licensed person during tracheostomy care for the first 72 hours after tracheostomy.)

Providing Bronchial and Oral Hygiene. Bronchial hygiene promotes a patent airway and prevents ***infection***. Turn and reposition the patient every 1 to 2 hours, support out-of-bed activities, and encourage ambulation to promote lung expansion and ***gas exchange*** and help remove secretions. Coughing and deep breathing, combined with chest percussion, vibration, and postural drainage, promote pulmonary hygiene (see Chapter 27).

Good oral hygiene keeps the airway patent, prevents ***infection*** from bacterial overgrowth, and promotes comfort. Avoid using glycerin swabs or mouthwash that contains alcohol for oral care because these products dry the mouth, change its pH, and promote bacterial growth. Instead use a sponge tooth cleaner or soft-bristle toothbrush moistened in water for mouth care. Diluted hydrogen peroxide solutions can help remove crusted matter but may break down healing tissue and should be used only if ordered. Chlorhexidine oral rinse has been shown to prevent ***infection*** in patients requiring mechanical ventilation, thus helping to decrease the incidence of ventilator-associated pneumonia (VAP). Help the patient rinse the mouth with normal saline every 4 hours while awake or as often as he or she desires.

Assess the mouth for reduced ***tissue integrity***. Ulcers and ***infection*** are treated medically. Apply lip balm or water-soluble jelly to prevent cracked lips and promote comfort. Mouth care promotes oral health and comfort. Offering an opportunity for the patient or family member to perform mouth care allows participation in care and increases self-esteem.

Oral secretions can move down the trachea and collect above the inflated cuff of the endotracheal tube. When the cuff is deflated, the secretions can move into the lungs. Some endotracheal tubes have an extra lumen open to the area above the cuff that allows suctioning of the airway above the cuff before deflating to reduce the risk for aspiration.

Ensuring Nutrition. Swallowing can be difficult with a tracheostomy tube in place (Mountain & Golles, 2017). In a normal swallow, the larynx lifts and moves forward to prevent food and saliva from entering (McCance et al., 2019). The tracheostomy tube sometimes tethers the larynx in place, making it unable to move effectively. The result is difficulty in swallowing. In addition, when the tracheostomy tube cuff is inflated, it can balloon backward and interfere with food passage in the esophagus because the wall between the trachea and esophagus is thin.

Instruct the patient to keep the head of the bed elevated for at least 30 minutes after eating. Use the techniques listed in the Best Practice for Patient Safety & Quality Care: Preventing Aspiration While Swallowing box to prevent aspiration during swallowing.

BEST PRACTICE FOR PATIENT SAFETY & QUALITY CARE (QSEN)

Preventing Aspiration While Swallowing

- Avoid serving meals when the patient is fatigued.
- Provide smaller and more frequent meals.
- Provide adequate time; do not "hurry" the patient.
- Closely supervise the self-feeding patient.
- Keep suctioning equipment close at hand and turned on.
- Avoid water and other "thin" liquids, as well as the use of straws.
- Thicken all liquids, including water.
- Thin liquids may be permitted after a swallowing evaluation by a speech-language pathologist.
- Avoid foods that generate thin liquids during the chewing process, such as fruit.
- Position the patient in the most upright position possible.
- When possible, completely (or at least partially) deflate the tube cuff during meals.
- Suction after cuff deflation to clear the airway and allow comfort during the meal.
- Feed each bite or encourage the patient to take each bite slowly.
- Encourage the patient to "dry swallow" after each bite ("double swallowing") to clear residue from the throat.
- Avoid consecutive swallows of liquids.
- Provide controlled small volumes of liquids, using a spoon.
- Tell the patient to "tuck" the chin down and move the forehead forward while swallowing.
- Allow the patient to indicate when he or she is ready for the next bite.
- If coughing occurs, stop the feeding until the patient indicates that the airway is clear.
- Assess respiratory rate, ease of swallowing, pulse oximetry, and heart rate during feeding.

Maintaining Communication. The patient can speak when there is a cuffless tube, when a fenestrated tracheostomy tube is in place, and when the fenestrated tube is capped or covered. Until natural speech is feasible, teach him or her and the family about other communication means. A writing tablet, a board with pictures and letters, communication "flash cards," hand signals, computer tablets, and smartphones are used to promote communication and decrease frustration from not being able to speak or be understood (Bell, 2016). Phrase questions for "yes" or "no" answers to help the patient respond easily. Mark the central call light system to indicate that he or she cannot speak. For any patient with a communication problem, including a speech-language pathologist as part of the interprofessional team promotes better outcomes.

! NATIONAL PATIENT SAFETY GOALS

The inability to talk is a stressor for the patient. Helping communication is an important nursing action and is required by The Joint Commission's National Patient Safety Goals. When the patient can tolerate cuff deflation, he or she places a finger over the tracheostomy tube on exhalation, forcing air up through the larynx and mouth for speech.

A device to facilitate speech for the patient with a tracheostomy is a one-way valve that fits over the tube and replaces the need for finger occlusion. The valve allows him or her to breathe in through the tracheostomy tube. On exhalation, the valve closes so air is forced through the vocal cords, allowing speech. For this valve to assist in speech, the patient must not be connected to a ventilator, must have the cuff deflated, and must be able to breathe around the tube. Some valves have a port for supplemental oxygen without impairing the ability to speak.

Supporting Psychosocial Needs and Self-Esteem. Addressing psychological concerns is an important aspect of nursing care for patients recovering from a tracheostomy and having an artificial airway. Acknowledge the patient's frustration with communication and allow sufficient time for communication. When speaking to him or her, use a normal tone of voice because hearing and understanding are not altered by the presence of a tube.

The patient may have a change in self-image because of the presence of a stoma or artificial airway, speech changes, a change in the method of eating, or difficulty with speech. Help him or her set realistic goals, starting with involvement in self-care.

Work with the family to ease the patient into a more normal social environment. Provide encouragement and positive reinforcement while demonstrating acceptance and caring behaviors. Assess the caregiver(s) for the need for counseling.

After surgery the patient may feel shy and socially isolated. He or she can wear loose-fitting shirts, decorative collars, or scarves to cover the tracheostomy tube.

Weaning. Weaning the patient from a tracheostomy tube entails a gradual decrease in the tube size and ultimate removal of the tube. Carefully monitor this process, especially after each change. The physician or advanced practice nurse performs the steps in the process.

First, the cuff is deflated as soon as the patient can manage secretions and does not need mechanical ventilation. This change allows him or her to breathe through the tube and through the upper airway. Next, the tube is changed to an uncuffed tube. If this is tolerated, the size of the tube is gradually decreased. When a small fenestrated tube is placed, the tube is capped so all air passes through the upper airway and the fenestrations, with none passing through the tube. Assess the patient to ensure adequate airflow around the tube when it is capped. The tube may be removed after he or she tolerates more than 24 hours of capping. Place a dry dressing over the stoma (which gradually heals on its own).

Another device used for the transition from tracheostomy to natural breathing is a *tracheostomy button*. The button maintains stoma patency and assists spontaneous breathing. The Kistner tracheostomy tube and Olympic tracheostomy button are examples of this type of device. To function, the button must fit properly. A disadvantage is the possibility of covert decannulation (i.e., the tube can dislodge from the trachea but remain in the neck tissues).

Care Coordination and Transition Management

At discharge the patient should be able to provide self-care, including tracheostomy care, nutrition care, suctioning, and communication. Although education begins before surgery, most self-care is taught in the hospital. Teach the patient and caregiver how to care for the tracheostomy tube. Review airway care, including cleaning and signs of ***infection*** or loss of ***tissue integrity***. Teach clean suction technique, and review the plan of care with the patient.

Instruct the patient to use a shower shield over the tracheostomy tube when bathing to prevent water from entering the airway. Teach him or her to cover the airway loosely with a small cotton cloth to protect it during the day. Covering the opening filters the air entering the stoma, keeps humidity in the airway, and enhances appearance. Attractive coverings are available as cotton scarves, decorative collars, and jewelry.

Teach the patient to increase humidity in the home. Instruct him or her to wear a medical alert bracelet that identifies the inability to speak.

The interprofessional health care team assesses specific discharge needs and makes referrals to home care agencies and durable medical equipment (DME) companies (for suction equipment and tracheostomy supplies). Follow-up visits occur early after discharge. The home care nurse initiates and coordinates the services of registered dietitian nutritionists, nurses, speech-language pathologists, and social workers, and identifies appropriate community resources.

PATIENT-CENTERED CARE: OLDER ADULT CONSIDERATIONS (QSEN)

The older patient who has vision problems or difficulty with upper arm movement may have difficulty self-managing tracheostomy care and oxygen therapy. Teach him or her to use magnifying lenses or glasses to ensure the proper setting on the oxygen gauge. Assess his or her ability to reach and manipulate the tracheostomy. If possible, work with a family member who can provide assistance during tracheostomy care.

GET READY FOR THE NEXT-GENERATION NCLEX® EXAMINATION!

Key Points

Review these Key Points for each NCLEX Examination Client Needs Category.

Safe and Effective Care Environment

- Never allow water condensation in an oxygen delivery system to drain back into the system. **QSEN: Safety**
- Use sterile technique when performing endotracheal or tracheal suctioning. **QSEN: Safety**
- Assess ***tissue integrity*** of the oral mucous membranes for injury or ***infection*** each shift for anyone who has an endotracheal tube. **QSEN: Safety**
- Keep a tracheostomy tube (and obturator) and tracheostomy insertion tray at the bedside, and ensure that tracheostomy care is performed with two licensed personnel for the first 72 hours after a tracheostomy has been created. **QSEN: Safety**
- Verify safe use of oxygen delivery systems and tracheostomy equipment. **QSEN: Safety**
- Keep the tracheal cuff pressure between 14 and 20 mm Hg to prevent loss of ***tissue integrity***. **QSEN: Safety**
- Teach the patient and caregivers about home management of oxygen therapy, including the avoidance of smoking or open flames in rooms in which oxygen is being used. **QSEN: Safety**
- Teach the patient and caregivers how to perform tracheostomy care. **QSEN: Safety**

Health Promotion and Maintenance

- Ensure that the patient and caregiver(s) know whom to contact about needed supplies and durable medical equipment (DME). **QSEN: Patient-Centered Care**

Psychosocial Integrity

- Allow the patient and family to express concerns about a change in breathing status or the possibility of intubation and mechanical ventilation. **QSEN: Patient-Centered Care**
- Teach caregivers and family members ways to communicate with a patient who is intubated or being mechanically ventilated. **QSEN: Patient-Centered Care**
- Reassure patients who are intubated that the loss of speech is temporary. **QSEN: Patient-Centered Care**

Physiological Integrity

- Apply oxygen to anyone who is hypoxemic. **QSEN: Evidence-Based Practice**
- Monitor arterial blood gases (ABGs) and oxygen saturation of all patients receiving oxygen therapy. **QSEN: Evidence-Based Practice**
- Assess the skin under the mask and under the plastic tubing every shift for patients receiving oxygen by mask. **QSEN: Patient-Centered Care**
- Assess the ***tissue integrity*** of the nares and under the elastic band every shift for patients receiving oxygen by nasal cannula. **QSEN: Patient-Centered Care**
- Assess patients receiving oxygen at a 50% concentration or higher for early indications of oxygen toxicity (i.e., dyspnea, nonproductive cough, chest pain, GI upset). **QSEN: Patient-Centered Care**
- Use a manual resuscitation bag to ventilate the patient if the tracheostomy tube has dislodged or become decannulated. **QSEN: Safety**
- Assess the new tracheostomy stoma site at least once per shift for purulent drainage, redness, pain, and swelling as indicators of ***infection*** or loss of ***tissue integrity***. **QSEN: Evidence-Based Practice**

MASTERY QUESTIONS

1. Which assessment finding for a client receiving oxygen therapy with a nonrebreather mask requires the nurse to intervene immediately?
   A. The oxygen flow rate is set at 12 L/min.
   B. The exhalation ports are open during exhalation.
   C. The exhalation ports are closed during inhalation.
   D. The reservoir bag is not inflated during inhalation.
2. Which statement made by a client prescribed oxygen therapy at home indicates to the nurse that more instruction is needed?
   A. "When I want to smoke, I will use the liquid oxygen reservoir instead of the compressed oxygen tank."
   B. "Using oxygen should help me have more breath and stamina when I eat, bathe, and take care of myself."
   C. "Even though they contain alcohol, I can still drink a glass of wine or can of beer while using oxygen."
   D. "If my shortness of breath becomes worse or if I have chest pain I will contact my primary health care provider immediately."
3. Which action does the nurse take care to **avoid** while suctioning a client's tracheostomy tube?
   A. Twirling the catheter while applying suction
   B. Applying suction only when withdrawing the catheter
   C. Performing oral suctioning before suctioning the artificial airway
   D. Lubricating the suction catheter with sterile saline before insertion

REFERENCES

Asterisk (*) indicates a classic or definitive work on this subject.

Bell, L. (2016). Caring for patients who are unable to speak. *American Journal of Critical Care, 25*(2), 109.

Dixon, L., Mascoli, S., Mixell, J., Gillin, T., Upchurch, C., & Bradley, K. (2018). Reducing tracheostomy-related pressure injuries. *AACN Advanced Critical Care, 29*(4), 426–431.

Dries, D. (2018). High-flow nasal cannula: Where does it fit? *Respiratory Care, 63*(1), 367–370.

Hernandez, G., Vaquero, C., Colina, L., Cuena, R., Gonzalez, P., Canabal, A., et al. (2016). Effect of postextubation high-flow nasal cannula vs noninvasive ventilation on reintubation and postextubation respiratory failure in high risk patients: A randomized clinical trial. *Journal of the American Medical Association, 316*(15), 1565–1574.

Lamb, K., Spilman, S., Oetting, T., Jackson, J., Trump, M., & Sahr, S. (2018). Proactive use of high-flow nasal cannula with critically ill subjects. *Respiratory Care, 63*(1), 259–266.

McCance, K., Huether, S., Brashers, V., & Rote, N. (2019). *Pathophysiology: The biologic basis for disease in adults and children* (8th ed.). St. Louis: Mosby.

Mountain, C., & Golles, K. (2017). Detecting dysphagia. *American Nurse Today, 12*(5), 22–23.

Mussa, A., Tonyan, L., Chen, Y.-F., & Vines, D. (2018). Perceived satisfaction with long-term oxygen delivery devices affects mobility and quality of life of oxygen-dependent individuals with COPD. *Respiratory Care, 63*(1), 11–19.

*Nishimura, M. (2015). High flow nasal cannula oxygen therapy in adults. *Journal of Intensive Care, 3*(15), 1–8. https://doi.org/10.1186/s40560-015-0084-5.

*Schreiber, M. (2015). Tracheostomy: Site care, suctioning, and readiness. *MEDSURG Nursing, 24*(2), 121–124.

Siela, D., & Kidd, K. (2017). Oxygen requirements for acutely and critically ill patients. *Critical Care Nurse, 37*(4), 58–69.

Smith, S., & Pietrantonio, T. (2016). Best method for securing an endotracheal tube. *Critical Care Nurse, 36*(2), 78–79.

Vo, H., Park, M., & Wang, S. (2017). Effective bag-valve-mask ventilation saves lives. *American Nurse Today, 12*(2), 6–9.

26

Concepts of Care for Patients With Noninfectious Upper Respiratory Problems

M. Linda Workman

http://evolve.elsevier.com/Iggy/

LEARNING OUTCOMES

1. Collaborate with the interprofessional team to coordinate high-quality care and promote ***gas exchange*** for patients who have upper respiratory problems.
2. Apply knowledge of anatomy, physiology, genetics, and pathophysiology to assess patients with upper respiratory problems affecting ***gas exchange***.
3. Use clinical judgment to prioritize evidence-based nursing care for patients with upper respiratory problems that decrease ***gas exchange***.
4. Teach all adults measures to take to protect the upper respiratory system from damage and cancer, including the avoidance of known environmental causative agents.
5. Implement nursing interventions to help the patient and family cope with the psychosocial impact caused by upper respiratory problems.
6. Teach the patient and family about common drugs and other management strategies used for upper respiratory problems.
7. Prioritize the nursing care needs of the patient and family experiencing head and neck cancer.

KEY TERMS

epistaxis Nosebleed.

gas exchange Oxygen transport to the cells and carbon dioxide transport away from cells through ventilation and diffusion.

hypopnea Lower than normal respiratory rate and depth insufficient for gas exchange.

inspissated secretions Thickly crusted oral and nasopharyngeal secretions that can cause an upper airway obstruction (also known as *mucoid impaction*).

laryngectomee An adult who has had a laryngectomy.

obstructive sleep apnea (OSA) A breathing disruption during sleep that lasts at least 10 seconds and occurs a minimum of five times in an hour.

polysomnography A formal and definitive overnight sleep study with direct observation of the patient while he or she wears a variety of monitoring equipment to evaluate depth of sleep, type of sleep, respiratory effort, oxygen saturation, carbon dioxide exhalation, and muscle movement.

rhinoplasty Surgical reconstruction of the nose.

upper airway obstruction Interruption of airflow through nose, mouth, pharynx, or larynx.

PRIORITY AND INTERRELATED CONCEPTS

The priority concept for this chapter is:
- ***Gas Exchange***

The ***Gas Exchange*** concept exemplar for this chapter is Obstructive Sleep Apnea.

The interrelated concept for this chapter is:
- ***Tissue Integrity***

The nose, sinuses, oropharynx, larynx, and trachea are the structures of the upper respiratory tract. These structures are the body's only entry site for the oxygen in atmospheric air. Keeping these structures patent, therefore, especially the oropharynx, larynx, and trachea, is essential for ***gas exchange***. (Recall from Chapter 3 that *gas exchange* is oxygen transport to the cells and carbon dioxide transport away from cells through ventilation and diffusion.) Problems that obstruct any of these airways can interfere with airflow and gas exchange. The nursing priority for patients with disorders of the upper respiratory tract is to promote gas exchange by ensuring a continuously patent airway.

UPPER AIRWAY OBSTRUCTION

Pathophysiology Review

Upper airway obstruction is the interruption of airflow through nose, mouth, pharynx, or larynx. When ***gas exchange*** is impaired, obstruction can be a life-threatening condition. Early recognition is essential to prevent complications, including respiratory arrest and death. Causes of upper airway obstruction include:

- Tongue edema (surgery, trauma, angioedema as an allergic response to a drug)
- Tongue occlusion (e.g., loss of gag reflex, loss of muscle tone, unconsciousness, coma)
- Laryngeal edema from any cause (e.g., smoke or toxin inhalation, local or generalized inflammation, allergic reactions, anaphylaxis)
- Peritonsillar and pharyngeal abscess
- Head and neck cancer
- Thick secretions
- Stroke and cerebral edema
- Facial, tracheal, or laryngeal trauma or burns
- Foreign-body aspiration

One preventable cause of airway obstruction leading to asphyxiation is thickly crusted oral and nasopharyngeal secretions, a condition formally called **inspissated secretions** or *mucoid impaction*. This condition often is caused by poor oral hygiene with thickened and hardened oral secretions that can completely block the airway and lead to death. Proper nursing care can eliminate this cause of airway obstruction. Patients at highest risk are those who have an altered mental status and level of consciousness, are dehydrated, are unable to communicate, are unable to cough effectively, or are at risk for aspiration.

! NURSING SAFETY PRIORITY QSEN

Action Alert

Assess the oral care needs of the patient with risk factors for thickly crusted secretions daily. Ensure that assistive personnel who provide oral care understand the importance and the correct techniques for preventing secretion buildup and airway obstruction.

❖ Interprofessional Collaborative Care

An acute airway obstruction from a foreign body may be managed in the community or emergency department. When chronic problems cause airway obstruction, more intensive interventions may be needed in an acute care setting.

◆ Assessment: Recognize Cues. Airway obstruction requires prompt care to prevent a partial obstruction from progressing to a complete obstruction. Partial obstruction produces general symptoms such as diaphoresis, tachycardia, anxiety, and elevated blood pressure. Persistent or unexplained symptoms must be evaluated even though vague. Diagnostic procedures include chest or neck x-rays, laryngoscopic examination, and CT.

Observe for hypoxia and hypercarbia, restlessness, increasing anxiety, sternal retractions, a "seesawing" chest motion, abdominal movements, or a feeling of impending doom from air hunger. Use pulse oximetry or end-tidal carbon dioxide ($ETco_2$ or $PETco_2$) for ongoing monitoring of ***gas exchange***. Continually assess for stridor, cyanosis, and changes in level of consciousness.

◆ Interventions: Take Action. Assess for the cause of the obstruction. When the obstruction is caused by the tongue falling back or excessive secretions, slightly extend the patient's head and neck and insert a nasal or an oral airway. Suction to remove obstructing secretions. If the obstruction is caused by a foreign body that cannot be removed by clearing the oral cavity manually, perform abdominal thrusts (Fig. 26.1).

! NURSING SAFETY ALERT QSEN

Action Alert

Abdominal thrust maneuver is performed on an unconscious patient instead of chest compressions *only* when a known obstruction is present and the patient has a palpable pulse. If no obstruction has been observed in an unconscious person, chest compressions are started instead of abdominal thrusts because many more unconscious adults have cardiac problems than have airway obstruction.

Upper airway obstruction may require emergency procedures such as cricothyroidotomy or tracheotomy to improve ***gas exchange*** if the object causing the obstruction cannot be removed quickly. When obstruction is not caused by a foreign object, endotracheal intubation may be needed. Laryngoscopy may be performed to determine the cause of obstruction or to remove foreign bodies.

Cricothyroidotomy is an emergency procedure performed by emergency medical personnel as a stab wound through the cricothyroid membrane between the thyroid cartilage and the cricoid cartilage (see Fig. 24.3). Any hollow tube—but preferably a tracheostomy tube—can be placed through the opening to hold this airway open until a tracheotomy can be performed. This procedure is used when it is the *only* way to secure an airway. Another emergency procedure to bypass an obstruction is the insertion of a 14-gauge needle or a very small endotracheal tube directly into the cricoid space to allow airflow into and out from the lungs.

Endotracheal intubation is performed by inserting a tube into the trachea via the nose *(nasotracheal)* or mouth *(orotracheal)* by a physician, anesthesia provider, or other specially trained personnel. When pharyngeal or laryngeal edema formation is expected or likely, an endotracheal tube is placed *before* swelling is severe enough to make insertion impossible.

Tracheotomy is a surgical procedure and takes about 5 to 10 minutes to perform. It is best performed in the operating room (OR) with the patient under local or general anesthesia but can be performed at the bedside. Local anesthesia is used if there is concern that the airway will be lost during the induction of anesthesia. A tracheotomy is reserved for the patient who cannot be easily intubated with an endotracheal tube. An emergency tracheotomy can establish an airway in less than 2 minutes. See Chapter 25 for a discussion of care of the patient with a tracheotomy.

Patients receiving mechanical ventilation for upper airway obstruction or respiratory failure may require a tracheostomy after 7 or more days of continuous endotracheal intubation. In such cases, a tracheotomy is performed to prevent laryngeal injury and loss of ***tissue integrity*** by the endotracheal tube.

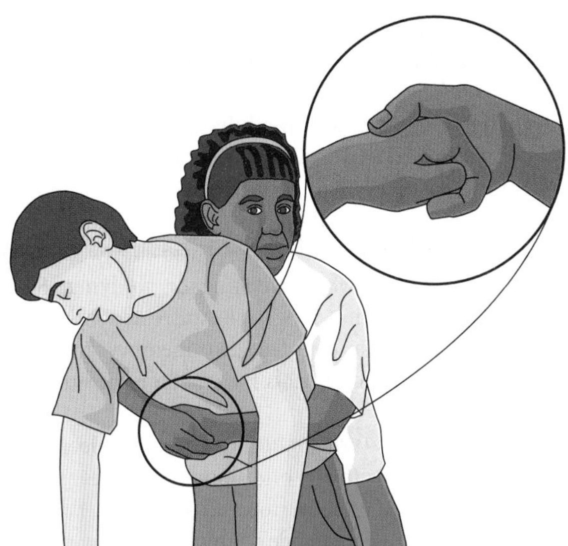

With the conscious victim standing or sitting, place your fist between the victim's lower rib cage and navel. Wrap the palm of your hand around your fist. A quick inward, upward thrust expels the air remaining in the victim's lungs, and with it the foreign body. If the first thrust is unsuccessful, repeat several thrusts in rapid succession until the foreign body is expelled or until the victim loses consciousness.

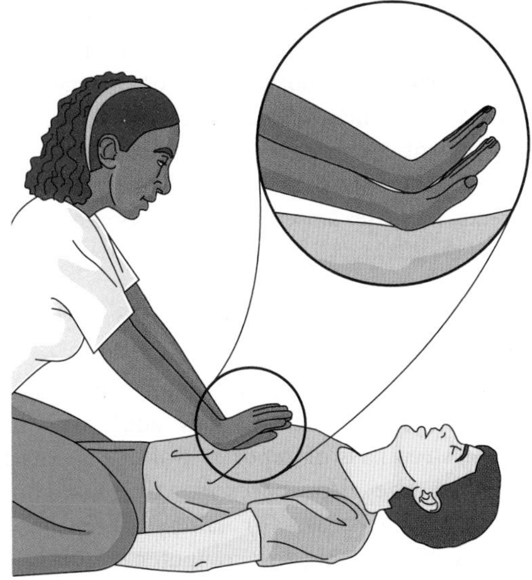

With the unconscious victim lying supine, straddle the victim's thighs. Place one hand on top of the other as shown, with the heel of the bottom hand just above the victim's navel. Quickly thrust inward and upward, toward the victim's head.

FIG. 26.1 Abdominal thrust maneuver (formerly known as the Heimlich maneuver) for relief of upper airway obstruction known to be caused by a foreign body.

NCLEX EXAMINATION CHALLENGE 26.1

Physiological Integrity

When answering the call light for a client on bedrest, the nurse finds the client's visitor unconscious on the floor with no discernable pulse and not breathing. The nurse estimates that at least 2 minutes have passed since the client's light first came on. What is the nurse's **priority action**?

A. Initiate CPR with chest compressions.
B. Perform an abdominal thrust maneuver.
C. Assess the visitor for the presence of a head injury.
D. Ask the client what event led up to the visitor's fall.

GAS EXCHANGE CONCEPT EXEMPLAR: OBSTRUCTIVE SLEEP APNEA

Pathophysiology Review

Sleep apnea can occur as a result of several different pathologic mechanisms, including dysfunction in central nervous system control over ventilation, poor circulation and oxygenation, and airway obstruction. This discussion focuses on the sleep apnea from obstructive causes.

Obstructive sleep apnea (OSA) is a type of breathing pattern disruption during sleep that lasts at least 10 seconds and occurs a minimum of five times in an hour (Miles et al., 2017; Nations & Mayo, 2016). OSA usually occurs with sleep time hypopnea (lower-than-normal respiratory rate and depth insufficient for effective *gas exchange*). During sleep the head and neck muscles relax, allowing the tongue, soft palate, and neck structures to be displaced. As a result, the upper airway is obstructed, but neural control of chest movement is unimpaired. The apnea decreases *gas exchange*, increases blood carbon dioxide levels, and decreases the pH. These blood gas changes then stimulate neural centers. The sleeper awakens after 10 seconds or longer of apnea and corrects the obstruction, and respiration resumes. After he or she goes back to sleep, the cycle begins again, sometimes as often as every 5 minutes.

This cyclic pattern of disrupted sleep and fragmented sleep prevents the deep sleep needed for best physiologic restoration. The apnea period can result in arterial blood oxygen saturation levels of significantly less than 80%. The adult with OSA usually has chronic excessive daytime sleepiness, an inability to concentrate, morning headache, and irritability. Long-term effects of chronic OSA include increased risk for hypertension, stroke, cognitive deficits, weight gain, diabetes, and pulmonary and cardiovascular disease (Senaratna et al., 2017). Hormonal energy balance regulation can lead to serious metabolic issues that ultimately affect overall health (Shechter, 2017).

Etiology and Genetic Risk. The most common cause of OSA is upper airway obstruction by the soft palate or tongue. Contributing factors include obesity, a large uvula, a short neck, smoking, enlarged tonsils or adenoids, and oropharyngeal edema. Adults with congenital variation in oral cavity structures, the pharynx, or the neck also are at increased risk for OSA. For example, adults who have the genetic disorder achondroplasia have a higher incidence of sudden infant death syndrome (SIDS) during the first year of life and OSA as older children and adults (Beery et al., 2018).

Incidence and Prevalence. The actual incidence of OSA is not known because it is an underreported health problem.

Adults may consider heavy snoring a minor normal issue and not understand what it may reflect. The prevalence of OSA among adults in affluent countries is estimated at between 9% and 38%. Men are affected more frequently than women, and the incidence greatly increases among both genders after age 65 years (Senaratna et al., 2017)

❖ Interprofessional Collaborative Care

◆ Assessment: Recognize Cues

History. Patients are often unaware that they have sleep apnea. The disorder is suspected for any adult who has persistent daytime sleepiness or reports "waking up tired," particularly if he or she also snores heavily. Ask about sensations of daytime sleepiness or falling asleep while performing tasks such as using the computer, reading, or driving. In extreme cases, patients may fall asleep while eating or any time they sit down. Ask whether the patient can recall ever being awakened by his or her own snoring and whether family members have noticed heavy snoring. Ask about the frequency of nightmares, which are associated with OSA. Also ask whether family members have ever observed the patient to have a disturbed breathing pattern while sleeping. A common pattern consists of breaths that become further apart followed by a period of no breathing *(apnea)*, which is then followed by chest and abdominal movements that lead to gasping and snorting with partial awakening to correct the obstruction temporarily. Also ask patients who may have OSA whether they have tried to induce a deeper sleep with over-the-counter sleep aids or increased evening alcohol consumption.

Many patients with OSA develop some degree of gastroesophageal reflux disease (GERD) at night. Possible causes include strong abdominal and chest movements during an apnea episode, overeating, eating or drinking close to bedtime, and lying flat while sleeping. Ask the patient whether he or she is awakened often with "heartburn," stomach contents in the mouth, or a burning, choking sensation with coughing. Determine the frequency of such episodes.

Physical Assessment/Signs and Symptoms. Assess the patient's general appearance including height and weight. Many adults with OSA are overweight, which can both cause OSA and be caused by this disorder. Examine the jaw, external neck, and chin. OSA is associated with a retracted lower jaw, smaller chin, and shorter neck. Examine the oral cavity and throat for size and shape of the pharynx, size and shape of the uvula, and tongue thickness and position, and determine whether other structures (e.g., tonsils, adenoids, pillars, soft palate) are swollen or enlarged.

Chronic OSA is associated with cardiovascular changes, especially hypertension that may not respond as expected to prescribed drug therapy. Assess the patient's blood pressure and heart rate and rhythm, as well as pulse oximetry. If the patient is being treated for hypertension, ask which drug(s) and drug dosages are used for its management. If the patient is not being treated for hypertension but blood pressure is elevated on assessment, retake the blood pressure later during the examination. Document persistent elevations.

Psychosocial Assessment. Irritability and personality changes are common in adults with persistent OSA, including depression, as is a general loss of interest in social activities. Family members can be helpful in determining the presence of these psychosocial changes. Ask the patient about problems with recall, concentration, perceived energy level, and the ability to stay on task when working or studying. Some clinicians have suggested that long-term untreated OSA with significant cerebral hypoxia can lead to memory loss and dementia, although no clinical trials have been performed to explore this possibility.

Diagnostic Assessment. Obstructive sleep apnea (OSA) is not diagnosed with any one blood test or imaging method. Some specific tests may be performed after OSA has been diagnosed to determine the presence of any anatomic variations and health problems that either predispose the adult to OSA or are made worse by it. Results can then be used to help determine the best intervention approach for the patient's specific cause of OSA.

A beginning assessment includes having the patient complete a questionnaire regarding perceived sleep quality and extent of daytime sleepiness. Examples of such questionnaires include the STOP-Bang Sleep Apnea Questionnaire, the Epworth Sleepiness Scale, the Pittsburgh Sleep Quality Index, and the Multiple Sleep Latency Test, among others. If the results of a questionnaire suggest OSA, the patient may then undergo a less intrusive "at-home" sleep study. The patient sleeps in his or her own bed with electronic monitoring of respiratory rate, heart rate, chest movement, eye movements, and other muscle activity. If results indicate a sleep apnea problem, the patient is referred for a more definitive overnight sleep study known as **polysomnography** in which he or she is directly observed during a full sleep time while wearing a variety of monitoring equipment to evaluate depth of sleep, type of sleep, respiratory effort, oxygen saturation, carbon dioxide exhalation, and muscle movement. Monitoring methods include an electroencephalogram (EEG), an electrocardiogram (ECG), pulse oximetry, and electromyography (EMG).

◆ Analysis: Analyze Cues and Prioritize Hypotheses. The primary collaborative problem for the patient with moderate-to-severe OSA is persistent poor ***gas exchange*** and hypoxia due to abnormal sleep pattern.

◆ Planning and Implementation: Generate Solutions and Take Action

Improving the Duration of Restorative Sleep

Planning Expected Outcomes. The patient is expected to achieve a sleep pattern consistent with adequate ***gas exchange*** and longer-duration restorative sleep.

Interventions. Management strategies for OSA vary with the severity of the problem and the patient's willingness to participate in the treatment process. Both nonsurgical and surgical management approaches are available to help correct the problem, depending on the cause and the severity. Far more patients are helped by nonsurgical procedures; surgical management is reserved for anatomic-related causes and severe OSA that remains resistant to nonsurgical approaches.

Nonsurgical Management. Collaborative management for patients with OSA focuses on reducing the obstruction and improving both the depth and the duration of restorative sleep patterns. Changes in sleeping position or weight loss may correct mild sleep apnea and improve ***gas exchange***. More severe OSA requires additional methods to prevent obstruction.

Position-fixing devices may prevent subluxation of the tongue and reduce obstruction. Use of an oral appliance, called *maxillomandibular advancement,* can improve airflow by supporting the lower jaw in a more forward position. These devices are especially helpful for adults who have a retracted lower jaw. Some devices also help prevent the tongue from slipping backward during sleep. These devices are bulky and some patients cannot tolerate their presence in the mouth. They may also increase the risk for loss of ***tissue integrity*** of the oral mucosa.

Noninvasive positive-pressure ventilation (NPPV) via continuous positive airway pressure (CPAP) to hold open the upper airways is the most commonly used form of nonsurgical management for OSA. CPAP delivers a set positive airway pressure continuously during each cycle of inhalation and exhalation with the use of a small electric compressor and some type of delivery device such as a nasal-oral facemask, nasal mask, or nasal pillows (with or without cushioned or gel prongs). Any type of delivery mask or pillow used requires a proper and relatively tight fit to form a seal over the nose and mouth or just over the nose for successful therapy. Fig. 25.9 in Chapter 25 shows a properly fitted standard nasal CPAP mask.

Older CPAP setups had machines that were noisy, were not always humidified, and used larger masks, all of which contributed to reduced patient adherence with the therapy. Newer machines are very quiet and humidify the air. Many patients find the use of small masks (with or without cushioned or gel prongs) such as that shown in Fig. 26.2, rather than a full or partial mask, less intrusive and more acceptable. Smaller masks can help maintain ***tissue integrity***. In addition, newer CPAP compressors are able to monitor many patient parameters (e.g., oxygen saturation, number and duration of apnea episodes, heart rate, air leaks, duration of correct usage, and other data) that can be sent electronically to the patient's smart phone and/or the health care provider's office as a way to measure therapy effectiveness.

Stress to the patient that adherence with the therapy is critical in reducing all the health problem risks associated with OSA. The equipment can be expensive and much of the cost is covered by Medicare for older adults if the patient uses it consistently for at least 6 hours daily. After a period of adjustment many patients who use CPAP therapy consistently sleep well and feel so much better that adherence is less of an issue. Other patients find the equipment and routine too intrusive or unacceptable and may not even try it. Providing accurate information and patient education is therefore essential for therapy success. Many sleep apnea clinics and practices provide in-depth educational materials and patient-assistance resources to help reduce patient anxiety and promote adherence.

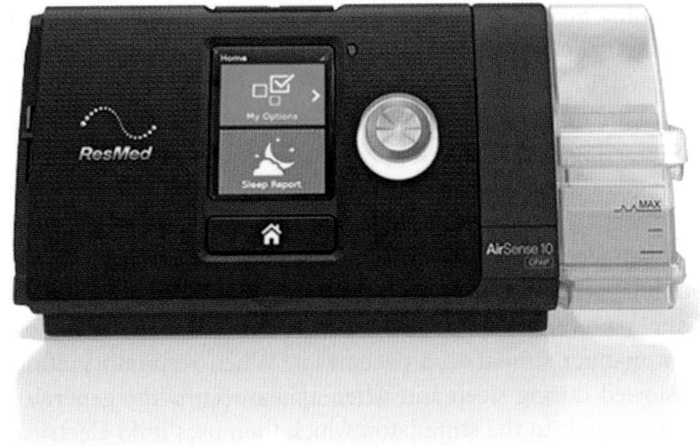

A

B

FIG. 26.2 (A) Automated CPAP machine and monitor. (B) Patient wearing the nasal "pillow" (without prongs) device (connecting to the CPAP tubing) to manage sleep apnea. (A ©ResMed. All rights reserved.)

Drug therapy for OSA has not been very successful. Sedatives to promote nighttime sleep may make OSA worse. Stimulants to help promote daytime wakefulness have many side effects and do not contribute to restorative sleep. Neither sedatives nor stimulants treat the cause of OSA.

Surgical Management. Surgical intervention is considered when patients are not able to tolerate CPAP or when its use does not improve OSA. Before surgery is planned, patients may first undergo a thorough endoscopic examination under deep sedation to determine which problem or problems cause the OSA. This examination can reveal variation in anatomic structures or changes in anatomic features that result from oral-pharyngeal muscle relaxation. Once a specific cause or problem has been identified, the correct specific surgery can be planned. Regardless of the specific type of surgery used, follow the standard preoperative and postoperative care procedures and nursing responsibilities presented in Chapter 9.

Implanted stimulators represent a minimally invasive surgery that can help patients with mild-to-moderate sleep apnea. This surgery involves placing an electrode in the neck that can stimulate the hypoglossal nerve (cranial nerve XII). The small battery-powered charge generator is implanted in the chest in a manner similar to a pacemaker. When respiratory effort is slowed during sleep and when apnea occurs, the generator sends signals to the stimulator, which then uses mild electrical shocks to cause contraction of appropriate airway muscles. The stimulatory shocks are of such a low intensity that the patient is not awakened and does not feel pain but are strong enough to keep the airway open. It is not strong enough to keep the airway open in patients whose OSA is caused by complete concentric collapse of the soft palate during sleep.

Tracheostomy is a possible but uncommon type of surgery to manage OSA. It is reserved as a last resort for very severe OSA that is not relieved by more moderate interventions.

Common minor surgical procedures that can correct some anatomic problems associated with mild-to-moderate OSA include simple tonsillectomy, adenoidectomy, uvulectomy, or repair of a deviated septum. When such procedures are performed individually, same-day surgery may be appropriate. If bleeding risk is increased or if airway swelling is significant, the patient may need to be observed overnight. Any or all of these procedures can be combined as part of more complex surgeries to manage OSA.

Uvulopalatopharyngoplasty (UPPP) is a collection of procedures that are more complex and intended to resolve OSA by remodeling the entire posterior oropharynx. Older UPPP procedures focused on significant removal of tissue in the oropharyngeal cavity. These older, more extensive procedures often were not successful in correcting OSA, leaving some patients no better off and sometimes worse than before surgery. Immediate complications included severe pain, bleeding, and oropharyngeal swelling. Long-term complications sometimes included permanent taste changes, changes in voice quality, and scar tissue formation.

Modified uvulopalatopharyngoplasty (modUPPP) is a more recent reconstructive approach with a variety of procedures that may be performed using conventional, robotic-assisted, or laser surgery techniques. The procedure is individualized by the surgeon for each patient. With modUPPP the focus is less on extensive tissue removal and more on repositioning and reinforcing oropharyngeal support structures to improve oropharyngeal airway flow. Although exact surgical techniques vary, the desired outcome is to change the pull of palatal and oropharyngeal muscles from central and downward to upward and toward the sides of the throat, thus making the oropharynx larger. Usually patients are hospitalized for 2 or more days, and recovery takes an average of 3 to 6 weeks. Complications in the immediate period after surgery include edema, infection, and bleeding. Pain and difficulty swallowing are common for the first week after surgery.

Postoperative Care. Specific nursing care needs for the patient after surgery to manage OSA focus on maintaining a patent airway, relieving pain, and preventing complications.

Maintaining a patent airway in the postoperative period is important because the tissue manipulation during surgery results in some degree of temporary swelling. Observe the patient for respiratory effort and effectiveness of ***gas exchange*** based on pulse oximetry or end-tidal carbon dioxide measurement. Assess the size and shape of the oropharynx. Assess whether the patient can swallow effectively, even if it is painful. Note whether he or she can swallow oral secretions or whether drooling is present. Assess voice quality and determine whether stridor or crowing is present; these conditions indicate a partial obstruction of the airway.

! NURSING SAFETY PRIORITY QSEN

Critical Rescue

Assess the patient at least every 2 hours during the first 24 hours after surgery for indications of airway narrowing or partial obstruction (e.g., increased respiratory effort, presence of stridor or crowing, drooling or an inability to swallow oral secretions, reduction in the size of the oropharynx, decreasing oxygen saturation, rising end-tidal carbon dioxide level). If any of these signs or symptoms are present, initiate the Rapid Response Team to prevent a partial obstruction from becoming a complete obstruction.

Relieving pain after surgery has a high priority because the oropharynx has a rich nerve supply and is extremely sensitive. Usually the patient receives pain control drugs parenterally for the first 24 hours because of the pain involved in swallowing. Pain is best managed when analgesics are given on a schedule rather than PRN. Aspirin and other NSAIDs are avoided during the first 24 hours to reduce the risk for excessive bleeding.

Preventing complications focuses on the potential for bleeding and potential for infection. The oropharynx has a rich blood supply and excessive bleeding is possible.

Infection risk after surgery for OSA is somewhat increased because the surgical area disrupts ***tissue integrity*** and is open to the environment, and the patient's microbiome is continually present. Many surgeons prescribe antibiotics in the intraoperative and postoperative periods. This operation cannot be a truly sterile procedure. Assess the oropharynx daily for indicators of infection including the presence of purulent exudate, foul-smelling breath, or a change in color of mucous membranes to beefy red. Document and report any of these changes.

The oropharynx and its associated structures have a rich blood supply and have the potential for excessive bleeding during and after surgery. Some bleeding or oozing after surgery is normal. Examine the oropharynx for the amount and color of bleeding from surgical sites every 2 to 4 hours the first day. Darker blood and blood mixed with secretions is considered normal. If the amount of blood increases or becomes bright red, notify the surgeon. Instruct the patient to tell nursing personnel if he or she perceives an increase in bleeding. Assess the patient for excessive swallowing or belching that could indicate blood dripping down the throat. Avoid the use of aspirin or NSAID-containing pain relievers until the risk for bleeding has passed. Instruct the patient to avoid trauma to the area by avoiding toothbrushes and using mouthwash and oral sponges to clean the teeth and gums until the surgeon indicates toothbrushing and flossing are permitted.

Care Coordination and Transition Management. Most patients who are prescribed to use CPAP for treatment of OSA are managed in the community. Usually follow-up with the primary health care provider or a sleep center is ongoing to determine treatment effectiveness. For those patients who require surgery for management of OSA, the patient is usually discharged home within 2 to 3 days. At the time of discharge pain is controlled with oral drugs and the patient should be able to swallow effectively.

Self-Management Education. An important issue with CPAP therapy for OSA management is appropriate maintenance of the compressor and the mask/tubular system. Keeping the system clean is critical to prevent infection and maintain ***tissue integrity***. With humidification, fungal infections are possible. Most setups require the use of distilled water in the humidifier. The mask device or pillows must be cleaned daily using agents recommended by the specific manufacturer. Instruct the patient to not share the mask, pillows, or tubing with other people to reduce the risk for infection.

Teach patients who had surgical interventions for OSA to assess the oropharynx for bleeding, swelling, or indications of infection. A small amount of blood mixed with saliva or mucus, particularly after coughing, is normal. However, new-onset bleeding, large clots, or bright red blood may indicate serious problems. Instruct the patient to notify the surgeon immediately or go to the emergency department if this should occur.

Teach the patient how to examine his or her throat with a mirror twice daily and assess its internal size (often by comparing it to coin sizes). A narrowing of the throat or an inability to swallow (with or without pain), and the presence of drooling are indicators of swelling that may obstruct the airway. Instruct the patient to go to the emergency room should these occur.

Pain is expected to decrease daily and swallowing should become increasingly more comfortable. Drinking cool liquids, keeping the environment humidified, gargling frequently with warm salt water, and eating soft foods can help reduce pain. Instruct the patient to report an increase in pain or increasingly greater difficulty swallowing to the surgeon.

Teach the patient the indications of infection and to notify the surgeon if they occur. Infection indications include an increase in swelling, the presence of pus in any area of the oropharynx, a change in color of the mucous membrane to a "beefy red," an increase in pain, the presence of fever, taste changes, and the presence of bad breath.

Activity restriction varies depending on the exact nature of the procedure performed. Obtain a list of surgeon-directed activity restrictions and educate the patient about why each restriction has been prescribed. The most common restrictions include lifting and performing the Valsalva maneuver (holding the breath and bearing down).

Psychosocial Preparation. Some patients using CPAP therapy for management of OSA may have anxiety about correct use of the equipment and possible disruption of nighttime routine. All patients require some period of adjustment to the therapy. Provide the patient with written and digital instructions for the use and care of CPAP. Also provide telephone resource numbers for health care professionals specializing in the management of OSA and for supplies needed for long-term use of CPAP.

After surgery the patient may have some anxiety about whether the surgical intervention was successful and about pain and swallowing issues. Remind him or her that pain and difficulty swallowing are expected but should rapidly improve in a week. Snoring or sleep apnea may continue for a short time after surgery until all swelling is gone.

◆ **Evaluation: Evaluate Outcomes.** Evaluate the care of the patient with obstructive sleep apnea (OSA) based on the priority patient problem. The expected outcomes are that the patient:

- Does not remain hypertensive or has hypertension that can be controlled with appropriate therapy
- Is adherent with prescribed nonsurgical interventions
- Has fewer sleep-time apnea periods of 10 seconds or longer
- Has improved ***gas exchange*** with greater duration of restorative sleep
- Reports less daytime sleepiness and has more energy
- Has an uneventful recovery from surgical intervention

NCLEX EXAMINATION CHALLENGE 26.2

Health Promotion and Maintenance

Which information is **most relevant** for the nurse to teach a client about CPAP therapy for OSA? **Select all that apply.**

A. Avoid alcoholic beverages or drugs that make you sleepy within 3 hours of bed time.
B. Clean the mask device daily.
C. Ensure your mask device fits tightly enough to prevent air leaks.
D. Keep open flames such as candles out of the room when CPAP is in use.
E. Seal the mask edges to your face with petroleum jelly.
F. Use only sterile water in the humidifier tank.
G. Use the CPAP during all sleep periods, especially in bed.
H. Do not share your mask or tubing system with others.

EPISTAXIS

Pathophysiology Review

Epistaxis (nosebleed) is a common problem because of the many capillaries within the nose. Nosebleeds occur as a result of loss of ***tissue integrity*** from trauma to the nasal mucosa, hypertension, blood dyscrasia (e.g., leukemia), inflammation, tumor, decreased humidity, nose blowing, nose picking, chronic cocaine use, and procedures such as nasogastric (NG) suctioning. Older adults tend to bleed most often from the posterior portion of the nose.

❖ Interprofessional Collaborative Care

The patient often reports that the bleeding started after sneezing or blowing the nose. Document the amount and color of the blood, and take vital signs. Ask about the number, duration, and causes of previous bleeding episodes.

BEST PRACTICE FOR PATIENT SAFETY & QUALITY CARE QSEN

Emergency Care for a Patient With an Anterior Nosebleed

- Maintain Standard Precautions or Body Substance Precautions.
- Position the patient upright and leaning forward to prevent blood from entering the larynx and possible aspiration.
- Reassure the patient and attempt to keep him or her quiet to reduce anxiety and blood pressure.
- Apply direct lateral pressure to the nose for 10 minutes and apply ice or cool compresses to the nose and face if possible.
- If nasal packing is necessary, loosely pack both nares with gauze or nasal tampons.
- To prevent rebleeding from dislodging clots, instruct the patient to not blow the nose for 24 hours after the bleeding stops.
- Instruct the patient to seek medical assistance if these measures are ineffective or if the bleeding occurs frequently.

Review the Best Practice for Patient Safety & Quality Care box for emergency care of the patient with an anterior nosebleed. An additional intervention for use at home or in the emergency department is a nasal plug that contains an agent to promote blood clotting and expands on contact with blood to compress mucosal blood vessels.

Medical attention is needed if the nosebleed does not respond to these interventions. In such cases, the affected capillaries may be cauterized with silver nitrate or electrocautery, and the nose packed. Anterior packing controls bleeding from the anterior nasal cavity.

Posterior nasal bleeding is an emergency because it cannot be easily reached and the patient may lose a lot of blood quickly. Posterior packing, epistaxis catheters (nasal pressure tubes), or gel tampons are placed through the nose within the posterior nasal region to stop the bleeding. Placement of these devices is uncomfortable; and the airway may be obstructed with reduced ***gas exchange*** if the pack slips (Schreiber, 2020).

Observe the patient for respiratory distress and for tolerance of the devices. Humidity, oxygen, bedrest, and antibiotics may be prescribed. Opioid drugs may be prescribed for pain. Assess patients receiving opioids at least hourly for gag and cough reflexes. Use pulse oximetry to monitor for hypoxemia. The tubes or packing is usually removed after 1 to 3 days.

For posterior bleeding that does not respond to packing or tubes, additional options include cauterizing or ligating the blood vessels or performing an embolization of the bleeding artery with interventional radiology. Potential complications of embolization include facial pain, loss of ***tissue integrity*** with necrosis of skin or nasal mucosa, facial nerve paralysis, and blindness.

After the tubes or packing has been removed, teach the patient and family these interventions to use at home for comfort and safety:

- Apply petroleum jelly sparingly to the nares for comfort.
- Use saline nasal sprays after healing to add moisture and prevent rebleeding.
- Avoid vigorous nose blowing, the use of aspirin or other NSAIDs, and strenuous activities such as heavy lifting for at least 1 month.

FRACTURES OF THE NOSE

Pathophysiology Review

Injury to the nose may result in loss of ***tissue integrity*** with nasal fractures that interfere with ***gas exchange***. If the bone or cartilage is not displaced and no complications are present, treatment may not be needed. However, displacement of either the bone or cartilage can cause airway obstruction or cosmetic deformity and is a potential source of infection.

❖ Interprofessional Collaborative Care

◆ Assessment: Recognize Cues. Document any nasal problem, including deviation, malaligned nasal bridge, a change in nasal breathing, crackling of the skin *(crepitus)* on palpation, bruising, and pain. Blood or clear fluid (cerebrospinal fluid [CSF]) may drain from one or both nares as a result of a simple nasal fracture. This is rare and, if present, indicates a serious injury (e.g., skull fracture). CSF can be differentiated from normal nasal secretions because CSF contains glucose that will test positive with a dipstick test for glucose. When CSF dries on a piece of filter paper, a yellow "halo" appears as a ring at the dried edge of the fluid.

◆ Interventions: Take Action. The primary health care provider performs a simple closed reduction (moving the bones by palpation to realign them) of the nasal fracture using local or general anesthesia within the first 24 hours after injury. After 24 hours the fracture is more difficult to reduce because of edema and scar formation. Then reduction may be delayed for several days until edema is gone. Management focuses on pain relief and cold compresses to decrease swelling.

Rhinoplasty. Reduction and surgery may be needed for severe fractures or for those that do not heal properly. **Rhinoplasty** is a surgical reconstruction of the nose performed to repair a fractured nose and also to change the shape of the nose for improved function or appearance. The patient returns from surgery with packing in both nostrils, which prevents bleeding and provides support for the reconstructed nose. As long as the packing is in place, the patient cannot breathe through the nose. A "moustache" dressing (or drip pad), often a folded 2 × 2 gauze pad, is usually placed under the nose (Fig. 26.3). A splint or cast may cover the nose for better alignment and protection. Change or teach the patient to change the drip pad as necessary.

After surgery, observe for edema and bleeding from loss of ***tissue integrity***. The patient with uncomplicated rhinoplasty usually is discharged the day of surgery. Instruct him or her and the family about the routine care described in the following paragraphs.

! NURSING SAFETY PRIORITY QSEN

Action Alert

Assessing how often the patient swallows after nasal surgery is a priority because repeated swallowing may indicate posterior nasal bleeding. Use a penlight to examine the throat for bleeding and notify the surgeon if bleeding is present.

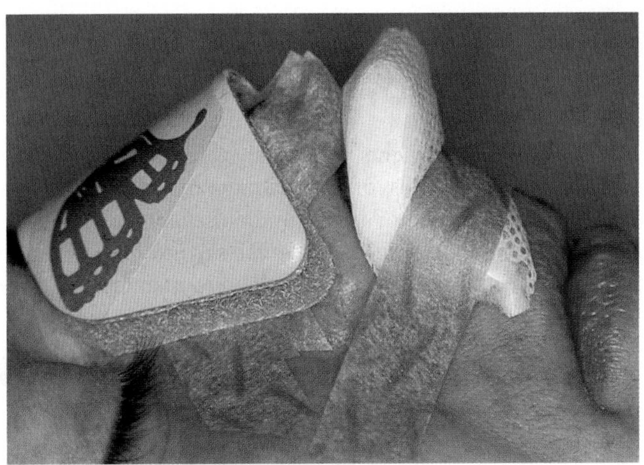

FIG. 26.3 Immediate postoperative appearance of a patient who has undergone rhinoplasty. Note the splint and gauze drip pad (moustache dressing). (From Tardy, M.E. [1997]. *Rhinoplasty: The art and science*. Philadelphia: Saunders. Used with permission.)

Instruct the patient to stay in a semi-Fowler position and to move slowly. Suggest that he or she rest and use cool compresses on the nose, eyes, and face to help reduce swelling and bruising. After the gag reflex has returned, urge the patient to drink at least 2500 mL/day.

To prevent bleeding, teach the patient to avoid forceful coughing or straining during a bowel movement, not to sniff upward or blow the nose, and not to sneeze with the mouth closed for the first few days after the packing is removed. Instruct him or her to avoid aspirin and other NSAIDs to prevent bleeding. Antibiotics may be prescribed to prevent infection. Explain that because of edema the final surgical result may require 6 to 12 months.

Nasoseptoplasty. Nasoseptoplasty, or submucous resection (SMR), may be needed to straighten a deviated septum when chronic symptoms or discomfort occurs. The deviated section of cartilage and bone is removed or reshaped as an ambulatory surgical procedure. Nursing care is similar to that for a rhinoplasty.

FACIAL TRAUMA

Pathophysiology Review

Facial trauma is described by the specific bones (e.g., mandibular, maxillary, orbital, nasal fractures) and the side of the face involved. Mandibular (lower jaw) fractures are the most common. *Le Fort I* is a nasoethmoid complex fracture. *Le Fort II* is a maxillary *and* nasoethmoid complex fracture. *Le Fort III* combines I and II plus an orbital-zygoma fracture, called *craniofacial disjunction* because the midface has no connection to the skull. The rich facial blood supply results in extensive bleeding and bruising with loss of ***tissue integrity***.

❖ Interprofessional Collaborative Care

◆ **Assessment: Recognize Cues.** *The priority action when caring for a patient with facial trauma is airway assessment for* ***gas exchange****.* Signs of airway obstruction are stridor, shortness of breath, dyspnea, anxiety, restlessness, hypoxia, decreased oxygen saturation, cyanosis, and loss of consciousness. After establishing the airway, assess the trauma site for bleeding and obvious fractures. Check for soft-tissue edema, facial asymmetry, pain, or leakage of spinal fluid through the ears or nose, indicating a skull fracture. Assess vision and eye movement because orbital and maxillary fractures can entrap the eye nerves and muscles. Check behind the ears (mastoid area) for extensive bruising, known as the "battle sign," which is often associated with skull fracture and brain trauma. Because facial trauma can occur with spinal trauma and skull fractures, cranial CT, facial series, and cervical spine x-rays are obtained.

◆ **Interventions: Take Action.** *The priority action is to establish and maintain an airway for adequate* ***gas exchange****.* Anticipate the need for emergency intubation, tracheotomy, or *cricothyroidotomy* (creation of a temporary airway by making a small opening in the throat between the thyroid cartilage and the cricoid cartilage). Care at first focuses on establishing an airway, controlling hemorrhage, and assessing for the extent of injury.

Time is critical in stabilizing the patient who has head and neck trauma. Early response and treatment by special interprofessional services (e.g., trauma team, maxillofacial surgeon, general surgeon, otolaryngologist, plastic surgeon, dentist) optimize the patient's recovery.

Stabilizing the fractured jaw allows the teeth to heal in proper alignment and involves *fixed occlusion* (wiring the jaws together with the mouth in a closed position). The patient remains in fixed occlusion for 6 to 10 weeks. Treatment delay, tooth infection, or poor oral care may cause jaw bone infection. This condition may then require surgical removal of dead tissue, IV antibiotic therapy, and a longer period with the jaws in a fixed position.

Extensive jaw fractures may require open reduction with internal fixation (ORIF) procedures. Compression plates and reconstruction plates with screws may be applied. Plates may be made of stainless steel, titanium, or a metal alloy. Usually these plates are permanent. Depending on the metal used, they may or may not interfere with MRI studies.

Facial fractures may be repaired with microplating surgical systems that involve bone substitutes or commercial bone graft material. Shaping plates hold the bone fragments in place until new bone growth occurs. The plates may remain in place permanently or may be removed after healing.

With inner maxillary fixation (IMF), the bones are realigned and then wired in place with the bite closed. Nondisplaced aligned fractures can be repaired in a clinic or office using local dental anesthesia. General anesthesia is used to repair displaced or complex fractures or fractures that occur with other facial bone fractures.

After surgery, teach the patient about oral care with an irrigating device such as a Water-Pik or Sonicare. If the patient has IMF, teach self-management with wires in place, including a dental liquid diet. If the patient vomits, watch for aspiration because of the patient's inability to open the jaws to allow ejection of the emesis. Teach him or her how to cut the wires if vomiting occurs to maintain ***gas exchange***. If the wires are cut, instruct the patient to return to the surgeon for rewiring as soon as possible to reinstitute fixation.

Nutrition is important and difficult for a patient with fractures because of oral fixation. Collaborate with the registered dietitian nutritionist for patient teaching and support.

> **! NURSING SAFETY PRIORITY (QSEN)**
>
> ***Action Alert***
>
> Instruct the patient to keep wire cutters with him or her at all times to prevent aspiration if vomiting occurs.

> **CLINICAL JUDGMENT CHALLENGE 26.1**
>
> ***Safety; Patient-Centered Care***
>
> The client is a 28-year-old social worker and former opioid addict who was a passenger in a car crash about an hour ago in which he was restrained but a heavy object came through the windshield and hit him in the face. He is bleeding heavily from facial trauma and has lost several front teeth. His face and neck have extensive bruising and lacerations. He is alert and aware of his surroundings and can talk. He is concerned about his girlfriend, who was driving the car when it was hit by a vehicle that swerved into her lane while trying to avoid a deer. He rates his pain as an 8 on a scale of 0 to 10. His admitting vital signs are:
>
> HR = 110 beats/min
> RR = 30 breaths/min
> BP = 108/50 mm Hg
> Oxygen saturation = 91%
>
> 1. **Recognize Cues:** What assessment information in this client situation is the most important and immediate concern for the nurse? (Hint: Identify the **relevant** information first to determine what is most important.)
> 2. **Analyze Cues:** What client conditions are consistent with the **most relevant** information? (Hint: Think about priority collaborative problems that support and contradict the information presented in this situation.)
> 3. **Prioritize Hypotheses:** Which possibilities or explanations are **most likely** to be present in this client situation? Which possibilities or explanations are the most serious? (Hint: Consider all possibilities and determine their urgency and risk for this client.)
> 4. **Generate Solutions:** What actions would most likely achieve the desired outcomes for this client? Which actions should be **avoided** or are **potentially harmful**? (Hint: Determine the desired outcomes first to decide which interventions are appropriate and those that should be avoided.)
> 5. **Take Action:** Which actions are the most appropriate and how should they be implemented? In what **priority order** should they be implemented? (Hint: Consider health teaching, documentation, requested health care provider orders or prescriptions, nursing skills, collaboration with or referral to health team members, etc.)
> 6. **Evaluate Outcomes:** What client assessment would indicate that the nurse's actions were **effective**? (Hint: Think about signs that would indicate an improvement, decline, or unchanged client condition.)

LARYNGEAL TRAUMA

Laryngeal trauma and damage occur with a crushing or direct-blow injury, fracture, or prolonged endotracheal intubation with loss of ***tissue integrity***. Symptoms include difficulty breathing, inability to produce sound *(aphonia)*, hoarseness, and subcutaneous emphysema (air present in the subcutaneous tissue). Bleeding from the airway *(hemoptysis)* may occur, depending on the location of the trauma. The primary health care provider performs a direct visual examination of the larynx by laryngoscopy or fiberoptic laryngoscopy to determine the extent of the injury.

Management of patients with laryngeal injuries consists of assessing the effectiveness of ***gas exchange*** and monitoring vital signs (including respiratory status and pulse oximetry) every 15 to 30 minutes. *Maintaining a patent airway is a priority.* Apply oxygen and humidification as prescribed to maintain adequate oxygen saturation.

> **! NURSING SAFETY PRIORITY (QSEN)**
>
> ***Critical Rescue***
>
> Assess the patient for signs of respiratory difficulty (tachypnea, nasal flaring, anxiety, sternal retraction, shortness of breath, restlessness, decreased oxygen saturation, decreased level of consciousness, stridor). If any signs are present, respond by staying with the patient and instructing other trauma team members or the Rapid Response Team to prepare for an emergency intubation or tracheotomy.

Surgical intervention is needed for lacerations of the mucous membranes, cartilage exposure, and cord paralysis. Laryngeal repair is performed as soon as possible to prevent laryngeal stenosis and to cover any exposed cartilage. An artificial airway may be needed temporarily.

> **NCLEX EXAMINATION CHALLENGE 26.3**
>
> ***Safe and Effective Care Environment***
>
> Which nursing action has the **highest priority** when caring for a client with any type of facial or laryngeal trauma?
>
> A. Managing pain
> B. Providing nutrition
> C. Assessing self-image
> D. Maintaining a patent airway

CANCER OF THE NOSE AND SINUSES

Tumors of the nasal cavities and sinuses result from the loss of cellular regulation. Malignant tumors are rare and are more common among adults with chronic exposure to wood dusts, dusts from textiles, leather dusts, flour, nickel and chromium dust, mustard gas, and radium. Cigarette smoking along with these exposures increases the risk (American Cancer Society [ACS], 2020).

The onset of sinus cancer is slow, and symptoms resemble sinusitis. These include persistent nasal obstruction, drainage, bloody discharge, and pain that persists after treatment of sinusitis. Lymph node enlargement often occurs on the side with tumor mass. Tumor location is identified with x-ray, CT, or MRI. A biopsy is performed to confirm the diagnosis.

Surgical removal of all or part of the tumor is the main treatment for nasopharyngeal cancers and often is combined with radiation therapy. Chemotherapy may be used in conjunction with surgery and radiation for some tumors. Problems after surgery include a change in body image or speech and changes in taste and smell.

Provide general postoperative care as described in Chapter 9, including maintaining a patent airway, monitoring for hemorrhage, providing wound care, assessing nutrition status, and performing tracheostomy care (if needed). (See Chapter 25 for tracheostomy care.) Perform careful mouth and sinus cavity care with saline irrigations using an electronic irrigation system (e.g., Water-Pik, Sonicare) or a syringe. Assess the patient for pain and infection.

HEAD AND NECK CANCER

Pathophysiology Review

Head and neck cancer is relatively common and its effect can have devastating consequences for ***gas exchange***, eating, facial appearance, self-image, speech, and communication. The care needs for patients with these problems are complex, requiring a coordinated interprofessional team approach. Common team members include an oncologist, surgeon, nurse, registered dietitian nutritionist, speech-language pathologist, dentist, respiratory therapist, social worker, wound care specialist, clergy, occupational and physical therapists, and psychosocial counselors (Janotha & Tamari, 2017).

Head and neck cancers are usually squamous cell carcinomas. These slow-growing tumors are curable when diagnosed and treated at an early stage. The prognosis for those who have more advanced disease at diagnosis depends on the extent and location of the tumors. Untreated, these cancers are often fatal within 2 years of diagnosis (ACS, 2020).

The cancer begins as a loss of cellular regulation when the mucosa is chronically irritated and becomes tougher and thicker. Eventually genes controlling cell growth are damaged, allowing excessive growth of these abnormal and malignant cells. Initial lesions first appear as white, patchy lesions *(leukoplakia)* or red, velvety patches *(erythroplakia)*. Head and neck cancer first spreads (metastasizes) into local lymph nodes, muscle, and bone. Later spread is systemic to distant sites, usually to the lungs or liver.

Most head and neck cancers arise from the mucous membrane and skin, but they also can start from salivary glands, the thyroid, tonsils, or other structures. Treatment is based on tumor cell type and degree of spread at diagnosis.

The two major risk factors for head and neck cancer are tobacco and alcohol use, especially in combination (McCance et al., 2019). Other risk factors include voice abuse, chronic laryngitis, exposure to chemicals or dusts, poor oral hygiene, long-term gastroesophageal reflux disease (GERD), and oral infection with human papillomavirus (HPV) (ACS, 2020; Gallagher et al., 2017; McKiernan & Thom, 2016). An interesting feature of HPV-positive head and neck cancers is that they have a much higher overall survival rate than do HPV-negative head and neck cancers at the same stage (Katz, 2017). About 68,000 new cases of oral, pharyngeal, and laryngeal cancers are diagnosed each year in North America and account for more than 14,000 deaths per year (ACS, 2020; Canadian Cancer Society, 2019). They affect men twice as often as women and are most common in adults older than 60 years.

❖ Interprofessional Collaborative Care

Adults with head and neck cancer may be treated on an outpatient basis with radiation for early-stage disease. When surgery is needed, care starts in an acute care environment and can involve a stay of 5 days or more. Chemotherapy is usually performed in an outpatient setting.

INTERPROFESSIONAL COLLABORATION

The Patient With Head and Neck Cancer

The three health care professionals who work with the nursing staff, patient, and family closely after surgery are the respiratory therapist (RT), registered dietitian nutritionist (RDN), and speech-language pathologist (SLP). These professionals help prevent complications and ensure desired long-term outcomes. While the patient is being mechanically ventilated, the RT is a valuable resource. He or she can ensure ventilator function and assist with teaching the patient how to perform tracheostomy care. All patients having extensive head and neck surgery are at high risk for weight loss and poor nutrition. On average, patients lose at least 20 lb after surgery, and some had nutrition deficits even before surgery. Most patients have difficulty swallowing and ingesting sufficient nutrients. The RDN makes individualized nutrition plans for each patient and participates in patient-family education about meeting the patient's nutritional needs at home. The SLP is critical in helping the patient manage communication when speech is diminished or lost. He or she also provides ongoing assessment of the patient's ability to swallow effectively (Clark & Ebersole, 2018).

◆ **Assessment: Recognize Cues.** Ask about tobacco and alcohol use, history of acute or chronic laryngitis or pharyngitis, oral sores, swallowing difficulty, and lumps in the neck. Calculate the patient's pack-years of smoking history (see Chapter 24). Ask about alcohol intake (how many drinks per day and for how many years). Also ask about oral exposure to HPV (Schiech, 2016), which has been recognized as an increasing cause of head and neck cancer.

Table 26.1 lists the warning signs of head and neck cancer. With laryngeal cancer, painless hoarseness may occur because of tumor size and an inability of the vocal cords to come together for normal speech. Any adult who has a history of hoarseness, mouth sores, or a lump in the neck for 3 to 4 weeks should be evaluated for laryngeal cancer.

Many types of imaging studies, including x-rays of the skull, sinuses, neck, and chest, are useful in diagnosing cancer spread and the extent of tumor invasion. Studies commonly included in diagnosis are CT with contrast medium; MRI; nuclear imaging, single-photon emission computed tomography (SPECT), and fluorodeoxyglucose positron emission tomography/CT (FDG-PET/CT) scans to locate metastatic sites (National Comprehensive Cancer Network [NCCN], 2019). Endoscopic examination under anesthesia may be used to define the extent of the tumor. Biopsy tissues taken at the time of endoscopy confirm the diagnosis, tumor type, cell features, location, and stage (see Chapter 19).

TABLE 26.1 Warning Signs of Head and Neck Cancer

- Pain
- Lump in the mouth, throat, or neck
- Difficulty swallowing
- Color changes in the mouth or tongue to red, white, gray, dark brown, or black
- Oral lesion or sore that does not heal in 2 weeks
- Persistent or unexplained oral bleeding
- Numbness of the mouth, lips, or face
- Change in the fit of dentures
- Burning sensation when drinking citrus juices or hot liquids
- Persistent, unilateral ear pain
- Hoarseness or change in voice quality
- Persistent or recurrent sore throat
- Shortness of breath
- Anorexia and weight loss

◆ **Interventions: Take Action.** The focus of treatment is to remove or eradicate the cancer while preserving as much function as possible. Surgery, radiation, chemotherapy, or biotherapy may be used alone or in combination, depending on the stage of the disease; the patient's general health, nutrition status, and age; and the patient's personal choice. Treatment for laryngeal cancer may range from radiation therapy (for a small specific area or tumor) to total laryngopharyngectomy with bilateral neck dissections followed by radiation therapy, depending on the extent and location of the lesion. Nursing care focuses on preoperative preparation, optimal in-hospital care, discharge planning and teaching, and extensive outpatient rehabilitation.

Radiation therapy for treatment of small cancers in specific locations has a cure rate of at least 40%. Radiation, particularly proton beam therapy (PBT) may be used alone or in combination with surgery and chemotherapy, and may be performed before or after surgery (see Chapter 20). Most patients have hoarseness, sore throat, dysphagia, skin problems, impaired taste, and dry mouth for weeks after radiation (NCCN, 2019).

The skin at the site of irradiation becomes red and tender and may peel during therapy. Instruct the patient to avoid exposing this area to sun, heat, cold, and abrasive actions such as shaving. Teach the patient to wear protective clothing made of soft cotton and to wash this area gently daily with a mild soap. Using appropriate skin care products (approved by the radiation oncology department) can reduce the intensity of skin reactions.

If the salivary glands are in the irradiation path, the mouth becomes dry *(xerostomia)*. This effect is long-term and may be permanent (Cullen et al., 2018). A dental consultation is needed because the risk for cavities is increased by both the radiation and the dry mouth. Moisturizing sprays, increased water intake, and humidification can help ease the discomfort.

Chemotherapy can be used alone or in addition to surgery or radiation for head and neck cancer. Chemotherapy and radiation therapy *(chemoradiation)* are often used at the same time. Although the exact drugs used may vary, depending on cancer cell features, most chemotherapy regimens for head and neck cancers include cisplatin (or another platinum-based drug) in combination with 5-FU. Chapter 20 discusses care needs of patients receiving chemotherapy.

Biotherapy (targeted therapy) with an epidermal growth factor receptor inhibitor (EGFRI) such as cetuximab is used for those patients whose tumors overexpress the receptor. Although it is a targeted therapy, this drug blocks epidermal growth factor receptors (EGFRs) in normal tissues as well as those in the tumor. As a result, severe skin reactions are common and difficult for the patient. Other biotherapies for head and neck cancer include some that are more specific for cancer caused by HPV types 16, 18, 31, and 33. These may include nivolumab and pembrolizumab (NCCN, 2019).

Surgical intervention is determined by tumor size, node number, and metastasis location. Very small, early-stage tumors may be removed with laser therapy or photodynamic therapy; however, most head and neck cancers require extensive traditional surgery. Examples of possible surgical procedures include laryngectomy (total and partial), tracheotomy, and oropharyngeal cancer resections. The major types of surgery for laryngeal cancer include cord stripping, removal of a vocal cord *(cordectomy)*, partial laryngectomy, and total laryngectomy. If cancer is in the lymph nodes in the neck, the surgeon performs a nodal neck dissection along with removal of the primary tumor ("radical neck").

Preoperative Care. Teach the patient and family about the tumor. Explain about self-management of the airway, suctioning, pain-control methods, the critical care environment (including ventilators and critical care routines), nutrition support, feeding tubes, and plans for discharge. The patient will need to learn new methods of speech, at least during the time that mechanical ventilation is used and, depending on surgery type, perhaps forever. Along with the SLP, help the patient prepare for this change before surgery and practice the use of the selected form of communication.

Operative Procedures. Table 26.2 lists specific information about the various surgical procedures for laryngeal cancer. When a partial or complete laryngectomy is performed a tracheostomy is needed. With a partial laryngectomy, the tracheostomy is temporary. With a total laryngectomy, the upper airway is separated from the throat and esophagus, and a permanent laryngectomy stoma in the neck is created.

Neck dissection includes the removal of lymph nodes, the sternocleidomastoid muscle, the jugular vein, the 11th cranial nerve, and surrounding soft tissue. Shoulder drop is expected after extensive surgery.

Postoperative Care. Head and neck surgery often lasts 8 hours or longer, and the patient spends the immediate period after surgery in an ICU. Monitor airway patency, vital signs, hemodynamic status, and comfort level. Take vital signs and monitor for hemorrhage and other general complication of anesthesia and surgery hourly for the first 24 hours and then according to agency policy until the patient is stable.

Complications after surgery include airway obstruction, hemorrhage, wound breakdown, and tumor recurrence. *The first priorities after head and neck surgery are airway maintenance and ensuring* ***gas exchange****.*

TABLE 26.2 Surgical Procedures for Laryngeal Cancer and Their Effect on Voice Quality

Procedure	Description	Resulting Voice Quality
Laser surgery	Tumor reduced or destroyed by laser beam through laryngoscope	Normal or hoarse
Transoral cordectomy	Tumor (early lesion) resected through laryngoscope	Normal or hoarse (high cure rate)
Laryngofissure	No cord removed (early lesion)	Normal (high cure rate)
Supraglottic partial laryngectomy	Hyoid bone, false cords, and epiglottis removed Neck dissection on affected side performed if nodes involved	Normal or hoarse
Hemilaryngectomy or vertical laryngectomy	One true cord, one false cord, and one half of thyroid cartilage removed	Hoarse
Total laryngectomy	Entire larynx, hyoid bone, strap muscles, one or two tracheal rings removed Nodal neck dissection if nodes involved	No natural voice

Maintaining the Airway and Gas Exchange. Immediately after surgery, the patient may need mechanical ventilation. During weaning, the patient usually uses a tracheostomy collar (over the artificial airway or open stoma) with oxygen and humidity to help move mucus secretions. Secretions may remain blood-tinged for 1 to 2 days. Use Standard Precautions, and report any increase in bleeding to the surgeon.

A laryngectomy tube is used for patients who have undergone a *total laryngectomy* and need an appliance to prevent scar tissue shrinkage of the skin-tracheal border. This tube is similar to a tracheostomy tube but is shorter and wider with a larger lumen. Care is similar to tracheostomy tube care (see Chapter 25) except that the patient can change the laryngectomy tube daily or as needed. A laryngectomy button is similar to a laryngectomy tube but is softer, has a single lumen, and is very short. Provide alternative communication techniques because the patient cannot speak.

Managing the Wound. Stoma care after a total laryngectomy is a combination of wound care and airway care. Inspect the stoma and clean the suture line with sterile saline (or a prescribed solution) to prevent secretions from forming crusts and obstructing the airway. Perform suture line care every 1 to 2 hours during the first few days after surgery and then every 4 hours. The mucosa of the stoma and trachea should be bright pink and shiny and without crusts, similar to the appearance of the oral mucosa.

Tissue "flaps" may be used to close the wound and improve appearance. Flaps are skin, subcutaneous tissue, and sometimes muscle, taken from other body areas and used for reconstruction after head and neck resection.

The first 24 hours after surgery are critical. Evaluate all grafts and flaps hourly for the first 72 hours. Monitor capillary refill, color, drainage, and Doppler activity of the major blood vessel to the area. Report changes to the surgeon immediately because surgical intervention may be needed. Position the patient so the surgical flaps are not dependent.

Wound breakdown with loss of ***tissue integrity*** is a common complication in patients after head and neck surgery, especially if radiation therapy occurred before surgery. Manage wound breakdown with packing and local care as prescribed to keep the wound clean and stimulate the growth of healthy granulation tissue. Wounds may be extensive, and the carotid artery may be exposed, which increases the risk for rupture and hemorrhage.

! NURSING SAFETY PRIORITY (QSEN)

Critical Rescue

Assess the patient hourly for the first several days after head and neck surgery to recognize a carotid artery leak. If you suspect a leak, respond by initiating the Rapid Response Team and *do not touch the area because additional pressure could cause an immediate rupture.* If the carotid artery actually ruptures because of drying or infection, immediately place constant pressure over the site and secure the airway. Maintain direct manual, continuous pressure on the carotid artery and immediately transport the patient to surgery for carotid resection. Do not leave the patient. Carotid artery rupture has a high risk for stroke and death.

Managing Pain. Pain after surgery has many causes and should be managed while still allowing the patient to be able to participate in care. Morphine often is given IV by a patient-controlled analgesia (PCA) pump for the first 1 to 2 days after surgery. As the patient progresses, liquid opioid analgesics can be given by feeding tube. Oral drugs for pain and discomfort are started only after the patient can tolerate oral intake.

Maintaining Nutrition. All patients are at risk for malnutrition during treatment for head and neck cancer. A nasogastric (NG), gastrostomy, or jejunostomy tube is placed during surgery for nutrition support while the head and neck heal and may remain in place for 7 to 10 days. It is removed when the patient is able to swallow safely. Aspiration *cannot* occur after a total laryngectomy because the airway is completely separated from the esophagus.

Promoting Communication. The patient's voice quality and speech are altered after surgery. This problem has enormous effects on the patient's social interactions, continued employment, and quality of life. In collaboration with an SLP, work with the patient and family toward developing an acceptable communication method during the inpatient period. Speech production varies with patient practice, amount of tissue removed, and radiation effects but can be very understandable.

The speech rehabilitation plan for patients who have a total laryngectomy at first consists of writing, using a picture board, smart phone, or computer. The patient then uses an artificial larynx and may eventually learn esophageal speech. He or she needs encouragement and support from the SLP, hospital team,

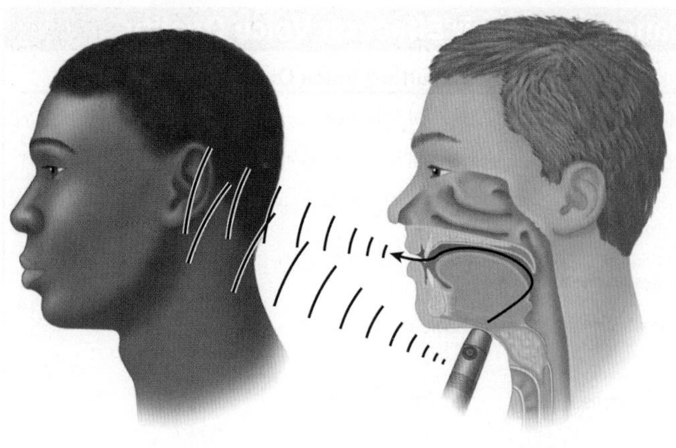

FIG. 26.4 An electrolarynx to generate speech after a laryngectomy.

and family while relearning to speak. Having a **laryngectomee** (an adult who has had a laryngectomy) from one of the local self-help organizations, such as the ACS Visitor Program or the International Association of Laryngectomees, visit the patient and family is often beneficial.

Esophageal speech is attempted by most patients who have a total laryngectomy. Sound can be produced this way by "burping" the air swallowed or injected into the esophageal pharynx and shaping the words in the mouth.

Mechanical devices, called *electrolarynges*, may be used for communication. Most are battery-powered devices placed against the side of the neck or cheek (Fig. 26.4). The air inside the mouth and throat is vibrated, and the patient moves his or her lips and tongue as usual. The quality of speech generated with mechanical devices is robotlike.

Tracheoesophageal puncture (TEP) may be used if esophageal speech is ineffective and if the patient meets strict criteria. A small surgical puncture is created between the trachea and the esophagus using a special catheter. After the puncture heals, a silicone prosthetic voice device is inserted in place of the catheter. The patient covers the stoma and the opening of the prosthesis with a finger or with a special valve to divert air from the lungs, through the trachea, into the esophagus, and out of the mouth where lip and tongue movement produces speech.

Preventing Aspiration. The surgical changes in the upper respiratory tract and altered swallowing mechanisms increase the patient's risk for aspiration. Aspiration can result in pneumonia, weight loss, and prolonged hospitalization.

A nasogastric (NG) feeding tube increases the risk for aspiration because it keeps the lower esophageal sphincter partially open. Most patients who need enteral feeding supplementation have a percutaneous endoscopic gastrostomy (PEG) tube placed rather than an NG tube. See Chapter 55 for care of patients receiving enteral nutrition by NG or PEG tube.

Swallowing can be a problem for the patient who has a tracheostomy tube. It can be normal if the cranial nerves and anatomic structures are intact. In a normal swallow, the larynx rises and moves forward to protect itself from the passing stream of food and saliva. The tracheostomy tube may fix the larynx in place, resulting in difficulty swallowing. An inflated tracheostomy tube cuff can balloon backward into the esophagus and interfere with the passage of food. The wall between the posterior trachea and the esophagus is very thin, which allows this pushing action. The patient who is cognitively intact may adapt to eating normal food when the tracheostomy tube is small and the cuff is not inflated.

The patient who has had a partial vertical or supraglottic laryngectomy *must* be observed for aspiration. It is critical to teach the patient to use alternate methods of swallowing without aspirating. The "supraglottic" method of swallowing, as listed in the Patient and Family Education: Preparing for Self-Management box, is used after a swallowing study has determined it is safe for the patient and is especially effective after a partial laryngectomy or base-of-tongue resection. This method exaggerates the normal protective mechanisms of cessation of respiration during the swallow. The double swallow helps clear food that may be pooling in the pharynx or throat structures.

PATIENT AND FAMILY EDUCATION: PREPARING FOR SELF-MANAGEMENT

The Supraglottic Method of Swallowing

1. Sit in an upright, preferably out-of-bed, position.
2. Clear your throat.
3. Take a deep breath.
4. Place ½ to 1 teaspoon of food into your mouth.
5. Hold your breath or "bear down" (Valsalva maneuver).
6. Swallow twice.
7. Release your breath and clear your throat.
8. Swallow twice again.
9. Breathe normally.

Supporting Self-Esteem. The patient with head and neck cancer usually has a change in self-concept and self-image resulting from issues such as the presence of a stoma or artificial airway, speech changes, and a change in the method of eating. Psychosocial issues may include guilt, regret, and uncertainty. He or she may not be able to speak at all or may have permanent speech deficits. Help the patient set realistic goals, starting with involvement in self-care. Reinforce the alternative communication methods suggested by the SLP so the patient can communicate in the hospital and after discharge.

After surgery, the patient may feel socially isolated because of the change in voice and facial appearance. Loose-fitting, high-collar shirts or sweaters, scarves, and jewelry can be worn to cover the laryngectomy stoma, tracheostomy tube, and other changes related to surgery. Cosmetics may aid in covering any facial or neck disfigurement.

Care Coordination and Transition Management. If no complications occur, the patient is usually discharged home or to an extended-care facility within 2 weeks. At the time of discharge, he or she or a family member should be able to perform tracheostomy or stoma care and participate in nutrition, wound care, and communication methods. Often the patient and family need referrals to support groups or a community health agency familiar with the care of patients recovering from head and neck cancer. Coordinate the efforts of

PATIENT AND FAMILY EDUCATION: PREPARING FOR SELF-MANAGEMENT

Home Laryngectomy Care

- Avoid swimming and use care when showering or shaving.
- Lean slightly forward and cover the stoma when coughing or sneezing.
- Wear a stoma guard or loose clothing to cover the stoma.
- Clean the stoma with mild soap and water. Lubricate the stoma with a non–oil-based ointment as needed.
- Increase humidity by using saline in the stoma as instructed, a bedside humidifier, pans of water, and houseplants.
- Obtain and wear a MedicAlert bracelet and emergency care card for life-threatening situations.

the interprofessional team in assessing the specific discharge needs and making the appropriate referrals to home care agencies.

Home Care Management. Extensive home care preparation is needed after a laryngectomy for cancer. The convalescence period is long, and airway management is complicated.

For the patient with severe respiratory problems, home changes to allow for one-floor living may be needed. Increased humidity is needed. A humidifier add-on to a forced-air furnace can be obtained, or a room humidifier or vaporizer may be used. Be sure to stress that meticulous cleaning of these items is needed to prevent spread of mold or other sources of infection.

A home care nurse is often an important resource for the patient and family. This nurse assesses the patient and home situation for problems in self-care, complications, adjustment, and adherence to the medical regimen.

Self-Management Education. Teach the patient and family how to care for the stoma or tracheostomy or laryngectomy tube, depending on the type of surgery performed, using the actions listed in the Patient and Family Education: Preparing for Self-Management: Home Laryngectomy Care box.

Stoma care teaching is focused on protection, which is needed as a result of the anatomic changes resulting from surgery. Instruct the patient to use a shower shield over the tube or stoma when bathing to prevent water from entering the airway. Suggest that the patient wear a protective cover or stoma guard to protect the stoma during the day.

Communication involves having the patient continue the selected communication method that began in the hospital. Instruct him or her to wear a medical alert (MedicAlert) bracelet and carry a special identification card. For patients with a laryngectomy, this card is available from the local chapters of the International Association of Laryngectomees. The card instructs the reader about providing an emergency airway or resuscitating someone who has a stoma.

Psychosocial Preparation. The many changes resulting from a laryngectomy influence physical, social, and emotional functioning for both the patient and his or her significant other (Sterba et al., 2016). The patient with a permanent stoma, tracheostomy tube, NG or PEG tube, and wounds has an altered body image. Stress the importance of returning to as normal a lifestyle as possible. Most patients can resume many of their usual activities within 4 to 6 weeks after surgery.

The patient with a total laryngectomy cannot produce sounds during laughing and crying. Mucus secretions may appear unexpectedly when these emotions arise or when coughing or sneezing occurs. The mucus can be embarrassing, and the patient needs to be prepared to cover the stoma with a handkerchief or gauze. The patient who has undergone composite resections has difficulty with speech *and* swallowing. He or she may need to deal with tracheostomy and feeding tubes in public places.

NCLEX EXAMINATION CHALLENGE 26.4

Psychosocial Integrity

A client who underwent radical neck surgery for head and neck cancer 5 days ago tells the nurse that he is worried because his right shoulder is lower than the left and does not go back into place when he tries to raise it. What is the nurse's best response?

A. "I will notify the surgeon right away because some leftover tumor must be pressing on the nerve."
B. "The nerve to the shoulder was removed during surgery. Physical therapy will help you to use other muscles to regain some motion."
C. "This problem is not related to your surgery. If it persists after you go home you will need to see your primary health care provider about it."
D. "Your time under anesthesia was long and you are not yet fully recovered. It is likely you will regain full motion in that shoulder by the end of the week."

GET READY FOR THE NEXT-GENERATION NCLEX® EXAMINATION!

Key Points

Review these Key Points fro each NCLEX Examination Client Needs Category.

Safe and Effective Care Environment

- Supervise care assigned or delegated to licensed practical nurses/licensed vocational nurses (LPNs/LVNs) or assistive personnel (AP) to patients who have risk factors for airway obstruction. **QSEN: Safety**
- Document any direct observations of obstructive sleep apnea (OSA). **QSEN: Safety**
- Instruct patients using CPAP to manage OSA to avoid sharing the mask device or tubing with others to prevent infection. **QSEN: Safety**
- Apply knowledge of anatomy to prevent aspiration in a patient with a tracheostomy. **QSEN: Safety**

Health Promotion and Maintenance

- Teach patients using CPAP how to correctly use and care for the equipment. **QSEN: Patient-Center Care**
- Remind patients using CPAP to use it daily whenever they sleep in a bed. **QSEN: Evidence-Based Practice**
- Assess the airway patency of any patient who experiences facial or nasal trauma. **QSEN: Safety**
- Assess the patient for risk factors for head and neck cancer. **QSEN: Patient-Centered Care**
- Encourage adults who smoke to quit smoking or using tobacco in any way. **QSEN: Patient-Centered Care**

- Teach patients who have had radiation therapy to the oral cavity to have dental examinations at least every 6 months. **QSEN: Patient-Centered Care**
- Teach the patient and family about home management of a laryngectomy stoma or tracheostomy. **QSEN: Patient-Centered Care**

Psychosocial Integrity

- Encourage patients prescribed CPAP therapy for OSA to use the equipment for at least 2 weeks to give them time to adjust to a new and somewhat intrusive sleep routine. **QSEN: Patient-Centered Care**
- Encourage patients with permanent tracheostomies or laryngectomies to become involved in self-care and to look at the wound and touch the affected area. **QSEN: Patient-Centered Care**
- Allow time to communicate with the patient who has voice loss. **QSEN: Patient-Centered Care**
- Teach family members ways to communicate with a patient who cannot speak after surgery for head and neck cancer. **QSEN: Patient-Centered Care**

Physiological Integrity

- Assess comatose, cognitively impaired, or noncommunicative patients every shift for the need for oral care to prevent a mucoid impaction. **QSEN: Patient-Centered Care**
- Remind patients that CPAP is only effective if the mask is tight enough to prevent air leaks. **QSEN: Patient-Centered Care**
- Perform a focused upper respiratory assessment and reassessment to determine adequacy of ***gas exchange*** and tissue perfusion. **QSEN: Patient-Centered Care**
- Check the airway and packing at least every hour for a patient who has posterior nasal packing placed after nasal surgery or posterior epistaxis. **QSEN: Evidence-Based Practice**
- Instruct patients who have had mandibular immobilization or fixation after a mandibular fracture to keep wire cutters with them at all times. **QSEN: Safety**
- Apply oxygen to any patient who develops stridor. **QSEN: Safety**
- Assess the incisions and wounds of a patient who has undergone radical neck surgery for indications of loss of ***tissue integrity***, graft perfusion insufficiency, and carotid artery leak or rupture. **QSEN: Patient-Centered Care**

MASTERY QUESTIONS

1. When making rounds, the nurse observes that a cognitively impaired client has a partial airway obstruction from inspissation. What is the nurse's **priority action**?
   A. Place the bed in reverse Trendelenburg position and apply humidified oxygen by nasal cannula.
   B. Check the flow sheet to assess for trends in the client's oxygen saturation patterns.
   C. Determine which assistive personnel (AP) provided this client's morning care today.
   D. Immediately provide complete oral care to this client.

2. A client with severe angioedema and tongue swelling from a drug allergy has stridor and an oxygen saturation of 60%. For which type of respiratory support does the nurse prepare?
   A. Nasal CPAP
   B. Tracheotomy
   C. Cricothyroidotomy
   D. Endotracheal intubation

3. A client has just come to the floor after undergoing inner maxillary fixation for a mandibular fracture with wiring of the jaws. As the nurse raises the head of the bed, the client starts to vomit a large amount of liquid vomitus. What is the nurse's **priority action**?
   A. Administer the prescribed antiemetic by the intravenous or rectal route.
   B. Immediately notify the surgeon, the anesthesiologist, or the rapid response team.
   C. Cut the wires holding his jaws together, and carefully remove them from the mouth.
   D. Reposition the client to the side and suction the mouth with a large-bore catheter.

4. In preparing a client with head and neck cancer (pharyngeal) for radiation therapy, which side effects does the nurse teach the client to expect? **Select all that apply.**
   A. Scalp and eyebrow alopecia
   B. Taste sensation loss or changes
   C. Bloody and purulent sinus drainage
   D. Increased risk for skin breakdown
   E. Moderate weight gain
   F. Increased risk for cavities
   G. Gastroesophageal reflux
   H. A persistent blue tinge to the skin and mucous membranes around the mouth

REFERENCES

American Cancer Society (ACS). (2020). *Cancer facts and figures-2020.* Report No. 00-300M-No. 500820. Atlanta: Author.

Beery, T., Workman, M., & Eggert, J. (2018). *Genetics and genomics in nursing and health care* (2nd ed.). Philadelphia: F.A: Davis.

Canadian Cancer Society, Statistics Canada. (2019). *Canadian cancer statistics, 2019.* Toronto, ON: Canadian Cancer Society.

Clark, S., & Ebersole, B. (2018). Understanding the role of speech language pathologists in managing dysphagia. *Nursing, 48*(12), 42–46.

Cullen, L., Baumler, S., Farrington, M., Dawson, C., Folkmann, P., & Brenner, L. (2018). Oral care for head and neck symptom management. *American Journal of Nursing, 118*(1), 24–34.

Gallagher, S., Deal, A., Ballard, D., & Mayer, D. (2017). Oropharyngeal cancer and HPV. *Clinical Journal of Oncology Nursing, 21*(3), 321–330.

Janotha, B., & Tamari, K. (2017). Oral squamous cell carcinoma: Focusing on interprofessional collaboration. *The Nurse Practitioner, 42*(4), 26–30.

Katz, A. (2017). Human papillomavirus-related oral cancers: The nurse's role in mitigating stigma and dispelling myths. *American Journal of Nursing, 117*(1), 34–39.

McCance, K., Huether, S., Brashers, V., & Rote, N. (2019). *Pathophysiology: The biologic basis for disease in adults and children* (8th ed.). St. Louis: Mosby.

McKiernan, J., & Thom, B. (2016). Human papillomavirus-related oropharyngeal cancer: A review of nursing considerations. *The American Journal of Nursing, 116*(8), 34–43.

Miles, H., Dols, J., & DiLeo, H. (2017). Improving provider AASM guideline adherence for adult obstructive sleep apnea. *Journal for Nurse Practitioners, 13*(6), e277–e281.

National Comprehensive Cancer Network (NCCN). (2019). *NCCN Practice Guidelines: Head and Neck Cancers—version 1.2019—March 6 2019.* https://www.nccn.org/professionals/physician_gls/pdf/head-and-neck.pdf.

Nations, R., & Mayo, A. (2016). Critique of the STOP-Bang sleep apnea questionnaire. *Clinical Nurse Specialist CNS, 30*(1), 11–14.

Schiech, L. (2016). Tonsillar cancer: What nurses need to know. *Nursing, 46*(7), 36–44.

Schreiber, M.L. (2020). Epistaxis: A closer look. *MEDSURG Nursing, 29*(2), 126–128.

Senaratna, C., Perret, J., Lodge, C., Lowe, A., Campbell, B., Matheson, M., et al. (2017). Prevalence of obstructive sleep apnea in the general population: A systematic review. *Sleep Medicine Reviews, 34*, 70–81.

Shechter, A. (2017). Obstructive sleep apnea and energy balance regulation: A systematic review. *Sleep Medicine Reviews, 34*, 59–69.

Sterba, K., Zapka, J., Cranos, C., Laursen, A., & Day, T. (2016). Quality of life in head and neck patient-caregiver dyads. *Cancer Nursing, 39*(3), 238–250.

27

Concepts of Care for Patients With Noninfectious Lower Respiratory Problems

M. Linda Workman

http://evolve.elsevier.com/Iggy/

LEARNING OUTCOMES

1. Collaborate with the interprofessional team to coordinate high-quality care and promote ***gas exchange*** in patients with chronic lower respiratory problems.
2. Protect patients with lower respiratory problems from injury or infection.
3. Apply knowledge of anatomy, physiology, pathophysiology, and genetics to assess patients with lower respiratory problems affecting ***gas exchange*** or ***perfusion***.
4. Teach the patient and family how to manage a chronic lower respiratory disorder and avoid complications.
5. Teach all adults measures to take to protect the respiratory system from damage and cancer, including the avoidance of known environmental causative agents.
6. Identify community resources for patients requiring assistance with long-term ***gas exchange*** issues related to chronic lower airway problems.
7. Implement nursing interventions to help the patient and family cope with the psychosocial impact of living with a chronic lower respiratory problem.
8. Teach the patient and caregiver(s) about common drugs and other management strategies used for acute or chronic lower respiratory problems.
9. Use clinical judgment to prioritize nursing care for the patient with chest tubes.

KEY TERMS

asthma A chronic disease in which acute reversible airway obstruction occurs intermittently, reducing airflow.

chronic bronchitis An inflammation of the bronchi and bronchioles caused by exposure to irritants, especially cigarette smoke.

chronic obstructive pulmonary disease (COPD) A collection of lower airway disorders that interfere with airflow and gas exchange.

control therapy drugs Asthma drugs used daily to reduce airway sensitivity (responsiveness) to prevent asthma attacks from occurring and to maintain gas exchange.

cor pulmonale Right-sided heart failure caused by pulmonary disease occurring with bronchitis or emphysema.

cystic fibrosis (CF) An autosomal recessive genetic disease that affects many organs with most impairment occurring to pancreatic and/or lung function.

dyspnea Perceived shortness of breath.

emphysema A destructive problem of lung elastic tissue that reduces its ability to recoil after stretching, leading to hyperinflation of the lung.

hypercapnia Higher than normal blood carbon dioxide levels. Also known as *hypercarbia*.

hypoxemia Low blood oxygen levels.

lobectomy Removal of a lobe of the lung.

orthopnea Breathlessness that is worse in a supine position.

pneumonectomy Surgical removal of an entire lung.

pulmonary artery hypertension (PAH) A condition in which pulmonary vessels and often other lung tissues undergo growth changes that greatly increase pressure in the lung circulatory system for unknown reasons (also known as *idiopathic pulmonary artery hypertension*).

reliever drugs Asthma drugs used to actually stop an asthma attack once it has started. Also known as *rescue drugs*.

PRIORITY AND INTERRELATED CONCEPTS

The priority concept for this chapter is:

- ***Gas Exchange***

The ***Gas Exchange*** concept exemplar for this chapter is Chronic Obstructive Pulmonary Disease.

The interrelated concepts for this chapter are:

- ***Perfusion***
- ***Inflammation***
- ***Cellular Regulation***

The lower respiratory tract is the tubular system of the trachea (below the larynx), two mainstem bronchi, five secondary bronchi, thousands of branching bronchi and bronchioles, and the alveolar ducts, which connect to the final portions of the tract, the alveoli. Air must flow through the entire tubular system for needed oxygen to reach the alveolar ducts and alveoli where primary ***gas exchange*** occurs. When the function of any of these structures is reduced, both gas exchange and systemic ***perfusion*** are impaired.

Many lower airway problems are chronic and progressive, requiring changes in lifestyle, especially for older adults (Touhy & Jett, 2020). The Patient-Centered Care: Older Adult Considerations box lists nursing accommodations to make when caring for an older patient with a respiratory problem.

PATIENT-CENTERED CARE: OLDER ADULT CONSIDERATIONS QSEN

Nursing Accommodations for an Older Adult With a Respiratory Problem

- Provide rest periods between activities such as bathing, meals, and ambulation.
- Have the patient sit in an upright position for meals to prevent aspiration.
- Encourage nutritional fluid intake after the meal to prevent an early sensation of fullness and promote increased calorie intake.
- Schedule drugs around routine activities to increase adherence to drug therapy.
- Arrange chairs in strategic locations to allow the patient with dyspnea to stop and rest while walking.
- Urge the patient to notify the primary health care provider promptly for any symptoms of infection.
- Encourage the patient to receive the pneumococcal vaccines and to have an annual influenza vaccination.
- For patients who are prescribed home oxygen, instruct them to keep tubing coiled when walking to reduce the risk for tripping.

Through its direct interaction with the environment during breathing of atmospheric air, the respiratory system may be one of the first areas of the body to experience a negative impact when changes occur (Cook et al., 2019). Air pollution, extremes of temperature, changes in the type and distribution of insect and microorganism populations, and periodic heavy flooding associated with climate change have the potential to increase the incidence and severity of chronic respiratory disorders, especially asthma, chronic obstructive pulmonary disease (COPD), pulmonary fibrosis, and lung cancer. A nursing responsibility consistent with climate action and health promotion with this possible health threat is to educate patients with chronic respiratory disorders how to adapt their ADLs and lifestyles to minimize the acute effects of such changes.

ASTHMA

Pathophysiology Review

One of the most common lower respiratory disorders that reduces ***gas exchange*** is asthma, which can lead to severe lower airway obstruction and death. **Asthma** is a chronic disease in which reversible acute airway obstruction occurs intermittently, reducing airflow (Fig. 27.1). Airway obstruction occurs by both ***inflammation*** and airway tissue sensitivity *(hyperresponsiveness)* with bronchoconstriction. Inflammation obstructs the airway *lumens* (i.e., the hollow insides) (Fig. 27.2). Airway hyperresponsiveness and constriction of bronchial smooth muscle narrow the tubular structure of the airways. Airway inflammation and sensitivity can trigger bronchiolar constriction, and many adults with asthma have both problems (McCance et al., 2019). More than 3300 deaths from acute asthma occur in the United States each year (Centers for Disease Control and Prevention [CDC], 2019a).

Etiology and Genetic Risk

Although asthma may be classified into types based on what triggers the attacks, the effect on ***gas exchange*** is the same. Inflammation of the mucous membranes lining the airways is a key event in triggering an asthma attack. It occurs in response to the presence of specific allergens; general irritants such as cold air, dry air, or fine airborne particles; microorganisms; and aspirin and other NSAIDs. Increased airway sensitivity (hyperresponsiveness) can occur with exercise or upper respiratory illness and for unknown reasons.

Inflammation associated with asthma can be triggered by different types of white blood cells (WBCs) within the epithelial lining of the lower respiratory tract. For some people, an overabundance of eosinophils makes these airways hyperresponsive, a condition known as *eosinophilic asthma*. The major mediator that activates eosinophils and increases inflammation leading to asthma attacks is interleukin 5 (IL-5). About 50% of adults with asthma have eosinophilic asthma (Muhrer, 2018). For other people, the WBC type most responsible for the inflammation is the neutrophil, a condition known as *neutrophilic asthma*. The major mediator that activates neutrophils and increases inflammation leading to asthma attacks is interleukin 17 (IL-17) (Abbas et al., 2018; McCance et al., 2019). The symptoms are the same; however, there are some differences in the long-term effects of the disease on the respiratory epithelium. In addition, some drugs are more specific for one type of asthma than the other.

PATIENT-CENTERED CARE: GENETIC/GENOMIC CONSIDERATIONS QSEN

Genetic studies indicate that more than 1000 gene variations are associated with asthma, although asthma is a disorder with both genetic and environmental input needed for expression (Online Mendelian Inheritance in Man [OMIM], 2019a; Wysocki, 2018). Variation in the gene that controls the activity of beta-adrenergic receptors also has an impact on drug therapy for asthma. Adults with this mutation do not respond as expected to beta agonist drugs. Teaching these adults about why their drug therapies are different from standard recommendations is a nursing responsibility that can assist with therapy adherence.

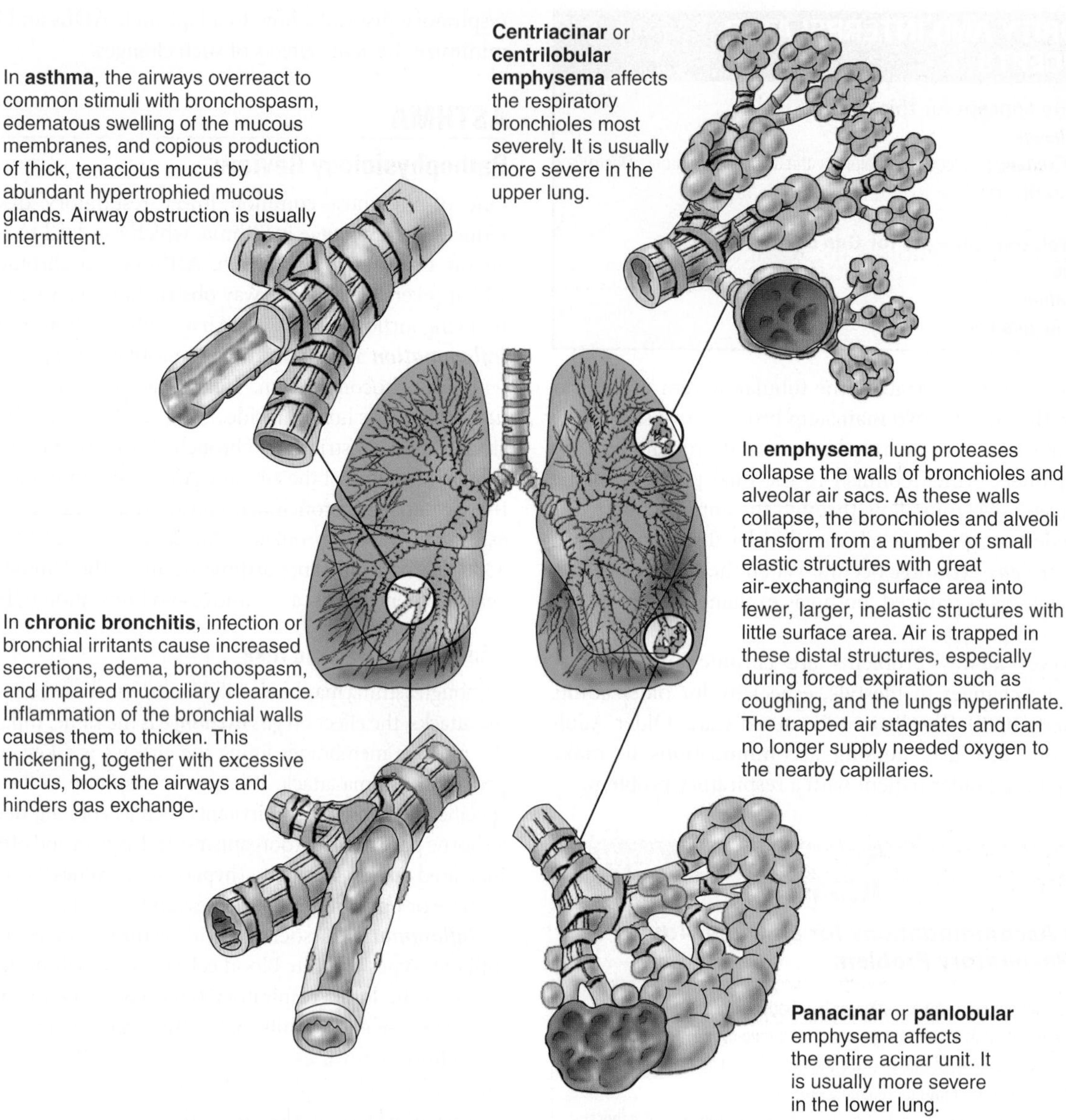

In **asthma**, the airways overreact to common stimuli with bronchospasm, edematous swelling of the mucous membranes, and copious production of thick, tenacious mucus by abundant hypertrophied mucous glands. Airway obstruction is usually intermittent.
Centriacinar or **centrilobular emphysema** affects the respiratory bronchioles most severely. It is usually more severe in the upper lung.
In **emphysema**, lung proteases collapse the walls of bronchioles and alveolar air sacs. As these walls collapse, the bronchioles and alveoli transform from a number of small elastic structures with great air-exchanging surface area into fewer, larger, inelastic structures with little surface area. Air is trapped in these distal structures, especially during forced expiration such as coughing, and the lungs hyperinflate. The trapped air stagnates and can no longer supply needed oxygen to the nearby capillaries.
In **chronic bronchitis**, infection or bronchial irritants cause increased secretions, edema, bronchospasm, and impaired mucociliary clearance. Inflammation of the bronchial walls causes them to thicken. This thickening, together with excessive mucus, blocks the airways and hinders gas exchange.
Panacinar or **panlobular** emphysema affects the entire acinar unit. It is usually more severe in the lower lung.

FIG. 27.1 Pathophysiology of chronic lower airway problems.

Surrounding smooth muscle layer
Cartilage ring
A
B
C
D
E
Mucous membrane lining
Lumen (open center where air moves freely)

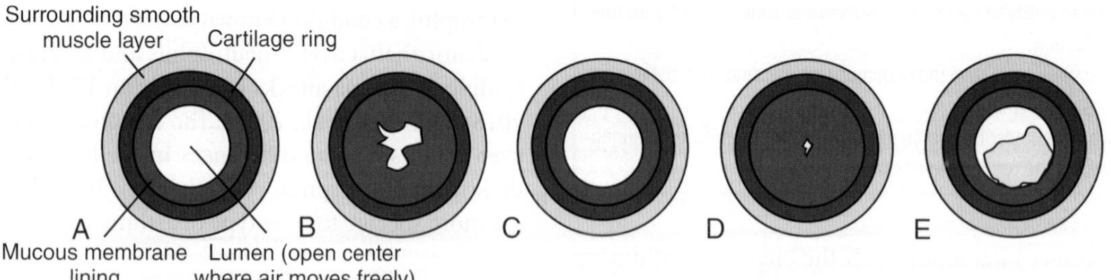

FIG. 27.2 Causes of narrowed airways. A, Cross-section of a small normal airway with tissue layers. B, Airway mucosal swelling. C, Constriction of smooth muscle. D, Mucosal swelling and constriction of smooth muscle. E, Mucus plug.

When asthma is well controlled, airway changes are temporary and reversible. With poor control, chronic ***inflammation*** leads to airway damage and altered ***cellular regulation*** with enlargement of the bronchial epithelial cells, including mucus-secreting cells, and changes in the bronchial smooth muscle. With frequent asthma attacks, even exposure to low levels of the triggering agent or event may stimulate an attack.

Inflammation triggers asthma for some adults when allergens bind to specific antibodies (especially immunoglobulin E [IgE]). These antibodies are attached to tissue *mast cells,* as well as the WBCs basophils, eosinophils, and neutrophils, which are filled with chemicals that can start local inflammatory responses (see Chapters 16 and 18). Some chemicals, such as histamine, start an immediate inflammatory response, which can be blocked by drugs such as diphenhydramine. Others, such as leukotriene and eotaxin, are slower and cause later, prolonged inflammatory responses, which can be blocked by drugs such as montelukast, zafirlukast, and zileuton. Chemicals also attract more WBCs to the area, which then continue the responses of blood vessel dilation and capillary leak, causing mucous membrane swelling and increased mucus production (McCance et al., 2019). These responses narrow the lumens even more, which then interferes with airflow and ***gas exchange***. Inflammation can also occur through general irritation rather than allergic responses.

Bronchospasm is narrowing of the bronchial tubes by constriction of the smooth muscle around and within the bronchial walls. It can occur when small amounts of pollutants or respiratory viruses stimulate nerve fibers, causing constriction of bronchial smooth muscle. If an inflammatory response is stimulated at the same time, the chemicals released during ***inflammation*** also trigger constriction. Severe bronchospasm alone, especially in smaller bronchioles, can profoundly limit airflow to the alveoli and greatly reduce ***gas exchange***.

Aspirin and other NSAIDs can trigger asthma in some adults, although this response is not a true allergy. It results from increased production of leukotriene when aspirin or NSAIDs suppress other pathways of inflammatory mediator production.

Gastroesophageal reflux disease (GERD) can trigger asthma in some adults and causes asthma symptoms at night (Global Initiative for Asthma [GINA], 2018). With GERD, highly acidic stomach contents enter the airway and make preexisting tissue sensitivity worse.

Incidence and Prevalence

Asthma can occur at any age. About half of adults with asthma also had the disease in childhood. Asthma affects over 22 million adults in the United States and Canada (19.9 million in the United States and 2.6 million in Canada) (CDC, 2018b; Statistics Canada, 2017). It is more common in urban settings than rural settings.

❖ Interprofessional Collaborative Care

As a treatable chronic disorder, asthma is generally managed in the community with health care oversight. Acute exacerbations may require management in emergency departments or ICUs. Because asthma is a common disorder, adults admitted to the hospital for other health problems or surgery may also have asthma. For optimal control, continuing the asthma management plan, including drug therapy, is a priority regardless of setting.

◆ Assessment: Recognize Cues

Asthma is classified on the basis of how well controlled the symptoms are on a consistent basis as defined by the Global Initiative for Asthma (GINA) (GINA, 2018). The Key Features: Asthma Symptoms and Control Level box outlines this classification.

History. The patient with asthma usually has a pattern of intermittent episodes of dyspnea (perceived shortness of breath), chest tightness, coughing, wheezing, and increased mucus production. Ask whether the symptoms occur continuously, seasonally, in association with specific activities or exposures, at work, or more frequently at night. Some patients have symptoms for 4 to 8 weeks after a cold or other upper respiratory infection. The patient with atopic (allergic) asthma also may have other allergic problems. Ask whether any family members have asthma or respiratory problems. Ask about current or previous smoking habits. If the patient smokes, use this opportunity to teach him or her about smoking cessation (see Chapter 24). Wheezing in nonsmokers is important in the diagnosis of asthma.

Physical Assessment/Signs and Symptoms. The patient with mild to moderate asthma may have no symptoms between asthma attacks. During an acute episode, common symptoms are an audible wheeze and increased respiratory rate. At first

PATIENT-CENTERED CARE: OLDER ADULT CONSIDERATIONS QSEN

Although often thought of as a disorder that develops most commonly in childhood, asthma also can occur as a new disorder in older adults. In addition, about 3% of adults older than 60 years have asthma as a continuing chronic disorder (CDC, 2018b). Lung and airway changes as a part of aging make breathing problems more serious in the older adult, and asthma-related deaths are highest in adults over age 65 years (Touhy & Jett, 2020). Another problem related to aging is a decrease in the sensitivity of beta-adrenergic receptors. When stimulated, these receptors relax smooth muscle and cause bronchodilation. As these receptors become less sensitive, they no longer respond as quickly or as strongly to agonists and beta-adrenergic drugs, which are often used as rescue therapy during an acute asthma attack. Thus teaching older patients how to avoid asthma attacks and how to correctly use preventive drug therapy is a nursing priority.

KEY FEATURES

Asthma Symptoms and Control Level

Symptoms

- Daytime symptoms of wheezing, dyspnea, coughing present more than twice weekly
- Waking from night sleep with symptoms of wheezing, dyspnea, coughing
- Reliever (rescue) drug needed more than twice weekly
- Activity limited or stopped by symptoms more than twice weekly

Control Level

Controlled: None of the above symptoms
Partly Controlled: 1 or 2 of the above symptoms
Uncontrolled: 3 to 4 of the above symptoms

Adapted from: Global Initiative for Asthma (GINA). (2018). *Pocket guide for asthma management and prevention.* https://ginasthma.org/wp-content/uploads/2018/03/wms-GINA-main-pocket-guide_2018-v1.0.pdf the wheeze is louder on exhalation. When ***inflammation*** occurs with asthma, coughing may increase.

The patient may use accessory muscles to help breathe during an attack. Observe for muscle retraction at the sternum and the suprasternal notch and between the ribs. The patient with long-standing, severe asthma may have a "barrel chest," caused by air trapping (Fig. 27.3). The anteroposterior (AP) diameter (diameter between the front and the back of the chest) increases with air trapping, giving the chest a rounded rather than an oval shape. The normal chest is about 1.5 times as wide as it is deep. In severe, chronic asthma, the AP diameter may equal or exceed the lateral diameter (Jarvis, 2020). Compare the chest AP diameter with the lateral diameter. Chronic air trapping also flattens the diaphragm and increases the space between the ribs.

Along with an audible wheeze, the breathing cycle is longer, with prolonged exhalation, and requires more effort. The patient may be unable to speak more than a few words between breaths. Hypoxia occurs with severe attacks. Pulse oximetry shows **hypoxemia** (poor blood oxygen levels). Examine the oral mucosa and nail beds for cyanosis. Other indicators of hypoxemia include changes in the level of cognition or consciousness and tachycardia.

Laboratory Assessment. Laboratory tests can determine asthma type and the degree of breathing impairment. Arterial blood gas (ABG) levels show the effectiveness of ***gas exchange*** (see Chapter 14 for discussion of ABGs). The arterial oxygen level ($Pa{O_2}$) may decrease during an asthma attack. Early in the attack, the arterial carbon dioxide level ($Pa{CO_2}$) may be decreased as the patient increases the breathing rate and depth. Later in an asthma episode, $Pa{CO_2}$ rises, as does the end-tidal carbon dioxide level, indicating carbon dioxide retention. Allergic asthma often occurs with elevated serum eosinophil counts and immunoglobulin E (IgE) levels. The sputum may contain eosinophils and mucus plugs with shed epithelial cells (Curschmann spirals).

Pulmonary Function Tests. The most accurate tests for measuring airflow in asthma are the pulmonary function tests (PFTs) using spirometry. Baseline PFTs are obtained for all patients diagnosed with asthma. The most important PFTs for a patient with asthma are the forced vital capacity (FVC), the forced expiratory volume in the first second (FEV_1), and the peak expiratory flow (PEF), sometimes called *peak expiratory rate flow* (PERF). Definitions of PFTs are listed in Chapter 24. A decrease in either the FEV_1 or the PEF (PERF) of 15% to 20% below the expected value for age, gender, and size is common for the patient with asthma (Durham et al., 2017). Asthma is diagnosed when these values increase by 12% or more after treatment with bronchodilators. Airway responsiveness is tested by measuring the PEF and FEV_1 before and after the patient inhales the drug *methacholine,* which induces bronchospasm in susceptible adults.

◆ Interventions: Take Action

The purposes of asthma therapy are to control and prevent episodes, improve airflow and ***gas exchange***, and relieve symptoms. Asthma is best controlled when the patient is an active partner in the management plan. Priority nursing actions focus on patient education about using his or her personal asthma action plan, which includes drug therapy and lifestyle management strategies to help him or her understand the disease and its management (GINA, 2018).

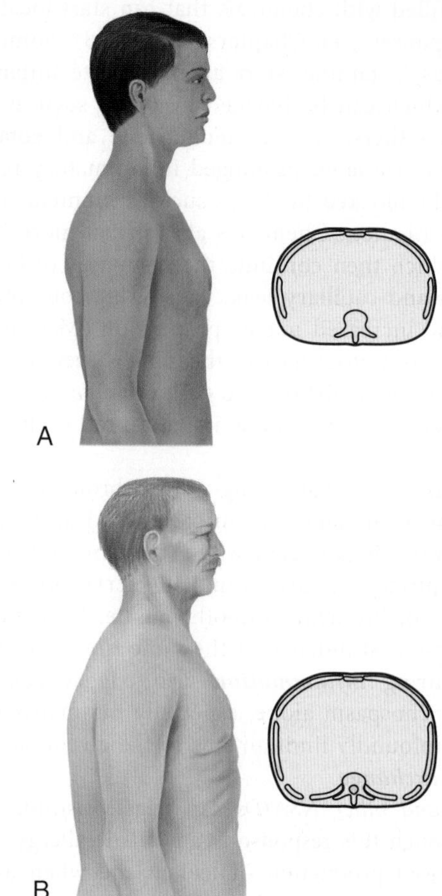

FIG. 27.3 A, Normal adult. The thorax has an oval shape with an anteroposterior-to-transverse diameter of 1:1.5 or 5:7. B, Barrel chest. Note equal anteroposterior-to-transverse diameter and that ribs are horizontal instead of the normal downward slope. This is associated with chronic obstructive pulmonary disease and severe asthma as a result of hyperinflation of the lungs. (From Jarvis, C. [2016]. Physical examination and health assessment [7th ed.]. Philadelphia: Saunders.)

Self-Management Education. Asthma often has intermittent overt symptoms. With guided self-care, patients can co-manage this disease, increasing symptom-free periods and decreasing the number and severity of attacks. Good management decreases hospital admissions and increases participation in patient-chosen work and leisure activities. Self-care requires extensive education for the patient to be able to self-assess respiratory status, self-manage (by adjusting the frequency and dosage of prescribed drugs), and know when to consult the primary health care provider (Keep et al., 2016).

Ideally a personal asthma action plan is developed by the primary health care provider and the patient. The plan is tailored to meet the patient's personal triggers, asthma symptoms, and drug responses. It includes:

- The prescribed daily controller drug(s) schedule and prescribed reliever drug directions
- Patient-specific daily asthma control assessment questions
- Directions for adjusting the daily controller drug schedule
- When to contact the primary health care provider (in addition to regularly scheduled visits)
- Emergency actions to take when asthma is not responding to controller and reliever drugs

At one time, patients were instructed to assess their asthma severity at least daily with a peak flow meter. However, this process is now only recommended for those patients whose asthma is not well controlled (GINA, 2018).

Teach the patient to keep a symptom and intervention diary to learn specific triggers of asthma, early cues for impending attacks, and personal response to drugs. Stress the importance of proper use of his or her personal asthma action plan for any severity of asthma, as described in the Patient and Family Education: Preparing for Self-Management: Asthma Management box.

Drug Therapy. Pharmacologic management of adults with asthma is based on the step category for severity and treatment as outlined in the Best Practice for Patient Safety & Quality Care : The Step System for Medication Use in Asthma Control box (GINA, 2018). **Control therapy drugs** are used to reduce airway sensitivity (responsiveness) to prevent asthma attacks from occurring and maintain ***gas exchange***. *They are used every day, regardless of symptoms.* **Reliever drugs** (also called *rescue drugs*) are used to actually stop an attack once it has started. Some patients may need drug therapy only during an asthma episode. For others, daily drugs are needed to keep asthma episodic rather than a more frequent problem. Therapy involves the use of bronchodilators and various drug types to reduce inflammation. Some drugs reduce the asthma response, and other drugs actually prevent it. Combination drugs are two or more agents from different classes combined together for better response.

With step therapy, drug therapy is prescribed at different levels, starting with step 1 and progressing up *(stepping up)*, until acceptable control is achieved. When the patient achieves control and maintains it for 3 months, the respiratory health care provider adjusts the drug regimen down a step *(stepping down)* at a time to reach and maintain a goal of good control at the lowest possible drug dosages.

BEST PRACTICE FOR PATIENT SAFETY & QUALITY CARE (QSEN)

The Step System for Medication Use in Asthma Control

Step 1	Step 2	Step 3	Step 4	Step 5
As-needed rapid-acting $beta_2$ agonist (relief inhaler)	As-needed rapid-acting $beta_2$ agonist (relief inhaler)	As-needed rapid-acting $beta_2$ agonist (relief inhaler)	As-needed rapid-acting $beta_2$ agonist (relief inhaler)	As-needed rapid-acting $beta_2$ agonist (relief inhaler)
No daily drugs needed	Daily treatment with the use of *one* of these two options:	Daily treatment with the use of *one* of these four options:	Daily treatment with Step 3 option that provided best control and tolerance along with one or more of these two options:	Daily treatment with Step 4 option(s) that provided best control and tolerance along with either of these two options:
	Low-dose ICS	Low-dose ICS *and* long-acting $beta_2$ agonist	Medium-dose or high-dose ICS *and* long-acting $beta_2$ agonist	Oral glucocorticosteroid (lowest dose)
	Leukotriene modifier[a]	Medium-dose or high-dose ICS Low-dose ICS and leukotriene modifier Low-dose ICS and sustained-release theophylline	Leukotriene modifier and sustained-release theophylline	IgE[b] antagonist Interleukin-5 antagonist Interleukin-17 antagonist

ICS, Inhaled corticosteroid.

[a] Leukotriene modifier = Leukotriene receptor antagonist or leukotriene synthesis inhibitor.

[b] IgE = Immunoglobulin E.

Data adapted from Global Initiative for Asthma (GINA). (2018). *Pocket guide for asthma management and prevention.* https://ginasthma.org/wp-content/uploads/2018/03/wms-GINA-main-pocket-guide_2018-v1.0.pdf

PATIENT AND FAMILY EDUCATION: PREPARING FOR SELF-MANAGEMENT

Asthma Management

- Avoid potential environmental asthma triggers, such as smoke, fireplaces, dust, mold, and weather changes of warm to cold.
- Avoid drugs that trigger your asthma (e.g., aspirin, NSAIDs, beta blockers).
- Avoid food that has been prepared with monosodium glutamate (MSG) or metabisulfite.
- If you have exercise-induced asthma, use your reliever bronchodilator inhaler 30 minutes before exercise to prevent or reduce bronchospasm.
- Be sure that you know the proper technique and correct sequence when you use metered dose inhalers.
- Get adequate rest and sleep.
- Reduce stress and anxiety; learn relaxation techniques; adopt coping mechanisms that have worked for you in the past.
- Wash all bedding with hot water to destroy dust mites.
- Seek immediate emergency care if you experience any of these:
  - Gray or blue fingertips or lips
  - Difficulty breathing, walking, or talking
  - Retractions of the neck, chest, or ribs
  - Nasal flaring
  - Failure of drugs to control worsening symptoms

The Common Examples of Drug Therapy: Asthma Prevention and Treatment box lists the most common preferred drugs in each class for control and relief therapy of asthma. The actions and interventions for most drugs within a single class are similar. Be sure to consult a drug handbook, electronic drug reference, or pharmacist for information on a specific drug.

Many of the drugs used for asthma control and relief are delivered using inhalers. Currently three types of inhalers are available: metered dose inhalers (MDIs), which deliver drugs as a fine liquid spray; dry powder inhalers (DPIs), which deliver drugs as a fine powder; and soft mist inhalers (SMIs), which deliver drugs as a very fine soft mist. The MDIs require a propellant to form an aerosol spray and may be used with a spacer (preferred) or without a spacer. DPIs rely on the negative pressure of inhalation to pull the drug into the respiratory tract. SMIs have a mechanical spring-loaded device that creates an aerosol cloud or mist, which is then pulled into the respiratory tract by patient inhalation. Neither DPIs nor SMIs use a spacer for drug delivery. An advantage of SMIs over MDIs and DPIs is that the speed of the drug particles within the mist increases the distance they travel, which increases the likelihood of reaching the lower airways (Burchum & Rosenthal, 2019).

Many patients do not get the full benefit of inhaled drugs because of incorrect device use. Often the inhaled drug stays in the mouth and throat or exits through the nose without ever reaching the lower airways. Ensuring that drug dosages reach the site of action requires strict attention to correct technique regardless of which type of inhaler is used (Chike-Harris & Kinyon-Munch, 2019). Teaching patients the correct techniques is often best accomplished by showing manufacturer-generated videos demonstrating the correct technique for the type of inhaler prescribed (Henrich & Logue, 2017). In addition, some videos also demonstrate proper care and cleaning of the device. Many of the videos are available to the patient for repeated review online. Most prescribed inhalers now have meters that indicate the number of doses left in the canister so that patients will know when to have the prescription refilled and not miss doses (Fig. 27.4).

COMMON EXAMPLES OF DRUG THERAPY

Asthma Prevention and Treatment

Drug	Nursing Implications
Bronchodilators	
Induce rapid bronchodilation through relaxing bronchiolar smooth muscle by binding to and activating pulmonary beta$_2$ receptors.	
Short-Acting Beta$_2$ Agonist (SABA)	
Primarily used as a fast-acting reliever (rescue) drug to be used either during an asthma attack or just before engaging in activity that usually triggers an attack.	
Albuterol (inhaled drug) Levalbuterol (inhaled drug)	Teach patients to carry drug with them at all times *because it can stop or reduce life-threatening bronchoconstriction.* Teach patient to monitor heart rate *because excessive use causes tachycardia and other systemic symptoms.* When taking any of these drugs with other inhaled drugs, teach patient to use them at least 5 minutes before the other inhaled drugs *to allow the bronchodilation effect to increase the penetration of other inhaled drugs.* Teach patient the correct technique for using the MDI or DPI *to ensure that the drug reaches the site of action.*
Long-Acting Beta$_2$ Agonist (LABA)	
Causes bronchodilation through relaxing bronchiolar smooth muscle by binding to and activating pulmonary beta$_2$ receptors. Onset of action is slow with a long duration. Primary use is prevention of an asthma attack.	
Salmeterol (inhaled drug) Indacaterol (COPD only) (inhaled drug) Formoterol Arformoterol (COPD only)	Teach patient to not use these drugs as reliever drugs *because they have a slow onset of action and do not relieve acute symptoms.* Teach patient the correct technique for using the MDI or DPI *to ensure that the drug reaches the site of action.*
Cholinergic Antagonist	
Causes bronchodilation by inhibiting the parasympathetic nervous system, allowing the sympathetic system to dominate, releasing norepinephrine that activates beta$_2$ receptors. Purpose is to prevent asthma attacks or COPD bronchospasms and improve ***gas exchange,*** although some are considered reliever drugs.	
Aclidinium (inhaled drug for prevention only) Ipratropium (inhaled drug for relief and prevention) Tiotropium (inhaled drug) Umeclidinium (inhaled drug for prevention only)	If patient is to use any of these as a reliever drug, teach him or her to carry it at all times *because it can stop or reduce life-threatening bronchoconstriction.* For drugs delivered by MDI, teach patient to shake the inhaler well before using *because the drugs separate easily.* Teach patient to increase daily fluid intake *because the drugs cause mouth dryness.* Teach patient to observe for and report blurred vision, eye pain, headache, nausea, palpitations, tremors, and inability to sleep *as these are systemic symptoms of overdose and require intervention.* Teach patient the correct technique for using the MDI or DPI *to ensure that the drug reaches the site of action.*

Continued

COMMON EXAMPLES OF DRUG THERAPY—CONT'D

Asthma Prevention and Treatment

Drug	Nursing Implications
Anti-Inflammatories	
All of these drugs help improve bronchiolar airflow and increase ***gas exchange*** by decreasing the inflammatory response of the mucous membranes in the airways. *They do not cause bronchodilation.*	
Corticosteroids	
Disrupt production pathways of inflammatory mediators. The main purpose is to prevent an asthma attack caused by inflammation or allergies (controller drug).	
Fluticasone (MDI inhaled drug) Beclomethasone (MDI inhaled drug) Budesonide (MDI inhaled drug)	Teach patient to use the drug daily, *even when no symptoms are present, because maximum effectiveness requires continued use for 48-72 hours and depends on regular use.* Teach patient to use good mouth care and to check mouth daily for lesions or drainage *because these drugs reduce local immunity and increase the risk for local infections, especially Candida albicans (yeast).* Teach patient to not use these drugs as reliever drugs *because they have a slow onset of action and do not relieve acute symptoms.* Teach patient the correct technique for using the MDI *to ensure that the drug reaches the site of action.*
Prednisone (oral drug)	Teach patient about expected side effects *because knowing which side effects to expect may reduce anxiety when they appear.* Teach patient to avoid anyone who has an upper respiratory infection *because the drug reduces all protective inflammatory responses, increasing the risk for infection.* Teach patient to avoid activities that lead to injury *because blood vessels become more fragile, leading to bruising and petechiae.* Teach patient to take drug with food *to help reduce the side effect of GI ulceration.* Teach patient not to suddenly stop taking the drug for any reason *because the drug suppresses adrenal production of corticosteroids, which are essential for life.*
Cromone	
Stabilizes the membranes of mast cells and prevents the release of inflammatory mediators. Purpose is to prevent asthma attack triggered by inflammation or allergens.	
Nedocromil (inhaled drug)	Teach patient to use the drug daily, *even when no symptoms are present, because maximum effectiveness requires continued use for 48-72 hours and depends on regular use.* Teach patient to not use this drug as a reliever drug *because it has a slow onset of action and does not relieve acute symptoms.* Teach patient the correct technique for using the MDI *to ensure that the drug reaches the site of action.*
Leukotriene Modifier	
Blocks the leukotriene receptor, preventing the inflammatory mediator from stimulating inflammation. Purpose is to prevent asthma attack triggered by inflammation or allergens.	
Montelukast (oral drug)	Teach patient to use the drug daily, *even when no symptoms are present, because maximum effectiveness requires continued use for 48-72 hours and depends on regular use.* Teach patient not to decrease the dose of or stop taking any other asthma drugs unless instructed by the health care professional *because this drug is for long-term asthma control and does not replace other drugs, especially corticosteroids and reliever (rescue) drugs.*
Monoclonal Antibodies	
Bind to and block the actions of proinflammatory cytokines (interleukin 5) or cell surface sites of IgE that trigger and maintain asthma attacks.	
Interleukin antagonists: Benralizumab (subcutaneous injection) Mepolizumab (subcutaneous injection) Reslizumab (slow IV infusion only)	Only for use in patients who have eosinophilic asthma *because these drugs block the actions of interleukin-5 (IL-5), which activates eosinophils and increases their numbers.* Do not administer these drugs as a reliever drug *because they do not relieve acute symptoms.* Monitor patient for at least 2 hours after injection for indications of severe hypersensitivity and anaphylaxis *because these drugs contain a foreign protein that has an increased risk for severe allergic reactions.*
IgE antagonist: Omalizumab (subcutaneous injection)	Used only for patients who have a known allergy that triggers asthma attacks *because the drug works by antagonizing IgE.* Monitor patient for at least 2 hours after injection for indications of severe hypersensitivity and anaphylaxis *because the drug contains a foreign protein that has an increased risk for severe allergic reactions.* Do not administer this drug as a reliever drug *because it does not relieve acute symptoms.*

COPD, Chronic obstructive pulmonary disease; *DPI,* dry powder inhaler; *MDI,* metered dose inhaler.

Data from Global Initiative for Asthma (GINA). (2018). *Pocket guide for asthma management and prevention.* https://ginasthma.org/wp-content/uploads/2018/03/wms-GINA-main-pocket-guide_2018-v1.0.pdf; and Burchum, J., & Rosenthal, L. (2019). *Lehne's pharmacology for nursing care* (10th ed.). St. Louis: Mosby.

Bronchodilators. Bronchodilators cause bronchiolar smooth muscle relaxation but have no effect on ***inflammation***. Thus for patients who have airflow obstruction by both bronchospasm and inflammation, at least two types of drug therapy are needed. Bronchodilators include beta$_2$ agonists and cholinergic antagonists.

Beta$_2$ agonists bind to and stimulate the beta$_2$-adrenergic receptors in the same way that epinephrine and norepinephrine do. This causes an increase in smooth muscle relaxation. Short-acting beta$_2$ agonists (SABAs) provide rapid but short-term relief. These inhaled drugs are most useful when an attack begins (as relief) or as premedication when the patient is about to begin an activity that is likely to induce an attack (GINA, 2018). Such agents include albuterol, levalbuterol, and terbutaline.

! NURSING SAFETY PRIORITY QSEN

Action Alert

Teach the patient with asthma to always carry the relief drug inhaler with him or her and to ensure that enough drug remains in the inhaler to provide a quick dose when needed.

Long-acting beta$_2$ agonists (LABAs) are also delivered by inhaler directly to the site of action—the bronchioles. Proper use of the long-acting agonists decreases the need to use reliever drugs as often. Unlike short-acting agonists, long-acting drugs need time to build up an effect, but the effects are longer lasting. These drugs are useful in *preventing* an asthma attack but cannot stop an acute attack. Therefore teach patients not to use LABAs alone to relieve symptoms of an attack or when wheezing is getting worse but, instead, to use a SABA. Examples of LABAs include formoterol and salmeterol. Both drugs are associated with increased asthma deaths when used as the only therapy for asthma and carry a black box warning from the Food and Drug Administration (FDA).

! NURSING SAFETY PRIORITY QSEN

Drug Alert

LABAs should never be prescribed as the **only** drug therapy for asthma and are not to be used during an acute asthma attack or bronchospasm. Teach the patient to use these control drugs daily as prescribed, even when no symptoms are present, and to use a SABA to relieve acute symptoms. Any patient using these drugs must be monitored closely.

Cholinergic antagonists, also called *anticholinergic drugs* or *long-acting muscarinic antagonists (LAMAs),* are similar to atropine and block the parasympathetic nervous system. This action increases bronchodilation and decreases pulmonary secretions. The most common drug in this class is ipratropium inhalant. Some cholinergic antagonists are short acting and are used several times a day. Long-acting agents such as tiotropium are used once daily.

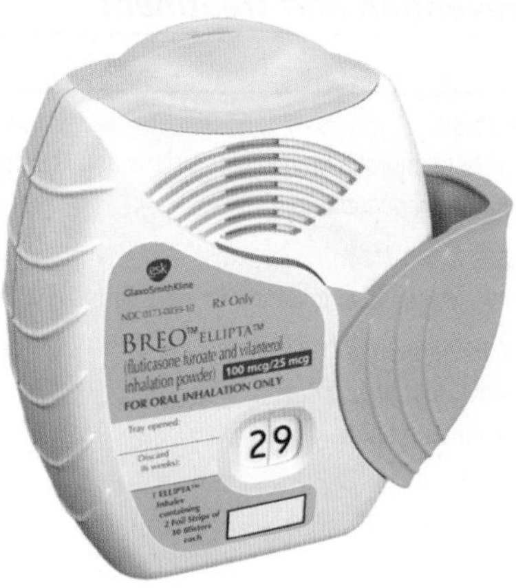

FIG. 27.4 Example of a dry powder inhaler with a counter. (Courtesy GlaxoSmithKline.)

Xanthines such as theophylline and aminophylline are used rarely, only when all other types of management are ineffective. These drugs are given systemically, and the dosage that is effective is close to the dosage that produces many dangerous side effects. Blood levels must be monitored closely to ensure that the drug level is within the therapeutic range.

Anti-inflammatory Agents. Anti-inflammatory agents decrease airway ***inflammation***. The inhaled forms have fewer systemic side effects than those taken systemically. *All of the anti-inflammatory drugs, whether inhaled or taken orally, are controller drugs only.*

! NURSING SAFETY PRIORITY QSEN

Drug Alert

Anti-inflammatory drug therapy for asthma is for prevention or control of asthma. They are **not** effective in reversing symptoms during an asthma attack and should not be used alone as reliever drugs. Teach patients to take anti-inflammatory asthma drugs on a scheduled basis, even when no symptoms are present.

Corticosteroids decrease ***inflammation*** in many ways, including by reducing the production of inflammatory chemicals. Inhaled corticosteroids (ICSs) can be helpful in controlling asthma symptoms and have overall fewer serious side effects than systemic corticosteroids (Penkalski, 2019). High-potency steroid inhalers, such as fluticasone, budesonide, and mometasone, may be used once per day for maintenance. Some drugs for asthma control include those that are combinations of an inhaled corticosteroid and an inhaled beta$_2$ agonist, such as Breo Elipta. This combination comes in different strengths and is used once daily.

Systemic corticosteroids, because of severe side effects, are avoided for mild-to-moderate intermittent asthma and are used on a short-term basis for moderate asthma. For some patients with severe asthma, daily oral corticosteroids may be needed.

Cromones, either inhaled or taken orally, are useful as *controller* asthma therapy when taken on a scheduled basis. These agents reduce airway inflammation by either inhibiting the release of inflammatory chemicals (nedocromil) or preventing mast cell membranes from opening when an allergen binds to IgE (cromolyn sodium).

Leukotriene modifiers are oral drugs that work in several ways to control asthma when taken on a scheduled basis. Montelukast and zafirlukast block the leukotriene receptor. Zileuton prevents leukotriene synthesis.

Monoclonal antibodies are newer drugs specifically for the management of eosinophilic asthma and include benralizumab, mepolizumab, and reslizumab. All of these drugs block the activity of IL-5. They are used as "add-on" drugs for patients whose eosinophilic asthma has not responded well to more standard therapies (Hussar, 2019).

Exercise and Activity. Regular exercise is a recommended part of asthma therapy to maintain cardiac health, strengthen muscles, and promote ***gas exchange*** and ***perfusion***. Teach patients to examine the conditions that trigger an attack and adjust the exercise routine as needed. Some may need to use an inhaled SABA before beginning activity. For others, adjusting the environment may be needed (e.g., changing from outdoor ice-skating in cold, dry air to indoor ice-skating).

Oxygen Therapy. Supplemental oxygen by mask or nasal cannula is often used during an acute asthma attack. High-flow delivery may be needed when bronchospasms are severe and limit flow of oxygen through the bronchiole tubes (see Chapter 25 for high-flow delivery systems).

! NURSING SAFETY PRIORITY (QSEN)

Action Alert

Ensure that no open flames (e.g., smoking, fireplaces, burning candles) or other combustion hazards are in rooms where oxygen is in use.

Status Asthmaticus. Status asthmaticus is a severe, life-threatening acute episode of airway obstruction that intensifies once it begins and often does not respond to usual therapy. The patient arrives in the emergency department with extremely labored breathing and wheezing. Use of accessory muscles for breathing and distention of neck veins are observed. *If the condition is not reversed, the patient may develop pneumothorax and cardiac or respiratory arrest.* IV fluids, potent systemic bronchodilators, steroids, epinephrine, and oxygen are given immediately to reverse the condition. Magnesium sulfate also may be used, although this practice is controversial. Prepare for emergency intubation. Sudden absence of wheezing along with a low oxygen saturation indicates complete airway obstruction and requires a tracheotomy. When breathing improves, management is similar to that for any patient with asthma.

NCLEX EXAMINATION CHALLENGE 27.1

Safe and Effective Care Environment

When performing a medication reconciliation for a newly admitted client before planned abdominal surgery, the nurse notes that the client is prescribed salmeterol and fluticasone daily for asthma control. What is the **priority action** for the nurse to take regarding this information to **prevent harm?**

A. Record and display the information in a prominent place within the client's medical record.
B. Ask the client how long the drugs have been prescribed and how well the asthma is controlled.
C. Collaborate with the surgeon to arrange for continuation of this therapy in the perioperative period.
D. Ensure that parenteral forms of these drugs are prescribed for use while the client remains NPO after surgery.

CLINICAL JUDGMENT CHALLENGE 27.1

Patient-Centered Care; Evidence-Based Practice

A 38-year-old mildly obese woman is brought to the emergency department by her older sister with a severe acute attack of her chronic asthma. The client has audible wheezes on inhalation and exhalation. Her admitting vital signs are blood pressure 172/100, pulse rate 114, respiratory rate 24, temperature 100° F (38° C); oxygen saturation 78%. When the nurse asks her if she took any asthma medications today, she nods yes but is too breathless to speak. Her lips and nailbeds are cyanotic, and she has an anxious expression on her face. The nurse notes that the client has a brace around her right knee. Her sister tells the nurse that the client called her about 30 minutes ago and asked to be taken to the hospital because several doses of her reliever inhaler were not helping her asthma attack. The sister has all of the client's prescribed medications in her purse, which include an albuterol inhaler, a salmeterol inhaler, and a fluticasone inhaler. When asked about the client's knee brace, the sister reports that the client has chronic knee pain and has been taking both acetaminophen and an NSAID daily to manage the discomfort.

1. **Recognize Cues:** What assessment information in this client situation is the most important and immediate concern for the nurse? (Hint: Identify the **relevant** information *first* to determine what is most important.)
2. **Analyze Cues:** What client conditions are consistent with the most **relevant** information? (Hint: Think about priority collaborative problems that support and contradict the information presented in this situation.)
3. **Prioritize Hypotheses:** Which possibilities or explanations are **most likely** to be present in this client situation? Which possibilities or explanations are the most serious? (Hint: Consider all possibilities and determine their urgency and risk for this client.)
4. **Generate Solutions:** What activities would most likely achieve the desired outcomes for this client? Which actions should be **avoided** or are **potentially harmful**? (Hint: Determine the desired outcomes first to decide which interventions are appropriate and those that should be avoided.)
5. **Take Action:** Which actions are the most appropriate and how should they be implemented? In what **priority order** should they be implemented? (Hint: Consider health teaching, documentation, requested health care provider orders or prescriptions, nursing skills, collaboration with or referral to health team members, etc.)
6. **Evaluate Outcomes:** What client assessment would indicate the nurse's actions were **effective**? (Hint: Think about signs that would indicate an improvement, decline, or unchanged patient condition.)

GAS EXCHANGE CONCEPT EXEMPLAR: CHRONIC OBSTRUCTIVE PULMONARY DISEASE

Pathophysiology Review

Chronic obstructive pulmonary disease (COPD) is a collection of lower airway disorders that interfere with airflow and ***gas exchange***. These disorders include emphysema and chronic bronchitis. Although these are separate disorders with different pathologic processes, many patients with emphysema also have chronic bronchitis (Fig. 27.5).

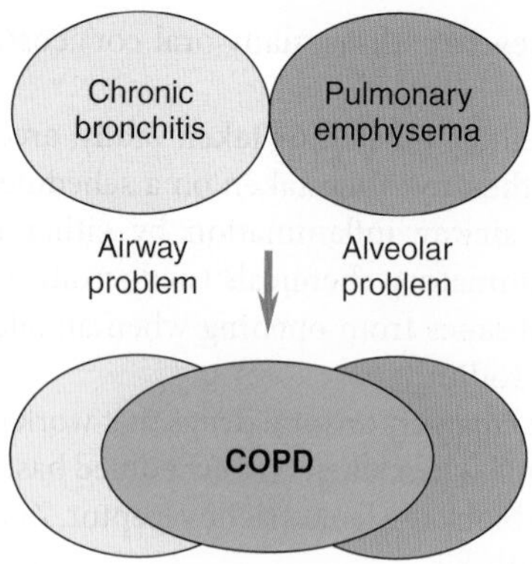

FIG. 27.5 Interaction of chronic bronchitis and emphysema in chronic obstructive pulmonary disease.

Emphysema

Emphysema is a destructive problem of lung elastic tissue that reduces its ability to recoil after stretching, leading to hyperinflation of the lung (see Fig. 27.1). These changes result in dyspnea with reduced ***gas exchange*** and the need for an increased respiratory rate.

In the healthy lung, enzymes called *proteases* are present to destroy and eliminate particulates inhaled during breathing. Cigarette smoking triggers increased synthesis of these enzymes to higher-than-normal levels, which then damage the alveoli and small airways by breaking down elastin. Over time, alveolar sacs lose their elasticity (recoil) and the small airways collapse or narrow. Some alveoli are destroyed, and others become large and flabby, with less area for gas exchange.

An increased amount of air is trapped in the lungs. Causes of air trapping are loss of elastic recoil in the alveolar walls, overstretching and enlargement of the alveoli into air-filled spaces called *bullae,* and collapse of small bronchioles. These changes greatly increase the work of breathing and interfere with airflow to the lungs. The hyperinflated lung flattens the diaphragm (Fig. 27.6), weakening the effectiveness of this muscle. As a result, the patient with emphysema needs to use accessory muscles in the neck, chest wall, and abdomen to inhale and exhale. This increased effort increases the need for oxygen, making the patient have an "air hunger" sensation. Inhalation starts before exhalation is completed, resulting in an uncoordinated breathing pattern.

Gas exchange is affected by the increased work of breathing and the loss of alveolar tissue. Although some alveoli enlarge, the functional area available for gas exchange is decreased. Often the patient adjusts by increasing the respiratory rate, so arterial blood gas (ABG) values may not show gas exchange problems until the patient has advanced disease. Then carbon dioxide is produced faster than it can be eliminated, resulting in carbon dioxide retention and chronic respiratory acidosis (see Chapter 14). The patient with late-stage emphysema also has a low arterial oxygen (Pao_2) level because it is difficult for oxygen to move from diseased alveoli into the blood.

Emphysema is classified as *panlobular, centrilobular,* or *paraseptal,* depending on the pattern of destruction and dilation of the gas-exchanging units (acini) (see Fig. 27.1). Each type can occur alone or in combination in the same lung. Most are associated with tobacco smoking (e.g., cigarettes, cigars, pipes), marijuana smoking, or other chronic inhaled particulate matter exposures (PME) such as wood smoke and biomass fuels (Global Initiative for Chronic Obstructive Lung Disease [GOLD], 2019).

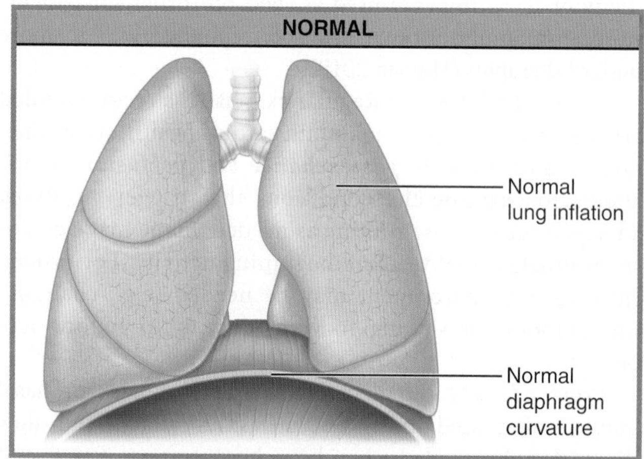

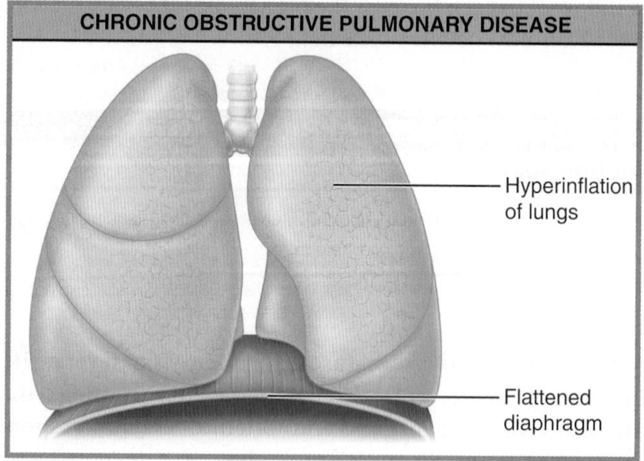

FIG. 27.6 Diaphragm shape and lung inflation in the normal patient and in the patient with chronic obstructive pulmonary disease.

Chronic Bronchitis

Chronic bronchitis is an inflammation of the bronchi and bronchioles *(bronchiolitis)* caused by exposure to irritants, especially cigarette smoke. The irritant triggers inflammation, vasodilation, mucosal edema, congestion, and bronchospasm. Bronchitis affects only the airways, not the alveoli.

Chronic ***inflammation*** increases the number and size of mucus-secreting glands, which produce large amounts of thick mucus. The bronchial walls thicken and impair airflow. This thickening, along with excessive mucus, blocks some of the smaller airways and narrows larger ones. The increased mucus provides a breeding ground for organisms and leads to chronic infection.

Chronic bronchitis impairs airflow and ***gas exchange*** because mucus plugs and inflammation narrow the airways. As a result, the Pao_2 level decreases *(hypoxemia),* and the arterial carbon dioxide ($Paco_2$) level increases (respiratory acidosis).

Etiology and Genetic Risk

Cigarette smoking is the greatest risk factor for COPD. The patient with a 20–pack-year history or longer often has early-stage COPD with changes in pulmonary function tests (PFTs).

The inhaled smoke triggers the release of excessive proteases in the lungs. These enzymes break down elastin, the major component of alveoli. By impairing the action of cilia, smoking also inhibits the cilia from clearing the bronchi of mucus, cellular debris, and fluid.

Alpha$_1$-antitrypsin deficiency is a less common but important risk factor for COPD, although it is often underrecognized (Southard et al., 2020). The enzyme alpha$_1$-antitrypsin (AAT) is normally present in the lungs. AAT inhibits excessive protease activity, so the proteases only break down inhaled pollutants and organisms and do not damage lung structures.

The production of normal amounts of AAT depends on the inheritance of a pair of normal gene alleles for this protein. The *AAT* gene is recessive. Thus if one of the pair of alleles is faulty and the other allele is normal, the adult makes enough AAT to prevent COPD unless there is significant exposure to cigarette smoke or other inhalation irritants. However, this adult is a carrier for AAT deficiency. When both alleles are faulty, COPD develops at a fairly young age even when the person is not significantly exposed to cigarette smoke or other irritants.

About 100,000 Americans have severe AAT deficiency, and many more have mild to moderate deficiencies (Southard et al., 2020). Although an AAT deficiency also can cause problems in the skin and liver, lung diseases are more common.

PATIENT-CENTERED CARE: GENETIC/GENOMIC CONSIDERATIONS QSEN

AAT deficiency is a single gene disorder with many known gene variations, and some increase the risk for emphysema. Different variations result in different levels of AAT deficiency, which is why the disease is more severe for some adults than for others (OMIM, 2019c). The most serious variation for emphysema risk is the Z mutation, although others also increase the risk but to a lesser degree. Table 27.1 shows the most common AAT mutations increasing the risk for emphysema. Urge patients who have any AAT deficiency to avoid smoking and other environmental pollutants.

In addition to genetic and environmental factors, asthma also appears to be a risk factor for COPD. The incidence of COPD is reported to be 12 times greater among adults with asthma than among adults without asthma after adjusting for smoking history (GOLD, 2019). Both disorders may be present at the same time, known as *asthma-COPD overlap syndrome* (Bradshaw & Kosnar, 2017).

TABLE 27.1 Characteristics Associated With the Most Common Alpha$_1$-Antitrypsin Gene Mutations

Mutation Genotype	Level of Serum Alpha$_1$-Antitrypsin (% of Normal)	Disease Severity
M/S	80%	No detectable disease
S/S	50%-60%	Minimal to no disease expression
M/Z	50%-55%	Minimal to no disease expression
S/Z	30%-35%	Pulmonary disease, early age
Z/Z	10%-15%	Severe COPD, extrapulmonary involvement

COPD, Chronic obstructive pulmonary disease.

Incidence and Prevalence

The prevalence of chronic bronchitis and emphysema in the United States has been estimated at about 15 million and 900,000 in Canada (CDC, 2018a; Statistics Canada, 2019). More than 10% of nursing home residents have COPD. COPD is the fourth leading cause of morbidity and mortality in the United States (GOLD, 2019).

Complications

COPD affects ***gas exchange*** and the oxygenation of all tissues. Complications include hypoxemia, acidosis, respiratory infection, cardiac failure, dysrhythmias, and respiratory failure.

Hypoxemia and acidosis occur because the patient with COPD has reduced gas exchange, leading to decreased oxygenation and increased carbon dioxide levels. These problems reduce cellular function.

Respiratory infection risk increases because of the increased mucus and poor ***gas exchange***. Bacterial infections are common and make COPD symptoms worse by increasing ***inflammation*** and mucus production and inducing more bronchospasm. Airflow becomes even more limited, the work of breathing increases, and dyspnea results.

Cardiac failure, especially **cor pulmonale** (right-sided heart failure caused by pulmonary disease), occurs with bronchitis or emphysema. Air trapping, airway collapse, and stiff alveolar walls increase the lung tissue pressure and narrow lung blood vessels, making blood flow more difficult. The increased pressure creates a heavy workload on the right side of the heart, which pumps blood into the lungs. To pump blood through the narrowed vessels, the right side of the heart generates high pressures. In response to this heavy workload, the right chambers of the heart enlarge and thicken, causing right-sided heart failure with backup of blood into the general venous system. The Key Features: Cor Pulmonale box lists the symptoms and problems of cor pulmonale.

Cardiac dysrhythmias are common in patients with COPD. They result from hypoxemia (from decreased oxygen to the heart muscle), other cardiac disease, drug effects, or acidosis.

KEY FEATURES

Cor Pulmonale

- Hypoxia and hypoxemia
- Increasing dyspnea
- Fatigue
- Enlarged and tender liver
- Warm, cyanotic hands and feet, with bounding pulses
- Cyanotic lips
- Distended neck veins
- Right ventricular enlargement (hypertrophy)
- Visible pulsations below the sternum
- GI disturbances such as nausea or anorexia
- Dependent edema
- Metabolic and respiratory acidosis
- Pulmonary hypertension

Health Promotion and Maintenance

The incidence and severity of COPD would be greatly reduced by smoking cessation. Urge all adults who smoke to quit smoking or vaping and to avoid particulate matter exposure using the I-PREPARE model as described in Chapter 24.

Interprofessional Collaborative Care

Although COPD is a life-limiting chronic disorder, most patients live decades in the community, although management is continuous. Acute infections and other complications often require hospital stays. Adults with COPD may be admitted to the hospital for other health problems or surgery and require continued COPD management.

COPD can affect every aspect of a patient's life, and care is best provided by an interprofessional team. Like many chronic disorders, COPD management is most effective when the patient and family are full partners with the health care team.

INTERPROFESSIONAL COLLABORATIVE CARE

The Patient With COPD

In addition to primary health care providers and nurses, other professionals important to ensuring optimal management include registered dietitian nutritionists, pharmacists, respiratory therapists, occupational therapists, physical therapists, social workers, patient navigators, community health workers, and mental health practitioners.

Assessment: Recognize Cues

History. Identifying patients with early-stage COPD is important in starting the appropriate management. Initiation of drug management together with reducing particulate matter exposures can help delay the pathologic consequences of the disorder and increase the patient's functional activity (GOLD, 2019; O'Dell et al., 2018). Although pulmonary function testing is needed for confirmation of COPD presence, the disorder should be suspected in any patient who has dyspnea, chronic cough or sputum production, recurrent lower respiratory infections, and/or a history of particulate matter exposures (GOLD, 2019).

Ask about risk factors such as age, gender, and occupational history. COPD is seen more often in older men. Some types of emphysema occur in families, especially those with alpha$_1$-antitrypsin (AAT) deficiency (Southard et al., 2020).

Obtain a thorough smoking history because tobacco use is a major risk factor. Ask about the length of time the patient has smoked and the number of packs smoked daily. Use these data to determine the pack-year smoking history. Also ask about the use of electronic cigarettes or vaping, including the type of product inhaled and the duration of the habit.

Ask the patient to describe the breathing problems and assess whether he or she has any difficulty breathing while talking. Does he or she speak in complete sentences, or is it necessary to take a breath between every one or two words? Ask about the presence, duration, or worsening of wheezing, coughing, and shortness of breath. Determine which activities trigger these problems. Assess any cough, and ask whether sputum is clear or colored and how much is produced each day. Ask about the time of day when sputum production is greatest. Smokers often have a productive cough when they get up in the morning; nonsmokers generally do not.

Ask the patient to compare the activity level and shortness of breath now with those of a month ago and a year ago. Ask about any difficulty with eating and sleeping. Many patients sleep in a semisitting position because breathlessness is worse when lying down (**orthopnea**). Ask about any difficulty with ADLs or sexual activity. Document this assessment to personalize the intervention plan.

Weigh the patient and compare this weight with previous weights. Unplanned weight loss is likely when COPD severity increases, because the work of breathing increases metabolic needs. Dyspnea and mucus production often result in poor food intake and inadequate nutrition. Ask the patient to recall a typical day's meals and fluid intake. When heart failure is present with COPD, general edema with weight gain may occur.

Physical Assessment/Signs and Symptoms. *General appearance* can provide clues about respiratory status and energy level. Observe weight in proportion to height, posture, mobility, muscle mass, and overall hygiene. The patient with increasingly severe COPD is thin, with loss of muscle mass in the extremities, although the neck muscles may be enlarged. He or she tends to be slow moving and slightly stooped. The patient often sits in a forward-bending posture with the arms held forward, a position known as the *orthopneic* or *tripod position* (Fig. 27.7). When dyspnea becomes severe, activity intolerance may be so great that bathing and general grooming are neglected.

Respiratory changes that occur as a result of obstruction include changes in chest size, and fatigue. Inspect the chest and assess the breathing rate and pattern. The patient with respiratory muscle fatigue breathes with rapid, shallow respirations and may have an abnormal breathing pattern in which the abdominal wall is sucked in during inspiration or may use accessory muscles in the abdomen or neck. During an acute exacerbation, the respiratory rate could be as high as 40 to 50 breaths/min and requires immediate medical attention. As respiratory muscles

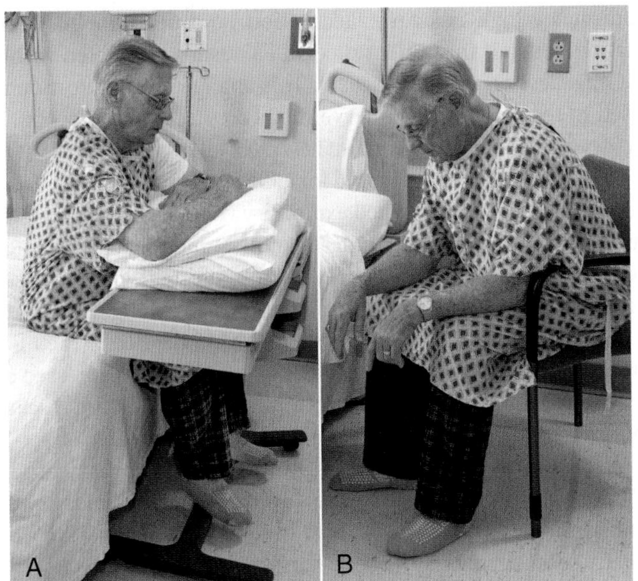

FIG. 27.7 Orthopnea positions that patients with chronic obstructive pulmonary disease often assume to ease the work of breathing.

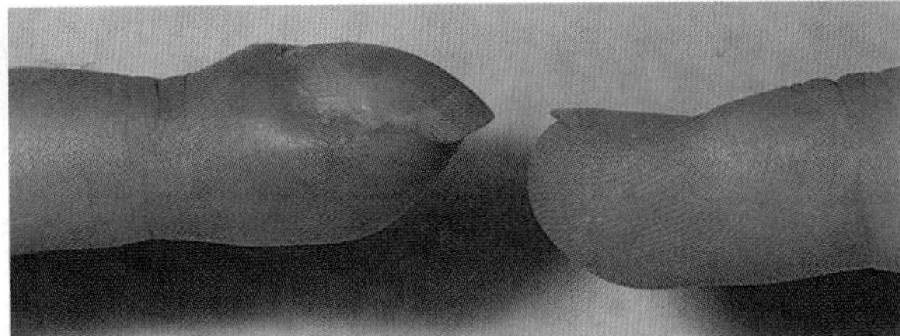

FIG. 27.8 Late digital clubbing (on left) compared with a normal digit (on right). (From Swartz, M. H. [2009]. *Textbook of physical diagnosis: History and examination* [6th ed.]. Philadelphia: Saunders.)

become fatigued, respiratory movement is jerky and appears uncoordinated.

Check the patient's chest for retractions and asymmetric chest expansion. The patient with emphysema has limited diaphragmatic movement *(excursion)* because the diaphragm is flattened and below its usual resting state. Chest vibration *(fremitus)* is often decreased, and the chest sounds hyperresonant on percussion because of trapped air (Jarvis, 2020).

Auscultate the chest to assess the depth of inspiration and any abnormal breath sounds. Wheezes and other abnormal sounds often occur on inspiration and expiration, although crackles are usually not present. Reduced breath sounds are common, especially with emphysema. Note the pitch and location of the sound and the point in the respiratory cycle at which the sound is heard. A silent chest may indicate serious airflow obstruction or pneumothorax.

Assess the degree of dyspnea using a Visual Analog Dyspnea Scale (VADS), as shown in Chapter 24, Fig. 24.8. Ask the patient to place a mark on the line to indicate his or her breathing difficulty. Document and use this scale to determine the therapy effectiveness and pace the patient's activities.

Examine the patient's chest for the presence of a "barrel chest" (see Fig. 27.3). With a barrel chest, the ratio between the anteroposterior (AP) diameter of the chest and its lateral diameter is 1:1 rather than the normal ratio of 1:1.5, as a result of lung overinflation and diaphragm flattening (Jarvis, 2020).

The patient with chronic bronchitis often has a cyanotic, or blue-tinged, dusky appearance and has excessive sputum production. Assess for cyanosis, delayed capillary refill, and finger clubbing (Fig. 27.8), which indicate chronically decreased arterial oxygen levels.

Cardiac changes occur as a result of the anatomic changes associated with COPD. Assess the patient's heart rate and rhythm. Check for swelling of the feet and ankles (dependent edema) or other signs of right-sided heart failure. Examine nail beds and oral mucous membranes. In late-stage emphysema the patient may have pallor or cyanosis and is usually underweight.

Psychosocial Assessment. COPD affects all aspects of a patient's life. He or she may be isolated because dyspnea causes fatigue or because of embarrassment from coughing and excessive sputum production.

Ask the patient about interests and hobbies to assess whether socialization has decreased or whether hobbies cause exposure to irritants. Ask about home conditions for exposure to smoke or crowded living conditions that promote transmission of respiratory infections.

Economic status may be affected by the disease through changes in income and health insurance coverage. Drugs delivered by inhalers are expensive, and many patients with limited incomes may use them only during exacerbations and not as prescribed on a scheduled basis.

Anxiety and fear from feelings of breathlessness may reduce the patient's ability to participate in a full life. Work, family, social, and sexual roles can be affected. Encourage the patient and family to express their feelings about disease progression and the limitations on lifestyle. Assess their use of support groups and community services.

Laboratory Assessment. Arterial blood gas (ABG) values identify abnormal ***gas exchange***, oxygenation, ventilation, and acid-base status. Compare repeated ABG values to assess changes in respiratory status. Once baseline ABG values are obtained, pulse oximetry can gauge treatment response. As COPD worsens, the amount of oxygen in the blood decreases (**hypoxemia**) and the amount of carbon dioxide increases (**hypercapnia**, also known as *hypercarbia*). Chronic respiratory acidosis (increased arterial carbon dioxide [$Paco_2$]) then results; metabolic alkalosis (increased arterial bicarbonate) occurs as compensation by kidney retention of bicarbonate. This change is seen on ABGs as an elevation of HCO_3-, although pH remains lower than normal. Not all patients with COPD are CO_2 retainers, even when hypoxemia is present, because CO_2 diffuses more easily across lung membranes than does oxygen. Hypercapnia is often chronically present in advanced emphysema (because the alveoli are affected) rather than in bronchitis (in which the airways are affected). Acute hypercapnia with rapid rises above the patient's usual CO_2 levels represents a serious decline in the patient's condition and can lead to respiratory failure (Dorman, 2016). Sputum samples are obtained for culture from hospitalized patients with an acute respiratory infection. The infection is treated on the basis of symptoms and the common bacterial organisms in

TABLE 27.2 Gold Classification of Chronic Obstructive Pulmonary Disease Severity

Class	Pulmonary Function Test Results
GOLD 1: Mild	FEV_1 ≥80% of predicted
GOLD 2: Moderate	FEV_1 50% to 79% of predicted
GOLD 3: Severe	FEV_1 30% to 49% of predicted
GOLD 4: Very severe	FEV_1 <30% of predicted

COPD, Chronic obstructive pulmonary disease; *FEV_1,* volume of air blown out as hard and fast as possible during the first second of the most forceful exhalation after the greatest full inhalation; *FVC,* functional vital capacity.
Data from Global Initiative for Chronic Obstructive Lung Disease (GOLD). (2019). *Global strategy for the diagnosis, management, and prevention of chronic obstructive pulmonary disease.* https://goldcopd.org/wp-content/uploads/2018/11/GOLD-2019-POCKET-GUIDE-FINAL_WMS.pdf

the local community. A WBC count helps confirm the presence of infection.

Other blood tests include hemoglobin and hematocrit to determine *polycythemia* (a compensatory increase in red blood cells [RBCs] and iron in the chronically hypoxic patient). Serum electrolyte levels are examined because acidosis can change electrolyte values. Low phosphate, potassium, calcium, and magnesium levels reduce muscle strength. In patients with a family history of COPD, serum AAT levels may be assessed.

Imaging Assessment. Chest x-rays are used to rule out other lung diseases and to check the progress of patients with respiratory infections or chronic disease. With advanced emphysema, chest x-rays show hyperinflation with widely spaced ribs and a flattened diaphragm.

Other Diagnostic Assessments. COPD is classified from mild to very severe on the basis of symptoms and pulmonary function test (PFT) changes (Table 27.2; see Table 24.6). Airflow rates and lung volume measurements help distinguish airway disease (obstructive diseases) from interstitial lung disease (restrictive diseases). PFTs determine lung volumes, flow volume curves, and diffusion capacity. Each test is performed before and after the patient inhales a bronchodilator agent. Explain the preparations for the procedures (if any), whether pain or discomfort will be involved, and any needed follow-up care.

Although the severity classification in Table 27.2 can help clinicians determine overall disease severity, it does not predict how well the patient can manage his or her activity on a daily basis and how likely an acute exacerbation could occur. So this classification was modified in 2017 to include the severity indications based on symptom scores obtained with the patient responses to the COPD Assessment Test (CAT) (GOLD, 2019). This 8-item test requires the patient to rate his or her specific symptoms on a 0 (no symptom) to a 5 (worst symptom) scale. Scores can range from 0 to 40, with lower scores indicating less severe problems. As a result, each of the GOLD classes also can contain an ABCD designation for actual symptom severity as an indicator of risk for exacerbation. An *A* designation indicates a low risk for exacerbation, even when the patient has a GOLD class of 4 (very severe disease), whereas a *D* designation indicates a high risk for exacerbation (and need for hospitalization), even if the patient meets PFT results associated with a GOLD class of 1 (mild disease). This change in classification is used to recognize when interventions are needed to prevent an acute exacerbation (Kaufman, 2017; O'Dell et al., 2018).

The lung volumes measured for COPD are vital capacity (VC), residual volume (RV), forced expiratory volume (FEV), and total lung capacity (TLC). Although all volumes and capacities change to some degree in COPD, the RV is most affected, with increases reflecting the trapped, stale air remaining in the lungs.

A diagnosis of COPD is based mostly on the FEV_1 (the FEV in the first second of exhalation). FEV_1 can also be expressed as a percentage of the forced vital capacity (FVC). As the disease progresses, the ratio of FEV_1 to FVC becomes smaller.

The diffusion test measures how well a test gas (carbon monoxide) diffuses across the alveolar-capillary membrane and combines with hemoglobin. In emphysema, alveolar wall destruction decreases the large surface area for diffusion of gas into the blood, leading to a decreased diffusion capacity. In bronchitis alone, the diffusion capacity is usually normal.

The patient with COPD has decreased oxygen saturation, often much lower than 90%. Changes in Spo_2 below the patient's usual saturation require medical attention. Patients who have been managing COPD for a long time often are aware of their usual Spo_2 values.

Peak expiratory flow meters are used to monitor the effectiveness of drug therapy to relieve obstruction. Peak flow rates increase as obstruction resolves. Teach the patient to self-monitor the peak expiratory flow rates at home and adjust drugs as needed.

◆ Analysis: Analyze Cues and Prioritize Hypotheses

The priority collaborative problems for patients with chronic obstructive pulmonary disease (COPD) include:

1. Decreased ***gas exchange*** due to alveolar-capillary membrane changes, reduced airway size, ventilatory muscle fatigue, excessive mucus production, airway obstruction, diaphragm flattening, fatigue, and decreased energy
2. Weight loss due to dyspnea, excessive secretions, anorexia, and fatigue
3. Anxiety due to a change in health status and situational crisis
4. Decreased endurance due to fatigue, dyspnea, and an imbalance between oxygen supply and demand
5. Potential for pneumonia or other respiratory infections

◆ Planning and Implementation: Generate Solutions and Take Action

Improving Gas Exchange and Reducing Carbon Dioxide Retention

Planning: Expected Outcomes. The patient with COPD is expected to attain and maintain ***gas exchange*** at his or her usual baseline level.

Interventions. Most patients with COPD use nonsurgical management to improve or maintain ***gas exchange***. Surgical management requires that the patient meet strict criteria.

Nursing care is most successful with helping the patient become a partner in COPD management by participating in all therapies to improve ***gas exchange***. Thus priority nursing management for patients with COPD focuses on ensuring consistent use of prescribed drug therapy and on airway maintenance, monitoring, breathing techniques, positioning, effective coughing, oxygen therapy, exercise conditioning, suctioning, and hydration.

Before any intervention, assess the breathing rate, rhythm, depth, and use of accessory muscles. The accessory muscles are less efficient than the diaphragm, and the work of breathing increases. Determine whether any factors are contributing to the increased work of breathing, such as respiratory infection. *Airway maintenance is the most important focus of interventions to improve **gas exchange**.*

Drug Therapy. Drug therapy is recommended at all levels of disease to delay progression and promote continued activity tolerance (GOLD, 2019; O'Dell et al., 2018). Drugs used to manage COPD are the same drugs as for asthma and include beta-adrenergic agents, cholinergic antagonists, xanthines, corticosteroids, and cromones (see the Common Examples of Drug Therapy: Asthma Prevention and Treatment box in the Asthma section). The focus is on long-term control therapy with longer-acting drugs, such as arformoterol, indacaterol, tiotropium, aclidinium bromide, olodaterol, and the combination drugs, such as fluticasone/vilanterol (e.g., BREO ELLIPTA), olodaterol/tiotropium, vilanterol/umeclidinium (e.g., ANORO ELLIPTA), and a newer triple combination of fluticasone/umeclidinium/vilanterol (e.g., TRELEGY ELLIPTA).

Just as for asthma management, a key issue for successful drug therapy for COPD management is the correct technique for inhaler use. Have the patient demonstrate or fully describe exactly how he or she uses the inhaler(s) at every new outpatient interaction. Reinforce correct technique use and apply a variety of interventions that can help the patient acquire the knowledge and skills needed to use the inhaler correctly (see the Systems Thinking and Quality Improvement: Reducing Critical Errors in Patient Inhaler Use box).

The patient with COPD is more likely to be taking systemic agents in addition to inhaled drugs. Another drug class for COPD is the mucolytics, which thin the thick secretions, making them easier to cough up and expel. Nebulizer treatments with normal saline or a mucolytic agent such as acetylcysteine or dornase alfa and normal saline help thin secretions. Guaifenesin is a systemic mucolytic that is taken orally. A combination of guaifenesin and dextromethorphan also raises the cough threshold.

Stepped therapy, which adds drugs as COPD progresses, is recommended for patients with chronic bronchitis or emphysema, although the patient's response to drug therapy is the best indicator of when drugs or their dosages need changing. Ideally the patient notices changes and participates in management strategies. Drugs are "stepped" up with disease exacerbations and decreased when the patient's symptoms return to his or her stable level. If the patient's symptoms decrease over time and remain stable, drug therapy can be "stepped down" to the lowest level that allows the disease severity to remain stable (O'Dell et al., 2018).

Monitoring. Monitoring for changes in respiratory status is key to providing prompt interventions to reduce complications. Assess the hospitalized patient with COPD at least every 2 hours, even when the purpose of hospitalization is not COPD management. Apply prescribed oxygen, assess the patient's response to therapy, and prevent complications.

SYSTEMS THINKING AND QUALITY IMPROVEMENT QSEN

Reducing Critical Errors in Patient Inhaler Use

Henrich, R., & Logue, M. (2017). Feasibility of using the test for adherence to inhalers tool and tailoring education to the individual with chronic obstructive pulmonary disease. *The Journal for Nurse Practitioners, 13*(10), e481–e483.

A key component for successful management of COPD and asthma is the use of correct technique for patient administration of inhaled drugs regardless of the type of inhaler used (GOLD, 2019). For each inhaler type, there are multiple steps that must be performed correctly and in proper order for drug dose delivery to the airways. Poor performance with critical errors in technique are common and contribute to reduced disease control and increased complications. Although brochures and pamphlets have been used along with teach-back demonstrations to help patients learn and use correct techniques, critical errors still occur.

The current project used the Test for Adherence to Inhalers (TAI) tool to identify critical errors in inhaler use by patients with COPD who had been using prescribed inhalers for some time. Results indicated that 40% of the participants made at least one critical error in technique that would result in inadequate drug reaching the site of action. The education intervention of manufacturer-generated videos demonstrating the correct techniques for the prescribed inhaler type were used by those participants who initially made critical errors. After viewing the videos, only 7% of participants made one or more critical errors, demonstrating reasonable efficacy of the intervention.

Commentary: Implications for Practice and Research

Results of this QI project are important to improving the overall and self-management of COPD, even though the number of subjects was small. Many literature reviews report up to 90% of patients do not correctly follow the recommended steps for effective use of inhalers, which has a negative impact on disease control, as well as quality of life. These manufacturer videos are available for free on YouTube sites and can be accessed by private computer or at public libraries. Most videos are also available in Spanish. Helping patients to actually see the correct techniques rather than just reading about them provides additional sensory input for learning. Having access to these videos allows patients to self-reinforce correct techniques. This teaching intervention represents low risk, positive outcomes, and minimal cost.

The article did not report the duration of the effect of the intervention for continued reduction of critical errors. Such information could be a subject of the "next step" research to help determine how often reinforcement may be needed. Other studies could be conducted to compare hospital admission rates for patients with COPD who use these videos compared with those who do not.

If the patient's condition worsens, as evidenced by a sudden sharp rise in CO_2 or severe decrease in PaO_2, more aggressive therapy is needed. Noninvasive ventilation (NIV) may be useful for patients with stable, very severe COPD and daytime hypercapnia (Dorman, 2016; GOLD, 2019). Intubation and mechanical ventilation may be needed for patients in respiratory failure.

Breathing Techniques. Diaphragmatic or abdominal and pursed-lip breathing may be helpful for managing dyspneic episodes. Teach the patient to use these techniques, shown in the Patient and Family Education: Preparing for Self-Management: Breathing Exercises box, during all activities to reduce the amount of stale air in the lungs and manage dyspnea. Teach these techniques when the patient has less dyspnea.

PATIENT AND FAMILY EDUCATION: PREPARING FOR SELF-MANAGEMENT

Breathing Exercises

Diaphragmatic or Abdominal Breathing

- If you can do so comfortably, lie on your back with your knees bent. If you cannot lie comfortably, perform this exercise while sitting in a chair.
- Place your hands or a book on your abdomen to create resistance.
- Begin breathing from your abdomen while keeping your chest still. You can tell if you are breathing correctly if your hands or the book rises and falls accordingly.

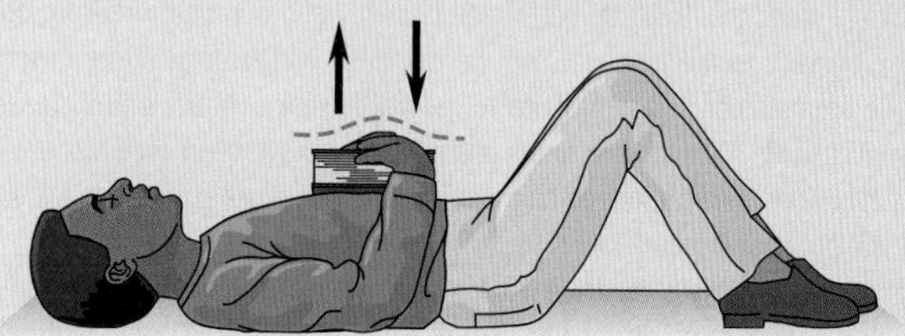

Pursed-Lip Breathing

- Close your mouth and breathe in through your nose.
- Purse your lips as you would to whistle. Breathe out slowly through your mouth, without puffing your cheeks. Spend at least twice the amount of time it took you to breathe in.
- Use your abdominal muscles to squeeze out every bit of air you can.
- Remember to use pursed-lip breathing during any physical activity. Always inhale before beginning the activity and exhale while performing it. Never hold your breath.

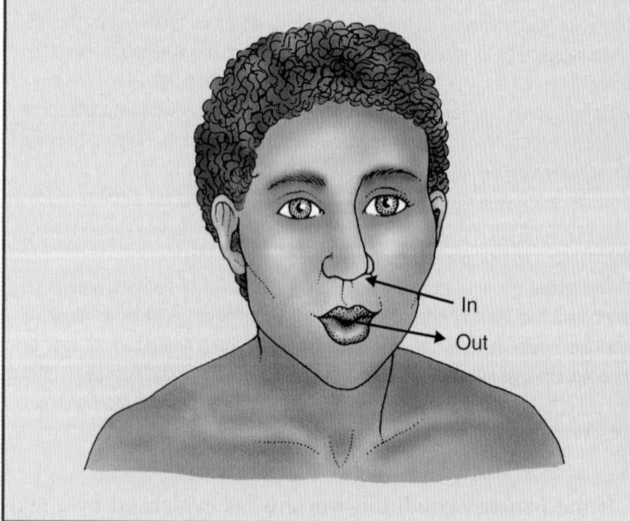

In diaphragmatic breathing, the patient consciously increases movement of the diaphragm. Lying on the back allows the abdomen to relax. Breathing through pursed lips creates mild resistance, which prolongs exhalation and increases airway pressure. This technique delays airway compression and reduces air trapping.

Positioning. Having the patient remain in an upright position with the head of the bed elevated can help alleviate dyspnea by increasing chest expansion and keeping the diaphragm in the proper position to contract. This position conserves energy by supporting the patient's arms and upper body. Help the patient who can tolerate sitting in a chair get out of bed for 1-hour periods two to three times a day.

Effective Coughing. Coughing effectively can improve ***gas exchange*** by helping increase airflow in the larger airways. The patient with COPD has difficulty removing secretions, which results in poor gas exchange. Excessive mucus increases the risk for infections.

Controlled coughing is helpful in removing excessive mucus. Teach the patient to cough on arising in the morning to eliminate mucus that collected during the night. Coughing to clear mucus before mealtimes may make meals more pleasant. Coughing before bedtime may help clear lungs for a less interrupted night's sleep.

For effective coughing, teach the patient to sit in a chair or on the side of a bed with feet placed firmly on the floor. Instruct him or her to turn the shoulders inward and to bend the head slightly downward, hugging a pillow against the stomach. The patient then takes a few breaths, attempting to exhale more fully. After the third to fifth breath (in through the nose, out through pursed lips), instruct him or her to take a deeper breath and bend forward slowly while coughing two or three times ("mini" coughs) from the same breath. On return to a sitting position, the patient takes a comfortably deep breath. The entire coughing procedure is repeated at least twice.

Oxygen Therapy. Oxygen is prescribed for relief of hypoxemia and hypoxia. The need for oxygen therapy and its effectiveness can be determined by arterial blood gas (ABG) values and oxygen saturation. The patient with COPD may need an oxygen flow of 2 to 4 L/min via nasal cannula or up to 40% via Venturi mask. Ensure that there are no open flames in rooms in which oxygen is in use. See Chapter 25 for information on oxygen therapy.

In the past, the patient with COPD was thought to be at risk for extreme hypoventilation with oxygen therapy because of a decreased drive to breathe as blood oxygen levels rose. However, this concern has not been shown to be evidence based and has been responsible for ineffective management of hypoxia in patients with COPD. *All hypoxic patients, even those with COPD and hypercarbia, should receive oxygen therapy at rates appropriate to reduce hypoxia and bring* SpO_2 *levels up between 88% and 92%.*

Exercise Conditioning. Exercise for conditioning and pulmonary rehabilitation can improve function and endurance in patients with COPD. Patients often respond to the dyspnea of COPD by limiting their activity, even basic ADLs (Lee et al., 2018). Over time, the muscles used in breathing weaken, resulting in increased dyspnea with lower activity levels.

Pulmonary rehabilitation involves education and exercise training to prevent muscle deconditioning. Each patient's exercise program is personalized to his or her current limitations and planned outcomes. The simplest plan is having the patient walk (indoors or outdoors) daily at a self-paced rate until symptoms limit further walking, followed by a rest period, and then continue walking until 20 minutes of actual walking has been accomplished. As the time during rest periods decreases, the patient can add 5 more minutes of walking time. Teach patients whose symptoms are severe to modify the exercise by using a walker with wheels or, if needed, to use oxygen while exercising. Exercise needs to be performed at least two or three times weekly for best improvement. Formal pulmonary rehabilitation programs can be beneficial even for patients who are severely impaired.

Additional exercise techniques to retrain ventilatory muscles include isocapneic hyperventilation and resistive breathing. Isocapneic hyperventilation, in which the patient hyperventilates into a machine that controls the levels of oxygen and carbon dioxide, increases endurance. In resistive breathing the patient breathes against a set resistance. Resistive breathing increases respiratory muscle strength and endurance.

Suctioning. Perform suctioning only when needed—not routinely. Nasotracheal suction is used only for patients with a weak cough, weak pulmonary muscles, and inability to expectorate effectively. Assess for dyspnea, tachycardia, and dysrhythmias during the procedure. Assess for improved breath sounds after suctioning. Suctioning is discussed in detail in Chapter 25.

Hydration. Maintaining hydration may thin the thick, tenacious (sticky) secretions, making them easier to remove by coughing. Unless hydration needs to be avoided for other health problems, teach the patient with COPD to drink at least 2 L/day. Humidifiers may be useful for those living in a dry climate or those who use dry heat during the winter.

Surgical Management. Lung transplantation and lung volume reduction surgery (LVRS) can improve ***gas exchange*** in the patient with COPD. Transplantation is a less common procedure because of cost and the scarce availability of donor lungs. The more common surgical procedure for patients with emphysema is LVRS.

The purpose of LVRS is to improve ***gas exchange*** through removal of hyperinflated lung tissues that are filled with stagnant air containing little, if any, oxygen. The level of carbon dioxide is the same as that in the capillary, and no gas exchange occurs. Successful lung volume reduction results in increased forced expiratory volume and decreased total lung capacity and residual volume. Activity tolerance increases, and oxygen therapy may no longer be needed.

Preoperative care involves careful patient selection and testing to determine which areas of the lungs should be reduced. Patients who are selected for this procedure have end-stage emphysema, minimal chronic bronchitis, and stable cardiac function. They also must be ambulatory; not ventilator dependent; free of pulmonary fibrosis, asthma, or cancer; and not have smoked for at least 6 months. The patient must be rehabilitated to the stage that he or she is able to walk, without stopping, for 30 minutes at 1 mile/hr and maintain a 90% or better oxygen saturation level.

In addition to standard preoperative testing, tests to determine the location of greatest lung hyperinflation and poorest lung blood flow are performed. These tests include pulmonary plethysmography, gas dilution, and perfusion scans.

Operative procedures for lung reduction are usually performed on both lungs, most often by the minimally invasive surgical technique of video-assisted thoracoscopic surgery (VATS) (GOLD, 2019). Each lung is examined for areas of hyperinflation. The surgeon removes as much of the hyperinflated tissue as possible.

Postoperative care after LVRS involves close patient monitoring for continuing respiratory problems, as well as for usual postoperative complications. Bronchodilator and mucolytic therapies are maintained. Pulmonary hygiene includes incentive spirometry 10 times per hour while awake, chest physiotherapy starting on the first day after surgery, and hourly pulmonary assessment.

Preventing Weight Loss

Planning: Expected Outcomes. The patient with COPD is expected to achieve and maintain a body weight within 10% of ideal.

Interventions. The patient with COPD often has nausea, *early satiety* (feeling too "full" to eat), poor appetite, and meal-related dyspnea. The work of breathing raises calorie and protein needs, which can lead to protein-calorie malnutrition. Malnourished patients lose muscle mass and strength, lung elasticity, and alveolar-capillary surface area, all of which reduce ***gas exchange***.

Identify patients at risk for or who have this complication and collaborate with a registered dietitian nutritionist (RDN) to perform a nutrition assessment. Monitor weight and other indicators of nutrition, such as serum prealbumin levels.

Dyspnea management is needed because shortness of breath interferes with eating. Teach the patient to plan the biggest meal of the day for the time when he or she is most hungry and well rested. Four to six small meals a day may be preferred to three larger ones. Remind patients to use pursed-lip and abdominal breathing and to use the prescribed bronchodilator 30 minutes before the meal to reduce bronchospasm.

Food selection can help prevent weight loss. Abdominal bloating and a feeling of fullness often prevent the patient from eating a complete meal. Collaborate with the RDN to teach about foods that are easy to chew and not gas forming. Advise the patient to avoid dry foods that stimulate coughing and caffeine-containing drinks that increase urine output and may lead to dehydration.

Urge the patient to eat high-calorie, high-protein foods. Some supplements are formulated for patients with COPD and provide nutrition with reduced carbon dioxide production. If early satiety is a problem, advise him or her to avoid drinking fluids before and during the meal and to eat smaller, more frequent meals.

Minimizing Anxiety

Planning: Expected Outcomes. The patient with COPD is expected to have decreased anxiety.

Interventions. Patients with COPD become anxious during acute dyspneic episodes, especially when excessive secretions are present. Anxiety also may cause dyspnea.

Help the patient understand that anxiety can increase dyspnea and have a plan for dealing with anxiety. Together with the patient, develop a written plan that states exactly what he or she should do if symptoms flare. Having a plan provides confidence and control in knowing what to do, which often helps reduce anxiety. Stress the use of pursed-lip and diaphragmatic breathing techniques during periods of anxiety or panic.

Family, friends, and support groups can be helpful. Recommend professional counseling, if needed, as a positive suggestion. Stress that talking with a counselor can help identify techniques to maintain control over dyspnea and panic.

Explore other approaches to help the patient manage dyspneic episodes and panic attacks, such as progressive relaxation, hypnosis therapy, and biofeedback. For some patients, antianxiety drug therapy may be needed for severe anxiety.

Improving Endurance

Planning: Expected Outcomes. The patient with COPD is expected to increase activity to a level acceptable to him or her.

Interventions. The patient with COPD often has chronic fatigue. During acute exacerbations, he or she may need extensive help with the ADLs of eating, bathing, and grooming. As the acute problem resolves, encourage the patient to pace activities and perform as much self-care as possible. Teach him or her to not rush through morning activities because rushing increases dyspnea, fatigue, and hypoxemia. As activity gradually increases, assess the patient's response by noting skin color changes, pulse rate and regularity, oxygen saturation, and work of breathing. Suggest the use of oxygen during periods of high energy use such as bathing or walking.

Energy conservation is the planning and pacing of activities for best tolerance and minimum discomfort. Ask the patient to describe a typical daily schedule. Help him or her divide each activity into its smaller parts to determine whether that task can be performed in a different way or at a different time. Teach about planning and pacing daily activities with rest periods between activities. Help the patient develop a chart outlining the day's activities and planned rest periods.

Encourage the patient to avoid working with the arms raised. Activities involving the arms decrease exercise tolerance because the accessory muscles are used to stabilize the arms and shoulders rather than to assist breathing. Many activities involving the arms can be done sitting at a table leaning on the elbows. Teach the patient to adjust work heights to reduce back strain and fatigue. Remind him or her to keep arm motions smooth and flowing to prevent jerky motions that waste energy. Work with the occupational therapist to teach about the use of adaptive tools for housework, such as long-handled dustpans, sponges, and dusters, to reduce bending and reaching.

Suggest organizing work spaces so that items used most often are within easy reach. Measures such as dividing laundry or groceries into small parcels that can be handled easily, using disposable plates to save washing time, and letting dishes dry in the rack also conserve energy. Teach the patient to not talk when engaged in other activities that require energy, such as walking. In addition, teach him or her to avoid breath holding while performing any activity.

Preventing Respiratory Infection

Planning: Expected Outcomes. The patient with COPD is expected to avoid serious respiratory infection.

Interventions. Pneumonia is a common complication of COPD, especially among older adults. Patients who have excessive secretions are at increased risk for respiratory tract infections. Teach patients to avoid crowds, and stress the importance of receiving a pneumonia vaccination and a yearly influenza vaccine.

NCLEX EXAMINATION CHALLENGE 27.2

Health Promotion and Maintenance

A client with COPD has just been reclassified for disease severity from a GOLD 2 to a GOLD 3. Which client statement about changes in management or lifestyle indicate to the nurse that more teaching is needed to **prevent harm**?

A. "This year I will get the pneumonia vaccination in addition to a flu shot."
B. "Now I will try to rest as much as possible and avoid any unnecessary exercise."
C. "Maybe drinking a supplement will help me retain weight and have more energy."
D. "Perhaps using a spacer with my metered dose inhaler will make the drug work better."

Care Coordination and Transition Management

Sustained transition to home or community management of COPD following acute exacerbation management can be difficult. Readmission within 30 to 60 days after discharge from acute care is high, and intensive care coordination is needed to reduce it (Saunier, 2017).

Home Care Management. Most patients with COPD are managed in the ambulatory care setting and cared for at home. When pneumonia or a severe exacerbation develops, the patient often returns home after hospitalization. For those with advanced disease, 24-hour care may be needed for ADLs and monitoring. If home care is not possible, placement in a long-term care setting may be needed.

Patients with hypoxemia may use oxygen at home either as needed or continually. Continuous, long-term oxygen therapy can reverse tissue hypoxia and improve cognition and well-being. For more information on home oxygen therapy, see Chapter 25.

Collaborate with the case manager to obtain the equipment needed for care at home. Patient needs may include oxygen therapy, a hospital-type bed, a nebulizer, a tub transfer bench or shower chair, and scheduled visits from a home care nurse for monitoring and evaluation.

The patient with COPD faces a lifelong disease with remissions and exacerbations. Explain to the patient and family that he or she may have periods of anxiety, depression, and ineffective coping.

Self-Management Education. Patients with COPD need to know as much about the disease as possible so that they can better manage it and themselves. Patients and families should be able to discuss drug therapy, correct use of inhalers, signs of infection, avoidance of respiratory irritants, the nutrition therapy regimen, and activity progression. Instruct them to identify and avoid stressors that can worsen the disease.

Reinforce the techniques of pursed-lip breathing, diaphragmatic breathing, positioning, relaxation therapy, energy conservation, and coughing and deep breathing. Teaching about all of the needed topics may require coordination with the home care or clinic staff.

Health Care Resources. Provide appropriate referrals as needed. Home care visits may be needed, especially when home oxygen therapy is first prescribed. The Home Care Considerations: The Patient with Chronic Obstructive Pumonary Disease box lists assessment areas for the patient

HOME CARE CONSIDERATIONS

The Patient With Chronic Obstructive Pulmonary Disease

Assess respiratory status and adequacy of ***gas exchange:***
- Measure rate, depth, and rhythm of respirations.
- Examine mucous membranes and nail beds for evidence of hypoxia.
- Determine use of accessory muscles.
- Examine chest and abdomen for paradoxical breathing.
- Count number of words patient can speak between breaths.
- Determine need and use of supplemental oxygen. (How many liters per minute is the patient using?)
- Determine level of consciousness and presence/absence of confusion.
- Auscultate lungs for abnormal breath sounds.
- Measure oxygen saturation by pulse oximetry.
- Determine sputum production, color, and amount.
- Ask about activity level.
- Observe general hygiene.
- Measure body temperature.

Assess cardiac status for adequate ***perfusion***:
- Measure rate, quality, and rhythm of pulse.
- Check dependent areas for edema.
- Check neck veins for distention with the patient in a sitting position.
- Measure capillary refill.

Assess nutrition status:
- Check weight maintenance, loss, or gain.
- Determine food and fluid intake.
- Determine use of nutritional supplements.
- Observe general condition of the skin.

Assess the patient's and caregiver's understanding of disease and adherence to management, including:
- Correct use of supplemental oxygen
- Correct technique and dosing schedule for use of inhalers
- Symptoms to report to the primary health care provider indicating the need for acute care
- Increasing severity of resting dyspnea
- Increasing severity of usual symptoms
- Development of new symptoms associated with poor ***gas exchange***
- Respiratory infection
- Failure to obtain the usual degree of relief with prescribed therapies
- Use of pursed-lip and diaphragmatic breathing techniques
- Scheduling of rest periods and priority activities
- Participation in rehabilitation activities

with COPD at home. Referral to assistance programs, such as Meals on Wheels, can be helpful. Provide a list of support groups and Better Breather clubs sponsored by the American Lung Association. If the patient wants to quit smoking, make the appropriate referrals.

◆ Evaluation: Evaluate Outcomes

Evaluate the care of the patient with COPD based on the identified priority patient problems. The expected outcomes of care are that the patient will:

- Attain and maintain ***gas exchange*** at a level within his or her chronic baseline values
- Cough and clear secretions effectively
- Maintain a respiratory rate and rhythm appropriate to his or her activity level
- Achieve an effective breathing pattern that decreases the work of breathing
- Maintain a patent airway
- Achieve and maintain a body weight within 10% of his or her ideal weight
- Have decreased anxiety
- Increase activity to a level acceptable to him or her
- Perform ADLs with no or minimal assistance
- Avoid serious respiratory infections
- Use prevention activities such as pneumonia and influenza vaccination and crowd avoidance

CYSTIC FIBROSIS

Pathophysiology Review

Cystic fibrosis (CF) is an autosomal recessive genetic disease that affects many organs with most impairment occurring to pancreatic and/or lung function. Although CF is present from birth and usually is first seen in early childhood, almost half of patients with CF in the United States are adults (Cystic Fibrosis Foundation [CFF], 2019 ; Lomas & Tran, 2020).

The underlying problem of CF is blocked chloride transport in the cell membranes. Poor chloride transport causes the formation of mucus that has little water content and is thick. The thick, sticky mucus causes problems in the lungs, pancreas, liver, salivary glands, and testes. The mucus plugs up the airways in the lungs and the glandular tissues in nonpulmonary organs, causing atrophy and organ dysfunction. Nonpulmonary problems include pancreatic insufficiency, malnutrition, intestinal obstruction, poor growth, male sterility, and cirrhosis of the liver. Additional problems of CF in young adults include osteoporosis and diabetes mellitus. Respiratory failure is the main cause of death. Improved management has increased life expectancy, even among those with severe disease, to about 47 years (CFF, 2019; Loas & Tran, 2020).

The pulmonary problems of CF result from the constant presence of thick, sticky mucus and are the most serious complications of the disease. The mucus narrows airways, reducing airflow and interfering with ***gas exchange***. The constant presence of mucus results in chronic respiratory tract infections, chronic bronchitis, and dilation of the bronchioles (bronchiectasis). Lung abscesses are common. Over time the bronchioles distend, and mucus-producing cells have increased numbers (hyperplasia) and increased size (hypertrophy). Complications include pneumothorax, arterial erosion and hemorrhage, and respiratory failure.

CF is most common among whites, and about 4% (1 in 29) are carriers (CFF, 2019). It is rarer among Hispanic Americans (1 in 46 are carriers), African Americans (1 in 65 are carriers), and Asian American (1 in 90 are carriers). Males and females are affected equally.

❖ Interprofessional Collaborative Care

◆ Assessment: Recognize Cues

Usually, but not always, CF is diagnosed in childhood. The major diagnostic test is sweat chloride analysis (Pagana & Pagana, 2018). The sweat chloride test is positive for CF when

PATIENT-CENTERED CARE: GENETIC/GENOMIC CONSIDERATIONS QSEN

CF is an autosomal-recessive disorder in which both gene alleles must be mutated for the disease to be expressed. The CF gene (*CTFR*) produces a protein that controls chloride movement across cell membranes. The severity of CF varies; however, life expectancy is always reduced, with an average of 47 years. Adults with one mutated allele are carriers and have few or no symptoms of CF but can pass the abnormal allele on to their children. More than 1700 different mutations have been identified, which is responsible for variation in disease severity (OMIM, 2019d). Help patients understand why their symptoms may be more or less severe than others with the disease.

NCLEX EXAMINATION CHALLENGE 27.3

Physiological Integrity

Which statement about the genetics of cystic fibrosis is true?

A. Recessive disorder affecting chloride transport
B. Recessive disorder affecting alpha$_1$-antitrypsin levels
C. Dominant disorder inhibiting alveoli formation
D. Dominant disorder increasing production of interleukin-5

the chloride level in the sweat ranges between 60 and 200 mEq/L (mmol/L), compared with the normal value of less than 40 mEq/L (mmol/L) (CFF, 2019). Values of 40 to 59 mEq/L (mmol/L) are considered borderline. Genetic testing can be performed to determine which specific mutation an adult may have. Different mutations result in different degrees of disease severity.

Nonpulmonary symptoms include abdominal distention, gastroesophageal reflux, rectal prolapse, foul-smelling stools, and *steatorrhea* (excessive fat in stools). The patient is often malnourished and has many vitamin deficiencies, especially of the fat-soluble vitamins (e.g., vitamins A, D, E, K). As pancreatic function decreases, diabetes mellitus develops with loss of insulin production. Diabetes is present in more than 50% of adults with CF (Frost et al., 2018). The adult with severe CF is usually smaller and thinner than average. Another problem seen in adults with CF is the early onset of osteoporosis and osteopenia, with a greatly increased risk for bone fracture (CFF, 2019).

Pulmonary symptoms caused by CF are progressive (McCance et al., 2019). Respiratory infections are frequent or chronic with exacerbations. Patients usually have chest congestion, limited exercise tolerance, cough, sputum production, use of accessory muscles, and decreased pulmonary function (especially forced vital capacity [FVC] and forced expiratory volume in the first second of exhalation [FEV$_1$]). Chest x-rays show infiltrate and an increased anteroposterior (AP) diameter.

During an acute exacerbation or when the disease progresses to end stage, the patient has increased chest congestion, reduced activity tolerance, increased crackles, increased cough, increased sputum production (often with hemoptysis), and severe dyspnea with fatigue. Arterial blood gas (ABG) studies show acidosis (low pH), greatly reduced arterial oxygen (PaO_2) levels, increased arterial carbon dioxide (PaCO_2) levels, and increased bicarbonate levels.

With infection, the patient has fever, an elevated white blood cell count, and decreased oxygen saturation. Other symptoms of infection include tachypnea, tachycardia, intercostal retractions, weight loss, and increased fatigue.

◆ Interventions: Take Action

The patient with CF needs daily therapy to slow disease progress and enhance ***gas exchange***. There is no cure for CF.

Nonsurgical Management. The management of the patient with CF is complex and lifelong. Nutrition management focuses on weight maintenance, vitamin supplementation, diabetes management, and pancreatic enzyme replacement (Razga & Handu, 2019). Pulmonary management focuses on preventive maintenance and management of exacerbations. Priority nursing interventions focus on teaching about drug therapy, infection prevention, pulmonary hygiene, nutrition, and vitamin supplementation.

Preventive/maintenance therapy involves the use of positive expiratory pressure, active cycle of breathing technique, and an individualized exercise program. Daily chest physiotherapy with postural drainage is beneficial for the patient with CF. This therapy uses chest percussion, chest vibration, and dependent drainage to loosen secretions and promote drainage. Increasingly, the use of a chest physiotherapy (CPT) vest is recommended (Fig. 27.9), although no specific evidence supports its use as superior to any other type of chest physiotherapy (Wilson, 2018). This system uses an inflatable vest that rapidly fills and deflates, gently compressing and releasing the chest wall up to 25 times per second, a process called high-frequency chest wall oscillation (HFCWO). The action creates minicoughs that dislodge mucus from the bronchial walls, increase mobilization, and move it toward central airways, where it can be removed by coughing or suctioning. HFCWO also thins secretions, making them easier to clear. Pulmonary function tests are monitored regularly. Daily drugs include bronchodilators, anti-inflammatories, mucolytics, and antibiotics.

Exacerbation therapy is needed when the patient with CF has increased chest congestion, reduced activity tolerance, increased or new-onset crackles, and a 10% decrease in FEV$_1$. Other symptoms include increased sputum production with bloody or purulent sputum, increased coughing, decreased appetite, weight loss, fatigue, decreased SpO_2, and chest muscle

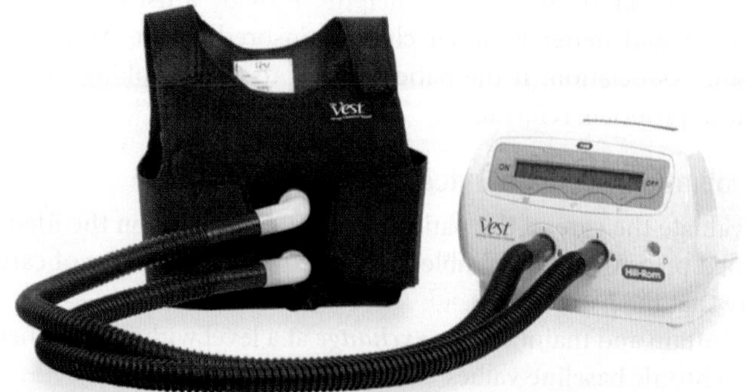

FIG. 27.9 Inflatable chest physiotherapy vest for high-frequency chest wall oscillation. (Modified ©2015 Hill-Rom Services, Inc. Reprinted with permission—all rights reserved.)

retractions. Often infection is present, with fever, increased lung infiltrate on x-ray, and an elevated white blood cell count.

Every attempt is made to avoid mechanical ventilation for the patient with CF. Bi-level positive airway pressure (BiPAP) may be a part of daily therapy for the patient with advanced disease (see Chapters 25 and 29 for information on BiPAP). Management focuses on airway clearance, increased ***gas exchange***, and antibiotic therapy. Supplemental oxygen is prescribed on the basis of Spo_2 levels. The respiratory therapist initiates airway clearance techniques four times a day. Bronchodilator and mucolytic therapies are intensified. Steroidal agents are started or increased.

Depending on the severity of the exacerbation, a 14- to 21-day course of oral antibiotics may be prescribed. Antibiotic choice is based on which bacteria are found in the patient's sputum. If antibiotics are not effective or if the exacerbation is very severe, IV antibiotics are used, usually an aminoglycoside such as tobramycin and colistin or meropenem.

The most common respiratory infection for patients with CF is *Pseudomonas aeruginosa* (CFF, 2019). Another serious bacterial infection for patients with CF is *Burkholderia cepacia*. The organism lives in the respiratory tracts of patients with CF and is often resistant to antibiotic therapy. It is spread by casual contact from one CF patient to another. It is possible for *B. cepacia* to be transmitted to a CF patient during clinic and hospital visits; thus special infection control measures that limit close contact between adults with CF are needed. These measures include separating infected CF patients from noninfected CF patients on hospital units and seeing them in the clinic on different days. Strict CFF-approved procedures are used to clean clinic rooms and respiratory therapy equipment. Drug therapy for this infection usually includes co-trimoxazole (a combination of trimethoprim and sulfamethoxazole) along with the usual drugs used for exacerbation therapy.

Teach patients about protecting themselves by not routinely shaking hands or kissing in social settings. Handwashing is critical because the organism also can be acquired indirectly from contaminated surfaces such as sinks and tissues.

As life span increases for patients with CF, other problems, such as bronchiole bleeding from lung arteries, may develop. Interventional radiology may be needed to embolize the bleeding arterial branches. Patients with CF may undergo this procedure repeatedly to control hemoptysis.

Other problems that occur with CF over time include severe gastroesophageal reflux disease (GERD), osteoporosis, and sensory hearing loss. Osteoporosis increases the risk for bone fractures.

Gene therapy for CF is available for use in patients with specific gene mutations. The drug ivacaftor, known as a CFTR modulator or potentiator, has been found to be of value to patients with CF who are heterozygous for any one of about 35 specific mutations in the *CFTR* gene alleles. It is of no benefit to patients who are homozygous for the mutations (Coulthard, 2018). This drug helps improve chloride transport by increasing the time that the ion channels are open. The combination drug ivacaftor/lumacaftor is effective as therapy for patients whose CF is caused by the *F508del* (also known as the *Phe508del*) mutation, the most common mutation involved in CF, even in patients who are homozygous for the mutation with both alleles being affected. This oral drug combination is considered a "corrector" rather than a modulator, by moving the activated CFTR to the membrane surface for improved function. Another newly approved corrector oral drug, tezacaftor, when combined with ivacaftor has some effect for patients with the *Phe508del* mutation and appears to have fewer adverse respiratory events than the other combination, although decreases in liver function have been found with the use of all of these drugs. The successful outcome for these agents is increased movement of chloride ions across epithelial membranes, resulting in reduced sodium and fluid absorption so that mucus is less thick and sticky. These drugs have no effect in patients whose *CFTR* gene does not have the specific mutations. A significant drawback to these therapies is the cost, which is about $250,000/year of treatment (Coulthard, 2018).

Surgical Management. Surgical management of the patient with CF is lung transplantation. The patient has greatly reduced symptoms but is at continuing risk for lethal pulmonary infections, especially with antirejection drug therapy. Nonpulmonary problems are not helped by this treatment. Transplantation extends life for 1 to 15 years with an average of 7 years, but the transplant rejection rate is high, possibly caused by poor GI absorption of antirejection drugs (CFF, 2019).

Fewer lung transplants are performed compared with transplantation of other solid organs because of the scarcity of available lungs. In addition, many patients who could benefit from lung transplantation have serious problems in other organs that make the procedure even more dangerous.

Lung transplant procedures include two lobes or a single lung transplantation, as well as double-lung transplantation. The type of procedure is determined by the patient's overall condition and the life expectancy after transplantation. Usually the patient with CF has a bilateral lobe transplant from either a cadaver donor or a living-related donor.

Preoperative Care. Many factors are considered before lung transplantation surgery. Recipient and donor criteria vary from one program to another, but some criteria are universal.

Recipient criteria for the patient with CF include that he or she must have severe, irreversible lung damage and still be well enough to survive the surgery. Common exclusion criteria include a cancer diagnosis, systemic infection, HIV/AIDS, and irreversible heart, kidney, or liver disease.

Donor criteria, regardless of whether the lung tissue is obtained from a cadaver or from a living-related donor, include that the donor be infection free and cancer free, have healthy lung tissue, be a close tissue match with the recipient, and have the same blood type as the recipient. When the donor is a living relative, additional criteria include an age restriction and that he or she has healthy organs and has not had previous chest surgery.

The two nursing priorities before surgery are teaching the patient the expected regimen of pulmonary hygiene to be used in the period immediately after surgery and assisting him or her in a pulmonary muscle strengthening/conditioning regimen.

Operative Procedure. The patient may or may not need to be placed on cardiopulmonary bypass, depending on the exact procedure. Those having single-lung or lobe transplantation usually do not need bypass; those having double-lung transplantation usually do.

The most common incision used for lung transplantation is a transverse thoracotomy ("clamshell"). The diseased lung or lungs are removed. The new lobes, lung, or lungs are placed in the chest cavity with proper connections made to the trachea, bronchi, and blood vessels. Usually lung transplantation surgery is completed within 4 to 6 hours.

Postoperative Care. The patient is usually intubated for at least 48 hours, and chest tubes and arterial lines are in place. The care needed is the same as that for any thoracic surgery.

Major problems after lung transplantation are bleeding, infection, and transplant rejection. The patient usually remains in the ICU for several days after transplantation. Postoperative chest physiotherapy often is performed with high-frequency chest wall oscillation (HFCWO) at this time.

Antirejection drug regimens are started immediately after surgery, which increases the risk for infection. Combination therapy with the antirejection drugs is used for the rest of the patient's life. Corticosteroids are avoided in the first 10 to 14 days after surgery because of their negative impact on the healing process.

After transplantation, patients have more energy and usually feel very good. The drug regimen for nonpulmonary CF problems is continued for the rest of the patient's life or until after a pancreatic transplant is performed. Exercise is gradually increased, and some patients even participate in intense activities, such as jogging, running, skiing, skating, swimming, etc.

PULMONARY ARTERIAL HYPERTENSION

Pathophysiology Review

Pulmonary hypertension is the chronic increase in pulmonary vascular pressures above 25 mm Hg, which makes the right side of the heart work much harder for lung ***perfusion*** to support proper ***gas exchange***. Normally the pulmonary vascular pressures are low, 15 to 18 mm Hg, allowing the pressures generated by the contraction of the less-muscled right ventricle to easily overcome them and move blood into the pulmonary artery (McCance et al., 2019). Over time, the higher lung vascular pressures lead to right-sided heart failure (cor pulmonale) that can be fatal. Many lung problems, such as chronic obstructive pulmonary disease and pulmonary fibrosis, can secondarily cause increased pulmonary pressures. For secondary pulmonary hypertension, good control of the condition causing it can delay or prevent cor pulmonale.

Primary **pulmonary artery hypertension (PAH)**, also known as idiopathic pulmonary artery hypertension, is a condition in which pulmonary vessels and often other lung tissues undergo growth changes that greatly increase pressure in the lung circulatory system for unknown reasons. Just as with secondary pulmonary hypertension, PAH progresses and leads to cor pulmonale with reduced ***perfusion*** and ***gas exchange***. The absolute cause of PAH is unknown, and it is diagnosed in the absence of other lung disorders (McCance et al., 2019). Genetic and environmental factors working together may increase the risk. For example, although it is a relatively rare problem, exposure to some drugs, such as fenfluramine/phentermine or dasatinib, increases the risk. The disorder occurs mostly in women between the ages of 20 and 40 years and occurs more often within some families, suggesting a possible genetic susceptibility. The familial PAH form appears to be transmitted in an autosomal dominant pattern with reduced penetrance (OMIM, 2018). Without treatment, death usually occurs within 2 years after diagnosis, most often from profound heart failure.

The pathologic problem in PAH is blood vessel constriction with increasing vascular resistance in the lung. The events that lead up to increasing resistance may include an imbalance between those factors that increase vascular resistance and those that induce blood vessel relaxation. Intrinsic agents that increases vascular resistance are endothelin-1, a very powerful vasoconstrictor that works by binding to endothelin receptors on vascular smooth muscle, and thromboxane, which induces arterial vasoconstriction and enhances clotting by activating platelets. Intrinsic factors that promote vascular relaxation are nitric oxide (NO) and prostacyclin-1. Many adults with primary PAH have a deficiency of prostacyclin 1.

PATIENT-CENTERED CARE: GENETIC/GENOMIC CONSIDERATIONS QSEN

About 50% of patients with pulmonary arterial hypertension have a genetic mutation in the *BMPR2* gene, which codes for a growth factor receptor. Excessive activation of this receptor allows increased growth of arterial smooth muscle in the lungs, making these arteries thicker. Many more adults have mutations in this gene than have PAH. It is thought that these mutations increase the susceptibility for PAH to occur when other, often unknown, environmental factors are also present. Mutations in other genes, such as the *PPH1* and the *SMAD9* gene, are also associated with thickening of lung arteries and increased risk for PAH (OMIM, 2018).

Often PAH is not diagnosed until late in the disease process when the lungs and heart have already been damaged significantly (McCance et al., 2019). Teach adults, especially women, who have a first-degree relative (parent or sibling) with PAH to have regular health checks and to consult a primary health care provider whenever pulmonary problems are present.

❖ Interprofessional Collaborative Care

◆ Assessment: Recognize Cues

The most common early symptoms are dyspnea and fatigue in an otherwise healthy adult. Some patients also have angina-like chest pain. Table 27.3 lists the classification of PAH.

Diagnosis is made from the results of right-sided heart catheterization showing elevated pulmonary pressures. Other test results suggesting PAH include abnormal ventilation-perfusion scans, pulmonary function tests (PFTs) showing reduced functional pulmonary volumes with reduced diffusion capacity, and an abnormal appearance on CT.

TABLE 27.3 Severity Classification for Primary Pulmonary Arterial Hypertension

Class	Symptoms
I	Pulmonary hypertension diagnosed by pulmonary function tests and right-sided cardiac catheterization No limitation of physical activity Moderate physical activity does not induce dyspnea, fatigue, chest pain, or light-headedness
II	No symptoms at rest Mild-to-moderate physical activity induces dyspnea, fatigue, chest pain, or light-headedness
III	No or slight symptoms at rest Mild (less than ordinary) activity induces dyspnea, fatigue, chest pain, or light-headedness
IV	Dyspnea and fatigue present at rest Unable to carry out any level of physical activity without symptoms Symptoms of right-sided heart failure apparent (dependent edema, engorged neck veins, enlarged liver)

◆ Interventions: Take Action

Drug therapy can reduce pulmonary pressures and slow the development of cor pulmonale by dilating pulmonary vessels and preventing clot formation (related to narrowed vessel lumens). Warfarin is taken daily to achieve an international normalized ratio (INR) of 1.5 to 2.0. Calcium channel blockers have been used to dilate blood vessels. The three classes of drugs that have been shown to be most effective in the treatment of PAH are the endothelin-receptor antagonists, prostacyclin agonists, and guanylate cyclase stimulators when used in combination (Hohsfield, 2018). Drug therapy is usually required until lung transplantation or disease progression to death.

Endothelin-receptor antagonists, such as bosentan, induce blood vessel relaxation and decrease pulmonary arterial pressure. However, these agents cause general vessel dilation and some degree of hypotension. Other endothelin receptor antagonist drugs include ambrisentan and macitentan. Teach patients to take the drug with a full glass of water, and teach them not to break, chew, or crush the tablet.

All drugs in this class increase the risk for birth defects and are contraindicated for women who are pregnant or breast-feeding. Instruct women who are sexually active and within child-bearing age to use two reliable methods of contraception while taking these drugs. In addition, the drugs are associated with some liver toxicity and patients should avoid drinking alcoholic beverages while taking any of them. Also teach patients the indications of liver problems (e.g., jaundice, nausea, pain or tenderness in the upper right abdominal quadrant, dark urine).

Natural and synthetic prostacyclin agonists provide specific dilation of pulmonary blood vessels. Continuous infusion of epoprostenol or treprostinil through a small IV pump reduces pulmonary pressures and increases lung blood flow. Treprostinil can also be delivered by continuous subcutaneous infusion. Continuous infusions of prostacyclin drugs can be performed by the patient at home and in other settings. These drugs are also continued when the patient is hospitalized for any reason. The unusual continuous infusion, the need to keep an IV line dedicated strictly to prostacyclin infusion, and the varied dosages of the different brands of prostacyclins contribute to a high drug error rate when infusing this drug. Newer oral formulations of prostacyclin agonists include selexipag and treprostinil are available (Hohsfield et al., 2018; Noel et al., 2017). Iloprost and treprostinil can be delivered by inhalation. A drug often given along with prostacyclins is oral or IV sildenafil.

Guanylate cyclase stimulators (also known as *phosphodiesterase 5 inhibitors*), trigger endothelial nitric oxide and increase the amount an intracellular substance (cGMP) in endothelial cells, which induces relaxation and vasodilation. Oral agents in this class include sildenafil and tadalafil. Another oral drug, riociguat, also stimulates guanylate cyclase without inhibiting phosphodiesterase. All of these drugs can cause general hypotension and significant postural hypotension. Riociguat is associated with birth defects and is contraindicated for use in pregnant or breast-feeding women.

! NURSING SAFETY PRIORITY (QSEN)

Action Alert

A critical nursing priority for a patient undergoing therapy with IV prostacyclin agents is to ensure that the drug therapy is never interrupted. Deaths have been reported if the drug delivery is interrupted even for a matter of minutes. Teach the patient to always have backup drug cassettes and battery packs. If these are not available or if the line is disrupted, the patient should go to the emergency department immediately.

Another critical priority is helping the patient receiving IV prostacyclin agents prevent sepsis. The central line IV setup provides an access for organisms to enter the bloodstream directly. Teach the patient to use strict aseptic technique for all aspects of the drug delivery system. Also teach him or her to notify the pulmonologist at the first sign of any infection. Even when sepsis is diagnosed early and appropriate therapy started, patients with PAH have an overall worse outcome (Tartavoulle, 2017).

Oxygen therapy is used when dyspnea is uncomfortable. This therapy improves function and reduces symptoms but does not cure or improve PAH.

Surgical management of PAH involves lung transplantation. When cor pulmonale is also present, the patient may need combined heart-lung transplantation.

NCLEX EXAMINATION CHALLENGE 27.4

Safe and Effective Care Environment

A client with primary pulmonary arterial hypertension (PAH) receiving treprostinil by continuous IV infusion now has a fever of 101.6°F (38.7°C). Which actions will the nurse perform to **prevent harm? Select all that apply**.

A. Administer the prescribed antipyretic
B. Ask the client whether a productive cough is present
C. Apply oxygen by nasal cannula
D. Culture the IV site
E. Determine whether a durable power of attorney has been signed
F. Increase the treprostinil flow rate
G. Initiate a second IV access and administer prescribed antibiotic
H. Place the client in protective isolation

IDIOPATHIC PULMONARY FIBROSIS

Pathophysiology Review

Idiopathic pulmonary fibrosis is a common restrictive lung disease. The patient is usually an older adult with a history of cigarette smoking, chronic exposure to inhalation irritants, or exposure to the drugs amiodarone or ambrisentan. Most patients have progressive disease with few remission periods. Even with proper treatment, most patients usually survive only 2 to 3 years after diagnosis (Vega-Olivo & Criner, 2018).

Pulmonary fibrosis is an example of excessive wound healing with loss of ***cellular regulation***. Once lung injury occurs, ***inflammation*** begins tissue repair. The inflammation continues beyond normal healing time, causing fibrosis and scarring. These changes thicken alveolar tissues, making ***gas exchange*** difficult.

❖ Interprofessional Collaborative Care

The onset is slow, with early symptoms of mild dyspnea on exertion. Pulmonary function tests show decreased forced vital capacity (FVC). High-resolution computed tomography (HRCT) shows a "honeycomb" pattern in affected lung tissue. As the fibrosis progresses, the patient becomes more dyspneic and hypoxemia becomes severe. Eventually he or she needs high levels of oxygen and is often still hypoxemic. Respirations are rapid and shallow.

Therapy focuses on slowing the fibrotic process and managing dyspnea. Drug therapy with nintedanib, a tyrosine kinase inhibitor, or pirfenidone, an antifibrotic agent, can help improve ***cellular regulation*** of fibrous cell growth and delay progression (Vega-Olivo & Criner, 2018). Immunosuppressant drugs include corticosteroids and cytotoxic drugs such as cyclophosphamide, azathioprine, chlorambucil, or methotrexate but have many side effects and shown limited benefit.

Starting any drug therapy early is critical, even though not all patients respond to therapy. Even among those who have a response to therapy, the disease eventually continues to progress and leads to death by respiratory failure. Lung transplantation is a curative therapy; however, the selection criteria, cost, and availability of organs make this option unlikely for most patients.

The patient and family need support and help with community resources. Nursing care focuses on helping the patient and family understand the disease process and maintaining hope for fibrosis control. It is important to prevent respiratory infections. Teach the patient and family about the symptoms of infection and to avoid respiratory irritants, crowds, and people who are ill.

Home oxygen is needed by the time the patient has dyspnea because significant fibrosis has already occurred and ***gas exchange*** is reduced. Teach about oxygen use as a continuous therapy. Fatigue is a major problem. Teach the patient and family about energy conservation measures (see the discussion of activity intolerance in the Chronic Obstructive Pulmonary Disease section). These measures and rest help reduce the work of breathing and oxygen consumption. Encourage the patient to pace activities and accept assistance as needed.

In the later stages of the disease, the focus is to reduce the sensation of dyspnea. This is often accomplished with the use of oral, parenteral, or nebulized morphine. Provide information about hospice, which supports and coordinates resources to meet the needs of the patient and family when the prognosis for survival is less than 6 months (see Chapter 8).

LUNG CANCER

Pathophysiology Review

Lung cancer is a leading cause of cancer-related deaths worldwide in affluent and less affluent countries. In North America, more deaths from lung cancer occur each year than from prostate cancer, breast cancer, and colon cancer combined, although the incidence has been decreasing somewhat for the past decade. In the United States, more than 228,000 new cases are diagnosed each year and more than 135,000 deaths occur from lung cancer annually (American Cancer Society [ACS], 2020). In Canada, more than 29,300 new cases are diagnosed each year and more than 21,000 deaths from lung cancer occur annually (Canadian Cancer Society, 2019). The overall 5-year survival for all patients with lung cancer is only about 19%. This poor long-term survival is because most lung cancers are diagnosed at a late stage, when metastasis is present. Only 15% of patients have small tumors and localized disease at the time of diagnosis. The 5-year survival rate for this population is 56% (ACS, 2020).

The prognosis for advanced lung cancer remains poor. Treatment often focuses on relieving symptoms or increasing survival time *(palliation)* rather than cure.

Most primary lung cancers arise as a result of failure of ***cellular regulation*** in the bronchial epithelium. Chapter 19 discusses the general mechanisms and processes of cancer development. Lung cancers are collectively called *bronchogenic carcinomas* and are classified as small cell lung cancer (SCLC) and non–small cell lung cancer (NSCLC). NSCLC has several subtypes that are managed in the same ways, although causes and locations in the lungs differ.

Metastasis (spread) of lung cancer occurs by direct extension, through the blood, and by invading lymph glands and vessels. Tumors in the lungs can grow and obstruct the bronchus partially or completely, interfering with ***gas exchange***. Tumors in other areas of lung tissue can grow so large that they can compress and obstruct the airway. Compression of the alveoli, nerves, blood vessels, and lymph vessels can occur and also interfere with ***gas exchange***. Lung cancer can spread to the lung lymph nodes, distant lymph nodes, and other tissues including bone, liver, brain, and adrenal glands.

Additional symptoms, known as *paraneoplastic syndromes,* complicate certain lung cancers. The paraneoplastic syndromes are caused by hormones secreted by tumor cells and occur most commonly with SCLC. Table 27.4 lists the endocrine paraneoplastic syndromes that may occur.

Staging of lung cancer is performed to assess the size and extent of the disease using the standard TNM system described in Chapter 19. Higher numbers represent later stages and less chance for cure or long-term survival.

TABLE 27.4 Endocrine Paraneoplastic Syndromes Associated With Lung Cancer

Ectopic Hormone	Symptoms
Adrenocorticotropic hormone (ACTH)	Cushing syndrome
Antidiuretic hormone	Syndrome of inappropriate antidiuretic hormone (SIADH) Weight gain General edema Dilution of serum electrolytes
Follicle-stimulating hormone (FSH)	Gynecomastia
Parathyroid hormone	Hypercalcemia
Ectopic insulin	Hypoglycemia

Incidence and Prevalence

Lung cancers occur as a result of repeated exposure to inhaled substances that cause chronic tissue irritation or ***inflammation*** interfering with ***cellular regulation*** of cell growth. Cigarette smoking is the major risk factor and is responsible for 81% of all lung cancer deaths (ACS, 2020).

Etiology and Genetic Risk

Nonsmokers exposed to "secondhand" or "thirdhand" smoke also have a greater risk for lung cancer than do nonsmokers who are minimally exposed to cigarette smoke. See Chapter 24 for a discussion of passive smoking risks.

Other lung cancer risk factors include chronic exposure to asbestos, beryllium, chromium, coal distillates, cobalt, iron oxide, mustard gas, petroleum distillates, radiation, tar, nickel, and uranium. Air pollution with benzopyrenes and hydrocarbons also increases the risk for lung cancer.

Lung cancer, especially the adenocarcinoma form of NSCLC, does occur in adults who are "never smokers" (Sherry, 2017), particularly among women. Possible contributing factors for lung cancer in this population include exposure to environmental carcinogens, second-hand smoke exposure, genetic differences, familial predisposition, and advancing age.

PATIENT-CENTERED CARE: GENETIC/GENOMIC CONSIDERATIONS QSEN

Lung cancer development varies among adults with similar smoking histories, suggesting that genetic factors can influence susceptibility. Genome-wide association studies have found specific variations in a variety of genes that increase the susceptibility to lung cancer development (OMIM, 2019b). Help patients understand that lung cancer susceptibility varies by both genetic issues and exposure to carcinogens.

Health Promotion and Maintenance

Primary prevention for lung cancer is directed at reducing tobacco smoking. Chapter 24 discusses strategies for helping adults reduce smoking and ways to protect lungs from other exposures to inhalation irritants linked to lung cancer development.

Secondary prevention by early detection involves screening adults at high risk for lung cancer development. Annual CT scans can detect cancers at stage I, when cure is probable and long-term survival (longer than 5 years) is very likely (ACS, 2020).

TABLE 27.5 Warning Signals Associated With Lung Cancer

- Hoarseness
- Change in respiratory pattern
- Persistent cough or change in cough
- Blood-streaked sputum
- Rust-colored or purulent sputum
- Frank hemoptysis
- Chest pain or chest tightness
- Shoulder, arm, or chest wall pain
- Recurring episodes of pleural effusion, pneumonia, or bronchitis
- Dyspnea
- Fever associated with one or two other signs
- Wheezing
- Weight loss
- Clubbing of the fingers

❖ Interprofessional Collaborative Care

◆ Assessment: Recognize Cues

History. Ask the patient about risk factors, including smoking, hazards in the workplace, and warning signals (Table 27.5). Calculate the pack-year smoking history as described in Chapter 24.

Ask about the presence of lung cancer symptoms, such as hoarseness, cough, sputum production, hemoptysis, shortness of breath, or change in endurance. Symptoms often have been present for years. Ask the patient to describe any recent symptom changes or if position affects them.

Assess for chest pain or discomfort, which can occur at any stage of tumor development. Chest pain may be localized or on just one side and can range from mild to severe. Ask about any sensation of fullness, tightness, or pressure in the chest, which may suggest obstruction. A piercing chest pain or pleuritic pain may occur on inspiration. Pain radiating to the arm results from tumor invasion of nerve plexuses in advanced disease.

Physical Assessment/Signs and Symptoms—Pulmonary. Symptoms of lung cancer are often nonspecific and appear late in the disease. Specific symptoms depend on tumor location. Chills, fever, and cough may be related to pneumonitis or bronchitis that occurs with obstruction. Assess sputum quantity and character. Blood-tinged sputum may occur with bleeding from a tumor. Hemoptysis is a later finding in the course of the disease. If infection or necrosis is present, sputum may be purulent and copious.

Breathing may be labored or painful. Obstructive breathing may occur as prolonged exhalation alternating with periods of shallow breathing. Rapid, shallow breathing occurs with pleuritic chest pain and an elevated diaphragm. Look for and document abnormal retractions, the use of accessory muscles, flared nares, stridor, and asymmetric diaphragmatic movement on inspiration. Dyspnea and wheezing may be present with airway obstruction. Ask about dyspnea severity at rest, with activity, and in the supine position. Assess how much the dyspnea interferes with the patient's participation in ADLs, work, recreational activities, and family responsibilities.

Increased vibrations felt on the chest wall when the patient speaks *(fremitus)* indicate areas of the lung where air spaces are replaced with tumor or fluid. Fremitus is decreased or absent when the bronchus is obstructed. The trachea may be displaced from midline if a mass is present in the area.

Breath sounds may change with the presence of a tumor. Wheezes indicate partial obstruction of airflow in passages narrowed by tumors. Decreased or absent breath sounds indicate complete obstruction of an airway by a tumor or fluid. A pleural friction rub may be heard when ***inflammation*** is present.

Physical Assessment/Signs and Symptoms—Nonpulmonary. Many other systems can be affected by lung cancer and have changes at the time of diagnosis. Heart sounds may be muffled by a tumor or fluid around the heart *(cardiac tamponade)*. Dysrhythmias may occur as a result of hypoxemia or direct pressure of the tumor on the heart. Cyanosis of the lips and fingertips or clubbing of the fingers may be present (see Fig. 27.8).

Bones lose density with tumor invasion and break easily with little pressure and without trauma. The patient may have bone pain or fragility fractures.

Late symptoms of lung cancer usually include fatigue, weight loss, anorexia, dysphagia, and nausea and vomiting. *Superior vena cava syndrome may result from tumor pressure in or around the vena cava. This syndrome is an emergency (see Chapter 20) and requires immediate intervention.* The patient may have confusion or personality changes from brain metastasis.

Psychosocial Assessment. The poor prognosis for lung cancer has made it a much-feared disease. Dyspnea and pain add to the patient's fear and anxiety. Encourage the patient and family to express their feelings about the possible diagnosis of lung cancer.

Diagnostic Assessment. Most commonly, lung lesions are first identified on chest x-rays. CT scans are then used to identify the lesions more clearly and guide biopsy procedures. The definitive diagnosis of lung cancer is made by examination of cancer cells from biopsy or from pleural effusion fluid (if present). A thoracoscopy to directly view lung tissue may be performed through a video-assisted thoracoscope entering the chest cavity via small incisions through the chest wall.

Other diagnostic studies may be needed to determine how widely the cancer has spread. Such tests include MRI and radionuclide scans of the liver, spleen, brain, and bone help. Positron emission tomography (PET) scanning is a thorough way to locate metastases. These tests help determine the extent of the cancer and the best methods to treat it.

◆ Interventions: Take Action

Interventions for the patient with lung cancer can have the purposes of curing the disease, increasing survival time, and enhancing quality of life through palliation. Both nonsurgical and surgical interventions are used to achieve these purposes. Cure is most likely for patients who undergo treatment for stage I or II disease. Cure is rare for patients who undergo treatment for stage III or IV disease, although survival time is increasing.

Nonsurgical Management. *Chemotherapy* is often the treatment of choice for lung cancers, especially small cell lung cancer (SCLC). It may be used alone or as adjuvant (add-on) therapy in combination with surgery for non–small cell lung cancer (NSCLC). The combination of drugs used depends on tumor response and the overall health of the patient; however, most include platinum-based agents.

Side effects of cancer chemotherapy include chemotherapy-induced nausea and vomiting (CINV), *alopecia* (hair loss), open sores on mucous membranes *(mucositis)*, immunosuppression with neutropenia, anemia, decreased numbers of platelets, and peripheral neuropathy. Consult Chapter 20 for discussion of the nursing care needs for patients who have these side effects.

Immunosuppression with neutropenia, which greatly increases the risk for infection, is the major dose-limiting side effect of chemotherapy for lung cancer. It can be managed by the use of growth factors to stimulate bone marrow production of immune system cells. Teach the patient and family about precautions to take to reduce the patient's risk for infection (see Chapter 20 for information about chemotherapy and associated nursing care).

Targeted therapy is common in the treatment of non–small cell lung cancer (NSCLC). These agents take advantage of one or more differences in cancer cell growth or metabolism that is either not present or only slightly present in normal cells. For lung cancer, usually these differences are identified as variations in two different genes, *EGFR* (which codes for epidermal growth factor receptors) and *ALK* (which codes for ALK receptor tyrosine kinases). Agents used as targeted therapies work to disrupt cancer cell division in one of several ways. However, these agents only work when the cancer cell has the particular target or specific genetic mutation. Therefore testing of the cancer cells is needed before therapy begins, and not all cancers of the same type express the target. These agents are increasing survival time for patients with NSCLC but do not lead to a cure. The Common Examples of Drug Therapy: Targeted Therapy and Immunotherapy of Lung Cancer box lists some targeted agents used in lung cancer therapy.

COMMON EXAMPLES OF DRUG THERAPY

Targeted Therapy and Immunotherapy of Lung Cancer

Agents	Approved For
Targeted Therapy Agents	
Afatinib	EGFR-positive metastatic NSCLC
Alectinib	ALK-positive metastatic NSCLC
Crizotinib	ALK-positive metastatic NSCLC
Erlotinib	EGFR-positive metastatic NSCLC
Immunotherapy Agents	
Atezolizumab	Stage IV NSCLC
Durvalumab	Stage III NSCLC
Nivolumab	Stage III or IV NSCLC and SCLC
Pembrolizumab	Stage IV NSCLC

NSCLC, Non–small-cell lung cancer; *SCLC*, small-cell lung cancer.

Immunotherapy for lung cancer is a type of targeted therapy designed to allow the patient's own immune system to better recognize and attack his or her cancer cells. Normally, certain immune system cells including T-cells, B-cells, monocytes, and natural killer (NK) cells recognize and attack foreign cells and unhealthy self cells. Many "checkpoints" are in place to ensure that these cells do not "go rogue" and attack normal healthy self cells. One type of checkpoint is activation of the PD-1 receptor on these cells. PD stands for "programmed death." When the PD-1 receptors are activated, the immune system cell stops dividing, stops its seek-and-destroy actions, and may die. Some lung cancer cells are able to evade detection as unhealthy self cells by having their cell surface proteins known as PD-L1 and PD-L2 bind to and activate the PD-1 receptors on immune system cells. (PD-L stands for programmed death ligand.) When the PD-1 receptors are activated by cancer cell PD-L proteins, the immune system cells' activity is suppressed and they fail to recognize the cancer cells and take no action against them. The immunotherapy drugs for lung cancer prevent the suppressive interaction between the cancer cells' PD-L1 or PD-L2 proteins and the immune system cells' PD-1 receptors. Some drugs do this by binding and covering the PD-L proteins so that they cannot interact with immune system cells' PD-1 receptors and other drugs essentially hide the PD-1 receptors. Either way, the result is that immune system cells remain active and able to seek and destroy cancer cells.

At present, immunotherapy does not replace traditional chemotherapy or radiation for first-line lung cancer treatment and is not used for cure. It may be used in combination with chemotherapy or as monotherapy for later-stage (III or IV) lung cancers. Use of immunotherapy, when lung cancer cells have large amounts of PD-L1 or PD-L2 on their surfaces, has significantly extended the lives of patients with NSCLC. One is also being used with later-stage small cell lung cancer. All are monoclonal antibodies administered by intravenous infusion. The Common Examples of Drug Therapy: Targeted Therapy and Immunotherapy of Lung Cancer box lists the most common approved immunotherapies for lung cancer.

Radiation therapy can be an effective treatment for locally advanced lung cancers confined to the chest. Best results are seen when radiation is used in addition to surgery or chemotherapy. Radiation may be performed before surgery to shrink the tumor and make resection easier.

Only the areas thought to have cancer are positioned in the radiation path. The immediate side effects of this treatment are skin irritation and peeling at the radiation site, fatigue, nausea, and taste changes. Some patients have esophagitis during therapy, making nutrition more difficult. Collaborate with a registered dietitian nutritionist to teach patients to eat foods that are soft, bland, and high in calories.

Skin care in the radiation-treated area can be difficult, and consultation with a wound care specialist may be needed. Because skin in the radiation path is more sensitive to sun damage, advise patients to avoid direct skin exposure to the sun during treatment and for at least 1 year after radiation is completed. See Chapter 20 for other nursing care issues associated with radiation therapy.

Photodynamic therapy (PDT) may be used to remove small bronchial tumors when they are accessible by bronchoscopy. This therapy first involves injecting the patient with an agent that sensitizes cells to light and remains in cancer cells longer than normal cells. After 48 to 72 hours, most of the drug has accumulated in the cancer cells. A laser light is focused on the tumor with the patient intubated and under anesthesia. The light activates a reaction that causes irreversible damage and death to cells retaining the sensitizing drug.

Surgical Management. Surgery is the main treatment for stage I and stage II NSCLC. Total tumor removal may result in a cure. If complete resection is not possible, the surgeon removes the bulk of the tumor. The specific surgery depends on the stage of the cancer and the patient's overall health. Lung cancer surgery may involve removal of the tumor only, removal of a lung segment, removal of a lobe (**lobectomy**), or removal of the entire lung (**pneumonectomy**). These procedures can be performed by open thoracotomy or by minimally invasive surgery in select patients.

Preoperative care is focused on relieving anxiety and promoting the patient's participation (see Chapter 9 for routine preoperative care). Reinforce the surgeon's explanation of the procedure, and provide education related to what is expected after surgery. Teach about the probable placement of the chest tube and drainage system (except after pneumonectomy).

Operative procedures for lung cancer may consist of a lobectomy, pneumonectomy, segmental resection, or wedge resection. A segmental resection is a lung resection that includes the bronchus, pulmonary artery and vein, and tissue of the involved lung segment or segments of a lobe. A wedge resection is removal of the peripheral portion of small, localized areas of disease.

A lobe or entire lung can be removed through video-assisted thoracoscopic surgery (VATS), which is minimally invasive, in select patients. The procedure involves making small incisions in the chest for placement of the instruments. The lung, section, or lobe is then isolated from its airway, which is surgically closed. The lobe or lung is closed off from the rest of the lung and sealed in a bag to prevent leakage of tumor tissue and possible seeding of the cancer. The bagged lung is then removed whole through one of the small incisions.

Postoperative care for patients who have undergone thoracotomy (except for pneumonectomy) requires closed-chest drainage to drain air and blood that collect in the pleural space. A chest tube drain placed in the pleural space allows lung re-expansion and prevents air and fluid from returning to the chest (Fig. 27.10). The drainage system consists of one or more chest tubes or drains, a collection container placed below the chest level, and a water seal to keep air from entering the chest. The drainage system may be a stationary, disposable, self-contained system (Fig. 27.11) or a smaller, portable, disposable, self-contained system that requires no connection to a vacuum source (Fig. 27.12). The nursing care priorities for the patient with a chest tube are to ensure the integrity of the system, promote comfort, ensure chest tube patency, and prevent complications (Sasa, 2019).

Chest Tube Placement and Care. The tip of the tube used to drain air is placed near the front lung apex (see Fig. 27.10).

The tube that drains liquid is placed on the side near the base of the lung. The wounds are covered with airtight dressings, most commonly silicone foam dressings (Wood et al., 2019).

The chest tube is connected by about 6 feet of tubing to a collection device placed below the chest, allowing gravity to drain the pleural space while the patient can turn and move without pulling on the chest tube. When two chest tubes are inserted, they are joined by a Y-connector close to the patient and the 6 feet of tubing is attached to the Y-connector.

Stationary chest tube drainage systems, such as the Pleur-evac system, use a water-seal mechanism that acts as a one-way valve to prevent air or liquid from moving back into the chest cavity. Disposable system use a one-piece disposable plastic unit with three chambers. The three chambers are connected to one another. The tube(s) from the patient is (are) connected to the first chamber in the series of three, which is the drainage collection container. The second chamber is the water seal to prevent air from moving back up the tubing system and into the chest. The third chamber, when suction is applied, is the suction regulator. Tubing from the patient penetrates chamber one shallowly, as does the tube connecting chamber one with chamber two.

The fluid in chamber one collected from the patient is measured hourly during the first 24 hours. *This drainage fluid must never fill to the point that it comes into contact with any tubes! If the tubing from the patient enters the fluid, drainage stops and can lead to a tension pneumothorax.*

Chamber two is the water seal that prevents air from re-entering the patient's pleural space. As the trapped air leaves the pleural space, it will pass through chamber one (collection chamber) before entering chamber two (the water-seal chamber), which should always contain at least 2 cm of water to prevent air from returning to the patient. As trapped air from the patient's pleural space passes through the water seal, which serves as a one-way valve, the water will bubble. Once all the air has been evacuated from the pleural space, bubbling of the water seal stops.

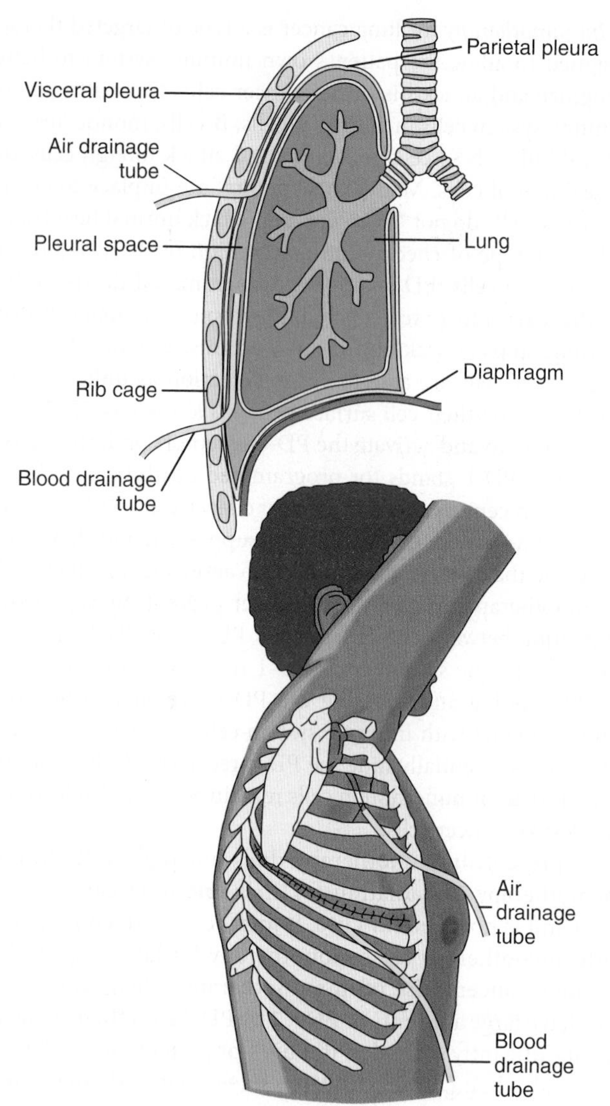

FIG. 27.10 Chest tube placement.

! NURSING SAFETY PRIORITY QSEN

Action Alert

For a water-seal chest tube drainage system, 2 cm of water is the minimum needed in the water seal to prevent air from flowing backward into the patient. Check the water level every shift and add sterile water to this chamber to the level marked on the indicator (specified by the manufacturer of the drainage system).

Bubbling of water in the water-seal chamber indicates air drainage from the patient. Bubbling is seen when intrathoracic pressure is greater than atmospheric pressure, such as when the patient exhales, coughs, or sneezes. When the air in the pleural space has been removed, bubbling stops. A blocked or kinked chest tube can also cause bubbling to stop. Excessive bubbling in the water-seal chamber may indicate an air leak. The water in the water-seal chamber column normally rises 2 to 4 inches during inhalation and falls during exhalation, a process called *tidaling*. Absence of tidaling may mean that the lung has fully re-expanded or that there is an obstruction in the chest tube.

Chamber three is the suction control of the system. There are different types of suction, most commonly wet or dry. With wet suction, the fluid level in chamber three is prescribed by the surgeon. The chamber is connected to wall suction, which is turned up until there is gentle bubbling in the chamber. With dry suction, the prescribed suction is dialed in on the device. When connected to wall suction, the regulator is set to the amount indicated by the device's manufacturer.

Check hourly to ensure the sterility and patency of the drainage system. Keep sterile gauze at the bedside to cover and occlude the insertion site immediately if the chest tube becomes dislodged. Also keep padded clamps at the bedside for use if the drainage system is interrupted.

Check the water-seal chamber for unexpected bubbling created by an air leak in the system. Bubbling is normal during forceful expiration or coughing because air in the chest is being expelled. Continuous bubbling indicates an air leak (Sasa,

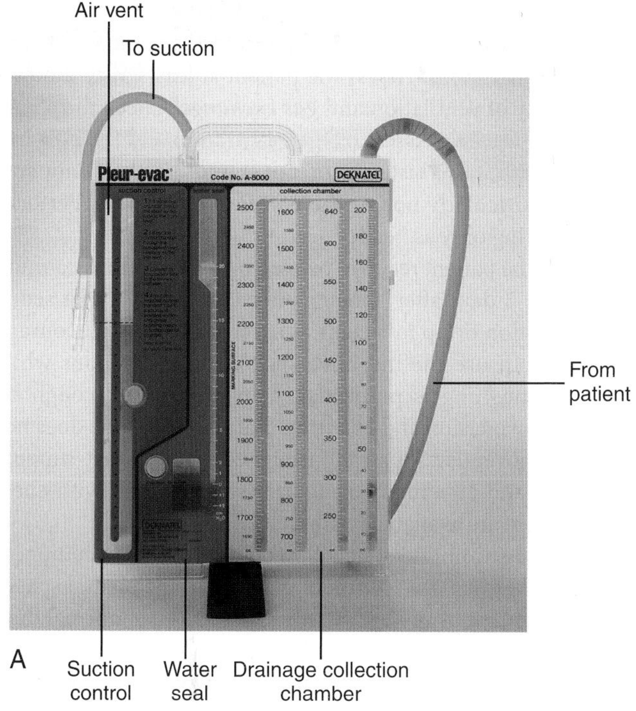

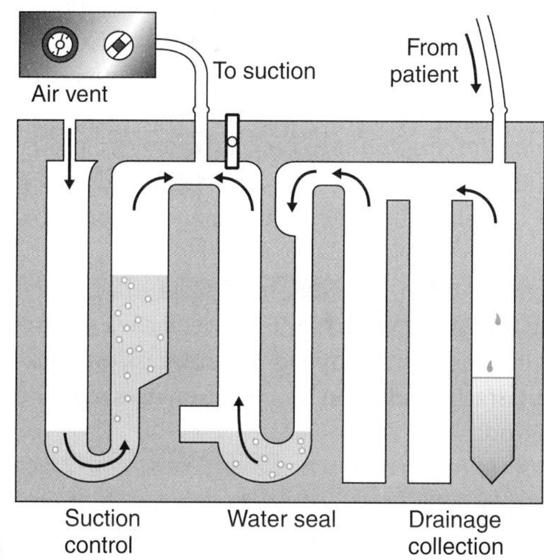

FIG. 27.11 A, Pleur-evac drainage system, a commercial three-chamber chest drainage device. B, Schematic of the drainage device.

2019). Notify the surgeon if bubbling occurs continuously in the water-seal chamber. See the Best Practice for Patient Safety & Quality Care: Management of Chest Tube Drainage System box for additional evidence-based actions to use when caring for a patient with a water-seal chest tube drainage system.

Mobile or portable chest tube drainage systems are "dry" chest drainage systems without a water seal to prevent air from re-entering the patient's lung through the chest tube. Instead, these lightweight devices use a dynamic control "flutter" valve that prevents backflow of air. When the patient exhales, air is forced from the chest cavity into the chest tube under pressure, the soft flutter valve opens, and air moves into the harder surrounding tube shell, where it is vented. Portable units allow the patient to ambulate and even go home with chest tubes still in place (Sasa, 2019).

BEST PRACTICE FOR PATIENT SAFETY & QUALITY CARE (QSEN)

Management of Chest Tube Drainage System

Patient

- Ensure that the dressing on the chest around the tube is tight and intact. Depending on agency policy and the surgeon's preference, reinforce or change loose dressings.
- Assess for difficulty breathing.
- Assess breathing effectiveness by pulse oximetry.
- Listen to breath sounds for each lung.
- Check alignment of trachea.
- Check tube insertion site for condition of the skin. Palpate area for puffiness or crackling that may indicate subcutaneous emphysema.
- Observe site for signs of infection (redness, purulent drainage) or excessive bleeding.
- Check to see if tube "eyelets" are visible (they should not be visible).
- Assess for pain and its location and intensity and administer drugs for pain as prescribed.
- Assist patient to deep breathe, cough, perform maximal sustained inhalations, and use incentive spirometry.
- Reposition the patient who reports a "burning" pain in the chest.

Drainage System

- Do not "strip" the chest tube; use a hand-over-hand "milking" motion.
- Keep drainage system lower than the level of the patient's chest.
- Keep the chest tube as straight as possible from the bed to the suction unit, avoiding kinks and dependent loops. Extra tubing can be loosely coiled on the bed.
- Ensure that the chest tube is securely taped to the connector and that the connector is taped to the tubing going into the collection chamber.
- Assess bubbling in the water-seal chamber; should be gentle bubbling on patient's exhalation, forceful cough, position changes.
- Assess for "tidaling" (rise and fall of water in chamber two with breathing).
- Check water level in the water-seal chamber and keep at the level recommended by the manufacturer.
- Check water level in the suction control chamber and keep at the level prescribed by the surgeon (unless dry suction system is used).
- Clamp the chest tube only for brief periods to change the drainage system or when checking for air leaks.
- Check and document amount, color, and characteristics of fluid in the collection chamber as often as needed according to the patient's condition and agency policy.
- Empty collection chamber or change the system before the drainage makes contact with the bottom of the tube.
- When a sample of drainage is needed for culture or other laboratory test, obtain it from the chest tube; after cleaning the chest tube, use a 20-gauge (or smaller) needle and draw up specimen into a syringe.

Immediately Notify Surgeon or Rapid Response Team for:

- Tracheal deviation from midline
- Sudden onset or increased intensity of dyspnea
- Oxygen saturation less than 90%
- Drainage greater than 70 mL/hr
- Visible eyelets on chest tube
- Chest tube falls out of the patient's chest (first, cover the area with dry, sterile gauze)
- Chest tube disconnects from the drainage system (first, put end of tube in a container of sterile water and keep below the level of the patient's chest)
- Drainage in tube stops (in the first 24 hours)

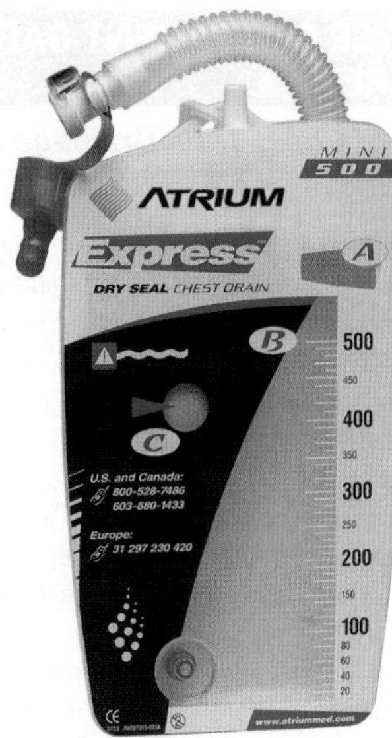

FIG. 27.12 Portable chest drainage system. (Courtesy Atrium Medical Corporation, Hudson, NH.)

Chest tube removal is performed when drainage is minimal and lung expansion is stable. Usually the surgeon removes the chest tube at the bedside, which causes a short period of procedural pain. After removal, the site is dressed and sealed with an occlusive dressing and observed for drainage. Assess the patient hourly for respiratory distress for the first few hours after chest tube removal. Respiratory distress may signal lung collapse and the need for chest tube reinsertion.

NCLEX EXAMINATION CHALLENGE 27.5

Safe and Effective Care Environment

The client, who is 24 hours postoperative after a right lower lobectomy for stage II lung cancer and has two chest tubes in place, reports intense burning pain in his lower chest. On assessment, the nurse notes there is no bubbling on exhalation in the water seal chamber. What action will the nurse perform **first?**

A. Immediately notify either the Rapid Response Team or the thoracic surgical resident.
B. Assist the client to a side-lying position and reassess the water seal chamber for bubbling.
C. Administer the prescribed opioid analgesic immediately, and then assess the chest tube system.
D. No action is needed because these responses are normal for the first postoperative day after lobectomy.

Pain Management. Pain control measures are needed regardless of whether surgery is performed as an open procedure or with minimally invasive techniques. Give the prescribed drugs for pain and assess the patient's responses to them. Teach patients using patient-controlled analgesia (PCA) devices to self-administer the drug before pain intensity becomes too severe. Monitor vital signs before and after giving opioid analgesics, especially for the patient who is not being mechanically ventilated.

Respiratory Management. Immediately after surgery the patient is mechanically ventilated. See Chapter 29 for nursing care of the patient receiving mechanical ventilation.

Once the patient is breathing on his or her own, the priorities are to maintain a patent airway, ensure adequate ventilation, and prevent complications. Assess the patient at least every 2 hours for adequacy of ventilation and ***gas exchange***. Check the alignment of the trachea. Assess oxygen saturation and the rate and depth of respiration. Listen to breath sounds on the nonoperative side, particularly noting the presence of crackles. Perform oral suctioning only as needed.

Usually the patient receives oxygen by mask or nasal cannula for the first 2 days after surgery. Assist the patient to a semi-Fowler position or up in a chair as soon as possible. Encourage him or her to use the incentive spirometer every hour while awake. If coughing is permitted, help him or her cough by splinting any incision and ensuring that the chest tube does not pull with movement. Specially designed walkers that support the patient and all equipment for early ambulation with chest tubes in place are available (Grondell et al., 2018).

Preventing Complications. Complications of a pneumonectomy include *empyema* (purulent material in the pleural space) and development of a bronchopleural *fistula* (an abnormal duct that develops between the bronchial tree and the pleura). Positioning of the patient after pneumonectomy varies according to surgeon preference and the patient's comfort. Some surgeons want the patient placed on the nonoperative side immediately after a pneumonectomy to reduce stress on the bronchial stump incision. Others prefer to place the patient on the operative side to allow fluids to fill in the now empty space.

Interventions for Palliation. *Oxygen therapy* is prescribed when the patient is hypoxemic and helps relieve dyspnea and anxiety. (See Chapter 25 for issues related to home oxygen therapy.)

Radiation therapy can help relieve hemoptysis, obstruction of the bronchi and great veins (superior vena cava syndrome), difficulty swallowing from esophageal compression, and pain from bone metastasis. Radiation for palliation uses higher doses for shorter periods.

Thoracentesis is performed when pleural effusion is a problem for the patient with lung cancer. The excess fluid increases dyspnea, discomfort, and the risk for infection. The purpose of treatment is to remove pleural fluid and prevent its formation. *Thoracentesis* is a procedure for fluid removal by suction after the placement of a large needle or catheter into the intrapleural space. Fluid removal temporarily relieves hypoxia; however, the fluid can rapidly re-form in the pleural space. When fluid development is continuous and uncomfortable, a tunneled pleural catheter that continuously drains may be placed into the intrapleural space to collect the fluid (Miller et al., 2018).

Dyspnea management is needed because the patient with lung cancer tires easily and is often most comfortable resting in a semi-Fowler position. Dyspnea is reduced with oxygen, use of a continuous morphine infusion, and positioning for comfort. The severely dyspneic patient may be most comfortable sitting and sleeping in a lounge chair or reclining chair.

Pain management is usually to help the patient be as pain free and comfortable as possible. Pharmacologic management with opioid drugs as oral, parenteral, or transdermal preparations is needed. Analgesics are most effective when given around the clock with additional PRN analgesics used for breakthrough pain.

Hospice care can be beneficial for the patient in the terminal phase of lung cancer. Hospice programs provide support to the terminally ill patient and the family, meet physical and psychosocial needs, adjust the palliative care regimen as needed, make home visits, and provide volunteers for errands and respite care. (See Chapter 8 for a more complete discussion of end-of-life issues.)

GET READY FOR THE NEXT-GENERATION NCLEX® EXAMINATION!

Key Points

Review these Key Points for each NCLEX Examination Client Needs Category.

Safe and Effective Care Environment

- Ensure there are no open flames or combustion hazards in rooms where oxygen is in use. **QSEN: Safety**
- Protect the patient with cystic fibrosis from hospital-acquired pulmonary infections. **QSEN: Safety**
- Ensure proper function of chest tube drainage equipment. **QSEN: Safety**

Health Promotion and Maintenance

- Teach patients who have particulate matter exposure (PME) by inhalation in workplaces or leisure-time activities to use a mask to protect the respiratory system. **QSEN: Safety**
- Teach patients with asthma to develop a management plan based on changes in their breathing patterns and responses to prescribed drug therapies. **QSEN: Patient-Centered Care**
- Teach all patients who smoke the warning signs of lung cancer. **QSEN: Evidence-Based Practice**

Psychosocial Integrity

- Encourage the patient and family to express their feelings regarding the diagnosis of a chronic respiratory disease or cancer and about management and treatment regimens. **QSEN: Patient-Centered Care**
- Explain all diagnostic procedures, restrictions, and follow-up care to the patient scheduled for tests. **QSEN: Patient-Centered Care**

Physiological Integrity

- Assess the airway and effectiveness of ***gas exchange*** for any patient who experiences shortness of breath or any change in mental status. **QSEN: Evidence-Based Practice**
- Assess the degree to which breathing problems interfere with the patient's ability to perform ADLs, work, and leisure-time activities. **QSEN: Patient-Centered Care**
- Apply oxygen to anyone who is hypoxemic. **QSEN: Evidence-Based Practice**
- Collaborate with respiratory therapists, registered dietitian nutritionists, social workers, and other members of the interprofessional team to meet the hospital and home care needs of patients with chronic lower respiratory problems. **Teamwork and Collaboration**
- Instruct patients who are prescribed to use inhalers how to use and care for them properly. **QSEN: Patient-Centered Care**
- Instruct patients with asthma to carry a reliever inhaler with them at all times. **QSEN: Safety**
- Teach patients receiving chemotherapy for lung cancer the signs and symptoms of infection. **QSEN: Patient-Centered Care**

MASTERY QUESTIONS

1. Which specific information will the nurse teach to the client with eosinophilic asthma newly prescribed benralizumab therapy?
   A. Avoid breathing into the inhaler or getting it wet.
   B. The drug can only be given by a health care professional.
   C. Do not chew, crush, or split the tablet containing this drug.
   D. The drug must be taken at bedtime because of the extreme drowsiness it causes.
2. A client with COPD has all of the following ABG changes from earlier today. Which change alerts the nurse to take immediate action to **prevent harm?**
   A. pH from 7.21 to 7.20
   B. HCO_3- remains the same at 31 mEq/L
   C. $Paco_2$ from 45 mm Hg to 68 mm Hg
   D. Pao_2 from 88 mm Hg to 86 mm Hg
3. Which precaution is a **priority** for the nurse to teach a client prescribed the gene therapy combination of ivacaftor/tezacaftor in order to **prevent harm** from this therapy?
   A. Examine your skin and the whites of your eyes daily for a yellow appearance.
   B. Apply ice to the injection site for 30 minutes after each dose to keep bleeding to a minimum.
   C. Wait at least 15 minutes after using other inhaled drugs before inhaling this drug combination.
   D. Go to your primary health care provider immediately if you develop a fever or other signs of infection.

4. The nurse teaching clients precautions to use with drug therapy for primary pulmonary arterial hypertension (PAH) instructs the female clients to use two reliable forms of contraception while taking which drugs? **Select all that apply.**
   A. ambrisentan
   B. bosentan
   C. epoprostenol
   D. iloprost
   E. macitentan
   F. riociguat
   G. selexipag
   H. sildenafil
   I. tadalafil
   J. treprostinil

5. A client newly diagnosed with stage I nonsmall cell lung cancer (NSCLC) who is getting ready for curative surgery asks the nurse whether the oncologist might consider this new drug he has seen on television, pembrolizumab, instead of surgery. What is the nurse's best response?
   A. "This drug will only work on those lung cancers that have the right target and your tumor does not have it."
   B. "This drug is approved for use in clients whose lung cancer has metastasized not for early-stage cancers."
   C. "Why would you want to take a drug for months when you may be cured by surgery alone?"
   D. "You need to talk about this with your oncologist and your surgeon."

REFERENCES

Abbas, A., Lichtman, A., & Pillai, S. (2018). *Cellular and molecular immunology* (8th ed.). Philadelphia: Elsevier.

American Cancer Society (ACS). (2020). *Cancer facts and figures-2020.* No. 01-300M-No. 500820. Atlanta: Author.

Bradshaw, M., & Kosnar, D. (2017). Asthma-COPD overlap: A new diagnostic consideration. *The Journal for Nurse Practitioners, 13*(1), e41–e42.

Burchum, J., & Rosenthal, L. (2019). *Lehne's pharmacology for nursing care* (10th ed.). St. Louis: Elsevier.

Canadian Cancer Society, Statistics Canada. (2019). *Canadian cancer Statistics, 2019.* Toronto, ON: Canadian Cancer Society.

Centers for Disease Control and Prevention (CDC). (2018a). *COPD.* https://www.cdc.gov/dotw/copd/.

Centers for Disease Control and Prevention (CDC). (2018b). *Most recent asthma data.* https://www.cdc.gov/asthma/most_recent_data.htm.

Chike-Harris, K., & Kinyon-Munch, K. (2019). Asthma 101: Teaching children to use metered dose inhalers. *Nursing, 49*(3), 56–60.

Cook, C., Demorest, S., & Schenk, E. (2019). Nurses and climate action. *American Journal of Nursing, 119*(4), 54–60.

Coulthard, K. (2018). Cystic fibrosis: Novel therapies, remaining challenges. *Journal of Pharmacy Practice and Research, 48*, 569–577.

Cystic Fibrosis Foundation (CFF). (2019). *About cystic fibrosis.* https://www.cff.org/.

Dorman, J. (2016). Recognizing acute hypercapnia. *American Nurse Today, 11*(11), 24.

Durham, C., Smith, W., & Sterrett, J. (2017). Adult asthma: Diagnosis and treatment. *The Nurse Practitioner, 42*(11), 16–24.

Frost, F., Dyce, P., Nazareth, D., Malone, V., & Walshaw, M. (2018). Continuous glucose monitoring guided insulin therapy is associated with improved clinical outcomes in cystic fibrosis-related diabetes. *Journal of Cystic Fibrosis, 17*(1), 798–803.

Global Initiative for Asthma (GINA). (2018). *Pocket guide for asthma management and prevention.* https://ginasthma.org/wp-content/uploads/2018/03/wms-GINA-main-pocket-guide_2018-v1.0.pdf.

Global Initiative for Chronic Obstructive Lung Disease (GOLD). (2019). *Global strategy for the diagnosis, management, and prevention of chronic obstructive pulmonary disease.* https://goldcopd.org/wp-content/uploads/2018/11/GOLD-2019-POCKET-GUIDE-FINAL_WMS.pdf.

Grondell, J., Holleran, C., Mintz, E., & Wiesel, O. (2018). Postoperative bedside critical care of thoracic surgery patients. *American Journal of Critical Care, 27*(4), 328–333.

Henrich, R., & Logue, M. (2017). Feasibility of using the test for adherence to inhalers tool and tailoring education to the individual with chronic obstructive pulmonary disease. *The Journal for Nurse Practitioners, 13*(10), e481–e483.

Hohsfield, R., Archer-Chicko, C., Housten, T., & Nolley, S. (2018). Pulmonary arterial hypertension emergency complications and evaluation. *Advanced Emergency Nursing Journal, 40*(4), 246–259.

Hussar, D. (2019). New drugs 2019: Part 1. *Nursing, 49*(2), 28–36.

Jarvis, C. (2020). *Physical examination & health assessment* (8th ed.). St. Louis: Elsevier.

Kaufman, J. (2017). Acute exacerbation of COPD: Diagnosis and management. *The Nurse Practitioner, 42*(6), 1–7.

Keep, S., Reiffer, A., & Bahl, T. (2016). Supporting self-management of asthma care. *Home Healthcare Now, 34*(3), 126–134.

Lee, J., Nguyen, H., Jarrett, M., Mitchell, P., Pike, K., & Fan, V. (2018). Effect of symptoms on physical performance in COPD. *Heart & Lung, 47*(2), 149–156.

Lomas, P., & Tran, Q. (2020). The changing face of cystic fibrosis. *American Nurse Journal, 15*(3), 28-32.

McCance, K., Huether, S., Brashers, V., & Rote, N. (2019). *Pathophysiology: The biologic basis for disease in adults and children* (8th ed.). St. Louis: Elsevier.

Miller, C., Bridges, E., Laxmanan, B., Cox-North, P., & Thompson, H. (2018). Tunneled pleural catheter: Treatment for recurrent pleural effusion. *AACN Advanced Critical Care, 29*(4), 432–441.

Muhrer, J. (2018). Update on diagnosis and management of severe asthma. *The Journal for Nurse Practitioners, 14*(7), 520–525.

Noel, Z., Kida, K., & Macaulay, T. (2017). Selexipag for treatment of pulmonary arterial hypertension. *American Journal of Health-System Pharmacists, 74*(15), 1135–1141.

Online Mendelian Inheritance in Man (OMIM). (2018). *Pulmonary hypertension.* primary www.omim.org/entry/178600.

Online Mendelian Inheritance in Man (OMIM). (2019a). *Asthma, susceptibility to.* www.omim.org/entry/600807.

Online Mendelian Inheritance in Man (OMIM). (2019b). *Adenocarcinoma of the lung.* www.omim.org/entry/211980.

Online Mendelian Inheritance in Man (OMIM). (2019c). *Alpha-1-antitrypsin deficiency.* www.omim.org/entry/613490.

Online Mendelian Inheritance in Man (OMIM). (2019d). *Cystic fibrosis.* CF. www.omim.org/entry/219700.

O'Dell, A., Diegel-Vacek, L., Burt, L., & Corbridge, S. (2018). Managing stable COPD: An evidence-based approach. *American Journal of Nursing, 118*(9), 36–47.

Pagana, K., & Pagana, T. (2018). *Mosby's manual of diagnostic and laboratory tests* (6th ed.). St. Louis: Elsevier.

Penkalski, M. (2019). Inhaled corticosteroids for asthma management. *Medsurg Nursing, 28*(2), 101–105.

Razga, M., & Handu, D. (2019). Nutrition care for patients with cystic fibrosis: An evidence analysis center scoping review. *Journal of the Academy of Nutrition and Dietetics, 119*(1), 137–151.

Sasa, R. (2019). Evidence-based update on chest tube management: Is your practice current? *American Nurse Today, 14*(4), 10–14.

Saunier, D. (2017). Creating and interprofessional team and discharge planning guide to decrease hospital readmissions for COPD. *Medsurg Nursing, 26*(4), 258–262.

Sherry, V. (2017). Lung cancer: Not just a smoker's disease. *American Nurse Today, 12*(2), 16–20.

Southard, E., Cannon, E., Bauer, R., & Heck, N. (2020). Lurking in the shadows: Alpha-1 antitrypsin deficiency. *MEDSURG Nursing, 29*(2), 96-100.

Statistics Canada. (2017). *Health fact sheets: Chronic conditions.* https://www150.statcan.gc.ca/n1/en/pub/82-625-x/2017001/article/54858-eng.pdf?st=SI_ORLtQ.

Statistics Canada. (2019). *Chronic obstructive pulmonary disease (COPD), 35 years and older.* https://www150.statcan.gc.ca/t1/tbl1/en/tv.action?pid=1310009619.

Taetavoulle, T. (2017). Management of sepsis in patients with pulmonary arterial hypertension in the intensive care unit. *Critical Care Clinics of North America, 29*(1), 15–23.

Touhy, T., & Jett, K. (2020). *Ebersole and hess' toward healthy aging: Human needs & nursing response* (10th ed.). St. Louis: Mosby.

Vega-Olivo, M., & Criner, G. (2018). Idiopathic pulmonary fibrosis: A guide for nurse practitioners. *The Nurse Practitioner, 43*(5), 48–54.

Wilson, A. (2018). Oscillating devices for airway clearance in people with cystic fibrosis: A Cochrane review summary. *International Journal of Nursing Studies, 88*, 165–166.

Wood, M., Powers, J., & Rechter, J. (2019). Comparative evaluation of chest tube insertion site dressings: A randomized controlled trial. *American Journal of Critical Care, 28*(6), 415–423.

Wysocki, K. (2018). Lung disease and genomics. *AACN Advanced Critical Care, 29*(1), 74–83.

28

Concepts of Care for Patients With Infectious Respiratory Problems

M. Linda Workman

http://evolve.elsevier.com/Iggy/

LEARNING OUTCOMES

1. Collaborate with the interprofessional team to coordinate high-quality, evidence-based care and promote ***gas exchange*** in patients with infectious respiratory problems.
2. Teach adults how to decrease the risk for development of respiratory ***infection***.
3. Implement actions to reduce the spread of respiratory ***infection***.
4. Implement nursing interventions to help the patient and family cope with the psychosocial impact caused by respiratory ***infection***.
5. Apply knowledge of anatomy, physiology, and pathophysiology to assess patients with common respiratory infections that impair ***gas exchange***.
6. Use clinical judgment to plan care for patients with respiratory ***infection*** and impaired ***gas exchange***.
7. Teach the patient and caregiver(s) about common drugs used for pneumonia, tuberculosis, and other respiratory ***infections***.

KEY TERMS

anergy Failure to have a skin response to TB skin testing because of reduced immunity even when ***infection*** is present.

consolidation An abnormal solidification with lack of air spaces in a segment of area of the lung.

COVID-19 A new coronavirus mutation (CO= corona; VI = virus; D = disease; 19 = 2019, the year the new virus was identified) that enabled this animal virus to infect humans and is responsible for the 2020 influenza pandemic.

empyema A collection of pus in the pleural cavity.

endemic infection Respiratory ***infection*** caused by organisms that are much more common within a geographic location but the actual incidence of the infection is relatively low.

gas exchange Oxygen transport to the cells and carbon dioxide transport away from cells through ventilation and diffusion.

immunity Protection from illness or disease that is maintained by the body's physiologic defense mechanisms.

induration Localized swelling with hardness of soft tissue.

infection Invasion of pathogens into the body that multiply and cause disease or illness.

inflammation A syndrome of normal tissue responses to cellular injury, allergy, or the invasion of pathogens.

miliary (hematogenous) TB Spread of TB throughout the body when a large number of organisms enter the blood.

pandemic infection An infection with an organism to which most humans have no ***immunity*** and that has the potential to spread globally.

tuberculosis (TB) A highly communicable disease caused by ***infection*** with *Mycobacterium tuberculosis*.

PRIORITY AND INTERRELATED CONCEPTS

The priority concepts for this chapter are:

- ***Gas Exchange***
- ***Infection***

The ***Gas Exchange*** concept exemplar for this chapter is Pneumonia.
The ***Infection*** concept exemplar for this chapter is Pulmonary Tuberculosis.

The interrelated concepts for this chapter are:

- ***Cognition***
- ***Immunity***
- ***Inflammation***

Infection, which is the invasion of pathogens into the body that multiply and cause disease or illness, is a common health problem of the respiratory tract and can greatly interfere with pulmonary gas exchange. (Recall from Chapters 3 and 24 that *gas exchange* is oxygen transport to the cells and carbon dioxide transport away from cells through ventilation and diffusion.) Some respiratory infections are relatively mild and self-limiting. Others are more serious and, if therapy is ineffective, can lead to death. The most common serious respiratory infections are influenza, pneumonia, and tuberculosis.

SEASONAL INFLUENZA

Pathophysiology Review

Seasonal influenza, or "flu," is a highly contagious acute viral respiratory infection that can occur at any age (Cannon et al., 2018). Influenza may be caused by different strains of one of several virus families, referred to as A, B, and C. Epidemics are common and lead to complications of pneumonia or death, especially in older adults, those with heart failure or chronic lung disorders, and immunocompromised patients. Most patients are treated at home, but hospitalization may be needed when symptoms are severe or the patient develops complications such as pneumonia. During the 2017–2018 influenza season, more than 30,000 patients were hospitalized for the infection with about 60% of these being older than 65 years (Centers for Disease Control and Prevention [CDC], 2018d).

The patient with influenza often has a rapid onset of severe headache, muscle aches, fever, chills, fatigue, and weakness. Adults are contagious 24 hours before symptoms occur and up to 5 days after they begin. Sore throat, cough, and watery nasal discharge can also occur. ***Infection*** with influenza strain B can lead to nausea, vomiting, and diarrhea. Most patients feel fatigued for 1 to 2 weeks after the acute episode has resolved.

Health Promotion and Maintenance

Seasonal influenza can be prevented or its severity reduced when adults receive an annual influenza vaccination. The vaccine is changed every year based on which specific viral strains are most likely to cause illness during the influenza season (i.e., late fall and winter in the Northern Hemisphere). Usually the vaccines contain antigens for the three (trivalent) or four (quadrivalent) viral strains expected to be prevalent that season. The recommended influenza vaccination for all adults is an IM injection. For adults age over 65 years, a new formulation is available, known as a "senior flu shot." This injection is a higher dose, trivalent or quadrivalent vaccine designed for more effective protection for adults with age-related reduced ***immunity***. For adults under age 50 years, a new formulation of a quadrivalent nasal mist using live attenuated viruses has been approved (Pfeifer, 2018). Although annual vaccination is not 100% effective at preventing influenza, it is especially important for adults who:

- Are older than 50 years
- Have chronic illness or immune compromise
- Reside in institutions
- Live with or care for others with health problems that put them at risk for severe complications of influenza
- Are health care personnel providing direct care to patients (CDC, 2018a)

Nurses have an opportunity to urge vaccination in the community and can show support for this action by receiving annual vaccinations themselves. This action not only helps practicing nurses avoid becoming infected, but it also reduces the risk for ***infection*** transmission from health care professional to patient. The influenza vaccination rate among health care personnel during the 2017–2018 flu season was 78% (by self-report) (Black et al., 2018).

> **! NATIONAL PATIENT SAFETY GOALS**
>
> Vaccinations for the prevention of influenza are widely available and are recommended for adults by The Joint Commission's National Patient Safety Goals.

Teach the patient who is sick to reduce the risk for spreading the flu by thoroughly washing hands, especially after nose blowing, sneezing, coughing, rubbing the eyes, or touching the face. Other precautions include staying home from work, school, or crowded places; covering the mouth and nose with a tissue when sneezing or coughing; disposing properly of used tissues immediately; and avoiding close contact with other people (social distancing) (CDC, 2018a). Although handwashing is a good way to prevent transmitting the virus, many people cannot wash their hands immediately after sneezing. The technique recommended by the CDC for controlling flu spread is to sneeze or cough into the upper sleeve rather than into the hand (CDC, 2018c). (Respiratory droplets on the hands can contaminate surfaces and be transmitted to others.)

❖ Interprofessional Collaborative Care

Tests for influenza are available; however, in a community that already has cases of the disease, the diagnosis is usually based on the patient's reported symptoms. The rapid influenza diagnostic test (RIDT) is common but has high false-negative rates, and the patient should be treated if influenza is suspected even if the RIDT is negative. Other tests, including cultures, are usually recommended only in specific situations.

Viral infections do not respond to antibiotic therapy. Neuraminidase inhibitor (NAI) antiviral drugs such as oseltamivir, zanamivir, and peramivir have been effective in the prevention and treatment of some strains of influenza A and B. They can be given to adults at high risk for complications who have been exposed to influenza but have not yet been vaccinated. These drugs also shorten the duration of influenza. The drugs prevent viral spread in the respiratory tract by inhibiting a viral enzyme that allows the virus to penetrate respiratory cells. To be most effective as treatment rather than for prevention, they must be taken within 24 to 48 hours after symptoms begin. Peramivir is only available as an IV drug. A newly approved antiviral drug with a different mechanism of action is baloxavir. This oral drug taken once daily prevents influenza viral gene transcription and reproduction. Patients older than 65 years should be treated with antiviral drugs as soon as possible to reduce their risks for hospitalization, complications, and disability (CDC, 2018a).

Instruct the patient to rest for several days and increase fluid intake unless another problem requires fluid restriction. Saline gargles may ease sore throat pain. Antihistamines may reduce the rhinorrhea. Other supportive measures are the same as those for rhinosinusitis.

NCLEX EXAMINATION CHALLENGE 28.1

Physiological Integrity

The spouse of a 78-year-old client who was discharged to home 1 day ago after hospitalization for seasonal influenza calls to report the fever has returned and is now 103.4°F (39.7°C). What is the nurse's **primary** concern for this client?

A. The client may not be taking the prescribed antiviral drug correctly
B. A second strain of influenza is likely
C. Pneumonia may be present
D. The client may be dehydrated

PANDEMIC RESPIRATORY INFECTIONS

Pathophysiology Review

Respiratory viral ***infections*** are common among humans and vary from mild colds to severe seasonal influenza that can lead to pneumonia, other complications, and death. These infections are considered *human disorders* and are not usually found in other animals. Respiratory infections caused by viruses are usually self-limiting because humans are able to mount some degree of an ***immunity*** response against the invading viruses. Part of adaptive immunity develops as a result of generations of ancestral exposures to common viral families such as rhinoviruses, respiratory syncytial viruses (RSV), and coronaviruses, among others. However, this immunity is not perfect. These viral strains change slightly every year so that the antibodies an adult makes against a specific strain one year are not completely effective against exposure to other strains of that same viral family later that year or another year. This is why adults can have several colds in the same year. It is also why influenza vaccinations are needed yearly to increase protection, as discussed in the Seasonal Influenza section.

Pandemic Influenza

A **pandemic** respiratory viral ***infection*** is one that has the potential to spread globally because the virus has previously infected only birds or other animals, so no human ancestral immunity is present. Most bird and animal viruses cannot be transmitted to humans. A few notable exceptions have occurred when these viruses mutated and became highly infectious to humans, causing pandemics. Example pandemics include the 1918 "Spanish" influenza and the 2009 H1N1 influenza A.

COVID-19 Infection

The coronavirus family, in addition to causing the common cold in humans, includes bird and animal strains that have caused severe respiratory influenzas. In 2002 and 2003, the coronavirus COVID-2 jumped species and was responsible for SARS (severe acute respiratory syndrome). In 2012 another coronavirus mutation was responsible for MERS-Cov (Middle East respiratory syndrome), which had a high but demographically confined mortality rate.

In December 2019 extending into 2020, the world experienced a coronavirus pandemic, COVID-19 (CO = coronavirus; VI = virus; D = disease; 19 = 2019). This strain of virus was first reported to have infected humans and rapidly spread in the fall of 2019 (McIntosh, 2020). Evidence shows that COVID-19 is spread via droplet transmission (CDC, 2020b; Palmore, 2020; WHO, 2020). It can also be transmitted during medical procedures that generate aerosols (WHO, 2020). Researchers continue to investigate whether airborne transmission can occur in the absence of a medical procedure, such as in poorly ventilated indoor settings (WHO, 2020). By the middle of September 2020 it infected almost 28 million people in 188 countries and territories, resulting in 905,181 deaths (Johns Hopkins University, 2020). At this same time in Canada, 136,565 cases were reported with 9208 deaths; in the United States 6.3 million people were infected, with 191,248 deaths (reflecting a death rate of 3%) (Johns Hopkins University, 2020). In comparison, 35.5 million people in the United States contracted seasonal influenza in the 2018-2019 influenza season, resulting in 34,200 deaths (death rate of about 0.1%) (CDC, 2019). COVID-19 statistics continue to change with increased testing and better understanding of care based upon evolving evidence.

Some patients who develop COVID-19 are asymptomatic or experience minimal symptoms. Others experience minor respiratory symptoms similar to a common cold, and recover with no apparent long-term effects. Others, particularly older adults and individuals with pre-existing chronic conditions, can develop a viral pneumonia that can lead to severe acute respiratory distress syndrome. See the Key Features: COVID-19 box for symptoms that are currently associated with the infection. Typically, symptoms appear 2 to 14 days after exposure to the virus.

KEY FEATURES

COVID-19

Most Common Symptoms

- Fever or chills
- Cough
- Shortness of breath or difficulty breathing
- Fatigue
- Muscle or body aches
- Headache
- New loss of taste or smell
- Sore throat
- Nausea or vomiting
- Diarrhea
- Abdominal pain

Unique Features in Some Patients

- Conjunctivitis
- Prothrombotic state (venous thromboembolic disease)
- Neurologic findings (encephalopathy with agitated delirium)
- Dermatologic findings, especially reddish nodules on distal digits (in young adults)

Indications for Emergency Interventions

- Trouble breathing
- Persistent pain or pressure in the chest
- New confusion
- Inability to wake or stay awake
- Bluish lips or face

Data from Centers for Disease Control and Prevention (CDC) (2020). *Coronavirus disease 19 (COVID-19): Symptoms of coronavirus.* https://www.cdc.gov/coronavirus/2019-ncov/symptoms-testing/symptoms.html; Cuker, A., & Peyvandi, F. (2020). Coronavirus disease 2019 (COVID-19): Hypercoagulability. In *UpToDate,* Leung, L. (Ed.). Waltham, MA; and McIntosh, K. (2020). Coronavirus disease 2019 (COVID-19): Clinical features. In *UpToDate,* Hirsch, M. (Ed.). Waltham, MA.

PATIENT-CENTERED CARE: CULTURAL/ SPIRITUAL CONSIDERATIONS QSEN

Although the effects of COVID-19 on the health of racial and ethnic minority groups are still emerging, current data indicate a disproportionate and substantially higher incidence of illness and a greater death rate among black and Hispanic adults (CDC, 2020a). The report also suggests that these disease differences appear to be more socioeconomic in origin rather than the result of an increased genetic or racial risk.

Health Promotion and Maintenance

The prevention of worldwide respiratory pandemics is the responsibility of everyone. Health officials at the global, national, and state levels monitor for outbreaks. The recommended approach for any potential or actual pandemic is early recognition of cases and implementation of community and personal quarantine. Social-distancing behaviors help to reduce viral exposure. When a cluster of cases is discovered in an area, stockpiled vaccines are made available for immunization.

Nonessential public activities in the area should be stopped, such as public gatherings, attendance at schools, religious services, shopping, and many types of employment. Adults should stay home and use the food, water, and medications they have stockpiled to last at least 2 weeks per person for disaster preparedness as described in Chapter 12. Travel to and from this area should be stopped.

Pandemic Influenza

Antiviral drugs such as oseltamivir are stockpiled in the event of a pandemic influenza. They can be used for prevention or to shorten the duration of the ***infection***. Distribution for treatment is made on a case-by-case basis, as the drug must be started within 48 hours of symptom onset. Infected patients in the hospital setting should be placed on Droplet Precautions for 7 days and placed in a private room.

COVID-19 Infection

Vaccines for the prevention of COVID-19 are currently in phase 3 clinical trials. Teach all people the need to properly wear a mask, engage in frequent handwashing, and practice social distancing to prevent the spread of COVID-19.

Nonintubated patients should wear a mask while hospitalized and should be placed in a standard, single-patient room with a private bathroom. The door to the room should be closed at all times. Those having aerosolized-generating interventions should be placed in an airborne infection isolation room (AIIR) (CDC, 2020b). Most inpatient agencies have designated certain wings or floors reserved for patients with COVID-19.

❖ Interprofessional Collaborative Care

Care priorities for the patient with any pandemic respiratory ***infection*** include supportive measures and preventing spread of the disease. Ask all patients about travel within the last 14 days to areas of the world affected by an outbreak. If such travel has occurred, have the patient don a mask and place him or her in isolation until further assessment is completed.

Pandemic Influenza

Until the specific type of potentially pandemic influenza is identified and its routes of transmission are known, patients must be isolated, and Airborne, Droplet, and Contact Precautions must be used. Rapid influenza diagnostic tests are available.

Treatment for influenza is often supportive in nature. Patients who are stable are instructed to recover at home and to avoid exposure to other individuals. Rest and fluids should be encouraged. If fever or myalgias are present, acetaminophen can be taken. The health care provider may prescribe an antiviral medication such as oseltamivir to be started within 48 hours of symptom onset. For influenzas with no effective treatment, interventions are supportive to allow the patient's own immune system to fight the ***infection***. Oxygen is given when hypoxia, breathlessness, or a change in ***cognition*** occurs. Respiratory treatments to dilate the bronchioles and move respiratory secretions are used. If hypoxemia is not improved with oxygen therapy, intubation and mechanical ventilation may be needed. Antibiotics are used to treat a bacterial pneumonia that may occur with influenza.

COVID-19 Infection

Viral and antibody tests for COVID-19 became available in summer 2020. Viral tests indicate if a person has the active (current) COVID-19 infection; the antibody test *might* indicate if the person previously had COVID-19 (CDC, 2020c). People who should be tested include those with symptoms, those who have been within 6 feet of an infected person for at least 15 minutes, and those referred by a health care provider or state health department.

Depending on the severity of symptoms, management ranges from supportive measures to critical care. Patients who are asymptomatic or have only mild symptoms must be taught to quarantine for 14 days. For severe cases, management may include noninvasive ventilation, intubation with mechanical ventilation, and extracorporeal membrane oxygenation (ECMO). A trial of self-proning may be recommended by the health care provider before intubation (Anesi, 2020). Trials of hyperbaric oxygen therapy (HBO) continue.

As of September 2020, no specific drug had received full approval for treatment. One new and not yet approved drug, the IV antiviral agent remdesivir, received emergency use authorization by the U.S. Food and Drug Administration (FDA, 2020). Mixed results have arisen regarding treatment with certain drugs used for other disorders; true and reliable efficacy cannot be determined without large, randomized, and controlled clinical trials. Current evidence shows that dexamethasone, other glucocorticoids, convalescent plasma, and other antibody-based therapies are used in treatment. Other new and existing antiviral drugs are in early-phase trials to measure activity against replication of COVID-19.

The highly contagious nature of the disease and the need for the use of techniques/interventions that more easily disperse droplets to others (e.g., suctioning, intubation) requires extraordinary containment measures during all aspects of care. When caring for a patient with COVID-19, it is critical that health care providers wear an N95 respirator mask (with a face shield whenever possible), gowns, shoe covers, gloves, and goggles (if no face shield is available).

Inhaled medications should be delivered by metered dose inhalers with spacer devices versus given by nebulizer to avoid aerosolization of COVID-19. Physical distancing between patients and among health care providers, when not providing direct care, is recommended (CDC, 2020b). Teach family members to monitor themselves for illness, especially respiratory infection, for at least 2 weeks after the last contact with the patient.

! NURSING SAFETY PRIORITY (QSEN)

Action Alert

When performing procedures that induce coughing or promote aerosolization of particles (e.g., suctioning, using a positive-pressure facemask, obtaining a sputum culture, or giving aerosolized treatments) for the patient with a potentially pandemic respiratory infection, protect yourself and other health care workers. Wear a gown, N95 mask, face shield, and protective eyewear during the procedures. Keep the door to the patient's room closed. Avoid touching your face. Wash your hands after removing personal protective equipment (PPE) and when you leave the patient's room. Wear gloves when disinfecting contaminated surfaces or equipment.

GAS EXCHANGE CONCEPT EXEMPLAR: PNEUMONIA

Pathophysiology Review

Pneumonia is a common disorder with many causes that reduce ***gas exchange***. Although all pneumonias have excess fluid in the lungs from an inflammatory process, pneumonia from respiratory ***infection*** is associated with the formation of thick exudate containing proteins and other particles that seriously reduce gas exchange.

Inflammation causing pneumonia can be triggered by infectious organisms and by inhaling irritating agents. ***Inflammation,*** which is the syndrome of normal tissue responses to cellular injury, allergy, or the invasion of pathogens, occurs in the interstitial spaces, the alveoli, and often the bronchioles. The process begins when pathogens penetrate the airway mucosa and multiply in the alveolar spaces. White blood cells (WBCs) move into the area of infection, causing local capillary leak, edema, and formation of exudates. The exudates collect in and around the alveoli, and the alveolar walls thicken. Both events seriously reduce ***gas exchange*** by interfering with diffusion in the lungs leading to hypoxemia, which can cause death. Red blood cells (RBCs) and fibrin move into the alveoli, and capillary leak spreads the ***infection*** to other lung areas. If organisms move into the bloodstream, septicemia and sepsis results (Giuliano & Baker, 2020). If the infection extends into the pleural cavity, **empyema** (a collection of pus in the pleural cavity) results.

The fibrin and edema stiffen the lung tissue, reducing compliance and decreasing the vital capacity. Alveolar collapse *(atelectasis)* reduces ***gas exchange*** even more. As a result, arterial oxygen levels fall, causing hypoxemia.

TABLE 28.1 Risk Factors for Pneumonia

Community-Acquired Pneumonia

- Is an older adult
- Has never received the pneumococcal vaccination or received it more than 5 years ago
- Did not receive the influenza vaccine in the previous year
- Has a chronic health problem or other coexisting condition that reduces ***immunity***
- Has recently been exposed to respiratory viral or influenza ***infection***
- Uses tobacco or alcohol or is exposed to high amounts of secondhand smoke

Health Care–Acquired Pneumonia

- Is an older adult
- Has a chronic lung disease
- Has presence of gram-negative colonization of the mouth, throat, and stomach
- Has an altered level of consciousness
- Has had a recent aspiration event
- Has presence of endotracheal, tracheostomy, or nasogastric tube
- Has poor nutritional status
- Has reduced ***immunity*** (from disease or drug therapy)
- Uses drugs that increase gastric pH (histamine [H_2] blockers, antacids) or alkaline tube feedings
- Is currently receiving mechanical ventilation (ventilator-associated pneumonia [VAP])

Pneumonia may occur as *lobar pneumonia* with **consolidation** (an abnormal solidification with lack of air spaces) in a segment or an entire lobe of the lung or as *bronchopneumonia* with diffusely scattered patches around the bronchi. The extent of lung involvement depends on the host defenses. Bacteria multiply quickly in a person whose immune system is compromised. Tissue necrosis results when an abscess forms and perforates the bronchial wall.

Etiology

Infectious pneumonia develops when a patient's ***immunity*** cannot overcome the invading organisms (Arsbad et al., 2016). Organisms from the environment (especially after natural disasters), invasive devices, equipment, and supplies or other people can invade the body. Risk factors are listed in Table 28.1. Pneumonia can be caused by any organism such as bacteria, viruses, mycoplasmas, fungi, rickettsiae, protozoa, and helminths (worms). Noninfectious causes of pneumonia include inhalation of toxic gases, chemical fumes, and smoke; and aspiration of water, food, fluid (including saliva), and vomitus. Infectious pneumonia can be categorized as community acquired (CAP), hospital acquired (HAP), health care acquired (HCAP) or ventilator-associated (VAP) (see Table 28.2).

Incidence and Prevalence

In the United States 2 to 5 million cases of pneumonia occur annually. About 1 million people are hospitalized for treatment, and more than 50,000 deaths result from the disease (CDC, 2018b). In Canada, influenza and pneumonia incidence and deaths are reported together and both disorders are common, accounting for about 6000 deaths annually (Statistics Canada, 2018). The rate of pneumonia is higher among older adults, nursing home residents, hospitalized patients, patients with neurologic problems or difficulty swallowing, and those being mechanically ventilated (Meehan & McKenna, 2020). CAP is

PATIENT AND FAMILY EDUCATION: PREPARING FOR SELF-MANAGEMENT

Preventing Pneumonia

- Know your risk for pneumonia (older than 65 years, have a chronic health problem [especially a respiratory problem], or have limited mobility and are confined to a bed or chair during your waking hours).
- Have the annual influenza vaccination after discussing appropriate timing of the immunization with your primary health care provider.
- Discuss the pneumococcal vaccine with your primary health care provider and have the vaccination as recommended.
- Avoid crowded public areas during flu seasons.
- If you have a mobility problem, cough, turn, move about as much as possible, and perform deep-breathing exercises.
- If you are using respiratory equipment at home, clean the equipment as you have been instructed by the manufacturer.
- Avoid indoor pollutants, such as dust, secondhand (passive) smoke, and aerosols.
- If you do not smoke, vape, or use tobacco in any form, do not start.
- If you smoke or vape, seek professional help on how to stop (or at least decrease) your habit.
- Get enough rest and sleep on a daily basis.
- Eat a healthy, balanced diet.
- Drink at least 3 L (quarts) of nonalcoholic fluids each day (unless fluid restrictions are needed because of another health problem).

more common than HAP and occurs most often in late fall and winter, frequently as a complication of influenza.

Health Promotion and Maintenance

Vaccination can help prevent pneumonia. Currently, there are two pneumonia vaccines: pneumococcal polysaccharide vaccine (PPSV23) and pneumococcal conjugate vaccine (PCV13) for prevention of pneumonia (Phillips & Swanson, 2016). The CDC recommends that adults older than 65 years be vaccinated with both, first with PCV13 followed by PPSV23 about 12 months later. Adults who have already received the PPSV23 should have PCV13 about a year or more later. These recommendations also apply to adults between 19 and 64 years of age who have specific risk factors such as chronic illnesses (CDC, 2018b). Because pneumonia often follows influenza, especially among older adults, urge all adults to receive the seasonal vaccination annually.

Patient education about vaccination and other means of pneumonia prevention is important. Teaching points are presented in the Patient and Family Education: Preparing for Self-Management: Preventing Pneumonia box.

! NATIONAL PATIENT SAFETY GOALS

The Joint Commission recommends that nurses especially encourage adults older than 65 years and those with a chronic health problem to receive immunization against pneumonia. For inpatients admitted for any condition, The Joint Commission recommends checking the pneumonia vaccination status and, if needed, offer the vaccination during the inpatient stay.

Other pneumonia prevention techniques include strict handwashing to avoid spreading organisms and avoiding crowds during cold and flu season. Teach the patient who has a cold or the flu to see his or her primary health care provider if fever lasts more than 24 hours, the problem lasts longer than 1 week, or symptoms worsen.

Respiratory therapy equipment must be well maintained and decontaminated or changed as recommended. Use sterile water rather than tap water in GI tubes and institute Aspiration Precautions as indicated, including screening patients for aspiration risk (Meehan & McKenna, 2020).

VAP is on the rise, but the risk can be reduced with conscientious assessment and meticulous nursing care. The preventive care for VAP is discussed in Chapter 29 and is listed in Table 28.2.

! NURSING SAFETY PRIORITY (QSEN)

Action Alert

Because pneumonia is a frequent cause of sepsis, use a sepsis screening tool to monitor patients who have pneumonia (see Chapter 34). For patients with pneumonia, always check oxygen saturation with vital signs.

❖ Interprofessional Collaborative Care

Depending on the patient's overall health status, specific cause of the pneumonia, and severity of hypoxemia, patients may be cared for in the home or other residential setting or may need acute hospital care. Signs and symptoms of pneumonia differ in older patients compared with younger patients.

◆ Assessment: Recognize Cues

History. Assess for the risk factors for respiratory ***infection*** (see Table 28.1). Document age; living, work, or school environment; diet, exercise, and sleep routines; swallowing problems; presence of a nasogastric tube; tobacco and alcohol use; and past and current use of or addiction to "street" drugs. Remember that often aspiration is "silent" with no signs or symptoms. Ask about past respiratory illnesses and whether the patient has been exposed to influenza or pneumonia or has had a recent viral infection. Using the I PREPARE model listed in Chapter 24, assess the patient for particulate matter exposure (PME). Even noninfectious exposures can result in respiratory ***inflammation***, which increases the risk for pneumonia development.

If the patient has chronic respiratory problems, ask whether respiratory equipment is used in the home. Assess whether the patient's cleaning routine for the equipment is adequate to prevent infection. Ask when he or she received the last influenza or pneumococcal vaccine. Ask family members whether they have noticed a change in the patient's ***cognition***.

Physical Assessment/Signs and Symptoms. Observe the general appearance. Many patients with pneumonia have flushed cheeks and an anxious expression. The patient may have chest pain or discomfort, myalgia, headache, chills, fever, cough, tachycardia, dyspnea, tachypnea, *hemoptysis* (bloody sputum), and sputum production. Severe chest muscle weakness may also be present from sustained coughing.

Observe the patient's breathing pattern, position, and use of accessory muscles. The patient with hypoxia and reduced ***gas exchange*** may be uncomfortable in a lying position and will sit

TABLE 28.2 Types of Pneumonia

Type of Pneumonia	Definition	Management Considerations
Community-acquired	Contracted outside a health care setting; acquired in the community	Most common bacterial agents: *Streptococcus pneumoniae, Haemophilus influenzae* Most common viral agents: influenza, respiratory syncytial virus (RSV) Antibiotics are often empirical based on multiple patient and environmental factors Treatment length: minimum of 5 days Prompt initiation of antibiotics required; in ED setting, first dose given before patient leaves unit for inpatient bed or within 6 hr of presentation to the ED
Health care–associated	Onset/diagnosis of pneumonia occurs <48 hr after admission in patient with specific risk factors: • In hospital for >48 hr in the past 90 days • Living in nursing home or assisted-living facility • Received IV therapy, wound care, antibiotics, chemotherapy in the past 30 days • Seen at a hospital or dialysis clinic within the past 30 days	May have multidrug-resistant organisms Hand hygiene critical
Hospital-acquired	Onset/diagnosis of pneumonia >48 hr after admission to hospital	Encourage pulmonary hygiene and progressive ambulation Provide adequate hydration Assess risk for aspiration using an evidence-based tool Monitor for early signs of sepsis Hands hygiene is critical Provide vigorous oral care
Ventilator-associated	Onset/diagnosis of pneumonia within 48-72 hr after endotracheal intubation	Presence of ET tube increases risk for pneumonia by bypassing protective airway mechanisms and allowing aspiration of secretions from the oropharynx and stomach; dental plaque also increases risk Initiate ventilator bundle order set, including: • Elevate HOB at least 30 degrees • Daily sedation "vacation" and weaning assessment • DVT prophylaxis • Oral care regimen • Stress ulcer prophylaxis • Suctioning, either as needed or continuous subglottal suction Hand hygiene is critical

DVT, Deep vein thrombosis; *ED,* emergency department; *ET,* endotracheal; *HOB,* head of bed.

upright, balancing with the hands ("tripod position"). Assess the cough and the amount, color, consistency, and odor of sputum produced.

Crackles are heard on auscultation when fluid is in interstitial and alveolar areas, and breath sounds may be diminished. Wheezing may be heard if ***inflammation*** or exudate narrows the airways. Bronchial breath sounds are heard over areas of density or consolidation. Fremitus is increased over areas of pneumonia, and percussion is dulled. Chest expansion may be diminished or unequal on inspiration.

In evaluating vital signs, compare the results with baseline values. A patient with pneumonia, especially an older adult, is often hypotensive with orthostatic changes because of vasodilation and dehydration. A rapid, weak pulse may indicate hypoxemia, dehydration, or impending sepsis and shock. Dysrhythmias may occur from cardiac tissue hypoxia. Common pneumonia signs and symptoms and their causes are listed in Table 28.3.

The primary health care provider uses one of several evidence-based pneumonia severity scales to determine whether the patient can be managed in the community or requires hospitalization. When pneumonia is uncomplicated by other health problems, it is often managed in the community.

TABLE 28.3 Pathophysiology of Common Signs and Symptoms of Pneumonia

Sign or Symptom	Pathophysiology
Increased respiratory rate/dyspnea	Stimulation of chemoreceptors Increased work of breathing as a result of decreased lung compliance Stimulation of J receptors Anxiety Pain
Hypoxemia	Alveolar consolidation Pulmonary capillary shunting
Cough	Fluid accumulation in receptors of the trachea, bronchi, and bronchioles
Purulent, blood-tinged, or rust-colored sputum	A result of the inflammatory process in which fluid from the pulmonary capillaries and red blood cells moves into the alveoli
Fever	Phagocytes release pyrogens that cause the hypothalamus to increase body temperature
Pleuritic chest discomfort	***Inflammation*** of the parietal pleura causes pain on inspiration

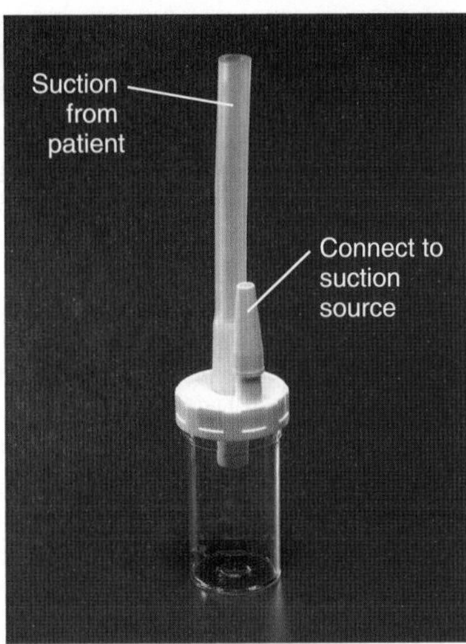

FIG. 28.1 Lukens tube for collection of sterile sputum/mucus specimens. (Courtesy Covidien, AG, Switzerland.)

> **PATIENT-CENTERED CARE: OLDER ADULT CONSIDERATIONS** QSEN
>
> The older adult with pneumonia has weakness, fatigue (which can lead to falls), lethargy, confusion, and poor appetite. Fever and cough may be absent, but hypoxemia is often present. The most common symptom of pneumonia in the older-adult patient is a change in ***cognition*** with acute confusion from hypoxia. The WBC count may not be elevated until the infection is severe. Waiting to treat the disease until more typical symptoms appear greatly increases the risk for sepsis and death (Touhy & Jett, 2020).

Psychosocial Assessment. The patient with pneumonia often has pain, fatigue, and dyspnea, all of which promote anxiety. Assess anxiety by looking at his or her facial expression and general tenseness of facial and shoulder muscles. Listen to the patient carefully, and use a calm approach. Because of airway obstruction and muscle fatigue, the patient with dyspnea speaks in broken sentences. Keep the interview short if severe dyspnea or breathing discomfort is present.

Laboratory Assessment. Sputum is obtained and examined by Gram stain, culture, and sensitivity testing; however, the responsible organism is often not identified. A sputum sample is easily obtained from the patient who can cough into a specimen container. Extremely ill patients may need suctioning to obtain a sputum specimen. In these situations, a specimen is obtained by sputum trap (Fig. 28.1) during suctioning. A complete blood count (CBC) is obtained to assess for an elevated WBC count, which is a common finding except in older adults. Blood cultures may be performed to determine whether the organism has entered the bloodstream.

In severely ill patients, arterial blood gases (ABGs) may be assessed to determine baseline arterial oxygen and carbon dioxide levels and to help identify a need for supplemental oxygen. Serum electrolyte, blood urea nitrogen (BUN), and creatinine levels are also assessed. A high BUN level may occur as a result of dehydration. Hypernatremia (high blood sodium levels) occurs with dehydration. A lactate level may be performed to help assess for sepsis. Because CAP often follows or is present with influenza, recommend that adults with CAP also have influenza testing (Esden, 2020).

Imaging Assessment. Chest x-ray is the most common diagnostic test for pneumonia but may not show changes until 2 or more days after symptoms are present. Pneumonia usually appears on chest x-ray as an area of increased density. It may involve a lung segment, a lobe, one lung, or both lungs. *In the older adult, the chest x-ray is essential for early diagnosis because other pneumonia symptoms are often vague* (Touhy & Jett, 2020).

Other Diagnostic Assessments. Pulse oximetry is used to assess for hypoxemia. Thoracentesis is used in patients who have an accompanying pleural effusion.

◆ Analysis: Analyze Cues and Prioritize Hypotheses

The priority interprofessional collaborative problems for patients with pneumonia include:

1. Decreased ***gas exchange*** due to decreased diffusion at the alveolar-capillary membrane
2. Potential for airway obstruction due to ***inflammation*** with excessive pulmonary secretions, fatigue, muscle weakness
3. Potential for sepsis due to the presence of microorganisms in a very vascular area and reduced ***immunity***
4. Potential for pulmonary empyema due to spread of infectious organisms from the lung into the pleural space

◆ Planning and Implementation: Generate Solutions and Take Action

Improving Gas Exchange

Planning: Expected Outcomes. The patient with pneumonia is expected to have adequate ***gas exchange*** and oxygenation.

Interventions. Interventions to improve ***gas exchange*** are similar to those for the patient with asthma or chronic obstructive pulmonary disease (see Chapter 27). Nursing priorities include delivery of oxygen therapy and assisting the patient with bronchial hygiene.

Oxygen therapy is usually delivered by nasal cannula or mask unless the hypoxemia does not improve with these devices. The patient who is confused may not tolerate a facemask. Check the skin under the device and under the elastic band, especially around the ears, for areas of redness or skin breakdown. Actions for oxygen therapy are listed in the Best Practice for Patient Safety & Quality Care: Oxygen Therapy box in Chapter 25.

Incentive spirometry is used to improve inspiratory muscle action and to prevent or reverse atelectasis (alveolar collapse). Instruct the patient to sit up if possible, exhale fully, place the mouthpiece in his or her mouth; take a long, slow, deep breath, raising the piston as high as possible, and then hold the breath for 2 to 4 seconds before slowly exhaling. Evaluate technique and record the volume of air inspired. Teach the patient to perform 5 to 10 breaths per session every hour while awake. This intervention may not be helpful to patients who are very fatigued and/or have severe dyspnea.

Preventing Airway Obstruction

Planning: Expected Outcomes. The patient with pneumonia is expected to maintain a patent airway.

Interventions. Interventions to improve ***gas exchange*** by avoiding airway obstruction in pneumonia are similar to those for chronic obstructive pulmonary disease (COPD) or asthma. Because of fatigue, muscle weakness, chest discomfort, and excessive secretions, the patient often has difficulty clearing secretions. Help him or her cough and deep breathe at least every 2 hours. The alert patient may use an incentive spirometer to facilitate deep breathing and stimulate coughing. Encourage the alert patient to drink at least 2 L of fluid daily to prevent dehydration and to thin secretions unless another health problem requires fluid restriction. Monitor intake and output, oral mucus membranes, and skin turgor to assess hydration status, especially when fever and tachypnea are present.

Bronchodilators, especially $beta_2$ agonists (see the Common Examples of Drug Therapy: Asthma Prevention and Treatment box in Chapter 27), are prescribed when bronchospasm is present. They can be given by nebulizer or metered-dose inhaler. Inhaled or IV steroids are used with acute pneumonia when ***inflammation*** and airway swelling are present. Expectorants such as guaifenesin may be used.

Preventing Sepsis

Planning: Expected Outcomes. The patient with pneumonia is expected to be free of the invading organism and to return to a pre-pneumonia health status.

Interventions. Eliminating the infecting organism is key to treating pneumonia and preventing sepsis. When sepsis occurs with pneumonia, the risk for death is high. Anti-infectives are given for all types of pneumonias except those caused by viruses. Selection of drugs and route of delivery is based on how the pneumonia was acquired (i.e., CAP, HAP, or HCAP), how ill the patient is, which organism is involved, and whether the patient has conditions that increase the risk for complications, especially reduced immunity. The primary health care provider must consider drug resistance in the specific geographic area and in that hospital setting. Drug resistance is becoming increasingly common, especially for ***infection*** with *Streptococcus pneumoniae* (drug resistant *S. pneumoniae* [DRSP]). Usually anti-infectives are used for 5 to 7 days for a patient with uncomplicated CAP and up to 21 days for a patient with severely impaired ***immunity*** or one with HAP (Connor, 2018; Esden, 2020).

For pneumonia caused by aspiration of food or stomach contents, interventions focus on preventing lung damage and treating the infection. Aspiration of acidic stomach contents can cause widespread ***inflammation***, leading to acute respiratory distress syndrome (ARDS) and permanent lung damage. See Chapter 29 for a discussion of ARDS.

Managing Empyema. When pulmonary empyema occurs as a result of pneumonia, further interventions are needed. Pulmonary empyema is a collection of pus in the pleural space most commonly caused by pulmonary ***infection***. When empyema is present, ***gas exchange*** can be impaired by both reduced lung diffusion and reduced effective ventilation.

Empyema is suspected when chest wall motion is reduced, fremitus is reduced or absent, percussion is flat, and breath sounds are decreased. Abnormal breath sounds, including bronchial breath sounds, egophony, and whispered pectoriloquy, may also be present. Diagnosis is made by chest x-ray or CT scan and a sample of the pleural fluid (obtained via thoracentesis). Empyema fluid is thick, opaque, exudative, and foul smelling.

Treatment includes draining the empyema cavity, re-expanding the lung, and controlling the ***infection***. Appropriate antibiotics are prescribed. A chest tube(s) to closed-chest drainage is used to promote lung expansion and drainage. The tube is removed when the lung is fully expanded and the infection is under control. Chest surgery may be needed for thick pus or excessive pleural thickening. Nursing interventions are similar to those for patients with a pleural effusion, pneumothorax, or infection. Chapters 27and 29 discuss these interventions in more detail.

SYSTEMS THINKING AND QUALITY IMPROVEMENT (QSEN)

Can 30-Day Hospital Readmissions Be Reduced for Patients Recovering From Pneumonia?

Goering, L. (2018). Pneumonia recovery: A plan can help. *MEDSURG Nursing, 27*(5), 305–309, 330.

Hospital re-admissions within 30 days after discharge for treatment of pneumonia, especially among older adults, are relatively high. Many of the problems and complications responsible for re-admission are preventable with appropriate transitional care, patient and family education, and consistent implementation of evidence-based interprofessional care interventions. One Midwestern hospital group developed a written interprofessional plan, known as the Pneumonia Recovery Plan (PRP), targeted to patients admitted for pneumonia. This tool for patients and families, which used both sides of a single sheet of paper, was given to patients on the first day of admission. It listed specific patient actions needed at admission and throughout the hospital stay, as well as for the weeks after discharge. Nurses were the primary explainers of the PRP for patients both initially and daily through discharge. Discharge planners and other interprofessional team members routinely reinforced the proscribed patient actions. No new interventions were introduced nor was nursing workload increased, just more consistent implementation of current evidence-based practices. Outcome measures for evaluation were reduction of length of stay (LOS), reduction of 20% for 30-day re-admission, and improvement of patient satisfaction to the 95th percentile in all categories.

As a result of this quality improvement project, LOS for patients with pneumonia was reduced an average of 1.29 days and re-admission rates dropped from 33.3% to 7.4%. Although patient satisfaction did not improve to the 95th percentile in all categories, patients indicated a high degree of satisfaction with the PRP and the communication of needed patient actions and medication information. Eventually, the PRP was a part of electronic medical records and successfully instituted at another hospital.

Commentary: Implications for Research and Practice

This project started with identifying where gaps in care for hospitalized patients with pneumonia were likely contributing to the need for re-admission within 30 days. The emphasis of making the patient a full partner in pneumonia recovery care and ensuring consistent actions recognized as important by all members of the interprofessional team contributed heavily to successful transitional care for patient benefit. Nurses were key to consistent implementation of the plan. This plan and its collaborative development processes could serve as a model to improve transitional care and promote an uncomplicated return to health for other common disorders.

FOCUSED ASSESSMENT

The Patient Recovering From Pneumonia

Ask whether the patient has had any of these problems:

- New-onset confusion
- Chills and fever
- Persistent cough
- Dyspnea
- Wheezing
- Hemoptysis
- Increased sputum production
- Chest discomfort
- Increasing fatigue
- Any other symptoms that have failed to resolve

Assess the patient for:

- Fever
- Diaphoresis
- Cyanosis, especially around the mouth or conjunctiva
- Dyspnea, tachypnea, or tachycardia
- Adventitious or abnormal breath sounds
- Weakness

Care Coordination and Transition Management

The patient needs to continue the anti-infective drugs as prescribed. An important nursing role is to reinforce, clarify, and provide information to the patient and family as needed. Unfortunately, the re-admission rate within 30 days after discharge is relatively high, especially among older adults (Goering, 2018). See the accompanying Systems Thinking and Quality Improvement box focusing on one group's successful method of reducing preventable re-admissions.

Home Care Management. No special changes are needed in the home. If the home has a second story, the patient may prefer to stay on one floor for a few weeks, because stair climbing can be tiring. Toileting needs may be met by using a bedside commode if a bathroom is not located on the level the patient is using. Home care needs depend on the patient's level of fatigue, dyspnea, and family and social support.

The long recovery phase, especially in the older adult, can be frustrating. Fatigue, weakness, and a residual cough can last for weeks. Some patients fear they will never return to a "normal" level of functioning. Prepare them for the disease course and offer reassurance that complete recovery will occur. After discharge a home nursing assessment may be helpful. Specific issues to assess for a patient recovering from pneumonia are presented in the Focused Assessment box.

Self-Management Education. Review all drugs with the patient and family and emphasize the importance of completing anti-infective therapy. Instruct the patient to notify the primary health care provider if chills, fever, persistent cough, dyspnea, wheezing, hemoptysis, increased sputum production, chest discomfort, or increasing fatigue returns or fails to go away completely. Instruct him or her to get plenty of rest and increase activity gradually.

An important aspect of education for the patient and family is avoiding upper respiratory tract ***infection*** and viruses. Teach him or her to avoid crowds (especially in the fall and winter when viruses are prevalent), people who have a cold or flu, and exposure to irritants such as smoke. A balanced diet and adequate fluid intake are essential.

Health Care Resources. Inform patients who smoke or vape that these activities are risk factors for pneumonia. Use the suggestions and interventions discussed in Chapter 24 to help the patient quit or reduce cigarette smoking and/or vaping. Teach about pneumonia, and urge the patient who has not already been vaccinated against influenza or pneumonia to get these vaccinations after the pneumonia has resolved.

◆ Evaluation: Evaluate Outcomes

Evaluate the care of the patient with pneumonia based on the identified priority patient problems. The expected outcomes are that he or she:

- Attains or maintains adequate ***gas exchange*** with Sao_2 of at least 95% or his or her normal level
- Maintains patent airways as evidenced by absence of crackles and wheezes on auscultation
- Is free from ***infection*** as evidenced by absence of fever and a WBC count within normal limits
- Avoids empyema
- Returns to his or her pre-pneumonia health status

NCLEX EXAMINATION CHALLENGE 28.2

Safe and Effective Care Environment

A nurse assessing an older adult client with pneumonia notes the client is now confused and the oxygen saturation has dropped since the last assessment 1 hour ago from 90% to 84%. The nurse also notes the respiratory rate has increased from 26 to 32. What is the nurse's **best first** action?

A. Encourage the client to use the incentive spirometer hourly.
B. Increase her O_2 flow rate by 2 L and reassess in 5 minutes.
C. Increase the flow rate of the IV antibiotic.
D. Document the changes as the only action.

INFECTION CONCEPT EXEMPLAR: PULMONARY TUBERCULOSIS

Pathophysiology Review

Tuberculosis (TB) is a highly communicable disease caused by ***infection*** with *Mycobacterium tuberculosis.* It is one of the most common bacterial infections worldwide and one of the top 10 causes of death (World Health Organization [WHO], 2019). The organism is transmitted via *aerosolization* (i.e., an airborne route) (Fig. 28.2). When a person with active TB coughs, laughs, sneezes, whistles, or sings, infected respiratory droplets become airborne and may be inhaled by others. Not all TB infections actually develop into active TB (American Lung Association [ALA], 2018). This is because the normal protection of immunity prevents full development of TB in the healthy person (McCance et al., 2019). (***Immunity*** is the protection from illness or disease that is maintained by the body's physiologic defense mechanisms.)

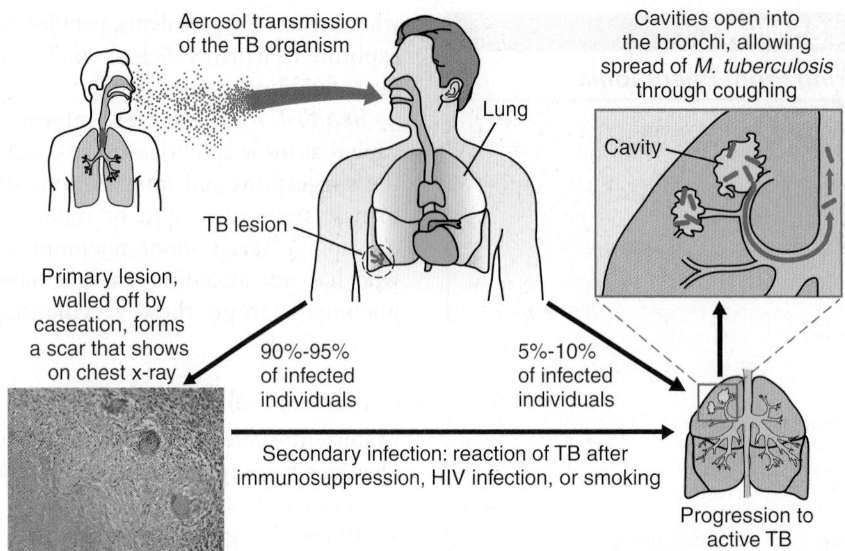

FIG. 28.2 Primary TB infection with progression to secondary infection and active disease. *HIV,* Human immune deficiency virus; *M. tuberculosis, Mycobacterium tuberculosis; TB,* tuberculosis. (Illustration from Workman, M. L., & LaCharity, L. [2016]. Understanding pharmacology [2nd ed.]. St. Louis: Saunders; photo from Kumar, V., Abbas, A., & Aster, J. [2015]. *Robbins and Cotran pathologic basis for disease* [9th ed.]. Philadelphia: Saunders.)

The bacillus multiplies freely when it reaches a susceptible site (bronchi or alveoli). An ***inflammation*** and exudative response occurs, causing pneumonitis. With the development of acquired immunity to TB, further growth of bacilli is controlled in most cases. The lesions usually resolve and leave little or no residual bacilli. *Only a small percentage of adults infected with the bacillus ever develop active TB.*

Cell-mediated ***immunity*** against TB develops 2 to 10 weeks after initial ***infection*** and is manifested by a positive reaction to a tuberculin test. The primary infection may be so small that it does not appear on a chest x-ray. The process of TB infection occurs in this order:

1. The granulomatous ***inflammation*** created by the TB bacillus in the lung becomes surrounded by collagen, fibroblasts, and lymphocytes.
2. *Caseation necrosis,* which is necrotic tissue being turned into a granular mass, occurs in the center of the lesion. If this area shows on x-ray, it is the *primary* lesion.

Areas of caseation then undergo resorption, degeneration, and fibrosis. These necrotic areas may calcify *(calcification)* or liquefy *(liquefaction).* If liquefaction occurs, this material then empties into a bronchus and the emptied area becomes a cavity *(cavitation).* Bacilli continue to grow in the necrotic cavity wall and spread the ***infection*** through the lymph channels into new areas of the lung.

A lesion also may grow by direct extension if bacilli multiply rapidly during ***inflammation***. The lesions can extend through the pleura, resulting in pleural or pericardial effusion. **Miliary** or **hematogenous TB** is the spread of TB throughout the body when a large number of organisms enter the blood. Many tiny nodules scattered throughout the lung are seen on chest x-ray. Other body areas can become infected as a result of this spread.

Initial infection is seen more often in the upper lobes of the lung. The local lymph nodes are infected and enlarged. An asymptomatic period usually follows the primary ***infection*** and can last for years or decades before clinical symptoms develop. This is called *latent TB. An infected person is not contagious to others until symptoms of disease occur.*

Secondary TB is a reactivation of the disease in a previously infected person. It is more likely to occur when ***immunity*** is reduced, especially among older adults, those with chronic diseases, and those with HIV disease.

Etiology

M. tuberculosis is a slow-growing, acid-fast rod transmitted via the airborne route. Adults most often infected are those having repeated close contact with an infectious person who has not yet been diagnosed with TB. The risk for ***infection*** transmission is reduced after an adult with active TB has received proper drug therapy for 2 to 3 weeks, clinical improvement occurs, and acid-fast bacilli (AFB) in the sputum are reduced.

Incidence and Prevalence

Worldwide, 10 million people were diagnosed and an additional 1.6 million people died from TB in 2017 (WHO, 2019). About 23% (1.7 billion) of the world's population has latent TB. In the United States, over 9100 new cases of TB were diagnosed in 2017 (CDC, 2018e). The incidence of TB has been steadily decreasing in North America. The world areas in which the incidence of TB continues to increase include many less affluent countries. In North America, the adults who are at greatest risk for development of TB are:

- Those in constant, frequent contact with an untreated infected person
- Those who have reduced ***immunity*** or HIV disease
- Adults who live in crowded areas such as long-term care facilities, prisons, homeless shelters, and mental health facilities
- Older homeless adults
- Users of injection drugs or alcohol
- Lower socioeconomic groups
- Foreign immigrants from less affluent countries

Health Promotion and Maintenance

Many adults who acquire TB have risk factors such as homelessness, living in very crowded conditions, or substance use with malnutrition. These risk factors are best managed on a societal level. Communities need to work toward providing adequate housing, substance-use programs that are accessible, and feeding centers or food banks for those in need. On a personal level, many health conditions make it more likely to contract TB if exposed. Adults with these health conditions should avoid people who are ill, stay well nourished, and practice good handwashing and social distancing. Any adult who works with people at high risk of having TB should be screened yearly.

❖ Interprofessional Collaborative Care

TB is a disorder with a long period of treatment and care. It can affect every aspect of a patient's life, and care is best provided by an interprofessional team.

INTERPROFESSIONAL COLLABORATION

The Patient With Tuberculosis

In addition to primary health care providers and nurses, other professionals important to ensuring optimal management include registered dietician nutritionists (RDNs), pharmacists, social workers, patient navigators, and community health workers. Just as for any chronic disorder, TB management is most effective when the patient and family are full partners with the health care team.

◆ Assessment: Recognize Cues

Early detection of TB depends on patient reports rather than observable indicators. TB has a slow onset, and patients are often not aware of problems until the disease is advanced. *TB is considered for any patient with a persistent cough and other symptoms, such as unintended weight loss, anorexia, night sweats, hemoptysis, shortness of breath, fever, or chills* (Johnson et al., 2017).

History. Assess the patient's past exposure to TB. Ask about his or her country of origin and travel to or from foreign countries where incidence of TB is high (Benkert & Rayford, 2018). It is important to ask about the results of any previous tests for TB. Also ask whether the patient has had bacille Calmette-Guérin (BCG) vaccine (often given in childhood overseas), which contains attenuated tubercle bacilli. *Anyone who has received BCG vaccine within the previous 10 years will have a positive skin test that can complicate interpretation for current TB* ***infection***. Usually the size of the skin response decreases each year after BCG vaccination. These patients should be evaluated for TB with a chest x-ray or an interferon-gamma release assay (IGRA), such as the QuantiFERON-TB Gold test (CDC, 2018e; WHO, 2019).

Physical Assessment/Signs and Symptoms. The patient with TB has progressive fatigue, lethargy, nausea, anorexia, weight loss, irregular menses, and a low-grade fever. Symptoms may have been present for weeks or months. Night sweats may occur with the fever. A cough with mucopurulent sputum, often streaked with blood, is present. Chest tightness and a dull, aching chest pain occur with the cough. Ask about, assess for, and document the presence of any of these symptoms to help with diagnosis, establish a baseline, and plan nursing interventions.

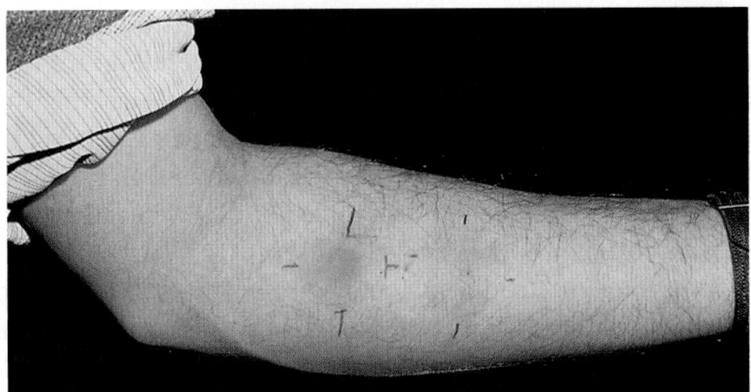

FIG. 28.3 Positive tuberculin skin test with induration on the left. The spot on the right is a negative control test site. (From Zitelli, B. J., McIntire, S. C., & Nowalk, A. J. [2012]. *Zitelli and Davis' atlas of pediatric physical diagnosis* [6th ed.]. Philadelphia: Saunders; courtesy Kenneth Schuitt, MD.)

When assessing the patient, you may note dullness with percussion over the involved lung fields, bronchial breath sounds, crackles, and increased transmission of spoken or whispered sounds. Partial obstruction of a bronchus from the disease or compression by lymph nodes may produce localized wheezing.

Psychosocial Assessment. Tuberculosis is a frightening diagnosis. Explain the disease to the patient and family, including the need to maintain good hygiene and avoid infecting others. The patient may feel isolated and shunned. Take time to listen to him or her and help to resolve any concerns. The family and friends of the patient may have similar concerns as well. Often close contacts will be afraid they have contracted the illness. Encourage all close contacts to get tested. Help the patient notify his or her employer, if needed, about required time off. Directly observed therapy may feel threatening. Explain how this helps improve adherence to the long treatment schedule.

Diagnostic Assessment. TB infection can be tested by methods. In addition to chest x-ray, sputum cultures of blood or respiratory secretions can be tested. Many fully automated nucleic acid amplification tests (NAATs) for TB are used on respiratory secretions. Results of these tests are available in less than 2 hours; however, they have limitations.

Tuberculin skin testing (TST), also known as the Mantoux test, is the most commonly used reliable screening test for TB. A small amount (0.1 mL) of purified protein derivative (PPD) is placed intradermally in the forearm. The test is "read" in 48 to 72 hours. An area of **induration** (localized swelling with hardness of soft tissue), not just redness, measuring 10 mm or greater in diameter, indicates exposure to and possible infection with TB (Fig. 28.3). In adults with reduced ***immunity***, induration of 5 mm is a positive result. If possible, the site is re-evaluated after 72 hours because false-negative readings occur more often after only 48 hours. *A positive reaction indicates exposure to TB or the presence of inactive (dormant) disease, not active disease. A reduced skin reaction or a negative skin test does not rule out TB disease or infection of the very old or anyone who has severely reduced* ***immunity***. Failure to have a skin response because of reduced immunity when infection is present is called **anergy**.

Blood analysis can be done with interferon-gamma release assays, or IGRAs. The first IGRA was the QuantiFERON-TB

Gold In-Tube test. IGRAs show how the patient's immune system responds to the TB bacterium. A positive result means that the person is infected with TB but does not indicate whether the ***infection*** is latent or active. Another blood test, the Xpert MTB/RIF Ultra, which can detect drug-resistant strains of TB and is also recommended for testing people with HIV infection, has been approved by both the CDC and WHO.

Sputum culture confirms the diagnosis and is also used to evaluate treatment effectiveness. Enhanced TB cultures take up to 4 weeks for a valid result. After drug therapy is started, sputum samples are obtained at specified intervals. Cultures are usually negative after 3 months of effective treatment.

Annual screening is needed for anyone who comes into contact with people who may be infected with TB, including some health care workers. Screening is very important for foreign-born adults and migrant workers. Participation in screening programs is higher when programs are delivered in a culturally sensitive and nonthreatening manner. Urge anyone who is considered high risk to have an annual TB screening test.

Imaging Assessment. Once a person's skin test is positive for TB, a chest x-ray is used to detect active TB or old, healed lesions. Calcifications usually indicate old, healed lesions. Caseation and ***inflammation*** may be seen on the x-ray if the disease is active (McCance et al., 2019). The chest x-rays of HIV-infected patients may be normal or may show infiltrates in any lung zone and lymph node enlargement.

◆ Analysis: Analyze Cues and Prioritize Hypotheses

The priority collaborative problems for patients with TB include:

1. Potential for airway obstruction due to thick secretions and weak cough effort
2. Potential for development of drug-resistant disease and spread of ***infection*** due to inadequate adherence to therapy regimen
3. Weight loss due to inadequate intake and nausea from therapy regimen
4. Fatigue due to lengthy illness, poor ***gas exchange,*** and increased energy demands

◆ Planning and Implementation: Generate Solutions and Take Action

Promoting Airway Clearance

Planning: Expected Outcomes. The patient with TB is expected to maintain a patent and adequate airway.

Interventions. Interventions to maintain a patent airway are similar to those for pneumonia and COPD. Instruct the patient to drink plenty of fluids unless another condition requires restriction. Teach him or her to take a deep breath before coughing. An incentive spirometer may facilitate effective coughing.

Reducing Drug-Resistance and Infection Spread

Planning: Expected Outcomes. The patient with TB is expected to become free of active disease and not spread the disease to others.

Interventions. Interventions to help the patient become free of active disease are focused on antimicrobial therapy and ***infection*** control measures.

Combination drug therapy is the most effective method of treating active TB and preventing transmission (Burchum & Rosenthal, 2019). Therapy continues until the disease is under control. Multiple-drug regimens kill or suppress the growth of organisms as quickly as possible and reduce the emergence of drug-resistant organisms. First-line therapy for non–drug-resistant (drug-susceptible) TB is listed in the Common Examples of Drug Therapy: First-Line Treatment for Tuberculosis box and uses isoniazid, rifampin, pyrazinamide, and ethambutol for the first 8 weeks (initial treatment phase). The continuation phase for most patients lasts another 18 weeks for drug-susceptible TB, and the patient takes isoniazid and rifampin either daily or twice a week (CDC, 2018e). (Some of the same drugs are also used for shorter time periods to treat latent TB infections.) Patients who remain culture positive after 8 weeks and those who are HIV positive but not taking antiretroviral therapy may require 7 months of continuation therapy. These drugs are now available in two- or three-drug combinations. Variations of the first-line drugs along with other drug types, such as fluoroquinolone and aminoglycoside antibiotics, are used when the patient does not tolerate the standard first-line therapy. Nursing interventions focus on patient teaching for drug therapy adherence and infection control.

Strict adherence to the prescribed drug regimen is crucial for suppressing the disease. Adherence is difficult because of the long duration of treatment. (Duration of therapy is often 26 weeks but can be as long as 2 years for multidrug-resistant [MDR] TB.) Thus your major role is educating the patient about drug therapy and stressing the importance of taking each drug regularly, exactly as prescribed, for as long as it is prescribed. Provide accurate information in multiple formats, such as pamphlets, videos, and drug-schedule worksheets. To determine whether the patient understands how to take the drugs, ask him or her to describe the treatment regimen, side effects, and when to call the health care agency and primary health care provider.

The patient with TB often has concerns about the disease prognosis. Offer a positive outlook for the patient who adheres to the drug regimen. *However, with current resistant strains of TB, emphasize that not taking the drugs as prescribed could lead to a drug-resistant* ***infection****.*

! NURSING SAFETY PRIORITY (QSEN)

Drug Alert

The first-line drugs used as therapy for TB all can damage the liver. Warn the patient to not drink any alcoholic beverages for the entire duration of TB therapy.

NCLEX EXAMINATION CHALLENGE 28.3

Health Promotion and Maintenance

A client who has been taking the four first-line drugs for tuberculosis treatment for a month reports all of the following changes. Which changes would cause the nurse to collaborate quickly with the health care provider? **Select all that apply.**

A. Blurry vision
B. Constipation
C. Difficulty sleeping
D. Nausea when drinking beer
E. Red-tinged urine
F. Sunburn with minimal sun exposure
G. Yellowing of the sclera

Some *multidrug-resistant TB* (MDR TB) strains are emerging as extensively drug-resistant (XDR TB). MDR TB is an infection that resists INH and rifampin. XDR TB is resistant not only to the first-line antituberculosis drugs but also to the second-line antibiotics, including the fluoroquinolones and at least one of the aminoglycosides. The WHO estimates that 4% to 5% of all TB cases are drug resistant (WHO, 2019). The most common cause of MDR TB and XDR TB is mismanagement of drug therapy, either from inappropriate selection or use of antibiotics. Patients with acquired immune deficiency syndrome (AIDS; HIV-III) also often have MDR TB (WHO, 2018). *Patients who contract TB from a person with a resistant strain will also have a resistant strain of TB.* So teaching patients to adhere to their drug regimens will also help them prevent the spread of the disease in both forms.

Drug therapy for MDR TB and XDR TB is limited and requires higher doses for longer periods. Bedaquiline is specifically targeted to multidrug-resistant TB. Side effects of this drug can be life threatening, so it is not used when other drugs will work. It should be given through directly observed therapy

! NURSING SAFETY PRIORITY (QSEN)

Drug Alert

Bedaquiline can prolong the QT interval, cause ventricular dysrhythmias, and lead to sudden death. Patients on this drug need to have regular ECGs and serum electrolyte evaluations.

! NURSING SAFETY PRIORITY (QSEN)

Action Alert

Warn patients with extensively drug-resistant TB that absolute adherence to therapy is critical for survival and cure of the disease. These patients should receive directly observed therapy (DOT) (described under the "Self-Management Education" section).

COMMON EXAMPLES OF DRUG THERAPY

First-Line Treatment for Tuberculosis

Drug and Action	Nursing Implications
Isoniazid Kills actively growing mycobacteria outside the cell and inhibits the growth of dormant bacteria inside macrophages and caseating granulomas	Instruct patients to avoid antacids and to take the drug on an empty stomach (1 hour before or 2 hours after meals) *to prevent slowing of drug absorption in the GI tract.* Teach patients to take a daily multiple vitamin that contains the B-complex vitamins while on this drug *because the drug can deplete the body of this vitamin.* Remind patients to avoid alcoholic beverages while on this drug *because the liver-damaging effects of this drug are potentiated by alcohol.* Tell patients to report darkening of the urine, a yellow appearance to the skin or whites of the eyes, and an increased tendency to bruise or bleed, *which are signs and symptoms of liver toxicity or failure.*
Rifampin Kills slower-growing organisms, even those that reside inside macrophages and caseating granulomas	Warn patients to expect an orange-reddish staining of the skin and urine and all other secretions to have a reddish-orange tinge; also, soft contact lenses will become permanently stained *because knowing the expected side effects decreases anxiety when they appear.* Instruct sexually active women using oral contraceptives to use an additional method of contraception while taking this drug and for 1 month after stopping it *because this drug reduces the effectiveness of oral contraceptives.* Remind patients to avoid alcoholic beverages while on this drug *because the liver-damaging effects of this drug are potentiated by alcohol.* Tell patients to report darkening of the urine, a yellow appearance to the skin or whites of the eyes, and an increased tendency to bruise or bleed, *which are signs and symptoms of liver toxicity or failure.* Ask patients about all other drugs in use *because this drug interacts with many other drugs.*
Pyrazinamide Can effectively kill organisms residing within the very acidic environment of macrophages (which is where the tuberculosis bacillus sequesters) Available only in combination with other anti-TB drugs	Ask patients if they have ever had gout *because the drug increases uric acid formation and will make gout worse.* Instruct patients to drink at least 8 ounces of water when taking this tablet and to increase fluid intake *to prevent uric acid from precipitating, making gout or kidney problems worse.* Teach patients to wear protective clothing, a hat, and sunscreen when going outdoors in the sunlight *because the drug causes photosensitivity and greatly increases the risk for sunburn.* Remind patients to avoid alcoholic beverages while on this drug *because the liver-damaging effects of this drug are potentiated by alcohol.* Tell patients to report darkening of the urine, a yellow appearance to the skin or whites of the eyes, and an increased tendency to bruise or bleed, *which are signs and symptoms of liver toxicity or failure.*
Ethambutol Inhibits bacterial RNA synthesis, thus suppressing bacterial growth Slow acting and bacteriostatic rather than bactericidal; thus it must be used in combination with other anti-TB drugs	Instruct patients to report any changes in vision, such as reduced color vision, blurred vision, or reduced visual fields, immediately to his or her primary health care provider *because the drug can cause optic neuritis, especially at high doses, and can lead to blindness.* Minor eye problems are usually reversed when the drug is stopped. Remind patients to avoid alcoholic beverages while on this drug *because the drug induces severe nausea and vomiting when alcohol is ingested.* Ask patients if they have ever had gout because the drug increases uric acid formation and will make gout worse. Instruct patients to drink at least 8 ounces of water when taking this drug and to increase fluid intake *to prevent uric acid from precipitating, making gout or kidney problems worse.*

(DOT). The drug delamanid has been approved by WHO and the regulatory bodies for other countries for use alone, in combination with bedaquiline, or following bedaquiline therapy with multidrug-resistant TB. It is currently in clinical trials with the U.S. Food and Drug Administration (FDA).

The hospitalized patient with active TB is placed on Airborne Precautions (see Chapter 21) in a well-ventilated room that has at least six exchanges of fresh air per minute. All health care workers must use a personal respirator when caring for the patient. Use Standard Precautions with appropriate protection as with all patients. Airborne Precautions are discontinued when the patient is no longer contagious.

Other care issues for the patient with TB include teaching about ***infection*** prevention and what to expect about disease monitoring and participating in activities. TB is often treated outside the acute care setting, with the patient convalescing at home. Airborne Precautions are not necessary in this setting because family members have already been exposed; however, all members of the household need to undergo TB testing. Teach the patient to cover the mouth and nose with a tissue when coughing or sneezing, to place used tissues in plastic bags, to wear a mask when in contact with crowds, and to use social distancing until the drugs suppress infection.

Tell the patient that sputum specimens are needed about every 4 weeks once drug therapy is initiated. When the results of three consecutive sputum cultures are negative, the patient is no longer infectious (contagious) and may return to former activities. Remind him or her to avoid exposure to any inhalation irritants because these can cause further lung damage.

Improving Nutrition

Planning: Expected Outcomes. The patient with TB is expected to have improved nutrition.

Interventions. The patient with TB often has a long-standing history of malnutrition. Conduct a nutrition assessment using an evidence-based tool. Determine patient likes/dislikes, the ability to buy healthy food, condition of teeth or dentures, weight and body mass index, and history of substance use. When inadequate nutrition is a problem, be sure to include a registered dietitian nutritionist (RDN) as part of the interprofessional team.

Drugs to treat TB often cause nausea. If this happens, instruct the patient to take once-a-day drugs at night. Antiemetics can also be prescribed. If food doesn't interfere with the drug absorption (check the label), taking pills with a small snack of simple carbohydrates may help. Refer the patient to Meals on Wheels or other meal-delivery service. Instruct him or her about good oral hygiene, which makes food taste better. Monitor weight weekly and document trends to determine the effectiveness of nutrition interventions.

For best healing, the patient needs a diet with quality proteins; iron; vitamins A, B, C, and E; and abundant fresh produce. Educate him or her about nutrition in collaboration with an RDN. Tell the patient to avoid alcohol. Alcohol can cause liver damage, and so can most of the antituberculosis drugs. Alcohol is also a source of "empty calories," and adults who drink alcohol to excess are often malnourished. An adult who gets a large number of calories from alcohol will not feel hungry. A special problem for this group of patients is lack of phosphorus, which is part of the cellular energy compound ATP. With low phosphorus, the patient will lack energy. Refer the patient to support groups if alcoholism or other substance abuse is present. Improved nutrition will help improve ***immunity***.

Managing Fatigue

Planning: Expected Outcomes. The patient with TB is expected to have improved stamina and less fatigue.

Interventions. Many of the interventions for fatigue will be the same as those for improving nutrition. Poor nutrition can lead directly to fatigue. Encourage the patient to resume activities slowly and get plenty of rest. Reassure him or her that the fatigue will improve as therapy progresses and the disease is controlled. Assess the patient's sleep-wake habits and encourage a full night's sleep with short daytime naps. Help him or her develop a healthy bedtime ritual if needed. Mental stamina may be decreased as a result of the lengthy convalescence. Reassure the patient that, by taking drugs as directed, the disease will be cured and energy levels will increase.

Care Coordination and Transition Management

Home Care Management. Most patients with TB are managed outside the hospital; however, patients may be diagnosed with TB while in the hospital for another problem. Discharge may be delayed if the living situation is high risk or if nonadherence to prescribed drug therapy is likely. Ensure collaboration with other members of the interprofessional team, including the case manager or social service worker in the hospital or the community health nursing agency, to ensure that the patient is discharged to the appropriate environment with continued supervision.

Self-Management Education. Teach the patient to follow the drug regimen exactly as prescribed and always to have a supply on hand. Teach about side effects and ways of reducing them to promote adherence. Remind him or her that the disease is usually no longer contagious after drugs have been taken for 2 to 3 consecutive weeks and clinical improvement is seen; however, *he or she must continue with the prescribed drugs for 6 months or longer as prescribed. Directly observed therapy,* in which a health care professional watches the patient swallow the drugs, may be indicated in some situations. This practice leads to more treatment successes, fewer relapses, and less drug resistance. More recently, DOT has been successfully performed using a video format (VDOT) in which patients use a phone or other real-time electronic device to demonstrate compliance with the drug regimen. This method helps patients "live their lives" without having to physically come to a place for DOT. Drawbacks to this method include whether the patient is willing and able to use such a device and how good the connectivity is for both the patient's device and the nurse's access to the video (Ingram, 2018).

The patient who has weight loss and severe lethargy should gradually resume usual activities. Proper nutrition is needed to prevent infection recurrence.

Provide the patient with information about how TB can be spread to others. A key to preventing ***infection*** transmission is identifying those in close contact with the infected person so that they can be tested and treated if needed. Multidrug therapy may be indicated to prevent TB in heavily exposed adults or for those who have other health problems that reduce ***immunity***.

Health Care Resources. Teach the patient to receive follow-up care by a primary health care provider for at least 1 year after active treatment. The American Lung Association (ALA) can provide free information to the patient about the disease and its treatment. In addition, Alcoholics Anonymous (AA) and other health care resources for patients with alcoholism are available if needed. Inform patients who smoke or vape that smoking and vaping further reduce breathing effectiveness. Use the suggestions and interventions discussed in Chapter 24 to help the patient quit or reduce cigarette smoking. Assist the patient who uses illicit drugs to locate a drug-treatment program.

◆ Evaluation: Evaluate Outcomes

Evaluate the care of the patient with TB based on the identified priority patient problems. The expected outcomes are that he or she:

- Effectively clears his or her airways as evidenced by absence of crackles and wheezes on auscultation
- Is free of active TB and does not spread the ***infection***
- Demonstrates improved nutrition as evidenced by weight maintenance or weight gain
- Reports decreased fatigue and increased energy and is able to participate in activities to the extent he or she desires
- Returns to his or her pretuberculosis health status

RHINOSINUSITIS

Pathophysiology Review

Rhinosinusitis is an ***inflammation*** of the mucous membranes of one or more of the sinuses and is usually seen with rhinitis, especially the common cold *(coryza)*. Anything that interferes with sinus drainage (e.g., deviated nasal septum, nasal polyps or tumors, inhaled air pollutants or cocaine, allergies, facial trauma, and dental infection) can lead to rhinosinusitis. Even when the problem starts with a noninfectious cause such as seasonal allergies, swelling and inflammation block the flow of secretions from the sinuses, which may then become infected.

Most episodes of rhinosinusitis are caused by viral ***infection*** and usually develop in the maxillary and frontal sinuses, although bacterial infection can also occur. Complications include cellulitis, abscess, and meningitis.

❖ Interprofessional Collaborative Care

Rhinosinusitis is usually managed as an outpatient problem. Even when sinus surgery is needed, it usually takes place in an ambulatory surgical setting.

Assess for signs and symptoms of rhinosinusitis, which include pain over the cheek radiating to the teeth, tenderness to percussion over the sinuses, referred pain to the temple or back of the head, and general facial pain that is worse when bending forward. In bacterial ***infection***, purulent nasal drainage with postnasal drip, sore throat, fever, erythema, swelling, fatigue, dental pain, and ear pressure may be present.

Management focuses on symptom relief and patient education. Teach him or her about correct use of the drug therapy prescribed. Also teach the patient to use the techniques described for reducing the transmission of influenza infection.

CLINICAL JUDGMENT CHALLENGE 28.1

Safety; Patient-Centered Care; Evidence-Based Practice

The client is a 66-year-old homeless Vietnam veteran admitted this morning for a compound fracture of the left femur with hemorrhaging sustained when he was hit by a motorcycle. He usually sleeps outdoors in warmer weather and uses a variety of shelters now that it is winter. Surgery is planned for later today. The bleeding is now under control and he has received three units of packed red blood cells. He received morphine 3 mg IV push in the emergency department just before coming to the unit and now reports his pain as a 4 on a 0 to 10 scale. The nurse performing the admission assessment records these vital signs: temperature 101.6°F (38.7°C), heart rate 102, respiratory rate 22, blood pressure 110/84, and oxygen saturation 92%. The nurse notes the client is quite dirty and gaunt appearing. He says he is 6 feet (1.83 m) tall and his admitting weight is 129 lb (58.5 kg). He reports being homeless for 5 years after losing his job as a welder, when he was found using IV drugs while at work. He tells the nurse that the shelter is noisy and he is always tired because he doesn't sleep well. During the assessment, he coughed frequently (without covering his mouth) and produced thick greenish sputum with bloody streaks.

1. **Recognize Cues:** What assessment information in this client situation is the most important and immediate concern for the nurse? (Hint: Identify the **relevant** information *first* to determine what is most important.)
2. **Analyze Cues:** What client conditions are consistent with the **most relevant** information? (Hint: Think about priority collaborative problems that support and contradict the information presented in this situation.)
3. **Prioritize Hypotheses:** Which possibilities or explanations are **most likely** to be present in this client situation? Which possibilities or explanations are the most serious? (Hint: Consider all possibilities and determine their urgency and risk for this client.)
4. **Generate Solutions:** What actions would most likely achieve the desired outcomes for this client? Which actions should be **avoided** or are **potentially harmful**? (Hint: Determine the desired outcomes first to decide which interventions are appropriate and those that should be avoided.)
5. **Take Action:** Which actions are the most appropriate and how should they be implemented? In what **priority order** should they be implemented? (Hint: Consider health teaching, documentation, requested health care provider orders or prescriptions, nursing skills, collaboration with or referral to health team members, etc.)
6. **Evaluate Outcomes:** What client assessment would indicate that the nurse's actions were **effective**? (Hint: Think about signs that would indicate an improvement, decline, or unchanged client condition.)

Drug therapy includes decongestants, antihistamines, and intranasal steroid spray to block or reduce the amount of chemical mediators in nasal and sinus tissues and relieve local ***inflammation***. Antipyretics are given for fever, and analgesics may be given for pain.

PATIENT-CENTERED CARE: OLDER ADULT CONSIDERATIONS (QSEN)

First-generation antihistamines may not be appropriate drugs for older adults because these patients often have reduced drug clearance, higher risk for confusion, and anticholinergic effects such as dry mouth and constipation. Common drugs to avoid in this category include chlorpheniramine, diphenhydramine, and hydroxyzine. Teach older adults why they should not self-medicate with these drugs.

Treatment for bacterial rhinosinusitis includes broad-spectrum antibiotics, decongestants, and antipyretics. In some cases, nasal steroids or systemic steroids may be prescribed.

! NURSING SAFETY PRIORITY QSEN

Action Alert

Instruct patients with any bacterial infection to complete the entire antibiotic prescription, even when symptoms improve or subside. This action will help eradicate the organism and prevent development of resistant bacterial strains.

Supportive therapy such as humidification, nasal irrigation, and applying hot wet packs over the sinus area can increase the patient's comfort and help prevent spread of the ***infection***. Instruct the patient about the importance of rest and increased fluid intake. Sleeping with the head of the bed elevated and avoiding cigarette smoke may reduce discomfort.

PERITONSILLAR ABSCESS

Peritonsillar abscess (PTA) is a rare complication of acute bacterial tonsillitis. ***Infection*** spreads from the tonsil to the surrounding tissue and forms an abscess that can become large enough to obstruct the airway.

Signs and symptoms include a collection of pus behind the tonsil causing swelling on one side of the throat, pushing the uvula toward the unaffected side. The patient may have severe throat pain radiating to the ear or teeth, a muffled voice, fever, and difficulty swallowing. He or she may also have spasms and pain of the muscles used in chewing *(trismus)* and difficulty breathing. Bad breath is present, and lymph nodes on the affected side are swollen.

Most patients can be treated as outpatients with antibiotics, although some may need steroids to reduce the swelling. Drainage of the abscess may be needed. *Stress the importance of completing the antibiotic regimen and coming to the emergency department quickly if symptoms of obstruction (drooling and stridor) appear.*

INHALATION ANTHRAX

Pathophysiology Review

Inhalation anthrax (respiratory anthrax) is a bacterial ***infection*** caused by the gram-positive organism *Bacillus anthracis.* This organism lives as a spore in soil where grass-eating animals live and graze. Most naturally occurring cases of anthrax are on the skin (cutaneous). Inhalation anthrax accounts for only about 5% of cases and is not spread by person-to-person contact. When infection occurs through the lungs, the disease is nearly 100% fatal without treatment (CDC, 2017). Although inhalation anthrax is an occupational hazard of veterinarians, farmers, and others who frequently contact animal wool, hides, bone meal, and skin, any occurrence in other adults is considered an intentional act of bioterrorism.

! NURSING SAFETY PRIORITY QSEN

Action Alert

Inhalation anthrax is rare; thus any occurrence in a person who does not have an occupational risk is considered an intentional act of bioterrorism. Report the presence of symptoms consistent with inhalation anthrax to hospital authorities immediately.

This organism first forms a *spore* (i.e., an encapsulated organism that is inactive). When many spores are inhaled deeply into the lungs, they enter white blood cells (WBCs), leave their capsules, and replicate. The active bacteria produce toxins that are released into the infected tissues and into the blood, making the infection worse. Massive edema occurs along with hemorrhage and destruction of lung cells. Infected WBCs spread the organisms rapidly to the lymph nodes and blood, causing bacteremia, sepsis, and meningitis. Lethal toxins produced by the bacteria are the most common cause of death.

Inhalation anthrax has two stages: *prodromal* (or incubation period) and *fulminant* (with active disease). Symptoms (listed in the Key Features: Inhalation Anthrax box) may take up to 8 weeks to develop after exposure.

The prodromal stage is early and difficult to distinguish from influenza or pneumonia. Symptoms include low-grade fever, fatigue, mild chest pain, and a dry, harsh cough. *A special feature of inhalation anthrax is that it is* ***not*** *accompanied by upper respiratory symptoms of sore throat or rhinitis.* Usually the patient starts to feel better and symptoms improve in 2 to 4 days. If the diagnosis is made and the patient begins appropriate antibiotic therapy at this stage, the likelihood of survival is high.

The fulminant stage begins after the patient feels a little better. Usually there is a sudden onset of severe illness, including respiratory distress, *hematemesis* (bloody vomit), dyspnea, diaphoresis, stridor, chest pain, and cyanosis. High fever, hemorrhagic mediastinitis, and pleural effusions develop. As the infection spreads through the blood, septic shock and hemorrhagic meningitis develop. Death often occurs within 24 to 36 hours even if antibiotics are started in this stage.

KEY FEATURES

Inhalation Anthrax

Prodromal Stage (Early)	Fulminant Stage (Late)
• Fever	• Diaphoresis
• Fatigue	• Stridor on inhalation and exhalation
• Mild chest pain	• Hypoxia
• Dry cough	• High fever
• No indications of upper respiratory infection	• Mediastinitis
• Mediastinal "widening" on chest x-ray	• Pleural effusion
	• Hypotension
	• Septic shock

TABLE 28.4 Common Organisms Associated With Endemic Respiratory Infection in North America

Disorder/Organism	Source	Geographic Area	Management for Moderate to Severe Disease or Special Populations
Hantavirus pulmonary syndrome (HPS) *Hantavirus*	Urine, droppings, and saliva of infected rodents	Southwest United States, Mexico, Central America	Supportive Oxygen Mechanical ventilation in severe cases (38% fatal)
Aspergillosis *Aspergillus*	Common mold found indoors and outside in damp areas; may be extensive in older buildings; moist soil and decomposing wood and leaves	Can occur in any indoor environment damp enough to support mold growth Outdoor growth in San Francisco, Canada & United States around the Great Lakes; Ohio and Mississippi River Valleys	Supportive care Prolonged course of antifungal drugs Surgery may be needed in severe cases
Blastomycosis (fungal) *Blastomyces*	Moist soil, decomposing wood and leaves	Canada & United States around the Great Lakes; Ohio and Mississippi River Valleys	Supportive care Prolonged course of antifungal drugs
Coccidioidomycosis *Coccidioides*	Soil	Southwest, far west United States, Mexico, Central and South America	Supportive care Prolonged course of antifungal drugs
Cryptococcosis *Cryptococcus gattii*	Trees and soil beneath trees	U.S. Pacific coast regions, mid to southern British Columbia	Supportive care Prolonged course of antifungal drugs
Histoplasmosis *Histoplasma*	Soil containing large amounts of bird and bat droppings; surfaces with bird droppings	Central and eastern United States, especially areas around the Ohio and Mississippi River Valleys	Supportive care Prolonged course of antifungal drugs

❖ Interprofessional Collaborative Care

Organisms grown for bioterrorism may have been altered to be resistant to standard antibiotics. Therefore the antibiotics used for suspected or diagnosed inhalation anthrax include combinations of the following that have proven effective. These drugs include ciprofloxacin, doxycycline, amoxicillin, rifampin, clindamycin, and vancomycin. One or more of the same drugs are used individually to prevent illness when adults have been exposed to inhalation anthrax but do not yet have symptoms. An antitoxin (obiltoxaximab) has been approved to be added to the drug regimen once symptoms begin and the diagnosis has been made. The drug has improved survival rates but has many severe side effects.

Teach patients with any type of lower respiratory infection to especially watch for changes after they think they are getting well. They need to seek medical attention immediately on having a setback that starts with breathlessness.

ENDEMIC/GEOGRAPHIC RESPIRATORY INFECTION

Any organism can cause a pulmonary ***infection*** if the exposure is high enough, if the adult has little or no acquired ***immunity*** to it, or if the adult's general immune responses are reduced by age, drugs, or other health problems. A variety of respiratory infections are endemic, meaning that the causative organism is much more common within a geographic location, but even then the incidence of the infection is relatively low. Adults living in these areas have often developed some immunity to the organism over time and usually only develop the infection if they come into contact with large numbers of the organism or have a severely reduced immune response. Most commonly, the organisms are spore-forming fungi, although some viral infections also have endemic tendencies. Table 28.4 lists common endemic respiratory infections in North America.

These organisms are part of the environment. Healthy adults in endemic areas who are most susceptible to infection are those who have intense exposures. For soil-borne organisms, adults who dig in the soil, farm, or work in construction in which soil is disturbed can be heavily exposed. Everyone can be exposed when the soil is disturbed by dust storms, tornados, flooding, and other types of natural disasters. Working and living in buildings in which demolition and/or reconstruction are occurring can release spores trapped within walls that then become airborne. Working with or camping in areas with organisms that live in soil or decomposing wood and leaves can result in significant exposures.

All of these respiratory infections resemble influenza or pneumonia with fever, cough, headache, muscle aches, chest pain, and night sweats and are often misdiagnosed. Also, these infections are not contagious from person to person. Identification of the specific organism is important for specific treatment and prevention of complications. *Always ask anyone with respiratory infection symptoms whether they have visited endemic regions to help identify possible sources, expected courses, and appropriate management strategies.*

Depending on the health and ***immunity*** of the infected person and the number of spores present in the respiratory tract, the resulting infection can be mild, moderate, severe, or widely disseminated to other major organs. Special populations, such as older adults, pregnant women, and others who are immunocompromised are at greater risk for more severe disease. With fungal infections, a chronic infection state is possible. Fungal infections are difficult to eradicate. With moderate severity, oral antifungal agents may be prescribed for weeks to months. For more severe disease, IV antifungal agents, including amphotericin, may be needed initially and followed by long-term oral agents. Supportive care is similar to that provided for patients with influenza and pneumonia.

GET READY FOR THE NEXT-GENERATION NCLEX® EXAMINATION!

Key Points

Review these Key Points for each NCLEX Examination Client Needs Category.

Safe and Effective Care Environment

- Limit transmission of respiratory ***infection*** by washing hands after blowing the nose or using a tissue. **QSEN: Safety**
- Receive a yearly influenza vaccination because you are more likely to care for infected people and because you could spread influenza to adults who have reduced ***immunity***. **QSEN: Safety**
- When caring for a patient suspected to have COVID-19, wear an N95 mask and face shield, gown, gloves, and shoe coverings to prevent transmission. **QSEN: Safety**
- Use Airborne Precautions and Isolation Precautions for any patient who has TB symptoms until proven otherwise. **QSEN: Safety**
- Keep the door to the room of any patient with a respiratory infection closed until the cause of the infection is identified. **QSEN: Safety**
- Teach adults living with patients who have TB to ensure good ventilation of the home with open windows whenever possible. **QSEN: Safety**

Health Promotion and Maintenance

- Urge all adults older than 50 years, anyone who has a chronic respiratory problem, anyone who has reduced ***immunity***, and anyone who lives with a person who is older or immunocompromised or has a chronic respiratory disease to receive the pneumonia vaccine and yearly influenza vaccinations. **QSEN: Evidence-Based Practice**
- Teach all adults to wear a mask, engage in frequent handwashing, and to social distance to prevent the spread of COVID-19. **QSEN: Evidence-Based Practice**

Psychosocial Integrity

- Assess older patients with acute confusion for pneumonia (cough and fever may not be present). **QSEN: Evidence-Based Practice**
- Inform patients who have a positive TB test that far more adults are infected with the bacillus than have active TB disease. **QSEN: Patient-Centered Care**

Physiological Integrity

- Assess the respiratory status of any adult suspected of having a respiratory ***infection*** by taking vital signs, noting color of nail beds and mucous membranes, measuring oxygen saturation, determining ease of ventilation, determining cognition, and auscultating lung fields. **QSEN: Evidence-Based Practice**
- Ask any patient with a respiratory ***infection*** if he or she is from a foreign country, has recently visited a foreign country, or has recently traveled to other areas of his or her home country. **QSEN: Patient-Centered Care**
- Educate the family and the patient with TB who lives at home about the side effects of anti-TB therapy and when to notify the primary health care provider. **QSEN: Patient-Centered Care**
- Assess the patient receiving first-line drug therapy for TB for any symptoms of liver impairment (dark urine, clay-colored stools, anorexia, jaundiced sclera or hard palate). **QSEN: Patient-Centered Care**

MASTERY QUESTIONS

1. A nurse interviewing an 82-year-old, somewhat confused client who is becoming a nursing home resident today asks the client's daughter if she would consent for the client to receive an influenza vaccination today. The daughter replies "she had one 2 years ago and doesn't need another." What is the nurse's best response?
   A. "Your mother is older now and is more fragile, so she should have one this year, too, as a booster."
   B. "The virus causing influenza often changes each year, and a new influenza vaccination is needed every flu season."
   C. "The "flu shot" she had 2 years ago will still protect her this year, but if she has not had a previous pneumonia vaccination, she should have one now."
   D. "If you are worried that she is afraid to have an injection, we could use the nasal mist vaccination this year."
2. A nursing home client who has completed a 2-week course of antibiotics for bacterial pneumonia asks whether he can go out to a restaurant to celebrate his grandson's high school graduation if he uses a wheelchair. What is the nurse's best response?
   A. "No, going out now before you have recovered your strength can cause a relapse of the pneumonia."
   B. "No, the risk that you could spread this disease to other people is much too high."
   C. "Yes, if you want to and feel that you could tolerate a couple of hours of sitting."
   D. "Yes, if you agree to wear a face mask to prevent spreading droplets."
3. Which adults are at higher risk for development of active tuberculosis? **Select all that apply.**
   A. 21-year-old college student living in a dorm at a Canadian university
   B. 38-year-old with HIV-III (AIDS) who stopped taking antiretroviral therapy
   C. 42-year-old injection drug user
   D. 50-year-old Guatemalan migrant farm worker
   E. 62-year-old incarcerated in prison for 20 years
   F. 70-year-old with moderate to severe chronic obstructive pulmonary disease (COPD)

REFERENCES

American Lung Association (ALA). (2018). *Tuberculosis.* http://www.lung.org/lung-health-and-diseases/lung-disease-lookup/tuberculosis/?referrer=.

Anesi, G. (2020). Coronavirus disease 2019 (COVID-19): Critical care and airway management issues. In *UpToDate,* Manaker S. (Ed.). Waltham, MA.

Arsbad, H., Fasanya, A., Cheema, T., & Singh, A. (2016). Acute pneumonia. *Critical Care Nursing Quarterly, 39*(2), 148–160.

Benkert, R., & Rayford, A. (2018). Understanding tuberculosis in an era of global travel. *The Nurse Practitioner, 43*(2), 47–54.

Black, C., Yue, X., Ball, S., Fink, R., de Perio, M., Laney, S., et al. (2018). Influenza vaccination coverage among health care personnel-United States, 2017-18 influenza season. *Morbidity and Mortality Weekly Report, 67*(38), 1050–1054.

Burchum, J., & Rosenthal, L. (2019). *Lehne's pharmacology for nursing care* (10th ed.). St. Louis, MO: Elsevier.

Cannon, E., Bauer, R., Weust, J., & Southard, E. (2018). Nursing management of influenza. *Medsurg Nursing, 27*(2), 83–85.

Centers for Disease Control and Prevention (CDC). (2017). *Anthrax.* https://www.cdc.gov/anthrax/index.html.

Centers for Disease Control and Prevention (CDC). (2018a). *Key facts about influenza.* https://www.cdc.gov/flu/protect/keyfacts.htm.

Centers for Disease Control and Prevention (CDC). (2018b). *Pneumonia.* https://www.cdc.gov/penumonia/prevention.htm.

Centers for Disease Control and Prevention (CDC). (2018c). *Preventing the flu: Good health habits can help stop germs.* www.cdc.gov/flu/protect/habits/index.htm.

Centers for Disease Control and Prevention (CDC). (2018d). *Summary of the 2017-2018 influenza season.* http://www.cdc.gov/flu/about/flu-season-2017-2018.htm.

Centers for Disease Control and Prevention (CDC). (2018e). *Treatment for TB disease.* http://www.cdc.gov/tb/topic/treatment/tbdisease.htm.

Centers for Disease Control and Prevention (CDC). (2018f). *Prevention strategies for seasonal influenza in healthcare settings.* https://www.cdc.gov/flu/professionals/infectioncontrol/healthcaresettings.htm?fbclid=IwAR3HHfak58eWBBO3j5YjLmWFA_4n6X2BmYAWaepgVmHbO_H1QbFF1zTC4b4.

Centers for Disease Control and Prevention (CDC). (2019). *Estimated influenza illnesses, medical visits, hospitalizations, and deaths in the United States: 2018–2019 influenza season.* https://www.cdc.gov/flu/about/burden/2018-2019.html.

Centers for Disease Control and Prevention (CDC). (2020a). *COVID-19 in racial and ethnic minority groups.* https://www.cdc.gov/coronavirus/2019-ncov/need-extra-precautions/racial-ethnic-minorities/html.

CDC. (2020b). *Interim infection prevention and control recommendations for healthcare personnel during the coronavirus disease 2019 (COVID-19) pandemic.* https://www.cdc.gov/coronavirus/2019-ncov/hcp/infection-control-recommendations.html.

Centers for Disease Control and Prevention (CDC). (2020c). *COVID-19 testing overview.* https://www.cdc.gov/coronavirus/2019-ncov/symptoms-testing/testing.html?fbclid=IwAR3HHfak58eWBBO3j5YjLmWFA_4n6X2BmYAWaepgVmHbO_H1QbFF1zTC4b4.

Connor, K. (2018). Management of nosocomial pneumonia. *AACN Advanced Critical Care, 29*(1), 5–10.

Esden, J. (2020). Treatment update: Outpatient management of community-acquired pneumonia. *The Nurse Practitioner, 45*(3), 16–25.

Food and Drug Administration (FDA). (2020). *COVID-19 update: FDA broadens emergency use authorization for Veklury (remdesivir) to include all hospitalized patients for treatment of COVID-19.* https://www.fda.gov/news-events/press-announcements/covid-19-update-fda-broadens-emergency-use-authorization-veklury-remdesivir-include-all-hospitalized.

Giuliano, K., & Baker, D. (2020). Sepsis in the context of nonventilator hospital-acquired pneumonia. *American Journal of Critical Care, 29*(1), 9–14.

Goering, L. (2018). Pneumonia recovery: A plan can help. *Medsurg Nursing, 27*(5), 305–309, 330.

Ingram, D. (2018). Video directly observed therapy: Enhancing care patterns for patients with active tuberculosis. *Nursing, 48*(5), 64–66.

Johns Hopkins University (2020). *Coronavirus resource center.* https://coronavirus.jhu.edu/map.html.

Johnson, C., Moore, A., & Patterson-Johnson, J. (2017). Tuberculosis: Still an emerging threat. *The Nurse Practitioner, 42*(7), 46–51.

Kim, A., & Gandhi, R. (2020). Coronavirus disease 2019 (COVID-19): Management in hospitalized adults. In *UpToDate,* Hirsch. M. (Ed.). Waltham, MA.

McCance, K., Huether, S., Brashers, V., & Rote, N. (2019). *Pathophysiology: The biologic basis for disease in adults and children* (8th ed.). St. Louis: Mosby.

McIntosh, K. (2020). Coronavirus disease 2019 (COVID-19): Epidemiology, virology, clinical features, diagnosis, and prevention. In *UpToDate,* Hirsch, M. (Ed.). Waltham, MA.

Meehan, C., & McKenna, C. (2020). Preventing hospital-acquired pneumonia. *American Nurse Journal, 15*(2), 16–20.

Palmore, T. (2020). Cornavirus disease 2019 (COVID-19): Infection control in health care and home settings. In *UpToDate,* Sexton, D. (Ed.). Waltham, MA.

Pfeifer, G. (2018). 2018 flu vaccine recommendations for adults and children. *American Journal of Nursing, 118*(120), 13.

Phillips, A., & Swanson, M. (2016). Which pneumococcal vaccine and when? A guide for nurses. *American Nurse Today, 11*(11), 10–12.

Statistics Canada. (2018). *Deaths by cause.* Chapter X: Diseases of the respiratory system. http://www150.statcan.gc.ca/t1/tbl1/en/action?pid=1310078201.

Touhy, T., & Jett, K. (2020). *Ebersole and Hess' toward healthy aging: Human needs & nursing response* (9th ed.). St. Louis: Mosby.

World Health Organization (WHO). (2019). *Global tuberculosis report.* https://apps.who.int/iris/bitstream/handle/10665/329368/9789241565714-eng.pdf?ua=1.

World Health Organization (WHO). (2020). *Coronavirus deases (COVID-2019) situation reports.* https://www.who.int/energencies/diseases/novel-coronavirus-2019/situation-reports.

29

Critical Care of Patients With Respiratory Emergencies

Harry Rees

http://evolve.elsevier.com/Iggy/

LEARNING OUTCOMES

1. Collaborate with the interprofessional team to coordinate high-quality care and promote ***gas exchange*** in critically ill patients with respiratory problems.
2. Teach the patient and caregiver(s) about how decreased ***gas exchange*** and impaired ***perfusion*** affect home safety.
3. Identify community resources for patients requiring assistance with long-term complications of severe respiratory problems.
4. Teach adults how to decrease the risk for severe respiratory damage or disease.
5. Implement patient- and family-centered nursing interventions to help people cope with the psychosocial impact of severe respiratory problems and reduced ***gas exchange***.
6. Apply knowledge of anatomy, physiology, and pathophysiology to assess critically ill patients with respiratory problems affecting ***gas exchange*** or ***perfusion***.
7. Teach the patient and caregiver(s) about common drugs and other management strategies used for respiratory problems.
8. Use clinical judgment to plan evidence-based nursing interventions to prevent complications of pulmonary embolism, mechanical ventilation, or any other critical respiratory problem.

KEY TERMS

acute respiratory distress syndrome (ARDS) A type of acute respiratory failure with hypoxemia that persists even when 100% oxygen is given, decreased pulmonary compliance, dyspnea, bilateral pulmonary edema, and dense pulmonary infiltrates on x-ray (ground-glass appearance). It often occurs after an acute lung injury as a result of other conditions such as sepsis, burns, pancreatitis, trauma, and transfusion.

atelectrauma Ventilator-induced trauma of shear injury to alveoli from opening and closing.

barotrauma Ventilator-induced damage to the lungs from positive pressure.

biotrauma Inflammatory response–mediated damage to alveoli.

dyspnea Perceived difficulty breathing.

embolism A blood clot or other object (e.g., air bubble, fatty deposit) that is carried in the bloodstream and lodges in another area.

extubation The removal of an endotracheal (ET) tube.

flail chest The result of fractures of at least two neighboring ribs in two or more places causing paradoxical chest wall movement (inward movement of the thorax during inspiration, with outward movement during expiration).

hemoptysis Bloody sputum.

hemothorax Bleeding into the chest cavity.

hypoventilation Poor respiratory movements.

hypoxemia Low arterial blood oxygen level.

lung compliance Elasticity and recoil of lung tissue.

pneumothorax Air in the pleural space causing a loss of negative pressure in the chest cavity, a rise in chest pressure, and a reduction in vital capacity, which can lead to lung collapse.

pulmonary embolism (PE) A collection of particulate matter (solids, liquids, or air) that enters venous circulation and lodges in the pulmonary vessels.

refractory hypoxemia Hypoxemia that persists even when 100% oxygen is given.

tension pneumothorax A life-threatening complication of pneumothorax in which air continues to enter the pleural space during inspiration and does not exit during expiration.

thrombus Blood clot.

ventilator-associated events (VAEs) Conditions that result in a significant and sustained deterioration in oxygenation (greater than 20% increase in the daily minimum fraction of inspired oxygen or an increase of at least 3 cm H_2O in the daily minimum positive end-expiratory pressure (PEEP) to maintain oxygenation) following a baseline period of at least 2 days of stability or improvement.

ventilator-associated lung injury/ventilator-induced lung injury (VALI/VILI) Damage from prolonged ventilation causing loss of surfactant, increased inflammation, fluid leakage, and noncardiac pulmonary edema).

volutrauma Ventilator-induced damage to the lung by excess volume delivered to one lung over the other.

weaning The process of going from ventilatory dependence to spontaneous breathing.

PRIORITY AND INTERRELATED CONCEPTS

The priority concept for this chapter is:
- ***Gas Exchange***

The ***Gas Exchange*** concept exemplar for this chapter is Pulmonary Embolism.

The interrelated concepts for this chapter are:
- ***Perfusion***
- ***Clotting***

Any type of respiratory problem can progress and cause rapid, life-threatening reductions in ***gas exchange*** and tissue ***perfusion*** that require emergency intervention and critical care. These emergencies include pulmonary embolism, acute respiratory failure (ARF), acute respiratory distress syndrome, and chest trauma.

GAS EXCHANGE CONCEPT EXEMPLAR: PULMONARY EMBOLISM

Pathophysiology Review

A **pulmonary embolism (PE)** is a collection of particulate matter (solids, liquids, or air) that enters venous circulation and lodges in the pulmonary vessels. (An **embolism** is a blood clot [**thrombus**] or other object [e.g., air, fatty deposit] that is carried in the bloodstream and lodges in another area.) Large emboli in the lung vessels obstruct pulmonary blood flow, leading to reduced ***gas exchange***, reduced oxygenation, pulmonary tissue hypoxia, decreased ***perfusion***, and potential death. Any substance can cause an embolism, but a blood clot is the most common (McCance et al., 2019; Moore, 2019). PE is common and may account for as many as 100,000 deaths each year in the United States (Centers for Disease Control and Prevention [CDC], 2018). It may be the most common cause of preventable death in hospitalized patients, but because symptoms can be vague it may be misdiagnosed, and patients at risk may not receive appropriate initial care.

Most often, a PE occurs when inappropriate blood ***clotting*** forms a *venous thromboembolism* (VTE) (or deep vein thrombosis [DVT]) in a vein in the legs or the pelvis and a clot breaks off and travels to the right side of the heart. The clot then lodges in the pulmonary artery or within one or more of its branches, obstructing the alveolar perfusion and outflow, which results in increased alveolar dead space and creating a ventilation-perfusion ($\dot{V}/\dot{Q}$) mismatch. Platelets collect on the embolus, triggering the release of substances that cause blood vessel constriction. Widespread pulmonary vessel constriction and pulmonary hypertension impair ***gas exchange*** and tissue ***perfusion***. Deoxygenated blood moves into arterial circulation, causing **hypoxemia** (low arterial blood oxygen level), although some patients with PE do *not* have hypoxemia.

Major risk factors for VTE leading to PE are:
- Prolonged immobility
- Central venous catheters
- Surgery
- Pregnancy
- Obesity
- Advancing age
- General and genetic conditions that increase blood ***clotting***
- History of thromboembolism

Smoking, estrogen therapy, heart failure, stroke, cancer (particularly lung or prostate), and trauma also increase the risk for VTE and PE (McCance et al., 2019).

Fat, oil, air, tumor cells, amniotic fluid and fetal debris, foreign objects (e.g., broken IV catheters), injected particles, and infected clots can enter a vein and cause PE. Fat emboli can occur with fracture of the femur, and oil emboli from diagnostic procedures. These have a mortality rate of about 10% (Fukumoto & Fukumoto, 2018; Moore, 2016). Fat emboli cause injury to pulmonary vessels and cause acute respiratory distress syndrome (ARDS) (discussed as a disorder later in this chapter) rather than directly disrupting blood flow. Septic clots may develop from a pelvic abscess, an infected IV catheter, and injections of illegal drugs. VTE and PE are also associated with heparin-induced thrombocytopenia (HIT) (Bethea et al., 2017).

Health Promotion and Maintenance

Prevention of conditions, especially venous stasis, that lead to VTE and PE is a major nursing concern. Preventive actions are outlined in the Best Practice for Patient Safety & Quality Care: Prevention of Pulmonary Embolism box.

Lifestyle changes can help reduce the risk for PE. Tobacco use and nicotine in any form narrow blood vessels and increase the risk for clot formation. Hormone-based contraceptives also increase blood ***clotting.*** Urge patients to stop smoking cigarettes, especially women who use hormone-based contraceptives.

BEST PRACTICE FOR PATIENT SAFETY & QUALITY CARE (QSEN)

Prevention of Pulmonary Embolism

- Start passive and active range-of-motion exercises for the extremities of immobilized and postoperative patients.
- Ambulate patients as soon as possible after surgery.
- Use pneumatic compression devices after surgery as prescribed.
- Evaluate patient for criteria indicating the need for anticoagulant therapy.
- Give prescribed prophylactic low-dose anticoagulant or antiplatelet drugs after specific surgical procedures as soon as surgical bleeding risk has subsided.
- Teach patients to avoid the use of tight garters, girdles, and constricting clothing.
- Prevent pressure under the popliteal space (e.g., do not place a pillow under the knee; instead, use an alternating pressure mattress).
- Perform a comprehensive assessment of peripheral circulation every 8 hours.
- Elevate the affected limb 20 degrees or more above the level of the heart to improve venous return, as appropriate.
- Change patient position every 2 hours or ambulate as tolerated.
- Refrain from massaging leg muscles.
- Instruct patients not to cross their legs.
- Teach the patient and family about precautions.
- Encourage smoking cessation.

Reducing weight and becoming more physically active can reduce risk for PE. Teach patients who are traveling for long periods to drink plenty of water, change positions often, avoid crossing their legs, and get up from the sitting position at least 5 minutes out of every hour to prevent stasis and clot formation.

For patients known to be at risk for PE, small doses of heparin or low-molecular-weight heparin, or an indirect thrombin inhibitor, may be prescribed. Oral direct thrombin inhibitors may be used instead of heparin for VTE prevention in patients who have nonvalvular atrial fibrillation (Burchum & Rosenthal, 2019).

For adults who have an ongoing risk for VTE and PE, prevention may include preoperative placement of a retrievable inferior vena cava (IVC) filter. This placement occurs before any surgery in which the patient is expected to be confined to bed for more than just a few days, and the filter is retrieved when the patient is fully ambulatory.

❖ Interprofessional Collaborative Care

The patient who has a pulmonary embolism (PE) is critically ill and at risk for life-threatening complications. Initial management occurs in an acute care environment, most often an ICU. In addition to medical and nursing care providers, pharmacists and respiratory therapists are key interprofessional team members at this time.

Some patients have ongoing issues or residual problems after the acute problems have resolved that continue to impair ***gas exchange*** and ***perfusion***. When these changes are permanent, continuing care occurs in the home or residential setting.

INTERPROFESSIONAL COLLABORATION

The Patient With Pulmonary Embolism Requiring Continuing Care

The interprofessional team for ongoing issues includes a variety of specialists for optimal patient function. A pulmonary health care provider in addition to a primary health care provider is needed for continual assessment and management of any reduced lung function. Respiratory therapists assist with prescribed oxygen therapy and delivery needs. Physical therapists can help the patient maintain muscle conditioning. Occupational therapists provide information and home setup suggestions to help patients conserve energy when endurance is affected. Registered dietitian nutritionists assess patients' caloric and protein needs and plan personalized interventions to meet these needs. Pastoral care workers and clergy may help patients who experience spiritual distress with this life-altering condition. Social workers together with home care nurses determine which types of home modifications and durable supplies would be most helpful in maintaining functional ability for self-management of ADLs. When significant lifestyle changes are needed, mental health professionals can help the patient and family cope with adjustments (Harmon, 2019).

◆ **Assessment: Recognize Cues.** Signs and symptoms range from vague, nonspecific discomforts to hemodynamic collapse and death. *It is important to remember that many patients with PE do not have the "classic" signs and symptoms, which often leads to PEs being overlooked.*

KEY FEATURES

Pulmonary Embolism (Classic Signs and Symptoms)

- Sudden onset of dyspnea
- Sharp, stabbing chest pain
- Apprehension, restlessness
- Feeling of impending doom
- Cough
- Hemoptysis
- Diaphoresis
- Increased respiratory rate
- Crackles
- Pleural friction rub
- Tachycardia
- S_3 or S_4 heart sound
- Fever, low grade
- Petechiae over chest and axillae (usually only associated with fat embolism syndrome [FES])
- Decreased arterial oxygen saturation (Sao_2)

Physical Assessment/Signs and Symptoms. *Respiratory symptoms* are outlined in the Key Features: Pulmonary Embolism (Classic Signs and Symptoms) box and are mostly related to decreased ***gas exchange*** (McCance et al., 2019). Assess the patient for dyspnea and *pleuritic chest pain* (sharp, stabbing-type pain on inspiration). Other symptoms vary depending on the size and type of embolism. Breath sounds may be normal or include crackles, wheezes, or a pleural friction rub. A dry or productive cough may be present; **hemoptysis** (bloody sputum) may result from pulmonary infarction but is not present in all patients.

Cardiac symptoms related to decreased tissue ***perfusion*** include tachycardia, distended neck veins, *syncope* (fainting or loss of consciousness), cyanosis, and hypotension. Systemic hypotension results from acute pulmonary hypertension and reduced forward blood flow. Abnormal heart sounds, such as an S_3 or S_4, may occur. ECG changes are nonspecific and transient. T-wave and ST-segment changes may occur, as may left-axis or right-axis deviations. Right ventricular dysfunction and failure are extreme complications. The patient may have cardiac arrest or frank shock.

! NURSING SAFETY PRIORITY QSEN

Critical Rescue

Monitor patients at risk to recognize signs and symptoms of PE (e.g., shortness of breath, chest pain, and/or hypotension without an obvious cause). If symptoms are present, respond by initiating the Rapid Response Team. If PE is strongly suspected, prompt categorization and management strategies are started before diagnostic studies have been completed.

Psychosocial Assessment. Symptoms of PE often occur abruptly, and the patient is anxious. Hypoxemia may trigger a sense of impending doom and cause increased restlessness. The life-threatening nature of PE and admission to an ICU increase the patient's anxiety and fear.

Laboratory Assessment. The hyperventilation triggered by hypoxia and pain first leads to respiratory alkalosis, indicated by low partial pressure of arterial carbon dioxide ($Paco_2$) on arterial blood gas (ABG) analysis. The Pao_2/Fio_2 (fraction of inspired oxygen) ratio falls as a result of "shunting" of blood from the right side of the heart to the left without picking up oxygen from the lungs. Shunting causes the $Paco_2$ level to rise, resulting in respiratory acidosis. Later, metabolic acidosis results from buildup of lactic acid caused by tissue hypoxia. (See Chapter 14 for a more detailed discussion of acidosis.)

Even if ABG studies and pulse oximetry show hypoxemia, these results alone are not sufficient for the diagnosis of PE (McCance et al., 2019; Moore, 2019). *A patient with a small embolus may not be hypoxemic, and PE is not the only cause of hypoxemia.*

Other laboratory studies performed when PE is suspected include a general metabolic panel, troponin, brain natriuretic peptide (BNP), and D-dimer levels. The D-dimer rises with fibrinolysis. When the value is normal or low, it can rule out a PE (McCance et al., 2019). However, even if the value is high, other diagnostic testing is needed to determine whether a PE has occurred (Pagana & Pagana, 2018).

PATIENT-CENTERED CARE: GENETIC/GENOMIC CONSIDERATIONS (QSEN)

Factor V Leiden (also known as activated protein C resistance) is an inherited abnormal tendency to develop blood clots. The gene coding for blood clotting factor V (the *F5* gene) has a mutation that changes the nature of the factor V produced. With this genetic alteration, factor V functions normally but is more slowly degraded, and ***clotting*** activity continues longer than usual, increasing the risk for clot development, VTE, PE, and thrombotic strokes, especially for smokers and those who use hormone-based contraceptives (Online Mendelian Inheritance in Man [OMIM], 2017). Other inherited disorders that increase clotting and the risk for PE include protein C deficiency, protein S deficiency, and mutations in the prothrombin gene. Always ask a patient with a PE who has no known risk factors whether other family members have ever had clots form. Such patients may require changes in initial management and in prevention strategies.

Imaging Assessment. Computed tomography pulmonary angiography (CTPA) or helical CT may be used for diagnosis. This type of imaging has the added advantage of revealing other pulmonary abnormalities causing the patient's symptoms. Magnetic resonance arteriography (MRA) is used in place of CTPA in some settings. A chest x-ray may be used to diagnose other conditions that mimic acute PE. Doppler ultrasound may be used to document the presence of VTE.

◆ Analysis: Analyze Cues and Prioritize Hypotheses.

The priority interprofessional collaborative problems for patients with PE are:

1. Hypoxemia due to mismatch of lung ***perfusion*** and alveolar ***gas exchange*** with oxygenation
2. Hypotension due to inadequate circulation to the left ventricle
3. Potential for excessive bleeding due to anticoagulation or fibrinolytic therapy causing inadequate ***clotting***
4. Anxiety due to hypoxemia and life-threatening illness

◆ Planning and Implementation: Generate Solutions and Take Action

Managing Hypoxemia. *When a patient has a sudden onset of dyspnea and chest pain, or other symptoms of respiratory impairment, immediately initiate the Rapid Response Team.* Apply oxygen, reassure the patient, and elevate the head of the bed. Prepare for blood gas analysis while continuing to monitor and assess for other changes.

Planning: Expected Outcomes. The patient with PE is expected to have adequate tissue perfusion in all major organs.

Interventions. Nonsurgical management of PE is most common. In some cases invasive procedures also may be needed. Nursing management involves using the care practices listed in the Best Practice for Patient Safety & Quality Care: Management of Pulmonary Embolism box. Rapid categorization of PE severity and prompt management are required (Table 29.1).

Nonsurgical Management. Management activities for PE focus on increasing ***gas exchange*** and oxygenation, improving lung ***perfusion***, reducing risk for further clot formation, and preventing complications. Priority nursing interventions include implementing oxygen therapy, administering anticoagulation or fibrinolytic therapy to improve tissue perfusion, monitoring the patient's responses to the interventions, and providing psychosocial support.

Oxygen therapy is critical for the patient with PE. The severely hypoxemic patient may need mechanical ventilation and close

BEST PRACTICE FOR PATIENT SAFETY & QUALITY CARE (QSEN)

Management of Pulmonary Embolism

- Apply oxygen by nasal cannula or mask.
- Reassure patient that the correct measures are being taken.
- Place patient in high-Fowler position.
- Apply telemetry monitoring equipment.
- Obtain venous access.
- Assess oxygenation continuously with pulse oximetry.
- Assess respiratory status at least every 30 minutes by:
  - Listening to lung sounds
  - Measuring the rate, rhythm, and ease of respirations
  - Checking skin color and capillary refill
  - Checking position of trachea
- Assess cardiac status by:
  - Comparing blood pressures in right and left arms
  - Checking pulse quality
  - Checking cardiac monitor for dysrhythmias
  - Checking for distention of neck veins
- Ensure that prescribed chest imaging and laboratory tests are obtained immediately (may include complete blood count [CBC] with differential, platelet count, prothrombin time, partial thromboplastin time, D-dimer level, arterial blood gases).
- Examine the chest for presence of petechiae.
- Give prescribed anticoagulants.
- Assess for bleeding.
- Handle patient gently.
- Institute Bleeding Precautions.

TABLE 29.1 **Pulmonary Embolism (PE) Severity and Management Options**

Category	Possible Symptoms	Management Options
Massive PE Mortality may be as high as 65%	Severe hypotension (SBP <90 mm Hg for at least 15 minutes) Cardiac arrest/cardiopulmonary collapse Severe bradycardia Shock Severe dyspnea/respiratory distress	CPR Inotropic and/or vasopressor support; fluids Fibrinolytic therapy Tissue plasminogen activator (tPA) Alteplase Unfractionated heparin initial treatment
Submassive PE	Normotension RV dysfunction on echocardiography RV dilation on echocardiography or CT Right bundle branch block ST elevation or depression T-wave inversion Elevated BNP or troponin	Treatment is controversial; some agents not approved for this group Must weigh benefits of thrombolytic therapy against risk for bleeding Fibrinolytics may be preferred if patient appears to be decompensating or if there is RV dysfunction (hypokinesis) or elevation in BNP or troponin LMWH (preferred agent) Fondaparinux Unfractionated heparin
Low-risk PE Mortality ranges from 1% to 8%	Normotension No RV dysfunction No elevation in BNP or troponin	Fibrinolytics not warranted because of risk for bleeding LMWH Direct thrombin inhibitor Inpatient hospitalization not usually required

BNP, Brain natriuretic peptide; *CPR,* cardiopulmonary resuscitation; *LMWH,* low–molecular-weight heparin; *RV,* right ventricular; *SBP,* systolic blood pressure.

Adapted from Jaff, M.R., McMurtry, M.S., & Archer, S.L. (2011). The use of fibrinolytics in patients with acute pulmonary embolism. *Circulation, 123,* 1788–1830.

monitoring with ABG studies. In less severe cases oxygen may be applied by nasal cannula or mask. Use pulse oximetry to monitor oxygen saturation and hypoxemia. See Chapter 25 for a detailed discussion of oxygen therapy.

Monitor the patient continually for any changes in status. Check vital signs, lung sounds, and cardiac and respiratory status at least every 1 to 2 hours. Document increasing dyspnea, dysrhythmias, distended neck veins, and pedal or sacral edema. Assess for crackles and other abnormal lung sounds along with cyanosis of the lips, conjunctiva, oral mucosa, and nail beds.

NCLEX EXAMINATION CHALLENGE 29.1

Safe and Effective Health Care Environment

A client who 3 days ago underwent extensive abdominal surgery for cancer reports having a difficult time "catching her breath" and feeling very scared. After assessing the client, what is the nurse's **best** action or response to prevent **harm**?

A. Ask the client about possible drug allergies
B. Apply oxygen and initiate the Rapid Response Team
C. Determine when she last received an opioid dose
D. Check the oxygen saturation and encourage her to cough

Drug therapy begins immediately with anticoagulants to prevent embolus enlargement and more ***clotting*** (Brien, 2019). Unfractionated heparin, low–molecular-weight heparin, or fondaparinux is used unless the PE is massive or occurs with hemodynamic instability. Review the patient's partial thromboplastin time (PTT)—also called activated partial thromboplastin time (aPTT)—before therapy is started and thereafter according to facility policy. Therapeutic PTT values usually range between 1.5 and 2.5 times the control value for this health problem. Factor anti-Xa levels may be used instead of PTT or aPTT if the response to unfractionated heparin is insufficient or inappropriate. (Heparin primarily acts on Factor Xa, making the anti-Xa assay more useful to guide treatment in some situations.)

Fibrinolytic drugs, such as alteplase, are used for treatment of PE when specific criteria are met such as shock, hemodynamic collapse, or instability. Fibrinolytic drugs are used to break up the existing clot.

Both heparin and fibrinolytic drugs are *high-alert drugs.* These drugs have an increased risk to cause harm if given at too high a dose, at too low a dose, or to the wrong patient. Because of the high risk for bleeding, patients receiving fibrinolytic therapy are monitored in an ICU setting.

! NATIONAL PATIENT SAFETY GOALS

Heparin comes in a variety of concentrations in vials that have differing amounts, which contributes to possible drug errors. In accordance with The Joint Commission's National Patient Safety Goals (NPSGs), check the prescribed dose carefully and ensure that the correct concentration is being used to prevent overdosing or underdosing.

Heparin therapy usually continues for 5 to 10 days. Most patients are started on an oral anticoagulant, such as warfarin, on day 1 or 2 of heparin therapy. Therapy with both heparin and warfarin continues until the international normalized ratio (INR) reaches 2.0 to 3.0. Heparin is usually infused for at least 5 days and continues for 24 hours after the INR is greater than 2. Monitor the platelet count and INR during this time. A low–molecular-weight heparin (e.g., dalteparin, enoxaparin) or a direct thrombin inhibitor (e.g., apixaban, dabigatran, rivaroxaban) is often used instead of warfarin. Oral anticoagulant use continues for 3 to 6 weeks, but patients at continuing risk for PE may take it indefinitely. These drugs, laboratory values to be monitored, and the associated nursing care are discussed in Chapters 33, 35, and 36.

PATIENT-CENTERED CARE: GENETIC/GENOMIC CONSIDERATIONS QSEN

Genetic variation in two specific genes can change patient responses to warfarin therapy. One gene, *VKORC1*, produces an enzyme that alters vitamin K so it can help activate the vitamin K–dependent clotting factors. Warfarin interferes with the activity of this enzyme. Patients who have one type of variation in this enzyme are resistant to the effects of warfarin, and much higher doses are needed to achieve coagulation. On the other hand, a different variation in the same gene increases the patient's sensitivity to the drug and much lower doses are needed.

The gene *CYP2C19* produces an enzyme that metabolizes warfarin and prepares it for elimination. Patients who have a variation in this gene do not metabolize warfarin well, so higher blood levels remain and more severe bleeding is possible. Warfarin dosage needs to be much lower in patients with this gene variation. When a patient's coagulation response to warfarin is either greater than expected or much less than expected, consider the possibility of a gene mutation.

Anticoagulation and fibrinolytic therapy can lead to excessive bleeding. The antidote for heparin is protamine sulfate; the antidote for warfarin is vitamin K_1, which is available as an injectable drug, phytonadione. Antidotes for fibrinolytic therapy include clotting factors, fresh-frozen plasma, and aminocaproic acid. Antidotes to anticoagulant drugs and fibrinolytic drugs should be readily available on the unit, from the pharmacy, or from the blood bank for patients undergoing these therapies.

Surgical Management. Two surgical procedures for the management of PE are embolectomy and inferior vena cava (IVC) filtration.

Embolectomy is the surgical or percutaneous removal of the embolus. It may be performed when fibrinolytic therapy cannot be used for a patient who has massive or multiple large pulmonary emboli with shock or bleeding complications.

Inferior vena cava filtration with placement of a retrievable vena cava filter prevents further emboli from reaching the lungs in patients with ongoing risk for PE. Patients for whom filter placement is considered less risky than drug therapy include those with recurrent or major bleeding while receiving anticoagulants, those with septic PE, and those undergoing pulmonary embolectomy. Placement of a vena cava filter is detailed in Chapter 33.

Managing Hypotension

Planning: Expected Outcomes. The patient with PE is expected to have adequate circulation and tissue ***perfusion***.

Interventions. In addition to the interventions used for hypoxemia, IV fluid therapy and drug therapy are used to increase cardiac output and maintain blood pressure.

IV fluid therapy involves giving crystalloid solutions to restore plasma volume and prevent shock (see Chapter 34). Continuously monitor the ECG and pulmonary artery and central venous/right atrial pressures of the patient receiving IV fluids because increased fluids can worsen pulmonary hypertension and lead to right-sided heart failure. Also monitor indicators of fluid adequacy, including urine output, skin turgor, and moisture of mucous membranes.

Drug therapy with vasopressors is used when hypotension persists despite fluid resuscitation. Commonly used agents include norepinephrine, epinephrine, or dopamine. Agents that increase myocardial contractility *(positive inotropic agents)*, including milrinone and dobutamine, may be used. Vasodilators, such as nitroprusside, may be used to decrease pulmonary artery pressure if it is impeding cardiac contractility. Assess the patient's cardiac status hourly during therapy with any of these drugs.

Minimizing Bleeding

Planning: Expected Outcomes. The patient with PE is expected to have appropriate ***clotting*** and remain free from bleeding.

Interventions. Drug therapy that disrupts clots or prevents their formation impairs the patient's ability to start and continue the blood clotting cascade when injured, increasing the risk for bleeding. Priority nursing actions are ensuring that specific antidotes are present on the nursing unit, protecting the patient from situations that could lead to bleeding, ensuring correct dosage and timing of drug therapy, assessing laboratory values, and monitoring the amount of bleeding that occurs.

Assess for evidence of bleeding (e.g., oozing around puncture sites or the gums, bruises that cluster, petechiae, or purpura) at least every 2 hours. Examine all stools, urine, drainage, and vomitus for gross blood, and test for occult blood. Measure any blood loss as accurately as possible. Assess the patient's abdomen for increasing distention or firmness. Consider measuring the abdominal girth every 8 hours (increasing girth can indicate internal bleeding).

Monitor laboratory values daily. Review the complete blood count (CBC) to determine the risk for impaired ***clotting*** and whether any blood loss has occurred. If the patient has severe blood loss, packed red blood cells and/or fresh-frozen plasma may be prescribed (see Transfusion Therapy in Chapter 37). Monitor the platelet count. A decreasing count may indicate ongoing ***clotting*** or heparin-induced thrombocytopenia (HIT) caused by the formation of anti-heparin antibodies. A platelet transfusion may be indicated.

Minimizing Anxiety

Planning: Expected Outcomes. The patient with PE is usually anxious and fearful as a result of the life-threatening nature of the problem and cerebral hypoxia. He or she is expected to have anxiety reduced to an acceptable level.

Interventions. The patient with PE is anxious and fearful and often has pain. Interventions for reducing anxiety in those with

PE include oxygen therapy (see Interventions discussion in the Managing Hypoxemia section), communication, and drug therapy.

Communication is critical in allaying anxiety. Acknowledge the anxiety and the patient's perception of a life-threatening situation. Stay with him or her and speak calmly and clearly, providing assurances that appropriate measures are being taken. Explain the rationale and share information when giving drugs, changing position, taking vital signs, or assessing the patient. Coordinate with pastoral care to help provide spiritual comfort.

Drug therapy with an antianxiety drug may be prescribed if the patient's anxiety interferes with diagnostic testing, management, or adequate rest. Unless he or she is mechanically ventilated, sedating agents are avoided to reduce the risk for hypoventilation and to reduce the risk for worsening delirium with older patients. Pharmacologic therapy is used for pain management. Care is taken to avoid suppressing the respiratory response.

Care Coordination and Transition Management. The patient with a PE is discharged when hypoxemia and hemodynamic instability have resolved and adequate anticoagulation has been achieved. Anticoagulation therapy usually continues after discharge.

Home Care Management. Some patients are discharged to home with minimal risk for recurrence and no permanent physiologic changes. Others have heart or lung damage that requires home and lifestyle changes.

Patients with extensive lung damage may have activity intolerance from reduced ***gas exchange*** and become fatigued easily. The living arrangements may need to be modified so patients can spend most of the time on one floor and avoid climbing stairs. Depending on the degree of impairment, patients may require varying amounts of assistance with ADLs. Coordinate with members of the interprofessional team as described earlier under the Interprofessional Collaborative Care section to ensure optimal patient function.

Self-Management Education. The patient with a PE may continue anticoagulation therapy for weeks, months, or years after discharge, depending on the risks for PE, and have impaired ***clotting***. Teach him or her and the family about Bleeding Precautions, activities to reduce the risk for VTE and recurrence of PE, complications, and the need for follow-up care as described in Chapter 33.

Health Care Resources. Patients using anticoagulation therapy with warfarin are usually seen in a clinic or primary health care provider's office frequently for blood tests. Those who are homebound may have a visit from a home care nurse to perform these tests. Enoxaparin and newer anticoagulation agents (dabigatran, rivaroxaban, and apixaban) do not require laboratory monitoring. Patients with severe dyspnea may need home oxygen therapy. Respiratory therapy treatments can be performed in the home. The nurse or case manager coordinates arrangements for oxygen and other respiratory therapy equipment to be available if needed at home. This person also helps ensure continuing follow-up with the variety of specialists and laboratory monitoring needed based on the degree of the patient's continuing health problems (Harmon, 2019). See the Home Care Considerations box for a home care assessment guide.

HOME CARE CONSIDERATIONS

Assessment of Patients Recovering from Pulmonary Embolism

Assess respiratory status:
- Observe rate and depth of ventilation.
- Auscultate lungs.
- Examine nail beds and mucous membranes for evidence of reduced ***gas exchange.***
- Take a pulse oximetry reading.
- Ask the patient if chest pain or shortness of breath is experienced in any position.
- Ask the patient about the presence of sputum and its color and character.

Assess cardiovascular status:
- Take vital signs, including apical pulse, pulse pressure; assess for presence or absence of orthostatic hypotension and quality and rhythm of peripheral pulses.
- Note presence or absence of peripheral edema.
- Examine neck vein filling in the recumbent and sitting positions.

Assess lower extremities for deep vein thrombosis (DVT):
- Examine lower legs and compare with each other for:
  - General edema and calf swelling
  - Surface temperature
  - Presence of red streaks or cordlike, palpable structure

Assess for evidence of bleeding:
- Examine the mouth and gums for oozing or frank bleeding.
- Examine all skin areas, especially old puncture sites and wounds, for bleeding, bruising, or petechiae.

Assess cognition and mental status:
- Check level of consciousness (LOC) and orientation.

Assess the patient's understanding and adherence to management:
- Symptoms to report to the primary health care provider.
- Drug therapy plan (correct timing and dose, adverse effects).
- Bleeding Precautions.
- Prevention of venous thromboembolism (VTE).

◆ **Evaluation: Evaluate Outcomes.** Evaluate the care of the patient with PE on the basis of the identified priority patient problems. The expected outcomes are that he or she:
- Attains and maintains adequate ***gas exchange*** and oxygenation
- Does not experience hypovolemia and shock
- Remains free from bleeding episodes
- States that the level of anxiety is reduced
- Uses effective coping strategies

ACUTE RESPIRATORY FAILURE

Pathophysiology Review

A near match in the lungs between air movement or ventilation ($\dot{V}$) and blood flow or ***perfusion*** ($\dot{Q}$) is needed for adequate pulmonary ***gas exchange.*** When either ventilation or perfusion is mismatched with the other in a lung or lung area, gas exchange is reduced, and respiratory failure can result (McCance et al., 2019; Lamba et al., 2016).

Acute respiratory failure (ARF) can be *ventilatory failure, oxygenation (**gas exchange**) failure,* or a *combination of both*

CLINICAL JUDGMENT CHALLENGE 29.1

Patient-Centered Care; Evidence-Based Practice

The client is a 51-year-old woman who is a grade school principal. She is brought to the emergency department on Sunday morning by her wife of 15 years. The client appears anxious and tells the nurse that she thinks she has the "flu" because she has been nauseated since she left school on Friday afternoon (but has not vomited), has a cough, is sweaty, and is very tired. For 2 days she has felt chest heaviness and now has sharp chest pain that seems to be getting worse and feels breathless. She is 5 feet 7 inches tall (1.7 m) and weighs about 196 lb (89 kg). She quit smoking 20 years ago. Her current medications include olmesartan daily for hypertension and meloxicam for chronic low back pain. Her mother and sister have type 2 diabetes mellitus. She drinks a glass of wine at dinner daily. She began menopause about 6 months ago. Her only hospitalization was 10 years ago for gallbladder surgery.

Her admitting vital signs and laboratory results are:

- Temperature = 100.6°F (38.1°C)
- HR = 116 beats/min, regular
- RR = 34 breaths/min, shallow
- BP = 122/60
- Oxygen saturation = 89%
- WBC count = 12,000/mm^3
- RBC count = 4.0 million/mcL (4.0×10^{12} cells/L)
- Hemoglobin = 10 g/dL (100 g/L)
- Hematocrit = 42% (0.42 volume fraction)
- Platelets = 180,000/mm^3 (180×10^9/L)
- D-dimer = 1.4 mcg/mL
- Blood glucose level (fasting) = 216 mg/dL

1. **Recognize Cues:** What assessment information in this client situation is the most important and immediate concern for the nurse? (Hint: Identify the **relevant** information *first* to determine what is most important.)
2. **Analyze Cues:** What client conditions are consistent with the **most relevant** information? (Hint: Think about priority collaborative problems that support and contradict the information presented in this situation.)
3. **Prioritize Hypotheses:** Which possibilities or explanations are **most likely** to be present in this client situation? Which possibilities or explanations are the most serious? (Hint: Consider all possibilities and determine their urgency and risk for this client.)
4. **Generate Solutions:** What activities would most likely achieve the desired outcomes for this client? Which actions should be **avoided** or are **potentially harmful**? (Hint: Determine the desired outcomes first to decide which interventions are appropriate and those that should be avoided.)
5. **Take Action:** Which actions are the most appropriate and how should they be implemented? In what **priority order** should they be implemented? (Hint: Consider health teaching, documentation, requested health care provider orders or prescriptions, nursing skills, collaboration with or referral to health team members, etc.)
6. **Evaluate Outcomes:** What client assessment would indicate the nurse's actions were **effective**? (Hint: Think about signs that would indicate an improvement, decline, or unchanged patient condition.)

ventilatory and oxygenation failure and is classified by abnormal blood gas values. The critical values are:

- Partial pressure of arterial oxygen (Pao_2) less than 60 mm Hg (hypoxemic/oxygenation failure)
- *or* Partial pressure of arterial carbon dioxide ($Paco_2$) more than 45 mm Hg occurring with acidemia (pH <7.35) (hypercapnia/ventilatory failure)
- *and* Arterial oxygen saturation (Sao_2) less than 90% in both cases

Whatever the underlying problem, the patient in ARF is always hypoxemic (has low arterial blood oxygen levels).

Ventilatory Failure. Ventilatory failure is a problem in oxygen intake (air movement or ventilation) and blood flow (***perfusion***) that causes a ventilation-perfusion ($\dot{V}/\dot{Q}$) mismatch in which blood flow (perfusion) is normal but air movement (ventilation) is inadequate. It occurs when the chest pressure does not change enough to permit air movement into and out of the lungs. As a result, too little oxygen reaches the alveoli, and carbon dioxide is retained. Perfusion is wasted in this area of no air movement from either inadequate oxygen intake or excessive carbon dioxide retention, leading to poor ***gas exchange*** and hypoxemia.

Ventilatory failure usually results from any of these problems: a physical problem of the lungs or chest wall; a defect in the respiratory control center in the brain; or poor function of the respiratory muscles, especially the diaphragm. The problem is defined by a $Paco_2$ level above 45 mm Hg plus acidosis (pH below 7.35) in patients who have otherwise healthy lungs.

Many disorders can result in ventilatory failure. Causes are either *extrapulmonary* (involving nonpulmonary tissues but affecting respiratory function) or *intrapulmonary* (disorders of the respiratory tract). Table 29.2 lists causes of ventilatory failure.

Oxygenation (Gas Exchange) Failure. In oxygenation (***gas exchange***) failure, chest pressure changes are normal, and air moves in and out without difficulty but does not oxygenate the pulmonary blood sufficiently. It occurs in the type of ($\dot{V}/\dot{Q}$) mismatch in which air movement and oxygen intake *(ventilation)* are normal but lung blood flow (***perfusion***) is decreased.

Many lung disorders can cause oxygenation failure. Problems include impaired diffusion of oxygen at the alveolar level, right-to-left shunting of blood in the pulmonary vessels, ($\dot{V}/\dot{Q}$) mismatch, breathing air with a low oxygen level, and abnormal hemoglobin that fails to bind oxygen. In one type of ($\dot{V}/\dot{Q}$) mismatch, areas of the lungs still have ***perfusion,*** but ***gas exchange*** does not occur, which leads to hypoxemia. An extreme example of ($\dot{V}/\dot{Q}$) mismatch is when systemic venous blood (oxygen poor) passes through the lungs without being oxygenated and is "shunted" to the left side of the heart and into the systemic arterial system. Normally, less than 5% of cardiac output contains venous blood that has bypassed oxygenation. With poor oxygenation in the lungs or a shunt that allows venous blood to bypass the lungs, even more arterial blood is not oxygenated, and applying 100% oxygen does not correct the problem. A classic cause of such a ($\dot{V}/\dot{Q}$) mismatch is acute respiratory distress syndrome (ARDS), which is discussed later in the chapter. Table 29.3 lists specific causes of oxygenation failure.

Combined Ventilatory and Oxygenation Failure. Combined ventilatory and oxygenation failure involves **hypoventilation** (poor respiratory movements). Impaired ***gas exchange*** at the alveolar-capillary membrane results in poor diffusion of oxygen into arterial blood and carbon dioxide retention.

TABLE 29.2 Common Causes of Ventilatory Failure

Extrapulmonary Causes	Intrapulmonary Causes

• Neuromuscular disorders
  • Myasthenia gravis
  • Guillain-Barré syndrome
  • Poliomyelitis
  • Spinal cord injuries affecting nerves to intercostal muscles
• Central nervous system dysfunction
  • Stroke
  • Increased intracranial pressure
  • Meningitis
• Chemical depression
  • Opioid analgesics, sedatives, anesthetics
• Kyphoscoliosis
• Massive obesity
• Sleep apnea
• External obstruction or constriction
	• Airway disease
	  • Chronic obstructive pulmonary disease (COPD), asthma
	• Ventilation-perfusion ($\dot{V}/\dot{Q}$) mismatch
	  • Pulmonary embolism
	  • Pneumothorax
	  • Acute respiratory distress syndrome (ARDS)
	  • Amyloidosis
	  • Pulmonary edema
	  • Interstitial fibrosis

The condition may or may not include poor lung perfusion. When lung ***perfusion*** is not adequate, ($\dot{V}/\dot{Q}$) mismatch occurs, and both ventilation and perfusion are inadequate. This type of respiratory failure leads to a more profound hypoxemia than either ventilatory failure or oxygenation failure alone.

A combination of ventilatory failure and oxygenation (***gas exchange***) failure occurs in patients who have abnormal lungs, such as those who have any form of chronic bronchitis, emphysema, or cystic fibrosis, or who are having an asthma attack. The bronchioles and alveoli are diseased (causing oxygenation failure), and the work of breathing increases until the respiratory muscles cannot function effectively, causing ventilatory failure leading to acute respiratory failure (ARF). ARF can also occur in patients who have cardiac failure along with ventilatory failure and is made worse because the cardiac system cannot adapt to the hypoxia by increasing the cardiac output.

❖ Interprofessional Collaborative Care

◆ **Assessment: Recognize Cues.** The symptoms of ARF are related to the systemic effects of hypoxia, hypercapnia, and acidosis. Assess for **dyspnea** (perceived difficulty breathing)—the hallmark of respiratory failure. Evaluate dyspnea on the basis of how breathless the patient becomes while performing common tasks. Depending on the nature of the underlying problem, the patient might not be aware of changes in the work of breathing.

Dyspnea is more intense when it develops rapidly. Slowly progressive respiratory failure may first be noticed as dyspnea on exertion (DOE) or when lying down. The patient may have *orthopnea,* finding it easier to breathe in an upright position.

TABLE 29.3 Common Causes of Oxygenation Failure

- High altitudes, closed spaces, smoke inhalation, carbon monoxide poisoning
- Pneumonia
- Congestive heart failure with pulmonary edema
- Pulmonary embolism (PE)
- Acute respiratory distress syndrome (ARDS)
- Interstitial pneumonitis-fibrosis
- Methemoglobinemia
- Hypovolemic shock
- Hypoventilation

With chronic respiratory problems, a minor increase in dyspnea may represent severe ***gas exchange*** problems.

Assess for a change in the patient's respiratory rate or pattern and changes in lung sounds. Pulse oximetry (Spo_2) may show decreased oxygen saturation, but end-tidal CO_2 ($ETco_2$ or $PETco_2$) monitoring may be more valuable for monitoring the patient with ARF. Pulse oximetry may show adequate oxygen saturation, but because of increased $ETco_2$ the patient may be close to respiratory failure. Review arterial blood gas (ABG) values to accurately identify the degree of hypoxia and hypercarbia.

Other symptoms of hypoxic respiratory failure include restlessness, irritability or agitation, confusion, and tachycardia. Symptoms of hypercapnic failure may include decreased level of consciousness (LOC), headache, drowsiness, lethargy, and seizures. The effects of acidosis may lead to decreased LOC, drowsiness, confusion, hypotension, bradycardia, and weak peripheral pulses.

◆ **Interventions: Take Action.** *Oxygen therapy is appropriate for any patient with acute hypoxemia.* It is used in ARF to keep the arterial oxygen (Pao_2) level above 60 mm Hg while treating the cause of the respiratory failure. Oxygen therapy is discussed in detail in Chapter 25. If oxygen therapy does not maintain acceptable Pao_2 levels indicating adequate ***gas exchange***, mechanical ventilation (invasive or noninvasive) may be needed.

Drugs given systemically, by nebulizer, or by metered dose inhaler (MDI) may be prescribed to dilate the bronchioles and decrease inflammation to promote ***gas exchange***. Corticosteroids may be used, but their benefit has not been demonstrated conclusively. Analgesics are needed if the patient has pain. If the patient requires mechanical ventilation, he or she may need neuromuscular blockade drugs for optimal ventilator effect. Other management strategies depend on the underlying condition(s) that predisposed the patient to ARF development, which may include diuretic therapy or antibiotic therapy.

Help the patient find a position of comfort that allows easier breathing (i.e., usually a more upright position). To decrease the anxiety occurring with dyspnea, help him or her to use relaxation, diversion, and guided imagery. Start energy-conserving measures, such as minimal self-care and no unnecessary procedures. Encourage deep breathing and other breathing exercises.

ACUTE RESPIRATORY DISTRESS SYNDROME

Pathophysiology Review

Acute respiratory distress syndrome (ARDS) is acute respiratory failure (ARF) with these features:

- Hypoxemia that persists even when 100% oxygen is given (**refractory hypoxemia**, a cardinal feature)
- Decreased pulmonary compliance
- Dyspnea
- Non–cardiac-associated bilateral pulmonary edema
- Dense pulmonary infiltrates on x-ray (ground-glass appearance)

Often ARDS occurs after an *acute lung injury (ALI)* in people who have no pulmonary disease as a result of other conditions such as sepsis, burns, pancreatitis, trauma, and transfusion. Other terms for ARDS include *adult respiratory distress syndrome, "stiff lungs," shock lung, and acute respiratory dysfunction syndrome*

Despite different causes of ALI in ARDS, the trigger is a systemic inflammatory response that activates a variety of proinflammatory cytokines that maintain a continuing inflammation in the alveoli and pulmonary vasculature. This response is known as a "cytokine storm" and, when prolonged, results in thick, swollen tissues that hinder gas exchange and promote the formation of scar tissue. As a result, ARDS symptoms are similar regardless of the cause. The main site of injury in the lung is the alveolar-capillary membrane, which normally is permeable only to small molecules. It can be injured during sepsis, pulmonary embolism, shock, aspiration, severe inflammation from COVID-19 infection, or inhalation injury (Mitchell & Seckel, 2018). When injured, this membrane becomes more permeable to large molecules, which allows debris, proteins, and fluid into the alveoli. Lung tissue normally remains relatively dry, but in patients with ARDS lung fluid increases and contains more proteins. In ARDS associated with COVID-19, the thick exudate inhibits gas exchange.

Other changes occur in the alveoli and respiratory bronchioles. Normally the type II pneumocytes produce surfactant, a substance that increases **lung compliance** (elasticity and recoil of lung tissue) and prevents alveolar collapse. Surfactant activity is reduced in ARDS because type II pneumocytes are damaged and because the surfactant is diluted by excess lung fluids. As a result, the alveoli become unstable and tend to collapse. These collapsed or fluid-filled alveoli cannot participate in ***gas exchange***. Edema then forms around terminal airways, which are compressed and closed and can be destroyed. Lung volume and compliance are further reduced. As fluid continues to leak in more lung areas, fluid, protein, and blood cells collect in the alveoli and in the spaces between the alveoli. Lymph channels are compressed, and more fluid collects. Poorly inflated alveoli receive blood but cannot oxygenate it, increasing the shunt. Hypoxemia and ventilation-perfusion ($\dot{V}/\dot{Q}$) mismatch result.

Transfusion-related acute lung injury (TRALI) is the sudden onset (within 6 hours of a transfusion) of hypoxemic lung disease along with infiltrates on x-ray without cardiac problems. TRALI is associated with the activation of the inflammatory response caused by a recent transfusion of plasma-containing blood products such as packed red blood cells (PRBCs), platelets, and fresh-frozen plasma. Other lung complications of transfusion include *transfusion-associated circulatory overload (TACO)* and *transfusion-related immunomodulation (TRIM)*. These conditions are discussed further in Chapter 37.

TABLE 29.4 Common Causes of Acute Lung Injury

- Shock
- Trauma
- Serious nervous system injury
- Pancreatitis
- Fat and amniotic fluid emboli
- Pulmonary infections
- Sepsis
- Excessive inflammation from COVID-19 pneumonia
- Inhalation of toxic gases (smoke, oxygen)
- Pulmonary aspiration (especially of stomach contents)
- Drug ingestion (e.g., heroin, opioids, aspirin)
- Hemolytic disorders
- Multiple blood transfusions
- Cardiopulmonary bypass
- Submersion in water with water aspiration (especially in fresh water)

Etiology and Genetic Risk. ALI leading to ARDS has many causes (Table 29.4), but sepsis is the most common (Mitchell & Seckel, 2018). Some causes result in direct injury to lung tissue; other causes do not directly involve the lungs. As a result of sepsis, pancreatitis, trauma, and other conditions, inflammatory mediators spread to the lungs, causing damage (McCance et al., 2019), another instance of "cytokine storm."

ARDS also can occur from direct lung injury. Aspiration of acidic gastric contents, pneumonia, near-drowning, or inhaling toxic fumes are examples of conditions causing direct lung injury. With such events, surfactant production is impaired and the remaining surfactant is diluted. This situation leads to atelectasis, decreased lung compliance, and *shunting* (movement of blood in the lungs without ***gas exchange*** and oxygenation) (McCance et al., 2019).

Incidence and Prevalence. The actual incidence of ARDS is unknown because it is part of other health problems and is not systematically reported as a separate disorder. According to the ARDS Foundation, about 150,000 cases of ARDS occur yearly in North America, although many health care professionals believe this estimate to be low. The mortality rate is estimated at 46% (ARDS Foundation, 2018; Mitchell & Seckel, 2018).

Health Promotion and Maintenance

The nursing priority in the prevention of ARDS is early recognition of patients at high risk for the syndrome. Because patients who aspirate gastric contents are at great risk, closely assess and monitor those receiving tube feedings (because the tube keeps the gastric sphincter open) and those with problems that impair swallowing and gag reflexes. To help prevent ARDS, follow meticulous infection control guidelines, including handwashing, invasive catheter and wound care, and Contact Precautions. Teach assistive personnel the importance of always adhering to infection control guidelines. Carefully observe patients who are being treated for any health problem associated with ARDS. For patients with swallowing problems or a poor gag reflex, use a suction toothbrush when providing oral care (Warren et al., 2019).

❖ Interprofessional Collaborative Care

ARDS is a life-threatening health problem that may result in permanent impairment of lung function requiring major changes in lifestyle (Eakin et al., 2017). For optimum patient function, a comprehensive interprofessional team approach is needed. Essential team members are the same as those for pulmonary embolism (see the exemplar earlier in this chapter).

◆ Assessment: Recognize Cues

Physical Assessment/Signs and Symptoms. Assess the breathing of any patient at increased risk for ARDS. Determine whether increased work of breathing is present, as indicated by hyperpnea, noisy respiration, cyanosis, pallor, and retraction *intercostally* (between the ribs) or *substernally* (beneath the ribs and sternum). Document sweating, respiratory effort, and any change in mental status. *Abnormal lung sounds are **not** heard on auscultation because the edema occurs first in the interstitial spaces and not in the airways.* Assess vital signs at least hourly for hypotension, tachycardia, and dysrhythmias.

Diagnostic Assessment. The diagnosis of ARDS is established by a lowered partial pressure of arterial oxygen (Pa_{O_2}) value (decreased ***gas exchange*** and oxygenation), determined by arterial blood gas (ABG) measurements. Because a widening alveolar oxygen gradient (i.e., increased fraction of inspired oxygen [Fi_{O_2}] does not lead to increased Pa_{O_2} levels) develops with increased shunting of blood, the patient has a progressive need for higher levels of oxygen. Another characteristic of ARDS is a P/F ratio (Pa_{O_2} divided by Fi_{O_2}) of less than 200 mm Hg. The patient develops refractory hypoxemia and often needs intubation and mechanical ventilation. Sputum cultures obtained by bronchoscopy and transtracheal aspiration are used to determine if a lung infection also is present. The chest x-ray may show diffuse haziness or a "whited-out" (ground-glass) appearance of the lung. An ECG rules out cardiac problems and usually shows no specific changes.

NCLEX EXAMINATION CHALLENGE 29.2

Physiological Integrity

Which condition, sign, or symptom does the nurse consider **most relevant** in assessing a client suspected to have ARDS? **Select all that apply.**

A. Dyspnea
B. Electrocardiogram shows ST elevation
C. Intercostal retractions
D. Pa_{O_2} 84% on oxygen at 6 L/min
E. Substernal pain or rubbing
F. Wheezing on exhalation

◆ Interventions: Take Action

Management Overview. General management of the patient with ARDS focuses on the three phases of ARDS. Timing of the phases varies from patient to patient.

Exudative phase. This phase includes early changes of dyspnea and tachypnea resulting from the alveoli becoming fluid filled and from pulmonary shunting and atelectasis. Early interventions focus on supporting the patient and providing oxygen.

Fibrosing alveolitis phase. Increased lung injury leads to pulmonary hypertension and fibrosis. The body attempts to repair the damage, and increasing lung involvement reduces ***gas exchange*** and oxygenation. Multiple organ dysfunction syndrome (MODS) can occur. Interventions focus on delivering adequate oxygen, preventing complications, and supporting the lungs.

Resolution phase. Usually occurring after 14 days, resolution of the injury is possible; if not, the patient either dies or has chronic disease. Fibrosis may or may not occur. Patients surviving ARDS often have neuropsychologic deficits.

Specific Management. The patient with ARDS often needs intubation and mechanical ventilation with positive end-expiratory pressure (PEEP) or continuous positive airway pressure (CPAP). Best practice involves using "open lung" and lung protective ventilation strategies. Low tidal volumes (6 mL/kg of body weight) have been shown to prevent lung injury. PEEP is started at 5 cm H_2O and increased to keep oxygen saturation adequate. PEEP levels may need to be high. Pressure-controlled ventilation is preferred over volume-controlled ventilation to promote the nonfunctional alveoli to participate in ***gas exchange***. Because one of the side effects of PEEP is tension pneumothorax, assess lung sounds hourly and suction as often as needed to maintain a patent airway.

Airway pressure release ventilation (APRV) and high-frequency oscillatory ventilation (HFOV) are alternative modes of mechanical ventilation that improve ***gas exchange*** with oxygenation and ventilation in patients with moderate-to-severe ARDS. The airway pressure with both APRV and HFOV is significantly higher than with conventional mechanical ventilation. Sedation and paralysis may be needed for adequate ventilation and to reduce tissue oxygen needs, especially with HFOV. Sedation and paralysis are not required with APRV but may be needed to prevent patient disruption of mechanical ventilation. This method can allow for spontaneous breathing between mandatory breaths (see the section Modes of Ventilation).

Positioning may be important in promoting ***gas exchange***, but the exact position is controversial. Some patients do better in the prone position, especially if it is started early in the disease course (Arias et al., 2017; Mitchell & Seckel, 2018; Schreiber, 2018) (see the Evidence-Based Practice box). Prone positioning may be achieved using a mechanical turning device, although the turning equipment is awkward and care in the prone position is more difficult. Automated kinetic beds are available to assist with turning. Manually turning the patient every 2 hours has been shown to improve ***perfusion***; however, this intervention often is not performed as frequently as needed. Early progressive mobility also has demonstrated benefit in reducing ventilator needs, days on the ventilator, and mortality. Automatic turning appears to have a slight advantage of decreasing some pulmonary complications but has not yet shown secondary benefits such as decreased lengths of stay, reduced ICU mortality, or decreased ventilator days.

For severe ARDS, extracorporeal membrane oxygenation (ECMO) using heart-lung bypass equipment has been a successful life-support technique when the patient does not improve with more traditional management (American Lung Association [ALA], 2018). Patients with severe COVID-19

EVIDENCE-BASED PRACTICE (QSEN)

Does Prone Positioning Improve Oxygenation or Survival for Patients With Acute Respiratory Distress Syndrome?

Arias, C., Pokharel, B., Papathanassoglou, E., Norris, C. (2017). Prone positioning for the treatment of adult respiratory distress syndrome. *CONNECT: The World of Critical Care Nursing, 11*(3), 49–54.

Multiple studies have shown that prone positioning for patients with ARDS resulted in clinical improvement but not always a difference in mortality. This study was a comprehensive literature review and meta-analysis of prone positioning as a treatment for ARDS to determine best practices. The systemized literature review used PubMed, CINAHL, and Scopus. The limit was set to clinical trials, and studies were excluded if they did not focus on prone positioning alone or were secondary studies. The review identified 10 studies with a total of 1891 ICU patients with ARDS. Main outcomes were oxygenation and morbidity and mortality. All the studies showed improved oxygenation with prone positioning compared with supine positioning; however, in some of the studies the differences did not reach statistical significance. One study with improved survival rates did not show a statistically significant difference between the prone group and the supine group. Among the studies, there was no consistent number of hours of prone positioning or duration of prone positioning. One study showed no difference between the onset of prone positioning at 48 hours and an onset at greater than 48 hours. A more recent study indicated that early prone positioning had the greatest impact for oxygenation and mortality. The results of the Proning Severe ARDS Patients (PROSEVA) trial demonstrated a 90-day mortality benefit, and its findings corroborated those of many other smaller studies. Patients in the PROSEVA trial used a mean duration of prone positioning of 17 hours and showed significant improvement in survival at 28 days and 90 days. Benefits of prone positioning during mechanical ventilation for ARDS appear to be related to a reduction of intrapulmonary shunting, increasing ventilation to larger areas of posterior lung structures by reducing compression of the dorsal lung structures, and improving lymphatic drainage to resolve pulmonary edema. Prone positioning was also found to minimize ventilator-induced lung injury (VILI) by reducing barotrauma and atelectrauma while halting the inflammatory cascade. Oxygen requirements also were reduced.

Level of Evidence: 1

This study is a meta-analysis of previous research studies of the use of prone positioning for ICU patients with ARDS. The methods used were appropriate for the purposes of the study, and the number of patients included added credible support to the results and recommendations.

Commentary: Implications for Practice and Research

The use of prone positioning has been shown to improve oxygenation through improved ventilation and perfusion and resolution of edema. Recent studies and the PROSEVA trial have also shown improved short- and long-term survival rates. However, this review was limited by the use of only three databases. No information was gathered or presented regarding any potential detrimental effects of prone positioning or the effect on nursing workflow. The PROSEVA investigators acknowledged the technical aspects required in positioning and noted that all participating centers were skilled in the turning process. The benefits of early prone positioning indicate that it is a viable treatment modality for patients with ARDS; however, further research is needed to determine the optimal duration of prone positioning and guidelines for managing potential adverse consequences, as well as nursing workflow issues.

infection may also be treated with ECMO if all other treatment methods fail (Fitzsimons & Crowley, 2020). However, the proper timing of ECMO and standardization of this therapy for best outcomes have not been established, and survival is more likely in younger patients who have no other health problems (Sahetya et al., 2018). In addition, it is often not available in many community hospitals.

Drug and Fluid Therapy. Antibiotics are used to treat infections when organisms are identified. Other drugs are used to manage any underlying cause. Currently no treatments reverse the pathologic changes in the lungs, although many interventions that modify the inflammatory responses and reduce oxidative stress are under investigation. These agents include vitamins C and E, *N*-acetylcysteine, and nitric oxide (Zhang et al., 2017).

Research shows that patients with ARDS who receive conservative fluid therapy have improved lung function and a shorter duration of mechanical ventilation and ICU length of stay compared with those who receive more liberal fluid therapy. Conservative fluid therapy involves infusing smaller amounts of IV fluid and using diuretics to maintain fluid balance, whereas liberal fluid therapy often results in an increasingly positive fluid balance and more edema. For those critically ill patients who are at risk for ARDS as a result of trauma, fluid management that involves slight hypotension is thought to help prevent ARDS (Kolarik & Roberts, 2017).

Nutrition Therapy. The patient with ARDS is at risk for malnutrition, which further reduces respiratory muscle function and the immune response. The interprofessional team must include a registered dietitian nutritionist. Enteral nutrition (tube feeding) or parenteral nutrition is started as soon as possible.

THE PATIENT REQUIRING INTUBATION AND VENTILATION

Pathophysiology Review

With mechanical ventilation, the patient who has severe problems of ***gas exchange*** may be supported until the underlying problem improves or resolves. Usually mechanical ventilation is a temporary life-support technique. The need for this support may be lifelong for those with severe restrictive lung disease or chronic progressive neuromuscular disease that reduces ventilation.

Mechanical ventilation is most often used for patients with hypoxemia and progressive alveolar hypoventilation with respiratory acidosis. The hypoxemia is usually caused by pulmonary shunting of blood when other methods of oxygen delivery do not provide a sufficiently high fraction of inspired oxygen (FiO_2). Mechanical ventilation may be used for patients who need temporary ventilatory support after surgery, those who expend too much energy with breathing and barely maintain adequate ***gas exchange***, or those who receive general anesthesia or heavy sedation.

❖ Interprofessional Collaborative Care

Assess the patient to be intubated in the same way as for other breathing problems. Once mechanical ventilation has been started, assess the respiratory system on an ongoing basis. Monitor and assess for problems related to the artificial airway or ventilator.

Endotracheal Intubation. The patient who needs mechanical ventilation must have an artificial airway. The most common type of airway for a short-term basis is the endotracheal (ET) tube.

Although there is no exact time frame, a tracheostomy is considered if an artificial airway is needed for longer than 10 to 14 days in order to reduce tracheal and vocal cord damage (see Chapter 25). Tracheostomy also is considered when a patient requires more than one intubation for respiratory failure. The expectations of intubation are to maintain a patent airway, provide a means to remove secretions, and provide ventilation and oxygen.

Endotracheal Tube. An ET tube is a long polyvinyl chloride tube that is passed through the mouth or nose and into the trachea (Fig. 29.1). When properly positioned, the tip of the ET tube rests about 2 cm above the *carina* (the point at which the trachea divides into the right and left mainstem bronchi). Oral intubation is a fast and easy way to establish an airway and is often performed as an emergency procedure. The nasal route is used for oral surgeries and when oral intubation is not possible, but is avoided with midface trauma or possible basilar skull fracture and is not used if the patient has a bleeding problem. An anesthesiologist, nurse anesthetist, or respiratory therapist usually performs the intubation.

When intubating a patient with COVID-19, all personnel involved must wear full protective gear, including eye protection, because this procedure has the highest risk for dispersion of infectious droplets. It is recommended that the intubation take place in an airborne infection isolation room (AIIR) (CDC, 2020).

The shaft of the tube has a radiopaque line running the length of the tube. This line shows on x-ray and is used to determine correct tube placement. Short horizontal lines (depth markings) are used to place the tube correctly at the naris or mouth (at the incisor tooth) and to identify how far the tube has been inserted.

The cuff at the distal end of the tube is inflated after placement and creates a seal between the trachea and the tube. The seal ensures delivery of a set tidal volume when mechanical ventilation is used. The cuff is inflated using a minimal-leak technique; when the cuff is inflated to an adequate sealing volume, a minimal amount of air can pass around it to the vocal cords, nose, or mouth. The patient cannot talk when the cuff is inflated.

The pilot balloon with a one-way valve permits air to be inserted into the cuff and prevents air from escaping. This balloon is a guide for determining whether air is present in the cuff, but it does not show how much or how little air is present, nor does it indicate how much pressure is exerted on the trachea from the cuff balloon.

The adapter connects the ET tube to the ventilator tubing or an oxygen delivery system. The ET tube size is listed on the shaft of the tube. Adult tube sizes range from 7 to 9 mm. Tube size selected is based on the size of the patient.

Preparing for Intubation. Know the proper procedure for summoning intubation personnel in the facility to the bedside in an emergency situation. Explain the procedure to the patient as clearly as possible. *Basic life-support measures, such as obtaining a patent airway and delivering 100% oxygen by a manual resuscitation bag with a facemask, are crucial to survival until help arrives.*

! NURSING SAFETY PRIORITY QSEN

Critical Rescue

Monitor patients at risk for airway obstruction and impaired ventilation. When you recognize the need for emergency intubation and ventilation, respond by bringing the code (or "crash") cart, airway equipment box, and suction equipment (often already on the code cart) to the bedside. Maintain a patent airway through positioning (head-tilt, chin-lift) and the insertion of an oral or nasopharyngeal airway until the patient is intubated. Delivering manual breaths with a bag-valve-mask may also be required.

During intubation, the nurse coordinates the rescue response and continuously monitors the patient for changes in vital signs, signs of hypoxia or hypoxemia, dysrhythmias, and aspiration. Ensure that each intubation attempt lasts no longer than 30 seconds, preferably less than 15 seconds. After 30 seconds, provide oxygen by means of a mask and manual resuscitation bag to prevent hypoxia and cardiac arrest. Suction as necessary.

Verifying Tube Placement. Immediately after an ET tube is inserted, placement is verified by checking end-tidal carbon dioxide levels and by chest x-ray (Barton et al., 2016). Assess for breath sounds bilaterally, sounds over the gastric area, symmetric chest movement, and air emerging from the ET tube. If breath sounds and chest wall movement are absent on the left side, the tube may be in the right mainstem bronchus. The respiratory health care provider intubating the patient should

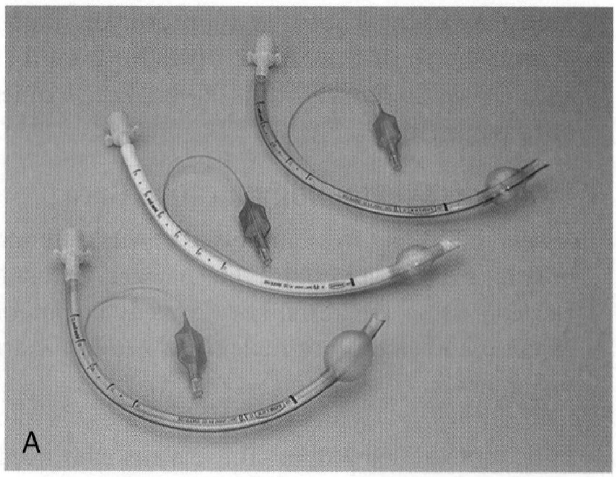

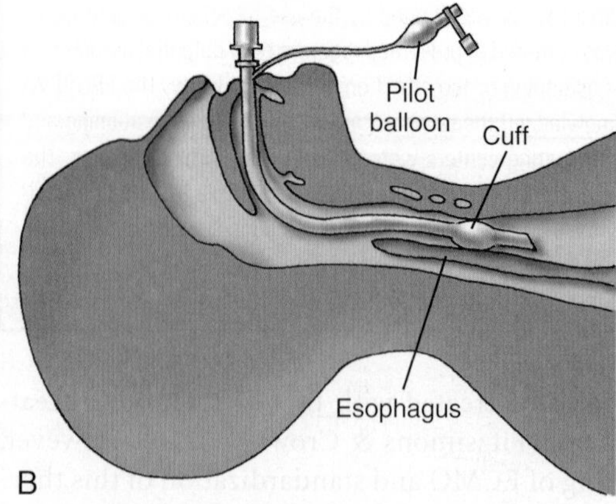

Fig. 29.1 (A) Endotracheal tubes. (B) Correct placement of an oral endotracheal tube. (A Courtesy Sims Porter, Inc.)

be able to reposition the tube without repeating the entire intubation procedure.

If the tube is in the stomach or esophagus, the abdomen may be distended and end-tidal carbon dioxide ($ETco_2$) monitoring would indicate the absence of carbon dioxide. In such a case, reintubation is necessary and the stomach must be decompressed with a nasogastric (NG) tube after the ET tube is properly placed. Monitor chest wall movement and breath sounds until tube placement is verified by chest x-ray.

Stabilizing the Tube. The nurse, respiratory therapist, or anesthesia provider stabilizes the ET tube at the mouth or nose. The tube is marked at the level where it touches the incisor tooth or naris. Two people working together use a head halter technique to secure the tube. An oral airway also may be inserted or a commercial bite block placed to keep the patient from biting an oral ET tube. One person stabilizes the tube at the correct position and prevents head movement while a second person applies the tube-holding device. After the procedure is completed, verify and document the presence of bilateral and equal breath sounds and the level of the tube.

Nursing Care. *The priority nursing action when caring for an intubated patient is maintaining a patent airway.* Assess tube placement, cuff leak, breath sounds, indications of adequate ***gas exchange*** and oxygenation, and chest wall movement regularly.

! NURSING SAFETY PRIORITY QSEN

Critical Rescue

Assess intubated patients to recognize indications of decreased ***gas exchange*** (cyanosis, decreased oxygen saturation, increased end-tidal CO_2, anxiety). When these indications are present, respond by checking for DOPE: *d*isplaced tube, *o*bstructed tube (most often with secretions), *p*neumothorax, and *e*quipment problems.

Prevent the patient from pulling or tugging on the tube to avoid tube dislodgment, and check the pilot balloon to ensure that the cuff is inflated. The most common causes of unplanned extubation in adults are confusion and agitation (Rojo et al., 2020). Monitor the pressure within the cuff to ensure that it is maintained between 20 to 30 cm H_2O to stabilize the tube without causing tracheal injury. Suctioning, coughing, and speaking can cause dislodgment. Neck flexion, neck extension, and rotation of the head also can cause the tube to move. In addition, cuff pressures may be affected by patient position changes and may require more frequent monitoring. Tongue movement also can change the tube's position. When other measures fail, obtain a prescription for soft wrist restraints and apply these for the patient who is pulling on the tube. *Restraints are used only as a last resort to prevent accidental extubation.*

! NATIONAL PATIENT SAFETY GOALS

To remain in compliance with The Joint Commission's National Patient Safety Goals (NPSGs), reassess the need for restraint use daily. If the need continues, a new prescription is needed daily. Adequate sedation (chemical restraint) may be needed to decrease agitation or prevent extubation. Obtain permission for restraints from the patient or family. More information on airway management is found in Chapter 25.

Complications of an ET or nasotracheal tube can occur during placement, while in place, during extubation, or after extubation (either early or late). Common complications include tube obstruction, tube dislodgment, pneumothorax, tracheal tears, bleeding, and infection. Trauma and other problems can occur to the face; eye; nasal and paranasal areas; oral, pharyngeal, bronchial, tracheal, and pulmonary areas; esophageal and gastric areas; and cardiovascular, musculoskeletal, and neurologic systems.

Mechanical Ventilation. Mechanical ventilation to support and maintain ***gas exchange*** is used in many settings, not just in critical care units. The nurse plays a pivotal role in the coordination of care and prevention of problems. The Best Practice for Patient Safety & Quality Care box: Care of the Patient Receiving Mechanical Ventilation box lists essential nursing care actions during mechanical ventilation.

The purposes of mechanical ventilation are to improve ***gas exchange*** and decrease the work needed for effective breathing. It is used to support the patient until lung function is adequate or until the acute episode has passed. *A ventilator does not cure diseased lungs; it provides ventilation until the patient can resume the process of breathing on his or her own.* Remember *why* the patient is using the ventilator so your management efforts also can focus on correcting the causes of the respiratory failure. If normal ***gas exchange*** with oxygenation, ventilation, and respiratory muscle strength is achieved, mechanical ventilation can be discontinued.

Types of Ventilators. Ventilators are available in two types. The most commonly used ventilators are positive-pressure ventilators. During inspiration, a pressure is generated that drives gas flow to push air into the lungs and expand the chest. Usually an endotracheal (ET) tube or tracheostomy is needed. Noninvasive positive-pressure ventilation systems use a mask or nasal prongs to deliver the gas flow. The nomenclature varies among ventilator manufacturers and sometimes between clinical areas (e.g., ICU, operating room). In general, ventilator settings are based on three components: trigger, gas delivery, and breath termination.

Inspiratory trigger is the initiation of the ventilator breath from the effort of the patient or as a set, timed breath from the ventilator. *Gas delivery* is achieved by setting the tidal volume, which is a specific target volume of gas, or setting a target pressure that delivers a variable volume of gas. *Breath termination* is the transition between inspiration and expiration. The inspiratory breath is terminated by a set volume, pressure, time, or flow. Volume-cycled ventilation pushes air into the lungs until a preset volume is delivered. A constant tidal volume is delivered, regardless of the pressure needed to deliver the tidal volume. However, a set pressure limit prevents excessive pressure from being exerted on the lungs. The advantage of this mode is that a constant tidal volume is delivered regardless of changes in lung or chest wall compliance or airway resistance. *Pressure-cycled ventilation* pushes air into the lungs until a preset airway pressure is reached. Tidal volumes and inspiratory time vary. *Time-cycled ventilations* push air into the lungs until a preset time has elapsed. Tidal volume and pressure vary. *Flow-cycled ventilation*

BEST PRACTICE FOR PATIENT SAFETY & QUALITY CARE QSEN

Care of the Patient Receiving Mechanical Ventilation

- Assess the patient's respiratory status and ***gas exchange*** at least every 4 hours for the first 24 hours and then as needed:
  - Take vital signs every 4 hours including oxygen saturation and lung auscultation (assess hourly or more often for patients in an ICU).
  - Be alert for the possibility of unintended extubation or self-extubation. If the patient requires sedation or restraints, follow institution guidelines for patient safety.
  - Assess color around the lips and nail beds, and observe for bilateral chest expansion.
  - Assess the placement of the endotracheal tube.
  - Evaluate ABGs as available.
- Maintain head of the bed more than 30 degrees when patient is supine to decrease the risk for aspiration and ventilator-associated pneumonia.
- Review ventilator settings at least every 8 hours, including alarm settings, with the respiratory therapist (RT).
- Review the patient information on the ventilator display to confirm that the patient is receiving the prescribed set tidal volume and that peak pressures are not elevated (indicator of obstruction or decreased lung compliance).
- Empty ventilator tubings when moisture collects.
- Be sure the cuff is adequately inflated to ensure tidal volume. If there is a concern for overinflation, have the RT check the cuff pressure.
- Assess the need for suctioning every 2 hours and suction only as needed (being sure to preoxygenate the patient before suctioning).
- Assess the patient's mouth around the ET tube for pressure injuries.
- Perform mouth care at least every 12 hours using standard ventilator bundles.
- Perform tracheostomy care at least every 8 hours, changing the ET tube holder or tape as needed, and moving the oral ET tube to the opposite side of the mouth daily to prevent ulcers.
- Assess ventilated patients for GI distress (diarrhea, constipation, tarry stools).
- Turn the patient at least every 2 hours and get him or her out of bed as prescribed to prevent complications of immobility.
- Monitor the patient's progress on current ventilator settings and promptly relay any concerns to the respiratory health care provider or RT.
- Monitor for adverse effects of mechanical ventilation: infection, barotrauma, reduced cardiac output.
- Position the patient to facilitate ventilation-perfusion ($\dot{V}/\dot{Q}$) matching ("good lung down"), as appropriate.
- Monitor the effects of ventilator changes on ***gas exchange,*** the patient's subjective responses, and readiness to wean.
- Provide a method of communication. Request consultation with a speech-language pathologist for assistance, if necessary.
- Administer muscle-paralyzing agents, sedatives, and narcotic analgesics, as prescribed, using the lowest possible dose to achieve patient comfort without oversedation.
- Include the patient and family whenever possible (especially during suctioning and tracheostomy care).

ABGs, Arterial blood gases; *ET,* endotracheal; *PEEP,* positive end-expiratory pressure.

is used with pressure support ventilation. It will terminate the breath when it reaches a preset flow rate derived as a percentage of the patient's maximum inspiratory flow.

Modes of Ventilation. The mode of ventilation is the way in which the patient receives breaths from the ventilator. The most common modes of ventilation—assist-control (AC) ventilation, synchronized intermittent mandatory ventilation (SIMV), and pressure support (PS) ventilation—are based on either the volume mode or pressure mode of gas delivery.

Assist-control (AC) ventilation is a full support mode. The ventilator takes over the work of breathing for the patient. The tidal volume and ventilatory rate are preset and referred to as *mandatory breaths.* If the patient does not trigger spontaneous breaths, a ventilatory pattern is established by the ventilator. This mode of ventilation can be used with either a pressure-regulated mode or a volume-regulated mode of gas delivery. It is programmed to respond to the patient's inspiratory effort if he or she begins a breath. In this case, the ventilator delivers the preset tidal volume whether the breath is mandatory or patient initiated. This mode allows the patient to increase the rate of breathing above the set rate.

A disadvantage of the AC mode is that the ventilator continues to deliver a preset tidal volume even when the patient's spontaneous breathing rate increases. This can cause hyperventilation and respiratory alkalosis. Investigate and correct causes of hyperventilation, such as pain, anxiety, or acid-base imbalances. Although AC is considered a full support mode, it is possible for the patient to be weaned directly from AC to a spontaneous mode such as pressure support ventilation.

Synchronized intermittent mandatory ventilation (SIMV) is similar to AC ventilation in that tidal volume and ventilatory rate are preset. This type of ventilation can be used in either pressure- or volume-regulated mode. If the patient does not breathe, a ventilatory pattern is established by the ventilator. Unlike the AC mode, SIMV allows spontaneous breathing at the patient's own rate and tidal volume between the ventilator breaths. It can be used as a main ventilatory mode or as a weaning mode. When used for weaning, the number of mechanical breaths (SIMV breaths) is gradually decreased (e.g., from 12 to 2) as the patient resumes spontaneous breathing. The mandatory ventilator breaths are delivered when the patient is ready to inspire. This action coordinates breathing between the ventilator and the patient.

Pressure support ventilation is used for spontaneously breathing patients. No tidal volume is set. It delivers the patient's own breath with assistance from a set airway pressure and PEEP. It is used as a step in the weaning process.

Continuous positive airway pressure (CPAP) and bi-level positive airway pressure (BiPAP) are noninvasive pressure support modes of ventilation (NIPPV) used for spontaneously breathing patients. They require the use of a nasal mask or facemask. CPAP applies positive airway pressure throughout the entire respiratory cycle, keeps the alveoli open during inspiration, and prevents alveolar collapse during expiration. This process increases functional residual capacity (FRC) and improves ***gas exchange*** and oxygenation. Normal levels of CPAP are 5 to 15 cm H_2O. BiPAP provides two levels of pressure: a higher inspiratory (IPAP) pressure, typically 10 to 20 cm H_2O, and a lower expiratory (EPAP) pressure, typically 4 to 8 cm H_2O, which make exhalation easier and improve ***gas exchange.*** Both machines can be used to treat patients with sleep apnea, but BiPAP may also be used for patients with chronic obstructive pulmonary disease (COPD), heart failure, respiratory muscle fatigue, or impending respiratory failure to avoid more invasive ventilation methods.

Other modes of ventilation, such as airway pressure release ventilation (APRV), proportional assist ventilation (PAV), and high-frequency oscillatory ventilation (HFOV), are alternative modes of ventilation for patients with severe hypoxemia, those needing improved ventilator synchrony, or those needing rescue therapy.

Ventilator Controls and Settings. Manufacturers of positive pressure ventilators may have various accessories and different terminology, but the basic settings are generally similar (Fig. 29.2). The pulmonologist, intensivist, or respiratory health care provider prescribes the ventilator settings, and usually the ventilator is readied or set up by the respiratory therapy department. The nurse assists in connecting the patient to the ventilator and monitors the ventilator settings in conjunction with respiratory therapy.

Tidal volume (V_T) is the volume of air the patient receives with each breath, as measured on either inspiration or expiration. The average prescribed V_T ranges between 6 and 8 mL/kg of body weight, based on ideal body weight (IBW) and an accurate measure of patient height.

Rate, or breaths/min, is the number of ventilator breaths delivered per minute. The rate is usually set between 10 and 14 breaths/min. Patient condition and ventilator mode can be factors in setting a rate above or below this range.

Fraction of inspired oxygen (Fio_2) is the oxygen level delivered to the patient. The prescribed Fio_2 is based on the ABG values and the patient's condition. The range is 21% to 100% oxygen.

The oxygen delivered to the patient is warmed to body temperature (98.6°F [37°C]) and humidified to 100%. This is needed because upper air passages of the respiratory tree, which normally warm and humidify air, are bypassed. Humidifying and warming prevent mucosal damage.

Peak airway (inspiratory) pressure (PIP) is the pressure used by the ventilator to deliver a set tidal volume at a given lung compliance. The PIP value appears on the display of the ventilator. It is the highest pressure reached during inspiration. Trends in PIP reflect changes in resistance of the lungs and resistance in the ventilator. An increased PIP reading means increased airway resistance in the patient or the ventilator tubing (bronchospasm or pinched tubing, patient biting the ET tube), increased secretions, pulmonary edema, or decreased pulmonary compliance (the lungs or chest wall is "stiffer" and harder to inflate). An upper pressure limit is set to prevent barotrauma. When the limit is reached, the high-pressure alarm sounds, and the remaining volume is not given.

Positive end-expiratory pressure (PEEP) is positive pressure exerted during expiration. PEEP improves oxygenation by enhancing ***gas exchange*** and preventing atelectasis. Most patients on mechanical ventilation will have a set PEEP of 5 to 6 cm H_2O in order to prevent alveolar collapse and improve arterial oxygenation. PEEP may be increased to 15 cm H_2O or greater when the arterial oxygen pressure (Pao_2) remains low despite increasing the Fio_2.

The need for increased PEEP indicates a severe **gas exchange** problem. It is important to lower the Fio_2 delivered whenever

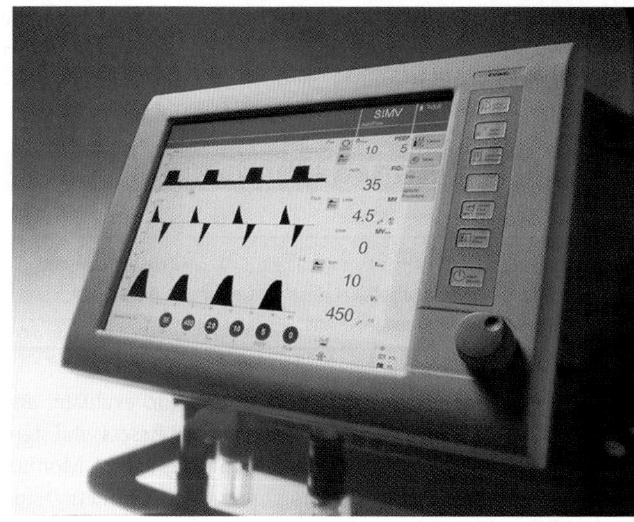

Fig. 29.2 Display signals, alarms, and control panel of a typical volume-cycled ventilator. (© Dräger Medical AG & Co. KG, Lübeck, Germany. All rights reserved. No portion hereof may be reproduced, saved or stored in a data processing system, electronically or mechanically copied or otherwise recorded by any other means without express prior written permission.)

possible because prolonged use of a high Fio_2 can damage lungs from the toxic effects of oxygen. PEEP prevents alveoli from collapsing because the lungs are kept partially inflated so alveolar-capillary gas exchange is promoted throughout the ventilatory cycle. The effect should be an increase in arterial blood oxygenation so the Fio_2 can be decreased.

Flow rate is how fast each breath is delivered and the range is usually set between 40 and 60 L/min. *If a patient is agitated or restless, has a widely fluctuating inspiratory pressure reading, or has other signs of air hunger, the flow may be set too low. Increasing the flow should be tried before using chemical restraints.*

Other settings may be used depending on the mode of ventilation and patient condition. These settings may include waveform, plateau, pressure-volume loop, trigger sensitivity, and alarm settings.

Nursing Management. The use of mechanical ventilation involves a collaborative and complex decision-making process for the patient, family, and interprofessional care team. Long-term use and its discontinuance has both ethical and legal consequences. Address the physical and psychological concerns of the patient and family because the mechanical ventilator often causes them anxiety. Explain the purpose of the ventilator and acknowledge the patient's and family's feelings. Encourage the patient and family to express their concerns. Act as the coach to help and support them through this experience. Patients undergoing mechanical ventilation in ICUs often experience delirium, or "ICU psychosis." These patients need frequent, repeated explanations and reassurance.

When caring for a ventilated patient, be concerned with the patient first and the ventilator second. If the ventilator alarm sounds, examine the patient for breathing, color, and oxygen saturation before assessing the ventilator. It is vital to understand *why* mechanical ventilation is needed. Some problems requiring ventilation, such as excessive secretions, sepsis, and trauma, require different interventions to successfully wean from the ventilator. Chronic health problems (e.g., COPD, left-sided heart failure, anemia, malnutrition) may slow weaning from mechanical ventilation and require close monitoring and intervention.

! NURSING SAFETY PRIORITY (QSEN)

Action Alert

The nursing priorities in caring for the patient during mechanical ventilation are monitoring and evaluating patient responses, managing the ventilator system safely, and preventing complications.

Monitoring the Patient's Response. Monitor, evaluate, and document the patient's response to the ventilator. Assess vital signs and listen to breath sounds every 30 to 60 minutes at first. Monitor respiratory parameters (e.g., capnography, pulse oximetry) and check ABG values. Monitoring provides information to guide the patient's activities, such as weaning, physical or occupational therapy, and self-care. Pace activities to ensure effective ventilation with adequate ***gas exchange*** and oxygenation. Interpret ABG values to evaluate the effectiveness of ventilation and determine whether ventilator settings need to be changed.

Assess the breathing pattern in relation to the ventilatory cycle to determine whether the patient is tolerating or fighting the ventilator. Patient asynchrony with mechanical ventilation has many causes and reduces the effectiveness of ***gas exchange***. Assess and record breath sounds, and confirm that breath sounds are equal bilaterally to ensure proper endotracheal (ET) tube placement. Determine the need for suctioning by observing secretions for type, color, and amount. The most common indicator of the need for suctioning is the presence of coarse crackles over the trachea. Assess the area around the ET tube or tracheostomy site at least every 4 hours for color, tenderness, skin irritation, and drainage, and document the findings.

The nurse spends the most time with the patient and is most likely to be the first person to recognize changes in vital signs or ABG values, fatigue, or distress. If the patient's condition does not respond to current intervention, promptly coordinate with the respiratory health care provider and respiratory therapist. The respiratory health care provider may change the prescribed management plan to prevent the patient's condition from deteriorating. The respiratory therapist can most accurately assess the function of the ventilation equipment and make appropriate adjustments or replacements.

! NURSING SAFETY PRIORITY (QSEN)

Critical Rescue

Always assess patients being mechanically ventilated for indications of respiratory distress and poor ***gas exchange***. When symptoms of respiratory distress develop during mechanical ventilation, respond by immediately removing the ventilator and providing ventilation with a bag-valve-mask device. This action allows quick determination of whether the problem is with the ventilator or the patient. If no ventilator problem is identified, reconnect the patient to the ventilator and request respiratory therapy assistance.

Serve as a resource for the psychological needs of the patient and family. Anxiety can reduce tolerance for mechanical ventilation. Skilled and sensitive nursing care promotes emotional well-being and synchrony with the ventilator. The patient cannot speak, and communication can be frustrating and produce anxiety. The patient and family may panic because they believe that the voice has been lost. Reassure them that the ET tube prevents speech only temporarily.

Plan methods of communication to meet the patient's needs, such as a picture board, pen and paper, alphabet board, electronic tablet computer, or programmable speech-generating device. Some patients who are alert are able to use text messaging on smart phones for communication with staff, relatives, and friends. Finding a successful means for communication is important because the patient often feels isolated by the inability to speak. Anticipate his or her needs, and provide easy access to frequently used belongings. The observation of facial expressions in noncommunicative patients may indicate pain, especially during suctioning. Visits from family, friends, and pets and keeping a call light within reach are some ways of giving patients a sense of control over the environment. Urge them to participate in self-care.

Managing the Ventilator System. Ventilator settings are prescribed by the respiratory health care provider in conjunction with the respiratory therapist. Settings include tidal volume, respiratory rate, fraction of inspired oxygen (FiO_2), and mode of ventilation (assist-control [AC] ventilation, synchronized intermittent mandatory ventilation [SIMV], and adjunctive therapies such as positive end-expiratory pressure [PEEP] or pressure support).

Perform and document ventilator checks according to the standards of the unit or facility (in many facilities this function is performed by respiratory therapists). Respond promptly to alarms. During a ventilator check, compare the prescribed ventilator settings with the actual settings and confirm these findings with the respiratory therapist. Check the level of water in the humidifier and the temperature of the humidifying system to ensure that they are not too high. Temperature extremes damage the airway mucosa. Remove any condensation in the ventilator tubing by draining water into drainage collection receptacles, and empty them every shift.

! NURSING SAFETY PRIORITY (QSEN)

Action Alert

To prevent bacterial contamination, do not allow moisture and water in the ventilator tubing to enter the humidifier.

Mechanical ventilators have alarm systems that warn of a problem with either the patient or the ventilator. *Alarms should never be turned off or ignored during mechanical ventilation.* The major alarms on a ventilator indicate either a high pressure or a low exhaled volume. Table 29.5 lists interventions for causes of ventilator alarms.

! NATIONAL PATIENT SAFETY GOALS

The Joint Commission requires that ventilator alarm systems be activated and functional at all times. If the cause of the alarm cannot be determined, ventilate the patient manually with a resuscitation bag until the problem is corrected by another health care professional.

TABLE 29.5 **Nursing Interventions for Various Causes of Ventilator Alarms**

Cause	Nursing Actions
High-Pressure Alarm (sounds when peak inspiratory pressure reaches the set alarm limit [usually set 10-20 mm Hg above the patient's baseline PIP])	
An increased amount of secretions or a mucus plug is in the airways.	Suction as needed.
The patient coughs, gags, or bites on the oral ET tube.	Insert oral airway to prevent biting on the ET tube. Provide adequate pain management and sedation as prescribed.
The patient is anxious or fights the ventilator.	Provide emotional support to decrease anxiety. Increase the flow rate. Explain all procedures to the patient. Provide sedation or paralyzing agent as prescribed.
Airway size decreases related to wheezing or bronchospasm.	Auscultate breath sounds. Collaborate with respiratory therapy department to provide prescribed bronchodilators.
Pneumothorax occurs.	Alert the pulmonary health care provider or Rapid Response Team about a new onset of decreased breath sounds or unequal chest excursion, which may be caused by pneumothorax. Auscultate breath sounds.
The artificial airway is displaced; the ET tube may have slipped into the right mainstem bronchus.	Assess the chest for unequal breath sounds and chest excursion. Obtain a chest x-ray as ordered to evaluate the position of the ET tube. After the proper position is verified, secure the tube in place.
Obstruction in tubing occurs because the patient is lying on the tubing or there is water or a kink in the tubing.	Assess the system, beginning with the artificial airway and moving toward the ventilator.
There is increased PIP associated with deliverance of a sigh.	Empty water from the ventilator tubing and remove any kinks. Coordinate with respiratory therapist or pulmonary health care provider to adjust the pressure alarm.
Decreased compliance of the lungs is noted; a trend of gradually increasing PIP is noted over several hours or a day.	Evaluate the reasons for the decreased compliance of the lungs. Increased PIP occurs in ARDS, pneumonia, or any worsening of pulmonary disease.
Low–Exhaled Volume (or Low-Pressure) Alarm (sounds when there is a disconnection or leak in the ventilator circuit or a leak in the patient's artificial airway cuff)	
A leak in the ventilator circuit prevents breath from being delivered.	Assess all connections and all ventilator tubing for disconnection.
The patient stops spontaneous breathing in the SIMV or CPAP mode or on pressure support ventilation.	Evaluate the patient's tolerance of the mode. Evaluate for overmedication with sedation or pain drugs.
A cuff leak occurs in the ET or tracheostomy tube.	Evaluate the patient for a cuff leak. A cuff leak is suspected when the patient can talk (air escapes from the mouth) or when the pilot balloon on the artificial airway is flat (see Tracheostomy Tubes section in Chapter 25).

ARDS, Acute respiratory distress syndrome; *CPAP,* continuous positive airway pressure; *ET,* endotracheal; *PIP,* peak inspiratory pressure; *SIMV,* synchronized intermittent mandatory ventilation.

Assess and care for the ET or tracheostomy tube. Maintain a patent airway by suctioning when any of these conditions are present:

- Secretions
- Increased peak airway (inspiratory) pressure (PIP)
- Rhonchi
- Decreased breath sounds

Proper care of the ET or tracheostomy tube also ensures a patent airway. Assess tube position at least every 2 hours, especially when the airway is attached to heavy ventilator tubing that may pull on the tube. Position the ventilator tubing so the patient can move without pulling on the ET or tracheostomy tube, possibly dislodging it. To detect changes in tube position, mark it where the tube touches the patient's teeth or nose. Give oral care per facility policy. Standardized oral care performed at least every 12 hours has been shown to reduce ventilator-associated pneumonia (VAP), although the exact solution remains controversial (Boltey et al., 2017; Parisi et al., 2016; Warren et al., 2019).

Special attention is needed for the patient being transported while receiving mechanical ventilation. Monitor Spo_2 during transport to assess adequacy of ventilation. Assess lung sounds each time the patient is moved, transferred, or turned. Consider the use of end-tidal carbon dioxide ($ETco_2$) monitoring, if available.

Preventing Complications. A wide variety of complications, now known as **ventilator-associated events (VAEs)**, are conditions that result in a sustained decrease in oxygenation (Baird, 2016). Specific indicators include greater than 20%

NCLEX EXAMINATION CHALLENGE 29.3

Safe and Effective Care Environment

The client, a woman who is 5 feet 11 inches tall and 176 lb (80 kg), has been mechanically ventilated at a tidal volume of 400 mL and a respiratory rate of 12 breaths/min for the past 24 hours. The most recent arterial blood gas (ABG) results for this client are pH = 7.32; Pa_{O_2} = 84 mm Hg; Pa_{CO_2} = 56 mm Hg. What is the nurse's interpretation of these results?

A. Ventilation adequate to maintain oxygenation.
B. Ventilation excessive; respiratory alkalosis present.
C. Ventilation inadequate; respiratory acidosis present.
D. Ventilation status cannot be determined from information presented.

increase in the daily minimum fraction of inspired oxygen or an increase of at least 3 cm H_2O in the daily minimum positive end-expiratory pressure (PEEP) to maintain oxygenation. Table 29.6 lists the tiers of VAEs. Other complications affecting many body systems are related to positive pressure from the ventilator.

TABLE 29.6 Tiers of Ventilator-Associated Events

Tier	Characteristics
1. Ventilator-associated condition (VAC)	Patient develops hypoxemia for a sustained period of more than 2 days, regardless of its etiology.
2. Infection-related ventilator-associated complication (IVAC)	Hypoxemia develops in the setting of generalized infection or inflammation, and antibiotics are instituted for a minimum of 4 days.
3. Ventilator-associated pneumonia (VAP)	There is additional laboratory evidence of white blood cells or Gram stain of material from a respiratory secretion specimen of acceptable quality and/or presence of respiratory pathogens on quantitative cultures from patients with IVAC.

Cardiac problems from mechanical ventilation include hypotension and fluid retention. Hypotension is caused by positive pressure that increases chest pressure and inhibits blood return to the heart. The decreased blood return reduces cardiac output, causing hypotension, especially in patients who are dehydrated or need high PIP for ventilation. Teach the patient to avoid a *Valsalva maneuver* (bearing down while holding the breath).

Fluid is retained because of decreased cardiac output. The kidneys receive less blood flow, which stimulates the renin-angiotensin-aldosterone system (RAAS) to retain fluid. Humidified air in the ventilator system contributes to fluid retention. Monitor the patient's fluid intake and output, weight, hydration status, and indications of hypovolemia.

Lung problems from mechanical ventilation include:

- **Barotrauma** (damage to the lungs by positive pressure)
- **Volutrauma** (damage to the lung by excess volume delivered to one lung over the other)
- **Atelectrauma** (shear injury to alveoli from opening and closing)
- **Biotrauma** (inflammatory response–mediated damage to alveoli)
- **Ventilator-associated lung injury/ventilator-induced lung injury (VALI/VILI)** (damage from prolonged ventilation causing loss of surfactant, increased inflammation, fluid leakage, and noncardiac pulmonary edema)
- Acid-base imbalance

Barotrauma includes pneumothorax, subcutaneous emphysema, and pneumomediastinum. Patients at highest risk for barotrauma have chronic airflow limitation (CAL), have blebs or bullae, are on PEEP, have dynamic hyperinflation, or require high pressures to ventilate the lungs (because of "stiff" lungs, as seen in acute respiratory distress syndrome [ARDS]). Ventilator-induced lung injury can be prevented by using low tidal volumes combined with moderate levels of PEEP, especially in patients with acute lung injury (ALI) or ARDS. Blood gas problems can be corrected by ventilator changes and adjustment of fluid and electrolyte imbalances.

GI and nutrition problems result from the stress of mechanical ventilation. Stress ulcers occur in many patients receiving mechanical ventilation. These ulcers complicate the nutrition status and, because the mucosa is not intact, increase the risk for systemic infection. Antacids and histamine blockers such as cimetidine or proton pump inhibitors such as esomeprazole may be prescribed as soon as the patient is intubated.

Because many other acute or life-threatening events occur at the same time, nutrition is often neglected. Malnutrition is an extreme problem for these patients and is a cause of failing to wean from the ventilator. In malnutrition, the respiratory muscles lose mass and strength. The diaphragm, the major muscle of inspiration, is affected early. When it and other respiratory muscles are weak, ineffective breathing results, fatigue occurs, and the patient cannot be weaned.

Balanced nutrition, whether by diet, enteral feedings, or parenteral feeding, is essential during ventilation and is often started within 48 hours of intubation in consultation with a registered dietitian nutritionist. Nutrition for the patient with chronic obstructive pulmonary disease (COPD) is more complicated because it requires a reduction of dietary carbohydrates. During metabolism, carbohydrates are broken down to glucose, which then produces energy, carbon dioxide, and water. Excessive carbohydrate loads increase carbon dioxide production, which the patient with COPD may be unable to exhale. Hypercarbic respiratory failure may result. Nutrition formulas with a higher fat content (e.g., Pulmocare, Nutren Pulmonary) are calorie sources to combat this problem.

Electrolyte replacement is also important because electrolytes influence muscle function. Monitor potassium, calcium, magnesium, and phosphate levels and replace them as prescribed.

Infections are part of two tiers of ventilator-associated events (VAEs) and are a threat for the patient using a ventilator, especially ventilator-associated pneumonia (VAP). The ET or tracheostomy tube bypasses the body's filtering process and provides direct access for bacteria to enter the lower respiratory system. The artificial airway is colonized with bacteria within 48 hours, which promotes pneumonia development and increases morbidity. Aspiration of colonized fluid from the mouth or stomach can be a source of infection. *Infection prevention through strict adherence to infection control, especially handwashing during suctioning and care of the tracheostomy or ET tube, is essential, as is meticulous oral care* (Warren et al., 2019).

To prevent VAP, implement "ventilator bundle" order sets, which typically include these actions (Parisi et al., 2016; Warren et al., 2019):

- Keeping the head of the bed elevated at least 30 degrees
- Performing oral care per agency policy (usually brushing teeth with a suction toothbrush at least every 12 hours and antimicrobial rinse)
- Ulcer prophylaxis
- Preventing aspiration
- Pulmonary hygiene, including chest physiotherapy, postural drainage, and turning and positioning

Using the ventilator bundle has greatly reduced the overall incidence of VAP. Vigilant oral care using a suction toothbrush is a key component of the VAP prevention strategy, although actual practice varies regarding timing, products used, and specific application methods (Wong et al., 2016). Additional information on pneumonia can be found in Chapter 28.

Most patients requiring mechanical ventilation, except those with ARDS, are placed in a supine position with the head of the bed elevated to at least 30 degrees. This backrest elevation does not appear to be associated with an increase in sacral skin breakdown when other skin protection practices are in place (Grap et al., 2018).

Muscle deconditioning and weakness can occur because of immobility. Getting the patient out of bed and having him or her ambulate with help and perform exercises not only improve muscle strength and help prevent pneumonia but also boost morale, enhance ***gas exchange***, and promote oxygen delivery to all muscles. Early progressive mobility decreases ventilator days and ICU stays, although it is an underused intervention, possible because of staff misconceptions. The Systems Thinking and Quality Improvement box demonstrates how education and engagement can help increase the implementation of this evidence-based intervention (Castro et al., 2015). Early passive exercise also may be beneficial.

Ventilator dependence is the inability to wean off the ventilator and can have both a physiologic and a psychological basis. The longer a patient uses a ventilator, the more difficult the weaning process is because the respiratory muscles fatigue and cannot assume breathing. Special units and facilities can maximize the rehabilitation and weaning of ventilator-dependent patients. The health care team uses every method of weaning before a patient is declared "unweanable." Long-term ventilator use and the decision to terminate ventilator use even when respiratory independence has not been achieved have both ethical and legal implications for the patient, family, and health care professionals. Some of these issues are presented in the Ethical/Legal Considerations box.

Weaning. Weaning is the process of going from ventilatory dependence to spontaneous breathing. The process is prolonged by complications. Many problems can be avoided with appropriate nursing care. For example, turning and positioning the patient not only promote comfort and prevent skin breakdown but also improve ***gas exchange*** and prevent pneumonia and atelectasis. Table 29.7 lists various weaning techniques.

Extubation. Extubation is the removal of the endotracheal (ET) tube. The tube is removed when the need for intubation has been resolved. Before removal, explain the procedure. Set up the prescribed oxygen delivery system at the bedside and bring in the equipment for emergency reintubation. Hyperoxygenate

SYSTEMS THINKING AND QUALITY IMPROVEMENT QSEN

Can the Mindset of Nursing Staff Be Changed Regarding the Mobilization of Patients Receiving Mechanical Ventilation?

Castro, E., Turcinovic, M., Platz, J., Law, I. (2015). Early mobilization: Changing the mindset. *Critical Care Nurse Online, 35*(4), e1–e6.

Patients in an ICU face prolonged periods of bedrest and immobility, leading to deconditioning and alterations in neuropsychological function. Increasing the frequency of physical and occupational therapy results in improved functional independence and decreased mechanical ventilation days. Staff of a surgical ICU (SICU) at an academic teaching center had concerns about mobilizing patients receiving mechanical ventilation. A quality improvement project was implemented with the goal of changing the mindset of the SICU staff toward mobilization of mechanically ventilated patients using a Plan-Do-Study-Act model. A questionnaire was developed to assess the mindset of the nurses and the strength of their concerns. It was administered 2 weeks before, 6 months after, and 1 year after the implementation of early mobilization. The SICU interdisciplinary team developed criteria and a protocol for early mobilization based on the findings of a previous study that demonstrated a decreased length of stay for the mobility group. Activity levels ranged from passive range of motion through leg-dangling at bedside to sitting in a chair to ambulating. Staff education addressing the adverse outcomes of immobility and the eligibility criteria was conducted by a nurse educator, physical therapist, respiratory therapist, and SICU attending physician to all unit nursing staff. Plans to remove barriers and promote mobilization included hiring of dedicated physical therapists, increasing physical therapy presence to 5 days weekly, and obtaining the necessary equipment needed to ambulate patients. The results of the quality improvement project showed an increase in the mindset of SICU nurses toward mobilizing patients during mechanical ventilation, which resulted greater implementation of the mobilization intervention.

Commentary: Implications for Practice and Research

Although this quality improvement project was performed a number of years ago, its nature and results remain important in helping identify paths to implementing evidence-based interventions by assisting nurses to be willing to dispel myths regarding a perceived "sacred cow" and promoting evidence-based changes for patient benefit. The project assessed nursing concerns, provided education about the importance and benefits of early mobilization, addressed safety concerns, and removed barriers to implementing an early mobilization program. The overall nursing mindset improved to acknowledge that it was safe to mobilize mechanically ventilated patients. However, one of the survey questions indicated that nurses did not agree with the shared responsibility for providing daily exercises for patients. Given the importance and accepted benefit of early mobility, this would be an area for further investigation to determine if there are additional barriers or ongoing lack of knowledge about the benefits of mobility. This project also indicated that length of stay, ventilator-associated pneumonia, and skin breakdown occurrence decreased. Data indicating the statistical significance of those outcomes were not specifically presented and remain an opportunity for additional research.

ETHICAL/LEGAL CONSIDERATIONS

When conditions indicate that a patient is likely to be permanently ventilator dependent, the patient and family are faced with decisions that require a clear understanding of possible alternatives regarding home ventilation, nursing home placement, or withdrawal of life support. The patient's family always have input into the decision to continue or withdraw ventilator support; however, the most ethical plans are ones that support the patient's verified wishes. Having advance directives in place help make such decisions easier on families and health care professionals. When the patient cannot give input and advance directives are not in place, the issues are more difficult and decisions must be based on the patient's quality of life, goals, and values. Collaboration with the hospital's ethics committee, pulmonology health care provider, social worker or psychologist, and clergy is needed to ensure the family have the most complete and accurate information (in a form they understand) in order to make a truly informed decision based on expert recommendations, as well as on the laws of the state with regard to withdrawal of life support. The role of the nurse is to help ascertain the family's understanding of the situation, ensure coercion is not present, and support the family during and after the decision-making process.

PATIENT-CENTERED CARE: OLDER ADULT CONSIDERATIONS QSEN

The older patient, especially one who has smoked or who has a chronic lung problem such as COPD, is at risk for ventilator dependence and failure to wean. Age-related changes, such as chest wall stiffness, reduced ventilatory muscle strength, and decreased lung elasticity, reduce the likelihood of weaning. The usual symptoms of ventilatory failure—hypoxemia and hypercarbia—may be less obvious in the older adult. Use other clinical measures of gas exchange and oxygenation, such as a change in mental status, to determine breathing effectiveness (Touhy & Jett, 2020; Stieff et al., 2017).

the patient and thoroughly suction both the ET tube and the oral cavity. Instruct the patient to inhale deeply and then rapidly deflate the cuff of the ET tube and remove the tube during exhalation. Immediately instruct the patient to cough. It is normal for large amounts of oral secretions to collect. Give oxygen by facemask or nasal cannula. The fraction of inspired oxygen (Fio_2) is usually prescribed at 10% higher than the level used while the ET tube was in place.

Monitor vital signs after extubation every 5 minutes at first and assess the ventilatory pattern for signs of respiratory distress. It is common for patients to be hoarse and have a sore throat for a few days after extubation. Teach the patient to sit in a semi-Fowler position, take deep breaths every half-hour, use an incentive spirometer every 2 hours, and limit speaking. These measures help improve ***gas exchange***, decrease laryngeal edema, and reduce vocal cord irritation. Observe closely for respiratory fatigue and airway obstruction.

Early symptoms of obstruction are mild dyspnea, coughing, and the inability to expectorate secretions. *Stridor* is a high-pitched, crowing noise during inspiration caused by laryngospasm or edema around the glottis. *It is a late sign of a narrowed airway*

! NURSING SAFETY PRIORITY QSEN

Critical Rescue

Monitor the patient frequently to recognize symptoms of obstruction. When stridor or other symptoms of obstruction occur after extubation, respond by immediately initiating the Rapid Response Team *before* the airway becomes completely obstructed.

TABLE 29.7 Weaning Methods

Synchronous Intermittent Mandatory Ventilation
- The patient breathes between the machine's preset breaths/min rate.
- The machine is initially set on an SIMV rate of 12, meaning that the patient receives a minimum of 12 breaths/min by the ventilator.
- The patient's respiratory rate will be a combination of ventilator breaths and spontaneous breaths.
- As the weaning process ensues, the pulmonary health care provider prescribes gradual decreases in the SIMV rate, usually at a decrease of 1 to 2 breaths/min.

T-Piece Technique
- The patient is removed from the ventilator for short periods (initially 5 to 10 minutes) and allowed to breathe spontaneously.
- The ventilator is replaced with a T-piece (see Chapter 25) or CPAP, which delivers humidified oxygen.
- The prescribed Fio_2 may be higher for the patient on the T-piece than on the ventilator.
- Weaning progresses as the patient can tolerate progressively longer periods off the ventilator.
- Nighttime weaning is not usually attempted until the patient can maintain spontaneous respirations for most of the day.

Pressure Support Ventilation
- The patient's respiratory rate and tidal volume are their own.
- PSV allows the patient's respiratory effort to be augmented by a predetermined pressure assist from the ventilator.
- As the weaning process ensues, the amount of pressure applied to inspiration is gradually decreased.

Daily Spontaneous Breathing Trials
- The patient remains on PSV but the PEEP and pressure support (PS) are both decreased.
- In some trials, the PEEP is decreased to 5 cm H_2O and the PS is decreased to 0.
- The patient's hemodynamic status is monitored as well as pulmonary status.
- After 30 to 60 minutes ABGs are obtained for analysis.
- SBT should be attempted daily to assess for readiness to liberate from mechanical ventilation.

ABG, Arterial blood gas; *CPAP*, continuous positive airway pressure; *Fio_2*, fraction of inspired oxygen; *PEEP*, positive end-expiratory pressure; *PSV*, pressure support ventilation; *SBT*, spontaneous breathing trial; *SIMV*, synchronized intermittent mandatory ventilation.

and requires prompt attention. Racemic epinephrine, a topical aerosol vasoconstrictor, is given, and reintubation may be needed.

CHEST TRAUMA

Unintentional traumatic injuries accounted for 161,371 deaths in the United States during 2016, with chest trauma as a contributing factor in about 50% of those deaths (CDC, 2019). Many of the injured die before arriving at the hospital. Few types of chest injuries require thoracotomy. Most can be treated with basic resuscitation, intubation, or chest tube placement. *The first emergency approach to all chest injuries is ABC (**airway, breathing, circulation**), a rapid assessment and treatment of life-threatening conditions.* See Chapter 10 for more information on care of the trauma patient.

Pulmonary Contusion

Pulmonary contusion, a potentially lethal injury, is a common chest injury and occurs most often by rapid deceleration during car crashes. After a contusion, respiratory failure can develop immediately or over time. Hemorrhage and edema occur in and between the alveoli, reducing both lung movement and the area available for ***gas exchange***. Local inflammation can cause further damage. The patient becomes hypoxemic and dyspneic.

Patients may be asymptomatic at first and can later develop various degrees of respiratory failure and possibly pneumonia. These patients often have decreased breath sounds or crackles and wheezes over the affected area. Other symptoms include bruising over the injury, dry cough, tachycardia, tachypnea, and dullness to percussion. If there is no disruption of the parenchyma, bruise resorption often occurs without treatment.

Management includes maintenance of ventilation and oxygenation. Provide oxygen, give IV fluids as prescribed, and place the patient in a moderate-Fowler position. If a high FiO_2 is needed, oxygen may be administered using a high-flow nasal cannula (HFNC). When side-lying, the "good lung down" position may be helpful. The patient in obvious respiratory distress may need noninvasive positive-pressure ventilation (NIPPV) or mechanical ventilation with positive end-expiratory pressure (PEEP) to inflate the lungs.

A vicious cycle occurs in which more muscle effort is needed for ventilating a lung with a contusion and the patient becomes progressively hypoxemic. This situation causes him or her to tire easily, have reduced ***gas exchange***, and become more fatigued and more hypoxemic. This condition often leads to acute respiratory distress syndrome (ARDS).

Rib Fracture

Rib fractures are a common injury to the chest wall, often resulting from direct blunt trauma to the chest. The force applied to the ribs fractures them and drives the bone ends into the chest. Thus there is a risk for deep chest injury such as pulmonary contusion, pneumothorax, and hemothorax.

The patient has pain on movement and splints the chest defensively. Splinting reduces breathing depth and clearance of secretions. If the patient has pre-existing lung disease, the risk for atelectasis and pneumonia increases. Those with injuries to the first or second ribs, flail chest, seven or more fractured ribs, or expired volumes of less than 15 mL/kg often have a deep chest injury and a poor prognosis.

Management of uncomplicated rib fractures is simple because the fractured ribs reunite spontaneously. The chest is usually not splinted by tape or other materials. The main focus is to decrease pain so adequate ventilation is maintained. An intercostal nerve block may be used if pain is severe. Opioids are effective analgesics that allow for coughing and effective incentive spirometry use; however, they can cause respiratory depression. NSAIDs, epidural anesthesia, and patient-controlled analgesia (PCA) are other available options.

Flail Chest

Flail chest is the result of fractures of three or more adjacent ribs in two or more places causing *paradoxical chest wall movement* (inward movement of the thorax during inspiration, with outward movement during expiration) (Fig. 29.3). It usually involves one side of the chest and results from blunt chest trauma—often high-speed car crashes. Because the force required to produce a flail chest is great, it is important to assess for other possible underlying injuries.

Flail chest can also occur from bilateral separations of the ribs from their cartilage connections to each other anteriorly, without an actual rib fracture. This condition can occur as a complication of cardiopulmonary resuscitation. Other injuries to the lung tissue under the flail segment may be present. ***Gas exchange***, coughing, and clearance of secretions are impaired. Splinting further reduces the patient's ability to exert the extra effort to breathe and may contribute later to failure to wean.

Assess the patient with a flail chest for paradoxical chest movement, dyspnea, cyanosis, tachycardia, and hypotension. The patient is often anxious, short of breath, and in pain. Work of breathing is increased from the paradoxical movement of the involved segment of the chest wall.

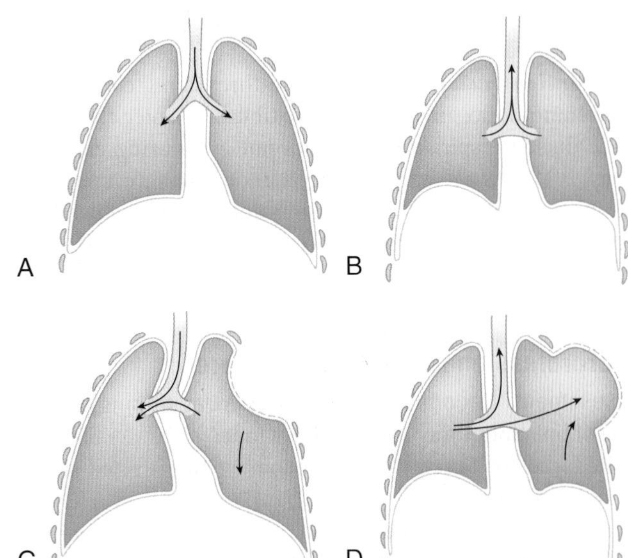

Fig. 29.3 Flail chest. Normal respiration: (A) Inspiration; (B) expiration. Paradoxical motion: (C) Inspiration—area of the lung underlying unstable chest wall sucks in on inspiration; (D) expiration—unstable area balloons out. Note movement of mediastinum toward opposite lung during inspiration.

Interventions include humidified oxygen, pain management, promotion of lung expansion through deep breathing and positioning, and secretion clearance by coughing and tracheal suction.

The patient with a flail chest may be managed with vigilant respiratory care. Mechanical ventilation is needed if respiratory failure or shock occurs. Monitor ABG values and vital capacity closely. With severe hypoxemia and hypercarbia, the patient is intubated and mechanically ventilated with PEEP. With lung contusion or an underlying pulmonary disease, the risk for respiratory failure increases. Usually flail chest is stabilized by positive-pressure ventilation. Surgical stabilization is used only in extreme cases of flail chest.

Monitor the patient's vital signs and fluid and electrolyte balance closely so hypovolemia or shock can be managed immediately. If he or she has a lung contusion, provide oxygen as needed and give IV fluids as prescribed. Assess for and relieve pain with prescribed analgesic drugs by IV, epidural, or nerve block route. Give psychosocial support to the anxious patient by explaining all procedures, talking slowly, and allowing time for expression of feelings and concerns.

PNEUMOTHORAX AND HEMOTHORAX

Pathophysiology Review

A **pneumothorax** is air in the pleural space causing a loss of negative pressure in the chest cavity, a rise in chest pressure, and a reduction in vital capacity, which can lead to lung collapse (Arsbad et al., 2016). It is often caused by blunt chest trauma and may occur with some degree of **hemothorax**, which is bleeding into the chest cavity. It can also occur as a complication of medical procedures. (A *simple* hemothorax is a blood loss of less than 1000 mL into the chest cavity; a *massive* hemothorax is a blood loss of more than 1000 mL.) The pneumothorax can be *open* (pleural cavity is exposed to outside air, as through an open wound in the chest wall) or *closed* (such as when a patient with chronic obstructive pulmonary disease has a spontaneous pneumothorax).

A ***tension pneumothorax*** is a life-threatening complication of pneumothorax in which air continues to enter the pleural space during inspiration and does not exit during expiration (Shay, 2017). As a result, air collects under pressure, completely collapsing the lung and compressing blood vessels, which limits blood return. This process leads to decreased filling of the heart and reduced cardiac output. *If not promptly detected and treated, tension pneumothorax is quickly fatal.*

❖ Interprofessional Collaborative Care

◆ **Assessment: Recognize Cues.** Assessment findings for any type of pneumothorax commonly include:

- Reduced (or absent) breath sounds of the affected side on auscultation
- Hyperresonance on percussion
- Prominence of the involved side of the chest, which moves poorly with respirations
- When severe, deviation of the trachea *away* from the midline and side of injury toward the *unaffected* side (indicating pushing of tissues to the unaffected side [a *mediastinal shift*] from increasing pressure within the injured side)

For tension pneumothorax, additional assessment findings also may include:

- Extreme respiratory distress and cyanosis
- Distended neck veins
- Hemodynamic instability

With a hemothorax, percussion on the involved side produces a dull sound.

In addition to symptoms, chest x-rays, CT scans, or ultrasonography may be used for diagnosis of any type of pneumothorax or hemothorax.

◆ **Interventions: Take Action.** For a stable patient with a small pneumothorax who has mild symptoms and no continuing air leak, no treatment may be needed. For more severe pneumothorax, tension pneumothorax, and hemothorax, chest tube therapy is essential. Chest tube management is discussed in Chapter 27.

Initial management of a tension pneumothorax is an immediate needle thoracostomy, with a large-bore needle inserted by the primary health care provider into the second intercostal space in the midclavicular line of the affected side. This intervention changes a tension pneumothorax to a simple pneumothorax and is only a temporary measure. More definitive treatment is mandatory, with chest tube placement into the fourth intercostal space, and the other end attached to a water seal drainage system until the lung reinflates. Interventions for hemothorax include chest tube placement to remove the blood in the pleural space to normalize breathing and prevent infection.

Closely monitor the chest tube drainage. Serial chest x-rays are used to determine treatment effectiveness. Other care includes pain control, pulmonary hygiene, and continued assessment for respiratory failure.

An open thoracotomy is needed when there is initial blood loss of 1000 mL from the chest or persistent bleeding at the rate of 150 to 200 mL/hr over 3 to 4 hours. Monitor the vital signs, blood loss, and intake and output. Assess the patient's response to the chest tubes and infuse IV fluids and blood as prescribed. The blood lost through chest drainage can be infused back into the patient after processing if needed.

NCLEX EXAMINATION CHALLENGE 29.4

Physiological Integrity

Which symptom or change in assessment of a client with four broken ribs on the right side indicates to the nurse the possibility of a tension pneumothorax?

A. Distended neck veins
B. Mediastinal shift toward the left side
C. Right-sided pain on deep inhalation
D. Right side of the chest more prominent than the left

GET READY FOR THE NEXT-GENERATION NCLEX® EXAMINATION!

Key Points

Review these Key Points for each NCLEX Examination Client Needs Category.

Safe and Effective Care Environment

- Use aseptic technique when caring for a patient requiring pulmonary suctioning. **QSEN: Safety**
- Identify patients in your setting who are at risk for developing a pulmonary embolism. **QSEN: Safety**
- Inspect the mouth and perform oral care every 2 hours for anyone who has an endotracheal tube or is being mechanically ventilated. **QSEN: Safety**
- Review ventilator settings with respiratory therapy at least every 4 hours and with any patient changes. **QSEN: Safety**
- Ensure that alarm systems on mechanical ventilators are activated and functional at all times. **QSEN: Safety**
- Ensure that bag-valve-mask device and suction equipment are at the bedside at all times. **QSEN: Safety**

Health Promotion and Maintenance

- Teach patients ways to prevent injury when taking drugs that reduce ***clotting***. **QSEN: Patient-Centered Care**

Psychosocial Integrity

- Allow the patient and family members the opportunity to express feelings and concerns about a change in breathing status or the possibility of intubation and mechanical ventilation. **QSEN: Patient-Centered Care**
- Use alternate ways to communicate with a patient who is intubated or being mechanically ventilated. **QSEN: Patient-Centered Care**
- Remember that patients who are receiving mechanical ventilation and are being chemically paralyzed usually can hear and can feel pain. **QSEN: Patient-Centered Care**

Physiological Integrity

- Use Aspiration Precautions, including maintaining an orogastric or nasogastric tube, for any patient with an altered level of consciousness (LOC), poor gag reflex, or neurologic impairment or who has an endotracheal tube. **QSEN: Evidence-Based Practice**
- Check the patient with ARDS hourly for oxygen saturation, vital sign changes, or any indication of increased work of breathing such as cyanosis, pallor, and retractions. **QSEN: Patient-Centered Care**
- Assess all patients with blunt chest trauma for tracheal position, chest wall movement, and bilateral breath sounds. **QSEN: Patient Centered Care**
- Notify the primary health care provider immediately for any patient who develops sudden-onset respiratory difficulty. **QSEN: Safety**
- Check oxygen saturation by pulse oximetry for any patient who has trouble breathing or who develops acute confusion. **QSEN: Patient-Centered Care**
- Apply oxygen to anyone who is hypoxemic. **QSEN: Evidence-Based Practice**
- Check all ventilator settings with the prescription at least once per shift. **QSEN: Safety**
- Administer appropriate analgesics to patients who have rib fractures, and encourage deep breaths. **QSEN: Patient-Centered Care**
- If a patient experiences respiratory distress during mechanical ventilation, remove him or her from the ventilator and provide ventilation by bag-valve-mask resuscitation device. **QSEN: Safety**

MASTERY QUESTIONS

1. An attempt by a primary health care provider to intubate a client for mechanical ventilation is unsuccessful after 45 seconds. What is the nurse's **priority action**?
   A. Placing a nasotracheal tube
   B. Assessing for bilateral breath sounds
   C. Assessing oxygen saturation by pulse oximetry
   D. Applying oxygen with a bag-valve-mask device
2. Which actions does the nurse ensure are performed for a client being mechanically ventilated to prevent ventilator-associated pneumonia (VAP)? **Select all that apply.**
   A. Assessing temperature every 4 hours
   B. Checking ventilator settings every 4 hours
   C. Getting the patient out of bed as soon as prescribed
   D. Keeping the head of the bed elevated to 30 degrees or above
   E. Maintaining the client in the prone position
   F. Providing adequate humidification
   G. Providing meticulous mouth care every 12 hours
   H. Suggesting that the pneumonia vaccine be prescribed
3. A client being mechanically ventilated has all of the following changes. Which changes are **most relevant** in helping the nurse determine whether suctioning is needed at this time? **Select all that apply.**
   A. Decreased Spo_2
   B. Elevated temperature
   C. Crackles auscultated over the trachea
   D. Crackles auscultated in the lung periphery
   E. High-pressure ventilator alarm sounds
   F. Presence of fluid within the endotracheal tube
   G. Presence of fluid within the ventilator tubing

REFERENCES

Asterisk (*) indicates a classic or definitive work on this subject.

American Lung Association. (2018). *Acute Respiratory Distress Syndrome (ARDS).* http://www.lung.org/lung-health-and-diseases/lung-disease-lookup/ards/.

ARDS Foundation. (2018). *Acute Respiratory Distress Syndrome.* http://ardsglobal.org/.

Arias, C., Pokharel, B., Papathanassoglou, E., & Norris, C. (2017). Prone positioning for the treatment of adult respiratory distress syndrome. *Connect: The World of Critical Care Nursing, 11*(3), 49–54.

Arsbad, H., Young, M., Adyrty, R., & Singh, A. (2016). Acute pneumothorax. *Critical Care Nursing Quarterly, 39*(2), 176–189.

Baird, H. (2016). Identifying and managing complications of mechanical ventilation. *Critical Care Nursing Clinics of North America, 28*(4), 451–462.

Barton, G., Vandespank-Wright, B., & Shea, J. (2016). Optimizing oxygenation in the mechanically ventilated patient: Nursing practice implications. *Critical Care Nursing Clinics of North America, 28*(4), 425–435.

Bethea, B., Elliot, J., Richardson, J., & Ahmed, M. (2017). Treatment of pulmonary embolism with argatroban and ultrasound-assisted catheter-directed thrombolysis with alteplase in a patient with heparin-induced thrombocytopenia. *American Journal of Health-System Pharmacy, 74*(15), 1153–1157.

Boltey, E., Yakusheva, O., & Costa, D. (2017). 5 nursing strategies to prevent ventilator-associated pneumonia. *American Nurse Today, 12*(6), 42–43.

Brien, L. (2019). Anticoagulant medications for the prevention and treatment of thromboembolism. *AACN Advanced Critical Care, 30*(2), 126–138.

Burchum, J., & Rosenthal, L. (2019). *Lehne's pharmacology for nursing care* (10th ed.). St. Louis: Elsevier.

*Castro, E., Turcinovic, M., Platz, J., & Law, I. (2015). Early mobilization: Changing the mindset. *Critical Care Nurse Online, 35*(4), e1–e6.

Centers for Disease Control and Prevention (CDC). (2018). *Venous thromboembolism (blood clots): Data & statistics.* http://www.cdc.gov/ncbddd/dvt/data.html.

Centers for Disease Control and Prevention (CDC). (2019). *National Center for health statistics: Deaths and morbidity.* https://www.cdc.gov/nchs/fastats/deaths.htm.

Centers for Disease Control and Prevention (CDC). (2020). Interim infection prevention and control recommendations for healthcare personnel during the coronavirus disease 2019 (COVID-19) pandemic. https://www.cdc.gov/coronavirus/2019-ncov/hcp/infection-control-recommendations.html.

Eakin, M., Patel, Y., Mendez-Tellez, P., Dinglas, V., Needham, D., & Turnbull, A. (2017). Patients' outcomes after acute respiratory failure: A qualitative study with the PROMIS framework. *American Journal of Critical Care, 26*(6), 456–465.

Fitzsimons, M., & Crowley, J. (2020). Coronavirus disease 2019 (COVID-19): Extracorporeal membrane oxygenation (ECMO). In O'Connor, M., & Mark, J. (Eds.), *UpToDate*, Waltham, MA.

Fukumoto, L., & Fukumoto, K. (2018). Fat embolism syndrome. *Nursing Clinics of North America, 53*, 335–347.

Grap, M. J., Munro, C., Schubert, C., Wetzel, P., Burk, R., Pepperi, A., et al. (2018). Lack of association of high backrest position with sacral tissue changes in adults receiving mechanical ventilation. *American Journal of Critical Care, 27*(2), 104–113.

Harmon, D. (2019). Pulmonary embolism response teams: Coordinating care beyond the hospital. *Medsurg Nursing, 28*(1), 63–65.

Kolarik, M., & Roberts, E. (2017). Permissible hypotension and trauma: Can fluid restriction reduce the incidence of ARDS? *Journal of Trauma Nursing, 24*(1), 19–24.

Lamba, T., Sharara, R., Singh, A., & Balaan, M. (2016). Pathophysiology and classification of respiratory failure. *Critical Care Nursing Quarterly, 39*(2), 85–93.

McCance, K., Huether, S., Brashers, V., & Rote, N. (2019). *Pathophysiology: The biologic basis for disease in adults and children* (8th ed.). St. Louis: Mosby.

Mitchell, D., & Seckel, M. (2018). Acute respiratory distress syndrome and prone positioning. *AACN Advanced Critical Care, 29*(4), 415–425.

Moore, D. (2016). Fat embolism threatens a patient's life. *American Nurse Today, 11*(5), 26.

Moore, D. (2019). Sudden onset of shortness of breath: Consider pulmonary embolism threatens. *American Nurse Today, 14*(3), 20–23.

Online Mendelian Inheritance in Man (OMIM). (2017). Coagulation factor V; F5. www.omim.org/entry/612309.

Pagana, K., & Pagana, T. (2018). *Mosby's manual of diagnostic and laboratory tests* (6th ed.). St. Louis: Elsevier.

Parisi, M., Gerovasili, V., Dimopoulos, S., Kampisiouli, E., Goga, C., Perivolioti, E., et al. (2016). Use of ventilator bundle and staff education to decrease ventilator-associated pneumonia in intensive care patients. *Critical Care Nursing, 36*(5), e1–e7.

Rojo, A., Lukyanova, V., Greenier, E., Kanowitz, A., & Berry, B. (2020). Unplanned extubation: Eliminating preventable deaths. *American Nurse Journal, 15*(5), 18–21.

Sahetya, S., Brower, R., & Stephens, S. (2018). Survival of patients with severe acute respiratory distress syndrome treated without extracorporeal membrane oxygenation. *American Journal of Critical Care, 27*(3), 220–227.

Schreiber, M. (2018). Acute respiratory distress syndrome. *Medsurg Nursing, 27*(1), 59–60 65.

Shay, A. (2017). When all signs point to tension pneumothorax. *American Nurse Today, 12*(6), 23.

Stieff, K., Lim, F., & Chen, L. (2017). Factors influencing weaning older adults from mechanical ventilation: An integrative review. *Critical Care Nursing Quarterly, 40*(2), 165–177.

Touhy, T., & Jett, K. (2020). *Ebersole and Hess' toward healthy aging: Human needs & nursing response* (10th ed.). St. Louis: Mosby.

Warren, C., Medei, M., Wood, B., & Schutte, D. (2019). A nurse-driven oral care protocol to reduce hospital-acquired pneumonia. *American Journal of Nursing, 119*(2), 44–51.

Wong, T., Schlichting, A., Stoltze, A., Fuller, B., Peacock, A., Harland, K., et al. (2016). No decrease in early ventilator-associated pneumonia after early use of chlorhexidine. *American Journal of Critical Care, 25*(2), 173–177.

Zhang, Y., Ding, S., Li, C., Wang, Y., Chen, Z., & Wang, Z. (2017). Effects of N-acetylcysteine treatment on acute respiratory distress syndrome: A meta-analysis. *Experimental and Therapeutic Medicine, 14*(4), 2863–2868.

30

Assessment of the Cardiovascular System

Nicole M. Heimgartner

http://evolve.elsevier.com/Iggy/

LEARNING OUTCOMES

1. Collaborate with the interprofessional team to perform a complete cardiovascular (CV) assessment, including ***perfusion*** status and ***fluid and electrolyte balance.***
2. Prioritize evidence-based care for patients having invasive CV diagnostic testing affecting ***perfusion.***
3. Teach evidence-based ways for adults to decrease their risk for CV health problems.
4. Explain how physiologic aging changes of the CV system affect ***perfusion*** and associated care of older adults.
5. Implement nursing interventions to decrease the psychosocial impact caused by a CV health problem.
6. Apply knowledge of anatomy and physiology to perform a patient-centered assessment for the patient with a CV health problem, including cultural and spiritual considerations.
7. Use clinical judgment to document the cardiovascular assessment in the electronic health record.
8. Interpret assessment findings for patients with a suspected or actual CV health problem.
9. Identify the CV assessment components that contribute to disparities in certain populations.

KEY TERMS

afterload The pressure or resistance that the ventricles must overcome to eject blood through the semilunar valves and into the peripheral blood vessels.

apical impulse The pulse located at the left fifth intercostal space in the midclavicular line (in the mitral area); also called the *point of maximal impulse* (PMI).

baroreceptors Sensory receptors in the arch of the aorta and at the origin of the internal carotid arteries that are stimulated when the arterial walls are stretched by an increased blood pressure.

blood pressure (BP) The *force* of blood exerted against the vessel walls.

bruit Swishing sound that may occur from turbulent blood flow in narrowed or atherosclerotic arteries; heard via auscultation or Doppler.

cardiac catheterization The most definitive but most invasive test in the diagnosis of heart disease; involves passing a small catheter into the heart and injecting contrast medium.

cardiac index A calculation of cardiac output requirements to account for differences in body size; determined by dividing the cardiac output by the body surface area.

cardiac output (CO) The volume of blood ejected by the heart each minute.

cholesterol Serum lipid that includes high-density lipoproteins and low-density lipoproteins.

diastole The phase of the cardiac cycle that consists of relaxation and filling of the atria and ventricles; normally about two-thirds of the cardiac cycle.

diastolic blood pressure The amount of pressure or force against the arterial walls during the relaxation phase of the cardiac cycle.

echocardiography The use of ultrasound waves to assess cardiac structure and mobility, particularly of the valves.

electrophysiologic study (EPS) An invasive procedure during which programmed electrical stimulation of the heart is used to cause and evaluate dysrhythmias and conduction abnormalities to permit accurate diagnosis and treatment.

exercise electrocardiography A test that assesses cardiovascular response to an increased workload; also called *exercise tolerance* or *stress test.*

exercise tolerance test See *exercise electrocardiography.*

heart rate (HR) Term referring to the number of times the ventricles contract each minute.

high-density lipoproteins (HDLs) Part of the total cholesterol value that should be more than 45 mm/dL (>0.75 mmol/L) for men and more than 55 mg/dL (>0.91 mmol/L) for women; "good" cholesterol.
highly sensitive C-reactive protein (hsCRP) A serum marker of inflammation and a common and critical component of the development of atherosclerosis.
homocysteine An amino acid that is produced when proteins break down; elevated values may be a risk factor for the development of cardiovascular disease.
low-density lipoproteins (LDLs) Part of the total cholesterol value that should be less than 130 mg/dL; "bad" cholesterol.
mean arterial pressure (MAP) The arterial blood pressure necessary (between 60 and 70 mm Hg) necessary to maintain perfusion of major body organs, such as the kidneys and the brain.
murmur Abnormal heart sound that reflects turbulent blood flow through normal or abnormal valves.
myocardial nuclear perfusion imaging (MNPI) The use of radionuclide techniques in cardiovascular assessment.
myocardium The heart muscle.
orthostatic hypotension A decrease in blood pressure that occurs the first few seconds to minutes after changing from a sitting or lying position to a standing position. Also called *postural hypotension.*
pack-years The number of packs of cigarettes per day multiplied by the number of years the patient has smoked; used to record a patient's smoking history.
palpitations A feeling of fluttering in the chest, an unpleasant awareness of the heartbeat, or an irregular heartbeat.
paradoxical blood pressure An exaggerated decrease in systolic pressure by more than 10 mm Hg during the inspiratory phase of the respiratory cycle; also known as paradoxical pulse and pulsus paradoxus.
pericardial friction rub An abnormal sound that originates from the pericardial sac and occurs with the movements of the heart during the cardiac cycle.
point of maximal impulse (PMI) See *apical impulse.*
preload The degree of myocardial fiber stretch at the end of diastole and just before contraction.
pulse pressure The difference between the systolic and diastolic pressures.
stress test See *exercise electrocardiography.*
stroke volume (SV) The amount of blood ejected by the left ventricle during each contraction.
systole The phase of the cardiac cycle that consists of the contraction and emptying of the atria and ventricles.
systolic blood pressure The amount of pressure or force generated by the left ventricle to distribute blood into the aorta with each contraction of the heart.
transesophageal echocardiography (TEE) A form of echocardiography performed through the esophagus that examines cardiac structure and function.
triglycerides Serum lipid profile that includes the measurement of cholesterol and lipoproteins.
troponin A myocardial muscle protein released into the bloodstream with injury to myocardial muscle.

PRIORITY AND INTERRELATED CONCEPTS

The priority concept for this chapter is:
- ***Perfusion***

The interrelated concept for this chapter is:
- ***Fluid and Electrolyte Balance***

Cardiovascular disease (CVD) continues to be the number-one cause of death in the United States. The disease kills more people each year than cancer and chronic lung disease combined (Benjamin et al., 2019). By the year 2035, it is projected that 45% of the U.S. population will have some form of CVD (Benjamin et al., 2019). In Canada, 1 in 12 adults (2.4 million) over the age of 20 live with diagnosed heart disease (Government of Canada, 2017).

The cardiovascular (CV) system is responsible for supplying oxygen to body organs and other tissues (***perfusion***). It is made up of the heart and blood vessels (both arteries and veins).

The heart muscle, called the **myocardium**, must receive sufficient oxygen to pump blood to other parts of the body. The arteries must be patent so the pumped blood can reach the rest of the body. Oxygen in the blood is required for cells to live and function properly. When diseases or other problems of the CV systems occur, gas exchange and ***perfusion*** decrease, often resulting in life-threatening events or a risk for these events. The CV system works with the respiratory and hematologic systems to meet the human need for gas exchange and tissue ***perfusion.*** Any problem in these systems requires the CV system to work harder to meet gas exchange and tissue perfusion needs.

ANATOMY AND PHYSIOLOGY REVIEW

Heart

Structure. The human heart is a fist-sized, muscular organ located in the mediastinum between the lungs (Fig. 30.1). Each beat of the heart pumps about 60 mL of blood, or 5 L/min. During strenuous physical activity, the amount of blood pumped can double to meet the body's increased gas exchange needs. A covering called the pericardium protects the heart. A muscular wall (septum) separates the heart into two halves: right and left. Each half has an atrium and a ventricle (Fig. 30.2).

The *right atrium (RA)* receives *deoxygenated* venous blood, which is returned from the body through the superior and inferior vena cava. It also receives blood from the heart muscle through the coronary sinus. Most of this venous return flows passively from the RA, through the opened tricuspid valve, and to the right ventricle during ventricular diastole, or filling. The RA actively propels the remaining venous return into the right ventricle during atrial systole, or contraction.

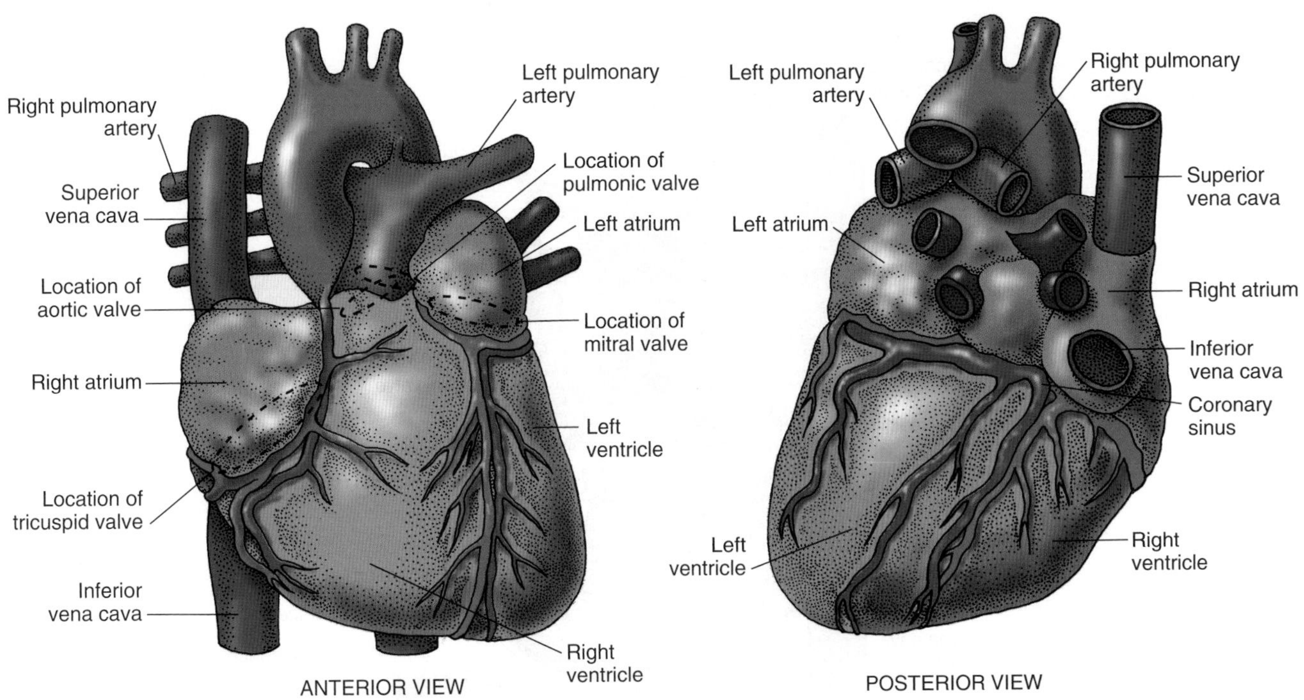

FIG. 30.1 Surface anatomy of the heart.

The *right ventricle (RV)* is a muscular pump located behind the sternum. It generates enough pressure to close the tricuspid valve, open the pulmonic valve, and propel blood into the pulmonary artery and the lungs.

After blood is *reoxygenated* in the lungs, it flows freely from the four pulmonary veins into the left atrium. Blood then flows through an opened mitral valve into the left ventricle during ventricular diastole. When the left ventricle is almost full, the *left atrium (LA)* contracts, pumping the remaining blood volume into the left ventricle. With systolic contraction, the *left ventricle (LV)* generates enough pressure to close the mitral valve and open the aortic valve. Blood is propelled into the aorta and the systemic arterial circulation. Blood flow through the heart is shown in Fig. 30.2.

Blood moves from the aorta throughout the systemic circulation to the various tissues of the body. The pressure of blood in the aorta of a young adult averages about 100 to 120 mm Hg, whereas the pressure of blood in the RA averages about 0 to 5 mm Hg. These differences in pressure produce a pressure gradient, with blood flowing from an area of higher pressure to an area of lower pressure. The heart and vascular structures are responsible for maintaining these pressures.

The four *cardiac valves* are responsible for maintaining the forward flow of blood through the chambers of the heart (see Fig. 30.2). These valves open and close when pressure and volume change within the heart's chambers. The cardiac valves are classified into two types: atrioventricular (AV) valves and semilunar valves.

The *AV valves* separate the atria from the ventricles. The *tricuspid valve* separates the RA from the RV. The *mitral (bicuspid) valve* separates the LA from the LV. During ventricular diastole, these valves act as funnels and help move the flow of blood from the atria to the ventricles. During systole, the valves close to prevent the backflow (valvular regurgitation) of blood into the atria.

The *semilunar valves* are the pulmonic valve and the aortic valve, which prevent blood from flowing back into the ventricles during diastole. The *pulmonic valve* separates the right ventricle from the pulmonary artery. The *aortic valve* separates the left ventricle from the aorta.

The heart muscle receives blood to meet its metabolic needs through the coronary arterial system (Fig. 30.3). The coronary arteries originate from an area on the aorta just beyond the aortic valve. All of the coronary arteries feeding the left side of the heart originate from the left main coronary artery (LMCA). The right coronary artery (RCA) branches from the aorta to perfuse the right side of the heart and inferior wall of the left side of the heart.

Coronary artery blood flow to the myocardium occurs primarily during diastole, when coronary vascular resistance is minimized. To maintain adequate blood flow through the coronary arteries, **mean arterial pressure (MAP)** must be *at least 60 mm Hg.* A MAP between 60 and 70 mm Hg is necessary to maintain ***perfusion*** of major body organs, such as the kidneys and brain.

The *left main artery* divides into two branches: the left anterior descending (LAD) branch and the left circumflex (LCX) branch. The LAD branch descends toward the anterior wall and the apex of the left ventricle. It supplies blood to portions of the left ventricle, ventricular septum, chordae tendineae, papillary muscle, and, to a lesser extent, the right ventricle.

The LCX branch descends toward the lateral wall of the left ventricle and apex. It supplies blood to the left atrium, the lateral and posterior surfaces of the left ventricle, and sometimes portions of the interventricular septum. In about half of people, the LCX branch supplies the sinoatrial (SA) node. In a very small number of people, it supplies the AV node. Peripheral branches

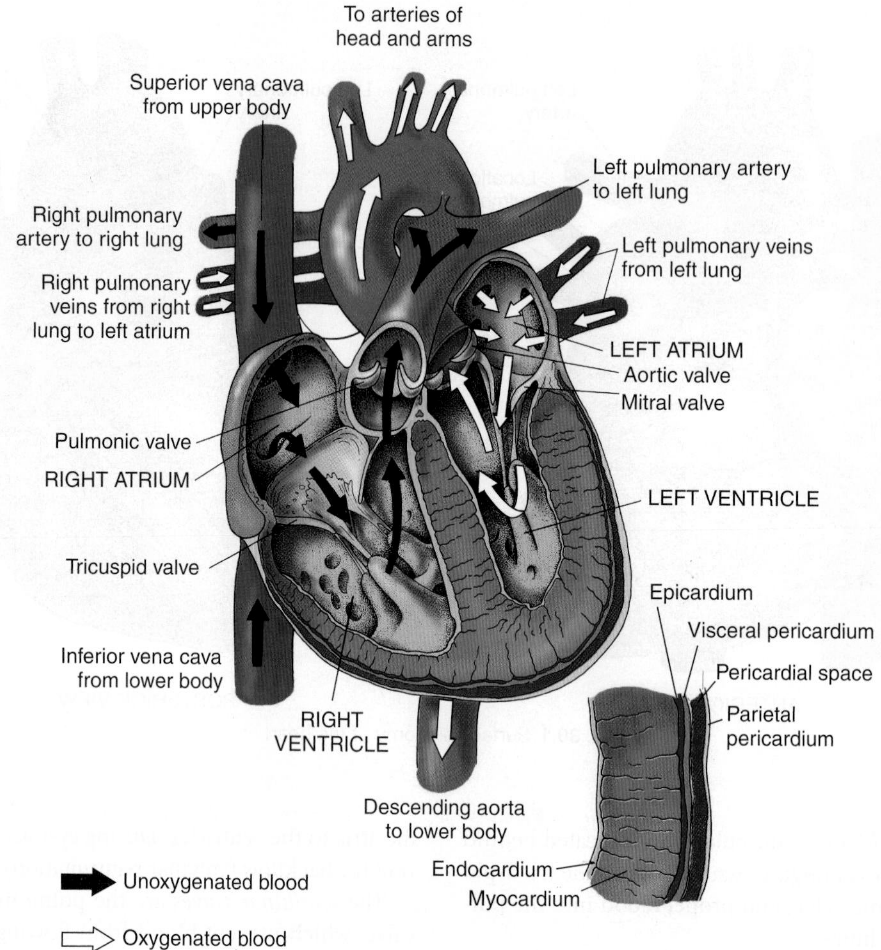

FIG. 30.2 Blood flow through the heart.

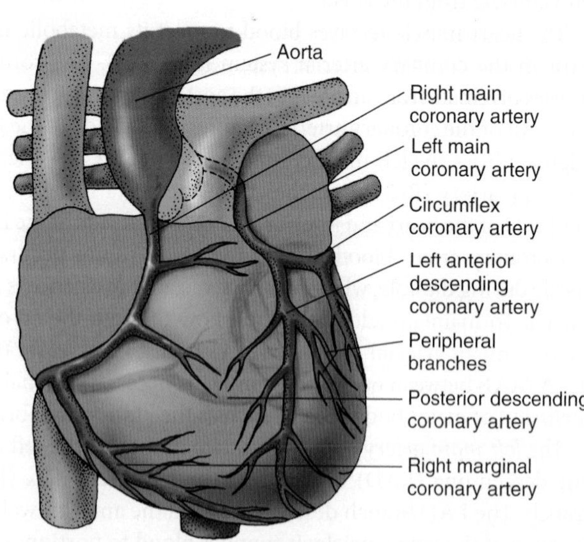

FIG. 30.3 Coronary arterial system.

arise from the LAD and LCX branches and form an abundant network of vessels throughout the entire myocardium.

The *right coronary artery (RCA)* originates from the right sinus of Valsalva, encircles the heart, and descends toward the apex of the right ventricle. The RCA supplies the RA, RV, and inferior portion of the LV. In about half of the people, the RCA supplies the SA node; and in almost everyone, it supplies the AV node.

Function. The electrophysiologic properties of heart muscle are responsible for regulating heart rate (HR) and rhythm. Cardiac muscle cells possess the characteristics of automaticity, excitability, conductivity, contractility, and refractoriness. Chapter 31 describes these properties and cardiac conduction in detail.

Sequence of Events During the Cardiac Cycle. The phases of the cardiac cycle are generally described in relation to changes in pressure and volume in the left ventricle during filling (diastole) and ventricular contraction (systole) (Fig. 30.4). **Diastole** consists of relaxation and filling of the atria and ventricles and comprises about two thirds of the cardiac cycle. **Systole** consists of the contraction and emptying of the atria and ventricles.

Myocardial contraction results from the release of large numbers of calcium ions from the sarcoplasmic reticulum and the blood. These ions diffuse into the myofibril sarcomere (the basic contractile unit of the myocardial cell). Calcium ions promote the interaction of actin and myosin protein filaments, causing these filaments to link and overlap (McCance et al., 2019). Cross-bridges, or linkages, are formed as the protein filaments slide over or overlap each other. These cross-bridges act as force-generating sites. The sliding of these protein filaments shortens the sarcomeres, producing myocardial contraction.

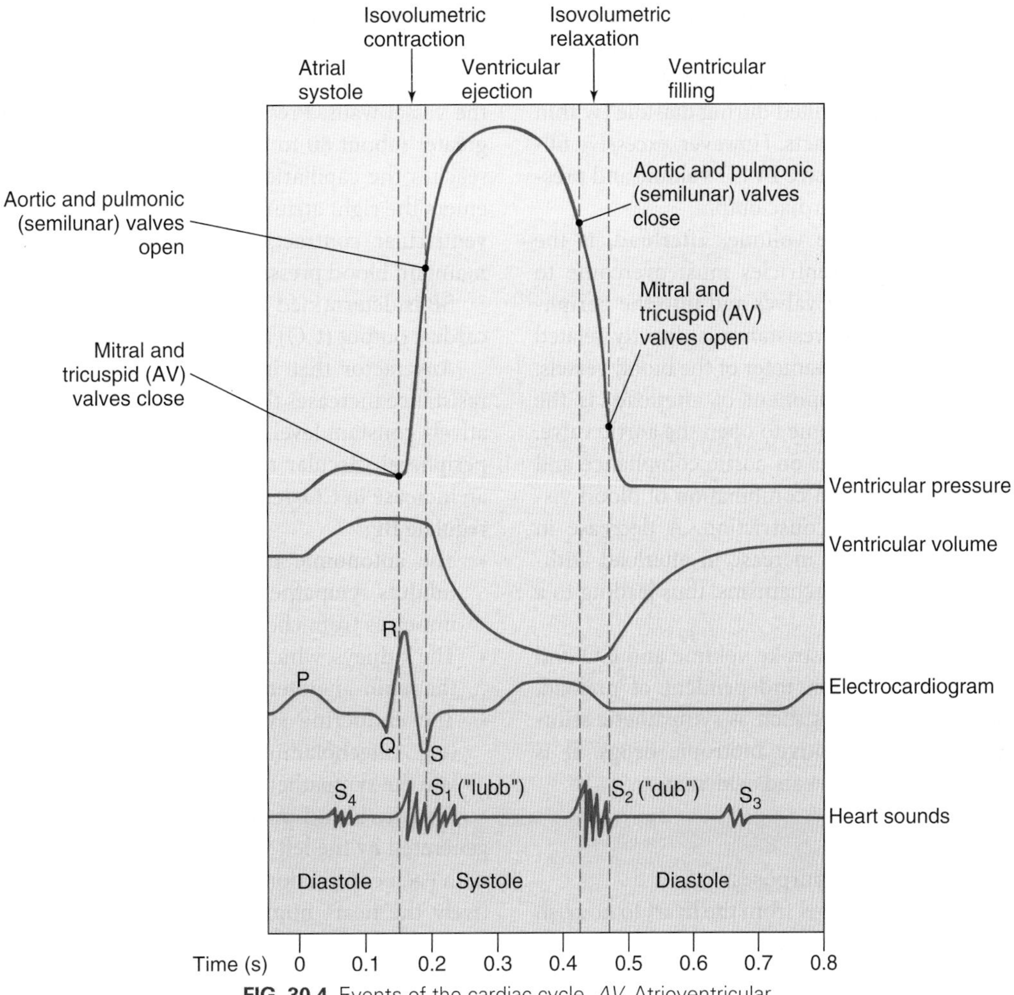

FIG. 30.4 Events of the cardiac cycle. *AV*, Atrioventricular.

Cardiac muscle relaxes when calcium ions are pumped back into the sarcoplasmic reticulum, causing a decrease in the number of calcium ions around the myofibrils. This reduced number of ions causes the protein filaments to disengage, the sarcomere to lengthen, and the muscle to relax.

Mechanical Properties of the Heart. The electrical and mechanical properties of cardiac muscle determine the function of the cardiovascular system. The healthy heart can adapt to various pathophysiologic conditions (e.g., stress, infections, hemorrhage) to maintain ***perfusion*** to the various body tissues. Blood flow from the heart into the systemic arterial circulation is measured clinically as cardiac output (CO), the amount of blood pumped from the left ventricle each minute. CO depends on the relationship between heart rate (HR) and stroke volume (SV); it is the product of these two variables:

Cardiac output = Heart rate × Stroke volume

In adults the CO ranges from 3 to 6 L/min. Because CO requirements vary according to body size, the cardiac index is calculated to adjust for differences in body size. The cardiac index can be determined by dividing the CO by the body surface area. The normal range is 2.8 to 4.2 L/min/m^2 (Pagana et al., 2019).

Heart rate (HR) refers to the number of times the ventricles contract each minute. The normal resting HR for an adult is between 60 and 100 beats/min. Increases in rate increase myocardial oxygen demand. The HR is extrinsically controlled by the autonomic nervous system (ANS), which adjusts rapidly when necessary to regulate cardiac output. The parasympathetic (vagus nerve) system *slows* the HR, whereas sympathetic stimulation *increases* the heart rate. An increase in circulating catecholamines (e.g., epinephrine and norepinephrine) usually causes an increase in HR and contractility. Many cardiovascular drugs, particularly beta blockers, block this sympathetic (fight-or-flight) pattern by decreasing the HR.

Stroke volume (SV) is the amount of blood ejected by the left ventricle during each contraction. Several variables influence SV and ultimately CO. These variables include HR, preload, afterload, and contractility.

Preload refers to the degree of myocardial fiber stretch at the end of diastole and just before contraction. The stretch imposed on the muscle fibers results from the volume contained within the ventricle at the end of diastole. Preload is determined by the amount of blood returning to the heart from both the venous system (right heart) and the pulmonary system (left heart) (left ventricular end-diastolic [LVED] volume).

An increase in ventricular volume increases muscle-fiber length and tension, thereby enhancing contraction and improving stroke volume. This statement is derived from Starling's law of the heart: The more the heart is filled during diastole (within limits), the more forcefully it contracts. However, excessive filling of the ventricles results in excessive LVED volume and pressure and may result in decreased cardiac output.

Another factor affecting stroke volume, **afterload**, is the pressure or resistance that the ventricles must overcome to eject blood through the semilunar valves and into the peripheral blood vessels. The amount of resistance is directly related to arterial blood pressure and the diameter of the blood vessels.

Impedance, the peripheral component of afterload, is the pressure that the heart must overcome to open the aortic valve. The amount of impedance depends on aortic compliance and total systemic vascular resistance, a combination of blood viscosity (thickness) and arteriolar constriction. A decrease in stroke volume can result from an increase in afterload without the benefit of compensatory mechanisms, thus leading to a decrease in cardiac output.

Myocardial contractility affects stroke volume and CO and is the force of cardiac contraction independent of preload. Contractility is increased by factors such as sympathetic stimulation, calcium release, and positive inotropic drugs. It is decreased by factors such as hypoxia and acidemia.

Vascular System

The vascular system serves several purposes:

- Provides a route for blood to travel from the heart to nourish the various tissues of the body
- Carries cellular wastes to the excretory organs
- Allows lymphatic flow to drain tissue fluid back into the circulation
- Returns blood to the heart for recirculation

The vascular system is divided into the arterial system and the venous system. In the arterial system, blood moves from the larger arteries to a network of smaller blood vessels, called *arterioles,* which meet the capillary bed. In the venous system, blood travels from the capillaries to the venules and to the larger system of veins, eventually returning in the vena cava to the heart for recirculation.

Arterial System. The primary function of the arterial system is to deliver oxygen and nutrients to various tissues in the body. Nutrients are carried through arteries to arterioles, then branch into smaller terminal arterioles, and finally join with capillaries and venules to form a capillary network. Within this network, nutrients are exchanged across capillary membranes by three primary processes: osmosis, filtration, and diffusion. (See Chapter 13 for detailed discussions of these processes.)

The arterial system delivers blood to various tissues for oxygen and nourishment. At the tissue level, nutrients, chemicals, and body defense substances are distributed and exchanged for cellular waste products, depending on the needs of the particular tissue. The arteries transport the cellular wastes to the excretory organs (e.g., kidneys and lungs) to be reprocessed or removed. These vessels also contribute to temperature regulation in the tissues. Blood can be either directed toward the skin to promote heat loss or diverted away from it to conserve heat.

Blood pressure (BP) is the *force* of blood exerted against the vessel walls. Pressure in the larger arterial blood vessels is greater (about 80 to 100 mm Hg) and decreases as blood flow reaches the capillaries (about 25 mm Hg). By the time blood enters the right atrium, the BP is about 0 to 5 mm Hg. Volume, ventricular contraction, and vascular tone are necessary to maintain blood pressure.

BP is determined primarily by the quantity of blood flow or cardiac output (CO) and by the resistance in the arterioles.

Any factor that increases CO or total peripheral vascular resistance increases the BP. In general, BP is maintained at a relatively constant level. Therefore an increase or decrease in total peripheral vascular resistance is associated with a decrease or an increase in CO, respectively. Three mechanisms mediate and regulate BP:

- The autonomic nervous system (ANS), which excites or inhibits sympathetic nervous system activity in response to impulses from chemoreceptors and baroreceptors
- The kidneys, which sense a change in blood flow and activate the renin-angiotensin-aldosterone mechanism
- The endocrine system, which releases various hormones (e.g., catecholamine, kinins, serotonin, histamine) to stimulate the sympathetic nervous system at the tissue level

Systolic blood pressure is the amount of pressure or force generated by the left ventricle to distribute blood into the aorta with each contraction of the heart. It is a measure of how effectively the heart pumps and is an indicator of vascular tone. **Diastolic blood pressure** is the amount of pressure or force against the arterial walls during the relaxation phase of the heart.

BP is regulated by balancing the sympathetic and parasympathetic nervous systems of the ANS. Changes in autonomic activity are responses to messages sent by the sensory receptors in the various tissues of the body. These receptors, including the baroreceptors, chemoreceptors, and stretch receptors, respond differently to the biochemical and physiologic changes of the body.

Baroreceptors in the arch of the aorta and at the origin of the internal carotid arteries are stimulated when the arterial walls are stretched by an increased BP. Impulses from these baroreceptors inhibit the vasomotor center, which is located in the pons and the medulla. Inhibition of this center results in a drop in BP.

Several 1- to 2-mm collections of tissue known as peripheral chemoreceptors have been identified in the carotid arteries and along the aortic arch. These receptors are sensitive primarily to hypoxemia (a decrease in the partial pressure of arterial oxygen [Pao_2]). When stimulated, these chemoreceptors send impulses along the vagus nerves to activate a vasoconstrictor response and raise BP.

The central chemoreceptors in the respiratory center of the brain are also stimulated by hypercapnia (an increase in partial pressure of arterial carbon dioxide [$Paco_2$]) and acidosis. However, the direct effect of carbon dioxide on the central nervous system (CNS) is 10 times stronger than the effect of hypoxia on the peripheral chemoreceptors.

Stretch receptors in the vena cava and the right atrium are sensitive to pressure or volume changes. When a patient is hypovolemic, stretch receptors in the blood vessels sense a reduced volume or pressure and send fewer impulses to the CNS. This reaction stimulates the sympathetic nervous system to increase the heart rate (HR) and constrict the peripheral blood vessels.

The kidneys also help regulate cardiovascular activity. When renal blood flow or pressure decreases, the kidneys retain sodium and water. BP tends to rise because of fluid retention and activation of the renin-angiotensin-aldosterone mechanism (see Fig. 13.7). This mechanism results in vasoconstriction and sodium retention (and thus fluid retention). Vascular volume is also regulated by the release of antidiuretic hormone (vasopressin) from the posterior pituitary gland (see Chapter 13).

Other factors can also influence the activity of the cardiovascular system. Emotional behaviors (e.g., excitement, pain, anger) stimulate the sympathetic nervous system to increase BP and HR. Increased physical activity such as exercise also increases BP and HR during the activity. Body temperature can affect the metabolic needs of the tissues, thereby influencing the delivery of blood. In hypothermia, tissues require fewer nutrients, and BP falls. In hyperthermia, the metabolic requirement of the tissues is greater, and BP and HR rise.

Venous System. The primary function of the venous system is to complete the circulation of blood by returning blood from the capillaries to the right side of the heart. It is composed of a series of veins that are located next to the arterial system. A second superficial venous circulation runs parallel to the subcutaneous tissue of the extremity. These two venous systems are connected by communicating veins that provide a means for blood to travel from the superficial veins to the deep veins. Blood flow is directed toward the deep venous circulation.

Veins have the ability to accommodate large shifts in volume with minimal changes in venous pressure. This flexibility allows the venous system to accommodate the administration of IV fluids and blood transfusions and to maintain pressure during blood loss and dehydration. Veins in the superficial and deep venous systems (except the smallest and the largest veins) have valves that direct blood flow back to the heart and prevent backflow. Skeletal muscles in the extremities provide a force that helps push the venous blood forward. The superior vena cava and inferior vena cava are valveless and large enough to allow blood flow to return easily to the heart.

Gravity exerts an increase in *hydrostatic pressure* in the capillaries when the patient is in an upright position, delaying venous return. Hydrostatic pressure is decreased in dependent areas such as the legs when the patient is lying down; thus there is less hindrance of venous return to the heart.

Cardiovascular Changes Associated With Aging

A number of physiologic changes in the cardiovascular system occur with advancing age (see the Patient-Centered Care: Older Adult Considerations: Changes in the Cardiovascular System Related to Aging box). Many of these changes result in a loss of cardiac reserve. These changes are usually not evident when the older adult is resting. They become apparent only when the person is physically or emotionally stressed and the heart cannot meet the increased metabolic demands of the body.

ASSESSMENT: RECOGNIZE CUES

Patient History

The focus of the patient history is on obtaining information about risk factors and symptoms of cardiovascular disease (CVD). Assess *nonmodifiable* (uncontrollable) risk factors, including the patient's age, gender, ethnic origin, and a family history of CVD. Ask about any chronic disease or illness that the patient may have. The incidence of conditions such as coronary artery disease (CAD) and valvular disease increases with age. The incidence of CAD also varies with the patient's gender. Men have a higher risk for CAD than women of all ages (Benjamin et al., 2019). Although risk factors are for CAD are similar for men and women, women have several gender-specific risks, such as disorders of pregnancy and menopause (Benjamin et al., 2019)

Heart disease is the leading cause of diabetes-related death for both men and women. Adults with diabetes have heart disease death rates two to four times higher than those without diabetes. The risk for stroke is also two to four times higher among people with diabetes.

Modifiable (controllable) risk factors should also be assessed. *Modifiable* risk factors are personal lifestyle habits, including cigarette smoking, physical inactivity, obesity, and psychological variables. Ask the patient about each of these common risk factors.

Cigarette smoking is a major risk factor for CVD, specifically coronary artery disease (CAD) and peripheral vascular disease (PVD). Three compounds in cigarette smoke have been implicated in the development of CAD: tar, nicotine, and carbon monoxide. The smoking history should include the number of cigarettes smoked daily, the duration of the smoking habit, and the age of the patient when smoking started. Record the smoking history in **pack-years,** which is the number of packs per day multiplied by the number of years the patient has smoked.

To foster smoking cessation, the Centers for Disease Control and Prevention (CDC) recommends that health care providers use the 5A algorithm developed by the World Health Organization (WHO). The 5A approach is a task-based approach to help guide tobacco screening and cessation (WHO, 2014).

1. *A*sk about tobacco use.
   - Assess the patient's desire to quit, past attempts to quit, and the methods used.
2. *A*dvise patients to quit.
   - Tobacco use is one of the largest preventable causes of death in the United States (Benjamin et al., 2019).
3. *A*ssess readiness for quitting.
4. *A*ssist by providing resources.
5. *A*rrange follow-up.

Evidence demonstrates successful outcomes with consistent use of the 5A approach, allowing nurses to create a lasting impact on the patient's health (Thomas et al., 2018). In 3 to 4 years after a patient has stopped smoking, his or her CVD risk appears to be similar to that of a person who has never smoked. Be sure to ask those who do not currently smoke whether they have ever smoked and when they quit. Passive smoke (or

PATIENT-CENTERED CARE: OLDER ADULT CONSIDERATIONS QSEN

Changes in the Cardiovascular System Related to Aging

Change	Nursing Interventions	Rationales
Cardiac Valves		
Calcification and mucoid degeneration occur, especially in mitral and aortic valves.	Assess heart rate and rhythm and heart sounds for murmurs. Question patients about dyspnea.	Murmurs may be detected before other symptoms. Valvular abnormalities may result in rhythm changes.
Conduction System		
Pacemaker cells decrease in number. Fibrous tissue and fat in the sinoatrial node increase. Few muscle fibers remain in the atrial myocardium and bundle of His. Conduction time increases.	Assess the electrocardiogram (ECG) and heart rhythm for dysrhythmias or a heart rate less than 60 beats/min.	The sinoatrial (SA) node may lose its inherent rhythm. Atrial dysrhythmias occur in many older adults; 80% of older adults experience premature ventricular contractions (PVCs).
Left Ventricle		
The size of the left ventricle increases. The left ventricle becomes stiff and less distensible. Fibrotic changes in the left ventricle decrease the speed of early diastolic filling by about 50%.	Assess the ECG for a widening QRS complex and a longer QT interval. Assess the heart rate at rest and with activity. Assess for activity intolerance.	Ventricular changes result in decreased stroke volume, ejection fraction, and cardiac output during exercise; the heart is less able to meet increased oxygen demands. Maximum heart rate with exercise is decreased.
Aorta and Other Large Arteries		
The aorta and other large arteries thicken and become stiffer and less distensible. Systolic blood pressure increases to compensate for the stiff arteries. Systemic vascular resistance increases as a result of less distensible arteries; therefore the left ventricle pumps against greater resistance, contributing to left ventricular hypertrophy.	Assess blood pressure. Note increases in systolic, diastolic, and pulse pressures. Assess for activity intolerance and shortness of breath. Assess the peripheral pulses.	Hypertension may occur and must be treated to avoid target organ damage.
Baroreceptors		
Baroreceptors become less sensitive.	Assess the patient's blood pressure with the patient lying and then sitting or standing. Assess for dizziness when the patient changes from a lying to a sitting or standing position. Teach the patient to change positions slowly.	Orthostatic (postural) and postprandial changes occur because of ineffective baroreceptors. Changes may include blood pressure decreases of 10 mm Hg or more, dizziness, and fainting.

secondhand smoke) significantly reduces blood flow in healthy young adults' coronary arteries. Exposure to secondhand smoke at home or work increases the risk of CVD in nonsmokers by 25% to 30% (Benjamin et al., 2019). See Chapter 24 for additional information regarding smoking cessation.

A *sedentary lifestyle* is also a major risk factor for heart disease. Regular physical activity promotes cardiovascular fitness and produces beneficial changes in blood pressure and levels of blood lipids and clotting factors. Unfortunately, few people in the United States follow the recommended exercise guidelines: 150 minutes of moderate exercise or 75 minutes of vigorous exercise per week (or a combination of the two) plus completing muscle-strengthening exercises at least 2 days per week (Benjamin et al., 2019). Only 22.5% of adults in the United States meet the guidelines for physical activity (Benjamin et al., 2019). Encourage increased physical exercise as part of a lifestyle change to reduce the risk for CAD. Ask patients about the type of exercise they perform, how long a period they have participated in the exercise, and the frequency and intensity of the exercise.

About two-thirds of American adults are overweight as defined by a body mass index (BMI) of 25 to 30. Obesity is defined as a BMI greater than 30 and is associated with hypertension, hyperlipidemia, and diabetes; all are known contributors to CVD.

The American Heart Association (AHA) provides guidelines to combat obesity and improve cardiac health, including ingesting more nutrient-rich foods that have vitamins, minerals, fiber, and other nutrients but are low in calories. To get the necessary nutrients, teach patients to choose foods such as vegetables, fruits, unrefined whole-grain products, and fat-free dairy products most often. Also teach patients to not eat more calories than they can burn every day (AHA, 2017).

A variety of *psychological factors* make people more vulnerable to the development of heart disease. Those who are highly competitive, overly concerned about meeting deadlines, and often hostile or angry are at higher risk for heart disease. Psychological stress, anger, depression, and hostility are all closely associated with risk for developing heart disease.

You might ask the patient, "How do you respond when you have to wait for an appointment?" Chronic anger and hostility appear to be closely associated with CVD. The constant arousal of the sympathetic nervous system as a result of anger may influence

BP, serum fatty acids and lipids, and clotting mechanisms. Observe the patient and assess his or her response to stressful situations.

Review the patient's medical history, noting any major illnesses such as diabetes mellitus, renal disease, anemia, high BP, stroke, bleeding disorders, connective tissue diseases, chronic pulmonary diseases, heart disease, and thrombophlebitis. These conditions can influence the patient's cardiovascular status.

Ask about previous treatment for CVD, identify previous diagnostic procedures (e.g., ECG, cardiac catheterization), and request information about any medical or invasive treatment of CVD. Ask specifically about recurrent tonsillitis, streptococcal infections, and rheumatic fever, because these conditions may lead to valvular abnormalities of the heart. In addition, inquire about any known congenital heart defects. Many patients with congenital heart problems live into adulthood because of improved treatment and surgeries.

Ask patients about their drug history, beginning with any current or recent use of prescription or over-the-counter (OTC) medications or herbal/natural products. Inquire about known sensitivities to any drug and the nature of the reaction (e.g., nausea, rash). Patients should be asked whether they have recently used cocaine or any IV "street" drugs, because these substances are often associated with heart disease.

NCLEX EXAMINATION CHALLENGE 30.1

Health Promotion and Maintenance

The nurse is conducting an admission assessment on a male client. Which assessment data does the nurse identify as a risk factor for cardiovascular disease? **Select all that apply.**

A. BMI of 26
B. BP of 120/66 mm Hg
C. Triglycerides 140 mg/dL
D. Moderate exercise for 20 to 30 minutes weekly
E. Exposure to secondhand cigarette smoke
F. History of repeated streptococcal tonsillitis
G. Family history of cardiovascular disease

PATIENT-CENTERED CARE: GENDER HEALTH CONSIDERATIONS (QSEN)

Research is clear that women frequently present with CAD differently than men. Assess women for nonspecific cardiovascular symptoms, such as fatigue, malaise, anxiety, and shortness of breath. Although knowledge of presentation in women is increasing, educational needs remain, because heart disease remains the leading cause of death in women in the United States (Centers for Disease Control and Prevention, 2019; Garcia et al., 2016).

The *social history* includes information about the patient's living situation, including having a domestic partner, other household members, environment, and occupation. Identification of support systems is especially important in exploring the possibility that the patient might have difficulty paying for medications or treatment. Ask about occupation, including the type of work performed and the requirements of the specific job. For instance, does the job involve physical exertion such as lifting heavy objects? Is the job emotionally stressful? What does a day's work entail? Does the patient's job require him or her to be outside in extreme weather conditions?

PATIENT-CENTERED CARE: VETERANS HEALTH CONSIDERATIONS (QSEN)

Past research indicated that the health requirements for active duty service members could reduce mortality later in life. These protective effects, referred to as the "healthy soldier effect," were reported to last 10 to 30 years after military service had ended. However, even with a reduction in mortality, evidence indicated that veterans experienced higher rates of CVD, mental health issues, and substance use disorders when compared with nonveterans (Assari, 2014). New evidence suggests that the healthy soldier effect may not be as relevant for the newest generation of veterans because of earlier reporting of the development of cardiovascular conditions (Hinojosa, 2019). Research suggests that targeted teaching interventions should be considered in veterans before the development of heart disease to decrease their risk for heart disease (Assari, 2014).

Nutrition History. A nutrition history includes the patient's recall of food and fluid intake during a 24-hour period, self-imposed or medically prescribed dietary restrictions or supplementations, and the amount and type of alcohol consumption. If needed, the registered dietitian nutritionist may review the type of foods selected by the patient for the amount of sodium, sugar, cholesterol, fiber, and fat. Cultural beliefs and economic status can influence the choice of food items and therefore are seriously considered. Family members or significant others who are responsible for shopping and cooking should be included in this screening.

Family History and Genetic Risk. Review the family history and obtain information about the age, health status, and cause of death of immediate family members. A positive family history for CAD in a first-degree relative (parent, sibling, or child) is a major risk factor. It is *more* important than other factors such as hypertension, obesity, diabetes, or sudden cardiac death.

PATIENT-CENTERED CARE: GENETIC/GENOMIC CONSIDERATIONS (QSEN)

Cardiovascular disease has many contributory factors, including a genetic tendency. A significant association between familial cardiac history and CVD is consistently demonstrated in the evidence from multiple large-scale prospective epidemiology studies (Benjamin et al., 2019). Although several genes have been reported to be associated with heart disease, stroke, and hypertension, the impact of each individual gene is not fully understood. Additional discussions about genetic factors related to specific CVDs are found in other chapters in this unit.

Current Health Problems. Ask the patient to describe his or her health concerns. Expand on the description of these concerns by obtaining information about their onset, duration, sequence, frequency, location, quality, intensity, associated symptoms, and precipitating, aggravating, and relieving factors. Major symptoms usually identified by patients with CVD include chest pain or discomfort, dyspnea, fatigue, palpitations, weight gain, syncope, and extremity pain.

Pain or discomfort, considered a traditional symptom of heart disease, can result from ischemic heart disease, pericarditis, and aortic dissection. Chest pain can also be caused by noncardiac conditions such as pleurisy, pulmonary embolus, hiatal hernia,

NURSING SAFETY PRIORITY (QSEN)

Action Alert

Thoroughly evaluate the nature and characteristics of the chest ***pain***. Because pain resulting from myocardial ischemia is life threatening and can lead to serious complications, its cause should be considered ischemic (reduced or obstructed blood flow to the myocardium) until proven otherwise. When assessing for symptoms, ask the patient if he or she has "discomfort," "heaviness," "pressure," and/or "indigestion." It is important to note that chest pain can occur in any setting. Proper assessment of the pain can decrease the potential for serious complications.

gastroesophageal reflux disease, neuromuscular abnormalities, and anxiety.

Ask the patient to identify when the symptoms were first noticed (onset):

- Did the symptoms begin suddenly or develop gradually (manner of onset)?
- How long did the symptoms last (duration)?

If he or she has repeated painful episodes, assess how often the symptoms occur (frequency). If pain is present, ask whether it is different from any other episodes of pain. Ask the patient to describe which activities he or she was doing when it first occurred, such as sleeping, arguing, or running (precipitating factors). If possible, the patient should point to the area where the chest pain occurred (location) and describe if and how the pain radiated (spread).

In addition, ask how the pain feels and whether it is sharp, dull, or crushing (quality of pain). To understand the severity of the pain, ask the patient to grade it from 0 to 10, with 10 indicating severe pain (intensity). He or she may also report other signs and symptoms that occur at the same time (associated symptoms), such as dyspnea, diaphoresis (excessive sweating), nausea, and vomiting. Other factors that need to be addressed are those that may have made the chest pain worse (aggravating factors) or less intense (relieving factors). Chest pain can arise from a variety of sources (Table 30.1). By obtaining the appropriate information, you can help identify the source of the discomfort.

PATIENT-CENTERED CARE: GENDER HEALTH CONSIDERATIONS (QSEN)

Some patients, especially women, do not experience ***pain*** in the chest but instead feel discomfort or indigestion. Women often present with a "triad" of symptoms. In addition to indigestion or a feeling of abdominal fullness, chronic fatigue despite adequate rest and feelings of an "inability to catch my breath" (dyspnea) are also common in heart disease. The patient may also describe the sensation as aching, choking, strangling, tingling, squeezing, constricting, or viselike. Others with severe neuropathy may experience few or no traditional symptoms except shortness of breath, despite major ischemia. Be aware that CVD also affects younger people. According to the American Heart Association (AHA, 2019), 44.7% of women over the age of 20 have some form of cardiovascular disease.

Dyspnea (difficult or labored breathing) can occur as a result of both cardiac and pulmonary disease. It is experienced by the patient as uncomfortable breathing or shortness of breath. When obtaining the history, ask which factors precipitate and relieve dyspnea, what level of activity produces dyspnea, and what the patient's body position was when dyspnea occurred.

Dyspnea that is associated with activity, such as climbing stairs, is referred to as *dyspnea on exertion* (DOE). This is usually an early symptom of heart failure and may be the *only* symptom experienced by women.

The patient with advanced heart disease may experience orthopnea (dyspnea that appears when he or she lies flat). Several pillows may be needed to elevate the head and chest, or a recliner may be used to prevent breathlessness. The number of pillows or the amount of head elevation needed to achieve restful sleep is often a measure of the severity of orthopnea. This symptom is usually relieved within a matter of minutes by sitting up or standing.

Paroxysmal nocturnal dyspnea (PND) develops after the patient has been lying down for several hours. In this position, blood from the lower extremities is redistributed to the venous system, which increases venous return to the heart. A diseased heart cannot compensate for the increased volume and is ineffective in pumping the additional fluid into the circulatory system. Pulmonary congestion results, and the patient awakens abruptly, often with a feeling of suffocation and panic. He or she sits upright and dangles the legs over the side of the bed to relieve the dyspnea. This sensation may last for 20 minutes.

Fatigue may be described as a feeling of tiredness or weariness resulting from activity. The patient may report that an activity takes longer to complete or that he or she tires easily after activity. Although fatigue in itself is not diagnostic of heart disease, many people with heart failure are limited by leg fatigue during exercise. Fatigue that occurs after mild activity and exertion usually indicates inadequate cardiac output (due to low stroke volume) and anaerobic metabolism in skeletal muscle. It can also accompany other symptoms or may be an early indication of heart disease in women.

Ask about the time of day the patient experiences fatigue and the activities that he or she can perform. Fatigue resulting from decreased cardiac output is often worse in the evening. Ask whether the patient can perform the same activities as he or she could perform a year ago or the same activities as others of the same age. Often he or she limits activities in response to fatigue and, unless questioned, is unaware how much less active he or she has become.

A feeling of fluttering or an unpleasant feeling in the chest caused by an irregular heartbeat is referred to as **palpitations**. They may result from a change in heart rate or rhythm or from an increase in the force of heart contractions. Rhythm disturbances that may cause palpitations include paroxysmal supraventricular tachycardia, premature contractions, and sinus tachycardia. Those that occur during or after strenuous physical activity, such as running and swimming, may indicate overexertion or possibly heart disease. Noncardiac factors that may precipitate palpitations include anxiety; stress; fatigue; insomnia; hyperthyroidism; and the ingestion of caffeine, nicotine, or alcohol. Ask the patient about specific factors that cause his or her palpitations.

A sudden weight increase of 2.2 lb (1 kg) can result from excess fluid (1 L) in the interstitial spaces. The *best indicator* of

TABLE 30.1 **Assessment of Chest Discomfort: How Various Types of Chest Pain Differ**

Onset	Quality and Severity	Location and Radiation	Duration and Relieving Factors
Angina			
Sudden, usually in response to exertion, emotion, or extremes in temperature	Squeezing, viselike pain	Usually the left side of chest without radiation Substernal; may spread across the chest and the back and/or down the arms	Usually lasts less than 15 min; relieved with rest, nitrate administration, or oxygen therapy
Myocardial Infarction			
Sudden, without precipitating factors, often in early morning	Intense stabbing, viselike pain or pressure, severe	Substernal; may spread throughout the anterior chest and to the arms, jaw, back, or neck	Pain is often continuous and is not relieved with rest or change in position; relieved with morphine and cardiac drugs
Pericarditis			
Sudden	Sharp, stabbing, moderate to severe	Substernal; usually spreads to the left side or the back	Intermittent; relieved with sitting upright, analgesia, or administration of anti-inflammatory agents
Pleuropulmonary			
Variable	Moderate ache, worse on inspiration	Lung fields	Continuous until the underlying condition is treated or the patient has rested
Esophageal-Gastric			
Variable	Squeezing, heartburn, variable severity	Substernal; may spread to the shoulders or the abdomen	Variable; may be relieved with antacid administration, food intake, or taking a sitting position
Anxiety			
Variable, may be in response to stress or fatigue	Dull ache to sharp stabbing; may be associated with numbness in fingers	Not well located and usually does not radiate to other parts of the body as pain	Usually lasts a few minutes

fluid balance is weight. Excess fluid accumulation is commonly known as *edema*. It is possible for weight gains of up to 10 to 15 lb (4.5 to 6.8 kg, or 4 to 7 L of fluid) to occur before edema is apparent. Ask whether the patient has noticed a tightness of shoes, indentations from socks, or tightness of rings.

Syncope refers to a brief loss of consciousness. The most common cause is decreased perfusion to the brain. Any condition that suddenly reduces cardiac output, resulting in decreased cerebral blood flow, can lead to a syncopal episode. Conditions such as cardiac rhythm disturbances, especially ventricular dysrhythmias, and valvular disorders such as aortic stenosis may trigger this symptom. *Near-syncope* refers to dizziness with an inability to remain in an upright position. Explore the circumstances that lead to dizziness or syncope.

PATIENT-CENTERED CARE: OLDER ADULT CONSIDERATIONS QSEN

Syncope in the aging person may result from hypersensitivity of the carotid sinus bodies in the carotid arteries. Pressure applied to these arteries while turning the head, shrugging the shoulders, or performing a Valsalva maneuver (bearing down during defecation) may stimulate a vagal response. A decrease in blood pressure and heart rate can result, which can produce syncope. This type of syncopal episode may also result from orthostatic (postural) or postprandial (after eating) hypotension.

Extremity pain may be caused by two conditions: ischemia from atherosclerosis and venous insufficiency of the peripheral blood vessels. Patients who report a moderate-to-severe cramping sensation in their legs or buttocks associated with an activity such as walking have intermittent claudication related to decreased arterial tissue ***perfusion.*** Resting or lowering the affected extremity to decrease tissue demands or to enhance arterial blood flow usually relieves claudication pain. Leg pain that results from prolonged standing or sitting is related to venous insufficiency from either incompetent valves or venous obstruction. Elevating the extremity may relieve this pain.

NCLEX EXAMINATION CHALLENGE 30.2

Physiological Integrity

The nurse is assessing a client with heart failure. Which assessment data are the **best** indicator of fluid balance?

A. Blood pressure 144/79 mm Hg
B. Urine output 200 mL in the last 4 hours
C. Weight increase of 9 lb in the past week
D. Generalized edema in the lower extremities

Functional History. After the history of the patient's cardiovascular status has been obtained, he or she may be classified according to the New York Heart Association Functional Classification (Table 30.2) or other system. The four classifications (I, II, III, and IV) depend on the degree to which ordinary physical activities (routine ADLs) are affected by heart disease. The Killip classification provides a more objective description of the hemodynamics of heart failure and is described in Chapter 35.

TABLE 30.2 New York Heart Association Functional Classification of Cardiovascular Disability

Class I

- Patients with cardiac disease but without resulting limitations of physical activity
- Ordinary physical activity does not cause undue fatigue, palpitation, dyspnea, or anginal pain

Class II

- Patients with cardiac disease resulting in slight limitation of physical activity
- Comfortable at rest
- Ordinary physical activity results in fatigue, palpitation, dyspnea, or anginal pain

Class III

- Patients with cardiac disease resulting in marked limitation of physical activity
- Comfortable at rest
- Less than ordinary physical activity causes fatigue, palpitation, dyspnea, or anginal pain

Class IV

- Patients with cardiac disease resulting in inability to carry out any physical activity without discomfort
- Symptoms of cardiac insufficiency or of the anginal syndrome may be present, even at rest
- If any physical activity is undertaken, discomfort is increased

Excerpt from The New York Heart Association. (1964). *Diseases of the heart and blood vessels: Nomenclature and criteria for diagnosis* (6th ed.). Boston: Little, Brown.

Physical Assessment

A thorough physical assessment is the foundation for the nursing database and the patient's priority problems. Any changes noted during the course of illness can be compared with this initial database. Evaluate the patient's vital signs on admission to the hospital or during the initial visit to the clinic or primary care provider's office.

General Appearance. Physical assessment begins with the patient's general appearance. Assess general build and appearance, skin color, distress level, level of consciousness, shortness of breath, position, and verbal responses.

Patients can have left- or right-sided heart failure, or both. They can also be diagnosed with systolic and/or diastolic heart failure. As a result, poor cardiac output and decreased cerebral ***perfusion*** may cause confusion, memory loss, and slowed verbal responses, especially in older adults. Patients with chronic heart failure may also appear malnourished, thin, and cachectic. Late signs of severe right-sided heart failure are ascites, jaundice, and anasarca (generalized edema) as a result of prolonged congestion of the liver. Heart failure may also cause fluid retention and may manifest with obvious generalized dependent edema. Chapter 35 differentiates right and left failure and systolic from diastolic heart failure in detail.

Skin. Skin assessment includes color and temperature. The best areas in which to assess circulation include the nail beds, mucous membranes, and conjunctival mucosa, because small blood vessels are located near the surface of the skin in those areas.

If there is normal blood flow or adequate perfusion to a given area in light-colored skin, it appears pink, perhaps rosy, and is warm. Decreased ***perfusion*** manifests as cool, pale, and moist skin. Pallor is characteristic of anemia and can be seen in areas such as the nail beds, palms, and conjunctival mucous membranes in any patient.

A bluish or darkened discoloration of the skin and mucous membranes in light-skinned adults is referred to as *cyanosis*. Dark-skinned adults may experience cyanosis as a graying of the same tissues. This condition results from an increased amount of deoxygenated hemoglobin. It is not an early sign of decreased perfusion but occurs later with other symptoms.

Central cyanosis involves decreased oxygenation of the arterial blood in the lungs and appears as a bluish tinge of the conjunctivae and the mucous membranes of the mouth and tongue. Central cyanosis may indicate impaired lung function or a right-to-left shunt found in congenital heart conditions. Because of impaired circulation, there is marked desaturation of hemoglobin in the peripheral tissues, which produces a bluish or darkened discoloration of the nail beds, earlobes, lips, and toes.

Peripheral cyanosis occurs when blood flow to the peripheral vessels is decreased by peripheral vasoconstriction. Constriction results from a low cardiac output or an increased extraction of oxygen from the peripheral tissues. Peripheral cyanosis localized in an extremity is usually a result of arterial or venous insufficiency. Rubor (dusky redness) that replaces pallor in a dependent foot suggests arterial insufficiency.

Skin *temperature* can be assessed for symmetry by touching different areas of the body with the dorsal (back) surface of the hand or fingers. Decreased blood flow results in decreased skin temperature. It is lowered in several clinical conditions, including heart failure, peripheral vascular disease (PVD), and shock.

Extremities. Assess the patient's hands, arms, feet, and legs for skin changes, vascular changes, clubbing, and edema. Skin mobility and turgor are affected by fluid status. Dehydration and aging reduce skin turgor, and edema decreases skin elasticity. Vascular changes in an affected extremity may include paresthesia, muscle fatigue and discomfort, numbness, pain, coolness, and loss of hair distribution from a reduced blood supply.

Clubbing of the fingers and toes is caused by long-term (chronic) oxygen deprivation in body tissues. It is common in patients with advanced chronic pulmonary disease, congenital heart defects, and cor pulmonale (right-sided heart failure). The angle of the normal nail bed is 160 degrees. With clubbing, the nail straightens out to an angle of 180 degrees and the base of the nail becomes spongy. Fig. 27.8 shows late clubbing.

Peripheral edema (fluid accumulation in the legs and feet) is a common finding in patients with cardiovascular problems. The location of edema helps determine its potential cause. Bilateral edema of the legs may be seen in those with heart failure or

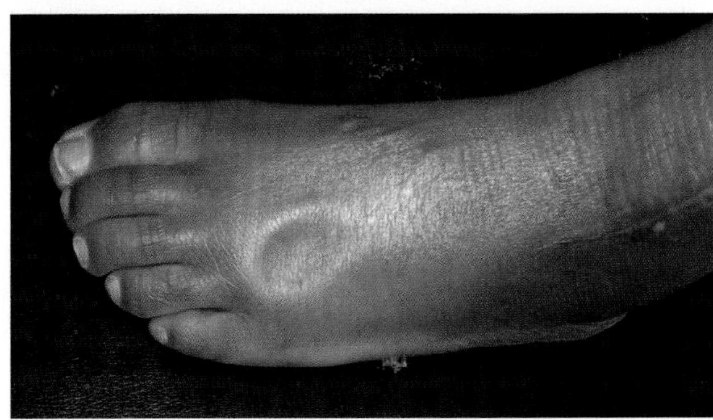

FIG. 30.5 Peripheral pitting edema. (From Sahrmann, S. [2011]. *Movement system impairment syndromes of the extremities, cervical and thoracic spines.* St. Louis: Mosby.)

chronic venous insufficiency. Abdominal and leg edema can be seen in patients with heart disease and cirrhosis of the liver. Localized edema in one extremity may be the result of venous obstruction (thrombosis) or lymphatic blockage of the extremity (lymphedema). Edema may also be noted in dependent areas, such as the sacrum, when a patient is confined to bed. In other patients, edema results from third spacing when plasma proteins decrease. Dependent foot and ankle edema is also a common side effect of certain antihypertensive drugs, such as amlodipine.

Document the location of edema as precisely as possible (e.g., midtibial or sacral) and the number of centimeters from an anatomic landmark. The extent of edema can be assessed as mild, moderate, or severe (or 1+, 2+, 3+, or 4+). However, these values are not precise and are very unreliable. Determine whether the edema is *pitting* (the skin can be indented) (Fig. 30.5) or nonpitting.

The finger is typically used for pulse oximetry as a noninvasive method for assessing oxygenation and ***perfusion*** of many medical-surgical nursing patients. Correct placement of the pulse oximetry sensor is essential for accurate readings. Oxygen saturation levels of above 90% are considered normal, depending on the patient's age. Detailed information about this assessment method can be found in Chapter 24.

Blood Pressure. Arterial blood pressure is measured *indirectly* by sphygmomanometry. This technique of measurement is described in detail in nursing skills textbooks.

The Eighth National High Blood Pressure Education Program Joint National Committee (JNC) on Prevention, Detection, Evaluation, and Treatment of High Blood Pressure (James et al., 2014) defines hypertension as a systolic pressure of 140 mm Hg or higher or a diastolic pressure of 90 mm Hg or higher or taking drugs to control blood pressure. The American Heart Association (AHA) and the American College of Cardiology (ACC) have suggested that blood pressure be below 130/80 mm Hg in all people, which is slightly lower than the widely accepted JNC guidelines (Whelton et al., 2017). Chapter 33 describes hypertension in detail.

A BP less than 90/60 mm Hg (hypotension) may not be adequate for providing enough oxygen and sufficient nutrition to body cells. In certain circumstances such as shock, the Korotkoff sounds are less audible or are absent. In these cases palpate the BP, use an ultrasonic device (Doppler device), or obtain a direct measurement by arterial catheter in the critical care setting. When BP is palpated, only the systolic pressure can be determined. Patients may report dizziness or light-headedness when they move from a flat, supine position to a sitting or a standing position at the edge of the bed. Normally these symptoms are transient and pass quickly; pronounced symptoms may be due to postural hypotension. **Orthostatic (postural) hypotension** occurs when the BP is not adequately maintained while moving from a lying to a sitting or standing position. It is defined as a decrease of more than 20 mm Hg of the systolic pressure or more than 10 mm Hg of the diastolic pressure and a 10% to 20% increase in heart rate. The causes of postural hypotension include cardiovascular drugs, blood volume decrease, prolonged bedrest, age-related changes, or disorders of the nervous system.

To detect orthostatic changes in BP, first measure the BP when the patient is supine. After remaining supine for at least 3 minutes, the patient changes position to sitting or standing. Normally systolic pressure drops slightly or remains unchanged as the patient rises, whereas diastolic pressure rises slightly. After the position change, wait for at least 1 minute before auscultating BP and counting the radial pulse. The cuff should remain in the proper position on the patient's arm. Observe and record any signs or symptoms of dizziness. If the patient cannot tolerate the position change, return him or her to the previous position of comfort.

Paradoxical blood pressure is an exaggerated decrease in systolic pressure by more than 10 mm Hg during the inspiratory phase of the respiratory cycle (normal it is 3 to 10 mm Hg). Certain clinical conditions that potentially alter the filling pressures in the right and left ventricles may produce a paradoxical BP. Such conditions include pericardial tamponade, constrictive pericarditis, and pulmonary hypertension. During inspiration, the filling pressures normally decrease slightly. However, decreased fluid volume in the ventricles resulting from these pathologic conditions produces a marked reduction in cardiac output. The difference between the systolic and diastolic values is referred to as **pulse pressure**. This value can be used as an indirect measure of cardiac output. Narrowed pulse pressure is rarely normal and results from increased peripheral vascular resistance or decreased stroke volume in patients with heart failure, hypovolemia, or shock. It can also be seen in those with mitral stenosis or regurgitation. An increased pulse pressure may occur in patients with slow heart rates, aortic regurgitation, atherosclerosis, hypertension, and aging.

The ankle-brachial index (ABI) can be used to assess the vascular status of the lower extremities. A BP cuff is applied to the lower extremity just above the malleolus. The systolic pressure is measured with Doppler ultrasound at both the dorsalis pedis and posterior tibial pulses. The higher of these two pressures is then divided by the higher of the two brachial pulses to obtain the ABI.

Normal values for the ABI are 1.00 or higher because BP in the legs is usually higher than BP in the arms. ABI values less than 0.9 usually indicate moderate vascular disease, whereas values less than 0.5 indicate severe vascular compromise.

A toe brachial pressure index (TBPI) may be performed instead of or in addition to the ABI to determine arterial perfusion in the feet and toes. TBPI is the toe systolic pressure divided by the brachial (arm) systolic pressure.

Venous and Arterial Pulses. Observe the venous pulsations in the neck to assess the adequacy of blood volume and central venous pressure (CVP). Specially educated or critical care nurses can assess jugular venous pressure (JVP) to estimate the filling volume and pressure on the right side of the heart. An increase in JVP causes jugular venous distention (JVD). Increases are usually caused by fluid volume overload and right ventricular failure (Urden et al., 2018). Other causes include tricuspid regurgitation or stenosis, pulmonary hypertension, cardiac tamponade, constrictive pericarditis, hypervolemia, and superior vena cava obstruction.

Assessment of *arterial pulses* provides information about vascular integrity and circulation. For patients with suspected or actual vascular disease, major peripheral pulses should be assessed for presence or absence, amplitude, contour, rhythm, rate, and equality. Palpate the peripheral arteries in a head-to-toe approach with a side-to-side comparison (Fig. 30.6).

A *hypokinetic* pulse is a weak pulse indicative of a narrow pulse pressure. It is seen in patients with hypovolemia, aortic stenosis, and decreased cardiac output. A *hyperkinetic* pulse is a large, "bounding" pulse caused by an increased ejection of blood. It occurs in patients with a high cardiac output (with exercise, sepsis, or thyrotoxicosis) and in those with increased sympathetic system activity (with pain, fever, or anxiety).

Auscultation of the major arteries (e.g., carotid and aorta) is necessary to assess for bruits. **Bruits** are swishing sounds that may occur from turbulent blood flow in narrowed or atherosclerotic arteries. Assess for the absence or presence of bruits by placing the bell of the stethoscope on the neck over the carotid artery while the patient holds his or her breath. Normally there are no sounds if the artery has uninterrupted blood flow. A bruit may develop when the internal diameter of the vessel is narrowed by 50% or more, but this does not indicate the severity of disease in the arteries. Once the vessel is blocked 90% or more, the bruit often cannot be heard.

Precordium. Assessment of the precordium (the area over the heart) involves inspection, palpation, percussion, and auscultation. In most settings, the medical-surgical nurse seldom performs precordial palpation and percussion. Critical care nurses and advanced practice nurses are qualified to perform the complete assessment. Therefore only inspection and auscultation are described here. Begin by placing the patient in a supine position, with the head of the bed slightly elevated for comfort. Some patients may require elevation of the head of the bed to 45 degrees for ease and comfort in breathing.

Inspection. A cardiac examination is usually performed in a systematic order, beginning with inspection. Inspect the chest from the side, at a right angle, and downward over areas of the precordium where vibrations are visible. Cardiac motion is of low amplitude, and sometimes the inward movements are more easily detected by the naked eye.

Examine the entire precordium (Fig. 30.7) and note any prominent pulses. Movement over the aortic, pulmonic, and tricuspid areas is abnormal. Pulses in the mitral area (the apex of the heart) are considered normal and are referred to as the **apical impulse**, or the **point of maximal impulse (PMI)**. The PMI should be located at the left fifth intercostal space (ICS) in the midclavicular line. If it appears in more than one ICS and has shifted lateral to the midclavicular line, the patient may have left ventricular hypertrophy.

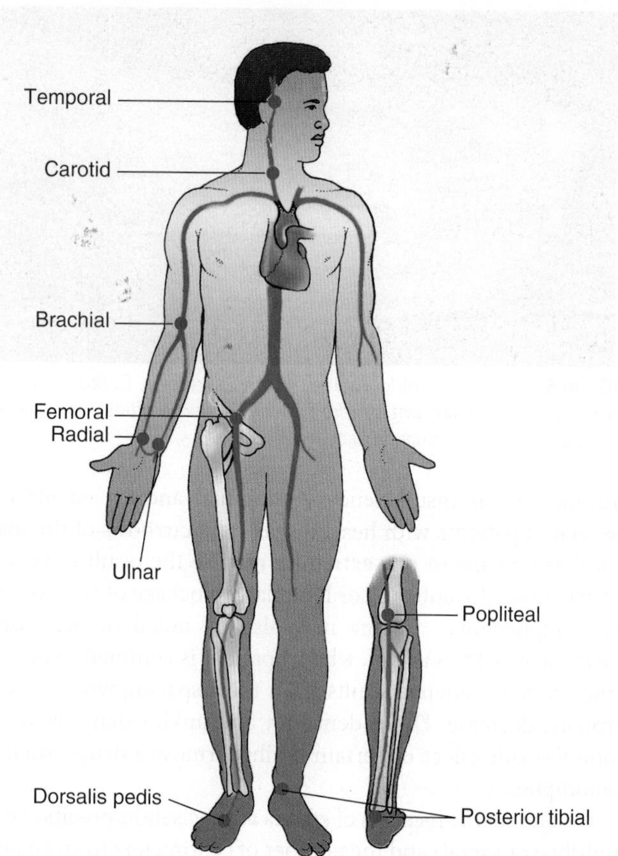

FIG. 30.6 Pulse points for assessment of arterial pulses.

Auscultation. Auscultation evaluates heart rate and rhythm, cardiac cycle (systole and diastole), and valvular function. The technique of auscultation requires a good-quality stethoscope and extensive clinical practice. Identifying specific abnormal heart sounds is most important in critical care and telemetry.

Listen to heart sounds in a systematic order. Examination usually begins at the aortic area and progresses slowly to the apex of the heart. The diaphragm of the stethoscope is pressed tightly against the chest to listen for high-frequency sounds and is useful in listening to the first and second heart sounds and high-frequency murmurs. Repeat the progression from the base to the apex of the heart using the bell of the stethoscope, which is held lightly against the chest. The bell can screen out high-frequency sounds and is useful in listening for low-frequency gallops (diastolic filling sounds) and murmurs.

Normal Heart Sounds. The *first heart sound* (S_1) is created by the closure of the mitral and tricuspid valves (atrioventricular valves) (see Fig. 30.4). When auscultated, S_1 is softer and longer; it is of a low pitch and is best heard at the lower left sternal border or the apex of the heart. Palpating the carotid pulse while listening may help to identify S_1. S_1 marks the beginning

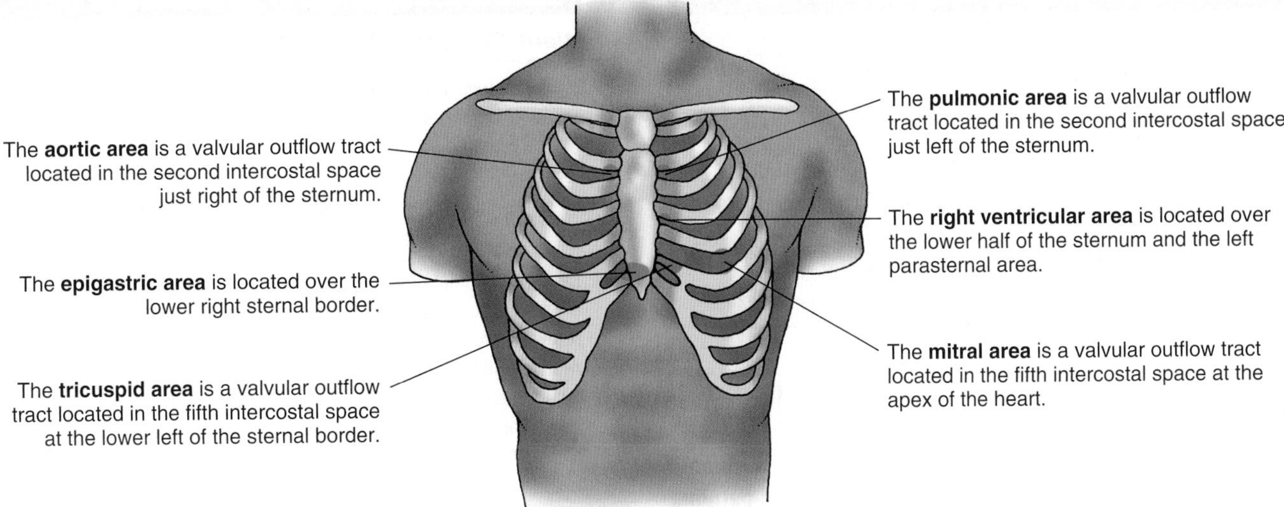

The aortic area is a valvular outflow tract located in the second intercostal space just right of the sternum.
The epigastric area is located over the lower right sternal border.
The tricuspid area is a valvular outflow tract located in the fifth intercostal space at the lower left of the sternal border.
The pulmonic area is a valvular outflow tract located in the second intercostal space just left of the sternum.
The right ventricular area is located over the lower half of the sternum and the left parasternal area.
The mitral area is a valvular outflow tract located in the fifth intercostal space at the apex of the heart.

FIG. 30.7 Areas for myocardial inspection and auscultation.

of ventricular systole and occurs right after the QRS complex on the ECG.

S_1 can be accentuated or intensified in conditions such as exercise, hyperthyroidism, and mitral stenosis. A decrease in sound intensity occurs in patients with mitral regurgitation and heart failure. If you have difficulty hearing heart sounds, have the patient lean forward or roll to his or her left side.

The *second heart sound (S_2)* is created by the closing of the aortic and pulmonic valves (semilunar valves) (see Fig. 30.4). S_2 is characteristically shorter. It is higher pitched and is heard best at the base of the heart at the end of ventricular systole.

The splitting of heart sounds is often difficult to differentiate from diastolic filling sounds (gallops). A splitting of S_1 (closure of the mitral valve followed by closure of the tricuspid valve) occurs physiologically because left ventricular contraction occurs slightly before right ventricular contraction. However, closure of the mitral valve is louder than closure of the tricuspid valve, so splitting is often not heard. Normal splitting of S_2 occurs because of the longer systolic phase of the right ventricle. Splitting of S_1 and S_2 can be accentuated by inspiration (due to increased venous return), and it narrows during expiration.

Abnormal Heart Sounds. Abnormal splitting of S_2 is referred to as *paradoxic splitting* and has a wider split heard on expiration. Paradoxic splitting of S_2 is heard in patients with severe myocardial depression that causes early closure of the pulmonic valve or a delay in aortic valve closure. Such conditions include myocardial infarction (MI), left bundle-branch block, aortic stenosis, aortic regurgitation, and right ventricular pacing.

Gallops and murmurs are common abnormal heart sounds that may occur with heart disease, but they can occur in some healthy people. Diastolic filling sounds (S_3 and S_4) are produced when blood enters a noncompliant chamber during rapid ventricular filling. The third heart sound (S_3) is produced during the rapid passive filling phase of ventricular diastole when blood flows from the atrium to a noncompliant ventricle. The sound arises from vibrations of the valves and supporting structures. The fourth heart sound (S_4) occurs as blood enters the ventricles during the active filling phase at the end of ventricular diastole.

S_3 is called a *ventricular gallop*, and S_4 is referred to as *atrial gallop*. These sounds can be caused by decreased compliance of either or both ventricles. Left ventricular diastolic filling sounds are best heard with the patient on his or her left side. The bell of the stethoscope is placed at the apex and at the left lower sternal border during expiration.

An S_3 heart sound is most likely to be a normal finding in those younger than 35 years. An S_3 gallop in patients older than 35 years is considered abnormal and represents a decrease in left ventricular compliance. It can be detected as an early sign of heart failure or as a ventricular septal defect.

An atrial gallop (S_4) may be heard in patients with hypertension, anemia, ventricular hypertrophy, MI, aortic or pulmonic stenosis, and pulmonary emboli. It may also be heard with advancing age because of a stiffened ventricle.

Murmurs reflect turbulent blood flow through normal or abnormal valves. They are classified according to their timing in the cardiac cycle: *systolic* murmurs (e.g., aortic stenosis and mitral regurgitation) occur between S_1 and S_2, whereas *diastolic* murmurs (e.g., mitral stenosis and aortic regurgitation) occur between S_2 and S_1. Murmurs can occur during presystole, midsystole, or late systole or diastole or can last throughout both phases of the cardiac cycle. They are also graded by the primary care provider according to their intensity, depending on their level of loudness (Table 30.3).

Although you are not expected to grade murmurs as a medical-surgical nurse, describe their location based on where they are best heard. Some murmurs transmit or radiate from their loudest point to other areas, including the neck, the back, and the axilla. The configuration is described as *crescendo* (increases in intensity) or *decrescendo* (decreases in intensity). The quality of murmurs can be further characterized as harsh, blowing, whistling, rumbling, or squeaking. They are also described by pitch—usually *high* or *low*.

TABLE 30.3 Grading of Heart Murmurs

Grade I	Very faint
Grade II	Faint but recognizable
Grade III	Loud but moderate in intensity
Grade IV	Loud; accompanied by a palpable thrill
Grade V	Very loud; accompanied by a palpable thrill; audible with the stethoscope partially off the patient's chest
Grade VI	Extremely loud; may be heard with the stethoscope slightly above the patient's chest; accompanied by a palpable thrill

A **pericardial friction rub** originates from the pericardial sac and occurs with the movements of the heart during the cardiac cycle. Rubs are usually transient and are a sign of inflammation, infection, or infiltration. They may be heard in patients with pericarditis resulting from MI or cardiac tamponade or after thoracotomy.

Psychosocial Assessment

To most people, the heart is a symbol of their ability to exist, survive, and love. A patient with a heart-related illness, whether acute or chronic, usually perceives it as a major life crisis. The patient and family confront not only the possibility of death but also fears about pain, disability, lack of self-esteem, physical dependence, and changes in family dynamics. Assess the meaning of the illness to the patient and family by asking, "What do you understand about what happened to you (or the patient)?" and "What does that mean to you?" When they perceive the stressor as overwhelming, formerly adequate support systems may no longer be effective. In these circumstances, the patient and family members attempt to cope to regain a sense or feeling of control.

Coping behaviors vary among patients and their families. Those who feel helpless to meet the demands of the situation may exhibit behaviors such as disorganization, fear, and anxiety. Ask them, "Have you ever encountered such a situation before?" "How did you manage that situation?" and "To whom can you turn for help?" The answers to these questions often reassure the patient and family that they have encountered difficult situations in the past and have the ability and resources to cope with them.

A common and normal response is *denial,* which is a defense mechanism that enables the patient to cope with threatening circumstances. He or she may deny the current cardiovascular condition, may state that it was present but is now absent, or may be excessively cheerful. Denial becomes maladaptive when the patient is noncompliant or does not adhere to the interdisciplinary plan of care.

Family members and significant others may be more anxious than the patient. Often they recall all events of the illness, are unprotected by denial, and are afraid of recurrence. Disagreements may occur between the patient and family members over adherence with appropriate follow-up care.

CLINICAL JUDGMENT CHALLENGE 30.1

Patient-Centered Care; Safety

A 52-year-old woman presents to the emergency department (ED) with reports of sweating, indigestion, and fatigue. The client reports occasional chest pressure. The client is alert and oriented; BP 90/50; HR 80; oxygen saturation 94% on room air. The client is diaphoretic and pale and appears apprehensive. The client states, "My mother had a heart attack when she was 50, so I'm worried."

1. **Recognize Cues:** What assessment information in this client situation is the most important and immediate concern for the nurse? (Hint: Identify the **relevant** information *first* to determine what is most important.)
2. **Analyze Cues:** What client conditions are consistent with the **most relevant** information? (Hint: Think about priority collaborative problems that support and contradict the information presented in this situation.)

Diagnostic Assessment

Laboratory Assessment. Assessment of the patient with cardiovascular dysfunction includes examination of the blood for abnormalities. The examination is performed to help establish a diagnosis, detect concurrent disease, assess risk factors, and monitor response to treatment. Normal values for serum cardiac enzymes and serum lipids are listed in the Laboratory Profile: Cardiovascular Assessment box.

Serum Markers of Myocardial Damage. Events leading to cellular injury cause a release of enzymes from intracellular storage, and circulating levels of these enzymes are dramatically elevated. Acute myocardial infarction (MI), also known as *acute coronary syndrome,* can be confirmed by abnormally high levels of certain proteins or isoenzymes.

Troponin is a myocardial muscle protein released into the bloodstream with injury to myocardial muscle. Troponins T and I are not found in healthy patients, so any rise in values indicates cardiac necrosis or acute MI. Specific markers of myocardial injury, troponins T and I, have a wide diagnostic time frame, making them useful for patients who present several hours after the onset of chest pain. Even low levels of troponin T are treated aggressively because of increased risk for death from cardiovascular disease (CVD). Obtaining cardiac markers at the bedside in the emergency department can be done as "point-of-care" (POC) testing for patients experiencing or at risk for acute MI, with results available within 15 to 20 minutes. These markers are evaluated in addition to clinical signs and symptoms and ECG changes when identifying at-risk patients. Following initial troponin assessment, levels should be assessed again in 3 to 6 hours. Before the development of highly sensitive troponin levels, providers relied on creatine kinase (CK), its isoenzyme (CK-MB), and myoglobin to assist with diagnosis of acute MI. Use of these cardiac markers is no longer recommended (Jaffe & Morrow, 2018).

Serum Lipids. Elevated lipid levels are considered a risk factor for coronary artery disease (CAD). **Cholesterol**, **triglycerides**, and the protein components of **high-density lipoproteins (HDLs)** and **low-density lipoproteins (LDLs)** are evaluated to

LABORATORY PROFILE

Cardiovascular Assessment

Normal Range	Significance of Abnormal Findings
Serum Lipids	
Cholesterol <200 mg/dL or <5.2 mmol/L (SI units)	Elevation indicates increased risk for CAD.
Triglycerides *Females:* 35-135 mg/dL or 0.40-1.52 mmol/L (SI units) *Males:* 40-160 mg/dL or 0.45-1.81 mmol/L (SI units)	Elevation indicates increased risk for CAD.
Plasma high-density lipoproteins (HDLs) *Females:* >55 mg/dL or >0.91 mmol/L (SI units) *Males:* >45 mg/dL or 0.75 mmol/L (SI units) *Older adults:* range increases with age	Elevations protect against CAD.
Plasma low-density lipoproteins (LDLs) <130 mg/dL or <3.4 mmol/L (SI units)	Elevation indicates increased risk for CAD.
HDL/LDL ratio 3:1	Elevated ratios may protect against CAD.
Very-low-density lipoprotein (VLDL) 7-32 mg/dL or 0.18-0.83 mmol/L (SI units)	Elevated level indicates risk for CAD.
C-reactive protein (CRP) <1.0 mg/dL or <10.0 mg/L (SI units)	Elevation may indicate tissue infarction or damage.
Serum Markers	
Troponins Cardiac troponin T <0.1 ng/mL Cardiac troponin I <0.03 ng/mL	Elevations indicate myocardial injury or infarction.

Data from Pagana, K., & Pagana, T. J. (2018). *Mosby's manual of diagnostic and laboratory tests* (6th ed.). St. Louis: Elsevier.

assess the risk for CAD. The desired ranges for lipids are (Pagana & Pagana, 2018):

- Total cholesterol less than 200 mg/dL
- Triglycerides between 40 and 160 mg/dL for men and between 35 and 135 mg/dL for women
- HDL more than 45 mg/dL for men; more than 55 mg/dL for women ("good" cholesterol)
- LDL less than 130 mg/dL

Each of the lipoproteins contains varying proportions of cholesterol, triglyceride, protein, and phospholipid. HDL contains mainly protein and 20% cholesterol, whereas LDL is mainly cholesterol. Elevated LDL levels are positively correlated with CAD, whereas elevated HDL levels are negatively correlated and appear to be protective for heart disease. LDL pattern size is of significant importance in determining risk for CVD. LDL pattern A is associated with non–insulin resistance; normal glucose, insulin, and HDL levels; and normal blood pressure. LDL pattern B is associated with insulin resistance; increased glucose, insulin, and triglyceride levels; and hypertension.

A fasting blood sample for the measurement of serum cholesterol levels is preferable to a nonfasting sample. If triglycerides are to be evaluated with cholesterol, the health care provider requests the specimen after a 12-hour fast.

Other Laboratory Tests. Homocysteine is an amino acid that is produced when proteins break down. A certain amount of homocysteine is present in the blood, but elevated values may be an independent risk factor for the development of CVD. Although the relationship between homocysteine and CVD remains controversial, elevated levels of homocysteine may increase the risk for disease as much as smoking and hyperlipemia, especially in women. High-risk patients who have a personal or family history of premature heart disease should be screened. A level less than 14 mmol/dL is considered optimal, but this level increases as one ages (Pagana & Pagana, 2018).

Inflammation is a common and critical component to the development of atherothrombosis. Highly sensitive C-reactive protein (hsCRP) has been the most studied marker of inflammation. Any inflammatory process can produce CRP in the blood. Elevations also are seen with hypertension, infection, and smoking. A level less than 1 mg/L is considered low risk; a level over 3 mg/L places the patient at high risk for heart disease (Pagana & Pagana, 2018). The CRP is very helpful in determining treatment outcomes in patients at risk for coronary disease and in managing statin therapy after an acute myocardial infarction (MI). The most useful time to measure CRP appears to be for risk assessment in middle-age or older persons.

Microalbuminuria, or small amounts of protein in the urine, has been shown to be a clear marker of widespread endothelial dysfunction in CVD (along with elevated CRP). It should be screened annually in all patients with hypertension, metabolic syndrome, or diabetes mellitus. Microalbuminuria has also been used as a marker for renal disease, particularly in patients with hypertension and diabetes.

Blood coagulation studies evaluate the ability of the blood to clot. They are important in patients with a greater tendency to form thrombi (e.g., those with atrial fibrillation, prosthetic valves, or infective endocarditis). These tests are also essential for monitoring patients receiving anticoagulant therapy (e.g., during cardiac surgery, during treatment of an established thrombus).

Prothrombin time (PT) and *international normalized ratio (INR)* are used when initiating and maintaining therapy with oral anticoagulants, such as sodium warfarin. They measure the activity of prothrombin, fibrinogen, and factors V, VII, and X. INR is the most reliable way to monitor anticoagulant status in warfarin therapy. The therapeutic ranges vary significantly based on the reason for the anticoagulation and the patient's history. The normal INR is 0.8 to 1.1 (Pagana & Pagana, 2018).

Partial thromboplastin time (PTT) is assessed in patients who are receiving heparin. It measures deficiencies in all coagulation factors except VII and XIII.

Arterial blood gas (ABG) determinations are often obtained in patients with CVD. Determination of tissue oxygenation, carbon dioxide removal, and acid-base status is essential to appropriate treatment. (See Chapter 14 for a complete discussion of ABGs.)

Fluid and electrolyte balance is essential for normal cardiovascular performance. Cardiac manifestations often occur when there is an imbalance in either fluids or electrolytes in the body. For example, the cardiac effects of hypokalemia (low serum potassium level) include increased electrical instability, ventricular dysrhythmias, and an increased risk for digitalis toxicity. The effects of hyperkalemia on the myocardium include slowed ventricular conduction, peaked T waves on the ECG, and contraction followed by asystole (cardiac standstill).

Cardiac manifestations of hypocalcemia are ventricular dysrhythmias, a prolonged QT interval, and cardiac arrest. Hypercalcemia shortens the QT interval and causes atrioventricular block, digitalis hypersensitivity, and cardiac arrest. Serum sodium values reflect fluid balance and may be decreased, indicating fluid excess in patients with heart failure (dilutional hyponatremia).

Because magnesium regulates some aspects of myocardial electrical activity, hypomagnesemia has been implicated in some forms of ventricular dysrhythmias known as *torsades de pointes*. Hypomagnesemia prolongs the QT interval, causing this specific type of ventricular tachycardia. Chapter 13 describes these electrolytes in more detail.

The *erythrocyte (red blood cell [RBC]) count* is usually decreased in rheumatic fever and infective endocarditis. It is increased in heart diseases as needed to compensate for decreased available oxygen.

Decreased *hematocrit and hemoglobin* levels (e.g., caused by hemorrhage or hemolysis from prosthetic valves) indicate anemia and can lead to angina or aggravate heart failure. Vascular volume depletion with hemoconcentration (e.g., hypovolemic shock and excessive diuresis) results in an elevated hematocrit.

The *leukocyte (white blood cell [WBC]) count* typically is elevated after an MI and in various infectious and inflammatory diseases of the heart (e.g., infective endocarditis and pericarditis).

Other Diagnostic Assessment. Posteroanterior (PA) and left lateral *x-ray* views of the chest are routinely obtained to determine the size, silhouette, and position of the heart. In acutely ill patients, a simple anteroposterior (AP) view may be obtained at the bedside. Cardiac enlargement, pulmonary congestion, cardiac calcifications, and placement of central venous catheters, endotracheal tubes, and hemodynamic monitoring devices are assessed by x-ray.

Angiography of the arterial vessels, or arteriography, is an invasive diagnostic procedure that involves fluoroscopy and the use of contrast media. This procedure is performed when an arterial obstruction, narrowing, or aneurysm is suspected. The interventional radiologist performs selective arteriography to evaluate specific areas of the arterial system. For example, coronary arteriography, which is performed during left-sided cardiac catheterization, assesses arterial circulation within the heart. It can also be performed on arteries in the extremities, mesentery, and cerebrum. Angiography is discussed under the appropriate associated diseases elsewhere in this text.

TABLE 30.4 Indications for Cardiac Catheterization

- To confirm suspected heart disorders, including congenital abnormalities, coronary artery disease, myocardial disease, valvular disease, and valvular dysfunction
- To determine the location and extent of the disease process
- To assess:
  - Stable, severe angina unresponsive to medical management
  - Unstable angina pectoris
  - Uncontrolled heart failure, ventricular dysrhythmias, or cardiogenic shock associated with acute myocardial infarction, papillary muscle dysfunction, ventricular aneurysm, or septal perforation
- To determine best therapeutic option (percutaneous transluminal coronary angioplasty, stents, coronary artery bypass graft, valvulotomy versus valve replacement)
- To evaluate effects of medical or invasive treatment on cardiovascular function, percutaneous transluminal coronary angioplasty, or coronary artery bypass graft patency

Cardiac Catheterization. The most definitive but most invasive test in the diagnosis of heart disease is cardiac catheterization. Cardiac catheterization may include studies of the right or left side of the heart and the coronary arteries. Some of the most common indications for cardiac catheterization are listed in Table 30.4.

Patient Preparation. Assess the patient's physical and psychosocial readiness and knowledge level about the procedure because many patients have anxiety and fear about cardiac catheterization. Review the purpose of the procedure, inform the patient about the length of the procedure, state who will be present, and describe the appearance of the catheterization laboratory. Tell the patient about the sensations that he or she may experience during the procedure, such as palpitations (as the catheter is passed up to the left ventricle), a feeling of heat or a hot flash (as the medium is injected into either side of the heart), and a desire to cough (as the medium is injected into the right side of the heart). Written, electronic, or illustrated materials or DVDs may be used to assist in understanding.

The cardiologist explains the risks of cardiac catheterization. The risks vary with the procedures to be performed and the patient's physical status (Table 30.5). Although not common, several serious complications may follow coronary arteriography, such as:

- Myocardial infarction (MI)
- Stroke
- Arterial bleeding
- Thromboembolism
- Lethal dysrhythmias
- Arterial dissection
- Death

The cardiologist or interventional radiologist obtains written informed consent from the patient or responsible party before the procedure.

The patient is admitted to the hospital on the day of the catheterization procedure. He or she may be admitted earlier if there is renal dysfunction. Fluids may be given 12 to 24 hours before

TABLE 30.5 Complications of Cardiac Catheterization

Right-Sided Heart Catheterization
- Thrombophlebitis
- Pulmonary embolism
- Vagal response

Left-Sided Heart Catheterization and Coronary Arteriography
- Myocardial infarction
- Stroke
- Arterial bleeding or thromboembolism
- Dysrhythmias

Right-Sided or Left-Sided Heart Catheterization[a]
- Cardiac tamponade
- Hypovolemia
- Pulmonary edema
- Hematoma or blood loss at insertion site
- Reaction to contrast medium

[a]In addition to those cited for each procedure.

the procedure for renal protection. Contrast-induced renal dysfunction can result from vasoconstriction and the direct toxic effect of the contrast agent on the renal tubules. Hydration before and after the study helps eliminate or minimize contrast-induced renal toxicity.

Standard preoperative tests are performed, which usually include a chest x-ray, complete blood count, coagulation studies, and 12-lead ECG. Patients may ingest clear liquids up to 2 hours prior; solids and other liquids are held 6 hours before the procedure. The catheterization site is antiseptically prepared with hairs clipped according to agency policy.

Before the procedure, take the patient's vital signs, auscultate the heart and the lungs, and assess the peripheral pulses. Question him or her about any history of allergy to iodine-based contrast agents. An antihistamine or steroid may be given to a patient with a positive history or to prevent a reaction. Be sure that the signed informed consent is completed, as required by The Joint Commission. A mild sedative is usually administered before the procedure. Certain medications, such as diuretics, may be held before the procedure. In addition, warfarin and other oral anticoagulants are held if it is anticipated that the femoral artery will be used for access. Analysis of electrolytes, blood urea nitrogen (BUN), creatinine, coagulation profile, and complete blood count (CBC) is essential before and after the procedure; abnormalities are discussed with the health care provider.

Procedure. The patient is taken to the cardiac catheterization laboratory (sometimes referred to as the *cath lab*), placed in the supine position on the x-ray table, and securely strapped to the table. The physician injects a local anesthetic at the insertion site. During the procedure, the patient is instructed to report any chest pain, pressure, or other symptoms to the staff.

The *right side of the heart* is catheterized first and may be the only side examined. The cardiologist inserts a catheter through the femoral vein to the inferior vena cava or through the basilic vein to the superior vena cava. The catheter is advanced through either the inferior or the superior vena cava and, guided by fluoroscopy, is advanced through the right atrium, through the right ventricle, and at times into the pulmonary artery. Intracardiac pressures (right atrial, right ventricular, pulmonary artery, and pulmonary artery occlusion pressures) and blood samples are obtained. A contrast medium is usually injected to detect any cardiac shunts or regurgitation from the pulmonic or tricuspid valves.

In a *left-sided heart catheterization,* the cardiologist advances the catheter against the blood flow from the femoral, brachial, or radial artery up the aorta, across the aortic valve, and into the left ventricle (Fig. 30.8). Radial artery access has recently become a common access site for diagnostic heart catheterization examinations. Because of the size of stent delivery catheters, radial artery access is not possible for all patients. Alternatively, the catheter may be passed from the right side of the heart through the atrial septum, using a special needle to puncture the septum. Intracardiac pressures and blood samples are obtained. The pressures of the left atrium, left ventricle, and aorta and mitral and aortic valve status are evaluated. The cardiologist injects contrast dye into the ventricle; digital subtraction angiography evaluates left ventricular motion. Calculations are made regarding end-systolic volume, end-diastolic volume, stroke volume, and ejection fraction.

The technique for *coronary arteriography* is the same as for left-sided heart catheterization. The catheter is advanced into the aortic arch and positioned selectively in the right or left coronary artery. Injection of a contrast medium permits viewing the coronary arteries. By assessing the flow of the medium through the coronary arteries, information about the site and severity of coronary lesions is obtained.

An alternative to injecting a medium into the coronary arteries is *intravascular ultrasonography (IVUS),* which introduces a flexible catheter with a miniature transducer at the distal tip to view the coronary arteries. The transducer emits sound waves, which reflect off the plaque and the arterial wall to create an image of the blood vessel. IVUS can be used in vessels as small as 2 mm to assess the nature of plaques or vessel condition following an intervention.

Fractional flow reserve (FFR) can also be assessed to determine if a blockage needs to be revascularized. FFR is an objective method to measure the flow across the stenosis in the coronary artery. A special pressure wire is passed through the area of stenosis, and measurements are taken proximal and distal to the area of stenosis. These two measurements are used to calculate the FFR. A measure of 0.8 or less indicates that the stenosis is clinically significant and the artery should be revascularized.

Follow-up Care. The patient recovers in a specialty area equipped with monitored beds. After cardiac catheterization, restrict the patient to bedrest and keep the insertion site extremity straight. A soft knee brace can be applied to prevent bending of the affected extremity. Some cardiologists allow the head of the bed to be elevated up to 30 degrees during the period of bedrest, whereas others prefer that the patient remain supine. Current practice is for patients to remain in bed for 2 to 6 hours depending on the type of vascular closure device used.

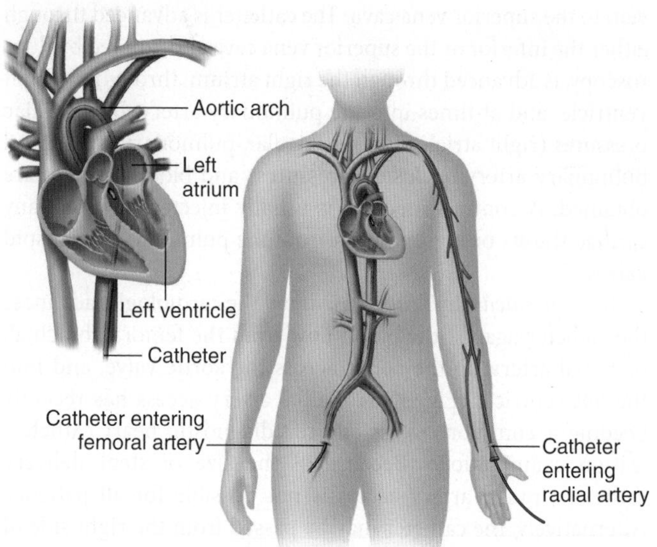

FIG. 30.8 Left-sided cardiac catheterization.

Various types of vascular closure devices are used to eliminate the need for manual compression after the catheterization. Examples include arteriotomy sutures and collagen plugs to seal the insertion site. Radial artery access is growing in popularity because it allows for a faster discharge (when compared with femoral access) and has fewer postdischarge restrictions on the patient than femoral or brachial artery access.

Monitor the patient's vital signs every 15 minutes for 1 hour, then every 30 minutes for 2 hours or until vital signs are stable, and then every 4 hours or according to agency policy. Assess the insertion site for bloody drainage or hematoma formation. Complications with vascular closure devices are not common but can be very serious. Assess peripheral pulses in the affected extremity and skin temperature and color with every vital sign check. Observe for complications of cardiac catheterization (see Table 30.5).

! NURSING SAFETY PRIORITY QSEN

Critical Rescue

If the patient experiences symptoms of cardiac ischemia such as chest ***pain***, dysrhythmias, bleeding, hematoma formation, or a dramatic change in peripheral pulses in the affected extremity, contact the Rapid Response Team or provider immediately to provide prompt intervention! Remain with the patient and obtain a 12-lead ECG for patients experiencing chest pain or dysrhythmias. For bleeding or hematoma formation, hold steady, firm pressure to the access site until the Rapid Response Team arrives. Neurologic changes indicating a possible stroke, such as visual disturbances, slurred speech, swallowing difficulties, and extremity weakness, should also be reported immediately.

Because the contrast medium acts as an osmotic diuretic, monitor urine output and ensure that the patient receives sufficient oral and IV fluids for adequate excretion of the medium. Pain medication for insertion site or back discomfort may be given as prescribed.

Review home instructions and risk factor modification with the patient before discharge. Remind the patient to:

- Limit activity for several days, including avoiding lifting and exercise.
- Leave the dressing in place for at least the first day at home.
- Observe the insertion site over the next few weeks for increased swelling, redness, warmth, and pain. (Bruising or a small hematoma is expected.)

NCLEX EXAMINATION CHALLENGE 30.3

Physiological Integrity

The nurse is caring for a client immediately following a cardiac catheterization. Which assessment data require immediate nursing intervention?

A. Blood pressure 146/70 mm Hg
B. Hematoma developing at insertion site
C. Client reports headache pain
D. Client reports extreme thirst

Electrocardiography. The electrocardiogram (ECG) is a routine part of every cardiovascular evaluation and is one of the most valuable diagnostic tests. Various forms are available: resting ECG, continuous ambulatory ECG (Holter monitoring), exercise ECG (stress test), signal-averaged ECG, and 30-day event monitoring. The resting ECG provides information about cardiac dysrhythmias, myocardial ischemia, the site and extent of MI, cardiac hypertrophy, electrolyte imbalances, and the effectiveness of cardiac drugs. The normal ECG pattern and a detailed discussion of the interpretation of abnormal patterns are discussed in Chapter 31.

Electrophysiologic Studies. An electrophysiologic study (EPS) is an invasive procedure during which programmed electrical stimulation of the heart is used to cause and evaluate lethal dysrhythmias and conduction abnormalities. Patients who have survived cardiac arrest, have recurrent tachydysrhythmias, or experience unexplained syncopal episodes may be referred for EPS. Induction of the dysrhythmia during EPS helps find an accurate diagnosis and aids in effective treatment. These procedures have risks similar to those for cardiac catheterization and are performed in a special catheterization laboratory, where conditions are strictly controlled and immediate treatment is available for any adverse effects.

Exercise Electrocardiography (Stress Test). The exercise electrocardiography test (also known as exercise tolerance test or stress test) assesses cardiovascular response to an increased workload. The stress test helps determine the functional capacity of the heart and screens for asymptomatic coronary artery disease. Dysrhythmias that develop during exercise may be identified, and the effectiveness of antidysrhythmic drugs can be evaluated.

Patient Preparation. Because risks are associated with exercising, the patient must be adequately informed about the purpose of the test, the procedure, and the risks involved. Written consent must be obtained. Anxiety and fear are common before stress testing. Therefore assure the patient that the procedure is performed in a controlled environment in which prompt nursing and medical attention are available.

Instruct the patient to get plenty of rest the night before the procedure. He or she may have a light meal 2 hours before the test but should avoid smoking or drinking alcohol or caffeine-containing beverages on the day of the test. The cardiologist decides whether the patient should stop taking any cardiac medications. Usually cardiovascular drugs such as beta blockers or calcium channel blockers are withheld on the day of the test to allow the heart rate to increase during the stress portion of the test. Patients are advised to wear comfortable, loose clothing and rubber-soled, supportive shoes. Remind them to tell the provider if symptoms such as chest pain, dizziness, shortness of breath, or an irregular heartbeat are experienced during the test.

Before the stress test, a resting 12-lead ECG, cardiovascular history, and physical examination are performed to check for any ECG abnormalities or medical factors that might interfere with the test. Check to see that all emergency supplies such as cardiac drugs, a defibrillator, and other necessary resuscitation equipment are available in the room in which the stress test is performed. It is important to be proficient in the use of resuscitation equipment when assisting the provider because chest pain, dysrhythmias, and other ECG changes may occur.

Procedure. The technician places electrodes on the patient's chest and attaches them to a multilead monitoring system. Note baseline blood pressure (BP), heart rate (HR), and respiratory rate. The two major modes of exercise available for stress testing are pedaling a bicycle ergometer and walking on a treadmill. A bicycle ergometer has a wheel operated by pedals that can be adjusted to increase the resistance to pedaling. The treadmill is a motorized device with an adjustable conveyor belt. It can reach speeds of 1 to 10 miles/hr and can also be adjusted from a flat position to a 22-degree incline.

After the patient has been shown how to use the bicycle or walk on the treadmill, he or she begins to exercise. During the test, the BP and ECG are closely monitored as the resistance to cycling or the speed and incline of the treadmill are increased (Fig. 30.9). The patient exercises until one of these findings occurs:

- A predetermined HR is reached and maintained.
- Signs and symptoms such as chest pain, fatigue, extreme dyspnea, vertigo, hypotension, and ventricular dysrhythmias appear.
- Significant ST-segment depression or T-wave inversion occurs.
- The 20-minute protocol is completed.

Follow-up Care. After the test, the nurse or other qualified health care team member monitors the ECG and BP until the patient has completely recovered. After recovery, he or she can return home if the test was performed on an ambulatory basis. Advise the patient to avoid a hot shower for 1 to 2 hours after the test because this may cause hypotension. If the patient does not recover but continues to have pain or ventricular dysrhythmias or appears medically unstable, admission to a telemetry unit for observation is needed.

For patients who cannot exercise because of conditions such as peripheral vascular disease (PVD) or arthritis, pharmacologic stress testing with inotropes such as dobutamine and a vasodilator such as adenosine, dipyridamole, or regadenoson may be indicated. The nursing considerations are similar to those for the patient who has undergone an exercise ECG.

Echocardiography. As a noninvasive, risk-free test, echocardiography is easily performed at the bedside or on an ambulatory care basis. **Echocardiography** uses ultrasound waves to assess cardiac structure and mobility, particularly of the valves. It helps assess and diagnose cardiomyopathy, valvular disorders, pericardial effusion, left ventricular function, ventricular aneurysms, and cardiac tumors.

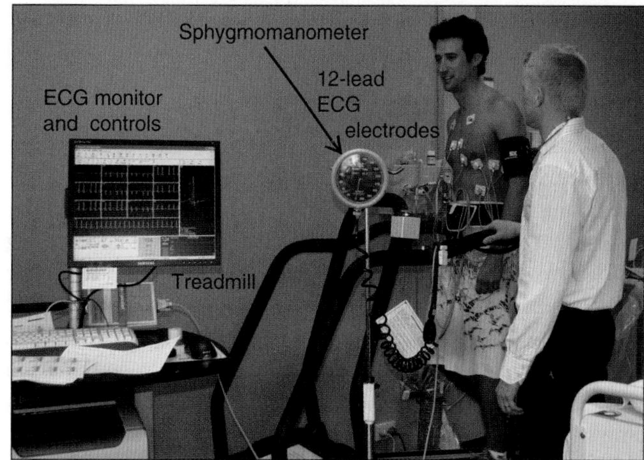

FIG. 30.9 Patient using a treadmill for a stress test. (From Baker, T., Nikolic, G., & O'Connor, S. [2008]. *Practical cardiology* [2nd ed.]. Sydney: Churchill Livingstone Australia.)

There is no special *preparation* for echocardiography. Inform the patient that the test is painless and takes 30 to 60 minutes to complete. The patient is instructed to lie quietly during the test and on his or her left side with the head elevated 15 to 20 degrees.

During an echocardiogram, a small transducer lubricated with gel to facilitate movement and conduction is placed on the patient's chest at the level of the third or fourth intercostal space (ICS) near the left sternal border. The transducer transmits high-frequency sound waves and receives them as they are reflected from different structures. These echoes are usually videotaped simultaneously with the echocardiogram and can be recorded on graph paper for a permanent record.

After the images are taped, cardiac measurements that require several images can be obtained. Routine measurements include chamber size, ejection fraction, and flow gradient across the valves. There is no specific *follow-up care* for a patient who has undergone an echocardiogram.

A slightly more aggressive form of echocardiogram is a *pharmacologic stress echocardiogram* using either dobutamine or dipyridamole. This test is usually used when patients cannot tolerate exercise. Dobutamine increases the heart's contractility; dipyridamole is a coronary artery dilator. Patients are required to be NPO for 3 to 6 hours before the test, except for sips of water with medications. The technician ensures that IV access is present before the procedure and monitors BP and pulse continuously throughout the procedure. After the procedure, vital signs are monitored until BP returns to baseline and the pulse rate slows to less than 100 beats/min.

Transesophageal Echocardiography. Echocardiograms may also be performed transesophageally (through the esophagus). **Transesophageal echocardiography (TEE)** examines cardiac structure and function with an ultrasound transducer placed immediately behind the heart in the esophagus or stomach.

The transducer provides especially detailed views of posterior cardiac structures such as the left atrium, mitral valve, and aortic arch. Preparation and follow-up are similar to those for an upper GI endoscopic examination (see Chapter 48).

Myocardial Nuclear Perfusion Imaging. The use of radionuclide techniques in cardiovascular assessment is called **myocardial nuclear perfusion imaging (MNPI)**. Cardiovascular abnormalities can be viewed, recorded, and evaluated using radioactive tracer substances. These studies are useful for detecting myocardial infarction (MI) and decreased myocardial blood flow and for evaluating left ventricular ejection. Conducting myocardial nuclear imaging tests, in conjunction with exercise or the administration of vasodilating agents, allows clearer identification of how the heart responds to stress.

Inform the patient that these tests are noninvasive. Because the amount of radioisotope is small, radiation exposure risks are minimal. If a dilating agent is to be used, advise the patient to avoid cigarettes and caffeinated food or drinks for 4 hours before administration of the vasodilator.

Common tests in nuclear cardiology include technetium (99mTc) pyrophosphate scanning, thallium imaging, and multigated cardiac blood pool imaging. Each test requires the injection of different types of radioactive isotopes into the antecubital vein. After the cells and tissues have time to take up the radioactive substances, usually 10 minutes to 2 hours, nuclear imaging can detect the difference between healthy and unhealthy tissue.

During the *technetium scan*, radioisotopes (^{99m}Tc pyrophosphate) accumulate in damaged myocardial tissue, which appears as a "hot spot" during the scan. This test helps detect the location and size of acute myocardial infarctions (MIs).

Alternatively, during the *thallium imaging scan*, necrotic or ischemic tissue does not absorb the radioisotope (thallium-201) and appears as "cold spots" on the scan. Thallium imaging is used to assess myocardial scarring and perfusion, to detect the location and extent of an acute or chronic MI, to evaluate graft patency after coronary bypass surgery, and to evaluate antianginal therapy, thrombolytic therapy, or balloon angioplasty.

Thallium imaging may be performed during an exercise test or with the patient at rest. Thallium imaging performed during an exercise test may demonstrate perfusion deficits not apparent at rest. First the stress test procedure is performed. After the patient reaches maximum activity level, a small dose of thallium-201 is injected IV. The patient continues to exercise for about 1 to 2 minutes, after which the scanning is performed. Nuclear cardiologists often compare the resting and stress images to differentiate between fixed and reversible defects in the myocardium.

If a patient cannot exercise on a bike or treadmill, dipyridamole or dobutamine hydrochloride is administered to simulate the effects of exercise. Tell the patient that these vasodilators may cause flushing, headache, dyspnea, and chest tightness for a few moments after injection.

Cardiac blood pool imaging is a noninvasive test for evaluating cardiac motion and calculating ejection fraction. It uses a computer to synchronize the patient's ECG with pictures taken by a special camera. The technician attaches the patient to an ECG and injects a small amount of 99mTc IV. The radioisotope is not taken up by tissue but remains "tagged" to red blood cells (RBCs) in the circulation. The camera may take pictures of the radioactive material as it makes its first pass through the heart.

During *multigated blood pool scanning*, the computer breaks the time between R waves on the ECG into fractions of a second, called *gates*. The camera records blood flow through the heart during each of these gates. By analyzing the information from multiple gates, the computer can evaluate the ventricular wall motion and calculate ejection fraction (percentage of the left ventricular volume that is ejected with each contraction) and ejection velocity. Areas of decreased, absent, or paradoxical movement of the left ventricle may also be identified.

Positron emission tomography (PET) scans are used to compare cardiac perfusion and metabolic function and differentiate normal from diseased myocardium. The technician administers the first radioisotope (nitrogen-13 ammonia) and then begins a 20-minute scan to detect myocardial perfusion. Next the technician administers a second radioisotope (fluoro-18-deoxyglucose). After a pause, a second scan is performed to detect the metabolically active myocardium, which is using glucose.

The two scans are compared. In a normal heart, performance and metabolic function will match. In an ischemic heart, there will be a mismatch (i.e., a reduction in perfusion and increased glucose uptake by the ischemic myocardium). The scanning procedure takes 2 to 3 hours, and the patient may be asked to use a treadmill or exercise bicycle in conjunction with the scan.

Depending on which test is performed, the patient may report fatigue or discomfort at the antecubital injection site. If a stress test was paired with the study, he or she will need follow-up care for the stress test.

CT Imaging. Cardiac CT imaging is a noninvasive option to evaluate calcium formation in the coronary arteries. This modality requires a low resting heart rate as images are taken during end systole and mid-diastole. Beta blockers or calcium channel blockers may be given to assist with slowing the heart rate. Coronary artery calcium (CAC) calculation is often performed during the CT and may help identify patients at risk for coronary artery disease. To identify areas of stenosis, iodinated contrast may be administered IV to visualize the coronary arteries. This is referred to as *CT angiography (CTA)*. Presence of coronary stents can make this test less reliable. Use of IV iodinated contrast puts the patient at risk for contrast-induced nephropathy (CIN) or renal damage. Assess renal function before and after the test and ensure adequate hydration by administering IV fluids as ordered. Encourage oral fluids after testing.

MRI. MRI is a noninvasive diagnostic option. An image of the heart or great vessels is produced through the interaction of magnetic fields, radio waves, and atomic nuclei showing hydrogen density. Simply put, the radio waves "bounce off" the body tissue being examined. Because each tissue has its own density, the computer image clearly differentiates between various types of tissues. MRI permits determination of cardiac wall thickness, chamber dilation, valve and ventricular function, and blood movement in the great vessels. Improved MRI techniques allow coronary artery blood flow to be mapped with nearly the accuracy of a cardiac catheterization.

Before an MRI, ensure that the patient has removed all metallic objects, including watches, jewelry, clothing with metal fasteners, and hair clips. Patients with pacemakers or implanted defibrillators may not be able to have an MRI because the magnetic fields can deactivate them. However, some newer MRI machines have eliminated this complication. A few patients may experience claustrophobia during the 15 to 60 minutes required to complete the scan.

GET READY FOR THE NEXT-GENERATION NCLEX® EXAMINATION!

Key Points

Review these Key Points for each NCLEX Examination Client Needs Category.

Safe and Effective Care Environment

- Assess patients for allergy to iodine-based contrast media before they undergo invasive diagnostic tests requiring an iodine-based contrast agent. **QSEN: Safety**
- After invasive cardiovascular diagnostic testing, such as angiography and cardiac catheterization, monitor the insertion site for bleeding and hematoma formation. **QSEN: Safety**
- Assess vital signs carefully in patients undergoing invasive cardiovascular testing; report and document any new dysrhythmias after testing. **QSEN: Informatics**

Health Promotion and Maintenance

- Identify patients at risk for cardiovascular disease, especially those with hyperlipidemia, hypertension, excess weight, physical inactivity, smoking, psychological stress, a positive family history, and diabetes. **QSEN: Evidence-Based Practice**
- Teach patients how to reduce the risk for heart disease through modifiable factors such as exercise, diet modification, smoking cessation, and medications, as needed. **QSEN: Patient-Centered Care**
- Inform patients that genetics and other nonmodifiable risk factors contribute to the development of coronary artery disease (CAD). **QSEN: Evidence-Based Practice**

Psychosocial Integrity

- Recognize that denial is a common and normal response to help patients cope with threatening circumstances. **QSEN: Patient-Centered Care**
- Allow the patient to express feelings about an actual or perceived loss of health or social status related to cardiovascular disease. **QSEN: Patient-Centered Care**

Physiological Integrity

- Assess the patient's report of pain to differentiate the pain of angina and myocardial infarction (MI) from other noncardiac causes; *discomfort, indigestion, squeezing, heaviness,* and *viselike* are common terms used to describe chest pain of cardiac origin. **Clinical Judgment**
- Be aware that gender differences in CVD exist; women often experience vaguer symptoms such as fatigue, indigestion, and shortness of breath. **Health Care Disparities**
- Be aware that the veteran population has increased risk for development of cardiovascular disease. **Health Care Disparities**
- Auscultate the heart for normal first and second sounds and for abnormalities such as an S_3, S_4, murmur, or gallop. **QSEN: Patient-Centered Care**
- Monitor serum markers of myocardial damage and other cardiac-related laboratory tests. **QSEN: Patient-Centered Care**
- Prepare patients having a cardiac catheterization for expectations of the procedure and postprocedure care. **QSEN: Patient-Centered Care**
- Assess patients having cardiac catheterizations for potential complications as listed in Table 30.5. **QSEN: Safety**
- Include all relevant findings of the patient's CV assessment in the electronic health record. **QSEN: Informatics**

MASTERY QUESTIONS

1. The nurse is teaching a class regarding reduction of risk factors for cardiovascular disease. Which teaching statement will the nurse include? **Select all that apply.**
   A. "If you tend to get angry easily, then your risk for heart disease is higher."
   B. "To reduce your overall risk, it is important to keep your BMI greater than 30."
   C. "Do not eat more calories on a daily basis that you are able to burn."
   D. "Decreasing the amount that you smoke will decrease your overall cardiovascular risk."
   E. "Secondhand smoke creates a significant risk to others for cardiovascular disease."
   F. "Exercise moderately at least 2 days per week for a total of 150 minutes."
2. The nurse is assessing the client's heart sounds. Which instruction will the nurse provide if there is difficulty in hearing heart sounds?
   A. "Please roll onto your left side."
   B. "Lay all the way down on your back."
   C. "Please hold your breath while I use my stethoscope."
   D. "I will just take your pulse instead."
3. Which statement made by the client on the way to the catheterization laboratory requires an **immediate** action by the nurse?
   A. "My allergies are bothering me, so I took some Benadryl last night before bed."
   B. "I was nervous last night, but I still remembered to take my warfarin."
   C. "I sure am hungry. I haven't had anything to eat since I went to bed last night."
   D. "I don't know what I will do if they find a blockage in my heart."

REFERENCES

Asterisk (*) indicates a classic or definitive work on this subject.

American Heart Association (AHA). (2017). *Diet and lifestyle recommendations* (reviewed August 15, 2017). www.heart.org/HEARTORG/GettingHealthy/Diet-and-Lifestyle-Recommendations_UCM_305855_Article.jsp.

American Heart Association (AHA). (2019). *Statistical fact sheet. 2019 update.* Retrieved from: https://www.heart.org/idc/groups/ahamah-public/@wcm/@sop/@smd/documents/downloadable/ucm_495090.pdf.

*Assari, S. (2014). Veterans and risk of heart disease in the United States: A cohort with 20 years of follow up. *International Journal of Preventative Medicine*, *5*(6), 703–709.

Benjamin, E. J., Muntner, P., Alonso, A., Bittencourt, M., Calloway, C., & Virani, S. (2019). Heart disease and stroke statistics—2019 update: A report from the American Heart Association. *Circulation*, *139*(12), e67–e492. Retrieved from https://www.ahajournals.org/doi/pdf/10.1161/CIR.0000000000000659.

Centers for Disease Control and Prevention. (2019). *Women and heart disease.* Retrieved from: https://www.cdc.gov/heartdisease/women.htm.

Garcia, M., Mulvagh, S., Merz, C., Buring, J., & Manson, J. (2016). Cardiovascular disease in women. Clinical perspectives. *Circulation Research.* Retrieved from: https://www.ahajournals.org/doi/pdf/10.1161/CIRCRESAHA.116.307547.

Government of Canada. (2017). *Heart disease in Canada.* Retrieved from: https://www.canada.ca/en/public-health/services/publications/diseases-conditions/heart-disease-canada.html.

Hinojosa, R. (2019). Veterans' likelihood of reporting cardiovascular disease. *The Journal of the American Board of Family Medicine*, *32*(1), 50–57. Retrieved from: https://www.jabfm.org/content/jabfp/32/1/50.full.pdf.

Jaffe, A., & Morrow, D. (2018). *Troponin testing: Clinical use. UpToDate.* Retrieved from: https://www.uptodate.com/contents/troponin-testing-clinical-use.

James, P. A., Oparil, S., Carter, B. L., Cushman, W. C., Dennison-Himmelfarb, C., Handler, J., et al. (2014). 2014 evidence-based guidelines for the management of high blood pressure in adults: Report from the panel members appointed to the Eighth Joint National Committee (JNC 8). *The Journal of the American Medical Association*, *311*(5), 507–520.

McCance, K., & Huether, S. (2019). *Pathophysiology: The biologic basis for disease in adults and children* (8th ed.). St. Louis: Elsevier.

Pagana, K., & Pagana, T. J. (2018). *Mosby's manual of diagnostic and laboratory tests* (6th ed.). St. Louis: Elsevier.

*The New York Heart Association. (1964). *Diseases of the heart and blood vessels: Nomenclature and criteria for diagnosis* (6th ed.). Boston: Little, Brown.

Thomas, M., Taha, A., & Greenberg, C. (2018). Tobacco cessation in hospitals: Updates for practice. *Medsurg Nursing*, *27*(5), 291–296.

Urden, L., Stacy, K., & Lough, M. (2018). *Critical care nursing. diagnosis and management* (8th ed.). St. Louis, MO: Elsevier.

Whelton, P. K., Carey, R. M., Aronow, W. S., et al. (2017). ACC/AHA/AAPA/ABC/ACPM/AGS/APhA/ASH/ASPC/NMA/PCNA Guideline for the Prevention, Detection, Evaluation, and Management of High Blood Pressure in Adults: Executive Summary. A Report of the American College of Cardiology/American Heart Association Task Force on Clinical Practice Guidelines. *Hypertension.* 2017. http://hyper.ahajournals.org/content/early/2017/11/10/HYP.0000000000000066.

31

Concepts of Care for Patients With Dysrhythmias

Nicole M. Heimgartner

http://evolve.elsevier.com/Iggy/

LEARNING OUTCOMES

1. Collaborate with the interprofessional team to coordinate high-quality care to promote ***perfusion*** in patients with dysrhythmias.
2. Provide a safe environment for patients and staff when using a cardiac defibrillator.
3. Teach the patient and caregiver(s) about drug therapy used for common dysrhythmias.
4. Teach the patient with a pacemaker or implantable cardioverter/defibrillator about self-management when in the community.
5. Implement patient and family-centered nursing interventions to decrease the psychosocial impact caused by life-threatening dysrhythmias and emergency care procedures.
6. Apply knowledge of pathophysiology to assess patients with common dysrhythmias.
7. Analyze an ECG rhythm strip to identify normal sinus rhythm and common or life-threatening dysrhythmias.
8. Use clinical judgment to plan care coordination and transition management for patients experiencing common dysrhythmias.
9. Plan evidence-based nursing care to promote ***perfusion*** to prevent complications in patients experiencing dysrhythmias.
10. Explain the need to perform evidence-based emergency care procedures, such as cardiopulmonary resuscitation (CPR) and automated external defibrillation.

KEY TERMS

artifact Interference seen on the monitor or rhythm strip, which may look like a wandering or fuzzy baseline; can be caused by patient movement, loose or defective electrodes, improper grounding, or faulty equipment.

atrial fibrillation (AF) A cardiac dysrhythmia in which multiple rapid impulses from many atrial foci, at a rate of 350 to 600 times per minute, depolarize the atria in a totally disorganized manner, with no P waves, no atrial contractions, a loss of the atrial kick, and an irregular ventricular response.

atrioventricular (AV) junction In the cardiac conduction system, the area consisting of a transitional cell zone, the atrioventricular (AV) node itself, and the bundle of His.

automaticity The ability of a cell to initiate an impulse spontaneously and repetitively; in cardiac electrophysiology, the ability of primary pacemaker cells (SA node, AV junction) to generate an electrical impulse.

bradycardia Slowness of the heart rate; characterized as a pulse rate less than 60 beats/min.

bradydysrhythmia An abnormal heart rhythm with a heart rate less than 60 beats/min; also known as bradyarrhythmia.

conductivity The ability of a cell to send an electrical stimulus from cell membrane to cell membrane.

contractility The ability of atrial and ventricular muscle cells to shorten their fiber length in response to electrical stimulation, causing sufficient pressure to push blood forward through the heart. Contractility is the mechanical activity of the heart.

defibrillation An asynchronous countershock, depolarizes a critical mass of myocardium simultaneously to stop the re-entry circuit, allowing the sinus node to regain control of the heart.

depolarization The ability of a cell to respond to a stimulus by initiating an impulse. Also called excitability.

dysrhythmia A disorder of the heartbeat involving a disturbance in cardiac rhythm; irregular heartbeat.

ECG caliper A measurement tool used in analysis of an electrocardiographic (ECG) rhythm strip.

electrocardiogram (ECG) A graphic representation of cardiac electrical activity.

excitability The ability of nonpacemaker heart cells to respond to an electrical impulse that begins in pacemaker cells. Also called depolarization.

isoelectric Having equal electric potentials, such as in the heart. In ECG interpretation, the isoelectric line is the baseline.

lead In an ECG, the provider of one view of the heart's electrical activity. Multiple leads, or views, can be obtained.

lead axis In ECG, the imaginary line that joins the positive and negative poles of the lead systems.

maze procedure An open chest surgical technique often performed with coronary artery bypass grafting for patients in atrial fibrillation with decompensation.

negative deflection In ECG, the flow of electrical current in the heart (cardiac axis) away from the positive pole and toward the negative pole.

normal sinus rhythm (NSR) The rhythm originating from the sinoatrial (SA) node (dominant pacemaker), with atrial and ventricular rates of 60 to 100 beats/min and regular atrial and ventricular rhythms.

P wave In an ECG, the deflection representing atrial depolarization.

PR interval The interval measured from the beginning of the P wave to the end of the PR segment; represents the time required for atrial depolarization, the impulse delay in the AV node, and the travel time to the Purkinje fibers.

PR segment The isoelectric line from the end of the P wave to the beginning of the QRS complex, when the electrical impulse is traveling through the atrioventricular (AV) node, where it is delayed.

premature complex An early complex that occurs when a cardiac cell or cell group other than the sinoatrial node becomes irritable and fires an impulse before the next sinus impulse is generated.

premature ventricular complexes (PVCs) Also called premature ventricular contractions; result from increased irritability of ventricular cells and are seen as early ventricular complexes followed by a pause.

positive deflection In ECG, the flow of electrical current in the heart (cardiac axis) toward the positive pole.

pulse deficit The difference between the apical and peripheral pulses.

Purkinje cells In the cardiac conduction system, the cells that make up the bundle of His, bundle branches, and terminal Purkinje fibers. These cells are responsible for the rapid conduction of electrical impulses throughout the ventricles, leading to ventricular depolarization and subsequent ventricular muscle contraction.

QRS complex Represents ventricular depolarization.

QRS duration Represents the time required for depolarization of both ventricles; measured from the beginning of the QRS complex to the J point (the junction where the QRS complex ends and the ST segment begins).

QT interval The time from the beginning of the QRS complex to the end of the T wave. It represents the total time required for ventricular depolarization and repolarization.

sinoatrial (SA) node The SA node is the heart's primary pacemaker. It can spontaneously and rhythmically generate electrical impulses at a rate of 60 to 100 beats/min.

sinus arrhythmia A variant of normal sinus rhythm that results from changes in intrathoracic pressure during breathing; heart rate increases slightly during inspiration and decreases slightly during exhalation. Atrial and ventricular rates are between 60 and 100 beats/min, and atrial and ventricular rhythms are slightly irregular.

sinus bradycardia A cardiac dysrhythmia caused by a decreased rate of sinus node discharge, with a heart rate that is less than 60 beats/min.

sinus tachycardia A cardiac dysrhythmia caused by an increased rate of sinus node discharge, with a heart rate that is more than 100 beats/min.

ST segment Normally an isoelectric line and represents early ventricular repolarization.

supraventricular tachycardia (SVT) A form of tachycardia that involves the rapid stimulation of atrial tissue at a rate of 100 to 280 beats/min.

T wave The deflection that follows the ST segment and represents ventricular repolarization.

tachycardia An excessively fast heart rate; characterized as a pulse rate greater than 100 beats/min.

tachydysrhythmia An abnormal heart rhythm with a heart rate greater than 100 beats/min.

telemetry In ECG, the use of a battery-powered transmitter system for monitoring an ambulatory patient; allows freedom of movement within a certain radius without losing transmission of the ECG.

temporary pacing A nonsurgical intervention for cardiac dysrhythmia that provides a timed electrical stimulus to the heart when either the impulse initiation or the intrinsic conduction system of the heart is defective.

torsades de pointes A life-threatening type of ventricular tachycardia that is related to a prolonged QT interval.

transcutaneous pacing Temporary pacing that is accomplished through the application of two large external electrodes.

U wave The deflection that may follow the T wave and may result from slow repolarization of ventricular Purkinje fibers. Abnormal prominence of the U wave suggests an electrolyte abnormality or other disturbance.

vagal maneuver Nonsurgical management of cardiac dysrhythmias that is intended to induce vagal stimulation of the cardiac conduction system, specifically the sinoatrial and atrioventricular nodes.

Vaughn-Williams classification System used to categorize antidysrhythmic agents according to their effects on the action potential of cardiac cells.

ventricular fibrillation (VF) A cardiac dysrhythmia that results from electrical chaos in the ventricles; impulses from many irritable foci fire in a totally disorganized manner so that ventricular contraction cannot occur; there is no cardiac output or pulse and therefore no cerebral, myocardial, or systemic perfusion. This rhythm is rapidly fatal if not successfully terminated within 3 to 5 minutes.

ventricular tachycardia (VT) An abnormal heart rhythm that occurs with repetitive firing of an irritable ventricular ectopic focus, usually at a rate of 140 to 180 beats/min or more.

PRIORITY AND INTERRELATED CONCEPTS

The priority concept for this chapter is:
- ***Perfusion***

The ***Perfusion*** concept exemplar for this chapter is Atrial Fibrillation.

The interrelated concepts for this chapter are:
- ***Fluid and Electrolyte Balance***
- ***Clotting***

Cardiac dysrhythmias are abnormal rhythms of the heart's electrical system that can affect its ability to effectively pump *oxygenated* blood throughout the body. Some dysrhythmias are life threatening, and others are not. They are the result of disturbances in cardiac electrical impulse formation, conduction, or both.

Many health problems, especially coronary artery disease (CAD), electrolyte imbalances, impaired gas exchange, and drug toxicity (both legal and illicit drugs), can cause abnormal heart rhythms. Dysrhythmias can occur in people of any age but occur most often in older adults. To provide collaborative patient-centered care using best practices, a *basic* understanding of cardiac electrophysiology, the conduction system of the heart, and the principles of electrocardiography is needed as a medical-surgical nurse. Specialty nurses and advanced practice nurses have a more in-depth knowledge because they manage patients with these cardiac problems in critical care and ambulatory care settings.

REVIEW OF CARDIAC CONDUCTION SYSTEM

Conduction begins with the **sinoatrial (SA) node** (also called the *sinus node*), located close to the surface of the right atrium near its junction with the superior vena cava. *The SA node is the heart's primary pacemaker.* It can spontaneously and rhythmically generate electrical impulses at a rate of 60 to 100 beats/min and therefore has the greatest degree of automaticity (pacing function). The SA node is richly supplied by the sympathetic and parasympathetic nervous systems, which increase and decrease the rate of discharge of the sinus node, respectively. This process results in changes in the heart rate.

Impulses from the sinus node move directly through atrial muscle and lead to atrial depolarization, which is *reflected in a P wave on the electrocardiogram (ECG).* Atrial muscle contraction should follow. Within the atrial muscle are slow and fast conduction pathways leading to the atrioventricular (AV) node.

The **atrioventricular (AV) junction** consists of a transitional cell zone, the AV node itself, and the bundle of His. The AV node lies just beneath the right atrial endocardium, between the tricuspid valve and the ostium of the coronary sinus. Here T-cells (transitional cells) cause impulses to slow down or be delayed in the AV node before proceeding to the ventricles. This delay is reflected in the *PR segment* on the ECG. This slow conduction provides a short delay, allowing the atria to contract and the ventricles to fill. The contraction is known as *atrial kick* and contributes additional blood volume for a greater cardiac output. The AV node is also controlled by both the sympathetic and parasympathetic nervous systems. The bundle of His connects with the distal portion of the AV node and continues through the interventricular septum.

The *bundle of His* extends as a right bundle branch down the right side of the interventricular septum to the apex of the right ventricle. On the left side, it extends as a left bundle branch, which further divides.

At the ends of both the right and the left bundle branch systems are the Purkinje fibers. These fibers are an interweaving network located on the endocardial surface of both ventricles, from apex to base. The fibers then partially penetrate into the myocardium. **Purkinje cells** make up the bundle of His, bundle branches, and terminal Purkinje fibers. These cells are responsible for the rapid conduction of electrical impulses throughout the ventricles, leading to ventricular depolarization and the subsequent ventricular muscle contraction. A few nodal cells in the ventricles also occasionally demonstrate automaticity, giving rise to ventricular beats or rhythms.

The cardiac conduction system consists of specialized myocardial cells (Fig. 31.1). The electrophysiologic properties of these cells regulate heart rate and rhythm and possess unique properties: automaticity, excitability, conductivity, and contractility.

Automaticity (pacing function) is the ability of cardiac cells to generate an electrical impulse spontaneously and repetitively. Normally only the sinoatrial (SA) node can generate an electrical impulse. However, under certain conditions, such as myocardial ischemia (decreased blood flow), electrolyte imbalance, hypoxia, drug toxicity, and infarction (cell death), any cardiac cell may produce electrical impulses independently and create dysrhythmias. Disturbances in automaticity may involve either an increase or a decrease in pacing function.

Excitability is the ability of nonpacemaker heart cells to respond to an electrical impulse that begins in pacemaker cells. **Depolarization** occurs when the normally negatively charged cells within the heart muscle develop a positive charge.

Conductivity is the ability to send an electrical stimulus from cell membrane to cell membrane. As a result, excitable cells depolarize in rapid succession from cell to cell until all cells have depolarized. The wave of depolarization causes the deflections in the ECG waveforms that are recognized as the P wave and the QRS complex. Disturbances in conduction result when conduction is too rapid or too slow, when the pathway is totally blocked, or when the electrical impulse travels an abnormal pathway.

Contractility is the ability of atrial and ventricular muscle cells to shorten their fiber length in response to electrical stimulation, causing sufficient pressure to push blood forward through the heart. In other words, *contractility is the mechanical activity of the heart.*

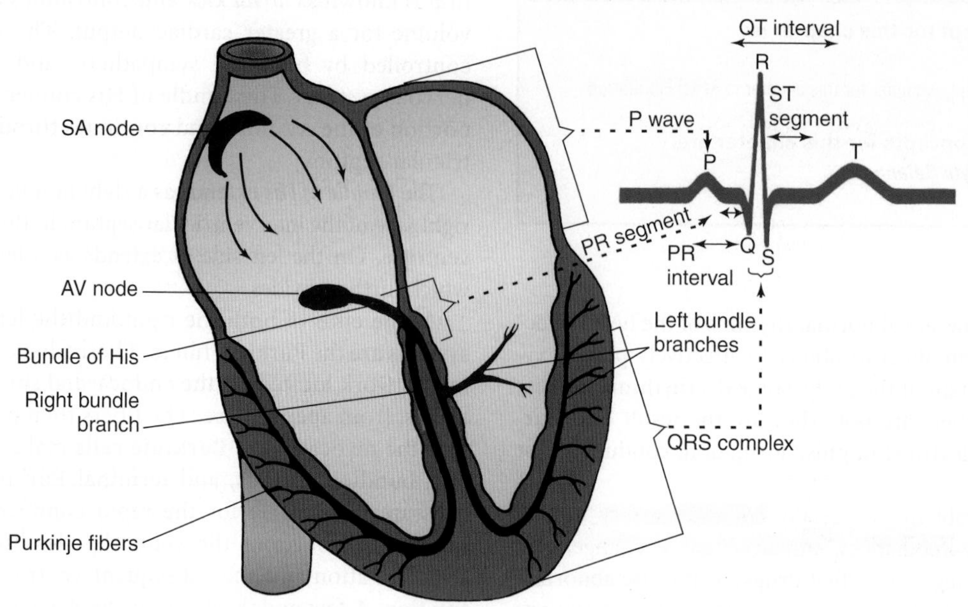

Fig. 31.1 The cardiac conduction system.

ELECTROCARDIOGRAPHY

The **electrocardiogram (ECG)** provides a graphic representation, or picture, of cardiac electrical activity. The cardiac electrical currents are transmitted to the body surface. Electrodes, consisting of a conductive gel on an adhesive pad, are placed on specific sites on the body and attached to cables connected to an ECG machine or a monitor. The cardiac electrical current is transmitted via the electrodes and through the lead wires to the machine or monitor, which displays the cardiac electrical activity. A **lead** provides one view of the heart's electrical activity. Multiple leads, or views, can be obtained. Electrode placement is the same for male and female patients.

Lead systems are made up of a positive pole and a negative pole. An imaginary line joining these two poles is called the *lead axis.* The direction of electrical current flow in the heart is the cardiac axis. The relationship between the cardiac axis, and the lead axis is responsible for the deflections seen on the ECG pattern:

- The baseline is the **isoelectric** line. It occurs when there is no current flow in the heart after complete depolarization and also after complete repolarization. Positive deflections occur above this line, and negative deflections occur below it. Deflections represent depolarization and repolarization of cells.
- If the direction of electrical current flow in the heart (cardiac axis) is toward the positive pole, a **positive deflection** (above the baseline) is viewed (Fig. 31.2A).
- If the direction of electrical current flow in the heart (cardiac axis) is moving away from the positive pole toward the negative pole, a **negative deflection** (below the baseline) is viewed (Fig. 31.2B).

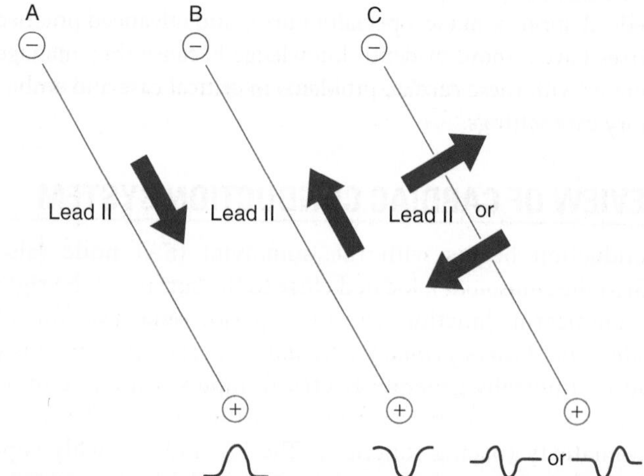

Fig. 31.2 A, The cardiac axis *(bold arrow)* is parallel to the lead axis *(the line between the negative and the positive electrodes)*, going toward the positive electrode; a positive deflection is inscribed. B, The cardiac axis is parallel to the lead axis, going toward the negative electrode; a negative deflection is inscribed. C, The cardiac axis is perpendicular to the lead axis, going toward neither the positive electrode nor the negative electrode; a biphasic deflection is inscribed.

- If the cardiac axis is moving neither toward nor away from the positive pole, a biphasic complex (both above and below baseline) will result (Fig. 31.2C).

Lead Systems

The standard 12-lead ECG consists of 12 leads (or views) of the heart's electrical activity. Six of the leads are called *limb leads* because the electrodes are placed on the four extremities in the frontal plane. The remaining six leads are called *chest (precordial) leads* because the electrodes are placed on the chest in the horizontal plane.

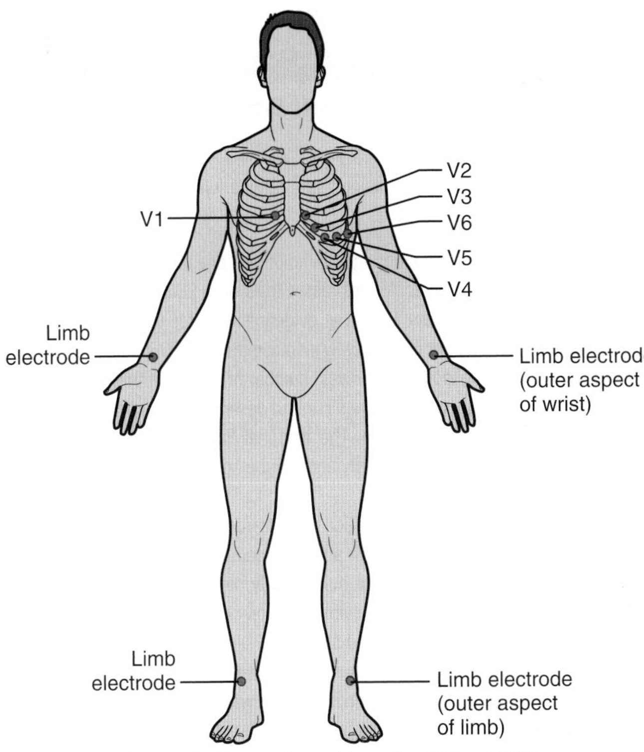

Fig. 31.3 Electrode positions for 12-lead ECG.

Standard bipolar *limb leads* consist of three leads (I, II, and III) that each measure the electrical activity between two points and a fourth lead (right leg) that acts as a ground electrode. Of the three measuring leads, the right arm is always negative, the left leg is always positive, and the left arm can be either positive or negative.

Other lead systems include the 18-lead ECG, which adds six leads placed on the horizontal plane on the right side of the chest to view the right side of the heart. This is sometimes referred to as a *right-sided ECG*. The extra leads are sometimes placed on the back. Unipolar limb leads consist of a positive electrode only. The unipolar limb leads are aVR, aVL, and aVF, with *a* meaning augmented; *V* is a designation for a unipolar lead. The third letter denotes the positive electrode placement: *R* for right arm, *L* for left arm, and *F* for foot (left leg). The positive electrode is at one end of the lead axis. The other end is the center of the electrical field, at about the center of the heart.

There are six unipolar (or V) *chest leads*, determined by the placement of the chest electrode. The four limb electrodes are placed on the extremities, as designated on each electrode (right arm, left arm, right leg, and left leg). The fifth (chest) electrode on a monitor system is the positive, or exploring, electrode and is placed in one of six designated positions to obtain the desired chest lead. With a 12-lead ECG, four leads are placed on the limbs and six are placed on the chest, eliminating the need to move any electrodes about the chest (Fig. 31.3).

Positioning of the electrodes is crucial in obtaining an accurate ECG. Comparisons of ECGs taken at different times will be valid only when electrode placement is accurate and identical at each test. Positioning is particularly important when working with patients with chest deformities or large breasts. Patients may be asked to move the breasts to ensure proper electrode placement. For serial ECGs, a surgical marker may be used to mark the electrode placement site to allow for accurate placement. It is important to remove the electrodes following the ECG because skin breakdown can occur.

While obtaining a 12-lead ECG, remind the patient to be as still as possible in a semireclined position, breathing normally. Any repetitive movement will cause an artifact and could lead to inaccurate interpretation of the ECG.

Nurses are sometimes responsible for obtaining 12-lead ECGs, but more commonly, technicians are trained to perform this skill. Remind the technician to notify the nurse or primary health care provider of any suspected abnormality. A nurse may direct a technician to take a 12-lead ECG on a patient experiencing chest pain to observe for diagnostic changes, but it is ultimately the primary health care provider's responsibility to definitively interpret the ECG.

Continuous Electrocardiographic Monitoring

For continuous ECG monitoring, the electrodes are not placed on the limbs because movement of the extremities causes "noise," or motion artifact, on the ECG signal. Place the electrodes on the trunk, a more stable area, to minimize such artifacts and to obtain a clearer signal. If the monitoring system provides five electrode cables, place the electrodes as follows:

- Right arm electrode just below the right clavicle
- Left arm electrode just below the left clavicle
- Right leg electrode on the lowest palpable rib, on the right midclavicular line
- Left leg electrode on the lowest palpable rib, on the left midclavicular line
- Fifth electrode placed to obtain one of the six chest leads

With this placement, the monitor lead-select control may be changed to provide lead I, II, III, aVR, aVL, aVF, or one chest lead. The monitor automatically alters the polarity of the electrodes to provide the lead selected.

The clarity of continuous ECG monitor recordings is affected by skin preparation and electrode quality. To ensure the best signal transmission and decrease skin impedance, clean the skin and clip hairs if needed. Make sure that the area for electrode placement is dry. The gel on each electrode must be moist and fresh. Attach the electrode to the lead cable and then to the contact site. The contact site should be free of any lotion, tincture, or other substance that increases skin impedance. Electrodes cannot be placed on irritated skin or over scar tissue. Electrodes may be applied by assistive personnel (AP), but the nurse determines which lead to select and checks for correct electrode placement. Assess the quality of the ECG rhythm transmission to the monitoring system.

The ECG cables can be attached directly to a wall-mounted monitor (a hard-wired system) if the patient's activity is restricted to bedrest and sitting in a chair, as in a critical care unit. For an ambulatory patient, the ECG cable is attached to a battery-operated transmitter (a **telemetry** system) held in a pouch. The ECG is transmitted to a remote monitor via antennae located in strategic places, usually in the ceiling. Telemetry allows freedom of movement within a certain area without losing transmission of the ECG.

Most acute care facilities have monitor technicians (monitor "techs") who are educated in ECG rhythm interpretation and are responsible for:

- Watching a bank of monitors on a unit
- Printing ECG rhythm strips routinely and as needed
- Interpreting rhythms
- Reporting the patient's rhythm and significant changes to the nurse

The technical support is particularly helpful on a telemetry unit that does not have monitors at the bedside. The nurse is responsible for accurate patient assessment and management. The use of telemetry monitors on medical-surgical units is increasing and nursing assessment is critical to initiate appropriate interventions (Nickasch et al., 2016).

Some units have full-disclosure monitors, which continuously store ECG rhythms in memory up to a certain amount of time. This system allows nurses and health care providers to access and print rhythm strips for more thorough patient assessment. Routine strips and any changes in rhythm are printed and documented in the patient's record.

The health care provider is responsible for determining when monitoring can be suspended, such as during showering. He or she also determines whether monitoring is needed during off-unit testing procedures and for transportation to other facilities. Clinical alarms, such as those associated with continuous ECG monitoring, have been identified as one of the top 10 technology hazards.

! NATIONAL PATIENT SAFETY GOAL

Reduce Harm Associated With Clinical Alarms

Clinical alarms, such as those associated with continuous ECG monitoring, were designed to protect patients. These alarms can alert health care providers to a patient problem; however, the alarms are only beneficial if they are used in an effective manner. This is a complex problem, as care units are often filled with numerous types of alarms, making individual alarms hard to distinguish and creating desensitization among the staff (The Joint Commission, 2020). As a result, alarm safety must be recognized as a priority. The National Patient Safety Goal to improve clinical alarm safety asks hospitals to implement specific policy and procedure regarding clinical alarm safety including:

- Clinically appropriate settings for alarms
- When alarm signals can be disabled
- What alarm parameters can be changed
- Monitoring and responding to alarm signals

Nurses must be proactive in the management of clinical alarms. Think carefully before suspending an alarm or adjusting alarm parameters and be informed regarding organization policy regarding alarm management.

Prehospital personnel, such as paramedics and emergency medical technicians (EMTs) with advanced training, frequently monitor ECG rhythms at the scene and on the way to a health care facility. They function under medical direction and protocols but may also be communicating with a nurse in the emergency department.

The ECG strip is printed on graph paper (Fig. 31.4), with each small block measuring 1 mm in height and width. ECG recorders and monitors are standardized at a speed of 25 mm/sec. Time is measured on the horizontal axis. At this speed, each small block represents 0.04 second. Five small blocks make up one large block, defined by darker bold lines and representing 0.20 second. Five large blocks represent 1 second, and 30 large blocks represent 6 seconds. Vertical lines in the top margin of the graph paper are usually 15 large blocks apart, representing 3-second segments (Fig. 31.5).

SYSTEMS THINKING AND QUALITY IMPROVEMENT (QSEN)

Solving Alarm Fatigue With Smartphone Technology

Short, K. & Chung, Y. (2019). Solving alarm fatigue with smartphone technology. *Nursing2019, 49*(1), 52–57.

Electrocardiogram (ECG) monitoring is common practice in the care of patients with cardiovascular disease. Alarms, associated with ECG monitoring, were developed to improve safety. However, evidence indicates that alarm fatigue in the clinical environment may actually increase the safety risk. Alarm fatigue has developed as a response to the vast number of alarms in the clinical setting. The sheer number of alarms has created desensitization, often resulting in delayed versus rapid response. The National Patient Safety Goals have established alarm safety as a priority and require agency guidelines for alarm management.

Based on an analysis at one 473-bed acute care facility, the existing beeper-based system was replaced with a new system designed to decrease the number of false alarms and allow more timely nursing response. The new system was developed as a multidisciplinary project incorporating information technology, nursing informatics, and clinical nursing departments. The newly developed system comprised four parts: the telemetry monitoring system, middleware software, smartphone alarm app, and a waveform app. The telemetry monitor would generate the alarm, sending it through the middleware software with built-in filters, carefully defined by the multidisciplinary team. The filtered alarms were then transmitted to the smartphone app, providing the patient's name, alarm type, time, and room number directly to the assigned nurse. The nurse could then acknowledge the alarm and with one swipe also launch a waveform app allowing the nurse to see the patient's real-time ECG.

This pilot study with the new system was conducted in one telemetry unit over 6 weeks. The pilot allowed the multidisciplinary team time to fine-tune the alarm filters. The pilot progressed to project implementation on the remaining five telemetry units over a 3-month period. When compared with the previous beeper-based alert system, the new app system decreased clinical alarms by 78%. Presurvey and postsurvey data were also collected to better understand the nursing perception of alarm fatigue and the new system. Postsurvey results indicate the perception of nuisance alarms decreased with the new system, while the perception of alarm adequacy within the unit increased. Nursing feedback was also used to better tailor the new app system to meet the needs at the bedside.

Commentary: Implications for Practice and Research

The Joint Commission's (TJC's) National Patient Safety Goal specific to alarm management requires alarm management strategies. These strategies include educating staff about alarms and developing policy and procedure for alarm management. This quality improvement study provides initial evidence that smartphone technology can be a useful tool in decreasing clinical alarms. Having real-time vital information, including ECGs on the smartphone at the point of care, allows the nurse to respond to the patient much quicker and promotes a more efficient workflow for alarms that are not critical in nature. This project clearly demonstrates implementation of TJC's National Patient Safety Goal. Additional research to address parameters for alarms, as well as response time to clinical alarms, is needed to determine best practice.

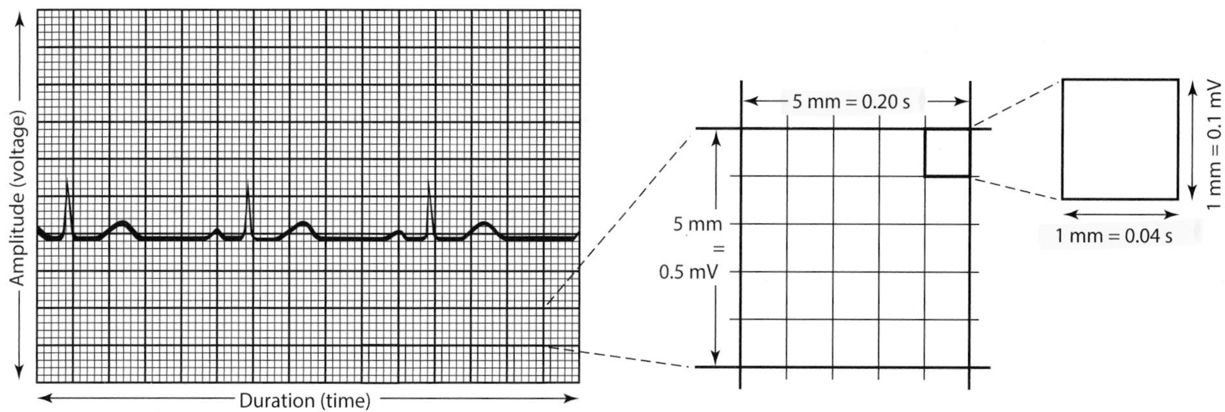

Fig. 31.4 Electrocardiographic waveforms are measured in amplitude (voltage) and duration (time).

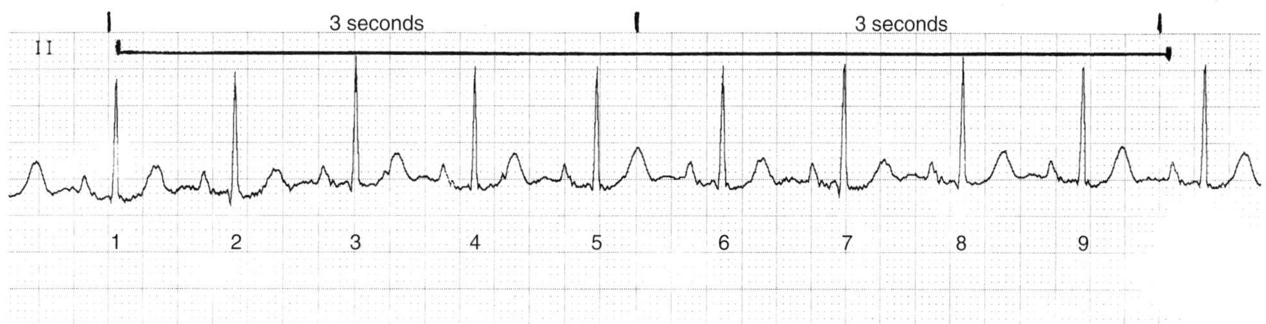

Fig. 31.5 Each segment between the dark lines *(above the monitor strip)* represents 3 seconds when the monitor is set at a speed of 25 mm/sec. To estimate the ventricular rate, count the QRS complexes in a 6-second strip and multiply that number by 10 to estimate the rate for 1 minute. In this example, there are 9 QRS complexes in 6 seconds. Therefore the heart rate can be estimated to be 90 beats/min.

Electrocardiographic Complexes, Segments, and Intervals

Complexes that make up a normal ECG consist of a P wave, a QRS complex, a T wave, and possibly a U wave. Segments include the PR segment, ST segment, and TP segment. Intervals include the PR interval, QRS duration, and QT interval (Fig. 31.6).

The **P wave** is a deflection representing atrial depolarization. The shape of the P wave may be a positive, negative, or biphasic (both positive and negative) deflection, depending on the lead selected. When the electrical impulse is consistently generated from the sinoatrial (SA) node, the P waves have a consistent shape in a given lead. If an impulse is then generated from a different (ectopic) focus, such as atrial tissue, the shape of the P wave changes in that lead, indicating that an ectopic focus has fired.

The **PR segment** is the isoelectric line from the end of the P wave to the beginning of the QRS complex, when the electrical impulse is traveling through the atrioventricular (AV) node, where it is delayed. It then travels through the ventricular conduction system to the Purkinje fibers.

The **PR interval** is measured from the beginning of the P wave to the end of the PR segment. It represents the time required for atrial depolarization, the impulse delay in the AV node, and the travel time to the Purkinje fibers. It normally measures from 0.12 to 0.20 second (five small blocks).

The **QRS complex** represents ventricular depolarization. The shape of the QRS complex depends on the lead selected. The Q wave is the first negative deflection and is not present in all leads. When present, it is small and represents initial ventricular septal depolarization. When the Q wave is abnormally present in a lead, it represents myocardial necrosis (cell death). The R wave is the first positive deflection. It may be small, large, or absent, depending on the lead. The S wave is a negative deflection following the R wave and is not present in all leads.

The **QRS duration** represents the time required for depolarization of both ventricles. It is measured from the beginning of the QRS complex to the J point (the junction where the QRS complex ends and the ST segment begins). It normally measures from 0.06 to 0.10 second (1 ½ to 2 ½ small blocks) (Urden et al., 2018; Prutkin, 2018).

The **ST segment** is normally an isoelectric line and represents early ventricular repolarization. It occurs from the J point to the beginning of the T wave. Its length varies with changes in the heart rate, the administration of medications, and electrolyte disturbances.

The **T wave** follows the ST segment and represents ventricular repolarization. It is usually positive, rounded, and slightly asymmetric. T waves may become tall and peaked, inverted (negative), or flat as a result of myocardial ischemia, potassium or calcium imbalances, medications, or autonomic nervous system effects.

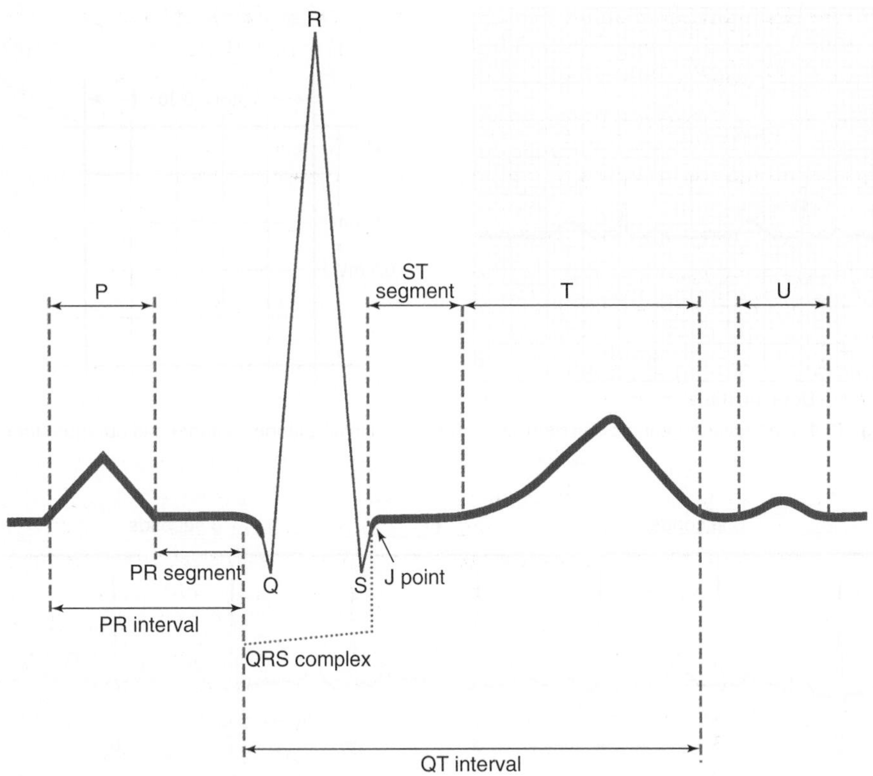

P wave:	Represents atrial depolarization.
PR segment:	Represents the time required for the impulse to travel through the AV node, where it is delayed, and through the bundle of His, bundle branches, and Purkinje fiber network, just before ventricular depolarization.
PR interval:	Represents the time required for atrial depolarization as well as impulse travel through the conduction system and Purkinje fiber network, inclusive of the P wave and PR segment. It is measured from the beginning of the P wave to the end of the PR segment.
QRS complex:	Represents ventricular depolarization and is measured from the beginning of the Q (or R) wave to the end of the S wave.
J point:	Represents the junction where the QRS complex ends and the ST segment begins.
ST segment:	Represents early ventricular repolarization.
T wave:	Represents ventricular repolarization.
U wave:	Represents late ventricular repolarization.
QT interval:	Represents the total time required for ventricular depolarization and repolarization and is measured from the beginning of the QRS complex to the end of the T wave.

Fig. 31.6 Components of a normal electrocardiogram.

The **U wave,** when present, follows the T wave and may result from slow repolarization of ventricular Purkinje fibers. It is of the same polarity as the T wave, although generally it is smaller. It is not normally seen in all leads and is more common in lead V_3. An abnormal U wave may suggest an electrolyte abnormality (particularly hypokalemia) or other disturbance. Correct identification is important so that it is not mistaken for a P wave. If in doubt, notify the primary health care provider and request that a potassium level be obtained.

The **QT interval** represents the total time required for ventricular depolarization and repolarization. The QT interval is measured from the beginning of the Q wave to the end of the T wave. This interval varies with the patient's age and gender and changes with the heart rate, lengthening with slower heart rates and shortening with faster rates. It may be prolonged by certain medications, electrolyte disturbances, or subarachnoid hemorrhage. A prolonged QT interval may lead to a unique type of ventricular tachycardia called *torsades de pointes*.

Artifact is interference seen on the monitor or rhythm strip, which may look like a wandering or fuzzy baseline. It can be caused by patient movement, loose or defective electrodes, improper grounding, or faulty ECG equipment such as broken wires or cables. Some artifacts can mimic lethal dysrhythmias such as ventricular tachycardia (with toothbrushing) or ventricular fibrillation (with tapping on the electrode). *Assess the patient to differentiate an artifact from actual lethal rhythms! Do not rely only on the ECG monitor.*

Electrocardiographic Rhythm Analysis

Analysis of an ECG rhythm strip requires a systematic approach using an eight-step method facilitated by use of a measurement tool called an **ECG caliper** (Prutkin, 2018; Palmer, 2011):

1. **Determine the heart rate.** The most common method is to count the number of QRS complexes in 6 seconds and multiply that number by 10 to calculate the rate for a full minute. This is called the *6-second strip method* and is a quick method to determine the mean or *average* heart rate. Normal heart rates fall between 60 and 100 beats/min. A rate less than 60 beats/min is called **bradycardia**. A rate greater than 100 beats/min is called **tachycardia**. Current monitoring systems will display a continuous heart rate and print it on the ECG strip. *Use caution and confirm that the rate is correct by assessing the patient's heart rate directly.* Many factors can incorrectly alter the rate displayed by the monitor.
2. **Determine the heart rhythm.** Assess for atrial and/or ventricular regularity. Heart rhythms can be either regular or irregular. Irregular rhythms can be regularly irregular, occasionally irregular, or irregularly irregular. Check the regularity of the atrial rhythm by assessing the PP intervals, placing one caliper point on a P wave and the other point on the precise spot on the next P wave. Then move the caliper from P wave to P wave along the entire strip ("walking out" the P waves) to determine the regularity of the rhythm. P waves of a different shape (ectopic waves), if present, create an irregularity and do not walk out with the other P waves. A slight irregularity in the PP intervals, varying no more than three small blocks, is considered essentially regular if the P waves are all of the same shape. This alteration is caused by changes in intrathoracic pressure during the respiratory cycle.

   Check the regularity of the ventricular rhythm by assessing the RR intervals, placing one caliper point on a portion of the QRS complex (usually the most prominent portion of the deflection) and the other point on the precise spot of the next QRS complex. Move the caliper from QRS complex to QRS complex along the entire strip (walking out the QRS complexes) to determine the regularity of the rhythm. QRS complexes of a different shape (ectopic QRS complexes), if present, create an irregularity and do not walk out with the other QRS complexes. A slight irregularity of no more than three small blocks between intervals is considered essentially regular if the QRS complexes are all of the same shape.
3. **Analyze the P waves.** Check that the P-wave shape is consistent throughout the strip, indicating that atrial depolarization is occurring from impulses originating from one focus, normally the SA node. Determine whether there is one P wave occurring before each QRS complex, establishing that a relationship exists between the P wave and the QRS complex. This relationship indicates that an impulse from one focus is responsible for both atrial and ventricular depolarization. The nurse may observe more than one P-wave shape, more P waves than QRS complexes, absent P waves, or P waves coming after the QRS, each indicating that a dysrhythmia exists. Ask these five questions when analyzing P waves:
   - Are P waves present?
   - Are the P waves occurring regularly?
   - Is there one P wave for each QRS complex?
   - Are the P waves smooth, rounded, and upright in appearance or are they inverted?
   - Do all P waves look similar?
4. **Measure the PR interval.** Place one caliper point at the beginning of the P wave and the other point at the end of the PR segment. The PR interval normally measures between 0.12 and 0.20 second. The measurement should be constant throughout the strip. The PR interval cannot be determined if there are no P waves or if P waves occur after the QRS complex. Ask these three questions about the PR interval:
   - Are PR intervals greater than 0.20 second?
   - Are PR intervals less than 0.12 second?
   - Are PR intervals constant across the ECG strip?
5. **Measure the QRS duration.** Place one caliper point at the beginning of the QRS complex and the other at the J point, where the QRS complex ends and the ST segment begins. The QRS duration normally measures between 0.06 and 0.10 second. The measurement should be constant throughout the entire strip. Check that the QRS complexes are consistent throughout the strip. When the QRS is narrow (0.10 second or less), it indicates that the impulse was not formed in the ventricles and is referred to as *supraventricular* or *above the ventricles*. When the QRS complex is wide (greater than 0.10 second), it indicates that the impulse is either of ventricular origin or of supraventricular origin with aberrant conduction, meaning deviating from the normal course or pattern. More than one QRS complex pattern or occasionally missing QRS complexes may be observed, indicating a dysrhythmia. Ask these questions to evaluate QRS intervals:
   - Are QRS intervals less than or greater than 0.10 second?
   - Are the QRS complexes similar in appearance across the ECG paper?
6. **Examine the ST segment.** The normal ST segment begins at the isoelectric line. ST elevation or depression is significant if displacement is 1 mm (one small box) or more above or below the line and is seen in two or more leads. ST *elevation* may indicate problems such as myocardial infarction, pericarditis, and hyperkalemia. ST *depression* is associated with hypokalemia, myocardial infarction, or ventricular hypertrophy.
7. **Assess the T wave.** Note the shape and height of the T wave for peaking or inversion. Abnormal T waves may indicate problems such as myocardial infarction and ventricular hypertrophy.
8. **Measure the QT interval.** A normal QT interval should be equal to or less than one-half the distance of the RR interval.

Using steps 1 through 8, you can interpret the cardiac rhythm and differentiate normal and abnormal cardiac rhythms (dysrhythmias).

Overview of Normal Cardiac Rhythms

Normal sinus rhythm (NSR) is the rhythm originating from the sinoatrial (SA) node (dominant pacemaker) that meets these ECG criteria (Fig. 31.7):

- *Rate:* Atrial and ventricular rates of 60 to 100 beats/min
- *Rhythm:* Atrial and ventricular rhythms regular
- *P waves:* Present, consistent configuration, one P wave before each QRS complex
- *PR interval:* 0.12 to 0.20 second and constant
- *QRS duration:* 0.06 to 0.10 second and constant

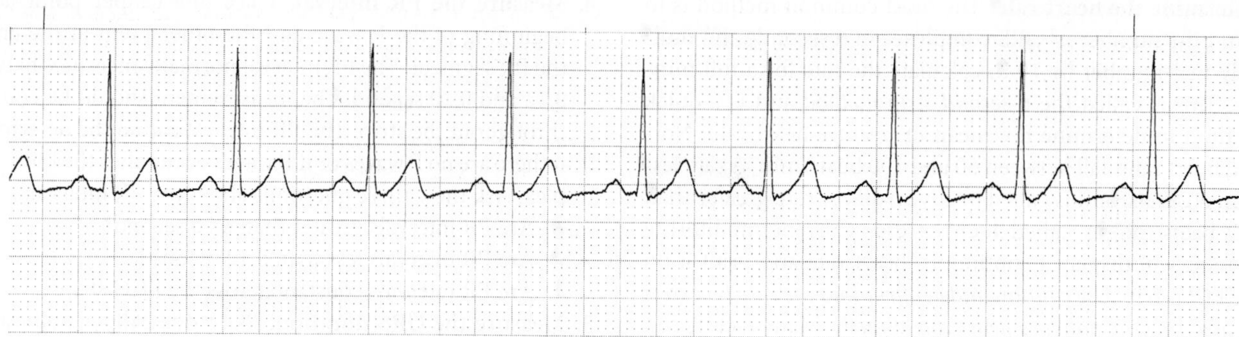

Fig. 31.7 Normal sinus rhythm. Both atrial and ventricular rhythms are essentially regular (a slight variation in rhythm is normal). Atrial and ventricular rates are both 87 beats/min. There is one P wave before each QRS complex, and all the P waves are of a consistent morphology, or shape. The PR interval measures 0.18 second and is constant; the QRS complex measures 0.06 second and is constant.

Sinus arrhythmia is a variant of NSR. It results from changes in intrathoracic pressure during breathing. In this context, the term *arrhythmia* does not mean an absence of rhythm, as the term suggests. Instead, the heart rate increases slightly during inspiration and decreases slightly during exhalation. This irregular rhythm is frequently observed in healthy adults.

Sinus arrhythmia has all the characteristics of NSR except for its irregularity. The PP and RR intervals vary, with the difference between the shortest and the longest intervals being greater than 0.12 second (three small blocks):

- *Rate:* Atrial and ventricular rates between 60 and 100 beats/min
- *Rhythm:* Atrial and ventricular rhythms irregular, with the shortest PP or RR interval varying at least 0.12 second from the longest PP or RR interval
- *P waves:* One P wave before each QRS complex; consistent configuration
- *PR interval:* Normal, constant
- *QRS duration:* Normal, constant

Sinus arrhythmias are occasionally due to nonrespiratory causes such as digoxin or morphine. These drugs enhance vagal tone and cause decreased heart rate and irregularity unrelated to the respiratory cycle.

COMMON DYSRHYTHMIAS

Any disorder of the heartbeat is called a **dysrhythmia**. Although the terms *arrhythmia* and *dysrhythmia* are often used interchangeably, *dysrhythmia* is more accurate. Although many dysrhythmias have no signs and symptoms, others have serious consequences if not treated.

Pathophysiology Review

Dysrhythmias are classified in several ways. As broad categories, they include premature complexes, bradydysrhythmias (bradycardias), and tachydysrhythmias (tachycardias).

Premature Complexes. **Premature complexes** are early rhythm complexes. They occur when a cardiac cell or cell group, other than the sinoatrial (SA) node, becomes irritable and fires an impulse before the next sinus impulse is produced. The abnormal focus is called an *ectopic focus* and may be generated by atrial, junctional, or ventricular tissue. After the premature complex, there is a pause before the next normal complex, creating an irregularity in the rhythm. The patient with premature complexes may be unaware of them or may feel palpitations or a "skipping" of the heartbeat. If premature complexes, especially those that are ventricular, become more frequent, the patient may experience symptoms of decreased cardiac output.

Premature complexes may occur repetitively in a rhythmic fashion:

- *Bigeminy* exists when normal complexes and premature complexes occur alternately in a repetitive two-beat pattern, with a pause occurring after each premature complex, so complexes occur in pairs.
- *Trigeminy* is a repeated three-beat pattern, usually occurring as two sequential normal complexes followed by a premature complex and a pause, with the same pattern repeating itself in triplets.
- *Quadrigeminy* is a repeated four-beat pattern, usually occurring as three sequential normal complexes followed by a premature complex and a pause, with the same pattern repeating itself in a four-beat pattern.

Bradydysrhythmias. **Bradydysrhythmias** occur when the heart rate is less than 60 beats/min. These rhythms can also be significant because:

- Myocardial oxygen demand is reduced from the slow heart rate, which can be beneficial.
- Coronary ***perfusion*** time may be adequate because of a prolonged diastole, which is desirable.
- Coronary perfusion pressure may decrease if the heart rate is too slow to provide adequate cardiac output and blood pressure; this is a serious consequence.

Therefore the patient may tolerate the bradydysrhythmia well if the blood pressure is adequate. If the blood pressure is not adequate, symptomatic bradydysrhythmias may lead to myocardial ischemia or infarction, dysrhythmias, hypotension, and heart failure.

Tachydysrhythmias. **Tachydysrhythmias** are heart rates greater than 100 beats/min. They are a major concern in the adult patient with coronary artery disease (CAD). Coronary artery blood flow occurs mostly during diastole when the aortic valve is closed and is determined by diastolic time and blood pressure in the root of the aorta. Tachydysrhythmias are serious because they:

- Shorten the diastolic time and therefore the coronary ***perfusion*** time (the amount of time available for blood to flow through the coronary arteries to the myocardium)
- Initially increase cardiac output and blood pressure (However, a continued rise in heart rate decreases the ventricular filling time because of a shortened diastole, decreasing the stroke volume. Consequently, cardiac output and blood pressure will begin to decrease, reducing aortic pressure and therefore coronary ***perfusion*** pressure.)
- Increase the work of the heart, increasing myocardial oxygen demand

The patient with a tachydysrhythmia may have:

- Palpitations
- Chest discomfort (pressure or pain from myocardial ischemia or infarction)
- Restlessness and anxiety
- Pale, cool skin
- Syncope ("blackout") from hypotension

Tachydysrhythmias may also lead to heart failure. Presenting symptoms of heart failure may include dyspnea, lung crackles, distended neck veins, fatigue, and weakness (see Chapter 32). See the Key Features box for signs and symptoms of sustained bradydysrhythmias and tachydysrhythmias.

Etiology

Dysrhythmias occur for many reasons, including myocardial infarction (MI), electrolyte imbalances (especially potassium and magnesium), hypoxia, drug toxicity, and hypovolemia (decreased blood volume). People who use cocaine and illicit inhalants are particularly at risk for potentially fatal dysrhythmias. Stress, fear, anxiety, and caffeine can cause an increased heart rate (tachycardia or premature ventricular contractions). Nicotine and alcohol excess can lead to an abnormal heart rate or heart rhythm such as atrial fibrillation. Specific etiologies are described for each common dysrhythmia discussed in this chapter.

❖ Interprofessional Collaborative Care

Dysrhythmias may also be classified by their site of origin in the heart. These include common sinus, atrial, and ventricular dysrhythmias. Although many specific dysrhythmias can occur, general assessment and interventions for patient care may be similar (see the Best Practice for Patient Safety & Quality Care: Care of the Patient With Dysrhythmias box). Assess the patient's apical and radial pulses for a full minute for any irregularity, which may occur with premature beats or atrial fibrillation. If the apical pulse differs from the radial pulse rate, a **pulse deficit** exists and indicates that the heart is not pumping adequately to achieve optimal ***perfusion*** to the body.

Dysrhythmias are often managed with antidysrhythmic drug therapy. Specific drugs and other treatments for common dysrhythmias are discussed later in this chapter.

SINUS DYSRHYTHMIAS

The sinoatrial (SA) node in the right atrium is the pacemaker in all sinus dysrhythmias. Innervation from sympathetic and parasympathetic nerves is normally in balance to ensure a normal sinus rhythm (NSR). An imbalance increases or decreases the rate of SA node discharge either as a normal response to activity

KEY FEATURES

Sustained Tachydysrhythmias and Bradydysrhythmias

- Chest discomfort, pressure, or pain, which may radiate to the jaw, back, or arm
- Restlessness, anxiety, nervousness, confusion
- Dizziness, syncope
- Palpitations (in tachydysrhythmias)
- Change in pulse strength, rate, and rhythm
- Pulse deficit
- Shortness of breath, dyspnea
- Tachypnea
- Pulmonary crackles
- Orthopnea
- S_3 or S_4 heart sounds
- Jugular venous distention
- Weakness, fatigue
- Pale, cool, skin; diaphoresis
- Nausea, vomiting
- Decreased urine output
- Delayed capillary refill
- Hypotension

BEST PRACTICE FOR PATIENT SAFETY & QUALITY CARE (QSEN)

Care of the Patient With Dysrhythmias

- Assess vital signs at least every 4 hours and as needed.
- Monitor patient for cardiac dysrhythmias.
- Evaluate and document the patient's response to dysrhythmias.
- Encourage the patient to notify the nurse when chest pain occurs.
- Assess chest pain (e.g., location, intensity, duration, radiation, precipitating and alleviating factors).
- Assess peripheral circulation (e.g., palpate for presence of peripheral pulses, edema, capillary refill, color, temperature of extremity).
- Provide antidysrhythmic therapy according to unit policy (e.g., antidysrhythmic medication, cardioversion, defibrillation), as appropriate.
- Monitor and document patient's response to antidysrhythmic medications or interventions.
- Monitor appropriate laboratory values (e.g., cardiac enzymes, electrolyte levels).
- Monitor the patient's activity tolerance and schedule exercise/rest periods to avoid fatigue.
- Observe for respiratory difficulty (e.g., shortness of breath, rapid breathing, labored respirations).
- Promote stress reduction.
- Offer spiritual support to the patient and/or family (e.g., contact clergy), as appropriate.

or physiologic changes or as a pathologic response to disease. Sinus tachycardia and sinus bradycardia are the two most common types of sinus dysrhythmias.

Sinus Tachycardia: Pathophysiology Review

Sympathetic nervous system stimulation or vagal (parasympathetic) inhibition results in an increased rate of SA node discharge, which increases the heart rate. When the rate of SA node discharge is more than 100 beats/min, the rhythm is called **sinus tachycardia** (Fig. 31.8A). From age 10 years to adulthood, the heart rate normally does not exceed 100 beats/min except in response to activity and then usually does not exceed 160 beats/min. Rarely does the heart rate reach 180 beats/min.

Sinus tachycardia initially increases cardiac output and blood pressure. However, continued increases in heart rate decrease coronary ***perfusion*** time, diastolic filling time, and coronary ***perfusion*** pressure while increasing myocardial oxygen demand.

Increased sympathetic stimulation is a normal response to physical activity but may also be caused by anxiety, pain, stress, fever, anemia, hypoxemia, and hyperthyroidism. Drugs such as epinephrine, atropine, caffeine, alcohol, nicotine, cocaine, aminophylline, and thyroid medications may also increase the heart rate. In some cases, sinus tachycardia is a compensatory response to decreased cardiac output or blood pressure, as occurs in dehydration, hypovolemic shock, myocardial infarction (MI), infection, and heart failure. Assess patients for signs and symptoms of hypovolemia and dehydration, including increased pulse rate, decreased urinary output, decreased blood pressure, and dry skin and mucous membranes.

❖ Interprofessional Collaborative Care

The patient may be asymptomatic except for an increased pulse rate. However, if the rhythm is not well tolerated, he or she may have symptoms of instability.

! NURSING SAFETY PRIORITY QSEN

Action Alert

For patients with sinus tachycardia, assess for fatigue, weakness, shortness of breath, orthopnea, decreased oxygen saturation, increased pulse rate, and decreased blood pressure. Also assess for restlessness and anxiety from decreased cerebral ***perfusion*** and for decreased urine output from impaired renal ***perfusion.*** The patient may also have anginal pain and palpitations. The ECG pattern may show T-wave inversion or ST-segment elevation or depression in response to myocardial ischemia.

The desired outcome is to decrease the heart rate to normal levels by treating the underlying cause. Remind the patient to remain on bedrest if the tachycardia is causing hypotension or weakness. Teach the patient to avoid substances that increase cardiac rate, including caffeine, alcohol, and nicotine. Help patients develop stress-management strategies or refer the patient to a mental health professional.

Sinus Bradycardia: Pathophysiology Review

Excessive vagal (parasympathetic) stimulation to the heart causes a decreased rate of sinus node discharge. It may result from carotid sinus massage, vomiting, suctioning, Valsalva maneuvers (e.g., bearing down for a bowel movement or gagging), ocular pressure, or pain. Increased parasympathetic stimuli may also result from hypoxia, inferior wall MI, and the administration of drugs such as beta-adrenergic blocking agents, calcium channel blockers, and digoxin. Lyme disease, ***electrolyte*** disturbances, neurologic disorders, and hypothyroidism may also cause bradycardia.

The stimuli slow the heart rate and decrease the speed of conduction through the heart. When the sinus node discharge rate is less than 60 beats/min, the rhythm is called **sinus bradycardia** (Fig. 31.8B) (Kusumoto et al., 2019). Sinus bradycardia increases coronary ***perfusion*** time, but it may decrease coronary perfusion pressure. However, myocardial oxygen demand is *decreased*. Well-conditioned athletes with bradycardia have a hypereffective heart in which the strong heart muscle provides an adequate stroke volume and a low heart rate to achieve a normal cardiac output.

❖ Interprofessional Collaborative Care

◆ **Assessment: Recognize Cues** The patient with sinus bradycardia may be asymptomatic except for the decreased pulse rate. In many cases, the cause of sinus bradycardia is unknown. Assess the electronic health record (EHR) to determine if the patient is receiving medications that slow the conduction through the SA or AV node. Assess the patient for:

- Syncope ("blackouts" or fainting)
- Dizziness and weakness
- Confusion
- Hypotension
- Diaphoresis (excessive sweating)
- Shortness of breath
- Chest pain

NCLEX EXAMINATION CHALLENGE 31.1

Physiological Integrity

The nurse is assessing the client's cardiac rhythm and notes the following: HR 64, regular rhythm, PR interval 0.20; QRS 0.10. How will the nurse document this rhythm interpretation in the electronic health record?

A. Sinus tachycardia
B. Sinus bradycardia
C. Normal sinus rhythm
D. Sinus arrhythmia

◆ **Interventions: Take Action.** If the patient is stable, treatment includes identification and treatment of the underlying cause. If the patient has any of these symptoms and the underlying cause cannot be determined, the treatment is to administer drug therapy with intravenous atropine, increase intravascular volume via IV fluids, and apply oxygen if oxygen saturation is below 94% or the patient is short of air. Drugs suspected of causing the bradycardia are discontinued. If beta-blocker overdose is suspected, administration of glucagon may help by increasing the heart rate and blood pressure. If the heart rate does not increase sufficiently,

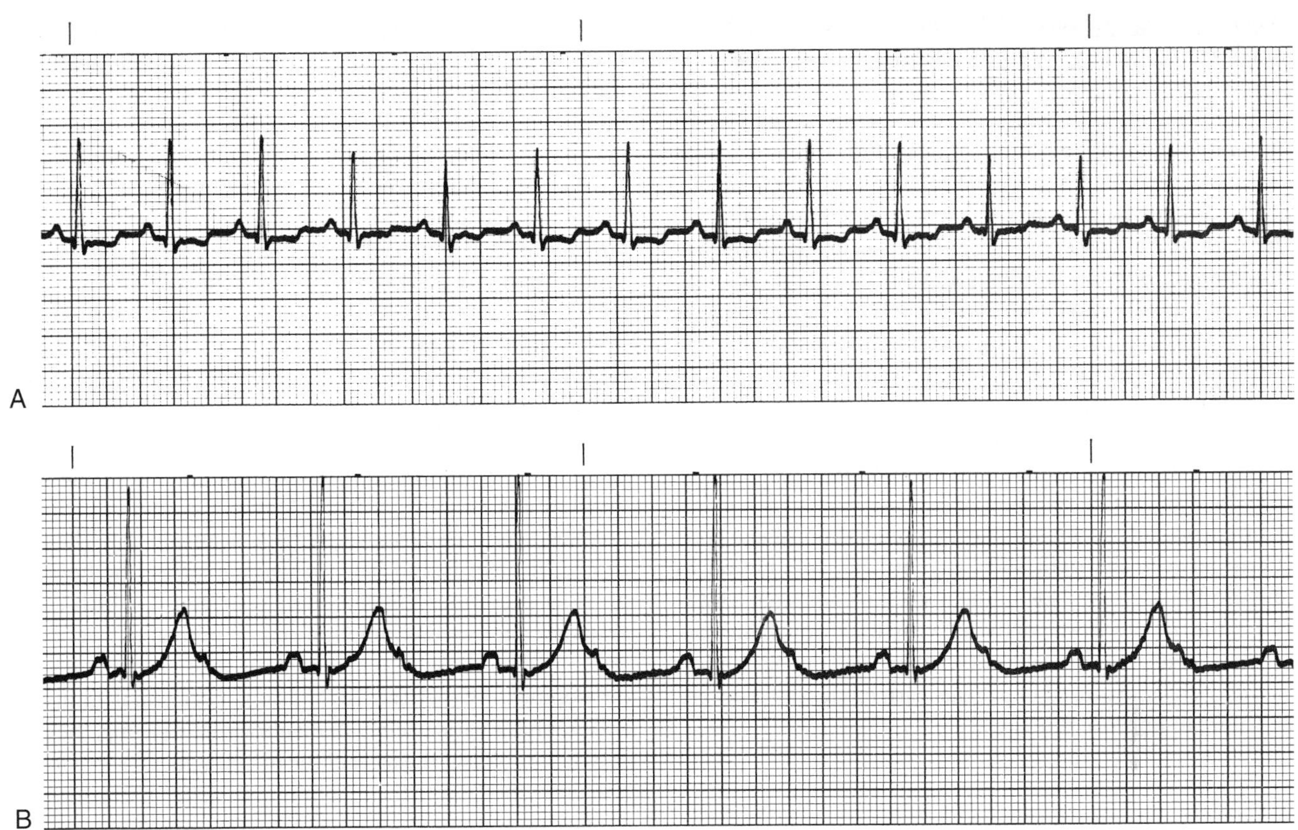

Fig. 31.8 Sinus rhythms. A, Sinus tachycardia (heart rate, 115 beats/min; PR interval, 0.12 second; QRS complex, 0.08 second). B, Sinus bradycardia (heart rate, 52 beats/min; PR interval, 0.18 second; QRS complex, 0.08 second).

prepare for transcutaneous or transvenous pacing to increase the heart rate. If treatment of the underlying cause does not restore normal sinus rhythm, the patient will require permanent pacemaker implantation.

Temporary Pacing. Temporary pacing is a nonsurgical intervention that provides a timed electrical stimulus to the heart when either the impulse initiation or the conduction system of the heart is defective. The electrical stimulus then spreads throughout the heart to depolarize the cells, which should be followed by contraction and cardiac output. Electrical stimuli may be delivered to the right atrium or right ventricle (single-chamber pacemakers) or to both (dual-chamber pacemakers).

Temporary pacing is used for patients with symptomatic bradydysrhythmias who do not respond to atropine or for patients with asystole. There are two types of temporary pacing: transcutaneous and transvenous.

Transcutaneous pacing is accomplished through the application of two large external electrodes. The electrodes are attached to an external pulse generator. The generator emits electrical pulses, which are transmitted through the electrodes and then transcutaneously to stimulate ventricular depolarization when the patient's heart rate is slower than the rate set on the pacemaker. Transcutaneous pacing is used as an *emergency* measure to provide demand ventricular pacing in a profoundly bradycardic or asystolic patient until invasive pacing can be used or the patient's heart rate returns to normal. This method of pacing is painful and may require administration of pain and sedative medications for the patient to tolerate the therapy. Transcutaneous pacing is used only as a temporary measure to maintain heart rate and ***perfusion*** until a more permanent method of pacing is used.

A temporary transvenous system can be inserted in an emergency as a bridge until a permanent pacemaker can be inserted. This system consists of an external battery-operated pulse generator and pacing electrodes, or lead wire. The wire attaches to the generator on one end and is threaded to the right ventricle via the subclavian or femoral vein (Fig. 31.9).

In pacemaker systems, electrical pulses, or stimuli, are emitted from the negative terminal of the generator, flow through a lead wire, and stimulate the cardiac cells to depolarize. The current seeks ground by returning through the other lead wire to the positive terminal of the generator, thus completing a circuit. The intensity of electrical current is set by selecting the appropriate current output, measured in milliamperes.

The two major modes of pacing are synchronous (demand) pacing and asynchronous (fixed-rate) pacing. Temporary pacing is *usually* done in the synchronous (demand) pacing mode. The pacemaker's sensitivity is set to sense the patient's own beats. When the patient's heart rate is above the rate set on the pulse generator, the pacemaker does not fire (inhibits itself). When the patient's heart rate is less than the generator setting, the pacemaker provides electrical impulses (paces).

When a pacing stimulus is delivered to the heart, a spike (or pacemaker artifact) is seen on the monitor or ECG strip. The spike should be followed by evidence of depolarization (i.e., a P wave, indicating atrial depolarization, or a QRS complex, indicating ventricular depolarization). This pattern is referred to as *capture,* indicating that the pacemaker has successfully depolarized, or captured, the chamber.

Permanent Pacemaker. Permanent pacemaker insertion is performed to treat conduction disorders that are not temporary, including complete heart block. These pacemakers are usually powered by a lithium battery and have an average life span of 10 years. After the battery power is depleted, the generator must be replaced by a procedure done with the patient under local anesthesia. Some pacemakers can be recharged externally. Combination pacemaker/defibrillator devices are also available.

A biventricular pacemaker may be used to coordinate contractions between the right and left ventricles. In addition to pacing used in the right side of the heart, an additional lead is placed in the left lateral wall of the left ventricle through the coronary sinus. This procedure allows synchronized depolarization of the ventricles and is used in patients with moderate-to-severe heart failure to improve functional ability.

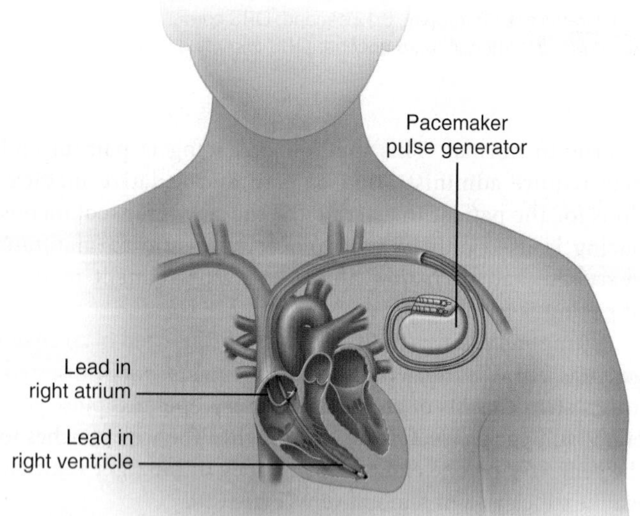

Fig. 31.9 Placement of pacemaker in chest and heart leads.

The electrophysiologist implants the pulse generator in a surgically made subcutaneous pocket at the shoulder in the right or left subclavicular area, which may create a visible bulge (see Fig. 31.9). The leads are introduced transvenously via the cephalic or the subclavian vein to the endocardium on the right side of the heart. A leadless pacing system has recently been developed where the pacemaker is a self-contained unit that is placed in the right ventricle via the femoral vein (Urden et al., 2018). Previous attempts with this approach have been associated with high complication rates; however, newer developments are showing promise. Further research regarding long-term use of leadless pacing systems is under way (Hayes, 2018).

After the procedure, monitor the ECG rhythm to check that the pacemaker is working correctly. Assess the implantation site for bleeding, swelling, redness, tenderness, and infection. The dressing over the site should remain clean and dry. The patient should be afebrile and have stable vital signs. The health care provider prescribes initial activity restrictions, which are then gradually increased. Complications of permanent pacemakers are similar to those of temporary invasive pacing and include development of pericardial effusion, pericardial tamponade, and diaphragmatic pacing. In diaphragmatic pacing, the patient may report pain at the level of the diaphragm. Observe for muscle contractions over the diaphragm that are synchronous with the heart rate.

Pacemaker checks are done on an ambulatory-care basis at regular intervals. Reprogramming may be needed if pacemaker problems develop. The pulse generator is interrogated using an electronic device to determine the pacemaker settings and battery life (Fig. 31.10). In addition, most pacemaker manufacturers offer wireless home transmitter devices. Data are then sent via landline telephone to a database, which is accessed by the device clinic or primary health care provider. Stress the need to keep follow-up appointments for more detailed pacemaker checks and reprogramming, if necessary, and for assessment.

Give written and verbal information to patients who have a *permanent pacemaker* about the type and settings of their pacemaker. Teach the patient to report any pulse rate lower than that set on the pacemaker. Review the proper care of the pacemaker insertion site and the importance of reporting any fever or any redness, swelling, or drainage at the pacemaker

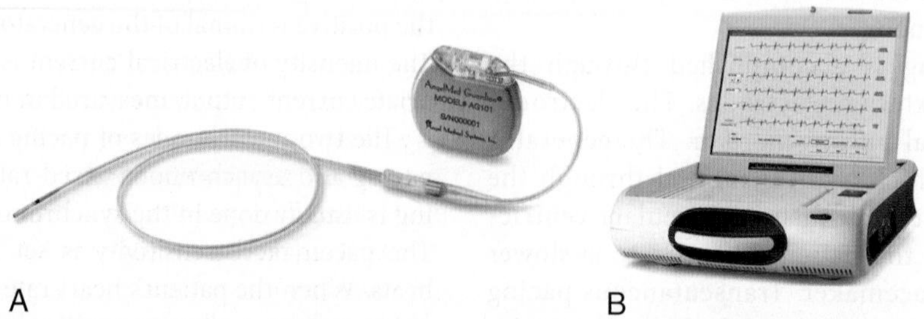

Fig. 31.10 Permanent pacemaker (A) and programmer (B). (From Fischell, T. A., et al. [2010]. Initial clinical results using intracardiac electrogram monitoring to detect and alert patients during coronary plaque rupture and ischemia, *Journal of the American College of Cardiology, 56*[14], 1089–1098.)

insertion site. If the surgical incision is near either shoulder, advise the patient to avoid lifting the arm over the head or lifting more than 10 lb for the next 4 weeks because this could dislodge the pacemaker wire. Encourage the patient that usual arm movement is encouraged to prevent shoulder stiffness.

! NURSING SAFETY PRIORITY (QSEN)

Action Alert

Teach patients who have permanent pacemakers to:

- Avoid sources of strong electromagnetic fields, such as magnets and telecommunications transmitters. (These may cause interference and could change the pacemaker settings, causing a malfunction. Magnetic resonance imaging (MRI) is usually contraindicated, depending on the machine's technology.)
- Carry a pacemaker identification card provided by the manufacturer and wear a medical alert bracelet at all times

Current evidence does not include special precautions with common household appliances (e.g. microwaves), with modern communication devices (e.g. cell phones), or with portable media players (Olshansky & Hayes, 2017).

See the Patient and Family Education: Preparing for Self-Management box for care after the insertion of a permanent pacemaker.

PATIENT AND FAMILY EDUCATION: PREPARING FOR SELF-MANAGEMENT

Permanent Pacemakers

- Follow the instructions for pacemaker site skin care that have been specifically prepared for you. Report any fever or redness, swelling, or drainage from the incision site to your physician.
- Do not manipulate the pacemaker generator site. Twisting or manipulation of the generator site can cause the leads to shift (lead dislodgement) (Townsend, 2018).
- Keep your pacemaker identification card in your wallet and wear a medical alert bracelet.
- Take your pulse for 1 full minute at the same time each day and record the rate in your pacemaker diary. Take your pulse any time you feel symptoms of a possible pacemaker failure and report your heart rate and symptoms to your primary health care provider.
- Know the rate at which your pacemaker is set and the basic functioning of your pacemaker. Know which rate changes to report to your primary health care provider.
- Do not apply pressure over your generator. Avoid tight clothing or belts.
- You may take baths or showers without concern for your pacemaker.
- Inform all health care providers that you have a pacemaker. Certain tests that they may wish to perform (e.g., magnetic resonance imaging) could affect or damage it.
- Know the indications of battery failure for your pacemaker as you were instructed and report these findings to your primary health care provider if they occur.
- Do not operate electrical appliances directly over your pacemaker site because this may cause your pacemaker to malfunction.
- Do not lean over electrical or gasoline engines or motors. Be sure that electrical appliances or motors are properly grounded.
- Avoid all transmitter towers for radio, television, and radar. Radio, television, other home appliances, and antennas do not pose a hazard.
- Be aware that antitheft devices in stores may cause temporary pacemaker malfunction. If symptoms develop, move away from the device.
- Inform airport personnel of your pacemaker before passing through a metal detector and show them your pacemaker identification card. The metal in your pacemaker will trigger the alarm in the metal detector device.
- Stay away from any arc welding equipment.
- Be aware that it is safe to operate a microwave oven unless it does not have proper shielding (old microwave ovens) or is defective.
- Report any of these symptoms to your primary health care provider if you experience them: difficulty breathing, dizziness, fainting, chest pain, weight gain, and prolonged hiccupping. If you have any of these symptoms, check your pulse rate and call your primary health care provider.
- If you feel symptoms when near any device, move 5 to 10 feet away from it and check your pulse. Your pulse rate should return to normal.
- Keep all of your health care provider and pacemaker clinic appointments.
- Take all medications prescribed for you as instructed.
- Follow your prescribed diet.
- Follow instructions about restrictions on physical activity, such as no sudden, jerky movement, for 8 weeks to allow the pacemaker to settle in place.

ATRIAL DYSRHYTHMIAS

In patients with atrial dysrhythmias, the focus of impulse generation shifts away from the sinus node to the atrial tissues. The shift changes the axis (direction) of atrial depolarization, resulting in a P-wave shape that differs from normal P waves. The most common atrial dysrhythmias are:

- Premature atrial complexes
- Supraventricular tachycardia
- Atrial fibrillation

Premature Atrial Complexes

A **premature atrial complex (contraction) (PAC)** occurs when atrial tissue becomes irritable. This ectopic focus fires an impulse before the next sinus impulse is due. The premature P wave may not always be clearly visible because it can be hidden in the preceding T wave. Examine the T wave closely for any change in shape and compare with other T waves. A PAC is usually followed by a pause.

The causes of atrial irritability include:

- Stress
- Fatigue
- Anxiety
- Inflammation
- Infection
- Caffeine, nicotine, or alcohol
- Drugs such as epinephrine, sympathomimetics, amphetamines, digoxin, or anesthetic agents

PACs may also result from myocardial ischemia, hypermetabolic states, electrolyte imbalance, or atrial stretch. Atrial stretch can result from congestive heart failure, valvular disease, and pulmonary hypertension with cor pulmonale.

The patient usually has no symptoms except for possible heart palpitations. No intervention is needed except to treat causes such as heart failure. If PACs occur frequently, they may lead to more serious atrial tachydysrhythmias and therefore may need treatment. Administration of prescribed antidysrhythmic drugs may be necessary (see the Common Examples of Drug Therapy: Antidysrhythmic Medication box). Teach the patient measures to manage stress and substances to avoid, such as caffeine and alcohol, that are known to increase atrial irritability.

Supraventricular Tachycardia: Pathophysiology Review

Supraventricular tachycardia (SVT) involves the rapid stimulation of atrial tissue at a rate of 100 to 280 beats/min in adults. During SVT, P waves may not be visible, especially if there is a 1:1 conduction with rapid rates, because the P waves are

COMMON EXAMPLES OF DRUG THERAPY

Antidysrhythmic Medication

Drug Category	Selected Nursing Implications
Class I: Sodium Channel Blockers	
There are 3 subgroups of class I drugs.	
Common examples of sodium channel blockers: Type IA • Disopyramide phosphate Type IB • Lidocaine • Mexiletine hydrochloride Type IC • Flecainide acetate • Propafenone hydrochloride	• Monitor BP and HR; *hypotension and bradycardia can occur.* • Monitor for arrhythmias; *these agents affect conduction patterns, sometimes increasing the frequency or severity of dysrhythmias.* • Monitor for CNS side effects such as dizziness, anxiety, ataxia, insomnia, confusion, seizures, and GI distress; *these side effects may require dose reduction or discontinuation of the drug.* • Monitor for signs of heart failure; *many class I agents can also cause HF.*
Class II: Beta Blockers	
Only 4 beta blockers are approved for the treatment of dysrhythmias (Burchum & Rosenthal, 2019).	

Common examples of beta blockers:
• Propranolol
• Acebutolol
• Esmolol
• Sotalol
  • Sotalol is a class II dysrhythmic and a class III drug because of its effect on the QT interval and delay of repolarization.
  • Assess ventricular arrhythmias because this drug can have proarrhythmic effects.
	• Monitor HR and BP; bradycardia and decreased BP are expected effects.
	• Assess for wheezing or shortness of breath; beta$_2$-blocking effects on the lungs can cause bronchospasm.
	• Assess for insomnia, fatigue, and dizziness; side effects may require a decrease in dosage or discontinuation of the drug.

Class III: Potassium Channel Blockers	
There are currently 5 class III agents. Each drug works to delay repolarization and prolongs the QT interval. Although their effects are similar, the side effects and mechanism of action vary greatly. **Selected examples** of drug-specific side effects with associated rationales are listed.	
• Sotalol • Used for atrial and ventricular dysrhythmias.	**For all class III potassium channel blockers:** • Monitor BP and HR; hypotension and bradycardia can occur. • Monitor for arrhythmias; these agents affect conduction patterns, sometimes increasing the frequency or severity of dysrhythmias.
• Amiodarone • Used for atrial and ventricular dysrhythmias.	For amiodarone: • Continually monitor ECG rhythm during infusion; *bradycardia and AV block can occur.* • This drug can cause serious toxicities (lung damage, visual impairment). As a result, *approval is limited to use for life-threatening dysrhythmias. However, because of efficacy, use remains very common* (Burchum & Rosenthal, 2019). • Corneal pigmentation occurs in most patients, but it generally does not interfere with vision.
• Dronedarone • Used for AF and atrial flutter.	For dronedarone: • Teach patient to take with meals and to avoid grapefruit juice; *this drug is better absorbed with food, and grapefruit juice alters the effect of the drug.* • Teach patient to notify provider with signs of HF; *this drug is contraindicated for patients with HF.*
• Ibutilide • Used for AF and atrial flutter.	For ibutilide: • Stop infusion as soon as the dysrhythmia is terminated or in the event of VT; *this drug may cause potentially fatal dysrhythmias.* • Assess potassium and magnesium levels before infusion *because electrolyte balance must be corrected prior to and during use.*
• Dofetilide • Used for AF and atrial flutter.	For dofetilide: • Teach patient to change positions slowly; *orthostatic hypotension is a common side effect.*

COMMON EXAMPLES OF DRUG THERAPY—cont'd

Antidysrhythmic Medication

Drug Category	Selected Nursing Implications
Class IV: Calcium Channel Blockers	
Only 2 calcium channel blockers are approved for use in the treatment of dysrhythmias.	
• Verapamil • Diltiazem	For all class IV calcium channel blockers: • Monitor HR and BP; bradycardia and hypotension are common side effects. • Teach patients to change position slowly when receiving oral therapy; *orthostatic hypotension can occur until tolerance develops.* • Used for AF and atrial flutter. • Teach patients to report dyspnea, orthopnea, distended neck veins, or swelling of the extremities; *HF can occur, necessitating a decrease in dosage or discontinuation of drug.*
Class: Other	
Other drugs used in the treatment of dysrhythmias fall outside of the previous categories. They are unclassified drugs for dysrhythmia treatment.	
Common examples of other dysrhythmia medications:	
• Digoxin • Used for AF and atrial flutter.	For digoxin: • Assess apical HR before administration; *decreased HR is an expected response.* • Teach patient to report nausea, vomiting, diarrhea, paresthesias, confusion, or visual disturbance; *these can indicate digoxin toxicity.*
• Atropine sulfate • Used for bradycardia.	• Monitor HR and rhythm after administration; *increased heart rate is expected.*
• Adenosine • Used for paroxysmal SVT.	• Have emergency equipment available *because a short period of asystole is common after administration; bradycardia and hypotension may occur.* • Facial flushing, shortness of breath, and chest pain are common side effects.

AF, Atrial fibrillation; *AV,* atrioventricular; *BP,* blood pressure; *BUN,* blood urea nitrogen; *CAD,* coronary artery disease; *CHF,* congestive heart failure; *CNS,* central nervous system; *ECG,* electrocardiogram; *HF,* heart failure; *HR,* heart rate; *SVT,* supraventricular tachycardia. (Burchum & Rosenthal, 2019.)

embedded in the preceding T wave. *SVT may occur in healthy young people, especially women.*

SVT is usually caused by a re-entry mechanism in which one impulse circulates repeatedly throughout the atrial pathway, restimulating the atrial tissue at a rapid rate. The term *paroxysmal supraventricular tachycardia (PSVT)* is used when the rhythm is intermittent. It is initiated suddenly by a premature complex such as a PAC and terminated suddenly with or without intervention.

❖ Interprofessional Collaborative Care

Signs and symptoms depend on the duration of the SVT and the rate of the ventricular response. In patients with a sustained rapid ventricular response, assess for palpitations, chest pain, weakness, fatigue, shortness of breath, nervousness, anxiety, hypotension, and syncope. Cardiovascular deterioration may occur if the rate does not sustain adequate blood pressure. In that case, SVT can result in angina, heart failure, and cardiogenic shock. With a *nonsustained* or slower ventricular response, the patient may be asymptomatic except for occasional palpitations.

If SVT occurs in a healthy person and stops on its own, no intervention may be needed other than eliminating identified causes. If it continues, the patient should be studied in the electrophysiology study (EPS) laboratory. The preferred treatment for recurrent SVT is radiofrequency catheter ablation, described later in this chapter with treatment of atrial fibrillation. In sustained SVT with a rapid ventricular response, the desired outcomes of treatment are to decrease the ventricular response, convert the dysrhythmia to a sinus rhythm, and treat the cause.

Vagal maneuvers induce vagal stimulation of the cardiac conduction system, specifically the SA and AV nodes. Although not as common today, vagal maneuvers may be attempted to treat supraventricular tachydysrhythmias and include carotid sinus massage and Valsalva maneuvers. However, the results of these interventions are often temporary and may cause "rebound" tachycardia or severe bradycardia. Further therapy must be initiated.

In *carotid sinus massage,* the health care provider massages over one carotid artery for a few seconds, observing for a change in cardiac rhythm. This intervention causes vagal stimulation, slowing SA and AV nodal conduction. Prepare the patient for the procedure. Instruct him or her to turn the head slightly away from the side to be massaged and observe the cardiac monitor for a change in rhythm. An ECG rhythm strip is recorded before, during, and after the procedure. After the procedure, assess vital signs and the level of consciousness. Complications include bradydysrhythmias, asystole, ventricular fibrillation (VF), and cerebral damage. Because of these risks, carotid massage is not commonly performed. *A defibrillator and resuscitative equipment must be immediately available during the procedure.*

To stimulate a *vagal reflex,* the health care provider instructs the patient to bear down as if straining to have a bowel movement. Assess the patient's heart rate, heart rhythm, and blood pressure. Observe the cardiac monitor and record an ECG rhythm strip before, during, and after the procedure to determine the effect of therapy.

Drug therapy is prescribed for some patients to convert SVT to a normal sinus rhythm (NSR). Adenosine is used to terminate the acute episode and is given rapidly (over several seconds) followed by a normal saline bolus.

! NURSING SAFETY PRIORITY (QSEN)

Drug Alert

Side effects of adenosine include significant bradycardia with pauses, nausea, and vomiting. When administering adenosine, be sure to have emergency equipment readily available!

AV nodal blocking agents, such as beta and calcium channel blockers, are also given to treat SVT. The Common Examples of Drug Therapy: Antidysrhythmic Medication box lists medications that may be used for SVT.

If symptoms of poor ***perfusion*** are severe and persistent, the patient may require synchronized cardioversion to immediately terminate the SVT. For long-term treatment, patients are referred to an electrophysiologist for radiofrequency catheter ablation. Synchronized cardioversion and catheter ablation are discussed later in this chapter with treatment of atrial fibrillation.

PERFUSION CONCEPT EXEMPLAR: ATRIAL FIBRILLATION

Atrial fibrillation (AF) is the most common dysrhythmia seen in clinical practice. AF can be encountered and treated in the ambulatory and acute care settings. It can impair quality of life and cause considerable morbidity and mortality, largely related to ***clotting*** concerns such as embolic stroke, deep venous thrombosis (DVT), or pulmonary embolism (PE).

Pathophysiology Review

In patients with AF, multiple rapid impulses from many atrial foci depolarize the atria in a totally disorganized manner at a rate of 350 to 600 times per minute; ventricular response is usually 120 to 200 beats/min. The result is a chaotic rhythm with no clear P waves, no atrial contractions, loss of atrial kick, and an irregular ventricular response (Fig. 31.11). The atria merely quiver in fibrillation (commonly called *A fib*). Often the ventricles beat with a rapid rate in response to the numerous atrial impulses. The rapid and irregular ventricular rate decreases ventricular filling and reduces cardiac output. This alteration in cardiac function allows for blood to pool, placing the patient at risk for ***clotting*** concerns such as DVT or PE. AF is frequently associated with underlying cardiovascular disease (Urden et al., 2018).

Etiology and Genetic Risk. AF is associated with atrial fibrosis and loss of muscle mass. These structural changes are common in heart diseases such as hypertension, heart failure, and coronary artery disease. For those without an underlying disorder leading to the development of AF, as many as 30 genetic mutations have been identified as the potential cause (Palatinus & Das, 2015). Investigation continues in the development of genetic testing to identify patients at risk and targeted treatment (Palatinus & Das, 2015). As AF progresses, cardiac output decreases by as much as 20% to 30%.

Incidence and Prevalence. Atrial fibrillation (AF) is the most common dysrhythmia in the developed world, currently affecting 2.7 to 6.1 million people in the United States (January et al., 2014; January et al., 2019). The incidence of AF increases with age. As such, it is predicted that this number will double in the next 25 years (Morillo et al., 2017). Atrial fibrillation causes serious problems in older people, leading to stroke and/or heart failure. Risk factors include hypertension (HTN), previous ischemic stroke, transient ischemic attack (TIA) or other thromboembolic event, coronary heart disease, diabetes mellitus, heart failure, obesity, hyperthyroidism, chronic kidney disease, excessive alcohol use, and mitral valve disease.

❖ Interprofessional Collaborative Care

◆ Assessment: Recognize Cues

History. When obtaining a history, assess for prior history of AF or other dysrhythmias. Recurrence of AF is common, and assessment of previous conduction issues can be helpful in developing the plan of care. Assess for history of cardiovascular disease. The risk of AF is much higher in patients with a history of hypertension, heart failure, obesity, or acute coronary syndrome (Urden et al., 2018).

Physical Assessment/Signs and Symptoms. On physical examination, the apical pulse may be irregular. Symptoms depend on the ventricular rate. Because of the loss of atrial kick, the patient in uncontrolled AF is at greater risk for inadequate cardiac output. Signs of poor ***perfusion*** may be observed. Assess the patient for fatigue, weakness, shortness of breath, dizziness, anxiety, syncope, palpitations, chest discomfort or pain, and hypotension. Some patients may be asymptomatic.

Psychosocial Assessment. Patients with AF, especially those with a high ventricular rate, can feel very anxious. With increased heart rate, cardiac output decreases, which can create dyspnea, contributing to feelings of anxiety. Assess patients who have chronic atrial fibrillation for methods of coping with a long-term conduction issue. Patients with chronic AF may have anxiety related to anticoagulation medications and the potential for emboli development.

Other Diagnostic Assessment. Definitive diagnosis occurs by obtaining a 12-lead ECG. AF is classified into five categories based on length of time in the rhythm: paroxysmal, persistent, long-standing persistent, permanent, and nonvalvular. AF is termed *paroxysmal* when the patient experiences an episode within 7 days that converts back to sinus rhythm. Episode lengths vary but do not continue beyond a week. *Persistent AF* is experienced as episodes that occur for longer than 7 days. AF sustained for more than 12 months is categorized as *long-standing persistent*. *Permanent AF* is defined as patients who remain in AF, and a decision is made not to restore or maintain sinus rhythm by either medical or surgical intervention. *Nonvalvular AF* occurs in the absence of mitral valve disease or repair.

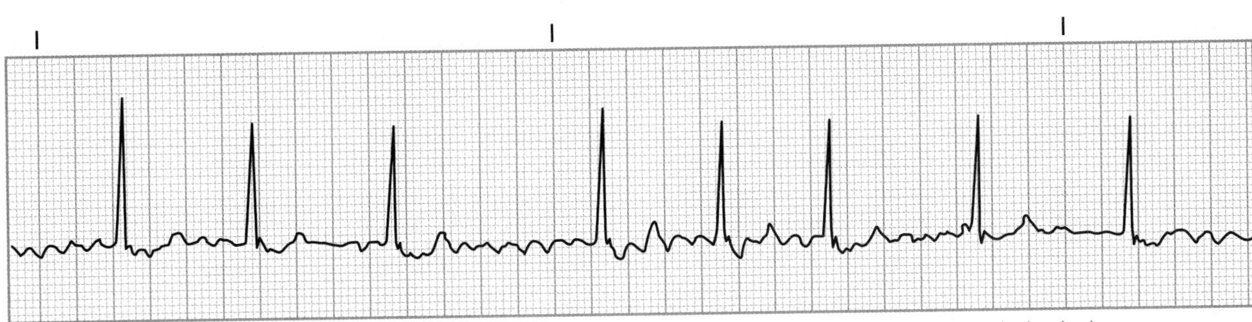

Fig. 31.11 Atrial fibrillation. Note wavy baseline with atrial electrical activity and irregular ventricular rhythm.

◆ **Analysis: Analyze Cues and Prioritize Hypotheses.** The priority collaborative problems for most patients with atrial fibrillation are:

1. Potential for embolus formation due to irregular cardiac rhythm
2. Potential for heart failure due to altered conduction pattern

◆ **Planning and Implementation: Generate Solutions and Take Action.** Interventions for AF depend on the severity of the problem and the patient's response. Be sure to individualize care based on the patient's values and preferences, your clinical expertise, and best current evidence. Drug therapy is often effective for treating AF.

Preventing Embolus Formation

Planning: Expected Outcomes The expected outcome is that the patient will remain free of embolus formation by restoring regular cardiac conduction.

Interventions. The purpose of collaborative care is to restore regular blood flow through the atrium when possible. Correcting the rhythm and controlling the rate of the rhythm restore blood flow, which helps prevent embolus formation and increases cardiac output. Drug therapy is often effective for treating AF.

! NURSING SAFETY PRIORITY QSEN

Action Alert

The loss of coordinated atrial contractions in AF can lead to pooling of blood, resulting in **clotting.** *The patient is at high risk for pulmonary embolism!* Thrombi may form within the right atrium and then move through the right ventricle to the lungs. If pulmonary embolism is suspected, remain with the patient and monitor for shortness of breath, chest pain, and/or hypotension. Initiate the Rapid Response Team and notify the provider.

In addition, the patient is at risk for systemic emboli, particularly an embolic stroke, which may cause severe neurologic impairment or death. Monitor patients carefully for signs of stroke. Initiate Rapid Response Team if stroke is suspected to facilitate timely diagnosis.

Patients with AF who have valvular disease are particularly at risk for venous thromboembolism (VTE). In VTE, the patient may report lower extremity pain and swelling. Anticipate ultrasound of vasculature and initiation of systemic anticoagulation.

Traditional interventions for AF include antidysrhythmic drugs to slow the ventricular conduction or to convert the AF to normal sinus rhythm (NSR). Examples of drugs to slow conduction are calcium channel blockers such as diltiazem or, for more difficult-to-control AF, amiodarone. Dronedarone is a medication similar to amiodarone, yet better tolerated by patients, for maintenance of sinus rhythm after cardioversion. However, dronedarone should not be used in patients with heart failure because it can cause an exacerbation of cardiac symptoms or with permanent AF because it increases the risk of stroke, myocardial infarction, or cardiovascular death.

Beta blockers, such as metoprolol and esmolol, may also be used to slow ventricular response. Digoxin is given for patients with heart failure and AF. It is useful in controlling the rate of ventricular response. However, it does not convert AF to sinus rhythm. Carefully monitor the pulse rate of patients taking these drugs.

Medications used for rhythm control of AF include flecainide, dofetilide, propafenone, and ibutilide. These medications are usually started within the acute care setting because of the risk of developing prolonged QT intervals and bradycardia. Continuous cardiac monitoring and frequent 12-lead ECGs are needed. Amiodarone is also used but does not require an acute care stay. If permanent AF is present, rhythm control antiarrhythmic medications should not be used. The medications used for rate and rhythm control are further discussed in the Common Examples of Drug Therapy: Antidysrhythmic Medication box.

Although the goal is to convert the patient from AF to SR, that may not be possible for many older adults (Urden et al., 2018). As such, these patients require long-term anticoagulation to prevent stroke and thrombus formation. See Chapter 33 for more on anticoagulant therapy.

Because of the unpredictable drug response and many food-drug interactions, laboratory test monitoring (e.g., international normalized ratio [INR]) is required when a patient is taking warfarin. Teach patients the importance of avoiding foods high in vitamin K and to avoid herbs such as ginger, ginseng, goldenseal, *Ginkgo biloba*, and St. John's wort, which could interfere with the drug's action.

Because of the problems associated with warfarin, direct oral anticoagulants (DOACs) such as dabigatran, rivaroxaban, apixaban, or edoxaban may be given on a long-term basis to prevent strokes associated with nonvalvular AF. Because these drugs achieve a steady state, there is no need for laboratory test monitoring. Prothrombin time (PT) and INR are not accurate predictors of bleeding time when DOACs are used.

Although the risk of bleeding is lower with DOACs, it is important to be aware of the reversal agents for these medications. Initially, dabigatran was the only DOAC with a reversal agent. Idarucizumab, an intravenous monoclonal antibody, binds to dabigatran, thereby preventing dabigatran from inhibiting thrombin. Side effects of idarucizumab include hypokalemia, confusion, constipation, fever, and pneumonia. Recently, the FDA has approved andexanet alfa as the reversal agent for rivaroxaban and apixaban (Garcia & Crowther, 2018). However, use of these reversal agents significantly increases the risk of ***clotting*** and stroke and should only be used in the event of life-threatening bleeding.

! NURSING SAFETY PRIORITY QSEN

Drug Alert

Teach patients taking any type of anticoagulant drug to report bruising, bleeding nose or gums, and other signs of bleeding to their primary health care provider immediately.

Preventing Heart Failure

Planning: Expected Outcomes The expected outcome is that the patient will remain free of heart failure by restoration of normal conduction with a controlled ventricular rate.

Interventions. Collaborative care to prevent heart failure and improve cardiac output generally begins with drug therapy; however, the patient may require other nonsurgical or surgical interventions if medication is not successful in meeting optimal outcomes.

Nonsurgical Interventions. Nonsurgical interventions most commonly include electrical cardioversion, left atrial appendage closure, radiofrequency catheter ablation, and pacing.

Electrical cardioversion. Electrical cardioversion is a *synchronized* countershock that may be performed to restore normal conduction in a hospitalized patient with *new-onset* AF. A cardioversion can also be scheduled electively for stable AF that is resistant to medical therapy. When the onset of AF is greater than 48 hours, the patient must take anticoagulants for at least 3 weeks (or until the INR is 2 to 3) before the procedure to prevent clots from moving from the heart to the brain or lungs (Urden et al., 2018). If the onset of AF is uncertain, a transesophageal echocardiogram (TEE) may be performed to assess for clot formation in the left atrium.

The shock depolarizes a large amount of myocardium during the cardiac depolarization. It is intended to stop the re-entry circuit and allow the sinus node to regain control of the heart. Emergency equipment must be available during the procedure. The physician, advanced practice nurse, or other qualified nurse explains the procedure to the patient and family. Help the patient sign a consent form unless the procedure is an emergency for a life-threatening dysrhythmia. Because he or she is usually conscious, a short-acting anesthetic agent is administered for sedation.

One electrode is placed to the left of the precordium, and the other is placed on the right next to the sternum and below the clavicle. The defibrillator should be set in the synchronized mode. A dot or line will be indicated over each QRS complex, confirming the synchronized mode. This avoids discharging the shock during the T wave, which may increase ventricular irritability, causing ventricular fibrillation (VF). Charge the defibrillator to the energy level requested, usually starting at a low rate of 120 to 200 joules for biphasic machines.

! NURSING SAFETY PRIORITY QSEN

Critical Rescue

For safety before cardioversion, turn oxygen off and remove from patient; fire could result. Shout "CLEAR" before shock delivery for electrical safety!

After cardioversion, assess the patient's response and heart rhythm. Therapy is repeated, if necessary, until the desired result is obtained or alternative therapies are considered. If the patient's condition deteriorates into VF after cardioversion, check to see that the synchronizer is turned off so immediate defibrillation can be administered.

Nursing care after cardioversion includes:

- Maintaining a patent airway
- Administering oxygen
- Assessing vital signs and the level of consciousness
- Administering antidysrhythmic drug therapy, as prescribed
- Monitoring for dysrhythmias
- Assessing for chest burns from electrodes
- Providing emotional support
- Documenting the results of cardioversion

Left atrial appendage closure. For patients who are at high risk for stroke and who are not candidates for long-term anticoagulation, the left atrial appendage (LAA) occlusion device may be an option (Hijazi & Saw, 2018; January et al., 2019). The LAA is a small sac in the wall of the left atrium. For those with nonvalvular AF, the LAA is the most common site of blood clot development leading to the risk of stroke. Inserted percutaneously via the femoral vein, a device to occlude the LAA is delivered via a transseptal puncture. In the United States, the Watchman (nitinol frame with fenestrated fabric) is the only device approved for use in atrial fibrillation patients. After insertion, anticoagulation with aspirin and warfarin is required. A repeat TEE is performed approximately 45 days after insertion to assess for leaks around the device. If no leak is detected, the warfarin is stopped and antiplatelet therapy is continued. Complications are similar to those for undergoing cardiac ablation procedure.

Radiofrequency catheter ablation. Radiofrequency catheter ablation (RCA) is an invasive procedure that may be used to destroy an irritable focus in atrial or ventricular conduction. The patient must first undergo electrophysiologic studies and mapping procedures to locate the focus. Then radiofrequency waves are delivered to abolish the irritable focus. When ablation is performed in the AV nodal or His bundle area, damage may also occur to the normal conduction system, causing heart blocks and requiring implantation of a permanent pacemaker.

In AF, pulmonary vein isolation and ablation create scar tissue that blocks impulses and disconnects the pathway of the abnormal rhythm. Patients with AF with a rapid ventricular rate not responsive to drug therapy may have AV nodal ablation performed to totally disconnect the conduction from the atria to the ventricles, which requires implantation of a permanent pacemaker. AF ablation should not be performed if long-term anticoagulation is contraindicated.

Biventricular pacing. This type of pacing may be another alternative for patients with heart failure and conduction disorders. Biatrial pacing, antitachycardia pacing, and implantable atrial defibrillators are other methods used to suppress or resolve AF. (See full pacing discussion earlier in this chapter.)

Surgical Interventions. Patients in AF with heart failure (discussed in Chapter 32) may benefit from the *surgical* **maze procedure**, an open-chest surgical technique often performed with coronary artery bypass grafting (CABG). Before this procedure, electrophysiologic mapping studies are done to confirm the diagnosis of AF. The surgeon places a maze of sutures in strategic places in the atrial myocardium, pulmonary artery, and possibly the superior vena cava to prevent electrical circuits from developing and continuing AF. Sinus impulses can then depolarize the atria before reaching the AV node and preserve the atrial kick. Postoperative care is similar to that after other open-heart surgical procedures (see Chapter 35).

The surgical MAZE procedure is being replaced by catheter procedures using a minimally invasive form. The *catheter* maze procedure is done by inserting a catheter through a leg vein into the atria and dragging a heated ablating catheter along the atria to create lines (scars) of conduction block. Patients having this minimally invasive form of the procedure have fewer complications, less pain, and a quicker recovery than those with the open, surgical maze procedure.

PATIENT-CENTERED CARE: OLDER ADULT CONSIDERATIONS (QSEN)

Older adults are at increased risk for dysrhythmias because of normal physiologic changes in their cardiac conduction system. The sinoatrial node has fewer pacemaker cells. There is a loss of fibers in the bundle branch system. Therefore older adults are at risk for sinus node dysfunction and may require pacemaker therapy. The most common dysrhythmias are premature atrial contractions, premature ventricular contractions, and atrial fibrillation. Dysrhythmias tend to be more serious in older patients because of underlying heart disease, causing cardiac decompensation. Consequently, blood flow to organs that may already be decreased because of the aging process may be further compromised, leading to multisystem organ dysfunction. See the Patient-Centered Care: Older Adult Considerations: Dysrhythmias box for special considerations for older adults receiving antidysrhythmic therapy.

PATIENT-CENTERED CARE: OLDER ADULT CONSIDERATIONS (QSEN)

Dysrhythmias

Special nursing considerations for the older patient with dysrhythmias are:

- Evaluate the patient with dysrhythmias immediately for the presence of a life-threatening dysrhythmia or hemodynamic deterioration.
- Assess the patient with a dysrhythmia for angina, hypotension, heart failure, and decreased cerebral and renal ***perfusion***.
- Consider these causes of dysrhythmias when taking the patient's history: hypoxia, drug toxicity, electrolyte imbalances, heart failure, and myocardial ischemia or infarction.
- Assess the patient's level of education, hearing, learning style, and ability to understand and recall instructions to determine the best approaches for teaching.
- Assess the patient's ability to read written instructions.
- Teach the patient the generic and trade names of prescribed antidysrhythmic drugs and their purposes, dosage, side effects, and special instructions for use.
- Provide clear written instructions in basic language and easy-to-read print.
- Provide a written drug dosage schedule for the patient, considering all the drugs the patient is taking and possible drug interactions.
- Assess the patient for possible side effects or adverse reactions to drugs, considering age and health status.
- Teach the patient to take his or her pulse and to report significant changes in heart rate or rhythm to the primary health care provider.
- Inform the patient of available resources for blood pressure and pulse checks, such as blood pressure clinics, home health agencies, and cardiac rehabilitation programs.
- Instruct the patient about the importance of keeping follow-up appointments with the primary health care provider and reporting symptoms promptly.
- Include the patient's family members or significant other in all teaching whenever possible.
- Teach the patient to avoid drinking caffeinated beverages, stop smoking, drink alcohol only in moderation, and follow his or her prescribed diet.

Care Coordination and Transition Management

Home Care. Patients discharged from the hospital may have considerable needs, often more related to their underlying chronic diseases than to their dysrhythmia. A case manager or care coordinator can assess the need for health care resources and coordinate access to services.

The focus of home care is often nursing assessment and health teaching. The community-based nurse provides the patient and family members with an opportunity to verbalize their concerns and fears. Provide emotional support and referrals for ongoing care in the community. Assess the patient for possible side effects of antidysrhythmic agents or anticoagulation therapy.

Self-Management Education. Patients and their families must have a thorough understanding of the prescribed *medication therapy*, including antidysrhythmic and anticoagulant agents. Pharmacies provide written instructions with filled prescriptions. Teach patients and families the generic and trade names of their drugs and the drugs' purposes, using basic terms that are easily understood. Clear instructions regarding dosage schedules and common side effects are important (see the Common Examples of Drug Therapy: Antidysrhythmic Medication box). Emphasize the importance of reporting these side effects and any dizziness, nausea, vomiting, chest discomfort, or shortness of breath to the primary care provider. Be sure to include education that medication should not be stopped abruptly unless instructed by the primary health care provider. Teach the patient the signs and symptoms of bleeding. Advise patients to call the provider if any signs of bleeding are identified.

Teach all patients and their family members how to take a pulse and blood pressure. Some patients may want to use technology to calculate and record their pulse rate. Several applications (apps) for handheld mobile devices (such as the iPhone) are available, but their accuracy varies. "Instant Heart Rate" and "Quick Heart Rate" are examples of apps used to calculate pulse rate. Recently, Apple released an update to the Apple watch that includes an ECG app specifically designed to detect atrial fibrillation. The device is FDA cleared for over-the-counter use to help identify (not diagnose) atrial fibrillation (U.S. Food and Drug Administration, 2018).

Remind patients to report any signs of a change in heart rhythm, such as a significant decrease in pulse rate, a rate more than 100 beats/min, or increased rhythm irregularity. Smart Blood Pressure (SmartBP) is a blood pressure and pulse-management system that records, tracks, and analyzes data to share via an iPhone or iPad. The patient can send these readings to his or her primary health care provider as needed to maintain frequent vital sign monitoring. See the Patient and Family Education: Preparing for Self-Management: How to Prevent or Decrease Dysrhythmias box for patient and family education.

Health Care Resources. The cardiac rehabilitation nurse typically provides written and oral information about dysrhythmias, antidysrhythmic drugs, and anticoagulant drugs. In addition, information about cardiac exercise programs, educational programs, and support groups is provided. The office or ambulatory care nurse may also provide information about resources. Teach the patient how to contact the local chapter of the American Heart Association (www.americanheart.org) or the provincial chapter of the Heart and Stroke Foundation in Canada (www.heartandstroke.ca) for information about dysrhythmias, pacemakers, and CPR training.

◆ **Evaluation: Evaluate Outcomes.** Evaluate the care of the patient with AF on the basis of the identified patient problems. The expected outcomes include that the patient will:

- Remain free of embolus formation associated with AF
- Remain free of heart failure with regular heart rate and rhythm

PATIENT AND FAMILY EDUCATION: PREPARING FOR SELF-MANAGEMENT

How to Prevent or Decrease Dysrhythmias

For Patients at Risk for Vasovagal Attacks Causing Bradydysrhythmias

- Avoid doing things that stimulate the vagus nerve, such as raising your arms above your head, applying pressure over your carotid artery, applying pressure on your eyes, bearing down or straining during a bowel movement, and stimulating a gag reflex when brushing your teeth or putting objects in your mouth.

For Patients With Premature Beats and Ectopic Rhythms

- Take the medications that have been prescribed for you and report any adverse effects to your health care provider.
- Stop smoking, avoid caffeinated beverages and energy drinks as much as possible, and drink alcohol only in moderation.
- Learn ways to manage stress and avoid getting too tired.

For Patients With Ischemic Heart Disease

- If you have an angina attack, treat it promptly with rest and nitroglycerin administration as prescribed by your health care provider. This decreases your chances of experiencing a dysrhythmia.
- If chest pain is not relieved after taking the amount of nitroglycerin that has been prescribed for you, seek medical attention promptly. Also seek prompt medical attention if the pain becomes more severe or you experience other symptoms, such as sweating, nausea, weakness, and palpitations.

For Patients at Risk for Potassium Imbalance

- Know the symptoms of decreased potassium levels, such as muscle weakness and cardiac irregularity.
- Eat foods high in potassium, such as tomatoes, beans, prunes, avocados, bananas, strawberries, and lettuce.
- Take the potassium supplements that have been prescribed for you.

VENTRICULAR DYSRHYTHMIAS

Ventricular dysrhythmias are potentially more life threatening than atrial dysrhythmias because the left ventricle pumps oxygenated blood throughout the body to perfuse vital organs and other tissues. The most common or life-threatening ventricular dysrhythmias include (Al-Khatib et al., 2018):

- Premature ventricular complexes
- Ventricular tachycardia
- Ventricular fibrillation
- Ventricular asystole

Premature Ventricular Complexes: Pathophysiology Review

Premature ventricular complexes (PVCs), also called *premature ventricular contractions,* result from increased irritability of ventricular cells and are seen as early ventricular complexes followed by a pause. When multiple PVCs are present, the QRS complexes may be unifocal or uniform, meaning that they are of the same shape (Fig. 31.12A), or multifocal or multiform, meaning that they are of different shapes (Fig. 31.12B). PVCs frequently occur in repetitive rhythms, such as bigeminy (two), trigeminy (three), and quadrigeminy (four). Two sequential PVCs are a pair, or couplet. Three or more successive PVCs are usually called *nonsustained ventricular tachycardia (NSVT).*

Premature ventricular contractions are common, and their frequency increases with age. They may be insignificant or may occur with problems such as myocardial infarction, chronic heart failure, chronic obstructive pulmonary disease (COPD), and anemia. PVCs may also be present in patients with hypokalemia or hypomagnesemia. Sympathomimetic agents, anesthesia drugs, stress, nicotine, caffeine, alcohol, infection, or surgery can also cause PVCs, especially in older adults. Postmenopausal women often find that caffeine causes palpitations and PVCs.

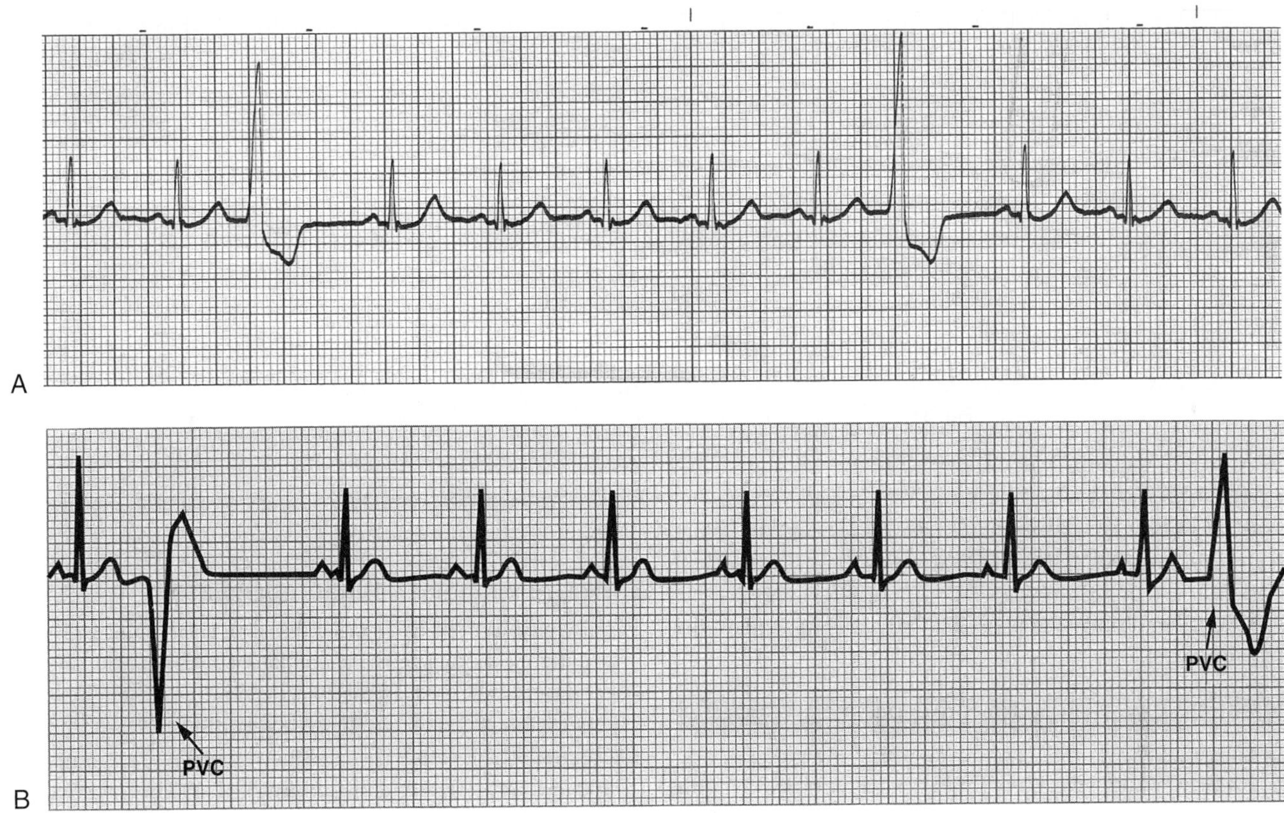

Fig. 31.12 Premature ventricular contractions. A, Normal sinus rhythm with unifocal premature ventricular complexes (PVCs). B, Normal sinus rhythm with multifocal PVCs (one negative and the other positive).

Interprofessional Collaborative Care

The patient may be asymptomatic or experience palpitations or chest discomfort caused by increased stroke volume of the normal beat after the pause. Peripheral pulses may be diminished or absent with the PVCs themselves because the decreased stroke volume of the premature beats may *decrease peripheral perfusion.*

NURSING SAFETY PRIORITY (QSEN)

Action Alert

Because other dysrhythmias can cause widened QRS complexes, assess whether the premature complexes perfuse to the extremities. Palpate the carotid, brachial, or femoral arteries while observing the monitor for widened complexes or auscultating apical heart sounds. With acute MI, PVCs may be considered a warning, possibly triggering life-threatening ventricular tachycardia (VT) or ventricular fibrillation (VF).

If there is no underlying heart disease, PVCs are not usually treated other than by eliminating or managing any contributing cause (e.g., caffeine, stress). Potassium or magnesium is given for replacement therapy if hypokalemia or hypomagnesemia is the cause. If the number of PVCs in a 24-hour period is excessive, the patient may be placed on beta-adrenergic blocking agents (beta blockers) (see the Common Examples of Drug Therapy: Antidysrhythmic Medication box).

NCLEX EXAMINATION CHALLENGE 31.2

Physiological Integrity

The nurse is caring for client who is experiencing occasional premature ventricular contractions. What assessment data are **most** concerning to the nurse?

A. Potassium 4.8 mEq/L
B. Magnesium 2 mEq/L
C. Heart rate 90
D. History of smoking

Ventricular Tachycardia: Pathophysiology Review

Ventricular tachycardia (VT), sometimes referred to as *V tach,* occurs with repetitive firing of an irritable ventricular ectopic focus, usually at a rate of 140 to 180 beats/min or more (Fig. 31.13). VT may result from increased automaticity or a re-entry mechanism. It may be intermittent (nonsustained VT) or sustained, lasting longer than 15 to 30 seconds. The sinus node may continue to discharge independently, depolarizing the atria but not the ventricles, although P waves are seldom seen in sustained VT.

Interprofessional Collaborative Care

Ventricular tachycardia may occur in patients with ischemic heart disease, MI, cardiomyopathy, hypokalemia, hypomagnesemia, valvular heart disease, heart failure, drug toxicity (e.g., steroids), or hypotension. Patients who use cocaine or

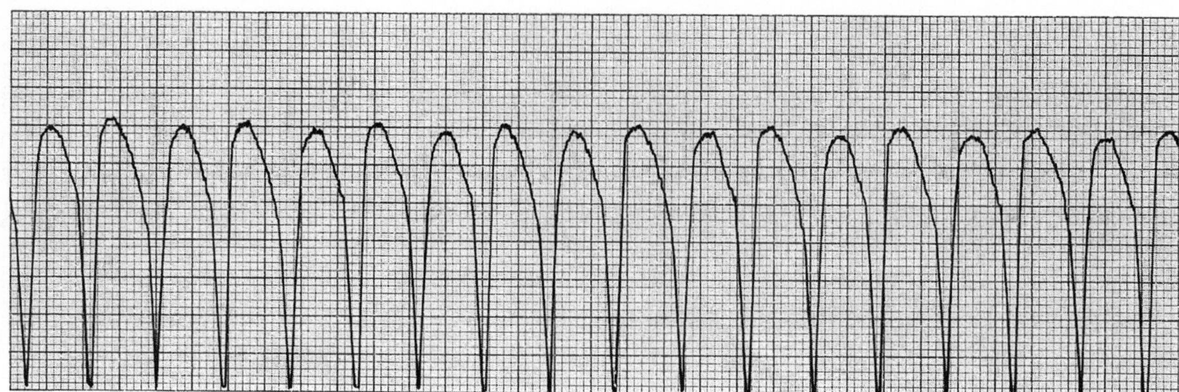

Fig. 31.13 Sustained ventricular tachycardia at a rate of 166 beats/min.

illicit inhalants are at a high risk for VT. *In patients who go into cardiac arrest, VT is commonly the initial rhythm before deterioration into ventricular fibrillation (VF) as the terminal rhythm!*

Signs and symptoms of sustained VT partially depend on the ventricular rate. Slower rates are better tolerated.

! NURSING SAFETY PRIORITY (QSEN)

Critical Rescue

In some patients, VT causes cardiac arrest. Assess the patient's circulation and airway, breathing, level of consciousness, and oxygenation level. For the *stable* patient with sustained VT, administer oxygen and confirm the rhythm via a 12-lead ECG. Amiodarone or lidocaine may be prescribed.

Current Advanced Cardiac Life Support (ACLS) guidelines state that elective cardioversion is highly recommended for stable VT. The primary health care provider may prescribe an oral antidysrhythmic agent to prevent further occurrences. If the patient has been taking digoxin, the drug is withheld for up to 48 hours before an elective cardioversion. Digoxin increases ventricular irritability and puts the patient at risk for VF after the countershock. Patients who persist with episodes of stable VT may require radiofrequency catheter ablation. *Unstable* VT without a pulse is treated the same way as ventricular fibrillation, as described in the following paragraphs.

Ventricular Fibrillation: Pathophysiology Review

Ventricular fibrillation (VF), sometimes called *V fib,* is the result of electrical chaos in the ventricles and is *life threatening!* Impulses from many irritable foci fire in a totally disorganized manner, so ventricular contraction cannot occur. There are no recognizable ECG deflections (Fig. 31.14A). The ventricles merely quiver, consuming a tremendous amount of oxygen. *There is no cardiac output or pulse and therefore no cerebral, myocardial, or systemic* ***perfusion.*** *This rhythm is rapidly fatal if not successfully ended within 3 to 5 minutes.*

VF may be the first manifestation of coronary artery disease (CAD). Patients with myocardial infarction (MI) are at great risk for VF. It may also occur in those with hypokalemia, hypomagnesemia, hemorrhage, drug therapy, rapid supraventricular tachycardia (SVT), or shock. Surgery or trauma may also cause VF.

❖ Interprofessional Collaborative Care

Emergency care for VF is critical for survival. When VF begins, the patient becomes faint, immediately loses consciousness, and becomes pulseless and apneic (no breathing). There is no blood pressure, and heart sounds are absent. Respiratory and metabolic acidosis develop. Seizures may occur. Within minutes, the pupils become fixed and dilated, and the skin becomes cold and mottled. *Death results without prompt intervention.*

The desired outcomes of collaborative care are to resolve VF promptly and convert it to an organized rhythm. *Therefore the priority is to defibrillate the patient immediately according to ACLS protocol.* If a defibrillator is not readily available, high-quality CPR must be initiated and continued until the defibrillator arrives. An automated external defibrillator (AED) is frequently used because it is simple for both medical and lay personnel. Defibrillation is discussed with cardiopulmonary resuscitation later in this chapter.

Drug therapy is used when dysrhythmias are sustained and/or life threatening. Drug therapy from one or more classes of antidysrhythmic agents is often used (see the Common Examples of Drug Therapy: Antidysrhythmic Medication box). The **Vaughn-Williams classification** is commonly used to categorize drugs according to their effects on the action potential of cardiac cells (classes I through IV). Other drugs also have antidysrhythmic effects but do not fit the Vaughn-Williams classification.

Class I antidysrhythmics are membrane-stabilizing agents used to decrease automaticity. The three subclassifications in this group include type IA drugs, which moderately slow conduction and prolong repolarization, prolonging the QT interval. These drugs are used to treat or prevent supraventricular and ventricular premature beats and tachydysrhythmias, but they are not as commonly used as other drugs. An example is procainamide hydrochloride. Type IB drugs shorten repolarization. These drugs are used to treat or prevent ventricular premature beats, ventricular tachycardia (VT), and ventricular fibrillation (VF). Examples include lidocaine and mexiletine hydrochloride. Type IC drugs markedly slow conduction and widen the QRS complex. These agents are used primarily to treat or prevent recurrent, life-threatening ventricular premature beats,

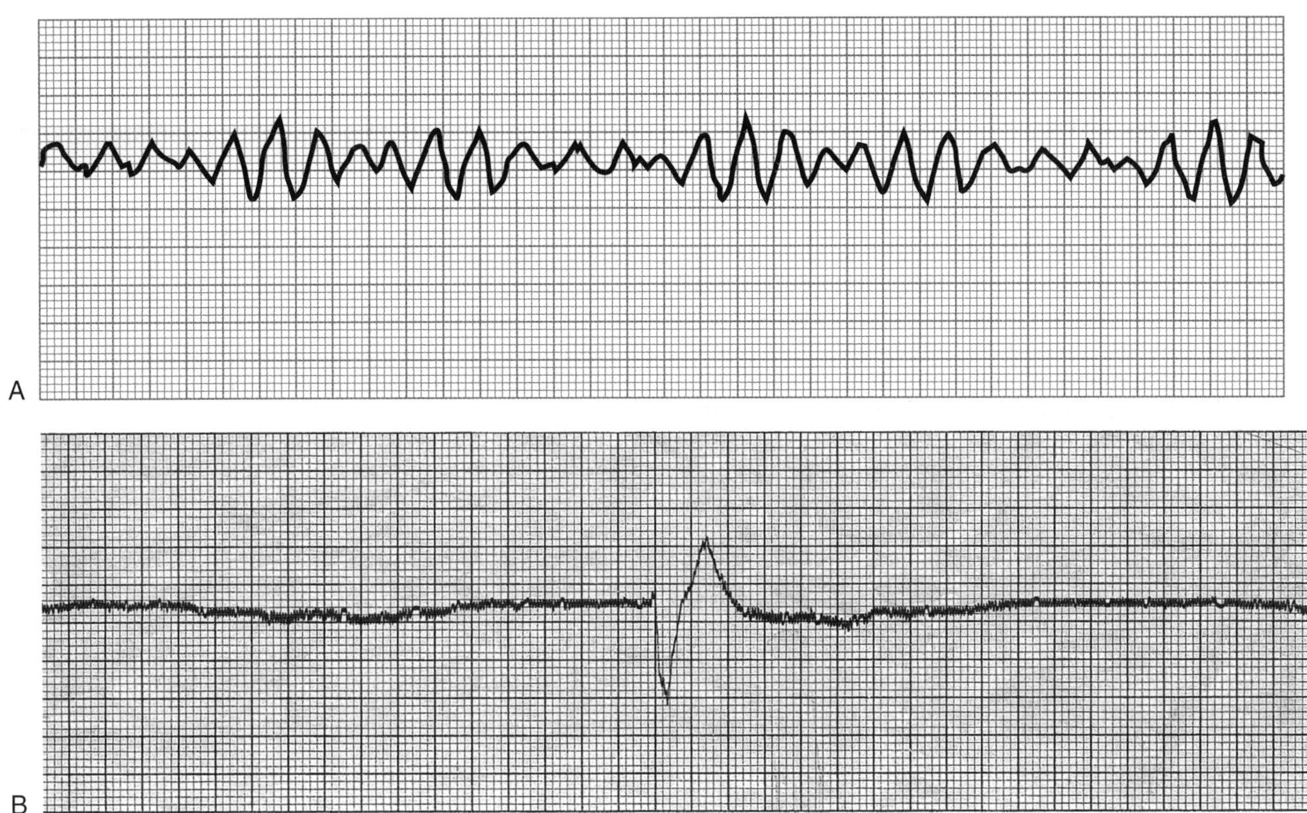

Fig. 31.14 Ventricular dysrhythmias. A, Coarse ventricular fibrillation. B, Ventricular asystole with one idioventricular complex.

VT, and VF. Examples include flecainide acetate and propafenone hydrochloride.

Class II antidysrhythmics control dysrhythmias associated with excessive beta-adrenergic stimulation by competing for receptor sites, thereby decreasing heart rate and conduction velocity. Beta-adrenergic blocking agents, such as propranolol and esmolol hydrochloride, are class II drugs. They are used to treat or prevent supraventricular and ventricular premature beats and tachydysrhythmias. Sotalol hydrochloride is an antidysrhythmic agent with both noncardioselective beta-adrenergic blocking effects (class II) and action potential duration prolongation properties (class III). It is an oral agent that may be used for the treatment of documented ventricular dysrhythmias, such as VT, that are life threatening.

Class III antidysrhythmics lengthen the absolute refractory period and prolong repolarization and the action potential duration of ischemic cells. Class III drugs include amiodarone and ibutilide and are used to treat or prevent ventricular premature beats, VT, and VF.

Class IV antidysrhythmics slow the flow of calcium into the cell during depolarization, thereby depressing the automaticity of the sinoatrial (SA) and atrioventricular (AV) nodes, decreasing the heart rate, and prolonging the AV nodal refractory period and conduction. Calcium channel blockers, such as verapamil hydrochloride and diltiazem hydrochloride, are class IV drugs. They are used to treat supraventricular tachycardia (SVT) and atrial fibrillation (AF) to slow the ventricular response.

Magnesium sulfate is an electrolyte administered to treat refractory VT or VF because these patients may be hypomagnesemic, with increased ventricular irritability. The drug is also used for a life-threatening VT called **torsades de pointes,** which can result from certain antidysrhythmics such as amiodarone.

Ventricular Asystole: Pathophysiology Review

Ventricular asystole, sometimes called *ventricular standstill,* is the complete absence of any ventricular rhythm (Fig. 31.14B). There are no electrical impulses in the ventricles and therefore *no* ventricular depolarization, no QRS complex, no contraction, no cardiac output, and no ***perfusion*** to the rest of the body.

❖ Interprofessional Collaborative Care

◆ **Assessment: Recognize Cues** The patient in ventricular asystole has no pulse, respirations, or blood pressure. *The patient is in full cardiac arrest.* In some cases, the sinoatrial (SA) node may continue to fire and depolarize the atria, with only P waves seen on the ECG. However, the sinus impulses do not conduct to the ventricles, and QRS complexes remain absent. In most cases, the entire conduction system is electrically silent, with no P waves seen on the ECG.

Ventricular asystole usually results from myocardial hypoxia, which may be a consequence of advanced heart failure. It may also be caused by severe hyperkalemia and acidosis. If P waves are seen, asystole is likely because of severe ventricular conduction blocks.

◆ **Interventions: Take Action.** *When cardiac arrest occurs, cardiac output stops.* The underlying rhythm is usually ventricular tachycardia (VT), ventricular fibrillation (VF), or asystole. Without cardiac output, the patient is pulseless and becomes unconscious because of inadequate cerebral ***perfusion*** and gas exchange. Shortly after cardiac arrest, respiratory arrest occurs. Therefore cardiopulmonary resuscitation is essential to prevent brain damage and death.

Cardiopulmonary Resuscitation and Defibrillation. Cardiopulmonary resuscitation (CPR), also known as *Basic Cardiac Life Support (BCLS),* must be initiated immediately when asystole occurs. When finding an unresponsive patient, confirm unresponsiveness and call 911 (in community or long-term care setting) or the emergency response team (in the hospital). Gather the AED or defibrillator *before initiating CPR.* Guidelines for CPR have changed from an ABC (airway-breathing-compressions) approach to the initial priorities of CAB (compressions-airway-breathing) (AHA, 2017; Craig-Brangan & Day, 2019).

- Check for a carotid pulse for 5 to 10 seconds.
- *If carotid pulse is absent,* start chest compressions of 100 to 120 compressions per minute and a compression depth of at least 2 inches with no more than 2.4 inches. Push hard and fast! Avoid leaning into the chest after each compression to allow for full chest wall recoil.
- Maintain a patent **a**irway.
- Ventilate (**b**reathing) with a mouth-to-mask device. Give rescue breaths at a rate of 10 to 12 breaths/min. If an advanced airway is in place, one breath should be given every 6 to 8 seconds (8 to 10 breaths/min).
- Ventilation-to-compression ratio should be maintained at 30 compressions to 2 breaths if advanced airway is not in place.
- Limit interruptions to compressions to less than 10 seconds.
- When possible, compressors should be changed every 2 minutes to maintain effective compressions.

Be sure to use Standard Precautions when administering CPR. Be aware that complications of CPR include:

- Rib fractures
- Fracture of the sternum
- Costochondral separation
- Lacerations of the liver and spleen
- Pneumothorax
- Hemothorax
- Cardiac tamponade
- Lung contusions
- Fat emboli

As soon as help arrives, place a board under the patient who is not on a firm surface. To make room for the resuscitation team and the crash cart, ask that the area be cleared of movable items and unnecessary personnel. When the AED or defibrillator arrives, *do not stop chest compressions while the defibrillator is being set up.* If trained to use the AED or defibrillator, apply hands-off defibrillator pads to the patient's chest and turn on the monitor. If the patient is in VF or pulseless VT, the immediate priority is to defibrillate! **Defibrillation,** an *asynchronous* countershock, depolarizes a critical mass of myocardium simultaneously to stop the re-entry circuit, allowing the sinus node to regain control of the heart. After defibrillation, CPR is resumed. CPR must continue at all times except during defibrillation.

! NURSING SAFETY PRIORITY (QSEN)

Critical Rescue

Early defibrillation is critical in resolving pulseless ventricular tachycardia (VT) or ventricular fibrillation (VF). It must not be delayed for any reason after the equipment and skilled personnel are present. The earlier defibrillation is performed, the greater the chance of survival! *Do not defibrillate ventricular asystole.* The purpose of defibrillation is disruption of the chaotic rhythm. allowing the SA node signals to restart. In ventricular asystole, no electrical impulses are present to disrupt.

Before defibrillation, loudly and clearly command all personnel to clear contact with the patient and the bed and check to see they are clear before the shock is delivered. Deliver shock and immediately resume CPR for 5 cycles or about 2 minutes. Reassess the rhythm every 2 minutes and if indicated. Charge the defibrillator to deliver an additional shock at the same energy level previously used. During the 2-minute intervals while high-quality CPR is being delivered, the Advanced Cardiac Life Support (ACLS) team administers medications and performs interventions to try and restore an organized cardiac rhythm (AHA, 2018). *Discussion of ACLS protocol is beyond the scope of this text.*

NCLEX EXAMINATION CHALLENGE 31.3

Safe and Effective Care

Upon entering a client's room, the nurse finds the client unresponsive. In what order will the nurse provide care?

A. Begin chest compressions
B. Check carotid pulse
C. Notify the Rapid Response Team
D. Get the crash cart/AED
E. Provide rescue breaths

After the ACLS team initiates interventions, the role of the medical-surgical nurse is to provide information about the patient. Specific nursing responsibilities include providing a brief summary of the patient's medical condition and the events that occurred up until the time of cardiac arrest. Report the patient's initial cardiac rhythm. Remain in the room to answer questions, document the event, and assist with compressions. If family is present, provide emotional support and explanation of events in the room.

An emerging clinical practice is allowing or encouraging family presence at resuscitation attempts. This can be a positive experience for family members and significant others because it promotes closure after the death of a loved one. Although there may be staff resistance and some limits to family presence, overall it is a beneficial practice that should be considered in all resuscitation attempts.

When spontaneous circulation resumes, the patient is transported to the intensive care unit. Be ready to hand off a report to the ICU nurse using SBAR communication or another agency system and assist with patient transport.

CLINICAL JUDGMENT CHALLENGE 31.1

Teamwork and Collaboration; Evidence-Based Practice; Safety

A 54-year-old male was found unresponsive at an outdoor concert. An AED was used on site and delivered a shock to the client. He was transferred via emergency medical services to the nearest hospital and admitted to the hospital following the event. Currently the client is in sinus rhythm with frequent PVCs and reports intermittent chest pain and dyspnea. HR is 112, BP 92/48, and oxygen saturation 92% on 2 L of oxygen via nasal cannula.

1. **Recognize Cues:** What assessment information in this client situation is the most important and immediate concern for the nurse? (Hint: Identify the **relevant** information *first* to determine what is most important.)
2. **Analyze Cues:** What client conditions are consistent with the **most relevant** information? (Hint: Think about priority collaborative problems that support and contradict the information presented in this situation.)
3. **Prioritize Hypotheses:** Which possibilities or explanations are **most likely** to be present in this client situation? Which possibilities or explanations are the most serious? (Hint: Consider all possibilities and determine their urgency and risk for this client.)
4. **Generate Solutions:** What activities would most likely achieve the desired outcomes for this client? Which actions should be **avoided** or are **potentially harmful**? (Hint: Determine the desired outcomes first to decide which interventions are appropriate and those that should be avoided.)
5. **Take Action:** Which actions are the most appropriate and how should they be implemented? In what **priority order** should they be implemented? (Hint: Consider health teaching, documentation, requested health care provider orders or prescriptions, nursing skills, collaboration with or referral to health team members, etc.)
6. **Evaluate Outcomes:** What client assessment would indicate the nurse's actions were **effective?** (Hint: Think about signs that would indicate an improvement, decline, or unchanged patient condition.)

Automated External Defibrillation. The American Heart Association promotes the use of automated external defibrillators (AEDs) for use by laypersons and health care professionals responding to cardiac arrest emergencies (Fig. 31.15). These devices are found in many public places such as malls, airports, and commercial jets. The patient in cardiac arrest must be on a firm, dry surface. The rescuer places two large adhesive-patch electrodes on the patient's chest in the same positions as for defibrillator electrodes. The rescuer stops CPR and commands anyone present to move away, ensuring that no one is touching the patient. This measure eliminates motion artifact when the machine analyzes the rhythm. The rescuer presses the "analyze" button on the machine. After rhythm analysis, which may take up to 30 seconds, the machine advises that a shock is either necessary or not indicated. *Shocks are recommended for VF or pulseless VT only.*

If a shock is indicated, issue a command to clear all contact with the patient and press the charge button. Once the AED is charged, press the shock button and the shock will be delivered. The shock is delivered through the patches, so it is hands-off defibrillation, which is safer for the rescuer. The rescuer then resumes CPR until the AED instructs to "stop CPR" to analyze the rhythm. If the rhythm is VF or VT and another shock is indicated, the AED will instruct the rescuer to charge and deliver another shock. Newer AEDs perform rhythm analysis and defibrillation without the need for a rescuer to press a button to analyze or shock the victim. It is essential that Advanced Cardiac Life Support (ACLS) be provided as soon as possible. Use of AEDs allows for earlier defibrillation. Therefore there is a greater chance of successful rhythm conversion and patient survival.

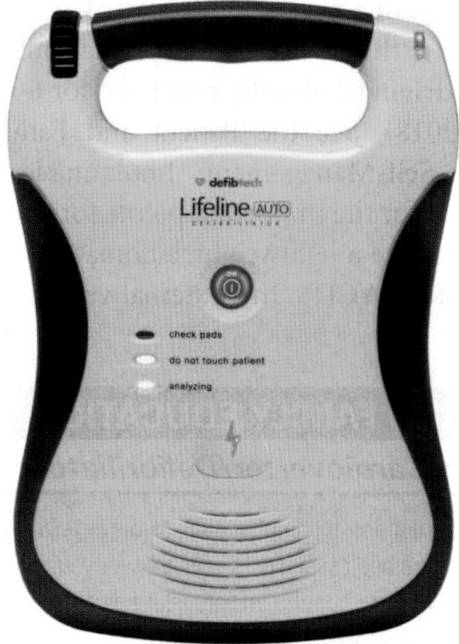

Fig. 31.15 Automated external defibrillator. (Courtesy Defibtech LLC, Guilford, CT.)

Implantable Cardioverter/Defibrillator. The implantable cardioverter/defibrillator (ICD) is indicated for patients who have experienced one or more episodes of spontaneous sustained ventricular tachycardia (VT) or ventricular fibrillation (VF) not caused by a myocardial infarction (MI). Collaborate with the physician and the electrophysiology nurse to prepare the patient for this procedure. A psychological profile is done to determine whether the patient can cope with the discomfort and fear associated with internal defibrillation from the ICD. Many patients report anxiety, depression, and decreased quality of life, which improves for the majority of patients after 12 months.

Two types of lead systems are available: transvenous and subcutaneous. In the traditional transvenous system, the leads are introduced via the subclavian vein and the generator is implanted in the left pectoral area, similar to a permanent pacemaker insertion. In the subcutaneous ICD, the leads are tunneled underneath the skin and placed to the left of the sternum to form a right angle just below the xiphoid, where they attach to the generator. The generator is implanted in the left midaxillary chest wall. The subcutaneous ICD is recommended for younger patients (<40 years), patients without venous access, and patients who do not require concomitant pacemaker therapy. This procedure is performed in the electrophysiology laboratory. If the patient experiences a VT or VF episode after ICD placement and the ICD therapies are not successful, the qualified nurse or health care provider promptly externally defibrillates and initiates high-quality CPR.

The generator may be activated or deactivated by the provider placing a magnet over the implantation site for a few moments. The patient requires close monitoring in the postoperative period for dysrhythmias and complications such as bleeding and cardiac tamponade. The nurse must know whether the ICD is activated or deactivated. Care of the patient is similar to that after implantation of a permanent pacemaker, discussed earlier in this chapter. If the device was implanted following sudden cardiac arrest, driving is usually restricted for 6 months (Brady & MacLeod, 2018). See the Patient and Family Education: Preparing for Self-Management: Implantable Cardioverter/Defibrillator box for the important points for health teaching.

Some patients use a lightweight, automated wearable cardioverter/defibrillator (WCD). This external vestlike device is worn 24 hours a day except when the patient showers or bathes. One popular brand is the Zoll Lifecore LifeVest, which is programmed to monitor for VT and VF. A family member must be present to call 911 and initiate CPR if the patient experiences pulseless VT or VF while in the shower. If the patient is conscious while experiencing VT, he or she can press a button to prevent a shock. This precaution is an advantage over implantable devices because ICDs are programmed to always deliver a shock when VT or VF occurs.

PATIENT AND FAMILY EDUCATION: PREPARING FOR SELF-MANAGEMENT

Implantable Cardioverter/Defibrillator

- Follow the instructions for implantable cardioverter/defibrillator (ICD) site skin care that have been specifically prepared for you.
- Report to your primary health care provider any fever or redness, swelling, soreness, or drainage from your incision site.
- Do not wear tight clothing or belts that could cause irritation over the ICD generator.
- Do not manipulate your generator site.
- Avoid activities that involve rough contact with the ICD implantation site. Activity more vigorous than bowling or golf should be avoided (Brady & MacLeod, 2018).
- Keep your ICD identification card in your wallet and consider wearing a medical alert bracelet.
- Know the basic functioning of your ICD device, its rate cutoff, and the number of consecutive shocks it can deliver.
- Avoid magnets directly over your ICD because they can inactivate the device. If beeping tones are coming from the ICD, move away from the electromagnetic field immediately (within 30 seconds) before the inactivation sequence is completed and notify your primary health care provider.
- Inform all health care providers caring for you that you have an ICD implanted, because certain diagnostic tests and procedures must be avoided to prevent ICD malfunction. These include diathermy, electrocautery, and nuclear magnetic resonance tests.
- Avoid other sources of electromagnetic interference, such as devices emitting microwaves (not microwave ovens); transformers; radio, television, and radar transmitters; large electrical generators; metal detectors, including handheld security devices at airports; antitheft devices; arc welding equipment; and sources of 60-cycle (Hz) interference. Also avoid leaning directly over the alternator of a running motor of a car or boat.
- Most modern wireless communication devices do not interfere with ICD function; however, cell phones should be used on the opposite side from the ICD (Brady & MacLeod, 2018).
- Report to your primary health care provider symptoms such as fainting, nausea, weakness, blackout, and rapid pulse rates.
- Take all medications prescribed as instructed.
- Follow instructions on restrictions on physical activity, such as not swimming, driving motor vehicles, or operating dangerous equipment. Driving is typically restricted for 1 week to allow for healing.
- Keep all health care provider and ICD clinic appointments.
- Sit or lie down immediately if you feel dizzy or faint to avoid falling if the ICD discharges.
- Know how to contact the local emergency medical services (EMS) in your community. Inform them in advance that you have an ICD so that they can be prepared if they need to respond to an emergency call for you.
- Encourage family members to learn how to perform CPR. Family members should know that if they touch you when the device discharges, they may feel a slight but not harmful shock.
- Follow instructions on what to do if the ICD successfully discharges. This may include maintaining a diary of the date, the time, activity preceding the shock, symptoms, the number of shocks delivered, and how you feel after the shock. The health care provider may want to be notified each time the device discharges.
- Avoid strenuous activities that may cause your heart rate to meet or exceed the rate cutoff of your ICD because this causes the device to discharge inappropriately.
- Notify your primary health care provider for information regarding access to health care if you are leaving town or relocating.

GET READY FOR THE NEXT-GENERATION NCLEX® EXAMINATION!

Key Points

Review these Key Points for each NCLEX Examination Client Needs Category.

Safe and Effective Care Environment

- Be very careful to protect patients and staff to prevent electrical injury when assisting with invasive pacemakers, cardioversion, and defibrillation. **QSEN: Safety**
- For safety during cardioversion, turn oxygen off and away from the patient to prevent a fire. Shout "CLEAR" before shock delivery for electrical safety. **QSEN: Safety**
- Teach patients who have permanent pacemakers to wear a medical alert bracelet at all times, and carry a pacemaker identification card. **QSEN: Safety**

Health Promotion and Maintenance

- Teach patients with dysrhythmias the correct drug, dose, route, time, and side effects of prescribed drugs and teach them to notify their primary care provider if adverse effects occur (see the Common Examples of Drug Therapy box).
- Teach patients taking anticoagulant therapy to report any signs of bruising or unusual bleeding immediately to their primary health care provider.
- Teach family members where to learn cardiopulmonary resuscitation (CPR) to decrease their anxiety while living with a patient with dysrhythmias or ICD/pacemaker. **QSEN: Patient-Centered Care**

- Teach patients the importance of adhering to their prescribed cardiac regimen, such as checking their pulse to ascertain pacemaker function.

Physiological Integrity

- Assess patients with dysrhythmias for a decrease in cardiac output resulting in inadequate gas exchange and ***perfusion*** to vital organs. **Clinical Judgment**
- Monitor patients with dysrhythmias, including conducting a physical assessment and health history and interpreting ECG rhythm strips. Report significant changes to the primary health care provider. **Clinical Judgment**
- Interpret common dysrhythmias, especially bradycardia, tachycardia, atrial fibrillation (AF) and ventricular fibrillation (VF), premature ventricular contractions (PVCs), and asystole, using the steps of ECG analysis.
- Identify and intervene in life-threatening situations by providing cardiopulmonary resuscitation, electrical therapy, or drug administration. **QSEN: Evidence-Based Practice**
- Do not perform CPR while the patient is being defibrillated. **QSEN: Safety**
- Educate patients who have permanent pacemakers or ICDs about self-management

MASTERY QUESTIONS

1. While suctioning a client with a tracheostomy, the client becomes diaphoretic and nauseous and the heart rate decreases to 37 beats/min. What is the priority nursing action?
   A. Continue to clear the airway.
   B. Stop suctioning the patient.
   C. Administer atropine.
   D. Call the health care provider immediately.
2. A client in the telemetry unit is on a cardiac monitor. The monitor technician alerts the nurse that there are no ECG complexes, and the alarm is sounding. What is the **first** action by the nurse?
   A. Suspend the alarm.
   B. Call the emergency response team.
   C. Press the record button to get an ECG strip.
   D. Assess the client and check lead placement.
3. The primary health care provider prescribes warfarin for a client with atrial fibrillation. Which client statement indicates that additional education is needed?
   A. "I need to go to the clinic once a week to have my blood level checked."
   B. "If my stools turn black, I will be sure to call my primary health care provider."
   C. "I'm glad I don't need to change my diet. Salads are my favorite food."
   D. "I need to stop taking my herbal supplement."

REFERENCES

Asterisk (*) indicates a classic or definitive work on this subject.

Al-Khatib, S. M., Stevenson, W. G., Ackerman, M. J., Bryant, W. J., Callans, D. J., Curtis, A. B., et al. (2018). 2017 AHA/ACC/HRS guideline for management of patients with ventricular arrhythmias and the prevention of sudden cardiac death: A report of the American College of Cardiology foundation/american heart association task force on clinical practice guidelines and the heart rhythm society. *Circulation, 138*, e272–e391. https://doi.org/10.1161/CIR.0000000000000549.

American Heart Association (AHA). (2017). *Highlights of the 2017 American Heart Association focused updates on adult and pediatric basic life support and cardiopulmonary resuscitation quality.* Retrieved from: https://eccguidelines.heart.org/wp-content/uploads/2017/11/2017-Focused-Updates_Highlights.pdf.

American Heart Association (AHA). (2018). *Highlights of the 2018 focused updates to the American Heart Association guidelines for CPR and ECG: Advanced cardiovascular life support and pediatric advanced life support.* Retrieved from: https://eccguidelines.heart.org/wp-content/uploads/2018/10/2018-Focused-Updates_Highlights.pdf.

Brady, D., & MacLeod, C. (2018). Implantable cardioverter-defibrillators in adults. *Nursing 2018 Critical Care, 13*(3), 34–38.

Burchum, J., & Rosenthal, L. (2019). *Lehne's pharmacology for nursing care* (10th ed.). St. Louis: Elsevier.

Craig-Brangan, K., & Day, M. (2019). Update: 2017/2018 AHA BLS, ACLS, and PALS guidelines. *Nursing 2019 Critical Care, 14*(1), 33–35.

Garcia, D., & Crowther, M. (2018). *Management of bleeding in patients receiving direct oral anticoagulants. UpToDate.* Retrieved from: https://www.uptodate.com/contents/management-of-bleeding-in-patients-receiving-direct-oral-anticoagulants.

Hayes, D. (2018). *Permanent cardiac pacing: Overview of devices and indications. UpToDate.* Retrieved from: https://www.uptodate.com/contents/permanent-cardiac-pacing-overview-of-devices-and-indications.

Hijazi, Z., & Saw, J. (2018). *Nonpharmacologic therapy to prevent embolization in patients with AF. UpToDate.* Retrieved from: https://www.uptodate.com/contents/nonpharmacologic-therapy-to-prevent-embolization-in-patients-with-atrial-fibrillation.

January, C., Wann, S., Alpert, J., Calkins, H., Cigarroa, J., Cleveland, J., et al. (2014). 2014 AHA/ACC/HRS Guideline for the management of patients with atrial fibrillation: Executive summary. *Journal of the American College of Cardiology, 64*(21), 2246–2280.

Kusumoto, F. M., Schoenfeld, M. H., Barrett, C., Lee, R., Edgerton, J. R., Marine, J. E., et al. (2019). 2018 ACC/AHA/HRS guideline on the evaluation and management of patients with bradycardia and cardiac conduction delay. *Heart Rhythm*, https://doi.org/10.1016/j.hrthm.2018.10.037.

Morillo, C. A., Banerjee, A., Perel, P., Wood, D., & Jouven, X. (2017). Atrial fibrillation: The current epidemic. *Journal of Geriatric Cardiology : JGC, 14*(3), 195–203.

Nickasch, B., Marnocha, S., Grebe, L., Scheelk, H., & Kuehl, C. (2016). 'What do I do next?' Nurses' confusion and uncertainty with ECG monitoring. *Medsurg Nursing, 25*(6), 418–422.

Olshansky, B., & Hayes, D. (2017). *Patient education: Pacemakers (Beyond the basics). UpToDate.* Retrieved from: https://www.uptodate.com/contents/pacemakers-beyond-the-basics.

Palatinus, J., & Das, S. (2015). Your father and grandfather's atrial fibrillation: A review of the genetics of the most common pathological cardiac dysrhythmia. *Current Genomics, 16*(2), 75–81.

*Palmer, B. (2011). Systematic cardiac rhythm strip analysis. *Medsurg Nursing, 20*(2), 96–97.

Prutkin, J. (2018). *ECG tutorial: Basic principles of ECG analysis. UpToDate.* Retrieved from https://www.uptodate.com/contents/ecg-tutorial-basic-principles-of-ecg-analysis.

Short, K., & Chung, Y. (2019). Solving alarm fatigue with smartphone technology. *Nursing, 49*(1), 52–57.

The Joint Commission. (2020). *National patient safety goals effective January 2019.* Retrieved from https://www.jointcommission.org/-/media/tjc/documents/standards/national-patient-safety-goals/npsg_chapter_hap_jan2020.pdf.

Townsend, T. (2018). Five common permanent cardiac pacemaker complications. *Nursing 2018 Critical Care, 13*(3).

Urden, L., Stacy, K., & Lough, M. (2018). *Priorities in critical care nursing* (8th ed.). St. Louis: Elsevier.

U.S. Food and Drug Administration. (2018). *De Novo request for classification of ECG device. Letter.* Retrieved from: https://www.accessdata.fda.gov/cdrh_docs/pdf18/DEN180044.pdf.

32

Concepts of Care for Patients With Cardiac Problems

Laura M. Dechant, Nicole M. Heimgartner

http://evolve.elsevier.com/Iggy/

LEARNING OUTCOMES

1. Collaborate with the interprofessional team to provide high-quality care for patients with cardiac problems that impact ***perfusion*** and ***gas exchange.***
2. Teach the patient and caregiver(s) about home safety affected by cardiac problems.
3. Prioritize evidence-based care for patients with common cardiac problems affecting ***perfusion.***
4. Plan care coordination and transition management for patients and caregiver(s) with cardiac problems.
5. Teach the patient and caregiver(s) about drug therapy used for cardiac problems.
6. Implement patient and family-centered nursing interventions to decrease the psychosocial impact of living with chronic cardiac problems.
7. Apply knowledge of anatomy and physiology to perform an evidence-based assessment for the patient with a cardiovascular problem.
8. Explain how common drug therapies improve cardiac output, enhance peripheral perfusion, and prevent worsening cardiovascular problems.
9. Plan nursing care to promote ***perfusion*** and prevent complications such as altered ***gas exchange, pain,*** and ***infection*** in patients with cardiovascular problems.
10. Use clinical judgment to assess laboratory data and signs and symptoms to prioritize nursing care for patients with a cardiovascular problem.
11. Plan postoperative care for patients requiring cardiovascular surgery.
12. Provide emergency care for patients experiencing life-threatening complications, such as cardiac tamponade and pulmonary edema.

KEY TERMS

acute pericarditis An inflammation or alteration of the pericardium, the membranous sac that encloses the heart; may be fibrous, serous, hemorrhagic, purulent, or neoplastic.

afterload The pressure or resistance that the ventricles must overcome to eject blood through the semilunar valves and into the peripheral blood vessels; the amount of resistance is directly related to blood pressure and blood vessel diameter.

aortic regurgitation The flow of blood from the aorta back into the left ventricle during diastole; occurs when the valve leaflets do not close properly during diastole and annulus (the valve ring that attaches to the leaflets) is dilated or deformed.

aortic stenosis Narrowing of the aortic valve orifice and obstruction of left ventricular outflow during systole.

B-type natriuretic peptide (BNP) A peptide produced and released by the ventricles when the patient has fluid overload as a result of heart failure.

cardiac resynchronization therapy (CRT) In patients with some types of heart failure, the use of a permanent pacemaker alone or in combination with an implantable cardioverter-defibrillation (ICD) to provide biventricular pacing.

cardiac tamponade Compression of the myocardium by fluid that has accumulated around the heart; this compresses the atria and the ventricles, prevents them from filling adequately, and reduces cardiac output.

cardiomegaly Enlargement of the heart.

cardiomyopathy A subacute or chronic disease of cardiac muscle; classified into four categories based on abnormalities in structure and function: dilated, hypertrophic, restrictive, and arrhythmogenic.

diastolic heart failure Heart failure that occurs when the left ventricle is unable to relax adequately during diastole, which prevents the ventricle from filling with enough blood to ensure adequate cardiac output.

dilated cardiomyopathy Inability of the heart to pump effectively due to enlargement (dilation) and weakening of the ventricles.

ejection fraction Percentage of blood ejected from the left ventricle with each contraction.

exertional dyspnea Breathlessness or difficulty breathing that develops during activity or exertion.

heart failure A general term for the inadequacy of the heart to pump blood throughout the body, causing insufficient perfusion of body tissues with vital nutrients and oxygen.

hemodynamic monitoring Continuous monitoring of the movement of blood and pressures within the veins, arteries, and chambers of the heart; invasive hemodynamic monitoring is the use of a specialized catheter inserted into the heart to continuously monitor pulmonary pressures, central venous pressure, and left atrial pressure.

high output heart failure Failure of the heart due to high peripheral demand with a cardiac output that is higher than normal.

hypertrophic cardiomyopathy Inability of the heart to pump blood effectively due to thickening (hypertrophy) of the heart muscle.

infective endocarditis A microbial infection (e.g., viruses, bacteria, fungi) involving the endocardium.

mitral regurgitation Inability of the mitral valve to close completely during systole, which allows the backflow of blood into the left atrium when the ventricle contracts.

mitral stenosis Thickening of the mitral valve due to fibrosis and calcification. The valve leaflets fuse and become stiff, and the valve opening narrows, which prevents normal blood flow from the left atrium to the left ventricle.

mitral valve prolapse Dysfunction of the mitral valve that occurs because the valvular leaflets enlarge and prolapse into the left atrium during systole.

myocardial hypertrophy Enlargement of the cardiac muscle.

orthopnea Shortness of breath that occurs when lying down but is relieved by sitting up.

paradoxical pulse An exaggerated decrease in systolic blood pressure by more than 10 mm Hg during the inspiratory phase of the respiratory cycle (normal is 3 to 10 mm Hg); indicative of cardiac tamponade, constrictive pericarditis, and pulmonary hypertension; also referred to as *pulsus paradoxus.*

paroxysmal nocturnal dyspnea In the patient with heart disease, shortness of breath that develops after lying down for several hours and causes the patient to awaken abruptly with a feeling of suffocation and panic.

pericardial effusion Accumulation of fluid in the pericardial space.

pericardiocentesis Withdrawal of pericardial fluid through a catheter inserted into the pericardial space to relieve the pressure on the heart.

petechiae Pinpoint, red or purple spots on the mucous membranes, palate, conjunctivae, or skin caused by bleeding within the dermal or submucosal layers.

pulsus alternans A type of pulse in which a weak pulse alternates with a strong pulse despite a regular heart rhythm; seen in patients with severely depressed cardiac function.

restrictive cardiomyopathy Inability of the heart to pump effectively due to restrictive filling of the ventricles.

right-sided heart (ventricular) failure The inability of the right ventricle to empty completely, resulting in increased volume and pressure in the systemic veins and systemic venous congestion with peripheral edema.

S3 gallop The third heart sound; an early diastolic filling sound that indicates an increase in left ventricular pressure and may be heard on auscultation in patients with heart failure.

splinter hemorrhage Black, longitudinal line or small red streak on the distal third of the nail bed; seen in patients with infective endocarditis.

systolic heart failure Heart failure that results when the heart is unable to contract forcefully enough during systole to eject adequate amounts of blood into circulation.

ventricular assist device (VAD) Mechanical pump that is surgically inserted with external power source that supports the function of the ventricles and heart.

PRIORITY AND INTERRELATED CONCEPTS

The priority concept for this chapter is:
- ***Perfusion***

The ***Perfusion*** concept exemplar for this chapter is Heart Failure.

The interrelated concepts for this chapter are:
- ***Gas Exchange***
- ***Comfort***
- ***Infection***

Heart failure is the most common reason for hospital stays in patients over 65 years of age in the United States. When the heart is diseased, it cannot effectively pump an adequate amount of arterial blood to the rest of the body. Arterial blood carries *oxygen* and nutrients to vital organs, such as the kidneys and brain, and to peripheral tissues. When these organs and other body tissues are not adequately *perfused,* they may not function properly. This chapter focuses on heart failure and its common causes in the adult population; coronary artery disease is discussed in Chapter 35.

PERFUSION CONCEPT EXEMPLAR: HEART FAILURE

Heart failure, also called *pump failure,* is a general term for the inability of the heart to work effectively as a pump. It results from a number of acute and chronic cardiovascular problems that are discussed in this chapter and within the cardiovascular unit.

Pathophysiology Review

Heart failure (HF) is a common *chronic* health problem, with acute episodes often causing hospitalization. Acute coronary disease and other structural or functional problems of the heart can lead to *acute* HF. Both acute and chronic HF can be life threatening if they are not adequately treated or if the patient does not respond to treatment.

Types of Heart Failure. The major types of heart failure are:

- Left-sided heart failure
- Right-sided heart failure
- High-output failure

Because the two ventricles of the heart represent two separate pumping systems, it is possible for one to fail by itself for a short period. *Most heart failure begins with failure of the left ventricle and progresses to failure of both ventricles.* Typical causes of **left-sided heart (ventricular) failure** include hypertension, coronary artery disease, and valvular disease. Decreased tissue ***perfusion*** from poor cardiac output and pulmonary congestion from increased pressure in the pulmonary vessels indicate left ventricular failure (LVF).

Left-sided heart failure was formerly referred to as *congestive heart failure (CHF);* however, not all cases of LVF involve fluid accumulation. In the clinical setting, though, the term *CHF* is still used. Left-sided failure may be acute or chronic and mild to severe. It can be further divided into two subtypes: systolic heart failure and diastolic heart failure.

Systolic heart failure (heart failure with reduced ejection fraction [HFrEF]) results when the heart cannot contract forcefully enough during systole to eject adequate amounts of blood into the circulation. Preload increases with decreased contractility, and afterload increases as a result of increased peripheral resistance (e.g., hypertension) (McCance & Huether, 2019). The **ejection fraction** (the percentage of blood ejected from the heart during systole) drops from a normal of 50% to 70% to below 40% with ventricular dilation. As it decreases, tissue ***perfusion*** diminishes and blood accumulates in the pulmonary vessels. Manifestations of systolic dysfunction may include symptoms of inadequate tissue ***perfusion*** or pulmonary and systemic congestion. Systolic heart failure is often called *forward failure* because cardiac output is decreased and fluid backs up into the pulmonary system. Because these patients are at high risk for sudden cardiac death, patients with an ejection fraction of less than 30% are considered candidates for an implantable cardioverter/defibrillator (ICD) (see Chapter 31).

In contrast, **diastolic heart failure** (heart failure with preserved left ventricular function [HFpEF]) occurs when the left ventricle cannot relax adequately during diastole. Inadequate relaxation or "stiffening" prevents the ventricle from filling with sufficient blood to ensure an adequate cardiac output. Although ejection fraction is more than 40%, the ventricle becomes less compliant over time because more pressure is needed to move the same amount of volume compared with a healthy heart. Diastolic failure represents about 20% to 40% of all heart failure, primarily in older adults and in women who have chronic hypertension and undetected coronary artery disease. Signs and symptoms and management of diastolic failure are similar to those of systolic dysfunction (McCance & Huether, 2019).

Right-sided heart (ventricular) failure may be caused by left ventricular failure, right ventricular myocardial infarction (MI), or pulmonary hypertension. In this type of heart failure (HF), the right ventricle cannot empty completely. Increased volume and pressure develop in the venous system, and peripheral edema results.

High-output heart failure can occur when cardiac output remains normal or above normal, unlike left- and right-sided heart failure, which are typically low-output states. High-output failure is caused by increased metabolic needs or hyperkinetic conditions, such as septicemia, high fever, anemia, and hyperthyroidism. This type of heart failure is not as common as other types.

Classification and Staging of Heart Failure. The American College of Cardiology (ACC) and American Heart Association (AHA) have developed evidence-based guidelines for staging and managing heart failure as a chronic, progressive disease. These guidelines do not replace the New York Heart Association (NYHA) functional classification system, which is used to describe symptoms that a patient may exhibit (see Table 30.2 in Chapter 30).

The ACC/AHA staging system when compared with the NYHA system categorizes patients as:

A. Patients at high risk for developing heart failure (Class I NYHA)
B. Patients with cardiac structural abnormalities or remodeling who have not developed HF symptoms (Class I NYHA)
C. Patients with current or prior symptoms of heart failure (Class II or III NYHA)
D. Patients with refractory end-stage heart failure (Class IV NYHA)

Another method for staging heart failure is the Killip classification system, which is based on the heart's hemodynamic ability. Table 35.5 in Chapter 35 outlines this system.

Compensatory Mechanisms. When cardiac output is insufficient to meet the demands of the body, compensatory mechanisms work to improve output (Fig. 32.1). Although these mechanisms may initially increase cardiac output, they eventually have a damaging effect on pump function. Major compensatory mechanisms include:

- Sympathetic nervous system stimulation
- Renin-angiotensin system (RAS) activation (also called *renin-angiotensin-aldosterone [RAAS] activation*)
- Other chemical responses
- Myocardial hypertrophy

In heart failure (HF), *stimulation of the sympathetic nervous system* (i.e., increasing catecholamines) as a result of tissue hypoxia represents the most immediate compensatory mechanism. Stimulation of the adrenergic receptors causes an increase in heart rate (beta adrenergic) and blood pressure from vasoconstriction (alpha adrenergic).

Because cardiac output (CO) is the product of heart rate (HR) and stroke volume (SV), an increase in HR results in an immediate *increase in CO.* The HR is limited, however, in its ability to compensate for decreased CO. If it becomes too rapid, diastolic filling time is limited and CO may start to decline. An increase in HR also significantly increases oxygen demand by the myocardium. If the heart is poorly perfused because of arteriosclerosis, HF may worsen.

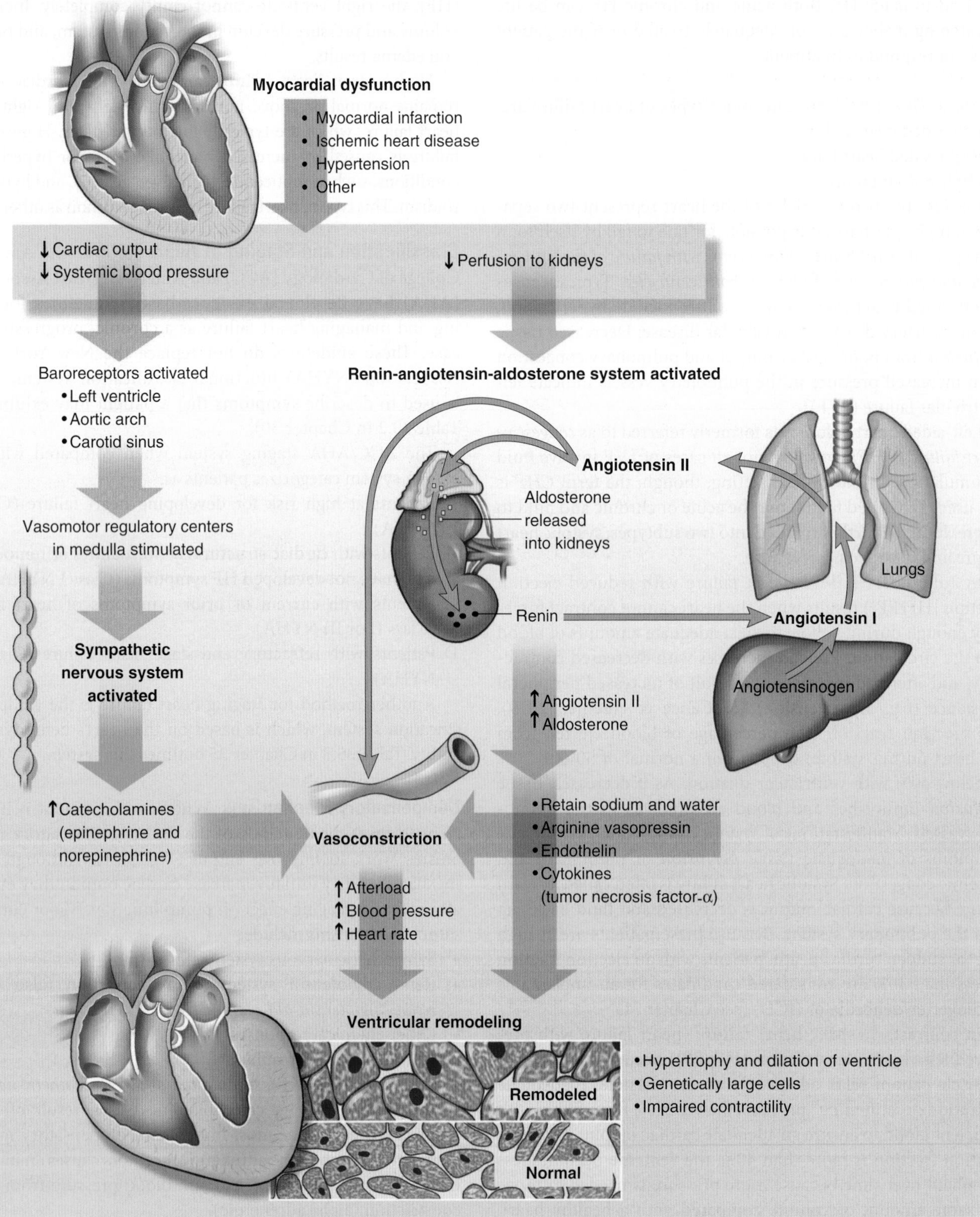

FIG. 32.1 Compensatory mechanisms in heart failure. Myocardial dysfunction activates the renin-angiotensin-aldosterone and sympathetic nervous systems, releasing neurohormones (angiotensin II, aldosterone, catecholamines, and cytokines). (From McCance, K. L., Huether S. E., Brashers, V., & Rote, N. [2019]. *Pathophysiology: The biologic basis for disease in adults and children* [8th ed.]. St. Louis: Mosby. Redrawn from Carelock, J., Clark, A. P. [2001]. *The American Journal of Nursing, 101*[12], 27.)

Stroke volume (SV) is also *improved* by sympathetic stimulation. Sympathetic stimulation increases venous return to the heart, which further stretches the myocardial fibers causing dilation. According to Starling's law, increased myocardial stretch results in more forceful contraction. More forceful contractions increase SV and CO. After a critical point is reached within the cardiac muscle, further volume and stretch reduce the force of contraction and cardiac output.

Sympathetic stimulation also results in *arterial vasoconstriction*. Vasoconstriction has the benefit of maintaining blood pressure and improving tissue ***perfusion*** in low-output states. However, constriction of the arteries increases **afterload**, the resistance against which the heart must pump. Afterload is the major determinant of myocardial oxygen requirements. As it increases, the left ventricle requires more energy to eject its contents and SV may decline.

Reduced blood flow to the kidneys, a common occurrence in low-output states, results in *activation of the renin-angiotensin system (RAS)*. Vasoconstriction becomes more pronounced in response to angiotensin II, and aldosterone secretion causes sodium and water retention. Preload and afterload increase. Angiotensin II contributes to *ventricular remodeling*, resulting in progressive myocyte (myocardial cell) contractile dysfunction over time (McCance & Huether, 2019).

In addition to the sympathetic nervous system and RAS responses, other mechanisms are activated when a patient experiences heart failure (HF). Most of these actions contribute to worsening of the condition.

For example, in those who have had an MI, heart muscle cell injury causes an *immune response*. Proinflammatory cytokines, such as tumor necrosis factor (TNF) and interleukins (IL-1 and IL-6), are released, especially with left-sided HF. These substances contribute to ventricular remodeling.

Natriuretic peptides are neurohormones that work to promote vasodilation and diuresis through sodium loss in the renal tubules. The **B-type natriuretic peptide (BNP)** is produced and released by the ventricles as they stretch in response to fluid overload from HF. BNP levels increase with age and are generally higher in healthy women than healthy men (Pagana & Pagana, 2018).

Low cardiac output (CO) causes decreased cerebral perfusion. As a result, the posterior pituitary gland secretes *vasopressin* (antidiuretic hormone [ADH]). The hormone causes vasoconstriction and fluid retention, which worsen HF.

Endothelin is secreted by endothelial cells when they are stretched. As the myocardial fibers are stretched in patients with HF, this potent vasoconstrictor is released, which increases peripheral resistance and hypertension. HF worsens as a result of these actions.

Myocardial hypertrophy (enlargement of the myocardium), with or without chamber dilation, is another compensatory mechanism. The walls of the heart thicken to provide more muscle mass, which results in more forceful contractions, further increasing CO. However, cardiac muscle may hypertrophy more rapidly than collateral circulation can provide adequate blood supply to the muscle. Often a hypertrophied heart is slightly oxygen deprived.

All the compensatory mechanisms contribute to an increase in the consumption of myocardial oxygen. When the demand for oxygen increases and the myocardial reserve has been exhausted, signs and symptoms of HF develop.

Etiology. Heart failure (HF) is caused by systemic hypertension in most cases. Some patients experiencing myocardial infarction (MI, "heart attack") also develop HF. The next most common cause is structural heart changes, such as valvular dysfunction, particularly pulmonic or aortic stenosis, which leads to pressure or volume overload on the heart. Common direct causes and risk factors for HF are listed in Table 32.1.

PATIENT-CENTERED CARE: OLDER ADULT CONSIDERATIONS QSEN

Heart failure is a common problem among older adults. The use of certain drugs can contribute to the development or exacerbation of the problem in this population. For example, long-term use of NSAIDs for arthritis and other persistent (chronic) pain can cause fluid and sodium retention. NSAIDs may cause peripheral vasoconstriction and increase the toxicity of diuretics and angiotensin-converting enzyme inhibitors (ACEIs). Thiazolidinediones (TZDs) (e.g., pioglitazone used for patients with diabetes) also cause fluid and sodium retention.

Right-sided HF in the absence of left-sided HF is usually the result of pulmonary problems such as chronic obstructive pulmonary disease (COPD) or pulmonary hypertension. Acute respiratory distress syndrome (ARDS) may also cause right-sided HF. These problems are discussed elsewhere in this text.

Incidence and Prevalence. Over 6.5 million people in the United States have HF, and it is projected that this number will increase to over 8 million people by 2030 (Benjamin et al., 2018). HF is the most common reason for hospital admission for people older than 65 years. Heart failure occurs in African Americans younger than age 50 more often than Euro-Americans because they have more risk factors that can lead to HF (Benjamin et al., 2018). The disease is a major cause of disability and death after MI, often because of nonadherence to the treatment plan and recommended lifestyle changes.

PATIENT-CENTERED CARE: OLDER ADULT CONSIDERATIONS QSEN

Heart failure has been referred to as a U.S. epidemic, although it is a major problem worldwide. One of the U.S. *Healthy People 2020* objectives is to reduce the number of hospitalizations of older adults with HF as the principal diagnosis. Patient and family education can help meet this objective (Table 32.2). As the "baby boomer" population reaches 65 years of age, the number of hospital stays and deaths from HF are likely to increase dramatically.

❖ Interprofessional Collaborative Care

◆ Assessment: Recognize Cues

History. When obtaining a history, keep in mind the many conditions that can lead to HF. Carefully question the patient about his or her medical history, including hypertension, angina (cardiac pain), MI, rheumatic heart disease, valvular disorders, endocarditis, and pericarditis. Ask about the patient's perception of his or her activity tolerance, breathing pattern,

TABLE 32.1 Common Causes and Risk Factors for Heart Failure

- Hypertension
- Coronary artery disease
- Cardiomyopathy
- Substance abuse (alcohol and illicit/prescribed drugs)
- Valvular disease
- Congenital defects
- Cardiac infections and inflammations
- Dysrhythmias
- Diabetes mellitus
- Smoking/tobacco use
- Family history
- Obesity
- Severe lung disease
- Sleep apnea
- Hyperkinetic conditions (e.g., hyperthyroidism)

TABLE 32.2 Meeting Healthy People 2020 Objectives

Cardiac Disease

To reduce hospitalizations of older adults with heart failure as the principal diagnosis:

- For patients hospitalized for heart failure, collaborate with the case manager for discharge planning, including adequate support in the community.
- Provide a continuing plan of care for patients and their families or other caregivers when the patient is discharged from the hospital.
- If the patient is discharged to home, call to check that he or she has no impending signs and symptoms of heart failure (the case manager may make calls).
- Teach the patient and family or other caregiver about when to call the health care provider for health changes so that the patient can be treated at home.
- Ensure that the interprofessional team provides the patient with follow-up care in the home or nursing home.

sleeping pattern, urinary pattern, and fluid volume status and his or her knowledge about HF.

Left-Sided Heart Failure. With left ventricular systolic dysfunction, cardiac output (CO) is diminished, leading to impaired tissue ***perfusion,*** anaerobic metabolism, and unusual fatigue. Assess activity tolerance by asking whether the patient can perform normal ADLs or climb flights of stairs without fatigue or dyspnea. Many patients with heart failure (HF) experience weakness or fatigue with activity or have a feeling of heaviness in their arms or legs. Ask about their ability to perform simultaneous arm and leg work (e.g., walking while carrying a bag of groceries). Such activity may place an unacceptable demand on the failing heart. Ask the patient to identify his or her most strenuous activity in the past week. Many people unconsciously limit their activities in response to fatigue or dyspnea and may not realize how limited they have become.

Perfusion to the myocardium is often impaired as a result of left ventricular failure, especially with cardiac hypertrophy. The patient may report *chest pain* or may describe palpitations, skipped beats, or a fast heartbeat.

As the amount of blood ejected from the left ventricle diminishes, hydrostatic pressure builds in the pulmonary venous system and results in fluid-filled alveoli and pulmonary congestion, which results in a *cough.* The patient in early HF describes the cough as irritating, nocturnal (at night), and usually nonproductive. *As HF becomes very severe, he or she may begin expectorating frothy, pink-tinged sputum—a sign of life-threatening pulmonary edema.*

Dyspnea also results from increasing pulmonary venous pressure and pulmonary congestion. Carefully question about the presence of dyspnea and how it developed. The patient may refer to dyspnea as "trouble catching my breath," "breathlessness," or "difficulty breathing."

As **exertional dyspnea** develops (also called *dyspnea upon* or *on exertion [DUE/DOE]),* the patient often stops previously tolerated levels of activity because of shortness of breath. Dyspnea at rest in the recumbent (lying flat) position is known as **orthopnea.** Ask how many pillows are used to sleep or whether the patient sleeps in an upright position in a bed, recliner, or other type of chair.

Patients who describe sudden awakening with a feeling of breathlessness 2 to 5 hours after falling asleep have **paroxysmal nocturnal dyspnea (PND).** Sitting upright, dangling the feet, or walking usually relieves this condition.

Right-Sided Heart Failure. Signs of systemic congestion occur as the right ventricle fails, fluid is retained, and pressure builds in the venous system. Edema develops in the lower legs and may progress to the thighs and abdominal wall. Patients may notice that their shoes fit more tightly, or their shoes or socks may leave indentations on their swollen feet. They may have removed their rings because of swelling in their fingers and hands. Ask about weight gain. An adult may retain 4 to 7 L of fluid (10 to 15 lb [4.5 to 6.8 kg]) before pitting edema occurs.

Reports of *nausea and anorexia* may be a direct consequence of liver engorgement (congestion) resulting from fluid retention. In *advanced* heart failure (HF), *ascites* and an increased abdominal girth may develop from severe liver congestion. Another common finding related to fluid retention is *diuresis at rest.* At rest, fluid in the peripheral tissue is mobilized and excreted, and the patient describes frequent awakening at night to urinate.

Obtain a careful nutritional history, questioning about the use of salt and the types of food consumed. Ask about daily fluid intake. Patients with HF may experience increased thirst and drink excessive fluid (4000 to 5000 mL/day) because of sodium retention.

Physical Assessment/Signs and Symptoms. Signs and symptoms of HF depend on the type of failure, the ventricle involved, and the underlying cause. Impaired tissue ***perfusion*** and pulmonary congestion are associated with *left* ventricular failure. (See the Key Features: Left Ventricular Failure box.)

Conversely, systemic venous congestion and peripheral edema are associated with *right* ventricular failure. (See the Key Features: Right Ventricular Failure box.)

KEY FEATURES

Left Ventricular Failure

Decreased Cardiac Output	Pulmonary Congestion
• Fatigue • Weakness • Oliguria during the day (nocturia at night) • Angina • Confusion, restlessness • Dizziness • Tachycardia, palpitations • Pallor • Weak peripheral pulses • Cool extremities	• Hacking cough, worse at night • Dyspnea/breathlessness • Crackles or wheezes in lungs • Frothy, pink-tinged sputum • Tachypnea • S_3/S_4 summation gallop

KEY FEATURES

Right Ventricular Failure

- Systemic congestion
- Jugular (neck vein) distention
- Enlarged liver and spleen
- Anorexia and nausea
- Dependent edema (legs and sacrum)
- Distended abdomen
- Swollen hands and fingers
- Polyuria at night
- Weight gain
- Increased blood pressure (from excess volume) or decreased blood pressure (from failure)

Left-Sided Heart Failure. Left ventricular failure is associated with decreased cardiac output and elevated pulmonary venous pressure. It may appear clinically as:

- Weakness
- Fatigue
- Dizziness
- Acute confusion
- Pulmonary congestion
- Breathlessness
- Oliguria (scant urine output)

Decreased blood flow to the major body organs can cause dysfunction, especially renal failure. Nocturia may occur when the patient is at rest.

The pulse may be tachycardic, or it may alternate in strength (**pulsus alternans**). Take the apical pulse for a full minute, noting any irregularity in heart rhythm. *An irregular heart rhythm resulting from premature atrial contractions (PACs), premature ventricular contractions (PVCs), or atrial fibrillation (AF) is common in HF* (see Chapter 31). The sudden development of an irregular rhythm may further compromise CO. Carefully monitor the patient's respiratory rate, rhythm, and character, as well as oxygen saturation. The respiratory rate typically exceeds 20 breaths/min.

Assess whether the patient is oriented to person, place, and time. A short mental status examination may be used if there are concerns about orientation. Objective assessment is important because many people are skillful at covering up memory loss. Older adults are frequently disoriented or confused when the heart fails as a result of brain hypoxia (decreased oxygen).

Increased heart size is common with a displacement of the apical impulse to the left. A third heart sound, **S3 gallop**, is an early diastolic filling sound indicating an increase in left ventricular pressure. This sound is often the first sign of HF. A fourth heart sound (S_4) can also occur; it is not a sign of failure but rather a reflection of decreased ventricular compliance.

Auscultate for crackles and wheezes of the lungs. Late inspiratory crackles and fine profuse crackles that repeat themselves from breath to breath and do not diminish with coughing indicate HF. *Crackles are produced by intra-alveolar fluid and are often noted first in the bases of the lungs and spread upward as the condition worsens.* Wheezes indicate a narrowing of the bronchial lumen caused by engorged pulmonary vessels. Identify the precise location of crackles and wheezes and whether the wheezes are heard on inspiration, expiration, or both.

Right-Sided Heart Failure. Right ventricular failure is associated with increased systemic venous pressures and congestion. On inspection, assess the neck veins for distention and measure abdominal girth. Hepatomegaly (liver engorgement), hepatojugular reflux, and ascites may also be assessed. Abdominal fluid can reach volumes of more than 10 L. When the fluid accumulates in the abdomen, pressure is placed on the stomach and intestines. This pressure can lead to early satiety and malnutrition.

Assess for dependent edema. In ambulatory patients, edema commonly presents in the ankles and legs. When patients are restricted to bedrest, the sacrum is dependent and fluid accumulates there.

! NURSING SAFETY PRIORITY (QSEN)

Action Alert

Edema is an extremely unreliable sign of HF. Be sure that accurate daily weights are taken to document fluid retention. Assessing weight at the same time of the morning using the same scale is important. *Weight is the most reliable indicator of fluid gain and loss!*

NCLEX EXAMINATION CHALLENGE 32.1

Physiological Integrity

A client is diagnosed with left-sided heart failure. Which client assessment findings will the nurse anticipate? **Select all that apply.**

A. Peripheral edema
B. Crackles in both lungs
C. Tachycardia
D. Ascites
E. Tachypnea
F. S_3 gallop

Psychosocial Assessment. Chronic heart failure (HF) typically is a slow, debilitating disease. Anxiety and frustration are common. Symptoms such as dyspnea increase the patient's anxiety level.

Patients with HF, especially those with advanced disease, are at high risk for depression. It is not certain whether the functional impairments contribute to the depression or depression affects functional ability. Older hospitalized patients may be depressed, particularly those who have been re-admitted for an acute episode of HF. Lifestyle changes and quality-of-life issues can also cause depression many months after the initial diagnosis of HF.

Assess patients and their families for anxiety and depression. Ask them about their usual methods of coping and any history of depression. If anxiety or depression is present, notify the primary health care provider for further assessment. Social workers, certified clinical chaplains, or psychologists may administer specific assessment tools to determine the extent of the problem. Some patients need drug therapy and nonpharmacologic modalities, such as cognitive behavior therapy, biofeedback, or relaxation training.

Hope is a major indicator of well-being for patients with HF. Those who are hopeful tend to feel better and are more socially involved. Ask patients about their daily activities and how often they interact with the significant people in their life to help determine patient and family coping strategies.

Laboratory Assessment. Electrolyte imbalance may occur from complications of HF or as side effects of drug therapy, especially diuretic therapy. Regular evaluations of a patient's serum electrolytes, including sodium, potassium, magnesium, calcium, and chloride, are essential. Any impairment of renal function resulting from inadequate perfusion causes elevated blood urea nitrogen and serum creatinine and decreased creatinine clearance levels. Hemoglobin and hematocrit tests should be performed to identify HF resulting from anemia. If the patient has fluid volume excess, the hematocrit levels may be low as a result of hemodilution.

B-type natriuretic peptide (BNP) is used for diagnosing HF (in particular, diastolic HF) in patients with acute dyspnea. As discussed earlier, it is part of the body's response to decreased cardiac output (CO) from either left or right ventricular dysfunction. An absence of elevation in BNP, in conjunction with history and physical, rules out HF as the cause of acute dyspnea and points to a primary lung dysfunction (Pagana & Pagana, 2018). In the ambulatory care setting, BNP trends may be used over time to guide ambulatory care treatment (Colucci & Chen, 2017).

Urinalysis may reveal proteinuria and high specific gravity. *Microalbuminuria* is an early indicator of decreased compliance of the heart and occurs before the BNP rises. It serves as an "early warning detector" that lets the primary health care provider know that the heart is experiencing early signs of decreased compliance long before symptoms occur.

PATIENT-CENTERED CARE: OLDER ADULT CONSIDERATIONS QSEN

Thyroxine (T_4) and thyroid-stimulating hormone (TSH) levels should be assessed in patients who are older than 65 years, have atrial fibrillation, or have evidence of thyroid disease. Heart failure (HF) may be caused or aggravated by hypothyroidism or hyperthyroidism.

Arterial blood gas (ABG) values often reveal hypoxemia (low blood oxygen level) because oxygen does not diffuse easily through fluid-filled alveoli. Respiratory alkalosis may occur because of hyperventilation; respiratory acidosis may occur because of carbon dioxide retention. Metabolic acidosis may indicate an accumulation of lactic acid.

Imaging Assessment. *Chest x-rays* can be helpful in diagnosing left ventricular failure. Typically the heart is enlarged (cardiomegaly), representing hypertrophy or dilation. Pleural effusions develop less often and generally reflect biventricular failure. *Echocardiography is considered the best tool in diagnosing heart failure.* Cardiac valvular changes, pericardial effusion, chamber enlargement, and ventricular hypertrophy can be diagnosed with this noninvasive technique. The test can also be used to determine ejection fraction.

Radionuclide studies (thallium imaging or technetium pyrophosphate scanning) can also indicate the presence and cause of HF. Multigated acquisition (MUGA) scans, also called *multigated blood pool scans,* provide information about left ventricular ejection fraction and velocity, which are typically low in patients with HF. These tests are discussed in Chapter 30.

Other Diagnostic Assessment. An *electrocardiogram* (ECG) is also performed. It may show ventricular hypertrophy, dysrhythmias, and any degree of myocardial ischemia, injury, or infarction. However, it is *not* helpful in determining the presence or extent of HF.

Invasive **hemodynamic monitoring** allows the direct assessment of cardiac function and volume status in acutely ill patients. Although medical-surgical nurses do not manage these systems on general hospital units, they should be familiar with the interpretation of some of the major hemodynamic pressures as they relate to patient assessment. These measurements can confirm the diagnosis and guide the management of HF. For example, right atrial pressure is either normal or elevated in left ventricular failure and elevated in right ventricular failure. Pulmonary artery pressure (PAP) and pulmonary artery occlusion pressure (PAOP) are elevated in left-sided HF because volumes and pressures are increased in the left ventricle. Hemodynamic monitoring is described in Chapter 35.

◆ **Analysis: Analyze Cues and Prioritize Hypotheses.** The priority collaborative problems for most patients with heart failure (HF) include:

1. Decreased ***gas exchange*** due to ventilation/perfusion imbalance
2. Potential for decreased ***perfusion*** due to inadequate cardiac output
3. Potential for pulmonary edema due to left-sided HF

◆ **Planning and Implementation: Generate Solutions and Take Action.** The patient-centered collaborative care that patients with HF need depends on their disease stage and severity of signs and symptoms. Be sure to individualize care based on the patient's values and preferences, your clinical expertise, and best current evidence.

Increasing Gas Exchange

Planning: Expected Outcomes. The expected outcome is that the patient will have an optimal spontaneous breathing pattern that increases ***gas exchange*** and maintains a serum carbon dioxide level that is within normal limits.

Interventions. The purpose of collaborative care is to help promote ***gas exchange.*** *Ventilation assistance* may be needed because the oxygen content of the blood is often decreased in patients who have pulmonary congestion. Monitor the patient's respiratory rate, rhythm, and quality every 1 to 4 hours. Auscultate breath sounds every 4 to 8 hours.

! NURSING SAFETY PRIORITY (QSEN)

Action Alert

Provide the necessary amount of supplemental oxygen within a range prescribed by the health care provider *to maintain oxygen saturation at 90% or greater.* If the patient has dyspnea, place in a high-Fowler's position with pillows under each arm to maximize chest expansion and improve ***gas exchange.*** Repositioning and performing coughing and deep-breathing exercises every 2 hours helps to improve gas exchange and prevents atelectasis. Interprofessional collaboration with the respiratory therapist is important to plan the most effective methods for assisting with ventilation.

Increasing Perfusion

Planning: Expected Outcomes. The expected outcome is that the patient will have increased perfusion with adequate cardiac output.

Interventions. Collaborative care begins with nonsurgical interventions, but the patient may need surgery if these are not successful in meeting optimal outcomes.

Nonsurgical Management. Nonsurgical management relies primarily on a variety of drugs (Table 32.3). If drug therapy is ineffective, other nonsurgical options are available. Drugs to improve stroke volume include those that reduce afterload, reduce preload, and improve cardiac muscle contractility. A major role of the nurse is to administer medications as prescribed, monitor for their therapeutic and adverse effects, and teach the patient and family about drug therapy.

Drugs that reduce afterload. By relaxing the arterioles, arterial vasodilators can reduce the resistance to left ventricular ejection (afterload) and improve cardiac output (CO). These drugs do not cause excessive vasodilation but reverse some of the inappropriate or excessive vasoconstriction common in HF.

Angiotensin-converting enzyme inhibitors and angiotensin-receptor blockers. Patients with even mild heart failure (HF) resulting from left ventricular dysfunction are given a trial of angiotensin-converting enzyme (ACE) inhibitors or angiotensin-receptor blockers (ARBs). Both ACE inhibitors (e.g., enalapril and captopril) and ARBs (e.g., valsartan, irbesartan, and losartan) improve function and quality of life for patients with HF. Because of the significant clinical experience with ACE inhibitors, this drug class is the drug of choice in the treatment of HF (Burchum & Rosenthal, 2019). ARBs are also effective and can be used as an initial agent for those who do not tolerate ACE inhibitors, usually due to a nagging dry cough. For patients with *acute* HF, the health care provider may prescribe an IV-push ACE inhibitor such as Vasotec IV.

TABLE 32.3 Commonly Used Drug Classifications for Patients With Systolic Heart Failure

Angiotensin-converting enzyme (ACE) inhibitors or angiotensin-receptor blockers (ARBs)

Diuretics:
- Loop
- Potassium-sparing

Nitrates

Inotropics:
- Beta-adrenergic agonists
- Phosphodiesterase inhibitors
- Calcium sensitizers
- Digoxin

Beta-adrenergic blockers

Angiotensin receptor neprilysin inhibitor (ARNI):
- Sacubitril/valsartan

Aldosterone antagonist

HCN channel blocker:
- Ivabradine

HCN, Hyperpolarization-activated cyclic nucleotide-gated.

The ACE inhibitors and ARBs suppress the renin-angiotensin system (RAS), which is activated in response to decreased renal blood flow. ACE inhibitors prevent conversion of angiotensin I to angiotensin II, resulting in arterial dilation and increased stroke volume. ARBs block the effect of angiotensin II receptors and thus decrease arterial resistance and arterial dilation. In addition, these drugs block aldosterone, which prevents sodium and water retention, thus decreasing fluid overload. *Both ACEIs and ARBs work more effectively for Euro-Americans than for African-American populations* (Paul & Page, 2016). Volume-depleted patients should receive a low starting dose, or the fluid volume should be restored before beginning the prescribed drug as the principle adverse effects of these drugs is hypotension. Monitor for hyperkalemia, a potential adverse drug effect in patients who have renal dysfunction. Be aware that there is a risk of angioedema as well; although the risk is low, angioedema is a potentially lethal side effect (Burchum & Rosenthal, 2019; Yancy et al., 2017).

Angiotensin receptor neprilysin inhibitor (ARNI). A newer combination drug, sacubitril/valsartan, has demonstrated a reduction in death and hospitalization in patients with chronic Class II to IV heart failure with a decreased ejection fraction. Valsartan is an ARB that is combined with sacubitril, which inhibits neprilysin. Together these drugs increase natriuretic peptides while suppressing the RAAS (Burchum & Rosenthal, 2019). Sucubitril/valsartan is used in place of an ACE inhibitor or ARB and should not be given within 36 hours of the last dose of an ACE inhibitor or in patients with a history of angioedema (Drazner, 2018; Yancy et al., 2017). Other side effects are similar to those of ACE inhibitors and include hypotension, hyperkalemia, cough, dizziness, and renal failure. Assess for orthostatic hypotension, acute confusion, poor peripheral perfusion, and reduced urine output in patients with low systolic blood pressure. Monitor serum potassium and creatinine levels to determine renal dysfunction.

! NURSING SAFETY PRIORITY (QSEN)

Drug Alert

ACEIs and ARBs are started slowly and cautiously. The first dose may be associated with a rapid drop in blood pressure (BP). Patients at risk for hypotension usually have an initial systolic BP less than 100 mm Hg, are older than 75 years, have a serum sodium level less than 135 mEq/L, or are volume depleted. Monitor BP every hour for several hours after the initial dose and each time the dose is increased. Immediately report to the health care provider and document a systolic blood pressure of less than 90 mm Hg (or designated protocol level). If this problem occurs, place the patient flat and elevate legs to increase cerebral perfusion and promote venous return.

Interventions that reduce preload. Ventricular fibers contract less forcefully when they are overstretched, such as in a failing heart. Interventions aimed at reducing preload attempt to decrease volume and pressure in the left ventricle, increasing ventricular muscle stretch and contraction. Preload reduction is appropriate for HF accompanied by congestion with total body sodium and water overload.

Nutrition therapy. In HF, nutrition therapy is aimed at reducing sodium and water retention to decrease the workload of the heart. The primary care provider may restrict sodium intake in an attempt to decrease fluid retention. Many patients need to omit table salt (no added salt) from their diet, thus reducing sodium intake to about 3 g daily.

If salt intake must be reduced further, the patient may need to eliminate high-sodium foods (e.g., ham, bacon, pickles) and all salt in cooking, thus reducing sodium intake to 2 g daily. If needed, collaborate with the dietitian to help the patient select foods that meet a restricted therapeutic diet. There is no strong evidence to suggest that less than 2 g of sodium daily is helpful; in fact, it may be harmful (Horwitz & Krumholz, 2018).

Few patients are placed on severe fluid restrictions. However, patients with excessive aldosterone secretion may experience thirst and drink 3 to 5 L of fluid each day. As a result, their fluid intake may be limited to a more normal 2 L daily. *Supervise assistive personnel (AP) to ensure that they limit the prescribed intake and accurately record intake and output.*

Weigh the patient daily or delegate this activity to UAP and supervise that it is done. Keep in mind that *1 kg of weight gain or loss equals 1 L of retained or lost fluid*. The same scale should be used every morning before breakfast for the most accurate assessment of weight. Monitor for an expected *decrease* in weight because excess fluid is excreted from the body.

Drug therapy. Common drugs prescribed to reduce preload are diuretics and venous vasodilators. *Morphine sulfate* is also given for patients in *acute* HF to reduce anxiety, decrease preload and afterload, slow respirations, and reduce pain associated with a myocardial infarction (MI).

The primary health care provider adds *diuretics* to the regimen when diet and fluid restrictions have not been effective in managing the symptoms of HF. Diuretics are the first-line drug of choice in older adults with HF and fluid overload. These drugs enhance the renal excretion of sodium and water by reducing circulating blood volume, decreasing preload, and reducing systemic and pulmonary congestion.

The type and dosage of diuretic prescribed depend on the severity of HF and renal function. Loop diuretics such as furosemide, torsemide, and bumetanide are most effective for treating fluid volume overload. For patients with *acute* HF, furosemide or bumetanide can be administered by IV push (IVP).

PATIENT-CENTERED CARE: OLDER ADULT CONSIDERATIONS (QSEN)

Loop diuretics continue to work even after excess fluid is removed. As a result, some patients, especially older adults, can become dehydrated. Observe for signs of dehydration in the older adult, especially acute confusion, decreased urinary output, and dizziness. Provide evidence-based interventions to reduce the risk for falls, as discussed in Chapter 4.

The health care provider may initially prescribe a thiazide diuretic, such as hydrochlorothiazide (HCTZ), for *older adults* with *mild* volume overload. Unlike loop diuretics, the action of thiazides is self-limiting (i.e., diuresis decreases after edema fluid is lost). Therefore the dehydration that may occur with loop diuretics is not common with these drugs. Patients also prefer thiazides because of the gradual onset of diuresis.

As HF progresses, many patients develop diuretic resistance with refractory edema. The health care provider may choose to manage this problem by prescribing both types of diuretics. Other strategies include IV continuous infusion of furosemide or bumetanide or rotating loop diuretics.

Monitor for and prevent potassium deficiency (hypokalemia) from diuretic therapy. The primary signs of hypokalemia are nonspecific neurologic and muscular symptoms, such as generalized weakness, depressed reflexes, and irregular heart rate. A potassium supplement may be prescribed for some patients. Other health care providers prescribe a potassium-sparing diuretic, such as spironolactone, for patients at risk for dysrhythmias from hypokalemia. Although not as effective as other diuretics, spironolactone helps retain potassium, which decreases the risk for ventricular dysrhythmias, and is usually used in stage III/IV heart failure. Monitor for hyperkalemia and renal failure and anticipate stopping the medication if potassium or creatinine levels rise.

Patients being managed with ACE inhibitors or ARBs and diuretics at the same time may not experience hypokalemia. However, if their kidneys are not functioning well, they may develop hyperkalemia (elevated serum potassium level). Review the patient's serum creatinine level. *If the creatinine is greater than 1.8 mg/dL, notify the health care provider before administering supplemental potassium.*

The health care provider may prescribe *venous vasodilators* (e.g., nitrates) for the patient with HF who has persistent dyspnea. Significant constriction of venous and arterial blood vessels occurs to compensate for reduced CO. Constriction reduces the volume of fluid that the vascular bed can hold and increases preload. Venous vasodilators may benefit by:

- Returning venous vasculature to a more normal capacity
- Decreasing the volume of blood returning to the heart
- Improving left ventricular function

Nitrates may be administered IV, orally, or topically. IV nitrates are used most often for *acute* HF. These drugs cause primarily venous vasodilation but also a significant amount of arteriolar vasodilation. Monitor the patient's blood pressure when starting nitrate therapy or increasing the dosage. Patients may initially report headache, but assure them that they will develop a tolerance to this effect and that the headache will cease or diminish. Acetaminophen can be given to help relieve discomfort.

Unfortunately, tolerance to the vasodilating effects develops when nitrates are given around the clock. To prevent this tolerance, the health care provider may prescribe at least one 12-hour nitrate-free period out of every 24 hours (usually overnight). Nitrates such as isosorbide are prescribed to provide nitrate-free periods and reduce the problem of tolerance. Chapter 35 discusses nitrates in more detail.

Drugs that enhance contractility. Contractility of the heart can also be enhanced with drug therapy. Positive inotropic drugs are most commonly used, but vasodilators and beta-adrenergic blockers may also be administered. For *chronic* HF, low-dose beta blockers are most commonly used. Digoxin may be prescribed to improve symptoms, thereby decreasing dyspnea and improving functional activity.

Digoxin. Although not as commonly used today, digoxin, a cardiac glycoside, has been demonstrated to provide symptomatic benefits for patients in *chronic* heart failure (HF) with sinus rhythm and atrial fibrillation. Digoxin (sometimes called *dig*) therapy reduces exacerbations of HF and hospitalizations when added to a regimen of ACE inhibitors or ARBs, beta blockers, and diuretics. However, it may increase mortality as a result of drug toxicity, especially in older adults. As a result, digoxin is considered a second-line agent (Burchum & Rosenthal, 2019).

The potential benefits of digoxin include:

- Increased contractility
- Reduced heart rate (HR)
- Slowing of conduction through the atrioventricular node
- Inhibition of sympathetic activity while enhancing parasympathetic activity

Digoxin is absorbed from the GI tract erratically. Many drugs, especially antacids, interfere with its absorption. It is eliminated primarily by renal excretion. Older patients, those with impaired renal function, and those with low lean body mass should be maintained on lower doses of the drug (McIlvennan & Page, 2016).

NCLEX EXAMINATION CHALLENGE 32.2

Physiological Integrity

The nurse is caring for a client with heart failure who is prescribed spironolactone. Which client statement requires further nursing education?

A. "I may need to take this drug every other day according to lab values."
B. "I need to take potassium supplements with this medication."
C. "I will try my best not to use table salt on my food."
D. "This medication will cause me to urinate more often."

! NURSING SAFETY PRIORITY (QSEN)

Drug Alert

Increased cardiac automaticity occurs with toxic digoxin levels or in the presence of hypokalemia, resulting in ectopic beats (e.g., premature ventricular contractions [PVCs]). Changes in potassium level, especially a decrease, cause patients to be more sensitive to the drug and cause toxicity.

The signs and symptoms of digoxin toxicity are often vague and nonspecific and include anorexia, fatigue, blurred vision, and changes in mental status, especially in older adults. Toxicity may cause nearly any dysrhythmia, but PVCs are most commonly noted. Assess for early signs of toxicity such as bradycardia, heart block, and loss of the P wave on the ECG. Carefully monitor the apical pulse rate and heart rhythm of patients receiving digoxin.

The health care provider determines the desirable heart rate (HR) to achieve. Current evidence indicates that a heart rate greater than 70 beats/min is a risk factor for increased morality and has negative clinical effects (see Fig. 32.2) (Prasun & Albert, 2018). Report the development of either an irregular rhythm in a patient with a previously regular rhythm or a regular rhythm in a patient with a previously irregular one. Monitor serum digoxin and potassium levels (hypokalemia potentiates digoxin toxicity) to identify toxicity. Older adults are more likely than other patients to become toxic because of decreased renal excretion.

Any drug that increases the workload of the failing heart also increases its oxygen requirement. Be alert for the possibility that the patient may experience angina (chest pain) in response to digoxin.

Other inotropic drugs. Patients experiencing *acute* heart failure are candidates for IV drugs that increase contractility. For example, *beta-adrenergic agonists,* such as dobutamine, are used for short-term treatment of *acute* episodes of HF. Dobutamine improves cardiac contractility and thus cardiac output and myocardial-systemic perfusion.

A more potent drug used for *acute* HF, milrinone, functions as a vasodilator/inotropic agent with phosphodiesterase activity. Also known as a *phosphodiesterase inhibitor,* this drug increases cyclic adenosine monophosphate (cAMP), which enhances the entry of calcium into myocardial cells to increase contractile function. Like the beta-adrenergic agonists, milrinone is given IV. Chapter 35 discusses inotropic drugs in more detail.

Beta-adrenergic blockers. Beta-adrenergic blockers (commonly referred to as *beta blockers*) improve the condition of some patients in HF. Prolonged exposure to increased levels of sympathetic stimulation and catecholamines worsens cardiac function. Beta-adrenergic blockade reverses this effect, improving morbidity, mortality, and quality of life for patients in HF.

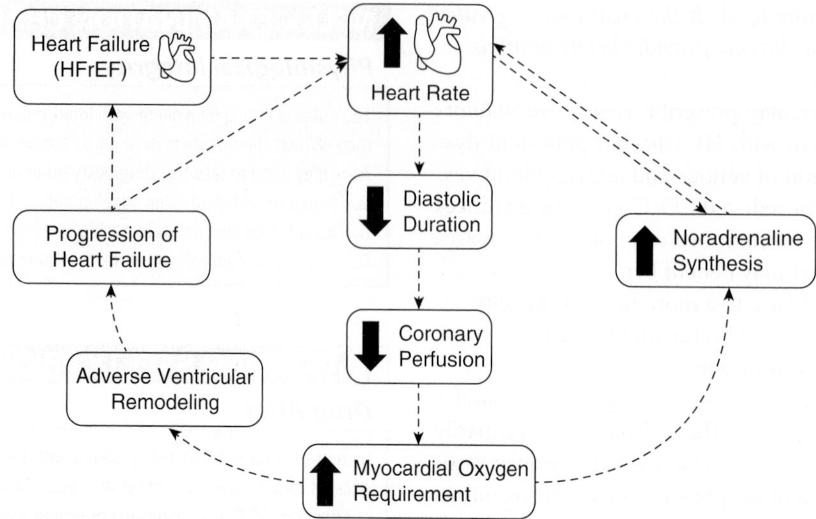

FIG. 32.2 Pathophysiologic mechanisms promoted by an increased heart rate. *HFrEF*, Heart failure with reduced ejection fraction. (From Prasun, M. & Albert, N. [2018]. The importance of heart rate in heart failure and reduced ejection fraction. *Journal of Cardiovascular Nursing, 33*(5), 453–459. Originally published by Arnold, J., Fitchett, D., Howlett, J., Lonn, E., & Tardif, J. [2008] Resting heart rate: a modifiable prognostic indicator of cardiovascular risk and outcome? *Canadian Journal of Cardiology, 24*[suppl A]: 3A–8A.)

Beta blockers must be started slowly for HF. Carvedilol, extended-release metoprolol succinate, and bisoprolol are approved for treatment of HF (Burchum & Rosenthal, 2019). ***Do not confuse metoprolol tartrate with metoprolol succinate.*** The first dose is extremely low. Monitor the patient in either the hospital or primary health care provider's office to assess for bradycardia or hypotension after the first dose is given. Do not stop taking beta blockers abruptly as this can cause an increased risk of clinical decompensation (McIlvennan & Page, 2016).

Instruct the patient to weigh daily and report any signs of worsening HF immediately. The primary health care provider gradually increases the drug dose if HF worsens. The patient is evaluated at least weekly for changes in BP, pulse, activity tolerance, and orthopnea. A modest drop in BP is acceptable if he or she remains asymptomatic and can stand without experiencing dizziness or a further drop in BP. The resting heart rate (HR) should remain between 55 and 60 and increase slightly with exercise. Activity tolerance improves, and less orthopnea is experienced. Most patients with mild and moderate HF demonstrate improved ejection fraction, decreased hospital admissions, and improvement in symptoms when beta blockers are added to their treatment regimens. The benefits of this therapy are seen over a long period rather than immediately.

Aldosterone antagonists. Aldosterone antagonists (spironolactone or eplerenone) can reduce symptoms associated with HF and may be added to HF therapy in patients who remain symptomatic while taking an ACE inhibitor and a beta blocker (Burchum & Rosenthal, 2019). As a potassium-sparing diuretic, aldosterone antagonists decrease the risk for dysrhythmias from hypokalemia. Aldosterone antagonists also block the effect of aldosterone, which decreases the amount of water and sodium retained. Monitor the patient for hyperkalemia and renal failure and anticipate stopping the medication if potassium or creatinine levels rise. Every-other-day dosing is an alternative for patients at risk of developing hyperkalemia.

HCN channel blocker. In 2015, ivabradine was approved by the Food and Drug Administration (FDA) for the treatment of symptomatic stabilized chronic heart failure. This medication is a first-in-class, hyperpolarization-activated cyclic nucleotide-gated (HCN) channel blocker, which slows the heart rate by inhibiting a specific channel in the sinus node. It has been shown to reduce the risk of hospitalization rate in HF patients. Ivabradine is used for HF patients who have an ejection fraction (EF) less than 35% who are in sinus rhythm with a resting heart rate of 70 beats/min or greater. This medication is used for patients who are on the maximally tolerated dose of beta-blocker therapy or have a contraindication to beta-blocker therapy. Side effects of ivabradine include bradycardia, hypertension, atrial fibrillation, and luminous phenomena (visual brightness) (Colucci, 2018). Advise the patient to take this medication with meals. Teach the patient how to check radial pulse and to report low heart rate or irregularity to the health care provider. Advise that visual changes associated with light may occur with initial treatment. These visual changes are usually transient and will disappear with time (Colucci, 2018). Patients should use caution when driving or using machines in situations where light intensity may change abruptly.

For patients with *diastolic* HF, drug therapy has not been as effective. Calcium channel blockers, ACE inhibitors, and beta blockers have been used with various degrees of success.

Other nonsurgical options. In addition to drug therapy, other nonsurgical options, both noninvasive and invasive, may be used and include:

- Continuous positive airway pressure (CPAP)
- Cardiac resynchronization therapy (CRT)
- CardioMEMS implantable monitoring system
- Investigative gene therapy

Continuous positive airway pressure (CPAP) is a respiratory treatment that improves obstructive sleep apnea in patients with HF. It also improves cardiac output (CO) and ejection fraction

(EF) by decreasing afterload and preload, blood pressure (BP), and dysrhythmias. Sleep apnea is directly correlated with coronary artery disease as a result of diminished oxygen supply to the heart during apneic episodes. This respiratory problem is discussed in detail in Chapter 26.

Cardiac resynchronization therapy (CRT), also called *biventricular pacing*, uses a permanent pacemaker alone or is combined with an implantable cardioverter/defibrillator. Electrical stimulation causes more synchronous ventricular contractions to improve EF, CO, and mean arterial pressure. This modality is indicated for patients with Class III or IV HF, an EF of less than 35%, and presence of a left bundle branch block. CRT improves the patient's ability to perform ADLs. Chapter 31 discusses pacing in more detail.

A *CardioMems implantable monitoring system* inserted into the pulmonary artery allows the patient to take a daily reading of the pulmonary artery pressure. These data are transmitted to the provider's office and allow for management and adjustment of medications. The device, about the size of the quarter, is implanted during a right heart catheterization and is permanent. The patient is provided a special pillow with an antenna and portable electronic unit. He or she turns the system on, places the pillow on the bed, and lies on top of the pillow. The device will advise if the position needs to be changed and when reading is complete. The CardioMEMS device can detect increases in pulmonary pressures, indicating fluid retention before the patient demonstrates symptoms. Therapy can be adjusted before symptoms, which may prevent readmission to the hospital and improve quality of life.

Gene therapy may be indicated for patients in end-stage HF who are not candidates for heart transplantation. This therapy replaces damaged genes with normal or modified genes by a series of injections of growth factor into the left ventricle. Although still investigative, this therapy may result in improved exercise tolerance and regrowth of cardiac cells.

Surgical Management. Heart transplantation is the most definitive surgical option for patients with refractory end-stage HF (see the Heart Transplantation section). However, donor availability is limited, and candidacy for heart transplantation is often complicated by comorbidities that exist in the HF patient. Several surgical procedures are available to improve CO in patients who are *not* candidates for a transplant or are awaiting transplant.

Ventricular assist devices. Patients with debilitating end-stage heart failure are often sent home on drug therapy and referred to hospice. However, ventricular assist devices (VADs) can dramatically improve the lives of many patients. In this procedure, a mechanical pump is implanted to work with the patient's own heart (Fig. 32.3). Both left and right VADs are available, depending on the type of HF the patient has. Those with end-stage kidney disease, severe chronic lung disease, clotting disorders, and infections that do not respond to antibiotics are not candidates for this surgery. Postoperative complications include bleeding, infective endocarditis, ventricular dysrhythmias, and stroke. Nursing care is similar to that described for cardiac surgery in Chapter 35.

VADs can be used in the short term while awaiting heart transplantation (a "bridge-to-transplant" procedure) or long term (destination therapy) (Broglio et al., 2015). Most patients survive with a VAD until a transplant is available.

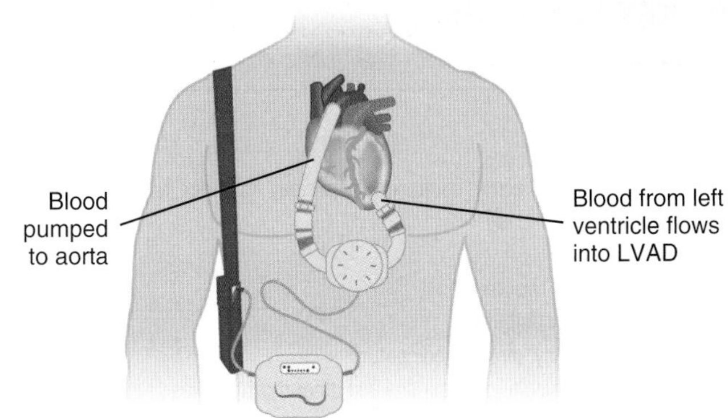

FIG. 32.3 An example of a left ventricular assist device. (From Urden, L., Stacy, K., & Lough, M. [2018]. *Critical care nursing: diagnosis and management* [8th ed.]. St. Louis: Elsevier.)

Other surgical therapies. HF causes ventricular remodeling, or dilation, which worsens as the disease progresses. Left ventricular surgical reconstruction can be done as an alternative to cardiac transplantation in an attempt to improve function of the left ventricle. However, potential impact and long-term survival rates have not been established (Fang, 2015). For example, in *endoventricular circular patch cardioplasty*, the surgeon removes portions of the cardiac septum and left ventricular wall and grafts a circular patch (synthetic or autologous) into the opening. This procedure provides a more normal shape to the left ventricle to improve the heart's ejection fraction (EF) and cardiac output (CO). Perioperative care is similar to that for the patient having a coronary artery bypass graft (CABG) (see Chapter 35).

Preventing or Managing Pulmonary Edema

Planning: Expected Outcomes. The most desirable outcome is that the patient will not develop pulmonary edema as a result of heart failure (HF). However, if the patient progresses to pulmonary edema, the expected outcome is that he or she will recover from this complication without other problems.

Interventions. Monitor for signs of acute pulmonary edema, a life-threatening event that can result from severe HF (with fluid overload), acute myocardial infarction (MI), mitral valve disease, and possibly dysrhythmias. In pulmonary edema, the left ventricle fails to eject sufficient blood and pressure increases in the lungs as a result. The increased pressure causes fluid to leak across the pulmonary capillaries and into the lung airways and tissues.

! NURSING SAFETY PRIORITY (QSEN)

Critical Rescue

Assess for and report early symptoms, such as crackles in the lung bases, dyspnea at rest, disorientation, and confusion, especially in older patients. Document the precise location of the crackles because the level of the fluid progresses from the bases to higher levels in the lungs as the condition worsens. The patient in acute pulmonary edema is typically extremely anxious, tachycardic, and struggling for air. As pulmonary edema becomes more severe, he or she may have a moist cough productive of frothy, blood-tinged sputum; and his or her skin may be cold, clammy, or cyanotic (see the Key Features: Pulmonary Edema box).

KEY FEATURES

Pulmonary Edema

- Crackles
- Dyspnea at rest
- Disorientation or acute confusion (especially in older adults as early symptom)
- Tachycardia
- Hypertension or hypotension
- Reduced urinary output
- Cough with frothy, pink-tinged sputum
- Premature ventricular contractions and other dysrhythmias
- Anxiety
- Restlessness
- Lethargy

NURSING SAFETY PRIORITY QSEN

Critical Rescue

If the patient is not hypotensive, place in a sitting (high-Fowler's) position with the legs down to decrease venous return to the heart. The *priority nursing action* is to administer oxygen therapy at 5 to 12 L/min by simple facemask or at 6 to 10 L/min by nonrebreathing mask with reservoir (which may deliver up to 100% oxygen) to promote ***gas exchange*** and ***perfusion*** (Urden et al., 2018). Apply a pulse oximeter and titrate the oxygen flow to keep the patient's oxygen saturation above 90%. If supplemental oxygen does not resolve the patient's respiratory distress, collaborate with the respiratory therapist, physician, advanced practice nurse, or physician assistant for more aggressive therapy, such as continuous positive airway pressure (CPAP) or bi-level positive airway pressure (BiPAP) ventilation. Intubation and mechanical ventilation may be needed for some patients.

The patient diagnosed with pulmonary edema is admitted to the acute care hospital, often in a critical care unit. Reassure the patient and family that his or her distress will decrease with proper management.

If the patient's systolic blood pressure is above 100, administer sublingual nitroglycerin (NTG) as prescribed to decrease afterload and preload every 5 minutes for three doses while establishing IV access for additional drug therapy. The health care provider prescribes rapid-acting diuretics, such as furosemide or bumetanide. Give furosemide IV push (IVP) over 1 to 2 minutes to avoid ototoxicity (Burchum & Rosenthal, 2019). Bumetanide may be administered IVP over 1 to 2 minutes to avoid ototoxicity or as a continuous infusion to provide consistent fluid removal over 24 hours. Monitor vital signs frequently, at least every 30 to 60 minutes.

If the patient's blood pressure is adequate, IV morphine sulfate may be prescribed to reduce venous return (preload), decrease anxiety, and reduce the work of breathing. Monitor respiratory rate and BP closely. Other drugs, such as IV NTG and drugs to treat HF, may be administered. Monitor the patient's vital signs closely (especially BP) while these drugs are being given.

In severe cases of fluid overload and renal dysfunction or diuretic resistance, ultrafiltration may be used. See Chapter 63 for a complete discussion of this procedure and nursing implications.

The benefits of ultrafiltration include:

- Decrease in cardiac filling pressures
- Decrease in pulmonary arterial pressure
- Increase in cardiac index
- Reduction in norepinephrine, renin, and aldosterone

Care Coordination and Transition Management. Patients who are not adequately prepared for discharge or do not have adequate community support and follow-up for self-management are at high risk for repeated hospital admissions for heart failure (HF). To decrease readmissions, National Quality Measures specific to heart failure, developed by the Joint Commission, have been established. (See the Core Measures: Advanced Certification of Heart Failure box.)

Care transition is an integral part of evidence-based care for heart failure. It is important to understand that even though the acute issues that caused inpatient care for the HF patient may have resolved, there is a high risk of readmission following discharge. Two interventions have been shown to reduce readmission rates: early and intensive nursing care (at least one visit on the day of discharge and at least three nursing visits in the first

CLINICAL JUDGMENT CHALLENGE 32.1

Safety; Patient-Centered Care; Evidence-Based Practice; Informatics

A 73-year-old woman is admitted to the telemetry unit with Class III left-sided heart failure, type 2 diabetes mellitus, and hypertension. When the client arrives to the unit, the nurse assesses that her color is pale, she is becoming increasingly dyspneic, and she appears restless. The client's husband is very concerned because he thinks his wife is slightly disoriented. The client has crackles in bilateral lung bases, and her oxygen saturation levels are 88% on oxygen at 2 L per nasal cannula.

1. **Recognize Cues:** What assessment information in this client situation is the most important and immediate concern for the nurse? (Hint: Identify the **relevant** information *first* to determine what is most important.)
2. **Analyze Cues:** What client conditions are consistent with the **most relevant** information? (Hint: Think about priority collaborative problems that support and contradict the information presented in this situation.)
3. **Prioritize Hypotheses:** Which possibilities or explanations are **most likely** to be present in this client situation? Which possibilities or explanations are the most serious? (Hint: Consider all possibilities and determine their urgency and risk for this client.)
4. **Generate Solutions:** What actions would most likely achieve the desired outcomes for this client? Which actions should be **avoided** or are **potentially harmful**? (Hint: Determine the desired outcomes first to decide which interventions are appropriate and those that should be avoided.)
5. **Take Action:** Which actions are the most appropriate and how should they be implemented? In what **priority order** should they be implemented? (Hint: Consider health teaching, documentation, requested health care provider orders or prescriptions, nursing skills, collaboration with or referral to health team members, etc.)
6. **Evaluate Outcomes:** What client assessment would indicate that the nurse's actions were **effective**? (Hint: Think about signs that would indicate an improvement, decline, or unchanged client condition.)

posthospital week) and follow-up with the health care provider within 1 week of discharge (Murtaugh et al., 2017). As the nurse is planning for discharge, it is critical that care transmission records are used to provide critical information to the home care agency. When reviewing discharge instructions, the nurse should go over the follow-up appointment and include verbal and written information including the date, time, and location of the appointment. Refer to the Systems Thinking and Quality Improvement box for discussion of the teach-back method to reduce readmissions associated with heart failure.

Collaborate with the case manager or care coordinator to assess the patient's needs for health care resources. An inability to obtain help in activities such as food shopping and obtaining medications is a major contributor to hospital readmission. If home support is available, the patient may be discharged home in the care of a family member or other caregiver. Home care nurses may direct the care and assess for adherence to the discharge plan; home health aides may provide assistance with ADLs for a short time. If the patient has multiple health problems or has been severely compromised by heart disease, he or she may require admission to a skilled unit for either transitional or long-term care.

Home Care Management. The home care nurse's interventions focus on assessment and health teaching, which are reimbursable by Medicare and other third-party payers. See the Home Care Considerations: The Patient With Heart Failure box for the major areas of home health assessment.

! CORE MEASURES

Advanced Certification of Heart Failure

Six core measures are associated with the interprofessional health care team's care of patients with heart failure (The Joint Commission, 2018). The six core measures for Advanced Certification of Heart Failure in acute care include:

- Beta-blocker prescribed at discharge
- Follow-up within 7 days after discharge
- Record of care transmitted to the next level of care within 7 days of discharge
- Documentation of advance care planning (advance directives) discussion with a health care provider
- Documentation of advance directives within the medical record
- Follow-up discharge evaluation of patient status and treatment adherence within 72 hours of discharge (can occur by phone, scheduled office visit, or home visit)

SYSTEMS THINKING AND QUALITY IMPROVEMENT QSEN

Almkuist, K. (2017). Using teach-back method to prevent 30-day readmissions in patients with heart failure: A systematic review. *Med-Surg Nursing, 26*(5), 309-351.

Heart failure accounts for one-fourth of all-cause readmissions in Medicare patients (Almkuist, 2017). To offset declining reimbursements due to readmission, many health care institutions focus on interventions to prevent heart failure readmissions. One of the most vulnerable times for a patient is the transition period from a hospital stay to the home environments. The teach-back method has been widely used as a method to assess patient understanding of condition, as well as discharge instructions. The teach-back method requires that the nurse ask the patient an open-ended question where the patient will explain the information that was provided to them during the teaching session. While the strategy is widely used, evidence for use varies. Almkuist (2017) reviewed existing literature from 2011 to 2016. In each of the studies, the teach-back method was utilized; however, length of education time and type of personnel providing the education varied. Some studies looked at more than one intervention, and as such it was difficult to tell which intervention was impacting readmission rates. The results of the studies were mixed; some found a significant reduction in readmission rates, but others found none. The teach-back process did increase patient knowledge base across all studies. Limitations of the studies include small sample sizes, no control group or limited ability to control this group, and inconsistency in education sessions.

Commentary: Implications for Practice

The teach-back methodology has gained momentum as a method to assess patient understanding of both disease process and treatment planning. Although the review by Almquist (2017) shows variability in evidence regarding the direct connection between teach-back methodology and a reduction in readmissions due to heart failure, the method is easy to implement and can have a positive effect on health outcomes. This method should be combined with other initiatives to reduce readmissions, and more research to establish direct connection to readmission rates with the use of the teach-back strategy is needed.

HOME CARE CONSIDERATIONS

The Patient With Heart Failure

Assess for signs of heart failure, including:

- Changes in vital signs (heart rate >100 beats/min at rest, new atrial fibrillation, blood pressure <90 or >150 systolic)
- Indications of poor tissue ***perfusion:***
  - Fatigue
  - Angina
  - Activity intolerance
  - Changes in mental status
  - Pallor or cyanosis
  - Cool extremities
  - Indications of congestion:
  - Presence of cough or dyspnea
  - Weight gain
  - Jugular venous distention and peripheral edema

Assess functional ability, including:

- Performance of ADLs
- Mobility and ambulation (review frequency and duration of walking, development of symptoms, and pulse rate)
- Cognitive ability

Assess nutritional status, including:

- Food and fluid intake
- Intake of sodium-rich foods
- Alcohol consumption
- Skin turgor

Assess home environment, including:

- Safety hazards, especially related to oxygen therapy
- Structural barriers affecting functional ability
- Social support (family, home health services)

Assess the patient's adherence and understanding of illness and its treatment, including:

- Signs and symptoms to report to primary health care provider
- Dosages, effects, and side or toxic effects of medications
- When to report for laboratory and health care provider visits
- Ability to accurately weigh self on scale
- Presence of advance directive
- Use of home oxygen, if appropriate

Assess patient and caregiver coping skills.

TABLE 32.4 Heart Failure Self-Management Health Teaching (MAWDS)

Medications:
- Take medications as prescribed and do not run out.
- Know the purpose and side effects of each drug.
- Avoid NSAIDs to prevent sodium and fluid retention.

Activity:
- Stay as active as possible but don't overdo it.
- Know your limits.
- Be able to carry on a conversation while exercising.

Weight:
- Weigh each day at the same time on the same scale to monitor for fluid retention.

Diet:
- Limit daily sodium intake to 2 to 3 g as prescribed.
- Limit daily fluid intake to 2 L.

Symptoms:
- Note any new or worsening symptoms and notify the health care provider immediately.

Patients with chronic HF need to make many adjustments in their lifestyles. They must adhere to the collaborative plan of care that includes dietary restrictions, activity, prescriptions, and drug therapy. They need careful, concise explanations of the self-management plan. The community-based nurse in any setting encourages the patient to verbalize fears and concerns about his or her illness and helps to explore coping skills. Patient participation in self-management can help alleviate and control symptoms.

Self-Management Education. Health teaching is essential for promoting self-management (also called *self-care*). Many patients are re-admitted to hospitals because they do not maintain their prescribed treatment plan, including lifestyle changes. Because of the need for extensive discharge instructions, most hospitals are using teaching packets with videos, CDs, and easy-to-read information about the importance of adhering to specific self-management strategies at home. One standardized and commonly used self-management plan called *MAWDS* is outlined in Table 32.4. Medication reconciliation is also important to be sure that similar drugs are not being prescribed and that patients meet the Core Measure requirements for HF. It is important to perform a learning needs assessment and tailor education to the patient's particular need to see changes in behavior and improved outcomes.

Ambulatory care clinics for HF patients are also becoming increasingly common. Their purpose is to offer assessments, drug therapy, and health teaching. Some nurses specialize in caring for patients with health failure.

Activity Schedule. Encourage patients with HF to stay as active as possible and to develop a regular exercise regimen (e.g., home walking program). However, teach the patient not to overdo it. Patients should be referred to cardiac rehabilitation programs. Medicare and third-party payers are now reimbursing for this service, but patients may need to wait 6 weeks to fully participate in the program. In addition to exercise programs, cardiac rehabilitation provides education on risk factor modification, medication adherence, and diet and weight management.

Remind patients with persistent crackles and uncontrolled edema to begin exercise after their condition stabilizes. When exercise is indicated, teach the patient to begin walking 200 to 400 feet per day. At home the patient should try to walk at least three times a week and should slowly increase the amount of time walked over several months. If chest pain or severe dyspnea occurs while exercising or the patient has fatigue the next day, he or she is probably advancing the activity too quickly and should slow down. Encourage the patient to keep a diary that documents the time and duration of each exercise session, heart rate, and any symptoms that occur with exercise.

Indications of Worsening or Recurrent Heart Failure. Many patients who are re-admitted to hospitals for treatment of HF fail to seek medical attention promptly when symptoms recur.

! NURSING SAFETY PRIORITY (QSEN)

Action Alert

Teach the patient and caregiver to immediately report to the primary health care provider the occurrence of *any* of these symptoms, which could indicate worsening or recurrent heart failure:
- Rapid weight gain (3 lb in a week or 1 to 2 lb overnight)
- Decrease in exercise tolerance lasting 2 to 3 days
- Cold symptoms (cough) lasting more than 3 to 5 days
- Excessive awakening at night to urinate
- Development of dyspnea or angina at rest or worsening angina
- Increased swelling in the feet, ankles, or hands

Drug Therapy. Provide oral, written, and video instructions about the drug regimen. Teach the caregiver and patient how to count a pulse rate, especially if the patient is taking digoxin, beta blockers, or ivabradine. See the Patient and Family Education: Preparing for Self-Management: Beta Blocker/Digoxin Therapy box for instructions for the patient taking beta blockers and digoxin.

Advise the patient taking diuretics to take them in the morning to avoid waking during the night for voiding. After determining whether he or she has a weight scale and can use it, emphasize the importance of weighing each morning at the same time. Daily weights indicate whether the patient is losing or retaining fluid. Some patients are taught to use a sliding scale to adjust their daily diuretic dose, depending on their daily weight, similar to the way a patient with diabetes adjusts an insulin dose based on the capillary glucose level.

Teach patients taking ACEIs, ARBs, or sacubitril/valsartan to move slowly when changing positions, especially from a lying to a sitting position. Remind them to report dizziness, light-headedness, and cough to the health care provider.

PATIENT AND FAMILY EDUCATION: PREPARING FOR SELF-MANAGEMENT

Beta Blocker/Digoxin Therapy

- Establish same time of day to take this medication every day.
- Continue taking this medication unless your health care provider tells you to stop.
- Do not take digoxin at the same time as antacids or cathartics (laxatives).
- Take your pulse rate before taking each dose of digoxin. Notify your health care provider of a change in pulse rate (60 to 100 beats/min is typically normal, depending on your baseline pulse rate) or rhythm and increasing fatigue, muscle weakness, confusion, or loss of appetite (signs of digoxin toxicity).
- If you forget to take a dose, it may be delayed a few hours. However, if you do not remember it until the next day, you should take only your usual daily dose.
- Report for scheduled laboratory tests (e.g., potassium and digoxin levels).
- If potassium supplements are prescribed, continue the dose until told to stop by your health care provider.

Serum potassium level and renal function are monitored at least every few months for patients taking diuretics and ACE inhibitors, ARBs, or sacubitril/valsartan. Diuretics, especially loop diuretics such as furosemide and bumetanide, deplete potassium and often cause hypokalemia. Conversely, ACE inhibitors, ARBs, sacubitril/valsartan, or potassium-sparing diuretics may result in potassium retention. If serum potassium levels drop below 4 mEq/L, the health care provider may prescribe potassium supplements or add a potassium-sparing diuretic such as spironolactone or eplerenone. Provide information about potassium-rich foods to include in the diet for patients at risk for hypokalemia (see Chapter 13).

Nutrition Therapy. Remind patients with chronic HF to restrict their dietary sodium. In collaboration with the home care nurse or dietitian, provide written instructions on low- or restricted-sodium diets. A 3-g sodium diet is recommended for *mild-to-moderate* disease. Remind the patient to avoid salty foods and table salt. Patients usually find this diet acceptable and fairly easy to follow. Teach patients how to read food labels, specifically ingredients that include sodium.

A 2-g sodium diet may be needed for patients with *severe* HF. They should not add salt during or after meal preparation, avoid milk and milk products, use few canned or prepared foods, and read food labels to determine sodium content. This diet is not easily tolerated by many patients, and the cost of low-sodium foods can be a financial burden.

Commercial salt substitutes typically contain potassium. Teach patients that their renal status and serum potassium level must be evaluated while using these products. Suggest that patients try lemon, spices, and herbs to enhance the flavor of low-salt foods.

Advance Directives. HF is a chronic, progressive debilitating disease. The only potential cure is transplantation. Early in the diagnosis stage, patients and families should be made aware of the progressive nature of this disease process. About 50% of deaths from HF are sudden—many without any warning or worsening of symptoms. Assess whether the patient has written advance directives. If not, provide information about them during the hospital stay. Because most of these deaths occur at home, it is important for the primary health care provider or home care nurse to discuss advance directives with the patient and family. Chapter 8 discusses advance directives in detail. The family should be prepared to act in agreement with the patient's wishes in the event of cardiac arrest. If resuscitation is desired, be sure that the family knows how to activate the emergency medical system (EMS) and how to provide cardiopulmonary resuscitation (CPR) until an ambulance arrives. If CPR is not desired, the patient, family, and nurse plan how the family will respond.

Palliative consultation can provide support to the patient and the family as condition progresses and the patient's conditions declines. Goals of palliative care are to improve the quality of life, manage symptoms, and provide support. As the patient approaches end of life, hospice consultation would be appropriate. Chapter 8 discusses hospice and end-of-life care in detail.

Health Care Resources. A home care nurse, ambulatory care clinic, or nurse-led follow-up program may be needed to assess the patient's adherence to drug and nutrition therapy and to monitor for worsening or recurrent HF. Many large hospitals use follow-up telephone calls or teleconferencing/videoconferencing devices to monitor patients at home. Teleconferencing can also assess the patient's heart and lung sounds. These follow-up processes have been very successful in decreasing repeated hospital stays for chronic HF patients.

In addition to home care support, other resources are available for patient education and family support. The American Heart Association (AHA) is an excellent community resource for educational information related to HF and heart disease. AHA (2019) has developed an app called HF Path to help patients manage heart failure. The app includes weight, symptom, and med tracking and can be used on android or IOS devices (https://www.heart.org/en/health-topics/heart-failure/heart-failure-tools-resources/hf-path-heart-failure-self-management-tool). Although the app is not a substitute for health care, it can be a valuable tool for record keeping and help patients remain alert to the progression of symptoms. AHA also provides referrals to various local support groups for patients and their caregivers.

For equipment needs (e.g., home oxygen therapy, hospital bed), medical supply companies provide setup and maintenance services. Chapter 25 provides a detailed description of home oxygen therapy.

◆ **Evaluation: Evaluate Outcomes.** Evaluate the care of the patient with HF on the basis of the identified patient problems. The expected outcomes include that the patient will:

- Have adequate pulmonary tissue ***perfusion***
- Have increased cardiac pump effectiveness
- Be free of pulmonary edema

 **KEY FEATURES**

Valvular Heart Disease

Mitral Stenosis	Mitral Regurgitation	Mitral Valve Prolapse	Aortic Stenosis	Aortic Regurgitation
Fatigue	Fatigue	Atypical chest pain	Dyspnea on exertion	Palpitations
Dyspnea on exertion	Dyspnea on exertion	Dizziness, syncope	Angina	Dyspnea
Orthopnea	Orthopnea	Palpitations	Syncope on exertion	Orthopnea
Paroxysmal nocturnal dyspnea	Palpitations	Atrial tachycardia	Fatigue	Paroxysmal nocturnal dyspnea
Hemoptysis	Atrial fibrillation	Ventricular tachycardia	Orthopnea	Fatigue
Hepatomegaly	Neck vein distention	Systolic click	Paroxysmal nocturnal dyspnea	Angina
Neck vein distention	Pitting edema		Harsh, systolic crescendo-decrescendo murmur	Sinus tachycardia
Pitting edema	High-pitched holosystolic murmur			Blowing, decrescendo diastolic murmur
Atrial fibrillation				
Rumbling, apical diastolic murmur				
S_1 S_2 S_1 S_2 S_1	S_1 S_2S_3 S_1 S_2S_3	click click S_1 S_2 S_1 S_2	S_1 S_2 S_1 S_2	S_1 S_2 S_1 S_2 S_1

VALVULAR HEART DISEASE

Pathophysiology Review

Acquired valvular dysfunctions include mitral stenosis, mitral regurgitation, mitral valve prolapse, aortic stenosis, and aortic regurgitation. The tricuspid valve is not affected often; however, dysfunction may occur following endocarditis in IV drug misuse. (See the Key Features: Valvular Heart Disease box.)

Mitral Stenosis. **Mitral stenosis** usually results from rheumatic carditis, which can cause valve thickening by fibrosis and calcification. Rheumatic fever is the most common cause of the problem. In mitral stenosis, the valve leaflets fuse and become stiff and the chordae tendineae contract and shorten. The valve opening narrows, preventing normal blood flow from the left atrium to the left ventricle. As a result of these changes, left atrial pressure rises, the left atrium dilates, pulmonary artery pressures increase, and the right ventricle hypertrophies.

Pulmonary congestion and right-sided heart failure occur first. Later, when the left ventricle receives insufficient blood volume, preload is decreased and cardiac output (CO) falls.

People with mild mitral stenosis are usually asymptomatic. As the valvular orifice narrows and pressure in the lungs increases, the patient experiences dyspnea on exertion, orthopnea, paroxysmal nocturnal dyspnea (sudden dyspnea at night), palpitations, and dry cough. Hemoptysis (coughing up blood) and pulmonary edema occur as pulmonary hypertension and congestion progress. Right-sided HF can cause hepatomegaly (enlarged liver), neck vein distention, and pitting dependent edema late in the disorder.

On palpation, the pulse may be normal, rapid, or irregular (as in atrial fibrillation). Because the development of atrial fibrillation indicates that the patient may decompensate, the health care provider should be notified immediately of changes to the heart rhythm. A rumbling, apical diastolic murmur is noted on auscultation.

Mitral Regurgitation (Insufficiency). The fibrotic and calcific changes occurring in **mitral regurgitation** (insufficiency) prevent the mitral valve from closing completely during *systole.* Incomplete closure of the valve allows the backflow of blood into the left atrium when the left ventricle contracts. During *diastole,* regurgitant output again flows from the left atrium to the left ventricle along with the normal blood flow. The increased volume must be ejected during the next systole. To compensate for the increased volume and pressure, the left atrium and ventricle dilate and hypertrophy.

The causes of primary mitral regurgitation are mitral valve prolapse, rheumatic heart disease, infective endocarditis, myocardial infarction (MI), connective tissue diseases such as Marfan syndrome, and dilated cardiomyopathy. (McCance & Huether, 2019). Secondary causes include ischemic and nonischemic heart disease that damage the valve. Rheumatic heart disease is the number-one cause in developing nations. When it results from rheumatic heart disease, it usually coexists with some degree of mitral stenosis.

Mitral regurgitation usually progresses slowly; patients may remain symptom free for decades. Symptoms begin to occur when the left ventricle fails in response to chronic blood volume overload. Symptoms include fatigue and chronic weakness as a result of reduced CO. Dyspnea on exertion and orthopnea develop later. A significant number of patients report anxiety, atypical chest pains, and palpitations. Assessment may reveal normal BP, atrial fibrillation, or changes in respirations characteristic of left ventricular failure.

When right-sided HF develops, the neck veins become distended, the liver enlarges (hepatomegaly), and pitting edema develops. A high-pitched systolic murmur at the apex, with radiation to the left axilla, is heard on auscultation. Severe regurgitation often exhibits a third heart sound (S_3).

Mitral Valve Prolapse. Mitral valve prolapse (MVP) occurs because the valvular leaflets enlarge and prolapse into the left atrium during systole. This abnormality is usually benign but may progress to pronounced mitral regurgitation in some patients.

The etiology of MVP is variable and has been associated with conditions such as Marfan syndrome and other congenital cardiac defects. MVP also has a familial tendency. Usually, however, no other cardiac abnormality is found.

Most patients with MVP are asymptomatic. However, some may report chest pain, palpitations, or exercise intolerance. Chest pain is usually atypical, with patients describing a sharp pain localized to the left side of the chest. Dizziness, syncope, and palpitations may be associated with atrial or ventricular dysrhythmias.

A normal heart rate and BP are usually found on physical examination. A midsystolic click and a late systolic murmur may be heard at the apex of the heart. The intensity of the murmur is not related to the severity of the prolapse.

Aortic Stenosis. Aortic stenosis is the most common cardiac valve dysfunction in the United States and is often considered a disease of "wear and tear." In aortic stenosis, the aortic valve orifice narrows and obstructs left ventricular outflow during systole. This increased resistance to ejection or afterload results in ventricular hypertrophy. As stenosis worsens, cardiac output becomes fixed and cannot increase to meet the demands of the body during exertion. Symptoms then develop. Eventually the left ventricle fails, blood backs up in the left atrium, and the pulmonary system becomes congested. Right-sided HF can occur late in the disease. *When the surface area of the valve becomes 1 cm or less, surgery is indicated on an urgent basis!*

Congenital bicuspid or unicuspid aortic valves are the primary causes for aortic stenosis in many patients. Rheumatic aortic stenosis occurs with rheumatic disease of the mitral valve and develops in young and middle-age adults. Atherosclerosis and degenerative calcification of the aortic valve are the major causative factors in older adults. *Aortic stenosis has become the most common valvular disorder in all countries with aging populations.*

The classic symptoms of aortic stenosis result from fixed cardiac output: dyspnea, angina, and syncope occurring on exertion. When cardiac output falls in the late stages of the disease, the patient experiences marked fatigue, debilitation, and peripheral cyanosis. A narrow pulse pressure is noted when the BP is measured. A diamond-shaped, systolic crescendo-decrescendo murmur is usually noted on auscultation.

Aortic Regurgitation (Insufficiency). In patients with aortic regurgitation, the aortic valve leaflets do not close properly during diastole; and the *annulus* (the valve ring that attaches to the leaflets) may be dilated, loose, or deformed. This allows flow of blood from the aorta back into the left ventricle during diastole. The left ventricle, in compensation, dilates to accommodate the greater blood volume and eventually hypertrophies.

Aortic insufficiency usually results from nonrheumatic conditions such as infective endocarditis, congenital anatomic aortic valvular abnormalities, hypertension, and Marfan syndrome (a rare, generalized, systemic connective tissue disease).

Patients with aortic regurgitation remain asymptomatic for many years because of the compensatory mechanisms of the left ventricle. As the disease progresses and left ventricular failure occurs, the major symptoms are exertional dyspnea, orthopnea, and paroxysmal nocturnal dyspnea. Palpitations may be noted with severe disease, especially when the patient lies on the left side. Nocturnal angina with diaphoresis often occurs.

On palpation, the nurse notes a "bounding" arterial pulse. The pulse pressure is usually widened, with an elevated systolic pressure and diminished diastolic pressure. The classic auscultatory finding is a high-pitched, blowing, decrescendo diastolic murmur.

❖ Interprofessional Collaborative Care

◆ **Assessment: Recognize Cues.** A patient with valvular disease may suddenly become ill or slowly develop symptoms over many years. Collect information about the patient's family health history, including valvular or other forms of heart disease to which he or she may be genetically predisposed. Ask about attacks of rheumatic fever and infective endocarditis, the specific dates when these occurred, and the use of antibiotics to prevent recurrence of these diseases. Also ask the patient about a history of IV drug misuse, a common cause of infective endocarditis. Discuss fatigue and tolerated activity levels, the presence of angina or dyspnea, and the occurrence of palpitations, if present.

As part of the physical assessment, obtain vital signs, inspect for signs of edema, palpate and auscultate the heart and lungs, and palpate the peripheral pulses. Assessment findings are summarized in the Key Features: Valvular Heart Disease box.

Echocardiography is the noninvasive diagnostic procedure of choice to visualize the structure and movement of the heart. The more invasive transesophageal echocardiography (TEE) or transthoracic echocardiography (TTE) is also performed to assess most valve problems. Exercise tolerance testing (ETT) and stress echocardiography are sometimes done to evaluate symptomatic response and assess functional capacity. With either mitral or aortic stenosis, cardiac catheterization may be indicated to assess the severity of the stenosis and its other effects on the heart.

In patients with mitral stenosis, the chest x-ray shows left atrial enlargement, prominent pulmonary arteries, and an enlarged right ventricle. In those with mitral regurgitation (insufficiency), the chest x-ray reveals an increased cardiac shadow, indicating left ventricular and left atrial enlargement.

In the later stages of aortic stenosis, the chest x-ray may show left ventricular enlargement and pulmonary congestion. Left atrial and left ventricular dilation appear on the chest x-ray of patients with aortic regurgitation (insufficiency). If HF is present, pulmonary venous congestion is also evident.

An ECG can be used to evaluate rhythm status in patients with mitral stenosis. Atrial fibrillation is a common finding in both mitral stenosis and mitral regurgitation and may develop in aortic stenosis because of left atrial dilation.

◆ **Interventions: Take Action.** Management of valvular heart disease depends on which valve is affected and the degree of valve impairment. Some patients can be managed with annual monitoring and drug therapy, whereas others require invasive procedures or heart surgery (Nishimura et al., 2017).

Nonsurgical Management. Nonsurgical management focuses on drug therapy and rest. During the course of valvular disease, left ventricular failure with pulmonary or systemic congestion may develop.

Drug Therapy. Diuretics, beta blockers, ACE inhibitors, digoxin, and oxygen are often administered to improve the symptoms of HF. Nitrates are administered cautiously to patients with aortic stenosis because of the potential for syncope associated with a reduction in left ventricular volume (preload). Vasodilators such as calcium channel blockers may be used to reduce the regurgitant flow for patients with aortic or mitral stenosis.

! NURSING SAFETY PRIORITY (QSEN)

Drug Alert

Teach patients with valve disease the importance of prophylactic antibiotic therapy before any invasive dental or oral procedure. This includes patients with a previous history of endocarditis and cardiac transplant or valve recipients. Have patients demonstrate appropriate oral hygiene because optimal oral health is the best intervention to prevent endocarditis.

Prophylactic antibiotics are *not* recommended before GI procedures such as upper GI endoscopy, colonoscopy, or procedures requiring genitourinary instrumentation.

A major concern in valvular heart disease is maintaining cardiac output (CO) if atrial fibrillation develops. With mitral valvular disease, left ventricular filling is especially dependent on atrial contraction. When atrial fibrillation develops, there is no longer a single coordinated atrial contraction. CO can decrease, and HF may occur. Ineffective atrial contraction may also lead to the stasis of blood and thrombi in the left atrium. Monitor the patient for the development of an irregular rhythm and notify the primary care provider if it develops. (See Chapter 31 for a detailed explanation of atrial fibrillation.)

The primary care provider usually starts drug therapy first to control the heart rate (HR) and maintain CO (HR < 100 is considered a controlled ventricular response). After these outcomes are met, drugs are used in an attempt to restore normal sinus rhythm (NSR). In some cases, the provider elects to convert a patient from atrial fibrillation to sinus rhythm using IV diltiazem or amiodarone. Monitor the patient on a unit where both cardiac rhythm and BP can be assessed closely. Synchronized countershock (cardioversion) may be attempted if atrial fibrillation is rapid, the patient's condition worsens, and the rhythm is unresponsive to medical treatment (see Chapter 31).

If the patient remains in atrial fibrillation, low-dose amiodarone is often prescribed to slow ventricular rate. Procainamide hydrochloride may be added to the regimen. A beta-blocking agent (e.g., metoprolol) may also be considered to slow the ventricular response.

For valvular heart disease and chronic atrial fibrillation, anticoagulation with warfarin is usually a part of the plan of care to prevent thrombus formation. Thrombi (clots) may form in the atria or on defective valve segments, resulting in systemic emboli. If a portion breaks off and travels to the brain, one or more strokes may occur. Assess the patient's baseline neurologic status and monitor for changes. A transesophageal echocardiography (TEE) is often done before synchronized cardioversion to ensure that thrombi that could embolize when this therapy is administered are not present. Direct oral anticoagulants (DOACs) *rivaroxaban, dabigatran, apixaban,* and *edoxaban* are *not recommended* to anticoagulate patients with atrial fibrillation related to valvular disease.

Rest is often an important part of treatment. Activity may be limited because CO cannot meet increased metabolic demands and angina or HF can result. A balance of rest and exercise is needed to prevent skeletal muscle atrophy and fatigue.

Nonsurgical Heart Valve Reparative Procedures. Reparative procedures are becoming more popular because of continuing problems with thrombi, endocarditis, and left ventricular dysfunction after valve replacement. Reparative procedures do not result in a normal valve, but they usually "turn back the clock," resulting in a more functional valve and an improvement in CO. Turbulent blood flow through the valve may persist, and degeneration of the repaired valve is possible.

Balloon valvuloplasty, an invasive nonsurgical procedure, is possible for stenotic mitral and aortic valves; however, careful selection of patients is needed. It may be the initial treatment of choice for people with noncalcified, mobile mitral valves. Patients selected for *aortic* valvuloplasty are usually older and are at high risk for surgical complications. The benefits of this procedure for aortic stenosis tend to be short lived, rarely lasting longer than 6 months. Aortic valvuloplasty may be beneficial as a bridge to either surgical or percutaneous aortic valve replacement.

When performing *mitral* valvuloplasty, the physician passes a balloon catheter from the femoral vein, through the atrial septum, and to the mitral valve. The balloon is inflated to enlarge the mitral orifice. For *aortic* valvuloplasty, the physician inserts the catheter through the femoral artery and advances it to the aortic valve, where it is inflated to enlarge the orifice. The procedure usually offers immediate relief of symptoms because the balloon has dilated the orifice and improved leaflet mobility. The results are comparable with those of surgical commissurotomy for appropriately selected patients.

Minimally invasive techniques have expanded. For patients who are not surgical candidates, *transcatheter aortic valve replacement (TAVR)* is an alternate option for treatment of aortic stenosis (Fig. 32.4). Interprofessional collaboration with the cardiologist, surgeon, patient, and the patient's family is often used to determine the best approach. A bioprosthetic valve is placed percutaneously over the damaged valve. This procedure is usually performed through a small incision in the groin allowing for bilateral transfemoral access (Karycki, 2019). One access

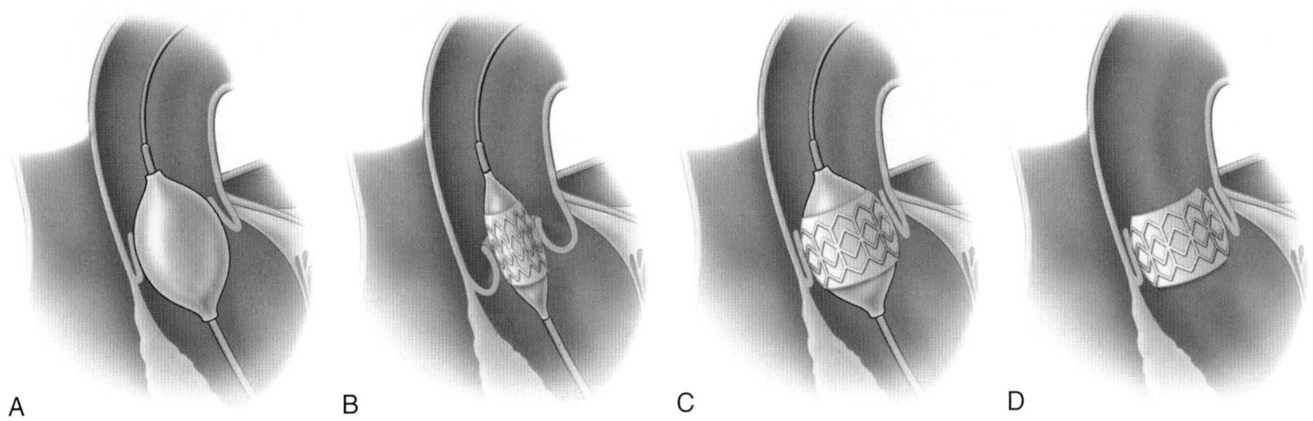

FIG. 32.4 Transcatheter aortic valve replacement (TAVR) procedure. **A**, Balloon aortic valvuloplasty. **B**, New valve placed around balloon. **C**, Balloon inflated, deploying valve. **D**, Catheter removed, valve in place.

is used to place the prosthetic valve while the other is used to place a temporary transvenous pacemaker. After initial balloon aortic valvuloplasty, the new valve is wrapped around a balloon on a large catheter that is inserted via the femoral artery (see Fig. 32.4A-B). The patient is then transvenously paced temporarily at a rate of about 200 beats/min to reduce cardiac output and cardiac motion. The balloon is then inflated, and the valve is deployed (see Fig. 32.4C-D). This procedure is performed by a heart valve team consisting of interventional cardiologists and cardiovascular surgeons. The team must be prepared to convert to an open or surgical aortic valve replacement (SAVR) if necessary. If SAVR is required, care of the patient is similar to that of the patient undergoing coronary artery bypass graft (CABG) (see Chapter 35). After the TAVR, patients remain on bedrest for 6 hours and are monitored overnight for complications (Karycki, 2019). This patient population requires antiplatelet therapy with lifelong daily aspirin and clopidogrel for the first 6 months (Karycki, 2019).

The pulmonary valve can also be replaced percutaneously by a device using a similar procedure to the TAVR. Transcatheter mitral valve repair is also available (Al-Lawati & Cheung, 2016). The MitraClip is used to repair the mitral valve in patients with mitral regurgitation. Under general anesthesia, access is gained percutaneously via the femoral vein, and the catheter and Mitraclip are advanced in the atria and then the left ventricle. The Mitraclip is then retracted and deployed to hold the leaflets of the valve together. Additional devices are currently in clinical trial.

! NURSING SAFETY PRIORITY (QSEN)

Action Alert

After valvuloplasty, observe the patient closely for bleeding from the catheter insertion site and institute postangiogram precautions. Bleeding is likely because of the large size of the catheter. Assess for signs of a regurgitant valve by closely monitoring heart sounds, CO, and heart rhythm. Because vegetations (thrombi) may have been dislodged from the valve, observe for any indication of systemic emboli (see the Infective Endocarditis section in this chapter).

Surgical Management. Surgeries for patients with valvular heart disease include invasive reparative procedures and replacement. These procedures are performed after symptoms of left ventricular failure have developed but before irreversible dysfunction occurs. Surgical therapy is the *only* definitive treatment of *aortic stenosis* and is recommended when angina, syncope, or dyspnea on exertion develops.

Heart Valve Reparative Procedures. *Direct (open) commissurotomy* is accomplished with cardiopulmonary bypass during open-heart surgery. The surgeon visualizes the valve, removes thrombi from the atria, incises the fused commissures (leaflets), and débrides calcium from the leaflets, widening the orifice.

Mitral valve annuloplasty (reconstruction) is the reparative procedure of choice for most patients with acquired mitral insufficiency. To make the annulus (the valve ring that attaches to and supports the leaflets) smaller, the surgeon may suture the leaflets to an annuloplasty ring or take tucks in the patient's annulus. Leaflet repair is often performed at the same time. Elongated leaflets may be shortened, and shortened leaflets may be repaired by lengthening the chordae that bind them in place. Perforated leaflets may be patched with synthetic grafts.

Annuloplasty and leaflet repair result in an annulus of the appropriate size and leaflets that can close completely. Thus regurgitation is eliminated or markedly reduced.

Heart Valve Replacement Procedures. The development of a wide variety of *prosthetic* (synthetic) and *biologic* (tissue) valves has improved the surgical therapy and prognosis of valvular heart disease. Each type has advantages and disadvantages. An aortic valve can be replaced only with a prosthetic valve for symptomatic adults with aortic stenosis and aortic insufficiency. A biologic valve cannot be used because of the high pressure within the aorta.

Biologic valve replacements may be *xenograft* (from other species), such as a porcine valve (from a pig) (Fig. 32.5) or a bovine valve (from a cow). Because tissue valves are associated with little risk for clot formation, long-term anticoagulation is *not* indicated. Xenografts are not as durable as prosthetic valves and usually must be replaced every 7 to 10 years. The durability of the graft is related to the age of the recipient. Calcium in the blood, which is present in larger quantities in younger patients, breaks down the valves. The older the patient, the longer the

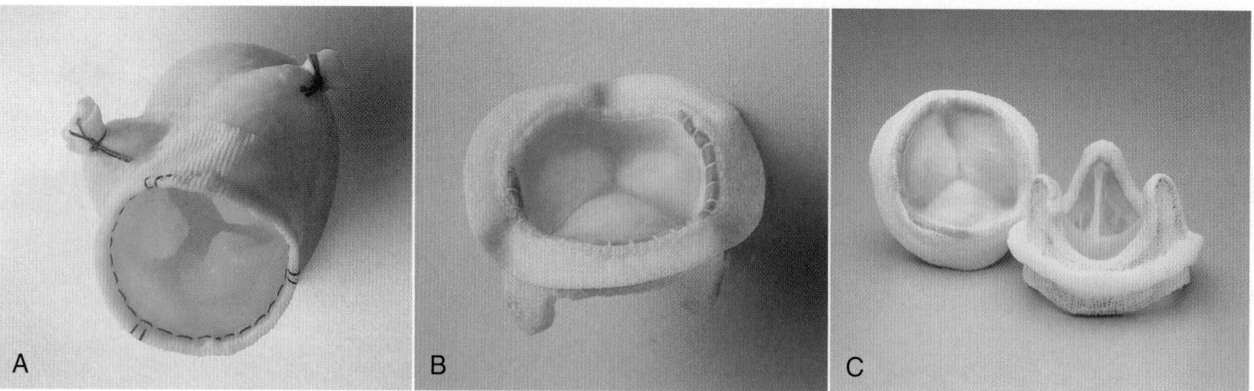

FIG. 32.5 Examples of biologic (tissue) heart valves. **A**, Freestyle, a stentless pig valve with no frame. **B**, Hancock II, a stented pig valve. **C**, Carpentier-Edwards pericardial bioprosthesis. (**A** and **B** courtesy Medtronic, Inc., Minneapolis, MN; **C** courtesy Baxter Healthcare Corporation, Edwards CVS Division, Santa Ana, CA.)

xenograft will last. Valves donated from human cadavers and *pulmonary autographs* (relocation of the patient's own pulmonary valve to the aortic position) are also used for valve replacement.

Patients having a valve replacement have open-heart surgery similar to the procedure for a CABG (see Chapter 35). Ideally surgery is an elective and planned procedure. Patients need to have a preoperative dental examination. If dental caries or periodontal disease is present, these problems must be resolved before valve replacement. Teach patients receiving oral anticoagulants to stop taking them before surgery, usually at least 72 hours before the procedure. Inform the patient and family about the management of postoperative pain, incision care, and strategies to prevent ***infection*** and respiratory complications. Postoperative nursing interventions for patients with valve replacement are similar to those for a CABG (see Chapter 35).

! NURSING SAFETY PRIORITY (QSEN)

Critical Rescue

Patients with mitral stenosis often have pulmonary hypertension and stiff lungs. Therefore monitor respiratory status closely during weaning from the ventilator. Be especially alert for bleeding in those with aortic valve replacements because of a higher risk for postoperative hemorrhage. If heart rate or blood pressure decreases, call the Rapid Response Team or other health care provider immediately!

Patients with valve replacements are also more likely to have significant reductions in cardiac output (CO) after surgery, especially those with aortic stenosis or left ventricular failure from mitral valve disease. Carefully monitor CO and assess for indications of heart failure. Report any indications of HF to the surgeon immediately, and prepare for collaborative management (see earlier discussion on HF in this chapter).

When a patient has a mechanical valve, lifelong anticoagulant therapy with warfarin is required. Teach the patient that the international normalized ratio (INR) will need to be monitored frequently. The therapeutic goal for patients with mechanical heart valves is 3.0 to 4.0 (Pagana & Pagana, 2018). However, therapy must be individualized to each patient. Low-dose aspirin is also recommended. Direct oral anticoagulants (DOACs) *are not recommended* in patients with valve replacement. Teach patients the signs and symptoms of bleeding and to report these symptoms to the primary health care provider.

Care Coordination and Transition Management. The patient with valvular heart disease may be discharged home on medical therapy or after valve repair or replacement surgery. Because fatigue is a common problem, ensure that the home environment can provide rest while moving the patient toward increased activity levels. Some older adults with aortic stenosis live in long-term care settings.

Home Care Management. A home care nurse may be needed to help the patient adhere to drug therapy and activity schedules and to detect any problems, particularly with anticoagulant therapy. Patients who have undergone surgery may require a nurse for help with incision care. A home care aide may assist with ADLs if the patient lives alone or is older.

Self-Management Education. The teaching plan for the patient with valvular heart disease includes:

- The disease process and the possibility of HF
- Drug therapy, including diuretics, vasodilators, beta blockers, calcium channel blockers, antibiotics, and anticoagulants
- The prophylactic use of antibiotics
- A plan of activity and rest to conserve energy

Because patients with defective or repaired valves are at risk for infective endocarditis, teach them to adhere to the precautions described for endocarditis. Remind them to inform all health care providers of the valvular heart disease history. Tell providers that they require antibiotic administration before all invasive dental procedures. See the Patient and Family Education: Preparing for Self-Management: Valvular Heart Disease box for a summary of health teaching.

Patients who have had valve replacements with prosthetic valves require lifetime prophylactic anticoagulation therapy to prevent thrombus formation. Teach patients taking anticoagulants how to manage their drug therapy successfully, including nutritional considerations (if taking warfarin) and the prevention of bleeding. For example, the patient should be taught to avoid foods high in vitamin K, especially dark green leafy

PATIENT AND FAMILY EDUCATION: PREPARING FOR SELF-MANAGEMENT

Valvular Heart Disease

- Notify all your health care providers that you have a defective heart valve.
- Remind the health care provider of your valvular problem when you have any invasive dental work (e.g., extraction).
- Request antibiotic prophylaxis before and after these procedures if the health care provider does not offer it.
- Clean all wounds and apply antibiotic ointment to prevent ***infection.***
- Notify your primary health care provider immediately if you experience fever, petechiae (pinpoint red dots on your skin), or shortness of breath.

vegetables, and to use an electric razor to avoid skin cuts. In addition, teach him or her to report any bleeding or excessive bruising to the primary health care provider.

For patients who have surgery, reinforce how to care for the sternal incision and instruct them to watch for and report any fever, drainage, or redness at the site. Most patients can usually return to normal activity after 6 weeks but should avoid heavy physical activity involving their upper extremities for 3 to 6 months to allow the incision to heal. Those who have had valvular surgery should also avoid invasive dental procedures for 6 months because of the potential for endocarditis. Those with prosthetic valves need to avoid any procedure using magnetic resonance unless the newest technology is available. Remind patients to obtain a medical alert bracelet, card, or necklace to indicate that they have a valve replacement and are taking anticoagulants.

Patients with valvular heart disease may have complicated medication schedules that can potentially lead to inadequate self-management. Provide clear, concise instructions about drug therapy and discuss the risks associated with nonadherence. Patients with a failed valve or those who do not follow the treatment plan are at high risk for heart failure. Teach them to report any changes in cardiovascular status, such as dyspnea, syncope, dizziness, edema, and palpitations.

The psychological response to valve surgery is similar to that after coronary artery bypass surgery. Patients may experience an altered self-image as a result of the required lifestyle changes or the visible medial sternotomy incision. In addition, those with prosthetic valves may need to adjust to a soft but audible clicking sound of the valve. Encourage patients to verbalize their feelings about the prosthetic heart valve. They may display a variety of emotions after surgery, especially after hospital discharge.

NCLEX EXAMINATION CHALLENGE 32.3

Physiological Integrity

A client who recently had a heart valve replacement is preparing for discharge. Which client statement indicates that the nurse will need to do additional health teaching?

A. "I need to brush my teeth at least twice daily and rinse with water."
B. "I will eat foods that are low in vitamin K, such as potatoes and iceberg lettuce."
C. "I need to take a full course of antibiotics prior to my colonoscopy."
D. "I will take my blood pressure every day and call if it is too high or low."

Health Care Resources. The American Heart Association's *Mended Hearts, Inc.* (www.mendedhearts.org) is a community resource that provides information about valvular heart disease. A wallet-size card can be obtained to identify the patient as needing prophylactic antibiotics. An identification bracelet or necklace that states the name of the drugs the patient is taking should also be worn.

INFLAMMATIONS AND INFECTIONS

INFECTIVE ENDOCARDITIS

Pathophysiology Review

Infective endocarditis (previously called *bacterial endocarditis*) is a microbial ***infection*** (e.g., viruses, bacteria, fungi) of the endocardium. The most common infective organism is *Streptococcus viridans* or *Staphylococcus aureus.*

Infective endocarditis occurs primarily in patients with injection drug use (IDU) and those who have had valve replacements, have experienced systemic alterations in immunity, or have structural cardiac defects. It is important to note that the incidence of infective endocarditis is rising in conjunction with the opioid epidemic in the United States. (See Chapter 5 for more on the opioid epidemic). With a cardiac defect, blood may flow rapidly from a high-pressure area to a low-pressure zone, eroding a section of endocardium. Platelets and fibrin adhere to the denuded endocardium, forming a vegetative lesion. During bacteremia, bacteria become trapped in the low-pressure "sinkhole" and are deposited in the vegetation. Additional platelets and fibrin are deposited, causing the vegetative lesion to grow. The endocardium and valve are destroyed. Valvular insufficiency may result when the lesion interferes with normal alignment of the valve. If vegetations become so large that blood flow through the valve is obstructed, the valve appears stenotic and then is very likely to *embolize* (i.e., cause the emboli to be released into the systemic circulation) (McCance & Huether, 2019).

Possible ports of entry for infecting organisms include:

- The oral cavity (especially if dental procedures have been performed)
- Skin rashes, lesions, or abscesses
- Infections (cutaneous, genitourinary, GI, systemic)
- Surgery or invasive procedures, including IV line placement

❖ Interprofessional Collaborative Care

◆ **Assessment: Recognize Cues.** Because the mortality rate remains high, early detection of infective endocarditis is essential. Without treatment, infective endocarditis is fatal. Unfortunately, many patients (especially older adults) are misdiagnosed. Signs and symptoms typically occur within 2 weeks of a bacteremia. See the Key Features: Infective Endocarditis box for key features of infective endocarditis.

Most patients have recurrent fevers from 99°F to 103°F (37.2°C to 39.4°C). However, as a result of physiologic changes associated with aging, older adults may be afebrile. The severity of symptoms may depend on the virulence of the infecting organism.

KEY FEATURES

Infective Endocarditis

- Fever associated with chills, night sweats, malaise, and fatigue
- Anorexia and weight loss
- Cardiac murmur (newly developed or change in existing)
- Development of heart failure
- Evidence of systemic embolization
- Petechiae
- Splinter hemorrhages
- Osler nodes (on palms of hands and soles of feet)
- Janeway lesions (flat, reddened maculae on hands and feet)
- Roth spots (hemorrhagic lesions that appear as round or oval spots on the retina)
- Positive blood cultures

Physical Assessment/Signs and Symptoms. Assess the patient's *cardiovascular status.* Almost all patients with infective endocarditis develop murmurs. Carefully auscultate the precordium, noting and documenting any new murmurs (usually regurgitant in nature) or any changes in the intensity or quality of an old murmur. An S_3 or S_4 heart sound also may be heard.

HF is the most common complication of infective endocarditis. Assess for right-sided HF (as evidenced by peripheral edema, weight gain, and anorexia) and left-sided HF (as evidenced by fatigue, shortness of breath, and crackles on auscultation of breath sounds). See the discussion of HF earlier in this chapter.

Arterial embolization is a major complication in up to half of patients with infective endocarditis. Fragments of vegetation (clots) break loose and travel randomly through the circulation. When the left side of the heart is involved, vegetation fragments are carried to the spleen, kidneys, GI tract, brain, and extremities. When the right side of the heart is involved, emboli enter the pulmonary circulation.

Splenic infarction with sudden abdominal pain and radiation to the left shoulder can also occur. When performing an *abdominal assessment,* note rebound tenderness on palpation. The classic symptom with renal infarction is flank ***pain*** that radiates to the groin and is accompanied by hematuria (red blood cells in the urine) or pyuria (white blood cells in the urine). Mesenteric emboli cause diffuse abdominal pain, often after eating, and abdominal distention.

About a third of patients have *neurologic changes;* others have signs and symptoms of pulmonary problems. Emboli to the central nervous system cause either transient ischemic attacks (TIAs) or a stroke. Confusion, reduced concentration, and aphasia or dysphagia may occur. Pleuritic chest pain, dyspnea, and cough are symptoms of pulmonary infarction related to embolization.

Petechiae (pinpoint red spots) occur in many patients with endocarditis. Examine the mucous membranes, the palate, the conjunctivae, and the skin above the clavicles for small, red, flat lesions. Assess the distal third of the nail bed for splinter hemorrhages (Fig. 32.6), which appear as black longitudinal lines or small red streaks.

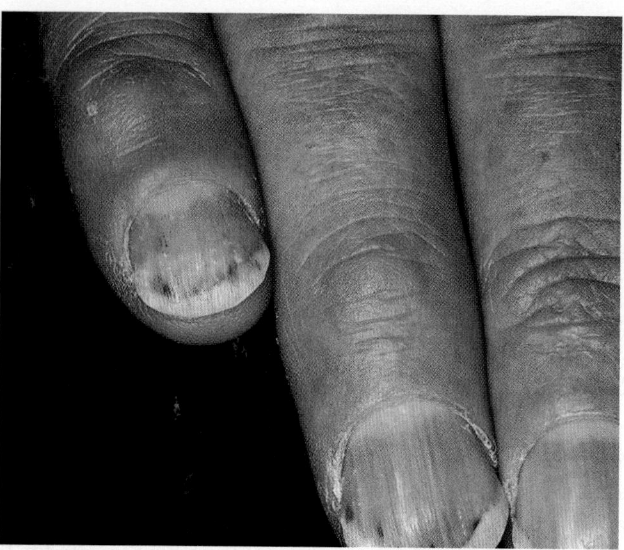

FIG. 32.6 Splinter hemorrhages on the nail bed of the fingers, hemorrhagic nodular lesions on the pad of the finger and left palm. (From Callen, J. P., Jorizzo, J. L., Zone, J. J., Piette, W. W., Rosenbach, M. A., & Vleugels, R. A. [2017]. *Dermatological signs of systemic disease* [5th ed.]. Philadelphia: Elsevier.)

Diagnostic Assessment. The most reliable criteria for diagnosing endocarditis include positive blood cultures, a new regurgitant murmur, and evidence of endocardial involvement by echocardiography.

A positive *blood culture* is a prime diagnostic test. Both aerobic and anaerobic specimens are obtained for culture. Some slow-growing organisms may take 3 weeks and require a specialized medium to isolate. Low hemoglobin and hematocrit levels may also be present.

Echocardiography has improved the ability to diagnose infective endocarditis accurately. Transesophageal echocardiography (TEE) allows visualization of cardiac structures that are difficult to see with transthoracic echocardiography (TTE) (see Chapter 30) (Baddour et al., 2015).

◆ **Interventions: Take Action.** Care of the patient with endocarditis usually includes antimicrobials, rest balanced with activity, and supportive therapy for HF. If these interventions are successful, surgery is usually not required.

Nonsurgical Management. The major component of treatment for endocarditis is drug therapy. Other interventions help prevent the life-threatening complications of the disease.

Antimicrobials are the main treatment, with the choice of drug depending on the specific organism involved. Because vegetations surround and protect the offending microorganism, an appropriate drug must be given in a sufficiently high dose to ensure its destruction. Antimicrobials are usually given IV, with the course of treatment lasting 4 to 6 weeks. For most bacterial cases, the ideal antibiotic is one of the penicillins or cephalosporins.

Patients may be hospitalized for several days to institute IV therapy and then are discharged for continued IV therapy at home. After hospitalization, most patients who respond to therapy may continue it at home when they become afebrile, have negative blood cultures, and have no signs of HF or embolization.

Anticoagulants do not prevent embolization from vegetations. Because they may result in bleeding, these drugs are avoided unless they are required to prevent thrombus formation (clotting) on a prosthetic valve.

The patient's activities are balanced with *adequate rest*. Consistently use appropriate aseptic technique to protect the patient from contact with potentially infective organisms. Continue to assess for signs of HF (e.g., rapid pulse, fatigue, cough, dyspnea) throughout the antimicrobial regimen and report significant changes.

NCLEX EXAMINATION CHALLENGE 32.4

Physiological Integrity

The nurse is caring for a hospitalized client with infective endocarditis who has been receiving antibiotics for 2 days. The client is now experiencing flank pain with hematuria. What complication will the nurse suspect?

A. Pulmonary embolus
B. Renal infarction
C. Transient ischemic attack
D. Splenic infarction

Surgical Management. The cardiac surgeon may be consulted if antibiotic therapy is ineffective in sterilizing a valve, if refractory HF develops secondary to a defective valve, if large valvular vegetations are present, or if multiple embolic events occur. Current surgical interventions for infective endocarditis include:

- Removing the infected valve (either biologic or prosthetic)
- Repairing or removing congenital shunts
- Repairing injured valves and chordae tendineae
- Draining abscesses in the heart

Preoperative and postoperative care of patients having surgery involving the valves is similar to that described earlier in this chapter for valve replacement.

Care Coordination and Transition Management. Community-based care for patients with infective endocarditis is essential to resolve the problem, prevent relapse, and avoid complications. Patients and families need to be willing and have the knowledge, physical ability, and resources to administer IV antibiotics at home. Collaborate with the home care nurse to complete health teaching started in the hospital and to monitor patient adherence and health status.

In collaboration with the case manager, the home care nurse and pharmacist arrange for appropriate supplies to be available to the patient at home. Supplies include the prepared antibiotic, IV pump with tubing, alcohol wipes, IV access device, normal saline solution, and a saline flush solution drawn up in syringes. A saline lock, peripherally inserted central catheter (PICC) line, or central catheter is positioned at a venous site that is easily accessible to the patient or a family member.

Teach the patient and family how to administer the antibiotic and care for the infusion site while maintaining aseptic technique. The patient or family member should demonstrate this technique before the patient is discharged from the hospital. Emphasize the importance of maintaining a blood level of the antibiotic by administering the antibiotics as scheduled. After stabilization at home, the case manager or other nurse contacts the patient every week to determine whether he or she is adhering to the antibiotic therapy and whether any problems have been encountered.

Encourage proper oral hygiene. Advise patients to use a soft toothbrush, to brush their teeth at least twice per day, and to rinse the mouth with water after brushing. They should not use irrigation devices or floss the teeth because bacteremia may result. Teach them to clean any open skin areas well and apply an antibiotic ointment.

! NURSING SAFETY PRIORITY (QSEN)

Action Alert

Patients must remind health care providers (including their dentists) of their endocarditis. Guidelines for antibiotic prophylaxis have been revised and are recommended only if the patient with a prosthetic valve, a history of infective endocarditis, or an unrepaired cyanotic congenital heart disease undergoes an invasive dental or oral procedure (Habib et al., 2015).

Instruct patients to note any indications of recurring endocarditis such as fever. Remind them to monitor and record their temperature daily for up to 6 weeks. Teach them to report fever, chills, malaise, weight loss, increased fatigue, sudden weight gain, or dyspnea to their primary care provider.

PERICARDITIS

Pathophysiology Review

Acute pericarditis is an inflammation or alteration of the pericardium (the membranous sac that encloses the heart). The problem may be fibrous, serous, hemorrhagic, purulent, or neoplastic. Acute pericarditis is most commonly associated with:

- Infective organisms (bacteria, viruses, or fungi) (usually respiratory)
- Post–myocardial infarction (MI) syndrome (Dressler syndrome)
- Postpericardiotomy syndrome
- Acute exacerbations of systemic connective tissue disease

Chronic constrictive pericarditis occurs when chronic pericardial inflammation causes a fibrous thickening of the pericardium. It is caused by tuberculosis, radiation therapy, trauma, renal failure, or metastatic cancer. In chronic constrictive pericarditis, the pericardium becomes rigid, preventing adequate filling of the ventricles and eventually resulting in cardiac failure.

❖ Interprofessional Collaborative Care

◆ Assessment: Recognize Cues. Assessment findings for patients with *acute pericarditis* include substernal precordial ***pain*** that radiates to the left side of the neck, the shoulder, or the back. The pain is classically grating and oppressive and is aggravated by breathing (mainly on inspiration), coughing, and swallowing. The pain is worse when the patient is in the supine position and may be relieved by sitting up and leaning forward. Ask specific questions to evaluate chest discomfort to differentiate it from the pain associated with an acute MI (see Chapter 35).

A pericardial friction rub may be heard with the diaphragm of the stethoscope positioned at the left lower sternal border. This scratchy, high-pitched sound is produced when the inflamed, roughened pericardial layers create friction as their surfaces rub together.

Patients with acute pericarditis may have an elevated white blood cell count and usually have a fever. Therefore blood culture and sensitivity may be analyzed in the laboratory. The ECG usually shows ST elevation in all leads, which returns to baseline with treatment. Atrial fibrillation is also common. Echocardiograms may be used to determine a pericardial effusion.

The proposed diagnostic criteria for acute pericarditis are two of the following:

- Pericardial chest pain
- Presence of pericardial rub
- New ST elevation in all ECG leads or PR-segment depression
- New or worsening pericardial effusion

Patients with *chronic constrictive pericarditis* (lasting longer than 3 months) have signs of right-sided HF, elevated systemic venous pressure with jugular distention, hepatic engorgement, and dependent edema. Exertional fatigue and dyspnea are common complications. Thickening of the pericardium is seen on echocardiography or a computed tomography (CT) scan.

◆ **Interventions: Take Action.** The focus of collaborative management is to relieve ***pain*** and treat the cause of pericarditis before severe complications occur. See the Best Practice for Patient Safety & Quality Care box for care of the patient with pericarditis.

BEST PRACTICE FOR PATIENT SAFETY & QUALITY CARE QSEN

Care of the Patient With Pericarditis

- Assess the nature of the patient's chest discomfort. (Pericardial pain is typically substernal. It is worse on inspiration and decreases when the patient leans forward.)
- Auscultate for a pericardial friction rub.
- Assist the patient to a position of ***comfort.***
- Provide anti-inflammatory agents as prescribed.
- Explain that anti-inflammatory agents usually decrease ***pain*** within 48 hours.
- Avoid the administration of aspirin and anticoagulants because these may increase the possibility of tamponade.
- Auscultate the blood pressure carefully to detect paradoxical blood pressure (pulsus paradoxus), a sign of tamponade:
  - Palpate the blood pressure and inflate the cuff above the systolic pressure.
  - Deflate the cuff gradually and note when sounds are first audible on expiration.
  - Identify when sounds are also audible on inspiration.
  - Subtract the inspiratory pressure from the expiratory pressure to determine the amount of pulsus paradoxus (>10 mm Hg is an indication of tamponade).
  - Inspect for other indications of tamponade, including jugular venous distention with clear lungs, muffled heart sounds, and decreased cardiac output.
  - Notify the health care provider if tamponade is suspected.

The health care provider usually prescribes NSAIDs for pain associated with pericarditis. Patients who do not obtain pain relief and who do not have bacterial pericarditis may receive corticosteroid therapy. Help the patient assume positions that promote ***comfort***—usually sitting upright and leaning slightly forward. If the pain is not relieved within 24 to 48 hours, notify the primary health care provider. Colchicine twice a day, orally, for 3 months has been shown to prevent pericarditis recurrence (Campbell et al., 2015).

The various causes of pericarditis require specific therapies. For example, bacterial pericarditis (acute) usually requires antibiotics and pericardial drainage. The usual clinical course of acute pericarditis is short term (2 to 6 weeks), but episodes may recur. Chronic pericarditis caused by malignant disease may be treated with radiation or chemotherapy, whereas uremic pericarditis is treated by hemodialysis. The definitive treatment for chronic constrictive pericarditis is surgical excision of the pericardium *(pericardiectomy).*

Monitor all patients for **pericardial effusion,** which occurs when the space between the parietal and visceral layers of the pericardium fills with fluid. This complication puts the patient at risk for **cardiac tamponade,** or excessive fluid within the pericardial cavity.

Emergency Care: Acute Cardiac Tamponade. **Acute cardiac tamponade** may occur when small volumes (20 to 50 mL) of fluid accumulate rapidly in the pericardium and cause a sudden decrease in cardiac output (CO). If the fluid accumulates slowly, the pericardium may stretch to accommodate several hundred milliliters of fluid. Cardiac tamponade can occur with pericarditis, as well as other conditions such as ventricular wall rupture from acute MI, cancer, aortic dissection, and as a complication from invasive cardiac (York et al., 2018). Report any suspicion of this complication to the health care provider immediately. Findings of cardiac tamponade include (Kaplow & Iyere, 2017):

- Jugular venous distention
- **Paradoxical pulse,** also known as *pulsus paradoxus.* See the earlier box, Best Practice for Patient Safety & Quality Care: Care of the Patient With Pericarditis, for more information on paradoxical pulse assessment.
- Tachycardia
- Muffled heart sounds
- Hypotension

Cardiac tamponade is an emergency! The health care provider may initially manage the decreased CO with increased fluid volume administration while awaiting an echocardiogram or x-ray to confirm the diagnosis. Unfortunately, these tests are not always helpful because the fluid volume around the heart may be too small to visualize. Hemodynamic monitoring in a specialized critical care unit usually demonstrates compression of the heart, with all pressures (right atrial, pulmonary artery, and wedge) being similar and elevated (plateau pressures).

The health care provider may elect to perform a **pericardiocentesis** to remove fluid and relieve the pressure on the heart. Under echocardiographic or fluoroscopic and hemodynamic monitoring, the cardiologist inserts an 8-inch (20.3-cm), 16- or 18-gauge pericardial needle into the pericardial space. When the needle is positioned properly, a catheter is inserted and all available pericardial fluid is withdrawn. A pericardial drain may be placed temporarily. Monitor the pulmonary artery, wedge, and right atrial pressures during the procedure. The pressures should return to normal as the fluid compressing the heart is removed, and the signs and symptoms of tamponade should resolve. In situations in which the cause of the tamponade is unknown, pericardial fluid specimens may be sent to the laboratory for culture and sensitivity tests and cytology.

! NURSING SAFETY PRIORITY (QSEN)

Action Alert

After the pericardiocentesis, closely monitor the patient for the recurrence of tamponade. Pericardiocentesis alone often does not resolve acute tamponade. Be prepared to provide adequate fluid volumes to increase CO and to prepare the patient for surgical intervention if tamponade recurs.

If the patient has a recurrence of tamponade or recurrent effusions or adhesions from chronic pericarditis, a portion or all of the pericardium may need to be removed to allow adequate ventricular filling and contraction. The surgeon may create a pericardial window, which involves removing a portion of the pericardium to permit excessive pericardial fluid to drain into the pleural space. In more severe cases, removal of the toughened encasing pericardium (pericardiectomy) may be necessary.

RHEUMATIC CARDITIS

Pathophysiology Review

Rheumatic carditis, also called *rheumatic endocarditis,* is a sensitivity response that develops after an upper respiratory tract ***infection*** with group A beta-hemolytic *Streptococci*. It occurs in almost half of patients with rheumatic fever. The precise mechanism by which the infection causes inflammatory lesions in the heart is not established; however, inflammation is evident in all layers of the heart. The inflammation results in impaired contractile function of the myocardium, thickening of the pericardium, and valvular damage.

Rheumatic carditis is characterized by the formation of Aschoff bodies (small nodules in the myocardium that are replaced by scar tissue). A diffuse cellular infiltrate also develops and may be responsible for the resulting heart failure (HF). The pericardium becomes thickened and covered with exudate, and a serosanguineous pleural effusion may develop. The most serious damage occurs to the endocardium, with inflammation of the valve leaflets developing. Hemorrhagic and fibrous lesions form along the inflamed surfaces of the valves, resulting in stenosis or regurgitation of the mitral and aortic valves (McCance & Huether, 2019).

❖ Interprofessional Collaborative Care

◆ **Assessment: Recognize Cues.** Rheumatic carditis is one of the major indicators of rheumatic fever. The common signs and symptoms are:

- Tachycardia
- Cardiomegaly (enlarged heart)
- Development of a new murmur or a change in an existing murmur
- Pericardial friction rub
- Precordial pain
- Electrocardiogram (ECG) changes (prolonged P-R interval)
- Indications of HF
- Evidence of an existing streptococcal infection

Primary prevention is extremely important. Teach all patients to remind their primary health care providers to provide appropriate antibiotic therapy if they develop the indications of streptococcal pharyngitis:

- Moderate-to-high fever
- Abrupt onset of a sore throat
- Reddened throat with exudate
- Enlarged and tender lymph nodes

◆ **Interventions: Take Action.** Penicillin is the antibiotic of choice for treatment. Erythromycin is the alternative for pen icillin-sensitive patients.

Once a diagnosis of rheumatic fever is made, antibiotic therapy is started immediately. Teach the patient to continue the antibiotic administration for the full 10 days to prevent reinfection. Suggest ways to manage fever, such as maintaining hydration and taking antipyretics. Encourage the patient to get adequate rest.

Explain to the patient and family that a recurrence of rheumatic carditis is most likely the result of reinfection by *Streptococcus*. Antibiotic prophylaxis is necessary for the rest of the patient's life to prevent infective endocarditis discussed earlier in this chapter (see the Infective Endocarditis section).

CARDIOMYOPATHY

Pathophysiology Review

Cardiomyopathy is a subacute or chronic disease of cardiac muscle, and the cause may be unknown. Cardiomyopathies are classified into four categories on the basis of abnormalities in structure and function: dilated cardiomyopathy, hypertrophic cardiomyopathy, restrictive cardiomyopathy, and arrhythmogenic right ventricular cardiomyopathy (Table 32.5). **Dilated cardiomyopathy (DCM)** is the structural abnormality most commonly seen. DCM involves extensive damage to the myofibrils and interference with myocardial metabolism. Ventricular wall thickness is normal, but both ventricles are dilated (left ventricle is usually worse) and systolic function is impaired. Causes may include alcohol abuse, chemotherapy, infection, inflammation, and poor nutrition. Decreased CO from inadequate pumping of the heart causes the patient to experience dyspnea on exertion (DOE), decreased exercise capacity, fatigue, and palpitations.

The cardinal features of **hypertrophic cardiomyopathy (HCM)** are asymmetric ventricular hypertrophy and disarray of the myocardial fibers. Left ventricular hypertrophy leads to a stiff left ventricle, which results in diastolic filling abnormalities. Obstruction in the left ventricular outflow tract is seen in most patients with HCM. Mitral valve structural abnormalities are commonly associated with HCM and contribute

TABLE 32.5 Pathophysiology, Signs and Symptoms, and Treatment of Common Cardiomyopathies

	HYPERTROPHIC CARDIOMYOPATHY	
Dilated Cardiomyopathy	**Nonobstructed**	**Obstructed**
Pathophysiology		
Fibrosis of myocardium and endocardium Dilated chambers Mural wall thrombi prevalent	Hypertrophy of all walls Hypertrophied septum Relatively small chamber size	Same as for nonobstructed except for obstruction of left ventricular outflow tract associated with the hypertrophied septum and mitral valve incompetence
Signs and Symptoms		
Fatigue and weakness Heart failure (left side) Dysrhythmias or heart block Systemic or pulmonary emboli S_3 and S_4 gallops Moderate to severe cardiomegaly	Dyspnea Angina Fatigue, syncope, palpitations Mild cardiomegaly S_4 gallop Ventricular dysrhythmias Sudden death common Heart failure	Same as for nonobstructed except with mitral regurgitation murmur Atrial fibrillation
Treatment		
Symptomatic treatment of heart failure Vasodilators Control of dysrhythmias Surgery: heart transplant	For both: Symptomatic treatment Beta blockers Conversion of atrial fibrillation Surgery: ventriculomyotomy or muscle resection with mitral valve replacement Nitrates and other vasodilators *contraindicated* with the obstructed form	

to the obstruction in ventricular outflow (Larkin et al., 2019). HCM is transmitted as a single-gene autosomal-dominant trait occurring in 1 in 500 people (McCance & Huether, 2019). Some patients die without any symptoms, whereas others have DOE, syncope, dizziness, and palpitations. Many athletes who die suddenly probably had hypertrophic cardiomyopathy.

Restrictive cardiomyopathy, the rarest of the cardiomyopathies, is characterized by stiff ventricles that restrict filling during diastole. Symptoms are similar to those of left or right HF or both. The disease can be primary or caused by endocardial or myocardial disease such as sarcoidosis or amyloidosis. The prognosis for this type of cardiomyopathy is poor.

Arrhythmogenic right ventricular cardiomyopathy (dysplasia) results from replacement of myocardial tissue with fibrous and fatty tissue. Although the name implies right ventricle disease, about a third of patients also have left ventricle (LV) involvement. This disease has a familial association and most often affects young adults. Some patients have symptoms, and others do not.

❖ Interprofessional Collaborative Care

◆ **Assessment: Recognize Cues.** Findings in cardiomyopathy depend on the structural and functional abnormalities. For example, left ventricular or biventricular failure is characteristic of *dilated* cardiomyopathy (DCM). Some patients with DCM are asymptomatic for months to years and have left and/or right ventricular dilation confirmed on x-ray examination or echocardiography. Others experience sudden, pronounced symptoms of left ventricular failure, such as progressive dyspnea on exertion, orthopnea, palpitations, and activity intolerance. Right-sided HF develops late in the disease and is associated with a poor prognosis. Atrial fibrillation occurs in some patients and is associated with embolism.

The clinical picture of *hypertrophic cardiomyopathy* (HCM) results from the hypertrophied septum causing a reduced stroke volume (SV) and cardiac output (CO). Most patients are asymptomatic until late adolescence or early adulthood. The primary symptoms of HCM are exertional dyspnea, angina, and syncope. The chest pain is atypical in that it usually occurs at rest, is prolonged, has no relation to exertion, and is not relieved by the administration of nitrates. A high incidence of ventricular dysrhythmias is associated with HCM. Sudden death occurs and may be the first manifestation of the disease (Cao & Zhang, 2017).

Echocardiography, radionuclide imaging, and angiocardiography during cardiac catheterization are performed to diagnose and differentiate cardiomyopathies.

◆ **Interventions: Take Action.** The treatment of choice for the patient with cardiomyopathy varies with the type of cardiomyopathy and may include both medical and surgical interventions.

Nonsurgical Management. The care of patients with dilated or restrictive cardiomyopathy is initially the same as that for HF. Drug therapy includes the use of diuretics, vasodilating agents, and cardiac glycosides to increase CO. Because patients are at risk for sudden death, teach them to report any palpitations, dizziness, or fainting, which might indicate a dysrhythmia. Antidysrhythmic drugs or implantable cardiac defibrillators may be used to control life-threatening dysrhythmias. To block inappropriate sympathetic stimulation and tachycardia, beta blockers (e.g., metoprolol) are used. If cardiomyopathy has developed in response to a toxin (such as alcohol), further exposure to that toxin must be avoided.

Management of obstructive HCM includes administering negative inotropic agents such as beta-adrenergic blocking agents (carvedilol) and calcium antagonists (verapamil). These drugs decrease the outflow obstruction that accompanies exercise. They also decrease heart rate (HR), resulting in less angina, dyspnea, and syncope. Vasodilators, diuretics, nitrates, and cardiac glycosides are contraindicated in patients with obstructive HCM because vasodilation and positive inotropic effects may worsen the obstruction. Strenuous exercise is also prohibited because it can increase the risk for sudden death. Excess alcohol intake and dehydration should also be avoided. Depending on risk stratification, an implantable cardioverter defibrillator (ICD) may be recommended to prevent sudden cardiac death. Patients with HCM are encouraged to seek genetic counseling. First-degree relatives should be screened for the presence of HCM, and echocardiography should be offered starting at age 12.

Surgical Management

Myectomy and Ablation. The type of surgery performed depends on the type of cardiomyopathy. The most commonly used surgical treatment for obstructive HCM involves excising a portion of the hypertrophied ventricular septum to create a wider outflow tract *(ventricular septal myectomy)*. This procedure results in long-term improvement in activity tolerance for most patients.

Percutaneous alcohol septal ablation is another option for patients with HCM. Absolute alcohol is injected into a target septal branch of the left anterior descending coronary artery to produce a small septal infarction. Over time this will result in remodeling of the area, reducing the obstruction.

The patient with arrhythmogenic right ventricular cardiomyopathy who does not respond to drug therapy may have a radiofrequency catheter ablation or placement of an implantable defibrillator (see Chapter 31 for discussion of these procedures).

Heart Transplantation. *Heart transplantation* (surgical replacement with a donor heart) is the treatment of choice for patients with severe DCM and may be considered for patients with restrictive cardiomyopathy. The procedure may also be done for end-stage heart disease caused by coronary artery disease, valvular disease, or congenital heart disease.

Preoperative Care. Criteria for candidate selection for heart transplantation include:

- Life expectancy less than 1 year
- Age generally younger than 65 years
- New York Heart Association (NYHA) Class III or IV
- Normal or only slightly increased pulmonary vascular resistance
- Absence of active infection
- Stable psychosocial status
- No evidence of current drug or alcohol misuse

Once the candidate is eligible and a heart is available, provide preoperative care as described in Chapter 9.

Operative Procedures. The surgeon transplants a heart from a donor with a comparable body weight and ABO compatibility into a recipient less than 6 hours after procurement. In the most common procedure *(bicaval technique)*, the intact right atrium of the donor heart is preserved by anastomoses at the patient's (recipient's) superior and inferior venae cavae. In the more traditional *orthotopic* technique, cuffs of the patient's right and left atria are attached to the donor's atria. Anastomoses are made between the recipient and donor atria, aorta, and pulmonary arteries (Fig. 32.7). Because the remaining remnant of the recipient's atria contains the sinoatrial (SA) node, two unrelated P waves are visible on the ECG.

Postoperative Care. The postoperative care of the heart transplant recipient is similar to that for conventional cardiac surgery (see Chapter 35). However, the nurse must be especially observant to identify occult bleeding into the pericardial sac with the potential for tamponade. The patient's pericardium has usually stretched considerably to accommodate the diseased, hypertrophied heart, predisposing the patient to concealed postoperative bleeding.

The transplanted heart is denervated (disconnected from the body's autonomic nervous system) and unresponsive to vagal stimulation. In the early postoperative phase, isoproterenol may be titrated to support the heart rate and maintain cardiac output. Atropine, digoxin, and carotid sinus pressure are not used because they do not have their usual effects on the new heart. Denervation of the heart may cause pronounced orthostatic hypotension in the immediate postoperative phase. Caution the patient to change position slowly to help prevent this complication. Some patients also require a permanent pacemaker that is rate responsive to his or her activity level. The purpose is to increase CO and improve activity tolerance.

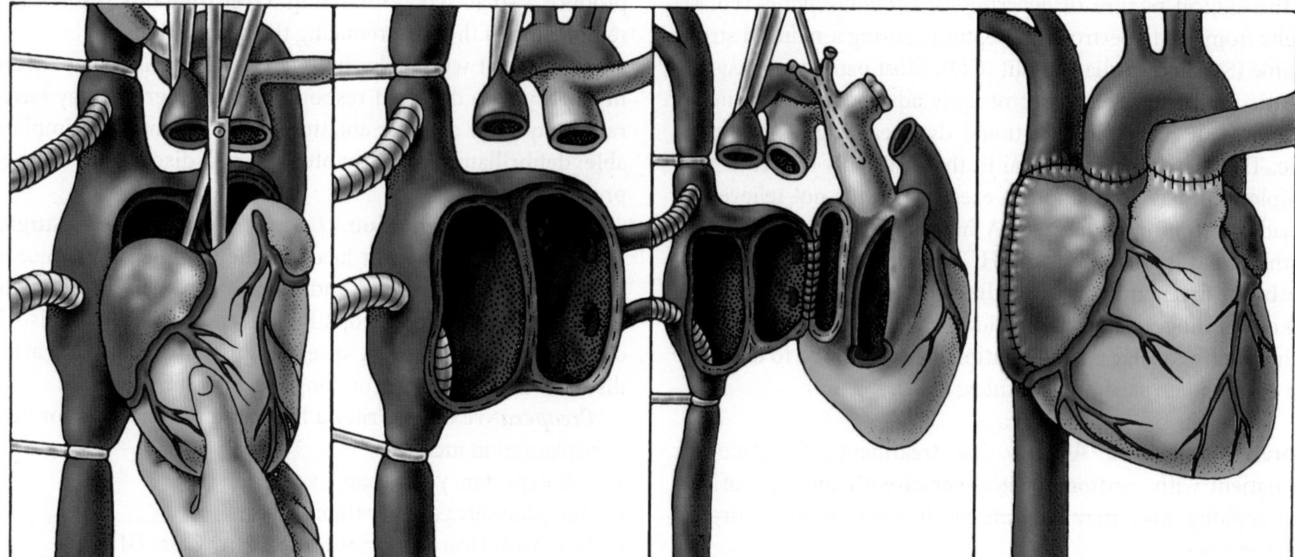

1. After the recipient is placed on cardiopulmonary bypass, the heart is removed.
2. The posterior walls of the recipient's left and right atria are left intact.
3. The left atrium of the donor heart is anastomosed to the recipient's residual posterior atrial walls, and the other atrial walls, the atrial septum, and the great vessels are joined.
POSTOPERATIVE RESULT

FIG. 32.7 One technique for heart transplantation.

To suppress natural defense mechanisms and prevent transplant rejection, patients require a combination of immunosuppressants for the rest of their lives. Chapter 16 describes transplant rejection and prevention in detail.

! NURSING SAFETY PRIORITY (QSEN)

Critical Rescue

After surgery, perform comprehensive cardiovascular and respiratory assessments frequently according to agency or heart transplant surgical protocol. See the Best Practice for Patient Safety & Quality Care box for the signs and symptoms of rejection that are specific to heart transplant. Report any of these manifestations to the surgeon immediately! To detect rejection, the surgeon performs right endomyocardial biopsies at regularly scheduled intervals and whenever symptoms occur.

BEST PRACTICE FOR PATIENT SAFETY & QUALITY CARE (QSEN)

Assessing for Signs and Symptoms of Heart Transplant Rejection

- Shortness of breath
- Fatigue
- Fluid gain (edema, increased weight)
- Abdominal bloating
- New bradycardia
- Hypotension
- Atrial fibrillation or flutter
- Decreased activity tolerance
- Decreased ejection fraction (late sign)

Be very careful about handwashing and aseptic technique because patients are immunosuppressed from drug therapy. ***Infection*** *is the major cause of death* and usually develops in the immediate post-transplant period or during treatment for acute rejection.

The median survival rate for adults following cardiac transplantation is 11 years and rising (Pham, 2018). Over time, many of these surviving patients are developing a form of coronary artery disease (CAD) called cardiac allograft vasculopathy (CAV), which presents as diffuse plaque in the arteries of the donor heart. The cause is thought to involve a combination of immunologic and nonimmunologic processes that result in vascular endothelial injury and an inflammatory response (Pham, 2018). Because the heart is denervated, patients do not usually experience angina. Regularly scheduled exercise tolerance tests and angiography are required to identify CAV. Only a small percentage of patients with CAV benefit from revascularization procedures such as balloon angioplasty or coronary artery bypass surgery. Stents are beginning to show some promise in managing these patients. Retransplantation may be done in select patients.

To delay the development of CAV, encourage patients to follow lifestyle changes similar to those with primary CAD (see Chapter 35). The provider may prescribe a calcium channel blocker such as diltiazem to prevent coronary spasm and closure. Stress the importance of strict adherence to nutritional modifications and drug regimens. Teach the patient the importance of participating in a regular exercise program. Collaborate with the physical therapist and the cardiac rehabilitation specialist to plan the most appropriate exercise plan for the patient.

Discharge planning involves a collaborative, interdisciplinary approach. Patients require extensive health teaching for self-management and community resources for support. Counseling and support groups can help patients cope with their fear of organ rejection. Drug therapy adherence is crucial to prevent this problem. Continuing community-based care for patients with a heart transplant is similar to that for heart failure discussed earlier in this chapter.

GET READY FOR THE NEXT-GENERATION NCLEX® EXAMINATION!

Key Points

Review these Key Points for each NCLEX Examination Client Needs Category.

Safe and Effective Care Environment

- Provide discharge information about continuing care for patients with heart failure (HF).
- Assess patients with end-stage HF for advance directives. If the patient does not have an advance directive, provide information about them.
- Collaborate with the health care team to develop and implement a plan of care for patients with HF. **QSEN: Teamwork and Collaboration**
- Teach patients about community support groups and resources.

Health Promotion and Maintenance

- Provide teaching about self-management for patients with HF (see Table 32.4).
- Monitor older adults who are taking digoxin for signs and symptoms of toxicity. Monitor for hypokalemia. **QSEN: Safety**
- Teach patients taking ACE inhibitors, ARBs, or sacubitril/valsartan to change positions slowly to avoid orthostatic hypotension. **QSEN: Safety**
- Teach the patient with valvular dysfunction, cardiac ***infection,*** or cardiomyopathy the necessity of taking preventive antibiotic therapy before any invasive dental procedure. **QSEN: Evidence-Based Practice**

Psychosocial Integrity

- Assess the patient for depression resulting from altered self-concept and anxiety.
- Assess the patient's coping skills. **QSEN: Patient-Centered Care**

Physiological Integrity

- Assess the patient for signs and symptoms of right- and left-sided HF.
- Weigh daily and record intake and output.
- Assess for early signs and symptoms of pulmonary edema. **QSEN: Safety**
- Assess for symptoms of worsening HF: rapid weight gain (3 lb in a week), a decrease in exercise tolerance lasting 2 to 3 days, cold symptoms (cough) lasting more than 3 to 5 days, nocturia, development of dyspnea or angina at rest, or unstable angina. **QSEN: Safety**
- Monitor the HF patient on beta blockers carefully for hypotension and bradycardia. **QSEN: Safety**
- Monitor the pulse of patients taking digoxin before administration and report to the health care provider a pulse that is not within the desired parameters.
- Monitor for signs and symptoms of pulmonary edema.
- Place the patient in a sitting position and provide oxygen therapy at a high flow rate (unless otherwise contraindicated) if pulmonary edema is suspected. **QSEN: Evidence-Based Practice**
- Monitor the patient with valvular dysfunction for atrial fibrillation. Monitor for an irregular cardiac rhythm and administer warfarin as prescribed.
- Document neurovascular status frequently because emboli from valvular disease may cause strokes. **QSEN: Informatics**
- Differentiate major types of cardiomyopathy as described in Table 32.5.

MASTERY QUESTIONS

1. The nurse is teaching a client with heart failure about a newly prescribed medication, ivabradine. What teaching will the nurse include? Select all that apply.
   A. "Visual changes with exposure to light are expected initially."
   B. "Be sure to take this medication with food."
   C. "Call your health care provider if your pulse rate is low or irregular."
   D. "Use caution when driving in the sunlight."
   E. "Check your BP regularly and notify the health care provider if elevated."
2. The nurse is caring for a client with heart failure who is on oxygen at 2 L per nasal cannula with an oxygen saturation of 90%. The client states, "I feel short of breath." Which action will the nurse take first?
   A. Contact respiratory therapy.
   B. Increase the oxygen to 4 L.
   C. Place the client in a high-Fowler position.
   D. Draw arterial blood for arterial blood gas analysis.
3. The nurse is admitting an 84-year-old client with heart failure to the emergency department with confusion, blurry vision, and an upset stomach. Which assessment data are most concerning?
   A. Digoxin therapy daily
   B. Daily metoprolol
   C. Furosemide twice daily
   D. Currently taking an antacid for upset stomach

REFERENCES

Al-Lawati, A., & Cheung, A. (2016). Transcatheter mitral valve replacement. *Interventional Cardiology Clinic, 5*, 109–115.

Almkuist, K. (2017). Using teach-back method to prevent 30-day readmissions in patients with heart failure: A systematic review. *Medsurg Nursing, 26*(5), 309–312.

American Heart Association. (2019). *HF Path self management tool.* Retrieved from: https://www.heart.org/en/health-topics/heart-failure/heart-failure-tools-resources/hf-path-heart-failure-self-management-tool.

Baddour, L., Wilson, W., Bayer, A., Fowler, V., Tleyjeh, I., Rybak, M., et al. (2015). Infective endocarditis in adults: Diagnosis, antimicrobial therapy, and management of complications: A scientific statement for healthcare professionals from the American heart association. *Circulation, 132*, 1435–1486.

Benjamin, E., Virani, S., Callaway, C., Cheng, A., Chiuve, S., Delling, F., et al. (2018). Heart disease and stroke statistics -2018 update: A report from the American heart association. *Circulation, 135*(10), e146–e603. https://doi.org/10.1161/CIR.0000000000000485.

Broglio, K., Eichholz-Heller, F., & Nakagawa, S. (2015). Left ventricular assist devices: When bridge to transplantation becomes destination. *Journal of Hospice and Palliative Nursing, 17*(5), 374–379.

Burchum, J., & Rosenthal, L. (2019). *Lehne's pharmacology for nursing care* (10th ed.). St. Louis, MO: Elsevier.

Campbell, K. B., Cicci, T. A., Vora, A. K., & Burgess, L. D. (2015). Beyond gout: Colchicine use in the cardiovascular patient. *Hospital Pharmacy, 50*(10), 859–867. https://doi.org/10.1310/hpj5010-859.

Cao, Y., & Zhang, P. Y. (2017). Review of recent advances in the management of hypertrophic cardiomyopathy. *European Review for Medical and Pharmacological Sciences, 21*, 5207–5210.

Colucci, W. (2018). *Use of beta blockers in heart failure with reduced ejection fraction. UpToDate.* Retrieved from: https://www.uptodate.com/contents/use-of-beta-blockers-in-heart-failure-with-reduced-ejection-fraction.

Colucci, W., & Chen, H. (2017). *Natriuretic peptide measurement in heart failure. UpToDate.* Retrieved from: https://www.uptodate.com/contents/natriuretic-peptide-measurement-in-heart-failure.

Drazner, M. (2018). *Use of angiotensin receptor-neprilysin inhibitor in heart failure with reduced ejection fraction. UpToDate.* Retrieved from: https://www.uptodate.com/contents/use-of-angiotensin-receptor-neprilysin-inhibitor-in-heart-failure-with-reduced-ejection-fraction.

Fang, J. (2015). *Surgical management of heart failure. UpToDate.* Retrieved from: https://www.uptodate.com/contents/surgical-management-of-heart-failure.

*Habib, G., Lancellotti, P., Antunes, M., Bongiorni, M., Casalta, J., Del Zotti, F., et al. (2015). 2015 ESC guidelines for the management of infective endocarditis. *European Heart Journal, 36*(44), 3075–3128.

Horwitz, L., & Krumholz, H. (2018). Heart failure self-management. *UpToDate.* Retrieved from: https://www.uptodate.com/contents/heart-failure-self-management.

Kaplow, R., & Iyere, K. (2017). When cardiac tamponade puts the pressure on. *Nursing 2017, 47*(2), 24–30.

Karycki, M. (2019). Transcatheter aortic valve replacement. *Nursing2019, 49*(6), 25–31.

Larkin, G., Bellomo, T., & Caze, L. (2019). Hypertrophic cardiomyopathy: New hope for an old disease. *Nursing2019, 49*(9), 24–31.

McCance, K., & Huether, S. (2019). *Pathophysiology: The biologic basis for disease in adults and children* (8th ed.). St. Louis: Mosby.

McIlvennan, C., & Page, R. (2016). Foundations of pharmacotherapy for heart failure with reduced ejection fraction: Evidence meets practice, part II. *Journal of Cardiovascular Nursing, 31*(6), 545–554.

Murtaugh, C., Deb, P., Zhu, C., Peng, T., Barron, Y., Shah, S., & Siu, A. (2017). Reducing readmissions among heart failure patients discharged to home health care: Effectiveness of early and intensive nursing services and early physician follow-up. *Heath Services Research, 54*(4), 1445–1472.

Nishimura, R., Otto, C., Bonow, R., Carabello, B., Erwin, J., Fleisher, L., & Thompson, A. (2017). 2017 AHA/ACC focused update on 2014 AHA/ACC guidelines for the management of patients with valvular heart disease: A report of the American College of Cardiology/American heart association task force on clinical practice guidelines. *Journal of the American College of Cardiology, 70*(2), 253–289.

Pagana, K., & Pagana, T. (2018). *Mosby's manual of diagnostic and laboratory tests* (6th ed.). St. Louis: Mosby.

Paul, S., & Page, R. (2016). Foundation of pharmacotherapy for heart failure with reduced ejection fraction: Evidence meets practice, part 1. *Journal of Cardiovascular Nursing, 31*(2), 101–113.

Pham, M. (2018). *Prognosis after cardiac transplantation in adults. UpToDate.* Retrieved from: https://www.uptodate.com/contents/prognosis-after-cardiac-transplantation-in-adults.

Prasun, M., & Albert, N. (2018). The importance of heart rate in heart failure and reduced ejection fraction. *Journal of Cardiovascular Nursing, 33*(5), 453–459.

The Joint Commission. (2018). *Specifications manual for Joint Commission national quality measures.* Retrieved from: https://manual.jointcommission.org/releases/TJC2017B2/.

Urden, L., Stacy, K., & Lough, M. (2018). *Critical care nursing: Diagnosis and management* (8th ed.). St. Louis: Elsevier.

Yancy, C., Jessup, M., Bozkurt, B., Butler, J., Casey, D., Colvin, M., et al. (2017). 2017 ACC/AHA/AFSA focused update of the 2013 ACCF/AHA guideline for the management of heart failure. *Journal of the American College of Cardiology, 70*(6), 776–803.

York, N., Kane, C., & Smith, C. (2018). Identification and management of acute cardiac tamponade. *Dimensions of Critical Care Nurse, 37*(3), 130–134.

33

Concepts of Care for Patients With Vascular Problems

Jonathon Rospierski, Nicole M. Heimgartner

http://evolve.elsevier.com/Iggy/

LEARNING OUTCOMES

1. Collaborate with the interprofessional team to provide high-quality care for patients with vascular problems that impact ***perfusion*** and ***clotting.***
2. Prioritize evidence-based care for patients with vascular problems affecting ***perfusion*** and ***clotting.***
3. Teach patients about lifestyle modifications to reduce the risk for vascular problems.
4. Teach patient and caregiver(s) about common drugs used for vascular problems, including anticoagulants to prevent ***clotting.***
5. Implement nursing interventions to decrease the psychosocial impact of living with chronic vascular disease.
6. Apply knowledge of anatomy and physiology to perform an evidence-based assessment for the patient with a vascular problem.
7. Plan nursing care to promote ***perfusion*** and prevent complications such as ***clotting*** or ***inflammation.***
8. Use clinical judgment to assess laboratory data and signs and symptoms to prioritize care for patients with vascular problems.

KEY TERMS

acute arterial occlusion The sudden blockage of an artery, typically in the lower extremity, in the patient with chronic peripheral arterial disease.

aneurysm A permanent localized dilation of an artery that enlarges the artery to at least two times its normal diameter.

aneurysmectomy A surgical procedure performed to excise an aneurysm.

ankle-brachial index (ABI) Measurement of arterial insufficiency based on the ratio of ankle systolic pressure to brachial systolic pressure.

arterial revascularization A surgical procedure most commonly used to increase arterial blood flow in the affected limb of a patient with peripheral arterial disease.

arterial ulcers Painful ulcers caused by diminished blood flow through an artery that develop on the toes (often the great toe), between the toes, or on the upper aspect of the foot.

arteriosclerosis A thickening or hardening of the arterial wall, often associated with aging.

arteriotomy A surgical opening into an artery.

atherectomy A invasive nonsurgical technique in which a high-speed, rotating metal burr uses fine abrasive bits to scrape plaque from inside an artery while minimizing damage to the vessel surface.

atherosclerosis A type of arteriosclerosis that involves the formation of plaque within the arterial wall; the leading contributor to coronary artery and cerebrovascular disease.

autogenous Belonging to the person; for example, when a person's vein is moved from one part of the body to another.

clotting A complex, multistep process by which blood forms a protein-based structure (clot) in an appropriate area of tissue injury to prevent excessive bleeding while maintaining whole-body blood flow (perfusion).

collateral circulation that provides blood to an area with altered tissue perfusion through smaller vessels that develop and compensate for the occluded vessels.

deep vein thrombosis (DVT) A blood clot that forms in one or more of the deep veins in the body, usually the legs.

embolus A blood clot or other object (e.g., air bubble, fatty deposit) that is carried in the bloodstream and lodges in another area.

endovascular stent grafts The repair of an abdominal aortic aneurysms using a stent made of flexible material.

essential hypertension The most common type of hypertension that is not caused by an existing health problem. Also called *primary hypertension.*

heparin-induced thrombocytopenia (HIT) A potentially devastating immune-mediated adverse drug reaction caused by the emergence of antibodies that activate platelets in the presence of heparin.

hyperlipidemia An elevation of serum lipid levels in the blood.

hypertensive crisis A severe elevation in blood pressure (greater than 180/120), which can cause damage to organs such as the kidneys or heart. Also called *malignant hypertension.*

inferior vena cava filtration A type of vascular filter inserted by a surgeon percutaneously into the inferior vena cava; indicated for deep vein thrombosis (DVT) or pulmonary embolism (PE) when anticoagulation therapy is contraindicated.

inflow disease Obstructions in the distal end of the aorta and the common, internal, and external iliac arteries that results in pain or discomfort in the lower back, buttocks, or thighs.

intermittent claudication Characteristic leg pain experienced by patients with chronic peripheral arterial disease. Typically, patients can walk only a certain distance before a cramping muscle pain forces them to stop. As the disease progresses, the patient can walk only shorter distances before pain occurs.

lipid Fat, including cholesterol and triglycerides, that can be measured in the blood.

malignant hypertension See *hypertensive crisis.*

orthostatic hypotension A decrease in blood pressure (20 mm Hg systolic and/or 10 mm Hg diastolic) that occurs when the patient changes position from lying or sitting to standing.

outflow disease Obstructions in the femoral, popliteal, and tibial arteries and below the superficial femoral artery (SFA) that cause burning or cramping in the calves, ankles, feet, and toes.

percutaneous vascular intervention A nonsurgical procedure used to treat blood vessels that are narrowed or closed because of vascular disease.

peripheral vascular disease (PVD) Disorders that change the natural flow of blood through the arteries and veins of the peripheral circulation, causing decreased perfusion to body tissues.

phlebitis Inflammation of a vein, which can predispose patients to thrombosis.

phlebothrombosis A thrombus in the vein without inflammation.

rubor Dusky red discoloration of the skin.

secondary hypertension Elevated blood pressure that is related to a specific disease (e.g., kidney disease) or medication.

stasis dermatitis In patients with venous insufficiency, discoloration of the skin along the ankles; may extend up to the calf.

stasis ulcers Associated with long-term venous insufficiency; ulcer formed as a result of edema or minor injury to the limb; typically occurs over the malleolus.

telangiectasias Vascular lesions with a red center and radiating branches. Commonly referred to as *spider veins* or *spider angiomas.*

thrombectomy A surgical procedure used to remove deep thrombosis, or blood clots that have formed in the deep veins.

thrombophlebitis A thrombus that is associated with inflammation.

thrombus A blood clot believed to result from an endothelial injury, venous stasis, or hypercoagulability.

Unna boot A wound dressing constructed of gauze moistened with zinc oxide; used to promote venous return in the ambulatory patient with a stasis ulcer and form a sterile environment for the ulcer.

varicose veins Distended, protruding veins that appear darkened and tortuous.

venous insufficiency Alteration of venous efficiency by thrombosis or defective valves; caused by prolonged venous hypertension, which stretches the veins and damages the valves, resulting in further venous hypertension, edema, and eventually venous stasis ulcers, swelling, and cellulitis.

venous thromboembolism (VTE) A term that refers to both deep vein thrombosis and pulmonary embolism; obstruction by a thrombus.

Virchow triad Describes the three factors that contribute to thrombosisstasis of blood flow, endothelial injury, and hypercoagulability.

PRIORITY AND INTERRELATED CONCEPTS

The priority concepts for this chapter are:

- ***Perfusion***
- ***Clotting***

The ***Perfusion*** concept exemplar for this chapter is Hypertension.

The ***Clotting*** concept exemplar for this chapter is Venous Thromboembolism.

The interrelated concept for this chapter is:

- ***Inflammation***

PERFUSION CONCEPT EXEMPLAR: HYPERTENSION

Hypertension, or high blood pressure (BP), is the most common health problem seen in primary care settings and can cause stroke, myocardial infarction (MI) (heart attack), kidney failure, and death if not treated early and effectively. Current guidelines from the American College of Cardiology (ACC) and the American Heart Association (AHA) recommend a BP below 130/80 mm Hg in all people. This BP recommendation is lower than the guidance provided by the Eighth Joint National Committee (JNC 8) on Prevention, Detection, Evaluation, and Treatment of High Blood Pressure. According to JNC 8, in the general population ages 60 years and older, the desired BP is below 150/90. For people younger than 60 years, the desired BP is below 140/90. Patients with a BP above these goals should be treatment with medication (James et al., 2014). The ACC/AHA guidelines suggest that patients with BP above the goal should be treated with drug therapy and lifestyle modifications (Whelton et al., 2017). Adult patients with specific risk factors for developing hypertension should be treated at any age, as described later under Drug Therapy.

Pathophysiology Review

To best understand the pathophysiology of hypertension, a review of normal BP and how it is normally maintained is essential.

Mechanisms That Influence Blood Pressure. The systemic arterial BP is a product of cardiac output (CO) and total peripheral vascular resistance (PVR). CO is determined by the stroke volume (SV) multiplied by heart rate (HR):

$$CO = SV \times HR$$

Control of PVR (i.e., vessel constriction or dilation) is maintained by the autonomic nervous system and circulating hormones, such as norepinephrine and epinephrine. Consequently, any factor that increases PVR, HR, or SV increases the systemic arterial pressure. Conversely, any factor that decreases PVR, HR, or SV decreases the systemic arterial pressure and can cause decreased ***perfusion*** to body tissues.

Stabilizing mechanisms exist in the body to exert an overall regulation of systemic arterial pressure and to prevent circulatory collapse. Four control systems play a major role in maintaining blood pressure:

- The arterial baroreceptor system
- Regulation of body fluid volume
- The renin-angiotensin-aldosterone system
- Vascular autoregulation

Arterial baroreceptors are found primarily in the carotid sinus, aorta, and wall of the left ventricle. They monitor the level of arterial pressure and counteract a rise in arterial pressure through vagally mediated cardiac slowing and vasodilation with decreased sympathetic tone. Reflex control of circulation therefore elevates the systemic arterial pressure when it falls and lowers it when it rises. Why baroreceptor control fails in hypertension is not clear (McCance & Huether, 2019).

Changes *in fluid volume* also affect the systemic arterial pressure. For example, if there is an excess of sodium and/or water in a person's body, the BP rises through complex physiologic mechanisms that change the venous return to the heart, producing a rise in cardiac output (CO). If the kidneys are functioning adequately, a rise in systemic arterial pressure produces diuresis (excessive voiding) and a fall in pressure. Pathologic conditions change the pressure threshold at which the kidneys excrete sodium and water, thereby altering the systemic arterial pressure.

The *renin-angiotensin-aldosterone* system also regulates BP (see discussion in Chapter 13). The kidney produces renin, an enzyme that acts on angiotensinogen to split off angiotensin I, which is converted by an enzyme in the lung to form angiotensin II. Angiotensin II has strong vasoconstrictor action on blood vessels and is the controlling mechanism for aldosterone release. Aldosterone then works on the collecting tubules in the kidneys to reabsorb sodium. Sodium retention inhibits fluid loss, thus increasing blood volume and subsequent BP.

Inappropriate secretion of renin may cause increased peripheral vascular resistance (PVR) in patients with hypertension. When the BP is high, renin levels should decrease because the increased renal arteriolar pressure usually inhibits renin secretion. However, for most people with essential hypertension, renin levels remain normal.

The process of vascular autoregulation, which keeps ***perfusion*** of tissues in the body relatively constant, appears to be important in causing hypertension. However, the exact mechanism of how this system works is poorly understood.

Classifications of Hypertension. Blood pressure is categorized into four levels: normal, elevated (or prehypertension), and stage 1 or 2 hypertension (Table 33.1). Hypertension, categorized as stage 1 or stage 2, can be classified as either essential (primary) or secondary (Whelton et al., 2017). **Essential hypertension** is the most common type and is not caused by an existing health problem. However, a number of risk factors can increase a person's likelihood of becoming hypertensive. Continuous BP elevation in patients with essential hypertension results in damage to vital organs by causing medial hyperplasia (thickening) of the arterioles. As the blood vessels thicken and ***perfusion*** decreases, body organs are damaged. These changes can result in myocardial infarctions (MIs), strokes, peripheral vascular disease (PVD), or kidney failure.

Specific disease states and drugs can increase a person's susceptibility to hypertension. A person with this type of elevation in BP has **secondary hypertension**.

Hypertensive crisis (or malignant hypertension) is a severe type of elevated BP that rapidly progresses and is considered a medical emergency. A person with this health problem usually has symptoms such as morning headaches, blurred vision, and dyspnea and/or symptoms of uremia (accumulation in the blood of substances ordinarily eliminated in the urine). Patients are often in their 30s, 40s, or 50s with their systolic BP greater than 200 mm Hg. The diastolic BP is greater than 150 mm Hg or greater than 130 mm Hg when there are pre-existing complications. Unless intervention occurs promptly, a patient with hypertensive crisis may experience kidney failure, left ventricular heart failure, or stroke.

Etiology and Genetic Risk. *Essential* hypertension can develop when a patient has any one or more of the risk factors listed in Table 33.2.

Kidney disease is one of the most common causes of *secondary* hypertension (see Table 33.2). Hypertension can develop when there is any sudden damage to the kidneys. Renovascular hypertension is associated with narrowing of one or more of the main arteries carrying blood directly to the kidneys, known as *renal artery stenosis (RAS)*. Many patients have been able to reduce the use of their antihypertensive drugs when the narrowed arteries are dilated through angioplasty with stent placement.

Dysfunction of the adrenal medulla or the adrenal cortex can also cause secondary hypertension. *Adrenal-mediated hypertension* is caused by primary excesses of aldosterone, cortisol, and catecholamines. In *primary aldosteronism,* excessive aldosterone causes hypertension and hypokalemia (low potassium levels). It usually arises from benign adenomas of the adrenal cortex. *Pheochromocytomas* are tumors that originate most commonly in the adrenal medulla and result in excessive

TABLE 33.1 Categories of Blood Pressure in Adults

Guidelines From Eighth Joint National Committee (JNC 8) on Prevention, Detection, Evaluation, and Treatment of High Blood Pressure Guidelines and From American College of Cardiology (ACC)/American Heart Association (AHA)

Blood Pressure Category	Systolic Blood Pressure		Diastolic Blood Pressure
Normal (ACC/AHA)	<120 mm Hg	and	<80 mm Hg
Elevated (ACC/AHA)	120-129 mm Hg	and	<80 mm Hg
Prehypertension (JNC-8)	120-139 mm Hg	or	80-89 mm Hg
Hypertension			
Stage 1			
ACC/AHA	130-139 mm Hg	or	80-89 mm Hg
JNC-8	140-159 mm Hg	or	90-99 mm Hg
Stage 2			
ACC/AHA	≥140 mm Hg	or	≥90 mm Hg
JNC-8	>160 mm Hg	or	>100 mm Hg

Data from Whelton, P.K., Carey, R.M., Aronow W.S., et al. (2017). CC/AHA/AAPA/ABC/ACPM/AGS/APhA/ASH/ASPC/NMA/PCNA guideline for the prevention, detection, evaluation, and management of high blood pressure in adults: executive summary. A report of the American College of Cardiology/American Heart Association Task Force on Clinical Practice Guidelines. *Hypertension,* Nov 13; and James, P.A., Oparil, S., Carter, B.L., Cushman, W.C., Dennison-Himmelfarb, C., Handler, J., et al. (2014). 2014 evidence-based guidelines for the management of high blood pressure in adults: Report from the panel members appointed to the Eighth National Committee (JNC 8). *JAMA: The Journal of the American Medical Association, 311*(5), 507–520.

TABLE 33.2 Etiology of Hypertension

Essential (Primary)	Secondary
Family history of hypertension	Kidney disease
African-American ethnicity	Primary aldosteronism
Hyperlipidemia	Pheochromocytoma
Smoking	Cushing disease
Older than 60 years or postmenopausal	Coarctation of the aorta
Excessive sodium and caffeine intake	Brain tumors
Overweight/obesity	Encephalitis
Physical inactivity	Pregnancy
Excessive alcohol intake	Drugs: • Estrogen (e.g., oral contraceptives) • Glucocorticoids • Mineralocorticoids • Sympathomimetics
Low potassium, calcium, or magnesium intake	
Excessive and continuous stress	

secretion of catecholamines, resulting in life-threatening high blood pressure. In *Cushing syndrome,* excessive glucocorticoids are excreted from the adrenal cortex. The most common cause of Cushing syndrome is either adrenocortical hyperplasia or adrenocortical adenoma (tumor).

Drugs that can cause secondary hypertension include estrogen, glucocorticoids, mineralocorticoids, sympathomimetics, cyclosporine, and erythropoietin. The use of estrogen-containing oral contraceptives is likely the most common cause of secondary hypertension in women. Drugs that cause hypertension are discontinued to reverse this problem.

Incidence and Prevalence. Hypertension is a worldwide epidemic. In the United States, it is estimated that 85.7 million adults 20 years of age and older have high blood pressure (Benjamin et al., 2018). The disease can shorten life expectancy.

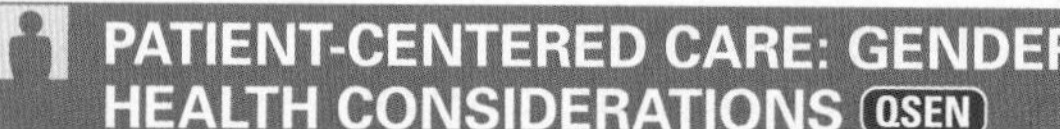

PATIENT-CENTERED CARE: GENDER HEALTH CONSIDERATIONS QSEN

A higher percentage of men than women have hypertension until 45 years of age. From ages 45 to 64, the percentages of men and women with hypertension are similar. After age 64, women have a higher percentage of the disease (Benjamin et al., 2018). The causes for these differences are not known.

PATIENT-CENTERED CARE: CULTURAL/ SPIRITUAL CONSIDERATIONS QSEN

The prevalence of hypertension in African Americans in the United States is among the highest in the world and is increasing. When compared with Euro-Americans, they develop high blood pressure earlier in life, making them much more likely to die from strokes, heart disease, and kidney disease (Benjamin et al., 2018). The exact reasons for these differences are not known. Because of the prevalence in the African-American population, JNC-8 guidelines as well as ACC/AHA guidelines offer population-specific recommendations for treatment (Whelton et al., 2017; James et al., 2014).

Health Promotion and Maintenance. Control of hypertension has resulted in major decreases in cardiovascular morbidity and mortality. The U.S. *Healthy People 2020* campaign includes a number of objectives related to hypertension to decrease cardiovascular mortality (Table 33.3). Many of these objectives remain goals in the projected development of *Healthy People 2030.*

Evidence-based dietary and exercise practices that can help lower blood pressure include:

- Achieve weight reduction through lifestyle changes using a combination of reduced caloric intake and increased physical activity.

TABLE 33.3 Meeting *Healthy People 2020* Objectives: Heart Disease and Stroke

Selected objectives retained from *Healthy People 2010:*

- Increase the proportion of adults with high blood pressure who are taking action to help control their blood pressure.
- Increase the proportion of adults who have had their blood pressure measured within the preceding 2 years and can state whether their blood pressure was normal or high.

Selected objectives retained but modified from *Healthy People 2010:*

- Reduce the proportion of people in the population with hypertension.
- Increase the proportion of adults with hypertension who meet the recommended guidelines for:
    a. Body mass index (BMI)
    b. Saturated fat consumption
    c. Sodium intake
    d. Physical activity
    e. Moderate alcohol consumption

New objectives for *Healthy People 2020:*

- Increase the proportion of adults with hypertension who are taking the recommended medications to decrease their blood pressure.

Leading Health Indicator and high-priority health issue:

- Increase the proportion of adults with hypertension whose blood pressure is controlled.

Data from Department of Health and Human Services. (2020). *Healthy People 2020*. Retrieved from: https://www.healthypeople.gov/2020/topics-objectives/topic/heart-disease-and-stroke/objectives.

- Implement Dietary Approaches to Stop Hypertension (DASH), a diet that is high in fruits, vegetables, and low-fat dairy products; enhance intake of potassium, calcium, magnesium, and fiber.
- Reduce the intake of dietary sodium. The optimal goal is less than 1500 mg of sodium per day.
- Increase physical activity that includes aerobic exercise, resistance training, and static isometric exercise.

In addition to following specific dietary and physical activity guidelines, teach patients ways to decrease other modifiable risk factors for hypertension, such as smoking cessation and stress reduction. Risk factor prevention and lifestyle changes are discussed in more detail in Chapter 35.

❖ Interprofessional Collaborative Care

◆ Assessment: Recognize Cues

History. Review the patient's risk factors for hypertension. Collect data on the patient's age; ethnic origin or race; family history of hypertension; average dietary intake of calories, sodium- and potassium-containing foods and alcohol; and exercise habits. Also assess any past or present history of kidney or cardiovascular disease (CVD) and current use of drug therapy or illicit drugs.

Physical Assessment/Signs and Symptoms. When a diagnosis of hypertension is made, most people have no symptoms. However, some patients experience headaches, facial flushing (redness), dizziness, or fainting as a result of the elevated blood pressure. Obtain blood pressure readings in both arms. Two or more readings may be taken at each visit (Fig. 33.1). Some patients have high blood pressure due to anxiety associated with visiting a health care provider. Be sure to take an accurate blood pressure by using an appropriate-size cuff.

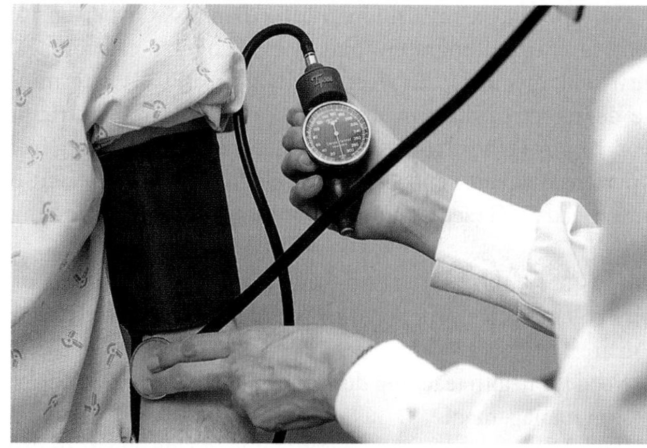

Fig. 33.1 Blood pressure screening during history and physical examination. (From Wilson S.F., Giddens J.F. [2017]. *Health assessment for nursing practice* [6th ed.]. St. Louis: Mosby.)

To detect postural (orthostatic) changes, take readings with the patient in the supine (lying) or sitting position and at least 3 minutes later when standing (McCance & Huether, 2019). **Orthostatic hypotension** is a decrease in blood pressure (20 mm Hg systolic and/or 10 mm Hg diastolic) when the patient changes position from lying to sitting.

Funduscopic examination of the eyes to observe vascular changes in the retina is done by a skilled health care practitioner. The appearance of the retina can be a reliable index of the severity and prognosis of hypertension. Physical assessment is also helpful in diagnosing several conditions that produce secondary hypertension. The presence of abdominal bruits is typical of patients with renal artery stenosis (RAS). Tachycardia, sweating, and pallor may suggest a pheochromocytoma (adrenal medulla tumor). Coarctation of the aorta is evidenced by elevation of blood pressure in the arms, with normal or low blood pressure in the lower extremities.

Psychosocial Assessment. Assess for psychosocial stressors that can worsen hypertension and affect the patient's ability to adhere to treatment. Evaluate job-related, economic, and other life stressors and the patient's response to these stressors. Some patients may have difficulty coping with the lifestyle changes needed to control hypertension. Be sure to assess past coping strategies.

Diagnostic Assessment. Although no laboratory tests are diagnostic of essential hypertension, several laboratory tests can assess possible causes of secondary hypertension. Kidney disease can be diagnosed by the presence of protein and red blood cells in the urine, elevated levels of blood urea nitrogen (BUN), and elevated serum creatinine levels. The creatinine clearance test directly indicates the glomerular filtration ability of the kidneys. The normal value is 107 to 139 mL/min for men and 87 to 107 mL/min for women (Pagana et al., 2018). Decreased levels indicate acute or chronic kidney disease.

Urinary test results are positive for the presence of catecholamines in patients with a pheochromocytoma (tumor of the adrenal medulla). An elevation in levels of serum corticoids and 17-ketosteroids in the urine is diagnostic of Cushing disease.

No specific x-ray studies can diagnose hypertension. Routine chest radiography may help recognize cardiomegaly (heart enlargement). An electrocardiogram (ECG) determines the degree of cardiac involvement. Left atrial and ventricular hypertrophy is the first ECG sign of heart disease resulting from hypertension. Left ventricular remodeling can be detected on the 12-lead ECG (see Chapter 35 for discussion of remodeling).

◆ **Analysis: Analyze Cues and Prioritize Hypotheses.** The priority collaborative problems for most patients with hypertension are:

1. Need for health teaching due to the plan of care for hypertension management
2. Potential for decreased adherence due to side effects of drug therapy and necessary changes in lifestyle

◆ Planning and Implementation: Generate Solutions and Take Action

Health Teaching

Planning: Expected Outcomes. The patient with hypertension is expected to verbalize his or her individualized plan of care for hypertension.

Interventions. Lifestyle changes are considered the foundation of hypertension control. If these changes are unsuccessful, the primary care provider considers the use of antihypertensive drugs. There is no surgical treatment for essential hypertension. However, surgery may be indicated for certain causes of secondary hypertension, such as kidney disease, coarctation of the aorta, and pheochromocytoma.

Lifestyle Changes. In collaboration with the health care team, teach the patient to (Whelton et al., 2017):

- Restrict dietary sodium according to ACC/AHA guidelines
- Reduce weight, if overweight or obese
- Implement a heart-healthy diet, such as the DASH diet
- Increase physical activity with a structured exercise program
- Abstain or decrease alcohol consumption (no more than one drink a day for women and two drinks a day for men)
- Stop smoking and tobacco use
- Use relaxation techniques to reduce stress

Strategies to help patients make these changes are discussed in Chapter 35.

Complementary and Integrative Health. Garlic, coenzyme Q_{10}, and fish oil have been used for a number of health problems, but evidence to support their use to prevent hypertension is controversial. Evidence by consensus and case reports do support garlic's cholesterol-lowering ability and its ability to decrease blood pressure in patients with hypertension (National Center for Complementary and Integrative Health, 2018). Garlic can increase the risk of bleeding in patients taking anticoagulants and can interfere with the effectiveness of some drugs. Teach patients to check with their primary health care provider before starting any herbal therapy because of possible side effects and interactions with other herbs, foods, or drugs.

Some patients have also had success with biofeedback, meditation, and acupuncture as part of their overall management plan. These methods may be most useful as adjuncts for patients who experience continuous and severe stress.

Drug Therapy. Drug therapy is individualized for each patient, with consideration given to culture, age, other existing illness, severity of blood pressure elevation, and cost of drugs and follow-up. Once-a-day drug therapy is best, especially for the older adult, because the more doses required each day, the higher the risk that a patient will not follow the treatment regimen. However, many patients with hypertension need two or more drugs to adequately control blood pressure.

In the largest hypertensive trial done to date, Antihypertensive and Lipid-Lowering Treatment to Prevent Heart Attack Trial (ALLHAT), the use of diuretics has been practically unmatched in preventing the cardiovascular complications of hypertension (ALLHAT, 2002). Current guidelines recommend use of one or more of these four classes of drugs: thiazide-type diuretics, calcium channel blockers (CCBs), angiotensin-converting enzyme inhibitors (ACEIs), and angiotensin II receptor blockers (ARBs). Using an ACEI, ARB, and/or renin inhibitor simultaneously is potentially harmful and is not recommended in the treatment of hypertension. Patients who do not respond to these first-line drugs may be placed on other diuretics, an aldosterone receptor antagonist (blocker), a beta-adrenergic blocker, or a renin inhibitor. Examples of commonly used drug classes for hypertension are listed in the Common Examples of Drug Therapy: Hypertension Management box.

Diuretics. Diuretics are the first type of drugs for managing hypertension. Three basic types of diuretics are used to decrease blood volume and lower blood pressure in the order of how commonly they are typically prescribed:

- Thiazide (low-ceiling) diuretics, such as hydrochlorothiazide, inhibit sodium, chloride, and water reabsorption in the distal tubules while promoting potassium, bicarbonate, and magnesium excretion. However, they decrease calcium excretion, which helps prevent kidney stones and bone loss. Because of the low cost and high effectiveness of thiazide-type diuretics, they are usually the drugs of choice for patients with uncomplicated hypertension. These drugs can be prescribed as a single agent or in combination with other classes of drugs.

! NURSING SAFETY PRIORITY QSEN

Drug Alert

Teach men that they may experience decreased libido (desire for sex) and decreased sexual performance when taking thiazide diuretics. Thiazide diuretics should be used with caution in patients with diabetes mellitus because they can interfere with serum glucose control. Caution is also indicated for patients with gout or a history of significant hyponatremia (decreased serum sodium level) because these problems can worsen when thiazides are taken.

- Loop (high-ceiling) diuretics, such as furosemide and torsemide, inhibit sodium, chloride, and water reabsorption in the ascending loop of Henle and promote potassium excretion.

COMMON EXAMPLES OF DRUG THERAPY

Hypertension Management

Drug Category	Nursing Implications
Diuretics Common examples of diuretics: • Potassium-sparing: spironolactone • Loop: furosemide; bumetanide • Thiazide: hydrochlorothiazide; chlorothiazide	Assess for weakness, dizziness, or a new onset of confusion *because these drugs can cause hypovolemia and dehydration.* Teach older adults to rise slowly *because the medication can cause orthostatic hypotension associated with diuresis.* For potassium-sparing agents: • Teach the patient to decrease intake of foods that are high in potassium and have follow-up laboratory tests for electrolyte levels *because these agents cause retention of* K^+ *in the body.* • Teach the patient to report weakness and irregular pulse to the primary health care provider *because these symptoms may indicate hyperkalemia.* For loop and thiazide agents: • Teach the patient to eat foods high in K^+ and to have follow-up laboratory tests to monitor electrolyte levels *because these agents cause* K^+ *and* Mg^{2+} *excretion.* • Use with caution in patients with diabetes *because glucose control can be affected.* • Use with caution in patients with gout *because uric acid retention can occur.*
Beta Blockers Common examples of beta blockers: • Atenolol • Metoprolol	Assess heart rate (HR) and blood pressure (BP) before administration *because beta blockers cause a decrease in HR and cardiac output and suppress renin activity.* • Do not administer if HR is <50-60 beats/min. • Hold for systolic <90-100 mm Hg and contact the health care provider. • Monitor for orthostatic hypotension *because this is a common adverse effect that can contribute to falls and confusion, especially in older adults.* Use with caution in patients with diabetes *because glucose production may be affected.* Teach the patient that these agents can cause fatigue, depression, and sexual dysfunction. These adverse effects should be reported to the primary health care provider.
Calcium Channel Blockers Common examples of calcium channel blockers: • Verapamil • Amlodipine • Diltiazem	Monitor pulse and BP before taking each day *because the drug slows SA and AV conduction, which decreases HR and vasodilation and causes decreased BP.* Teach patients to avoid grapefruit juice and grapefruit while taking calcium channel blockers *because grapefruit and its juice can enhance the action of the drug, causing organ dysfunction or death.*
Angiotensin-Converting Enzyme (ACE) Inhibitors Common examples of ACE inhibitors: • Lisinopril • Enalapril • Captopril	Report persistent, dry cough to the primary health care provider *because this is a common and annoying side effect, and another type of antihypertensive medication may be necessary.* Monitor BP carefully, especially orthostatic pressures, *because these agents result in vasodilation and decreased BP.* • Do not give the drug without checking with the health care provider if systolic BP is below 100. Assess for hyperkalemia *because ACE inhibitors reduce the excretion of potassium.*
Angiotensin II Receptor Blockers (ARBs) Common examples of ARBs: • Valsartan • Losartan	Teach patients to avoid foods high in potassium *because ARBs can cause hyperkalemia, especially when combined with other hypertensive agents.* Monitor BP carefully, especially orthostatic pressures, *because these agents result in vasodilation and decreased BP.* • Do not give the drug without checking with the health care provider if systolic BP is below 100.

AV, Atrioventricular; *SA*, sinoatrial.

NURSING SAFETY PRIORITY QSEN

Drug Alert

The most frequent side effect associated with *thiazide and loop diuretics* is hypokalemia (low potassium level). Monitor serum potassium levels and assess for irregular pulse, dysrhythmias, and muscle weakness, which may indicate hypokalemia. Teach patients taking potassium-depleting diuretics to eat foods high in potassium, such as bananas, potatoes, and orange juice. Most people also need a potassium supplement to maintain adequate serum potassium levels.

Assess for hyperkalemia (high potassium level) in patients taking potassium-sparing diuretics such as spironolactone. Like hypokalemia, an increased potassium level can also cause weakness, irregular pulse, and cardiac dysrhythmias. In some cases, patients may have painful muscle spasms (cramping) in their legs. These electrolyte imbalances are described in detail in Chapter 13.

Monitor renal function prior to administration because renal failure is a side effect of *thiazide and loop diuretics.* Tinnitus and hearing loss may occur when high doses are given over an extended period of time or when given as a rapid infusion.

PATIENT-CENTERED CARE: OLDER ADULT CONSIDERATIONS QSEN

Loop diuretics are not used commonly for older adults because they can cause dehydration and orthostatic hypotension. These complications increase the patient's risk for falls. Teach families to monitor for and report patient dizziness, falls, or confusion to the primary health care provider as soon as possible and discontinue the drug.

Potassium-sparing diuretics, such as spironolactone, triamterene, and amiloride, act on the distal renal tubule to inhibit reabsorption of sodium ions in exchange for potassium, thereby *retaining* potassium in the body. When used, they are typically in combination with another diuretic or antihypertensive drug to *conserve* potassium.

Frequent voiding caused by any type of diuretic may interfere with daily activities. Teach patients to take their diuretic in the morning rather than at night to prevent nocturia (voiding during the night).

Other Antihypertensive Drugs. *Calcium channel blockers (CCBs),* such as verapamil hydrochloride and amlodipine, lower blood pressure by interfering with the transmembrane flux of calcium ions. This results in vasodilation, which *decreases* blood pressure. These drugs also block sinoatrial (SA) and atrioventricular (AV) node conduction, resulting in a decreased heart rate (HR). Calcium channel blockers, in combination withthiazide diuretics, are first-line drug therapy for African Americans (Whelton et al., 2017).

Some CCBs, especially felodipine and nifedipine, react with grapefruit and grapefruit juice. Teach the patient to avoid grapefruit juice to prevent complications such as kidney failure, heart failure, GI bleeding, or even death. A newer CCB, clevidipine butyrate, is available only in IV form and must be administered using an infusion pump. This drug, indicated when oral therapy is not possible, is used for severe hypertension. The most common side effects are headache and nausea. Notify the health care provider immediately if neurologic symptoms, visual changes, or symptoms of heart failure occur (Skidmore-Roth, 2018)

Angiotensin-converting enzyme inhibitors (ACE inhibitors or ACEIs), known as the *"-pril" drugs,* are also used as single or combination agents in the treatment of hypertension. These drugs block the action of angiotensin-converting enzyme (ACE) as it attempts to convert angiotensin I to angiotensin II, one of the most powerful vasoconstrictors in the body. This action also decreases sodium and water retention and lowers peripheral vascular resistance (PVR), both of which lower blood pressure. ACEIs include capto*pril,* lisino*pril,* and enala*pril. The most common side effect of this group of drugs is a nagging, dry cough.* Teach patients to report this problem to their primary health care provider as soon as possible. If a cough develops, the drug is discontinued.

! NURSING SAFETY PRIORITY (QSEN)

Drug Alert

Instruct the patient receiving an ACEI for the first time to get out of bed slowly to avoid the severe hypotensive effect that can occur with initial use. Orthostatic hypotension may occur with subsequent doses, but it is usually less severe. If dizziness continues or there is a significant decrease in the systolic blood pressure (more than a change of 20 mm Hg), notify the health care provider or teach the patient to notify the health care provider. *The older patient is at the greatest risk for orthostatic hypotension because of the cardiovascular changes associated with aging.*

Angiotensin II receptor antagonists, also called *angiotensin II receptor blockers (ARBs)* or the *-sartan drugs,* make up a group of drugs that selectively block the binding of angiotensin II to receptor sites in the vascular smooth muscle and adrenal tissues by competing directly with angiotensin II but not inhibiting ACE. Examples of drugs in this group are cande*sartan,* val*sartan,* lo*sartan,* and azil*sartan.* ARBs can be used alone or in combination with other antihypertensive drugs. These drugs are excellent options for patients who report a nagging cough associated with ACEIs. In addition, they do not require initial adjustment of the dose for older adults or for any patient with renal impairment. Like the ACEs, the ARBs are not as effective in African Americans unless they are taken with diuretics or another category such as a beta blocker or calcium channel blocker (CCB) (Whelton et al., 2017). In 2018 the U.S. Food and Drug Administration (FDA) found that there were impurities that presented a safety concern in some ARBs, most notably valsartan. This recall expanded in 2019 to include certain manufacturers of losartan and irbesartan (FDA, 2019). It is important to note that the FDA recalled certain lots of the drugs, and formulations with the known impurities are no longer on the U.S. market. Unaffected ARBs remain on the market and continue to be used safely (FDA, 2018; FDA, 2019).

Beta-adrenergic blockers, identified by the ending *-olol,* are categorized as cardioselective (working on only the cardiovascular system) and noncardioselective. Cardioselective beta blockers, affecting only beta$_1$ receptors, may be prescribed to lower blood pressure by blocking beta receptors in the heart and peripheral vessels. By blocking these receptors, the drug decreases heart rate (HR) and myocardial contractility. Teach patients about common side effects of beta blockers, including fatigue, weakness, depression, and sexual dysfunction. The potential for side effects depends on the "selective" blocking effects of the drug. Aten*olol,* bisopr*olol,* and metopr*olol* are cardioselective beta blockers given for hypertension.

Patients with diabetes who take beta blockers may not have the usual manifestations of hypoglycemia because the sympathetic nervous system is blocked. The body's responses to hypoglycemia such as gluconeogenesis may also be inhibited by certain beta blockers.

Beta blockers are often the drug of choice for hypertensive patients with ischemic heart disease because the heart is the most common target of end-organ damage with hypertension. If this drug is not tolerated, a long-acting CCB can be used. In patients with unstable angina or myocardial infarction (MI), beta blockers or CCBs should be used initially in combination with ACEIs or ARBs, with addition of other drugs if needed to control the blood pressure (see Chapter 35). It is important to teach patients that beta blockers should not be stopped abruptly. Tapering off of these medications over a 2-week period is recommended because abrupt cessation can lead to angina or MI.

NCLEX EXAMINATION CHALLENGE 33.1

Health Promotion and Maintenance

The nurse is caring for a diabetic client who will be discharged on hydrochlorothiazide (HCTZ). What information will the nurse include in the discharge teaching? **Select all that apply.**

A. "This drug may cause a dry, nagging cough."
B. "Take this drug with a snack, right before bed."
C. "Try to increase your intake of potassium in your diet."
D. "This drug can affect your glucose control."
E. "Increased urination is expected with this drug.

Promoting Adherence to the Plan of Care

Planning: Expected Outcomes. The patient with hypertension is expected to adhere to the plan of care, including making necessary lifestyle changes.

Interventions. Patients who require medications to control essential hypertension usually need to take them for the rest of their lives. Some patients stop taking them because they have no symptoms and have troublesome side effects.

In the hospital setting, interprofessional collaboration with the pharmacist to discuss the outcomes of therapy with the patient, including potential side effects, can help the patient tailor the therapeutic regimen to his or her lifestyle and daily schedule.

Patients who do not adhere to antihypertensive treatment are at a high risk for target organ damage and hypertensive crisis, a severe elevation in blood pressure (>180/120) that can cause organ damage in the kidneys or heart (target organs) (see the Best Practice for Patient Safety & Quality Care: Emergency Care of Patients With Hypertensive Crisis box).

Patients in hypertensive crisis are admitted to critical care units, where they receive IV antihypertensive therapy such as nitroprusside, nicardipine, fenoldopam, or labetalol. For adults without a compelling condition, systolic BP should be reduced by no more than 25% within the first hour; then, if stable, to 160/100 mm Hg within the next 2 to 6 hours; and then cautiously to normal during the following 24 to 48 hours (Whelton et al., 2017). A gradual reduction in blood pressure is preferred because rapid reduction can cause cerebral ischemia, MI, and renal failure. Provide oxygen to the patient and monitor oxygen saturation levels. When the patient's blood pressure stabilizes, oral antihypertensive drugs are given.

BEST PRACTICE FOR PATIENT SAFETY & QUALITY CARE (QSEN)

Emergency Care of Patients With Hypertensive Crisis

Assess:
- Severe headache
- Extremely high blood pressure (BP)
- Dizziness
- Blurred vision
- Shortness of breath
- Epistaxis (nosebleed)
- Severe anxiety

Intervene:
- Place patient in semi-Fowler position.
- Administer oxygen.
- Administer IV beta blocker or nicardipine or other infusion drug as prescribed; when stable, switch to oral antihypertensive drug.
- Monitor BP every 5 to 15 minutes until the diastolic pressure is below 90 and not less than 75; then monitor BP every 30 minutes to ensure that BP is not lowered too quickly.
- Observe for neurologic or cardiovascular complications, such as seizures; numbness, weakness, or tingling of extremities; dysrhythmias; or chest pain (possible indicators of target organ damage).

Care Coordination and Transition Management

Home Care Management. Hypertension is a chronic illness. Allow patients to verbalize feelings about the disease and its treatment. Emphasize that their involvement in the collaborative plan of care can lead to control of the disease and can prevent complications.

Some patients do not adhere to their drug therapy regimen at home because they have no symptoms or they simply forget to take their drugs. Others may think they are not sick enough to need medication. Some patients may assume that once their blood pressure (BP) returns to normal levels, they no longer need treatment. They may also stop taking their drugs because of side effects or cost. Develop a plan with the patient and family and identify ways to encourage adherence to the plan of care.

Self-Management Education. Health teaching is essential to help patients become successful in managing their BP. Provide oral and written information about the indications, dosage, times of administration, side effects, and drug interactions for antihypertensives. Stress that medication must be taken as prescribed; when all of it has been consumed, the prescription must be renewed on a continual basis. Suddenly stopping drugs such as beta blockers can result in angina (chest pain), myocardial infarction (MI), or rebound hypertension. Urge patients to report unpleasant side effects such as excessive fatigue, cough, or sexual dysfunction. In many instances, an alternative drug can be prescribed to minimize certain side effects.

Teach the patient to obtain an ambulatory BP monitoring (ABPM) device for use at home so the pressure can be checked. Evaluate the patient's and family's ability to use this device. If weight reduction is a desired outcome, suggest having a scale in the home for weight monitoring. For patients who do not want to self-monitor, are not able to self-monitor, or have "white-coat" syndrome when they go to their primary health care provider (causing elevated BP), continuous ABPM may be used. The monitor is worn for 24 hours or longer while patients perform their normal daily activities. BP is automatically taken every 15 to 30 minutes and recorded for review later. The advantage of this technique is that the primary health care provider can view the changes in BP readings throughout the 24-hour period to get a picture of a true BP value. Research strongly supports 24-hour ambulatory BP monitoring as a first-line procedure to determine the need for antihypertensive therapy (U.S. Preventive Services Task Force, 2017).

Instruct the patient about sodium restriction, weight maintenance or reduction, alcohol restriction, stress management, and exercise. If necessary, also explain about the need to stop using tobacco, especially smoking.

Health Care Resources. A home care nurse may be needed for follow-up to monitor the BP. Evaluate patient or family ability to obtain accurate BP measurements and assess adherence with treatment. The American Heart Association, the Red Cross, or a local pharmacy may be used for free BP checks if patients cannot buy equipment to monitor their BP. Health fairs and BP screening programs located in faith-based centers are also available in most locations.

◆ **Evaluation: Evaluate Outcomes.** Evaluate the care of the patient with hypertension on the basis of the identified patient problems. The expected outcomes are that the patient will:

- Verbalize understanding of the plan of care, including drug therapy and any necessary lifestyle changes
- Report adverse drug effects, such as coughing, dizziness, or sexual dysfunction, to the primary health care provider immediately
- Consistently adhere to the plan of care, including regular follow-up with the primary health care provider

CLINICAL JUDGMENT CHALLENGE 33.1

Patient-Centered Care; Teamwork and Collaboration; Evidence-Based Practice

The nurse is performing an assessment in the outpatient clinic on a 63-year-old male client. His initial blood pressure is 189/113 mm Hg, heart rate is 94 beats/min, and respiration rate is 26 breaths/min. The client reports a smoking history of 25 cigarettes per day and an average of two alcoholic drinks per day. The client also informs the nurse that he recently lost his job as the director of sales at a local company and is worried about providing for his family. The client exercises once a week by walking with his family in the park. The client does not take any prescription or herbal medications.

1. **Recognize Cues:** What assessment information in this client situation is the most important and immediate concern for the nurse? (Hint: Identify the **relevant** information *first* to determine what is most important.)
2. **Analyze Cues:** What client conditions are consistent with the **most relevant** information? (Hint: Think about priority collaborative problems that support and contradict the information presented in this situation.)
3. **Prioritize Hypotheses:** Which possibilities or explanations are **most likely** to be present in this client situation? Which possibilities or explanations are the most serious? (Hint: Consider all possibilities and determine their urgency and risk for this client.)
4. **Generate Solutions:** What actions would most likely achieve the desired outcomes for this client? Which actions should be **avoided** or are **potentially harmful**? (Hint: Determine the desired outcomes first to decide which interventions are appropriate and those that should be avoided.)
5. **Take Action:** Which actions are the most appropriate and how should they be implemented? In what **priority order** should they be implemented? (Hint: Consider health teaching, documentation, requested health care provider orders or prescriptions, nursing skills, collaboration with or referral to health team members, etc.)
6. **Evaluate Outcomes:** What client assessment would indicate that the nurse's actions were **effective**? (Hint: Think about signs that would indicate an improvement, decline, or unchanged client condition.)

ARTERIOSCLEROSIS AND ATHEROSCLEROSIS

Pathophysiology Review

Arteriosclerosis is a thickening, or hardening, of the arterial wall that is often associated with aging. **Atherosclerosis**, a type of arteriosclerosis, involves the formation of plaque within the arterial wall and is the leading risk factor for cardiovascular disease (CVD). Usually the disease affects the larger arteries, such as coronary artery beds; aorta; carotid and vertebral arteries; renal, iliac, and femoral arteries; or any combination of these.

The exact pathophysiology of atherosclerosis is not known, but the condition is thought to occur from blood vessel damage that causes ***inflammation*** (Fig. 33.2). ***Inflammation*** occurs in response to cellular injury. After the vessel becomes inflamed, a fatty streak appears on the intimal surface (inner lining) of the artery. Through the process of cellular proliferation, collagen migrates over the fatty streak, forming a fibrous plaque. The fibrous plaque is often elevated and protrudes into the vessel lumen, partially or completely obstructing blood flow through the artery. Plaques are either stable or unstable. Unstable plaques are prone to rupture and are often clinically silent until they rupture (McCance & Huether, 2019).

In the final stage, the fibrous plaques become calcified, hemorrhagic, ulcerated, or thrombosed and affect all layers of the vessel. The rate of progression of the process may be influenced by genetic factors; certain chronic diseases (e.g., diabetes mellitus); and lifestyle habits, including smoking, eating habits, and level of exercise.

When *stable* plaque ruptures, thrombosis (blood clot) and constriction obstruct the vessel lumen, causing inadequate ***perfusion*** and oxygenation to distal tissues. *Unstable* plaque rupture causes more severe damage. After the rupture occurs, the exposed underlying tissue causes platelet adhesion and rapid thrombus formation. The thrombus may suddenly block a blood vessel, resulting in ischemia and infarction (e.g., myocardial infarction [MI]).

Endothelial (intimal) injury of the major arteries of the body can be caused by many factors. Elevated levels of **lipids** (fats) such as low-density lipoprotein cholesterol (LDL-C) and decreased levels of high-density lipoprotein cholesterol (HDL-C) can cause chemical injuries to the vessel wall. (Chapter 30 discusses lipids in detail.) Chemical injury can also be caused by elevated levels of toxins in the bloodstream, which may occur with renal failure or by carbon monoxide circulating in the bloodstream from cigarette smoking. The vessel wall can be weakened by the natural process of aging or by diseases such as hypertension.

Genetic predisposition and diabetes have a major effect on the development of atherosclerosis. Some patients have familial **hyperlipidemia**, an elevation of serum lipid levels. In these people, the liver makes excessive cholesterol and other fats. However, some people with hereditary atherosclerosis have a normal blood cholesterol level. The reason for the development and progression of plaque in these patients is not understood (McCance & Huether, 2019).

Adult patients of any age with severe diabetes mellitus frequently have premature and severe atherosclerosis from microvascular damage. The premature atherosclerosis occurs because diabetes promotes an increase in LDL-C and triglycerides (TGs) (lipids) in plasma. In addition, arterial damage may result from the effect of hyperglycemia.

Other factors are indirectly related to atherosclerosis development. A list of risk factors is found in Table 33.4.

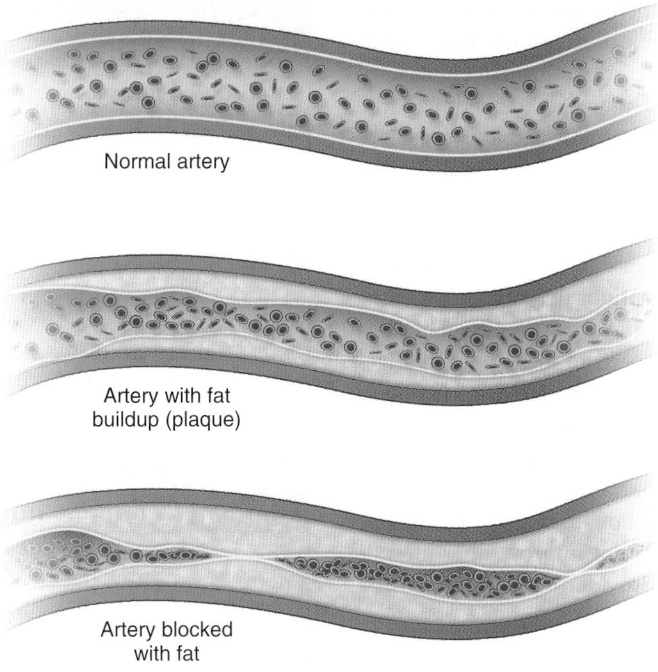

Fig. 33.2 Pathophysiology of atherosclerosis.

TABLE 33.4 Risk Factors for Atherosclerosis

- Low HDL-C
- High LDL-C
- Increased triglycerides
- Genetic predisposition
- Diabetes mellitus
- Obesity
- Hypertension
- Sedentary lifestyle
- Smoking
- Stress
- African-American or Hispanic ethnicity
- Older adult
- Diet high in saturated and *trans* fats, cholesterol, sodium, and sugar

HDL-C, High-density lipoprotein cholesterol; *LDL-C,* low-density lipoprotein cholesterol.

It is not known exactly how many people have atherosclerosis, but small plaques are almost always present in the arteries of young adults. The incidence can be better quantified by assessing the number of cardiovascular diseases (CVDs) that result from atherosclerosis. An estimated 92.1 million U.S. adults have one or more types of CVD (Benjamin et al., 2018). About half of those with CVD are older than 60 years, and many more are middle-age. The number of people affected by atherosclerosis is likely to increase as the population ages.

Interprofessional Collaborative Care

Assessment: Recognize Cues. The assessment of a patient with atherosclerosis includes a complete cardiovascular assessment because associated heart disease is often present. Because of the high incidence of hypertension in patients with atherosclerosis, assess the blood pressure in both arms.

Palpate pulses at all the major sites on the body and note any differences. *Palpate each carotid artery separately to prevent blocking blood flow to the brain!* Also feel for temperature differences in the lower extremities and check capillary filling. Prolonged capillary filling (>3 seconds in young-to-middle-age adults; >5 seconds in older adults) generally indicates poor circulation, *although this is not the most reliable indicator of* ***perfusion.*** With severe atherosclerotic disease, the extremity may be cool or cold with a diminished or absent pulse.

Many patients with vascular disease have a bruit in the larger arteries, which can be heard with a stethoscope or Doppler probe. A *bruit* is a turbulent, swishing sound, which can be soft or loud in pitch. It is heard as a result of blood trying to pass through a narrowed artery. A bruit is considered abnormal, but it does not indicate the severity of disease. Bruits often occur in the carotid, aortic, femoral, and popliteal arteries.

! NURSING SAFETY PRIORITY QSEN

Critical Rescue

A decrease in intensity or a complete loss of a pulse in a patient with atherosclerosis may indicate an arterial occlusion (blockage) in the area supplied by the artery. If a pulse is not palpable, use a Doppler to further assess the pulse. Immediately report pulselessness to the health care provider and document for emergency management (described later in this chapter under Acute Peripheral Arterial Occlusion).

Patients with atherosclerosis often have elevated lipids, including cholesterol and triglycerides (TGs). Elevated cholesterol levels are confirmed by HDL and LDL measurements. Increased low-density lipoprotein cholesterol (LDL-C) ("bad" cholesterol) levels and low high-density lipoprotein cholesterol (HDL-C) ("good" cholesterol) indicate that a person is at an increased risk for atherosclerosis. The *triglyceride* level may also be elevated with atherosclerosis. Elevated TGs are considered a marker for other lipoproteins. They also suggest metabolic syndrome, which increases the risk for coronary disease (see Chapter 30 for in-depth serum lipid information).

◆ **Interventions: Take Action.** Atherosclerosis progresses for years before signs and symptoms occur. Adults who are at risk for the disease can often be identified through cholesterol screening and history. Because of the high incidence in the United States, low-risk people 20 years of age and older are advised to have their total serum cholesterol level evaluated at least once every 4 to 6 years. More frequent measurements are suggested for people with multiple risk factors and those older than 40 years. People with multiple risk factors are grouped into high-risk patient categories. Interventions for patients with atherosclerosis or those at high risk for the disease focus on lifestyle changes. Teach patients about the need to make daily changes by avoiding or minimizing modifiable risk factors. *Modifiable risk factors* are those that can be changed or controlled by the patient, such as smoking, weight management, and exercise. Nutrition is one of the most important parts of the risk-reduction plan. Chapter 35 describes how to manage modifiable risk factors. If lipoprotein levels do not improve after lifestyle changes, the primary health care provider may prescribe drug therapy to lower cholesterol and/or TGs.

Nutrition Therapy. The ACC and AHA publish dietary recommendations for lowering LDL-C levels (Grundy et al., 2018). These recommendations are based on the best current evidence from randomized controlled trials and include:

- Consume a dietary pattern that emphasizes intake of vegetables, fruits, and whole grains.
- Consume low-fat dairy products, poultry (without the skin), fish, legumes, nontropical (e.g., canola) vegetable oils, and nuts.
- Limit intake of sweets, sugar-sweetened beverages, and red meats.
- Aim for a dietary pattern that includes 5% to 6% of calories from saturated fat; limiting *trans* fats.

These guidelines are similar to the Dietary Approaches to Stop Hypertension (DASH), which also recommend daily sodium, potassium, and fiber amounts (National Heart, Lung, and Blood Institute, 2018). Interprofessional collaboration with the registered dietitian nutritionist to teach the patient about the types of fat content in food is encouraged. Meats and eggs contain mostly saturated fats and are high in cholesterol. Instruct patients about increasing dietary fiber to 30 g each day, which is consistent with DASH guidelines.

Physical Activity. The ACC/AHA guidelines also recommend that adults engage in aerobic physical activity three or four times a week to reduce LDL-C levels. Each session should last for 40 minutes on average and involve moderate-to-vigorous physical activity (Grundy et al., 2018).

Drug Therapy. For patients with elevated total and LDL-C levels that do not respond adequately to dietary intervention, the primary health care provider prescribes a cholesterol-lowering agent. Drug choice and dosing depend on the serum cholesterol level, the degree to which the level needs to be decreased, and the patient's age (Grundy et al., 2018). Because most of these drugs can produce side effects, they are generally given only when nonpharmacologic management has been unsuccessful.

A class of drugs known as *3-hydroxy-3-methylglutaryl coenzyme A (HMG-CoA) reductase inhibitors (statins)* successfully reduces total cholesterol in most patients when used for an extended period. Examples include lovastatin, simvastatin, and pitavastatin, which lower both LDL-C and triglyceride levels (Table 33.5).

TABLE 33.5 Commonly Used Drugs for Lowering LDL-C Levels

HMG-CoA Reductase Inhibitors (Statins)	Combination Drugs
• Lovastatin	• Ezetimibe and simvastatin (Vytorin)
• Atorvastatin	• Amlodipine and atorvastatin (Caduet)
• Simvastatin	• Aspirin and pravastatin (Pravigard)
• Fluvastatin	
• Rosuvastatin	
• Pravastatin	
• Pitavastatin	

HMG-CoA, 3-hydroxy-3-methylglutaryl coenzyme A; *LDL-C,* low-density lipoprotein cholesterol.

TABLE 33.6 Selected 2018 Cholesterol Clinical Practice Guidelines

Physical activity	Engage in aerobic physical activity consisting of three to four sessions per week, lasting 40 minutes per session. Physical activity should involve moderate-to vigorous intensity.
Diet	Reduced-calorie diet consisting of fruits and vegetables (combined five or more servings per day), grains (primarily whole grains), fish, and lean meats. Intake of saturated fats, *trans* fats, and cholesterol should be limited; LDL-C–lowering macronutrient intake should include plant stanols/sterols (~2 g/ day) and soluble fiber.
Tobacco cessation	Tobacco cessation should be strongly encouraged and facilitated. Current smoking is a high-risk condition for future atherosclerotic cardiovascular disease (ASCVD).
Pharmacologic therapy	Statin drugs are the drug of choice for decreasing lipids. People within high-risk and very-high-risk categories may also be treated with combination therapy, which may include ezetimibe, bile acid sequestrants, or PCSK9 inhibitors.

LDL-C, Low-density lipoprotein cholesterol.
Data from Grundy, S., Stone, N., Bailey, A., Beam, C., Birtcher, K.K., Blumenthal, R.S., et al. (2018). 2018 AHA/ACC guideline on the management of blood cholesterol: a report of the American College of Cardiology/American Heart Association Task Force on Clinical Practice Guidelines. *Circulation,* 10 Nov.

The American College of Cardiology (ACC)/American Heart Association (AHA) publishes recommendations for treatment of high cholesterol to reduce atherosclerotic cardiovascular disease (ASCVD) in adults (Grundy et al., 2018). Selected evidence-based recommendations are highlighted in Table 33.6. It is important to note that although these guidelines support regular monitoring of laboratory data, the focus of care is based on patient risk and the modification of that risk versus just reduction of the laboratory value. Statin therapy should be used as an adjunct therapy to lifestyle modification (i.e., adherence to a heart-healthy diet, regular exercise habits, avoidance of tobacco products, and maintenance of a healthy weight) for risk reduction versus simply a medication to modify cholesterol levels (Lloyd-Jones et al., 2017).

! NURSING SAFETY PRIORITY (QSEN)

Drug Alert

Statins reduce cholesterol synthesis in the liver and increase clearance of LDL-C from the blood. Therefore they are contraindicated in patients with active liver disease or during pregnancy because they can cause muscle myopathies and marked decreases in liver function. Statins also have the potential for interactions with other drugs, such as warfarin, cyclosporine, and selected antibiotics. They are discontinued if the patient has muscle cramping or elevated liver enzyme levels. Some patients also report abdominal bloating, flatulence, diarrhea, and/or constipation as side effects of these drugs. Remind patients to have laboratory testing follow-up as prescribed by their primary health care provider.

Teach patients taking statin drugs, especially those taking atorvastatin, lovastatin, and simvastatin, to *limit grapefruit (no more than half a grapefruit) and grapefruit juice (no more than 8 ounces) in their diet* (Rosenson & Baker, 2018). Grapefruit contains a group of chemicals called *furanocoumarins* that bind to and inactivate the enzyme CYP3A4. This enzyme is important for metabolism of many drugs, including statins. If it is inactivated, too much of the statin drug can remain in the patient's bloodstream, causing adverse interactions or muscle injury.

A different type of lipid-lowering agent, ezetimibe, may be used in place of or in combination with statin-type drugs. This drug inhibits the absorption of cholesterol through the small intestine, leading to a decrease in the delivery of intestinal cholesterol to the liver, and increases the clearance of cholesterol from the blood. Vytorin is a combination drug containing ezetimibe and simvastatin. This drug works two ways—by reducing the absorption of cholesterol and by decreasing the amount of cholesterol synthesis in the liver. Amlodipine and atorvastatin are combined as Caduet to decrease blood pressure while decreasing triglycerides (TGs), increasing HDL, and lowering LDL. Combining drugs may improve adherence for the patient who is often taking multiple drugs.

The U.S. Food and Drug Administration (FDA) approved the drug class PCSK9 inhibitors for use in patients with familial hypercholesterolemia or for those in whom existing therapies are unable to reduce LDLs. These potent drugs inhibit PCSK9, which is a protease produced primarily in the liver that can cause elevations in LDLs. Alirocumab and evolocumab are administered by subcutaneous injection on a monthly or bimonthly basis for patients who are on maximally tolerated doses of statins.

Complementary and Integrative Health. Nicotinic acid or niacin, a B vitamin, may lower LDL-C and very-low-density lipoprotein (VLDL) cholesterol levels and increase HDL-C levels in some patients. The use of nicotinic acid is limited by poor tolerability (Rosenson & Kastelein, 2018). Low doses are recommended because many patients experience flushing and a very warm feeling all over. Higher doses can result in an elevation of hepatic enzymes. In statin-intolerant patients, niacin can be useful to help lower LDL cholesterol levels in combination with other drugs.

Lovaza (omega-3 ethyl esters) is approved by the FDA as an adjunct to diet to reduce TGs that are greater than 500 mg/dL (Burchum & Rosenthal, 2019).

NCLEX EXAMINATION CHALLENGE 33.2

Health Promotion and Maintenance

Which assessment finding will the nurse anticipate in a client with severe atherosclerotic disease?

A. Carotid artery bruit
B. HDL 60 mg/dL
C. Palpable peripheral pulses
D. BP 120/58 mm Hg

PERIPHERAL ARTERIAL DISEASE

Pathophysiology Review

Peripheral vascular disease (PVD) includes disorders that change the natural flow of blood through the arteries and veins of the peripheral circulation, causing decreased ***perfusion*** to body tissues. It affects the legs much more frequently than the arms. In general, a diagnosis of PVD implies arterial disease (peripheral arterial disease [PAD]) rather than venous involvement. Some patients have both arterial and venous disease. The cost of the disease is very high and is expected to increase as "baby boomers" age and obesity in the United States continues to be a major health problem.

PAD is a result of systemic atherosclerosis. It is a chronic condition in which partial or total arterial occlusion (blockage) decreases ***perfusion*** to the extremities. The tissues below the narrowed or obstructed arteries cannot live without an adequate *oxygen* and nutrient supply. PAD in the legs is sometimes referred to as *lower extremity arterial disease (LEAD)*.

Obstructions are classified as inflow or outflow, according to the arteries involved and their relationship to the inguinal ligament (Fig. 33.3). *Inflow* obstructions involve the distal end of the aorta and the common, internal, and external iliac arteries. They are located above the inguinal ligament. *Outflow* obstructions involve the femoral, popliteal, and tibial arteries and are below the superficial femoral artery (SFA). Gradual inflow occlusions may not cause significant tissue damage. Gradual outflow occlusions typically do.

Atherosclerosis is the most common cause of chronic arterial obstruction; therefore the risk factors for atherosclerosis apply to PAD as well (see Table 33.4). Advancing age also increases the risk for disease related to atherosclerosis. Patients with PAD have an increased risk for developing chronic angina, MI, or stroke. PAD is a marker for systemic atherosclerotic disease, making people with PAD more likely to have atherosclerosis in other vascular beds such as the coronary, carotid, and renal arteries and the abdominal aorta (Benjamin et al., 2018). About 8.5 million people in the United States age 40 and older have PAD. African Americans are affected more often than any other group, most likely because they have many risk factors such as diabetes and hypertension (Benjamin et al., 2018).

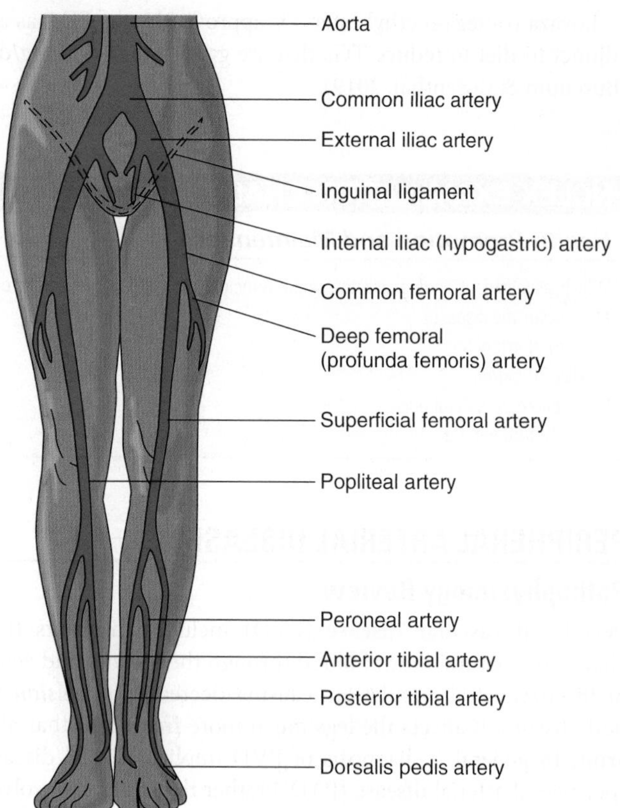

Fig. 33.3 Common locations of inflow and outflow lesions.

Interprofessional Collaborative Care

Assessment: Recognize Cues. The clinical course of chronic PAD can be divided into four stages (see the Key Features: Chronic Peripheral Arterial Disease box). Patients do not experience symptoms in the early stages of disease. Many patients are not diagnosed until they develop leg pain.

KEY FEATURES

Chronic Peripheral Arterial Disease

Stage I: Asymptomatic
- No claudication is present.
- Bruit or aneurysm may be present.
- Pedal pulses are decreased or absent.

Stage II: Claudication
- Muscle pain, cramping, or burning occurs with exercise and is relieved with rest.
- Symptoms are reproducible with exercise.

Stage III: Rest Pain
- Pain while resting commonly awakens the patient at night.
- Pain is described as numbness, burning, toothache-type pain.
- Pain usually occurs in the distal part of the extremity (toes, arch, forefoot, or heel), rarely in the calf or the ankle.
- Pain is relieved by placing the extremity in a dependent position.

Stage IV: Necrosis/Gangrene
- Ulcers and blackened tissue occur on the toes, forefoot, and heel.
- Distinctive gangrenous odor is present.

Most patients initially seek medical attention for a classic leg pain known as **intermittent claudication** (a term derived from a word meaning "to limp"). Usually they can walk only a certain distance before discomfort, such as cramping or burning muscular pain, forces them to stop. The pain stops with rest. When patients resume walking, they can walk the same distance before it returns. Thus the pain is considered reproducible. As the disease progresses, they can walk only shorter and shorter distances before pain recurs. Ultimately it may occur even while at rest.

Rest pain, which may begin while the disease is still in the stage of intermittent claudication, is a numb or burning sensation, often described as feeling like a toothache that is severe enough to awaken patients at night. It is usually located in the toes, the foot arches, the forefeet, the heels, and rarely in the calves or ankles. Patients can sometimes alleviate pain by keeping the limb in a dependent position (below the heart). Those with rest pain often have advanced disease that may result in limb loss.

Patients with **inflow disease** have discomfort in the lower back, buttocks, or thighs. Patients with *mild* inflow disease have discomfort after walking about two blocks. This discomfort is not severe but causes them to stop walking. It is relieved with rest. Patients with *moderate* inflow disease experience pain in these areas after walking about one or two blocks. The discomfort is described as being more like pain, but it eases with rest most of the time. *Severe* inflow disease causes severe pain after walking less than one block. These patients usually have rest pain.

Patients with **outflow disease** describe burning or cramping in the calves, ankles, feet, and toes. Instep or foot discomfort indicates an obstruction below the popliteal artery. Those with *mild* outflow disease experience discomfort after walking about five blocks. Rest relieves this discomfort. Patients with *moderate* outflow disease have pain after walking about two blocks. Intermittent rest pain may be present. Those with *severe* outflow disease usually cannot walk more than one-half block. They may hang their feet off the bed at night for comfort and report more frequent rest pain than patients with inflow disease.

Specific findings for PAD depend on the severity of the disease. Observe for loss of hair on the lower calf, ankle, and foot; dry, scaly, dusky, pale, or mottled skin; and thickened toenails. With severe arterial disease, the extremity is cold and gray-blue (cyanotic) or darkened. Pallor may occur when the extremity is elevated. Dependent **rubor** (redness) may occur when the extremity is lowered (Fig. 33.4). Muscle atrophy can result from prolonged chronic arterial disease.

PATIENT-CENTERED CARE: CULTURAL/SPIRITUAL CONSIDERATIONS QSEN

Only severe cyanosis is evident in the skin of patients with dark skin. To detect cyanosis, assess the skin and nail beds for a dull, lifeless color. The soles of the feet and the toenails are less pigmented and allow detection of cyanosis or duskiness in the lower extremities.

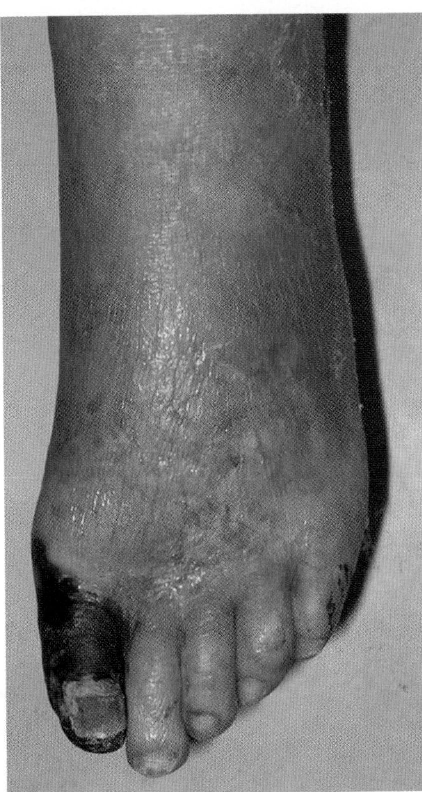

Fig. 33.4 Dependent rubor in the left leg of a patient with peripheral arterial disease. (From Brooks, M., & Jenkins, M.P. [2008]. Acute and chronic ischaemia of the limb. *Surgery 26*[1], 17–20.)

Palpate all pulses in both legs. The most sensitive and specific indicator of arterial function is the quality of the posterior tibial pulse because the pedal pulse is not palpable in a small percentage of people. The strength of each pulse should be compared bilaterally.

Note early signs of ulcer formation or complete ulcer formation, a complication of PAD. Arterial and venous stasis ulcers differ from diabetic ulcers (see the Key Features: Chronic Peripheral Arterial Disease box). Initially, **arterial ulcers** are painful and develop on the toes (often the great toe), between the toes, or on the upper aspect of the foot. With prolonged occlusion, the toes can become gangrenous. Typically, the ulcer is small and round with a hollow appearance and well-defined borders. Skin lesions are discussed in further detail in Chapter 23.

Magnetic resonance angiography (MRA) is commonly used to assess blood flow in the peripheral arteries. A contrast medium is used to help visualize blood flow through these arteries. This test is often the only one used to diagnose PAD, although computed tomography angiography (CTA) may also be performed.

Using a Doppler probe, *segmental systolic blood pressure measurements* of the lower extremities at the thigh, calf, and ankle are an inexpensive, noninvasive method of assessing PAD. Normally, blood pressure readings in the thigh and calf are higher than those in the upper extremities. With the presence of arterial disease, these pressures are lower than the brachial pressure.

With *inflow* disease, pressures taken at the thigh level indicate the severity of disease. Mild inflow disease may cause a difference of only 10 to 30 mm Hg in pressure on the affected side compared with the brachial pressure. Severe inflow disease can cause a pressure difference of more than 40 to 50 mm Hg. The ankle pressure is normally equal to or more than the brachial pressure.

To evaluate *outflow* disease, compare ankle pressure with the brachial pressure, which provides a ratio known as the **ankle-brachial index (ABI)**. The value can be derived by dividing the ankle blood pressure by the brachial blood pressure. *An ABI of less than 0.90 in either leg is diagnostic of PAD. Patients with diabetes are known to have a falsely elevated ABI.*

Exercise tolerance testing (by chemical stress test or treadmill) may give valuable information about claudication (muscle pain). The technician obtains resting pulse volume recordings and asks the patient to walk on a treadmill until the symptoms are reproduced. At the time of symptom onset or after about 5 minutes, the technician obtains another pulse volume recording. Normally, there may be an increased waveform with minimal, if any, drop in the ankle pressure. In patients with arterial disease, the waveforms are decreased (dampened), and there is a decrease in the ankle pressure of 40 to 60 mm Hg for 20 to 30 seconds in the affected limb. If the return to normal pressure is delayed (longer than 10 minutes), the results suggest abnormal arterial flow in the affected limb.

Plethysmography can also be performed to evaluate arterial flow in the lower extremities. The measurement provides graphs or tracings of arterial flow in the limb. If an occlusion is present, the waveforms are decreased to flattened, depending on the degree of occlusion.

◆ **Interventions: Take Action.** Collaborative management of PAD may include nonsurgical interventions and/or surgery. The patient must first be assessed to determine if the altered tissue ***perfusion*** is caused by arterial disease, venous disease, or both.

Nonsurgical Management. Exercise, positioning, promoting vasodilation, drug therapy, and invasive nonsurgical procedures are used to increase *arterial* flow to the affected leg(s).

Using Exercise and Positioning. *Exercise* may improve arterial blood flow to the affected leg through buildup of the collateral circulation. **Collateral circulation** provides blood to the affected area through smaller vessels that develop and compensate for the occluded vessels. Exercise is individualized for each patient, but people with severe rest pain, venous ulcers, or gangrene should not participate. Others with PAD can benefit from exercise that is started gradually and slowly increased. Instruct the patient to walk until the point of claudication, stop and rest, and then walk a little farther. Eventually, he or she can walk longer distances as collateral circulation develops. Collaborate with the primary health care provider and physical therapist in determining an appropriate exercise program. Exercise rehabilitation has been used to relieve symptoms but requires a motivated patient. The cost of supervised sessions generally is not reimbursed by health care insurance.

Positioning to promote circulation has been somewhat controversial. Some patients have swelling in their extremities. Teach them to avoid raising their legs above the heart level because extreme elevation slows arterial blood flow to the feet.

KEY FEATURES

Lower Extremity Ulcers

Feature	Arterial Ulcers	Venous Ulcers	Diabetic Ulcers
History	Patient reports claudication after walking about one to two blocks Rest pain usually present Pain at ulcer site Two or three risk factors present	Chronic nonhealing ulcer No claudication or rest pain Moderate ulcer discomfort Patient reports of ankle or leg swelling	Diabetes Peripheral neuropathy No reports of claudication
Ulcer location and appearance	End of the toes Between the toes Deep Ulcer bed pale, with even edges Little granulation tissue	Ankle area Brown pigmentation Ulcer bed pink Usually superficial, with uneven edges Granulation tissue present	Plantar area of foot Metatarsal heads Pressure points on feet Deep Pale, with even edges Little granulation tissue
Other assessment findings	Cool or cold foot Decreased or absent pulses Atrophy of skin Hair loss Pallor with elevation Dependent rubor Possible gangrene When acute, neurologic deficits noted	Ankle discoloration and edema Full veins when leg slightly dependent No neurologic deficit Pulses present May have scarring from previous ulcers	Pulses usually present Cool or warm foot Painless
Treatment	Treat underlying cause (surgical, revascularization) Prevent trauma and infection Patient education, stressing foot care	Long-term wound care (Unna boot, damp-to-dry dressings) Elevate extremity Patient education Prevent infection	Rule out major arterial disease Control diabetes Patient education regarding foot care Prevent infection

Photograph of arterial ulcer from Bonow, R.O., Mann, D.L., Zipes, D.P., & Libby, P. (2011). *Braunwald's heart disease: A textbook of cardiovascular medicine* (9th ed.). Philadelphia: Saunders. Photograph of venous ulcer from Bryant, R., & Nix, D. (2012). *Acute and chronic wounds: Current management concepts* (4th ed.). Philadelphia: Saunders. Photograph of diabetic ulcer from Bryant, R., & Nix, D. (2007). *Acute and chronic wounds: Current management concepts* (3rd ed.). Philadelphia: Saunders.

In severe cases, patients with PAD and swelling may sleep with the affected leg hanging from the bed or sit upright in a chair for comfort.

NURSING SAFETY PRIORITY QSEN

Action Alert

Instruct all patients with the disease to avoid crossing their legs and avoid wearing restrictive clothing (e.g., garters to hold up nylon stockings, particularly common among older women), which interfere with blood flow. Teach them the importance of inspecting their feet daily for color or other changes.

Promoting Vasodilation. Vasodilation can be achieved by providing warmth to the affected extremity and preventing long periods of exposure to cold. Encourage the patient to maintain a warm environment at home and to wear socks or insulated shoes at all times. *Caution the patient to avoid the application of direct heat to the limb with heating pads or extremely hot water. Sensitivity is decreased in the affected limb. Burns may result.*

Encourage patients to prevent exposure of the affected limb to the cold because cold temperatures cause vasoconstriction (decreasing of the diameter of the blood vessels) and therefore decrease arterial ***perfusion.***

Emotional stress, caffeine, and nicotine also can cause vasoconstriction. *Emphasize that complete abstinence from smoking or chewing tobacco is essential to prevent vasoconstriction.* The vasoconstrictive effects of each cigarette may last up to 1 hour after the cigarette is smoked.

NCLEX EXAMINATION CHALLENGE 33.3

Health Promotion and Maintenance

The nurse is caring for a client with intermittent claudication due to peripheral arterial disease. Which client statement indicates understanding of proper self-management?

A. "I need to reduce the number of cigarettes that I smoke each day."
B. "I'll elevate my legs above the level of my heart."
C. "I'll use a heating pad to promote circulation."
D. "I'll start to exercise gradually, stopping when I have pain."

Drug Therapy. For patients with chronic PAD, prescribed drugs include hemorheologic and antiplatelet agents. Pentoxifylline is a hemorheologic agent that increases the flexibility of red blood cells. It decreases blood viscosity by inhibiting platelet aggregation and decreasing fibrinogen and thus increases blood flow in the extremities. Many patients report limited improvement in their daily lives after taking pentoxifylline, and evidence indicates minimal benefit. However, those with extremely limited endurance for walking have reported improvement to the point that they can perform some activities (e.g., walk to the mailbox or dining room) that were previously impossible.

Antiplatelet agents, such as aspirin and clopidogrel, are commonly used. If there are no contraindications to antiplatelet therapy, patients with symptomatic PAD should receive aspirin or clopidogrel to reduce MI, stroke, and vascular death (Gerhard-Herman et al., 2017). Some patients receive both drugs (dual antiplatelet therapy). Evidence suggests that dual antiplatelet therapy is reasonable to reduce the risk of limb-related events in patients with symptomatic PAD after lower extremity revascularization (Gerhard-Herman et al., 2017). Patients who are taking clopidogrel should not eat grapefruit or drink grapefruit juice because of risk of kidney failure, GI bleeding, heart failure, or even death.

Patients who experience disabling intermittent claudication may also benefit from phosphodiesterase inhibitors such as cilostazol because it can help improve symptoms and increasing walking distance. This drug can also increase HDL-C levels. Teach patients taking the drug that it may cause headaches and GI disturbances, especially flatulence (gas) and diarrhea.

Controlling hypertension can improve tissue ***perfusion*** by maintaining pressures that are adequate to perfuse the periphery but not constrict the vessels. Teach about the effect of blood pressure on the circulation and instruct in methods of control. For example, patients taking beta blockers may have drug-related claudication or a worsening of symptoms. The primary health care provider closely monitors those who are receiving beta blockers. If the patient has high serum lipids, lipid-lowering drugs such as statins are used (see discussion of statins earlier in this chapter).

Invasive Nonsurgical Procedures. A nonsurgical but invasive approach for improving arterial flow is the use of **percutaneous vascular intervention.** This procedure requires an arterial puncture in the patient's groin. One or more arteries are dilated with a balloon catheter advanced through a cannula, which is inserted into or above an occluded or stenosed artery. When the procedure is successful, it opens the vessel and improves arterial blood flow. Patients who are candidates for percutaneous procedures must have occlusions or stenoses that are accessible to the catheter. Reocclusion may occur, and the procedure may be repeated. Some patients are occlusion free for up to 3 to 5 years, whereas others may experience reocclusion within a year.

During percutaneous vascular intervention, intravascular stents (wire meshlike devices) are usually inserted to ensure adequate blood flow in a stenosed vessel. Candidates for stents are patients with stenosis of the common or external iliac arteries. Stents are also available to effectively treat superficial femoral artery (SFA) disease. Patients have these procedures in same-day surgery or ambulatory care centers.

Another arterial technique to improve blood flow to ischemic legs in people with PAD is mechanical rotational abrasive **atherectomy.** The Rotablator device is designed to scrape plaque from inside the artery while minimizing damage to the vessel surface and is useful at the popliteal artery and below.

! NURSING SAFETY PRIORITY (QSEN)

Critical Rescue

The priority for nursing care following a percutaneous vascular intervention or atherectomy is to observe for bleeding at the arterial puncture site, which is sealed with a special collagen plug. Monitor for manifestations of impending hypovolemic shock, including a decrease in blood pressure, increased pulse rate, and decreased urinary output. Related complications can include: hematoma, retroperitoneal bleeding, pseudoaneurysm, arteriovenous fistula, nerve compression, and atheroembolism. Perform frequent checks of the arterial puncture site and distal pulses in both legs to ensure adequate ***perfusion.***

Most patients receive anticoagulant or antiplatelet therapy such as heparin or clopidogrel, before and/or during the procedure. An antiplatelet drug may also be prescribed after the procedure to prevent arterial *clotting*. The most common time frame for the administration of the antiplatelet is 1 to 3 months following the procedure. However, this time frame is highly variable (Singh et al., 2017).

Surgical Management. Patients with severe rest pain or claudication that interferes with the ability to work or threatens loss of a limb become surgical candidates. **Arterial revascularization** is the surgical procedure most commonly used to increase arterial blood flow in an affected limb.

Surgical procedures are classified as *inflow* or *outflow.* Inflow procedures involve bypassing arterial occlusions above the superficial femoral arteries (SFAs). Outflow procedures involve surgical bypassing of arterial occlusions at or below the SFAs. For those who have both inflow and outflow problems, the inflow procedure (for larger arteries) is done before the outflow repair.

Inflow procedures include aortoiliac, aortofemoral, and axillofemoral bypasses. Outflow procedures include femoropopliteal and femorotibial bypasses. Inflow procedures are more successful, with less chance of reocclusion or postoperative ischemia. Outflow procedures are less successful in relieving ischemic pain and are associated with a higher incidence of reocclusion.

Graft materials for bypasses are selected on an individual basis. For outflow procedures, the preferred graft material is the patient's own (**autogenous**) saphenous vein. However, some patients experience coronary artery disease and may need this vein for coronary artery bypass. When the saphenous vein is not usable, the cephalic or basilic arm veins may be used. Grafts made of synthetic materials have also been used when autogenous veins were not available.

Preoperative Care. Preparing the patient for surgery is similar to procedures described for general or epidural anesthesia (see Chapter 9). Documentation of vital signs and peripheral pulses provides a baseline of information for comparison during the postoperative phase. Depending on the surgical procedure, the patient may have one or more IV lines, urinary catheter, central venous catheter, and/or arterial line. To prevent postoperative infection, antibiotic therapy is typically given before the procedure.

Operative Procedures. The anesthesia provider places the patient under general, epidural, or spinal anesthesia. Epidural or spinal induction is preferred for older adults to decrease the risk for cardiopulmonary complications in this age-group. If arterial bypass is to be accomplished by autogenous grafts, the surgeon removes the veins through an incision. The blocked artery is then exposed through an incision, and the replacement vein or synthetic graft material is sutured above and below the occlusion to increase blood flow around the occlusion.

For conventional open *aortoiliac* and *aortofemoral* bypass (AFB) surgery, the surgeon makes a midline incision into the abdominal cavity to expose the abdominal aorta, with additional incisions in each groin (Fig. 33.5). Graft material is tunneled from the aorta to the groin incisions, where it is sutured in place.

In an open *axillofemoral* bypass (Fig. 33.6), the surgeon makes an incision beneath the clavicle and tunnels graft material subcutaneously with a catheter from the chest to the iliac crest, into a groin incision, where it is sutured in place. Neither the thoracic nor the abdominal cavity is entered. For that reason, the axillofemoral bypass is used for high-risk patients who cannot tolerate a procedure requiring abdominal surgery.

Minimally invasive surgical techniques are beginning to be performed by vascular surgeons using robotic-assisted laparoscopic procedures. These newer surgical techniques require extensive training and further research data to determine their usefulness.

Postoperative Care. Thorough and ongoing nursing assessment for postoperative arterial revascularization patients is crucial to detect complications. Deep breathing every 1 to 2 hours and using an incentive spirometer are essential to prevent respiratory complications.

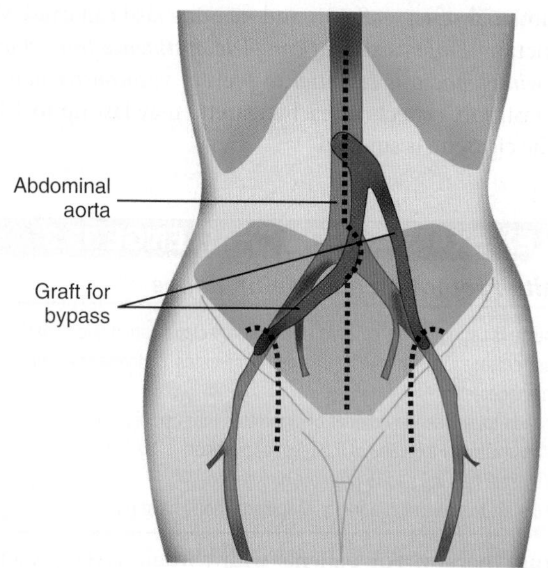

Fig. 33.5 In aortoiliac and aortofemoral bypass surgery, a midline incision into the abdominal cavity is required, with an additional incision in each groin.

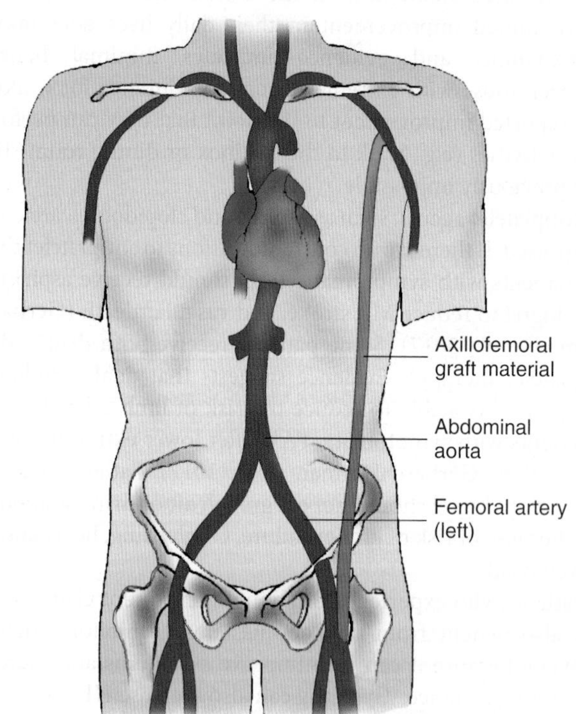

Fig. 33.6 An axillofemoral bypass graft.

Patients who have undergone conventional aortoiliac or aortofemoral bypass are NPO status for at least 1 day after surgery to prevent nausea and vomiting, which could increase intra-abdominal pressure. Those who have undergone bypass surgery of the lower extremities not involving the aorta or abdominal wall (femoropopliteal or femorotibial bypass) may remain NPO until the first postoperative day, when they are allowed clear liquids.

Warmth, redness, and edema of the affected extremity are often expected outcomes of surgery as a result of increased arterial ***perfusion.***

! NATIONAL PATIENT SAFETY GOALS

Improve Staff Communication

Immediately after surgery, the operating suite or postanesthesia care unit (PACU) nurse marks the site where the distal (dorsalis pedis or posterior tibial) pulse is best palpated or heard by Doppler ultrasonography. This information and other critical assessment information are communicated to the nursing staff on the critical care unit where the patient will be sent. *Hand-off reporting* provides accurate information about a patient's care, treatment, current condition, and any recent or anticipated changes. This process also includes an opportunity to ask and respond to questions. Hand-off reporting is essential to promote safety and is a standard of high-quality care (The Joint Commission, 2017a).

To promote graft patency, monitor the patient's blood pressure and notify the surgeon if the pressure increases or decreases beyond the patient's baseline. Hypotension may indicate hypovolemia, which can increase the risk for ***clotting.*** Range of motion of the operative leg is usually limited, with no bending of the hip and knee. Consult with the surgeon on a case-by-case basis regarding limitations of movement, including turning. Patients having open procedures may be restricted to bedrest for 24 hours or longer after surgery to prevent disruption of the suture lines. Patients having minimally invasive surgery (MIS) may be ambulatory and eat within the day of surgery. Pain and surgical complications tend to occur less often in patients who have MIS procedures.

! NURSING SAFETY PRIORITY (QSEN)

Critical Rescue

Graft occlusion (blockage) is a postoperative emergency that can occur within the first 24 hours after arterial revascularization. Monitor the patient for and report severe continuous and aching pain, which may be the first indicator of postoperative graft occlusion and ischemia. Many people experience a throbbing pain caused by the increased blood flow to the extremity. Because this alteration in comfort is different from that of ischemic pain, be sure to assess the type of pain that is experienced. Pain from occlusion may be masked by patient-controlled analgesia (PCA). Some patients have ischemic pain that is not relieved by PCA.

Monitor the patency of the graft by checking the extremity every 15 minutes for the first hour and then hourly for changes in color, temperature, and pulse intensity. Compare the operative leg with the unaffected one. *If the operative leg feels cold; becomes pale, ashen, or cyanotic; or has a decreased or absent pulse, contact the surgeon immediately!*

Emergency **thrombectomy** (removal of the clot), which the surgeon may perform at the bedside, is the most common treatment for acute graft occlusion. Thrombectomy is associated with excellent results in prosthetic grafts. Results of thrombectomy in autogenous vein grafts are not as successful and often necessitate graft revision and even replacement.

Local intra-arterial thrombolytic (clot-dissolving) therapy with an agent such as tissue plasminogen activator (t-PA) or an infusion of a platelet inhibitor such as abciximab may be used for acute graft occlusions. This therapy is provided in select settings in which health care providers are experts in its use. Other antiplatelet drugs such as the glycoprotein IIb/IIIa inhibitors *tirofiban* and *eptifibatide* may be used as alternatives. The health care provider considers these therapies when the surgical alternative (e.g., thrombectomy with or without graft revision or replacement) carries high morbidity or mortality rates or when surgery for this type of occlusion has traditionally yielded poor results. Closely assess the patient for manifestations of bleeding if thrombolytics are used.

Graft or wound infections can be life threatening. Use sterile technique when providing incisional care and observe for symptoms of infection. Assess the area for induration, erythema, tenderness, warmth, edema, or drainage. Also monitor for fever and leukocytosis (increased serum white blood cell count). Notify the surgeon promptly if any of these symptoms occur. Patients having conventional open bypass procedures are usually hospitalized for 5 to 7 days. Those having MIS procedures usually have shorter stays of 2 or 3 days.

Peripheral arterial disease (PAD) is a chronic, long-term problem with frequent complications. Patients may benefit from a case manager who can follow them across the continuum of care. The desired outcome is that the patient can be maintained in the home.

Management at home often requires an interprofessional team approach, including several home care visits. See the Home Care Considerations: The Patient With Peripheral Vascular Disease box for home care of patients with peripheral vascular disease.

Instruct patients on methods to promote vasodilation. Teach them to avoid raising their legs above the level of the heart unless venous stasis is also present. Provide written and

HOME CARE CONSIDERATIONS

The Patient With Peripheral Vascular Disease

Assess tissue ***perfusion*** to affected extremity(ies), including:

- Distal circulation, sensation, and motion
- Presence of pain, pallor, paresthesias, pulselessness, paralysis, poikilothermy (coolness)
- Ankle-brachial index

Assess adherence to therapeutic regimen, including:

- Following foot care instructions
- Quitting smoking
- Maintaining heart-healthy diet low in saturated fat
- Participating in exercise regimen
- Avoiding exposure to cold and constrictive clothing

Assess ability to manage wound care and prevent further injury, including:

- Use of compression stockings or compression pumps as directed
- Use of various dressing materials
- Signs and symptoms to report to nurse

Assess coping ability of patient and family members.

Assess home environment, including:

- Safety hazards, especially related to falls

PATIENT AND FAMILY EDUCATION: PREPARING FOR SELF-MANAGEMENT

Foot Care for the Patient With Peripheral Vascular Disease

- Keep your feet clean by washing them with a mild soap in room-temperature water.
- Keep your feet dry, especially the ankles and between the toes.
- Avoid injury to your feet and ankles. Wear comfortable, well-fitting shoes. Never go without shoes.
- Keep your toenails clean and filed. Have someone cut them if you cannot see them clearly. Cut your toenails straight across.
- To prevent dry, cracked skin, apply a lubricating lotion to your feet.
- Prevent exposure to extreme heat or cold. Never use a heating pad on your feet.
- Avoid constricting garments.
- Avoid extended pressure on your feet or ankles, such as occurs when you lean against something.
- Inspect your feet daily for injuries.
- See your health care provider at the first sign of a sore or injury to your skin.

oral instructions on foot care and methods to prevent injury and ulcer development. See the Patient and Family Education: Preparing for Self-Management: Foot Care for the Patient With Peripheral Vascular Disease box.

Patients who have had surgery require additional instruction on incision care (see Chapter 9). Encourage all patients to avoid smoking, limit dietary fat intake, and increase protein intake (Jellinger et al., 2017). Remind them to drink adequate fluids to prevent dehydration.

Patients with chronic arterial obstruction may fear recurrent occlusion or further narrowing of the artery. They often fear that they might lose a limb or become debilitated in other ways. Indeed, chronic PAD may worsen, especially in those with diabetes mellitus. Reassure them that participation in prescribed exercise, nutrition therapy, and drug therapy, along with cessation of smoking, can limit further formation of atherosclerotic plaques.

Patients with arterial compromise or surgery may need assistance from the family, another caregiver, or a home care aide with ADLs if activity is limited by pain. They may need to limit or avoid stair climbing, depending on the severity of disease. Those who have undergone surgery may require a home care nurse to help with incision care. In collaboration with the case manager, arrange for home care resources before discharge.

ACUTE PERIPHERAL ARTERIAL OCCLUSION

Pathophysiology Review

Although chronic peripheral arterial disease (PAD) progresses slowly, the onset of **acute arterial occlusion** is sudden and dramatic. An **embolus** (piece of a clot that travels and lodges in a new area) is the most common cause of peripheral occlusions, although a local thrombus may be the cause. Occlusion may affect the upper extremities, but it is more common in the lower extremities. Emboli originating from the heart are the most common cause of acute arterial occlusions. Most patients with an embolic occlusion have had an acute myocardial infarction (MI) and/or atrial fibrillation within the previous weeks.

❖ Interprofessional Collaborative Care

Patients with an acute arterial occlusion describe severe pain below the level of the occlusion that occurs even at rest. The affected extremity is cool or cold, pulseless, and mottled. Small areas on the toes may be blackened or gangrenous due to lack of ***perfusion.*** *Those with acute arterial insufficiency often present with the "six Ps" of ischemia:*

- Pain
- Pallor
- Pulselessness
- Paresthesia
- Paralysis
- Poikilothermy (coolness)

The primary health care provider must initiate treatment promptly to avoid permanent damage or loss of an extremity. Anticoagulant therapy with unfractionated heparin (UFH) is usually the first intervention to prevent further clot formation. The patient may undergo angiography.

A surgical *thrombectomy* or *embolectomy* with local anesthesia may be performed to remove the occlusion. The health care provider makes a small incision, which is followed by an **arteriotomy** (a surgical opening into an artery). A catheter is inserted into the artery to retrieve the embolus. It may be necessary to close the artery with a synthetic or autologous (patient's own blood vessel) patch graft.

! NURSING SAFETY PRIORITY QSEN

Critical Rescue

After an arterial thrombectomy, observe the affected extremity for improvement in color, temperature, and pulse every hour for the first 24 hours or according to the postoperative surgical protocol. Monitor patients for manifestations of new thrombi or emboli, especially pulmonary emboli (PE). Chest pain, dyspnea, and acute confusion (older adults) typically occur in patients with PE. Notify the health care provider or Rapid Response Team immediately if these symptoms occur.

Alterations in comfort should significantly diminish after the surgical procedure, although mild incisional pain remains. Watch closely for complications caused by reperfusing the artery after thrombectomy or embolectomy, either of which includes spasms and swelling of the skeletal muscles. Swelling of the skeletal muscles can result in compartment syndrome.

Compartment syndrome occurs when tissue pressure within a confined body space becomes elevated and restricts blood flow. The resulting ischemia can lead to tissue damage and eventually tissue death. Assess the motor and sensory function of the affected extremity. Monitor for increasing pain, swelling, and tenseness. Report any of these symptoms to the health care provider immediately. Fasciotomy (surgical opening into the tissues) may be necessary to prevent further injury and save the limb.

The use of *systemic thrombolytic therapy* for acute arterial occlusions has been disappointing because bleeding complications often outweigh the benefits obtained. Catheter-directed intra-arterial thrombolytic therapy with *fibrinolytics,* such as alteplase or t-PA, has emerged as an alternative to surgical treatment in selected settings. A catheter is placed percutaneously (through the skin) into the artery with or without ultrasound guidance by the vascular surgeon or interventional radiologist. The tip of the catheter is embedded in the clot to directly deliver the thrombolytic infusion until the clot dissolves, which can take 24 to 36 hours.

During infusion, monitor the patient for complications such as bleeding and hemorrhagic stroke. Maintaining a normal blood pressure is essential in preventing a potential stroke. As the clot dissolves, the patient typically experiences severe pain due to reperfusion that requires patient-controlled analgesia (PCA).

! NURSING SAFETY PRIORITY QSEN

Drug Alert

When *fibrinolytics* are given, assess for signs of bleeding, bruising, or hematoma. For patients receiving any *platelet inhibitor,* monitor platelet counts for the first 3, 6, and 12 hours after the start of the infusion or per agency protocol. If the platelet count decreases to below 100,000/mm^3, the infusion needs to be readjusted or discontinued. If any of these complications occur, notify the health care provider or Rapid Response Team immediately.

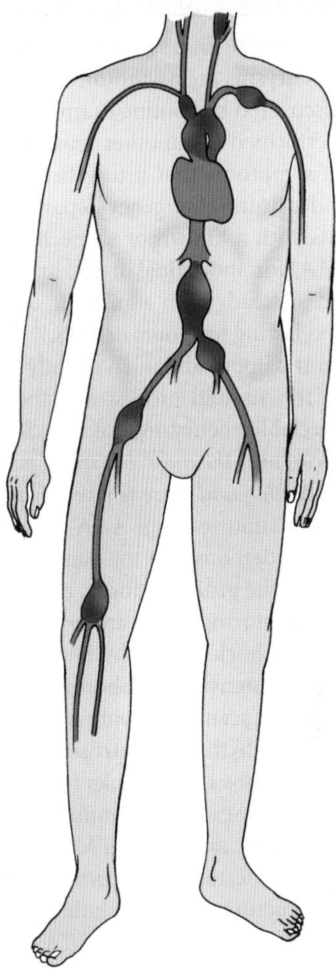

Fig. 33.7 Common anatomic sites of arterial aneurysms.

ANEURYSMS OF THE CENTRAL ARTERIES

Pathophysiology Review

An **aneurysm** is a permanent localized dilation of an artery, which enlarges the artery to at least two times its normal diameter. It may be described as *fusiform* (a diffuse dilation affecting the entire circumference of the artery) or *saccular* (an outpouching affecting only a distinct portion of the artery). Aneurysms may also be described as *true* or *false.* In true aneurysms, the arterial wall is weakened by congenital or acquired problems. False aneurysms occur as a result of vessel injury or trauma to all three layers of the arterial wall. *Dissecting aneurysms* differ from aneurysms in that they are formed when blood accumulates in the wall of an artery.

Aneurysms tend to occur at specific anatomic sites (Fig. 33.7), most commonly in the abdominal aorta. They often occur at a point where the artery is not supported by skeletal muscles or on the lines of curves or flexion in the arterial tree. This chapter discusses aneurysms of the central arteries. Brain aneurysms are discussed in Chapter 41.

An aneurysm forms when the middle layer (media) of the artery is weakened, producing a stretching effect in the inner layer (intima) and outer layers of the artery. As the artery widens, tension in the wall increases; and further widening occurs, thus enlarging the aneurysm and increasing the risk for arterial rupture. Elevated blood pressure can also increase the rate of aneurysmal enlargement and risk for early rupture. When *dissecting* aneurysms occur, the aneurysm enlarges, blood is lost, and blood flow to organs is diminished.

Abdominal aortic aneurysms (AAAs) account for most aneurysms, are commonly asymptomatic, and frequently rupture. Most of these are located between the renal arteries and the aortic bifurcation (dividing area).

Thoracic aortic aneurysms (TAAs) are not quite as common and are frequently misdiagnosed. They are typically discovered when advanced imaging is used to assess other conditions. TAAs commonly develop between the origin of the left subclavian artery and the diaphragm. They are located in the descending, ascending, and transverse sections of the aorta. They can also occur in the aortic arch and are very difficult to manage surgically.

Aneurysms can cause symptoms by exerting pressure on surrounding structures or by rupturing. *Rupture is the most frequent complication and is life threatening because abrupt and massive hemorrhagic shock results.* Thrombi within the wall of an aneurysm can also be the source of emboli in distal arteries below the aneurysm.

Atherosclerosis is the most common cause of aneurysms, with hypertension, hyperlipidemia, and cigarette smoking being contributing factors. Age, gender, and family history also play a role (McCance & Huether, 2019).

❖ Interprofessional Collaborative Care

◆ **Assessment: Recognize Cues.** Most patients with abdominal or thoracic aneurysms are asymptomatic when their aneurysms are first discovered by routine examination or during an imaging study performed for another reason. However, a few patients do have symptoms that bring them to their primary health care provider or the emergency department.

Assess patients with a known or suspected *abdominal aortic aneurysm (AAA)* for abdominal, flank, or back pain. Pain is usually described as steady with a gnawing quality, unaffected by movement, and lasting for hours or days.

A pulsation in the upper abdomen slightly to the left of the midline between the xiphoid process and the umbilicus may be present. A detectable aneurysm is at least 5 cm in diameter. *Auscultate for a bruit over the mass, but avoid palpating the mass because it may be tender, and there is risk for rupture!* If expansion and impending rupture of an AAA are suspected, assess for severe pain of sudden onset in the back or lower abdomen, which may radiate to the groin, buttocks, or legs.

Patients with a rupturing AAA are *critically ill* and are at risk for hypovolemic shock caused by hemorrhage. Signs and symptoms include hypotension, diaphoresis, decreased level of consciousness, oliguria (scant urine output), loss of pulses distal to the rupture, and dysrhythmias. Retroperitoneal hemorrhage manifests with hematomas in the flanks (lower back). Rupture into the abdominal cavity causes abdominal distention.

When a *thoracic aortic aneurysm* (TAA) is suspected, assess for back pain and manifestations of compression of the aneurysm on adjacent structures. Signs include shortness of breath, hoarseness, and difficulty swallowing. TAAs are not often detected by physical assessment, but occasionally a mass may be visible above the suprasternal notch. Assess the patient with suspected rupture of a thoracic aneurysm for sudden and excruciating back or chest pain. Hypovolemic shock also occurs with TAA.

Computed tomography (CT) scanning with contrast is the standard tool for assessing the size and location of an abdominal or thoracic aneurysm. *Ultrasonography* is also used.

◆ **Interventions: Take Action.** The size of the aneurysm and the presence of symptoms determine patient management. The nurse's role is to perform frequent patient assessments, including blood pressure, pulse, and peripheral circulation checks.

Nonsurgical Management. The desired outcome of nonsurgical management is to monitor the growth of the aneurysm and maintain the blood pressure at a normal level to decrease the risk for rupture. Patients with hypertension are treated with antihypertensive drugs to decrease the rate of enlargement and the risk for early rupture.

For those with small or asymptomatic aneurysms, frequent ultrasound or CT scans are necessary to monitor the growth of the aneurysm. Emphasize the importance of following through with scheduled tests to monitor the growth. Also explain the signs and symptoms of aneurysms that need to be promptly reported.

Surgical Management. Surgical management of an aneurysm may be an elective or an emergency procedure. *For patients with a rupturing abdominal aortic or a thoracic aneurysm, emergency surgery is performed.* Patients with smaller aneurysms that are producing symptoms are advised to have elective surgery. Those with smaller aneurysms that are not causing symptoms are treated nonsurgically until symptoms occur or the aneurysm enlarges.

The most common surgical procedure for AAA has traditionally been a resection or repair (**aneurysmectomy**). However, the mortality rate for elective resection is high and markedly increases for emergency surgery. Endovascular stent grafts have improved mortality rates and shortened the hospital stay for select patients who need AAA repair.

The repair of AAAs with **endovascular stent grafts** is the procedure of choice for almost all patients on an elective or emergent basis. Stents (wirelike devices) are inserted percutaneously (through the skin), avoiding abdominal incisions and therefore decreasing the risk for a prolonged postoperative recovery. Postoperative care is similar to care required after an arteriogram (angiogram).

Different designs of endovascular stent grafts are used, depending on the anatomic involvement of the aneurysm. The stent graft is flexible with either Dacron or polytetrafluoroethylene (PTFE) material. It is inserted through a skin incision into the femoral artery by way of a catheter-based system. The catheter is advanced to a level above the aneurysm away from the renal arteries. The graft is released from the catheter, and the stent graft is placed with a series of hooks. This procedure is done in collaboration with the vascular surgeon, interventional radiologist, operating suite team, and at some centers the vascular medicine physician.

Complications of stent repair include:

- Conversion to open surgical repair
- Bleeding
- Aneurysm rupture
- Peripheral embolization
- Misplacement of the stent graft
- Endoleak
- Infection

The endovascular repair of AAAs has decreased the length of hospital stay for patients requiring repair of abdominal aneurysms. However, the patient needs to be closely monitored, in the hospital and at home, for the development of complications after the procedure. Expert nursing care is required to allow for early identification of problems, and complications require timely surgical intervention. In addition, coordination and interprofessional collaboration with the health care team are required for discharge planning and follow-up care for patients at home.

Most patients are discharged to home after aneurysm repair. However, in the absence of family or other support systems, the postoperative patient may be discharged to a transitional care or long-term care facility for rehabilitation.

If discharged to home, the patient must follow instructions regarding activity level and incisional care. Because stair climbing may be restricted initially, he or she may need a bedside commode if the bathroom is inaccessible. Teach the patient who has undergone surgical repair about activity restrictions, wound care, and pain management. Patients may not perform activities that involve lifting heavy objects (usually more than 15 to 20 lb [6.8 to 9.1 kg]) for 6 to 12 weeks after surgery. Advise them to use caution for activities that involve pulling, pushing, or straining. Most patients are restricted from driving a car for several weeks after discharge.

For patients who have not undergone surgical aneurysm repair, the teaching plan emphasizes the importance of compliance with the schedule of frequent ultrasound scanning to monitor the size of the aneurysm.

! NURSING SAFETY PRIORITY (QSEN)

Action Alert

Teach patients receiving treatment for hypertension about the importance of continuing to take prescribed drugs. Instruct them about the signs and symptoms that must be reported promptly to the primary health care provider, which include:

- Abdominal fullness or pain or back pain
- Chest or back pain
- Shortness of breath
- Difficulty swallowing or hoarseness

In collaboration with the case manager or social worker, assess the availability of transportation to and from appointments for patients needing ultrasound monitoring. Those who have undergone surgery may require the services of a home care nurse for initial assistance with dressing changes. A home care aide may be needed to assist with ADLs, depending on the patient's support system.

ANEURYSMS OF THE PERIPHERAL ARTERIES

Although femoral and popliteal aneurysms are not common, they may be associated with an aneurysm in another location of the arterial tree (see Fig. 33.7). To detect a popliteal aneurysm, assess for a pulsating mass in the popliteal space. To detect a femoral aneurysm, observe a pulsatile mass over the femoral artery. *To prevent its rupture, do not palpate the mass!* Evaluate both extremities because more than one femoral or popliteal aneurysm may be present.

The patient may have symptoms of limb ischemia (decreased ***perfusion***), including diminished or absent pulses, cool to cold skin, and pain. Alterations in comfort may be present if an adjacent nerve is compressed. The recommended treatment for either type of aneurysm, regardless of size, is surgery because of the risk for thromboembolic complications.

To treat a femoral aneurysm, the surgeon removes the aneurysm and restores circulation using a synthetic or an autogenous saphenous vein graft-stent repair. Most surgeons prefer to bypass rather than resect a popliteal aneurysm.

After surgery, monitor for lower-limb ischemia. Palpate pulses below the graft to assess graft patency. Often Doppler ultrasonography is necessary to assess blood flow when pulses are not palpable. *Report sudden development of pain or discoloration of the extremity immediately to the surgeon because it may indicate graft occlusion.*

AORTIC DISSECTION

Pathophysiology Review

Aortic dissection was previously referred to as a *dissecting aneurysm*. However, because this condition is more accurately described as a *dissecting hematoma*, the term *aortic dissection* is more commonly used. Aortic dissection is not common but is a life-threatening problem.

Aortic dissection is thought to be caused by a sudden tear in the aortic intima, allowing blood to enter the aortic wall. Degeneration of the aortic media may be the primary cause for this condition, with hypertension being an important contributing factor. It is often associated with genetic connective tissue disorders such as Marfan syndrome. It occurs also in middle-age and older people, peaking in adults in their 50s and 60s. Men are more commonly affected than women.

The circulation of any major artery arising from the aorta can be impaired in patients with aortic dissection; therefore this condition is highly lethal and represents an emergency situation. Although the ascending aorta and descending thoracic aorta are the most common sites, dissections can also occur in the abdominal aorta and other arteries.

❖ Interprofessional Collaborative Care

◆ **Assessment: Recognize Cues.** The most common symptom is pain. It is described as "sharp," "tearing," "ripping," and "stabbing" and tends to move from its point of origin. Depending on the site of dissection, the patient may feel pain in the anterior chest, back, neck, throat, jaw, or teeth at a level of 10 on a 0-to-10 pain intensity scale.

Diaphoresis (excessive sweating), nausea, vomiting, faintness, pallor, a rapid and weak pulse, and apprehension are also common. Blood pressure is usually elevated unless complications such as cardiac tamponade or rupture have occurred. In these cases, the patient becomes rapidly hypotensive. A decrease or absence of peripheral pulses is common, as is aortic regurgitation, which is characterized by a musical murmur best heard along the right sternal border. Neurologic deficits such as an altered level of consciousness, paraparesis, and strokes also can occur.

If the patient is medically stable, computed tomographic angiography (CTA) is the test of choice to confirm diagnosis. However, the patient is often too unstable to be transported, and transesophageal echocardiography (TEE) may be performed at the bedside to confirm diagnosis (Black & Manning, 2018).

◆ **Interventions: Take Action.** The expected outcomes for emergency care for a patient with an aortic dissection are increased comfort and reduction of systolic blood pressure to 100 to 120 mm Hg. Make sure that the patient has two large-bore IV catheters to infuse 0.9% sodium chloride and give medication. Insert an indwelling urinary catheter. The health care provider prescribes IV morphine sulfate to relieve pain and an IV beta blocker, such as esmolol, to lower heart rate and blood pressure (Black & Manning, 2018). If this regimen is not effective, nitroprusside or nicardipine hydrochloride may be used.

TABLE 33.7 Interprofessional Collaborative Care for Other Arterial Health Problems

Assessment: Recognize Cue	Interventions: Take Action	Nursing Implications
Buerger Disease		
Claudication in feet and lower extremities, worse at night; causes ischemia and fibrosis of vessels in extremities with increased sensitivity to cold; ulcerations and gangrene on digits; cause unknown but is associated with smoking.	Vasodilating drugs, such as nifedipine (Procardia); management of ulceration and gangrene; chronic pain management modalities.	Teach patient about smoking cessation, avoiding cold by wearing gloves and warm clothes, managing stress, avoiding caffeine; teach patient taking nifedipine to avoid grapefruit and grapefruit juice to prevent severe adverse effects, including possible death; teach patients on vasodilators about side effects such as facial flushing, hypotension, headaches.
Raynaud Phenomenon/Disease		
Painful vasospasms of arteries and arterioles in extremities, especially digits; causes red-white-blue skin color changes on exposure to cold or stress; cause unknown, occurs more in women, and may be an autoimmune disorder because it is associated with many rheumatic diseases such as systemic lupus erythematosus.	Same as for Buerger disease.	Same as for Buerger disease.
Subclavian Steal		
Occurs in upper extremities as result of subclavian artery occlusion or stenosis causing ischemia in the arm and pain; paresthesias and dizziness are also common; blood pressure difference in arms and presence of subclavian bruit on the affected side.	Surgical interventions for cyanosis or unrelenting pain, such as endarterectomy, bypass, or dilation of subclavian artery.	Monitor patient closely for new signs and symptoms; postoperatively, check pulses and observe for ischemic changes, including severe pain or color changes (e.g., cyanosis).
Thoracic Outlet Syndrome		
Compression of subclavian artery by rib or muscle that is more common in women and those who have to keep arms moving or above their heads (e.g., golfers, swimmers); also present with trauma; causes neck, arm, and shoulder pain with numbness and possible cyanosis.	Physical therapy for exercise program; avoiding aggravating positions; surgery as last resort for severe pain.	Health teaching about avoiding activities and positions that aggravate pain; monitor for new signs and symptoms; neurovascular assessments; postoperative care if needed.

Subsequent treatment depends on the location of the dissection. Patients receive continued medical treatment for uncomplicated distal dissections and surgical treatment for proximal dissections. For long-term medical treatment, the recommended target for blood pressure is less than 120/80 mm Hg (Black & Manning, 2018). Beta blockers (e.g., propranolol) and calcium channel antagonists (e.g., amlodipine) are prescribed to assist with blood pressure maintenance once the patient is stabilized. Patients having surgical intervention for a proximal dissection typically require cardiopulmonary bypass (CPB) (see Chapter 35). The surgeon removes the intimal tear and sutures edges of the dissected aorta. Usually a synthetic graft is used.

Other Arterial Health Problems

Less common health problems affecting peripheral and central arteries are summarized in Table 33.7.

PERIPHERAL VENOUS DISEASE

To function properly, veins must be patent (open) with competent valves. Vein function also requires the assistance of the surrounding muscle beds to help pump blood toward the heart. If one or more veins are not operating properly, they become distended, and signs and symptoms occur.

Three health problems alter the blood flow in veins:

- Thrombus formation *(venous thrombosis)* can lead to pulmonary embolism (PE), a life-threatening complication. **Venous thromboembolism (VTE)** is the current term that includes both deep vein thrombosis (DVT) and PE.
- Defective valves lead to *venous insufficiency* and *varicose veins,* which are not life threatening but are problematic.
- Skeletal muscles do not contract to help pump blood in the veins. This problem can occur when weight bearing is limited or muscle tone decreases.

CLOTTING CONCEPT EXEMPLAR: VENOUS THROMBOEMBOLISM

Pathophysiology Review

Venous thromboembolism (VTE) is one of health care's greatest challenges and includes both thrombus and embolus complications. A **thrombus** (also called a *thrombosis*) is a blood clot believed to result from an endothelial injury, venous stasis, or hypercoagulability. The thrombosis may be specifically attributable to one element, or it may involve all three elements. It is often associated with an inflammatory process. When a thrombus develops, immunity is altered, causing ***inflammation*** to occur around the clot, thickening of the vein wall, and possible embolization (the formation of an embolus). Pulmonary embolism (PE) is the most common type of embolus and is discussed in detail in Chapter 29.

Phlebothrombosis is a thrombus without inflammation. **Thrombophlebitis** refers to a thrombus that is associated with ***inflammation.*** Thrombophlebitis can occur in superficial veins. However, it most frequently occurs in the deep veins of the lower extremities.

Deep vein thrombophlebitis, commonly referred to as **deep vein thrombosis (DVT)**, is the most common type of thrombophlebitis. It is more serious than superficial thrombophlebitis because it presents a greater risk for PE. With PE, a dislodged blood clot travels to the pulmonary artery—*a medical emergency!* DVT develops most often in the legs but can also occur in the upper arms as a result of increased use of central venous devices.

Etiology. Thrombus formation has been associated with stasis of blood flow, endothelial injury, and/or hypercoagulability, known as the **Virchow triad**. The precise cause of these events remains unknown; however, a few predisposing factors have been identified.

The highest incidence of clot formation occurs in patients who have undergone hip surgery, total knee replacement, or open prostate surgery. Other conditions that seem to promote thrombus formation are ulcerative colitis, heart failure, cancer, oral contraceptives, and immobility. Complications of immobility occur during prolonged bedrest such as when a patient is confined to bed for an extensive illness. People who sit for long periods (e.g., on an airplane or at a computer) are also at risk. **Phlebitis** (vein ***inflammation***) associated with invasive procedures such as IV therapy can also predispose patients to thrombosis.

Incidence and Prevalence. Millions of people in the United States are affected by DVT each year, and many die from pulmonary embolism. The largest number of deaths occurs in older adults. Among patients who have a DVT, over half will have long-term complications, and one-third will have a recurrence within 10 years (Benjamin et al., 2018).

Interprofessional Collaborative Care

Assessment: Recognize Cues

History. Assess the patient for a history of any type of VTE. In addition, assess him or her for risks that may be associated with the development of VTE such as prolonged periods of sitting or bedrest, recent surgical procedures, or any factors that may affect coagulation.

The Padua Prediction Score (PPS) has been suggested as the best available model for the assessment of the risk of VTE in hospitalized medical patients (Germini et al., 2016). The PPS is meant to assess risk for VTE, not to diagnose VTE. During the nursing assessment, one point is given for each of the characteristics, which include:

- Active cancer
- Previous VTE (excluding superficial vein thrombosis)
- Reduced mobility
- Known thrombophilic condition
- Recent (≤1 month) trauma and/or surgery
- Older adult (≥70 years)
- Cardiac and/or respiratory failure
- Acute MI and/or ischemic stroke
- Acute infection and/or rheumatologic disorder
- Obesity (body mass index [BMI] ≥30)
- Ongoing hormonal treatment

A score of 4 or more indicates that a DVT is likely to occur.

Physical Assessment/Signs and Symptoms. People with DVT may have symptoms or may be asymptomatic. The classic signs and symptoms of DVT are calf or groin tenderness and pain and sudden onset of unilateral swelling of the leg. Pain in the calf on dorsiflexion of the foot (positive Homans sign) appears in only a small percentage of patients with DVT, and

TABLE 33.8 Venous Thromboembolism (VTE) Core Measure Set

Core Measure	Assessment of Measure
VTE-1	**VTE Prophylaxis:** Number of patients who received VTE prophylaxis or have documentation regarding why no VTE prophylaxis was given the day of or the day after hospital admission or surgery
VTE-2	**ICU VTE:** Number of patients who received VTE prophylaxis on ICU admission or have documentation regarding why no VTE prophylaxis was given the day of admission, transfer, or surgery
VTE-6	**Hospital-Acquired Potentially Preventable VTE:** Number of patients who developed VTE while hospitalized

Data from The Joint Commission. (2017). *Venous thromboembolism.* https://www.jointcommission.org/venous_thromboembolism/.

CORE MEASURES

Venous Thromboembolism (VTE)

The Joint Commission's (TJC) VTE Core Measure Set required hospitals to report data on six areas related to VTE prophylaxis and management. In 2017, VTE-1 and VTE-2 became electronic clinical quality measures (eCQM) available for selection by hospitals to meet hospital accreditation program requirements (The Joint Commission, 2017b). Electronic quality measures reduce the burden of manual data collection and extraction and allow hospitals and providers to use real time data to improve the provision of quality care (Centers for Medicare and Medicaid Services, 2018). VTE-6, which is specific to hospital-acquired VTE, is the remaining measure required for chart abstracted measures (Table 33.8). If VTE is not prevented or adequately managed, the hospital may not be paid by the third-party payer (e.g., Medicare) for the patient's care. In the *inpatient setting,* all patients must be assessed for risk for VTE on admission.

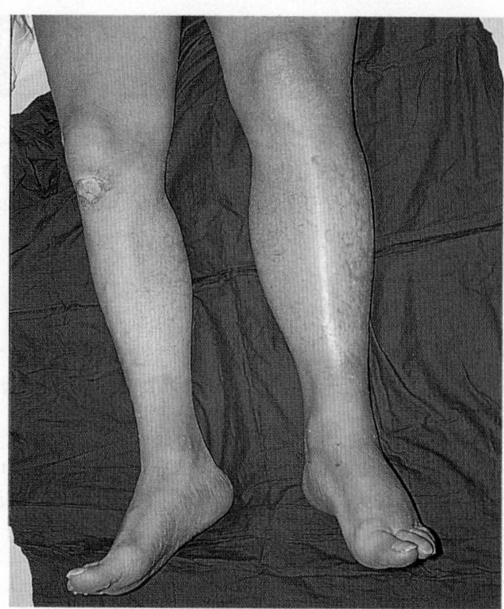

Fig. 33.8 Deep vein thrombosis (DVT) of lower left leg. (From Forbes, C.D., & Jackson, W.F. [2003]. *Colour atlas and text of clinical medicine* [3rd ed.]. London: Mosby.)

false-positive findings are common. Therefore checking a Homans sign is not advised because it is an unreliable tool! Examine the area described as painful, comparing this site with the other limb. Gently palpate the site, observing for induration (hardening) along the blood vessel and for warmth and edema. Redness may also be present (Fig. 33.8).

Other Diagnostic Assessments. If a definitive diagnosis is lacking from physical assessment findings alone, diagnostic tests may be performed. The preferred diagnostic test for DVT is *venous duplex ultrasonography,* a noninvasive ultrasound that assesses the flow of blood through the veins of the arms and legs. *Doppler flow studies* may also be useful in the diagnosis, but they are more sensitive in detecting proximal rather than distal DVT. Normal venous circulation creates audible signals, whereas thrombosed veins produce little or no sound. The accuracy of the scanning depends on the technical skill of the health care professional performing the test. If the test is negative but a DVT is still suspected, a venogram may be needed to make an accurate diagnosis.

Impedance plethysmography assesses venous outflow and can detect most DVTs that are located above the popliteal vein. It is not helpful in locating clots in the calf and is less sensitive than Doppler studies.

Magnetic resonance direct thrombus imaging, another noninvasive test, is useful in finding a DVT in the proximal deep veins and is better than traditional venography in finding DVT in the inferior vena cava or pelvic veins.

A D-dimer test is a global marker of coagulation activation and measures fibrin degradation products produced from fibrinolysis (clot breakdown). The test is used for the diagnosis of DVT when the patient has few clinical signs and stratifies patients into a high-risk category for recurrence. Useful as an adjunct to noninvasive testing, a negative D-dimer test can exclude a DVT without an ultrasound.

Physical and diagnostic assessment of patients with pulmonary embolism is described in Chapter 29.

◆ **Analysis: Analyze Cues and Prioritize Hypotheses.** The priority collaborative problem for most patients with venous thromboembolism (VTE) is: Potential for Injury due to complications of VTE and anticoagulation therapy.

◆ Planning and Implementation: Generate Solutions and Take Action

Preventing Injury

Planning: Expected Outcomes. The patient with VTE is expected to remain free of injury from VTE complications and the use of anticoagulant therapy.

Interventions. The focus of managing thrombophlebitis is to prevent complications such as pulmonary emboli, further thrombus formation, and an increase in size of the thrombus. Patients with deep vein thrombosis (DVT) may be hospitalized for treatment, although this practice is changing as a result of the use of newer drugs.

Nonsurgical Management. DVT is usually treated medically with a combination of rest and drug therapy. Prevention of DVT and other types of VTE is crucial for patients at risk. For those at moderate-to-high risk, initiate these interventions to prevent VTE:

- Patient education
- Leg exercises
- Early ambulation
- Adequate hydration
- Graduated compression stockings
- Intermittent pneumatic compression, such as sequential compression devices (SCDs)
- Venous plexus foot pump
- Anticoagulant therapy

Supportive therapy for DVT has typically included bedrest and elevation of the extremity. However, research shows that ambulation does not increase the risk for pulmonary embolus (Lip & Hull, 2018). The risk of pulmonary embolism (PE) associated with more aggressive activity is unknown. The accepted approach is a gradual increase in ambulation as tolerated by the patient. Allowing patients to ambulate may decrease their fear and anxiety about dislodging the clot and life-threatening complications.

Teach the patient to elevate his or her legs when in the bed and chair. To help prevent chronic venous insufficiency, instruct patients with active and resolving DVT to wear knee- or thigh-high sequential or graduated compression stockings for an extended period. Be sure to select the correct stocking size for the patient according to the sizing chart provided.

Some health care providers prescribe intermittent or continuous warm, moist soaks to the affected area to promote circulation and reduce pain. *To prevent the thrombus from dislodging and becoming an embolus, do not massage the affected extremity.* Monitor all patients for signs and symptoms of PE, which include shortness of breath, chest pain, and acute confusion (in older adults). Emboli may also travel to the brain or heart, but these complications are not as common as PE. Chapter 29 describes PE manifestations in detail.

Drug therapy. *Anticoagulants are the drugs of choice for actual DVT and for patients at risk for DVT. However, these* *drugs are known to cause medical complications and even death.* The Joint Commission's National Patient Safety Goals (NPSGs) include elements of performance to reduce the likelihood of patient harm associated with the use of anticoagulant therapy (TJC, 2018).

! NATIONAL PATIENT SAFETY GOALS

Anticoagulants

Reduce the likelihood of patient harm associated with the use of anticoagulants by (The Joint Commission, 2019):

- Using approved protocols for initiation and maintenance of anticoagulant therapy
- Using approved protocols for reversal of anticoagulation and bleeding events
- Using established protocols for perioperative patients on anticoagulants
- Establishing policy for ongoing laboratory tests to monitor and adjust anticoagulant therapy
- Consistently addressing safety and evaluating anticoagulation safety practices
- Providing education to patients and families on anticoagulants including:
    - Adherence to medication dose and schedule
    - Importance of follow-up appointments
    - Nutritional support including foods to avoid
    - Information about drug reactions or interactions (e.g., bleeding, bruising)
- Using only unit-dose products and prefilled syringes, or premixed infusion bags when these types of products are available
- Using programmable pumps when administering heparin intravenously and continuously in order to provide consistent and accurate dosing

The conventional treatment has been IV unfractionated heparin (UFH) followed by oral anticoagulation with warfarin (Coumadin). However, UFH can be problematic because each patient's response to the drug is unpredictable and hospital admission is usually required for laboratory monitoring and dose adjustments. The use of low-molecular-weight heparin (LMWH) and the development of novel direct oral anticoagulants (DOACs, also referred to as *novel oral anticoagulants [NOACs]*) has changed the management of both DVT and PE. Regardless of the approach to anticoagulation, all patients should be assessed before and during anticoagulant therapy for bleeding risk.

Unfractionated heparin therapy. Some patients with a confirmed diagnosis of an existing blood clot are started on a regimen of IV UFH therapy. The health care provider prescribes UFH to prevent further ***clotting,*** which often develops in the presence of an existing clot, and to prevent enlargement of the existing clot. Over a long period of time, the body slowly absorbs the existing clot.

Before UFH administration, a baseline prothrombin time (PT), activated partial thromboplastin time (APTT or aPTT), international normalized ratio (INR), complete blood count (CBC) with platelet count, urinalysis, stool for occult blood, and creatinine level are required. Notify the primary health care provider if the platelet count is below 100,000 to 120,000/mm^3, depending on agency protocol.

UFH is initially given in a bolus IV dose followed by continuous infusion via pump (Hull et al., 2018). The infusion is regulated by a reliable electronic pump that protects against accidental free flow of solution. The health care provider or clinical pharmacist prescribes concentrations of UFH (in 5% dextrose in water) and the number of units or milliliters per hour needed to maintain a therapeutic aPTT. aPTT is measured at least daily, 6 hours after initiation, and 6 hours after any dose change, and the results are reported to the health care provider as soon as they are available to allow adjustment of heparin dosage. Therapeutic levels of aPTT are usually 1.5 to 2.5 times normal control levels. While most patients who receive UFH are monitored using the aPTT value, the heparin anti-factor Xa (anti-Xa) is sometimes used to monitor and adjust therapy (Zehnder, 2019). The therapeutic range of the anti-Xa factor for UFH is 0.3 to 0.7 IU/mL (Pagana & Pagana, 2018). There is no evidence to suggest that one value is better for monitoring than another, and the aPTT and anti-factor Xa may be used together. Refer to specific agency policy for monitoring protocols.

! NURSING SAFETY PRIORITY QSEN

Critical Rescue

Notify the health care provider if the aPTT value is greater than 70 seconds or follow hospital protocol for reporting critical laboratory values. Assess patient for signs and symptoms of bleeding, which include hematuria, frank or occult blood in the stool, ecchymosis (bruising), petechiae, an altered level of consciousness, or pain. **If bleeding occurs, stop the anticoagulant immediately and call the health care provider or Rapid Response Team**!

UFH can also decrease platelet counts. Mild reductions are common and are resolved with continued heparin therapy. Severe platelet reductions, although rare, result from the development of antiplatelet bodies within 6 to 14 days after the beginning of treatment. Platelets aggregate into "white clots" that can cause thrombosis, usually in the form of an acute arterial occlusion. The health care provider discontinues heparin administration if severe **heparin-induced thrombocytopenia (HIT)** (platelet count <150,000), or "white clot syndrome," occurs. Low-molecular-weight heparin (LMWH) is used more commonly today because of the complications involved with UFH.

Dabigatran is a *direct thrombin inhibitor* that may be used as an alternative to heparin or for patients who have had HIT. Like heparin, these drugs increase the risk for bleeding. Monitor hemoglobin, hematocrit, aPTT, platelet count, urinalysis, fecal occult blood test, and blood pressure for indications of this complication. An oral anticoagulant such as warfarin (Coumadin) may also be substituted for heparin if necessary.

Ensure that protamine sulfate, the antidote for heparin, is available if needed for excessive bleeding. The Best Practice for Patient Safety & Quality Care: The Patient Receiving Anticoagulant Therapy box highlights information important to nursing care and patient education associated with anticoagulant therapy.

BEST PRACTICE FOR PATIENT SAFETY & QUALITY CARE (QSEN)

The Patient Receiving Anticoagulant Therapy

- Carefully check the dosage of anticoagulant to be administered, even if the pharmacy prepared the drug.
- Monitor the patient for signs and symptoms of bleeding, including hematuria, frank or occult blood in the stool, ecchymosis, petechiae, altered mental status (indicating possible cranial bleeding), or pain (especially abdominal pain, which could indicate abdominal bleeding).
- Monitor vital signs frequently for decreased blood pressure and increased pulse (indicating possible internal bleeding).
- Have antidotes available as needed (e.g., protamine sulfate for heparin; vitamin K for warfarin).
- Monitor activated partial thromboplastin time (aPTT) for patients receiving unfractionated heparin. Monitor prothrombin time (PT)/international normalized ratio (INR) for patients receiving warfarin or low–molecular-weight heparin (LMWH).
- Apply prolonged pressure over venipuncture and injection sites.
- When administering *subcutaneous* heparin, apply pressure over the site and do not massage.
- Teach the patient going home while taking an anticoagulant to:
- Use only an electric razor
- Take precautions to avoid injury (e.g., do not use tools such as hammers or saws, with which accidents commonly occur)
- Report signs and symptoms of bleeding, such as blood in the urine or stool, nosebleeds, ecchymosis, or altered mental status
- Take the prescribed dosage of drug at the precise time that it was prescribed to be taken
- Do not stop taking the drug abruptly; the health care provider usually tapers the anticoagulant gradually

To *prevent* DVT, UFH may be given in low doses subcutaneously for high-risk patients, especially after orthopedic surgery.

Alternatives to UFH include:

- Low–molecular-weight heparin (LMWH; e.g., enoxaparin) (drug class of choice after orthopedic surgery)
- Novel oral anticoagulants (dabigatran, rivaroxaban, apixaban, edoxaban)
- Warfarin

Low-molecular-weight heparin. Subcutaneous LMWHs such as enoxaparin or dalteparin have a consistent action and are preferred for prevention and treatment of DVT. LMWHs bind less to plasma proteins, blood cells, and vessel walls, resulting in a longer half-life and more predictable response. These drugs inhibit thrombin formation because of reduced factor IIa activity and enhanced inhibition of factor Xa and thrombin.

Some patients taking LMWH may be safely managed at home with visits from a home care nurse. Candidates for home therapy must have stable DVT or PE, low risk for bleeding, adequate renal function, and normal vital signs. They must be willing to learn self-injection or have a family member, friend, or home care nurse administer the subcutaneous injections.

Some health care providers place the patient on a regimen of IV unfractionated heparin (UFH) for several days and then follow up with an LMWH. In this case, the UFH is discontinued at least 30 minutes before the first LMWH injection. Assess all stools for occult blood. The aPTTs are not checked on an ongoing basis because the doses of LMWH are not routinely adjusted. The anti-Xa factor can be assessed to monitor the effect of the LMWH. Therapeutic range of the anti-Xa factor for LMWH therapy is 0.5 to 1.2 IU/mL (Pagana & Pagana, 2018).

Warfarin therapy. If the patient is receiving continuous UFH, warfarin (Coumadin), an oral anticoagulant, may be *added.* This anticoagulant drug overlap is necessary because heparin and warfarin work differently. Warfarin works in the liver to inhibit synthesis of the four vitamin K–dependent ***clotting*** factors and takes 3 to 4 days before it can exert therapeutic anticoagulation. The heparin continues to provide therapeutic anticoagulation until this effect is achieved. IV heparin is then discontinued. Patients receiving LMWH are placed on the oral drug after the first dose.

! NATIONAL PATIENT SAFETY GOALS

Warfarin

According to the National Patient Safety Goals, therapeutic levels of warfarin must be monitored by measuring the international normalized ratio (INR) at frequent intervals. Because prothrombin times are often inconsistent and misleading, the INR was developed. Most laboratories report both results. Most patients receiving warfarin should have an INR between 1.5 and 2.0 to prevent future DVT and to minimize the risk for stroke or hemorrhage (Pagana & Pagana, 2018). For patients with additional cardiovascular problems or pulmonary embolus, the desired INR is higher, up to 3.5 or 4.0. The health care provider specifies the desired INR level to obtain. Be aware of the critical value for INR according to agency policy (usually greater than 5). Notify the health care provider immediately if your patient's INR is at a critical value.

After obtaining the patient's baseline INR, warfarin therapy should be started with low doses and gradually titrated up according to the INR. Patients usually receive this drug for at least 3 months or longer after an episode of DVT if no precipitating factors were discovered, with recurrence, or if there are continuing risk factors.

! NURSING SAFETY PRIORITY (QSEN)

Drug Alert

For patients taking warfarin, assess for any bleeding, such as hematuria or blood in the stool. *Ensure that vitamin K, the antidote for warfarin, is available in case of excessive bleeding.* Report any bleeding to the health care provider and document in the patient's health record. Teach patients to avoid foods with high concentrations of vitamin K, especially dark green leafy vegetables. These foods interfere with the action of warfarin, which is a vitamin K synthesis inhibitor.

Direct oral anticoagulants (DOACs). The latest development in anticoagulation is the use of DOACs (also referred to as novel oral anticoagulants [NOACs]). These medications (dabigatran, rivaroxaban, apixaban, edoxaban, betrixaban) were developed to have fewer drug interactions and a wide therapeutic index to allow for fixed dosing without the need for frequent laboratory monitoring (Di Minno et al., 2017). Current research suggests that efficacy with DOACs is similar to that of warfarin therapy in the treatment of VTE (Coleman et al., 2018). Prothrombin time (PT) and INR are not accurate predictors of bleeding time when DOACs are used.

Dabigatran has been the only DOAC with a reversal agent (idarucizumab); however, in 2018 the FDA approved andexanet alfa for the reversal of rivaroxaban and apixaban (Garcia & Crowther, 2018). It is important to note that although these antidotes are now available, the side effects and risk of ***clotting*** are significant. Therefore the use of the antidote is suggested only in the event of life-threatening bleeding that presents an imminent risk of death.

Patients should be informed that this medication should not be stopped prematurely because of a significant risk of ***clotting.*** Initial laboratory values, including PT and aPTT, are suggested. However, recurrent laboratory monitoring is not required with this medication. Dosage is decreased when renal insufficiency is present. The same teaching specific to all anticoagulants, with the exception of repeat laboratory testing, applies to patients taking NOACs.

Thrombolytic therapy. Thrombolytic therapy using a catheter-directed approach can be used. However, anticoagulant therapy is preferred for most patients with an uncomplicated DVT, reserving thrombolytic therapy for extensive DVT.

NCLEX EXAMINATION CHALLENGE 33.4

Physiological Integrity

A client who is receiving heparin therapy is started on warfarin. Which nursing explanation is appropriate?

A. "You will need both drugs long-term to provide long-term anticoagulation."
B. "Warfarin is easier on your stomach so you can take it long-term."
C. "It takes several days for warfarin to begin working, so both drugs are required for a shorttime."
D. "These drugs work the same, but one is taken by mouth, so it is easier to take at home."

Surgical Management. A deep vein thrombus is rarely removed surgically unless there is a massive occlusion that does not respond to medical treatment and the thrombus is of recent (1 to 2 days) onset. Thrombectomy is a surgical procedure for clot removal. Preoperative and postoperative care of patients undergoing thrombectomy is similar to the care for those undergoing arterial surgery (see the Peripheral Arterial Disease section).

For patients with recurrent deep vein thrombosis (DVT) or pulmonary emboli that do not respond to medical treatment and for patients who cannot tolerate anticoagulation, **inferior vena cava filtration** may be indicated. The surgeon or interventional radiologist inserts a filter device into the femoral vein or jugular vein. The device is meant to trap emboli in the inferior vena cava before they progress to the lungs. Holes in the device allow blood to pass through, without interfering with the return of blood to the heart. Several new filter brands are available that are designed for removal if and when DVT risks diminish.

SYSTEMS THINKING AND QUALITY IMPROVEMENT QSEN

Increasing Nurse-Driven Heparin Infusion Administration Safety

Johnson, C., Miltner, R., & Wilson, M. (2018). Increasing nurse-driven heparin infusion administration safety: A quality improvement initiative. *MedSurg Nursing, 27*(4), 243–246.

Intravenous heparin therapy is one of the highest-risk medications used commonly in the inpatient health care setting. National Patient Safety Goals call for measures to reduce patient harm associated with the use of anticoagulants in the clinical setting. In this quality improvement (QI) initiative, the existing protocol for the titration of heparin infusions was evaluated. This evaluation found multiple inconsistencies in adherence to the process. Because the laboratory assessments were based on the time of the heparin rate titration by the nurse, there were no standardized times for assessment. Therefore it was difficult for nurses to remember when to complete the laboratory assessment requirements.

To address the issues, a quality initiative was developed through an interprofessional team that worked to establish a standardized process for all patients receiving intravenous heparin therapy. The team identified two main tasks: (1) developing a standardized tool for nursing shift report that included details of the heparin infusion; and (2) scheduled times for laboratory testing (this facility used anti-Xa for titration) for patients receiving intravenous heparin. Scheduling the test eliminated the nurse forgetting, decreased the time between testing, and eliminated the danger of allowing too much time to pass between testing.

Nurses were educated on the new process and the report tool. After the new process was put into place, nurses were given a week to become more comfortable with the new process. After the week, times between laboratory testing for patients on intravenous heparin were evaluated. Results showed much more consistency and more consistent monitoring after implementation of the scheduled laboratory testing. This pilot project demonstrated that standardization of shift report as well as a standardized schedule for laboratory monitoring with heparin administration improved the safe nursing administration of heparin. The pilot results were then used to promote hospital-wide changes to the nurse-driven heparin protocol.

Commentary: Implications for Research and Practice

This project was successful at improving the clinical nursing practice and demonstrates action associated with The Joint Commission's National Patient Safety Goal to decrease harm associated with the use of anticoagulants. The results of this QI project demonstrate that standardization can improve the consistency of nursing care. This project could be used in other hospitals to improve standardization and safety in the administration of therapeutic heparin.

Preoperative care is similar to that provided for patients receiving local anesthesia (see Chapter 9). If they have recently been taking anticoagulants, collaborate with the health care provider about interrupting this therapy in the preoperative period to avoid hemorrhage.

After surgery, inspect the groin insertion site for bleeding and signs or symptoms of infection. Other postoperative nursing care is similar to that for any patient undergoing local anesthesia (see Chapter 9).

Care Coordination and Transition Management

Home Care Considerations. Patients recovering from thrombophlebitis or DVT are ambulatory when they are discharged from the hospital. The primary focus of planning for discharge is to educate the patient and family about anticoagulation therapy. Patients who have experienced DVT may fear recurrence of a thrombus. They may also be concerned about treatment with warfarin and the risk for bleeding. Assure them that the prescribed treatment will help resolve this problem and that ongoing assessment of prothrombin times and INR values decreases the risks for bleeding.

Self-Management Education. Teach patients recovering from DVT to stop smoking and avoid the use of oral contraceptives to decrease the risk for recurrence. Alternative forms of birth control may be used. Most patients are discharged on a regimen of warfarin (Coumadin) or low-molecular-weight heparin (LMWH). Patients receiving subcutaneous LMWH injections at home need instruction on self-injection (see the National Patient Safety Goals: Anticoagulants box). Teach the appropriate caregiver and family members or friends, if necessary, to administer the injections.

Instruct patients and their families to avoid potentially traumatic situations, such as participation in contact sports. Provide written and oral information about the signs and symptoms of bleeding (see the Best Practice for Patient Safety & Quality Care: The Patient Receiving Anticoagulant Therapy box). Reinforce the need to report any of these manifestations to the primary health care provider immediately. The anticoagulant effect of warfarin may be reversed by omitting one or two doses of the drug or by the administration of vitamin K. In case of injury, teach patients to apply pressure to bleeding wounds and to seek medical assistance immediately. Encourage them to carry an identification card or wear a medical alert bracelet that states that they are taking warfarin or any other anticoagulant.

Instruct patients to tell their dentist and other health care providers that they are taking warfarin before receiving treatment or prescriptions. Prothrombin times are affected by many prescription and over-the-counter drugs such as NSAIDs. Teach patients to avoid high-fat and vitamin K–rich foods (see the Patient and Family Education: Preparing for Self-Management: Food and Drugs That Interfere With Warfarin [Coumadin] box). Remind them to drink adequate fluids to stay well hydrated, avoid alcohol (which can cause dehydration), and avoid sitting for prolonged periods.

Health Care Resources. Collaborate with the case manager or office nurse to arrange for the patient to obtain a device to self-monitor INR at home. Some insurance companies do not pay for the INR monitoring device. Clinical studies show that self-monitoring the INR and self-adjusting anticoagulation therapy result in better anticoagulation control, improve patient satisfaction, and improve quality of life (Heneghan et al., 2017). The device used to self-monitor is similar to a glucometer for glucose testing and requires a finger stick blood sample. If the patient cannot use a monitoring device, teach a family member or other caregiver how to perform the procedure. If the patient lives alone, collaborate with the case manager to arrange for follow-up laboratory appointments to have blood drawn at frequent intervals—usually every week until the patient's values are stabilized. Communication with the primary health care provider is essential while patients are receiving warfarin.

PATIENT AND FAMILY EDUCATION: PREPARING FOR SELF-MANAGEMENT

Foods and Drugs That Interfere With Warfarin (Coumadin)

Eat only small amounts of foods rich in vitamin K each day, including any of these:
- Broccoli
- Cauliflower
- Spinach
- Kale
- Other green leafy vegetables
- Brussels sprouts
- Cabbage
- Beef liver
- Parsley
- Soybeans

If possible, avoid:
- Allopurinol
- NSAIDs
- Acetaminophen
- Vitamin E
- Histamine blockers
- Cholesterol-reducing drugs
- Antibiotics
- Oral contraceptives
- Antidepressants
- Thyroid drugs
- Antifungal agents
- Other anticoagulants
- Corticosteroids
- Herbs, such as St. John's wort, garlic, ginseng, *Ginkgo biloba*

◆ **Evaluation: Evaluate Outcomes.** Evaluate the care of the patient with VTE on the basis of the identified priority problem. The expected outcome is that he or she:
- Remains free of injury associated with VTE complications such as pulmonary embolism and bleeding associated with anticoagulation therapy.

VENOUS INSUFFICIENCY

Pathophysiology Review

Venous insufficiency occurs as a result of prolonged venous hypertension that stretches the veins and damages the valves. Valvular damage can lead to a backup of blood and further venous hypertension, resulting in edema and decreased tissue ***perfusion.*** With time, this stasis (stoppage) results in venous stasis ulcers, swelling, and cellulitis.

The veins cannot function properly when thrombosis occurs or when valves are not working correctly. Venous hypertension can occur in people who stand or sit in one position for long periods (e.g., teachers, office personnel). Obesity can also cause chronically distended veins, which lead to damaged valves. Thrombus formation can contribute to valve destruction. Chronic venous insufficiency also often occurs in patients who have had thrombophlebitis. In severe cases, venous ulcers develop.

Venous leg ulcers are a major cause of pain, death, and health care costs. Most venous ulcer care is delivered in the community setting by home care nurses or through self-management.

❖ Interprofessional Collaborative Care

◆ Assessment: Recognize Cues. Venous insufficiency may result in edema of both legs. There may be **stasis dermatitis** or reddish-brown discoloration along the ankles, extending up to the calf. In people with long-term venous insufficiency, **stasis ulcers** often form. They can result from the edema or from minor injury to the limb. Ulcers typically occur over the malleolus, more often medially (inner ankle) than laterally (outer ankle). The ulcer usually has irregular borders. In general, these ulcers are chronic and difficult to heal (see the Key Features: Lower Extremity Ulcers box). Many people live with ulcers for years, and recurrence is common. Some may lose one or both legs if ulcers are not controlled.

◆ Interventions: Take Action. The focus of treating venous insufficiency is to decrease edema and promote venous return from the affected leg. Patients are not usually hospitalized for venous insufficiency alone unless it is complicated by an ulcer or another disorder is occurring at the same time.

Treatment of chronic venous insufficiency is nonsurgical unless it is complicated by a venous stasis ulcer that requires surgical débridement. The desired outcomes of managing venous stasis ulcers are to heal the ulcer, prevent infection, and prevent stasis with recurrence of ulcer formation. Interprofessional collaboration with the wound care nurse or wound, ostomy, and continence nurse (WOCN) is essential in providing ulcer care. A registered dietitian nutritionist can suggest dietary supplements such as zinc and vitamins A and C, high-protein foods, and sufficient caloric intake to promote wound healing.

Patients with chronic venous insufficiency wear graduated compression stockings, which fit from the middle of the foot to just below the knee or to the thigh. Stockings should be worn during the day and evening. Explain the purpose and importance of wearing the compression stockings. Be sure to use the sizing chart that comes with the stockings to select the best fit. Teach patients to not roll them down and to report if they become too tight or uncomfortable.

Teach the patient to elevate his or her legs for at least 20 minutes four or five times per day. When the patient is in bed, remind him or her to elevate the legs above the level of the heart (see the Patient and Family Education: Preparing for Self-Management: Venous Insufficiency box).

Coordinate with the health care provider about the use of intermittent sequential pneumatic compression or foot plexus pumps for patients with past or present venous stasis ulcers. If an open venous ulcer is present, the device may be applied over a dressing such as an Unna boot. Instruct the patient to apply the pump as directed during the period of healing. Because of the high incidence of venous ulcer recurrence, encourage patients with chronic venous insufficiency whose ulcers have healed to continue compression therapy for life.

PATIENT AND FAMILY EDUCATION: PREPARING FOR SELF-MANAGEMENT

Venous Insufficiency

Graduated Compression Stockings (GCSs)

- Wear stockings as prescribed, usually during the day and evening.
- Put the stockings on upon awakening and before getting out of bed.
- When applying the stockings, do not "bunch up" and apply like socks. Instead, place your hand inside the stocking and pull out the heel. Then place the foot of the stocking over your foot and slide the rest of the stocking up. Be sure that rough seams on the stocking are on the outside, not next to your skin.
- Do not push stockings down for comfort because they may function like a tourniquet and further impair venous return.
- Put on a clean pair of stockings each day. Wash them by hand (not in a washing machine) with a gentle detergent and warm water.
- If the stockings seem to be "stretched out," replace them with a new pair.
- Be sure to assess sizing if the patient has gained or lost weight.

Dos and Don'ts

- Elevate your legs for at least 20 minutes 4 or 5 times a day. When in bed, elevate your legs above the level of your heart.
- Avoid prolonged sitting or standing.
- Do not cross your legs. Crossing at the ankles is acceptable for short periods.
- Do not wear tight, restrictive pants. Avoid girdles and garters.

Venous stasis ulcers are slightly more manageable than ulcers resulting from arterial disease. They are chronic in nature, with some patients having the same ulcer for years. Ulcers often heal, only to recur in the same area several years later.

Two types of occlusive dressings are used for venous stasis ulcers: oxygen-permeable dressings and oxygen-impermeable dressings. Because the role of atmospheric oxygen in wound healing is controversial, opinions vary with regard to which type of dressing is preferred. An oxygen-permeable polyethylene film and an oxygen-impermeable hydrocolloid dressing (e.g., DuoDERM) are common. Hydrocolloid dressings are left in place for a minimum of 3 to 5 days for best effect. Use medical aseptic technique when changing dressings. If the wound is infected, use Contact Precautions in addition to Standard Precautions.

Artificial skin products can be used for difficult-to-heal venous leg ulcers. These first-generation products are very expensive but are laying the foundation in the field, with costs anticipated to come down in the future. Except for cultured epithelial autografts, artificial skins are only temporary. Artificial skin serves as a biologic cover to secrete growth factors to promote more growth factor secretion from the patient's own skin to speed the wound healing process.

If the patient is ambulatory, an **Unna boot** may be used. An Unna boot dressing is constructed of gauze that has been moistened with zinc oxide. Apply the boot to the affected limb, from the toes to the knee, after the ulcer has been cleaned with normal saline solution. It is then covered with an elastic wrap and hardens like a cast. This promotes venous return and prevents stasis. The Unna boot also forms a sterile environment for the ulcer. The health care provider changes the boot about once a week. Instruct the patient to report increased pain, which indicates that the boot may be too tight.

The primary health care provider may prescribe topical agents, such as Accuzyme, to chemically débride the ulcer, eliminating necrotic tissue and promoting healing. Remind patients that they may temporarily feel a burning sensation when the agent is applied. If an infection or cellulitis develops, systemic antibiotics are necessary.

Surgery for chronic venous insufficiency is not usually performed because it is not successful. Attempts at transplanting vein valves have had limited success. Surgical débridement of venous ulcers is similar to that performed for arterial ulcers.

NCLEX EXAMINATION CHALLENGE 33.5

Physiological Integrity

The nurse is admitting a client with an ulcer on the right foot. Which client statement indicates venous insufficiency to the nurse? **Select all that apply.**

A. "My ankles swell up all the time."
B. "My leg hurts after I walk about a block."
C. "My feet are always really cold."
D. "My veins really stick out in my legs."
E. "My ankles have been discolored for years."

The desired outcome for the patient with chronic venous insufficiency is to be managed in the home. For patients with frequent acute complications and repeated hospital admissions, case management can help meet appropriate clinical and cost outcomes. Help patients plan for opportunities and facilities that allow for elevation of the lower extremities in and outside the home. In addition, collaborate with the wound specialist to plan care of the ulcers at home.

If the primary health care provider prescribes graduated compression stockings, teach patients to apply these stockings before they get out of bed in the morning and to remove them just before going to bed at night. Also advise them that they will probably need to wear these stockings for the rest of their lives.

To improve circulation and aid in weight reduction, collaborate with the physical therapist to prescribe an exercise program on an individual basis. Encourage all patients to maintain an optimal weight and consult with the registered dietitian nutritionist to plan a weight-reduction diet.

Patients with venous stasis disease, especially those with venous stasis ulcers, may require long-term emotional support to help them meet long-term needs. They may also need help to cope with necessary lifestyle adjustments, such as possible changes in occupation. Patients with venous stasis ulcers may need the assistance of a home care nurse to perform dressing changes. Those with Unna boots need weekly transportation to their primary health care provider for dressing changes. Collaborate with the case manager to arrange for a sequential compression device (SCD) in the home if the primary health care provider prescribes one.

VARICOSE VEINS

Pathophysiology Review

Varicose veins are distended, protruding veins that appear darkened and tortuous. They can occur in anyone, but they are common in adults older than 30 years whose occupations require prolonged standing or heavy physical activity. Varicose veins are also frequently seen in patients with systemic problems (e.g., heart disease), obesity, high estrogen states, and a family history of varicose veins.

As the vein wall weakens and dilates, venous pressure increases, and the valves become incompetent (defective), causing venous reflux. The incompetent valves enhance the vessel dilation, and the veins become tortuous and distended. The severity of the disease depends on the extent of the distention and reflux. **Telangiectasias** (spider veins) are dilated *intradermal* veins less than 1 to 3 mm in diameter that are visible on the skin surface. Most patients are not bothered by them but may consider them unattractive. Most telangiectasias do not develop into the more severe varicose vein disease.

More advanced disease causes venous distention (bulging), edema, a feeling of fullness in the legs, and pruritus (itching). As a result, signs and symptoms of venous insufficiency may occur, including venous stasis ulcers, brown pigmentation from extravasated red blood cells (also called *skin staining*), and pain. Varicose veins and reflux are diagnosed by simple or duplex ultrasonography.

❖ Interprofessional Collaborative Care

The overall purpose of management for patients with varicose veins is to improve and maintain optimal venous return to the heart and prevent disease progression. Conservative measures are the treatment of choice, including the three *E*s: *e*lastic compression hose, *e*xercise, and *e*levation. Graduated compression stockings (GCSs) rely on graduated external pressure to improve venous return by applying pressure to the muscles. They are available in many grades or strengths, ranging from 8 to 50 mm Hg pressure. Exercise increases venous return by helping the muscles pump blood back to the heart. Teach patients to avoid high-impact exercises such as horseback riding and running. Daily walks and ankle flexion exercises while sitting are common exercises that are helpful in promoting circulation. Elevating the extremities as much as possible allows gravity to work with the valves in promoting venous return and preventing reflux.

Patients who continue to have pain or unsightly veins despite using the three *E*s may opt for more invasive approaches. Surgical ligation and/or removal of veins ("stripping") were the procedures of choice for many years. Sclerotherapy to occlude the affected vessel is also an option.

However, newer, less-invasive treatments are more common today. They are less painful and have a shorter recovery time. A common procedure is an endovenous ablation, which occludes the varicose vein, most commonly the saphenous vein. Using ultrasound guidance, the clinician advances a catheter into the vein and injects an anesthetic agent. Then the vessel is ablated (occluded) while the catheter is slowly removed.

After the procedure, teach the patient the importance of using a GCS or other form of compression (such as elastic compression bandages) for 24 hours a day, except for showers, for at least the first week. Follow-up ultrasonography ensures that the treated vein is closed. The patient is monitored carefully for the first 6 to 8 weeks to determine how healing has progressed. Some patients require continued use of the three *E*s for many years, depending on the severity of their disease.

Assess the affected limb for vascular status, including any changes in color or temperature of the leg. Monitor for pain, edema, and paresthesias that could indicate complications such as DVT or nerve damage. Nerve damage is usually temporary and minimal; it usually resolves within a few months (Witte et al., 2017).

GET READY FOR THE NEXT-GENERATION NCLEX® EXAMINATION!

Key Points

Review these Key Points for each NCLEX Examination Client Needs Category.

Safe and Effective Care Environment

- Plan care for the patient with atherosclerosis and hypertension in collaboration with the health care team. **QSEN: Teamwork and Collaboration**
- To reduce the risk for injury, caution patients about orthostatic hypotension when taking antihypertensive drugs. **QSEN: Safety**
- Monitor blood pressure carefully to prevent a hypertensive crisis (see the Best Practice for Patient Safety & Quality Care: Emergency Care of Patients With Hypertensive Crisis box). **QSEN: Safety**

Health Promotion and Maintenance

- In collaboration with the registered dietitian nutritionist, help the patient incorporate healthy eating behaviors such as the DASH diet. **QSEN: Teamwork and Collaboration**
- Teach patients to engage in 40 minutes of moderate-to-vigorous physical activity three or four times a week to lower blood pressure and LDL-C levels.
- Assess for and teach the patient and family about modifiable and nonmodifiable risk factors for vascular disease (see Table 33.4). **QSEN: Patient-Centered Care**

Physiological Integrity

- Risk factors such as smoking increase the pathophysiologic process of atherosclerosis, preventing adequate ***perfusion*** (see Table 33.4).
- Monitor total cholesterol, HDL-C, and LDL-C levels to assess risk for atherosclerosis.
- Teach patients taking any of the statins in Table 33.5 to report any adverse effects, including muscle cramping, to their primary health care provider. Monitor the patient's liver enzymes carefully.
- Teach patients to decrease saturated and *trans* fats in their diet; instruct them to consume a diet rich in fruits, vegetables, and whole grains; and instruct them to include legumes, poultry, fish, and low-fat dairy products. **QSEN: Evidence-Based Practice**
- Hypertension is categorized as either essential or secondary; the risk factors and causes for each type are described in Table 33.1.
- Closely observe the patient receiving anticoagulants or fibrinolytics for signs of bleeding and monitor appropriate laboratory values (see the Best Practice for Patient Safety & Quality Care: The Patient Receiving Anticoagulant Therapy box). **QSEN: Safety**
- Monitor for decreased serum potassium levels when patients are taking thiazide or loop diuretics to prevent life-threatening cardiac dysrhythmias (see the Common Examples of Drug Therapy box). **QSEN: Safety**
- Teach patients to move slowly when changing position if taking any of the antihypertensive drugs listed in the Common Examples of Drug Therapy box. **QSEN: Safety**
- Recognize the signs and symptoms of peripheral vascular disease (see the Key Features: Chronic Peripheral Arterial Disease box).
- Deep vein thrombosis (DVT) is the most common type of peripheral vascular problem, with symptoms of swelling, redness, localized pain, and warmth.
- DVT can lead to pulmonary embolism, a life-threatening emergency! **Clinical Judgment**
- Teach patients to prevent VTE with leg exercises, early ambulation, adequate hydration, graduated compression stockings (GCSs), sequential compression devices (SCDs), and anticoagulant therapy.
- Monitor aPTT values for patients receiving unfractionated heparin; monitor INR for patients receiving warfarin (Coumadin). **QSEN: Safety**
- Assess for venous and arterial ulcers as described in the Key Features: Lower Extremity Ulcers box.
- Teach foot care for patients with PVD as outlined in the Patient and Family Education: Preparing for Self-Management: Foot Care of the Patient With PVD box.
- Teach patients about precautions for anticoagulant therapy as described in the Best Practice for Patient Safety & Quality Care: The Patient Receiving Anticoagulant Therapy box.
- Teach about food and drugs that interfere with warfarin as listed in the Patient and Family Education: Preparing for Self-Management: Foods and Drugs That Interfere With Warfarin (Coumadin) box. **QSEN: Evidence-Based Practice**
- Monitor for indications of aneurysm rupture: diaphoresis, nausea, vomiting, pallor, hypotension, tachycardia, severe pain, and decreased level of consciousness. **QSEN: Safety**
- Varicose veins require the three *E*s: *e*lastic compression hose, *e*xercise, and *e*levation.

MASTERY QUESTIONS

1. The nurse is teaching a client with stage 1 hypertension. Which client statement indicates understanding of dietary modifications?
   A. "I will reduce my sodium intake to 2500 mg per day."
   B. "I will restrict my intake of daily dietary lean protein."
   C. "I am only going to drink one cup of coffee to start my day."
   D. "I will drink a glass of low-fat milk with my breakfast."
2. A client is admitted to the hospital with an abdominal aortic aneurysm. Which assessment data would cause the nurse to suspect that the aneurysm has ruptured?
   A. Shortness of breath and hemoptysis
   B. Sudden, severe low back pain and bruising along the flank
   C. Gradually increasing substernal chest pain and diaphoresis
   D. Rapid development of patchy blue mottling on feet and toes
3. The nurse is caring for a client receiving intravenous heparin for treatment of DVT who begins to begins to vomit blood. What action should the nurse be prepared to take?
   A. Administer vitamin K
   B. Stop the infusion of heparin
   C. Administer an antiemetic
   D. Insert a nasogastric tube

REFERENCES

Asterisk (*) indicates a classic or definitive work on this subject.

*ALLHAT Officers and Coordinators for the ALLHAT Collaborative Research Group. (2002). Major outcomes in high-risk hypertensive patients randomized to angiotensin-converting enzyme inhibitor or calcium channel blocker vs diuretic. The Antihypertensive and Lipid-Lowering Treatment to Prevent Heart Attack Trial (ALLHAT). *Journal of the American Medical Association, 288*(23), 2981–2997.

Benjamin, E. J., Virani, S. S., Callaway, C. W., Chamberlain, A. M., Chang, A. R., Cheng, S., et al. (2018). Heart disease and stroke statistics—2018 update: A report from the American heart association. *Circulation, 137*(12), e67–e492.

Black, J. H., & Manning, W. (2018). *Management of acute aortic dissection. UpToDate.* Retrieved from https://www.uptodate.com/contents/management-of-acute-aortic-dissection.

Burchum, J., & Rosenthal, L. (2019). *Lehne's pharmacology for nursing care* (9th ed.). St. Louis: Elsevier.

Centers for Medicare and Medicaid Services (CMS). (2018). *eCQMs.* Retrieved from https://ecqi.healthit.gov/ecqms.

Coleman, C. I., Turpie, A. G., Bunz, T. J., Baker, W. L., & Beyer-Westendorf, J. (2018). Effectiveness and safety of outpatient rivaroxaban versus warfarin for treatment of venous thromboembolism in patients with a known primary hypercoagulable state. *Thrombosis Research, 163*, 132–137.

Department of Health and Human Services. (2019). *Proposed objectives for inclusion in healthy people 2030.* Retrieved from https://www.healthypeople.gov/sites/default/files/ObjectivesPublicComment508_1.17.19.pdf.

Di Minno, A., Frigerio, B., Spadarella, G., Ravani, A., Sansaro, D., Amato, M., et al. (2017). Old and new oral anticoagulants: Food, herbal medicines and drug interactions. *Blood Reviews, 31*(4), 193–203.

Garcia, D., & Crowther, M. (2018). *Management of bleeding in patients receiving direct oral anticoagulants. UpToDate.* Retrieved from https://www.uptodate.com/contents/management-of-bleeding-in-patients-receiving-direct-oral-anticoagulants.

Gerhard-Herman, M. D., Gornik, H. L., Barrett, C., Barshes, N. R., Corriere, M. A., Drachman, D. E., et al. (2017). 2016 AHA/ACC guideline on the management of patients with lower extremity peripheral artery disease: Executive summary: A report of the American College of Cardiology/American heart association task force on clinical practice guidelines. *Journal of the American College of Cardiology, 69*(11), 1465–1508.

Germini, F., Agnelli, G., Fedele, M., Galli, M. G., Giustozzi, M., Marcucci, M., et al. (2016). Padua prediction score or clinical judgment for decision making on antithrombotic prophylaxis: A quasi-randomized controlled trial. *Journal of Thrombosis and Thrombolysis, 42*(3), 336–339.

Grundy, S., Stone, N., Bailey, A., Beam, C., Birtcher, K. K., Blumenthal, R. S., et al. (2018). 2018 AHA/ACC guideline on the management of blood cholesterol: A report of the American College of Cardiology/American heart association task force on clinical practice guidelines. *Circulation.* https://doi.org/10.1161/CIR.0000000000000625.

Heneghan, C. J., Spencer, E. A., & Mahtani, K. R. (2017). Cochrane corner: Self-monitoring and self-management of oral anticoagulation. *British Medical Journal, 103*(12).

Hull, R., Garcia, D., & Burnett, A. (2018). *Heparin and LMW heparin: Dosing and adverse effects. UpToDate.* Retrieved from https://www.uptodate.com/contents/heparin-and-lmw-heparin-dosing-and-adverse-effects.

*James, P. A., Oparil, S., Carter, B. L., Cushman, W. C., Dennison-Himmelfarb, C., Handler, J., et al. (2014). 2014 evidence-based guidelines for the management of high blood pressure in adults: Report from the panel members appointed to the Eighth National Committee (JNC 8). *Journal of the American Medical Association, 311*(5), 507–520. http://jama.jamanetwork.com/article.aspx?articleid=1791497.

Jellinger, P. S., Handelsman, Y., Rosenblit, P. D., Bloomgarden, Z. T., Fonseca, V. A., Garber, A. J., et al. (2017). American Association of Clinical Endocrinologists and American College of Endocrinology guidelines for management of dyslipidemia and prevention of cardiovascular disease. *Endocrine Practice, 23*(s2), 1–87.

Johnson, C., Miltner, R., & Wilson, M. (2018). Increasing nurse-drive heparin infusion administration safety: A quality improvement initiative. *Medsurg Nursing, 27*(4), 243–246.

Lip, G., & Hull, R. (2018). *Overview of the treatment of lower extremity deep venous thrombosis (DVT). UpToDate.* www.uptodate.com.

Lloyd-Jones, D. M., Morris, P. B., Ballantyne, C. M., Birtcher, K. K., Daly, D. D., DePalma, S. M., et al. (2017). 2017 focused update of the 2016 ACC expert consensus decision pathway on the role of non-statin therapies for LDL-cholesterol lowering in the management of atherosclerotic cardiovascular disease risk: A report of the American College of Cardiology task force on expert consensus decision pathways. *Journal of the American College of Cardiology, 70*(14), 1785–1822.

McCance, K., & Huether, S. (2019). *Pathophysiology: The biologic basis for disease in adults and children* (8th ed.). St. Louis: Elsevier.

National Center for Complementary and Integrative Health. (2018). *Complementary health approaches for hypertension: What the science saysClinical digest for health professionals.* Retrieved from: https://nccih.nih.gov/health/providers/digest/Hypertension-science.

National Heart, Lung, and Blood Institute. (2018). *Description of the DASH eating plan.* https://www.nhlbi.nih.gov/health-topics/dash-eating-plan.

Pagana, K., & Pagana, T. J. (2018). *Mosby's manual of diagnostic and laboratory tests* (6th ed.). St. Louis: Elsevier.

Rosenson, R., & Baker, S. (2018). *Statin muscle-related adverse events. UpToDate.* Retrieved from: https://www.uptodate.com/contents/statin-muscle-related-adverse-events.

Rosenson, R., & Kastelein, J. (2018). *Low density lipoprotein cholesterol lowering with drugs other than statins and PCSK9 inhibitors. UpToDate.* Retrieved from: https://www.uptodate.com/contents/low-density-lipoprotein-cholesterol-lowering-with-drugs-other-than-statins-and-pcsk9-inhibitors.

Singh, P., Harper, Y., Oliphant, C. S., Morsy, M., Skelton, M., Askari, R., et al. (2017). Peripheral interventions and antiplatelet therapy: Role in current practice. *World Journal of Cardiology, 9*(7), 583–593.

Skidmore-Roth, L. (2018). *Mosby's 2018 nursing drug reference* (31st ed.). Elsevier Health Sciences.

The Joint Commission. (2017a). Inadequate hand-off communication. *Sentinel Event Alert, 58*, 2. Retrieved from: https://www.jointcommission.org/assets/1/18/SEA_58_Hand_off_Comms_9_6_17_FINAL_(1).pdf.

The Joint Commission. (2017b). *Venous thromboembolism.* Retrieved from: https://www.jointcommission.org/venous_thromboembolism/.

The Joint Commission. (2018). *National patient safety goal for anticoagulant therapy.* R3 Report. Retrieved from: https://www.jointcommission.org/assets/1/18/R3_19_Anticoagulant_therapy_FINAL2.PDF.

The Joint Commission. (2019). *National patient safety goals effective january 2019: Hospital accreditation program.* Retrieved from: https://www.jointcommission.org/assets/1/6/NPSG_Chapter_HAP_Jan2019.pdf.

U.S. Food and Drug Administration. (2018). *FDA announces voluntary recall of several medicines containing valsartan following detection of an impurity.* Retrieved from: https://www.fda.gov/newsevents/newsroom/pressannouncements/ucm613532.htm.

U.S. Food and Drug Administration. (2019). *FDA updates and press announcements on angiotensin II receptor blocker (ARB) recalls (valsartan, losartan, and irbesartan).* Retrieved from: https://www.fda.gov/drugs/drug-safety-and-availability/fda-updates-and-press-announcements-angiotensin-ii-receptor-blocker-arb-recalls-valsartan-losartan.

U.S. Preventive Services Task Force. (2017). *Final recommendation statement: High blood pressure in adults: Screening.* https://www.uspreventiveservicestaskforce.org/Page/Document/RecommendationStatementFinal/high-blood-pressure-in-adults-screening.

Whelton PK, Carey RM, Aronow WS, et al. (2017). ACC/AHA/AAPA/ABC/ACPM/AGS/APhA/ASH/ASPC/NMA/PCNA Guideline for the prevention, detection, evaluation, and management of high blood pressure in adults: Executive summary. A Report of the American College of Cardiology/American Heart Association Task Force on Clinical Practice Guidelines. *Hypertension.* 2017 Nov 13. http://hyper.ahajournals.org/content/early/2017/11/10/HYP.0000000000000066.

Witte, M. E., Zeebregts, C. J., de Borst, G. J., Reijnen, M. M., & Boersma, D. (2017). Mechanochemical endovenous ablation of saphenous veins using the ClariVein: A systematic review. *Phlebology, 32*(10), 649–657.

Zehnder, J. (2019). *Clinical use of coagulation tests. UpToDate.* Retrieved from: https://www.uptodate.com/contents/clinical-use-of-coagulation-tests.

34

Critical Care of Patients With Shock

Nicole M. Heimgartner, Maureen Bishop

http://evolve.elsevier.com/Iggy/

LEARNING OUTCOMES

1. Collaborate with the interprofessional team to coordinate high-quality care and promote ***perfusion*** in patients who are experiencing shock.
2. Teach adults how to decrease the risk for sepsis and shock.
3. Implement nursing interventions to help the patient and family cope with the psychosocial impact caused by shock or its complications.
4. Apply knowledge of anatomy and physiology to assess critically ill patients with respiratory problems affecting ***perfusion*** or ***infection.***
5. Implement evidence-based nursing interventions to prevent complications of sepsis and shock.

KEY TERMS

anaphylaxis An extreme type of allergic reaction.

multiple organ dysfunction syndrome (MODS) Progressive organ dysfunction in an acutely ill patient, such that homeostasis cannot be maintained without intervention.

sepsis A life-threatening organ dysfunction caused by simultaneous systemic inflammation and coagulation in response to microbial infection.

septic shock A subset of sepsis in which circulatory, cellular, and metabolic alterations are associated with a higher mortality rate than sepsis alone.

shock Widespread abnormal cellular metabolism occurring when oxygenation and tissue perfusion needs do not maintain cell function.

sympathetic tone A state of partial blood vessel constriction caused when nerves from the sympathetic division of the autonomic nervous system continuously stimulate vascular smooth muscle.

PRIORITY AND INTERRELATED CONCEPTS

The priority concepts for this chapter are:
- ***Perfusion***
- ***Infection***

The ***Perfusion*** concept exemplar for this chapter is Hypovolemic Shock.
The ***Infection*** concept exemplar for this chapter is Sepsis and Septic Shock.

The interrelated concepts for this chapter are:
- ***Clotting***
- ***Gas Exchange***
- ***Immunity***

OVERVIEW

All organs, tissues, and cells need a continuous supply of oxygen to function properly. The lungs first bring oxygen into the body through ventilation and ***gas exchange,*** and the cardiovascular system (heart, blood, and blood vessels) delivers oxygen by ***perfusion*** to all tissues and removes cellular wastes. **Shock** is widespread abnormal cellular metabolism that occurs when gas exchange with oxygenation and tissue perfusion needs are not met sufficiently to maintain cell function (McCance & Huether, 2019). It is a condition rather than a disease and is the "whole-body" response that occurs when too little oxygen is delivered to the tissues. All body organs are affected by shock and either work harder to adapt and compensate for reduced gas exchange or perfusion or fail to function because of hypoxia. Shock is a "syndrome" because the problems resulting from it occur in a predictable sequence.

*Any problem that impairs **perfusion** and **gas exchange** to tissues and organs can start the syndrome of shock and lead to a life-threatening emergency.* Shock is often a result of cardiovascular problems. Patients in acute care settings are at higher risk, but shock can occur in any setting. For example, older patients in long-term care settings are at risk for sepsis and septic shock related to urinary tract infections and pneumonia. When the body's adaptive adjustments (compensation) or health care interventions are not effective or exhausted and shock progresses, it can lead to cell loss, multiple organ dysfunction syndrome (MODS), and death.

Shock is classified by the type of impairment causing it into the categories of hypovolemic shock, cardiogenic shock,

KEY FEATURES

Shock

Cardiovascular Symptoms
- Decreased cardiac output
- Increased pulse rate
- Thready pulse
- Decreased blood pressure
- Narrowed pulse pressure
- Postural hypotension
- Low central venous pressure
- Flat neck and hand veins in dependent positions
- Slow capillary refill in nail beds
- Diminished peripheral pulses

Respiratory Symptoms
- Increased respiratory rate
- Shallow depth of respirations
- Decreased $Paco_2$ initially then progressing to increased $Paco_2$
- Decreased Pao_2
- Cyanosis, especially around lips and nail beds

Gastrointestinal Symptoms
- Decreased motility
- Diminished or absent bowel sounds
- Nausea and vomiting
- Constipation

Neuromuscular Symptoms

Early
- Anxiety
- Restlessness
- Increased thirst

Late
- Decreased central nervous system activity (lethargy to coma)
- Generalized muscle weakness
- Diminished or absent deep tendon reflexes
- Sluggish pupillary response to light

Kidney Symptoms
- Decreased urine output
- Increased specific gravity
- Sugar and acetone present in urine

Integumentary Symptoms
- Cool to cold
- Pale to mottled to cyanotic
- Moist, clammy
- Mouth dry; pastelike coating present
- Decreased capillary refill

$Paco_2$, Partial pressure of arterial carbon dioxide; *Pao_2*, partial pressure of arterial oxygen.

distributive shock (which includes septic shock, neurogenic shock, and anaphylactic shock), and obstructive shock. Table 34.1 describes this classification and common causes of shock.

Most signs and symptoms of shock are similar regardless of what starts the process or which tissues are affected first. Symptoms result from physiologic adjustments *(compensatory mechanisms)* that the body makes in the attempt to ensure continued ***perfusion*** of vital organs. Compensatory actions are triggered by the sympathetic nervous system's stress response activating the endocrine and cardiovascular systems. Symptoms unique to any one type of shock result from specific tissue dysfunction. The common features of shock are listed in in the Key Features: Shock box.

Review of Gas Exchange and Tissue Perfusion

Gas exchange and ***perfusion*** depend on how much oxygen from arterial blood perfuses the tissue. Perfusion is related to mean arterial pressure (MAP). The factors that influence MAP include:

- Total blood volume (viscosity)
- Cardiac output (heart rate × stroke volume)
- Size and integrity of the vascular bed, especially capillaries

Total blood volume and cardiac output are directly related to MAP, so increases in either total blood volume or cardiac output *raise* MAP. Decreases in either total blood volume or cardiac output *lower* MAP.

The size of the vascular bed is inversely (negatively) related to MAP. This means that increases in the size of the vascular bed *lower* MAP and decreases *raise* MAP (Fig. 34.1). The small arteries and veins connected to capillaries can increase in diameter by relaxing the smooth muscle in vessel walls *(dilation)* or decrease in diameter by contracting the muscle *(vasoconstriction)*. When blood vessels dilate and total blood volume remains the same, blood pressure decreases and blood flow is slower. When blood vessels constrict and total blood volume remains the same, blood pressure increases and blood flow is faster.

Blood vessels are innervated by the sympathetic nervous system. Some nerves continuously stimulate vascular smooth muscle so the blood vessels are normally partially constricted, a condition called **sympathetic tone**. Increases in sympathetic stimulation constrict smooth muscle even more, raising MAP. Decreases in sympathetic tone relax smooth muscle, dilating blood vessels and lowering MAP.

Perfusion to organs adjusts to changes in tissue oxygen needs. The body can selectively increase blood flow to some areas while reducing flow to others. The skin and skeletal muscles can tolerate low levels of oxygen for hours without dying or being damaged. Other organs (e.g., heart, brain, liver, pancreas) do not tolerate hypoxia, and a few minutes without oxygen results in serious damage and cell death.

Types of Shock

Types of shock vary because shock is a problem caused by a pathologic condition rather than a disease state (see Table 34.1). *More than one type of shock can be present at the same time.* For example, trauma caused by a car crash may trigger hemorrhage (leading to hypovolemic shock) and a myocardial infarction (leading to cardiogenic shock).

Hypovolemic shock occurs when too little circulating blood volume decreases MAP, resulting in inadequate total body ***perfusion*** and ***gas exchange.*** Common problems leading to hypovolemic shock are dehydration and poor ***clotting*** with hemorrhage. A complete discussion of the pathophysiology and management of hypovolemic shock begins with the ***perfusion*** concept exemplar.

Cardiogenic shock occurs when the heart muscle is unhealthy and pumping is impaired. Cardiogenic shock is most often associated with acute myocardial infarction (McCance & Huether, 2019). Other causes are listed in Table 34.1. Any type of pump failure decreases cardiac output and MAP. Chapter 35 discusses the pathophysiology and care for the adult with shock from myocardial infarction.

Distributive shock occurs when blood volume is not lost from the body but is distributed to the interstitial tissues where it cannot perfuse organs. It can be caused by blood vessel dilation, pooling of blood in venous and capillary beds, and increased capillary leak. All these factors decrease MAP and may be started either by nerve changes *(neural induced)* or by the presence of some chemicals *(chemical induced)*. Septic shock is the most common cause of distributive shock (Gaieski & Mikkelsen, 2018).

Anaphylaxis is an extreme type of allergic reaction. It begins within seconds to minutes after exposure to a specific

TABLE 34.1 Causes and Types of Shock by Functional Impairment

Hypovolemic Shock

Overall Cause

Total body fluid decreased (in all fluid compartments)

Specific Cause or Risk Factors

- Hemorrhage
- Trauma
- GI ulcer
- Surgery
- Inadequate ***clotting***
- Hemophilia
- Liver disease
- Cancer therapy
- Anticoagulation therapy
- Dehydration
- Vomiting
- Diarrhea
- Heavy diaphoresis
- Diuretic therapy
- Nasogastric suction
- Diabetes insipidus

Cardiogenic Shock

Overall Cause

Direct pump failure (fluid volume not affected)

Specific Cause or Risk Factors

- Myocardial infarction
- Cardiac arrest
- Ventricular dysrhythmias
- Cardiomyopathies
- Myocardial degeneration
- Cardiac tamponade

Distributive Shock

Overall Cause

Fluid shifted from central vascular space (total body fluid volume normal or increased)

Specific Cause or Risk Factors

- Neural induced
- Pain
- Anesthesia
- Stress
- Spinal cord injury
- Head trauma
- Chemical induced
- Anaphylaxis
- Sepsis
- Capillary leak
- Burns
- Extensive trauma
- Liver impairment
- Hypoproteinemia

Obstructive Shock

Overall Cause

Cardiac function decreased by noncardiac factor (indirect pump failure); total body fluid not affected, although central volume is decreased

Specific Cause or Risk Factors

- Cardiac tamponade
- Arterial stenosis
- Pulmonary embolus
- Pulmonary hypertension
- Constrictive pericarditis
- Thoracic tumors
- Tension pneumothorax

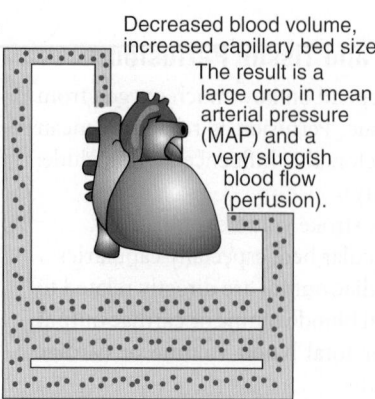

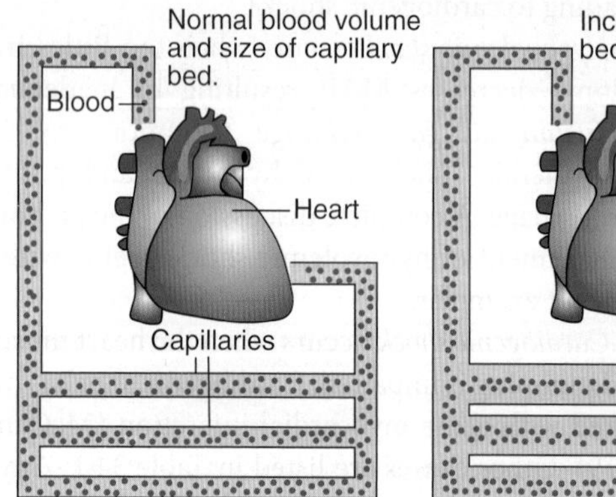

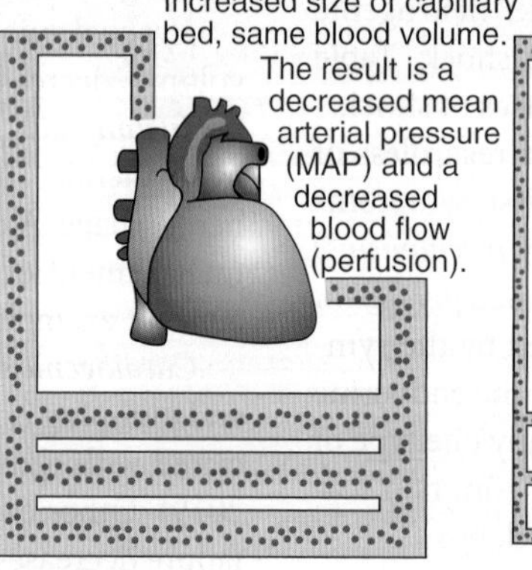

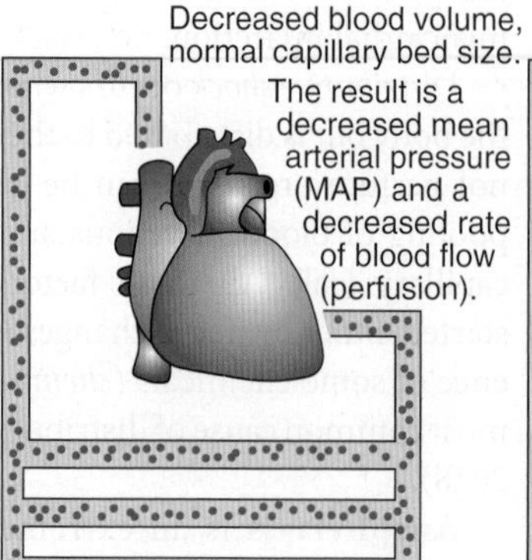

Decreased blood volume, normal capillary bed size.
The result is a decreased mean arterial pressure (MAP) and a decreased rate of blood flow (perfusion).

Decreased blood volume, increased capillary bed size.
The result is a large drop in mean arterial pressure (MAP) and a very sluggish blood flow (perfusion).

Fig. 34.1 Interaction of blood volume and the size of the capillary bed affecting mean arterial pressure (MAP).

allergen in a susceptible adult. The result is widespread loss of blood vessel tone, with decreased blood pressure and cardiac output. Chapter 18 describes the pathophysiology, prevention, and care of the patient with anaphylactic shock.

Sepsis is life-threatening organ dysfunction brought on by a dysregulated response to infection (Singer et al., 2016). Septic shock is a subset of sepsis in which circulatory, cellular, and metabolic abnormalities substantially increase the risk of death over that associated with sepsis alone (Singer et al., 2016). A complete discussion of the pathophysiology, prevention, and care for the patient with sepsis and septic shock is located later in the chapter in the ***infection*** concept exemplar.

Obstructive shock is caused by problems that impair the ability of the normal heart to pump effectively. The heart itself remains normal, but conditions outside the heart prevent either adequate filling of the heart or adequate contraction of the healthy heart muscle. The most common cause of obstructive shock is cardiac tamponade (see Table 34.1). Care of the adult with cardiac tamponade is presented in Chapter 32 (pericarditis) and Chapter 35.

Although the causes and initial signs and symptoms associated with the different types of shock vary, eventually the effects of hypotension and *anaerobic cellular metabolism* (metabolism without oxygen) result in the common key features of shock as indicated in the Key Features: Shock box.

PERFUSION CONCEPT EXEMPLAR: HYPOVOLEMIC SHOCK

Pathophysiology Review

The basic problem of hypovolemic shock is a loss of vascular volume, resulting in a decreased mean arterial pressure (MAP) (see Fig. 34.1) and, in some cases, a loss of circulating red blood cells (RBCs). The reduced MAP slows blood flow, decreasing tissue perfusion. The loss of RBCs decreases the ability of the blood to oxygenate the tissue it does reach. These ***gas exchange*** and ***perfusion*** problems lead to anaerobic cellular metabolism.

The main trigger leading to hypovolemic shock is a sustained decrease in MAP from decreased circulating blood volume. A decrease in MAP of 5 to 10 mm Hg below the patient's normal baseline value is detected by pressure-sensitive nerve receptors *(baroreceptors)* in the aortic arch and carotid sinus. This information is transmitted to brain centers, which stimulate compensatory mechanisms to help ensure continued blood flow and oxygen delivery to vital organs while limiting blood flow to less vital areas. The movement of blood into selected areas while bypassing others ("shunting") results in some shock symptoms.

If the events that caused the initial decrease in MAP are halted now, compensatory mechanisms provide adequate ***gas exchange*** and ***perfusion*** without intervention. If events continue and MAP decreases further, some tissues function under anaerobic conditions. This condition increases lactic acid levels and other harmful metabolites (e.g., protein-destroying enzymes, oxygen free radicals) (McCance & Huether, 2019). These substances cause acidosis with tissue-damaging effects and depressed heart muscle activity. The effects are temporary and reversible if the cause of shock is corrected within 1 to 2 hours after onset. When shock conditions continue for longer periods without help, the resulting increased metabolites cause so much cell damage in vital organs that they are unable to perform their critical functions. When this problem, known as *multiple organ dysfunction syndrome (MODS),* occurs to the extent that vital organs die, recovery from shock is no longer possible (see the section Refractory Stage and Multiple Organ Dysfunction Syndrome). Table 34.2 summarizes the progression of shock.

TABLE 34.2 Adaptive Responses and Events During Hypovolemic Shock

Initial Stage
- Decrease in mean arterial pressure (MAP) of 5-10 mm Hg from baseline value
- Increased sympathetic stimulation
- Mild vasoconstriction
- Increased heart rate

Compensatory Stage
- Decrease in MAP of 10-15 mm Hg from baseline value
- Continued sympathetic stimulation
- Moderate vasoconstriction
- Increased heart rate
- Decreased pulse pressure
- Chemical compensation
- Renin, aldosterone, and antidiuretic hormone secretion
- Increased vasoconstriction
- Decreased urine output
- Stimulation of the thirst reflex
- Some anaerobic metabolism in nonvital organs
- Mild acidosis
- Mild hyperkalemia

Progressive Stage
- Decrease in MAP of >20 mm Hg from baseline value
- Anoxia of nonvital organs
- Hypoxia of vital organs
- Overall metabolism is anaerobic
- Moderate acidosis
- Moderate hyperkalemia
- Tissue ischemia

Refractory Stage
- Severe tissue hypoxia with ischemia and necrosis
- Release of myocardial depressant factor from the pancreas
- Buildup of toxic metabolites
- Multiple organ dysfunction syndrome (MODS)
- Death

Stages of Shock. The syndrome of shock progresses in four stages when the conditions that cause shock remain uncorrected and poor cellular oxygenation continues. These stages are:

1. Initial stage
2. Compensatory stage
3. Progressive stage
4. Refractory stage

Initial Stage. The initial stage is present when the patient's baseline MAP is decreased by less than 10 mm Hg. Compensatory mechanisms are effective at returning systolic pressure to normal at this stage; thus oxygen ***perfusion*** to vital organs is maintained. Cellular changes include increased anaerobic metabolism in some tissues with production of lactic acid, although overall metabolism is still aerobic. The compensation responses of vascular constriction and increased heart rate are effective, and both cardiac output and MAP are maintained within the normal range. Because vital organ function is not disrupted, the indicators of shock are difficult to detect at this stage.

! NURSING SAFETY PRIORITY (QSEN)

Action Alert

Be aware that increased heart and respiratory rates or a slight *increase* in diastolic blood pressure may be the only sign of this stage of shock.

Compensatory Stage. The compensatory stage of shock occurs when MAP decreases by 10 to 15 mm Hg from baseline. Kidney and hormonal compensatory mechanisms are activated because cardiovascular responses alone are not enough to maintain MAP and supply oxygen to vital organs.

The ongoing decrease in MAP triggers the release of renin, antidiuretic hormone (ADH), aldosterone, epinephrine, and norepinephrine to start kidney compensation. Urine output decreases, sodium reabsorption increases, and widespread blood vessel constriction occurs. ADH increases water reabsorption in the kidney, further reducing urine output, and increases blood vessel constriction in the skin and other less vital tissue areas. Together these actions compensate for shock by maintaining the fluid volume within the central blood vessels.

Tissue hypoxia occurs in nonvital organs (e.g., skin, GI tract) and in the kidney, but it is not great enough to cause permanent damage. Buildup of metabolites from anaerobic metabolism causes acidosis (low blood pH) and increased blood potassium levels.

Signs and symptoms of this stage include changes resulting from decreased tissue ***perfusion.*** Subjective changes include thirst and anxiety. Objective changes include restlessness, tachycardia, increased respiratory rate, decreased urine output, falling systolic blood pressure, rising diastolic blood pressure, narrowing pulse pressure, cool extremities, and a decrease in oxygen saturation. *Comparing these changes with the values and observations obtained earlier is critical to identifying this stage of shock.*

If the patient is stable and compensatory mechanisms are supported by interventions, he or she can remain in this stage for hours without having permanent damage. *Stopping the conditions that started shock and providing supportive interventions can prevent the shock from progressing.* The effects of this stage are reversible when nurses recognize the problem and coordinate the interprofessional health care team to start appropriate interventions.

Progressive Stage. The progressive stage of shock occurs when there is a sustained decrease in MAP of more than 20 mm Hg from baseline. Compensatory mechanisms are functioning but can no longer deliver sufficient oxygen, even to vital organs. Vital organs develop hypoxia, and less vital organs become *anoxic* (no oxygen) and *ischemic* (cell dysfunction or death from lack of oxygen). As a result of poor ***perfusion*** and a buildup of metabolites, some tissues die.

Indications of the progressive stage include a *worsening* of changes resulting from decreased tissue ***perfusion.*** The patient may express a sense of "something bad" (impending doom) about to happen. He or she may be confused, and thirst increases. Objective changes are a rapid, weak pulse; low blood pressure; pallor to cyanosis of oral mucosa and nail beds; cool and moist skin; anuria; and a 5% to 20% decrease in oxygen saturation. Laboratory data may show a low blood pH, along with rising lactic acid and potassium levels.

! NURSING SAFETY PRIORITY (QSEN)

Action Alert

The progressive stage of shock is a life-threatening emergency. Vital organs tolerate this situation for only a short time before development of multiple organ dysfunction syndrome (MODS) with permanent damage. Immediate interventions are needed to reverse the effects of this stage of shock. The patient's life usually can be saved if the conditions causing shock are corrected within 1 hour or less of the onset of the progressive stage. Continuously monitor and compare with earlier findings to assess therapy effectiveness and determine when therapy changes are needed.

NCLEX EXAMINATION CHALLENGE 34.1

Safe and Effective Care Environment

A client in the progressive stage of hypovolemic shock has all of the following signs, symptoms, or changes. Which signs will the nurse attribute to ongoing compensatory mechanisms? **Select all that apply.**

A. Increasing pallor
B. Increasing thirst
C. Increasing confusion
D. Increasing heart rate
E. Increasing respiratory rate
F. Decreasing systolic blood pressure
G. Decreasing blood pH
H. Decreasing urine output

Refractory Stage and Multiple Organ Dysfunction Syndrome. The refractory stage of shock occurs when too much cell death and tissue damage result from too little oxygen reaching the tissues. Vital organs have extensive damage and cannot respond effectively to interventions, and shock continues. So much damage has occurred with release of metabolites and enzymes that damage to vital organs continues despite interventions.

The sequence of cell damage caused by the massive release of toxic metabolites and enzymes is termed **multiple organ dysfunction syndrome (MODS)**. Once the damage has started, the sequence becomes a vicious cycle as more dead cells open and release metabolites. These trigger small clots *(microthrombi)* to form, which block tissue ***perfusion*** and damage more cells, continuing the devastating cycle. Liver, heart, brain, and kidney functions are lost first. The most profound change is damage to the heart muscle.

Signs are a rapid loss of consciousness; nonpalpable pulse; cold, dusky extremities; slow, shallow respirations; and unmeasurable oxygen saturation. *Therapy, including fluid replacement, is not effective in saving the patient's life, even if the cause of shock is corrected and MAP temporarily returns to normal.*

Etiology. Hypovolemic shock occurs when too little circulating blood volume causes a MAP decrease that prevents total body ***perfusion*** and adequate ***gas exchange.*** Problems leading to hypovolemic shock are listed in Table 34.1.

Hypovolemic shock from hemorrhage is common after trauma or surgery; and internal hemorrhage occurs with blunt trauma, GI ulcers, and poor control of surgical bleeding. Hemorrhage leading to hypovolemia also can be caused by any problem that reduces the levels of ***clotting*** factors (see Table 34.1). Hypovolemia from dehydration can be caused by any problem that decreases fluid intake or increases fluid loss (see Table 34.1).

Incidence and Prevalence. The exact incidence of hypovolemic shock is not known because it is a response rather than a disease. It is a common complication among hospitalized patients in emergency departments and after surgery or invasive procedures.

Health Promotion and Maintenance. Recognizing hypovolemic shock is a major nursing responsibility. Identify patients at risk for dehydration and assess for early signs and symptoms. This is especially important for those who have reduced cognition or mobility or who are on NPO status.

Assess all patients with invasive procedures or trauma for obvious or occult bleeding from impaired ***clotting.*** Compare pulse quality and rate with baseline. Compare urine output with fluid intake; this includes monitoring trends in intake and output as well as changes in daily weight. Check vital signs of patients who have persistent thirst. Assess for shock in any patient who develops a change in mental status, an increase in pain, or an increase in anxiety.

Teach patients who have invasive procedures about the signs and symptoms of shock. Stress the importance of seeking immediate help for obvious heavy bleeding, persistent thirst, decreased urine output, light-headedness, or a sense of impending doom.

❖ Interprofessional Collaborative Care

Hypovolemic shock is an emergent problem that is usually managed in an acute care setting. If complications from the problem or its treatment are ongoing, patients may be cared for in a variety of community settings.

◆ Assessment: Recognize Cues

History. Ask about risk factors related to hypovolemic shock. If the patient is alert, question him or her directly. If the patient is not alert, collect information from family members. Ask about recent illness, trauma, procedures, or chronic health problems that may lead to shock (e.g., GI ulcers, general surgery, hemophilia, liver disorders, prolonged vomiting or diarrhea). Ask about the use of drugs such as aspirin, other NSAIDs, diuretics, and herbal supplements that may cause changes leading to hypovolemic shock.

Ask about fluid intake and output during the previous 24 hours. *Information about urine output is especially important because urine output is reduced during the first stages of shock, even when fluid intake is normal.*

Assess the patient for factors that can lead to shock. Areas to examine for poor ***clotting*** and hemorrhage include the gums, wounds, and sites of dressings, drains, and vascular accesses. Also check *under* the patient for blood. Observe for any swelling or skin discoloration that may indicate an internal hemorrhage.

Physical Assessment/Signs and Symptoms. Most signs and symptoms of hypovolemic shock are caused by the changes resulting from compensatory efforts. Shock may first be evident as changes in cardiovascular function. As shock progresses, changes in the renal, respiratory, integumentary, musculoskeletal, and central nervous systems become evident. Ensure that vital sign measurements are accurate, and monitor for trends indicating shock. A trend is indicated when any or all of the vital signs or other assessment findings move in a downward or upward direction over a period of 1 to 4 hours.

! NURSING SAFETY PRIORITY (QSEN)

Action Alert

Assign a registered nurse (RN) rather than a licensed practical nurse/licensed vocational nurse (LPN/LVN) or assistive personnel (AP) to assess the vital signs of a patient who is suspected of having hypovolemic shock. The rapid progression associated with shock requires the interpretation of vital signs, which is included in the RN scope of practice. Remember to watch for trends in vital signs and in all other assessment parameters.

Cardiovascular changes that occur with hypovolemic shock start with decreased mean arterial pressure (MAP) leading to compensatory responses. Assess the central and peripheral pulses for rate and quality. In the initial stage of shock, the pulse rate increases above the patient's baseline to keep cardiac output and MAP at normal levels, even though the actual stroke volume (amount of blood pumped out from the heart) per beat is decreased. *Increased heart rate is often the first sign of shock.* Because stroke volume is decreased, the peripheral pulses are difficult to palpate and easily blocked. As shock progresses, peripheral pulses may not be palpable, and a Doppler may be needed.

! NURSING SAFETY PRIORITY (QSEN)

Action Alert

Because changes in systolic blood pressure are not always present in the initial stage of shock, use changes in pulse rate and quality as the main indicators of shock presence or progression.

With vasoconstriction, diastolic pressure increases but systolic pressure remains the same. As a result, the difference between the systolic and diastolic pressures *(pulse pressure)* is smaller or "narrower." Monitor blood pressure for changes from baseline levels and for changes from the previous measurement. For accuracy, use the same equipment on the same extremity. Validate an abnormal electronic blood pressure reading with a manual blood pressure reading.

Systolic pressure decreases as shock progresses and cardiac output decreases. A reduced systolic pressure narrows the pulse pressure even further. When shock continues and interventions are not adequate, compensation fails, both systolic and diastolic pressures decrease, and blood pressure is difficult to hear. Palpation or a Doppler device may be needed to detect the systolic blood pressure.

Oxygen saturation is assessed through pulse oximetry. Pulse oximetry values between 90% and 95% occur with the compensatory stage of shock, and values between 75% and 80% occur with the progressive stage of shock. *Any value below 70% is considered a life-threatening emergency and may signal the refractory stage of shock.*

Respiratory changes with shock are an adaptive response to help maintain *gas exchange* when tissue *perfusion* is decreased. Assess the rate and depth of respiration. Respiratory rate increases during shock to ensure that oxygen intake is increased so it can be delivered to critical tissues.

Kidney and urinary changes occur with shock to compensate for decreased mean arterial pressure (MAP) by saving body water through decreased filtration and increased water reabsorption. Assess urine for volume, color, specific gravity, and the presence of blood or protein. *Decreased urine output (less than 30 mL/hr or 0.5 mL/kg/hr) is a sensitive indicator of early shock. Measure urine output at least every hour. In severe shock, urine output may be absent.* When hypoxia or anoxia persists beyond about an hour, patients are at risk for acute kidney injury (AKI) and kidney failure.

Skin changes occur because of reduced blood flow in the skin. An early compensatory mechanism is skin blood vessel constriction, which reduces skin *perfusion.* This allows more blood to perfuse the vital organs, which cannot tolerate low oxygen levels.

Assess the skin for temperature, color, and moisture. With shock, it feels cool or cold to the touch and is moist. Color changes appear first in oral mucous membranes and in the skin around the mouth. In dark-skinned patients, pallor or cyanosis is best assessed in the oral mucous membranes. Other color changes are noted first in the skin of the extremities and then in the central trunk area. The skin feels clammy or moist to the touch, not because sweating increases but because the normal fluid lost through the skin does not evaporate well on cool skin. As shock progresses, skin becomes mottled. Lighter-skinned patients have an overall grayish-blue color; and darker-skinned patients appear darker, without an underlying reddish glow.

Evaluate capillary refill time by pressing on the patient's fingernail until it blanches and then observing how fast the nail bed resumes color when pressure is released. Normally capillaries resume color as soon as pressure is released. With shock, capillary refill is slow or may be absent. Capillary refill is not a reliable indicator for peripheral blood flow in older patients or those with anemia, diabetes, or peripheral vascular disease.

Central nervous system (CNS) changes with shock first manifest as thirst. Thirst is caused by stimulation of the thirst centers in the brain in response to decreased blood volume.

Assess the patient's level of consciousness (LOC) and orientation, which are sensitive to cerebral hypoxia. In the initial and nonprogressive stages, patients may be restless or agitated and may be anxious or have a feeling of impending doom. As hypoxia progresses, confusion and lethargy occur, which progress to loss of consciousness as cerebral hypoxia worsens.

Skeletal muscle changes during shock include weakness and pain in response to tissue hypoxia and anaerobic metabolism, which are later indications. Weakness is generalized and has no specific pattern. Deep tendon reflexes are decreased or absent.

Psychosocial Assessment. *Changes in mental status and behavior occur early in shock.* Assess mental status by evaluating LOC and noting whether the patient is asleep or awake. If the patient is asleep, attempt to awaken him or her and document how easily he or she is aroused. If the patient is awake, determine whether he or she is oriented to person, place, and time. Avoid asking questions that can be answered with a "yes" or a "no" response. Consider these points during assessment:

- Is it necessary to repeat questions to obtain a response?
- Does the response answer the question asked?
- Does the patient have difficulty making word choices?
- Is the patient irritated or upset by the questions?
- Can the patient concentrate on a question long enough to answer, or is the attention span limited?

Talk with the family to determine whether the patient's behavior and cognition are typical or represent a change.

Laboratory Assessment. Although no single test confirms or rules out shock, changes in laboratory data may support the diagnosis. The Laboratory Profile: Hypovolemic Shock box lists laboratory changes occurring with hypovolemic shock.

LABORATORY PROFILE

Hypovolemic Shock

Test	Normal Range for Adults	Significance of Abnormal Findings
pH (arterial)	7.35-7.45	Decreased: insufficient tissue oxygenation causing anaerobic metabolism and acidosis
Pao_2	80-100 mm Hg	Decreased: anaerobic metabolism
$Paco_2$	35-45 mm Hg	Increased: anaerobic metabolism
Lactic acid (lactate) (arterial)	3-7 mg/dL 0.3-0.8 mmol/L	Increased: anaerobic metabolism with buildup of metabolites
Hematocrit	*Females:* 37%-47% (0.37-0.47 volume fraction) *Males:* 42%-52% (0.42-0.52 volume fraction)	Increased: fluid shift, dehydration Decreased: hemorrhage
Hemoglobin	*Females:* 12-16 g/dL (120-160 g/L) *Males:* 14-18 g/dL (140-180 g/L)	Increased: fluid shift, dehydration Decreased: hemorrhage
Potassium	3.5-5.0 mEq/L or mmol/L	Increased: dehydration, acidosis

$Paco_2$, Partial pressure of arterial carbon dioxide; *Pao_2,* partial pressure of arterial oxygen.

Data from Pagana, K., & Pagana, T. (2018). *Mosby's manual of diagnostic and laboratory tests* (6th ed.). St. Louis: Elsevier; and Pagana, K., Pagana, T., & Pike-MacDonald, S. (2019). *Mosby's Canadian manual of diagnostic and laboratory tests* (2nd ed.). St. Louis: Elsevier.

BEST PRACTICE FOR PATIENT SAFETY & QUALITY CARE (QSEN)

The Patient in Hypovolemic Shock

- Ensure a patent airway.
- Insert an IV catheter or maintain an established catheter. A large-bore catheter is suggested.
- Administer oxygen to maintain O_2 saturation at 92% to 96%; supplemental oxygen is no longer recommended if saturation is normal (Chu et al., 2018).
- Elevate the patient's feet, keeping his or her head flat or elevated to no more than a 30-degree angle.
- Examine the patient for overt bleeding.
- If overt bleeding is present, apply direct pressure to the site.
- Administer drugs as prescribed.
- Increase the rate of IV fluid delivery.
- Do not leave the patient.

As shock progresses, arterial blood gas values become abnormal. The pH decreases, the partial pressure of arterial oxygen ($Pa{O_2}$) decreases, and the partial pressure of arterial carbon dioxide ($Pa{CO_2}$) increases. Other laboratory changes occur with specific causes of hypovolemic shock.

Hematocrit and hemoglobin levels decrease if shock is caused by hemorrhage from poor ***clotting*** or large open wounds. When shock is caused by dehydration or a fluid shift, hematocrit and hemoglobin levels are elevated.

◆ **Analysis: Analyze Cues and Prioritize Hypotheses.** The priority collaborative problem for patients with hypovolemic shock is:

- Inadequate ***perfusion*** due to active fluid volume loss and hypotension

◆ **Planning and Implementation: Generate Solutions and Take Action.** Interventions for patients in hypovolemic shock focus on reversing the shock, restoring fluid volume to the normal range, and preventing complications. Monitoring is critical to determine whether the patient is responding to therapy or whether shock is progressing and a change in intervention is needed. Surgery may be needed to correct some causes of shock. The Best Practice for Patient Safety & Quality Care: The Patient in Hypovolemic Shock box lists best practices for patients in hypovolemic shock.

NCLEX EXAMINATION CHALLENGE 34.2

Safe and Effective Care Environment

The nurse is reviewing the laboratory profile of a client with hypovolemic shock. What laboratory value will the nurse anticipate?

A. pH 7.51
B. $Pa{O_2}$ 106 mm Hg
C. $Pa{CO_2}$ 49 mm Hg
D. Lactate 0.4 mmol/L

Nonsurgical Management. The purposes of shock management are to maintain ***perfusion,*** increase vascular volume, and support compensatory mechanisms. Oxygen therapy, fluid replacement therapy, and drug therapy are useful.

Oxygen therapy is used at any stage of shock and is delivered by mask, hood, nasal cannula, endotracheal tube, or tracheostomy tube. Maintain O_2 saturations at 94% to 96%. Supplemental oxygen with normal oxygen saturations is no longer recommended, because it may be associated with increased mortality risk (Chu et al., 2018). Chapter 25 describes oxygen-delivery methods.

IV therapy for fluid resuscitation is a primary intervention for hypovolemic shock. However, the type and amount of solution remain the subject of debate. Accordingly, the type of solution that is used is generally situation specific (Urden et al., 2018). Crystalloids and colloids are often used for volume replacement. Crystalloid solutions contain nonprotein substances (e.g., minerals, salts, sugars). Colloid solutions contain large molecules of proteins or starches (see Chapter 13).

Crystalloid fluids help maintain an adequate fluid and electrolyte balance. Two common solutions are normal saline and Ringer's lactate. Normal saline (0.9% sodium chloride in water) is a replacement solution used to increase plasma volume and can be infused with any blood product. Ringer's lactate is considered a balanced salt solution containing sodium, chloride, calcium, potassium, and lactate. This isotonic solution expands volume, and the lactate buffers acidosis. Selection of specific fluid is based on the patient's fluid and electrolyte status, acid-base status, and organ function (Procter, 2018; Urden et al., 2018).

! NURSING SAFETY PRIORITY (QSEN)

Action Alert

Use only normal saline for infusion with blood or blood products because the calcium in Ringer's lactate induces ***clotting*** of the infusing blood.

Protein-containing colloid fluids help restore osmotic pressure and fluid volume. Blood products are used when shock is caused by blood loss. These fluids most often include packed red blood cells (PRBCs) and plasma. PRBCs increase hematocrit and hemoglobin levels along with some fluid volume. See Chapter 37 for nursing care during transfusion therapy.

Drug therapy is used in addition to fluid therapy when volume loss is severe and the patient does not respond sufficiently to fluid replacement and blood products. Drugs for shock increase venous return, improve cardiac contractility, or improve cardiac ***perfusion*** by dilating the coronary vessels. See Common Examples of Drug Therapy: Hypovolemic Shock box for common drugs used to treat hypovolemic shock.

Monitoring vital signs and level of consciousness is a major nursing action to determine the patient's condition and the effectiveness of therapy. Monitor these patient responses:

- Pulse (rate, regularity, and quality)
- Blood pressure
- Pulse pressure
- Central venous pressure (CVP)
- Respiratory rate
- Skin and mucosal color
- Oxygen saturation
- Cognition
- Urine output

COMMON EXAMPLES OF DRUG THERAPY

Hypovolemic Shock

Drug Category	Nursing Implications
Vasoconstrictors	
Improve mean arterial pressure by increasing peripheral resistance, increasing venous return, and increasing myocardial contractility.	
Norepinephrine Phenylephrine HCl	Assess patient for chest pain *because these drugs increase myocardial consumption and can cause angina or ischemia.* Monitor urine output hourly *because higher doses decrease kidney perfusion and urine output.* Assess blood pressure every 15 min *because hypertension is a symptom of overdose.* Assess patient for headache *because headache is an early symptom of drug excess.* Assess every 30 min for extravasation; check extremities for color and perfusion *because if the drug gets into the tissues, it can cause severe vasoconstriction, tissue ischemia, and tissue necrosis.* Assess for chest pain *because the drug can cause rapid onset of vasoconstriction in the myocardium and impair cardiac oxygenation.*
Inotropic Agents	
Directly stimulate beta-adrenergic receptors on the heart muscle, improving contractility.	
Dobutamine Milrinone	Assess for chest pain *because these drugs increase myocardial oxygen consumption and can cause angina or infarction.* Monitor for transient hypotension as *both drugs may cause vascular dilation.* Assess blood pressure every 15 min *because hypertension is a symptom of overdose.*
Agents That Enhance Myocardial Perfusion	
Improve myocardial perfusion by dilating coronary arteries rapidly for a short time.	
Sodium nitroprusside Nitroglycerin	Protect drug container from light *because light degrades the drug quickly.* Assess blood pressure at least every 15 min *because the drug can cause systemic vasodilation and hypotension, especially in older adults.*

NURSING SAFETY PRIORITY (QSEN)

Drug Alert

Monitor the patient closely because drugs that dilate coronary blood vessels, such as nitroprusside and nitroglycerin, can cause systemic vasodilation and increase shock if the patient is volume depleted. Drugs that increase heart muscle contraction increase heart oxygen consumption and can cause angina or infarction.

Assess these parameters at least every 15 minutes until the shock is controlled and the patient's condition improves. Hemodynamic monitoring in critical care settings includes intra-arterial monitoring, mixed venous oxygen saturation (Svo_2), and pulmonary artery monitoring.

Insertion of a CVP catheter allows pressure to be monitored in the patient's right atrium or superior vena cava while providing venous access. A decrease in CVP from baseline levels reflects hypovolemic shock with reduced venous return to the right atrium.

Intra-arterial catheters allow continuous blood pressure monitoring and are an access for arterial blood sampling. They are inserted into an artery (radial, brachial, or femoral). The catheter is attached to pressure tubing and a transducer, which converts arterial pressure into an electrical signal seen as a waveform on an oscilloscope and as a numeric value.

NCLEX EXAMINATION CHALLENGE 34.3

Safe and Effective Care Environment

The nurse is caring for a client with hypovolemic shock who is bleeding from a traumatic injury to the upper chest wall. What is the **priority** nursing action?

A. Insert a large-bore IV catheter.
B. Administer supplemental oxygen.
C. Elevate the client's feet, keeping the head flat.
D. Apply direct pressure to the area of overt bleeding.

Surgical Management. Surgical intervention in addition to nonsurgical management may be needed to correct the cause of shock. Such procedures include vascular repair, surgical hemostasis of major wounds, closure of bleeding ulcers, and chemical scarring (chemosclerosis) of varicosities.

Care Coordination and Transition Management. Hypovolemic shock is a complication of another condition and is resolved before patients are discharged from the acute care setting. Because surgery and many other invasive procedures now occur on an ambulatory care basis, more patients at home are at increased risk for hypovolemic shock. Teach patients and family members the early indicators of shock (increased thirst, decreased urine output, light-headedness, sense of apprehension) and to seek immediate medical attention if they appear.

◆ **Evaluation: Evaluate Outcomes.** Evaluate the care of the patient with hypovolemic shock. The expected outcome is that the patient's vascular volume will be restored with normal tissue perfusion.

INFECTION CONCEPT EXEMPLAR: SEPSIS AND SEPTIC SHOCK

Pathophysiology Review

Sepsis is an extreme response to ***infection*** that can cause tissue damage, organ failure, and death if not treated promptly and appropriately. Septic shock is a subset of sepsis that is associated with a much higher risk of death than is sepsis alone (Lester et al., 2018). Septic shock is associated with both systemic inflammatory response syndrome (SIRS) and sepsis with multiple organ dysfunction syndrome (MODS) (Urden et al., 2018).

Infection. When infection is confined to a local area, it should not lead to sepsis and shock. In the adult whose ***immunity*** and inflammatory responses are effective, the presence of organism invasion first starts a helpful, local response of inflammation to confine and eliminate the organism and prevent the infection from becoming worse or widespread.

The white blood cells (WBCs) in the area of invasion secrete cytokines to trigger local inflammation and bring more WBCs to kill the invading organisms. The results of this response constrict the small veins and dilate the arterioles in the area, which increases ***perfusion*** to locally infected tissues.

Capillary leak occurs, allowing plasma to leak into the tissues. This response causes swelling (edema). The duration of inflammation depends on the size and severity of the infection, but usually it subsides within a few days, when the infection has been managed by these responses. A benefit of inflammation is that it is limited only to the area of infection and stops as soon as it is no longer needed. The patient does not have fever, tachycardia, decreased oxygen saturation, or reduced urine output.

Sepsis and Septic Shock. In 2016, the Third International Consensus Definitions for Sepsis and Septic Shock (Sepsis-3) were introduced. Sepsis-3 defines sepsis as life-threatening organ dysfunction brought on by a dysregulated response to infection, and *septic shock* is a term used to describe a subset of sepsis in which circulatory, cellular, and metabolic abnormalities substantially increase the risk of death over that associated with sepsis alone (Singer et al., 2016).

Etiology. The syndrome of sepsis and septic shock is a complex systemic response that begins when an infectious organism enters the bloodstream and causes an infection (McCance & Huether, 2019). If the infection escapes local control, sepsis develops. As the bacteria increases, widespread inflammation, known as *systemic inflammatory response syndrome (SIRS),* is triggered. SIRS criteria are not used to diagnose sepsis anymore, because SIRS can present with infectious and noninfectious pathologies (McCance & Huether, 2019). However, the inflammatory response is associated with sepsis and septic shock. With the organisms and their toxins in the bloodstream and entering other body areas, inflammation becomes an enemy, leading to extensive hormonal, tissue, and vascular changes and oxidative stress that further impair ***gas exchange*** and ***tissue perfusion***.

The patient often has mild hypotension, a low urine output, and an increased respiratory rate. These responses result in a hypodynamic state with decreased cardiac output. Body temperature varies depending on the duration of the sepsis and on WBC function. Some patients have a low-grade fever and others have a high fever. Still others may have a below-normal body temperature. The reduced urine output and increased respiratory rate are the compensatory responses to impaired ***gas exchange*** and ***perfusion.*** Often the patient has the elevated WBC count expected with a systemic infection.

Inappropriate ***clotting*** with microthrombi forming in some organ capillaries causes hypoxia and reduces organ function. This problem is hard to detect, but if sepsis is stopped at this point, the organ damage is reversible. The microthrombi increase hypoxic conditions, which then generate more toxic metabolites, which can amplify inflammation and create a vicious repeating cycle of poor ***gas exchange*** and ***perfusion.*** Although these signs are subtle, they indicate sepsis and will progress unless intervention begins immediately.

Unfortunately, this early hypodynamic state has a relatively short duration, and indicators are so subtle that the condition is often missed or misdiagnosed. When early sepsis is identified and treated aggressively, the cycle of progression can be stopped, and the outcome is good. When sepsis is not identified and treated at this stage, it becomes much harder to control. Nurses and all other health care professionals have a responsibility to identify cues that indicate sepsis before it progresses to organ failure. The Sepsis-3 task force recommends the use of the Sequential Organ Failure Assessment (SOFA) score in critical care settings and use of the quick SOFA (qSOFA) in non–intensive care settings (Lester et al., 2018). Although the qSOFA score is not a defining tool for sepsis, it is a predictor of mortality, and a positive score requires further assessment for organ failure (Makic & Bridges, 2018). See Table 34.3.

! NURSING SAFETY PRIORITY (QSEN)

Critical Rescue

Monitor the patient at risk for sepsis to recognize symptoms indicating sepsis and septic shock. If *any* of these are present, respond by notifying the health care provider or the Rapid Response Team.

When sepsis becomes amplified, all tissues are involved and are hypoxic to some degree. Some organs are experiencing cell death and dysfunction at this time. Microthrombi formation is widespread, with clots forming where they are not needed. This process uses up (consumes) many of the available platelets and clotting factors, a condition known as *disseminated intravascular coagulation (DIC).* Anaerobic metabolism continues, and cell uptake of oxygen is poor. The continued stress response triggers the continued release of glucose from the liver and causes hyperglycemia. The more severe the response, the higher the blood glucose level (Kleinpell et al., 2016).

Despite the severity of the pathophysiology, some of the signs and symptoms of sepsis may be missed. One of the reasons it may be missed is that the cardiac function is hyperdynamic in this phase. The pooling of blood and the widespread capillary leak stimulate the heart, and cardiac output is *increased* with a more rapid heart rate and an elevated systolic blood pressure. In addition, the patient's extremities may feel warm, and there is little or no cyanosis. Even though the patient may "look" better, the pathologic changes occurring at the tissue level are serious and have caused significant damage. The WBC count at this time may no longer be elevated because prolonged sepsis may have exceeded

TABLE 34.3 Sequential Organ Failure Assessment (SOFA)[a] and Quick Sequential Organ Failure Assessment (qSOFA)

To calculate the SOFA score, the following laboratory values are needed: bilirubin, creatinine, coagulation studies, and arterial blood gases. These laboratory values combined with clinical assessment data are then scored from 0 (normal function) to 4 (organ failure). The higher the cumulative score, the greater the patient's risk. A score of 2 or higher in any system indicates an increased risk for organ failure, poor outcome, or death (Makik & Bridges, 2018). The following parameters are considered abnormal, and each would receive a score of 2 or higher:

- Respiratory: Pa_{O_2}/Fi_{O_2} <300 mm Hg
- Coagulation: Platelets <100 × $10^3/mm^3$
- Liver: Bilirubin ≥2 mg/dL
- Cardiovascular: Hypotension requiring vasopressor support
- Central nervous system: Glasgow Coma Scale score ≤12
- Renal: Creatinine ≥2 mg/dL, or urine output <500 mL/day

Quick Sequential Organ Failure Assessment (qSOFA)[a]

The qSOFA can quickly alert clinicians to the need for further assessment for organ dysfunction (Makik & Bridges, 2018). There are three parameters, and patients are assigned 1 point for each abnormal parameter. Abnormal parameters include:

- Systolic blood pressure ≤100 mm Hg
- Respiratory rate ≥22 breaths/min
- Any change in mental status

Non-ICU patients with a score of 2 or 3 require additional assessment using the SOFA and are at risk for an extended ICU stay or death.

Fi_{O_2}, Fraction of inspired oxygen; *Pa_{O_2}*, partial pressure of oxygen

[a]Adapted from Makic, M., & Bridges, E. (2018). Managing sepsis and septic shock: current guidelines and definitions. *The American Journal of Nursing, 118*(2), 34–39 and Singer, M., Deutschman, C.S., Seymour, C.W., Shankar-Hari, M., Annane, D., Bauer, M., et al. (2016). The Third International Consensus Definitions for Sepsis and Septic Shock (Sepsis-3). *JAMA: The Journal of the American Medical Association, 315*(8), 801–810.

the bone marrow's ability to keep producing and releasing new mature neutrophils and other WBCs. The WBC count may be extremely low, especially the segmented neutrophils (segs).

Signs and symptoms include a lower oxygen saturation, rapid respiratory rate, decreased-to-absent urine output, and a change in the patient's cognition and affect. Appropriate and aggressive interventions at this stage can still prevent septic shock, although mortality after a patient reaches this stage is much higher than for sepsis. *At this point, the downhill course leading to septic shock is extremely rapid.*

Septic shock is a subset of *sepsis*, a term used to describe the circulatory, cellular, and metabolic abnormalities occurring that substantially increase the risk of death over that of sepsis alone (Singer et al., 2016). Septic shock can be identified in patients who (Singer et al., 2016):

- Require vasopressor therapy to maintain a mean arterial pressure (MAP) of at least 65 mm Hg

  or
- Have a serum lactate level greater than 2 mmol/L (18 mg/dL), despite adequate fluid resuscitation

Septic shock is the stage of sepsis when multiple organ dysfunction syndrome (MODS) with organ failure is evident and poor ***clotting*** with uncontrolled bleeding can occur. Severe hypovolemic shock and hypodynamic cardiac function are present as a result of an inability of the blood to clot because the platelets and clotting factors were consumed earlier in response to sepsis. Vasodilation and capillary leak continue from vascular endothelial cell disruption, and cardiac contractility is poor from cellular ischemia. The signs and symptoms resemble the late stage of hypovolemic shock.

Incidence and Prevalence. According to the Centers for Disease Control and Prevention (CDC), each year one in three patients who die in a hospital have sepsis (CDC, 2018). Sepsis affects more than 1.7 million adults annually and is the cause of death of nearly 270,000 Americans per year (CDC, 2018). Patients especially at risk for sepsis are those who have any type of reduced ***immunity*** and those who have central lines. Central lines in place even for short periods create a potential direct access point for microorganisms and can lead to central line–associated bloodstream infections (CLABSIs). Table 34.4 lists some of the health problems that increase the risk for sepsis and septic shock.

Health Promotion and Maintenance. Prevention is the best management strategy for sepsis and septic shock. Evaluate all patients for their risk for sepsis, especially older adults, because the death rate from sepsis in adults older than 65 years is nearly twice that in younger adults. Use aseptic technique during invasive procedures and when working with nonintact skin and mucous membranes in patients. Remove indwelling urinary catheters and IV access lines as soon as they are no longer needed. Ensure that patients receiving mechanical ventilation are weaned from the ventilator as soon as possible (Kleinpell et al., 2016).

Because sepsis can be a complication of many conditions found in acute care settings, always consider its possibility. *Early detection of sepsis before progression to septic shock is a major nursing responsibility.* The nurse is the health care professional most in contact with the patient and is in a unique position to detect subtle changes in appearance and behavior that can indicate sepsis. See Table 34.3 to review the quick SOFA score, which is recommended in non–intensive care settings to screen for progression of sepsis. The higher the score, the greater the patient's risk of morbidity and mortality.

The Modified Early Warning Score (MEWS) was developed to identify hospitalized patients at risk for clinical deterioration

(Fig. 34.2). All components of the qSOFA are incorporated into the MEWS, in addition to heart rate and temperature. Scores of 5 or greater are associated with a higher risk of death and ICU admission. Scores can be calculated by the nurse, or many of these screening tools have been integrated into many electronic health records to aid in prompt recognition and treatment of sepsis. When used appropriately, the MEWS can reduce the number of codes in the hospital setting by as much as 50% (Lester et al., 2018). These screening tools, combined with astute nursing assessment, lead to early detection, which can significantly alter the prognosis for a patient with sepsis or septic shock.

Early detection can also be made by patients and families. This is especially important for patients discharged to home after invasive procedures or surgery. Teach patients and families the signs and symptoms of local infection (local redness, pain, swelling, purulent drainage, loss of function) and early sepsis (fever, urine output less than intake, light-headedness). Teach them how to use a thermometer and to take the temperature twice a day and whenever they are not feeling well. Urge those with symptoms of early sepsis to immediately contact their health care provider. Teach them that if antibiotics are prescribed, they should take these drugs as prescribed and should complete the entire course.

TABLE 34.4 Conditions Predisposing to Sepsis and Septic Shock

- Malnutrition
- Immunosuppression
- Large, open wounds
- Mucous membrane fissures in prolonged contact with bloody or drainage-soaked packing
- GI ischemia
- Exposure to invasive procedures
- Cancer
- Age above 80 years
- Infection with resistant microorganisms
- Receiving cancer chemotherapy
- Alcoholism
- Diabetes mellitus
- Chronic kidney disease
- Transplant recipient
- Hepatitis
- HIV/AIDS (HIV-III)

AIDS, Acquired immune deficiency syndrome; *HIV*, human immune deficiency virus.

Interprofessional Collaborative Care

Sepsis and septic shock may occur in any setting. Successful outcomes from management usually require intensive interventions in an acute care setting.

Assessment: Recognize Cues. Early detection of sepsis is a key component of saving lives. Nursing assessment plays a critical role in the detection of subtle changes that can occur indicating sepsis or a progression to septic shock. When sepsis is recognized and treated quickly, chances of recovery are good. Once a patient progresses to septic shock in which circulatory, cellular, and metabolic abnormalities are occurring, the risk of death substantially increases (Lester et al., 2018).

History. Age is important because sepsis develops more easily in older, debilitated patients. (Abbas et al., 2015; Englert & Ross, 2015; Umberger et al., 2015). The Patient-Centered Care: Older Adult Considerations: Risk Factors for Shock box lists factors that increase the older adult's risk for shock. Ask about the patient's medical history, including recent illness, trauma, invasive procedures, or chronic conditions that may lead to sepsis. Check which drugs the patient has used in the past week. Some drugs may directly cause changes leading to shock. A drug regimen may also indicate a disorder or problem that can contribute to sepsis (e.g., drugs that include aspirin, corticosteroids, antibiotics, and cancer drugs).

MEWS (Modified Early Warning System)

	3	2	1	0	1	2	3
Respiratory rate per minute		Less than 8		9–14	15–20	21–29	More than 30
Heart rate per minute		Less than 40	40–50	51–100	101–110	111–129	More than 129
Systolic blood pressure	Less than 70	71–80	81–100	101–199		More than 200	
Conscious level (AVPU)	**U**nresponsive	Responds to **P**ain	Responds to **V**oice	**A**lert	New agitation Confusion		
Temperature (°C)		Less than 35.0	35.1–36	36.1–38	38.1–38.5	More than 38.6	
Hourly urine for 2 hours	Less than 10 mL/hr	Less than 30 mL/hr	Less than 45 mL/hr				

Early warning scoring system for detecting adult patients who have or are developing critical illness:
Is the score for your patient 1–2? Perform 2 hourly observations and inform nurse in charge
Is the score for your patient 3? Perform 1–2 hourly observations and inform nurse in charge
If the MEWS score is deteriorating: The ward S.H.O. or duty doctor MUST attend
Is the score for your patient 4 or more? Perform observations at least 1/2 hourly. Ensure medical advice is sought and contact outreach team.

Fig. 34.2 Modified Early Warning System (MEWS). (Used with permission from Glan Clwyd Hospital, Rhyl, Denbighshire, Wales.)

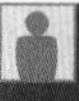

PATIENT-CENTERED CARE: OLDER ADULT CONSIDERATIONS QSEN

Risk Factors for Shock

Hypovolemic Shock
- Diuretic therapy
- Diminished thirst reflex
- Immobility
- Use of aspirin-containing products
- Use of complementary therapies such as *Ginkgo biloba*
- Anticoagulant therapy

Cardiogenic Shock
- Diabetes mellitus
- Presence of cardiomyopathies

Distributive Shock
- Diminished immune response
- Reduced skin integrity
- Presence of cancer
- Peripheral neuropathy
- Strokes
- Being in a hospital or extended-care facility
- Malnutrition
- Anemia

Obstructive Shock
- Pulmonary hypertension
- Presence of cancer

Physical Assessment/Signs and Symptoms. Signs and symptoms of sepsis and septic shock occur over many hours, and some change during the progression. Some signs and symptoms of sepsis are nonspecific and present similarly to other conditions such as pancreatitis or acute respiratory failure.

Cardiovascular changes differ in the progression of sepsis and septic shock. Cardiac output and blood pressure are low in early sepsis and very low in septic shock. As sepsis progresses, cardiac output is higher, as are heart rate and blood pressure, although this is an indication of a worsening condition rather than an improvement. Increased cardiac output is reflected by tachycardia, increased stroke volume, a normal systolic blood pressure, and a normal central venous pressure (CVP). Increased cardiac output and vasodilation make the skin color appear normal with pink mucous membranes, and the skin is warm to the touch. This situation is temporary, and eventually the cardiac output is greatly reduced.

With progression, disseminated intravascular coagulation (DIC) occurs as a result of excessive ***clotting,*** with formation of thousands of small clots in the tiny capillaries of the liver, kidney, brain, spleen, and heart. DIC reduces ***perfusion*** and ***gas exchange*** and decreases oxygen saturation, causing widespread hypoxia and ischemia.

The huge number of small clots uses clotting factors and fibrinogen faster than they can be produced, which eventually leads to poor ***clotting.*** This leads to hemorrhage, which occurs in septic shock. Coupled with continued capillary leak, bleeding causes hypovolemia and a dramatic decrease in cardiac output, blood pressure, and pulse pressure. The signs and symptoms of this phase are the same as those of the later stages of hypovolemic shock.

Respiratory changes are first caused by compensatory mechanisms that try to maintain oxygenation with a rate increase. The lungs are susceptible to damage, and the complication of acute respiratory distress syndrome (ARDS) may occur in septic shock. ARDS in septic shock is caused by the continued systemic inflammatory response syndrome (SIRS) increasing the formation of oxygen free radicals, which damage lung cells. *ARDS in a patient with septic shock has a high mortality rate.*

Skin changes differ as sepsis progresses. In the hyperdynamic stage, the skin is warm and no cyanosis is evident. With progression to septic shock and compromised circulation, it is cool and clammy with pallor, mottling, or cyanosis. In DIC, petechiae and ecchymoses can occur anywhere. Blood may ooze from the gums, other mucous membranes, and venipuncture sites and around IV catheters.

A kidney/urinary change of low urine output compared with fluid intake indicates shock. When a patient who has no known kidney problems suddenly starts having a low urine output, be suspicious of sepsis or septic shock. Reduced output is caused by low circulating volume and hormonal changes. Kidney function decreases, and serum creatinine levels rise.

As sepsis and sepsis shock progress, they can lead to multiple organ dysfunction syndrome (MODS). *Multiple organ dysfunction syndrome* refers to progressive organ dysfunction in two or more separate organ systems in an acutely ill patient, such that homeostasis cannot be maintained without intervention (Singer et al., 2016). MODS is at the severe end of the illness spectrum of both infectious (sepsis, septic shock) and noninfectious (acute pancreatitis) conditions (Urden et al., 2018; Neviere, 2019).

Psychosocial Assessment. An indicator that patients may be progressing in sepsis is often a change in affect or behavior. Compare the patient's current behavior, verbal responses, and general affect with those assessed earlier in the day or the day before. They may seem just slightly different in their reactions to greetings, comments, or jokes. They may be less patient than usual or act restless or fidgety. Patients may make statements such as, "I feel as if something is wrong, but I don't know what." If behavior is changed from prior assessments, consider the possibility of progressing sepsis and shock.

Laboratory Assessment. No single laboratory test confirms the presence of sepsis and septic shock, although hallmarks of sepsis are a rising serum procalcitonin level, an increasing serum lactate level, a normal or low total white blood cell (WBC) count, and a decreasing segmented neutrophil level with a rising band neutrophil level (left shift; see Chapter 16). The presence of bacteria in the blood supports the diagnosis of sepsis, although this finding may not be present. Obtain specimens of urine, blood, sputum, and any drainage for culture to identify the causative organisms. Blood culture specimens should be taken before antibiotic therapy is started, provided that this action does not delay antibiotic therapy by more than 45 minutes (Dellinger et al., 2013). Other abnormal laboratory findings that occur with septic shock include changes in the white blood cell (WBC) count; the differential leukocyte count may show a left shift. Hematocrit and hemoglobin levels usually do not change until late in septic shock. At that point, the hematocrit and hemoglobin levels, fibrinogen levels, and platelet count are low from disseminated intravascular coagulation (DIC). The serum lactate level is above normal, and the serum bicarbonate levels are lower than normal.

Because the results of blood cultures may not be available until the patient's condition has progressed to sepsis or septic shock, other biomarkers for sepsis and septic shock are needed to help identify the condition when it can be managed and cured. One such marker is serum lactate, which is measured to assess patients who are not yet hypotensive but are at risk for septic shock. Lactate levels of 4 mmol/L or higher are associated with a 30% mortality rate (Lester et al., 2018).

The actual diagnosis of sepsis is difficult to make, yet the best outcome depends on an early diagnosis and the implementation of appropriate aggressive interventions.

NCLEX EXAMINATION CHALLENGE 34.4

Safe and Effective Care Environment

The nurse is teaching a client's family regarding the diagnosis of septic shock. Which teaching will the nurse include? **Select all that apply.**

A. "The blood cultures will tell us for sure if your loved one has septic shock."
B. "The client's change in behavior and lethargy may be associated with septic shock."
C. "Antibiotics, as prescribed, will be started within the hour to treat the sepsis."
D. "An insulin drip has been started to keep the client's glucose as low as possible."
E. "Septic shock is easily treated with multiple antibiotics."

◆ Analysis: Analyze Cues and Prioritize Hypotheses.

The priority collaborative problems for patients with sepsis and septic shock are:

1. Widespread ***infection*** due to altered immunity
2. Potential for organ dysfunction due to inappropriate ***clotting,*** poor ***perfusion,*** and poor ***gas exchange*** from widespread ***infection***

◆ Planning and Implementation: Generate Solutions and Take Action

Planning: Expected Outcomes. With appropriate interventions, the patient with sepsis or septic shock is expected to have normal aerobic cellular metabolism. Indicators include:

- Arterial blood gases (pH, Pao_2, and $Paco_2$) within the normal range
- Maintenance of a urine output of at least 20 mL/hr
- Maintenance of mean arterial blood pressure within 10 mm Hg of baseline
- Absence of multiple organ dysfunction syndrome (MODS)

Interventions. Interventions for sepsis and septic shock focus on identifying the problem as early as possible, correcting the conditions causing it, and preventing complications. The use of a sepsis resuscitation bundle for treatment of sepsis within 1 hour is now the standard of practice. A *bundle* is a group of two or more specific interventions that have been shown to be effective when applied together or in sequence. The Surviving Sepsis Campaign (SSC) is a national initiative that was started to standardize sepsis care and promote early recognition of patients with sepsis and septic shock. In 2004, SSC care bundle guidelines were developed to reduce sepsis-related deaths. These bundles were previously incorporated into 3- and 6-hour time periods. However in 2018, in order to treat sepsis as a medical emergency with the same degree of urgency as trauma and stroke, the SSC combined the 3- and 6-hour bundles into a 1-hour bundle, which is now the standard of care (Lester et al., 2018). Table 34.5 details the bundle updated by the SSC.

TABLE 34.5 Hour-1 Bundle for Management of Sepsis

Within 1 hour:
1. Measure lactate level.[a]
2. Obtain blood cultures before administering antibiotics.
3. Administer broad-spectrum antibiotics.
4. Begin rapid administration of 30 mL/kg crystalloid for hypotension or lactate ≥4 mmol/L.
5. Apply vasopressors if hypotensive during or after fluid resuscitation to maintain a mean arterial pressure ≥65 mm Hg.

[a]Remeasure lactate if initial lactate elevated (>2 mmol/L). Data from Surviving Sepsis Campaign. (2019). http://www.survivingsepsis.org/Bundles/Pages/default.aspx.

Oxygen therapy is useful whenever poor tissue ***perfusion*** and poor ***gas exchange*** are present. The patient with septic shock is more likely to be mechanically ventilated. Care of the patient being mechanically ventilated is discussed in detail in Chapter 29.

Drug therapy to enhance cardiac output and restore vascular volume is essentially the same as that used in hypovolemic shock (see the Common Examples of Drug Therapy: Hypovolemic Shock box). In addition, drug therapy is needed to combat sepsis, adrenal insufficiency, hyperglycemia, and clotting problems.

Multiple antibiotics with broad-spectrum activity are prescribed, based on the site of infection and the most common geographic infections, until the actual causative organism is known (Droege et al., 2016). The goal, using the Hour-1 Sepsis Bundle, is to start antibiotics as prescribed within 1 hour of recognizing sepsis (see Table 34.5).

The stress of sepsis can cause adrenal insufficiency. Adrenal support may involve providing the patient with low-dose corticosteroids during the treatment period. Drugs used for this purpose are IV hydrocortisone and oral fludrocortisone.

Patients with sepsis or septic shock usually have elevated blood glucose levels (>180 mg/dL or >10 mmol/L), which is associated with a poor outcome. Insulin therapy is used to maintain blood glucose levels between 140 mg/dL (7.7 mmol/L) and 180 mg/dL (10 mmol/L) (Stapleton & Heyland, 2018). Keeping the blood glucose level below 110 mg/dL (6.1 mmol/L) is associated with increased mortality.

During severe sepsis, patients have microvascular abnormalities and form many small clots. Heparin therapy with fractionated heparin is used to limit inappropriate ***clotting*** and prevent the excessive consumption of clotting factors.

Blood replacement therapy is used when poor ***clotting*** with hemorrhage occurs and may include clotting factors, platelets, fresh-frozen plasma (FFP), or packed red blood cells. Chapter 37 discusses in detail the care of the patient during blood replacement. The use of platelet transfusion is recommended ahead of other blood products for patients with septic shock to improve ***clotting*** (Dellinger et al., 2013).

CLINICAL JUDGMENT CHALLENGE 34.1

Safety; Patient-Centered Care; Teamwork and Collaboration

A 54-year-old obese male with a history of type 2 diabetes and previous deep vein thrombosis of the left leg presents to the emergency department with an enlarged abdomen, nausea, and a blood glucose level of 278 mg/dL (15.4 mmol/L). The client reports feeling tired for 2 days and has not eaten or taken any of his usual medications (rivaroxaban 20 mg, losartan 50 mg, and metformin 850 mg). Your initial assessment findings include pale skin and mucous membranes, abdominal tenderness, an irregular pulse of 118 beats/min, an oral temperature of 96.4°F (35.8°C), a blood pressure of 102/40 mm Hg, and a pulse oximetry reading of 89%. Immediate orders are to draw blood for a complete blood count with differential, serum electrolytes, and serum lactate; start an IV of lactated Ringers at 200 mL/hr, and apply oxygen by nasal cannula at 4 L/min.

1. **Recognize Cues:** What assessment information in this client situation is the most important and immediate concern for the nurse? (Hint: Identify the **relevant** information *first* to determine what is most important.)
2. **Analyze Cues:** What client conditions are consistent with the **most relevant** information? (Hint: Think about priority collaborative problems that support and contradict the information presented in this situation.)
3. **Prioritize Hypotheses:** Which possibilities or explanations are **most likely** to be present in this client situation? Which possibilities or explanations are the most serious? (Hint: Consider all possibilities and determine their urgency and risk for this client.)
4. **Generate Solutions:** What actions would most likely achieve the desired outcomes for this client? Which actions should be **avoided** or are **potentially harmful**? (Hint: Determine the desired outcomes first to decide which interventions are appropriate and those that should be avoided.)
5. **Take Action:** Which actions are the most appropriate and how should they be implemented? In what **priority order** should they be implemented? (Hint: Consider health teaching, documentation, requested health care provider orders or prescriptions, nursing skills, collaboration with or referral to health team members, etc.)
6. **Evaluate Outcomes:** What client assessment would indicate that the nurse's actions were **effective**? (Hint: Think about signs that would indicate an improvement, decline, or unchanged client condition.)

Care Coordination and Transition Management. Identified sepsis should be resolved before patients are discharged from the acute care setting. Because more patients are receiving treatment on an ambulatory care basis and are being discharged earlier from acute care settings, more patients at home are at increased risk for sepsis.

HOME CARE CONSIDERATIONS

The Patient at Risk for Sepsis

Assess the patient for any signs and symptoms of infection, including:

- Temperature, pulse, respiration, and blood pressure
- Color of skin and mucous membranes
- The mouth and perianal area for fissures or lesions
- Any nonintact skin area for the presence of exudates, redness, increased warmth, swelling
- Any pain, tenderness, or other discomfort anywhere
- Cough or any other symptoms of a cold or the flu
- Urine; or ask patient whether urine is dark or cloudy, has an odor, or causes pain or burning during urination

Assess patient's and caregiver's adherence to and understanding of infection prevention techniques.

Assess home environment, including:

- General cleanliness
- Kitchen and bathroom facilities, including refrigeration
- Availability and type of soap for handwashing
- Presence of pets, especially cats, rodents, or reptiles

Home Care Management. Evaluate the home environment for safety regarding infection hazards. Note the general cleanliness, especially in the kitchen and bathrooms. See the Home Care Considerations: The Patient at Risk for Sepsis box for focused patient and environmental assessment data to obtain during a home visit.

Self-Management Education. Protecting frail patients from infection and sepsis at home is an important nursing function. Teach about the importance of self-care strategies, such as good hygiene, handwashing, balanced diet, rest and exercise, skin care, and mouth care. If patients or family members do not know how to take a temperature or read a thermometer, teach them and obtain a return demonstration. Teach patients and families to notify the primary health care provider immediately if fever or other signs of infection appear. General recommendations for Infection Precautions for patients at risk for sepsis are listed in the Patient and Family Education: Preparing for Self-Management: Prevention of Infection box in Chapter 20.

◆ **Evaluation: Evaluate Outcomes.** Evaluate the care of the patient with sepsis or septic shock. The expected outcome is that the patient will maintain normal aerobic cellular metabolism.

GET READY FOR THE NEXT-GENERATION NCLEX® EXAMINATION!

Key Points

Review these Key Points for each NCLEX Examination Client Needs Category.

Safe and Effective Care Environment

- Ensure that vital sign measurements are accurate and monitor them for changes or trends indicating the presence of shock. **QSEN: Safety**
- Identify patients at high risk for infection caused by age, disease, or the environment. **QSEN: Safety**
- Use the recommended criteria to assess for the presence of sepsis (see Table 34.3). **QSEN: Safety**
- Use strict aseptic techniques when performing invasive procedures, administering IV drugs, changing dressings, and handling nonintact skin. **QSEN: Safety**
- Use good handwashing techniques before providing any care to a patient. **QSEN: Safety**
- Assign a registered nurse rather than a licensed practical nurse/licensed vocational nurse (LPN/LVN) or assistive personnel (AP) to assess the vital signs of a patient who is suspected of having hypovolemic shock. **QSEN: Safety**

Health Promotion and Maintenance

- Teach all adults the importance of handwashing to prevent infection. **QSEN: Patient-Centered Care**
- Teach all patients who have a local infection to seek medical attention when signs of systemic infection appear. **QSEN: Patient-Centered Care**

Psychosocial Integrity

- Assess all patients at risk for shock for a change in affect, reduced cognition, altered level of consciousness, and increased anxiety. **QSEN: Patient-Centered Care**
- Stay with the patient in shock. **QSEN: Patient-Centered Care**
- Reassure patients who are in shock that the appropriate interventions are being instituted. **QSEN: Patient-Centered Care**

Physiological Integrity

- Assess the immunocompromised patient every shift for infection. **QSEN: Safety**
- Assess the skin integrity of the patient with reduced ***immunity*** at least every shift. **QSEN: Patient-Centered Care**
- Immediately assess vital signs of patients who have a change in level of consciousness, increased thirst, or anxiety. **QSEN: Evidence-Based Practice**
- Assess for changes in pulse rate and quality or a decrease in urine output rather than blood pressure as an indicator of shock. **QSEN: Evidence-Based Practice**
- Use early identification tools such as qSOFA and MEWS to identify sepsis early. **QSEN: Evidence-Based Practice**
- Assess hourly urine output to evaluate the adequacy of treatment for hypovolemic shock. **QSEN: Evidence-Based Practice**
- Before administering prescribed antibiotics, obtain blood cultures and cultures of urine, wound drainage, and sputum for any patient suspected to have sepsis. **QSEN: Evidence-Based Practice**
- Administer prescribed antibiotics within 1 hour of a diagnosis of sepsis. **QSEN: Evidence-Based Practice**

MASTERY QUESTIONS

1. The nurse is caring for a client with hypovolemic shock. Which new assessment finding indicates to the nurse that interventions are currently effective?
   A. Oxygen saturation remains unchanged.
   B. Core body temperature has increased to 99°F (37.2°C).
   C. The client correctly states the month and year.
   D. Serum lactate and serum potassium levels are declining.
2. The nurse is caring for a patient in the initial stage of hypovolemic shock. What assessment data will the nurse anticipate?
   A. Heart rate 118 beats/min
   B. 2+ pedal pulses
   C. Bilateral fine crackles in lung bases
   D. BP change from 100/60 to 100/40 mm Hg
3. The nurse is assessing a client with septic shock. What assessment data indicate a progression of shock? **Select all that apply.**
   A. BP change from 86/50 to 100/64 mm Hg
   B. Heart rate change from 98 to 76 beats/min
   C. Cool and clammy skin
   D. Petechiae along the gum line
   E. Urine output 45 mL/hr

REFERENCES

Asterisk (*) indicates a classic or definitive work on this subject.

*Dellinger, R. P., Levy, M., Rhodes, A., Annane, D., Gerlach, H., Opal, S. M., et al. (2013). Surviving sepsis campaign: International guidelines for management of severe sepsis and septic shock: 2012. *Critical Care Medicine, 41*(2), 580–637.

Abbas, A., Lichtman, A., & Pillai, S. (2015). *Cellular and molecular immunology* (8th ed.). Philadelphia: Saunders.

Centers for Disease Control and Prevention. (2018). *Sepsis: Data and reports*. Retrieved from: https://www.cdc.gov/sepsis/datareports/index.html.

Chu, D., et al. (2018). *Mortality and morbidity in acutely ill adults treated with liberal versus conservative oxygen therapy (IOTA): A systematic review and meta-analysis*. 391, p1693–1705.

Droege, M., Van Fleet, S., & Mueller, E. (2016). Application of pharmacodynamics and dosing principles in patients with sepsis. *Critical Care Nurse, 36*(2), 22–32.

Englert, N., & Ross, C. (2015). The older adult experiencing sepsis. *Critical Care Nursing Quarterly, 38*(2), 175–181.

Gaieski, D., & Mikkelsen, M. (2018). *Definition, classification, etiology, and pathophysiology of shock in adults. UpToDate*. Retrieved from https://www.uptodate.com/contents/definition-classification-etiology-and-pathophysiology-of-shock-in-adults.

Kleinpell, R., Schorr, C., & Balk, R. (2016). The new sepsis definitions: Implications for critical care practitioners. *American Journal of Critical Care, 25*(5), 457–464.

Lester, D., Hartjes, T., & Bennett, A. (2018). A review of the revised sepsis care bundles. *American Journal of Nursing*, 40–49.

Makic, M., & Bridges, E. (2018). Managing sepsis and septic shock: Current guidelines and definitions. *American Journal of Nursing, 118*(2), 34–39.

McCance, K. H., & Huether, S. (2019). *Pathophysiology: The biologic basis for disease in adults and children* (8th ed.). St. Louis: Elsevier.

Neviere, R. (2019). *Sepsis syndromes in adults: Epidemiology, definitions, clinical presentation, diagnosis, and prognosis. UpToDate*. Retrieved from https://www.uptodate.com/contents/sepsis-syndromes-in-adults-epidemiology-definitionsclinical-presentation-diagnosis-and-prognosis.

Pagana, K., & Pagana, T. J. (2018). *Mosby's manual of diagnostic and laboratory tests* (6th ed.). St. Louis: Elsevier.

Pagana, K., Pagana, T., & Pike-MacDonald, S. (2019). *Mosby's Canadian manual of diagnostic and laboratory tests* (2nd ed.). St. Louis: Elsevier.

Procter, L. (2018). *Merck manual/professional version/critical care medicine/shock and fluid resuscitation*. Retrieved from Merck Manuals: https://www.merckmanuals.com/professional/critical-care-medicine/shock-and-fluid-resuscitation/intravenous-fluid-resuscitation.

Singer, M., et al. (2016). The third international Consensus definitions for sepsis and septic shock (Sepsis-3). *Journal of the American Medical Association, 315*(8), 801–810.

Stapleton, R., & Heyland, D. (2018). *Glycemic control and intensive insulin therapy in critical illness. UpToDate*. Retrieved from: https://www.uptodate.com/contents/glycemic-control-and-intensive-insulin-therapy-in-critical-illness.

Surviving Sepsis Campaign. (2019). *Hour-1 bundle*. Retrieved from: http://www.survivingsepsis.org/Bundles/Pages/default.aspx.

Umberger, R., Callen, B., & Brown, M. (2015). Severe sepsis in older adults. *Critical Care Nursing Quarterly, 38*(3), 259–270.

Urden, L., Stacy, K., & Lough, M. (2018). *Critical care nursing: Diagnosis and management* (9th ed.). St. Louis: Elsevier.

35

Critical Care of Patients With Acute Coronary Syndromes

Laura M. Dechant, Nicole M. Heimgartner

http://evolve.elsevier.com/Iggy/

LEARNING OUTCOMES

1. Collaborate with the interprofessional team to provide high-quality care for patients with acute coronary syndromes that affect ***perfusion*** and cause ***pain.***
2. Prioritize evidence-based care for patients with acute coronary syndromes affecting ***perfusion.***
3. Teach patients about lifestyle modifications to reduce modifiable and nonmodifiable risk factors for acute coronary syndromes.
4. Teach the patient and caregiver(s) about common drugs used for acute coronary syndromes.
5. Implement nursing interventions to decrease the psychosocial impact of acute coronary events, especially myocardial infarction (MI).
6. Apply knowledge of anatomy and physiology to provide evidence-based nursing care for patients with stable angina, unstable angina, and MI.
7. Use clinical judgment to prioritize nursing care to promote ***perfusion*** and prevent complications in patients with chest pain.
8. Use laboratory data and signs and symptoms to prioritize care for the patient with acute coronary syndrome.
9. Develop a plan of care using quality improvement measures for the patient who requires percutaneous or surgical coronary intervention to promote ***perfusion.***

KEY TERMS

acute coronary syndrome (ACS) Disorder including unstable angina and myocardial infarction; results from obstruction of the coronary artery by ruptured atherosclerotic plaque and leads to platelet aggregation, thrombus formation, and vasoconstriction.

angina pectoris Chest pain caused by a temporary imbalance between the coronary arteries' ability to supply oxygen and the cardiac muscle's demand for oxygen.

atypical angina Angina with vague presentation such as indigestion, pain between the shoulders, an aching jaw, or choking sensation that occurs with exertion.

cardiac rehabilitation The process of actively assisting the patient with coronary disease to achieve and maintain a productive life while remaining within the limits of the heart's ability to respond to increases in activity and stress.

cardiogenic shock Post–myocardial infarction heart failure in which necrosis of more than 40% of the left ventricle has occurred; also called *Class IV heart failure.*

chronic stable angina (CSA) Type of angina characterized by chest discomfort that occurs with moderate-to-prolonged exertion and in a pattern that is familiar to the patient.

coronary artery bypass graft (CABG) Surgical procedure in which occluded arteries are bypassed with the patient's own venous or arterial blood vessels or synthetic grafts.

coronary artery disease (CAD) Disease affecting the arteries that provide blood, oxygen, and nutrients to the myocardium; also known as *coronary heart disease* or simply *heart disease.*

infarction Necrosis, or cell death.

intra-aortic balloon pump (IABP) Specialized catheter and balloon inserted into aorta that inflates and deflates with the cardiac cycle in order to decrease afterload and increase coronary perfusion.

ischemia Blockage of blood flow through a blood vessel, resulting in a lack of oxygen.

metabolic syndrome Collection of related health problems with insulin resistance as a main feature; increases the risk for cardiovascular disease.

myocardial infarction (MI) Injury and necrosis of myocardial tissue that occurs when the tissue is abruptly and severely deprived of oxygen.

new-onset angina Cardiac chest pain that occurs for the first time.

non–ST-elevation myocardial infarction (NSTEMI) Myocardial infarction in which the patient typically has ST- and T-wave changes on a 12-lead ECG; this indicates myocardial ischemia.

percutaneous coronary intervention (PCI) Nonsurgical method of improving arterial flow by opening the vessel lumen. A balloon is inserted in the coronary artery and inflated to open blood vessels; procedure may include insertion of a coronary stent.

pulmonary artery occlusion pressure (PAOP) Measurement of pressure in the left atrium using a balloon-tipped catheter introduced into the pulmonary artery.

ST-elevation myocardial infarction (STEMI) Myocardial infarction in which the patient typically has ST elevation in two contiguous leads on a 12-lead ECG; this indicates myocardial infarction (necrosis).

vasospastic angina Angina caused by coronary artery vasospasm that often occurs at rest or during the early morning hours; also called *variant* or *Prinzmetal angina.*

ventricular remodeling After a myocardial infarction, permanent changes in the size and shape of the left ventricle due to scar tissue; such remodeling can decrease left ventricular function and cause heart failure.

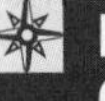

PRIORITY AND INTERRELATED CONCEPTS

The priority concept for this chapter is:

- ***Perfusion***

The ***Perfusion*** concept exemplar for this chapter is Acute Coronary Syndrome.

The interrelated concept for this chapter is:

- ***Pain***

Coronary artery disease (CAD) is a broad term that includes chronic stable angina and acute coronary syndrome (ACS). It affects the arteries that provide blood, oxygen, and nutrients to the myocardium. When blood flow through the coronary arteries is partially or completely blocked, ischemia and infarction of the myocardium may result. **Ischemia** occurs when *insufficient oxygen* is supplied to meet the requirements of the myocardium. **Infarction** (necrosis, or cell death) occurs when severe ischemia is prolonged and decreased ***perfusion*** causes irreversible damage to tissue.

CAD, also called *coronary heart disease (CHD)* or simply *heart disease,* is the single largest killer of American men and women in all ethnic groups. When the arteries that supply the myocardium are diseased, the heart cannot pump blood effectively to adequately perfuse vital organs and peripheral tissues. The organs and tissues need oxygen in arterial blood for survival. When ***perfusion*** is impaired, the patient can have life-threatening signs and symptoms and possibly death.

The death rate from CAD has declined over the past decade (Benjamin et al., 2018). This decline is due to many factors, including increasingly effective treatment and an increased awareness and emphasis on reducing major cardiovascular (CV) risk factors (e.g., hypertension, smoking, high cholesterol). However, some coronary events occur in patients without common risk factors.

CHRONIC STABLE ANGINA PECTORIS

Angina pectoris is chest pain caused by a temporary imbalance between the coronary arteries' ability to supply oxygen and the cardiac muscle's demand for oxygen. Ischemia (lack of oxygen) that occurs with angina is limited in duration and does not cause permanent damage of myocardial tissue.

Angina may be of two main types: stable angina and unstable angina. **Chronic stable angina (CSA)** is chest discomfort that occurs with moderate-to-prolonged exertion in a pattern that is familiar to the patient. The frequency, duration, and intensity of symptoms remain the same over several months. CSA results in only slight limitation of activity and is usually associated with a *fixed* atherosclerotic plaque. It is usually relieved by nitroglycerin (NTG) or rest and often is managed with drug therapy. Rarely does CSA require aggressive treatment. *Unstable* angina is discussed in the Acute Coronary Syndrome section.

PERFUSION CONCEPT EXEMPLAR: ACUTE CORONARY SYNDROME

Pathophysiology Review

The term **acute coronary syndrome (ACS)** is used to describe patients who have either *unstable* angina or an acute myocardial infarction (MI). In ACS, it is believed that the atherosclerotic plaque in the coronary artery *ruptures,* resulting in platelet aggregation ("clumping"), thrombus (clot) formation, and vasoconstriction (Fig. 35.1). The amount of disruption of the atherosclerotic plaque determines the degree of coronary artery obstruction (blockage) and the specific disease process. Once the artery reaches 50% occlusion, blood flow is impaired, creating myocardial ischemia when myocardial demand is increased (McCance & Huether, 2019).

Unstable angina (UA) is chest pain or discomfort that occurs at rest or with exertion and causes severe activity limitation. An increase in the number of attacks and in the intensity of the pressure indicates UA. The pressure may last longer than 15 minutes or may be poorly relieved by rest or nitroglycerin. Unstable angina can include *new-onset angina, vasospastic angina,* and *pre-infarction angina. Patients with unstable angina may present with ST changes on a 12-lead ECG but do not have changes in troponin levels.* Ischemia is present but is not severe enough to cause detectable myocardial damage or cell death. As the assays for troponins become more sensitive, the diagnosis of UA is decreasing.

New-onset angina describes the patient who has his or her first angina symptoms, usually after exertion or other increased demands on the heart. **Vasospastic angina** (also called *variant* or *Prinzmetal angina*) is chest pain or discomfort resulting from coronary artery spasm and typically occurs after rest. Pre-infarction angina refers to chest pain that occurs in the days or weeks before a myocardial infarction.

The most serious acute coronary syndrome is myocardial infarction (MI), often referred to as *acute MI* or *AMI.* Undiagnosed or untreated angina can lead to this very serious health problem. **Myocardial infarction (MI)** occurs when myocardial tissue is abruptly and severely deprived of oxygen.

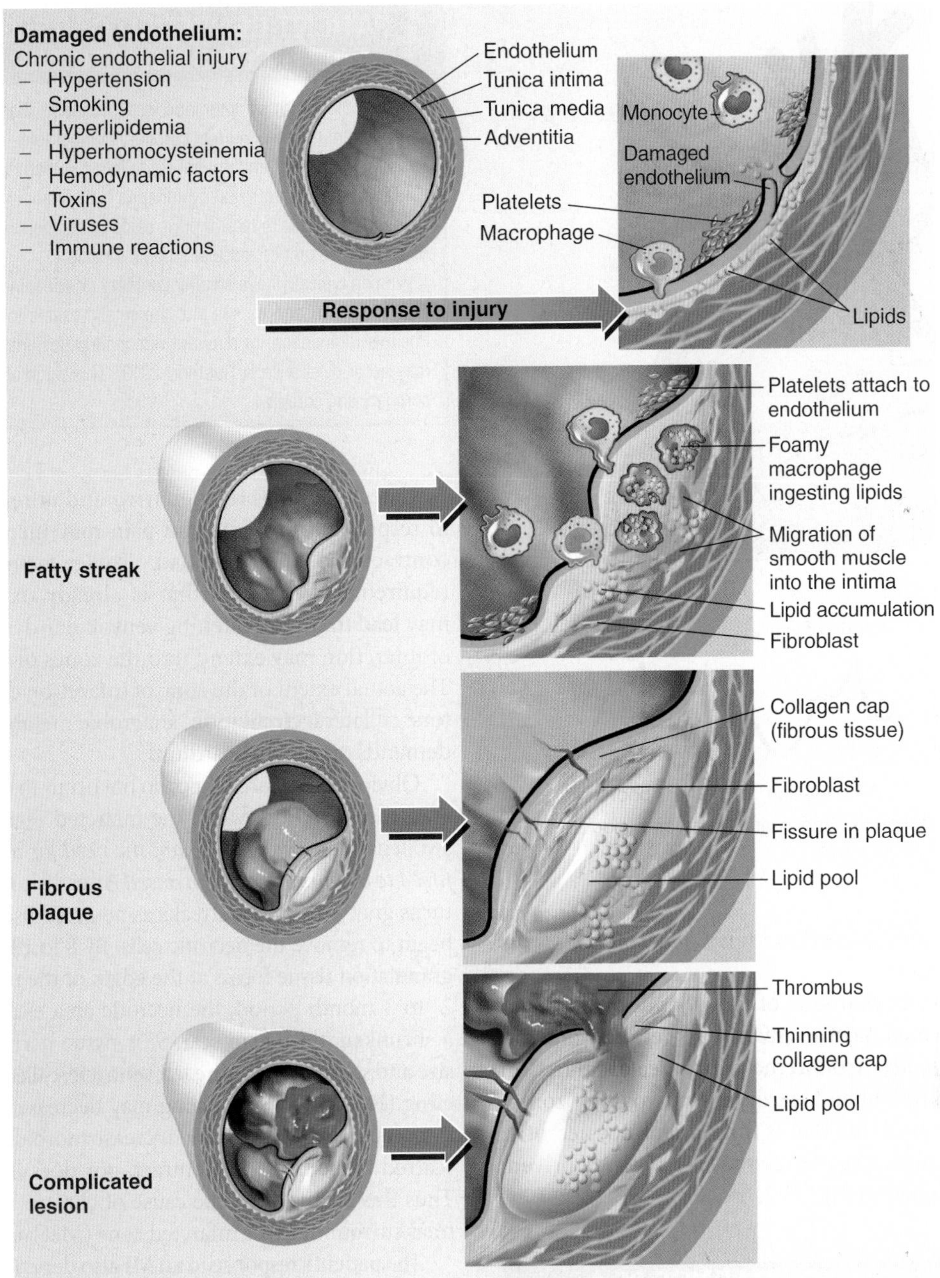

Fig. 35.1 A cross-section of an atherosclerotic coronary artery. (From Huether S.E., McCance, K.L., Brashers, V.L., & Rote, N.S. [2014]. *Understanding pathophysiology* [6th ed.]. St. Louis: Mosby.)

When blood flow is quickly reduced by 80% to 90%, ischemia develops. Ischemia can lead to injury and necrosis of myocardial tissue if blood flow is not restored. There are two types of MI: **non–ST-segment elevation myocardial infarction (NSTEMI)** and **ST-elevation myocardial infarction (STEMI)**.

Patients presenting with *NSTEMI* typically have ST segment and T-wave changes on a 12-lead ECG. These changes include ST depression and T-wave inversion. This indicates myocardial ischemia. Initially troponin may be normal, but it elevates over the next 3 to 12 hours. The combination of changes on the ECG and elevation in cardiac troponin indicates myocardial cell death or necrosis (Amsterdam et al., 2014). Causes of NSTEMI include coronary vasospasm, spontaneous dissection, and sluggish blood flow due to narrowing of the coronary artery. It is important to note that changes in ECG along with elevation of troponin should always be assessed in conjunction with the clinical presentation and history of the patient. Patients with elevated troponin and ECG changes without typical symptoms of acute coronary syndrome (i.e., chest discomfort, shortness of breath, nausea) typically have a condition other than CAD (such as sepsis), causing the imbalance between myocardial oxygen supply and demand.

Patients presenting with *STEMI* typically have ST elevation in two contiguous leads on a 12-lead ECG. This indicates MI/necrosis (O'Gara et al., 2013). STEMI is attributable to rupture of the fibrous atherosclerotic plaque leading to platelet aggregation and thrombus formation at the site of rupture (McCance & Huether, 2019). *The thrombus causes an abrupt 100% occlusion to the coronary artery; this is a medical*

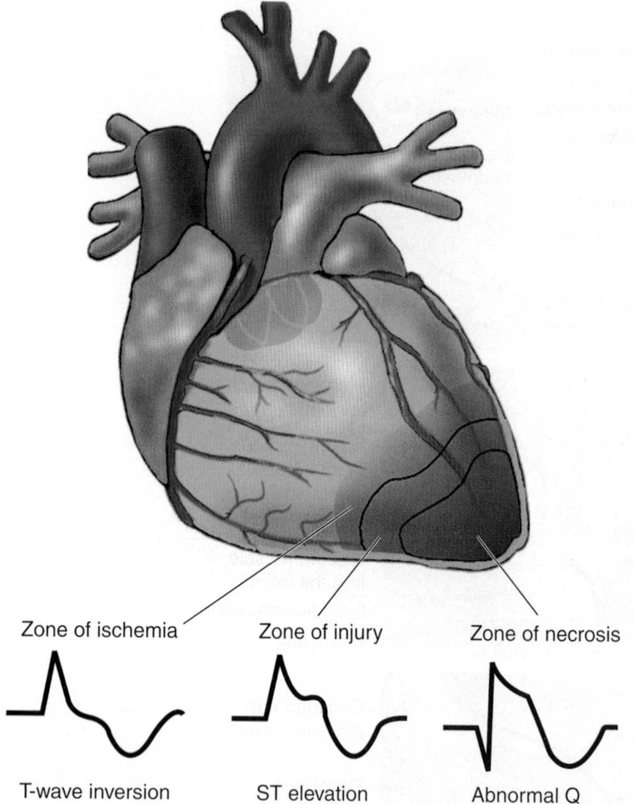

Fig. 35.2 Electrocardiographic changes and patterns associated with myocardial infarction.

emergency and requires immediate revascularization of the blocked coronary artery.

Often MIs begin with infarction of the subendocardial layer of cardiac muscle, which has the *greatest* oxygen *demand* and the *poorest* oxygen *supply.* Around the initial area of infarction (zone of necrosis) in the subendocardium are two other zones: (1) the zone of injury—tissue that is injured but not necrotic; and (2) the zone of ischemia—tissue that is oxygen deprived. This pattern is illustrated in Fig. 35.2.

NCLEX EXAMINATION CHALLENGE 35.1

Safe and Effective Care Environment

The nurse is caring for a client with chest pain. What assessment data would cause the nurse to suspect unstable angina? **Select all that apply.**

A. ST changes
B. Troponin T 0.6 ng/mL
C. Pain lasts 15 to 25 minutes
D. Increased number of angina attacks
E. The intensity of the chest pain has increased

Infarction is a dynamic process that does not occur instantly. Rather, it evolves over a period of several hours. Hypoxemia from ischemia may lead to local vasodilation of blood vessels and acidosis. Potassium, calcium, and magnesium imbalances, as well as acidosis at the cellular level, may cause changes in normal conduction and contractile functions.

PATIENT-CENTERED CARE: GENDER HEALTH CONSIDERATIONS QSEN

Many women with symptomatic ischemic heart disease or abnormal stress testing do not have abnormal coronary angiography. Studies implicate microvascular disease or endothelial dysfunction or both as the causes for risk for CAD in women. Endothelial dysfunction is the inability of the arteries and arterioles to dilate due to lack of nitric oxide production by the endothelium. Nitric oxide is a relaxant of vascular smooth muscle.

Women typically have smaller coronary arteries and frequently have plaque that breaks off and travels into the small vessels to form an embolus (clot). Positive remodeling, or outward remodeling (lesions that protrude outward), may occur (McCance & Huether, 2019). This outpouching may be missed on coronary angiography.

Catecholamines (epinephrine and norepinephrine) released in response to hypoxia and pain may increase the heart's rate, contractility, and afterload. These factors increase *oxygen* requirements in tissue that is already oxygen deprived. This may lead to life-threatening ventricular dysrhythmias. The area of infarction may extend into the zones of injury and ischemia. The actual extent of the zone of infarction depends on three factors: collateral circulation, anaerobic metabolism, and workload demands on the myocardium.

Obvious physical changes do not occur in the heart until 6 hours after the infarction, when the infarcted region appears blue and swollen. *These changes explain the need for intervention within the first 4 to 6 hours of symptom onset!* After 48 hours, the infarcted area turns gray with yellow streaks as neutrophils invade the tissue and begin to remove the necrotic cells. By 8 to 10 days after infarction, granulation tissue forms at the edges of the necrotic tissue. Over a 2- to 3-month period, the necrotic area eventually develops into a shrunken, thin, firm scar. Scar tissue permanently changes the size and shape of the entire left ventricle, called **ventricular remodeling** (Fig. 35.3). Remodeling may decrease left ventricular function, cause heart failure, and increase morbidity and mortality. The scarred tissue does not contract, nor does it conduct electrically. Thus this area is often the cause of chronic ventricular dysrhythmias surrounding the infarcted zone (McCance & Huether, 2019).

The patient's response to an MI also depends on which coronary artery or arteries were obstructed and which part of the ventricle wall was damaged: anterior, septal, lateral, inferior, or posterior. Fig. 30.3 in Chapter 30 shows the location of the major coronary arteries.

Obstruction of the left anterior descending (LAD) artery causes *anterior* or *septal* MIs because it perfuses the anterior wall and most of the septum of the left ventricle. Patients with anterior wall MIs (AWMIs) have the highest mortality rate because they are most likely to have left ventricular failure and dysrhythmias from damage to the left ventricle.

The circumflex artery supplies the lateral wall of the left ventricle and possibly portions of the posterior wall or the sinoatrial (SA) and atrioventricular (AV) nodes. Patients with obstruction of the circumflex artery may experience a *posterior* wall MI (PWMI) or a *lateral* wall MI (LWMI) and sinus dysrhythmias.

In most people, the right coronary artery (RCA) supplies most of the SA and AV nodes, as well as the right ventricle and inferior or

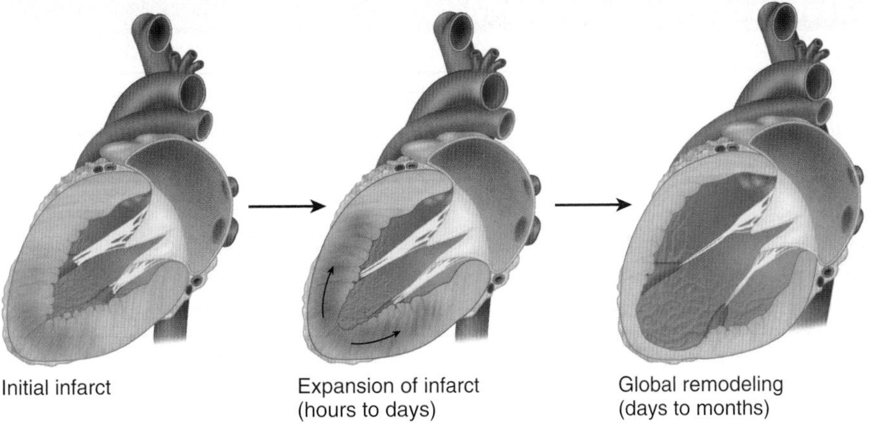

Fig. 35.3 Ventricular remodeling after myocardial infarction.

diaphragmatic portion of the left ventricle. Patients with obstruction of the RCA often have *inferior* wall MIs (IWMIs). About half of all IWMIs are associated with an occlusion of the RCA, causing significant damage to the right ventricle. *Thus it is important to obtain a "right-sided" ECG to assess for right ventricular involvement.*

Etiology and Genetic Risk

Atherosclerosis is the primary factor in the development of CAD. Numerous risk factors, both nonmodifiable and modifiable, contribute to atherosclerosis and subsequently to CAD. Atherosclerosis is described in Chapter 33. Nonmodifiable and modifiable risk factors are described in detail in Chapter 30. The Patient and Family Education: Preparing for Self-Management: Prevention of Coronary Artery Disease box discusses risk factors for CAD.

Metabolic syndrome, also called insulin resistance syndrome or syndrome X, is a risk factor for cardiovascular (CV) disease. Patients who have three of the factors in Table 35.1 are diagnosed with **metabolic syndrome**. This health problem increases the risk for developing diabetes and CAD. The presence of central obesity, high blood pressure, and hyperglycemia when diagnosed with metabolic syndrome presents the highest risk for development of cardiovascular disease. Females have a higher prevalence of metabolic syndrome, and overall prevalence increases with age (Benjamin et al., 2018). The incidence of metabolic syndrome continues to increase. This increase is likely a result of physical inactivity and the current obesity epidemic. Management is aimed at reducing risks, managing hypertension, and preventing complications.

PATIENT-CENTERED CARE: CULTURAL/SPIRITUAL CONSIDERATIONS QSEN

Several groups have a higher genetic risk for CAD than others. Nearly half of all non-Hispanic black adults have some form of cardiovascular disease, affecting 47% of black females and 46% of males (Benjamin et al., 2018). Currently, the highest death rates attributable to CAD occur in non-Hispanic black males, followed by non-Hispanic white males, Hispanic males, non-Hispanic black females, non-Hispanic white females, and Hispanic females (Benjamin et al., 2018).

NCLEX EXAMINATION CHALLENGE 35.2

Safe and Effective Care Environment

A 45-year-old male client having an annual physical asks the nurse about his risk for developing a myocardial infarction (MI). Which modifiable risk factors will the nurse assess to guide the client's teaching plan? **Select all that apply.**

A. Age
B. Tobacco use
C. Gender
D. Diet
E. Family history
F. Weight

PATIENT-CENTERED CARE: GENDER HEALTH CONSIDERATIONS QSEN

Age is the most important risk factor for developing CAD in women. The older a woman is, the more likely it is that she will have the disease. When compared with men, women are usually 10 years older when they have CAD. Only 56% of women are aware that heart disease is the leading cause of death in women, and even fewer can identify the symptoms of a heart attack (Benjamin et al., 2018). Women who have MIs have a greater risk for dying. More women than men die within a year after a MI (Mehta et al., 2016). For those who survive, more women develop associated complications such as heart failure or stroke. Women are also less likely to participate in cardiac rehabilitation programs (Benjamin et al, 2018).

Incidence and Prevalence

The average age of a person having a first MI is 65 years for men and 72 years for women (Benjamin et al., 2018). Every 40 seconds, a person in the United States has a major coronary event, and every 84 seconds an American will die from CAD (Benjamin et al., 2018). Many people die from CAD without being hospitalized. Most of these are sudden deaths caused by cardiac arrest.

TABLE 35.1 Indicators of Risk Factors for Metabolic Syndrome

Risk Factor	Indicator
Hypertension	Either blood pressure of 130/85 mm Hg or higher OR taking antihypertensive drug(s)
Decreased HDL-C (usually with high LDL-C) level	Either HDL-C <40 mg/dL for men or <50 mg/dL for women OR taking an anticholesterol drug
Increased level of triglycerides	Either 150 mg/dL or higher OR taking an anticholesterol drug
Increased fasting blood glucose (caused by diabetes, glucose intolerance, or insulin resistance)	Either 100 mg/dL or higher OR taking antidiabetic drug(s)
Large waist size (excessive abdominal fat causing central obesity)	40 inches (102 cm) or greater for men or 35 inches (88 cm) or greater for women

HDL-C, High-density lipoprotein cholesterol; *LDL-C,* low-density lipoprotein cholesterol.
Data from Meigs, J. (2019). *The metabolic syndrome (insulin resistance syndrome or syndrome X). UpToDate.* https://www.uptodate.com/contents/the-metabolic-syndrome-insulin-resistance-syndrome-or-syndrome-x; and Grundy, S.M., Cleeman, J.I., Daniels, S.R., Donato, K.A., Eckel, R.H., Franklin, B.A., et al. (2005). Diagnosis and management of the metabolic syndrome: An American Heart Association/National Heart, Lung, and Blood Institute scientific statement. *Circulation, 112*(17), 2735–2752.

PATIENT AND FAMILY EDUCATION: PREPARING FOR SELF-MANAGEMENT

Prevention of Coronary Artery Disease

Smoking/Tobacco Use
- If you smoke or use tobacco, quit.
- If you don't smoke or use tobacco, don't start.

Diet
- Consume sufficient calories for your body to include:
  - 5% to 6% from saturated fats
  - Avoiding *trans* fatty acids
- Limit your cholesterol intake to less than 200 mg/day.
- Limit your sodium intake as specified by your health care provider, or under 1500 mg/day, if possible.

Cholesterol
- Have your lipid levels checked regularly.
- If your cholesterol and LDL-C levels are elevated, follow your health care provider's advice, including taking statin medications as indicated.

Physical Activity
- If you are middle-age or older or have a history of medical problems, check with your health care provider before starting an exercise program.
- Exercise periods should be at least 40 minutes long with 10-minute warm-up and 5-minute cool-down periods.
- If you cannot exercise moderately three to four times each week, walk daily for 30 minutes at a comfortable pace.
- If you cannot walk 30 minutes daily, walk any distance you can (e.g., park farther away from a site than necessary; use the stairs, not the elevator, to go one floor up or two floors down).

Diabetes Mellitus
- Manage your diabetes with your health care provider.

Hypertension
- Have your blood pressure checked regularly.
- If your blood pressure is elevated, follow your health care provider's advice.
- Continue to monitor your blood pressure at regular intervals.

Obesity
- Avoid severely restrictive or fad diets.
- Restrict intake of saturated fats, sweets, sweetened beverages, and cholesterol-rich foods.
- Increase your physical activity.

LDL-C, Low-density lipoprotein cholesterol.

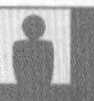

PATIENT-CENTERED CARE: GENDER HEALTH CONSIDERATION QSEN

Premenopausal women have a lower incidence of MI than men. However, for postmenopausal women in their 70s or older, the incidence of MI equals that of men. Family history is also a risk factor for women; those whose parents had CAD are more susceptible to the disease. Women with abdominal obesity (androidal shape) and metabolic syndrome are also at increased risk for CAD. Although studies are limited, research indicates that LGBT adults have an increased risk of cardiovascular disease related to increased incidence of modifiable risk factors such as smoking, alcohol use, and drug use (Caceres et al, 2016).

Many patients who survive MIs are not able to return to work. CAD is the leading cause of premature, permanent disability in the United States and the world.

Health Promotion and Maintenance

Ninety percent of sudden cardiac arrest victims die before reaching the hospital, and many of these deaths are attributed to ventricular fibrillation ("v fib") (Benjamin et al., 2018). To help combat this problem, automatic external defibrillators (AEDs) are found in many public places, such as in shopping centers and on airplanes. Employees are taught how to use these devices if a sudden cardiac arrest occurs. Some patients with diagnosed CAD have AEDs in their homes or at work. The procedure for using this device is described in Chapter 31.

Health promotion efforts are directed toward controlling or altering modifiable risk factors for CAD. For patients at risk for coronary artery disease (CAD), especially MI, assess specific risk factors and implement an individualized health teaching

KEY FEATURES
Angina and Myocardial Infarction

Angina	Myocardial Infarction
• Substernal chest discomfort: • Radiating to the left arm • Precipitated by exertion or stress (or rest in vasospastic angina) • Relieved by nitroglycerin or rest • Lasting less than 15 minutes • Few, if any, associated symptoms	• Pain or discomfort: • Substernal chest pain/pressure radiating to the left arm • Pain or discomfort in jaw, back, shoulder, or abdomen • Occurring without cause, usually in the morning • Relieved only by opioids • Lasting 30 minutes or more • Frequent associated symptoms: • Nausea/vomiting • Diaphoresis • Dyspnea • Feelings of fear and anxiety • Dysrhythmias • Fatigue • Palpitations • Epigastric distress • Anxiety • Dizziness • Disorientation/acute confusion • Feeling "short of breath"

plan. Teach people who have one or more of these risk factors the importance of modifying or eliminating them to decrease their chances of CAD. Chapter 33 describes health teaching and evidence-based interventions for preventing and managing atherosclerosis and hypertension. Smoking cessation is discussed in Chapter 24.

Interprofessional Collaborative Care

Assessment: Recognize Cues

History. If symptoms of CAD are present at the time of the interview, delay collecting data until interventions are started to relieve symptoms. If the patient has pain, ask how he or she has managed the discomfort and other symptoms and which drugs he or she may be taking. When the patient is pain free, obtain information about family history and modifiable risk factors, including eating habits, lifestyle, and physical activity levels. Ask about a history of smoking and how much alcohol is consumed each day. Collaborate with the registered dietitian nutritionist (RDN) to assess current body mass index (BMI) and weight as needed.

Physical Assessment/Signs and Symptoms. *Rapid assessment of the patient with chest pain or other presenting symptoms is crucial.* It is important to differentiate among the types of chest ***pain*** and identify the source. Question the patient to determine the characteristics of the pain. However, patients may deny pain and report that they feel "pressure." Appropriate questions to ask concerning the discomfort include onset, location, radiation, intensity, duration, and precipitating and relieving factors.

If ***pain*** is present, ask the patient if the pain is in the chest, epigastric area, jaw, back, shoulder, or arm. Ask the patient to rate the pain on a scale of 0 to 10, with 10 being the highest level of pain. Some patients describe the discomfort as tightness, a burning sensation, pressure, or indigestion. A complete pain assessment is described in Chapter 5.

PATIENT-CENTERED CARE: GENDER HEALTH CONSIDERATIONS QSEN

Many women of any age experience atypical angina. **Atypical angina** manifests as indigestion, pain between the shoulders, an aching jaw, or a choking sensation that occurs with exertion. Other symptoms may include unusual fatigue, shortness of breath, dizziness, palpitations, generalized anxiety or weakness and flulike symptoms (Mehta et al., 2016). These symptoms typically manifest during stressful circumstances or ADLs. Women may curtail activity as a result of angina, and health care providers need to ask about changes in routine. Symptoms in women typically include chest discomfort, unusual fatigue, and dyspnea (Mehta et al., 2016).

The Key Features: Angina and Myocardial Infarction box provides a comparison of angina and infarction pain. Because angina pain is ischemic pain, it usually improves when the imbalance between oxygen supply and demand is resolved. For example, rest reduces tissue demands, and nitroglycerin improves oxygen supply. Discomfort from a myocardial infarction (MI) does not usually resolve with these measures. Ask about any associated symptoms, including *nausea, vomiting, diaphoresis, dizziness, weakness, palpitations,* and *shortness of breath.*

PATIENT-CENTERED CARE: OLDER ADULT CONSIDERATIONS QSEN

The presence of associated symptoms without chest discomfort is significant. Older adults are more likely to have atypical symptoms. These patients often present with associated symptoms instead of the typical chest pain or pressure (Reeder & Kennedy, 2019). Some older patients may think they are having indigestion and therefore not recognize that they are having an MI. Others report shortness of breath as the only symptom. Because of the ambiguity of symptoms, the older adult is more likely to wait before seeking treatment. The major manifestation of MI in people older than 80 years may be disorientation or acute confusion because of poor cardiac output and inadequate coronary perfusion.

In some older adults with MI, absence of chest pain may be caused by cognitive impairment or inability to verbalize pain sensation. However, in most cases it is probably the result of increased collateral circulation. Silent myocardial ischemia increases the incidence of new coronary events and should be treated aggressively.

Assess *blood pressure* and *heart rate.* Interpret the patient's cardiac rhythm and presence of *dysrhythmias.* Sinus tachycardia with premature ventricular contractions (PVCs) frequently occurs in the first few hours after an MI.

Next assess *distal peripheral pulses* and *skin temperature.* The skin should be warm with all pulses palpable. In the patient with unstable angina or MI, poor cardiac output may manifest with cool, diaphoretic ("sweaty") skin and diminished or absent pulses. *Auscultate for an S_3 gallop, which often indicates heart failure—a serious and common complication of MI.* In adults, the S_3 heart sound is heard with the bell of the stethoscope over the apex of the heart (Jarvis, 2020).

Assess the *respiratory rate* and breath sounds for signs of heart failure. An increased respiratory rate is common because of anxiety and pain, but *crackles or wheezes* may indicate *left-sided* heart failure. Assess for the presence of jugular venous distention and peripheral edema.

The patient with MI may experience a *temperature elevation* for several days after infarction. Temperatures as high as 102°F (38.9°C) may occur in response to myocardial necrosis, indicating the inflammatory response.

Psychosocial Assessment. Assess the patient's current coping mechanisms. The most common are denial, anger, and depression. *Denial* is a common early reaction to chest ***pain*** associated with angina or MI. On average, the patient with an acute MI waits more than 2 hours before seeking medical attention. Often he or she rationalizes that symptoms are caused by indigestion or overexertion. In some situations, denial is a normal part of adapting to a stressful event. However, denial that interferes with identifying a symptom such as chest pain can be harmful. Explain the importance of reporting any pain to the health care provider.

Fear, depression, anxiety, and anger are other common reactions of many patients and their families. Assist in identifying these feelings. Encourage them to explain their understanding of the event and clarify any misconceptions.

Laboratory Assessment. Although there is no single test to diagnose MI, the most common laboratory tests include troponins T and I. Troponin is specific for MI and cardiac necrosis. Troponins T and I rise quickly. These tests are described in more detail in Chapter 30. If serial troponins are negative, the patient has a nuclear medicine test such as those described in the next section.

SYSTEMS THINKING AND QUALITY IMPROVEMENT

Stanfield, L. (2018). Improvement of door-to-electrocardiogram time using the first-nurse role in the ED setting. Journal of Emergency Nursing, 44(5), 466–471.

When a patient presents with chest pain, it is imperative that assessment and intervention occur as quickly as possible. The national guidelines recommend that an initial ECG be obtained within the first 10 minutes of arrival to the emergency department. For patients who are experiencing a myocardial infarction, a delay in acquiring an ECG could lead to a delay in treatment, costing the patient increased damage to the heart muscle. In this quality improvement (QI) project, a community hospital emergency department initiated the use of a "first nurse" role in an attempt to decrease the overall door-to-ECG time. The first nurse role was designated to a nurse who remained in the lobby of the emergency department to quickly and effectively assess patients on arrival. The QI initiative also included education for the first nurse role, as well as interventions to promote a positive attitude toward the potential impacts of the role, in terms of patient safety. Data regarding door-to-ECG times were compared before and after the initiation of the first nurse role by using data that are reported through the Acute Coronary Treatment and Interventions Outcomes Network (ACTION) Registry. Although the data did suggest improvement in door-to-ECG times, statistical significance was not achieved.

Commentary: Implications for Practice

Although statistical significance within this project was not achieved, the monthly data do indicate that the first nurse role made a difference in the treatment times. In addition, patient satisfaction scores increased with the addition of the first nurse role in the emergency department. The implications of this project show that further study is warranted and that the first nurse role could be beneficial in providing care more quickly to populations that need rapid intervention.

Imaging Assessment. Unless there is associated cardiac dysfunction (e.g., valve disease) or heart failure, a chest x-ray is not diagnostic for angina or MI. A chest x-ray may be performed to help rule out aortic dissection, which may mimic an MI. If the x-ray demonstrates a widened mediastinum, further testing for aortic dissection with either transesophageal echography (TEE) or CT scan is needed.

Thallium scans use radioisotope imaging to assess for ischemia or necrotic muscle tissue related to angina or MI. Areas of decreased or absent ***perfusion,*** referred to as *cold spots,* identify ischemia or infarction. Thallium may be used with the exercise tolerance test. Dipyridamole thallium scanning (DTS) may also be used.

Contrast-enhanced cardiovascular magnetic resonance (CMR) imaging may also be done as a noninvasive approach to detect CAD. *Echocardiography* may be used to visualize the structures of the heart.

Use of 64-slice computed tomography coronary angiography (CTCA) has been found to be helpful in diagnosing CAD. The high-speed CT scanner is a highly reliable, noninvasive way to evaluate calcified plaque. This plaque is then quantified into the calcium score. Those with a calcium score (also called the Agatston score) higher than 400 have a higher risk of developing myocardial infarction and death within the next 2 to 5 years (Pagana & Pagana, 2018).

Other Diagnostic Assessment. *Twelve-lead ECGs* allow the health care provider to examine the heart from varying perspectives. By identifying the lead(s) in which ECG changes are occurring, the health care provider can identify both the occurrence and the location of ischemia (angina) or necrosis (infarction). In addition to the traditional 12-lead ECG, the health care provider may request a "right-sided" or 18-lead ECG to determine whether ischemia or infarction has occurred in the right ventricle. *The ECG should be obtained within 10 minutes of patient presentation with chest discomfort!*

An ischemic myocardium does not repolarize normally. Thus 12-lead ECGs obtained during an angina episode reveal ST depression, T-wave inversion, or both. Vasospastic angina, caused by coronary vasospasm (vessel spasm), usually causes elevation of the ST segment during angina attacks. These ST and T-wave changes usually subside when the ischemia is resolved and pain is relieved. However, the T wave may remain flat or inverted for a period of time. If the patient is not experiencing angina at the moment of the test, the ECG is usually normal unless he or she has evidence of an old MI.

When infarction occurs, one of two ECG changes is usually observed: ST-elevation MI (STEMI), or non–ST-elevation MI (NSTEMI). An abnormal Q wave (wider than 0.04 second or more than one-third the height of the QRS complex) may develop, depending on the amount of myocardium that has necrosed. Women having an MI often present with NSTEMI.

The Q wave may develop because necrotic cells do not conduct electrical stimuli. Hours to days after the MI, the ST-segment and T-wave changes return to normal. However, when the Q wave exists, it may become permanent. The Q waves may disappear after a number of years, but their absence does not necessarily mean that the patient has not had an MI.

After the acute stages of an unstable angina episode, the health care provider often requests an *exercise tolerance test (stress test)* on a treadmill to assess for ECG changes consistent with ischemia, evaluate medical therapy, and identify those who might benefit from invasive therapy. Pharmacologic stress-testing agents such as dobutamine may be used instead of the treadmill. Treadmill exercise testing is only moderately accurate for women compared with men. The results are also not as reliable in tall, obese men when compared with short, thinner men. In women with suspected CAD, stress echocardiography or single-photon emission CT (SPECT) should be performed.

Cardiac catheterization may be performed to determine the extent and exact location of coronary artery obstructions. It allows the cardiologist and cardiac surgeon to identify patients who might benefit from percutaneous coronary intervention (PCI) or from coronary artery bypass graft (CABG). Each of these diagnostic tests is described in detail in Chapter 30.

◆ **Analysis: Analyze Cues and Prioritize Hypotheses.** The patient with coronary artery disease (CAD) may have either stable angina or acute coronary syndrome (ACS). If ACS is suspected or cannot be completely ruled out, the patient is admitted to a telemetry unit for continuous monitoring or to a critical care unit if hemodynamically unstable.

The priority collaborative problems for most patients with ACS include:

1. Acute ***pain*** due to an imbalance between myocardial oxygen supply and demand
2. Decreased myocardial tissue ***perfusion*** due to interruption of arterial blood flow
3. Potential for dysrhythmias due to ischemia and ventricular irritability
4. Potential for heart failure due to left ventricular dysfunction

◆ **Planning and Implementation: Generate Solutions and Take Action.** Astute assessment skills, timely analysis of troponin, and analysis of the 12-lead ECG (or 18-lead ECG for a suspected right ventricular infarction) are essential to ensure appropriate patient care management. This is particularly important given that the average time a patient waits before seeking treatment is over 2 hours. This delay lessens the 4- to 6-hour window of opportunity for the most advantageous treatment with percutaneous intervention.

Managing Acute Pain

Planning: Expected Outcomes. The expected outcome is that the patient will verbalize decreased ***pain*** as a result of prompt collaborative interventions to increase ***perfusion***.

Interventions. The purpose of interprofessional collaborative care is to decrease ***pain,*** decrease myocardial oxygen demand, and increase ***perfusion*** (myocardial oxygen supply). Pain relief helps increase the oxygen supply and decrease myocardial oxygen demand. Evaluate any reports of pain, obtain vital signs, ensure IV access, and notify the health care provider of the patient's condition. The Best Practice for Patient Safety & Quality Care: Emergency Care of the Patient With Chest Discomfort box summarizes emergency interventions for the patient with chest pain.

Drug Therapy. At home or in the hospital, the patient may take nitroglycerin to relieve episodic anginal pain.

BEST PRACTICE FOR PATIENT SAFETY & QUALITY CARE (QSEN)

Emergency Care of the Patient With Chest Discomfort

- Assess airway, breathing, and circulation (ABCs). Defibrillate as needed.
- Provide continuous ECG monitoring.
- Obtain the patient's description of pain or discomfort.
- Obtain the patient's vital signs (blood pressure, pulse, respiration).
- Assess/provide vascular access.
- Consult chest pain protocol or notify the health care provider or Rapid Response Team for specific intervention.
- Obtain a 12-lead ECG within 10 minutes of report of chest pain.
- Provide pain relief medication and aspirin (non–enteric coated) as prescribed.
- Administer supplemental oxygen therapy to maintain an oxygen saturation greater than 90%.
- Remain calm. Stay with the patient if possible.
- Assess the patient's vital signs and intensity of pain 5 minutes after administration of medication.
- Remedicate with prescribed drugs (if vital signs remain stable) and check the patient every 5 minutes.
- Notify the health care provider if vital signs deteriorate.

! NURSING SAFETY PRIORITY (QSEN)

Drug Alert

Before administering NTG, ensure that the patient has not taken any phosphodiesterase inhibitors for erectile dysfunction, such as sildenafil, tadalafil, avanafil, or vardenafil, within the past 24 to 48 hours. Concomitant use of NTG with these inhibitors can cause profound hypotension. Remind patients not to take these medications within 24 to 48 hours of one another.

Some phosphodiesterase inhibitors are also used in the treatment of pulmonary arterial hypertension (PAH). Patients with PAH cannot stop taking the phosphodiesterase inhibitor. As a result, NTG is contraindicated in this patient population.

Nitroglycerin (NTG), a nitrate often referred to as "nitro," increases collateral blood flow, redistributes blood flow toward the subendocardium, and dilates the coronary arteries. In addition, it decreases myocardial oxygen demand by peripheral vasodilation, which decreases both preload and afterload.

Teach the patient to hold the NTG tablet under the tongue and drink 5 mL (1 teaspoon) of water, if necessary, to allow the tablet to dissolve. NTG spray is also available and is more quickly absorbed. Pain relief should begin within 1 to 2 minutes and should be clearly evident in 3 to 5 minutes. After 5 minutes, recheck the patient's pain intensity and vital signs. If the blood pressure (BP) is less than 100 mm Hg systolic or 25 mm Hg lower than the previous reading, lower the head of the bed and notify the health care provider.

If the patient is experiencing some but not complete relief and vital signs remain stable, another NTG tablet or spray may be used. In 5-minute increments, a total of three doses may be administered in an attempt to relieve angina pain. If the patient uses NTG spray instead of the tablet, teach him or her to sit upright and spray the dose under the tongue.

Angina usually responds to NTG. The patient typically states that the pain is relieved or markedly diminished. When simple measures, such as taking three sublingual nitroglycerin tablets, in timed increments, one after the other, do not relieve chest discomfort, the patient may be experiencing an MI.

NURSING SAFETY PRIORITY QSEN

Critical Rescue

If the patient is experiencing an MI, prepare him or her for transfer to a specialized unit where close monitoring and appropriate management can be provided. If the patient is at home or in the community, call 911 for transfer to the closest emergency department.

When ischemia persists, the health care provider may prescribe IV NTG for management of the chest pain. Begin the drug infusion slowly, checking the blood pressure (BP) and pain level every 3 to 5 minutes. The NTG dose is increased until the pain is relieved, the BP falls excessively, or the maximum prescribed dose is reached (see the Common Examples of Drug Therapy: Acute Coronary Syndrome [Nitrates, Beta Blockers, Antiplatelets] box).

When the pain or other symptoms have subsided and the patient is stabilized, the health care provider may change the drug to an oral or topical nitrate. During administration of long-term oral and topical nitrates, an 8- to 12-hour nitrate-free period should be maintained to prevent tolerance. The patient may initially report a headache. Give acetaminophen before the nitrate to ease some of this discomfort.

COMMON EXAMPLES OF DRUG THERAPY

Acute Coronary Syndrome (Nitrates, Beta Blockers, Antiplatelets)

Drug Category	Selected Nursing Implications
Nitrates Common examples of nitrates: • Sublingual tablets: Nitrostat, Nitroquick • Sublingual spray: Nitrolingual • Transdermal nitroglycerin: Minitran, Nitro-Dur, Nitrek • Isosorbide dinitrate • Isosorbide mononitrate	Monitor blood pressure (BP) and pay close attention to orthostatic changes *because a decrease in BP occurs with vasodilation.* • Dizziness can occur with drop in BP. Monitor for headache *because vasodilation is generalized.* **Do not administer to patients taking drugs used to treat sexual dysfunction or pulmonary arterial hypertension (e.g., sildenafil, tadalafil, vardenafil) *because very serious, possibly fatal interactions can occur.*** Always assess for pain relief *because additional medication may be required.* With sublingual tablets or spray: • Instruct patient to lie down when taking *because the hypotensive response can be dramatic.* • Tablets can be taken every 5 minutes for pain relief, up to 3 tablets. • Be sure to allow the tablet to dissolve *because it is absorbed through the mucous membranes.* • Check expiration date *because the efficacy decreases over time and the drug should be replaced every 3-5 months.* With transdermal nitroglycerin: • Apply the patch to a clean, dry, hairless area *because the medication will be better absorbed.* • Rotate application sites *to prevent skin irritation.* • Remove the patch before defibrillation *to prevent burns.* • Remove patch after 12-14 hours each day *to prevent drug tolerance.*
Beta Blockers Common examples of beta blockers: • Carvedilol • Metoprolol, a cardioselective beta-adrenergic blocker	Assess HR and BP before administration *because beta blockers cause a decrease in HR and cardiac output and suppress renin activity.* • Do not administer if heart rate is <50-60 beats/min. • Hold for systolic BP <90-100 mm Hg. Observe for signs of heart failure such as cough, edema, shortness of breath, and weight gain *because this can occur with a decrease in cardiac output.* Assess for wheezing and shortness of breath *because $beta_2$-blocking effects in the lungs can cause bronchoconstriction.*

Antiplatelets
Common examples of antiplatelets:
• Aspirin
• P2Y12 Inhibitors:
  • Clopidogrel
  • Prasugrel
  • Ticagrelor
  • Cangrelor
• PAR-1 inhibitor:
  • Vorapaxar sulfate
	Inform patients to report any unusual bleeding or bruising *because bleeding is a side effect for all medications in this category.*
	Avoid over-the-counter pain medications that contain additional aspirin.
	With aspirin therapy:
	• Take with food *because gastric irritation may occur.*
	• Assess for ringing in ears *because this can be a sign of aspirin toxicity.*
	• Teach patient that aspirin is an important cardiac medication that should not be stopped unless indicated by the provider *as studies indicate better survival rates for patients with CAD who receive aspirin.*
	With P2Y12 platelet inhibitors:
	• Take with food *because drug can cause diarrhea and GI upset.*
	• Do not confuse Plavix with Paxil.

The health care provider may prescribe *morphine sulfate (MS)* to relieve discomfort that is unresponsive to nitroglycerin. Morphine decreases pain, decreases myocardial oxygen demand, relaxes smooth muscle, and reduces circulating catecholamines. For persistent cardiac pain, morphine is administered in doses of 2 to 4 mg using slow IV push every 5 to 15 minutes (Reeder & Kennedy, 2019). Monitor for adverse effects of morphine, which include respiratory depression, hypotension, bradycardia, and severe vomiting.

If hypoxemia is present, the health care provider may prescribe oxygen at a flow rate of 2 to 4 L/min to maintain an arterial oxygen saturation of 90% or higher. The use of oxygen in the absence of hypoxemia has been shown to increase coronary vascular resistance, decrease coronary blood flow, and increase mortality. Monitor the patient's vital signs and cardiac rhythm every few minutes. If the BP is stable, help the patient assume any position of comfort. Placing the patient in semi-Fowler position often enhances comfort and tissue oxygenation. A quiet, calm environment and explanations of interventions often reduce anxiety and help relieve chest pain. If needed, remind the patient to take several deep breaths to increase oxygenation.

For the patient experiencing a myocardial infarction, combining pain relief strategies with interventions to increase myocardial perfusion is essential.

PATIENT-CENTERED CARE: OLDER ADULT CONSIDERATIONS (QSEN)

Coronary Artery Disease

- Recognize that chest pain may not be evident in the older patient. Examples of associated symptoms are unexplained dyspnea, confusion, or GI symptoms.
- Although older adults have a greater reduction in mortality rate from myocardial infarction (MI) with the use of fibrinolytic therapy, they also have the most severe side effects.
- Dysrhythmia may be a normal age-related change rather than a complication of MI. Determine whether the dysrhythmia is causing significant symptoms. Then notify the health care provider.
- If beta blockers are used, assess the patient carefully for the development of side effects. Exacerbation of the depression some older adults have is a significant problem with beta blockade.
- Plan slow, steady increases in activity. Older adults with minimal previous exercise show particular benefit from a gradual increase in activity.
- Older adults should plan longer warm-up and cool-down periods when participating in an exercise program. Their pulse rates may not return to baseline until 30 minutes or longer after exercise.

Increasing Myocardial Tissue Perfusion

Planning: Expected Outcomes. The primary outcome is that the patient will have increased myocardial ***perfusion*** as evidenced by adequate cardiac output, normal sinus rhythm, and vital signs within normal limits.

Interventions. Because myocardial infarction (MI) is a dynamic process, restoring ***perfusion*** to the injured area (usually within 4 to 6 hours for NSTEMI and 60 to 90 minutes for STEMI) often limits the amount of extension and improves left ventricular function. Complete, sustained reperfusion of coronary arteries after an acute coronary syndrome (ACS) has decreased mortality rates. Drug therapy as well as percutaneous coronary intervention (PCI) are used to restore cardiac perfusion.

Drug Therapy. *Aspirin (ASA)* therapy is recommended by the American College of Cardiology (ACC) and the American Heart Association (AHA). It inhibits both platelet aggregation and vasoconstriction, thereby decreasing the likelihood of thrombosis. *If the patient has new-onset angina at home, teach him or her to chew aspirin 325 mg (4 "baby aspirins" that are 81 mg each) immediately and call 911!* The antiplatelet effect of ASA begins within 1 hour of use and continues for several days. In the hospital setting, aspirin should be given on arrival to the emergency department or when an MI occurs in the hospital. If the patient is unable to swallow the aspirin, the dose can be administered by rectal suppository. All patients with suspected CAD should receive low–dose, non–enteric-coated aspirin daily unless absolutely contraindicated (Levine et al., 2016). Instruct the patient to chew and swallow the drug and continue taking it as prescribed unless adverse effects occur.

$P2Y_{12}$ platelet inhibitors such as clopidogrel or ticagrelor, may be given with an initial loading dose followed by a daily dose for up to 12 months after diagnosis. These oral agents work to prevent platelets from aggregating (clumping) together to form clots. When dual antiplatelet therapy is used, evidence shows a significant reduction in associated mortality (Cutlip & Lincoff, 2018).

CLINICAL JUDGMENT CHALLENGE 35.1

Patient-Centered Care; Evidence-Based Practice; Clinical Judgment; Informatics

A 50-year-old man presents to the emergency department with reports of intermittent chest pain occurring over the past 2 hours. The client reports nausea, vomiting, and diaphoresis. The client has a history of hypertension, anxiety, and erectile dysfunction. The client is alert and oriented and currently reports pain in his chest, rated as a 6 on a scale of 0 to 10, described as "aching pressure." The client's BP is currently 186/100 mm Hg, HR 120 beats/min, RR 26 breaths/min, with oxygen saturation 89% on room air.

1. **Recognize Cues:** What assessment information in this client situation is the most important and immediate concern for the nurse? (Hint: Identify the **relevant** information *first* to determine what is most important.)
2. **Analyze Cues:** What client conditions are consistent with the **most relevant** information? (Hint: Think about priority collaborative problems that support and contradict the information presented in this situation.)
3. **Prioritize Hypotheses:** Which possibilities or explanations are **most likely** to be present in this client situation? Which possibilities or explanations are the most serious? (Hint: Consider all possibilities and determine their urgency and risk for this client.)
4. **Generate Solutions:** What actions would most likely achieve the desired outcomes for this client? Which actions should be **avoided** or are **potentially harmful**? (Hint: Determine the desired outcomes first to decide which interventions are appropriate and those that should be avoided.)
5. **Take Action:** Which actions are the most appropriate and how should they be implemented? In what **priority order** should they be implemented? (Hint: Consider health teaching, documentation, requested health care provider orders or prescriptions, nursing skills, collaboration with or referral to health team members, etc.)
6. **Evaluate Outcomes:** What client assessment would indicate that the nurse's actions were **effective?** (Hint: Think about signs that would indicate an improvement, decline, or unchanged client condition.)

NURSING SAFETY PRIORITY QSEN

Drug Alert

Dual antiplatelet therapy (DAPT) is suggested for all patients with ACS, incorporating aspirin with a $P2Y_{12}$ receptor blocker, such as clopidogrel or ticagrelor (Lincoff & Cutlip, 2018). The major side effect for *each* of these agents is bleeding. Observe for bleeding tendencies, such as nosebleeds or blood in the stool. Medications will need to be discontinued if evidence of bleeding occurs. Teach patients signs of bleeding and when to contact the health care provider. While receiving DAPT, patients with high risk for GI bleeding may be prescribed a proton pump inhibitor, such as omeprazole (Levine et al., 2016).

Glycoprotein (GP) IIb/IIIa inhibitors such as abciximab, eptifibatide, or tirofiban may be administered IV to prevent fibrinogen from attaching to activated platelets at the site of a thrombus. These medications are used in unstable angina and NSTEMI. They are also given before and during percutaneous coronary intervention (PCI) to maintain patency of an artery with a large clot and are given with fibrinolytic agents after STEMI.

NURSING SAFETY PRIORITY QSEN

Drug Alert

When giving GP IIb/IIIa inhibitors, assess the patient closely for bleeding or hypersensitivity reactions. If either occurs, notify the health care provider or Rapid Response Team immediately. Monitor the platelet level 4 hours after starting the drug and daily thereafter. Notify the cardiologist if the patient develops a significant decrease in platelet count per agency protocol.

Another antiplatelet, a *protease-activated receptor inhibitor (PAR-1)*, vorapaxar, is shown to decrease the risk of recurrent MI when added to the regimen of aspirin and clopidogrel (Burchum & Rosenthal, 2019). The main side effect is bleeding, including an increased risk of intracranial hemorrhage.

In addition to antiplatelet therapy, *anticoagulation therapy* may also be used to prevent clot formation. Choice of anticoagulant is determined by provider preference because national guidelines do not currently recommend one agent over another. Anticoagulation is stopped before cardiac catheterization and is usually not continued following coronary intervention unless a high risk for clot reformation exists following the intervention. See Chapter 33 for full discussion of anticoagulation therapy.

Once-a-day *beta-adrenergic blocking agents* (e.g., metoprolol XL, carvedilol CR), sometimes just called *beta blockers (BBs)*, decrease the size of the infarct, the occurrence of ventricular dysrhythmias, and mortality rates in patients with MI. The provider usually prescribes a cardioselective beta-blocking agent within the first 1 to 2 hours after an MI if the patient is hemodynamically stable. Beta blockers slow the heart rate and decrease the force of cardiac contraction (see the Common Examples of Drug Therapy: Acute Coronary Syndrome [Nitrates, Beta Blockers, Antiplatelets] box). Thus these agents prolong the period of diastole and increase myocardial ***perfusion*** while reducing the force of myocardial contraction. With beta blockade, the heart can perform more work without ischemia. During beta-blocking therapy, monitor for:

- Bradycardia
- Hypotension
- Decreased level of consciousness (LOC)
- Chest discomfort

Assess the lungs for crackles (indicative of heart failure) and wheezes (indicative of bronchospasm). Hypoglycemia, depression, nightmares, and forgetfulness are also problems with beta blockade, especially in older patients. Many of these side effects decrease with time. Unless contraindicated, all patients experiencing NSTEMI and STEMI should be discharged on beta-blocker therapy. If the patient has a history or new onset of heart failure, extended release metoprolol succinate, carvedilol, or bisoprolol should be used because these agents have been shown to reduce mortality in patients with heart failure.

NURSING SAFETY PRIORITY QSEN

Drug Alert

Do not give beta blockers if the pulse is below 50 beats/min or the systolic BP is below 100 mm Hg without first checking with the health care provider. The beta-blocking agent may lead to persistent bradycardia or further reduction of systolic BP, leading to poor peripheral and coronary perfusion.

Health care providers frequently prescribe *angiotensin-converting enzyme inhibitors (ACEIs)* or *angiotensin receptor blockers (ARBs)* within 24 hours of ACS to prevent ventricular remodeling and the development of heart failure. After STEMI, all patients in the absence of contraindications should receive either an ACEI or an ARB as both ACEIs and ARBs increase survival after an MI. Monitor the patient for decreased urine output, hypotension, and cough. Check for changes in serum potassium, creatinine, and blood urea nitrogen. If ACEIs or ARBs are initiated, they should be continued on discharge indefinitely. Chapter 33 provides a more detailed discussion of ACEIs and ARBs.

For patients with angina, the health care provider may prescribe *calcium channel blockers* (CCBs) to promote vasodilation and myocardial ***perfusion.*** These drugs are indicated for patients with vasospastic angina or for those who are hypertensive and continue to have angina despite therapy with beta blockers (unstable angina). They are *not* indicated after an acute MI unless beta blockade is contraindicated. Monitor the patient for hypotension and peripheral edema and review the frequency of angina episodes. Calcium channel blockers are also used for chronic stable angina (CSA). When they are not successful in managing CSA, *ranolazine* may be added to the drug regimen. This drug has antiangina and anti-ischemic properties and is often effective in relieving the pain associated with CSA.

Statin therapy reduces the risk of developing recurrent MI, mortality, and stroke. Before discharge, all patients diagnosed with ACS should be started on high-intensity statin therapy despite results of lipid panel testing. High-intensity statins include atorvastatin and rosuvastatin.

Reperfusion Therapy. As time passes, myocardial tissue can become increasingly ischemic and necrotic. Therefore based on the location and skill set within the health care institution, one of two reperfusion strategies are used to open a blocked artery in a patient experiencing acute MI: thrombolytic therapy or percutaneous coronary intervention (PCI). PCI is the treatment of choice for most patients with STEMI.

Fibrinolytic therapy. *Fibrinolytic therapy* (also called *thrombolytic therapy*) dissolves thrombi in the coronary arteries and restores myocardial blood flow. Examples of these agents, which target the fibrin component of the coronary thrombosis, include:

- Tissue plasminogen activator (tPA, alteplase)
- Reteplase
- Tenecteplase

Patients who cannot receive timely PCI with indications of STEMI should be considered for fibrinolytic therapy. The benefit of fibrinolytic therapy declines as the time between onset of symptoms to therapy increases (Gibson & Corbalan, 2017). The goal is to administer fibrinolytic therapy within 30 minutes of arrival to the hospital. It is *not* indicated for the NSTEMI patient population. Absolute contraindications include previous intracranial hemorrhage, active bleeding, and significant trauma within 3 months. Table 35.2 lists the current contraindications to thrombolytic therapy.

! NURSING SAFETY PRIORITY (QSEN)

Drug Alert

During and after thrombolytic administration, immediately report any indications of bleeding to the health care provider or Rapid Response Team. Observe for signs of bleeding by:

- Documenting the patient's neurologic status (in case of intracranial bleeding)
- Observing all IV sites for bleeding and patency
- Monitoring clotting studies
- Observing for signs of internal bleeding (monitor hemoglobin, hematocrit, and blood pressure)
- Testing stools, urine, and emesis for occult blood

Patients who receive fibrinolytics require percutaneous coronary intervention (PCI) for more definitive treatment such as stent placement. Therefore if criteria for PCI are met, it is more advantageous to go directly to the catheterization laboratory where definitive treatment, not just clot resolution, can be performed.

Monitor the patient for indications that the clot has been lysed (dissolved) and the artery reperfused. These indications include:

- Abrupt cessation of pain or discomfort
- Sudden onset of ventricular dysrhythmias
- Resolution of ST-segment depression/elevation or T-wave inversion
- A peak at 12 hours of markers of myocardial damage

TABLE 35.2 Contraindications to Thrombolytic Therapy

Absolute

- Any prior intracranial hemorrhage
- Known structural cerebral vascular lesion (e.g., arteriovenous malformations)
- Known malignant intracranial neoplasm (primary or metastatic)
- Ischemic stroke within 3 months EXCEPT acute ischemic stroke within 3 hours
- Suspected aortic dissection
- Active bleeding or bleeding diathesis (excluding menses)
- Significant closed-head or facial trauma within 3 months

Relative

- History of chronic, severe, poorly controlled hypertension
- Severe uncontrolled hypertension on presentation (SBP >180 mm Hg)
- History of prior ischemic stroke within 3 months, dementia, or known intracranial pathology not covered in contraindications
- Traumatic or prolonged (≥10 minutes) CPR or major surgery (within 3 weeks)
- Recent (within 2-4 weeks) internal bleeding
- Noncompressible vascular puncture
- For streptokinase: prior exposure (>5 days ago) or prior allergic reaction to these agents
- Pregnancy
- Active peptic ulcer
- Current use of anticoagulants; the higher the INR, the higher risk for bleeding

CPR, Cardiopulmonary resuscitation; *INR,* international normalized ratio; *SBP,* systolic blood pressure.

After clot lysis with fibrinolytics, large amounts of thrombin are released into the system, increasing the risk for vessel reocclusion. To maintain the patency of the coronary artery after thrombolytic therapy, the health care provider usually prescribes aspirin and IV heparin, a *high-alert drug.* Maintain the heparin infusion via pump to maintain an activated partial thromboplastin time (aPTT) between 50 and 70 seconds (which is 1½ to 2 times the control) (Urden et al., 2018). The heparin drip is continued for a minimum of 48 hours or until revascularization. Low–molecular-weight heparin (LMWH) (enoxaparin) may be substituted for IV heparin. Therapeutic dosing of LMWH in this patient population should be based on weight. Chapter 33 describes in detail the care of the patient receiving heparin or LMWH.

Percutaneous coronary intervention. **Percutaneous coronary intervention (PCI)** is an invasive but nonsurgical technique that is the treatment of choice to reopen the clotted coronary artery and restore perfusion. The goal is to perform PCI within 90 minutes of an acute STEMI diagnosis. This procedure is associated with excellent return of blood flow through the coronary artery and, when intervention is timely, can decrease the extent of myocardial damage. In addition, this procedure can also reduce the frequency and severity of discomfort for patients with angina and serve as a bridge for patients to CABG surgery.

Percutaneous coronary intervention is performed in the cardiac catheterization laboratory and combines clot retrieval,

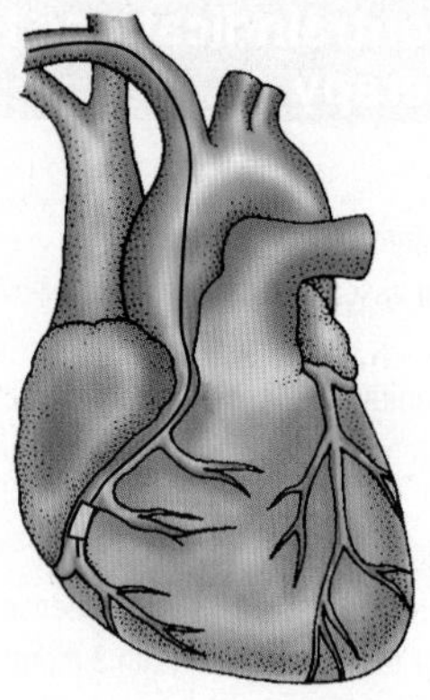

1. The balloon-tipped catheter is positioned in the artery.

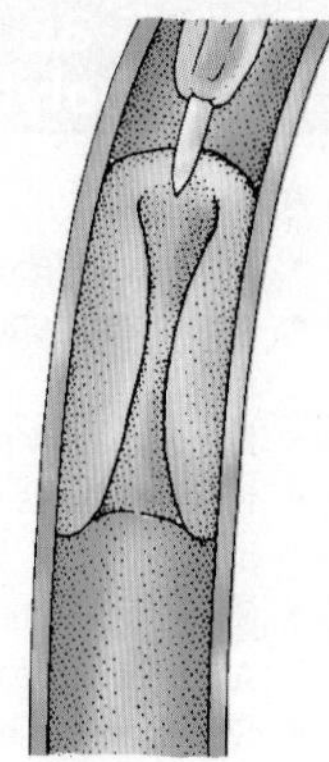

2. The uninflated balloon is centered in the obstruction.

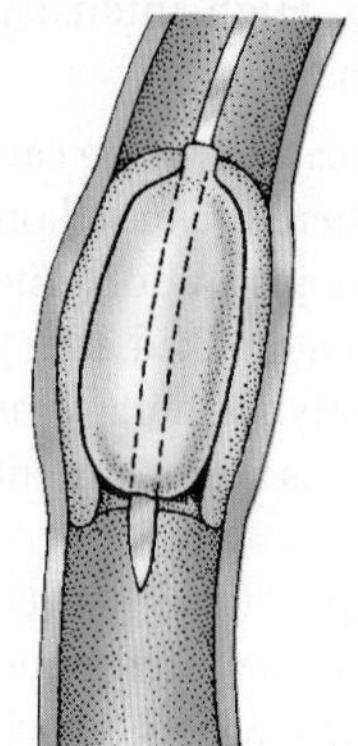

3. The balloon is inflated, which flattens plaque against the artery wall.

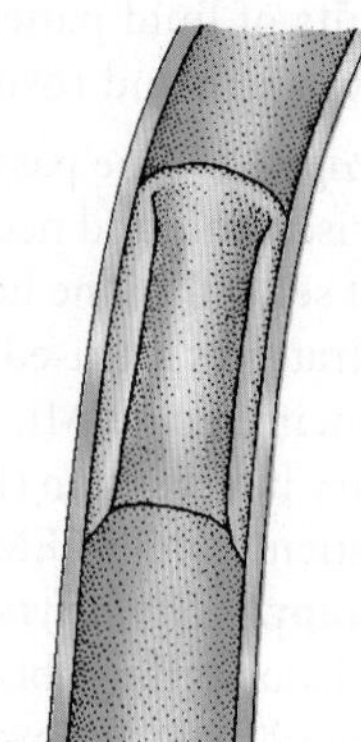

4. The balloon is removed, and the artery is left unoccluded.

Fig. 35.4 Percutaneous coronary intervention.

coronary angioplasty, and stent placement. Under fluoroscopic guidance, the cardiologist performs initial coronary angiography, inserting an arterial sheath and advancing a catheter in a retrograde manner through the aorta (Urden et al., 2018). See Chapter 30 for full discussion of cardiac catheterization. In the STEMI patient, if a clot is seen, a clot retrieval device is inserted over the guidewire, and the clot is removed. Once the clot is removed in the STEMI patient or area of narrowing is identified in the NSTEMI patient, a balloon-tipped catheter is introduced through a guidewire to the coronary artery occlusion. The physician activates a compressor that inflates the balloon (angioplasty) to force the plaque against the vessel wall, thus dilating the wall, and reduces or eliminates the occluding clot. Balloon inflation may be repeated until angiography indicates a decrease in the stenosis (narrowing) to less than 50% of the vessel's diameter (Fig. 35.4). The balloon catheter is then withdrawn, and a balloon catheter with stent is introduced. Once the stent and balloon are in position, the stent is deployed by the balloon inflation. The balloon is deflated and the stent stays in place, acting as scaffolding to hold the diseased artery open. *Stents* are expandable metal mesh devices that are used to maintain the patent lumen created by angioplasty or atherectomy. Bare metal or drug-eluting stents (DESs) (drug coated) may be used. By providing a supportive scaffold, these devices prevent closure of the vessel from arterial dissection or vasospasm. Fig. 35.5 shows a stent positioned in a coronary artery.

During the procedure, the patient may receive boluses of IV heparin or a continuous infusion of bivalirudin (direct thrombin inhibitor). Heparin is used to maintain an elevated activated clotting time and prevent clotting on wires and catheters during the procedure. Heparin or other anticoagulants are usually stopped immediately after the procedure, allowing the access sheath to be removed once the clotting time returns to normal. PCI initially reopens the vessel in most patients. However, within the first 24 hours, a small percentage of patients have restenosis. At 6 months, a larger

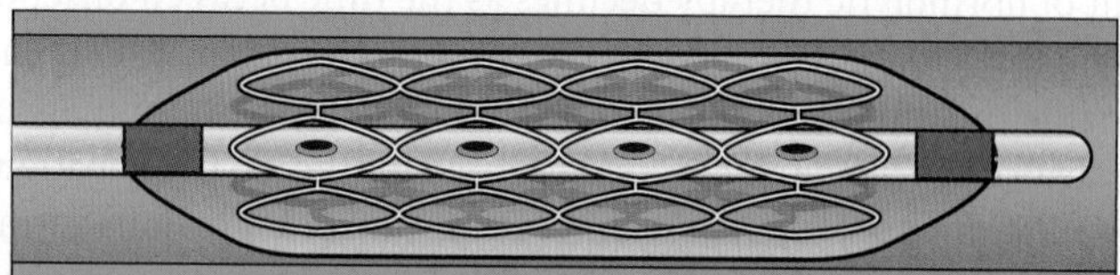

Fig. 35.5 A coronary stent open after balloon inflation.

number have one or more blockages. Without stent placement, the artery often reoccludes because of its normal elasticity and memory.

Patients who are most likely to benefit from PCI have single- or double-vessel disease with discrete, proximal, noncalcified lesions or clots. This procedure often does not work for complex lesions. When identifying which lesions are treatable with PCI, the cardiologist considers the clot's complexity and location and the amount of myocardium at risk. Although treating lesions located in the left main artery places a large amount of myocardial tissue at risk if the vessel closes quickly, these lesions are now being treated more with PCI. In the past, CABG was the intervention used for these patients. PCI can be used for a patient with an evolving acute MI, either alone or with thrombolytic therapy or glycoprotein (GP) IIb/IIIa inhibitor, to reperfuse the damaged myocardium.

Patients who undergo PCI are required to take dual antiplatelet therapy (DAPT) consisting of aspirin and a platelet inhibitor (see the Common Examples of Drug Therapy: Acute Coronary Syndrome [Nitrates, Beta Blockers, Antiplatelets] box). The health care provider also prescribes a long-term nitrate and beta blocker, and an ACEI or ARB is added for patients who have had primary angioplasty after an MI. Some patients may experience hypokalemia after the procedure and require careful monitoring and potassium supplements. The nursing interventions for patients receiving these drugs are described in the Common Examples of Drug Therapy: Acute Coronary Syndrome [Nitrates, Beta Blockers, Antiplatelets] box. Provide careful explanations of drug therapy and any recommended lifestyle changes.

! NURSING SAFETY PRIORITY (QSEN)

Critical Rescue

After PCI, monitor for potential problems, including acute closure of the vessel (causes chest pain and potential ST elevation on 12-lead ECG), bleeding from the insertion (sheath) site, and reaction to the contrast medium used in angiography. Also monitor for and document hypotension, hypokalemia, and dysrhythmias. Document and report any of these findings to the health care provider or Rapid Response Team immediately!

Other Procedures. Other techniques being used to ensure continued patency of the vessel are laser angioplasty (the laser breaks up the clot) and atherectomy. *Atherectomy* devices can either excise and retrieve plaque or emulsify it. One of the advantages of this procedure is that it creates a less bulky vessel with better elastic recoil. However, evidence indicates that atherectomy did not significantly alter the rate of restenosis. Therefore the use of this procedure has declined dramatically (Urden et al., 2018).

For some patients, coronary artery bypass graft (CABG) surgery is required for revascularization. This surgical procedure is discussed in detail later in the chapter.

Identifying and Managing Dysrhythmias

Planning: Expected Outcomes. The desired outcome for the patient is that he or she will be free of dysrhythmias. If dysrhythmias occur, they will be identified and managed early to prevent complications or death.

Interventions. *Dysrhythmias are the leading cause of prehospital death in most patients with ACS.* Even in the early period of hospitalization, most patients with ACS experience some abnormal cardiac rhythm. When a dysrhythmia develops:

- Identify the dysrhythmia.
- Assess hemodynamic status.
- Evaluate for discomfort.

Dysrhythmias are treated when they cause hemodynamic compromise, increase myocardial oxygen requirements, or predispose the patient to lethal ventricular dysrhythmias.

Typical dysrhythmias for the patient with an *inferior* ACS are bradycardias and second-degree atrioventricular (AV) blocks resulting from ischemia of the AV node. These rhythms tend to be intermittent. Monitor the cardiac rhythm and rate and the hemodynamic status. If the patient becomes hemodynamically unstable, a temporary pacemaker may be necessary.

The patient with an *anterior* ACS is likely to exhibit premature ventricular contractions (PVCs) caused by ventricular irritability. Third-degree or bundle branch block is a serious complication in this patient because it indicates that a large portion of the left ventricle is involved. The health care provider may insert a pacemaker. Observe the patient closely to detect the development of heart failure. Appropriate interventions for dysrhythmias are described in Chapter 31.

Monitoring for and Managing Heart Failure

Planning: Expected Outcomes. The desired outcome for the patient is that he or she will be free of heart failure. However, if it occurs, the outcome is that the heart failure will be identified and treated early to prevent further complications.

Interventions. Decreased cardiac output due to heart failure is a relatively common complication after an MI resulting from left ventricular dysfunction, rupture of the intraventricular septum, papillary muscle rupture with valvular dysfunction, or right ventricular infarction. The most severe form of acute heart failure, *cardiogenic shock,* discussed later in this chapter, causes most in-hospital deaths after an ACS. The type of management used to increase cardiac output depends on the location of the ACS and the type of heart failure that resulted from the infarction.

Managing Left Ventricular Failure. When a patient with ACS experiences damage to the left ventricle, rupture of the intraventricular septum, or tear of a papillary muscle, the amount of blood that the heart can eject is reduced. When volume and pressure are markedly increased in the pulmonary vasculature, pulmonary complications can develop.

Assess for manifestations of left ventricular failure and pulmonary edema by listening for crackles and identifying their location in the lung fields. Wheezing, tachypnea, and frothy sputum may also occur with pulmonary edema. Auscultate the heart, paying particular attention to the presence of an S_3 heart sound.

! NURSING SAFETY PRIORITY (QSEN)

Critical Rescue

Monitor for, report, and document these signs of inadequate organ ***perfusion*** that may result from decreased cardiac output:

- A change in orientation or mental status
- Urine output less than 0.5 to 1 mL/kg/hr
- Cool, clammy extremities with decreased or absent pulses
- Unusual fatigue
- Recurrent chest pain

Hemodynamic monitoring. *Hemodynamic monitoring* is a term that refers to a variety of monitoring techniques designed to provide quantitative information about vascular capacity, blood volume, pump effectiveness, and tissue ***perfusion.*** The type of monitoring can vary from noninvasive to highly invasive. Historically, hemodynamic monitoring was always invasive; however, newer technology is fostering the development of noninvasive and less invasive methodology. For example, the finger cuff hemodynamic monitoring systems provide noninvasive continuous monitoring of stroke volume, cardiac output, and blood pressure (Urden et al., 2018).

Invasive hemodynamic monitoring directly measures pressures in the heart and great vessels. These procedures are usually performed for more seriously ill patients and can provide more accurate measurements of blood pressure, heart function, and volume status. Although medical-surgical nurses do not manage these systems on general hospital units, they should be familiar with the interpretation of some of the major hemodynamic pressures as they relate to patient assessment.

Invasive hemodynamic monitoring does involve significant risks; informed consent is therefore required. After obtaining consent, the critical care nurse prepares a pressure-monitoring system. The components of this system are a catheter with an infusion system, a transducer, and a monitor. The catheter receives the pressure waves (mechanical energy) from the heart or the great vessels. The transducer converts the mechanical energy into electrical energy, which is displayed as waveforms or numbers on the monitor. Patency of the catheter is maintained with a slow continuous flush of normal saline, usually infused at 3 to 4 mL/hr under pressure to prevent the backup of blood and occlusion of the catheter.

Because this system is designed to measure pressure, it is important to account for atmospheric pressure (calibration) and hydrostatic pressure associated with the level of the transducer. To prepare the transducer, balance and calibrate it according to hospital policy and the manufacturer's specifications. Finally, identify the phlebostatic axis, a physical reference point on the chest, and level the transducer to this point. See the Best Practice for Patient Safety & Quality Care box for identification of the phlebostatic axis.

For intra-arterial blood pressure monitoring, a catheter is usually inserted into the radial artery. After the catheter is inserted, it is attached to pressure tubing. A normal saline flush solution is infused constantly under pressure to maintain the integrity of the system. A transducer attached to the tubing allows continuous direct monitoring of the arterial BP. Direct measurements of BP are usually 10 to 15 mm Hg greater than indirect (cuff) measurements. The arterial catheter may also be used to obtain blood samples for arterial blood gas values and other blood tests.

BEST PRACTICE FOR PATIENT SAFETY & QUALITY CARE (QSEN)

Identification of the Phlebostatic Axis

1. Position the patient supine.
2. Palpate the fourth intercostal space at the sternum.
3. Follow the fourth intercostal space to the side of the patient's chest.
4. Determine the midway point between anterior and posterior.
5. Find the intersection between the midway point and the line from the fourth intercostal space and mark it with an X in indelible ink. This is the phlebostatic axis.

Because the arterial vasculature is a high-pressure system, frequent assessment of the arterial site and infusion system is essential. *Note any bleeding around the intra-arterial catheter or any loose connections and correct the situation immediately.* Collateral circulation must be assessed by Doppler before and while the arterial catheter is in place. Carefully monitor color, pulse, and temperature distal to the insertion site for any early signs of circulatory compromise. Complications of intra-arterial monitoring include pain, infection, arteriospasm, or obstruction at the site with the potential for distal infarction, air embolism, and hemorrhage.

A more invasive form of hemodynamic monitoring is catheter placement within the central veins (central venous catheter) or catheters that pass through the heart chambers (Urden et al., 2018). The central venous catheter is used for the critically ill patient to monitor the central venous pressure (CVP). The CVP is an indicator of fluid volume status. Normal CVP is 2 to 5 mm Hg (Urden et al., 2018).

The most invasive form of hemodynamic monitoring is the pulmonary artery (PA) catheter (sometimes referred to as a Swan-Ganz catheter). This is a multilumen catheter with the capacity to measure right atrial pressures, pulmonary artery pressures (PAPs), pulmonary artery occlusion pressure (PAOP; also called *wedge pressure*), and cardiac output. The physician inserts a balloon-tipped catheter percutaneously through a large vein, usually the internal jugular or subclavian, and directs it to the right atrium (RA). When the catheter tip reaches the RA, the balloon is inflated. The catheter advances with the flow of blood through the tricuspid valve, into the right ventricle, past the pulmonic valve, and into a branch of the pulmonary artery. The balloon is deflated after the catheter tip reaches the pulmonary artery. Waveforms are viewed on the monitor as the pulmonary artery catheter is advanced (Fig. 35.6). A chest x-ray is used to check the location of the catheter.

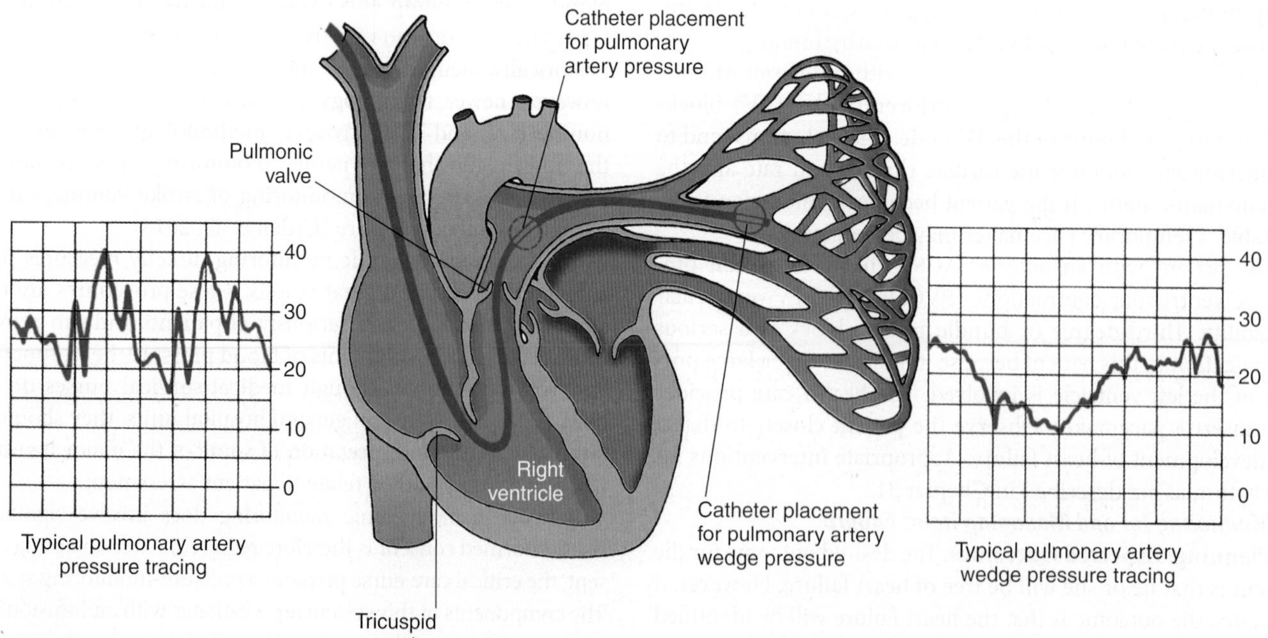

Fig. 35.6 Cardiac pressure waveforms can be seen on the monitor.

Right atrial pressure is measured by a pressure sensor on the catheter inside the right atrium (RA). Normal RA pressure ranges from 0 to 8 mm Hg (McCance & Huether, 2019). Increased RA pressures may occur with right ventricular failure, whereas low RA pressures usually indicate hypovolemia. Pulmonary artery pressure (PAP) is also assessed and is constantly visible on most hemodynamic monitors. Normal PAP ranges from 15 to 30 mm Hg systolic to 3 to 12 mm Hg diastolic (McCance & Huether, 2019). When the balloon at the catheter tip is inflated, the catheter advances and wedges in a branch of the pulmonary artery. The tip of the catheter can sense pressures transmitted from the left atrium, which reflect left ventricular end-diastolic pressure (LVEDP). The pressure measured during balloon inflation is called the **pulmonary artery occlusion pressure (PAOP),** also referred to as a *wedge pressure* because the balloon is wedged within the small vessel (Urden et al., 2018). Normal PAOP ranges from 5 to 12 mm Hg (Urden et al., 2018). Elevated PAOP measurements may indicate left ventricular failure, hypervolemia, mitral regurgitation, or intracardiac shunting. A decreased PAOP is seen with hypovolemia or afterload reduction.

The critical care nurse obtains and records RA pressure, PAP, and PAOP at appropriate intervals (usually every 1 to 4 hours). Single values of these measurements are less significant than the trend of values combined with the patient's signs and symptoms. Change the occlusive sterile dressing over the catheter according to hospital policy. Inspect the insertion site for redness, induration, swelling, drainage, and intactness of the sutures. Detailed discussion of the management and care of patients with pulmonary artery catheters can be found in textbooks on critical care nursing.

Historically, the PA catheter has been a routine approach for critically ill patients. However, evidence now indicates that the risk associated with the invasive nature of the PA catheter does not correlate with increased survival or better patient outcomes. As a result, the use of the PA catheter has dramatically decreased in practice, with routine use occurring only during and immediately after coronary surgery (Urden et al., 2018). Be sure to assess for risks and complications associated with pulmonary artery catheters. For example, pulmonary infarction or pulmonary rupture can occur if the catheter remains in the wedge position. Air embolism is possible if the balloon has ruptured and repeated inflation attempts are made. Ventricular dysrhythmias may occur during insertion or if the catheter tip slips back into the right ventricle and irritates the myocardium. Thrombus and embolus formation may occur at the catheter site. Infection may result, and bleeding may be pronounced if the infusion system becomes disconnected.

Classification of post–myocardial infarction heart failure. Several classification systems may be used to categorize heart failure after an MI. For example, the classic Killip system identifies four classes based on prognosis (Table 35.3). This system complements the ACC/AHA heart failure classification of function assessment discussed in Chapter 32.

Patients with *class I* heart failure often respond well to reduction in preload with IV nitrates and diuretics. Monitor the urine output hourly, check vital signs hourly, continue to assess for signs of heart failure, and review the serum potassium level.

Patients with *class II* and *class III* heart failure may require diuresis and more aggressive medical intervention, such as afterload reduction and/or enhancement of contractility. IV nitroprusside or nitroglycerin may be used to decrease both preload and afterload. These drugs are given as continuous infusions in specialized units where hemodynamic monitoring can occur. Intra-arterial BP monitoring is preferred for nitroprusside administration (Colucci, 2019).

Patients in *classes II* and *III* are usually started on once-a-day beta blockers. Dosing is titrated, depending on goal achievement and drug tolerance. Other drugs, including ACEIs and ARBs, are commonly prescribed to inhibit ventricular remodeling (see Fig 35.3). These drugs are described in the Common Examples of Drug Therapy: Commonly Used Intravenous Vasodilators and Inotropes box and Chapter 32.

! NURSING SAFETY PRIORITY (QSEN)

Drug Alert

Use caution when giving positive inotropes because of the potential risk for increasing myocardial oxygen consumption and further decreasing cardiac output. Monitor the patient frequently, paying particular attention to the development of chest pain.

Class IV heart failure is cardiogenic shock. In cardiogenic shock, necrosis of more than 40% of the left ventricle occurs. Most patients have a stuttering pattern of chest pain, resulting in extension of the ACS.

! NURSING SAFETY PRIORITY (QSEN)

Critical Rescue

Monitor for, report, and document manifestations of cardiogenic shock immediately. These signs and symptoms include:

- Tachycardia
- Hypotension
- Systolic BP less than 90 mm Hg or 30 mm Hg less than the patient's baseline
- Urine output less than 0.5-1 mL/kg/hr
- Cold, clammy skin with poor peripheral pulses
- Agitation, restlessness, or confusion
- Pulmonary congestion
- Tachypnea
- Continuing chest discomfort

Early detection is essential because undiagnosed cardiogenic shock has a high mortality rate!

TABLE 35.3 Killip Classification of Heart Failure

Class	Description
I	Absent crackles and S_3
II	Crackles in the lower half of the lung fields and possible S_3
III	Crackles more than halfway up the lung fields and frequent pulmonary edema
IV	Cardiogenic shock

COMMON EXAMPLES OF DRUG THERAPY

Commonly Used Intravenous Vasodilators and Inotropes

Drug Category	Selected Nursing Implications
Nitrates	
Nitroprusside sodium	This agent is a potent, rapidly reversible vasodilator acting on both peripheral venous and arterial musculature. • Monitor BP every 2-5 minutes when initiating therapy. • Monitor PAOP, SVR, BP, heart rate, urine output frequently. Titrate medication to obtain the desired effect. Protect from light *because this medication is light sensitive.* Administered in micrograms per kilograms per minute (mcg/kg/min). Higher doses are associated with thiocyanate or cyanide toxicity. • Monitor for metabolic acidosis, confusion, and hyperreflexia, *which are symptoms of toxicity.*
Nitroglycerin	This agent produces systemic vasodilation and dilates coronary arteries rapidly. • Monitor BP every 1-3 minutes when initiating therapy *because BP may drop in 1 minute.* • Monitor RAP, PAOP, SVR, BP, HR, and urine output frequently. • Assess for headache *because this is a frequent side effect of initial therapy.* • Tolerance to this agent can develop with continued administration.
Milrinone Fenoldopam	Assess BP and HR every 5 minutes *because hypotension is a common adverse effect.* • If systolic BP drops 30 mm Hg, stop infusion and call the health care provider. Monitor I&O and weight *because this drug causes diuresis.*
Sympathomimetics	
Dopamine	This agent is a dose-dependent activator of alpha, beta, and dopaminergic receptors. • Assess reason for use and expected result. • Observe HR, BP, PAOP, SVR, cardiac output, and urine output every 5 minutes to 1 hour. • Titrate dosage to maintain dose range and obtain the desired effect. • Infuse through central line *because extravasation can cause tissue necrosis and sloughing.* • Monitor for ectopy and angina.
Dobutamine	Observe patients continuously during administration *because this agent is a very strong beta$_1$-receptor activator and a moderately strong beta$_2$-receptor activator.* • Titrate the drug on the basis of adequate tissue perfusion: mentation, skin temperature, peripheral pulses, PAOP, cardiac output, SVR, and urine output. Monitor for atrial and ventricular ectopy *because dysrhythmias are an adverse effect.*

BP, Blood pressure; *HR,* heart rate; *I&O,* input and output; *PAOP,* pulmonary artery occlusion pressure; *RAP,* right atrial pressure; *SVR,* systemic vascular resistance.

Drug therapy. Medical interventions aim to relieve pain and decrease myocardial oxygen requirements through preload and afterload reduction. The health care provider prescribes IV morphine, which is used to decrease pulmonary congestion and relieve pain. Oxygen is administered. Intubation and mechanical ventilation may be necessary.

Use the information gained from hemodynamic monitoring to titrate drug therapy. Preload reduction may be attempted cautiously with diuretics or nitroglycerin, as described for patients with Killip class III heart failure. (See Chapter 32 for a complete discussion of preload and afterload.) Monitor systolic pressure continuously because vasodilation may result in a further decline in BP. Vasopressors and positive inotropes may be used to maintain organ perfusion, but these drugs increase myocardial oxygen consumption and can worsen ischemia. Use extreme caution in giving drug therapy.

Other interventions for left-sided heart failure. When patients do not respond to drug therapy with improved tissue perfusion, decreased workload of the heart, and increased cardiac contractility, mechanical circulatory support, such as an **intra-aortic balloon pump (IABP)** may be inserted. The IABP is a temporary, invasive, percutaneous intervention that is used to improve myocardial ***perfusion*** during an acute MI, reduce preload and afterload, and facilitate left ventricular ejection.

The health care provider can insert the device percutaneously. Inflation of the IABP during diastole augments the diastolic pressure and improves coronary perfusion by increasing blood flow to the arteries. Deflation of the balloon just before systole reduces afterload at the time of systolic contraction. This action facilitates emptying of the left ventricle and improves cardiac output. The balloon catheter is attached to a pump console, which is triggered by an ECG tracing and arterial waveform.

In patients undergoing high-risk percutaneous coronary intervention (PCI) or those at risk for cardiogenic shock, a *percutaneous ventricular assist device* may be used. These devices are used temporarily to decrease the myocardial workload and oxygen consumption of the heart and increase cardiac output and peripheral perfusion.

Immediate reperfusion is an invasive intervention that shows some promise for managing cardiogenic shock. The patient is taken to the cardiac catheterization laboratory, and an emergency left-sided heart catheterization is performed. If he or she has a treatable occlusion or occlusions, the interventional cardiologist performs a

PCI in the catheterization laboratory, or the patient is transferred to the operating suite for a coronary artery bypass graft (CABG).

Managing Right Ventricular Failure. Conditions other than left ventricular failure may result in decreased cardiac output after an ACS. In about a third of patients with inferior MIs, right ventricular infarction and failure develop. In this instance, the right ventricle fails independently of the left. Decreased cardiac output with a paradoxical pulse, clear lungs, and jugular venous distention occurs when the patient is in semi-Fowler position.

The desired outcome of management is to improve right ventricular stroke volume by increasing right ventricular fiber stretch or preload. To enhance right ventricular preload, give sufficient fluids to increase right atrial pressure to 20 mm Hg. In the critical care unit, *monitor the pulmonary artery occlusion pressure (PAOP), and auscultate the lungs to assess for left-sided heart failure. If symptoms of this complication occur, notify the health care provider immediately.* If medical therapy is not sufficient to support the right ventricle and reverse the shock state, a *right percutaneous ventricular assist device* may be needed. This is a temporary measure to support the failing heart while treating the cardiogenic shock with medical therapy.

Coronary Artery Bypass Graft Surgery. While the traditional coronary artery bypass graft (CABG) surgery has declined somewhat due to newer options in percutaneous coronary interventions, there are still over 371,000 traditional open CABG surgeries performed in the United States each year (Benjamin et al., 2018). It is the most common type of cardiac surgery and the most common procedure for older adults. Almost half of all CABGs are done for patients older than 65 years. The occluded coronary arteries are bypassed with the patient's own venous or arterial blood vessels or synthetic grafts. The internal thoracic artery (also referred to as the internal mammary artery [IMA]) is often the graft of choice because it has an excellent patency rate many years after the procedure. Arterial grafts are generally more durable than venous grafts.

CABG is indicated when patients do not respond to medical management of CAD or when disease progression is evident. Because of the development of drug-eluting stents (DESs), patients who previously had no option other than CABG have been able to have their vessels revascularized without surgery. The decision for surgery is based on the patient's symptoms and the results of cardiac catheterization. Candidates for surgery are patients who have:

- Angina with greater than 50% occlusion of the left main coronary artery that cannot be stented
- Unstable angina with severe two-vessel disease, moderate three-vessel disease, or small-vessel disease in which stents could not be introduced
- Ischemia with heart failure
- Acute MI with cardiogenic shock
- Signs of ischemia or impending MI after angiography or percutaneous coronary intervention
- Valvular disease
- Coronary vessels unsuitable for PCI

CABG is most effective when adequate ventricular function remains and the ejection fraction is close to or greater than 50%. Patients with lower ejection fractions are subject to develop more complications. For most patients, the risk is low, and the benefits of bypass surgery are clear. Surgical treatment of CAD does not appear to affect the life span. Left ventricular function is the most important long-term indicator of survival. CABG improves the quality of life for most patients. Most are pain free 1 year after surgery and remain so 5 years after the procedure. The percentage of patients experiencing some pain increases sharply after 5 years.

Preoperative care. CABG surgery may be planned as an elective procedure or performed as an emergency. It may be done as a *traditional* operative technique or as *minimally invasive surgery (MIS),* discussed later in this chapter. Patients undergoing elective surgery are admitted on the morning of surgery. Preoperative preparations and teaching are completed during prehospitalization interviews. Teach patients that their drugs will be changed after surgery. Ensure that the necessary drugs have been administered before surgery.

One potential complication of CABG is sternal wound infection. To decrease risk, have the patient shower with 4% chlorhexidine gluconate (CHG). This decreases the number of microorganisms on the skin. Surgical sites are prepared by clipping hair and applying CHG with isopropyl alcohol (either 0.5% or 2%). In addition, IV antibiotics are administered 1 hour before the surgical procedure.

Familiarize the patient and family with the cardiac surgical–critical care unit (sometimes referred to as the *open heart unit*) and prepare them for postoperative care. If the procedure is elective, demonstrate and have the patient return a demonstration of how to splint the chest incision, cough, deep breathe, and perform arm and leg exercises. Stress that:

- The patient should report any ***pain*** to the nursing staff.
- Most of the pain will be in the site where the vessel was harvested. (With the use of endovascular vessel harvesting [EVH] and one or two small incisions, the pain and edema are less than for previously performed procedures.)
- Analgesics will be given to decrease pain.
- Coughing and deep breathing are essential to prevent pulmonary complications.
- Early ambulation is important to decrease the risk for venous thrombosis and possible embolism.

For the traditional surgical procedure, explain that the patient will have a sternal incision; possibly a large leg incision; one, two, or three chest tubes; an indwelling urinary catheter; pacemaker wires; and invasive hemodynamic monitoring. An endotracheal tube will be connected to a ventilator during surgery. The endotracheal tube is removed as soon as the patient is awake and stable. Tell the patient and family that the patient will not be able to talk while the endotracheal tube is in place. When describing the postoperative course, emphasize that close monitoring and the use of sophisticated equipment are standard treatment.

Preoperative anxiety is common and can negatively affect postoperative outcomes. An appropriate nursing assessment should identify the level of anxiety and the coping methods that patients have used successfully in the past. Some patients may find it helpful to define their fears. Common sources of fear

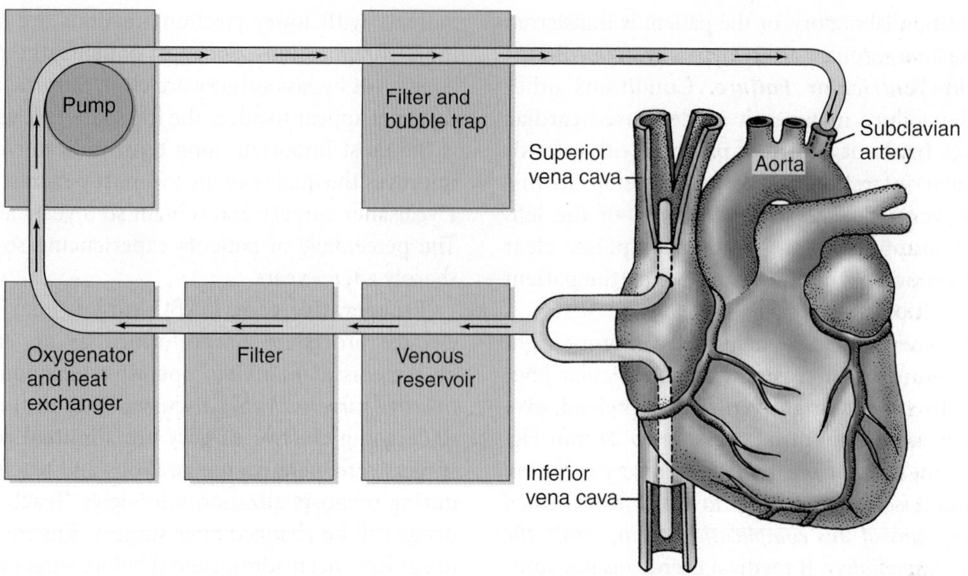

Fig. 35.7 Heart-lung bypass circuitry used during cardiopulmonary bypass.

include fear of the unknown, fear of bodily harm, and fear of death.

In elective procedures, patients may benefit from detailed information about the surgery, depending on individual preferences and cultural practices. Others may feel overwhelmed by so much material. Some patients need to discuss their feelings in detail or describe the experiences of people they know who have undergone CABG. Assess patients' anxiety level and help them cope.

Operative procedures. Coronary artery bypass surgery is performed with the patient under general anesthesia for both cardiopulmonary bypass (CPB) and off-pump surgery. For the *traditional operative procedure,* the cardiac surgical team begins the procedure with a median sternotomy incision and visualization of the heart and great vessels. Another surgical team may begin harvesting the vein if it is to be used for the graft. Synthetic grafts may be used instead.

Cardiopulmonary bypass (CPB) is used to provide oxygenation, circulation, and hypothermia during induced cardiac arrest. Blood is diverted from the heart to the bypass machine, where it is heparinized, oxygenated, and returned to the circulation through a cannula placed in the ascending aortic arch or femoral artery (Fig. 35.7). During bypass, the patient's core temperature remains between 95°F (35°C) (cold cardioplegia) and normal temperature (warm cardioplegia). Although cooling decreases the rate of metabolism and demand for oxygen, keeping the heart "warm" decreases postoperative complications that were more common when cold cardioplegia was used. The heart is perfused with a potassium solution, which decreases myocardial oxygen consumption and causes the heart to stop during diastole. This process ensures a motionless operative field and prevents myocardial ischemia.

Once the heart is arrested, the grafting procedure can begin. The surgeon uses the internal mammary artery (IMA), a saphenous vein, and/or a radial artery to bypass blockages in the coronary arteries (Fig. 35.8). The distal end of the vessel graft is dissected and attached below the clot in the coronary artery. If the surgeon uses a venous graft or the radial artery, it is anastomosed (sutured) proximally to the aorta and distally to the coronary artery just beyond the occlusion, thus improving myocardial perfusion. After flow rates through the grafts are measured, the heart is rewarmed slowly. The cardioplegic solution is flushed from the heart. The heart regains its rate and rhythm, or it may be defibrillated to return it to a normal rhythm. When the procedure is completed, the patient may be rewarmed (if cold cardioplegia was used) and weaned from the bypass machine while the grafts are observed for patency and leakage. The surgeon may place atrial and ventricular pacemaker wires and mediastinal and pleural chest tubes. Finally the surgeon closes the sternum with wire sutures.

Postoperative care. After traditional surgery, the patient is transported to a post–open heart surgery unit. He or she requires highly skilled nursing care from a nurse qualified to provide post–cardiac surgery care, including routine postoperative care described in Chapter 9. *Be sure to use sterile technique when changing sternal or donor-site dressings.* Interventions to prevent surgical site infections are listed in Box 35.1.

Connect the mediastinal tubes to water-seal drainage systems and ground the epicardial pacing wires by connecting them to the pacemaker generator. The cardiac nurse will monitor pulmonary artery and arterial pressures, as well as the heart rate and rhythm, which are displayed on a hemodynamic cardiac monitor.

Closely assess the patient for dysrhythmias, such as bradydysrhythmias, atrial fibrillation, or heart block. Manage symptomatic dysrhythmias according to unit protocol or the health care provider's prescription. Hypoxemia and hypokalemia are frequent causes of ventricular dysrhythmias. If the patient has symptomatic bradydysrhythmias or heart block, turn on the pacemaker and adjust the pacemaker settings as prescribed. Monitor for, report, and document other complications of CABG, including:

- Fluid and electrolyte imbalance
- Hypotension
- Hypothermia
- Hypertension
- Bleeding

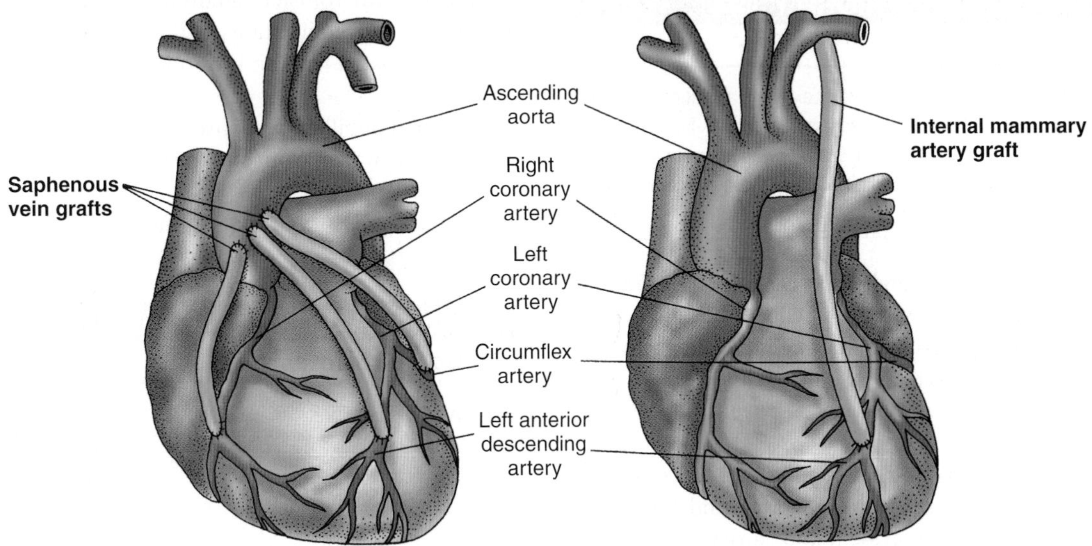

Fig. 35.8 Two methods of coronary artery bypass graft. The procedure used depends on the nature of the coronary artery disease, the condition of the vessels available for grafting, and the patient's health status.

- Cardiac tamponade
- Decreased level of consciousness
- Anginal pain

Managing fluid and electrolyte imbalance. *Assessing fluid and electrolyte balance is a high priority in the early postoperative period.* Edema is common. However, decisions concerning fluid administration are made on the basis of BP, pulmonary artery occlusion pressure (PAOP), right atrial pressure, cardiac output, cardiac index, systemic vascular resistance, blood loss, and urine output. An experienced specialized nurse interprets the assessment findings and adjusts fluid administration on the basis of standing unit policies or specific prescription from the health care provider.

Serum electrolytes (especially calcium, magnesium, and potassium) may be decreased after surgery and are monitored carefully. Because the serum potassium level can fluctuate dramatically, electrolyte levels are checked frequently, since imbalances can cause dysrhythmias. Potassium and magnesium depletions are common and may result from hemodilution or diuretic therapy.

Managing other complications. Hypotension (systolic BP <90 mm Hg) is a major problem because it may result in the collapse of the coronary graft. Decreased preload can result from hypovolemia or vasodilation. If the patient is hypovolemic, it might be appropriate to increase fluid administration or administer blood. The health care provider may manage the patient with volume replacement followed by vasopressor therapy to increase the BP. However, if hypotension is the result of left ventricular failure, IV inotropes might be needed.

Hypothermia is a common problem after surgery. Although warm cardioplegia is now the usual operative procedure used, it is not uncommon for the body temperature to drift downward after the patient leaves the surgical suite. Monitor the body temperature and institute rewarming procedures if the temperature drops below 96.8°F (36°C). Rewarming may be accomplished with warm blankets, lights, or thermal blankets. The danger of rewarming patients too quickly is that they may begin shivering, resulting in metabolic acidosis, increased myocardial oxygen consumption, and hypoxia. To prevent shivering, rewarming should proceed at a rate no faster than 1.8°F (1°C) per hour. Discontinue the procedure when the body temperature approaches 98.6°F (37°C) and the patient's extremities feel warm.

Hypothermia is a significant risk for the patient after CABG surgery because it promotes vasoconstriction and *hypertension.* Other factors contributing to hypertension in the CABG patient include CPB, drug therapy, and increased sympathetic nervous system activity.

After surgery, many patients experience *hypertension* (hypertension is defined as a systolic BP greater than 140 to 150 mm Hg). Hypertension is dangerous because increased pressure promotes leakage from suture lines and may cause bleeding. Drugs such as nitroprusside or fenoldopam may be given to decrease afterload, ease the workload of the heart, and prevent heart failure.

BOX 35.1 Interventions to Reduce Surgical Site Infections

- If possible, treat any underlying infections prior to surgical procedure.
- Have patient shower or bathe with soap or antiseptic agent the night before surgery. Chlorhexidine gluconate for skin preparation is recommended (Seifert, 2017).
- If hair removal is necessary, clip hair immediately prior to the procedure.
- Preoperative antibiotics or antimicrobials are used prior to skin incision.
- Use an alcohol-based antiseptic agent to prepare skin prior to incision.
- Antimicrobial agents should not be applied to incision sites.
- Maintain perioperative glucose levels <200 mg/dL even in those patients without a history of diabetes mellitus.
- Maintain normothermia.

Data from Berrios-Torres, S., Umscheid, C., Bratzler, D., Leas, B., Stone, E., Kelz, R., et al. (2017). Centers for Disease Control and Prevention guidelines for the prevention of surgical site infections, 2017. *JAMA: The Journal of the American Medical Association, 152*(8), 784–791; and Seifert, P. (2017). Reducing readmissions after coronary artery bypass grafting. *AORN Journal, 106*(4), 332–337.

! NURSING SAFETY PRIORITY QSEN

Action Alert

Bleeding after CABG surgery occurs to a limited extent in all patients. Measure mediastinal and pleural chest tube drainage at least hourly. Report drainage amounts over 150 mL/hr to the surgeon. Patients with internal mammary artery (IMA) grafts may have more chest drainage than those with saphenous vein grafts (from the leg).

To access the IMA, the pleural space has to be entered and requires a pleural chest tube with the mediastinal tubes, making pulmonary assessment crucial. Maintain the patency of the mediastinal and pleural chest tubes. One effective way of promoting chest tube drainage is to prevent a dependent loop from forming in the tubing.

If the patient is bleeding and the mediastinal tubes are not kept patent, fluid (blood) may accumulate around the heart. The myocardium is then compressed, and cardiac tamponade results. The fluid compresses the atria and ventricles, preventing them from filling adequately and thus reducing cardiac output.

! NURSING SAFETY PRIORITY QSEN

Critical Rescue

Assess for, document, and report manifestations of cardiac tamponade immediately, including:

- Sudden cessation of previously heavy mediastinal drainage
- Beck triad:
  - Jugular venous distention but clear lung sounds
  - Distant, muffled heart sounds
  - Hypotension
- Pulsus paradoxus (BP more than 10 mm Hg higher on expiration than on inspiration)
- An equalizing of PAOP and right atrial pressure
- Cardiovascular collapse

Prepare the patient for echocardiogram or chest x-ray to confirm the diagnosis. Pericardiocentesis (withdrawal of fluid from the pericardium via a large needle) may not be appropriate for tamponade after CABG because the blood in the pericardium may have clotted. Volume expansion and emergency sternotomy with drainage are the treatments of choice.

The patient may also demonstrate *changes in level of consciousness,* which may be permanent or transient (temporary, short-term). Transient changes related to anesthesia, cardiopulmonary bypass (CPB), air emboli, or hypothermia occur in many patients. Assess for neurologic deficits, which may include slowness to arouse, memory loss, and new-onset confusion.

! NURSING SAFETY PRIORITY QSEN

Action Alert

After a CABG, check the patient's neurologic status every 30 to 60 minutes until he or she has awakened from anesthesia. Then check every 2 to 4 hours or per agency policy.

Patients with transient neurologic deficits usually return to baseline neurologic status within 4 to 8 hours. *Permanent* deficits associated with an intraoperative stroke may manifest with:

- Abnormal pupillary response
- Failure to awaken from anesthesia
- Seizures
- Absence of sensory or motor function

NCLEX EXAMINATION CHALLENGE 35.3

Physiological Integrity

The nurse is assessing a client who had a coronary artery bypass graft yesterday. Which assessment finding indicates the client is at risk for decreased perfusion?

A. Heart rate of 50 beats/min
B. Potassium level of 4.2 mEq/L
C. Systolic blood pressure of 120 mm/Hg
D. 50 mL of bloody drainage in chest tube over 4 hours

Managing pain. Differentiate between *sternotomy pain,* which is expected after CABG, and *anginal pain,* which might indicate graft failure. Typical sternotomy pain is localized, does not radiate, and often becomes worse when the patient coughs or breathes deeply. He or she may describe the pain as sharp, aching, or burning. Pain may stimulate the sympathetic nervous system, which increases the heart rate and vascular resistance while decreasing cardiac output. Administer enough of the prescribed analgesic in adequate doses to control ***pain.*** However, during the process of weaning the patient from mechanical ventilation, it may be necessary to use short-acting analgesics and limit pain medication because of the respiratory depressant effects of analgesia.

Transfer from the special care unit. Mechanical ventilation is continued until the patient is breathing adequately and is hemodynamically stable (usually 3 to 6 hours after surgery). During the first day, the patient usually has pacemaker wires, hemodynamic monitoring lines, and mediastinal tubes removed. He or she is then transferred to an intermediate care unit. *All CABG patients, especially those with IMA grafts, are at high risk for atelectasis, the number-one complication.* Encourage the patient to splint, cough, turn, and deep breathe to expectorate secretions. Early ambulation after surgery is essential. Two hours after extubation (removal of the endotracheal tube), patients should be dangled at the bedside as tolerated and turned side to side. Within 4 to 8 hours after extubation, help patients out of bed into a chair. By the first day after surgery, they should be out of bed in a chair and ambulating 25 to 100 feet three times a day as tolerated. Continue to monitor for decreased cardiac output, pain, dysrhythmias, decreased oxygen saturation, and infection during these activities. Older adults may progress more slowly and are subject to additional risks. The Patient-Centered Care: Older Adult Considerations: Coronary Artery Bypass Graft Surgery box focuses on care of the older-adult population following CABG.

PATIENT-CENTERED CARE: OLDER ADULT CONSIDERATIONS QSEN

Coronary Artery Bypass Graft Surgery

- Be aware that perioperative mortality rates are higher for the older patient than for the patient younger than 60 years.
- Monitor neurologic and mental status carefully because older adults are more likely to have transient neurologic deficits after coronary artery bypass graft (CABG) surgery than younger adults are.
- Observe for side effects of cardiac drugs because older patients are more likely to develop toxic effects from positive inotropes (dobutamine) and potent antihypertensives (nitroglycerin or nitroprusside).
- Monitor the patient closely for dysrhythmias because older adults are more likely to have dysrhythmias such as atrial fibrillation or supraventricular tachycardia after CABG surgery.
- Be aware that recuperation after CABG surgery is slower for older patients and that their average hospital stay is longer.
- Teach the patient and family that during the first 2 to 5 weeks after discharge, fatigue, chest discomfort, and lack of appetite may be particularly bothersome for older adults.

NURSING SAFETY PRIORITY QSEN

Action Alert

With each increase in patient activity, assess the patient's heart rate, blood pressure (BP), respiratory rate, and level of fatigue. Decreases greater than 20 mm Hg in the systolic BP, changes of 20 beats/min in the pulse rate, and/or reports of dyspnea or chest pain indicate intolerance of activity. If these manifestations develop, notify the health care provider and do not advance the patient to the next level.

NURSING SAFETY PRIORITY QSEN

Action Alert

Monitor the neurovascular status of the donor arm of patients whose radial artery was used as a graft in CABG (usually the nondominant arm is used). Assess the hand color, temperature, pulse (both ulnar and radial), and capillary refill every hour initially. In addition, check the fingertips, hand, and arm for sensation and mobility at least every 4 hours. IV nitroglycerin is often given for the first 24 hours after surgery to promote vasodilation in the donor arm and therefore maintain circulation.

Many patients have supraventricular dysrhythmias (especially atrial fibrillation) during the postoperative period, usually on the second or third postoperative day. Examine the monitor pattern for atrial fibrillation. When auscultating the heart, listen for an irregular rhythm.

Sternal wound infections develop between 5 days and several weeks after surgery in a small number of patients and are responsible for increased costs and longer hospital stays. Be alert for mediastinitis (infection of the mediastinum) by observing for:

- Fever continuing beyond the first 4 days after CABG
- Instability (bogginess) of the sternum
- Redness, induration, swelling, or drainage from suture sites
- An increased white blood cell count

The health care provider may perform a needle biopsy to confirm a sternal infection. Surgical débridement, antibiotic wound irrigation, and IV antibiotics are usually indicated. If sternal osteomyelitis has developed, 4 to 6 weeks of IV antibiotics are required. Prophylactic use of mupirocin intranasally may be prescribed to decrease the incidence of sternal wound infection.

Postpericardiotomy syndrome is a source of chest discomfort for some post–cardiac surgery patients. The syndrome is characterized by pericardial and pleural pain, pericarditis, a friction rub, elevated temperature and white blood cell count, and dysrhythmias. Postpericardiotomy syndrome may occur days to weeks after surgery and seems to be associated with blood remaining in the pericardial sac. Observe for the development of pericardial or pleural ***pain.*** For most patients, the syndrome is mild and self-limiting. However, the patient may require treatment similar to that for pericarditis. Be prepared to detect acute cardiac (pericardial) tamponade.

Minimally invasive direct coronary artery bypass. The minimally invasive direct coronary artery bypass (MIDCAB) may be indicated for patients with a lesion of the left anterior descending (LAD) artery. In the most common MIDCAB procedure, a left thoracotomy incision is made, and the rib retraction is required. Then the left internal mammary artery (IMA) is dissected and attached to the still-beating heart below the level of the lesion. Cardiopulmonary bypass (CPB) is not required.

After surgery, assess for chest pain and ECG changes (Q waves and ST-segment and T-wave changes in leads V_2 to V_6) because occlusion of the IMA graft occurs acutely in only a small percentage of patients. *If there is any question of acute graft closure, immediately notify the health care provider.* Patients tend to have more incisional pain after MIDCAB than after traditional CABG surgery, due to the thoracotomy incision and the required rib retraction. Because they have a thoracotomy incision and a chest tube or smaller-lumen vacuum chest device, patients are encouraged to cough, deep breathe, and use an incentive spirometer for a week after surgery. Most patients spend less than 6 hours in a critical care unit and are discharged in 2 or 3 days.

Endovascular (endoscopic) vessel harvesting. Regardless of whether the traditional CABG or the MIDCAB is performed, the donor vessel may be obtained using an endoscope rather than a large surgical incision. The radial artery or a vein in the leg may be taken with this method. Instead of a large, painful incision, the patient has one or two very small incisions in the leg or arm. This procedure has decreased hospital length of stay, postoperative complications, and pain.

Off-pump coronary artery bypass. Off-pump coronary artery bypass (OPCAB) is a procedure in which open-heart surgery is performed without the use of a heart-lung bypass machine. Advantages include shorter hospital stays and decreased mortality rate, risk for infection, and cost. The disadvantage of OPCAB is that it requires cardiac surgeons to have increased skill to master the technique.

Robotic-assisted heart surgery. Robotic-assisted heart surgery is a step toward less invasive open-heart surgery. Surgeons operate endoscopically through very small incisions in the chest wall. Use of robotics provides surgeons with capabilities that simplify the surgical process, eliminate tremors that can exist with human hands, increase the ability to reach otherwise inaccessible sites, and improve depth perception and visual acuity.

Other advantages of robotic-assisted procedures include shorter hospital stays (average stay is 2 to 3 days), less pain because of smaller incisions, no need for heart-lung bypass machine, less anxiety for the patient, and greater patient acceptance. The use of robotics also allows surgeons to perform telesurgery, performing heart procedures over long distances.

Disadvantages include computer failure, limited numbers of surgeons skilled in these techniques, and the length of surgery time (the time is about 50 minutes longer than the conventional surgery).

Care Coordination and Transition Management

Home Care Management. Case management is most appropriate for patients who meet high-cost, high-volume, and high-risk criteria. Patients with coronary artery disease (CAD) clearly meet all these criteria. Evidence-based care and case-management programs for those with CAD are used in most U.S. hospitals. By focusing on cardiovascular risk reduction and improving the continuity of care, health care professionals have reduced the length and cost of hospital stays. Posthospital case management should reduce hospital readmission rates and improve patient health.

Patients who have experienced a myocardial infarction (MI), angina, or coronary artery bypass graft (CABG) surgery are usually discharged to home or to a transitional care setting with drug therapy and specific activity prescriptions. Depending on the procedure, hospital stays may be 3 to 5 days for patients with MI or those undergoing CABG and only 1 to 2 days for those undergoing percutaneous coronary intervention (PCI) or newer surgeries. Therefore patients are still recovering when they are discharged from the hospital and need continuing care.

Patients should not be discharged to home alone. Assess whether the patient has family or friends to provide assistance. In some cases, a home care nurse may be needed. Home care for the patient who has had an MI are discussed in the Home Care Considerations: The Patient Who Has Had a Myocardial Infarction box.

Older adults are often living alone when coronary events occur and may have a greater need for home assistance after CABG surgery. A patient who was a resident in a long-term care facility may be returned there after hospitalization for unstable angina, MI, or CABG surgery.

Cardiac rehabilitation is available in most communities for patients after an MI or CABG surgery, but only a small

HOME CARE CONSIDERATIONS
The Patient Who Has Had a Myocardial Infarction

Assess cardiovascular function, including:
- Current vital signs (compare with previous to identify changes)
- Recurrence of ***pain*** (characteristics, frequency, onset)
- Indications of heart failure (weight gain, crackles, cough, dyspnea)
- Adequacy of tissue ***perfusion*** (mentation, skin temperature, peripheral pulses, urine output)
- Indications of dysrhythmia (irregular pulse, palpitations with fainting or near fainting)

Assess coping skills, including:
- Is the patient displaying anxiety, denial, anger, or depression?
    - Assess the patient's level of anxiety while allowing expression of any apprehension, and attempt to define its origin. Simple, repeated explanations of therapies, expectations, and surroundings, as well as patient progress, may help relieve anxiety.
    - Denial allows the patient to decrease a threat and use problem-focused coping mechanisms. Some denial can help allay anxiety; however, *denial that results in a patient who refuses to follow treatment regimens can be harmful.* Because this behavior is usually caused by extreme anxiety or fear, threats only worsen the behavior. Remain calm and avoid confronting the patient. Clearly indicate when a behavior is not acceptable and is potentially harmful as a result of nonadherence to the plan of care.
    - Anger can be an attempt to regain control. Encourage the patient to verbalize the source of frustration, and provide opportunities for decision making and control.
    - Depression may be a response to grief and loss of function. Listen as the patient verbalizes feelings of loss, being careful not to offer false or general reassurances. Acknowledge depression, but encourage the patient to perform ADLs and other activities within restrictions.
- Is caregiver providing adequate support?
- Are patient and caregiver disagreeing about treatment?

Assess functional ability, including:
- Activity tolerance (examine the patient's activity diary; review distance, duration, frequency, and symptoms occurring during exercise)
- ADLs (Is any assistance needed?)
- Household chores (Who performs them?)
- Does patient plan to return to work? When?

Assess nutritional status, including:
- Food intake (review patient's intake of fats and cholesterol)

Assess patient's understanding of illness and treatment, including:
- How to treat chest pain
- Signs and symptoms to report to health care provider
- Dosage, effects, and side effects of medications
- How to advance and when to limit activity
- Modification of risk factors for coronary artery disease

percentage participate in structured rehabilitation programs. The most frequently cited reasons for nonparticipation are lack of insurance coverage, a health care provider's decision that it is unnecessary, and the patient's decision that it is not necessary. Those who participate in these programs report greater improvement in exercise tolerance and improved ability to control stress. (See the Interprofessional Collaboration: The Patient with ACS box.)

INTERPROFESSIONAL COLLABORATION

The Patient With ACS

A planned program of cardiac rehabilitation increases functional ability and tolerance to activity. Cardiac rehabilitation is implemented primarily by the nurse and cardiac rehabilitation specialist and is continued after discharge. **Cardiac rehabilitation** is the process of actively assisting the patient with cardiac disease in achieving and maintaining a vital and productive life while remaining within the limits of the heart's ability to respond to increases in activity and stress. It can be divided into three phases. *Phase 1* begins with the acute illness and ends with discharge from the hospital. *Phase 2* begins after discharge and continues through convalescence at home. *Phase 3* refers to long-term conditioning. All patients with ACS should be referred to a cardiac rehabilitation program on discharge from the hospital. According to the Interprofessional Education Collaborative (IPEC) Expert Panel's Competency of Roles and Responsibilities, using the unique and complementary abilities of other team members optimizes health and patient care (IPEC, 2016; Slusser et al., 2019).

Self-Management Education. The need for health teaching depends in part on the treatment plan or type of procedure that the patient received. Because hospital stays are short and patients are quite ill during hospitalization, most in-hospital education programs concentrate on the skills essential for self-care after discharge.

As part of home visits or a cardiac rehabilitation program, identify the additional educational needs of the patient and family and their readiness to learn. Develop a teaching plan, which usually includes education about the normal anatomy and physiology of the heart, the pathophysiology of angina and MI, risk factor modification, activity and exercise protocols, cardiac drugs, and when to seek medical assistance. Teach patients that myocardial healing after an MI begins early and is usually complete in 6 to 8 weeks. Remind those who have undergone traditional CABG that the sternotomy should heal in about 6 to 8 weeks, but upper body exercise needs to be limited for several months.

Patients who have undergone CABG require instruction on incision care for the sternum and the graft site. Teach them to inspect the incisions daily for any redness, swelling, or drainage. The leg of a saphenous vein donor site is often edematous. Instruct patients to avoid crossing legs, to wear elastic stockings until the edema subsides, and to elevate the surgical limb when sitting in a chair. Teach patients who have had a radial artery graft to open and close the hand vigorously 10 times every 2 hours.

Risk Factor Modification. Modification of risk factors is a necessary part of a patient's management and involves changing his or her health maintenance patterns. Such modifications may include tobacco cessation, altered dietary patterns, regular exercise, BP control, and blood glucose control.

For patients who use tobacco, explain its negative effects, especially cigarette smoking. Many patients choose to quit smoking soon after an MI. Additional information on smoking cessation can be found in Chapter 24.

The mainstays of cholesterol control are nutritional therapy and antihyperlipidemic agents, as described in Chapter 33. Teach patients to avoid adding salt when beginning a meal. A reduction of 80 mg/day of sodium can reduce the systolic blood pressure (SBP) by 5 mm Hg, and the diastolic blood pressure (DBP) by 3 mm Hg. Maintain adequate dietary potassium, calcium, and magnesium intake. Increasing potassium may reduce the SBP by 8 mm Hg. Booklets and cookbooks that can help the patient learn to cook with reduced fats, oils, and salt are available from the American Heart Association (AHA).

Collaborate with the cardiac rehabilitation specialist to establish an activity and exercise schedule as part of rehabilitation, depending on the cardiac procedure that was performed (see the Interprofessional Collaboration: The Patient With ACS box). Instruct the patient to remain near home during the first week after discharge and to continue a walking program. Patients may engage in light housework or any activity done while sitting and that does not precipitate angina. During the second week, they are encouraged to increase social activities and possibly to return to work part-time. By the third week, they may begin to lift objects as heavy as 15 lb (e.g., 2 gallons of milk) but should avoid lifting or pulling heavier objects for the first 6 to 8 weeks. Suggested activity discussed in the Patient and Family Education: Preparing for Self-Management: Activity for the Patient With Coronary Artery Disease box.

Patients may begin a simple walking program by walking 400 feet twice a day at the rate of 1 mile/hr the first week after discharge and increasing the distance and rate as tolerated,

PATIENT AND FAMILY EDUCATION: PREPARING FOR SELF-MANAGEMENT

Activity for the Patient With Coronary Artery Disease

- Begin by walking the same distance at home as in the hospital (usually 400 feet) three times each day.
- Carry nitroglycerin with you.
- Check your pulse before, during, and after the exercise.
- Stop the activity for a pulse increase of more than 20 beats/min, shortness of breath, angina, or dizziness. Make gradual increases in walking distance.
- Exercise outdoors when the weather is good.
- After an exercise tolerance test and with your health care provider's approval, walk at least three times each week, increasing the distance every other week until the total distance is 1 mile.
- Avoid straining (lifting, push-ups, pull-ups, and straining at bowel movements).

usually weekly, until they can walk 2 miles at 3 to 4 miles/hr. Teach them to take their pulse reading before, halfway through, and after exercise. Teach the patient to stop exercising if the target pulse rate is exceeded or if dyspnea or angina develops.

After a limited exercise tolerance test, the cardiac rehabilitation specialist or nurse encourages the patient to join a formal exercise program, ideally one that helps him or her monitor cardiovascular progress. The program should include 5- to 7-minute warm-up and cool-down periods and 30 minutes of aerobic exercise. The patient should engage in aerobic exercise a minimum of three (and preferably five) times a week.

Complementary and Integrative Health. Additional therapies can aid in reducing the patient's anxiety about progressive activity both in the immediate postoperative period and during the rehabilitation phase. Many patients who have had cardiac surgery or other invasive procedures use complementary and integrative therapy practices. However, they often do not share with their health care providers that they use these practices. Techniques such as progressive muscle relaxation, guided imagery, music therapy, pet therapy, and therapeutic touch may decrease anxiety, reduce depression, and increase adherence with activity and exercise regimens after heart surgery.

Teach patients that adding omega-3 fatty acids from fish and plant sources has been effective for some patients in reducing lipid levels, stabilizing atherosclerotic plaques, and reducing sudden death from an MI. The preferred source of omega-3 acids is from fish rich in long-chain n-3 polyunsaturated fatty acids two times a week (Rimm et al., 2018) or a daily fish oil nutritional supplement (1 to 2 g/day) (Siscovick et al., 2017). Patients often take a number of other supplements, such as vitamin E, coenzyme Q_{10}, Pantesin, and vitamin B complex to decrease the risk for heart disease. However, studies do not show that these substances are helpful in reducing coronary artery disease.

Sexual Activity. Sexual activity is often a subject of great concern to patients and their partners. Inform the patient and his or her partner that engaging in their usual sexual activity is unlikely to damage the heart. Patients can resume sexual intercourse on the advice of the health care provider, usually after an exercise tolerance assessment. In general, those who can walk one block or climb two flights of stairs without symptoms can usually safely resume sexual activity.

Suggest that initially these patients have intercourse after a period of rest. They might try having intercourse in the morning when they are well rested or wait 1½ hours after exercise or a heavy meal. The position selected should be comfortable for both the patient and his or her partner so no undue stress is placed on the heart or suture line.

Drug Therapy. Assess patients with diabetes mellitus for their ability to control hyperglycemia. Review the prescribed dosage of insulin or oral antidiabetic drugs with the patient and family. The patient and/or family should demonstrate accurate testing of blood for glucose levels and the technique for insulin administration, if used. Teach patients that some medications, such as beta blockers, may block symptoms of hypoglycemia.

Teach the patient about the type of prescribed cardiac drugs, the benefit of each drug, potential side effects, and the correct dosage and time of day to take each drug. Drug regimens vary considerably. Many patients with angina are discharged while taking aspirin, a beta blocker, a calcium channel blocker, a statin agent, and a nitrate. Those who have experienced an MI may require dual antiplatelet therapy with aspirin and a P2Y12 inhibitor, a beta blocker, a statin drug, and, if the ejection fraction is below 40%, an ACEI and/or an ARB. It is recommended that all patients with cardiovascular disease receive an annual influenza vaccine and that patients over age 56 also receive the pneumococcal vaccine. Determine whether the patient can afford the medication and adhere to the instructions.

! NURSING SAFETY PRIORITY (QSEN)

Drug Alert

Use of NSAIDs is associated with an increased risk of cardiovascular events. This risk includes heart failure, heart attack, and stroke (Solomon, 2019). This risk of heart attack or stroke can occur early in treatment and may increase with length of treatment. Those with CVD have the greatest risk for adverse cardiovascular events. Teach the patient that NSAIDs are commonly available over the counter, so it is very important to read box labels. Acetaminophen products provide an alternative for pain relief and fever reduction.

! NURSING SAFETY PRIORITY (QSEN)

Drug Alert

Use of sublingual or spray nitroglycerin (NTG) deserves special attention. *Teach the patient to carry NTG at all times.* Keep the tablets in a glass, light-resistant container. The drug should be replaced every 3 to 5 months before it loses its potency or stops producing a tingling sensation when placed under the tongue. The Patient and Family Education: Preparing for Self-Management box gives instructions for management of chest pain at home.

Health Care Resources. The American Heart Association (AHA) is an excellent source for booklets, films, CDs, DVDs, cookbooks, and professional service referrals for the patient with coronary artery disease (CAD). Many local chapters have their own cardiac rehabilitation programs. Specifically for women, the AHA has established the Go Red for Women campaign.

Within the community, cardiac rehabilitation programs may be affiliated with local hospitals, community centers, or other facilities such as clinics. Many shopping malls open before shopping hours to allow a measured walking program indoors. This opportunity is particularly popular with older patients because it provides a good support group and allows for an appropriate place to exercise in inclement weather.

Mended Hearts is a nationwide program with local chapters that provides education and support to coronary artery bypass graft (CABG) patients and their families. Smoking-cessation programs and clinics and weight-reduction programs are located within the community. Many hospitals and places of worship also sponsor health fairs, BP screening, and risk-factor modification programs.

PATIENT AND FAMILY EDUCATION: PREPARING FOR SELF-MANAGEMENT

Management of Chest Pain at Home

- Keep fresh nitroglycerin available for immediate use.
- At the first indication of chest discomfort, cease activity and sit or lie down.
- Place one nitroglycerin tablet or spray under your tongue, allowing the tablet to dissolve.
- Wait 5 minutes for relief.
- If no relief results, call 911 for transportation to a health care facility.
- While waiting for emergency medical services (EMS), repeat the nitroglycerin and wait 5 more minutes.
- If there is no relief, repeat and wait 5 more minutes.
- Carry a medical identification card or wear a bracelet or necklace that identifies a history of heart problems.

Seeking Medical Assistance

Teach patients to notify their health care provider if they have:

- Heart rate remaining less than 50 after arising
- Wheezing or difficulty breathing
- Weight gain of 3 lb in 1 week or 1 to 2 lb overnight
- Persistent increase in NTG use
- Dizziness, faintness, or shortness of breath with activity

Remind them to always call 911 for transportation to the hospital if they **have**:

- Chest discomfort that does not improve after 5 minutes or 1 sublingual NTG tablet or spray
- Extremely severe chest or epigastric pain with weakness, nausea, or fainting
- Other associated symptoms that are particular to the patient, such as fatigue or nausea

◆ **Evaluation: Evaluate Outcomes.** Evaluate the care of the patient with CAD based on the identified priority patient problems. The expected outcomes are that the patient will:

- State that pain is alleviated
- Have adequate myocardial perfusion
- Be free of complications such as dysrhythmias and heart failure

GET READY FOR THE NEXT-GENERATION NCLEX® EXAMINATION!

Key Points

Review these Key Points for each NCLEX Examination Client Needs Category.

Safe and Effective Care Environment

- with members of the interprofessional health care team when caring for patients participating in cardiac rehabilitation. **QSEN: Teamwork and Collaboration**

Health Promotion and Maintenance

- Assess and teach the patient about risk factors for coronary artery disease (CAD).

Psychosocial Integrity

- Allow patients to verbalize and express feelings regarding their CAD. **QSEN: Patient-Centered Care**
- Address the needs of the family and significant others and provide teaching and information regarding the disease process. Clarify any misconceptions.

Physiological Integrity

- Teach patients that angina is the pain associated with decreased blood flow to the heart muscle.
- Identify and interpret troponin levels. **Clinical Judgment**
- Monitor patients receiving fibrinolytics or anticoagulants and those undergoing invasive cardiac procedures, for bleeding and bruising. **QSEN: Safety**
- Interpret and assess the patient with CAD for dysrhythmias.
- Evaluate the patient for pain characteristics.
- Teach patients and their families about drug therapy, including how to use nitroglycerin if they have chest or other cardiac-related pain (see Table 35.3).
- After percutaneous coronary intervention, monitor the patient for potential complications such as chest pain, bleeding from the insertion site, hypotension, hypokalemia, and dysrhythmias. Report and document any of these findings immediately. **QSEN: Safety**
- For patients having coronary artery bypass graft (CABG) surgery, be sure to manage pain adequately, assess fluid and electrolyte balance, and monitor for potential complications. Examples of complications include fluid and electrolyte imbalances (especially hypokalemia), hypothermia, hypertension, bleeding, sternal wound infections, and neurologic deficits. **Clinical Judgment; QSEN: Evidence-Based Practice, Quality Improvement**

MASTERY QUESTIONS

1. The nurse is providing community education regarding myocardial infarction. What teaching will the nurse include? **Select all that apply.**
   A. Denial is common reaction to chest pain.
   B. A myocardial infarction can occur in minutes.
   C. Exercise at least 20 minutes three to four times per week.
   D. Age is a significant risk factor in the development of CAD.
   E. Women are more likely to experience atypical chest pain.
   F. Atherosclerosis is a primary factor in the development of CAD.
2. A client who is 9 days post–coronary artery bypass graft presents to a follow-up appointment. Which client statement requires nursing action?
   A. "My chest hurts when I sneeze or cough."
   B. "If I get tired when I walk, then I stop and rest for a bit."
   C. "I have a bandage on my sternum to collect the drainage."
   D. "I haven't had my normal appetite since the surgery."
3. The nurse is preparing to discharge a client who recently experienced a STEMI. Which client statement indicates understanding of nitroglycerin use?
   A. "The nitroglycerin should tingle when I put it in my mouth."
   B. "I will keep nitroglycerin in the glove compartment of my car."
   C. "Since the pills are small, they won't be hard to swallow."
   D. "The nitroglycerin should relieve the pain immediately."
4. The nurse assesses a client who had a coronary artery bypass graft yesterday. Which assessment finding will cause the nurse to suspect cardiac tamponade?
   A. Incisional pain with decreased urine output
   B. Muffled heart sounds with the presence of JVD
   C. Sternal wound drainage with nausea
   D. Increased blood pressure and decreased heart rate

REFERENCES

Asterisk (*) indicates a classic or definitive work on this subject.

*Amsterdam, E., Wenger, N., Brindis, R., Casey, D., Ganiats, T., Holmes, D., et al. (2014). 2014 AHA/ACC guideline for the management of patients with non–ST-elevation acute coronary syndromes. *Journal of the American College of Cardiology, 64*(4), e139–e228.

Ascheim, D., Casey, D., Chung, M., de Lemos, J., Kushner, F., *O'Gara, P., et al. (2013). 2013 ACCF/AHA guideline for the management of ST-elevation myocardial infarction. *Circulation, 127*, e362–e425.

Bailey, S., Bates, E., Blankenship, J., Kushner, F., Levine, G., O'Gara, P., et al. (2015). 2015 ACC/AHA/SCAI Focused Update on primary percutaneous coronary intervention for patients with ST-elevation myocardial infarction: An update of the 2011 ACCF/AHA/SCAI guideline for percutaneous coronary intervention and the 2013 ACF/AHA guideline for the management of ST-elevation myocardial infarction. *Journal of the American College of Cardiology.* https://doi.org/10.1016/.jacc.2015.10.005.

Benjamin, E., Virani, S., Callaway, C., Cheng, A., Chiuve, S., Delling, F., & Muntner, P. (2018). Heart disease and stroke statistics -2018 update: A report from the American heart association. *Circulation, 135*(10), e146–e603. https://doi.org/10.1161/CIR.0000000000000485.

Berrios-Torres, S., Umscheid, C., Bratzler, D., Leas, B., Stone, E., Kelz, R., & Schecter, W. (2017). Centers for disease control and prevention guidelines for the prevention of surgical site infections, 2017). *Journal of the American Medical Association, 152*(8), 784–791.

Burchum, J., & Rosenthal, L. (2019). *Lehne's pharmacology for nursing care* (10th ed.). St. Louis: Elsevier.

Caceres, B., Brody, A., & Chyun, D. (2016). Recommendations for cardiovascular disease research with lesbian, gay, and bisexual adults. *Journal of Clinical Nursing, 25*(23–24), 3728–3742.

Colucci, W. (2019). *Treatment of acute decompensated heart failure: Components of therapy. UpToDate.* Retrieved from: https://www.uptodate.com/contents/treatment-of-acute-decompensated-heart-failure-components-of-therapy.

Cutlip, D., & Lincoff, M. (2018). *Antiplatelet agents in acute non-ST elevation acute coronary syndromes. UpToDate.* Retrieved from: https://www.uptodate.com/contents/antiplatelet-agents-in-acute-non-st-elevation-acute-coronary-syndromes.

Gibson, M., & Corbalan, R. (2017). *Fibrinolysis for ST elevation myocardial infarction: Initiation of therapy. UpToDate.* Retrieved from: https://www.uptodate.com/contents/fibrinolysis-for-acute-st-elevation-myocardial-infarction-initiation-of-therapy.

*Grundy, S. M., Cleeman, J. I., Daniels, S. R., Donato, K. A., Eckel, R. H., Franklin, B. A., et al. (2005). Diagnosis and management of the metabolic syndrome: An American heart Association/national heart, lung, and blood institute scientific statement. *Circulation, 112*(17), 2735–2752.

Interprofessional Education Collaborative. (2016). *Core competencies for interprofessional collaborative practice:* 2016 update. Retrieved from https://nebula.wsimg.com/2f68a39520b03336b-41038c370497473?AccessKeyId=DC06780E69ED19E2B3A5&disposition=0&alloworigin=1.

Jarvis, C. (2020). *Physical examination & health assessment* (8th ed.). St. Louis: Elsevier.

Levine, G., Bates, E., Bittl, J., Brindis, R., Finn, S., Fleisher, L., & Smith, S. (2016). 2016 ACC/AHA guideline focused update on the duration of dual antiplatelet therapy in patients with coronary artery disease: A report of the American College of Cardiology/American heart association task force on clinical practice guidelines. *Journal of the American College of Cardiology, 68*(10), 1082–1115.

Lincoff, A. M., & Cutlip, D. (2018). *Antiplatelet agents in acute ST elevation myocardial infarction. UpToDate.* Retrieved from: https://www.uptodate.com/contents/antiplatelet-agents-in-acute-st-elevation-myocardial-infarction.

McCance, K., & Huether, S. (2019). *Pathophysiology: The biologic basis for disease in adults and children* (8th ed.). St. Louis: Elsevier.

Mehta, L., Beckie, T., DeVon, H., Grines, C., Krumholz, H., Johnson, M., & Wenger, N. (2016). Acute myocardial infarction in women: A scientific statement from the American heart association. *Circulation, 133*, 916–947. https://doi.org/10.1161/CIR0000000000000351.

Meigs, J. (2019). *The metabolic syndrome (insulin resistance syndrome or syndrome X). UpToDate.* Retrieved from: https://www.uptodate.com/contents/the-metabolic-syndrome-insulin-resistance-syndrome-or-syndrome-x.

Pagana, K., & Pagana, T. (2018). *Mosby's manual of diagnostic and laboratory tests* (6th ed.). St. Louis: Elsevier.

Reeder, G., & Kennedy, H. (2019). *Overview of the acute management of ST-elevation myocardial infarction. UpToDate.* Retrieved from: https://www.uptodate.com/contents/overview-of-the-acute-management-of-st-elevation-myocardial-infarction/print.

Rimm, E., Appel, L., Chiuve, S., Djousse, L., Engler, M., Kris-Etherton, P., et al. (2018). Seafood long-chain n-3 polyunsaturated fatty acids and cardiovascular disease: A science advisory form the American heart association. *Circulation, 137.* https://doi.org/10.1161/CIR0000000000000574.

Seifert, P. (2017). Reducing readmissions after coronary artery bypass grafting. *AORN Journal, 106*(4), 332–337.

Siscovick, D., Barringer, T., Fretts, A., Wu, J., Lichtenstein, A., Costello, R., & Mozaffarian, D. (2017). Omega-3 polyunsaturated fatty acid (fish oil) supplementation and the prevention of clinical cardiovascular disease: A science advisory from the American heart association. *Circulation, 135,* e867–e884.

Slusser, M., et al. (2019). *Foundations of interprofessional collaborative practice* (1st ed.). St. Louis: Elsevier .

Solomon, D. (2019). *NSAIDs: Adverse cardiovascular effects. UpToDate.* Retrieved from: https://www.uptodate.com/contents/nsaids-adverse-cardiovascular-effects.

Stanfield, L. (2018). Improvement of door-to-electrocardiogram time using the first-nurse role in the ED setting. *Journal of Emergency Nursing, 44*(5), 466–471.

Urden, L., Stacy, K., & Lough, M. (2018). *Critical care nursing: Diagnosis and management* (8th ed.). St. Louis: Elsevier.

36

Assessment of the Hematologic System

M. Linda Workman

http://evolve.elsevier.com/Iggy/

LEARNING OUTCOMES

1. Collaborate with the interprofessional team to perform a complete hematologic assessment, including the effectiveness of ***clotting*** and ***perfusion,*** by applying knowledge of anatomy and physiology, genetics, and pathophysiology.
2. Explain how physiologic aging changes the hematologic functions of ***clotting*** and ***perfusion*** and how these changes may affect the associated care of older adults.
3. Teach all adults how to protect the hematologic system.
4. Teach the patient and caregivers about diagnostic procedures associated with hematologic assessment.
5. Implement patient-centered nursing interventions to help the patient and family cope with the psychosocial impact of a possible hematologic health problem.
6. Use clinical judgment to prioritize nursing care for the patient before, during, and after bone marrow aspiration or biopsy.

KEY TERMS

blood stem cells Unspecialized (undifferentiated) cells that are capable of becoming any type of blood cell.

clotting A complex, multistep process by which blood forms a protein-based structure (clot) in an appropriate area of tissue injury to prevent excessive bleeding while maintaining whole-body blood flow (*perfusion*).

erythrocytes Mature red blood cells (RBCs).

erythropoiesis Selective growth of bone marrow stem cells into mature erythrocytes.

fibrinolysis The process that dissolves fibrin clot edges with special enzymes to prevent overenlargement of a clot beyond the area where it is needed.

hemostasis The multistep process of controlled blood *clotting*, resulting in localized blood clotting in damaged blood vessels to prevent excessive blood loss while continuing blood *perfusion* to all other areas.

perfusion The total arterial blood flow through the tissues (peripheral perfusion) and blood that is pumped by the heart (central perfusion).

petechiae Reddish-purple pinpoint hemorrhagic lesions in the skin.

PRIORITY CONCEPTS

The priority concepts for this chapter are:
- ***Clotting***
- ***Perfusion***

The hematologic system involves all the components and organs responsible for blood formation, circulation, function, storage, and recycling. These components include blood cells, lymph, and lymph nodes, along with the bone marrow, spleen, liver, and thymus. Formation and circulation of normal blood are critical to tissue ***perfusion*** and gas exchange (oxygenation) because the blood is the oxygen delivery system. *Perfusion* is the total arterial blood flow through the tissues *(peripheral perfusion)* and blood that is pumped by the heart *(central perfusion)*. Because all tissues and organs depend on liquid blood for perfusion and oxygen delivery, any problem of the hematologic system affects total body health. Part of maintaining adequate whole-body perfusion is ensuring that liquid blood remains circulating to deliver oxygen to all cells, tissues, and organs; however, the concept of ***clotting*** also is a critical function of this system. *Clotting* is a complex, multistep process by which blood forms a protein-based structure (clot) in an appropriate area of tissue injury to prevent excessive bleeding while maintaining whole-body blood flow (perfusion). This chapter, together with Chapter 16, reviews the normal physiology of the hematologic system and assessment of hematologic status.

ANATOMY AND PHYSIOLOGY REVIEW

Bone Marrow

Bone marrow is the functional site of blood formation in adults and produces red blood cells (RBCs, *erythrocytes*), white blood cells (WBCs, *leukocytes*), and platelets *(thrombocytes)*. Bone marrow also is involved in the immune responses (see Chapter 16).

About 2.5 billion RBCs, 2.5 billion platelets, and 1 billion WBCs per kilogram of body weight are released from the bone marrow daily. The cell-producing part of the marrow in adults is present only in flat bones (sternum, skull, pelvic and shoulder girdles) and the ends of long bones. With aging, fatty tissue replaces active red bone marrow, and only a small portion of the remaining marrow continues to produce blood in older adults (Touhy & Jett, 2020).

Bone marrow first produces immature **blood stem cells**, which are unspecialized (undifferentiated) cells that are capable of becoming any type of blood cell, depending on the body's needs (Fig. 36.1) (McCance et al., 2019). The next stage in blood cell production is the *committed stem cell* (or *precursor* cell). A committed stem cell enters one growth pathway and can at that point specialize *(differentiate)* into only one cell type. Committed stem cells actively divide but require the presence of a specific growth factor for specialization. For example, erythropoietin is a growth factor specific for the RBC. Other growth factors control WBC and platelet growth (see Chapters 16 and 37 for discussion of growth factors and cytokines).

Blood Components

Plasma is the liquid portion of the blood that contains the cells. It is an extracellular fluid similar to the interstitial fluid found between tissue cells, but containing much more protein. The three major types of plasma proteins are albumin, globulins, and fibrinogen.

Albumin maintains the osmotic pressure of the blood, preventing the plasma from leaking into the tissues (see Chapter 13). *Globulins* have many functions, such as transporting other substances and, as antibodies, protecting the body against infection. *Fibrinogen* is activated to form fibrin, which is critical in the blood ***clotting*** process.

Differentiated blood cells include RBCs, WBCs, and platelets. These cells differ in structure, site of maturation, and function.

Red blood cells (**erythrocytes**) are the largest proportion of blood cells. Mature RBCs have a biconcave disk shape and no nucleus. Together with a flexible membrane, this feature allows RBCs to change their shape without breaking as they pass through narrow, winding capillaries. The number of RBCs an adult has varies with gender, age, and general health, but the normal range is from 4.2×10^6/mcL to 6.1×10^6/mcL (4.2 to 6.1×10^{12}/L).

As shown in Figs. 36.1 and 36.2, RBCs start out as stem cells, enter the myeloid pathway, and progress in stages to mature erythrocytes. Healthy, mature, circulating RBCs have a life span of about 120 days. As RBCs age, their membranes become more fragile and are easily destroyed when trapped in the tissues, spleen, and liver. Some parts of destroyed RBCs (e.g., iron, hemoglobin [Hgb]) are recycled and used to make new RBCs.

The RBCs produce hemoglobin (Hgb). Each normal mature RBC contains millions of hemoglobin molecules. Iron is an essential part of hemoglobin because iron is the cellular substance to which oxygen binds. Each complete hemoglobin molecule can transport up to four molecules of oxygen. Hemoglobin molecules also carry carbon dioxide but at a different site from oxygen.

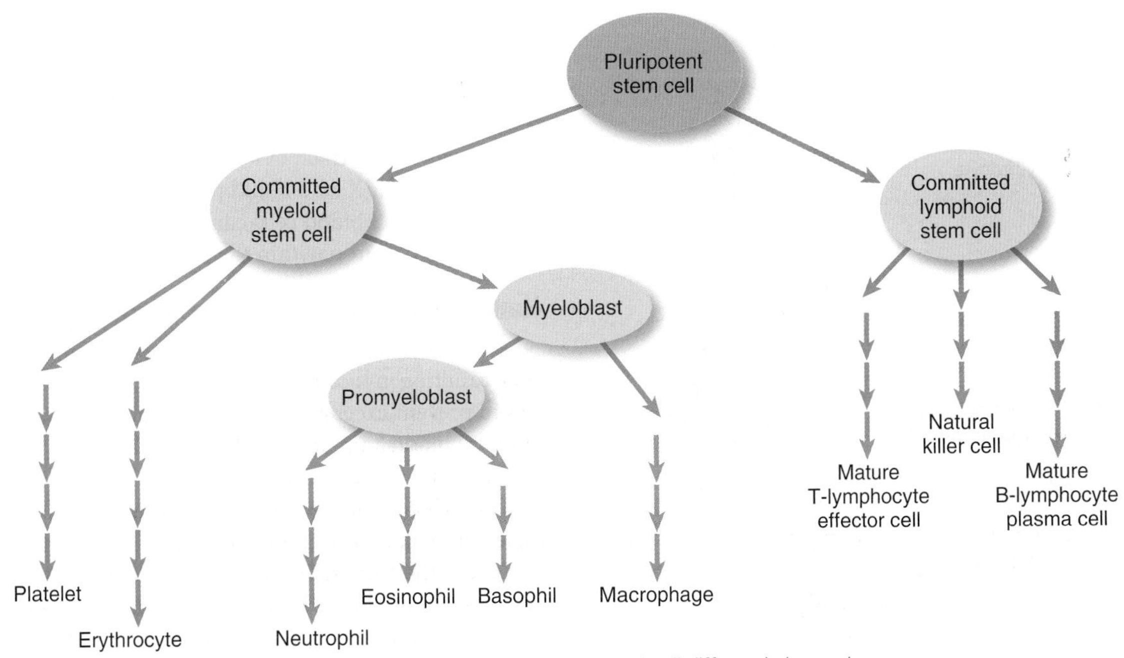

Fig. 36.1 Bone marrow cell growth and blood cell differentiation pathways.

The most important feature of hemoglobin is its ability to combine loosely with oxygen. Only a small drop in tissue oxygen levels increases the transfer of oxygen from hemoglobin to tissues, known as *oxygen dissociation.* See Chapter 24 for a discussion of oxygen dissociation.

An adult's total number of RBCs is carefully controlled to ensure that enough are present for good oxygen ***perfusion*** and for ***clotting*** without having too many cells that could "thicken" the blood and slow flow. RBC production or **erythropoiesis** (selective growth of bone marrow stem cells into mature erythrocytes) must be properly balanced with RBC destruction or loss. When balanced, this process helps tissue perfusion by ensuring adequate delivery of oxygen. The trigger for RBC production and maturation is an increase in the tissue need for oxygen. The kidney produces the RBC growth factor *erythropoietin* at the same rate as RBC destruction or loss occurs to maintain a constant normal level of circulating RBCs. When tissue oxygen is less than normal *(hypoxia),* the kidney releases more erythropoietin, which then increases marrow production of RBCs. When the tissue oxygen level is normal or high, erythropoietin levels fall, slowing RBC production. Synthetic erythrocyte-stimulating agents (ESAs) have the same effect on bone marrow as the naturally occurring erythropoietin.

Many substances are needed to form hemoglobin and RBCs, including iron, vitamin B_{12}, folic acid, copper, pyridoxine, cobalt, and nickel. A lack of any of these substances can lead to *anemia* (reduced numbers of function of RBCs), which results in unmet tissue oxygen needs because of a reduction in the number or function of RBCs.

White blood cells (WBCs, leukocytes) also are formed in the bone marrow. The many types of WBCs all have specialized functions that provide protection through inflammation and immunity, as presented in Chapter 16.

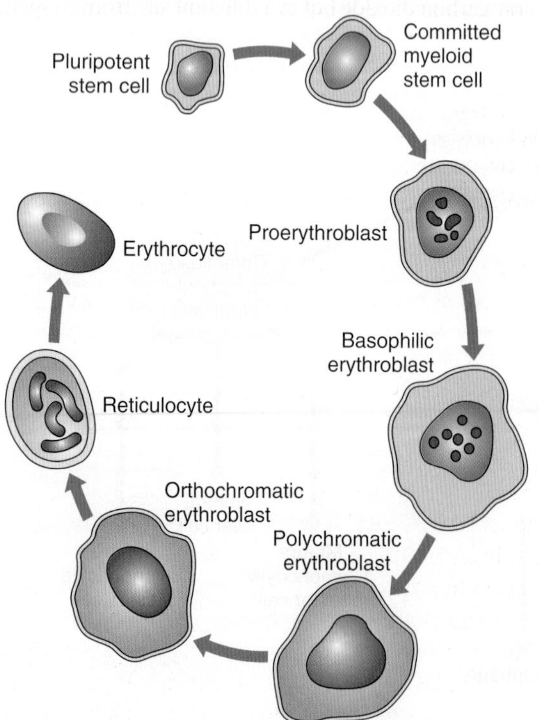

Fig. 36.2 Erythrocyte (red blood cell) growth pathway.

Platelets, also called *thrombocytes,* are the third type of blood cells. They are the smallest blood cells, formed in the bone marrow from megakaryocyte precursor cells. When activated, platelets stick to injured blood vessel walls and form platelet plugs that can stop the flow of blood at the injured site. They also produce substances important to blood ***clotting*** and aggregate (clump together) to perform most of their functions. Platelets help keep small blood vessels intact by initiating repair after damage.

Production of platelets is controlled by the growth factor *thrombopoietin.* After platelets leave the bone marrow, they are stored in the spleen and then released slowly to meet the body's needs. Normally 80% of platelets circulate and 20% are stored in the spleen.

Accessory Organs of Blood Formation

The spleen and liver are important accessory organs for blood production. They help regulate the growth of blood cells and form factors that ensure proper blood ***clotting.*** Problems with either the spleen or the liver result in impaired hematologic function, which usually decreases adequate ***perfusion*** or clotting to some degree.

The *spleen* contains three types of tissue: white pulp, red pulp, and marginal pulp. These tissues help balance blood cell production with blood cell destruction and assist with immunity. White pulp is filled with white blood cells (WBCs) and is a major site of antibody production. As whole blood filters through the white pulp, bacteria and old RBCs are removed. Red pulp is the storage site for RBCs and platelets. Marginal pulp contains the ends of many blood vessels.

The spleen destroys old or imperfect RBCs, breaks down the hemoglobin released from these destroyed cells for recycling, stores platelets, and filters antigens. Anyone who has had a splenectomy has reduced immune functions and an increased risk for infection and sepsis.

The *liver* produces prothrombin and other blood clotting factors. Also, proper liver function is important in forming vitamin K in the intestinal tract. (Vitamin K is needed to produce clotting factors VII, IX, and X and prothrombin.) Large amounts of whole blood and blood cells can be stored in the liver. The liver also stores extra iron within the protein *ferritin.*

Hemostasis and Blood Clotting

Hemostasis is the multistep process of controlled blood ***clotting,*** resulting in localized blood clotting in damaged blood vessels to prevent excessive blood loss while continuing ***perfusion*** of liquid blood and individual cells to all other areas. This complex function balances blood clotting actions with anticlotting actions. When injury occurs, hemostasis starts the formation of a platelet plug and continues with a series of steps that eventually cause the formation of a fibrin clot. Three sequential processes result in blood clotting: platelet aggregation with platelet plug formation, the blood clotting cascade, and the formation of a complete fibrin clot.

Platelet aggregation begins forming a platelet plug by having platelets clump together, a process essential for blood ***clotting***. Platelets normally circulate as individual small cells that do not clump together until activated. Activation causes platelet membranes to become sticky, allowing them to clump together. When platelets clump, they form large, semisolid plugs in blood vessels, disrupting local blood flow. *These platelet plugs are **not** clots and last only a few hours. Thus they cannot provide complete hemostasis but only trigger the start of the hemostatic process.*

Substances that activate platelets and cause clumping include adenosine diphosphate (ADP), calcium, thromboxane A_2 (TXA_2), and collagen. Platelets secrete some of these substances (making platelets able to continue self-activation), and other activating substances are external to the platelet. Platelet plugs start the cascade action that ends with local blood ***clotting*** and are important at all steps within the cascade. When too few platelets are present, clotting is impaired, increasing the risk for excessive bleeding.

Blood clotting is a cascade triggered by platelet aggregation and the formation of a platelet plug, which then rapidly amplifies the cascade. The final result is much larger than the triggering event. Thus the cascade works like a landslide—a few stones rolling down a steep hill can eventually dislodge large rocks, trees, and soil, causing an enormous movement of earth. Just like landslides, cascade reactions are hard to stop once they are set into motion. Normal blood clotting is triggered initially by conditions that activate either of two distinct pathways: the *extrinsic clotting pathway* (outside the blood vessels) and the *intrinsic clotting pathway*, which begins with changes in the blood rather than with trauma (Fig. 36.3). These pathways merge later in the cascade, forming a common path to result in a stable clot for hemostasis.

Triggering of the extrinsic pathway is generally a protective function in which factors outside of the blood or that are abnormally present in the body activate platelets. The most common extrinsic event is trauma that damages blood vessels and exposes the collagen within vessel walls. Collagen then activates platelets to form a platelet plug within seconds. The blood clotting cascade is started sooner by this pathway because some intrinsic pathway steps are bypassed. Other conditions or substances that can activate platelets in the extrinsic pathway include inflammation, bacterial toxins, or the presence of foreign proteins.

Triggering of the intrinsic pathway occurs through more internal conditions, such as impaired blood flow *(venous stasis)* or the presence of excessive amounts of substances that promote blood clotting within the blood itself that can activate platelets and trigger the blood clotting cascade (see Fig. 36.3). Thus the intrinsic pathway is less of a protective response and results from problems that promote abnormal ***clotting***.

Whether the platelet plugs are formed because of abnormal blood (intrinsic factors) or by exposure to inflamed or damaged blood vessels (extrinsic factors), the end result of the cascade is the same: *formation of a fibrin clot and local blood clotting (coagulation)*. The cascade, from the formation of a platelet plug to the formation of a fibrin clot, depends on the presence of specific clotting factors, calcium, and more platelets at every step.

Clotting factors (Table 36.1) are inactive enzymes that become activated in sequence. At each step, the activated enzyme from the previous step activates the next enzyme. (Although clotting factors are identified by number, the numbers only indicate the order in which the factors were discovered and not the order of their actions within the cascade.) Insufficient amounts of any clotting factor can interfere with normal ***clotting*** and hemostasis. The last two critical steps in the cascade are the activation of thrombin from prothrombin and the conversion (by thrombin) of fibrinogen into fibrin. Only fibrin molecules can begin the formation of a true clot.

Fibrin clot formation is the last phase of blood clotting. Fibrinogen is an inactive protein made in the liver. The activated enzyme *thrombin* removes the end portions of fibrinogen, converting it to active fibrin molecules that can link together to form fibrin threads. Fibrin threads make a meshlike base to form a blood clot.

After the fibrin mesh is formed, clotting factor XIII tightens up the mesh, making it dense and more stable. More platelets stick to the threads of the mesh and attract other blood cells and proteins to form an actual blood clot. As this clot tightens (retracts), the serum is squeezed out, and clot formation is complete.

Anticlotting Forces

Because ***clotting*** occurs through a rapid cascade process, in theory it keeps forming fibrin clots whenever the cascade is set into motion until all blood throughout the entire body has coagulated and ***perfusion*** stops. Obviously this action would be lethal. Thus whenever the clotting cascade is started, anticlotting forces are also started to limit clot formation only to damaged areas so normal perfusion is maintained everywhere else. When blood proclotting and anticlotting actions are balanced, clotting occurs only where it is needed, and normal perfusion is maintained. The anticlotting forces both ensure that activated clotting factors are present only in limited amounts and also cause fibrinolysis to prevent overenlargement of the fibrin clot. **Fibrinolysis** is the process that dissolves fibrin clot edges with special enzymes (Fig. 36.4). The process starts by activating plasminogen to plasmin. Plasmin, an active enzyme, then digests fibrin, fibrinogen, and prothrombin, controlling the size of the fibrin clot (McCance et al., 2019).

When the blood clotting cascade is activated, additional anticlotting substances are also activated, such as protein C, protein S, and antithrombin III. Protein C and protein S increase the breakdown of clotting factors V and VIII. Antithrombin III inactivates thrombin and clotting factors IX and X. These actions prevent clots from becoming too large or forming in an area where ***clotting*** is not needed. Deficiency of any anticlotting factor increases the risk for venous thromboembolism (VTE) such as pulmonary embolism, myocardial infarction (MI), and strokes.

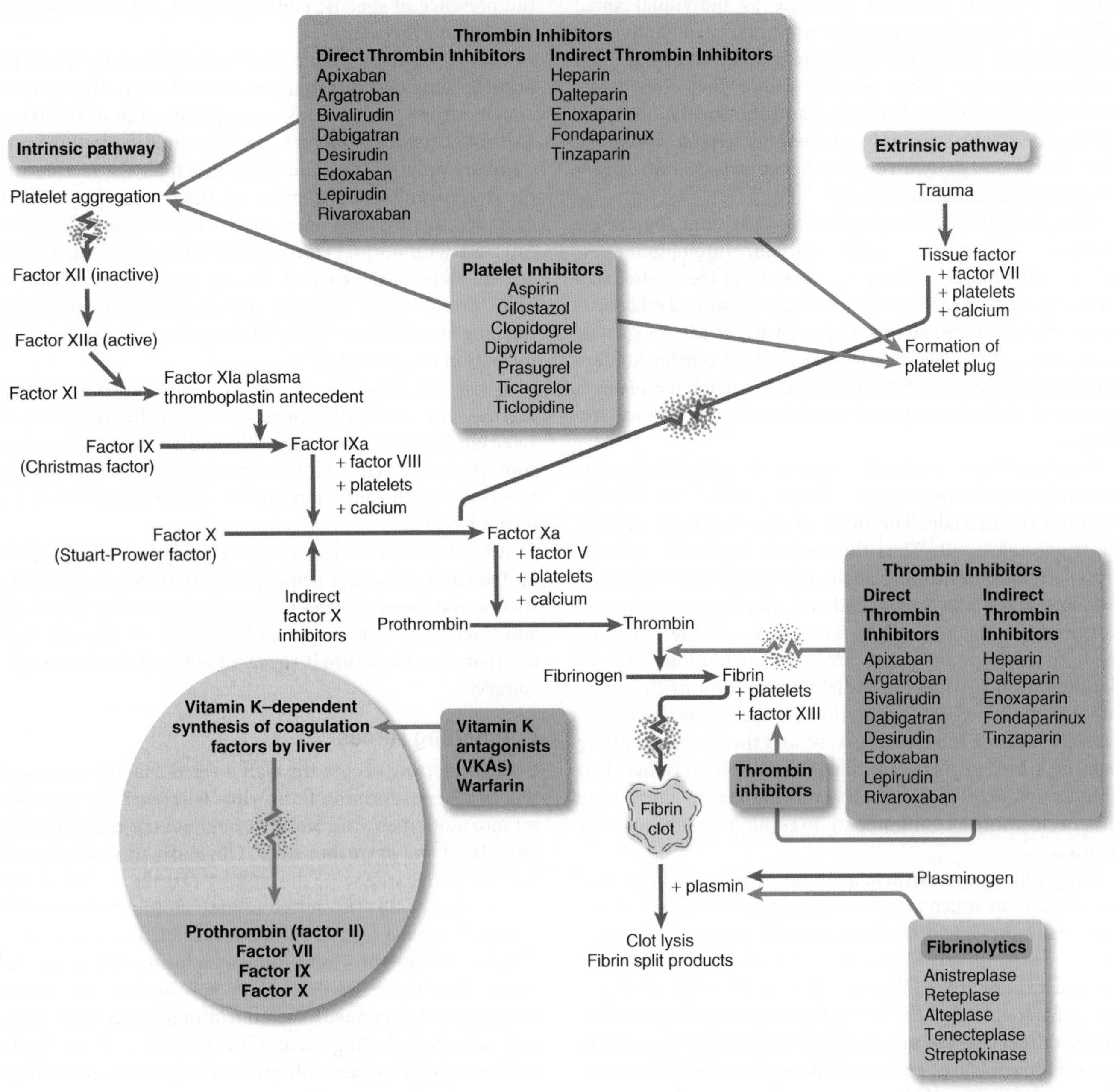

Fig. 36.3 Summary of the blood clotting cascade.

Hematologic Changes Associated With Aging

Aging changes the blood components, necessitating adaptations in techniques for assessment as described in the Patient-Centered Care: Older Adult Considerations: Adaptations for Hematologic Assessment box (Touhy & Jett, 2020). The older adult has a decreased blood volume with lower levels of plasma proteins. The lower plasma protein level may be related to a low dietary intake of proteins and to reduced protein production by the older liver.

As bone marrow ages, it produces fewer blood cells. Total red blood cell (RBC) and white blood cell (WBC) counts are lower among older adults, although platelet counts do not change. Lymphocytes become less reactive to antigens and lose immune function. Antibody levels and responses are lower and slower in older adults. The WBC count does not rise as high in response to infection in older adults as it does in younger adults.

Hemoglobin levels in men and women fall after middle age. Iron-deficient diets may play a role in this reduction.

PATIENT-CENTERED CARE: OLDER ADULT CONSIDERATIONS QSEN

Adaptations for Hematologic Assessment

Usual Indicators of Hematologic Disorders	Normal Changes in Older Adults	Assessment Adaptation
Nail Bed Capillary Refill		
Pallor or cyanosis indicates reduced ***perfusion*** or oxygenation.	Thickened or discolored nails make assessing the nail beds impossible.	Use another body area, such as the lip, to assess central capillary refill and ***perfusion***.
Hair Distribution		
Thin or absent hair on the trunk or extremities may indicate poor ***perfusion*** to a particular area.	Progressive loss of body hair, especially on the extremities, is a normal facet of aging.	A relatively even pattern of hair loss that has occurred over an extended period is not significant and cannot be used as an indicator of inadequate ***perfusion***.
Skin Moisture		
Skin dryness is associated with many hematologic disorders.	Skin dryness and loss of turgor is a normal part of aging.	Do not use skin moisture as a reliable indicator of an underlying hematologic problem in the older adult.
Skin Color		
Skin color changes, especially pallor and jaundice, are associated with some hematologic disorders.	Pigment loss and skin yellowing are common changes associated with aging.	Use laboratory test results to confirm anemia or jaundice rather than skin color changes in older adults.

ASSESSMENT: RECOGNIZE CUES

Patient History

Age and gender are important to consider when assessing the patient's hematologic status. Bone marrow function and immune activity decrease with age.

PATIENT-CENTERED CARE: GENDER HEALTH CONSIDERATIONS QSEN

Women have lower red blood cell counts than do men. This difference is greater during menstrual years because menstrual blood loss may occur faster than blood cell production. This difference also is related to blood dilution caused by fluid retention from female hormones. Always assess for RBC adequacy in a woman hospitalized for any reason.

Liver function, the presence of known immunity or hematologic disorders, current drug use, dietary patterns, and socioeconomic status are important to assess. Because the liver is important in producing ***clotting*** factors, ask about symptoms that may indicate liver problems, such as jaundice, anemia, and gallstones. Previous radiation therapy for cancer may impair hematologic function if marrow-forming bones were in the radiation path.

TABLE 36.1 The Clotting Factors

Factor	Action
I: Fibrinogen	Factor I is converted to fibrin by the enzyme *thrombin*. Individual fibrin molecules form fibrin threads, which are the mesh for clot formation and wound healing.
II: Prothrombin	Factor II is the inactive thrombin. Prothrombin is activated to thrombin by clotting factor X. Activated thrombin converts fibrinogen (clotting factor I) into fibrin and activates factors V and VIII. Synthesis is vitamin K dependent.
III: Tissue thromboplastin	Factor III interacts with factor VII to initiate the extrinsic clotting cascade.
IV: Calcium	Calcium (Ca^{2+}), a divalent cation, is a cofactor for most of the enzyme-activated processes required in blood clotting. Calcium enhances platelet aggregation and makes red blood cells clump together.
V: Proaccelerin	Factor V is a cofactor for activated factor X, which is essential for converting prothrombin to thrombin.
VI: Is an artifact	No factor VI is involved in blood clotting.
VII: Proconvertin	Factor VII activates factors IX and X, which are essential in converting prothrombin to thrombin. Synthesis is vitamin K dependent.
VIII: Antihemophilic factor	Factor VIII together with activated factor IX activates factor X. Factor VIII combines with von Willebrand factor to help platelets adhere to capillary walls in areas of tissue injury. A lack of factor VIII results in classic hemophilia (hemophilia A).
IX: Plasma thromboplastin component (Christmas factor)	Factor IX, when activated, activates factor X to convert prothrombin to thrombin. A lack of factor IX causes hemophilia B. Synthesis is vitamin K dependent.
X: Stuart-Prower factor	Factor X, when activated, converts prothrombin into thrombin. Synthesis is vitamin K dependent.
XI: Plasma thromboplastin antecedent	Factor XI, when activated, assists in the activation of factor IX. However, a similar factor must exist in tissues. People who are deficient in factor XI have mild bleeding problems.
XII: Hageman factor	Factor XII is critically important in the intrinsic pathway for the activation of factor XI.
XIII: Fibrin-stabilizing factor	Factor XIII assists in forming cross-links among the fibrin threads to form a strong fibrin clot.

Ask about the patient's occupation and hobbies and whether the home is located near an industrial setting. This information may identify exposure to agents that affect bone marrow and hematologic function.

Check all drugs the patient is using or has used in the past 3 weeks. Ask about the use of drugs listed in Table 36.2 that are known to change hematologic function. Check with a pharmacist or a comprehensive drug reference to determine whether other drugs the patient takes can affect hematologic function.

Ask the patient about use of anticoagulation agents and NSAIDs, which change blood ***clotting*** activity. Many patients

TABLE 36.2 Examples of Drugs Impairing the Hematologic System

Drugs Causing Bone Marrow Suppression	Drugs Causing Hemolysis	Drugs Disrupting Platelet Action
• Altretamine	• Acetohydroxamic acid	• Aspirin
• Amphotericin B	• Amoxicillin	• Carbenicillin
• Azathioprine	• Chlorpropamide	• Carindacillin
• Chemotherapeutic agents	• Doxapram	• Dipyridamole
• Chloramphenicol	• Glyburide	• Ibuprofen
• Chromic phosphate	• Mefenamic acid	• Meloxicam
• Colchicine	• Menadiol diphosphate	• Naproxen
• Didanosine	• Methyldopa	• Oxaprozin
• Eflornithine	• Nitrofurantoin	• Pentoxifylline
• Foscarnet sodium	• Penicillin G benzathine	• Sulfinpyrazone
• Ganciclovir	• Penicillin V	• Ticarcillin
• Interferon alfa	• Primaquine	• Ticlopidine
• Pentamidine	• Procainamide hydrochloride	• Valproic acid
• Sodium iodide	• Quinidine polygalacturonate	
• Zalcitabine	• Quinine	
• Zidovudine	• Sulfonamides	
	• Tolbutamide	
	• Vitamin K	

refer to anticoagulants as "blood thinners," although they do not change blood thickness *(viscosity)*. Fig. 36.4 shows where in the blood clotting cascade different types of anticoagulants work.

Anticoagulant drugs work by interfering with one or more steps involved in the blood clotting cascade. Thus these agents *prevent* new clots from forming and limit or prevent extension of formed clots. *Anticoagulants do not break down existing clots.* These drugs are classified as platelet inhibitors (antiplatelet drugs), direct thrombin inhibitors, indirect thrombin inhibitors, and vitamin K antagonists (VKAs).

Fibrinolytic drugs (also known as *thrombolytic drugs* or "clot busters") selectively break down fibrin threads present in formed blood clots. The mechanism starts with activation of the inactive tissue protein *plasminogen* to its active form, *plasmin*. Plasmin directly attacks and degrades the fibrin molecule. Fibrinolytic drugs include the IV agents alteplase, reteplase, tenecteplase, and urokinase. Urokinase is approved for use only in patients who have a massive pulmonary embolism.

NCLEX EXAMINATION CHALLENGE 36.1

Health Promotion and Maintenance

What is the **most important** precaution **to prevent** harm that a nurse will teach a client who is prescribed to take the anticoagulant drug warfarin?

A. Apply an ice pack to any body area that you bump or otherwise injure to reduce bleeding.
B. Check with your primary health care provider before taking any vitamin supplements.
C. Always take your medication within an hour of the same time every day and never with meals.
D. Avoid taking aspirin or any aspirin-containing product unless prescribed.

Nutrition Status

Food intake and diet can alter cell quality and affect ***clotting***. Ask patients to recall what they have eaten during the past week. Use this information to collaborate with a registered dietitian nutritionist (RDN) to assess possible iron, protein, mineral, or vitamin deficiencies. Diets high in fat and carbohydrates and low in protein, iron, and vitamins can cause many types of anemia and decrease the functions of all blood cells. Diets high in vitamin K, found in leafy green vegetables, may increase the rate of blood clotting. Assess the amount of salads and other raw vegetables that the patient eats and whether supplemental vitamins and calcium are used. Ask about alcohol consumption because chronic alcoholism causes nutrition deficiencies and impairs the liver, both of which reduce blood ***clotting***.

Ask about personal resources, such as finances and social support. An adult with a low income may have a diet deficient in iron and protein because foods containing these substances are more expensive.

Family History and Genetic Risk

Assess family history because many disorders affecting blood and blood ***clotting*** are inherited, especially those affecting the production of clotting factors and anticlotting substances. Ask whether anyone in the family has had hemophilia, frequent nosebleeds, postpartum hemorrhages, excessive bleeding after tooth extractions, or heavy bruising after mild trauma. Ask whether any family member has sickle cell disease or sickle cell trait. Although sickle cell disease is seen most often among African Americans, anyone can have the trait. Asking whether conditions with excessive clotting are common within the family is also important in identifying a possible genetic problem triggering the intrinsic clotting pathway.

Current Health Problems

Ask about lymph node swelling, excessive bruising or bleeding, and whether the bleeding was spontaneous or induced by trauma. Ask about the amount and duration of bleeding after routine dental work. Have women estimate the number of pads or tampons used during the most recent menstrual cycle and determine whether this amount represents a change from the usual pattern of flow. Ask whether clots are present in menstrual blood. If menstrual clots occur, ask women to estimate clot size using coins or fruit for comparison.

Assess and record whether the patient has shortness of breath on exertion, palpitations, frequent infections, fevers, recent weight loss, headaches, or paresthesias. Any or all of these symptoms may occur with hematologic disease.

The most common symptom of anemia is fatigue as a result of decreased oxygen delivery to cells. Cells use oxygen to produce the high-energy chemical *adenosine triphosphate (ATP)* needed to perform most cellular work. When oxygen delivery to cells is reduced, cellular work decreases, and fatigue increases. Ask patients about feeling tired, needing more rest, or losing endurance during normal activities. Ask them to compare their activities during the past month with those of the same month a year ago. Determine whether other symptoms of anemia, such as vertigo, tinnitus, and a sore tongue, are present.

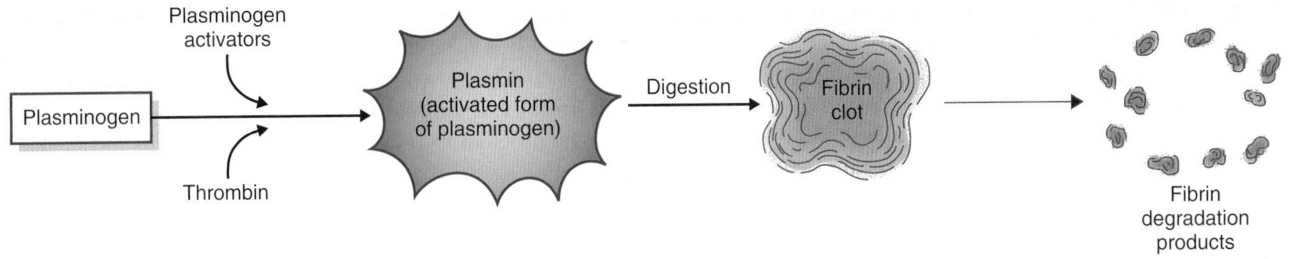

Fig. 36.4 The process of fibrinolysis.

NCLEX EXAMINATION CHALLENGE 36.2

Safe and Effective Care Environment

Which client history information is **most relevant** for the nurse to document when assessing for a possible hematologic problem? **Select all that apply.**

A. Eats a vegan diet
B. Participates in basketball twice weekly
C. Mother has pernicious anemia
D. Has a sister with Down syndrome
E. Sprays fertilizers and weed killers for a lawn care company
F. Takes aspirin or NSAIDs occasionally for minor muscle pain
G. Has used a vaping device instead of cigarette smoking for the past 2 years

Physical Assessment

Assess the whole body because blood problems may reduce oxygen delivery and tissue ***perfusion*** to all systems (Jarvis, 2020; McCance et al., 2019). Some assessment findings associated with hematologic problems are less reliable when seen in the older adult as described earlier in the section Hematologic Changes Associated With Aging. Equipment needed for hematologic assessment includes gloves, a stethoscope, a blood pressure (BP) cuff, and a penlight. Remember to gently handle the patient suspected of having a hematologic problem to avoid causing bruising, petechiae, or excessive bleeding.

Skin Assessment. Inspect the skin and mucous membranes for pallor or jaundice. Assess nail beds for pallor or cyanosis. Pallor of the gums, conjunctivae, and palmar creases (when the palm is stretched) indicates decreased hemoglobin levels and poor tissue oxygenation. Assess the gums for active bleeding in response to light pressure or brushing the teeth with a soft-bristled brush, and assess any lesions or draining areas. Inspect for petechiae and large bruises (*ecchymoses*). Petechiae are reddish-purple pinpoint hemorrhagic lesions in the skin. Bruises may cluster together. For hospitalized patients, determine whether there is bleeding around nasogastric tubes, endotracheal tubes, central lines, peripheral IV sites, or Foley catheters. Check the skin turgor and ask about itching because dry skin from poor perfusion itches. Assess body hair patterns. Areas with poor circulation, especially the lower legs and toes, may have sparse or absent hair, although this may be a normal finding in an older adult (Jarvis, 2020; Touhy & Jett, 2020).

Head and Neck Assessment. Check for pallor or ulceration of the oral mucosa. The tongue is smooth in pernicious anemia and iron deficiency anemia or smooth and beefy red in other nutrition deficiencies (McCance et al., 2019). These symptoms may occur with fissures at the corners of the mouth. Assess for scleral jaundice.

PATIENT-CENTERED CARE: CULTURAL/SPIRITUAL CONSIDERATIONS QSEN

Pallor and cyanosis are more easily detected in adults with darker skin by examining the oral mucous membranes and the conjunctiva of the eye. Jaundice can be seen more easily on the roof of the mouth. Petechiae may be visible only on the palms of the hands, the soles of the feet, the oral mucous membranes, and the conjunctiva. Bruises can be seen as darker areas of skin and palpated as slight swellings or irregular skin surfaces. Ask the patient about pain when skin surfaces are touched lightly or palpated.

Inspect and palpate all lymph node areas. Document any lymph node enlargement, including whether palpation of the enlarged node causes pain and whether the enlarged node moves or remains fixed with palpation.

Respiratory Assessment. When blood problems reduce oxygen delivery, the lungs work harder to maintain tissue perfusion. Assess the rate and depth of respiration while the patient is at rest and during and after mild physical activity (e.g., walking 20 steps in 10 seconds). Note whether the patient can complete a 10-word sentence without stopping for a breath. Assess whether he or she is fatigued easily, has shortness of breath at rest or on exertion, or needs extra pillows to breathe well at night. Anemia can cause these problems as a result of respiratory changes made as adjustments to the reduced tissue oxygen levels (McCance et al., 2019).

Cardiovascular Assessment. When blood problems reduce oxygen delivery, the heart works harder to help maintain tissue ***perfusion***. Pulses may become weak and thready. Observe for distended neck veins, edema, or indications of phlebitis. Use a stethoscope to listen for abnormal heart sounds and irregular rhythms. Assess blood pressure (BP). Systolic BP tends to be lower than normal in patients with anemia and higher than normal when the patient has excessive red blood cells.

Kidney and Urinary Assessment. The kidneys have many blood vessels, and bleeding problems may cause hematuria (blood in the urine). Inspect urine for color. Hematuria may be seen as grossly bloody red or dark-brownish gold urine. Test the urine for proteins with a urine test dipstick because blood contains protein and blood in the urine increases its protein content. Keep in mind that the adult with chronic kidney disease (CKD) produces less natural erythropoietin and often is anemic.

Musculoskeletal Assessment. Rib or sternal tenderness may occur with leukemia (blood cancer) when the bone marrow overproduces cells, increasing the pressure in the bones. Examine the skin over superficial bones, including the ribs and sternum, by applying firm pressure with the fingertips. Assess the range of joint motion and document any swelling or joint pain.

Abdominal Assessment. The normal adult spleen is usually not palpable, but an enlarged spleen occurs with many hematologic problems. An enlarged spleen may be detected by palpation, but this is usually performed by the primary health care provider because an enlarged spleen is tender and can rupture easily.

! NURSING SAFETY PRIORITY (QSEN)

Action Alert

Do not palpate the splenic area of the abdomen for any patient with a suspected hematologic problem. An enlarged spleen ruptures easily, which can lead to hemorrhage and death.

Palpating the edge of the liver in the right upper quadrant of the abdomen can detect enlargement, which often occurs with hematologic problems. The normal liver may be palpable as much as 4 to 5 cm below the right costal margin but is usually not palpable in the epigastrium.

A common cause of anemia among older adults is a chronically bleeding GI ulcer or intestinal polyp. If the ulcer is located in the stomach or the small intestine, obvious blood may not be visible in the stool, or such a small amount is passed each day that the patient is not aware of it. Obtain a stool specimen for occult blood testing.

Central Nervous System Assessment. Assessing cranial nerves and testing neurologic function are important in hematologic assessment because some problems cause specific changes. Vitamin B_{12} deficiency impairs nerve function, and severe chronic deficiency may cause permanent neurologic degeneration. Many neurologic problems can develop in patients who have leukemia, because leukemia can cause bleeding, infection, or tumor spread within the brain. When the patient with a suspected bleeding disorder has any head trauma, expand the assessment to include frequent neurologic checks and checks of cognitive function (see Chapter 38).

Psychosocial Assessment

Regardless of the type of hematologic problem, each patient brings his or her own coping style to the illness. Develop a rapport with the patient and learn which coping mechanisms he or she has used successfully in the past.

Diagnostic Assessment

Laboratory Tests. Laboratory test results provide definitive information about hematologic problems. The Laboratory Profile: Hematologic Assessment: Normal Ranges and Significance of Changes box lists laboratory data used to assess hematologic function. When a venipuncture is necessary, apply pressure to the site for at least 5 minutes on a patient suspected of having a hematologic problem to prevent harm from bleeding and hematoma formation.

Tests of Cell Number and Function. A *peripheral blood smear* is made by taking a drop of blood and spreading it over a slide. It can be read by an automated calculator or a technologist with a microscope. This rapid test provides information on the sizes, shapes, and proportions of different blood cell types within the peripheral blood.

A *complete blood count (CBC)* includes a number of studies: red blood cell (RBC) count, white blood cell (WBC) count, hematocrit, and hemoglobin level. The RBC count measures circulating RBCs in 1 mm^3 (or 1 L) of blood. The WBC count measures all leukocytes present in 1 mcL (or 1 L) of blood. To determine the percentages of different types of leukocytes circulating in the blood, a WBC count with differential leukocyte count is performed (see Chapter 16). The hematocrit (Hct) is the percentage of RBCs in the total blood volume (also known as *volume fraction*). The hemoglobin (Hgb) level is the total amount of hemoglobin in blood and is measured in grams per deciliter (g/dL) (or grams per liter [g/L]).

The CBC can measure other features of the RBCs. The mean corpuscular volume (MCV) measures the average volume or size of individual RBCs and is useful for classifying anemias. When the MCV is elevated, the cell is larger than normal *(macrocytic),* as seen in megaloblastic anemias. When the MCV is decreased, the cell is smaller than normal *(microcytic),* as seen in iron deficiency anemia. The mean corpuscular hemoglobin (MCH) is the average amount of hemoglobin by weight in a single RBC. The mean corpuscular hemoglobin concentration (MCHC) measures the average amount of hemoglobin by percentage in a single RBC. When the MCHC is decreased, the cell has a hemoglobin deficiency and is *hypochromic* (a lighter color), as in iron deficiency anemia. These three tests can help determine possible causes of low RBC counts that are not related to blood loss.

Reticulocyte count is helpful in determining bone marrow function. A reticulocyte is an immature RBC that still has its nucleus. An elevated reticulocyte count indicates that RBCs are being produced and released by the bone marrow before they mature. Normally only about 2% of circulating RBCs are reticulocytes. An elevated reticulocyte count is desirable in an anemic patient or after hemorrhage because this indicates that the bone marrow is responding to a decrease in the total RBC level. An elevated reticulocyte count without a precipitating cause usually indicates health problems, such as polycythemia vera (a malignant condition in which the bone marrow overproduces RBCs).

A *platelet count,* also known as a thrombocyte count, reflects the number of platelets in circulation. The normal range is 150,000 to 400,000/mm^3 (150 to 400 $\times$ 10^9/L). When this value is low

LABORATORY PROFILE

Hematologic Assessment: Normal Ranges and Significance of Changes

Test	Normal Range (SI Units)	Significance of Changes From Normal
Red blood cell (RBC) count	*Females:* 4.2-5.4 × 10^6/mcL (4.2-5.4 × 10^{12} cells/L) *Males:* 4.7-6.1 × 10^6/mcL (4.7-6.1 × 10^{12} cells/L)	*Decreased levels:* possible anemia or hemorrhage *Increased levels:* possible chronic hypoxia or polycythemia vera
Hemoglobin (Hgb)	*Females:* 12-16 g/dL (7.4-9.9 mmol/L) *Males:* 14-18 g/dL (8.7-11.2 mmol/L)	Same as RBC count
Hematocrit (Hct)	*Females:* 37%-47% (0.37-0.47 volume fraction) *Males:* 42%-52% (0.42-0.52 volume fraction)	Same as RBC count
Mean corpuscular volume (MCV)	80-95 fL	*Increased levels:* macrocytic cells, possible anemia *Decreased levels:* microcytic cells, possible iron deficiency anemia
Mean corpuscular hemoglobin (MCH)	27-31 pg	Same as MCV
Mean corpuscular hemoglobin concentration (MCHC)	32-36 g/dL or 32%-36%	*Increased levels:* spherocytosis or anemia *Decreased levels:* iron deficiency anemia or a hemoglobinopathy
White blood cell (WBC) count	5000-10,000/mm³ (5.0-10.0 × 10^9 cells/L)	*Increased levels:* associated with infection, inflammation, autoimmune disorders, and leukemia *Decreased levels:* prolonged infection or bone marrow suppression
Reticulocyte count	0.5%-2.0% of RBCs	*Increased levels:* possible chronic blood loss or recovery from anemia *Decreased levels:* possible inadequate RBC production
Total iron-binding capacity (TIBC)	250-460 mcg/dL (45-82 mcmol/L)	*Increased levels:* iron deficiency *Decreased levels:* anemia, hemorrhage, hemolysis
Iron (Fe)	*Females:* 60-160 mcg/dL (11-29 mcmol/L) *Males:* 80-180 mcg/dL (14-32 mcmol/L)	*Increased levels:* iron excess, liver disorders, hemochromatosis, megaloblastic anemia *Decreased levels:* possible iron deficiency anemia, hemorrhage
Serum ferritin	*Females:* 10-150 ng/mL (10-150 mcg/L) *Males:* 12-300 ng/mL (12-300 mcg/L)	Same as iron
Platelet count	150,000-400,000/mm³ (150-400 × 10^9/L)	*Increased levels:* polycythemia vera or malignancy *Decreased levels:* bone marrow suppression, autoimmune disease, hypersplenism
Hemoglobin electrophoresis	Hgb A_1: 95%-98% Hgb A_2: 2%-3% Hgb F: 0.8%-2% Hgb S: 0% Hgb C: 0% Hgb E: 0%	*Variations:* hemoglobinopathies
Direct and indirect Coombs test	Negative	*Positive findings:* antibodies to RBCs
International normalized ratio (INR)	0.8-1.1 times the control value	*Increased values:* longer clotting times (desirable for therapy with warfarin) *Decreased values:* hypercoagulation and increased risk for VTE
Prothrombin time (PT)	11-12.5 sec 85%-100%	*Increased time* indicates possible deficiency of clotting factors V and VII *Decreased time* may indicate vitamin K excess

fL, Femtoliter; *pg,* picograms; *VTE,* venous thromboembolism.
From Pagana, K., & Pagana, T. (2018). *Mosby's manual of diagnostic and laboratory tests* (6th ed.). St. Louis: Elsevier.

(thrombocytopenia), the patient is at greater risk for bleeding because platelets are critical for blood clotting. Patients who have values between 40,000/mm³ (40 × 10^9/L) and 80,000/mm³ (800 × 10^9/L) may have prolonged bleeding from trauma, dental work, and surgery. With platelet values below 20,000/mm³ (20 × 10^9/L) the patient may have spontaneous bleeding that is very difficult to stop.

Hemoglobin electrophoresis detects abnormal forms of hemoglobin, such as hemoglobin S in sickle cell disease. Hemoglobin A is the major type of hemoglobin in an adult.

Leukocyte alkaline phosphatase (LAP) is an enzyme produced by normal mature neutrophils. Elevated LAP levels occur during episodes of infection or stress. An elevated neutrophil count without an elevation in LAP level occurs with some types of leukemia.

Coombs tests, both direct and indirect, are used for blood typing. The direct test detects antibodies against RBCs that may be attached to a patient's RBCs. Although healthy adults can make these antibodies, in certain diseases (e.g., systemic lupus erythematosus, mononucleosis) these antibodies are directed against the patient's own RBCs. Excessive amounts of these antibodies can cause hemolytic anemia (Pagana & Pagana, 2018).

The indirect Coombs test detects the presence of circulating antiglobulins. The test is used to determine whether the patient has serum antibodies to the type of RBCs that he or she is about to receive by blood transfusion (Pagana & Pagana, 2018).

Serum ferritin, transferrin, and the total iron-binding capacity (TIBC) tests measure iron levels. Abnormal levels of iron and TIBC occur with problems such as iron deficiency anemia.

The serum ferritin test measures the amount of free iron present in the plasma, which represents 1% of the total body iron stores. Therefore the serum ferritin level provides a means to assess total iron stores. Adults with serum ferritin levels of at least 10 ng/100 mL have adequate iron stores; adults with levels less than 10 ng/100 mL have inadequate iron stores and have difficulty recovering from any blood loss.

Transferrin is a protein that transports dietary iron from the intestines to cell storage sites. Measuring the amount of iron that can be bound to serum transferrin indirectly determines whether an adequate amount of transferrin is present. This test is the total iron-binding capacity (TIBC) test. Normally, only about 30% of the transferrin is bound to iron in the blood. TIBC increases when a patient is deficient in serum iron and stored iron levels. Such a value indicates that an adequate amount of transferrin is present but less than 30% of it is bound to serum iron.

Tests Measuring Bleeding and Coagulation. Tests that measure bleeding and coagulation provide information that reflects the effectiveness of different aspects of blood ***clotting***. These tests are used to diagnose specific hematologic health problems, determine drug therapy effectiveness, and identify risk for excessive bleeding or clotting.

Prothrombin time (PT) measures how long blood takes to clot, reflecting the level of clotting factors II, V, VII, and X and how well they are functioning. When enough of these clotting factors are present and functioning, the PT shows blood clotting between 11 and 12.5 seconds or within 85% to 100% of the time needed for a control sample of blood to clot. PT is prolonged when one or more of these clotting factors are deficient.

The PT test is now used less often to assess how fast blood clots, because control blood is taken from different adults and may not be the same even in one laboratory from one day to the next. To reduce PT errors as a result of control blood variation or in some of the chemicals used in the test, the international normalized ratio (INR) is used to assess clotting time.

International normalized ratio (INR) measures the same process as the PT by establishing a normal mean or standard for PT. The INR is calculated by dividing the patient's PT by the established standard PT. A normal INR ranges between 0.8 and 1.2 (Pagana & Pagana, 2018). When using the INR to monitor warfarin therapy, the desired outcome is usually to maintain the patient's INR between 2.0 and 3.0 regardless of the actual PT in seconds. However, the desired INR range for any patient is individualized for specific patient factors and medical conditions.

The *partial thromboplastin time (PTT)* assesses the intrinsic ***clotting*** cascade and the action of factors II, V, VIII, IX, XI, and XII. PTT is prolonged whenever any of these factors is deficient, such as in hemophilia or disseminated intravascular coagulation (DIC). Because factors II, IX, and X are vitamin K dependent and are produced in the liver, liver disease can prolong the PTT. Desired therapeutic ranges for anticoagulation are usually between 1.5 and 2.0 times normal values but can be greater depending on the reason the adult is receiving anticoagulation therapy.

The *anti-factor Xa test* measures the amount of anti-activated factor X (anti-Xa) in blood, which is affected by heparin. It is used mainly to monitor heparin levels in patients treated with either standard unfractionated heparin or low–molecular-weight heparin. For adults not receiving heparin in any form, the reference range is less than 0.1 IU/mL. The usual therapeutic range for patients receiving standard heparin is 0.5 to 1.0 IU/mL, and the usual therapeutic range for patients receiving low–molecular-weight heparin is 0.3 to 0.7 IU/mL. Test results are affected by age, gender, health history, and the specific laboratory technique used for the test.

Platelet aggregation, or the ability to clump, is tested by mixing the patient's plasma with an agonist substance that should cause clumping. The degree of clumping is noted. Aggregation can be impaired in von Willebrand disease and during the use of drugs such as aspirin, anti-inflammatory agents, psychotropic agents, and platelet inhibitors.

NCLEX EXAMINATION CHALLENGE 36.3

Safe and Effective Care Environment

When reviewing the laboratory results for a client in the emergency department, which finding does the nurse report **immediately** to **prevent harm**?

A. International normalized ratio (INR) is 5.2
B. Platelet count of 180,000/mm^3 (180 × 10^9/L)
C. Hematocrit of 27% (0.27 volume fraction)
D. Reticulocyte value of 4%

Imaging Assessment. Assessment of the patient with a suspected hematologic problem can include radioisotopic imaging. Isotopes are used to evaluate the bone marrow for sites of active blood cell formation and iron storage. Radioactive colloids are used to determine organ size and liver and spleen function.

The patient is given an IV radioactive isotope about 3 hours before the procedure. Once in the nuclear medicine department, he or she must lie still for about an hour during the scan. No special patient preparation or follow-up care is needed for these tests.

Standard x-rays may be used to diagnose some hematologic problems. For example, multiple myeloma causes classic bone destruction, with a "Swiss cheese" appearance on x-ray. Long term sickle cell disease can result in bony destruction of the top of the skull showing as a "crew-cut" appearance on x-ray.

Bone Marrow Aspiration and Biopsy. Bone marrow aspiration and biopsy, which are similar invasive procedures, help evaluate the patient's hematologic status when other tests show abnormal findings that indicate a possible problem in blood cell production or maturation. Results provide information about bone marrow function, including the production of all blood cells and platelets. In a bone marrow aspiration, cells and fluids are suctioned from the bone marrow. In a bone marrow biopsy, solid tissue and cells are obtained by coring out an area of bone marrow with a large-bore needle.

A primary health care provider's prescription and a signed informed consent form are obtained before either procedure is performed. Bone marrow aspiration may be performed by a physician, an advanced practice nurse, or a physician assistant, depending on the agency's policy and regional law. The procedure may be performed at the patient's bedside, in an examination room, or in a laboratory.

After learning which specific tests will be performed on the marrow, check with the hematology laboratory to determine how to handle the specimen. Some tests require that heparin or other solutions be added to the specimen.

Patient Preparation. Most patients are anxious before a bone marrow aspiration, even those who have had one in the past. You can help reduce anxiety and allay fears by providing accurate information and emotional support. Some patients like to have their hand held during the procedure.

Explain the procedure and reassure the patient that you will stay during the entire procedure. Tell the patient that the local anesthetic injection will feel like a stinging or burning sensation. Tell him or her to expect a heavy sensation of pressure and pushing while the needle is being inserted. Sometimes a crunching sound can be heard or scraping sensation felt as the needle punctures the bone. Explain that a brief sensation of painful pulling will be experienced as the marrow is being aspirated by mild suction in the syringe. If a biopsy is performed, the patient may feel more discomfort as the needle is rotated into the bone.

Help the patient onto an examining table and expose the site (usually the iliac crest). If this site is not available or if more marrow is needed, the sternum may be used. If the iliac crest is used, place the patient in the prone or side-lying position. Depending on the tests to be performed on the specimen, a laboratory technician may be present to ensure its proper handling.

Procedure. The procedure usually lasts from 5 to 15 minutes. A local anesthetic agent is injected into the skin around the site. The patient may also receive a mild tranquilizer or a rapid-acting sedative, such as midazolam, lorazepam, or etomidate. Some patients do well with guided imagery or autohypnosis.

! NURSING SAFETY PRIORITY (QSEN)

Action Alert

Aspiration or biopsy procedures are invasive, and sterile technique must be observed.

The skin over the site is cleaned. For an aspiration, the needle is inserted with a twisting motion, and the marrow is aspirated by pulling back on the plunger of the syringe. When sufficient marrow has been aspirated to ensure accurate analysis, the needle is withdrawn rapidly while the tissues are supported. For a biopsy, a small skin incision is made and the biopsy needle is inserted. Pressure and several twisting motions are needed to ensure coring and loosening of an adequate amount of marrow tissue. Apply external pressure to the site until hemostasis is ensured. A pressure dressing or sandbags may be applied to reduce bleeding at the site.

Follow-up Care. The nursing priority after a bone marrow aspiration or biopsy is prevention of excessive bleeding. Cover the site with a dressing after bleeding is controlled, and closely observe it for 24 hours for signs of bleeding and infection. A mild analgesic (aspirin-free) may be given for discomfort, and ice packs can be placed over the site to limit bruising. If the patient goes home the same day as the procedure, instruct him or her to inspect the site every 2 hours for the first 24 hours to assess for active bleeding or bruising. Advise the patient to avoid any activity that might result in trauma to the site for 48 hours.

Information obtained from bone marrow aspiration or biopsy reflects the degree and quality of bone marrow activity present. The counts made on a marrow specimen can indicate whether different cell types are present in the expected quantities and proportions. In addition, bone marrow aspiration or biopsy can confirm the spread of cancer cells from other tumor sites.

CLINICAL JUDGMENT CHALLENGE 36.1

Patient-Centered Care; Safety

A 74-year-old woman is seen by her primary health care provider because she "just doesn't feel good." For about 2 months she has been feeling too tired to work in her garden or even make jewelry, her two main hobbies. Yesterday she fell asleep sitting up while providing after-school care for her two school-age grandchildren. She also reports heart palpitations on rising to a standing position and whenever she exerts herself. She says she is worried because her father died of chronic lymphocytic leukemia and his first symptoms were fatigue and heart palpitations. She is 5 feet 5 inches tall (1.65 m) and weighs 140 lb (63.3 kg). Her only medications are travoprost drops twice daily for glaucoma, aspirin 650 mg twice daily for mild-to-moderate joint pain, and a calcium-containing multiple vitamin once daily. She is allergic to mold and penicillin. She has three large bruises and explains that all three resulted from several different mild traumas (bumping the back of her hand on a door handle, dropping a casserole dish and trying to stop it with her foot, being hit on the leg by a car door opening next to her in a parking lot).

Vital signs are:

- T = 98.0°F (36.7°C)
- P = 112 beats/min
- BP = 96/50 mm Hg
- R = 24 breaths/min

Results of complete blood count with differential are:

- RBC count = 2.2×10^6/mcL ($2.2\text{-}5.4 \times 10^{12}$ cells/L)
- Hgb = 7.5 g/dL (4.6 mmol/dL)
- Hct = 22% (0.22 volume fraction)
- MCV = 52 fL
- Reticulocyte count = 7%
- TIBC = 160 mcg/dL (30 mcmol/L)
- Fe = 25 mcg/dL (4.5 mcmol/L)
- Platelets = 300,000/mm^3 (300×10^9/L)
- WBC count = 6600/mm^3 (6.6×10^9/L)

Differential:

- Neutrophils = 4488/mm^3 (4.48×10^9/L)
- Bands = 330/mm^3 (3.0×10^9/L)
- Lymphocytes = 1584/mm^3 (1.584×10^9/L)
- Basophils = 66/mm^3 (0.066×10^9/L)
- Eosinophils = 132/mm^3 (0.132×10^9/L)

1. **Recognize Cues:** What assessment information in this client situation is the most important and immediate concern for the nurse? (Hint: Identify the **relevant** information *first* to determine what is most important.)
2. **Analyze Cues:** What client conditions are consistent with the **most relevant** information? (Hint: Think about priority collaborative problems that support and contradict the information presented in this situation.)

GET READY FOR THE NEXT-GENERATION NCLEX® EXAMINATION!

Key Points

Review these Key Points for each NCLEX Examination Client Needs Category.

Safe and Effective Care Environment

- Handle patients with suspected hematologic problems gently to avoid bleeding or bruising. **QSEN: Safety**
- Do not palpate the splenic area of any patient suspected of having a hematologic problem. **QSEN: Safety**
- Maintain pressure over a venipuncture site for at least 5 minutes to prevent excessive bleeding. **QSEN: Safety**

Health Promotion and Maintenance

- Teach adults to avoid unnecessary contact with environmental chemicals or toxins. If contact cannot be avoided, teach them to use safety precautions.
- Instruct patients about the importance of eating a diet with adequate amounts of foods that are good sources of iron, folic acid, and vitamin B_{12}. **QSEN: Patient-Centered Care**

Psychosocial Integrity

- Support the patient during a bone marrow aspiration or biopsy. **QSEN: Patient-Centered Care**

Physiological Integrity

- Interpret blood cell counts and clotting test results to assess hematologic status. **QSEN: Evidence-Based Practice**
- Use the lip rather than nail beds to assess capillary refill on older adults. **QSEN: Evidence-Based Practice**
- Rely on laboratory tests rather than skin color changes in older adults to assess anemia or jaundice. **QSEN: Evidence-Based Practice**
- Teach patients and family members about what to expect during procedures to assess hematologic function, including restrictions, drugs, and follow-up care. **QSEN: Patient-Centered Care**
- Apply an ice pack to the needle site after a bone marrow aspiration or biopsy. **QSEN: Patient-Centered Care**
- Instruct patients to avoid activities that may traumatize the site after a bone marrow aspiration or biopsy. **QSEN: Evidence-Based Practice**

MASTERY QUESTIONS

1. Which statement regarding erythrocytes is true?
   A. Reticulocytes represent the final stage of mature erythrocytes.
   B. The lack of a nucleus in a mature erythrocyte increases its life span.
   C. Each erythrocyte can carry up to a maximum of four molecules of oxygen.
   D. The main trigger for erythrocyte production is the secretion of thrombopoietin.
2. Which response or health problem does the nurse expect to be present in a client who has a lifelong deficiency of antithrombin III?
   A. Chronic fatigue resulting from reduced production of normal hemoglobin
   B. Failure to produce and maintain normal circulating levels of platelets
   C. Prolonged bleeding and hematoma formation at sites of tissue injury
   D. Increased risk for clot formation and disruption of perfusion
3. Which precaution has the **highest priority for prevention of harm** when the nurse teaches the client about home care after a bone marrow aspiration?
   A. Clean the suture line daily with soap and water.
   B. Drink at least 4 L of fluid to ensure adequate hydration.
   C. Avoid taking any aspirin or aspirin-containing products.
   D. Stay in bed and get up only to use the bathroom for the next 2 days.

REFERENCES

Jarvis, C. (2020). *Physical examination & health assessment* (8th ed.). St. Louis: Elsevier.

McCance, K., Huether, S., Brashers, V., & Rote, N. (2019). *Pathophysiology: The biologic basis for disease in adults and children* (8th ed.). St. Louis: Elsevier.

Pagana, K., & Pagana, T. J. (2018). *Mosby's manual of diagnostic and laboratory tests* (6th ed.). St. Louis: Elsevier.

Touhy, T., & Jett, K. (2020). *Ebersole and Hess' toward healthy aging* (10th ed.). St. Louis: Elsevier.

37

Concepts of Care for Patients With Hematologic Problems

Katherine Byar

http://evolve.elsevier.com/Iggy/

LEARNING OUTCOMES

1. Collaborate with the interprofessional team to coordinate high-quality care to patients who have a hematologic problem affecting ***clotting***, ***immunity***, ***perfusion***, or ***gas exchange***.
2. Teach the patient and caregiver(s) about how impaired ***immunity***, impaired ***clotting***, and other changes caused by hematologic problems or their management affect home safety.
3. Use clinical judgment to prioritize evidence-based care for patients with common complications of hematologic problems affecting ***clotting***, ***immunity***, ***perfusion***, or ***gas exchange***.
4. Teach the patient and caregiver(s) about common drugs used as therapy for hematologic problems and their complications, including ***pain***, impaired ***immunity***, and impaired ***clotting***.
5. Teach the patient and family with a chronic hematologic problem about self-care management when in the community.
6. Teach adults undergoing therapy for a hematologic problem how to reduce the risk for ***infection*** and bleeding related to impaired ***immunity*** and impaired ***clotting***.
7. Implement patient- and family-centered nursing interventions to help people cope with the psychosocial impact of chronic or life-threatening hematologic problems and their therapies.
8. Apply knowledge of anatomy, physiology, pathophysiology, and genetics to assess patients with common complications caused by hematologic problems and their therapies.
9. Prioritize nursing responsibilities during transfusion therapy.

KEY TERMS

anemia A reduction in the number of red blood cells (RBCs), the amount of hemoglobin, or the *hematocrit* (percentage of packed RBCs per deciliter of blood).

apheresis The withdrawal of whole blood and removal of some of the patient's blood components followed by reinfusion of the plasma back into the patient.

blast phase cells Immature white cells that are dividing rapidly.

engraftment The successful "take" of the stem cells transplanted into the recipient.

erythrocytes Red blood cells (RBCs).

glossitis A smooth, beefy-red tongue.

hemoglobin A (HbA) Normal adult hemoglobin with two normal A chains and two normal B chains.

hemoglobin F (HbF) The main type of hemoglobin in the fetus, having two normal A chains and two normal gamma chains that bind oxygen more tightly than does hemoglobin A or S.

hemoglobin S (HbS) The hemoglobin of sickle cell disease in which there are two normal A chains and two abnormal beta chains that fold poorly, causing the red blood cell to assume a sickle shape under low-oxygen conditions.

hemolytic Blood destroying.

hypercellularity Cellular excess in the peripheral blood.

indolent Slow growing or slow to progress.

intrinsic factor A substance normally secreted by the gastric mucosa that is needed for intestinal absorption of vitamin B12.

leukemia Blood cancer that results from a loss of normal ***cellular regulation***, leading to uncontrolled production of immature WBCs ("blast" cells) in the bone marrow.

leukocytes White blood cells (WBCs).

leukopenia Reduction in the circulating number of white blood cells (WBCs).

lymphomas Cancers of the lymphoid cells and tissues with loss of ***cellular regulation*** and abnormal overgrowth of lymphocytes.

malignant Cancerous.

multiple myeloma (MM) A white blood cell cancer of mature B-lymphocytes called plasma cells that secrete antibodies.

nadir The period after chemotherapy in which bone marrow suppression is the most severe.

pancytopenia A condition of low circulating numbers of all blood cell types.

perfusion Adequate arterial blood flow through the tissues *(peripheral perfusion)* and blood that is pumped by the heart *(central perfusion)* to oxygenate body tissues.

peripheral blood stem cells (PBSCs) Stem cells that have been released from the bone marrow and circulate within the peripheral blood.

pernicious anemia Anemia resulting from failure to absorb vitamin B_{12}, caused by a deficiency of intrinsic factor (a substance normally secreted by the gastric mucosa), which is needed for intestinal absorption of vitamin B_{12}.

Philadelphia chromosome An abnormal chromosome often associated with chronic myelogenous leukemia caused by a translocation of the *ABL* gene from chromosome 9 onto the *BCR* gene of chromosome 22.

polycythemia vera (PV) One of the chronic myeloproliferative neoplasms (MPNs) in which there is loss of ***cellular regulation*** and excessive proliferation of specific groups of abnormal myeloid cells that have decreased function.

SCD crises Episodes of extensive cellular sickling that obstruct ***perfusion***, causing tissue hypoxia and severe pain.

sickle cell disease (SCD) A genetic disorder in which a mutation in the gene for the beta chains of hemoglobin causes chronic anemia, pain, disability, organ damage, increased risk for ***infection***, and early death as a result of poor blood ***perfusion***.

stomatitis Mouth sores.

teratogen An agent that can cause birth defects.

thrombocytopenia A reduction in the number of circulating platelets from reduced platelet production.

thrombocytopenic purpura The destructive reduction of circulating platelets after normal platelet production.

PRIORITY AND INTERRELATED CONCEPTS

The priority concepts for this chapter are:

- ***Perfusion***
- ***Immunity***

The ***Perfusion*** exemplar for this chapter is Sickle Cell Disease.

The ***Immunity*** exemplar for this chapter is Leukemia and Preleukemia.

The interrelated concepts for this chapter are:

- ***Cellular Regulation***
- ***Gas Exchange***
- ***Clotting***
- ***Pain***
- ***Infection***

As discussed in Chapter 36, the most important function of the hematologic system is the production of blood cells and blood cell products that are critical for the vital activities of ***perfusion***, ***immunity***, ***clotting***, and ***gas exchange***. Red blood cells (RBCs) deliver oxygen and, together with platelets, participate in clotting. White blood cells (WBCs) and their many products protect the body from ***infection*** and initiate wound healing after any type of injury. Any hematologic problem interfering with the production, function, and maintenance of blood cells can also impair the processes of perfusion, immunity, clotting and gas exchange. This chapter discusses the interprofessional care issues for common chronic and acute hematologic disorders.

PERFUSION CONCEPT EXEMPLAR: SICKLE CELL DISEASE

Pathophysiology Review

Several genetic hemoglobin problems can cause chronic anemia and other problems. These include sickle cell disease (SCD), hemoglobin C disease, and several types of thalassemia. Of these, SCD is more common in North America and tends to be more severe than the other hemoglobin disorders (Tanabe et al., 2019). **Sickle cell disease (SCD)** is a genetic disorder in which a mutation in the gene for the beta chains of hemoglobin causes chronic anemia, pain, disability, organ damage, increased risk for ***infection***, and early death as a result of poor blood perfusion.

As discussed in Chapter 3, **perfusion** is adequate arterial blood flow through the tissues *(peripheral perfusion)* and blood that is pumped by the heart *(central perfusion)* to oxygenate body tissues.

The SCD genetic mutation results in the formation of abnormal hemoglobin chains. In adults without SCD, the normal adult hemoglobin (**hemoglobin A [HbA]**) molecule has two alpha chains and two beta chains of amino acids. Normal adult RBCs usually contain 98% to 99% HbA, with a small percentage of a fetal form of hemoglobin (HbF).

In SCD, at least 40% (and often much more) of the total hemoglobin is composed of two normal alpha chains and two abnormal beta chains (**hemoglobin S [HbS]**) that fold poorly. HbS is sensitive to low oxygen content of RBCs, which causes them to fold even more, distorting the cells into sickle shapes. Sickled cells become rigid and clump together, causing the RBCs to become "sticky" and fragile. The clumped masses of sickled RBCs block blood flow and ***perfusion*** (Fig. 37.1), known as a *vaso-occlusive event (VOE)*. VOE leads to further tissue *hypoxia* (reduced oxygen supply) and more sickle-shaped cells, which then leads to more blood vessel obstruction, inadequate perfusion, and ischemia in the affected tissues. Conditions that cause sickling include hypoxia, dehydration, ***infection***, venous stasis, pregnancy, alcohol consumption, high altitudes, low or high environmental or body temperatures, acidosis, strenuous exercise, emotional stress, nicotine use (especially cigarettes), and anesthesia.

Sickled cells usually go back to normal shape when the precipitating condition is removed and the blood oxygen level is normalized, which allows tissue ***perfusion*** to resume. Although the cells then appear normal, some of the hemoglobin remains twisted, decreasing cell flexibility. The cell membranes are damaged over time, and cells are permanently sickled. The membranes of cells with HbS are more fragile and more easily broken. The average life span of an RBC containing 40% or more of HbS is about 10 to 20 days, much less than the 120-day life span of normal RBCs (McCance et al., 2019). This reduced RBC life span causes **hemolytic** (blood cell–destroying) anemia in patients with SCD.

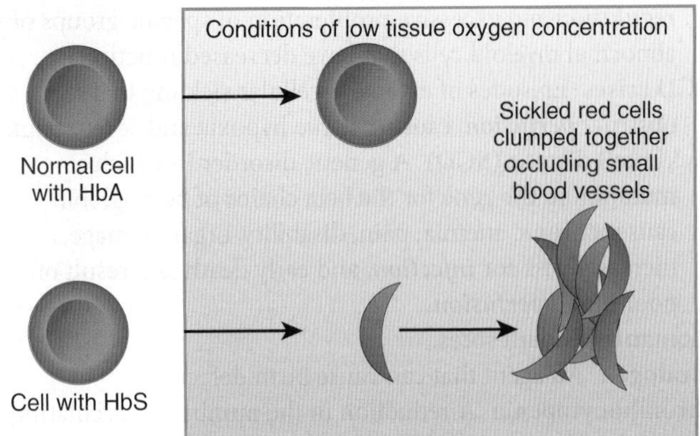

Fig. 37.1 Red blood cell actions under conditions of low tissue oxygenation. *HbA,* Hemoglobin A; *HbS,* hemoglobin S.

The patient with SCD has periodic episodes of extensive RBC sickling, called **SCD crises** or *vaso-occlusive crises (VOC).* The crises have a sudden onset and can occur as often as weekly or as seldom as once a year. Many patients are in good health much of the time, with crises occurring only in response to conditions that cause local or systemic *hypoxemia* (deficient oxygen in the blood).

Repeated VOEs and impaired ***perfusion*** cause long-term damage to tissues and organs. Most damage results from tissue hypoxia, anoxia, ischemia, and cell death. Organs develop small infarcted areas and scar tissue formation, and eventually organ failure results. The spleen, liver, heart, kidney, brain, joints, bones, and retina are affected most often. The average life expectancy of adult men with SCD is 42 years and for women with SCD is 48 years (Tanabe et al., 2019)

Etiology and Genetic Risk. *Sickle cell disease* (SCD) is a genetic disorder with an autosomal recessive pattern of inheritance (see Chapter 6). A specific mutation in the hemoglobin gene alleles on chromosome 11 leads to the formation of HbS instead of HbA (Online Mendelian Inheritance in Man [OMIM], 2019b). In SCD, the patient has two HbS gene alleles, one inherited from each parent, usually resulting in 80% to 100% of his or her hemoglobin being HbS. Because both hemoglobin alleles are S, SCD is sometimes abbreviated "SS." Patients with SCD often have severe symptoms and greatly impaired ***perfusion*** even when triggering conditions are mild. If a patient with SCD has children, each child will inherit one of the two abnormal gene alleles and at least have sickle cell trait.

Sickle cell trait occurs when one normal gene allele and one abnormal gene allele for hemoglobin are inherited and only about half of the hemoglobin chains are abnormal. Sickle cell trait is abbreviated "AS." The patient is a carrier of the HbS gene allele and can pass the trait on to his or her children. However, the patient usually has only mild symptoms of the disease when precipitating conditions are present because less hemoglobin is abnormal.

Incidence and Prevalence. Sickle cell trait and different forms of SCD occur in people of all races and ethnicities but are most common among African Americans in the United States. About 100,000 people have SCD, which occurs in 1 in 500 African Americans. About 1 in 13 (8%) African Americans are carriers of one sickle cell gene allele and have AS (Centers for Disease Control and Prevention [CDC], 2017; Tanabe et al., 2019).

❖ Interprofessional Collaborative Care

SCD is a chronic disease that reduces ***perfusion***, and complications become worse over time. Patients must self-manage continually at home or in other residential settings. When crises or other acute complications occur, patients are cared for in an acute care environment, usually in a medical-surgical setting.

◆ Assessment: Recognize Cues

History. An adult with SCD usually has a long-standing diagnosis of the disorder. Those with sickle cell trait usually have no symptoms or abnormal laboratory findings other than the presence of hemoglobin S. Patients with sickle cell trait may be unaware that they have a hematologic problem until an acute illness is present or when anesthesia is administered.

Ask about previous crises, what led to the crises, severity, and usual management. Explore recent contact with ill people and activities to determine what caused the current crisis. Ask about signs and symptoms of infection.

Review all activities and events during the past 24 hours, including food and fluid intake, exposure to temperature extremes, drugs taken, exercise, trauma, stress, recent airplane travel, and use of alcohol, tobacco, or other recreational drugs. Ask about changes in sleep and rest patterns, ability to climb stairs, and any activity that induces shortness of breath. Assess the patient's perceived energy level using a scale ranging from 0 to 10 (0 = not tired with plenty of energy; 10 = total exhaustion) to assess the degree of fatigue.

Physical Assessment/Signs and Symptoms. ***Pain*** *is the most common symptom of SCD crisis.* Others vary with the site of reduced ***perfusion*** and the tissue damaged.

Cardiovascular changes, including the risk for high-output heart failure, occur because of the anemia. Assess the patient for shortness of breath and general fatigue or weakness. Other problems may include murmurs, the presence of an S_3 heart sound, and increased jugular-venous pulsation or distention (Jarvis, 2020). Assess the cardiovascular status by comparing peripheral pulses, temperature, and capillary refill in all extremities. Extremities distal to blood vessel occlusion are cool to the touch with slow capillary refill and may have reduced or absent pulses, which indicate reduced ***perfusion***. Heart rate may be rapid, and blood pressure may be low to normal with anemia.

Respiratory system changes occur over time. Many patients with SCD develop pulmonary hypertension, and all are at risk for recurrent pneumonia. Further assessment with pulmonary function testing of the adult with SCD who has symptoms of pulmonary disease is recommended (U.S. Department of Health and Human Services [USDHHS], 2017). (See Chapter 24 for a discussion of pulmonary function testing.)

Acute chest syndrome is a common reason for hospitalization and is the most common cause of death (Taylor, 2019; USDHHS, 2014). This life-threatening condition is usually associated with respiratory ***infection*** and can also be caused by fat embolism and debris from sickled cells. Symptoms are similar to pneumonia with cough, shortness of breath, abnormal breath sounds, and an infiltrate on chest x-ray. Fever may or may not be present. This complication can lead to respiratory failure and multiple organ dysfunction syndrome (MODS).

Priapism is a prolonged penile erection that can occur in men who have SCD. The cause is excessive vascular engorgement in erectile tissue. The condition causes severe ***pain*** and can last for hours. During the priapism episode, the patient usually cannot urinate.

Skin changes include pallor or cyanosis because of poor ***gas exchange*** from decreased ***perfusion*** and anemia. Assess the lips, tongue, nail beds, conjunctivae, palms, and soles of the feet at least every 8 hours for subtle color changes. With cyanosis, the lips and tongue are gray; and the palms, soles, conjunctivae, and nail beds have a bluish tinge.

Another skin sign of SCD is jaundice. Jaundice results from RBC destruction and release of bilirubin. To assess for jaundice in patients with darker skin, inspect the roof of the mouth for a yellow appearance (Jarvis, 2020). Examine the sclera closest to the cornea to assess jaundice more accurately. Jaundice often causes intense itching.

Many adults with SCD have ulcers on the lower legs that are caused by poor ***perfusion***, especially on the outer sides and inner aspect of the ankle or the shin. These lesions often become necrotic or infected, requiring débridement and antibiotic therapy. Inspect the legs and feet for ulcers or darkened areas that may indicate necrotic tissue.

Abdominal changes include damage to the spleen and liver, which often occurs early from many episodes of hypoxia and ischemia. In crisis, abdominal pain from reduced ***perfusion*** is diffuse and steady, also involving the back and legs. The liver and spleen may feel firm and enlarged with a nodular or "lumpy" texture in later stages of the disease.

Kidney and urinary changes are common as a result of poor ***perfusion*** and decreased tissue ***gas exchange***. Chronic kidney disease occurs as a result of anoxic damage to the kidney nephrons (USDHHS, 2017). Early damage makes the kidneys less effective at filtration and reabsorption. The urine contains protein, and the patient may not concentrate urine. Eventually the kidneys fail, resulting in little or no urine output.

Musculoskeletal changes occur because arms and legs are often sites of blood vessel occlusion. Joints may be damaged from hypoxic episodes and have necrotic degeneration. Inspect the arms and legs and record any areas of swelling, temperature, or color difference. Ask patients to move all joints. Record the range of motion and any pain with movement.

Central nervous system (CNS) changes may occur in SCD. During crises patients may have a low-grade fever. Long-term effects of reduced ***perfusion*** to the CNS may result in infarcts with repeated episodes of hypoxia, causing the patient to have seizures or symptoms of a stroke (USDHHS, 2017). Assess for the presence of "pronator drift," bilateral hand grasp strength, gait, and coordination. See Chapter 38 for details of neurologic assessment.

Psychosocial Assessment. Often cognitive and behavioral changes are early indications of cerebral hypoxia from poor ***perfusion***. Assess the patient and document mental status examination results. Ask family members whether the current behavior and mental status are usual for the patient. Assess the patient and family for knowledge and understanding of SCD and how to live with the disease to the highest level of wellness possible.

SCD is a painful, life-limiting disorder that can be passed on to one's children. When assessing psychosocial needs, keep in mind new factors that might contribute to a crisis. Also assess established support systems, use of coping patterns, disease progression, and the impact that all of these have on the patient and family.

Laboratory Assessment. The diagnosis of SCD is based on the percentage of hemoglobin S (HbS) on electrophoresis (Pagana & Pagana, 2018). A person who has AS usually has less than 40% HbS, and the patient with SCD may have 80% to 100% HbS. This percentage does not change during crises. Another indicator of SCD is the number of RBCs with permanent sickling. This value is less than 1% among people with no hemoglobin disease, 5% to 50% among people with AS, and up to 90% among patients with SCD.

Other laboratory tests can indicate complications of the disease, especially during crises. The hematocrit of patients with SCD is low (between 20% and 30% [0.2 and 0.3 volume fraction]) because of RBC shortened life span and destruction. This value decreases even more during crises or stress (aplastic crisis). The reticulocyte count is high, indicating anemia of long duration. The total bilirubin level may be high because damaged RBCs release iron and bilirubin.

The WBC count is usually high in patients with SCD. This elevation is related to chronic inflammation caused by tissue hypoxia and ischemia.

Imaging Assessment. Bone changes occur as a result of chronically stimulated marrow and low bone oxygen levels. The skull may show changes on x-ray as a result of bone surface cell destruction and new growth, giving the skull a "crew cut" appearance on x-ray. X-rays of joints may show necrosis and destruction. Ultrasonography, CT, positron emission tomography (PET), and MRI may show soft-tissue and organ changes from poor ***perfusion*** and chronic inflammation.

Other Diagnostic Assessment. ECG changes indicate cardiac infarcts and tissue damage. Specific ECG changes are related to the area of the heart damaged. Echocardiograms may show cardiomyopathy and decreased cardiac output (low ejection fraction).

◆ Analysis: Analyze Cues and Prioritize Hypotheses. The priority collaborative problems for the patient with sickle cell disease include:

1. ***Pain*** due to poor tissue ***perfusion*** and joint destruction with low oxygen levels
2. Potential for ***infection***, sepsis, multiple organ dysfunction syndrome (MODS), and death

◆ Planning and Implementation: Generate Solutions and Take Action

Managing Pain

Planning: Expected Outcomes. ***Pain*** associated with sickle cell disease may be acute during crises and persistent as a result of complications. Acute pain episodes have a sudden onset usually involving the chest, back, abdomen, and extremities. Complications of SCD can cause severe, persistent pain, requiring large doses of opioid analgesics. Regardless of the pain type, expected outcomes include that the pain is controlled to a level acceptable to the patient (e.g., a 3 or less on a pain intensity rating scale of 0 to 10) and that will allow him or her to participate in self-care or other activities to the degree he or she wishes (Lentz & Kautz, 2017).

Interventions. ***Pain*** with sickle cell crisis is the result of tissue injury caused by poor ***perfusion*** and tissue ***gas exchange*** from RBC clumping that obstructs blood flow. Pain is often severe enough to require hospitalization and opioid analgesics.

Ask whether the pain is typical of past pain episodes. If not, other pain causes or disease complications must be explored. Ask the patient to rate pain on a scale ranging from 0 to 10 and evaluate the effectiveness of interventions based on the ratings.

Concerns about substance abuse can lead to inadequate pain treatment in these patients. Opioid addiction is rare in patients with SCD. Because the pain of crisis has no objective signs, pain management is based on past pain history, previous drug use, disease complications, and current pain assessment. Many patients have had negative interactions with nurses and other members of the interprofessional team who suggest that the pain is not a problem and that patients with SCD may be "drug seekers." Health care professionals must be aware of their own attitudes when caring for this population. If substance abuse occurs, management of addiction is incorporated into the overall treatment plan. *Addicted patients in acute pain crisis still need opioids.*

Drug therapy for patients in acute sickle cell crisis and ***pain*** often starts with at least 48 hours of IV analgesics. (See the Best Practice for Patient Safety & Quality Care: Care of the Patient in Sickle Cell Crisis Care box.) Morphine and hydromorphone are given IV on a routine schedule or by infusion pump using patient-controlled analgesia (PCA). Once relief is obtained the IV dose can be tapered, and the drug given orally. Avoid "as needed" (PRN) schedules because they do not provide adequate relief. Moderate pain may be managed with oral doses of opioids or NSAIDs. (See Chapter 5 for more information on pain management.)

BEST PRACTICE FOR PATIENT SAFETY & QUALITY CARE (QSEN)

Care of the Patient in Sickle Cell Crisis

- Administer oxygen.
- Administer prescribed pain medication.
- Hydrate the patient with normal saline IV and with beverages of choice (without caffeine) orally.
- Remove any constrictive clothing.
- Encourage the patient to keep extremities extended to promote venous return.
- Do not raise the knee position of the bed.
- Elevate the head of the bed no more than 30 degrees.
- Keep room temperature at or above 72°F (22.2°C).
- Avoid taking blood pressure with a standard or automatic external arm cuff.
- Check circulation in extremities every hour:
  - Pulse oximetry of fingers and toes
  - Peripheral pulses
  - Capillary refill

Hydroxyurea may reduce the number of sickling and ***pain*** episodes by stimulating fetal hemoglobin (**hemoglobin F [HbF]**) production, which is the main type of hemoglobin present during fetal life. It has two normal alpha chains and two gamma chains instead of beta chains. The gamma chains keep oxygen bound to hemoglobin molecules more tightly than do beta chains even when tissue oxygen levels are lower. By maintaining oxygen binding, increased levels of HbF increase tissue ***gas exchange*** and reduce sickling of red blood cells. Hydroxyurea produces this effect in some but not all patients with sickle cell disease (Vaçca & Blank, 2017). However, this drug increases the risk for leukemia. Long-term complications should be discussed with the patient before this therapy is started. Hydroxyurea also suppresses bone marrow function, including ***immunity***, and regular follow-up to monitor complete blood counts (CBCs) for drug toxicity is important.

! NURSING SAFETY PRIORITY (QSEN)

Action Alert

Hydroxyurea is a ***teratogen*** (agent that can cause birth defects). Teach sexually active women of childbearing age using hydroxyurea to adhere to strict contraceptive measures while taking it and for 1 month after it is discontinued.

A newer drug used for SCD is Endari, which is composed of the amino acid glutamine. Higher levels of glutamine in RBCs appears to lower oxidative stress in these cells. This cellular response to glutamine both decreases sickling rates and increases RBC lifespans, thus reducing or delaying complications of SCD. With longer life spans, the circulating percentage of mature erythrocytes increases and the percentage of reticulocytes decreases. The drug is a powder that is mixed with 8 ounces of liquid and taken orally. Common side effects include constipation, nausea, headache, abdominal pain, cough, pain in extremity, back pain, and chest pain.

Another newly approved drug for SCD is crizanlizumab, which is a monoclonal antibody that binds to platelets and inhibits selectin. Normally selectin helps platelets, RBCs, and endothelial cells adhere together. This new drug prevents adhesion and reduces vaso-occlusive crises. Crizanlizumab is a once-monthly infusion, and side effects include nausea, back pain, muscle pain, and fever.

Hydration by the oral or IV route helps reduce the duration of ***pain*** episodes. Urge the patient to drink water or juices. Because the patient is often dehydrated and his or her blood is hypertonic, hypotonic fluids are usually infused at 250 mL/hr for 4 hours. Once the patient's blood osmolarity is reduced to the normal range of 270 to 300 mOsm, the IV rate is reduced to 125 mL/hr if more hydration is needed.

Integrative therapies and other measures, such as keeping the room warm, using distraction and relaxation techniques, positioning with support for painful areas, aromatherapy, therapeutic touch, and warm soaks or compresses, all help reduce ***pain*** perception.

Preventing Sepsis, Multiple Organ Dysfunction Syndrome (MODS), and Death

Planning: Expected Outcomes. The patient with SCD is expected to remain free from ***infection*** and sepsis.

Interventions. The patient with SCD is at high risk for bacterial ***infection*** because of reduced ***immunity*** from anoxic damage to the spleen. Interventions focus on preventing ***infection***, controlling infection, and starting drug therapy early when infection is present. The patient with a fever should have diagnostic testing for sepsis, including CBC with differential WBC count, blood cultures, reticulocyte count, urine culture, and a chest x-ray. Usually these patients are started on prophylactic antibiotics.

Prevention and early detection strategies are used to protect the patient in sickle cell crisis from infection. Frequent, thorough handwashing is especially important. Any person with an upper respiratory tract infection who enters the patient's room must wear a mask. Strict aseptic technique is used for all invasive procedures.

Continually assess the patient for ***infection*** and monitor the daily CBC with differential WBC count. Inspect the mouth every 8 hours for lesions indicating fungal or viral infection. Listen to the lungs every 8 hours for crackles, wheezes, or reduced breath sounds. Inspect urine for odor and cloudiness and ask about urgency, burning, or pain on urination. Take vital signs at least every 4 hours to assess for fever, or supervise this action when performed by others.

Drug therapy by prophylaxis with twice-daily oral penicillin reduces the number of pneumonia and other streptococcal infections. Urge the patient to receive a pneumonia vaccination and an annual influenza vaccination. Drug therapy for an actual ***infection*** depends on the sensitivity of the specific organism and the extent of the infection.

Continued blood vessel occlusion by clumping of sickled cells increases the risk for multiple organ dysfunction syndrome (MODS). Acute chest syndrome, in which a vaso-occlusive event (VOE) causes infiltration and damage to the pulmonary system, is a major cause of death in adults with SCD. Thus preventing heart and lung damage is a priority. Management focuses on prevention of VOEs and promotion of ***perfusion***.

Assess the patient admitted in sickle cell crisis for adequate perfusion to all body areas. Remove restrictive clothing and instruct the patient to avoid keeping the knees and hips flexed.

Hydration is needed because dehydration increases cell sickling and must be avoided. Help the patient maintain adequate hydration. The patient in acute crisis needs an oral or IV fluid intake of at least 200 mL/hr.

Oxygen is given during crises because lack of oxygen is the main cause of sickling. Ensure that oxygen therapy is nebulized to prevent dehydration. Monitor oxygen saturation. If saturation is low, evaluation of arterial blood gases (ABGs) and a chest x-ray may be needed.

Transfusion with RBCs can be helpful to increase HbA levels and dilute HbS levels, although they must be prescribed cautiously to prevent iron overload from repeated transfusions (Martin & Haines, 2016). Transfusion therapy in some centers is a mainstay of SCD management to reduce sickling and the risk for stroke. Monitor the patient for transfusion complications (discussed in the Acute Transfusion Reactions section).

Hematopoietic stem cell transplantation (HSCT) may correct abnormal hemoglobin permanently during childhood. However, HSCT is expensive and may result in life-threatening complications. At this time HSCT is not approved as therapy for adults with SCD (Vacca & Blank, 2017). A recent experiment in which gene therapy was combined with autologous HSCT for an adult with SCD resulted in a 15-month span of time with expression of 50% HbA and no crisis episodes (Ribeil et al., 2017). Although promising, this combination therapy approach requires more testing before acceptance as an approved treatment for SCD.

NCLEX EXAMINATION CHALLENGE 37.1

Physiological Integrity

Which change in laboratory test results of a client with sickle cell disease who was started on therapy with Endari 2 months ago indicates to the nurse that the therapy is effective?

A. Increased HbF from 2% to 10%
B. Increased HbA from 3% to 5%
C. Decreased reticulocyte count from 12% to 4%
D. Decreased white blood cells from 8200/mm^3 to 7000/mm^3 (8.2 × 10^9/L to 7.0 × 10^9/L)

Care Coordination and Transition Management. Care focuses on teaching the patient and family how to prevent crises and complications. This care is summarized in the Patient and Family Education: Preparing for Self-Management: Prevention of Sickle Cell Crisis box. The patient with SCD may receive care in acute care, subacute care, extended or assistive care, and home care settings.

PATIENT AND FAMILY EDUCATION: PREPARING FOR SELF-MANAGEMENT

Prevention of Sickle Cell Crisis

- Drink at least 3 to 4 liters of liquids every day.
- Avoid alcoholic beverages.
- Avoid smoking cigarettes or using tobacco or nicotine in any form.
- Contact your primary health provider at the first sign of illness or infection.
- Be sure to get a "flu shot" every year.
- Ask your primary health care provider about receiving the pneumonia vaccine.
- Avoid hot and cold temperature extremes.
- Be sure to wear socks and gloves when going outside on cold days.
- Avoid airplanes with unpressurized passenger cabins.
- Avoid travel to areas at high altitudes (e.g., Denver, Flagstaff, Santa Fe, Lake Louise).
- Be sure all your health care providers know that you have sickle cell disease, especially the anesthesia provider and radiologist.
- Consider genetic counseling before becoming sexually active.
- Avoid strenuous physical exercise.
- When you are not in crisis, perform mild, low-impact exercise three times a week.

Self-Management Education. Having patients be partners in the lifelong management of SCD is essential for best outcomes. Self-management education is extensive and must be reinforced by all members of the interprofessional team at every health care encounter with a patient who has SCD.

Teach the patient to avoid specific activities that lead to reduced ***gas exchange*** from hypoxia and hypoxemia. Stress the recognition of the early symptoms of crisis or ***infection*** so interventions can be started early to prevent ***pain***, complications, and permanent tissue damage. Teach the patient and family the correct use of opioid analgesics at home.

Health Care Resources. Refer patients who are unaware of the genetic aspects of SCD to genetic counselors. These professionals can provide information about genetic transmission, birth control methods, and pregnancy options.

Many patients and family members can be helped by local support groups. Provide information about the closest local chapter of the Sickle Cell Foundation. Often local children's hospitals have sickle cell support groups that include adults with the disease.

PATIENT-CENTERED CARE: GENDER HEALTH CONSIDERATIONS (QSEN)

Pregnancy in women with SCD may be life threatening. Barrier methods of contraception (cervical cap, diaphragm, or condoms with or without spermicides) are often recommended for women with SCD who are sexually active. The use of combination hormone drugs for contraception may increase ***clotting***, especially among smokers, predisposing them to impaired ***perfusion*** and crises. The use of progestin-only hormonal contraception is recommended to reduce the risk for venous thrombotic events (VTEs) (Binette et al., 2017). Urge women using any hormone-based contraceptives not to smoke.

◆ **Evaluation: Evaluate Outcomes.** Evaluate the care of the patient with SCD based on the identified priority patient problems. The expected outcomes include that the well-informed patient will:

- Report ***pain*** to be maintained at an acceptable level
- Maintain ***perfusion*** and ***gas exchange*** to extremities and vital organs
- Remain free of ***infection***, sepsis, and multiple organ dysfunction syndrome (MODS)

ANEMIA

Anemia is a reduction in the number of RBCs, the amount of hemoglobin, or the *hematocrit* (percentage of packed RBCs per deciliter of blood). It is a clinical indicator, not a specific disease, and occurs with many health problems. For men a hemoglobin level of less than 13.5 g/dL (8.5 mmol/L) indicates anemia, and a level less than 12.0 g/dL (7.2 mmol/L) indicates anemia in women. The many causes of anemia include dietary problems, genetic disorders, bone marrow disease, or excessive bleeding. GI bleeding is a common reason for anemia in adults.

There are many types and causes of anemia (Table 37.1). Some are caused by a deficiency in one of the components needed to make fully functional RBCs. Others are caused by decreased RBC production, increased RBC destruction, or chronic RBC loss. Despite the many causes, the symptoms (see the Key Features: Anemia box) and the nursing interventions are similar for all types of anemia.

TABLE 37.1 Common Causes of Anemia

Type of Anemia	Common Causes
Sickle cell disease	Autosomal-recessive inheritance of two defective gene alleles for hemoglobin synthesis
Glucose-6-phosphate dehydrogenase (G6PD) deficiency anemia	X-linked recessive deficiency of the enzyme G6PD
Autoimmune hemolytic anemia	Abnormal immune function in which a person's immune reactive cells fail to recognize his or her own red blood cells as self-cells
Iron deficiency anemia	Inadequate iron intake caused by: • Iron-deficient diet • Chronic alcoholism • Malabsorption syndromes • Partial gastrectomy Rapid metabolic (anabolic) activity caused by: • Pregnancy • Adolescence • Infection
Vitamin B_{12} deficiency anemia	Dietary deficiency Failure to absorb vitamin B_{12} from intestinal tract as a result of: • Partial gastrectomy • Pernicious anemia • Malabsorption syndromes
Folic acid deficiency anemia	Dietary deficiency Malabsorption syndromes Drugs: • Oral contraceptives • Anticonvulsants • Methotrexate
Aplastic anemia	Exposure to myelotoxic agents: • Radiation • Benzene • Chloramphenicol • Alkylating agents • Antimetabolites • Sulfonamides • Insecticides Viral infection (unproven): • Epstein-Barr virus • Hepatitis B • Cytomegalovirus

Pathophysiology Review

Iron deficiency anemia is the most common anemia worldwide, especially among women, older adults, and people with poor diets. It is a decreased iron supply that results from blood loss, poor GI absorption of iron, and an inadequate diet (Cadet, 2018; McCance et al., 2019). *Any adult with iron deficiency should be evaluated for abnormal bleeding, especially from the GI tract.*

Healthy adults usually have between 2 and 6 total-body grams of iron, depending on size and the amount of hemoglobin in the

CLINICAL JUDGMENT CHALLENGE 37.1

Ethical and Legal; Patient-Centered Care

A 21-year-old college student is admitted to a medical-surgical nursing unit in sickle-cell crisis and has a urinary tract infection. Her temperature is now 102.8°F (39.3°C), which is increased from the 101.2°F (38.4°C) assessed in the emergency department. Her pulse oximetry is 88%. Her total white blood cell count is 14,500/mm^3 (14.5 × 10^9/L). She has orders for an IV with normal saline at 125 mL/hr, a broad-spectrum IV antibiotic, morphine IV push, and oxygen at 6 L/min by nasal cannula. She rates her pain as an 8 on a 0 to 10 scale and appears calm. Her parents live about an hour away and are on their way to the hospital.

While reviewing her health record the nurse notes that the client's number of crisis episodes has increased dramatically during the past 6 months. When asked if there is anything different in her life, at first she says no but looks away from the nurse. The nurse then asks if she feels stressed by her classes or exams and she responds that college is going well. Then she reports that some things have changed. She is now a member of a sorority and has a steady boyfriend. The nurse asks her if she is drinking alcohol or taking drugs and whether she is now sexually active. She then tells the nurse that she is sexually active and is using oral contraceptives prescribed at an off-campus health clinic where she and her other health problems are not known. She then shakes her head a little and reports that she also began vaping to "fit in" with her sorority sisters. She begs the nurse not to tell her parents or her primary health care provider about either her sexual activity or her new nicotine use habit.

1. **Recognize Cues:** What assessment information in this client situation is the most important and immediate concern for the nurse? (Hint: Identify the **relevant** information *first* to determine what is most important.)
2. **Analyze Cues:** What client conditions are consistent with the **most relevant** information? (Hint: Think about priority collaborative problems that support and contradict the information presented in this situation.)
3. **Prioritize Hypotheses:** Which possibilities or explanations are **most likely** to be present in this client situation? Which possibilities or explanations are the most serious? (Hint: Consider all possibilities and determine their urgency and risk for this client.)
4. **Generate Solutions:** What actions would most likely achieve the desired outcomes for this client? Which actions should be **avoided** or are **potentially harmful**? (Hint: Determine the desired outcomes first to decide which interventions are appropriate and those that should be avoided.)
5. **Take Action:** Which actions are the most appropriate and how should they be implemented? In what **priority order** should they be implemented? (Hint: Consider health teaching, documentation, requested health care provider orders or prescriptions, nursing skills, collaboration with or referral to health team members, etc.)
6. **Evaluate Outcomes:** What client assessment would indicate that the nurse's actions were **effective**? (Hint: Think about signs that would indicate an improvement, decline, or unchanged client condition.)

cells. With chronic iron deficiency, RBCs are small *(microcytic)* and the patient has mild symptoms of anemia, including weakness and pallor. Other symptoms include fatigue, reduced exercise tolerance, and fissures at the corners of the mouth. Serum ferritin values are less than 10 ng/mL (normal range is 10 to 300 ng/mL [10 to 300 mcg/L]).

Vitamin B_{12} deficiency anemia is caused by conditions that fail to activate enzymes needed to move folic acid into precursor RBCs for cell division and growth into functional RBCs. These precursor cells then undergo improper DNA synthesis

KEY FEATURES

Anemia

Skin Signs and Symptoms

- General pallor (more noticeable on the ears, nail beds, palm creases, and around the mouth)
- Cool to the touch
- Patient does not tolerate cooler temperatures
- When chronic, nails become brittle and concave

Cardiovascular Signs and Symptoms

- Continuous rapid heartbeat that increases after meals and with activity
- With severe anemia, abnormal heart sounds (murmurs and gallops) may be heard
- Orthostatic hypotension

Respiratory Signs and Symptoms

- Breathless on exertion
- Decreased oxygen saturation levels

Neurologic Signs and Symptoms

- Fatigue
- Increased need for sleep
- Reduced energy levels

and increase in size. This anemia is described as *megaloblastic* or *macrocytic* anemia because of the large size of the abnormal cells.

Causes of vitamin B_{12} (also known as cobalamin) deficiency include vegan diets or other diets lacking proteins, small bowel resection, chronic diarrhea, diverticula, tapeworm, or overgrowth of intestinal bacteria. Anemia resulting from failure to absorb vitamin B_{12} (**pernicious anemia**) is caused by a deficiency of **intrinsic factor** (a substance normally secreted by the gastric mucosa), which is needed for intestinal absorption of vitamin B_{12}. Pernicious anemia is a type of autoimmune disorder. All autoimmune problems may have a genetic predisposition and may be present in other family members. Pernicious anemia is more common among older adults who may have reduced gastric absorption of many nutrients (Jarvis, 2020).

Vitamin B_{12} deficiency anemia may be mild or severe and usually develops slowly. Specific symptoms include pallor and jaundice, **glossitis** (a smooth, beefy-red tongue) (Fig. 37.2), fatigue, and weight loss. Patients may also have *paresthesias* (abnormal nerve sensations) in the feet and hands and poor balance because vitamin B_{12} helps maintain nerve function.

Folic acid deficiency anemia may have symptoms similar to those of vitamin B_{12} deficiency. However, paresthesias do not occur because folic acid deficiency alone does not affect nerve function. This disease develops slowly.

Common causes of folic acid deficiency are poor nutrition, malabsorption, and drugs. Poor nutrition, especially a diet lacking green leafy vegetables, liver, yeast, citrus fruits, dried beans, and nuts, is the most common cause. Malabsorption syndromes, such as Crohn's disease, are the second most common cause. Anticonvulsants and oral contraceptives can contribute to folic acid deficiency and anemia.

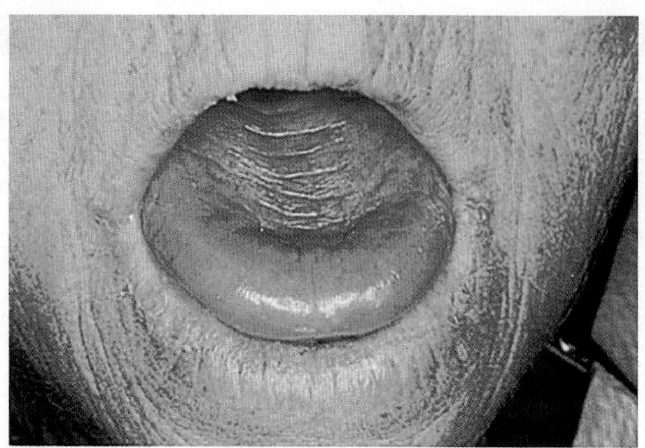

Fig. 37.2 Glossitis, a smooth tongue as a result of vitamin B_{12} deficiency anemia. (From Feldman, M., Friedman, L., & Brandt, L. [2010]. *Sleisenger and Fordtran's gastrointestinal and liver disease* [9th ed.]. Philadelphia: Saunders.)

PATIENT-CENTERED CARE: OLDER ADULT CONSIDERATIONS QSEN

Older patients often have poor diets or chewing difficulties and thus are at risk for anemias that result from deficiency (Mangels, 2018). Ask about a family history of anemia. B_{12} deficiency anemia often occurs in patients 50 to 80 years of age (Touhy & Jett, 2020). Because symptoms are vague, the disorder can easily be overlooked.

Aplastic anemia is a deficiency of circulating red blood cells (RBCs) because of impaired ***cellular regulation*** of the bone marrow, which then fails to produce these cells. It is caused by an injury to the immature precursor cell for RBCs. Although aplastic anemia sometimes occurs alone, it usually occurs with **leukopenia** (a reduction in white blood cells [WBCs]) and **thrombocytopenia** (a reduction in the number of circulating platelets from reduced platelet production), a condition known as **pancytopenia**. Disease onset may be slow or rapid.

Often aplastic anemia is caused by long-term exposure to toxic agents, drugs (see Table 36.2), ionizing radiation, or infection, but many times the cause is unknown. The disease also may follow a viral infection. The most common hereditary form of the disease is Fanconi anemia. These problems all result in loss of normal ***cellular regulation***.

The patient has symptoms of severe anemia. A complete blood count (CBC) shows severe macrocytic anemia, leukopenia, and thrombocytopenia. A bone marrow biopsy may show replacement of the red, cell-forming marrow with fat. Infection is common.

Glucose-6-phosphate dehydrogenase deficiency (G6PD) anemia is a genetic problem in which there is a deficiency of the enzyme G6PD. This disease is inherited as an X-linked recessive disorder, with severe expression in males and mild expression in carrier females. It affects about 10% of all African Americans and also is more common in adults from the Middle East and Asia (McCance et al., 2019).

G6PD stimulates reactions in glucose metabolism important for energy in RBCs because they contain no other way to produce adenosine triphosphate (ATP). Cells with reduced amounts of G6PD break more easily during exposure to some drugs (e.g., sulfonamides, aspirin, quinine derivatives, chloramphenicol, dapsone, high doses of vitamin C, and thiazide diuretics) and benzene and other toxins.

New RBCs have some G6PD, but the enzyme diminishes as the cells age. The patient usually does not have symptoms until exposed to triggering agents or until a severe ***infection*** develops. After exposure to a precipitating cause, acute RBC breakage begins and lasts 7 to 12 days. During this acute phase, anemia and jaundice develop. The hemolytic reaction is limited because only older RBCs, containing less G6PD, are destroyed.

Immunohemolytic anemia, also referred to as *autoimmune hemolytic anemia* (McCance et al., 2019), is caused by ***immunity*** problems that, for unknown reasons, allow a person to form antibodies that attack and destroy his or her own RBC membranes *(lysis).* This destruction is then followed by accelerated production of abnormal RBCs.

The two types of immunohemolytic anemia are warm antibody anemia and cold antibody anemia. *Warm antibody anemia* occurs with immunoglobulin G (IgG) antibody excess. These antibodies are most active at 98.6°F (37°C) and may be triggered by drugs, chemicals, or other autoimmune problems. *Cold antibody anemia* has complement protein fixation on immunoglobulin M (IgM) and occurs most often at body temperatures around 86°F (30°C). This problem often occurs with a Raynaud-like response in which the arteries in the hands and feet constrict completely in response to cold temperatures or stress.

NCLEX EXAMINATION CHALLENGE 37.2

Physiological Integrity

With which types of anemia does the nurse ask the client about the presence of the disorder in other family members? **Select all that apply.**

A. Sickle cell anemia
B. Folic acid deficiency anemia
C. Glucose-6-phosphate dehydrogenase deficiency anemia
D. Iron deficiency anemia
E. Pernicious anemia
F. Vitamin B_{12} deficiency anemia

❖ Interprofessional Collaborative Care

Iron deficiency anemia management involves increasing the oral intake of iron from food sources (e.g., red meat, organ meat, egg yolks, kidney beans, leafy green vegetables, and raisins). If iron losses are mild, oral iron supplements are started until the hemoglobin level returns to normal (Cadet, 2018). If the supplements cause GI distress, they can be taken with meals. When iron deficiency anemia is severe, iron solutions (iron dextran; ferumoxytol) can be given parenterally.

Vitamin B_{12} deficiency anemia is managed by teaching the patient to increase his or her intake of foods rich in vitamin B_{12} (animal proteins, fish, eggs, nuts, dairy products, dried beans, citrus fruit, and leafy green vegetables). Vitamin supplements

! NURSING SAFETY PRIORITY QSEN

Drug Alert

Ferumoxytol has a black box warning for an increased risk for life-threatening anaphylaxis that can occur during or within 5 minutes after receiving the infusion. Stay with the patient during the infusion and for 10 to 15 minutes after the infusion is complete.

may be prescribed when anemia is severe. Patients who have pernicious anemia are given vitamin B_{12} injections weekly at first and then monthly for the rest of their lives. Oral B_{12} preparations and nasal spray or sublingual cobalamin preparations may be used to maintain vitamin levels after the patient's deficiency has first been corrected by the traditional injection method.

Folic acid deficiency anemia is best managed by identifying adults at risk and preventing the deficiency. High-risk adults include older, debilitated patients with alcoholism; malnourished patients; and those with increased folic acid requirements. A diet rich in foods containing folic acid and vitamin B_{12} prevents deficiency. This anemia is managed with scheduled folic acid replacement therapy.

Aplastic anemia is managed differently depending on the absolute cause. For transient or drug-induced aplastic anemia, short-term management may include blood transfusions along with discontinuing the responsible drug. Blood transfusions are used when the anemia causes debility or when bleeding is life threatening because of low platelet counts. Unnecessary transfusions increase the chance for developing immune reactions to platelets and shorten the life span of transfused cells. This therapy is discontinued as soon as the bone marrow begins to produce RBCs if the problem is transient.

Immunosuppressive therapy helps patients who have the types of aplastic anemia with a disease course similar to that of autoimmune problems. Drugs such as prednisone, antithymocyte globulin (ATG), and cyclosporine have resulted in partial or complete remissions. For moderate aplastic anemia, daclizumab has improved both blood counts and transfusion requirements. Splenectomy may be needed for patients with an enlarged spleen that is either destroying normal RBCs or suppressing their development.

Hematopoietic stem cell transplantation with donor cells is the most successful method of treatment for aplastic anemia that does not respond to other therapies. Cost, availability, and complications limit this treatment. For patients who are unable to undergo such treatment or lack a suitable donor, immunosuppressive therapy remains the treatment of choice.

Glucose-6-phosphate dehydrogenase deficiency anemia management has prevention as the most important strategy. Patients, especially men, who belong to the high-risk groups should be tested for this problem before receiving drugs that can cause the hemolytic reaction.

Hydration is important during an episode of hemolysis to prevent debris and hemoglobin from collecting in the kidney tubules, which can lead to acute kidney injury (AKI). Osmotic diuretics, such as mannitol, help prevent this complication. Transfusions are needed when anemia is present and kidney function is normal (see the Transfusion Therapy section).

Immunohemolytic anemia management depends on disease severity. Steroid therapy to suppress ***immunity*** is temporarily effective in many patients. Immunotherapy with rituximab (a monoclonal antibody), splenectomy, and more intense immunosuppressive therapy with chemotherapy are used if steroid therapy fails (Zanella & Barcelleini, 2016).

POLYCYTHEMIA VERA

Pathophysiology Review

Polycythemia vera (PV) is one of the chronic myeloproliferative neoplasms (MPNs) in which there is loss of ***cellular regulation*** with excessive expansion of specific groups of abnormal myeloid cells with decreased function. PV differs from other MPNs by polycythemia in which the number of RBCs in the blood is *greater* than normal. The blood of a patient with polycythemia is *hyperviscous* (thicker than normal blood). The problem may be temporary because of other conditions or chronic.

The blood hemoglobin levels in PV are sustained at greater than 18 g/dL (11.2 mmol/L) in men or greater than 16.5 g/dL (9.9 mmol/L) in women, with an RBC count of 6 million/mm^3 (6×10^{12}), or with a hematocrit of 55% (0.55 volume fraction) or greater. PV is actually a cancer of the RBCs with three major hallmarks: massive production of RBCs, excessive leukocyte production, and excessive production of platelets. This cellular excess in the peripheral blood is known as **hypercellularity**. More than 90% of patients with PV have a mutation of the *JAK2* kinase gene in the affected cells; this mutation causes a loss of ***cellular regulation*** over blood cells (McCance et al., 2019).

❖ Interprofessional Collaborative Care

◆ **Assessment: Recognize Cues.** The patient's facial skin and mucous membranes have a dark, purple or cyanotic, flushed *(plethoric)* appearance with distended veins (Jarvis, 2020). Intense itching caused by dilated blood vessels and poor ***perfusion*** is common. The thick blood moves more slowly and causes hypertension. Blood flow may be so slow in some areas that stasis occurs. Vascular stasis causes *thrombosis* (clot formation) within the smaller vessels, occluding them, which interferes with ***perfusion*** and leads to tissue hypoxia, anoxia, and, later, infarction and necrosis. Tissues most at risk are the heart, spleen, and kidneys, although damage can occur in any organ.

Because the actual number of cells in the blood is greatly increased and the cells are not completely normal, cell life spans are shorter. The shorter life spans and increased cell production cause a rapid turnover of circulating blood cells. This rapid turnover increases cell debris (released when cells die) in the blood, which further thickens it. This debris includes uric acid and potassium, which cause the symptoms of gout and hyperkalemia (elevated serum potassium level).

Even though the number of RBCs is greatly increased, their oxygen-carrying capacity is reduced, and patients have poor ***gas exchange*** with severe hypoxia. Bleeding problems are common because of platelet impairment with poor ***clotting***.

PATIENT AND FAMILY EDUCATION: PREPARING FOR SELF-MANAGEMENT

Polycythemia Vera

- Drink at least 3 liters of liquids each day.
- Avoid tight or constrictive clothing, especially garters and girdles.
- Wear gloves when outdoors in temperatures lower than 50°F (10°C).
- Keep all health care–related appointments.
- Contact your primary health care provider at the first sign of infection.
- Take anticoagulants as prescribed.
- Wear support hose or stockings while you are awake and up.
- Elevate your feet whenever you are seated.
- Exercise slowly and only on the advice of your primary health care provider.
- Stop activity at the first sign of chest pain.
- Use an electric shaver.
- Use a soft-bristle toothbrush to brush your teeth.
- Do not floss between your teeth.
- If you are a smoker, strongly consider smoking cessation.

◆ **Interventions: Take Action.** PV is a malignant disease that progresses in severity over time. If left untreated, few people with PV live longer than 2 years after diagnosis. When managed by repeated phlebotomy with apheresis (two to five times per week), the patient may live 10 to 15 years or longer. (**Apheresis** is the withdrawal of whole blood and removal of some of the patient's blood components, in this case RBCs. The plasma is then reinfused back into the patient.) Increasing hydration and promoting venous return help prevent clot formation. Drug therapy for PV includes anticoagulants. The Patient and Family Education: Preparing for Self-Management: Polycythemia Vera box lists health tips for patients with PV.

Aspirin therapy may be used to decrease ***clotting*** but increases the risk for GI bleeding. Hydroxyurea, an oral chemotherapy drug, may be prescribed for severe disease symptoms. Pegylated interferon has also shown some benefit in controlling RBC production.

IMMUNITY CONCEPT EXEMPLAR: LEUKEMIA AND PRELEUKEMIA

Leukocytes (white blood cells [WBCs]), when present in the blood within normal numbers and maturation ratios, protect us from ***infection*** and cancer development (see Chapter 16). When any one type of WBC is present in either abnormal amounts (too high or too low), ***immunity***, ***gas exchange***, and ***clotting*** are affected, increasing patients' risks for many complications.

Pathophysiology Review

Leukemia is an actual blood cancer that results from a loss of normal ***cellular regulation***, leading to uncontrolled production of immature WBCs ("blast" cells) in the bone marrow. As a result, the bone marrow becomes overcrowded with immature, nonfunctional cells, and production of other normal blood cell types is greatly decreased. Leukemia may be *acute*, with a sudden onset, or *chronic*, with a slow onset and symptoms that persist for years. In addition, a group of precancerous or preleukemic disorders that can progress to leukemia are the myelodysplastic syndromes (MDSs) that also result from the formation of abnormal cells in the bone marrow. These abnormal cells are usually destroyed shortly after they are released into the blood, so most patients with MDS have a decrease in all circulating blood cell types. About 30% of all patients with MDS eventually develop acute leukemia (McCance et al., 2019).

Leukemia is classified by cell type. Leukemic cells coming from the lymphoid pathways (see Fig. 16.4) are classified as *lymphocytic* or *lymphoblastic*. Leukemic cells coming from the myeloid pathways are classified as *myelocytic, myelogenous,* or *myeloblastic*. Several subtypes exist for each of these diseases, which are classified according to the degree of maturity of the abnormal cell and the specific cell type involved. Treatment may differ based on subtype. *Biphenotypic leukemia* is acute leukemia that shows both lymphocytic and myelocytic features.

With leukemia, cancer most often occurs in the stem cells or early precursor leukocyte cells, causing excessive growth of one specific type of immature leukocyte. In some chronic leukemias, the cancerous cells may be more mature. These cells are abnormal, and their excessive production in the bone marrow stops normal bone marrow production, leading to anemia, **thrombocytopenia** (reduced circulating platelet numbers), and **leukopenia** (reduced circulating WBC numbers). Often the number of immature, abnormal WBCs ("blasts") in the blood is greatly elevated, but these cells do not provide infection protection. Leukemic cells may also be in the spleen, liver, lymph nodes, and central nervous system. With acute leukemia these changes occur rapidly and, without intervention, progress to cause death from ***infection*** or hemorrhage. Chronic leukemia and myelodysplastic syndromes (MDSs) may be present for years before changes appear. With MDS anemia is the most common problem initially; leukopenia and thrombocytopenia are present later in the course of the disorder.

Etiology and Genetic Risk. The exact causes of leukemia and MDS are unknown, although many genetic and environmental factors are involved in their development. The basic problem involves damage to genes controlling cell growth, resulting in a loss of normal ***cellular regulation***. This damage then changes cells from normal to **malignant** (cancerous). Bone marrow analysis shows abnormal chromosomes about 50% of the time (McCance et al., 2019). Possible risk factors for leukemia development include exposure to ionizing radiation, viral ***infection***, exposure to chemicals and drugs, genetic factors, ***immunity*** factors, and the interaction of these factors.

Ionizing radiation exposures such as radiation therapy for cancer treatment or heavy accidental exposures increase the risk for leukemia development, particularly acute myelogenous leukemia (AML). Chemicals and drugs have been linked to leukemia and MDS development because of their ability to damage DNA and disrupt normal ***cellular regulation***. Previous treatment for cancer with some chemotherapy drugs increases the risk for leukemia or MDS development about 5 to 8 years after treatment. Table 36.2 lists chemicals and drugs that damage the hematologic system.

Genetic and ***immunity*** factors influence leukemia development. There is an increased incidence of the disease among patients with genetic conditions such as Down syndrome, Bloom syndrome, Klinefelter syndrome, and Fanconi anemia. Immune deficiencies may promote the development of leukemia. Chronic lymphocytic leukemia often has a familial predisposition.

Incidence and Prevalence. Leukemia accounts for 3% to 4% of all new cases of cancer and of all deaths from cancer (American Cancer Society [ACS], 2020). In Canada, leukemia accounts for 6.3% of new cancer cases and 6.9% of all deaths from cancer (Canadian Cancer Society [CCS], 2019). The incidence depends on many factors, including the type of WBC affected, age, gender, race, and geographic locale.

About 70,000 new cases of leukemia occur each year in North America (ACS, 2020; CCS, 2019). Table 37.2 lists different leukemia types and MDSs based on the cell type and how fast the disease progresses.

❖ Interprofessional Collaborative Care

Leukemia can be cured; but the acute phase of treatment is long, affects every aspect of a patient's life, and is best managed by an interprofessional team. Like many disorders, leukemia management is most effective when the patient and family are full partners with the health care team.

INTERPROFESSIONAL COLLABORATIVE CARE

The Patient With Acute Leukemia

In addition to hematology oncologists and oncology nurses, other professionals important to ensuring optimal management include registered dietitian nutritionists (RDNs), pharmacists, occupational therapists, social workers, patient navigators, community health workers, mental health practitioners, and spiritual care advisors.

The only potentially curative treatment for MDS is hematopoietic stem cell transplantation (HSCT), which is often not an option because of the advanced age of many patients. Alternative management strategies with antitumor immunomodulating agents have demonstrated some promise based on specific MDS cell characteristics. Just as for leukemia, supportive care for MDS includes blood transfusions for anemia and platelet transfusions when platelet levels are very low. Erythrocyte-stimulating agents (ESAs) such as epoetin alfa or darbepoetin alfa may be given in addition to transfusions for supportive care.

Initial care for leukemia usually occurs in an inpatient setting, as does care for treatment complications such as ***infection***. Some therapy is provided on an outpatient basis; even HSCT recipients may be managed as outpatients in some health centers. Care coordination is extensive, and patient and family education is an ongoing process.

TABLE 37.2 Classification of Leukemia Types

Leukemia Type	Features
Acute myelogenous leukemia (AML)	Most common in adults Has eight subtypes
Acute promyelocytic leukemia (APL)	Subtype of AML Most curable of adult leukemias
Acute lymphocytic leukemia (ALL)	Forms about 10% of adult-onset leukemias Often is Philadelphia chromosome positive
Chronic myelogenous leukemia (CML)	Forms about 20% of adult-onset leukemias Occurs most often after age 50 years Usually is Philadelphia chromosome positive Has three phases: • *Chronic:* slow growing with mild manifestations that respond to therapy • *Accelerated:* more rapid growing with more severe manifestations, increased blast cells, and failure to respond to therapy • *Blast:* very aggressive leukemia with high percentage of blast cells and promyelocytes that spread to other organs
Chronic lymphocytic leukemia (CLL)	Most common chronic leukemia in adults; occurs most often after age 50 years Is associated with a genetic predisposition Survival time can extend to 10 years or more in patients diagnosed with early-stage disease

◆ Assessment: Recognize Cues

History. Ask the patient about exposure to risk factors and related genetic factors. Age is important because the risk for some leukemias and MDSs increases with age. Occupation, hobbies, and the medical history may reveal exposure to chemicals, drugs, or ionizing radiation agents that increase the risk for bone marrow injury.

Changes in ***immunity*** increase the risk for infection in the patient with leukemia or MDS. Even when the blood count shows a normal or high level of WBCs, these cells are immature and cannot protect the patient from ***infection***. Ask about the frequency and severity of infections, such as colds, influenza, pneumonia, bronchitis, or unexplained fevers, during the past 6 months.

Platelet function is reduced with leukemia, interfering with ***clotting***. Ask about any excessive bleeding episodes, such as:

- A tendency to bruise easily or longer after minor trauma
- Nosebleeds
- Increased menstrual flow
- Bleeding from the gums
- Rectal bleeding
- Hematuria (blood in the urine)

If the patient has a bleeding episode, ask whether the type and extent of bleeding is his or her usual response to injury or represents a change.

The patient with leukemia or MDS often has weakness and fatigue from anemia. The increased metabolism of leukemic cells causes fatigue for those with leukemia. Ask whether any of these problems have occurred:

- Headaches
- Behavior changes
- Decreased alertness, fatigue, increased need for sleep
- Decreased attention span
- Loss of appetite
- Weight loss

Ask about activity intolerance, changes in behavior, and unexplained fatigue. Assess how long the patient has had any of these debilitating problems.

Physical Assessment/Signs and Symptoms. Leukemia and MDS affect the function of all organs and systems. Thus the signs and symptoms are widespread as indicated in the Key Features: Acute Leukemia box. These problems occur with acute leukemia, chronic leukemia in the blast phase, and severe MDS.

Cardiovascular changes are related to adjustments that occur when ***perfusion*** and ***gas exchange*** are reduced from anemia. Heart rate is increased and blood pressure is decreased. *Murmurs* (abnormal blood flow sounds in the heart) and *bruits* (abnormal blood flow sounds over arteries) may be heard because less viscous blood results in more turbulent flow. Capillary refill is slow. When the WBC count is greatly elevated and blood is highly *viscous* (thicker), blood pressure is elevated with a bounding pulse.

 **KEY FEATURES**

Acute Leukemia

Integumentary Signs and Symptoms
- Ecchymoses
- Petechiae
- Open infected lesions
- Pallor of the conjunctivae, the nail beds, the palmar creases, and around the mouth

GI Signs and Symptoms
- Bleeding gums
- Anorexia
- Weight loss
- Enlarged liver and spleen

Renal Signs and Symptoms
- Hematuria

Musculoskeletal Signs and Symptoms
- Bone pain
- Joint swelling and pain

Cardiopulmonary Signs and Symptoms
- Tachycardia at basal activity levels
- Orthostatic hypotension
- Palpitations
- Dyspnea on exertion

Neurologic Signs and Symptoms
- Fatigue
- Headache
- Fever

Respiratory changes result from reduced ***gas exchange*** with anemia and ***infection***. Respiratory rate increases as anemia becomes more severe. A respiratory infection may cause coughing and dyspnea. Abnormal breath sounds are heard on auscultation.

Skin changes include pallor and coolness to the touch with the reduced ***perfusion*** from anemia. Pallor is seen on the face, around the mouth, and in the nail beds. The conjunctiva is pale, as are the creases on the palms. Petechiae not caused by trauma may be present on any area of skin surface, especially the legs and feet. Inspect for skin infections or injured areas that have failed to heal. Inspect the mouth for gum bleeding and any sore or lesion.

Intestinal changes include weight loss, nausea, and anorexia. Examine the rectal area for fissures, and test stool for occult blood. Many patients with leukemia have reduced bowel sounds and are constipated because reduced intestinal blood flow decreases peristalsis. Liver and spleen enlargement and abdominal tenderness are caused by leukemic cells trapped in these organs.

Central nervous system (CNS) changes include cranial nerve problems, headache, and papilledema from leukemic invasion of the CNS. Seizures and coma also may occur.

Miscellaneous changes can include bone and joint tenderness as the marrow is damaged and the bone reabsorbs. Leukemic cells invade lymph nodes, causing enlargement.

Psychosocial Assessment. The patient and family with newly diagnosed leukemia or MDS are anxious and fearful. Assess what the diagnosis means to the patient and family and what they expect in the future.

A diagnosis of leukemia or MDS results in major changes in the patient's lifestyle. For leukemia, hospitalization for initial treatment often lasts weeks and may result in boredom, loneliness, isolation, and financial stress. Assess coping patterns, including activities that the patient finds enjoyable and methods that help him or her relax. After initial therapy, the patient may resume work, depending on the occupation. Often the patient must adjust to changes in functional status. He or she may be hospitalized repeatedly for complications.

Laboratory Assessment. The patient usually has decreased hemoglobin and hematocrit levels, a low platelet count, and an abnormal WBC count. The count may be low, normal, or elevated. The patient with leukemia who has a high WBC count of mostly blast cells at diagnosis has a poorer prognosis.

The definitive test for leukemia and MDS is an examination of cells obtained from bone marrow aspiration and biopsy (Fig. 37.3). In leukemia the bone marrow is full of leukemic **blast phase cells** (immature white cells that are dividing). The proteins (antigens) on the surfaces of the leukemic cells are "markers" to diagnose the type of leukemia and indicate prognosis. These include the T11 protein, terminal deoxynucleotidyl transferase (TDT), the common acute lymphoblastic leukemia antigen (CALLA), and the CD33 antigen. In MDS, peripheral blood smears are used to assess the maturation and proportion of abnormal cells in circulation.

Blood ***clotting*** times and factors are usually abnormal with acute leukemia and MDS with thrombocytopenia. Reduced levels of clotting factors are common. Whole-blood clotting time is prolonged, as is the activated partial thromboplastin time (aPTT).

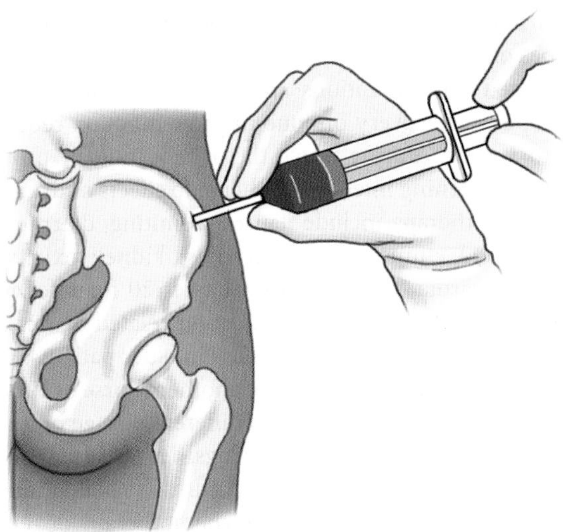

Fig. 37.3 Bone marrow aspiration from the posterior iliac crest. (From Leonard, P.C. [2012]. *Building a medical vocabulary: With Spanish translations* [8th ed.]. St. Louis: Saunders.)

Chromosome analysis (cytogenetic studies) of the leukemic and MDS cells may identify marker chromosomes to help diagnose the type of leukemia, predict the prognosis, and determine therapy effectiveness. An example is the Philadelphia chromosome, which is important in the diagnosis and treatment of some types of chronic myelogenous leukemia (CML) and adult acute lymphocytic leukemia (ALL). The **Philadelphia chromosome** is an abnormal chromosome caused by a translocation of the *ABL* gene from chromosome 9 onto the *BCR* gene of chromosome 22. The new protein produced by this mutation causes loss of normal ***cellular regulation*** by inhibiting cell apoptosis and DNA repair (Jorde et al., 2016; OMIM, 2019a).

Imaging Assessment. Imaging is based on specific signs and symptoms. In a patient with dyspnea, a chest x-ray may show leukemic infiltrates in the lung. Skeletal x-rays help determine bone density loss.

◆ **Analysis: Analyze Cues and Prioritize Hypotheses.** The priority collaborative problems for patients with acute myelogenous leukemia (AML), the most common type of acute leukemia seen in adults, or advanced MDS include:

1. Potential for ***infection*** due to reduced ***immunity*** and chemotherapy
2. Potential for injury due to poor ***clotting*** from thrombocytopenia and chemotherapy
3. Fatigue due to reduced ***gas exchange*** and increased energy demands

◆ Planning and Implementation: Generate Solutions and Take Action

Preventing Infection

Planning: Expected Outcomes. With appropriate interventions, the patient with leukemia is expected to remain free from ***infection***.

Interventions. *Infection is a major cause of death in the patient with leukemia* because the WBCs are immature and nonfunctional or are depleted, leading to sepsis. ***Infection*** occurs through *autocontamination* (normal flora overgrows and penetrates the internal environment) and *cross-contamination* (organisms from another person are transmitted to the patient). The most common sources of infection are the skin, respiratory tract, and intestinal tract.

Interventions aim to halt infection and control infections early. A controversial practice is the use of antibiotic prophylaxis to prevent infection for patients receiving high-dose chemotherapy. Although some differences in infection rates have been noted, the differences have not reached statistical significance (Ganti et al., 2017) (see the Evidence-Based Practice box). The Focused Assessment: Patients at Risk for Infection box lists areas to assess for infection.

EVIDENCE-BASED PRACTICE (QSEN)

Does Prophylactic Antibiotic Therapy Reduce Bacterial Infections in Patients Undergoing Reinduction Chemotherapy for Relapsed or Refractory Acute Myeloid Leukemia?

Ganti, B.R., Marini, B.L., Nagel, J., Bixby, D., & Perissinotti, A.J. (2017). Impact of antibacterial prophylaxis during reinduction chemotherapy for relapsed or refractory acute myeloid leukemia. *Supportive Care in Cancer, 25,* 541–547.

The risk for infection is always high during induction chemotherapy for leukemia and is even greater in those adults with leukemia who are undergoing reinduction. This retrospective cohort comparison study evaluated the effects of prophylaxis with levofloxacin over a 9-year period in relapsed or refractory acute myeloid leukemia (AML) receiving reinduction chemotherapy. Data were obtained from medical records of patients (N = 145) with relapsed or refractory AML admitted at a single institution. Standard levofloxacin prophylaxis was started with 500 mg once daily on day 1 of chemotherapy and continued until neutrophil recovery (defined as absolute neutrophil count [ANC] greater than 500 cells/mm^3 [0.5×10^9/L]). The rate and type of infections for the cohort of 48 patients who received levofloxacin were compared with those in the cohort of 98 patients who did not receive prophylaxis.

A lower rate of bacteremia occurred in the prophylaxis group, but the difference did not reach statistical significance. Time to onset of bacteremia from onset of neutropenia was delayed in the prophylaxis group compared with the control cohort (P = .012). No differences in drug-resistant organisms was found between cohorts, nor were any differences in the incidence of febrile neutropenia found. In the prophylaxis cohort the frequency of gram-negative organism–related infections was lower.

Level of Evidence: 4

The study was confined to a single center and was retrospective.

Commentary: Implications for Practice and Research

The results of this study minimally support the practice of prophylactic antibiotic use for patients undergoing reinduction chemotherapy for relapsed or refractive acute myeloid leukemia. Limitations of the study include its retrospect nature, the length of the study period (9 years), and the fact that all patients were treated at a single institution. Although the profound neutropenia experienced by patients undergoing intensive chemotherapy has the potential to lead to sepsis and death, prophylactic antibiotic therapy has not shown a consistent benefit and may contribute to increasing drug-resistant organisms. Larger prospective studies incorporating data from multiple institutions representing wider geographic areas are needed before prophylactic antibiotic therapy can become a standard of care. Nurses are often asked by patients and families why antibiotics are not routinely prescribed to prevent infection in this very vulnerable population. Results of this study can be used to help nurses explain to patients and families the rationale against routine prophylactic antibiotic use.

FOCUSED ASSESSMENT

Patients at Risk for Infection

General Condition

- Age and mobility status
- Allergies
- Previous chemotherapy, radiotherapy, or other any immunosuppressive therapy
- Chronic diseases
- Previous febrile neutropenia and associated symptoms
- Nutrition status
- Use of alcohol, tobacco products, or recreational drug
- Prescribed and over-the-counter drug use
- Baseline and ongoing vital signs—blood pressure, heart rate, respiratory rate, and temperature

Skin and Mucous Membranes

- Inspect all skin surfaces with attention to axillae, anorectal area, and under breasts; check for color, bleeding, lesions, edema, moist areas, open areas, irritation, erythema; condition of hair and nails, pressure areas, swelling, pain, tenderness, biopsy or surgical sites, enlarged lymph nodes, catheters, or other devices
- Inspect the mouth cavity, including lips, tongue, mucous membranes, gingiva, and teeth for color, moisture, bleeding, lesions, exudate, mucositis, stomatitis, plaque, swelling, pain, tenderness, taste changes, amount and character of saliva, ability to swallow, changes in voice, dental caries, patient's oral hygiene routine

Head, Eyes, Ears, Nose

- Pain, tenderness, exudate, crusting, enlarged lymph nodes

Cardiopulmonary

- Respiratory rate and pattern, breath sounds, quantity and characteristics of sputum, shortness of breath, use of accessory muscles, dysphagia, diminished gag reflex, tachycardia, blood pressure

Gastrointestinal

- Pain, diarrhea, bowel sounds, character and frequency of bowel movements, rectal bleeding, hemorrhoids, change in bowel habits, sexual practices, erythema, ulceration

Genitourinary

- Dysuria, frequency, urgency, hematuria, pruritus, pain, vaginal or penile discharge, vaginal bleeding, burning, lesions, ulcerations, characteristics of urine

Neuromuscular

- Cognition, level of consciousness, personality, behavior
- Bone tenderness, pain, loss of joint function

Drug Therapy for Acute Leukemia. Drug therapy for patients with AML is divided into three distinctive phases: induction, consolidation, and maintenance.

Induction therapy is intense combination chemotherapy started at the time of diagnosis. The purpose of this therapy is to achieve a rapid, complete remission of all disease symptoms. Agencies and oncologists differ in drug combinations used and the treatment schedule. Regardless of the agents used or duration of therapy, the result is severe bone marrow suppression with neutropenia and reduced ***immunity***, making the patient even more at risk for ***infection***. Different chemotherapy regimens are used for specific types of leukemia.

Prolonged hospitalizations are common while the patient is neutropenic. Recovery of bone marrow function requires at least 2 to 3 weeks, during which the patient must be protected from life-threatening infection. Other side effects of drugs used for induction therapy include nausea, vomiting, diarrhea, *alopecia* (hair loss), **stomatitis** (mouth sores), kidney toxicity, liver toxicity, and cardiac toxicity. (See Chapter 20 for information on effects of anticancer agents.) Infection-related deaths occur more often during the induction phase in older patients.

Consolidation therapy consists of another course of either the same drugs used for induction at a different dosage or a different combination of chemotherapy drugs. This treatment occurs early in remission, and its intent is to cure. Consolidation therapy may be either a single course of chemotherapy or repeated courses. Hematopoietic stem cell transplantation also may be considered, depending on the disease subtype and the patient's response to induction therapy.

Maintenance therapy may be prescribed for months to years after successful induction and consolidation therapies for some types of acute leukemia. The purpose is to maintain the remission achieved through induction and consolidation.

Drug Therapy for Chronic Leukemia. Imatinib mesylate is a common first-line drug therapy for CML that is Philadelphia chromosome positive. This oral drug has been effective at inducing remission for early stages of CML. Other drugs approved for first-line therapy or for patients whose disease is resistant to imatinib are dasatinib and bosutinib. Other drugs used to treat CML include interferon alfa, which slows the growth of leukemic cells.

Chronic lymphocytic leukemia (CLL) is the most prevalent form of leukemia in adults, affecting women more often than men. Treatment of CLL with standard chemotherapy, monoclonal antibody therapy (e.g., rituximab, ofatumumab, alemtuzumab, obinutuzumab), or targeted therapy such as ibrutinib (a Bruton tyrosine kinase [BTK] inhibitor), idelalisib (a highly selective inhibitor of the delta isoform of PI3K, which plays a critical role in B-cell function through BCR signaling), or venetoclax (a selective BCL2 inhibitor), can cause remissions but does not cure the disease (Glode & Babiker, 2017; Paradis et al., 2017). The decision to initiate therapy is based on disease stage, symptoms, and disease activity. Monoclonal antibody therapy is often combined with standard chemotherapy drugs or used as a single agent.

Allogeneic hematopoietic stem cell transplantation in patients with CLL is an option for cure or increased survival at time of relapse, but has considerable risk for mortality and is not an appropriate alternative for all patients. Therefore many other alternative options are offered to patients such as other chemotherapies or second-line targeted therapies.

Drug Therapy for Myelodysplastic Syndrome. Drug therapy can be used to improve blood counts for patients with MDS. Antitumor immunomodulating agents have improved blood counts in patients who have less severe MDS, especially those whose abnormal cells have a specific chromosome aberration. For higher-grade MDS, azacitidine and decitabine have been approved, although positive responses usually require 3 to 6 months of therapy and not every patient responds.

Drug Therapy for Infection. Drug therapy is the main defense against actual ***infection*** that develops in patients undergoing therapy for acute leukemia. Drugs used depend on the sensitivity of the organism causing the infection, as well as on infection severity. Drugs for infection include antibacterial, antiviral, and antifungal agents.

Infection Protection. A major focus in caring for the patient with leukemia is protection from ***infection***. All personnel must use extreme care during all procedures. Frequent, thorough handwashing is of the utmost importance. Anyone with an upper respiratory tract infection who enters the patient's room must wear a mask. Observe strict asepsis when changing dressings or accessing a central venous catheter. Maintain strict aseptic technique in the care of these catheters at all times.

If possible, ensure that the patient is in a private room to reduce cross-contamination. Other precautions are used, such as not allowing standing water in vases, denture cups, or humidifiers in the patient's room, because they are breeding grounds for organisms.

Continually assess the patient for signs of ***infection***. This task is difficult because symptoms are not obvious in the patient with leukopenia. He or she may have a severe infection without pus and with only a low-grade fever.

Monitor the patient's daily complete blood count (CBC) with differential WBC count and absolute neutrophil count (ANC). Inspect the mouth during every shift for lesions and mucosa breakdown. Assess the lungs every 8 hours for crackles, wheezes, and reduced breath sounds that indicate reduced ***gas exchange***. Assess urine for odor and cloudiness. Ask about any urgency, burning, or pain on urination. Take vital signs at least every 4 hours to assess for fever.

! NURSING SAFETY PRIORITY (QSEN)

Critical Rescue

A temperature elevation of even 1°F (or 0.5°C) above baseline is an indication of *infection* for a patient with reduced *immunity*. Monitor patients closely to recognize signs of infection. When any temperature elevation is present in a patient with leukemia, respond by reporting it to the oncology health care provider immediately and implement standard infection protocols.

Many hospital units that specialize in the care of patients with neutropenia have specific protocols for antibiotic therapy if *infection* is suspected. Usually the hematology oncologist is notified immediately, and specific specimens are obtained for culture. Obtain blood for bacterial and fungal cultures from peripheral IV sites and the central venous catheter. Obtain urine specimens, sputum specimens, and specimens from open lesions for culture. Chest x-rays are taken. After the specimens are obtained, the patient begins IV antibiotics.

Skin care is important for preventing ***infection*** in the patient with leukemia and reduced ***immunity*** because the skin may be the only intact defense. Teach him or her about hygiene and urge daily bathing. Turn immobile patients every hour and apply skin lubricants.

Perform pulmonary hygiene every 2 to 4 hours. Listen to the lungs for crackles, wheezes, and reduced breath sounds. Urge the patient to cough and deep breathe or to use an incentive spirometer every hour while awake to promote ***gas exchange***.

Hematopoietic Stem Cell Transplantation. Hematopoietic stem cell transplantation (HSCT), is standard treatment for the patient with acute leukemia who has a closely matched donor and who is in temporary remission after induction therapy. It can also be used for some forms of chronic leukemia, MDS, lymphoma, multiple myeloma, aplastic anemia, sickle cell disease, and many solid tumors. Stem cells for transplantation can be obtained directly from the donor's bone marrow or, more often, from his or her peripheral blood.

The bone marrow is the actual site of leukemic and MDS cell production. It can be difficult to ensure that all leukemic cells have been eradicated during induction therapy. Before HSCT, therefore, additional chemotherapy with or without total-body irradiation (TBI) is given to *purge* (clear) the marrow of leukemic cells (Koniarczyk & Ferraro, 2016). *These treatments are lethal to the bone marrow, and without replacement of stem cells by HSCT, the patient would die of* ***infection*** *or hemorrhage.*

After conditioning, new healthy stem cells are given to the patient. The new cells go to the marrow and then begin the process of hematopoiesis, which results in normal, properly functioning blood cells and ideally a permanent cure.

Many hospitals have transplant units. With long-term survival increasing after HSCT, nurses can expect to be caring for these people—if not during the actual transplantation or recovery period, then after the recovery period—in a variety of health care settings.

HSCT with the use of bone marrow or stem cells from a sibling or matched unrelated donor, or human leukocyte antigen (HLA)–matched stem cells from the umbilical cords of unrelated donors is a standard treatment for some leukemia types. HSCT is classified by the source of stem cells (Table 37.3). Stem cells may be obtained by bone marrow harvest, peripheral stem cell apheresis,

TABLE 37.3 Classification of Transplants

Type of Transplant	Sources of Stem Cells
Autologous	
Self-donation	Bone marrow harvest Peripheral stem cell apheresis Umbilical cord blood
Syngeneic	
Patient's HLA identical twin or other identical sibling	Bone marrow harvest Peripheral stem cell apheresis
Allogeneic	
HLA-matched relative	Bone marrow harvest
Unrelated HLA-matched donor	Peripheral stem cell apheresis
Mismatched or partially HLA-matched family member or unrelated donor (donor registries)	Umbilical cord blood

HLA, Human leukocyte antigen.

or umbilical cord blood stem cell banking. Transplantation has five phases: stem cell obtainment, conditioning regimen, transplantation, engraftment, and posttransplantation recovery.

Obtaining the stem cells. Stem cells are taken from the patient directly *(autologous stem cells)*, an HLA-identical twin *(syngeneic stem cells)*, or an HLA-matched person *(allogeneic stem cells)*. For allogeneic HSCT, best results occur when the donor is an HLA-identical sibling; however, transplant also can be successful between closely but not perfectly matched HLA types. The chance of matching with any given sibling is 25%. Donor registries list potential donors who can provide stem cells for patients who do not have a family member match. The chance of matching with an unrelated donor is 1 in 5000. Regardless of whether HSCT is autologous, syngeneic, or allogeneic, complications of the procedure are often life threatening (Young & Mansfield, 2017). This is not a benign procedure.

Patients often believe that a donor's blood type must be a match to theirs. Although the tissue type must be a close match for a successful stem cell transplant, the blood type is not related to tissue type, and blood-type compatibility is not included in donor criteria.

PATIENT-CENTERED CARE: CULTURAL/SPIRITUAL CONSIDERATIONS QSEN

Tissue types can vary among different racial and ethnic groups. Disparities exist regarding the availability of diverse donors. As such, it is important for the nurse to encourage more people of all races and ethnicities to become donors (National Marrow Donor Program, 2020).

Bone marrow harvesting occurs after a matching donor has been identified by tissue typing. The procedure occurs in the operating room, where marrow is removed through multiple aspirations from the iliac crests, although this technique is used less often today. About 500 to 1000 mL of marrow is aspirated, and the donor's marrow regrows within a few weeks. The marrow is then filtered and, if autologous, is treated to rid the marrow of any remaining cancer cells. It is usually frozen for later use. Allogeneic marrow is transfused into the recipient immediately.

Monitor the donor for fluid loss, assess for complications of anesthesia, and manage ***pain***. During surgery, donors may lose a large amount of fluid in addition to the volume of marrow taken. Donors are hydrated with saline infusions before and immediately after surgery. Assess harvest sites to ensure that the dressings are dry and intact, and that bleeding is not excessive.

Marrow donation is usually a same-day surgical procedure. Instruct the donor to inspect the harvest sites for bleeding and take analgesics for pain. ***Pain*** at harvest sites (hips) is common and is managed with oral non–aspirin-containing analgesics. Some donors may require opioid analgesics for pain control.

Peripheral blood stem cell harvesting requires three phases: mobilization, collection by apheresis, and reinfusion. **Peripheral blood stem cells (PBSCs)** are stem cells that have been released from the bone marrow and circulate within the blood. Although there are fewer stem cells in peripheral blood than in bone marrow, their numbers can be stimulated in the patient for autologous transplantation or in the donor for an allogeneic transplantation. Stimulation increases the numbers of stem cells and WBCs in the peripheral blood. Artificially stimulating stem cells before donation can decrease the number of apheresis collections needed.

After stimulation is successful, stem cells are collected by **apheresis** (withdrawing whole blood, filtering out the cells, and returning the plasma to the patient). One to five apheresis procedures, each lasting 2 to 4 hours, are needed to obtain enough stem cells for transplantation. Cells are frozen and stored for infusion after the patient's conditioning regimen is completed.

Monitor the patient or donor closely during apheresis. Complications include catheter clotting and hypocalcemia (caused by anticoagulants). Low calcium levels may cause numbness or tingling in the fingers and toes, abdominal or muscle cramping, or chest pain. Oral calcium supplements may be used to manage these symptoms. Monitor vital signs at least every hour during apheresis. The patient may become hypotensive from fluid loss during the procedure.

Cord blood harvesting obtains stem cells from umbilical cord blood of newborns, which has a high concentration of stem cells. These cells are obtained through a simple blood draw from the placenta after birth and before the placenta detaches. The blood is sent to the Cord Blood Registry for processing and storage. Stem cells may be used later for an unrelated recipient or stored in case the infant develops a serious illness later in life and needs them.

Conditioning regimen. Fig. 37.4 outlines the timing and steps involved in transplantation. The day the patient receives the stem cells is day T–0. Before transplantation, the conditioning

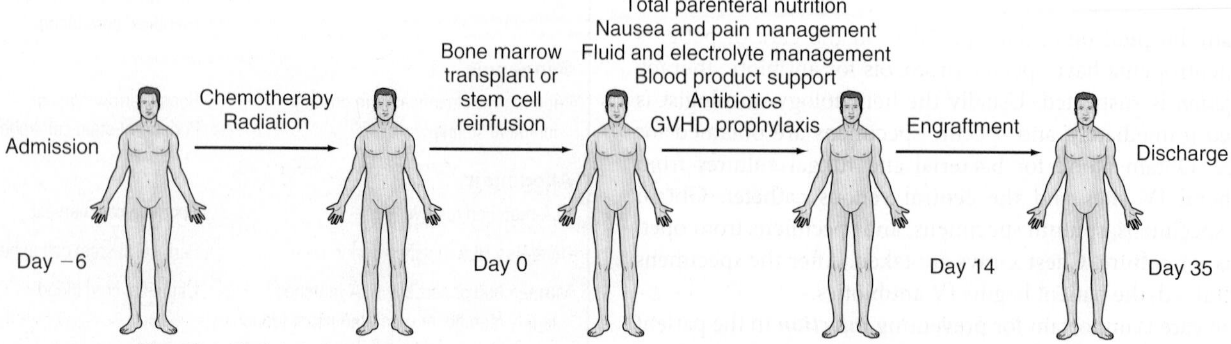

Fig. 37.4 Timing and steps of allogeneic bone marrow transplantation. *GVHD*, Graft-versus-host disease.

days are counted in reverse order from T–0, just like a rocket countdown. After transplantation, days are counted in order from the day of transplantation.

The patient first undergoes a conditioning regimen, which varies with the diagnosis and type of transplant to be received. The conditioning regimen serves two purposes: (1) to "wipe out" the patient's own bone marrow, thus preparing him or her for replacement by a new immune system; and (2) to give high doses of chemotherapy and/or radiotherapy to rid the patient of cancer cells *(myeloablation)*. Usually a period of 5 to 10 days is required. The regimen usually includes high-dose chemotherapy and, less often, total-body irradiation (TBI). Each regimen is tailored to the patient's specific disease, overall health, and previous treatment.

Because of the problems and risk for death with conditioning regimens, a *nonmyeloablative* approach may be used instead. This approach uses lower doses of chemotherapy and/or a lower dose of TBI that allows for recovery of the patient's own immune system. Nonmyeloablative conditioning regimens decrease the chemotherapy side effects but rely on the development of graft-versus-host disease (GVHD) for the control of the cancer.

During conditioning, bone marrow and normal tissues respond immediately to the chemotherapy and radiation. The patient has all of the side effects associated with both therapies (see Chapter 20). When chemotherapy is given in high doses, these side effects are more intense than those seen with standard doses.

Late effects from the conditioning regimen may occur as long as 3 to 10 years later. These effects include sinusoidal obstructive syndrome (SOS) (previously termed *veno-occlusive disease* [VOD]), skin problems, cataracts, lung fibrosis, second cancers, cardiomyopathy, endocrine complications, and neurologic changes.

Transplantation. Day T–0 is the day of transplantation. The transplantation itself is very simple. Frozen marrow, PBSCs, or umbilical cord blood cells are thawed and infused through the patient's central catheter as in an ordinary blood transfusion.

! NURSING SAFETY PRIORITY (QSEN)

Action Alert

Do not use blood administration tubing to infuse stems cells because the cells may be trapped in the filter, resulting in the patient receiving fewer stem cells. Usually standard, larger-bore, IV administration tubing is used.

Side effects of stem cell transfusions may include fever and hypertension in response to the preservative used in stem cell storage. To prevent these reactions, acetaminophen, hydrocortisone, and diphenhydramine are given before the infusion. Antihypertensives or diuretics may be needed to treat fluid volume changes.

Engraftment. The transfused PBSCs and marrow cells circulate briefly in the peripheral blood. The stem cells then "home in" on the marrow-forming sites of the patient's bones and establish residency there.

Engraftment, the successful "take" and growth of the transplanted cells in the patient's bone marrow, is key to the whole transplantation process. For the stem cells to "rescue" the patient after his or her own bone marrow has been "wiped out," the stem cells must survive and grow in the patient's bone marrow sites. The average time to engraftment ranges from 14 to 21 days. Growth factors may be given to aid engraftment. When engraftment occurs, the patient's WBC, RBC, and platelet counts begin to rise. Engraftment syndrome (ES) with fever and weight gain may occur at this time.

Monitoring engraftment involves checking the patient's blood for *chimerism*, which is the presence of blood cells that show a genetic profile or marker different from those of the patient. *Mixed chimerism* is the presence of both the patient's cells and those from the donor. *Progressive chimerism* with increasing percentages of donor cells indicates engraftment. *Regressive chimerism* with increasing percentages of the patient's cells indicates graft failure. When engraftment is successful, only the donor's cells are present.

Prevention of complications. The period after transplantation is difficult. ***Infection*** and poor ***clotting*** with bleeding are severe problems because the patient remains without any ***immunity*** until the transfused cells grow and engraft. Care for this patient is the same as that for the patient during induction therapy for acute leukemia. Helping the patient maintain hope through this long recovery period is challenging. Complications are often severe and life threatening. Help the patient have a positive attitude and be involved in his or her own recovery. Encourage the patient to express his or her feelings and concerns while maintaining a supportive presence and trusting nurse-patient relationship.

In addition to the problems related to the period of **pancytopenia** (low levels of all circulating blood cells), other complications of HSCT include failure to engraft, development of graft-versus-host disease (GVHD), and sinusoidal obstructive syndrome (SOS).

Failure to engraft occurs when the donated stem cells fail to grow and function in the bone marrow. This issue is discussed in advance with the patient and donor. Failure to engraft occurs more often with allogeneic HSCT than with autologous HSCT. The causes include too few cells transplanted, attack or rejection of donor cells by the recipient's remaining immune system cells, ***infection*** of transplanted cells, and unknown biologic factors. *If the transplanted cells fail to engraft, the patient will die unless another HSCT procedure is successful.*

GVHD occurs mostly in allogeneic transplants but also can occur in autologous transplants (rarely). The immunocompetent cells of the donated marrow recognize the patient's (recipient) cells, tissues, and organs as foreign and start an immunologic attack against them. The graft is actually trying to destroy the host tissues and cells.

Although all host tissues can be attacked and harmed, the tissues usually damaged are the skin, eyes, intestinal tract, liver, genitalia, lungs, immune system, and musculoskeletal system. Fig. 37.5 shows the typical skin appearance of GVHD. About 25% to 50% of all allogeneic HSCT recipients have some degree of GVHD, and about 15% of patients who develop GVHD die

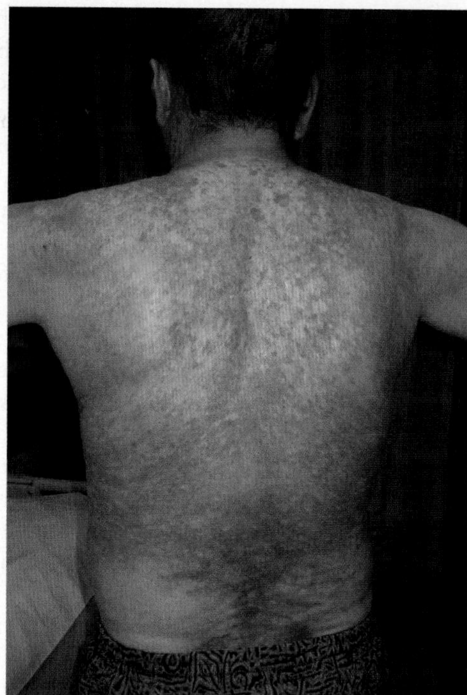

Fig. 37.5 Typical skin manifestations of graft-versus-host disease.

of its complications. The presence of some GVHD indicates engraftment.

Management of GVHD involves limiting the activity of donor T-cells by using drugs to suppress ***immunity*** such as cyclosporine, tacrolimus, methotrexate, corticosteroids, mycophenolate mofetil, and antithymocyte globulin (ATG). Care is taken to avoid suppressing the new immune system to prevent increasing infection risk or stopping new cell engraftment.

Sinusoidal obstructive syndrome (SOS) is the blockage of liver blood vessels by ***clotting*** and inflammation *(phlebitis)* and occurs in about one-fifth of patients with HSCT. Problems usually begin within the first 30 days after transplantation. Patients who received high-dose chemotherapy with alkylating agents are at risk for life-threatening liver problems. Symptoms include jaundice, pain in the right upper quadrant, ascites, weight gain, and liver enlargement.

Because there is no way of opening the liver vessels, treatment is supportive. Early detection improves the chance for survival. Fluid management is also crucial. Assess the patient daily for weight gain, fluid retention, ascites, and hepatomegaly.

Minimizing Injury. Bone marrow production of platelets is severely limited with acute leukemia, leading to thrombocytopenia. The patient is at great risk for poor ***clotting*** with excessive bleeding in response to minimal trauma. Thrombocytopenia can also be caused by induction therapy or high-dose chemotherapy for transplantation.

Planning: Expected Outcomes. The patient is expected to remain free from bleeding.

Interventions. The platelet count is decreased as a side effect of chemotherapy. During the period of greatest bone marrow suppression (the **nadir**), the platelet count may be less than 10,000/mm^3 (10 × 10^9/L). The patient is at extreme risk for bleeding once the platelet count falls below 50,000/mm^3 (50 × 10^9/L), and spontaneous bleeding may occur when the count is lower than 20,000/mm^3 (20 × 10^9/L).

Bleeding Precautions are used to protect the patient at increased risk for injury from impaired ***clotting***. Assess at least every 4 hours for evidence of bleeding: oozing, enlarging bruises, petechiae, or purpura. Inspect all stools, urine, drainage, and vomit for obvious blood and test for occult blood. Measure any blood loss as accurately as possible and measure the abdominal girth daily. Increases in abdominal girth can indicate internal hemorrhage. Institute the Bleeding Precautions listed in the Best Practice for Patient Safety & Quality Care: The Patient With Thrombocytopenia box in Chapter 20. Platelet levels return to normal more slowly than do either WBCs or RBCs, and the patient remains at bleeding risk for weeks after discharge.

Monitor laboratory values daily, especially CBC results, to assess bleeding risk and actual blood loss. The patient with a platelet count below 10,000/mm^3 (10 × 10^9/L) may need a platelet transfusion. For the patient with severe blood loss, packed RBCs may be prescribed (see the section Red Blood Cell Transfusions).

Conserving Energy. Production of RBCs is limited in leukemia and in MDS, causing anemia and fatigue. In addition, leukemic cells have high rates of metabolism, increasing fatigue in the anemic patient. Anemia may also occur as a side effect of chemotherapy.

Planning: Expected Outcomes. The patient is expected to have no increase in fatigue.

Interventions. Interventions to reduce fatigue focus on conserving energy and improving RBC counts.

Nutrition therapy is needed to help the patient eat enough calories to meet at least basal energy requirements. However, increasing food intake can be difficult with fatigue. Collaborate with a registered dietitian nutritionist to provide small, frequent meals high in protein and carbohydrates.

Blood transfusions are sometimes indicated for the patient with fatigue. Transfusions with packed RBCs increase the blood's oxygen-carrying capacity and replace missing RBCs. (See the Best Practice for Patient Safety & Quality Care: Transfusion Therapy box later in the chapter for nursing care during transfusions.)

Drug therapy with colony-stimulating growth factors may reduce the severity and duration of anemia and neutropenia after intensive chemotherapy. For anemia, erythropoiesis-stimulating agents (ESAs) that boost production of RBCs may be used.

! NURSING SAFETY PRIORITY QSEN

Drug Alert

ESAs have a warning for causing hypertension and increasing the risk for myocardial infarction. They must be given with care and are avoided in patients with myeloid malignancies. ESAs are not used unless the hemoglobin level is lower than 10 mg/dL (6.2 mmol/L) and are stopped when this level is reached. Assess for side effects such as hypertension, headaches, fever, myalgia (muscle aches), and rashes. (See Chapter 20 for information on hematopoietic growth factors.)

BEST PRACTICE FOR PATIENT SAFETY & QUALITY CARE (QSEN)

Conserving Energy

- Reassure the patient that fatigue is temporary and energy levels will improve over a period of weeks to months. Stress that a return to pre-illness energy levels may take as long as a year.
- Teach the patient that shortness of breath and palpitations are symptoms of overactivity.
- Instruct the patient to stop activity when shortness of breath or palpitations are present.
- Space care activities at least an hour apart and avoid the time right before or right after meals.
- Schedule care activities at times when the patient has more energy (e.g., immediately after naps).
- Perform complete bed bath only every other day. Between complete baths, ensure cleansing of face, hands, axillae, and perineum.
- In collaboration with other members of the health care team, cancel or reschedule nonessential tests and activities.
- Provide four to six small, easy-to-eat meals instead of three larger ones.
- Urge the patient to drink small amounts of protein shakes or other nutritional supplements.
- During periods of extreme fatigue, encourage the patient to allow others to perform personal care.
- Help the patient identify one or two lead visitors (those designated as allowed to visit at any time and who do not disturb the patient).
- Selectively limit nonlead visitors when the patient is resting or sleeping.
- Remind families that although independence is important, independence in ADLs during extreme fatigue can be detrimental to the patient's health.
- Monitor oxygen saturation and respiratory rate during any activity to determine patient responses and activity tolerance.

Activity management helps conserve the patient's energy using the interventions listed in the Best Practice for Patient Safety & Quality Care: Conserving Energy box. Examine the patient's schedule of prescribed and routine activities. Assess activities that do not have a direct positive effect on the patient's condition in terms of their usefulness. If the benefit of an activity is less than its worsening of fatigue, coordinate with other interprofessional team members about eliminating or postponing it. Activities that may be postponed include physical therapy and invasive diagnostic tests not needed for assessment or treatment of current problems.

Care Coordination and Transition Management. The patient with acute leukemia is discharged after induction chemotherapy and recovery of blood cell production. Follow-up care continues on an ambulatory care basis. Although many transplant centers discharge patients after engraftment, some centers give high-dose chemotherapy and stem cell infusion on an ambulatory care basis. This plan involves daily clinic visits and frequent follow-up by nurses in the home care setting.

Home Care Management. Planning for home care for the patient with leukemia begins as soon as remission is achieved. Assess the available support systems. Many patients need a visiting nurse to assist with dressing changes for central venous catheters and infusions and to answer questions. Home transfusion therapy for blood components may be needed.

PATIENT AND FAMILY EDUCATION: PREPARING FOR SELF-MANAGEMENT

Home Care of the Central Venous Catheter

- To keep the catheter open, flush it quickly with saline once a day and after completing infusions.
- Change the Luer-Lok cap on each catheter lumen weekly.
- Change the dressing as often as prescribed.
- Use clean technique with thorough handwashing.
- Clean the exit site with alcohol and povidone-iodine or with chlorhexidine.
- Apply antibacterial ointment to the site, if prescribed.
- Cover the site with dry sterile gauze dressing, taped securely, or with transparent adherent dressing.
- To prevent pulling, always tape the catheter to yourself.
- Look for and report any signs of infection (redness, swelling, or drainage at the exit site).
- In case of a break or puncture in the catheter lumen, immediately clamp the catheter between yourself and the opening. Notify your oncology health care provider immediately.

Coordination of the home care team is critical for the patient receiving stem cell transplantation in the home setting. Criteria for use of this setting include a knowledgeable caregiver, a clean home environment, location near the hospital, telephone access, and emotional stability of the patient and caregiver.

Home care nurses give chemotherapy and monitor for complications. Nurses visit the patient once or twice per day and spend between 4 and 8 hours per day in the home. The patient receives the stem cell infusion in the ambulatory care clinic. Nursing care is similar to that provided in the hospital. If complications such as ***infection***, sepsis, or sinusoidal obstructive syndrome (SOS) occur, the patient is admitted to the inpatient facility.

Self-Management Education. Instruct the patient and family about the importance of continuing therapy and follow-up. Many patients go home with a central venous catheter in place and need instructions about its care. Teach the patient and family the guidelines for central venous catheter care at home listed in the Patient and Family Education: Preparing for Self-Management: Home Care of the Central Venous Catheter box. These guidelines may be altered depending on the home setting, assistance available, and agency policy.

Protecting the patient from ***infection*** at home is just as important as it was during hospitalization. (See the Focused Assessment: Patients at Risk for Infection box.) Teach about proper hygiene and the need to avoid crowds or others with infections. Neither the patient nor any household member should receive live virus immunization (poliomyelitis, measles, or rubella) for 2 years after transplantation. In general, the patient receives no vaccinations for the first year after transplantation because his or her immune function has not returned sufficiently to generate antibodies in response to vaccination. Instruct the patient to continue mouth care regimens at home. Stress to the patient that he or she should immediately notify the oncology health care provider if a fever or any other signs of infection develop. Teach the patient and family the guidelines listed in the Patient and Family Education: Preparing for Self-Management: Prevention of Infection box in Chapter 17 for infection prevention among patients with reduced ***immunity***.

NCLEX EXAMINATION CHALLENGE 37.3

Physiological Integrity

A client returning to the clinic 7 weeks after hematopoietic stem cell transplantation for leukemia has a total white blood cell (WBC) count of 5200/mm^3 (5.2 × 10^9/L) and a neutrophil count of 3000/mm^3 (3 × 10^9/L). What is the nurse's **priority action** in view of these values?

A. Notify the oncology health care provider immediately.
B. Assess the client for other symptoms of infection.
C. Document the laboratory report as the only action.
D. Obtain a urine specimen, sputum specimen, and chest x-ray.

Many patients return home still at risk for bleeding because platelet recovery is slower than recovery of other cells and ***clotting*** remains slow. Reinforce safety and bleeding precautions and emphasize that these precautions must be followed until the platelet count remains above 50,000/mm^3 (50 × 10^9/L). Teach the patient and family to assess for petechiae, avoid trauma and sharp objects, apply pressure to wounds for 10 minutes, and report blood in the stool or urine or headache that does not respond to acetaminophen. Teach the patient and family about guidelines for patients with reduced ***clotting*** listed in the Patient and Family Education: Preparing for Self-Management: Preventing Injury or Bleeding box in Chapter 20.

Psychosocial Preparation. A diagnosis of acute leukemia changes the patient's sense of self and his or her role within the family. The possibility of death and the intense treatment often cause the patient to have major changes in self-image, body image, level of independence, and lifestyle. Some feel threatened by the environment, seeing everything as infectious. Patients who are cared for in protective isolation may feel lonely and isolated. Help the patient and family define priorities, understand the illness and its treatment, and find hope. Make referrals and urge patients and families to use support groups sponsored by organizations such as the American Cancer Society or the Leukemia and Lymphoma Society.

One problem that lasts for a long time after transplantation is severe fatigue. Although the acute period after transplantation requires energy conservation with reduced activity, in the later recovery period, exercise provides benefits and fatigue reduction. Help the patient and family understand the benefits of low-impact exercise and encourage them to organize their day with exercise included.

Health Care Resources. The patient with limited social support may need help at home until strength and energy return. A home care aide may suffice for some patients, whereas for others a visiting nurse may be needed for more skilled care and evaluation. The patient may also need equipment for ADLs and ambulation. Assess financial resources. Cancer treatment is expensive, and coordination with the social services department is needed to ensure that insurance is adequate. If the patient is uninsured, other sources, such as drug company-sponsored compassionate aid programs and local cancer center foundations, are explored. The Leukemia and Lymphoma Society also offers limited financial help.

Prolonged outpatient contact and follow-up are necessary, and patients need transportation to the outpatient facility. Many local units of the American Cancer Society and the Canadian Cancer Society offer free transportation to patients with cancer or leukemia.

◆ **Evaluation: Evaluate Outcomes.** Evaluate the care of the patient with leukemia based on the identified priority patient problems. The expected outcomes include that with appropriate interventions and support the patient will:

- Remain free of ***infection*** and sepsis
- Not experience episodes of bleeding
- Be able to balance activity and rest
- Use energy conservation techniques

MALIGNANT LYMPHOMAS

Lymphomas are cancers of the lymphoid cells and tissues with abnormal overgrowth of lymphocytes. They are cancers of committed lymphocytes rather than immature cells (as in leukemia). This growth occurs as solid tumors in lymphoid tissues scattered throughout the body, especially the lymph nodes and spleen, rather than in the bone marrow. The two major adult forms of lymphoma are Hodgkin lymphoma (HL) and non-Hodgkin's lymphoma (NHL).

Pathophysiology Review

Hodgkin's lymphoma (HL) is a cancer that can affect any age-group. However, it appears to peak in two different age-groups: (1) teens and young adults, and (2) adults in their 50s and 60s (McCance et al., 2019). HL affects younger men and women equally, but the disease is more prevalent in men in the older group. About 9000 cases are diagnosed in North America each year (ACS, 2020; CCS, 2019).

The exact cause of HL is uncertain. Possible causes include viral infections (e.g., Epstein-Barr virus [EBV], human T-cell leukemia/lymphoma virus [HTLV], and human immune deficiency virus [HIV]) and exposure to chemicals. However, most cases of the disease occur in people without known risk factors.

This cancer usually starts in a single lymph node or a single chain of nodes. These nodes contain a specific cancer cell type, the *Reed-Sternberg cell,* a marker for HL. HL often spreads predictably from one group of lymph nodes to the next, unlike non-Hodgkin lymphoma.

Non-Hodgkin lymphoma (NHL) includes all lymphoid cancers that do not have the Reed-Sternberg cell. The over 60 subtypes of NHL are classified as either indolent or aggressive lymphomas. NHL spreads through the lymphatic system in a less orderly fashion than HL. About 82,500 new cases occur each year in North America (ACS, 2020; CCS, 2019). NHL is more common in men and older adults.

The exact cause of NHL is unknown, although the incidence is higher among patients with solid organ transplantation, immunosuppressive drug therapy, and HIV disease. Chronic infection from *Helicobacter pylori* is associated with a type of NHL called mucosa-associated lymphoid tissue (MALT) lymphoma, and Epstein-Barr viral ***infection*** has been associated with Burkitt lymphoma. There is an increased incidence of NHL among people exposed to pesticides, insecticides, and dust.

NHL is a group of disorders, not a single disease. The specific subtype of lymphoma must be classified because management varies with the subtype. Classification is based on histology, immunophenotyping by flow cytometry, and genetic (chromosomal changes and molecular rearrangements) and clinical features. NHLs are classified as B-cell or T-cell lymphomas, depending on the cell type that gave rise to the cancer. B-cell lymphomas are more common.

Patients with **indolent** (slow-growing, slow to progress) lymphomas often have painless lymph node swelling at diagnosis. Those with more aggressive B-cell lymphomas may have large masses at diagnosis and *constitutional symptoms,* which are specific whole-body symptoms as seen in HL. These occur in about one-third of patients with aggressive NHL. Bone marrow involvement in indolent lymphomas is common.

❖ Interprofessional Collaborative Care

◆ Assessment: Recognize Cues. The major assessment finding for any lymphoma is a large, painless lymph node or nodes. The patient may also have constitutional symptoms ("B symptoms") that include fevers (temperature >101.5°F [>38.6°C]), drenching night sweats, and unplanned weight loss (>10% of normal body weight). These symptoms often mean a poorer prognosis. Many patients have no symptoms except lymph node swelling at time of diagnosis. Other symptoms depend on the site and extent of disease.

Diagnosis and subtype of HL are established when biopsy reveals Reed-Sternberg cells (McCance et al., 2019). HL is then classified into one of several different subtypes. The diagnosis of NHL is made only after the biopsy of an involved lymph node is reviewed by a hematopathologist.

After diagnosis of HL, staging is performed to determine extent of disease. This process is detailed and must be accurate because it determines the treatment regimen. Staging includes a history and physical examination; CBC; electrolyte panel; kidney and liver function tests; erythrocyte sedimentation rate (ESR); bone marrow aspiration and biopsy; and CT of the neck, chest, abdomen, and pelvis. Positron emission tomography (PET) is used to stage the disease and monitor response to therapy. After testing is complete, the disease is staged according to the Lugano Modification of the Ann Arbor Staging System for primary lymphoma. Just as with other types of cancer, the higher the staging number, the more widespread the disease (see Chapter 19).

Classification of NHL is more complicated and is based on the World Health Organization (WHO) classification system. Additional tests to measure tumor growth and calculate prognosis include lactate dehydrogenase (LDH) levels and beta$_2$-microglobulin levels, higher levels of which are associated with a poorer prognosis. Cerebrospinal fluid is evaluated when lymphoma is present in the CNS or around the spinal cord, brain, or testes and when HIV-related lymphoma is diagnosed.

◆ Interventions: Take Action. HL is a type of cancer that responds well to aggressive therapy, and long-term survival for decades is now the normal expectation (Xin & Corcoran, 2019). For earlier disease stages, the treatment is external radiation of involved lymph node regions. With more extensive disease, radiation and combination chemotherapy are used to achieve remission. (See Chapter 20 on general care of patients receiving radiation and chemotherapy.) An important issue is that when the disease is in the inguinal area, radiation therapy usually results in permanently reduced fertility or sterility in men. Sperm banking before therapy begins is an option to assist in future reproductive plans.

Although the regimens for treatment of HL are often effective, they can result in complications years and even decades later from both radiation and chemotherapy. The "late effects" include cardiovascular disease, which is a major noncancer cause of death for NL survivors; secondary malignancies from radiation (especially breast cancer and lung cancer); restrictive lung disease; and endocrine dysfunction that includes female infertility, hypothyroidism, and premature menopause (Xin & Corcoran, 2019).

Treatment options for patients with NHL vary based on the tumor subtype, prognosis, disease stage, performance status, and overall tumor burden. Special consideration for patients with additional health problems is important, especially among older-adult patients. Many new therapies have evolved over the past decade for various subtypes of NHL. These therapies include combinations of chemotherapy drugs alone or in combination with other therapies, depending on the stage of the disease. Therapies include monoclonal antibodies (e.g., rituximab, obinutuzumab, ofatumumab, pembrolizumab); localized radiation therapy; radiolabeled antibodies (iodine-131 [^{131}I] tositumomab and yttrium-90 [^{90}Y] ibritumomab tiuxetan); chimeric antigen receptor (CAR) T-cell therapy (e.g., axicabtagene ciloleucel and tisagenlecleucel); targeted therapies (e.g., acalabrutinib, ibrutinib); novel therapies used in other malignancies but also effective in lymphoma (e.g., lenalidomide, bortezomib; and investigational agents) (Harvey, 2018; McConville & Harvey, 2016).

CAR T-cell therapy is designed to enhance a patient's own immune system cell killing of cancer cells. It is known as "adoptive cell therapy" and dates back to the late 1980s. A patient's T-cells (T-lymphocytes) are extracted from his or her blood and placed into culture with artificial cancer receptors known as *chimeric antigen receptors.* These receptors integrate into the T-cell's membrane and modify its activity specifically against cancer cells. After modification, these CAR-T cells are infused back into the patient's blood, where their numbers increase. CAR T-cells then serve as guided missiles that seek out cancer cells and attack them (Callahan et al., 2017).

A general response to CAR-T therapy is to charge up the entire immune system with release of many inflammatory cytokines, a problem known as cytokine release syndrome (CRS) or "cytokine storm." This is an intense but limited (5 to 7 days) response involving flulike symptoms with high fever, fatigue, body aches, hypotension, edema, and decreased urine output. Some patients also become confused and have nausea and vomiting. CAR T-cell therapy is given as a single infusion, and all side effects are gone in about 2 weeks. At present, CAR T-cell therapy is approved for use with some specific types of NHL and is showing some promise with other hematologic malignancies.

Nursing management of the patient undergoing treatment for HL or NHL focuses on the acute side effects of therapy, especially:

- Drug-induced pancytopenia with increased risk for ***infection***, anemia, and bleeding from impaired ***immunity*** and ***clotting***
- Severe nausea and vomiting
- Skin problems at the radiation site
- Constipation or diarrhea
- Permanent sterility for male patients receiving radiation to the lower abdomen or pelvic region in combination with specific chemotherapy drugs (The patient is informed and given the option to store sperm in a sperm bank *before* treatment.)
- Secondary cancer development from drug-induced impaired ***cellular regulation*** and the need for long-term follow-up

With the use of biotherapy for NHL, close monitoring for infusion-related reactions is needed during and after the delivery of monoclonal antibodies. (See Chapter 20 for general care of patients undergoing treatment with biotherapy.)

MULTIPLE MYELOMA

Pathophysiology Review

Multiple myeloma (MM) is a white blood cell (WBC) cancer of mature B-lymphocytes called *plasma cells* that secrete antibodies. These cancer cells produce excessive antibodies (gamma globulins) and the disorder is a *gammopathy*. Myeloma cells also produce excess *cytokines* (see Chapter 16) that increase cancer cell growth and destroy bone. The excess antibodies are in the blood, increasing the serum protein levels and clogging blood vessels in the kidney and other organs. Excessive myeloma cell proliferation reduces production of red blood cells (RBCs), WBCs, and platelets, leading to anemia and increased risk for ***infection*** and bleeding. Without treatment, the disease quickly causes progressive bone destruction, kidney failure, reduced ***immunity***, and death. Although few patients with MM are cured of the disorder, with current management methods life expectancy can exceed 10 years (Faiman, 2017; Rajkumar, 2016).

Multiple myeloma accounts for about 13,500 deaths per year in North America (ACS, 2020; CCS, 2019). The disease is most common in people older than 65 years. The incidence is higher in African Americans than in white Americans and is much higher in men.

The cause of MM is unknown. Possible risk factors include radiation exposure, chemical exposure, and infection with human herpesvirus 8 (HHV-8). This cancer can be identified early by changes in immunoglobulin structure that begin in some bone marrow cells even before actual cancer develops. When the abnormal immunoglobulin is present in a high enough quantity, the type can be recognized as a unique "spike" pattern on serum electrophoresis of plasma proteins. The abnormal immunoglobulin produced by these cells is a *monoclonal paraprotein*.

Major complications of the disease occur in the renal, cardiac, and pulmonary systems. Damage to the kidneys is associated with the protein burden of excessive antibody production. In addition, the disorder occurs most often among older adults who may already have experienced age-related decreases in kidney function. These factors increase the risk for both acute kidney injury and chronic kidney disease in the patient with multiple myeloma (Faiman et al., 2017).

Cardiopulmonary complications of MM are related to the increased blood viscosity, which increases the risk for the formation of venous thromboembolism (VTE) anywhere in any vascular organ. Problems most often occur in the lower extremities and lungs. Many of the drugs used to manage the disorder also increase the risk for these complications (Noonan et al., 2017).

❖ Interprofessional Collaborative Care

◆ **Assessment: Recognize Cues.** Some patients have no symptoms at time of the diagnosis. An elevation of serum total protein or paraprotein in the blood or urine may be the only finding. Other symptoms include fatigue, anemia, bone pain, fractures, recurrent bacterial ***infection***, and kidney problems.

A positive finding of a serum paraprotein is not sufficient alone for the diagnosis of MM. About 1% of the population produces some paraprotein in the blood but does not have multiple myeloma. This condition is labeled ***m****onoclonal* ***g****ammopathy of* ***u****ndetermined* ***s****ignificance* or MGUS, which is a premalignant condition. Follow-up of patients with MGUS is important because a small percentage eventually will develop multiple myeloma. MM is distinguished from MGUS by having more than 10% of the bone marrow infiltrated with plasma cells, paraprotein in the serum or urine, and osteolytic bone lesions.

The staging system for MM divides patients into stages and prognostic groups based on the serum beta$_2$-microglobulin and albumin levels. Other factors that help determine prognosis include age, performance status, serum creatinine, serum albumin, serum calcium, lactate dehydrogenase (LDH) level, C-reactive protein, hemoglobin level, platelet count, quantitative immunoglobulins, beta$_2$-microglobulin, serum free light chains, serum protein electrophoresis (SPEP) with immunofixation, 24-hour urine for SPEP, and cytogenetic abnormalities found in the bone marrow biopsy specimen.

The patient usually first notices fatigue, easy bruising, and bone ***pain***. Bone fractures, hypertension, infection, hypercalcemia, and fluid imbalance may occur as the disease progresses. Diagnosis is made by x-ray findings of bone thinning with areas of bone loss that resemble Swiss cheese, high immunoglobulin and plasma protein levels, and the presence of Bence Jones protein (protein composed of incomplete antibodies) in the urine. A bone marrow biopsy is performed to diagnose the disease and to determine chromosome changes. An abnormality of chromosome 11 predicts a longer survival, and absence of chromosome 13 is a poor prognostic factor.

◆ **Interventions: Take Action.** ***Pain***, particularly bone pain, is common in MM and must be addressed as soon as possible.

Pain reduces mobility and greatly interferes with quality of life (Rome et al., 2017). Early detection of MM and initiation of treatment can greatly reduce pain, but this is not an immediate result. Drugs, such as bisphosphonates, can reduce bone pain by reducing bone destruction. When changes in the spinal column result from bone involvement, emergency treatment is needed to prevent nerve damage (see Chapter 20 for oncologic emergencies).

Treatment options vary. For minimal disease, watchful waiting may be an option instead of chemotherapy. Standard treatment for MM is the use of proteasome inhibitors and immunomodulating drugs (Gleason & Kaufman, 2017). These agents, which are types of targeted cancer therapy (see Chapter 20), may be used alone or in combination with steroids. Drug selection is based on whether the patient is eligible for an autologous stem cell transplant. If eligible, drug therapy is used to reduce tumor burden before transplantation. For patients who are not eligible for autologous stem cell transplantation, standard chemotherapy drugs are usually effective in controlling but not curing the disease.

Side effects and severe toxicities can occur with these agents. Myelosuppression is an expected side effect of many myeloma therapies. A nursing priority is to teach the patient about the symptoms. The risk for thromboembolic events is increased with the use of thalidomide and lenalidomide. Other side effects, such as peripheral neuropathy, nausea, vomiting, diarrhea, and constipation, are managed as described in Chapter 20.

Despite therapy, MM remains largely incurable (McCance et al., 2019). Best outcomes are seen with hematopoietic stem cell transplantation, although few patients can pursue this option. Because most patients with MM have bone ***pain***, analgesics and alternative approaches for pain management, such as relaxation techniques, aromatherapy, or hypnosis, are used. Bone loss is treated with bisphosphonates (pamidronate, zoledronic acid, denosumab), which inhibit bone resorption and can help reduce skeletal complications (Rome et al., 2017).

THROMBOCYTOPENIC PURPURA

Pathophysiology Review

Thrombocytopenic purpura is the destructive reduction of circulating platelets after normal platelet production. Two common types are *autoimmune thrombocytopenia purpura* (ATP), (formerly called *idiopathic thrombocytopenic purpura*) and *thrombotic thrombocytopenia purpura (TTP)*. A common additional type is *heparin-induced thrombocytopenia (HIT)*. Although symptoms are similar, the causes and managements vary.

Autoimmune thrombocytopenia purpura is an autoimmune disease in which the patient's immune system begins making antibodies against his or her own platelet membranes (an antiplatelet antibody). When these antibodies attach to platelets, white blood cells attack and destroy the circulating platelets and those stored in the spleen faster than new platelets are produced. As the number of circulating platelets decreases, ***clotting*** is impaired. This disorder is most common among women between the ages of 20 and 50 years and among people who have other autoimmune disorders (McCance et al., 2019; Vacca, 2019). (See Chapter 18 for a discussion of the pathophysiology of autoimmune diseases.)

Thrombotic thrombocytopenic purpura (TTP) is also thought to be an autoimmune disorder, with the reaction occurring in small blood vessel cells (endothelial cells) and triggering abnormal platelet clumping in these vessels. As a result, too few platelets remain in circulation. The patient's blood forms clots and platelet plugs where they are not needed, yet the blood fails to clot when trauma occurs. Tissues become ischemic, leading to kidney failure, myocardial infarction, and stroke. Untreated, this disorder is often fatal within 3 months.

Heparin-induced thrombocytopenia (HIT) is a serious immune-mediated ***clotting*** disorder with an unexplained drop in platelet count after heparin treatment. The problem is increasing because of the increased use of heparin. HIT is an immune-mediated drug reaction that is caused by heparin-dependent platelet-activating antibodies that allow heparin to bind with platelet factor 4 (PF4). (The antibodies are directed against the heparin rather than patient's own cells.) Heparin binding to PF4 creates an immune complex that activates the platelets, causing the formation of many microclots that use up circulating platelets, leading to thrombocytopenia. HIT can occur in patients receiving any type of heparin, although it is more common after exposure to unfractionated heparin. The incidence is higher among female patients who are treated with unfractionated heparin for longer than 1 week.

❖ Interprofessional Collaborative Care

◆ **Assessment: Recognize Cues.** Symptoms of all types of thrombocytopenia are first seen in the skin and mucous membranes and result from excessive bleeding in these tissues. Changes include large ecchymoses (bruises) or purpura (a reddish-purple fine petechial rash) on the arms, legs, upper chest, and neck. Mucous membranes bleeding easily. If the patient has had significant blood loss, anemia may also be present.

For TTP and HIT, in addition to excessive bleeding problems, small microclots can block capillaries in major organs, causing tissue ischemia. This problem increases the risk for kidney damage, myocardial infarction, and stroke. Other problems associated with HIT include venous thromboembolism and pulmonary embolism.

Platelet levels are low in all three types of thrombocytopenia. If the patient has any episodes of bleeding, hematocrit and hemoglobin levels may be low. ATP can be distinguished from TTP by the presence of antiplatelet antibodies in the blood. Diagnosis of HIT is made by the clinical symptoms and a history of heparin therapy within the previous 100 days.

◆ **Interventions: Take Action.** The decreased platelet count increases the patient's risk for poor ***clotting*** and excessive bleeding. Interventions include protection from bleeding episodes and therapy for the different underlying condition.

Platelet transfusions are used when platelet counts are less than 10,000/mm^3 (10 × 10^9/L) or when the patient has an acute life-threatening bleeding episode. (See the discussion in the Platelet Transfusions section.)

Maintaining a safe environment helps protect the patient from bleeding. Closely monitor the amount of bleeding that is occurring. (For nursing care actions, see the discussion of Minimizing Injury in the Leukemia section.)

Drug therapy to control ATP and TTP includes drugs that suppress immune function. Drugs such as corticosteroids, azathioprine, eltrombopag, rituximab, and romiplostim are used to inhibit production of antibodies directed against platelets or endothelial cells. For ATP, IV immunoglobulin and IV anti-Rho can help prevent the destruction of antibody-coated platelets. Aggressive therapy involves low doses of chemotherapy drugs.

Drug management of TTP and HIT also includes anticoagulants. For TTP, drug therapy includes platelet inhibitors such as aspirin, alprostadil, and plicamycin. Plasma removal and the infusion of fresh-frozen plasma (plasma exchange) reduce the clumping caused by elements in the patient's blood. This therapy for autoimmune TTP has been responsible for dramatically increasing the survival rate (Vacca, 2019). Drug management for HIT includes a direct thrombin inhibitor such as argatroban or lepirudin (Greenberg, 2017).

Surgical management of ATP may involve a splenectomy for those patients who do not respond to drug therapy (Greenberg, 2017). (In ATP the spleen is the site of excessive platelet destruction.) Splenectomy is usually not performed for TTP or HIT.

Depending on the size of the spleen and the risk for bleeding, splenectomy may be performed as an open abdominal surgical procedure or as minimally invasive surgery by laparoscopy. Nursing care after surgery is the same as for any other abdominal surgery (see Chapter 9). After splenectomy, the patient is at increased risk for ***infection*** because the spleen performs many protective immune functions, especially antibody generation. For this reason, vaccinations against pneumococcal and meningococcal disorders and *Haemophilus influenzae* are recommended either 2 weeks before a planned splenectomy or 2 weeks after the surgery. Teaching patients about their increased risk for infection, avoiding crowds and people who are ill, and when to consult with the primary health care provider is a nursing priority.

TRANSFUSION THERAPY

Any blood component may be removed from a donor and transfused into a recipient. Blood components may be transfused individually or collectively, with varying degrees of benefit to the recipient. The associated risks of bloodborne disease transmission and other complications of transfusion therapy have resulted in fewer transfusion with more limited indications of the need for this practice (Frazier et al., 2017). Table 37.4 lists indications for transfusion therapy.

Pretransfusion Responsibilities

Nursing actions during transfusions focus on prevention or early recognition of transfusion reactions. Preparation of the patient for transfusion is critical, and blood product administration procedures must be followed carefully. Before infusing any blood product, review the agency's policies and procedures, as well as the Best Practices for Patient Safety & Quality Care: Transfusion Therapy box.

TABLE 37.4 Indications for Treatment With Blood Components

Component	Volume	Infusion Time	Indications
Packed red blood cells (PRBCs)	200-250 mL	2-4 hr	Anemia; hemoglobin <6 g/dL (<60 g/L), 6-10 g/dL (60-100 g/L), depending on symptoms
Washed red blood cells (WBC-poor PRBCs)	200 mL	2-4 hr	History of allergic transfusion reactions Hematopoietic stem cell transplant patients
Platelets			
Pooled	About 300 mL	15-30 min	Thrombocytopenia, platelet count <20,000 (<20 × 10^9/L) Patients who are actively bleeding with a platelet count <50,000 (<50 × 10^9/L)
Single donor	200 mL	30 min	History of febrile or allergic reactions
Fresh-frozen plasma	200 mL	15-30 min	Deficiency in plasma coagulation factors Prothrombin or partial thromboplastin time 1.5 times normal
White blood cells (WBCs)	400 mL	1 hr	Sepsis, neutropenic infection not responding to antibiotic therapy

A primary health care provider's prescription is needed to administer blood components. The prescription specifies the type of component, the volume, and any special conditions. In many hospitals, a separate consent form is obtained from the patient before a transfusion is performed.

A blood specimen is obtained for type and crossmatch (testing of the donor's blood and the recipient's blood for compatibility). The procedures for obtaining this specimen are specified by hospital policy. Usually a new type and crossmatch specimen is required every 72 hours.

Both Y-tubing and straight tubing sets are used for blood component infusion. A blood filter (about 170 microns) to remove sediment from the stored blood products is included with blood administration sets and must be used to transfuse most, but not all, blood products (Fig. 37.6).

Use normal saline as the solution to administer with blood products, although this practice is not evidence based. Ringer's lactate and dextrose in water are not used for infusion with blood products because they may cause clotting or hemolysis of blood cells, although there is not sufficient evidence of hemolysis when using hypotonic fluids.

Examine the blood bag label, the attached tag, and the requisition slip to ensure that the ABO and Rh types are compatible with those of the patient. Check the expiration date and inspect the product for discoloration, gas bubbles,

BEST PRACTICE FOR PATIENT SAFETY & QUALITY CARE (QSEN)

Transfusion Therapy

Before Infusion

- Assess laboratory values *to ensure agency guidelines for blood transfusions are followed.*
- Verify the primary health care provider's prescription for type of product, dose, and duration of transfusion *because the therapy legally requires a prescription.*
- Assess the patient's vital signs, urine output, skin color, and history of transfusion reactions *to establish a baseline for identifying possible reactions during and after the procedure.*
- Establish or use a venous access with a 19-gauge needle or catheter *to prevent catheter occlusion or damage to red blood cells.*
- Transfuse blood products (after all safety checks) soon after receiving them from the blood bank *to suppress bacterial growth and prevent product deterioration.*
- With another registered nurse, verify the patient by name and number, check blood compatibility, and note expiration time *because human error is the most common cause of incompatibility reactions.*

During Infusion

- Administer the blood product using the appropriate filtered tubing *to remove aggregates and possible contaminants.*
- Unless directed otherwise. infuse blood products only with IV normal saline solutions *because some other IV solutions can cause hemolysis.*
- Stay with the patient for the first 15 to 30 minutes of the infusion *because this is the time when hemolytic transfusion reactions occur.*
- Infuse the blood product at the prescribed rate for the transfusion type *to avoid the possible complication of fluid overload.*
- Monitor vital signs at least as often as agency policy and the patient's condition indicates *to identify early indications of adverse transfusion reactions.*

After Infusion

- When the transfusion is completed, discontinue the infusion and dispose of the bag and tubing according to agency and blood-bank policies *to prevent the spread of bloodborne pathogens.*
- Document all aspects of the transfusion (e.g., type of product, product number, volume infused, duration of infusion, vital signs, and any adverse reactions) *to identify patient responses to the transfusion as part of the permanent record.*

! NURSING SAFETY PRIORITY (QSEN)

Action Alert

Never add to or infuse other drugs with blood products because they may clot the blood during transfusion.

or cloudiness, which are all indicators of bacterial growth or hemolysis.

Transfusion Responsibilities

Before starting the transfusion, explain the procedure to the patient. Assess vital signs and temperature immediately before starting the infusion. Begin the infusion slowly. *Remain with the patient for the first 15 to 30 minutes.* Any severe reaction usually occurs with infusion of the first 50 mL of blood. Ask the patient to report unusual sensations such as chills, shortness of breath, hives, itching, or back pain. Assess vital signs 15 minutes after

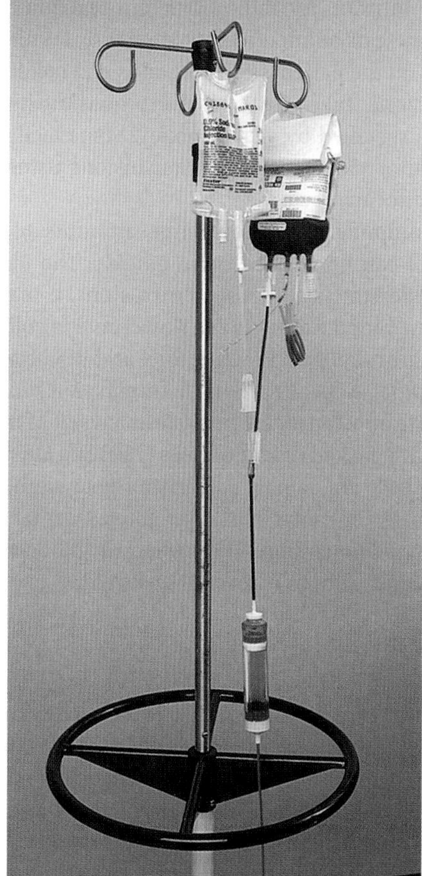

Fig. 37.6 Blood administration setup. (From deWit, S.C., & O'Neill, P. [2014]. *Fundamental concepts and skills for nursing* [4th ed.]. St. Louis: Saunders.)

! NATIONAL PATIENT SAFETY GOALS

In compliance with recommendations by The Joint Commission's National Patient Safety Goals and before the transfusion, the priority actions are to determine that the blood component delivered is correct and that identification of the patient is correct. Check the health care provider's prescription together with another registered nurse to determine the patient's identity and whether the hospital identification band name and number are identical to those on the blood component tag. According to The Joint Commission's National Patient Safety Goals, *the patient's room number is not an acceptable form of identification* (2017). Some facilities use a bar code–point of care (BC-POC) system, similar to drug-dispensing systems, in an attempt to improve patient safety and reduce identification errors.

! NURSING SAFETY PRIORITY (QSEN)

Action Alert

The nurse who will infuse the blood products *must* be one of the two professionals comparing the patient's identification with the information on the blood component bag.

starting the infusion for indications of a reaction. If there are none, the rate can be increased to transfuse 1 unit in 2 hours (depending on the patient's cardiac status and facility policy for rate of infusion). Take vital signs every hour during the transfusion or as specified by agency policy. Some facilities continuously monitor patients during transfusions using a wireless remote monitoring device.

Blood components without large amounts of red blood cells (RBCs) can be infused more quickly. The identification checks are the same as for RBC transfusions. It may be necessary to infuse blood products at a slower rate for older patients as described in the Best Practice for Patient Safety & Quality Care: The Older Adult Receiving a Transfusion box.

Electrolyte imbalances are possible as a result of transfusions, especially with packed red blood cells (PRBCs). During transfusions, some cells are damaged, releasing potassium and raising the patient's serum potassium level above normal *(hyperkalemia)*. This problem is more likely when the blood being transfused has been frozen or is several weeks old.

Types of Transfusions

At one time transfusion with whole blood was a common form of transfusion therapy. Today whole-blood transfusions are rare (Carson et al., 2016), except for military conditions in which banked blood components are not available (Goforth et al., 2016). When a whole-blood donation is made, it is most commonly centrifuged on arrival at the blood-banking facility and separated into various components. These components are transfused according to patients' specific needs.

BEST PRACTICE FOR PATIENT SAFETY & QUALITY CARE (QSEN)

The Older Adult Receiving a Transfusion

- Assess the patient's circulatory, kidney, and fluid status before starting the transfusion.
- Use no larger than a 19-gauge needle.
- Try to use blood that is less than 1 week old. (Older blood cell membranes are more fragile, break easily, and release potassium into the circulation.)
- Take vital signs (especially pulse, blood pressure, and respiratory rate) every 15 minutes throughout the transfusion. Changes in these parameters can indicate fluid overload and may also be the only indicators of adverse transfusion reactions:
  - Rapid bounding pulse
  - Hypertension
  - Swollen superficial veins
  - Transfusion reaction:
    - Hypotension
    - Rapid thready pulse
    - Increased pallor, cyanosis
- Infuse blood slowly, taking 2 to 4 hours for each unit of whole blood, packed red blood cells, or plasma.
- Avoid concurrent fluid administration into any other IV site.
- If possible, allow 2 full hours after infusing 1 unit of blood before infusing the next unit.

Red Blood Cell Transfusions. RBCs are given to replace cells lost from trauma or surgery. Patients with problems that destroy RBCs or impair RBC maturation also may receive RBC transfusions. PRBCs, supplied in 250-mL bags, are a concentrated source of RBCs and are the most common component given to RBC-deficient patients.

Blood transfusions are transplants of tissue from one person to another. Therefore the donor and recipient blood must be checked carefully for compatibility to prevent lethal reactions (Table 37.5). Compatibility is determined by two different antigen systems (cell surface proteins): the ABO system antigens and the Rh antigen, present on the membranes of RBCs.

RBC antigens are inherited. For the ABO system, a person inherits one of these:

- A antigen (type A blood)
- B antigen (type B blood)
- Both A and B antigens (type AB blood)
- Neither A nor B antigens (type O blood)

People develop circulating antibodies against the blood type antigens they did not inherit. For example, a person with type A blood forms antibodies against type B blood. A person with type O blood has not inherited either A or B antigens and will form antibodies against RBCs with either A or B antigens. If RBCs that have an antigen are infused into a recipient who does not share that antigen, the infused blood is recognized by the recipient's antibodies as non-self, and the recipient then has a reaction to the transfused products.

The Rh antigen system is slightly different. An Rh-negative person is born without the Rh-antigen on his or her RBCs and does not form antibodies unless specifically sensitized to it. Sensitization can occur with RBC transfusions from an Rh-positive person or from exposure during pregnancy and birth. Once an Rh-negative person has been sensitized and antibodies develop, any exposure to Rh-positive blood can cause a transfusion reaction. Antibody development can be prevented by giving anti-Rh immunoglobulin as soon as exposure to the Rh antigen is suspected. *Adults who have Rh-positive blood can receive an RBC transfusion from an Rh-negative donor, but Rh-negative adults must not receive Rh-positive blood.*

Platelet Transfusions. Platelets are given to patients with platelet counts below 10,000/mm^3 (10×10^9/L) and to patients with thrombocytopenia who are actively bleeding or are scheduled for an invasive procedure. Platelet transfusions are pooled from as many as 10 donors and do not have to be of the same blood type as the patient has. For patients who are having

TABLE 37.5 Compatibility Chart for Red Blood Cell Transfusions

	RECIPIENT			
Donor	**A**	**B**	**AB**	**O**
A	X		X	
B		X	X	
AB			X	
O	X	X	X	X

hematopoietic stem cell transplantation (HSCT) or who need multiple platelet transfusions, platelets from a single donor may be prescribed, which reduces the chances of allergic reactions.

Platelet infusion bags contain about 300 mL for pooled platelets and 200 mL for single-donor platelets. Platelets are fragile and must be infused immediately after being brought to the patient's room, usually over a 15- to 30-minute period. A special transfusion set with a smaller filter and shorter tubing is used. Platelet filters help remove WBCs from the platelets for patients who have a history of febrile reactions or who need multiple platelet transfusions.

! NURSING SAFETY PRIORITY QSEN

Action Alert

When infusing platelets, do not use the standard blood administration set because the longer tubing increases platelet adherence to the lumen, which reduces the number of platelets the patient actually receives.

At a minimum take the vital signs before the infusion, 15 minutes after the infusion starts, and at its completion. A patient who has had a transfusion reaction in the past may be given diphenhydramine and acetaminophen before the transfusion to reduce the fever and severe chills (rigors) that often occur during platelet transfusions.

Plasma Transfusions. Plasma infusions may be given fresh to replace blood volume and clotting factors. More often, plasma is frozen immediately after donation, *forming fresh-frozen plasma (FFP)*. Infuse FFP immediately after thawing while the clotting factors are still active.

ABO compatibility is required for transfusion of plasma products because the plasma contains the donor's ABO antibodies, which could react with the recipient's RBC antigens. The infusion bag contains about 200 mL. Infuse FFP as rapidly as the patient can tolerate, generally over a 30- to 60-minute period, through a regular Y-set or straight filtered tubing.

Granulocyte (White Blood Cell) Transfusions. Rarely, neutropenic patients with infections receive white blood cell (WBC) replacement transfusions. WBC surfaces have many antigens that can cause severe reactions when infused into a patient whose immune system recognizes these antigens as non-self.

WBCs are suspended in 400 mL of plasma and are infused slowly, usually over a 45- to 60-minute period, depending on the concentration of cells being infused. Agency policies often require stricter monitoring during WBC infusions because reactions are more common. A physician may need to be present in the hospital unit, and vital signs may need to be taken every 15 minutes throughout the transfusion. Amphotericin B infusion should be separated from WBC transfusions by 4 to 6 hours because this drug can hemolyze the blood cells. In addition, amphotericin B has so many side effects that these may mask a transfusion reaction.

Massive Transfusion Protocol. Although packed red blood cell (PRBC) transfusions are the therapy of choice when hematocrit and hemoglobin levels are low, this transfusion type does not contain clotting factors or platelets that may be needed when continuing heavy blood loss and hemorrhage are present. For many years PRBCs were used in massive transfusion situations, using precious resources and not necessarily having a good outcome. Now, in massive transfusion protocols (MTPs) in which large amounts of blood products are needed to counteract hemorrhage, all blood components are used to restore volume, clotting ability, and oxygen-carrying capacity. Often the protocols call for balanced delivery of components, with PRBCs, plasma, and platelets infused in an order and proportion that mimic whole blood (Adams, 2019; Passerini, 2019). The exact protocols differ slightly from one institution to another, from 1:1:1 to those that provide twice as much plasma and PRBCs compared with platelets. Regardless of specific protocols, this balanced approach has resulted in better patient survival with less consumption and wastage of blood products and fewer transfusion-related complications. Although administration of transfusions by MTPs generally occurs more rapidly than infusion of blood products by standard protocols, all required safety precautions remain and the risk for transfusion reactions is increased by the volume of products transfused.

Acute Transfusion Reactions

Although complications and acute transfusion reactions can occur with any type of RBC component therapy, reactions are more common when components are more than 30 days old and when multiple transfusions are administered (Jones & Frazier, 2017). Patients can develop any of these transfusion reactions: febrile, hemolytic, allergic, or bacterial reactions; circulatory overload; or transfusion-associated graft-versus-host disease (TA-GVHD). To prevent complications, remain alert during transfusions to detect early reactions and initiate appropriate management. Instructing the patient to immediately report any change in physical or emotional status, such as new-onset joint, back, chest, or abdominal pain; chills; nausea; feeling unwell; or feeling uneasy, may help identify a possible transfusion reaction (Frazier et al., 2017; Menendez & Edwards, 2016).

Febrile transfusion reactions occur most often in the patient with anti-WBC antibodies, which can develop after multiple transfusions, WBC transfusions, and platelet transfusions. The patient develops chills, tachycardia, fever, hypotension, and tachypnea. Giving leukocyte-reduced blood or single-donor HLA-matched platelets reduces the risk for this type of reaction. WBC filters may be used to trap WBCs and prevent their infusion into the patient.

Hemolytic transfusion reactions are caused by blood type or Rh incompatibility. When blood containing antigens different from the patient's own antigens is infused, antigen-antibody complexes are formed in his or her blood. These complexes destroy the transfused cells and start inflammatory responses in the blood vessel walls and organs. The reaction may be mild, with fever and chills, or life threatening, with disseminated intravascular coagulation

(DIC) and circulatory collapse (McCance et al., 2019). Other symptoms include:

- Apprehension
- Headache
- Chest pain
- Low back pain
- Tachycardia
- Tachypnea
- Hypotension
- Hemoglobinuria
- A sense of impending doom ("I feel like something's wrong, but I don't know what.")

The onset of a hemolytic reaction may be immediate or may not occur until subsequent units have been transfused.

Allergic transfusion reactions (anaphylactic transfusion reactions) are most often seen in patients with other allergies. They may have urticaria, itching, bronchospasm, or anaphylaxis. Onset usually occurs during or up to 24 hours after the transfusion. Patients with an allergy history can be given leukocyte-reduced or washed RBCs, in which the WBCs, plasma, and immunoglobulin A have been removed, reducing the risk for an allergic reaction.

Bacterial transfusion reactions occur from infusion of contaminated blood products, especially those contaminated with a gram-negative organism. Symptoms include tachycardia, hypotension, fever, chills, and shock. The onset of a bacterial transfusion reaction is rapid. (See Chapter 34 for care of the patient with septic shock.)

Transfusion-related acute lung injury (TRALI) is a life-threatening event that occurs most often when donor blood contains antibodies against the recipient's neutrophil antigens, HLA, or both. Common symptoms are a rapid onset of dyspnea and hypoxia within 6 hours of the transfusion (Carman et al., 2018). Early recognition is key to survival. Most patients require intubation and mechanical ventilation for respiratory support.

Transfusion-associated circulatory overload (TACO) can occur when a blood product is infused too quickly, especially in an older adult. It is a pulmonary reaction that may be difficult at first to differentiate from TRALI. This is most common with whole-blood transfusions or when the patient receives multiple packed RBC transfusions. Symptoms include:

- Hypertension
- Bounding pulse
- Distended jugular veins
- Dyspnea
- Restlessness
- Confusion

Manage and prevent this complication by monitoring intake and output, infusing blood products more slowly, and giving diuretics. (See Chapter 13 for management of fluid overload.)

Transfusion-associated graft-versus-host disease (TA-GVHD) is a rare but life-threatening problem that occurs more often in an immunosuppressed patient. Its cause in immunosuppressed patients is similar to that of GVHD that occurs with allogeneic stem cell transplantation, discussed in the interventions section of Leukemia and Preleukemia, in which donor T-cell lymphocytes attack host tissues.

PATIENT-CENTERED CARE: CULTURAL/SPIRITUAL CONSIDERATIONS (QSEN)

Interestingly, the incidence of TRALI and TACO is increased when the donor and recipient are from different ethnicities even though ABO and Rh compatibility are matched (MacIntyre, 2017). These reactions may occur within 24 hours to 21 days after the transfusion. These reactions are thought to arise from differences in other red blood cell antigens that are not usually a part of screening. These antigens vary considerably among ethnicities. A more diverse donor population could help to reduce the incidence of severe transfusion reactions (Yazer et al., 2017).

Symptoms usually occur within 1 to 2 weeks and include thrombocytopenia, anorexia, nausea, vomiting, chronic hepatitis, weight loss, and recurrent ***infection***. TA-GVHD has an 80% to 90% mortality rate but can be prevented by using irradiated blood products. Irradiation destroys most T-cells and their cytokine products.

Acute pain transfusion reaction or APTR is a rare event with an unknown cause that can occur during or shortly after transfusion of any blood product. Symptoms are severe chest ***pain***, back pain, joint pain, hypertension, anxiety, and redness of the head and neck. The reaction does not appear to be life threatening, and most patients respond well with drugs for pain and rigors. Although symptoms are general, diagnosis can be supported with a positive direct antibody test (DAT), indicating that some degree of hemolysis has occurred but is not widespread. APTR management focuses on patient support and drugs to control or reduce symptoms.

Interventions for reactions occurring during transfusion (hemolytic reactions, allergic reactions, and bacterial reactions) begin with stopping the transfusion and removing the blood tubing. (For hemolytic and suspected bacterial reactions, return the component bag, labels, and all tubing to the blood bank or laboratory.) Initiate the Rapid Response Team. If the patient has no other IV access, keep the access and flush with normal saline. *Do not flush the contents of the blood transfusion tubing, which would allow more of the reaction-causing blood to enter the patient.* Usually oxygen is applied, and diphenhydramine is given by IV push. If shock is present, fluid resuscitation and hemodynamic monitoring are needed. Blood pressure support with vasopressors may be needed (see Chapter 34). Other drug therapy is supportive, such as antipyretics for fever, antibiotics for possible bacterial contamination, and meperidine for rigors.

NCLEX EXAMINATION CHALLENGE 37.4

Psychosocial Integrity

The family of a client receiving a blood transfusion report with distress to the nurse that although the blood bag hanging has the client's name on it, the bag label says B negative and the client's blood type is B positive. What is the nurse's **priority action**?

A. Alert the blood bank and Rapid Response Team about a potential error.
B. Thank the family for being alert and preventing a serious complication.
C. Explain that a person who is Rh positive can receive Rh negative blood.
D. Immediately go and stop the infusion but keep the IV line open with normal saline.

Autologous Blood Transfusions

Autologous blood transfusions involve collection and infusion of the patient's own blood. This type of transfusion eliminates compatibility problems and reduces the risk for transmitting bloodborne diseases. The four types of autologous blood transfusions are preoperative autologous blood donation, acute normovolemic hemodilution, intraoperative autologous transfusion, and postoperative blood salvage.

Self-blood donation before surgery is the most common type of autologous blood transfusion (Frazier et al., 2017). It involves collecting whole blood from a qualified patient, dividing it into components, and storing them for later use. If hematocrit and hemoglobin levels remain within a safe range, the patient can donate blood on a weekly basis until the prescribed amount of blood is obtained. Fresh packed RBCs may be stored for 40 days. For patients with rare blood types, blood may be frozen for up to 10 years.

Acute normovolemic hemodilution involves withdrawal of a patient's RBCs and volume replacement just before a surgical procedure. The goal is to decrease RBC loss during surgery. The blood is stored at room temperature for up to 6 hours and reinfused after surgery. This type of autologous transfusion is not used with anemic patients or those with poor kidney function.

Intraoperative autologous transfusion and blood salvage after surgery are the recovery and reinfusion of a patient's own blood from an operative field or from a bleeding wound. Special devices collect, filter, and drain the blood into a transfusion bag. This blood is used for trauma or surgical patients with severe blood loss. The salvaged blood must be reinfused within 6 hours.

Transfuse autologous blood products using the guidelines previously described. Although the patient receiving autologous blood is not at risk for some types of transfusion reactions, circulatory overload or bacterial transfusion reactions can still occur and are managed in the same way that these complications are managed in transfusions derived from donors.

GET READY FOR THE NEXT-GENERATION NCLEX® EXAMINATION!

Key Points

Review these Key Points for each NCLEX Examination Client Needs Category.

Safe and Effective Care Environment

- Use aseptic technique during all central line dressing changes or any invasive procedure. **QSEN: Safety**
- Use Bleeding Precautions for any patient with ***clotting*** problems from thrombocytopenia or pancytopenia. **QSEN: Safety**
- Verify with another registered nurse prescriptions for transfusion of blood products. **QSEN: Safety**
- Use at least two forms of identification for the patient who is to receive a blood product transfusion (e.g., name, birthdate, identification number). **QSEN: Safety**
- Teach patients with sickle cell disease to avoid conditions that are known to trigger crises. **QSEN: Patient-Centered Care**
- Teach the patient and family the symptoms of ***infection*** and when to seek medical advice. **QSEN: Patient-Centered Care**
- Teach precautions to take to avoid injury to patients at risk for poor ***clotting*** and increased bleeding. **QSEN: Patient-Centered Care**
- Report any temperature over 100°F (37.8°C) in a patient with neutropenia. **QSEN: Evidence-Based Practice**

Health Promotion and Maintenance

- Make referrals to support groups sponsored by organizations such as local chapters of the Sickle Cell Foundation, American Cancer Society, and the Leukemia and Lymphoma Society. **QSEN: Teamwork and Collaboration**

Psychosocial Integrity

- Allow the patient and family the opportunity to express their feelings about the diagnosis of leukemia or lymphoma or the treatment regimen. **QSEN: Patient-Centered Care**
- Explain all procedures, restrictions, drugs, and follow-up care to the patient and family. **QSEN: Patient-Centered Care**

Physiological Integrity

- Pace nonurgent health care activities to reduce the risk for fatigue in patients with anemia or pancytopenia. **QSEN: Patient-Centered Care**
- Assess patients with neutropenia every 8 hours for indicators of ***infection***. **QSEN: Evidence-Based Practice**
- Administer analgesics on a schedule rather than PRN. **QSEN: Evidence-Based Practice**
- Transfuse blood products more slowly to older patients or those who have a cardiac problem. **QSEN: Patient-Centered Care**
- Remain with the patient during the first 15 minutes of infusion of any blood product. **QSEN: Safety**
- Do not administer any drugs in the same line with infusing blood products. **QSEN: Evidence-Based Practice**

MASTERY QUESTIONS

1. Which new symptoms in a client who is being managed for sickle cell crisis does the nurse report immediately to **prevent harm? Select all that apply.**
   A. Decreased handgrip strength on one side
   B. Diffuse abdominal pain
   C. Fever of 102.2°F (39°C)
   D. Increased urine output
   E. Shortness of breath
   F. Sore throat
2. Which intervention is a **priority** for the nurse to teach the client with polycythemia vera to **prevent harm** related to injury as a result of impaired platelet function?
   A. Wear gloves and socks outdoors in cool weather.
   B. Elevate your feet whenever you are seated.
   C. Drink at least 3 L of liquids per day.
   D. Use a soft-bristle toothbrush.
3. A client who is 5 weeks posttransplant after an allogeneic stem cell transplantation for acute lymphocytic leukemia comes to the clinic with a swollen belly and weight gain. Which additional assessment data support the nurse's suspicion of possible sinusoidal obstructive syndrome (SOS)? **Select all that apply.**
   A. Jaundiced skin and sclera
   B. Platelet count is 28,000/mm^3
   C. Skin peeling on the hands and feet
   D. Mixed chimerism by laboratory finding
   E. Body temperature slightly below normal
   F. Pain in the upper right abdominal quadrant

REFERENCES

Asterisk (*) indicates a classic or definitive work on this subject.

Adams, A. (2019). Massive blood transfusion protocols. *American Nurse Today, 14*(7), 18–20.

American Cancer Society (ACS). (2020). *Cancer facts and figures 2020. Report No. 01-300M-No. 500820.* Atlanta: Author.

Binette, A., Howatt, K., Waddington, A., & Reid, R. (2017). Ten challenges in contraception. *Journal of Women's Health, 26*(1), 44–49.

Cadet, M. (2018). Iron deficiency anemia: A clinical case study. *Medsurg Nursing, 27*(2), 108–109 120.

Callahan, C., Baniewicz, D., & Ely, B. (2017). CAR-T cell therapy. *Clinical Journal of Oncology Nursing, 21*(Suppl. 2), 22–28.

Canadian Cancer Society, Statistics Canada. (2019). *Canadian cancer statistics, 2019.* Toronto, ON: Canadian Cancer Society.

Carman, M., Schreferle, J., & McClintock, S. (2018). Emergency: A review of current practice in transfusion therapy. *American Journal of Nursing, 118*(5), 36–44.

Carson, J., Guyatt, G., Heddle, N., Grossman, B., Cohn, C., Fung, M., et al. (2016). Clinical practice guidelines from the AABB: Red blood cell transfusion thresholds and storage. *Journal of the American Medical Association, 316*(19), 2025–2035.

Centers for Disease Control and Prevention (CDC). (2017). *Sickle cell disease: Data & statistics.* www.cdc.gov/ncbddd/sicklecell/data.html.

Faiman, B. (2017). Disease and symptom care: A focus on specific needs of patients with multiple myeloma. *Clinical Journal of Oncology Nursing, 5*(Suppl. 21), 3–6.

Faiman, B., Doss, D., Colson, K., Mangan, P., King, T., Tariman, J., & the International Myeloma Foundation Leadership Board (2017). Renal, GI, and peripheral nerves: Evidence-based recommendations for eh management of symptoms and care for patients with multiple myeloma. *Clinical Journal of Oncology Nursing, 5*(Suppl. 21), 19–36.

Frazier, S., Higgins, J., Bugajski, A., Jones, A., & Brown, M. (2017). Adverse reactions to transfusion of blood products and best practices for prevention. *Critical Care Nursing Clinics of North America, 29*(3), 271–290.

Ganti, B. R., Marini, B. L., Nagel, J., Bixby, D., & Perissinotti, A. J. (2017). Impact of antibacterial prophylaxis during reinduction chemotherapy for relapse/refractory acute myeloid leukemia. *Supportive Care in Cancer, 25*, 541–547.

Gleason, C., & Kaufman, J. (2017). New treatment strategies making an impact in multiple myeloma. *Journal of Advanced Practitioner in Oncology, 8*(3), 285–290.

Glode, A., & Babiker, H. (2017). Emerging therapies in chronic lymphocytic leukemia: Current trials. *Journal of Advanced Practitioner in Oncology, 8*(7), 71–86.

Goforth, C., Tranberg, J., Boyer, P., & Silvestri, P. (2016). Fresh whole blood transfusion: Military and civilian implications. *Critical Care Nurse, 36*(3), 50–57.

Greenberg, E. (2017). Thrombocytopenia: A destruction of platelets. *Journal of Infusion Nursing, 40*(1), 41–50.

Harvey, D. (2018). New drug updates in hematologic malignancies: CAR-T, targeted therapeutics, and other agents. *Journal of Advanced Practitioner in Oncology, 9*(3), 282–286.

Jarvis, C. (2020). *Physical examination & health assessment* (8th ed.). St. Louis: Elsevier.

Jones, A., & Frazier, S. (2017). Consequences of transfusing blood components in patients with trauma: A conceptual model. *Critical Care Nurse, 37*(2), 18–29.

Jorde, L., Carey, J., & Bamshad, M. (2016). *Medical genetics* (5th ed.). Philadelphia: Elsevier.

Koniarczyk, H., & Ferraro, C. (2016). Transplant preparative regimens, cellular infusion, acute complications, and engraftment. In B. Faiman (Ed.), *BMTCN® Certification review Manual* (pp. 37–67). Pittsburgh, PA: Oncology Nursing Society.

Lentz, M., & Kautz, D. (2017). Acute vaso-occlusive crisis in patients with sickle cell disease. *Nursing 2017, 47*(1), 67–68.

MacIntyre, L. (2017). The growing need for diverse blood donors. *American Journal of Nursing, 117*(7), 44–48.

Mangels, A. R. (2018). Malnutrition in older adults. *American Journal of Nursing, 118*(3), 34–41.

Martin, M., & Haines, D. (2016). Clinical management of patients with thalassemia syndromes. *Clinical Journal of Oncology Nursing, 20*(3), 310–317.

McCance, K., Huether, S., Brashers, V., & Rote, N. (2019). *Pathophysiology: The biologic basis for disease in adults and children* (7th ed.). St. Louis: Mosby.

McConville, H., & Harvey, M. (2016). A review of chimeric antigen receptor T-cell therapy. *Oncology Nurse Advisor, March/April*, 22–28.

Menendez, J., & Edwards, B. (2016). Early identification of acute hemolytic transfusion reactions: Realistic implications for best practice in patient monitoring. *Medsurg Nursing, 25*(2), 88–90 109.

National Marrow Donor Program. (2020). *How does a patient's ethnic background affect matching?* https://bethematch.org/transplant-basics/matching-patients-with-donors/how-does-a-patients-ethnic-background-affect-matching.

Noonan, K., Rome, S., Faiman, B., Verina, D., & the International Myeloma Foundation Nurse Leadership Board (2017). Heart and lung complications: Assessment and prevention of venous thromboembolism and cardiovascular disease in patients with multiple myeloma. *Clinical Journal of Oncology Nursing, 5*(Suppl. 21), 37–46.

Online Mendelian Inheritance in Man (OMIM). (2019a). *Leukemia, chronic myeloid.* CML. https://www.omim.org/entry/608232.

Online Mendelian Inheritance in Man (OMIM). (2019b). *Sickle cell anemia.* https://www.omim.org/entry/603903.

Pagana, K., & Pagana, T. (2018). *Mosby's manual of diagnostic and laboratory tests* (6th ed.). St. Louis: Mosby.

Paradis, H., Alter, D., & Lierandi, D. (2017). Venetoclax. *Clinical Journal of Oncology Nursing, 21*(5), 604–610.

Passerini, H. (2019). Contemporary transfusion science and challenges. *AACN Advanced Critical Care, 30*(2), 139–150.

Rajkumar, S. (2016). Multiple myeloma: 2016 update on diagnosis, risk-stratification, and management. *American Journal of Hematology, 91*, 719–734.

Ribeil, J., Abina, S., Payen, M., Magnami, A., Semeraro, M., et al. (2017). Gene therapy in a patient with sickle cell disease. *New England Journal of Medicine, 376*(9), 848–855.

Rome, S., Noonan, K., Bertolotto, P., Tariman, J., Miceli, T., & the International myeloma foundation nurse Leadership board (2017). bone health, pain, and mobility: Evidence-based recommendations for patients with multiple myeloma. *Clinical Journal of Oncology Nursing, 5*(Suppl. 21), 47–59.

Tanabe, P., Spratling, R., Smith, D., Grissom, P., & Hulihan, M. (2019). Understanding the complications of sickle cell disease. *American Journal of Nursing, 119*(6), 26–35.

Taylor, J. (2019). A case of acute chest syndrome. *American Nurse Today, 14*(4), 8–9.

The Joint Commission (TJC). (2017). *Implementation guide for the Joint Commission patient blood management performance measures.* www.jointcommission.org/patient_blood_management_performance_measures_project/.

Touhy, T., & Jett, K. (2020). *Ebersole and Hess' toward healthy aging* (10th ed.). St. Louis: Mosby.

*U.S. Department of Health and Human Services (USDHHS). (2014). *National Institutes of Health: Evidence-based management of sickle cell disease-Expert panel report, 2014.* https://www.nhlbi.nih.gov/health-topics/all-publications-and-resources/evidence-based-management-sickle-cell-disease-expert-0.

U.S. Department of Health and Human Services (USDHHS). (2017). *Sickle cell disease.* https://www.nhlbi.nih.gov/health-topics/sickle-cell-disease.

Vacca, V. (2019). Acquired autoimmune thrombotic thrombocytopenic purpura. *Nursing 2019, 49*(1), 22–29.

Vacca, V., & Blank, L. (2017). Sickle cell disease: Where are we now? *Nursing 2017, 47*(4), 26–34.

Xin, L., & Corcoran, S. (2019). Caring for survivors of Hodgkin lymphoma. *American Journal of Nursing, 119*(2), 32–41.

Yazer, M. H., Delaney, M., Germain, M., Karafin, M. S., Sayers, M., Vassallo, R., Ziman, A., & Shaz, B. (2017). Trends in U.S. minority red blood cell unit donations. *Transfusion*, 57(5), 1226–1234. doi: 10.1111/trf.14039.

Young, L., & Mansfield, B. (2017). Nursing care of adult hematopoietic stem cell transplant patients and families in the intensive care unit: An evidence-based review. *Critical Care Nursing Clinics of North America, 29*(3), 341–352.

Zanella, A., & Barcelleini, W. (2016). Treatment of autoimmune hemolytic anemias. *Haematologica, 99*(10), 1547–1554. http://www.cancer.ca/~/media/cancer.ca/CW/publications/Canadian%20Cancer%20Statistics/Canadian-Cancer-Statistics-2019-EN.pdf.

38

Assessment of the Nervous System

Donna D. Ignatavicius

http://evolve.elsevier.com/Iggy/

LEARNING OUTCOMES

1. Apply knowledge of anatomy and physiology to perform a rapid/focused neurologic assessment based on the patient's history and presenting signs and symptoms.
2. Identify behaviors or lifestyle choices that place patients at risk for neurologic health problems.
3. Provide patient-centered health teaching for preparation and follow-up care for selected neurologic diagnostic testing to assess ***perfusion*** status.
4. Apply knowledge of common physiologic changes associated with aging to accurately interpret neurologic assessment findings and plan interventions to ensure patient safety.
5. Document findings from the neurologic nursing assessment to identify changes in ***cognition, mobility,*** and ***sensory perception.***
6. Describe evidence-based precautions for the use of iodine-based or gadolinium contrast for diagnostic testing to ensure patient safety.
7. Identify potential complications that may result from selected invasive neurologic diagnostic testing.

KEY TERMS

autonomic nervous system (ANS) Part of the nervous system that is composed of two parts: the sympathetic nervous system (SNS) and the parasympathetic nervous system.

Babinski sign Dorsiflexion of the great toe and fanning of the other toes that is abnormal in anyone older than 2 years and represents the presence of central nervous system (CNS) disease.

Bell palsy A peripheral nervous system disorder in which the patient has paralysis of all facial muscles on the affected side (also called facial paralysis). The patient cannot close his or her eye, wrinkle the forehead, smile, whistle, or grimace. Tearing may stop or become excessive. The face appears masklike and sags.

clonus (also called *myoclonus*) The sudden, brief, jerking contraction of a muscle or muscle group often seen in seizures.

decerebration Abnormal movement with rigidity characterized by extension of the arms and legs, pronation of the arms, plantar flexion, and opisthotonos (body spasm in which the body is bowed forward).

decortication Abnormal motor movement seen in the patient with lesions that interrupt the corticospinal pathways.

electroencephalography (EEG) A diagnostic test that records the electrical activity of the cerebral hemispheres of the brain. The frequency, amplitude, and characteristics of the brain waves are recorded.

electromyography A diagnostic test used to identify nerve and muscle disorders, such as myasthenia gravis, as well as spinal cord disease.

Glasgow Coma Scale (GCS) A tool used in many acute care settings to establish baseline data in each of these areas: eye opening, motor response, and verbal response. The patient is assigned a numeric score for each of these areas. The lower the score, the lower the patient's neurologic function.

Guillain-Barré syndrome (GBS) A rare acute inflammatory disorder that affects the axons and/or myelin of the peripheral nervous system resulting in ascending muscle weakness or paralysis.

level of consciousness (LOC) The degree of alertness or amount of stimulation needed to engage a patient's attention and can range from alert to comatose.

magnetoencephalography (MEG) A noninvasive imaging technique used to measure the magnetic fields produced by electrical activity in the brain via extremely sensitive devices such as superconducting quantum interference devices.

myasthenia gravis A rare progressive autoimmune disease characterized by muscle weakness as a result of impaired acetylcholine receptors.

neurotransmitter A chemical (e.g., acetylcholine and serotonin) within the nervous system that can either enhance or inhibit the neurologic impulse but not do both.
PERRLA Pupils are equal in size, round and regular in shape, and react to light and accommodation (a desired normal finding for most individuals).
proprioception Awareness of body position.
single-photon emission computed tomography (SPECT) A diagnostic imaging study that uses a radiopharmaceutical agent to enable radioisotopes to cross the blood-brain barrier.
trigeminal neuralgia A persistently painful and debilitating disorder that involves the trigeminal cranial nerve (CN V) and affects women more often than men.

PRIORITY AND INTERRELATED CONCEPTS

The priority concepts for this chapter are:
- ***Cognition***
- ***Mobility***
- ***Sensory Perception***

The interrelated concept for this chapter is:
- ***Perfusion***

The major divisions of the nervous system are the central nervous system (CNS) (brain and spinal cord), peripheral nervous system (PNS), and autonomic nervous system (ANS). The divisions of the nervous system work together to control ***cognition, mobility,*** and ***sensory perception***. See Chapter 3 for review of these health concepts. Health problems usually affect the CNS more often than other divisions of the nervous system and are the primary focus of this textbook unit.

ANATOMY AND PHYSIOLOGY REVIEW

Nervous System Cells: Structure and Function

The basic unit of the nervous system, the neuron, transmits impulses, or "messages." Some neurons are *motor* (causing purposeful physical movement or ***mobility***), and some are *sensory* (resulting in the ability to perceive stimulation through one's sensory organs or ***sensory perception***). Some process information and some retain information (***cognition***). When a neuron receives an impulse from another neuron, the effect may be excitation (increasing action) or inhibition (decreasing action). Each neuron has a *cell body,* or *soma;* short, branching processes called *dendrites;* and a single *axon* (Fig. 38.1).

Afferent neurons, also known as *sensory neurons,* are specialized to send impulses toward the CNS, away from the PNS. *Efferent* neurons are motor nerve cells that carry signals away from the CNS to the cells in the PNS. Each dendrite synapses with another cell body, axon, or dendrite and sends impulses along the efferent and afferent neuron pathways.

Many axons are covered by a myelin sheath—a white, lipid covering. Myelinated axons appear whitish and therefore are also called *white matter.* Nonmyelinated axons have a grayish cast and are called *gray matter.* Myelinated axons have gaps in the myelin called *nodes of Ranvier.* The nodes of Ranvier play a major role in impulse conduction (see Fig. 38.1). When the myelin is impaired, the impulses cannot travel from the brain to the rest of the body, such as in patients with multiple sclerosis (see Chapter 40).

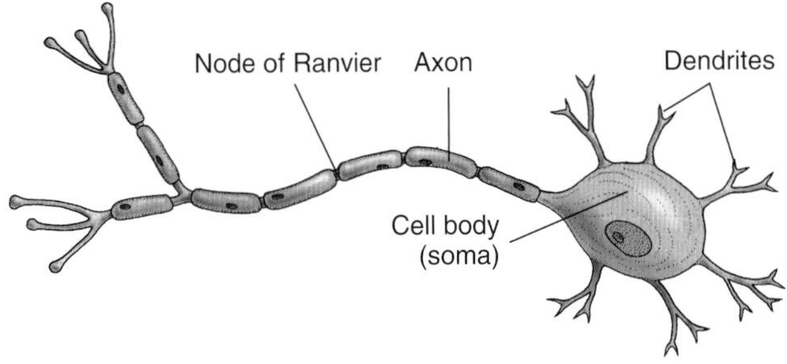

FIG. 38.1 Structure of a typical neuron.

The enlarged distal end of each axon is called the *synaptic* or *terminal knob.* Within the synaptic knobs are the mechanisms for manufacturing, storing, and releasing a transmitter substance. Each neuron produces a specific **neurotransmitter** chemical (e.g., acetylcholine and serotonin) that can either enhance or inhibit the impulse, but it cannot do both.

Impulses are transmitted to their eventual destination through synapses, or spaces between neurons. There are two distinct types of synapses: *neuron to neuron* and *neuron to muscle* (or gland). Between the terminal knob and the next cell is a small space called the *synaptic cleft.* The knob, the cleft, and the portion of the cell to which the impulse is being transmitted make up the *synapse.*

Neuroglia cells (sometimes referred to as glial cells), which vary in size and shape, provide protection, structure, and nutrition for the neurons. They are classified into four types: astroglial cells, ependymal cells, oligodendrocytes, and microglial cells. These cells are also part of the blood-brain barrier and help regulate cerebrospinal fluid (CSF) (McCance et al., 2019). Malignant tumors that affect glial cells are very aggressive and typically have a poor outcome.

Central Nervous System: Structure and Function

The central nervous system (CNS) is composed of the *brain,* which directs the regulation and function of the nervous system and all other systems of the body, and the *spinal cord,* which starts reflex activity and transmits impulses to and from the brain.

Brain. The **meninges** form the protective covering of the brain and the spinal cord. The outside layer is the *dura mater.* The *subdural space* is located between the dura mater and the middle layer, the *arachnoid.* The *pia mater* is the most inner layer. Situated between the arachnoid and pia mater is the *subarachnoid space,* where CSF circulates. The *epidural space* is located between the skull and the outer layer of the dura mater. This

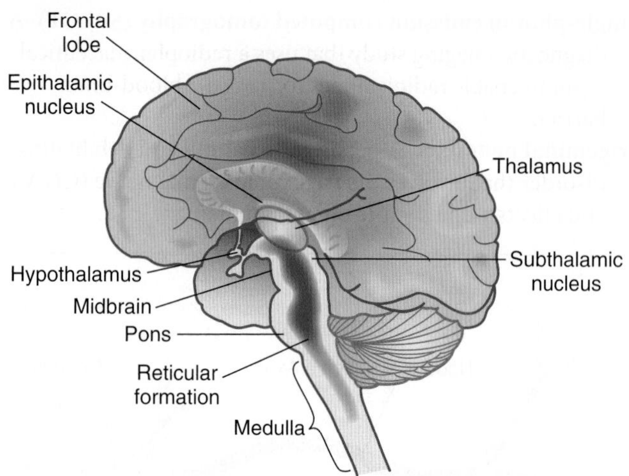

FIG. 38.2 Structures of the brainstem and diencephalon.

area also extends down the spinal cord and is used for the delivery of epidural analgesia and anesthesia.

The dura mater also lies between the cerebral hemispheres and the cerebellum and is called the *tentorium.* It helps decrease or prevents the transmission of force from one hemisphere to another and protects the lower brainstem when head trauma occurs. Clinical references may be made to a lesion (e.g., a tumor) as being supratentorial (above the tentorium) or infratentorial (below the tentorium).

Major Parts of the Brain. The brain consists of three main areas—the forebrain, cerebellum, and brainstem. The *forebrain* lies above the brainstem and cerebellum and is the most advanced in function complexity. This area of the brain is further divided into three areas—the diencephalon, cerebrum, and cerebral cortex.

The *diencephalon,* which lies below the cerebrum, includes the thalamus, hypothalamus, and epithalamus (Fig. 38.2). The *thalamus* is the major "relay station," or "central switchboard," for the CNS. The *hypothalamus* plays a major role in autonomic nervous system control (controlling temperature and other functions) and ***cognition***. The *epithalamus* connects the pathways to regulate emotion and contribute to smooth voluntary motor function.

The *cerebrum* is the largest part of the brain and controls intelligence, creativity, and memory. The "gray matter" of the cerebrum is the central cortex—the center that receives information from the thalamus and all the lower areas of the brain. The cerebrum consists of two halves, referred to as the *right hemisphere* and the *left hemisphere,* which are joined by the corpus callosum. The *left* hemisphere is the dominant hemisphere in most people (even in many left-handed people). Within the deeper structures of the cerebrum are the right and left lateral ventricles. At the base of the cerebrum near the ventricles is a group of neurons called the *basal ganglia,* which help regulate motor function.

The *cerebral cortex* is part of the cerebrum and is involved with almost all of the higher functions of the brain. This part of the brain processes and communicates all information coming from the peripheral nervous system (PNS). It also translates the impulses into understandable feelings and thoughts. The cerebral cortex is so complex that it is further divided into four lobes: the frontal lobe, parietal lobe, temporal lobe, and occipital lobe. Table 38.1 summarizes the major functions of each lobe.

TABLE 38.1 Cerebral Lobe Main Functions

Frontal Lobe
- Primary motor area (also known as the *motor "strip"* or *cortex*) (***mobility***)
- Broca speech center on the dominant side
- Voluntary eye movement
- Access to current sensory data (***sensory perception***)
- Access to past information or experience
- Affective response to a situation
- Behavior regulation
- Cognition
  - Judgment
  - Ability to develop long-term goals
  - Reasoning, concentration, abstraction

Parietal Lobe
- Understanding sensory input such as texture, size, shape, and spatial relationships
- Three-dimensional (spatial) perception
- Needed for singing, playing musical instruments, and processing nonverbal visual experiences
- Perception of body parts and body position awareness
- Taste impulses for interpretation

Temporal Lobe
- Auditory center for sound interpretation
- Complicated memory patterns
- Wernicke area for language comprehension

Occipital Lobe
- Primary visual center

The *cerebellum* receives immediate and continuous information about the condition of the muscles, joints, and tendons. Cerebellar function enables a person to:
- Keep an extremity from overshooting an intended target
- Move from one skilled movement to another in an orderly sequence
- Predict distance or gauge the speed with which one is approaching an object
- Control voluntary movement
- Maintain equilibrium

Unlike the motor cortex, cerebellar control of the body is *ipsilateral* (situated on the same side). The right side of the cerebellum controls the right side of the body, and the left cerebellum controls the left side of the body.

The *brainstem* includes the midbrain, pons, and medulla. The functions of these structures are presented in Table 38.2. Throughout the brainstem are special cells that constitute the reticular activating system (RAS), which controls awareness and alertness. For example, this tissue awakens a person from sleep when presented with a stimulus such as loud noise or pain or when it is time to awaken. The RAS has many connections with the cerebrum, the rest of the brainstem, and the cerebellum.

TABLE 38.2 Brainstem Functions

Medulla

- Cardiac-slowing center
- Respiratory center
- Cranial nerve nuclei IX (glossopharyngeal), X (vagus), XI (accessory), and XII (hypoglossal) and parts of cranial nerves VII (facial) and VIII (vestibulocochlear)

Pons

- Cardiac acceleration and vasoconstriction centers
- Pneumotaxic center that helps control respiratory pattern and rate
- Cranial nerve nuclei V (trigeminal), VI (abducens), VII (facial), and VIII (vestibulocochlear)

Midbrain

- Contains the cerebral aqueduct or aqueduct of Sylvius
- Location of periaqueductal gray, which may abolish pain when stimulated
- Cranial nerve nuclei III (oculomotor) and IV (trochlear)

Circulation in the Brain. Circulation in the brain originates from the carotid and vertebral arteries. The internal carotid arteries branch into the anterior cerebral artery (ACA) and middle cerebral artery (MCA), the largest ones. The two posterior vertebral arteries become the basilar artery, which then divides into two posterior cerebral arteries. The anterior, middle, and posterior cerebral arteries are joined together by small communicating arteries to form a ring at the base of the brain known as the *circle of Willis.*

The *middle* cerebral artery supplies the lateral surface of the cerebrum from about the midtemporal lobe upward (i.e., the area for hearing and upper body motor and sensory neurons). The *anterior* cerebral artery supplies the midline, or medial, aspect of the same area (i.e., the lower body motor and sensory neurons). The *posterior* cerebral arteries supply the area from the midtemporal region down and back (occipital lobe), as well as much of the brainstem. When blood flow is interrupted in any of these arteries (e.g., by a clot), ***perfusion*** to the area of the brain being supplied is affected and may not function as it should.

The *blood-brain barrier (BBB)* seems to exist because the endothelial cells of the cerebral capillaries are joined tightly together. This barrier keeps some substances in the bloodstream out of the cerebrospinal circulation and out of brain tissue. Substances that can pass through the BBB include oxygen, glucose, carbon dioxide, alcohol, anesthetics, and water. Large molecules such as albumin, any substance bound to albumin, and many antibiotics are prevented from crossing the barrier.

Cerebrospinal fluid (CSF) also circulates, surrounds, and cushions the brain and spinal cord. While moving through the subarachnoid space, the fluid is continuously produced by the choroid plexus, reabsorbed by the arachnoid villi, and then channeled into the superior sagittal sinus. Expanded areas of subarachnoid space, where there are large amounts of CSF, are called *cisterns.* The largest one is the lumbar cistern, the site of lumbar puncture, from the level of the second lumbar vertebra to the second sacral vertebra (L2-S2) (Jarvis, 2020).

Spinal Cord. The spinal cord controls ***mobility;*** regulates organ function; processes ***sensory perception*** information from the extremities, trunk, and many internal organs; and transmits information to and from the brain. It contains H-shaped *gray matter* (neuron cell bodies) that is surrounded by *white matter* (myelinated axons). Groups of cells in the white matter (ascending and descending tracts) have been fairly well identified. These tracts carry impulses from the spinal cord to the brain (ascending tracts, such as the spinothalamic tract) or from the brain to the spinal cord (descending tracts, such as the corticospinal tract).

Peripheral Nervous System: Structure and Function

The peripheral nervous system (PNS) is composed of the spinal nerves, cranial nerves, and autonomic nervous system.

There are 31 pairs of spinal nerves (8 cervical, 12 thoracic, 5 lumbar, 5 sacral, and 1 coccygeal) exiting from the spinal cord. Each of the nerves has a posterior and an anterior branch. The posterior branch carries ***sensory perception*** information to the cord *(afferent pathway).* The anterior branch transmits motor impulses to the muscles of the body to allow ***mobility*** *(efferent pathway).*

Each spinal nerve is responsible for the muscle innervation and sensory reception of a given area of the body. The cervical and thoracic spinal nerves are relatively close to their areas of responsibility, whereas the lumbar and sacral spinal nerves are some distance from theirs. Because the spinal cord ends between L1 and L2, the axons of the lumbar and sacral cord extend downward before exiting at the appropriate intervertebral foramen. The area controlled by each spinal nerve is roughly reflected in the dermatomes. *Dermatomes* represent sensory input from spinal nerves to specific areas of the skin (Fig. 38.3). For example, the patient with an injury to cervical spinal nerves C6 and C7 has sensory changes in the thumb, index finger, middle finger, middle of the palm, and back of the hand.

Sensory receptors throughout the body monitor and transmit impulses of pain, temperature, touch, vibration, pressure, visceral sensation, and proprioception. Sensory receptors also monitor and transmit the sensory perceptions of the special senses (i.e., vision, taste, smell, and hearing).

The cell bodies of the anterior spinal nerves are located in the anterior gray matter (anterior horn) of each level in the spinal cord. The anterior motor neurons are also referred to as *lower motor neurons.* As each nerve axon leaves the spinal cord, it joins other spinal nerves to form plexuses (clusters of nerves). Plexuses continue as trunks, divisions, and cords and finally branch into individual peripheral nerves.

The reflex arc is a closed circuit of spinal and peripheral nerves and therefore requires no control by the brain (Fig. 38.4).

Reflexes consist of sensory input from:

- Skeletal muscles, tendons, skin, organs, and special senses
- Small cells in the spinal cord lying between the posterior and anterior gray matter (interneurons)
- Anterior motor neurons, along with the muscles they innervate

There are 12 *cranial nerves.* Their number, name, origin, type, and function are summarized in Table 38.3. Cranial nerve function is an important part of the complete neurologic assessment (Jarvis, 2020).

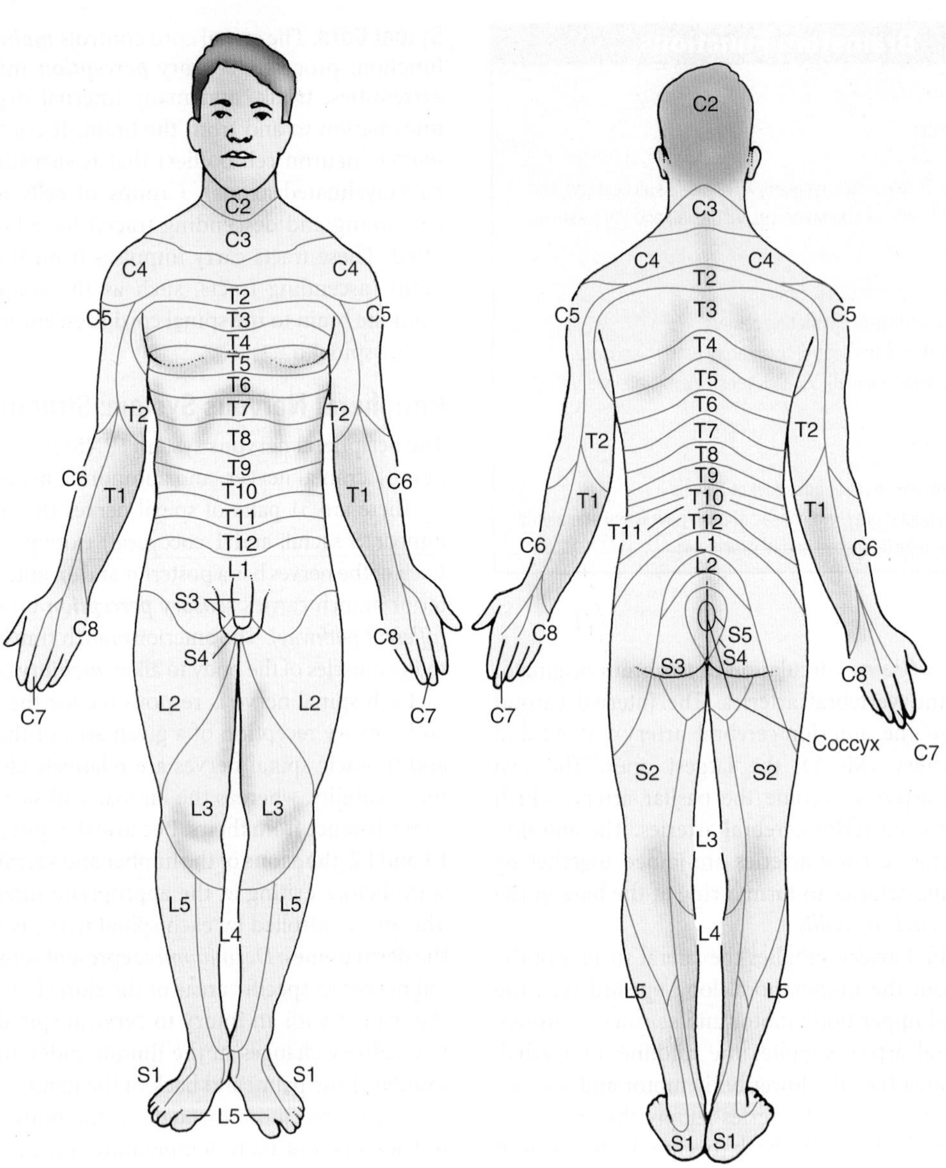

FIG. 38.3 Dermatomes (cutaneous innervation of spinal nerves). *C*, Cervical; *L*, lumbar; *S*, sacral; *T*, thoracic.

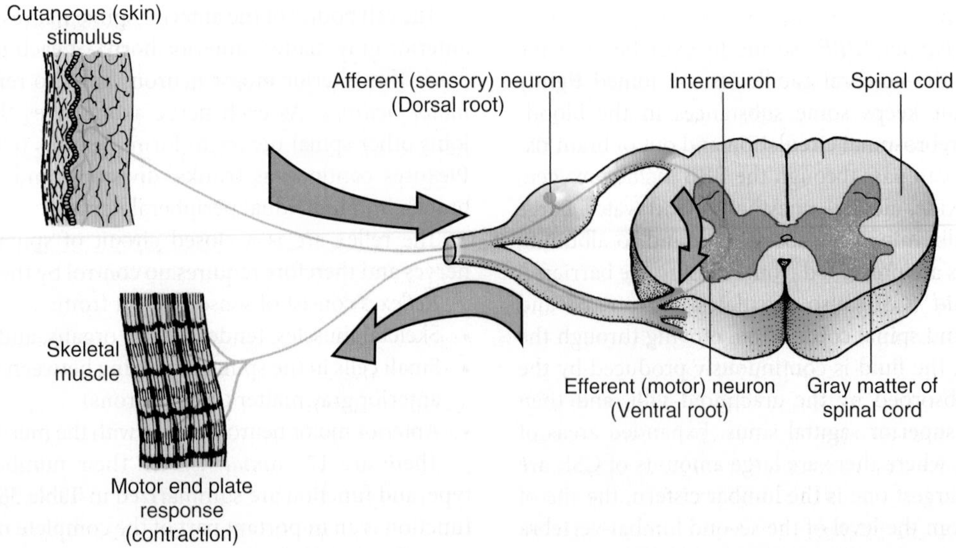

FIG. 38.4 An example of reflex activity. Stimulation of skin results in involuntary muscle contraction (reflex arc).

TABLE 38.3 **Origins, Types, and Functions of Cranial Nerves**

Cranial Nerve	Origin	Type	Function
I: Olfactory	Olfactory bulb	Sensory	Smell
II: Optic	Midbrain	Sensory	Central and peripheral vision
III: Oculomotor	Midbrain	Motor to eye muscles	Eye movement via medial and lateral rectus and inferior oblique and superior rectus muscles; lid elevation via the levator muscle
		Parasympathetic-motor	Pupil constriction; ciliary muscles
IV: Trochlear	Lower midbrain	Motor	Eye movement via superior oblique muscles
V: Trigeminal	Pons	Sensory	Sensory perception from skin of face and scalp and mucous membranes of mouth and nose
		Motor	Muscles of mastication (chewing)
VI: Abducens	Inferior pons	Motor	Eye movement via lateral rectus muscles
VII: Facial	Inferior pons	Sensory	Pain and temperature from ear area; deep sensations from the face; taste from anterior two thirds of the tongue
		Motor	Muscles of the face and scalp
		Parasympathetic-motor	Lacrimal, submandibular, and sublingual salivary glands
VIII: Vestibulocochlear	Pons-medulla junction	Sensory	Hearing Equilibrium
IX: Glossopharyngeal	Medulla	Sensory	Pain and temperature from ear; taste and sensations from posterior one third of tongue and pharynx
		Motor	Skeletal muscles of the throat
		Parasympathetic-motor	Parotid glands
X: Vagus	Medulla	Sensory	Pain and temperature from ear; sensations from pharynx, larynx, thoracic and abdominal viscera
		Motor	Muscles of the soft palate, larynx, and pharynx (swallowing)
		Parasympathetic-motor	Thoracic and abdominal viscera; cells of secretory glands; cardiac and smooth muscle innervation to the level of the splenic flexure
XI: Accessory	Medulla (anterior gray horn of the cervical spine)	Motor	Skeletal muscles of the pharynx and larynx and sternocleidomastoid and trapezius muscles (swallowing)
XII: Hypoglossal	Medulla	Motor	Skeletal muscles of the tongue (swallowing)

Autonomic Nervous System: Structure and Function

The **autonomic nervous system (ANS)** is composed of two parts: the sympathetic nervous system (SNS) and the parasympathetic nervous system. ANS functions are not usually under conscious control but may be altered in some people by using biofeedback and other methods.

The SNS cells originate in the gray matter of the spinal cord from T1 through L2 or L3. This part of the ANS is considered *thoracolumbar* because of its anatomic location. The SNS stimulates the functions of the body needed for "fight or flight" (e.g., heart and respiratory rate). It also inhibits certain functions not needed in urgent and stressful situations.

The parasympathetic cells originate in the gray matter of the sacral area of the spinal cord (from S2 through S4) plus portions of cranial nerves III, VII, IX, and X *(craniosacral)*. The parasympathetic nervous system can slow body functions when needed and contribute to digestion and reproduction ("feed and breed").

Parasympathetic fibers to the organs have some sensory ability in addition to motor function. Sensory perceptions of irritation, stretching of an organ, or a decrease in tissue oxygen are transmitted to the thalamus through pathways not yet fully understood. Because pain from internal organs is often felt below the body wall innervated by the spinal nerve, it is presumed that there are connections between the viscera and body structure that relay pain sensation.

Neurologic Changes Associated With Aging

Neurologic changes associated with aging often affect ***mobility*** and ***sensory perception***. Mobility changes in late adulthood can cause slower movement and response time and decreased sensory perception as outlined in the Patient-Centered Care: Older Adult Considerations: Changes in the Nervous System Related to Aging box. Any problems that affect the nerves, bones, muscles, or joints also affect motor and ADL ability. Determining functional status is a recommended quality indicator for patients with complex chronic conditions.

Sensory changes in older adults can also affect their ADLs. Pupils decrease in size, which restricts the amount of light entering the eye, and adapt more slowly. Older adults need increased lighting to see. Chapter 43 describes collaborative care for people with hearing loss. Touch sensation decreases, which may lead to falls because the older person may not feel small objects or a step underfoot (Touhy & Jett, 2018). Vibration sense may be lost in the ankles and feet. These changes can contribute to falls. (See the discussion on fall prevention in Chapter 4.)

PATIENT-CENTERED CARE: OLDER ADULT CONSIDERATIONS QSEN

Changes in the Nervous System Related to Aging

Physiologic Changes	Nursing Implications	Rationales
Slower cognitive processing time	Provide sufficient time for the affected older adult to respond to questions and/or direction.	Allowing adequate time for processing helps differentiate normal findings from neurologic deterioration.
Recent memory loss	Reinforce teaching by repetition, using written teaching and memory aids such as electronic alarms or applications for electronic devices that provide frequent alerts.	Greatest loss of brain weight is in the white matter of the frontal lobe. Repetition helps the patient learn new information and recall it when needed.
Decreased sensory perception of touch	Remind the patient to look where his or her feet are placed when walking. Instruct the patient to wear shoes that provide good support when walking. If the patient is unable, change his or her position frequently (every hour) while he or she is in the bed or chair. Teach the patient to check water temperature with a thermometer due to decreased lower extremity sensation caused by decreased circulation.	Decreased sensory perception may cause the patient to fall. Decreased lower extremity sensation can cause burns if water is too hot.
Possible change in perception of pain	Ask the patient to describe the nature and specific characteristics of pain. Monitor additional assessment variables to detect possible health problems.	Accurate and complete nursing assessment ensures that the interventions will be appropriate for the older adult (see Chapter 4 and 5).
Change in sleep patterns	Ascertain sleep patterns and preferences. Ask if sleep pattern interferes with ADLs. Adjust the patient's daily schedule to his or her sleep pattern and preference as much as possible (e.g., evening vs. morning bath).	Older adults require as much sleep as younger adults. It is more common for older adults to fall asleep early and arise early. Daytime napping is especially common in older adults of advanced age.
Altered balance and/or decreased coordination	Instruct the patient to move slowly when changing positions. If needed, advise the patient to hold on to handrails when ambulating. Assess the need for an ambulatory aid, such as a cane or walker.	The patient may fall if moving too quickly. Assistive and adaptive aids provide support and prevent falls.
Increased risk for infection	Monitor the patient carefully for signs and symptoms of infection.	Older adults often have structural deterioration of microglia, the cells responsible for cell-mediated immune response in the central nervous system (CNS).

Cognitive functions of perceiving, registering, storing, and using information often change as a normal part of aging. *Intellect does not decline as a result of aging.* However, a person with certain health problems may have a decrease in ***cognition.*** *Cognitive decline is frequently caused by drug interactions or toxicity or by an inadequate oxygen supply to the brain (hypoxia).* Some older adults may need more time than a younger person to process questions, learn and process new information, solve problems, or complete analogies.

Subtle memory changes can occur for many older people. Long-term memory often seems better than recall (recent) or immediate (registration) memory. Older adults may need more time to retrieve information. These changes may be partly caused by the loss of cerebral neurons, which is associated with the aging process.

Biorhythms vary among people. Circadian responses are reduced in older adults, and the sleep-wake cycle may become less responsive to stimuli that signal patterns of sleep. Older adults may experience changes in sleep habits and sleeping patterns (Touhy & Jett, 2018). For example, older adults are more likely to go bed earlier and experience an earlier awakening compared with younger adults. They are also more likely to experience more periods of wakefulness lasting 30 or more minutes during the night. On average, an older person needs as much sleep as a younger person but is more likely to nap in the afternoon.

Sleep deprivation, common in many inpatient settings, is related to both the earlier onset and greater severity of delirium (acute confusion) in older adults. Lack of sleep can worsen symptoms of dementia (chronic confusion). Sleep deprivation can also interfere with normal immune function and wound healing.

Mental status may be impaired as a result of infection, hypoxia, and hypoglycemia or hyperglycemia in the older adult. These conditions are usually easily assessed and managed. During an acute change in mental status, assess the adult for peripheral oxygenation saturation (Spo_2), serum glucose (fingerstick), and potential infection (e.g., fever, urine with sediment or odor, sputum production, red or draining wound). *Often a decrease or change in mental status (e.g., acute confusion) is a key early sign of an infectious process in the older patient, such as a urinary tract infection.*

Health Promotion and Maintenance

Prevention of neurologic health problems includes avoiding risky behaviors and practicing a healthy lifestyle. Young adults, especially men, are particularly at risk for engaging in risky physical activities, such as motorcycle or car racing without wearing a helmet or taking other safety precautions or diving into shallow water. Unfortunately, these activities often lead to serious spinal cord or traumatic brain injuries and should be avoided. Remind adults of any age to avoid excessive alcohol or other substances that can impair judgment and cause an accident.

PATIENT-CENTERED CARE: VETERANS HEALTH CONSIDERATIONS QSEN

Active military men and women who are in or near combat areas are also at risk for neurologic problems, especially traumatic brain injury (TBI). The most common cause of TBI in this population is a blast from an improvised explosive device (IED). Continued improvements in IED detection and protective headgear may help decrease these injuries. TBI in veterans is discussed later in Chapter 41.

Practicing a healthy lifestyle can help promote nervous system health. For example, smoking constricts blood vessels and can lead to decreased ***perfusion*** to the brain, resulting in a brain attack or stroke. Teach these patients the importance of smoking cessation as discussed elsewhere in this text.

Sleep deprivation at any age can lead to significant changes in ***cognition***. Interrupted sleep and sleep deprivation can also impair physical function and self-management. Sleep and rest are both necessary to promote health. Teach patients that proper nutrition and regular exercise are also important to prevent neurologic impairment. For example, the brain requires adequate glucose to function properly. Decreased blood glucose can cause light-headedness and dizziness, leading to falls, especially among older adults. Skipping meals or poor nutrition can affect the function of the body's neurons.

NCLEX EXAMINATION CHALLENGE 38.1

Health Promotion and Maintenance

The nurse performs an initial neurologic assessment on an older client. Which assessment findings would the nurse expect to be the result of **normal** physiologic aging? **Select all that apply.**

A. Decreased coordination
B. Hearing loss
C. Long-term memory loss
D. Recent memory loss
E. Decreased balance control

ASSESSMENT: RECOGNIZE CUES

Patient History

Obtain information from the patient about health problems, drug therapy history, smoking and substance abuse history, occupation, and current lifestyle. During your introduction, note the patient's appearance and assess his or her speech, affect, and movement. If he or she seems to have ***cognition*** deficits or has trouble speaking or hearing, ask a family member or significant other to stay during the interview to help obtain an accurate history. If the patient is not English-speaking, obtain an interpreter to ensure accuracy of patient information. Be sure that glasses, contact lenses, and hearing aids are available if the patient wears any of these devices.

Ask the patient about his or her medical history to determine its association with the current health problem. Inquire about the ability to perform ADLs. Knowing the level of daily activity helps establish a baseline for later comparison as the patient improves or worsens. Ask whether the patient is right handed or left handed. This information is important for several reasons:

- The patient may be somewhat stronger on the dominant side, which is expected.
- The effects of cerebral injury or disease may be more pronounced if the dominant hemisphere is involved.

Ask about family neurologic history such as stroke. Some diseases occur more often in certain groups of people and may be caused by a genetic influence or other reason. Many neurologic diseases have a genetic basis, such as migraine headaches and epilepsy. These genetic risks are described with specific neurologic health problems found later in this unit.

Physical Assessment

Compare each assessment with the patient's baseline, between right and left sides, and between upper and lower extremities. *Two types of neurologic assessments may be performed: a complete assessment and a focused assessment.* Some focused assessments are specifically designed to be rapid to ease repetition when frequent neurologic assessments are needed to monitor the patient's condition over time. The type chosen depends on the information needed, the time available with the patient, and your clinical skill level. Advanced practice registered nurses (APRNs) and other primary health care providers usually perform the *complete* assessment, with selected parts done by the nurse generalist or staff nurse. Collaborate with the interprofessional health care team to determine which components each member will perform. It is important to understand each component of the assessment and what the results might indicate.

Complete Neurologic Assessment. A complete neurologic assessment includes a history and evaluation of mental status, cranial nerves (see Table 38.3), ***mobility*** and motor system function, deep tendon reflexes, ***sensory perception,*** and cerebellar function. Although not all components of a complete assessment are performed by the nurse generalist or staff nurse, noting abnormalities at baseline or with disease progression is important. During any neurologic assessment, look for asymmetry, such as subtle unequal movement in the facial muscles. For example, patients with Bell palsy, a peripheral nervous system disorder, have paralysis of all facial muscles on the affected side (also called *facial paralysis*). The patient cannot close his or her eye, wrinkle the forehead, smile, whistle, or grimace. Tearing may stop or become excessive; the face appears masklike and sags. Taste is usually impaired to some degree, but this symptom seldom persists beyond the second week of paralysis.

The complete neurologic assessment is performed by the primary health care provider to consider whether a single lesion or more than one site in the nervous system may be contributing to abnormal physical assessment findings. If the lesion or injury is in the CNS, the assessment can further help the provider determine if abnormalities are in the cortex, below the cortex, or multifocal. These findings, along with patient history, help determine the urgency of treatment. For example, a sudden unilateral (one side of the body) loss in motor function and sensation is an emergency requiring a stroke center and staff with expertise to diagnose and intervene during a "brain attack." Generally, the nurse completes a *focused* or *rapid assessment* to detect major changes in signs and symptoms and determine indications of patient deterioration.

Assessment of Mental Status. Mental status assessment is generally divided into assessment of *consciousness* and *cognition*. Consciousness is the ability to be aware of the environment, an object, and oneself; it is often documented as one's level of consciousness. **Level of consciousness (LOC)** refers to the degree of alertness or amount of stimulation needed to engage a patient's attention and can range from *alert* to *comatose*.

The patient who is described as *alert* is awake, engaged, and responsive. A patient may be alert but not oriented to person, place, or time. Patients who are less than alert are labeled *lethargic, stuporous,* or *comatose.* A *lethargic* patient is drowsy but easily awakened. One who is arousable only with vigorous or painful stimulation is *stuporous*. The *comatose* patient is unconscious and cannot be aroused despite vigorous or noxious simulation.

! NURSING SAFETY PRIORITY (QSEN)

Critical Rescue

Be aware that a change in level of consciousness and orientation is the earliest and most reliable indication that central neurologic function has declined! If a decline occurs, contact the Rapid Response Team or primary health care provider immediately. Perform a focused neurologic assessment as described later in this chapter to determine if additional changes are present.

After determining alertness, the next step is to evaluate *orientation*. Once the patient's attention is engaged, ask questions to determine orientation. Varying the sequence of questioning on repeated assessments prevents the patient from memorizing the answers. Responses that indicate orientation include ability to answer questions about person, place, and time such as:

- The patient's ability to relate the onset of symptoms
- The name of the primary health care provider or nurse
- The year and month
- Home address
- The name of the health care agency

Time of day, drug therapy, and the need for sleep, glucose, or oxygen may affect these responses. Be sure to link any changes in orientation with respiratory status, changes in drug regimens or use of intermittent drugs, time of day/sleep deprivation, or current serum glucose values. Education, occupation, interest, culture, anxiety, and depression affect performance during assessment of mental status. What is considered "normal" may not be so for a particular patient, so adaptation of questions suggested for mental status assessment may be necessary. Be alert to both *sudden* and *subtle* changes, particularly when changes are noted by family members or others who know the patient.

NCLEX EXAMINATION CHALLENGE 38.2

Physiological Integrity

During a client's neurologic assessment, the nurse finds that the client is arousable only with vigorous or painful stimulation. How does the nurse document this client's level of consciousness?

A. Stuporous
B. Lethargic
C. Comatose
D. Alert

Cognition is typically evaluated in a rapid or focused manner using tests of memory and attention that require verbal or written ability as outlined in the Best Practice for Patient Safety & Quality Care: Assessment of Cognition box. *Loss of memory, especially recent memory, tends to be an early sign of neurologic problems, especially in older adults.*

Many *speech and language* skills can be assessed during the initial interview. Language skills include understanding the spoken or written word and being able to speak or write. The patient demonstrates understanding by following directions on admission (e.g., getting undressed). If he or she hesitates, it may be that he or she does not understand the vocabulary or word. When speech hesitation or performance hesitation occurs, point to objects and ask the patient to name them, such as the door or bed. Speech is assessed as being normal, slow, garbled,

BEST PRACTICE FOR PATIENT SAFETY & QUALITY CARE (QSEN)

Assessment of Cognition

Perform assessment during the following care interactions:

- On admission to and discharge from an institutional care setting
- On transfer from one care setting to another
- Every 4 to 8 hours throughout hospitalization or per agency protocol
- Following major changes in pharmacotherapy
- With behavior that is unusual for the person and/or inappropriate to the situation

Assess and document (noting "sometimes," "frequently," or "always" as observed):

- Does the patient respond to voice; require being shaken awake to communicate; doze off during a conversation or when no activities occur; or not respond to voice or touch?
- Is speech clear and understandable; disoriented to person, place, or time; inappropriate; or incomprehensible/garbled?
- Can the patient name the place, reason for admission or visit, month, and age?
- Can the patient follow one-step commands: open/close eyes; make fist/let go?
- Can the patient switch to a different topic or activity versus lose the thread of the conversation or be easily distracted (inattention)?
- Can the patient recognize a familiar object and its purpose or a familiar person and name relationship?
- Can the patient respond relevantly and quickly?
- Does the patient have unrealistic thoughts or act distrustful of others (e.g., does not dare to take his/her medicine; says that people are "listening")?
- Is the patient cooperative, euphoric, hostile, anxious, withdrawn, or guarded?
- Is the patient's appearance, behavior, or facial expression appropriate for the situation?

difficult to find words, or other impairments. If the change in speech is new and represents a deterioration from a previous ability to communicate, this change must be urgently reported to the primary health care provider because it may indicate a stroke, new onset of confusion, or other serious neurologic condition. The speech-language pathologist (SLP) completes additional language tests such as reading comprehension.

PATIENT-CENTERED CARE: CULTURAL/SPIRITUAL CONSIDERATIONS QSEN

Remember that some patients cannot read or write or may speak a language different from that of the clinician. In this case, modify the examination accordingly such as having the patient copy something that has been drawn (e.g., a cross, circle, diamond, or square). In some cases, an interpreter may be needed.

Several ***cognition*** screening tests are used by nurses in clinical settings to assess for delirium (acute confusion) or dementia (chronic confusion). Chapter 4 describes common tests for assessing delirium; Chapter 39 describes tests for dementia in the Alzheimer's disease section.

Assessment of Cranial Nerves. Cranial nerves are typically tested to establish a baseline from which to compare progress or deterioration. However, they are not routinely tested unless the patient has a suspected problem affecting one or more of them (see Table 38.3). For example, if the patient reports severe, intermittent facial pain, he or she may have trigeminal neuralgia. **Trigeminal neuralgia** is a persistently painful and debilitating disorder that involves the trigeminal cranial nerve (CN V) and affects women more often than men. Adding the specific cranial nerves to be tested to the documentation record of a patient with a problem affecting them helps to ensure continued comparison and assessment.

Testing pupils is a common cranial nerve test performed by nurses. Pupil constriction is a function of cranial nerve III, the oculomotor nerve. **P**upils should be **e**qual in size, **r**ound and **r**egular in shape, and react to **l**ight and **a**ccommodation (**PERRLA**). Estimate the size of both pupils using a millimeter ruler or a pupillometer. Patients who have had eye surgery for cataracts or glaucoma often have irregularly shaped pupils. Those using eyedrops for either cataracts or glaucoma may have unequal pupils if only one eye is being treated, and the pupillary response may be altered.

To test for pupil constriction, ask the patient to close his or her eyes and dim the room lights. Bring a penlight in from the side of the patient's head and shine the light in the eye being tested as soon as the patient opens his or her eyes. The pupil being tested should constrict (direct response). The other pupil should also constrict slightly (consensual response). To test accommodation, relight the room and ask the patient to focus on a distant object and then immediately look at an object 4 to 5 inches from the nose. The eyes should converge, and the pupils should constrict. Pinpoint or severely dilated nonreactive pupils are usually late signs of neurologic deterioration (Jarvis, 2020).

Assessment of Motor Function. Throughout the physical assessment, observe the patient for involuntary tremors or movements. Describe these movements as accurately as possible, such as "pill-rolling with the thumbs and fingers at rest" or "intention tremors of both hands" (tremors that occur when the patient tries to do something). These abnormalities can indicate certain diseases, such as multiple sclerosis, or the effects of selected psychotropic drugs. In addition, assess the patient for motor movements that indicate irritability, hyperactivity, or slowed movements. Measure the patient's hand *strength* by asking him or her to grasp and squeeze two fingers of each of your hands. Then compare the grasps for equality of strength. As another means of evaluating strength, try to withdraw the fingers from the patient's grasp and compare the ease or difficulty. He or she should release the grasps on command—another assessment of consciousness and the ability to follow commands.

Collaborate with the physical therapist to test the patient's strength. To test strength against resistance, ask the patient to resist the examiner's bending or straightening of the arm, hand, leg, or foot being tested. A five-point rating scale is commonly used (see Chapter 44). Always evaluate and compare strength on each side. Compare previous results with current findings and report all decreases to the primary health care provider.

Cerebral motor or *brainstem* integrity may also be assessed. Ask the patient to close his or her eyes and hold the arms perpendicular to the body with the palms up for 15 to 30 seconds. If there is a cerebral or brainstem reason for muscle weakness, the arm on the weak side will start to fall, or "drift," with the palm pronating (turning inward). This is called a *pronator drift*. The same can be done for the lower extremities, with the patient lying on his or her stomach with the legs bent upward at the knees. However, it is easier for most patients to sit on the side of the bed and extend the legs outward.

Decortication is abnormal motor movement seen in the patient with lesions that interrupt the corticospinal pathways (Fig. 38.5A). The patient's arms, wrists, and fingers are flexed with internal rotation and plantar flexion of the legs. **Decerebration** is abnormal movement with rigidity characterized by extension of the arms and legs, pronation of the arms, plantar flexion, and opisthotonos (body spasm in which the

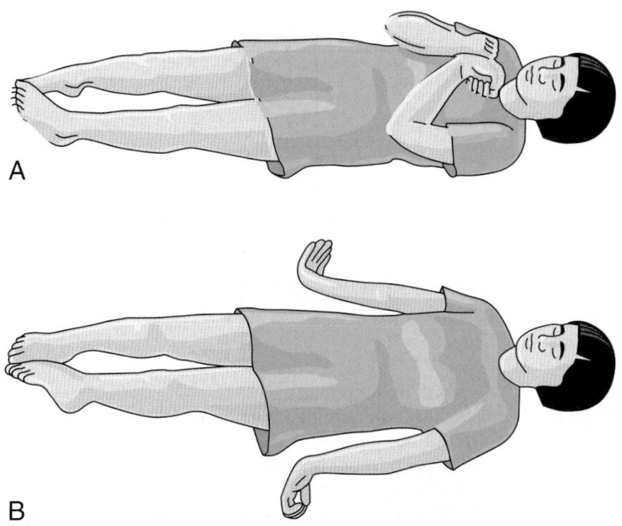

FIG. 38.5 Posturing. A, Decorticate posturing. B, Decerebrate posturing.

body is bowed forward) (Fig. 38.5B). Decerebration is usually associated with dysfunction in the brainstem area.

Assessment of Reflex Activity. The primary health care provider, including the APRN, may assess deep tendon reflexes (DTRs) and superficial (cutaneous) reflexes. The *deep tendon reflexes* of the biceps, triceps, brachioradialis, and quadriceps muscles and of the Achilles tendon can be tested as part of the complete neurologic assessment (Jarvis, 2020). Striking the tendon with the reflex hammer should cause contraction of the muscle. The appropriate muscle contraction indicates an intact reflex arc.

The *cutaneous (superficial) reflexes* usually tested are the plantar reflexes and sometimes the abdominal reflexes. The plantar reflex is tested with a pointed (but not sharp) object, such as the handle end of the reflex hammer or the rounded end of bandage scissors. The normal response is plantar flexion of all toes. **Babinski sign**, a dorsiflexion of the great toe and fanning of the other toes, is abnormal in anyone older than 2 years and represents the presence of central nervous system (CNS) disease. The terms *positive Babinski sign* (abnormal response) and *negative Babinski sign* (normal response) are clinically used terms but are not technically accurate. Health care team members may also use the terms *upgoing* or *downgoing* to refer to the toes of the stimulated foot. Upgoing toes are an abnormal response that indicates the presence of pathology in the CNS. Babinski sign can occur with drug and alcohol intoxication, after a seizure, or in patients with multiple sclerosis or severe liver disease.

Hyperactive reflexes indicate possible upper motor neuron disease (damage to the brain or upper spinal cord). *Hypoactive* reflexes may result from lower motor neuron disease (damage to the lower spinal cord) or neuromuscular diseases.

Asymmetry of reflexes is an important finding because it probably indicates a disease process or injury. The results of reflex testing are recorded by use of a stick figure and a scale of 0 to 4 (Fig. 38.6). A score of 2 is considered normal, although scores of 1 (hypoactive) or 3 (stronger than normal) may be normal for a particular patient. **Clonus** (also called *myoclonus*) is the sudden, brief, jerking contraction of a muscle or muscle group often seen in seizures.

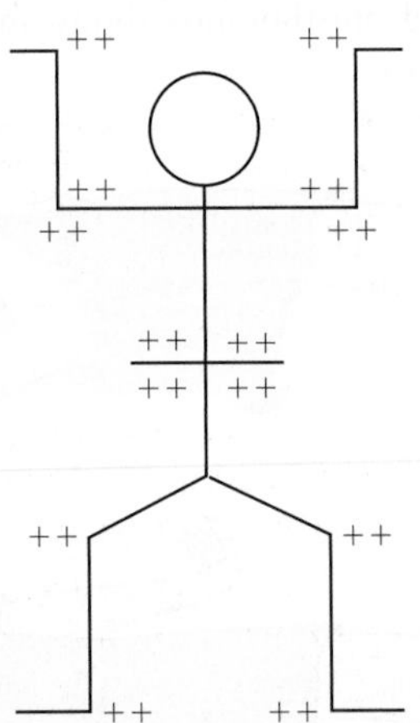

0	Absent, no response
1 (+)	Weaker than normal, hypoactive
2 (++)	Normal
3 (+++)	Stronger or more brisk than normal
4 (++++)	Hyperactive
	(Note: 1 and 3 may be normal for some individuals.)

FIG. 38.6 Stick figure and scale for recording reflex activity.

Assessment of Sensory Function. The acuity level of the patient determines how often the sensory assessment is done. For example, patients with acute spinal cord trauma or ascending Guillain-Barré syndrome are assessed every hour until stable and then every 4 hours. **Guillain-Barré syndrome (GBS)** is a rare acute inflammatory disorder that affects the axons and/or myelin of the PNS resulting in ascending muscle weakness or paralysis. As the condition improves, neurologic assessment may be needed only once each shift. Findings are documented according to agency protocol. A special spinal cord assessment flow sheet may be used to document sensory and/or motor findings for the patient with a spinal cord injury. If GBS does not improve, respiratory failure may result in death.

Pain and temperature sensation are transmitted by the same nerve endings. Therefore if one sensation is tested and found to be intact, it can safely be assumed that the other is intact. Testing temperature sensation can usually be accomplished using a cold reflex hammer and the warm touch of the hand for patients with known or suspected spinal problems.

Assess for *pain perception* with any sharp or dull object, such as the tips of a cotton-tipped applicator. While the patient's eyes are open, demonstrate what will be done. Then ask him or her to keep eyes closed and indicate whether the touch is sharp or dull. The sharp and dull ends should be changed at random so that he or she does not anticipate the next type of stimulus for ***sensory perception***. Not all areas need to be tested unless a spinal cord injury has occurred. If testing begins on the hands and feet, there is no need to test the other parts of the extremities because the tracts transmitting pain and temperature sensations are intact. Compare reactions on each side. A sensation reported as dull when the stimulus was actually sharp requires further testing. A patient with sensory loss as a result of diabetes mellitus or peripheral vascular disease may or may not be aware of the loss until tested. Some patients with chronic illness may report that they have had sensory losses for a long time. Before testing for pain, the nurse must check to determine whether the patient is on anticoagulant therapy. If the patient is on anticoagulant therapy, avoid any testing with a sharp object because it can cause bleeding.

Light touch discrimination is likely to be normal if pain and temperature sensory tracts are intact. Touch discrimination and two-point discrimination may be assessed as part of a complete neurologic examination by the primary health care provider.

For testing *touch discrimination*, the patient closes his or her eyes. The practitioner touches the patient with a finger and asks that he or she point to the area touched. This procedure is repeated on each extremity at random rather than at sequential points. Next, the practitioner touches the patient on each side of the body on corresponding sites at the same time. The patient should be able to point to both sites.

The clinician then touches the patient in two places on the same extremity with two objects, such as cotton-tipped applicators. A person can normally identify two points fairly close together, depending on the location of the stimuli. When an area is heavily innervated, the *two-point discrimination will feel closer.*

Abnormal sensory findings may have a CNS or a peripheral nervous system (PNS) cause. The neuropathies of diabetes, malnutrition, and vascular problems have a PNS cause. Damage to a specific spinal nerve may not result in significant sensory loss because the spinal nerves overlap. Injury to several nearby spinal nerves is manifested as decreased or absent ***sensory perception*** in the dermatomes of those nerves.

CNS problems in the brainstem, thalamus, and cortex generally result in loss of sensation on the *contralateral* (opposite) side of the body. Cerebellar lesions result in sensory deficits on the *same* side of the body.

Assessment of Cerebellar Function. Most of the assessment of cerebellar function can be performed with the patient sitting on the side of the bed or examining table. Fine *coordination* of muscle activity is tested. If cerebellar problems are suspected or diagnosed, ask the patient to perform these tasks with his or her eyes closed:

- Run the heel of one foot down the shin of the other leg and repeat with the other leg (the patient should be able to do this smoothly and keep the heel on the shin).
- Place the hands palm up and then palm down on each thigh, repeating as fast as possible (this can normally be done rapidly).
- With arms out at the side, touch the finger to the nose two or three times, with eyes open and then with eyes closed (this can be done with alternating arms or with each arm individually).

For the last part of the cerebellar assessment, the *ambulatory* patient stands for testing of *gait and equilibrium.* Gait and equilibrium are usually tested at the end or beginning of the entire neurologic assessment. Ask the patient to walk across the room, turn, and return. Observe for uneven steps, difficulty walking, and so forth. To evaluate balance, ask him or her to stand on one foot and then on the other. Tiptoe and heel-to-toe walking can also demonstrate gait problems. For patients with sciatic nerve involvement, pain may worsen when they walk on their toes or heels.

To test equilibrium, ask the patient to stand with arms at the sides, feet and knees close together, and eyes open. Check for swaying and then ask him or her to close his or her eyes and maintain position. The examiner should be close enough to prevent falling if the patient cannot stay erect. If he or she sways with the eyes closed but not when the eyes are open (the Romberg sign), the problem is probably related to **proprioception** (awareness of body position). If the patient sways with the eyes both open and closed, the neurologic disturbance is probably *cerebellar* in origin (Jarvis, 2020).

If the patient cannot perform any of these activities smoothly, the problem is manifested on the same side as the cerebellar lesion. If both lobes of the cerebellum are involved, the incoordination affects both sides of the body (bilateral).

Rapid/Focused Neurologic Assessment. A rapid/focused neurologic assessment, or "neuro check," is completed when the patient is admitted to a health care facility on an emergent basis. It is also a major part of frequent ongoing patient assessment

GLASGOW COMA SCALE*

Eye Opening	
Spontaneous	4
To sound	3
To pain	2
Never	1
Motor Response	
Obeys commands	6
Localizes pain	5
Normal flexion (withdrawal)	4
Abnormal flexion	3
Extension	2
None	1
Verbal Response	
Oriented	5
Confused conversation	4
Inappropriate words	3
Incomprehensible sounds	2
None	1

* The highest possible score is 15.

FIG. 38.7 The Glasgow Coma Scale.

and performed in the event of a sudden change in neurologic status. The typical record contains data related to alertness, orientation, movement of arms and legs, and pupil size and reaction to light. *Be sure to document all aspects of the rapid neurologic assessment frequently in the designated or standardized part of the electronic record as needed per agency protocol or primary health care provider request.*

An example of a standard rapid neurologic assessment tool is the **Glasgow Coma Scale (GCS)** (Fig. 38.7). The GCS is used in many acute care settings to establish baseline data in each of these areas: eye opening, motor response, and verbal response. The patient is assigned a numeric score for each of these areas. The lower the score, the lower the patient's neurologic function. For patients who are intubated and cannot talk, record their score with a "t" after the number for verbal response.

The GCS is easy to teach and has demonstrated a consistent score among trained assessors. The reliability of the GCS is based on recording the patient's "best" response. If the patient does not follow commands or is unresponsive to voice, the nurse proceeds to increasingly noxious (painful) stimuli to elicit an eye and motor response. Typically the patient's response to central pain (brain response) is assessed first. On the basis of this response, peripheral pain may then be assessed. Failure to apply painful stimuli appropriately may lead to an incorrect conclusion about the patient's neurologic status. If the patient responds fully to voice or light touch, there is no need to progress to more vigorous or painful stimuli.

Start with the least noxious irritation or pressure and proceed to more painful stimulation if the patient does not respond. Begin each phase of the assessment by speaking in a normal voice. If no response is obtained, use a loud voice. If the patient does not respond, gently shake him or her. The shaking should be similar to that used in attempting to wake up a child. If that is unsuccessful, apply painful stimuli using one of these methods:

- Supraorbital (above eyes) pressure by placing a thumb under the orbital rim in the middle of the eyebrow and pushing upward (Do not use this technique if the patient has orbital or facial fractures.)
- Trapezius muscle squeeze by pinching or squeezing the trapezius muscle located at the angle of the shoulder and neck muscle
- Mandibular (jaw) pressure to the jaw by using your index and middle fingers to pinch the lower jaw
- Sternal (breastbone) rub by making a fist and rubbing/twisting your knuckles against the sternum

The tissue in these areas is tender, and bruising is not unusual. Therefore do not use this technique for older adults or for patients who may experience severe bruising (e.g., those taking anticoagulant therapy). Peripheral pain is assessed with pressure at the base of the nail on one finger or one toe, both on the right and left.

The patient may respond to painful stimuli in several ways. Although the initial response to pain may be abnormal flexion or extension, continued application of pain for no more than 20 to 30 seconds may demonstrate that he or she can localize or withdraw. If the patient does not respond after 20 to 30 seconds, stop applying the painful stimulus.

NURSING SAFETY PRIORITY QSEN

Critical Rescue

A decrease of 2 or more points in the Glasgow Coma Scale total is clinically significant and should be communicated to the primary health care provider immediately. Other findings requiring urgent communication with the primary health care provider include a new finding of abnormal flexion or extension, particularly of the upper extremities (decerebrate or decorticate posturing); pinpoint or dilated nonreactive pupils; and sudden or subtle changes in mental status. *Remember, a change in level of consciousness is the earliest sign of neurologic deterioration!* Communicate early recognition of neurologic changes to the Rapid Response Team or primary health care provider for the best opportunity to prevent complications and preserve CNS function.

Psychosocial Assessment

Patients vary in their responses to a suspected or actual health problem, often depending on whether it is acute or chronic. Response is also influenced by the patient's ***mobility***, ***sensory perception***, and/or ***cognition***. These abilities can be temporarily or permanently altered as a result of neurologic disease or injury. For example, patients who have a mild stroke and no lasting neurologic deficits are less likely to be severely depressed than patients who experience a loss of independent movement or impaired communication as a result of a stroke.

CLINICAL JUDGMENT CHALLENGE 38.1

Safety

A 64-year-old man awakened with an episode of new-onset weakness in his left leg and dizziness. His wife called their family nurse practitioner, who recommended that she call 911 to take her husband to the closest emergency department (ED) for evaluation. By the time he was admitted to the ED, his condition improved. He stated that he had a headache but otherwise felt fine now. The nurse collects this information based on admission assessment:

Client History

- Has a history of hypertension for the past 15 years
- Has a history of diabetes mellitus type 2 for the past 3 years, which is controlled by diet
- Had a left total knee replacement 6 months ago
- Has been married for 42 years
- Has no children or other close family members in the area
- Has been independent with ADLs
- Works part-time for a large retail store in the area

Current Assessment

- Reported height = 6 feet (1.83 meters)
- Current weight = 258 lb (117 kilograms)
- Oral temperature = 98.6° F (37° C)
- Apical pulse = 84 beats/min; respiratory rate = 20 breaths/min
- Blood pressure = 180/98
- Reports a headache pain of 8/10

1. **Recognize Cues:** What assessment information in this client situation is the most important and immediate concern for the nurse? (Hint: Identify the **relevant** information *first* to determine what is most important.)
2. **Analyze Cues:** What client conditions are consistent with the **most relevant** information? (Hint: Think about priority collaborative problems that support and contradict the information presented in this situation.)

PATIENT-CENTERED CARE: CULTURAL/SPIRITUAL CONSIDERATIONS QSEN

Age may also be a factor in how a patient accepts the illness. For instance, a young adult who has a motorcycle crash causing a traumatic brain injury (TBI) may react differently from an older adult who has a spinal injury. In some cases, the patient's emotional responses result from the health problem itself, especially for TBI patients.

Men may feel differently about their illness than women. Male patients who have had strokes are typically depressed more often than women who have had strokes. Discussions of these response differences can be found in the following chapters on specific neurologic health problems.

Regardless of what the health problem is, do not assume that everyone reacts the same way to his or her illness or injury. Consider the cultural and spiritual background of the patient because this will influence his or her reaction. Patients experiencing the grieving process may fluctuate among denial, anger, and depression. Encourage patients to express their feelings and have hope. Refer them to the appropriate support services as needed, including counseling, social work, or clergy, depending on patient preference and service availability. Assess the patient's support systems, including family members and friends, if available. Be sure to document your assessment and interventions.

Depression can result in cognitive and behavioral changes that are similar to delirium or dementia. Depression is a common mental health disorder that is often missed in a variety of health care settings, especially in settings that care for older adults

(Touhy & Jett, 2018). Consider using a depression screening tool such as the Center for Epidemiological Studies Depression-Revised (CESD-R) or the Geriatric Depression Scale (short form) to identify patients with depressive symptoms. Refer patients to the appropriate provider (both primary care and mental health care) if the screening is positive. Chapter 4 briefly discusses depression in older adults. More information on depression can be found in mental/behavioral health resources.

Diagnostic Assessment

Laboratory Assessment. Fluid, electrolyte, and glucose abnormalities can cause neurologic impairment. The basic metabolic panel (BMP) and serum calcium, phosphorus, and magnesium are evaluated. Both anemia and malnutrition can contribute to neurologic disorders, so a complete blood count and serum levels of prealbumin, albumin, and minerals/vitamins (particularly B vitamins) are collected.

Arterial blood to evaluate pH, oxygen, and carbon dioxide levels may be collected because these three results, when either too high or too low, can alter neurologic status. For patients with a neurologic problem resulting from an infection, cultures are necessary to identify the pathogen. Although the cause of infection must be determined for any patient, this is especially true for those with existing CNS disease. The blood-brain barrier is often not intact in neurologic disease; and the patient is more likely to get an infection of the nervous system, such as meningitis or encephalitis.

Imaging Assessment. In general, for any image that involves being placed in a scanner, the nurse needs to be aware of special circumstances that can either prevent the procedure from taking place or interfere with it. If the patient is alert and claustrophobic, two options are available: a mild sedative to calm the patient or an open scanner. The nurse must determine whether the patient has any metal prosthetics, such as joint arthroplasty or shrapnel (often found in veterans) in the part of the body to be scanned. If he or she does have any type of metal object in the body part to be examined, the nurse must notify the radiology department immediately because the procedure may need to be cancelled. The nurse should ask the patient or significant other if he or she carries a medical alert card from a medical device manufacturer. Medical device manufacturers issue cards to primary health care providers for their patients to carry with the device number and instructions if radiologic diagnostic testing is needed.

Plain X-Rays. Plain *x-rays* of the skull and spine are used to determine bony fractures, curvatures, bone erosion, bone dislocation, and possible calcification of soft tissue, which can damage the nervous system. Several views are taken (i.e., anteroposterior, lateral, oblique, and, when necessary, special views of the facial bones). *In head trauma and multiple injuries, after assessing the ABCs (airway, breathing, and circulation), one of the first priorities is to rule out cervical spine fracture.*

Explain that the x-ray procedure for the skull and spine is similar to that for a chest x-ray. The patient must remain still during the procedure. Remind him or her that the exposure to radiation is minimal. If the patient is in traction and a portable x-ray unit is not available, the nurse may need to accompany him or her to help with positioning. Any patient who cannot walk from a wheelchair to the x-ray table should be transferred to the radiology department on a stretcher. Hospitals may have specific procedures for transferring patients in wheelchairs or on stretchers. Check with your hospital on this procedure. For example, with a patient who is confused or disoriented, the hospital radiology department staff may require two or more hospital personnel to assist with the transfer. The patient is positioned for each of the desired views and is asked to not move just before each x-ray. Follow-up care is not required.

Cerebral Angiography. Cerebral angiography (arteriography) is done to visualize the cerebral circulation to detect blockages in the arteries or veins in the brain, head, or neck that impair ***perfusion***. It remains the gold standard for the diagnosis of intracranial vascular disease and is required for any transcatheter therapy or for surgical intervention. Angiography may be used to identify aneurysms, traumatic injuries, strictures/occlusions, tumors, blood vessel displacement from edema, and arteriovenous (AV) malformations.

Patient Preparation. Risk factors for adverse events must be determined before scheduling the test. Patients sensitive to iodine may be sensitive to iodinated contrast agents. Patients with a history of hypersensitivity in general (e.g., multiple food allergies or asthma) are more likely to have an adverse reaction than the general population. Seafood allergies are no longer considered an indicator of iodinated contrast allergy. Patients with known contrast sensitivity are pretreated with steroids. The Best Practice for Patient Safety & Quality Care: Precautions for Use of Iodine-Based or Gadolinium Contrast for Diagnostic Testing box summarizes the precautions that must be taken for patients having any test using contrast agents.

To minimize the risk for aspiration during the procedure, assess for the presence of nausea or recent vomiting and medicate as needed before the test. Ensure that the patient is NPO 4 to 6 hours before the test. Assess and document neurologic signs, vital signs, and neurovascular checks.

Reinforce these important points:

- Your head is immobilized during the procedure.
- Do not move during the procedure.
- Contrast dye is injected through a catheter placed in the femoral artery. You will feel a warm or hot sensation when the dye is injected; this is normal.
- You will be able to talk to health care professionals during the procedure; let them know if you are in pain or have any concerns.

Procedure. The patient is placed on an examining table and made as comfortable as possible. At this time, dentures and hearing aids must be removed. He or she is then connected to cardiac monitoring throughout the procedure. Deep or moderate sedation is usually not used, although the patient may be given medication for relaxation.

The interventional radiologist or other specially trained physician numbs the area at the groin and inserts a catheter into the femoral artery. Under fluoroscopic guidance, the catheter is advanced into a carotid or vertebral artery. Then the physician injects contrast material into each vessel while recording images from different angles over the head and neck. After all the vessels have been imaged, the radiologist reviews all the images and consults with the referring physician to decide whether the

BEST PRACTICE FOR PATIENT SAFETY & QUALITY CARE QSEN

Precautions for Use of Iodine-Based or Gadolinium Contrast for Diagnostic Testing

Special precautions are taken for patients who will receive an iodinated or high-osmolar contrast agent (e.g., gadolinium) as part of their diagnostic test. These measures include:

- Following agency guidelines regarding informed consent.
- Screening patients at risk for developing contrast-induced kidney damage:
  - Ask the patient about all allergies (food, drug, environmental antigens), asthma, and prior reaction to contrast agents.
  - Review for the presence of these conditions:
    - Preexisting renal disease such as a diagnosis of chronic kidney disease
    - Diabetic nephropathy
    - Heart failure
    - Dehydration
    - Older age
    - Drugs that interfere with renal perfusion such as metformin or NSAIDs
    - Administration of contrast media in the previous 72 hours
- Evaluating current kidney function. Patients with a serum creatinine greater than or equal to 1.5 mg/dL *or* a calculated glomerular filtration rate (GFR) of less than 60 mL/min are at highest risk for kidney damage from contrast media.
- Communicating with the primary health care provider before diagnostic testing when risk factors and allergic reaction to iodinated contrast are present:
  - Consider including a discussion of the patient's serum creatinine as a component of the "time-out" process before a diagnostic procedure.
  - Document the date, time, and name of the primary health care provider with whom communication of risk occurred and which actions were prescribed, if any.
  - Hold drugs that are associated with kidney damage for 24 to 48 hours before *and* after the test.
- Providing adequate hydration before and after contrast administration:
  - Collaborate with the primary health care provider to determine whether hydration before the diagnostic test, typically with IV normal saline, is needed. Bicarbonate with normal saline or an IV dose of *N*-acetylcysteine may be used in a high-risk patient.
  - Determine the optimal postdiagnostic intake and output. Provide sufficient hydration to flush out the contrast with oral or IV fluids over the 4 to 5 hours following the test.
- Re-evaluating serum creatinine and glomerular filtration rate (GFR) 24 to 48 hours after the diagnostic test. Report an increase of serum creatinine 0.5 mg/dL above baseline and a decrease in GFR greater than 25% to the primary health care provider. Document SBAR communication and follow-up interventions, if any. Generally the peak creatinine rise is at 48 to 72 hours after the administration of contrast.

patient could benefit from a therapeutic radiologic procedure or surgery to treat the problem. An arterial closure device is typically used to seal the artery and prevent bleeding.

The x-ray images are stored on a computer. With older equipment, a two-dimensional picture of the vessels is produced. Most radiographic systems now come with software to create three-dimensional images of the blood vessels in the head and/or neck. These systems can also display a "subtracted image" made from two images—one just before the contrast was injected and one with the contrast in the artery.

Follow-up Care. Follow agency policy regarding nursing care of the injection site, which includes:

- Check the dressing for bleeding and swelling around the site.
- Apply an ice pack to site.
- Keep the extremity straight and immobilized.
- Maintain the pressure dressing for 2 hours.

Check the extremity for adequate circulation to include skin color and temperature, pulses distal to the injection site, and capillary refill. Be sure to monitor for the risks of the procedure, including contrast reaction (usually manifested by hives and flushing), thrombosis (clotting), and bleeding from the entry site. *If bleeding is present, maintain manual pressure on the site and notify the primary health care provider or Rapid Response Team immediately!* Assess vital signs and neurologic status. Increase oral or IV fluid intake unless contraindicated. Document all nursing assessments and interventions.

Computed Tomography. Computed tomography (CT) scanning is accurate, quick, easy, noninvasive, painless, and the least expensive method of diagnosing neurologic problems. Using x-rays (i.e., ionizing radiation), pictures are taken at many horizontal levels, or slices, of the brain or spinal cord. A computer then generates three-dimensional detailed anatomic pictures of tissues, typically the brain, spinal cord, or peripheral neuromuscular system in neurologic testing. A contrast medium may be used to enhance the image. CT scans distinguish bone, soft tissue (e.g., the brain, vascular system, ventricular system), and fluids such as cerebrospinal fluid (CSF) or blood. Tumors, infarctions, hemorrhage, hydrocephalus, and bone malformations can also be identified.

The patient is placed on a movable table in a head-holding device. He or she must remain completely still during the test, which may be difficult. The table is positioned in the machine—a large, donut-shaped structure. Depending on the scan, the patient may be completely enclosed or in a more open situation. A noncontrast series of pictures are taken first. Then, if needed, the patient is withdrawn from the scanner and given an injection of the iodinated contrast medium. The scan is then repeated. Each set of head scans takes less than 5 minutes in newer scanners. Spinal studies take about 10 minutes per body section (cervical, thoracic, lumbar) and are less likely to require contrast injection.

Most patients with new cranial neurologic symptoms have both a precontrast and postcontrast study of the head. Contrast-enhanced CT is especially useful in locating and identifying tumor types and abscesses. For situations in which bleeding is the only concern (e.g., in trauma patients), contrast scans are not usually required.

After a standard CT scan, imaging software digitally removes images of soft tissue so that only images of bone remain. Through the use of this technology, bone deformities, trauma, and birth defects are more easily identified.

CT angiography involves administering contrast dye IV before the CT scan. It is used to identify blockages or narrowing of blood vessels, aneurysms, and other blood vessel abnormalities.

A *CT perfusion study* is an important tool in the evaluation of patients with acute strokelike symptoms. These symptoms have several causes, and the cause must be determined as quickly as possible so that the correct treatment can begin for optimal outcomes. Perfusion CT is performed using an advanced CT scanner with a special software system. For the patient, though, it will seem like a standard CT examination.

An *intrathecal contrast-enhanced CT* scan is performed to diagnose disorders of the spine and spinal nerve roots. A lumbar puncture is performed so that a small amount of spinal fluid can be removed and mixed with contrast dye and injected. The patient is positioned to allow for the contrast medium to move around the spinal cord and nerve roots as needed. He or she may have a headache after the procedure. Follow facility policy regarding patient positioning after the procedure.

NCLEX EXAMINATION CHALLENGE 38.3

Physiological Integrity

The nurse is teaching a client about what to expect immediately after a cerebral angiographic examination. Which statement by the client indicates a need for **further** teaching?

A. "I'll have a pressure dressing on my groin for a couple of hours."
B. "I'll have to keep my leg straight for a while after the procedure."
C. "The nurses will check circulation in my injected leg frequently."
D. "I can use heat on my groin to decrease any discomfort."

Magnetic Resonance Imaging. Magnetic resonance imaging (MRI or MR) has advantages over CT in the diagnostic imaging of the brain, spinal cord, and nerve roots. It does not use ionizing radiation but instead relies on magnetic fields. Multiple sets of images are taken to determine normal and abnormal anatomy. Images may be enhanced with the use of gadolinium, a non–iodine-based contrast medium. MRIs of the spine have largely replaced CT scans and myelography for evaluation. Bony structures cannot be viewed with MRI; CT scans are the best way to see bones. Some facilities have a *functional MRI (fMRI)* machine that can assess blood flow to the brain rather than merely show its anatomic structure.

In addition to the traditional MRI, *magnetic resonance angiography (MRA), magnetic resonance spectroscopy (MRS),* or *diffusion imaging (DI)* may be requested. MRA is used to evaluate ***perfusion*** and blood vessel abnormalities such as an arterial blockage, intracranial aneurysms, and AV malformations. MRS is used to detect abnormalities in the brain's biochemical processes, such as that which occurs in epilepsy, Alzheimer's disease, and brain attack (stroke). Diffuse imaging uses MRI techniques to evaluate ischemia in the brain to determine the location and severity of a stroke.

Open-sided units ("open MRI") produce adequate images for patients who are claustrophobic or do not want standard MRI scanners. However, image quality from these scanners is not as good as that from long-bore traditional scanners. Traditional scanners have higher magnetic field strength and provide better resolution, especially for patients with neurologic health problems.

In the past, MRI has been contraindicated for patients with cardiac pacemakers, other implanted pumps or devices, and ion-containing metal aneurysm clips. However, newer pacemakers and internal defibrillators may be scanned depending on the type of device. Other implanted devices, such as vascular stents, intravascular catheter (IVC) filters, and metal antiembolic devices, may be scanned immediately or after a certain period of time, depending on manufacturer recommendations. MRI may also be contraindicated in patients who are confused or agitated, have unstable vital signs, are on continuous life support, or have older tattoos (which contain lead). New physiologic monitoring systems made specifically for the scanner allow some patients who are unstable to be scanned. A comprehensive online list of medical devices tested for MRI safety and compatibility can be found at *www.mrisafety.com.* Medical personnel must remove any medical devices they are carrying or wearing and ensure that only approved devices are allowed in the MRI room.

Computed Tomography–Positron Emission Tomography. Single positron emission tomography (PET) machines are no longer commonly used or available. Instead, the newest PET machines are combination CT-PET scanners that fuse images together to produce better information about the type and location of neurologic dysfunction. They are particularly useful in staging brain, spinal cord, and other primary cancers.

The physician or nuclear medicine technologist injects the patient with IV deoxyglucose, which is tagged to an isotope. The isotope emits activity in the form of positrons, which are scanned and converted into a color image by computer. The more active a given part of the brain, the greater the glucose uptake. This test is used to evaluate drug metabolism and detect areas of metabolic alteration that occur in dementia, epilepsy, psychiatric and degenerative disorders, neoplasms, and Alzheimer's disease. The level of radiation is equivalent to that of five or six x-rays but much less than exposure during CT.

Teach the patient that he or she will be NPO the night before morning testing and 4 hours before afternoon testing. Patients with diabetes have their test in the morning before taking their antidiabetic drugs. During this 2- to 3-hour procedure, the patient may be blindfolded and have earplugs inserted for all or part of the test. He or she is asked to perform certain mental functions to activate different areas of the brain. Older adults and patients with mental health/behavioral health problems may be too anxious to have a CT-PET scan.

Single-Photon Emission Computed Tomography. The **single-photon emission computed tomography (SPECT)** uses a radiopharmaceutical agent to enable radioisotopes to cross the blood-brain barrier. The agent is administered by IV injection. Gamma-emitting radionuclides have longer half-lives, therefore eliminating the need for a cyclotron near the scanner. Although SPECT is less expensive than PET, the resolution of the images is limited. SPECT is particularly useful in studying cerebral blood flow, amnesia, neoplasms, head trauma, or persistent vegetative state. The test is contraindicated in women who are breast-feeding.

The patient is injected with the material about 1 hour before the actual scan by the radiologist, certified nuclear medicine technologist, or specially trained RN. The patient is positioned on an x-ray table in a quiet dark room for the actual scans. Several gamma cameras scan his or her head. When completed, the images are downloaded to a computer.

Magnetoencephalography. **Magnetoencephalography (MEG)** is a noninvasive imaging technique used to measure the magnetic fields produced by electrical activity in the brain via extremely sensitive devices such as superconducting quantum interference devices (SQUIDs). MEG is somewhat similar to electroencephalography (EEG). The advantage is greater accuracy because of the minimal distortion of the signal. This allows for more usable and reliable localization of brain function. The brain can be observed "in action" rather than just from viewing a still magnetic resonance image. These machines are not widely available because of their extremely high cost.

Other Diagnostic Assessment

Electromyography. Electromyography (EMG) is used to identify nerve and muscle disorders, as well as spinal cord disease. During EMG, recording electrodes are placed onto skeletal muscles to monitor their electrical activity. A progressive decrease in the amplitude of the electrical waveform is a classic sign of several neuromuscular diseases, such as myasthenia gravis, a rare progressive autoimmune disease characterized by muscle weakness as a result of impaired acetylcholine receptors. Electromyography and electroneurography or nerve-conduction studies are usually used together and are referred to as *electromyoneurography.*

Electroencephalography. Electroencephalography (EEG) records the electrical activity of the cerebral hemispheres. The frequency, amplitude, and characteristics of the brain waves are recorded. Certain illnesses or health problems can cause changes in brain waves. For example, a cerebral tumor or infarct may have abnormally slow waveforms.

Fasting is avoided before EEG testing because hypoglycemia can alter the test results. Ensure that hair is clean and without conditioners, hair creams, lotions, sprays, or styling gels. Teach the patient to avoid the use of sedatives or stimulants in the 12 to 24 hours preceding the EEG. Ensure a quiet room with signage to inform visitors of EEG recording in progress. Instruct the patient or family members about the reasons for periodic or continuous monitoring. The reasons for EEG monitoring include:

- Determining the general activity of the cerebral hemispheres
- Determining the origin of seizure activity (such as epilepsy)
- Determining cerebral function in epilepsy and other pathologic conditions such as tumors, abscesses, cerebrovascular disease, hematomas, injury, metabolic diseases, degenerative brain disease, and drug intoxication
- Differentiating between organic and hysterical blindness or deafness
- Monitoring cerebral activity during surgical anesthesia or sedation in the intensive care unit
- Diagnosing sleep disorders (If the EEG is related to a sleep disorder diagnosis, the patient may be asked to sleep less the night before the EEG.)
- Assisting in the determination of brain death

The patient is placed on a reclining chair or bed. Multiple electrodes are applied to the scalp with a jellylike substance and connected to the machine. The physician or EEG technician places glue over the electrodes to prevent slippage. The patient must lie still with his or her eyes closed during the initial recording. The rest of the test engages the patient in certain activities: hyperventilation, photic stimulation, and sleep. A portable EEG may be performed at the bedside if necessary, but the preference is for the EEG to be done in a very quiet room.

Hyperventilation produces cerebral vasoconstriction and alkalosis, which increase the likelihood of seizure activity. The patient is asked to breathe deeply 20 times per minute for 3 minutes. In *photic stimulation,* a flashing bright light is placed in front of the patient. Frequencies of 1 to 20 flashes per second are used with the patient's eyes open and then closed. If the patient's seizures are photosensitive in origin, seizure activity may be seen on the EEG. A *sleep* EEG may be performed to aid in the detection of abnormal brain waves that are seen only when the patient is sleeping, such as with frontal lobe epilepsy.

During an EEG test, which takes 45 to 120 minutes, the recording can be stopped about every 5 minutes to allow the patient to move. If he or she moves during the recording, movement creates a change in the brain waves and the technician will note movements on the graph. Examples of unintentional movement that can affect the recordings are tongue movement, eye blinking, and muscle tensing. The technician may induce or request certain movements or sensory stimulation and record these events on the EEG record to link changes in brain waves with motor activity or sensory stimulation; these intentional movements are also documented on the EEG recording.

The gel and glue used for placing electrodes can be washed out immediately after the test ends. Acetone or witch hazel will dissolve the paste. Advise the patient who has had a sleep-deprived EEG to have someone drive the patient home.

Evoked Potentials. Evoked potentials (also called *evoked response*) measure the electrical signals to the brain generated by sound, touch, or light. These tests are used to assess sensory nerve problems and confirm neurologic conditions, including multiple sclerosis, brain tumor, acoustic neuroma (small tumors of the inner ear), and spinal cord injury. Evoked potentials are also used to monitor brain activity in comatose patients and confirm brain death. During evoked potentials, a second set of electrodes is attached to the part of the body that will experience sensation. A stimulus is applied, and the amount of time it takes for the impulse generated by the stimulus to reach the brain is recorded. Under normal circumstances, the process of signal transmission is instantaneous.

Auditory evoked potentials (also called *brainstem auditory evoked response*) are used to assess high-frequency hearing loss, diagnose any damage to the acoustic nerve and auditory pathways in the brainstem, and detect acoustic neuromas. The patient sits in a soundproof room and wears headphones. Clicking sounds are delivered one at a time to one ear while a masking sound is sent to the other ear.

Visual evoked potentials detect loss of vision from optic nerve damage (in particular, damage caused by multiple sclerosis). The patient sits close to a screen and is asked to focus on the center of a shifting checkerboard pattern. Only one eye is tested at a time. The other eye is either kept closed or covered with a patch.

Somatosensory evoked potentials measure response from stimuli to the peripheral nerves and can detect nerve or spinal cord damage or nerve degeneration from multiple sclerosis and other degenerating diseases. Tiny electrical shocks are delivered by electrode to a nerve in an arm or leg.

Lumbar Puncture. Lumbar puncture (spinal tap) is the insertion of a spinal needle into the subarachnoid space between the third and fourth (sometimes the fourth and fifth) lumbar vertebrae. A lumbar puncture (LP) is used to:

- Obtain cerebrospinal fluid (CSF) pressure readings with a manometer
- Obtain CSF for analysis

- Check for spinal blockage caused by a spinal cord lesion
- Inject contrast medium or air for diagnostic study
- Inject selected drugs

Because of the danger of sudden release of CSF pressure, a lumbar puncture is not done for patients with symptoms indicating severely increased intracranial pressure (ICP). The procedure is also not performed in patients with skin infections at or near the puncture site because of the danger of introducing infective organisms into the CSF.

! NURSING SAFETY PRIORITY (QSEN)

Action Alert

It is very important that the patient not move during a lumbar puncture. If the patient is restless or cannot cooperate, two people may need to assist instead of one. The patient may need a sedative to reduce movement. Consider patient needs for additional assistance or sedation before beginning the procedure.

In preparation for the procedure, position the patient in a fetal side-lying position to separate the vertebrae and move the spinal nerve roots away from the area to be accessed. The primary health care provider then cleans the skin site thoroughly. The injection site is determined, and a local anesthetic is injected. In a few minutes, a spinal needle is inserted between the third and fourth lumbar vertebrae. Instruct the patient to inform the primary health care provider if there is shooting pain or a tingling sensation. After determining proper placement in the subarachnoid space by removing the stylet and seeing CSF, the patient is asked to relax as much as possible so that the pressure reading will be accurate. Opening and closing pressure readings are taken and recorded. The normal opening pressure should be no more than 20 cm H_2O; the CSF should be clear and colorless and contain only a few cells. Three to five test tubes of CSF are usually collected and numbered sequentially. After specimen collection, the needle is withdrawn, slight pressure is applied, and an adhesive bandage strip is placed over the insertion site.

Examination of CSF has been a useful diagnostic tool for some time. Recent technical advances are increasing the number of analyses that can be done on CSF. Gram stain smears can test for particular types of meningitis, such as tubercular meningitis. CSF can be cultured, and sensitivity studies determine the best choice of antibiotic if an infection is diagnosed. A specific test for neurosyphilis is the fluorescent treponemal antibody absorption (FTA-ABS) test. Cytologic studies of CSF can identify tumor cells.

Obtain vital signs and perform frequent neurologic checks as directed by agency protocol. Follow agency policy regarding how long the patient should be on bedrest and remain flat. Encourage the patient to increase fluid intake unless contraindicated. Monitor for complications, especially increased ICP (severe headache, nausea, vomiting, photophobia, and change in level of consciousness). Serious complications of lumbar puncture, although not common, include brainstem herniation (discussed in Chapter 41), infection, CSF leakage, and hematoma formation. Observe the needle insertion site for leakage and notify the primary health care provider if it occurs. Provide the prescribed medication for patient report of headache. Be sure to notify the health care provider if the medication does not relieve pain.

Transcranial Doppler Ultrasonography. Intracranial hemodynamics can be evaluated through the use of transcranial Doppler (TCD), which uses sound waves to measure blood flow through the arteries. The test is particularly valuable in evaluating cerebral vasospasm or narrowing of arteries. TCD is safe, can be used repeatedly for the same patient, and is an inexpensive alternative to angiography.

GET READY FOR THE NEXT-GENERATION NCLEX® EXAMINATION!

Key Points

Review these Key Points for each NCLEX Examination Client Needs Category.

Safe and Effective Care Environment

- Coordinate with the primary health care provider, physical therapist, and speech-language pathologist to establish priorities in neurologic assessment based on the patient's history and presenting signs and symptoms. **QSEN: Teamwork and Collaboration**

Health Promotion and Maintenance

- Identify risk factors that place patients at risk for neurologic health problems such as behaviors that result in serious harm (e.g., driving recklessly) and lifestyle choices. **QSEN: Patient-Centered Care**
- Teach patients how to prepare for selected neurologic diagnostic tests, including what to expect during and after the test. **QSEN: Patient-Centered Care**
- Be sure to be aware of the normal neurologic changes that occur in older adults when interpreting assessment data. **QSEN: Patient-Centered Care**
- Recognize that older adults do not normally experience significant deterioration in ***Cognition*** and memory but do experience physical and physiological changes that affect ***mobility*** and ***sensory perception***. **QSEN: Patient-Centered Care**
- Provide a safe environment when memory loss is part of the older adult's health status by using memory aids and assistive technology to meet teaching or self-care goals. **QSEN: Safety**
- Provide safe opportunities for ***mobility***, including physical activity such as walking, when caring for older adults. **QSEN: Safety**

Psychosocial Integrity

- Assess the reaction of the person to neurologic disease. The psychological responses to neurologic health problems can vary by age, gender, and cultural background. **QSEN: Patient-Centered Care**

Physiological Integrity

- Take a patient history before performing a rapid/focused neurologic assessment if the situation is not emergent. **Clinical Judgment**
- Detect neurologic changes early with health screening and physical assessment strategies that reflect the prioritized assessment. Recall that a deterioration in level of consciousness (e.g., from alert to lethargic) is the most sensitive and reliable indicator of an adverse neurologic change. **QSEN: Evidence-Based Practice; Clinical Judgment**
- Apply knowledge of anatomy and physiology to perform a rapid/focused neurologic assessment as determined by patient needs. **Clinical Judgment**
- Use the Glasgow Coma Scale for patients with traumatic brain injury. **QSEN: Evidence-Based Practice**
- Include assessment of gait, balance, and coordination to determine risk for falls. **QSEN: Safety**
- Check cranial nerve III by examining pupils for size, shape, and reaction to light. Pupils should be equal in size and round and regular in shape and become smaller in bright light. Changes in eye signs can indicate new neurologic deterioration in nonverbal patients. **QSEN: Evidence-Based Practice**
- Be sure to monitor for potentially life-threatening complications after invasive diagnostic testing to assess ***perfusion*** to the brain. For example, monitor for bleeding in patients who have cerebral angiography. If bleeding is observed, call the radiologist or primary physician immediately. Monitor for cerebrospinal fluid (CSF) leakage after a lumbar puncture; CSF should be clear and colorless. **QSEN: Safety; Clinical Judgment**
- Use serum creatinine or estimated glomerular filtration rate to identify patients with reduced kidney function. Older adults and patients with chronic kidney disease, diabetes, or heart failure are at high risk for kidney damage from iodinated and gadolinium contrast media. Provide adequate fluid intake before and after diagnostic testing to flush contrast after a diagnostic test. **QSEN: Evidence-Based Practice**
- Before MRI, check for implanted devices such as pacemakers, vascular stents, pumps, and aneurysm clips. **QSEN: Safety**
- Remember that decerebrate or decorticate posturing and pinpoint or dilated nonreactive pupils are late signs of neurologic deterioration. **Clinical Judgment**

MASTERY QUESTIONS

1. The nurse is preparing to conduct a focused neurologic assessment for a client who had a traumatic brain injury. Which assessment finding is the immediate concern of the nurse?
A. Disorientation
B. Numbness in both arms
C. Decreased level of consciousness
D. Report of headache

2. The nurse is caring for a client following a cerebral angiography. Which assessment finding will the nurse report immediately to the primary health care provider?
A. Discomfort at the injection site
B. Bleeding from the injection site
C. Fatigue and weakness
D. Mild headache

REFERENCES

Jarvis, C. (2020). *Physical examination & health assessment* (8th ed.). St. Louis: Elsevier Saunders.

McCance, K., Huether, S., Brashers, V., & Rote, N. (2019). *Pathophysiology: The biologic basis for disease in adults and children* (8th ed.). St. Louis: Mosby.

Touhy, T. A., & Jett, K. F. (2018). *Geronotological nursing and healthy aging* (5th ed.). St. Louis: Mosby.

Concepts of Care for Patients With Problems of the Central Nervous System: The Brain

Donna D. Ignatavicius

http://evolve.elsevier.com/Iggy/

LEARNING OUTCOMES

1. Collaborate with the interprofessional team to coordinate high-quality care for patients with Alzheimer's disease (AD) or Parkinson disease (PD).
2. Teach patients about health promotion strategies to prevent and manage migraine headaches and meningitis, a potentially fatal ***infection.***
3. Implement nursing interventions to help the patient and family cope with the psychosocial impact caused by commonly occurring brain disorders.
4. Plan care for patients with PD and AD to ensure safety and promote optimum functioning and ***mobility.***
5. Prioritize evidence-based care for patients with commonly occurring brain disorders that affect ***cognition*** and ***mobility.***
6. Plan care coordination and transition management for patients with commonly occurring brain disorders.
7. Plan interventions to prevent or reduce the risk for common complications that contribute to functional decline, ***pain,*** and decreased quality of life in adults with AD and PD.

KEY TERMS

Alzheimer's disease (AD) The most common type of dementia that typically affects people older than 65 years.

agnosia Loss of sensory comprehension, including facial recognition.

amnesia Loss of memory.

anomia An inability to find words.

aphasia Problems with speech (expressive aphasia) and/or language (receptive aphasia).

apraxia Inability to use words or objects correctly.

aura A sensation (e.g., visual changes) that signals the onset of a migraine headache or seizure.

bradykinesia/akinesia Slow movement/no movement.

clonus Rhythmic jerking of all extremities during a seizure.

dementia (sometimes referred to as a *chronic confusional state* or *syndrome*) A general term for progressive loss of brain function and impaired cognition; there are many types of dementia.

dyskinesia The inability to perform voluntary movement.

encephalitis An infection (usually viral) of brain tissue and often the surrounding meninges.

epilepsy (as defined by the National Institute of Neurological Disorders and Stroke) A chronic disorder in which repeated unprovoked seizure activity occurs.

Huntington disease A rare hereditary disorder that is characterized by progressive dementia and choreiform movements (uncontrollable rapid, jerky movements) in the limbs, trunk, and facial muscles.

meningitis An infection of the meninges of the brain and spinal cord, specifically the pia mater and arachnoid.

migraine headache A common clinical syndrome characterized by recurrent episodic attacks of head pain that serve no protective purpose.

nystagmus An involuntary condition in which the eyes make repetitive uncontrolled movements.

Parkinson disease (PD)(also referred to as *Parkinson's disease* and *paralysis agitans*) A progressive neurodegenerative disease that affects mobility and is characterized by four cardinal symptoms (also referred to as *Parkinson's disease* and *paralysis agitans*) A progressive neurodegenerative disease that affects mobility and is characterized by four cardinal symptomstremor, muscle rigidity, bradykinesia/akinesia (slow movement/no movement), and postural instability.

phonophobia A sensitivity to sound.

photophobia A sensitivity to light.

seizure An abnormal, sudden, excessive, uncontrolled electrical discharge of neurons within the brain that may result in a change in level of consciousness (LOC), motor or sensory ability, and/or behavior.

status epilepticus A medical emergency and is a prolonged seizure lasting longer than 5 minutes or repeated seizures over the course of 30 minutes.

validation therapy Recognition and acknowledgement of a patient's feelings and concerns.

vascular dementia The second most common type of dementia caused by disorders that decrease blood flow to parts of the brain.

PRIORITY AND INTERRELATED CONCEPTS

The priority concepts for this chapter are:
- ***Cognition***
- ***Mobility***

The ***Cognition*** concept exemplar for this chapter is Alzheimer's Disease.
The ***Mobility*** concept exemplar for this chapter is Parkinson Disease.

The interrelated concepts for this chapter are:
- ***Pain***
- ***Infection***

Neurologic disorders can interfere with self-management and functional ability; many of them cause impaired ***cognition,*** decreased ***mobility,*** and persistent ***pain. Infection*** can also cause neurologic problems. Chapter 3 briefly reviews these health concepts. Care of patients with health problems affecting the brain requires coordination by nurses and interprofessional collaboration.

COGNITION CONCEPT EXEMPLAR: ALZHEIMER'S DISEASE

Pathophysiology Review

Dementia, sometimes referred to as a *chronic* confusional state or syndrome, is a general term for progressive loss of brain function and impaired ***cognition;*** there are many types of dementia. **Alzheimer's disease (AD)** is the most common type of dementia that typically affects people older than 65 years. **Vascular dementia,** such as *multi-infarct dementia,* results from strokes or other vascular disorders that decrease blood flow to parts of the brain. Table 39.1 compares AD with vascular dementia, the second most common type of dementia.

Any type of dementia affects a person's ability to learn new information and eventually impairs language, judgment, and behavior. As the disease progresses, the patient's functional ability declines and death occurs as a result of complications of decreased ***mobility.***

Dementia is not a normal physiologic change of aging. The brain of the older adult usually weighs less and occupies less space in the cranium than does the brain of a younger person. Other changes in the brain that occur with aging include widening of the cerebral sulci, narrowing of the gyri, and enlargement of the ventricles. In the presence of AD and other types of dementia, these normal changes are greatly accelerated. Brain weight is reduced further. Marked atrophy of the cerebral cortex and loss of cortical neurons occur.

Microscopic changes of the brain found in people with AD include neurofibrillary tangles, amyloid-rich senile or neuritic plaques, and vascular degeneration. *Neurofibrillary tangles* are composed of fibrous tissue that impairs the ability of impulses from being transmitted from neuron to neuron (McCance et al., 2019).

Neuritic plaques are composed of degenerating nerve terminals and are found particularly in the hippocampus, an important part of the limbic system. Deposited within the plaques are increased amounts of an abnormal protein called *beta amyloid.* These proteins have a tendency to accumulate and form the neurotoxic plaques found in the brain that impair neuronal transmission (McCance et al., 2019).

Although *vascular degeneration* occurs in the normally aging brain, its presence is significantly increased in patients with dementia. Vascular degeneration accounts for at least partial loss of the ability of nerve cells to function properly. This pathologic change contributes to the cognitive decline and mortality associated with AD.

In addition to the structural changes in the brain associated with this disorder, abnormalities in the neurotransmitters (acetylcholine [ACh], norepinephrine, dopamine, and serotonin) may occur. High levels of beta amyloid can reduce the amount of acetyltransferase in the hippocampus. This loss is important

TABLE 39.1 Comparison of the Two Major Types of Dementia: Alzheimer's Disease and Vascular Dementia

	Alzheimer's Disease	Vascular Dementia
Cause	Genetic and environmental factors; possibly viral	Strokes or other vascular disorders that decrease blood flow to the brain
Pathophysiologic changes	Chronic, terminal disease that is characterized by formation of neuritic plaques, neurofibrillary tangles, and vascular degeneration in the brain	Impaired blood flow to the brain, causing ischemia or necrosis of brain neurons
Course of dementia	Steady and gradual decline of cognitive, mobility, and ADL function from mild through severe stages; patients usually die from complications of immobility	Stepwise progression of dementia symptoms that get significantly worse after each vascular event, such as a stroke or series of ministrokes; symptoms may improve as collateral circulation to vital neurons develops
Risk factors	Female Over 65 years of age Down syndrome Traumatic brain injury	Male Over 65 years of age History of diabetes mellitus (DM), high cholesterol, myocardial infarction, atherosclerosis, hypertension, smoking, obesity
Management	Safety measures to prevent injury, wandering, or falls Cholinesterase inhibitors Behavior management ADL and mobility assistance as needed based on stage	Identification of risk factors and management of the risk for or actual vascular event (e.g., antidiabetes drugs for DM, antihypertensive drugs, low-fat diet, smoking cessation, weight loss) Safety measures to prevent injury or falls Behavior management

because the decrease in Ach interferes with cholinergic innervation to the cerebral cortex. This change results in impaired ***cognition,*** recent memory, and the ability to acquire new memories.

Etiology and Genetic Risk. The exact cause of AD is unknown. It is well established that *age, gender, and genetics are the most important risk factors.* Age is strongly linked to the incidence of AD for people older than 65, and women are more likely to develop the disease than men (McCance et al., 2019). As older adults age further, they become more at risk for the disease. Although not commonly occurring, when AD is diagnosed in people in their 40s and 50s, it is referred to as *early dementia, Alzheimer's type,* or *presenile dementia.* Other risk factors for AD have been studied, including chemical imbalances, environmental agents, immunologic changes, excessive stress, and ethnicity/race. There is also a high incidence of AD in people who have Down syndrome (Alzheimer's Association, 2018).

PATIENT-CENTERED CARE: VETERANS HEALTH CONSIDERATIONS QSEN

Veterans who have experienced a traumatic brain injury (TBI) or repeated head trauma causing chronic traumatic encephalopathy (CTE) are more at risk for AD and at an earlier age than others. Those who have a diagnosis of post-traumatic stress disorder (PTSD) are twice as likely to develop dementia than veterans without PTSD. Rural veterans have an increased risk of dementia from PTSD and often have difficulty accessing Veterans Affairs (VA) and other support services. To add to this problem, health professionals working in rural areas may lack the specialized knowledge in how to care for these patients (Tasseff & Nies, 2017).

PATIENT-CENTERED CARE: GENETIC/GENOMIC CONSIDERATIONS QSEN

There is little doubt that many patients with AD had a genetic predisposition to the development of the disease. The most well-established genetic factor for AD in Euro-Americans is apolipoprotein E *(APOE),* a protein that transports cholesterol. Individuals who have one or more of the e4 forms of the protein are at high risk for AD; however, they may not actually develop the disease (Alzheimer's Association, 2018).

PATIENT-CENTERED CARE: CULTURAL/SPIRITUAL CONSIDERATIONS QSEN

African Americans and Hispanics have a greater risk for developing AD when compared with non-Hispanic whites (Euro-Americans) (Alzheimer's Association, 2018). The exact reason for these differences is not known, but factors that may influence these differences include increased body mass index (obesity), smoking, and depression, which occur more commonly in minority groups when compared with non-Hispanic whites.

Incidence and Prevalence. There is a significant increase in both the incidence and prevalence of AD after 65 years of age, although it may affect anyone older than 40 years. The number of people in the United States with AD is estimated at over 5.7 million. One in 10 people in the United States over 65 years of age has the disease. Eight-one percent are over 75 years of age (Alzheimer's Association, 2018). AD has a significant impact on health care costs, including direct (such as drug therapy and primary health care provider visits) and indirect medical costs (such as home care or nursing home care). Millions of informal caregivers, most often spouses/partners or other family members, provide care at home for years for most patients with AD. Many of these individuals are at risk for physical and psychosocial problems as a result of the burden of caregiving.

Health Promotion and Maintenance. There are no proven ways to prevent AD; however, research is ongoing. Many patients with AD have other chronic health problems, such as diabetes mellitus, strokes, and atherosclerosis. Maintaining a healthy lifestyle helps to prevent these problems, such as eating a well-balanced diet, and consuming sufficient amounts of nutrients. Walking, swimming, and other exercise not only increase tone and muscle strength but also may decrease cognitive decline. Potentially harmful lifestyle habits that increase the individual's risk of stroke and cardiovascular disease should be avoided, such as smoking and excessive alcohol intake.

❖ Interprofessional Collaborative Care

◆ Assessment: Recognize Cues

History. A thorough history and physical assessment are necessary to differentiate AD from other, possibly reversible causes of impaired ***cognition.*** Some patients experience cognitive impairment as acute confusion (delirium) as discussed in Chapter 4. Table 3.1 in Chapter 3 compares dementia and delirium. Patients who have dementia are at an increased risk of delirium when hospitalized or admitted to a long-term care (LTC) setting.

Obtain information from family members or significant others because the patient may be unaware of the problems, denying their existence or covering them up. Some family members often do not recognize or may deny early changes in their loved one as well. Others may recognize subtle changes early in the disease process.

The most important information to be obtained is the onset, duration, progression, and course of the symptoms. Question the patient and the family about changes in memory or increasing forgetfulness and about the ability to perform ADLs. Ask about current employment status; work history; military history; and ability to fulfill household responsibilities, including cleaning, grocery shopping, and preparing meals. Inquire about changes in driving ability, ability to handle routine financial transactions, and language and communication skills. In addition, document any changes in personality and behavior. *Assessing functional status for complex chronic conditions such as dementia is a recommended core measure by the Centers for Medicare and Medicaid Services.*

Physical Assessment/Signs and Symptoms

Stages of Alzheimer's Disease. The National Institute of Aging in the United States recognizes three phases of AD:

- Asymptomatic preclinical phase
- Symptomatic predementia phase (mild impaired ***cognition***)
- Dementia phase

The signs and symptoms associated with the dementia phase can be grouped into three broad stages based on the progress of the disease, as outlined in the Key Features: Alzheimer's Disease box.

KEY FEATURES

Alzheimer's Disease

Early (Mild), or Stage I (First Symptoms up to 4 Years)
- Independent in ADLs
- Denies presence of symptoms
- Forgets names; misplaces household items
- Has short-term memory loss and difficulty recalling new information
- Shows subtle changes in personality and behavior
- Loses initiative and is less engaged in social relationships
- Has mild impaired *cognition* and problems with judgment
- Demonstrates decreased performance, especially when stressed
- Unable to travel alone to new destinations
- Often has decreased sense of smell

Middle (Moderate), or Stage II (2 to 3 Years)
- Has impairment of all cognitive functions
- Demonstrates problems with handling or unable to handle money and finances
- Is disoriented to time, place, and event
- Is possibly depressed and/or agitated
- Is increasingly dependent in ADLs
- Has visuospatial deficits: has difficulty driving and gets lost
- Has speech and language deficits: less talkative, decreased use of vocabulary, increasingly nonfluent, and eventually aphasic
- Incontinent
- Psychotic behaviors, such as delusions, hallucinations, and paranoia
- Has episodes of wandering; trouble sleeping

Late (Severe), or Stage III
- Completely incapacitated; bedridden
- Totally dependent in ADLs
- Has loss of *mobility* and verbal skills
- Possibly has seizures and tremors
- Has **agnosia**

The patient does not necessarily progress from one stage to the next in an orderly fashion. A stage may be bypassed, or he or she may exhibit symptoms of one or several stages. Each patient exhibits different disease stages and signs and symptoms. Consequently, most authorities now use broader terms such as *early (mild), middle (moderate),* and *late (severe)* stages, although other staging systems exist.

Changes in Cognition. As defined in Chapter 3, ***cognition*** is the complex integration of mental processes and intellectual function for the purposes of reasoning, learning, and memory. Therefore assess patient for deficits in these abilities:
- Attention and concentration
- Judgment and perception
- Learning and memory
- Communication and language
- Speed of information processing

One of the first symptoms of AD is short-term memory impairment. New memory and defects in information retrieval result from dysfunction in the hippocampal, frontal, or parietal region. Alterations in communication abilities, such as **apraxia** (inability to use words or objects correctly), **aphasia** (inability to speak or understand), **anomia** (inability to find words), and **agnosia** (loss of sensory comprehension, including facial recognition), are due to dysfunction of the temporal and parietal lobes. Frontal lobe impairment causes problems with judgment, an inability to make decisions, decreased attention span, and a decreased ability to concentrate. As the disease progresses to a later stage, the patient loses all cognitive abilities, is totally unable to communicate, and becomes less aware of the environment.

To more clearly identify the nature and extent of the patient's impaired ***cognition,*** the neurologist or psychologist administers several neuropsychological tests. The tests selected depend on clinician preference and the ability of the patient to participate in testing. All of the tests focus on cognitive ability and may be repeated over time to measure changes. Folstein's Mini-Mental State Examination (MMSE) is an example of a tool used to determine the onset and severity of cognitive impairment. The MMSE is also known as the "mini-mental exam." The MMSE assesses five major areas—orientation, registration, attention and calculation, recall, and speech-language (including reading). The patient performs certain cognitive tasks that are scored and added together for a total score of 0 to 30. The lower the score is, the greater the severity of the dementia. It is not unusual for a patient with advanced AD to score below 5.

Another sensitive tool used by health professionals to screen for dementia is the Montreal Cognitive Assessment Test (MoCA). Although the MMSE and MoCA are used frequently, they require that the patient be able to read. For the patient who cannot read or for a quicker screening test, the "set test" can be used. The patient is asked to name 10 items in each of four sets or categories: fruits, animals, colors, and towns (FACT). Other categories can be used, if needed. The patient receives 1 point for each item for a possible maximum score of 40. Patients who score above 25 do not have dementia. Although this assessment is easy to administer, it should not be used for patients with hearing impairments or speech and language problems.

The Clock Drawing Test does not require that the patient can read and is nonthreatening to perform. In LTC settings, the federally required Brief Interview for Mental Status (BIMS) is included as part of the Minimum Data Set 3.0 for Nursing Homes (see Chapter 4).

Changes in Behavior and Personality. One of the most difficult aspects of AD and other types of dementia with which families and caregivers cope is the behavioral changes that can occur in advanced disease. Assess the patient for:
- Aggressiveness, especially verbal and physical abusive tendencies
- Rapid mood swings
- Increased confusion at night or when light is not adequate ("sundowning") or in excessively fatigued patients

The patient may wander and become lost or may go into other rooms to rummage through another's belongings. Hoarding or hiding objects is also common. For example, patients may hoard washcloths in the long-term care setting.

For some patients with dementia, emotional and behavioral problems occur with the primary disease. They may experience paranoia (suspicious behaviors), delusions, hallucinations, and depression. Document these behaviors and ensure the patient's safety. (Refer to a mental health/behavior health nursing textbook for a complete discussion of these psychotic disorders.)

Changes in Self-Management Skills. Observe for changes in the patient's self-management skills that decline over time, such as:

- Decreased interest in personal appearance
- Selection of clothing that is inappropriate for the weather or event
- Loss of bowel and bladder control
- Decreased appetite or ability to eat (often due to forgetting how to chew food and swallow in late dementia)

Over time, the patient becomes less mobile, and complications of impaired ***mobility*** develop. These potential complications are listed in Table 3.3 in Chapter 3 of this textbook. The patient eventually becomes totally immobile and requires total physical care.

Psychosocial Assessment. In people with dementia, the cognitive changes and biochemical and structural dysfunctions affect personality and behavior. In the early stage, patients often recognize that they are experiencing memory or cognitive changes and may attempt to hide the problems. They begin the grieving process because of anticipated loss, experiencing denial, anger, bargaining, and depression at varying times.

When the patient and family receive the diagnosis, one or more family members may desire genetic testing. Support the patient's/family's decisions regarding testing and help them find credible resources for testing and professional genetics counseling.

As the disease progresses, patients begin to display major changes in emotional and behavioral affect. Of particular importance is the need for an assessment of the patients' reactions to changes in routine or environment. For example, a hospital admission is very traumatic for most patients with dementia. It is not unusual for them to exhibit a catastrophic response or overreact to any change by becoming excessively aggressive or abusive. This is referred to as *traumatic relocation syndrome.*

Sexual disinhibition is one of the most challenging symptoms for both family and staff members. Sexually inappropriate behaviors may include masturbating publicly, attempting sexual acts on staff or other patients, disrobing or exposing the genital area, and/or making sexualized comments to staff or other patients. Assess a history of or current manifestation of these behaviors to include into the patient's plan of care.

Neuropsychiatric symptoms are common in patients with AD and increase as the disease progresses and aphasia increases. The patient's emotions are often displayed as nonverbal behaviors, including hitting, yelling, and agitation. Any new hospital procedure may cause anxiety and fear as a trigger for these behaviors.

As patients become unaware of their behavior, the focus of the psychosocial assessment shifts to the family or significant others. The interprofessional health care team assesses their ability to cope with the chronicity and progression of the disease and identifies possible support systems.

Laboratory and Imaging Assessment. No laboratory test can confirm the diagnosis of AD. Definitive diagnosis is made on the basis of brain tissue examination at autopsy, which confirms the presence of neurofibrillary tangles and neuritic plaques.

Genetic testing, specifically for *apolipoprotein E4 (APOE 4),* may be helpful as an ancillary test (not a predictive test) for the differential diagnosis of AD. *Amyloid beta protein precursor (soluble)* (sBPP) may be measured for patients to diagnose AD and other types of dementia. A decrease in the patient's sBPP in the cerebrospinal fluid (CSF) supports the diagnosis because the amyloid tends to deposit in the brain and is not circulating in the CSF (Pagana & Pagana, 2018).

A variety of imaging tests (CT or MRI) may be performed to rule out other treatable causes of dementia or delirium. The CT scan typically shows cerebral atrophy, vascular degeneration, ventricular enlargement, wide sulci, and shrunken gyri in the later stages of the disease.

NCLEX EXAMINATION CHALLENGE 39.1

Psychosocial Integrity

The nurse assesses a client with a diagnosis of **early-stage** Alzheimer's disease. Which assessment findings would the nurse expect for this client? **Select all that apply.**

A. Forgetfulness
B. Hallucinations
C. Wandering
D. Urinary incontinence
E. Difficulty eating
F. Personality changes

◆ **Analysis: Analyze Cues and Prioritize Hypotheses.** The priority collaborative problems for patients with Alzheimer's disease (AD) include:

1. Decreased memory and ***cognition*** due to neuronal changes in the brain
2. Potential for injury or falls due to wandering or inability to ambulate independently
3. Potential for elder abuse by caregivers due to the patient's prolonged progression of disability and the patient's increasing care needs

◆ **Planning and Implementation: Generate Solutions and Take Action.** *The priority for interprofessional care is safety! Chronic confusion and physical deficits place the patient with AD at a high risk for injury, accidents, and elder abuse.*

Managing Memory and Cognitive Dysfunction

Planning: Expected Outcomes. In the very early stages of the disease, the patient with AD is expected to maintain the ability to perform basic mental processes. As the disease progresses, patients cannot meet this outcome. Instead, the desired outcome is to maintain memory and ***cognition*** for as long as possible to keep patients safe and increase their quality of life.

Interventions. Although drug therapy may be used for patients with AD, nonpharmacologic interventions are the main focus of nursing teamwork and interprofessional collaboration. Teach family members and significant others about the importance of being consistent in following the individualized plan of care.

Nonpharmacologic Management

Behavioral management in a structured environment. The primary health care provider should answer the patient's questions truthfully concerning the diagnosis of AD. In this way, the patient and family can more fully participate in the interprofessional plan of care. Interventions are the same whether he or she is cared for at home, in an adult day-care center, in an assisted-living center, in an LTC facility, or in a hospital. *The patient with memory problems benefits best from a structured and consistent environment.* Training in communication can help nurses and health care team members interact with better affect and compassion.

Many factors, including physical illness and environmental factors, can exacerbate (worsen) the signs and symptoms of AD. The patient with dementia frequently has other health problems such as cardiovascular disease, arthritis, renal insufficiency, and pulmonary disease. Changes in vision and hearing also may be present. Managing these problems often improves the patient's functional ability.

Approaches to managing the patient who has AD include:

- Cognitive stimulation and memory training
- Structuring the environment
- Orientation or validation therapy
- Promoting self-management
- Promoting bowel and bladder continence
- Promoting communication

The purpose of *cognitive stimulation and memory training* is to reinforce or promote desirable cognitive function and facilitate memory. Cognitive-stimulation therapy programs and mindfulness provide some benefit for patients. An example of cognitive stimulation is to show a video of family members to the patient with dementia to manage behaviors or help improve memory. Interactive animal-assisted therapy can help patients with mild-to-moderate impaired cognition to decrease disruptive or psychotic behaviors (see the Evidence-Based Practice box).

EVIDENCE-BASED PRACTICE

Does Animal-Assisted Therapy Help Patients With Dementia?

Yakimicki, M. L., Edwards, N. E., Richards, E., & Beck, A. M. (2018). Animal-assisted intervention and dementia: A systematic review. *Clinical Nursing Research, 28*(1), 9–29.

The authors conducted a systematic review of the literature to determine the effectiveness, if any, of animal-assisted therapy as an intervention for patients with dementia. After a complete appraisal, 32 studies were selected for review. As a result of pet therapy, findings included:

- 27 of the 32 studies used dogs as an intervention.
- 9 of 15 studies demonstrated an improvement in agitation and aggression.
- 11 of 12 studies showed that patients had increased social interaction.
- 3 of 4 studies revealed an improved quality of life.
- All of the studies showed that patients with dementia increased their social and physical activities.

Level of Evidence: 1

The research was a systematic review of the literature that included multiple studies to summarize best practices for a specific intervention for patients with dementia.

Implications for Nursing Practice and Research:

This research provides evidence for using animal-assisted interventions to help patients with dementia manage behaviors and improve social and physical activity. Nurses need to explore how this intervention can be used in both health care and community settings. Although this research did not limit its search to studies of patients with Alzheimer's disease, all patients with dementia, regardless of type, may exhibit disruptive behaviors and socially withdraw. Additional systematic reviews for other interventions need to be conducted as the population ages and the incidence of dementia is expected to increase.

As the disease progresses, the patient may experience an inability to recognize oneself and other familiar faces. Encourage the family to provide pictures of family members and close friends that are labeled with the person's name on the picture. In addition, advise the family to reminisce with the patient about pleasant experiences from the past. Use *reminiscence therapy* while assisting the patient with ADLs or performing a treatment or assessment. Refer to personal items in the room to help the patient begin to talk about its meaning in the present and in the past.

It is not unusual for the patient to talk to his or her image in the mirror. This behavior should be allowed as long as it is not harmful. If the patient becomes frightened by the mirror image, remove or cover the mirror. In some long-term care or memory-care units, a picture of the patient is placed on the room door to help with facial recognition and to help the patient locate his or her room. This picture also helps the staff locate the patient in case of wandering or elopement.

Teach the family to keep environmental distractions and noise to a minimum. The patient's home, hospital room, or nursing home room should not have pictures on the wall or other decorations that could be misinterpreted as people or animals that could harm the patient. An abstract painting or wallpaper might look like a fire or an explosion and scare the patient. The room should have adequate, nonglare lighting and no potentially frightening shadows.

In addition to disturbed sleep, other negative effects of high noise levels include decreased nutritional intake, changes in blood pressure and pulse rates, and feelings of increased stress and anxiety. The patient with AD is especially susceptible to these changes and needs to have as much undisturbed sleep at night as possible. Fatigue increases confusion and behavioral manifestations such as agitation and aggressiveness.

! NURSING SAFETY PRIORITY (QSEN)

Action Alert

When a patient with Alzheimer's disease is in a new setting or environment, collaborate with the staff and admitting department to select a room that is in the quietest area of the unit and away from obvious exits, if possible. A private room may be needed if the patient has a history of agitation or wandering. The television should remain off unless the patient turns it on or requests that it be turned on.

Objects such as furniture, a hairbrush, and eyeglasses should be kept in the same place. Establish a daily routine and follow it as much as possible. Arrange for a communication board or digital handheld device for scheduled activities and other information to promote orientation such as the day of the week, the month, and the year. Pictures of people familiar to the patient can also be placed on this board.

Explain changes in routine to the patient before they occur, repeating the explanation immediately before the changes take place. Clocks and single-date calendars also help the patient maintain day-to-day orientation to the environment in the early stages of the disease process. *For the patient with early disease, reality orientation is usually appropriate.* Teach family members and health care staff to frequently reorient the patient to the environment. Remind the patient what day and time it is, where he or she is, and who you are.

For the patient in the later stages of AD or dementia, reality orientation does not work and often increases agitation. *The interprofessional health care team uses validation therapy for the patient with moderate or severe AD. In* **validation therapy**, *the staff member recognizes and acknowledges the patient's feelings and concerns.* For example, if the patient is looking for his or her mother, ask him or her to talk about what Mother looks like and what she might be wearing. This response does not argue with the patient but also does not reinforce the patient's belief that Mother is still living.

As the disease progresses, altered thought processes affect the *ability to perform ADLs.* Encourage the patient to perform as much self-care as possible and to maintain independence in daily living skills as long as possible. For example, in the home setting, complete clothing outfits that can be easily placed on a single hanger are preferred for patient selection. When possible, the patient should participate in meal preparation, grocery shopping, and other household routines.

NCLEX EXAMINATION CHALLENGE 39.2

Psychosocial Integrity

A client with **moderate** dementia asks the nurse to find her son who is deceased. What is the nurse's **most appropriate** response?

A. "We can call him in a little while if you want."
B. "Your son died over 20 years ago."
C. "What did your son look like?"
D. "I'll ask your husband to find him when he visits."

INTERPROFESSIONAL COLLABORATION

Care of Patients with Alzheimer's Disease

Collaborate with the occupational and physical therapists to provide a complete evaluation and assistance in helping the patient remain as independent as possible. Adaptive devices, such as grab bars in the bathtub or shower area, an elevated commode, and adaptive eating utensils, may enable him or her to maintain independence in grooming, toileting, and feeding. The physical therapist prescribes an exercise program to improve physical health and functionality.

According to the Interprofessional Education Collaborative (IPEC) Expert Panel's Competency of Roles and Responsibilities, using the unique and complementary abilities of other team members optimizes health and patient care (IPEC, 2016; Slusser et al., 2019).

The patient may remain continent of bowel and bladder for long periods if taken to the bathroom or given a bedpan or urinal every 2 hours. Toileting may be needed more often during the day and less frequently at night. Assistive personnel (AP) or home caregivers should encourage the patient to drink adequate fluids to promote optimal voiding. A patient may refuse to drink enough fluids because of a fear of incontinence. Assure the patient that he or she will be toileted on a regular schedule to prevent incontinent episodes.

When patients with dementia are in the hospital or another unfamiliar place, avoid the use of restraints, including side rails. Serious injury can occur when a patient with dementia attempts to get out of bed with either limb restraints or side rail use. Use frequent surveillance, toileting every 2 hours, and other strategies to prevent falls. In some cases, sitters may be used to help prevent patient injury. Chapter 4 discusses fall prevention in detail.

Maintain a clear path between the bed and bathroom at all times. For patients who are too weak to walk to the bathroom, a bedside commode may be used. Some patients may void in unusual places, such as the sink or a wastebasket. As a reminder of where they should toilet, place a picture of the commode on the bathroom door.

Complementary and integrative health. If culturally appropriate and if the patient allows being touched by staff, teach AP to provide a massage before bedtime to promote sleep or at other times to reduce stress and promote relaxation. Use some type of oil or lotion if the patient does not have allergies to these substances. Slow, rhythmic massage strokes on the upper back, neck, and shoulders can be very relaxing and calming (Westman & Blaisdell, 2016). Essential oils such as lavender and bergamot may also produce a calming effect and promote relaxation (Allard & Katseres, 2016).

Use **redirection** by attracting the patient's attention to promote communication. Keep the environment as free from distractions as possible. Speak directly to the patient in a distinct manner. Sentences should be clear and short. Remind the patient to perform one task at a time and allow sufficient time for completion. It may be necessary to break each task down into many small steps and limit choices. The Best Practice for Patient Safety & Quality Care: Promoting Communication With the Patient With Alzheimer's Disease box lists other tips for communicating with patients who have AD.

As the disease progresses, the patient is unable to perform tasks when asked. Show the patient what needs to be done, or provide cues to remind him or her how to perform the task. When possible, explain and demonstrate the task that the patient is asked to perform.

BEST PRACTICE FOR PATIENT SAFETY & QUALITY CARE (QSEN)

Promoting Communication With the Patient With Alzheimer's Disease

- Ask simple, direct questions that require only a "yes" or "no" answer if the patient can communicate.
- Provide instructions with pictures in a place that the patient will see if he or she can read them.
- Use simple, short sentences and one-step instructions.
- Use gestures to help the patient understand what is being said.
- Validate the patient's feelings as needed.
- Limit choices; too many choices cause frustration and increased confusion.
- Never assume that the patient is totally confused and cannot understand what is being communicated.
- Try to anticipate the patient's needs and interpret nonverbal communication.

Patients with dementia disorders typically have specific speech and language problems. Recognize that emotional and physical behaviors may be a form of communication. Interpret the meaning of these behaviors to address them. For example, restlessness may indicate urinary retention, pain, infection, or hypoxia (lack of oxygen to the brain). Collaborate with the speech-language pathologist to assist with communication ability.

Drug Therapy. There are no drugs that can cure or slow the progression of Alzheimer's disease, but a few drugs may improve symptoms associated with the disease for some patients. Psychotropic drugs may be prescribed to help control the signs and symptoms of associated mental/behavioral health problems (e.g., depression, anxiety, paranoia).

Cholinesterase inhibitors are drugs approved for treating AD symptoms. They work to improve cholinergic neurotransmission in the brain by delaying the destruction of acetylcholine (ACh) by the enzyme *cholinesterase*. This action may slow the onset of cognitive decline in some patients, but none of these drugs alters the course of the disease. In some cases, cholinesterase inhibitors can improve functional ADL ability. Examples include donepezil, galantamine, and rivastigmine (Burchum & Rosenthal, 2019).

! NURSING SAFETY PRIORITY QSEN

Drug Alert

Teach the family to monitor the patient's heart rate and report dizziness or falls because cholinesterase inhibitors can cause bradycardia. Therefore they are used cautiously for patients who have a history of heart disease.

Memantine is the first of a new class of drugs that is a low-to-moderate affinity **N-methyl-d-aspartate (NMDA) receptor antagonist**. Overexcitation of NMDA receptors by the neurotransmitter *glutamate* may play a role in AD. This drug blocks excess amounts of glutamate that can damage nerve cells. It is indicated for advanced AD and has been shown in some patients to slow the pace of deterioration (Burchum & Rosenthal, 2019). Memantine may help maintain patient function for a few months longer. Some patients also have improved memory and thinking skills. This drug can be given with donepezil, a cholinesterase inhibitor.

Some patients with AD develop depression and may be treated with *antidepressants*. Selective serotonin reuptake inhibitors (SSRIs), such as paroxetine and sertraline, are typically prescribed.

Psychotropic drugs, also called *antipsychotic* or *neuroleptic drugs,* should be reserved for patients with psychoses that sometimes accompany dementia, such as hallucinations and delusions. However, in clinical practice, these drugs are sometimes incorrectly used for agitation, combativeness, or restlessness. Psychotropic drugs are considered chemical restraints because they decrease ***mobility*** and patients' self-management ability. Therefore most geriatricians recommend that they be used as a last resort and with caution in low doses for a specific mental/behavioral health problem. The specific drug prescribed depends on side effects, the condition of the patient, and expected outcomes. *Follow agency policy and The Joint Commission standards concerning the use of chemical restraints.*

BEST PRACTICE FOR PATIENT SAFETY & QUALITY CARE QSEN

Approaches to Prevent and Manage Wandering in Hospitalized Patients

- Identify the patients most at risk for wandering through observation and history provided by family.
- Provide appropriate supervision, including frequent checks (especially at shift-change times).
- Place the patient in an area that provides maximum observation but not in the nurses' station.
- Use family members, friends, volunteers, and sitters as needed to monitor the patient.
- Keep the patient away from stairs or elevators.
- Do not change rooms to prevent increasing confusion.
- Avoid physical or chemical restraints.
- Assess and treat pain.
- Use reorientation methods or validation therapy, as appropriate.
- Provide frequent toileting and incontinence care as needed.
- Use bed and/or chair alarms, as available.
- If possible, prevent overstimulation, such as excessive noise.
- Use soft music and nonglare lighting if possible.

Preventing Injuries or Falls

Planning: Expected Outcomes. The patient with dementia is expected to remain free from physical harm and not injure anyone else.

Interventions. Many patients with dementia tend to wander and may easily become lost. In later stages of the disease, some patients may become severely agitated and physically or verbally abusive to others. Teach the family the importance of a patient identification badge or bracelet. The badge should include how to contact the primary caregiver. In an inpatient setting, check the patient frequently and place him or her in a room that can be monitored easily. The room should be away from exits and stairs. Some health care agencies place large stop signs or red tape on the floor in front of exits. Others have installed alarm systems to indicate when a patient is opening the door or getting out of a bed or chair.

Restlessness may be decreased if the patient is taken for frequent walks. If the patient begins to wander, redirect him or her. For example, if the patient insists on going shopping for clothes, he or she is redirected to his or her closet to select clothing that will not be recognized as his or her own. This type of activity can be repeated a number of times because the patient has lost short-term memory. Interventions for preventing and managing wandering are listed in the Best Practice for Patient Safety & Quality Care: Approaches to Prevent and Manage Wandering in Hospitalized Patients box.

In any setting, keep the patient busy with structured activities. In a health care agency, an activity therapist or volunteer may work with patients as a group or individually to determine the type of activity that is appropriate for the stage of the disease. Puzzles, board games, art supplies, and computer games are often appropriate. Music and art therapy are also helpful activities to keep patients with AD busy while stimulating ***cognition.*** These activities allow patients to be engaged and promote their creativity.

NURSING SAFETY PRIORITY (QSEN)

Action Alert

In inpatient health care agencies, use the least restrictive physical restraints, such as waist belts and geri-chairs with lapboards, only as a last resort because they often increase patient restlessness and cause agitation. Federal regulations in long-term care facilities in the United States mandate that all residents have the right to be free of both physical and chemical restraints. *All health care agencies accredited by The Joint Commission are required to use alternatives to restraints before resorting to any physical or chemical restraint.*

Patients with dementia may be injured because they cannot recognize objects or situations as harmful. Remove or secure all potentially dangerous objects (e.g., knives, drugs, cleaning solutions). Patients are often unaware that their driving ability is impaired and usually want to continue this activity even if their driver's license has been suspended or they are unsafe. Automobile keys must be secured, but the patient should be told why they were taken. (See Chapter 4 for more discussion on older-adult driving.)

Late in the disease process, the patient may experience seizure activity. If he or she is cared for at home, teach caregivers what action to take when a seizure occurs to prevent injury. (See the discussion of Interventions in the Seizures and Epilepsy section.)

Talking calmly and softly and attempting to redirect the patient to a more positive behavior or activity are effective strategies when he or she is agitated. For example, some patients refuse to take a bath or are unable to bathe. Bathing disability predicts decline for patients with dementia and, combined with safety issues, often leads the family to place them in long-term care (LTC) settings. LTC staff may label these patients as "difficult" when they aggressively refuse to bathe.

Use calm, positive statements and reassure the patient that he or she is safe. Statements such as, "I'm sorry that you are upset," "I know it's hard," and "I will have someone stay with you until you feel better" may help. Actions to *avoid* when the patient is agitated include raising the voice, confronting, arguing, reasoning, taking offense, or explaining. Teach the caregiver to not show alarm or make sudden movements out of the person's view. If the patient remains agitated, ensure his or her safety and leave the room after explaining that you will return later. Frequent visual checks must be done during this time. If the patient is connected to any type of tubing or other device, he or she may try to disconnect it or pull it out. These devices should be used cautiously in the patient with dementia. For example, if IV access is needed, the catheter or cannula is placed in an area that the patient cannot easily see, or it should be covered.

Another way to manage this problem is to provide a diversion. For example, if the patient is doing an activity or holding an item such as a stuffed animal or other special item, he or she might be less likely to pay attention to medical devices. Additional strategies to minimize behavioral problems, especially at home, are listed in Table 39.2.

Patients who are cared for at home are at high risk for neglect or abuse. *The Joint Commission requires all patients to be assessed for neglect and abuse on admission to a health care facility.* Patients with mild dementia may not report these concerns for fear of retaliation. Those with severe dementia may not have the ability to report the abuse. Asking questions such as, "Who cooks for you?" "Do you get help when you need it?" or "Do you wait long for help to the bathroom?" may be less stressful for the patient to answer.

TABLE 39.2 Minimizing Behavioral Problems for Patients With Alzheimer's Disease at Home

- Carefully evaluate the patient's environment to ensure it is safe:
  - Remove small area rugs.
  - Consider replacing tile floors with nonslippery floors.
  - Arrange furniture and room decorations to maximize the patient's safety when walking.
  - Minimize clutter in all rooms in and outside of the house.
  - Install nightlights in patient's room, bathroom, and hallway.
  - Install and maintain smoke alarms, fire alarms, and natural gas detectors.
  - Install safety devices in the bathroom such as handles for changing position (sit-to-stand).
  - Install alarm system or bells on outside doors; place safety locks on doors and gates.
  - Ensure that door locks cannot be easily opened by the patient.
- Help the patient with mild-stage disease remain oriented to the extent possible:
  - Place single-date calendars in patient's room and in kitchen.
  - Use large-face clocks with a neutral background.
- Communicate with the patient based on his or her ability to understand:
  - Explain activity immediately before the patient needs to carry it out.
  - Break complex tasks down to simple steps.
- Allow and encourage the patient to be as independent as possible in ADLs:
  - Place complete outfits for the day on hangers; have the patient select one to wear.
  - Develop and maintain a predictable routine (e.g., meals, bedtime, morning routine).
- When a problem behavior occurs, divert patient to another activity; minimize excessive stimulation:
  - Take the patient on outings when crowds are small.
  - If crowds cannot be avoided, minimize the amount of time the patient is present in a crowd. For example, at family gatherings, provide a quiet room for the patient to rest throughout the visit.
  - Arrange for a day-care program to maintain interaction and provide respite for home caregiver.
- In the United States (www.alz.org); in Canada, register the patient with the Alzheimer Society of Canada Medic Alert Safely Home program (www.alzheimer.ca).

Preventing Elder Abuse

Planning: Expected Outcomes. The family or other caregivers of the patient with dementia are expected to plan time to care for themselves to promote a reasonable quality of life and satisfaction, which should help prevent patient abuse.

Interventions. AD is a chronic, progressive condition that eventually leaves the patient completely dependent on others for all aspects of care. The patient with moderate or severe dementia requires continual 24-hour supervision and caregiving. Severe cognitive changes leave the patient unable to manage finances, property, or personal care. The family needs to seek legal counsel regarding the patient's competency and the need to obtain guardianship or a durable medical power of attorney when necessary.

Millions of family caregivers provide direct care for patients with impaired ***cognition***. Family caregivers include relatives, significant others, and neighbors who provide the majority of home health care. A qualitative study by Czekanski (2017) examined the experience of transitioning of family members, usually spouses and daughters, to the role of caregiver for patients with AD or related dementias. As a result of the study, the researcher identified common themes experienced by family caregivers, which included losses and challenges, seeking knowledge and support, and preserving themselves without guilt.

Teach family caregivers to be aware of their own health and stress levels. Signs of stress include anger, social withdrawal, anxiety, depression, lack of concentration, sleepiness, irritability, and physical health problems. When signs of stress and strain occur, the caregiver should be referred to his or her primary health care provider or seek one on his or her own. It is not unusual for the caregiver to refuse to accept help from others, even for a few brief hours. Initially, the caregiver may be more comfortable accepting help for just a few minutes a day so that he or she could shower, enjoy a cup of tea, or take a brief walk. Some caregivers find that eventually they need to place their loved one into a respite setting or unit so they can re-energize and prevent or manage spiritual distress.

PATIENT-CENTERED CARE: CULTURAL/SPIRITUAL CONSIDERATIONS QSEN

Both religion and spirituality can help family caregivers give meaning to the work they provide for patients with AD. Spirituality is considered an important part of holistic patient care; it may or may not include religion. Spirituality and religion may decrease the incidence of caregiver depression and anxiety. Assess the patient's and family caregiver's cultural beliefs and values related to spirituality and religion. The Patient and Family Education: Preparing for Self-Management: Reducing Family/Informal Caregiver Stress box lists strategies for reducing caregiver stress and includes interventions to promote spirituality and prevent spiritual distress.

PATIENT AND FAMILY EDUCATION: PREPARING FOR SELF-MANAGEMENT

Reducing Family/Informal Caregiver Stress

- Maintain realistic expectations for the person with Alzheimer's disease (AD).
- Take each day one at a time.
- Try to find the positive aspects of each incident or situation.
- Use humor with the person who has AD.
- Use the resources of the Alzheimer's Association in the United States (or Alzheimer Society of Canada), including attending local support group meetings and using the AD toll-free hotline when needed.
- Explore alternative care settings early in the disease process for possible use later.
- Establish advance directives with the AD patient early in the disease process.
- Set aside time each day for rest or recreation away from the patient, if possible.
- Seek respite care periodically for longer periods of time.
- Take care of yourself by watching your diet, exercising, and getting plenty of rest.
- Be realistic about what you or they can do and accept help from family, friends, and community resources.
- Use relaxation techniques, including meditation and massage.
- Seek out clergy or other spiritual counselor as needed.

As stated earlier, African Americans and Hispanics have a greater risk for developing AD and often earlier and typically live longer than non-Hispanic whites (Euro-Americans). These ethnic groups are known to be very family centered and tend to care for their family members at home as needed. As a result of these values and beliefs, an increase in family caregivers is expected as the number of older ethnic minority adults increases dramatically within the next 20 to 30 years. More research that focuses on older adults from these populations is needed to better provide essential care and support.

Care Coordination and Transition Management

Home Care Management. In the early stages of AD, patients may be cared for at home with little need for outside intervention. Whenever possible, the patient and family should be assigned a case manager who can assess their needs for health care resources and find the best placement throughout the continuum of care.

The patient usually begins to withdraw from friends and social events as memory impairment and personality and behavior changes progress. The family may begin to decrease their own social activities as the demands of the patient's care take more of their time. Emphasize to the family the importance of maintaining their own social contacts and leisure activities.

In most areas of the United States and Canada, respite care is available for families. The patient may be placed in a respite facility or nursing home for the weekend or for several weeks to give the family a rest from the constant care demands. The family may also be able to obtain respite care in the home through a home care agency or assisted-living facility. Remind the family that respite care is for a short period; it is not permanent placement. Some health care agencies have opened adult medical day-care centers or memory care units for patients with AD. In the day-care center, patients spend all or part of the day at the facility and participate in activities as their condition permits. Although these centers are usually open only on weekdays, this arrangement allows the caregiver to work or participate in other activities. If patients require 24-hour care, they may be placed in a memory-care unit of a long-term care or assisted-living facility.

Teach the family how to be prepared in case the patient becomes restless, agitated, abusive, or combative. In addition, the family can learn how to use reality orientation or validation therapy, depending on the stage of the disease.

Self-Management Education. Usually patients with AD and dementia are cared for in the home until late in the disease process unless they can afford private-pay care. Because health insurance coverage in the United States and family finances may not be sufficient to cover the services of a private duty nurse or home care aide, family members typically provide the care. The patient plan of care developed by the nurse or case manager, in conjunction with the family, must be reasonable and realistic for the family to implement.

Provide information to the family on what to do in the event of a seizure and how to protect the patient from injury. Instruct them to notify the primary health care provider if the seizure is prolonged or if the patient's seizure pattern changes.

Review with the family or other caregiver the name, time, and route of administration; the dosage; and the side effects of all drugs. Remind the family to check with the health care provider before using any over-the-counter drugs or herbs because they may interact with prescribed drug therapy.

Emphasis is placed on the need for the patient to have an established exercise program to maintain ***mobility*** for as long as possible and to prevent complications of immobility. In collaboration with the family, the physical therapist (PT) may develop an individualized exercise program. The PT may continue to work with the patient at home until goals are achieved, depending on the payer source.

Remind the family or other caregiver to take special precautions to maintain the patient safely at home. The environment must be uncluttered, consistent, and structured. All hazardous items (e.g., cooking range and oven, power tools) are removed, secured, or "locked out." All electrical sockets not in use should be covered with safety plugs. Teach families to install handrails and grab bars in the bathroom. Handrails should be along all stairways, and a guardrail should be placed around porches or open stairwells. Because the patient may have a tendency to wander, especially at night, the family may want to install alarms to all outside doors, the basement, and the patient's bedroom. All outside and basement doors should have deadbolt locks to prevent the patient from going outside unsupervised. Remind the family to adjust the temperature of the water to prevent accidental burns. Nightlights should be used in the patient's bedroom, hallway, and bathroom to prevent fear and to help with orientation.

Health Care Resources. Refer all families to their local chapter of the Alzheimer's Association (www.alz.org) in the United States or to the Alzheimer Society of Canada (www.alzheimer.ca). These organizations provide information and support services to patients and their families, including seminars, audiovisual aids, and publications. In most locations, caregiver telephone or email support is available.

Teach the family to enroll the patient in the Safe Return Program, a U.S. government-funded program of the Alzheimer's Association that assists in the identification and safe, timely return of people with dementia. The program includes registration of the patient and a 24-hour hotline to be called to assist in finding a lost patient. If a patient wanders and becomes lost, the family (or health care institution) should immediately notify the police department. An up-to-date picture of the patient makes it easier for local authorities, the public, and neighbors to identify the missing patient. Devices using radio-wave beacons and a global positioning system (GPS) have been developed to help families and law enforcement officials find a lost patient more easily. These devices include shoes with a GPS unit implanted, jewelry that is hard to remove, and bracelets. Caution families that these devices are not foolproof. Just like cell phones, there are some areas where the signal from the patient may not be picked up easily if at all.

When the patient can no longer be cared for at home, referral to an assisted-living or long-term care facility may be needed. Early in the course of the disease, advise the family that placement might be needed in the late stages of the disease or sooner. This allows the family to begin to search for an appropriate facility before a crisis develops and immediate placement is needed. The national office of the Alzheimer's Association publishes an outline of criteria for a memory-care unit. In the advanced stage of the disease, the patient may need referral to palliative and hospice services for total care. (See the discussion of end-of-life and hospice care in Chapter 8.)

PATIENT-CENTERED CARE: VETERANS HEALTH CONSIDERATIONS (QSEN)

For veterans who have AD, help families locate the closest Veterans Administration (VA) for support and services. Services may include home-based primary care, homemaker and home health aides, respite care, adult day health care, outpatient clinics, inpatient hospital services, nursing home, or hospice care. Caregiver support is an essential part of all of these services.

◆ **Evaluation: Evaluate Outcomes.** Evaluate the care of the patient with AD based on the identified priority patient problems. The expected outcomes include that the patient and/or family will:

- Maintain memory and ***cognition*** for as long as possible and increase their quality of life
- Remain free from injury and accidents and have a safe environment
- Manage caregiver stress and strain to prevent elder abuse

MOBILITY CONCEPT EXEMPLAR: PARKINSON DISEASE

Pathophysiology Review

Parkinson disease (PD), also referred to as *Parkinson's disease* and *paralysis agitans,* is a progressive neurodegenerative disease that is one of the most common neurologic disorders of older adults. It is a debilitating disease affecting ***mobility*** and is characterized by four cardinal symptoms: tremor, muscle rigidity, **bradykinesia** or **akinesia** (slow movement/no movement), and postural instability. Changes in ***cognition,*** including dementia and psychoses, can occur in some patients with late-stage PD.

Young and middle-age adults with these signs and symptoms may be misdiagnosed as having **Huntington disease**, a rare hereditary disorder that is characterized by progressive dementia and choreiform movements (uncontrollable rapid, jerky movements) in the limbs, trunk, and facial muscles. Table 39.3 briefly compares Parkinson and Huntington diseases.

Most people have *primary,* or idiopathic, disease. A few patients have *secondary* parkinsonian symptoms from conditions such as brain tumors and certain antipsychotic drugs.

Normally, motor activity occurs as a result of integrating the actions of the cerebral cortex, basal ganglia, and cerebellum. The basal ganglia are a group of neurons located deep within the cerebrum at the base of the brain near the lateral ventricles. When the basal ganglia are stimulated, muscle tone in the body is inhibited and voluntary movements are refined. The secretion of two major neurotransmitters accomplishes this process: dopamine and acetylcholine (ACh).

Dopamine is produced in the substantia nigra and the adrenal glands and is transmitted to the basal ganglia along a connecting neural pathway for secretion when needed. *ACh* is produced and secreted by the basal ganglia and in the nerve endings in the

TABLE 39.3 Comparison of Parkinson Disease and Huntington Disease

	Parkinson Disease	Huntington Disease
Cause	*Primary disease:* Cause not known, but could be a combination of genetic and environmental factors *Secondary disease:* Caused by antipsychotic drugs or another condition such as brain tumor or trauma	Hereditary disease transmitted by an autosomal-dominant trait at conception
Pathophysiologic changes	Chronic, terminal disease caused by degeneration of substantia nigra cells in the basal ganglia of the brain causing decreased dopamine, which normally functions to promote voluntary muscle and sympathetic nervous system control	Chronic, terminal disease caused by alterations in amounts of dopamine, gamma-aminobutyric acid (GABA), and glutamate from the basal ganglia
Course of disease	Steady and gradual decline (typically 10-20 years) of cognitive, mobility, and ADL function from mild through severe stages; patients usually die from complications of immobility	Gradual decline (typically about 15 years) of cognitive and neuromuscular symptoms; characterized by progressive dementia and choreiform movements (uncontrollable rapid, jerky movements) in the limbs, trunk, and facial muscles; patients usually die from complications of impaired ***mobility***
Risk factors	**Primary:** Male Over 40 years of age Family history (particularly first-degree relatives (e.g., parent, sibling) **Secondary:** Traumatic brain injury Brain tumor or other lesion	Dominant inheritance 30-50 years of age equally in men and women (when symptoms typically begin)
Management	Safety measures to prevent injury or falls Anti-Parkinson drugs Symptom management ADL and mobility assistance as needed based on stage	Safety measures to prevent injury or falls Supportive care Behavior management ADL and mobility assistance as needed based on stage

periphery of the body. ACh-producing neurons transmit *excitatory* messages throughout the basal ganglia. Dopamine *inhibits* the function of these neurons, allowing control over voluntary movement. This usual system of checks and balances usually allows for refined, coordinated movement, such as picking up a pencil and writing.

In PD, widespread degeneration of the *substantia nigra* leads to a decrease in the amount of dopamine in the brain. When dopamine levels are decreased to 70% to 80% of usual levels, a person becomes symptomatic and loses the ability to refine voluntary movement (Vacca, 2019). The large numbers of excitatory ACh-secreting neurons remain active, creating an imbalance between excitatory and inhibitory neuronal activity. The resulting excessive excitation of neurons prevents a person from controlling or initiating voluntary movement (McCance et al., 2019).

PD interferes with movement as a result of dopamine loss in the brain, but it also reduces the sympathetic nervous system influence on the heart, blood vessels, and other areas of the body. This loss results in the orthostatic hypotension, drooling, nocturia (voiding at night), and other autonomic symptoms frequently seen in the patient with PD.

PD is separated into stages according to the symptoms and degree of disability. Stage 1 is mild disease with unilateral limb involvement, whereas the patient with stage 5 disease is completely dependent in all ADLs. Other classifications refer simply to mild, moderate, and severe disease (Box 39.1).

BOX 39.1 Stages of Parkinson Disease

Stage 1: Initial Stage
- Unilateral limb involvement
- Minimal weakness
- Hand and arm trembling

Stage 2: Mild Stage
- Bilateral limb involvement
- Masklike face
- Slow, shuffling gait

Stage 3: Moderate Disease
- Postural instability
- Increased gait disturbances

Stage 4: Severe Disability
- Akinesia
- Rigidity

Stage 5: Complete ADL Dependence

Etiology and Genetic Risk. Although the exact cause of PD is not known, it is probably the result of environmental and genetic factors. Exposure to pesticides, herbicides, and industrial chemicals and metals and being older than 40 years are known risk factors for the development of PD.

Primary Parkinson disease (PD) often has a familial tendency. The disease is associated with a variety of mitochondrial DNA (mtDNA) variations that often involve deletions in the genetic sequences that are used in central nervous system (CNS) mitochondria, the energy powerhouses of cells. These variations ultimately cause destruction of neurons that produce dopamine in the substantia nigra (McCance et al., 2019).

Incidence and Prevalence. In the United States, about 60,000 new cases of PD are diagnosed each year, most in people older than 50 years of age. As many as 1 million patients live with the disease. As the population ages, the number of people affected by PD is expected to dramatically increase. About 50% more men than women currently have the disease, but the exact reason for this difference is not known (Parkinson's Foundation, 2019).

❖ Interprofessional Collaborative Care

◆ Assessment: Recognize Cues

History. Collect data related to the time and progression of symptoms noticed by the patient or family. The older adult may assume that these behaviors are normal changes associated with aging and therefore ignore early signs and symptoms such as *resting* tremors, bradykinesia, fatigue, and problems with muscular rigidity.

Physical Assessment/Signs and Symptoms. In Stage 1 of Parkinson disease (PD), unilateral resting tremors are usually noticed in one arm. Slow voluntary movements and reduced automatic movements may also occur. In Stage 2, signs and symptoms begin to worsen and become bilateral. In mid-stage PD (Stage 3), loss of balance and slow movement (bradykinesia) occur and the patient is at higher risk for falls (Vacca, 2019). Some patients report "freezing" because they feel that they are stuck to the floor. Assess the patient for *rigidity,* or resistance to passive movement of the extremities. Rigidity is present early in the disease process and progresses over time. Observe the patient's ability to relax a muscle or move a selected muscle group. Observe the patient's gait, posture (often unstable), and ability to ambulate with or without ambulatory aids.

Due to increased muscle stiffness, patients in Stage 4 require a walker to ambulate and assistance with ADLs (Vacca, 2019). Changes in facial expression or a *masklike face* with wide-open, fixed, staring eyes is caused by rigidity of the facial muscles (Fig. 39.1). In late-stage advanced disease, or Stage 5, this rigidity can lead to difficulties in chewing and swallowing, particularly if the pharyngeal muscles are involved. As a result, the patient may have inadequate nutrition. Uncontrolled drooling may occur. Some patients develop dementia later as the disease progresses and can experience psychotic events, such as delusions, paranoia, and/or hallucinations. In addition to changes in voluntary movement, many patients experience autonomic nervous system symptoms, such as excessive perspiration and orthostatic hypotension. Orthostatic hypotension is likely related to loss of sympathetic innervation in the heart and blood vessel response.

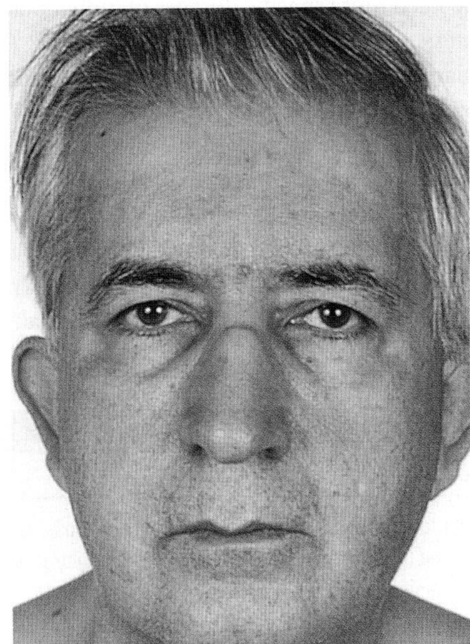

Fig. 39.1 The masklike facial expression typical of patients with Parkinson disease.

Patients can also develop emotional changes such as depression, irritability, apathy, anxiety, and insecurity. These symptoms may develop because patients fear that they will not be able to cope with new situations.

Changes in speech pattern are common in PD patients. They may speak very softly, slur or repeat their words, use a monotone voice or a halting speech, hesitate before speaking, or exhibit a rapid speech pattern.

Bowel and bladder problems are commonly seen in PD as a result of malfunction of the autonomic nervous system, which regulates smooth muscle activity. Patients can exhibit symptoms of either urinary incontinence or difficulty urinating. Constipation can occur because of slow motility of the GI tract, lack of adequate nutritional and fluid intake, and/or impaired ***mobility***.

Laboratory and Imaging Assessment. The diagnosis of PD is made based on clinical findings after other neurologic diseases are eliminated as possibilities. There are no specific diagnostic tests. Analysis of cerebrospinal fluid (CSF) may show a decrease in dopamine levels, although the results of other studies are usually normal. Other diagnostic tests may be done, such as a single-photon emission computed tomography (SPECT), to rule out other CNS health problems. A SPECT can also detect a loss of dopamine-producing neurons. Diffusion-weighted imaging is a type of MRI that can differentiate PD from other types of neurodegenerative disorders (Vacca, 2019).

A newer imaging test called a dopamine transporter (DaT) scan may be performed via SPECT to confirm abnormalities in dopamine transmission in the basal ganglia. This scan uses a radioactive agent that binds to DaT proteins in the substantia nigra and is used to monitor neuronal degeneration (Vacca, 2019).

◆ Analysis: Analyze Cues and Prioritize Hypotheses. The priority collaborative problems for patients with PD include:

1. Decreased ***mobility*** (and possible self-care deficit) due to muscle rigidity, resting tremors, and postural/gait changes
2. Impaired ***cognition*** due to neurotransmitter changes in the brain

◆ Planning and Implementation: Generate Solutions and Take Action

Promoting Mobility

Planning: Expected Outcomes. The expected outcome is that the patient will maintain optimal ***mobility*** to promote safety and not experience complications of decreased ***mobility***.

Interventions

Nonsurgical Management. Care for the patient with PD includes drug therapy, exercise programs or physical therapy,

BEST PRACTICE FOR PATIENT SAFETY & QUALITY CARE (QSEN)

Care of the Patient With Parkinson Disease

- Allow the patient extra time to respond to questions.
- Administer medications promptly on schedule to maintain continuous therapeutic drug levels.
- Provide drug therapy for pain and/or tingling in limbs, as needed.
- Monitor for drug side effects, especially orthostatic hypotension, hallucinations, and acute confusional state (delirium).
- Place the patient on Fall Precautions according to agency protocol.
- Collaborate with physical and occupational therapists to keep the patient as mobile and independent as possible in ADLs.
- Allow the patient time to perform ADLs and *mobility* skills; provide assistance only as needed.
- Implement interventions to prevent complications of impaired *mobility*, such as constipation, pressure injuries, and contractures.
- Schedule appointments and activities late in the morning to prevent rushing the patient or schedule them at the time of the patient's optimal level of functioning.
- Teach the patient to speak slowly and clearly. Use alternative communication methods, such as a communication board or handheld mobile device. Refer to the speech-language pathologist.
- Monitor the patient's ability to eat and swallow. Monitor actual food and fluid intake.
- Collaborate with the registered dietitian nutritionist to provide high-protein, high-calorie foods or supplements to maintain weight.
- Recognize that Parkinson disease can affect the patient's self-esteem. Focus on the patient's strengths.
- Assess for depression, anxiety, and impaired *cognition*.
- Assess for insomnia or sleeplessness.

and interprofessional collaboration to promote ***mobility*** and self-care and prevent falls or other injuries. The Best Practice for Patient Safety & Quality Care: Care of the Patient With Parkinson Disease box summarizes best practices for nursing management of the patient with PD.

Drug therapy. Drugs are prescribed to treat the symptoms of PD with the purpose of increasing the patient's ***mobility*** and self-care abilities. An equally important desired outcome is that drugs used for the disease have minimal long-term side effects. Many controversies remain about which drugs to use, when to start therapy, and how to prevent complications. Drug administration is closely monitored, and the primary health care provider adjusts the dosage or changes therapy as the patient's condition requires. Teach the patient and family how to monitor for and report adverse effects of drug therapy.

Dopamine agonists mimic dopamine by stimulating dopamine receptors in the brain. They are typically the most effective during the first 3 to 5 years of use. The benefit of these agents is fewer incidents of dyskinesias (problems with movement) and "wearing off" phenomenon (loss of response to the drug) when compared with other drugs. This problem is characterized by periods of good mobility ("on" periods) alternating with periods of altered ***mobility*** ("off" periods). Patients report that their most distressing symptom is the "off time."

Examples of dopamine agonists are apomorphine (a morphine derivative), pramipexol, and ropinirole. Another drug in

! NURSING SAFETY PRIORITY (QSEN)

Drug Alert

Dopamine agonists are associated with adverse effects, such as orthostatic (postural) hypotension, hallucinations, sleepiness, and drowsiness, and can be mistaken for signs and symptoms of PD. Remind patients to avoid operating heavy machinery or driving if they have any of these symptoms. Teach them to change from a lying or sitting position to standing by moving slowly. The primary health care provider should not prescribe drugs in this class to older adults because of their severe adverse drug effects.

this class, rotigotine, is available as a continuous transdermal patch to maintain a consistent level of dopamine.

Almost all patients are on levodopa or a combination *levodopa-carbidopa* drug at some point in their disease. It may be the initial drug of choice if the patient's presenting symptoms are severe or interfere with daily life. Both an immediate-release (IR) and controlled-release (CR) form in varying doses are available. Levodopa agents are less expensive than dopamine agonists and are better at improving motor function. An inhaled form of levodopa has been approved recently for "off" periods (Parkinson's Foundation, 2019). Safinamide is an adjunct drug to levodopa combination agents when these drugs do not work alone.

Long-term use of levodopa preparations can lead to **dyskinesia** (inability to perform voluntary movement). Teach the patient and family to give the drug before meals to increase absorption and transport across the blood-brain barrier. Keep in mind that long-term use of levodopa preparations can cause the same adverse effects as dopamine agonists, including orthostatic hypotension and psychotic episodes.

Catechol O–methyltransferases (COMTs) are enzymes that inactivate dopamine. Therefore COMT *inhibitors* block this enzyme activity, thus prolonging the action of levodopa. One example is entacapone, which is often used in combination with levodopa. The benefit of these combinations is that the disease is treated in several ways with one drug. However, they are not beneficial for patients who need more specific dosages of individual drugs.

Monoamine oxidase type B (MAO-B) inhibitors (MAOIs) are more popular for use in patients with early or mild symptoms of PD. Entacapone and selegiline are often given with levodopa for early or mild disease. A newer MAOI-B for PD is rasagiline mesylate, which can be given as a single drug or with levodopa. The MAOI-B drugs work by slowing the main type (B) of monoamine oxidase in the brain, increasing dopamine concentrations, and helping reduce the signs and symptoms of PD. They may also protect neurons in the brain (Burchum & Rosenthal, 2019).

! NURSING SAFETY PRIORITY (QSEN)

Drug Alert

Teach patients taking MAOIs about the need to avoid foods, beverages, and drugs that contain tyramine, including cheese and aged, smoked, or cured foods and sausage. Remind them to also avoid red wine and beer to prevent severe headache and life-threatening hypertension (Burchum & Rosenthal, 2019). Patients should continue these restrictions for 14 days after the drug is discontinued.

When other drugs are no longer effective, bromocriptine mesylate, a *dopamine receptor agonist,* may be prescribed to promote the release of dopamine. It may be used alone or in combination with carbidopa/levodopa. Some providers may prescribe bromocriptine early in the course of treatment. It is especially useful in the patient who has experienced side effects such as dyskinesias or orthostatic hypotension while receiving levodopa or a combination drug.

Amantadine is an *antiviral drug* that has anti-Parkinson benefits. It may be given early in disease to reduce symptoms. It is also prescribed with levodopa-carbidopa preparations to reduce dyskinesias. Rivastigmine is a *cholinesterase inhibitor* that is used only when patients with PD have dementia. This drug works to improve the transmission of acetylcholine in the brain by delaying its destruction by the enzyme *acetylcholinesterase.*

For severe motor symptoms such as tremors and rigidity, one of the older *anticholinergic* drugs may be prescribed, but they are rarely used as primary drugs of choice for PD. Examples are benztropine, trihexyphenidyl HCl, and procyclidine. *These drugs should be avoided in older adults because they can cause acute confusion, urinary retention, constipation, dry mouth, and blurred vision. Newer and safer drugs are available for this age-group.*

A recently approved drug for PD during "off times" is istradefylline, an adenosine A2A antagonist. This drug blocks the release of adenosine in the brain, triggering dopamine signals, and is used when other drug classes are ineffective in controlling PD signs and symptoms.

For the patient on any long-term drug therapy regimen, drug tolerance or *drug toxicity* often develops. Drug toxicity may be evidenced by changes in ***cognition*** such as delirium (acute confusion) or hallucinations and decreased effectiveness of the drug. Delirium may be difficult to assess in the patient who is already suffering from chronic dementia as a result of PD or another disease. If possible, compare the patient's current cognitive and behavioral status with his or her baseline before drug therapy begins.

When drug tolerance is reached, the drug's effects do not last as long as previously. The treatment of PD drug toxicity or tolerance includes:

- A reduction in drug dosage
- A change of drug or in the frequency of administration
- A drug holiday (particularly with levodopa therapy)

During a *drug holiday,* which typically lasts up to 10 days, the patient receives no drug therapy for PD. Carefully monitor the patient for symptoms of PD during this time and document assessment findings.

Many patients are on additional drugs to help relieve symptoms associated with the disease. For example, muscle spasms may be relieved by baclofen, drooling can be minimized by sublingual atropine sulfate, and insomnia may require a sleeping aid such as zolpidem tartrate.

Medical marijuana. Medical marijuana, also called cannabis, has been legalized in Canada and most states in the United States. Although there is inadequate evidence that medical marijuana is effective in managing symptoms associated with PD, many patients report its ability to help relieve tremors, dyskinesias, pain, insomnia, and depression (Maxwell & Farmer, 2018). Large studies are needed to provide strong evidence that marijuana is an appropriate drug to prescribe to patients with PD.

Other interventions. *A freezing gait and postural instability are major problems for patients with PD.* Nontraditional exercise programs, such as yoga and tai chi, may help elevate mood and improve ***mobility*** in the early stage of the disease. Early in the disease process, collaborate with physical and occupational therapists to plan and implement a program to keep the patient flexible, prevent falling, and retain mobility by incorporating active and passive range-of-motion (ROM) exercises, muscle stretching, and out-of-bed activity. Remind the patient to avoid concentrating on his or her feet when walking to prevent falls. *If the patient is hospitalized for any reason, be sure that he or she is placed on Fall Precautions according to agency policy.*

In collaboration with the rehabilitation team, encourage the patient to participate as much as possible in self-management, including ADLs. The team makes the environment conducive to independence in activity and as stress free and safe as possible. Occupational and physical therapists provide training in ADLs and the use of adaptive devices, as needed, to facilitate independence. The occupational therapist (OT) evaluates the patient for the need for adaptive devices (e.g., special utensils for eating).

Patients with PD tend to not sleep well at night because of drug therapy and the disease itself. Some patients nap for short periods during the day and may not be aware that they have done so. This sleep misperception may put the patient at risk for injury. For example, he or she may fall asleep while driving an automobile. Therefore teach the patient and family to monitor the patient's sleeping pattern and discuss whether he or she can operate machinery or perform other potentially high-risk tasks safely.

Collaborate with the registered dietitian nutritionist, if needed, to evaluate the patient's food intake and ability to eat. The patient's intake of nutrients is evaluated, especially in the patient who has difficulty swallowing or is susceptible to injury from falling. The dietitian considers the patient's bowel habits and adjusts the diet if constipation occurs. If the patient has trouble swallowing, collaborate with the speech-language pathologist (SLP) for an extensive swallowing evaluation. Based on these findings and the patient interview, an individualized nutritional plan is developed. Usually a soft diet and thick, cold fluids, such as milk shakes, are tolerated more easily.

Small, frequent meals or a commercial powder, such as Thick-It, added to liquids may assist the patient who has difficulty swallowing. Elevate the patient's head to allow easier swallowing and prevent aspiration. Remind AP and teach the family to be careful when serving or feeding the patient. The SLP can be very helpful in recommending specific feeding strategies. Be sure that AP record food intake daily or as needed. The patient often loses weight because of altered food intake and the increased number of calories burned secondary to muscle rigidity. Teach the family to weigh the patient once a week so that adjustments to the diet can be made as indicated. As the disease progresses and swallowing becomes more of a problem, supplemental feedings become the main source of nutrition to maintain weight, with meals and other foods taken as the patient can tolerate.

Collaborate with the SLP if the patient has speech difficulties. Together with the interprofessional health care team, patient, and family, develop a communication plan. The SLP teaches exercises to strengthen muscles used for breathing, speech, and swallowing. Remind the patient to speak slowly and clearly and to pause and take deep breaths at times during each sentence. Teach the family the importance of avoiding unnecessary environmental noise to increase the listener's ability to hear and understand the patient. Ask the patient to repeat words that the listener does not understand. Have the listener watch the patient's lips and nonverbal expressions for cues to the meaning of conversation. Remind the patient to organize his or her thoughts before speaking and use facial expression and gestures, if possible, to assist with communication. In addition, he or she should exaggerate words to increase the listener's ability to understand. If the patient cannot communicate verbally, he or she can use alternative methods of communication, such as a communication board, mechanical voice synthesizer, computer, or handheld mobile device. The SLP assesses the ability to use these devices before a decision is made about which method to use. Some older patients may not want to use electronic methods to communicate.

NCLEX EXAMINATION CHALLENGE 39.3

Physiological Integrity

The nurse is preparing to teach a client who has been prescribed a levodopa-carbidopa preparation for Parkinson disease. What health teaching will the nurse include for the client and family? **Select all that apply.**

A. "Move slowly when changing positions from sitting to standing."
B. "Take your medication after meals to help prevent nausea."
C. "Report any hallucinations that the client may have."
D. "Note any changes in mental or emotional status."
E. "Pay attention to whether your tremors improve or worsen."

Surgical Management. Several options are available if surgery for the patient with PD is needed. Surgery is a last resort when drugs are not effective in symptom management. The most common surgeries are stereotactic pallidotomy and deep brain stimulation, although newer surgical procedures are being tried. Deep brain stimulation has largely replaced the older thalamotomy procedure.

Stereotactic pallidotomy (opening into the pallidum within the corpus striatum) can be a very effective treatment for controlling the symptoms associated with PD. First, the target area within the pallidum is identified by a CT or MRI scan. Next, the stereotactic head frame is placed on the patient. IV sedation is given, and a burr hole is made into the cranium. An electrode or cylindric rod is inserted into the target area. The target area receives a mild electrical stimulation, and the patient's reaction is assessed for reduction of tremor and rigidity. If this result does not occur or if unexpected visual, motor, or sensory symptoms appear, the probe is repositioned. When the probe is in the ideal location, a permanent lesion (scarring) is made to destroy the tissue. The patient is monitored in the postanesthesia care unit (PACU) for about 1 hour and is then returned to the inpatient unit for continuing observation.

Deep brain stimulation (DBS) is approved as a treatment for PD. In DBS, electrodes are implanted into the brain and connected to a small electrical device called a *pulse generator* that delivers electrical current. The generator is placed under the skin similar to a cardiac pacemaker device. It is externally programmed to deliver an electrical current to decrease involuntary movements known as dyskinesias, resulting in a reduced need for levodopa and related drugs. DBS also helps to alleviate fluctuations of symptoms and reduce tremors, slowness of movements, and gait problems (National Institute of Neurological Disorders and Stroke [NINDS], 2019).

Fetal tissue transplantation is an experimental and highly controversial ethical and political treatment. Fetal substantia nigra tissue, either human or pig, is transplanted into the caudate nucleus of the brain. Preliminary reports suggest that patients show clinical improvement in motor symptoms without dyskinesias after receiving the transplanted tissue. Long-term results are yet to be seen or studied (NINDS, 2019).

Managing Cognitive Dysfunction

Planning: Expected Outcomes. The expected outcome is that the patient with PD will maintain memory and ***cognition*** for as long as possible. For patients experiencing cognitive dysfunction, the expected outcome is to keep them safe and increase their quality of life.

Interventions. About 50% of patients with PD have cognitive dysfunction. Pimavanserin is a new drug that is only used for Parkinson disease–related hallucinations and delusions (psychoses).

! NURSING SAFETY PRIORITY QSEN

Drug Alert

Patients who have been diagnosed with cardiac dysrhythmias should not take pimavanserin because it can prolong the Q-T interval. Teach patients and their families to report any irregular heart rhythm to their primary health care provider immediately. In addition, the concurrent use of strong CYP3A4 inhibitors, such as ketoconazole, clarithromycin, and itraconazole, can increase the activity of pimavanserin. In this case, the primary health care provider should prescribe pimavanserin in a very low dose.

Although not all patients with PD have dementia, impaired ***cognition*** and memory deficits are common. Some patients also experience changes in gait and tremors that are uncontrollable. In the late stages of the disease, they cannot move without assistance, have difficulty talking, have minimal facial expression, and may drool. Patients often state that they are embarrassed and tend to avoid social events or groups of people. They should not be forced into situations in which they feel ashamed of their appearance. Many patients become depressed as a result of their disease. If patients are moderately to severely depressed, an antidepressant such as short-acting venlafaxine may be prescribed.

A small qualitative study by Sjödahl Hammarlund et al. (2018) found that patients in the community with Parkinson disease identified four changes that resulted from their disease:

- Changing plans for managing day-to-day demands due to the unpredictability of the disease; some days they would experience fatigue, mood swings, or ***pain,*** which determined their physical functioning
- Loss of identify and dignity
- Compromised social participation
- Use of practical psychosocial strategies, including compensatory mechanisms and accepting support from family and others

Teach the family to emphasize the patient's abilities or strengths and provide positive reinforcement when he or she meets expected outcomes. The patient, family or significant other, and rehabilitation team mutually set realistic expected outcomes that can be achieved.

Care Coordination and Transition Management

Home Care Preparation. The long-term management of PD presents a special challenge in the home care setting. A case manager may be required to coordinate interprofessional care and provide support for the patient and family. Impaired ***mobility*** and ***cognition*** can affect the patient's daily lifestyle and self-concept, including sexuality. The case manager or home care nurse uses a holistic approach to ensure that both psychosocial and physical needs are addressed.

Self-Management Education. Teach patients and their families about the need to follow instructions regarding the safe administration of drug therapy. Remind them to immediately report adverse effects of medication such as dizziness, falls, acute confusion (delirium), and hallucinations. For patients who had surgery, review discharge instructions about when to resume activity and contact the surgeon.

Teach family members or other caregivers the importance of maintaining or improving the patient's quality of life by helping to alleviate or manage symptoms. For example, constipation can be prevented or managed by encouraging adequate fluids, a high-fiber diet, and a regular bowel-training program with suppositories and bulk-forming laxatives. Sleep disorders may be managed with a good sleep-hygiene program, including avoiding alcohol and caffeine, darkening the bedroom, and bedtime rituals.

Neuropsychiatric health problems, such as impulse control disorders, altered ***cognition,*** anxiety, and depression can be very difficult for both the patient and family. Remind families and other caregivers that the patient cannot control these symptoms. Caregiver role strain can be a major problem when caring for patients with PD (see earlier discussion under Alzheimer's disease for caregiver stress management).

Health Care Resources. Collaborate with the social worker or case manager to help the family with financial and health insurance issues, as well as respite care or permanent placement if needed. Refer the patient and family to social and state agencies, support groups, and information as needed. Examples in the United States are the National Parkinson Foundation (www.parkinson.org), American Parkinson Disease Association (www.apdaparkinson.org), and the Parkinson Disease Foundation (www.pdf.org). The Michael J. Fox Foundation for Parkinson's Research (www.michaeljfox.org) provides an extensive list of resources about living with PD. Patients and families in Canada can access Parkinson Canada (www.parkinson.ca) for information about the disease and support groups.

As the disease progresses and drug effectiveness decreases, refer the family to a palliative care organization or hospice. Referral sources can be obtained from the Center to Advance Palliative Care (www.capc.org), which advocates applying the principles of palliative care to chronic disease. Chapter 8 discusses palliative and hospice care in detail.

CLINICAL JUDGMENT CHALLENGE 39.1

Patient-Centered Care; Safety QSEN

A 78-year-old man who has had Parkinson disease (PD) for over 15 years is admitted to the emergency department. His wife and caretaker states that he fell after trying to stand up from a chair because he refused to use his walker. He has several new and older bruises on both arms. Although his wife indicates that he can communicate and does not have dementia, he seems reluctant to answer the nurse's questions. His admission data include:

- Oral temperature = 98° F (36.7° C)
- Pulse = 90 beats/min
- Respiratory rate = 18
- Blood pressure (reclined position) = 98/50
- Oxygen saturation = 94%
- Resting hand tremors of both arms, right worse than left
- Facial expressions stay constant when communicating
- When asked about whether he has been abused, patient refuses to answer
- Stated that he got dizzy at home when he stood up
- Is currently taking levodopa-carbidopa 25-100 mg XR twice a day for PD
- One episode last week of seeing bugs crawl on a vase (but no bugs were actually there) (no history of hallucinations before that event)

1. **Recognize Cues:** What assessment information in this client situation is the most important and immediate concern for the nurse? (Hint: Identify the **relevant** information *first* to determine what is most important.)
2. **Analyze Cues:** What client conditions are consistent with the **most relevant** information? (Hint: Think about priority collaborative problems that support and contradict the information presented in this situation.)
3. **Prioritize Hypotheses:** Which possibilities or explanations are **most likely** to be present in this client situation? Which possibilities or explanations are the most serious? (Hint: Consider all possibilities and determine their urgency and risk for this client.)
4. **Generate Solutions:** What actions would most likely achieve the desired outcomes for this client? Which actions should be **avoided** or are **potentially harmful**? (Hint: Determine the desired outcomes first to decide which interventions are appropriate and those that should be avoided.)
5. **Take Action:** Which actions are the most appropriate and how should they be implemented? In what **priority order** should they be implemented? (Hint: Consider health teaching, documentation, requested health care provider orders or prescriptions, nursing skills, collaboration with or referral to health team members, etc.)
6. **Evaluate Outcomes:** What client assessment would indicate that the nurse's actions were **effective**? (Hint: Think about signs that would indicate an improvement, decline, or unchanged client condition.)

◆ **Evaluation: Evaluate Outcomes.** Evaluate the care of the patient with PD based on the identified priority patient problems. The expected outcomes include that the patient and/or family will:

- Improve ***mobility*** to provide self-care and not experience complications of impaired mobility
- Maintain safety and an acceptable quality of life

MIGRAINE HEADACHE

Pathophysiology Review

Most individuals experience some type of headache during their lifetime from a variety of causes, such as low blood sugar, sinus infection, alcohol, and stress. These headaches are acute and temporary and often resolve by managing the cause of the headache and/or mild analgesics such as acetaminophen. Some adults have specific types of headache that cause severe, debilitating ***pain*** and recur. The most common type is migraine headache. This type of headache is most likely to affect quality of life when compared with other less common types.

A **migraine headache** is a common clinical syndrome characterized by recurrent episodic attacks of head pain that serve no protective purpose. Migraine headache ***pain*** is usually described as throbbing and unilateral. Migraines are often accompanied by associated symptoms such as nausea or sensitivity to light, sound, or head movement and can last 4 to 72 hours. They tend to be familial, and women are affected more commonly than men. Women diagnosed with migraines are more likely to have major depressive disorder. Migraine sufferers are also at risk for stroke and epilepsy (McCance et al., 2019).

The cause of migraine headaches is not clear but includes a combination of neuronal hyperexcitability and vascular, genetic, hormonal, and environmental factors. In general, experts suggest that migraines are a neurogenic process with secondary cerebral vasodilation followed by a sterile brain tissue inflammation. Patients may inherit a condition of neuronal hyperexcitability from ion channel variations, particularly calcium and sodium-potassium pump channels, as well as from genetic variations in serotonin and dopamine receptors. Following stimulation of these hyperexcitable neuronal pathways, vascular changes occur. Pain-sensing cells in the blood vessels of the brain initiate the attack. Activation of the trigeminal nerve pathways contributes to the cascade of events that activate nociceptors. Substances that increase sensitivity to pain such as glutamate are synthesized through the trigeminal pathway (McCance et al., 2019). As cerebral arteries dilate, prostaglandins are released (chemicals that cause inflammation and swelling). Vasodilation, in turn, allows prostaglandins and other intravascular molecules to leak (extravasate), contributing to widespread tissue swelling and the sensation of throbbing pain.

Many patients find that certain factors, or *triggers,* such as caffeine, red wine, and monosodium glutamate (MSG), tend to cause migraine headache attacks. Each patient is different regarding which environmental factors trigger headaches. For some patients, high-intensity light, stress, excessive fatigue, or a change in weather can lead to an attack. These stimuli are thought to initiate the cascade of events that cause migraines by activating hyperexcitable neurons. Neurons involved in the initiation and propagation of migraines may have an early sensitization to neurotransmitters such that patients become increasingly susceptible to triggers and to the cascade of events that culminate in migraine pain. Thus care includes not only managing pain but also disrupting the migraine cascade to decrease sensitization and recurrent attacks.

❖ Interprofessional Collaborative Care

◆ Assessment: Recognize Cues. Migraines fall into three categories: migraines with aura, migraines without aura, and atypical migraines. An **aura** is a sensation (e.g., visual changes) that signals the onset of a migraine headache or seizure. In a migraine, the aura occurs immediately before the migraine episode. *Most headaches are migraines without aura.* The key features of migraines are listed by stage in the Key Features: Migraine Headaches box.

KEY FEATURES
Migraine Headaches

Phases of Migraine With Aura (Classic Migraine)

First, or Prodromal, Phase

- Aura that develops over a period of several minutes and lasts no longer than 1 hour
- Well-defined transient focal neurologic dysfunction
- Pain may be preceded by:
  - Visual disturbances
  - Flashing lights
  - Lines or spots
  - Shimmering or zigzag lights
- A variety of neurologic changes, including:
  - Numbness, tingling of the lips or tongue
  - Acute confusional state
  - Aphasia
  - Vertigo
  - Unilateral weakness
  - Drowsiness

Second Phase

- Headache accompanied by nausea and vomiting
- Unilateral, frontotemporal, *throbbing* pain in the head that is often worse behind one eye or ear within an hour

Third Phase

- Pain changing from throbbing to dull
- Headache, nausea, and vomiting usually lasting from 4 to 72 hours (Older patients may have aura without pain, known as a *visual migraine.*)

Migraine Without Aura (Common Migraine)

- Migraine beginning without an aura before the onset of the headache
- Pain aggravated by performing routine physical activities
- Pain that is unilateral and pulsating
- One of these symptoms is present:
  - Nausea and/or vomiting
  - **Photophobia** (light sensitivity)
  - **Phonophobia** (sound sensitivity)
  - Headache lasting 4 to 72 hours
  - Migraine often occurring in the early morning, during periods of stress, or in those with premenstrual tension or fluid retention

Atypical Migraine

- Status migrainosus:
  - Headache lasting longer than 72 hours
- Migrainous infarction:
  - Neurologic symptoms not completely reversible within 7 days
  - Ischemic infarct noted on neuroimaging
- Unclassified:
  - Headache not fulfilling all of the criteria to be classified a migraine

The diagnosis of migraine headache is based on the patient's history and on physical, neurologic, and psychological assessment. Patients tend to have the same signs and symptoms each time they have a migraine headache. Some may have to refrain from regular activities for several days if they cannot control or relieve the ***pain*** in its early stage.

Neuroimaging such as MRI may be indicated if a migrainous infarction is suspected or if the patient has other neurologic findings, a history of seizures, findings not consistent with a migraine, or a change in the severity of the symptoms or frequency of the attacks. Neuroimaging is also recommended in patients older than 50 years with a new onset of headaches, especially women. Women with a history of migraines with visual symptoms may have an increased risk for stroke, particularly if a migraine with visual symptoms occurred in the past year. Teach women older than 50 years who have migraines about the risk factors for cardiovascular disease. *Encourage them or their family to call 911 if they experience symptoms such as facial drooping, arm weakness, or difficulties with speech!*

◆ **Interventions: Take Action.** *The priority for care of the patient having migraines is* ***pain*** *management.* This outcome may be achieved by abortive and preventive therapy. Drug therapy, trigger management, and complementary and integrative therapies are the major approaches to care. Provide detailed patient and family education regarding the collaborative plan of care. Effective health care provider/patient communication is increasingly important in managing the symptoms of migraines.

Abortive Therapy. Abortive therapy is aimed at alleviating ***pain*** during the aura phase (if present) or soon after the headache has started. Some of the drugs used have major side effects, contraindications, and nursing implications. The primary health care provider must consider any other medical conditions that the patient has when prescribing drug therapy. In general, the patient is started on a low dose that is increased until the desired clinical effect is obtained. Many new drugs are being investigated for this painful and often debilitating health problem.

Mild migraines may be relieved by acetaminophen (APAP). NSAIDs such as ibuprofen and naproxen may also be prescribed. In the United States and Canada, several over-the-counter (OTC) NSAID drugs combined with caffeine for migraines are available. Caffeine narrows blood vessels by blocking adenosine, which dilates vessels and increases inflammation. Antiemetics may be prescribed to relieve nausea and vomiting. Metoclopramide may be administered with NSAIDs to promote gastric emptying and decrease vomiting.

For more *severe* migraines, drugs such as triptans, ditans, ergotamine derivatives, and isometheptene combinations are often needed. A potential side effect of these drugs is *rebound* headache, also known as *medication overuse headache,* in which another headache occurs after the drug relieves the initial migraine.

Triptan preparations relieve the headache and associated symptoms by activating the 5-HT (serotonin) receptors on the cranial arteries, the basilar artery, and the blood vessels of the dura mater to produce a vasoconstrictive effect. Examples are sumatriptan, eletriptan, naratriptan, and almotriptan. The older drug sumatriptan is available as an oral agent, injection, and nasal spray (Burchum & Rosenthal, 2019). For many patients, these drugs are highly and quickly effective for pain, nausea, vomiting, and light and sound sensitivity with few side effects. However, sumatriptan is most likely to cause chest pain after one or more doses. Therefore most triptans are contraindicated in patients with actual or suspected ischemic heart disease, cerebrovascular ischemia, hypertension, and peripheral vascular disease and in those with Prinzmetal angina because of the potential for coronary vasospasm. Patients respond differently to drugs, and several types or combinations may be tried before the headache is relieved (Burchum & Rosenthal, 2019).

! NURSING SAFETY PRIORITY (QSEN)

Drug Alert

Teach patients taking triptan drugs to take them as soon as migraine symptoms develop. Instruct patients to report angina (chest pain) or chest discomfort to their primary health care providers immediately to prevent cardiac damage from myocardial ischemia. Remind them to use contraception (birth control) while taking the drugs because the drugs may not be safe for women who are pregnant. Teach them to expect common side effects that include flushing, tingling, and a hot sensation. These annoying sensations tend to subside after the patient's body gets used to the drug. Triptan drugs should not be taken with selective serotonin reuptake inhibitor (SSRI) antidepressants or St. John's wort, an herb used commonly for depression (Burchum & Rosenthal, 2019).

Ditans, such as the recently approved lasmiditan, are a newer group of abortive drugs that block only one specific serotonin receptor without constricting blood vessels. Therefore this class of drugs tends to be safer and work more effectively than triptans.

A new type of *calcitonin gene–related peptide receptor (CGRP-R) antagonist* is ubrogepant. This oral drug is used only for acute treatment of migraines and should not be taken with strong CYP3A4 inhibitors such as ketoconazole, itraconazole, and clarithromycin (Burchum & Rosenthal, 2019).

Ergotamine preparations such as Cafergot may be taken at the start of the headache. The patient may take up to six tablets in 24 hours or use a rectal suppository. Dihydroergotamine (DHE) may be given IV, IM, or as a nasal spray with an antiemetic if pain control and relief of nausea are not achieved with other drugs. It should not be given within 24 hours of a triptan drug.

A combination drug containing APAP, isometheptene, and dichloralphenazone is the most common *isometheptene combination* given for treating migraines and is an excellent option when ergotamine preparations are not tolerated or do not work.

Preventive Therapy. Prevention drugs and other strategies are used when a migraine occurs more than twice per week, interferes with ADLs, or is not relieved with acute treatment. Unless otherwise contraindicated, the primary health care provider may initially prescribe an NSAID, a beta-adrenergic blocker, a calcium channel blocker, or an antiepileptic drug (AED). Propranolol and timolol are common *beta blockers* approved for migraine prevention. Verapamil, a *calcium channel blocking agent,* may also be used for some patients. The calcium channel and beta blockers are thought to reduce the activity of hyperexcitable neurons and act on the neurogenic causes of migraine. Both calcium channel blockers and beta blockers interfere with vasodilation, a contributing cause of migraine pain. Both beta-adrenergic blockers and calcium channel blocking drugs can lower blood pressure and decrease pulse rate (Burchum & Rosenthal, 2016).

! NURSING SAFETY PRIORITY (QSEN)

Drug Alert

Teach patients who take beta-adrenergic blockers or calcium channel blockers how to take their pulse. Encourage them to report bradycardia or adverse reactions such as fatigue and shortness of breath to their primary health care provider as soon as possible.

Topiramate is one of the most common *antiepileptic drugs (AEDs)* used for migraines, but it should be used in low doses of 25 to 100 mg daily. The mechanism of action is not clear, but this drug may inhibit the sodium channels, channels that may be hyperexcitable in patients with migraine. Reports of suicides have been associated with this drug when it is used in larger doses of 400 mg daily, most often with patients who have bipolar disorder.

Nortriptyline is a tricyclic *antidepressant* that is often effective as a drug to prevent or reduce migraine episodes. The drug is started in a low dose, usually 10 mg, and may be increased to 30 mg or more, depending on the patient's needs. Side effects include dry mouth, urinary retention, and constipation. This anticholinergic drug is not used for older adults because it can also cause delirium or acute confusion (Burchum & Rosenthal, 2019).

Some patients experience chronic migraine, which is defined as having 15 or more migraine headaches in a month. For chronic migraine, *onabotulinumtoxinA* was approved in 2010. Monthly treatments for up to five treatment cycles are considered safe and effective.

The newest drugs for chronic migraine are in a monoclonal antibody drug class known as *calcitonin gene–related peptide receptor (CGRP-R) antagonists.* Examples of these drugs administered by injection subcutaneously every 1 to 3 months include erenumab, fremanezumab and, most recently, galcanezumab. Galcanezumab has also been recently approved for treatment of cluster headaches. Side effects of this class of drugs are not common, but teach the patient receiving any of them to report pain, redness, or swelling at the injection site.

Encourage patients to keep a headache diary to help identify the type of headache they are experiencing and the response to preventive medication or other intervention. Teach them to notify their primary health care provider if the quality, intensity, or nature of the headache increases or changes. Encourage them to report whether the headache is associated with new or unusual visual changes and if the prescribed drug is no longer effective.

In addition to drug therapy, *trigger avoidance* and *management* are important interventions for preventing migraine episodes. For example, some patients find that *avoiding* tyramine-containing products, such as pickled products, aged cheeses, smoked sausages, and beer; caffeine; wine; preservatives; and artificial sweeteners reduces their headaches. Others have identified specific factors that trigger an attack for them. Help patients identify triggers that could cause migraine episodes and teach them to avoid them once identified. For example, at the beginning of a migraine attack, the patient may be able to reduce pain by lying down and darkening the room. He or she may want both eyes covered and a cool cloth on the forehead. If the patient falls asleep, he or she should remain undisturbed until awakening.

Medical Marijuana. Some patients get relief of pain or have less migraine episodes each month by smoking marijuana, also known as *cannabis.* Cannabis contains two natural compounds called cannabinoids: tetrahydrocannabinol (THC) and cannabidiol (CBD). THC is a mind-altering and intoxicating substance; CBD does not alter the mind or cause intoxication. CBD is the most effective in easing the pain of migraines. A study of 121 patients who had frequent migraines showed that marijuana significantly decreased the monthly number of migraine episodes (Rhyne et al., 2016). More clinical evidence is needed to replicate this study and include larger numbers of subjects.

External Trigeminal Nerve Stimulator. A certified medical device called the Cefaly is available in the United States, Europe, and Canada by prescription for the primary health care provider to prevent migraines. This *external trigeminal nerve stimulator (E-TNS)* is a wearable headband that stimulates several branches of the trigeminal nerve associated with migraine attacks and pain. Teach the patient to use the device no more than 20 minutes a day as recommended by its manufacturer. For more information, teach the patient to visit either www.cefaly.us or www.cefaly.ca for a video about how to use this nondrug alternative to preventive medications.

Complementary and Integrative Health. Many patients use complementary and integrative therapies as adjuncts to drug therapy. Yoga, meditation, massage, exercise, and biofeedback are helpful in preventing or treating migraines for some patients. Vitamin B_{12} (riboflavin) and magnesium supplements to maintain normal serum values may have a role in migraine prevention (National Center for Complementary and Integrative Health [NCCIH], 2019). A number of herbs are also used for headaches, for both prevention and pain management. Teach patients that all herbs and nutritional remedies should be approved by their primary health care provider before use because they could interact with prescribed medication.

NCLEX EXAMINATION CHALLENGE 39.4

Health Promotion and Maintenance

The nurse is preparing a teaching plan for a client with migraine headaches. Which of these foods or food additives that may trigger a migraine and should be avoided will the nurse include in the teaching? **Select all that apply.**

A. Sugar
B. Beer
C. Smoked sausage
D. Pickles
E. Caffeine
F. Wine

Acupuncture and acupressure may be effective in relieving pain for some patients (NCCIH, 2019). Some plastic surgeons have resected the trigeminal nerve to relieve chronic migraine pain.

SEIZURES AND EPILEPSY

Pathophysiology Review

A **seizure** is an abnormal, sudden, excessive, uncontrolled electrical discharge of neurons within the brain that may result in a change in level of consciousness (LOC), motor or sensory ability, and/or behavior. A single seizure may occur for no known reason. Some seizures are caused by a pathologic condition of the brain, such as a tumor. In this case, once the underlying problem is treated, the patient is often asymptomatic.

Epilepsy is defined by the National Institute of Neurological Disorders and Stroke as a chronic disorder in which repeated unprovoked seizure activity occurs. It may be caused by an abnormality in electrical neuronal activity; an imbalance of neurotransmitters, especially gamma aminobutyric acid (GABA); or a combination of both (McCance et al., 2019).

Types of Seizures. The International Classification of Epileptic Seizures recognizes three broad categories of seizure disorders: generalized seizures, partial seizures, and unclassified seizures.

Five types of *generalized seizures* may occur in adults and involve *both* cerebral hemispheres. The *tonic-clonic seizure* lasting 2 to 5 minutes begins with a tonic phase that causes stiffening or rigidity of the muscles, particularly of the arms and legs, and immediate loss of consciousness. *Clonic* or rhythmic jerking (**clonus**) of all extremities follows. The patient may bite his or her tongue and become incontinent of urine or feces. Fatigue, acute confusion, and lethargy may last up to an hour after the seizure.

Occasionally only tonic or clonic movement may occur. A *tonic seizure* is an abrupt increase in muscle tone, loss of consciousness, and autonomic changes lasting from 30 seconds to several minutes. The *clonic seizure* lasts several minutes and causes muscle contraction and relaxation.

The *myoclonic seizure* causes a brief jerking or stiffening of the extremities that may occur singly or in groups. Lasting for just a few seconds, the contractions may be symmetric (both sides) or asymmetric (one side).

In an *atonic (akinetic) seizure,* the patient has a sudden loss of muscle tone, lasting for seconds, followed by *postictal* (after the seizure) confusion. In most cases, these seizures cause the patient to fall, which may result in injury. This type of seizure tends to be most resistant to drug therapy.

Partial seizures, also called *focal* or *local* seizures, begin in a part of *one* cerebral hemisphere. They are further subdivided into two main classes: complex partial seizures and simple partial seizures. In addition, some partial seizures can become generalized tonic-clonic, tonic, or clonic seizures. Partial seizures are most often seen in adults and generally are less responsive to medical treatment when compared with other types.

Complex partial seizures may cause loss of consciousness (syncope), or "blackout," for 1 to 3 minutes. Characteristic automatisms may occur as in absence seizures. The patient is unaware of the environment and may wander at the start of the seizure. In the period after the seizure, he or she may have **amnesia** (loss of memory). Because the area of the brain most often involved in this type of epilepsy is the temporal lobe, complex partial seizures are often called *psychomotor* seizures or *temporal lobe* seizures.

> **PATIENT-CENTERED CARE: OLDER ADULT CONSIDERATIONS** QSEN
>
> Complex partial seizures are most common among older adults. These seizures are difficult to diagnose because symptoms appear similar to those of dementia, psychosis, or other neurobehavioral disorders, especially in the postictal stage (after the seizure). New-onset seizures in older adults typically are associated with conditions such as hypertension, cardiac disease, diabetes mellitus, stroke, dementia, and recent brain injury (McCance et al., 2019).

The patient with a *simple partial seizure* remains conscious throughout the episode. He or she often reports an **aura** (unusual sensation) before the seizure takes place. This may consist of a "déjà vu" (already seen) phenomenon, perception of an offensive smell, or sudden onset of pain. During the seizure, the patient may have one-sided movement of an extremity, experience unusual sensations, or have autonomic symptoms. Autonomic changes include a change in heart rate, skin flushing, and epigastric discomfort.

Unclassified or *idiopathic seizures* account for about half of all seizure activity. They occur for no known reason and do not fit into the generalized or partial classifications.

Etiology and Genetic Risk. Primary or *idiopathic epilepsy* is not associated with any identifiable brain lesion or other specific cause; however, genetic factors most likely play a role in its development. *Secondary seizures* result from an underlying brain lesion, most commonly a tumor or trauma. They may also be caused by:

- Metabolic disorders
- Acute alcohol withdrawal
- Electrolyte disturbances (e.g., hyperkalemia, water intoxication, hypoglycemia)
- High fever
- Stroke
- Head injury
- Substance abuse
- Heart disease

Seizures resulting from these problems are not considered epilepsy. Various risk factors can trigger a seizure, such as increased physical activity, emotional stress, excessive fatigue, alcohol or caffeine consumption, or certain foods or chemicals.

Interprofessional Collaborative Care

Assessment: Recognize Cues. Question the patient or family about how many seizures the patient has had, how long they last, and any pattern of occurrence. Ask the patient or family to describe the seizures that the patient has had. Signs and symptoms vary, depending on the type of seizure experienced, as described earlier. Ask about the presence of an aura before seizures begin *(preictal phase)*. Question whether the patient is taking any prescribed drugs or herbs or has had head trauma or high fever. Assess any alcohol and/or illicit drug history. Ask about any other medical condition such as a previous stroke or hypertension.

If the seizure is a new symptom, ask the patient or family if any loss of consciousness or brain injury has occurred, in both the recent and distant past. Often patients may have had a head or brain injury sufficient to cause a loss of consciousness but may not remember this at the time of the seizure, especially if it was during their childhood.

Diagnosis is based on the history and physical examination. A variety of diagnostic tests are performed to rule out other causes of seizure activity and to confirm the diagnosis of epilepsy. Typical diagnostic tests include an electroencephalogram (EEG), CT scan, MRI, or SPECT/PET scan. These tests are described elsewhere in this textbook. Laboratory studies are performed to identify metabolic or other disorders that may cause or contribute to seizure activity.

◆ **Interventions: Take Action.** Removing or treating the underlying condition or cause of the seizure manages *secondary* epilepsy and seizures that are not considered epileptic. In most cases, primary epilepsy is successfully managed through drug therapy.

Nonsurgical Management. Most seizures can be completely or almost completely controlled through the administration of *antiepileptic drugs (AEDs),* sometimes referred to as *anticonvulsants,* for specific types of seizures.

Drug Therapy. Drug therapy is the major component of management (Box 39.2). The primary health care provider introduces one antiepileptic drug (AED) at a time to achieve control for the type of seizure that the patient has. If the chosen drug is not effective, the dosage may be increased, or another drug introduced. At times, seizure control is achieved only through a combination of drugs. The dosages are adjusted to achieve therapeutic blood levels without causing major side effects. Because of these potential side effects, teach patients to:

- Follow up on laboratory test appointments to monitor the patient's complete blood count (CBC) and liver enzymes and assess for therapeutic drug levels. Most AEDs can cause leukopenia and liver dysfunction.
- Observe for and report beginning gingival hyperplasia and perform frequent oral care to prevent permanent gingival damage.

PATIENT-CENTERED CARE: GENDER HEALTH CONSIDERATIONS QSEN

Management of women with epilepsy is often challenging. Hormonal changes from menstrual cycling and the interaction of oral contraceptives with antiepileptic drugs (AEDs) require the primary health care provider and patient to be aware of a variety of guidelines and to more frequently monitor drug effectiveness. AEDs can also contribute to osteoporosis in menopausal women. As a result, coordination among the neurologist, the woman's primary health care provider, and the patient is required for safe, effective care. Nurses can facilitate patient education, communication, and collaboration to promote safe, effective care.

Teach patients to take their drugs on time to maintain therapeutic blood levels and maximum effectiveness. Emphasize the importance of taking their AEDs as prescribed. Instruct patients that they can build up sensitivity to the drugs as they age. If sensitivity occurs, tell them they will need to have blood levels of this drug checked frequently to adjust the dose. In some cases, the antiseizure effects of drugs can decline and lead to an increase in seizures. Because of this potential for "drug decline and sensitivity," patients need to keep their scheduled laboratory appointments to check serum drug levels.

BOX 39.2 Examples of Drug Therapy Epilepsy and Seizure Prevention

- Phenytoin
- Fosphenytoin
- Carbamazepine
- Oxcarbazepine
- Felbamate
- Lamotrigine
- Valproic acid
- Primidone
- Gabapentin
- Pregabalin
- Levetiracetam
- Brivaracetam
- Topiramate
- Ezogabine (first approved potassium channel opener drug approved for adjunctive management of partial-onset seizures)
- Cenobamate

Be aware of drug-drug and drug-food interactions. For instance, warfarin should not be given with phenytoin (Dilantin). Document side and adverse effects of the prescribed drugs and report to the health care provider. Teach patients that some citrus fruits, such as grapefruit juice, can interfere with the metabolism of these drugs. This interference can raise the blood level of the drug and cause the patient to develop drug toxicity.

Seizure Precautions. Precautions are taken to prevent the patient from injury if a seizure occurs. Specific seizure precautions vary, depending on health care agency policy.

! NURSING SAFETY PRIORITY QSEN

Action Alert

Seizure precautions include ensuring that oxygen and suctioning equipment with an airway are readily available. If the patient does not have an IV access, insert a saline lock, especially if he or she is at significant risk for generalized tonic-clonic seizures. The saline lock provides ready access if IV drug therapy must be given to stop the seizure.

Side rails are rarely the source of significant injury, and the effectiveness of the use of padded side rails to maintain safety is debatable. Padded side rails may embarrass the patient and the family. Follow agency policy about the use of side rails because they may be classified as a restraint device.

Padded tongue blades do not belong at the bedside and should NEVER be inserted into the patient's mouth because the jaw may clench down as soon as the seizure begins! Forcing a tongue blade or airway into the mouth is more likely to chip the teeth and increase the risk for aspirating tooth fragments than prevent the patient from biting the tongue. Furthermore, improper placement of a padded tongue blade can obstruct the airway.

BEST PRACTICE FOR PATIENT SAFETY & QUALITY CARE (QSEN)

Care of the Patient During a Tonic-Clonic or Complex Partial Seizure

- Protect the patient from injury.
- Do not force anything into the patient's mouth.
- Turn the patient to the side to prevent aspiration and keep the airway clear.
- Remove any objects that might injure the patient.
- Suction oral secretions if possible without force.
- Loosen any restrictive clothing the patient is wearing.
- Do not restrain or try to stop the patient's movement; guide movements if necessary.
- Record the time the seizure began and ended.
- At the completion of the seizure:
  - Take the patient's vital signs.
  - Perform neurologic checks.
  - Keep the patient on his or her side.
  - Allow the patient to rest.
- Document the seizure:
  - How often the seizures occur: date, time, and duration of the seizure
  - Whether more than one type of seizure occurs
- Observations during the seizure:
  - Changes in pupil size and any eye deviation
  - Level of consciousness
  - Presence of apnea, cyanosis, and salivation
  - Incontinence of bowel or bladder during the seizure
  - Eye fluttering or blinking
  - Movement and progression of motor activity
  - Lip smacking or other automatism
  - Tongue or lip biting
  - How long the seizure lasts
  - When the last seizure took place
  - Whether the seizure was preceded by an aura
  - What the patient does after the seizure
  - How long it takes for the patient to return to pre-seizure status

Seizure Management. The actions taken during a seizure should be appropriate for the type of seizure, as outlined in the Best Practice for Patient Safety & Quality Care: Care of the Patient During a Tonic-Clonic or Complex Partial Seizure box.

It is not unusual for the patient to become cyanotic during a generalized tonic-clonic seizure. The cyanosis is generally self-limiting, and no treatment is needed. Some primary health care providers prefer to give the high-risk patient (e.g., older adult, critically ill, or debilitated patient) oxygen by nasal cannula or facemask during the postictal phase. For any type of seizure, carefully observe the seizure and document assessment findings.

Emergency Care: Acute Seizure and Status Epilepticus Management. Seizures occurring in greater intensity, number, or length than the patient's usual seizures are considered *acute.* They may also appear in clusters that are different from the patient's typical seizure pattern. Treatment with lorazepam or diazepam may be given to stop the clusters to prevent the development of status epilepticus. IV phenytoin or fosphenytoin may be added (Burchum & Rosenthal, 2019).

Status epilepticus is a medical emergency and is a prolonged seizure lasting longer than 5 minutes or repeated seizures over the course of 30 minutes. It is a potential complication of all types of seizures. *Seizures lasting longer than 10 minutes can cause death!* Common causes of status epilepticus include:

- Sudden withdrawal from antiepileptic drugs
- Infection
- Acute alcohol or drug withdrawal
- Head trauma
- Cerebral edema
- Metabolic disturbances

! NURSING SAFETY PRIORITY (QSEN)

Critical Rescue

Convulsive status epilepticus must be treated promptly and aggressively! Establish an airway and notify the primary health care provider or Rapid Response Team immediately if this problem occurs! *Establishing an airway is the priority for this patient's care.* Intubation by an anesthesia provider or respiratory therapist may be necessary. Administer oxygen as indicated by the patient's condition. If not already in place, establish IV access with a large-bore catheter and start 0.9% sodium chloride. The patient is usually placed in the intensive care unit for continuous monitoring and management.

Brain damage and death may occur in the patient with tonic-clonic status epilepticus. Left untreated, metabolic changes result, leading to hypoxia, hypotension, hypoglycemia, cardiac dysrhythmias, or lactic (metabolic) acidosis. Further harm to the patient occurs when muscle breaks down and myoglobin accumulates in the kidneys, which can lead to renal failure and electrolyte imbalance. *This is especially likely in the older adult.*

The drugs of choice for treating status epilepticus are IV-push lorazepam or diazepam. Diazepam rectal gel may be used instead. Lorazepam is usually given as 4 mg over a 2-minute period. This procedure may be repeated, if necessary, until a total of 8 mg is reached.

! NURSING SAFETY PRIORITY (QSEN)

Drug Alert

To prevent additional tonic-clonic seizures or cardiac arrest, a loading dose of IV phenytoin is given and oral doses are administered as a follow-up after the emergency is resolved. Initially give phenytoin at no more than 50 mg/min using an infusion pump. If the drug is piggybacked into an existing IV line, use only normal saline as the primary IV fluid to prevent drug precipitation. Be sure to flush the line with normal saline before and after phenytoin administration (Burchum & Rosenthal, 2019).

An alternative to phenytoin is fosphenytoin, a water-soluble phenytoin prodrug. It is compatible with most IV solutions. It also causes fewer cardiovascular complications than phenytoin and can be given in an IV dextrose solution. After administration, fosphenytoin converts to phenytoin in the body. Therefore the FDA requires the dosage to be written as a phenytoin equivalent (PE) (e.g., 150 mg of fosphenytoin converts to 100 mg of phenytoin). If given IV, infuse fosphenytoin at a rate of no more than 150 PE/min (Burchum & Rosenthal, 2019).

Teach the patient and family that serum drug levels are checked every 6 to 12 hours after the loading dose and then 2 weeks after oral phenytoin has started. The desired serum therapeutic range

PATIENT AND FAMILY EDUCATION: PREPARING FOR SELF-MANAGEMENT

Health Teaching for the Patient With Epilepsy

- Know drug therapy information:
  - Name, dosage, time of administration
  - Actions to take if side effects occur
  - Importance of taking drug as prescribed and not missing a dose
  - What to do if a dose is missed or cannot be taken
- Understand importance of having blood drawn for therapeutic or toxic levels as requested by the primary health care provider.
- Do not take any drug, including over-the-counter drugs, without asking your primary health care provider.
- Wear a medical alert bracelet or necklace or carry an identification card indicating epilepsy.
- Follow up with your neurologist or other primary health care provider as directed.
- Be sure that a family member or significant other knows how to help you in the event of a seizure and knows when your primary health care provider or emergency medical services should be called.
- Investigate and follow state laws concerning driving and operating machinery.
- Avoid alcohol and excessive fatigue.
- Contact the Epilepsy Foundation (www.epilepsy.com) or other organized epilepsy group for additional information. Epilepsy Canada (www.epilepsy.ca) also provides resources and support.

is 10 to 20 mcg/mL (Burchum & Rosenthal, 2019). Drug levels of more than 30 mg/mL are considered an indicator of drug toxicity.

Surgical Management. Patients who cannot be managed effectively with drug therapy may be candidates for surgery, including vagal nerve stimulation (VNS). VNS has been very successful for many patients with epilepsy and is sometimes referred to as the "pacemaker for the brain" (Shafer & Dean, 2018).

VNS may be performed for control of continuous simple or complex partial seizures. Patients with generalized seizures are not candidates for surgery because VNS may result in severe neurologic deficits. The stimulating device (much like a cardiac pacemaker) is surgically implanted in the left chest wall. An electrode lead is attached to the left vagus nerve, tunneled under the skin, and connected to a generator. The procedure usually takes 2 hours with the patient under general anesthesia. The stimulator is activated by the primary health care provider either in the operating room or, more commonly, 2 weeks after surgery. Programming is adjusted gradually over a period of time. The pattern of stimulation is individualized to the patient's tolerance. The generator runs continuously, stimulating the vagus nerve according to the programmed schedule.

The patient can activate the VNS with a handheld magnet when experiencing an aura, thus aborting the seizure. Patients experience a change in voice quality, which signifies that the vagus nerve has been stimulated. They usually report a relief in intensity and duration of seizures and an improved quality of life (Shafer & Dean, 2018).

Observe for complications after the procedure such as hoarseness (most common), cough, dyspnea, neck pain, or dysphagia (difficulty swallowing). Teach the patient to avoid MRIs, microwaves, shortwave radios, and ultrasound diathermy (a physical therapy heat treatment).

Care Coordination and Transition Management. Provide self-management education for the patient and family (see the Patient and Family Education: Preparing for Self-Management: Health Teaching for the Patient With Epilepsy box). Ask them what they understand about the disorder and correct any misinformation. As new information is presented, be sure that the patient and family can understand it.

Emphasize that AEDs must not be stopped even if the seizures have stopped. Discontinuing these drugs can lead to the recurrence of seizures or the life-threatening complication of status epilepticus (discussed earlier). Some patients may stop therapy because they do not have the money to purchase the drugs. Refer limited-income patients to the social services department for assistance or to a case manager to locate other resources.

A balanced diet, proper rest, and stress-reduction techniques usually minimize the risk for breakthrough seizures. Encourage the patient to keep a seizure diary to determine whether there are factors that tend to be associated with seizure activity.

All states prohibit discrimination against people who have epilepsy. Patients who work in occupations in which a seizure might cause serious harm to themselves or others (e.g., construction workers, operators of dangerous equipment, pilots) may need other employment. They may need to decrease or modify strenuous or potentially dangerous physical activity to avoid harm, although this varies with each person. Various local, state, and federal agencies can help with finances, living arrangements, and vocational rehabilitation.

MENINGITIS

Pathophysiology Review

Meningitis is an ***infection*** of the meninges of the brain and spinal cord, specifically the pia mater and arachnoid. Bacterial and viral organisms are most often responsible for meningitis, although fungal and protozoal meningitis also occur. Cancer and some drugs, notably NSAIDs, antibiotics, and IV immunoglobulins, can also cause sterile meningitis. Regardless of cause of meningitis, the symptoms are similar.

The organisms responsible for meningitis enter the central nervous system (CNS) via the bloodstream or are directly introduced into the CNS. Direct routes of entry occur as a result of penetrating trauma, surgical procedures on the brain or spine, or a ruptured brain abscess. A basilar skull fracture may lead to meningitis as a result of the direct communication of cerebrospinal fluid (CSF) with the ear or nasal passages, manifested by otorrhea (ear discharge) or rhinorrhea (nasal discharge, or "runny nose") that is actually CSF. The infecting organisms follow the tract created by skull damage to enter the CNS and circulate in the CSF. The patient with an infection in the head (i.e., eye, ear, nose, mouth) or neck/throat has an increased risk for meningitis because of the proximity of anatomic structures. Infections linked to meningitis include otitis media, acute or chronic sinusitis, and tooth abscess; there are also reports of rare infection from a tongue piercing leading to meningitis. The immunocompromised patient (e.g., one without a spleen receiving treatment for cancer, taking immunosuppressant drugs to manage autoimmune disease or solid organ transplant, and older adults) is also at increased risk for meningitis. The infecting organism may spread to both cranial and spinal nerves, causing irreversible neurologic damage. Increased intracranial pressure (ICP) may occur as a result of blockage of the flow of CSF, change in cerebral blood flow, or thrombus (blood clot) formation (McCance et al., 2019).

Viral meningitis, the most common type, is sometimes referred to as *aseptic meningitis* because no organisms are typically isolated from culture of the CSF. Common viral organisms causing meningitis are enterovirus, herpes simplex virus–2 (HSV-2), varicella zoster virus (VZV) (also causes chickenpox and shingles), mumps virus, and the human immune deficiency virus (HIV) (McCance et al., 2019). The severity of symptoms can vary by the infecting viral agent. For example, the herpes simplex virus alters cellular metabolism, which quickly results in necrosis of the cells. HSV-2 meningitis may be accompanied by genital infections. Other viruses cause an alteration in the production of enzymes or neurotransmitters. Although these alterations result in cell dysfunction, neurologic defects are more likely to be temporary, and a full recovery occurs as the inflammation resolves.

Cryptococcus neoformans meningitis is the most common *fungal* infection that affects the CNS of patients with acquired immune deficiency syndrome (AIDS [HIV-III]). Fulminant invasive fungal sinusitis is also a recognized cause of fungal meningitis. The signs and symptoms vary because the compromised immune system affects the inflammatory response. For example, some patients have fever and others do not.

The most frequently involved organisms responsible for *bacterial meningococcal meningitis* are *Streptococcus pneumoniae* (pneumococcal disease) and *Neisseria meningitidis. N. meningitidis* meningitis is also known as *meningococcal meningitis. Meningococcal meningitis is a medical emergency with a fairly high mortality rate, often within 24 hours.* Unlike other types, this disorder is highly contagious. Outbreaks of meningococcal meningitis are most likely to occur in areas of high population density, such as college dormitories, military barracks, and crowded living areas.

NURSING SAFETY PRIORITY QSEN

Action Alert

People ages 16 through 21 years have the highest rates of infection from life-threatening *N. meningitidis* meningococcal infection. The Centers for Disease Control and Prevention (CDC) recommends an initial meningococcal vaccine between ages 11 and 12 years with a booster at age 16 years (www.cdc.gov). Adults are advised to get an initial or a booster vaccine if living in a shared residence (residence hall, military barracks, group home) or traveling or residing in countries in which the disease is common or if they are immunocompromised as a result of a damaged or surgically removed spleen or a serum complement deficiency. If the patient's baseline vaccination status is unclear and the immediate risk for exposure to *N. meningitidis* infection is high, the CDC recommends vaccination. It is safe to receive a booster as early as 8 weeks after the initial vaccine.

KEY FEATURES

Meningitis

- Decreased level of consciousness
- Disorientation to person, place, and time
- Pupil reaction and eye movements:
  - **Photophobia** (sensitivity to light)
  - **Nystagmus** (involuntary condition in which the eyes make repetitive uncontrolled movements)
- Motor response:
  - Normal early in disease process
  - Hemiparesis (weakness on one side of the body), hemiplegia (paralysis on one side of the body), and decreased muscle tone possible later
  - Cranial nerve dysfunction, especially CN III, IV, VI, VII, VIII
- Memory changes:
  - Attention span (usually short)
  - Personality and behavior changes
- Severe, unrelenting headaches
- Generalized muscle aches and pain (myalgia)
- Nausea and vomiting
- Fever and chills
- Tachycardia
- Red macular rash (meningococcal meningitis)

Interprofessional Collaborative Care

Assessment: Recognize Cues. Perform a complete neurologic and neurovascular assessment to detect signs and symptoms associated with a diagnosis of meningitis or suspected meningitis as outlined in the Key Features: Meningitis box.

Although the classic nuchal rigidity (stiff neck) and positive Kernig and Brudzinski signs have been traditionally used to diagnose meningitis, these findings occur in only a small percentage of patients with a definitive diagnosis. Older adults, patients who are immunocompromised, and those who are receiving antibiotics may not have fever. Assess the patient for complications, including increased ICP. Left untreated, increased ICP can lead to herniation of the brain and death (see Chapter 41).

Seizure activity may occur when meningeal inflammation and ***infection*** spreads to the cerebral cortex. Inflammation can also result in abnormal stimulation of the hypothalamic area where excessive amounts of antidiuretic hormone (ADH) (vasopressin) are produced. Excess vasopressin results in water retention and dilution of serum sodium caused by increased sodium loss by the kidneys. This syndrome of inappropriate antidiuretic hormone (see SIADH discussion elsewhere in this textbook) may lead to further increases in ICP.

Meningitis may be misdiagnosed as **encephalitis**, an ***infection*** (usually viral) of brain tissue and often the surrounding meninges. Diagnostic testing is needed to differentiate these two diseases.

The most significant laboratory test used in the diagnosis of meningitis is the analysis of the *cerebrospinal fluid (CSF).* Patients older than 60 years, those who are immunocompromised, or those who have signs of increased ICP usually have a CT scan before the lumbar puncture. If there will be a delay in obtaining the CSF, blood is drawn for culture and sensitivity. A broad-spectrum antibiotic should be given before the lumbar

BEST PRACTICE FOR PATIENT SAFETY & QUALITY CARE (QSEN)

Care of the Patient With Meningitis

- Prioritize care to maintain airway, breathing, and circulation.
- Take vital signs and perform neurologic checks every 2 to 4 hours, as needed.
- Perform cranial nerve assessment, with particular attention to cranial nerves III, IV, VI, VII, and VIII, and monitor for changes.
- Manage pain with drug and nondrug methods.
- Perform vascular assessment and monitor for changes.
- Give drugs and IV fluids as prescribed and document the patient's response.
- Record intake and output carefully to maintain fluid balance and prevent fluid overload.
- Monitor body weight to identify fluid retention early.
- Monitor laboratory values closely; report abnormal findings to the physician or nurse practitioner promptly.
- Position carefully to prevent pressure injuries.
- Perform range-of-motion exercises every 4 hours as needed.
- Decrease environmental stimuli:
  - Provide a quiet environment.
  - Minimize exposure to bright lights from windows and overhead lights.
- Maintain bedrest with head of bed elevated 30 degrees.
- Maintain Transmission-Based Precautions per hospital policy (for bacterial meningitis).
- Monitor for complications:
  - Increased intracranial pressure
  - Vascular dysfunction
  - Fluid and electrolyte imbalance
  - Seizures
  - Shock

puncture. The CSF is analyzed for cell count, differential count, and protein. Glucose concentrations are determined, and culture, sensitivity, and Gram stain studies are performed.

Counterimmunoelectrophoresis (CIE) may be performed to determine the presence of viruses or protozoa in the CSF. CIE is also indicated if the patient has received antibiotics before the CSF was obtained. To identify a bacterial source of infection, specimens for Gram stains and culture are obtained from the urine, throat, and nose when indicated.

A complete blood count (CBC) is performed. The white blood cell (WBC) count is usually elevated well above the normal value. Serum electrolyte values are also checked to assess and maintain fluid and electrolyte balance.

X-rays of the chest, air sinuses, and mastoids are obtained to determine the presence of ***infection.*** A CT or MRI scan may be performed to identify increased ICP, hydrocephalus, or the presence of a brain abscess.

◆ **Interventions: Take Action.** *Prevent meningitis by teaching people to obtain vaccination.* Vaccines are available to protect against *Haemophilus influenzae* type B (Hib), pneumococcal, mumps, varicella, and meningococcal organisms. Although many of these vaccines were developed to prevent respiratory illness, they have also reduced CNS infections. Mandatory vaccination programs for school enrollment and proof of vaccination as a prerequisite for group home or dormitory experiences have significantly reduced the incidence of meningitis.

The most important nursing interventions for patients with meningitis are accurate monitoring of and documenting their neurologic status. Best practices for nursing care are listed in the Best Practice for Patient Safety & Quality Care: Care of the Patient With Meningitis box.

! NURSING SAFETY PRIORITY (QSEN)

Action Alert

For the patient with meningitis, assess his or her neurologic status and vital signs at least every 4 hours or more often if clinically indicated. *The priority for care is to monitor for early neurologic changes that may indicate increased ICP, such as decreased level of consciousness (LOC).* The patient is also at risk for seizure activity. Care should be provided as discussed in Interventions in the Seizures and Epilepsy section.

Cranial nerve testing is included as part of the routine neurologic assessment because of possible cranial nerve involvement. *A sixth cranial nerve defect (inability to move the eyes laterally) may indicate the development of* **hydrocephalus** *(excessive accumulation of CSF within the brain's ventricles).* Other indicators of hydrocephalus include signs of increased ICP and urinary incontinence. Urinary incontinence results from decreasing LOC.

To avoid life-threatening complications from bacterial meningitis, the primary health care provider prescribes a broad-spectrum antibiotic until the results of the culture and Gram stain are available. After this information is available, the appropriate anti-infective drug to treat the specific type of meningitis is given. Treatment of bacterial meningitis generally requires a 2-week course of IV antibiotics. Drug therapy should begin within 1 to 2 hours after it is prescribed. Monitor and document the patient's response.

Drugs may be used to treat increased ICP or seizures, including mannitol, a hyperosmolar agent for ICP, and antiepileptic drugs (AEDs). Controversy exists as to whether adjuvant steroids are helpful in the treatment of adults with acute bacterial meningitis. However, they may be used for some patients with *S. pneumoniae* meningitis, although more evidence is needed to support this treatment (Smyth, 2016).

People who have been in close contact with a patient with *N. meningitidis* should have prophylaxis (preventive) treatment with rifampin, ciprofloxacin, or ceftriaxone. Preventive treatment with rifampin may be prescribed for those in close contact with a patient with *H. influenzae* meningitis (Burchum & Rosenthal, 2019).

Perform a complete vascular assessment every 4 hours or more often, if indicated, to detect early vascular compromise. Thrombotic or embolic complications are most often seen in circulation to the hand. Assess the patient's temperature, color, pulses, and capillary refill in the fingernails. If vascular compromise is not noticed and left untreated, gangrene can develop quickly, possibly leading to

! NURSING SAFETY PRIORITY (QSEN)

Action Alert

Place the patient with bacterial meningitis that is transmitted by droplets on Droplet Precautions *in addition to* Standard Precautions. When possible, place the patient in a private room. Stay at least 3 feet from the patient unless wearing a mask. Patients who are transported outside of the room should wear a mask (see Chapter 21). Teach visitors about the need for these precautions and how to follow them.

loss of the involved arm. The health care team monitors the patient for other complications, including septic shock, coagulation disorders, acute respiratory distress syndrome, and septic arthritis. These health problems are discussed elsewhere in this textbook.

Standard Precautions are appropriate for all patients with meningitis unless the patient has a bacterial type that is transmitted by droplets, such as *N. meningitides* and *H. influenzae.*

GET READY FOR THE NEXT-GENERATION NCLEX® EXAMINATION!

Key Points

Review these Key Points for each NCLEX Examination Client Needs Category.

Safe and Effective Care Environment

- Implement best practices for fall prevention and wandering behaviors that are typically seen in patients with impaired ***cognition,*** such as those with AD). **QSEN: Safety**
- Collaborate with the health care team in discharge planning and health teaching for patients who have chronic seizures or neurodegenerative diseases such as AD and PD. **QSEN: Teamwork and Collaboration**

Health Promotion and Maintenance

- Teach patients with migraine headaches about triggers that could cause an attack, such as tyramine in pickled products and aged cheeses; wine; and caffeine; and other dietary or environmental triggers. **QSEN: Patient-Centered Care**
- In addition to prescribed drug therapy, encourage patients with headaches to use complementary and integrative therapies to help relieve ***pain,*** such as ice, darkened room, and relaxation techniques. **QSEN: Patient-Centered Care**
- Teach the patient with epilepsy to maintain seizure-free health or reduced seizure activity through using prescribed antiepileptic drugs (AEDs) and follow-up medical care. **QSEN: Evidence-Based Practice**
- Teach the importance of vaccination to prevent some types of infectious meningitis, particularly meningococcal vaccination, to people who are in areas of high population density, such as university residences, military barracks, and crowded living areas. **QSEN: Evidence-Based Practice; Safety**

Psychosocial Integrity

- Remind caregivers of patients with chronic neurologic diseases, such as dementia, to find ways to cope with their own stress to remain physically and psychologically healthy. **QSEN: Patient-Centered Care**
- Teach caregivers of patients with dementia to use validation therapy rather than reality orientation. Acknowledge the patient's feelings and concerns. **QSEN: Patient-Centered Care; Evidence-Based Practice**
- Emphasize the strengths of patients with PD rather than focus on their limitations; provide positive reinforcement when tasks are completed. Provide encouragement for the patient to promote self-concept. **QSEN: Patient-Centered Care**

Physiological Integrity

- Adults at risk for AD and other dementias include older adults and those who experience a traumatic brain injury (TBI), including war veterans. **QSEN: Patient-Centered Care**
- Ensure a safe environment for a patient with seizure precautions by ensuring that suction and oxygen are available and that frequent observation occurs to detect seizure activity early. **QSEN: Safety**
- Patients with status epilepticus have a life-threatening complication. Lorazepam and diazepam are the major drugs used for this emergency. **QSEN: Evidence-Based Practice**
- During a seizure, document the patient's body movements and other assessments. **QSEN: Informatics**
- Monitor for side and adverse effects of antiepileptic drugs (AEDs). **QSEN: Safety**
- For patients who have had one or more seizures, place on "seizure precautions," which includes having oxygen delivery and suctioning equipment available and starting or maintaining IV access. **QSEN: Safety**
- For patients with meningitis, carefully monitor neurologic status, including vital signs and neurologic and vascular checks. Observe for signs and symptoms of increased intracranial pressure (ICP) and communicate changes in level of consciousness immediately to the health care provider. **QSEN: Safety**
- Monitor for drug toxicity when patients are taking medications for PD, especially levodopa combinations. Delirium and decreased drug effectiveness are the most common indicators of toxicity. **QSEN: Safety**
- Document cognitive and functional abilities of the patient with dementia, recognizing that it is a progressive condition. **QSEN: Informatics**
- For patients with dementia, recall that a few drugs improve function and cognition (cholinesterase inhibitors, such as donepezil) or slow the disease process but do not cure the disease. **QSEN: Evidence-Based Practice**

MASTERY QUESTIONS

1. The nurse is caring for a client who is diagnosed with early-stage Alzheimer's disease who has periods of lucidity. What is the **best** principle for the nurse to use when communicating with this client?
   A. Use validation therapy to prevent upsetting the client.
   B. Encourage pet therapy to help allay the client's anxiety.
   C. Use aromatherapy and other integrative therapies to relax the client.
   D. Reorient the client frequently to foster reality.
2. A client experiences a seizure that is observed by the nurse. What will the nurse document in the client's medical record? **Select all that apply.**
   A. Time that seizure began and ended
   B. Whether the seizure was preceded by an aura
   C. What the client does after the seizure
   D. How long it takes for the client to return to preseizure status
   E. The drugs that are administered during the seizure
3. The nurse is admitting a client with a probable diagnosis of meningitis. What signs and symptoms might the nurse expect when assessing this client? **Select all that apply.**
   A. Photophobia
   B. Nystagmus
   C. Decreased level of consciousness
   D. Decreased movement, such as hemiparesis
   E. Disorientation to person, place, and time

REFERENCES

Allard, M. E., & Katseres, J. (2016). Using essential oils to enhance nursing practice and for self-care. *American Journal of Nursing, 116*(2), 42–50.

Alzheimer's Association. (2018). 2018 Alzheimer's disease facts and figures. *Alzheimer's and Dementia, 14*(3), 367–429.

Burchum, J. L. R., & Rosenthal, L. D. (2019). *Lehne's pharmacology for nursing care* (10th ed.). St. Louis: Elsevier.

Czekanski, K. (2017). The experience of transitioning to a caregiving role for a family member with Alzheimer's disease or related dementia. *AJN, 117*(9), 24–33.

Interprofessional Education Collaborative Expert Panel. (2016). *Core competencies for interprofessional collaborative practice: Report of an expert panel* (2nd ed.). Washington, D.C: Interprofessional Education Collaborative.

Maxwell, C. R., & Farmer, J. (2018). Medical marijuana and Parkinson's disease. *Practical Neurology,* 52–71.

McCance, K., Huether, S., Brashers, V., & Rote, N. (2019). *Pathophysiology: The biologic basis for disease in adults and children* (8th ed.). St. Louis: Mosby.

National Center for Complementary and Integrative Health (NCCIH). (2019). Headaches: In depth. https://nccih.nih.gov/health/pain/headachefacts.htm#hed3.

National Institute of Neurological Disorders and Stroke (NINDS). (2019). *Parkinson's disease.* www.ninds.nih.gov/disorders/parkinsons_disease/parkinsons_disease.htm.

Pagana, K. D., & Pagana, T. J. (2018). *Manual of diagnostic and laboratory tests* (6th ed.). St. Louis: Mosby.

Parkinson's Foundation. (2019). *Understanding Parkinson's disease.* https://www.parkinson.org/understanding-parkinson-disease.

Rhyne, D. N., Gedde, M., Anderson, S. L., & Borgelt, L. M. (2016). Effects of medical marijuana on migraine headache frequency in an adult population. *Pharmacotherapy, 36*(5), 505–510.

Shafer, P. O., & Dean, P. M. (2018). *Vagus nerve stimulation (VNS).* https://www.epilepsy.com/learn/treating-seizures-and-epilepsy/devices/vagus-nerve-stimulation-vns.

Sjödahl Hammarlund, C., Westergren, A., Astrom, I., Edberg, A. K., & Hagell, P. (2018). The impact of living with Parkinson's disease: Balancing within a web of needs and demands. *Parkinson's Disease,* https://doi.org/10.1155/2018/4598651.

Slusser, M. M., Garcia, L. I., Reed, C.-R., & McGinnis, P. Q. (2019). *Foundations of interprofessional collaborative practice in health care.* St. Louis: Elsevier.

Tasseff, T. L., & Nies, M. A. (2017). Alzheimer's and dementia: The next war for rural veterans and their families? *AJN, 117*(11), 11.

Vacca, V. M. (2019). Parkinson's disease: Enhance nursing knowledge. *Nursing2020, 49*(11), 24–32.

Westman, K. F., & Blaisdell, C. (2016). Many benefits, little risk: The use of massage in nursing practice. *American Journal of Nursing, 116*(1), 34–40.

Yakimicki, M. L., Edwards, N. E., Richards, E., & Beck, A. M. (2018). Animal-assisted intervention and dementia: A systematic review. *Clinical Nursing Research, 28*(1), 9–29.

40

Concepts of Care for Patients With Problems of the Central Nervous System: The Spinal Cord

Donna D. Ignatavicius

http://evolve.elsevier.com/Iggy/

LEARNING OUTCOMES

1. Collaborate with the interprofessional health care team to manage quality care for patients with multiple sclerosis (MS) and SCI.
2. Identify community resources for patients with MS and SCI, including resources for patients having problems with ***sexuality.***
3. Develop an evidence-based teaching plan on how to prevent back injury.
4. Prioritize care for patients with spinal cord–related problems of ***mobility, sensory perception,*** and ***pain.***
5. Apply knowledge of the pathophysiology of MS to identify common assessment findings affecting ***mobility, sensory perception, cognition,*** and ***immunity.***
6. Plan care coordination and transition management for patients with commonly occurring spinal cord–related problems.
7. Develop an evidence-based postoperative plan of care for patients having back surgery, including monitoring for complications.

KEY TERMS

amyotrophic lateral sclerosis (ALS) A progressive neurodegenerative disease that affects neurons in the brain and spinal cord that is likely caused by genetic mutations.

autonomic dysreflexia (AD) (sometimes referred to as *autonomic hyperreflexia*) A potentially life-threatening condition in which noxious visceral or cutaneous stimuli cause a sudden, massive, uninhibited reflex sympathetic discharge in people with high-level spinal cord injury.

cough assist A technique in which an assistant places his or her hands on the patient's upper abdomen over the diaphragm and below the ribs. Hands are placed one over the other, with fingers interlocked and away from the skin while the patient takes a breath and coughs during expiration. The assistant locks his or her elbows and pushes inward and upward as the patient coughs.

diplopia Double vision.

dysarthria Difficulty speaking due to slurred speech.

dysmetria The inability to direct or limit movement.

dysphagia Difficulty swallowing.

ergonomics An applied science in which the workplace is designed to increase worker comfort (thus reducing injury) while increasing efficiency and productivity.

heterotopic ossification (HO) Bony overgrowth, often into muscle; a complication of immobility.

hyperesthesia Increased ***sensory perception.***

hypoalgesia A decreased sensitivity to pain.

hypoesthesia Decreased ***sensory perception.***

intention tremor A tremor, usually of the arm and hand, that occurs while performing an activity.

log rolling A position change in which the patient turns as a unit while his or her back is kept as straight as possible.

multiple sclerosis (MS) A chronic disease caused by immune, genetic, and/or infectious factors that affects the myelin and nerve fibers of the brain and spinal cord.

nystagmus An involuntary condition in which the eyes make repetitive uncontrolled movements.

paraparesis Weakness that affects only the lower extremities, as seen in lower thoracic and lumbosacral injuries or lesions.

paraplegia Paralysis that affects only the lower extremities, as seen in lower thoracic and lumbosacral injuries or lesions.

progressive multifocal leukoencephalopathy (PML) An opportunistic viral infection of the brain that leads to death or severe disability.

quadriparesis Weakness involving all four extremities, as seen with cervical cord and upper thoracic injury.

radiculopathy Spinal nerve root involvement.

scotomas Changes in peripheral vision, often in patients with multiple sclerosis.

spinal cord stimulation An invasive technique that provides pain relief by applying an electrical field over the spinal cord.

spinal shock A syndrome that occurs immediately as the cord's response to the injury in which the patient has complete but temporary loss of motor, sensory, reflex, and autonomic function. It typically lasts less than 48 hours but may continue for several weeks.

spinal stenosis Narrowing of the spinal canal, nerve root canals, or intervertebral foramina typically seen in people older than 50 years of age.

tetraplegia (also called quadriplegia) Paralysis of all four extremities, as seen with cervical cord and upper thoracic cord injury.

tinnitus Ringing in the ears.

vertigo Dizziness.

PRIORITY AND INTERRELATED CONCEPTS

The priority concepts for this chapter are:

- ***Immunity***
- ***Mobility***

The ***Immunity*** concept exemplar for this chapter is Multiple Sclerosis.
The ***Mobility*** concept exemplar for this chapter is Spinal Cord Injury.

The interrelated concepts for this chapter are:

- ***Pain***
- ***Sensory Perception***
- ***Cognition***
- ***Sexuality***

The spinal cord relays messages to and from the brain. Besides injuries, the spinal cord can develop inflammatory and autoimmune diseases, such as multiple sclerosis (MS) and tumors, both benign and malignant. The spinal cord itself may be damaged, or the spinal nerves leading from the cord to the extremities may be affected. In some cases, both the spinal cord and the nerves are involved. Signs and symptoms of spinal cord health problems vary but often include problems with ***immunity, mobility, pain, sensory perception, cognition,*** and ***sexuality.*** Interprofessional health care team members with expertise in symptom management collaborate to improve quality of life, promote a safe environment, and prevent complications from spinal cord health problems. Chapter 3 briefly reviews each of these nursing and health concepts in detail.

IMMUNITY CONCEPT EXEMPLAR: MULTIPLE SCLEROSIS

Pathophysiology Review

Multiple sclerosis (MS) is a chronic disease caused by immune, genetic, and/or infectious factors that affects the myelin and nerve fibers of the brain and spinal cord. It is one of the leading causes of neurologic disability in young and middle-age adults. MS is characterized by periods of remission and exacerbation (flare). Patients progress at different rates and over different lengths of time. However, as the severity and duration of the disease progress, the periods of exacerbation become more frequent. Patients with MS can have a normal life expectancy as long as the effects of the disease are managed effectively.

MS is characterized by demyelination (loss of myelin sheaths). Diffuse random or patchy areas of *plaque* in the white matter of the central nervous system (CNS) are the definitive finding (McCance et al., 2019). Initially, remyelination takes place to some degree, and clinical symptoms decrease. However, over time, new lesions develop and neuronal injury and muscle atrophy occur. Myelin is responsible for the electrochemical transmission of impulses between the brain and spinal cord and the rest of the body; demyelination can result in slowed or stopped impulse transmission. The white fiber tracts that connect the neurons in the brain and spinal cord are also usually involved in MS. The areas particularly affected include optic nerves, spinal pyramidal tracts, spinal posterior columns, brainstem nuclei, and the ventricular region of the brain. The four major types of MS include (McCance et al., 2019):

- Relapsing-remitting
- Primary progressive
- Secondary progressive
- Progressive-relapsing

The classic picture of *relapsing-remitting multiple sclerosis (RRMS)* occurs in most cases of MS. The course of the disease may be mild or moderate, depending on the degree of disability. Symptoms develop and resolve in a few weeks to months, and the patient returns to baseline. During the relapsing phase, the patient reports loss of function and the continuing development of new symptoms.

Primary progressive multiple sclerosis (PPMS) involves a steady and gradual neurologic deterioration without remission of symptoms. The patient has progressive disability with no acute attacks. Patients with this type of MS tend to be between 40 and 60 years of age at onset of the disease.

Secondary progressive multiple sclerosis (SPMS) begins with a relapsing-remitting course that later becomes steadily progressive. About half of all people with RRMS develop SPMS within 10 years. The current addition of disease-modifying drugs as part of disease management may decrease the development of SPMS.

Progressive-relapsing multiple sclerosis (PRMS) is characterized by frequent relapses with partial recovery but not a return to baseline. This type of MS is seen in only a small percentage of patients. Progressive, cumulative symptoms and deterioration occur over several years.

Etiology and Genetic Risk. The cause of MS is very complex and involves multiple immune, genetic, and/or infectious factors, although changes in ***immunity*** are the most likely etiology. The environment may also contribute to its development. For example, the disease is seen more often in the colder climates of the northeastern, Great Lakes, and Pacific northwestern states and in Canada. MS is common in areas inhabited by people of northern European ancestry (National Multiple Sclerosis Society, 2020).

PATIENT-CENTERED CARE: GENETIC/GENOMIC CONSIDERATIONS QSEN

Large genome studies of families have helped identify familial patterns of multiple sclerosis (MS). For example, having a first-degree relative such as a parent or sibling with MS increases a person's risk for developing the disease. Research also confirms the association of MS with over 100 gene variants, including interleukin (IL)-7 and IL-2 receptor genes (McCance et al., 2019; National Multiple Sclerosis Society, 2020). These findings have helped guide the development of targeted drug therapies that are important in current disease management.

Incidence and Prevalence. MS usually occurs in people between the ages of 20 and 50 years, but cases may occur at any age. About 400,000 people in the United States have MS. The disease affects over 2.3 million people worldwide (National Multiple Sclerosis Society, 2020). About 100,000 Canadians have MS (MS Society of Canada, 2019). Although it tends to occur more frequently among whites of Northern European ancestry, it affects people of all races and ethnicity.

PATIENT-CENTERED CARE: GENDER HEALTH CONSIDERATIONS QSEN

MS affects women two to three times more often than men, suggesting a possible hormonal role in disease development. Some studies show that the disease occurs up to four times more often in women than men. However, the exact reason for this difference is not known (National Multiple Sclerosis Society, 2020).

❖ Interprofessional Collaborative Care

◆ Assessment: Recognize Cues

History. Multiple sclerosis (MS) often looks like other neurologic diseases, such as **amyotrophic lateral sclerosis (ALS)**, which can make the diagnosis difficult and prolonged. ALS is also a progressive neurodegenerative disease that affects neurons in the brain and spinal cord and that is likely caused by genetic mutations. Unlike MS, there is no established treatment or cure for ALS, which is 100% fatal. Table 40.1 compares these two neurologic health problems.

Patients often visit many primary health care providers and undergo a variety of diagnostic tests and treatments to obtain the correct diagnosis. Obtaining a thorough history is essential for accurate diagnosis. Ask the patient about a history of vision, ***mobility,*** and ***sensory perception*** changes, all of which are early indicators of MS. Symptoms are often vague and nonspecific in the early stages of the disease and may disappear for months or years before returning. Many patients have a single isolated clinical episode that lasts for 24 hours or more. These neurologic symptoms then disappear and occur later.

Ask about the progression of symptoms. Pay particular attention to whether they are intermittent or are becoming progressively worse. Document the date (month and year) when the patient first noticed these changes.

Next, ask about factors that aggravate the symptoms, such as fatigue, stress, overexertion, temperature extremes, or a hot shower or bath. Ask the patient and the family about any personality or behavioral changes that have occurred (e.g., euphoria [very elated mood], poor judgment, attention loss). In addition, determine whether there is a family history of MS or autoimmune disease.

Physical Assessment/Signs and Symptoms. MS produces a wide variety of signs and symptoms, as described in the Key Features: Multiple Sclerosis box.

Some patients with the RRMS also report ***pain.*** Perform a complete pain assessment for all patients with MS as described in Chapter 5.

Psychosocial Assessment. A major concern reported by most patients is how long it takes to establish a diagnosis of MS. Many patients go to several primary health care providers, are given varying diagnoses and treatment, and/or are told that their symptoms are related to stress and anxiety. Often, young adults present with weakness, fatigue, or changes in vision and are diagnosed with exhaustion and advised to get more sleep. The patient and family are often relieved to have a definite diagnosis but may express anger and frustration that it took a long time to start appropriate treatment. Therefore establish open and honest communication with the patient and allow him or her to share frustrations, anger, and anxiety.

After the initial diagnosis of MS, the patient is often anxious. Apathy and emotional lability are common problems that occur later. Depression may occur at the time of diagnosis and can also occur later with disease progression. The patient may be

KEY FEATURES

Multiple Sclerosis

- Muscle weakness and spasticity
- Fatigue (usually with continuous sensitivity to temperature)
- **Intention tremors** (tremor when performing an activity)
- Flexor muscle spasms
- **Dysmetria** (inability to direct or limit movement)
- Numbness or tingling sensations (paresthesia)
- **Hypoalgesia** (decreased sensitivity to pain)
- Ataxia (decreased motor coordination)
- **Dysarthria** (difficulty speaking due to slurred speech)
- **Dysphagia** (difficulty swallowing)
- **Diplopia** (double vision)
- **Nystagmus** (an involuntary condition in which the eyes make repetitive uncontrolled movements)
- **Scotomas** (changes in peripheral vision)
- Decreased visual and hearing acuity
- **Tinnitus** (ringing in the ears), **vertigo** (dizziness)
- Bowel and bladder dysfunction (flaccid or spastic)
- Alterations in sexual function, such as impotence
- Cognitive changes, such as memory loss, impaired judgment, and decreased ability to solve problems or perform calculations
- Depression

TABLE 40.1 **Comparison of Multiple Sclerosis and Amyotrophic Lateral Sclerosis**

	Multiple Sclerosis (MS)	Amyotrophic Lateral Sclerosis (ALS)
Pathophysiology and etiology	Chronic neurologic disease that affects the brain and spinal cord due to immune-mediated demyelination and nerve injury; characterized by remissions and exacerbations	Chronic neurologic disease of unknown cause (genetic and environmental factors identified) causing progressive muscle weakness and wasting, leading to paralysis of respiratory muscles
Populations affected	Commonly occurring disease that affects people (women twice as often as men) between the ages of 20 and 50 yr; most often affects whites of Northern European ancestry	Uncommon disease that affects people (more men than women) between the ages of 40 and 60 yr; incidence increases with each decade of life
Signs and symptoms	Fatigue Muscle spasticity Blurred or double vision (diplopia) Scotomas Nystagmus Paresthesias Areflexic (flaccid) or spastic bladder Decreased sexual function Intention tremors Gait changes	Fatigue Muscle atrophy (including tongue) Muscle weakness Twitching of face and tongue Dysarthria Dysphagia Stiff and clumsy gait Abnormal reflexes
Interprofessional collaborative care	Multiple immunomodulating and antineoplastic drugs available Collaborative care to promote and maintain optimal functioning Symptom management to achieve maximal function Psychosocial support	One approved drug to slow disease (riluzole [Rilutek]) Supportive care to promote optimal function Palliative care for symptom management at end of life Psychosocial support

euphoric either as a result of the disease itself or because of the drugs used to treat it. Assess the patient's previously used coping and stress-management skills in preparing him or her for a chronic, potentially debilitating disease. Secondary depression is the most frequent mental health disorder diagnosed in patients with MS.

Assess the patient for mental status changes. Changes in ***cognition*** are usually seen late in the course of the disease and can include decreased short-term memory, concentration, and ability to perform calculations; inattentiveness; and impaired judgment (Maloni, 2018).

Assess the impact of bowel and bladder problems. Managing fecal incontinence or constipation can be time-consuming and embarrassing.

Sexuality can be affected in people with MS, and sexual dysfunction can have a major impact on quality of life. Assess the patient's fatigue level and pattern, since fatigue contributes to sexual dysfunction. Be sensitive when asking about the patient's sexual practices and orientation. Women often report impaired genital sensation, diminished orgasm, and loss of sexual interest. Men most often report difficulty in achieving and maintaining an erection and delayed ejaculation.

Laboratory Assessment. No single specific laboratory test is definitively diagnostic for MS. However, the collective results of a variety of tests are usually conclusive. Abnormal cerebrospinal fluid (CSF) findings include elevated proteins (oligoclonal bands) and an increase in the white blood cell (WBC) count. CSF electrophoresis reveals an increase in the myelin basic protein and the presence of increased immunoglobulins, especially immunoglobulin G (IgG) (Pagana & Pagana, 2018). Newer tests are being developed to identify biomarkers for MS.

Other Diagnostic Assessment. *MRI* of the brain and spinal cord demonstrates the presence of plaques in at least two areas, which is considered diagnostic for MS. MRI with contrast shows active plaques and reveals older lesions not associated with current symptoms (Fig. 40.1).

Evoked potential testing, usually the visual evoked response (VER), is commonly performed for patients suspected of having MS. This noninvasive test can identify impaired transmission along the optic nerve pathway. Chapter 38 discusses this test in more detail.

NCLEX EXAMINATION CHALLENGE 40.1

Physiologic Integrity

A nurse is assessing a client with a suspected diagnosis of multiple sclerosis. Which assessment findings will the nurse expect? **Select all the apply.**

A. Resting tremors
B. Memory loss
C. Muscle spasticity
D. Fatigue
E. Diplopia
F. Dysarthria

◆ **Analysis: Analyze Cues and Prioritize Hypotheses.** The priority collaborative problems for patients with multiple sclerosis include:

1. Impaired ***immunity*** due to the disease and drug therapy for disease management
2. Decreased or impaired ***mobility*** due to muscle spasticity, intention tremors, and/or fatigue
3. Decreased visual acuity and ***cognition*** due to dysfunctional brain neurons

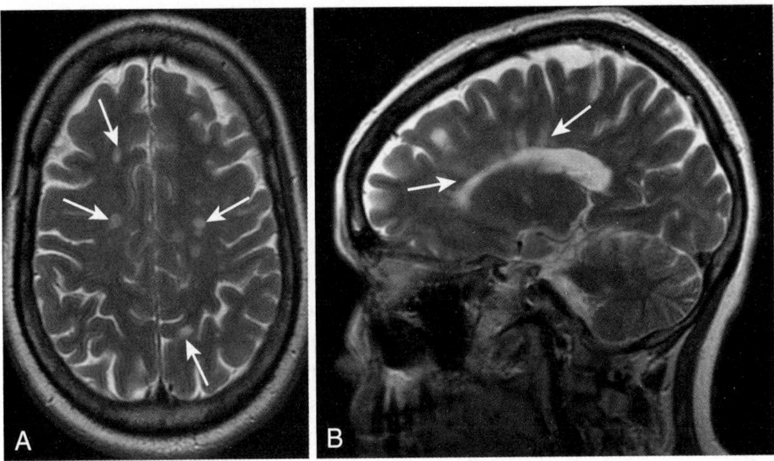

FIG. 40.1 Typical plaques *(arrows)* seen in brain CT images of patient with multiple sclerosis. (From Herring W. [2020]. *Learning radiology* [4th ed.]. St. Louis: Saunders.)

◆ **Planning and Implementation: Generate Solutions and Take Action.** The purpose of management is to modify the disease's effects on the immune system, prevent exacerbations, manage symptoms, improve function, and maintain quality of life. As with other spinal cord diseases, care of the patient with MS requires the collaborative efforts of the interprofessional health care team.

Managing Impaired Immunity

Planning: Expected Outcomes. The patient with MS is expected to be free from episodes of secondary infection due to impaired ***immunity*** from the disease or from drug therapy used to manage the illness.

Interventions. As with any chronic disease, the client who has been diagnosed with MS is at an increased risk for infection. Teach the patient to avoid large crowds and children, who develop many infections from their classmates in school. Remind them to wash their hands frequently and use hand sanitizer when soap and water are not readily available.

Drug Therapy. The patient with MS is treated with a variety of drugs that are used to treat and control the disease progression. Many of these drugs are immunomodulators or anti-inflammatory medications that can alter ***immunity*** and place patients at risk for secondary infection. Teach patients receiving drug therapy for MS to avoid crowds and anyone with an infection. If signs and symptoms of an infection occur, remind them to contact their primary health care provider for prompt management and medical observation.

Examples of drugs used for treatment of relapsing types of MS include (Burcham & Rosenthal, 2019):

- Interferon-beta preparations (interferon beta-1a and beta-1b drugs), immunomodulators that *modify* the course of the disease and also have antiviral effects
- Glatiramer acetate, a synthetic protein that is similar to myelin-based protein
- Mitoxantrone, an IV antineoplastic anti-inflammatory agent used to resolve relapses but with risks for leukemia and cardiotoxicity
- Natalizumab, the first IV monoclonal antibody approved for MS that binds to white blood cells (WBCs) to prevent further damage to the myelin

! NURSING SAFETY PRIORITY (QSEN)

Drug Alert

The interferons and glatiramer acetate are subcutaneous injections that patients can self-administer. Teach patients how to give and rotate the site of interferon-beta and glatiramer acetate injections because local injection site (skin) reactions are common. The first dose of these drugs is given under medical supervision to monitor for allergic response, including anaphylactic shock. Teach patients receiving them to avoid crowds and people with infections because these drugs can cause bone marrow suppression. Remind them to report any sign or symptom associated with infection immediately to their primary health care provider.

Instruct patients about flulike reactions that are very common for patients receiving any of the interferons. These symptoms can be minimized by starting at a low drug dose and giving acetaminophen or ibuprofen. Adverse effects of glatiramer are not common (Burcham & Rosenthal, 2019).

- Fingolimod, teriflunomide, and dimethyl fumarate, newer *oral* immunomodulating drugs

Natalizumab, a humanized monoclonal antibody, can cause many adverse events. It is usually given as an IV infusion in a specialty clinic under careful supervision. The patient is monitored carefully for allergic or anaphylactic reaction when each dose is given because the drug tends to build up in the body. *Patients receiving this drug are at risk for* **progressive multifocal leukoencephalopathy (PML)**. This opportunistic viral infection of the brain leads to death or severe disability. Monitor for neurologic changes, especially changes in mental state, such as disorientation or acute confusion. PML is confirmed by MRI and by examining the cerebrospinal fluid for the causative pathogen (Burcham & Rosenthal, 2019). Natalizumab also causes damage to hepatic cells. Carefully monitor liver enzymes and teach patients to have frequent laboratory tests to assess for changes.

Mitoxantrone, a chemotherapy drug, has been shown to be effective in reducing neurologic disability. It also decreases the frequency of clinical relapses in patients with secondary progressive, progressive-relapsing, or worsening relapsing-remitting MS.

Fingolimod was the first oral immunomodulator approved for the management of MS. The capsules may be taken with or without food. Teach patients to monitor their pulse every day because the drug can cause bradycardia, especially within the first 6 hours after taking it. Two other immunomodulating drugs have been approved for MS: teriflunomide and dimethyl fumarate. Like fingolimod, these drugs inhibit immune cells and have antioxidant properties that protect brain and spinal cord cells. Teach the patient that the two most common side effects of all the oral drugs are facial flushing and GI disturbances (Burcham & Rosenthal, 2019). Remind the patient to keep follow-up appointments for laboratory monitoring of the WBC count because the oral drugs can cause a decrease in WBCs, which can predispose the patient to infection.

Medical Marijuana (Cannabis). The National Multiple Sclerosis Society supports the use of medical marijuana (cannabis) for symptom management. Studies have shown that cannabis may reduce pain, muscle stiffness, and spasticity for some patients with MS. However, it may worsen cognitive function and cause dizziness and intoxication, depending on the form used (Cameron & Rice, 2018).

Improving Mobility

Planning Expected Outcomes. The patient with MS will have optimal ***mobility*** as a result of successful interprofessional management and self-care interventions.

Interventions. The symptoms of MS that affect ***mobility*** include spasticity, tremor, pain, and fatigue. Referral to rehabilitative services, such as physical and occupational therapy, can help manage functional deficits from MS symptoms. An interprofessional team approach is important to attain patient-centered outcomes for care.

To lessen muscle spasticity (which often contributes to pain), the primary health care provider may prescribe baclofen or tizanidine (Bhimani et al., 2018). Severe muscle spasticity may also be treated with intrathecal baclofen (ITB) administered through a surgically implanted pump. Paresthesia may be treated with carbamazepine or tricyclic antidepressants. Propranolol hydrochloride and clonazepam have been used to treat cerebellar ataxia.

In collaboration with physical and occupational therapists, plan an exercise program that includes range-of-motion (ROM) exercises and stretching and strengthening exercises to manage spasticity and tremor. If needed as a last resort, neurosurgery (e.g., thalamotomy or deep brain stimulation) may provide some relief from tremors.

Emphasize the importance of avoiding rigorous activities that increase body temperature. Increased body temperature may lead to increased fatigue, diminished motor ability, and decreased visual acuity resulting from changes in the conduction abilities of the injured axons.

In collaboration with the case manager and occupational therapist, assess the patient's home before discharge for any hazards. Any items that might interfere with ***mobility*** (e.g., scatter rugs) are removed. In addition, care must be taken to prevent injury resulting from vision problems. Teach the patient and family to keep the home environment as structured and free from clutter as possible. As the disease progresses, the home may need to be adapted for wheelchair accessibility. Adaptation in the kitchen, bedroom, and bathroom may also be needed to promote self-management. Any necessary assistive-adaptive device should be readily available before discharge from the hospital.

The patient with MS is often weak and easily fatigued. Teach the patient the importance of planning activities and allowing sufficient time to complete activities. For example, he or she should check that all items needed for work are gathered before leaving the house. Items used on a daily basis should be easily accessible.

If the patient experiences **dysarthria** as a result of muscle weakness, refer him or her to the speech-language pathologist (SLP) for evaluation and treatment. It is not unusual for the patient with dysarthria also to have **dysphagia**. The SLP performs a swallowing evaluation, but further diagnostic testing may be indicated. Monitor the patient to determine if there are problems swallowing at meal time that increase the risk of aspiration. Thickened liquids may be necessary.

Managing Decreased Visual Acuity and Cognition

Planning: Expected Outcomes. The patient with MS will maintain optimal visual acuity and ***cognition*** with use of available drug treatment and supportive services.

Interventions. Alterations in visual acuity and cognition can occur at any time during the course of the disease process. Areas affected include attention, memory, problem solving, auditory reasoning, handling distractions, and visual perception.

! NURSING SAFETY PRIORITY (QSEN)

Action Alert

For the patient with MS who has impaired *cognition*, assist with orientation by using a single-date calendar. Give or encourage the patient to use written lists or recorded messages. To maintain an organized environment, encourage him or her to keep frequently used items in familiar places. Applications for handheld devices such as mobile phones and electronic tablets can also be used for reorientation, reminders, and behavioral cues.

An eye patch that is alternated from eye to eye every few hours usually relieves **diplopia**. For peripheral visual deficits, teach scanning techniques by having the patient move his or her head from side to side. Changes in visual acuity may be helped by corrective lenses.

Complementary and Integrative Health. Patients with MS often report that complementary therapies are successful in decreasing their symptoms. Some of the integrative therapies used by patients with MS are:

- Reflexology
- Massage
- Yoga
- Relaxation and meditation
- Acupuncture
- Aromatherapy

Care Coordination and Transition Management

Home Care Management. To help the patient maintain maximum strength, function, and independence, continuity of care by an interprofessional team in the rehabilitation and/or home setting is necessary. Admission to a rehabilitation center may be needed to improve functional ability.

Self-Management Education. The primary health care provider explains to the patient and family the development of MS and the factors that may exacerbate the symptoms. Emphasize the importance of avoiding overexertion, stress, extremes of temperatures (fever, hot baths, use of sauna baths and hot tubs, overheating, and excessive chilling), humidity, and people with infections. Explain all medications to be taken on discharge, including the time and route of administration, dosage, purpose, and side effects. Teach the patient how to differentiate expected side effects from adverse or allergic reactions and provide the name of a resource person to call if questions or problems occur. Provide written instructions as a resource for the patient and caregivers at home.

The physical therapist develops an exercise program appropriate for the patient's tolerance level at home. The patient is instructed in techniques for self-care, daily living skills, and the use of required adaptive equipment such as walkers and electric carts. Include information related to bowel and bladder management, skin care, nutrition, and positioning techniques. Chapter 7 describes in detail these aspects of chronic illness and rehabilitation.

Teach patients about conservation strategies that balance periods of rest and activity, including regular social interactions. Remind them to use assistive devices and modify the environment to avoid fatigue. Explore strategies to manage stress and avoid undue stress. Often patients are anxious and worry about how long the remission will last or when the disease will progress.

MS affects the entire family because of the unpredictability and uncertainty of the course of the disease. Chronic fatigue may also prevent the patient from participating in family and community activities. Assess coping strategies of family members or other caregivers and help them identify support systems that can assist them as they live with the patient with MS.

Because personality changes are not unusual, teach the family or significant others strategies to enable them to cope with these changes. For example, the family may develop a nonverbal signal to alert the patient to potentially inappropriate behavior. This action avoids embarrassment for the patient.

Sexual dysfunction may occur as a result of fatigue, nerve involvement, and/or psychological reasons. Therefore some patients may benefit from counseling. If able, answer the patient's questions or refer him or her to a counselor or urologist with experience in the field of ***sexuality,*** intimacy, and disability.

Prostaglandin-5 inhibitors (sildenafil, vardenafil, tadalafil) can be used to help men with erectile dysfunction. Penile prostheses are also used for men. The EROS Clitoral Therapy Device is a U.S. Food and Drug Administration (FDA)–approved therapy for women with impaired sexual response.

Health Care Resources. Resources required by the patient depend on the course of the disease and the complications that occur. Patients usually are able to live independently, but they may need some assistance. In severe disease, placement in an assisted-living or long-term care facility may be the best alternative. The population of young and middle-age residents in these settings is increasing as people with chronic, disabling diseases live longer. Refer the patient and family members or significant others to the local chapter of the National Multiple Sclerosis Society (www.nationalmssociety.org) or the MS Society of Canada (https://mssociety.ca). Other community resources include meal-delivery services (e.g., Meals on Wheels), transportation services for the disabled, and homemaker services.

◆ **Evaluation: Evaluate Outcomes.** Evaluate the care of the patient with MS on the basis of the identified priority problems. The expected outcomes are that he or she:

- Remains free of infection as a result of drug therapy affecting ***immunity*** or the disease process
- Maintains optimal ***mobility*** and function as a result of managing fatigue and pain
- Maintains adequate visual acuity and ***cognition*** to function independently

MOBILITY CONCEPT EXEMPLAR: SPINAL CORD INJURY

Pathophysiology Review

Spinal cord injuries (SCIs) are classified as complete or incomplete. A *complete* SCI is one in which the spinal cord has been damaged in a way that eliminates all innervation below the level of the injury. Injuries that allow some function or movement below the level of the injury are described as an *incomplete* SCI. Incomplete injuries are more common than complete SCIs. Loss of or decreased ***mobility, sensory perception,*** and bowel and bladder control often result from an SCI.

Mechanisms of Injury. When enough force is applied to the spinal cord, the resulting damage causes many neurologic deficits. Sources of force include direct injury to the vertebral column (fracture, dislocation, and subluxation [partial dislocation]) or penetrating injury from violence (gunshot or knife wounds). Although in some cases the cord itself may remain intact, at other times it undergoes a destructive process caused by a contusion (bruise), compression, laceration, or transaction (severing of the cord, either complete or incomplete).

The causes of SCI can be divided into primary and secondary mechanisms of injury. Five *primary* mechanisms may result in an SCI:

- *Hyperflexion:* a sudden and forceful acceleration (movement) of the head forward, causing extreme flexion of the neck (Fig. 40.2). This is often the result of a head-on motor vehicle collision or diving accident. Flexion injury to the lower thoracic and lumbar spine may occur when the trunk is suddenly flexed on itself, such as occurs in a fall on the buttocks.
- *Hyperextension* occurs most often in vehicle collisions in which the vehicle is struck from behind or during falls when the patient's chin is struck (Fig. 40.3). The head is suddenly accelerated and then decelerated. This stretches or tears the anterior longitudinal ligament, fractures or subluxates the vertebrae, and perhaps ruptures an intervertebral disk. As with flexion injuries, the spinal cord may easily be damaged.

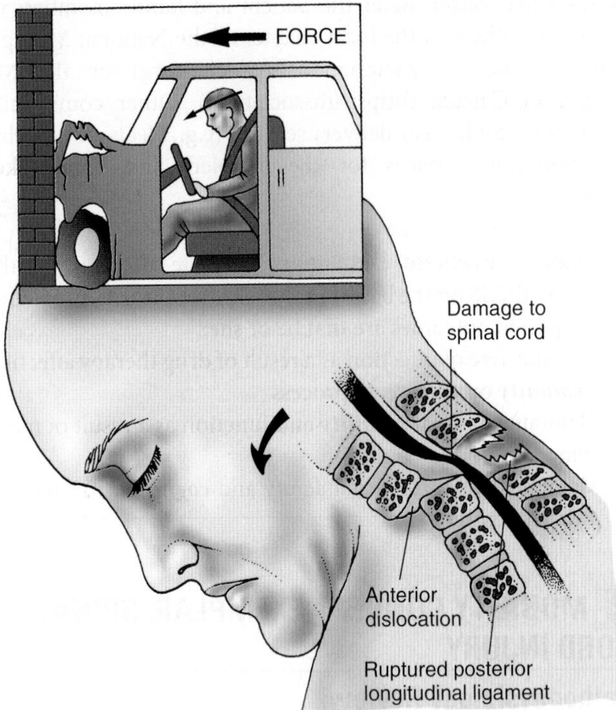

FIG. 40.2 Hyperflexion injury of the cervical spine.

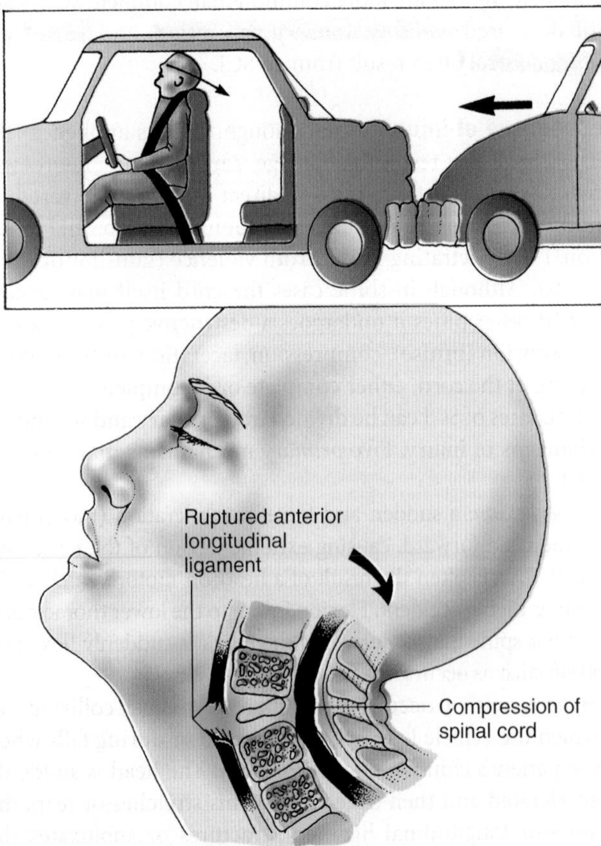

FIG. 40.3 Hyperextension injury of the cervical spine.

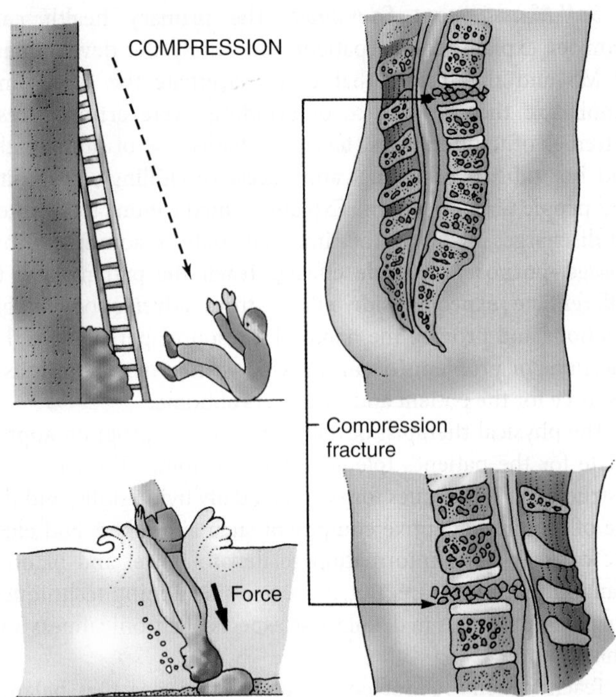

FIG. 40.4 Axial loading (vertical compression) injury of the cervical spine and the lumbar spine.

- *Axial loading or vertical compression* injuries resulting from diving accidents, falls on the buttocks, or a jump in which a person lands on the feet can cause many of the injuries attributable to *axial loading* (vertical compression) (Fig. 40.4). A blow to the top of the head can cause the vertebrae to shatter. Pieces of bone enter the spinal canal and damage the cord.
- *Excessive rotation* results from injuries that are caused by turning the head beyond the normal range.
- *Penetrating trauma* is classified by the speed of the object (e.g., knife, bullet) causing the injury. Low-speed or low-impact injuries cause damage directly at the site or local damage to the spinal cord or spinal nerves. In contrast, high-speed injuries that occur from gunshot wounds (GSWs) cause both direct and indirect damage.

Secondary injury worsens the primary injury. Secondary injuries include:

- Hemorrhage
- Ischemia (lack of oxygen, typically from reduced/absent blood flow)
- Hypovolemia (decreased circulating blood volume)
- Impaired tissue perfusion from neurogenic shock *(a medical emergency)*
- Local edema

Hemorrhage into the spinal cord may manifest with contusion or petechial leaking into the central gray matter and later into the white matter. Systemic hemorrhage can result in shock and decrease perfusion to the spinal cord. Edema occurs with both primary and secondary injuries, contributing to capillary compression and cord ischemia. In neurogenic shock, loss of blood vessel tone (dilation) after *severe* cord injury may result in hypoperfusion (McCance et al., 2019).

Patients who have SCI have a decreased life expectancy owing to complications of immobility or, more often, some type of infection. The major causes of death are pneumonia and septicemia (National Spinal Cord Injury Statistical Center, 2018).

Etiology. Trauma is the leading cause of spinal cord injuries (SCIs), with more than a third resulting from vehicle crashes. Other leading causes are falls, acts of violence (usually gunshot wounds [GSWs]), and sports- or recreation-related accidents (National Spinal Cord Injury Statistical Center, 2018). SCIs from falls are particularly likely among older adults. Spinal cord damage in adults can also result from nontraumatic vertebral fracture and diseases such as benign or malignant tumors.

PATIENT-CENTERED CARE: VETERANS HEALTH CONSIDERATIONS QSEN

Be aware that veterans who experience an SCI typically have other major injuries, including traumatic brain injury and amputation of one or more limbs. These additional injuries may take priority over attending to the problems related to the SCI.

Incidence and Prevalence. According to the National Spinal Cord Injury Statistical Center (2018), about 18,000 *new* SCIs occur every year in the United States. Almost 80% of all SCIs occur in young males, with the majority being Euro-American. Cervical cord injuries are more common than thoracic or lumbar cord injuries. The most common neurologic level of injury is C5. In paraplegia, T12 and L1 are the most common levels. The average age of patients who have SCI is 43 years (National Spinal Cord Injury Statistical Center, 2018).

Health Promotion and Maintenance. Because trauma is the leading cause of SCI, teach people to avoid taking risks, such as ensuring adequate protective measures (e.g., padding and helmets) for sports and recreation. Remind them to wear seat belts at all times when driving and avoid impaired driving caused by alcohol, marijuana, and other substances. Instruct them on the danger of diving into shallow pools or other water when the depth is not known. Water should be at least 9 feet deep before diving is attempted.

❖ Interprofessional Collaborative Care

◆ Assessment: Recognize Cues

History. When obtaining a history from a patient with an acute SCI, gather as much data as possible about how the accident occurred and the probable mechanism of injury once the patient is stabilized. Questions include:

- Location and position of the patient immediately after the injury
- Symptoms that occurred immediately with the injury
- Changes that have occurred subsequently
- Type of immobilization devices used and whether any problems occurred during stabilization and transport to the hospital
- Treatment given at the scene of injury or in the emergency department (ED) (e.g., medications, IV fluids)
- Medical history, including osteoporosis or arthritis of the spine, congenital deformities, cancer, and previous injury or surgery of the neck or back
- History of any respiratory problems, especially if the patient has experienced a cervical SCI

Physical Assessment/Signs and Symptoms

Initial Assessment. *The initial and priority assessment focuses on the patient's ABCs (airway, breathing, and circulation).* After an airway is established, assess the patient's breathing pattern. The patient with a cervical SCI is at high risk for respiratory compromise because the cervical spinal nerves (C3-5) innervate the phrenic nerve controlling the diaphragm.

Evaluate pulse, blood pressure, and peripheral perfusion such as pulse strength and capillary refill. Multiple injuries may contribute to circulatory compromise from hemorrhagic hypovolemic shock. Assess for indications of *hemorrhage.* All symptoms of circulatory compromise or hypovolemic shock must be treated aggressively to preserve tissue perfusion to the spinal cord. Shock is discussed in detail in Chapter 34.

Use the Glasgow Coma Scale (see Chapter 38) or other agency-approved assessment tool to assess the patient's *level of consciousness (LOC).* Cognitive impairment as a result of an associated traumatic brain injury (TBI) or substance use disorder can occur in patients with traumatic SCIs.

Spinal shock, also called *spinal shock syndrome,* occurs immediately as the cord's response to the injury. The patient has complete but temporary loss of motor, sensory, reflex, and autonomic function that often lasts less than 48 hours but may continue for several weeks (McCance et al., 2019). Spinal shock is *not* the same as neurogenic shock.

Sensory Perception and Mobility Assessment. Perform a detailed assessment of the patient's ***mobility*** and ***sensory perception*** status to determine the level of injury and establish baseline data for future comparison. The level of injury is the lowest neurologic segment with intact or normal motor and sensory function. **Tetraplegia** (also called *quadriplegia*) (paralysis) and **quadriparesis** (weakness) involve all four extremities, as seen with cervical cord and upper thoracic injury. **Paraplegia** (paralysis) and **paraparesis** (weakness) involve only the lower extremities, as seen in lower thoracic and lumbosacral injuries or lesions.

Neurologic level defined by the American Spinal Injury Association (ASIA) refers to the highest neurologic level of normal function and is not the same as the *anatomic* level of injury. The neurologic level is determined by evaluation of the zones of sensory and motor function, known as *dermatomes* and *myotomes.* Follow the sensory distribution of the skin dermatomes (see Fig. 38.3 in Chapter 38), with the examination beginning in the area of reported loss of ***sensory perception*** and ending where sensory perception becomes normal. For example, sensation of the top of the foot and calf of the leg is spinal skin segment (dermatome) levels L3, L4, and L5. The area at the level of the umbilicus is T10, the clavicle (collarbone) is C3 or C4, and finger sensation is C7 and C8. The patient may report a complete sensory loss,

hypoesthesia (decreased ***sensory perception***), or **hyperesthesia** (increased ***sensory perception***).

The primary health care provider may also test deep tendon reflexes (DTRs), including the biceps (C5), triceps (C7), patella (L3), and ankle (S1). It is not unusual for these reflexes, as well as all ***mobility*** or ***sensory perception,*** to be absent immediately after the injury because of spinal shock. After spinal shock has resolved, the reflexes may return.

! NURSING SAFETY PRIORITY (QSEN)

Critical Rescue

In *acute* SCI, monitor for a decrease in *sensory perception* from baseline, especially in a proximal (upward) dermatome and/or new loss of motor function and *mobility.* The presence of these changes is considered an emergency and requires immediate communication with the primary health care provider using SBAR or other agency-approved protocol for notification. Document these assessment findings in the electronic health record.

Cardiovascular and Respiratory Assessment. *Cardiovascular* dysfunction results from disruption of sympathetic fibers of the autonomic nervous system (ANS), especially if the injury is above the sixth thoracic vertebra. Bradycardia, hypotension, and hypothermia occur because of loss of sympathetic input. These changes may lead to cardiac dysrhythmias. *A systolic blood pressure below 90 mm Hg requires treatment because lack of perfusion to the spinal cord could worsen the patient's condition.*

A patient with a cervical SCI is at risk for *breathing* problems resulting from an interruption of spinal innervation to the respiratory muscles. In collaboration with the respiratory therapist (RT), if available, perform a complete respiratory assessment, including pulse oximetry for arterial oxygen saturation, every 8 to 12 hours. An oxygen saturation of 92% or less and adventitious breath sounds may indicate a complication such as atelectasis or pneumonia.

Autonomic dysreflexia (AD), sometimes referred to as *autonomic hyperreflexia,* is a potentially life-threatening condition in which noxious visceral or cutaneous stimuli cause a sudden, massive, uninhibited reflex sympathetic discharge in people with high-level SCI. The signs and symptoms of AD are listed in the Key Features: Autonomic Dysreflexia box. Severely elevated blood pressure can cause a hemorrhagic stroke, discussed in Chapter 41.

KEY FEATURES

Autonomic Dysreflexia

- Sudden, significant rise in systolic and diastolic blood pressure, accompanied by bradycardia
- Profuse sweating above the level of lesion—especially in the face, neck, and shoulders; rarely occurs below the level of the lesion because of sympathetic cholinergic activity
- Goose bumps above or possibly below the level of the lesion
- Flushing of the skin above the level of the lesion—especially in the face, neck, and shoulders
- Blurred vision
- Spots in the patient's visual field
- Nasal congestion
- Onset of severe, throbbing headache
- Flushing about the level of the lesion with pale skin below the level of the lesion
- Feeling of apprehension

The causes of AD are typically GI, gynecologic-urologic (GU), and vascular stimulation. Specific risk factors are bladder distention, urinary tract infection, epididymitis or scrotal compression, bowel distention or impaction from constipation, or irritation of hemorrhoids. Pain; circumferential constriction of the thorax, abdomen, or an extremity (e.g., tight clothing); contact with hard or sharp objects; and temperature fluctuations can also cause AD. Patients with altered ***sensory perception*** are at great risk for this complication (McCance et al., 2019).

Gastrointestinal and Genitourinary Assessment. Assess the patient's *abdomen* for symptoms of internal bleeding, such as abdominal distention, pain, or paralytic ileus. Hemorrhage may result from the trauma, or it may occur later from a stress ulcer or the administration of steroids. Monitor for abdominal pain and changes in bowel sounds. Paralytic ileus may develop within 72 hours of hospital admission. During the period of spinal shock, peristalsis decreases, leading to a loss of bowel sounds and to gastric distention. This disruption of the autonomic nervous system may lead to a hypotonic bowel.

After the first few days, when edema subsides, the spinal reflexes that innervate the bowel and bladder usually begin to establish function, depending on the level of the injury. Patients with cervical or high thoracic SCIs have upper motor neuron damage that spares lower spinal reflexes, causing a *spastic* bowel and bladder. Patients with lower thoracic and lumbosacral injuries usually have damage to their lower spinal nerves and therefore have a *flaccid* bowel and bladder.

Assessment of Patients for Long-Term Complications. Patients with complete SCI are at a high risk for complications that result from prolonged impaired ***mobility,*** including *pressure injuries* and *venous thromboembolism (VTE).* Assess skin integrity with each turn or repositioning. Monitor for signs of VTE with vital signs, including lower extremity deep vein thrombosis (DVT). More detailed information on prevention and management of these complications may be found elsewhere in this text.

Bones can become *osteopenic* and *osteoporotic* without weight-bearing exercise, placing the long-term SCI patient at risk for fractures. Another complication of prolonged immobility is **heterotopic ossification (HO)** (bony overgrowth, often into muscle). Assess for swelling, redness, warmth, and decreased range of motion (ROM) of the involved extremity. The hip is the most common place where HO occurs. Changes in the bony structure are not visible until several weeks after initial symptoms appear.

Chapters 3 and 7 describe additional nursing assessments and interventions to help prevent and monitor for complications of decreased ***mobility.***

Psychosocial Assessment. Patients experiencing an SCI may have significant behavior and emotional reactions as a result of changes in functional ability, body image, role performance, and self-concept. Many of these patients are young men who may feel guilty for engaging in high-risk behaviors such as diving into shallow water or racing a vehicle that caused the injury. Some patients with SCI are war veterans. Assess patients for their reaction to the injury and provide opportunities to listen to their concerns. Be realistic about their abilities and projected function, but offer hope and encouragement. Aggressive rehabilitation can help most patients live productive and independent lives.

Laboratory and Imaging Assessment. The primary health care provider may request basic laboratory studies for the patient with an SCI to establish baseline data. A spine CT and MRI are performed to determine the degree and extent of damage to the spinal cord and detect the presence of blood and bone within the spinal column. In addition, patients may have a series of x-rays of the spine to identify vertebral fractures, subluxation, or dislocation.

◆ **Analysis: Analyze Cues and Prioritize Hypotheses.** The priority collaborative problems for patients with an *acute* spinal cord injury (SCI) include:

1. Potential for respiratory distress/failure due to aspiration, decreased diaphragmatic innervation, and/or decreased ***mobility***
2. Potential for cardiovascular instability (e.g., shock and autonomic dysreflexia) due to loss or interruption of sympathetic innervation or hemorrhage
3. Potential for secondary spinal cord injury due to hypoperfusion, edema, or delayed spinal column stabilization
4. Decreased ***mobility*** and ***sensory perception*** due to spinal cord damage and edema

In addition, the patient with a long-term SCI is at risk for multiple problems caused by prolonged immobility or decreased ***mobility.*** These problems are discussed in fundamentals textbooks.

◆ **Planning and Implementation: Generate Solutions and Take Action.** Caring for a patient with an SCI requires both a patient- a and family-centered collaborative approach and involves every health care team member to help meet the patient's expected outcomes. Optimally, patients with a new SCI are quickly transported to an SCI Model System Center. Because of the complexity of an SCI, discharge planning, including the rehabilitation team, needs to begin the day of admission.

The desired outcomes of patient-centered collaborative care following acute SCI are to stabilize the vertebral column, manage damage to the spinal cord, and prevent secondary injuries.

Managing the Airway and Improving Breathing

Planning: Expected Outcomes. The patient with an SCI is expected to not experience respiratory distress as evidenced by a patent airway and adequate ventilation.

Interventions. *Airway management is the priority for a patient with cervical spinal cord injury!* Patients with injuries at or above T6 are especially at risk for respiratory distress and pulmonary embolus during the first 5 days after injury. These complications are caused by impaired functioning of the intercostal muscles and disruption in the innervation to the diaphragm. Depending on the level of injury, intubation or tracheotomy with mechanical ventilation may be needed.

Respiratory secretions are managed with manually assisted coughing, pulmonary hygiene, and suctioning. Implement strategies to prevent ventilator-associated pneumonia (VAP) when the patient needs continuous mechanical ventilation as discussed in Chapter 29. Encourage the non–mechanically ventilated patient to use an incentive spirometer. The nurse and respiratory therapist perform a respiratory assessment at least every 8 hours to determine the effectiveness of these strategies. In some cases, it may be necessary to perform oral or nasal suctioning if the patient cannot clear the airway of secretions effectively.

Teach the patient who is tetraplegic to coordinate his or her cough effort with an assistant. The nurse, or other assistant, places his or her hands on the upper abdomen over the diaphragm and below the ribs. Hands are placed one over the other, with fingers interlocked and away from the skin (Fig. 40.5). If the patient is obese, an alternate hand placement is one hand on either side of the rib cage. Have the patient take a breath and cough during expiration. The assistant locks his or her elbows and pushes inward and upward as the patient coughs. This technique is sometimes called *assisted coughing, quad cough,* or cough assist. Repeat the coordinated effort, with rest periods as needed, until the airway is clear.

! NURSING SAFETY PRIORITY (QSEN)

Action Alert

Assess breath sounds every 2 to 4 hours during the first few days after SCI and document and report any adventitious or diminished sounds. Monitor vital signs with pulse oximetry. Watch for changes in respiratory pattern or airway obstruction. Intervene per agency or primary health care provider protocol when there is a decrease in oxygen saturation (Spo_2) to below 95%.

Monitoring for Cardiovascular Instability

Planning: Expected Outcomes. The patient is expected to not develop neurogenic or hypovolemic shock due to hemorrhage; he or she is expected to be free from episodes of autonomic dysreflexia (AD). If any of these potentially life-threatening complications occur, the patient is expected to receive prompt interventions.

Interventions. Maintain adequate hydration through IV therapy and oral fluids as appropriate, depending on the patient's overall condition. Carefully observe for manifestations of *neurogenic shock,* which may occur within 24 hours after injury, most commonly in patients with injuries above T6. This potentially life-threatening problem results from disruption in the communication pathways between upper motor neurons and lower motor neurons.

Dextran, a plasma expander, may be used to increase capillary blood flow within the spinal cord and prevent or treat

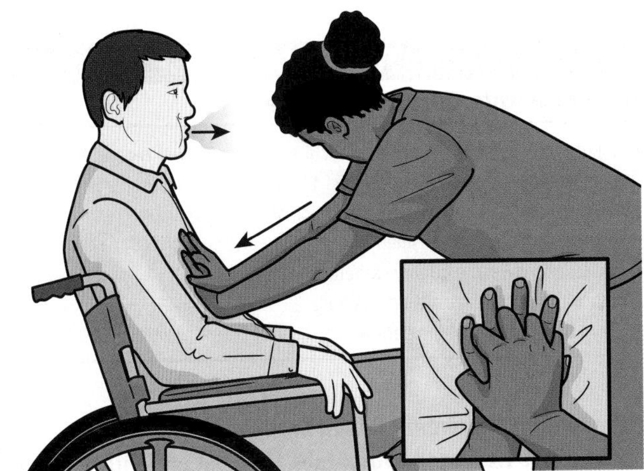

FIG. 40.5 "Cough assist" technique for patient with high spinal cord injury.

! NURSING SAFETY PRIORITY QSEN

Critical Rescue

Monitor the patient with acute spinal cord injury at least hourly for indications of neurogenic shock:

- Pulse oximetry (Spo_2) <95% or symptoms of aspiration (e.g., stridor, garbled speech, or inability to clear airway)
- Symptomatic bradycardia, including reduced level of consciousness and deceased urine output
- Hypotension with systolic blood pressure (SBP) <90 or mean arterial pressure (MAP) <65 mm Hg

Notify the Rapid Response Team or primary health care provider immediately if these symptoms occur because this problem is an emergency! Respiratory compromise from aspiration may be treated with intubation or bronchial endoscopy. Similar to interventions for any type of shock, neurogenic shock is treated symptomatically by providing fluids to the circulating blood volume, adding vasopressor IV therapy, and providing supportive care to stabilize the patient.

hypotension. *Atropine sulfate* is used to treat bradycardia if the pulse rate falls below 50 to 60 beats/min. Hypotension, if severe, is treated with continuous IV sympathomimetic agents such as *dopamine* or other vasoactive agent. Chapter 34 discusses in detail the care of patients experiencing or at risk for shock.

In addition to observing the patient for shock or hypotension, monitor the patient who has a high-level SCI injury for the additional risk of autonomic dysreflexia (AD). *AD is a neurologic emergency and must be promptly treated to prevent a hypertensive stroke!* Be sure to reduce potential causes for this complication by preventing bladder and bowel distention, managing pain and room temperature, and monitoring for early vital sign changes.

! NURSING SAFETY PRIORITY QSEN

Critical Rescue

If the patient experiences AD, raise the head of the bed *immediately* to help reduce the blood pressure as the first action. Notify the Rapid Response Team or primary health care provider immediately for drug therapy to quickly reduce blood pressure as indicated. Determine the cause of AD and manage it promptly as described in the Best Practice for Patient Safety & Quality Care: Emergecy Care of the Patient Experiencing Autonomic Dysreflexia: Immediate Interventions box.

NCLEX EXAMINATION CHALLENGE 40.2

Safe Effective Care Environment

A client who sustained a recent cervical spinal cord injury reports having a throbbing headache and feeling flushed. The client's blood pressure is 190/110 mm Hg. What is the nurse's **priority** action at this time?

A. Perform a bladder assessment.
B. Insert an indwelling urinary catheter.
C. Place the patient in a sitting position.
D. Turn on a fan to cool the patient.

Preventing Secondary Spinal Cord Injury

Planning: Expected Outcomes. The patient with an *acute* SCI is expected to have adequate spinal cord stabilization as evidenced by no further deterioration in neurologic status.

BEST PRACTICE FOR PATIENT SAFETY & QUALITY CARE QSEN

Emergency Care of the Patient Experiencing Autonomic Dysreflexia: Immediate Interventions

- Place patient in a sitting position (first priority!), or return to a previous safe position.
- Assess for and remove/manage the cause:
  - Check for urinary retention or catheter blockage.
  - Check the urinary catheter tubing (if present) for kinks or obstruction.
  - If a urinary catheter is not present, check for bladder distention and catheterize immediately if indicated. (Consider using anesthetic ointment on tip of catheter before catheter insertion to reduce urethral irritation.)
- Determine if a urinary tract infection or bladder calculi (stones) are contributing to genitourinary irritation.
- Check the patient for fecal impaction or other colorectal irritation, using anesthetic ointment at rectum. Disimpact if needed.
- Examine skin for new or worsening pressure injury symptoms.
- Monitor blood pressure every 10 to 15 minutes.
- Give nifedipine or nitrate as prescribed to lower blood pressure as needed. (Patients with recurrent autonomic dysreflexia may receive clonidine or other centrally acting alpha-agonist agent prophylactically [Burchum & Rosenthal, 2019].)

Interventions. If the patient has a fractured vertebra, the primary concern of the health care team is to reduce and immobilize the fracture to prevent further damage to the spinal cord from bone fragments. Nonsurgical techniques include external fixation or orthotic devices, but surgery is often needed to stabilize the spine and prevent further spinal cord damage.

Assess the patient's neurologic status, particularly focusing on ***mobility*** (motor) and ***sensory perception*** function, vital signs, pulse oximetry, and ***pain*** level, at least every 1 to 4 hours, depending on his or her overall condition. *Document your assessments carefully and in detail, particularly changes in motor or sensory function. Failure to do so may prevent other staff members from quickly recognizing deterioration in neurologic status.*

Regardless of the level of SCI, keep the patient in proper body alignment to prevent further cord injury or irritability. Devices such as traction, orthoses, or collars may be used to keep the spine immobilized during healing and rehabilitation.

Spinal Immobilization and Stabilization. During the immediate care of the patient with a suspected or confirmed cervical spine injury, a hard cervical collar, such as the Miami J or Philadelphia collar, is placed immediately and maintained until a specific order indicates that it can be removed (Fig. 40.6). A daily inspection of skin beneath the collar is recommended while a primary health care provider helps to maintain neck alignment when the collar is removed. Padding at pressure points beneath and at the edges of the collar, particularly at the occiput, may be necessary to sustain skin integrity. Until the spinal column is stabilized, a jaw-thrust maneuver is preferable to a head-tilt maneuver to open the airway should the patient need an airway intervention. Maintain spinal alignment at all times with log rolling to change position from supine to side-lying.

The patient may be placed in fixed skeletal traction to realign the vertebrae, facilitate bone healing, and prevent further injury, often after surgical stabilization. The most commonly used device for immobilization of the cervical spine is the *halo fixator* device, also called a *halo crown,* which is worn for 6 to 12 weeks. This static device is affixed by four pins (or screws) into the outer aspect of the skull and is connected to a vest or jacket (Fig. 40.7). For patients not having surgery, the addition of traction helps reduce the fracture.

Nonsurgical treatment of *thoracic and lumbosacral injuries* is often challenging. Most primary health care providers choose to refer the patient for surgery and then immobilize

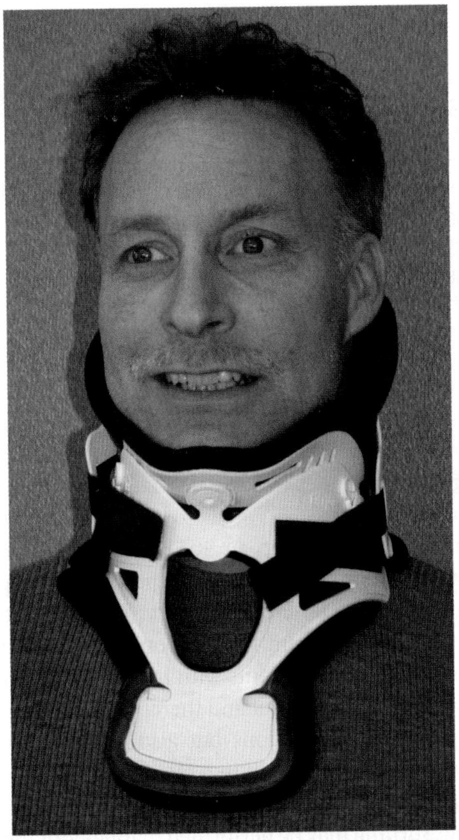

FIG. 40.6 Patient with spinal cord injury wearing a hard cervical (Miami J) collar. (From Garfin, S.R., Eismont, F.J., Bell, G.R., et al. [2018]. *Rothman-Simeone and Herkowitz's the spine.* [7th ed.]. Philadelphia: Elsevier.)

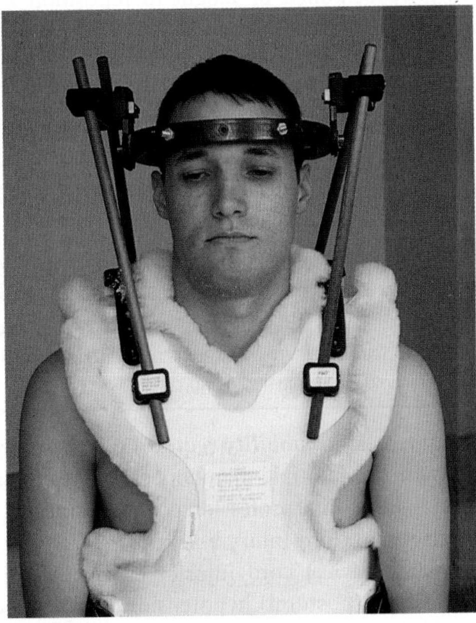

FIG. 40.7 Halo fixation device with jacket.

! NURSING SAFETY PRIORITY (QSEN)

Action Alert

Never move or turn the patient by holding or pulling on the halo device. Do not adjust the screws holding it in place. Check the patient's skin frequently to ensure that the jacket is not causing pressure. Pressure is avoided if one finger can be inserted easily between the jacket and the patient's skin. Monitor the patient's neurologic status for changes in movement or decreased strength. A special wrench is needed to loosen the vest in emergencies such as cardiopulmonary arrest. Tape the wrench to the vest for easy and consistent accessibility. Do not use sharp objects (e.g., coat hangers, knitting needles) to relieve itching under the vest; skin damage and infection will slow recovery.

Common complications of the halo device are pin loosening, local infection, and scarring. More serious but less common complications include osteomyelitis (cranial bone infection), subdural abscess, and instability. Hospital policy is followed for pin-site care, which may specify the use of solutions such as saline. Vaseline dressings may also be used. *Monitor vital signs for indications of possible infection (e.g., fever, purulent drainage from the pin sites) and report any changes to the primary health care provider immediately.*

Discharge teaching related to halo fixator management is described in the Patient and Family Education: Preparing for Self-Management: Use of a Halo Fixator With Vest box.

PATIENT AND FAMILY EDUCATION: PREPARING FOR SELF-MANAGEMENT

Use of a Halo Fixator With Vest

- Be aware that the weight of the halo device alters balance. Be careful when leaning forward or backward.
- Wear loose clothing, preferably with hook and loop (Velcro) fasteners or large openings for head and arms.
- Bathe in the bathtub or take a sponge bath. (Some primary health care providers allow showers.)
- Wash under the liner of the vest to prevent rashes or sores; use powders or lotions sparingly under the vest.
- Have someone change the liner if it becomes odorous.
- Support the head with a small pillow when sleeping to prevent unnecessary pressure and discomfort.
- Try to resume usual activities to the extent possible; keep as active as possible. (The weight of the device may cause fatigue or weakness.) However, avoid contact sports and swimming.
- Do not drive because vision is impaired with the device.
- Keep straws available for drinking fluids.
- Cut meats and other food into small pieces to facilitate chewing and swallowing.
- Before going outside in cold temperatures, wrap the pins with cloth to prevent the metal from getting cold.
- Have someone clean the pin sites as recommended by the primary health care provider or hospital protocol.
- Observe the pin sites daily for redness, drainage, or loosening; report changes to the primary health care provider.
- Increase fluids and fiber in the diet to prevent constipation.
- Use a position of comfort during sexual activity.

the spine with lightweight, custom-fit thoracic-lumbar sacral orthoses (TLSOs) to prevent prolonged periods of immobility.

NCLEX EXAMINATION CHALLENGE 40.3

Physiological Integrity

A nurse is caring for a client who has a halo fixator device with vest for a complete cervical spinal cord injury. Which assessment finding will the nurse report to the primary health care provider?

A. Purulent drainage from the pin sites on the client's forehead
B. Painful pressure injury under the collar
C. Inability to move legs or feet
D. Oxygen saturation of 95% on room air

Drug Therapy. Because SCI is a physical trauma, the patient is started on a proton pump inhibitor, such as pantoprazole, to help prevent the development of stress ulcers. This drug may be administered IV or orally. Oral doses may be taken with our without food (Burcham & Rosenthal, 2019).

Centrally acting skeletal muscular relaxants, such as tizanidine, may help control severe muscle spasticity. However, these drugs cause severe drowsiness and sedation in most patients and may not be effective in reducing spasticity. As an alternative to these drugs, intrathecal baclofen (ITB) therapy may be prescribed in a lower dose (Bhimani et al., 2018). This drug is administered through a programmable, implantable infusion pump and intrathecal catheter directly into the cerebrospinal fluid. The pump is surgically placed in a subcutaneous pouch in the lower abdomen. Monitor for common adverse effects, which include sedation, fatigue, headache, hypotension, and changes in mental status (Bhimani et al., 2018). *Seizures and hallucinations may occur if ITB is suddenly withdrawn.*

Other drugs to prevent or treat complications of immobility may be needed *later* during the rehabilitative phase. For example, celecoxib may be prescribed to prevent or treat **heterotopic ossification** (bony overgrowth). However, recall that the adverse effects of this drug include an increased risk of myocardial infarction and stroke. Calcium and bisphosphonates may prevent the osteoporosis that results from lack of weight-bearing or resistance activity. Osteoporosis can cause fractures in later years. Early and continued exercise may help decrease the incidence of these complications.

Surgical Management. Surgery within 24 hours of injury to stabilize the vertebral spinal column, particularly if there is evidence of spinal cord compression, results in decreased secondary complications. Emergent surgery also removes bone fragments, hematomas, or penetrating objects such as a bullet. Typical procedures include wiring and spinal fusion for cervical injuries and the insertion of steel or metal rods (e.g., Harrington rods) to stabilize thoracic and lumbar spinal injuries. During a cervical fusion, the surgeon reduces the fracture by placing the bone ends in proper alignment. Metal wiring is then used to secure bone chips taken from the patient's hip or other source of bone grafting. The patient wears a halo vest to immobilize the spine during the healing process. For thoracic and lumbar fusions, metal or steel rods (e.g., Harrington rods) are used to keep the bone ends in alignment after fracture reduction. After surgery the patient usually wears a molded plastic support (cervical or thoracic-lumbar or both) to keep the injured and operative areas immobilized during recovery. Postoperative care is similar to that described in Chapter 9.

! NURSING SAFETY PRIORITY QSEN

Action Alert

After surgical spinal fusion, assess the patient's neurologic status and vital signs at least every hour for the first 4 to 6 hours and then, if the patient is stable, every 4 hours. Assess for complications of surgery, including worsening of motor or sensory function at or above the site of surgery.

Managing Decreased Mobility

Planning: Expected Outcomes. The patient with an SCI is expected to be free from complications of decreased ***mobility*** and perform ADLs as independently as possible with or without assistive-adaptive devices.

Interventions. Patients with an SCI are especially at risk for pressure injuries due to altered ***sensory perception*** of pressure areas on skin below the level of the injury. They are also at risk for venous thromboembolism (VTE), contractures, orthostatic hypotension (especially in patients with high SCI), and fractures related to osteoporosis. Frequent and therapeutic positioning not only helps prevent complications but also provides alignment to prevent further SCI or irritability. Assess the condition of the patient's skin, especially over pressure points, with each turn or repositioning. Turning may be performed manually, or the patient may be placed on an automatic rotating bed. Reduce pressure on any reddened area and monitor it with the next turn. Reposition patients frequently (every 1 to 2 hours). When sitting in a chair, the patient is repositioned or taught to reposition himself or herself more often than every hour. Paraplegic patients usually perform frequent "wheelchair push-ups" to relieve skin pressure. Use a pressure-reducing mattress and wheelchair or chair pad to help prevent skin breakdown. Prevent pressure injuries using best practices as described in Chapter 22. Prevent VTE, including using interventions of intermittent pneumatic compression stockings and low–molecular-weight heparin (LMWH).

! CORE MEASURES

Document pressure injury and VTE prophylaxis in accordance with Core Measures developed by the Centers for Medicare and Medicaid Services and The Joint Commission (www.jointcommision.org).

Managing decreased ***mobility*** requires communication and coordination among multiple members of the health care team as described in the Interprofessional Collaboration: Care of Patients With Spinal Cord Injury box.

Patients with cervical cord injuries especially are at high risk for orthostatic (postural) hypotension, but anyone who is

INTERPROFESSIONAL COLLABORATION

Care of Patients With Spinal Cord Injury

In collaboration with the rehabilitation team, teach or reinforce teaching for bed *mobility* skills and bed-to-chair transfers. Patients with paraplegia are usually able to transfer from the bed to chair or wheelchair with minimal or no assistance unless balance is a problem (seen in patients with high thoracic injuries). Techniques to improve balance are usually taught by occupational therapists. Tetraplegic patients may learn how to transfer using a slider, also called a *sliding board*. This simple boardlike device allows the patient to move from the bed to chair or vice versa by creating a bridge. When using the slider, remind patients to lift the buttocks while moving incrementally and slowly across the board. Patients with severe muscle spasticity have more challenges when learning transfer skills, and contractures are common.

Contractures may be prevented or minimized with splints and range-of-motion exercises. Consult with the physical therapist (PT) and occupational therapist (OT) for optimal scheduling for placing and removing splints (typically individually molded to the patient's extremity), applying pressure to trigger points to relieve spasticity, and positioning to maintain joint function.

According to the Interprofessional Education Collaborative (IPEC) Expert Panel's Competency of Interprofessional Communication, be sure to use language that is easily understood by the patient when coordinating care. Avoid discipline-specific terminology when possible (IPEC, 2016; Slusser et al., 2019).

immobilized may have this problem. If the patient changes from a lying position to a sitting or standing position too quickly, he or she may experience hypotension, which could result in dizziness and falls. Because of interrupted sympathetic innervation caused by the SCI, the blood vessels do not constrict quickly enough to push blood up into the brain. The resulting vasodilation causes dizziness or light-headedness and possible falls with syncope ("blackout").

All patients with an SCI require bowel and bladder retraining, including adequate fluids and stool softeners to prevent constipation from immobility and the injury itself. Those with *upper* motor neuron lesions (usually cervical and high thoracic injuries) have *spastic* bowel and bladder function with an intact spinal reflex for elimination. However, voiding patterns may be uncontrollable and require long-term indwelling or external catheters. Rectal suppositories are often successful to promote regular bowel elimination.

The patient with a *lower* motor neuron lesion has a *flaccid* bowel and bladder. Intermittent urinary catheterizations, manual pressure over the bladder area, and bowel impaction on a regular basis help to establish a routine. Chapter 7 describes bowel and bladder training in more detail.

In patients with established or long-term SCI, assess baseline ability and encourage their participation in self-care and management. Encourage family participation in care, and support their effort to keep the patient engaged in family life.

Care Coordination and Transition Management. Case managers are ideal care coordinators to act as SCI patient advocates. In some settings, case managers begin working with patients in the emergency department to establish a positive image of SCI rehabilitation. The primary purpose of rehabilitation is to

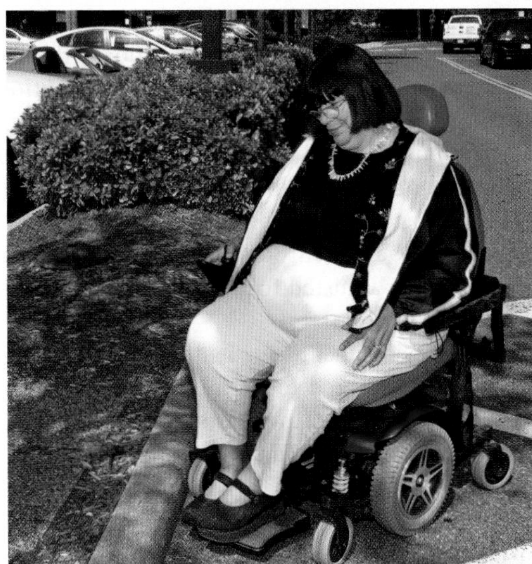

FIG. 40.8 Community physical barrier example: A curb prevents the patient in a wheelchair from getting onto the sidewalk.

enable patients to function independently in their communities. However, many physical barriers still exist in some communities that prevent the patient in a wheelchair from finding a parking place, using sidewalks, and attending activities or using resources (Fig. 40.8).

Rehabilitation begins in the acute or critical care unit when patients are hemodynamically stable. They are usually transferred from the acute care setting to a rehabilitation setting, where they learn more about self-care, mobility skills, and bladder and bowel retraining.

Psychosocial adaptation is one of the critical factors in determining the success of rehabilitation. The case manager or acute care nurse can help the patient and family members prepare for discharge or transfer to a rehabilitation hospital. Assist in verbalizing feelings and fears about body image, self-concept, role performance, self-esteem, and sexuality. The patient should be told about the expected reactions of those outside the security of the hospital environment. Role playing or anticipating responses to potential problems is helpful. For example, the patient can practice answering questions from children about why he or she is in a wheelchair or cannot move certain parts of the body.

For young men with SCI, sexuality is a major issue. Many patients are concerned about their ability to have sexual intercourse and have children. Most hospitals do not have psychological social workers or counselors to discuss sexuality issues. By contrast, rehabilitation programs often include a ***sexuality***/intimacy counselor as part of the interprofessional team approach to patient care.

Many patients with previous SCIs are admitted to the acute care or long-term care setting for complications of immobility, such as pressure injuries or fractures resulting from osteoporosis. Pressure injuries contribute to local infection, including osteomyelitis and septicemia. Priorities in care may need to be reevaluated as complications occur and resolve.

Home Care Management. If the patient is discharged home or returns home for a weekend visit from the rehabilitation setting, the environment must be assessed to ensure that it is free from hazards and can accommodate the patient's special needs (e.g., a wheelchair). The occupational or physical therapist, in collaboration with rehabilitation and the home care nurse, usually assesses the patient's temporary or permanent home environment. Ease of accessibility is particularly important at the entrance of the home and in the bathroom, kitchen, and bedroom. The height of the patient's bed may need to be adjusted to allow a smooth transfer into and out of the bed.

All adaptive devices that the patient will use at home should be requested and delivered to the rehabilitation facility. This enables the nurse and other therapists to ensure that the items fit correctly and that the patient and family know how to use them correctly.

Self-Management Education. The teaching plan for the patient with an SCI includes:

- *Mobility* skills
- Pressure injury prevention
- ADL skills
- Bowel and bladder program
- Education about *sexuality* and referral for counseling to promote sexual health
- Prevention of autonomic dysreflexia with appropriate bladder, bowel, and skin-care practices and recognition of early signs or symptoms of autonomic dysreflexia

This information should be reinforced with written handouts, CDs, DVDs, or other patient-education material that the patient and family members can use after discharge to the home. The Patient-Centered Care: Older Adult Considerations: What Patients Need to Know About Aging With Spinal Cord Injury box provides information about aging for middle-age and older adults with an SCI.

A full-time caregiver or personal assistant is sometimes required if the patient with tetraplegia returns home. The caregiver may be a family member or a nursing assistant employed to help provide care and companionship. A patient who is paraplegic is often able to function without assistance after an appropriate rehabilitation program.

ADL and mobility training for the patient with an SCI includes a structured exercise program to promote strength and endurance. One promising therapy in rehabilitation is functional electrical stimulation (FES). FES uses small electrical pulses to paralyzed muscles to restore or improve their function. It is commonly used for exercise; but it is also used to assist with breathing, grasping, transferring, standing, and walking. The occupational therapist instructs the patient in the correct use of all adaptive equipment and therapies. In collaboration with the therapists, instruct family members or the caregiver in transfer skills, feeding, bathing, dressing, positioning, bowel and bladder training, and skin care as discussed briefly in this chapter and in more detail in Chapter 7.

Sexuality is associated with sexual and reproductive function. Sexual function after SCI depends on the level and extent of injury. Incomplete lesions allow some control over ***sensory perception*** and ***mobility.*** Complete lesions disconnect the messages from the brain to the rest of the body and vice versa. However, men with injuries above T6 are often able to have erections by stimulating reflex activity. For example, stroking the penis will cause an erection. Ejaculation is less predictable and may be mixed with urine. However, urine is sterile, so the patient's partner will not get an infection. To prevent autonomic

PATIENT-CENTERED CARE: OLDER ADULT CONSIDERATIONS QSEN

What Patients Need to Know About Aging With Spinal Cord Injury

Nursing Intervention	Rationales
Follow guidelines for adult vaccination, particularly influenza and pneumococcus vaccination recommendations.	Respiratory complications are the most common cause of death after spinal cord injury (SCI).
For women, have Papanicolaou (Pap) smears and mammograms as recommended by the American Cancer Society or your primary health care provider.	Limitations in movement may make breast self-awareness difficult.
Take measures to prevent osteoporosis, such as increasing calcium and vitamin D intake, avoiding caffeine, and not smoking. Exercise against resistance can maintain muscle strength and slow bone loss.	Women older than 50 years often lose bone density, which can result in fractures. Men can also have osteoporotic fractures as a result of immobility.
Practice meticulous skin care, including frequent repositioning, using pressure-reduction surfaces in bed and chairs/wheelchairs, and applying skin protective products.	As a person ages, skin becomes dry and less elastic, predisposing the patient to pressure injuries.
Take measures to prevent constipation, such as drinking adequate fluids, eating a high-fiber diet, adding a stool softener or bowel stimulant daily, and establishing a regular time for bowel elimination.	Constipation is a problem for most patients with SCI, and bowel motility can slow, contributing to constipation later in life.
Modify activities if joint pain occurs; use a powered rather than a manual wheelchair. Ask the primary health care provider about treatment options.	Arthritis occurs in more than half of people older than 65 years. Patients with SCI are more likely to develop arthritis as a result of added stress on the upper extremities when using a wheelchair.

NURSING SAFETY PRIORITY QSEN

Drug Alert

Teach the SCI patient and his or her family or other caregiver about the name, purpose, dosage, timing of administration, and side effects of all *drugs.* Make sure they understand the possible interaction of prescribed drugs with over-the-counter drugs or alcohol and illegal drugs.

dysreflexia (AD), prophylactic administration of a vasodilator may be needed before intercourse.

Women with an SCI have a different challenge because they have indwelling urinary catheters more commonly than men. However, some women do become pregnant and have full-term children. For others, ovulation stops in response to the injury. In this case, alternate methods for pregnancy, such as *in vitro* fertilization, may be an option. Some women also report vaginal dryness. Recommend a water-soluble lubricant for both partners to promote comfort.

For patients who choose not to have intercourse, intimate pleasure can be achieved in other ways, including kissing, hugging, fondling, masturbation, and oral sex. Variations in positioning may be needed to accommodate weak or paralyzed parts of the body. An understanding partner can help the patient adjust to his or her physical changes.

Health Care Resources. Refer the patient and family to local, state or province, and national organizations for more information and support for patients with SCI. These organizations include the United Spinal Association (www.unitedspinal.org) in the United States and Spinal Cord Injury Canada (www.sci-can.ca). Many excellent consumer-oriented books, journals, and DVDs are also available. Support groups may help the patient and family adjust to a changed lifestyle and provide solutions to commonly encountered problems.

PATIENT-CENTERED CARE: VETERANS HEALTH CONSIDERATIONS QSEN

Young male and female veterans may experience an SCI as a result of an explosion or vehicular accident during war or other military operations. In addition to the U.S. Veterans Health Administration services offered in inpatient units and outpatient clinics, the Paralyzed Veterans of America (PVA) (www.pva.org) can assist with educational materials, caregiver services, medical equipment, and support groups. The PVA also sponsors spinal cord research and raises money to help veterans with a variety of needs. It also supports wheelchair-sports teams composed of veterans with an SCI or diseases that affect the spinal cord.

◆ **Evaluation: Evaluate Outcomes.** Evaluate the care of the patient with an SCI based on the identified priority patient problems. The expected outcomes are that the patient:

- Exhibits no deterioration in neurologic status
- Maintains a patent airway, a physiologic breathing pattern, and adequate ventilation
- Does not experience a cardiovascular event (e.g., shock, hemorrhage, autonomic dysreflexia) or receives prompt treatment if an event occurs
- Does not experience secondary spinal cord injury, including VTE and heterotopic ossification
- Is free from complications of decreased ***mobility***
- Performs ***mobility*** skills and basic ADLs as independently as possible with or without the use of assistive-adaptive devices

LOW BACK PAIN (LUMBOSACRAL BACK PAIN)

Pathophysiology Review

Back ***pain*** affects most adults at some time in their life. It can be recurrent, and subsequent episodes tend to increase in severity. The lumbosacral (lower back) and cervical (neck) vertebrae are most commonly affected because these are the areas where the vertebral column is the most flexible. *Acute* back pain is usually self-limiting and lasts less than 4 weeks. *Subacute* back pain lasts from 4 to 12 weeks. If the ***pain*** continues for 12 weeks (3 months) or more, the patient has *chronic persistent* back pain (Qaseem et al., 2017).

Low back pain (LBP) occurs along the lumbosacral area of the vertebral column. Acute pain is caused by muscle strain or spasm, ligament sprain, disk (also spelled "disc") degeneration (osteoarthritis), or herniation of the center of the disk, the nucleus pulposus, past the lateral vertebral border. A herniated nucleus pulposus (HNP) in the lumbosacral area can press on the adjacent spinal nerve (usually the sciatic nerve), causing burning or stabbing pain down into the leg or foot, which in some cases can be severe (Fig. 40.9). Herniated disks occur most often between the fourth and fifth lumbar vertebrae (L4-L5) but may occur at other levels. The specific area of symptoms depends on the level of herniation.

In addition to acute or persistent ***pain,*** there may be both muscle spasm and numbness and tingling (paresthesia) in the affected leg because spinal nerves have both motor and sensory fibers. The HNP may press on the spinal cord itself, causing leg weakness. Bowel and bladder incontinence or retention may occur with motor nerve involvement and because sacral spinal nerves have parasympathetic nerve fibers that help control bowel and bladder function. This can further alter the patient's pain level.

Back pain may also be caused by spinal stenosis, which is a narrowing of the spinal canal, nerve root canals, or intervertebral foramina typically seen in people older than 50 years. This narrowing may be caused by infection, trauma, herniated disk, arthritis, and disk degeneration. Most adults older than 50 years have some degree of degenerative disk disease, although they may not be symptomatic.

LBP is most prevalent during the third to sixth decades of life but can occur at any time. Women have a higher incidence of LBP compared with men (Pfieffer, 2020). *Acute* and *subacute* back pain usually result from injury or trauma such as during a fall or vehicular crash or when lifting a heavy object. The mechanisms of injury include repetitive flexion and/or extension and hyperflexion or hyperextension with or without rotation. Obesity places increased stress on the vertebral column and back muscles, contributing to risk for injury. Smoking has been linked to disk degeneration, possibly caused by constriction of blood vessels that supply the spine. Congenital spinal conditions such as scoliosis (an abnormal lateral curvature of the spine) can also lead to LBP at any age.

PATIENT-CENTERED CARE: OLDER ADULT CONSIDERATIONS QSEN

Older adults are at high risk for acute, subacute, and chronic LBP. Vertebral fracture from osteoporosis contributes to LBP. Petite, older Euro-American women are at high risk for both bone loss and subsequent vertebral fractures. The Patient-Centered Care: Older Adult Considerations: Factors Contributing to Low Back Pain box provides a list of specific factors that can cause LBP in the older adult. Vertebral compression fractures are discussed in Chapter 47.

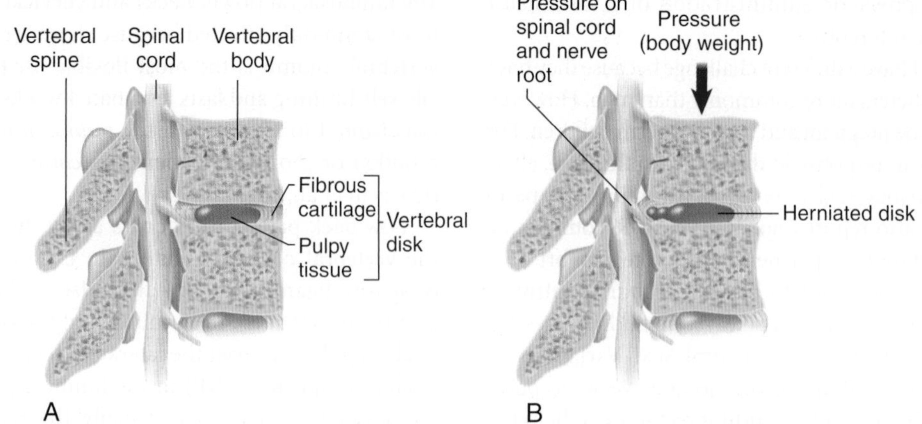

FIG. 40.9 Sagittal section of vertebrae showing a normal disk (A) and a herniated disk (B). (From Patton, K.T., & Thibodeau, G.A. [2018]. *The human body in health and disease.* [7th ed.]. St. Louis: Mosby.)

PATIENT-CENTERED CARE: OLDER ADULT CONSIDERATIONS (QSEN)

Factors Contributing to Low Back Pain

- Changes in support structures
- Spinal stenosis
- Hypertrophy of the intraspinal ligaments
- Osteoarthritis
- Osteoporosis
- Changes in vertebral support and malalignment with deformity
- Scoliosis
- Lordosis (an inward abnormal curvature of the lumbar spinal area)
- Vascular changes
- Diminished blood supply to the spinal cord or cauda equina caused by arteriosclerosis
- Blood dyscrasias
- Intervertebral disk degeneration

Health Promotion and Maintenance. Many of the problems related to back pain can be prevented by recognizing the factors that contribute to tissue injury and taking appropriate preventive measures to prevent ***pain.*** For example, proper posture and exercise can significantly decrease the incidence of LBP. The U.S. Occupational Safety and Health Administration (OSHA) has mandated that all industries develop and implement a plan to decrease musculoskeletal injuries among their workers. One way to meet this requirement is to develop an ergonomic plan for the workplace. Ergonomics is an applied science in which the workplace is designed to increase worker comfort (thus reducing injury) while increasing efficiency and productivity. An example is a ceiling lift designed to help nurses assist patients to get out of bed. A variety of equipment can be used to decrease injury related to moving patients. Professional guidelines and legislative rules promote safe patient handling for health care workers (www.nursingworld.org/rnnoharm). The Patient and Family Education: Preparing for Self-Management: Prevention of Low Back Pain and Injury box summarizes various ways to help prevent LBP related to lifting objects and handling patients.

PATIENT AND FAMILY EDUCATION: PREPARING FOR SELF-MANAGEMENT

Prevention of Low Back Pain and Injury

- Use safe manual handling practices, with specific attention to bending, lifting, and sitting.
- Assess the need for assistance with your household chores or other activities.
- Participate in a regular exercise program, especially one that promotes back strengthening, such as swimming and walking.
- Do not wear high-heeled shoes.
- Use good posture when sitting, standing, and walking.
- Avoid prolonged sitting or standing. Use a footstool and ergonomic chairs and tables to lessen back strain. Be sure that equipment in the workplace is ergonomically designed to prevent injury.
- Keep weight within 10% of ideal body weight.
- Ensure adequate calcium intake. Consider vitamin D supplementation if serum levels are low.
- Stop smoking. If you are not able to stop, cut down on the number of cigarettes or decrease the use of other forms of tobacco.

❖ Interprofessional Collaborative Care

◆ Assessment: Recognize Cues

Physical Assessment/Signs and Symptoms. *The patient's primary concern is continuous pain.* Some patients have so much ***pain*** that they walk in a stiff, flexed posture or they may be unable to bend at all. They may walk with a limp, indicating possible sciatic nerve impairment. Walking on the heels or toes often causes severe pain in the affected leg, the back, or both.

Conduct a complete ***pain*** assessment as discussed in Chapter 5. Record the patient's current pain score and the worst and best score since the pain began. Ask about precipitating or relieving factors such as symptoms at night or during rest. Determine if a recent injury to the back has occurred. It is not unusual for the patient to say, "I just moved to do something and felt my back go out."

Inspect the patient's back for vertebral alignment and tenderness. Examine the surrounding anatomy and lower extremities for secondary injury. Patients will often describe ***pain*** as stabbing and continuous in the muscle closest to the affected disk. They often describe a sharp, burning posterior thigh or calf pain that may radiate to the ankle or toes along the path of one or more spinal nerves. Pain usually does not extend the entire length of the limb. Patients may also report the same type of pain in the middle of one buttock or hip. The pain is often aggravated by sneezing, coughing, or straining. Driving a vehicle is particularly painful.

Ask whether *paresthesia* (tingling sensation) or numbness is present in the involved leg. Both extremities may be checked for ***sensory perception*** by using a cotton ball and a paper clip for comparison of light or dull and sharp touch. The patient may feel sensation in both legs but may experience a stronger sensation on the unaffected side. Ask about urinary and fecal continence and difficulty with urination or having new-onset constipation.

If the sciatic nerve is compressed, severe ***pain*** usually occurs when the patient's leg is held straight and lifted upward. Foot, ankle, and leg weakness may accompany LBP. To complete the neurologic assessment, evaluate the patient's muscle tone and strength. Muscles in the extremity or lower back can atrophy as a result of severe persistent back pain. The patient has difficulty with movement, and certain movements create more pain than others.

Ask patients if they have frequent feelings of sadness or have considered suicide. For many patients, persistent pain can cause a depression and/or suicidal ideation.

Imaging Assessment. Imaging studies for patients who report mild nonspecific back ***pain*** may not be done, depending on the nature of the pain. Patients with severe or progressive motor or ***sensory perception*** deficits or who are thought to have other underlying conditions (e.g., cancer, infection) require complete diagnostic assessment. To determine the exact cause of the pain, a number of diagnostic tests may be used, including:

- Plain x-rays (show general arthritis changes and bony alignment)
- CT scan (shows spinal bones, nerves, disks, and ligaments)
- MRI (provides images of the spinal tissue, bones, spinal cord, nerves, ligaments, musculature, and disks)
- Bone scan (shows bone changes after injection of radioactive tracers, which attach to areas of increased bone production or show increased vascularity associated with tumor or infection)

Electrodiagnostic testing, such as electromyography (EMG) and nerve-conduction studies, may help distinguish motor neuron diseases from peripheral neuropathy and **radiculopathy** (spinal nerve root involvement). These tests are especially useful in chronic diseases of the spinal cord or associated nerves. Chapters 38 and 44 describe these tests in more detail.

◆ **Interventions: Take Action.** Management of patients with low back ***pain*** varies with the severity and chronicity of the problem. If acute pain is not treatment or managed effectively, persistent neuropathic ***pain*** may occur. Most patients with acute LBP experience a spontaneous resolution of pain and other symptoms over the short term in less than 3 months.

Some patients need only a brief treatment regimen of at-home exercise or physical therapy to manage pain. In general, return to work, if safe, is beneficial for recovery and well-being. Some patients have continuous or intermittent chronic pain that must be managed for an extended period. Referral to an interprofessional team that specializes in ***pain*** or back pain can provide expert long-term management.

Nonsurgical Management. A recently published evidence-based clinical practice guideline recommends interprofessional nonpharmacologic interventions as first-line management for all types of LBP (Qaseem et al., 2017). For *acute* and *subacute* LBP, these interventions may include massage, spinal manipulation, heat, and acupuncture. If these measures are not successful in reducing acute ***pain,*** NSAIDs are recommended; acetaminophen is not helpful (Qaseem et al., 2017).

The Williams position is typically more comfortable and therapeutic for the patient with *acute* LBP from a bulging or herniated disk. In this position, the patient lies in the semi-Fowler position with a pillow under the knees to stay flexed or sits in a recliner chair. This position relaxes the muscles of the lower back and relieves pressure on the spinal nerve root. Most patients also find that they need to change position frequently. Prolonged standing, sitting, or lying down increases back pain. If the patient must stand for a long time for work or other reason, shoe insoles or special floor pads may help decrease pain. However, bedrest should also be limited, and patients should begin stretching exercises and resume normal daily activities as soon as possible after an injury.

Patients having *persistent* LBP are also initially managed with nonpharmacologic interventions. In addition to the measures described earlier, patients often benefit from complementary and integrative therapies such as stress reduction, mindfulness, progressive muscle relaxation, and yoga. If these measures with NSAIDs are not effective in relieving persistent LBP, tramadol, a mild opioid drug, or duloxetine, a selective serotonin-norepinephrine reuptake inhibitor (SNRI), is recommended as second-line drug therapy (Qaseem et al., 2017). Duloxetine is an especially good choice for patients with both persistent LBP and depression (Pfieffer, 2020). The use of stronger drugs such as opioids is not recommended owing to the risk of abuse and addiction (see Chapter 5).

If muscle spasms are present, skeletal muscle relaxants such as tizanidine and cyclobenzaprine may be used as adjunctive therapy. Older adults should avoid these drugs because dizziness and sedation are common side effects (Burchum & Rosenthal, 2019; Pfieffer, 2020).

Other adjunctive therapies, such as over-the-counter (OTC) topical creams, sprays, and gels, may provide temporary feelings of warmth or cold to dull the sensation of all types of low back pain. Some patients use a transcutaneous electrical nerve stimulation (TENS) unit at home to help decrease pain. Chapter 5 discusses the use of this device.

Ziconotide is a centrally acting analgesic that can be given for severe persistent back pain as a last resort. It is given by intrathecal (spinal) infusion with a surgically implanted pump. It is the first available drug in a new class called *N-type calcium channel blockers (NCCBs).* NCCBs seem to selectively block calcium channels on nerves that usually transmit pain signals to the brain. Common side effects of ziconotide include drowsiness, headache, GI distress, loss of balance, and urinary retention. Older adults are not candidates for this drug therapy. Ziconotide can also cause muscle injury resulting in high levels of creatine kinase (Burcham & Rosenthal, 2019). As a result of the invasive route of drug administration, common side effects, and adverse drug events, the drug is not practical as a treatment for most patients.

! NURSING SAFETY PRIORITY (QSEN)

Drug Alert

Ziconotide can be taken with opioid analgesics but should *not* be given to patients with severe mental health/behavioral health problems because it can cause psychosis. *If symptoms such as hallucinations and delusions occur, teach patients to stop the drug immediately and notify their primary health care provider.*

A physical therapist (PT) works with the patient to develop an individualized exercise program. The type of exercises prescribed depends on the location and nature of the injury and the type of pain. The patient does not begin exercises until acute pain is reduced by other means. Water therapy combined with exercise is helpful for some patients with chronic pain. The water also provides muscle resistance during exercise to prevent atrophy.

Weight reduction may help reduce persistent LBP by decreasing the strain on the vertebrae caused by excess weight. If the patient's weight exceeds the ideal by more than 10%, caloric restriction is recommended. Weight reduction can improve back ***pain.*** Health care professionals must be sensitive when reinforcing the need for patients to lose weight to prevent or lessen chronic back pain. Behavioral approaches to weight loss and positive reinforcement are important for the nutrition plan.

Surgical Management. Surgery may be performed if conservative measures fail to relieve persistent back pain or if neurologic deficits continue to progress. An orthopedic surgeon and/or neurosurgeon perform these surgeries. Two general surgical methods are used, depending on the severity and exact location of pain: minimally invasive surgery (MIS) and conventional open surgical procedures. MIS is not done if the disk is pressing into the spinal cord (central cord involvement).

Preoperative Care. Preoperative care for the patient preparing for lumbar spinal surgery is similar to that for any patient undergoing surgery (see Chapter 9). Teach the patient about postoperative expectations depending on surgical method, including:

- Techniques to get into and out of bed
- Turning and moving in bed
- Reporting immediately new ***sensory perception,*** such as numbness and tingling, or new motor impairment that may occur in the affected leg or in both legs
- Home care activities and restrictions, if any

As part of preoperative teaching, make sure patients understand the type of procedure they are having and the postoperative care that will be needed. A recent randomized controlled trial found that the knowledge of patients about their surgical procedure was inadequate. There was no significant difference between the knowledge of patients who had routine preoperative education and of patients who had specific preoperative education their spinal surgical procedure (Kesanen et al., 2019).

Newer surgical procedures allow many patients to have same-day surgery. Other patients are discharged to home within 23 to 48 hours after surgery. Therefore before surgery, teach family members or other caregiver how to assist the patient and what restrictions the patient must follow at home.

A bone graft is done if the patient has a large traditional *spinal fusion* that involves multiple vertebra. The surgeon explains from where the bone for grafting will be obtained. The patient's own bone is used whenever possible, but additional bone from a bone bank may be needed. The surgeon provides verbal and written information about the type and source of bone for surgery. Informed consent is obtained. While the bone graft heals, the patient may wear a back orthotic device for 4 to 6 weeks after surgery. Provide information about the importance of wearing the brace as instructed during the healing process, how to take it off and put it on while maintaining spinal alignment, and how to clean it.

Operative Procedures. *Minimally invasive surgery (MIS)* using endoscopy or percutaneous instrumentation results in minimal muscle injury, decreased blood loss, and decreased postoperative pain. Therefore the primary advantages of MIS procedures are a shortened hospital stay, less pain, and the possibility of an ambulatory care (same-day) procedure. Spinal cord and nerve complications are also less likely. Several specific procedures are commonly performed.

A *microdiskectomy* involves microscopic surgery directly through a 1-inch incision using an endoscope. This procedure allows easier identification of anatomic structures, improved precision in removing small fragments, and decreased tissue trauma and pain. A special cutting tool or laser probe is threaded through the cannula for removal or destruction of the *disk pieces* that are compressing the nerve root. This process is also called a *percutaneous endoscopic diskectomy (PED).* A newer procedure combines the PED with *laser thermodiskectomy* to also shrink the herniated disk before removal. Inpatient hospitalization is not necessary for this procedure.

Laser-assisted laparoscopic lumbar diskectomy combines a laser with modified standard disk instruments inserted through the laparoscope using an umbilical ("belly button") incision. The procedure may be used to treat herniated disks that are bulging but do not involve the vertebral canal. The primary risks of this surgery are infection and nerve root injury. The patient is typically discharged in 23 hours but may go home sooner.

The newest addition to MIS procedures is robot-assisted spinal surgery. This procedure requires additional training and experience for the surgeon and is currently limited to assistance with hardware placement (Staub & Sadrameli, 2019).

The most common *open surgical procedures* are diskectomy, laminectomy, and/or spinal fusion. Artificial disk replacement may also be part of this type of surgery. These procedures involve a surgical incision to expose anatomic landmarks for extensive muscle and soft-tissue dissection. The location and length of incision depends on the procedure and on surgeon preference and training.

BEST PRACTICE FOR PATIENT SAFETY & QUALITY CARE QSEN

Assessing and Managing the Patient With Major Complications of Open Traditional Lumbar Spinal Surgery

Complication	Assessment and Interventions
Cerebrospinal fluid (CSF) leakage	Observe for clear fluid on or around the dressing. If leakage occurs, place patient flat. Report CSF leakage immediately to the surgeon. (The patient is usually kept on flat bedrest for several days while the dural tear heals.)
Fluid volume deficit	Monitor intake and output; assess for dehydration, including vital signs and skin turgor. Monitor vital signs carefully for hypotension and tachycardia.
Acute urinary retention	Assist the patient to the bathroom or a bedside commode as soon as possible after surgery. Help male patients stand at the bedside as soon as possible after surgery.
Paralytic ileus	Monitor for flatus or stool. Assess for abdominal distention, nausea, and vomiting.
Fat embolism syndrome (FES) (more common in people with traditional open spinal fusion)	Observe for and report chest pain, dyspnea, anxiety, and mental status changes (more common in older adults). Note petechiae around the neck, upper chest, buccal membrane, and conjunctiva. Monitor arterial blood gas values for decreased Pao_2.
Persistent or progressive lumbar radiculopathy (nerve root pain)	Report pain not responsive to analgesics. Document the location and nature of pain. Administer analgesics as prescribed.
Infection (e.g., wound, diskitis, hematoma)	Monitor the patient's temperature carefully (a slight elevation is normal). Increased temperature elevation or a spike after the second postoperative day may indicate infection. Report increased pain or swelling at the wound site or in the legs. Give antibiotics as prescribed if infection is confirmed.

As the name implies, a *diskectomy* is removal of a herniated disk. A *laminectomy* involves removal of part of the laminae and facet joints to obtain access to the disk space. A *spinal fusion* connects two or more vertebra to stabilize the spine and release compression on spinal nerves. In an interbody cage fusion surgery, a titanium mesh device is implanted into the space where the disk was removed, and several screws ensure stabilization.

When repeated laminectomies are performed or the spine is unstable, the surgeon may perform a spinal fusion (arthrodesis) with bone graft to stabilize the affected area. Chips of bone are grafted between the vertebrae for support and to strengthen the back. Metal implants (usually titanium pins, screws, plates, or rods) may be required to ensure the fusion of the spine. The surgeon may give an intrathecal (spinal) or epidural dose of long-acting morphine to decrease postoperative pain.

Postoperative Care. Postoperative care depends on the surgical method and procedure that was performed. In the postanesthesia care unit (PACU), vital signs and level of consciousness are monitored frequently, as for any surgery. Best practices for PACU nursing care are discussed in Chapter 9. Patients who have a *minimally invasive spinal surgery* go home the same day or the day after surgery with one or more wound closure tapes over the small incision. Those having a microdiskectomy may also have a clear or gauze dressing over the bandage. Most patients notice less pain immediately after surgery, but mild oral analgesics are needed while nerve tissue heals over the next few weeks to promote patient comfort. Teach the patient to follow the prescribed exercise program, which begins immediately after discharge. Patients should start walking routinely every day. Complications of MIS are rare.

Early postoperative nursing care focuses on preventing and assessing complications that might occur in the first 24 to 48 hours for patients having conventional open surgeries. Major complications for open traditional lumbar spinal surgery include nerve injuries, diskitis (disk inflammation), and dural tears (tears in the dura covering the spinal cord). Additional complications are outlined in the Best Practice for Patient Safety & Quality Care: Assessing and Managing the Patient With Major Complications of Open Traditional Lumbar Spinal Surgery box.

As for any patient undergoing surgery, take vital signs at least every 4 hours during the first 24 hours to assess for fever, hypotension, or severe pain. Perform a neurologic assessment every 4 hours. Of particular importance are movement, strength, and ***sensory perception*** in the lower extremities.

Carefully check the patient's ability to void. Acute back ***pain*** and a flat position in bed make voiding difficult, especially for men. An inability to void may indicate damage to the sacral spinal nerves, which control the detrusor muscle in the bladder. The patient with an open traditional diskectomy, laminectomy, and/or traditional open spinal fusion typically gets out of bed with assistance on the evening of surgery, which may help with voiding.

! NURSING SAFETY PRIORITY QSEN

Critical Rescue

For the patient after back surgery, inspect the surgical dressing for blood or any other type of drainage. Clear drainage may mean cerebrospinal fluid (CSF) leakage. Blood and CSF may be mixed on the dressing, with the CSF being visible as a "halo" around the outer edges of the dressing. The loss of a large amount of CSF may cause the patient to report having a sudden headache. *If a CSF leak is suspected, keep the patient on bedrest and lower the head of the bed immediately to slow the loss of fluid! Report signs of any drainage on the dressing to the surgeon or Rapid Response Team. Bulging at the incision site may be due to a CSF leak or a hematoma, both of which should also be reported immediately.*

Correct turning of the patient in bed who is recovering from open traditional lumbar spinal injury is especially important. Do not place an overhead trapeze on the bed to assist the patient with ***mobility*** skills. This apparatus can cause more back pain and damage the surgical area. Teach the patient to log roll every 2 hours from side to back and vice versa. In **log rolling**, the patient turns as a unit while his or her back is kept as straight as possible. A turning sheet may be used for obese patients. Either turning method may require additional assistance, depending on how much the patient can assist and on his or her weight. Instruct the patient to keep his or her back straight when getting out of bed. He or she should sit in a straight-back chair with the feet resting comfortably on the floor. As with all surgical patients, prevent atelectasis and hypostatic pneumonia with deep breathing and incentive spirometry.

! CORE MEASURES

Follow best practices to avoid venous thromboembolism (VTE) after surgery with early *mobility*, intermittent sequential compression or pneumatic devices, and an anticoagulant/antiplatelet drug per The Joint Commission's Core Measures.

When a lumbar spinal fusion is performed in addition to a laminectomy, more care is taken with positioning. The nurse or assistive personnel (AP) assist with log rolling the patient every 2 hours. For conventional fusion with bone grafting, inspect both the iliac and spinal incision dressings for drainage and make sure they are intact. Remind the patient to avoid prolonged sitting or standing. Be sure to check with the surgeon or surgeon's prescription regarding whether to place the orthotic device or brace on the patient before or after getting the patient out of bed.

Care Coordination and Transition Management. The patient with back pain who does not undergo surgery is typically managed at home. If back surgery is performed, the patient is usually discharged to home with support from family or significant others. For older adults without a community support system, a short-term stay in a nursing home or transitional care unit may be needed. Collaborate with the case manager or discharge planner, patient, and family to determine the most appropriate placement.

Home Care Management. Patients having any of the *MIS procedures* or a lumber interbody fusion may resume normal activities within a few days up to 3 weeks after surgery, depending on the specific procedure and the condition of the patient. He or she may take a shower on the third or fourth day after surgery. Teach the patient to leave the wound closure tapes in place for removal by the surgeon or until they fall off. Instruct the patient to contact the primary health care provider immediately if clear drainage seeps from the incision. Clear drainage usually indicates a meningeal tear and that cerebrospinal fluid is leaking.

BEST PRACTICE FOR PATIENT SAFETY & QUALITY CARE (QSEN)

Prevention of Musculoskeletal Injuries

- Avoid lifting objects of more than 5 to 10 lb (2.3 to 4.5 kg) without assistance or aid.
- Push objects rather than pulling them.
- Do not twist your back during movement.
- Use handles or grips to prevent unintended shifting of the object during movement.
- Avoid prolonged sitting or standing. Use a footstool to lessen back strain.
- Sit in chairs with good support.
- Avoid shoulder stooping; maintain proper posture.
- Avoid wearing high-heeled shoes.

After *conventional open lumbar surgery,* the patient may have activity restrictions for the first 4 to 6 weeks, such as:

- Limit daily stair climbing.
- Restrict or limit driving.
- Do not lift objects heavier than 5 lb.
- Restrict pushing and pulling activities (e.g., dog walking).
- Avoid bending and twisting at the waist.
- Take a daily walk.

The duration of home-based recovery depends on the nature of the job and the extent and type of surgery. Most patients return to work after 2 to 6 weeks; some patients having more complex open spinal procedures may not return for several months if their jobs are physically strenuous.

Self-Management Education. The patient with an *acute* episode of back pain typically returns to his or her usual activities but may fear a recurrence. Remind the patient that he or she may never have another episode if caution is used. However, continuous or episodic ***pain*** can be frustrating and tiring. Encourage the patient and family members to plan short-term goals and take steps toward recovering each day.

After surgery, in collaboration with the physical therapist, instruct the patient to:

- Continue with a weight-reduction diet, if needed
- Stop smoking, if applicable
- Perform strengthening exercises as instructed

The physical therapist reviews and demonstrates the principles of body mechanics and muscle-strengthening exercises. The patient is then asked to demonstrate these principles as described in the Best Practice for Patient Safety & Quality Care: Prevention of Musculoskeletal Injuries box. Teach him or her the importance of keeping all appointments and following the prescribed exercise plan.

The primary health care provider may want the patient to continue taking anti-inflammatory drugs or, if muscle spasm is present, to take muscle relaxants. Remind the patient and family about the possible side effects of drugs and what to do if they occur.

In a few patients, back surgery is not successful. This situation, referred to as *failed back surgery syndrome (FBSS),* is a complex combination of organic, psychological, and socioeconomic factors. Repeated surgical procedures often discourage these patients, who must continue aggressive pain management after multiple operations. Nerve blocks, implantable spinal cord stimulators (neurostimulators), and other modalities may be needed on a long-term basis to help with persistent ***pain.***

Spinal cord stimulation is an *invasive* technique that provides persistent pain relief by applying an electrical field over the spinal cord. A trial with a percutaneous spinal cord stimulator is conducted to determine whether or not permanent placement is appropriate. If the trial is successful, electrodes are surgically placed internally in the epidural space and connected to an external or implanted programmable generator. The patient is taught to program and adjust the device to maximize comfort. Spinal cord stimulation can be extremely effective in select patients, but it is reserved for intractable (unrelenting continuous) neuropathic pain syndromes that have been unresponsive to other treatments.

! NURSING SAFETY PRIORITY QSEN

Critical Rescue

For patients who have a spinal cord stimulator implanted in the epidural space, assess neurologic status below the level of insertion frequently. Monitor for early changes in ***sensory perception,*** movement, and muscle strength. Ensure that the patient can void without difficulty. *If any changes occur, document and report them immediately to the surgeon!*

Health Care Resources. Help the patient identify support systems (e.g., family, church groups, clubs) after back surgery. For example, a spouse may help the patient with exercises or perform the exercises with the patient. Members of a church group may run errands and do household chores. The patient with back pain may continue physical therapy on an ambulatory basis after discharge. In some cases, the patient may be referred to a pain specialist or clinic. A case manager may be assigned to the patient to help with resource management and utilization.

CERVICAL NECK PAIN

Pathophysiology Review

Cervical neck pain most often results from a bulging or herniation of the nucleus pulposus (HNP) in a cervical intervertebral disk, illustrated in Fig. 40.1. The disk tends to herniate laterally where the annulus fibrosus is weakest and the posterior longitudinal ligament is thinned. The result is spinal nerve root compression, with resulting motor and sensory manifestations and moderate to severe ***pain,*** typically in the neck, upper back (over the shoulder), and down the affected arm. The disk between the fifth and sixth cervical vertebrae (C5-C6) is affected most often.

If the disk does not herniate, nerve compression may be caused by osteophyte (bony spur) formation from osteoarthritis. The osteophyte presses on the intervertebral foramen, which results in a narrowing of the disk and pressure on the nerve root. As with sciatic nerve compression, the patient with cervical nerve compression may have either continuous or intermittent chronic pain. When the disk herniates centrally, pressure on the spinal cord occurs.

Cervical ***pain***—acute or persistent—may also occur from muscle strain, ligament sprain resulting from aging, poor posture, lifting, tumor, rheumatoid arthritis, osteoarthritis, or infection. The typical history of the patient includes a report of pain when moving the neck, which radiates to the shoulder and down the arm. The ***pain*** may interrupt sleep and may be accompanied by a headache or numbness and tingling in the affected arm. To determine the exact cause, plain x-rays, and imaging studies may be used. Electromyography/nerve conduction

CLINICAL JUDGMENT CHALLENGE 40.1

Safety; Clinical Judgment

A 52-year-old woman married to a veteran fell down a flight of stairs 10 years ago and sustained an acute herniated disk at the L4-L5 spinal level. A laminectomy and diskectomy relieved her pain for about 3 years. Two additional surgeries later, including a recent spinal fusion, failed to provide pain relief, but she could ambulate with a cane. The client was admitted to surgical unit yesterday to implant a spinal nerve simulator as a last resort for pain management. On admission from the postanesthesia care unit yesterday afternoon, she reported that her legs were still "numb" because of her epidural anesthetic. Her vital signs were within her baseline, and her pain level was a 2 on a 0-to-10 pain scale. During the night, the client was unable to void and required a straight urinary catheterization. The night nurse documented that her legs were still numb from the epidural she had received during surgery. She reported increased pain during most of the night.

This morning, the surgeon stated that she could be discharged to home in the care of her very attentive husband. The client received an oral dose of codeine with acetaminophen about an hour ago. Upon assessment, the nurse documents the following assessment findings:

- Blood pressure = 166/88 mm Hg
- Pulse rate = 86 beats/min
- Respiratory rate = 28 breaths/min
- Pain level = 8 (on a 0-10 scale)
- Reports that she remains unable to void more than "a few dribbles," although she has been drinking water frequently
- Reports numbness from her waist down to her toes
- Is barely able to move her legs
- Requires maximum assistance to get out of bed into a chair

1. **Recognize Cues:** What assessment information in this client situation is the most important and immediate concern for the nurse? (Hint: Identify the **relevant** information *first* to determine what is most important.)
2. **Analyze Cues:** What client conditions are consistent with the **most relevant** information? (Hint: Think about priority collaborative problems that support and contradict the information presented in this situation.)
3. **Prioritize Hypotheses:** Which possibilities or explanations are **most likely** to be present in this client situation? Which possibilities or explanations are the most serious? (Hint: Consider all possibilities and determine their urgency and risk for this client.)
4. **Generate Solutions:** What actions would most likely achieve the desired outcomes for this client? Which actions should be **avoided** or are **potentially harmful**? (Hint: Determine the desired outcomes first to decide which interventions are appropriate and those that should be avoided.)
5. **Take Action:** Which actions are the most appropriate and how should they be implemented? In what **priority order** should they be implemented? (Hint: Consider health teaching, documentation, requested health care provider orders or prescriptions, nursing skills, collaboration with or referral to health team members, etc.)
6. **Evaluate Outcomes:** What client assessment would indicate that the nurse's actions were **effective**? (Hint: Think about signs that would indicate an improvement, decline, or unchanged client condition.)

studies are used to help differentiate cervical radiculopathy, ulnar or radial neuropathy, carpal tunnel syndrome, or other peripheral nerve problems.

❖ Interprofessional Collaborative Care

Conservative treatment for acute neck ***pain*** is the same as described for low back pain except that exercises focus on the shoulders and neck. The physical therapist teaches the patient the correct techniques for performing "shoulder shrug," "shoulder squeeze," and "seated rowing." Some primary health care providers prescribe a soft collar to stabilize the neck, especially at night. Using the collar for longer than 10 days can lead to decreased muscle strength and range of motion. For that reason, some primary health care providers do not recommend collars for cervical disk problems. Therapeutic manipulation (chiropractic interventions) alone or in combination with other interventions does not appear to cause harm for most patients but does not consistently reduce pain or disability.

If conservative treatment is ineffective, surgery may be required—either *minimally invasive surgery* or *conventional open surgery.* A neurosurgeon usually performs this surgery because of the complexity of the nerves and other structures in that area of the spine. For open procedures and depending on the cause and the location of the disk herniation, either an anterior or a posterior surgical approach is used.

One of the most common procedures performed today is the anterior or lateral interbody cervical fusion (AICF or LICF). In these procedures, a titanium mesh device is implanted into the space where the cervical disk was removed, and several screws ensure stabilization. For clients who have multiple cervical disk herniations, a traditional anterior cervical diskectomy and fusion (ACDF) with bone grafting may be performed. This surgery is much more complex and causes more postoperative complications than the AICF or LICF. The patient having the more traditional ACDF may be fitted with a large neck brace before surgery. General preoperative and postoperative care nursing interventions are the same as described in Chapter 9.

! NURSING SAFETY PRIORITY (QSEN)

Critical Rescue

The priority for care in the immediate postoperative period after an ACDF is maintaining an airway and ensuring that the patient has no problem with breathing. Swelling from the surgery can narrow the trachea, causing a partial obstruction. Surgery can also interfere with cranial innervation for swallowing, resulting in a compromised airway or aspiration. If these changes occur, open the patient's airway, sit the patient upright, suction if needed, and provide supplemental oxygen. Promptly notify the surgeon or rapid response team using SBAR and document your assessment and interventions.

The Best Practice for Patient Safety & Quality Care: Care of the Patient After a Traditional Anterior Cervical Diskectomy and Fusion box summarizes best practices for postoperative care and discharge planning.

BEST PRACTICE FOR PATIENT SAFETY & QUALITY CARE (QSEN)

Care of the Patient After a Traditional Anterior Cervical Diskectomy and Fusion

Postoperative Interventions

- Assess *a*irway, *b*reathing, and *c*irculation (first priority!).
- Check for bleeding and drainage at the incision site.
- Monitor vital signs and neurologic status frequently.
- Check for swallowing ability.
- Monitor intake and output.
- Assess the patient's ability to void (may be a problem secondary to opiates or anesthesia).
- Manage *pain* adequately.
- Assist the patient with ambulation within a few hours of surgery, if he or she is able.

Discharge Teaching

- Be sure that someone stays with the patient for the first few days after surgery.
- Review drug therapy.
- Teach care of the incision.
- Review activity restrictions:
  - No lifting
  - No driving until surgeon permission received
  - No strenuous activities
- Walk every day.
- Call the primary health care provider if symptoms of pain, numbness, and tingling worsen or if swallowing becomes difficult.
- Wear brace or collar per the primary health care provider's prescription.

Complications of ACDF can occur from the brace or the surgery itself. The initial brace is usually worn for 4 or more weeks. When it is removed, a soft collar may be worn for several more weeks.

Some patients are candidates for minimally invasive surgery (MIS), such as percutaneous cervical diskectomy (PCD) through an endoscope, with or without laser thermodiskectomy, to shrink the herniated portion of the disk. The care for these patients is very similar to that for the patient with low back pain who has MIS (see discussion of surgical management of patients with low back pain earlier in this chapter).

Many patients have positive clinical outcomes after interbody fusion (ADIF or LDIF) procedures, which has reduced the need for more complex fusions with bone grafting. The patient has a small incision and is able to return to work in 2 weeks. Complications of these procedures are not common.

Patients may also benefit from the placement of an artificial disk, a surgical option that preserves movement of the vertebrae. Artificial disks are approved by the FDA. Although there is evidence of their safety, the long-term effects on patient health are not yet established.

GET READY FOR THE NEXT-GENERATION NCLEX® EXAMINATION!

Key Points

Review these Key Points for each NCLEX Examination Client Needs Category.

Safe and Effective Care Environment

- Assess airway and breathing *first* for patients with an acute SCI. **QSEN: Evidence-Based Practice; Safety**
- Collaborate with members of the interprofessional health care team when caring for patients with spinal cord problems; assist with transition management to rehabilitation settings and home care. **QSEN: Teamwork and Collaboration**

Health Promotion and Maintenance

- Use safe object- and patient-handling practices to prevent back injury. **QSEN: Safety**
- Include community resources in discharge planning and teaching for patients with MS and SCI. There are specialty organizations for each of these spinal conditions. **QSEN: Patient-Centered Care**
- Apply knowledge of older-adult development to outline special care for older adults with spinal cord injury. **Clinical Judgment**

Psychosocial Integrity

- Refer patients to appropriate resources, such as a sexual counselor, for sexual dysfunction resulting from illness or disease. Counsel them as needed about ***sexuality.*** **QSEN: Teamwork and Collaboration; Patient-Centered Care**
- Recognize that spinal cord injury and progressive neurologic diseases, such as MS, require the patient and family to make major adjustments to roles and goals. **QSEN: Patient-Centered Care**
- Determine patient and family coping strategies to help patients adjust to spinal trauma or disease. **QSEN: Patient-Centered Care**

Physiological Integrity

- Assess ***pain*** level in patients with back injury, including the nature of the pain and location. **QSEN: Patient-Centered Care**
- Implement effective drug and nondrug interventions for back pain, including NSAIDs, anticonvulsants, and adjunctives such as heat/cold and exercise. **Clinical Judgment**
- Implement interventions to prevent complications associated with decreased ***mobility,*** including turning; VTE prophylaxis; early ambulation or transfers out of bed; and airway and breathing management such as bedside suctioning equipment, incentive spirometry, and Aspiration Precautions. **QSEN: Safety**
- Monitor patients with cervical spinal injuries for manifestations of autonomic dysreflexia. Provide a bowel and bladder regimen to prevent retention of stool and urine because these common problems can initiate autonomic dysreflexia. **QSEN: Evidence-Based Practice**
- Provide emergency care for patients who experience autonomic dysreflexia. **QSEN: Safety; Clinical Judgment**
- Assess patients with MS for signs and symptoms, including complications of impaired ***Immunity.*** **QSEN: Safety**
- For patients who have surgery to manage vertebral or spinal cord conditions, observe the incision site for bleeding and cerebrospinal fluid leakage (clear fluid) and document findings. **QSEN: Informatics; Clinical Judgment**
- Log roll during repositioning, especially during acute SCI or following surgical fusion of vertebrae. **QSEN: Safety**
- Reinforce health teaching for exercises for low back pain; teach principles of body mechanics and lifting to prevent back injury. **QSEN: Safety**
- Provide evidence-based postoperative care and discharge teaching for patients having cervical neck surgery. **QSEN: Evidence-Based Practice**

MASTERY QUESTIONS

1. The primary health care provider started a client with multiple sclerosis on mitoxantrone therapy. Which statement will the nurse **include** in teaching the client about this drug?
   A. "Report changes in urinary and bowel elimination immediately."
   B. "Follow up for annual lab testing to monitor for liver toxicity."
   C. "Rotate the sites for your self-administered injections."
   D. "Avoid crowded places such as malls and large public gatherings."
2. A client is admitted with a suspected cervical spinal cord injury. What is the nurse's **priority** action for this client?
   A. Assess cardiac sounds.
   B. Manage the client's airway.
   C. Check oxygen saturation level.
   D. Perform a neurologic assessment.
3. Which statement by the client indicates a **need for further teaching** by the nurse about preventing back injuries?
   A. "I need to lose weight because I'm too big."
   B. "I should not stand or sit for a long period of time."
   C. "It would be best if I could get ergonomic office furniture."
   D. "Exercise is not going to help my back very much."

REFERENCES

Bhimani, R., Medina, F., & Carney,-Anderson, L. (2018). Managing movement disorders: A clinical review. *The American Journal of Nursing.*, *118*(12), 34–40.

Burcham, J. L. R., & Rosenthal, L. D. (2019). *Lehne's pharmacology for nursing care* (10th ed.). St. Louis: Elsevier.

Cameron, M., & Rice, J. (2018). *Cannabis for multiple sclerosis symptoms.* https://www.NationalMSSociety/media/MSNationalFiles/Professionals/Cannabis-and-Multiple-Sclerosis.pdf.

Interprofessional Education Collaborative Expert Panel. (2016). *Core competencies for interprofessional collaborative practice: Report of an expert panel* (2nd ed.). Washington, D.C: Interprofessional Education Collaborative.

Kesänen, J., Leino-Kilpi, H., Lund, T., Montin, L., Puukka, P., & Valkeapää, K. (2019). Spinal stenosis patients' visual and verbal description of the comprehension of their surgery. *Orthopaedic Nursing*, *38*(4), 253–261.

Maloni, H. (2018). Cognitive impairment in multiple sclerosis. *Journal of Neuroparasitology: The Journal for Nurse Practitioners*, *14*(3), 172–177.

McCance, K., Huether, S., Brashers, V., & Rote, N. (2019). *Pathophysiology: The biologic basis for disease in adults and children* (8th ed.). St. Louis: Mosby.

MS Society of Canada. (2019). *What is multiple sclerosis?* https://ms-society.ca/about-ms-what-is-ms.

National Multiple Sclerosis Society. (2020). *Who gets MS.* www.nationalmssociety.org/about-multiple-sclerosis/what-we-know-about-ms/index.aspx.

National Spinal Cord Injury Statistical Center. (2018). *Spinal cord injury facts and figures at a glance.* www.nscisc.uab.edu/PublicDocuments/fact_figures_docs/Facts2018.pdf.

Pagana, K. D., & Pagana, T. J. (2018). *Manual of diagnostic and laboratory tests* (6th ed.). St. Louis: Mosby.

Pfieffer, M. L. (2020). How to care for adults with low back pain in the primary care setting. *Nursing 2020*, *50*(2), 48–53.

Qaseem, A., Wilt, T. J., McLean, R. M., & Forciea, M. A. (2017). Non-invasive treatments for acute, subacute, and chronic low back pain: A clinical practice guideline from the American college of physicians. *Annals of Medicine.* annals.org/aim/article/2603228/noninvasive-treatment-acute-subacute-chronic-low-back-pain-clinical-practice.

Slusser, M. M., Garcia, L. I., Reed, C.-R., & McGinnis, P. Q. (2019). *Foundations of interprofessional collaborative practice in health care.* St. Louis: Elsevier.

Staub, B. N., & Sadrameli, S. S. (2019). The use of robotics in minimally invasive spinal surgery. *Journal of Spine Surgery*, *5*(Suppl. 1), S31–S40.

41

Critical Care of Patients With Neurologic Emergencies

Donna D. Ignatavicius

http://evolve.elsevier.com/Iggy/

LEARNING OUTCOMES

1. Collaborate with the interprofessional team to manage quality care for patients with impaired ***perfusion*** and/or ***cognition*** caused by neurologic emergencies, such as traumatic brain injury (TBI) and stroke.
2. Develop a teaching plan about managing risk factors for stroke or TBI and prevention of secondary brain injury.
3. Identify community resources for families and patients recovering from neurologic emergencies.
4. Apply knowledge of pathophysiology of stroke and TBI to identify common assessment findings, including actual or risk for impaired ***mobility, sensory perception,*** and ***perfusion.***
5. Prioritize nursing care for patients having a stroke and TBI, including monitoring for, preventing, and managing ***perfusion*** to the brain.

KEY TERMS

acalculia The inability to perform math calculations.

acute ischemic stroke (AIS) A stroke caused by the occlusion (blockage) of a cerebral or carotid artery by either a thrombus or an embolus.

agnosia The inability to use an object correctly.

agraphia The inability to write.

alexia The inability to read.

amnesia Loss of memory.

aphasia Problems with speech (expressive aphasia) and/or language (receptive aphasia).

apraxia Inability to perform previously learned motor skills or commands; may be verbal or motor.

ataxia Lack of muscle control and coordination that affects gait, balance, and the ability to walk.

atherosclerotic plaque A buildup of fat and other substances that adhere to the arterial wall and obstruct or restrict blood flow.

bruit A sound heard over an artery through a stethoscope that indicates turbulent blood flow usually due to a narrowed or partially obstructed blood vessel.

carotid stenosis The hardening and narrowing of the artery, which decreases blood flow to the brain.

chronic traumatic encephalopathy (CTE) An uncommon degenerative brain disease that occurs most often in military veterans, athletes, and others who experienced repetitive trauma to the brain.

concussion A traumatic injury to the brain caused by a blow to the head; may or may not result in some period of unconsciousness.

craniotomy Surgical incision to open the cranium and allow access to the brain.

Cushing triad A classic but late sign of increased intracranial pressure that manifests with severe hypertension, a widened pulse pressure (increasing difference between systolic and diastolic values), and bradycardia.

diplopia A condition in which the client has double vision.

dysarthria Slurred speech caused by muscle weakness or paralysis.

dysphagia Difficulty swallowing.

embolectomy Surgical blood clot (thrombosis) removal.

embolic stroke A stroke caused by an embolus (dislodged clot).

emotional lability An uncontrollable emotional state that can occur in patients who have had a stroke or other brain injury.

epidural hematoma An accumulation of blood (clot) that results from arterial bleeding into the space between the dura and the inner skull.

expressive (Broca or motor) aphasia Aphasia that is the result of damage in the Broca area of the frontal lobe. It is a motor speech problem in which the patient generally understands what is said but cannot speak.

hemianopsia A condition in which the vision of one or both eyes is affected.

hemiparesis One-sided weakness of the body affecting the arm and/or leg.

hemiplegia One-sided paralysis of the body affecting the arm and/or leg.

homonymous hemianopsia Blindness in the same side of both eyes.

hydrocephalus A condition in which there is increased cerebrospinal fluid in the brain.

hyperbaric oxygen therapy (HBOT) An intervention that is used to provide high-dose oxygen to treat ischemia and hypoxia.

impaired airway defense An inability to clear one's airway.

infratentorial tumor A tumor that is located beneath the tentorium (the area of the brainstem structures and cerebellum).

intracerebral hemorrhage (ICH) The accumulation of blood within the brain tissue caused by the tearing of small arteries and veins in the subcortical white matter.

nystagmus Involuntary movements of the eyes that can be vertical or horizontal.

organ procurement The process of donating an organ from a person who is designated as an organ donor and has been declared brain dead.

papilledema Edema and hyperemia (increased blood flow) of the optic disc; a sign of increasing intracranial pressure.

photophobia Sensitivity to light.

postconcussion syndrome The most common secondary injury resulting from mild traumatic brain injury (TBI) in which the patient reports that headaches, impaired cognition, and dizziness continue to occur for weeks to months after the initial brain injury.

proprioception Body position sense.

ptosis Eyelid drooping.

receptive (Wernicke or sensory) aphasia Aphasia that is caused by injury involving the Wernicke area in the temporoparietal area. The patient cannot understand the spoken or written word. Although he or she may be able to talk, the language is often meaningless.

stroke A neurologic health problem caused by an interruption of perfusion to any part of the brain that results in infarction (cell death).

stroke center An agency that is designated by The Joint Commission (TJC) or other body for its ability to rapidly recognize and effectively treat strokes.

subdural hematoma (SDH) An accumulation of blood (clot) that results from venous bleeding into the space beneath the dura and above the arachnoid.

supratentorial tumor A tumor that is within the cerebral hemispheres above the tentorium (dural fold).

thrombotic stroke A stroke that is caused by a thrombus (clot).

transient ischemic attack (TIA) A temporary neurologic dysfunction resulting from a brief interruption in cerebral blood flow.

traumatic brain injury (TBI) Damage to the brain from an external mechanical force and not caused by neurodegenerative or congenital conditions.

unilateral neglect (or inattention) A client's inability to recognize his or her physical impairment, especially on one side of the body.

vertigo A feeling of spinning or dizziness.

PRIORITY AND INTERRELATED CONCEPTS

The priority concepts for this chapter are:

- ***Perfusion***
- ***Cognition***

The ***Perfusion*** concept exemplar for this chapter is Stroke.

The ***Cognition*** concept exemplar for this chapter is Traumatic Brain Injury.

The interrelated concepts for this chapter are:

- ***Mobility***
- ***Sensory Perception***

Many acute neurologic problems are associated with high mortality and severe morbidity and create significant and enduring impact on patients, their families, and society. Early recognition and comprehensive care of adult patients with acute neurologic compromise by the nurse and interprofessional health care team can reduce mortality and disability. Acute neurologic problems from stroke, brain trauma, and malignancy cause varying degrees of impaired ***perfusion, cognition, mobility,*** and ***sensory perception.*** Chapter 3 reviews each of these health concepts for nursing practice.

TRANSIENT ISCHEMIC ATTACK

Acute ischemic strokes often follow warning signs such as a **transient ischemic attack (TIA)**. A TIA is a temporary neurologic dysfunction resulting from a *brief* interruption in cerebral blood flow. The symptoms of TIA are easy to ignore or miss, particularly if symptoms resolve by the time the patient reaches the emergency department (ED). Typically, symptoms of a TIA resolve within 30 to 60 minutes but may last as long as 24 hours (see the Key Features: Transient Ischemic Attack box).

KEY FEATURES

Transient Ischemic Attack

Visual Symptoms

- Blurred vision
- **Diplopia** (a condition in which the client has double vision)
- **Hemianopsia** (a condition in which the vision of one or both eyes is affected)
- Tunnel vision

Mobility (Motor) Symptoms

- Weakness (facial droop, arm or leg drift, hand grasp)
- **Ataxia** (lack of muscle control and coordination that affects gait, balance, and the ability to walk)

Sensory Perception Symptoms

- Numbness (face, hand, arm, or leg)
- **Vertigo** (a feeling of spinning or dizziness)

Speech Symptoms

- **Aphasia** (problems with speech and/or language)
- **Dysarthria** (slurred speech caused by muscle weakness or paralysis)

On admission to the ED, a complete neurologic assessment is performed. The interprofessional health care team administers the National Institutes of Health Stroke Scale (NIHSS; see later discussion under Stroke) and other agency-specific assessment tools. Routine laboratory tests, including coagulation tests (prothrombin time [PT], international normalized ratio [INR], activated partial thromboplastin time [aPTT]) and lipids, ECG, and imaging scans are performed. The initial scan is typically a head CT, followed by MRI brain scan without contrast. Depending on agency protocol and the patient's assessment, computed tomography angiography (CTA) or magnetic resonance angiography (MRA) of the brain and neck is also performed to determine the patency of the carotid arteries, which provide ***perfusion*** to the brain, and arterial circulation within the brain.

Common causes of a TIA or stroke are **carotid stenosis** (hardening and narrowing of the artery, which decreases blood flow to the brain), often with atherosclerotic plaque buildup, and atrial fibrillation. **Atherosclerotic plaque** consists of fat and other substances that adhere to the arterial wall and obstruct or restrict blood flow.

In addition to the NIH score, patients are often evaluated using the ABCD assessment tool to determine their risk of having a stroke in the days and weeks after the TIA. The following factors are scored:

- Age greater than or equal to 60 (stroke risk increases with age)
- Blood pressure (BP) greater than or equal to 140/90 mm Hg (either systolic or diastolic or both)
- Clinical TIA features (unilateral [one-sided] weakness increases stroke risk)
- Duration of symptoms (the longer the TIA symptoms last, the greater the risk of stroke)

Patients diagnosed with TIA may or may not be admitted, depending on their neurologic and cardiovascular status. For example, a patient who has a new onset of atrial fibrillation with the TIA or a TIA and carotid artery stenosis of greater than 70% will most likely be admitted, depending on agency protocol. Some agencies have a dedicated TIA unit. Management of the patient who had a TIA includes treating the cause, if determined. Depending on the patient, collaborative interventions may include:

- Performing traditional or minimally invasive surgery to remove atherosclerotic plaque buildup within the carotid artery and increase ***perfusion*** to the brain
- Performing a carotid angioplasty with stenting to increase ***perfusion*** to the brain (see discussion of arterial stenting under Endovascular Interventions discussion for stroke later in this chapter)
- Prescribing antiplatelet drugs, typically aspirin or clopidogrel, to prevent thrombotic or embolic strokes (may be placed on a combination of both drugs)
- Reducing high blood pressure (the most common risk factor for stroke) by adding or adjusting drugs to lower blood pressure

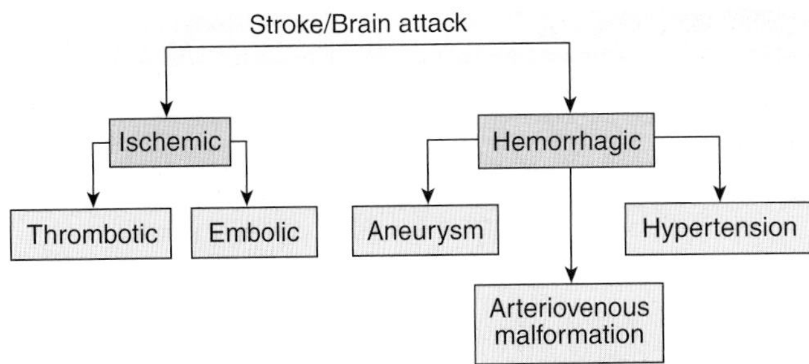

Fig. 41.1 Types of stroke or brain attack.

- Controlling diabetes (if present) and keeping glucose levels within a target range, typically 100 to 180 mg/dL
- Promoting lifestyle changes, such as smoking cessation, eating more heart-healthy foods, and increasing ***mobility*** and physical activity

In collaboration with the interprofessional health team, teach patients about how to achieve a healthier lifestyle to prevent more TIAs or a major stroke. Provide them with information about community resources that can help them meet this desired outcome.

PERFUSION CONCEPT EXEMPLAR: STROKE

Pathophysiology Review

A **stroke** is caused by an interruption of ***perfusion*** to any part of the brain that results in infarction (cell death). Chapter 3 reviews the concept of ***perfusion.*** The National Stroke Association uses the term "brain attack" to convey the urgency for acute stroke care similar to that provided for acute myocardial infarction (MI; heart attack). *A stroke is a medical emergency and should be treated immediately to reduce or prevent permanent disability.*

The brain cannot store oxygen or glucose and therefore must receive a constant flow of blood to provide these substances for normal function. In addition, blood flow is important for the removal of metabolic waste (e.g., carbon dioxide, lactic acid). If ***perfusion*** to any part of the brain is interrupted for more than a few minutes, infarction occurs. Brain metabolism and blood flow after a stroke can be affected around the infarction and in the contralateral (opposite side) hemisphere. Effects of a stroke on the *nonaffected* side may be the result of brain edema or global changes in brain ***perfusion.*** As a result of brain edema, patients may develop increased intracranial pressure (ICP) and secondary brain damage. These secondary changes most commonly occur following a severe traumatic brain injury (TBI) and are discussed in that section of this chapter in detail.

Types of Strokes. Strokes are generally classified as ischemic (occlusive) or hemorrhagic (Fig. 41.1). Acute ischemic strokes are either thrombotic or embolic in origin (Table 41.1). Most strokes are ischemic.

Acute Ischemic Stroke. An **acute ischemic stroke (AIS)** is caused by the occlusion (blockage) of a cerebral or carotid artery by either a thrombus or an embolus. A stroke that is caused by

TABLE 41.1 **Differential Features of the Types of Stroke**

	ISCHEMIC		
Feature	**Thrombotic**	**Embolic**	**Hemorrhagic**
Evolution	Intermittent or stepwise improvement between episodes of worsening symptoms Completed stroke	Abrupt development of completed stroke Steady progression	Usually abrupt onset
Onset	Gradual (minutes to hours)	Sudden	Sudden; may be gradual if caused by hypertension
Level of consciousness	Preserved (patient is awake)	Preserved (patient is awake)	Deepening lethargy/stupor or coma
Contributing associated factors	Hypertension Atherosclerosis	Cardiac disease	Hypertension Vessel disorders Genetic factors
Prodromal symptoms	Transient ischemic attack (TIA)	TIA	Headache
Neurologic deficits	May be deficits during the first few weeks Slight headache Speech deficits Visual problems Confusion	Maximum deficit at onset Paralysis Expressive aphasia	Focal deficits Severe, frequent
Cerebrospinal fluid	Normal; possible presence of protein	Normal	Bloody
Seizures	No	No	Usually
Duration	Improvements over weeks to months Permanent deficits possible	Usually rapid improvements	Variable Permanent neurologic deficits possible

a *thrombus* (clot) is referred to as a **thrombotic stroke**, whereas a stroke caused by an *embolus* (dislodged clot) is referred to as an **embolic stroke**.

Thrombotic strokes account for more than half of all strokes and are commonly associated with the development of atherosclerosis in either intracranial or extracranial arteries (usually the carotid arteries). Atherosclerosis is the process by which fatty plaques develop on the inner wall of the affected arterial vessel. Chapter 33 describes this health problem in detail.

Rupture of one or more atherosclerotic plaques can promote clot formation. When the clot is of sufficient size, it interrupts blood flow to the brain tissue supplied by the vessel, causing an ischemic (occlusive) stroke. The bifurcation (point of division) of the common carotid artery with the internal carotid artery and the vertebral arteries at their junction with the basilar artery are the most common sites involved in **atherosclerotic plaque** formation because of turbulent blood flow. Because of the gradual nature of clot formation when atherosclerotic plaque is present, thrombotic strokes tend to have a *slow* onset, evolving over minutes to hours.

An *embolic stroke* is caused by a thrombus or a group of thrombi that break off from one area of the body and travel to the cerebral arteries via the carotid artery or vertebrobasilar system. The usual source of emboli is the heart. Emboli can occur in patients with atrial fibrillation, heart valve disease, mural thrombi after a myocardial infarction (MI), a prosthetic heart valve, or endocarditis (infection within the wall of the heart). Another source of emboli may be atherosclerotic plaque or clot that breaks off from the carotid sinus or internal carotid artery. Emboli tend to become lodged in the smaller cerebral blood vessels at their point of bifurcation or where the lumen narrows.

As the emboli block the vessel, ischemia develops, and the patient experiences the signs and symptoms of the stroke. The occlusion (blockage) may be temporary if the embolus breaks into smaller fragments, enters smaller blood vessels, and is absorbed. For these reasons, embolic strokes are characterized by the *sudden* development and rapid occurrence of neurologic deficits. The symptoms may resolve over a few days. Conversion of an occlusive stroke to a hemorrhagic stroke may occur because the arterial vessel wall is also vulnerable to ischemic damage from blood supply interruption. Sudden hemodynamic stress may result in vessel rupture, causing bleeding directly within the brain tissue.

Hemorrhagic Stroke. The second major classification of stroke is hemorrhagic stroke. In this type of stroke, vessel integrity is interrupted, and bleeding occurs into the brain tissue or into the subarachnoid space.

Intracerebral hemorrhage (ICH) describes bleeding into the brain tissue generally resulting from severe or sustained hypertension. Elevated blood pressure (BP) leads to changes within the arterial wall that leave it likely to rupture. Damage to the brain occurs from bleeding, causing edema, irritation, and displacement, which cause pressure on brain tissue. Cocaine use is one example of a trigger for sudden, dramatic BP elevation leading to hemorrhagic stroke.

Subarachnoid hemorrhage (SAH) is much more common and results from bleeding into the subarachnoid space—the space between the pia mater and arachnoid layers of the meninges covering the brain. This type of bleeding is usually caused by a ruptured aneurysm or arteriovenous malformation (AVM).

An *aneurysm* is an abnormal ballooning or blister along a normal artery commonly developing in a weak spot on the artery wall. Larger aneurysms are more likely to rupture than smaller ones (see Chapter 33).

An *arteriovenous malformation (AVM)* is an angled collection of malformed, thin-walled, dilated vessels without a capillary network. This uncommon abnormality occurs during embryonic development. Vasospasm may occur as a result of a sudden and periodic constriction of a cerebral artery, often following an SAH or bleeding from an aneurysm or AVM rupture. This constriction interrupts blood flow to distal areas of the brain. Reduced ***perfusion*** from vasospasm contributes to secondary cerebral ischemia and further neurologic dysfunction.

Etiology and Genetic Risk. As with many health problems, the causes of stroke are likely a combination of genetic and environmental risk factors. The leading causes of stroke include smoking, obesity, hypertension, diabetes mellitus, and elevated cholesterol (Centers for Disease Control and Prevention [CDC], 2020a). Many of these risk factors have a familial or genetic predisposition and are discussed elsewhere in this text.

For example, first-degree relative (mother, father, sister, brother) stroke risk increases with a strong family history of hypertension, atherosclerotic disease, and a diagnosis of aneurysm (McCance et al., 2019). Relatives of a patient with an aneurysm, regardless of vessel location, may be at higher risk for intracranial aneurysms and should consider diagnostic testing and follow-up. Other risk factors for stroke include substance use disorder (especially cocaine and heavy alcohol consumption) and use of oral contraceptives by women who are at risk for cardiovascular adverse effects.

Incidence and Prevalence. Stroke is the fifth leading cause of death in the United States and is considered a major cause of disability worldwide. According to the U.S. Centers for Disease Control and Prevention (CDC), more than 800,000 people experience new or recurrent stroke; about 130,000 Americans die each year from stroke (CDC, 2020a). About 13,000 Canadians die each year from stroke (Heart and Stroke Foundation, 2019). Women have a higher incidence of strokes than men, most likely because they tend to live longer (CDC, 2020a).

Eight southeastern states in the United States are known as the "stroke belt" because they have a mortality rate that is 20% higher than the rest of the nation. The coastal plains of North Carolina, South Carolina, and Georgia have a 40% higher mortality rate. Possible factors influencing these differences include income, education, dietary habits, and access to health care (Bowen, 2016).

It is estimated that there are more than 4.7 million stroke survivors in the United States (CDC, 2020a) and 400,000 stroke survivors in Canada living with long-term disability (Heart and Stroke Foundation, 2019). Deaths from stroke have declined over the past 15 years as a result of advances in prompt and effective medical treatment. However, the number of strokes occurring in the younger-adult and middle-age population is increasing (CDC, 2020a). In this group, strokes are associated with illicit drug use because many street drugs cause hypercoagulability, vasospasm, or hypertensive crisis.

Health Promotion and Maintenance

Most strokes are preventable. The CDC and other cardiovascular professional organizations recommend to apply the ABCS of heart health to prevent strokes:

- **A**spirin use when appropriate
- **B**lood pressure control
- **C**holesterol management
- **S**moking cessation

Lifestyle changes include smoking cessation, if needed; a heart-healthy diet rich in fruits and vegetables and low in saturated fats (including red meats); and regular activity, including planned exercise. Teach patients about the importance of identifying and managing risk factors such as hypertension, obesity, substance use disorder, and diabetes mellitus that contribute to the potential for a major stroke.

PATIENT-CENTERED CARE: CULTURAL/SPIRITUAL CONSIDERATIONS QSEN

American Indian and Alaskan Native groups have the highest prevalence of stroke when compared with other populations. Black men and women have more strokes twice as often as white men and women, especially hemorrhagic strokes caused by hypertension. Hispanic or Latino men have more strokes than non-Hispanic men. All of these groups tend to be at a higher risk for hypertension than the Euro-American population. Socioeconomic factors, such as lifestyle (e.g., diet), health care disparities, and genetic or familial factors, may also play a role in stroke risk among these minority groups (CDC, 2020a).

NCLEX EXAMINATION CHALLENGE 41.1

Health Promotion and Maintenance

Which statement by a client who had a transient ischemic attack (TIA) and is at risk for stroke indicates a need for **further** health teaching by the nurse?

A. "I'm glad I can keep eating protein like red meat."
B. "I'll try to walk at least 20 to 30 minutes each day."
C. "I'm going to talk to my doctor about a weight loss plan."
D. "I plan to include more fruits and vegetables in my diet."

❖ Interprofessional Collaborative Care

◆ Assessment: Recognize Cues

History. Although an accurate history is important in the diagnosis of a stroke, *the first priority is to ensure that the patient is transported to a stroke center.* A **stroke center** is designated by The Joint Commission (TJC) or other organization for its ability to rapidly recognize and effectively treat strokes. TJC designates two distinct levels of stroke-center certification. The *primary certified* stroke center is required to provide diagnostic testing (imaging), stroke therapy with IV fibrinolytic therapy, and a stroke team. The *comprehensive* stroke center provides timely and advanced diagnostics and lifesaving measures such as endovascular interventions that can prevent long-term disability. Obtaining a history should not delay the patient's arrival to either the stroke center or interventional radiology within the comprehensive stroke center. A focused history to determine if the patient has had a recent bleeding event or is taking an anticoagulant is an important part of the rapid stroke assessment protocol.

Several important parts of the history should be collected:

- When did symptoms begin? The time of onset of symptoms is essential for making treatment decisions.
- What was the patient doing when the stroke began? Hemorrhagic strokes tend to occur during activity. Ischemic strokes tend to occur early in the morning.
- How did the symptoms progress? Symptoms of a hemorrhagic stroke tend to occur abruptly, whereas thrombotic strokes generally have a more gradual progression.
- Did the symptoms worsen after the initial onset, or did they begin to improve?
- What is the patient's medical history (with specific attention directed toward a history of head trauma, diabetes, hypertension, heart disease, anemia, and obesity)?
- What are the patient's current medications, including prescribed drugs, over-the-counter (OTC) drugs, herbal and nutritional supplements, and recreational (illicit) drugs?
- What is the patient's social history, including education, employment, travel, leisure activities, and personal habits (e.g., smoking, diet, exercise pattern, drug and alcohol use)?

During the interview, observe the patient's level of consciousness (LOC) and assess for indications of impaired ***cognition, mobility,*** and ***sensory perception.*** Question the patient or family member about the presence of sensory deficits or motor changes, visual problems, problems with balance or gait, communication problems, and changes in reading or writing abilities.

When LOC is suddenly decreased or altered, immediately determine if hypoglycemia or hypoxia is present because these conditions may mimic emergent neurologic disorders! Hypoglycemia and hypoxia are easily treated and reversed, unlike brain injury from inadequate **perfusion** or trauma.

The patient with an SAH, particularly when the hemorrhage is from a ruptured (leaking) aneurysm, often reports the onset of a sudden, severe headache described as "the worst headache of my life." Additional symptoms of SAH or cerebral aneurysmal and AVM bleeding are nausea and vomiting, **photophobia** (sensitivity to light), cranial nerve deficits, stiff neck, and change in mental status. There may also be a family history of aneurysms (see Chapter 33).

Physical Assessment/Signs and Symptoms. First-responder personnel (e.g., paramedics, emergency medical technicians) perform an initial neurologic examination using well-established stroke assessment tools.

! NURSING SAFETY PRIORITY (QSEN)

Critical Rescue

In the ED, assess the stroke patient within 10 minutes of arrival. This same standard applies to patients already hospitalized for other medical conditions who have a stroke. The priority is assessment of ABCs—*a*irway, *b*reathing, and *c*irculation. Many hospitals have designated stroke teams and centers that are expert in acute stroke assessment and management.

Nurses also perform a complete neurologic assessment on arrival to the ED. The National Institutes of Health Stroke Scale (NIHSS) is a commonly used valid and reliable assessment tool that nurses complete as soon as possible after the patient arrives in the ED. This tool is used as one assessment to determine eligibility for IV fibrinolytics (Table 41.2) (Powers et al., 2018).

Although the NIHSS is the standard tool for assessing neurologic status after an acute stroke, there is no standard for when and how often to use the tool. Wells-Pittman and Gullicksrud (2020) implemented a quality improvement (QI) project to determine the minimum use of the NIHSS across their large health care system (see the Systems Thinking and Quality Improvement Box).

As the patients are transitioned from the ED to other settings, the most important area to assess is the patient's LOC. Use the Glasgow Coma Scale (GCS; see Chapter 38) or a modified NIHSS to frequently monitor for changes in LOC throughout the patient's acute care.

Strokes and other neurologic injuries, including brain tumors or traumatic brain injury, can cause an **impaired airway defense**, or an inability to clear one's airway. This impairment can cause inadequate cough and **dysphagia** (difficulty swallowing), which can lead to aspiration (causing aspiration pneumonia) or death. Therefore assess the client's ability to effectively cough. Some agencies also allow nurses to use a one of a variety of screening tools to assess for the presence of dysphagia (Miller et al., 2017).

Stroke symptoms can appear at any time of the day or night. In general, the five most common symptoms are (CDC, 2020a):

- Sudden confusion or trouble speaking or understanding others
- Sudden numbness or weakness of the face, arm, or leg
- Sudden trouble seeing in one or both eyes
- Sudden dizziness, trouble walking, or loss of balance or coordination
- Sudden severe headache with no known cause

More specific stroke symptoms depend on the extent and location of the ischemia and the arteries involved as described in the Key Features: Stroke box.

The *right* cerebral hemisphere is more involved with visual and spatial awareness and proprioception (sense of body position). A person who has a stroke involving the right cerebral hemisphere is often unaware of any deficits and may be disoriented to time and place. Personality changes include

SYSTEMS THINKING AND QUALITY IMPROVEMENT QSEN

Is There a Standard for Using the NIHSS After Acute Stroke?

Wells-Pittman, J., & Gullicksrud, A. (2020). Standardizing the frequency of neurologic assessment after acute stroke. *American Journal of Nursing, 120*(3), 48-54.

The authors of this study were employed in a large health care system that has four Joint Commission–certified primary stroke centers and two Joint Commission–certified comprehensive stroke centers. Each center determined when and how often to assess stroke patients using the National Institutes of Health Stroke Scale (NIHSS). A QI nursing team was formed to review the literature and collect data on national best practices regarding the use of the NIHSS. A six-item questionnaire was sent to 22 stroke centers across the United States. Examples of questions included:

- Do you use the full NIHSS or the modified NIHSS?
- How frequently is the NIHSS being completed?
- Do you do other neurologic assessment on your stroke patients as well?

The QI nursing team analyzed the data and developed guidelines that allowed nurses to use clinical judgment about when the NIHSS would be used for patient assessment. These guidelines were based on national best practices, available evidence, and nursing expertise.

Commentary: Implications for Practice and Research

The system in this QI project was the health system stroke centers. The QI team worked to develop standardized guidelines to establish consistency but still allow nurses to use clinical judgment about when and how often to assess stroke patients using the NIHSS.

impulsivity (poor impulse control) and poor judgment. The *left* cerebral hemisphere, the dominant hemisphere in all but about 15% to 20% of the population, is the center for speech, language, mathematic skills, and analytic thinking. Therefore problems in these areas are expected for patients who have a left-sided stroke.

Patients with *embolic* strokes may have a heart murmur, dysrhythmias (most often atrial fibrillation), and/or hypertension. It is not unusual for the patient to be admitted to the hospital with a blood pressure greater than 180 to 200/110 to 120 mm Hg, especially if he or she has hypertensive bleeding. Although a somewhat higher blood pressure of 150/100 mm Hg is needed to maintain cerebral ***perfusion*** after an acute ischemic stroke, pressures above this reading may lead to extension of the stroke.

Psychosocial Assessment. Assess the patient's reaction to the illness, especially in relation to changes in body image, self-concept, and ability to perform ADLs. In collaboration with the patient's family and friends, identify any problems with coping or personality changes.

Ask about the patient's financial status and occupation, because they may be affected by the residual neurologic deficits of the stroke and the potential long recovery. Patients who do not have disability or health insurance may worry about how their family will cope financially with the disruption in their lives. Early involvement of social services,

KEY FEATURES

Stroke

Middle Cerebral Artery Strokes (most common)

- Contralateral (opposite side) **hemiparesis** (one-sided weakness) or **hemiplegia** (one-sided paralysis); typically the arm is flaccid and the leg is spastic if both extremities are affected
- **Dysphagia**
- Contralateral sensory perception deficit (numbness, tingling, unusual sensations)
- **Ptosis**
- **Nystagmus**
- **Homonymous hemianopsia**
- **Unilateral neglect or inattention**
- **Dysarthria**
- **Aphasia**
- **Anomia**
- **Apraxia**
- **Agnosia**
- **Alexia**, **agraphia**, and/or **acalculia**
- Impaired vertical sensation
- Visual and spatial deficits
- Memory loss (**amnesia**)
- Altered level of consciousness: drowsy to comatose

Posterior Cerebral Artery Strokes

- Perseveration (word or action repetition)
- **Aphasia**, **amnesia**, **alexia**, **agraphia**, visual **agnosia**, and **ataxia**
- Loss of deep sensation
- Decreased touch sensation
- Increased lethargy/stupor, coma

Internal Carotid Artery Strokes

- Contralateral **hemiparesis**
- Sensory perception deficit
- **Hemianopsia**, blurred vision, blindness
- **Aphasia** (dominant side)
- Headache
- Carotid **bruit**

Anterior Cerebral Artery Strokes

- Contralateral **hemiparesis**: leg more than arm
- Bladder incontinence
- Personality and behavior changes
- **Aphasia** and **amnesia**
- Positive grasp and sucking reflex
- ***Sensory perception*** deficit (lower extremity)
- Memory impairment
- Ataxic gait

Vertebrobasilar Artery Strokes

- Headache and vertigo
- Possible coma
- Memory loss and confusion
- Flaccid paresis or paralysis (quadriparesis affecting all four extremities)
- **Ataxia**
- **Vertigo**
- Cranial nerve dysfunction (such as dysphagia from cranial nerve IX involvement)
- Visual deficits (one eye) or **homonymous hemianopsia**
- Sensory loss: numbness

TABLE 41.2 National Institutes of Health Stroke Scale (NIHSS)

Category and Measurement	Score[a]
1a. Level of Consciousness (LOC) 0 = Alert; keenly responsive 1 = Not alert; but arousable by minor stimulation to obey, answer, or respond 2 = Not alert; requires repeated stimulation to attend or is obtunded and requires strong or painful stimulation to make movements (not stereotyped) 3 = Responds only with reflex motor or autonomic effects or totally unresponsive, flaccid, and areflexic	____
1b. LOC Questions 0 = Answers two questions correctly 1 = Answers one question correctly 2 = Answers neither question correctly	____
1c. LOC Commands 0 = Performs two tasks correctly 1 = Performs one task correctly 2 = Performs neither task correctly	
2. Best Gaze 0 = Normal 1 = Partial gaze palsy; gaze abnormal in one or both eyes, but forced deviation or total gaze paresis not present 2 = Forced deviation, or total gaze paresis not overcome by the oculocephalic maneuver	____
3. Visual 0 = No visual loss 1 = Partial hemianopia 2 = Complete hemianopia 3 = Bilateral hemianopia (blind, including cortical blindness)	____
4. Facial Palsy 0 = Normal symmetric movements 1 = Minor paralysis (flattened nasolabial fold, asymmetry on smiling) 2 = Partial paralysis (total or near-total paralysis of lower face) 3 = Complete paralysis of one or both sides (absence of facial movement in the upper and lower face)	____
5. Motor (Arm) 0 = No drift; limb holds 90 (or 45) degrees for full 10 seconds 1 = Drift; limb holds 90 (or 45) degrees, but drifts down before full 10 seconds; does not hit bed or other support 2 = Some effort against gravity; limb cannot get to or maintain (if cued) 90 (or 45) degrees; drifts down to bed but has some effort against gravity 3 = No effort against gravity; limb falls 4 = No movementUntestable = Amputation or joint fusion	Right arm: ____ Left arm: ____
6. Motor (Leg) 0 = No drift; leg holds 30-degree position for full 5 seconds 1 = Drift; leg falls by the end of the 5-second period but does not hit bed 2 = Some effort against gravity; leg falls to bed by 5 seconds but has some effort against gravity 3 = No effort against gravity; leg falls to bed immediately 4 = No movementUntestable = Amputation or joint fusion	Right leg: ____ Left leg: ____
7. Limb Ataxia 0 = Absent 1 = Present in one limb 2 = Present in two limbsUntestable = Amputation or joint fusion	____
8. Sensory 0 = Normal; no sensory loss 1 = Mild-to-moderate sensory loss; patient feels pinprick less sharp or dull on the affected side; or loss of superficial pain with pinprick, but patient aware of being touched 2 = Severe-to-total sensory loss; patient not aware of being touched in the face, arm, and leg	____
9. Best Language 0 = No aphasia; normal 1 = Mild-to-moderate aphasia; some obvious loss of fluency or facility of comprehension, without significant limitation on ideas expressed or form of expression 2 = Severe aphasia; all communication is through fragmentary expression; great need for inference, questioning, and guessing by the listener 3 = Mute, global aphasia; no usable speech or auditory comprehension	____

TABLE 41.2 National Institutes of Health Stroke Scale (NIHSS)—cont'd

Category and Measurement	Score[a]
10. Dysarthria	___
0 = Normal	
1 = Mild-to-moderate dysarthria; patient slurs at least some words and, at worst, can be understood with some difficulty	
2 = Severe dysarthria; patient's speech so slurred as to be unintelligible in the absence of or out of proportion to any dysphasia or is mute/anarthricUntestable = Intubated or other physical barrier	
11. Extinction and Inattention (Neglect)	___
0 = No abnormality	
1 = Visual, tactile, auditory, spatial, or personal inattention or extinction to bilateral simultaneous stimulation in one of the sensory modalities	
2 = Profound hemi-inattention or extinction to more than one modality; does not recognize own hand or orients to only one side of space	

[a]The patient can have a score of 0 to 40, with 0 indicating no neurologic deficits and 40 indicating the most deficits.
Adapted from *National Institutes of Health Stroke Scale (NIHSS), 2013.* www.stroke.nih.gov/documents/NIH_Stroke_Scale.pdf.

certified hospital chaplain, or psychological counseling may enhance coping skills.

Assess for **emotional lability** (uncontrollable emotional state), especially if the frontal lobe or right side of the brain has been affected. In such cases the patient often laughs and then cries unexpectedly for no apparent reason. Explain the cause of uncontrollable emotions to the family or significant others so they do not feel responsible for these reactions.

Laboratory Assessment. Clinical history, physical assessment, and a National Institutes of Health Stroke Scale (NIHSS) score are usually enough to identify a stroke once it has occurred. No definitive laboratory tests confirm its diagnosis. Elevated hematocrit and hemoglobin levels are often associated with a severe or major stroke as the body attempts to compensate for lack of oxygen to the brain. An elevated white blood cell (WBC) count may indicate the presence of an infection or a response to physiologic stress or inflammation. Blood glucose and hemoglobin A1C levels are used to evaluates whether the client has diabetes and whether it is controlled.

In addition to other routine lab oratory testing, the primary health care provider typically requests a prothrombin time (PT), an international normalized ratio (INR), and an activated partial thromboplastin time (aPTT) to establish baseline information before fibrinolytic or anticoagulation therapy may be started.

Imaging Assessment. For definitive evaluation of a suspected stroke, a *computed tomography perfusion (CTP) scan* and/or *computed tomography angiography (CTA)* is used to assess the extent of ischemia of brain tissue. Cerebral aneurysms or AVM may also be identified. *Magnetic resonance angiography (MRA)* and multimodal techniques such as perfusion-weighted imaging enhance the sensitivity of the MRI to detect early changes in the brain, including confirming blood flow. *Ultrasonography* (carotid duplex scanning) may also be performed.

◆ **Analysis: Analyze Cues and Prioritize Hypotheses.** Depending on stroke severity and/or response to immediate management, the priority collaborative problems for patients with a stroke may include:

1. Inadequate ***perfusion*** to the brain due to interruption of arterial blood flow and a possible increase in ICP
2. Decreased ***mobility*** and possible need for assistance to perform ADLs due to neuromuscular or impaired ***cognition***
3. Aphasia and/or dysarthria due to decreased circulation in the brain (aphasia) or facial muscle weakness (dysarthria)
4. ***Sensory perception*** deficits due to altered neurologic reception and transmission

◆ Planning and Implementation: Generate Solutions and Take Action

Improving Cerebral Perfusion

Planning: Expected Outcomes. The patient with a stroke is expected to have improved cerebral ***perfusion*** to maintain adequate brain function and prevent further brain injury.

Interventions. Most strokes are treatable. Improvements in acute stroke management have helped to decrease deaths from stroke. Almost all large hospitals in the United States have designated stroke centers; however, community and rural acute care settings may not have access to a neurologist or other resources needed to manage an acute stroke. As a result, teleneurology using two-way video technology is a growing strategy to provide acute stroke consultation with a board-certified neurologist (Bowen, 2016; Powers et al., 2018).

Interventions for patients experiencing strokes are determined primarily by the type and extent of the stroke. Nursing interventions are initially aimed at monitoring for neurologic changes or complications associated with stroke and its treatment. The two major treatment modalities for patients with acute ischemic stroke are IV fibrinolytic therapy and endovascular interventions. Regardless of the immediate management approach used, once the patient is stable, provide ongoing supportive care. Provide interventions to prevent and/or monitor for early signs of complications. Implement interventions to prevent patient falls. These health problems are discussed in appropriate chapters in this textbook.

Fibrinolytic Therapy. For selected patients with acute ischemic strokes, early intervention with IV fibrinolytic therapy ("clot-busting drug") is the standard of practice to improve blood flow to viable tissue around the infarction or through the brain. The success of fibrinolytic therapy for a stroke depends on the interval between the time that symptoms begin and treatment is available. IV (systemic) fibrinolytic therapy (also called *thrombolytic therapy*) for an acute ischemic stroke dissolves the cranial artery occlusion to re-establish blood flow and prevent cerebral infarction. *IV alteplase is the only drug approved at this time for the treatment of acute ischemic stroke.* The most important factor in determining whether or not to give alteplase is the time between symptom onset and time seen in the stroke center. Currently, the U.S. Food and Drug Administration (FDA) approves administration of alteplase within 3 hours of stroke onset. The American Stroke Association endorses extension of that time frame to 4.5 hours to administer this fibrinolytic for patients *unless* they fall into one or more of these categories (Powers et al., 2018):

- Age older than 80 years
- Anticoagulation regardless of international normalized ratio (INR)
- Imaging evidence of ischemic injury involving more than one-third of the brain tissue supplied by the middle cerebral artery
- Baseline National Institutes of Health Stroke Scale (NIHSS) score greater than 25
- History of both stroke and diabetes
- Evidence of active bleeding

Fibrinolytic therapy is explained to the patient and/or family member, and informed consent is obtained. The dosage of alteplase is based on the patient's actual weight at 0.9 mg/kg. The 2018 Clinical Practice Guidelines for management of patients with acute ischemic stroke recommend IV alteplase 90 mg over 60 minutes, with the initial 10% of that dose given as a bolus over the first minute. The newest recommendation for door-to-needle time (ED admission to fibrinolytic therapy start) is 45 minutes (Powers et al., 2018).

Each hospital has strict protocols for mixing and administering the fibrinolytic drug and for monitoring the patient before and after fibrinolytic drug administration. In some cases, the patient's blood pressure may be too high to give the medication. In this instance, the patient receives a rapid-acting antihypertensive drug until the blood pressure is below 185/110 mm Hg (Powers et al., 2018). This level must be maintained during fibrinolytic therapy.

! NURSING SAFETY PRIORITY QSEN

Drug Alert

In addition to frequent monitoring of vital signs, carefully observe for signs of intracerebral hemorrhage and other signs of bleeding during administration of fibrinolytic drug therapy. Additional best practice nursing interventions are listed in the Best Practice for Patient Safety & Quality Care: Evidence-Based Nursing Interventions During and After IV Administration of Alteplase box.

NCLEX EXAMINATION CHALLENGE 41.2

Physiological Integrity

The nurse is caring for a client treated with alteplase following a stroke. Which assessment finding is the **highest priority** for the nurse to report to the primary health care provider?

A. Client has a new-onset mild headache.
B. Client's blood pressure is 194/120 mm Hg.
C. Client has left hemiparesis.
D. Client continues to be drowsy.

Endovascular Interventions. Endovascular procedures to improve ***perfusion*** include intra-arterial thrombolysis using drug therapy, mechanical **embolectomy** (surgical blood clot [thrombosis] removal), and carotid stent placement. *Intra-arterial thrombolysis* has the advantage of delivering the fibrinolytic agent directly into the thrombus within 6 hours of the stroke onset. It is particularly beneficial for some patients who have an occlusion of the middle cerebral artery or those who arrive in the ED after the window for IV alteplase. Patients having either fibrinolytic therapy or endovascular interventions are admitted to the critical care setting for intensive monitoring.

Carotid artery angioplasty with stenting is common to prevent or, in some cases, help manage an acute ischemic stroke. This interventional radiology procedure is usually done under moderate sedation. It may be performed by a cardiovascular surgeon or interventional radiologist. A technique using a distal/embolic protection device has made this procedure very safe. The device is placed beyond the stenosis through a catheter

BEST PRACTICE FOR PATIENT SAFETY & QUALITY CARE QSEN

Evidence-Based Nursing Interventions During and After IV Administration of Alteplase

- Admit the patient to a critical care or specialized stroke unit.
- Perform a double check of the drug dose. Use a programmable pump to deliver the initial dose of 0.9 mg/kg (maximum dose 90 mg) over 60 minutes, with 10% of the dose given as a bolus over 1 minute. Do not manually push this drug.
- Perform neurologic assessments, including vital signs, every 10 to 15 minutes during infusion and every 30 minutes after that for at least 6 hours; monitor hourly for 24 hours after treatment. Be consistent regarding the device used to obtain blood pressures because blood pressures can vary when switching from a manual to a noninvasive automatic to an intra-arterial device.
- If systolic blood pressure is 185 mm Hg or greater or diastolic is 110 mm Hg or greater during or after alteplase, give antihypertensive drugs, such as labetalol, as prescribed (IV is recommended for faster response).
- To prevent bleeding, do not place invasive tubes, such as nasogastric (NG) tubes or indwelling urinary catheters, until the patient is stable (usually for 24 hours).
- Discontinue the infusion if the patient reports severe headache or has severe hypertension, bleeding, nausea, and/or vomiting; notify the primary health care provider immediately.
- Obtain a follow-up CTA or CTP scan after fibrinolytic therapy and before starting antiplatelet or anticoagulant drugs.

inserted into the femoral artery (groin). The device catches any clot debris that breaks off during the procedure. Placement of a carotid stent is performed to open a blockage in the carotid artery typically at the division of the common carotid artery into the internal and external carotid arteries. Throughout the procedure, carefully assess the patient's neurologic and cardiovascular status.

! NURSING SAFETY PRIORITY (QSEN)

Action Alert

Before discharge after carotid stent placement, teach the patient and family to report these symptoms to the primary health care provider immediately:

- Severe headache
- Change in LOC or *cognition* (e.g., drowsiness, new-onset confusion)
- Muscle weakness or motor dysfunction
- Severe neck pain
- Swelling at neck incisional site
- Hoarseness or dysphagia (due to nerve damage)

When the stroke is hemorrhagic and the cause is related to an AVM or cerebral aneurysm, the patient is evaluated for the optimal procedure to stop bleeding. Some procedures can be used to prevent bleeding in an AVM or aneurysm that is discovered *before* symptom onset or SAH. Procedures occur in the interventional radiology suite or operating room.

Monitoring for increased intracranial pressure. The patient is most at risk for increased ICP resulting from edema during the first 72 hours after onset of the stroke. Some patients may have worsening of their neurologic status starting within 24 to 48 hours after their endovascular procedure from increased ICP (see the Key Features: Increased Intracranial Pressure (ICP) box).

KEY FEATURES

Increased Intracranial Pressure (ICP)

- Decreased level of consciousness (LOC) (earliest sign)
- Behavior changes: restlessness, irritability, and confusion
- Headache
- Nausea and vomiting (may be projectile)
- **Aphasia**
- Change in speech pattern/**dysarthria**
- Change in sensorimotor status:
    - Pupillary changes: dilated and nonreactive pupils ("blown pupils") or constricted and nonreactive pupils (very late sign)
    - Cranial nerve dysfunction
- **Ataxia**
- Seizures (usually within first 24 hours after stroke)
- **Cushing triad** (very late sign):
    - Severe hypertension
    - Widened pulse pressure
    - Bradycardia
- Abnormal posturing (very late sign) (see Chapter 38):
    - Decerebrate
    - Decorticate

Reassess patients with acute stroke and after endovascular treatment of stroke symptoms every 1 to 4 hours, depending on severity of the condition. Use the approved agency assessment strategy and documentation tools.

! NURSING SAFETY PRIORITY (QSEN)

Critical Rescue

Be alert for symptoms of increased ICP in the stroke patient and report any deterioration in the patient's neurologic status to the primary health care provider or Rapid Response Team immediately! *The first sign of increased ICP is a declining level of consciousness (LOC).*

Best practices for preventing or managing increasing ICP for patients experiencing a stroke include:

- Elevate the head of the bed per agency or primary health care provider protocol to improve ***perfusion*** pressure.
- Provide oxygen therapy to prevent hypoxia for patients with oxygen saturation less than 95% or per agency or primary health care provider protocol or prescription.
- Maintain the head in a midline, neutral position to promote venous drainage from the brain.
- Avoid sudden and acute hip or neck flexion during positioning. Extreme hip flexion may increase intrathoracic pressure, leading to decreased cerebral venous outflow and elevated ICP. Extreme neck flexion also interferes with venous drainage from the brain and intracranial dynamics.
- Avoid the clustering of nursing procedures (e.g., giving a bath followed immediately by changing the bed linen). When multiple activities are clustered in a narrow time period, the effect on ICP can be dramatic elevation.
- Hyperoxygenate the patient before and after suctioning to avoid transient hypoxemia and resultant ICP elevation from dilation of cerebral arteries.
- Provide airway management to prevent unnecessary suctioning and coughing that can increase ICP.
- Maintain a quiet environment for the patient experiencing a headache, which is common with cerebral hemorrhage or increased ICP.
- Keep the room lights low to accommodate any **photophobia** the patient may have.
- Closely monitor blood pressure, heart rhythm, oxygen saturation, blood glucose, and body temperature to prevent secondary brain injury and promote positive outcomes after stroke.

! NURSING SAFETY PRIORITY (QSEN)

Critical Rescue

For ischemic strokes, if the stroke patient's systolic BP is more than 185 mm Hg, notify the Rapid Response Team or primary health care provider immediately and anticipate possible prescription of an IV antihypertensive medication. Monitor the patient's BP and mean arterial pressure (MAP) (normal MAP is 70 to 100 mm Hg; at least 60 mm Hg is necessary to perfuse major organs) every 5 minutes until the systolic BP is adequate to maintain brain ***perfusion.*** Avoid a sudden systolic BP drop to less than 120 mm Hg with drug administration, which may cause brain ischemia.

Ongoing drug therapy. Ongoing drug therapy depends on the type of stroke and the resulting neurologic dysfunction. In general, the purposes of drug therapy are to prevent further thrombotic or embolic episodes (with antithrombotics and anticoagulation) and to protect the neurons from hypoxia.

Antiplatelet drugs such as aspirin and clopidogrel are the standard of care for treatment following acute ischemic strokes and for preventing future strokes (Powers et al., 2018). Sodium heparin and other anticoagulants, such as warfarin, are reserved for use in patients who have cardiopulmonary issues such as atrial fibrillation. *Anticoagulants are high-alert drugs that can cause bleeding, including intracerebral hemorrhage in the area of the ischemia.* Therefore a newer trend is to use heparinoids, such as low–molecular-weight heparin (LMWH), rather than unfractionated heparin for patients with acute ischemic stroke. However, a systematic review of nine randomized controlled trials showed no significant difference in clinical outcomes when comparing LMWH and sodium heparin (Sandercock & Leong, 2017).

An *initial* low dose of aspirin is safer and recommended within 24 to 48 hours after stroke onset (CDC, 2020a; Sandercock & Leong, 2017). Aspirin should not be given within 24 hours of fibrinolytic administration. Aspirin is an antiplatelet drug that prevents further clot formation by reducing platelet adhesiveness (clumping or "stickiness"). It can cause bruising, hemorrhage, and liver disease over a long-term period. Teach the patient to report any unusual bruising or bleeding to the primary health care provider or call 911 if bleeding is severe or does not stop.

A calcium channel blocking drug that crosses the blood-brain barrier such as nimodipine may be given to treat or prevent cerebral vasospasm after a subarachnoid hemorrhage. Vasospasm, which usually occurs between 4 and 14 days after the stroke, slows blood flow to the area and causes ischemia. Nimodipine works by relaxing the smooth muscles of the vessel wall and reducing the incidence and severity of the spasm. In addition, this drug dilates collateral vessels to ischemic areas of the brain.

Stool softeners, analgesics for pain, and antianxiety drugs may also be prescribed as needed for symptom management. Stool softeners also prevent the Valsalva maneuver during defecation to prevent increased ICP.

Promoting Mobility and ADL Ability

Planning: Expected Outcomes. The patient with a stroke is expected to ambulate and provide self-care independently, with or without one or more assistive-adaptive devices.

Interventions. In collaboration with the rehabilitation therapists, assess the patient's functional ability for bed ***mobility*** skills, ambulation with or without assistance, and ADL ability, including feeding, bathing, and dressing. Patients who have had a stroke are at risk for aspiration due to impaired swallowing as a result of muscle weakness. *Therefore the best practice for all suspected and diagnosed stroke patients is to maintain NPO status until their swallowing ability is assessed!* Follow agency guidelines for screening or use an evidence-based bedside swallowing screening tool to determine if **dysphagia** is present. Refer the patient to the speech-language pathologist (SLP) for a swallowing evaluation per stroke protocol as needed. If dysphagia is present, develop a collaborative plan of care to prevent aspiration and support nutrition. Collaborate with the registered dietitian nutritionist to ensure that nutritional needs are met. Monitor the patient's weight daily and serum prealbumin levels to detect any decrease from baseline.

Many patients who have an untreated stroke often have flaccid or spastic paralysis. It is not unusual for the patient to eventually have a flaccid arm and spastic leg on the affected side because the affected leg often regains function more quickly than the arm. Be sure to support the affected flaccid arm of the stroke patient, and teach assistive personnel (AP) to avoid pulling on it. Position the arm on a pillow while the patient is sitting to prevent it from hanging freely, which could cause shoulder subluxation. The physical therapist or occupational therapist provides a slinglike device to support the arm during ambulation. Chapter 7 describes interventions for rehabilitation, including improving ***mobility*** and promoting self-care.

Patients begin rehabilitation as soon as possible to regain function and prevent complications of immobility, such as pneumonia, atelectasis, and pressure injuries. Another major complication of impaired ***mobility*** is the development of venous thromboembolism (VTE), especially deep vein thrombosis (DVT), which can lead to a pulmonary embolism (PE). This risk is highest in older patients and those with a severe stroke.

> **! CORE MEASURES**
>
> Per The Joint Commission's Core Measures for VTE (2019), provide care to prevent this complication by applying intermittent sequential pneumatic (or compression) devices, changing the patient's position frequently, and ambulating the patient if possible. Report any indications of DVT to the primary health care provider and document assessments in the patient's record. Chapter 33 discusses VTE prevention in detail.

Promoting Effective Communication

Planning: Expected Outcomes. The patient with a stroke is expected to receive, interpret, and express spoken, written, and nonverbal messages, if possible. However, some patients may need to develop strategies for alternative methods of communication, such as pictures, images, or nonverbal language.

Interventions. Language or speech problems are usually the result of a stroke involving the dominant hemisphere. The left cerebral hemisphere is the speech center in most patients. Speech and language problems may be the result of aphasia or dysarthria. **Aphasia** is caused by cerebral hemisphere damage; **dysarthria** is the result of a loss of motor function to the tongue or the muscles of speech, causing facial weakness and slurred speech.

TABLE 41.3 Types of Aphasia

Expressive
- Referred to as Broca, or motor, aphasia
- Difficulty speaking
- Difficulty writing

Receptive
- Referred to as Wernicke, or sensory, aphasia
- Difficulty understanding spoken words
- Difficulty understanding written words
- Speech often meaningless
- Made-up words

Mixed
- Combination of difficulty understanding words and speech
- Difficulty with reading and writing

Global
- Profound speech and language problems
- Often no speech or sounds that cannot be understood

Aphasia can be classified in a number of ways. Most commonly, it is classified as expressive, receptive, or mixed (Table 41.3). **Expressive (Broca or motor) aphasia** is the result of damage in the Broca area of the frontal lobe. It is a motor speech problem in which the patient generally understands what is said but cannot speak. He or she also has difficulty writing but may be able to read. Rote speech and automatic speech such as responses to a greeting are often intact. The patient is aware of the deficit and may become frustrated and angry.

Receptive (Wernicke or sensory) aphasia is caused by injury involving the Wernicke area in the temporoparietal area. The patient cannot understand the spoken or written word. Although he or she may be able to talk, the language is often meaningless.

Usually the patient has some degree of dysfunction in the areas of both expression and reception. This is known as *mixed* or *global aphasia*. Reading and writing ability are equally affected. Few patients have only expressive *or* receptive aphasia. In most cases, however, one type is dominant.

To help communicate with the patient with aphasia, use these guiding principles:

- Present one idea or thought in a sentence (e.g., "I am going to help you get into the chair.").
- Use simple one-step commands rather than asking patients to do multiple tasks.
- Speak slowly but not loudly; use cues or gestures as needed.
- Avoid "yes" and "no" questions for patients with expressive aphasia.
- Use alternative forms of communication if needed, such as a computer, handheld mobile device, communication board, or flash cards (often with pictures).
- Do not rush the patient when speaking.

For more specific communication strategies for the patient with aphasia or dysarthria, collaborate with the speech-language pathologist.

INTERPROFESSIONAL COLLABORATION

Care of Patients With Aphasia

For patients with moderate-to-severe aphasia or dysarthria, consult with the speech-language pathologist (SLP), who can complement your patient care with specialized knowledge of speech and language problems. The SLP may identify additional patient problems that could trigger the need for other team members to achieve positive outcomes for the patient who experienced a stroke. According to the Interprofessional Education Collaborative (IPEC) Expert Panel's Competency of Roles and Responsibilities, using the unique and complementary abilities of other team members optimizes health and patient care (IPEC, 2016; Slusser et al., 2019).

NCLEX EXAMINATION CHALLENGE 41.3

Physiological Integrity

The nurse is caring for an older client with receptive (sensory) aphasia. Which nursing action is **most appropriate** for communicating with the client?
A. Refer the client to the speech-language pathologist (SLP).
B. Speak loudly to help the client interpret what is being said.
C. Provide pictures to help the client understand.
D. Ask the client to read messages on a whiteboard.

Managing Changes in Sensory Perception

Planning: Expected Outcomes. The major concern of patients with ***sensory perception*** deficits is adapting to neurologic deficits. The patient with a stroke is expected to adapt to sensory perception changes in vision, **proprioception** (body position sense), and/or peripheral sensation and to be free from injury.

Interventions. Patients with right hemisphere brain damage typically have difficulty with visual-perceptual or spatial-perceptual tasks. They often have problems with depth and distance perception and with discrimination of right from left or up from down. Because of these problems, patients can have difficulty performing routine ADLs. Caregivers can help the patient adapt to these disabilities by using frequent verbal and tactile cues and by breaking down tasks into discrete steps. *Always approach the patient from the unaffected side, which should face the door of the room!*

Unilateral neglect (or inattention), occurs most commonly in patients who have had a right cerebral stroke. However, it can occur in any patient who experiences **hemianopsia**, in which the vision of one or both eyes is affected (Fig. 41.2). This problem places the patient at additional risk for injury, especially falls, because of an inability to recognize his or her physical impairment on one side of the body or because of a lack of **proprioception**.

- Teach the patient to touch and use both sides of the body.
- When dressing, remind the patient to dress the affected side first.
- If **homonymous hemianopsia** is present, teach the patient to turn his or her head from side to side to expand the visual field because the same half of each eye is affected. This scanning technique is also useful when the patient is eating or ambulating.

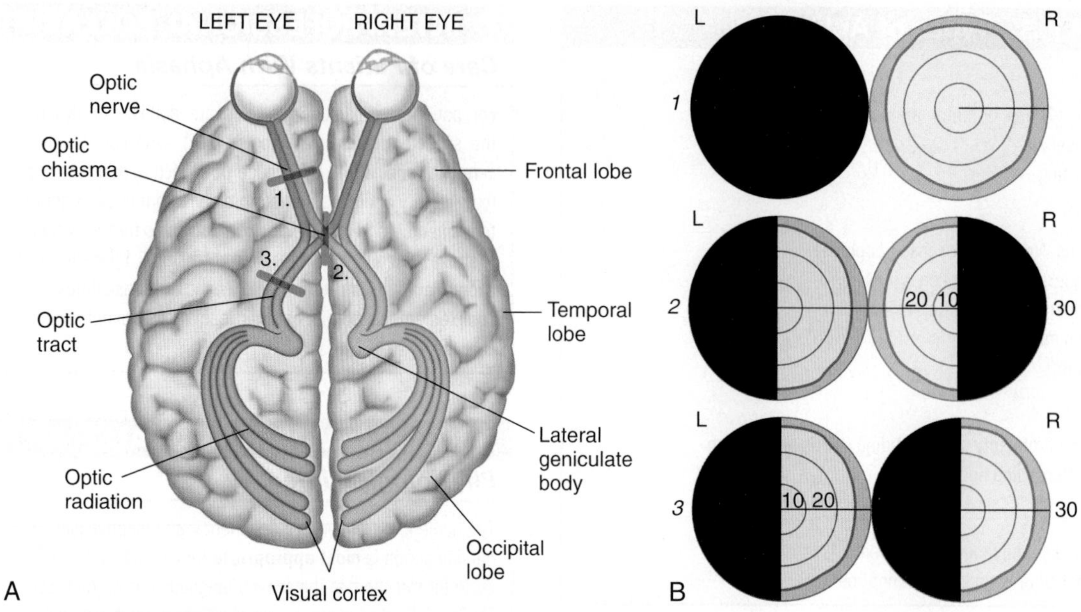

Fig. 41.2 (A) Site of lesions causing visual loss. 1, Total blindness left eye. 2, Bitemporal hemianopia. 3, Left homonymous hemianopia. (B) Visual fields corresponding to lesions shown in (A) 1, Total blindness left eye. 2, Bitemporal hemianopia. 3, Left homonymous hemianopia. (A from Ball, J.W., Dains, J.E., Flynn, J.A., Solomon, B.S., & Stewart, R.W. [2015]. *Seidel's guide to physical examination* [8th ed.]. St. Louis: Mosby. B modified from Stein, H.A., Slatt, B.J., & Stein, R.M. [1994]. *The ophthalmic assistant* [6th ed.]. St. Louis: Mosby.)

Place objects within the patient's field of vision. A mirror may help visualize more of the environment. If the patient has **diplopia**, a patch may be placed over the affected eye and changed every 2 to 4 hours.

The patient with a left hemisphere lesion generally has memory deficits and may show significant changes in the ability to carry out simple tasks, such as eating and grooming. Help with ADLs but encourage the patient to do as much as possible independently. To assist with memory problems, reorient the patient to the month, year, day of the week, and circumstances surrounding hospital admission. Establish a routine or schedule that is as structured, repetitious, and consistent as possible. Provide information in a simple, concise manner. **Apraxia** may be present. Typically the patient with apraxia exhibits a slow, cautious, and hesitant behavior style. The physical therapist helps the patient compensate for loss of position sense.

! CORE MEASURES

Eight core measures and quality indicators are associated with the care of stroke patients by the interprofessional health care team (TJC, 2017). Certification as a primary stroke center or a comprehensive stroke center is tied to consistent performance in achieving satisfactory core measures. The core measures may have additional implications in terms of reimbursement in the future. The eight core measures for ischemic stroke care for all patients include:

- Venous thromboembolism (VTE) prophylaxis
- Discharge with antithrombotic therapy
- Discharge with anticoagulation therapy for atrial fibrillation/flutter
- Thrombolytic therapy as indicated
- Antithrombotic therapy re-evaluated by end of hospital day 2
- Discharge on statin medication
- Stroke education provided and documented
- Assessment for rehabilitation

Care Coordination and Transition Management. The patient with a stroke may be discharged to home, a rehabilitation center, or a skilled nursing facility (SNF). Some patients have no significant neurologic dysfunction and are able to return home and live independently or with minimal support. Other patients are able to return home but require ongoing assistance with ADLs and supervision to prevent accidents or injury. The case manager (CM) coordinates speech-language, physical, and/or occupational therapy services to continue in the home or on an ambulatory care basis. Patients admitted to an inpatient rehabilitation unit or facility or SNF require continued or more complex nursing care and extensive physical, occupational, recreational, speech-language, or cognitive therapy. The expected outcome for rehabilitation is to maximize the patient's abilities in all aspects of life.

Nurses not only provide direct care to patients with stroke but also contribute to the peer review process to evaluate and monitor the care provided to patients with stroke who are planning transition from the hospital for continued care. According to the Centers for Medicare and Medicaid, stroke and preventable complications are in the top 10 causes of hospital readmission (https://www.cms.gov/medicare/medicare).

Many hospitals have developed transition-of-care systems to improve patient and family education, patient and family satisfaction, and 30-day hospital readmission rates. For example, Ross et al. (2017) implemented a nurse-driven quality

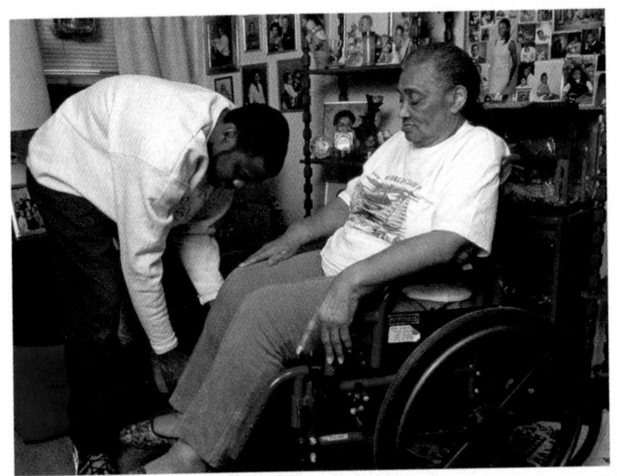

Fig. 41.3 Son adjusting his mother's wheelchair as part of caregiving responsibilities.

improvement (QI) project to improve patient education and reduce readmissions by:

- Using a teach-back method for patient and family education
- Conducting a follow-up phone call to the patient and family at 72 hours after discharge

The QI project did not improve patient satisfaction scores but did improve the 30-day readmission rate and the patient's perception of discharge education.

Home Care Management. Collaborate with the case manager to plan the patient's discharge. Coordinate with rehabilitation therapists to identify needs for assistive or adaptive and safety equipment. The extent of this assessment depends on the patient's disabilities, if any. Teach the patient and family to ensure that the home is free from scatter rugs or other obstacles in the walking pathways. The bathtub/shower and toilet should be equipped with grab bars, and the toilet may need an elevated seat. Antiskid patches or strips should be placed in the bathtub to prevent slipping. The physical therapist or occupational therapist works with the patient and the family or significant others to obtain all needed assistive devices and home modifications *before* the patient is discharged from the hospital, rehabilitation setting, or SNF. Appointments for ambulatory care speech, physical, and occupational therapy, if needed, are arranged before discharge for seamless transition management and care coordination.

Self-Management Education. The three areas that should be included in patient and family education are disease prevention, disease-specific information, and self-management. The teaching plan may include lifestyle changes, drug therapy, ambulation and transfer skills, communication skills, safety precautions, nutritional management, activity levels, and self-management skills. Health teaching should focus on tasks that must be performed by the patient and the family after hospital discharge. Return demonstrations help to evaluate the family members' competency in tasks required for the patient's care (Fig. 41.3). Provide both written and verbal instruction in all these areas. Specific teaching for stroke patients (and their families) includes:

- Provide information about prescribed drugs to prevent another stroke and control hypertension. Instruct the patient and the family in the name of each drug, the dosage, the timing of administration, how to take it, and possible side effects.
- Teach the patient how to climb stairs safely, if he or she is able; transfer from the bed to a chair; get into and out of a car; and use any aids for ***mobility.***
- Provide important information regarding what to do in an emergency and who to call for nonemergency questions.

As part of the discharge process, teach the family about the signs and symptoms of depression that may occur within 3 months after a stroke. The strongest predictors of poststroke depression (PSD) are a history of depression, severe stroke, and poststroke physical or cognitive impairment. Patients may not exhibit typical signs of depression because of their cognitive, physical, and emotional impairments. PSD is associated with increased morbidity and mortality, especially in older men.

Patients who have had a TIA or stroke are at risk for a new stroke. Teach family members to observe for and act on signs of a new stroke using the *FAST* mnemonic:

- *F*ace drooping
- *A*rm weakness
- *S*peech or language difficulty
- *T*ime to call 911

Families may feel overwhelmed by the continuing demands placed on them. Depending on the location of the lesion, the patient may be anxious, slow, cautious, and hesitant and lack initiative (left hemisphere lesions). As a result of right hemisphere lesions, he or she may be impulsive and seemingly unaware of any deficit. Family member caregivers are often uncertain about the progress of the patient and can become depressed the longer they care for him or her. Therefore family members need to spend time away from the patient on a routine basis to continue to provide full-time care without sacrificing their own physical and emotional health. Refer the family to social services or other community resources for further support, counseling, and possible respite care.

Health Care Resources. Available resources include a variety of publications from the American Heart Association (www.americanheart.org), including *Stroke: A Guide for Families* and *Stroke: Why Do They Behave That Way?* The National Stroke Association (www.stroke.org) also provides publications and videotapes for caregivers and patients. *Recovering After a Stroke: A Patient and Family Guide* is available from the Agency for Healthcare Research and Quality (www.ahrq.gov). A good resource for stroke information and family support in Canada is the Heart and Stroke Foundation of Canada (www.heartandstroke.com). Refer the patient and family members or significant others to local stroke support groups.

For patients who require long-term symptom management or end-of-life care, refer the family to palliative care or hospice services. Chapter 8 gives a detailed description of end-of-life care and advance directives.

◆ **Evaluation: Evaluate Outcomes.** Evaluate the care of the patient with stroke based on the identified priority patient problems. The expected outcomes are that the patient:

- Has adequate cerebral ***perfusion*** to avoid long-term disability
- Maintains blood pressure and blood glucose within a safe, prescribed range

- Performs self-care and ***mobility*** activities independently, with or without assistive devices
- Learns to adapt to ***sensory perception*** changes, if present
- Communicates effectively or develops strategies for effective communication as needed
- Has adequate nutrition and avoids aspiration

COGNITION CONCEPT EXEMPLAR: TRAUMATIC BRAIN INJURY

Pathophysiology Review

Traumatic brain injury (TBI) is damage to the brain from an external mechanical force and not caused by neurodegenerative or congenital conditions. TBI can lead to temporary and permanent impairment in ***cognition, mobility, sensory perception,*** and/or psychosocial function.

Various terms are used to describe the brain injuries that occur when a mechanical force is applied either directly or indirectly to the brain. A force produced by a blow to the head is a *direct* injury, whereas a force applied to another body part with a rebound effect to the brain is an *indirect* injury. The brain responds to these forces by movement within the rigid cranial vault. It may also rebound or rotate on the brainstem, causing diffuse nerve axonal injury (shearing injuries). The brain may be contused (bruised) or lacerated (torn) as it moves over the inner surfaces of the cranium, which are irregularly shaped and sharp.

Movement or distortion within the cranial cavity is possible because of multiple factors. The first factor is how the brain is supported by cerebrospinal fluid (CSF) within the cranial cavity. When external force is applied to the head, the brain can be injured by the internal surfaces of the skull. The second factor is the consistency of brain tissue, which is very fragile, gel-like, and prone to injury. Brain injury occurs both from initial forces on the cranium and brain and as a result of secondary injury related to mechanical pressure or cerebral edema.

The type of force and the mechanism of injury contribute to TBI. An *acceleration* injury is caused by an external force contacting the head, suddenly placing the head in motion. A *deceleration* injury occurs when the moving head is suddenly stopped or hits a stationary object (Fig. 41.4). These forces may be sufficient to cause the cerebrum to rotate about the brainstem, resulting in shearing, straining, and distortion of the brain tissue, particularly of the axons in the brainstem and cerebellum. Small areas of hemorrhage (contusion, intracranial hemorrhage) may develop around the blood vessels that sustain the impact of these forces (stress), with destruction of adjacent brain tissue. Particularly affected are the basal nuclei and the hypothalamus, which are located deep in the brain.

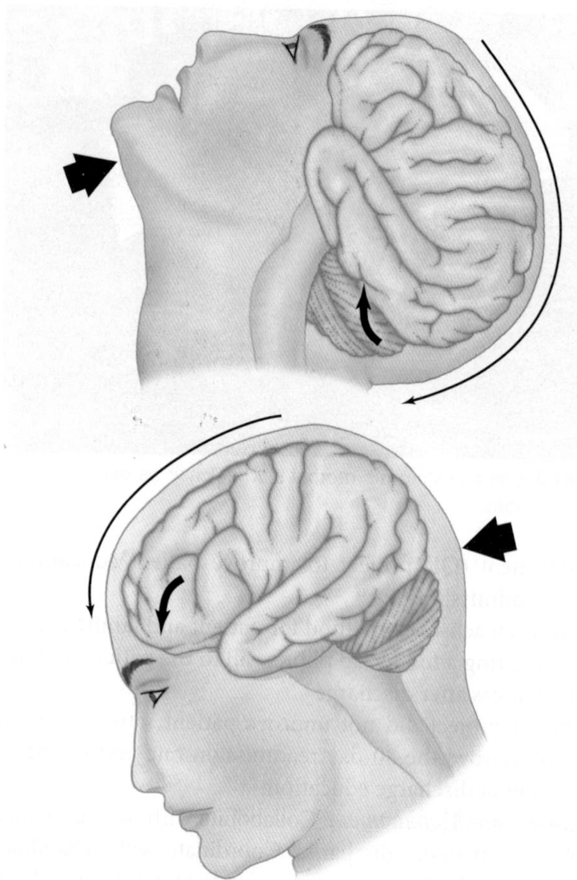

Fig. 41.4 Head movement during acceleration-deceleration injury, which is typically seen in motor vehicle crashes.

Primary Brain Injury. Primary brain damage occurs at the time of injury and results from the physical stress (force) within the tissue caused by blunt or penetrating force. A primary brain injury may be categorized as focal or diffuse. A *focal* brain injury is confined to a specific area of the brain and causes localized damage that can often be detected with a CT scan or MRI. *Diffuse* injuries are characterized by damage throughout many areas of the brain. They begin at a microscopic level and are not initially detectable by CT scan. MRI has greater ability to detect microscopic damage, but these areas may not be imaged until necrosis occurs.

Primary brain injuries are also classified as either open or closed. An *open* traumatic brain injury occurs when the skull is fractured or when it is pierced by a penetrating object. The integrity of the brain and the dura is violated, and there is exposure to environmental contaminants. Damage may occur to the underlying vessels, dural sinuses, brain, and cranial nerves. In a *closed* traumatic brain injury, the integrity of the skull is intact, but damage to the brain tissue still occurs as a result of increased intracranial pressure.

TBI is further defined as mild, moderate, or severe. Generally, the determination of severity of TBI is the result of the Glasgow Coma Scale (GCS) score immediately following resuscitation, the presence (or absence) of brain damage imaged by CT or MRI following the trauma, an estimation of the force of the trauma, and symptoms in the injured person.

One type of mild TBI is a concussion. A **concussion** is a traumatic injury to the brain caused by a blow to the head and may or may not result in some period of unconsciousness. Military personnel and people who participate in recreational or professional sports are especially at risk for concussions. Some patients report no immediate symptoms until later, which typically include impaired ***cognition*** (such as memory or thinking processes) and headache.

Secondary Brain Injury. Secondary injury to the brain includes any processes that occur *after* the initial injury and worsen or negatively influence patient outcomes. Secondary injuries result from physiologic, vascular, and biochemical events that are an extension of the primary injury.

The most common secondary injury from mild TBI, such as a concussion, is postconcussion syndrome. In this syndrome, the patient reports that headaches, impaired ***cognition,*** and dizziness continue to occur for weeks to months after the initial brain injury. Other patients who have been diagnosed with concussions may experience only posttraumatic headaches or posttraumatic vertigo (feeling of spinning or dizziness) for weeks to months after the initial injury.

Some patients may not have been diagnosed as having a TBI because they are not symptomatic. However, later they may be diagnosed with chronic traumatic encephalopathy (CTE), an uncommon degenerative brain disease that occurs most often in military veterans, athletes, and others who experienced repetitive trauma to the brain. CTE can lead to dementia, depression, suicidal thinking, and substance use disorder. Although the disease is usually diagnosed by history and clinical presentation, it can only be confirmed at autopsy when the classic tau neurofibrillary tangles are evident (McCance et al., 2019).

For patients with moderate or severe TBI, the most common secondary injuries result from hypotension and hypoxia, intracranial hypertension, and cerebral edema. Damage to the brain tissue occurs primarily because the delivery of oxygen and glucose to the brain is interrupted from cerebral edema and increasing pressure. Each of these problems is discussed in the following sections.

Hypotension and Hypoxia. Both hypotension, defined as a mean arterial pressure less than 70 mm Hg, and hypoxemia, defined as a partial pressure of arterial oxygen ($Pa{O_2}$) less than 80 mm Hg, restrict the flow of blood to vulnerable brain tissue. Hypotension may be related to shock (see Chapter 34) or other states of reduced ***perfusion*** to the brain such as that caused by clot formation. Hypoxia can be caused by respiratory failure, asphyxiation, or loss of airway and impaired ventilation (see Chapter 29). These problems may occur as a direct result of moderate-to-severe brain injury or secondary to systemic injuries and comorbidities. Low blood flow and hypoxemia contribute to cerebral edema, creating a cycle of deteriorating ***perfusion*** and hypoxic damage. Patients with hypoxic damage related to moderate or severe brain injury face a poor prognosis and eventually experience impaired ***cognition.***

Increased Intracranial Pressure. The cranial contents include brain tissue, blood, and cerebrospinal fluid (CSF). These components are encased in the relatively rigid skull. Within this space, there is little room for any of the components to expand or increase in volume. *A normal level of intracranial pressure (ICP) is 10 to 15 mm Hg.* Periodic increases in pressure occur with straining during defecation, coughing, or sneezing but do not harm the uninjured brain. A sustained ICP of greater than 20 mm Hg is considered detrimental to the brain because neurons begin to die.

As a result of brain injury, the increase in the volume of one component must be compensated for by a decrease in the volume of one of the other components. As a first response to an increase in the volume of any of these components, the CSF is shunted or displaced from the cranial compartment to the spinal subarachnoid space, or the rate of CSF absorption is increased. An additional response, if needed, is a decrease in cerebral blood volume by movement of cerebral venous blood into the sinuses or jugular veins. As long as the brain can compensate for the increase in volume and remain compliant, increases in ICP are minimal.

Increased ICP is the leading cause of death from head trauma in patients who reach the hospital alive. It occurs when compliance no longer takes place and the brain cannot accommodate further volume changes. As ICP increases, cerebral ***perfusion*** decreases, leading to brain tissue ischemia and edema. If edema remains untreated, the brainstem may herniate downward through the foramen of Monro or laterally from a unilateral lesion within one cerebral hemisphere, causing irreversible brain damage and possibly death (from brain herniation syndromes discussed later) (McCance et al., 2019).

Hemorrhage. Hemorrhage, which causes a brain hematoma (collection of blood) or clot, may occur as part of the primary injury and begin at the moment of impact. It may also arise later from vessel damage. Classically, bleeding is caused by vascular damage from the shearing force of the trauma or direct physical damage from skull fractures or penetrating injury. *All hematomas are potentially life threatening because they act as space-occupying lesions and are surrounded by edema.* Three major types of hemorrhage after TBI are epidural, subdural, and intracerebral hemorrhage. Subarachnoid hemorrhage may also occur.

An epidural hematoma results from arterial bleeding into the space between the dura and the inner skull (Fig. 41.5). It is often caused by a fracture of the temporal bone, which houses the middle meningeal artery. Patients with epidural hematomas have "lucid intervals" that last for minutes, during which time the patient is awake and talking. This follows a momentary unconsciousness that can occur within minutes of the injury (McCance et al., 2019).

! NURSING SAFETY PRIORITY QSEN

Critical Rescue

After the initial interval, symptoms of neurologic impairment from hemorrhage can progress very quickly, with potentially life-threatening ICP elevation and irreversible structural damage to brain tissue. Monitor the patient suspected of epidural bleeding frequently (every 5 to 10 minutes) for changes in neurologic status. The patient can become quickly and increasingly symptomatic. *A loss of consciousness from an epidural hematoma is a neurosurgical emergency!* Notify the primary health care provider or Rapid Response Team immediately if these changes occur. Carefully document your assessments and identify any trends.

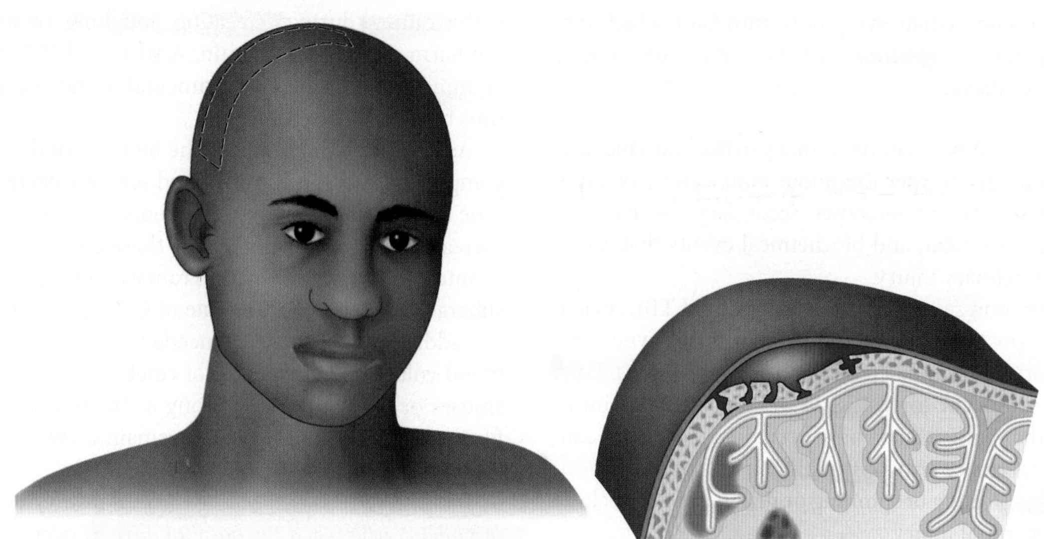

Fig. 41.5 Epidural hematoma (outside the dura mater of the brain), subdural hematoma (under the dura mater), and intracerebral hemorrhage (within the brain tissue).

A **subdural hematoma (SDH)** results from venous bleeding into the space beneath the dura and above the arachnoid (see Fig. 41.5). It occurs most often from a tearing of the bridging veins within the cerebral hemispheres, from a laceration of brain tissue. *Bleeding from this injury occurs more slowly than from an epidural hematoma.* SDHs are subdivided into acute, subacute, and chronic. Acute SDH presents within 48 hours after impact; subacute SDH between 48 hours and 2 weeks, and chronic SDH from 2 weeks to several months after injury. SDHs have the highest mortality rate because they often are unrecognized until the patient presents with severe neurologic compromise.

The incidence of chronic SDHs (sometimes written as cSDH) nearly doubles when people are between 65 and 75 years of age and continues to increase in patients over 80 years old. Common causes of chronic SDHs in older adults include head trauma resulting from a fall and anticoagulant or antiplatelet therapy. Typical signs and symptoms include worsening headaches, paresis, acute confusion, and seizures. In some cases, patients may experience a decreased level of consciousness, including coma (Vacca & Argenti, 2018).

Traumatic **intracerebral hemorrhage (ICH)** is the accumulation of blood within the brain tissue caused by the tearing of small arteries and veins in the subcortical white matter (see Fig. 41.5). It often acts as a space-occupying lesion (e.g., a tumor) and may be potentially devastating, depending on its location. ICH may also produce significant brain edema and ICP elevations. A traumatic brainstem hemorrhage occurs as a result of a blow to the back of the head, fractures, or torsion injuries to the brainstem (vital sign center). *Brainstem injuries have a very poor prognosis.*

Brain Herniation Syndromes. In the presence of increased ICP, the brain tissue may shift and herniate downward. Of the several types of herniation syndromes (Fig. 41.6), *uncal herniation* is one of the most clinically significant because it is life threatening. It is caused by a shift of one or both areas of the temporal lobe, known as the uncus. This shift creates pressure on the third cranial nerve (oculomotor). Late findings include dilated and nonreactive pupils, **ptosis** (eyelid drooping), and a rapidly deteriorating level of consciousness. *Central herniation* is caused by a downward shift of the brainstem and the diencephalon from a supratentorial lesion. It manifests clinically with Cheyne-Stokes respirations, pinpoint and nonreactive pupils, and potential hemodynamic instability. *All herniation syndromes are potentially life threatening, and the Rapid Response Team or primary health care provider must be notified immediately when they are suspected!*

Hydrocephalus. **Hydrocephalus** is an abnormal increase in CSF volume in the brain. It may be caused by impaired reabsorption of CSF at the arachnoid villi (from subarachnoid hemorrhage or meningitis), called a *communicating hydrocephalus.* It may also be caused by interference or blockage with CSF outflow from the ventricular system (from cerebral edema, tumor, or debris) (called a *noncommunicating hydrocephalus*). The ventricles may dilate from the relative increase in CSF volume. Ultimately, if not treated, this increase may lead to increased ICP.

Etiology. The most common causes of TBI in the United States are falls and motor vehicle crashes, followed by colliding with a stationary or moving object (CDC, 2020b). Alcohol and illicit drugs are significant contributing factors to the causes of TBI. Summer and spring months, evenings, nights, and weekends are associated with the greatest number of injuries. Young males are more likely than young females to have a TBI. Men tend to play more sports, enroll in the military service, take more risks when driving, and consume larger amounts of alcohol than women. Falls are the most common cause of TBI in older adults.

PATIENT-CENTERED CARE: VETERANS HEALTH CONSIDERATIONS QSEN

The United States is seeing increasing numbers of survivors of brain injury from wartime blast injuries. As a result, TBI has become a major health problem among veterans of war and active military personnel. **Chronic traumatic encephalopathy** is also becoming more recognized as a TBI from repetitive brain injuries among active duty military personnel and veterans.

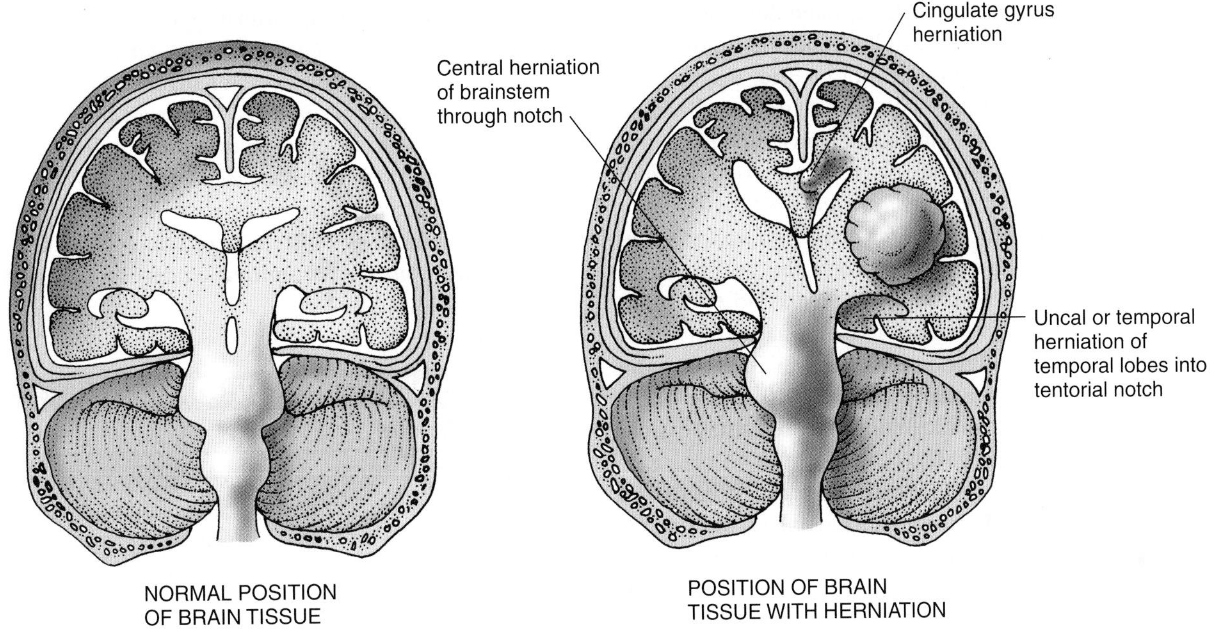

Fig. 41.6 Herniation syndromes.

Incidence and Prevalence. Annually, at least 1.7 million people sustain a TBI in the United States. Of these, about 52,000 die, 275,000 are hospitalized, and 1.4 million are treated and released from an emergency department because of mild TBI (CDC, 2020b). In Canada, statistics are calculated for acquired brain injuries (ABIs), which include both traumatic *and* nontraumatic brain injuries, such as strokes.

Health Promotion and Maintenance

Nurses can educate the public on ways to decrease the incidence of TBI by using safe driving practices such as not driving while impaired and wearing seat belts. Teach people at risk about how alcohol and illicit drug use, including marijuana, affect driving ability. Promote the use of helmets for skateboarding and bicycle and motorcycle riding. Help prevent falls by providing a safe environment, especially for older adults. People need to be aware of environmental factors that may increase the likelihood of falls such as inadequate lighting and loose rugs. When possible, install safety equipment in bathtubs and showers. Evaluate balance and coordination as part of a fall prevention strategy inside the hospital and at home. Chapter 4 discusses fall prevention for older adults in detail.

❖ Interprofessional Collaborative Care

◆ Assessment: Recognize Cues

History. Obtaining an accurate history from a patient who has sustained a TBI may be difficult because of changes in the patient's ***cognition.*** The seriousness of the injury can cause amnesia (loss of memory). It is not unusual for the patient to experience amnesia for events before or after the injury. The patient with a moderate or severe brain injury may be unconscious or in a confused and combative state. If the patient cannot provide information, the history can be obtained from first responders or witnesses to the injury. Always ask when, where, and how the injury occurred. Did the patient lose consciousness; if so, for how long? Has there been a change in the level of consciousness (LOC)? If trauma is related to drug or alcohol consumption, it may be difficult to differentiate neurologic changes caused by head trauma from those produced by intoxication.

Determine whether the patient had fluctuating consciousness or seizure activity and whether there is a history of a seizure disorder. Obtain precise information about the circumstances of falls, particularly in the older patient. Recognize that many factors can contribute to death in older adults from TBI (see the Patient-Centered Care: Older Adult Considerations: Traumatic Brain Injury box).

PATIENT-CENTERED CARE: OLDER ADULT CONSIDERATIONS QSEN

Traumatic Brain Injury

- Brain injury is the fifth leading cause of death in older adults (CDC, 2020b).
- The 65- to 75-year age-group has the second highest incidence of brain injury of all age-groups (CDC, 2020b).
- Falls and motor vehicle crashes are the most common causes of brain injury (CDC, 2020b).
- Factors that contribute to high mortality are:
  - Falls causing subdural hematomas (closed head injuries), especially chronic subdural hematomas
  - Poorly tolerated systemic stress, which is increased by admission to a high-stimulus environment
  - Medical complications, such as hypotension, hypertension, and cardiac problems
  - Decreased protective mechanisms, which make patients susceptible to infections (especially pneumonia)
  - Decreased immunologic competence, which is further diminished by brain injury

Other pertinent information includes hand dominance, any diseases of or injuries to the eyes, and any allergies to drugs or food. Inquire about a history of alcohol or drug use because these substances may interfere with the neurologic baseline assessment. Consider whether the patient is a victim of violence if he or she lives in residential care or has a caregiver. *The Joint Commission and the Centers for Medicare and Medicaid Services require that all patients be screened for abuse and neglect when they are admitted to any type of health care facility.*

Physical Assessment/Signs and Symptoms. No two brain injuries are alike. The patient with a TBI may have a variety of signs and symptoms depending on the severity of injury and the resulting increase in intracranial pressure (ICP) (Table 41.4). The Key Features: Mild Traumatic Brain Injury box lists possible signs and symptoms of *mild* TBI.

For any patient having a TBI, assess for signs of increased ICP, hypotension, hypoxemia (decreased blood level of oxygen), hypercarbia ($Paco_2$ greater than 40 to 45 mm Hg or increased partial pressure of carbon dioxide in arterial blood), or hypocarbia ($Paco_2$ less than 40 to 45 mm Hg or decreased partial pressure of carbon dioxide in arterial blood). *Hypercarbia* can cause cerebral vasodilation and contribute to elevated ICP. *Hypocarbia* is caused by hyperventilation and can lead to profound vasoconstriction with resulting ischemia. Carbon dioxide levels in an intubated patient can be determined with an end-tidal carbon dioxide ($ETco_2$) monitor, or capnography. The early detection of changes in the patient's neurologic status enables the health care team to prevent or treat potentially life-threatening complications. *Be aware that subtle changes in blood pressure, consciousness, and pupillary reaction to light can be very informative about neurologic deterioration!*

Airway and Breathing Pattern Assessment. *The first priority is the assessment of the patient's ABCs—airway, breathing, and circulation!* Because TBI is occasionally associated with cervical spinal cord injuries, all patients with head trauma are treated as though they have cord injury until radiography proves otherwise. *Older adults are especially prone to cervical injuries at the first or second vertebral level, a life-threatening problem.* Assess for indicators of spinal cord injury, such as loss of ***mobility*** and ***sensory perception,*** tenderness along the spine, and abnormal head tilt.

! NURSING SAFETY PRIORITY (QSEN)

Critical Rescue

The upper cervical spinal nerves innervate the diaphragm to control breathing. Monitor all TBI patients for respiratory problems and diaphragmatic breathing, as well as for diminished or absent reflexes in the airway (cough and gag). Hypoxia and hypercapnia are best detected through arterial oxygen levels (partial pressure of arterial oxygen [Pao_2]), oxygen saturation (Spo_2), and end-tidal volume carbon dioxide measurement ($ETco_2$). Observe chest wall movement and listen to breath sounds. Provide respiratory support including oxygen therapy and bed positioning. Report any sign of respiratory problems immediately to the Rapid Response Team or primary health care provider!

Injuries to the brainstem may cause a major life-threatening change in the patient's breathing pattern, such as Cheyne-Stokes respirations and/or apnea. In the unconscious patient, an artificial airway provides protection from aspiration and a route for oxygenation. Mechanical ventilation is often needed to support inadequate client respiratory effort.

TABLE 41.4 Differences Among Mild, Moderate, and Severe Traumatic Brain Injury

Type	Caused By	Symptoms
Mild traumatic brain injury (MTBI)	Characterized by a blow to the head, transient confusion or feeling dazed or disoriented, and one or more of these conditions: (1) possible loss of consciousness for up to 30 minutes, (2) loss of memory for events immediately before or after the accident, and (3) focal neurologic deficit(s) that may or not be transient. Loss of consciousness does not have to occur for a person to be diagnosed with MTBI. No evidence of brain damage on a CT or MRI scan.	Includes a wide array of physical and cognitive problems that range from headache and dizziness to changes in behavior. Symptoms usually resolve within 72 hours. Symptoms may persist and last days, weeks, or months. Persistent symptoms following MTBI are also referred to as *postconcussion syndrome.*
Moderate	A moderate TBI is characterized by a period of loss of consciousness (LOC) for 30 minutes to 6 hours and a GCS score of 9 to 12. Often but not always, focal or diffuse brain injury can be seen with a diagnostic CT or MRI scan. Posttraumatic *amnesia* (memory loss) may last up to 24 hours. May occur with either closed or open brain injury.	A short acute or critical care stay may be needed for close monitoring and to prevent secondary injury from brain edema, intracranial bleeding, or inadequate cerebral ***perfusion.***
Severe	A severe TBI is defined by a Glasgow Coma Scale (GCS) score of 3 to 8 and loss of consciousness for longer than 6 hours. Focal and diffuse damage to the brain, cerebrovascular vessels, and/or ventricles is common. Both open and closed head injuries can cause severe TBI, and injury can be focal or diffuse. CT and MRI scans can capture images of tissue damage quite early in the course of this illness.	Patients with severe TBI require management in critical care, including monitoring of hemodynamics, neurologic status, and possibly intracranial pressure (ICP). Patients with severe TBI are also at high risk for secondary brain injury from cerebral edema, hemorrhage, reduced ***perfusion,*** and the biomolecular cascade.

KEY FEATURES
Mild Traumatic Brain Injury

Physical Findings
- Appears dazed or stunned
- Loss of consciousness (if any) <30 minutes
- Headache
- Nausea
- Vomiting
- Balance or gait problems
- Dizziness
- Visual problems
- Fatigue
- Sensitivity to light
- Sensitivity to noise

Cognitive Findings
- Feeling mentally foggy
- Feeling slowed down
- Difficulty concentrating
- Difficulty remembering
- **Amnesia** about the events around the time of injury

Sleep Disturbances
- Drowsiness
- Sleeping less than usual
- Sleeping more than usual
- Trouble falling asleep

Emotional Changes
- Irritability
- Sadness
- Nervousness
- More "emotional"
- Depression

Spine Precautions. Patients with blunt trauma to the head or neck are typically transported from the scene of the injury to the hospital with a rigid cervical collar and a long spine board. *The expected outcome is to prevent new and secondary spine injury.* Spine precautions require placing the patient supine and aligning the spinal column in a neutral position so there is no rotation, flexion, or extension. The long spine board is removed as soon as possible on arrival at the emergency department (ED) or ICU. The rigid cervical collar is maintained until definitive diagnostic studies to rule out cervical spine injury are completed.

Once the spine board is removed, spinal precautions are maintained until the primary health care provider indicates that it is safe to bend or rotate the cervical, thoracic, and lumbar spine. Spinal precautions include: (1) bedrest; (2) no neck flexion with a pillow or roll; (3) no thoracic or lumbar flexion; (4) manual control of the cervical spine anytime the rigid collar is removed; and (5) use of a "log-roll" procedure to reposition the patient. A hard, rigid cervical collar is used to maintain cervical spine ("C-spine") precautions and immobilization with a confirmed cervical injury. If the collar is ill-fitting or soiled, it may be changed according to hospital guidelines while a second qualified person maintains C-spine immobilization. Frequent assessment of the skin under the collar is important to monitor for skin breakdown.

Spine clearance is a clinical decision made by the primary health care provider, often in collaboration with the radiologist. Spine clearance includes determining the absence of acute bony, ligamentous, and neurologic abnormalities of the cervical spine based on history, physical examination, and/or negative radiologic studies.

Vital Signs Assessment. The mechanisms of autoregulation are often impaired as the result of a TBI. The more serious the injury, the more severe is the impact on *autoregulation* or the ability of cerebral vasculature to modify systemic pressure such that blood flow to the brain is sufficient. Monitor the patient's blood pressure and pulse frequently based on agency protocol and patient status. The patient may have hypotension or hypertension. **Cushing triad,** a classic but very late sign of increased ICP, consists of severe hypertension, a widened pulse pressure (increasing difference between systolic and diastolic values), and bradycardia. This triad of cardiovascular changes usually indicates imminent death.

Neurologic Assessment. Many hospitals use the Glasgow Coma Scale (GCS) to document neurologic status (see Chapter 38). A change of 2 points is considered clinically important; notify the primary health care provider if the change is a 2-point or more deterioration of GCS values.

The most important variable to assess with any brain injury is LOC! A decrease or change in LOC is typically the *first* sign of deterioration in neurologic status. A decrease in arousal, increased sleepiness, and increased restlessness or combativeness are all signs of declining neurologic status. *Early* indicators of a change in LOC include behavior changes (e.g., restlessness, irritability) and disorientation, which are often subtle in nature. *Report any of these signs and symptoms immediately to the primary health care provider or Rapid Response Team!*

Use a bright light to assess pupillary size and reaction to light. Facial trauma may swell eyelids, making this assessment difficult. Consider whether drugs that affect pupillary dilation and constriction, such as anticholinergics or adrenergics, have been used recently.

NURSING SAFETY PRIORITY QSEN
Critical Rescue

Check pupils of TBI patients for size and reaction to light, particularly if the patient is unable to follow directions, to assess changes in level of consciousness. *Document any changes in pupil size, shape, and reactivity and notify the Rapid Response Team or primary health care provider immediately because they could indicate an increase in ICP!*

Pupillary changes or eye signs differ depending on which areas of the brain are damaged. *Pinpoint and nonresponsive pupils are indicative of brainstem dysfunction at the level of the pons.* The *ovoid* pupil is regarded as the mid-stage between a normal-size and a dilated pupil. Asymmetric (uneven) pupils, loss of light reaction, or unilateral or bilateral dilated pupils are treated as herniation of the brain from increased ICP until proven differently. *Pupils that are fixed (nonreactive) and dilated are a poor prognostic sign. Patients with this problem are sometimes referred to as having "blown" pupils.*

Check gross vision if the patient's condition permits. Have the patient read any printed material (e.g., your name tag) or count the number of fingers that you hold within his or her visual field. Loss of vision is usually caused by either direct injury to the eye or injury to the occipital lobe.

Monitor for additional late signs of increased ICP. These manifestations include severe headache, nausea, vomiting (often projectile), and seizures. The primary health care provider may evaluate for papilledema (seen by ophthalmoscopic examination). Papilledema is edema and hyperemia (increased blood flow) of the optic disc. *It is always a sign of increased ICP.* Headache and seizures are a response to the injury and may or may not be associated with increased ICP. Always remember that the patient with a brain injury is at risk for potentially devastating ICP elevations during the first hours after the event and up to 3 to 4 days after injury when cerebral edema can occur.

Assess for bilateral *motor* responses. The patient's motor loss or dysfunction usually appears contralateral (opposite side) to the site of the lesion, similar to that of a stroke. For example, a left-sided hemiparesis reflects an injury to the right cerebral hemisphere. Deterioration in ***mobility*** or the development of abnormal posturing or flaccidity is another indicator of progressive brain injury (see Chapter 38). These changes are the result of dysfunction within the pyramidal (motor) tracts of the spinal cord. Assess for brainstem or cerebellar injury, which may cause ataxia, decreased or increased muscle tone, and weakness. Remember that absence of motor function may also be an indicator of a spinal cord injury.

Carefully observe the patient's ears and nose for any signs of cerebrospinal fluid (CSF) leaks that result from a basilar skull fracture. Suspicious ear or nose fluid can be analyzed by the laboratory for glucose and electrolyte content. CSF placed on a white absorbent paper or linen can be distinguished from other fluids by the *"halo" sign,* a clear or yellowish ring surrounding a spot of blood. Although other body fluids can be used, a halo sign is most reliable when blood is in the center of the absorbent material because tears and saliva can also cause a clear ring in some conditions.

Palpate the patient's head gently to detect the presence of fractures or hematomas. Look for areas of ecchymosis (bruising), tender areas of the scalp, and lacerations. *Raccoon's eyes* are purplish discoloration around eyes that can follow fracture of the skull's base. When CT scans are used with head and brain injury, these fractures are often visualized before bruising appears.

Psychosocial Assessment. Patients with any level of TBI usually have varying degrees of psychosocial changes that may persist for a year or for a lifetime, depending on the severity of the injury and the person's response. Emotional lability and/or personality changes manifesting with temper outbursts, depression, risk-taking behavior, and denial of disability can occur. The patient may become talkative and develop a very outgoing personality. Memory, especially recent or short-term memory, is often affected. The patient may report difficulties in ***cognition,*** such as concentrating or the ability to learn new information, and may have problems with insight and planning. Aggressive behavior, agitation, and sleep disorders may interfere with the ability to return to work or school. The ability to communicate and understand spoken and written language may be altered. Changes in ***mobility*** and ***sensory perception*** may require rehabilitation or use of assistive devices. All these changes in health status may lead to difficulties within the family structure and with social and work-related interactions.

Imaging Assessment. The primary health care provider immediately requests CT of the brain to identify the extent and scope of injury. This diagnostic test can identify the presence of an injury that requires surgical intervention, such as an epidural or subdural hematoma. An *MRI* may be done to detect subtle changes in brain tissue and show more specific detail of the brain injury. MRI is particularly useful in the diagnosis of diffuse axonal injury, but it is not recommended for patients with ICP-monitoring devices. A functional MRI may be done to more specifically detect anoxic injury to the brain.

◆ **Analysis: Analyze Cues and Prioritize Hypotheses.** The priority collaborative problems for patients with traumatic brain injury (TBI) vary greatly, depending on the severity of the event. The most common problems include:

1. Potential for decreased cerebral tissue ***perfusion*** due to primary event and/or secondary brain injury
2. Potential for decreased ***cognition, sensory perception,*** and/or ***mobility*** due to primary or secondary brain injury

◆ Planning and Implementation: Generate Solutions and Take Action

Maintaining Cerebral Tissue Perfusion

Planning: Expected Outcomes. The expected outcome is that the patient will maintain adequate cerebral tissue ***perfusion*** with no evidence of secondary brain injury from cerebral edema and increased ICP.

Interventions. The patient with a *severe* TBI is admitted to the critical care unit or trauma center. Patients with *moderate* TBI are admitted to either the general nursing unit or the critical care unit, where they are closely observed for at least 24 hours. Those with *mild* TBI are usually sent home from the emergency department with instructions for home-based observation and primary health care provider follow-up. In some cases, the patient is hospitalized for 23-hour observation by staff. Cerebral ***perfusion*** is *not* typically affected by a mild TBI.

As with any critically injured patient, priority is given to maintaining a patent airway, breathing, and circulation. Specific nursing interventions for the patient with a TBI are directed toward preventing or detecting secondary brain injury or the conditions that contribute to secondary brain injury such as increased ICP, promoting fluid and electrolyte balance, and monitoring the effects of treatments and drug therapy. Providing health teaching and emotional support for the patient and family are vital parts of the plan of care.

Preventing and Detecting Secondary Brain Injury. Take and record the patient's *vital signs* every 1 to 2 hours or more often based on patient acuity. The primary health care provider may prescribe IV fluids or drug therapy to prevent severe hypertension or hypotension. Dysrhythmias and nonspecific ST-segment or T-wave changes may occur, possibly in response to stimulation of the autonomic nervous system or an increase in the level of circulating catecholamines (such as epinephrine) from the stress of trauma. *Document and report the presence of cardiac dysrhythmias, hypotension, and hypertension to the primary* *health care provider.* Obtain the target range for blood pressure and heart rate from the provider and monitor parameters.

The patient with a brain injury may develop a fever as a result of systemic trauma, blood in the cranium, or a generalized inflammatory response to the injury. Fever from any cause is associated with higher morbidity and mortality rates. Therapeutic hypothermia may be started, regardless of the presence of fever. The purpose of therapeutic hypothermia is to rapidly cool the patient to a core temperature of 89.6°F to 93.2°F (32°C to 34°C) for 24 to 48 hours after the primary injury. Rewarming to a normal core temperature requires specialized knowledge and skill because rapid fluid and electrolyte shifts can cause cardiac dysrhythmias and changes to systemic and cerebral pressures. The rationale for therapeutic hypothermia is to reduce brain metabolism and prevent the cascade of molecular and biochemical events that contribute to secondary brain injury in moderate-to-severe TBI.

Arterial blood gas (ABG), oxygen saturation (Spo_2), and end-tidal carbon dioxide ($ETco_2$) values are all used to evaluate respiratory status and guide mechanical ventilation therapy. *Hyperventilation* for the intubated patient during the first 24 hours after brain injury is usually avoided because it may produce ischemia by causing cerebral vasoconstriction. *Carbon dioxide is a very potent vasodilator that can contribute to increases in ICP.*

Prevent intermittent and sustained hypoxemia. Monitor peripheral oxygen saturation continuously in moderate-to-severe TBI. Hypoxemia damages brain tissue and contributes to cerebral vasodilation and increased ICP. Arterial oxygen levels (Pao_2) are maintained between 80 and 100 mm Hg to prevent secondary injury. If available, hyperbaric oxygen therapy (HBOT) may be used to provide high-dose oxygen to treat ischemia and hypoxia. HBOT may be used as part of early management of TBI or in the chronic stage of the injury (Dang et al., 2017).

If the patient is intubated, provide 100% oxygen before and after each pass of the endotracheal suction catheter. Avoid overly aggressive hyperventilation with endotracheal suctioning because of the potential for hypocarbia. Cerebral ischemia caused by even transiently decreased oxygen and either high or low carbon dioxide levels contributes to secondary brain injury. Lidocaine given IV or endotracheally may be used to suppress the cough reflex; coughing increases ICP.

! NURSING SAFETY PRIORITY (QSEN)

Action Alert

Position the TBI patient to avoid extreme flexion or extension of the neck and to maintain the head in the midline, neutral position. Log roll him or her during turning to avoid extreme hip flexion ,and keep the head of the bed (HOB) elevated at least 30 degrees or as prescribed by the primary health care provider.

Generally, HOB elevation in patients with TBI is at 30 to 45 degrees to prevent aspiration. However, if increasing head elevation significantly lowers systemic blood pressure, the patient does not benefit from drainage of venous blood or CSF out of the skull from this position. If hypotension accompanies an elevated backrest position, the patient may be harmed. Avoid sudden vertical changes of the HOB in the older patient because the dura is tightly adhered to the skull and may pull away from the brain, leading to a subdural hematoma.

Patients with *severe* TBI often die. As the physiologic deterioration begins, keep in mind that the patient may be a potential organ donor. *Before* brain death is declared, contact the local organ-procurement organization. Determine if the patient consented to be an organ donor. This information is typically on a driver's license or other state-issued card or advance directive. The patient's wishes should be followed unless he or she has a medical condition that prevents organ donation. The organ donor agency representative or primary health care provider discusses the possibility of organ procurement with the family. Some families may not agree with the patient's decision, which can cause an ethical dilemma. Many health care agencies have an ethics specialist or committee members who can help with these situations.

Determining Brain Death. In 2010, the American Academy of Neurology guidelines for determining brain death were updated and remain the standard in the United States today. Four classic prerequisites must be met to establish a brain death diagnosis (Wijdicks et al., 2010):

- Coma of known cause as established by history, clinical examination, laboratory testing, and neuroimaging
- Normal or near-normal core body temperature (higher than 96.8°F (36°C)
- Normal systolic blood pressure (higher than or equal to 100 mm Hg)
- At least one neurologic examination (many U.S. states and health care systems require two)

No consensus has been reached on who is qualified to perform head-to-toe brain-death neurologic examinations, but neurologists and critical care intensivists typically do them. Neuroimaging tests are not required to confirm brain death in some states or provinces, but are desirable. Examples of tests that may be done include cerebral angiography, bedside electroencephalography (EEG), cerebral computed tomography angiography (CTA), and/or transcranial Doppler ultrasonography (Milliken & Uveges, 2020; Russell et al., 2020).

Drug Therapy. Mannitol, an osmotic diuretic, is often used to treat cerebral edema by pulling water out of the extracellular space of the edematous brain tissue. It is most effective when given in boluses rather than as a continuous infusion. Furosemide, a loop diuretic, is often used as adjunctive therapy to reduce the incidence of rebound from mannitol. It also enhances the therapeutic action of mannitol, reduces edema and blood volume, decreases sodium uptake by the brain, and decreases the production of CSF at the choroid plexus. Although mannitol decreases intracranial pressure, research suggests that it does not improve mortality from TBI (see the Evidence-Based Practice box).

Administer *mannitol* through a filter in the IV tubing or, if given by IV push, draw it up through a filtered needle to eliminate microscopic crystals. For the patient receiving either osmotic or loop diuretics, monitor for intake and output, severe dehydration, and indications of acute renal failure, weakness, edema, and changes in urine output. Serum electrolyte and osmolarity levels are measured every 6 hours. Mannitol is used to obtain a serum osmolarity of 310 to 320 mOsm/L, depending on primary health care provider preference and the desired

EVIDENCE-BASED PRACTICE QSEN

Does Mannitol Reduce Mortality From Traumatic Brain Injury (TBI)?

Gottlieb, M., & Bailitz, J. (2016). Does mannitol reduce mortality from traumatic brain injury? *Annals of Emergency Medicine, 67*(1), 83–85.

Traumatic brain injury (TBI) results in more than 4.5% of all injury-related emergency department visits and 15% of annual hospitalizations. Extensive research has been conducted on prevention and treatment of TBI, including administration of mannitol. Mannitol is an osmotic diuretic that produces an initial reduction of the intracellular volume of brain tissue, resulting in transient improvement in cerebral blood flow and oxygenation. With an improvement in *perfusion,* mortality may decrease. However, there is little evidence of the effect of mannitol on mortality in patients with TBI.

In this systematic review, the researchers found four studies that met inclusion criteria to examine the effect of mannitol on mortality after severe TBI. Two of the studies compared mannitol with nonmannitol intracranial pressure (ICP)–lowering agents. Although all four trials were randomized, in only three was blinding in the methodology. The review found that there was limited evidence that mannitol alone is sufficient to reduce mortality of severe TBI. Other agents, such as hypertonic saline, may be as effective as mannitol in decreasing ICP.

Level of Evidence: 1

The evidence in this paper was obtained in a systematic review of studies about head injury in which patients sustained severe brain injury with a Glasgow Coma Scale score of less than 8.

Commentary: Implications for Practice and Research

This research questions whether traditional treatment with mannitol is sufficient for decreasing ICP while reducing mortality from severe TBI. Although staff nurses do not prescribe medications, these findings may explain a beginning shift in ICP management. More research is needed to improve survival of patients experiencing moderate-to-severe TBI.

outcome of therapy. Insert an indwelling urinary catheter to maintain strict measurement of output every hour. Check the patient's serum and urine osmolarity daily.

Opioids such as fentanyl may be used with ventilated patients to decrease pain and control restlessness if the agitation is caused by pain. Fentanyl has fewer effects on blood pressure and heart rate than morphine and therefore may be a safer agent to manage pain for the TBI patient. Propofol and midazolam (GABA-receptor agonists) provide sedation to decrease ICP but are not as effective for pain control. Most mechanically ventilated patients receive a combination of these drugs.

Maintaining Cognition, Sensory Perception, and Mobility

Planning: Expected Outcomes. The desired outcome is that the patient will not experience long-term decreased or altered ***cognition, sensory perception,*** and/or ***mobility.*** If alterations occur, the patient will receive rehabilitation to achieve optimal functioning.

Interventions. An overwhelming majority of brain injury survivors have altered ***cognition,*** including decreased memory and impaired judgment and reasoning ability. Cognitive impairments may interfere with the brain-injured patient's ability to function effectively in school, at work, and in his or her personal life. *Cognitive rehabilitation* is a way of helping brain-injured patients regain function in areas that are essential for a return to independence and a reasonable quality of life.

If a large lesion of the parietal lobe is present, the patient may experience a loss of ***sensory perception*** for pain, temperature, touch, and **proprioception**, which prevents an appropriate response to environmental stimuli. A hazard-free environment is necessary to prevent injury (e.g., from burns if the patient's coffee is too hot). In collaboration with the rehabilitation therapist, integrate a sensory stimulation program into the comatose or stuporous patient's routine care activities. Sensory stimulation is done to facilitate a meaningful response to the environment. Present visual, auditory, or tactile stimuli one at a time, and explain the purpose and the type of stimulus presented. For example, show a picture of the patient's mother and say, "This is a picture of your mother." The picture is shown several times, and the same words are used to describe the picture. If auditory tapes or DVDs are used, they should be played no longer than 10 to 15 minutes. If the stimulus is presented for a longer period, it simply becomes "white noise" (meaningless background noise).

Some patients with TBI experience seizure activity as a result of primary or secondary brain injury. Be sure to initiate Seizure Precautions according to your agency's policy and procedure. Nursing care for patients with seizures is described in Chapter 39.

Patients with a mild brain injury may be disoriented and have short-term memory loss. Always introduce yourself before any interaction. Keep explanations of procedures and activities short and simple, and give them immediately before and throughout patient care. To the extent possible, maintain a sleep-wake cycle with scheduled rest periods. Orient the patient to time (day, month, and year) and place, and explain the reason for the hospitalization. Reassure the patient that he or she is safe. If the client is hospitalized, ask the family to bring in familiar objects, such as pictures. Provide orientation cues within the environment, such as a large clock with numbers or a single-date calendar.

Care Coordination and Transition Management. The patient with a *mild* brain injury recovers at home after discharge from the emergency department (ED) or hospital (see the Patient and Family Education: Preparing for Self-Management: Mild Brain Injury box).

The patient with a severe brain injury requires long-term case management and ongoing rehabilitation after hospitalization. Behavioral interventions are used by cognitive and brain injury rehabilitation specialists to help both the patient and family members develop adaptive strategies. A number of specialized brain injury rehabilitation facilities are available in the United States and Canada. Some facilities offer noninvasive magnetic or electrical brain stimulation to provide neuronal excitability (Dang et al., 2017). Chapter 7 discusses interprofessional collaborative rehabilitative care in detail.

PATIENT AND FAMILY EDUCATION: PREPARING FOR SELF-MANAGEMENT

Mild Brain Injury

- For a headache, give acetaminophen every 4 hours as needed.
- Avoid giving the person sedatives, sleeping pills, or alcoholic beverages for at least 24 hours after TBI unless the primary health care provider instructs otherwise.
- Do not allow the person to engage in strenuous activity for at least 48 hours.
- Teach the caregiver to be aware that balance disturbances cause safety concerns and that he or she should provide for monitored or assisted movement.
- If any of these symptoms occur, take the person back to the emergency department or call 911 *immediately*:
  - Seizure
  - Severe, or worsening, headache
  - Persistent or severe nausea or vomiting
  - Blurred vision
  - Clear drainage from the ear or nose
  - Increasing weakness
  - Slurred speech
  - Progressive sleepiness
  - Unequal pupil size
- Keep follow-up appointments with the primary health care provider.

Communicate the patient's plan of care, including drug therapy, to the receiving nurse or provider during each transition in care. Many patients continue on antiepileptic drugs (AEDs) to control seizure activity. Other drugs may be prescribed to help stabilize emotional behaviors or manage depression.

Home Care Management. The major overall desired outcome for rehabilitation after brain injury is to maximize the patient's ability to return to his or her highest level of functioning. Activities such as occupational therapy, physical therapy, and speech-language therapy may continue in the home after discharge from the hospital or rehabilitation facility. Adaptation of the home environment to accommodate the patient safely may be needed. For example, smoke and fire alarms must function properly because the patient with a brain injury often loses the sense of smell. Home evaluations and referrals to outside agencies are completed before discharge. Be sure to refer the patient and family to the registered dietitian nutritionist for health teaching regarding healthy nutrition to prevent weight gain from decreased activity or stress eating. Many patients with TBI gain significant weight within a year of their injury, most likely because of inactivity.

Self-Management Education. Collaborate with the case manager (CM) to provide the patient and family with both written and verbal instructions for discharge. The teaching plan includes a review of safety at home and strategies to adapt to sensory dysfunction. Discuss issues related to personality or behavior problems that may arise and how to cope with them. Explain the purpose, dosage, schedule, and route of administration of drug therapy. Teach the family to encourage the patient to participate in activities as tolerated. Demonstrations and return demonstrations of care activities help family members become more skillful. Stress the importance of regular follow-up visits with therapists and other health care providers.

Patients with personality and behavior problems respond best to a structured and consistent environment. Instruct the family to develop a home routine that provides structure, repetition, and consistency. Remind the family about the importance of reinforcing positive behaviors rather than negative behaviors.

! NURSING SAFETY PRIORITY (QSEN)

Action Alert

Teach the patient who has sustained a *mild* brain injury that symptoms that disturb sleep; affect enjoyment of daily activities, work performance, mood, memory, and ability to learn new material; and cause changes in personality require follow-up care. Provide the patient and family with education materials that will alert them to symptoms and management options. A good source of written instructions is available from the CDC (see document "What To Expect After a Concussion" [CDC, 2020c]).

Most patients with *moderate-to-severe* TBI are discharged with varied long-term physical and cognitive disabilities. Changes in personality and behavior are very common. A qualitative study by Kivunja et al. (2018) identified six themes that summarized the experiences of patients living with TBI:

- Seeking personhood to determine who they are after the injury
- Navigating challenging behaviors
- Valuing the skills and competence that one has
- Struggling with changed family responsibilities
- Maintaining productive and successful relationships
- Reflecting on workplace culture

As evident in the study, the patient and family must learn to cope with the patient's increased fatigue, irritability, temper outbursts, depression, loneliness, and memory problems. These patients often require constant supervision at home, and families may feel socially isolated. Provide support and encouragement for the family and patient to help them get through each day.

Teach the family about the importance of regular respite care, either in a structured day-care respite program for the patient or through relief provided by a friend or neighbor. Family members, particularly the primary caregiver, may become depressed and have feelings of loneliness. In addition, they may feel angry with the patient because of the physical, financial, and emotional responsibilities that his or her care has placed on them. To help the family cope with these problems, suggest that they join and actively participate in a local brain-injury support group.

Health Care Resources. Collaborate with the case manager to refer families and patients to local chapters of the Brain Injury Association of America (BIAA) (www.biausa.org) for information and support. The Brain Injury Association of Canada (www.braininjurycanada.ca) is available as a resource for patients in Canada. All of these organizations have a number of helpful publications on preventing and living with TBI. Other resources include religious, spiritual, and cultural leaders.

PATIENT-CENTERED CARE: VETERANS HEALTH CONSIDERATIONS QSEN

The incidence of TBI in young veterans has increased in the past 20 years as a result of concussive blast injuries. Spouses of veterans often have the responsibility of caring for the patient at home following rehabilitation. Expert case management is needed to ensure transitions and continuity of care.

A classic qualitative study by Saban et al. (2015) found that veterans with TBI in the United States also experience depression, anxiety, and posttraumatic stress disorder (PTSD). The researchers found that family caregivers fear the anger and agitation displayed by their loved ones with TBI. In addition, the patient's children are often negatively affected by the veterans' change in personality and emotional behaviors as a result of these health problems.

Suggest that the spouse or other family caregiver contact the U.S. Defense and Veterans Brain Injury Center for support groups and information. The Veterans Health Administration has case-management services to assist with transition management and care coordination in support of both the veteran and family.

◆ **Evaluation: Evaluate Outcomes.** Evaluate the care of the patient with TBI based on the identified priority problems. Expected outcomes are that the patient:

- Maintains cerebral tissue ***perfusion***
- Learns to adapt to altered ***mobility*** and ***sensory perception*** changes, if any
- Has minimal alterations in ***cognition*** or understands how to compensate for ***cognition*** changes when necessary

CLINICAL JUDGMENT CHALLENGE 41.1

Safety; Clinical Judgment; Evidence-Based Practice

A 38-year-old veteran returns home from his third tour of duty from the Middle East. He is married and has three young children. His history reveals use of opioids from a previous lower back injury, two depressive episodes, and a suicide attempt during his first tour in Iraq. Since then he has become a believer in God and attends church as often as he can. He tells you that his deep faith and spirituality have helped him "turn his life around." Today he was admitted from the emergency department (ED) to the 23-hour observation unit with suspected mild traumatic brain injury as a result of a motor vehicle crash. On assessment for this shift, the nurse notes the following assessment findings:

- Reports increasing headache pain from a 3 on admission to a 5 on a 0-10 pain scale
- More drowsy than on admission (alert on admission)
- Oxygen saturation = 92% (decreased from 96% on admission)
- Oriented to person, place, and time
- Heart rate = 86 beats/min
- Blood pressure = 118/74 mm Hg

1. **Recognize Cues:** What assessment information in this client situation is the most important and immediate concern for the nurse? (Hint: Identify the **relevant** information *first* to determine what is most important.)
2. **Analyze Cues:** What client conditions are consistent with the **most relevant** information? (Hint: Think about priority collaborative problems that support and contradict the information presented in this situation.)
3. **Prioritize Hypotheses:** Which possibilities or explanations are **most likely** to be present in this client situation? Which possibilities or explanations are the most serious? (Hint: Consider all possibilities and determine their urgency and risk for this client.)
4. **Generate Solutions:** What actions would most likely achieve the desired outcomes for this client? Which actions should be **avoided** or are **potentially harmful?** (Hint: Determine the desired outcomes first to decide which actions are appropriate and those that should be avoided.)
5. **Take Action:** Which actions are the most appropriate and how should they be implemented? In what **priority order** should they be implemented? (Hint: Consider health teaching, documentation, requested health care provider orders or prescriptions, nursing skills, collaboration with or referral to health team members, etc.)
6. **Evaluate Outcomes:** What client assessment would indicate that the nurse's actions were **effective?** (Hint: Think about signs that would indicate an improvement, decline, or unchanged client condition.)

BRAIN TUMORS

Pathophysiology Review

Brain tumors can arise anywhere within the brain structures and are named according to the cell or tissue where they originate; however, cerebral tumors are the most common. *Primary* tumors originate within the central nervous system (CNS) and rarely metastasize (spread) outside this area. *Secondary* brain tumors result from metastasis from other areas of the body, such as the lung, breast, kidney, and GI tract.

Regardless of location, tumors can expand and invade, infiltrate, compress, and displace normal brain tissue. Similar to the pathophysiologic changes that occur in patients with TBI, these changes can lead to cerebral edema or brain tissue inflammation, increased intracranial pressure (ICP), and neurologic deficits (focal or diffuse). In some cases, pituitary dysfunction can result. (See the Pathophysiology Review for TBI earlier in this chapter.)

Cerebral edema (vasogenic edema) results from changes in capillary endothelial tissue permeability that allows plasma to seep into the extracellular spaces. This leads to *increased ICP* and, depending on the location of the tumor, brain herniation syndromes. A variety of *neurologic deficits* result from edema, infiltration, distortion, and compression of surrounding brain tissue. The cerebral blood vessels may become compressed because of edema and increased ICP. This compression leads to ischemia (decreased blood flow) of the area supplied by the vessel. In addition, the tumor may enter the walls of the vessel, causing it to rupture and hemorrhage into the tumor bed or other brain tissue. Many patients who have brain tumors have headaches and seizures from interference with the brain's normal electrical activity.

Pituitary dysfunction may occur as the tumor compresses the pituitary gland and causes the syndrome of inappropriate antidiuretic hormone (SIADH) or diabetes insipidus (DI). These disorders result in severe fluid and electrolyte imbalances and can be life threatening. (See Chapter 57 for a complete description of these disorders.)

Brain tumors are usually classified as benign, malignant, or metastatic. They may or may not be treated, depending on their location. Benign (noncancerous) tumors, such as meningiomas, can usually be removed and are generally associated with a positive outcome. Malignant or metastatic tumors, such as astrocytomas, require more aggressive intervention, including surgery, radiation, and/or chemotherapy.

A second classification system is based on location. **Supratentorial tumors** are located within the cerebral hemispheres above the tentorium (dural fold). Located beneath the tentorium is the infratentorial area (the area of the brainstem structures and cerebellum) where tumors may also occur (**infratentorial tumors**).

The exact cause of brain tumors is unknown. Several areas under investigation include genetic mutations and a variety of environmental factors. The use of cellular phones has been investigated as a cause of brain tumors, but findings are not confirmed. Brain tumors account for a small percentage of all cancer deaths. Primary brain tumors are relatively uncommon, but many more patients have metastatic lesions. Malignant brain tumors are seen primarily in patients 40 to 70 years of age, and the survival rate is low compared with that of other cancers (McCance et al., 2019).

❖ Interprofessional Collaborative Care

◆ **Assessment: Recognize Cues.** When possible, obtain a history from both the patient and family, including current signs and symptoms. A complete neurologic assessment is needed to establish baseline data and determine the nature and extent of neurologic deficits.

The signs and symptoms of brain tumors vary with the site of the tumor and are similar to those seen in patients with traumatic brain injury (TBI). In general, assess for these *common* symptoms of a brain tumor:

- Headaches that are usually more severe on awakening in the morning
- Nausea and vomiting
- Seizures (also called convulsions)
- Impaired ***sensory perception,*** such as facial numbness or tingling and visual changes
- Loss of balance or dizziness
- Weakness or paralysis in one part or one side of the body (hemiparesis or hemiplegia)
- Difficulty thinking, speaking, or articulating words
- Changes in ***cognition,*** mentation, or personality

Neurologic deficits result from the destruction, distortion, or compression of brain tissue. *Supratentorial (cerebral)* tumors usually result in paralysis, seizures, memory loss, cognitive impairment, language impairment, or vision problems. *Infratentorial* tumors produce **ataxia**, autonomic nervous system dysfunction, vomiting, drooling, hearing loss, and vision impairment. As the tumor grows, ICP increases, and the symptoms become progressively more severe.

Diagnosis is based on the history, neurologic assessment, clinical examination, and results of neurodiagnostic testing. Noninvasive diagnostic studies such as *CT* and *MRI* are conducted first. These tests identify the size, location, and extent of the tumor. The MRI may be used for initial diagnostic evaluation and is a more sensitive diagnostic study, whereas CT is often used for follow-up during the course of illness. Skull x-rays may be done to determine any bone involvement caused by the tumor.

◆ **Interventions: Take Action.** Interventions depend on the type, size, and location of the tumor. For example, a small benign tumor may be monitored through CT and MRI scanning to assess its growth.

Nonsurgical Management. The desired outcomes of brain tumor management are to remove the tumor or decrease tumor size, improve quality of life, and improve survival time. The type of treatment selected depends on the tumor size and location, patient symptoms and general condition, and whether the tumor has recurred. In addition to traditional interventions, a number of experimental treatment modalities are being investigated. These include blood-brain barrier disruption, recombinant DNA, monoclonal antibodies, new chemotherapeutic drugs, and immunotherapy. Traditional *radiation therapy* may be used alone, after surgery, or in combination with chemotherapy and surgery. Chapter 20 discusses radiation treatment for patients with cancer.

Drug Therapy. The primary health care provider may prescribe a variety of drugs to treat the malignant or metastatic tumor, manage the patient's symptoms, and prevent complications. *Chemotherapy* may be given alone, in combination with radiation and surgery, and with tumor progression. Although these drugs may control tumor growth or decrease tumor burden, the benefit does not last. Chemotherapy usually involves more than one agent that may be given orally, IV, intra-arterially, and/or intrathecally through an Ommaya reservoir placed in a cranial ventricle. When given systemically, the drug must be lipid soluble to cross the blood-brain barrier.

Commonly used oral drugs are lomustine, temozolomide, procarbazine, and methotrexate. Vincristine may be given IV in combination with other drugs. Monitor for side effects of these drugs, which are similar to those of any chemotherapeutic drug. Chapter 20 describes general nursing implications for care of a patient receiving chemotherapy.

Direct drug delivery to the tumor is another treatment option. Disk-shaped drug wafers, such as carmustine, may be placed directly into the cavity created during surgical tumor removal (interstitial chemotherapy). This therapy is usually given for newly diagnosed high-grade malignant tumors, but recurrent tumors may also be treated with this method. Other drugs used are molecularly targeted. Examples include erlotinib, gefitinib, and bevacizumab (Burchum & Rosenthal, 2019).

Analgesics, such as codeine and acetaminophen, are given for headache. Dexamethasone is given to control cerebral edema. Phenytoin or other antiepileptic drugs (AEDs) may be given to prevent seizure activity (see Chapter 39 for discussion of AEDs). Proton pump inhibitors are given to decrease gastric acid secretion and prevent the development of stress ulcers.

Stereotactic Radiosurgery. Stereotactic radiosurgery (SRS) is an alternative to traditional surgery. Several techniques are used, including the modified linear accelerator (LINAC) using accelerated x-rays, a particle accelerator using beams of protons (cyclotron), and isotope seeds implanted in the tumor (brachytherapy).

The Gamma Knife is a device used in an SRS procedure in which a single high dose of ionized radiation is used to focus

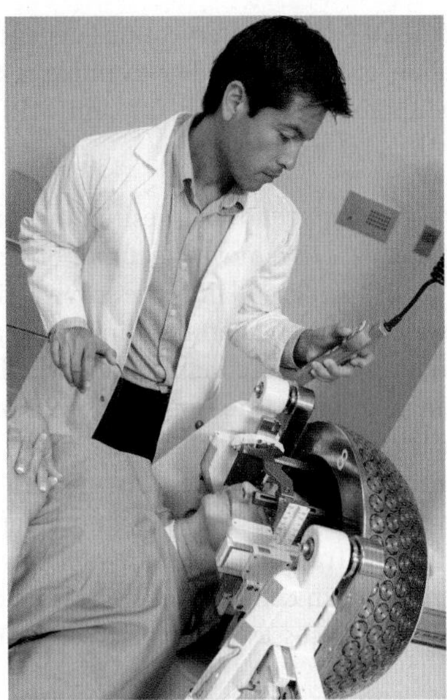

Fig. 41.7 A Gamma Knife treatment. The treatment beams are widely dispersed over the surface of the head to prevent damage to healthy brain tissue. The beams are intense only at the point of target. (© Getty Images. In Lampignano, J.P., & Kendrick, L.E. [2018]. *Bontrager's textbook of radiographic positioning and related anatomy* [9th ed.]. St. Louis: Elsevier.)

multiple beams of gamma radiation produced by the radioisotope *cobalt-60* to destroy intracranial lesions selectively without damaging surrounding healthy tissue (Fig. 41.7). Combining neurodiagnostic imaging tools, including MRI, CT, magnetic resonance angiography (MRA), and angiography, with the Gamma Knife allows for precise localization of deep-seated or anatomically difficult lesions. Treatment usually takes less than an hour, and patients require only overnight hospitalization.

A disadvantage is that the device requires an uncomfortable rigid head frame. In another system, called the *CyberKnife,* no frame is needed. Both procedures are used primarily for brain tumors or arteriovenous malformations (AVMs) that are in a difficult location and therefore not removable by craniotomy. These procedures may also be used with patients who decline conventional surgery, for patients whose age and physical condition do not allow general anesthesia, as an adjunct to radiation therapy, and for recurrent or residual AVMs or tumors after embolization or craniotomy.

Surgical Management. A craniotomy (surgical incision into the cranium to access the brain) may be performed to remove the tumor, improve symptoms related to the lesion, or decrease the tumor size (debulk). The challenge for the neurosurgeon is to remove the tumor as completely as possible without damaging normal tissue. Complete removal is possible with some benign tumors, which results in a "surgical cure." After surgery the patient is often admitted to the critical care unit or neurosurgical unit for frequent observation.

Preoperative Care. The patient having a craniotomy is typically very anxious about having his or her head opened and the brain exposed. Concerns are centered on the possibility of increased neurologic deficits after the surgery and the patient's self-image when part or all of the head is shaved. Provide reassurance that the surgeon will spare vital parts of the brain while removing or decreasing the size of the tumor. Teach the patient and family about what to expect immediately after surgery and throughout the recovery period. Some patients require short-term or long-term rehabilitation.

Other preoperative care is similar to that for any patient having surgery, as described in Chapter 9.

Operative Procedures. Surgery is performed under local or general anesthesia or sedation. Small tumors that are easily located may be removed by *minimally invasive surgery (MIS).* For example, the transnasal approach using endoscopy can be performed for pituitary tumors. The patient has a short hospital stay and few complications after surgery. Stereotactic surgery using a rigid head frame can be done for tumors that are easily reached. This procedure requires only burr holes and local anesthesia because the brain has no sensory neurons for pain. Laser surgery can also be done.

For an *open traditional* craniotomy, the surgeon makes an incision along or behind the hairline after placing the patient's head in a skull fixation device. Several burr holes are drilled into the skull, and a saw is used to remove a piece of bone (bone flap) to expose the tumor area. The flap is stored carefully until the end of the procedure or for a later time. The tumor is located using imaging technology and removed or debulked (partially removed). After the tumor removal, the bone flap is replaced and held by small screws or bolts. A drain or monitoring device may be inserted. The surgeon creates a soft dressing "cap" over the top of the head to keep the surgical area clean and prevent the patient from touching the incision site.

Postoperative Care. The focus of postoperative care is to monitor the patient to detect changes in status and prevent or minimize complications, especially increased intracranial pressure (ICP).

! NURSING SAFETY PRIORITY QSEN

Action Alert

Assess neurologic and vital signs every 15 to 30 minutes for the first 4 to 6 hours after a craniotomy and then every hour. If the patient is stable for 24 hours, the frequency of these checks may be decreased to every 2 to 4 hours, depending on agency policy and the patient's condition. *Report immediately and document new neurologic deficits, particularly a decreased level of consciousness (LOC), motor weakness or paralysis, aphasia, decreased* ***sensory perception,*** *and sluggish pupil reaction to light!* Personality changes such as agitation, aggression, or passivity can also indicate worsening neurologic status.

Managing the Patient in the Immediate Postoperative Period. Periorbital edema and ecchymosis (bruising) around one or both eyes are not unusual and are treated with cold compresses to decrease swelling. Irrigate the affected eye(s) with warm saline solution or artificial tears to improve patient comfort. The patient in the critical care unit has routine cardiac monitoring because dysrhythmias may occur as a result of brain–autonomic nervous system–cardiac interactions or fluid and electrolyte imbalance.

Regardless of setting, ensure recording of the patient's intake and output for the first 24 hours. Anticipate fluid restriction to 1500 mL daily if there is pituitary involvement in either the tumor or surgical site and SIADH develops (see Chapter 57). Reposition the patient, being careful not to cause pressure on the operative site. Delegate or provide repositioning and deep breathing every 2 hours. To prevent the development of venous thromboembolism (VTE), maintain intermittent sequential pneumatic devices until the patient ambulates.

For patients who have undergone *supratentorial* surgery, elevate the head of the bed 30 degrees or as tolerated to promote venous drainage from the head. *Position the patient to avoid extreme hip or neck flexion and maintain the head in a midline, neutral position to prevent increased ICP.* Turn the patient side to side or supine to prevent pressure injury and pneumonia.

Keep the patient with an *infratentorial* (brainstem) craniotomy flat or at 10 degrees, depending on the primary health care provider's prescription. Position the patient side-lying, alternating sides every 2 hours, for 24 to 48 hours or until ambulatory. This position prevents pressure on the neck-area incision site. It also prevents pressure on the internal tumor excision site from higher cerebral structures. Make sure that the patient remains NPO status until awake and alert because edema around the medulla and lower cranial nerves may also cause vomiting and aspiration.

Check the head dressing every 1 to 2 hours for signs of drainage. Mark the area of drainage once during each shift for baseline comparison, although this practice varies by health care agency. A small or moderate amount of drainage is expected. Some patients may have a Hemovac or Jackson-Pratt drain in place for 24 to 72 hours after surgery. Measure the drainage every 8 hours and record the amount and color. A typical amount of drainage is 30 to 50 mL every 8 hours. Follow the manufacturer's and neurosurgeon's instructions to maintain suction within the drain.

! NURSING SAFETY PRIORITY (QSEN)

Critical Rescue

After craniotomy, monitor the patient's dressing for excessive amounts of drainage. Report a saturated head dressing or drainage greater than 50 mL/8 hr immediately to the surgeon! *Monitor frequently for signs of increasing ICP!*

The usual laboratory studies monitored after surgery include complete blood count (CBC), serum electrolyte levels and osmolarity, and coagulation studies. The patient's hematocrit and hemoglobin concentration may be abnormally low from blood loss during surgery, diluted from large amounts of IV fluids given during surgery, or elevated if the blood was replaced. Hyponatremia (low serum sodium) may occur as a result of fluid volume overload, syndrome of inappropriate antidiuretic hormone (SIADH), or steroid administration.

Hypokalemia (low serum potassium) may cause cardiac irritability. Weakness, a change in LOC, and confusion are symptoms of hyponatremia and hypokalemia. Hypernatremia may be caused by meningitis, dehydration, or diabetes insipidus (DI). It manifests with muscle weakness, restlessness, extreme thirst, and dry mouth (see Chapter 57). Additional signs of dehydration such as decreased urinary output, thick lung secretions, and hypotension may be present. *Untreated hypernatremia can lead to seizure activity. DI should be considered if the patient voids large amounts of very dilute urine with an increasing serum osmolarity and electrolyte concentration.*

The patient may be mechanically ventilated for the first 24 to 48 hours after surgery to help manage the airway and maintain optimal oxygen levels. If the patient is awake or attempting to breathe at a rate other than that set on the ventilator, drugs such as propofol and fentanyl are given to treat pain and anxiety and promote rest and comfort. Suction the patient as needed. *Remember to hyperoxygenate the patient carefully before, during, and after suctioning!*

Drugs routinely given after surgery include antiepileptic drugs, histamine blockers or proton pump inhibitors for stress ulcer prevention, and glucocorticoids such as dexamethasone to reduce cerebral edema. Give acetaminophen for fever or mild pain. Antibiotics are typically prescribed to prevent infection for several days after surgery.

NCLEX EXAMINATION CHALLENGE 41.4

Physiological Integrity

A client returns from the postanesthesia care unit (PACU) after a surgical removal of a frontal lobe tumor. In what position will the nurse place the client **at this time**?

A. Turn the client from side to side to prevent aspiration.
B. Elevate the head of the bed to at least 30 degrees at all times.
C. Keep the client flat in bed or up 10 degrees and reposition from side to side.
D. Keep the client in a high-Fowler position in bed at all times.

Preventing and Managing Postoperative Complications. Postoperative complications are listed in Table 41.5. The major complications of *supratentorial* surgery are increased ICP from cerebral edema or hydrocephalus and hemorrhage.

Symptoms of *increased ICP* include severe headache, deteriorating LOC, restlessness, and irritability. Dilated or pinpoint pupils that are slow to react or nonreactive to light are late signs of increased ICP. Management of increased ICP is the same as that described under Interventions in the Traumatic Brain Injury section.

Hydrocephalus (increased CSF in the brain) is caused by obstruction of the normal CSF pathway from edema, an expanding lesion such as a hematoma, or blood in the subarachnoid space. Rapidly progressive hydrocephalus produces the classic symptoms of increased ICP. Slowly progressive hydrocephalus manifests with headache, decreased LOC, irritability, blurred vision, and urinary incontinence. An intraventricular catheter may be placed to drain CSF during surgery or emergently after surgery for rapidly deteriorating neurologic function (ventriculostomy). If long-term treatment is required for chronic hydrocephalus, a surgical shunt is inserted to drain CSF to another area of the body. Additional information about shunts may be found in neuroscience nursing textbooks. Other complications

TABLE 41.5 Postoperative Complications of Craniotomy

Early	Late
• Increased intracranial pressure (ICP)	• Wound infection
• Hematomas	• Meningitis
• **Subdural hematoma**	• Fluid and electrolyte imbalances
• **Epidural hematoma**	• Dehydration
• **Subarachnoid hemorrhage**	• Hyponatremia
• Hypovolemic shock	• Hypernatremia
• Hydrocephalus	• Seizures
• Respiratory complications	• Cerebrospinal fluid (CSF) leak
• Atelectasis	• Cerebral edema
• Hypoxia	
• Pneumonia	
• Neurogenic pulmonary edema	

listed in Table 41.5 are discussed in detail elsewhere in this chapter or this text.

Care Coordination and Transition Management. The patient with a brain tumor is managed at home if possible. Maintaining a reasonable quality of life is an important outcome for recovery and rehabilitation. Unless the patient has a significant degree of disability, no special preparation for home care is needed. Patients with hemiparesis need assistance to ensure that their home is accessible according to their method of ***mobility*** (e.g., cane, walker, or wheelchair). The environment should be made safe to prevent falls. For example, teach caregivers to remove scatter rugs and to place grab bars in the bathroom.

Information about the selection of rehabilitation or chronic care facility, if needed, can be obtained from the case manager (CM) or discharge planner. The selected facility should have experience in providing care for neurologically impaired patients. A psychologist should be available to provide input in the evaluation of the cognitive disabilities that the patient may have.

Seizures are a potential complication that can occur at any time for as long as 1 year or more after surgery. Provide the patient and family with information about seizure precautions and what to do if a seizure occurs. Teach the need for follow-up appointments to monitor for therapeutic levels of antiepileptic drugs (AEDs).

PATIENT-CENTERED CARE: CULTURAL/SPIRITUAL CONSIDERATIONS QSEN

Be sure that the patient and family have access to resources for support. Discuss ways that they have coped with crisis in the past, such as spiritual counselors or clergy. Provide hope and help them feel empowered to make the best decisions for their care and future. Listen to the patient's concerns and offer ideas for other community resources, depending on the patient's specific needs. Psychological support is essential because of potential changes in self-esteem, decreased ADL ability, and prognosis.

Refer the patient and the family or significant others to the American Brain Tumor Association (www.abta.org) or the National Brain Tumor Foundation (www.braintumor.org). The American Cancer Society (www.cancer.org) is also an appropriate community resource for patients with malignant tumors. In Canada, the Brain Tumor Foundation of Canada (www.braintumour.ca) can be very useful for providing information and support to patients and their families who live there. Home care agencies are available to provide both the physical and rehabilitative care that the patient may need at home. Hospice services and palliative care may be needed if he or she is terminally ill. (See Chapter 8 for additional information about end-of-life care.) Brain tumor support groups may also be a valuable asset to the patient and family.

GET READY FOR THE NEXT-GENERATION NCLEX® EXAMINATION!

Key Points

Review these Key Points for each NCLEX Examination Client Needs Category.

Safe and Effective Care Environment

- When caring for a patient with a stroke or traumatic brain injury (TBI), assess airway, breathing, and circulation status first and implement interventions to maintain them. **QSEN: Safety**
- Collaborate with the interprofessional team members, including primary health care providers, physical therapists, respiratory therapists, occupational therapists, social workers, and registered dietitian nutritionists to ensure optimal patient function and quality of life. **QSEN: Teamwork and Collaboration**

Health Promotion and Maintenance

- Identify risk factors for new or recurrent stroke and teach patients and families about modifiable risk factors. **QSEN: Evidence-Based Practice**
- Prevent secondary brain injury by protecting the airway, promoting an appropriate range of blood pressure and mean arterial pressure, maintaining fluid and electrolyte balance, promptly treating fever, avoiding sustained hypoglycemia and hyperglycemia, addressing hypoxia and hypercarbia, positioning the patient appropriately, and managing intracranial hypertension with prescribed interventions. **Clinical Judgment; QSEN: Safety**
- Teach patients and families about community organizations, such as the National Stroke Association and the Brain Injury Association of America. **QSEN: Patient-Centered Care**

Psychosocial Integrity

- Assess the emotional reactions of families to a TBI, stroke, or brain cancer diagnosis and help them cope by providing information and including them in planning for care. **QSEN: Patient-Centered Care**

Physiological Integrity

- Perform a comprehensive, rapid, or focal neurologic assessment at regular intervals to identify changes in status. **QSEN: Evidence-Based Practice**
- Recall that decreased level of consciousness is the most sensitive indicator of adverse outcome or complication from stroke, TBI, brain tumor, or craniotomy due to decreased ***perfusion*** from cerebral edema or hemorrhage. **QSEN: Evidence-Based Practice**
- Monitor patients with critical neurologic health problems for manifestations of increasing intracranial pressure (ICP). **Clinical Judgment**
- Assess the patient's ability to swallow before providing oral intake if a stroke is suspected or diagnosed. **QSEN: Safety**
- Assess patients with strokes for ***sensory perception*** changes such as unilateral neglect and impaired vision; help patients adapt to these changes, such as turning their head from side to side to see the entire meal tray. **QSEN: Patient-Centered Care**
- Provide alternative means of communication, in consultation with the speech-language expert, when expressive and/or receptive aphasia is present in patients who have had a stroke or brain injury. **QSEN: Teamwork and Collaboration**
- Monitor the patient on fibrinolytic therapy or anticoagulants for bleeding and abnormal coagulation studies. **QSEN: Safety**
- Teach patients with mild TBI and their families to monitor for neurologic changes. **QSEN: Safety**
- Recognize that the desired outcome for the patient with a brain tumor is to remove it if possible. Other methods may be used to decrease its size, including chemotherapy and radiation. **QSEN: Evidence-Based Practice**
- Monitor patients having a craniotomy for potential complications. **QSEN: Safety**

MASTERY QUESTIONS

1. The nurse reassesses a client who was admitted 8 hours after stroke symptoms began and documents the following findings. Which assessment findings would the nurse report immediately to the primary health care provider? **Select all that apply.**
   A. Blood pressure increase to 196/100 mm Hg
   B. Heart rate of 88 beats/min
   C. Respiratory rate of 22 breaths/min
   D. New-onset headache reported as 8/10 pain intensity
   E. Increased drowsiness and dozing frequently
   F. Urine output of 360 mL since admission
2. A client was admitted to the hospital unit a few minutes ago with a new diagnosis of right hemiparesis and aphasia, which resulted from a traumatic brain injury. Which of the following interventions is a **priority for the client at this time**?
   A. Contact the physical therapist (PT) to plan care to increase the client's mobility.
   B. Contact the occupational therapist (OT) to assess the client's ADL ability.
   C. Contact the unit social worker (SW) to talk with the family about the client's discharge.
   D. Contact the speech-language pathologist (SLP) to schedule a swallowing study.

REFERENCES

Asterisk (*) indicates a classic or definitive work on this subject.

*Bowen, P. (2016). Early identification, rapid response, and effective treatment of acute stroke. *Medsurg Nursing, 25*(4), 241–243.

Burchum, J. L. R., & Rosenthal, L. D. (2019). *Lehne's pharmacology for nursing care* (10th ed.). St. Louis: Elsevier.

Centers for Disease Control and Prevention (CDC). (2020a). *Stroke.* www.cdc.gov/stroke/.

Centers for Disease Control and Prevention (CDC). (2020b). *Injury prevention & control: Traumatic brain injury.* www.cdc.gov/TraumaticBrainInjury.

Centers for Disease Control and Prevention (CDC). (2020c). *What to expect after a concussion.* www.cdc.gov/headsup/pdfs/providers/TBI_Patient_Instructions-a.pdf.

Dang, B., Chen, W., He, W., & Chen, G. (2017). *Rehabilitation treatment and progression of traumatic brain injury dysfunction. Neural Plasticity.* Retrieved from https://doi.org/10.1155/2017/1582182.

Gottlieb, M., & Bailitz, J. (2016). Does mannitol reduce mortality from traumatic brain injury? *Annals of Emergency Medicine, 67*(1), 83–85.

Heart and Stroke Foundation. (2019). *Statistics.* www.hands.com/site.c.ikIQLcMWJtE/b.3483991/k.34A8/Statistics.htm.

Interprofessional Education Collaborative Expert Panel. (2016). *Core competencies for interprofessional collaborative practice: Report of an expert panel* (2nd ed.). Washington, D.C: Interprofessional Education Collaborative.

Kivunja, S., River, J., & Gullick, J. (2018). Experiences of giving and receiving care in traumatic brain injury. *Journal of Clinical Nursing, 27*(7–8), 1304–1328.

McCance, K., Huether, S., Brashers, V., & Rote, N. (2019). *Pathophysiology: The biologic basis for disease in adults and children* (9th ed.). St. Louis: Mosby.

Miller, S., Silverman, E., & Hoffman-Ruddy, B. (2017). Assessment of airway defenses in the neurologically impaired patient. *Medsurg Nursing, 26*(2), 113–117.

Milliken, A., & Uveges, M. (2020). Brain death: History, updates, and implications for nurses. *American Journal of Nursing, 120*(3), 32–38.

Powers, W. J., Rabinstein, A. A., Ackerson, T., Adeoye, O. M., Bambakidid, N. C., Becker, K., et al. (2018). *American Heart Association/American Stroke Association Guideline: 2018 guidelines for the early management of patients with acute ischemic stroke—A guideline for healthcare professionals from the American Heart Association/American Stroke Association*. Retrieved from https://strokeassociation.org/idc/groups/stroke-public/@wcm/@hcm/@sta/documents/downloadable/ucm_499252.pdf.

Ross, S. Y., Roberts, S., Taggart, H., & Patronas, C. (2017). Stroke transitions of care. *Medsurg Nursing*, *26*(2), 119–125.

Russell, J. A., Epstein, L. G., Greer, D. M., Kirschen, M., Rubin, M. A., & Lewis, A. (2019). Brain death, the determination of brain death, and member guidance for brain accommodation requests: AAN position statement. *Neurology*, *92*, 228–232.

*Saban, K. L., Hogan, N. S., Hogan, T. P., & Pape, T. L. -B. (2015). He looks normal but…Challenges of family caregivers of veterans diagnosed with a traumatic brain injury. *Rehabilitation Nursing*, *40*(5), 277–283.

Sandercock, P. A. G., & Leong, T. S. (2017). Low-molecular-weight heparins or heparinoids versus standard unfractionated heparin for cute ischemic stroke. *Cochrane Database Systematic Review*, *4*(CD000119).

Slusser, M., Garcia, L. I., Reed, C.-R., & McGinnis, P. Q. (2019). *Foundations of interprofessional collaborative practice in health care*. St. Louis: Elsevier.

The Joint Commission. (2017). *Stroke*. http://www.jointcommission.org/specifications_manual_for_national_hospital_inpatient_quality_measures.aspx.

Vacca, V. M., & Argenti, I. (2018). Chronic subdural hematoma: A common complexity. *Nursing*, *48*(5), 25–31 2018.

Wells-Pittman, J., & Gullicksrud, A. (2020). Standardizing the frequency of neurologic assessment after acute stroke. *American Journal of Nursing*, *120*(3), 48–54.

*Wijdicks, E. F., Varelas, P. N., Gronseth, G. S., Greer, D. M., & American Academy of Neurology. (2010). Evidence-based guideline update: Determining brain death in adults: Report of the quality standards subcommittee of the American Academy of Neurology. *Neurology*, *74*(23), 1911–1918.

42

Assessment and Concepts of Care for Patients With Eye and Vision Problems

Cherie R. Rebar, Samuel A. Borchers, Andrea A. Borchers

http://evolve.elsevier.com/Iggy/

LEARNING OUTCOMES

1. Collaborate with the interprofessional team to perform assessments of eyes and vision.
2. Prioritize evidence-based care for patients having an eye assessment or treatment for eye or vision problems that affect **sensory perception.**
3. Teach evidence-based way for adults to protect their eyes from injury or infection to preserve **sensory perception.**
4. Explain how physiologic aging changes of the eyes and vision affect **sensory perception.**
5. Teach patients who need vision assistive devices how to use them.
6. Implement nursing interventions to decrease the psychosocial impact for the patient undergoing eye assessment or treatment for eye or vision problems.
7. Apply knowledge of anatomy and physiology, genetic risk, and principles of aging to perform a focused assessment of the eyes and vision.
8. Use clinical judgment to analyze assessment findings and diagnostic data in the care of patients with an eye or vision problem.
9. Plan care coordination and transition management for patients with an eye or vision problem.

KEY TERMS

arcus senilis An opaque, bluish-white ring within the outer edge of the cornea.

cataract A lens opacity that distorts the image projected onto the retina.

enucleation Surgical removal of the entire eyeball.

glaucoma A condition in the eye that occurs with increased pressure and resulting hypoxia of photoreceptors and their synapsing nerve fibers.

hyperopia Farsightedness.

keratitis Inflammation of the cornea.

keratoconus Degeneration of the cornea.

keratoplasty Corneal transplant. The surgical removal of diseased corneal tissue and replacement with tissue from a human donor cornea.

myopia Nearsightedness.

nystagmus An involuntary and rapid twitching of the eyeball.

photophobia Sensitivity to light.

primary angle-closure glaucoma (PACG) A form of glaucoma that can have a sudden onset and is an emergency; it is characterized by a forward displacement of the iris, which presses against the cornea and closes the chamber angle, suddenly preventing outflow of aqueous humor. Also called *closed-angle glaucoma, narrow-angle glaucoma,* or *acute glaucoma.*

primary open-angle glaucoma (POAG) The most common form of primary glaucoma; characterized by reduced outflow of aqueous humor through the chamber angle. Because the fluid cannot leave the eye at the same rate it is produced, intraocular pressure gradually increases.

retinal detachment The separation of the retina from the epithelium.

retinal hole a break in the retina, often caused by trauma or aging.

retina tear A jagged and irregularly shaped break in the retina, which can result from traction on the retina.

PRIORITY AND INTERRELATED CONCEPTS

The priority concept for this chapter is:
- ***Sensory Perception***

The ***Sensory Perception*** concept exemplars for this chapter are Cataract and Glaucoma.

Sensory perception is the ability to perceive and interpret sensory input into one or more meaningful responses (see Chapter 3). Many adults think of vision as their most important sense because it assesses surroundings, allows independence, warns of danger, appreciates beauty, and helps them work, play, and interact with others. Changes in the eye and vision can provide information about the patient's general health status and problems that might occur in self-care.

ANATOMY AND PHYSIOLOGY REVIEW

Visual ***sensory perception*** takes place when the eye and brain work together. Vision begins when light is changed into nerve impulses in the eye and the impulses are sent on to the brain to fully perceive images (McCance et al., 2019). Systemic conditions and eye problems can change vision temporarily or permanently.

Structure

The eyeball, a round, ball-shaped organ, is located in the front part of the eye orbit. The orbit is the bony socket of the skull that surrounds and protects the eye along with the attached muscles, nerves, vessels, and tear-producing glands.

Layers of the Eyeball. The eye has three layers (Fig. 42.1). The external layer is the sclera (the "white" of the eye) and the transparent cornea on the front of the eye.

The middle layer, or **uvea,** is heavily pigmented and consists of the choroid, the ciliary body, and the iris. The choroid, a dark brown membrane between the sclera and the retina, lines most of the sclera. It has many blood vessels that supply nutrients to the retina.

The ciliary body connects the choroid with the iris and secretes aqueous humor. The **iris** is the colored portion of the external eye; its center opening is the *pupil.* The muscles of the iris contract and relax to control pupil size and the amount of light entering the eye.

The innermost layer is the *retina,* a thin, delicate structure made up of sensory photoreceptors that begin the transmission of impulses to the optic nerve (McCance et al., 2019). The retina contains blood vessels and two types of photoreceptors called *rods* and *cones.* The rods work at low light levels and provide peripheral vision. The cones are active at bright light levels and provide color and central vision.

The *optic fundus* is the area at the inside back of the eye that can be seen with an ophthalmoscope. This area contains the *optic disc,* a pinkish-orange or white depressed area where the nerve fibers that synapse with the photoreceptors join together to form the optic nerve and exit the eyeball. The optic disc contains only nerve fibers and no photoreceptor cells. To one side of the optic disc is a small, yellowish pink area called the *macula lutea.* The center of the macula is the *fovea centralis,* where vision is most acute.

Refractive Structures and Media. Light waves pass through the cornea, aqueous humor, lens, and vitreous humor on the way to the retina. Each structure bends *(refracts)* the light waves to focus images on the retina. Together these structures are the eye's *refracting media.*

The *cornea* is the clear layer that forms the external bump on the front of the eye (see Fig. 42.1). The *aqueous humor* is a clear,

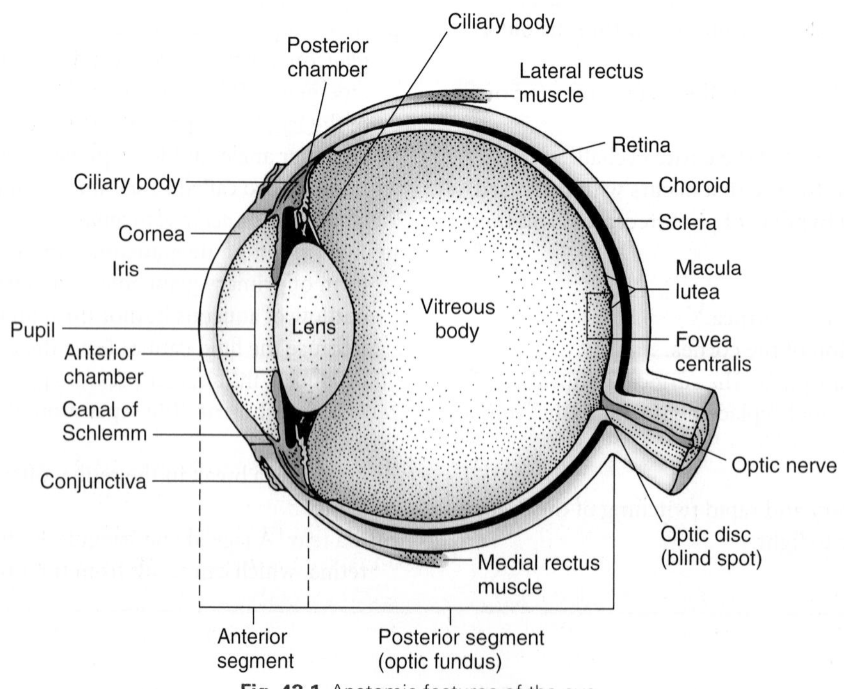

Fig. 42.1 Anatomic features of the eye.

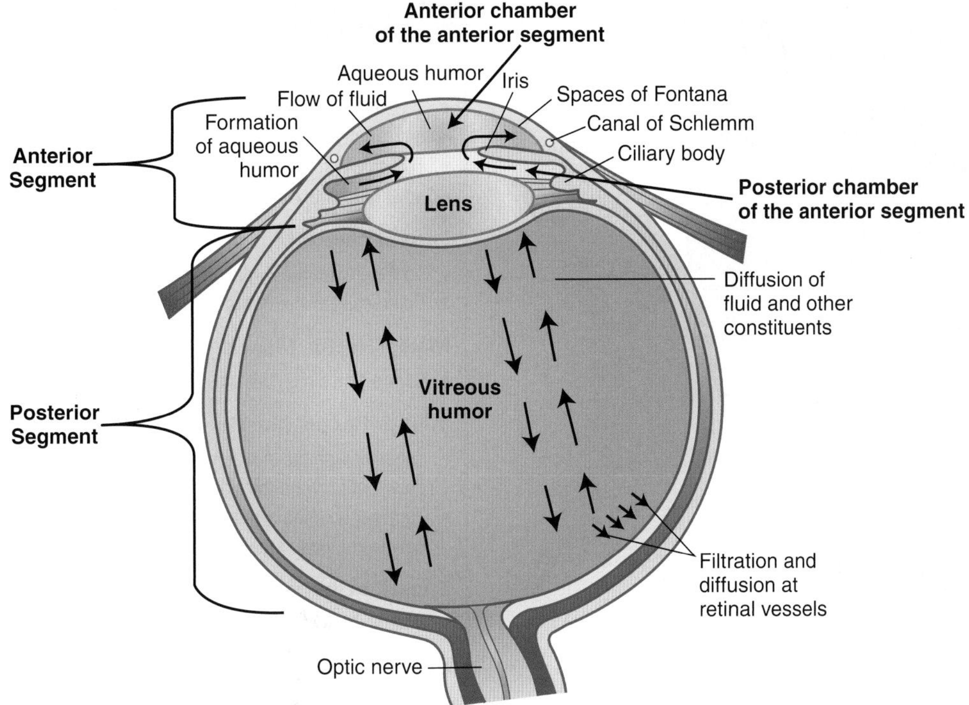

Fig. 42.2 Flow of aqueous humor.

watery fluid that fills the anterior and posterior chambers of the eye. This fluid is continually produced by the ciliary processes and passes from the posterior chamber, through the pupil, and into the anterior chamber. This fluid drains through the canal of Schlemm into the blood to maintain a balanced intraocular pressure (IOP), the pressure within the eye (Fig. 42.2).

The *lens* is a circular, convex structure that lies behind the iris and in front of the vitreous body. It is transparent and bends the light rays entering through the pupil to focus properly on the retina. The curve of the lens changes to focus on near or distant objects. A cataract is a lens opacity that distorts the image projected onto the retina.

The *vitreous body* is a clear, thick gel that fills the large vitreous chamber (the space between the lens and the retina). This gel transmits light and maintains eye shape.

The eye is a hollow organ and must be kept in the shape of a ball for vision to occur. To maintain this shape, the vitreous humor gel in the posterior segment and the aqueous humor in the anterior segment must be present in set amounts that apply pressure inside the eye to keep it inflated. This pressure is the *intraocular pressure* or *IOP*. IOP has to be precisely accurate. If the pressure is too low, the eyeball is soft and collapses, preventing light from getting to the photoreceptors on the retina in the back of the eye. If the pressure becomes too high, the extra pressure compresses capillaries in the eye and nerve fibers. Pressure on retinal blood vessels prevents blood from flowing through them; therefore, the photoreceptors and nerve fibers become hypoxic. Compression of the fine nerve fibers prevents intracellular fluid flow, which also reduces nourishment to the distal portions of these thin nerve fibers. Glaucoma occurs with increased pressure and resulting hypoxia of photoreceptors and their synapsing nerve fibers. Continued retinal hypoxia results in necrosis and death of photoreceptors, as well as permanent nerve fiber damage. When extensive photoreceptor and nerve fiber loss occur, vision is lost, and the person is permanently blind (Bagheri & Wajda, 2017).

External Structures. The eyelids are thin, movable skinfolds that protect the eyes and keep the cornea moist. The *canthus* is the place where the two eyelids meet at the corner of the eye.

The *conjunctivae* are the mucous membranes of the eye. The palpebral conjunctiva is a thick membrane with many blood vessels that lines the undersurface of each eyelid. The thin, transparent bulbar conjunctiva covers the entire front of the eye.

A small *lacrimal gland,* which is located in the upper outer part of each orbit (Fig. 42.3), produces tears. Tears flow across the front of the eye, toward the nose, and into the inner canthus. They drain through the *punctum* (an opening at the nasal side of the lid edges) into the lacrimal duct and sac and then into the nose through the nasolacrimal duct.

Muscles, Nerves, and Blood Vessels. Six voluntary muscles rotate the eye and coordinate eye movements (Fig. 42.4 and Table 42.1). Coordinated eye movements ensure that both eyes receive an image at the same time so that only a single image is seen.

The muscles around the eye are innervated by cranial nerves (CNs) III (oculomotor), IV (trochlear), and VI (abducens). The *optic nerve* (CN II) is the nerve of sight, connecting the optic disc to the brain. The trigeminal nerve (CN V) stimulates the blink reflex when the cornea is touched. The facial nerve (CN VII) innervates the lacrimal glands and muscles for lid closure.

The ophthalmic artery brings oxygenated blood to the eye and the orbit. It branches to supply blood to the retina. The ciliary arteries supply the sclera, choroid, ciliary body, and iris.

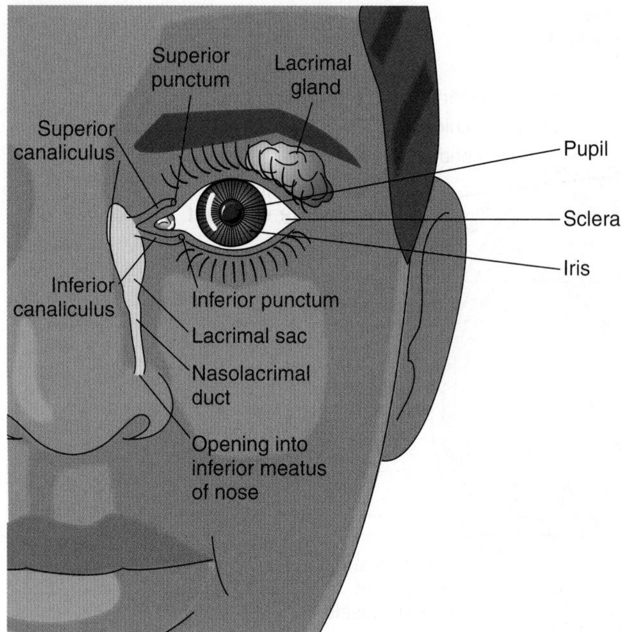

Fig. 42.3 Front view of the eye and adjacent structures.

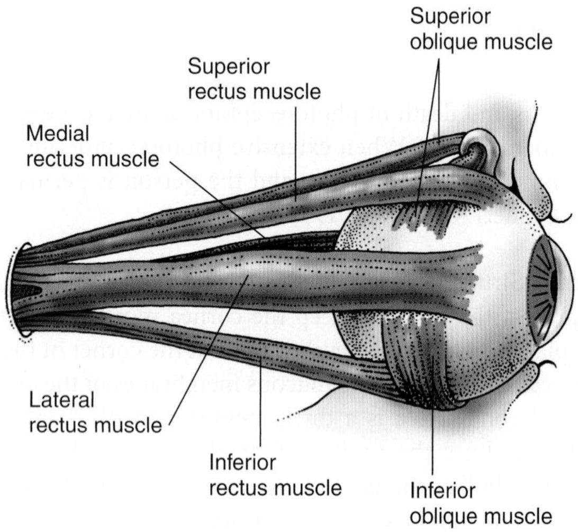

Fig. 42.4 Extraocular muscles.

Outflow moves through several venous pathways that empty into the superior ophthalmic vein.

Function

The four eye functions that provide clear images and vision are refraction, pupillary constriction, accommodation, and convergence.

Refraction bends light rays from the outside into the eye through curved surfaces and refractive media and finally to the retina. Each surface and media bend (refract) light differently to focus an image on the retina. *Emmetropia* is the perfect refraction of the eye in which light rays from a distant source are focused into a sharp image on the retina. Fig. 42.5 shows the normal refraction of light within the eye. Images fall on the retina inverted and reversed left to right. For example, an object in the lower nasal visual field strikes the upper outer area of the retina.

TABLE 42.1 Functions of Ocular Muscles

Superior Rectus Muscle

- Together with the lateral rectus, this muscle moves the eye diagonally upward toward the side of the head.
- Together with the medial rectus, this muscle moves the eye diagonally upward toward the middle of the head.

Lateral Rectus Muscle

- Together with the medial rectus, this muscle holds the eye straight.
- Contracting alone, this muscle turns the eye toward the side of the head.

Medial Rectus Muscle

- Contracting alone, this muscle turns the eye toward the nose.

Inferior Rectus Muscle

- Together with the lateral rectus, this muscle moves the eye diagonally downward toward the side of the head.
- Together with the medial rectus, this muscle moves the eye diagonally downward toward the middle of the head.

Superior Oblique Muscle

- Contracting alone, this muscle pulls the eye downward.

Inferior Oblique Muscle

- Contracting alone, this muscle pulls the eye upward.

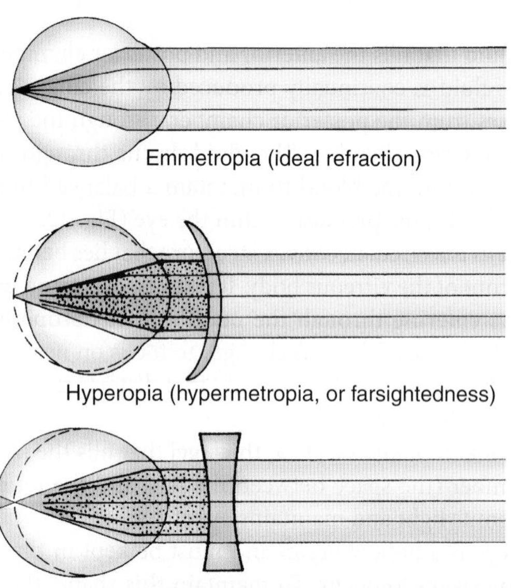

Fig. 42.5 Refraction and correction in emmetropia, hyperopia, and myopia.

Errors of refraction are common. **Hyperopia** (farsightedness) occurs when the eye does not refract light enough. As a result, images actually converge behind the retina (see Fig. 42.5). In hyperopia, distant vision is normal, but near vision is poor. It is corrected with a convex lens in eyeglasses or contact lenses.

Myopia (nearsightedness) occurs when the eye overbends the light and images converge in front of the retina (see Fig. 42.5). Near vision is normal, but distance vision is poor. Myopia is corrected with a concave lens in eyeglasses or contact lenses.

Astigmatism is a refractive error caused by unevenly curved surfaces on or in the eye, especially the cornea. These uneven surfaces distort vision.

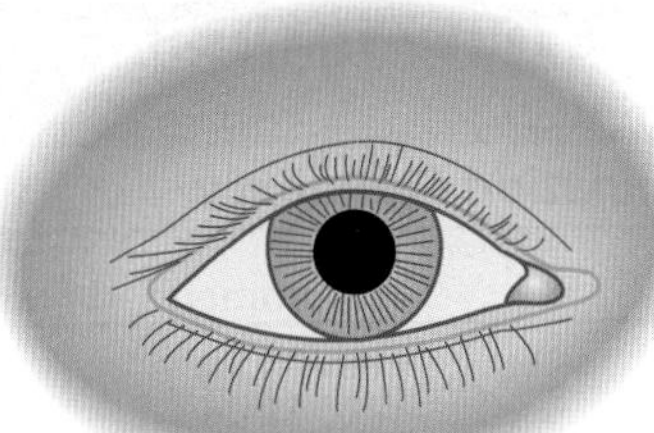
Normal pupil slightly dilated for moderate light

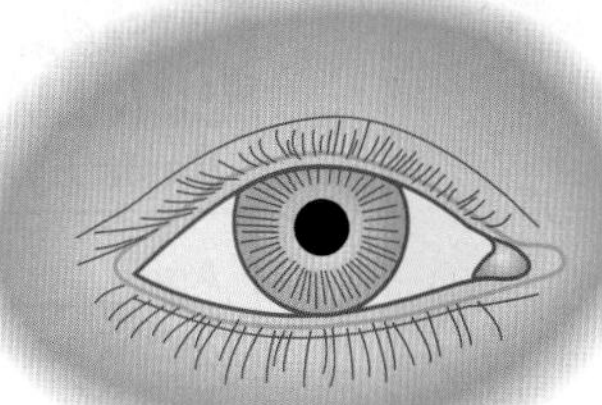
Miosis—pupil constricted when exposed to increased light or close work, such as reading

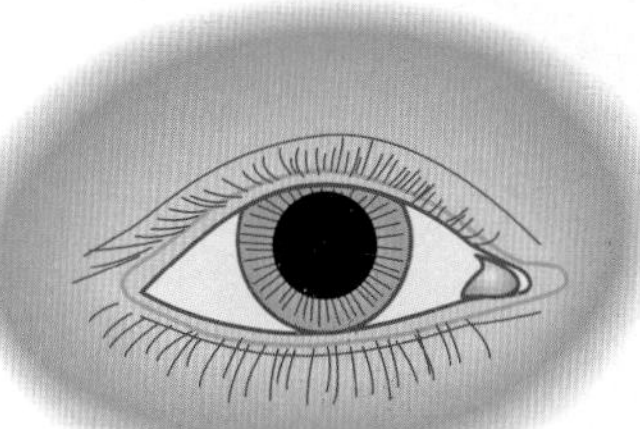
Mydriasis—pupil dilated when exposed to reduced light or when looking at a distance

Fig. 42.6 Miosis and mydriasis.

PATIENT-CENTERED CARE: OLDER ADULT CONSIDERATIONS (QSEN)

Changes in the Eye and Vision Related to Aging

Structure/ Function	Change	Implication
Appearance	Eyes appear "sunken." Arcus senilis forms. Sclera yellows or appears blue.	Do not use eye appearance as an indicator for hydration status. Reassure patient that this change does not affect vision. Do not use sclera to assess for jaundice.
Cornea	Cornea flattens, which blurs vision and can cause or worsen astigmatism.	Encourage older adults to have regular eye examinations and wear prescribed corrective lenses for best vision.
Ocular muscles	Muscle strength is reduced, making it more difficult to maintain an upward gaze or a focus on a single image.	Reassure patient that this is a normal finding and to refocus gaze frequently to maintain a single image.
Lens	Elasticity is lost, increasing the near point of vision (making the near point of best vision farther away). Lens hardens, compacts, and forms a cataract.	Encourage use of corrective lenses for reading. Emphasize the importance of annual vision checks and monitoring.
Iris and pupil	Decrease in ability to dilate results in small pupil size and poor adaptation to darkness.	Teach that good lighting is needed to avoid bumping into objects, tripping, and falling.
Color vision	Discrimination among greens, blues, and violets decreases.	The patient may not be able to use color-indicator monitors of health status.
Tears	Tear production is reduced, resulting in dry eyes, discomfort, and increased risk for corneal damage or eye infections.	Teach the proper use of saline eyedrops to reduce dryness. Teach to increase humidity in the home.

Pupillary constriction (miosis) and pupillary dilation (mydriasis) (Fig. 42.6) control the amount of light that enters the eye. If the level of light to one or both eyes is increased, both pupils constrict (become smaller). The amount of constriction depends on how much light is available and how well the retina can adapt to light changes. Certain drugs can alter pupillary constriction.

The process of maintaining a clear visual image when the gaze is shifted from a distant to a near object is known as *accommodation.* The healthy eye can adjust its focus by changing the curve of the lens.

Convergence is the ability to turn both eyes inward toward the nose at the same time. This action helps ensure that only a single image of close objects is seen.

Eye Changes Associated With Aging

Visual acuity decreases with age due to changes inside the eye (Touhy & Jett, 2018). Age-related changes of the nervous system and in the eye support structures also reduce visual function (see the Patient-Centered Care: Older Adult Considerations: Changes in the Eye and Vision Related to Aging box).

Structural changes occur with aging, including decreased eye muscle tone that reduces the ability to keep the gaze focused on a single object. The lower eyelid may relax and fall away from the eye *(ectropion),* leading to dry eye signs and symptoms.

Arcus senilis, an opaque, bluish-white ring within the outer edge of the cornea, is caused by fat deposits (Fig. 42.7). This change does not affect vision.

Fatty deposits cause the sclera to develop a yellowish tinge. A bluish color may be seen as the sclera thins. With age, the iris has less ability to dilate, which leads to difficulty in adapting to dark environments. Older adults may benefit from additional light for reading and other "close-up" work and to avoid tripping over objects.

Functional changes also occur with aging. The lens yellows, hardens, shrinks, and loses elasticity, which reduces accommodation. The **near point of vision** (i.e., the closest distance at which the eye can see an object clearly) increases. Near objects,

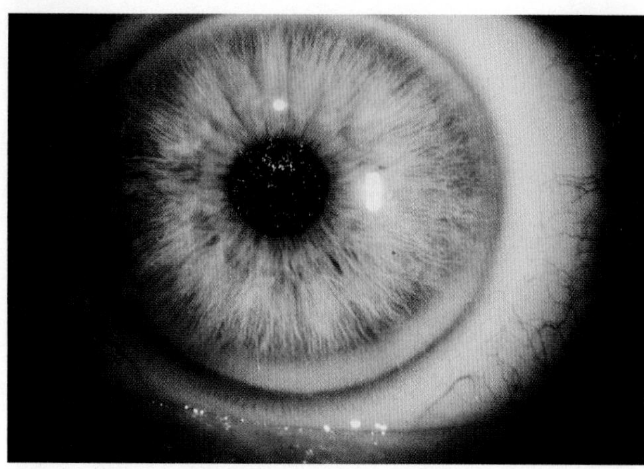

Fig. 42.7 Arcus senilis of the iris.

especially reading material, must be placed farther from the eye to be seen clearly (**presbyopia**). The **far point** (i.e., the farthest point at which an object can be distinguished) decreases. Together these changes narrow the visual field of an older adult.

General color perception decreases, especially for green, blue, and violet. More light is needed to stimulate the visual receptors. Intraocular pressure (IOP) is slightly higher in older adults.

Health Promotion and Maintenance

Impairment of vision impacts physical and psychological well-being and is identified as one of the top 10 disabilities in the United States (Quaranta et al., 2016). Many vision and eye problems can be avoided, and others can be corrected or managed if found early. Teach adults about eye-protection methods, adequate nutrition that supports eye health, and the importance of regular eye examinations.

The risks for cataract formation and for cancer of the eye (ocular melanoma) increase with exposure to ultraviolet (UV) light. Teach adults to protect the eyes by using sunglasses that filter UV light whenever they are outdoors, at tanning salons, and when work involves UV exposure.

Vision can be affected by eye injury, which increases the risk for cataract formation and glaucoma. Teach adults to wear eye and head protection when working with particulate matter, fluid or blood spatter, high temperatures, or sparks. Protection should also be worn during participation in sports or any activity that increases the risk for the eye being hit by objects in motion. Teach adults to avoid rubbing the eyes to avoid trauma to outer eye surfaces.

Eye infections can lead to vision loss. Although the eye surface is not sterile, the sclera and cornea have no separate blood supply and thus are at risk for infection. Teach adults to wash their hands before touching the eye or eyelid. Teach patients who use eyedrops about the proper technique to use these drugs and to not share eyedrops with others. If an eye has a discharge, teach the patient to use a separate eyedrop bottle for this eye and to wash the unaffected eye before washing the affected eye.

Other health problems, especially diabetes and hypertension, can seriously affect visual ***sensory perception.*** Teach patients with these conditions about the importance of controlling blood glucose levels and managing blood pressure to reduce the risk for vision loss. Annual evaluation by an eye care provider is needed prevent eye complications and detect problems early. See the Best Practice for Patient Safety & Quality Care: Basic Eye Examination Frequency box for specific recommendations about how often patients should be seen by an eye care provider for a general eye examination.

Eye care providers may recommend that adults older than 40 years have an eye examination annually that includes assessment of intraocular pressure and visual fields because the risk for both glaucoma and cataract formation increases with age.

BEST PRACTICE FOR PATIENT SAFETY & QUALITY CARE (QSEN)

Basic Eye Examination Frequency

Age	Recommended Frequency
20-39 African-American	Every 2-4 years
20-39 Caucasian	Every 3-5 years
40-64 (any race)	Every 2-4 years
65 years and over (of any race)	Every 1-2 years
People with special risks (e.g., diabetes, eye surgery or trauma, glaucoma)	As recommended by the eye care provider (may be more frequent)

Adapted from American Academy of Ophthalmology. (2019). Eye exam and vision testing basics. Retrieved from https://www.aao.org/eye-health/tips-prevention/eye-exams-101; and PreventBlindness.org. (2020). How often should I have an eye examination? Retrieved from https://www.preventblindness.org/how-often-should-i-have-eye-exam.

! NURSING SAFETY PRIORITY (QSEN)

Action Alert

Teach adults to see a health care provider immediately when an eye injury occurs or an eye infection is suspected.

NCLEX EXAMINATION CHALLENGE 42.1

Health Promotion and Maintenance

What is the appropriate nursing response when a 66-year-old healthy client asks how often a visit to the eye care provider is recommended?

A. "Annually."
B. "Every 6 months."
C. "Only if you have vision problems."
D. "Every 1-2 years if you have no eye problems."

◆ ASSESSMENT: RECOGNIZE CUES

Patient History

Collect information to determine whether problems with the eye or vision have an impact on ADLs or other daily functions.

Age is an important factor to consider when assessing visual ***sensory perception*** and eye structure. The incidence of glaucoma and cataract formation increases with aging. Presbyopia commonly begins in the 40s.

TABLE 42.2 Systemic Conditions and Common Drugs Affecting the Eye and Vision

Systemic Conditions and Disorders	Drugs
• Diabetes mellitus • Hypertension • Lupus erythematosus • Sarcoidosis • Thyroid problems • HIV-III (acquired immune deficiency syndrome) • Cardiac disease • Multiple sclerosis • Pregnancy	• Antihistamines[a] • Decongestants[a] • Antibiotics • Opioids • Anticholinergics • Cholinergic agonists • Adrenergic agonists • Adrenergic antagonists (beta blockers) • Oral contraceptives • Chemotherapy agents • Corticosteroids[a]

[a]Prescription and over-the-counter.

Gender may be important. Retinal detachments occur more often in men, and dry eye syndromes occur more often in women.

Occupation and leisure activities can affect visual ***sensory perception.*** Ask about how the eyes are used at work, because those who frequently use computers may experience eyestrain. Machine operators are at risk for injury because of high speeds at which particles can be thrown at the eye. Chronic exposure to infrared or UV light may cause photophobia and cataract formation. A blow to the face or head near the eye when playing sports such as baseball can damage external structures, the eye, the connections with the brain, or the area of the brain where vision is perceived. Teach all people to wear eye protection that is in keeping with their chosen occupation or sport.

Social habits such as smoking or vaping can be a significant risk factor for developing eye problems. Specifically, airborne formaldehyde can cause burning and watering of the eyes. Inquire about whether a patient smokes or vapes, and collect pertinent history regarding this practice.

Systemic health problems can affect vision. Check whether the patient has any condition listed in Table 42.2. Ask about past accidents, injuries, surgeries (including laser surgeries), or blows to the head that may have led to the present problem.

Drugs can also affect vision and the eye (see Table 42.2). Ask about the use of any prescription or over-the-counter drugs, especially decongestants and antihistamines, which cause eye dryness and may increase intraocular pressure. Document the name, strength, dose, and scheduling for all drugs the patient uses. Ocular effects from drugs include itching, foreign body sensation, redness, tearing, photophobia (sensitivity to light), and development of cataracts or glaucoma.

Nutrition History. Some eye problems are caused or worsened by vitamin deficiencies, so ask the patient about food choices. Vitamin A deficiency can cause eye dryness, keratomalacia, and blindness. Some nutrients and antioxidants, such as lutein, zeaxanthin, and beta carotene, help maintain retinal function (Eisenhauer, Natoli, Liew, & Flood, 2017). A diet rich in fruit and red, orange, and dark green vegetables is important to eye health.

NCLEX EXAMINATION CHALLENGE 42.2

Health Promotion and Maintenance

Which supplement will the nurse recommend to a client who wants to enhance eye health?

A. Lutein
B. Vitamin D
C. Magnesium
D. Saw palmetto

Family History and Genetic Risk. Ask about a family history of eye problems because some conditions have a familial tendency and some genetic problems lead to visual impairment.

Current Health Problems. Ask the patient about the onset of visual changes. Question whether the change occurred rapidly or slowly. Determine whether the signs and symptoms are present to the same degree in both eyes. If eye injury or trauma is involved, also ask:

- How long ago did the injury occur?
- What was the patient doing when it happened?
- If a foreign body was involved, what was its source?
- Was any first aid administered at the scene? If so, what kind, and what other actions were taken?

! NURSING SAFETY PRIORITY (QSEN)

Critical Rescue

Recognize that a sudden or persistent loss of visual ***sensory perception*** within the past 48 hours, eye trauma, a foreign body in the eye, or sudden ocular pain is an emergency. Respond by notifying the eye care provider immediately.

Physical Assessment

Inspection. Look for head tilting, squinting, or other actions that indicate that the patient is trying to attain clear vision. For example, patients with double vision may cock the head to the side to focus the two images into one, or they may close one eye to see clearly.

Assess for symmetry in the appearance of the eyes. Determine whether they are equally distant from the nose, are the same size, and have the same degree of prominence. Assess for their placement in the orbits and for symmetry of movement. *Exophthalmos (proptosis)* is protrusion of the eye. *Enophthalmos* is the sunken appearance of the eye.

Examine the eyebrows and eyelashes for hair distribution and determine the direction of the eyelashes. Eyelashes normally point outward and away from the eyelid. Assess the eyelids for ptosis (drooping), redness, lesions, or swelling. The lids normally close completely, with the lid edges touching. When the eyes are open, the upper lid covers a small portion of the iris. The edge of the lower lid lies at the iris. No sclera should be visible between the eyelid and the iris.

Scleral and corneal assessment require a penlight. Examine the sclera for color; it is usually white. In patients with light skin, a yellow color may indicate jaundice or systemic problems. In adults with dark skin, the normal sclera may appear yellow; and small, pigmented dots may be visible (Jarvis, 2020).

The cornea is best seen by directing a light at it from the side. It should be transparent, smooth, shiny, and bright. Any cloudy areas or specks may indicate injury.

Assess the blink reflex by bringing a hand quickly toward the patient's face. Use extreme caution when performing this maneuver, especially with confused patients. Patients with vision will blink.

Pupillary assessment involves examining each pupil separately and comparing the results. The pupils are usually round and of equal size, between 3 and 5 mm in diameter. About 20% of adults normally have a noticeable difference in the size of their pupils, which is known as **anisocoria** (Merck Manual, 2019). Pupil size varies in adults exposed to the same amount of light. Pupils are smaller in older adults, which reduces vision in low light conditions. Patients with myopia have larger pupils, whereas those with hyperopia have smaller pupils.

Observe pupils for response to light. Increasing light causes constriction, whereas decreasing light causes dilation. Constriction of both pupils is the normal response to direct light and to accommodation. Assess pupillary reaction to light by asking the patient to look straight ahead while you quickly bring the beam of a penlight in from the side and direct it at the right pupil. Constriction of the right pupil is a direct response to shining the penlight into that eye. Constriction of the left pupil when light is shined at the right pupil is known as a *consensual response*. Assess the responses for each eye. (You may see the abbreviation "PERRLA" in the electronic health record, which stands for **p**upils **e**qual, **r**ound, **r**eactive to **l**ight, and **a**ccommodation.)

Evaluate each pupil for speed of reaction. The pupil should immediately constrict when a light is directed at it (i.e., a *brisk* response). If the pupil takes more than 1 second to constrict, the response is *sluggish*. Pupils that fail to react are *nonreactive* or *fixed*. Compare the reactivity speed of right and left pupils and document any difference.

Assess for accommodation by holding your finger about 18 degrees cm from the patient's nose and move it toward the nose. The patient's eyes normally converge during this movement, and the pupils constrict equally.

Vision Testing. Visual ***sensory perception*** is measured by first testing each eye separately and then testing both eyes together. Patients who wear corrective lenses are tested without and with their lenses. The eye care provider usually conducts this type of testing, which includes:

- Visual acuity testing to measure distance and near vision
- Use of the *Snellen eye chart* to assess distance vision
- Use of the Rosenbaum Pocket Vision Screener or Jaeger card to assess near vision
- Testing for light perception
- Testing the visual field for degree of peripheral vision
- Assessment of extraocular muscle function (Fig. 42.8) and eye alignment, and assessment of color vision via *Ishihara color plates* (Fig. 42.9).

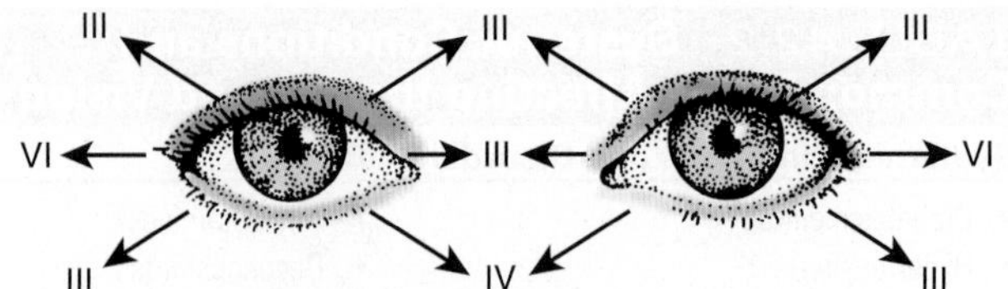

Fig. 42.8 Checking extraocular movements in the six cardinal positions indicates the functioning of cranial nerves III, IV, and VI.

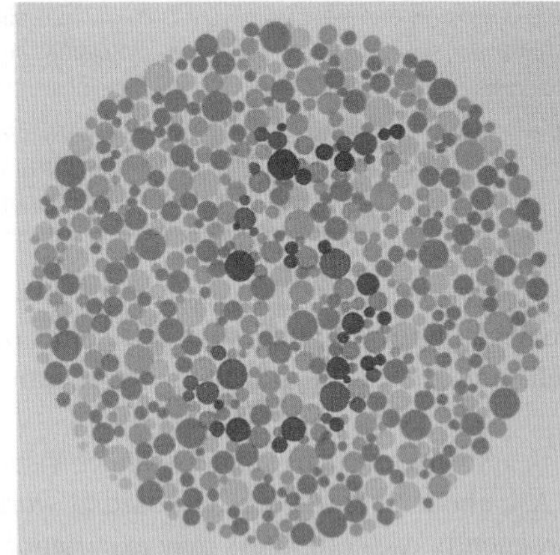

Fig. 42.9 An Ishihara color plate for testing color vision.

Psychosocial Assessment

A patient with changes in visual ***sensory perception*** may be anxious about possible vision loss. Patients with severe visual defects may be unable to perform ADLs. Dependency from reduced vision can affect self-esteem. Ask the patient how he or she feels about vision changes. Assess available family support, and the patient's coping techniques. Provide information about local resources and services as needed.

Diagnostic Assessment

Laboratory Assessment. Results of corneal cultures or conjunctival swabs and scrapings can help diagnose infections. If a culture is ordered, obtain a sample of the exudate from the conjunctiva or an ulcerated or inflamed area before antibiotics or topical anesthetics are instilled.

Imaging Assessment. *CT* is useful for assessing the eyes, the bony structures around the eyes, and the extraocular muscles. It can also detect tumors in the orbital space. A contrast agent is used unless trauma is suspected.

MRI is often used to examine the orbits and optic nerves and to evaluate ocular tumors. It cannot be used to evaluate injuries involving metal in the eyes. *Metal in the eye is an absolute contraindication for MRI.*

Radioisotope scanning is used to locate tumors and lesions. This test requires that the patient sign an informed consent, and sedation may be used for those who are very anxious. A tracer dose of the radioactive isotope is given orally or by injection, and then the patient must lie still. The scanner measures the radioactivity emitted by the radioactive atoms concentrated in the area being studied. No special follow-up care is required.

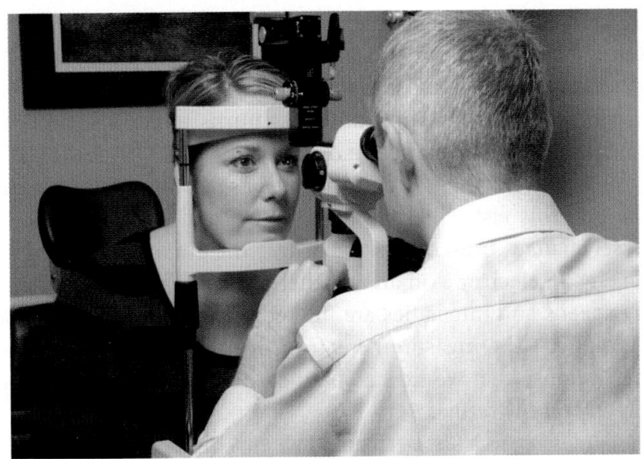

Fig. 42.10 Slit-lamp ocular examination. (From deWit, S. C., Stromberg, H. K., & Dallred, C. V. [2017]. *Medical-surgical nursing* [3rd ed.]). St. Louis: Elsevier.)

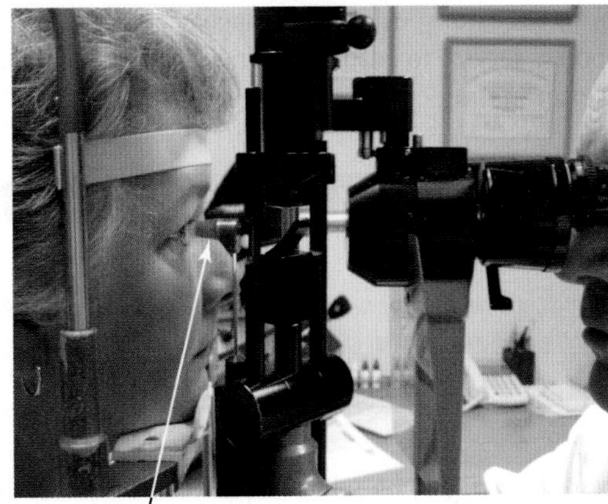

Fig. 42.11 Use of Goldmann applanation tonometer and a slit lamp to measure intraocular pressure.

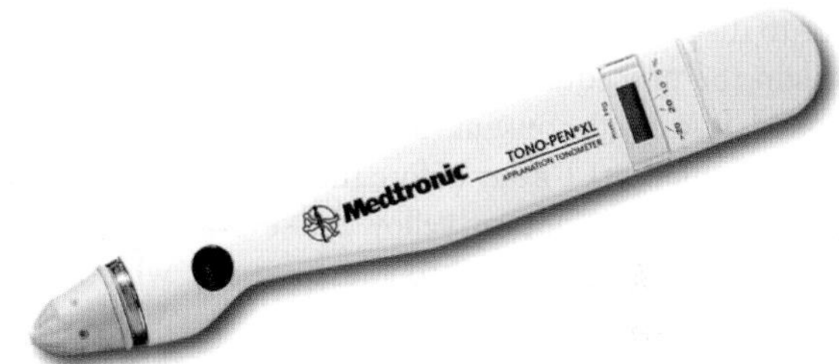

Fig. 42.12 The Tono-Pen XL. (Courtesy Medtronic Ophthalmics, Minneapolis, Minn.)

Ultrasonography is used to examine the orbit and eye with high-frequency sound waves. This noninvasive test helps diagnose trauma, intraorbital tumors, proptosis, and choroidal or retinal detachments. It is also used to determine the length of the eye and any gross outline changes in the eye and the orbit in patients with cloudy corneas or lenses that reduce direct examination of the fundus.

Inform the patient that this test is painless. It is performed with the eyes closed or, when the eyes must remain open, with anesthetic eyedrops instilled first. The patient is usually positioned upright with the chin in the chin rest, although the test can be done with the patient lying back. The probe is touched against the patient's anesthetized cornea, and sound waves are bounced through the eye. The sound waves create a reflective pattern on a computer screen that can be examined for abnormalities. No special follow-up care is needed. Remind the patient not to rub or touch the eye until the anesthetic agent has worn off.

Other Diagnostic Assessment. Many tests are used to examine specific eye structures when patients have risks, signs and symptoms, or exposures. These tests are performed only by health care providers.

Slit-lamp examination magnifies the anterior eye structures (Fig. 42.10). The patient leans on a chin rest to stabilize the head. A narrow beam (slit) of light is aimed so that only a segment of the eye is brightly lit. The eye care provider can then locate the position of any abnormality in the cornea, lens, or anterior vitreous humor.

Corneal staining consists of placing fluorescein or other topical dye into the conjunctival sac, and then the eye is viewed through a blue filter. The procedure is noninvasive and is performed under aseptic conditions. The dye outlines corneal surface irregularities in a bright green color. This test is used to assess corneal trauma, problems caused by a contact lens, or the presence of foreign bodies, abrasions, ulcers, or other corneal disorders.

Tonometry measures intraocular pressure (IOP) using a tonometer, which applies pressure to the outside of the eye until it equals the pressure inside the eye. The thickness of the cornea affects how much pressure must be applied before indentation occurs. Tonometer readings are indicated for all patients older than 40 years of age. Adults with a family history of glaucoma should have their IOP measured once or twice a year. Normal readings range from 10 to 20 mm Hg (Gudgel, 2018). IOP varies throughout the day and typically peaks at certain times of the day. Therefore always document the type and time of measurement.

The most common instrument used by eye care providers to measure IOP is the Goldmann applanation tonometer used with a slit lamp (Fig. 42.11). This method involves direct eye contact. Another instrument, the Tono-Pen XL (Fig. 42.12), is designed for use by eye care providers in extended care or long-term care facilities or for other patients unable to be positioned behind a slit lamp. Evidence shows that the Goldmann tonometer remains the most reliable method of IOP assessment (Wong et al., 2018).

Ophthalmoscopy allows viewing of the eye's external and interior structures with an *ophthalmoscope*. The health care provider positions the ophthalmoscope to see the patient's eye through the sight hole (Fig. 42.13). A *red reflex* is usually seen in the pupil as a reflection of the light off of the retina. An absent red reflex in an adult may indicate a lens opacity or cloudiness of the vitreous. The provider can also examine the retina, optic disc, optic vessels, fundus, and macula with this tool. Table 42.3 lists the features that can be observed in each structure.

The use of an ophthalmoscope may raise anxiety in some patients. When working with a patient with confusion or a patient who does not speak the language used at the agency, use an interpreter service to ensure understanding and cooperation with the examination.

! NURSING SAFETY PRIORITY (QSEN)

Action Alert

Avoid using an ophthalmoscope with a confused patient or one who does not understand the language spoken at the facility to prevent accidental injury to the eye.

Fluorescein angiography, which is performed by a health care provider, provides a detailed image of eye circulation. Digital pictures are taken in rapid succession after the dye is given IV. This test helps to assess problems of retinal circulation (e.g., diabetic retinopathy, retinal hemorrhage, and macular degeneration) or to diagnose intraocular tumors.

Explain the procedure to the patient, check that the patient has signed informed consent, and instill mydriatic eyedrops (cause pupil dilation) 1 hour before the test. Teach that the dye may cause the skin to appear yellow for several hours after the test. The stain is eliminated through the urine, which may be green in appearance.

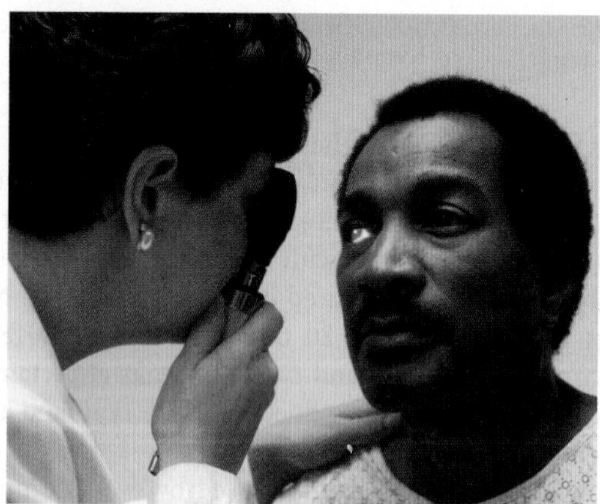

Fig. 42.13 Proper technique for direct ophthalmoscopic visualization of the retina.

TABLE 42.3 Structures Assessed by Direct Ophthalmoscopy

Red Reflex	**Fundus**
• Presence or absence	• Color
Optic Disc	• Tears or holes
• Color	• Lesions
• Margins (sharp or blurred)	• Bleeding
• Cup size	**Macula**
• Presence of rings or crescents	• Presence of blood vessels
Optic Blood Vessels	• Color
• Size	• Lesions
• Color	• Bleeding
• Kinks or tangles	
• Light reflection	
• Narrowing	
• Nicking at arteriovenous crossings	

Encourage patients to drink fluids to help eliminate the dye. Remind them that any staining of the skin will disappear in a few hours. Instruct the patient to wear dark glasses and avoid direct sunlight until pupil dilation returns to normal because the bright light will cause eye discomfort.

Electroretinography graphs the retina's response to light stimulation. This test is helpful in detecting and evaluating blood vessel changes from disease or drugs. The graph is obtained by placing an electrode on an anesthetized cornea. Lights at varying speeds and intensities are flashed, and the neural response is graphed. The measurement from the cornea is identical to the response that would be obtained if electrodes were placed directly on the retina.

Gonioscopy is a test performed when a high IOP is found and determines whether open-angle or closed-angle glaucoma is present. It uses a special lens that eliminates the corneal curve, is painless, and allows visualization of the angle where the iris meets the cornea.

Ultrasonic imaging of the retina and optic nerve (ocular coherence tomography) creates a three-dimensional view of the back of the eye. It is often used for patients with ocular hypertension or who are at risk for glaucoma because of other health problems.

SENSORY PERCEPTION CONCEPT EXEMPLAR: CATARACT

Pathophysiology Review

The lens is a transparent, elastic structure suspended behind the iris that focuses images onto the retina. A **cataract** is a lens opacity that distorts the image (Fig. 42.14). As people age, the lens gradually loses water and increases in density (Touhy & Jett, 2018). Lens density increases with drying and compression of older lens fibers and production of new fibers and lens crystals. With time, as lens density increases and transparency is lost, visual ***sensory perception*** is greatly reduced. Both eyes may have cataracts, but the rate of progression is different in each eye.

Etiology and Genetic Risk. Cataracts may be present at birth or develop at any time. They may be age related or caused by

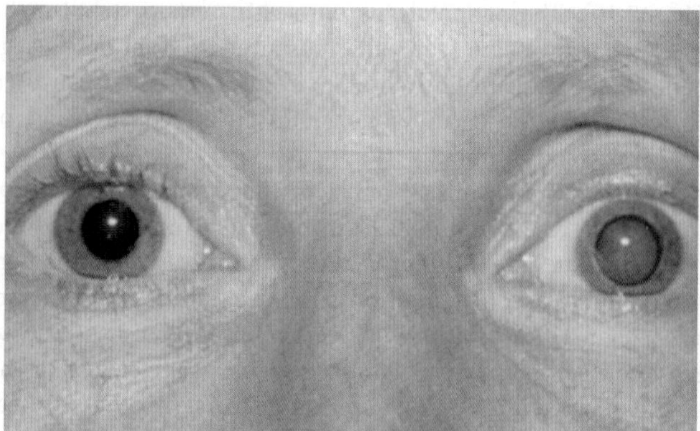

Fig. 42.14 Appearance of an eye with a mature cataract. (From Patton, K. T., & Thibodeau, G. A. [2016]. *Anatomy and physiology* [9th ed.]. St. Louis: Mosby.)

TABLE 42.4 Common Causes of Cataracts

Age	**Health Conditions**
• Lens water loss and fiber compaction	• Diabetes mellitus
Trauma	• Hypoparathyroidism
• Blunt injury to eye or head	• Down syndrome
• Penetrating eye injury	• Chronic sunlight exposure
• Intraocular foreign bodies	**Complications**
• Radiation exposure, therapy	• Retinitis pigmentosa
Toxin Exposure	• Glaucoma
• Corticosteroids	• Retinal detachment
• Phenothiazine derivatives	
• Miotic agents	

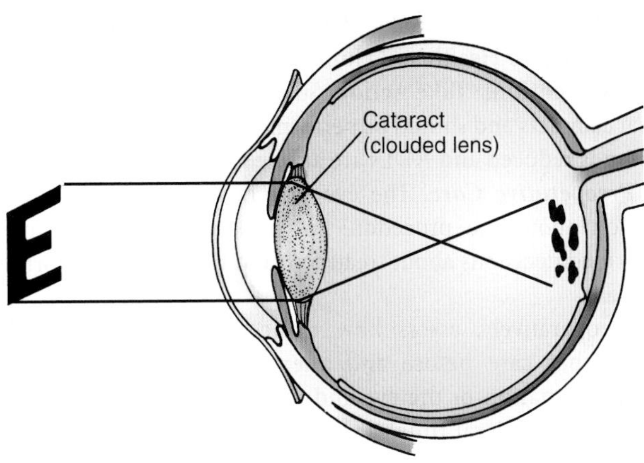

Fig. 42.15 Visual impairment produced by the presence of a cataract.

trauma or exposure to toxic agents. They also occur with other diseases and eye disorders (Table 42.4).

Incidence and Prevalence. The age-related cataract is the most common type. By age 75, more than half of all Americans have had a cataract (American Academy of Ophthalmology, 2020).

Health Promotion and Maintenance

Although most cases of cataracts in North America are age related, the onset of cataract formation occurs earlier with heavy sun exposure or exposure to other sources of ultraviolet (UV) light. Teach adults to reduce the risk for cataracts by wearing sunglasses that limit exposure to UV light whenever they are outdoors in the daytime. Cataracts also may result from direct eye injury. Urge adults to wear eye and head protection during sports, such as baseball, or any activity that increases the risk for the eye being hit. Individuals who smoke are at higher risk for development of cataracts versus nonsmokers (Boyd, 2020).

❖ Interprofessional Collaborative Care

Care for the patient with cataracts occurs in the community, with the exception of the surgical procedure, which takes place in an ambulatory surgical setting.

◆ Assessment: Recognize Cues

History. Age is important because cataracts are most prevalent in the older adult. Ask about these other predisposing factors:

- Recent or past trauma to the eye
- Exposure to radioactive materials, x-rays, or UV light
- Prolonged use of corticosteroids, chlorpromazine, or beta blockers
- Presence of intraocular disease (e.g., recurrent uveitis)
- Presence of systemic disease (e.g., diabetes mellitus, hypoparathyroidism, hypertension)
- Previous cataract, or family history of cataracts
- History of smoking

Ask the patient to describe his or her vision. For example, you might say, "Tell me what you can see well and what you have difficulty seeing."

Physical Assessment/Clinical Signs and Symptoms. Early signs and symptoms of cataracts are slightly blurred vision and decreased color perception. At first the patient may think that his or her glasses are smudged, or contacts are not fitting correctly. As lens cloudiness continues, blurred and/or double vision occurs and the patient may have difficulty with ADLs. Patients commonly report increasing difficulty seeing at night, especially while driving. Without surgical intervention, visual impairment progresses to blindness. *No pain or eye redness is associated with age-related cataract formation.*

Unless a cataract has matured, it is not always visible to the naked eye upon examination. Visual ***sensory perception*** is tested using an eye chart and brightness acuity testing. The health care provider will examine the lens with an ophthalmoscope and note any observed densities by size, shape, and location. A slit lamp can also be used to visualize the cornea, iris (and space between the cornea and iris), and lens. A retinal examination will also likely be performed to clearly see the back of the eye. As a cataract matures, the opacity makes it difficult to see the retina, and the red reflex may be absent. When this occurs, the pupil is bluish white (Fig. 42.15).

Psychosocial Assessment. Loss of vision is gradual, and the patient may not be aware of it until reading or driving is affected. The patient may have anxiety about loss of independence. Encourage the patient and family to express concerns about reduced vision.

◆ Analysis: Analyze Cues and Prioritize Hypotheses. The priority collaborative problem for patients with cataracts is:

1. Impaired visual ***sensory perception*** due to cataracts

◆ Planning and Implementation: Generate Solutions and Take Action. The priority problem for the patient with cataracts is impaired visual ***sensory perception,*** which is a safety risk. Patients often live with reduced vision for years before the cataract is removed.

Improving Vision

Planning: Generate Solutions. As long as a patient does not have cognitive deficits, he or she is expected to recognize when ADLs cannot be performed safely and independently due to cataracts. At that time, surgery is indicated. For patients on Medicare, coverage is provided for an intraocular lens that is implanted during cataract surgery; the cost of the facility, provider, and supplies needed to perform the surgery; and one pair of eyeglasses or contact lenses after cataract surgery (U.S. Department of Health and Human Services, 2018).

Interventions: Take Action. Surgery is the only treatment to treat cataracts and should be performed as soon as possible after vision is reduced and ADLs are affected.

Preoperative Care. The eye care provider provides information about the procedure so that the patient can make informed decisions about treatment and then obtains informed consent.

Preoperatively, assess how reduced vision affects ADLs. Teach that care before and after surgery requires regular self-examination of the eye and instillation of different types of eyedrops several times a day for 2 to 4 weeks. In very rare cases, an ophthalmologist will not prescribe eyedrops before surgery; advise the patient to clarify with the ophthalmologist whether there is a need, or lack of need, to use them before the procedure (American Academy of Ophthalmology, 2017). If the patient is unable to instill the drops, help him or her make arrangements for this care.

Ask whether the patient takes any drugs that affect blood clotting, such as aspirin, warfarin, clopidogrel, and dabigatran. Communicate this information to the surgeon because, for some patients, these drugs may need to be discontinued before cataract surgery.

A series of ophthalmic drugs are instilled just before surgery to dilate the pupils and cause vasoconstriction. Other eyedrops are instilled to induce paralysis to prevent lens movement. When the patient is in the surgical area, a local anesthetic is injected into the muscle cone behind the eye for anesthesia and eye paralysis.

Operative Procedures. The lens is often extracted by *phacoemulsification* (Fig. 42.16), in which a probe is inserted through the capsule and high-frequency sound waves break the lens into small pieces, which are then removed by suction. The replacement intraocular lens (IOL) is placed inside the capsule to be positioned so that light rays are focused in the retina. The IOL is a small, clear, plastic lens. Different types are available, and one is selected by the surgeon and patient to allow correction of a specific refractive error. Some patients have distant vision restored to 20/20 and may need glasses only for reading or close work. Some replacement lenses have multiple focal planes and may correct vision to the extent that glasses or contact lenses may not be needed.

CLINICAL JUDGMENT CHALLENGE 42.1

Patient-Centered Care

A 66-year-old female client is taking part in a community health fair, which offers free vision screenings. The nurse takes a brief history, noting that the client reports having type 2 diabetes, hypertension, and a history of seasonal allergies related to pollen and mold. She lives in a one-bedroom apartment in a city. Social history reveals that the client smokes one pack of cigarettes per day and consumes an occasional glass of wine at celebratory events two to three times per year. The client reports that over the past few months, she has noticed that it is becoming harder to see clearly out of her right eye and difficult to see at night when she drives. She finds herself squinting in an attempt to clear her vision, yet the field does not seem to change. While performing an assessment, the nurse does not observe any unusual findings in either eye.

1. **Recognize Cues:** What assessment information in this client situation is the most important and immediate concern for the nurse? (Hint: Identify the **relevant** information *first* to determine what is most important.)
2. **Analyze Cues:** What client conditions are consistent with the **most relevant** information? (Hint: Think about priority collaborative problems that support and contradict the information presented in this situation.)
3. **Prioritize Hypotheses:** Which possibilities or explanations are **most likely** to be present in this client situation? Which possibilities or explanations are the most serious? (Hint: Consider all possibilities and determine their urgency and risk for this client.)
4. **Generate Solutions:** What interventions would most likely achieve the desired outcomes for this client? Which interventions should be **avoided** or are **potentially harmful**? (Hint: Determine the desired outcomes first to decide which interventions are appropriate and those that should be avoided.)
5. **Take Action:** Which interventions are the most appropriate, and how should they be implemented? In what **priority order** should they be implemented? (Hint: Consider health teaching, documentation, requested health care provider orders or prescriptions, nursing skills, collaboration with or referral to health team members, etc.)
6. **Evaluate Outcomes:** What client assessment would indicate that the nurse's interventions were **effective**? (Hint: Think about signs that would indicate an improvement, decline, or unchanged client condition.)

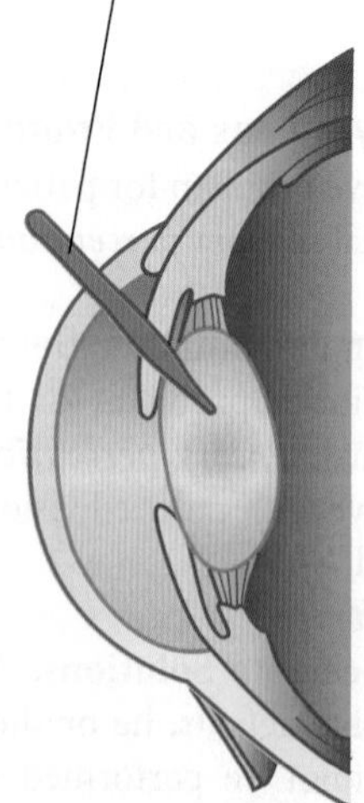
Sound wave and suctioning probe
Sound waves break up the lens, pieces are sucked out, and the capsule remains largely intact

Fig. 42.16 Cataract removal by phacoemulsification.

Postoperative Care. Immediately after surgery, antibiotic and steroid ointments are instilled. The patient is usually discharged within an hour after surgery, after stabilization and monitoring. Instruct him or her to wear dark glasses outdoors or in brightly lit environments until the pupil responds to light. Teach the patient and family members how to instill the prescribed eyedrops. Help them create a written schedule for the timing and the order of eyedrops administration. Remind the patient that vision in that eye will be blurred and to not drive or operate heavy machinery until the ointment is removed. Stress the importance of keeping all follow-up appointments.

TABLE 42.5 Activities That Increase Intraocular Pressure

- Bending from the waist
- Lifting objects weighing more than 10 lb.
- Sneezing, coughing
- Blowing the nose
- Straining to have a bowel movement
- Vomiting
- Having sexual intercourse
- Keeping the head in a dependent position
- Wearing tight shirt collars

Remind the patient that mild eye itching is normal, as is a "bloodshot appearance." The eyelid may be slightly swollen. However, significant swelling or bruising is abnormal. Cool compresses may be beneficial. Discomfort at the site is controlled with acetaminophen or acetaminophen with oxycodone as prescribed. Aspirin is avoided because of its effects on blood clotting.

Pain early after surgery may indicate increased intraocular pressure (IOP) or hemorrhage. Instruct patients to contact the surgeon if pain occurs with nausea or vomiting.

To prevent increases in IOP, teach the patient and family about activity restrictions. Activities that can cause a sudden rise in IOP are listed in Table 42.5.

Infection is a potential and serious complication. Teach the patient and family to observe for increasing eye redness, a decrease in vision, or an increase in tears and photophobia. Creamy white, dry, crusty drainage on the eyelids and lashes is normal. However, yellow or green drainage indicates infection and must be reported. Stress the importance of proper handwashing to reduce the potential for infection.

Patients usually experience a dramatic improvement in vision within a day of surgery. Remind them that final best vision will not occur until 4 to 6 weeks after surgery.

! NURSING SAFETY PRIORITY (QSEN)

Action Alert

Instruct the patient who has had cataract surgery to immediately report any reduction of vision in the eye that just had the cataract removed.

Care Coordination and Transition Management. Because the patient is usually discharged within an hour after cataract surgery, nursing interventions focus on helping the patient and family plan the eyedrop schedule and daily home eye examination.

Home Care Management. If the patient has difficulty instilling eyedrops, a supportive neighbor, friend, or family member can be taught the procedure. Adaptive equipment that positions the bottle of eyedrops directly over the eye can also be purchased (Fig. 42.17).

Self-Management Education. To achieve best results of cataract removal, the patient must be taught to closely adhere to the eyedrop regimen after surgery. Providing the patient or family with accurate information and demonstration of needed skills are nursing priorities. Before discharge, review these complications with the patient and family. Although complications are not anticipated, teach the patient to immediately report any of these symptoms following cataract surgery:

- Sharp, sudden pain in the eye
- Bleeding or increased discharge from the eye
- Green or yellow, thick drainage from the eye
- Eyelid swelling of the eye
- Reappearance of a bloodshot sclera after the initial appearance has cleared
- Decreased vision in the eye that had surgery
- Flashes of light or floating shapes seen in the eye

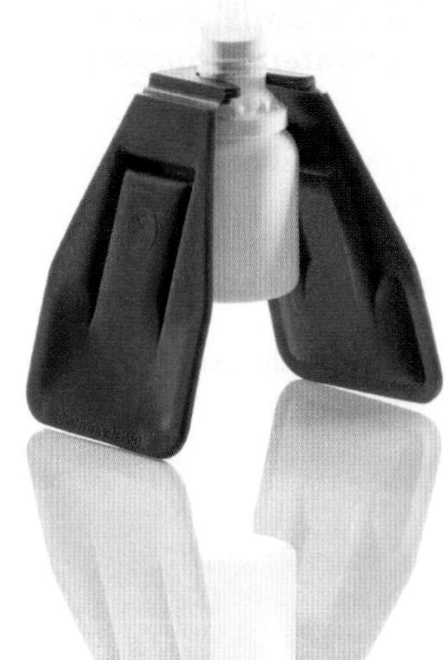

Fig. 42.17 Autosqueeze, a mechanism for self-administering eyedrops. (Courtesy Owen Mumford, Marietta, Ga.)

Remind the patient to avoid activities that can increase IOP (see Table 42.5). Some patients are prescribed to wear a light eye patch at night to prevent accidental rubbing. Instruct the patient to avoid getting water in the eye for 3 to 7 days after surgery.

Teach the patient about activity restrictions. Cooking and light housekeeping are permitted, but vacuuming should be avoided for several weeks because of the forward flexion involved and the rapid, jerky movements required. Advise the patient to refrain from driving until vision is clear. The Home Care Considerations: The Patient After Cataract Surgery box lists items to cover in the focused assessment of a patient at home after cataract surgery.

Health Care Resources. If the patient lives alone and has no support, arrange for a home care nurse to assess him or her and the home situation.

◆ Evaluation: Evaluate Outcomes. Evaluate the care of the patient with cataracts on the basis of improving visual ***sensory perception.*** The expected outcomes include that the patient will have improved visual ***sensory perception*** following surgery and recognize signs and symptoms of complications.

HOME CARE CONSIDERATIONS

The Patient After Cataract Surgery

Assess:
- Visual acuity in both eyes using a handheld eye chart
- Visual fields of both eyes
- Presence or absence of redness, tearing, and/or draining in the operative eye in comparison with the nonoperative eye

Ask the patient:
- If there is pain in or around the operative eye
- If there have been any changes in vision (decreased or improved) in the operative eye
- Whether any of these have been noticed in the operative eye:
  - Dark spots
  - Increase in the number of floaters
  - Bright flashes of light

Assess the home environment for:
- Safety hazards (especially tripping and falling hazards)
- Level of room lighting

Assess patient adherence to, and understanding of, treatment and limitations, such as:
- Signs and symptoms to report
- Drug regimen
- Activity restrictions
- Ability to perform ADLs

NCLEX EXAMINATION CHALLENGE 42.3

Physiological Adaptation: Reduction of Risk Potential

Which client statement affirms that nurse teaching about instillation of multiple different eyedrops has been effective? **Select all that apply.**

A. "It will be very easy for me to instill all of the drops at one time."
B. "A schedule will help me remember when to instill the eyedrops."
C. "If I have trouble instilling the drops, there are devices that can be helpful."
D. "I can label the eyedrops by color to help me easily distinguish which one is which."
E. "I will not touch the droppers to my eyes as this can cause contamination and infection."

SENSORY PERCEPTION CONCEPT EXEMPLAR: GLAUCOMA

Pathophysiology Review

Glaucoma is a group of eye disorders resulting in increased intraocular pressure (IOP). As described earlier in this chapter, the eye is a hollow organ. For proper eye function, the gel in the posterior segment (vitreous humor) and the fluid in the anterior segment (aqueous humor) must be present in set amounts that apply pressure inside the eye to keep it ball shaped.

In adults, the volume of the vitreous humor does not change. However, the aqueous humor is continuously made from blood plasma by the ciliary bodies located behind the iris and just in front of the lens (see Fig. 42.2). The fluid flows through the pupil into the bulging area in front of the iris. At the outer edges of the iris beneath the cornea, blood vessels collect fluid and return it to the blood. Usually about 1 mL of aqueous humor is always present, but it is continuously made and reabsorbed at a rate of about 5 mL daily. A normal IOP requires a balance between production and outflow of aqueous humor (McCance et al., 2019). If the IOP becomes too high, the extra pressure compresses retinal blood vessels and photoreceptors and their synapsing nerve fibers. This compression results in poorly oxygenated photoreceptors and nerve fibers. These sensitive nerve tissues become ischemic and die. When too many have died, vision is lost permanently. Tissue damage starts in the periphery and moves inward toward the fovea centralis. Untreated, glaucoma can lead to complete loss of visual ***sensory perception.*** Glaucoma is usually painless, and the patient may be unaware of gradual vision reduction.

TABLE 42.6 Common Causes of Glaucoma

Primary Glaucoma	Secondary Glaucoma
• Aging	• Uveitis
• Heredity	• Iritis
Associated Glaucoma	• Neovascular disorders
• Diabetes mellitus	• Trauma
• Hypertension	• Ocular tumors
• Severe myopia	• Degenerative disease
• Retinal detachment	• Eye surgery
	• Central retinal vein occlusion

There are several causes and types of glaucoma (Table 42.6), classified as primary, secondary, or associated. The most common type is primary glaucoma. Primary open-angle glaucoma (POAG), the most common form of primary glaucoma, usually affects both eyes and has no signs or symptoms in the early stages. It develops slowly, with gradual loss of visual fields that may go unnoticed because central vision at first is unaffected. At times, vision is foggy and the patient has mild eye aching or headaches. Late signs and symptoms occur after irreversible damage to optic nerve function and include seeing halos around lights, losing peripheral vision, and having decreased visual ***sensory perception*** that does not improve with eyeglasses. Outflow of aqueous humor through the chamber angle is reduced. Because the fluid cannot leave the eye at the same rate that it is produced, IOP gradually increases. Primary angle-closure glaucoma (PACG) or *acute glaucoma* has a sudden onset and is an emergency. The problem is a forward displacement of the iris, which presses against the cornea and closes the chamber angle, suddenly preventing outflow of aqueous humor.

Etiology and Genetic Risk. Anyone can develop glaucoma, although some adults are at higher risk, such as African Americans or Hispanic/Latino Americans over 40 years of age, any individual over 60 years of age, those who have a family history of glaucoma, and adults who have high eye pressure, corneal thinness, and abnormality of the optic nerve (National Eye Institute, 2020).

Incidence and Prevalence. Glaucoma is a common cause of blindness in North America. It is usually age related, occurring in about 3 million adults in the United States (Centers for Disease Control and Prevention, 2018a).

Health Promotion and Maintenance

At this time, there are no known ways to prevent glaucoma. The best prevention against damage that glaucoma can cause is for adults to have eye examinations with glaucoma checks done every 2 to 4 years before age 40, every 1 to 3 years between ages 40 and 54, every 1 to 2 years between ages 55 and 64, and every 6 to 12 months over the age of 65 (Glaucoma Research Foundation, 2017).

❖ Interprofessional Collaborative Care

Care for the patient with glaucoma generally takes place in the community setting. Members of the interprofessional team who collaborate most closely to care for this patient include the eye care provider and the nurse. For patients who experience psychosocial concerns related to decreased visual ***sensory perception,*** collaborate with the mental health provider (see the Interprofessional Collaboration: The Patient With Glaucoma box).

INTERPROFESSIONAL COLLABORATION

The Patient With Glaucoma

The possibility or reality of the loss of vision can be distressing for patients. Numerous studies have identified a connection between glaucoma and anxiety and depression (Quaranta et al., 2016). For patients who experience anxiety or depression related to changes in their sight, collaborate with a mental health professional. You can support the patient at regular visits, and the mental health professional can provide ongoing counseling and support to the patient during this time of transition. According to the Interprofessional Education Collaborative (IPEC) Expert Panel's Competency of Roles and Responsibilities, using the unique and complementary abilities of other team members optimizes health and patient care (IPEC, 2016; Slusser et al., 2019).

◆ Assessment: Recognize Cues

History. Ask about visual symptoms that have developed suddenly or over time. Symptoms of acute angle-closure glaucoma include a sudden visual loss, pain, conjunctival erythema, and corneal edema (Jacobs, 2019). In POAG, patients are often asymptomatic in the early stages. The visual fields first show a small loss of peripheral vision that gradually progresses to a larger loss.

Physical Assessment/Clinical Signs and Symptoms. Ophthalmoscopic examination shows cupping and atrophy of the optic disc. It becomes wider and deeper and turns white or gray. The sclera may appear reddened, and the cornea foggy. Ophthalmoscopic examination reveals a shallow anterior chamber, a cloudy aqueous humor, and a moderately dilated, nonreactive pupil.

Diagnostic Assessment. An elevated intraocular pressure (IOP) is measured by tonometry. In open-angle glaucoma, the tonometry reading is often between 22 and 32 mm Hg (normal is 10 to 20 mm Hg [Gudgel, 2018]). In angle-closure glaucoma, the tonometry reading may be 30 mm Hg or higher. Visual field testing by perimetry is performed, as is visualization by gonioscopy to determine whether the angle is open or closed. Usually the optic nerve is imaged to determine to what degree nerve damage is present.

◆ **Analysis: Analyze Cues and Prioritize Hypotheses.** The priority collaborative problems for patients with glaucoma include:

1. Impaired visual ***sensory perception*** due to glaucoma
2. Need for health teaching due to treatment regimen for glaucoma

◆ Planning and Implementation: Generate Solutions and Take Action

Supporting Visual Acuity via Health Teaching

Planning: Generate Solutions. With proper intervention, the patient is expected to maintain optimum visual acuity as long as possible by adhering to the treatment regimen.

Interventions: Take Action

Nonsurgical Management. Teach the patient that loss of visual *sensory perception* from glaucoma can be prevented by early detection, lifelong treatment, and close monitoring. Use of ophthalmic drugs that reduce ocular pressure can delay or prevent damage. The Patient-Centered Care: Older Adult Considerations: Promote Independent Living in Patients With Impaired Vision box lists ways to help the older-adult patient with reduced visual *sensory perception* to remain as independent as possible. The Best Practice for Patient Safety & Quality Care: Care of the Patient With Reduced Vision box provides a list of interventions to care for any patient who has reduced vision. These interventions can be very helpful when you care for hospitalized patients who have other disorders yet also have sight problems.

Drug therapy for glaucoma works to reduce IOP in several ways. Eyedrops can reduce the production of or increase the absorption of aqueous humor or constrict the pupil so that the ciliary muscle is contracted, allowing better circulation of the aqueous humor to the site of absorption. These drugs do not improve lost vision but prevent further damage by decreasing IOP. Close adherence to the prescribed dosage schedule is essential to receiving the maximum therapeutic effect of the eyedrops, so teach the patient to be dedicated to the regular timing of administration.

The prostaglandin agonist drugs reduce IOP by dilating blood vessels in the trabecular mesh, which then collects and drains aqueous humor at a faster rate. The adrenergic agonists and beta-adrenergic blockers reduce IOP by limiting the production of aqueous humor and by dilating the pupil, which improves the flow of the fluid to its absorption site. Cholinergic agonists reduce IOP by limiting the production of aqueous humor and making more room between the iris and the lens, which improves fluid outflow. Carbonic anhydrase inhibitors directly and strongly inhibit production of aqueous humor. They do not affect the flow or absorption of the fluid. Most eyedrops cause tearing, mild burning, blurred vision, and a reddened sclera for a few minutes after instilling the drug. Specific nursing implications related to drug therapy for glaucoma are listed in the Common Examples of

PATIENT-CENTERED CARE: OLDER ADULT CONSIDERATIONS QSEN

Promote Independent Living in Patients With Impaired Vision

Drugs

- Having a neighbor, relative, friend, or home health nurse visit weekly to organize the proper drugs for each day may be helpful.
- If the patient is to take drugs more than once each day, use a container of a different shape (with a lid) each time. For example, if the patient is to take drugs at 9 AM, 3 PM, and 9 PM, the 9 AM drugs would be placed in a round container, the 3 PM drugs in a square container, and the 9 PM drugs in a triangular container.
- Place each day's drug containers in a separate box with raised letters on the side of the box spelling out the day.
- "Talking clocks" are available for the patient with low vision.
- Some drug boxes have alarms that can be set for different times.

Communication

- Telephones with large, raised block numbers are helpful. Those with black numbers on a white phone or white numbers on a black phone are most easily seen by a patient with low vision.
- Telephones that recognize vocal commands or have programmable automatic dialing feature ("speed dial") are very helpful. Programmed numbers should include those for the fire department, police, relatives, friends, neighbors, and 911.

Safety

- It is best to leave furniture the way the patient wants it and not move it.
- Throw rugs should be eliminated, as these increase the risk for falls.
- Appliance cords should be short and kept out of walkways.
- Chairs with built-in footrests are preferable to footstools.
- Unbreakable dishes, cups, and glasses are preferable to breakable ones.
- Cleansers and other toxic agents should be labeled with large, raised letters.

Food Preparation

- Meals on Wheels America is a service that many older adults appreciate. This service is delivered at the local level and brings food at mealtime, cooked and ready to eat. The cost of this service varies, depending on the patient's ability to pay. Some seniors do not have to pay anything to receive this valuable service.
- Many grocery stores offer a delivery service. Customers can create a cart online or shop by telephone. The store gathers the ordered food and either has it ready for pick-up when a customer arrives or gives it to others who provide a delivery service to the patient's door. Costs vary for this service; some stores charge for each delivery, while others are more affordable by offering an annual subscription fee.
- A microwave oven is a safer means of cooking than a standard stove, although some older patients are afraid of microwave ovens. If the patient has and will use a microwave oven, others can prepare and label meals ahead of time and freeze them for later use. Also, many complete frozen dinners that comply with a variety of dietary restrictions are available to warm in the microwave.
- Friends or relatives may be able to help with food preparation. Often relatives do not know what to give an older adult for birthdays or other gift-giving occasions. One suggestion is a homemade prepackaged frozen dinner that the patient enjoys.

Personal Care

- Handgrips should be installed in bathrooms.
- The tub floor should have a nonskid surface.
- Patients who shave should use an electric shaver rather than a razor.
- Have the patient choose a hairstyle that is becoming but easy to care for; this promotes self-care.
- Home hair-care services are available in some areas.

Diversional Activity

- Some patients can read large-print books, newspapers, and magazines (available through local libraries and vision services).
- Books, magazines, and some newspapers are available on audiotape or by streaming.
- Card games, dominoes, and some board games are available in large, high-contrast print.

BEST PRACTICE QSEN PATIENT SAFETY & QUALITY CARE

Care of the Patient With Reduced Vision

- Always knock or announce your entrance into the patient's room or area and introduce yourself.
- Ensure that all members of the health care team also use this courtesy of announcement and introduction.
- Ensure that the patient's reduced vision is noted in the electronic health record, communicated to all staff, marked on the call board, and identified on the door of the patient's room.
- Determine to what degree the patient can see.
- Orient the patient to the environment, counting steps with him or her to the bathroom.
- Help the patient place objects on the bedside table and do not move them without the patient's permission.
- Remove all obstacles and clutter between the patient's bed and the bathroom.
- Ask the patient what type of assistance is preferred for grooming, toileting, eating, and ambulating; communicate these preferences with staff.
- Describe food placement on a plate in terms of a clock face.
- Open milk cartons; open salt, pepper, and condiment packages; and remove lids from cups and bowls.
- Unless the patient also has a hearing problem, use a normal tone of voice when speaking.
- When walking with the patient, offer him or her your arm and walk a step ahead.

Drug Therapy (Eyedrops): Glaucoma box. It is important to teach the patient about potential interactions that may exist between medications and systemic effects that may occur when using these drugs.

The priority nursing intervention for the patient with glaucoma is teaching. Teach the patient that the benefit of drug therapy occurs only when the drugs are used on the prescribed schedule; therefore, patients must instill drops on time and not skip doses. When more than one drug is prescribed, teach the patient to wait 5 to 10 minutes between drug instillations to prevent one drug from diluting another drug. Stress the need for good handwashing, keeping the eyedrop container

COMMON EXAMPLES OF DRUG THERAPY (EYEDROPS)

Glaucoma

Drug Category	Nursing Implications
Prostaglandin Agonists	
Bimatoprost Latanoprost Travoprost	Teach the patient to check the cornea for abrasions or trauma. *Drugs should not be used when the cornea is not intact.* Teach the patient that eye color darkens, and eyelashes elongate, over time in the eye receiving the drug. *Knowing the side effects in advance reassures the patient that their presence is expected and normal.* If only one eye is to be treated, teach the patient *not* to place drops in the other eye to try to make the eye colors similar. *Using the drug in an eye with normal IOP can cause a* ***lower****-than-normal IOP, which reduces vision.* Warn the patient that using more drops than prescribed reduces drug effectiveness. *Drug action is based on blocking receptors, which can increase in number when the drug is overused.*
Adrenergic Agonists	
Apraclonidine Brimonidine tartrate	Ask whether the patient is taking any antidepressants from the MAO inhibitor class. *These enzyme inhibitors increase blood pressure, as do the adrenergic agonists. When taken together, the patient may experience hypertensive crisis.* Teach the patient to wear dark glasses outdoors and also indoors when lighting is bright. *The pupil dilates (mydriasis) and remains dilated, even when there is plenty of light, causing discomfort.* Teach the patient not to use the eyedrops with contact lenses in place and to wait 15 minutes after using the drug to put in contact lenses, if worn. *These drugs are absorbed by the contact lens, which can become discolored or cloudy.*
Beta-Adrenergic Blockers	
Betaxolol hydrochloride Carteolol Levobunolol Timolol	Ask whether the patient has moderate-to-severe asthma or COPD. *If these drugs are absorbed systemically, they constrict pulmonary smooth muscle and narrow airways.* Teach patients with diabetes to check their blood glucose levels more often when taking these drugs. *These drugs induce hypoglycemia and can mask the hypoglycemic symptoms.* Teach patients who also take oral beta blockers to check their pulse at least twice per day and to notify the primary health care and eye care providers if the pulse is consistently below 60 beats/min. *These drugs potentiate the effects of systemic beta blockers and can cause an unsafe drop in heart rate and blood pressure.*
Cholinergic Agonists	
Carbachol Echothiophate Pilocarpine	Teach the patient not to administer more eyedrops than are prescribed and to report increased salivation or drooling to the primary health care and eye care providers. *These drugs are readily absorbed by conjunctival mucous membranes and can cause systemic side effects of headache, flushing, increased saliva, and sweating.* Teach the patient to use good light when reading and to turn lights on in rooms. *The pupil of the eye will not open more to let in more light, and it may be harder to see objects in dim light. This can increase the risk for falls.*
Carbonic Anhydrase Inhibitors	
Brinzolamide Dorzolamide	Ask whether the patient has an allergy to sulfonamide antibacterial drugs. *Drugs are similar to the sulfonamides; if a patient is allergic to the sulfonamides, an allergy is likely with these drugs.* Teach the patient to shake the drug before applying. *Drug separates on standing.* Teach the patient not to use the eyedrops with contact lenses in place and to wait 15 minutes after using the drug to put in the lenses. *These drugs are absorbed by the contact lens, which can become discolored or cloudy.*
Combination Drug	
Brimonidine tartrate and timolol maleate	Same as for each drug alone.

COPD, Chronic obstructive pulmonary disease; *IOP,* intraocular pressure; *MAO,* monoamine oxidase.

tip clean, and avoiding touching the tip to any part of the eye. Also teach the technique of punctal occlusion (placing pressure on the corner of the eye near the nose) immediately after eyedrop instillation to prevent systemic absorption of the drug (Fig. 42.18).

! NURSING SAFETY PRIORITY (QSEN)

Drug Alert

Most eyedrops used for glaucoma therapy can be absorbed systemically and cause systemic problems. It is critical to teach punctal occlusion to patients using eyedrops for glaucoma therapy (see Fig. 42.18).

Systemic osmotic drugs like IV mannitol may be given for angle-closure glaucoma to rapidly reduce IOP.

Surgical Management. Surgery can be performed when drugs for open-angle glaucoma are not effective at controlling IOP. Two common procedures are laser trabeculoplasty and trabeculectomy. A *laser trabeculoplasty* burns the trabecular meshwork, scarring it and causing the meshwork fibers to tighten. Tight fibers increase the size of the spaces between the fibers, improving outflow of aqueous humor and reducing IOP. *Trabeculectomy* is a surgical procedure that creates a new channel for fluid outflow. Both are ambulatory surgery procedures.

If glaucoma fails to respond to common approaches, an implanted shunt procedure may be used. A small tube or

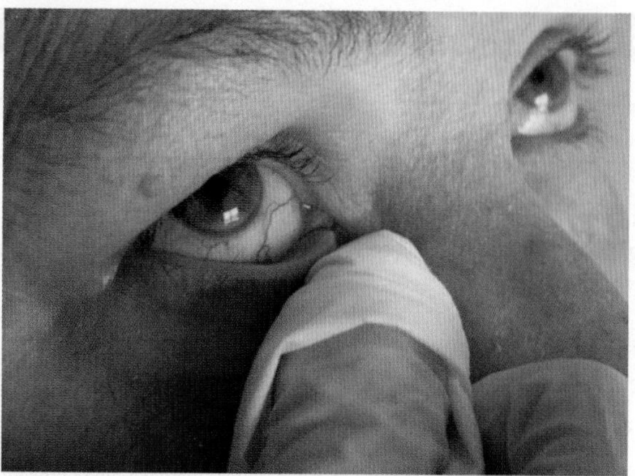

Fig. 42.18 Applying punctal occlusion to prevent systemic absorption of eyedrops. (From Workman, M. L., & LaCharity, L. [2016]. *Understanding pharmacology* [2nd ed.]. St. Louis: Saunders.)

filament is connected to a flat plate that is positioned on the outside of the eye in the eye orbit. The open part of the fine tube is placed into the front chamber of the eye. The fluid then drains through or around the tube into the area around the flat plate, where it collects and is reabsorbed into the bloodstream. Potential complications of glaucoma surgery include choroidal hemorrhage and choroidal detachment.

Care Coordination and Transition Management

Home Care Management. Similar to management of cataracts, the patient with glaucoma will need to instill eyedrops regularly as part of home care. If the patient is unable or resistant to instilling his or her own eyedrops, teach the caregiver the proper technique or recommend adaptive equipment (see Fig. 42.17).

Self-Management Education. The patient with glaucoma is usually managed in the outpatient setting and seen every 1 to 3 months, depending on how well controlled their IOP is. Teach the importance of good handwashing and keeping the tip of the eyedrop container clean. Remind the patient to instill eyedrops on time as recommended by the eye care provider and not to skip doses.

For the patient who has had surgical management, teach the signs and symptoms of choroidal detachment and hemorrhage. These can occur during or after coughing, sneezing, straining at stools, or Valsalva maneuver. Serous detachment involves some degree of vision loss yet is usually painless. Hemorrhagic detachment involves an immediate loss of vision with sudden, excruciating, throbbing pain. Any vision loss, particularly when accompanied by pain, should be reported immediately to the eye care provider.

Health Care Resources. If needed, refer the patient and family to care services that can assist in the home. Support groups for individuals with vision impairment may also be helpful.

NCLEX EXAMINATION CHALLENGE 42.4

Physiological Integrity

What finding does the nurse anticipate when assessing a client with a new diagnosis of glaucoma?

A. Seeing "shooting stars"
B. Decrease in central vision
C. Gradual loss of visual fields
D. Abrupt onset of excruciating pain

◆ **Evaluation: Evaluate Outcomes.** Evaluate the care of the patient with glaucoma based on the identified priority patient problem. The primary expected outcome is that the patient will have optimum visual acuity as long as possible as demonstrated by adherence to the treatment regimen.

CORNEAL DISORDERS

For a sharp retinal image, the cornea must be transparent and intact. Corneal problems may be caused by inflammation of the cornea (keratitis), degeneration of the cornea *(keratoconus)*, or deposits in the cornea. All corneal problems reduce visual ***sensory perception,*** and some can lead to blindness.

CORNEAL ABRASION, ULCERATION, AND INFECTION

Pathophysiology Review

A corneal abrasion is a scrape or scratch injury of the cornea. This painful condition can be caused by a small foreign body, trauma, contact lens use, malnutrition, dry eye syndromes, and certain cancer therapies. The abrasion allows organisms to enter, leading to corneal infection. Bacterial, protozoal, and fungal infections can lead to *corneal ulceration,* a deeper injury. This problem is an emergency because the cornea has no separate blood supply and infections that can permanently impair vision develop rapidly.

❖ Interprofessional Collaborative Care

The patient with a corneal disorder has pain, reduced vision, photophobia, and eye secretions. Cloudy or purulent fluid may be present on the eyelids or lashes. Care for patients with a corneal disorder usually takes place in the community setting. Members of the interprofessional team who collaborate most closely to care for this patient include the eye care provider and the nurse.

◆ **Assessment: Recognize Cues.** Wear gloves when examining the eye. Anticipate the cornea to look hazy or cloudy with a patchy area of ulceration. When fluorescein stain is used, the patchy area appears green. Corneal scrapings (done by an eye care provider after anesthetizing the cornea with a topical agent) and microbial cultures are used to determine the causative organism. For culture, obtain swabs from the ulcer and its edges.

◆ **Interventions: Take Action.** Anti-infective therapy is started before the organism is identified because of the high risk for vision loss. A broad-spectrum antibiotic is prescribed first and may be changed when culture results are known. Steroids may be used with antibiotics to reduce the eye inflammation. Drugs can be given topically as eyedrops or injected subconjunctivally or intravenously. The nursing priorities are to begin the drug therapy, to ensure patient understanding of the drug-therapy regimen, and to prevent infection spread.

Often the anti-infective therapy involves instilling eyedrops *every hour* for the first 24 hours. Teach the patient or family member how to instill the eyedrops correctly.

If the eye infection occurs only in one eye, teach the patient not to use the drug in the unaffected eye. Reinforce the importance of handwashing after touching the affected eye and before touching or doing anything to the healthy eye. If both eyes are infected, separate bottles of drugs are needed for each eye. Teach the patient to clearly label the bottles "right eye" and "left eye" and not to switch the drugs from eye to eye. Remind the patient not to wear contact lenses during the entire time that these drugs are being used because the eye is more vulnerable to infection or injury, and the drugs can cloud or damage the contact lenses.

! NURSING SAFETY PRIORITY QSEN

Action Alert

Teach the importance of applying the drug as often as prescribed, even at night, and to complete the entire course of antibiotic therapy. Treating the infection can save the vision in the infected eye. Remind the patient to make and keep all follow-up appointments.

Drug therapy may continue for weeks to ensure eradication of the infection. Teach patients to avoid using makeup around the eye until the infection has cleared. Instruct them to discard all open containers of contact lens solutions and bottles of eyedrops because these may be contaminated. Patients should not wear contact lenses for weeks to months until the infection is gone and the ulcer is healed.

! NURSING SAFETY PRIORITY QSEN

Drug Alert

Check the route of administration for ophthalmic drugs. Most are administered by the eye instillation route, not orally. Administering these drugs orally can cause systemic side effects and will not therapeutically treat the eye condition. Be sure to reinforce the correct route when teaching the patient.

KERATOCONUS

Pathophysiology Review

The cornea can permanently lose it shape, become scarred or cloudy, or become thinner, reducing useful visual ***sensory perception***. Keratoconus, the degeneration of corneal tissue resulting in abnormal corneal shape, can occur with trauma or may be an inherited disorder (Fig. 42.19). Inadequately treated corneal infection and severe trauma can scar the cornea and lead to severe visual impairment that can be improved only by surgical interventions.

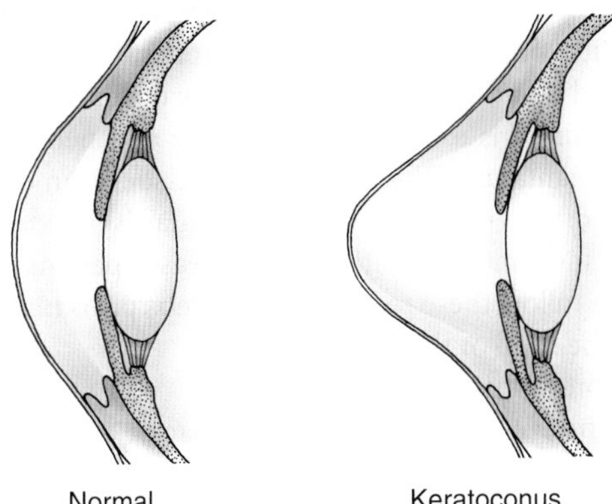

Fig. 42.19 Profile of a normal cornea and one with keratoconus.

❖ Interprofessional Collaborative Care

Keratoplasty (corneal transplant) is a surgical procedure to improve clarity for a permanent corneal disorder that obscures vision. The diseased corneal tissue is removed and replaced with tissue from a cornea donated by a human who has passed away.

Postoperative care involves comprehensive patient teaching. Local antibiotics are injected or instilled. Usually the eye is covered with a pressure patch and a protective shield until the patient returns to the surgeon.

Instruct the patient to lie on the nonoperative side to reduce intraocular pressure (IOP). If a patch is to be used for more than a day, teach application processes. Instruct the patient to wear the shield at night for the first month after surgery and whenever around small children or pets to avoid injury. Instruct him or her *not* to use an ice pack on the eye. Complications after surgery include bleeding, wound leakage, infection, and graft rejection. Teach the patient how to instill eyedrops. Teach him or her to examine the eye (or have a family member examine it) daily for the presence of infection or graft rejection. Stress that the presence of purulent discharge, a continuous leak of clear fluid from around the graft site (not tears), or excessive bleeding needs to be reported immediately to the surgeon. Other complications include decreased vision, increased reddening of the eye, pain, increased sensitivity to light, and the presence of light flashes or "floaters" in the field of vision. These concerns should be reported to the surgeon if they develop after the first 48 hours and persist for more than 6 hours.

The eye should be protected from any activity that can increase the pressure on, around, or inside the eye. Teach the patient to avoid jogging, running, dancing, and any other activity that promotes rapid or jerky head motions for several weeks after surgery. Other activities that may raise IOP and should be avoided are listed in Table 42.5.

Graft rejection can occur and starts as inflammation in the cornea near the graft edge that moves toward the center. Vision is reduced, and the cornea becomes cloudy. Topical corticosteroids and other immunosuppressants are used to stop the rejection process. If rejection continues, the graft becomes opaque and blood vessels branch into the opaque tissue.

Eye donation is a common procedure and needed for corneal transplantation. The Eye Banking Association of America (EBAA, n.d.) has published medical standards that detail donor eligibility and contraindications. If a deceased patient is a known eye donor, follow these recommended steps prior to donation:

- Raise the head of the bed 30 degrees.
- Instill prescribed antibiotic eyedrops.
- Close the eyes and apply a *small* ice pack.

RETINAL DISORDERS

MACULAR DEGENERATION

Pathophysiology Review

Macular degeneration, also known as *age-related macular degeneration* (AMD), is the deterioration of the macula (the area of central vision) and can be age related or exudative. It is the leading cause of blindness in individuals in the United States who are 65 years of age and older (Centers for Disease Control and Prevention, 2018b). There are two types of age-related macular degeneration (AMD): *dry* and *wet.*

Dry AMD is the more common type of this condition. It is caused by a slow and gradual blockage of retinal capillaries by pigmented residue and photoreceptor waste products in the retina, allowing retinal cells in the macula to become ischemic and necrotic. Central vision declines, and patients describe mild blurring and distortion at first. Night vision is impacted, and the ability to see clearly when reading is impaired. Eventually the patient loses all central vision.

Dry AMD progresses at a faster rate among smokers than among nonsmokers. Individuals with diabetes, hypertension, and high cholesterol are at risk for developing this condition. Other risk factors include being older than 60 years old, being Caucasian, and having a family history of AMD (National Eye Institute, 2019).

Wet (exudative) AMD progresses quickly. Patients experience a sudden decrease in vision after a detachment of pigment epithelium in the macula. Newly formed blood vessels, which have very thin walls, invade this injured area and cause fluid and blood to collect under the macula (like a blister), with scar formation and visual distortion. Wet (exudative) AMD can occur at any age, in only one eye or in both eyes. The patient with dry AMD can also develop wet (exudative) macular degeneration.

❖ Interprofessional Collaborative Care

◆ **Assessment: Recognize Cues.** An eye care provider will likely conduct indirect ophthalmoscopy to assess for gross macular changes, opacities, retinal concerns, and hemorrhage (Rebar & Rebar, 2019). IV fluorescein angiography may be performed by the eye care provider to locate leaking vessels, and Amsler's grid test may be conducted to demonstrate central visual field loss (Rebar & Rebar, 2019).

◆ **Interventions: Take Action.** Dry AMD has no cure. Management in the community setting is focused on slowing the progression of the vision loss and helping the patient maximize remaining vision and quality of life. The risk for dry AMD can be reduced by increasing long-term dietary intake of the carotenoids *lutein* and *zeaxanthin* (American Optometric Association, 2020).

Central vision loss reduces the ability to read, write, recognize safety hazards, and drive. Suggest alternatives (e.g., large-print books, public transportation) and refer to community resources that provide adaptive equipment.

Management of patients with wet (exudative) AMD involves slowing the process and identifying further changes in visual perception. Fluid and blood may reabsorb in some patients. Laser therapy to seal the leaking blood vessels can limit the extent of the damage. Ocular injections with the vascular endothelial growth factor inhibitors (VEGFIs), such as bevacizumab or ranibizumab, can improve vision for the patient with wet AMD.

NCLEX EXAMINATION CHALLENGE 42.5

Physiological Integrity

Which patient does the nurse identify at **highest** risk for development of dry age-related macular degeneration (AMD)?

A. 55-year-old client who recently began wearing glasses
B. 59-year-old client who has controlled hypertension
C. 62-year-old client with hypothyroidism
D. 65-year-old client with diabetes

RETINAL HOLES, TEARS, AND DETACHMENTS

Pathophysiology Review

A **retinal hole** is a break in the retina caused by trauma or that occurs with aging. A **retinal tear** is a jagged and irregularly shaped break in the retina, which can result from traction on the retina. A **retinal detachment** is the separation of the retina from the epithelium. Detachments are classified by the type and cause of their development.

One common cause of retinal holes, tears, and detachments is a *posterior vitreous detachment* (PVD). With aging, the vitreous gel often shrinks or thickens, causing it to pull away from the retina. The patient may experience small flashes of light seen as "shooting stars" or thin "lightning streaks" in one eye, most visible in a dark environment. These flashes of light may be accompanied by "floaters." In addition to aging, risk factors for PVD include extreme myopia, inflammation inside the eye, and cataract or eye laser surgery. When the PVD does not cause a retinal tear or detachment, no treatment is needed.

❖ Interprofessional Collaborative Care

◆ **Assessment Recognize Cues.** The onset of a retinal detachment is usually sudden and painless. Patients may report suddenly seeing bright flashes of light (*photopsia*) or floating dark spots in the affected eye. During the initial phase of the detachment or if the detachment is partial, the patient may describe the sensation of a curtain being pulled over part of the visual field. The visual field loss corresponds to the area of detachment. Patients who report this type of concern to a telehealth triage nurse should be cautioned to have another individual drive them to their eye care provider of choice.

The eye care provider will perform an ophthalmoscopic examination. Detachments are seen as gray bulges or folds in the retina. Sometimes a hole or tear may be seen at the edge of the detachment.

◆ **Interventions: Take Action.** If a retinal hole or tear is discovered before it causes a detachment, the defect may be closed or sealed. Closure prevents fluid from collecting under the retina and reduces the risk for a detachment. Treatment involves creating a scar with laser photocoagulation or a freezing probe *(cryopexy)* that will bind the retina and choroid together around the break.

Spontaneous reattachment of a totally detached retina is rare. Surgical repair—called *scleral buckling*—is needed to place the retina in contact with the underlying structures.

Preoperative Care. Most patients are anxious and fearful about the possible permanent loss of vision. Nursing priorities include providing information and support.

Instruct the patient to restrict activity and head movement before surgery to prevent further tearing or detachment. An eye patch is placed over the affected eye to reduce eye movement. Topical drugs are given before surgery to inhibit pupil constriction and accommodation.

Operative Procedures. Surgery is performed with the patient under general anesthesia. In scleral buckling, the eye surgeon repairs wrinkles or folds in the retina and indents the eye surface to relieve the tugging pressure on the retina. The indentation or "buckling" is performed by placing a small piece of silicone against the outside of the sclera and holding it in place with an encircling band. This device keeps the retina in contact with the choroid for reattachment. Any fluid under the retina is drained.

Silicone oil or gas is placed inside the eye to promote retinal reattachment. These agents float up and against the retina to hold it in place until healing occurs.

Postoperative Care. After surgery an eye patch and shield are usually applied. Monitor the patient's vital signs, and check the eye patch and shield for drainage.

Activity after surgery varies. If oil or gas has been placed in the eye, teach the patient to keep his or her head in the position instructed by the surgeon to promote reattachment. Teach the patient to report sudden increase in pain or pain occurring with nausea to the surgeon immediately. Remind him or her to avoid activities that increase intraocular pressure (IOP) (see Table 42.5).

Instruct the patient to avoid reading, writing, and work that requires close vision in the first week after surgery because these activities cause rapid eye movements and detachment. Teach the signs and symptoms of infection and detachment (sudden reduced visual acuity, eye pain, pupil that *does not constrict* in response to light) and to notify the surgeon immediately if these symptoms occur.

REFRACTIVE ERRORS

Pathophysiology Review

The ability of the eye to focus images on the retina depends on the length of the eye from front to back and the refractive power of the lens system. **Refraction** is the bending of light rays. Problems in either eye length or refraction can result in refractive errors.

Myopia is nearsightedness, in which the eye overrefracts the light and the bent images fall in front of, not on, the retina. **Hyperopia**, also called *hypermetropia,* is farsightedness, in which refraction is too weak, causing images to be focused behind the retina. **Presbyopia** is the age-related problem in which the lens loses its elasticity and is less able to change shape to focus the eye for close work. As a result, images fall behind the retina. This problem usually begins in adults in their 40s. **Astigmatism** occurs when the curve of the cornea is uneven. Because light rays are not refracted equally in all directions, the image does not focus on the retina.

❖ Interprofessional Collaborative Care

◆ **Assessment: Recognize Cues.** Refractive errors are diagnosed through a refraction test. The patient is asked to view an eye chart while lenses of different strengths are systematically placed in front of the eye. With each lens strength, he or she is asked whether the lenses sharpen or worsen vision. The strength of the lens needed to focus the image on the retina is expressed in measurements called *diopters.*

◆ **Interventions: Take Action**

Nonsurgical Management. Refractive errors are corrected with eyeglasses or contact lenses that focus light rays on the retina (see Fig. 42.5). Hyperopic vision is corrected with a convex lens that moves the image forward. Myopic vision is corrected with a concave lens that moves the image back to the retina.

Surgical Management. Surgery can correct some refractive errors and enhance vision. The most common vision-enhancing surgery is laser in-situ keratomileusis (LASIK). This procedure can correct nearsightedness, farsightedness, and astigmatism. The superficial layers of the cornea are lifted temporarily as a flap, and powerful laser pulses reshape the deeper corneal layers. After reshaping is complete, the corneal flap is placed back into its original position.

Usually both eyes are treated at the same time, which is convenient for the patient, although this practice has risks. Many patients have improved vision within an hour after surgery, and complete healing takes up to 4 weeks. The outer corneal layer is not damaged, and pain is minimal.

Complications of LASIK include infection, corneal clouding, chronic dry eyes, and refractive errors. Some patients have developed blurred vision, halos around lights, and other refractive errors months to years after this surgery as a result of excessive laser-thinning of the cornea. The cornea then becomes unstable and does not refract appropriately.

Aher procedure, corneal ring placement, can enhance vision for nearsightedness, although this procedure is usually performed for keratoconus.

TRAUMA

Trauma to the eye or orbital area can result from almost any activity. Care varies, depending on the area of the eye affected, whether the globe of the eye has been penetrated, and the mechanism of trauma.

Foreign Bodies

Eyelashes, dust, dirt, and airborne particles can come in contact with the conjunctiva or cornea and irritate or abrade the surface. If nothing is seen on the cornea or conjunctiva, the eyelid is everted to examine the conjunctivae. The patient usually has a feeling of something being in the eye and may have blurred vision. Pain occurs if the corneal surface is injured. Tearing and photophobia may be present.

Visual ***sensory perception*** is assessed before treatment. The eye is examined with fluorescein, followed by irrigation with normal saline (0.9%) to gently remove the particles. Ocular irrigation is discussed in the Best Practice for Patient Safety & Quality Care: Ocular Irrigation box. Remember, if both eyes are affected, irrigate them simultaneously using separate personnel and equipment.

If an eye dressing or patch is applied after the foreign body is removed, tell the patient how long this must be left in place. Follow-up as directed by the eye care provider is needed to confirm that appropriate healing is taking place.

Lacerations

Lacerations are caused by sharp objects and projectiles. The injury occurs most commonly to the eyelids and cornea, although any part of the eye can be lacerated. The patient with a laceration should receive medical attention right away. *Corneal lacerations are an emergency because eye contents may prolapse through the laceration.* Symptoms include severe eye pain, photophobia, tearing, decreased vision, and inability to open the eyelid. If the laceration is the result of a penetrating injury, an object may be seen protruding from the eye.

Minor lacerations of the eyelid can be sutured in an emergency department, an urgent care center, or an eye care provider's office. A microscope is needed in the operating room if the patient has a laceration that involves the eyelid margin, affects the lacrimal system, involves a large area, or has jagged edges.

Antibiotics are given to reduce the risk for infection. Depending on the depth of the laceration, scarring may develop. If the scar alters vision, a corneal transplant may be needed later. If the eye contents have prolapsed through the laceration or if the injury is severe, **enucleation** (surgical eyeball removal) may be indicated.

Penetrating Injuries

A penetrating eye injury often leads to permanent loss of visual ***sensory perception.*** Glass, high-speed metal or wood particles, BB pellets, and bullets are common causes of penetrating injuries. The particles can enter the eye and lodge in or behind the eyeball. A wound may be visible. Depending on where the object enters and rests within the eye, vision may be affected. Never remove an object protruding from the eye; the health care provider will assess the immediate condition and determine how to proceed.

X-rays and CT scans of the orbit are usually performed. MRI is contraindicated because the procedure may move any metal-containing projectile and cause more injury.

Surgery is usually needed to remove the foreign object, and sometimes vitreal removal is needed. IV antibiotics are started before surgery, and a tetanus booster is given if necessary.

BEST PRACTICE FOR PATIENT SAFETY & QUALITY CARE (QSEN)

Ocular Irrigation

1. Assemble equipment:
   - Normal saline IV (1000-mL bag)
   - Macrodrip IV tubing
   - IV pole
   - Eyelid speculum
   - Topical anesthetic (as prescribed)
   - Gloves
   - Collection receptacle (emesis basin works well)
   - Towels
   - pH paper
2. Quickly obtain a history from the patient while flushing the tubing with normal saline, including:
   - Nature and time of the injury
   - Type of irritant or chemical (if known)
   - Type of first aid administered at the scene
   - Any allergies to the "caine" family of medications
3. Evaluate the patient's visual acuity *before* treatment:
   - Ask the patient to read your name tag with the affected eye while covering the good eye.
   - Ask the patient to "count fingers" with the affected eye while covering the good eye.
4. Wash hands and don gloves.
5. Remove contact lenses, if worn, before irrigation.
6. Place a strip of pH paper in the cul-de-sac of the patient's affected eye to test the pH of the agent splashed into the eye and to know when it has been washed out.
7. Instill topical anesthetic eyedrops as prescribed.
8. Place the patient in a supine position with the head turned slightly toward the affected eye.
9. Have the patient hold the affected eye open or position an eyelid speculum.
10. Direct the flow of normal saline across the affected eye from the nasal corner of the eye toward the outer corner of the eye.
11. Assess the patient's comfort during the procedure.

Data from Gwenhure, T. (2020). Procedure for eye irrigation to treat ocular chemical injury. *Nursing Times [online], 116*(2), 46-48.

! NURSING SAFETY PRIORITY (QSEN)

Action Alert

An object protruding from the eye is removed only by an eye care provider because it may be holding the eye structures in place. Improper removal can cause structures to prolapse out of the eye.

GET READY FOR THE NEXT-GENERATION NCLEX® EXAMINATION!

Key Points

Review these Key Points for each NCLEX Examination Client Needs Category.

Safe and Effective Care Environment

- Wash hands and don gloves before touching a patient's eyes or lids or instilling eyedrops. **QSEN: Safety**
- If a patient has discharge from one eye, examine the eye without the discharge first. **QSEN: Safety**
- Avoid performing an ophthalmoscopic examination on a patient with confusion. **QSEN: Safety**
- Use and teach aseptic technique when instilling drugs into the eye. **QSEN: Safety**
- Orient the patient with reduced vision to immediate surroundings. **QSEN: Safety**
- Identify the room of a patient with reduced vision with a sign. **QSEN: Safety**

Health Promotion and Maintenance

- Teach patients to avoid rubbing their eyes. **QSEN: Safety**
- Identify patients at risk for eye injury as a result of occupation or leisure activities. **QSEN: Safety**
- Teach adults to wear eye protection in any environment in which drops or particulate matter is airborne. **QSEN: Safety**
- Teach adults to wear sunglasses that filter UV light outdoors in sunlight. **QSEN: Evidence-Based Practice**
- Teach patients to wash their hands before and after touching the eyes. **QSEN: Safety**
- Encourage adults older than 40 years of age and patients with chronic disorders to have an eye examination with measurement of intraocular pressure (IOP) at least annually. **QSEN: Safety**

Psychosocial Integrity

- Fully explain diagnostic and therapeutic procedures, restrictions, and follow-up care. **QSEN: Patient-Centered Care**
- Provide opportunities for expression of concerns about a change in visual ***sensory perception.*** **Ethics**
- Refer the patient with reduced visual ***sensory perception*** to local services, resources, and support groups for those with impaired vision. **QSEN: Patient-Centered Care**

Physiological Integrity

- Ask about a family history of vision problems because some conditions have a genetic component. **QSEN: Evidence-Based Practice**
- Test the vision of both eyes immediately if a patient has experienced an eye injury or any sudden change in vision. **QSEN: Safety**
- Stress the importance of completing an antibiotic regimen for an eye infection. **QSEN: Evidence-Based Practice**
- Teach patients who are at risk for increased IOP which activities to avoid and how to use glaucoma drops exactly as prescribed. **QSEN: Safety**
- Instruct the patient who had cataract surgery to immediately report any vision reduction after surgery. **QSEN: Safety**
- Never attempt to remove any object protruding from the eye. **QSEN: Safety**
- Collaborate with the interprofessional team to increase the patient's independence and safety within the home and community. **QSEN: Teamwork and Collaboration**

MASTERY QUESTIONS

1. Which symptom will the nurse teach the client who just had surgery to correct a retinal detachment to immediately report to the eye care provider? **Select all that apply.**
   A. Pain in the affected eye
   B. Pus in the affected eye
   C. Decreased visual acuity
   D. Temperature of 99.0°F
   E. Pupil that constricts in response to light

2. Which assessment data do the nurse anticipate when a client presents to the emergency department reporting the sensation of a foreign body in the eye? **Select all that apply.**
   A. Pain
   B. Fever
   C. Tearing
   D. Photophobia
   E. Blurred vision

REFERENCES

American Academy of Ophthalmology. (2017). *Are eye drops always necessary before cataract surgery?*. Retrieved from https://www.aao.org/eye-health/ask-ophthalmologist-q/are-eye-drops-always-necessary-before-cataract-sur.

American Academy of Ophthalmology. (2020). *Eye health statistics*. Retrieved from https://www.aao.org/newsroom/eye-health-statistics#_edn1.

American Optometric Association. (2020). *Lutein & zeaxanthin*. Retrieved from https://www.aoa.org/patients-and-public/caring-for-your-vision/diet-and-nutrition/lutein.

Bagheri, N., & Wajda, B. N. (Eds.). (2017). *The Wills eye manual: Office and emergency room diagnosis and treatment of eye disease* (7th ed.) Philadelphia: Lippincott Williams & Wilkins.

Boyd, K. (2020). *Smoking and eye disease. American Academy of Ophthalmology*. Retrieved from https://www.aao.org/eye-health/tips-prevention/smokers.

Centers for Disease Control and Prevention. (2018a). *Don't let glaucoma steal your sight!*. Retrieved from https://www.cdc.gov/features/glaucoma-awareness/index.html.

Centers for Disease Control and Prevention. (2018b). *Learn about age-related macular degeneration*. Retrieved from https://www.cdc.gov/features/healthyvisionmonth/index.html.

Eisenhauer, B., Natoli, S., Liew, G., & Flood, V. M. (2017). Lutein and zeaxanthin: Food sources, bioavailability and dietary variety in age-related macular degeneration protection. *Nutrition*, *9*(120), 1–14. https://doi.org/10.3390/nu9020.

Eye Banking Association of America (EBAA). (n.d.). Medical standards/procedures manual. http://restoresight.org/what-we-do/publications/medical-standards-procedures-manual/.

Glaucoma Research Foundation. (2017). What can I do to prevent glaucoma? http://www.glaucoma.org/gleams/what-can-i-do-to-prevent-glaucoma.php.

Gudgel, D. (2018). *Eye pressure*. Retrieved from https://www.aao.org/eye-health/anatomy/eye-pressure.

Gwenhure, T. (2020). Procedure for eye irrigation to treat ocular chemical injury. *Nursing Times [online]*, *116*(2), 46–48.

Interprofessional Education Collaborative. (2016). Core competencies for interprofessional collaborative practice: 2016 update. Retrieved from https://nebula.wsimg.com/2f68a39520b03336b41038c370497473?AccessKeyId=DC06780E69ED19E2B3A5&disposition=0&alloworigin=1.

Jacobs, D. (2019). *Open-angle glaucoma: Epidemiology, clinical presentation, and diagnosis*. In *UpToDate*, M. Gardiner (Ed.). Waltham, MA.

Jarvis, C. (2020). *Physical examination & health assessment* (8th ed.). St. Louis: Elsevier.

McCance, K., Huether, S., Brashers, V., & Rote, N. (2019). *Pathophysiology: The biologic basis for disease in adults and children* (8th ed.). St. Louis: Mosby.

Merck Manual. (2019). *Professional version*. Anisocoria. Retrieved from https://www.merckmanuals.com/professional/eye-disorders/symptoms-of-ophthalmologic-disorders/anisocoria.

National Eye Institute of the National Institutes of Health. (2019). *Facts about age-related macular degeneration*. Retrieved from https://nei.nih.gov/health/maculardegen/armd_facts.

National Eye Institute of the National Institutes of Health. (2020). *Facts about glaucoma*. https://nei.nih.gov/health/glaucoma/glaucoma_facts.

PreventBlindnessorg. (2020). How often should I have an eye examination? . Retrieved from https://www.preventblindness.org/how-often-should-i-have-eye-exam.

Quaranta, L., et al. (2016). Quality of life in glaucoma: A review of the literature. *Advanced Therapies*, *33*, 959–981. https://doi.org/10.1007/s12325-016-0333-6.

Rebar, C., & Rebar, M. (2019). *L. Willis's Professional Guide to Pathophysiology* (4th ed.). Philadelphia, PA: Wolters Kluwer. Authors for Chapter 15: Sensory System.

Slusser, M., et al. (2019). *Foundations of interprofessional collaborative practice* (1st ed.). St. Louis: Elsevier.

Touhy, T., & Jett, K. (2018). *Ebersole and Hess' gerontological nursing and healthy aging* (5th ed.). St. Louis: Mosby.

U.S. Department of Health and Human Services. (2018). *Medicare Learning Network: Medicare vision services*. Retrieved from https://www.cms.gov/outreach-and-education/medicare-learning-network-mln/mlnproducts/downloads/visionservices_factsheet_icn907165.pdf.

Wong, B., et al. (2018). Comparison of Disposable Goldmann applanation tonometer, ICare ic100, and Tonopen XL to standards of care Goldmann Nondisposable applanation tonometer for measuring intraocular pressure. *Journal of Glaucoma*, *27*(12), 1119–1124.

43

Assessment and Concepts of Care for Patients With Ear and Hearing Problems

Cherie R. Rebar, Andrea A. Borchers

http://evolve.elsevier.com/Iggy/

LEARNING OUTCOMES

1. Collaborate with the interprofessional team to perform assessments of ears and hearing.
2. Prioritize evidence-based care for patients having assessment or treatment for ear or hearing problems that affect ***sensory perception.***
3. Teach evidence-based ways for adults to protect their ears from injury or infection to preserve ***sensory perception.***
4. Explain how physiologic aging changes of the ears and hearing affect ***sensory perception.***
5. Teach patients who need hearing assistive devices how to use them.
6. Implement nursing interventions to decrease the psychosocial impact on the patient undergoing ear assessment or treatment for ear or hearing problems.
7. Apply knowledge of anatomy and physiology, genetic risk, and principles of aging to perform a focused assessment of the ears and hearing.
8. Use clinical judgment to analyze assessment findings and diagnostic data in the care of patients with an ear or hearing problem.
9. Plan care coordination and transition management for patients with an ear or hearing problem.

KEY TERMS

cerumen The wax produced by glands within the external ear canal; helps protect and lubricate the ear canal.

conductive hearing loss Hearing loss that results from any physical obstruction of sound wave transmission (e.g., a foreign body in the external canal, a retracted or bulging tympanic membrane, or fused bony ossicles).

external otitis A painful irritation or infection of the skin of the external ear, with resulting allergic response or inflammation. When it occurs in patients who participate in water sports, external otitis is called *swimmer's ear.*

frequency The highness or lowness of tones (expressed in hertz). The greater the number of vibrations per second, the higher the frequency (pitch) of the sound; the lower the number of vibrations per second, and the lower the pitch.

grommet A polyethylene tube that is surgically placed through the tympanic membrane to allow continuous drainage of middle ear fluids in the patient with otitis media.

intensity A quality of sound expressed in decibels (dB).

labyrinthectomy Surgical removal of the labyrinth.

mastoiditis An acute or chronic infection of the mastoid air cells caused by progressive otitis media.

Ménière disease Tinnitus, one-sided sensorineural hearing loss, and vertigo that is related to overproduction or decreased reabsorption of endolymphatic fluid, causing a distortion of the entire inner canal system.

mixed conductive-sensorineural hearing loss A profound hearing loss that results from a combination of both conductive and sensorineural types of hearing loss.

myringoplasty Simple surgical reconstruction of the eardrum.

myringotomy The surgical creation of a hole in the eardrum; performed to drain middle ear fluids and relieve pain in the patient with otitis media (middle ear infection).

nystagmus Involuntary eye movements.

ossiculoplasty Replacement of the ossicles within the middle ear.

otoscope An instrument used to examine the ear; consists of a light, a handle, a magnifying lens, and a pneumatic bulb for injecting air into the external canal to test eardrum mobility.

ototoxic Having a toxic effect on the inner ear structures.

presbycusis Sensorineural hearing loss, especially for high-pitched sounds; occurs as a result of aging.

sensorineural hearing loss Hearing loss that results from damage to the inner ear or auditory nerve (cranial nerve VIII).

swimmer's ear See *external otitis.*

threshold The lowest level of intensity at which pure tones and speech are heard by a patient about 50% of the time.

tinnitus A continuous ringing or noise perception in the ear.

vertigo A sense of whirling or turning in space.

PRIORITY AND INTERRELATED CONCEPTS

The priority concept for this chapter is:
- ***Sensory Perception***

The ***Sensory Perception*** concept exemplar for this chapter is Hearing Loss.

The interrelated concepts for this chapter are:
- ***Infection***
- ***Pain***

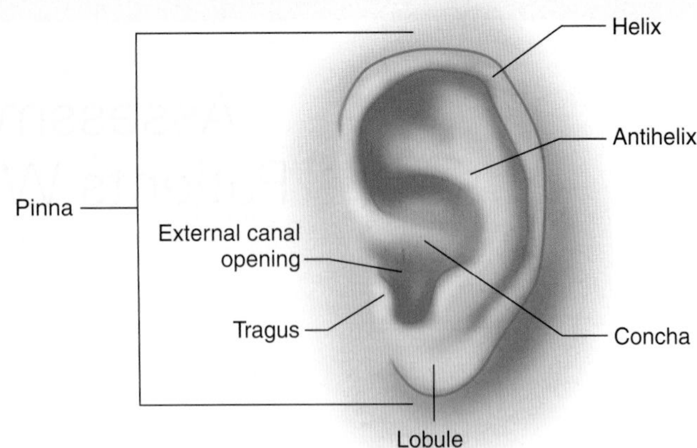

FIG. 43.1 Anatomic features of the external ear.

Used to assess surroundings, promote independence, warn of danger, appreciate music, and communicate with others, hearing is one of the five senses that allow ***sensory perception.*** Because ear and hearing problems are common in adults, assessment is an important skill for nurses practicing in any environment of care. Certain hearing problems develop over long periods and may be affected by drugs or systemic health problems; others occur suddenly, and immediately affect auditory ***sensory perception.*** These problems reduce the ability to fully communicate with the world and can lead to confusion, mistrust, and social isolation.

ANATOMY AND PHYSIOLOGY REVIEW

Structure

The external ear, the middle ear, and the inner ear make up the ear's three divisions.

External Ear. The external ear develops in the embryo at the same time as the kidneys and urinary tract. Any adult with a defect of the external ear should be examined for possible problems of the kidney and urinary systems, also.

The *pinna* is the part of the external ear that is composed of cartilage covered by skin and attached to the head at about a 10-degree angle at the level of the eyes. The external ear extends from the pinna through the external ear canal to the *tympanic membrane* (eardrum) (Fig. 43.1). It includes the *mastoid process,* which is the bony ridge located over the temporal bone behind the pinna. The ear canal is slightly S shaped and is lined with cerumen-producing glands, oil glands, and hair follicles. Cerumen (ear wax) helps protect and lubricate the ear canal. The distance from the opening of the ear canal to the eardrum in an adult is 1 to 1½ inches (2.5 to 3.75 cm).

Middle Ear. The eardrum separates the external ear and the middle ear. The middle ear consists of a compartment called the *epitympanum.* Located in the epitympanum are the top opening of the eustachian tube and three small bones known as the *bony ossicles,* which are the *malleus* (hammer), the *incus* (anvil), and the *stapes* (stirrup) (Fig. 43.2). The bony ossicles are joined loosely, thereby moving with vibrations created when sound waves hit the eardrum.

The eardrum is a thick sheet of tissue; is transparent, opaque, or pearly gray; and moves when air is injected into the external canal. The landmarks on the eardrum include the *annulus,* the *pars flaccida,* and the *pars tensa.* These correspond to the parts of the malleus that can be seen through the transparent eardrum. The eardrum is attached to the first bony ossicle, the malleus, at the umbo (Fig. 43.3). The umbo is seen through the eardrum membrane as a white dot and is one end of the long process of the malleus. The pars flaccida is that portion of the eardrum above the short process of the malleus. The pars tensa is that portion surrounding the long process of the malleus.

The middle ear is separated from the inner ear by the round window and the oval window. The eustachian tube begins at the floor of the middle ear and extends to the throat. The tube opening in the throat is surrounded by adenoid lymphatic tissue (Fig. 43.4). The eustachian tube allows the pressure on both sides of the eardrum to equalize. Secretions from the middle ear drain through the tube into the throat.

Inner Ear. The inner ear is on the other side of the oval window and contains the semicircular canals, the cochlea, the vestibule, and the distal end of the eighth cranial nerve (see Fig. 43.2). The *semicircular canals* are tubes made of cartilage and contain fluid and hair cells. These canals are connected to the sensory nerve fibers of the vestibular portion of the eighth cranial nerve. The fluid and hair cells within the canals help maintain the sense of balance.

The *cochlea,* the spiral organ of hearing, is divided into the scala tympani, the scala media, and the scala vestibuli. The scala media is filled with *endolymph,* and the scala tympani and scala vestibuli are filled with *perilymph.* These fluids protect the cochlea and the semicircular canals by allowing these structures to "float" in the fluids and be cushioned against abrupt head movements.

The *organ of Corti* is the receptor of hearing located on the membrane of the cochlea. The cochlear hair cells detect vibration from sound and stimulate the eighth cranial nerve.

The *vestibule* is a small, oval, bony chamber between the semicircular canals and the cochlea. It contains the utricle and the saccule, organs that are important for balance.

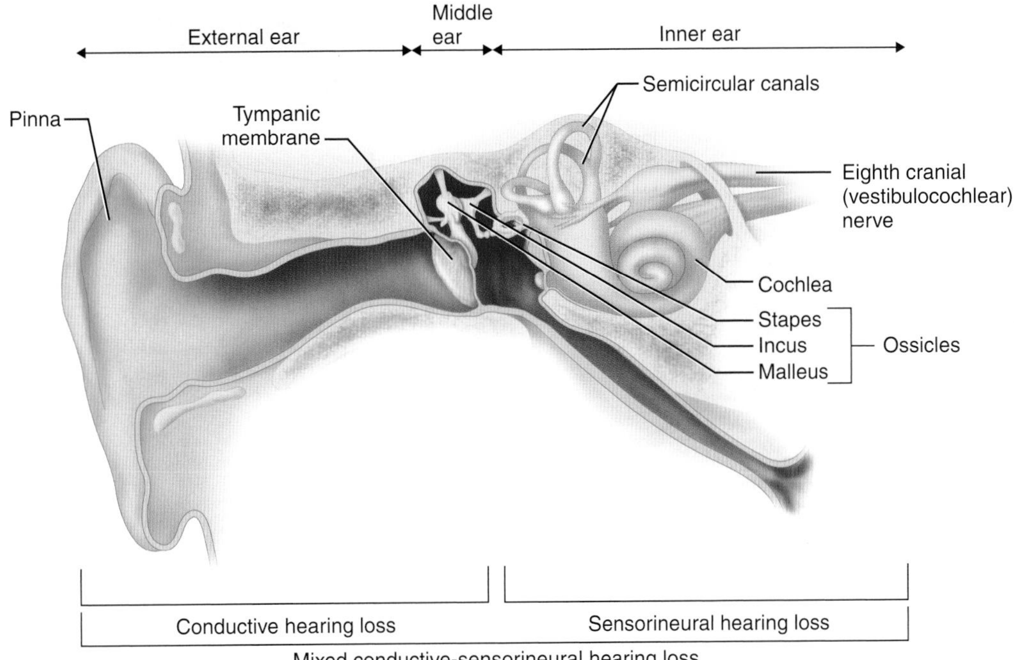

FIG. 43.2 Anatomic features of the middle and inner ear and areas involved in the three types of hearing loss.

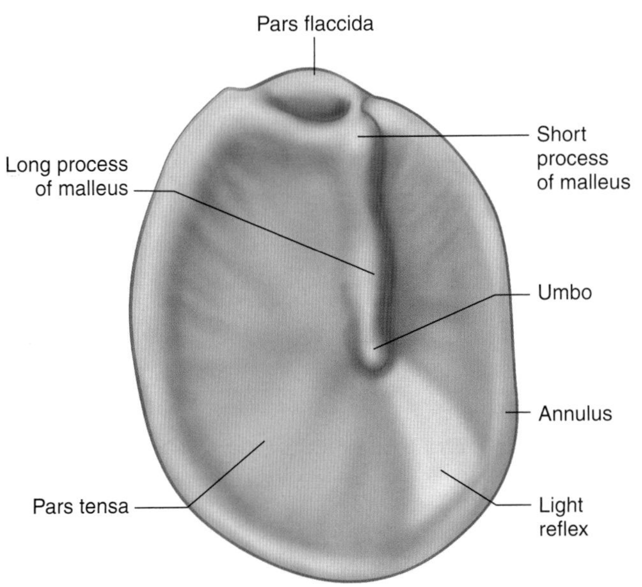

FIG. 43.3 Landmarks on the tympanic membrane.

Function

The ear's function is to promote auditory ***sensory perception,*** which occurs when sound is delivered through the air to the external ear canal. The sound waves strike the movable eardrum, creating vibrations. The eardrum is connected to the first bony ossicle, which allows the sound wave vibrations to be transferred from the eardrum to the malleus, the incus, and the stapes. From the stapes, the vibrations are transmitted to the cochlea. Receptors at the cochlea transduce (change) the vibrations into action potentials. The action potentials are conducted to the brain as nerve impulses by the cochlear portion of the eighth cranial (auditory) nerve. The nerve impulses are processed and interpreted as sound by the brain in the auditory cortex of the temporal lobe.

Ear and Hearing Changes Associated With Aging. All older adults should be screened for hearing acuity. Ear and hearing changes related to aging, and associated nursing adaptations and actions, are listed in the Patient Centered Care: Older Adult Considerations: Age-Related Changes in the Ear and Hearing box. Some of the ear changes do not cause harm; others affect the hearing ability of older adults.

SENSORY PERCEPTION CONCEPT EXEMPLAR: HEARING LOSS

Pathophysiology Review

Loss of auditory ***sensory perception*** is common and may be conductive, sensorineural, or a combination of the two (see Fig. 43.2). **Conductive hearing loss** results from obstruction of sound wave transmission such as a foreign body in the external canal, a retracted or bulging tympanic membrane, or fused bony ossicles. Tumors, scar tissue, and overgrowth of soft bony tissue (**otosclerosis**) on the ossicles from previous middle ear surgery also lead to conductive hearing loss.

Sensorineural hearing loss occurs when the inner ear or auditory nerve (cranial nerve VIII) is damaged. Prolonged exposure to loud noise damages the hair cells of the cochlea.

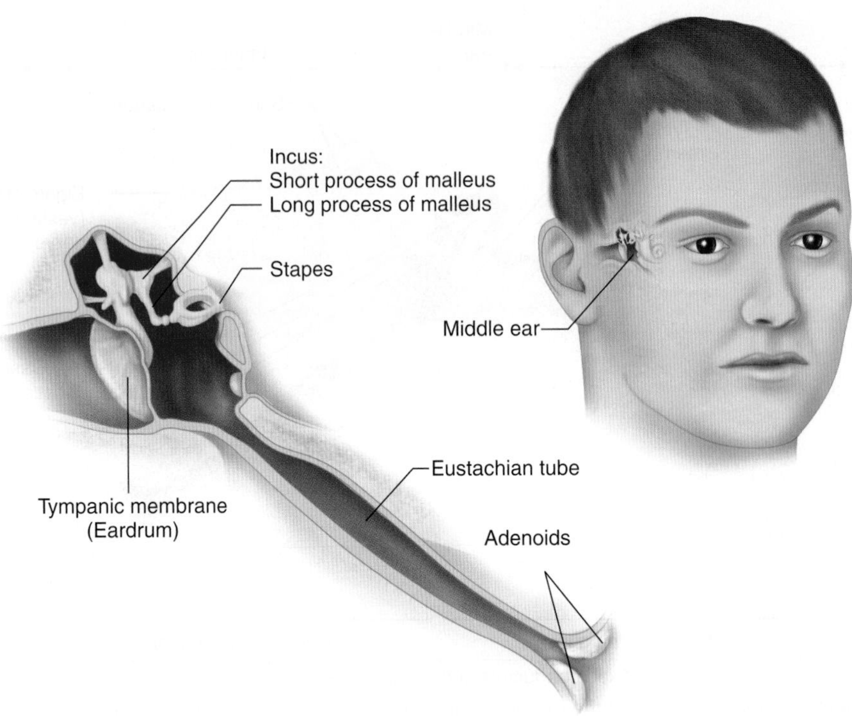

Fig. 43.4 Anatomic features and attached structures of the middle ear.

TABLE 43.1 Comparison of Features of Conductive and Sensorineural Hearing Loss

Conductive Hearing Loss	Sensorineural Hearing Loss
Causes	***Causes***
Cerumen	Prolonged exposure to noise
Foreign body	Presbycusis
Perforation of the tympanic membrane	Ototoxic substance
Edema	Ménière disease
Infection of the external ear or middle ear	Acoustic neuroma
Tumor	Diabetes mellitus
Otosclerosis	Labyrinthitis
	Infection
	Myxedema
Assessment Findings	***Assessment Findings***
Evidence of obstruction with otoscope	Normal appearance of external canal and tympanic membrane
Abnormality in tympanic membrane	Tinnitus common
Speaking softly	Occasional dizziness
Hearing best in a noisy environment	Speaking loudly
Rinne test: air conduction greater than bone conduction	Hearing poorly in loud environment
Weber test: lateralization to affected ear	Rinne test: air conduction less than bone conduction
	Weber test: lateralization to unaffected ear

Many drugs are toxic to the inner ear structures, and their effects on hearing can be transient or permanent.

The differences in conductive and sensorineural hearing loss are listed in Table 43.1. Disorders that cause conductive hearing loss are often corrected with minimal or no permanent damage. Sensorineural hearing loss is often permanent.

Presbycusis is a sensorineural hearing loss that occurs with aging (McCance et al., 2019). It is caused by degeneration of cochlear nerve cells, loss of elasticity of the basilar membrane, or a decreased blood supply to the inner ear. Deficiencies of vitamin B_{12} and folic acid increase the risk for presbycusis (Curhan et al., 2018).

PATIENT-CENTERED CARE: OLDER ADULT CONSIDERATIONS QSEN

Age-Related Changes in the Ear and Hearing

Ear or Hearing Change	Nursing Adaptations and Actions
Pinna becomes elongated because of loss of subcutaneous tissues and decreased elasticity.	Reassure the patient that this is normal. When positioning a patient on the side, do not "fold" the ear under the head.
Hair in the canal becomes coarser and longer, especially in men.	Reassure the patient that this is normal. More frequent ear irrigation may be needed to prevent cerumen attaching to hairs.
Cerumen is drier and becomes impacted more easily, reducing hearing function.	Teach the patient and caregiver to irrigate the ear canal weekly or whenever he or she notices a change in hearing.
Tympanic membrane loses elasticity and may appear dull and retracted.	Although this can indicate otitis media, do not use this as the only sign of this condition in older adults.
Hearing acuity decreases (in some people).	Assess hearing with the voice test or the watch test. If a deficit is present, refer the patient to a specialist to further assess hearing loss and recommend appropriate intervention. Do not assume that all older adults have a hearing loss!
The ability to hear high-frequency sounds is lost first. Older adults may have particular problems hearing the *f, s, sh,* and *pa* sounds.	Provide a quiet environment when speaking (close the door to the hallway) and face the patient. Avoid standing or sitting in front of bright lights or windows, which may interfere with the patient's ability to see your lips move. If the patient wears glasses, be sure that he or she is using them to enhance speech understanding. Speak slowly, clearly, and in a deeper voice and emphasize beginning word sounds. Some patients with an uncorrected hearing loss may benefit from wearing a stethoscope while listening to you speak.

Data from Touhy, T., & Jett, K. (2018). *Ebersole and Hess' gerontological nursing healthy aging* (5th ed.). St. Louis: Mosby.

Any type of hearing loss can impact quality of life, as noted in the Evidence-Based Practice box.

Etiology and Genetic Risk. Family history is important in determining genetic risk for hearing loss. Although most hearing loss resulting from a genetic mutation is noticed in childhood, some genetic problems can lead to progressive hearing loss in adults. For example, most people with Down syndrome develop hearing loss as adults. Assess who in the family experienced hearing problems (and whether problems were present in one gender versus another), at what age the hearing loss was diagnosed, and whether both ears were affected.

EVIDENCE-BASED PRACTICE QSEN

Hearing Loss and Its Impact on Residents of Long-Term Care Facilities

Punch, R., & Horstmanshof, L. (2019). Hearing loss and its impact on residents in long term care facilities: A systematic review of literature. *Geriatric Nursing, 40*(2), 138-147.

With the desire to maximize quality of life for older adults living in long-term care facilities, this systematic review was conducted to determine:

- If there was an association between residents' hearing and quality of life
- Barriers to and facilitators for achieving optimal hearing for these residents
- Barriers to and facilitators for using hearing aids or other assistive devices in long-term care
- Interventions that have been tried or implemented to improve residents' ability to hear

After initial consideration of more than 200 original articles, 22 articles were determined to be useful for this systematic review. Most studies were quantitative in nature; only three were purely qualitative, and four studies used mixed methods. Correlation was demonstrated between hearing loss and quality of life related to communication, social interaction, and psychological well-being. It was noted in many studies that the physical and social environment of the long-term care facility had significant bearing on the residents' abilities to communicate and engage socially.

Very few locations had sound-absorbent materials, quiet rooms, or optimal placement of furniture to facilitate communication. Even in the presence of locations attempting to provide a hearing-friendly environment, background noises including television, music, and loud staff contributed to communication difficulty for residents. Hearing loss was underestimated or unrecognized by staff in some patients, particularly those with dementia. Furthermore, in articles that indicated hearing aids were used by residents, staff members reported having a lack of training to implement and maintain these devices.

Level of Evidence: 1

This research was designed as a systematic review.

Commentary: Implications for Practice and Research

It is important for nurses to recognize hearing difficulties in all patients, especially older adults who may live in residential facilities where noise is not always controlled. The authors of this systematic review noted that the findings strongly suggest the need for environmental optimization with a focus placed on reducing background noises. When possible, sound-absorbent materials should be put in place, and quiet areas should be identified where people can talk together without the distraction of background sounds. Staff need greater training in the use and care of hearing aids and assistive hearing devices; without such, they may not engage residents (or patients) in the ongoing use of these items, which can greatly improve communication and therefore quality of life.

PATIENT-CENTERED CARE: GENETIC/GENOMIC CONSIDERATIONS QSEN

Mutations in several different genes are associated with hearing loss. One type of hearing loss among adults has a genetic basis with a mutation in gene *GJB2* (Online Mendelian Inheritance in Man [OMIM], 2016). This mutation causes poor production of the protein connexin 26, which has a role in the function of cochlear hair cells. Other genetic variations in some of the genes for drug-metabolizing enzymes (cytochrome P-450 family) slow the metabolism and excretion of drugs, including ototoxic drugs. This allows ototoxic drugs to remain in the body longer, thus increasing the risk for hearing loss.

Incidence/Prevalence. Because hearing loss may be gradual and affect only some aspects of hearing, many adults are unaware that their hearing is impaired. The prevalence of adult hearing loss in the United States is estimated to be approximately 15% of the adult population between 20 and 69 years of age; this amount increases among people in their 70s and 80s (National Institute on Deafness and Other Communication Disorders, 2016).

Health Promotion and Maintenance. When the ears are properly cared for, hearing can be preserved to the greatest extent possible. Encourage patients to have simple hearing testing performed as part of their annual health assessment.

Teach adults the danger in using objects such as hairpins, ear candles, cotton swabs, or toothpicks to clean the ear canal. These can scrape the skin of the canal, push cerumen up against the eardrum, and puncture the eardrum. If cerumen buildup is a problem, teach the patient the adhere only to the method of removal recommended by the primary health care provider.

Teach about the use of protective ear devices, such as over-the-ear headsets or foam ear inserts, when exposed to persistent loud noises. To prevent infections, suggest using earplugs when engaging in water sports and using an over-the-counter product such as Swim-Ear to help dry the ears after swimming.

❖ Interprofessional Collaborative Care

You will care for many patients with hearing loss who are seeking treatment for other conditions in a variety of inpatient and outpatient settings. Use the best practices strategies listed in the Best Practice for Patient Safety & Quality Care: Communicating With a Patient Who Is Hearing-Impaired box.

◆ Assessment: Recognize Cues

History. During the interview, sit in adequate light and face the patient to allow him or her to see you speak. The patient's posture and responses can provide information about hearing acuity. Tilting the head to one side or leaning forward when listening to another person speak may indicate the presence of a hearing problem. Other indicators of hearing difficulty include asking the speaker to repeat statements or frequently saying, "What?" or "Huh?" Note whether the patient responds to whispered questions or startles when an unexpected sound occurs in the environment. Assess whether the patient's responses match the question asked. For example, when you ask, "How old are you?" does the patient respond with an age or state, "No, I am not cold."

Obtain data on age, demographics, personal and family history, socioeconomic status, occupational history, current health problems, and the use of remedies for ear problems. The patient's gender is important as some hearing disorders such as otosclerosis are more common in women.

Personal history includes past or current signs and symptoms of ear pain or discharge, **vertigo** (spinning sensation), **tinnitus** (ringing), decreased hearing, and difficulty understanding others when they talk. Ask about:

- Changes in hearing, and when these began
- Head or ear trauma or surgery
- Past ear infections or perforations
- Excessive cerumen
- Type and pattern of ear hygiene
- Drugs used (for any condition), as some are **ototoxic** (having a toxic effect on the inner ear structures), such as NSAIDs, certain antibiotics (e.g., aminoglycosides), diuretics, quinine-based medications, and certain cancer medications (American Tinnitus Association, 2019)
- Exposure to loud noise or music during work or leisure activities
- Air travel (especially in unpressurized aircraft)
- Social or occupational habits that may affect hearing
- Health history of allergies, upper respiratory infections, cancer, hypothyroidism, atherosclerosis, human immune deficiency virus (HIV) disease, or diabetes.

Physical Assessment/Signs and Symptoms. Techniques for assessment of patients with suspected loss of auditory ***sensory perception*** are found in the Focused Assessment: The Patient With Suspected Hearing Loss box. Remember to use Contact Precautions when assessing the ear because drainage may be present.

BEST PRACTICE FOR PATIENT SAFETY & QUALITY CARE (QSEN)

Communicating With a Patient Who Is Hearing-Impaired

- Position yourself directly in front of the patient.
- Ensure that you are not sitting or standing in front of a bright light or window, which can interfere with the patient's ability to see your lips move.
- Make sure that the room is well lighted.
- Get the patient's attention before you begin to speak.
- Move closer to the better-hearing ear.
- Speak clearly and slowly.
- Do not shout (shouting often makes understanding more difficult).
- Keep hands and other objects away from your mouth when talking to the patient.
- Have conversations in a quiet room with minimal distractions.
- Have the patient repeat your statements, not just indicate assent.
- Rephrase sentences and repeat information to aid understanding.
- Use appropriate hand motions.
- Write messages on paper if the patient is able to read.
- Obtain the assistance of an interpreter if needed, and ensure that all members of the interprofessional team use this service.

FOCUSED ASSESSMENT

The Patient With Suspected Hearing Loss

Assess the ability to hear high-frequency consonants (*s, sh, f, th,* and *ch* sounds)

Assess visible ear structures:

- Position, size, and condition of the pinna; abnormalities include redness, excessive warmth, crusting, scaling, nodules, and pain (Jarvis, 2020).
- Patency of the external canal; presence of cerumen or foreign bodies, edema, or inflammation
- Condition of the tympanic membrane: intact, edema, fluid, inflammation
- Mastoid process, which should be free from pain, redness and swelling

Assess functional ability, including:

- Frequency of asking people to repeat statements
- Withdrawal from social interactions or large groups
- Shouting in conversation
- Failing to respond when not looking in the direction of the sound
- Answering questions incorrectly

Assess hearing aids (if present) for cracks, debris, proper fit

Tuning fork tests performed by the primary health care provider can help diagnose hearing loss. *Otoscopic examination,* performed by the primary health care provider with an otoscope, is used to assess the ear canal, eardrum, and middle ear structures that can be seen through the eardrum. Findings vary depending on the cause of the hearing loss. The purpose of a brief otoscopic examination is to assess the patency of the external canal, identify lesions or excessive cerumen in the canal, and assess whether the tympanic membrane (eardrum) is intact or inflamed (Jarvis, 2020).

! NURSING SAFETY PRIORITY (QSEN)

Action Alert

Do not use an otoscope to examine the ears of any patient who is unable to hold his or her head still during the examination or who is confused.

Psychosocial Assessment. For patients with a loss of auditory ***sensory perception,*** communication can be a struggle. They may isolate themselves because of the difficulty in talking, listening, and interpreting what is said to them. Social and work isolation can lead to depression. Encourage the patient and family to express their feelings and concerns about an actual or potential hearing loss.

NCLEX EXAMINATION CHALLENGE 43.1

Safe and Effective Care Environment

When caring for four clients, which client does the nurse report to the health care provider who should **not** receive an otoscopic examination?

A. 25-year-old with throat and ear pain
B. 39-year-old experiencing dizziness
C. 46-year-old who has type 2 diabetes
D. 60-year-old experiencing delirium

Imaging Assessment. Imaging assessment can determine some problems affecting hearing ability. Skull x-rays determine bony involvement in otitis media and the location of otosclerotic lesions. CT and MRI are used to determine soft-tissue involvement and the presence and location of tumors.

Other Diagnostic Assessment. Diagnostic assessments of hearing and balance can be useful in isolating the degree of hearing loss and, in some cases, the cause (Table 43.2).

Audiometry. Audiometry, performed by an audiologist, is the most reliable method of measuring the acuity of auditory ***sensory perception.*** Frequency is the highness or lowness of tones (expressed in hertz). The greater the number of vibrations per second, the higher the frequency (pitch) of the sound. The fewer the vibrations per second, the lower the frequency (pitch).

Intensity of sound is expressed in decibels (dB). Threshold is the lowest level of intensity at which pure tones and speech are heard by a patient about 50% of the time. The lowest intensity at which a healthy ear can detect sound about 50% of the time is 0 dB. Conversational speech is around 60 dB, and a soft whisper is around 20 dB (Table 43.3). Sound at 110 dB is so intense (loud) that it can be painful for most people with normal hearing; this type of sound is akin to being near the speakers at a loud rock concert. With a hearing loss of 45 to 50 dB, a hearing aid may be necessary to hear normal speech. Someone with a hearing loss of 90 dB may not be able to hear speech even with a hearing aid.

◆ Analysis: Analyze Cues and Prioritize Hypotheses.

The priority collaborative problems for the patient with any degree of hearing impairment include:

1. Decreased hearing ability due to obstruction, ***infection,*** damage to the middle ear, or damage to the auditory nerve
2. Decreased communication due to difficulty hearing

◆ Planning and Implementation: Generate Solutions and Take Action

Increasing Hearing. Nursing care priorities focus on teaching the patient about the use of any prescribed drug therapy and appropriate assistive devices, helping the patient and family to maintain or increase communication, and helping patients find community agency support.

Nonsurgical Management. Interventions include early detection of impaired auditory ***sensory perception,*** use of appropriate therapy, and use of assistive devices to augment the patient's usable hearing.

Early detection helps correct the problem causing the hearing loss. Assess for indications of hearing loss as covered in the Focused Assessment: The Patient With Suspected Hearing Loss box.

Drug therapy, if appropriate, is focused on correcting the underlying problem or reducing the side effects of problems occurring with hearing loss. Antibiotic therapy is used to manage external otitis and other ear infections. Teach the patient the importance of taking the drug or drugs exactly as prescribed. Caution him or her to not stop the drug just because signs and symptoms have improved. By treating the ***infection,*** antibiotics reduce local edema and improve hearing. When ***pain*** is also present, analgesics are used. Many ear disorders induce vertigo and dizziness with nausea and vomiting. Antiemetic, antihistamine, and antivertiginous drugs can be prescribed to reduce these problems.

Assistive devices are useful for patients with permanent hearing loss. Amplifiers increase telephone volume, allowing the caller to speak in a normal voice. Some phones also have a video display of words that are being spoken by the caller. Flashing lights activated by a ringing telephone or doorbell provides a visual alert. Video doorbell systems allow visualization of people outside. Some patients may have a service dog to alert them to sounds. Personal sound amplification products (PSAPs) offer solutions to situational activities that require a sound boost when a patient does not wish to have a hearing aid. These devices can help amplify sounds from a television or voices from people sitting at a table. Some devices are accessible via a headset or earpiece with Bluetooth capability, allowing a patient to take calls or listen to music directly through their smartphone.

A hearing aid is a small electronic amplifier that assists patients with conductive hearing loss but is less effective for sensorineural hearing loss (Fig. 43.5). The styles vary by size, placement, and the degree to which they amplify sound. Most common hearing aids are small. Some are attached to the wearer's glasses and are visible to other people. Another type fits into the ear and is less noticeable. Newer devices fit completely in the canal with only a fine, clear filament visible. The cost of smaller hearing aids varies with size and quality. The audiologist will teach the patient how to wear and acclimate to the hearing aid that is selected.

TABLE 43.2 Diagnostic Studies and Associated Nursing Care

Test	Purpose	Associated Nursing Care
Audiometry	*Pure tone audiometry* is used to assess hearing acuity (and demonstrates hearing loss). The test is done in a soundproof area and requires the patient to respond when a sound is heard. Speech audiometry is used to assess how intense (or loud) a simple speech stimulus must be before the patient can hear it well enough to repeat it correctly at least 50% of the time.	Describe procedure and confirm that no special preparation is needed.
Auditory brainstem evoked response (ABR)	Used to assess hearing in patients who are unable to indicate their recognition of sound stimuli during standard hearing tests. Can be used to diagnose conductive and sensorineural hearing losses.	Describe procedure. Teach that electrodes will be placed on the scalp, so no lotions, moisturizers, or oils should be on the face. Small red spots may remain on the areas where the electrodes were placed, but these will resolve. Teach that that hair should be cleaned afterward to remove electrode gel.
Auditory evoked potential (AEP)	Used to detect and estimate a patient's hearing level or degree of impairment.	Describe procedure, explaining that it is similar to an electroencephalogram (EEG). Teach that electrodes will be placed on the scalp, and that hair should be cleaned afterward to remove electrode gel.
Computerized dynamic posturography (CDP)	Used to measure whether a person can maintain steady balance as conditions (such as a visual field or the platform on which the patient stands) are manipulated.	Describe test and confirm that no special preparation is needed. Teach that a body sling may be used to promote safety.
Electronystagmography (ENG)	Used to assess for central and peripheral disease of the vestibular system in the ear by detecting and recording **nystagmus**.	Describe test. Remind to confirm which medications should be taken (or avoided) the day of the test. Teach that water and air will be introduced into the ear as part of caloric testing; cold water may be uncomfortable. Teach that dizziness, nausea, and vomiting during the test may occur. Teach to have an adult present after testing to drive home.
Imaging assessment	CT (with or without contrast)—used to assess ear structures in great detail; very helpful in diagnosing acoustic tumors. MRI—used to assess soft tissue changes.	Describe test. Teach to report claustrophobia prior to testing, as a mild sedative may be prescribed. Open MRI is an option for those who need this test.
Laboratory tests	Used to assess whether an infection is present; microbial culture and antibiotic sensitivity can be performed for specific causative organism and the antibiotic that will best manage the infection.	Describe test and confirm that no special preparation is needed.
Tympanometry	Used to assess eardrum mobility by changing air pressure in the external air canal. Used to assess middle ear problems (and recovery after treatment and/or surgery), eustachian tube patency, eardrum perforation, and/or fluid and wax accumulation.	Describe procedure and confirm that no special preparation is needed. Teach that there may be some discomfort while a probe is in the ear, and that sounds heard during the procedure may be loud.

TABLE 43.3 Decibel Intensity and Safe Exposure Time for Common Sounds

Sound	Decibel Intensity (dB)	Safe Exposure Time[a]
Threshold of hearing	0	
Whispering	20	
Average residence or office	40	
Conversational speech	60	
Car traffic	70	>8hr
Motorcycle	90	8hr
Chain saw	100	2hr
Rock concert, front row	120	3min
Jet engine	140	Immediate danger
Rocket launching pad	180	Immediate danger

[a]For every 5-dB increase in intensity, the safe exposure time is cut in half.

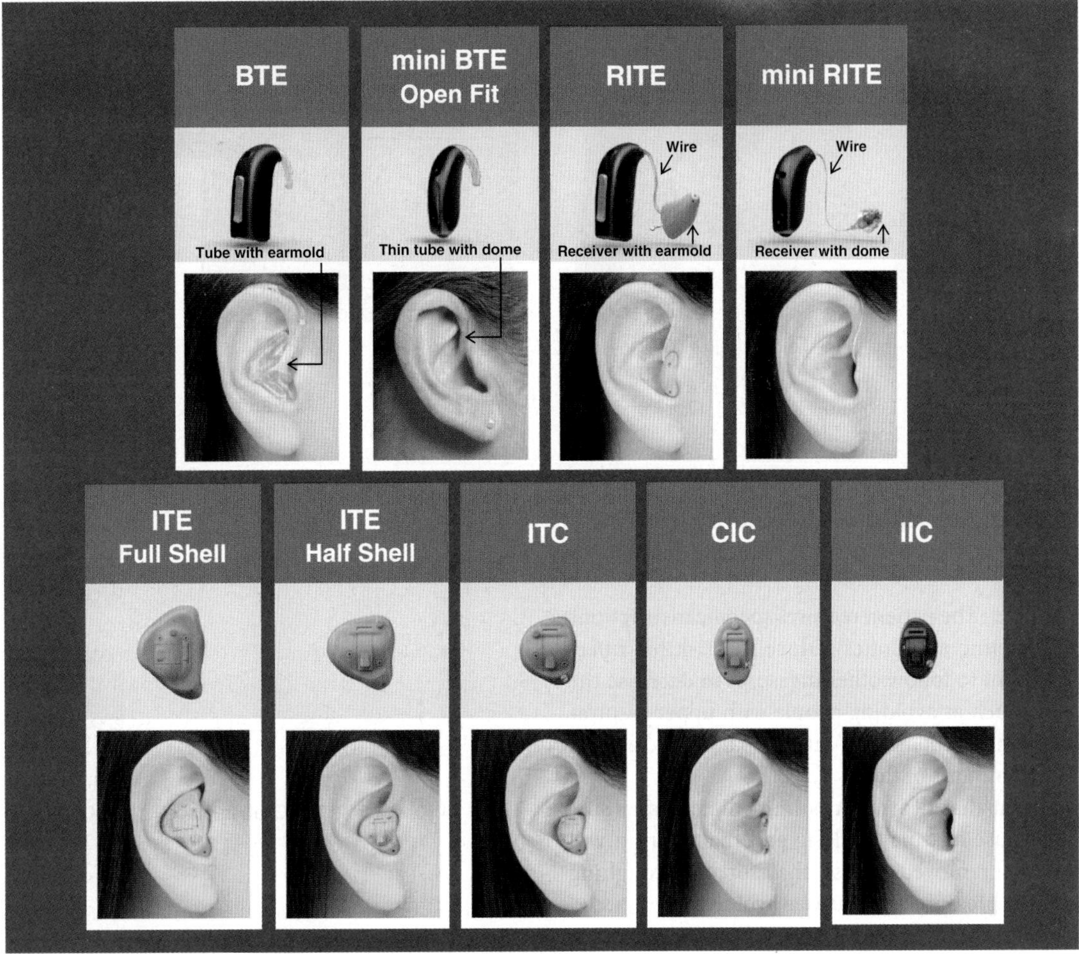

FIG. 43.5 Types of hearing aids. (From Oticon, Inc., Somerset, NJ. In Cifu, D.X., Lew, H.L., & Oh-Park, M. [2018]. *Geriatric rehabilitation.* Philadelphia: Elsevier.)

Teach the patient how to care for the hearing aid (see the Patient and Family Education: Preparing for Self-Management: Hearing Aid Care box). Hearing aids are delicate devices that should be handled only by people who know how to care for them properly.

Cochlear implantation may help patients with sensorineural hearing loss. Although a superficial surgical procedure is needed to implant the device, the procedure does not enter the inner ear and thus is not considered a surgical correction for hearing impairment (Fig. 43.6). A small computer converts sound waves into electronic impulses. Electrodes are placed near the internal ear, with the computer attached to the external ear. The electronic impulses then directly stimulate nerve fibers.

! NURSING SAFETY PRIORITY QSEN

Action Alert

Teach patients the safe way to clean their ears, stressing that nothing smaller than his or her own fingertip should be inserted into the canal.

Surgical Management. If nonsurgical management is not effective, various surgical interventions are available for patients with specific disorders that have contributed to hearing loss.

Tympanoplasty. Tympanoplasty (Fig. 43.7) reconstructs the middle ear to improve conductive hearing loss. The procedures

PATIENT AND FAMILY EDUCATION: PREPARING FOR SELF-MANAGEMENT

Hearing Aid Care

- Keep the hearing aid dry.
- Clean the ear mold with mild soap and water while avoiding excessive wetting.
- Using a soft toothbrush or the brush that came with the device, clean debris from the hole in the middle of the part that goes into your ear.
- Turn off the hearing aid when not in use.
- Check and replace the battery frequently.
- Keep extra batteries on hand.
- Keep the hearing aid in a safe place.
- Avoid dropping the hearing aid or exposing it to temperature extremes.
- Adjust the volume to the lowest setting that allows you to hear to prevent feedback squeaking.
- Avoid using hair spray, cosmetics, oils, or other hair and face products that might come into contact with the receiver.
- Check with your audiology provider to determine whether you can swim with your particular hearing aid(s). Some are water-resistant (and do not tolerate submersion), others are waterproof (and can be used while swimming).
- If the hearing aid does not work:
  - Change the battery.
  - Check the connection between the ear mold and the receiver.
  - Check the on/off switch.
  - Clean the sound hole.
  - Adjust the volume.
  - Take the hearing aid to an authorized service center for repair.

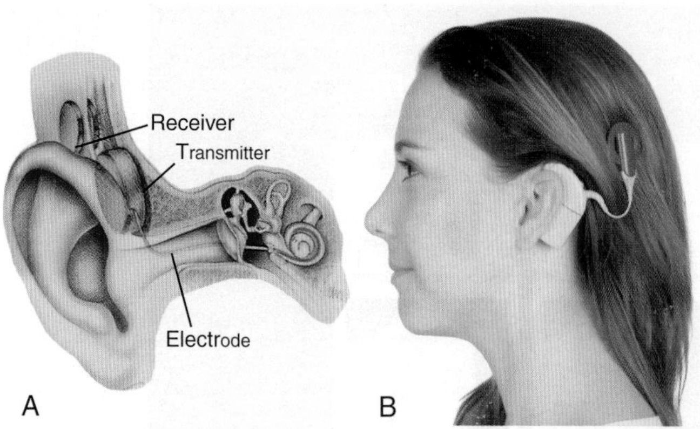

FIG. 43.6 Cochlear implant. (From Leonard, P.C. [2020]. *Quick and easy medical terminology.* [9th ed.]. St. Louis: Elsevier.)

vary from simple reconstruction of the eardrum (**myringoplasty**) to replacement of the ossicles within the middle ear (**ossiculoplasty**).

Preoperative care. The patient requires specific instructions before surgery. Systemic antibiotics reduce the risk for ***infection.*** Teach the patient to follow other measures to decrease the risks for infection, such as avoiding people with upper respiratory infections, getting adequate rest, eating a balanced diet, and drinking adequate amounts of fluid.

Assure the patient that hearing loss immediately after surgery is normal because of canal packing and that hearing will improve when it is removed. Stress that forceful coughing increases middle ear pressure and must be avoided.

Operative procedures. Surgery is performed only when the middle ear is free of infection. If an infection is present, the graft is more likely to become infected and not heal. Surgery of the eardrum and ossicles requires the use of a microscope and is a delicate procedure. Local anesthesia can be used, although general anesthesia is often used to prevent the patient from moving.

The surgeon can repair the eardrum with many materials, including tissue from a vein or muscle sheath. If the ossicles are damaged, more extensive surgery is needed for repair or replacement. The ossicles can be reached in several ways—through the ear canal, with an endaural incision, or by an incision behind the ear (Fig. 43.8).

The surgeon removes diseased tissue and cleans the middle ear cavity. The patient's cartilage or bone, cadaver ossicles, stainless steel wire, or special polymers (Teflon) are used to repair or replace the ossicles.

Postoperative care. Iodoform gauze, which is soaked in antiseptic, is packed in the ear canal. If a skin incision is used, a dressing is placed over it. Keep the dressing clean and dry, using sterile technique for changes. Keep the patient flat, with the head turned to the side and the operative ear facing up for at least 12 hours after surgery. Give prescribed antibiotics to prevent ***infection.***

Patients often report hearing improvement after removal of the canal packing. Until that time, communicate as with a patient who is hearing impaired, directing conversation to the unaffected ear. Instruct the patient in

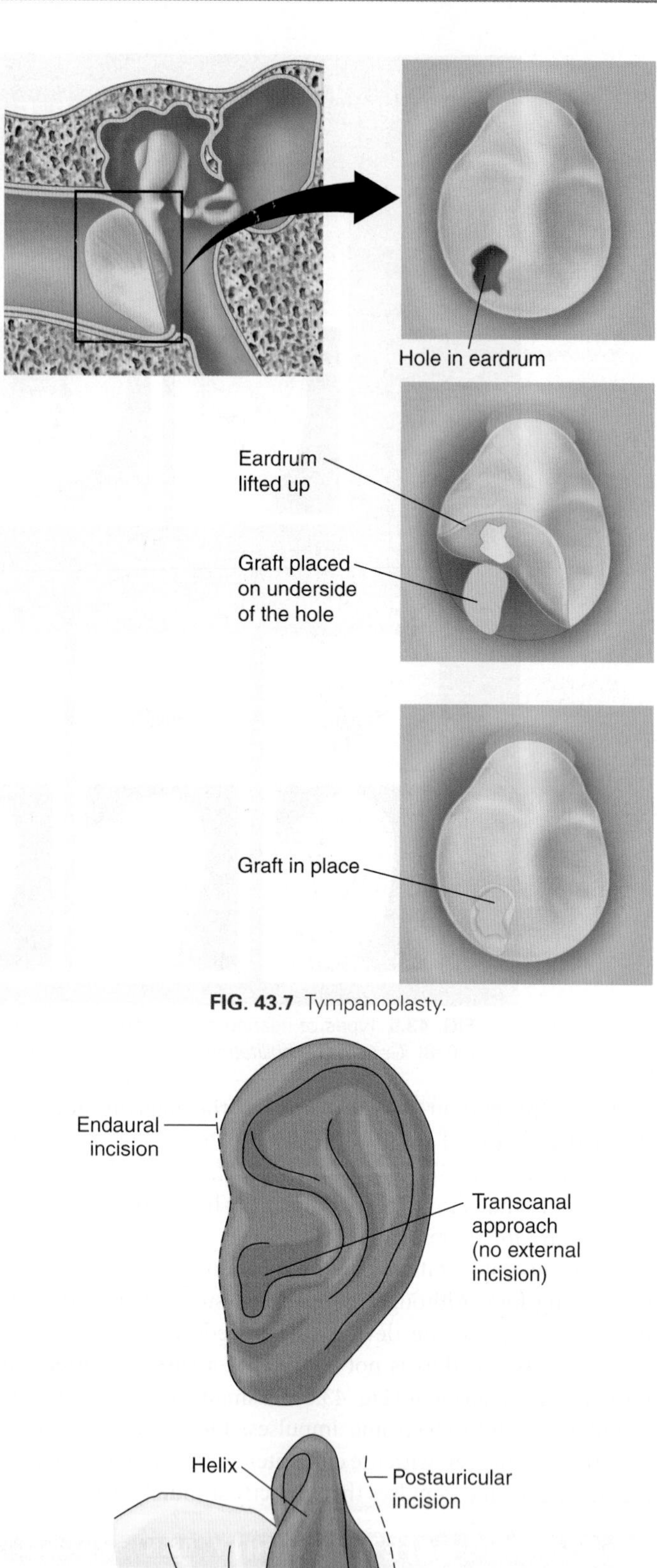

FIG. 43.7 Tympanoplasty.

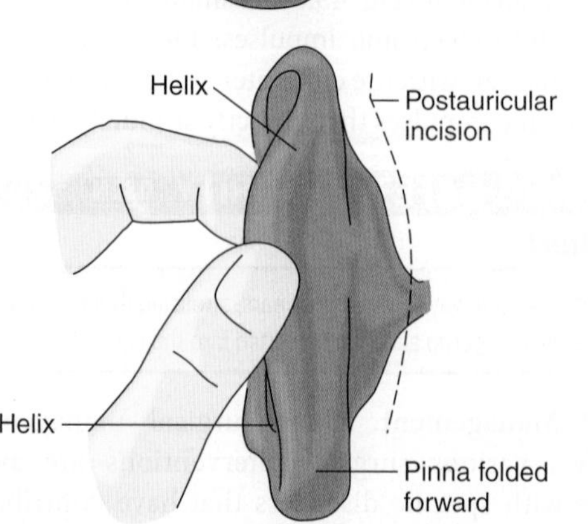

FIG. 43.8 Surgical approaches for repair of the ear and hearing structures.

care and activity restrictions (see the Patient and Family Education: Preparing for Self-Management: Recovery From Ear Surgery box).

Stapedectomy. A partial or complete stapedectomy with a prosthesis can correct some hearing loss, especially in patients with hearing loss related to otosclerosis. Although hearing usually improves after primary stapes surgery, some patients redevelop conductive hearing loss after surgery, and revision surgery is needed.

Preoperative care. To prevent ***infection***, the patient must be free from external otitis at surgery. Teach the patient to follow measures that prevent middle ear or external ear infections as noted in the Patient and Family Education: Preparing for Self-Management: Prevention of Ear Infection or Trauma box.

The surgeon will review the expected outcomes and possible complications of the surgery with the patient. The success rate of this procedure is high. However, there is always a risk for failure that might lead to total deafness on the affected side. Surgery is performed first on the ear with the greater hearing loss. If the surgery does not improve hearing, patients must decide to either attempt surgical correction of the other ear or continue to use an amplification device.

Other possible complications include vertigo, infection, and facial nerve damage. Remind the patient that hearing is initially worse after a stapedectomy.

Operative procedures. A stapedectomy is usually performed through the external ear canal with the patient under local anesthesia. After removal of the affected ossicles, a piston-shaped prosthesis is connected between the incus and the footplate (Fig. 43.9). Because the prosthesis vibrates with sound as the stapes did, most patients have restoration of functional hearing.

Postoperative care. Remind the patient that improvement in hearing may not occur until 6 weeks after surgery. Drugs for ***pain*** help reduce discomfort, and antibiotics are used to prevent infection. Teach the patient about the precautions in the Patient and Family Education: Preparing for Self-Management: Recovery From Ear Surgery box.

The surgical procedure is performed in an area where cranial nerves VII, VIII, and X can be damaged by trauma or by swelling after surgery. *Assess for facial nerve damage or muscle weakness. Indications include an asymmetric appearance or drooping of features on the affected side of the face. Ask the patient about changes in facial perception of touch and in taste.* Vertigo, nausea, and vomiting usually occur after surgery because of the nearness to inner ear structures.

Antivertiginous drugs (such as meclizine) and antiemetic drugs (such as ondansetron) may be prescribed. Prevent falls by assisting as needed and instructing the patient to move slowly from a sitting to a standing position.

PATIENT AND FAMILY EDUCATION: PREPARING FOR SELF-MANAGEMENT

Recovery From Ear Surgery

- Avoid straining when you have a bowel movement.
- Avoid drinking through a straw for 2 to 3 weeks.
- Avoid air travel for 2 to 3 weeks.
- Avoid excessive coughing for 2 to 3 weeks.
- Avoid people with respiratory infections.
- When blowing your nose, blow gently, without blocking either nostril, and with your mouth open.
- Avoid getting your head wet or washing your hair for several days.
- You may shower; before doing so, place a ball of cotton coated with petroleum jelly (e.g., Vaseline) in the ear, or use a waterproof earplug.
- Avoid rapidly moving the head, bouncing, and bending over for 3 weeks.
- If you have a dressing, change it every 24 hours or as directed.
- Report excessive drainage immediately to your primary health care provider.

PATIENT AND FAMILY EDUCATION: PREPARING FOR SELF-MANAGEMENT

Prevention of Ear Infection or Trauma

- Do not use small objects, such as cotton-tipped applicators, matches, toothpicks, keys, or hairpins, to clean your external ear canal.
- Wash your external ear and canal daily in the shower or while washing your hair.
- Blow your nose gently.
- Do not block one nostril while blowing your nose.
- Sneeze with your mouth open.
- Wear sound protection around loud or continuous noises.
- Avoid or wear head and ear protection during activities with high risk for head or ear trauma, such as wrestling, boxing, motorcycle riding, and skateboarding.
- Keep the volume on head receivers at the lowest setting that allows you to hear.
- Frequently clean objects that come into contact with your ear (e.g., headphones, telephone receivers).
- Avoid environmental conditions with rapid changes in air pressure.

! NURSING SAFETY PRIORITY (QSEN)

Action Alert

Prevent injury by assisting the patient with ambulation during the first 1 to 2 days after stapedectomy. Keep top bed side rails up and remind the patient to move the head slowly to avoid vertigo.

Totally Implanted Devices. Totally implanted devices, such as the Esteem, can improve bilateral moderate-to-severe sensorineural hearing loss without any visible part (Envoy Medical, 2020). These devices have three totally implanted components: a sound processor, a sensor, and a computer. Vibrations of the eardrum and ossicles are picked up by the sensor and converted to electric signals that are processed by the sound processor. The processor is programmed to the patient's specific hearing pathology. The processor filters out some background noise and amplifies the desired sound signal. The signal is transferred to the computer, which then converts the processed signal into

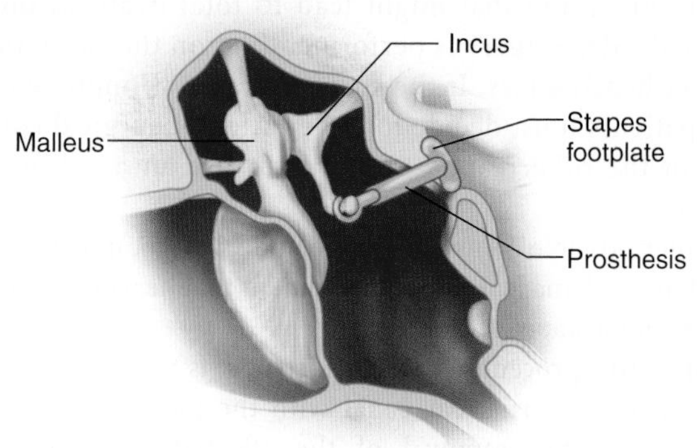

FIG. 43.9 Prosthesis used with stapedectomy. The stapes is removed, leaving the footplate. A metal or plastic prosthesis is connected to the incus and inserted through the hole to act as an artificial stapes.

vibrations that are transmitted to the inner ear for auditory ***sensory perception.***

Patient criteria for totally implantable devices include:

- Bilateral stable sensorineural hearing loss
- Speech discrimination score of 40% or higher
- Healthy tympanic membrane, eustachian tube, and ossicles of the middle ear
- Large enough ear cavity to fit the device components
- At least 30 days of experience with an appropriate hearing aid
- Absence of middle ear, inner ear, or mastoid infection
- Absence of Ménière disease or recurring vertigo
- Absence of sensitivity to device materials

The devices and the surgery may lead to possible complications, including temporary facial paralysis, changes in taste sensation, and ongoing or new-onset tinnitus. Unlike cochlear implants, the middle ear is entered, and it is considered a surgical procedure. Care before and after surgery is similar to that required with stapedectomy. The cost of the implant and procedure can be very high; currently this type of implantable device is not covered by Medicare or Medicaid, and only by select private insurers.

Maximizing Communication

Nonsurgical Management. Nursing priorities focus on facilitating communication and reducing anxiety. For communicating, use best practices that are listed in the Best Practice for Patient Safety & Quality Care: Communicating With a Patient Who Is Hearing-Impaired box. Do not shout at the patient because the sound may be projected at a higher frequency, making him or her less able to understand. Communicate by writing (if he or she is able to see, read, and write) or with pictures of familiar phrases and objects. Many television programs are now closed captioned or video described (subtitled).

Collaborate with members of the interprofessional team, such as the audiologist, who can help with maximizing hearing, which can improve communication.

ETHICAL/LEGAL CONSIDERATIONS

Remember that you have a legal and ethical responsibility to make sure that you communicate effectively so that the patient receives the best care possible (National Association of the Deaf, 2020). Use all appropriate resources, based on the individual patient's abilities and needs, to ensure proper communication.

Lip-reading and *sign language* can increase communication. Patients are taught special cues to look for when lip-reading and how to understand body language. However, the best lip-reader still misses more than half of what is being said. Because even minimal lip-reading assists hearing, urge patients to wear their eyeglasses when talking with someone to see lip movement.

Sign languages, such as American Sign Language (ASL), combine speech with hand movements that signify letters, words, and phrases. These languages take time and effort to learn, and many people are unable to use them effectively.

Managing anxiety can increase the effectiveness of communication efforts. One source of anxiety is the possibility of permanent hearing loss. Provide accurate information about the likelihood of hearing returning. When the hearing impairment is likely to be permanent, reassure patients that communication and social interaction can be maintained with some practical modification.

Help patients use resources and communication to make social contact satisfying. Identify the patient's most satisfying activities and social interactions and determine the effort necessary to continue them. The patient can alter activities to improve satisfaction. Instead of large gatherings, the patient might choose smaller groups. A meal at home with friends can substitute for dining out, or consider requesting a table in a quiet area of a restaurant.

Care Coordination and Transition Management. Lengthy hospitalization is rare for ear and hearing disorders. If surgery is needed and the procedure is completed without complications, it may be performed in an ambulatory surgery center.

Home Care Management. Patients who have persistent vertigo are in danger of falling. Assess the home for potential hazards and to determine whether family or significant others are available to assist with meal preparation and other ADLs.

Self-Management Education. Provide written instructions to the patient and family about how to take drugs and when to return for follow-up care, if needed. Follow-up hearing tests may be scheduled routinely or are scheduled when surgical lesions are well healed in about 6 to 8 weeks. Audiograms done before and after treatment are compared, and evaluation for further intervention to improve hearing begins.

Teach patients how to instill eardrops and irrigate the ears and obtain a return demonstration.

To prevent ***infection*** after surgery, instruct patients to follow the information located in the Patient and Family Education: Preparing for Self-Management: Prevention of Ear Infection or Trauma box. Teach patients who use a hearing aid and their caregivers how to use it effectively.

Health Care Resources. A nurse case manager can coordinate with the patient, caregiver, and home care nurse to determine how to best maintain adequate self-care abilities, maintain a safe environment, decide about assistance needs, and obtain needed care. Support groups organized for patients with hearing problems can also be most helpful.

Costs to the patient with a hearing impairment can be extensive. Information and support can come from public and private agencies that specialize in counseling patients with disorders affecting auditory ***sensory perception.***

◆ **Evaluation: Evaluate Outcomes.** Evaluate the care of the patient with hearing loss based on the identified priority patient problems. The expected outcomes include that the patient will:
- Maintain as much hearing as possible and/or use appropriate hearing compensation behaviors
- Successfully use (a) method(s) of communication that works best for the individual
- Successfully use assistive devices as needed

OTITIS MEDIA

Pathophysiology Review

The common forms of otitis media are acute otitis media, chronic otitis media, and serous otitis media. Each type affects the middle ear but has different causes and pathologic changes. If otitis progresses or is untreated, permanent conductive hearing loss may occur.

Acute otitis media and chronic otitis media are similar. An infecting agent in the middle ear causes inflammation of the mucosa, leading to swelling and irritation of the ossicles within the middle ear, followed by purulent inflammatory exudate. The acute form has a sudden onset and lasts 3 weeks or less. Chronic otitis media often follows repeated acute episodes, has a longer duration, and causes greater middle ear injury. It may be a result of the continuing presence of a biofilm in the middle ear. A *biofilm* is a community of bacteria working together to overcome host defense mechanisms to continue to survive and proliferate (see Chapter 21 for more information about biofilms). Therapy for complications associated with chronic otitis media usually involves surgical intervention.

The eustachian tube and mastoid, connected to the middle ear by a sheet of cells, are also affected by the ***infection.*** If the eardrum membrane perforates, the infection can thicken and scar the eardrum and middle ear if left untreated. Necrosis of the ossicles destroys middle ear structures and causes hearing loss.

❖ Interprofessional Collaborative Care

◆ **Assessment: Recognize Cues.** The patient with acute or chronic otitis media has ear ***pain.*** Acute otitis media causes more intense pain from increased pressure in the middle ear. Conductive hearing is reduced and distorted as sound-wave transmission is obstructed. The patient may notice tinnitus in the form of a low hum or a low-pitched sound. Headaches, malaise, fever, nausea, and vomiting can occur. As the pressure on the middle ear pushes against the inner ear, the patient may have dizziness.

Otoscopic examination findings vary, depending on the stage of the condition. The eardrum is initially retracted, which allows landmarks of the ear to be seen clearly. At this early stage, the patient may only have vague ear discomfort. As the condition progresses, the eardrum's blood vessels dilate and appear red (Fig. 43.10). Later the eardrum becomes red, thickened, and bulging, with loss of landmarks. Decreased eardrum mobility is evident on inspection with a pneumatic otoscope. Pus may be seen behind the membrane.

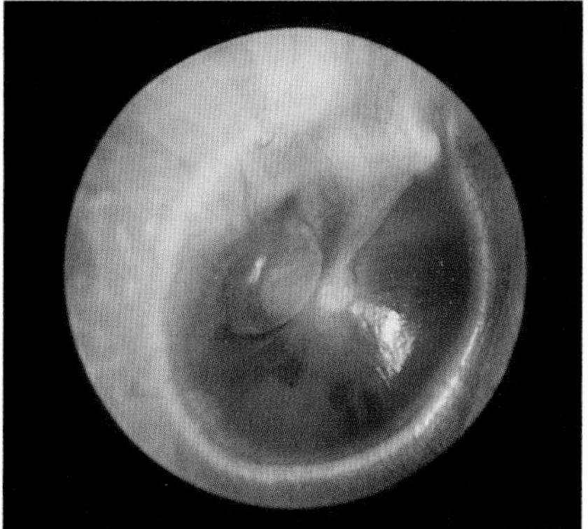

FIG. 43.10 Otoscopic view of otitis media.

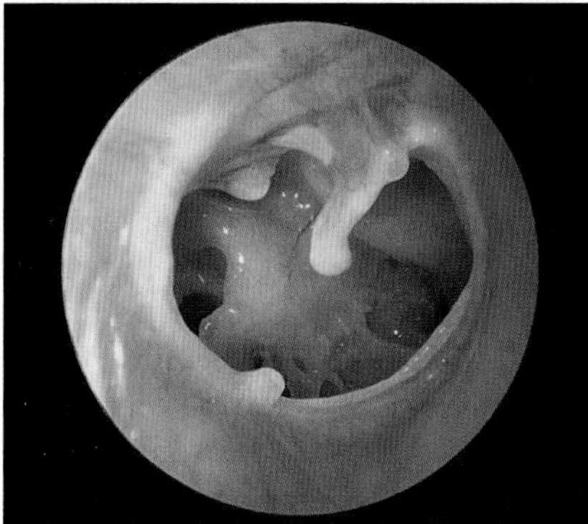

FIG. 43.11 Otoscopic view of a perforated tympanic membrane.

With progression, the eardrum spontaneously perforates, and pus or blood drains from the ear (Fig. 43.11). The patient usually has a marked decrease in pain as the pressure on middle ear structures is relieved. Eardrum perforations often heal if the underlying problem is controlled. Simple central perforation does not interfere with hearing unless the ossicles are damaged or the perforation is large. Repeated perforations with extensive scarring cause hearing loss.

◆ **Interventions: Take Action**

Nonsurgical Management. Bedrest limits head movements that intensify the ***pain.*** Application of low heat may help reduce pain. Systemic antibiotic therapy is needed to address the ***infection.*** Teach the patient to complete the antibiotic therapy as prescribed and to not stop taking the drug even when he or she begins to feel better. Analgesics such as ibuprofen and acetaminophen can be used to relieve pain and reduce fever. For severe pain, opioid analgesics may be prescribed. Antihistamines and decongestants can also be prescribed to decrease fluid in the middle ear.

Surgical Management. If ***pain*** persists after antibiotic therapy and the eardrum continues to bulge, a **myringotomy** (surgical opening of the eardrum) may be performed. This procedure drains middle ear fluids and immediately relieves pain.

The procedure requires only a small surgical incision, which is often performed in an office or clinic under local anesthesia, yet can also be done in a surgical suite under general anesthesia. The incision heals rapidly. For relief of pressure caused by

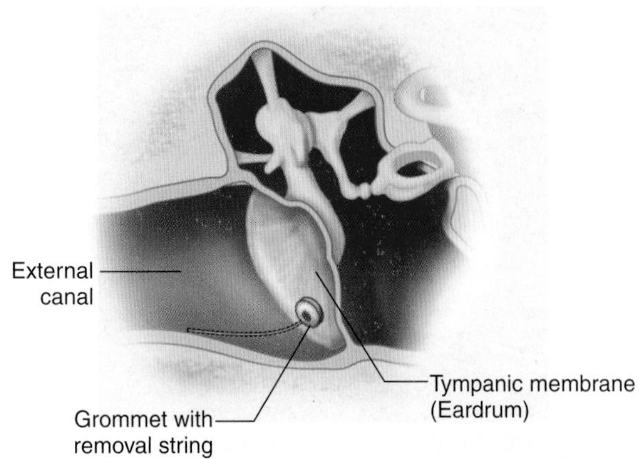

FIG. 43.12 Grommet through the tympanic membrane. A small grommet is placed through the tympanic membrane away from the margins, which allows prolonged drainage of fluids from the middle ear.

serous otitis media and for patients who have repeated episodes of otitis media, a small **grommet** (polyethylene tube) may be surgically placed through the eardrum to allow continuous drainage of middle ear fluids (Fig. 43.12).

Priority care after surgery includes teaching the patient to keep the external ear and canal clean and dry while the incision is healing. Hair-washing and showering should be avoided for several days so that water and chemicals are not introduced into the ear. Other instructions after surgery are listed in the Patient and Family Education: Preparing for Self-Management: Recovery from Ear Surgery box earlier in this chapter.

EXTERNAL OTITIS

Pathophysiology Review

External otitis (Fig. 43.13) is a painful condition caused when irritating or infective agents come into contact with the skin of the external ear. The result is an allergic response or inflammation with or without ***infection.*** Affected skin becomes red, swollen, and tender to touch or movement. Swelling of the ear canal can lead to temporary hearing loss from obstruction. Allergic external otitis is often caused by contact with cosmetics, hair sprays, earphones, earrings, or hearing aids. The most common infectious organisms are *Pseudomonas aeruginosa, Proteus vulgaris, Staphylococcus aureus,* and *Escherichia coli* (Kesser, 2019).

External otitis occurs more often in hot, humid environments, especially in the summer, and is known as **swimmer's ear** because it often occurs in people involved in water sports. Patients who have traumatized their external ear canal with sharp or small objects (e.g., hairpins, cotton-tipped applicators) or with headphones also are more susceptible to external otitis. Others at risk include people with general allergies, psoriasis, eczema, and seborrheic dermatitis (Kesser, 2019).

Necrotizing or *malignant otitis* is the most virulent form of external otitis. This extremely rare condition occurs most often in patients who are immunocompromised. Organisms spread beyond the external ear canal into the ear and skull. Death from complications such as meningitis, brain abscess, and destruction of cranial nerve VII is possible.

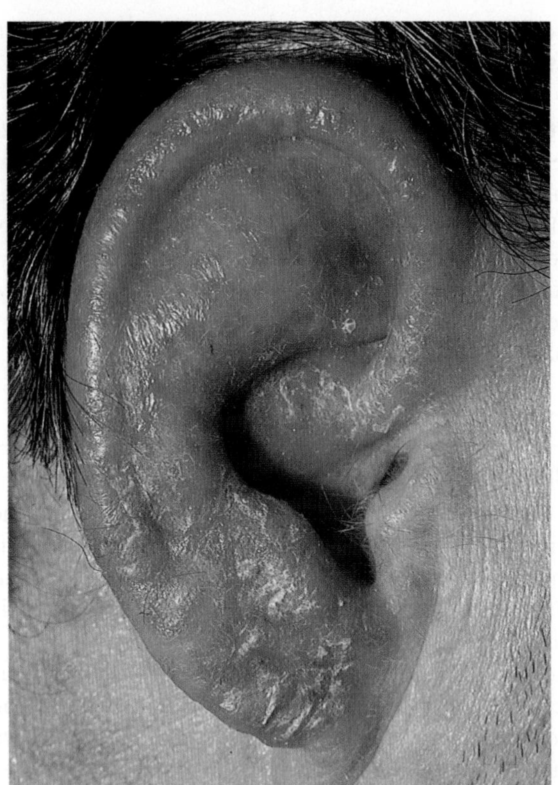

FIG. 43.13 External otitis. (From Habif, T.P. [2016]. *Clinical dermatology* [6th ed.]. Philadelphia: Elsevier.)

❖ Interprofessional Collaborative Care

◆ **Assessment: Recognize Cues.** Signs and symptoms of external otitis range from mild itching to ***pain*** with movement of the pinna or tragus, particularly when upward pressure is applied to the external canal. Patients report feeling as if the ear is plugged and hearing is reduced. The temporary hearing loss can be severe when inflammation obstructs the canal and prevents sounds from reaching the eardrum.

◆ **Interventions: Take Action.** Treatment focuses on reducing inflammation, edema, and ***pain.*** Cleaning is the first step, as cerumen, desquamated skin, and other purulent material must be removed from the ear canal (Goguen, 2019). The primary health care provider will conduct the cleaning through an otoscope. Once the ear canal is clean, eardrops will be much more effective.

Nursing priorities include enhancing comfort measures, such as applying heat to the ear for 20 minutes three times a day. This can be accomplished by using towels warmed with water and then wrapped in a plastic bag or by using a heating pad placed on the lowest setting. Teach the patient that minimizing head movements reduces pain.

Topical antibiotic and steroid therapies are generally prescribed to decrease inflammation and pain. Watch the patient or caregiver administer the eardrops to make sure that proper technique is used. Oral or IV antibiotics are used in severe cases, especially when ***infection*** spreads to surrounding tissue or when area lymph nodes are enlarged.

Analgesics, including opioids, may be needed for ***pain*** relief during the initial days of treatment. Ibuprofen or acetaminophen can relieve less severe pain. Teach the patient to place a cotton ball coated with petroleum jelly into the ear when showering. The patient must be taught to avoid water sports, ear buds, and hearing aid for at least 7 to 10 days. People who swim should be taught to wear earplugs when swimming. Finally, teach the patient to use preventive measures for minimizing ear canal moisture, trauma, or exposure to materials that lead to local irritation or contact dermatitis.

CERUMEN OR FOREIGN BODIES

Pathophysiology Review

Cerumen (earwax) is the most common cause of an impacted ear canal. Foreign bodies, such as small vegetables, beads, pencil erasers, and insects, can also be impacting. Although uncomfortable, cerumen or foreign bodies are rarely emergencies and can be removed carefully by a health care professional. Cerumen impaction in the older adult is common, and removal of the cerumen from older adults often improves hearing.

❖ Interprofessional Collaborative Care

◆ **Assessment: Recognize Cues.** Patients may report a sensation of fullness in the ear, with or without hearing loss, and may have ear ***pain,*** itching, dizziness, or bleeding from the ear. Cerumen or the foreign body may be visible with direct inspection.

◆ **Interventions: Take Action.** When the occluding material is cerumen, management options include watchful waiting, manual removal, or the use of ceruminolytic agents followed by manual removal or irrigation.

If the cerumen is thick and dry or cannot be removed easily, the primary health care provider may recommend use of a ceruminolytic product such as Cerumenex or Debrox to soften the wax before removal. Another recommendation may include adding 2 or 3 drops of mineral oil to the ear at bedtime. After a few days of this practice, a curette or cerumen spoon may then be used by the health care professional to remove the wax. In some cases, irrigation may be considered, only if the patient does not have an eardrum perforation or otitis media. Caution patients to avoid self-treatment without consultation with the primary health care provider.

Insects are killed before removal unless they can be coaxed out by a flashlight. A topical anesthetic can be placed in the ear canal for pain relief. Mineral oil or diluted alcohol instilled into the ear can suffocate the insect, which is then removed by the primary health care provider with ear forceps. If a foreign body cannot be removed in the outpatient setting, surgical removal under general anesthetic may be required.

! NURSING SAFETY PRIORITY (QSEN)

Action Alert

Do not irrigate an ear with an eardrum perforation or otitis media because this may spread the ***infection*** to the inner ear. Also, do not irrigate the ear when the foreign object is vegetable matter because this material expands when wet, making the impaction worse. An experienced health care professional performs removal of vegetable matter.

MASTOIDITIS

Pathophysiology Review

The lining of the middle ear is continuous with the lining of the mastoid air cells, which are embedded in the temporal bone. Mastoiditis is an ***infection*** of the mastoid air cells caused by progressive otitis media. Antibiotic therapy is used to treat the middle ear infection before it progresses to mastoiditis. If mastoiditis is not managed appropriately, it can lead to brain abscess, meningitis, and death.

❖ Interprofessional Collaborative Care

◆ **Assessment: Recognize Cues.** The signs and symptoms of mastoiditis include swelling behind the ear and ***pain*** when moving the ear or the head. Pain is *not* relieved by myringotomy. Cellulitis develops on the skin or external scalp over the mastoid process, pushing the ear sideways and down. The eardrum is red, dull, thick, and immobile. Perforation may or may not be present. Lymph nodes behind the ear are tender and enlarged. Patients may have low-grade fever, malaise, and ear drainage. Hearing loss occurs, and CT scans show fluid in the air cells of the mastoid process. If intracranial complications are anticipated, an MRI will be ordered instead of a CT scan (Lustig et al., 2018).

◆ **Interventions: Take Action.** Interventions focus on halting the ***infection*** before it spreads to other structures. IV antibiotics are used but do not easily penetrate the infected bony structure of the mastoid. Cultures of the ear drainage determine which antibiotics should be most effective. Surgical removal of the infected tissue is needed if the infection does not respond to antibiotic therapy within a few days. A simple or modified radical mastoidectomy with tympanoplasty is the most common treatment. All infected tissue must be removed so the infection does not spread to other structures. A tympanoplasty is then performed to reconstruct the ossicles and the eardrum to restore hearing (see the Tympanoplasty section).

TINNITUS

Tinnitus (continuous ringing or noise perception in the ear) is a common ear problem that can occur in one or both ears. Diagnostic testing cannot confirm tinnitus; however, testing is performed to assess hearing and rule out other disorders. A Tinnitus and Hearing Survey (Henry et al., 2015) may be used to help patients and clinicians determine whether intervention for tinnitus is warranted.

Signs and symptoms range from mild ringing, which can go unnoticed during the day, to a loud roaring in the ear, which can seriously interfere with thinking and attention span. Factors that contribute to tinnitus include age, sclerosis of the ossicles, Ménière disease, certain drugs (aspirin, NSAIDs, high-ceiling diuretics, quinine, aminoglycoside antibiotics), exposure to loud noise, and other inner ear problems.

The problem and its management vary with the underlying cause. When no cause can be found or the disorder is untreatable, therapy focuses on ways to mask the tinnitus with background sound, noisemakers, and music during sleeping hours. Ear-mold hearing aids can amplify sounds to dampen tinnitus during the day. A drug that is helpful to some patients is pramipexole, an antiparkinson drug. The American Tinnitus Association helps patients cope with tinnitus. Refer patients with tinnitus to local and online support groups as needed.

PATIENT-CENTERED CARE: VETERANS HEALTH CONSIDERATIONS QSEN

Veterans who have served are often exposed to noise, particularly if they have been around gunfire, detonation of weapons, explosives, or aircraft. Tinnitus and hearing loss are the top two compensated service-related disabilities and affect over 3.1 million veterans (U.S. Department of Veterans Affairs, 2018). Nurses must remember to assess patients for veteran status and inquire about occupational exposure (Elliott, 2019). Provide a quiet and private environment for care, be mindful of coexisting conditions that the veteran may have, and communicate with a multimodal approach using visual handouts and demonstrations (Elliott, 2019).

NCLEX EXAMINATION CHALLENGE 43.2

Physiological Integrity

Which client statement regarding a new diagnosis of tinnitus requires nursing teaching? **Select all that apply.**

A. "I am so glad this condition will go away permanently."
B. "It is important that I do not drive when I have tinnitus."
C. "Watching my diet will make a difference in my condition."
D. "Surgery is the only treatment that is available for tinnitus."
E. "I have found a couple of support groups that I like to attend."

MÉNIÈRE DISEASE

Pathophysiology Review

Ménière disease is a condition that includes a classic trio of symptoms—episodic **vertigo**, tinnitus, and hearing loss (Moskowitz & Dinces, 2020). Symptoms usually occur in adults between the ages of 20 and 60 years (Moskowitz & Dinces, 2020; National Institute on Deafness and Other Communication Disorders, 2017). Episodes, also called "attacks," can last several days, although some patients report ongoing symptoms of varying intensity at all times. Patients can be almost to totally incapacitated during an attack, and recovery can take hours to days. Although most patients have a window of forewarning when an attack is beginning, others experience Tumarkin otolithic crises, known as *sudden drop attacks* in which the patient falls to the ground with no warning (Wu et al., 2019).

The pathophysiology leading to this condition is not fully understood. However, it is known that Ménière disease is progressive, leading to an excess of endolymphatic fluid that builds up within the inner ear (Pullen, 2017) causing distortion and distention of portions of the labyrinth system (Moskowitz & Dinces, 2020). This distortion decreases hearing by dilating the cochlear duct, causes vertigo because of damage to the vestibular system, and stimulates tinnitus. At first, hearing loss is reversible, but repeated damage to the cochlea from increased fluid pressure can lead to permanent hearing loss.

❖ Interprofessional Collaborative Care

◆ **Assessment: Recognize Cues.** Signs and symptoms include vertigo, hearing loss, and tinnitus. Vertigo is often accompanied by nausea, vomiting, headache, and nystagmus (rapid eye movements). Blood pressure, pulse, and respirations may be elevated. Hearing loss occurs first with the low-frequency tones; in some patients, it progresses to include all levels and eventually becomes permanent. Patients may describe the tinnitus as having variable pitch and intensity, which may fluctuate or remain continuous.

◆ **Interventions: Take Action.** Nonpharmacologic treatment for Ménière disease includes diet and lifestyle adjustments, as some patients with this condition are sensitive to triggers such as high salt intake, caffeine, monosodium glutamate (MSG), alcohol, nicotine, stress, and allergens (Moskowitz & Dinces, 2020). Teach patients how to modify their diet accordingly. It is also important to teach the client to avoid activities that place them at risk of experiencing vertigo, such as standing on chairs or ladders. Patients with sudden drop attacks should not drive, and may be subject to having a driver's license suspended for safety purposes (Wu et al., 2019).

Teach patients to move the head slowly to prevent worsening of the vertigo. Institute and teach fall precautions to all patients with Ménière disease.

Vestibular rehabilitation therapy uses exercise activities to improve balance, which can be helpful. Pharmacologic treatment is used to reduce symptoms. Betahistine (in Canada) or diuretics can be prescribed to decrease endolymph volume, which reduces vertigo, hearing loss, tinnitus, and aural fullness. Other drugs, such as vestibular suppressants and antiemetics, may be used to address symptoms that occur during attacks. For patients who do not respond to pharmacologic intervention, systemic glucocorticoids may be used; if this fails, intratympanic glucocorticoid therapy or intratympanic gentamicin may be attempted (Moskowitz & Dinces, 2020).

When drug therapy is not effective in controlling symptoms or attacks, other procedures may be considered. Decompression and/or shunting of the endolymphatic sac has been shown to have favorable outcomes in controlling vertigo. Finally, **labyrinthectomy** can be done in extreme cases in which the patient already has significant hearing loss or continuous disabling vertigo. This surgical procedure destroys the bony and membranous labyrinth by removal of the neuroepithelium, resulting in total hearing loss on the operative side.

NCLEX EXAMINATION CHALLENGE 43.3

Physiological Integrity

What teaching will the nurse provide to a client who continues to experience more frequent episodes associated with Ménière disease? **Select all that apply.**

A. Reducing activity can reduce frequency of episodes.
B. Episodes will eventually decrease in severity and number.
C. Reducing sodium, caffeine, and alcohol intake can be beneficial.
D. The only treatment that is effective is to undergo labyrinthectomy.
E. When moving from sitting to standing, be cautious and take your time.

CLINICAL JUDGMENT CHALLENGE 43.1

Safety; Patient-Centered Care

A 45-year-old female client has been admitted for observation after coming to the emergency department reporting dizziness, nausea, and vomiting. She states, "I can't seem to get rid of the flu. This is the third time I've had it recently." She reports being at home earlier in the day and having a sensation of spinning come over her suddenly. When she fell to the floor, her partner brought her immediately to the emergency department. Now, several hours later, she reports feeling somewhat better but still has the spinning sensation and is nauseated. She says that she also has ringing in her ears. On assessment, vital signs include BP 140/90 mm Hg, pulse 100 beats/min, and respirations 20 breaths/min. Nystagmus is noted. When someone stands on the left side of the client, she does not respond to questions or dialogue.

1. **Recognize Cues:** What assessment information in this client situation is the most important and immediate concern for the nurse? (Hint: Identify the **relevant** information *first* to determine what is most important.)
2. **Analyze Cues:** What client conditions are consistent with the **most relevant** information? (Hint: Think about priority collaborative problems that support and contradict the information presented in this situation.)
3. **Prioritize Hypotheses:** Which possibilities or explanations are **most likely** to be present in this client situation? Which possibilities or explanations are the most serious? (Hint: Consider all possibilities and determine their urgency and risk for this client.)
4. **Generate Solutions:** What actions would most likely achieve the desired outcomes for this client? Which actions should be **avoided** or are **potentially harmful**? (Hint: Determine the desired outcomes first to decide which interventions are appropriate and those that should be avoided.)
5. **Take Action:** Which actions are the most appropriate and how should they be implemented? In what **priority order** should they be implemented? (Hint: Consider health teaching, documentation, requested health care provider orders or prescriptions, nursing skills, collaboration with or referral to health team members, etc.)
6. **Evaluate Outcomes:** What client assessment would indicate that the nurse's actions were **effective**? (Hint: Think about signs that would indicate an improvement, decline, or unchanged client condition.)

ACOUSTIC NEUROMA

An *acoustic neuroma* is a benign tumor of the vestibulocochlear nerve (cranial nerve VIII) that often damages other structures as it grows. Depending on the size and exact location of the tumor, damage to hearing, facial movements, and sensation can occur. An acoustic neuroma can cause neurologic signs and symptoms as the tumor enlarges in the brain.

Signs and symptoms begin with tinnitus and progress to gradual sensorineural hearing loss. Later, patients have constant mild-to-moderate vertigo. As the tumor enlarges, nearby cranial nerves are damaged.

The tumor is diagnosed with an MRI. If the patient cannot tolerate an MRI, high-resolution CT with or without contrast can be used (Park, 2020). Treatment involves surgery, radiation, or watchful observation. If surgery is performed, risks include hearing loss, facial weakness, persistent headaches, and/or vestibular disturbances (Park, 2020). Because these tumors grow very slowly, even patients who have had surgery need prolonged follow-up.

GET READY FOR THE NEXT-GENERATION NCLEX® EXAMINATION!

Key Points

Review these Key Points for each NCLEX Examination Client Needs Category.

Safe and Effective Care Environment

- Use Contact Precautions with any patient who has ear drainage. **QSEN: Safety**
- Do not perform an otoscopic examination on a patient who is confused. **QSEN: Safety**
- Protect the patient with vertigo or dizziness from injury by assisting with ambulation. **QSEN: Safety**
- Raise upper side rails for the patient experiencing dizziness or vertigo. **QSEN: Safety**
- Teach patients to move the head slowly after ear surgery to prevent dizziness or vertigo. **QSEN: Safety**

Health Promotion and Maintenance

- Identify adults at risk for hearing impairment based on occupational and leisure activities. **QSEN: Safety**
- Teach adults ways to protect hearing before loss occurs. **QSEN: Safety**
- Use best practices to enhance communication with a patient who is hearing-impaired. **QSEN: Patient-Centered Care**
- Ensure that all members of the interprofessional team use a medical interpreter as needed for the patient who cannot hear. **QSEN: Patient-Centered Care**
- Teach patients the proper way to clean their ears and safely remove cerumen. **QSEN: Evidence-Based Practice**
- If ordered, teach patients and caregivers the proper techniques for self-instillation of eardrops. **QSEN: Evidence-Based Practice**
- Teach patients and caregivers how to properly care for hearing aids. **QSEN: Safety**

Psychosocial Integrity

- Allow the patient the opportunity to express fear or anxiety about hearing concerns. **QSEN: Patient-Centered Care**

- Assess the degree to which hearing problems interfere with the patient's ability to interact with others. **Clinical Judgment**
- Refer patients newly diagnosed with hearing impairment to appropriate local resources and support groups. **QSEN: Teamwork and Collaboration**

Physiological Integrity

- Perform a thorough family history because some hearing problems have a genetic component. **QSEN: Evidence-Based Practice**
- Ask the patient about current and past drug use (prescribed, over-the-counter) and evaluate for the possibility of ototoxicity. **QSEN: Safety**
- Avoid ear canal irrigation if the eardrum is perforated or if the canal contains vegetable matter. **QSEN: Safety**
- Stress the importance of completing an antibiotic regimen for an ear ***infection***. **QSEN: Evidence-Based Practice**
- Remind patients having ear surgery that hearing in the affected ear may be reduced because of packing, swelling, or surgical manipulation. **QSEN: Patient-Centered Care**

MASTERY QUESTIONS

1. Which communication method is appropriate when the nurse is interacting with a client who is deaf?
   A. Use pictures and writing
   B. Speak with enunciated words
   C. Ask client to read the nurse's lips
   D. Dialogue with the client's caregivers
2. When teaching a community group of older adults, what information will the nurse include regarding normal hearing changes associated with aging? **Select all that apply.**
   A. Hair in the ear thins and falls out
   B. Hearing acuity changes in all older adults
   C. Cerumen dries and becomes impacted more easily
   D. The ability to hear low-frequency pitches diminishes first
   E. Sounds such as *f, s, sh,* and *pa* may be more difficult to discern
3. What teaching will the nurse provide to a client who has just been fitted for new hearing aids?
   A. Turn off the hearing aid when not using it.
   B. Immerse the ear mold in alcohol to fully clean it.
   C. Store the hearing aid in a warm, humid bathroom when not in use.
   D. Avoid using hair spray, makeup, and personal care products around the device.

REFERENCES

American Tinnitus Association. (2019). Causes. https://www.ata.org/understanding-facts/causes.

Curhan, S. G., Wang, M., Eavey, R. D., Stampfer, M. J., & Curhan, G. C. (2018). Adherence to healthful dietary patterns is associated with lower risk of hearing loss in women. *Journal of Nutrition, 143*(6), 944–951.

Elliott, B. (2019). Tinnitus and hearing impairment in the veteran population. *MedSurg Matters!, 38*(3), 8–10.

Envoy Medical. (2020). *Esteem*. http://esteemhearing.com/.

Goguen, L. (2019). External otitis: Treatment. In D. Deschler, & M. Edwards (Eds.), *UpToDate*. Waltham, MA.

Henry, J. A., Griest, S., Zaugg, T. L., Thielman, E., Kaelin, C., Galvez, G., et al. (2015). Tinnitus and hearing survey: A screening tool to differentiate bothersome tinnitus from hearing difficulties. *American Journal of Audiology, 24*, 66–77.

Jarvis, C. (2020). *Physical examination & health assessment* (8th ed.). St. Louis: Saunders.

Kesser, B. (2019). *External otitis (acute). Merck manual: Professional version*. Retrieved from https://www.merckmanuals.com/professional/ear,-nose,-and-throat-disorders/external-ear-disorders/external-otitis-acute.

Lustig, L., et al. (2018). Chronic otitis media, cholesteatoma, and mastoiditis in adults. In D. Descher (Ed.), *UpToDate*. Waltham, MA.

McCance, K., Huether, S., Brashers, V., & Rote, N. (2019). *Pathophysiology: The biologic basis for disease in adults and children* (8th ed.). St. Louis: Mosby.

Moskowitz, H., & Dinces, E. (2020). Meniere disease: Evaluation, diagnosis and management. In D. Deschler (Ed.), *UpToDate*. Waltham, MA.

National Association of the Deaf. (2020). *Hospitals and other health care facilities*. Retrieved from https://www.nad.org/resources/health-care-and-mental-health-services/health-care-providers/hospitals-and-other-health-care-facilities/.

National Institute Deafness and Other Communication Disorders (NIDCD). (2016). *Quick statistics about hearing*. http://www.nidcd.nih.gov/health/statistics/Pages/quick.aspx.

National Institute Deafness and Other Communication Disorders (NIDCD). (2017). *Meniere's disease*. Retrieved from https://www.nidcd.nih.gov/health/menieres-disease.

Online Mendelian Inheritance in Man (OMIM). (2020). *Gap junction proteins, beta-2*. GJB2. www.omim.org/entry/121011.

Park, J., et al. (2020). Vestibular schwannoma (acoustic neuroma). In Loeffler, J., & Wen, P. (Eds.). *UpToDate*. Waltham, MA.

Pullen, R. (2017). Navigating the challenges of Ménière disease. *Nursing 2017*, 38–45.

Touhy, T., & Jett, K. (2018). *Ebersole and Hess' gerontological nursing healthy aging* (5th ed.). St. Louis: Mosby.

U.S. Department of Veterans Affairs. (2018). *Veterans benefits administration annual benefits report: Fiscal year 2018*. Retrieved from https://www.benefits.va.gov/reports/abr.

Wu, V., et al. (2019). Approach to Ménière disease management. *Canadian Family Physician, 65*(7), 463–467.

44

Assessment of the Musculoskeletal System

Donna D. Ignatavicius

http://evolve.elsevier.com/Iggy/

LEARNING OUTCOMES

1. Identify evidence-based health promotion activities to help prevent musculoskeletal health problems or trauma.
2. Apply knowledge of common physiologic changes associated with aging to accurately interpret musculoskeletal assessment findings and plan interventions to ensure patient safety.
3. Identify potential patient reactions to musculoskeletal health problems or injuries.
4. Apply knowledge of anatomy and physiology for a focused musculoskeletal assessment to assess patients for ***mobility, pain***, and ***sensory perception.***
5. Use clinical judgment to interpret assessment findings in a patient with a musculoskeletal health problem.
6. Plan patient-centered health teaching for preparation and follow-up care for selected musculoskeletal diagnostic testing.

KEY TERMS

arthralgias Joint aches and discomfort.
arthritis Joint inflammation.
arthrogram An x-ray study of a joint after contrast medium (air or solution) has been injected to enhance its visualization.
arthroscopy A diagnostic or surgical procedure in which a fiberoptic tube is inserted into a joint for direct visualization of the ligaments, menisci, and articular surfaces of the joint.
bone scan A radionuclide test in which radioactive material is injected for viewing the entire skeleton.
bursitis Inflammation of bursae, which are small sacs lined with synovial membrane located at joints and bony prominences to prevent friction between bone and structures next to bone.
dermatomyositis Polymyositis which occurs with a purplish skin rash.
effusion Fluid accumulation, such as in a joint.
fascia Dense fibrous tissue that surrounds skeletal muscle, which contains the muscle's blood, lymph, and nerve supply.
goniometer A tool that may be used by rehabilitation therapists or nurses to provide an exact measurement of joint flexion and extension or joint range of motion.
gout A genetically linked arthritis caused by an inborn error of purine metabolism.
kyphosis Outward curvature of the thoracic spine causing a "humped back."
lordosis An inward abnormal curvature of the lumbar spine.
muscle atrophy Skeletal muscle deterioration that results when muscles are not regularly exercised and they deteriorate from disuse.
muscular dystrophy A group of genetically linked diseases that cause chronic skeletal muscle weakness and organ dysfunction due to smooth muscle involvement.
myopathy A problem in muscle tissue often resulting in weakness.
neuropathy A problem in nerve tissue often resulting in weakness and decreased *sensory perception.*
neurovascular assessment (also called a *circ check*) An assessment that includes palpation of pulses in the extremities below the level of injury and assessment of sensation, movement, color, temperature, and pain in the injured part.
osteoblasts Bone-forming cells.
osteoclasts Bone-destroying cells.
osteomalacia Softening of bone in adults due to inadequate vitamin D.
osteopenia Decreased bone density (bone loss) that occurs as one ages.
osteoporosis A chronic disease of *cellular regulation* in which bone loss causes significant decreased density and possible fracture.

Paget disease A chronic metabolic disorder that causes bone to become fragile and misshapen.
polymyositis An uncommon chronic rheumatic disease that is characterized by inflammation of multiple muscles.
scoliosis An abnormal lateral curvature of the spine.
synovial joints Body joints that are lined with synovium, a membrane that secretes synovial fluid for lubrication and shock absorption.

PRIORITY AND INTERRELATED CONCEPTS

The priority concepts for this chapter are:
- ***Mobility***
- ***Pain***

The interrelated concept for this chapter is:
- ***Sensory Perception***

The musculoskeletal system is the second largest body system. It includes the bones, joints, and skeletal muscles, as well as the supporting structures needed to move them. ***Mobility*** is a basic human need that is essential for performing ADLs. When a patient cannot move to perform ADLs or other daily routines, self-esteem and a sense of self-worth can be diminished. Chapter 3 reviews this concept.

Disease, surgery, and trauma can affect one or more parts of the musculoskeletal system, often leading to decreased mobility. When ***mobility*** is impaired for a long time, other body systems are affected. For example, prolonged immobility can lead to skin breakdown, constipation, and venous thromboembolism. If nerves are damaged by trauma or disease, patients may also have both impaired ***sensory perception*** and ***pain*** (see Chapter 3 for a review of these health concepts).

ANATOMY AND PHYSIOLOGY REVIEW

Skeletal System

The skeletal system consists of 206 bones and multiple joints. The growth and development of these structures occur during childhood and adolescence and are not discussed in this text. Common physical skeletal differences among selected racial/ethnic groups are listed in Table 44.1.

Bones

Types and Structure. Bone can be classified in two ways: by *shape* and by structure. For example, *long bones,* such as the femur, are cylindric with rounded ends and often bear weight. *Short bones,* such as the phalanges, are small and bear little or no weight.

The second way bone is classified is by *structure* or composition. As shown in Fig. 44.1, the outer layer of bone, or cortex, is composed of dense, compact bone tissue. The inner layer, in the medulla, contains spongy, cancellous tissue. Almost every bone has both tissue types but in varying quantities.

The structural unit of the cortical compact bone is the haversian system, which is detailed in Fig. 44.1. The haversian

TABLE 44.1 Musculoskeletal Differences in Selected Ethnic Groups

Group	Musculoskeletal Differences
African Americans	Greater bone density than Europeans, Asians, and Hispanics Accounts for decreased incidence of osteoporosis
Amish	Greater incidence of dwarfism than in other populations
Chinese Americans	Bones shorter and smaller with less bone density Increased incidence of osteoporosis
Egyptian Americans	Shorter in stature than Euro-Americans and African Americans
Filipino/Vietnamese	Short in stature; adult height about 5 feet
Irish Americans	Taller and broader than other Euro-Americans Less bone density than African Americans
Navajo American Indians	Taller and thinner than other American Indians

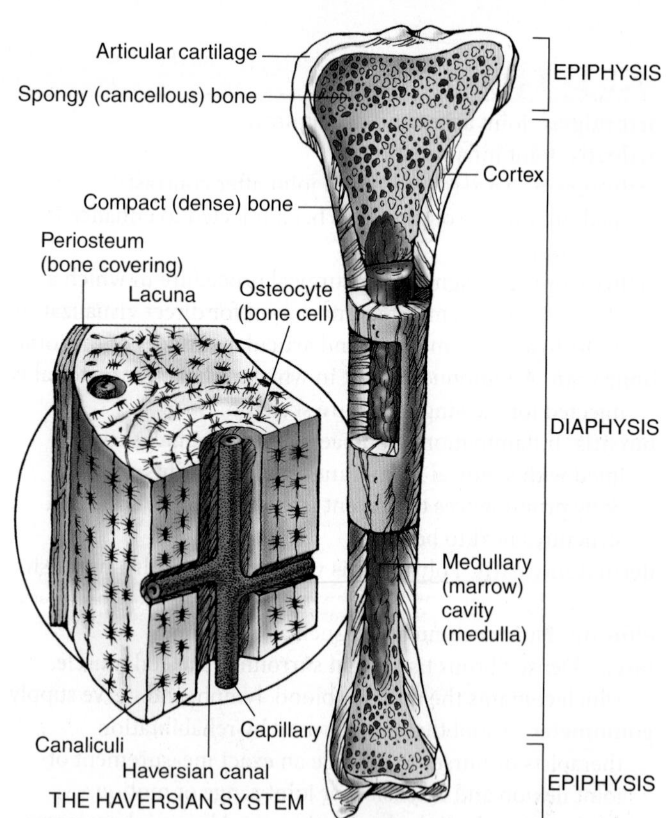

FIG. 44.1 Structure of a typical long bone. The cortex, or outer layer, is composed of dense, compact tissue. The microscopic structure of this compact cortical tissue is the haversian system.

system is a complex canal network containing microscopic blood vessels that supply nutrients and oxygen to bone and lacunae, which are small cavities that house osteocytes (bone cells). The canals run vertically within the hard cortical bone tissue.

The softer cancellous tissue contains large spaces, or trabeculae, which are filled with red and yellow marrow. Hematopoiesis (production of blood cells) occurs in the red marrow. The yellow marrow contains fat cells, which can be dislodged and enter the bloodstream to cause *fat embolism syndrome (FES)*, a life-threatening complication. Volkmann canals connect bone marrow vessels with the haversian system and periosteum, the outermost covering of the bone. In the deepest layer of the periosteum are osteogenic cells, which later differentiate into **osteoblasts** (bone-forming cells) and **osteoclasts** (bone-destroying cells) (McCance et al., 2019).

Bone is a very vascular tissue. Each bone has a main nutrient artery, which enters near the middle of the shaft and branches into ascending and descending vessels. These vessels supply the cortex, the marrow, and the haversian system. Very few nerve fibers are connected to bone. Sympathetic nerve fibers control dilation of blood vessels. Sensory nerve fibers transmit pain signals experienced by patients who have primary lesions of the bone, such as bone tumors.

Function. The skeletal system:

- Provides a framework for the body and allows the body to be weight bearing, or upright
- Supports the surrounding tissues (e.g., muscle and tendons)
- Assists in movement through muscle attachment and joint formation
- Protects vital organs, such as the heart and lungs
- Manufactures blood cells in red bone marrow
- Provides storage for mineral salts (e.g., calcium and phosphorus)

After puberty, bone reaches its maturity and maximum growth. Bone is a dynamic tissue. It undergoes a continuous process of formation and resorption, or destruction, at equal rates until the age of 35 years. In later years, bone resorption increases, decreasing bone mass and predisposing patients to injury, especially older women.

Bone accounts for about 99% of the *calcium* in the body and 90% of the *phosphorus*. In healthy adults, the serum concentrations of calcium and phosphorus maintain an inverse relationship. As calcium levels rise, phosphorus levels decrease. When serum levels are altered, calcitonin and parathyroid hormone (PTH) work to maintain equilibrium. If the calcium in the blood is decreased, the bone, which stores calcium, releases calcium into the bloodstream in response to PTH stimulation. Chapter 13 describes these electrolytes in more detail.

Calcitonin is produced by the thyroid gland and *decreases* the serum calcium concentration if it is increased above its normal level. Calcitonin inhibits bone resorption and increases renal excretion of calcium and phosphorus as needed to maintain balance in the body.

Vitamin D and its metabolites are produced in the body and transported in the blood to promote the absorption of calcium and phosphorus from the small intestine. They also seem to enhance PTH activity to release calcium from the bone. A decrease in the body's vitamin D level can result in **osteomalacia** (softening of bone) in the adult.

When serum calcium levels are lowered, *parathyroid hormone* (PTH, or parathormone) secretion increases and stimulates bone to promote osteoclastic activity and *release* calcium to the blood. PTH reduces the renal excretion of calcium and facilitates its absorption from the intestine. If serum calcium levels increase, PTH secretion diminishes to preserve the bone calcium supply. This process is an example of the feedback loop system of the endocrine system.

Growth hormone secreted by the anterior lobe of the pituitary gland is responsible for increasing bone length and determining the amount of bone matrix formed before puberty. During childhood, an increased secretion results in gigantism, and a decreased secretion results in dwarfism. In the adult, an increase causes acromegaly, which is characterized by bone and soft-tissue deformities.

Adrenal glucocorticoids regulate protein metabolism, either increasing or decreasing catabolism to reduce or intensify the organic matrix of bone. They also aid in regulating intestinal calcium and phosphorus absorption.

Estrogens stimulate osteoblastic activity and inhibit PTH. When estrogen levels decline at menopause, women are susceptible to low serum calcium levels with increased bone loss (osteoporosis). *Androgens,* such as testosterone in men, promote anabolism (body tissue building) and increase bone mass.

Thyroxine (T_4) is one of the principal hormones secreted by the thyroid gland. Its primary function is to increase the rate of protein synthesis in all types of tissue, including bone. *Insulin* works together with growth hormone to build and maintain healthy bone tissue. More information about these hormones can be found in the endocrine health problem chapters of this text.

Joints. A *joint* is a space in which two or more bones come together. This is also referred to as articulation of the joint. The major function of a joint is to provide movement and flexibility in the body.

There are three types of joints in the body:

- Synarthrodial, or completely immovable, joints (e.g., in the cranium)
- Amphiarthrodial, or slightly movable, joints (e.g., in the pelvis)
- Diarthrodial (synovial), or freely movable, joints (e.g., the elbow and knee)

Although any of these joints can be affected by disease or injury, the synovial joints are most commonly involved, as discussed in Chapter 46. The diarthrodial, or synovial, joint is

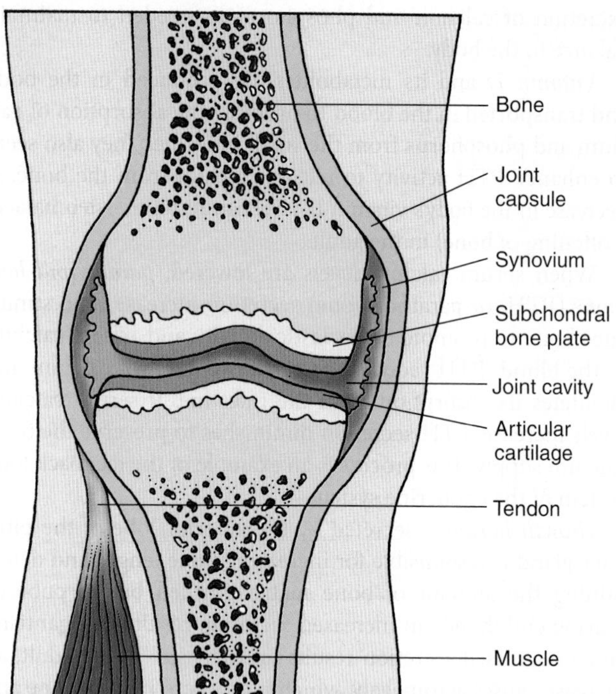

FIG. 44.2 Structure of a synovial joint. Synovium lines the joint capsule but does not extend into the articular cartilage.

the most common type of joint in the body. **Synovial joints** are the only type lined with synovium, a membrane that secretes synovial fluid for lubrication and shock absorption. As shown in Fig. 44.2, the synovium lines the internal portion of the joint capsule but does not normally extend onto the surface of the cartilage at the spongy bone ends. Articular cartilage consists of a collagen fiber matrix impregnated with a complex ground substance. Patients with **arthritis** (joint inflammation) often have synovitis (synovial inflammation) and breakdown of the cartilage. Bursae, small sacs lined with synovial membrane, are located at joints and bony prominences to prevent friction between bone and structures next to bone. These structures can also become inflamed, causing painful **bursitis**.

Synovial joints are described by their anatomic structures. For example, *ball-and-socket* joints (shoulder, hip) permit movement in any direction. *Hinge* joints (elbow) allow motion in one plane—flexion and extension. The knee is often classified as a hinge joint, but it rotates slightly, as well as flexes and extends. It is best described as a *condylar* type of synovial joint.

Muscular System

There are three types of muscle in the body: smooth muscle, cardiac muscle, and skeletal muscle. Smooth, or nonstriated, involuntary muscle is responsible for contractions of organs and blood vessels and is controlled by the autonomic nervous system. Cardiac or striated involuntary muscle is also controlled by the autonomic nervous system. The smooth and cardiac muscles are discussed in the assessment chapters, along with the body systems to which they belong.

In contrast to smooth and cardiac muscle, skeletal muscle is striated voluntary muscle controlled by the central and peripheral nervous systems. The junction of a peripheral motor nerve and the muscle cells that it supplies is sometimes referred to as a *motor end plate.* Muscle fibers are held in place by connective tissue in bundles, or fasciculi. The entire muscle is surrounded by dense fibrous tissue, or **fascia**, which contains the muscle's blood, lymph, and nerve supply.

The main function of skeletal muscle is *movement* of the body and its parts. When bones, joints, and supporting structures are adversely affected by injury or disease, the adjacent muscle tissue is often involved, limiting ***mobility.*** During the aging process, muscle fibers decrease in size and number, even in well-conditioned adults. **Muscle atrophy** results when muscles are not regularly exercised, and they deteriorate from disuse.

Supporting structures for the muscular system are very susceptible to injury. They include tendons (bands of tough, fibrous tissue that attach muscles to bones) and ligaments, which attach bones to other bones at joints.

Musculoskeletal Changes Associated With Aging

Osteopenia, or decreased bone density (bone loss), occurs as one ages. Many older adults, especially white, thin women, have *severe* osteopenia, a disease called **osteoporosis**. This condition can cause **kyphosis** (outward curvature of the thoracic spine causing a "humped back") and gait changes, which predispose the person to fractures (Jarvis, 2020). Chapter 45 discusses this health problem in detail.

Synovial joint cartilage can become less elastic and compressible as a person ages. As a result of these cartilage changes and continued use of joints, the joint cartilage becomes damaged, leading to osteoarthritis (OA). Genetic defects in cartilage may also contribute to joint disease. The most common joints affected are the weight-bearing joints of the hip, knee, and cervical and lumbar spine, but joints in the shoulder and upper extremity, feet, and hands also can be affected. Refer to Chapter 46 for a complete discussion of OA.

As one ages, muscle tissue atrophies. Increased activity and exercise can slow the progression of atrophy and restore muscle strength. Musculoskeletal changes cause decreased coordination, loss of muscle strength, gait changes, and a risk for falls with injury. (See Chapter 4 for discussion on fall prevention.) The Patient-Centered Care: Older Adult Considerations: Changes in the Musculoskeletal System Related to Aging box lists the major anatomic and physiologic changes and related nursing interventions to ensure patient safety.

Health Promotion and Maintenance

Many health problems of the musculoskeletal system can be prevented through health promotion strategies and avoidance

PATIENT-CENTERED CARE: OLDER ADULT CONSIDERATIONS QSEN

Changes in the Musculoskeletal System Related to Aging

Physiologic Change	Nursing Interventions	Rationales
Decreased bone density	Teach safety tips to prevent falls (see Chapter 4).	Porous bones are more likely to fracture.
	Reinforce need to exercise, especially weight-bearing exercise.	Exercise slows bone loss.
Increased bone prominence	Prevent pressure on bone prominences.	There is less soft tissue to prevent skin breakdown.
Kyphosis and widened gait, shift in the center of gravity, which could cause imbalance and falls	Teach proper body mechanics; instruct the patient to sit in supportive chairs with arms. Assess need for ambulatory device, such as cane or walker; ensure use of supportive shoes.	Correction of posture problems prevents further deformity; the patient should have support to ensure improved balance.
Cartilage degeneration (osteoarthritis [OA]) (see Chapter 46)	Provide moist heat, such as a shower or warm, moist compresses or heating pad.	Moist heat increases blood flow to the area and promotes ***mobility.***
Decreased range of motion (ROM)	Assess the patient's ability to perform ADLs and ***mobility***.	The patient may need assistance with ADLs and ambulation.
Muscle atrophy, decreased strength	Teach isometric and isotonic exercises.	Exercises increase muscle strength.
Slowed movement	Do not rush the person; be patient.	The patient may become frustrated if hurried or sustain a fall.

of risky lifestyle behaviors. For example, women can slow the process of bone loss by taking vitamin D and calcium supplements and increasing these nutrients in their diet. Weight-bearing activities, such as walking and strengthening exercises, can reduce risk factors for **osteoporosis** and maintain muscle strength (McCance et al., 2019).

Accidents, illnesses, lifestyle, and substance abuse can contribute to the occurrence of musculoskeletal injury. Young men are at the greatest risk for trauma related to motor vehicle or scooter crashes. Older adults are at the greatest risk for falls that result in fractures and soft-tissue injury. High-impact sports, such as excessive jogging or running, can cause musculoskeletal injury to soft tissues and bone.

Tobacco smoking also has negative effects on the musculoskeletal system (see the Evidence-Based Practice box). The nicotine in tobacco is the primary cause of these effects (Smith & Jackson, 2018).

EVIDENCE-BASED PRACTICE QSEN

What Is the Effect of Smoking on Musculoskeletal Health?

AL-Bashaireh, A.M., Haddad, L.G., Weaver, M., Kelly, D.L., Chengguo, X., & Yoon, S. (2018). The effect of tobacco smoking on musculoskeletal health: A systematic review. *Journal of Environmental and Public Health, July 11.* Doi:10.1155/2018/4184190.

The authors conducted a systematic study to determine the effect of tobacco smoking on the health of the musculoskeletal system. After a thorough review of the literature, 243 research articles were selected for inclusion and used for data abstraction. Findings of the systematic review include that the nicotine in cigarettes is associated with negative musculoskeletal effects, including:

- Decreased bone mineral density, which could lead to fractures
- Decreased immunity, which could delay fracture healing
- Muscle atrophy
- Deterioration in joint cartilage, especially in the knees

Level of Evidence: 1

The research was a systematic review of the literature that included multiple studies to determine the negative effects of tobacco smoking on musculoskeletal health.

Commentary: Implications for Practice and Research

This research provides evidence that not only does smoking cause cardiovascular and pulmonary health problems, but cigarette nicotine has negative effects on the musculoskeletal and immune systems. Nurses need to provide information on smoking cessation to help patients quit and improve health.

Excessive alcohol intake can decrease vitamins and nutrients that the person needs for bone and muscle tissue growth. Develop a patient-centered health promotion plan for each patient to help promote bone health and prevent musculoskeletal injury. Additional health promotion strategies can be found in other chapters of this unit related to specific health problems of the musculoskeletal system.

NCLEX EXAMINATION CHALLENGE 44.1

Health Promotion and Maintenance

A nurse is performing a musculoskeletal assessment on an older adult. What normal physiologic changes of aging does the nurse expect? **Select all that apply.**

A. Muscle atrophy
B. Slowed movement
C. Kyphosis
D. Arthritis
E. Widened gait
F. Decreased joint range of motion

ASSESSMENT: RECOGNIZE CUES

Patient History

In the assessment of a patient with an actual or potential musculoskeletal problem, a detailed and accurate history is helpful in identifying priority problems and nursing interventions. The history reveals information about the patient that can direct the physical assessment.

When taking a personal health history, question the patient about any traumatic injuries and sports activities, no matter when they occurred. An injury to the lumbar spine 30 years ago may have caused a patient's current low back pain. A motor vehicle crash or sports injury can cause osteoarthritis years after the event. Ask the patient if he or she is following a pain management plan, including the use of opioids or other substances such as cannabis (marijuana).

Previous or current illness or disease may affect musculoskeletal status. For example, a patient with diabetes who is treated for a foot ulcer is at high risk for acute or chronic osteomyelitis (bone infection). In addition, diabetes slows the healing process. Ask the patient about any previous hospitalizations and illnesses or complications. Inquire about his or her ability to perform ADLs independently or if assistive-adaptive devices are used.

Current lifestyle also contributes to musculoskeletal health. When assessing a patient with a possible musculoskeletal alteration, inquire about occupation or work life. A person's occupation can cause or contribute to an injury. For instance, fractures are not uncommon in patients whose jobs require manual labor, such as housekeepers, mechanics, and industrial workers. Certain occupations, such as computer-related jobs, may predispose a person to carpal tunnel syndrome (entrapment of the median nerve in the wrist) or neck pain.

Ask about allergies, particularly allergy to dairy products, and previous and current use of drugs (prescribed, over-the-counter, and illicit). Allergy to dairy products could cause decreased calcium intake. Some drugs, such as steroids, can negatively affect calcium metabolism and promote bone loss. Other drugs may be taken to relieve musculoskeletal pain. Inquire about herbs, vitamin and mineral supplements, or biologic compounds that may be used for arthritis and other musculoskeletal problems, such as glucosamine and chondroitin. These integrative therapies are commonly used by patients with various types of arthritis and **arthralgias** (joint aches and discomfort).

Nutrition History. A brief review of the patient's nutrition history helps determine any risks for inadequate nutrient intake. For example, most people, especially women, do not get enough calcium in their diet. Determine if the patient has had a significant weight gain or loss and whether the weight change was expected.

Ask the patient to recall a typical day of food intake to help identify deficiencies and excesses in the diet. Lactose intolerance is a common problem that can cause inadequate calcium intake. People who cannot afford to buy food are especially at risk for undernutrition. Some older adults and others are not financially able to buy the proper foods for adequate nutrition.

Inadequate protein or insufficient vitamin C or D in the diet slows bone and tissue healing. Obesity places excess stress and strain on bones and joints, with resulting trauma to joint cartilage. In addition, obesity inhibits ***mobility*** in patients with musculoskeletal problems, which predisposes them to complications such as respiratory and circulatory problems. People with eating disorders such as anorexia nervosa and bulimia nervosa are also at risk for osteoporosis related to decreased intake of calcium and vitamin D.

Family History and Genetic Risk. Obtaining a family history helps to identify disorders that have a familial or genetic tendency. For example, **osteoporosis** and **gout** (a genetically linked arthritis caused by an inborn error of purine metabolism) often occur in several generations of a family. Positive family history of these types of disorders can increase risks to the patient. Chapters 45 and 46 provide a more complete description of musculoskeletal problems that have strong genetic links.

Current Health Problems. The most common reports of people with a musculoskeletal problem are ***pain*** and/or weakness, either of which can impair ***mobility.*** Collect data pertinent to the patient's presenting health problem:

- Date and time of onset
- Factors that cause or exacerbate (worsen) the problem
- Course of the problem (e.g., intermittent or continuous)
- Signs and symptoms (as expressed by the patient) and the pattern of their occurrence
- Measures that improve signs and symptoms (e.g., heat, ice)

Assessment of pain can present many challenges. ***Pain*** can be related to bone, muscle, or joint problems. It may be described as acute or chronic, depending on the onset and duration. Pain with movement could indicate a fracture and/or muscle or joint injury. Assess the intensity of pain by using a pain scale and asking the patient to rate the level that he or she is experiencing. Quality of pain may be described as dull, burning, aching, or stabbing. Determine the location of pain and areas to which it radiates. With any assessment, it is always best if the patient describes the pain in his or her own words and points to its location, if possible. Chapter 5 describes acute and persistent pain in detail.

Weakness may be related to individual muscles or muscle groups. Determine if weakness occurs in proximal or distal muscles or muscle groups. Proximal weakness (near trunk of body) may indicate **myopathy** (a problem in muscle tissue), whereas distal weakness and impaired ***sensory perception*** (especially in lower extremities) may indicate **neuropathy** (a problem in nerve tissue). Muscle weakness in the lower extremities may increase the risk for falls and injury. Weakness in the upper extremities may interfere with ***mobility*** and functional ability.

Assessment of the Skeletal System

Although bones, joints, and muscles are usually assessed during a head-to-toe approach, each subsystem is described separately for emphasis and understanding. For physical assessment of the musculoskeletal system, use inspection, palpation, and range of motion (ROM). A general assessment is described in this chapter. More specific assessment techniques are discussed in the musculoskeletal problem chapters in this unit.

General Inspection. Observe the patient's posture, gait, and general ***mobility*** for gross deformities and impairment. Note unusual findings and coordinate with the physical or occupational therapist for an in-depth physical assessment.

Posture and Gait. *Posture* includes the person's body build and alignment when standing and walking. Assess the curvature of the spine and the length, shape, and symmetry of extremities. Fig. 44.3 illustrates several common spinal deformities. **Lordosis** (an inward abnormal curvature of the lumbar spine) is a common finding in adults who have abdominal obesity. During screening for **scoliosis** (an abnormal lateral curvature of the spine), ask the patient to flex forward from the hips and

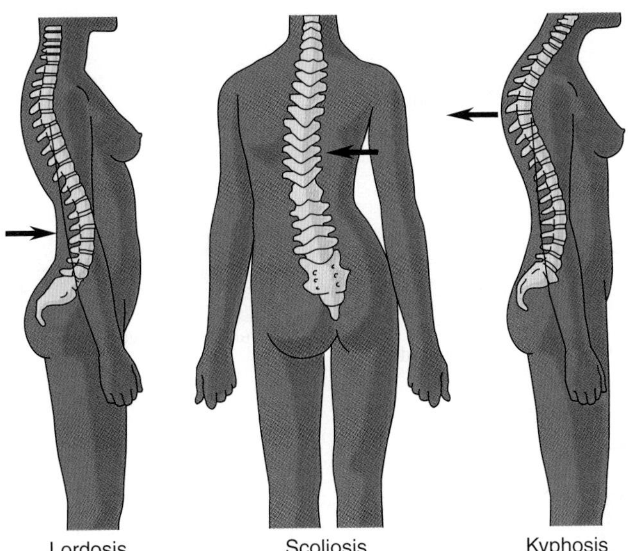

FIG. 44.3 Common spinal deformities.

inspect for the classic lateral curve in the spine. Inspect muscle mass for size and symmetry (Jarvis, 2020).

Most patients with musculoskeletal problems eventually have a problem with *gait.* The nurse or therapist evaluates the patient's balance, steadiness, and ease and length of stride. Any limp or other asymmetric leg movement or deformity is noted.

If the extremities are affected by a musculoskeletal problem, assess arms or legs at the same time for side-to-side comparisons. For example, inspect and palpate both shoulders for size, swelling, deformity, poor alignment, tenderness or pain, and ***mobility.*** A shoulder injury may prevent the patient from combing his or her hair with the affected arm, but severe arthritis may inhibit movement in both arms. Assess the elbows and wrists in a similar way.

Because the hand has multiple joints in a single digit, assessment of hand function is perhaps the most critical part of the examination. If the hands are affected, inspect and palpate the metacarpophalangeal (MCP), proximal interphalangeal (PIP), and distal interphalangeal (DIP) joints (Fig. 44.4). The same digits are compared on the right and left hands. Determine the range of motion (ROM) for each joint by observing active movement. If movement is not possible, evaluate passive motion. For a quick and easy assessment of ROM, ask the patient to make a fist and then appose each finger to the thumb. If he or she can perform these maneuvers, ROM of the hand is not seriously restricted.

Mobility and Functional Assessment. In collaboration with the physical or occupational therapist, assess the patient's need for ambulatory devices, such as canes and walkers, during transfer from bed to chair and while walking and climbing stairs. Observe his or her ability to perform ADLs, such as dressing and bathing. ***Pain***, deformity, and/or impaired ***sensory perception*** may limit physical ***mobility*** and function. Coordinate with the physical and occupational therapists to assess the patient's functional status. A discussion of functional assessment is found in Chapter 7.

Assess major bones, joints, and muscles by inspection, palpation, and determination of ROM. Pay special attention to areas that are affected or may be affected, according to the patient's history or current problem.

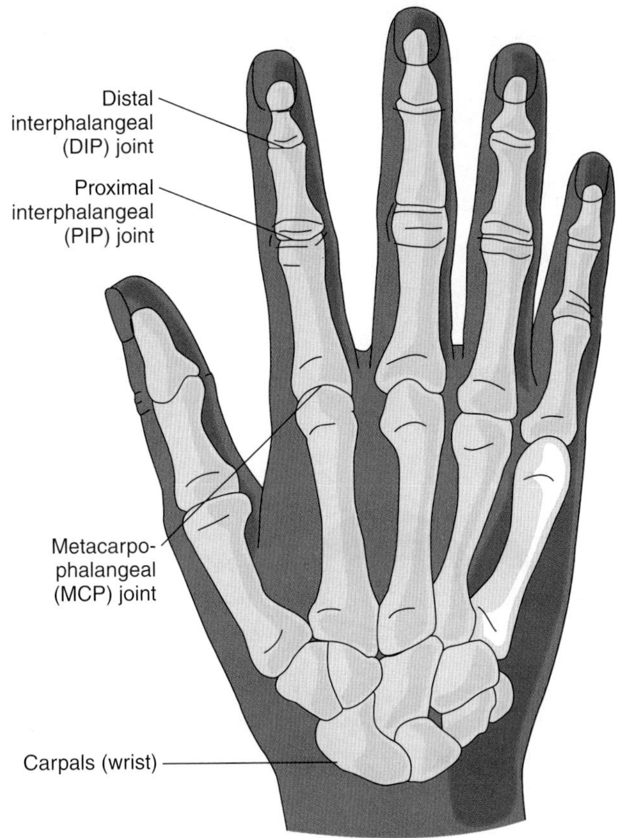

FIG. 44.4 Small joints of the hand.

A **goniometer** is a tool that may be used by rehabilitation therapists or nurses to provide an exact measurement of flexion and extension or joint ROM. Active range of motion (AROM) can be evaluated by asking the patient to move each joint through the ROM himself or herself. If the patient cannot actively move a joint through ROM, ask him or her to relax the muscles in the extremity. Hold the part with one hand above and one hand below the joint to be evaluated and allow passive range of motion (PROM) to evaluate joint ***mobility.*** Movements shown in Fig. 44.5 may be used to evaluate AROM and PROM. Circumduction is a movement that can also be evaluated in the shoulder by having the patient move the arm in circles from the shoulder joint. As long as the patient can function to meet personal needs, a limitation in ROM may not be significant. For each anatomic location, observe the skin for color, elasticity, and lesions that may relate to musculoskeletal dysfunction. For instance, redness or warmth may indicate an inflammatory process and/or pressure injury to skin.

Evaluation of the hip joint relies primarily on determination of its degree of mobility because the joint is deep and difficult to inspect or palpate. *The patient with hip joint pain usually experiences it in the groin or has pain that radiates to the knee or lower back.* The knee is readily accessible for physical assessment, particularly when the patient is sitting and the knee is flexed. Fluid accumulation, or **effusion**, is easily detected in the knee joint. Limitations in movement with accompanying pain are common findings. The knees may be poorly aligned, as in genu valgum ("knock-knee") or genu varum ("bowlegged") deformities (Jarvis, 2020).

The ankles and feet are often neglected in the physical examination. However, they contain multiple bones and joints that can

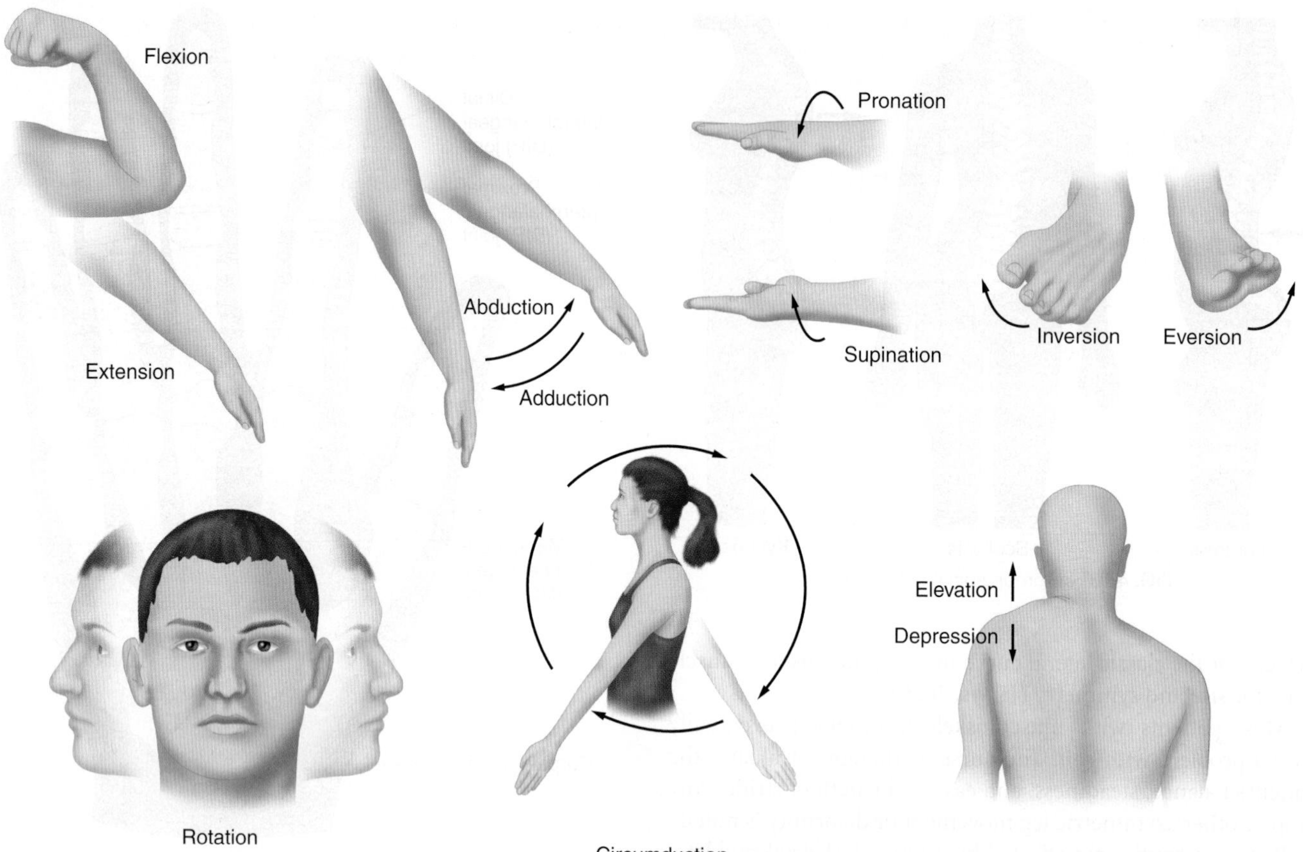

FIG. 44.5 Movements of the skeletal muscles.

be affected by disease and injury. Observe and palpate each joint and test for ROM if feet are affected by musculoskeletal problems.

Neurovascular Assessment. While completing a physical assessment of the musculoskeletal system, perform an assessment of peripheral vascular and nerve integrity. Beginning with the injured side, always compare one extremity with the other.

! NURSING SAFETY PRIORITY (QSEN)

Action Alert

Perform a complete neurovascular assessment (also called a *circ check*), which includes palpation of pulses in the extremities below the level of injury and assessment of sensation, movement, color, temperature, and pain in the injured part. If pulses are not palpable, use a Doppler to find pulses in the extremities.

Assessment of the Muscular System

During the skeletal assessment, note the size, shape, tone, and strength of major skeletal muscles. The circumference of each muscle may be measured and compared for symmetry for an estimation of muscle mass if abnormalities are observed.

Ask the patient to demonstrate muscle strength. Apply resistance by holding the extremity and asking the patient to move against resistance. As an option, place your hands on the patient's upper arms and ask him or her to try to raise the arms. Although movement against resistance is not easily quantified, several scales used by nurses and therapists are available for grading the patient's strength. A commonly used scale is shown in Table 44.2.

TABLE 44.2 Common Scale for Grading Muscle Strength

Rating	Description
5	Normal: ROM unimpaired against gravity with full resistance
4	Good: can complete ROM against gravity with some resistance
3	Fair: can complete ROM against gravity
2	Poor: can complete ROM with gravity eliminated
1	Trace: no joint motion and slight evidence of muscle contractility
0	Zero: no evidence of muscle contractility

ROM, Range of motion.

Psychosocial Assessment

The data from the history and physical assessment provide clues for anticipating psychosocial problems. For instance, prolonged absence from employment or permanent disability may cause job or career loss. Further stress may be experienced if chronic pain continues and the patient cannot cope with numerous stressors. Anxiety and depression are common when patients have chronic pain. Deformities resulting from musculoskeletal disease or injury, such as an amputation, can affect a person's body image and self-concept. Help the patient identify support systems and coping mechanisms that may be useful if he or she has long-term musculoskeletal health problems. Encourage him or her to verbalize feelings related to loss and body image changes. Refer the patient and family for psychological or spiritual counseling if needed and if it is culturally appropriate.

Diagnostic Assessment

Laboratory Assessment. The common laboratory tests used in assessing patients with musculoskeletal disorders are outlined in the Laboratory Profile: Musculoskeletal Assessment box (Pagana & Pagana, 2018; Pagana et al., 2019). There is no special patient preparation or follow-up care for any of these tests. Teach the patient about the purpose of the test and the procedure that can be expected. Additional tests performed for patients with connective tissue diseases, such as rheumatoid arthritis, are described in Chapter 46.

Disorders of bone and the parathyroid gland are often reflected in an alteration of the serum calcium or phosphorus level. Therefore these electrolytes, especially calcium, are monitored. A decrease in serum calcium could indicate bone density loss.

Alkaline phosphatase (ALP) is an enzyme normally present in blood. The concentration of ALP increases with bone or liver damage. In metabolic bone disease and bone cancer, the enzyme concentration rises in proportion to the osteoblastic activity, which indicates bone formation. The level of ALP is normally slightly increased in older adults (Pagana & Pagana, 2018).

The major *muscle enzymes* affected in skeletal muscle disease or injuries are:

- Creatine kinase (CK-MM)
- Lactate dehydrogenase (LDH)
- Aspartate aminotransferase (AST)
- Aldolase (ALD)

LABORATORY PROFILE

Musculoskeletal Assessment

Test	Normal Range for Adults	Significance of Abnormal Findings
Serum calcium	9.0-10.5 mg/dL (2.10-2.50 mmol/L) *Older adults:* decreased	*Hypercalcemia* (increased calcium) • Metastatic cancers of the bone • Paget disease • Bone fractures in healing stage *Hypocalcemia* (decreased calcium) • **Osteoporosis** • **Osteomalacia**
Serum phosphorus (phosphate)	3.0-4.5 mg/dL (0.97-1.45 mmol/L) *Older adults:* decreased	*Hyperphosphatemia* (increased phosphorus) • Bone fractures in healing stage • Bone tumors *Hypophosphatemia* (decreased phosphorus) • **Osteomalacia**
Alkaline phosphatase (ALP)	30-120 units/L (40-160 IU/L) *Older adults:* slightly increased	*Elevations* may indicate: • Metastatic cancers of the bone or liver • **Paget's disease** (a chronic metabolic disorder that causes bone to become fragile and misshapen) • **Osteomalacia**
Serum muscle enzymes Creatine kinase (CK-MM)	Total CK: *Men:* 55-170 units/L (20-215 IU/L) *Women:* 30-135 units/L (20-160 IU/L) CK-MM: 96%-100%	*Elevations* may indicate: • Muscle trauma • **Muscular dystrophy** (a group of genetically linked diseases that cause chronic skeletal muscle weakness and organ dysfunction due to smooth muscle involvement) • Effects of electromyography
Lactate dehydrogenase (LDH)	Total LDH: 100-190 units/L (45-90 IU/L) *Older adults:* slightly increased LDH_1: 17%-27% LDH_2: 27%-37% LDH_3: 18%-25% LDH_4: 3%-8% LDH_5: 0%-5%	*Elevations* may indicate: • Skeletal muscle necrosis (cell death) • Extensive cancer • **Muscular dystrophy**
Aspartate aminotransferase (AST)	0-35 units/L 97-40 IU/L *Older adults:* slightly increased	*Elevations* may indicate: • Skeletal muscle trauma • **Muscular dystrophy**
Aldolase (ALD)	3.0-8.2 units/dL (less than 8 U/L)	*Elevations* may indicate: • **Polymyositis** (an uncommon chronic rheumatic disease that is characterized by inflammation of multiple muscles) and **dermatomyositis** (polymyositis which occurs with a purplish skin rash) • **Muscular dystrophy**

As a result of damage, the muscle tissue releases additional amounts of these enzymes, which increases serum levels.

CLINICAL JUDGMENT CHALLENGE 44.1

Patient-Centered Care

A 33-year-old woman visits her primary health care provider with concerns about new-onset muscle weakness in her left arm. She also reports numbness and tingling in both hands and occasional pain in some of her finger joints. Currently she states that her pain is a 3/10 (3 on a 1-10 pain intensity scale). The nurse records this additional assessment.

- Works full-time as the main teller in a bank requiring long hours using the computer and other machines
- Client's mother has a history of osteoarthritis and carpal tunnel syndrome
- Has two small children (ages 1 and 3) who attend day care while the client is at work
- Single mother with little support from family or friends
- Has health insurance through her work
- Has been taking ibuprofen with some relief of pain

1. **Recognize Cues:** What assessment information in this client situation is the most important and immediate concern for the nurse? (Hint: Identify the **relevant** information *first* to determine what is most important.)
2. **Analyze Cues:** What client conditions are consistent with the **most relevant** information? (Hint: Think about priority collaborative problems that support and contradict the information presented in this situation.)

Imaging Assessment. The skeleton is very visible on *standard x-rays.* Anteroposterior and lateral projections are the initial screening views used most often. Other approaches, such as oblique or stress views, depend on the part of the skeleton to be evaluated and the reason for the x-ray.

Radiography. Bone density, alignment, swelling, and intactness can be seen on x-ray. The conditions of joints can be determined, including the size of the joint space, the smoothness of articular cartilage, and synovial swelling. Soft-tissue involvement may be evident but not clearly differentiated.

Inform the patient that the x-ray table is hard and cold, and instruct him or her to remain still during the filming process. Coordinate with the radiology department or clinic to keep older adults and those at risk for hypothermia as warm as possible (e.g., by using blankets).

CT has gained wide acceptance for detecting musculoskeletal problems, particularly those of the vertebral column and joints. The scanned images can be used to create additional images from other angles or to create three-dimensional images and view complex structures from any position. The nurse or radiology technologist should ask the patient about iodine-based contrast allergies.

Nuclear Scans. The bone scan is a radionuclide test in which radioactive material is injected for viewing the entire skeleton. It may be used primarily to detect tumors, arthritis, osteomyelitis (bone infection), osteoporosis, vertebral compression fractures, and unexplained bone ***pain.*** Bone scans are used less commonly today as more sophisticated MRI equipment becomes more available. However, it may be very useful for detecting hairline fractures in patients with unexplained bone pain and diffuse metastatic bone disease. Gallium citrate (^{67}Ga) is the radioisotope most commonly used. This substance also migrates to the brain, liver, and breast tissue and therefore is used in examination of these structures when disease is suspected.

For patients with osteosarcoma (type of primary bone cancer), thallium (^{201}Tl) is better than gallium or technetium for diagnosing the extent of the disease. Thallium has traditionally been used for the diagnosis of myocardial infarctions but can be used for additional evaluation of cancers of the bone.

Because bone takes up gallium slowly, the nuclear medicine physician or technician administers the isotope 4 to 6 hours before scanning. Other tests that require contrast media or other isotopes cannot be given during this time.

Instruct the patient that the radioactive material poses no threat because it readily deteriorates in the body. Because gallium is excreted through the intestinal tract, it tends to collect in feces after the scanning procedure.

Depending on the tissue to be examined, the patient is taken to the nuclear medicine department 4 to 6 hours after injection. The procedure takes 30 to 60 minutes, during which time the patient must lie still for accurate test results to be achieved. The scan may be repeated at 24, 48, and/or 72 hours. Mild sedation may be necessary to facilitate relaxation and cooperation during the procedure for confused older adults or those in severe pain.

No special care is required after the test. The radioisotope is excreted in stool and urine, but no precautions are taken in handling the excreta. Remind the patient to push fluids to facilitate urinary excretion.

Magnetic Resonance Imaging. MRI, with or without the use of contrast media, is commonly used to diagnose musculoskeletal disorders. It is more accurate than CT for many spinal and knee problems. MRI is most appropriate for joints, soft tissue, and bony tumors that involve soft tissue. CT is still the test of choice for injuries or pathology that involves only bone.

The image is produced through the interaction of magnetic fields, radio waves, and atomic nuclei showing hydrogen density. Simply put, the radio waves "bounce" off the body tissues being examined. Because each tissue has its own density, the computer image clearly distinguishes normal and abnormal tissues. For some tissues, the cross-sectional image is better than that produced by radiography or CT. The lack of hydrogen ions in cortical bone makes it easily distinguishable from soft tissues. The test is particularly useful in identifying problems with muscles, tendons, and ligaments.

Ensure that the patient removes all metal objects and checks for clothing zippers and metal fasteners. Many large facilities and those focused on sports medicine have orthopedic-type MRI machines that have an open design and are vertically oriented (upright) to make the examination more comfortable. The Best Practice for Patient Safety & Quality Care: Preparing the Patient for Magnetic Resonance Imaging box lists questions that the nurse or technician should consider in preparing the patient for MRI.

BEST PRACTICE FOR PATIENT SAFETY & QUALITY CARE (QSEN)

Preparing the Patient for Magnetic Resonance Imaging

- Is the patient pregnant?
- Does the patient have ferromagnetic fragments or implants, such as an older-style aneurysm clip?
- Does the patient have a cardiac pacemaker, metal stent, or electronic implant, such as a medication pump?
- Does the patient have chronic kidney disease? (Gadolinium contrast agents may cause severe systemic complications if the kidneys do not function.)
- Can the patient lie still in the supine position for 45 to 60 minutes (unless using an upright or vertically oriented machine)?
- Does the patient need life-support equipment available?
- Can the patient communicate clearly and understand verbal communication?
- Does the patient have a cochlear implant?
- Is the patient claustrophobic? (Ask this question for closed MRI units; open MRI units do not cause claustrophobia.)

MR arthrography combines arthrography and MRI. It is particularly useful for diagnosing problems of the shoulder and the type and degree of rotator cuff tears. The patient's shoulder is injected with gadolinium contrast medium under fluoroscopy. Then the patient is taken for an MRI, where the shoulder is examined.

Ultrasonography. Sound waves produce an image of the tissue in ultrasonography. An ultrasound procedure may be used to view:

- Soft-tissue disorders, such as masses and fluid accumulation
- Traumatic joint injuries
- Osteomyelitis (bone infection)
- Surgical hardware placement

A jelly-like substance applied to the skin over the site to be examined promotes the movement of a metal probe. No special preparation or posttest care is necessary. A quantitative ultrasound (QUS) may be done for determining fractures or bone density. Bone-density testing is discussed in Chapter 46.

Other Diagnostic Assessment

Biopsies. In a bone biopsy, the physician extracts a specimen of the bone tissue for microscopic examination. This invasive test may confirm the presence of infection or neoplasm, but it is not commonly done today. One of two techniques may be used to retrieve the specimen: needle (closed) biopsy or incisional (open) biopsy.

! NURSING SAFETY PRIORITY (QSEN)

Action Alert

After a bone biopsy, watch for bleeding from the puncture site and for tenderness, redness, or warmth that could indicate infection. Mild analgesics may be used.

Muscle biopsy is done for the diagnosis of atrophy (as in muscular dystrophy) and inflammation (as in polymyositis). The procedure and care for patients undergoing muscle biopsy are the same as those for patients undergoing bone biopsy.

Arthroscopy. Arthroscopy may be used as a diagnostic test or a surgical procedure. An arthroscope is a fiberoptic tube inserted into a joint for direct visualization of the ligaments, menisci, and articular surfaces of the joint. The knee and shoulder are most commonly evaluated. In addition, synovial biopsy and surgery to repair traumatic injury can be done through the arthroscope as an ambulatory care or same-day surgical procedure.

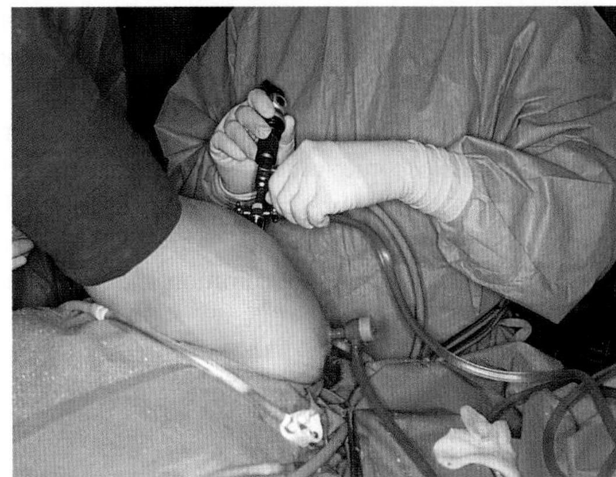

FIG. 44.6 An arthroscope is used in the diagnosis of pathologic changes in the joints. This patient is undergoing arthroscopy of the shoulder.

Patient Preparation. Arthroscopy is performed on an ambulatory care basis or as same-day surgery. The patient must have ***mobility*** in the joint being examined. Those who cannot move the joint or who have an infected joint are not candidates for the procedure.

If the procedure is done for surgical repair, the patient may have a physical therapy consultation before arthroscopy to learn the exercises that are necessary after the test. ROM exercises are also taught but may not be allowed immediately after arthroscopic surgery. The nurse in the surgeon's office or at the surgical center can teach these exercises or reinforce the information provided by the physical therapist. The nurse also reinforces the explanation of the procedure and posttest care and ensures that the patient has signed an informed consent form.

Procedure. The patient is usually given local, light general, or epidural anesthesia, depending on the purpose of the procedure. As shown in Fig. 44.6, the arthroscope is inserted through a small incision shorter than ¼ inch (0.6 cm). Multiple incisions may be required to allow inspection at a variety of angles. After the procedure, a dressing may be applied, depending on the amount of manipulation during the test or surgery.

Follow-up Care. The immediate care after arthroscopy is the same for patients having the procedure for diagnostic purposes as for those having it for surgical intervention.

! NURSING SAFETY PRIORITY (QSEN)

Action Alert

The priority for postprocedure care after arthroscopy is to assess the neurovascular status of the patient's affected limb every hour or according to agency or surgeon protocol. Monitor and document distal pulses, warmth, color, capillary refill, ***pain,*** movement, and sensation of the affected extremity.

Encourage the patient to perform exercises as taught before the procedure, if appropriate. For the mild discomfort experienced after the diagnostic arthroscopy, the primary health care provider prescribes a mild analgesic, such as acetaminophen. If postoperative, the patient may have short-term activity restrictions, depending on the musculoskeletal problem. Ice is often used for 24 hours, and the extremity should be elevated for 12 to 24 hours. When arthroscopic surgery is performed, the primary health care provider usually prescribes a short-term opioid-analgesic combination, such as oxycodone and acetaminophen.

Although complications are not common, monitor and teach the patient to observe for:

- Swelling
- Increased joint pain attributable to mechanical injury
- Thrombophlebitis
- Infection

Severe joint or limb pain after discharge may indicate a possible complication. Teach the patient to immediately contact the primary health care provider, who usually sees the patient about 1 week after the procedure to check for complications.

NCLEX EXAMINATION CHALLENGE 44.2

Safe and Effective Care Environment

A client returns to the postanesthesia care unit (PACU) after an arthroscopy to repair a shoulder injury. What is the nurse's **priority** when caring for this client?

A. Keep the affected arm elevated and immobilized.
B. Ensure that the client uses the patient-controlled analgesia (PCA) pump.
C. Check the neurovascular status of the affected arm.
D. Instruct the client to stay in bed for 24 hours.

GET READY FOR THE NEXT-GENERATION NCLEX® EXAMINATION!

Key Points

Review these Key Points for each NCLEX Examination Client Needs Category.

Safe and Effective Care Environment

- Perform a focused musculoskeletal assessment, including gait, muscle strength, ***pain***, and ***mobility*** status as indicated by the patient's signs and symptoms. **Clinical Judgment**

Health Promotion and Maintenance

- Be aware that older adults have physiologic changes that affect their musculoskeletal system, such as decreased bone density and joint cartilage degeneration; plan nursing interventions to ensure patient safety. **QSEN: Patient-Centered Care; Safety**

Psychosocial Integrity

- Recall that potential patient reactions to musculoskeletal trauma or disease can include anxiety, depression, and/or altered body image and self-concept. **QSEN: Patient-Centered Care**

Physiological Integrity

- Perform a thorough ***pain*** assessment, including pain intensity, quality, duration, and location. **Clinical Judgment**
- Interpret the patient's laboratory values that are related to musculoskeletal disease. **Clinical Judgment**
- Instruct the patient to report swelling, infection, and increased pain after an arthroscopy. **QSEN: Safety**
- Ask the patient questions to ensure safety before an MRI. **QSEN: Safety**
- Ask the patient about allergy to contrast media before diagnostic testing such as CT scans. **QSEN: Safety**
- Evaluate the neurovascular status of the patient's affected extremity after an arthroscopic procedure as the *priority for care*. **QSEN: Safety**

MASTERY QUESTIONS

1. The nurse is preparing to teach a client about how to promote musculoskeletal health. Which statements will the nurse include in the teaching plan? **Select all that apply.**
   A. "If you smoke, you need a smoking cessation plan."
   B. "Avoid drinking excessive alcohol."
   C. "Be sure to take in enough calcium and vitamin D."
   D. "Avoid high-risk activities that could cause an accident."
   E. "Include weight-bearing exercise like walking on a regular basis."

2. Which serum laboratory finding is of concern for the nurse and should be reported to the primary health care provider?
   A. Calcium = 9 mg/dL (2.10 mmol/L)
   B. Phosphorus = 4.5 mg/dL (1.45 mmol/L)
   C. Lactate dehydrogenase = 150 units/L (150 IU/L)
   D. Alkaline phosphatase = 210 units/L (210 IU/L)

REFERENCES

AL-Bashaireh, A. M., Haddad, L. G., Weaver, M., Kelly, D. L., Chengguo, X., & Yoon, S. (2018). The effect of tobacco smoking on musculoskeletal health: A systematic review. *Journal of Environmental and Public Health*. https://doi.org/10.1155/2018/4184190. July 11.

Jarvis, C. (2020). *Physical examination & health assessment* (8th ed.). St. Louis: Elsevier Saunders.

McCance, K., Huether, S., Brashers, V., & Rote, N. (2019). *Pathophysiology: The biologic basis for disease in adults and children* (8th ed.). St. Louis: Mosby.

Pagana, K. D., & Pagana, T. J. (2018). *Mosby's manual of diagnostic and laboratory tests* (6th ed.). St. Louis: Mosby.

Pagana, K. D., Pagana, T. J., & Pike-MacDonald, S. A. (2019). *Mosby's Canadian manual of diagnostic and laboratory tests* (2nd ed.). St. Louis: Mosby.

Smith, M. A., & Jackson, A. (2018). Tobacco use, tobacco cessation, & musculoskeletal health. *Orthopaedic Nursing, 37*(5), 280–284.

45

Concepts of Care for Patients With Musculoskeletal Problems

Donna D. Ignatavicius

http://evolve.elsevier.com/Iggy/

LEARNING OUTCOMES

1. Prioritize collaborative evidence-based care for patients with common musculoskeletal problems affecting mobility, perfusion, and cellular regulation.
2. Identify community resources for patients with common musculoskeletal problems.
3. Teach adults how to decrease the risk for osteoporosis.
4. Assess the psychosocial impact for patients experiencing common musculoskeletal health problems.
5. Apply knowledge of pathophysiology to assess patients with common musculoskeletal problems caused by impaired ***cellular regulation*** and ***infection.***
6. Plan health teaching for the patient and caregiver(s) about common drugs used for common musculoskeletal problems, including those used for ***pain*** control.

KEY TERMS

bone mineral density (BMD) The amount of mineral in bone that determines bone strength and peaks between 25 and 30 years of age.

bunionectomy Surgical removal of the first metatarsal bony overgrowth and bursa with realignment to manage *Pain*.

dual x-ray absorptiometry (DXA) A noninvasive radiographic scan to assess bone mineral density.

Dupuytren contracture (or deformity) A slowly progressive thickening of the palmar fascia, resulting in flexion contracture of the fourth (ring) and fifth (little) fingers of the hand.

fragility fracture A fracture caused by osteoporosis.

ganglion A round, benign cyst, often found on a wrist or foot joint or tendon.

hallux valgus deformity A common foot problem in which the great toe drifts laterally at the first metatarsophalangeal (MTP) joint.

kyphosis Outward curvature of the thoracic spine causing a "humped back."

osteomalacia Loss of bone related to lack of vitamin D, which causes bone softening.

osteomyelitis *Infection* in bone caused by bacteria (most often), viruses, parasites, or fungi; the infection may be acute or chronic.

osteonecrosis (also known as *avascular necrosis*); bone death secondary to lack of or disruption in blood supply to the affected bone, usually from trauma or chronic steroid therapy.

osteopenia Loss of bone mass.

osteoporosis A chronic disease of ***cellular regulation*** in which bone loss causes significant decreased density and possible fracture.

plantar fasciitis An inflammation of the plantar fascia, which is located in the area of the arch of the foot, causing pain.

PRIORITY AND INTERRELATED CONCEPTS

The priority concepts for this chapter are:
- ***Mobility***
- ***Infection***
- ***Cellular Regulation***

The ***Cellular Regulation*** concept exemplar for this chapter is Osteoporosis.

The interrelated concepts for this chapter are:
- ***Pain***
- ***Perfusion***

Musculoskeletal disorders include diseases of ***cellular regulation*** (e.g., osteoporosis), bone tumors, bone ***infection,*** and a variety of deformities and syndromes. Older adults are at the greatest risk for most of these problems, although *primary* bone cancer is most often found in adolescents and young adults.

Almost all musculoskeletal health problems result in decreased ***mobility,*** acute or persistent (chronic) ***pain,*** and/or impaired ***perfusion.*** These concepts are reviewed in Chapter 3. This chapter focuses on selected adult musculoskeletal health disorders not covered in Chapter 46 on arthritis and Chapter 47 on musculoskeletal trauma. Musculoskeletal problems that are seen most often in children, such as scoliosis and progressive muscular dystrophies, are not included in this chapter because they are included in pediatric textbooks.

CELLULAR REGULATION CONCEPT EXEMPLAR: OSTEOPOROSIS

Pathophysiology Review

Osteoporosis is a chronic disease of ***cellular regulation*** in which bone loss causes significant decreased density and possible fracture. It is often referred to as a *silent disease* or *silent thief* because the first sign of osteoporosis in most people follows some kind of a fracture.

Euro-American postmenopausal women have a 50% chance of having a **fragility fracture** (fracture caused by osteoporosis; sometimes referred to as a "bone attack") in their lifetime (National Osteoporosis Foundation [NOF], 2018). A woman who experiences a hip fracture has a greater risk for a second fracture. Fractures as a result of osteoporosis and falling can decrease a patient's ***mobility*** and quality of life. The mortality rate for older patients with hip fractures is very high, especially within the first 6 to 12 months, and the debilitating effects can be devastating (also see Chapter 47 on fractures).

Osteoporosis is a major global health problem. In less affluent or famine countries, many people have both osteoporosis *and* osteomalacia as a result of dietary deficiencies. **Osteomalacia** is loss of bone related to lack of vitamin D, which causes bone softening. Vitamin D is needed for calcium absorption in the small intestine. As a result of vitamin D deficiency, normal bone building is disrupted, and calcification does not occur to harden the bone. Table 45.1 compares these two bone diseases.

Bone is a living, changing tissue that is constantly undergoing changes in a process referred to as *bone remodeling*, a type of ***cellular regulation.*** Osteoporosis and **osteopenia** (loss of bone mass) occur when osteoclastic (bone resorption) activity is greater than osteoblastic (bone-building) activity. The result is a decreased **bone mineral density (BMD)**. BMD is the amount of mineral that determines bone strength and peaks between 25 and 30 years of age. Before and during the peak years, osteoclastic activity and osteoblastic activity work at the same rate. After the peak years, osteoclastic activity exceeds bone-building activity, and bone density decreases. BMD decreases most rapidly in postmenopausal women as serum estrogen levels diminish. Although estrogen does not build bone, it helps prevent bone loss. *Trabecular,* or *cancellous* (spongy), bone is lost first, followed by loss of *cortical* (compact) bone. The hip, wrist, and spinal column have the highest amount of cancellous bone and are therefore the most likely to fracture first.

Standards for the diagnosis of osteoporosis are based on BMD testing that provides a T-score for the patient. A T-score represents the number of standard deviations above or below (designated with a minus sign) the average BMD for young, healthy adults. The T-score in a healthy 30-year-old adult is 0. *Osteopenia is present when the T-score is at −1 and above −2.5. Osteoporosis is diagnosed in a person who has a T-score at or lower than −2.5* (NOF, 2018). *Severe or established osteoporosis is defined as the presence of osteoporosis plus one or more fractures.*

Osteoporosis can be classified as generalized or regional. *Generalized* osteoporosis involves many structures in the skeleton and is further divided into two categories: primary and secondary. *Primary* osteoporosis is more common and occurs in postmenopausal women and in men in their seventh or eighth decade of life. *Secondary* osteoporosis may result from other medical conditions, such as hyperparathyroidism; long-term drug therapy, such as with corticosteroids; or prolonged decreased ***mobility,*** such as that seen with spinal cord injury (Table 45.2). Treatment of the secondary type is directed toward the cause of the osteoporosis when possible.

Regional (localized) osteoporosis, an example of secondary disease, can occur when a limb is immobilized related to a fracture, injury, or paralysis. Decreased ***mobility*** for longer than 8 to 12 weeks can result in this type of osteoporosis. Bone loss also

TABLE 45.2 Common Causes of Secondary Osteoporosis

Diseases and Conditions	Drugs (Chronic Use)
• Diabetes mellitus	• Corticosteroids
• Hyperthyroidism	• Antiepileptic drugs (AEDs) (e.g., phenytoin)
• Hyperparathyroidism	• Barbiturates (e.g., phenobarbital)
• Cushing syndrome	• Ethanol (alcohol)
• Growth hormone deficiency	• Drugs that induce hypogonadism (decreased levels of sex hormones)
• Metabolic acidosis	• High levels of thyroid hormone
• Female hypogonadism	• Cytotoxic agents
• Rheumatoid arthritis	• Immunosuppressants
• Prolonged immobilization	• Loop diuretics
• Bone cancer	• Aluminum-based antacids
• Cirrhosis	
• HIV infection	

TABLE 45.1 Differential Features of Osteoporosis and Osteomalacia

Characteristic	Osteoporosis	Osteomalacia
Definition	Decreased bone mass caused by multiple factors	Bone softening caused by lack of calcification
Primary etiology	Lack of calcium and estrogen or testosterone	Lack of vitamin D
Radiographic findings	Osteopenia (bone loss), fractures	Fractures
Calcium level	Low or normal	Low or normal
Phosphate level	Normal	Low or normal
Parathyroid hormone	Normal	High or normal
Alkaline phosphatase	Normal	High

occurs when people spend prolonged time in a gravity-free or weightless environment (e.g., astronauts).

Etiology and Genetic Risk. Primary osteoporosis is caused by a combination of genetic, lifestyle, and environmental factors. The Best Practice for Patient Safety & Quality Care: Assessing Risk Factors for Primary Osteoporosis box lists the major modifiable and nonmodifiable risk factors that contribute to the development of this disease (Capriotti & Scanlon, 2018).

PATIENT-CENTERED CARE: GENETIC/ GENOMIC CONSIDERATIONS QSEN

The genetic and immune factors that cause osteoporosis are very complex. Strong evidence demonstrates that genetics is a significant factor. Many genetic changes have been identified as possible causative factors, but there is no agreement about which ones are most important or constant in all patients. For example, changes in the vitamin D_3 receptor *(VDR)* gene and calcitonin receptor *(CTR)* gene have been found in some patients with the disease. Receptors are essential for the uptake and use of these substances by the cells (McCance et al., 2019).

The bone morphogenetic protein 2 *(BMP-2)* gene has a key role in bone formation and maintenance. Some osteoporotic patients who had fractures have changes in their *BMP-2* gene. Alterations in the growth hormone 1 *(GH-1)* gene have been discovered in petite Asian-American women (i.e., those who are predisposed to developing osteoporosis.)

Hormones, tumor necrosis factor (TNF), interleukins, and other substances in the body help control osteoclasts in a very complex pathway. The identification of the importance of the cytokine receptor activator of nuclear factor kappa-B ligand (RANKL), its receptor RANK, and its decoy receptor osteoprotegerin (OPG) has helped researchers understand more about the activity of osteoclasts in metabolic bone disease. Disruptions in the RANKL, RANK, and OPG system can lead to increased osteoclast activity in which bone is rapidly broken down (McCance et al., 2019). Knowledge of these physiologic changes has contributed to the development of new drugs to manage osteoporosis (see the Drug Therapy section later in this chapter).

BEST PRACTICE FOR PATIENT SAFETY & QUALITY CARE QSEN

Assessing Risk Factors for Primary Osteoporosis

Assess for these *nonmodifiable* risk factors:

- Older age (over 50 years of age)
- Menopause or history of total hysterectomy, including removal of ovaries
- Parental history of osteoporosis, especially mother
- Euro-Caucasian or Asian ethnicity
- Eating disorders, such as anorexia nervosa
- Rheumatoid arthritis
- History of low-trauma fracture after age 50 years

Assess for these *modifiable* risk factors:

- Low body weight, thin build
- Chronic low calcium and/or vitamin D intake
- Estrogen or androgen deficiency
- Current smoking (active or passive)
- High alcohol intake (two or more drinks a day)
- Drug therapy, such as chronic steroid therapy (also see Table 45.2)
- Poor nutrition
- Lack of physical exercise or prolonged decreased ***mobility***

PATIENT-CENTERED CARE: GENDER HEALTH CONSIDERATIONS QSEN

Primary osteoporosis most often occurs in women after menopause or removal of both ovaries as a result of decreased estrogen levels. Obese women can store estrogen in their tissues for use as necessary to maintain a normal level of serum calcium better than thinner women and are therefore less likely to develop osteoporosis and resulting fractures.

Men also develop osteoporosis as they age because their testosterone levels decrease. Testosterone is the major sex hormone that builds bone tissue. Older men are often underdiagnosed.

The relationship of osteoporosis to nutrition is well established. For example, excessive caffeine in the diet can cause calcium loss in the urine. A diet lacking enough calcium and vitamin D stimulates the parathyroid gland to produce parathyroid hormone (PTH). PTH triggers the release of calcium from the bony matrix. Activated vitamin D is needed for calcium uptake in the body. Malabsorption of nutrients in the small intestine also contributes to low serum calcium levels. Institutionalized or homebound patients who are not exposed to sunlight may be at a higher risk because they do not receive adequate vitamin D for the metabolism of calcium (NOF, 2018).

Calcium loss occurs at a more rapid rate when phosphorus intake is high. (Chapter 13 describes the usual relationship between calcium and phosphorus in the body.) People who drink large amounts of carbonated beverages each day (over 40 ounces [1200 mL]) are at high risk for calcium loss and subsequent osteoporosis, regardless of age or gender.

Protein deficiency may also affect ***cellular regulation.*** Because 50% of serum calcium is protein bound, protein is needed to use calcium. However, excessive protein intake may increase calcium loss in the urine. For example, people who are on high-protein, low-carbohydrate diets, such as the Atkins diet, may consume too much protein to replace other foods that are not allowed.

Incidence and Prevalence. Osteoporosis is a health problem for more than 44 million Americans. About 10 million people in the United States have the disease, and about 34 million people

PATIENT-CENTERED CARE: CULTURAL/ SPIRITUAL CONSIDERATIONS QSEN

Body build, weight, and race/ethnicity seem to influence who gets the disease. Osteoporosis occurs most often in older, lean-built Euro-American and Asian women, particularly those who do not exercise regularly. However, African Americans are at risk for decreased vitamin D, which is needed for adequate calcium absorption in the small intestines. Dietary preferences or intolerances, sun avoidance, or the inability to afford high-nutrient food may influence anyone's rate of bone loss. For example, many blacks have lactose intolerance and cannot drink regular milk or eat other dairy-based foods (NOF, 2018). As an alternative, lactose-free milk, almond milk, or soy milk provides calcium. Milk and cheese are good sources of protein, a nutrient needed to bind calcium for use by the body.

50 years of age and older have osteopenia and are at risk for development of osteoporosis (NOF, 2018). As "baby boomers" age, these numbers are expected to increase dramatically.

Health Promotion and Maintenance

Peak bone mass is achieved by about 30 years of age in most women. *Building strong bone as a young person may be the best defense against osteoporosis in later adulthood.* Young women need to be aware of appropriate health and lifestyle practices that can prevent this potentially disabling disease. Patient-centered teaching should begin with young women because they begin to lose bone after 30 years of age. Nurses can play a vital role in patient education for women of any age to prevent and manage osteoporosis (Evenson & Sanders, 2016).

The focus of evidence-based osteoporosis prevention is to decrease modifiable risk factors to promote patient safety. For example, teach patients who do not include enough dietary calcium which foods to eat, such as dairy products and dark green leafy vegetables. Teach them to read food labels for sources of calcium content. Explain the importance of sun exposure (but not so much as to get sunburned) and adequate vitamin D in the diet. The National Osteoporosis Foundation recommends that all adults take a vitamin D_3 supplement, but strong evidence to support this recommendation is lacking or controversial (NOF, 2018; Reid, 2017).

Teach people at high risk for bone loss the importance of smoking cessation (if needed), weight loss (if needed), and avoidance of excessive alcohol use. Teach them the need to limit the amount of carbonated beverages consumed each day. Remind patients who have sedentary lifestyles about the importance of exercise and which types of exercise build bone tissue. Weight-bearing exercises, such as regularly scheduled walking, are preferred. Teach people at high risk to avoid activities that cause jarring, such as horseback riding and jogging, to prevent potential vertebral compression fractures.

❖ Interprofessional Collaborative Care

◆ Assessment: Recognize Cues

History. A complete health history with assessment of risk factors is important in the prevention, early detection, and treatment of osteoporosis. Patients who have risk factors for osteoporosis are at increased risk for fractures when falls occur. In some cases, the fracture occurs before the fall. Include a fall risk assessment in the health history, especially for older adults. Assess for fall risk factors as described in Chapter 4.

Physical Assessment/Signs and Symptoms. When performing a musculoskeletal assessment, inspect the vertebral column. The classic "dowager's hump," or kyphosis (outward curvature of the thoracic spine causing a "humped back"), is often present (Fig. 45.1). The older patient may state that he or she has gotten shorter, perhaps as much as 2 to 3 inches (5 to 7.5 cm), within the previous 20 years. Take or delegate the taking of height and weight measurements and compare with previous measurements if they are available (Jarvis, 2020).

> **! NATIONAL PATIENT SAFETY GOALS**
>
> The Joint Commission's National Patient Safety Goals (NPSGs) specify the need to reduce risk for harm to patients resulting from falls. Hospitals and long-term care facilities have risk management programs to assess for the risk for falls. For patients at high risk, communicate this information to other members of the health care team, using colored armbands, posted signs, or other easy-to-recognize methods. Chapter 4 discusses fall prevention in health care agencies and at home in more detail.

The patient may have back pain, which often occurs after lifting, bending, or stooping. The pain may be sharp and acute or persistent (chronic). ***Pain*** is worse with activity and is often reduced by rest. Back pain accompanied by tenderness and voluntary restriction of spinal movement suggests one or more compression vertebral fractures (i.e., one of the most common types of osteoporotic or fragility fracture). Movement restriction and spinal deformity may result in constipation, abdominal distention, reflux esophagitis, and respiratory compromise in severe cases. The most likely area for spinal fracture is between T8 and L3, the most movable part of the vertebral column.

Fractures are also common in the distal end of the radius (wrist) and the upper third of the femur (hip). Ask the patient to locate all areas that are painful and observe for signs and symptoms of fractures, such as swelling and malalignment. Signs and symptoms of fractures are discussed in Chapter 47.

> **NCLEX EXAMINATION CHALLENGE 45.1**
>
> ***Physiological Integrity***
>
> Which assessment data are factors that increase the risk for osteoporosis for an older Euro-American female? **Select all that apply.**
>
> A. Drinks 3 to 4 glasses of wine each day
> B. Sits at a desk all day at her job
> C. Smokes a pack of cigarettes a day
> D. Takes a mile-long walk 5 days a week
> E. Takes 1000 mg acetaminophen for arthritis daily
> F. Weighs 110 lb (50 kg)

Psychosocial Assessment. Women associate osteoporosis with menopause, getting older, and becoming less independent. The disease can result in decreased ***mobility,*** deformity, and disability that can affect the patient's well-being and life satisfaction. Quality of life may be further affected by persistent (chronic) ***pain,*** insomnia, depression, and fear of falling (Touhy & Jett, 2018).

Assess the patient's concept of body image, especially if he or she is severely kyphotic. For example, the patient may have difficulty finding clothes that fit properly. Social interactions may be avoided because of a change in appearance or the physical limitations of being unable to sit in chairs in restaurants, movie theaters, and other places. Changes in sexuality may occur as a result of poor self-esteem or the discomfort caused by positioning during intercourse.

Because osteoporosis poses a risk for fractures, teach the patient to be extremely cautious about activities. As a result, the

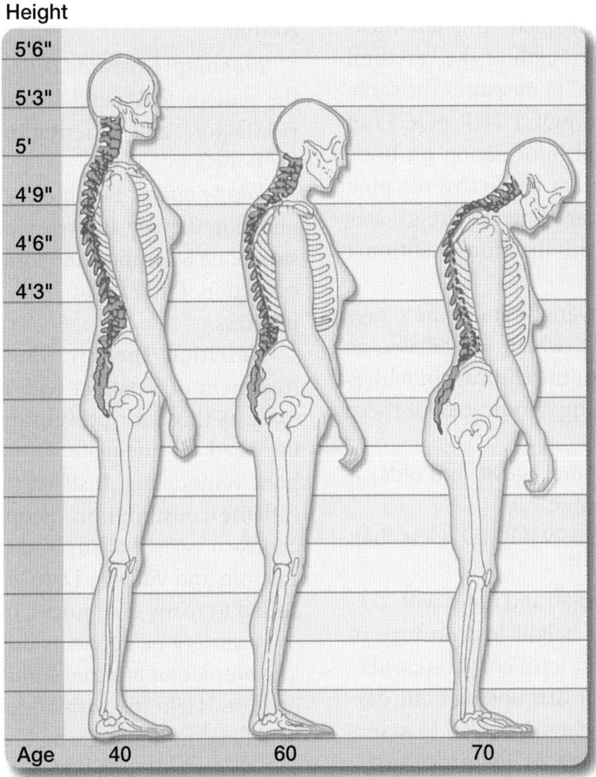

FIG. 45.1 Normal spine at age 40 years and osteoporotic changes at ages 60 and 70 years. These changes can cause a loss of as much as 6 inches in height and can result in the so-called *dowager's hump (far right)* in the upper thoracic vertebrae.

threat of fracture can create anxiety and fear and result in further limitation of social or physical activities. Assess for these feelings to assist in treatment decisions and health teaching. For example, the patient may not exercise as prescribed for fear that a fracture will occur.

Laboratory Assessment. Serum calcium and vitamin D_3 levels should be routinely monitored (at least once a year) for all women and for men older than 50 years who are at a high risk for the disease. Serum calcium should be between 9.0 and 10.5 mg/dL (2.10 and 2.50 mmol/L). Total 25-hydroxyvitamin D (D_2 plus D_3) levels should be between 25 and 80 ng/mL (75 and 200 nmol/L) (Pagana & Pagana 2018; Pagana et al., 2019). These results can help determine the need for supplements and preventive measures to slow bone loss. No definitive laboratory tests confirm a diagnosis of primary osteoporosis, although a number of *bone turnover markers* can provide information about bone resorption and formation activity. Although not commonly tested, these markers are sensitive to bone changes and can be used to monitor effectiveness of treatment for osteoporosis or to detect bone changes early in the disease process. Examples of these markers are osteocalcin and bone-specific alkaline phosphatase (BSAP).

Imaging Assessment. Conventional x-rays of the spine and long bones show decreased bone density, but only after a large amount of bone loss has occurred. Fractures can also be seen on x-rays. According to the National Osteoporosis Foundation (NOF, 2018), all postmenopausal women and men age 50 and older should be evaluated for osteoporosis risk to determine the need for BMD testing and/or vertebral imaging.

The most commonly used screening and diagnostic radiographic test for measuring bone mineral density (BMD) is **dual x-ray absorptiometry (DXA)**. The spine and hip are most often assessed when central DXA (cDXA) scan is performed. If spinal deformity is present, the wrist may also be assessed. Many primary health care providers recommend that women in their 40s have a baseline screening DXA scan so later bone changes can be detected and compared. DXA is a noninvasive, painless scan that emits less radiation than a chest x-ray. It is the most common test currently used but has limitations. First, BMD alone explains only part of the bone change and provides no information on cellular activity. Second, there are variations among different DXA systems. In addition, DXA is not useful for very tall or very obese patients.

Tell patients that their height is measured before a DXA scan. The patient stays dressed but is asked to remove any metallic objects such as belt buckles, coins, keys, or jewelry that might interfere with the test. The results are displayed on a computer graph, and a T-score is calculated. No special follow-up care for the test is required. However, the patient needs to discuss the results with the primary health care provider for any decisions about possible preventive or management interventions. Patients who have osteopenia usually have follow-up DXA scans every 2 years.

For some patients, *CT-based absorptiometry* (qualitative computed tomography [QCT]) may be performed. This test measures the volume of bone density and strength of the vertebral spine and hip. The peripheral QCT (pQCT) measures the same at the forearm or tibia. High-resolution pQCT (HR-pQCT) of the radius and tibia provides additional information on bone structure and architecture. These tests are predictive of spine and/or hip fractures in women; however, they require greater amounts of radiation when compared with the more traditional DXA.

Vertebral imaging can be performed using lateral spine x-rays or lateral vertebral fracture assessment, which is available as part of most DXA systems. According to the clinical guidelines outlined by NOF (2018), vertebral imaging is indicated for these groups:

- All women age 70 and older and all men age 80 and older if BMD is less than or equal to a T-score of 1.0
- Women age 65 to 69 and men age 70 to 79 if BMD is less than or equal to a T-score of 1.5
- Postmenopausal women and men age 50 and older with certain risk factors, such as significant height loss, history of low-trauma fracture, or being on long-term corticosteroids

The most promising imaging test for diagnosing bone disease is the use of *magnetic resonance imaging (MRI)* to assess bone marrow composition (see Chapter 44 for procedure). MRI does not involve radiation and can be used to view bone in ways that other techniques cannot. To determine the presence of osteoporosis, quantitative MRI procedures provide information about yellow bone marrow content, diffusion, and perfusion to the bone. ***Perfusion*** to osteoporotic bone is lower than to bone of normal bone density. Fat marrow content, sometimes referred to as *bone marrow adipose tissue (BMAT),* is higher in patients with bone loss compared with those with normal BMD (Xiaojuan & Schwartz, 2020). These tests are more reliable and offer more information about bone change than BMD measurements alone but are very expensive and not widely used.

Several imaging tests are available for community-based screening because these devices are more portable. However, they lack the preciseness and reliability of the previously discussed imaging procedures. Examples include the peripheral DXA (pDXA) and the peripheral quantitative ultrasound densitometry (pQUS). The *pDXA scan* assesses BMD of the heel, forearm, or finger. It is often used for large-scale screening purposes. The *pQUS* is an effective and low-cost screening tool that can detect osteoporosis and predict risk for hip fracture. The heel, tibia, and patella are most commonly tested. This procedure requires no special preparation, is quick, and has no radiation exposure or specific follow-up care (Pagana & Pagana, 2018). Both tests are commonly used for screening at community health fairs, skilled nursing facilities, and women's health centers.

◆ Analysis: Analyze Cues and Prioritize Hypotheses

The priority problem for patients with osteoporosis or osteopenia is *Potential for fractures due to weak, porous bone tissue.*

◆ Planning and Implementation: Generate Solutions and Take Action

Planning: Expected Outcomes. The expected outcome is that the patient will avoid fractures by preventing falls, managing risk factors, and adhering to preventive or treatment measures for bone loss.

Interventions. Because the patient is predisposed to fractures, nutrition therapy, lifestyle changes, and drug therapy are used to slow bone resorption and form new bone tissue. Self-management education (SME) can help prevent osteoporosis or slow the progress.

Nutrition Therapy. The nutritional considerations for the treatment of a patient with a diagnosis of osteoporosis are the same as those for preventing the disease. Teach patients about the need for adequate amounts of calcium and vitamin D for bone remodeling. Instruct them to avoid excessive alcohol and caffeine consumption. People who are lactose intolerant can choose a variety of soy and rice products that are fortified with calcium and vitamin D. In addition, calcium and vitamin D are added to many fruit juices, bread, and cereal products.

A variety of nutrients are needed to maintain bone health. *The promotion of a single nutrient will not prevent or treat osteoporosis.* Help the patient develop a nutrition plan that is most beneficial in maintaining bone health; the plan should emphasize fruits and vegetables, low-fat dairy and protein sources, increased fiber, and moderation in alcohol and caffeine (NOF, 2018).

Lifestyle Changes. Exercise is important in the prevention and management of osteoporosis. It also plays a vital role in ***pain*** management, cardiovascular function, and an improved sense of well-being.

In collaboration with the primary health care provider, the physical therapist may prescribe exercises for strengthening the abdominal and back muscles for those at risk for vertebral fractures. These exercises improve posture and support for the spine. Abdominal muscle tightening, deep breathing, and pectoral stretching are stressed to increase lung capacity. Exercises for the extremity muscles include muscle-tightening, resistive, and range-of-motion (ROM) exercises to improve ***mobility.*** Muscle strengthening also helps to prevent falls and promote balance. Swimming and yoga provides overall muscle exercise.

In addition to exercises for muscle strengthening, a general weight-bearing exercise program should be implemented. Teach patients that walking for 30 minutes three to five times a week is the single most effective exercise for osteoporosis prevention. Remind them to avoid any activity that would cause jarring of the body, such as jogging and horseback riding. These activities can cause compression fractures of the vertebral column.

In addition to nutrition and exercise, other lifestyle changes may be needed. Teach the patient to avoid tobacco in any form, especially active or passive cigarette smoking (NOF, 2018). Remind women not to consume more than one alcoholic drink per day (5 ounces each); instruct men not to have more than two alcoholic drinks per day.

Drug Therapy. The evidence shows that drug therapy should be used for postmenopausal women and men age 50 and older when the BMD T-score for the hip or lumbar spine is below or equal to −2.5 with no other risk factors, or when the T-score is below −1.5 with risk factors or previous fracture. Anyone age 50 or older who had a hip or vertebral fracture should also be treated (NOF, 2018). The primary health care provider may prescribe calcium and vitamin D_3 supplements, bisphosphonates, estrogen agonist/antagonists (formerly called *selective estrogen receptor modulators* [SERMS]), parathyroid hormone (PTH), RANKL inhibitor, or a combination of several drugs to treat or prevent osteoporosis (see the Common Examples of Drug Therapy: Osteoporosis box).

Calcium and Activated Vitamin D (D_3). Intake of *calcium* alone is not a treatment for osteoporosis, but calcium is an important part of any program to promote bone health. Many people cannot or do not have enough calcium in their diet; therefore calcium supplements may be needed. NOF (2018) supports the National Academy of Medicine's research recommendation of 1000 mg daily for all postmenopausal women and men between ages 50 and 70, and 1200 mg for both women and men 71 years of age and older (NOF, 2018). Teach women to start taking supplements in young adulthood to help maintain peak bone mass. Because vitamin D is needed for calcium absorption by the body, vitamin D_3 supplementation is also indicated. Laboratory tests to measure serum calcium and vitamin D_3 may be done to monitor the effectiveness of these supplements.

Bisphosphonates. Bisphosphonates slow bone resorption by binding with crystal elements in bone, especially spongy, cancellous bone tissue. They are the most common drugs used for osteoporosis, but some are also approved for Paget disease and hypercalcemia caused by cancer. Three Food and Drug Administration (FDA)–approved bisphosphonates (alendronate, ibandronate, and risedronate) are commonly used for the *prevention and treatment* of osteoporosis (Burchum & Rosenthal, 2019). These drugs are available as oral preparations; ibandronate is also available as an IV preparation.

COMMON EXAMPLES OF DRUG THERAPY

Osteoporosis

Drug Category	Nursing Implications
Calcium (With Vitamin D)	
Calcium and vitamin D_3 may be taken separately or in combination	Take a third of the daily dose at bedtime *because no weight-bearing activity to build bone occurs while sleeping.* Encourage increased fluids, unless medically contraindicated, *to help prevent urinary calculi (stones).* Teach patient to take the drugs with 6-8 ounces of water *to help dissolve them.* Assess for a history of urinary stones before giving calcium. Monitor calcium level to determine drug effectiveness. Observe for signs of hypercalcemia, such as calcium deposits under the skin, cardiac dysrhythmias, changes in skeletal muscle tone, and urinary stones, *which may indicate calcium excess.* Teach patients to check with their primary health care providers about recommended doses to take.
Bisphosphonates	
Common examples of bisphosphonates: • Alendronate • Ibandronate • Risedronate • Pamidronate (IV) • Zoledronic acid (IV)	Teach patients to take drug on an empty stomach first thing in the morning with a full glass of water *to help prevent esophagitis, esophageal ulcers, and gastric ulcers.* Remind patients to take drug 30 minutes before food, drink, and other drugs *to prevent interactions.* Instruct the patient to remain upright, sitting or standing, for 30 minutes after taking the drug *to help prevent esophagitis (esophageal inflammation).* Instruct the patient to have a dental examination before starting the drug because it can cause jaw and maxillary osteonecrosis, particular if oral hygiene is poor. Do not give the drug to patients who are sensitive to aspirin *because bronchoconstriction may occur.* For IV drug, infuse over 15-30 min to prevent rare complications such as atrial fibrillation. For IV drugs, check the patient's serum creatinine before and after administering the medication *because it can cause renal insufficiency or acute kidney injury.*
Estrogen Agonists/Antagonists	
Example of estrogen agonist/antagonists: • Raloxifene	Teach the patient the signs and symptoms of venous thromboembolism (VTE), especially in the first 4 months of therapy, *because these drugs can cause VTE.* Monitor liver function tests (LFTs) in collaboration with the primary health care provider *because the drug can increase LFT values.*
RANKL Inhibitors	
Common examples of RANKL inhibitors: • Denosumab • Romosozumab	Teach patients to report new musculoskeletal pain, especially in the back, and skin reactions, not just at the injection site. Teach patients to report signs and symptoms of infection, *a common adverse effect.* Monitor levels of calcium, magnesium, and phosphorus *because the drug can cause severe hypocalcemia;* patients with impaired renal function are especially at risk. Instruct the patient to have a dental examination before starting the drug *because it can cause jaw and maxillary osteonecrosis, particularly if oral hygiene is poor.*

The most recent additions to the bisphosphonates are IV zoledronic acid and IV pamidronate. For management of osteoporosis, zoledronic acid is needed only once a year, and pamidronate is given every 3 to 6 months. Both drugs have been linked to a complication called jaw **osteonecrosis** (also known as *avascular necrosis*, or *bone death*), in which infection and necrosis of the mandible or maxilla occur (Burchum & Rosenthal, 2019). The incidence of this serious problem is low, but it can be a complication of this infusion therapy.

! NURSING SAFETY PRIORITY (QSEN)

Drug Alert

Do not confuse Fosamax (U.S. trade name for alendronate) with Flomax (U.S. trade name for tamsulosin), a selective alpha-adrenergic blocker used for benign prostatic hyperplasia (BPH). To promote safety, teach patients to take bisphosphonates early in the morning with 8 ounces of water and wait 30 to 60 minutes in an upright position before eating. If chest discomfort (a symptom of esophageal irritation) occurs, instruct patients to discontinue the drug and contact their health care provider. Patients with poor renal function, hypocalcemia, or gastroesophageal reflux disease (GERD) should not take bisphosphonates. *Teach patients to have an oral assessment and preventive dentistry before beginning any bisphosphonate therapy.* To promote safety, instruct them to inform any dentist who is planning invasive treatment, such as a tooth extraction or implant, that they are taking a bisphosphonate drug.

Teach patients that they should not take bisphosphonates continuously as lifelong management owing to long-term adverse effects such as esophageal cancer, atrial fibrillation, jaw osteonecrosis, and severe musculoskeletal pain. The decision to continue the drug after 2 years is made based on follow-up DXA scan results. If bone loss is maintained or bone density increases, the bisphosphonate is discontinued. If bone loss continues to occur, the drug can be continued for up to 5 years (Burchum & Rosenthal, 2019).

Other Drugs. Formerly called the *selective estrogen receptor modulators (SERMs)*, estrogen agonist/antagonists are a class of drugs designed to mimic estrogen in some parts of the body while blocking its effect elsewhere. Raloxifene is currently the only approved drug in this class and is used for *prevention and treatment* of osteoporosis in postmenopausal women. Raloxifene increases bone mineral density (BMD), reduces bone resorption, and reduces the incidence of osteoporotic vertebral fractures. The drug should not be given to women who have a history of venous thromboembolism (VTE) because it can cause deep vein thrombosis and pulmonary embolism.

A newer drug class is *RANKL (receptor activator of nuclear factor kappa-B ligand) inhibitors*, such as denosumab and romosozumab. These drugs are approved for treatment of osteoporosis when other drugs are not effective (Burchum & Rosenthal, 2019). By preventing the protein from activating its receptor, the drug decreases bone loss. The drug is given subcutaneously twice a year by a health care professional.

Teriparatide and abaloparatide are *parathyroid hormone–related protein drugs* that build bone and may not be used long-term. These drugs are available as daily subcutaneous injections and are indicated for patients who had a previous fracture or have multiple risk factors. After the drug is stopped, the patient is usually started on a bisphosphonate (NOF, 2018).

Salmon *calcitonin* (Miacalcin or Fortical) is approved for osteoporosis in women who are at least 5 years postmenopausal when alternative drug therapy is not appropriate. Two preparations are available: an intranasal spray or a subcutaneous injection. Intranasal calcitonin can cause rhinitis and epistaxis (nosebleeds). In a few patients, malignancies have been attributed to the use of calcitonin. For others, allergic responses to salmon may prevent the drug from being used or continued. Patients are usually tested for this allergy before they begin the drug. Calcitonin is less commonly used than other drugs to prevent bone loss and fractures (Burchum & Rosenthal, 2019).

Care Coordination and Transition Management

Home Care Management. Patients with osteoporosis are usually managed at home unless they have major fragility fractures. Some patients do not know that they have osteoporosis until they experience a fall and have one or more fractures.

Remind patients to have follow up DXA scans as prescribed to determine the effectiveness of drug therapy. For example, some patients maintain or gain bone mass and can discontinue their prescribed drug as directed by their primary health care provider. After discontinuation of medication, follow-up scans determine whether drug therapy needs to be restarted or another drug prescribed. This process helps to reduce the potential adverse effects that are associated with certain drug classifications.

Part of your responsibility is to collaborate with members of the interprofessional health team to ensure that the patient's home is safe and hazard free to help prevent falling. In some cases, home modifications may be needed, such as ramps instead of stairs or handrails near toilets and bathtubs and showers. Teach patients to prevent clutter in the home for clear pathways, avoid slippery floors, wear rubber-soled shoes, and avoid scatter rugs. Chapter 4 describes fall prevention in detail.

Self-Management Education. Teach patients about lifestyle practices that can help prevent additional bone loss. For example, to help prevent vitamin D deficiency, daily sun exposure (at least 5 minutes each day) is the most important source of vitamin D. If vitamin D levels remain low, teach patients to take their vitamin D_3 and calcium supplements as described earlier. Increase calcium and vitamin D sources in the diet.

Some people are lactose intolerant or do not use dairy products because of their vegan diets. However, many products are available for people who avoid dairy products. Soy and rice milk, tofu, and soy products are substitutes, but they are expensive. Teach patients to choose products that are fortified with vitamin D. Other foods rich in the vitamin are eggs, swordfish, chicken, liver, and enriched cereals and bread products.

If the patient is on drug therapy for osteopenia or osteoporosis, teach him or her to adhere to the medication regimen and take the prescribed drug(s) as instructed. Lack of adherence to long-term therapy for osteoporosis and bone health promotion practices is a major problem that results in increased fractures, hospital stays, and health care costs.

Health Care Resources. Refer patients to the National Osteoporosis Foundation (www.nof.org) in the United States for information regarding the disease and its treatment. The Osteoporosis Society of Canada (www.osteoporosis.ca) has similar services. Large health care systems often have osteoporosis specialty clinics and support groups for patients with osteoporosis.

◆ Evaluation: Evaluate Outcomes

Evaluate the care of the patient with osteoporosis or at risk for osteoporosis based on the identified priority patient problem. Expected outcomes are that the patient:

- Continues to follow up with DXA screenings as recommended to assess ongoing bone health
- Makes necessary changes in lifestyle to help prevent further bone loss
- Does not experience a fragility fracture due to bone loss

OSTEOMYELITIS

Pathophysiology Review

Infection in bony tissue can be a severe and difficult-to-treat problem. Bone infection can result in chronic recurrence, loss of function, persistent (chronic) ***pain,*** amputation, or even death due to sepsis.

Bacteria (most common), viruses, parasites, or fungi can cause ***infection*** in bone, known as **osteomyelitis**. Invasion by one or more pathogenic microorganisms stimulates the inflammatory response in bone tissue. The inflammation produces an increased vascular leak and edema, often involving the surrounding soft tissues. Once inflammation is established, the vessels in the area become thrombosed and release exudate (pus) into bony tissue. Ischemia of bone tissue follows and results in necrotic bone. This area of necrotic bone separates from surrounding bone tissue, and *sequestrum* is formed. The presence of sequestrum prevents bone healing and causes superimposed infection, often in the form of bone abscess which can lead to chronic osteomyelitis (McCance et al., 2019). As shown in Fig. 45.2, the cycle repeats itself as the new infection leads to further inflammation, vessel thromboses, and necrosis. Because bone is a dynamic tissue and attempts to heal itself, osteoblasts often lay new bone tissue over the infected tissue, making it difficult for drug therapy to penetrate into the infected bone.

Osteomyelitis may be categorized as *exogenous,* in which infectious organisms enter from outside the body as in an open fracture or after surgery, or *endogenous (hematogenous),* in which organisms are carried by the bloodstream from other areas of infection in the body. A third category is *contiguous,* in which bone infection results from skin infection of adjacent tissues. Osteomyelitis can be further divided into two major types: acute and chronic (McCance et al., 2019).

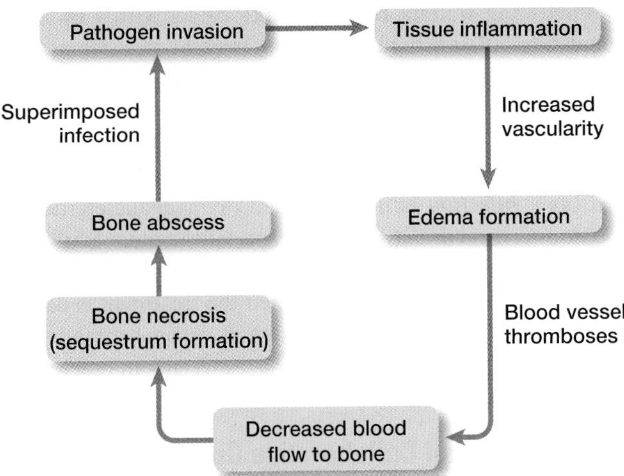

FIG. 45.2 Infection cycle of osteomyelitis.

Each type of bone infection has its own causative factors. Pathogenic microbes favor bone that has a rich blood supply and a marrow cavity. *Acute hematogenous infection* results from bacteremia, underlying disease, or nonpenetrating trauma. Urinary tract infections, particularly in older men, tend to spread to the lower vertebrae. Long-term IV catheters can be primary sources of infection. Patients undergoing long-term hemodialysis and IV drug users are also at risk for osteomyelitis. *Salmonella* infections of the GI tract may spread to bone. Patients with sickle cell disease and other hemoglobinopathies often have multiple episodes of salmonellosis, which can cause bone infection (McCance et al., 2019).

Poor dental hygiene and periodontal (gum) infection can be causative factors in *contiguous* osteomyelitis in facial bones. Minimal nonpenetrating trauma can cause hemorrhages or small-vessel occlusions, leading to bone necrosis. Regardless of the source of infection, many infections are caused by *Staphylococcus aureus.* Treatment of infection may be complicated further by the presence of *methicillin-resistant Staphylococcus aureus* (MRSA) or other multidrug-resistant organisms (MDROs), which are very common in hospitalized and other institutionalized patients as discussed in Chapter 21. The most common causes of MRSA in patients with musculoskeletal health problems are postoperative surgical site infections (SSIs) and infections from surgically implanted devices, such as an open reduction, internal fixation device.

PATIENT-CENTERED CARE: OLDER ADULT CONSIDERATIONS (QSEN)

Malignant external otitis media involving the base of the skull is sometimes seen in older adults with diabetes. However, the most common cause of contiguous spread in older adults is found in those who have slow-healing foot ulcers. Multiple organisms tend to be responsible for the resulting osteomyelitis (McCance et al., 2019).

Penetrating trauma leads to acute osteomyelitis by direct inoculation. A soft-tissue ***infection*** may be present as well. Animal bites, puncture wounds, skin ulcerations, and bone surgery can result in osteomyelitis. The most common offending organism is *Pseudomonas aeruginosa,* but other gram-negative bacteria may be found.

If bone ***infection*** is misdiagnosed or inadequately treated, *chronic osteomyelitis* may develop, especially in older adults who have foot ulcers. Inadequate care management results when the treatment period is too short or when the treatment is delayed or inappropriate. About half of cases of chronic osteomyelitis are caused by gram-negative bacteria, especially in older adults (McCance et al., 2019).

❖ Interprofessional Collaborative Care

◆ Assessment: Recognize Cues

Bone ***pain,*** with or without other signs and symptoms, is a common concern of patients with osteomyelitis. The pain is often described as a constant, localized, pulsating sensation that worsens with movement. Perform a complete pain assessment as described in Chapter 5.

The patient with acute osteomyelitis has fever, usually with temperature higher than 101°F (38.3°C). Older adults may not have an extreme temperature elevation because of a lower core body temperature and compromised immune system that occur with normal aging. The area around the infected bone swells and is tender when palpated. Erythema (redness) and heat may also be present. Fever, swelling, and erythema are less common in those with chronic osteomyelitis (see the Key Features: Acute Versus Chronic Osteomyelitis box). When vascular compromise is severe, patients may not experience **pain** because of nerve damage from lack of adequate **perfusion.**

When vascular insufficiency is suspected, assess circulation in the distal extremities. Ulcerations may be present on the feet or hands, indicating inadequate healing ability as a result of impaired ***perfusion.***

The patient with osteomyelitis may have an elevated white blood cell (leukocyte) count, which may be double the normal value. The erythrocyte sedimentation rate (ESR) may be normal early in the course of the disease but may rise as the condition progresses. It may remain elevated for as long as 3 months after drug therapy is discontinued.

If bacteremia (bacteria in the bloodstream that could lead to septic shock) is present, a blood culture identifies the offending organisms to determine which antibiotics should be used in treatment. Both aerobic and anaerobic blood cultures are collected before drug therapy begins. Further diagnostic testing using a variety of radionuclide scans or MRI may be performed to assess the extent of the infection and ***perfusion*** in the affected area.

◆ Interventions: Take Action

The specific treatment for osteomyelitis depends on the type and number of microbes present in the infected tissue. If other measures fail to resolve the infectious process, surgical management may be needed.

Nonsurgical Management. The primary health care provider typically prescribes at least 4 to 6 weeks of antimicrobial therapy as soon as possible for *acute* osteomyelitis based on the wound culture and sensitivity results. In the presence of copious wound drainage, follow Contact Precautions to prevent the spread of the offending organism to other patients and health care personnel. Teach patients, visitors, and staff members how to use these precautions. (See Chapter 21 for a discussion of Contact Precautions.)

More than one antimicrobial agent may be needed to combat multiple types of organisms. The hospital or home care nurse gives the drugs at specifically prescribed times so therapeutic serum levels are achieved. Observe for the actions, side effects, and toxicity of these drugs. Teach family members or other caregivers in the home setting how to administer drug therapy if they are continued after hospital discharge or are used only at home. Some patients may need to be admitted to a skilled nursing facility (SNF) for IV drug therapy. For patients with MRSA infection, IV vancomycin or linezolid (IV or oral) may be used. Oral linezolid allows older patients to remain at home or in assisted living rather than being admitted to an SNF (Burchum & Rosenthal, 2019).

The optimal drug regimen for patients with *chronic* osteomyelitis is not well established. Prolonged therapy for more than 3 months is typically needed to eliminate the ***infection.*** Patients are usually cared for in the home or skilled care setting with long-term vascular access catheters, such as a peripherally inserted central catheter (PICC). After discontinuation of IV drugs, oral therapy may be needed. Patients and families must understand the complications of inadequate treatment or failure to follow up with their primary health care provider.

KEY FEATURES

Acute Versus Chronic Osteomyelitis

Acute Osteomyelitis

- Fever; temperature usually above 101°F (38.3°C)
- Swelling around the affected area
- Possible erythema and heat in the affected area
- Tenderness of the affected area
- Bone pain that is constant, localized, and pulsating; worsens with movement

Chronic Osteomyelitis

- Foot ulcer(s) or bone surgery (most commonly)
- Sinus tract formation
- Localized ***pain***
- Drainage from the affected area (usually due to bone abscess)

! NURSING SAFETY PRIORITY (QSEN)

Drug Alert

Even when symptoms of osteomyelitis appear to be improved, teach the patient and family that the full course of IV and/or oral antimicrobials must be completed to ensure that the ***infection*** is resolved.

In addition to systemic drug therapy, if a wound is present it may be irrigated, either continuously or intermittently, with one or more antimicrobial solutions. A medical technique in which beads made of bone cement are impregnated with an antibiotic and packed into the wound can provide direct contact of the antibiotic with the offending organism.

Drugs are also needed to manage ***pain.*** Patients often experience acute and persistent (chronic) pain and must receive a regimen of drug therapy for control. Chapter 5 describes pharmacologic and nonpharmacologic interventions for both acute and persistent (chronic) pain.

A treatment to increase tissue ***perfusion*** for patients with chronic, unremitting osteomyelitis is the use of a hyperbaric chamber or portable device to administer hyperbaric oxygen (HBO) therapy. These devices are usually available in large tertiary care centers and may not be accessible to all patients who might benefit from them. With HBO therapy, the affected area is exposed daily to a high concentration of oxygen that diffuses into the tissues to promote healing. In conjunction with high-dose drug therapy and surgical débridement, HBO has proven very useful in treating a number of anaerobic infections. Other wound-management therapies are described in Chapter 23.

Surgical Management. Antimicrobial therapy alone may not meet the desired outcome of treatment. Surgical techniques include incision and drainage of skin and subcutaneous infection, wound débridement, and bone excision.

Because bone cannot heal in the presence of necrotic tissue, a *sequestrectomy* may be performed to remove the necrotic bone and allow revascularization of tissue. The excision of dead and infected bone often results in a sizable cavity, or bone defect. Bone *grafts* to repair bone defects are also widely used.

When infected bone is extensively resected, reconstruction with *microvascular bone transfers* or bone graft from donor bone may be done. This procedure is reserved for larger skeletal defects. The most common donor sites are the patient's fibula and iliac crest. Nursing care of the patient after surgery is similar to that for any postoperative patient (see Chapter 9). However, the important difference is that neurovascular assessments must be done frequently because the patient experiences increased swelling after the surgical procedure. Elevate the affected extremity to increase venous return and thus control swelling. Assess and document the patient's neurovascular status, including:

- Pain
- Movement
- Sensation
- Warmth
- Temperature
- Distal pulses
- Capillary refill (not as reliable as the above indicators)

When the previously described surgical procedures are not appropriate or successful and as a last resort, the affected limb may need to be amputated. The physical and psychological care for a patient who has undergone an amputation is discussed in Chapter 47.

CLINICAL JUDGMENT CHALLENGE 45.1

Patient-Centered Care; Safety

A 25-year-old obese man has received 2 weeks of a 6-week course of IV antibiotic therapy for acute osteomyelitis resulting from three knee surgeries for a sports injury. He visits his nurse practitioner but is initially assessed by the office nurse, who documents the following physical assessment changes:

- Reports increased difficulty when climbing stairs to his third-floor apartment when compared with last week (no elevator in building)
- States that the affected knee pain has increased from a 3 to a 7 on a 0-10 pain scale regardless of when he takes his analgesic
- States that he has noticed purulent, odorous drainage present when he changes his knee dressings daily
- Reports that he feels hot every evening but does not own a thermometer
- Reports increased fatigue and inability to concentrate while working remotely on his computer
- Oral temperature = 100.8°F (38.2°C)
- Radial pulse = 88 beats/min
- Blood pressure = 124/76 mm Hg
- WBCs = 18,500/mm^3 (drawn 3 days ago)

1. **Recognize Cues:** What assessment information in this client situation is the most important and immediate concern for the nurse? (Hint: Identify the **relevant** information *first* to determine what is most important.)
2. **Analyze Cues:** What client conditions are consistent with the **most relevant** information? (Hint: Think about priority collaborative problems that support and contradict the information presented in this situation.)
3. **Prioritize Hypotheses:** Which possibilities or explanations are **most likely** to be present in this client situation? Which possibilities or explanations are the most serious? (Hint: Consider all possibilities and determine their urgency and risk for this client.)
4. **Generate Solutions:** What actions would most likely achieve the desired outcomes for this client? Which actions should be **avoided** or are **potentially harmful**? (Hint: Determine the desired outcomes first to decide which interventions are appropriate and those that should be avoided.)
5. **Take Action:** Which actions are the most appropriate and how should they be implemented? In what **priority order** should they be implemented? (Hint: Consider health teaching, documentation, requested health care provider orders or prescriptions, nursing skills, collaboration with or referral to health team members, etc.)
6. **Evaluate Outcomes:** What client assessment would indicate that the nurse's actions were **effective**? (Hint: Think about signs that would indicate an improvement, decline, or unchanged client condition.)

BONE TUMORS

Pathophysiology Review

Benign Bone Tumors

Bone tumors may be classified as benign (noncancerous) or malignant (cancerous). *Benign* bone tumors are often asymptomatic and may be discovered on routine x-ray examination or as the cause of pathologic fractures. The cause of benign bone tumors is not known. Tumors may arise from several types of tissue. The major classifications include *chondrogenic* tumors (from cartilage), *osteogenic* tumors (from bone), and *fibrogenic* tumors (from fibrous tissue and found most often in children).

The most common benign bone tumor is the *osteochondroma.* Although its onset is usually in childhood, the tumor grows until skeletal maturity and may not be diagnosed until adulthood. The tumor may be a single growth or multiple growths and can occur in any bone. The femur and the tibia are most often involved (McCance et al., 2019).

Malignant Bone Tumors

Malignant (cancerous) bone tumors may be primary (those that begin in bone) or secondary (those that originate in other tissues and metastasize [spread] to bone). *Primary tumors* occur most often in people between 10 and 30 years of age and make up a small percentage of bone cancers. As with other forms of cancer, the exact cause of bone cancer is unknown, but genetic and environmental factors are likely causes. *Metastatic lesions* most often occur in the older age-group and account for most bone cancers in adults (McCance et al., 2019).

Osteosarcoma, or osteogenic sarcoma, is the most common type of *primary* malignant bone tumor. More than 50% of cases occur in the distal femur, followed in decreasing order of occurrence by the proximal tibia and humerus. The tumor is relatively large, causing acute ***pain*** and swelling. The involved area is usually warm because the blood flow to the site increases. The center of the tumor is sclerotic from increased osteoblastic activity. The periphery is soft, extending through the bone cortex in the classic sunburst appearance associated with the neoplasm (which is visible on x-ray). Osteosarcoma typically metastasizes (spreads), which results in death.

Although *Ewing sarcoma* is not as common as other tumors, it is the most malignant. Like other primary tumors, it causes ***pain*** and swelling. In addition, systemic signs and symptoms, particularly low-grade fever, leukocytosis, and anemia, are common. The pelvis and the lower extremity are most often affected. Pelvic involvement is a poor prognostic sign. It often extends into soft tissue. Death results from metastasis to the lungs and other bones. Although the tumor can be seen in patients of any age, it usually occurs in children and young adults in their 20s. Men are affected more often than women (McCance et al., 2019). The reason for this pattern is not known.

In contrast to the patient with osteosarcoma, the patient with *chondrosarcoma* experiences dull ***pain*** and swelling for a long period. The tumor typically affects the pelvis and proximal femur near the diaphysis. Arising from cartilaginous tissue, it destroys bone and often calcifies. The patient with this type of tumor has a better prognosis than one with osteogenic sarcoma. Chondrosarcoma occurs in middle-age and older people, with a slight predominance in men.

Arising from fibrous tissue, *fibrosarcomas* can be divided into subtypes, of which malignant fibrous histiocytoma (MFH) is the most malignant. Usually the clinical presentation of MFH is gradual, without specific symptoms. Local tenderness, with or without a palpable mass, occurs in the long bones of the lower extremity. As with other bone cancers, the lesion can metastasize to the lungs (McCance et al., 2019).

Primary tumors of the prostate, breast, kidney, thyroid, and lung are called *bone-seeking* cancers because they spread to the bone more often than other primary tumors. The vertebrae, pelvis, femur, and ribs are the bone sites commonly affected. Simply stated, primary tumor cells, or seeds, are carried to bone through the bloodstream. *Fragility fractures caused by metastatic bone are a major concern in patient care management.*

❖ Interprofessional Collaborative Care

◆ Assessment: Recognize Cues

Assess for ***pain,*** the most common symptom of most bone tumors. Pain can range from mild to severe. It can be caused by direct tumor invasion into soft tissue, compressed peripheral nerves, or a resulting pathologic or fragility fracture. Perform a complete pain assessment for the patient as a baseline to plan care as described in Chapter 5.

In addition, observe and palpate the suspected involved area. When the tumor affects the lower extremities or the small bones of the hands and feet, local swelling may be detected as the tumor enlarges. In some cases, muscle atrophy or muscle spasm may be present. Marked disability and impaired ***mobility*** may occur in those with advanced metastatic bone disease.

In performing a musculoskeletal assessment, inspect the involved area and palpate the mass, if possible, for size and tenderness. In collaboration with the physical and occupational therapists, assess the patient's ability to perform ***mobility*** tasks and ADLs.

In a patient with Ewing sarcoma, a low-grade fever may occur because of the systemic features of the neoplasm. For this reason, it may be confused with osteomyelitis. Fatigue and pallor resulting from anemia are also common.

Patients with malignant bone tumors may be young adults whose productive lives are just beginning. They need strong support systems to help cope with the diagnosis and its treatment. Family, significant others, and health care professionals are major components of the needed support. Determine which systems or resources are available.

Patients often experience a loss of control over their lives when a diagnosis of cancer is made. As a result, they become anxious and fearful about the outcome of their illness. Coping with the diagnosis becomes a challenge. As patients progress through the grieving process, there may be initial denial. Identify the anxiety level and assess the stage or stages of the grieving process. Explore any maladaptive behavior, indicating ineffective coping mechanisms. Chapter 20 further describes the psychosocial assessment for patients with cancer.

Routine x-rays are used to find bone tumors and bone metastasis. CT and MRI are useful for complex anatomic areas, such as the spinal column and sacrum. These tests are particularly helpful in evaluating the extent of soft-tissue involvement. Metastatic lesions may increase or decrease bone density, depending on the amount of osteoblastic and osteoclastic activity.

In some cases a needle bone biopsy may be performed, usually under fluoroscopy to guide the surgeon. Needle biopsy is an ambulatory care procedure with rare complications. After biopsy, the cancer is staged for size and degree of spread. One popular method is the TNM system, based on tumor size and number (T), the presence of cancer cells in lymph nodes (N), and metastasis (spread) to distant sites (M) (see Chapter 19 for further discussion).

The patient with a *malignant* bone tumor typically shows elevated serum alkaline phosphatase (ALP) levels, indicating the body's attempt to form new bone by increasing osteoblastic activity. The patient with Ewing sarcoma or metastatic bone cancer often has anemia and leukocytosis (increased white blood cells). The progression of Ewing sarcoma may be evaluated by elevated serum lactic dehydrogenase (LDH) levels.

In some patients with bone metastasis from the breast, kidney, or lung, the serum calcium level is elevated. Massive bone destruction stimulates release of the mineral into the bloodstream. In patients with Ewing sarcoma and bone metastasis, the erythrocyte sedimentation rate (ESR) may be elevated because of secondary tissue inflammation (Pagana & Pagana, 2018).

◆ Interventions: Take Action

Because ***pain*** is often due to direct primary tumor invasion, treatment is aimed at reducing the size of or removing the tumor. *Benign* or small primary malignant bone tumors are usually completely removed for a potential cure. The expected outcome of treating *metastatic* bone tumors is palliative rather than curative. Palliative therapies may prevent further bone destruction and improve patient function. A combination of nonsurgical and surgical management is used for bone cancer. Collaborate with members of the interprofessional health care team to plan high-quality care to achieve positive patient outcomes. The following discussion focuses on interventions for patients with malignant bone tumors or metastatic bone cancer.

Nonsurgical Management. In addition to analgesics for local ***pain*** relief, chemotherapy and radiation therapy are often given to shrink the malignant tumor. For patients with painful metastatic spinal involvement, bracing and short-term immobilization may be appropriate.

The primary health care provider may prescribe *chemotherapy* to be given alone or in combination with radiation or surgery. Certain proliferating tumors, such as Ewing sarcoma, are sensitive to cytotoxic drugs. Others, such as chondrosarcomas, are often totally drug resistant. Chemotherapy seems to work best for small, metastatic tumors and may be administered before or after surgery. In most cases the primary health care provider prescribes a combination of agents. The drugs selected are determined in part by the primary source of the cancer in metastatic disease. For example, when metastasis occurs from breast cancer, estrogen and progesterone blockers may be used. Chapter 20 describes the general nursing care of patients who receive chemotherapy. *Remember that all chemotherapeutic agents are categorized as high-alert medications* (Institute for Safe Medication Practices, 2020).

Other drugs are given for specific metastatic cancers, depending on the location of the primary site. For example, biologic agents, such as cytokines, are given to stimulate the immune system to recognize and destroy cancer cells, especially in patients with renal cancer. Zoledronic acid and pamidronate are two IV bisphosphonates that are approved for bone metastasis from the breast, lung, and prostate (Burchum & Rosenthal, 2019). These drugs help protect bones and prevent fractures. Although rare, inform patients that osteonecrosis of the jaw may also occur, especially in those who have invasive dental procedures. Monitor associated laboratory tests, such as serum creatinine and electrolytes, because these drugs can be toxic to the kidneys and cause acute kidney injury (AKI). Bisphosphonates are described earlier in the Osteoporosis section.

Denosumab is a RANKL inhibitor that is also approved for metastatic bone disease (Burchum & Rosenthal, 2019). The drug binds to a protein that is essential for the formation, function, and survival of osteoclasts. By preventing the protein from activating its receptor, the drug decreases bone loss and increases bone mass and strength.

Radiation therapy, either brachytherapy or external radiation, is used for selected types of malignant tumors. For patients with Ewing sarcoma and early osteosarcoma, radiation may be the treatment of choice in reducing tumor size and thus pain.

For patients with metastatic disease, radiation is given primarily for palliation. The therapy is directed toward the painful sites to provide a better quality of life. One or more treatments are given, depending on the extent of disease. With precise planning, radiation therapy can be used with minimal complications. The general nursing care for patients receiving radiation therapy is described in Chapter 20.

Interventional radiologists can perform several noninvasive procedures to help relieve ***pain*** in the patient with metastasis to the spinal column. For example, *microwave ablation (MWA)* can be done under moderate sedation or general anesthesia to kill the targeted tissue with heat using microwaves. Most patients have pain relief or control after this ambulatory care procedure.

Surgical Management. Primary malignant bone tumors are usually reduced or removed with surgery, and surgery may be combined with radiation or chemotherapy.

In addition to the nature, progression, and extent of the tumor, the patient's age and general health state are considered. Chemotherapy may be administered before surgery. As for any patient preparing for cancer surgery, the patient with bone cancer needs psychological support from the nurse and other members of the health care team.

PATIENT-CENTERED CARE: CULTURAL/SPIRITUAL CONSIDERATIONS QSEN

Assess the level of the patient's and family's understanding about the surgery and related treatments. Be present to establish a trusting relationship with the patient and be available for listening. As an advocate, encourage the patient and family to discuss concerns and questions and provide information regarding hospital routines and procedures. Provide hope but be realistic and accurate with information. Assess the patient to determine if religious and/or spiritual support is important. Contact a member of the clergy or a spiritual leader or talk with a clergy member affiliated with the hospital based on the patient's preferences.

Anticipate postoperative needs as much as possible before the patient undergoes surgery. Remind him or her what to expect after surgery and how to help ensure adequate recovery.

Wide or radical resection procedures are used for patients with bone sarcomas to salvage the affected limb. Wide excision is removal of the lesion surrounded by an intact cuff of normal tissue and leads to cure of low-grade tumors only. A radical resection includes removal of the lesion, the entire muscle, bone, and other tissues directly involved. It is the procedure used for high-grade tumors.

Large bone defects that result from tumor removal may require either:

- Total joint replacements with prosthetic implants, either whole or partial
- Custom metallic implants
- Allografts from the iliac crest, rib, or fibula

As an alternative to total replacement, an allograft may be implanted with internal fixation for patients who do not have metastases. This is a common procedure for sarcomas of the proximal femur. Allograft procedures for the knee are also performed, particularly in young adults. Preoperative chemotherapy is given to enhance the likelihood of success. Allografts with adjacent tendons and ligaments are harvested from cadavers and can be frozen or freeze-dried for a prolonged period. The graft is fixed with a series of bolts, screws, or plates.

The surgical incision for a limb salvage procedure is often extensive. A pressure dressing with wound suction is typically maintained for several days. The patient who has undergone a limb salvage procedure has some degree of impaired physical ***mobility*** and a self-care deficit. The nature and extent of the alterations depend on the location and extent of the surgery.

! NURSING SAFETY PRIORITY (QSEN)

Action Alert

For patients who have allografts, monitor for signs of hemorrhage, infection, and fracture. After ensuring that the patient is safe, report these complications to the Rapid Response Team or surgeon immediately.

After upper extremity surgery, the patient can engage in active-assistive exercises by using the opposite hand to help achieve motions such as forward flexion and abduction of the shoulder. Continuous passive motion (CPM) using a CPM machine may be initiated as early as the first postoperative day for either upper extremity or lower extremity procedures.

After lower extremity surgery, the emphasis is on strengthening the quadriceps muscles by using passive and active motion when possible. Maintaining muscle tone is an important prerequisite to weight bearing, which progresses from toe touch or partial weight bearing to full weight bearing by 2 to 3 months after surgery. Coordinate the patient's plan of care for ambulation and muscle strengthening with the physical therapist.

The patient who has had a bone graft may have a cast or other supportive device for several months. Weight bearing is prohibited until there is evidence that the graft is incorporated into the adjacent bone tissue.

During the recovery phase, the patient may also need assistance with ADLs, particularly if the surgery involves the upper extremity. Assist if needed but, at the same time, encourage the patient to do as much as possible unaided. Some patients need assistive-adaptive devices for a short period while they are healing. Coordinate the patient's plan of care for promoting independence in ADLs with the occupational therapist.

Surrounding tissues, including nerves and blood vessels, may be removed during surgery. Vascular grafting is common, but the lost nerve(s) is (are) usually not replaced. Assess the neurovascular status of the affected extremity and hand or foot every 1 to 2 hours immediately after surgery. Splinting or casting of the limb may also cause neurovascular compromise and needs to be checked for proper placement.

In addition to needing emotional support to cope with physical disabilities, the patient may need help coping with the surgery and its effects. Help identify available support systems as soon as possible.

As a result of most of the surgical procedures, the patient experiences an altered body image. Suggest ways to minimize cosmetic changes. For example, a lowered shoulder can be covered by a custom-made pad worn under clothing. The patient can cover lower extremity defects with pants.

NCLEX EXAMINATION CHALLENGE 45.2

Physiological Integrity

The nurse assesses a client recently diagnosed with metastatic vertebral bone cancer. Which intervention is the **priority** when caring for this client?

A. Consultation with rehabilitative therapy
B. Referral to hospice care
C. Drug therapy to manage persistent pain
D. Oxygen therapy to prevent dyspnea

Care Coordination and Transition Management

Home Care Management. After medical treatment for any type of primary bone tumor, the patient is usually managed at home with follow-up care. Hospice care at home is often needed for patients with metastatic disease. When home support is not available, the patient may be admitted to a long-term care facility for extended or hospice care. Coordinate the patient's transition and continuity of care with the case manager and other interprofessional health team members, depending on the patient's needs.

In collaboration with the occupational therapist, evaluate the patient's home environment for structural barriers that may hinder ***mobility.*** The patient may be discharged with a cast, walker, crutches, or a wheelchair. Assess his or her support system for availability of assistance if needed.

Accessibility to eating and toileting facilities is essential to promote ADL independence. Because the patient with metastatic disease is susceptible to pathologic fractures, potential hazards that may contribute to falls or injury should be removed.

For the patient receiving intermittent chemotherapy or radiation on an ambulatory care basis, emphasize the importance of keeping appointments. Review the expected side and toxic effects of the drugs with the patient and family. Teach how to treat less serious side effects and when to contact the primary health care provider. If the drugs are administered at home via long-term IV catheter, explain and demonstrate the care involved with daily dressing changes and potential catheter complications. Chapter 15 describes the health teaching required for a patient receiving infusion therapy at home.

If the patient has undergone surgery, he or she has a wound and the potential for impaired ***mobility.*** Teach the patient, family, and/or significant others how to care for the wound. Help the patient learn how to perform ADLs and mobility activities independently for self-management. Coordinate with the occupational therapist to assist in ADL teaching and provide or recommend assistive and adaptive devices, if necessary. The physical therapist can teach the proper use of any needed ambulatory aids, such as a walker or cane, and routine exercises.

Pain management can be a major challenge, particularly for the patient with metastatic bone disease. Discuss the various options for persistent pain relief, including relaxation and music therapy. Emphasize the importance of techniques that worked during hospitalization. See Chapter 5 for cancer pain assessment and management.

The patient with bone cancer may fear that the malignancy will return. Acknowledge this fear but reinforce confidence in the health care team and medical treatment chosen. Mutually establish realistic outcomes regarding returning to work and participating in recreational activities. Encourage the patient to resume a functional lifestyle but caution that it should be gradual. Certain activities, such as participating in sports, may be prohibited.

Help the patient with advanced metastatic bone disease prepare for death. The nurse and other support personnel assist the patient through the stages of death and dying. Identify resources that can help the patient write a will, visit with distant family members, or do whatever he or she thinks is needed for a peaceful death. Chapter 8 describes end-of-life care in detail.

In addition to family and significant others, cancer support groups are helpful to the patient with bone cancer. Some organizations, such as *I Can Cope,* provide information and emotional support. Others, such as *CanSurmount,* are geared more toward patient and family education. The American Cancer Society (www.cancer.org) and the Canadian Cancer Society (www.cancer.ca) can also provide education and resources for patients and families.

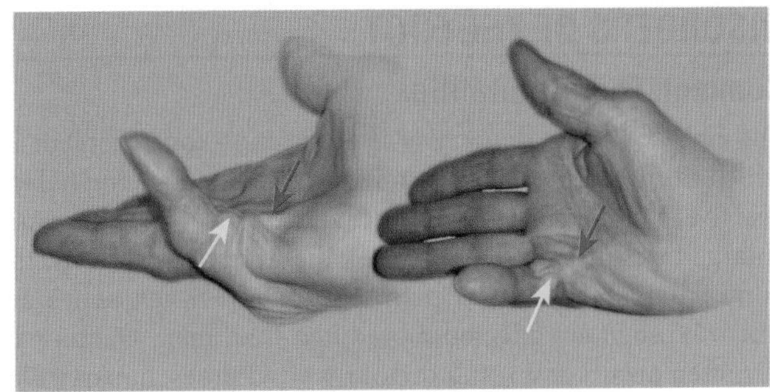

FIG. 45.3 Dupuytren contracture. (Courtesy of School of Medicine, SUNY Stony Brook, NY. In Wolfe, S.W., Hotchkiss, R.N., Pederson, W.C., & Kozin, S.H. [2011]. *Green's operative hand surgery* [6th ed.]. Philadelphia: Churchill Livingstone.)

DISORDERS OF THE HAND

Specific localized health problems affecting the hand or part of the hand may affect the musculoskeletal system. Two of these problems are discussed here. **Dupuytren contracture or deformity** is a slowly progressive thickening of the palmar fascia, resulting in flexion contracture of the fourth (ring) and fifth (little) fingers of the hand (Fig. 45.3). The third or middle finger is occasionally affected. Although Dupuytren contracture is a common problem, the cause is unknown. It usually occurs in older Euro-American men, tends to occur in families, is most common in people with diabetes, and can be bilateral.

When function becomes impaired, surgical release is required. A partial or selective fasciectomy (cutting of fascia) is performed. After removal of the surgical dressing, a splint may be used. Nursing care is similar to that for the patient with carpal tunnel repair (see Chapter 47).

A **ganglion** is a round, benign cyst, often found on a wrist or foot joint or tendon. The synovium surrounding the tendon degenerates, allowing the tendon sheath tissue to become weak and distended. Ganglia are painless on palpation, but they can cause joint discomfort after prolonged joint use or minor trauma or strain. The lesion can rapidly disappear and then recur. Ganglia are most likely to develop in people between 15 and 50 years of age. With local or regional anesthesia in a primary health care provider's office or clinic, the fluid within the cyst can be aspirated through a small needle. A cortisone injection may follow. If the cyst is very large, it is removed using a small incision. Teach patients to avoid strenuous activity for 48 hours after surgery and report any signs of inflammation to their primary health care provider.

DISORDERS OF THE FOOT

Common Foot Deformities

The **hallux valgus deformity** is a common foot problem in which the great toe drifts laterally at the first metatarsophalangeal (MTP) joint (Fig. 45.4). The first metatarsal head becomes enlarged, resulting in a *bunion*. As the deviation worsens, the bony enlargement causes pain, particularly when shoes are worn. Women are affected more often than men. Hallux valgus often occurs as a result of poorly fitted shoes, in particular those with narrow toes and high heels. Other causes include osteoarthritis, rheumatoid arthritis, foot and ankle surgery, and family history.

For some patients who are of advanced age or are not surgical candidates, custom-made shoes can be made to fit the deformed feet and provide comfort and support. A plaster mold is made to conform to each foot; shoes can be made from these molds. Teach the patient to consult with a podiatrist or foot clinic to be evaluated for custom shoes.

The surgical procedure, a simple **bunionectomy**, involves removal of the bony overgrowth and bursa and realignment to manage ***pain***. When other toe deformities accompany the condition or if the bony overgrowth is large, several *osteotomies*, or bone resections, may be performed. Fusions may also be performed. Screws or wires are often inserted to stabilize the bones in the great toe and first metatarsal during the healing process. If both feet are affected, one foot is usually treated at a time. Surgery usually is performed as a same-day procedure. Be sure to assess neurovascular status and pain control before allowing the patient to be discharged.

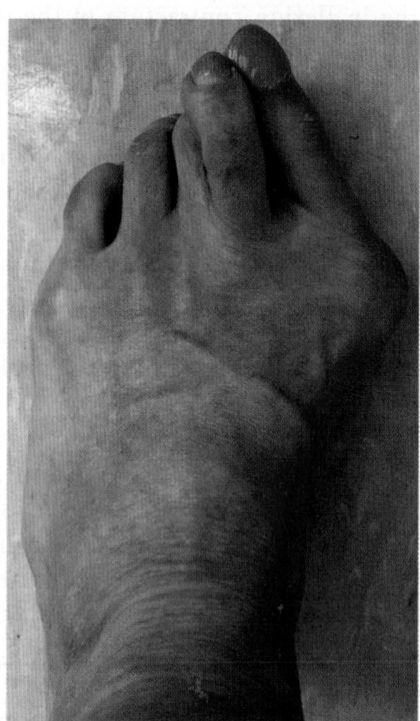

FIG. 45.4 Appearance of hallux valgus with a bunion and hammertoes. (From Federer, A.E., Tainter, D.M., Adams, S.B., & Schweitzer, K.M. [2018]. Conservative management of metatarsalgia and lesser toe deformities. *Foot and Ankle Clinics, 23*[1], 9–20. doi.org/10.1016/j.fcl.2017.09.003.)

Most patients are allowed partial weight bearing while wearing an orthopedic boot or shoe. Walking is difficult because the feet bear body weight. The healing time after surgery may be more than 6 to 12 weeks because the feet receive less blood flow than other parts of the body as a result of their distance from the heart.

Often patients have hammertoes and hallux valgus deformities at the same time. As shown in Fig. 45.4, a *hammertoe* is the dorsiflexion of any MTP joint with plantar flexion of the proximal interphalangeal (PIP) joint next to it. The second toe is most often affected. As the deformity worsens, uncomfortable corns may develop on the dorsal side of the toe, and calluses may appear on the plantar surface. Patients are uncomfortable when wearing shoes and walking.

Hammertoe may be treated by surgical correction of the deformity with osteotomies (bone resections) and the insertion of wires or screws for fixation. The postoperative course is similar to that for the patient with hallux valgus repair.

> **NCLEX EXAMINATION CHALLENGE 45.3**
>
> ***Physiological Integrity***
>
> The nurse is caring for a client immediately after a bunionectomy. What is the nurse's **priority** action?
>
> A. Relieve or reduce the client's pain.
> B. Maintain the client's airway.
> C. Assess neurovascular status in the surgical foot.
> D. Apply a hot compress to the surgical area.

Plantar Fasciitis

Plantar fasciitis is an inflammation of the plantar fascia, which is located in the area of the arch of the foot. It is often seen in middle-age and older adults, as well as in athletes, especially runners. Obesity is also a contributing factor. Patients report severe ***pain*** in the arch of the foot, especially when getting out of bed. The pain is worsened with weight bearing. Although most patients have unilateral plantar fasciitis, the problem can affect both feet (McCance et al., 2019).

Most patients respond to conservative management, which includes rest, ice, stretching exercises, strapping of the foot to maintain the arch, shoes with good support, and orthotics. NSAIDs or steroids may be needed to control ***pain*** and inflammation. If conservative measures are unsuccessful, endoscopic surgery to remove the inflamed tissue may be required. Teach the patient about the importance of adhering to the treatment plan and to follow the physical therapist's instruction regarding exercise.

GET READY FOR THE NEXT-GENERATION NCLEX® EXAMINATION!

Key Points

Review these Key Points for each NCLEX Examination Client Needs Category.

Safe and Effective Care Environment

- Collaborate with interprofessional team members when assessing patients with osteoporosis for risk for falls. **QSEN: Teamwork and Collaboration**
- Teach the patient with ***cellular regulation*** problems (e.g., osteoporosis) and his or her family about evidence-based home safety modifications and the need to create a hazard-freeenvironment. **QSEN: Safety; Evidence-Based Practice**

Health Promotion and Maintenance

- Develop a teaching plan for patients at risk for osteoporosis to minimize risk factors, such as stopping smoking, decreasing alcohol intake, exercising regularly, and increasing dietary calcium and vitamin D foods. **QSEN: Patient-Centered Care**
- Remind patients at risk for osteoporosis to have regular screening tests, such as the DXA scan, as needed. **QSEN: Evidence-Based Practice; Safety**
- Refer patients with musculoskeletal problems to appropriate community resources, such as the National Osteoporosis Foundation (NOF). **QSEN: Patient-Centered Care**

Psychosocial Integrity

- Assess the patient's and family's responses to a diagnosis of bone disorders and treatment options. Be aware that they may experience fear and require referral. **QSEN: Teamwork and Collaboration**

Physiological Integrity

- Osteoporosis and osteomalacia cause bone loss and fragility fractures (see Table 45.1); recognize that osteoporosis can be primary or secondary (see Table 45.2). **QSEN: Safety**
- Remind patients taking bisphosphonates to take them early in the morning, at least 30 to 60 minutes before breakfast, with a full glass of water, and to remain sitting upright during that time to prevent esophagitis, a common complication of bisphosphonate therapy. **QSEN: Safety**
- Recall that most patients are unaware that they have osteoporosis until they experience a fracture, the most common complication of the disease. **QSEN: Safety**
- Assess for signs and symptoms of osteomyelitis, which differ based on type (acute versus chronic). **QSEN: Patient-Centered Care**
- Use clinical judgment to prioritize care for patients with osteomyelitis, including maintaining Contact Precautions for open wounds. For patients having surgical intervention, assess the affected extremity for neurovascular status to ensure adequate tissue ***perfusion***. **Clinical Judgment**
- For patients who have surgery to remove benign or malignant bone tumors, report and document postoperative signs and symptoms of ***infection***, dislocation, or neurovascular compromise to the surgeon promptly. **QSEN: Safety; Informatics**
- Remember that severe persistent ***pain*** is a priority for patients with metastatic bone disease. **QSEN: Patient-Centered Care; Evidence-Based Practice**
- In collaboration with the health care team (physical therapist, occupational therapist, neurologist), provide supportive care for patients with bone cancer to improve ***mobility*** and function. **QSEN: Teamwork and Collaboration**
- Foot disorders can be treated with custom-made shoes or surgery to repair deformities and promote ***mobility***. QSEN: **Evidence-Based Practice; Safety**

MASTERY QUESTIONS

1. The nurse is teaching a client who has osteopenia about alendronate. Which statement by the client indicates a **need for further teaching?**
   A. "I will take this drug at night to prevent nausea."
   B. "I need a dental checkup before taking the drug."
   C. "I need to sit up for 30 minutes after taking the drug."
   D. "I will drink plenty of water after I take the drug."

2. The nurse is caring for a client who was admitted with a draining diabetic ulcer on the lower extremity. What personal protective equipment will the nurse teach the staff to use? **Select all that apply.**
   A. Gown
   B. Gloves
   C. Mask
   D. Foot covers
   E. Goggles

REFERENCES

Burchum, J. L. R., & Rosenthal, L. D. (2019). *Lehne's pharmacology for nursing care* (10th ed.). St. Louis: Elsevier.

Capriotti, T., & Scanlon, M. (2018). Osteoporosis: A clinical update for home healthcare clinicians. *Home Healthcare Now, 36*(4), 216–224.

Evenson, A. L., & Sanders, G. F. (2016). Educational intervention impact on osteoporosis knowledge, health beliefs, self-efficacy, dietary calcium, and vitamin D intakes in young adults. *Orthopaedic Nursing, 35*(1), 30–38.

Institute for Safe Medication Practices. (2020). *ISMPs list of high-alert medications*. www.ismp.org/Tools/highalertmedications.pdf.

Jarvis, C. (2020). *Physical examination & health assessment* (8th ed.). St. Louis: Elsevier Saunders.

McCance, K., Huether, S., Brashers, V., & Rote, N. (2019). *Pathophysiology: The biologic basis for disease in adults and children* (8th ed.). St. Louis: Mosby.

National Osteoporosis Foundation (NOF). (2018). *Clinician's guide to prevention and treatment of osteoporosis*. Washington, DC: Author.

Pagana, K. D., & Pagana, T. J. (2018). *Manual of diagnostic and laboratory tests* (6th ed.). St. Louis: Mosby.

Pagana, K. D., Pagana, T. J., & Pike-MacDonald, S. A. (2019). *Mosby's Canadian manual of diagnostic and laboratory tests* (2nd ed.). Toronto, ON: Elsevier.

Reid, I. R. (2017). Vitamin D effect on bone mineral density and fractures. *Endocrinology and Metabolism Clinics of North America, 46*(4), 935–945.

Touhy, T. A., & Jett, K. F. (2018). *Ebersole and Hess' gerontological nursing and healthy aging* (5th ed.). St. Louis: Elsevier.

Xiaojuan, L., & Schwartz, A. V. (2020). MRI assessment of bone marrow composition in osteoporosis. *Current Osteoporosis Reports, 18*, 57–66.

46

Concepts of Care for Patients With Arthritis and Total Joint Arthroplasty

Donna D. Ignatavicius

http://evolve.elsevier.com/Iggy/

LEARNING OUTCOMES

1. Collaborate with interprofessional team to coordinate high-quality care for patients with arthritis.
2. Use clinical judgment to prioritize collaborative interventions for patients with arthritis to promote ***mobility,*** reduce ***inflammation,*** and manage ***pain.***
3. Describe the psychosocial impact for patients experiencing arthritis.
4. Teach the patient and caregiver(s) about common drugs used for rheumatoid arthritis (RA), including those used for ***immunity*** suppression.
5. Plan evidence-based preoperative and postoperative care for the patient having a total hip or knee arthroplasty.
6. Plan care coordination and transition management for patients with arthritis.

KEY TERMS

arthritis Inflammation of one or more joints.

arthrocentesis An invasive diagnostic procedure performed at the bedside or in a primary health care provider's office to aspirate a sample of synovial fluid for analysis and to relieve pressure caused by excess fluid.

arthrofibrosis The buildup of excessive scar tissue that restricts joint motion and functional ability.

crepitus A grating sound caused by loosened bone and cartilage in a synovial joint.

exacerbations Flare-ups of disease (that typically alternate with disease remissions).

gout A systemic disease in which urate crystals (the result of errors in purine metabolism) deposit in joints causing severe joint inflammation.

joint coach A care partner who can help the patient having a total joint arthroplasty through the perioperative period and assist with discharge needs.

joint effusion The presence of excess joint fluid, especially common in the knee.

osteoarthritis The progressive deterioration and loss of articular (joint) cartilage and bone in one or more joints.

osteonecrosis Bone death secondary to lack of or disruption in blood supply to the affected bone, usually from trauma or chronic steroid therapy.

osteophytes Bone spurs caused by irregular bony overgrowth.

paresthesias Burning and tingling sensations, especially in the extremities.

peripheral nerve block (PNB) A single injection or continuous infusion by a portable pump (e.g., continuous femoral nerve blockade or CFNB) to provide regional/local anesthesia during and/or after surgery.

primary arthroplasty First-time joint arthroplasty.

quadriceps-setting exercises ("quad sets") Postoperative exercises designed to decrease the risk of deep vein thrombosis by straightening the legs and pushing the back of the knees into the bed.

regenerative therapies Minimally invasive treatment modalities, such as stem cell therapy and platelet-rich plasma, that are used to repair joint cartilage.

revision arthroplasty An arthroplasty done to replace an implant that has loosened or failed.

Sjögren syndrome A condition in which the patient has dry eyes (keratoconjunctivitis sicca [KCS], or the sicca syndrome), dry mouth (xerostomia), and dry vagina (in some cases). This health problem may occur as a separate condition or be associated with late-stage rheumatoid arthritis or other autoimmune arthritis-related disease.

subcutaneous nodules Soft, round, movable nodules that often occur along the ulnar side of the arm in patients with advanced rheumatoid arthritis.

subluxation Partial joint dislocation.

synovitis Joint inflammation.

total joint arthroplasty (TJA) The surgical creation of a functional (synovial) joint using implants, also sometimes called a *total joint replacement (TJR).*

vasculitis Inflammation of blood vessel walls that can decrease arterial blood flow.

PRIORITY AND INTERRELATED CONCEPTS

The priority concepts for this chapter are:
- ***Mobility***
- ***Immunity***

The ***Mobility*** concept exemplar for this chapter is Osteoarthritis.
The ***Immunity*** concept exemplar for this chapter is Rheumatoid Arthritis.

The interrelated concepts for this chapter are:
- ***Pain***
- ***Clotting***
- ***Infection***
- ***Inflammation***

Arthritis means ***inflammation*** of one or more joints. However, in clinical practice arthritis is categorized as either noninflammatory or inflammatory. Although there are many types of arthritis and diseases in which arthritis occurs as a symptom, the two most common types are osteoarthritis and rheumatoid arthritis and are the focus of this chapter.

The major exemplar for the concept of ***mobility*** is osteoarthritis (OA), a noninflammatory, localized disorder. The major exemplar for ***immunity*** is rheumatoid arthritis (RA), a systemic, autoimmune inflammatory disorder. Both of these health problems can cause joint ***pain*** and stiffness. These priority concepts are reviewed briefly in Chapter 3. Other autoimmune disorders causing arthritis are discussed elsewhere in this text.

MOBILITY CONCEPT EXEMPLAR: OSTEOARTHRITIS

Pathophysiology Review

Osteoarthritis is the most common arthritis and a major cause of impaired ***mobility,*** persistent ***pain,*** and disability among adults in the United States and the world. It is sometimes referred to as *osteoarthrosis* or *degenerative joint disease (DJD)*.

Osteoarthritis is the progressive deterioration and loss of articular (joint) cartilage and bone in one or more joints. Articular cartilage contains water and a matrix of:

- Proteoglycans (glycoproteins containing chondroitin, keratin sulfate, and other substances)
- Collagen (elastic substance)
- Chondrocytes (cartilage-forming cells)

As people age or experience joint injury, proteoglycans and water decrease in the joint. The production of synovial fluid, which provides joint lubrication and nutrition, also declines because of the decreased synthesis of hyaluronic acid and less body fluid in older adults when compared with younger adults (McCance et al., 2019).

In patients of any age with OA, enzymes such as stromelysin break down the articular matrix. In early disease the cartilage changes from its normal bluish-white, translucent color to an opaque and yellowish-brown appearance. As cartilage and the bone beneath the cartilage begin to erode, the joint space narrows and **osteophytes** (bone spurs caused by irregular bony overgrowth) form (Fig. 46.1). As the disease progresses, fissures, calcifications, and ulcerations develop and the cartilage thins.

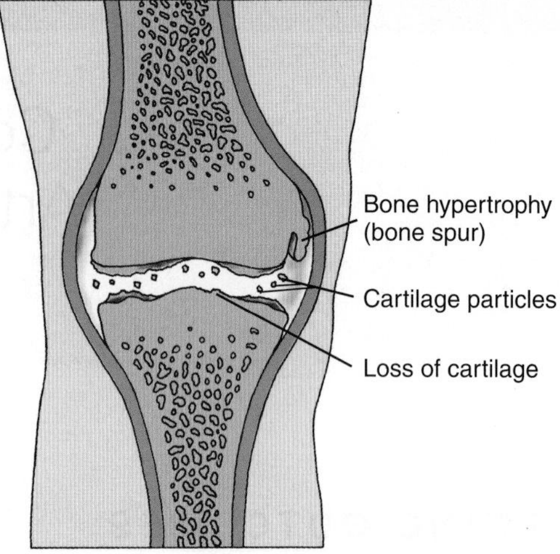

FIG. 46.1 Joint changes in osteoarthritis.

Inflammatory cytokines (enzymes) such as interleukin-1 (IL-1) may enhance this deterioration. The body's normal repair process cannot overcome the rapid process of degeneration (McCance et al., 2019). Secondary joint ***inflammation*** can occur when joint involvement is severe. Joint inflammation, also called **synovitis,** is evident when the joint is red, warm, painful, and swollen.

Eventually the cartilage disintegrates, and pieces of bone and cartilage "float" in the diseased joint, causing **crepitus,** a grating sound caused by the loosened bone and cartilage in a synovial joint. The resulting joint ***pain*** and stiffness can lead to decreased ***mobility*** and muscle atrophy. Muscle tissue helps support joints, particularly those that bear weight (e.g., hips, knees).

Etiology and Genetic Risk. The cause of OA is a combination of many factors. For patients with *primary* OA, the disease is caused by aging and genetic factors. Weight-bearing joints (hips and knees), the shoulders, the vertebral column, and the hands are most commonly affected, probably because they are used most often or bear the mechanical stress of body weight and many years of use.

Secondary OA occurs less often than primary disease and can result from joint injury and obesity. Injury to the joints from excessive use, trauma, or other joint disease (e.g., rheumatoid arthritis) predisposes a person to OA. Heavy manual occupations (e.g., carpet laying, construction, farming) cause high-intensity or repetitive stress to the joints. The risk for hip and knee OA is increased in professional and amateur athletes, especially football players, runners, and gymnasts. Fractures or other joint tissue injuries can lead to OA years after the trauma. Certain metabolic diseases (e.g., diabetes mellitus, Paget disease of the bone) and blood disorders (e.g., hemophilia, sickle cell disease) can also cause joint degeneration.

OA occurs in people who are obese much more commonly than in those who are not obese (Arthritis Foundation, 2019). Weight-bearing joints such as hips and knees are most often affected in obese individuals.

Incidence and Prevalence. The prevalence of OA varies among different populations but is a universal problem. Most people older than 60 years have joint changes that can be seen on x-ray examination, although not all of these adults actually develop the disease. According to the Arthritis Foundation (2019) estimates, 31 million people in the United States have symptomatic OA. By 2050, 40 million people worldwide are expected to be severely disabled by OA and 130 million will have the disease (Saccomano, 2018). OA is the fifth most common cause of disability worldwide (Arthritis Foundation, 2019).

PATIENT-CENTERED CARE: GENDER HEALTH CONSIDERATIONS QSEN

More men than women younger than 55 years old have OA caused by athletic injuries. After age 55 women have the disease more often than men. Although the cause for this difference is not known, contributing factors may include increased obesity in women after having children and broader hips in women than men (Arthritis Foundation, 2019). Be sure to assess all patients in the hospital or community-based setting, particularly those who are older and obese, for signs and symptoms of OA.

PATIENT-CENTERED CARE: VETERANS HEALTH CONSIDERATIONS QSEN

Almost all OA that occurs among the military population is the result of combat injury. OA occurs twice as often among the military who are younger than 40 years of age compared with the general population (Arthritis Foundation, 2019).

Health Promotion and Maintenance. Based on the etiology of OA, teach adults to:

- Maintain proper nutrition to prevent obesity.
- Take care to avoid injuries, especially those that can occur from professional or amateur sports.
- Take adequate work breaks to rest joints in jobs where repetitive motion or joint stress is common.
- Stay active and maintain a healthy lifestyle.

❖ Interprofessional Collaborative Care

◆ Assessment: Recognize Cues

History. Patients with OA usually seek medical attention in ambulatory care settings for their joint pain. However, you will also care for those who have OA as a secondary diagnosis in acute and chronic care facilities. Ask the patient about the course of the disease. Collect information specifically related to OA such as the nature and location of joint pain and how much pain and suffering he or she is experiencing. *Remember that older patients may underreport pain, resulting in inadequate management.* Use a 0-to-10 scale or other assessment tool to assess pain intensity. Chapter 5 discusses pain assessment in detail.

Other questions to ask include:

- If joint stiffness has occurred, where and for how long?
- When and where has any joint swelling occurred?
- How much discomfort are you having?
- How much is your ***pain*** disrupting your daily life?
- What do you do to control the discomfort, ***pain,*** or stiffness?
- Do you have any loss of ***mobility*** or difficulty in performing ADLs?

Because this disease occurs more often in older women, age and gender are important factors for the nursing history. Ask patients about their occupation, nature of work, history of injury (including falls), weight history, and current or previous involvement in sports. A history of obesity is significant, even for those currently within the ideal range for body weight. Document any family history of arthritis. Determine whether the patient has a current or previous medical condition that may cause joint symptoms.

Physical Assessment/Signs and Symptoms. In the early stage of the disease the signs and symptoms of OA may appear similar to those of rheumatoid arthritis (RA) (discussed later in this chapter) or other types of arthritis. The distinction between OA and RA becomes more evident as the disease progresses. Table 46.1 compares the major characteristics of both diseases and their common drug therapy. Some patients have both types of arthritis or an additional type, such as gout. **Gout** is a systemic disease in which urate crystals (the result of errors in purine metabolism) deposit in joints, causing severe joint inflammation. Common joints typically affected are the smaller joints of the body (especially the great toe). This type of arthritis is usually well controlled with drug therapy.

The typical patient with OA is a middle-age or older woman who reports *persistent (chronic) joint **pain** and stiffness.* Early in the course of the disease, these symptoms are relieved after rest or sleep and worsen after extended activity. Later, they may occur with slight motion or even when at rest. Because cartilage has no nerve supply, the ***pain*** is caused by joint and soft-tissue involvement and spasms of the surrounding muscles, or secondary joint ***inflammation***. During the joint examination the patient may have tenderness on palpation or when putting the joint through range of motion. **Crepitus** (a coarse grating sound caused by loosened bone and cartilage) may be felt or heard as the joint goes through range of motion. One or more joints may be affected. The patient may also report joint stiffness that usually lasts *less than* 30 minutes after a period of inactivity (McCance et al., 2019).

On inspection the joint is often enlarged because of bony hypertrophy (overgrowth) and osteophytes may be present. The joint feels hard on palpation. The presence of ***inflammation*** in patients with OA indicates a secondary synovitis. About half of patients with hand involvement have *Heberden nodes* (bony nodules at the distal interphalangeal [DIP] joints) and *Bouchard nodes* (bony nodules at the proximal interphalangeal [PIP] joints) (Fig. 46.2). Although OA is *not* typically a bilateral, symmetric disease, these large bony nodes appear on both hands, especially in women. The nodes may be painful and red. Some patients experience ***pain*** when developing nodes or when nodes are palpated. These deformities tend to be familial and are often a cosmetic concern to patients.

Joint effusions (excess joint fluid) are common when the knees are inflamed. Observe any *atrophy of skeletal muscle* from disuse. The vicious cycle of the disease discourages the movement of painful joints, which may result in contractures, muscle atrophy, and further ***pain***. *Loss of function* or decreased ***mobility*** may result, depending on which joints are involved. Hip or knee pain may cause the patient to limp and restrict walking distance.

TABLE 46.1 Differential Features of Rheumatoid Arthritis and Osteoarthritis

Characteristic	Rheumatoid Arthritis	Osteoarthritis
Typical onset (age)	35-45 yr	Older than 60 yr
Gender affected	Female (2-3:1)	Female (2:1)
Risk factors or cause	Autoimmune (genetic basis) Emotional stress (triggers exacerbation) Environmental factors	Aging Genetic factor (possible) Obesity Trauma Occupation
Disease process	Inflammatory	Likely degenerative with secondary ***inflammation***
Disease pattern	Bilateral, symmetric, multiple joints Usually affects upper extremities first Distal interphalangeal joints of hands spared Systemic	May be unilateral, single joint Affects weight-bearing joints and hands, spine Metacarpophalangeal joints spared Nonsystemic
Laboratory findings	Elevated rheumatoid factor, antinuclear antibody, and ESR	Normal or slightly elevated ESR
Common drug therapy	NSAIDs (short-term use) Methotrexate Leflunomide Biological response modifiers Other immunosuppressive agents	NSAIDs (short-term use) Acetaminophen Other analgesics

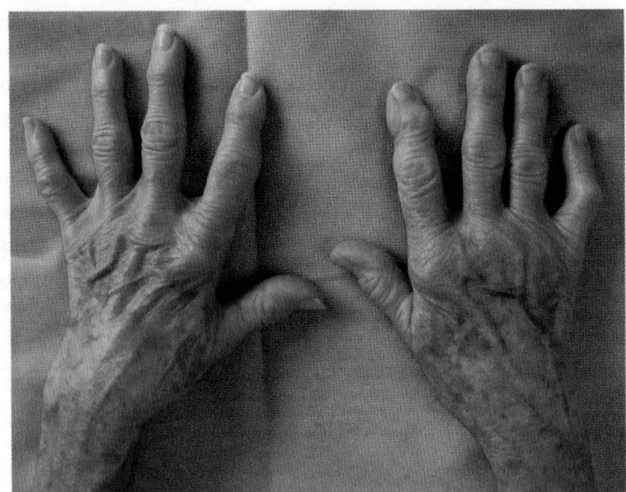

FIG. 46.2 Heberden and Bouchard nodes are enlarged bony nodules affecting the joints of the hand. (From Firestein, G.S., Budd, R.C., Gabriel, S.E., McInnes, I.B., & O'Dell, J.R. [2017]. *Kelley and Firestein's textbook of rheumatology* [10th ed.]. Philadelphia: Elsevier.)

OA can affect the spine, especially the lumbar region at the L3-4 level or the cervical region at C4-6 (neck). Compression of spinal nerve roots may occur as a result of vertebral facet bone spurs. The patient typically reports radiating pain, stiffness, and muscle spasms in one or both extremities (McCance et al., 2019).

Severe ***pain*** and deformity often interfere with ambulation and self-care. In addition to performing a musculoskeletal assessment, collaborate with the physical and occupational therapists to assess functional ability. Assess the patient's ***mobility*** and ability to perform ADLs. Chapter 7 describes functional assessment.

Psychosocial Assessment. OA is a chronic condition that may cause permanent changes in lifestyle. An inability to care for oneself in advanced disease can result in role changes and other losses. Persistent ***pain*** interferes with quality of life, including sexuality. Patients may not have the energy for sexual intercourse or may find positioning uncomfortable.

Patients with continuous ***pain*** from arthritis may develop depression or anxiety. The patient may also have a role change in the family, workplace, or both. To identify changes that have been or need to be made, ask about his or her roles before the disease developed. Identify coping strategies to help live with the disease. Ask the patient about his or her expectations regarding treatment for OA.

In addition to role changes, joint deformities and bony nodules often alter body image and self-esteem. Observe the patient's response to body changes. Does he or she ignore them or seem overly occupied with them? Ask patients directly how they perceive their body image. Document your assessment findings in the interprofessional health record per agency policy.

Laboratory Assessment. The primary health care provider uses the history and physical examination to make the diagnosis of OA. The results of routine laboratory tests are usually normal but can be helpful in screening for associated conditions. For example, an examination of aspirated joint fluid can show urate crystals, which indicates gout. The erythrocyte sedimentation rate (ESR) and high-sensitivity C-reactive protein (hsCRP) may be slightly elevated when secondary synovitis occurs. The ESR also tends to rise with age and ***infection.***

Imaging Assessment. Routine x-rays are useful in determining structural joint changes. Specialized views are obtained when the disease cannot be visualized on standard x-ray film but is suspected. Magnetic resonance imaging (MRI) may be used to determine vertebral or knee involvement.

◆ **Analysis: Analyze Cues and Prioritize Hypotheses.** The priority collaborative problems for patients with osteoarthritis (OA) include:

1. Persistent ***pain*** due to joint swelling, cartilage deterioration, and/or secondary joint ***inflammation***
2. Potential for decreased ***mobility*** due to joint ***pain*** and muscle atrophy

◆ **Planning and Implementation:Generate Solutions and Take Action.** In 2010 the Osteoarthritis Research Society International (OARSI) committee updated its evidence-based expert consensus guidelines for patients with knee, hand, and hip OA (Zhang et al., 2010). These interprofessional best practice guidelines remain the most current except for nonsurgical management for OA of the knee, which were updated in 2014 (McAlindon et al., 2014). The OARSI clinical guidelines have major implications for nursing care as described in the following section.

Managing Persistent Pain

Planning: Expected Outcomes. The patient with OA is expected to have a ***pain*** level that is acceptable to the patient (e.g., at a 3 or less on a pain intensity scale of 0 to 10).

Interventions. No drug therapy can influence the course of OA. Optimal management of patients with OA requires a multimodal approach (combination of therapies) to manage persistent ***pain***. Perform a pain assessment before and after implementing interventions (see Chapter 5).

Nonsurgical Management. Management of persistent joint ***pain*** can be challenging for both the patient and the health care professional. Drug therapy and a variety of nonpharmacologic therapies are used to manage the patient with OA. Chapter 5 elaborates on interventions for persistent noncancer pain.

Drug therapy. The purpose of drug therapy is to reduce ***pain*** and ***inflammation*** caused by cartilage destruction, muscle spasm, and/or synovitis. The American Pain Society, American Geriatrics Society, and OARSI committee recommend regular *acetaminophen* as the primary drug of choice because OA is not a primary anti-inflammatory disorder (Burchum & Rosenthal, 2019).

! NURSING SAFETY PRIORITY (QSEN)

Drug Alert

The standard ceiling dose of acetaminophen is 4000 mg each day. However, patients may be at risk for liver damage if they take more than 3000 mg daily, have alcoholism, or have liver disease. *Older adults are particularly at risk because of normal changes of aging such as slowed excretion of drug metabolites.* Remind patients to read the labels of over-the-counter (OTC) or prescription drugs that could contain acetaminophen before taking them. Teach them that their liver enzyme levels may be monitored while taking this drug.

Topical drug applications may help with temporary relief of mild ***pain***. Prescription lidocaine 5% patches have been approved by the U.S. Federal Drug Administration (FDA) for postherpetic neuralgia (nerve pain) but may also relieve joint pain (especially the knee) for some patients. Teach the patient to apply the patch on clean, intact skin for 12 hours each day. Up to three patches may be applied to painful joints at one time, but skin irritation may result. Teach the patient that the lidocaine patch is contraindicated in patients taking class I antidysrhythmics. Topical salicylates, such as OTC patches, gels, or creams, are useful for some patients as a temporary pain reliever, especially for knee pain.

If acetaminophen or topical agents do not relieve discomfort, other oral *NSAIDs* may be prescribed if the patient can tolerate them. These traditional drugs supported by OARSI guidelines include oral COX-2 nonselective and selective NSAIDs.

Before beginning oral NSAID therapy, baseline laboratory information is obtained, including a complete blood count (CBC) and complete metabolic panel (CMP). Celecoxib, a COX-2 inhibitor, is the preferred drug choice unless the patient has hypertension, kidney disease, or cardiovascular disease.

! NURSING SAFETY PRIORITY (QSEN)

Drug Alert

All of the COX-2 inhibiting drugs are thought to cause cardiovascular disease, such as myocardial infarction and hypertension, due to vasoconstriction and increased platelet aggregation (clumping). All NSAIDs can cause GI side effects, bleeding, and acute kidney injury if used long term (Burchum & Rosenthal, 2019). Therefore they are prescribed at the lowest effective dose. Remind patients to take celecoxib with food to decrease GI distress. Teach your patient about potential adverse effects and the need to report them to his or her primary health care provider. Examples include having dark, tarry stools; shortness of breath; edema; frequent dyspepsia; hematemesis (bloody vomitus); and changes in urinary output.

Topical NSAIDs are considered to be safer and effective nonsystemic drugs for pain relief. For example, the diclofenac-epolamine patch and diclofenac 1% gel may be used for patients with signs and symptoms associated with knee OA. However, diclofenac has the same two *black box warnings* as other NSAIDs in that they can cause cardiovascular or gastrointestinal adverse effects.

Weak opioid drugs such as tramadol may also be given for patients with OA. This drug should be used with caution in older adults because it can cause acute confusion. Remind any patient not to drive or operate dangerous machinery when taking any type of opioid. Chapter 5 discusses drug therapy for **pain** relief in more detail.

Nonpharmacologic interventions. In addition to analgesics, many nonpharmacologic measures can be used for patients with OA, such as rest balanced with exercise, joint positioning, heat or cold applications, weight control, and a variety of complementary and integrative therapies. Minimally invasive *regenerative therapies*, such as stem cell

NCLEX EXAMINATION CHALLENGE 46.1

Physiological Integrity

The primary health care provider prescribes daily celecoxib for a client experiencing persistent joint pain in both knees. Which health teaching will the nurse provide for the client regarding this drug for long-term pain control? **Select all that apply.**

A. "Take the prescribed drug before breakfast each day."
B. "Report any sign of bleeding, including bloody or dark, tarry stool."
C. "Do not take other NSAIDs while on celecoxib."
D. "Report any major changes in the amount of urine you excrete each day."
E. "Follow up with lab tests to assess liver function."

therapy and platelet-rich plasma (PRP), are being used for knee OA to delay surgery. PRP has shown very effective results in treating knee OA because it is rich in growth factor, which stimulates regeneration of knee cartilage, reduces pain, and improves joint function (Mogoi et al., 2019). More studies are needed to provide additional evidence for the use of regenerative therapies in clients who have OA (Zhao et al., 2018).

Teach the patient to *position joints in their functional position.* For example, when in a supine position (recumbent), he or she should use a small pillow under the head or neck but avoid the use of other pillows. The use of large pillows under the knees or head may result in flexion contractures. Remind him or her to use proper posture when standing and sitting to reduce undue strain on the vertebral column. Teach the patient to wear supportive shoes; foot insoles may help relieve pressure on painful metatarsal joints. Collaborate with the physical therapist (PT) to plan a program for muscle-strengthening exercises to better support the joints.

Many patients apply *heat* or *cold* for temporary relief of ***pain.*** Heat may help decrease the muscle tension around the tender joint and thereby decrease pain and stiffness. Suggest hot showers and baths, hot packs or compresses, and moist heating pads. *Regardless of treatment, teach him or her to check that the heat source is not too heavy or so hot that it causes burns.* A temperature just above body temperature is adequate to promote comfort.

If needed, collaborate with the PT to provide special heat treatments, such as paraffin dips, diathermy (using electrical current), and ultrasonography (using sound waves). A 15- to 20-minute application is usually sufficient to temporarily reduce pain, spasm, and stiffness. Cold packs or gels that feel hot and cold at the same time may also be used.

Cold therapy has limited use for most patients in promoting comfort. Cold works by numbing nerve endings and decreasing secondary joint ***inflammation,*** if present.

Gradual *weight loss* for obese patients may lessen the stress on weight-bearing joints, decrease ***pain,*** and perhaps slow joint degeneration. If needed, collaborate with the registered dietitian nutritionist to provide more in-depth teaching and meal planning or make referrals to community resources for weight reduction.

Complementary and integrative health. Some patients with OA report that a variety of integrative therapies are useful. However, the evidence supporting their effectiveness is often inconsistent and inconclusive.

Topical *capsaicin* products are safe over-the-counter (OTC) drugs. They work by blocking or modifying substance P and other neurotransmitters for ***pain.*** Tell the patient using capsaicin to expect a burning sensation for a short time after applying it. Recommend the use of plastic gloves for application. To prevent burning of eyes or other body areas, wash hands immediately after applying the substance.

Dietary supplements may complement traditional drug therapies. Glucosamine and chondroitin are widely used and are the most effective nonprescription supplements taken to decrease pain and improve functional ability. However, the evidence to support their use is inconsistent (Arthritis Foundation, 2019). These natural products are found in and around bone cartilage for repair and maintenance. Glucosamine may decrease ***inflammation,*** and chondroitin may play a role in strengthening cartilage. However, most national medical guidelines do not currently recommend these supplements (Gourdine, 2019).

Medical marijuana (cannabis). Medical marijuana (cannabis) has been used for many years to assist in pain management. Patients with osteoarthritis pain have reported the effectiveness of cannabinoids, and there is a growing body of scientific evidence that supports these reports. Both plant-based and man-made cannabinoids may be effective for pain control (O'Brien & McDougall, 2018).

Surgical Management. Surgery may be indicated when conservative measures and/or drug therapy no longer provide ***pain*** control, when ***mobility*** becomes so restricted that the patient cannot participate in activities he or she enjoys, and when he or she cannot maintain the desired quality of life. The most common surgical procedure for OA is **total joint arthroplasty (TJA)** (surgical creation of a functional [synovial] joint using implants), also known as *total joint replacement (TJR).* Almost any synovial joint of the body can be replaced with a prosthetic system that consists of at least two implants—one for each joint surface. The hip and knee are most often replaced, but shoulder and ankle arthroplasties are becoming increasingly common as a result of advances in technology. TJAs are expected to increase as baby boomers age over the next 20 years.

TJA is a procedure used most often to manage the pain of OA and improve ***mobility,*** although other conditions causing cartilage and bone destruction may require the surgery. These disorders include rheumatoid arthritis (RA), congenital anomalies, trauma, and osteonecrosis (Bodden & Coppola, 2018). **Osteonecrosis** is bone death secondary to lack of or disruption in blood supply to the affected bone, usually from trauma or chronic steroid therapy. The affected bone site is most commonly the femoral or humeral head, distal femur, and proximal tibia.

The *contraindications* for TJA are active ***infection*** anywhere in the body and rapidly progressive ***inflammation.*** An active infection elsewhere in the body or from the joint being replaced can result in an infected TJA and subsequent prosthetic failure. Severe medical problems, such as uncontrolled diabetes or hypertension, put the patient at risk for major postoperative complications and possible death. Therefore these problems should be stabilized before surgery (Hohler, 2018).

Total hip arthroplasty. The number of total hip arthroplasty (THA) procedures (also known as *total hip replacement [THR]*) has steadily increased over the past 40 years. If the patient has a joint replacement for the first time, it is referred to as **primary arthroplasty.** If the implant loosens or fails for any reason, **revision arthroplasty** may be performed to replace the previous one. Availability of improved joint implant materials and better custom design features allow longer life of a THA. Although adult patients of any age can undergo THA, the procedure is performed most often in those older than 60 years. *The special needs and normal physiologic changes of older adults often complicate the perioperative period and may result in additional postoperative complications.*

Preoperative care. As with any surgery, preoperative care begins with assessing the patient's level of understanding about the surgery and his or her ability to participate in the postoperative plan of care. Identifying a **joint coach** (care partner) can help the patient through the perioperative period and assist with discharge needs. The surgeon explains the procedure and postoperative expectations (including possible complications) during the office visit, but this *patient education* may have occurred weeks or months before the scheduled elective surgery. Research is needed to determine the best time for preoperative education (Bodden & Coppola, 2018). Information may be provided in a notebook, pamphlet, DVD format, or online so that the patient can review it at home and share with the joint coach and other family members. This review is particularly useful to patients with inadequate reading skills or poor memory.

PATIENT-CENTERED CARE: CULTURAL/ SPIRITUAL CONSIDERATIONS QSEN

Written materials or other media provided in the language appropriate for the patient's educational level and culture are essential. If an interpreter is needed to be sure that the information is understood, one needs to be provided at each appointment, while in the hospital, and when discharged with home or inpatient rehabilitation services.

Preoperative rehabilitation, or "prehab," is essential to prevent functional decline after surgery and provide a quicker functional recovery. As part of prehab, the patient and joint coach learn postoperative exercises, transfer and positioning techniques, and ambulation with a walker or crutches, depending on the patient's age and stability. Other best practices for preoperative patient and family education are summarized in the Patient and Family Education: Preparing for Self-Management: Preoperative Care and Education for Patients Having a Total Hip Arthroplasty box (Bodden & Coppola, 2018).

In addition to the care and patient education outlined in the Patient and Family Education: Preparing for Self-Management box, patients preparing for elective orthopedic surgery may be screened for their risk of postoperative *delirium.* Jones and Taylor (2019) described a quality improvement initiative for identifying delirium risk to anticipate the need for safety sitters to prevent patient falls. Delirium is discussed in Chapter 3 and in mental health textbooks.

PATIENT AND FAMILY EDUCATION: PREPARING FOR SELF-MANAGEMENT

Preoperative Care and Education for Patients Having a Total Hip Arthroplasty

Teaching Area	Health Teaching
Nutrition Assessment	Stress the need for preoperative assessment for clinical malnutrition, which is associated with prolonged postoperative rehabilitation and surgical complications. Collaborate with the registered dietitian nutritionist for nutritional assessment.
Pain Assessment and Management	Assess for use of opioids for persistent pain before surgery. Teach the patient and joint coach about multimodal pain management options.
Venous Thromboembolism (VTE) Prevention	Teach the need for anticoagulant drug therapy, which should start within 24 hours after surgery and continue for at least 14 days after surgery. For patients taking anticoagulants or antiplatelet drugs before surgery, plan for interruption of these drugs for several days before surgery. Teach the need for frequent mobilization after surgery; early mobility also helps to prevent constipation. Teach the need for compression stockings and/or sequential compression devices during the hospital stay.
Infection Prevention	Teach the patient that he or she will receive an IV antibiotic before surgery and possibly up to 24 hours after surgery. Teach the importance of screening for nares (nose) colonization of *Staphylococcus aureus* 2-4 weeks before surgery. Teach the need to use nasal mupirocin ointment twice a day for 1 week (or longer depending on the nasal culture) before surgery. Teach the need to bathe with chlorhexidine gluconate solution (CHG) for at least the night before and the morning of surgery (a longer period of time may be needed depending on agency or surgeon protocol). Teach the patient to sleep on clean linens and not use lotions or powders after the CHG baths; remind the patient to avoid sleeping with pets in the bed.

For patients not at risk for delirium, *Enhanced Recovery After Surgery (ERAS) programs,* also called "fast track," "accelerated track," or "rapid recovery" programs, are common in Total Joint Replacement Centers to improve patient outcomes, such as a shortened hospital length of stay (LOS), improved patient experiences, and enhanced functional outcomes. Patients who participate in this type of program also have fewer hospital readmissions (Bodden & Coppola, 2018).

In addition to usual preoperative laboratory tests and x-rays, the surgeon may ask the patient with RA to have a cervical spine x-ray if he or she is having general anesthesia. Those with RA often have cervical spine disease that can lead to **subluxation** (partial joint dislocation) during intubation. A CT scan and/or MRI may be done to assess the operative joint and surrounding soft tissues, especially if the patient is undergoing a robotic-assisted THA. Chapter 9 discusses general preoperative care in detail.

Operative procedures. Similar to other orthopedic surgeries, the patient receives an *IV antibiotic,* usually a cephalosporin such as cefazolin or cefuroxime, within an hour before the initial surgical incision per the Surgical Care Improvement Project (SCIP) Core Measures to help prevent infection. If the patient has a beta-lactum allergy, vancomycin or clindamycin is administered 2 hours before the initial incision (Bodden & Coppola, 2018).

Several different types of anesthesia are used for THA surgeries and are administered by an anesthesiologist or nurse anesthetist. These options include general anesthesia, neuraxial (spinal or epidural) anesthesia, regional nerve blocks, or a combination of these agents. Patients receiving neuraxial or regional anesthetics may also be given IV moderate sedation to keep them unaware of their environment during the procedure. The benefit of a regional block is that the patient may receive extended ***pain*** relief, often up to 24 hours after surgery. Chapter 9 describes complications and nursing implications associated with varying types of anesthesia.

For most patients, *tranexamic acid (TXA)* is used to reduce blood loss during the THA surgical procedure. TXA is an antifibrinolytic agent that improves postoperative hemoglobin and hematocrit and decreases the need for blood transfusions (Hohler, 2018). Preventing hypothermia is another important goal during THA surgery because it is associated with increased blood loss, increased risk for infection, and increased risk for a cardiac event. Patients with a low body mass index (BMI) are at the highest risk for hypothermia (Bodden & Coppola, 2018).

Some patients are candidates for *minimally invasive surgery (MIS)* using a small incision (usually 4 inches [10.16 cm] instead of 6 to 12 inches [15.24 to 30.48 cm] for traditional surgery) with special instruments, cameras, and computers to reduce muscle cutting and stretching. This newer technique cannot be used for patients who are obese or those with osteoporosis. It is done only for primary THAs, not for revision surgeries. Like those of any MIS, the benefits of minimally invasive THA are decreased soft tissue damage, blood loss, and postoperative ***pain.*** Patients usually have a shorter hospital stay and quicker recovery. They are generally satisfied with the cosmetic appearance of the incision because there is less scarring. Postoperative complications are not as common in patients having minimally invasive ("mini") hip arthroplasty compared with those having the traditional technique.

Hip resurfacing is an alternative to total hip replacement surgery. This procedure is most often performed for younger patients or for those with early-stage cartilage loss of the weight-bearing surface of the femoral head. Instead of completely removing the femoral head and inserting the stem into the femoral canal, the surgeon removes the cartilage from the surface and an artificial cap is placed over the existing natural femoral head.

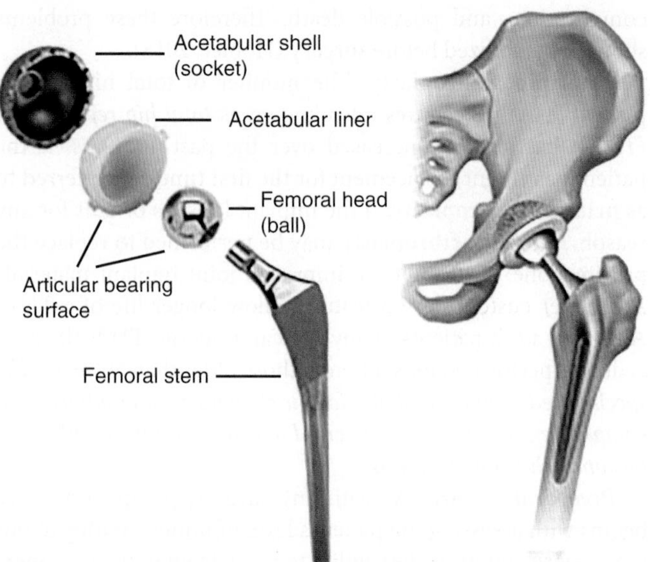

FIG. 46.3 Two major components of total hip arthroplasty. (From Zhang, Y., Zhu, J., Wang, Z., Zhou, Y., & Zhang, X. [2015]. Constructing a 3D-printable, bioceramic sheathed articular spacer assembly for infected hip arthroplasty. *Journal of Medical Hypotheses and Ideas, 9*[1], 13–19.)

Two components are used in the THA—the acetabular implant and the femoral implant (Fig. 46.3). A noncemented prosthesis is commonly used for younger patients. Bone surfaces are smoothed as they are prepared to receive the artificial implants. The noncemented components are press-fitted into the prepared bone. The acetabular cup may be placed using computer- or robotic-assisted guidance. For cemented prostheses, polymethyl methacrylate (an acrylic fixating substance) is typically used. It often contains an antibiotic to reduce the risk of ***infection.*** The hybrid surgical technique usually involves a cemented femoral component and a noncemented acetabular component. A closed wound drainage system is not commonly used today for a THA because it can contribute to increased blood loss and cause hematoma formation (Bodden & Coppola, 2018). A surgical pressure dressing is applied before the patient is discharged to the postanesthesia care unit (PACU).

Considerations of a noncemented prosthesis include protection of weight-bearing status to allow bone to grow into the prosthesis and decreased problems with loosening of the prosthesis. With a cemented prosthesis, cement can fracture or deteriorate over time, leading to loosening of the prosthesis. These problems cause ***pain*** and can lead to the need for a revision arthroplasty. In revision arthroplasty the old prosthesis is removed and new implants are placed. Bone graft may be added if bone loss is significant. Outcomes from revision arthroplasty may not be as positive as with primary arthroplasty, particularly for obese patients.

Three surgical approaches are commonly used to perform a THA. Nursing care and patient education differ slightly depending on which approach is used. Be sure to confirm the surgeon's surgical method for each patient. For the *anterior approach,* the hip joint can be exposed without detaching surrounding muscles. Therefore this approach has the least likely chance of postoperative hip dislocation and may have the quickest postoperative recovery.

Both of the other surgical methods, *direct lateral* and *posterolateral approaches,* require detaching and/or cutting into large skeletal muscles, which can cause severe postoperative ***pain*** and a high risk for hip dislocation. The posterolateral approach has the highest risk for dislocation and is therefore used less commonly today (Hohler, 2018).

Postoperative care. The typical hospital stay for the patient having a traditional THA is 3 days unless the patient participates in an ERAS program. Some younger patients only stay in the hospital overnight. The goal for rapid recovery programs is for the patients to have same-day THA surgery.

In addition to providing the routine postoperative care discussed in Chapter 9, assess for and help prevent possible postoperative complications. One of the most common complications after a THA is hip dislocation. Other complications include venous thromboembolism, ***infection,*** and complications of decreased ***mobility.***

Preventing Hip Dislocation. As described earlier, the risk for hip dislocation depends on the operative approach used by the surgeon.

NURSING SAFETY PRIORITY QSEN

Action Alert

Teach patients to maintain correct positioning of the hip joint and leg at all times. When the patient returns from the postanesthesia care unit (PACU), place him or her in a supine position with the head slightly elevated. One or two regular bed pillows are used in most cases to remind patients to keep their legs abducted if they had one of the two lateral surgical approaches. *For abduction devices with straps, be sure to loosen the straps every 2 hours and check the patient's skin for irritation or breakdown.* Place and support the affected leg in neutral rotation. The procedure for postoperative turning is not universal and is specified by agency policy or surgeon preference. Turning the patient to the operative side provides "splinting" of the operative hip but may be too painful for some patients. If the patient is turned to the nonoperative side, the operative leg needs to be fully supported with pillows to prevent slipping of the leg into an adducted position that can lead to dislocation. Teach the patient and family about other precautions to prevent hip dislocation.

Older adults may have difficulty understanding health teaching because they often become acutely confused after a THA as a result of surgery, anesthesia, and/or unfamiliar environments. The Patient Centered Care: Older Adult Considerations: Special Postoperative Care of the Older Adult With a Total Hip Arthroplasty box highlights special nursing care of older adults in the postoperative period.

Observe the patient carefully for signs and symptoms of hip dislocation, including report of sudden intense ***pain*** or sudden agitation for the patient who is unable to communicate, affected leg rotation, and/or leg shortening. If the surgical hip becomes dislocated, the surgeon may be able to manipulate and relocate it after the patient receives moderate sedation. If the hip does not reduce into position, the patient may have surgical reduction in the operating room (OR). Following reduction, the hip is usually immobilized by an abduction splint or other device until healing occurs—usually in about 6 weeks.

PATIENT-CENTERED CARE: OLDER ADULT CONSIDERATIONS QSEN

Special Postoperative Care of the Older Adult With a Total Hip Arthroplasty

- For patients who had a *posterolateral or direct lateral surgical approach,* use an abduction pillow or splint (rather than bed pillows) to keep their legs apart and prevent adduction, especially if the patient is very restless or has an altered mental state. Hip adduction can cause the surgical hip to become partially or completely dislocated.
- Keep the patient's heels off the bed to prevent pressure injuries.
- Do not rely on fever as a sign of ***infection;*** older patients often have infection without fever. Be alert to decreasing mental status and/or elevated white blood cell count as indicators of infection.
- When assisting the patient out of bed, move him or her slowly to prevent orthostatic (postural) hypotension. Allow the patient to sit on the side of the bed for a brief period of time before standing; have him or her stand for a brief period before beginning ambulation.
- Encourage the patient to deep breathe and cough and to use the incentive spirometer every 2 hours to prevent atelectasis and pneumonia.
- As soon as permitted, get the patient out of bed to a recliner chair to prevent complications of decreased ***mobility.***
- Anticipate the patient's need for pain medication, especially if he or she cannot verbalize the need for ***pain*** control. For patients on a multimodal pain protocol, assess the need to medicate for breakthrough pain (see Chapter 5).
- Expect a temporary change in mental state immediately after surgery as a result of the anesthetic and unfamiliar sensory stimuli. Reorient the patient frequently.

NURSING SAFETY PRIORITY QSEN

Action Alert

As with other musculoskeletal surgery, *monitor neurovascular assessments* frequently for a possible compromise in circulation to the affected distal extremity following a THA. Check and document color, temperature, distal pulses, capillary refill, movement, and sensation. The procedure for performing a thorough lower-extremity neurovascular assessment is described in detail in Chapter 44. Remember to compare the operative leg with the nonoperative leg. These assessments are performed at the same time the vital signs are checked. Report any changes in neurovascular assessment to the surgeon and carefully monitor for changes. Early detection of changes in neurovascular status can prevent permanent tissue damage.

Preventing Postoperative Complications. The most potentially life-threatening and commonly occurring complication after THA is venous thromboembolism (VTE), which includes deep venous thrombosis (DVT) and pulmonary embolism (PE). *Older patients are especially at increased risk for VTE because of age and decreased circulation before surgery. Obese patients, patients who currently smoke, and those with a history of VTE are also at high risk for thrombi.*

Preventive evidence-based postoperative interventions include a combination of ***p***harmacology, ***a***mbulation, and ***c***ompression (PAC) (Tubog, 2019; Wilson et al., 2018). *Anticoagulants* such as subcutaneous low-molecular-weight heparin (LMWH) or factor Xa inhibitors are effective drugs in preventing VTE to patients having a THA. Patients are usually on anticoagulants for 10 days to several weeks after surgery, depending on surgeon preference and the patient's response and risk factors.

The use of subcutaneous LMWH, such as enoxaparin and dalteparin, is common for patients with total hip or knee arthroplasty. As an alternative to LMWH, subcutaneous fondaparinux, a factor Xa inhibiting agent, may be prescribed for some patients undergoing these surgeries. A newer Xa inhibitor, rivaroxaban, can be given orally once a day. Recently oral apixaban has received FDA approval for VTE prophylaxis in patients having a THA. You do not need to monitor the PT or INR for patients receiving these drugs because they do not affect coagulation values. However, for other older anticoagulants such as warfarin, patients are at risk for bleeding due to impaired ***clotting.*** A complete discussion of nursing care associated with patients taking anticoagulants is found in Chapter 33.

Early *ambulation* and exercise also help prevent VTE. Wilson et al. (2018) reported the results of establishing best practices for VTE prevention, which included a requirement for ambulation at least three times a day for all patients who were allowed to be out of bed. Teach the patient about leg exercises, which should begin in the immediate postoperative period and continue through the rehabilitation period. These exercises include plantar flexion and dorsiflexion (heel pumping), circumduction (circles) of the feet, gluteal and quadriceps muscle setting, and straight-leg raises (SLRs). Teach the patient to perform gluteal exercises by pushing the heels into the bed and achieve **quadriceps-setting exercises** ("quad sets") by straightening the legs and pushing the back of the knees into the bed. In addition to preventing clots, these exercises improve muscle tone, which helps restore the function of the extremity.

Intermittent pneumatic *compression* devices, also called bilateral sequential compression devices (SCDs), are also important in preventing VTE by increasing venous blood flow during periods of inactivity (Wilson et al., 2018). However, clients often report that these devices are hot and bulky to wear, which affects their willingness to use them. Some surgeons prescribe antiembolism stockings, which are not as effective but are more widely accepted by clients.

Monitor the surgical incision and vital signs carefully—every 4 hours for the first 24 hours and every 8 to 12 hours thereafter, following facility and surgeon protocols. Observe for signs of ***infection,*** such as an elevated temperature, increased redness around the incision, and excessive or foul-smelling drainage from the incision. These signs and symptoms may be seen as early as 2 to 3 days after surgery. *An older patient may not have a fever with infection but instead may experience an altered mental state, especially delirium.* If you suspect this problem, obtain a sample of any drainage for culture and sensitivity to determine the causative organisms and the antibiotics that may be needed for treatment.

Managing Postoperative Pain. Although hip arthroplasty is performed to relieve joint ***pain,*** patients experience varying levels of pain related to the surgical procedure. Pain control protocols vary, depending on the region of the country, anesthesiologist/nurse anesthetist, and surgeon. Many patients equate pain control with opioids (Morland, 2019). However, in view of the opioid crisis, a *multimodal pain management* approach is best practice for patients having a major joint arthroplasty.

Immediate pain control may be achieved by short-term patient-controlled analgesia (PCA), or IV push, typically with morphine or hydromorphone. Pizzi et al. (2020) demonstrated that oral patient-controlled analgesia with oxycodone is effective in managing pain for patients having total joint arthroplasty. Nonopioid drugs are used as part of the multimodal analgesic approach because they act at different pain receptor sites. Examples of these drugs include (Bodden & Coppola, 2018; Goode et al., 2019):

- Continuous peripheral nerve block (e.g., bupivacaine, ropivacaine)
- NSAIDs (e.g., ketorolac, celecoxib)
- NMDA receptor antagonists (e.g., ketamine)
- Gabapentinoids (e.g., gabapentin, pregabalin)

Chapter 5 contains information on the nursing care associated with these medications.

Nonpharmacologic methods for acute and chronic pain control, such as cryotherapy and music therapy, can also be used to decrease the amount of drug therapy used. Chapter 5 describes these methods in detail. Also see the Evidence-Based Practice box in the section on total knee arthroplasty (TKA) later in this chapter.

Promoting Postoperative Mobility and Activity. Depending on the time of day that the surgery is performed, the patient with a THA gets out of bed with assistance the night of surgery to prevent problems related to decreased ***mobility*** (e.g., atelectasis, pneumonia), especially in older adults.

! NURSING SAFETY PRIORITY (QSEN)

Action Alert

Be sure to assist the patient the first time he or she gets out of bed to prevent falls and observe for dizziness. When getting the patient out of bed, put a gait belt on him or her and then stand on the same side of the bed as the affected leg. After the patient sits on the side of the bed, remind him or her to stand on the unaffected leg and pivot to the chair with guidance. *To avoid injury, do not lift the patient!*

The surgeon, type of prosthesis, and surgical procedure determine the amount of weight bearing that can be applied to the affected leg. A patient with a cemented implant is usually allowed immediate weight bearing as tolerated (WBAT). Typically only "toe-touch" or minimal weight bearing is initially permitted for patients with noncemented prostheses. When x-ray evidence of bony ingrowth can be seen, the patient can progress to partial weight bearing (PWB) and then to full weight bearing (FWB) over a period of weeks.

In collaboration with the physical therapist (PT), teach the patient how to follow weight-bearing restrictions. Most patients use a walker, but younger adults may use crutches. They are usually advanced to a single cane or crutch if they can walk without a severe limp 4 to 6 weeks after surgery. When the limp disappears, they no longer need an ambulatory/assistive device and may be permitted to sit in chairs of normal height, use regular toilets, and drive a car. Timing of driving may be slightly longer in a patient who has had surgery on the right hip because of patient safety concerns.

NCLEX EXAMINATION CHALLENGE 46.2

Physiological Integrity

A client had a left noncemented posterolateral total hip arthroplasty 2 days ago. Which statements will the nurse include in health teaching for the client? **Select all that apply.**

A. "Practice leg exercises each day as instructed."
B. "Take deep breaths and use incentive spirometry every 2 hours."
C. "Be sure to cross your legs to be more comfortable in a chair."
D. "Report sudden increased hip pain or rotation immediately to the nurse."
E. "Stand on your right leg and pivot into the chair when getting out of bed."

Promoting Postoperative Self-Management. With the increase in ERAS programs that emphasize a structured approach and rapid recovery, the length of stay in the acute care hospital is typically less than 3 days if there are no postoperative complications. McCann-Spry et al. (2016) reported a quality improvement project in which the patient's length of stay was reduced to 2.5 days for a 2-night stay rather than the typical 3-night stay (see the Systems Thinking and Quality Improvement box). Patients experiencing postoperative complications often stay longer. Medicare patients need a 3-day qualifying hospital stay to receive rehabilitation in a skilled inpatient unit. Discharge from the acute care facility may be to the home, a rehabilitation unit, a transitional care unit, or a skilled unit or long-term care facility for continued rehabilitation before discharge to home. The interprofessional team provides written instructions for posthospital care and reviews them with patients and their joint coaches. Be sure to provide a copy of these instructions for the patient.

Acute rehabilitation usually takes several weeks, depending on the patient's age and progress and the type of prosthesis used. However, it often takes 6 weeks or longer for complete recovery. Patients who are discharged to their home are able to attend physical therapy sessions in an office or ambulatory care setting. Others have no means or cannot use community resources and need physical therapy in the home, depending on their health insurance coverage. *Collaborate with the case manager to determine which option is best for your patient.* The Patient and Family Education: Preparing for Self-Management: Care of Patients With Total Hip Arthroplasty After Hospital Discharge box outlines the most important health teaching for you to provide to the patient being discharged after a THA.

SYSTEMS THINKING AND QUALITY IMPROVEMENT (QSEN)

Can Hospital Length of Stay Be Shortened for Patients Having Joint Replacements?

McCann-Spry, L., Pelton, J., Grandy, G., & Newell, D. (2016). An interdisciplinary approach to reducing length of stay in joint replacement patients. *Orthopaedic Nursing, 35*(5), 279–300.

Demand for total joint replacement surgeries is increasing as baby boomers become older adults. One large hospital in a northern U.S. state developed a process for decreasing postoperative hospital length of stay (LOS) using an interprofessional collaborative approach. Four interventions were implemented: (1) improve communication for primary health care providers (surgeons), including a letter explaining the goal of reducing LOS from 3 nights to 2 nights; (2) develop a script for staff conversations with the patient and family for each hospital day; (3) standardize the risk assessment and prediction for reducing LOS; and (4) initiate physical therapy the day of surgery. As a result of this quality improvement project, patient LOS was reduced an average of 0.5 days per patient for primary hip and knee replacement surgeries. This reduction was very cost-effective without negatively affecting patient and family satisfaction.

Commentary: Implications for Research and Practice

This QI project was very successful at improving financial outcomes and increasing collaboration and communication among interprofessional health care team members and improving staff-patient communication. Nurses play a major role in care coordination and discharge teaching for patients and their families. More QI projects and interventions are needed in additional joint replacement centers to achieve these positive outcomes and promote systems thinking.

Hospital readmission after THA. The most common complications of THA surgery that cause readmission to the hospital include thromboembolic problems, such as DVT and stroke; surgical site infection (SSI); and systemic infections, including pneumonia and sepsis. Men of advanced age and those with comorbidities, such as heart failure and diabetes, are at the highest risk for hospital re-admission after a THA (Bodden & Coppola, 2018).

Total knee arthroplasty. As the population ages, more adults are undergoing total knee arthroplasty (TKA, also known as *total knee replacement [TKR]*). The increased demand for TKA in the United States is due to the osteoarthritis and obesity, a contributing factor to OA in weight-bearing joints. Osteoarthritis is discussed earlier in this chapter. Patients who have rheumatoid arthritis or posttraumatic arthritis caused by a physical injury may also need a TKA (Mori & Ribsam, 2018). Similar to the THA, patients who experience a failed primary TKA have revision arthroplasty.

TKAs are most often performed as unilateral procedures, meaning that *one* knee is replaced during surgery. However, a growing number of patients chose to have *both* knees done at one time or within 3 months of each other. This procedure is referred to as bilateral total knee arthroplasty (BTKA). BTKA is sometimes done for patients who have moderate to severe arthritis in both knees. Two types of BTKA may be performed—a one-stage or two-stage procedure. In a one-stage procedure, both knees are replaced during the same surgery. This surgery is most

PATIENT AND FAMILY EDUCATION: PREPARING FOR SELF-MANAGEMENT

Care of Patients With Total Hip Arthroplasty After Hospital Discharge

Hip Precautions
- Do not sit or stand for prolonged periods.
- Do not cross your legs beyond the midline of your body.
- For *posterolateral or direct lateral surgical approach* patients: Do not bend your hips more than 90 degrees.
- For *anterior surgical approach* patients: Do not hyperextend your operative leg behind you.
- Do not twist your body when standing.
- Use the prescribed ambulatory aid such as a walker when walking.
- Use assistive/adaptive devices as needed (e.g., sock aids, shoehorns, dressing sticks, extenders [also see Chapter 7]).
- Do not put more weight on your affected leg than allowed and instructed.
- Call 911 if you experience any signs and symptoms of hip dislocation, including sudden difficulty bearing weight on the surgical leg, leg shortening or rotation, or a feeling that the hip has "popped" with immediate intense ***pain.***
- Resume sexual intercourse as usual on the advice of your surgeon.

Pain Management
- Report increased hip or anterior thigh pain to the surgeon immediately.
- Take oral analgesics as prescribed and only as needed.
- Do not overexert yourself; take frequent rests.
- Use ice as needed to operative hip to decrease or prevent swelling and minimize pain.

Incisional Care
- Follow the instructions provided regarding dressing changes, if needed. Some surgeons use specialty clear dressings that do not need to be changed. No dressing may be needed if a skin sealant was used.
- Inspect your hip incision every day for redness, heat, or drainage; if any of these are present, call your surgeon immediately.
- Do not bathe the incision or apply anything directly to the incision unless instructed to do so. Shower according to the surgeon's instructions.

Other Care
- Continue walking and performing the leg exercises as you learned them in the hospital. Do not increase the amount of activity unless instructed to do so by the therapist or surgeon.
- Do not cross your legs to help prevent blood clots.
- Report pain, redness, or swelling in your legs to your surgeon immediately.
- Call 911 for acute chest pain or shortness of breath (could indicate pulmonary embolus).
- If you are taking an anticoagulant, follow the precautions learned in the hospital to prevent bleeding; avoid using a straight razor, avoid injuries, and report bleeding or excessive bruising to your surgeon immediately.
- Be sure to follow up with outpatient physical therapy for your exercise and ambulation program to build strength, ***mobility,*** and endurance.
- Follow up with visits to the surgeon's office as instructed.

commonly performed for *younger* patients. In a two-stage procedure, two surgeries are done either during the same hospital stay or within 3 months of each other (Pietsch et al., 2018).

Partial knee replacements are used for patients with minimal cartilage loss in specified areas of the involved knee and are typically done more often in younger patients. Minimally invasive surgery (MIS) is also an option for either partial or total knee arthroplasty for this population. Severe bone loss, obesity, and previous knee surgeries are contraindications for this type of surgery. Patients who have MIS procedures have less ***pain*** and blood loss and greater range of motion to promote a faster postoperative recovery.

Preoperative care. TKA is performed when joint ***pain*** can no longer be managed by conservative measures. When limited ***mobility*** severely prevents patients from participating in work or activities they enjoy, this procedure can restore a high quality of life. The preoperative care and teaching for patients undergoing a TKA are similar to that for THA. However, precautions for positioning are not the same because joint dislocation is not a common complication. Differences in patient and family teaching depend on the procedure used by the orthopedic surgeon and established best practices.

The use of Enhanced Recovery After Surgery (ERAS) programs for many types of surgery has improved outcomes for patients having a TKA. As part of this program, patients have a screening to determine their *nutritional status,* including identifying those who are malnourished and/or obese. Obesity is linked to health problems, such as heart disease, diabetes, hypertension, and stroke, and can impair bone and wound healing. Patients who have had bariatric surgery may have chronic anemia and bone loss due to insufficient nutrients. Bone health is a concern for adults of any age who have a history of bariatric surgery (Chicoski, 2018). Chapter 55 discusses obesity and bariatric surgery in detail.

Planning for postdischarge *transitions of care* begins before surgery, including identifying a **joint coach** (care partner) who plays an active role in patient care through the perioperative care (Mori & Ribsam, 2018). *Preoperative rehabilitation* ("prehab") is important to enhance functional ability and provide a quicker postoperative recovery. All patients are given verbal and either written or video preoperative instructions, which include the activity protocol to follow after surgery. The PT and OT provide information about transfers, ambulation, postoperative exercises, and ADL assistance. Patients should practice walking with walkers or crutches to prepare them for ambulation after TKA. Teach patients about the possible need for assistive/adaptive devices to assist with ADLs, including an elevated toilet seat, safety handrails, and dressing devices like a long-handled shoehorn. Some third-party payers may cover these devices, depending on the patient's condition and age. Teach the patient and family how and where this equipment can be obtained to have it available after surgery. Case managers or social workers may arrange for needed items to be delivered to the patient's room before discharge.

A *pain management* assessment and plan before surgery are essential to promote a satisfactory postoperative patient experience. Patients with persistent preoperative pain may have mental health problems, such as anxiety, depression, and/or substance use disorder. Some patients have been treated with long-term analgesics, including opioids, for many years before surgery. These factors place patients having major joint arthroplasty at high risk for severe postoperative pain that can be challenging to manage (Mori & Ribsam, 2018; Jackman, 2019).

Best practices for postoperative management of persistent pain patients include to (Jackman, 2019):

- Identify at-risk patients preoperatively.
- Establish trust and discuss the postoperative pain management plan.
- Perform a comprehensive preoperative and postoperative assessment of pain and reassessment.
- Use multimodal and alternative pain management modalities.
- Consult the pain management team if needed and available.
- Manage mental health/psychological disorders that may be present.
- Plan continuing pain management for and after discharge.

Teach patients that they will need to shower with a chlorhexidine gluconate (CHG) body wash the night before and the morning of surgery to decrease bacteria on the skin that could cause ***infection.*** Remind them to wear clean nightwear, sleep on clean linen, and avoid having pets in their bed. All patients having a TKA should be treated for at least a week with nasal mupirocin ointment to prevent surgical site infection from *Staphylococcus aureus* (Mori & Ribsam, 2018).

Ask patients to check with their surgeon about which drugs they can take the morning of surgery with a small amount of water, including antihypertensives, thyroid hormone supplements, and antidiabetic agents. Some drugs, such as NSAIDs and anticoagulant/antiplatelets, are discontinued 5 to 10 days before surgery to prevent surgical bleeding. See Chapter 9 for additional general preoperative care interventions and teaching.

Operative procedures. As with the hip, the knee can be replaced with the patient under a variety of anesthetic agents, including general or neuraxial (epidural or spinal) anesthesia. One of the more recent advances in postoperative pain management for TKA is the use of a **peripheral nerve block (PNB)**, most commonly a femoral nerve block (FNB) using a local anesthetic. An IV moderate sedation agent is used in addition to the neuraxial or PNB drug. PNB may be either a single injection or continuous infusion by a portable pump (e.g., continuous femoral nerve blockade or CFNB). In addition, other local medications may be injected into the knee or surrounding tissues to assist in the reduction of severe pain that usually occurs after knee surgery and to minimize perioperative bleeding. Sasse et al. (2020) reported that adding a ketorolac periarticular injection decreased pain and improved postoperative mobility for patients having a TKS.

An antibiotic, usually an IV cephalosporin (cefazolin or cefuroxime), is given within 60 minutes before the surgical incision and proximal tourniquet inflation per the SCIP Core Measures to aid in the prevention of ***infection.*** If giving a fluoroquinolone or vancomycin, the infusion should begin 2 hours (120 minutes) before the incision and tourniquet inflation (Mori & Ribsam, 2018). In the *traditional surgery,* the surgeon makes a central longitudinal incision about 6 to 8 inches (15.24 to 20.32 cm) long. Osteotomies of the femoral and tibial condyles and of the posterior patella are performed, and the surfaces are prepared for the prosthesis. The femoral prosthesis is often noncemented (using a press-fit) with the tibial component being cemented.

Total knee arthroplasties require multiple bone incisions and extensive soft tissue involvement, which can result in significant blood loss. Interventions that may reduce blood loss include:

- Tourniquet use during surgery
- Surgical drains (used less commonly today)
- Fibrin sealants
- Transexamic acid (TXA), an antifibrinolytic agent

While these interventions may be effective, most of them also have disadvantages. For example, using an operative tourniquet can increase postoperative pain. The strongest evidence supports TXA use during surgery for blood loss reduction (Mori & Ribsam, 2018). This drug improves postoperative hemoglobin and hematocrit and decreases the need for blood transfusions. The surgeon also applies a compression (pressure) dressing from the toes to the thigh to decrease edema and bleeding.

Minimally invasive TKA may be performed using a shorter incision and special instruments to spare muscle and other soft tissue. Computer-guided or robotic equipment may be used to ensure accurate positioning of the knee implants.

Postoperative care. Provide the usual postoperative care needed for any patient who has surgery (see Chapter 9). Specific nursing care of the patient with a TKA is similar to that for the patient with a total hip arthroplasty as described in the previous section.

! NURSING SAFETY PRIORITY QSEN

Critical Rescue

If the patient has a continuous femoral nerve blockade (CFNB), perform and document neurovascular assessment every 2 to 4 hours, or according to hospital protocol. Be sure that patients can perform dorsiflexion and plantar flexion motions of the affected foot without pain in the lower leg. In addition, monitor these patients for signs and symptoms that indicate absorption of the local anesthetic into the patient's system, including:

- Metallic taste
- Tinnitus
- Nervousness
- Slurred speech
- Bradycardia
- Hypotension
- Decreased respirations
- Seizures

Document and report these new-onset signs and symptoms to the surgeon, anesthesiologist/nurse anesthetist, or Rapid Response Team immediately and carefully continue to monitor the patient for any changes.

Since joint dislocation is rare after TKA, there are no special positioning precautions required to prevent adduction. Maintain the operative leg in a neutral position, avoiding both internal and external rotation. Do not place a pillow under the replaced knee or hyperextend the knee.

Although not as commonly used today, the surgeon may prescribe a continuous passive motion (CPM) machine, which can be applied in the postanesthesia care unit (PACU) or soon after the patient is admitted to the postoperative unit (Fig. 46.4). For some patients, the CPM is prescribed for home use after the patient is discharged. The CPM machine keeps the prosthetic knee in motion

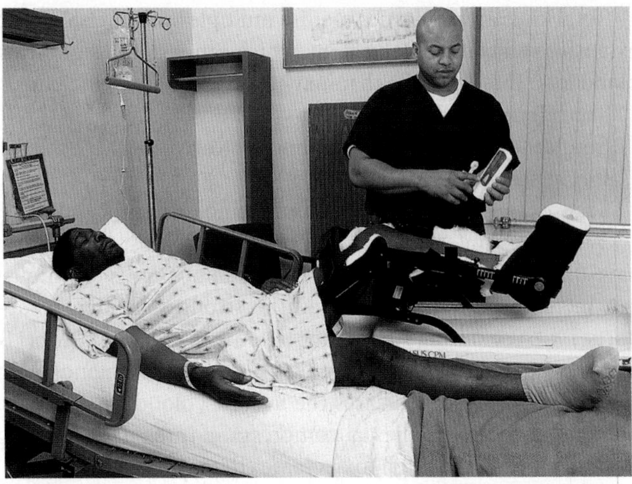

FIG. 46.4 A continuous passive motion (CPM) machine in use.

BEST PRACTICE FOR PATIENT SAFETY & QUALITY CARE QSEN

The Patient Using a Continuous Passive Motion (CPM) Machine

- Ensure that the machine is well padded.
- Check the cycle and range-of-motion settings at least once every 8 hours.
- Ensure that the joint being moved is properly positioned on the machine.
- If the patient is confused, place the controls to the machine out of his or her reach.
- Assess the patient's response to the machine.
- Turn off the machine while the patient is having a meal in bed.
- When the machine is not in use, do not store it on the floor.

and may prevent the formation of scar tissue, which could decrease knee ***mobility*** and increase postoperative pain. Observe and document the patient's response to the device and follow the surgeon's protocol for settings. The Best Practice for Patient Safety & Quality Care: The Patient Using a Continuous Passive Motion (CPM) Machine box outlines your responsibility when caring for a patient using the CPM machine. This device may also be used for other types of orthopedic surgery, including toe, ankle, and shoulder ligament and cartilage repair.

Managing Postoperative Pain. In the immediate postoperative period, the surgeon prescribes some form of cryotherapy (cold application) to decrease swelling, hematoma formation, and ***pain*** at the surgical site. The affected knee is typically very swollen and discolored for a number of weeks after surgery. These problems are more common with this type of surgery than with hip surgery. Several types of cryotherapy are used, including ice/gel pack compression and circulating cold water cryotherapy devices. A recent study comparing these two cryotherapy methods for 100 randomized subjects found that the less expensive ice-gel packs were as effective as the circulating cold water devices in managing pain and swelling. Patient satisfaction was the same for both study groups (Schinsky et al., 2016).

In general, ***pain*** control measures for patients with TKA are similar to those with total hip arthroplasty. Many patients report high ratings on the pain intensity scale and require

EVIDENCE-BASED PRACTICE QSEN

Is Music Therapy Effective to Promote Comfort for Patients Having a Total Joint Arthroplasty?

Gallagher, L.M., Gardner, V., Bates, D., Mason, S., Nemecek, J., DiFiore, D.B., et al. (2018). Impact of music therapy on hospitalized patients post-elective orthopaedic surgery: A randomized controlled trial. *Orthopaedic Nursing, 37*(2), 124-135.

The purpose of this randomized controlled study was to determine the impact of music therapy (MT) sessions on promoting comfort for patients who had total joint arthroplasty. Comfort outcomes included pain, mood, nausea, anxiety, and use of opioids. Data on hospital length of stay were also collected. The majority of the 163 subjects had either hip or knee arthroplasties and were randomly assigned to either a control or experimental group. The patients in the experimental group received an MT session by a board-certified music therapist each hospital day. The patients in the control group received the usual postarthroplasty care.

Results showed that the experimental group had better outcomes related to pain, anxiety, and mood on Day 1. By Day 2, all comfort measures were better for the experimental group when compared with the control group. The researchers concluded that structured music therapy was effective in improving pain, mood, nausea, anxiety, and use of opioids. However, no significant differences were noted between groups related to hospital length of stay and opioid use.

Level of Evidence: 1

The study was a randomized controlled trial with multiple subjects.

Commentary: Implications for Practice and Research

This study demonstrated that music therapy can be an effective nonpharmacologic modality for improving patient comfort after total joint arthroplasty. More research is needed to focus more specifically on the role of nonpharmacologic interventions on pain management and the use of analgesic medications.

analgesic medications longer than patients with THA, particularly if they have had bilateral knee surgery. Similar to best practices for managing pain in patients having a THA, a multimodal analgesic approach including a variety of opioid and nonopioid drugs is used (see earlier discussion in this chapter). For some younger patients, IV acetaminophen may be effective in managing TKA pain.

Nonpharmacologic pain modalities are becoming an integral part of the comprehensive pain management plan. For example, music therapy has been found to be an effective strategy for postoperative patients having a TKA (see the Evidence-Based Practice box).

Preventing Postoperative Complications. Some complications that affect patients with THA may also affect those having unilateral or bilateral TKA, such as venous thromboembolism (VTE) and ***infection***. Complications generally depend on the overall health of the patient.

Average-risk patients begin anticoagulant therapy within 24 hours after surgery and continue for at least 14 days. Common drugs used include fondaparinux, apixaban, dabigatran, rivaroxaban, low-dose unfractionated heparin, and low-molecular-weight heparin. Mechanical VTE prevention includes pneumatic or sequential compression devices and/or compression stockings that are applied before surgery and worn during the hospital stay.

A recent integrative literature review to determine evidence-based nursing practices to prevent complications for patients with bilateral TKA found a lack of clinical practice guidelines for both nursing and surgeon care (Pietsch et al., 2018). Assessments and interventions associated with impaired ***clotting*** and ***infection*** are described in the Postoperative Care section of the discussion of Total Hip Arthroplasty.

Promoting Postoperative Self-Management. The desired outcome for discharge from the acute hospital unit is that the patient can walk with crutches or a walker and has adequate flexion in the operative knee for ambulation, including walking up and down stairs. Patients are able to bear weight as tolerated unless the prosthesis is not cemented. Patients may be discharged to their home or to an acute rehabilitation unit, transitional care unit, or skilled unit in a long-term care facility for therapy after 1 to 3 days in acute care. Patients participating in enhanced recovery (ERAS) programs have a shorter hospital length of stay and fewer complications or readmissions.

For some patients, home care services may provide physical therapy and nursing care for 1 to 2 weeks followed by outpatient therapy. *Collaborate with the case manager to determine which option is best for your patient.* During the home rehabilitation phase, the use of a stationary bicycle or CPM machine may help gain flexion. These patients typically return to work and other usual activities in 6 weeks, depending on their age, type of surgery, and other health status factors. Total recovery from a TKA surgery takes 6 weeks or longer, especially for those older than 75 years.

Hospital readmission after TKA. The primary causes of readmission after a TKA are ***infection,*** DVT, and arthrofibrosis. **Arthrofibrosis** is the buildup of excessive scar tissue that restricts joint motion and functional ability (Cheuy et al., 2017). Women who had a longer postoperative hospital stay and were discharged to an inpatient rehabilitation facility or skilled nursing facility are at the greatest risk for these complications (Causey-Upton et al., 2019).

NCLEX EXAMINATION CHALLENGE 46.3

Safe and Effective Care Environment

Assistive personnel (AP) are assigned to care for a client who had a cemented total knee arthroplasty yesterday. Which observation by the AP indicates a need for follow-up by the nurse?

A. "The client's surgical knee is very swollen and discolored."
B. "The client states that the surgical knee is very painful when moving it."
C. "The client's lower leg on the surgical side is painful and red."
D. "The client needs assistance with walking to the bathroom."

Other joint arthroplasties. The shoulder and other upper-extremity joints do not bear weight and therefore tend to have less degeneration and subsequent pain. Preoperative teaching for patients having any of these surgeries depends on the surgeon's technique and postoperative protocols.

Total shoulder arthroplasty (TSA) has gained popularity as newer prostheses and technology have been developed. This procedure usually decreases arthritic or traumatic pain and increases the patient's ability to perform ADLs. Because the shoulder joint is complex and has many articulations (joint surfaces), **subluxation** or complete dislocation is a major potential complication. Usually the glenohumeral joint, created by the glenoid cavity of the shoulder blade (scapula) and the head of the humerus, is replaced because it moves the most and is therefore most affected by arthritis. A cemented or noncemented hemiarthroplasty (replacement of part of the joint), typically the humeral component, may be performed as an alternative to TSA.

After surgery the patient may be placed in an abduction immobilizer or pillow device to protect the joint from excessive motion until rehabilitation therapy begins. *Do not remove these devices unless instructed to do so by the surgeon.*

In addition to the potential for dislocation, postoperative complications are similar to those for other total joint replacements and include infection and neurovascular compromise. *As for any other total joint arthroplasty, perform frequent neurovascular assessments at least every 4 to 8 hours.* The procedure for performing a thorough upper-extremity neurovascular assessment is described in detail in Chapter 44. Document and report any significant changes to the surgeon immediately. The hospital stay for TSA is shorter than for a total hip or knee replacement and may be performed as a same-day procedure. Rehabilitation with an OT generally takes several months.

Improving Mobility

Planning: Expected Outcomes. The patient with osteoarthritis (OA) is expected to maintain or improve a level of ***mobility*** and activity that allows him or her to function independently with or without an assistive ambulatory device.

Interventions. Management of the patient with OA often requires an interprofessional health team effort. If needed, consult and collaborate with the physical therapist (PT) and occupational therapist (OT) to meet the outcome of independent function and ***mobility.*** Major interventions include therapeutic exercise and the promotion of ADLs and ambulation by teaching about health and the use of assistive devices.

Certain recreational activities may also be therapeutic, such as swimming to enhance chest and arm muscles. Aerobic exercises (e.g., walking, biking, swimming, aerobic dance) are also recommended. Exercises may be prescribed by rehabilitation therapists for the patient with OA, but you will need to reinforce their techniques and principles. The ideal time for exercise is immediately after the application of heat. To prevent further joint damage, teach patients to carefully follow the instructions for exercise outlined in the Patient and Family Education: Preparing for Self-Management: Exercises for Patients With Osteoarthritis box.

Collaborate with the PT to evaluate the patient's need for ambulatory aids, such as canes or walkers. Although some patients do not like to use these aids or may forget how to use them, they can help prevent further joint deterioration and pain. Collaborate with the OT, if needed, to provide suggestions and devices for assistance for ADLs. Chapter 7 discusses rehabilitation therapies in more detail.

PATIENT AND FAMILY EDUCATION: PREPARING FOR SELF-MANAGEMENT

Exercises for Patients With Osteoarthritis

- Follow the exercise instructions that have been prescribed specifically for you. There are no universal exercises; your exercises have been specifically tailored to your needs.
- Do your exercises on both "good" and "bad" days. Consistency is important.
- Respect pain. Reduce the number of repetitions when the inflammation is severe and you have more pain.
- Use active rather than active-assist or passive exercise whenever possible.
- Do not substitute your normal activities or household tasks for the prescribed exercises.
- Avoid resistive exercises when your joints are severely inflamed.

Care Coordination and Transition Management. The patient with OA is not usually hospitalized for the disease itself but may be admitted for surgical management. Expect that any patient older than 60 years will have some degree of arthritis and possibly persistent ***pain*** that needs to be managed.

Home Care Management. If weight-bearing joints are severely involved, the patient may have difficulty going up or down stairs. Making arrangements to live on one floor with accessibility to all rooms is often the best solution. A home care nurse or case manager may collaborate with a rehabilitation therapist to assess the need for structural alterations to the home to accommodate ambulatory aids and enable the patient to perform ADLs. For example, a kitchen counter may need to be lowered, or a seat and handrails may need to be installed in the shower. If the patient has undergone a total hip or knee arthroplasty, an elevated toilet seat is necessary for several weeks after surgery to prevent excessive hip flexion. Throw rugs and other environmental hazards should be removed to prevent tripping and falls.

Self-Management Education. Self-management education (SME) is an effective psychosocially focused nonpharmacologic intervention. Learning how to protect joints is the most important part of patient and family education. Preventing further damage to joints slows the progression of OA and minimizes ***pain.*** Explain the general principles of joint protection and give practical examples as outlined in the Patient and Family Education: Preparing for Self-Management: Evidence-Based Instructions for Joint Protection box.

As with other diseases in which drugs and nutrition therapy are used, teach the patient and family the drug therapy protocol, desired effects and potential side effects, and toxic effects. Emphasize the importance of reducing weight and eating a well-balanced diet to promote tissue healing.

Many patients with arthritis look for a cure after becoming frustrated and desperate about the course of the disease and treatment. Better control of arthritis is possible, but cure is not yet available. Unfortunately, tabloids, books, media, and the Internet often report "curative" remedies. People spend billions of dollars each year on quackery, including liniments, special diets, and copper bracelets. More hazardous substances such as snake oil and industrial cleaners are also advertised as remedies.

PATIENT AND FAMILY EDUCATION: PREPARING FOR SELF-MANAGEMENT

Evidence-Based Instructions for Joint Protection

- Use large joints instead of small ones; for example, place your purse strap over your shoulder instead of grasping the purse with your hand.
- Do not turn a doorknob clockwise. Turn it counterclockwise to avoid twisting your arm and promoting ulnar deviation (especially for patients who also have rheumatoid arthritis).
- Use two hands instead of one to hold objects.
- Sit in a chair that has a high, straight back.
- When getting out of bed, do not push off with your fingers; use the entire palm of both hands.
- Do not bend at your waist; instead, bend your knees while keeping your back straight.
- Use long-handled devices, such as a hairbrush with an extended handle.
- Use assistive/adaptive devices, such as Velcro closures and built-up utensil handles to protect your joints.
- Do not use pillows in bed except a small one under your head.
- Avoid twisting or wringing your hands; use a device or rubber grip to open jars or bottles.

Refer the patient to the Arthritis Foundation for up-to-date information about these "cures." The practice of wearing a copper bracelet will not cure arthritis, but it will not cause harm. However, if the patient is using a potentially harmful substance or method, reinforce the need to avoid the unproven remedy and explain why it should not be used. Respect the patient's preferences, values, and beliefs for using benign remedies that do not cause harm.

With most types of arthritis, patients must live with a persistent, unpredictable, and painful disorder. Their roles, self-esteem, and body image may be affected by these diseases. Body image is usually not as devastating in OA as in the inflammatory arthritic diseases such as RA. The psychosocial component associated with having arthritis is discussed in more detail later in this chapter in the Rheumatoid Arthritis section.

Health Care Resources. The patient who has undergone surgery may need help from community resources. After an arthroplasty, he or she may need assistance with ***mobility.*** The patient may be discharged to home or an inpatient rehabilitation unit. Collaborate with the case manager and surgeon to determine the best placement. If the patient is discharged to home, home care nurses may be approved for third-party payment for several visits, depending on the presence of any existing systemic diseases. A home care aide may visit the home to help with hygiene-related needs, and a PT may work with ambulatory and ***mobility*** skills. For older patients, a family member, significant other, or other caregiver should be in the home for at least the first few weeks when the patient needs the most assistance. Emphasize the need for patient safety, especially interventions to prevent falls as described in Chapter 4.

Provide written instructions about the required care, regardless of whether the patient goes home or to another inpatient facility. *As required by The Joint Commission's National Patient Safety Goals (NPSGs) and other health care accrediting organizations, hand-off communication with the new care provider is essential for seamless continuity of care and care coordination.*

The Arthritis Foundation (www.arthritis.org) is an important community resource for all patients with all types of arthritis. This organization provides information to lay people and health care professionals and refers patients and their families to other resources as needed. Local support groups can help them cope with these diseases.

◆ **Evaluation: Evaluate Outcomes.** Evaluate the care of the patient with OA on the basis of the identified priority problems. The expected outcomes are that he or she:

- Achieves pain control to a pain intensity level of 2 to 3 on a scale of 0 to 10 or at a level that is acceptable to the patient
- Does not experience complications associated with total joint arthroplasty (if performed)
- Moves and functions in his or her own environment independently with or without assistive devices

IMMUNITY CONCEPT EXEMPLAR: RHEUMATOID ARTHRITIS

Pathophysiology Review

Rheumatoid arthritis (RA) is a chronic, progressive, systemic inflammatory autoimmune disease process that affects primarily the synovial joints. *Systemic* means this disease can affect any or all parts of the body while affecting many joints.

In patients with RA, transformed autoantibodies (rheumatoid factors [RFs]) that attack healthy tissue, especially synovium, are formed, causing ***inflammation.*** The disease then begins to involve the articular cartilage, joint capsule, and surrounding ligaments and tendons. ***Immunity*** and inflammatory factors cause cartilage damage in patients with RA (McCance et al., 2019):

- CD4 helper T-cells and other immune cells in synovial fluid promote cytokine release, especially interleukin-1 (IL-1) and tumor necrosis factor–alpha (TNFA), which attack cartilage.
- Neutrophils and other inflammatory cells in the joint are activated and break down the cartilage.
- Immune complexes deposit in synovium, and osteoclasts are activated.
- B- and T-lymphocytes of the immune system are stimulated and increase the inflammatory response. (Also see Chapter 16 for a complete discussion of the inflammatory response.)

The synovium then thickens and becomes hyperemic, fluid accumulates in the joint space, and a pannus forms. The pannus is vascular granulation tissue composed of inflammatory cells; it erodes articular cartilage and eventually destroys bone. As a result, in late disease, fibrous adhesions, bony ankyloses (abnormal fusion of bones in the joint), and calcifications occur. Bone loses density, and secondary osteoporosis exists.

Permanent joint changes may be avoided if RA is diagnosed early. Early and aggressive treatment to suppress synovitis may lead to a remission. RA is a disease characterized by natural remissions and exacerbations (flare-ups). Interprofessional health care team management helps control the disease to decrease the intensity and number of exacerbations. Preventing flares helps prevent joint erosion and permanent joint damage.

Because RA is a systemic disease, areas of the body besides the synovial joints can be affected. Inflammatory responses similar to those occurring in synovial tissue may occur in any organ or body system in which connective tissue is prevalent. If blood vessel ***inflammation*** (vasculitis) occurs, the organ supplied by that vessel can be affected, leading to eventual failure of the organ or system in late disease.

Etiology and Genetic Risk. The etiology of RA remains unclear, but research suggests a *combination of environmental and genetic factors.* Some researchers also suspect that female reproductive hormones influence the development of RA because it affects women more often than men—usually young to middle-age women. Others suspect that infectious organisms may play a role, particularly the Epstein-Barr virus (McCance et al., 2019). Physical and emotional stresses have been linked to exacerbations of the disorder and may be contributing factors or "triggers" to its development.

PATIENT-CENTERED CARE: GENETIC/GENOMIC CONSIDERATIONS QSEN

Research has shown that there is a strong association between RA and several human leukocyte antigen (HLA)–*DR* alleles. The cause of this association is not clear, but most HLA diseases are autoimmune (McCance et al., 2019). *DR* alleles, especially *DR4* and *DRB1*, are the primary genetic factors contributing to the development of RA. *DR4* is associated with more severe forms of the disease. Other contributing factors are being researched.

Incidence and Prevalence. RA affects over 1.5 million people, and Euro-Americans have the disease more often than other groups. Women are two to three times more likely to have RA compared with men (Arthritis Foundation, 2019). The cause for these trends is not known.

❖ Interprofessional Collaborative Care

◆ **Assessment: Recognize Cues.** The onset of rheumatoid arthritis (RA) may be acute and severe or slow and progressive; patients may have vague symptoms that last for several months before diagnosis. The onset of the disease is more common in the winter months than in the warmer months. The signs and symptoms of RA can be categorized as early or late disease and as joint (articular) or systemic (extra-articular), as summarized in the Key Features: The Patient With Rheumatoid Arthritis box.

Physical Assessment/Signs and Symptoms

Early Signs and Symptoms. In the early stage of RA the patient typically reports joint *inflammation,* generalized weakness, and fatigue. Anorexia, weight loss of about 2 to 3 lb (1 kg), and persistent low-grade fever are common. In patients with early disease, the upper-extremity joints are involved initially—often the proximal interphalangeal (PIP) and metacarpophalangeal (MCP) joints of the hands. These

KEY FEATURES

The Patient With Rheumatoid Arthritis

Early Signs and Symptoms (Early Disease)	Late Signs and Symptoms (Advanced Disease)
Joint • Inflammation **Systemic** • Low-grade fever • Fatigue • Weakness • Anorexia • Paresthesias	**Joint** • Deformities (e.g., swan neck or ulnar deviation) • Moderate-to-severe ***pain*** and morning stiffness **Systemic** • Osteoporosis • Severe fatigue • Anemia • Weight loss • Subcutaneous nodules • Peripheral neuropathy • Vasculitis • Pericarditis • Fibrotic lung disease • Sjögren syndrome • Kidney disease • Felty syndrome

joints may be slightly reddened, warm, stiff, swollen, and tender or painful, particularly on palpation (caused by synovitis). The typical pattern of joint involvement in RA is bilateral and symmetric (e.g., both wrists). The number of joints involved usually increases as the disease progresses.

The presence of only *one* hot, swollen, painful joint (out of proportion to the other joints) may mean that the joint is infected. *Refer the patient to the primary health care provider (generally the rheumatologist) immediately if this is the case.* Single hot, swollen joints are considered infected until proven otherwise and require immediate long-term antibiotic treatment.

Late Signs and Symptoms. As the disease advances, the joints become progressively inflamed and very painful. The patient usually has frequent morning stiffness, which can last for several hours after awakening. On palpation the joints feel soft and look puffy because of synovitis and effusions. The fingers often appear spindle-like. Note any muscle atrophy (which can result from disuse secondary to joint pain) and a decreased range of motion in the affected joints.

Most or all synovial joints are eventually affected. The temporomandibular joint (TMJ) may be involved in severe disease, but such involvement is uncommon. When the TMJ is affected, the patient may have pain when chewing or opening the mouth.

When the spinal column is involved, the cervical joints are most likely to be affected. During clinical examination, gently palpate the posterior cervical spine and identify it as cervical pain, tenderness, or loss of motion.

NURSING SAFETY PRIORITY (QSEN)

Critical Rescue

Cervical RA may result in **subluxation**, especially of the first and second vertebrae. This complication may be life threatening because branches of the phrenic nerve that supply the diaphragm are restricted and respiratory function may be compromised. The patient is also in danger of becoming quadriparetic (weak in all extremities) or quadriplegic (paralyzed in all extremities). If cervical pain (may radiate down one arm) or loss of range of motion is present in the cervical spine, keep the neck straight in a neutral position to prevent permanent damage to the spinal cord or spinal nerves. *Notify the primary health care provider immediately about these neurologic changes!*

Joint deformity occurs as a late, articular manifestation, and secondary osteoporosis can cause bone fractures. Observe common deformities, especially in the hands and feet (Fig. 46.5). Extensive wrist involvement can result in carpal tunnel syndrome (see Chapter 47 for assessment and management of carpal tunnel syndrome).

Gently palpate the tissues around the joints to elicit pain or tenderness associated with other rheumatoid complications, unless the patient is having severe joint ***pain.*** For example, Baker cysts (enlarged popliteal bursae behind the knee) may occur and cause tissue compression and pain. Tendon rupture is also possible, particularly rupture of the Achilles tendon.

Numerous extra-articular signs and symptoms are associated with advanced disease. Assess the patient to ascertain systemic involvement. In addition to increased joint swelling and tenderness, *moderate-to-severe weight loss, fever,* and *extreme fatigue* are common in late disease **exacerbations,** often called *flare-ups.* Some patients have the characteristic soft, round, movable **subcutaneous nodules,** which usually appear on the ulnar surface of the arm, on the fingers, or along the Achilles tendon. These nodules can disappear and reappear at any time and are associated with severe, destructive disease. Rheumatoid nodules are usually not a problem themselves; however, they occasionally open and become infected and may interfere with ADLs. Accidentally bumping the nodules may cause discomfort. Occasionally nodules occur in the lungs.

Inflammation of the blood vessels results in **vasculitis,** particularly of small to medium-size vessels. When arterial involvement occurs, major organs can become ischemic and malfunction. Assess for ischemic skin lesions that appear in groups as small, brownish spots, most commonly around the nail bed. Monitor the number of lesions, note their location each day, and report vascular changes to the health care provider. Increased lesions indicate increased vasculitis, and a decreased number indicates decreased vasculitis. Also carefully assess any larger lesions that appear on the lower extremities. These lesions can lead to ulcerations, which heal slowly as a result of decreased circulation. Peripheral neuropathy associated with decreased circulation can cause footdrop and **paresthesias** (burning and tingling sensations), usually in older adults.

Respiratory complications may manifest as *pleurisy, pneumonitis, diffuse interstitial fibrosis,* and *pulmonary hypertension.* Cardiac complications include *pericarditis* and *myocarditis.* These health problems are discussed elsewhere in this text.

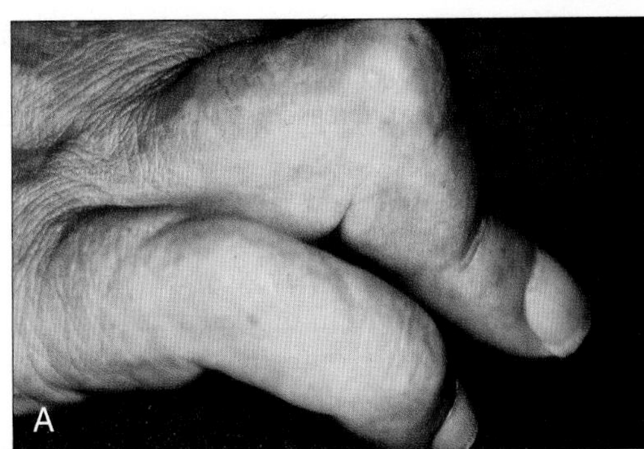

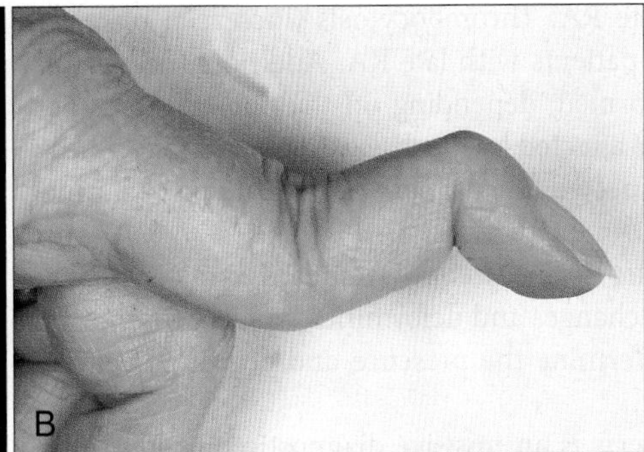

FIG. 46.5 Common joint deformities seen in rheumatoid arthritis. **A,** Boutonniere deformity; **B,** Swan neck deformity. (From Hochberg, M. C., Gravallese, E. M., Silman, A. J., et al. [2019]. *Rheumatology* [7th ed.]. Philadelphia: Elsevier.)

Assess for eye involvement, which typically manifests as *iritis* and *scleritis.* If either of these complications is present, the sclera of one or both eyes is reddened and the pupils have an irregular shape. Visual disturbances may occur.

Several syndromes are seen in patients with advanced RA. The most common is Sjögren syndrome, which includes a triad of:

- Dry eyes (keratoconjunctivitis sicca [KCS], or the sicca syndrome)
- Dry mouth (xerostomia)
- Dry vagina (in some cases)

Note the patient's report of dry mouth or dry eyes. Some patients state that their eyes feel "gritty," as if sand is in their eyes. Inspect the mouth for dry, sticky membranes and the eyes for redness and lack of tearing.

Psychosocial Assessment. Rheumatoid arthritis (RA) and other inflammatory types of arthritis are chronic diseases that can be disabling if not well controlled. Fear of becoming dependent, uncertainty about the disease process, altered body image, devaluation of self, frustration, and depression are common psychosocial problems. Physical limitations and persistent ***pain*** may limit the patient's ***mobility.*** These limitations can result in role changes in the family and society. For example, the person may not be able to cook for the family or be an active sexual partner. In addition, extreme fatigue often causes patients to desire an early bedtime and napping and may result in a reluctance to socialize.

Body changes caused by joint changes and drug therapy (if used) may also cause poor self-esteem and body image. Because many societies value people with physically fit, attractive bodies, the patient with RA may be embarrassed to be seen in public places. The patient may grieve or experience degrees of depression. He or she may have feelings of helplessness caused by a loss of control over a disease that can "consume" the body. Fortunately, newer drugs have improved the treatment of RA and provide the patient with hope and better disease control. Only a small percentage of patients with RA become wheelchair dependent.

Living with a chronic disease and its associated ***pain*** is difficult for the patient and family. Chronic suffering and pain affect quality of life. Assess the patient's emotional and mental status in relation to the disease and its problems. Evaluate his or her support systems and resources. Patients who are knowledgeable about their disease and treatment options feel emotionally stronger to cope with their disease and better able to discuss treatment options with their primary health care provider.

Laboratory Assessment. Laboratory tests help support a diagnosis of RA, but no single test or group of tests can confirm it. The test for *rheumatoid factor (RF)* measures the presence of unusual antibodies of the immunoglobulins G (IgG) and M (IgM) types that develop in a number of connective tissue diseases. Many patients with RA have a positive titer (greater than 1:80), *especially in older adults* (Pagana & Pagana, 2018). However, the presence of RF is not diagnostic for RA.

The newest laboratory test called the *anticyclic citrullinated peptide (anti-CCP)* is very specific and sensitive in detecting early RA. The presence of anti-CCP is also a marker for aggressive and erosive late-stage disease.

The *antinuclear antibody (ANA)* test measures the titer of a group of antibodies that destroy the nuclei of cells and cause tissue death in patients with autoimmune disease. The fluorescent method is sometimes referred to as *FANA.* If this test result is positive (a value higher than 1:40), various subtypes of this antibody are identified and measured.

An elevated *erythrocyte sedimentation rate (ESR),* or "sed rate," (greater than 20 mm/hr) can confirm ***inflammation*** or infection anywhere in the body. An elevated ESR helps support a diagnosis of an unspecified inflammatory disease. The test is most useful to monitor the course of a disease, especially for inflammatory autoimmune diseases. In general the more severe the disease gets, the higher the ESR rises; as the disease improves or goes into remission, the ESR level decreases.

The *high-sensitivity C-reactive protein,* or *hsCRP,* is another useful test to measure ***inflammation*** and may be done with or instead of the ESR. As the name implies, it is more sensitive to inflammatory changes than the ESR. It is also very useful for detecting ***infection*** anywhere in the body.

The presence of most chronic diseases usually causes mild-to-moderate anemia, which contributes to the patient's fatigue. Therefore monitor the patient's complete blood count (CBC) for a low hemoglobin, hematocrit, and red blood cell (RBC) count. An increase in white blood cell (WBC) count is consistent with an inflammatory response. A decrease in the WBC count may indicate Felty syndrome, a pulmonary complication associated with late RA. Thrombocytosis (increased platelets) can also occur in patients with late RA. Additional laboratory tests may be performed, depending on the body systems and organs that may be affected by the disease. For example, if heart involvement is suspected, the primary health care provider may request cardiac enzyme testing.

Other Diagnostic Assessment. A standard x-ray is used to visualize the joint changes and deformities typical of RA. A CT scan may help determine the presence and degree of cervical spine involvement.

An arthrocentesis is an invasive diagnostic procedure that may be used for patients with joint swelling caused by excess synovial fluid (effusion). It may be performed at the bedside or in a health care provider's office or clinic. After administering a local anesthetic, the provider inserts a large-gauge needle into the joint (usually the knee) to aspirate a sample of synovial fluid and to relieve pressure caused by excess fluid. The fluid is analyzed for inflammatory cells and immune complexes, including RF. Fluid from patients with RA typically reveals increased WBCs, cloudiness, and volume.

Teach the patient to use ice and rest the affected joint for 24 hours after arthrocentesis. Often the primary health care provider will recommend acetaminophen as needed for discomfort. If increased pain or swelling occurs, teach the patient or family to notify the primary health care provider immediately.

! NURSING SAFETY PRIORITY (QSEN)

Action Alert

After an arthrocentesis, monitor the insertion site for bleeding or leakage of synovial fluid. Notify the primary health care provider if either of these problems occurs.

A bone scan or joint scan can also assess the extent of joint involvement. MRI may be performed to assess spinal column disease or other joint involvement.

Because RA can affect multiple body systems, tests to diagnose specific systemic manifestations are performed as needed. For example, nerve conduction studies help confirm peripheral neuropathy. Pulmonary function tests help determine the presence of lung involvement.

NCLEX EXAMINATION CHALLENGE 46.4

Physiological Integrity

Which assessment findings will the nurse expect for the client with **early-stage** rheumatoid arthritis? **Select all that apply.**

A. Joint inflammation
B. Subcutaneous nodules
C. Severe weight loss
D. Fatigue
E. Thrombocytosis
F. Anorexia

◆ **Analysis: Analyze Cues and Prioritize Hypotheses.** The priority collaborative problems for patients with rheumatoid arthritis (RA) include:

1. Chronic ***inflammation*** and persistent ***pain*** due to systemic autoimmune disease process
2. Potential for decreased ***mobility*** due to joint deformity, muscle atrophy, and fatigue
3. Potential for decreased self-esteem image due to joint deformity

◆ **Planning and Implementation: Generate Solutions and Take Action.** Patients who have RA are managed in the community under the supervision of a qualified primary health care provider. The expected outcome for management is that the disease goes into remission and its progression slows to decrease ***pain,*** prevent joint destruction, and increase ***mobility.*** When patients with RA are admitted to the inpatient acute care or long-term care facility, it is usually for health problems other than for complications of arthritis. Whether the patient is in a facility or community, be sure to plan interventions to manage his or her persistent ***pain*** and ***inflammation***, as well as the potential for decreased ***mobility*** and decreased self-esteem.

Managing Chronic Inflammation and Pain

Planning: Expected Outcomes. The patient with RA is expected to have a ***pain*** level that is acceptable to the patient (e.g., at a 3 on a pain intensity scale of 0 to 10). A major focus of pain management is drug therapy to modify or prevent the progression of the disease, thereby decreasing joint and systemic ***inflammation.***

Interventions. As in other types of arthritis, the interprofessional health care team manages ***pain*** by using a combination of pharmacologic and nonpharmacologic measures. A synovectomy to remove inflamed synovium may be needed for joints such as the knee or elbow. Total joint arthroplasty (TJA) may be indicated when other measures fail to relieve pain. TJA is discussed in the Osteoarthritis section of this chapter.

Drug Therapy. Some drugs prescribed for RA have anti-inflammatory and/or analgesic actions. For example, NSAIDs are sometimes used for RA to help and decrease pain and inflammation. The choice of which one to prescribe depends on the patient's needs and tolerance and the scientific evidence supporting the drug therapy. To decrease GI problems, the NSAID may be given with an H2-blocking agent such as famotidine. If there is no clinical change after 6 to 8 weeks, the primary health care provider may discontinue the current NSAID and try another one or change to a different drug class.

It was once thought that celecoxib, a COX-2 inhibiting NSAID, should be given rather than the older NSAIDs such as ibuprofen. However, all COX-2 inhibiting drugs have recently been associated with cardiovascular disease such as myocardial infarction, and some have been taken off the market. The risk for GI bleeding is also high in patients taking celecoxib, and the drug cannot be given to those who have had recent open-heart surgery.

Other drugs affect ***immunity*** through immunosuppression, thus modifying the progress of the disease. As a result, these drugs may cause remission of the illness and prevent erosive joint changes. *Biological response modifiers* make up the newest class of disease-modifying drugs that help reduce signals for the immune system to cause ***inflammation.*** Patients with inflammatory diseases other than RA are also using various biological response–modifying drugs successfully. Although

RA is a chronic disease and no cure is yet available, drugs now used can better control the disease and prevent further deterioration. Adjustments in drug therapy are recommended every 3 to 6 months until the expected outcome or disease remission is met.

The primary health care provider, often a rheumatologist, makes decisions about appropriate drug therapy for patients with rheumatoid disease based on the severity of the disease. Initially most patients are managed with *disease-modifying antirheumatic drugs (DMARDs)*. As the name implies, these drugs are given to slow the progression of the disease. For best results, they should be started early in the disease process.

First-line disease-modifying antirheumatic drugs. Methotrexate (MTX), an immunosuppressive medication, in a low, once-a-week dose is the mainstay of therapy for RA because it is effective and relatively inexpensive. It is a slow-acting drug, taking 4 to 6 weeks to begin to control joint ***inflammation*** (Burchum & Rosenthal, 2019). Observe for desired therapeutic drug effects such as a decrease in joint ***pain*** and swelling.

Monitor patients for potential adverse effects such as decreasing WBCs and platelets (as a result of bone marrow suppression) or elevations in liver enzymes or serum creatinine.

! NURSING SAFETY PRIORITY QSEN

Drug Alert

Patients taking MTX are at risk for *infection* caused by impaired or decreased drug-induced ***immunity.*** Teach them to avoid crowds and people who are ill. Remind patients to avoid alcoholic beverages while taking MTX to prevent liver toxicity. Teach them to observe and report other side and toxic effects, which include mouth sores and acute dyspnea from pneumonitis. Although not commonly occurring, lymph node tumor (lymphoma) and pneumonitis (lung ***inflammation***) have been associated in those who have RA and are taking MTX. Folic acid, one of the B vitamins, is often given to those who are taking MTX to help decrease some of the drug's side effects.

Pregnancy is not recommended while taking methotrexate because birth defects are possible. *Strict birth control is recommended for childbearing women who are in need of MTX to control their RA.* If pregnancy is ever desired, instruct the patient to consult the rheumatologist and an obstetric/gynecologic (OB/GYN) health care provider. Generally the primary health care provider will discontinue the drug at least 3 months before planned pregnancy. MTX may be restarted after birth if the patient does not breast-feed (Burchum & Rosenthal, 2019).

Leflunomide may be prescribed for some patients. It is a slow-acting immune-modulating drug that helps diminish inflammatory symptoms of joint swelling and stiffness and improves ***mobility.*** The drug is generally prescribed as a loading dose for 3 days followed by a lower dose daily thereafter. Inform the patient that leflunomide takes 4 to 6 weeks and sometimes up to 3 months before maximum benefit is realized.

! NURSING SAFETY PRIORITY QSEN

Drug Alert

Leflunomide is a potent drug that is generally tolerated, but side effects of hair loss, diarrhea, decreased WBCs and platelets, or increased liver enzymes have been reported.

Teach patients to report these changes and monitor laboratory results carefully. Remind them to avoid alcohol. Inform them that leflunomide can cause birth defects; therefore recommend strict birth control to women of childbearing age. Tell patients to contact their primary health care provider immediately if pregnancy occurs while taking the drug.

Another DMARD sometimes used for RA is hydroxychloroquine. This drug slows the progression of mild rheumatoid disease before it worsens. It is an antimalarial drug that helps suppress the immune response to decrease joint and muscle ***pain.*** Patients generally tolerate hydroxychloroquine quite well. In a few cases mild stomach discomfort, light-headedness, or headache has been reported. The drug should not be used for patients who have known cardiac disease or dysrhythmias (Burchum & Rosenthal, 2019).

! NURSING SAFETY PRIORITY QSEN

Drug Alert

The most serious adverse effect of hydroxychloroquine is retinal damage. Teach patients to report blurred vision or headache. Remind them to have an eye examination before taking the drug and every 6 months to detect changes in the cornea, lens, or retina. If this rare complication occurs, the primary health care provider discontinues the drug (Burchum & Rosenthal, 2019).

Biological response modifiers. As a group, *biological response modifiers (BRMs)*, sometimes called biologics, are one of the newest classes of DMARDs. Most BRMs neutralize the biologic activity of tumor necrosis factor–alpha (TNFA) by inhibiting its binding with TNF receptors. Any one of the BRMs may be tried. If one drug is not effective, the primary health care provider prescribes another drug in the same class. All these drugs are extremely expensive, and insurance companies may not completely pay for their use.

Teach patients receiving any one of the BRMs that they are at a high risk for developing impaired ***immunity*** and subsequent ***infection.*** Instruct them to stay away from people with infections and to avoid large crowds if possible. Remind patients with multiple sclerosis (MS), tuberculosis (TB), or a positive TB test that they should not receive TNF inhibitors because they make patients susceptible to flare-ups of these diseases. Determine whether the patient has had a recent negative purified protein derivative (PPD) test for TB. If not, a PPD skin test is typically administered and the selected BRM is not started until a negative test result is confirmed (Burchum & Rosenthal, 2019). Collaborate with the primary health care provider to ensure that this process is complete. The Common Examples of Drug Therapy: Biological Response Modifiers Used for Rheumatoid Arthritis and Other Chronic Autoimmune Diseases box provides specific examples of BRMs and associated nursing implications. Most of these drugs are given parenterally and require health teaching for self-administration.

COMMON EXAMPLES OF DRUG THERAPY

Biological Response Modifiers Used for Rheumatoid Arthritis and Other Chronic Autoimmune Diseases

Common Drugs	Purpose of Drug/Drug Classification	Nursing Implications
For *all* biological response modifiers (BRMs) (also called *biologics*)	Neutralize biologic activity of tumor necrosis factor–alpha (TNFA), interleukins (IL), T-lymphocytes, or tyrosine kinase (TK) to decrease immune response and inflammation	Do not give BRMs if patient has a serious ***infection,*** TB, or MS *because they may exacerbate these health problems.* Teach patients taking BRMs to avoid getting live vaccines. Teach patient to avoid crowds and people with infections *because serious infections, especially respiratory infections, can lead to hospitalization or cause death.*
Etanercept	TNFA inhibitor	Teach patient to report site reaction, *which may indicate a local allergic response and cause pain.* Teach patient how to self-administer drug.
Infliximab	TNFA inhibitor	Refrigerate all BRMs, except infliximab, *to prevent drug decomposition.* Teach patient to report chest pain or difficulty breathing during infusion, *which could indicate a severe allergic response;* monitor blood pressure and infusion site.
Adalimumab	TNFA inhibitor	Teach patient to report site reaction, *which may indicate local allergic response.*
Anakinra	IL-1 receptor antagonist	Teach patient to monitor site for reaction (occurs more commonly when compared with other BRMs). Monitor WBC count *because the drug can cause a severe decrease in WBC count and make the patient very susceptible to infection.* Teach the patient to report respiratory symptoms, such as cough and fever. Teach him or her that malignancies can result from taking this drug.
Abatacept	Selective T-lymphocyte co-stimulator modulator (T-cell inhibitor)	Report cough, dizziness, and sore throat; do not receive live vaccines while taking the drug. Monitor for dyspnea, wheezing, flushing, itching, *which may indicate a mild-to-moderate allergic reaction.*
Rituximab	Monoclonal antibody	Observe for infusion reaction as for etanercept. *Drug has a* ***black box warning*** *about serious infections from opportunistic pathogens that can lead to hospitalizations or death.*
Golimumab	TNFA inhibitor	Teach patient to report signs and symptoms of ***infection,*** including fever and malaise; teach patient to avoid live vaccines while taking drug. Teach patient about adverse drug effects, including hypertension, GI distress, and ***infection*** from opportunistic pathogens; report signs and symptoms of these problems to the primary health care provider.
Tocilizumab	IL-6 inhibitor	Teach patient the importance of having frequent WBC, platelet, and liver enzyme testing. *This drug can cause decreased WBCs and platelets and liver dysfunction.*

MS, Multiple sclerosis; *TB,* tuberculosis; *TNF,* tumor necrosis factor; *WBC,* white blood cell.

Other drugs. A few drugs may be given in combination with or instead of the previously described drugs. It is not unusual for a patient to be taking several disease-modifying drugs such as methotrexate, a BRM, and an adjunct medication. Each drug works differently to relieve symptoms and slow the progression of the disease. For example, sulfasalazine, a sulfa drug, may be given in combination with other drugs to reduce inflammation and pain. Be aware that this drug should not be used for patients who have a sulfa allergy. Common side effects of sulfasalazine include nausea, vomiting, and skin rash (Burchum & Rosenthal, 2019).

Glucocorticoids (steroids)—usually prednisone—may be given for their fast-acting anti-inflammatory and immunosuppressive effects. Prednisone may be given in high dose for short duration (pulse therapy) or as a low chronic dose. Moderate-dose short-term tapering bridge therapy may be used when inflammation is symptomatic and other RA medications are insufficient or have not yet had an effect.

Chronic steroid therapy can result in numerous complications such as:

- Diabetes mellitus
- Impaired or decreased ***immunity***

- Fluid and electrolyte imbalances
- Hypertension
- Osteoporosis
- Glaucoma

Some drug effects are dose related, whereas others are not. Observe the patient for complications associated with chronic steroid therapy and report them to the primary health care provider. For example, if blood pressure becomes elevated or significant laboratory values change, notify the primary health care provider.

Patients with RA may experience one or a few joints that have more ***pain*** and ***inflammation*** than the others. Cortisone injections in single joints may be used to temporarily relieve local ***pain*** and ***inflammation***. Have the patient ice and rest the joint for 24 hours after the procedure. Oral analgesics are also sometimes needed during that time.

Nonpharmacologic Interventions. Adequate rest, proper positioning, and ice and heat applications are important in pain management. If acute inflammation is present, ice packs may be applied to "hot" joints for pain relief until the inflammation lessens. The ice pack should not be too heavy. At home the patient can use a small bag of frozen peas or corn as an ice pack.

Heated paraffin (wax) dips may help increase comfort of arthritic hands. Finger and hand exercises are often done more easily after paraffin treatment. To relieve morning stiffness or the pain of late-stage disease, recommend a hot shower rather than a sponge bath or a tub bath. It is often difficult for the patient with RA to get into and out of a bathtub, although special hydraulic lifts, tub chairs, and walk-in bathtubs are available to allow him or her to bathe. Safety (grab) bars and nonskid tread in the tub or shower floor are important safety features to discuss with all patients. Some older adults prefer using shower chairs and a walk-in shower that does not have a ledge that could cause falls.

Hot packs applied directly to involved joints may be beneficial. Most physical therapy departments have machines that keep hot packs ready anytime they are needed. Teach patients to use the microwave or stovetop heating instructions to warm heat packs at home. Remind them to follow the instructions given with each heating device used.

Plasmapheresis (sometimes called *plasma exchange*) is an in-hospital procedure prescribed by a primary health care provider in which the patient's plasma is treated to remove the antibodies causing the disease. Although not commonly done, this procedure may be combined with steroid pulse therapy for patients with severe, life-threatening disease.

Complementary and Integrative Health. Some patients may have ***pain*** relief from hypnosis, acupuncture, imagery, music therapy, or other techniques. Stress management is also popular as a pain relief intervention. Chapter 5 discusses these therapies in more detail.

Adequate nutrition is an important part of the management of RA. Obesity should be avoided or treated if present. The inflammatory state may place a greater burden on the metabolism of some essential nutrients. This catabolic state may be related to increased cytokine production, specifically tumor necrosis factor.

According to the Arthritis Foundation (2019), no one food causes or cures RA; however, healthy nutrition in general is important. Refer the patient to the Arthritis Foundation's publications regarding diet and arthritis. Refer him or her to the registered dietitian nutritionist for vitamin- and nutrition-specific questions or recommendations. Teach patients to take any herbal or nutrition supplement under the supervision of a qualified health care provider to prevent adverse events and drug-food or drug-drug interactions.

Other integrative therapies are safe and have been scientifically proven to be effective to help control RA ***pain*** for most people. Examples include mind-body therapies such as relaxation techniques, imagery, and spiritual practices. For information about these techniques, see Chapter 5.

Promoting Mobility

Planning: Expected Outcomes. Patients with RA often have decreased ***mobility*** related to multiple joint deformities and muscle atrophy. Fatigue and generalized weakness also contribute to decreased mobility. The expected outcome is that the patient will be able to independently perform ADLs with or without ambulatory and assistive devices.

Interventions. Although the physical appearance of a patient with severe RA may create the image that ADL independence is not possible, a number of alternative and creative methods can be used to perform these activities. *Do not perform these activities for the patient unless asked. Those with RA do not want to be dependent.* For example, hand deformities often prevent a patient from opening packages of food such as a box of crackers; however, he or she may prefer to use the teeth to open the crackers rather than depend on someone else.

In the hospital or long-term care facility, a patient may not eat because of the barriers of heavy plate covers, milk cartons, small packages of condiments, and heavy containers. Styrofoam or paper cups may bend and collapse as he or she attempts to hold them. A china or heavy plastic cup with handles may be easier to manipulate. Collaborate with the registered dietitian nutritionist to help with access to food and total independence in eating.

When fine-motor activities (e.g., squeezing a tube of toothpaste) become impossible, larger joints or body surfaces can substitute for smaller ones. For example, teach how to use the palm of the hand to press the paste onto the brush. Devices such as long-handled brushes can help patients brush their hair; dressing sticks can assist with putting on pants. These examples illustrate the need to assess the problem area, suggest alternative methods, and refer the patient to an OT or PT for special assistive and adaptive devices if necessary.

Additional nursing interventions depend in part on identifying the factors contributing to fatigue. For example, persistent ***pain,*** sleep disturbances, and weakness are associated with increased fatigue. Anemia may also be a contributing factor and may be treated with iron (if an iron deficiency anemia is present), folic acid, or vitamin supplements prescribed by the primary health care provider. Chronic normochromic or chronic hypochromic anemia often occurs in most chronic systemic diseases. Assess for drug-related blood loss such as that caused by NSAIDs by checking the stool for gross or occult blood. *Older white women are the most likely to experience GI bleeding as a result of taking these medications* (Burchum & Rosenthal, 2019).

PATIENT AND FAMILY EDUCATION: PREPARING FOR SELF-MANAGEMENT

Energy Conservation for the Patient With Arthritis

- Balance activity with rest. Take one or two naps each day.
- Pace yourself; do not plan too much for one day.
- Set priorities. Determine which activities are most important and do them first.
- Delegate responsibilities and tasks to your family and friends.
- Plan ahead to prevent last-minute rushing and stress.
- Learn your own activity tolerance and do not exceed it.

If fatigue and decreased ***mobility*** result from muscle atrophy, the primary health care provider prescribes an aggressive physical therapy program to strengthen muscles and prevent further atrophy. Patients also experience increased fatigue when ***pain*** prevents them from getting adequate rest and sleep. Measures to facilitate sleep include promoting a quiet environment, giving warm beverages, and administering hypnotics or relaxants as prescribed if necessary.

In addition to identifying and managing specific reasons for fatigue, determine the patient's usual daily activities and teach principles of *energy conservation,* including:

- Pacing activities
- Allowing rest periods
- Setting priorities
- Obtaining assistance when needed

The Patient and Family Education: Preparing for Self-Management: Energy Conservation for the Patient With Arthritis box provides specific suggestions for conserving energy and thus increasing activity tolerance and ***mobility.***

Enhancing Self Esteem

Planning: Expected Outcome. The patient with RA often has multiple joints that are inflamed or deformed, causing a potential for decreased self-esteem. Therefore the expected outcome is that the patient will verbalize a positive perception of self as a result of interprofessional interventions.

Interventions. Body image and self-esteem may be affected by the disease process. Determine the patient's perception of these changes and the impact of the reactions of family and significant others. The most important intervention is communicating acceptance of the patient. When a trusting relationship is established, encourage him or her to express personal feelings.

As a reaction to body changes and joint deformity and the presence of a chronic, painful disease, some patients display behaviors indicative of loss. They may use coping strategies that range from denial or fear to anger or depression. In an attempt to regain control over the effects of the disease process, they may appear to be "manipulative and demanding" and sometimes may be referred to as having an "arthritis personality." *This personality, which represents a negative label, is a myth; avoid using these terms.* Patients are trying to cope with the effects of their illness and should be treated with patience and understanding. Continually assess and accept these behaviors but remain realistic in discussing goals to improve self-esteem and body image. Emphasize their strengths and help them identify

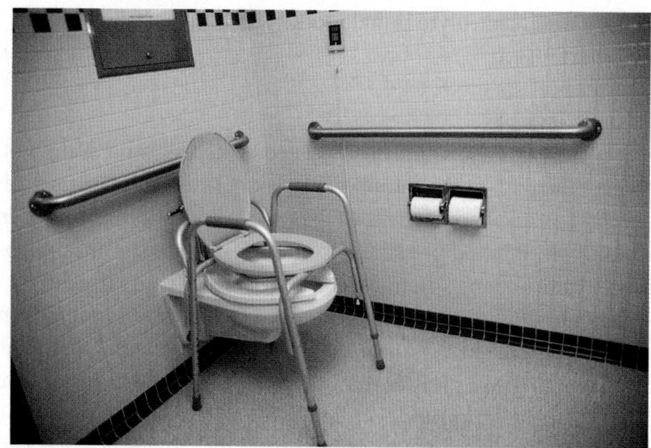

FIG. 46.6 Handrails and an elevated toilet seat make transfers easier for the patient.

previously successful coping strategies. If needed, consult with mental health professionals or religious/spiritual leaders to help patients cope with this potentially debilitating chronic disease.

Care Coordination and Transition Management. Patients with rheumatoid arthritis (RA) are usually managed at home but in a few cases may be institutionalized in a long-term care facility if they become restricted to bed or a wheelchair. Some patients may be transferred to a rehabilitation facility for several weeks to help develop strategies, techniques, and skills for independent living at home. Chapter 7 discusses the rehabilitation process in detail.

Home Care Management. The amount of home care preparation depends on the severity of the disease. Structural changes may be necessary if there are deficits in performing ADLs or ***mobility.*** Doors must be wide enough to accommodate a wheelchair or walker if one is used. Ramps are needed to prevent the patient in a wheelchair from becoming homebound. If the person cannot use stairs, he or she must have access to facilities for all ADLs on one floor. Handrails should be available in the bathroom and halls.

To promote continued homemaking functions, countertops and appliances may require structural changes. The patient may also require handrails and elevated chairs and toilet seats, which facilitate transfers (Fig. 46.6). *These devices are especially important for older adults with arthritis.*

Self-Management Education. Self-management education (SME) is a vital role for nurses in collaborative management of arthritis. Many people have signs and symptoms of joint ***inflammation*** but do not seek medical attention. Teach them to seek professional health care to reduce ***pain*** and prevent disability.

Teach patients to discuss any questions with their primary health care provider before trying any over-the-counter or home remedies. Some remedies may be harmful. Check with the Arthritis Foundation for the latest information on arthritis myths and quackery (www.arthritis.org).

Provide information to the patient and family about drug therapy, joint protection, energy conservation, rest, and exercise as summarized in the boxes presented earlier in the RA section.

Assess the patient's coping strategies. The patient with RA often reports being on an "emotional roller coaster" from coping with a chronic illness every day. Control over one's life is an important human need. The patient with an unpredictable chronic disease may lose this control, and this lowers self-esteem. Health care providers must allow the patient to make decisions about care. Families and significant others must also include him or her in decision making. Although the patient's behavior may be perceived as demanding or manipulative, his or her self-esteem cannot be improved without this important aspect of interpersonal relationships.

Increased dependency also affects a sense of control and self-esteem. Some people ignore their health needs and portray a tough image for others by insisting that they need no assistance. Emphasize to the patient and family that asking for help may be the best decision at times to prevent further joint damage and disease progression.

RA may also affect work and social roles. The patient may have physical difficulty doing tasks that require lifting, climbing, grasp, or gross- or fine-motor activities. The severity of RA disease may cause difficulty with total number of hours worked. Some people with RA can do their jobs well without problem; others may have varying degrees of difficulty. Those who can no longer do their job at work may need to discuss with their employer having a lighter workload, but some may need to file for disability with their company and U.S. Social Security office.

Health Care Resources. The need for health care resources for the patient with RA is similar to that for the patient with osteoarthritis. A home care nurse or aide, physical therapist, or occupational therapist may be needed during severe exacerbations or as the disease progresses. In collaboration with the case manager, identify these resources and make sure that they are available as needed. The Arthritis Foundation is an excellent source of information and support.

Arthritis support groups and self-help courses provide the education and support that patients, families, and friends need. Refer the patient to a psychological counselor or religious or spiritual leader for emotional support and guidance during times of crisis or as needed. Identify and recommend other support systems within the family and community when necessary.

◆ **Evaluation: Evaluate Outcomes.** Evaluate the care of the patient with RA on the basis of the identified priority problems. The expected outcomes are that he or she:

- Achieves ***pain*** control to a pain intensity level of 2 to 3 or less on a scale of 0 to 10 or at a level that is acceptable to the patient
- Moves and functions in his or her own environment independently with or without assistive devices
- Verbalizes increased self-esteem and positive perception of self

CLINICAL JUDGMENT CHALLENGE 46.1

Safety; Teamwork and Collaboration

A 70-year-old woman is admitted to the hospital with suspected streptococcal pneumonia. She continues to have an occasional cough, mild dyspnea, and a fever over 100° F (37.8° C) after a week of treatment with amoxicillin at home. The hospitalist prescribes IV levofloxacin 750 mg daily. The admitting nurse documents the following history and physical assessment data:

- Has a 25-year history of rheumatoid arthritis (RA) and osteoarthritis
- Was diagnosed with diabetes mellitus type 2 last year, which is controlled by diet
- Has a history of atrial fibrillation
- Is retired and lives alone in a senior housing apartment
- Volunteers twice a week in the local library
- Current medications include:
  - Etanercept 50 mg subcutaneously each week (self-administered) for RA
  - Leflunomide 10 mg orally each day for RA
  - Clopidogrel 75 mg orally each day for atrial fibrillation
  - Acetaminophen 500 mg orally as needed twice a day for OA pain
- Has two children who live locally
- Is able to perform ADLs independently, although she has ulnar deviation and finger deformities in both hands
- Uses a cane when not at home
- Drives short distances to the grocery store and bank
- Is alert and oriented
- Reports occasional constipation
- Reports current joint pain level is a 5 on a 0-10 pain scale; most painful joints are her feet and knees (states that her usual pain level is a 1-2 before hospital admission)
- Reports occasional paresthesias in both feet
- Has 1+ nonpitting edema in both feet
- Current oral temperature = 100.8° F (38.2° C)
- Current apical pulse = 82
- Resting respiratory rate = 32 breaths/min
- Current blood pressure = 138/88
- Admitting WBC = 15,500/mm^3

1. **Recognize Cues:** What assessment information in this client situation is the most important and immediate concern for the nurse? (Hint: Identify the **relevant** information *first* to determine what is most important.)
2. **Analyze Cues:** What client conditions are consistent with the **most relevant** information? (Hint: Think about priority collaborative problems that support and contradict the information presented in this situation.)
3. **Prioritize Hypotheses:** Which possibilities or explanations are **most likely** to be present in this client situation? Which possibilities or explanations are the most serious? (Hint: Consider all possibilities and determine their urgency and risk for this client.)
4. **Generate Solutions:** What actions would most likely achieve the desired outcomes for this client? Which actions should be **avoided** or are **potentially harmful**? (Hint: Determine the desired outcomes first to decide which interventions are appropriate and those that should be avoided.)
5. **Take Action:** Which actions are the most appropriate and how should they be implemented? In what **priority order** should they be implemented? (Hint: Consider health teaching, documentation, requested health care provider orders or prescriptions, nursing skills, collaboration with or referral to health team members, etc.)
6. **Evaluate Outcomes:** What client assessment would indicate that the nurse's actions were **effective**? (Hint: Think about signs that would indicate an improvement, decline, or unchanged client condition.)

GET READY FOR THE NEXT-GENERATION NCLEX® EXAMINATION!

Key Points

Review these Key Points for each NCLEX Examination Client Needs Category.

Safe and Effective Care Environment

- Collaborate with the health care team to manage chronic pain and increase ***mobility*** for patients with arthritis. **QSEN: Teamwork and Collaboration**
- Prioritize care for patients having a total joint arthroplasty to prevent complications, such as dislocation, ***infection,*** and venous thromboembolism. **QSEN: Safety**

Health Promotion and Maintenance

- Provide information about community resources for patients with arthritis, especially professional organizations such as the Arthritis Foundation. **QSEN: Patient-Centered Care**
- Teach patients to prevent joint trauma and reduce weight as needed to help prevent osteoarthritis. **QSEN: Evidence-Based Practice**
- Recall that a combination of environmental, genetic, and immune risk factors can cause rheumatoid arthritis (RA). **QSEN: Patient-Centered Care**
- Reinforce the importance of good health practices, such as adequate sleep, proper nutrition, regular exercise, and stress-management techniques for patients with arthritis. **QSEN: Patient-Centered Care**
- Provide patients and their families with discharge instructions to prevent complications and promote ***mobility*** after total hip or knee arthroplasty. **QSEN: Safety, Evidence-Based Practice**
- Teach patients with arthritis about appropriate exercises, joint protection techniques, and energy conservation guidelines. **QSEN: Evidence-Based Practice**

Psychosocial Integrity

- Recognize that patients with rheumatoid arthritis (RA) may have body image disturbance as a result of potentially deforming joint involvement and nodules. **QSEN: Patient-Centered Care**
- Encourage patients with arthritis to discuss their chronic illness and identify coping strategies that have previously been successful. **QSEN: Patient-Centered Care**
- Be aware that chronic, painful diseases affect the patient's quality of life and role performance. **QSEN: Patient-Centered Care**

Physiological Integrity

- Differentiate OA as primarily a joint problem that can affect one or more joints and RA as a systemic disease that presents as a bilateral symmetric joint ***inflammation.*** Both diseases can impact the patient's ***mobility.*** **Clinical Judgment**
- Realize that older patients have OA more than younger patients; younger patients have RA more than older adults. Both diseases cause persistent joint ***pain*** that needs to be managed. **Clinical Judgment**
- Teach patients who have osteoarthritis (OA) or are prone to the disease to lose weight (if obese), avoid trauma, and limit strenuous weight-bearing activities. **QSEN: Evidence-Based Practice**
- Instruct patients with arthritic pain to use multiple modalities for ***pain*** relief, including ice/heat, rest, positioning, integrative therapies, and drug therapy as prescribed. **QSEN: Evidence-Based Practice**
- Teach patients to monitor and report side and adverse effects of drugs used to treat OA and RA. **QSEN: Safety**
- Teach patients who are taking hydroxychloroquine to have frequent (every 6 months) eye examinations to monitor for retinal changes. **QSEN: Safety**
- Remind patients to avoid crowds and other possible sources of infection when they are taking drugs that decrease ***immunity.*** **QSEN: Safety**
- Implement interventions for patients having total joint arthroplasty (TJA) to prevent venous thromboembolism (e.g., anticoagulants, exercises, sequential compression devices); observe the patient for bleeding when he or she is taking anticoagulants. **Clinical Judgment**
- Be careful when positioning a patient after a total hip arthroplasty (THA) to prevent dislocation; do not hyperflex the hips or adduct the legs, especially for patients who had a posterolateral surgical approach. **QSEN: Safety**
- Recognize the surgical site for a TKA is typically very swollen and discolored for several weeks after surgery; teach the patient to use cold applications to reduce swelling. **QSEN: Patient-Centered Care**
- Be aware that disease-modifying antirheumatic drugs (DMARDs) and biological response modifiers (BRMs) slow the progression of autoimmune diseases such as RA. **QSEN: Evidence-Based Practice**
- Teach patients receiving BRMs and other disease-modifying agents to avoid crowds and people with infections; opportunistic pathogens may cause serious infections or death. Check the patient's PPD test or history of tuberculosis before starting any of these drugs. **QSEN: Safety**

MASTERY QUESTIONS

1. The nurse is caring for a client with severe osteoarthritis. What will the nurse anticipate as the client's **priority** problem?
   A. Joint pain
   B. ADL dependence
   C. Risk for falls
   D. Muscle stiffness

2. The nurse is caring for a client who had an anterior total hip arthroplasty yesterday. For which **commonly occurring** postoperative complication will the nurse monitor for this client?
   A. Pneumonia
   B. Paralytic ileus
   C. Wound dehiscence
   D. Venous thromboembolism

3. The nurse is assessing a client who has **late-stage** rheumatoid arthritis. Which assessment findings would the nurse expect for this client? **Select all that apply.**
   A. Joint inflammation
   B. Severe weight loss
   C. Bony nodules
   D. Joint deformities
   E. Sjögren syndrome

REFERENCES

Asterisk (*) indicates a classic or definitive work on this subject.

Arthritis Foundation. (2019). *Arthritis by the numbers: Book of trusted facts and figures*. Atlanta, GA: Arthritis Foundation.

Bodden, J., & Coppola, C. (2018). *Best practice guideline: Total hip replacement (arthroplasty)*. Chicago, IL: SmithBucklin (for the National Association of Orthopaedic Nursing).

Burchum, J. L. R., & Rosenthal, L. D. (2019). *Lehne's pharmacology for nursing care* (9th ed.). St. Louis: Elsevier.

Causey-Upton, R., Howell, D. M., Kitzman, P. H., Custer, M. G., & Dressler, E. V. (2019). Factors influencing discharge readiness after total knee replacement. *Orthopaedic Nursing, 38*(1), 6–14.

Cheuy, V. A., Foran, J. R. H., Paxton, R. J., Bade, M. J., Zeni, J. A., & Stevens-Lapsley, J. E. (2017). Arthrofibrosis associated with total knee arthroplasty. *The Journal of Arthroplasty, 32*, 2604–2611.

Chicoski, A. S. (2018). Caring for the orthopaedic patient with a history of bariatric surgery. *Orthopaedic Nursing, 37*(2), 106–112.

Gallagher, L. M., Gardner, V., Bates, D., Mason, S., Nemecek, J., DiFiore, D. B., et al. (2018). Impact of music therapy on hospitalized patients post-elective orthopaedic surgery: A randomized controlled trial. *Orthopaedic Nursing, 37*(2), 124–135.

Goode, V. M., Morgan, B., Muckler, V. C., Cary, M. P., Jr., Zbed, C. E., & Zychowicz, M. (2019). Multimodal pain management for major joint replacement surgery. *Orthopaedic Nursing, 38*(2), 150–156.

Gourdine, J. (2019). Review of nonsurgical treatment guidelines for lower extremity osteoarthritis. *Orthopaedic Nursing, 38*(5), 303–308.

Hohler, S. E. (2018). Walk patients through total hip arthroplasty. *Nursing, 48*(9), 24–31.

Jackman, C. (2019). Perioperative pain management for the chronic pain patient with long-term opioid use. *Orthopaedic Nursing, 38*(2), 159–163.

Jones, L., & Taylor, T. (2019). Identifying acute delirium on acute care units. *Medsurg Nursing, 28*, 172–175 181.

*McAlindon, T. E., Bannuru, R. R., Sullivan, M. C., Arden, N. K., Berenbaum, F., Bierma-Zeinstra, S. M., et al. (2014). OARSI guidelines for the non-surgical management of knee osteoarthritis. *Osteoarthritis and Cartilage, 22*, 363–388.

McCance, K., Huether, S., Brashers, V., & Rote, N. (2019). *Pathophysiology: The biologic basis for disease in adults and children* (8th ed.). St. Louis: Mosby.

McCann-Spry, L., Pelton, J., Grandy, G., & Newell, D. (2016). An interdisciplinary approach to reducing length of stay in joint replacement patients. *Orthopaedic Nursing, 35*(5), 279–300.

Mogoi, V., Elder, B., Hayes, K., & Huhman, D. (2019). Effectiveness of platelet-rich plasma in management of knee osteoarthritis in a rural clinic. *Orthopaedic Nursing, 38*(3), 193–198.

Mori, C., & Ribsam, V. (2018). *Best practice guideline: Total knee replacement (arthroplasty)*. SmithBucklin (for the National Association of Orthopaedic Nursing).

Morland, R. (2019). Evolution of the national opioid crisis. *Nursing2019, 39*(5), 51–56.

O'Brien, M., & McDougall, J. J. (2018). Cannabis and joints: Scientific evidence for the alleviation of osteoarthritis pain. *Current Opinion in Pharmacology, 40*, 104–109.

Pietsch, T., David, J., & Vergara, F. (2018). Integrative review for patients with bilateral total knee replacement: A call for nursing practice guidelines. *Orthopaedic Nursing, 37*(4), 237–243.

Pizzi, L. J., Bates, M., Chelly, J. E., & Goodrich, C. J. (2020). A prospective randomized trial of an oral patient-controlled analgesia deice versus usual care following total hip arthroplasty. *Orthopaedic Nursing, 39*(1), 37–46.

Saccomano, S. J. (2018). Osteoarthritis treatment: Decreasing pain, increasing mobility. *The Nurse Practitioner, 43*(9), 49–55.

Sasse, L., Laessig-Stary, B., & Abitz, T. (2020). Periarticular ketorolac improves outcomes for patients with joint replacements. *Orthopaedic Nursing, 39*(1), 47–50.

Schinsky, M. F., McCune, C., & Bonomi, J. (2016). Multifaceted comparison of two cryotherapy devices used after total knee arthroplasty: Cryotherapy device comparison. *Orthopaedic Nursing, 35*(5), 317–324.

Tubog, T. D. (2019). Combined intermittent pneumatic leg compression and pharmacological prophylaxis for prevention of venous thromboembolism. *Orthopaedic Nursing, 38*(4), 270–272.

Wilson, K., Devito, D., Zavotsky, K. E., Rusay, M., Allen, M., & Huang, S. (2018). Keep it moving and remember to P.A.C. (Pharmacology, Ambulation, and Compression) for venous thromboembolism prevention. *Orthopeadic Nursing, 37*(6), 339–345.

*Zhang, W. W., Nuki, G., Moskowitz, R., Abramson, S., Altman, R. D., Arden, N. K., et al. (2010). OARSI recommendations for the management of hip and knee osteoarthritis, Part III: Changes in evidence following systematic cumulative update of research published through January 2009. *Osteoarthritis and Cartilage, 18*(4), 476–499.

Zhao, L., Kaye, A. D., & Abd-Elsayed, A. (2018). Stem cells for the treatment of knee osteoarthritis: A comprehensive review. *Pain Physician, 21*(3), 229–242.

47

Concepts of Care for Patients With Musculoskeletal Trauma

Donna D. Ignatavicius

http://evolve.elsevier.com/Iggy/

LEARNING OUTCOMES

1. Collaborate with the interprofessional team to manage quality care for patients with impaired ***mobility*** caused by caused by musculoskeletal trauma, including fractures and amputation.
2. Identify community resources for families and patients recovering from musculoskeletal trauma.
3. Apply knowledge of pathophysiology of fracture and amputation to identify common assessment findings, including actual or risk for impaired ***sensory perception***, ***tissue integrity***, and ***perfusion.***
4. Prioritize evidence-based nursing interventions for patients with musculoskeletal trauma to promote ***mobility,*** maintain ***perfusion,*** manage ***pain,*** and protect ***tissue integrity.***
5. Plan transition management and care coordination for patients with fractures and amputations, including health teaching about complications such as ***infection*** and altered ***sensory perception.***

KEY TERMS

acute compartment syndrome (ACS) A serious but uncommon limb-threatening condition in which increased pressure within one or more compartments (that contain muscle, blood vessels, and nerves) reduces circulation to the lower leg or forearm.

amputation The removal of a part of the body.

ankle-brachial index A measure of blood flow in the lower extremities. It is calculated by dividing ankle systolic pressure by brachial systolic pressure. A normal ABI is 0.9 or higher.

avascular necrosis (also known as *osteonecrosis*) The death of bone tissue.

bone reduction Realignment of the bone ends for proper healing that is accomplished by a *closed* (nonsurgical) method or an *open* (surgical) procedure.

cast A rigid device (synthetic, or less commonly, plaster) that immobilizes the affected body part while allowing other body parts to move.

closed (simple) fracture A fracture that does not extend through the skin (no visible wound).

complex regional pain syndrome (CRPS) A poorly understood dysfunction of the central and peripheral nervous systems that leads to severe, persistent ***pain.***

ergonomics The study of how equipment and furniture can be arranged so that people can do work or other activities more efficiently and comfortably without injury.

external fixation A surgical procedure in which pins or wires are inserted through the skin and affected bone and then connected to a rigid external frame outside the body to immobilize the fracture during healing.

fascia iliaca compartment block (FICB) A regional anesthetic technique to manage pain for patients who have a fractured hip. The anesthetic agent (such as levobupivacaine) blocks the femoral, lateral cutaneous, and obturator nerves while avoiding the risk of injury to the femoral artery and vein.

fasciotomy A procedure for acute compartment syndrome in which the surgeon cuts through fascia to relieve pressure and tension on vital blood vessels and nerves.

fat embolism syndrome (FES) A serious but uncommon complication of fractures in which fat globules are released from the yellow bone marrow into the bloodstream within 12 to 48 hours after injury. These globules clog small blood vessels that supply vital organs, most commonly the lungs, and impair organ *perfusion.*

fracture A break or disruption in the continuity of a bone that often affects *mobility* and causes *pain.*

fragility fracture A fracture caused by osteoporosis or other disease that weakens bone.

internal fixation A surgical procedure in which metal pins, screws, rods, plates, or prostheses are inserted inside the body to immobilize a fracture during healing.

neuroma A sensitive tumor consisting of damaged nerve cells that forms most often in patients with amputations of the upper extremity but can occur anywhere.

open (compound) fracture A fracture that extends through the skin, causing a visible wound.

opioid-induced constipation (OIC) Constipation that can result from taking opioids for a long period of time.

phantom limb pain (PLP) A persistent altered *sensory perception* in the amputated body part that is unpleasant or painful.

repetitive stress injury (RSI) A fast-growing occupational injury, which occurs in people whose jobs require repetitive hand activities, such as pinching or grasping during wrist flexion; carpal tunnel syndrome (CTS) is the most common RSI.

subcutaneous emphysema The appearance of bubbles under the skin because of air trapping.

traction The application of a pulling force to a part of the body to provide bone alignment or relief of muscle spasm.

PRIORITY AND INTERRELATED CONCEPTS

The priority concepts for this chapter are:

- ***Mobility***
- ***Perfusion***

The ***Mobility*** concept exemplar for this chapter is Fracture.
The ***Perfusion*** concept exemplar for this chapter is Amputation.

The interrelated concepts for this chapter are:

- ***Pain***
- ***Tissue Integrity***
- ***Sensory Perception***
- ***Infection***

Musculoskeletal trauma accounts for about two thirds of all injuries and is one of the primary causes of disability in the United States. It includes health problems that range from simple muscle strain to multiple bone fractures with severe soft-tissue damage. This chapter focuses on the most common types of musculoskeletal trauma.

Fractures and other musculoskeletal trauma impair a patient's ***mobility*** in varying degrees, depending on the severity and extent of the injury. These injuries can also result in severe ***pain,*** altered ***sensory perception,*** and ***infection.*** Amputations result in impaired ***tissue integrity*** and are often performed because of inadequate arterial ***perfusion*** caused by chronic disease. These health concepts are reviewed in Chapter 3 of this text. In some cases, bleeding from traumatic injuries can lead to hemorrhage and hypovolemic shock, described elsewhere in this text.

MOBILITY CONCEPT EXEMPLAR: FRACTURE

Pathophysiology Review

A **fracture** is a break or disruption in the continuity of a bone that often affects ***mobility*** and causes ***pain***. It can occur anywhere in the body and at any age. All fractures have the same basic pathophysiologic mechanism and require similar patient-centered, interprofessional collaborative care, regardless of fracture type or location.

Classification of Fractures. A fracture can be classified by the extent of the break:

- *Complete fracture.* The break is across the entire width of the bone in such a way that the bone is divided into two distinct sections. If bone alignment is altered or disrupted, the fracture is also referred to as a *displaced* fracture. The ends of bone sections of a displaced fracture are more likely to damage surrounding nerves, blood vessels, and other soft tissues.

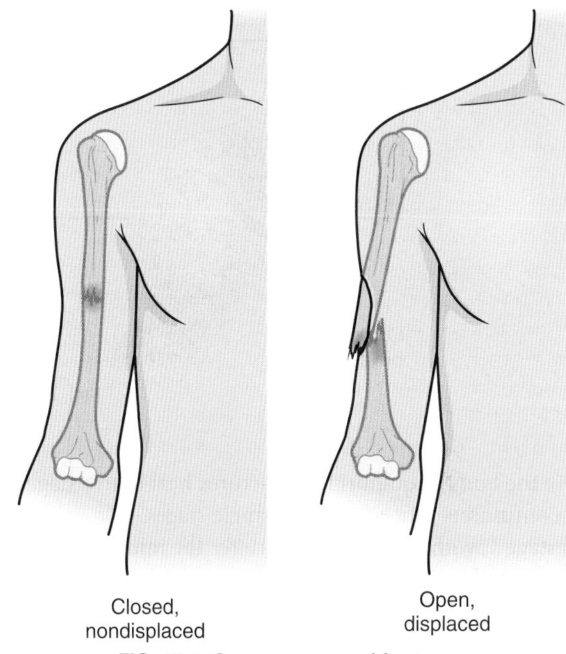

FIG. 47.1 Common types of fractures.

- *Incomplete fracture.* The fracture does not divide the bone into two portions because the break is through only part of the bone. This type of fracture is not typically displaced.

A fracture can also be described by the extent of associated soft-tissue damage: **open** (or **compound**) or **closed** (or **simple**) (Fig. 47.1). The skin surface over the broken bone is disrupted in a *compound* fracture, which causes an external wound. These fractures are often graded to define the extent of tissue damage. A *simple* fracture does not extend through the skin and therefore has no visible wound.

In addition to being identified by type, fractures are described by their cause. A *fragility fracture* (also known as a *pathologic* or *spontaneous fracture*) occurs after minimal trauma to a bone that has been weakened by disease. For example, a patient with bone cancer or osteoporosis can easily have a fragility fracture (see Chapter 45 for a discussion of these disorders). A *fatigue (stress) fracture* results from excessive strain and stress on the bone. This problem is commonly seen in recreational and professional athletes. *Compression fractures* are produced by a loading force applied to the long axis of cancellous bone. They commonly occur in the vertebrae of older patients with osteoporosis and are extremely painful.

Stages of Bone Healing. When a bone is fractured, the body immediately begins the healing process to repair the injury and

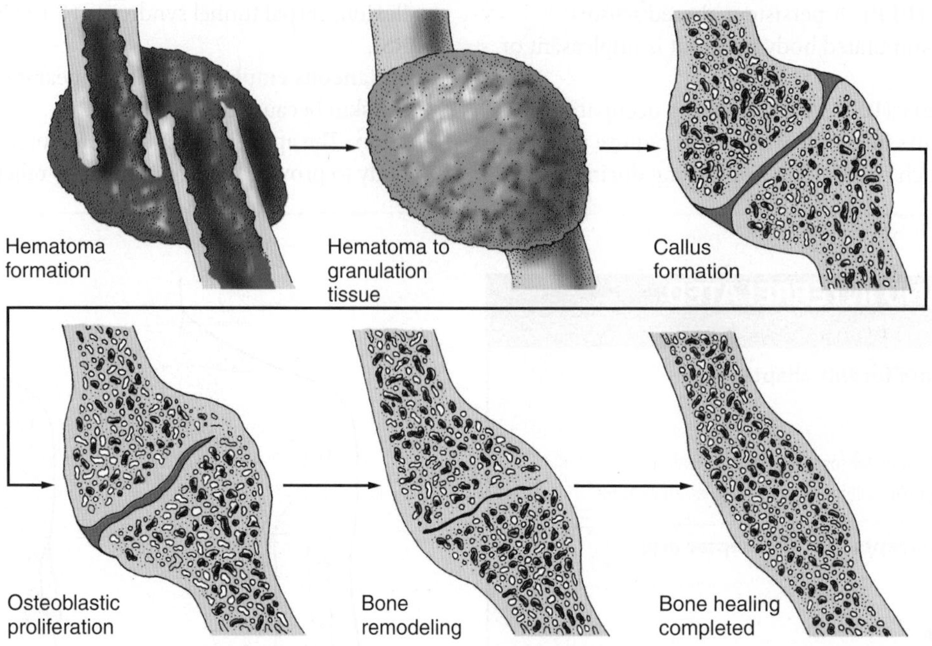

FIG. 47.2 Stages of bone healing.

restore the body's equilibrium. Fractures heal in five stages that are a continuous process and not single stages.

- In stage 1, within 24 to 72 hours after the injury, a hematoma forms at the site of the fracture because bone is extremely vascular.
- Stage 2 occurs in 3 days to 2 weeks when granulation tissue begins to invade the hematoma. This then prompts the formation of fibrocartilage, providing the foundation for bone healing.
- Stage 3 of bone healing occurs as a result of vascular and cellular proliferation. The fracture site is surrounded by new vascular tissue known as a *callus* (within 3 to 6 weeks). *Callus* formation is the beginning of a nonbony union.
- As healing continues in stage 4, the callus is gradually resorbed and transformed into bone. This stage usually takes 3 to 8 weeks.
- During the fifth and final stage of healing, consolidation and remodeling of bone continue to meet mechanical demands. This process may start as early as 4 to 6 weeks after fracture and can continue for up to 1 year, depending on the severity of the injury and the age and health of the patient. Fig. 47.2 summarizes the stages of bone healing.

In young, healthy adult bone, healing takes about 4 to 6 weeks. In the older person who has reduced bone mass, healing time is lengthened. Complete healing may take 3 months or longer in people who are older than 70 years. Other factors, such as the severity of the trauma, the type of bone injured, how the fracture is managed, and/or the presence of infection or avascular necrosis (AVN), also called *osteonecrosis,* can also impact healing.

Complications of Fractures. Regardless of the type or location of the fracture, several limb- and life-threatening acute and chronic complications can result from the injury. Signs and symptoms of beginning complications must be treated early to prevent serious consequences. In some cases, careful monitoring and assessment by the nurse can prevent these complications from occurring or worsening.

PATIENT-CENTERED CARE: OLDER ADULT CONSIDERATIONS QSEN

Bone healing is often affected by the aging process. Bone formation and strength rely on adequate nutrition. Calcium, phosphorus, vitamin D, and protein are necessary for the production of new bone (see Chapter 45). For women, the loss of estrogen after menopause decreases the body's ability to form new bone tissue. Chronic diseases can also affect the rate at which bone heals. For instance, peripheral vascular diseases, such as arteriosclerosis, reduce arterial circulation to bone. Thus the bone receivesfless oxygen and fewer nutrients, both of which are needed for repair.

Acute Complications of Fractures. Common acute complications of fractures include venous thromboembolism (VTE) and bone or soft tissue ***infection***. *Venous thromboembolism (VTE)* includes deep vein thrombosis (DVT) and its major complication, pulmonary embolism (PE). It is the most common complication of lower-extremity surgery or trauma and the most often fatal complication of musculoskeletal surgery. Chapter 33 discusses VTE, including prevention and management, in detail.

Whenever there is trauma to tissues, the body's defense system is disrupted. Wound infections are the most common type of ***infection*** resulting from orthopedic trauma. They range from superficial skin infections to deep wound abscesses. Infection can also be caused by implanted hardware used to repair a fracture surgically, such as screws, pins, plates, or rods. Clostridia infections can result in gas gangrene or tetanus and can prevent the bone from healing properly.

Bone ***infection,*** or osteomyelitis, is most common with open fractures in which ***tissue integrity*** is altered and after surgical repair of a fracture (see Chapter 45 for discussion of osteomyelitis). For patients experiencing this type of trauma, the risk for health care agency–acquired infections is increased. These infections are common, and many result from multidrug-resistant organisms, such as methicillin-resistant *Staphylococcus aureus* (MRSA). Reducing MRSA infection is a primary desired outcome for all health care agencies. Chapter 21 discusses prevention and management of ***infection*** in detail.

Several complications of fractures are more rare but are potentially life-threatening, including acute compartment syndrome and fat embolism syndrome. **Acute compartment syndrome (ACS)** is a serious, limb-threatening condition in which increased pressure within one or more compartments (that contain muscle, blood vessels, and nerves) reduces circulation to the lower leg or forearm.

The pathophysiologic changes of increased compartment pressure are sometimes referred to as the *ischemia-edema cycle.* Capillaries within the muscle dilate, which raises capillary (arterial) and venous pressure. Capillaries become more permeable because of the release of histamine by the ischemic muscle tissue, and venous drainage decreases. As a result, plasma proteins leak into the interstitial fluid space and edema occurs. Edema increases pressure on nerve endings and causes severe pain. The pain experienced is greater than expected for the nature of the injury. ***Perfusion*** to the area is reduced, and further ischemia results. ***Sensory perception*** deficits or paresthesia generally appears before changes in vascular or motor signs. The color of the tissue pales, and pulses begin to weaken but rarely disappear. The affected area is usually palpably tense, and acute severe ***pain*** occurs with passive motion of the extremity. If the condition is not treated, cyanosis, tingling, numbness, paresis, and necrosis can occur. The Key Features: Acute Compartment Syndrome box summarizes the sequence of pathophysiologic events in compartment syndrome and the associated clinical assessment findings.

KEY FEATURES
Acute Compartment Syndrome

Physiologic Change	Clinical Findings
Increased compartment pressure	No change
Increased capillary permeability	Edema
Release of histamine	Increased edema
Increased blood flow to area	Pulses present Pink tissue
Pressure on nerve endings	Acute pain
Increased tissue pressure	Referred pain to compartment(s)
Decreased tissue perfusion	Increased edema
Decreased oxygen to tissues	Pallor
Increased production of lactic acid	Unequal pulses Flexed posture
Anaerobic metabolism	Cyanosis
Vasodilation	Increased edema
Increased blood flow	Tense muscle swelling
Increased tissue pressure	Tingling Numbness
Increased edema	Paresthesia
Muscle ischemia	Severe pain unrelieved by drugs
Tissue necrosis	Paresis/paralysis

The pressure to the compartment can be from an external or internal source, but fracture is present in most cases of ACS. Tight, bulky dressings and casts are examples of *external* pressure causes. Blood or fluid accumulation in the compartment is a common source of *internal* pressure. ACS is not limited to patients with musculoskeletal problems. It can also occur in those with severe burns, extensive insect bites or snakebites, or massive infiltration of IV fluids. In these situations, edema increases internal pressure in one or more compartments. Patients with ACS may need a surgical procedure known as a **fasciotomy**. In this procedure, the surgeon cuts through the fascia to relieve pressure and tension on vital blood vessels and nerves. The wound remains open and requires care to begin to heal from the inside out. The surgeon usually closes the wound with a skin graft in several days. Wound care is described in Chapter 23 and in basic nursing fundamentals textbooks.

Long-term problems resulting from compartment syndrome include ***infection,*** persistent motor weakness in the affected extremity, contracture, and myoglobinuric renal failure. In extreme cases, amputation becomes necessary.

Fat embolism syndrome (FES) is another serious complication of fractures in which fat globules are released from the yellow bone marrow into the bloodstream within 12 to 48 hours after an injury. These globules clog small blood vessels that supply vital organs, most commonly the lungs, and impair organ ***perfusion***. FES usually results from fractures or fracture repair but may also occur, although less often, in patients experiencing pancreatitis, osteomyelitis, blunt trauma, or sickle cell disease.

The earliest signs and symptoms of FES are a low arterial oxygen level (hypoxemia), dyspnea, and tachypnea (increased respirations). Headache, lethargy, agitation, confusion, decreased level of consciousness, seizures, and vision changes may follow. Nonpalpable, red-brown *petechiae*—a macular, measles-like rash—may appear over the neck, upper arms, and/or chest. This rash is a classic manifestation but is usually the last sign to develop (McCance et al., 2019).

Abnormal laboratory findings include:

- Decreased Pao_2 level (often below 60 mm Hg)
- Increased erythrocyte sedimentation rate (ESR)
- Decreased serum calcium levels
- Decreased red blood cell and platelet counts
- Increased serum level of lipids

These changes in blood values are poorly understood, but they aid in diagnosis of the condition.

The chest x-ray often shows bilateral infiltrates but may be normal. The chest CT often reveals a patchy distribution of opacities. An MRI of the brain can show evidence of neurologic deficits from hypoxemia. FES can result in respiratory failure or death, often from pulmonary edema. When the lungs are affected, the complication may be misdiagnosed as a pulmonary embolism from a blood clot (Table 47.1).

Chronic Complications of Fractures. Avascular necrosis, delayed bone healing, and chronic regional pain syndrome are later chronic complications of musculoskeletal trauma. Blood supply to the bone may be disrupted, causing decreased ***perfusion***

TABLE 47.1 Fat Embolism Versus Blood Clot (Pulmonary) Embolism

Fat Embolism	Blood Clot Embolism
Definition	
Obstruction of the pulmonary (or other organ) vascular bed by fat globules	Obstruction of the pulmonary artery by a blood clot or clots
Origin	
Most from fractures of the long bones; occurs usually within 48 hr of injury	Most from deep vein thrombosis in the legs or pelvis; can occur anytime
Assessment Findings	
Altered mental status (earliest sign) Increased respirations, pulse, temperature Chest pain Dyspnea Crackles Decreased Sa_{O_2} Petechiae (not present in all patients) Mild thrombocytopenia	Same as for fat embolism, except no petechiae
Treatment	
Bedrest Gentle handling Oxygen Hydration (IV fluids) Possibly steroid therapy Fracture immobilization	Preventive measures (e.g., leg exercises, antiembolism stockings, SCDs) Bedrest Oxygen Possibly mechanical ventilation Anticoagulants Thrombolytics Possible surgery: pulmonary embolectomy, vena cava umbrella

Sa_{O_2}, Arterial oxygen saturation; *SCD*, sequential compression device.

and death of bone tissue, or **avascular necrosis**. This problem is most often a complication of hip fractures or any fracture in which there is displacement of bone. Surgical repair of fractures also can cause necrosis because the hardware can interfere with circulation. Patients on long-term corticosteroid therapy, such as prednisone, are also at high risk for ischemic necrosis.

Delayed union is a fracture that has not healed within 6 months of injury. Some fractures never achieve union; that is, they never completely heal *(nonunion)*. Others heal incorrectly *(malunion)*. These problems are most common in patients with tibial fractures, fractures that involve many treatment techniques (e.g., cast, traction), and pathologic fractures. Union may also be delayed or not achieved in the older patient due to poor bone health. If bone does not heal, he or she typically has persistent ***pain*** and decreased ***mobility*** from deformity.

Complex regional pain syndrome (CRPS), formerly called *reflex sympathetic dystrophy (RSD)*, is a poorly understood dysfunction of the central and peripheral nervous systems that leads to severe, persistent ***pain*** and other symptoms. Genetic factors may play a role in the development of this devastating complication. CRPS most often results from fractures or other traumatic musculoskeletal injury and commonly occurs in the feet and hands (Thurlow & Gray, 2018). In some cases, specific nerve injuries are present, but in others no injury can be identified. To facilitate soft tissue healing and *prevent* CRPS, the physical therapist asks the patient to frequently apply a variety of objects with varying surface types directly to the skin to desensitize it. These objects can be rough, smooth, hard, soft, sharp (but not enough to damage the skin), or dull.

When CRPS is present, a triad of signs and symptoms is present, including (Thurlow & Gray, 2018):

- Abnormalities of the autonomic nervous system (changes in color, temperature, and sensitivity of skin over the affected area, excessive sweating, edema)
- Motor symptoms (paresis, muscle spasms, loss of function)
- Altered ***sensory perception*** symptoms (intense burning pain that becomes intractable [unrelenting])

Etiology and Genetic Risk. The primary cause of a fracture is trauma from a motor vehicle crash or fall, especially in older adults. The trauma may be a direct blow to the bone or an indirect force from muscle contractions or pulling forces on the bone. Sports, vigorous exercise, and malnutrition are contributing factors. Bone diseases, such as osteoporosis, increase the risk for a fracture in older adults (see Chapter 45). Genetic factors that increase risk for fracture are discussed with these specific health problems throughout this text.

Incidence and Prevalence. The incidence of fractures depends on the location of the injury. Rib fractures are the most common type in the adult population. Femoral shaft fractures occur most often in young and middle-age adults.

PATIENT-CENTERED CARE: OLDER ADULT CONSIDERATIONS (QSEN)

The incidence of proximal femur (hip) fractures is highest in older adults. Humeral fractures are also common in older adults; the older the person, usually the more proximal is the fracture. Wrist (Colles) fractures are typically seen in middle and late adulthood and usually result from a fall. These fractures are sometimes referred to as *FOSH fractures* (fall out-stretched hand). Middle-age and older adults, especially women, have a higher incidence of osteoporosis, which increases the risk for fragility fractures.

Health Promotion and Maintenance

Airbags and seat belts have decreased the number of severe injuries and deaths, but they have *increased* the number of leg and ankle fractures, especially in older adults. Focus health teaching on risks for musculoskeletal injury, including:

- Osteoporosis screening and self-management education (see Chapter 45)
- Fall prevention (see Chapter 4)
- Home safety assessment and modification, if needed
- Dangers of substance use and driving
- Preventing overuse injuries for recreational and professional athletes
- Helmet use when riding bicycles, motorcycles, and other small motorized vehicles/devices

❖ Interprofessional Collaborative Care

◆ Assessment: Recognize Cues

History. The patient with a new fracture typically reports moderate-to-severe ***pain.*** Delay the detailed interview for a nursing history until he or she is more comfortable, and then ask about the cause of the fracture. Certain types of force (e.g., incisional, crush, acceleration, or deceleration), shearing, and friction lead to most musculoskeletal injuries. As a result, several body systems are often affected.

Incisional injuries, as from a knife wound, and *crush* injuries cause hemorrhage and decreased ***perfusion*** to major organs. *Acceleration or deceleration* injuries cause direct trauma to the spleen, brain, and kidneys when these organs are moved from their fixed locations in the body. *Shearing and friction* damage ***tissue integrity*** and cause a high level of wound contamination.

Asking about the events leading to the injury helps identify which forces were experienced and therefore which body systems or parts of the body to assess. For example, a forward fall often results in Colles fracture of the wrist because the person tries to catch himself or herself with an outstretched hand. Knowing the mechanism of injury also helps determine whether other types of injury, such as head and spinal cord injury, might be present.

Obtain a substance use history regardless of the patient's age. For example, a young adult may have had an excessive amount of alcohol and/or drugs, which contributed to a motor vehicle crash or a fall at the work site. Many older adults also consume alcohol and an assortment of prescribed and over-the-counter drugs, which can cause dizziness and loss of balance. *Assess adults of all ages about opioid use for persistent pain before the fracture. This information is essential for developing a pain management plan for the patient.*

Ask about the patient's occupation and recreational activities. Some occupations are more hazardous than others. For instance, construction work is potentially more physically dangerous than office work. Certain hobbies and recreational activities are also extremely hazardous, such as skiing. Contact sports, such as football and ice hockey, often result in musculoskeletal injuries, including fractures. Other activities do not have such an obvious potential for injury but can cause fractures nonetheless. For instance, daily jogging or running can lead to fatigue (stress) fractures.

Physical Assessment/Signs and Symptoms. The patient with a fracture often has trauma to other body systems. Therefore assess all major body systems *first* for life-threatening complications, especially when patients have head, chest, and/or abdominal trauma. Some fractures can cause internal organ damage resulting in hemorrhage. When a pelvic fracture is suspected, assess vital signs, skin color, and level of consciousness for indications of possible hypovolemic shock from internal blood loss. Remember that if there is one pelvic fracture, there is usually another fracture in the pelvis, even if it is small or hairline. Check the urine for blood, which indicates possible damage to the urinary system, often the bladder. If the patient cannot void, suspect that the bladder or urethra has been damaged. Complete assessment of organ function is described elsewhere in this text.

Patients with severe or multiple fractures of the arms, legs, or pelvis have severe ***pain.*** Vertebral compression fractures are also extremely painful. Patients *with a fractured hip may have groin pain or pain referred to the back of the knee or lower back.* ***Pain*** is usually caused by muscle spasm and edema that result from the fracture.

! NURSING SAFETY PRIORITY (QSEN)

Action Alert

Patients with one or more fractured ribs have severe pain when they take deep breaths. Monitor respiratory status, which may be severely compromised from pain or pneumothorax (air in the pleural cavity). Assess the patient's ***pain*** level and manage pain *before* continuing the physical assessment.

For fractures of the shoulder and upper arm, the physical assessment is best done with the patient in a sitting or standing position, if possible, so shoulder drooping or other abnormal positioning can be seen. Support the affected arm and flex the elbow to promote comfort during the assessment. For more distal areas of the arm, perform the assessment with the patient in a supine position so that the extremity can be elevated to reduce swelling.

Place the patient in a supine position for assessment of the legs and pelvis. A patient with an impacted hip fracture may be able to walk for a short time after injury, although this is not recommended.

When inspecting the site of a possible fracture, look for a change in bone alignment. The bone may appear deformed, a limb may be internally or externally rotated, and/or one or more bones may also be dislocated (out of their joint capsules). Observe for extremity shortening or a change in bone shape.

If the skin is intact (closed fracture), the area over the fracture may be ecchymotic (bruised) from bleeding into the underlying soft tissues. **Subcutaneous emphysema**, the appearance of bubbles under the skin because of air trapping, may be present but is usually seen later.

! NURSING SAFETY PRIORITY (QSEN)

Action Alert

Swelling at the fracture site is rapid and can result in marked neurovascular compromise as a result of decreased arterial ***perfusion.*** *Gently perform a thorough neurovascular assessment and compare extremities.* Assess skin color and temperature, ***sensory perception, mobility, pain,*** and pulses distal to the fracture site. If the fracture involves an extremity and the patient is not in severe pain, check the nails for capillary refill by applying pressure to the nail and observing for the speed of blood return (usually 3 to 5 seconds, depending on the patient's age). If nails are brittle or thick, assess the skin next to the nail. Checking for capillary refill is not as reliable as other indicators of ***perfusion.***

The Best Practice for Patient Safety & Quality Care: Assessment of Neurovascular Status in Patients With Musculoskeletal Injury box describes the procedure for a neurovascular assessment, which evaluates circulation, movement, and sensation (CMS function).

BEST PRACTICE FOR PATIENT SAFETY & QUALITY CARE (QSEN)

Assessment of Neurovascular Status in Patients With Musculoskeletal Injury

Assessment Method	Normal Findings
Skin Color	
Inspect the area distal to the injury.	No change in pigmentation compared with other parts of the body.
Skin Temperature	
Palpate the area distal to the injury (the dorsum of the hands is most sensitive to temperature).	The skin is warm.
Movement	
Ask the patient to move the affected area or the area distal to the injury (active motion).	The patient can move without discomfort.
Move the area distal to the injury (passive motion).	No difference in comfort compared with active movement.
Sensation	
Ask the patient if numbness or tingling is present (paresthesia).	No numbness or tingling.
Palpate with a paper clip (especially the web space between the first and second toes or the web space between the thumb and forefinger).	No difference in sensation in the affected and unaffected extremities. (Loss of sensation in these areas indicates peroneal nerve or median nerve damage.)
Pulses	
Palpate the pulses distal to the injury.	Pulses are strong and easily palpated; no difference in the affected and unaffected extremities.
Capillary Refill (Least Reliable)	
Press the nail beds distal to the injury until blanching occurs (or the skin near the nail if nails are thick and brittle).	Blood returns (return to usual color) within 3 sec (5 sec for older patients).
Pain	
Ask the patient about the location, nature, and frequency of the pain.	Pain is usually localized and is often described as stabbing or throbbing. (Pain out of proportion to the injury and unrelieved by analgesics might indicate compartment syndrome.)

Psycosocial Assessment. The psychosocial status of a patient with a fracture depends on the extent of the injury, possible complications, coping ability, and availability of support systems. Hospitalization is not required for a single, uncomplicated fracture, and the patient returns to usual daily activities within a few days. Examples include a single fracture of a bone in the finger, wrist, foot, or toe.

In contrast, a patient suffering severe or multiple traumas may be hospitalized for weeks and may undergo many surgical procedures, treatments, and prolonged rehabilitation. These disruptions in lifestyle can create a high level of stress, anxiety, and/or depression.

PATIENT-CENTERED CARE: CULTURAL/SPIRITUAL CONSIDERATIONS (QSEN)

For patients experiencing long-term recovery from fractures and other trauma, stress, anxiety, and depression can affect relationships between the patient and family members or friends. Assess the patient's feelings and ask how he or she coped with previously experienced stressful events. Body image and sexuality may be altered by deformity, treatment modalities for fracture repair, or long-term immobilization. Establish a trusting relationship and determine the patient's spiritual beliefs and practices. Assess the availability of love and support systems, such as family, friends, church or temple, or community groups, who can help patients during the acute and rehabilitation phases when multiple or severe fractures occur.

Active patients of any age or those who are older and live alone may become depressed during the healing process, especially if experiencing persistent ***pain*** that can decrease energy levels. Patients who were previously active and otherwise healthy often feel vulnerable and can become very anxious when they are not able to return to their usual level of activity. Provide hope that appropriate pain management will improve their comfort level and restore energy to return to their usual life habits. Some patients may benefit from counseling or psychotherapy services to help them with symptoms of depression and/or anxiety.

Laboratory Assessment. No special laboratory tests are available for assessment of fractures. Hemoglobin and hematocrit levels may often be low because of bleeding caused by the injury. If extensive soft-tissue damage is present, the erythrocyte sedimentation rate (ESR) may be elevated, which indicates the expected inflammatory response. If this value and the white blood cell (WBC) count increase during fracture healing, the patient may have a bone or soft tissue ***infection.*** During the healing stages, serum calcium and phosphorus levels may increase as the affected bone releases these elements into the blood.

Imaging Assessment. The primary health care provider requests standard *x-rays* to confirm a diagnosis of fracture, which often reveals bone disruption, malalignment, or deformity. If the x-ray does not show a fracture but the patient is symptomatic, the x-ray is usually repeated with additional views.

The *CT* scan is useful in detecting fractures of complex structures, such as the hip and pelvis. It also identifies compression fractures of the spine. *MRI* is useful in determining the amount of soft-tissue damage that may have occurred with the fracture.

◆ **Analysis: Analyze Cues and Prioritize Hypotheses.** The priority collaborative problems for patients with fractures include:

1. Acute ***pain*** due to fractured bone(s), soft-tissue damage, muscle spasm, and edema
2. Decreased ***mobility*** due to ***pain,*** muscle spasm, and soft-tissue damage
3. Potential for neurovascular compromise due to impaired tissue ***perfusion***
4. Potential for ***infection*** due to impaired ***tissue integrity*** caused by an open fracture and/or extensive soft tissue damage

◆ Planning and Implementation: Generate Solutions and Take Action

Managing Acute Pain

Planning: Expected Outcomes. The patient with a fracture is expected to state that he or she has adequate ***pain*** control (a 2 to 3 on a pain scale of 0 to 10) after fracture reduction and immobilization.

Interventions. A fracture can happen anywhere and may be accompanied by multiple injuries to vital organs or major vessels (e.g., thoracic aorta dissection or tear). Interprofessional collaborative care depends on the severity and extent of the injury and the number of fractures the patient has.

Emergency Care: Fracture. For any patient who experiences trauma in the community, first call 911 and assess for **a**irway, **b**reathing, and **c**irculation (ABCs, or primary survey). Then provide lifesaving care if needed before being concerned about the fracture. If cardiopulmonary resuscitation (CPR) is needed, ensure circulation first, followed by airway and breathing (see the Best Practice for Patient Safety & Quality Care: Emergency Care of the Patient With an Extremity Fracture box).

After a head-to-toe assessment (secondary survey) and patient stabilization by the prehospital team, pain is often managed with short-term IV opioids such as fentanyl, hydromorphone, or morphine sulfate. Depending on the severity of the injury, other drugs to decrease opioid use, such as NSAIDs and regional nerve blocks, are also administered. Cardiac monitoring for patients who are older than 50 years is established before drug administration. In the emergency department (ED), primary health care provider office, or urgent care center, fracture management begins with reduction and immobilization of the fracture while attending to continued ***pain*** assessment and management.

Bone reduction, or realignment of the bone ends for proper healing, is accomplished by a closed method or an open (surgical) procedure. In some cases, dislocated bones are also reduced, such as when the distal tibia and fibula are dislocated with a fractured ankle. Immobilization is achieved by the use of bandages, casts, traction, internal fixation, or external fixation.

The primary health care provider selects the treatment method based on the type, location, and extent of the fracture. These interventions prevent further injury and reduce ***pain.***

Nonsurgical Management. Nonsurgical management includes closed reduction and immobilization with a bandage, splint, boot, cast, or less commonly, traction. For some small, closed incomplete or "hairline" bone fractures in the hand or foot, reduction is not required. Immobilization with an orthotic device or special orthopedic shoe or boot may be the only management needed for healing to occur.

For each modality, the primary nursing concern is assessment and prevention of neurovascular dysfunction or compromise. Assess and document the patient's neurovascular status every hour for the first 24 hours and every 1 to 4 hours thereafter, depending on the injury and agency/primary health care provider protocol. Elevate the fractured extremity higher than the heart and apply ice for the first 24 to 48 hours as needed to reduce edema.

Closed reduction and immobilization. *Closed* reduction is the most common nonsurgical method for managing a simple fracture. While applying a manual pull, or traction, on the bone, the primary health care provider moves the bone ends so that they realign. Moderate sedation is used during this procedure for patient comfort. The nurse monitors the patient's oxygen saturation (and possibly end-tidal carbon dioxide [$ETCO_2$] level) to ensure adequate rate and depth of respirations during the procedure. *If the $ETCO_2$ becomes too low (30 mm Hg) and the respiratory rate falls to 10 breaths/min, rub the patient's sternum and encourage him or her to breathe.* An x-ray confirms that the bone ends are approximated (aligned) before the bone is immobilized, and a splint or other device is applied to keep the bone in alignment.

Splints and orthopedic boots/shoes. For certain areas of the body, such as the scapula (shoulder) and clavicle (collarbone), a commercial immobilizer may be used to keep the bone in place during healing. Because upper-extremity bones do not bear weight, splints may be sufficient to keep bone fragments in place for a closed fracture. Thermoplastic, a durable, flexible material for splinting, allows custom fitting to the patient's body part. Splints for lower extremities are also custom fitted using flexible materials and held in place with elastic bandages. When possible, splints are preferred over casts to prevent the complications that can occur with casting. Splints also allow room for extremity swelling without causing decreased arterial ***perfusion.***

For foot or toe fractures, orthopedic shoes may be used to support the injured area during healing. For ankles or the lower part of the leg, padded orthopedic boots supported by multiple Velcro straps to hold the boot in place may be used (Fig. 47.3). These devices are especially useful when the patient is allowed to bear weight on the affected leg.

Casts. For more complex fractures or fractures of the lower extremity, the primary health care provider or orthopedic technician may apply a cast to hold bone fragments in place after reduction. A **cast** is a rigid device that immobilizes the affected body part while allowing other body parts to move. It also

BEST PRACTICE FOR PATIENT SAFETY & QUALITY CARE (QSEN)

Emergency Care of the Patient With an Extremity Fracture

- Assess the patient's **a**irway, **b**reathing, and **c**irculation; establish any ABC that is affected by the injury.
- Perform a quick head-to-toe assessment.
- Remove the patient's clothing (cut if necessary) to inspect the affected area while supporting the area above and below the injury. Do not remove shoes because this can cause increased trauma unless the foot or ankle is injured.
- Apply direct pressure on the area if there is bleeding and pressure over the proximal artery nearest the fracture.
- Remove jewelry on the affected extremity in case of swelling.
- Keep the patient warm and in a supine position.
- Check the neurovascular status of the area distal to the fracture, including temperature, color, sensation, movement, and capillary refill. Compare affected and unaffected limbs.
- Immobilize the extremity by splinting; include joints above and below the fracture site. Recheck circulation after splinting.
- Cover any open areas with a dressing (preferably sterile).

allows early ***mobility*** and reduces ***pain***. Although its most common use is for fractures, a cast may be applied for correction of deformities (e.g., clubfoot) or for prevention of deformities (e.g., those seen in some patients with rheumatoid arthritis).

Fiberglass, a waterproof synthetic casting material, is used most often for fracture immobilization (Fig. 47.4). Fiberglass can dry and become rigid within minutes and decreases the risk for impaired ***tissue integrity.*** *Plaster* was the traditional material used for casts but is used less often today. When first applied, a plaster cast feels hot because an immediate chemical reaction occurs; it soon becomes damp and cool. This type of cast takes at least 24 hours to dry, depending on the size and location of the cast. A wet cast feels cold, smells musty, and is grayish. The cast is dry when it feels hard and firm, is odorless, and has a shiny white appearance.

If ***tissue integrity*** under the cast is impaired, the primary health care provider, orthopedic technician, or specially educated nurse cuts a window in the cast so that the wound can be observed and cared for. The piece of cast removed to make the window must be retained and replaced after wound care to prevent localized edema in the area. This is most important when a window is cut from a cast on an extremity. Tape or elastic bandage wrap may be used to keep the "window" in place. A window is also an access for taking pulses, removing wound drains, or preventing abdominal distention when the patient is in a body or spica cast.

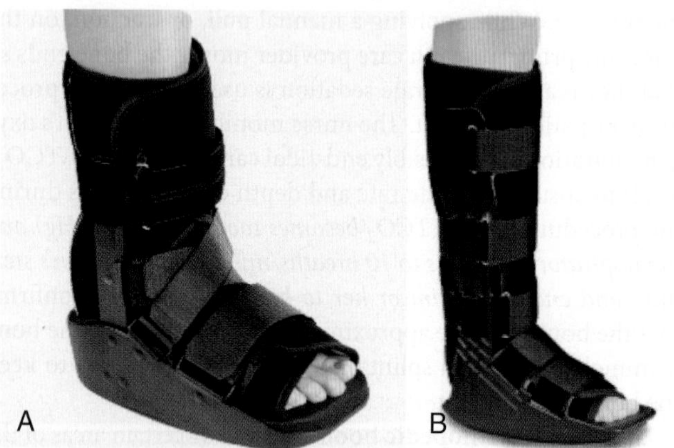

FIG. 47.3 A, Short boot. B, Long boot. (From Rizzone, K., & Gregory, A. [2013]. Using casts, splints, and braces in the emergency department. *Clinical Pediatric Emergency Medicine, 14*[4], 340–348. doi:10.1016/j.cpem.2013.11.003.)

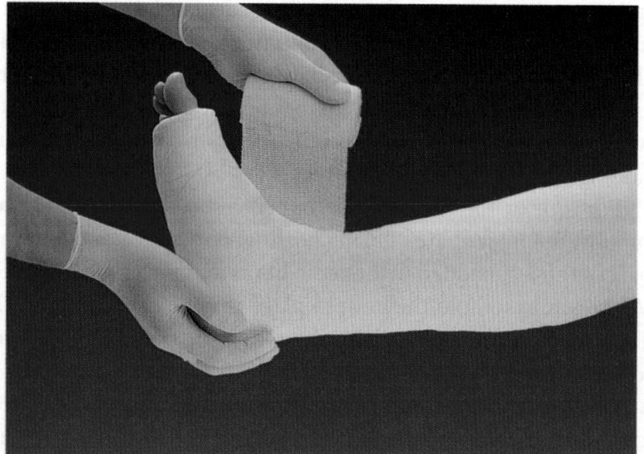

FIG. 47.4 Application of a fiberglass synthetic cast. (From Perry, A. G., Potter, P. A., & Elkin, M. K. [2012]. *Nursing interventions & clinical skills* [5th ed.]. St. Louis: Mosby.)

If the cast is too tight, it may be cut with a cast cutter to relieve pressure or allow tissue swelling. The primary health care provider may choose to bivalve the cast (i.e., cut it lengthwise into two equal pieces). Either half of the cast can be removed for inspection or for provision of care. The two halves are then held in place by an elastic bandage wrap.

When a patient has an *arm cast,* teach him or her to elevate the arm above the heart to reduce swelling. The hand should be higher than the heart. Ice may be prescribed for the first 24 to 48 hours. When the patient is walking or standing, the arm is supported with a sling placed around the neck to alleviate fatigue caused by the weight of the cast. The sling should distribute the weight over a large area of the shoulders and trunk, not just the neck. Some primary health care providers prefer that the patient not use a sling after the first few days in an arm cast, particularly a short-arm cast. This encourages normal movement of the mobile joints and enhances bone healing. For many wrist fractures, a splint is used to immobilize the area instead of a cast to accommodate for edema formation.

A *leg cast* allows ***mobility*** and requires the patient to use ambulatory aids such as crutches or a walker. A cast shoe, sandal, or boot that attaches to the foot or a rubber walking pad attached to the sole of the cast assists in ambulation (if weight bearing is allowed) and helps prevent damage to the cast. Teach the patient to elevate the affected leg on several pillows to reduce swelling and to apply ice for the first 24 hours or as prescribed.

Before the cast is applied, explain its purpose and the procedure for its application. With a *plaster* cast, warn the patient about the heat that will be felt immediately after the wet cast is applied. *Do not cover a new plaster cast.* Allow for air-drying and handle the cast with the palms of the hand to prevent damage.

! NURSING SAFETY PRIORITY QSEN

Action Alert

Check to ensure that any type of cast is not too tight and frequently monitor and document neurovascular status—usually every hour for the first 24 hours after application if the patient is hospitalized. You should be able to insert a finger between the cast and the skin. Teach the patient to apply ice for the first 24 to 36 hours to reduce swelling and inflammation.

Inspect the cast at least once every 8 to 12 hours for drainage, alignment, and fit. Plaster casts act like sponges and absorb drainage, whereas synthetic casts act like a wick pulling drainage away from the drainage site. Document the presence of any drainage on the cast. However, the evidence is not clear on whether drainage should be circled on the cast because it may increase anxiety and is not a reliable indicator of drainage amount. *Immediately report to the primary health care provider any sudden increases in the amount of drainage or change in the integrity of the cast.* After swelling decreases, it is not uncommon for the cast to become too loose and need replacement. If the patient is not admitted to the hospital, provide instructions regarding cast care.

During hospitalization, assess for other complications resulting from casting that can be serious and life threatening, such as infection, circulation impairment, and peripheral nerve damage. If the patient returns home after cast application, teach him or her how to monitor for these complications and when to notify the primary health care provider.

Infection most often results from impaired ***tissue integrity*** under the cast (pressure necrosis). If pressure necrosis occurs, the patient typically reports a very painful "hot spot" under the cast, and the cast may feel warmer in the affected area. Teach the patient or family to smell the area for mustiness or an unpleasant odor that would indicate infected material. If the infection progresses, a fever may develop. Teach the patient to never put anything down inside the cast, such as a hanger or pencil, to scratch an itch because this action can cause significant skin damage.

Circulation impairment causing decreased ***perfusion*** and ***peripheral nerve damage*** can result from tightness of the cast. Teach the patient to assess for circulation at least daily, including the ability to move the area distal to the extremity, numbness, and increased ***pain***. Remind the patient to wiggle his or her toes and move them up and down.

The patient with a cast may be immobilized for a prolonged period, depending on the extent of the fracture and the type of cast. In this case, assess for complications of decreased ***mobility***, such as skin breakdown, pneumonia, atelectasis, venous thromboembolism, and constipation. Before the cast is removed, inform the patient that the cast cutter will not injure the skin but that heat may be felt during the procedure.

Because of prolonged immobilization, a joint may become contracted, usually in a fixed state of flexion. Osteoarthritis and osteoporosis may develop from lack of weight bearing. Muscle can also atrophy from lack of exercise during prolonged immobilization of the affected body part, usually an extremity.

NCLEX EXAMINATION CHALLENGE 47.1

Physiological Integrity

A client has a new synthetic leg cast for a right fractured tibia. What health teaching will the nurse include before discharge to home? **Select all that apply.**

A. "Elevate your right leg as often as possible to reduce swelling."
B. "Report increased pain or burning sensation under your cast."
C. "Use ice on the affected leg for the first 24-36 hours."
D. "Do not bear weight on the affected leg until instructed to do so."
E. "Do not cover the cast when you are in bed; keep it open to air to dry."

Traction. Traction is the application of a pulling force to a part of the body to provide bone reduction or as a last resort to decrease muscle spasm (thus reducing ***pain***). A patient in traction is often hospitalized, but in some cases home care is possible even for skeletal traction.

Although not used as often today, the two major types of traction are skin and skeletal traction. *Skin traction* involves the use of a Velcro boot (Buck traction) (Fig. 47.5), belt, or halter, which is usually secured around the affected leg. The primary purpose of skin traction is to decrease painful muscle spasms

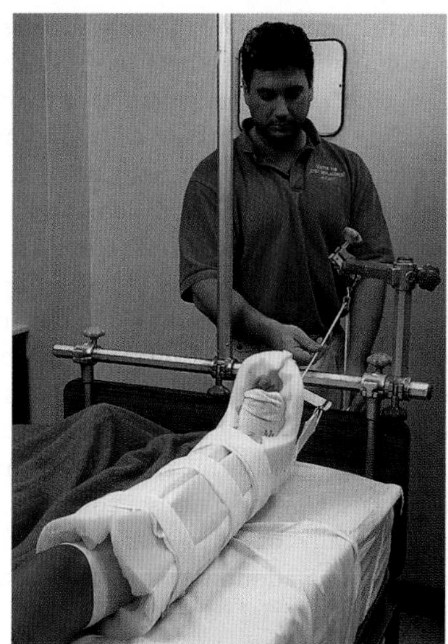

FIG. 47.5 Skin traction with a hook-and-loop fastener (Velcro) boot, commonly used for hip fractures. (Courtesy Smith & Nephew, Inc., Orthopaedics Divisions, Memphis, TN.)

that accompany hip and proximal femur fractures. A weight is used as a pulling force, which is limited to 5 to 10 lb (2.3 to 4.5 kg) to prevent injury to the skin (Duperouzel et al., 2018).

In *skeletal traction,* screws are surgically inserted directly into bone (e.g., femoral condyles for distal femur fractures). These allow the use of longer traction time and heavier weights, usually 15 to 30 lb (6.8 to 13.6 kg). Skeletal traction aids in bone realignment but impairs the patient's ***mobility***. Use pressure-reduction measures and monitor for indications of impaired ***tissue integrity***. Pin site care is also an important part of nursing management to prevent infection. Keep pin sites clean and document the nature of any drainage. Follow the agency's or primary health care provider's protocol for pin care.

! NURSING SAFETY PRIORITY (QSEN)

Action Alert

When patients are in traction, weights are not removed without a prescription. They should not be lifted manually or allowed to rest on the floor. Weights should be freely hanging at all times. Teach this important point to assistive personnel on the unit, to other personnel such as those in the radiology department, and to visitors. Inspect the skin at least every 8 hours for signs of irritation or inflammation. When possible, remove the belt or boot that is used for skin traction every 8 hours to inspect under the device. Assess neurovascular status of the affected body part per agency or primary health care provider protocol to detect impaired ***perfusion*** and ***tissue integrity***. The patient's circulation is usually monitored every hour for the first 24 hours after traction is applied and every 4 hours thereafter (Duperouzel et al., 2018).

Drug therapy. After fracture treatment, the patient often has ***pain*** for a prolonged time during the healing process. The primary health care provider commonly prescribes opioid and nonopioid analgesics, NSAIDs, and possibly, muscle relaxants.

For patients with severe persistent ***pain***, opioid and nonopioid drugs are alternated or given together to manage pain both centrally in the brain and peripherally at the site of injury. For severe or multiple fractures, short-term patient-controlled analgesia (PCA) with morphine, fentanyl, or hydromorphone is used. Oxycodone and oxycodone with acetaminophen or hydrocodone with acetaminophen are common oral opioid drugs that are very effective for most patients with fracture pain. NSAIDs and other drugs are given to decrease associated tissue inflammation; however, they can slow bone healing.

For patients who have less severe injury, the analgesic may be given on an as-needed basis. Collaborate with the patient regarding the best times for the strong analgesics to be given (e.g., before a complex dressing change, after physical therapy sessions, or at bedtime). Assess the effectiveness of the analgesic and its side effects. Constipation is a common side effect of opioid therapy, especially for older adults. Assess for frequency of bowel movements and administer stool softeners or laxatives as needed for **opioid-induced constipation (OIC)**. Encourage fluids, high-fiber foods, and activity as tolerated. Be aware that other drugs, such as anticholinergics, calcium channel blockers, antidepressants, and diuretics, may cause medication-induced constipation (MIC) (Turkowski, 2018).

Physical therapy. Collaborate with the physical therapist (PT) to assist with pain control and edema reduction by using ice/heat packs, electrical muscle stimulation ("e-stim"), and special treatments such as dexamethasone iontophoresis. Iontophoresis is a method for absorbing dexamethasone, a synthetic steroid, through the skin near the painful area to decrease inflammation and edema. A small device delivers a minute amount of electricity via electrodes that are placed on the skin. The patient may describe the sensation as a pinch or slight sting. The electrical current increases the ability of the skin to absorb the drug from a topical patch into the affected soft tissue.

When acute ***pain*** is not adequately controlled, some patients experience a chronic, intense burning pain and edema that are associated with **complex regional pain syndrome (CRPS)**. This syndrome often results from fractures and other musculoskeletal trauma as described earlier in this chapter.

Surgical Management. For some types of fractures, closed reduction is not sufficient. Surgical intervention may be needed to realign the bone to enhance the healing process.

Preoperative care. Teach the patient and family what to expect during and after the surgery. The preoperative care for a patient undergoing orthopedic surgery is similar to that for anyone having surgery with general or epidural anesthesia. Some patients may also receive a regional nerve blockade, which promotes comfort immediately after surgery. (See Chapter 9 for a thorough discussion of general preoperative nursing care.)

Operative procedures. Open reduction with internal fixation (ORIF) is one of the most common methods of reducing and immobilizing a fracture. **External fixation** with closed reduction is used when patients have soft-tissue injury (open fracture). Although nurses do not decide which surgical technique is used, understanding the procedures enhances patient teaching and care.

Because ORIF permits early ***mobility,*** it is often the preferred surgical method. *Open* reduction allows the surgeon to directly view the fracture site. **Internal fixation** uses metal pins, screws, rods, plates, or prostheses inside the body to immobilize a fracture during healing. The surgeon makes one or more incisions to gain access to the broken bone(s) and implants one or more devices into bone tissue after each fracture is reduced. A cast, boot, or splint is placed to maintain immobilization during the healing process, depending on the body part affected.

After the bone achieves union, the metal hardware may be removed, depending on the location and type of fracture. Hardware is removed most frequently in ankle fractures, depending on the severity of the injury. If the metal implants are not bothersome, they may remain in place. Examples of internal fixation devices for fractured hips are discussed later in this chapter.

An alternative modality for the management of fractures is the external fixation apparatus, as shown in Fig. 47.6. **External fixation** is a surgical procedure in which pins or wires are inserted through the skin and affected bone and then connected to a rigid external frame outside the body to stabilize the fracture during healing (Georgiades, 2018). The system may be used for upper- or lower-extremity fractures or for fractures of the pelvis, especially for open fractures when wound management is needed. After a fixator is removed, the patient may be placed in a cast, boot, or splint until healing is complete or have internal fixation.

External fixation has several advantages over other surgical techniques:

- There is minimal blood loss compared with internal fixation.
- The device allows early ambulation and exercise of the affected body part while relieving pain.
- The device maintains alignment in closed fractures that will not maintain position in a cast and stabilizes comminuted fractures that require bone grafting.

A disadvantage of external fixation is an increased risk for pin-site ***infection.*** Pin-site infections can lead to osteomyelitis, which is serious and difficult to treat (see Chapter 45).

Postoperative care. The postoperative care for a patient undergoing ORIF or external fixation is similar to that provided for any patient undergoing surgery (see Chapter 9). Because bone is a vascular, dynamic body tissue, the patient is at risk

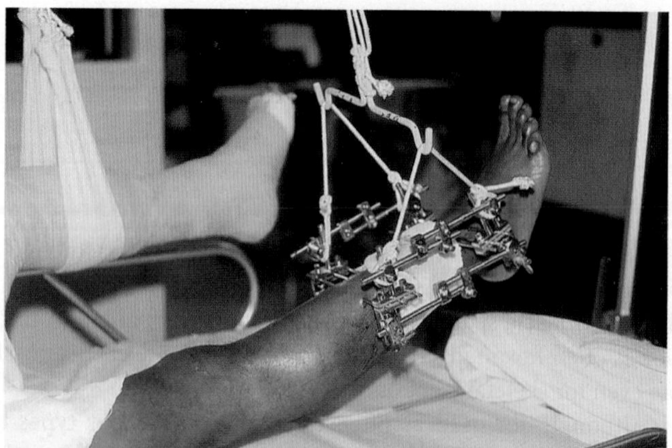

FIG. 47.6 Example of an external fixation device on the right leg. The left leg is in a splint. (From McCance, K. L., Huether, S. E., Brashers, V. L., & Rote, N. S. [2019]. *Pathophysiology: The biologic basis for disease in adults and children* [8th ed.]. St. Louis: Elsevier.)

for complications specific to fractures and musculoskeletal surgery. IV ketorolac is often given in the postanesthesia care unit (PACU) or soon after discharge to the postsurgical area to reduce inflammation and ***pain.*** Aggressive pain management starts as soon as possible after surgery to prevent the development of chronic pain and promote early ***mobility.*** Patients who had a regional nerve blockade typically have little or no pain immediately after surgery for about 18 to 24 hours. However, when the anesthetic begins to wear off, be sure that the patient is medicated to prevent severe pain. Use nonpharmacologic measures for pain management, such as imagery, distraction, music therapy, and other measures that the patient prefers and are allowed by agency policy to promote comfort.

Additional information about postoperative care may be found in the Selected Fractures of Specific Sites section later in this section. Depending on the fractures that are repaired, some ORIF procedures are performed as same-day surgeries. Patients stay in the hospital up to 23 hours after surgery.

For patients with an *external fixator,* assess the pin sites every 8 to 12 hours for drainage, color, odor, and severe redness, which indicate inflammation and possible ***infection***. In the first 48 to 72 hours, *clear* fluid drainage or weeping is expected, which creates crusting around the pins. Although no standardized method or evidence-based protocol for pin-site care has been established, recommendations have been made based on current evidence. A systematic review of pin site care found that pin site crusts should not be removed because they protect the patient from infection (Georgiades, 2018).

The patient with an external fixator may have a disturbed body image. The frame may be large and bulky, and the affected area may have massive tissue damage with dressings. Be sensitive to this possibility in planning care. Teach about alterations to clothing that may be required while the fixator is in place.

Procedures for Nonunion. Some management techniques are not successful because the bone does not heal. Several additional options are available to the primary health care provider to promote bone union, such as electrical bone stimulation, bone grafting, and ultrasound fracture treatment.

For selected patients, *electrical bone stimulation* may be successful. This procedure is based on research showing that bone has electrical properties that are used in healing. The exact mechanism of action is unknown. A noninvasive, external system delivers a small continuous electrical charge directed toward the nonhealed bone. There are no known risks with this system, although patients with pacemakers cannot use this device on an arm. Implanted direct-current stimulators are placed directly in the fracture site and have no external apparatus. Both systems require several months of treatment.

Another method of treating nonunion is *bone grafting.* In most cases, chips of bone are taken from the iliac crest or other site and are packed or wired between the bone ends to facilitate union. Allografts from cadavers may also be used. These grafts are frozen or freeze-dried and stored under sterile conditions in a bone bank.

Bone banking from living donors is becoming increasingly popular. If qualified, patients undergoing total hip arthroplasty may donate their femoral heads to the bank for later use as bone grafts for others. Careful screening ensures that the bone is healthy and that the donor has no communicable disease. The bone cannot be donated without written consent.

One of the newest modalities for fracture healing is *low-intensity pulsed ultrasound.* Used for slow-healing fractures or for new fractures as an alternative to surgery, ultrasound treatment has had excellent results. The patient applies the treatment for about 20 minutes each day. It has no contraindications or adverse effects.

Increasing Mobility

Planning: Expected Outcomes. The patient with a fracture is expected to increase physical ***mobility*** and be free of complications associated with immobility. The patient is also expected to move purposefully in his or her own environment independently with or without an ambulatory device unless restricted by traction or other modality.

Interventions. The interventions necessary for this patient problem can be grouped into two types: those that help increase and promote ***mobility*** and those that prevent complications of decreased ***mobility.*** Interventions to prevent complications of decreased mobility are briefly summarized in Chapter 3. Additional information may be found in nursing fundamentals textbooks.

Many patients with musculoskeletal trauma, including fractures, are referred by their primary health care provider for rehabilitation therapy with a physical therapist (PT) (usually for lower-extremity injuries) and/or occupational therapist (OT) (usually for upper-extremity injuries). The timing for this referral depends on the nature, severity, and treatment modality of the fracture(s) or other musculoskeletal trauma.

For example, some patients who have an ORIF for an ankle fracture begin therapy when the incisional staples or wound closure strips are removed and an orthopedic boot is fitted. Based on the initial evaluation, the PT performs gentle manipulative exercises to increase range of motion. The therapist may also begin to help the patient with *laterality,* a concept to help the brain identify the injured foot from the uninjured foot. Computer programs and mirror-box therapy can help reprogram the brain as part of *cognitive retraining.* In mirror-box therapy for an injured foot, the patient covers his or her affected foot while looking at and moving the uninjured foot in front of the mirror. The brain often perceives the foot in the mirror as the injured foot.

Stimulation by touch also helps the brain acknowledge the injured foot. The PT teaches the patient to frequently touch the injured area and use various materials and objects against the skin to desensitize it. These interventions improve ***mobility*** and decrease the risk for **complex regional pain syndrome**, discussed earlier in this chapter.

The success of rehabilitation is affected by the patient's motivation and willingness to perform prescribed exercises and activities between PT visits. For example, rehabilitation for ankle surgery may take several months, depending on the severity of the injury and the age and general health of the patient.

When weight bearing begins for lower-extremity fractures about 6 weeks after surgery, the PT teaches the patient how to begin with toe-touch or partial weight bearing using crutches or a walker. Muscle-strengthening exercises of the affected leg help with ambulation because atrophy begins shortly after injury.

The use of crutches, knee-walker scooter, or a walker increases ***mobility*** and assists in ambulation. The patient may progress to a cane after the bone heals. *Crutches* are the most commonly used ambulatory aid for many types of lower-extremity musculoskeletal trauma (e.g., fractures, sprains, amputations). In most agencies, the physical therapist or emergency department/ambulatory care nurse fits the patient for crutches and teaches him or her how to ambulate with them. Reinforce those instructions and evaluate whether the patient is using the crutches correctly.

Walking with crutches or a knee-walker scooter requires strong arm muscles, balance, and coordination. For this reason, these ambulatory aids are not often used for older adults; traditional walkers and canes are preferred. Crutches can cause upper-extremity bursitis or axillary nerve damage if they are not fitted or used correctly. For that reason, the top of each crutch is padded. To prevent pressure on the axillary nerve, there should be two to three finger-breadths between the axilla and the top of the crutch when the crutch tip is at least 6 inches (15 cm) diagonally in front of the foot. The crutch is adjusted so that the elbow is flexed no more than 30 degrees when the palm is on the handle (Fig. 47.7). The distal tips of each crutch are rubber to prevent slipping.

There are several types of gaits for walking with crutches. The most common one for musculoskeletal injury is the three-point gait, which allows little weight bearing on the affected leg. The procedure for these gaits is discussed in fundamentals of nursing books.

A *walker* is most often used by the older patient who needs additional support for balance. The physical therapist assesses the strength of the upper extremities and the unaffected leg. Strength is improved with prescribed exercises as needed.

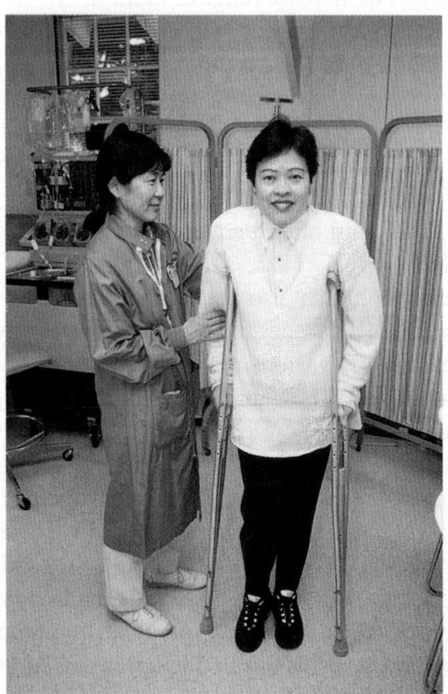

FIG. 47.7 Assisting the patient with crutch walking. Note how the therapist guards the patient and how the patient's elbows are at no more than 30 degrees of flexion.

A *cane* is sometimes used if the patient needs only minimal support for an affected leg. The straight cane offers the least support. A hemi-cane or quad-cane provides a broader base for the cane and therefore more support. The cane is placed on the *unaffected* side and should create no more than 30 degrees of flexion of the elbow. The top of the cane should be parallel to the greater trochanter of the femur or stylus of the wrist. Chapter 7 and fundamentals textbooks describe these ambulatory devices in more detail.

Preventing and Monitoring for Neurovascular Compromise

Planning: Expected Outcomes. The patient with a fracture is expected to have no compromise in neurovascular status as evidenced by adequate ***perfusion*** (circulation), ***mobility*** (movement), and ***sensory perception*** (sensation) (CMS). If severe compromise occurs, the patient is expected to have early and prompt emergency treatment to prevent severe tissue damage.

Interventions. Perform neurovascular (NV) assessments (also known as *"circ checks"* or *CMS assessments*) frequently before and after fracture treatment. Patients who have extremity casts, splints with elastic bandage wraps, and open reduction with internal fixation (ORIF) or external fixation are especially at risk for NV compromise. If ***perfusion*** to the distal extremity is impaired, the patient reports increased ***pain,*** impaired ***mobility,*** and decreased ***sensory perception.*** If these symptoms are allowed to progress, patients are at risk for acute compartment syndrome (ACS), as described earlier in this chapter.

! NURSING SAFETY PRIORITY (QSEN)

Critical Rescue

Monitor for and document early signs of ACS. Assess for the "six Ps" (i.e., **p**ain, **p**ressure, **p**aralysis, **p**aresthesia, **p**allor, and **p**ulselessness) (rare or late stage). ***Pain*** is increased even with passive motion and may seem out of proportion to the degree of injury. Analgesics that had controlled pain become less effective or noneffective. *Numbness and tingling (paresthesia) is often one of the first signs of the problem.* The affected extremity then becomes pale and cool as a result of decreased arterial perfusion to the affected area.

If ACS is suspected, notify the primary health care provider immediately and, if possible, implement interventions to relieve the pressure. For example, for the patient with tight, bulky dressings, loosen the bandage or tape. If the patient has a cast, follow agency protocol about who may cut the cast. Do not elevate or ice the extremity because that could compromise blood flow.

In some cases, compartment pressure may be monitored on a one-time basis with a handheld device with a digital display, or pressure can be monitored continuously. Monitoring is recommended for comatose or unresponsive high-risk patients with multiple trauma and fractures.

Preventing Infection

Planning: Expected Outcomes. The patient with a fracture is expected to be free of wound or bone ***infection*** as evidenced by no fever, no increase in white blood cell count, and negative wound culture (if wound is present).

Interventions. When caring for a patient with an open fracture, use aseptic technique for dressing changes and wound irrigations. Check agency policy for specific protocols. *Immediately notify the primary health care provider if you observe inflammation and purulent drainage.* Other infections, such as pneumonia and urinary tract infection, may occur several days after the fracture.

Monitor the patient's vital signs every 4 to 8 hours because increases in temperature and pulse often indicate systemic ***infection.***

PATIENT-CENTERED CARE: OLDER ADULT CONSIDERATIONS QSEN

Older adults may not have a temperature elevation even in the presence of severe infection. An acute onset of confusion (delirium) often suggests an infection in the older-adult patient.

For most patients with an open fracture, the primary care provider prescribes one or more broad-spectrum antibiotics prophylactically and performs surgical débridement of any wounds as soon as possible after the injury. First-generation cephalosporins, clindamycin, and gentamycin are commonly used. In addition to systemic antibiotics, local antibiotic therapy through wound irrigation is commonly prescribed, especially during débridement.

A very effective treatment is negative-pressure wound therapy (e.g., vacuum-assisted closure [VAC] system) as a method of increasing the rate of wound healing for open fractures. This device allows quicker wound closure, which decreases the risk for ***infection.***

Care Coordination and Transition Management. The patient with an *uncomplicated* fracture is usually discharged to home from the emergency department or urgent care center. Older adults with hip or other fractures or patients with multiple traumas are hospitalized and then transferred to home, a rehabilitation setting, or a long-term care facility for rehabilitation. Collaborate with the case manager or the discharge planner in the hospital to ensure care coordination. Be sure to communicate the plan of care clearly to the health care agency receiving the patient using situation-background-assessment recommendation or other communication method.

Home Care Management. If the patient is discharged to home, the nurse, rehabilitation therapist, or case manager (CM) may assess the home environment for structural barriers to ***mobility*** such as stairs. Be sure that the patient has easy access to the bathroom. Ask about small pets, scatter rugs, waxed floors, and walkway areas that could increase the risk for falls. If the patient needs to use a wheelchair or ambulatory aid, make sure that he or she can use it safely and that there is room in the house to ambulate with these devices. The physical therapist may teach the patient how to use stairs, but older adults or those using crutches may experience difficulty performing this task. Depending on the age and condition of the patient, a home health care nurse may make one or two visits to check that the home is safe and that the patient and family are able to follow the interprofessional plan of care.

Self-Management Education. The patient with a fracture may be discharged from the hospital, emergency department, office, or clinic with a bandage, splint, boot, or cast. Provide verbal and written instructions on the care of these devices.

The patient may also need to continue wound care at home. Instruct the patient and family about how to assess and dress the wound to promote healing and prevent ***infection.*** Teach them how to recognize complications and when and where to seek professional health care if complications occur. Additional educational needs depend on the type of fracture and fracture repair.

CLINICAL JUDGMENT CHALLENGE 47.1

Evidence-Based Practice; Safety

A 24-year-old woman was a passenger in her boyfriend's car when their car was in a motor vehicle crash. The damage to her side of the car caused her right leg and arm to be severely injured. She was admitted yesterday to the hospital with a fracture of her tibia and fibula ("tib-fib" fracture), massive soft tissue and leg muscle damage, and a right wrist fracture. She also has multiple contusions and superficial lacerations. Both her leg and wrist are in temporary splints and elevated on pillows with ice packs until she is cleared for surgery. The client is right-handed. The night nurse reported that her parents are staying with her and that the client has been crying most of the night. The day nurse performs a shift assessment and notes the following:

- Reports that her pain level has increased from a 5 to a 9 even though she recently received morphine via IV push
- Reports numbness and tingling in her injured leg and foot
- Toes on her right foot are colder and more pale than those on the left foot
- Right pedal pulse not palpable or located via Doppler
- Oral temperature = 98.4° F (36.9° C)
- Apical pulse = 88 beats/min
- Respiratory rate = 28 breaths/min
- Blood pressure = 132/84 mm Hg
- States that she wish she had died in the accident
- Has difficulty answering questions because she is very emotional and crying
- Refuses to eat, stating that she is not hungry
- Has a urinary catheter in place, which is draining amber urine

1. **Recognize Cues:** What assessment information in this client situation is the most important and immediate concern for the nurse? (Hint: Identify the **relevant** information *first* to determine what is most important.)
2. **Analyze Cues:** What client conditions are consistent with the **most relevant** information? (Hint: Think about priority collaborative problems that support and contradict the information presented in this situation.)
3. **Prioritize Hypotheses:** Which possibilities or explanations are **most likely** to be present in this client situation? Which possibilities or explanations are the most serious? (Hint: Consider all possibilities and determine their urgency and risk for this client.)
4. **Generate Solutions:** What actions would most likely achieve the desired outcomes for this client? Which actions should be **avoided** or are **potentially harmful**? (Hint: Determine the desired outcomes first to decide which interventions are appropriate and those that should be avoided.)
5. **Take Action:** Which actions are the most appropriate and how should they be implemented? In what **priority order** should they be implemented? (Hint: Consider health teaching, documentation, requested health care provider orders or prescriptions, nursing skills, collaboration with or referral to health team members, etc.)
6. **Evaluate Outcomes:** What client assessment would indicate that the nurse's actions were **effective**? (Hint: Think about signs that would indicate an improvement, decline, or unchanged client condition.)

Encourage patients and their families to ensure adequate foods high in protein and calcium that are needed for bone and tissue healing. For patients with lower-extremity fractures, less weight bearing on long bones can cause anemia. The red bone marrow needs weight bearing to simulate red blood cell production. Encourage foods high in iron content. Teach the patient to take a daily iron-added multivitamin (take with food to prevent possible nausea) and a stool softener with a stimulant to prevent opioid-induced constipation.

PATIENT AND FAMILY EDUCATION: PREPARING FOR SELF-MANAGEMENT

Care of the Extremity After Cast Removal

- Remove scaly, dead skin carefully by soaking; do not scrub.
- Move the extremity carefully. Expect smaller circumference, discomfort, weakness, and decreased range of motion.
- Support the extremity with pillows or your orthotic device until strength and movement return.
- Exercise slowly as instructed by your physical therapist.
- Wear support stockings or elastic bandages to prevent swelling (for lower extremity).

Teach patients about the need for follow-up visits to the primary health care provider to assess bone healing and determine when casts or other devices can be discontinued. The Patient and Family Education: Preparing for Self-Management box describes care of the affected extremity after removal of the cast.

NCLEX EXAMINATION CHALLENGE 47.2

Physiological Integrity

A client had an open reduction internal fixation (ORIF) of the right wrist. What health teaching is appropriate for the nurse to provide for this client before returning home? **Select all that apply.**

A. "Keep your right arm below the level of your heart as often as possible."
B. "Use an ice pack for the first 24 hours to decrease tissue swelling."
C. "Report coolness or discoloration of your right hand to your doctor."
D. "Don't place any device under the cast to scratch the skin if it itches."
E. "Move the fingers of the right hand frequently to promote blood flow."

Health Care Resources. Arrange for follow-up care at home if needed. A social worker may need to help the patient apply for funds to pay medical bills. If there is severe bone and tissue damage, be realistic and help the patient and family understand the long-term nature of the recovery period. Multiple treatment techniques and surgical procedures required for complications can be mentally and emotionally draining for the patient and family. A vocational counselor may be needed to help the patient find a different type of job, depending on the extent of the fracture.

An older or incapacitated patient may need assistance with ADLs, which can be provided by home care aides if family or other caregivers are not available. In collaboration with the case manager, anticipate the patient's needs and arrange for these services.

◆ **Evaluation: Evaluate Outcomes.** Evaluate the care of the patient with one or more fractures based on the identified priority patient problems. The expected outcomes include that the patient:

- States that he or she has adequate ***pain*** control (a 2 to 3 on a 0 to 10 pain scale) to accomplish ADLs
- Ambulates independently with or without an assistive device (if not restricted by traction or other device)
- Is free of physiologic consequences of decreased ***mobility***
- Has adequate blood flow to maintain tissue ***perfusion*** and function
- Is free of ***infection*** or other complication

LOWER EXTREMITY FRACTURES

Hip Fracture

Hip fracture is the most common injury in older adults and one of the most frequently seen injuries in any health care setting or community. It has a high mortality rate as a result of multiple complications related to surgery, depression, and decreased ***mobility.*** Over half of older adults experiencing a hip fracture are unable to live independently, and many die within the first year.

Hip fractures include those involving the upper third of the femur and are classified as *intracapsular* (within the joint capsule) or *extracapsular* (outside the joint capsule) (Hohler, 2018). These types are further divided according to fracture location (Fig. 47.8). In the area of the femoral neck, disruption of the blood supply to the head of the femur is a concern, which can result in ischemic or avascular necrosis (AVN) of the femoral head. AVN causes death and necrosis of bone tissue and results in pain and decreased ***mobility.*** This problem is most likely in patients with displaced fractures.

Osteoporosis is the biggest risk factor for hip fractures (see Chapter 45). This disease weakens the upper femur (hip), which causes it to break and lead to a fall. In some cases, a fall causes the fracture of the weakened hip, often referred to as a **fragility fracture**. The number of people with hip fracture is expected to continue to increase as the population ages, and the associated health care costs will be tremendous (Conley et al., 2020).

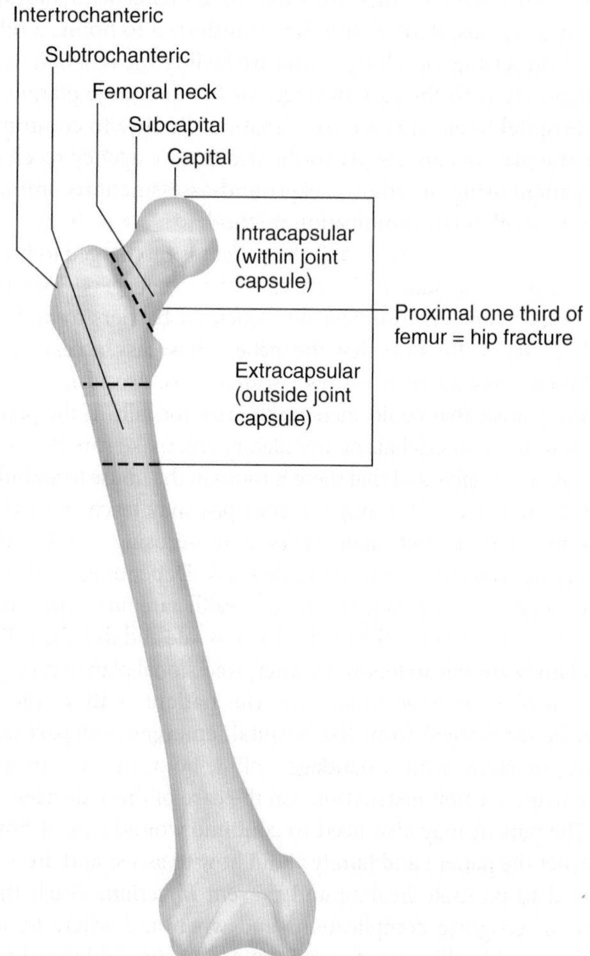

FIG. 47.8 Types of hip fractures.

PATIENT-CENTERED CARE: OLDER ADULT CONSIDERATIONS QSEN

Teach older adults about the risk factors for fragility hip fractures, including physiologic aging changes, disease processes, drug therapy, and environmental hazards. Physiologic changes include sensory changes such as diminished visual acuity and hearing; changes in gait, balance, and muscle strength; and joint stiffness. Disease processes such as osteoporosis, foot disorders, bony metastases, and changes in cardiac function increase the risk for fracture. These diseases are discussed elsewhere in this textbook. Drugs, such as diuretics, antihypertensives, antidepressants, sedatives, opioids, and alcohol, are factors that increase the risks for falling in older adults. Use of three or more drugs at the same time drastically increases the risk for falls. Throw rugs, loose carpeting, floor clutter, inadequate lighting, uneven walking surfaces or steps, and pets are environmental hazards that also cause falls.

The older adult with hip fracture usually reports groin pain or pain behind the knee on the affected side. In some cases, the patient has pain in the lower back or no pain at all. However, the patient is not able to stand without pain. X-ray or other imaging assessment confirms the diagnosis.

Preoperative Care. Patients usually receive IV morphine or hydromorphone after admission to the emergency department and may receive morphine or hydromorphone PCA or epidural analgesia after surgery. However, an integrative review of 38 research articles by Wennberg et al. (2018) found that first responders and emergency department staff do not adequately assess or manage pain among older adults who experience hip fracture. The authors recommended that nurses and other health professionals should continuously assess and better manage pain, which could improve cognition and patient satisfaction.

A major desired outcome for older adults experiencing a hip fracture is to achieve effective preoperative and postoperative pain management while avoiding adverse drug effects. A preoperative alternative to opioid administration is **fascia iliaca compartment block (FICB)**, a regional anesthetic technique using levobupivacaine or other drug to block femoral, lateral cutaneous, and obturator nerves. This procedure avoids the risk of injury to the femoral artery and vein. The benefits of FICB include effective pain relief without opioids and minimal cost (Williams et al., 2019).

Postoperative Care. The treatment of choice is surgical repair by ORIF, when possible, to reduce pain and allow the older patient to be out of bed and ambulatory. While not common, skin (Buck) traction may be applied before surgery to help decrease ***pain*** associated with muscle spasm. Depending on the exact location of the fracture, an ORIF may include an intramedullary rod, pins, prostheses (for femoral head or femoral neck fractures, also known as a *hemiarthroplasty*), or a compression screw. Figs. 47.9 and 47.10 illustrate examples of these devices. Epidural, spinal, or general anesthesia is used. Occasionally a patient will be so debilitated that surgery cannot be done. In these cases, nonsurgical options include pain management and bedrest to allow natural fracture healing.

Before and after a hip repair, older adults frequently experience acute confusion (delirium) (see Chapter 3). They may pull at tubes or the surgical dressing or attempt to climb out of bed, possibly falling and causing self-injury. Other patients stay awake all night and sleep during the day. Keep in mind that some patients have a quiet delirium. Monitor the patient frequently to prevent falls. Use evidence-based fall prevention strategies and ask the family or other visitors to let staff know if the patient is attempting to get out of bed. Chapter 4 describes fall prevention strategies and delirium management in detail.

NURSING SAFETY PRIORITY QSEN

Action Alert

Patients who have a *hemiarthroplasty* are at risk for hip dislocation or subluxation. Be sure to prevent hip adduction and rotation to keep the operative leg in proper alignment. Regular pillows or abduction devices can be used for patients who are confused or restless. If straps are used to hold the device in place, make sure that they are not too tight and check the skin every 2 hours for signs of pressure. Perform neurovascular assessments to ensure that the device is not interfering with arterial circulation or peripheral nerve conduction.

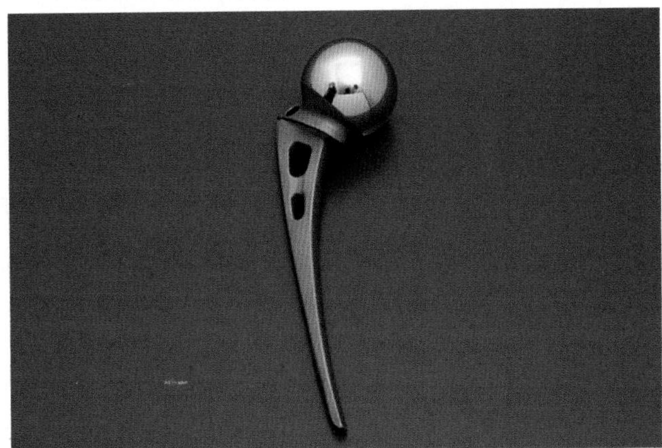

FIG. 47.9 Hip prosthesis used for femoral head or neck fractures (hemiarthroplasty). (Courtesy Smith & Nephew, Inc., Orthopaedics Divisions, Memphis, TN.)

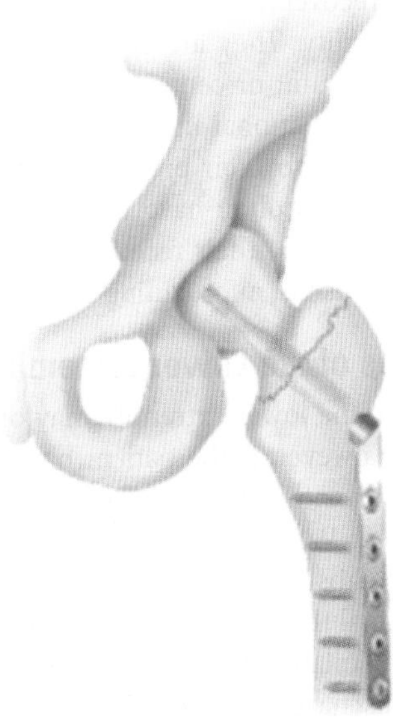

FIG. 47.10 Compression hip screw used for open reduction with internal fixation (ORIF) of the hip.

BEST PRACTICE FOR PATIENT SAFETY AND QUALITY CARE QSEN

Quality Indicators for Postoperative Nursing Care of Older Adults With Fragility Hip Fractures

Nursing Quality Indicator	Nursing Care Best Practice
Timing of Surgery	Ensure that the patient has surgery within 24-48 hours of the fracture, depending on the patient's condition.
Early and Frequent Mobility	Assist the patient to get out of the bed to stand, walk, or sit on the side of the bed on the day of surgery. Walk the patient 1-2 times a day on the first postoperative day.
Malnutrition Prevention	Conduct a nutritional screening on admission. Provide a diet as tolerated with daily oral nutritional supplements postoperatively.
Catheter-Associated Urinary Tract Infection (CAUTI) Prevention	Avoid the use of an indwelling urinary catheter, if possible. If a urinary catheter must be used, the catheter should be removed within 24 hours, if possible.
Pain Management	Use a multimodal pain management approach based on frequent pain assessments. Use geriatric drug dosing and regional nerve blocks if feasible.
Delirium	Complete cognitive screening on admission. Screen the patient each day for delirium.
Pneumonia Prevention	Keep the head of the patient's bed elevated to at least 30 degrees. Perform dysphagia screening and provide frequent mouth care.
Constipation Prevention	Assess daily for bowel movement. Implement an evidence-based bowel protocol, including preventive stool softeners and laxatives.
Venous Thromboembolism (VTE) Prevention	Implement an evidence-based VTE prevention protocol.
Pressure Injury Prevention	Perform a valid pressure injury risk assessment on admission. Perform daily skin assessments. Follow an evidence-based pressure injury prevention protocol/plan of care, including the need to keep the patient's heels off the bed to prevent breakdown.
Care Transitions/Preparing for Home	Provide patient self-management health teaching. Teach the need to follow up with the primary health care provider in 4-6 weeks after discharge.
Bone Health	Teach the patient the need to follow up on his or her bone health to prevent future fractures.

Best practices for care of patients with fragility hip fractures can be summarized by reviewing the 12 internationally accepted nursing quality indicators (MacDonald et al., 2018). These indicators and associated postoperative nursing care are outlined in the Best Practice for Patient Safety & Quality Care: Quality Indicators for Postoperative Nursing Care of Older Adults With Fragility Hip Fractures box.

Many patients recover fully from hip fracture repair and regain their functional ability. They are typically discharged to their home, rehabilitation unit or center, or a skilled nursing facility for physical and occupational therapy. However, some patients are not able to return to their prefracture ADLs and ***mobility*** level. Family caregivers often have unexpected responsibilities caring for patients during their recovery. Hip fracture resource centers can be very useful in providing caregiver support.

Other Fractures of the Lower Extremity

Other fractures of the lower extremity may or may not require hospitalization. However, if the patient has severe or multiple fractures, especially with soft-tissue damage, hospital admission is usually required. Patients who have surgery to repair their injury may also be hospitalized. Coordinate care with the physical and occupational therapists regarding transfers, positioning, and ambulation. Collaborate with the case manager regarding placement after discharge. Most patients go home unless there is no support system or additional rehabilitation is needed. Health teaching and ensuring continuity of care are essential.

Fractures of the *lower two thirds of the femur* usually result from trauma, often from a motor vehicle crash. A femur fracture is seldom immobilized by casting because the powerful muscles of the thigh become spastic, which causes displacement of bone ends and significant pain. Extensive hemorrhage can occur with femur fracture.

Surgical treatment is ORIF with plates, nails, rods, or a compression screw. In a few cases in which extensive bone fragmentation or severe tissue trauma is found, external fixation may be used. Healing time for a femur fracture may be 6 months or longer. Skeletal traction, followed by a full-leg brace or cast, may be used in nonsurgical treatment.

Trauma to the lower leg most often causes fractures of both the *tibia* and the *fibula,* particularly the lower third, and is often referred to as a *tib-fib* fracture. The major treatment techniques are closed reduction with casting, internal fixation, and external fixation. If closed reduction is used, the patient may wear a cast for 6 to 10 weeks. Because of poor ***perfusion*** to parts of the tibia and fibula, delayed union is not unusual with this type of fracture. Internal fixation with nails or a plate and screws, followed by a long-leg cast for 4 to 6 weeks, is another option. Since the fibula is a non–weight-bearing bone, occasionally no fixation is required.

When the fractures cause extensive skin and soft-tissue damage, the initial treatment may be external fixation, often for 6 to 10 weeks, usually followed by application of a cast until the fracture is completely healed. The patient is typically non–weight bearing and uses ambulatory aids such as crutches.

Ankle fractures are described by their anatomic place of injury. For example, a bimalleolar (Pott) fracture involves the medial malleolus of the tibia and the lateral malleolus of the fibula. The small talus that makes up the rest of the ankle joint may also be broken. An ORIF is usually performed using two incisions: one on the medial (inside) aspect of the ankle and one on the lateral (outer) side. Several screws or nails are placed into the tibia, and a compression plate with multiple screws keeps the fibula in alignment. Weight bearing is restricted until the bone heals.

Treatment of fractures of the foot or phalanges (toes) is similar to that of other fractures. Phalangeal fractures may be more painful but are not as serious as most other types of fractures. Crutches are used for ambulation if weight bearing is restricted, but many patients can ambulate while wearing an orthopedic shoe or boot while the bone heals.

FRACTURES OF THE CHEST AND PELVIS

Chest trauma may cause fractures of the ribs or sternum. The major concern with rib and sternal fractures is the potential for puncture of the lungs, heart, or arteries by bone fragments or ends. *Assess airway, breathing, and circulation status **first** for any patient having chest trauma!* Fractures of the lower ribs may damage underlying organs, such as the liver, spleen, or kidneys. These fractures tend to heal on their own without surgical intervention. Patients are often uncomfortable during the healing process and require analgesia. They also have a high risk for pneumonia because of shallow breathing caused by ***pain*** on inspiration. Encourage them to breathe normally if possible and ensure that their pain is well managed.

Because the pelvis is very vascular and is close to major organs and blood vessels, associated internal damage is the major focus in fracture management. After head injuries, pelvic fractures are the second most common cause of death from trauma. In young adults, pelvic fractures typically result from motor vehicle crashes or falls from buildings. Falls are the most common cause in older adults. The major concern related to pelvic injury is venous oozing or arterial bleeding. Loss of blood volume leads to hypovolemic shock.

Assess for internal abdominal trauma by checking for blood in the urine and stool and by monitoring the abdomen for the development of rigidity or swelling. The trauma team may use peritoneal lavage, CT scanning, or ultrasound for assessment of hemorrhage. Ultrasound is noninvasive, rapid, reliable, and cost-effective, and it can be done at the bedside.

There are many classification systems for pelvic fractures. A system that is particularly useful divides fractures of the pelvis into two broad categories: non–weight-bearing fractures and weight-bearing fractures.

When a *non–weight-bearing* part of the pelvis is fractured, such as one of the pubic rami or the iliac crest, treatment can be as minimal as bedrest on a firm mattress or bed board. This type of fracture can be quite painful, and the patient may need stool softeners to facilitate bowel movements because of hesitancy to move. Well-stabilized fractures usually heal in 2 months.

A *weight-bearing* fracture, such as multiple fractures of the pelvic ring creating instability or a fractured acetabulum, necessitates external fixation or ORIF or both. Progression to weight bearing depends on the stability of the fracture after fixation. Some patients can fully bear weight within days of surgery, whereas others managed with traction may not be able to bear weight for as long as 12 weeks. For complex pelvic fractures with extensive soft-tissue damage, external fixation may be required.

COMPRESSION FRACTURES OF THE SPINE

Most vertebral fractures are caused by osteoporosis or metastatic bone cancer. Compression fractures result when trabecular or cancellous bone within the vertebra becomes weakened and causes the vertebral body to collapse. The patient has *severe **pain*** (especially when moving), deformity (kyphosis), and possible neurologic compromise. As discussed in the Osteoporosis section of Chapter 45, the patient's quality of life is reduced by the impact of this problem.

Nonsurgical management includes bedrest, analgesics, nerve blocks, and physical therapy to maintain muscle strength. Vertebral compression fractures (VCFs) that remain painful and impair ***mobility*** may be treated with **vertebroplasty** or kyphoplasty. These procedures are minimally invasive techniques in which bone cement is injected through the skin (percutaneously) directly into the fracture site to provide stability and immediate pain relief. In addition to vertebroplasty, radiologists and orthopedic surgeons may do a kyphoplasty (using a balloon) or the preferred vertebral augmentation (using a different cavity-creating device) to partially re-expand a compressed vertebral body.

Minimally invasive procedures can be done in an operating or interventional radiology suite by a surgeon or interventional radiologist. They can be done with moderate sedation or general anesthesia. IV ketorolac may be given before the procedure to reduce inflammation. Large-bore needles are placed into the fracture site using fluoroscopy or CT guidance. Then the deflated balloon is inserted through the needles and inflated in the fracture site, and the cement is injected.

Patients may have the procedures in an ambulatory care setting and return home after 2 to 4 hours or be admitted to the hospital for an overnight stay. The Best Practice for Patient Safety & Quality Care: Nursing Care for Patients Having Vertebroplasty or Kyphoplasty box outlines the preprocedure and postprocedure care for percutaneous interventions for vertebral compression fractures.

Before discharge, teach the patient to report any signs or symptoms of ***infection*** from puncture sites. Remind him or

BEST PRACTICE FOR PATIENT SAFETY & QUALITY CARE (QSEN)

Nursing Care for Patients Having Vertebroplasty or Kyphoplasty

Provide *preprocedure care,* including:

- Check the patient's coagulation laboratory test results; platelet count should be more than 100,000/mm^3 (100×10^9/L).
- Make sure that all anticoagulant drugs were discontinued as requested by the surgeon or interventional radiologist.
- Assess and document the patient's neurologic status, especially extremity movement and sensation.
- Assess the patient's pain level.
- Assess the patient's ability to lie prone for at least 1 hour.
- Establish an IV line in a size suitable for surgery and take vital signs.

Provide *postprocedure care,* including:

- Place the patient in a flat supine position for 1 to 2 hours or as requested by the surgeon or interventional radiologist.
- Monitor and record vital signs and frequent neurologic assessments; report any change immediately to the physician.
- Apply an ice pack to the puncture site if needed to relieve pain.
- Assess the patient's pain level and compare it with the preoperative level; give mild analgesic as needed.
- Monitor for complications, such as bleeding at the puncture site or shortness of breath; report these findings immediately if they occur.
- Assist the patient with ambulation.

Before discharge, teach the patient and family the following:

- Avoid driving or operating machinery for the first 24 hours because of drugs used during the procedure.
- Monitor the puncture site for signs of infection, such as redness, pain, swelling, or drainage.
- Keep the dressing dry and remove it the next day.
- Begin usual activities, including walking, the next day and should slowly increase activity level over the next few days.

her to not soak in a bath for 1 week, use analgesics as needed, resume activity, and contact the primary health care provider for questions or concerns. Surgery generally reduces preoperative pain significantly.

PERFUSION CONCEPT EXEMPLAR: AMPUTATION

An **amputation** is the removal of a part of the body. Advances in microvascular surgical procedures, better use of antibiotic therapy, and improved surgical techniques for traumatic injury and bone cancer have reduced the number of elective amputations. The psychosocial aspects of the procedure are as devastating as the physical impairments that result. The loss is complete and permanent and causes a change in body image and self-esteem. Collaborate with members of the interprofessional team, including prosthetists, rehabilitation therapists, psychologists, case managers, and physiatrists (rehabilitation physicians), when providing care to the patient who has an amputation.

Pathophysiology Review

Types of Amputation. Amputations may be elective or traumatic. Most are *elective* and are related to complications of peripheral vascular disease (PVD) that result in decreased ***perfusion*** (ischemia) to distal areas of the lower extremity (Schrieber, 2017). Diabetes mellitus is often an underlying cause. Trauma to a limb is the second leading cause of amputation. Amputation is considered only after other interventions have not restored circulation to the lower extremity, sometimes referred to as *limb salvage procedures* (e.g., percutaneous transluminal angioplasty [PTA]). These procedures are discussed elsewhere in this text.

Traumatic amputations most often result from accidents or war and are the primary cause of *upper-extremity* amputation. A person may clean lawn mower blades or a snow blower without disconnecting the machine. A motor vehicle crash or industrial machine accident may also cause an amputation.

PATIENT-CENTERED CARE: VETERANS HEALTH CONSIDERATIONS (QSEN)

The number of traumatic amputations also increases during war as a result of hidden land mines (IEDs), bombs, and motor vehicle accidents (e.g., in Iraq and Afghanistan). Multiple limbs or parts of limbs may be amputated as a result of these devices. Thousands of veterans of war in the United States are amputees and have had to adjust to major changes in their lifestyles. Many veterans have multiple amputations that affect ***mobility,*** ADL functional ability, and psychosocial health.

Levels of Amputation. Elective lower-extremity (LE) amputations are performed much more frequently than upper-extremity amputations. Several types of LE amputations may be performed.

The loss of any or all of the small toes presents a minor disability. Loss of the great toe is significant because it affects balance, gait, and "push-off" ability during walking. Midfoot amputations and the Syme amputation are common procedures for peripheral vascular disease. In the Syme amputation, most of the foot is removed, but the ankle remains. The advantage of this surgery over traditional amputations below the knee is that weight bearing can occur without the use of a prosthesis and with reduced pain.

An intense effort is made to preserve knee joints with below-the-knee amputation (BKA). When the cause for the amputation extends beyond the knee, above-knee or higher amputations are performed. Hip disarticulation, or removal of the hip joint, and hemipelvectomy (removal of half of the pelvis with the leg) are more common in younger patients than in older ones who cannot easily handle the cumbersome prostheses required for ambulation. The higher the level of amputation, the more energy is required for ***mobility.*** These higher-level procedures are sometimes done for cancer of the bone, osteomyelitis, or trauma as a last resort.

An amputation of any part of the upper extremity is generally more incapacitating than one of the leg. The arms and hands are necessary for ADLs such as feeding, bathing, dressing, and driving a car. In the upper extremity, as much length as possible is saved to maintain function. Early replacement with a prosthetic device is vital for the patient with this type of amputation.

PATIENT-CENTERED CARE: CULTURAL/ SPIRITUAL CONSIDERATIONS QSEN

The incidence of lower-extremity amputations is greater in black populations than white populations, especially in men who have diabetes mellitus (McCance et al., 2019). Limited access to health care, lack of health insurance, and health care belief systems may play a major role in limb loss from long-term diseases in this population.

Complications of Amputation. The most common complications of amputations are:

- Hemorrhage leading to hypovolemic shock
- ***Infection***
- Phantom limb ***pain***
- Neuroma
- Flexion contractures

When a person loses part or all of an extremity either by surgery or by trauma, major blood vessels are severed, which causes *hemorrhage*. If the bleeding is uncontrolled, the patient is at risk for hypovolemic shock and possibly death.

As with any surgical procedure or trauma, infection can occur in the wound or the bone (osteomyelitis). The older adult who is malnourished and confused is at the greatest risk because excreta may soil the wound or he or she may remove the dressing and pick at the incision. Preventing ***infection*** is a major emphasis in hospitals and other health care settings.

Persistent ***pain*** is a frequent complication of amputation. This sensation is felt in the amputated part immediately after surgery and usually diminishes over time. When it persists and is unpleasant or painful, it is referred to as **phantom limb pain (PLP)**. PLP is more common in patients who had chronic limb pain before surgery and less common in those who have traumatic amputations. The patient reports pain in the removed body part shortly after surgery, usually after an above-the-knee amputation (AKA). The ***pain*** is often described as intense burning, crushing, or cramping. Some patients report that the removed part is in a distorted, uncomfortable position. They experience numbness and tingling, referred to as *phantom limb sensation,* and pain. Others state that the most distal area of the removed part feels as if it is retracted into the residual limb end. For most patients, the pain is triggered by touching the residual limb or by temperature or barometric pressure changes, concurrent illness, fatigue, anxiety, or stress. Routine activities such as urination can trigger the pain. If ***pain*** is long-standing, especially if it existed before the amputation, any stimulus can cause it, including touching any part of the body.

Neuroma, a sensitive tumor consisting of damaged nerve cells, forms most often in amputations of the upper extremity but can occur anywhere. The patient may or may not have pain. It is diagnosed by sonography and can be treated either surgically or nonsurgically. Surgery to remove the neuroma may be performed, but it often regrows and is more painful than before the surgery. Nonsurgical modalities include peripheral nerve blocks, steroid injections, and cognitive therapies such as hypnosis.

Flexion contractures of the hip or knee are most frequently seen in patients with amputations of the lower extremity. This complication must be avoided so that the patient can ambulate with a prosthetic device. Proper positioning and active range-of-motion exercises in the early postoperative period help prevent this complication.

Health Promotion and Maintenance

The typical patient undergoing elective amputation is a middle-age or older man with diabetes and a lengthy history of smoking. He most likely has not cared for his feet properly, which has resulted in a nonhealing, infected foot ulcer and possibly gangrene. Therefore adherence to the disease management plan may help prevent the need for later amputation. Lifestyle habits such as maintaining a healthy weight, regular exercise, and avoiding smoking can help prevent chronic diseases such as diabetes and poor blood circulation.

The second largest group who has amputations consists of young men who have motorcycle or other vehicular crashes, are injured by industrial equipment, or have been in combat or accidents in war. These men may either experience a traumatic amputation or undergo a surgical amputation because of a severe crushing injury and massive soft-tissue damage. Teach young male adults the importance of taking safety precautions to prevent injury at work and to avoid speeding or driving while drinking alcohol. An increasing number of young women also tend to speed and drive while drinking, which endangers themselves and others around them.

❖ Interprofessional Collaborative Care

◆ Assessment: Recognize Cues

Physical Assessment/Signs and Symptoms. Monitor neurovascular status in the affected extremity that will be electively amputated. When the patient has peripheral vascular disease, check circulation in both legs. Assess skin color, temperature, sensation, and pulses in both affected and unaffected extremities. Capillary refill can be difficult to determine in the older adult related to thickened and opaque nails. In this situation, the skin near the nail bed can be used. Capillary refill is not as reliable as other indicators. Observe and document any discoloration of the skin, edema, ulcerations, presence of necrosis, and hair distribution on the lower extremities.

Psychosocial Assessment. People react differently to the loss of a body part. Be aware that an amputation of only a portion of one finger, especially the thumb, can be traumatic to the patient. The thumb is needed for hand activities. Therefore the loss must not be underestimated. Patients undergoing amputation face a complete, permanent loss. Evaluate their psychological preparation for a planned amputation and expect them to go through the grieving process. Adjusting to a traumatic, unexpected amputation is often more difficult than accepting a planned one.

PATIENT-CENTERED CARE: VETERANS HEALTH CONSIDERATIONS QSEN

The young veteran may be bitter, hostile, and depressed. In addition to loss of a body part, he or she may lose a job, the ability to participate in favorite recreational activities, or a social relationship if other people cannot accept the body change.

The patient having one or more amputations has an altered self-concept. The physical alterations that result affect body image and self-esteem. For example, a young male may think that an intimate relationship with a partner is no longer possible or desirable. An older adult may feel a loss of independence. Assess the patient's feelings about himself or herself to identify areas in which he or she needs emotional support. Consult with the certified hospital chaplain, other spiritual leader, or hospital social worker if the patient is hospitalized. Counseling resources are also available in the community and the Veterans' Administration health system in the United States.

Attempt to determine the patient's willingness and motivation to withstand prolonged rehabilitation after the amputation. Asking questions about how he or she has dealt with previous life crises can provide clues. Adjustment to the amputation and rehabilitation is less difficult if the patient is willing to make needed changes.

PATIENT-CENTERED CARE: CULTURAL/ SPIRITUAL CONSIDERATIONS QSEN

In addition to assessing the patient's psychosocial status, assess the family's reaction to the surgery or trauma. Their response usually correlates directly with the patient's progress during recovery and rehabilitation and his or her values and beliefs. Expect the family to grieve for the loss and allow them time to adjust to the change. Establish a trusting relationship and reassure the patient and family that you are available to listen to their concerns and needs.

Assess the patient's and family's coping abilities and help them identify personal strengths and weaknesses. Assess the patient's religious, spiritual, and cultural beliefs. Some groups (e.g., Jewish) require that the amputated body part be stored for later burial with the rest of the body or buried immediately. Other cultural customs and rituals may apply, depending on the group with which the patient associates.

Diagnostic Assessment. The surgeon determines which tests are performed to assess for viability of the limb based on blood flow. A large number of noninvasive techniques are available for this evaluation. For complete accuracy, the surgeon does not rely on any single test.

One procedure is measurement of segmental limb blood pressures, which can also be used by the nurse at the bedside. In this test, an **ankle-brachial index (ABI)** is calculated by dividing ankle systolic pressure by brachial systolic pressure. A normal ABI is 0.9 or higher.

Blood flow in an extremity can also be assessed by other noninvasive tests, including *Doppler* ultrasonography or laser Doppler flowmetry and transcutaneous oxygen pressure ($TcPO_2$). The ultrasonography and laser Doppler measure the speed of blood flow in the limb. The $TcPO_2$ measures oxygen pressure to indicate blood flow in the limb and has proven reliable for predicting healing.

◆ Analysis: Analyze Cues and Prioritize Hypotheses

The collaborative problems for patients with amputations include:

1. Potential for decreased tissue ***perfusion*** in residual limb due to soft tissue damage, edema, and/or bleeding
2. Acute and/or persistent ***pain*** due to soft-tissue damage, muscle spasm, and edema
3. Decreased ***mobility*** due to pain, muscle spasm, soft-tissue damage, and/or lack of balance due to a missing body part
4. Decreased self-esteem due to one or more ADL deficits, disturbed self-concept and body image, and/or lack of support systems

◆ Planning and Implementation: Generate Solutions and Take Action

Monitoring for Decreased Tissue Perfusion

Planning: Expected Outcomes. The patient with one or more amputations is expected to have adequate peripheral ***perfusion*** to the residual (surgical) limb(s) as evidenced by warm, usual-color skin.

Interventions. A *traumatic* amputation requires rapid emergency care to possibly save the severed body part for reattachment to promote ***perfusion*** and prevent hemorrhage.

Emergency Care: Traumatic vs. Elective Amputation. For a person who has a *traumatic amputation* in the community, first call 911. Assess the patient for airway or breathing problems. Examine the amputation site and apply direct pressure with layers of dry gauze or other cloth, using clean gloves if available. Many nurses carry gloves and first-aid kits for this type of emergency. Elevate the extremity above the patient's heart to decrease the bleeding. Do not remove the dressing to prevent dislodging the clot.

The fingers are the most likely part to be amputated and replanted. The current recommendation for prehospital care is to wrap the completely severed finger in dry sterile gauze (if available) or a clean cloth. Put the finger in a watertight, sealed plastic bag. *Place the bag in ice water, never directly on ice, at 1 part ice and 3 parts water.* Avoid contact between the finger and the water to prevent tissue damage. Do not remove any semidetached parts of the digit. Be sure that the part goes with the patient to the hospital.

For patients with a *planned surgical amputation,* the nurse's primary focus is to monitor for signs indicating that there is sufficient tissue ***perfusion*** and no hemorrhage. The skin flap at the end of the residual (remaining) limb should be pink in a light-skinned person and not discolored (lighter or darker than other usual skin pigmentation) in a dark-skinned patient. The area should be warm but not hot. Assess the closest proximal pulse for presence and strength and compare it with that in the other extremity. However, if the patient has bilateral vascular disease, comparison of limbs may not be an accurate way of measuring blood flow. Use a Doppler device to determine if the affected side is being perfused. Monitor vital signs per agency protocol.

! NURSING SAFETY PRIORITY (QSEN)

Critical Rescue

If the patient has decreased tissue **perfusion**, notify the surgeon or Rapid Response Team immediately to communicate your assessment findings! If the patient's blood pressure drops and the pulse increases, suspect covert (hidden) bleeding. To check for the presence of overt (obvious) bleeding, be sure to lift the residual limb and feel under the pressure dressing for dampness or drainage. If bleeding occurs, apply direct pressure and notify the Rapid Response Team or primary health care provider immediately. Continue to monitor the patient until help arrives.

Managing Acute and/or Persistent Pain

Planning: Expected Outcomes. The patient with an amputation is expected to state that he or she has adequate ***pain*** control after appropriate management.

Interventions. All patients experience ***pain*** as a result of either a traumatic or surgical (elective) amputation. Some patients also report pain in the missing body part (phantom limb pain [PLP]). Be sure to determine which type the patient has, because they are managed very differently.

! NURSING SAFETY PRIORITY (QSEN)

Action Alert

If the patient reports PLP, recognize that the ***pain*** is real and should be managed promptly and completely! It is *not* therapeutic to remind the patient that the limb cannot be hurting because it is missing. To prevent increased pain, handle the residual limb carefully when assessing the site or changing the dressing (Schreiber, 2017).

Opioid analgesics are not as effective for PLP as they are for residual limb pain. IV infusions of calcitonin during the week after amputation can reduce PLP. The primary health care provider prescribes other drugs on the basis of the type of PLP the patient experiences. For instance, beta-blocking agents such as propranolol are used for constant, dull, burning pain. Antiepileptic drugs such as pregabalin and gabapentin may be used for knifelike or sharp burning (neuropathic) pain. Antispasmodics such as baclofen may be prescribed for muscle spasms or cramping. Some patients improve with antidepressant drugs as adjuvant therapy.

Other pain management modalities are described in Chapter 5. Incorporate them into the plan of care if agreeable with the patient by collaborating with specialists who are trained to perform them. For example, physical therapists often use massage, heat, transcutaneous electrical nerve stimulation (TENS), mirror therapy, and ultrasound therapy for pain control. Yildirim & Sen (2020) found that mirror therapy, in which the patient regularly practices exercises with the affected and unaffected extremity in front of a mirror, helps to decrease phantom limb pain.

Consult with the certified hospital chaplain or social worker to provide emotional support based on the patient's preferences and beliefs. A psychologist may be needed to provide diagnostic assessment and/or psychotherapy.

NCLEX EXAMINATION CHALLENGE 47.3

Psychosocial Integrity

A client who had an elective below-the-knee amputation (BKA) reports pain in the foot that was amputated last week. What is the nurse's **most appropriate** response to the client's pain?

A. "The pain will go away after the swelling decreases."
B. "That's phantom limb pain, and every amputee has that."
C. "Your foot has been amputated, so it's in your head."
D. "On a scale of 0 to 10, how would you rate your pain?"

Promoting Mobility

Planning: Expected Outcomes. The patient with an amputation is expected to have adequate ***Mobility*** and be free of complications associated with decreased mobility.

Interventions. Collaborate with the physical and/or occupational therapists to begin exercises as soon as possible after surgery. If the amputation is planned, the therapist may work with the patient before surgery to start muscle-strengthening exercises and evaluate the need for ambulatory aids, such as crutches. If the patient can practice with these devices before surgery, learning how to ambulate after surgery is much easier.

INTERPROFESSIONAL COLLABORATION

Care of Patients Who Have an Amputation

Interprofessional collaborative care depends on the type and location of the amputation. For example, an above-the-knee amputation (AKA) has the potential for more postoperative complications than does a partial foot amputation. Regardless of where the amputation occurs, collaborate with the rehabilitation therapists to improve ambulation and/or enable the patient to be independent in ADLs. For many amputations, prostheses can be used to substitute for the missing body part.

According to the Interprofessional Education Collaborative (IPEC) Expert Panel's Competency of Roles and Responsibilities, using the unique and complementary abilities of other team members optimizes health and patient care (Slusser et al., 2019).

For patients with AKAs or BKAs, teach range-of-motion (ROM) exercises for prevention of flexion contractures, particularly of the hip and knee. A trapeze and an overhead frame aid in strengthening the arms and allow the patient to move independently in bed. Teach the patient how to perform ROM exercises. Be sure to turn the patient every 2 hours or teach him or her to turn independently. Move the patient slowly to prevent muscle spasms.

A firm mattress is essential for preventing contractures with a leg amputation. Assist the patient into a prone position every 3 to 4 hours for 20- to 30-minute periods if tolerated and not contraindicated. This position may be uncomfortable initially but helps prevent hip flexion contractures. Instruct the patient to pull the residual limb close to the other leg and contract the gluteal muscles of the buttocks for muscle strengthening. After staples are removed, the physical therapist may begin resistive exercises, which should also be done at home.

For above- and below-the-knee amputations, teach the patient how to push the residual limb down toward the bed while supporting it on a soft pillow at first. Then instruct him or her to continue this activity using a firmer pillow and then progress to a harder surface. This activity helps prepare the residual limb for prosthesis and reduces the incidence of phantom limb ***pain*** and sensation.

Elevation of a lower-leg residual limb on a pillow while the patient is in a supine position is controversial. Some practitioners advocate avoiding this practice at all times because it promotes hip or knee flexion contracture. Others allow elevation for the first 24 to 48 hours to reduce swelling and subsequent ***pain.*** Inspect the residual limb daily to ensure that it lies completely flat on the bed.

Before an elective amputation, the patient often sees a certified prosthetist-orthotist (CPO) so that planning can begin for the postoperative period. Arrangements for replacing an arm part are especially important for the patient to achieve self-management. Some patients are fitted with a temporary prosthesis at the time of surgery. Others, particularly older patients with vascular disease, are fitted after the residual limb has healed.

The patient being fitted for a leg prosthesis should bring a sturdy pair of shoes to the fitting. The prosthesis will be adjusted to that heel height.

Several devices help shape and shrink the residual limb in preparation for the prosthesis. Rigid, removable dressings are preferred because they decrease edema, protect and shape the limb, and allow easy access to the wound for inspection. An air splint, a plastic inflatable device, is sometimes used for this purpose. One of its disadvantages is air leakage and loss of compression. Wrapping with elastic bandages can also be effective in reducing edema, shrinking the limb, and holding the wound dressing in place.

For wrapping to be effective, reapply the bandages every 4 to 6 hours or more often if they become loose. *Figure-eight wrapping prevents restriction of blood flow. Decrease the tightness of the bandages while wrapping in a distal-to-proximal direction.* After wrapping, anchor the bandages to the highest joint, such as above the knee for BKAs.

The design of and materials for prostheses have improved dramatically over the years. Computer-assisted design and manufacturing (CAD-CAM) is used for a custom fit. One of the most important developments in lower-extremity prosthetics is the ankle-foot prosthesis, such as the Flex-Foot for more active amputees.

Promoting Self-Esteem

Planning: Expected Outcomes. The patient with an amputation is expected to adapt to the amputation to achieve a positive self-esteem and have an active and productive life.

Interventions. The patient often experiences feelings of inadequacy as a result of losing a body part, especially the older adult who was in poor health before surgery and men who are often the main providers for their families. If the patient is not able to adapt psychologically to the amputation, he or she may have difficulty adapting to a possible lifestyle change. If possible, arrange for him or her to meet with a rehabilitated, active amputee who is about the same age as the patient.

Freysteinson et al. (2016) studied a technique to help amputees get used to their body change as part of rehabilitation therapy. The authors asked the patients to view themselves in a mirror for repeated viewings. Four key themes emerged as a result of the study: mirror shock, mirror anguish, recognizing self, and acceptance as a new "normal." These themes are similar to other loss and grieving responses (see Chapter 8).

Use of the word *stump* for referring to the remaining portion of the limb (residual limb) continues to be controversial. Patients have reported feeling as if they were part of a tree when the term was used. However, some rehabilitation specialists who routinely work with amputees believe the term is appropriate because it forces the patient to realize what has happened and promotes adjustment to the amputation. *Assess the patient to determine which term he or she prefers.*

Assess the patient's verbal and nonverbal references to the affected area. Some patients behave euphorically (extremely happy) and seem to have accepted the loss. *Do not jump to the conclusion that acceptance has occurred.* Ask the patient to describe his or her feelings about changes in body image and self-esteem. He or she may verbalize acceptance but refuse to look at the area during a dressing change. This inconsistent behavior is not unusual and should be documented and shared with other health care team members.

With advancements in prostheses and surgical techniques, most patients can return to their jobs and other activities. Professional athletes who use prostheses are often quite successful in sports. Patients with amputations ski, hike, golf, bowl, and participate in other physically demanding activities. Many amputees participate actively in organized and recreational sports.

If a job or career change is necessary, collaborate with a social worker or vocational rehabilitation specialist to evaluate the patient's skills. A supportive family or significant other is important for the adjustment to this change. The patient may also think that an intimate relationship is no longer possible because of physical changes. Discuss sexuality issues with the patient and his or her partner as needed. Professional assistance from a sex therapist, intimacy coach, or psychologist may be needed.

Help the patient and family set realistic desired outcomes and take one day at a time. Help them recognize personal strengths. If the desired outcomes are not realistic, frustration and disappointment may decrease motivation during rehabilitation. Basic principles of rehabilitation are discussed in Chapter 7.

Care Coordination and Transition Management. The patient is discharged directly to home or to a skilled facility or rehabilitation facility, depending on the extent of the amputation. When rehabilitation is not feasible, as in the debilitated or demented older adult, he or she may be discharged to a long-term care facility. Coordinate this transfer with the case manager or discharge planner to ensure continuity of care.

Home Care Management. At home, the patient with a leg amputation needs to have enough room to use a wheelchair if the prosthesis is not yet available. He or she must be able to use toileting facilities and have access to areas necessary for self-management, such as the kitchen. Structural home modifications may be required before the patient goes home.

Self-Management Education. After the sutures or staples are removed, the patient begins residual limb care. A home care nurse may be needed to teach the patient and/or family how to care for the limb and the prosthesis if it is available (see the Home Care Considerations: The Patient With a Lower-Extremity Amputation in the Home box).

HOME CARE CONSIDERATIONS

The Patient With a Lower-Extremity Amputation in the Home

Assess the residual limb for:
- Adequate circulation
- ***Infection***
- Healing
- Flexion contracture
- Dressing/elastic wrap

Assess the patient's ability to perform ADLs in the home.
- Evaluate the patient's ability to use ambulatory aids and care for the prosthetic device (if available).
- Assess the patient's pain level (intensity and quality).
- Assess the patient's nutritional status.
- Assess the patient's ability to cope with body image change.

The limb should be rewrapped several times a day with an elastic bandage applied in a figure-eight manner. For many patients, a shrinker stocking or sock is easier to apply. After the limb is healed, it is cleaned each day with the rest of the body during bathing with soap and water. Teach the patient and/or family to inspect it every day for signs of inflammation or skin breakdown.

NURSING SAFETY PRIORITY QSEN

Action Alert

Collaborate with the prosthetist to teach the patient about prosthesis care after amputation to ensure its reliability and proper function. These devices are custom made, taking into account the patient's level of amputation, lifestyle, and occupation. Proper teaching regarding correct cleansing of the socket and inserts, wearing the correct liners, and assessing shoe wear and a schedule of follow-up care are essential before discharge. This information may need to be reviewed by the home care nurse.

Health Care Resources. A patient who seems to adjust to the amputation during hospitalization may realize that it is difficult to cope with the loss after discharge from the hospital. Teach the patient and family about available resources and support from organizations such as the Amputee Coalition of America (ACA) (www.amputee-coalition.org) and the National Amputation Foundation (NAF) (www.nationalamputation.org). The NAF was originally started for veterans but has since expanded to offer services to civilians.

PATIENT-CENTERED CARE: VETERANS HEALTH CONSIDERATIONS QSEN

Teach patients who are veterans about the many resources that can help them adjust to one or more amputations. In addition to specialty clinics and other services offered by the Veterans Administration in the United States, many other community and military services exist to help veterans adapt their lifestyle and remain active. Many of these services also assist families of veterans who have been injured (Table 47.2).

◆ **Evaluation: Evaluate Outcomes.** Evaluate the care of the patient with one or more amputations based on the identified priority patient problems. The expected outcomes include that the patient:
- Have adequate ***perfusion*** to the residual limb
- State that ***pain*** is controlled to between a 2 and 3 or as acceptable to the patient on a 0 to 10 pain intensity assessment scale
- Perform ***mobility*** skills independently and not experience complications of decreased mobility
- Be free of surgical site ***infection***
- Have a positive self-esteem and lifestyle adaptation to live a productive, high-quality life

CARPAL TUNNEL SYNDROME

Pathophysiology Review

Carpal tunnel syndrome (CTS) is a common condition in which the median nerve in the wrist becomes compressed, causing pain and numbness (Durham & VanRavenstein, 2017). The carpal tunnel is a rigid canal that lies between the carpal bones and a fibrous tissue sheet. A group of tendons surround the synovium and share space with the median nerve in the carpal tunnel. When the synovium becomes swollen or thickened, this nerve is compressed.

The median nerve supplies motor, sensory, and autonomic function for the first three fingers of the hand and the palmar aspect of the fourth (ring) finger. Because the median nerve is close to other structures, wrist flexion causes nerve impingement and extension causes increased pressure in the lower portion of the carpal tunnel.

CTS is the most common type of repetitive stress injury (RSI). RSIs are the fastest-growing type of occupational injury. People whose jobs require repetitive hand activities, such as pinching or grasping during wrist flexion (e.g., factory workers, computer operators, jackhammer operators), are predisposed to CTS. In more recent years, young adults have an increased incidence of CTS due to texting and other cell phone use. It can also result from overuse in sports activities such as golf, tennis, or racquetball.

CTS usually presents as a chronic problem. Acute cases are rare. Excessive hand exercise, edema or hemorrhage into the carpal tunnel, or thrombosis of the median artery can lead to acute CTS. *Patients with hand burns or a Colles fracture of the wrist are particularly at risk for this problem.* In most cases, the cause may not result in nerve deficit for years.

TABLE 47.2 Examples of Military and Community Resources for Veterans With Amputations in the United States

Resource	Website Address
Hope for the Warriors™	www.hopeforthewarriors.org
Military OneSource	www.militaryonesource.com
U.S. Army Wounded Warrior Program	www.aw2.army.mil
Veterans Administration	www.va.gov
Amputee Coalition of America	www.amputee-coalition.org
Wounded Warrior Project	www.woundedwarriorproject.org
American Amputee Foundation	www.americanamputee.org
Amputee Resources for Canada	www.amputee.ca

CTS is also a common complication of certain metabolic and connective tissue diseases. For example, synovitis (inflammation of the synovium) occurs in patients with rheumatoid arthritis (RA). The hypertrophied synovium compresses the median nerve. In other chronic disorders such as diabetes mellitus, inadequate blood supply can cause median nerve neuropathy or dysfunction, resulting in CTS.

In a few cases, CTS may be a familial or congenital problem that manifests in adulthood. Space-occupying growths such as ganglia, tophi, and lipomas can also result in nerve compression.

PATIENT-CENTERED CARE: GENDER HEALTH CONSIDERATIONS QSEN

Women, especially those older than 50 years, are much more likely than men to experience CTS, probably due to the higher prevalence of diseases such as RA in women. The problem usually affects the dominant hand but can occur in both hands simultaneously. CTS is beginning to be found in children and adolescents as a result of the increased use of cell phones and other handheld mobile devices (Durham & VanRavenstein, 2017).

Health Promotion and Maintenance

Most businesses recognize the hazards of repetitive motion as a primary cause of occupational injury and disability. Both men and women in the labor force are experiencing increasing numbers of RSIs. Occupational health nurses have played an important role in ergonomics and in the development of ergonomically designed furniture and various aids to decrease CTS and other musculoskeletal injuries. **Ergonomics** is the study of how equipment and furniture can be arranged so that people can do work or other activities more efficiently and comfortably without injury.

U.S. federal and state legislation has been passed to ensure that all businesses, including health care organizations (HCOs), provide *ergonomically appropriate workstations* for their employees (Occupational Safety and Health Administration [OSHA]). The Joint Commission also requires that hospitals and other HCOs provide a safe work environment for all staff. In Canada, each province requires the work setting to have joint health and safety committees in which employees are actively involved in setting safety standards (Canadian Centre for Occupational Health and Safety). The Best Practice for Patient Safety & Quality Care: Health Promotion Activities to Prevent Carpal Tunnel Syndrome box lists best practices for preventing CTS in the health care setting.

BEST PRACTICE FOR PATIENT SAFETY & QUALITY CARE QSEN

Health Promotion Activities to Prevent Carpal Tunnel Syndrome

- Become familiar with federal and state laws regarding workplace requirements to prevent repetitive stress injuries such as carpal tunnel syndrome (CTS).
- When using equipment or computer workstations that can contribute to developing CTS, assess that they are ergonomically appropriate, including:
  - Specially designed wrist rest devices
  - Geometrically designed computer keyboards
  - Chair height that allows good posture
- Take regular short breaks away from activities that cause repetitive stress, such as working at computers and using cell phones and other handheld devices.
- Stretch fingers and wrists frequently during work hours.
- Stay as relaxed as possible when using equipment that causes repetitive stress.

❖ Interprofessional Collaborative Care

◆ **Assessment: Recognize Cues.** A diagnosis is often made based on the patient's history and report of hand pain and numbness and without further assessment. Ask about the nature, intensity, and location of the pain. Patients often state that the pain is worse at night as a result of flexion or direct pressure during sleep. The pain may radiate to the arm, shoulder and neck, or chest.

In addition to reports of numbness, patients with carpal tunnel syndrome (CTS) may also have paresthesia (painful numbness and tingling). *Sensory* changes usually occur weeks or months before *motor* manifestations.

The primary health care provider performs several tests for abnormal sensory findings. The Phalen wrist test, sometimes called **Phalen maneuver**, produces paresthesia in the median nerve distribution (palmar side of the thumb, index and middle fingers, and half of the ring finger) within 60 seconds as a result of increased internal carpal pressure. The patient is asked to relax the wrist into flexion or to place the back of the hands together and flex both wrists at the same time. The Phalen test is positive in most patients with CTS (Jarvis, 2018).

Motor changes in CTS begin with a weak pinch, clumsiness, and difficulty with fine movements. These changes progress to muscle weakness and wasting, which can impair self-management. If desired, test for pinching ability and ask the patient to perform a fine-movement task, such as threading a needle. Strenuous hand activity worsens the pain and numbness (McCance et al., 2019).

In addition to inspecting for muscle atrophy and task performance, observe the wrist for swelling. Gently palpate the area and note any unusual findings. Autonomic changes may be evidenced by skin discoloration, nail changes (e.g., brittleness), and increased or decreased hand sweating.

◆ **Interventions: Take Action.** The primary health care provider uses conservative measures before surgical intervention. However, CTS can recur with either type of treatment. Management depends on the patient, but established best practices have not been determined.

Nonsurgical Management. Aggressive drug therapy and immobilization of the wrist are the major components of nonsurgical management. Teach the patient the importance of these modalities in the hope of preventing surgical intervention.

NSAIDs are the most commonly prescribed drugs for the relief of ***pain*** and inflammation, if present, but they do not slow the progression of CTS (Blevins, 2020). In addition to or instead of systemic medications, the primary health care provider may inject corticosteroids directly into the carpal tunnel. If the patient responds to the injection, several additional weekly or monthly injections are given. Teach him or her to take NSAIDs with or after meals to reduce gastric irritation.

A splint or hand brace may be used to immobilize the wrist during the day, during the night, or both. Many patients experience temporary relief with these devices. The occupational therapist places the wrist in the neutral position or in slight extension.

Laser or ultrasound therapy may also be helpful. Some patients report fewer symptoms after beginning yoga or another exercise routine. For some patients, wrist-stretching exercises are recommended, including wrist extension and flexion stretches (Blevins, 2020).

Surgical Management. Surgery can relieve the pressure on the median nerve by providing nerve decompression to prevent irreversible damage for patients with extended cases of CTS. Major surgical complications are rare after CTS surgery.

The nurse in the surgeon's office or same-day surgical center reinforces the teaching provided by the surgeon regarding the nature of the surgery. Postoperative care is reviewed so that the patient knows what to expect. Chapter 9 describes general preoperative care in detail.

Whatever the cause of nerve compression, the surgeon removes it by either cutting or laser. The most common surgery is the endoscopic carpal tunnel release (ECTR). In this procedure, the surgeon makes a very small incision (less than ½ inch [1.2 cm]) through which the endoscope is inserted. He or she then uses special instruments to free the trapped median nerve. Although ECTR is less invasive and costs less than the open procedure, the patient may have a longer period of postoperative pain and numbness compared with recovery from open carpal tunnel release (OCTR). Surgical treatment seems to be more effective than conservative measures over the long term. However, there is no evidence that one type of procedure, open or endoscopic, is more effective than the other; it is basically surgeon preference (Durham & VanRavenstein, 2017).

After surgery, monitor vital signs and check the dressing carefully for drainage and tightness. If ECTR has been performed, the dressing is very small. The surgeon may require that the patient's affected hand and arm be elevated above heart level for several days to reduce postoperative swelling. Check the neurovascular status of the fingers every hour during the immediate postoperative period and encourage the patient to move them frequently. Offer pain medication and assure him or her that a prescription for analgesics will be provided before discharge. Discomfort should not last more than 24 to 72 hours (Blevins, 2020).

Hand movements, including lifting heavy objects, may be restricted for 4 to 6 weeks after surgery. The patient can expect weakness for weeks or perhaps months. Teach him or her to report any changes in neurovascular status, including increased pain, bleeding, or infection, to the surgeon's office immediately.

Remind the patient and family that the surgical procedure might not be a cure. For example, synovitis may recur with rheumatoid arthritis and may recompress the median nerve. Multiple surgeries and other treatments are common with CTS.

The patient may need help with self-management activities during recovery. Ensure that assistance in the home is available before discharge; this is usually provided by the family or significant others.

BEST PRACTICE FOR PATIENT SAFETY & QUALITY CARE (QSEN)

Emergency Care of Patients With Sports-Related Injuries

- Do not move the victim until spinal cord injury is ascertained (see Chapter 40 for assessment of spinal cord injury).
- Use RICE:
  - **Rest** the injured part; immobilize the joint above and below the injury by applying a splint if needed.
  - Apply **ice** intermittently for the first 24 to 48 hours (heat may be used thereafter).
  - Use **compression** for the first 24 to 48 hours (e.g., elastic wrap).
  - **Elevate** the affected limb to decrease swelling.
- Always assume that the area is fractured until x-ray studies are done.
- Assess neurovascular status in the area distal to the injury.

NCLEX EXAMINATION CHALLENGE 47.4

Safe and Effective Care Environment

What is the nurse's **priority** when doing an admission for a client who returned directly from the operating suite after a carpal tunnel repair?

A. Monitor vital signs, including pulse oximetry.
B. Check the surgical dressing to ensure that it is intact.
C. Assess neurovascular assessment in the affected arm.
D. Monitor intake and output.

KNEE INJURIES

In addition to the bone and muscle problems already discussed, trauma can cause cartilage, ligament, and tendon injury. Many musculoskeletal injuries are the result of playing sports (professional and recreational) or doing other strenuous physical activities. The popularity of all-terrain vehicles (ATVs) and skateboarding has increased injuries in younger patients. Sports injuries have become so common that large metropolitan hospitals have sports medicine clinics and physicians who specialize in this field.

The principles of injury to one part of the body are similar to those of other sports injuries and accidents. For example, a tendon rupture in a knee is cared for in the same manner as a tendon rupture in the wrist. The Best Practice for Patient Safety & Quality Care box lists general emergency measures for sports-related injuries.

Because the knee is most often injured, it is discussed as a typical example of other areas of the body. Trauma to the knee results in *internal derangement,* a broad term for disturbances of an injured knee joint. When surgery is required to resolve the problem, most surgeons prefer to perform the procedure through an arthroscope when possible. A description of arthroscopy is presented in Chapter 44. Postoperative care for knee surgeries generally includes analgesics, physical therapy, and bracing or splinting, often using a knee immobilizer (Fig. 47.11). All patients require frequent neurovascular monitoring. Table 47.3 lists examples of common knee injuries and their interprofessional management.

ROTATOR CUFF INJURIES

The musculotendinous, or rotator, cuff of the shoulder functions to stabilize the head of the humerus in the glenoid cavity during shoulder abduction. Young adults usually sustain a tear of the cuff by substantial trauma, such as may occur during a fall, while throwing a ball, or with heavy lifting. Older adults tend to have small tears related to aging, repetitive motions, or falls, and the tears are usually painless.

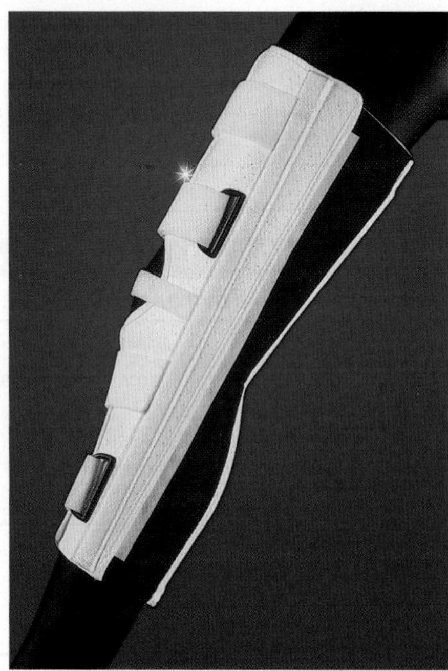

FIG. 47.11 Knee immobilizer. (Courtesy Zimmer, Inc., Warsaw, IN.)

The patient with a torn rotator cuff has shoulder ***pain*** and cannot easily abduct the arm at the shoulder. When the arm is abducted, he or she usually drops it because abduction cannot be maintained (drop arm test). Pain is more intense at night and with overhead activities. Partial-thickness tears are more painful than full-thickness tears, but full-thickness tears result in more weakness and loss of function. Muscle atrophy is commonly seen, and ***mobility*** is reduced. Diagnosis is confirmed with x-rays, MRI, ultrasonography, and/or CT scans.

The primary health care provider usually treats the patient with partial-thickness tears conservatively with NSAIDs, intermittent steroid injections, physical therapy, and activity limitations while the tear heals. Physical therapy treatments may include ultrasound, electrical stimulation, ice, and heat.

For patients who do not respond to conservative treatment in 3 to 6 months or for those who have a complete (full-thickness) tear, the surgeon repairs the cuff using mini-open or arthroscopic procedures. An interscalene nerve block may be used to extend analgesia for an open repair. If a peripheral nerve block is used, remind the patient that the arm will feel numb and cannot be moved for up to 20 or more hours after surgery. Observe, report, and document complications of respiratory distress and neurovascular compromise.

After surgery, the affected arm is usually immobilized for several weeks. Pendulum exercises are started on the third or fourth postoperative day and progress to active exercises in about 2 weeks. Patients then begin rehabilitation in the ambulatory-care occupational therapy department. Teach them that they may not have full function for several months.

TABLE 47.3 Examples of Acute Soft-Tissue Musculoskeletal Injuries

Acute Injury/Description	Management
Sprain: excessive stretching of a ligament	Immobilization, RICE, possible surgery if severe
Strain: excessive stretching of a muscle or tendon	Heat/cold, activity limitations, NSAIDs, muscle relaxants, possible tendon repair
Ligament tear (such as anterior cruciate ligament in knee): damage to ligament most often caused by sports or vehicular crash	RICE, surgery if does not heal or is severe (usually arthroscopic)
Meniscus tear: damage to knee cartilage caused by sports or other trauma	RICE, bracing, splinting, NSAIDs, surgery (usually arthroscopic)
Tendon rupture (such as the Achilles tendon in heel): often caused by sports or wearing high-heeled shoes; in some cases can occur after taking fluoroquinolones such as ciprofloxacin (Cipro)	RICE, NSAIDs, orthotic devices, ultrasound, surgery if severe or does not heal
Patellofemoral pain syndrome (PFPS): knee pain caused by overuse of the knee joint; also called *runner's knee*	Rest, splinting, bracing, NSAIDs, possibly surgery as last resort
Joint dislocation: displacement of a bone from its usual position in a synovial joint	Manual joint relocation; possible surgery

GET READY FOR THE NEXT-GENERATION NCLEX® EXAMINATION!

Key Points

Review these Key Points for each NCLEX Examination Client Needs Category.

Safe and Effective Care Environment

- Collaborate with physical and occupational therapists for care of patients with fractures to improve ***mobility*** and muscle strength. **QSEN: Teamwork and Collaboration**
- Remember that the priority care for patients with fractures and amputations is to maintain perfusion, reduce ***pain,*** and prevent decreased ***mobility.*** **QSEN: Evidence-Based Practice**
- Monitor for potentially life-threatening complications of fractures, including hemorrhage, venous thromboembolism, fat embolism syndrome, acute compartment syndrome, and ***infection.*** **Clinical Judgment**

Health Promotion and Maintenance

- Teach people to avoid musculoskeletal injury by treating or preventing osteoporosis (see Chapter 45), being cautious when walking to prevent a fall, wearing supportive shoes, avoiding dangerous sports or activities, and decreasing time spent doing repetitive stress activities, such as using a computer keyboard or cell phone. **QSEN: Safety**
- Several community organizations, such as the Amputee Coalition of America, are available to help patients and their families cope with the loss of a body part. **QSEN: Patient-Centered Care**
- Teach patients and their family members and significant others how to care for casts or other orthopedic devices at home. **QSEN: Safety**
- In collaboration with the interprofessional health team, reinforce teaching for ambulating with crutches, walkers, or canes and teach exercises to patients with leg amputation to prevent hip flexion contractures. **QSEN: Teamwork and Collaboration**
- Provide special care for older adults with hip fractures, including preventing heel pressure injuries and promoting early ambulation to prevent complications of immobility. **QSEN: Patient-Centered Care**

Psychosocial Integrity

- For patients with severe trauma or amputation, assess coping skills and encourage verbalization. **QSEN: Patient-Centered Care**
- Recognize that the patient having an amputation may need to adjust to an altered lifestyle but can be active and productive. **QSEN: Patient-Centered Care**

Physiological Integrity

- Be aware that open fractures cause a higher risk for infection than do closed fractures; use strict aseptic technique when providing wound management. **QSEN: Evidence-Based Care**
- Recognize that fat embolism syndrome is different from pulmonary (blood clot) embolism. **Clinical Judgment**
- Provide emergency care of the patient with a fracture. **Clinical Judgment**
- Identify the patient at risk for acute compartment syndrome; loosen bandages or request that the patient's cast be cut if neurovascular compromise is assessed; notify the health care provider immediately. **QSEN: Evidence-Based Practice**
- As a priority, document neurovascular status frequently in patients with musculoskeletal injury, traction, or cast and manage ***pain*** adequately. **QSEN: Informatics**
- Provide evidence-based appropriate cast care, depending on the type of cast (plaster or synthetic); check for pressure necrosis under the cast by feeling for heat, assessing the patient's pain level, and smelling the cast for an unpleasant odor. **QSEN: Evidence-Based Practice**
- Provide pin care for patients with skeletal traction or external fixation; assess for signs and symptoms of infection at the pin sites. **QSEN: Evidence-Based Practice**
- Provide postoperative care for the patient having a fracture repair, including promoting ***mobility*** and monitoring for complications of immobility. **QSEN: Safety**
- Provide emergency care for a patient having a traumatic amputation in the community. Call 911, assess the patient for ABCs, apply direct pressure on the amputation site, and elevate the extremity above the patient's heart to decrease bleeding. For finger parts, wrap the amputated part with a clean cloth and place in a sealed bag, which is lowered into ice water. **QSEN: Evidence-Based Practice**
- After surgery, assess for and promptly manage phantom limb ***pain*** in the patient who has an amputation; collaborate with specialists to incorporate complementary and integrative therapies and drug therapy into the patient's plan of care. **QSEN: Patient-Centered Care**
- Assess and document neurovascular status frequently after an endoscopic carpal tunnel release. **QSEN: Safety**
- Provide emergency care for patients with a sports-related injury using RICE (Rest, Ice, Compression, Elevation). **QSEN: Evidence-Based Practice**
- Recall that carpal tunnel syndrome (CTS) is the most common type of repetitive stress injury (RSI) caused by certain occupations such as computer operators and factory workers. **QSEN: Evidence-Based Practice**
- Many acute musculoskeletal injuries are initially treated by RICE: *r*est, *i*ce, *c*ompression, and *e*levation. **QSEN: Evidence-Based Practice**

MASTERY QUESTIONS

1. The nurse is assigned to care for a postoperative client who had an open reduction, internal fixation of the right tibia yesterday. The client reports increased right leg pain, numbness, and tingling. What would be the nurse's **first** action at this time?
   A. Elevate the surgical leg on a pillow.
   B. Perform a neurovascular assessment.
   C. Administer pain medication.
   D. Call the primary health care provider.
2. The nurse teaches assistive personnel (AP) how to position a client who had an above-the-knee amputation (AKA) last week. Which statement by the AP indicates **understanding** of the teaching?
   A. "We should keep the surgical leg elevated on two pillows at all times."
   B. "We should keep the client in a sitting position as long as possible."
   C. "We should keep the surgical leg as flat on the bed as possible."
   D. "We should keep the client in a prone position most of the day."
3. The nurse is caring for a client who was admitted to the emergency department (ED) with report of left knee pain and swelling after playing baseball with friends. Which nursing actions are appropriate when caring for the client? **Select all that apply.**
   A. Apply heat to the affected area.
   B. Assess the severity and quality of pain.
   C. Perform a neurovascular assessment.
   D. Elevate the affected extremity.
   E. Immobilize the injured knee joint.

REFERENCES

Blevins, S. (2020). Carpal tunnel syndrome. *Medsurg Nursing, 29*(1), 53–55.

Conley, R.B., Adib, G., Adler, R.A., Akesson, K.E., Alexander, I.M., Amenta, K.C., et al. (2020). Secondary fracture prevention: Consensus clinical recommendations from a multistakeholder coalition. *Orthopaedic Nursing, 39*(3), 145-161.

Duperouzel, W., Gray, B., & Santy-Tomlinson, J. (2018). The principles of traction and the application of lower limb skin traction. *International Journal of Orthopaedic and Trauma Nursing, 29*, 54–57.

Durham, C. O., & VanRavenstein, K. (2017). It's all in the wrist: Diagnosis and management of carpal tunnel syndrome. *Orthopaedic Nursing, 36*(5), 323–327.

Freysteinson, W., Thomas, L., Sebastian-Deutsch, A., Douglas, D., Meltom, D., Celia, T., et al. (2016). A study of the amputee experience of viewing self in the mirror. *Rehabilitation Nursing*. https://doi.org/10.1002/mj.256. [Epub ahead of print].

Georgiades, D. S. (2018). A systematic integrative review of pin site crusts. *Orthopaedic Nursing, 37*(1), 36–42.

Hohler, S. E. (2018). Providing evidence-based practices for patients with hip fractures. *Nursing, 48*(6), 52–57.

Jarvis, C. (2018). *Physical examination & health assessment* (8th ed.). St. Louis: Elsevier Saunders.

MacDonald, V., Maher, A. B., Mainz, H., Meehan, A. J., Brent, L., Hommel, A., et al. (2018). Developing and testing an international audit of quality indicators for older adults with fragility fractures. *Orthopaedic Nursing, 37*(2), 115–121.

McCance, K., Huether, S., Brashers, V., & Rote, N. (2019). *Pathophysiology: The biologic basis for disease in adults and children* (8th ed.). St. Louis: Mosby.

Schreiber, M. L. (2017). Lower limb amputation: Postoperative nursing care and considerations. *Medsurg Nursing, 26*(4), 274–279.

Slusser, M. M., Garcia, L. I., Reed, C.-R., & McGinnis, P. Q. (2019). *Foundations of interprofessional collaborative practice in health care.* St. Louis: Elsevier.

Thurlow, G., & Gray, B. (2018). Complex regional pain syndrome. *International Journal of Orthopaedic and Trauma Nursing, 30*, 44–47.

Turkowski, B. B. (2018). "I can't poop": Medication-induced constipation. *Orthopaedic Nursing, 37*(3), 192–196.

Wennberg, P., Andersson, H., & Sundstrom, B. W. (2018). Patients with suspected hip fractures in the chain of emergency care: An integrative review of the literature. *International Journal of Orthopaedic and Trauma Nursing, 29*, 16–31.

Williams, M. G., Jeffery, Z., Corner, H. W., Charity, J., Quantick, M., & Sartin, N. (2019). A robust approach to implementing fascia iliaca compartment nerve blocks in hip fracture patients. *Orthopaedic Nursing, 37*(3), 185–189.

Yildirim, M., & Sen, S. (2020). Mirror therapy in the management of phantom limb pain. *AJN, 120*(3), 41–46.

48

Assessment of the Gastrointestinal System

Charity Hacker

http://evolve.elsevier.com/Iggy/

LEARNING OUTCOMES

1. Collaborate with the interprofessional team to perform a gastrointestinal (GI) assessment.
2. Prioritize evidence-based care for patients having invasive diagnostic testing affecting ***nutrition, elimination,*** and GI ***pain.***
3. Teach evidence-based ways for adults to prevent GI problems.
4. Explain how physiologic aging changes of the gastrointestinal system affect ***nutrition*** and ***elimination.***
5. Implement nursing interventions to decrease the psychosocial impact caused by GI problems.
6. Apply knowledge of anatomy and physiology, genetic risk, and principles of aging to perform a focused GI assessment.
7. Use clinical judgment to document the GI assessment in the electronic health record.
8. Interpret assessment findings for patients with a suspected or actual GI problem.

KEY TERMS

amylase An enzyme that converts starch and glycogen into simple sugars; found most commonly in saliva and pancreatic fluids.

borborygmus High-pitched bowel sounds that are proximal (above) an obstruction.

bruit An audible swishing sound produced when the volume of blood or the diameter of the blood vessel changes.

colonoscopy An endoscopic examination of the entire large bowel.

digestion The mechanical and chemical process in which complex foodstuffs are broken down into simpler forms that can be used by the body.

dyspepsia An epigastric burning sensation, often referred to as "heartburn."

endoscope A tube that allows viewing and manipulation of internal body areas.

endoscopic retrograde cholangiopancreatography (ERCP) A procedure in which the bile ducts, pancreatic duct, and gallbladder are visualized through endoscopy.

endoscopy The direct visualization of the gastrointestinal tract by means of a flexible fiberoptic endoscope.

enteroscopy Visualization of the small intestine.

esophageal stricture Narrowing of the esophageal opening.

esophagogastroduodenoscopy (EGD) The visual examination of the esophagus, stomach, and duodenum by means of a fiberoptic endoscope.

flatulence Gas in the lower gastrointestinal tract.

guaiac-based fecal occult blood test (gFOBT) A diagnostic test that measures the presence of blood in the stool from gastrointestinal bleeding—a common finding associated with colorectal cancer.

lipase An enzyme secreted by the pancreas that facilitates the breakdown of triglycerides into fatty acids.

NPO (nothing by mouth) No eating, drinking (including water), or smoking.

PQRST A mnemonic (memory device) that may help in the assessment of abdominal pain. The letters represent these areas: P, precipitating or palliative (What brings it on? What makes it better or worse?); Q, quality or quantity (How does it look, feel, or sound?); R, region or radiation (Where is it? Does it spread anywhere?); S, severity scale (How bad is it [on a scale of 0 to 10]? Is it getting better, worse, or staying the same?); T, timing (Onset, duration, and frequency?).

reflux Reverse or backward flow.

sigmoidoscopy An endoscopic examination of the rectum and sigmoid colon using a flexible scope.

steatorrhea Fatty stools.

virtual colonoscopy Three-dimensional images of the colon and rectum created by use of an abdominal and pelvic CT scan.

PRIORITY AND INTERRELA CONCEPTS

The priority concepts for this chapter are:

- ***Nutrition***
- ***Elimination***
- ***Pain***

The *alimentary canal,* known as the GI tract, consists of the mouth, esophagus, stomach, small and large intestines, and rectum. The GI system is formed when the salivary glands, liver, gallbladder, and pancreas secrete substances into this tract (Fig. 48.1). The main functions of the GI tract, with the aid of organs such as the pancreas and the liver, are the digestion of food to adequately meet the body's ***nutrition*** needs, and the ***elimination*** of waste resulting from digestion. The GI tract is susceptible to numerous health problems, including structural or mechanical alterations, impaired motility, infection, inflammation or autoimmune disease, and cancer.

ANATOMY AND PHYSIOLOGY REVIEW

Structure

The lumen, or inner wall, of the GI tract consists of four layers: mucosa, submucosa, muscularis, and serosa. The *mucosa,* the innermost layer, includes a thin layer of smooth muscle and specialized exocrine gland cells. It is surrounded by the *submucosa,* which is made up of connective tissue. The *submucosa* layer is surrounded by the muscularis. The *muscularis* is composed of both circular and longitudinal smooth muscles, which work to keep contents moving through the tract. The outermost layer, the *serosa,* is composed of connective tissue. Although the GI tract is continuous from the mouth to the anus, it is divided into specialized regions. The mouth, pharynx, esophagus, stomach, and small and large intestines each perform a specific function. In addition, the secretions of the salivary, gastric, and intestinal glands; liver; and pancreas empty into the GI tract to aid digestion.

Function

The functions of the GI tract include secretion, digestion, absorption, motility, and ***elimination.*** Food and fluids are ingested, swallowed, and propelled along the lumen of the GI tract to the anus for elimination. The smooth muscles contract to move food from the mouth to the anus. Before food can be absorbed, it must be broken down to a liquid, called *chyme.* **Digestion** is the mechanical and chemical process in which complex foodstuffs are broken down into simpler forms that can be used by the body. During digestion, the stomach secretes hydrochloric acid, the liver secretes bile, and digestive enzymes are released from accessory organs, aiding in food breakdown. After the digestive process is complete, absorption takes place. *Absorption* is carried out as the nutrients produced by digestion move from the lumen of the GI tract into the body's circulatory system for uptake by individual cells (McCance & Huether, 2019).

Oral Cavity. The oral cavity (mouth) includes the buccal mucosa, lips, tongue, hard palate, soft palate, teeth, and salivary glands. The buccal mucosa is the mucous membrane lining the inside of the mouth. The tongue is involved in speech, taste, and *mastication* (chewing). Small projections called *papillae* cover the tongue and provide a roughened surface, permitting the movement of food in the mouth during chewing. The hard palate and the soft palate together form the roof of the mouth.

Adults have 32 permanent teeth: 16 each in upper and lower arches. The different types of teeth function to prepare food for digestion by cutting, tearing, crushing, or grinding the food. Swallowing begins after food is taken into the mouth and chewed. Saliva is secreted in response to the presence of food in the mouth and begins to soften the food. Saliva contains mucin and an enzyme called *salivary alpha-amylase* (McCance & Huether, 2019) (also known as *ptyalin*), which begins the breakdown of carbohydrates.

Esophagus. The *esophagus* is a muscular canal that extends from the pharynx (throat) to the stomach and passes through the center of the diaphragm. Its primary function is to move food and fluids from the pharynx to the stomach. At the upper end of the esophagus is a sphincter referred to as the upper esophageal sphincter (UES). When at rest, the UES is closed to prevent air into the esophagus during respiration. The portion of the esophagus just above the gastroesophageal (GE) junction is referred to as the lower esophageal sphincter (LES). When at rest, the LES is normally closed to prevent **reflux** of gastric contents into the esophagus. If the LES does not work properly, gastroesophageal reflux disease (GERD) can develop.

Stomach. The *stomach* is located in the midline and left upper quadrant (LUQ) of the abdomen and has three functional regions: the fundus, body, and antrum (McCance & Huether, 2019). Anatomically, the *cardia* is the narrow portion of the stomach that is below the gastroesophageal (GE) junction. The *fundus* is the area nearest to the cardia. The main area of the stomach is referred to as the *body* or *corpus.* The *antrum* (pylorus) is the distal (lower) portion of the stomach and is separated from the duodenum by the pyloric sphincter. Both ends of the stomach are guarded by sphincters (cardiac [LES] and pyloric), which aid in the transport of food through the GI tract and prevent backflow.

Smooth muscle cells that line the stomach are responsible for gastric motility. The stomach is also richly innervated with intrinsic and extrinsic nerves. Parietal cells lining the wall of the stomach secrete hydrochloric acid, whereas chief cells secrete pepsinogen (a precursor to pepsin, a digestive enzyme). Parietal cells also produce intrinsic factor, a substance that aids in the absorption of vitamin B_{12}. Absence of intrinsic factor causes pernicious anemia.

After ingestion of food, the stomach functions as a food reservoir where the digestive process begins, using mechanical movements and chemical secretions. The stomach mixes or churns the food, breaking apart the large food molecules and mixing them with gastric secretions to form chyme, which then empties into the duodenum. The *intestinal phase* begins as the chyme passes from the stomach into the duodenum, causing distention. It is assisted by secretin and cholecystokinin,

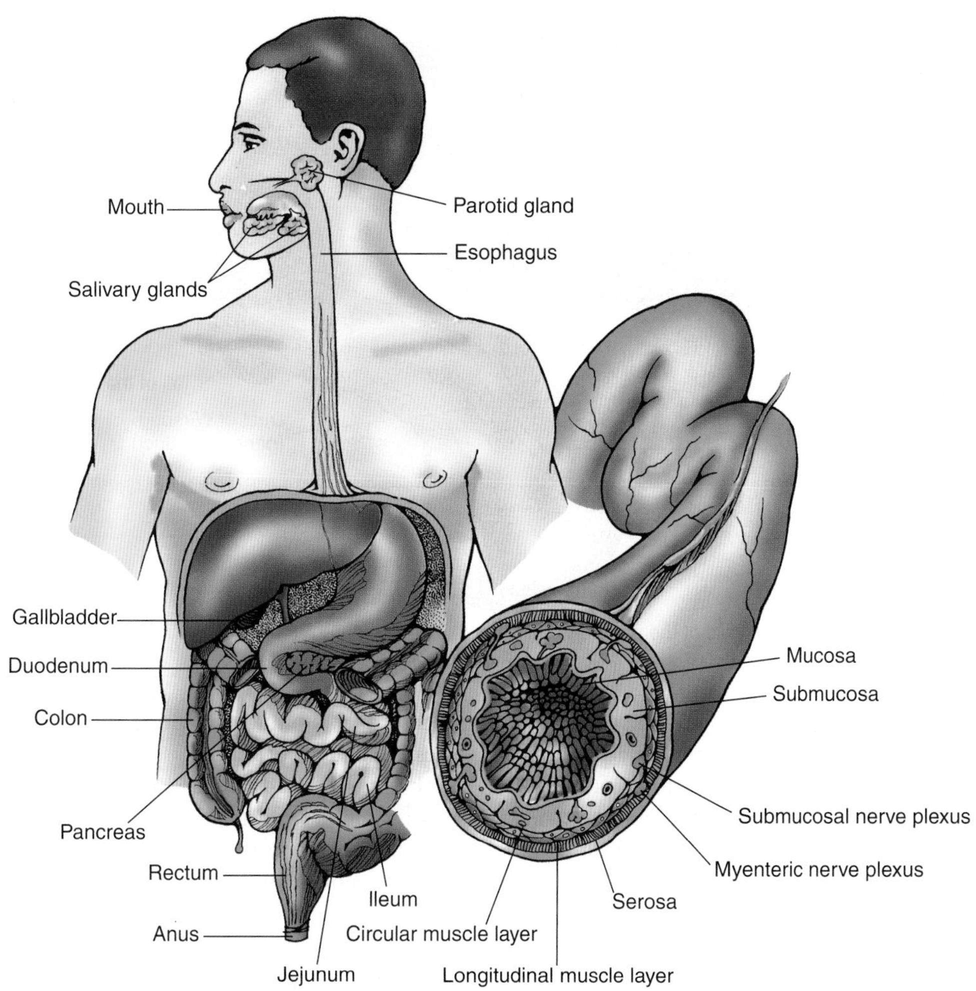

FIG. 48.1 The GI system (GI tract) can be thought of as a tube (with necessary structures) extending from the mouth to the anus for a 25-foot length. The structure of this tube *(shown enlarged)* is basically the same throughout its length.

hormones that inhibit further acid production and decrease gastric motility (Peate & Nair, 2016).

Pancreas. The *pancreas* is a fish-shaped gland that lies behind the stomach and extends horizontally from the duodenal C-loop to the spleen (McCance & Huether, 2019). The pancreas is divided into portions known as the head, the body, and the tail (Fig. 48.2).

Two major cellular bodies (exocrine and endocrine) within the pancreas have separate functions. The exocrine part consists of cells that secrete enzymes needed for digestion of carbohydrates, fats, and proteins (proteases, amylase, and lipase). The endocrine part of the pancreas is made up of the *islets of Langerhans,* with alpha cells producing glucagon and beta cells producing insulin, as well as delta and f (or PP) cells (McCance & Huether, 2019). The hormones produced are essential in the regulation of metabolism.

Liver and Gallbladder. The liver is the largest organ in the body (other than skin) and is located mainly in the right upper quadrant (RUQ) of the abdomen. The right and left hepatic ducts transport bile from the liver. It receives its blood supply from the hepatic artery and portal vein, resulting in approximately 1200 mL of blood flow through the liver every minute.

The liver performs more than 400 functions in three major categories: storage, protection, and metabolism. It stores many minerals and vitamins, such as iron; magnesium; fat-soluble vitamins A, D, E, and K; and water-soluble vitamin B_{12} (McCance & Huether, 2019).

The protective function of the liver involves phagocytic *Kupffer cells,* which are part of the body's reticuloendothelial system. They engulf harmful bacteria and anemic red blood cells. The liver also detoxifies potentially harmful compounds (e.g., drugs, chemicals, alcohol). Therefore the risk for drug toxicity increases with aging because of decreased liver function.

The liver functions in the metabolism of proteins that are vital for survival. It breaks down amino acids to remove ammonia, which is then converted to urea and is excreted via the kidneys as urine (McCance & Huether, 2019). It synthesizes several plasma proteins, including albumin, prothrombin, and fibrinogen. The liver's role in carbohydrate metabolism involves storing and releasing glycogen as the body's energy requirements change. The organ also synthesizes, breaks down, and temporarily stores fatty acids and triglycerides.

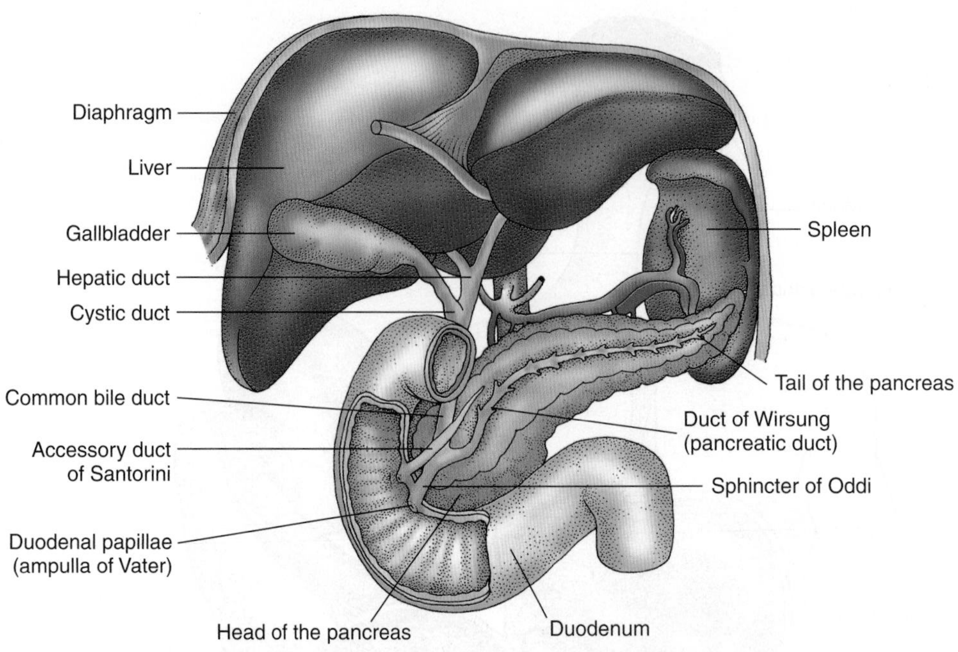

FIG. 48.2 Anatomy of the pancreas, liver, and gallbladder.

The liver forms and continually secretes bile, which is essential for the breakdown of fat. The secretion of bile increases in response to gastrin, secretin, and cholecystokinin. Bile is secreted into small ducts that empty into the common bile duct (CBD) and into the duodenum at the *sphincter of Oddi.* However, if the sphincter is closed, the bile goes to the gallbladder for storage.

The *gallbladder* is a pear-shaped, bulbous sac that is located underneath the liver. It is drained by the cystic duct, which joins with the hepatic duct from the liver to form the CBD. The gallbladder collects, concentrates, and stores the bile that has come from the liver. It releases the bile into the duodenum via the CBD when fat is present.

Small Intestine. The small intestine is the longest and most convoluted portion of the digestive tract, measuring an average of 9 to 16 feet (3 to 5 m) in length in an adult (Collins & Badireddy, 2020). It is composed of three different regions: duodenum, jejunum, and ileum. The *duodenum* is the first 8 to 10 inches (20 to 25 cm) of the small intestine and is attached to the distal end of the pylorus (Collins & Badireddy, 2020). The common bile duct and pancreatic duct join to form the ampulla of Vater, emptying into the duodenum at the duodenal papilla. This papillary opening is surrounded by muscle known as the sphincter of Oddi. The 8-foot (2.5-m) portion of the small intestine that follows the sphincter of Oddi is the *jejunum.* The last 10 feet (3 m) of the small intestine is called the *ileum* (Collins & Badireddy, 2020). The ileocecal valve separates the entrance of the ileum from the cecum of the large intestine (Peate & Nair, 2016).

The inner surface of the small intestine has a velvety appearance because of numerous mucous membrane finger-like projections. These projections are called *intestinal villi.* In addition to the intestinal villi, the small intestine has circular folds of mucosa and submucosa, which increase the surface area for digestion and absorption.

The small intestine has three main *functions*: movement (mixing and peristalsis), digestion, and absorption. Because the intestinal villi increase the surface area of the small intestine, it is the major organ of absorption of the digestive system. The small intestine mixes and transports the chyme to combine with many digestive enzymes. It takes an average of 3 to 6 hours for the contents to be passed by peristalsis through the small intestine (Peate & Nair, 2016). Intestinal enzymes aid the body in the digestion of proteins, carbohydrates, and lipids.

Large Intestine. The large intestine extends about 5 to 6 feet in length from the ileocecal valve to the anus and is lined with columnar epithelium that has absorptive and mucous cells. It begins with the *cecum,* a dilated, pouchlike structure that is inferior to the ileocecal opening. At the base of the cecum is the vermiform appendix, which has been discovered to play a role in intestinal immunity (Girard-Madoux et al., 2018). The large intestine then extends upward from the cecum as the colon. The colon consists of four divisions: ascending colon, transverse colon, descending colon, and sigmoid colon (McCance & Huether, 2019). The sigmoid colon empties into the rectum.

Beyond the sigmoid colon, the large intestine bends downward to form the rectum. The last 1 to 1½ inches (3 to 4 cm) of the large intestine are called the *anal canal,* which opens to the exterior of the body through the anus. The internal and external sphincter muscles surround the anal canal and control defecation.

The large intestine's *functions* are movement, absorption, and ***elimination.*** Movement in the large intestine consists mainly of segmental contractions, such as those in the small intestine, to allow enough time for the absorption of water and electrolytes. In addition, peristaltic contractions are triggered by colonic distention to move the contents toward the rectum, where the material is stored until the urge to defecate occurs. Absorption of water and some electrolytes occurs in the large intestine to reduce the fluid volume of the chyme. This process creates a more solid material, the feces, for ***elimination.***

Gastrointestinal Changes Associated With Aging

As people age, and especially after 65 years of age, physiologic changes occur in the GI system. Common digestive and ***elimination*** changes can affect ***nutrition*** (Terrery & Nicoteri, 2016). The Patient-Centered Care: Older Adult Considerations: Changes in the Gastrointestinal System Associated With Aging box lists common GI changes in older adults.

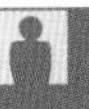

PATIENT-CENTERED CARE: OLDER ADULT CONSIDERATIONS QSEN

Changes in the Gastrointestinal System Associated With Aging

Physiologic Change	Disorders Related to Change
Atrophy of the gastric mucosa leads to decreased hydrochloric acid levels (hypochlorhydria).	Decreased absorption of iron and vitamin B_{12} and proliferation of bacteria. Atrophic gastritis occurs as a consequence of bacterial overgrowth.
Peristalsis decreases, and nerve impulses are dulled.	Decreased sensation to defecate can result in postponement of bowel movements, which leads to constipation and impaction.
Distention and dilation of pancreatic ducts change. Calcification of pancreatic vessels occurs with a decrease in lipase production.	Decreased lipase level results in decreased fat absorption and digestion. Steatorrhea (fatty stool) occurs because of decreased fat digestion.
A decrease in the number and size of hepatic cells leads to decreased liver weight and mass. This change and an increase in fibrous tissue lead to decreased protein synthesis and changes in liver enzymes. Enzyme activity and cholesterol synthesis are diminished.	Decreased enzyme activity depresses drug metabolism, which leads to accumulation of drugs—possibly to toxic levels.
The delicate microbial balance of good anaerobic and aerobic flora is disrupted over time, negatively affecting the immune response (Vemuri et al., 2018).	Dysfunctional microbial activity contributes to obesity, inflammatory disease, and reduced immunity.

ASSESSMENT: RECOGNIZE CUES

Patient History

The purpose of the health history is to determine the events related to the current health problem (see the Best Practice for Patient Safety & Quality Care: Questions for Gastrointestinal Health History box). Ask questions about changes in appetite, weight, and stool. Determine the patient's experience with ***pain,*** if that is one of his or her concerns.

Collect data about the patient's age, gender, and culture. This information can be helpful in assessing who is likely to have particular GI system disorders. For instance, older adults are more at risk for stomach cancer than are younger adults. Younger adults are at higher risk for inflammatory bowel disease (IBD). The exact reasons for these differences continue to be studied. Colon cancer, once a disease that affected older adults, has become more common among young people with obesity (Colorectal Cancer Alliance, 2019).

NCLEX EXAMINATION CHALLENGE 48.1

Physiological Integrity

Which daily behavior of a client with GI problems requires **further** nursing assessment? **Select all that apply.**

A. Smokes a pack of cigarettes
B. Uses Fleet enemas frequently to assist with bowel movements
C. Practices intentional relaxation
D. Eats multiple servings of fruits
E. Takes 325 mg of aspirin at night for arthritic pain
F. Exercises for 30 minutes three times weekly
G. Travels extensively across the world

Finally, investigate the patient's travel history. Ask whether he or she has traveled outside of the country recently or has been camping near lakes and streams in his or her country of residence. This information may provide clues about the cause of symptoms such as diarrhea.

BEST PRACTICE FOR PATIENT SAFETY & QUALITY CARE QSEN

Questions for Gastrointestinal Health History

- What is your typical daily food intake?
- What medications are you taking? (Obtain name, dose, and frequency)
- Do you take any vitamins, minerals, or herbal supplements? If so, what are they?
- How is your appetite? Has there been a recent change?
- Have you lost or gained weight recently? If so, was the weight loss or gain intentional?
- Are you on a special diet? If so, what kind, and for what purpose?
- Do you have difficulty chewing or swallowing?
- Do you wear dentures? If so, how well do they fit?
- Do you experience indigestion or "heartburn"? If so, how often? What seems to cause it? What helps it?
- Have you had GI disorders or surgeries in the past? If so, what are they and when did they occur?
- Is there a family history of GI health problems?
- Do you smoke (or vape), or have you ever smoked (vaped) in the past?
- Do you chew or have you ever chewed tobacco?
- Do you drink alcoholic beverages? If so, what kind, how much, and how many each week?
- Do you have pain, diarrhea, constipation, or gas? Do any specific foods accompany the problem?
- Have you traveled out of the country recently? If so, where and when?
- What is your usual bowel ***elimination*** pattern? Frequency? Character?
- Do you use laxatives to produce a bowel movement? If so, how frequently?
- Do you have any pain or bleeding associated with bowel movements?
- Have you experienced changes in your usual bowel pattern or stool?
- Have you ever had an endoscopy or a colonoscopy? If so, which one, and when?

Nutrition History. A ***nutrition*** history is important when assessing GI system function. Many conditions arise as a result of alterations in intake and absorption of nutrients. The purpose of a nutrition assessment is to gather information about how well the patient's needs are being met. Inquire about any special diet and whether there are any known food allergies. Ask the patient to describe the usual foods that are eaten daily and the times that meals are taken.

PATIENT-CENTERED CARE: CULTURAL/SPIRITUAL CONSIDERATIONS QSEN

Cultural and spiritual patterns are important in obtaining a complete ***nutrition*** history. Ask if certain foods pose a problem for the patient. For example, spices or hot pepper used in cooking can aggravate or precipitate GI tract symptoms such as indigestion. Note spiritual observations such as fasting or abstinence.

Many non-white Americans and those of Asian and South American heritage are lactose intolerant as a result of having insufficient amounts of the enzyme *lactase* or producing a less active form of the enzyme (Bass, 2017). A much smaller percentage of Caucasian people also have this problem. Lactase is needed to convert lactose in milk and other dairy products to glucose and galactose. Lactose intolerance causes bloating, cramping, and diarrhea as a result of lack of lactase.

Health problems can also affect ***nutrition***; therefore explore changes that have occurred in eating habits as a result of illness. Assess for *anorexia* (loss of appetite for food), changes in taste, and any difficulty or ***pain*** with swallowing (dysphagia) that could be associated with esophageal disorders. Also ask if abdominal ***pain*** or discomfort occurs with eating and whether the patient has experienced nausea, vomiting, or **dyspepsia** (an epigastric burning sensation, often referred to as "heartburn"). Unknown food allergies may be a cause of these symptoms. Inquire about unintentional weight loss because some GI cancers may present in this manner. Assess for alcohol and caffeine consumption because both substances are associated with many GI disorders, such as gastritis and peptic ulcer disease.

The patient's socioeconomic status may have a profound impact on ***nutrition.*** People who have limited budgets, such as some older adults or the unemployed, may not be able to purchase foods required for a balanced diet. They may substitute less expensive and less effective OTC medications or herbs for prescription drugs. People who live in "food deserts" (i.e., places with little access to fresh fruits and vegetables [U.S. Department of Agriculture, 2019] and other healthy foods) may also be affected by lack of ***nutrition.*** Necessary medical care may be delayed, and patients may not seek health care until conditions are well advanced.

Family History and Genetic Risk. Ask about a family history of GI disorders. Some GI health problems have a genetic predisposition. For example, familial adenomatous polyposis (FAP) is an inherited autosomal dominant disorder that predisposes the patient to colon cancer (Simonson, 2018). Pertinent genetic risks are discussed with the GI problems in later chapters.

Current Health Problems. Because GI signs and symptoms are often vague and difficult for the patient to describe, it is important to obtain a chronologic account of the current problem, symptoms, and any treatments taken. If a patient has kept a diary of dates, symptoms, and treatments used, this can be helpful to establish patterns. Ask about the location, quality, quantity, and timing of each symptom (onset, duration), and factors that may aggravate or alleviate it (see the Best Practice for Patient Safety and Quality Care: Questions for Gastrointestinal Health History box).

Changes in bowel habits are common assessment findings. Obtain this information from the patient:

- Pattern of bowel movements
- Color and consistency of the feces
- Occurrence of diarrhea or constipation
- Effective action taken to relieve diarrhea or constipation
- Presence of frank blood or tarry stools
- Presence of abdominal distention or gas
- Weight gain or loss that has been unintentional

Assess the patient's:

- Normal weight
- Weight gain or loss
- Period of time for weight change
- Changes in appetite or oral intake

Pain is a common concern of patients with GI tract disorders. Abdominal pain is often vague and difficult to evaluate. The mnemonic **PQRST** may be helpful in conducting a pain assessment (Jarvis, 2020):

P: Provocation or palliation
- What were you doing when the pain started?
- What caused it?
- What makes it better or worse?
- What seems to trigger it (e.g., stress, position, certain activities)?

Q: Quality or quantity
- Describe the feeling (e.g., sharp, dull, stabbing, burning, crushing, throbbing, nauseating, shooting, twisting, or stretching).

R: Region or radiation
- Where is the pain located?
- Does it radiate? (Where?)
- Does it feel as if it travels or moves around?
- Did it start elsewhere and is now localized to one spot?

S: Severity scale
- How severe is the pain on a scale of 0 to 10, with 0 being no pain and 10 being the worst pain ever?
- Does it interfere with activities?
- How bad is it at its worst?
- Does it force you to sit down, lie down, slow down?
- How long does an episode last?

T: Timing
- When or at what time did the pain start?
- How long did it last?
- How often does it occur (e.g., hourly, daily, weekly, monthly)?
- Is it sudden or gradual?

- What were you doing when you first experienced it?
- When do you usually experience it (e.g., daytime, night, early morning)?
- Are you ever awakened by it?
- Does it lead to anything else?
- Is it accompanied by other signs and symptoms?
- Does it ever occur before, during, or after meals?
- Does it occur seasonally?

Skin changes may result from GI tract disorders such as liver and biliary system *obstruction*. Ask whether these clinical signs and symptoms have occurred in the past or are currently present:

- Skin discolorations or rashes
- Itching
- *Jaundice* (yellowing of skin caused by bilirubin pigments)
- Increased bruising or tendency to bleed

Physical Assessment

Physical assessment involves a comprehensive examination of the patient's ***nutrition*** status, mouth, and abdomen. Nutrition assessment is discussed in detail in Chapter 55. Oral assessment is described in Chapter 49.

In preparation for assessment of the abdomen, ask the patient to empty his or her bladder and then to lie in a supine position with knees bent, keeping the arms at the sides to prevent tensing of the abdominal muscles.

The abdomen is assessed by using the four techniques of examination in a specific order. Nurse generalists perform inspection, auscultation, and light palpation. Health care providers perform inspection, auscultation, percussion, and deep palpation. These sequences are preferred so percussion and palpation do not increase intestinal activity and bowel sounds. If appendicitis or an abdominal aneurysm is suspected, palpation is not done.

Inspection. The abdominal examination usually begins with inspection of the patient's right side and proceeds in a systematic fashion (Fig. 48.3):

- Right upper quadrant (RUQ)
- Left upper quadrant (LUQ)
- Left lower quadrant (LLQ)
- Right lower quadrant (RLQ)

Table 48.1 lists the organs that lie in each of these areas.

If areas of ***pain*** or discomfort are noted from the history, they are cautiously assessed last in the examination sequence. This sequence should prevent the patient from tensing abdominal muscles because of the pain, which can make the examination difficult.

Inspect the skin and note any of these findings:

- Overall asymmetry of the abdomen
- Discoloration or scarring
- Abdominal distention
- Bulging flanks
- Taut, glistening skin
- Skin folds
- Subcutaneous fat noted
- Location, size, and description of any pressure injuries

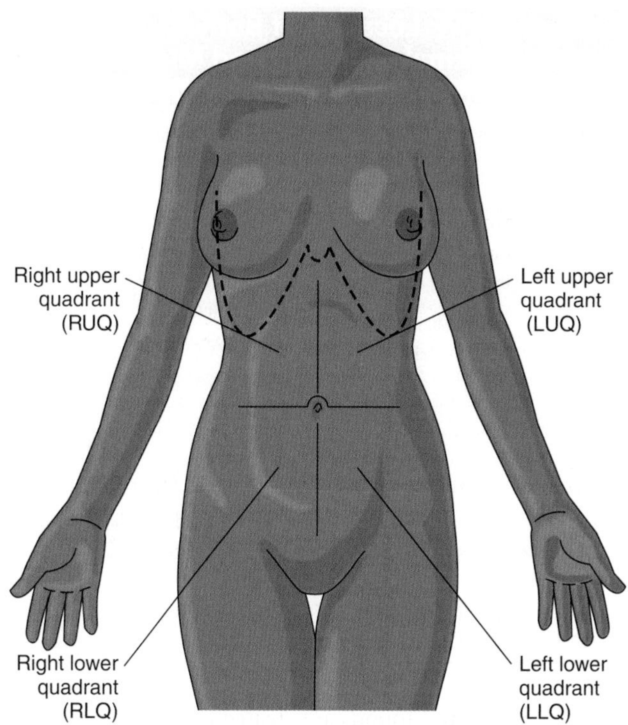

FIG. 48.3 Topographic division of the abdomen into quadrants.

Observe the contour and symmetry of the abdomen, which can be rounded, flat, concave, or distended. It is best determined when standing at the side of the bed or treatment table and looking down on the abdomen. View the abdomen at eye level from the side. Asymmetry of the abdomen can indicate problems affecting the underlying body structures (see Table 48.1). Note the shape and position of the umbilicus for any deviations.

! NURSING SAFETY PRIORITY (QSEN)

Action Alert

Peristaltic movements are rarely seen unless the patient is thin and has increased peristalsis. If these movements are observed, note the quadrant of origin and the direction of peristaltic flow. Report this finding to the health care provider because it may indicate an intestinal obstruction.

Finally, observe abdominal movements, including the normal rising and falling with inspiration and expiration, and note any distress during movement. Occasionally pulsations may be visible, particularly in the area of the abdominal aorta.

! NURSING SAFETY PRIORITY (QSEN)

Action Alert

If a bulging, pulsating mass is present during assessment of the abdomen, **do not touch** the area because the patient may have an abdominal aortic aneurysm, a life-threatening problem. Notify the health care provider of this finding immediately!

TABLE 48.1 Location of Body Structures in Each Abdominal Quadrant and Midline

Right Upper Quadrant (RUQ)	Left Upper Quadrant (LUQ)
• Most of the liver	• Left lobe of the liver
• Gallbladder	• Stomach
• Duodenum	• Spleen
• Head of the pancreas	• Body and tail of the pancreas
• Hepatic flexure of the colon	• Splenic flexure of the colon
• Part of the ascending and transverse colon	• Part of the transverse and descending colon
Midline	
• Abdominal aorta	
• Uterus (if enlarged)	
• Bladder (if distended)	
Right Lower Quadrant (RLQ)	**Left Lower Quadrant (LLQ)**
• Cecum	• Part of the descending colon
• Appendix	• Sigmoid colon
• Right ureter	• Left ureter
• Right ovary and fallopian tube	• Left ovary and fallopian tube
• Right spermatic cord	• Left spermatic cord

Auscultation. Bowel sounds are created as air and fluid move through the GI tract. They are normally heard as relatively high-pitched, irregular gurgles with a normal frequency range of 5 to 30 per minute (Jarvis, 2020). They are characterized as normal, hypoactive, or hyperactive. They are diminished or absent after abdominal surgery or in the patient with peritonitis or paralytic ileus. The most reliable method for assessing the return of peristalsis after abdominal surgery is to ask the patient if he or she has passed flatus within the past 8 hours or had a stool within the past 12 to 24 hours.

Increased high-pitched bowel sounds, especially loud, gurgling sounds, result from increased motility of the bowel (**borborygmus**). These sounds are usually heard in the patient with diarrhea or gastroenteritis or are heard above a complete intestinal obstruction.

Auscultation of the abdomen is performed with the diaphragm of the stethoscope because bowel sounds are usually high pitched. Place the stethoscope lightly on the abdominal wall, beginning in the RLQ in the area of the ileocecal valve, where bowel sounds are normally present (Jarvis, 2020). Proceed with listening to other quadrants.

During auscultation, also listen for vascular sounds or **bruits** ("swooshing" sounds) over the abdominal aorta, the renal arteries, and the iliac arteries. A bruit heard over the aorta usually indicates the presence of an aneurysm. *If this sound is heard, do not percuss or palpate the abdomen. Notify the health care provider immediately of your findings!*

Percussion. Percussion may be done by the **health care provider** to determine the size of solid organs; to detect the presence of masses, fluid, and air; and to estimate the size of the liver and spleen. The percussion notes heard in the abdomen are termed *tympanic* (the high-pitched, loud, musical sound of an air-filled intestine) or *dull* (the medium-pitched, softer, thudlike sound over a solid organ, such as the liver).

The liver and spleen can be percussed. An enlarged liver is called *hepatomegaly*. Dullness heard in the left anterior axillary line indicates enlargement of the spleen (*splenomegaly*). Mild-to-moderate splenomegaly can be detected by percussion before the spleen becomes palpable.

Palpation. The purpose of palpation is to determine the size and location of abdominal organs and to assess for the presence of masses or tenderness. Palpation of the abdomen consists of two types: light and deep. Nurse generalists perform light palpation. The technique of *light palpation* is used to detect large masses and areas of tenderness. Place the first four fingers of the palpating hand close together and then place them lightly on the abdomen and proceed smoothly and systematically from quadrant to quadrant. Depress the abdomen to a depth of ½ to 1 inch (1.25 to 2.5 cm). Proceed with a rotational movement of the palpating hand. Note any areas of tenderness or guarding because these areas will be examined last and cautiously during deep palpation. While performing light palpation, note signs of rigidity, which, unlike voluntary guarding, is a sign of peritoneal inflammation. Only health care providers, such as physicians, physician assistants, and advance practice nurses, should perform deep palpation. Deep palpation is used to further determine the size and shape of abdominal organs and masses.

NCLEX EXAMINATION CHALLENGE 48.2

Physiological Integrity

While performing an abdominal assessment on a client, the nurse notes a bruit over the aorta. What is the appropriate nursing action?

A. Consult another nurse to verify the bruit.
B. Auscultate each quadrant for 5 minutes each.
C. Notify the health care provider of the findings.
D. Perform light palpation to further assess the pulsation.

Psychosocial Assessment

Psychosocial assessment focuses on how the GI health problem affects the patient's life and lifestyle. Remember that patients are often reluctant to discuss ***elimination*** problems, which may be very personal and embarrassing. The interview focus is on whether usual daily activities and/or employment have been interrupted or disturbed. Ask about recent stressful events, as stress has been associated with the development or exacerbation (flare-up) of irritable bowel syndrome (IBS) and other GI disorders. If the patient is diagnosed with cancer, he or she is likely to experience the stages of the grieving process. Patients may be depressed, angry, or in denial.

Diagnostic Assessment

Laboratory Assessment. To make an accurate assessment of the many possible causes of GI system abnormalities, laboratory testing of blood, urine, and stool specimens may be performed.

Serum Tests. A *complete blood count (CBC)* aids in the diagnosis of anemia and infection. It also detects changes in the blood's formed elements. In adults, GI bleeding is the most frequent cause of anemia. It is associated with GI cancer, peptic ulcer disease, diverticulitis, and inflammatory bowel disease.

Prothrombin time (PT) is useful in evaluating levels of clotting factors. PT measures the rate at which prothrombin is converted to thrombin, a process that depends on vitamin K–associated clotting factors. Hepatocellular liver disease leads to a prolonged PT secondary to impaired synthesis of clotting proteins (Pagana & Pagana, 2018).

Many *electrolytes* are altered in GI tract dysfunction. For example, calcium is absorbed in the GI tract and may be measured to detect malabsorption. Excessive vomiting or diarrhea causes sodium or potassium depletion, thus requiring replacement.

Assays of serum enzymes are important in the evaluation of liver damage. *Aspartate aminotransferase (AST)* and *alanine aminotransferase (ALT)* are two enzymes found in the liver and other organs. These enzymes are elevated in most liver disorders, but they are highest in conditions that cause necrosis, such as hepatitis and cirrhosis.

Elevations in serum amylase and lipase may indicate acute pancreatitis, a serious inflammation of the pancreas characterized by a sudden onset of abdominal pain, nausea, and vomiting. In this disease, serum amylase levels begin to elevate within 24 hours of onset and remain elevated for up to 5 days. Serum amylase and lipase are not elevated when extensive pancreatic necrosis is present because there are few pancreatic cells manufacturing the enzymes.

Bilirubin is the primary pigment in bile, which is normally conjugated and excreted by the liver and biliary system. It is measured as total serum bilirubin, conjugated (direct) bilirubin, and unconjugated (indirect) bilirubin. These measurements are important in the evaluation of jaundice and liver and biliary tract functioning. Elevations in direct and indirect bilirubin levels and/or gamma-glutamyl transferase (GGT) can indicate impaired excretion.

The serum level of *ammonia* may also be measured to evaluate hepatic function. Ammonia is normally used to rebuild amino acids or is converted to urea for excretion. Elevated levels are seen in conditions that cause hepatocellular injury, such as pancreatitis, cholecystitis, and gastrointestinal disease (Pagana & Pagana, 2018).

Two primary *oncofetal antigens—CA19-9* and *CEA*—are evaluated to monitor the efficacy of cancer therapy and assess for the recurrence of cancer in the GI tract. These antigens may also be increased in benign GI conditions. The Laboratory Profile: Gastrointestinal Assessment box lists blood tests commonly used by the health care provider in the diagnosis of GI disorders. Additional serum tests are described in other GI chapters within this text.

Urine Tests. Amylase can be detected in the urine. In acute pancreatitis, renal clearance of amylase is increased. Amylase levels in the urine remain elevated 5 to 7 days after onset of disease processes, even after serum levels return to normal within 1 to 2 days (Pagana & Pagana, 2018). This becomes an important finding in patients who are symptomatic for several days or longer.

Urine *urobilinogen* is a form of bilirubin that is converted by the intestinal flora and excreted in the urine. Its measurement is useful in the evaluation of hepatic and biliary obstruction, because the presence of bilirubin in the urine often occurs before jaundice is seen.

Stool Tests. The American Cancer Society (ACS) recommends regular screening to detect colorectal cancer early when it can most effectively be treated (ACS, 2018). Options include an annual high-sensitivity fecal immunochemical test (FIT), an annual guaiac-based fecal occult blood test (gFOBT) (such as the Hemoccult II Sensa), or a FIT-DNA test performed every 3 years. These tests use a take-home, multisample method rather than having the test done during a digital rectal examination. These tests use a take-home, multisample method rather than having the test done during a digital rectal examination.

The traditionally used gFOBT (e.g., Hemoccult II Sensa) requires an active component of guaiac and is therefore more likely than the FIT (e.g., HemeSelect) to yield false-positive results. In addition, patients having the guaiac-based test must avoid NSAIDs for 7 days prior to and during the collection period, as well as red meat, citrus fruits and juices, and vitamin C in excess of 250 mg/day for 3 days prior to and during the test period (CliaWaived, 2019). Patient adherence is likely to be higher with the FIT method because drugs and food do not interfere with the test results.

As an alternate to the gFOBT or FIT, a stool DNA test (sDNA) can be completed every 3 years (American Cancer Society [ACS], 2018). Available only by prescription, this type of at-home diagnostic kit (such as Cologuard) is shipped directly to the patient after the health care provider has ordered the testing. Although less specific in detection than a colonoscopy, this type of testing can be encouraging to patients who may be fearful of undergoing a traditional colonoscopy or have concerns about financial coverage.

The cost for Cologuard testing is covered by Medicare and Medicare Advantage, with no additional cost to the patient (Exact Sciences Corporation, 2020). It also should be covered, based on the Affordable Care Act, by most private insurances; Cologuard reports that 94% of users have no out-of-pocket expenditures for this type of screening (Exact Sciences Corporation, 2020).

Once received in the mail, the test is easy to complete. The patient does not have to undergo any special preparation, such as the bowel cleansing that is required prior to a traditional colonoscopy. The patient collects one stool sample and returns it via a prepaid postage container. Although false-negative or false-positive results are possible, Cologuard reports identifying 92% of colon cancers and 42% of high-risk precancers per 10,000 samples (Imperiale et al., 2014).

Teach patients to talk openly with their health care provider to determine if a home screening test is appropriate. People who have a personal or family history of colon cancer, who have a condition that places them at risk (such as inflammatory bowel disease or Crohn's disease), or who have had previous positive results from another type of colon cancer screening test should be taught that a traditional colonoscopy is preferred over a home test. Emphasize the need to promptly follow up with the health care provider after the test to discuss results and possible subsequent actions that need to be taken.

LABORATORY PROFILE

Gastrointestinal Assessment

Test (Serum)	Normal Range for Adults	Significance of Abnormal Findings
Alanine aminotransferase (ALT)	4-36 units/L (may be slightly higher in older adults) Canadian: 5-35 mU/mL	*Increased* values indicate possible: • Liver disease • Hepatitis • Cirrhosis
Albumin	3.5-5.0 g/dL Canadian: 3.5-5.5 g/L	*Decreased* values indicate possible: • Hepatic disease • Undernutrition
Alkaline phosphatase	30-120 units/L (may be slightly higher in older adults) Canadian: 40-160 units/L	*Increased* values indicate possible: • Cirrhosis • Biliary obstruction • Liver tumor
Ammonia	10-80 mg/dL Canadian: 6-47 mcmol/L (10-80 mcg/dL)	*Increased* values indicate possible: • Hepatic disease such as cirrhosis
Aspartate aminotransferase (AST)	0-35 units/L (may be slightly higher in older adults; women may have slightly lower levels than men) Canadian: 7-40 units/L (may be slightly higher in older adults; women may have slightly lower levels than men)	*Increased* values indicate possible: • Liver disease • Hepatitis • Cirrhosis
Bilirubin (total)	0.3-1.0 mg/dL Canadian: 3-22 mcmol/L (0.2-1.3 mg/dL)	*Increased* values indicate possible: • Hemolysis • Biliary obstruction • Hepatic damage
Calcium (total)	9.0-10.5 mg/dL (values decrease in older adults) Canadian: 8.4-10.6 mg/dL	*Decreased* values indicate possible: • Malabsorption • Kidney failure • Acute pancreatitis
Cancer antigen 19-9 (CA19-9)	<37 units/mL Canadian: <37 kU/L	*Increased* values indicate possible: • Cancer of the pancreas, stomach, colon, gallbladder • Acute pancreatitis • Inflammatory bowel disease
Carcinoembryonic antigen (CEA)	<5 ng/mL Canadian: <5 mcg/L (<5 ng/mL)	*Increased* values indicate possible: • Colorectal, stomach, pancreatic cancer • Ulcerative colitis • Crohn's disease • Hepatitis • Cirrhosis
Cholesterol	<200 mg/dL Canadian: Same	*Increased* values indicate possible: • Pancreatitis • Biliary obstruction *Decreased* values indicate possible: • Liver cell damage
Conjugated (direct) bilirubin	0.1-0.3 mg/dL Canadian: 1.7-5.1 mcmol/L (0.1-0.3 mg/dL)	*Increased* values indicate possible: • Biliary obstruction
Potassium	3.5-5.0 mEq/L or 3.5-5.0 mmol/L Canadian: 3.5-5.1 mmol/L	*Decreased* values indicate possible: • Vomiting • Gastric suctioning • Diarrhea • Drainage from intestinal fistulas
Serum amylase	30-220 units/L Canadian: 25-125 units/L	*Increased* values indicate possible: • Acute pancreatitis
Serum lipase	0-160 units/L Canadian: Same	*Increased* values indicate possible: • Acute pancreatitis
Unconjugated (indirect) bilirubin	0.2-0.8 mg/dL Canadian: 3.4-12.0 mcmol/L (0.2-0.8 mg/dL)	*Increased* values indicate possible: • Hemolysis • Hepatic damage

LABORATORY PROFILE—cont'd

Gastrointestinal Assessment

Test (Serum)	Normal Range for Adults	Significance of Abnormal Findings
Xylose absorption	20-57 mg/dL (60-min plasma) 30-58 mg/dL (120-min plasma) Canadian: >1.3 mmol/L (>20 mg/dL) (60-min plasma) >1.6 mmol/L (>25 mg/dL) (120-min plasma)	*Decreased* values in blood and urine indicate possible: • Malabsorption in the small intestine

Data from Pagana, K., & Pagana, T. (2018). *Mosby's manual of diagnostic and laboratory tests* (6th ed.). St. Louis: Mosby; and Pagana, K., Pagana, T., & Pike-MacDonald, S. (2019). *Mosby's Canadian manual of diagnostic and laboratory tests* (2nd ed.). St. Louis: Mosby.

Stool samples may also be collected to test for *ova and parasites* to aid in the diagnosis of parasitic infection. They may also be tested for *fecal fats* when **steatorrhea** (fatty stools) or malabsorption is suspected. Fat is normally absorbed in the small intestine in the presence of biliary and pancreatic secretions; in malabsorption, fat is abnormally excreted in the stool. Stool samples can also be tested to detect the presence of infectious agents, such as *Clostridium difficile,* a common cause of diarrhea in older adults and patients on prolonged antibiotic therapy.

Imaging Assessment. Radiographic examinations and similar diagnostic procedures are useful in detecting structural and functional disorders of the GI system. Provide information about preparation for the examination, provide an explanation of the procedure, and teach the required postprocedure care.

A *plain film of the abdomen* may be the first x-ray study that the health care provider requests when diagnosing a GI problem. This film can reveal masses, tumors, and strictures or obstructions. Patterns of bowel gas appear light on the abdominal film and can be useful in detecting an obstruction (ileus). No preparation is required except to wear a hospital gown and remove any jewelry or belts, which may interfere with the film.

When abdominal ***pain*** is severe or bowel perforation is suspected, an *acute abdomen series* may be requested. This procedure consists of a chest x-ray, a supine abdomen film, and an upright abdomen film. The chest x-ray may reveal a hiatal hernia, and an upright abdomen film may show air in the peritoneum from a bowel perforation. Although x-rays are helpful, CT, MRI, and ultrasound scans are used more often (Gangadhar et al., 2016).

The 2019 American Cancer Society screening guidelines include the following tests as options to determine the presence of colorectal cancer and polyps in adults older than 45 years (ACS, 2019):

- Flexible sigmoidoscopy every 5 years, *or*
- CT colonography (**virtual colonoscopy**) every 5 years, *or*
- Colonoscopy every 10 years

CT, also referred to as a *CT scan,* provides a noninvasive cross-sectional x-ray view that can detect tissue densities and abnormalities in the abdomen, including the liver, pancreas, spleen, and biliary tract. It may be performed with or without contrast medium. If contrast medium is to be used, ask about allergies to seafood and iodine. The patient is to remain **NPO**, which means "nothing by mouth," for at least 4 hours before the test if a contrast medium is to be used. IV access is required for injection of the contrast medium. Advise the patient that on injection he or she may feel warm and flushed or experience a metallic taste. The patient who has claustrophobia may require a mild sedative to tolerate the study. The radiologic technician instructs the patient to lie still and to hold his or her breath when asked, as a series of images are taken. The test takes about 10 minutes.

Like other parts of the body, the abdomen and its organs may also be evaluated by *MRI,* such as *magnetic resonance cholangiopancreatography (MRCP).* Because of the use of powerful magnets, a special questionnaire is used and special precautions are taken to ensure that the patient meets requirements for this type of testing. Although this type of imaging takes longer than a CT scan, it does not expose patients to radiation.

NCLEX EXAMINATION CHALLENGE 48.3

Health Promotion and Maintenance

Which teaching will the nurse provide to a community group about early detection of colorectal cancer? **Select all that apply.**

A. Home testing kits are available with a prescription.
B. Sigmoidoscopy should be performed every 10 years.
C. People over 40 years old should be tested for colon cancer.
D. Bowel preparation is necessary prior to performance of a colonoscopy.
E. Virtual colonoscopies (CT colonography) can be performed every 5 years.

Other Diagnostic Assessment

Endoscopy. **Endoscopy** is direct visualization of the GI tract using a flexible fiberoptic **endoscope**, a tube that allows viewing and manipulation of internal body areas. It is commonly prescribed to evaluate bleeding, ulceration, inflammation, tumors, and cancer of the esophagus, stomach, biliary system, or bowel. Specimens for biopsy and cell studies (e.g., *Helicobacter pylori*) can be obtained through the endoscope. There are several types of endoscopic examinations, and the patient must sign an informed consent form before having any of these invasive studies performed.

Esophagogastroduodenoscopy. Esophagogastroduodenoscopy (EGD) is a visual examination of the esophagus, stomach, and duodenum by means of a fiberoptic endoscope. If GI bleeding is found during an EGD, the health care provider can use clips, thermocoagulation, injection therapy, or a topical hemostatic agent (National Institute of Diabetes and Digestive and Kidney Diseases [NIDDK], 2017). If the patient has an esophageal stricture, a narrowing of the esophageal opening, it can be dilated during EGD. Gastric lesions can be visualized using this procedure, and suspicion for celiac disease can be affirmed.

Usually patients are asked to avoid anticoagulants, aspirin, or other NSAIDs for several days before EGD unless it is absolutely necessary. The patient can take regularly prescribed medications the morning of the test unless otherwise instructed by the health care provider. Patients with diabetes should consult their primary health care provider for special instructions. Teach the patient to remain NPO for 6 to 8 hours before the procedure. If the patient has dentures, they are removed. Tell the patient that a flexible tube will be passed down the esophagus while he or she is under moderate sedation. Midazolam, fentanyl, or propofol is commonly used for sedation (Cohen, 2020). *These drugs can depress the rate and depth of the patient's respirations.* Atropine may be administered to dry secretions. A local anesthetic is sprayed to inactivate the gag reflex and facilitate passage of the tube. Explain that this anesthetic will depress the gag reflex and that swallowing will be difficult.

After the drugs are given, the patient is placed in a position with the head of the bed elevated. A bite block is inserted to prevent biting down on the endoscope and to protect the teeth. The health care provider passes the tube through the mouth and into the esophagus (Fig. 48.4). The procedure takes about 20 to 30 minutes.

During the test, the endoscopy nurse monitors the patient's respirations for rate and depth. Oxygenation saturation level is measured via pulse oximetry and ventilation is measured via capnography, capnometry, or mass spectroscopy (American Society of Anesthesiologists, 2015). Shallow respirations decrease the amount of carbon dioxide that the patient exhales. *If the patient's respiratory rate is below 10 breaths/min or the exhaled carbon dioxide level falls below 20%, the nurse typically uses a stimulus such as a sternal rub to encourage deeper and faster respirations.*

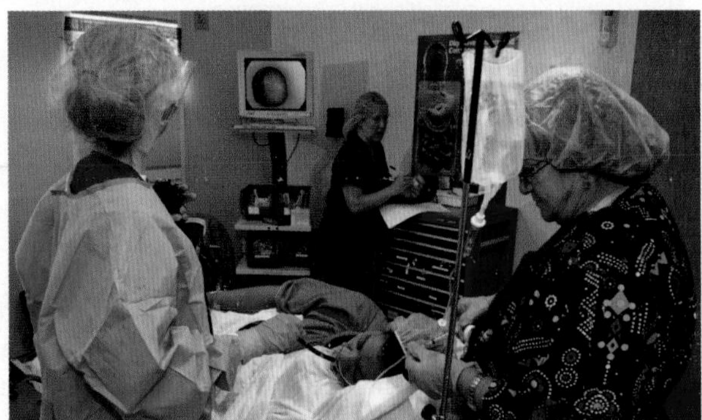

FIG. 48.4 Esophagogastroduodenoscopy allows visualization of the esophagus, the stomach, and the duodenum. If the esophagus is the focus of the examination, the procedure is called *esophagoscopy*. If the stomach is the focus, the procedure is called *gastroscopy*.

After the test, check vital signs frequently (usually every 15 to 30 minutes) until the sedation begins to wear off. The side rails of the bed are raised during this time. Keep the patient NPO until the gag reflex returns (usually in 30 to 60 minutes). IV fluids that were started before the procedure can be discontinued when the patient is able to tolerate oral fluids without nausea or vomiting.

! NURSING SAFETY PRIORITY (QSEN)

Action Alert

The priority for care to promote patient safety after esophagogastroduodenoscopy is to prevent aspiration. Do not offer fluids or food by mouth until you are sure that the gag reflex is intact! Monitor for signs of perforation, such as ***pain,*** bleeding, or fever.

Because EGD is most often performed as an ambulatory care (outpatient) procedure requiring moderate sedation, be sure that the patient has someone to drive him or her home. Remind the patient to not drive for at least 12 to 18 hours after the procedure because of sedation. Teach him or her that a hoarse voice or sore throat may persist for several days after the test. Throat lozenges can be used to relieve throat discomfort.

Endoscopic Retrograde Cholangiopancreatography. Endoscopic retrograde cholangiopancreatography (ERCP) includes visual and radiographic examination of the liver, gallbladder, bile ducts, and pancreas to identify the cause and location of obstruction. It is commonly used today for therapeutic purposes rather than for diagnosis. After a cannula is inserted into the common bile duct, a radiopaque dye is instilled, and several x-ray images are obtained. The health care provider may perform a *papillotomy* (a small incision in the sphincter around the ampulla of Vater) to remove gallstones. If a biliary duct stricture is found, plastic or metal stents may be inserted to keep the ducts open. Biopsy samples of tissue are also frequently taken during this test.

The patient prepares for this test in the same manner as for an EGD. Perform medication reconciliation to determine if the patient is taking anticoagulants, NSAIDs, antiplatelet drugs, or antihyperglycemic agents. The health care provider will determine whether drugs are safe to take and whether any will need to be stopped before the test.

The patient must be NPO for 6 to 8 hours before the test. If the patient has dentures, they are removed. Ask about prior exposure to x-ray contrast media and any sensitivities or allergies. IV access is required to administer drugs that cause moderate sedation. Ask the patient about any implantable medical devices, such as a cardiac pacemaker. Modern pacemakers generally are not affected by electrocautery; however, it is recommended that implantable defibrillators be deactivated, if possible, when electrocautery is used (Association of periOperative Registered Nurses [AORN], 2017).

The endoscopic procedure and nursing care for a patient having an ERCP are similar to those for the EGD procedure, except that the endoscope is advanced farther into the duodenum and into the biliary tract. Once the cannula is in the common duct, contrast medium is injected, and x-rays are taken to view the biliary tract. A tilt table assists in distributing the contrast medium to all areas to be assessed. The patient is placed in a left lateral position for viewing the common bile duct. Once the cannula is placed, he or she is put in a prone position. After examination of the biliary tree, the cannula is directed into the pancreatic duct for examination. The ERCP lasts from 30 minutes to 2 hours, depending on the treatment that may be done.

After the test, assess vital signs frequently, usually every 15 minutes, until the patient is stable. To prevent aspiration, check to ensure that the gag reflex has returned before offering fluids or food. Discontinue IV fluids that were started before the procedure when the patient is able to tolerate oral fluids without nausea or vomiting.

! NURSING SAFETY PRIORITY QSEN

Action Alert

Teach the patient and family to monitor for severe postprocedure complications at home, including cholecystitis or cholangitis (gallbladder inflammation or infection), bleeding, perforation, sepsis, and pancreatitis (Lee et al., 2018). The patient has severe ***pain*** if any of these complications occur. Fever is present in sepsis. These problems do not occur immediately after the procedure; they may take several hours to 2 days to develop.

Colicky abdominal ***pain*** and flatulence can result from air instilled during the procedure. Instruct the patient to report abdominal pain, fever, nausea, or vomiting that fails to resolve after returning home. Be sure that the patient has someone to drive him or her home if the test was done on an ambulatory care basis. Remind the patient to not drive for at least 12 to 18 hours after the procedure because of sedation.

Small Bowel Capsule Endoscopy. Small bowel endoscopy, or enteroscopy, provides a view of the small intestine. Video capsule endoscopy (VCE) is a procedure that uses a small-bowel enteroscopy device to visualize the entire small bowel (Keuchel et al., 2015), including the distal ileum. These devices are used to evaluate and locate the source of GI bleeding. Before the development of the VCE capsule endoscopes, viewing the small intestine was inadequate. The capsule battery lasts around 10 hours, so it is not used to view the colon.

Prepare the patient by explaining the procedure, the purpose, and what to expect during the testing. The patient must not eat or drink, including water, for 12 hours before the test and be NPO for the first 2 hours of the testing. The patient may drink clear liquids after 2 hours and have a light lunch after 4 hours (American Society for Gastrointestinal Endoscopy, 2020).

At the time of the procedure, the patient's abdomen is marked for the location of the sensors, and the sensors are applied. The patient wears an abdominal belt that houses a data recorder to capture the transmitted images. After the capsule is swallowed with a glass of water, the patient may return to normal activity, but should try to avoid vigorous activity and remain calm for the remainder of the study. At the end of the procedure, the patient returns the capsule equipment to the facility for downloading to a central computer. The procedure lasts about 8 hours or until the capsule is passed from the body.

Because the capsule endoscope is a single-use device that moves through the GI tract by peristalsis and is excreted naturally, explain to the patient that the capsule will be seen in the stool and is discarded after ***elimination.*** No other follow-up is necessary. The patient should report to the health care provider any signs or symptoms of GI obstruction, fever, chest pain, or difficulty breathing or if the capsule is not passed within 2 weeks.

Colonoscopy. Colonoscopy is an endoscopic examination of the entire large bowel. Be sure to fully assess all patients who may need a colonoscopy. The American Cancer Society recommends that beginning at age 45 years all healthy men and women should have a colonoscopy every 10 years or choose another equally effective recommended screening option (ACS, 2018). Evidence currently shows that younger adults with obesity are developing colon cancer, possibly due to chronic low-level inflammation that leads to cancer over a period of time (National Cancer Institute, 2017). Those at high risk for cancer (e.g., family history) or those who had polyps removed should have the test more often.

The health care provider can obtain tissue biopsy specimens or remove polyps through the colonoscope during this procedure. A colonoscopy can also evaluate the cause of chronic diarrhea or locate the source of GI bleeding. Topical hemostatic agents or other methods may be used to manage the bleeding.

Patient Preparation. Patients who have their first colonoscopy are often very anxious. Provide information about the procedure, level of sedation, and possibility of ***pain*** (Kartin et al., 2017). Reassure them that pain will be controlled with medication as needed.

Remind patients to avoid aspirin, anticoagulants, and antiplatelet drugs for several days before the procedure. Patients with diabetes should check with their primary health care provider about drug therapy requirements on the day of the test because they are NPO.

The health care provider will prescribe the specific method of preparation of the bowel, which begins the night before the procedure. Drinkable solutions can be chilled to improve taste. Teach the patient to partake of a clear liquid diet the day before the scheduled colonoscopy. Gatorade or other sports drinks will be recommended by the health care provider to replace electrolytes that are lost during bowel preparation. Instruct him or her to avoid red, orange, or purple (grape) beverages or gelatin. The patient should be NPO for several hours before the procedure, based on the health care provider's instructions.

Watery diarrhea usually begins in about an hour after starting the bowel preparation process. In some cases, the patient may also require laxatives, suppositories (e.g., bisacodyl), or one or more small-volume cleansing enemas (e.g., Fleet).

The failure to achieve adequate bowel preparation prior to this procedure can lead to decreased visualization of adenoma or unsuccessful colonoscopy. Patient education and type of bowel preparation solution are critical to a successful procedure (Writers, 2018).

Procedure. IV access is necessary for the administration of moderate sedation. The health care provider prescribes drugs to aid in relaxation, usually IV midazolam, fentanyl, or propofol (Cohen, 2020). Alternate therapies, such as using music, can improve the person's experience with a colposcopy, although it is not a substitute for sedation or pain medication (Kartin et al., 2017).

Initially the patient is placed on the left side with the knees drawn up while the endoscope is placed into the rectum and moved to the cecum. Air or carbon dioxide may be instilled for better visualization. Research indicates that the use of carbon dioxide is associated with decreased patient ***pain*** and distention (Lee & Salzman, 2020). The entire procedure lasts about 30 to 60 minutes. Atropine sulfate is kept available in case of bradycardia resulting from vasovagal response.

During the test, monitor the patient's respirations for rate and depth, and the oxygen saturation level via pulse oximetry. Shallow respirations decrease the amount of carbon dioxide that the patient exhales. If the patient's respiratory rate is below 10 breaths/min or the exhaled carbon dioxide level falls below 20%, use a stimulus such as a sternal rub to encourage deeper and faster respirations.

Follow-up Care. Check vital signs every 15 minutes until the patient is stable. Keep the side rails up until the patient is fully alert, and maintain NPO status. Ask the patient to lie on his or her left side to promote comfort and encourage passing flatus. Observe for signs of perforation (severe ***pain***) and hemorrhage, such as a rapid drop in blood pressure. Reassure the patient that a feeling of fullness, cramping, and passage of flatus is expected for several hours after the test. Fluids are permitted after the patient passes flatus to indicate that peristalsis has returned. Discontinue IV fluids that were started before the procedure when the patient is able to tolerate oral fluids without nausea or vomiting.

If a polypectomy or tissue biopsy was performed, there may be a small amount of blood in the first stool after the colonoscopy. Complications of colonoscopy are not common. *Report excessive bleeding or severe **pain** to the health care provider immediately* (see the Best Practice for Patient Safety & Quality Care: Care of the Patient After a Colonoscopy box).

BEST PRACTICE FOR PATIENT SAFETY & QUALITY CARE (QSEN)

Care of the Patient After a Colonoscopy

- Do not allow the patient to take anything by mouth until sedation wears off
- Take vital signs every 15 to 30 minutes until the patient is alert.
- Keep patient in left lateral position to promote passing of flatus.
- Keep the top side rails up until the patient is alert.
- Assess for rectal bleeding or severe pain.
- Remind the patient that fullness and mild abdominal cramping are expected for several hours.
- Assess for signs and symptoms of bowel perforation, including severe abdominal pain and guarding. Fever may occur later.
- Assess for signs and symptoms of hypovolemic shock, including dizziness, light-headedness, decreased blood pressure, tachycardia, pallor, and altered mental status (this may be the first sign in older adults).
- If the procedure is performed in an ambulatory care setting, arrange for another person to drive the patient home.
- Teach the patient to refrain from driving, making legal decisions, or carrying out other work that requires focus for the rest of the day.

As with other endoscopic procedures, the patient will need someone to provide transportation home if the procedure was done in an ambulatory care setting. Remind the patient to avoid driving and making important or legal decisions for the rest of the day after the procedure because of the effects of sedation.

Virtual Colonoscopy. A noninvasive imaging procedure to obtain multidimensional views of the entire colon is the *CT colonography,* known as virtual colonoscopy (Fig. 48.5). The bowel preparation and dietary restrictions are similar to those for traditional colonoscopy. However, if a polyp is detected during a virtual colonoscopy or bleeding is found, the patient must have

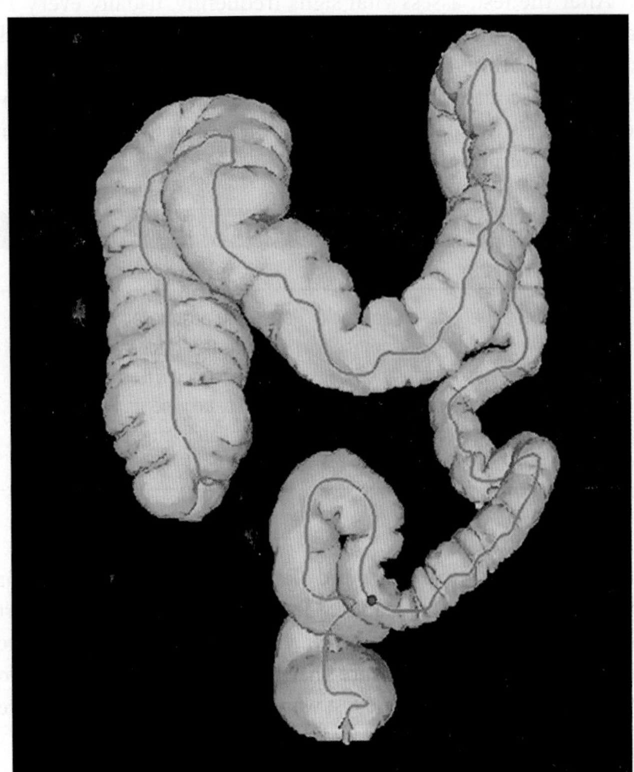

FIG. 48.5 Virtual colonoscopy. (From Pickhardt, P. J., & Kim, D. H. [2007]. CT colonography (virtual colonoscopy): A practical approach for population screening. *Radiologic Clinics of North America, 45*[2], 361-375.)

CLINICAL JUDGMENT CHALLENGE 48.1

Safety; Evidence-Based Practice

The nurse is providing preprocedure education to a 55-year-old client who is scheduled for an initial screening colonoscopy in 1 week. The electronic health record indicates a personal history of Crohn's disease and a family history of colon cancer. The client does not wish to go through the preparation process for a traditional colonoscopy, and voices a preference to have a home screening test performed.

1. **Recognize Cues:** What assessment information in this client situation is the most important and immediate concern for the nurse? (Hint: Identify the **relevant** information *first* to determine what is most important.)
2. **Analyze Cues:** What client conditions are consistent with the **most relevant** information? (Hint: Think about priority collaborative problems that support and contradict the information presented in this situation.)

a follow-up invasive colonoscopy for treatment. Therefore the advantage of the traditional colonoscopy is that both diagnostic testing and minor surgical procedures can be done at the same time.

Sigmoidoscopy. Proctosigmoidoscopy, referred to as a sigmoidoscopy, is an endoscopic examination of the rectum and sigmoid colon using a flexible scope. This procedures screens for colon cancer, investigates the source of GI bleeding, and can be used to diagnose or monitor inflammatory bowel disease. If sigmoidoscopy is used as an alternative to colonoscopy for colorectal cancer screening, it is recommended that screening begin at 45 years of age and be done every 5 years thereafter (ACS, 2018). Patients at high risk for cancer may require more frequent screening.

As with similar tests, the health care provider will determine which medicines, such as NSAIDs and anticoagulants, should be discontinued prior to the procedure. Teach the patient to consume a clear liquid diet for a period of time determined by the health care provider before the test. A laxative may be prescribed for the night before the test. A cleansing enema or sodium biphosphate (Fleet) enema is usually required the morning of the procedure.

The patient is placed on the left side in the knee-chest position. Moderate sedation is not required. The endoscope is lubricated and inserted into the anus to the required depth for viewing. Tissue biopsy may be performed during this procedure, but the patient cannot feel it. The examination usually lasts between 5 and 15 minutes.

Inform the patient that mild gas ***pain*** and flatulence may be experienced from air instilled into the rectum during the examination. If a biopsy specimen was obtained, a small amount of bleeding may be observed. Instruct the patient that excessive bleeding should be reported immediately to the health care provider.

Ultrasonography. Ultrasonography is a technique in which high-frequency, inaudible vibratory sound waves are passed through the body via a transducer. The echoes created by the sound waves are then recorded and converted into images for analysis. Ultrasonography is commonly used to view soft tissues, such as the liver, spleen, pancreas, and biliary system. The advantages of this test are that it is painless, is noninvasive, requires no radiation, and requires no specific preparation.

The patient may be fasting, depending on the abdominal organs to be examined. Inform him or her that it will be necessary to lie still during the study.

The patient is usually placed in a supine position. The technician applies insulating gel to the end of the transducer and on the area of the abdomen under study. This gel allows airtight contact of the transducer with the skin. The technician moves the transducer back and forth over the skin until the desired images are obtained. The study takes about 15 to 30 minutes. No follow-up care is necessary.

Endoscopic Ultrasonography. Endoscopic ultrasonography (EUS) provides images of the GI wall and high-resolution images of the digestive organs. The ultrasonography is performed through the endoscope. This procedure is useful in diagnosing the presence of lymph node tumors; mucosal tumors; and tumors of the pancreas, stomach, and rectum. The patient preparation and follow-up care are similar to those for both endoscopy and ultrasonography.

Liver-Spleen Scan. A liver-spleen scan uses IV injection of a radioactive material that is taken up primarily by the liver and secondarily by the spleen. The scan evaluates the liver and spleen for tumors or abscesses, organ size and location, and blood flow.

Teach the patient about the need to lie still during the scanning. Assure him or her that the injection has only small amounts of radioactivity and is not dangerous. Ask female patients of child-bearing age if they may be pregnant or are currently breast-feeding. The radionuclide can be found in breast milk, and radiation from x-rays or scans should be avoided in pregnancy.

The technician or the health care provider gives the radioactive injection through an IV line, and a wait of about 15 minutes is necessary for uptake. The patient is placed in many different positions while the scanning takes place. Tell the patient that the radionuclide is eliminated from the body through the urine in 24 hours. Careful handwashing after toileting decreases the exposure to any radiation present in the urine.

GET READY FOR THE NEXT-GENERATION NCLEX® EXAMINATION!

Key Points

Review these Key Points for each NCLEX Examination Client Needs Category.

Safe and Effective Care Environment

- Remind the patient to have someone available to drive him or her home after an endoscopic procedure because of the effects of moderate sedation. **QSEN: Safety**
- Check for the return of the gag reflex after an upper endoscopic procedure before offering fluids or food; aspiration may occur if the gag reflex is not intact. **QSEN: Safety**

Health Promotion and Maintenance

- Teach patients to carefully follow instructions for bowel preparation before diagnostic testing; the bowel must be clear to visualize the colon. **QSEN: Evidence-Based Practice**
- Instruct the patient to avoid vigorous activity, and follow the health care provider's instructions for eating, following a video capsule endoscopy. **QSEN: Evidence-Based Practice**

Psychosocial Integrity

- Remember that GI health problems markedly affect lifestyle and may cause anger, denial, and depression. **QSEN: Patient-Centered Care**
- Recall that GI testing may cause anxiety, fear, and/or embarrassment. **QSEN: Patient-Centered Care**

Physiological Integrity

- Recognize age-related changes in the GI system. **QSEN: Patient-Centered Care**
- Perform a focused abdominal assessment using inspection, auscultation, and light palpation. **QSEN: Evidence-Based Practice**

- Do not palpate or auscultate any abdominal pulsating mass because it could be a life-threatening aortic aneurysm. **QSEN: Safety**
- Assess and report major complications of GI testing to the health care provider. **QSEN: Safety**
- Review and interpret laboratory results and report abnormal findings to the health care provider. **Clinical Judgment**
- Monitor vital signs, and assess for bleeding, fever, and pain, for the patient having an endoscopic procedure. **QSEN: Safety**
- Do not allow foods or fluids for the patient who has had a colonoscopy until sedation wears off. **QSEN: Safety**

MASTERY QUESTIONS

1. Immediately following a colonoscopy, which client behavior will the nurse report to the health care provider? **Select all that apply.**
   A. Passing of flatus
   B. Blood pressure 128/80 mm Hg
   C. Abdominal guarding
   D. Change in mental status
   E. Report of mild abdominal cramping
2. Which teaching will the nurse include when educating a client who is scheduled to have an esophagogastroduodenoscopy (EGD)? **Select all that apply.**
   A. "Anesthesia will be used for sedation."
   B. "The procedure takes about 20 to 30 minutes to complete."
   C. "Informed consent will be needed prior to the procedure."
   D. "A separate test will be required to obtain any needed biopsies."
   E. "You will need to refrain from eating for at least 6 to 8 hours before the EGD."

REFERENCES

American Cancer Society (ACS). (2018). *Colorectal cancer screening test*. www.cancer.org/cancer/colon-rectal-cancer/detection-diagnosis-staging/screening-tests-used.html.

American Cancer Society (ACS). (2019). *American Cancer Society guidelines for the early detection of cancer*. https://www.cancer.org/healthy/find-cancer-early/cancer-screening-guidelines/american-cancer-society-guidelines-for-the-early-detection-of-cancer.html.

American Society of Anesthesiologists (ASA). (2015). *Standards for basic anesthetic monitoring*. www.asahq.org/quality-and-practice-management/standards-guidelines-and-related-resources/standards-for-basic-anesthetic-monitoring.

American Society for Gastrointestinal Endoscopy. (2020). *Understanding capsule endoscopy*. www.asge.org/home/for-patients/patient-information/understanding-capsule-endoscopy.

Association of periOperative Registered Nurses. (2017). Guideline summary: Energy-generating devices, Part 1--electrosurgery. (2017). *AORN Journal, 105*(3), 311–315. https://doi.org/10.1016/j.aorn.2016.12.021.

Bass, P. F., III. (2017). Lactose intolerance diagnosis and diet strategies. *Contemporary Pediatrics, 34*(6), 17–20.

CliaWaived. (2019). *Hemoccult II sensitive (fecal occult blood) tests*. https://www.cliawaived.com/hemoccult-ii-sensa-fecal-occult-blood-tests.html.

Cohen, J. (2020). Gastrointestinal endoscopy in adults: Procedural sedation administered by endoscopists. In Salzman, J., & Joshi, G. (Eds.), *UpToDate*, Waltham, MA.

Collins, J., & Badireddy, M. (2020). *StatPearls:Anatomy, abdomen and Pelvis, small intestine*. Treasure Island, FL: StatPearls Publishing.

Colorectal Cancer Alliance. (2019). Young onset. https://www.ccalliance.org/colorectal-cancer-information/young-onset.

Exact Sciences Corporation. (2020). *The easy Cologuard experience*. https://www.cologuardtest.com/meet-cologuard/easy-cologuard-experience.

Gangadhar, K., Kielar, A., Dighe, M. K., O'malley, R., Wang, C., Gross, J. A., et al, (2016). Multimodality approach for imaging of non-traumatic acute abdominal emergencies. *Abdominal Radiology, 41*(1), 136–148. https://doi.org/10.1007/s00261-015-0586-6.

Girard-Madoux, M., Gomez de Aguero, M., Ganal-Vonarburg, S., Mooser, C., Belz, G., Macpherson, A., et al. (2018). The immunological functions of the Appendix: An example of redundancy? *Seminars in Immunology, 36*, 31–44. https://doi.org/10.1016/j.smim.2018.02.005.

Imperiale, T. F., Ransohoff, D. F., Itzkowitz, S. H., et al. (2014). Multitarget stool DNA testing for colorectal-cancer screening. *New England Journal of Medicine, 370*(14), 1287–1297.

Jarvis, C. (2020). *Physical examination & health assessment* (8th ed.). St. Louis: Saunders.

Kartin, P., Bulut, F., Ceyhan, O., Tasci, S., Gursoy, S., & Isik, N. (2017). The effect of meditation and music listening on the anxiety level, operation tolerance and pain perception in people who were performed colonoscopy. *International Journal of Caring Sciences, 10*(3), 1587–1594.

Keuchel, M., Kurniawan, N., Baltes, P., Bandorski, D., & Koulaouzidis, A. (2015). Quantitative measurements in capsule endoscopy. *Computers in Biology and Medicine, 65*, 333–347.

Lee, H. S., Moon, J. C., Park, J. Y., Bang, S., Seung, W. P., Si, Y. S., et al. (2018). Urgent endoscopic retrograde cholangiopancreatography is not superior to early ERCP in acute biliary pancreatitis with biliary obstruction without cholangitis. *PloS One, 13*(2). https://doi.org/10.1371/journal.pone.0190835.

Lee, L., & Salzman, J. (2020). Overview of colonoscopy in adults. In Howell, D. (Ed.), *UpToDate*, Waltham, MA.

McCance, K. L., & Huether, S. E. (2019). *Pathophysiology: The biologic basis for disease in adults and children* (8th ed.). St. Louis: Elsevier.

National Cancer Institute at the National Institutes of Health. (2017). *Obesity and cancer.* www.cancer.gov/about-cancer/causes-prevention/risk/obesity/obesity-fact-sheet#q4.

National Institute of Diabetes and Digestive and Kidney Diseases (NIDDK). (2017). *Upper GI endoscopy.* www.niddk.nih.gov/health-information/diagnostic-tests/upper-gi-endoscopy.

Pagana, K., & Pagana, T. (2018). *Mosby's manual of diagnostic and laboratory tests* (6th ed.). St. Louis: Mosby.

Peate, I., & Nair, M. (2016). *Fundamentals of anatomy and physiology: For nursing and healthcare students* (2nd ed.). Hoboken, NJ: John Wiley & Sons.

Simonson, C. (2018). Colorectal cancer—an update for primary care nurse practitioners. *The Journal for Nurse Practitioners, 14*(4), 344–350. https://doi.org/10.1016/j.nurpra.2017.12.030.

Terrery, C. L., & Nicoteri, J. A. L. (2016). The 2015 American Geriatric Society beers criteria: Implications for nurse practitioners. *The Journal for Nurse Practitioners, 12*(3), 192–200. https://doi.org/10.1016/j.nurpra.2015.11.027.

U.S. Department of Agriculture. (2019). *Food access research atlas.* https://www.ers.usda.gov/data-products/food-access-research-atlas/documentation/.

Vemuri, R., Gundamaraju, R., Shastri, M. D., Shukla, S. D., Kalpurath, K., Ball, M., et al. (2018). Gut microbial changes, interactions, and their implications on human lifecycle: An ageing perspective. *BioMed Research International,* 1–13. https://doi.org/10.1155/2018/4178607.

Writers, A. M. (2018). Rates of adequate bowel preparation for colonoscopy may be improved by individualized treatment, education and support. *Drugs & Therapy Perspectives, 34*(1), 29–33. https://doi.org/10.1007/s40267-017-0454-2.

49

Concepts of Care for Patients With Oral Cavity and Esophageal Problems

Keelin C. Cromar, Cherie R. Rebar

http://evolve.elsevier.com/Iggy/

LEARNING OUTCOMES

1. Collaborate with the interprofessional team to coordinate high-quality care for patients with oral cavity or esophageal problems.
2. Describe factors that place a patient at high risk for oral cavity or esophageal problems and refer to the health care provider.
3. Implement patient-centered nursing interventions to decrease the psychosocial impact of living with an oral cavity or esophageal problem.
4. Apply knowledge of anatomy, physiology, and pathophysiology to assess patients with an oral cavity or esophageal problem.
5. Use clinical judgment to analyze assessment findings and diagnostic data in the care of patients with an oral cavity or esophageal problem.
6. Prioritize evidence-based care for patients with an oral cavity or esophageal problem affecting ***tissue integrity***, ***nutrition***, or ***gas exchange*** or that induces ***pain***.
7. Plan care coordination and transition management for patients with an oral cavity or esophageal problem.

KEY TERMS

aphthous stomatitis Noninfectious stomatitis.

Barrett epithelium Columnar epithelium (instead of the normal squamous cell epithelium) that develops in the lower esophagus during the process of healing from gastroesophageal reflux disease. It is considered premalignant and is associated with an increased risk of cancer in patients with prolonged disease.

candidiasis An infection caused by the fungus *Candida albicans.*

dysphagia Difficulty swallowing.

erythroplakia A velvety red mucosal lesion, most often occurring in the oral cavity.

esophageal stricture Narrowing of the esophageal opening.

esophagogastroduodenoscopy (EGD) The visual examination of the esophagus, stomach, and duodenum by means of a fiberoptic endoscope.

gastroesophageal reflux (GER) Condition that occurs as a result of backward flow of stomach contents into the esophagus.

gastroesophageal reflux disease (GERD) An upper gastrointestinal disease caused by the backward flow (reflux) of gastrointestinal contents into the esophagus.

hiatal hernia A condition, also called a diaphragmatic hernia, that involves the protrusion of the stomach through the esophageal hiatus of the diaphragm into the chest.

leukoplakia White, patchy lesions on a mucous membrane.

minimally invasive esophagectomy (MIE) A laparoscopic surgical procedure to remove part of the esophagus; may be performed in patients with early-stage cancer.

reflux esophagitis Damage to the esophageal mucosa, often with erosion and ulceration, in patients with gastroesophageal reflux disease.

regurgitation Backward flow of stomach contents into the esophagus.

sialadenitis Inflammation of a salivary gland.

stomatitis Inflammation of the oral mucosa; characterized by painful single or multiple ulcerations that impair the protective lining of the mouth. The ulcerations are commonly referred to as "canker sores."

upper endoscopy See *esophagogastroduodenoscopy.*

volvulus Obstruction of the bowel caused by twisting of the bowel.

xerostomia Very dry mouth caused by a severe reduction in saliva flow.

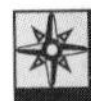

PRIORITY AND INTERRELATED CONCEPTS

The priority concepts for this chapter are:

- ***Tissue Integrity***
- ***Nutrition***

The ***Tissue Integrity*** concept exemplar for this chapter is Stomatitis.

The ***Nutrition*** concept exemplar for this chapter is Gastroesophageal Reflux Disease (GERD).

The interrelated concepts for this chapter are:

- ***Gas Exchange***
- ***Pain***

A HEALTHY ORAL CAVITY

Oral and esophageal problems can compromise ***tissue integrity,*** impair ***nutrition*** status and ***gas exchange,*** and induce ***pain***. This chapter discusses the most common oral and esophageal health problems. The nurse plays an important role in maintaining and restoring oral and esophageal health through nursing interventions, including provision of patient and family education to restore optimal ***nutrition*** comfort.

Inside the mouth, teeth tear, grind, and crush food into small particles to promote swallowing, beginning the process of digestion. Saliva enzymes begin carbohydrate breakdown. The esophagus moves partially digested food from the mouth to the stomach. Oral cavity disorders can severely affect physiologic well-being, speech, body image, and self-esteem. Those at highest risk include people who (Fischer et al., 2017):

- Have developmental delays or mental health disorders
- Have limited access to care due to homelessness or health disparities
- Reside in institutions
- Use tobacco and/or alcohol
- Consume an unhealthy diet
- Have a type of oral cancer
- Consume dietary excess

TISSUE INTEGRITY CONCEPT EXEMPLAR: STOMATITIS

Pathophysiology Review

Stomatitis is a broad term that refers to inflammation within the oral cavity. Painful, inflamed ulcerations (called *aphthous ulcers* or *canker sores*) (Fig. 49.1) that erode ***tissue integrity*** of the mouth are one of the most common forms of stomatitis. The sores cause ***pain*** and place the patient at risk for bleeding and infection. Treatment ranges from topical applicants to opioid analgesics and/or antifungal medication, depending on the source and degree of inflammation. Stomatitis is classified according to the cause of the inflammation.

Etiology and Genetic Risk. *Primary stomatitis,* the most common type, includes **aphthous stomatitis** (noninfectious stomatitis), herpes simplex stomatitis, and traumatic ulcers. *Secondary stomatitis* generally results from infection by opportunistic viruses, fungi, or bacteria in patients who are immunocompromised or as a result of chemotherapy, radiation, or steroid drug therapy.

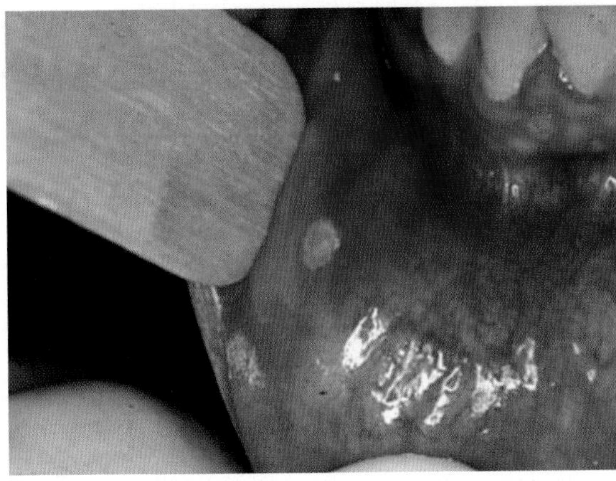

FIG. 49.1 Aphthous ulcer. (From Auerbach, P.S., Cushing, T.A., & Stuart H.N. [2017]. *Auerbach's wilderness medicine* [7th ed.]. Philadelphia: Elsevier.)

A common type of secondary stomatitis is caused by *Candida albicans,* which is sometimes present in small amounts in the mouth, especially in older adults. Long-term antibiotic therapy can destroy normal flora, which allows *Candida* to overgrow. The result can be **candidiasis**, *(moniliasis),* a painful fungal infection.

PATIENT-CENTERED CARE: OLDER ADULT CONSIDERATIONS (QSEN)

Older adults are at high risk for candidiasis because the immune system naturally declines during aging. The risk increases for those with diabetes or malnourishment, or those under great stress. Taking multiple medications can contribute to oral dryness and decreased salivation. Teach proper mouth care to preserve ***tissue integrity,*** as prevention is much easier than treatment of this painful kind of stomatitis.

Stomatitis can result from infection, allergy, vitamin or mineral deficiency (complex B vitamins, folate, zinc, iron), systemic disease, and irritants such as tobacco and alcohol. Certain foods such as coffee, potatoes, cheese, nuts, citrus fruits, and gluten may trigger allergic responses that cause aphthous ulcers. Evidence suggests that activation of the cell-mediated immune system in some patients may be related to a genetic predisposition (Plewa & Chatterjee, 2020).

Incidence and Prevalence. The most common type of stomatitis, recurrent aphthous stomatitis (RAS), affects approximately 20% of the general population and is more commonly found in females (Plewa & Chatterjee, 2020).

Health Promotion and Maintenance. Proper oral hygiene can decrease the frequency and severity of stomatitis. The Patient and Family Education: Preparing for Self-Management: Maintaining a Healthy Oral Cavity box contains important teaching points to provide to all adults, which will also help them to improve and maintain oral health.

PATIENT AND FAMILY EDUCATION: PREPARING FOR SELF-MANAGEMENT

Maintaining a Healthy Oral Cavity

- Eat a well-balanced diet and stay hydrated by drinking water.
- Manage stress by using healthy coping mechanisms; stress can increase inflammation.
- Perform a weekly self-examination of your mouth; report changes or unusual findings to the primary health care provider or dentist.
- Report occlusion of teeth, mouth ***pain***, or swelling to the primary health care provider.
- If you wear dentures, make sure that they are in good repair and fit properly.
- Thoroughly brush and floss your teeth (or brush dentures) consistently twice daily.
- Avoid mouthwashes that contain alcohol, which can damage ***tissue integrity***.
- Avoid drugs that increase inflammation of the mouth or reduce saliva flow.
- See your dentist regularly; have dental problems addressed as soon as they are noted.

❖ Interprofessional Collaborative Care

Care for the patient with stomatitis usually takes place in the community setting. The interprofessional team that collaborates to care for this patient includes the primary health care provider and nurse; a dentist and dental hygienist to provide care for the teeth, gums, and oral cavity; and an ear, nose, and throat specialist if needed.

◆ Assessment: Recognize Cues

History. Ask about a history of recent infections, ***nutrition*** changes, oral hygiene habits, oral trauma, and stress. Also collect a drug history, including over-the-counter (OTC) drugs and nutrition and herbal supplements. Document the course of the current symptoms, and determine if stomatitis has occurred in the past. Ask if the lesions interfere with swallowing, eating, or communicating. Severe stomatitis and edema have the potential to obstruct the airway. In cases of oral candidiasis, white plaquelike lesions appear on the tongue, palate, pharynx (throat), and buccal mucosa (inside the cheeks) (Fig. 49.2). When these patches are wiped away, the underlying surface is red, sore, and painful, and ***tissue integrity*** is compromised.

Physical Assessment/Signs and Symptoms. Assess for lesions, coating, and cracking. Document characteristics of the lesions, including location, size, shape, odor, color, and drainage. If lesions are seen along the pharynx and the patient reports dysphagia (difficulty with swallowing) or throat ***pain***, they might extend down the esophagus. To establish a definitive diagnosis, the primary health care provider may prescribe additional swallowing studies.

Psychosocial Assessment. Severe stomatitis can be very painful, which can cause distress. Assess the patient's ability to cope with pain. Also determine if the presence of stomatitis has an effect on the patient's body image or self-image.

◆ Analysis: Analyze Cues and Prioritize Hypotheses.

The priority collaborative problems for the patient with stomatitis include:

1. Impaired ***tissue integrity*** due to oral and/or esophageal lesions
2. ***Pain*** due to oral and/or esophageal lesions

! NURSING SAFETY PRIORITY (QSEN)

Action Alert

Airway obstruction, aspiration pneumonia, and malnutrition can result from dysphagia. Assess for signs and symptoms such as coughing or choking when swallowing, a sensation of food "sticking" in the pharynx, or difficulty swallowing. If dysphagia is suspected, use the PASS acronym for quick assessment: Is it **P**robable that the patient will have swallowing difficulty? **A**ccount for previous swallowing problems. **S**creen for signs and symptoms. Obtain a **S**peech-language pathologist (SLP) referral (Mountain & Golles, 2017). Report signs and symptoms to the primary health care provider, and institute aspiration prevention interventions.

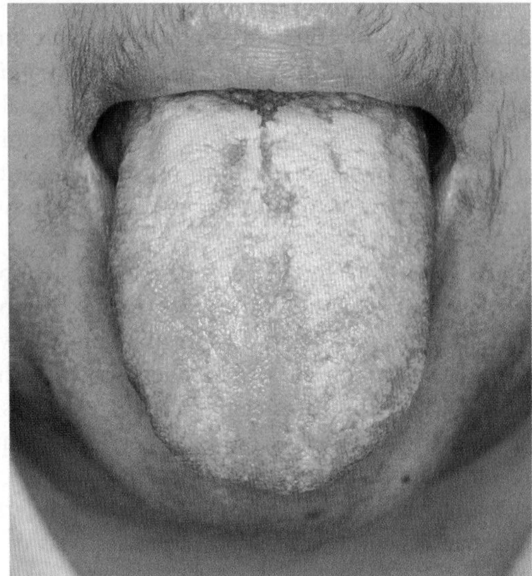

FIG. 49.2 Oral candidiasis. (From Millsop, J.W., & Fazel, N. [2016]. Oral candidiasis. *Clinics in Dermatology, 34*[4], 487–494. https://doi.org/10.1016/j.clindermatol.2016.02.022.)

◆ Planning and Implementation: Generate Solutions and Take Action

Preserving Tissue Integrity

Planning: Expected Outcomes. The patient with stomatitis is expected to regain a healthy oral cavity with intact ***tissue integrity***.

Interventions. Interventions for stomatitis are targeted toward health promotion and reduced risk for infection through careful *oral hygiene* and food selection. Delegate oral care to assistive personnel (AP), as this task falls within an AP's skill set, and inspect the patient's oral cavity when the AP is done. Follow the procedures described in the Best Practice for Patient Safety & Quality Care: Care of the Patient With Problems of the Oral Cavity box for best oral care.

Drug therapy used for stomatitis includes solutions to address pain and infection. Commonly used drugs to address infection include (Brice, 2019):

- Clotrimazole troches
- Nystatin suspension (swish and spit)
- Chlorhexidine (swish and spit)

BEST PRACTICE FOR PATIENT SAFETY & QUALITY CARE (QSEN)

Care of the Patient With Problems of the Oral Cavity

- Remove dentures if the patient has severe stomatitis or oral ***pain***.
- Encourage the patient who is able to do so to perform oral hygiene twice daily, after meals, and as often as needed. If the patient is unable, provide mouth care.
- Increase oral care frequency to every 2 hours or more if stomatitis is not controlled.
- Teach patient to use a soft toothbrush or gauze, to use toothpaste free of sodium lauryl sulfate (SLS), and to avoid commercial mouthwashes and lemon-glycerin swabs, which can irritate mucosa.
- Encourage frequent rinsing of the mouth with warm saline, sodium bicarbonate (baking soda) solution, or a combination of these solutions.
- Help the patient select soft, bland, and nonacidic foods.
- Apply topical analgesics or anesthetics as prescribed by the primary health care provider and document effectiveness.

Minimizing Pain

Planning: Expected Outcomes. The patient with stomatitis is expected to experience minimized discomfort or absence of ***pain***.

Interventions. Dietary changes may help decrease discomfort. Cool or cold liquids can be very soothing, whereas hard, spicy, salty, and acidic foods or fluids can further irritate the ulcers. Include foods high in protein to promote healing. Vitamin C may be recommended as a supplement; eating citrus fruits rich in vitamin C may be painful.

Over-the-counter (OTC) oral anesthetics can be recommended. Prescription drugs used as "swish and spit" agents for pain management include (Brice, 2019):

- Viscous lidocaine
- Diphenhydramine liquid
- Aluminum hydroxide, magnesium hydroxide, and simethicone suspension

! NURSING SAFETY PRIORITY (QSEN)

Drug Alert

Teach patients to use viscous lidocaine with extreme caution. Lidocaine causes a topical anesthetic effect, so patients may not easily feel burns from hot liquids. As sensation in the mouth and throat decreases, the risk for aspiration raises.

NCLEX EXAMINATION CHALLENGE 49.1

Physiological Integrity

A nurse is caring for a client with recurrent aphthous stomatitis (RAS) who asks about food choices while healing. Which food will the nurse suggest?

A. Half of an orange
B. Chocolate pudding
C. Chips with hummus
D. Glass of tomato juice

Care Coordination and Transition Management

Home Care Management. Remind the patient to take all medications as prescribed, especially antibiotics, even if he or she begins to feel better. If the patient has been prescribed medication for ***pain***, teach about possible side effects and discourage driving and activities that require concentration. Teach which drugs should be used to swish and swallow, which are to be used only as a rinse, and which are taken orally.

Self-Management Education. Teach about dietary choices that will not irritate the oral cavity and how to gently brush to promote good oral hygiene while preserving ***tissue integrity*** and minimizing ***pain***.

Health Care Resources. Although most cases of stomatitis are self-limiting, some patients may experience persistent pain (e.g., for stomatitis related to ongoing treatment with chemotherapy and/or radiation). These patients may benefit from a support group related to their underlying illness or a group designated for those who are coping with persistent pain.

◆ **Evaluation: Evaluate Outcomes.** Evaluate the care of the patient with stomatitis based on the identified priority patient problems. The expected outcomes include that the patient will:

1. Have healthy oral mucosa without inflammation or infection
2. Experience minimized discomfort or absence of ***pain***

ORAL CAVITY DISORDERS

ORAL TUMORS: PREMALIGNANT LESIONS

Tumors of the mouth, whether benign, precancerous, or cancerous, can affect swallowing, chewing, and speaking. ***Pain*** can also limit daily activities and self-care. Oral tumors affect body image, especially if treatment involves removal of the tongue or part of the mandible (jaw) or requires a tracheostomy.

ERYTHROPLAKIA

Erythroplakia, which is considered precancerous, appears as red, velvety mucosal lesions on the floor of the mouth, tongue, palate, and mandibular mucosa. It can be difficult to distinguish from inflammatory or immune reactions.

LEUKOPLAKIA

Leukoplakia causes thickened, white, firmly attached patches on the oral mucosa that cannot easily be scraped off. These common oral lesions appear slightly raised and sharply rounded. Most of these lesions are benign; however, lesions on the lips or tongue can progress to cancer. Tobacco use increases the chance of development of leukoplakia.

! CORE MEASURES

Always ask patients about current or historical tobacco use. The Joint Commission's Tobacco Treatment Measures (TOB) (2020b) requires offering practical counseling and treatment to people who use tobacco.

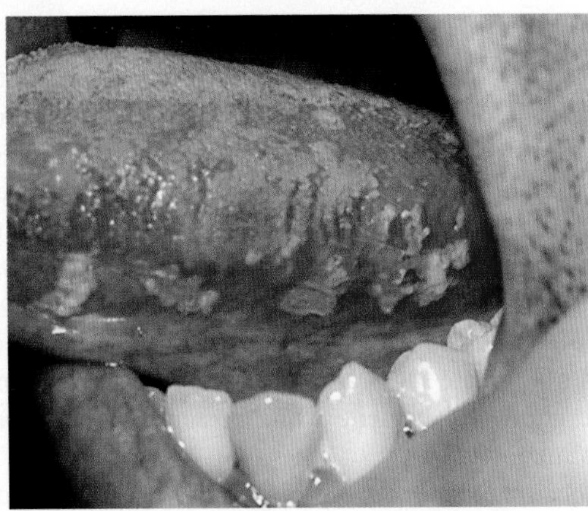

FIG. 49.3 Hairy leukoplakia. (From Sapp, J.P., Eversole, L.R., & Wysocki, G.P. [2004]. *Contemporary oral and maxillofacial pathology* [2nd ed.]. St. Louis: Elsevier.)

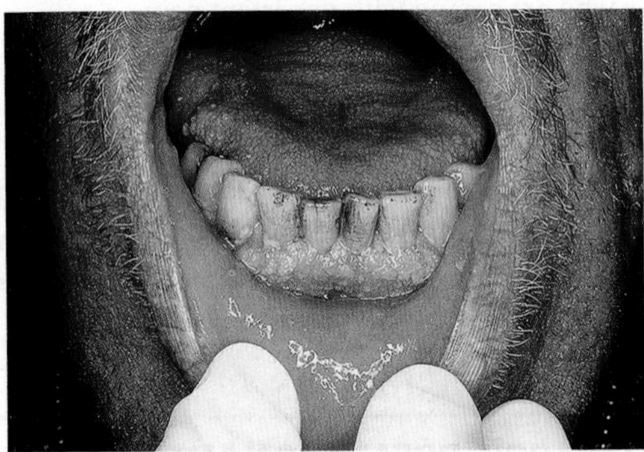

FIG. 49.4 Oral cancer. (From Salvo, S.G. [2014]. *Mosby's pathology for massage therapists* [3rd ed.]. St. Louis: Mosby.)

Long-term oral mucous membrane irritation (poorly fitting dentures, cheek chewing, broken teeth) can precede development of leukoplakia.

Oral hairy leukoplakia (Fig. 49.3) develops in people with immune compromise. It is often found in those with human immune deficiency virus (HIV) (as an early symptom) or Epstein-Barr virus (EBV).

ORAL CANCER

Teach adults to visit a dentist at least twice a year for professional dental hygiene and an oral cancer screening, which includes inspecting and palpating the mouth for lesions (Fig. 49.4). Prevention strategies including stopping use of tobacco and alcohol, avoiding sun exposure to lips, and avoiding exposure to human papillomavirus (HPV), a sexually transmitted infection (see Chapter 69).

Textile workers, plumbers, and coal and metal workers, who have prolonged exposure to polycyclic aromatic hydrocarbons (PAHs), are at high risk for development of oral cancer, particularly if they have exposure to HPV (Zhang et al., 2019). People with *periodontal disease* (gum disease) (Fig. 49.5) in which mandibular (jaw) bone loss has occurred are also at risk.

Teach adults to follow the guidelines in the Patient and Family Education: Preparing for Self-Management: Maintaining a Healthy Oral Cavity box to maintain oral health.

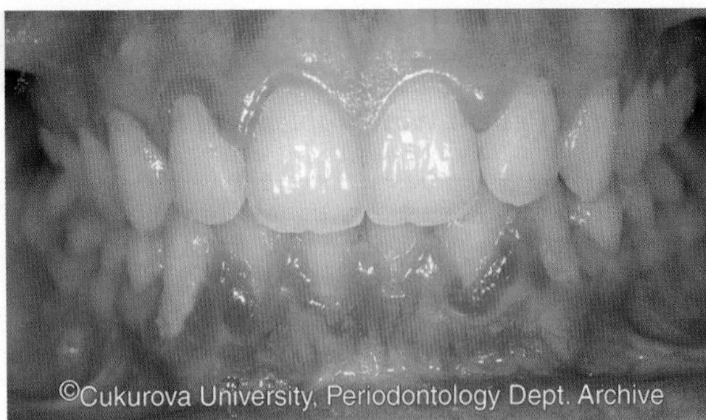

FIG. 49.5 Periodontal (gum) disease. (From Newman, M.G., Takei, H., Klokkevold, P.R., & Carranza, F.A. [2019]. *Newman and Carranza's Clinical Periodontology* [13th ed.]. Philadelphia: Elsevier.)

Pathophysiology Review

Most oral cancers are squamous cell carcinomas that begin on the lips, tongue, buccal mucosa, and oropharynx in people over the age of 40. Oral lesions that are red, raised, and eroded are suspicious for cancer. A lesion that does not heal within 2 weeks or a lump or thickening in the cheek warrants further assessment (Oral Cancer Foundation [OCF], 2019a).

Basal cell carcinoma of the mouth occurs primarily on the lips and is related most closely to sunlight exposure. The lesion is asymptomatic and resembles a raised scab. With time, it evolves into a characteristic ulcer with a raised, pearly border. Basal cell carcinomas do not metastasize but can aggressively involve the skin of the face.

Kaposi sarcoma is a vascular tumor, appearing as a raised, purple, reddish, or brownish nodule or plaque, which is usually painless. It can be found on the hard palate, gums, tongue, or tonsils. It is most often associated with acquired immune deficiency syndrome (AIDS [HIV-III]) (see Chapter 17).

PATIENT-CENTERED CARE: GENETIC/GENOMIC CONSIDERATIONS QSEN

Ask about history of any cancer in patients who are at risk for, or may have, oral cancer. Genetic variations in patients with oral cancer have been found, especially the mutation of the *TP53* gene (McCance et al., 2019). The tumor protein p53 is essential for cell division regulation and prevention of tumor formation (National Institutes of Health, 2020).

NCLEX EXAMINATION CHALLENGE 49.2

Health Promotion and Maintenance

A nurse is caring for four clients. Which individual does the nurse identify as being at the **highest** risk for development of oral cancer?

A. 28-year-old with human papillomavirus (HPV) infection
B. 30-year-old with recurrent aphthous stomatitis (RAS)
C. 55-year-old who quit chewing tobacco 5 years ago
D. 76-year-old who is sometimes negligent in denture care

KEY FEATURES
Oral Cancer

- Bleeding from the mouth
- Poor appetite, compromised ***nutrition*** status
- Difficulty chewing or swallowing
- Unplanned weight loss
- Thick or absent saliva
- Painless oral lesion that is red, raised, or eroded
- Thickening or lump in cheek

Interprofessional Collaborative Care

Care of the patient with oral cancer takes place in a variety of settings from the hospital to the community, depending on the degree of treatment needed. The interprofessional team that treats and cares for a patient with oral cancer may include the primary health care provider, dentist, surgeon, oncologist, nurse, speech therapist, registered dietitian nutritionist, social worker, and spiritual leader of the patient's choosing.

Assessment: Recognize Cues. Assess the patient's oral hygiene regimen and use of dentures or oral appliances. Ask about oral bleeding; alcohol or tobacco use; difficulty eating, chewing, or swallowing; and whether there has been unplanned recent weight loss (see the Key Features: Oral Cancer box). Assess for educational, cultural, and/or spiritual needs that might affect health teaching or treatment, as well as the patient's self-image. Evaluate for presence of a support system.

Thoroughly inspect the oral cavity for any lesions, ***pain,*** or restriction of movement; using gloves, a tongue blade, and penlight, examine all areas of the mouth. The primary health care provider will palpate for cervical nodes (Fig. 49.6).

A needle biopsy or an incisional biopsy of the abnormal tissue will be performed by the provider to assess for malignant or premalignant changes. In very small lesions, an excisional biopsy can permit complete tumor removal (OCF, 2019a). CT or MRI may be performed to determine if there is metastasis (or if staging is needed), and MRI is useful in detecting perineural involvement and evaluating thickness in cancers of the tongue.

Interventions: Take Action. Oral cavity lesions can be treated by surgical excision; radiation and surgery; or radiation, surgery, and chemotherapy. Multimodal therapy is most effective for more major oral cancers (OCF, 2019a). Airway maintenance to facilitate ***gas exchange*** is the priority of care for patients with oral cancer. Other nursing interventions focus on restoring and maintaining oral health to the best degree possible.

Nonsurgical Management. Implement interventions targeted to promote ***gas exchange,*** remove secretions, and prevent aspiration. Assess for dyspnea resulting from obstruction or excessive secretions. Assess the quality, rate, and depth of respirations. Auscultate the lungs for adventitious sounds, such as wheezes caused by aspiration. Listen for stridor caused by partial airway obstruction. Promote deep breathing to help produce an effective cough to mobilize secretions.

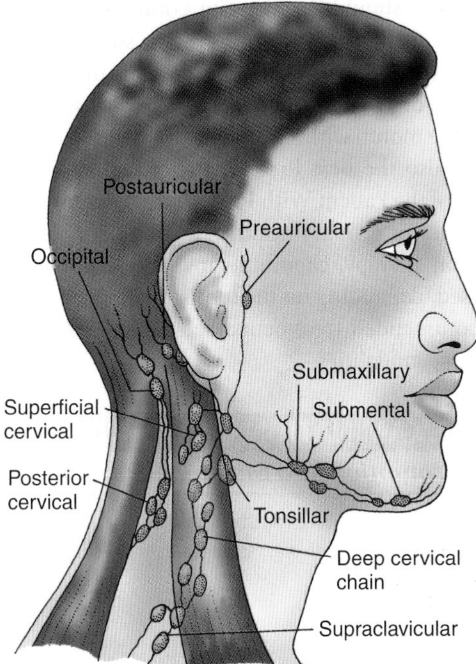

FIG. 49.6 The lymph nodes of the cervical region.

Place the patient in semi-Fowler or high-Fowler position. If the patient is able to swallow and the gag reflex is intact, it is beneficial to encourage fluids to liquefy secretions for easier removal. Chest physiotherapy, often performed by the respiratory therapist, can be helpful. If needed, use oral suction equipment with a dental tip or a tonsil tip (Yankauer) to remove secretions. Teach the patient and family to use suction catheters as appropriate.

Steroids, which reduce inflammation, may be prescribed for edema associated with oral cavity lesions. Antibiotics may be prescribed for infection. A cool mist supplied by a face tent may help with oxygen transport and edema control.

NURSING SAFETY PRIORITY QSEN
Action Alert

Aspiration precautions must be instituted for patients with oral cancer. Assess the patient's level of consciousness (LOC), gag reflex (especially before giving fluids), and ability to swallow. Place the patient in a semi-Fowler or high-Fowler position and keep suction equipment nearby. Remind assistive personnel to feed patients at risk for aspiration in small amounts. All family and visitors should be instructed to speak with the nurse before offering any type of food or drink to the patient. Thickened liquids may be needed; collaborate with the speech-language pathologist, who may recommend a swallow study.

Perform oral hygiene every 2 hours. Use a soft-bristle toothbrush or an ultrasoft "chemobrush," especially for patients with a low platelet count. Do not use oral swabs or disposable foam brushes, which do not adequately control bacteremia-promoting plaque and may further dry the oral mucosa. Water-based lubricant can be applied to moisten the lips and oral mucosa as needed.

The patient should avoid using commercial mouthwashes that contain alcohol and lemon-glycerin swabs owing to their acidity. These substances can cause a burning sensation and contribute to dry oral mucous membranes. Encourage frequent rinsing of the mouth with sodium bicarbonate solution or warm saline (see also the Best Practice for Patient Safety & Quality Care: Care of the Patient With Problems of the Oral Cavity box). Follow agency or primary health care provider protocol.

Radiation therapy, chemotherapy, and/or targeted therapy may be used, depending on the tumor type, location, stage, and other recommended treatments. See Chapter 20 for information on these modalities.

NCLEX EXAMINATION CHALLENGE 49.3

Health Promotion and Maintenance

When providing discharge teaching about mouth care, which substance will the nurse teach the client with oral cancer to avoid? **Select all that apply.**

A. Mouthwash
B. Lip lubricant
C. Warm saline rinses
D. Ultrasoft toothbrush
E. Disposable foam brushes
F. Bicarbonate mouth rinse

Surgical Management. Depending on the type and stage of cancer, a different surgery may be recommended. Common surgeries for oral cancer include (Cancer Treatment Centers of America, 2020):

- Scalpel, laser, or cryoprobe removal (of erythroplakia or leukoplakia, depending on type)
- Glossectomy—removal of the tongue
- Laryngectomy—removal of the larynx and tumor
- Mandible resection (full or partial)—removal of part or all of the mandible
- Maxillectomy—removal of part or all of the hard palate
- Microsurgery—reconstruction of the mouth, throat, or mandible with body tissue from the patient (e.g., from the intestine, arm, abdomen)
- Mohs micrographic surgery—removal of cancer on the lip by taking of thin slices until no cancer is left
- Neck dissection (partial, modified radical, or radical)—removal of lymph nodes in the neck, with or without muscle, nerve tissue, and veins
- Pedicle or free flap reconstruction—repair of the mouth, throat, or neck after a tumor is removed (often with the use of a skin graft)
- Tumor resection—removal of an entire oral tumor, with some surrounding normal tissue

Preoperative Care. Preoperative care for patients undergoing significant head and neck cancer is discussed in Chapter 26. For patients undergoing same-day procedures on an ambulatory basis, such as the scalpel, laser, or cryoprobe removal of erythroplakia or leukoplakia, document the patient's level of understanding of the disease process, the rationale for the procedure, and the planned intervention. Evidence shows that preoperative oral health reduces postoperative inflammation and complications, so provide teaching and encourage starting proper oral care before any procedure takes place.

PATIENT AND FAMILY EDUCATION: PREPARING FOR SELF-MANAGEMENT

Care of the Patient With Oral Cancer at Home

- Inspect the mouth daily for changes, such as redness or lesions, or signs of infection.
- Continue meticulous oral hygiene at home.
- Use an ultrasoft toothbrush or chemobrush; clean brush after every use.
- Keep all follow-up appointments.
- Use a thickening agent for liquids if dysphagia is present.
- Eat soft foods if stomatitis occurs.
- Use saliva substitute as prescribed, if needed.

Operative Procedures. The procedure chosen for isolated tumors is dependent on size, stage, and location. Removal may be done by scalpel, laser, or cryoprobe. Operative procedures for patients undergoing significant head and neck cancer are described in Chapter 26.

Postoperative Care. For small, local excisions, postoperative teaching includes planning for liquid diet for a day, and then advancing as tolerated. Activity can resume as tolerated, and ***pain*** is managed on a case-by-case basis. Remind the patient to keep any follow-up appointments, and to continue meticulous oral care. Postoperative care for patients undergoing significant head and neck cancer is located in Chapter 26.

Care Coordination and Transition Management. Continuing care for the patient with an oral tumor depends on the severity of the tumor and the degree of treatment. Teach the patient who underwent a minor procedure for localized oral cancer about ***nutrition*** therapies to best restore oral and systemic health, drug therapy (if prescribed), and symptoms of infection to report. See the Patient and Family Education: Preparing for Self-Management: Care of the Patient With Oral Cancer at Home box for more information. Also see Chapter 26 for care of the patient who underwent significant head and neck cancer surgery.

SIALADENITIS

Pathophysiology Review

Acute sialadenitis, inflammation of a salivary gland, can be associated with:

- Bacteria or viruses (commonly associated with cytomegalovirus)
- •Immunologic compromise (e.g., HIV infection, Sjögren syndrome)
- Decrease in saliva production (especially in patients undergoing radiation for head and neck, or thyroid, cancer)
- Systemic drugs (phenothiazines, tetracyclines)

Acute sialadenitis most commonly affects the parotid or submandibular gland in adults. Although there is not a defining timeline to mark the transition, sialadenitis can become chronic if swelling persists over weeks to months (Hoffman, 2019).

Untreated infections of the salivary glands can evolve into an abscess, which can rupture and spread infection into the tissues of the neck and the mediastinum. The best prevention for acute sialadenitis is adherence to routine oral hygiene, which prevents infection from ascending to the salivary glands.

❖ Interprofessional Collaborative Care

Assess for any predisposing factors for sialadenitis, such as ionizing radiation to the head or neck area. Collect a thorough drug history and ask about systemic illnesses, especially ones where immunity is compromised.

Assess the oral cavity for dryness, ***pain,*** and swelling of the face in the area of the affected gland. Purulent drainage can sometimes be massaged from the affected area. Assess facial function, as the branches of cranial nerve VII (the facial nerve) are near the salivary glands. The patient may also report fever and general malaise.

Conservative care is directed at treating the underlying cause and increasing the flow of saliva. Teach the patient to stay hydrated, apply moist heat, and massage the gland by sweeping the fingers along the course of the gland with gentle pressure. ***Pain*** and inflammation can be managed with NSAIDs, and antibiotics will be prescribed if infection is suspected. *Sialagogues* (substances that stimulate the flow of saliva) may be recommended if saliva production has decreased.

The salivary glands are sensitive to ionizing radiation, such as from radiation therapy or radioactive iodine treatment of thyroid cancers. Radiation of the salivary glands can cause ***pain*** and edema, which generally subside after several days. Exposure of the glands to radiation produces a type of sialadenitis known as **xerostomia** (very dry mouth caused by a severe reduction in the flow of saliva) within 24 hours.

Xerostomia may be temporary or permanent, depending on the radiation dose and percentage of total salivary gland tissue irradiated. Frequent sips of water and frequent mouth care, especially before meals, are the most effective interventions to address xerostomia. After the course of radiation therapy has been completed, saliva substitutes may provide moisture for short periods of time. Over-the-counter solutions are available.

NUTRITION CONCEPT EXEMPLAR: GASTROESOPHAGEAL REFLUX DISEASE (GERD)

Pathophysiology Review

Gastroesophageal reflux disease (GERD), the most common upper gastrointestinal disorder in the United States, occurs most often in middle-age and older adults. **Gastroesophageal reflux (GER)** occurs as a result of backward flow of stomach contents into the esophagus, known as **regurgitation**. GERD is the chronic and more serious condition that arises from persistent GER.

Patients who are overweight or have obesity are at highest risk for GERD because increased weight increases intra-abdominal pressure, which contributes to reflux. *Helicobacter pylori* may contribute to reflux (McCance et al., 2019) by causing gastritis and thus poor gastric emptying. This increases frequency of GER events and acid exposure to the esophagus.

TABLE 49.1 Factors Contributing to Decreased Lower Esophageal Sphincter Pressure

- Caffeinated beverages
- Coffee, tea, and cola
- Chocolate
- Nitrates
- Citrus fruits
- Tomatoes and tomato products
- Alcohol
- Peppermint, spearmint
- Smoking and use of other tobacco products
- Calcium channel blockers
- Anticholinergic drugs
- High levels of estrogen and progesterone
- Nasogastric tube placement

Etiology and Genetic Risk. There is not a single causative agent for GERD. Reflux produces symptoms by exposing the esophageal mucosa to the irritating effects of gastric or duodenal contents, resulting in inflammation. A patient with acute symptoms of inflammation is often described as having mild or severe **reflux esophagitis** (McCance et al., 2019). When the lower esophageal sphincter (LES) is compromised (relaxed), gastric contents reflux into the esophagus. Eating large meals or certain foods, taking certain drugs, smoking, and using alcohol influence the tone function of the LES (Table 49.1). Reflux is generally sour or bitter. Although rare, a reflex salivary hypersecretion known as ***water brash*** can occur in response to reflux. Water brash is different from regurgitation. The patient reports a sensation of fluid in the throat, but unlike with regurgitation, there is no bitter or sour taste.

Patients who have a nasogastric (NG) tube have decreased esophageal sphincter function. The tube keeps the cardiac sphincter open and allows acidic contents from the stomach to enter the esophagus. Other factors that increase intra-abdominal and intragastric pressure (e.g., pregnancy, wearing tight belts or abdominal binders, bending over, ascites) overcome the gastroesophageal pressure gradient maintained by the LES and allow reflux to occur. Many patients with obstructive sleep apnea report frequent episodes of GERD. Nighttime reflux causes prolonged exposure of the esophagus to acid because the patient is usually in supine position, and secretions do not drain back down with gravity.

Twin and family studies have demonstrated an approximate 31% heritability of GERD (Argyrou et al., 2018). As with many disorders, lifestyle choices contribute very significantly to this condition.

During the process of healing, the body may substitute **Barrett epithelium** (columnar epithelium) for the normal squamous cell epithelium of the lower esophagus; this becomes known as Barrett esophagus. Although this new tissue is more resistant to acid and supports esophageal healing, it is premalignant and is associated with an increased risk for cancer in patients with prolonged GERD. The fibrosis and scarring that accompany the healing process can produce **esophageal stricture** (narrowing of the esophageal opening), which leads to progressive difficulty swallowing. Uncontrolled esophageal reflux also increases the risk for other complications such as asthma, laryngitis, dental decay, and cardiac disease, as well as serious concerns for hemorrhage and aspiration pneumonia.

Incidence and Prevalence. The population affected by GERD continues to get younger. The greatest recent rise in proportion of people with GERD, as well as those using proton pump inhibitor (PPI) therapy, is seen in the 30- to 39-year-old demographic (Yamasaki et al., 2018). Prevalence in North America is 18.1% to 27.8% (Yamasaki et al., 2018).

Health Promotion and Maintenance. Adults with gastroesophageal reflux (GER) may initially be asymptomatic. Teach patients to engage in healthy eating habits that include consuming small, frequent meals and limiting intake of fried, fatty, and spicy foods, and caffeine. Sitting upright for at least 1 hour after eating can promote proper digestion and reduce the risk for reflux.

NCLEX EXAMINATION CHALLENGE 49.4

Health Promotion and Maintenance

Which client statement about GERD triggers requires further nursing teaching? **Select all that apply.**

A. "I will decrease my alcohol intake."
B. "Smoking one or two cigarettes a day won't hurt."
C. "My plan is to eat six small meals daily."
D. "Tomato-based foods should be avoided."'
E. "I love soda but I'm going to stop drinking it."
F. "Our family eats tacos and burritos several times weekly."

❖ Interprofessional Collaborative Care

Care for the patient with GERD usually takes place in the community setting. Seldom is surgery needed to correct the problem. The interprofessional team that collaborates to care for this patient typically includes the primary health care provider, nurse, and registered dietitian nutritionist (RDN).

◆ Assessment: Recognize Cues

History. Ask the patient about a history of heartburn or atypical chest pain associated with the reflux of GI contents. Ask whether he or she has been newly diagnosed with asthma, has experienced morning hoarseness, or has coughing or wheezing, especially at night. These symptoms may indicate severe reflux reaching the pharynx or mouth or pulmonary aspiration.

Ask about dysphagia and odynophagia (painful swallowing), which can accompany chronic GERD.

Physical Assessment/Signs and Symptoms. Dyspepsia, also known as *indigestion,* and regurgitation are the main symptoms of GERD, although symptoms may vary in severity (see the Key Features: Gastroesophageal Reflux Disease box). With severe GERD, this sensation generally occurs after each meal and lasts for 20 minutes to 2 hours. Discomfort may worsen when the patient lies down. Drinking fluids, taking antacids, or maintaining an upright posture usually provides prompt relief.

Other symptoms may include abdominal discomfort, feeling uncomfortably full, nausea, flatulence, eructation (belching), and bloating. Because indigestion might not be viewed as a serious concern, patients often delay seeking treatment. The symptoms typically worsen when the patient bends over, strains, or lies down. If the indigestion is severe, the ***pain*** may be felt in the chest and may radiate to the neck, jaw, or back, mimicking cardiac pain.

KEY FEATURES

Gastroesophageal Reflux Disease

- Dyspepsia (indigestion)
- Regurgitation (may lead to aspiration or bronchitis)
- Water brash (hypersalivation)
- Dental caries (severe cases)
- Dysphagia
- Odynophagia (painful swallowing)
- Globus (feeling of something in back of throat)
- Pharyngitis
- Coughing, hoarseness, or wheezing at night
- Chest pain
- Pyrosis (heartburn)
- Epigastric ***pain***
- Generalized abdominal ***pain***
- Belching
- Flatulence
- Nausea

In addition to performing a gastrointestinal assessment, auscultate the patient's lung fields, assessing for crackles, which can be an indication of associated aspiration.

Psychosocial Assessment. Patients may come to the emergency department (ED) fearing that they are having a myocardial infarction. Stay with the patient as much as possible until a diagnosis is made, as worrying can create intense anxiety. Assess the client's ability to cope with stress and fear, and provide referrals as necessary.

PATIENT-CENTERED CARE: OLDER ADULT CONSIDERATIONS QSEN

Older adults are at risk for developing severe complications associated with GERD caused by age-related physiologic changes, comorbidities, increased prevalence of obesity, and polypharmacy (Commisso & Fidelindo, 2019). Instead of the typical symptoms related to GERD, this population experiences more severe complications of the disease such as atypical chest pain; ear, nose, and throat infections; and pulmonary problems, such as aspiration pneumonia, sleep apnea, and asthma. Barrett esophagus and esophageal erosions are also more common in older adults.

Diagnostic Assessment. A definitive diagnostic test for GERD does not exist; however, the primary health care provider may use a clinical history and diagnostic tests to establish a diagnosis when GERD is suspected (Gyawali et al., 2018). Usually, patients with classic GERD symptoms are diagnosed on the basis of clinical symptoms and history alone (Kahrilas, 2020). Those with atypical symptoms may benefit from an upper endoscopy (also called esophagogastroduodenoscopy [EGD]). This procedure involves insertion of an endoscope (a flexible plastic tube equipped with a light and lens) down the throat, which shows the esophagus and any associated abnormalities. A biopsy can be performed at the same time (see Chapter 48) (Gyawali et al., 2018). This test requires the use of moderate sedation during the procedure, and patients must have someone drive them home after recovery.

Ambulatory esophageal pH monitoring is the most accurate method of diagnosing GERD. In this procedure, a transnasally placed catheter or wireless, capsule-like device is affixed to the distal esophageal mucosa (Kahrilas, 2020). The patient is asked to keep a diary of activities and symptoms over 24 to 48 hours (depending on diagnostic method), and the pH is continuously monitored and recorded.

Although not as common, *esophageal manometry,* or motility testing, may be performed. Water-filled catheters are inserted in the patient's nose or mouth and slowly withdrawn while measurements of LES pressure and peristalsis are recorded. When used alone, manometry cannot establish a diagnosis of GERD (Gyawali et al., 2018); it is used to rule out an esophageal motility disorder before considering surgery for GERD (Kahrilas, 2020).

◆ Analysis: Analyze Cues and Prioritize Hypotheses

The priority collaborative problems for the patient with gastroesophageal reflux disease (GERD) include:

1. Potential for compromised ***nutrition*** status due to dietary selection
2. Acute ***pain*** due to reflux of gastric contents

◆ Planning and Implementation: Generate Solutions and Take Action

Balancing Nutrition

Planning: Expected Outcomes. The patient with imbalanced ***nutrition*** is expected to have improvement in nutrition status while esophagitis heals.

Interventions. Interventions are designed to optimize ***nutrition*** status, decrease symptoms experienced with GERD, and prevent complications. Nursing care priorities focus on teaching the patient about proper dietary selections that provide optimum nutrients and that do not contribute to reflux.

Nonsurgical Management. For most patients, GERD can be controlled with ***nutrition*** therapy, lifestyle changes, and drug therapy. The most important role of the nurse is patient and caregiver education. Teach the patient that GERD is a chronic disorder that requires ongoing management. The disease should be treated more aggressively in older adults.

Ask about the patient's basic meal patterns and food preferences. Coordinate with the registered dietitian nutritionist (RDN), patient, and caregiver to adopt changes in eating that may decrease reflux symptoms.

Teach the patient to limit or eliminate foods that decrease LES pressure. Foods that irritate inflamed tissue and cause heartburn, such as peppermint, chocolate, fatty foods (especially fried), caffeine, and carbonated beverages, should be avoided. The patient should also restrict spicy and acidic foods (e.g., orange juice, tomatoes) until esophageal healing occurs. Recommend applications ("apps") that can help the patient follow a healthier diet, such as MyFitnessPal (www.myfitnesspal.com) or MyPlate (www.livestrong.com).

Explain that large meals increase volume and pressure within the stomach and delay gastric emptying. Recommend eating four to six small meals each day rather than three large ones. Advise the patient to eat slowly and chew thoroughly to facilitate digestion and prevent eructation (belching). Teach to avoid eating at least 3 hours before going to bed, because reflux episodes are most damaging at night. The risk for aspiration is increased if regurgitation occurs when the patient is lying down. Remind the patient to sleep propped up to promote ***gas exchange***. This can be done by placing blocks under the head of the bed or by using a large, wedge-style pillow instead of a standard pillow.

Teach that alcohol and tobacco should be avoided, and make referrals to cessation groups and programs if needed. If weight management is needed, refer to the appropriate resources and community support groups.

Minimizing Pain

Planning: Expected Outcomes. The patient is expected to have relief of ***pain*** associated with GERD.

Interventions. Interventions are designed to minimize the patient's ***pain.*** Nursing care priorities focus on teaching the patient about lifestyle modifications that will improve comfort.

Nonsurgical Management. In addition to appropriate dietary selections that promote ***nutrition*** and allow esophageal tissues to heal, the patient should be encouraged to adhere to other methods of controlling symptoms to minimize ***pain.***

Lifestyle changes. In addition to nutrition modifications, teach the patient about other lifestyle changes that decrease symptoms of GERD. Discourage heavy lifting, straining, and working in a position in which the patient bends at the abdomen. Encourage comfortable, nonrestrictive clothing.

Emphasize that these general adaptations are an essential and effective part of disease management and can produce prompt results in uncomplicated cases.

Patients with obesity often have obstructive sleep apnea in addition to GERD. Those who receive continuous positive airway pressure (CPAP) treatment report improved sleeping and decreased episodes of reflux at night. See Chapter 26 for a discussion of CPAP.

Drug therapy. Some drugs lower LES pressure and cause reflux; these include oral contraceptives, anticholinergic agents, sedatives, NSAIDs (e.g., ibuprofen), nitrates, and calcium channel blockers. Although not always possible, the elimination of drugs causing reflux should be explored with the primary health care provider.

Drug therapy for GERD management includes three major types: antacids, histamine blockers, and proton pump inhibitors (PPIs). These drugs, which are also used for peptic ulcer disease, have one or more of these functions:

- Inhibit gastric acid secretion
- Accelerate gastric emptying
- Protect the gastric mucosa

The stomach responds to these actions, and the ***pain*** that a patient experiences should decrease. See Table 50.1 in Chapter 50 for drug therapy used for GERD management.

Some PPIs, such as esomeprazole and pantoprazole, may be administered in IV form for short-term use to treat or prevent stress ulcers that can result from surgery. PPIs promote rapid tissue healing, but recurrence is common when the drug is stopped. Long-term use may mask reflux symptoms, and stopping the drug determines if reflux has been resolved. Recent research has linked long-term PPI use to community-acquired pneumonia, *Clostridium difficile,* bone fractures, chronic kidney injury, and vitamin and mineral deficiencies. Evidence is still being gathered regarding several of these adverse effects, but it is important to acknowledge the need for monitoring during extended PPI use (Nehra et al., 2018).

PATIENT-CENTERED CARE: OLDER ADULT CONSIDERATIONS QSEN

Research has found that long-term use of proton pump inhibitors (PPIs) may increase the risk for hip fracture, especially in older adults. PPIs can interfere with calcium absorption and protein digestion and therefore reduce available calcium to bone tissue. Decreased calcium makes bones more brittle and likely to fracture, especially as adults get older (Maes et al., 2017).

Endoscopic therapies. The Stretta procedure, a nonsurgical method, can replace surgery for GERD when other measures are not effective. In the Stretta procedure, the health care provider applies radiofrequency (RF) energy through the endoscope using needles placed near the gastroesophageal junction. The RF energy decreases vagus nerve activity, thus reducing discomfort for the patient. Patients with obesity or those who have severe symptoms may not be candidates for this procedure. Postoperative instructions for patients who have undergone the Stretta procedure can be found in the Patient and Family Education: Preparing for Self-Management box.

Surgical Management. A very small percentage of patients with GERD require antireflux surgery. It is usually indicated for patients who have not responded to medical treatment, have high-volume reflux, and have severe esophagitis; in some cases, it is also beneficial for patients with upper respiratory symptoms associated with GERD (Schwaitzberg, 2019). Various surgical procedures may be used through conventional open or laparoscopic techniques.

PATIENT AND FAMILY EDUCATION: PREPARING FOR SELF-MANAGEMENT

Postoperative Instructions for Patients Having the Stretta Procedure

- Remain on clear liquids for 24 hours after the procedure.
- After the first day, consume a soft diet, such as custard, pureed vegetables, mashed potatoes, and applesauce.
- Avoid NSAIDs and aspirin for 10 days.
- Continue drug therapy as prescribed, usually proton pump inhibitors.
- Use liquid medications whenever possible.
- Do not allow nasogastric tubes to be inserted for at least 1 month because the esophagus could be perforated.
- Contact the primary health care provider immediately if these problems occur:
  - Abdominal ***pain***
  - Bleeding
  - Chest ***pain***
  - Dysphagia
  - Nausea or vomiting
  - Shortness of breath

Laparoscopic Nissen fundoplication (LNF) is minimally invasive surgery (MIS) and is the standard surgical approach for treatment of severe GERD (Mermelstein et al., 2018). Information about this procedure can be found in the next section (Hiatal Hernias) in the Surgical Management discussion. Patients who have surgery are encouraged to continue following the basic antireflux regimen of antacids and ***nutrition*** therapy because the rate of recurrence is high.

The LINX Reflux Management System is a device that augments the LES with a ring composed of rare earth magnets (Schwaitzberg, 2020). The magnets attract to increase the closure pressure of the LES, yet still allow food passage with swallowing. The LINX can be effective for patients with typical GERD symptoms who have an abnormal pH study, only partially respond to daily PPI therapy, and do not have a hiatal hernia or severe esophagitis (Schwaitzberg, 2020). *Teach patients who have had LINX to talk with all health care providers before having an MRI.* Older LINX devices should *never* be in the presence of MRI, as serious injury could occur; newer devices, called MR Conditional, can undergo scanning under *certain* conditions (Schwaitzberg, 2020).

For patients having surgery for GERD, follow preoperative and postoperative interventions presented in Chapter 9.

! NURSING SAFETY PRIORITY QSEN

Safety Alert

When caring for a patient who has had LINX device insertion, emphasize the importance of telling each health care provider about this procedure. If an MRI is recommended, only certain patients with more recent LINX devices *may* be eligible to undergo scanning. Patients with older LINX devices (which contain magnets) should *never* undergo MRI scanning. The health care provider can determine whether MRI is acceptable for the patient, given the date of LINX device insertion.

Care Coordination and Transition Management. Patients with GERD that does not require surgical intervention are usually managed in the community setting. Nursing interventions focus on helping the patient and family with current treatment and reducing risk for continuing symptoms and complications.

Home Care Management. Remind the patient to make appropriate dietary selections that enhance ***nutrition*** and decrease symptoms associated with GERD. Teach how to properly adhere to drug therapy to minimize GERD-related ***pain.***

Self-Management Education. For patients with nonsurgical GERD, teach about signs and symptoms of more serious complications such as esophageal stricture and Barrett esophagus.

Health Care Resources. Patients may find it helpful to work with a registered dietitian nutritionist (RDN) or a support group for meal-planning purposes. Give the patient information about local support groups for people with GERD and direct toward online communities that provide credible information and discussion for ongoing management of this condition.

◆ **Evaluation: Evaluate Outcomes.** Evaluate the care of the patient with GERD based on the identified priority patient problem. The expected outcomes include that the patient will:

- Adhere to appropriate dietary selections, medication therapy, and lifestyle modifications, which decrease signs and symptoms of GERD
- Experience minimized or absence of ***pain***

HIATAL HERNIAS

Hiatal hernias, also called *diaphragmatic hernias,* involve the protrusion of the stomach through the esophageal hiatus of the diaphragm into the chest. The esophageal hiatus is the opening in the diaphragm through which the esophagus passes from the thorax to the abdomen.

CLINICAL JUDGMENT CHALLENGE 49.1

Patient-Centered Care; Evidence-Based Practice

The nurse is caring for a 33-year-old male client who is seeing the primary health care provider for several months of "heartburn" after lunch and dinner. He reports that these episodes last about an hour after eating, and are much worse if he lays down for sleep after a meal. Most of the time, he also experiences belching and bloating with the "heartburn". He has been taking over-the-counter antacids with minimal relief. He says that his wife sent him today because she was getting concerned about the amount of antacids he has been using. Reading in the electronic health record, the nurse notes a medical history of mild hypertension controlled with amlodipine, and a social history of smoking a pack of cigarettes daily and drinking 4 to 5 alcoholic beverages weekly. Further data collected today include: height 5'9" tall, weight 203 lb. The patient confirms that this information is still current.

1. **Recognize Cues:** What assessment information in this client situation is the most important and immediate concern for the nurse? (Hint: Identify the **relevant** information *first* to determine what is most important.)
2. **Analyze Cues:** What client conditions are consistent with the **most relevant** information? (Hint: Think about priority collaborative problems that support and contradict the information presented in this situation.)
3. **Prioritize Hypotheses:** Which possibilities or explanations are **most likely** to be present in this client situation? Which possibilities or explanations are the most serious? (Hint: Consider all possibilities and determine their urgency and risk for this client.)
4. **Generate Solutions:** What actions would most likely achieve the desired outcomes for this client? Which actions should be **avoided** or are **potentially harmful**? (Hint: Determine the desired outcomes first to decide which interventions are appropriate and those that should be avoided.)
5. **Take Action:** Which actions are the most appropriate and how should they be implemented? In what **priority order** should they be implemented? (Hint: Consider health teaching, documentation, requested health care provider orders or prescriptions, nursing skills, collaboration with or referral to health team members, etc.)
6. **Evaluate Outcomes:** What client assessment would indicate that the nurse's actions were **effective**? (Hint: Think about signs that would indicate an improvement, decline, or unchanged client condition.)

Pathophysiology Review

Hiatal hernias are classified as type I (*sliding* hernias, which are most common) or types II through IV (paraesophageal, or *rolling,* hernias). In a type I (sliding) hernia, the esophagogastric junction and a portion of the fundus of the stomach slide upward through the esophageal hiatus into the chest, usually as a result of weakening of the diaphragm (Fig. 49.7). The hernia generally moves freely and slides into and out of the chest during changes in position or intra-abdominal pressure. Although **volvulus** (twisting of a GI structure) and obstruction do occur rarely, the major concern for a sliding hernia is the development of esophageal reflux and associated complications (see the section Nutrition Concept Exemplar: Gastroesophageal Reflux Disease [GERD]earlier in this chapter).

Types II through IV (paraesophageal) hernias are characterized as follows (Kahrilas, 2019):

- Type II—The gastroesophageal junction remains in its normal intra-abdominal location, but the fundus (and possibly portions of the stomach's greater curvature) rolls through the esophageal hiatus and into the chest beside the esophagus (see Fig. 49.7).
- Type III—The gastroesophageal junction and the fundus both herniate through the hiatus, with the fundus lying above the gastroesophageal junction.
- Type IV—The colon, spleen, pancreas, or small intestine is found in the hernia sac (instead of the stomach).

The risks for volvulus (twisting of a GI structure), obstruction (blockage), and strangulation (stricture) are high. The development of iron deficiency anemia is common because slow bleeding from venous obstruction causes the gastric mucosa to become engorged and ooze. Significant bleeding or hemorrhage is rare.

❖ Interprofessional Collaborative Care

Care for the patient with a hiatal hernia usually takes place in the community setting, unless surgery is needed to correct the problem. The interprofessional health care team includes the primary health care provider, nurse, surgeon, registered dietitian nutritionist, and spiritual leader of the patient's choice.

◆ **Assessment: Recognize Cues.** Most patients with hiatal hernias are asymptomatic, but some experience symptoms similar to those with GERD (McCance et al., 2019) as listed in the Key Features: Hiatal Hernias box. Symptoms usually worsen after a meal or when the patient is supine. Obtain a history and perform a physical assessment as you would for a patient with GERD (covered earlier in this chapter).

The *barium swallow study with fluoroscopy* is the most specific diagnostic test for identifying hiatal hernia. Rolling hernias are usually clearly visible, and sliding hernias can often be observed when the patient moves through a series of positions that increase intra-abdominal pressure. To visualize sliding hernias, an esophagogastroduodenoscopy (EGD) may be performed to view both the esophagus and gastric lining (see Chapter 48). High-resolution manometry (HRM) with esophageal pressure topography (EPT) is used to identify larger sliding hiatal hernias (Kahrilas, 2020).

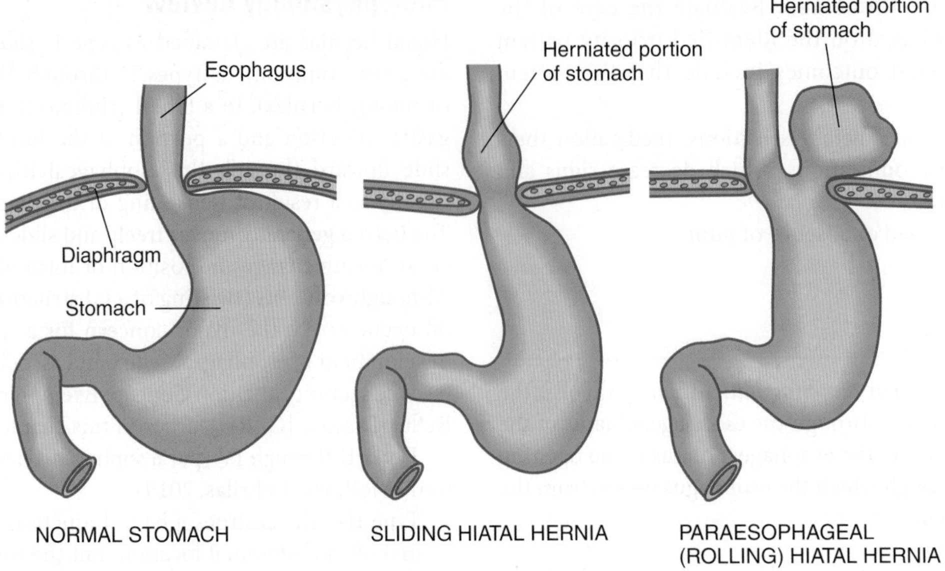

FIG. 49.7 Comparison of the normal stomach and sliding and paraesophageal (rolling) hiatal hernias.

KEY FEATURES
Hiatal Hernias

Sliding Hiatal Hernias	Paraesophageal Hernias
• Heartburn • Regurgitation • Chest pain • Dysphagia • Belching	• Feeling of fullness (after eating) • Breathlessness (after eating) • Feeling of suffocation (after eating) • Chest pain that mimics angina • Worsening of symptoms in a recumbent position

◆ **Interventions: Take Action.** Type I (sliding) hiatal hernias are usually treated medically. Treatment of types II through IV (paraesophageal) hiatal hernias are treated based on type, the severity of symptoms, and the risk for serious complications. When possible, medical management is favored. For patients at risk for, or who experience, volvulus, bleeding, obstruction, strangulation, perforation, or airway obstruction, surgery is performed (Kahrilas, 2020).

Nonsurgical Management. Interventions for patients with a type I (sliding) hiatal hernia are similar to those for GERD. These include drug therapy, ***nutrition*** therapy, and lifestyle changes. The primary health care provider typically recommends antacids or a proton-pump inhibitor in an attempt to control reflux and its symptoms. ***Nutrition*** therapy is also important and follows the guidelines discussed earlier for GERD.

! NURSING SAFETY PRIORITY (QSEN)
Action Alert

When caring for a patient with hiatal hernia, education is one of the most important parts of nursing care. Follow health teaching as described for patients with GERD.

Surgical Management. Surgery may be required when the risk for complications is high or when damage from chronic reflux becomes severe.

Preoperative Care. If the surgery is not urgent, the surgeon may instruct a patient who is overweight to lose weight before surgery. Any patient who is to undergo surgery for hiatal hernia is advised to quit smoking. As part of preoperative teaching, reinforce the surgeon's instructions and prepare the patient for what to expect after surgery. See Chapter 9 for preoperative intervention.

Operative Procedures. Surgical repair can be done transabdominally or transthoracically. The transabdominal approach can be done as an open procedure or laparoscopically (Rosen & Blatnik, 2019). Surgery involves fundoplication, in which the stomach fundus is wrapped around the distal esophagus. The wrap is then closed with sutures to anchor the lower esophagus below the diaphragm (Fig. 49.8).

Laparoscopic Nissen fundoplication (LNF) is a minimally invasive surgical procedure commonly used for hiatal hernia repair. Complications after LNF occur less frequently compared with those seen in patients having the more traditional open surgical approach. A small percentage of patients are not candidates for LNF and therefore require a conventional open fundoplication.

Prepare the patient undergoing a transthoracic approach for a chest tube and a nasogastric tube, which will be present after surgery. These will be inserted during surgery and remain in place for several days.

Postoperative Care. Patients having the *LNF procedure* or paraesophageal repair via laparoscope are at risk for bleeding and infection, although these problems are not common. The nursing care priority is to observe for these complications and provide health teaching. See specific education in the Patient and Family Education: Preparing for Self-Management: Postoperative Instructions for Patients Having Laparoscopic

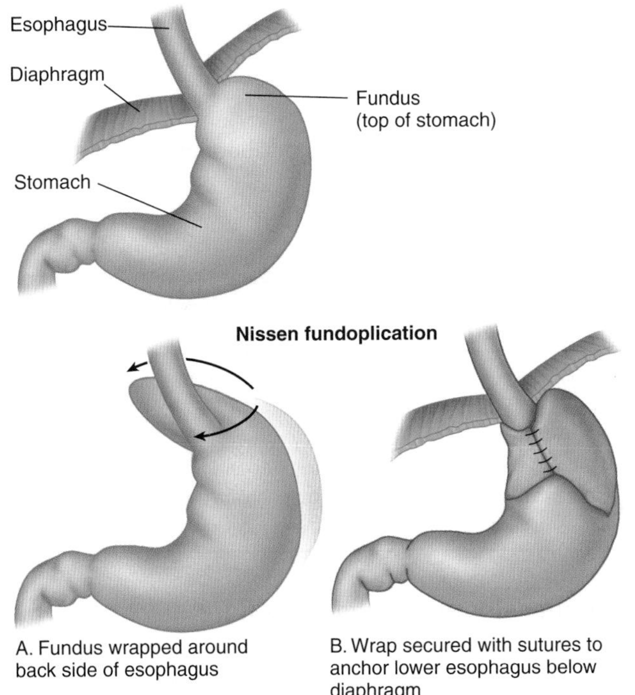

FIG. 49.8 Open surgical approach for Nissen fundoplication for gastroesophageal reflux disease or hiatal hernia repair.

Nissen Fundoplication (LNF) or Paraesophageal Repair via Laparoscope box.

Postoperative care after *open repair* closely follows that required after any esophageal surgery. Carefully assess for complications of open surgery as shown in the Best Practice for Patient Safety & Quality Care: Assessment of Postoperative Complications Related to Fundoplication Procedures box. Report any unusual assessment findings to the surgeon.

NURSING SAFETY PRIORITY (QSEN)

Action Alert

The primary focus of care after conventional surgery for a hiatal hernia repair is the prevention of respiratory complications. Elevate the head of the patient's bed at least 30 degrees to lower the diaphragm and promote lung expansion. Help the patient out of bed and begin ambulation as soon as possible. Be sure to support the incision during coughing to reduce ***pain*** and prevent excessive strain on the suture line, especially in patients with obesity.

For the patient who has undergone an open procedure, provide postoperative interventions presented in Chapter 9 regarding incentive spirometry, deep breathing, and prevention of venous thromboembolism. Patients with large hiatal hernias are at the highest risk for developing respiratory complications. The patient will have a large-bore (diameter) nasogastric (NG) tube to prevent the fundoplication wrap from becoming too tight around the esophagus. Initially the NG drainage should be dark brown with old blood. The drainage should become normal yellowish green within the first 8 hours after surgery. Check the NG tube every 4 to 8 hours for proper placement in the stomach. It should be properly anchored so it does not become displaced, because reinsertion could perforate the fundoplication. Follow the surgeon's recommendations for care of the patient with an NG tube.

Monitor patency of the NG tube to keep the stomach decompressed. This prevents retching or vomiting, which can strain or rupture the stomach sutures. The NG tube is irritating, so provide frequent oral hygiene to minimize ***pain.*** Assess hydration status regularly, and document accurate measures of intake and output. Adequate fluid replacement helps thin respiratory secretions.

Beginning with clear fluids, the patient gradually progresses to a near-normal diet during the first 4 to 6 weeks. Some foods, especially caffeinated or carbonated beverages and alcohol, are either restricted or eliminated. The food storage area of the stomach is reduced by the surgery, and meals need to be smaller and more frequent. *Carefully supervise the first oral feedings because temporary dysphagia is common.* Continuous dysphagia

PATIENT AND FAMILY EDUCATION: PREPARING FOR SELF-MANAGEMENT

Postoperative Instructions for Patients Having Laparoscopic Nissen Fundoplication (LNF) or Paraesophageal Repair via Laparoscope

- Consume a soft diet for about a week; avoid carbonated beverages, tough foods, and raw vegetables that are difficult to swallow.
- Remain on antireflux medications as prescribed for at least a month or per your health care provider's recommendation.
- Do not drive for a week after surgery; do not drive if taking opioid pain medication.
- Walk every day but do not do any heavy lifting.
- Remove small dressings 2 days after surgery and shower; do not remove wound closure strips until 10 days after surgery.
- Wash incisions with soap and water, rinse well, and pat dry; report any redness or drainage from the incisions to your surgeon.
- Report fever above 101°F (38.3°C), nausea, vomiting, or uncontrollable bloating or ***pain.*** For patients older than 65 years, report temperature elevations above 100°F (37.8°C).
- Keep your follow-up appointment with your surgeon, usually 3 to 4 weeks after surgery.

BEST PRACTICE FOR PATIENT SAFETY & QUALITY CARE (QSEN)

Assessment of Postoperative Complications Related to Fundoplication Procedures

Complication	Assessment Findings
Temporary dysphagia	Difficulty swallowing when oral feeding begins
Gas bloat syndrome	Difficulty belching to relieve distention
Atelectasis, pneumonia	Dyspnea, chest pain, or fever
Obstructed nasogastric tube	Nausea, vomiting, or abdominal distention, and/or a nondraining nasogastric tube

usually indicates that the fundoplication is too tight, and dilation may be required.

Other patients have *aerophagia* (air swallowing) from attempting to reverse or clear acid reflux. Teach them to relax consciously before and after meals, to eat and drink slowly, and to chew all food thoroughly. Air in the stomach that cannot be removed by belching can be extremely uncomfortable.

Some patients develop *gas bloat syndrome,* in which patients cannot voluntarily eructate (belch). The syndrome is usually temporary but may persist. Teach the patient to avoid drinking carbonated beverages and eating gas-producing foods (especially high-fat foods), chewing gum, and drinking with a straw. Frequent position changes and ambulation are often effective interventions for eliminating air from the GI tract. If gas ***pain*** is still present, it may be recommended that patients take simethicone, which relieves gas pressure.

Care Coordination and Transition Management. Patients undergoing open surgical repair require activity restrictions for 3 to 6 weeks postoperatively. For those who have undergone laparoscopic surgery, activity is typically restricted for a shorter time, and the patient can return to his or her usual lifestyle more quickly, usually in about a week.

For long-term management, educate the patient on:

- Appropriate ***nutrition*** modifications
- Use of stool softeners or bulk laxatives to prevent constipation and straining
- Daily incisional inspection
- Conditions that require notification of the health care provider, including swelling, redness, tenderness, discharge, or fever
- Avoidance of people with a respiratory infections; development of a respiratory infection with coughing can cause the incision or the fundoplication to dehisce

ESOPHAGEAL TUMORS

Pathophysiology Review

Although esophageal tumors can be benign, most are malignant (cancerous), and the majority develop from the epithelium. Squamous cell carcinomas of the esophagus are located in the upper two-thirds of the esophagus. Adenocarcinomas are more commonly found in the distal third and at the gastroesophageal junction and are now the most common type of esophageal cancer (McCance et al., 2019). Esophageal tumors grow rapidly because there is no serosal layer to limit their extension. Because the esophageal mucosa is richly supplied with lymph tissue, there is typically early spread of tumors to lymph nodes. Esophageal tumors can protrude into the esophageal lumen and can cause thickening or invade deeply into surrounding tissue. In rare cases, the lesion may be confined to the epithelial layer (in situ). In most cases, the tumor is large and well established at diagnosis. More than half of esophageal cancers metastasize throughout the body.

Primary risk factors associated with the development of esophageal cancer include:

- Alcohol intake
- Diets chronically deficient in fresh fruits and vegetables
- Diets high in nitrates and nitrosamines (found in pickled and fermented foods)
- Malnutrition
- Obesity (especially with increased abdominal pressure)
- Smoking
- Untreated GERD

NCLEX EXAMINATION CHALLENGE 49.5

Health Promotion and Maintenance

A community health nurse is screening clients for esophageal cancer. Which client is identified as being at **highest** risk?

A. 22-year-old who drinks a glass of beer weekly
B. 44-year-old who smokes a pack of cigarettes daily
C. 50-year-old who takes over-the-counter omeprazole
D. 63-year-old who uses protein supplements regularly

❖ Interprofessional Collaborative Care

Care of the patient with esophageal tumors usually takes place in the hospital, followed by the community setting. The interprofessional team that collaborates to care for this patient generally includes the primary health care provider, nurse, surgeon, registered dietitian nutritionist (RDN), respiratory therapist, social worker, and spiritual leader of the patient's choice.

◆ Assessment: Recognize Cues. Assess for risk factors related to the development or symptoms of esophageal cancer. Men, regardless of race or ethnicity, have higher incidence and mortality rates associated with esophageal cancer (American Cancer Society [ACS], 2020a).

Cancer of the esophagus is a silent tumor in its early stages, with few observable signs. By the time the tumor causes symptoms, it usually has spread extensively. One of the most common symptoms of esophageal cancer is dysphagia. This symptom may not be present until the esophageal opening has narrowed. Weight loss often accompanies progressive dysphagia and can exceed 20 lb over several months. See the Key Features: Esophageal Tumors box for more common clinical symptoms of esophageal tumors.

KEY FEATURES

Esophageal Tumors

- Persistent and progressive dysphagia (most common feature)
- Feeling of food sticking in the throat
- Odynophagia (painful swallowing)
- Halitosis
- Chronic hiccups
- Chronic cough with increasing secretions
- Hoarseness
- Severe, persistent chest or abdominal pain or discomfort
- Anorexia
- Regurgitation
- Nausea and vomiting
- Weight loss (often more than 20 lb)
- Changes in bowel habits (diarrhea, constipation, bleeding)

The diagnosis of esophageal cancer may cause significant anxiety. The disease is accompanied by distressing symptoms and is often terminal. The fear of choking can create unusual stress, especially at mealtimes. The loss of pleasure and social aspects of eating may affect relationships. Assess the patient's response to the diagnosis and prognosis. Ask about usual coping strengths and resources. Determine the availability of support systems and the potential impact of the disease and its treatment. Refer to psychological counseling, pastoral care, and/or the social worker or case manager as needed. Chapter 8 describes end-of-life care for patients in the terminal stage of the disease.

NCLEX EXAMINATION CHALLENGE 49.6

Psychosocial Integrity

The nurse is caring for a client with esophageal cancer who is scheduled for surgery. When the client asks, "Is this treatment going to cure me?" which nursing response is appropriate? **Select all that apply.**

A. "The surgery has been useful for many patients so it should work for you."
B. "You can beat this disease if you just put your mind to it and do not give up."
C. "Yes, and you have the best surgeon around who specializes in cancer treatment."
D. "Your surgeon can give more information about the effectiveness of this treatment."
E. "It sounds like you are concerned about surgical outcomes; let's talk about your feelings."

Diagnostic Assessment. An esophagogastroduodenoscopy (EGD) with biopsy is performed to inspect the esophagus and obtain tissue specimens for cell studies and disease staging. A complete cancer staging workup is performed, often by endoscopic ultrasound, to determine the extent of the disease and plan appropriate therapy.

Positron emission tomography (PET) may identify metastatic disease with more accuracy than a CT scan. PET can also help evaluate response to chemotherapy to treat the cancer.

◆ **Interventions: Take Action.** Treatment of patients with esophageal cancer depends on staging at diagnosis. Multimodal therapy is often necessary to treat esophageal cancer, as it is often advanced at diagnosis. Along with treatment of the cancer itself, patients with cancer of the esophagus experience many physical problems, and symptom management becomes essential.

Nonsurgical Management. Nonsurgical treatment options for cancer of the esophagus that can assist in disease and ***nutrition*** management may include:

- Nutrition and swallowing therapy
- Chemotherapy, radiation, and chemoradiation
- Photodynamic therapy and porfimer sodium
- Other therapies

Nutrition and Swallowing Therapy. Conduct a screening assessment to provide information about the patient's ***nutrition*** status. The registered dietitian nutritionist (RDN) determines the caloric needs of the patient to meet daily requirements. Perform weights daily before breakfast on the same scale each day. To keep the esophagus patent, position the patient upright for several hours after meals, and avoid allowing the patient to lay completely flat. Remind assistive personnel (AP) and other health care team members to keep the head of the bed elevated to a 30-degree angle or more to prevent reflux.

Semisoft foods and thickened liquids are preferred because they are easier to swallow. Document the amount of food and fluid intake every day to monitor progress in meeting desired ***nutrition*** outcomes. Liquid supplements are used between feedings to increase caloric intake. Ongoing efforts are made to preserve the ability to swallow, but enteral feedings (tube feedings) may be needed temporarily when dysphagia is severe. In patients with complete esophageal obstruction or life-threatening fistulas, the surgeon may create a gastrostomy or jejunostomy for feeding. Chapter 55 describes care for patients receiving enteral feeding.

Collaborate with the speech-language pathologist (SLP) to help the patient with oral exercises to improve swallowing *(swallowing therapy)* and with the occupational therapist (OT) for feeding techniques.

! NURSING SAFETY PRIORITY QSEN

Critical Rescue

When the patient with an esophageal tumor is eating or drinking, recognize that you must monitor for signs and symptoms of aspiration, which can cause airway obstruction, pneumonia, or both, especially in older adults. In coordination with the SLP, respond by teaching caregivers how to feed the patient, how to monitor for aspiration, and how to respond quickly if choking occurs.

Chemotherapy and Radiation. *Chemotherapy* may be given preoperatively or in concurrence with other treatments. *Radiation therapy* can also be used alone but is used most frequently in combination with other treatments. *Chemoradiation* is a treatment for esophageal cancer that involves the use of chemotherapy at the same time as radiation therapy.

Photodynamic Therapy and Porfimer Sodium. *Photodynamic therapy (PDT)* is used as palliative treatment for patients with advanced esophageal cancer; it can relieve pain or make swallowing somewhat easier. PDT is sometimes used with *porfimer sodium* (Photofrin), a light-sensitive drug that collects in cancer cells, for palliation. Chapter 20 describes these approaches to care in detail.

Other Therapies. *Esophageal dilation* may be performed as necessary throughout the course of the disease to achieve temporary but immediate relief of dysphagia. It is usually performed in an ambulatory care setting. Dilators are used to tear soft tissue, thereby widening the esophageal lumen (opening). In most cases, malignant tumors can be dilated safely, but perforation remains a significant risk. Large metal stents may be used to keep the esophagus open for longer periods. A stent covered with graft material can be used to seal a perforation. Bacteremia may also occur. To reduce the risk for sepsis and endocarditis, antibiotics are given. The treatment is repeated as often as needed to preserve the patient's ability to swallow. Prolonged stent embedment into benign esophageal tissue can cause ulceration, bleeding, fistula, dysphagia, and formation of a new stricture if the stent is not removed (Vermeulen & Siersema, 2018).

Endoscopic therapies like stenting can be offered as palliative care for patients who are not surgical candidates. Stenting can be performed with metal, plastic, or biodegradable mechanisms that are intended to relieve obstruction.

Targeted therapies such as trastuzumab, which targets the HER2 protein, may be given IV every 3 weeks; at this time the optimal length of treatment is not known (ACS, 2020b). This treatment can be used with chemotherapy, or alone if chemotherapy has not been effective.

Surgical Management. The purposes of different types of surgical resection vary from cure to palliation. *Esophagectomy* is the removal of all or part of the esophagus, and is usually selected as the initial surgical approach to esophageal cancer (Swanson, 2020). For patients with early-stage cancer, a laparoscopic-assisted **minimally invasive esophagectomy (MIE)** may be performed. However, most patients require conventional open surgery because of tumor size and metastasis by the time they are diagnosed with the disease.

Preoperative Care. Preoperative preparation for patients undergoing esophagectomy can be quite extensive. Advise the patient to stop smoking 2 to 4 weeks before surgery to enhance pulmonary function. Intensive preoperative respiratory rehabilitation may be prescribed to strengthen the pulmonary system, which has been shown to decrease postoperative pulmonary complications (Swanson, 2020). Patient preparation may include lengthy ***nutrition*** support to decrease the risk for postoperative complications. Ideally this supplementation is given orally, but some patients require tube feeding or parenteral nutrition. Teach the patient and caregiver to monitor the patient's weight and intake and output. A preoperative evaluation may be required to treat dental disease. Instruct the patient to practice meticulous oral care four times daily to decrease the risk for postoperative infection.

Preoperative nursing care focuses on teaching and psychological support regarding the surgical procedure and preoperative and postoperative instructions. See Chapter 9 for specific preoperative teaching. On the day of surgery, the surgeon usually prescribes prophylactic antibiotics and supplemental oxygen.

Operative Procedures. There are numerous types of esophagectomies that can be performed based on the tumor location, length, extension, and protrusion into surrounding structures (Swanson, 2020). The extent of lymphadenectomy needed and the surgeon's preferences also influence surgical approach. Surgery may be minimally invasive, or open. Carefully review the specific type of procedure performed in order to optimize postprocedure nursing care.

Postoperative Care. Intensive postoperative care is necessary for the patient who has had an esophagectomy, because of the risk for multiple serious complications. Follow postoperative care as outlined in Chapter 9.

Remind all staff to keep the patient in a semi-Fowler or high-Fowler position to support ventilation and prevent reflux. *Ensure the patency of the chest tube drainage system and monitor for changes in the volume or color of the drainage.*

! NURSING SAFETY PRIORITY QSEN

Action Alert

Respiratory care is the highest postoperative priority for patients having an esophagectomy. For those who had traditional surgery, intubation with mechanical ventilation is necessary for at least the first 16 to 24 hours. Pulmonary complications include atelectasis and pneumonia. The risk for postoperative pulmonary complications is increased in the patient who has received preoperative radiation. Once the patient is extubated, support deep breathing, turning, and coughing every 1 to 2 hours. Assess the patient for decreased breath sounds and shortness of breath every 1 to 2 hours. Provide incisional support and adequate analgesia to enhance effective coughing.

Cardiovascular complications, particularly hypotension during surgery, can occur as a result of pressure placed on the posterior heart. Carefully monitor cardiovascular and pulmonary statuses in the postoperative period. See the Nursing Safety Priority box.

! NURSING SAFETY PRIORITY QSEN

Action Alert

Monitor for symptoms of fluid volume overload, particularly in older patients and those who have undergone lymph node dissection. Assess for edema, crackles in the lungs, and increased jugular venous pressure. In the immediate postoperative phase, the patient is often admitted to the intensive care unit. Critical care nurses assess hemodynamic parameters such as cardiac output, cardiac index, and systemic vascular resistance every 2 hours to monitor for myocardial ischemia. Observe for atrial fibrillation, which can result from irritation of the vagus nerve during surgery, and manage according to agency protocol.

Wound management is a major postoperative concern with conventional surgery because the patient typically has multiple incisions and drains. *Provide direct support to the incision during turning and coughing to prevent dehiscence.* Wound infection can occur 4 to 5 days after surgery. Leakage from the site of anastomosis is a dreaded complication that can appear 2 to 10 days after surgery. If an anastomotic leak occurs, all oral intake is discontinued and does not resume until the site of the leak has healed. *Mediastinitis* (inflammation of the mediastinum) resulting from an anastomotic leak can lead to fatal sepsis.

! NURSING SAFETY PRIORITY QSEN

Critical Rescue

After esophageal surgery, recognize fever, fluid accumulation, signs of inflammation, and symptoms of early shock (e.g., tachycardia, tachypnea). Respond immediately by reporting any of these findings to the surgeon *and* the Rapid Response Team!

A nasogastric (NG) tube is placed intraoperatively to decompress the stomach to prevent tension on the suture line. Monitor the NG tube for patency and carefully secure the tube to prevent dislodgment, which can disrupt the sutures at the anastomosis. *Do not irrigate or reposition the NG tube in patients who have undergone esophageal surgery unless prescribed by the surgeon.* See the Best Practice for Patient Safety & Quality Care:

BEST PRACTICE FOR PATIENT SAFETY & QUALITY CARE (QSEN)

Managing the Patient With a Nasogastric Tube After Esophageal Surgery

- Check for tube placement every 4 to 8 hours.
- Ensure that the tube is patent (open) and draining; drainage should turn from bloody to yellowish green by the end of the first postoperative day.
- Secure the tube well to prevent dislodgment.
- Do not irrigate or reposition the tube without a health care provider's order.
- Provide meticulous oral and nasal hygiene every 2 to 4 hours.
- Keep the head of the bed elevated to at least 30 degrees.
- When the patient is permitted to have a small amount of water, place him or her in an upright position and observe for dysphagia (difficulty swallowing).
- Observe for leakage from the anastomosis site (indicated by fever, fluid accumulation, and symptoms of early shock [tachycardia, tachypnea, altered mental status]).

Managing the Patient With a Nasogastric Tube After Esophageal Surgery box for specific interventions.

Nutrition management of the patient who has undergone esophageal surgery is an early postoperative concern. After conventional surgery, on the second postoperative day, initial feedings usually begin through the jejunostomy tube (J tube). Do not aspirate for residual because this increases the risk for mucosal tearing. Feedings are slowly increased over the next several days through the fifth postoperative day. A barium swallow is performed on the seventh postoperative day; if no anastomotic leaks are seen, the NG tube is discontinued (Swanson, 2020). A minimal liquid diet should be continued for the following 2 weeks. Further oral intake should be prescribed by the surgeon at the time of follow-up.

Care Coordination and Transition Management. Patients with esophageal cancer have many challenges to face once they are discharged home. Treatment regimens cause long-lasting side effects, such as fatigue and weakness. These complex treatments also require the patient and caregiver to be knowledgeable about symptom management and to know when to report concerns.

Once the patient is discharged to home, ongoing respiratory care remains a priority. Give the patient and caregiver instructions for ambulation and incentive spirometer use. Encourage the patient to be as active as possible and avoid excessive bed rest because this can lead to complications of immobility.

Nutrition support is important. Encourage the patient to continue increasing oral feedings as prescribed by the surgeon. Remind him or her to eat small, frequent meals containing high-calorie, high-protein foods that are soft and easily swallowed. Teach the value of using supplemental shakes. Emphasize the importance of sitting upright to eat, and remaining upright after meals. Patients who have undergone esophageal resection can lose up to 10% of their body weight. Teach the patient to monitor his or her weight at home and to report a weight loss of 5 lb or more in 1 month. If sufficient oral intake is not possible, tube feedings or parenteral nutrition at home at home may be needed.

Teach the patient that dysphagia or odynophagia may recur because of stricture, reflux, or cancer recurrence. These symptoms should be reported to the health care provider promptly.

Despite radical surgery, the patient with cancer of the esophagus often still has a terminal illness and a relatively short life expectancy. This can cause significant anxiety and depression in some patients (see the Evidence-Based Practice box). Emphasis is placed on maximizing quality of life. Realistic planning is important. Help family members in exploring sources of support and in arranging for hospice care when it becomes necessary. Chapter 8 describes end-of-life care.

! NATIONAL PATIENT SAFETY GOALS

In accordance with The Joint Commission National Patient Safety Goals for 2020 (The Joint Commission, 2020a), teach the family to protect the patient from infection by following the World Health Organization (WHO) or the Centers for Disease Control and Prevention (CDC) handwashing guidelines and to contact the health care provider immediately if signs of respiratory infection develop. Patients should stay away from people with infections and avoid large crowds.

EVIDENCE-BASED PRACTICE (QSEN)

Anxiety and Depression Among Esophageal Cancer Patients

Hellstadius, Y., Lagergren, J., Zylstra, J., Gossage, J., Davies, A., Hultman, C.M., et al. (2017). Prevalence and predictors of anxiety and depression among esophageal cancer patients prior to surgery. *Diseases of the Esophagus, 30*(8), 1-7.

This study aimed to establish the prevalence and predictors of anxiety and depression in 106 esophageal cancer patients after diagnosis but before surgical intervention. The researchers collected information about prevalence and predictor variables in hospital records and self-report questionnaires from patients with esophageal cancer at one hospital in London, England from 2011 to 2014. The research focused on clinical and sociodemographic characteristics and how they related to each patient's results on the Hospital Anxiety and Depression Scale (HADS). The study found that a significant number of patients reported anxiety and depression following an esophageal cancer diagnosis. The two groups that reported anxiety and depression most often were woman and those who had limitations to their physical activity. Overall, they found that 40% of all patients in this study reported anxiety or depression immediately on being diagnosed with esophageal cancer.

Level of Evidence: 4

The research design was a cross-sectional study.

Commentary: Implications for Practice and Research

The observations made by this study have important implications for those caring for patients who have an esophageal cancer diagnosis. Due to the poor prognosis in patients with esophageal cancer, emotional assessment and supportive care are imperative. This study also helps health care providers to identify specific sociodemographic groups that are at higher risk for anxiety and depression during treatment. This information can assist the interprofessional health care team in providing patient-centered mental health interventions throughout esophageal cancer treatment. Because this study is of a cross-sectional design, no direct correlations can be made, but it does present significant trends that can guide future research and aid in improving care of those diagnosed with esophageal cancer.

Refer patients to community or home care organizations for in-home care. Teach about services available through the American Cancer Society (www.cancer.org), including support groups and transportation. Coordinate resource referrals with the case manager or home care agency as needed.

ESOPHAGEAL TRAUMA

Trauma to the esophagus can result from blunt injuries, chemical burns, surgery or endoscopy (although rare), or the stress of continuous severe vomiting. Trauma may affect the esophagus directly or it may create problems in the lungs or mediastinum. When excessive force is exerted on the esophageal mucosa, it may perforate or rupture, allowing the caustic acid secretions to enter the mediastinal cavity. These tears are associated with a high mortality rate related to shock, respiratory impairment, or sepsis.

Common causes of esophageal perforation include:

- Straining
- Seizures
- Trauma
- Foreign objects
- Instruments or tubes
- Chemical injury
- Complications of esophageal surgery
- Ulcers

Chemical injury is usually a result of the accidental or intentional ingestion of caustic substances. The damage to the mouth and esophagus is rapid and severe. Acid burns tend to affect the superficial mucosal lining, whereas alkaline substances cause deeper penetrating injuries. Strong alkalis can cause full perforation of the esophagus within 1 minute. Additional complications may include aspiration pneumonia and hemorrhage. Esophageal strictures may develop as scar tissue forms.

Patients with esophageal trauma are initially evaluated and treated in the emergency department. Assessment focuses on the nature of the injury and the circumstances surrounding it. *Assess for airway patency, breathing, chest pain, dysphagia, vomiting, and bleeding as the priorities for patient care.* If the risk for extending the damage is not excessive, an endoscopic study may be requested to evaluate tears or perforation. A CT scan of the chest can be done to assess for the presence of mediastinal air.

After the injury, keep the patient NPO to prevent further leakage of esophageal secretions. Esophageal and gastric suction can be used for drainage and to rest the esophagus. Esophageal rest is maintained for more than a week after injury to allow for initial healing of the mucosa. Total parenteral nutrition (TPN) is prescribed to provide calories and protein for wound healing while the patient is not eating.

To prevent sepsis, the health care provider prescribes broad-spectrum antibiotics. High-dose corticosteroids may be administered to suppress inflammation and prevent strictures (esophageal narrowing). Opioid and nonopioid analgesics may be prescribed for ***pain*** management. When caustic burns involve the mouth, topical agents such as viscous lidocaine may be used.

If nonsurgical management is not effective in healing injured esophageal tissue, the patient may need surgery to remove the damaged tissue. Those with severe injuries may require resection of part of the esophagus with a gastric pull-through and repositioning or replacement by a bowel segment. A gastrostomy tube (G-tube) placement may be needed to meet ***nutrition*** needs while healing.

GET READY FOR THE NEXT-GENERATION NCLEX® EXAMINATION!

Key Points

Review these key points for each NCLEX Examination Client Needs Category.

Safe and Effective Care Environment

- Check the gag reflex and implement airway management interventions for patients having oral or esophageal surgery. **QSEN: Safety**
- Collaborate with the registered dietitian nutritionist (RDN) to plan ***nutrition*** modifications for patients with GERD. **QSEN: Teamwork and Collaboration**
- Assess for complications and provide postoperative care for patients having surgical procedures for oral and esophageal problems. **QSEN: Safety**
- Teach the patient and caregiver to recognize dysphagia symptoms. **QSEN: Safety**

Health Promotion and Maintenance

- Teach oral hygiene techniques and remind adults to visit their dentist twice a year. **QSEN: Patient-Centered Care**
- Teach patients with nonhealing oral wounds to contact their primary health care provider or dentist. **QSEN: Safety**
- Teach adults to avoid tobacco, alcohol, and sun exposure to decrease risk for oral cancer. **QSEN: Evidence-Based Practice**

Psychosocial Integrity

- Assess the patient's response to an oral or esophageal cancer diagnosis, and refer to psychological and community resources as needed. **QSEN: Patient-Centered Care**
- Explain all procedures, restrictions, drug therapy, and follow-up care. **Ethics**

Physiological Integrity

- Assess all patients for oral lesions or tumors. **Clinical Judgment**
- Provide gentle oral care for patients with oral lesions to preserve ***tissue integrity***. **QSEN: Safety**
- Monitor the ***nutrition*** status of patients with GERD, hiatal hernia, and oral or esophageal cancer. **Clinical Judgment**
- Stress the importance of controlling reflux through ***nutrition*** and drug therapy. **QSEN: Evidence-Based Practice**
- Teach the patient with GERD to elevate the head of the bed or sleep propped up. **QSEN: Evidence-Based Practice**
- Teach the patient with esophageal cancer to report weight loss. **QSEN: Patient-Centered Care**
- Collaborate with the interprofessional team to design a plan of care for the patient with impaired swallowing and/or impaired ***nutrition***. **QSEN: Teamwork and Collaboration**

MASTERY QUESTIONS

1. A nurse is caring for a 34-year-old client newly diagnosed with GERD. Which lifestyle change will the nurse suggest? **Select all that apply.**
   A. Lose weight if needed.
   B. Do not eat before bed.
   C. Elevate the foot of your bed by 6 to 12 inches.
   D. Avoid pants with a tight waistband or belt.
   E. Eat fatty foods to minimize ongoing hunger.
2. A client who had the Stretta procedure to treat severe GERD is being discharged. Which client statement requires further nursing teaching? **Select all that apply.**
   A. "Dysphagia after this procedure is normal."
   B. "It's important to stop my proton pump inhibitor."
   C. "I will not take NSAIDs and aspirin for at least 10 days."
   D. "I might cough up some blood following this procedure."
   E. "Today I will drink clear liquids and tomorrow I can eat soft food."
3. A public health nurse is assessing community clients for oral health disorders. Which client is identified at highest risk?
   A. 23-year-old with three dental fillings
   B. 34-year-old with schizophrenia
   C. 55-year-old with stable angina
   D. 62-year-old with irritable bowel syndrome

REFERENCES

American Cancer Society (ACS). (2020a). *Esophageal cancer risk factors*. https://www.cancer.org/cancer/esophagus-cancer/causes-risks-prevention/risk-factors.html.

American Cancer Society (ACS). (2020b). *Targeted therapy for esophageal cancer*. https://www.cancer.org/cancer/esophagus-cancer/treating/targeted-therapy.html.

Argyrou, A., Legaki, E., et al. (2018). Rick factors for gastroesophageal reflux disease and analysis of genetic contributors. *World Journal of Clinical Cases*, *6*(8), 176–182.

Brice, S. (2019). Recurrent aphthous stomatitis. In Dellavalle, R. (Ed.), *UpToDate*. Waltham, MA.

Cancer Treatment Centers of America. (2020). *Surgery for oral cancer*. https://www.cancercenter.com/cancer-types/oral-cancer/treatments/surgery.

Commisso, A., & Fidelindo, L. (2019). Lifestyle modifications in adults and older adults with chronic gastroesophageal reflux disease (GERD). *Critical Care Nursing Quarterly*, *42*(1), 64–74. https://doi.org/10.1097/CNQ.0000000000000239.

Fischer, D. J., O'Hayre, M., Kusiak, J. W., Somerman, M. J., & Hill, C. V. (2017). Oral health disparities: A perspective from the national institute of dental and craniofacial research. *American Journal of Public Health*, *107*(S1), S36–S38. https://doi.org/10.2105/AJPH.2016.303622.

Gyawali, C. P., Kahrilas, P. J., Savarino, E., Zerbib, F., Mion, F., Smout, A., et al. (2018). Modern diagnosis of GERD: The lyon consensus. *Gut*, *67*, 1351–1362. https://doi.org/10.1136/gutjnl-2017-314722.

Hellstadius, Y., Lagergren, J., Zylstra, J., Gossage, J., Davies, A., Hultman, C. M., et al. (2017). Prevalence and predictors of anxiety and depression among esophageal cancer patients prior to surgery. *Diseases of the Esophagus*, *30*(8), 1–7. https://doi.org/10.1111/dote.12437.

Hoffman, H. (2019). Salivary gland swelling: Evaluation and diagnostic approach. In Deschler, D. (Ed.), *UpToDate*. Waltham, MA.

Kahrilas, P. (2020). Clinical manifestations and diagnosis of gastroesophageal reflux in adults. In Talley, N. (Ed.), *UpToDate*. Waltham, MA.

Kahrilas, P. (2019). Hiatus hernia. In Talley, N. (Ed.), *UpToDate*. Waltham, MA.

Maes, M., Fixen, D., & Linnebur, S. (2017). Adverse effects of proton-pump inhibitor use in older adults: A review of the evidence. *Therapeutic Advances in Drug Safety*, *8*(9), 273–297.

McCance, K., Huether, S., Brashers, V., & Rote, N. (2019). *Pathophysiology: The biologic basis for disease in adults and children* (8th ed.). St. Louis: Elsevier.

Mermelstein, J., Chait-Mermelstein, A., & Chait, M. M. (2018). Proton pump inhibitor-refractory gastroesophageal reflux disease: Challenges and solutions. *Clinical and Experimental Gastroenterology*, *11*, 119–134. https://doi.org/10.2147/CEG.S121056.

Mountain, C., & Golles, K. (2017). Detecting dysphagia. *American Nurse Today*, *12*(5). https://www.americannursetoday.com/detecting-dysphagia/.

National Institutes of Health. (2020). *Genetics home reference: TP53*. www.ghr.nlm.nih.gov/gene/TP53.

Nehra, A. K., Alexander, J. A., Loftus, C. G., & Nehra, V. (2018). Proton pump inhibitors: Review of emerging concerns. *Mayo Clinic Proceedings*, *93*(2), 240–246. https://doi.org/10.1016/j.mayocp.2017.10.022.

Oral Cancer Foundation (OCF). (2020). *April is oral cancer awareness month*. https://oralcancerfoundation.org/april-is-oral-cancer-awareness-month/.

Plewa, M. C., & Chatterjee, K. (2020). *Aphthous stomatitis. StatPearls. Treasure island (FL)*. StatPearls Publishing. https://www.ncbi.nlm.nih.gov/books/NBK431059/.

Rosen, M., & Blatnik, J. (2019). Surgical management of paraesophageal hernia. In Friedberg, J., & Talley, N. (Eds.), *UpToDate*. Waltham, MA.

Schwaitzberg, S. (2020). Surgical management of gastroesophageal reflux in adults. In Friedberg, J., & Talley, N. (Eds.), *UpToDate*. Waltham, MA.

Swanson, S. (2020). Surgical management of resectable esophageal and esophagogastric junction cancers. In Tanabe, K. (Ed.), *UpToDate*. Waltham, MA.

The Joint Commission. (2020a). *National patient safety Goals*, 2020. https://www.jointcommission.org/standards/national-patient-safety-goals/.

The Joint Commission. (2020b). *Core measures*. https://www.jointcommission.org/measurement/measures/.

Vermeulen, B. D., & Siersema, P. D. (2018). Esophageal stenting in clinical practice: An overview. *Current Treatment Options in Gastroenterology*, *16*(2), 260–273. https://doi.org/10.1007/s11938-018-0181-3.

Yamasaki, T., et al. (2018). The changing epidemiology of gastroesophageal reflux disease: Are patients getting younger? *Journal of Neurogastroenterology and Motility*, *24*(4), 559–569.

Zhang, C., et al. (2019). Role of polycyclic aromatic hydrocarbons as a co-factor in human papillomavirus–mediated carcinogenesis. *BMC Cancer*, *19*, 138.

50

Concepts of Care for Patients With Stomach Disorders

Lara Carver, Jennifer Powers, Donna D. Ignatavicius

http://evolve.elsevier.com/Iggy/

LEARNING OUTCOMES

1. Collaborate with the interprofessional team to manage quality care for patients with ***inflammation*** and ***pain*** caused by caused by stomach disorders.
2. Identify community resources for families and patients recovering from stomach disorders.
3. Apply knowledge of pathophysiology of stomach disorders to identify common assessment findings, including actual or risk for impaired ***nutrition.***
4. Prioritize evidence-based nursing interventions for patients with stomach disorders to promote ***nutrition*** and manage ***infection.***
5. Plan transition management and care coordination for the patient who has stomach disorders, including health teaching.

KEY TERMS

dumping syndrome A postgastrectomy condition that refers to a group of vasomotor symptoms that occur after eating.

dyspepsia An epigastric burning sensation, often referred to as "heartburn."

gastrectomy Surgical removal of all (total gastrectomy) or part (subtotal gastrectomy) of the stomach.

gastritis The ***inflammation*** of gastric mucosa (stomach lining).

hematemesis Vomiting bright red or coffee-ground blood.

melena Dark, "tarry" (sticky) stool, indicating occult blood caused by digestion of blood within the small intestine.

peptic ulcer disease A condition that results when GI mucosal defenses become impaired and no longer protect the epithelium from the effects of acid and pepsin.

peritonitis An abdominal ***infection*** in which the abdomen is tender, rigid, and boardlike.

stress ulcer Acute gastric mucosal lesion occurring after an acute medical crisis or trauma, such as sepsis or a head injury, or surgery.

PRIORITY AND INTERRELATED CONCEPTS

The priority concept for this chapter is:

- ***Infection***

The ***Infection*** concept exemplar for this chapter is Peptic Ulcer Disease (PUD).

The interrelated concepts for this chapter are:

- ***Inflammation***
- ***Nutrition***
- ***Pain***

The stomach is part of the upper GI system that is responsible for a large part of the digestive process. It is affected by only a few diseases, including gastritis, peptic ulcer disease (PUD), and cancer, yet these conditions can be very serious and sometimes life threatening. Each of these health problems can result in impaired or altered ***nutrition. Inflammation*** and ***infection*** can cause ***pain*** and discomfort. Chapter 3 briefly reviews each of these health concepts.

GASTRITIS

Gastritis is the ***inflammation*** of gastric mucosa (stomach lining) (see complete discussion of inflammation in Chapter 16). It can be classified according to cause, cellular changes, or distribution of the lesions, and can be erosive (causing ulcers) or nonerosive. Although the mucosal changes that result from *acute* gastritis typically heal after several months, this is not true for *chronic* gastritis.

Pathophysiology Review

Prostaglandins provide a protective mucosal barrier that prevents the stomach from digesting itself. If there is a break in the protective barrier, mucosal injury can occur. The resulting injury is worsened by histamine release and vagal nerve stimulation. Hydrochloric acid can then diffuse back into the mucosa and injure small vessels. This back-diffusion can cause edema, bleeding, and erosion of the stomach's lining.

Inflammation of the gastric mucosa or submucosa after exposure to local irritants or other causes can result in *acute gastritis.* The early pathologic manifestation of gastritis is a thickened, reddened mucous membrane with prominent rugae, or folds. Various degrees of mucosal necrosis and inflammation occur in acute disease. The diagnosis cannot be based solely on clinical symptoms. If the stomach muscle is not involved, complete recovery usually occurs in a few days with no residual evidence of gastric ***inflammation.*** If the muscle is affected, bleeding or hemorrhage may occur during an episode of acute gastritis.

Long-term NSAID use creates a high risk for acute gastritis. NSAIDs inhibit prostaglandin production in the mucosal barrier. Other risk factors include use of alcohol, coffee, and caffeine. Stress and cigarette smoking are considered risk factors for the development of acute gastritis (Ankita et al., 2017). Local irritation from radiation therapy and accidental or intentional ingestion of corrosive substances, including acids or alkalis (e.g., lye and drain cleaners), can also cause acute gastritis. Use of drugs such as steroids, aldosterone antagonists, and selective serotonin reuptake inhibitors can contribute to gastroduodenal ***inflammation*** and ulceration.

Chronic gastritis appears as a patchy, diffuse (spread out) ***inflammation*** of the mucosal lining of the stomach. As the disease progresses, the walls and lining of the stomach thin and atrophy. With progressive gastric atrophy from chronic mucosal injury, the function of the parietal (acid-secreting) cells decreases, and the source of intrinsic factor is lost. Intrinsic factor is critical for absorption of vitamin B_{12}. When body stores of vitamin B_{12} are eventually depleted, pernicious anemia results. The amount and concentration of acid in stomach secretions gradually decrease until the secretions consist of only mucus and water.

The most common form of chronic gastritis is type B gastritis, caused by *Helicobacter pylori* ***infection***. A direct correlation exists between the number of organisms and the degree of cellular abnormality present. The host response to the *H. pylori* infection is activation of lymphocytes and neutrophils. Release of inflammatory cytokines, such as interleukin (IL)-1, IL-8, and tumor necrosis factor–alpha (TNF-α), damages the gastric mucosa (McCance et al., 2019).

Chronic gastritis is associated with an increased risk for gastric cancer. The persistent ***inflammation*** extends deep into the mucosa, causing gastric gland destruction and cellular changes (McCance et al., 2019). Chronic local irritation and toxic effects caused by alcohol ingestion, radiation therapy, and smoking have been linked to chronic gastritis. Surgical procedures that involve the pyloric sphincter, such as pyloroplasty, can lead to gastritis by causing reflux of alkaline secretions into the stomach. Other systemic disorders such as Crohn's disease, graft-versus-host disease, and uremia can also precipitate the development of chronic gastritis (McCance et al., 2019).

Health Promotion and Maintenance

Gastritis is a very common health problem in the United States. A balanced diet, regular exercise, and stress-reduction techniques can help prevent it (see the Patient and Family Education: Preparing for Self-Management: Gastritis Prevention box).

PATIENT AND FAMILY EDUCATION: PREPARING FOR SELF-MANAGEMENT

Gastritis Prevention

- Eat a well-balanced diet and exercise regularly.
- Avoid drinking excessive amounts of alcoholic beverages.
- Do not take large doses of aspirin, other NSAIDs (e.g., ibuprofen), or corticosteroids.
- Avoid excessive intake of coffee (even decaffeinated).
- Be sure that foods and water are safe to avoid contamination.
- Manage stress levels using complementary and integrative therapies such as relaxation and meditation techniques.
- Stop smoking and/or using other forms of tobacco.
- Protect yourself against exposure to toxic substances in the workplace such as lead and nickel.
- Seek medical treatment if you are experiencing symptoms of gastroesophageal reflux (see Chapter 49).

A balanced diet includes following the recommendations of the U.S. Department of Agriculture (USDA) and limiting intake of foods and spices that can cause gastric distress, such as caffeine, chocolate, mustard, pepper, and other strong or hot spices. Alcohol and tobacco should also be avoided. Regular exercise maintains peristalsis, which helps prevent gastric contents from irritating the gastric mucosa. Stress-reduction techniques can include aerobic exercise, meditation, and/or yoga, depending on individual preferences.

❖ Interprofessional Collaborative Care

Care of the patient with gastritis usually takes place in the community setting. However, if symptoms are severe, the patient may be hospitalized.

◆ **Assessment: Recognize Cues.** Symptoms of *acute gastritis* range from mild to severe. Clients typically report a rapid onset of epigastric ***pain*** and **dyspepsia** (an epigastric burning sensation, often referred to as "heartburn"). In some cases, gastric bleeding may occur and manifest as **hematemesis** (vomiting bright red or coffee-ground blood), or **melena** (dark, "tarry" [sticky] stool, indicating occult blood caused by digestion of blood within the small intestine).

Gastritis or food poisoning caused by endotoxins, such as staphylococcal endotoxin, has an abrupt onset. Severe nausea and vomiting often occur within 5 hours of ingestion of the contaminated food. *In some cases gastric hemorrhage is the presenting symptom, which is a life-threatening emergency.*

Chronic gastritis causes few symptoms unless ulceration occurs. Patients may report nausea, vomiting, or upper abdominal discomfort. Periodic epigastric ***pain*** may occur after a meal. Some patients have anorexia.

Esophagogastroduodenoscopy (EGD) via an endoscope with biopsy is the gold standard for diagnosing gastritis. (See Chapter 48 for discussion of nursing care associated with this diagnostic procedure.) The primary health care provider performs a biopsy to establish a definitive diagnosis of the type of gastritis. If lesions are patchy and diffuse, biopsy of several suspicious areas may be necessary to avoid misdiagnosis. A *cytologic examination* of the biopsy specimen is performed to confirm or rule out gastric cancer. Tissue samples can also be taken to detect *H. pylori* ***infection*** using *rapid urease testing.* The results of these tests are more reliable if the patient has discontinued taking antacids and proton pump inhibitors (PPIs) for at least a week (Pagana & Pagana, 2018; Pagana et al., 2019).

◆ **Interventions: Take Action.** Patients with gastritis are not often seen in the acute care setting unless they have an exacerbation ("flare-up") of acute or chronic gastritis that results in fluid and electrolyte imbalance, bleeding, or increased ***pain.*** Collaborative care is directed toward supportive care for relieving the symptoms and removing or reducing the cause of discomfort.

Acute gastritis is treated symptomatically and supportively because the healing process is spontaneous, usually occurring within a few days. When the cause is removed, ***pain*** and discomfort usually subside. If bleeding occurs, a blood transfusion and fluid replacement may be given. Surgery, such as partial gastrectomy, pyloroplasty, and/or vagotomy, may be needed for patients with major bleeding or ulceration. (See discussion of gastric surgery procedures in this chapter later under Gastric Cancer.)

Eliminating the causative factor(s) is the primary treatment approach for *acute* gastritis. ***Nutrition*** and drug therapy may also be used. Teach the patient to limit intake of any foods and spices that cause distress, such as those that contain caffeine or high acid content (e.g., tomato products, citrus juices) or those that are heavily seasoned with strong or hot spices. Bell peppers and onions are also commonly irritating foods. Most patients seem to progress better with a bland, nonspicy diet and smaller, more frequent meals. Alcohol and tobacco should also be avoided.

The primary health care provider often prescribes drugs that block and buffer gastric acid secretions to relieve ***pain.*** *H_2-receptor antagonists,* such as famotidine and nizatidine, are typically used to block gastric secretions. Sucralfate, a *mucosal barrier fortifier,* may also be prescribed. Antisecretory agents *(proton pump inhibitors [PPIs]),* such as omeprazole or pantoprazole, may be prescribed to suppress gastric acid. *Antacids* used as buffering agents include aluminum hydroxide combined with magnesium hydroxide and aluminum hydroxide combined with simethicone and magnesium hydroxide (see the Common Examples of Drug Therapy: Gastritis and Peptic Ulcer Disease box). Calcium carbonate (chewable or liquid) is also a potent antacid, but it triggers gastrin release, causing rebound acid secretion.

Teach the patient about various techniques that reduce stress and ***pain,*** such as progressive relaxation, cutaneous stimulation, guided imagery, and distraction. Table 50.1 lists commonly used complementary and integrative therapies for gastritis and peptic ulcer disease.

Treatment of *chronic* gastritis varies with the cause. The approach to management includes the elimination of causative agents, treatment of any underlying disease (e.g., chronic kidney disease, Crohn's disease), avoidance of toxic substances (e.g., alcohol, tobacco), and health teaching.

Patients with *chronic* gastritis may require vitamin B_{12} for prevention or treatment of pernicious anemia. If *H. pylori* is found, the primary health care provider treats the ***infection.*** Current practice for infection treatment is described in the Drug Therapy discussion in the Peptic Ulcer Disease section.

TABLE 50.1 Commonly Used Complementary and Integrative Therapies for Gastritis and Peptic Ulcer Disease (PUD)

Herbs and Vitamins	Homeopathy
• Cranberry	• Carbo vegetabilis
• Deglycyrrhizinated licorice (DGL)	• Ipecacuanha
• Zinc	• Nux vomica
• Ginger	• Pulsatilla
• Glutamine	
• Acidophilus	
• Probiotics	
• Slippery elm	
• Vitamin A	
• Vitamin C	

INFECTION CONCEPT EXEMPLAR: PEPTIC ULCER DISEASE (PUD)

Peptic ulcer disease (PUD) results when GI mucosal defenses become impaired and no longer protect the epithelium from the effects of acid and pepsin.

Pathophysiology Review

Types of Ulcers. Three types of peptic ulcers may occur: duodenal ulcers, gastric ulcers, and stress ulcers (less common). Many ulcers are caused by *H. pylori* ***infection*** (National Institute of Diabetes and Digestive and Kidney Diseases, 2020). The most common route of *H. pylori* infection transmission is either oral-to-oral (stomach contents are transmitted from mouth to mouth) or fecal-to-oral (from stool to mouth) contact.

As a response to the bacteria, cytokines, neutrophils, and other substances are activated and cause epithelial cell necrosis. Urease produced by *H. pylori* breaks down urea into ammonia, which neutralizes the acidity of the stomach. In addition, the helical shape of *H. pylori* allows the bacterium to burrow into the mucus layer of the stomach and become undetectable by the body's immune cells. Although this bacterium does not cause illness in most people, it is a major risk factor for peptic ulcers and gastric cancer (McCance et al., 2019).

Duodenal ulcers occur more often than other types. Most duodenal ulcers present in the upper portion of the duodenum. They are deep, sharply demarcated lesions that penetrate through the mucosa and submucosa into the muscularis propria (muscle layer). The floor of the ulcer consists of a necrotic area residing on granulation tissue and surrounded by areas of fibrosis (McCance et al., 2019) (Fig. 50.1).

The main feature of a duodenal ulcer is high gastric acid secretion, although a wide range of secretory levels are found. In patients with duodenal ulcers, pH levels are low (excess acid) in the duodenum for long periods. Protein-rich meals, calcium, and vagus nerve excitation stimulate acid secretion. Combined with hypersecretion, a rapid emptying of food from the stomach reduces the buffering effect of food and delivers a large acid bolus to the duodenum. Inhibitory secretory mechanisms and pancreatic secretion may be insufficient to control the acid load.

COMMON EXAMPLES OF DRUG THERAPY

Gastritis and Peptic Ulcer Disease

Class and Common Examples	Selected Nursing Implications
Antacids Increase pH of gastric contents by deactivating pepsin	
Magnesium hydroxide with aluminum hydroxide	Give 2 hr after meals and at bedtime. *Hydrogen ion load is high after ingestion of foods.* Use liquid rather than tablets. *Suspensions are more effective than chewable tablets.* Do not give other drugs within 1-2 hr of antacids. *Antacids interfere with absorption of other drugs.* Assess patients for a history of chronic kidney disease. *Hypermagnesemia may result, especially in patients with poorly functioning kidneys, thus causing toxicity.* Assess the patient for a history of heart failure. *Inadequate renal perfusion from heart failure decreases the ability of the kidneys to excrete magnesium, thus causing toxicity.* Observe the patient for the side effect of diarrhea. *Magnesium often causes diarrhea.*
Aluminum hydroxide	Give 1 hr after meals and at bedtime. *Hydrogen ion load is high after ingestion of food.* Use liquid rather than tablets if palatable. *Suspensions are more effective than chewable tablets.* Do not give other drugs within 1-2 hr of antacids. *Antacids interfere with absorption of other drugs.* Observe patients for the side effect of constipation. If constipation occurs, consider alternating with magnesium antacid. *Aluminum causes constipation, and magnesium has a laxative effect.* Use for patients with chronic kidney disease. *Aluminum binds with phosphates in the GI tract. This antacid does not contain magnesium.*
H_2 Antagonists (Blockers) Decrease gastric acid secretions by blocking histamine receptors in parietal cells	
Famotidine Nizatidine **Note:** IV famotidine may also be given to prevent surgical stress ulcers.	Give single dose at bedtime for treatment of heartburn and PUD. *Bedtime administration suppresses nocturnal acid production.*
Mucosal Barrier Fortifiers Protect stomach mucosa	
Sucralfate	Give 1 hr before and 2 hr after meals and at bedtime. *Food may interfere with drug's adherence to mucosa.* Do not give within 30 min of giving antacids or other drugs. *Antacids may interfere with effect.*
Bismuth subsalicylate	Remind patient to refrain from taking aspirin while on this drug. *Aspirin is a salicylic acid and can lead to overdose.*
Proton Pump Inhibitors Suppress HK–ATPase enzyme system of gastric acid secretion to suppress acid	
Omeprazole	Have patients take capsule whole; do not crush. *Delayed-release capsules allow absorption after granules leave the stomach.* Give 30 min before the main meal of the day. *The proton pump is activated by the presence of food. Therefore the drug needs a chance to work before the patient eats.*
Lansoprazole	Give 30 min before the main meal of the day. *The proton pump is activated by the presence of food. Therefore the drug needs a chance to work before the patient eats.*
Rabeprazole	Take after the morning meal. *This drug promotes healing and symptom relief of duodenal ulcers.* Do not crush capsule. *This drug is a sustained-release capsule.*
Pantoprazole	Do not crush. *This drug is enteric coated.* IV form must be given on a pump with a filter and in a separate line. *Given IV, this drug precipitates easily.* Do not give IV pantoprazole with other IV drugs. Monitor for adverse drug interactions if patient is on other medications. *The IV form is not compatible with most other drugs. This drug will alter how other drugs are metabolized, either increasing or decreasing their effectiveness.*
Esomeprazole	Assess for hepatic impairment. *Patients with severe hepatic problems need a low dose.* Do not give Nexium IV with other IV drugs. *The IV form is not compatible with most other drugs.* Monitor for adverse drug interactions if patient is on other medications. *This drug will alter how other drugs are metabolized, either increasing or decreasing the effectiveness.*

Continued

COMMON EXAMPLES OF DRUG THERAPY—cont'd

Gastritis and Peptic Ulcer Disease

Class and Common Examples	Selected Nursing Implications
Prostaglandin Analogs	
Stimulate mucosal protection and decrease gastric acid secretions	
Misoprostol	Not commonly given, but used for clients receiving NSAIDs to *protect the stomach mucosa.* Avoid magnesium-containing antacids. *Misoprostol and magnesium-containing antacids can cause diarrhea.* Do not administer to pregnant women. *This drug can cause abortion, premature birth, or birth defects.*
Antimicrobials	
Treat *H. pylori* infection	
Clarithromycin	Give with caution to patients with renal impairment; monitor renal function laboratory values. *This drug can increase the patient's BUN level and should be monitored.*
Amoxicillin	Teach patients to take the drug with food or immediately after a meal. *This drug can cause GI disturbances, including nausea, vomiting, and diarrhea.*
Tetracycline	Teach patients to take the drug at least 1 hr before meals or 2 hr after meals. *Dairy products and other foods may interfere with drug absorption.* Teach patients to avoid direct sunlight and wear sunscreen when outdoors. *This drug can cause the skin to burn as a result of photosensitivity.*
Metronidazole	Teach patients to take the drug with food. *This drug can cause GI disturbances, especially nausea.* Teach patients to avoid alcohol during drug therapy and for at least 3 days after therapy is completed. *The patient can experience a drug-alcohol reaction, including severe nausea, vomiting, and headache.*

BUN, Blood urea nitrogen; *PUD,* peptic ulcer disease.

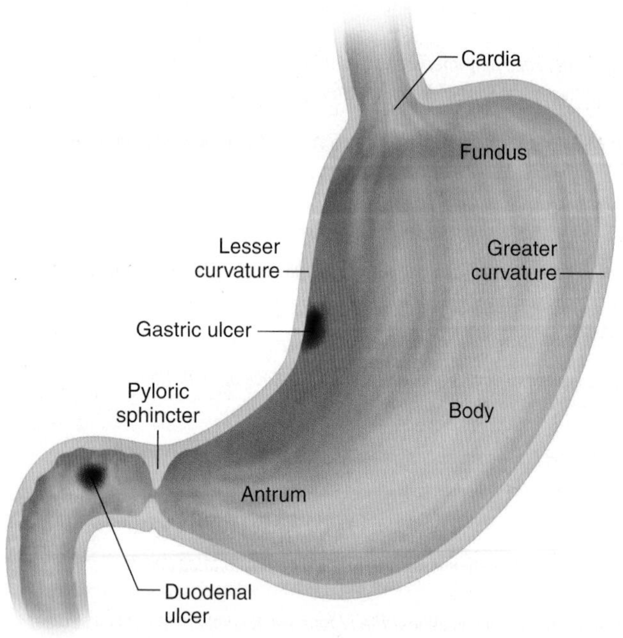

FIG. 50.1 Most common sites for peptic ulcers.

Gastric ulcers usually develop in the antrum of the stomach near acid-secreting mucosa (see Fig. 50.1). When a break in the mucosal barrier occurs (such as that caused by *H. pylori* ***infection***), hydrochloric acid injures the epithelium. Gastric ulcers may then result from back-diffusion of acid or dysfunction of the pyloric sphincter. Without normal functioning of the pyloric sphincter, bile refluxes (backs up) into the stomach. This reflux of bile acids may break the integrity of the mucosal barrier, which leads to mucosal ***inflammation.*** Toxic agents and bile then destroy the membrane of the gastric mucosa.

Gastric emptying is often delayed in patients with gastric ulceration. This causes regurgitation of duodenal contents, which worsens the gastric mucosal injury. Decreased blood flow to the gastric mucosa may also alter the defense barrier and thereby allow ulceration to occur.

Stress ulcers are acute gastric mucosal lesions occurring after an acute medical crisis or trauma, such as sepsis or a head injury. In the patient who is NPO for major surgery, gastritis may lead to stress ulcers. Patients who are critically ill, especially those with extensive burns (Curling ulcer), sepsis (ischemic ulcer), or increased intracranial pressure (Cushing ulcer), are also susceptible to these ulcers. Stress ulcers are associated with lengthened hospital stay and increased mortality rates. Therefore most patients who have major trauma or surgery receive IV drug therapy (e.g., PPIs) to prevent stress ulcer development.

Bleeding caused by gastric erosion is the main manifestation of acute stress ulcers. Multifocal lesions associated with stress ulcers occur in the stomach and proximal duodenum. These lesions begin as areas of ischemia and evolve into erosions and ulcerations that may progress to massive hemorrhage.

Complications of Ulcers. The most common complications of PUD are hemorrhage, perforation, pyloric obstruction, and intractable disease. *Hemorrhage is the most serious complication.* It tends to occur more often in patients with *gastric* ulcers and in older adults. Many patients have a second episode of bleeding if underlying ***infection*** with *H. pylori* remains untreated

KEY FEATURES

Upper GI Bleeding

- Bright red or coffee-ground vomitus (hematemesis)
- Melena (tarry or dark sticky stools)
- Decreased hemoglobin and hematocrit
- Decreased blood pressure
- Increased heart rate
- Weak peripheral pulses
- Acute confusion (in older adults)
- Vertigo
- Dizziness or light-headedness
- Syncope (loss of consciousness)

or if therapy does not include an H_2 antagonist. With massive bleeding the patient vomits bright red or coffee-ground blood (**hematemesis**). Gastric acid digestion of blood typically results in the coffee-ground appearance. Hematemesis usually indicates bleeding at or above the duodenojejunal junction (upper GI bleeding). Other signs and symptoms are listed in the Key Features: Upper GI Bleeding box.

Minimal bleeding from ulcers manifests with occult blood in a dark, "tarry" stool (**melena**). Melena may occur in patients with gastric ulcers but is more common in those with duodenal ulcers.

Gastric and duodenal ulcers can perforate and bleed (Fig. 50.2). *Perforation* occurs when the ulcer becomes so deep that the entire thickness of the stomach or duodenum is worn away. The stomach or duodenal contents can then leak into the peritoneal cavity. Sudden, sharp ***pain*** begins in the mid-epigastric region and spreads over the entire abdomen. The amount of pain correlates with the amount and type of GI contents spilled. The classic pain causes the patient to be apprehensive. The abdomen is tender, rigid, and boardlike as a result of this ***infection*** (**peritonitis**). The patient often assumes a "fetal" position to decrease the tension on the abdominal muscles. He or she can become severely ill within hours. Bacterial septicemia and hypovolemic shock can follow. Peristalsis diminishes, and paralytic ileus develops. *Peptic ulcer perforation is a surgical emergency and can be life threatening!*

NCLEX EXAMINATION CHALLENGE 50.1

Safe and Effective Care Environment

The nurse is caring for a client diagnosed with peptic ulcer disease (PUD). For which potential complications will the nurse monitor? **Select all that apply.**

A. Pneumonia
B. Peritonitis
C. Anemia
D. Stroke
E. Hypotension
F. Cirrhosis

Pyloric (gastric outlet) obstruction (blockage) occurs in a small percentage of patients and manifests with vomiting caused by stasis and gastric dilation. Obstruction occurs at the pylorus (the gastric outlet) and is caused by scarring, edema, inflammation, or a combination of these factors. Symptoms of obstruction include abdominal bloating, nausea, and vomiting. When vomiting persists, the patient may have *metabolic alkalosis* from loss of large quantities of acid gastric juice (hydrogen and chloride ions) in the vomitus. *Hypokalemia* may also result from the vomiting or metabolic alkalosis.

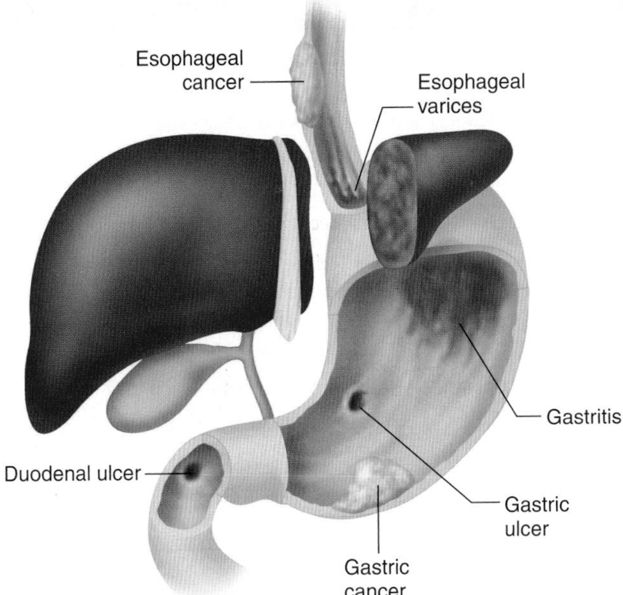

FIG. 50.2 Common causes of upper GI bleeding.

Many patients with ulcers have a single episode with no recurrence. However, *intractability* may develop from complications of ulcers, excessive stressors in the patient's life, or an inability to adhere to long-term therapy. He or she no longer responds to conservative management, or recurrences of symptoms interfere with ADLs. In general, the patient continues to have recurrent pain despite treatment. Those who fail to respond to traditional treatments or who have a relapse after discontinuation of therapy are referred to a gastroenterology practitioner.

Etiology and Genetic Risk. Peptic ulcer disease is caused most often by bacterial ***infection*** with *H. pylori* and long-term use of NSAIDs such as ibuprofen. NSAIDs break down the mucosal barrier and disrupt the mucosal protection mediated systemically by cyclooxygenase (COX) inhibition. Other risk factors for PUD are the same as for gastritis (see discussion earlier in this chapter). Patients with duodenal ulcers often have a positive family history of the disease.

Incidence and Prevalence. PUD affects millions of adults across the world. In the United States, the prevalence of PUD is over 15 million (McCance et al., 2019). However, primary health care provider visits, hospitalizations, and the mortality rate for PUD have decreased in the past few decades, in part because of the use of proton pump inhibitors and earlier treatment for *H. pylori.*

❖ Interprofessional Collaborative Care

Care of the patient with PUD generally takes place in the community setting, unless the patient develops a more serious condition such as upper GI bleeding, which requires acute management.

TABLE 50.2 Differential Features of Gastric and Duodenal Ulcers

Feature	Gastric Ulcer	Duodenal Ulcer
Age	50-70 yr	20-50 yr
Gender	Affects males and females equally	Affects males and females equally
Blood group	No differentiation	Most often type O
General nourishment	May be malnourished	Usually well nourished
Stomach acid production	Normal secretion or hyposecretion	Hypersecretion
Occurrence	Mucosa exposed to acid-pepsin secretion	Mucosa exposed to acid-pepsin secretion; positive family history
Clinical course	Healing and recurrence	Healing and recurrence
Upper abdominal pain	Occurs 30-60 min after a meal; at night, rarely Worsened by ingestion of food	Occurs 1½-3 hr after a meal; at night: often awakens patient between 1 and 2 a.m. Relieved by ingestion of food
Response to treatment	Healing with appropriate therapy	Remissions and exacerbations
Hemorrhage	Hematemesis more common than melena	Melena more common than hematemesis
Cancer risk	Increased, but in less than 10%	Not increased
Recurrence	Tends to heal and recurs often in the same location	60% recur within 1 yr; 90% recur within 2 yr
Surrounding mucosa	Atrophic gastritis	No gastritis

◆ Assessment: Recognize Cues

History. A history of current or past medical conditions focuses on GI problems, particularly any history of diagnosis or treatment for *H. pylori* ***infection.*** Review all prescription and OTC drugs the patient is taking. Specifically inquire whether the patient is taking corticosteroids, chemotherapy, or NSAIDs. Also ask whether he or she has ever undergone radiation treatments. Assess whether the patient has had any GI surgeries, especially a partial gastrectomy, which can cause chronic gastritis.

Collect data related to the causes and risk factors for peptic ulcer disease (PUD). Question the patient about factors that can influence the development of PUD, including alcohol intake and tobacco use. Note if certain foods such as tomatoes or caffeinated beverages precipitate or worsen symptoms. Information regarding actual or perceived daily stressors should also be obtained.

A history of GI upset, pain and its relationship to eating and sleep patterns, and actions taken to relieve pain are also important. Inquire about any changes in the character of the pain because this may signal the development of complications. For example, if ***pain*** that was once intermittent and relieved by food and antacids becomes constant and radiates to the back or upper quadrant, the patient may have ulcer perforation. However, many adults with active duodenal or gastric ulcers report having no ulcer symptoms.

Physical Assessment/Signs and Symptoms. Physical assessment findings may reveal epigastric tenderness and ***pain***, usually located at the midline between the umbilicus and the xiphoid process. *If perforation into the peritoneal cavity is present, the patient typically has a rigid, boardlike abdomen accompanied by rebound tenderness and intense pain* (peritonitis). Initially, auscultation of the abdomen may reveal hyperactive bowel sounds, but these may diminish with progression of the ***infection.*** Perform a comprehensive pain assessment.

Dyspepsia is the most commonly reported symptom associated with PUD. It is typically described as sharp, burning, or gnawing pain. Some patients may perceive discomfort as a sensation of abdominal pressure or of fullness or hunger. Specific differences between gastric and duodenal ulcers are listed in Table 50.2 (McCance et al., 2019).

To assess for fluid volume deficit that may occur from a bleeding ulcer, take orthostatic blood pressures and monitor for signs and symptoms of dehydration. Also assess for dizziness, especially when the patient is upright, because this is a symptom of fluid volume deficit. *Older adults often experience dizziness when they get out of bed and are at risk for falls.*

Psychosocial Assessment. Assess the impact of ulcer disease on the patient's lifestyle, occupation, family, and social and leisure activities. Evaluate the impact that lifestyle changes will have on the patient and family. This assessment may reveal information about the patient's ability to adhere to the prescribed treatment regimen and obtain the needed social support to alter his or her lifestyle.

Laboratory Assessment. There are three simple, noninvasive tests to detect *H. pylori* in the patient's blood, breath, or stool. Although the breath and stool tests are considered more accurate, *serologic testing* for *H. pylori* antibodies is the most common method to confirm *H. pylori* infection. The *urea breath test* involves swallowing a capsule, liquid, or pudding that contains urea with a special carbon atom. After a few minutes the patient exhales; and, if the special carbon atom is found, the bacterium is present. The *stool antigen test* is performed on a stool sample provided by the patient, which is tested for *H. pylori* antigens. Patients who have bleeding from a peptic ulcer may have *decreased hemoglobin and hematocrit* values. The *stool* may also be positive for occult (not seen) blood if bleeding is present (Pagana & Pagana, 2018; Pagana et al., 2019).

Other Diagnostic Assessment. *The major diagnostic test for PUD is esophagogastroduodenoscopy (EGD), which is the most accurate means of establishing a diagnosis.* Direct visualization of the ulcer crater by EGD allows the primary health care provider to take specimens for *H. pylori* testing and biopsy and cytologic studies for ruling out gastric cancer. The *rapid urease test* can confirm a quick diagnosis because urease is produced by the bacteria in the gastric mucosa. EGD may be repeated at 4- to 6-week intervals while the primary health care provider evaluates the progress of healing in response to therapy. Chapter 48 describes this test in more detail.

GI bleeding may be tested using a *nuclear medicine scan.* No special preparation is required for this scan. The patient is injected with a contrast medium (usually technetium [^{99m}Tc]), and the GI system is scanned for the presence of bleeding after a waiting period. A second scan may be done 1 to 2 days after treatment for the bleeding to determine if the interventions were effective.

◆ **Analysis: Analyze Cues and Prioritize Hypotheses.** The priority collaborative problems for patients with peptic ulcer disease (PUD) include:

1. Acute or persistent ***pain*** due to gastric and/or duodenal ulceration
2. Potential for upper GI bleeding due to gastric and/or duodenal ulceration or perforation

◆ **Planning and Implementation: Generate Solutions and Take Action**

Managing Acute or Persistent Pain

Planning: Expected Outcomes. The patient with PUD is expected to report pain control as evidenced by no more than a 3 on a 0 to 10 pain intensity scale.

Interventions. PUD causes significant discomfort that affects many aspects of daily living. Interventions to manage pain focus on drug therapy and dietary changes.

Drug Therapy. The primary purposes of drug therapy in the treatment of PUD are to (1) provide ***pain*** relief, (2) eliminate *H. pylori* ***infection,*** (3) heal ulcerations, and (4) prevent recurrence. Several different regimens can be used. Although numerous drugs have been evaluated for the treatment of *H. pylori* infection, no single agent has been used successfully against the organism. A common drug regimen for *H. pylori* infection is PPI–triple therapy, which includes a proton pump inhibitor (PPI), such as lansoprazole, plus two antibiotics such as metronidazole and tetracycline or clarithromycin and amoxicillin for 10 to 14 days. Some primary health care providers may prefer to use quadruple therapy, which contains a combination of a proton pump inhibitor (PPI), any two commonly used antibiotics as described previously, and the addition of bismuth. Bismuth therapy is often used in patients who are allergic to penicillin-based medications.

Bismuth subsalicylate inhibits *H. pylori* from binding to the mucosal lining and stimulates mucosal protection and prostaglandin production. Teach patients that they cannot take aspirin while on this drug because aspirin is a salicylic acid and could cause an overdose of salicylates. Patients should also be taught that bismuth may cause the stools and/or tongue to be discolored black. This discoloration is temporary and harmless.

> **PATIENT-CENTERED CARE: OLDER ADULT CONSIDERATIONS** QSEN
>
> Many older adults have *H. pylori infection* that is undiagnosed because of vague symptoms associated with physiologic changes of aging and comorbidities that mask **dyspepsia**. Because the average age of gastric cancer diagnosis is 70 years, it is important to teach older adults about the symptoms of PUD and to consider *H. pylori* screening. Early detection and aggressive treatment can prevent PUD and gastric cancer.

Hyposecretory drugs reduce gastric acid secretions and are therefore used for both peptic ulcer disease (PUD) and gastritis management. The primary prescribed drugs include proton pump inhibitors and H_2-receptor antagonists (see the Common Examples of Drug Therapy: Gastritis and Peptic Ulcer Disease box).

A proton pump inhibitor (PPI) is the drug class of choice for treating patients with acid-related disorders. Omeprazole, lansoprazole, and esomeprazole are each available as delayed-release capsules designed to release their contents after they pass through the stomach. Omeprazole and lansoprazole may be dissolved in a sodium bicarbonate solution and given through any feeding tube. Bicarbonate protects the dissolved omeprazole and lansoprazole granules in gastric acid. Therefore the drugs are still absorbed correctly. These capsules can also be opened. The enteric-coated capsules can be put in apple juice or orange juice and given through a large-bore feeding tube. Rabeprazole and pantoprazole are enteric-coated tablets that quickly dissolve after the tablet has moved through the stomach and should not be crushed before they are taken. Several of the PPIs, such as pantoprazole, are also available in an IV form, which is useful for patients who are NPO (Burchum & Rosenthal, 2019).

Some patients use PPIs for years and perhaps a lifetime; these patients should be assessed periodically to determine the necessity of PPI use. Some studies have suggested there may be an increased risk of osteoporotic fractures related to long-term PPI use, yet current research is ongoing to determine if there is a definitive link (Burchum & Rosenthal, 2019). Omeprazole reduces the effect of clopidogrel, an antiplatelet drug. Teach patients to tell their primary health care provider if they are taking clopidogrel. PPIs should not be discontinued abruptly, to prevent rebound activation of the proton pump; a step-down approach over several days is recommended (Burchum & Rosenthal, 2019).

Nutrition Therapy. The role of diet in the management of ulcer disease is controversial. There is no evidence that dietary restriction reduces gastric acid secretion or promotes tissue healing, although a bland diet may assist in relieving symptoms. Food itself acts as an antacid by neutralizing gastric acid for 30 to 60 minutes. An increased rate of gastric acid secretion, called *rebound,* may follow.

> **! NURSING SAFETY PRIORITY** QSEN
>
> ***Action Alert***
>
> Teach the patient with peptic ulcer disease to follow healthy *nutrition* habits and avoid substances that increase gastric acid secretion. This includes caffeine-containing beverages (coffee, tea, cola). Both caffeinated and decaffeinated coffees should be avoided because coffee contains peptides that stimulate gastrin release (Priyanka et al., 2016).

Teach the patient to exclude any foods that cause discomfort. A bland, nonirritating diet is recommended during the acute symptomatic phase. Bedtime snacks are avoided because they may stimulate gastric acid secretion. Eating six smaller meals daily may help, but this regimen is no longer a regular part of therapy. No evidence supports the theory that eating six meals daily promotes healing of the ulcer. This practice may actually stimulate gastric acid secretion. Patients should avoid alcohol and tobacco because of their stimulatory effects on gastric acid secretion.

Complementary and Integrative Health. Teach patients about complementary and integrative therapies that can reduce stress, including hypnosis and imagery. For example, the use of yoga and meditation techniques has demonstrated a beneficial effect on anxiety disorders. Many have suggested that GI disorders result from the dysfunction of both the GI tract itself and the brain. This means that emotional stress is thought to worsen GI disorders such as peptic ulcer disease. Yoga may alter the activities of the central and autonomic nervous systems.

Herbs and other supplements may be used by some patients as discussed earlier in this chapter under Gastritis.

Managing Upper GI Bleeding

Planning: Expected Outcomes. The patient with upper GI bleeding (often called *upper GI hemorrhage* or *UGH*) is expected to have bleeding promptly and effectively controlled and vital signs within normal limits.

Interventions. Blood loss from PUD results in high morbidity and mortality. Fluid volume loss secondary to vomiting can lead to dehydration and electrolyte imbalances. Interventions aimed at managing complications associated with PUD include prevention and/or management of bleeding, perforation, and gastric outlet obstruction. In some cases surgical treatment of complications becomes necessary.

Nonsurgical Management. Because prevention or early detection of complications is needed to obtain a positive clinical outcome, monitor the patient carefully and immediately report changes to the Rapid Response Team or primary health care provider.

Emergency: upper GI bleeding. The patient who is actively bleeding has a life-threatening emergency and needs supportive therapy to prevent hypovolemic shock and possible death (Farrar, 2018).

! NURSING SAFETY PRIORITY QSEN

Critical Rescue

Recognize that your priority for care of the patient with upper GI bleeding is to maintain airway, breathing, and circulation (ABCs). Respond to these needs by providing oxygen and other ventilatory support as needed, starting two large-bore IV lines for replacing fluids and blood, and monitoring vital signs, hematocrit, and oxygen saturation.

The purpose of managing hypovolemia is to expand intravascular fluid in a patient who is volume depleted. Carefully monitor the patient's fluid status, including intake and output. *Fluid replacement in older adults should be closely monitored to prevent fluid overload.* Serum electrolytes are also assessed because depletions from vomiting or nasogastric suctioning must be replaced. Volume replacement with isotonic solutions (e.g., 0.9% normal saline solution, lactated Ringer's solution) should be started immediately. The primary health care provider may prescribe blood products such as packed red blood cells (PRBCs) to expand volume and correct a low hemoglobin and hematocrit. For patients with active bleeding, fresh frozen plasma may be given if the prothrombin time is 1.5 times higher than the midrange control value (Farrar, 2018).

Continue to monitor the patient's hematocrit, hemoglobin, and coagulation studies for changes from the baseline measurements. With mild bleeding (less than 500 mL), slight feelings of weakness and mild perspiration may be present. When blood loss exceeds 1 L/24 hr, manifestations of hypovolemic shock may occur, such as hypotension, chills, palpitations, diaphoresis, and a weak, thready pulse (see Chapter 34 for management of shock).

A combination of several different treatments, including nasogastric tube (NGT) placement and lavage, endoscopic therapy, interventional radiologic procedures, and acid suppression, can be used to control acute bleeding and prevent rebleeding. If the patient is actively bleeding at home, he or she is usually admitted to the emergency department. After the bleeding has stopped, H_2-receptor antagonists and proton pump inhibitors are the primary drugs used.

Nasogastric tube placement and lavage. Upper GI bleeding or obstruction often requires the primary health care provider or nurse to insert a large-bore NGT to:

- Determine the presence or absence of blood in the stomach
- Assess the rate of bleeding
- Prevent gastric dilation
- Administer lavage

Although not performed as commonly today, *gastric lavage* requires the insertion of a large-bore NGT with instillation of a room-temperature solution in volumes of 200 to 300 mL. There is no evidence that sterile saline or sterile water is better than tap water for this procedure. Follow agency protocol for the solution that is required. The solution and blood are repeatedly withdrawn manually until returns are clear or light pink and without clots. Instruct the patient to lie on the left side during this procedure. The NGT may remain in place for a few days or be removed after lavage.

Treatment of pyloric obstruction is directed toward restoring fluid and electrolyte balance and decompressing the dilated stomach. Obstruction related to edema and spasm generally responds to medical therapy. First, the stomach must be decompressed with nasogastric suction. Next, interventions are directed at correcting metabolic alkalosis and dehydration. The NGT is typically clamped after about 72 hours. Check the patient for retention of gastric contents. If the amount retained is not more than 50 mL in 30 minutes or other prescribed parameters, the primary health care provider may allow oral fluids. In some cases, surgical intervention may be required to treat PUD.

Endoscopic therapy. Endoscopic therapy via an esophagogastroduodenoscopy (EGD) can assist in achieving homeostasis during an acute hemorrhage by isolating the bleeding artery to embolize (clot) it. The endoscopist can insert instruments through the endoscope during the procedure to stop bleeding in three different ways: (1) inject chemicals into the bleeding site; (2) treat the bleeding area with heat, electric current, or laser; or (3) close the affected blood vessels with a band or clip. During the EGD, a specialized endoscopy nurse and technician assist the physician with the procedure.

Pre-EGD nursing care involves inserting one or two large-bore IV catheters if they are not in place. A large catheter allows the patient to receive IV moderate sedation (e.g., midazolam [Versed] and an opioid) and possibly a blood transfusion. Keep the patient NPO for 4 to 6 hours before the procedure. This prevents the risk for aspiration and allows the endoscopist to view and treat the ulcer. A patient must sign a consent form before the EGD *after* the primary health care provider informs him or her about the procedure.

! NURSING SAFETY PRIORITY QSEN

Action Alert

After esophagogastroduodenoscopy (EGD), monitor vital signs, heart rhythm, and oxygen saturation frequently per agency protocol until they return to baseline. In addition, frequently assess the patient's ability to swallow saliva. The patient's gag reflex may initially be absent after EGD because of anesthetizing (numbing) of the throat with a spray before the procedure. *After the procedure, do not allow the patient to have food or liquids until the gag reflex has returned!*

Endoscopic therapy is beneficial for most patients with active bleeding. However, ulcers that continue to bleed or continue to rebleed despite endoscopic therapy may require an interventional radiologic procedure or surgical repair.

Interventional radiologic procedures. For patients with persistent, massive upper GI bleeding or those who are not surgical candidates, catheter-directed embolization may be performed. This endovascular procedure is usually done if endoscopic procedures are not successful or available. A femoral approach is most often used, but brachial access may be used. An arteriogram is performed to identify the arterial anatomy and find the exact location of the bleeding. The radiologist injects medication or other material into the blood vessels to stop the bleeding. Care of the patient following an arteriogram is similar to care following a percutaneous vascular intervention, which is described in Chapters 30 and 33. Postarteriogram nursing care should be provided after the procedure.

CLINICAL JUDGMENT CHALLENGE 50.1

Safety; Teamwork and Collaboration

A 52-year-old woman was admitted after vomiting bright red blood last night. She states that she has a history of gastritis and hypertension and takes medication for both. She cannot provide the names of the medications she is taking. This morning's nursing assessment findings include:

- States that she has been taking ibuprofen 1600 mg every day for over a year for osteoarthritis in her hands and feet
- Blood pressure = 112/68 mm Hg (down from 150/90 mm Hg last night)
- Apical pulse = 108 beats/min
- Respirations = 22 breaths/min
- Has dry, pale skin
- Has a slightly distended abdomen with mid-epigastric moderate pain (5 out of 10)
- Is alert and oriented × 3
- Has adequate bowel sounds × 4

1. **Recognize Cues:** What assessment information in this client situation is the most important and immediate concern for the nurse? (Hint: Identify the **relevant** information *first* to determine what is most important.)
2. **Analyze Cues:** What client conditions are consistent with the **most relevant** information? (Hint: Think about priority collaborative problems that support and contradict the information presented in this situation.)
3. **Prioritize Hypotheses:** Which possibilities or explanations are **most likely** to be present in this client situation? Which possibilities or explanations are the most serious? (Hint: Consider all possibilities and determine their urgency and risk for this client.)
4. **Generate Solutions:** What actions would most likely achieve the desired outcomes for this client? Which actions should be **avoided** or are **potentially harmful**? (Hint: Determine the desired outcomes first to decide which interventions are appropriate and those that should be avoided.)
5. **Take Action:** Which actions are the most appropriate and how should they be implemented? In what **priority order** should they be implemented? (Hint: Consider health teaching, documentation, requested health care provider orders or prescriptions, nursing skills, collaboration with or referral to health team members, etc.)
6. **Evaluate Outcomes:** What client assessment would indicate that the nurse's actions were **effective**? (Hint: Think about signs that would indicate an improvement, decline, or unchanged client condition.)

Drug therapy. *Aggressive acid suppression is used to prevent rebleeding.* When acute bleeding is stopped and clot formation has taken place within the ulcer crater, the clot remains in contact with gastric contents. Acid-suppressive agents are used to stabilize the clot by raising the pH level of gastric contents. Several types of drugs are used. H_2-receptor antagonists prevent acid from being produced by parietal cells. Proton pump inhibitors prevent the transport of acid across the parietal cell membrane (Burchum & Rosenthal, 2019).

Surgical Management. Evidence-based guidelines for the treatment of PUD that include *H. pylori* treatment and the development of nonsurgical means of controlling bleeding have led to a decline in the need for surgical intervention. In PUD, surgical intervention may be used to:

- Treat patients who do not respond to medical therapy or other nonsurgical procedures
- Treat a surgical emergency that develops as a complication of PUD, such as perforation

Two general surgical approaches are available for PUD: minimally invasive surgery and conventional open surgery.

Minimally invasive surgery (MIS) via laparoscopy may be used to remove a chronic gastric ulcer or treat hemorrhage from perforation. Several small incisions allow access to the stomach and duodenum. The patient may have partial stomach removal (subtotal gastrectomy), pyloroplasty (to open the pylorus), and/or a vagotomy (vagus nerve cutting) to control acid secretion. Acid-reduction surgery may not be necessary because of the increased use of PPIs and endoscopic procedures in the treatment of PUD. The advantages of MIS over traditional open surgical procedures include a shorter hospital stay, fewer complications, less pain, and better, quicker recovery. Care of patients having gastric surgery is discussed later in this chapter under Gastric Cancer.

Care Coordination and Transition Management. Patients may be discharged from the hospital if there is no evidence of ongoing bleeding, orthostatic changes, or cardiopulmonary distress or compromise. Those discharged after treatment for peptic ulcer disease (PUD) and/or complications secondary to the disease face several challenges to manage the disease successfully. Long-term adherence to drug therapy may require the patient to take several drugs each day. Permanent lifestyle alterations in ***nutrition*** habits must also be made.

Home Care Management. Most patients are discharged to home to continue their recovery. Those who have had major surgery or complications, such as hemorrhage, may require one or two visits from a home care nurse to assess clinical progress, especially if the patient is an older adult (see the Home Care Considerations: The Patient with Peptic Ulcer Disease box).

Self-Management Education. The primary focus of home care preparation is patient and family teaching regarding risk factors for the recurrence of PUD. Teach them how to recognize new complications and what to do if they occur.

Help the patient plan ways to make needed lifestyle changes. For postsurgical patients, especially those who have undergone partial stomach removal, smaller meals may be required. Other postoperative ***nutrition*** changes are described in the Self-Management Education discussion in the Gastric Cancer section.

HOME CARE CONSIDERATIONS

The Patient With Peptic Ulcer Disease

Assess gastrointestinal and cardiovascular status, including:
- Vital signs, including orthostatic vital signs
- Skin color
- Presence of abdominal pain (location, severity, character, duration, precipitating factors, and relief measures)
- Character, color, and consistency of stools
- Changes in bowel elimination pattern
- Hemoglobin and hematocrit
- Bowel sounds; palpate for areas of tenderness

Assess nutritional status, including:
- Dietary patterns and habits
- Intake of coffee and alcohol
- Relationship of food ingestion to symptoms

Assess medication history:
- Use of steroids
- Use of NSAIDs
- Use of over-the-counter medications

Assess patient's coping style:
- Recent stressors
- Past coping style

Assess patient's understanding of illness and ability to adhere to the therapeutic regimen:
- Symptoms to report to the primary health care provider
- Expected and side effects of medications
- Food and drug interactions
- Need for smoking cessation

NURSING SAFETY PRIORITY QSEN

Action Alert

Teach the patient who has peptic ulcer disease to seek immediate medical attention if experiencing any of these symptoms:
- Sharp, sudden, persistent, and severe epigastric or abdominal pain
- Bloody or black stools
- Bloody vomit or vomit that looks like coffee grounds

NURSING SAFETY PRIORITY QSEN

Action Alert

Teach the patient who has had surgery for PUD to avoid any OTC product containing aspirin or other NSAIDs. Emphasize the importance of following the treatment regimen for *H. pylori* infection and healing the ulcer and of keeping all follow-up appointments. Help the patient identify situations that cause stress, describe feelings during stressful situations, and develop a plan for coping with stressors.

Health Care Resources. If needed, refer the patient and family to the National Institute of Diabetes and Digestive and Kidney Diseases Health Information Center (www.digestive.niddk.nih.gov/) in the United States or to the Canadian Digestive Health Foundation (https://cdhf.ca/). These groups provide information and support to patients who have digestive disorders.

◆ **Evaluation: Evaluate Outcomes.** Evaluate the care of the patient with peptic ulcer disease (PUD) based on the identified priority patient problems. The expected outcomes are that the patient:

- Does not have active PUD or *H. pylori* ***infection***
- Verbalizes relief or control of ***pain***
- Adheres to the drug regimen and lifestyle changes to prevent recurrence and heal the ulcer
- Does not experience upper GI bleeding; if bleeding occurs, it will be promptly and effectively managed

GASTRIC CANCER

Most cancers of the stomach are adenocarcinomas. This type of cancer develops in the mucosal cells that form the innermost lining of any portion or all of the stomach. In general, gastric cancer is more common in males than in females, and there is a sharp increase in adults over 50 years of age (American Cancer Society, 2020). *Often there are no symptoms in the early stages, and the disease is advanced when detected.*

Pathophysiology Review

Gastric cancer usually begins in the glands of the stomach mucosa. Atrophic gastritis and intestinal metaplasia (abnormal tissue development) are precancerous conditions. Inadequate acid secretion in patients with atrophic gastritis creates an alkaline environment that allows bacteria (especially *H. pylori*) to multiply. This ***infection*** causes mucosa-associated lymphoid tissue (MALT) lymphoma, which starts in the stomach (McCance et al., 2019).

Gastric cancers spread by direct extension through the gastric wall and into regional lymphatics, which carry tumor deposits to lymph nodes. Direct invasion of and adherence to adjacent organs (e.g., the liver, pancreas, and transverse colon) may also result. Hematogenous spread via the portal vein to the liver and via the systemic circulation to the lungs and bones is the most common mode of metastasis. Peritoneal seeding of cancer cells from the tumor areas to the omentum, peritoneum, ovary, and pelvic cul-de-sac can also occur.

In adults with *advanced* gastric cancer, there is invasion of the muscularis (stomach muscle) or beyond. These lesions are not cured by surgical resection. The overall 5-year survival rate of adults with stomach cancer in the United States is poor because most patients have no symptoms until the disease advances.

Infection with *H. pylori* is the largest risk factor for gastric cancer because it carries the cytotoxin-associated gene A *(CagA)* gene. Patients with pernicious anemia, gastric polyps, chronic atrophic gastritis, and achlorhydria (absence of secretion of hydrochloric acid) are two to three times more likely to develop gastric cancer.

The disease also seems to be positively correlated with eating excessive pickled foods, nitrates from processed foods, and salt added to food. The ingestion of these foods over a long period can lead to atrophic gastritis, a precancerous condition. A low intake of fruits and vegetables is also a risk factor for cancer (McCance et al., 2019).

Gastric surgery seems to increase the risk for gastric cancer because of the possible development of atrophic gastritis, which results in changes to the mucosa. Patients with Barrett esophagus from prolonged or severe gastroesophageal reflux disease (GERD) have an increased risk for cancer in the cardia (at the point where the stomach connects to the esophagus). Chapter 49 discusses GERD and esophageal cancer in detail.

❖ Interprofessional Collaborative Care

Care of the patient with gastric cancer takes place in all settings, ranging from the home and community environment to the inpatient setting, depending on the stage of disease and the immediate course of treatment.

◆ **Assessment: Recognize Cues.** Although patients with *early* gastric cancer may be asymptomatic, **dyspepsia** and abdominal discomfort are the *most* common symptoms. However, these symptoms are often ignored, or a change in diet or use of antacids relieves them. As the tumor grows, these symptoms become more severe and do not respond to ***nutrition*** changes or drug therapy (see the Key Features: Early versus Advanced Gastric Cancer box).

In patients with advanced disease, anemia is evidenced by *low hematocrit* and hemoglobin values. Patients may have macrocytic or microcytic anemia associated with decreased iron or vitamin B_{12} absorption. *The stool may be positive for occult blood. Hypoalbuminemia* and *abnormal results of liver tests* (e.g., bilirubin and alkaline phosphatase) occur with advanced disease and hepatic metastasis. The level of carcinoembryonic antigen (CEA) is elevated in advanced cancer of the stomach (Pagana & Pagana, 2018; Pagana et al., 2019).

The primary health care provider uses esophagogastroduodenoscopy (EGD) with biopsy for definitive diagnosis of gastric cancer. (See Chapter 48 for a discussion of nursing care associated with this diagnostic test.) The lesion can be viewed directly, and biopsies of all visible lesions can be performed to determine the presence of cancer cells. During the endoscopy, an endoscopic (endoluminal) ultrasound (EUS) of the gastric mucosa can also be performed. This technology allows the primary health care provider to evaluate the depth of the tumor and the presence of lymph node involvement, which permits more accurate staging of the disease. CT, positron emission tomography (PET), and MRI scans of the chest, abdomen, and pelvis are used in determining the extent of the disease and planning therapy.

KEY FEATURES
Early Versus Advanced Gastric Cancer

Early Gastric Cancer
- **Dyspepsia**
- Abdominal discomfort initially relieved with antacids
- Feeling of fullness
- Epigastric, back, or retrosternal pain

Advanced Gastric Cancer
- Nausea and vomiting
- Iron deficiency anemia
- Palpable epigastric mass
- Enlarged lymph nodes
- Weakness and fatigue
- Progressive weight loss

◆ **Interventions: Take Action.** Management of gastric cancer includes drug therapy, radiation, and/or surgery. Drug therapy and radiation may be used instead of surgery or as an adjunct before and/or after surgery.

Nonsurgical Management. The treatment of gastric cancer depends highly on the stage of the disease. Radiation and chemotherapy commonly prolong survival of patients with advanced gastric disease.

Combination *chemotherapy* with multiple cycles of drugs such as cisplatin and epirubicin before and after surgery may be given. Bone marrow suppression, nausea, and vomiting are common adverse drug effects. Chapter 20 discusses the general nursing care of patients receiving chemotherapy.

Although gastric cancers are somewhat sensitive to the effects of radiation, the use of this treatment is limited because the disease is often widely spread to other abdominal organs at diagnosis. Organs such as the liver, kidneys, and spinal cord can endure only a limited amount of radiation. Intraoperative radiotherapy (IORT) is available in large tertiary care health care systems.

Surgical Management. *Surgical resection by removing the tumor is the preferred method for treating gastric cancer.* The primary surgical procedures for the treatment of gastric cancer are total and subtotal (partial) gastrectomy. In early stages, laparoscopic surgery (minimally invasive surgery [MIS]) plus adjuvant chemotherapy or radiation may be curative. Patients having MIS have less pain, shorter hospital stays, rare postoperative complications, and quicker recovery. However, MIS is performed less often in the United States than in Europe because very few patients are diagnosed in the early stage of the disease. A recent study in a U.S. cancer center examined outcomes of MIS and an Enhanced Recovery After Surgery protocol. In addition to expected outcomes associated with laparoscopic surgery, patients in the study advanced their diets more quickly, experienced less weight loss, and increased their physical activity more quickly within the first week after the procedure when compared with patients having open traditional surgery (Desiderio et al., 2018).

Most patients with advanced disease are candidates for palliative surgical treatment. Metastasis in the supraclavicular lymph nodes, inguinal lymph nodes, liver, umbilicus, or perirectal wall indicates that the opportunity for cure by resection has been lost. Palliative resection may significantly improve the quality of life for a patient with obstruction, hemorrhage, or pain.

Preoperative Care. Before conventional open-approach surgery, a nasogastric tube (NGT) is often inserted and connected to suction to remove secretions and empty the stomach. This allows surgery to take place without contamination of the peritoneal cavity by gastric secretions. The NGT remains in place for a few days *after surgery* to prevent the accumulation of secretions, which may lead to vomiting or GI distention and pressure on the incision. Patients having laparoscopic surgery (minimally invasive surgery [MIS]) do not require an NGT.

Because weight loss is problematic for patients with gastric cancer, ***nutrition*** therapy is a vital aspect of preoperative and postoperative management. Before surgery, compression by the tumor can prevent adequate nutritional intake. To correct malnutrition before surgery, if present, the primary health care provider may prescribe enteral supplements to the diet and/or total parenteral nutrition (TPN). Vitamin, mineral, iron, and protein supplements are essential to correct nutritional deficits.

Other preoperative nursing measures for the patient undergoing open gastric surgery are the same as those for any patient undergoing abdominal surgery and general anesthesia (see Chapter 9).

Operative Procedures. The surgeon usually removes part or all of the stomach to take out the tumor. When the tumor is located in the mid-portion or distal (lower) portion of the stomach, a subtotal (partial) gastrectomy is typically performed. The omentum and relevant lymph nodes are also removed. The surgery may be performed as an MIS procedure or as an open conventional surgical technique, with or without robotic assistance.

For the patient with a removable growth in the proximal (upper) third of the stomach, a total gastrectomy is typically performed (Fig. 50.3). In this procedure the surgeon removes the entire stomach along with the lymph nodes and omentum. The surgeon sutures the esophagus to the duodenum or jejunum to reestablish continuity of the GI tract. More radical surgery involving removal of the spleen and distal pancreas is controversial, although the Whipple procedure may be used to prolong life. The complications of this drastic surgery are very serious and common (see Chapter 54). For patients with advanced disease, total gastrectomy is performed when gastric bleeding or obstruction is present.

Patients with tumors at the gastric outlet who are not candidates for subtotal or total gastrectomy may undergo gastroenterostomy for palliation. The surgeon creates a passage between the body of the stomach and the small bowel, often the duodenum.

Postoperative Care. Provide evidence-based postoperative care for patients who have had general anesthesia to prevent atelectasis, paralytic ileus, wound ***infection,*** and peritonitis (see Chapter 9). Document and report any signs and symptoms of these complications immediately to the surgeon.

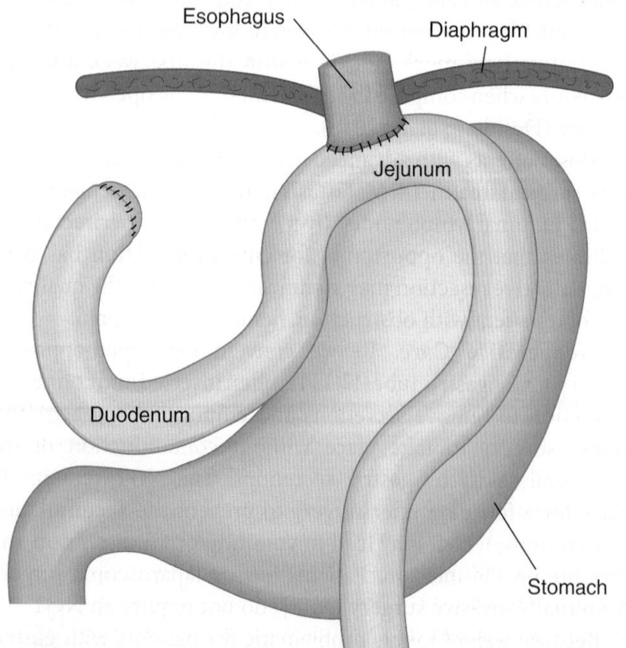

FIG. 50.3 Total gastrectomy with anastomosis of the esophagus to the jejunum (esophagojejunostomy) is the principal surgical intervention for extensive gastric cancer.

Auscultate the lungs for adventitious sounds (crackles or reduced breath sounds) and monitor for the return of bowel sounds. Take vital signs as appropriate to detect signs of infection or bleeding. Aggressive pulmonary exercises and early ambulation can help prevent respiratory complications and deep vein thrombosis. Also inspect the operative site every 8 to 12 hours for the presence of redness, swelling, or drainage, which indicate wound infection. Keep the head of the bed elevated to prevent aspiration from reflux.

Decreased patency caused by a clogged NGT can result in *acute gastric dilation* after surgery. This problem is characterized by epigastric pain and a feeling of fullness, hiccups, tachycardia, and hypotension. Notify the surgeon to obtain an order for irrigation or replacement of the NGT to relieve these symptoms.

Dumping syndrome is a term that refers to a group of vasomotor symptoms that occur after eating in patients who have had a gastrectomy. This syndrome is believed to occur as a result of the rapid emptying of food contents into the small intestine, which shifts fluid into the gut, causing abdominal distention. Observe for *early* manifestations of this syndrome, which typically occur within 30 minutes of eating. Symptoms include vertigo, tachycardia, syncope, sweating, pallor, palpitations, and the desire to lie down. Report these manifestations to the surgeon, and encourage the patient to lie down. Monitor the patient for late symptoms.

Late dumping syndrome, which occurs 90 minutes to 3 hours after eating, is caused by a release of an excessive amount of insulin. The insulin release follows a rapid rise in the blood glucose level that results from the rapid entry of high-carbohydrate food into the jejunum. Observe for manifestations, including dizziness, light-headedness, palpitations, diaphoresis, and confusion.

Dumping syndrome is managed by ***nutrition*** changes that include decreasing the amount of food taken at one time and eliminating liquids ingested with meals. In collaboration with the registered dietitian nutritionist, teach the patient to eat a high-protein, high-fat, low- to moderate-carbohydrate diet (Table 50.3). Acarbose may be used to decrease carbohydrate absorption. A somatostatin analog, octreotide, 50 mcg subcutaneously two or three times daily 30 minutes before meals, may be prescribed in severe cases. This drug decreases gastric and intestinal hormone secretion and slows stomach and intestinal transit time.

Delayed gastric emptying is often present after gastric surgery and usually resolves within 1 week. Edema at the anastomosis (surgical connection areas) or adhesions (scar tissue) obstructing the distal loop may cause mechanical blockage. Metabolic causes (e.g., hypokalemia, hypoproteinemia, or hyponatremia) should be considered. The edema usually resolves with nasogastric suction, maintenance of fluid and electrolyte balance, and proper ***nutrition.***

Several problems related to ***nutrition*** develop as a result of partial removal of the stomach, including deficiencies of vitamin B_{12}, folic acid, and iron; impaired calcium metabolism; and reduced absorption of calcium and vitamin D. These problems are caused by a reduction of intrinsic factor. The decrease results from the resection and from inadequate absorption because of rapid entry of food into the bowel. In the absence of intrinsic

TABLE 50.3 Diet for Dumping Syndrome

Food Group	Foods Allowed or Encouraged	Foods to Use With Caution	Foods That Must Be Excluded
Soups		Fluids 1 hr before and after meals	Spicy soups
Meat and meat substitutes	8 ounces or more per day: fish, poultry, beef, pork, veal, lamb, eggs, cheese, peanut butter		Spicy meats or meat substitutes
Potatoes	Potato, rice, pasta, starchy vegetables (small amount)		Highly spiced potatoes or potato substitutes
Bread and cereal	White bread, rolls, muffins, crackers, and cereals (small amount)	Whole-grain bread, rolls, crackers, and cereals	Breads with frosting or jelly, sweet rolls, and coffee cake
Vegetables	Two or more cooked vegetables	Gas-producing vegetables, such as cabbage, onions, broccoli, or raw vegetables	
Fruits	Limit three per day: unsweetened cooked or canned fruits	Unsweetened juice or fruit drinks 30-45 min after meals; fresh fruit	Sweetened fruit or juice
Beverages	Dietetic drinks	Limit to 1 hr after meals; caffeine-containing beverages, such as coffee, tea, and cola; if tolerated, diet carbonated beverages	Milk shakes, malts, and other sweet drinks; regular carbonated beverages and alcohol
Fats	Margarine, oils, shortening, butter, bacon, and salad dressings	Mayonnaise	Any milk products with fat
Desserts	Fruit (see Fruits)	Sugar-free gelatin, pudding, and custard	All sweets, cakes, pies, cookies, candy, ice cream, and sherbet
Seasonings and miscellaneous	Diet jelly, diet syrups, sugar substitutes	Excessive amounts of salt	Excessive amounts of spices, sugar, jelly, honey, syrup, or molasses

General Principles for Patients to Follow

- Several small meals daily
- Relatively high fat and protein content
- Low roughage
- Relatively low carbohydrate content
- No milk, sweets, or sugars
- Liquid between meals *only*

factor, signs and symptoms of pernicious anemia may occur. Assess for the development of atrophic glossitis secondary to vitamin B_{12} deficiency. In atrophic glossitis, the tongue takes on a shiny, smooth, and "beefy" appearance. The patient may also have signs of anemia secondary to folic acid and iron deficiency. Monitor the complete blood count (CBC) for signs of megaloblastic anemia (low red blood cell [RBC] level) and leukopenia (low white blood cell [WBC] level). These manifestations are corrected by the administration of vitamin B_{12}. The primary health care provider may also prescribe folic acid or iron preparations. Anemias are discussed elsewhere in this textbook.

Care Coordination and Transition Management. Patients who have undergone total gastrectomy and those who are debilitated with advanced gastric cancer are discharged to home with maximal assistance and support or to a transitional care unit or skilled nursing facility. Patients who have undergone subtotal gastrectomy and are not debilitated may be discharged to home with partial assistance for ADLs. Recurrence of cancer is common, and patients need regular follow-up examinations and imaging assessments. Collaborate with the case manager to ensure continuity of care and thorough follow-up with diagnostic testing.

Home Care Management. Gastric cancer is a life-threatening illness. Therefore the patient and family members require physical and emotional care. Assess their ability to cope with the disease and the possible need for end-of-life care. The adverse effects of gastric cancer treatment can be debilitating, and patients need to learn symptom-management strategies. Hospice programs can help both the patient and the family cope with these physical and emotional needs.

Patients may fear returning home because of their inability for self-management. Enlisting family and health care resources for the patient may ease some of this anxiety. Provide the family with adequate information about community support systems to make the transition to home care easier. If the prognosis is poor, they need continued professional support from case managers, social workers, and/or nurses to cope with death and dying. (See Chapter 8 for a discussion of end-of-life care.)

Self-Management Education. Educate the patient and family about any continuing needs, drug therapy, and nutrition therapy. If patients are discharged to home with surgical dressings, teach the patient and family how to change them. Review the manifestations of incisional infection (e.g., fever, redness, and drainage) that they should report to their surgeon.

Patients who will be receiving radiation therapy or chemotherapy require instructions related to the side effects of these treatments. Nausea and vomiting are common side effects of chemotherapy, and instruction in the use of prescribed antiemetics may be needed. (See Chapter 20 for health teaching for patients receiving chemotherapy or radiation therapy.)

In collaboration with the registered dietitian nutritionist, teach the patient and family about the type and quantity of foods that will provide optimal nutritional value. Interventions to minimize dumping syndrome and decrease gastric stimulants are also emphasized (see Table 50.3). Remind the patient to:

- Eat small, frequent meals
- Avoid drinking liquids with meals
- Avoid foods that cause discomfort
- Eliminate caffeine and alcohol consumption
- Begin a smoking-cessation program, if needed
- Receive B_{12} injections, as prescribed
- Lie flat for a short time after eating

Health Care Resources. A home care referral provides continued assessment, assistance, and encouragement to the patient and family. A home care nurse can help with care procedures and provide valuable psychological support. Additional referrals to a registered dietitian nutritionist, professional counselor, or clergy/spiritual leader may be necessary. Referral to a hospice agency can be of great assistance for the patient with advanced disease. Hospice care may be delivered in the home or in an institutional setting. Appropriate support groups (e.g., I Can Cope, provided by the American Cancer Society [http://www.cancer.org/treatment/index]) can be a major resource.

NCLEX EXAMINATION CHALLENGE 50.2

Psychosocial Integrity

Which client statement regarding diet and nutrition after a total gastrectomy requires **further teaching** by the nurse?

A. "I should stay sitting up for an hour after I eat."
B. "I will avoid liquids with my meals."
C. "I need to eat small frequent meals."
D. "I need to stay away from concentrated sweets."

GET READY FOR THE NEXT-GENERATION NCLEX® EXAMINATION!

Key Points

Review these Key Points for each NCLEX Examination Client Needs Category.

Safe and Effective Care Environment

- When caring for patients with gastric health problems, collaborate with the members of the interprofessional team, including the pharmacist, registered dietitian nutritionist, health care provider, and/or case manager. **QSEN: Teamwork and Collaboration**

Health Promotion and Maintenance

- Refer the patient with gastric cancer to the American Cancer Society. **QSEN: Patient-Centered Care**
- Identify patients at risk for gastritis and PUD, especially those with *H. pylori* and older adults who take large amounts of NSAIDs. **QSEN: Safety**
- Teach adults to prevent PUD by avoiding excess consumption of caffeine, alcohol, coffee, aspirin, NSAIDs, and contaminated food and water and by avoiding smoking. **QSEN: Evidence-Based Practice**
- Teach patients the importance of adhering to *H. pylori* treatment to prevent development of gastric cancer. **QSEN: Evidence-Based Practice**

Psychosocial Integrity

- Allow patients with gastric cancer to express feelings of grief, fear, and anxiety. **QSEN: Patient-Centered Care**
- For patients with advanced gastric cancer, identify end-of-life care needs, including referral to hospice care. **Ethics**

Physiological Integrity

- Recall that *acute* gastritis causes a rapid onset of epigastric pain and dyspepsia; *chronic* gastritis causes vague epigastric pain (usually relieved with food) and intolerance to fatty and spicy foods. **QSEN: Patient-Centered Care**
- Remember that patients with gastric ulcers may be malnourished and have pain that is worsened by ingestion of food; patients with duodenal ulcers are usually well nourished, have pain that is relieved by ingestion of food, and awaken with pain during the night. **QSEN: Patient-Centered Care**
- For patients who have undergone a gastrectomy, collaborate with the registered dietitian nutritionist and instruct the patient regarding diet changes to avoid abdominal distention and dumping syndrome. **QSEN: Teamwork and Collaboration**
- Teach patients with abnormal abdominal symptoms to consult with their health care provider immediately. **QSEN: Safety**
- Teach that hematemesis is a medical emergency and refer to the emergency department for prompt treatment. **QSEN: Safety**
- Teach the proper administration of antacids (one or two after meals), reminding patients that antacids can interfere with the effectiveness of certain drugs, such as phenytoin (Dilantin). **QSEN: Evidence-Based Practice**
- Teach the proper administration of H_2 antagonists and explain that they should be taken at bedtime (see the Common Examples of Drug Therapy: Gastritis and Peptic Ulcer Disease box.). **QSEN: Evidence-Based Practice**
- Teach the proper administration of antisecretory agents, noting that most cannot be crushed because they are sustained-release or enteric-coated tablets. **QSEN: Evidence-Based Practice**
- Monitor patients with ulcers for signs and symptoms of upper GI bleeding, such as hematemesis, melena, and low blood pressure. Report any of these symptoms to the primary health care provider immediately. **QSEN: Safety; Clinical Judgment**
- After EGD, monitor vital signs, heart rhythm, and oxygen saturation frequently until they return to baseline. To prevent aspiration, assess the gag reflex and ensure that it is intact before giving the patient food or fluids. **QSEN: Safety; Clinical Judgment**
- Observe for signs and symptoms of dumping syndrome after gastric surgery; teach characteristics and management of this syndrome. **QSEN: Evidence-Based Practice**

MASTERY QUESTIONS

1. The primary health care provider prescribes bismuth subsalicylate for a client as part of treating *H. pylori* infection. What health teaching will the nurse include for the client about this drug?
   A. "Do not crush this drug before taking."
   B. "The drug may cause your tongue and stool to turn black."
   C. "Take the drug at night only."
   D. "The drug may cause you to have diarrhea."

2. What health teaching will the nurse include to promote gastric health for an adult client? **Select all that apply.**
   A. "Stop smoking or using tobacco of any form."
   B. "Do not drink excessive amounts of alcohol."
   C. "Consume high-fat foods and decrease carbohydrates."
   D. "Avoid excessive amounts of pickled or smoked food."
   E. "Avoid taking large amounts of NSAIDs."

REFERENCES

American Cancer Society. (2020). *Stomach cancer.* http://www.cancer.org/cancer/stomachcancer/detailedguide/stomach-cancer-key-statistics.

Ankita, C., Nehal, G., Komal, K., Lambole, V., & Shah, D. P. (2017). A review: Peptic ulcer disease. *Pharma Science Monitor: An International Journal of Pharmaceutical Sciences, 8*(2), 210–218.

Benmassaoud, A., McDonald, E. G., & Lee, T. C. (2016). Potential harms of proton pump inhibitor therapy: Rare adverse effects of commonly used drugs. *Canadian Medical Association Journal, 188*(9), 657–662.

Burchum, J. L. R., & Rosenthal, L. D. (2019). *Lehne's pharmacology for nursing care* (10th ed.). St. Louis: Elsevier.

Desiderio, J., Stewart, C. L., Sun, V., Melstrom, L., Warner, S., Lee, B., et al. (2018). Enhanced recovery after surgery for gastric cancer improves clinical outcomes at a U.S. cancer center. *Journal of Gastric Cancer, 18*(3), 230–241.

Farrar, F. C. (2018). Management of acute gastrointestinal bleeding. *Critical Care Nursing Clinics of North America, 30*(1), 55–66.

McCance, K., Huether, S., Brashers, V., & Rote, N. (2019). *Pathophysiology: The biologic basis for disease in adults and children* (8th ed.). St. Louis: Mosby.

National Institute of Diabetes and Digestive and Kidney Diseases. (2020). *Definitions and facts for peptic ulcers (stomach ulcers).* https://www.niddk.nih.gov/health-information/health-topics/digestive-diseases/peptic-ulcer/pages/definition-facts.aspx.

Pagana, K. D., & Pagana, T. J. (2018). *Manual of diagnostic and laboratory tests* (6th ed.). St. Louis: Mosby.

Pagana, K. D., Pagana, T. J., & Pike-MacDonald, S. A. (2019). *Mosby's Canadian manual of diagnostic and laboratory tests* (2nd ed.). Toronto, ON: Elsevier.

Priyanka, C., Jenish, R., Gajera, V., Lambole, V., & Shah, D. P. (2016). Peptic ulcer: A review on epidemiology, etiology, pathogenesis and management strategies. *Pharma Science Monitor: An International Journal of Pharmaceutical Sciences, 7*(2), 139–147.

51

Concepts of Care for Patients With Noninflammatory Intestinal Disorders

Keelin Cromar

http://evolve.elsevier.com/Iggy/

LEARNING OUTCOMES

1. Collaborate with the interprofessional team to manage quality care for patients with impaired ***elimination*** caused by noninflammatory bowel disorders.
2. Identify community resources for families and patients recovering from noninflammatory bowel disorders.
3. Apply knowledge of pathophysiology of noninflammatory bowel disorders to identify common assessment findings, including actual or risk for impaired ***nutrition*** and ***fluid and electrolyte balance.***
4. Prioritize evidence-based nursing interventions for patients with noninflammatory bowel disorders to promote ***nutrition,*** maintain ***fluid and electrolyte balance,*** and manage ***pain.***
5. Plan transition management and care coordination for the patient who has a colostomy, including health teaching.

KEY TERMS

abdominoperineal (AP) resection Surgical removal of the sigmoid colon, rectum, and anus through combined abdominal and perineal incisions.

borborygmi High-pitched bowel sounds that are proximal (above) an obstruction.

colectomy Surgical removal of the entire colon.

colon resection Surgical removal of part of the colon and regional lymph nodes.

colostomy The surgical creation of an opening of the colon (stoma) onto the surface of the abdomen to allow passage of stool.

exploratory laparotomy A surgical opening of the abdominal cavity.

fecal occult blood test [FOBT] A laboratory test to determine the presence of occult (microscopic) blood in the stool.

flatulence Excessive gas (flatus) in the intestines.

hemorrhoidectomy Surgical removal of hemorrhoids.

hemorrhoids Unnaturally swollen or distended veins in the anorectal region.

hernia A weakness in the abdominal muscle wall through which a segment of the bowel or other abdominal structure protrudes.

hernioplasty A surgical hernia repair procedure performed to reinforce the weakened outside abdominal muscle wall with a mesh patch.

herniorrhaphy Surgical repair of a hernia.

intussusception Telescoping of a segment of the intestine within itself.

irreducible (incarcerated) hernia A hernia that cannot be reduced or placed back into the abdominal cavity. Any hernia that is not reducible requires immediate surgical evaluation.

irritable bowel syndrome A functional GI disorder that causes chronic or recurrent diarrhea, constipation, and/or abdominal pain and bloating.

mechanical obstruction A condition in which the bowel is physically blocked by problems outside the intestine (e.g., adhesions), in the bowel wall (e.g., Crohn's disease), or in the intestinal lumen (e.g., tumors).

minimally invasive inguinal hernia repair (MIIHR) Surgical hernia repair through a laparoscope.

nonmechanical obstruction A condition in which peristalsis is decreased or absent because of neuromuscular disturbance, resulting in a slowing of the movement or a backup of intestinal contents; also known as *paralytic ileus.*

obstipation No passage of stool.

polyps In the intestinal tract, small growths covered with mucosa and attached to the surface of the intestine; although most are benign, they are significant because some have the potential to become malignant.

reducible hernia A hernia that can be reduced or placed back into the abdominal cavity.

strangulated obstruction Bowel obstruction or hernia that has compromised blood flow (can be life-threatening).

volvulus Twisting of the intestine.

PRIORITY AND INTERRELATED CONCEPTS

The priority concept for this chapter is:

- ***Elimination***

The ***Elimination*** concept exemplar for this chapter is Intestinal Obstruction.

The interrelated concepts for this chapter are:

- ***Nutrition***
- ***Pain***
- ***Fluid and Electrolyte Balance***

If not diagnosed and managed early, some intestinal problems can lead to inadequate absorption of vital nutrients and affect ***nutrition*** and ***elimination.*** If these disorders become severe or progress, ***pain*** and problems with ***fluid and electrolyte balance*** may occur. Chapter 3 briefly reviews each of these health concepts. Intestinal health problems may be classified as inflammatory or noninflammatory; this chapter focuses on disorders that are noninflammatory in origin.

ELIMINATION CONCEPT EXEMPLAR: INTESTINAL OBSTRUCTION

Pathophysiology Review

Intestinal obstructions can be partial or complete and are classified as mechanical or nonmechanical. With either condition, ***elimination*** is compromised by this common and serious disorder.

Types of Intestinal Obstructions. In **mechanical obstruction**, the bowel is physically blocked by problems outside the intestine (e.g., adhesions), in the bowel wall (e.g., Crohn's disease), or in the intestinal lumen (e.g., tumors). **Nonmechanical obstruction** (also known as paralytic ileus or *functional obstruction*) does not involve a physical obstruction in or outside the intestine. Instead, peristalsis is decreased or absent because of neuromuscular disturbance, resulting in a slowing of the movement or a backup of intestinal contents (McCance et al., 2019).

Intestinal contents are composed of ingested fluid, food, and saliva; gastric, pancreatic, and biliary secretions; digestive enzymes; and swallowed air. In both mechanical and nonmechanical obstructions, the intestinal contents accumulate at and above the area of obstruction. Abdominal distention results from the intestine's inability to absorb the contents and move the waste down through the intestinal tract. To compensate for the delay, peristalsis increases in an effort to move the intestinal contents forward. This increase stimulates more secretions, which then leads to additional distention. The bowel then becomes edematous and increased capillary permeability results. Plasma leaking into the peritoneal cavity and fluid trapped in the intestinal lumen decrease the absorption of fluid and electrolytes into the vascular space. Reduced circulatory blood volume (hypovolemia) and electrolyte imbalances typically occur. Hypovolemia ranges from mild to extreme (hypovolemic shock).

Complications of Intestinal Obstruction. Specific problems related to ***fluid and electrolyte balance*** and acid-base balance result, depending on the part of the intestine that is blocked. An obstruction high in the small intestine causes a loss of gastric hydrochloric acid, which can lead to *metabolic alkalosis.* Obstruction below the duodenum but above the large bowel results in a loss of both acids and bases, so acid-base balance is usually not compromised. Obstruction at the end of the small intestine and lower in the intestinal tract causes loss of alkaline fluids, which can lead to *metabolic acidosis* (McCance et al., 2019).

If hypovolemia is severe, acute kidney injury or even death can occur. Bacterial peritonitis with or without actual perforation can also result. Bacteria in the intestinal contents lie stagnant in the obstructed intestine. This is not a problem unless the blood flow to the intestine is compromised. However, with *closed-loop obstruction* (blockage in two different areas) or a **strangulated obstruction** (obstruction with compromised blood flow that can be life threatening), the risk for peritonitis (infection) is greatly increased. Bacteria without blood supply can form and release endotoxins into the peritoneal or systemic circulation and cause septic shock. The same process occurs when gangrene results from intestinal ischemia caused by mesenteric arterial occlusion.

With a strangulated obstruction, major blood loss into the intestine and the peritoneum can occur. Sepsis and bleeding can result in an increased intra-abdominal pressure (IAP) or acute compartment syndrome.

Etiology. Intestinal obstruction is caused by a variety of conditions and is associated with significant morbidity. It can occur anywhere in the intestinal tract, although the ileum in the small intestine (the narrowest part of the intestinal tract) is the most common site.

Mechanical obstruction can result from:

- Adhesions (scar tissue from surgeries or pathology)
- Benign or malignant tumor
- Complications of appendicitis
- Hernias
- Fecal impactions (especially in older adults)
- Strictures due to Crohn's disease (a chronic inflammatory bowel disease) or previous radiation therapy
- **Intussusception** (telescoping of a segment of the intestine within itself) (Fig. 51.1)
- **Volvulus** (twisting of the intestine) (see Fig. 51.1)
- Fibrosis due to disorders such as endometriosis

In people ages 60 years or older, diverticulitis, tumors, and fecal impaction are the most common causes of obstruction (McCance et al., 2019).

Postoperative ileus (POI) (paralytic ileus), or *nonmechanical* obstruction, is most commonly caused by handling of the intestines during abdominal surgery. In patients with POI, intestinal function is lost for a few hours to several days. Electrolyte disturbances, especially hypokalemia, predispose the patient to this problem. The ileus can also be a consequence of peritonitis because leakage of colonic contents causes severe irritation and triggers an inflammatory response and infection (see Peritonitis in Chapter 52). Vascular insufficiency to the bowel, also referred to as *intestinal ischemia,* is another potential cause of an ileus.

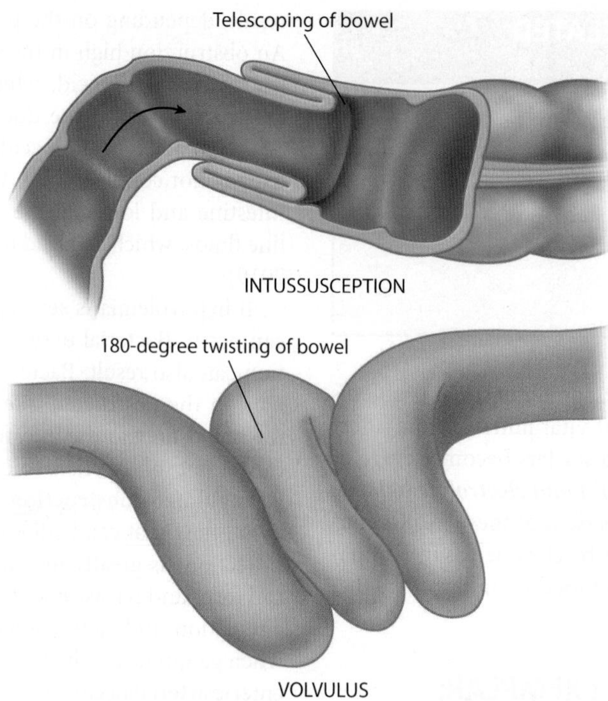

Fig. 51.1 Two major types of mechanical obstruction.

It results when arterial or venous thrombosis or an embolus decreases blood flow to or in the mesenteric blood vessels surrounding the intestines. Severe insufficiency of blood supply can result in infarction of surrounding organs (e.g., bowel infarction), gangrene, and eventually sepsis and septic shock.

Incidence and Prevalence. Because there are many causes of intestinal obstruction, the incidence and prevalence is not well known. However, it occurs much more commonly in patients who have had bowel surgery and those with intestinal tumors. Older adults are the most likely group to have a bowel obstruction.

❖ Interprofessional Collaborative Care

Care for the patient with an intestinal obstruction takes place in the hospital setting. The interprofessional team that primarily collaborates to care for this patient generally includes the primary health care provider, nurse, and registered dietitian nutritionist.

◆ Assessment: Recognize Cues

History. Collect information about a history of GI disorders, surgeries, and treatments. Question the patient about recent nausea and vomiting and the color of emesis, noting if vomitus is described as greenish-yellow, bilious, or hematemesis. Perform a thorough pain assessment with particular attention to the onset, aggravating factors, alleviating factors, and patterns or rhythms of the ***pain.*** Severe pain that then stops and changes to tenderness on palpation may indicate perforation; this finding should be reported promptly to the primary health care provider. Ask about ***elimination*** patterns, including the passage of flatus and the time, character, and consistency of the last bowel movement. Singultus (hiccups) is common with all types of intestinal obstruction. When an obstruction is suspected, keep the patient NPO and contact the primary health care provider promptly for further direction.

Assess for a family history of colorectal cancer (CRC) and ask about blood in the stool or a change in bowel pattern. Body temperature with uncomplicated obstruction is rarely higher than 100°F (37.8°C). A temperature higher than this, with or without guarding and tenderness, and a sustained elevation in pulse could indicate a strangulated obstruction, peritonitis, or intestinal ischemia. A fever, tachycardia, hypotension, increasing abdominal pain, abdominal rigidity, or change in color of skin overlying the abdomen should be reported to the health primary health care provider immediately.

Physical Assessment/Signs and Symptoms. The patient with *mechanical* obstruction in the *small intestine* often has mid-abdominal ***pain*** or cramping. The pain can be sporadic, and the patient may feel comfortable between episodes. If strangulation is present, the pain becomes more localized and steady. Vomiting often accompanies obstruction and is more profuse with obstructions in the proximal small intestine. The vomitus may contain bile and mucus or be orange-brown and foul smelling because of bacterial overgrowth with low ileal obstruction. Prolonged vomiting can result in a disruption in ***fluid and electrolyte balance.*** Obstipation (no passage of stool) and failure to pass flatus are associated with complete obstruction; diarrhea may be present in partial obstruction.

Mechanical colonic obstruction causes a milder, more intermittent colicky abdominal ***pain*** than is seen with small-bowel obstruction. Lower abdominal distention and obstipation may be present, or the patient may have ribbon-like stools if obstruction is partial. Alterations in bowel patterns and blood in the stools may accompany the obstruction if colorectal cancer or diverticulitis is the cause.

KEY FEATURES

Small-Bowel and Large-Bowel Obstructions

Small-Bowel Obstructions	Large-Bowel Obstructions
Abdominal discomfort or pain possibly accompanied by visible peristaltic waves in upper and middle abdomen	Intermittent lower abdominal cramping
Upper or epigastric abdominal distention	Lower abdominal distention
Nausea and early, profuse vomiting (may contain fecal material)	Minimal or no vomiting
Obstipation	Obstipation or ribbon-like stools
Severe fluid and electrolyte imbalances	No major fluid and electrolyte imbalances
Metabolic alkalosis (not always present)	Metabolic acidosis (not always present)

On examination of the abdomen, observe for abdominal distention, which is common in all forms of intestinal obstruction. Peristaltic waves may also be visible. Auscultate for proximal (above the obstruction) high-pitched bowel sounds (**borborygmi**), which are associated with cramping early in the obstructive process as the intestine tries to push the mechanical obstruction forward. In later stages of mechanical obstruction, bowel sounds are absent, especially distal to the obstruction. Abdominal tenderness and rigidity are usually minimal. The presence of a tense, fluid-filled bowel loop mimicking a palpable abdominal mass may signal a closed-loop, strangulating small-bowel obstruction.

In most types of *nonmechanical* obstruction, the pain is described as a constant, diffuse discomfort. Colicky cramping is not characteristic of this type of obstruction. ***Pain*** associated with obstruction caused by vascular insufficiency or infarction is usually severe and constant. On inspection, abdominal distention is typically present. On auscultation of the abdomen, note and document decreased bowel sounds in early obstruction and absent bowel sounds in later stages. Vomiting of gastric contents and bile is frequent, but the vomitus rarely has a foul odor and is rarely profuse. Obstipation may or may not be present. A comparison of small- and large-bowel obstructions is outlined in the Key Features: Small-Bowel and Large-Bowel Obstructions box.

Laboratory Assessment. There is no definitive laboratory test to confirm a diagnosis of mechanical or nonmechanical obstruction. *White blood cell (WBC) counts* are normal unless there is a strangulated obstruction, infarction, and/or gangrene. *Hemoglobin, hematocrit,* and *blood urea nitrogen (BUN)* values are often elevated, indicating dehydration. Serum sodium, chloride, and potassium are decreased. Elevations in serum amylase levels may occur with strangulating obstructions, which can damage the pancreas (Pagana & Pagana, 2018).

Other Diagnostic Assessment. The primary health care provider obtains imaging information from an *abdominal CT scan* or MRI as soon as an obstruction is suspected. Distention with fluid and gas in the small intestine with the absence of gas in the colon indicates an obstruction in the small intestine.

The diagnostic examination chosen depends on the suspected location of the obstruction. As an initial assessment, the primary health care provider may request an *abdominal ultrasound* to evaluate the potential cause of the obstruction. An endoscopy (sigmoidoscopy or colonoscopy) may also be performed to determine the cause of the obstruction, except when perforation or complete obstruction is suspected.

◆ **Analysis: Analyze Cues and Prioritize Hypotheses.** The priority collaborative problem for patients with intestinal obstruction is *Potential for life-threatening complications due to reduced flow or blocked flow of intestinal contents.*

◆ **Planning and Implementation: Generate Solutions and Take Action.** Interventions are aimed at uncovering the cause and relieving the obstruction. Relieving the obstruction decreases the potential for medical complications and reduces ***pain.*** Intestinal obstructions can be relieved by nonsurgical or surgical means.

Reducing the Risk of Life-Threatening Complications

Planning: Expected Outcomes. The expected outcome is that the patient's obstruction will resolve to restore normal bowel ***elimination,*** prevent potentially life-threatening complications, and relieve ***pain.***

Interventions. Collaborative and nursing interventions depend on the location, cause, type, and severity of the bowel obstruction. Therefore a nonsurgical or surgical approach may be used.

Nonsurgical Management. If the obstruction is partial and there is no evidence of strangulation or ischemia, nonsurgical management may be the treatment of choice, as summarized in the Best Practice for Patient Safety & Quality Care: Nursing Care of Patients Who Have an Intestinal Obstruction box. Once the obstruction has been addressed effectively, ***elimination*** patterns are expected to resume.

BEST PRACTICE FOR PATIENT SAFETY & QUALITY CARE (QSEN)

Nursing Care of Patients Who Have an Intestinal Obstruction

- Monitor vital signs, especially blood pressure and pulse, for indications of fluid balance.
- Assess the patient's abdomen at least twice a day for bowel sounds, distention, and passage of flatus.
- Monitor ***fluid and electrolyte balance*** status, including laboratory values.
- Manage the patient who has a nasogastric tube (NGT):
  - Monitor drainage.
  - Ensure tube patency.
  - Check tube placement.
  - Irrigate tube as prescribed.
  - Maintain the patient on NPO status.
  - Provide frequent mouth and nares care.
  - Maintain the patient in a semi-Fowler position.
- Give analgesics for ***pain*** as prescribed.
- Maintain IV therapy for fluid and electrolyte replacement.
- Give alvimopan as prescribed for patients with a postoperative ileus.
- Maintain parenteral ***nutrition*** if prescribed.

Paralytic ileus responds very well to nonsurgical methods of relieving obstruction. Nonsurgical approaches are also preferred in the treatment of patients with terminal disease associated with bowel obstruction. In addition to being NPO, patients typically have a nasogastric tube (NGT) inserted to decompress the bowel by draining fluid and air. The tube is attached to suction.

Nasogastric tubes. Most patients with an obstruction have an NGT unless the obstruction is mild. A Salem sump tube is inserted through the nose and placed into the stomach. It is attached to low *continuous* suction. This tube has a vent ("pigtail") that prevents the stomach mucosa from being pulled away during suctioning. Levin tubes do not have a vent and therefore should be connected only to low *intermittent* suction. They are used far less often than the Salem sump tubes.

! NURSING SAFETY PRIORITY (QSEN)

Action Alert

At least every 4 hours, assess the patient with an NGT for proper placement of the tube, tube patency, and output (quality and quantity). Monitor the nasal skin around the tube for irritation. Use an approved device that secures the tube to the nose to prevent accidental removal. Assess for peristalsis by auscultating for bowel sounds with the suction disconnected (suction masks peristaltic sounds).

Monitor any NGT for proper functioning. Occasionally, NGTs move out of optimal drainage position or become plugged. In this case, note a decrease in gastric output or stasis of the tube's contents. Assess the patient for nausea, vomiting, increased abdominal distention, and placement of the tube. If the NGT is repositioned or replaced, confirmation of proper placement may be obtained by x-ray before use. After appropriate placement is established, aspirate the contents and irrigate the tube with 30 mL of normal saline every 4 hours or as requested by the primary health care provider.

Other nonsurgical interventions. Most types of nonmechanical obstruction respond to nasogastric decompression with medical treatment of the primary disorder. Incomplete mechanical obstruction can sometimes be treated successfully without surgery. Obstruction caused by lower fecal impaction usually resolves after disimpaction and enema administration. Intussusception may respond to hydrostatic pressure changes during a barium enema.

For patients with a postoperative ileus (POI), alvimopan may be given for short-term use. This drug is an oral, peripherally acting mu opioid receptor antagonist that increases GI motility (Al-Mazrou et al., 2017).

IV fluid replacement and maintenance are indicated for all patients with intestinal obstruction because the patient is NPO and ***fluid and electrolyte balance*** is altered (particularly potassium and sodium) as a result of vomiting and nasogastric suction. On the basis of serum electrolytes and blood urea nitrogen (BUN) levels, the primary health care provider prescribes aggressive fluid replacement with 2 to 4 L of an isotonic solution (normal saline or lactated Ringer's solution) with potassium added. Use care with patients who are susceptible to fluid overload (e.g., older adults with a history of heart or chronic kidney disease). Monitor lung sounds, weight, and intake and output daily. *Weight is the most reliable indicator of fluid balance!* Blood replacement may be indicated in strangulated obstruction because of blood loss into the bowel or peritoneal cavity.

Monitor vital signs and other measures of fluid status (e.g., urine output, skin turgor, mucous membranes) every 2 to 4 hours, depending on the severity of the patient's symptoms. In collaboration with the registered dietitian nutritionist, the primary health care provider may prescribe parenteral ***nutrition*** (PN), especially if the patient has had chronic nutritional problems and has been NPO for an extended period. Chapter 55 discusses the nursing care of patients receiving PN.

The patient with intestinal obstruction is usually thirsty, although some older adults have a decreased thirst response. Remind assistive personnel (AP) to provide frequent mouth care to help maintain moist mucous membranes. A few ice chips may be allowed if the patient is not having surgery. Follow agency protocol or the primary health care provider's request regarding ice chips.

Abdominal distention can cause severe ***pain.*** The colicky, crampy pain that comes and goes with mechanical obstruction, as well as the nausea, vomiting, dry mucous membranes, and thirst, contribute to the patient's discomfort. Continually assess the character and location of the pain and immediately report any ***pain*** that significantly increases or changes from colicky and intermittent to a constant discomfort. These changes can indicate perforation of the intestine or peritonitis.

Analgesics may be temporarily withheld in the diagnostic workup period so that signs and symptoms of perforation or peritonitis are not masked. Explain to the patient and family the rationale for not giving analgesics. In addition, if analgesics such as morphine are given, they may slow intestinal motility and can cause vomiting. Be alert to this side effect because nausea and vomiting are also signs of NGT obstruction or worsening bowel obstruction. Consider the importance of nonpharmacologic pain control measures when withdrawing this type of medication (see Chapter 5 for detailed description of pain management).

Help the patient achieve a position of comfort, with frequent position changes to promote increased peristalsis. A semi-Fowler position helps alleviate the pressure of abdominal distention on the chest and promotes thoracic excursion to facilitate breathing.

Pain is generally less with nonmechanical obstruction than with mechanical obstruction. With both types of obstruction, food or oral fluids aggravate the GI tract and increase pain (McCance et al., 2019).

If strangulation is thought to be likely, the primary health care provider prescribes IV broad-spectrum antibiotics. In addition, in cases of partial obstruction or paralytic ileus, drugs that enhance gastric motility (prokinetic agents) such as metoclopramide may be used.

Surgical Management. In patients with complete mechanical obstruction and in some cases of incomplete mechanical obstruction, surgical intervention is necessary to relieve the obstruction. A strangulated obstruction is complete, and surgical intervention is always required. If surgery is needed, an exploratory laparotomy (a surgical opening of the abdominal cavity) to investigate the cause of the obstruction is performed. More specific surgical procedures depend on the cause of the obstruction.

Provide general preoperative teaching for both the patient and family as discussed in Chapter 9. In cases of complete obstruction, the patient may feel too ill to understand the information. In this case, reinforce the information with the family or other caregiver. Depending on the cause and severity of the obstruction and the expertise of the surgeon, patients have either minimally invasive surgery (MIS) via laparoscopy or a conventional open approach.

In the *conventional open surgical approach,* the surgeon makes a large incision, enters the abdominal cavity, and explores for obstruction and its cause, if possible (exploratory laparotomy). If adhesions are found, they are lysed (cut and released). Obstruction caused by a tumor or diverticulitis requires a colon resection with primary anastomosis or a temporary or permanent colostomy. If obstruction is caused by intestinal infarction, an embolectomy, thrombectomy, or resection of the gangrenous small or large bowel may be necessary. In severe cases a colectomy (surgical removal of the entire colon) may be needed.

Most patients today have laparoscopic surgery (MIS) for mechanical intestinal obstructions and do *not* have an NGT. For the *MIS* approach, the specially trained surgeon makes several small incisions in the abdomen and places a video camera to view the abdominal contents to determine the extent of the obstruction. This procedure takes longer than the open approach, but blood loss is less, and healing is faster. Robotic assistance may be used, depending on the experience of the surgeon and available equipment.

General postoperative care for the patient undergoing an *exploratory laparotomy* is similar to that described in Chapter 9. In addition, patients who had an open surgical approach have an NGT in place until peristalsis resumes. A clear liquid diet may be prescribed to encourage return of peristalsis. As liquids are started, the NGT can be disconnected from suction and capped for 1 to 2 hours after the patient has taken clear liquids to determine if he or she is able to tolerate them. If the patient vomits after liquids, the suction is resumed. When the patient has return of peristalsis, the NGT suction is discontinued, and the tube is clamped for a scheduled amount of time. If the patient does *not* experience nausea while the NGT is clamped, the tube is removed.

The hospital stay for a patient having MIS to remove tumors, adhesions, and other obstructions may be as short as 1 to 2 days compared with 3 days or longer for the patients undergoing the conventional open surgical approach. Recovery is much quicker because there is less ***pain*** and there are fewer postoperative complications among those who had laparoscopic surgery.

Care Coordination and Transition Management. All patients with intestinal obstruction are hospitalized for monitoring and treatment. The length of stay varies according to the type of obstruction, the treatment, and the presence of complications. Patients who have complicated obstruction, such as strangulation or incarceration, are at greater risk for peritonitis, sepsis, and shock.

Patients with nonmechanical (functional) intestinal obstruction are less likely to require a lengthy hospitalization because of the obstruction alone. Nonmechanical obstruction generally responds to nasogastric suction and possible drug therapy within a few days. However, if an ileus occurs as a complication of an abdominal surgery, the hospital stay could be lengthy.

Home Care Management. Preparation for home care depends on the cause of the obstruction and the treatment

CLINICAL JUDGMENT CHALLENGE 51.1

Patient-Centered Care; Teamwork and Collaboration; Informatics

A 45-year-old woman is transferred to a medical-surgical unit after having been admitted from the emergency department for a bowel obstruction. She has a history of Crohn's disease and a bowel resection for this disease. When the client arrives, she has a Salem sump nasogastric tube (NGT) in place that is attached to NGT suction and draining greenish drainage. She also has IV normal saline running at 150 mL/hr. The client's vital signs are stable, except for her blood pressure, which remains low at 95/50 mm Hg. She reports a pain score of 5/10 in her upper abdomen.

Additional nursing assessment data include:

- Abdominal distention present
- Reports mild nausea
- No bowel sounds in lower quadrants
- Distant bowel sounds in upper quadrants
- Apical pulse = 96 beats/min
- Oxygen saturation = 95% (on room air)

Lab results include:

- Serum sodium = 129 mEq/L (129 mmol/L)
- Serum chloride – 92 mEq/L (92 mmol/L)
- Serum potassium = 3.3 mEq/L (3.3 mmol/L)

1. **Recognize Cues:** What assessment information in this client situation is the most important and immediate concern for the nurse? (Hint: Identify the **relevant** information *first* to determine what is most important.)
2. **Analyze Cues:** What client conditions are consistent with the **most relevant** information? (Hint: Think about priority collaborative problems that support and contradict the information presented in this situation.)
3. **Prioritize Hypotheses:** Which possibilities or explanations are **most likely** to be present in this client situation? Which possibilities or explanations are the most serious? (Hint: Consider all possibilities and determine their urgency and risk for this client.)
4. **Generate Solutions:** What actions would most likely achieve the desired outcomes for this client? Which actions should be **avoided** or are **potentially harmful**? (Hint: Determine the desired outcomes first to decide which interventions are appropriate and those that should be avoided.)
5. **Take Action:** Which actions are the most appropriate and how should they be implemented? In what **priority order** should they be implemented? (Hint: Consider health teaching, documentation, requested health care provider orders or prescriptions, nursing skills, collaboration with or referral to health team members, etc.)
6. **Evaluate Outcomes:** What client assessment would indicate that the nurse's actions were **effective**? (Hint: Think about signs that would indicate an improvement, decline, or unchanged client condition.)

required. Those who have resolution of obstruction without surgical intervention are assessed for their knowledge of strategies to avoid recurrent obstruction. For example, if fecal impaction in an older adult was the cause of the obstruction, assess the patient's ability to carry out a bowel regimen independently (see the Patient-Centered Care: Older Adult Considerations box).

PATIENT-CENTERED CARE: OLDER ADULT CONSIDERATIONS (QSEN)

Preventing Fecal Impaction

- Teach the patient to eat high-fiber foods, including plenty of raw fruits and vegetables and whole-grain products.
- Encourage the patient to drink adequate amounts of fluids, especially water.
- Do not routinely take a laxative; teach the patient that laxative abuse decreases abdominal muscle tone and contributes to an atonic colon.
- Encourage the patient to exercise regularly, if possible. Walking every day is an excellent exercise for promoting intestinal motility.
- Use natural foods to stimulate peristalsis, such as warm beverages and prune juice.
- Take bulk-forming products to provide fiber and stool softeners to ease bowel *elimination.*

For those who have had surgery, evaluate their ability to function at home with the added tasks of incision care and possibly colostomy care (see later discussion of colostomy care in the Colorectal Cancer section).

Self-Management Education. Instruct the patient to report any abdominal ***pain*** or distention, nausea, or vomiting, with or without constipation, because these symptoms might indicate recurrent obstruction. However, the patient should be reassured that recurrent paralytic ileus is not common.

Teach the patient who has had surgery about incision care, drug therapy, and activity limitations. Drug therapy consists of an oral opioid analgesic, such as oxycodone hydrochloride with acetaminophen, to be taken as needed for incisional discomfort. As with any opioid therapy, an over-the-counter laxative with a softener (e.g., docusate with senna) may be added to prevent constipation and possible recurrent obstruction.

Health Care Resources. The need for follow-up appointments depends on the cause of the obstruction and the treatment required. In collaboration with the case manager, make arrangements for a home care nurse if the patient needs help with incision or colostomy care, discussed later in this chapter.

◆ **Evaluation: Evaluate Outcomes.** Evaluate the care of the patient with intestinal obstruction based on the identified priority patient problems. The expected outcomes are that the patient will:

- Have relief from the obstruction and no evidence of life-threatening complications.
- Report that he or she has returned to having usual bowel ***elimination.***

COLORECTAL CANCER

Pathophysiology Review

Colorectal refers to the colon and rectum, which together make up the large intestine, also known as the *large bowel.* Colorectal cancer (CRC) is cancer of the colon or rectum. In the United States, it is the third most common malignancy among adults (American Cancer Society [ACS], 2019a). Patients often consider a diagnosis of cancer as a "death sentence," but colon cancer is highly curable for many patients, especially if diagnosed early.

Tumors occur in different areas of the colon, with about two-thirds occurring within the rectosigmoid region as shown in Fig. 51.2. Most CRCs are adenocarcinomas, which are tumors that arise from the glandular epithelial tissue of the colon. Abnormal cellular regulation develops as a multistep process affecting immunity, resulting in a number of molecular changes. These changes include loss of key tumor suppressor genes and activation of certain oncogenes that alter colonic mucosa cell division. The increased proliferation of the colonic mucosa forms polyps that can transform into malignant tumors. Most CRCs are believed to arise from adenomatous polyps that present as small growths covered with mucosa and attached to the surface of the intestine (McCance et al., 2019).

CRC can metastasize by direct extension or by spreading through the blood or lymph. The tumor may spread locally into the four layers of the bowel wall and into neighboring organs. It may enlarge into the lumen of the bowel or spread through the lymphatics or the circulatory system. CRC enters the circulatory system directly from the primary tumor through blood vessels in the bowel or via the lymphatic system. The liver is the most common site of metastasis from circulatory spread. Metastasis to the lungs, brain, bones, and adrenal glands may also occur. Colon tumors can also spread by peritoneal seeding during surgical resection of the tumor. Seeding may occur when a tumor is excised and cancer

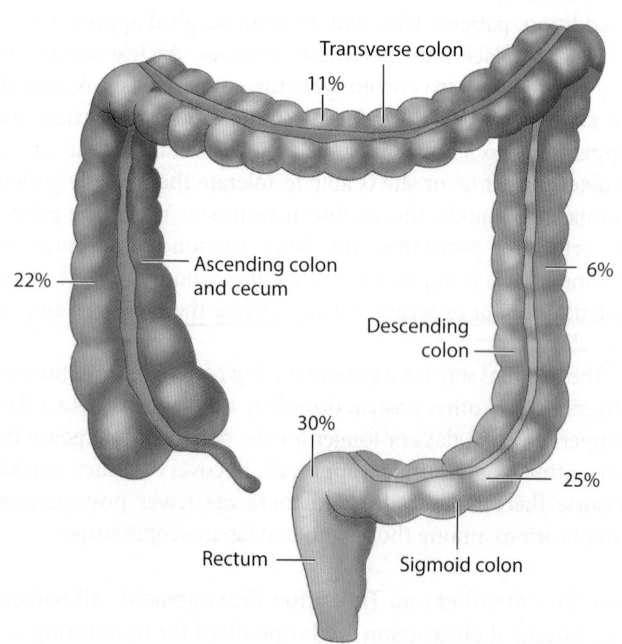

Fig. 51.2 Incidence of cancer in relation to colorectal anatomy.

cells break off from the tumor into the peritoneal cavity. Chapter 19 discusses cancer pathophysiology in more detail.

The major risk factors for the development of colorectal cancer (CRC) include age older than 50 years, genetic predisposition, and/or personal or family history of cancer. However, increasing numbers of adults under 45 years of age are being diagnosed with CRC. Some diseases also predispose the patient to cancer, such as familial adenomatous polyposis (FAP), Crohn's disease, and ulcerative colitis (McCance et al., 2019).

PATIENT-CENTERED CARE: GENETIC/GENOMIC CONSIDERATIONS QSEN

People with a first-degree relative (parent, sibling, or child) diagnosed with colorectal cancer (CRC) have three to four times the risk for developing the disease. Many genes are associated with CRC. An autosomal dominant inherited genetic disorder known as *familial adenomatous polyposis (FAP)* accounts for 1% of CRCs. FAP is the result of one or more mutations in the adenomatous polyposis coli *(APC)* gene. In very young patients, thousands of adenomatous polyps develop over the course of 10 to 15 years and have nearly a 100% chance of becoming malignant (McCance, et al., 2019). By 20 years of age, most patients require surgical intervention, usually a colectomy with ileostomy or ileoanal pull-through, to prevent cancer.

Lynch syndrome, also known as hereditary nonpolyposis colorectal cancer (HNPCC), is another autosomal dominant disorder and accounts for approximately 3% of all CRCs. Lynch syndrome is also caused by gene mutations, including mutations in *MLH1* and *MLH2*. People with these mutations have an 80% chance of developing CRC at an average of 45 years of age. They also tend to have a higher incidence of endometrial, ovarian, stomach, small bowel, brain, and ureteral cancers (McCance et al., 2019). Genetic testing is available for both of these familial CRC syndromes. Refer patients for genetic counseling and testing if the patient prefers.

The role of infectious agents in the development of colorectal and anal cancer continues to be investigated. Some lower GI cancers are related to *Helicobacter pylori, Streptococcus bovis,* and human papillomavirus (HPV) infections.

There is also strong evidence that long-term smoking, obesity, physical inactivity, and heavy alcohol consumption are risk factors for CRC (ACS, 2019b). A high-fat diet, particularly animal fat from red meats, increases bile acid secretion and anaerobic bacteria, which are thought to be carcinogenic for the bowel. Diets with large amounts of refined carbohydrates that lack fiber decrease bowel transit time.

NCLEX EXAMINATION CHALLENGE 51.1

Health Promotion and Maintenance

The nurse is talking with a group of older clients about colorectal cancer (CRC) risk factors. Which of the following factors are considered to be common CRC risk factors? **Select all that apply.**

A. High-fat diet
B. Crohn's disease
C. Smoking
D. Alcoholism
E. Family history of cancer
F. Obesity

Health Promotion and Maintenance. People at risk can take action to decrease their chance of getting CRC and/or increase their chance of surviving it. For example, those whose family members have had hereditary CRC should be genetically tested for FAP and Lynch syndrome. If gene mutations are present, the person at risk can collaborate with the health care team to decide which prevention or treatment plan to implement.

Teach adults about the need for diagnostic screening. When an adult turns 40 years of age, he or she should discuss with the primary health care provider the need for colon cancer screening. The interval depends on level of risk. Adults of average risk who are 45 years of age and older and without a family history should undergo regular CRC screening as recommended by the American Cancer Society (ACS). The ACS screening options include fecal occult blood testing (FOBT) every year, colonoscopy every 10 years, or flexible sigmoidoscopy or CT colonography every 5 years. Adults who have a personal or family history of the disease should begin screening earlier and more frequently.

Teach adults, regardless of risk, to modify their diets as needed to decrease fat, refined carbohydrates, and low-fiber foods. Obesity is a major risk factor for most types of cancer. Encourage baked or broiled foods, especially those high in fiber and low in animal fat. Remind adults to eat increased amounts of brassica vegetables, including broccoli, cabbage, cauliflower, and sprouts.

Educate about the hazards of smoking, excessive alcohol, and physical inactivity. Refer patients as needed for smoking- or alcohol-cessation programs and recommend ways to increase regular physical exercise.

❖ Interprofessional Collaborative Care

Care for the patient with CRC usually takes place in a variety of health care settings. The interprofessional team that collaborates to care for this patient generally includes the surgeon, oncologist, and nurse and may include the registered dietitian nutritionist, psychologist, social worker, and spiritual leader of the patient's choice.

◆ Assessment: Recognize Cues

Physical Assessment/Signs and Symptoms. Ask whether vomiting and changes in bowel ***elimination*** habits, such as constipation or change in shape of stool with or without blood, have been noted. The patient may also report fatigue (related to anemias), abdominal fullness, vague abdominal pain, or unintentional weight loss. These symptoms suggest advanced disease.

Additional signs and symptoms of CRC depend on the location of the tumor. *However, the most common signs are rectal bleeding, anemia, and a change in stool consistency or shape.* Stools may contain microscopic amounts of blood that are occult (hidden), or the patient may have mahogany (dark)-colored or bright red stools (Fig. 51.3). Gross blood is not usually detected with tumors of the right side of the colon, but it is common (but not massive) with tumors of the left side of the colon and the rectum.

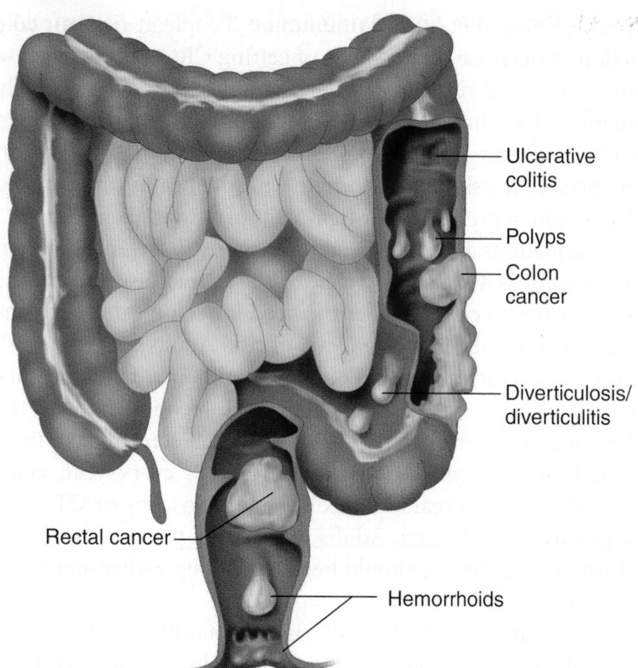

Fig. 51.3 Common causes of lower gastrointestinal bleeding.

Tumors in the transverse and descending colon result in symptoms of obstruction as growth of the tumor blocks the passage of stool. The patient may report "gas pains," cramping, or incomplete evacuation. Tumors in the rectosigmoid colon are associated with hematochezia (the passage of red blood via the rectum), straining to pass stools, and narrowing of stools. Patients may report dull pain. Right-sided tumors can grow quite large without disrupting bowel patterns or appearance because the stool consistency is more liquid in this part of the colon. These tumors ulcerate and bleed intermittently; consequently stools can contain mahogany (dark)-colored blood. A mass may be palpated in the lower right quadrant, and the patient often has anemia secondary to blood loss (McCance et al., 2019).

Laboratory Assessment. A positive test result for occult (microscopic) blood in the stool (**fecal occult blood test [FOBT]** or fecal immunochemical test [FIT]) indicates bleeding in the GI tract. These tests can yield false-positive results if certain vitamins or drugs are taken before the test. Depending on the type of test being used, the patient may need to avoid aspirin, vitamin C, iron, and red meat for 48 hours before giving a stool specimen. Also assess whether the patient is taking anti-inflammatory drugs (e.g., ibuprofen, corticosteroids, or salicylates). These drugs should be discontinued for a designated period before the test. For the FOBT two or three separate stool samples should be tested on 3 consecutive days. Negative results do not completely rule out the possibility of CRC; for this reason additional testing may be suggested (Pagana & Pagana, 2018).

Carcinoembryonic antigen (CEA), an oncofetal antigen, is elevated in many people with CRC. The normal value is less than 5 ng/mL (Pagana & Pagana, 2018). This protein is not specifically associated with the CRC, and it may be elevated in the presence of other benign or malignant diseases and in smokers. CEA is often used to monitor the effectiveness of treatment and to identify disease recurrence.

Other Diagnostic Assessment. *CT-guided virtual colonoscopy* is growing in popularity. This test is noninvasive and includes a CT scan of the rectum and colon. It is thought to be more thorough than traditional invasive colonoscopy. However, treatments, biopsies, or surgeries cannot be performed when a virtual colonoscopy is used.

A *sigmoidoscopy* provides visualization of the lower colon using a fiberoptic scope. Polyps can be visualized, and tissue samples can be taken for biopsy. Polyps are usually removed during the procedure. A *colonoscopy* provides views of the entire large bowel from the rectum to the ileocecal valve. As with sigmoidoscopy, polyps can be seen and removed, and tissue samples can be taken for biopsy. *Colonoscopy is the definitive test for the diagnosis of colorectal cancer.* These procedures and associated nursing care are discussed in Chapter 48.

◆ **Interventions: Take Action.** The primary approach to treating CRC is to remove the entire tumor or as much of the tumor as possible to prevent or slow metastatic spread of the disease. A patient-centered collaborative care approach is essential to meet the desired outcomes.

Although surgical resection is the primary method used to control the disease, several adjuvant (additional) therapies are used. Adjuvant therapies are administered before or after surgery to achieve a cure and prevent recurrence, if possible.

Nonsurgical Management. The type of therapy used is based on the pathologic staging of the disease. The staging system used most often in colorectal cancer is the TNM (tumor, nodes, metastasis) classification; more information on the use of this system can be found in Chapter 19.

The administration of preoperative *radiation therapy* has not improved overall survival rates for colon cancer, but it has been effective in providing local or regional control of the disease. Postoperative radiation has not demonstrated any consistent improvement in survival or recurrence. However, as a palliative measure, radiation therapy may be used to control pain, hemorrhage, bowel obstruction, or metastasis to the lung in advanced disease. For rectal cancer, unlike colon cancer, radiation therapy is often a part of the treatment plan. Reinforce information about the radiation therapy procedure to the patient and family and monitor for possible side effects (e.g., diarrhea, fatigue). Chapter 20 describes the general nursing care of patients undergoing radiation therapy.

Adjuvant *chemotherapy* after primary surgery is recommended for patients with stage II or stage III disease to interrupt the DNA production of cells and destroy them. The drugs of choice are IV 5-fluorouracil with leucovorin (5-FU/LV), capecitabine, and irinotecan hydrochloride (Burchum & Rosenthal, 2019). These drugs can be used individually but are generally used in combination for the greatest treatment benefit. As with other chemotherapeutic drugs, these agents cannot discriminate between cancer and healthy cells. Therefore, common side effects are diarrhea, mucositis, leukopenia, mouth ulcers, and peripheral neuropathy (Benson et al., 2017).

Bevacizumab is an antiangiogenesis drug, also known as a *vascular endothelial growth factor (VEGF) inhibitor,* approved for metastatic CRC. This drug reduces blood flow to the growing tumor cells, thereby depriving them of necessary nutrients needed to grow (Seow et al., 2016). A VEGF inhibitor is usually given in combination with other chemotherapeutic agents.

Cetuximab and panitumumab are monoclonal antibodies known as *epidermal growth factor receptor (EGFR) inhibitors (EGFRIs),* and may also be given in combination with other drugs for metastatic disease (Seow et al., 2016). These drugs work by blocking factors that promote cancer cell growth.

Intrahepatic arterial chemotherapy, often with 5-FU, may be administered to patients with liver metastasis. Patients with CRC also receive drugs for relief of symptoms, such as opioid analgesics and antiemetics. Chapter 20 describes care of patients receiving chemotherapy in detail.

Surgical Management. Surgical removal of the tumor with margins free of disease is the best method of ensuring removal of CRC. The size of the tumor, its location, the extent of metastasis, the integrity of the bowel, and the condition of the patient determine which surgical procedure is performed for colorectal cancer. Many regional lymph nodes are removed and examined for presence of cancer. The number of lymph nodes that contain cancer is a strong predictor of prognosis. The most common surgeries performed are **colon resection** (removal of the part of the colon and regional lymph nodes) with reanastomosis, partial **colectomy** with a *colostomy (temporary or permanent)* or total colectomy with an *ileostomy/ileoanal pull-through,* and *abdominoperineal resection.* A **colostomy** is the surgical creation of an opening (stoma) of the colon onto the surface of the abdomen to allow passage of stool. An **abdominoperineal (AP) resection** is performed when rectal tumors are present. In this procedure, the surgeon removes the sigmoid colon, rectum, and anus through combined abdominal and perineal incisions.

For patients having a colon resection, minimally invasive surgery (MIS) via laparoscopy is commonly performed today. This procedure results in shorter hospital stays, less pain, fewer complications, and quicker recovery compared with the conventional open surgical approach (Papageorge et al., 2016).

Preoperative Care. Reinforce the surgeon's explanation of the planned procedure. The patient is told as accurately as possible what anatomic and physiologic changes will occur with surgery. The location and number of incision sites and drains are also discussed.

Before evaluating the tumor and colon during surgery, the surgeon may not be able to determine whether a colostomy (or less commonly, an ileostomy) will be necessary. The patient is told that a colostomy is a possibility. If a colostomy is planned, the surgeon consults a certified wound, ostomy, and continence nurse (CWOCN, sometimes referred to as the WOC nurse) to recommend optimal placement of the ostomy. The CWOCN teaches the patient about the rationale and general principles of ostomy care. In many settings, the CWOCN marks the patient's abdomen to indicate a potential ostomy site that will decrease the risk for complications such as interference from undergarments or a prosthesis with the ostomy appliance. Table 51.1 describes the preoperative role of the CWOCN.

TABLE 51.1 Preoperative Assessment by the CWOCN Before Ostomy Surgery

Key Points of Psychosocial Assessment

- Patient's and family's level of knowledge of disease and ostomy care
- Patient's educational level
- Patient's physical limitations (particularly sensory)
- Support available to patient
- Patient's type of employment
- Patient's involvement in activities such as hobbies
- Financial concerns regarding purchase of ostomy supplies

Key Points of Physical Assessment

Before marking the placement for the ostomy, the nurse specialist considers:

- Contour of the abdomen in lying, sitting, and standing positions
- Presence of skinfolds, creases, bony prominences, and scars
- Location of belt line
- Location that is easily visible to the patient
- Possible location in the rectus muscle

CWOCN, Certified wound, ostomy, and continence nurse.

The patient who requires low rectal surgery (e.g., abdominoperineal resection) is faced with the risk for postoperative sexual dysfunction and urinary incontinence after surgery as a result of nerve damage during surgery. The surgeon discusses the risk for these problems with the patient before surgery and allows him or her to verbalize concerns and questions related to this risk before he or she gives informed consent. Reinforce teaching about abdominal surgery performed for the patient under general anesthesia and review the routines for turning and deep breathing (see Chapter 9). Teach the patient about the method of ***pain*** management to be used after surgery such as IV patient-controlled analgesia (PCA), epidural analgesia, or other method.

If the bowel is not obstructed or perforated, elective surgery is planned. The patient may be instructed to thoroughly clean the bowel, or perform "bowel prep," to minimize bacterial growth and prevent complications. Mechanical cleaning is accomplished with laxatives and enemas or with "whole-gut lavage." The use of bowel preps is controversial, and some surgeons do not recommend it. For example, older adults may become dehydrated from this process.

To reduce the risk for infection, the surgeon may prescribe one dose of oral or IV antibiotics to be given before the surgical incision is made. Teach patients that a nasogastric tube (NGT) may be placed for decompression of the stomach after conventional open surgery. A peripheral IV or central venous catheter is also placed for fluid and electrolyte replacement while the patient is NPO after surgery. Patients having minimally invasive surgeries do not need an NGT.

The patient with colorectal cancer faces a serious illness with long-term consequences of the disease and treatment. A case manager or social worker can be very helpful in identifying patient and family needs and ensuring continuity of care and support.

Operative Procedures. For the conventional open surgical approach, the surgeon makes a large incision in the abdomen and explores the abdominal cavity to determine whether the tumor can be removed. For a colon resection, the portion of the colon with the tumor is excised, and the two open ends of

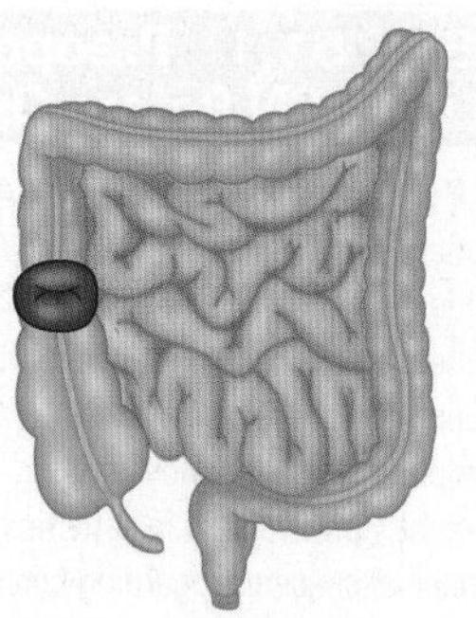

The **ascending colostomy** is done for right-sided tumors.

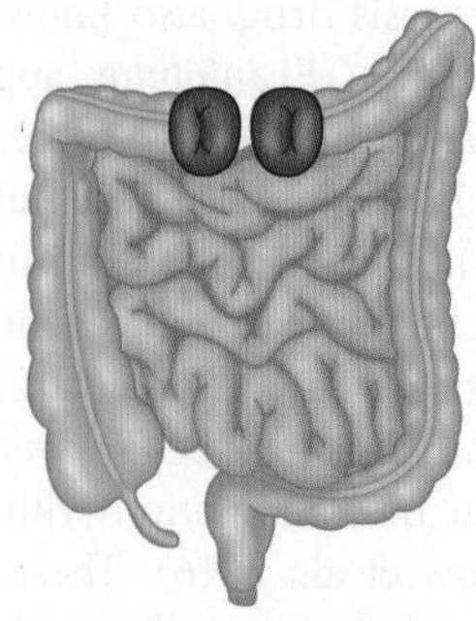

The **transverse (double-barrel) colostomy** is often used in such emergencies as intestinal obstruction or perforation because it can be created quickly. There are two stomas. The proximal one, closest to the small intestine, drains feces. The distal stoma drains mucus.

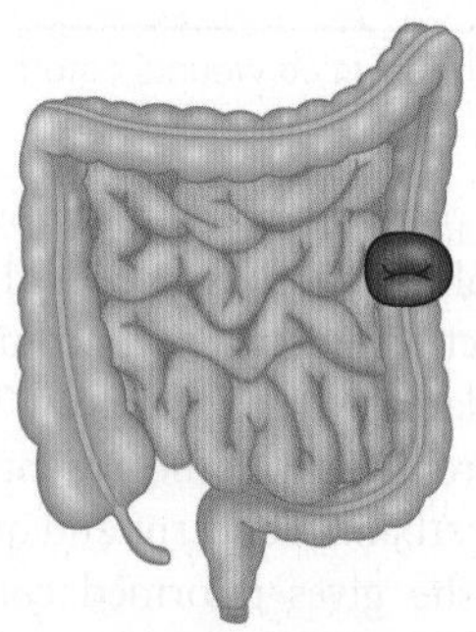

The **descending colostomy** is done for left-sided tumors.

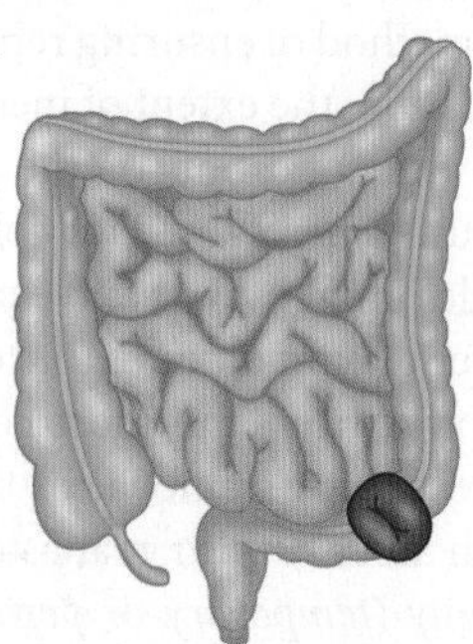

The **sigmoid colostomy** is done for rectal tumors.

Fig. 51.4 Different locations of colostomies in the colon.

the bowel are irrigated before anastomosis (reattachment) of the colon. If an anastomosis is not feasible because of the location of the tumor or inflammation of the bowel, a colostomy is created.

A temporary or permanent colostomy may be created in the ascending, transverse, descending, or sigmoid colon (Fig. 51.4). One of several techniques is used to construct a colostomy. A loop stoma (surgical opening) is made by bringing a loop of colon to the skin surface, severing and everting the anterior wall, and suturing it to the abdominal wall. Loop colostomies are usually performed in the transverse colon and are usually temporary. An external rod may be used to support the loop until the intestinal tissue adheres to the abdominal wall. Care must be taken to avoid displacing the rod, especially during appliance changes.

An end stoma is often constructed, usually in the descending or sigmoid colon, when a colostomy is intended to be permanent. It may also be done when the surgeon oversews the distal stump of the colon and places it in the abdominal cavity, preserving it for future reattachment. An end stoma is constructed by severing the end of the proximal portion of the bowel and bringing it out through the abdominal wall.

The least common colostomy is the *double-barrel stoma,* which is created by dividing the bowel and bringing both the proximal and distal portions to the abdominal surface to create two stomas. The proximal stoma (closest to the patient's head) is the functioning stoma and eliminates stool. The distal stoma (farthest from the head) is considered nonfunctioning, although it may secrete some mucus. The distal stoma is sometimes referred to as a *mucous fistula.*

Laparoscopic (MIS) colon resection or total colectomy allows complete tumor removal with an adequate surgical margin and removal of associated lymph nodes. Several small incisions are made, and a miniature video camera is placed within the abdomen to help see the area that is involved. This technique takes longer than the conventional procedure and requires specialized training. However, blood loss and postoperative pain are reduced.

Postoperative Care. Patients who have an *open colon resection* without a colostomy receive care similar to that of those having any abdominal surgery (see Chapter 9). Other patients have surgeries that also require colostomy management. They typically have a nasogastric tube (NGT) after open surgery and receive IV PCA for the first 24 to 36 hours. After NGT removal, the diet is slowly progressed from liquids to solid foods as tolerated. The care of patients with an NGT is found in the Interventions discussion in the Intestinal Obstruction section earlier in this chapter.

By contrast, patients who have *laparoscopic surgery* (MIS) can eat solid foods very soon after the procedure. Because they usually have less ***pain*** and are at risk for fewer postoperative complications, they are able to ambulate and heal earlier than those who have the conventional approach. The hospital stay is usually shorter for the patient with MIS—typically 1 to 2 days, depending on the patient's age and general condition.

Colostomy Management. The patient who has a colostomy may return from surgery with a clear ostomy pouch system in place. A clear pouch allows the health care team to observe the stoma. If no pouch system is in place, a petrolatum gauze dressing is usually placed over the stoma to keep it moist. This is covered with a dry, sterile dressing. In collaboration with the CWOCN, place a pouch system as soon as possible. The colostomy pouch system, also called an *appliance,* allows more convenient and suitable collection of stool than a dressing does. Pouches are available in both one and two-piece systems and ae held in place by adhesive barriers or wafers.

Assess the color and integrity of the stoma frequently. *A healthy stoma should be reddish pink (or dark red to pink) and moist and protrude about 1 to 3 cm from the abdominal wall but most commonly about ¾ inch (2 cm)* (Fig. 51.5). During the initial postoperative period, the stoma may be slightly edematous. A small amount of bleeding at the stoma is common. These minor problems tend to resolve within 6 to 8 weeks (Stelton, 2019).

! NURSING SAFETY PRIORITY (QSEN)

Action Alert

Report any of these early postoperative stoma problems to the surgeon:
- Stoma ischemia and necrosis (dark red, purplish, or black color; dry)
- Continuous heavy bleeding
- Mucocutaneous separation (breakdown of the suture line securing the stoma to the abdominal wall)

Also assess the condition of the peristomal skin (skin around the stoma) and frequently check the pouch system for proper fit and signs of leakage. The skin should be intact, smooth, and without redness or excoriation. The most common peristomal skin complications are irritant dermatitis (from fecal content), skin stripping (from the adhesive barrier or wafer), and candidiasis (fungal infection under the barrier or wafer) (Stelton, 2019).

The colostomy should start functioning 2 to 3 days after surgery. When it begins to function, the pouch may need to be emptied frequently because of excess gas collection. It should be emptied when it is one-third to one-half full of stool. Stool is liquid immediately after surgery but becomes more solid, depending on where in the colon the stoma was placed. For example, stool from an ascending colon colostomy continues to be liquid, stool from a transverse colon colostomy becomes pasty, and stool from a descending colon colostomy becomes more solid (similar to stool expelled from the rectum).

Wound Management. For an AP resection, the perineal wound is generally surgically closed, and two bulb suction drains such as Jackson-Pratt drains are typically placed in the wound or through stab wounds near the wound. The drains help prevent drainage from collecting within the wound and are

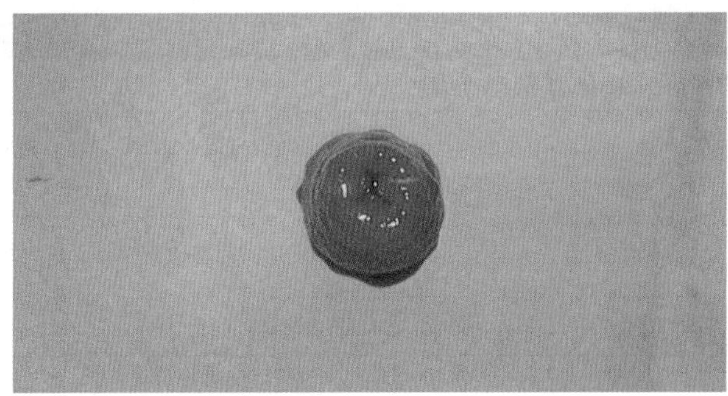

Fig. 51.5 Mature colostomy. (From Evans, S. [2009]. *Surgical pitfalls.* Philadelphia: Saunders.)

usually left in place for several days, depending on the character and amount of drainage. These drains are described in more detail in Chapter 9.

Monitoring drainage from the perineal wound and cavity is important because of the possibility of infection and abscess formation. Serosanguineous drainage from the perineal wound may be observed for 1 to 2 months after surgery. Complete healing of the perineal wound may take 6 to 8 months. This wound can be a greater source of ***pain*** than the abdominal incision and ostomy, and more care may be required. The patient may experience phantom rectal sensations because sympathetic innervation for rectal control has not been interrupted. Rectal pain and itching may occasionally occur after healing. Interventions may include use of antipruritic drugs, such as benzocaine, and warm compresses. Continually assess for signs of infection, abscess, or other complications and implement methods for promoting wound drainage and comfort (see the Best Practice for Patient Safety & Quality Care: Perineal Wound Care box).

BEST PRACTICE FOR PATIENT SAFETY & QUALITY CARE (QSEN)

Perineal Wound Care

Wound Care
- Place an absorbent dressing (e.g., abdominal pad) over the wound.
- Instruct the patient that he or she may:
  - Use a feminine napkin as a dressing
  - Wear jockey-type shorts rather than boxers

Comfort Measures
- If prescribed, soak the wound area in a sitz bath for 10 to 20 minutes three or four times per day or use warm/hot compresses or packs.
- Administer an analgesic as prescribed and assess its effectiveness.
- Instruct the patient about permissible activities. The patient should:
  - Assume a side-lying position in bed; avoid sitting for long periods
  - Use foam pads or a soft pillow on which to sit whenever in a sitting position
  - Avoid the use of air rings or rubber donut devices

Prevention of Complications
- Maintain ***fluid and electrolyte balance*** by monitoring intake and output and output from the perineal wound.
- Observe incision integrity and monitor wound drains; watch for erythema, edema, bleeding, drainage, unusual odor, and excessive or constant ***pain.***

NCLEX EXAMINATION CHALLENGE 51.2

Physiological Integrity

A client had an open partial colectomy and colostomy placement 6 hours ago. Which assessment would **concern** the nurse?

A. Purple, moist stoma
B. Stoma edema
C. Liquid stool collecting in the drainage bag
D. Serosanguineous fluid draining from the drain(s)

Care Coordination and Transition Management. The patient and family are faced with a possible alteration in body functions. Medical and surgical interventions for the treatment of colorectal cancer may result in cure, disease control, or palliation. Nursing interventions are designed to help the patient and family plan effective strategies for expressing feelings of grief and developing coping skills.

Collaborate with the case manager to help patients and their families cope with the immediate postoperative phase of recovery. After hospitalization for surgery, the patient is usually managed at home. Radiation therapy or chemotherapy is typically administered on an ambulatory care basis. For the patient with advanced cancer, hospice care may be an option (see Chapter 8).

Home Care Management. Assess all patients for their ability for self-management within limitations. For those requiring assistance with care, home care visits by nurses or assistive nursing personnel can be provided.

For the patient who has undergone a colostomy, review the home situation to help the patient arrange for care. Ostomy products should be kept in an area (preferably the bathroom) where the temperature is neither hot nor cold (skin barriers may become stiff or melt in extreme temperatures) to ensure proper functioning.

Self-Management Education. Before discharge, teach the patient to avoid lifting heavy objects or straining on defecation to prevent tension on the anastomosis site. If he or she had the open surgical approach, the patient should avoid driving and vigorous physical activity for 4 to 6 weeks while the incision heals. Patients who have had laparoscopy can usually return to all usual activities in 1 to 2 weeks.

! NURSING SAFETY PRIORITY (QSEN)

Action Alert

A stool softener may be prescribed to keep stools soft in consistency for ease of passage. Teach patients to note the frequency, amount, and character of the stools. In addition to this information, teach those with colon resections to watch for and report signs and symptoms of intestinal obstruction and perforation (e.g., cramping, abdominal pain, nausea, vomiting). Advise the patient to avoid gas-producing foods and carbonated beverages. The patient may require 4 to 6 weeks to establish the effects of certain foods on bowel patterns.

Ongoing Colostomy Care. Rehabilitation after surgery requires that patients and family members or other caregivers learn how to perform colostomy care. Provide adequate opportunity before discharge for patients to learn the psychomotor skills involved in this care. Plan sufficient practice time for learning how to handle, assemble, and apply all ostomy equipment. Teach patients and families or other caregivers about:

- Appearance of a normal stoma
- Signs and symptoms of complications
- Measurement of the stoma
- Choice, use, care, and application of the appropriate appliance to cover the stoma
- Measures to protect the skin adjacent to the stoma
- ***Nutrition*** changes to control gas and odor
- What to expect in terms of stool consistency
- Resumption of normal activities, including work, travel, and sexual intercourse

The appropriate pouch system must be selected and fitted to the stoma. Patients with flat, firm abdomens may use either flexible (bordered with paper tape) or nonflexible (full skin barrier wafer) pouch systems. A firm abdomen with lateral creases or folds requires a flexible system. Patients with deep creases, flabby abdomens, a retracted stoma, or a stoma that is flush or concave to the abdominal surface can benefit from a convex appliance with a stoma belt. This type of system presses into the skin around the stoma, causing the stoma to protrude. This protrusion helps tighten the skin and prevents leaks around the stoma opening onto the peristomal skin.

Measurement of the stoma is necessary to determine the correct size of the stoma opening on the appliance. The opening should be large enough not only to cover the peristomal skin but also to avoid stoma trauma. The stoma shrinks within 6 to 8 weeks after surgery. Therefore it needs to be measured at least once weekly during this time to gauge appliance fit and comfort. Measurements are also necessary if the patient gains or loses weight. Teach the patient and family caregiver to trace the pattern of the stoma area on the wafer portion of the appliance and to cut an opening about ⅛ to 1/16 inch larger than the stoma pattern to ensure that stoma tissue will not be constricted.

Skin preparation may include clipping peristomal hair or shaving the area (moving from the stoma outward) to achieve a smooth surface, prevent unnecessary discomfort when the wafer is removed, and minimize the risk for infected hair follicles. Advise the patient to clean around the stoma with mild soap and water before putting on an appliance. He or she should avoid using moisturizing soaps to clean the area because the lubricants can interfere with adhesion of the appliance.

! NURSING SAFETY PRIORITY (QSEN)

Action Alert

Teach the patient and family to apply a skin sealant (preferably without alcohol) and allow it to dry before application of the appliance (colostomy pouch) to facilitate less painful removal of the tape or adhesive. If peristomal skin becomes raw (skin stripping), stoma powder or paste or a combination may also be applied. The paste or other filler cream is also used to fill in crevices and creases to create a flat surface for the flange of the colostomy bag. If the patient develops a fungal rash (candidiasis), an antifungal cream or powder should be used.

Control of gas and odor from the colostomy is often an important outcome for patients with new ostomies. Although a leaking or inadequately closed pouch is the usual cause of odor, flatus can also contribute to it. Remind the patient with an ostomy that although, in general, no foods are forbidden, certain foods (such as vegetables) can cause flatus or contribute to odor when the pouch is open. Charcoal filters, pouch deodorizers, or placement of a breath mint in the pouch helps eliminate odors. The patient should be cautioned to not put aspirin tablets in the pouch because they may cause ulceration of the stoma. Vents that allow release of gas from the ostomy bag through a deodorizing filter are available and may decrease the patient's level of self-consciousness about odor.

The patient with a sigmoid colostomy may benefit from colostomy irrigation to regulate ***elimination***. However, most patients with a sigmoid colostomy can become regulated through diet. Irrigation is similar to an enema but is administered through the stoma rather than the rectum.

In addition to teaching the patient about the signs and symptoms of obstruction and perforation, ask him or her to report any fever or sudden onset of pain or swelling around the stoma. Other home care assessment is listed in the Home Care Considerations: The Patient With A Colostomy box.

Psychosocial Concerns. The diagnosis of cancer can be emotionally immobilizing for the patient and family or significant others, but treatment may be welcomed because it may provide hope for control of the disease. Explore reactions to the illness and perceptions of planned interventions.

The patient's reaction to ostomy surgery may include:

- Fear of not being accepted by others
- Feelings of grief related to disturbance in body image
- Concerns about sexuality

HOME CARE CONSIDERATIONS

The Patient With a Colostomy

Assess gastrointestinal status, including:

- Dietary and fluid intake and habits
- Presence or absence of nausea and vomiting
- Weight gain or loss
- Bowel ***elimination*** pattern and characteristics and amount of effluent stool
- Bowel sounds

Assess condition of stoma at least weekly, including:

- Location, size, protrusion, color, and integrity (check for stoma retraction, prolapse or stenosis)
- Presence of peristomal hernia
- Signs of ischemia, such as dull coloring or dark or purplish bruising

Assess peristomal skin for:

- Presence or absence of excoriated skin, leakage underneath drainage system
- Presence of folliculitis (inflammation of hair follicles) or dermatitis (inflammation of skin)
- Fit of appliance and effectiveness of skin barrier and appliance

Assess the patient's and family's coping skills, including:

- Self-care abilities in the home
- Acknowledgment of changes in body image and function
- Sense of loss

Encourage the patient and family to verbalize their feelings. Education about how to physically manage the ostomy will empower both the family and patient to begin restoration of self-esteem and improvement of body image. Inclusion of family and significant others in the rehabilitation process may help preserve relationships and raise self-esteem. Anticipatory instruction includes information on leakage accidents, odor control measures, and adjustments to resuming sexual relationships.

Health Care Resources. Several resources are available to maintain continuity of care in the home environment and provide for patient needs that the nurse is not able to meet. Make referrals to community-based case managers or social workers who can provide further emotional counseling, aid in managing financial concerns, or arrange for services in the home or long-term care facility as needed.

Provide information about the United Ostomy Associations of America (www.ostomy.org), a self-help group of people with ostomies. This group has literature, online resources, and information about local chapters. The organization conducts a visitor program that sends specially trained visitors (who have an ostomy ["ostomate"]) to talk with patients. After obtaining consent, make a referral to the visitor program so the volunteer ostomate can see the patient both before and after surgery. A primary health care provider's consent for visitation may be necessary.

The local division or unit of the American Cancer Society (ACS) (www.cancer.org) can help provide necessary medical equipment and supplies, home care services, travel accommodations, and other resources for the patient who is having cancer treatment or surgery. Inform the patient and family of the programs available through the local division or unit. Other excellent Internet resources include Cancer Care (www.cancercare.org), the Colorectal Cancer Alliance (www.ccalliance.org), and the National Cancer Institute (www.cancer.gov). The Canadian Cancer Society (www.cancer.ca) is an excellent resource for patients who live in Canada.

Because of short hospital stays, patients with new ostomies receive much health teaching from nurses working for home health care agencies. This resource also helps provide physical care needs, medication management, and emotional support. If the patient has advanced colorectal cancer, a referral for hospice services in the home, nursing home, or other long-term care setting may be appropriate. The home health care nurse informs the patient and family about which ostomy supplies are needed and where they can be purchased. Price and location are considered before recommendations are made.

IRRITABLE BOWEL SYNDROME

Pathophysiology Review

Irritable bowel syndrome (IBS) is a functional GI disorder that causes chronic or recurrent diarrhea, constipation, and/or abdominal ***pain*** and bloating. It is sometimes referred to as *spastic colon, mucous colon,* or *nervous colon.* IBS is the most common digestive disorder seen in clinical practice and may affect as many as one in five people in the United States (McCance et al., 2019).

In patients with IBS, GI motility changes, and increased or decreased bowel transit times result in changes in the normal ***elimination*** pattern to one of these classifications: diarrhea (IBS-D), constipation (IBS-C), alternating diarrhea and constipation (IBS-A), or a mix of diarrhea and constipation (IBS-M). Symptoms of the disease typically begin to appear in young adulthood and continue throughout the patient's life.

The etiology of IBS remains unclear. Research suggests that a combination of environmental, immunologic, genetic, hormonal, and stress factors play a role in the development and course of the disorder. Examples of environmental factors include foods and fluids such as caffeinated or carbonated beverages and dairy products. Infectious agents have also been identified. Several studies have found that patients with IBS often have small-bowel bacterial overgrowth, which causes bloating and abdominal distention. Multiple normal flora and pathogenic agents have been identified, including *Pseudomonas aeruginosa*. Researchers believe that these agents are less causative and serve as measurable biomarkers for the disease (Derkacz et al., 2018).

Immunologic and genetic factors have also been associated with IBS, especially cytokine genes, including proinflammatory interleukins (ILs), such as IL-6 and IL-8, and tumor necrosis factor–alpha (TNF-α). These findings may provide the basis of targeted drug therapy for the disease (McCance et al., 2019).

In the United States, women are two times more likely to have IBS than are men. This difference may be the result of hormonal differences. However, in other areas of the world, this distribution pattern may not occur.

Considerable evidence relates the role of stress and mental or behavioral illness, especially anxiety and depression, to IBS. Many patients diagnosed with IBS meet the criteria for at least one primary mental health disorder. However, the ***pain*** and other chronic symptoms of the disease may lead to secondary mental health disorders. For example, when diarrhea is predominant, patients fear that there will be no bathroom facilities available and can become very anxious. As a result, they may not want to leave their homes or travel on trips where bathrooms are not available at all times. The long-term nature of dealing with a chronic disease for which there is no cure can lead to secondary depression in some patients (McCance et al., 2019).

❖ Interprofessional Collaborative Care

Care for the patient with IBS usually takes place in the outpatient setting, although patients with severe cases of IBS may be hospitalized for a period of time.

◆ **Assessment: Recognize Cues.** Ask the patient about a history of fatigue, malaise, abdominal ***pain,*** changes in the bowel pattern (constipation, diarrhea, or an alternating pattern of both) or consistency of stools, and the passage of mucus. Patients with IBS do not usually lose weight. Ask whether the patient has had any GI infections. Collect information on all drugs that the patient is taking because some can cause symptoms similar to those of IBS. Ask about the ***nutrition*** history, including the use of caffeinated drinks or beverages sweetened with sorbitol or fructose, which can cause bloating or diarrhea.

The course of the illness is specific to each patient. Most patients can identify factors that cause exacerbations, such as diet, stress, or anxiety. Food intolerance may be associated with IBS. Dairy products (e.g., for those with lactose intolerance or milk protein), raw fruits, and grains can contribute to bloating, **flatulence** (excessive gas [flatus] in the intestines), and abdominal distention. Patients may keep a food diary to record possible triggers for IBS symptoms.

A flare-up of worsening cramps, abdominal ***pain,*** and diarrhea and/or constipation may bring the patient to the primary health care provider. One of the *most common concerns of patients with IBS is pain in the left lower quadrant of the abdomen, although it is not always present.* Assess the location, intensity, and quality of the ***pain.*** Some patients have internal visceral (organ) hypersensitivity that can cause or contribute to it. Nausea may be associated with mealtime and defecation. The constipated stools are small and hard and are generally followed by several softer stools. The diarrheal stools are soft and watery, and mucus is often present. Patients with IBS often report belching, gas, anorexia, and bloating.

The patient generally appears well, with a stable weight, and nutritional and fluid status is within normal ranges. Inspect and auscultate the abdomen. Bowel sounds vary but are generally within normal range. With constipation, bowel sounds may be hypoactive; with severe diarrhea, they may be hyperactive.

Routine laboratory values (including a complete blood count [CBC], serum albumin, erythrocyte sedimentation rate [ESR], and stools for occult blood) remain normal in IBS. Some health care providers request a *hydrogen breath test* or small-bowel bacterial overgrowth breath test (Ghoshal et al., 2017). When small-intestinal bacterial overgrowth or malabsorption of nutrients is present, an excess of hydrogen is produced. Some of this hydrogen is absorbed into the bloodstream and travels to the lungs, where it is exhaled. Patients with IBS often exhale an increased amount of hydrogen.

Teach the patient that he or she will need to be NPO (may have water) for at least 12 hours before the hydrogen breath test. At the beginning of the test, the patient blows into a hydrogen analyzer. Then, small amounts of test sugar are ingested, depending on the purpose of the test, and additional breath samples are taken every 15 minutes for 1 to 5 hours (Pagana & Pagana, 2018).

◆ **Interventions: Take Action.** The patient with IBS is usually managed on an ambulatory care basis and learns self-management strategies. Interventions include health teaching, drug therapy, and stress reduction. Some patients also use complementary and integrative therapies. A holistic approach to patient care is essential for positive outcomes (Sultan & Malhotra, 2017).

Dietary fiber and bulk help produce bulky, soft stools and establish regular bowel ***elimination*** habits. The patient should ingest about 30 to 40 g of fiber each day. Eating regular meals, drinking 8 to 10 glasses of water each day, and chewing food slowly help promote normal bowel function.

Drug therapy depends on the main symptom of IBS. The primary health care provider may prescribe bulk-forming or antidiarrheal agents and/or newer drugs to control symptoms.

For the treatment of *constipation-predominant IBS (IBS-C)*, bulk-forming laxatives, such as psyllium hydrophilic mucilloid, are generally taken at mealtimes with a glass of water. The hydrophilic properties of these drugs help prevent dry, hard, or liquid stools. Lubiprostone is an oral laxative approved for women with IBS-C, which increases fluid in the intestines to promote bowel ***elimination.*** Teach the patient to take the drug with food and water. Linaclotide is the newest drug for IBS-C, which works by simulating receptors in the intestines to increase fluid and promote bowel transit time. The drug also helps relieve ***pain*** and cramping that are associated with IBS. Teach patients to take this drug once a day about 30 minutes before breakfast.

Diarrhea-predominant IBS (IBS-D) may be treated with antidiarrheal agents, such as loperamide and psyllium (a bulk-forming agent). Alosetron, a selective serotonin (5-HT3) receptor antagonist, may be used with caution in *women* with IBS-D as a last resort when they have not responded to conventional therapy (Lacy et al., 2018). Patients taking this drug must agree to report symptoms of colitis or constipation early because it is associated with potentially life-threatening bowel complications, including ischemic colitis (lack of blood flow to the colon).

! NURSING SAFETY PRIORITY (QSEN)

Drug Alert

Before the patient begins alosetron, take a thorough drug history (including alternative treatments), both prescribed and over the counter, because it interacts with many drugs in a variety of classes. Remind patients that they should not take psychoactive drugs and antihistamines while taking alosetron. Teach patients to report severe constipation, fever, increasing abdominal ***pain,*** increasing fatigue, darkened urine, bloody diarrhea, or rectal bleeding as soon as it occurs and to stop the drug immediately (Burchum & Rosenthal, 2019).

Many patients with IBS who have bloating and abdominal distention *without constipation* have success with rifaximin, an antibiotic that works locally with little systemic absorption. The U.S. Food and Drug Administration (FDA) originally approved this drug for "traveler's diarrhea," and it now has been approved for use in IBS-D (Lembo et al., 2016).

For IBS in which ***pain*** is the predominant symptom, tricyclic antidepressants such as amitriptyline have also been used successfully. It is unclear whether their effectiveness is the result of the antidepressant or anticholinergic effects of the drugs. If patients have postprandial (after eating) ***pain,*** they should take these drugs 30 to 45 minutes before mealtime.

Complementary and Integrative Health. For patients with increased intestinal bacterial overgrowth, recommend daily probiotic supplements. *Probiotics* have been shown to be effective for reducing bacteria and successfully alleviating GI symptoms of IBS. There is also evidence that peppermint oil capsules may be effective in reducing symptoms for patients with IBS (Currò et al., 2017).

Stress management is also an important part of holistic care. Relaxation techniques, meditation, and/or yoga may help the patient decrease GI symptoms. If the patient has a stressful work or family situation, personal counseling may be helpful. Based on patient preference, make appropriate referrals or assist in making appointments if needed. The opportunity to discuss problems and attempt creative problem solving is often helpful. Teach the patient that regular exercise is important for managing stress and promoting regular bowel ***elimination.***

HERNIATION

Pathophysiology Review

A **hernia** is a weakness in the abdominal muscle wall through which a segment of the bowel or other abdominal structure protrudes. Hernias can also penetrate through any other defect in the abdominal wall, through the diaphragm, or through other structures in the abdominal cavity.

The most important elements in the development of a hernia are congenital or acquired muscle weakness and increased intra-abdominal pressure. The most significant factors contributing to increased intra-abdominal pressure are obesity, pregnancy, and lifting heavy objects.

The most common types of abdominal hernias are indirect, direct, femoral, umbilical, and incisional (McCance et al., 2019).

- An *indirect inguinal hernia* is a sac formed from the peritoneum that contains a portion of the intestine or omentum. The hernia pushes downward at an angle into the inguinal canal. In males, indirect inguinal hernias can become large and often descend into the scrotum.
- *Direct inguinal hernias,* in contrast, pass through a weak point in the abdominal wall.
- *Femoral hernias* protrude through the femoral ring. A plug of fat in the femoral canal enlarges and eventually pulls the peritoneum and often the urinary bladder into the sac.
- *Umbilical hernias* are congenital or acquired. Congenital umbilical hernias appear in infancy. Acquired umbilical hernias directly result from increased intra-abdominal pressure. They are most commonly seen in people who are obese.
- *Incisional,* or *ventral, hernias* occur at the site of a previous surgical incision. These hernias result from inadequate healing of the incision, which is usually caused by postoperative wound infections, inadequate ***nutrition,*** and obesity.

Hernias may also be classified as reducible, irreducible (incarcerated), or strangulated. A **reducible hernia** is one in which the contents of the hernial sac can be placed back into the abdominal cavity by application of gentle pressure. An **irreducible (incarcerated) hernia** cannot be reduced or placed back into the abdominal cavity. *Any hernia that is not reducible requires immediate surgical evaluation.*

A hernia is strangulated when the blood supply to the herniated segment of the bowel is cut off by pressure from the hernial ring (the band of muscle around the hernia). If a hernia is strangulated, there is ischemia and obstruction of the bowel loop. *This can lead to necrosis of the bowel, sepsis, and possibly bowel perforation. Signs of strangulation are abdominal distention, nausea, vomiting, pain, fever, and tachycardia.*

Indirect inguinal hernias, the most common type, occur mostly in men because they follow the tract that develops when the testes descend into the scrotum before birth. Direct hernias occur more often in older adults. Femoral and adult umbilical hernias are most common in pregnant women or those with obesity. Incisional hernias can occur in people who have undergone abdominal surgery.

❖ Interprofessional Collaborative Care

Care for the patient with a hernia usually takes place in the ambulatory outpatient setting. Patients with inguinal hernias often need surgery in a same-day surgical facility.

◆ Assessment: Recognize Cues. The patient with a hernia typically comes to the primary health care provider's office, clinic, or the emergency department with a report of a "lump" or protrusion felt at the involved site. The development of the hernia may be associated with straining or lifting.

Perform an abdominal assessment, inspecting the abdomen when the patient is lying and again when he or she is standing. If the hernia is reducible, it may disappear when the patient is lying flat. The primary health care provider asks the patient to strain or perform the Valsalva maneuver and observes for bulging. Auscultate for active bowel sounds. *Absent bowel sounds may indicate obstruction and strangulation, which are considered medical emergencies.*

To palpate an inguinal hernia, the primary health care provider gently examines the ring and its contents by inserting a finger in the ring and noting any changes when the patient coughs. *The hernia is never forcibly reduced; this maneuver could cause strangulated intestine to rupture.*

If a male patient suspects a hernia in his groin, the primary health care provider has him stand for the examination. Using the right hand for the patient's right side and the left hand for the patient's left side, the examiner pushes in the loose scrotal skin with the index finger, following the spermatic cord upward to the external inguinal cord. At this point, the patient is asked to cough, and any palpable herniation is noted.

◆ Interventions: Take Action. The type of treatment selected depends on patient factors such as age and the type and severity of the hernia.

Nonsurgical Management. If the patient is not a surgical candidate (often an older man with multiple health problems), the primary health care provider may prescribe a truss for an inguinal hernia, usually for men. A truss is a pad made with firm material. It is held in place over the hernia with a belt to help keep the abdominal contents from protruding into the hernial sac. If a truss is used, it is applied only after the primary health care provider has reduced the hernia if it is not incarcerated. The patient usually applies the truss on awakening. Teach him to assess the skin under the truss daily and to protect it with a light layer of powder.

Surgical Management. Most hernias are inguinal, and surgical repair is the treatment of choice. Surgery is usually performed on an ambulatory care basis for patients who have no pre-existing health conditions that would complicate the operative course. In same-day surgery centers, anesthesia may be regional or general, and the procedure is typically laparoscopic. If bowel strangulation and tissue death occur, more extensive surgery, such as a bowel resection or temporary colostomy, may be necessary. Patients undergoing this extensive surgery are hospitalized for a longer period.

Surgical repair of a hernia is called **herniorrhaphy**. A **minimally invasive inguinal hernia repair (MIIHR)** through a laparoscope is the surgery of choice. A conventional open herniorrhaphy may be performed when laparoscopy is not appropriate. Patients having minimally invasive surgery (MIS) recover more quickly, have less pain, and develop fewer postoperative complications compared with those having a conventional open surgery.

In addition to patient education about the procedure, the most important preoperative preparation is to teach the patient to remain NPO for the number of hours before surgery that the surgeon specifies. If same-day surgery is planned, remind the patient to arrange for someone to take him or her home and for that adult to be available for the rest of the day at home. For patients having a conventional open approach, provide general preoperative care as described in Chapter 9.

During an MIIHR, the surgeon makes several small incisions, identifies the defect, and places the intestinal contents back into the abdomen. During a conventional open herniorrhaphy, the surgeon makes an abdominal incision to perform this procedure. When a **hernioplasty** is also performed, the surgeon reinforces the weakened outside abdominal muscle wall with a mesh patch.

The patient who has had MIIHR is discharged from the surgical center in 3 to 5 hours, depending on recovery from anesthesia. Teach the patient to avoid strenuous activity for several days before returning to work and a normal routine. A stool softener may be needed to prevent constipation. Caution patients who are taking oral opioids for pain management to not drive or operate heavy machinery. Teach them to observe incisions for redness, swelling, heat, drainage, and increased pain and promptly report their occurrence to the surgeon. Remind patients that soreness and discomfort (rather than severe, acute pain) are common after MIIHR. Be sure to make a follow-up telephone call on the day after surgery to check on the patient's status.

General postoperative care of patients having a hernia repair is the same as that described in Chapter 9 *except that they should avoid coughing.* To promote lung expansion, encourage deep breathing and ambulation. With repair of an indirect inguinal hernia, the primary health care provider may suggest a scrotal support and ice bags applied to the scrotum to prevent swelling, which often contributes to pain. Elevation of the scrotum with a soft pillow helps prevent and control swelling.

In the immediate postoperative period, male patients who have had an inguinal hernia repair may experience difficulty voiding. Encourage them to stand to allow a more natural position for gravity to facilitate voiding and bladder emptying. Urine output of less than 30 mL/hr should be reported to the surgeon. Techniques to stimulate voiding such as allowing water to run may also be used. A fluid intake of at least 1500 to 2500 mL daily prevents dehydration, maintains urinary function, and minimizes constipation. A "straight" or intermittent ("in and out") catheterization is required if the patient cannot void. The Best Practice for Patient Safety & Quality Care: Nursing Care of the Postoperative Patient Having a Minimally Invasive Inguinal Hernia Repair (MIIHR) box summarizes best nursing practices for postoperative care after an MIIHR.

Most patients have uneventful recoveries after a hernia repair. Surgeons generally allow them to return to their usual activities after surgery, with avoidance of straining and lifting for several weeks while subcutaneous tissues heal and strengthen.

On discharge, provide oral instructions and a written list of symptoms to be reported, including fever, chills, wound drainage, redness or separation of the incision, and increasing incisional pain. Teach the patient to keep the wound dry and clean with antibacterial soap and water. Showering is usually permitted in a few days.

NCLEX EXAMINATION CHALLENGE 51.3

Physiological Integrity

A nurse provides discharge teaching for a male client who had a minimally invasive hernia repair this morning. Which statement by the client indicates a need for **further** teaching?

A. "I should avoid coughing if at all possible."
B. "I can shower in a day or two after I remove my surgical bandage."
C. "I can't go back to work for at least 6 weeks."
D. "I should use an ice pack to help relieve my pain."

BEST PRACTICE FOR PATIENT SAFETY & QUALITY CARE (QSEN)

Nursing Care of the Postoperative Patient Having a Minimally Invasive Inguinal Hernia Repair (MIIHR)

- Monitor vital signs, especially blood pressure and pulse, for indications of internal bleeding.
- Assess and manage incisional pain with oral analgesics; report and document severe ***pain*** that does not respond to drug therapy immediately.
- Encourage deep breathing and use of incentive spirometry after surgery; *teach the patient to avoid excessive coughing!*
- Encourage ambulation with assistance as soon as possible after surgery (within the first few hours).
- Apply ice packs as prescribed to the surgical area.
- Help the patient to void by standing the first time after surgery.
- Teach patients at discharge to:
  - Rest for several days after surgery.
  - Observe the incision sites for redness or drainage and report these findings to the surgeon.
  - Shower after 24 to 36 hours after removing any bandage, but do not remove wound closure strips; be aware that the strips will fall off in about a week.
  - Monitor temperature for the first few days and report the occurrence of a fever.
  - Do not lift more than 10 lb (4.5 kg) until allowed by the surgeon.
  - Avoid constipation by eating high-fiber foods and drinking extra fluids.
  - Return to work when allowed by the surgeon, usually in 1 to 2 weeks, depending on the patient's work responsibilities.

HEMORRHOIDS

Pathophysiology Review

Hemorrhoids are unnaturally swollen or distended veins in the anorectal region. The veins involved in the development of hemorrhoids are part of the normal structure of the anal region. With limited distention, the veins function as a valve overlying the anal sphincter that assists in continence. Increased intra-abdominal pressure causes elevated systemic and portal venous pressure, which is transmitted to the anorectal veins. Arterioles in the anorectal region shunt blood directly to the distended anorectal veins, which increases the pressure. With repeated elevations in pressure from increased intra-abdominal pressure and engorgement from arteriolar shunting of blood, the distended veins eventually separate from the smooth muscle surrounding them. The result is prolapse of the hemorrhoidal vessels.

Hemorrhoids can be internal or external (Fig. 51.6). *Internal hemorrhoids,* which cannot be seen on inspection of the perineal area, are above the anal sphincter. *External hemorrhoids* lie below the anal sphincter and can be seen on inspection of the anal region. *Prolapsed hemorrhoids* can become thrombosed or inflamed, or they can bleed (McCance et al., 2019).

Hemorrhoids are common and not significant unless they cause prolonged ***pain*** or bleeding. Because of the increase in abdominal pressure, the condition worsens during pregnancy, or with constipation with straining, obesity, heart failure, prolonged sitting or standing, and strenuous exercise and weight lifting. Decreased fluid intake can also cause hemorrhoids because of the development of hard stool and subsequent constipation. Straining while evacuating stool causes hemorrhoids to enlarge.

Health Promotion and Maintenance. Prevention of constipation is the most essential measure to prevent hemorrhoids. Constipation can be prevented by increasing fiber in the diet, such as eating more whole grains and raw vegetables and fruits. Encourage patients to drink plenty of water unless otherwise contraindicated (e.g., kidney disease, heart disease). Remind the patient to avoid straining at stool. Remind him or her to exercise regularly with a gradual buildup in intensity. Maintaining a healthy weight also helps prevent hemorrhoids.

❖ Interprofessional Collaborative Care

Care of the patient with hemorrhoids usually takes place in the ambulatory care setting and is provided by the primary health care provider and nurse. If surgery is required, the patient will be admitted to a same-day surgical center.

The most common symptoms of hemorrhoids are bleeding, swelling, and prolapse (bulging). Blood is characteristically bright red and is present on toilet tissue or streaked in the stool. ***Pain*** is a common symptom and is often associated with

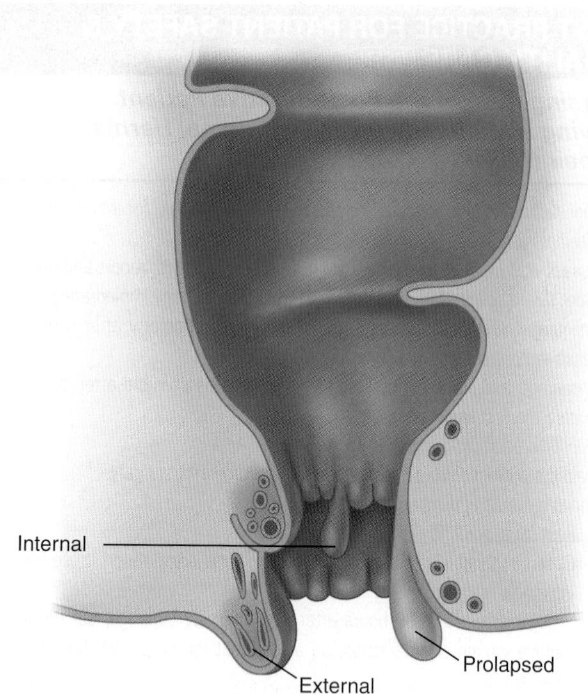

Fig. 51.6 Internal, external, and prolapsed hemorrhoids. *Internal hemorrhoids* lie above the anal sphincter and cannot be seen on inspection of the anal area. *External hemorrhoids* lie below the anal sphincter and can be seen on inspection of the anal region. Hemorrhoids that enlarge, fall down, and protrude through the anus are called *prolapsed hemorrhoids.*

thrombosis, especially if thrombosis occurs suddenly. Other symptoms include itching and a mucous discharge. Diagnosis is usually made by inspection and digital examination.

Interventions are typically conservative and are aimed at reducing symptoms with minimal discomfort, cost, and time lost from usual activities. Cold packs applied to the anorectal region for a few minutes at a time beginning with the onset of pain and tepid sitz baths three or four times per day are often enough to relieve discomfort, even if the hemorrhoids are thrombosed.

Topical anesthetics, such as lidocaine, are useful for severe pain. Dibucaine ointment and similar products are available over the counter and may be applied for mild-to-moderate ***pain*** and itching. However, this ointment should be used only temporarily, because it can mask worsening symptoms and delay diagnosis of a severe disorder. If itching or inflammation is present, the primary health care provider may prescribe a steroid preparation, such as hydrocortisone. Cleansing the anal area with moistened cleansing tissues rather than standard toilet tissue helps avoid irritation. The anal area should be cleansed gently by dabbing rather than wiping.

Diets high in fiber and fluids are recommended to promote regular bowel movements without straining. Stool softeners, such as docusate sodium, can be used temporarily. Irritating laxatives are avoided, as are foods and beverages that can make hemorrhoids worse. Spicy foods, nuts, coffee, and alcohol can be irritating. Remind patients to avoid sitting for long periods. The primary health care provider may prescribe mild oral analgesics for pain if the hemorrhoids are thrombosed.

Conservative treatment should alleviate symptoms in 3 to 5 days. If symptoms continue or recur frequently, the patient may require surgical intervention.

The surgeon can perform several procedures in an ambulatory care setting to remove symptomatic hemorrhoids (**hemorrhoidectomy**). The type of surgery (e.g., ultrasound or laser removal) depends on the degree of prolapse, whether there is thrombosis, and the overall condition of the patient. Complications of these procedures include ***pain,*** thrombosis of other hemorrhoids, infection, bleeding, and abscess formation. If the hemorrhoid is prolapsed, a circular stapling device may be used to excise a band of mucosa above the prolapse and restore the hemorrhoidal tissue back into the anal canal.

Teach patients with hemorrhoids about the need to eat high-fiber, high-fluid diets to promote regular bowel patterns before and after surgery. Advise them to avoid stimulant laxatives, which can be habit forming.

For patients who undergo any type of surgical intervention, monitor for bleeding and ***pain*** after surgery and teach them to report these problems to their health care provider. Using moist heat (e.g., sitz baths or warm compresses) three or four times per day can help promote comfort.

! NURSING SAFETY PRIORITY (QSEN)

Action Alert

Tell the patient who has had surgical intervention for hemorrhoids that the first postoperative bowel movement may be very painful. Be sure that someone is with or near the patient when this happens. Some patients become lightheaded and diaphoretic and may have syncope (temporary loss of consciousness) related to a vasovagal response.

The primary health care provider usually prescribes stool softeners such as docusate sodium to begin before surgery and continue after surgery. Analgesics and anti-inflammatory drugs are prescribed. A mild laxative should be administered if the patient has not had a bowel movement by the third postoperative day.

GET READY FOR THE NEXT-GENERATION NCLEX® EXAMINATION!

Key Points

Review these Key Points for each NCLEX Examination Client Needs Category.

Safe and Effective Care Environment

- Collaborate with the certified wound, ostomy, and continence nurse (CWOCN) when a patient is scheduled for or has a new colostomy. **QSEN: Teamwork and Collaboration**
- Collaborate with the case manager/discharge planner, health care provider, and CWOCN to plan care for the patient with colorectal cancer (CRC). **QSEN: Teamwork and Collaboration**

Health Promotion and Maintenance

- Refer patients with familial CRC syndromes for genetic counseling and testing. **QSEN: Evidence-Based Practice**
- Refer ostomy patients to the United Ostomy Associations of America and the American Cancer Society for additional information and support groups. **QSEN: Patient-Centered Care**
- Teach patients with irritable bowel syndrome (IBS) to avoid GI stimulants, such as caffeine, alcohol, and milk and milk products, and to manage stress. **QSEN: Evidence-Based Practice**
- Instruct patients on dietary modifications to decrease the occurrence of CRC, such as eating a diet high in fiber and avoiding red meat. **QSEN: Evidence-Based Practice**
- Teach adults age 45 years and older to have routine screening for CRC; people with genetic predispositions should have earlier and more frequent screening. **QSEN: Evidence-Based Practice**
- Teach patients to prevent or manage constipation to help avoid hemorrhoids; teach patients the importance of maintaining a healthy weight to decrease the risk for hemorrhoids. **QSEN: Evidence-Based Practice**
- Teach patients and caregivers how to provide colostomy care, including dietary measures, skin care, and ostomy products. **QSEN: Patient-Centered Care**

Psychosocial Integrity

- Assist the patient with CRC with the grieving process. **QSEN: Patient-Centered Care**
- Be aware that having a colostomy is a life-altering event that can severely impact one's body image; issues related to sexuality and fear of acceptance should be discussed. **QSEN: Patient-Centered Care**

Physiological Integrity

- Be aware that minimally invasive inguinal hernia repair is an ambulatory care procedure done via laparoscopy; postoperative management requires health teaching regarding rest for a few days and inspection of incisions for signs of infection. **QSEN: Evidence-Based Practice**
- Be aware that a strangulated hernia can cause ischemia and bowel obstruction, requiring immediate intervention. **QSEN: Safety**
- Monitor patients who have conventional open herniorrhaphy for ability to void. **QSEN: Safety**
- Recall that changes in bowel habits or stool characteristics and/or rectal bleeding are often associated with a diagnosis of CRC. **QSEN: Safety**
- Keep the peristomal skin clean and dry; observe for leakage around the pouch seal. **QSEN: Evidence-Based Practice**
- Provide meticulous perineal wound care for patients having an abdominoperineal resection. **QSEN: Safety**
- Recognize characteristics of the colostomy stoma, which should be reddish pink and moist; report abnormalities such as ischemia and necrosis (purplish or black) or unusual bleeding to the surgeon. **Clinical Judgment**
- Recall that bowel sounds are altered in patients with obstruction; absent bowel sounds imply total obstruction. **QSEN: Safety**
- Assess the patient's nasogastric tube (NGT) for proper placement, patency, and output at least every 4 hours. **QSEN: Safety**
- Monitor patients with bowel obstruction for signs and symptoms of fluid, electrolyte, and acid-base imbalances; patients with small bowel obstruction are at greater risk for problems with ***fluid and electrolyte balance.*** **QSEN: Safety**
- Teach patients having hemorrhoid surgery to take stool softeners before and after surgery to decrease discomfort during ***elimination.*** **QSEN: Evidence-Based Practice**
- Provide comfort measures for the patient who has chronic diarrhea associated with malabsorption. **QSEN: Patient-Centered Care**
- Reinforce teaching regarding supplements or dietary restrictions needed for malabsorption management. **QSEN: Evidence-Based Practice**

MASTERY QUESTIONS

1. The nurse is caring for a client with a complete large bowel obstruction. What assessment findings would the nurse expect? **Select all that apply.**
   A. Obstipation
   B. Dehydration
   C. Metabolic alkalosis
   D. Abdominal distention
   E. Abdominal pain
   F. Profuse vomiting
2. A client has a new diagnosis of irritable bowel syndrome (IBS) with diarrhea. What health teaching by the nurse is **appropriate** for this client?
   A. "Take a stool softener every day to ease defecation."
   B. "Avoid high-fiber foods in your diet."
   C. "Avoid dairy products and caffeinated beverages."
   D. "Ask your primary health care provider for an antidepressant."

REFERENCES

Al-Mazrou, A. M., Baser, O., & Pokala, R. K. (2017). Alvimopan, regardless of ileus risk, significantly impacts ileus, length of stay, and Readmission after intestinal surgery. *Journal of the American College of Surgeons*, *225*(4), S37.

American Cancer Society (ACS). (2019a). *Cancer facts and figures*. Atlanta: ACS.

American Cancer Society (ACS). (2019b). *Colorectal cancer risk factors*. Atlanta: ACS.

Benson, A. B., Venook, A. P., Cederquist, L., Chan, E., Chen, Y., Cooper, H. S., et al. (2017). Colon cancer: Clinical practice guidelines in oncology. *Journal of the National Comprehensive Cancer Network*, *15*(3), 370–398.

Burchum, J. L. R., & Rosenthal, L. D. (2019). *Lehne's pharmacology for nursing care* (10th ed.). St. Louis: Elsevier.

Currò, D., Ianiro, G., Pecere, S., Bibbò, S., & Cammarota, G. (2017). Probiotics, fibre and herbal medicinal products for functional and inflammatory bowel disorders. *British Journal of Pharmacology*, *174*(11), 1426–1449. https://doi.org/10.1111/bph.13632.

Derkacz, A., Olczyk, P., & Komosinska-Vassev, K. (2018). Diagnostic markers for Nonspecific inflammatory bowel diseases. *Disease Markers*, *2018*, 7451946. https://doi.org/10.1155/2018/7451946.

Ghoshal, U. C., Shukla, R., & Ghoshal, U. (2017). Small intestinal bacterial overgrowth and irritable bowel syndrome: A Bridge between functional organic Dichotomy. *Gut and Liver*, *11*(2), 196–208. https://doi.org/10.5009/gnl16126.

Lacy, B. E., Nicandro, J. P., Chuang, E., & Earnest, D. L. (2018). Alosetron use in clinical practice: Significant improvement in irritable bowel syndrome symptoms evaluated using the US food and drug administration composite endpoint. *Therapeutic Advances in Gastroenterology*, 111756284818771674. https://doi.org/10.1177/1756284818771674.

Lembo, A., Pimentel, M., Rao, S. S., Schoenfeld, P., Cash, B., Weinstock, L. B., et al. (2016). Repeat treatment with rifaximin is Safe and effective in patients with diarrhea-predominant irritable bowel syndrome. *Gastroenterology*, *151*(6), 1113–1121. https://doi.org/10.1053/j.gastro.2016.08.003.

McCance, K., Huether, S., Brashers, V., & Rote, N. (2019). *Pathophysiology: The biologic basis for disease in adults and children* (8th ed.). St. Louis: Elsevier.

Pagana, K. D., & Pagana, T. J. (2018). *Mosby's manual of diagnostic and laboratory tests* (*6th* ed.). St. Louis: Mosby.

Papageorge, C. M., Zhao, Q., Foley, E. F., Harms, B., Heise, C. P., Carchman, E. H., et al. (2016). Short-term outcomes of minimally invasive versus open colectomy for colon cancer. *Journal of Surgical Research*, *204*(1), 89–93.

Seow, H. F., Yip, W. K., & Fifis, T. (2016). Advances in targeted and immunobased therapies for colorectal cancer in the genomic era. *OncoTargets and Therapy*, *9*, 1899–1920.

Stelton, S. (2019). Stoma and peristomal skin care: A clinical review. *AJN*, *119*(6), 38–45.

Sultan, S., & Malhotra, A. (2017). Irritable bowel syndrome. *Annals of Internal Medicine*, *166*(11), ITC81–ITC96. https://doi.org/10.7326/AITC201706060.

52

Concepts of Care for Patients With Inflammatory Intestinal Disorders

Keelin Cromar

http://evolve.elsevier.com/Iggy/

LEARNING OUTCOMES

1. Collaborate with the interprofessional team to manage quality care for patients with impaired ***elimination*** caused by chronic inflammatory bowel disorders.
2. Identify community resources for families and patients recovering from inflammatory bowel disorders.
3. Apply knowledge of pathophysiology of inflammatory bowel disorders to identify common assessment findings, including actual or risk for impaired ***nutrition*** and ***fluid and electrolyte balance.***
4. Prioritize evidence-based nursing interventions for patients with inflammatory bowel disorders to promote ***nutrition,*** maintain ***fluid and electrolyte balance,*** and manage ***pain, infection,*** and/or ***inflammation.***
5. Plan transition management and care coordination for the patient who has an ileostomy, including health teaching.

KEY TERMS

abscess A localized infection in which there is a collection of pus.

appendectomy The removal of the inflamed appendix by one of several surgical approaches.

appendicitis An acute inflammation of the vermiform appendix that occurs most often among young adults.

celiac disease A chronic inflammation of the small intestinal mucosa that can cause bowel wall atrophy, malabsorption, and diarrhea.

Crohn's disease (CD) A chronic inflammatory disease of the small intestine (most often), the colon, or both; the terminal ileum is most often affected.

diverticulitis The inflammation or infection of diverticula.

diverticulosis The presence of many abnormal pouchlike herniations (diverticula) in the wall of the intestine.

effluent Drainage.

fissure A tear, crack, or split in skin and underlying tissue.

fistula Abnormal opening (tract) between two organs or structures.

gastroenteritis A very common health problem worldwide that causes diarrhea and/or vomiting related to inflammation of the mucous membranes of the stomach and intestinal tract.

ileostomy A procedure in which a loop of the ileum is placed through an opening in the abdominal wall (stoma) for drainage of fecal material into a pouching system worn on the abdomen.

intestinal malabsorption (malabsorption syndrome) The inability of essential nutrients to be absorbed through a diseased intestinal wall, causing anemia and malnutrition (most common in Crohn's disease).

laparoscopy A minimally invasive surgery (MIS) with one or more small incisions near the umbilicus through which a small endoscope and tools are placed.

laparotomy An open surgical approach requiring a large abdominal incision.

ostomate A person who has an ostomy.

peritonitis A life-threatening, acute inflammation and infection of the visceral/parietal peritoneum and endothelial lining of the abdominal cavity.

progressive multifocal leukoencephalopathy (PML) A deadly infection that affects the brain.

steatorrhea Fatty diarrheal stools.

tenesmus An unpleasant and urgent sensation to defecate.

toxic megacolon Massive dilation of the colon and subsequent colonic ileus that can lead to gangrene and peritonitis.

ulcerative colitis (UC) A disease that creates widespread chronic inflammation of the rectum and rectosigmoid colon but can extend to the entire colon when the disease is extensive.

PRIORITY AND INTERRELATED CONCEPTS

The priority concepts for this chapter are:
- ***Infection***
- ***Inflammation***

The ***Infection*** concept exemplar for this chapter is Peritonitis.
The ***Inflammation*** concept exemplar for this chapter is Ulcerative Colitis.

The interrelated concepts for this chapter are:
- ***Nutrition***
- ***Elimination***
- ***Pain***
- ***Fluid and Electrolyte Balance***

The *intestinal tract* is made up of the small intestine and large intestine (colon). Continued digestion of food and absorption of nutrients occurs primarily in the small intestine to meet the body's needs for energy. Water is reabsorbed in the large intestine to help maintain a fluid balance and promote the passage of waste products. When the intestinal tract and its nearby structures become acutely inflamed, ***pain*** and ***infection*** can occur. Chronic bowel ***inflammation*** can affect ***nutrition, elimination,*** and ***fluid and electrolyte balance.*** Chapter 3 briefly reviews each of these health concepts.

Appendicitis, gastroenteritis, and peritonitis are the most common *acute* inflammatory bowel disorders (IBDs). These disorders can be potentially life threatening and can have major systemic complications if not treated promptly. Ulcerative colitis and Crohn's disease are the two most common *chronic* IBDs that affect adults.

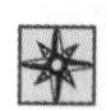

INFECTION CONCEPT EXEMPLAR: PERITONITIS

Pathophysiology Review

Peritonitis is a life-threatening, acute ***inflammation*** and ***infection*** of the visceral/parietal peritoneum and endothelial lining of the abdominal cavity. The peritoneal cavity normally contains about 50 mL of sterile fluid (transudate), which prevents friction in the abdominal cavity during peristalsis. When the peritoneal cavity is contaminated by bacteria, the body begins an inflammatory reaction, walling off a localized area to fight the infection. Vascular dilation and increased capillary permeability occur, allowing transport of leukocytes and subsequent phagocytosis of the offending organisms. If the process of walling off fails, the ***inflammation*** spreads and contamination becomes massive, resulting in diffuse (widespread) ***infection.***

Peritonitis is most often caused by contamination of the peritoneal cavity by bacteria or chemicals. Bacteria gain entry into the peritoneum by perforation (from appendicitis, diverticulitis, peptic ulcer disease) or from an external penetrating wound, a gangrenous gallbladder or bowel segment, bowel obstruction, or ascending infection through the genital tract. Less common causes include invasive tumors, leakage or contamination during surgery, or ***infection*** by skin pathogens in patients undergoing continuous ambulatory peritoneal dialysis (CAPD) (McCance et al., 2019).

When diagnosis and treatment of peritonitis are delayed, blood vessel dilation continues. The body responds to the continuing infectious process by shunting extra blood to the area of inflammation (hyperemia). Fluid is shifted from the extracellular fluid compartment into the peritoneal cavity, connective tissues, and GI tract *("third spacing")*. This shift of fluid can result in a significant decrease in circulatory volume and *hypovolemic shock.* Severely decreased circulatory volume can result in insufficient perfusion of the kidneys, leading to acute kidney injury with impaired ***fluid and electrolyte balance*** (McCance et al., 2019).

Peristalsis slows or *stops* in response to severe peritoneal ***inflammation*** and ***infection,*** and the lumen of the bowel becomes distended with gas and fluid. Fluid that normally flows to the small bowel and the colon for reabsorption accumulates in the intestine in volumes of 7 to 8 L daily. The toxins or bacteria responsible for the peritonitis can also enter the bloodstream from the peritoneal area and lead to bacteremia, or septicemia (bacterial invasion of the blood), a life-threatening condition that can lead to systemic sepsis and septic shock (see Chapter 34 on ***infection.***)

Respiratory problems can occur as a result of increased abdominal pressure against the diaphragm from intestinal distention and fluid shifts to the peritoneal cavity. Also, ***pain*** can interfere with respirations at a time when the patient has an increased oxygen demand because of the infectious process.

Etiology. Common bacteria responsible for peritonitis include *Escherichia coli, Streptococcus, Staphylococcus, Pneumococcus,* and *Gonococcus.* Chemical peritonitis results from leakage of bile, pancreatic enzymes, and gastric acid (McCance et al., 2019).

Incidence and Prevalence. Peritonitis is the dominant cause of death from surgical infections, with a mortality rate of up to 20% (Ross et al., 2018). It occurs most commonly in young adults who have appendicitis and older adults whose immunity is often decreased.

❖ Interprofessional Collaborative Care

Patients with peritonitis are hospitalized because of the severe nature of the illness. If complications are extensive, the patients are often admitted to a critical care unit.

◆ Assessment: Recognize Cues

History. Ask the patient about abdominal ***pain*** and determine the character of the pain (e.g., cramping, sharp, aching), location of the pain, and whether the pain is localized or generalized. Ask about a history of a low-grade fever or recent spikes in temperature.

Physical Assessment/Signs and Symptoms. Physical findings of peritonitis depend on several factors: the stage of the disease, the ability of the body to localize the process by walling off the ***infection,*** and whether the ***inflammation*** has progressed to generalized peritonitis (see the Key Features: Peritonitis box).

The patient most often appears acutely ill, lying still, possibly with the knees flexed. Movement is guarded, and he or she may report and show signs of ***pain*** (e.g., facial grimacing) with coughing or movement of any type. During inspection, observe for progressive abdominal distention, often seen when the

KEY FEATURES

Peritonitis

- Rigid, board-like abdomen (classic)
- Abdominal *pain* (localized, poorly localized, or referred to the shoulder or chest)
- Distended abdomen
- Nausea, anorexia, vomiting
- Diminishing bowel sounds
- Inability to pass flatus or feces
- Rebound tenderness in the abdomen
- High fever
- Tachycardia
- Dehydration from high fever (poor skin turgor)
- Decreased urine output
- Hiccups
- Possible compromise in respiratory status

inflammation and ***infection*** markedly reduce intestinal motility. Auscultate for bowel sounds, which usually disappear with progression of the inflammation.

*The cardinal signs of peritonitis are abdominal **pain**, tenderness, and distention.* In the patient with *localized* peritonitis, the abdomen is tender on palpation in a well-defined area with rebound tenderness in this area. With *generalized* peritonitis, tenderness is widespread.

Psychosocial Assessment. The patient with peritonitis may be very fearful and anxious about the implications of a diagnosis of peritonitis and may be distressed regarding the physical ***pain*** that he or she feels. Provide a calm, nonanxious presence and reassure the patient that you will be there (presence) to help him or her during this time. Allow the patient to express feelings of fear and anxiety, and provide nonjudgmental listening and presence.

Laboratory Assessment. *White blood cell (WBC) counts* are often elevated to 20,000/mm^3 with a high neutrophil count (leukocytosis). *Blood culture* studies may be done to determine whether septicemia has occurred and to identify the causative organism to determine appropriate antibiotic therapy. The primary health care provider may request laboratory tests to assess ***fluid and electrolyte balance*** and renal status, including blood urea nitrogen (BUN), creatinine, hemoglobin, and hematocrit. Oxygen saturation and arterial blood gases may be obtained to assess respiratory function and acid-base balance.

Imaging Assessment. *Abdominal x-rays* can assess for free air or fluid in the abdominal cavity, indicating perforation. The x-rays may also show dilation, edema, and ***inflammation*** of the small and large intestines. An *abdominal ultrasound* or *computerized tomography (CT) scan* may also be performed.

◆ **Analysis: Analyze Cues and Prioritize Hypotheses.** The priority collaborative problems for patients with peritonitis include:

1. Acute ***pain*** due to abdominal ***inflammation*** and ***infection***
2. Potential for fluid volume shift due to fluid moving into interstitial or peritoneal space

◆ **Planning and Implementation: Generate Solutions and Take Action.** The collaborative plan of care for the patient diagnosed with peritonitis focuses on treating the cause of the infection and managing the infectious process. Nonsurgical and/or surgical modalities may be required to resolve the ***infection.***

Managing Pain

Planning: Expected Outcomes. The patient is expected to report pain of 2 to 3 on a 0 to 10 pain intensity scale as the ***inflammation*** and ***infection*** resolve.

Interventions. Interventions for peritonitis are usually nonsurgical, but surgery may be required to remove abscesses or other infectious material.

Nonsurgical Management. Assess vital signs frequently, noting any change that may indicate septic shock, such as unresolved or progressive hypotension, decreased pulse pressure, tachycardia, fever, skin changes, and/or tachypnea. Monitor mental status changes for any sign of confusion or altered level of consciousness. Practice proper handwashing and maintain strict asepsis when caring for wounds, drains, and dressings to decrease chance of superimposed ***infection***. If the patient has or requires a urinary catheter, maintain strict sterile technique and provide appropriate catheter care. Observe and document wound drainage; report any changes immediately to the primary health care provider. Administer broad-spectrum antibiotics as prescribed to treat known or potential pathogens. Provide oxygen as prescribed and according to the patient's respiratory status and oxygen saturation via pulse oximetry.

Surgical Management. Abdominal surgery may be needed to identify and repair the cause of the peritonitis. If the patient is critically ill and surgery could be life threatening, it may be delayed. Surgery focuses on controlling the contamination, removing foreign material from the peritoneal cavity, and draining collected fluid.

An exploratory laparotomy (an open surgical approach requiring a large abdominal incision) or laparoscopy is used to remove or repair an inflamed or perforated organ (e.g., appendectomy for an inflamed appendix; a colon resection, with or without a colostomy, for a perforated diverticulum). Before the incision(s) is closed, the surgeon irrigates the peritoneum with antibiotic solutions. Several catheters may be inserted to drain the cavity and provide a route for irrigation after surgery.

If an *open* conventional surgical procedure is needed, the ***infection*** may slow healing of an incision or the incision may be partially open to heal by second or third intention. These wounds require special care involving manual irrigation or packing as prescribed by the surgeon. If the surgeon requests peritoneal irrigation through a drain, *maintain sterile technique during manual irrigation* to prevent further risk for infection. Chapter 9 describes general preoperative and postoperative care.

! NURSING SAFETY PRIORITY QSEN

Action Alert

Monitor the patient's level of consciousness, vital signs, respiratory status (respiratory rate and breath sounds), and intake and output at least hourly immediately after abdominal surgery. Maintain the patient in a semi-Fowler position to promote drainage of peritoneal contents into the lower region of the abdominal cavity. This position also helps increase lung expansion.

Restoring Fluid Volume Balance

Planning: Expected Outcomes. The patient will experience restoration of fluid volume balance.

Interventions. The primary health care provider prescribes hypertonic IV fluids and broad-spectrum antibiotics immediately after establishing the diagnosis of peritonitis. Remind assistive personnel to take a daily weight using the same scale each morning, and record intake and output carefully. A nasogastric tube (NGT) is inserted to decompress the stomach and the intestine if a laparotomy is anticipated.

Multisystem complications can occur with peritonitis. Loss of fluids and electrolytes from the extracellular space to the peritoneal cavity, NGT suctioning, and NPO status require that the patient receives IV fluid replacement. Fluid rates may be changed frequently on the basis of laboratory values, assessment findings, and patient condition.

Assess whether the patient retains fluid used for irrigation by comparing and recording the amount of fluid returned with the amount of fluid instilled. Fluid retention could cause abdominal distention or pain.

Care Coordination and Transition Management

Home Care Management. The length of hospitalization for a patient with peritonitis depends on the extent and severity of the infectious process. Patients who have a localized abscess (a localized ***infection*** in which there is a collection of pus) drained and who respond to antibiotics and IV fluids without multisystem complications are discharged in several days. Others may require mechanical ventilation or hemodialysis with longer hospital stays. Some patients may be transferred to a transitional care unit to complete their antibiotic therapy and recovery. Convalescence is often longer than other surgeries because of multisystem involvement.

Self-Management Education. Before being discharged home, assess the patient's ability for self-management. Provide the patient and family with written and oral instructions to report the following problems to the primary health care provider immediately:

- Unusual or foul-smelling drainage
- Swelling, redness, or warmth or bleeding from the incision site
- A temperature higher than 101° F (38.3° C)
- Abdominal ***pain***
- Signs of wound dehiscence or ileus

Patients with large incisions that are left open heal by secondary or tertiary intention and require dressings, solution, and catheter-tipped syringes to irrigate the wound. A home care nurse may be needed to assess, irrigate, or pack the wound and change the dressing as needed until the patient and family feel comfortable with the procedure. If the patient needs assistance with ADLs, a home care aide or temporary placement in a skilled care facility may be indicated.

Review information about antibiotics and analgesics. For patients taking short-term oral opioid analgesics such as oxycodone with acetaminophen, a stool softener such as docusate sodium may be prescribed with a laxative. Older adults are especially at risk for constipation from codeine-based drugs. Remind patients to avoid taking additional acetaminophen to prevent liver toxicity.

Teach patients to refrain from any lifting for *at least* 6 weeks after an open surgical procedure. Other activity limitations are based on individual need and the primary health care provider's recommendation. Patients who have laparoscopic surgery can resume activities within a week or two and may not have any major restrictions.

NCLEX EXAMINATION CHALLENGE 52.1

Safe and Effective Care Environment

A client had an exploratory laparotomy to treat the cause of peritonitis and has a large incision that is closed with staples and two abdominal drains. Which finding(s) would the nurse report **immediately** to the surgeon? **Select all that apply.**

A. Serosanguineous drainage
B. Increased abdominal distention
C. Fever and chills
D. Pain level 2 on a scale of 0 to 10
E. Passing flatus

Health Care Resources. Patients with peritonitis may benefit from a social services consultation. Social workers can help patients locate the most appropriate and affordable supplies that will be needed for ongoing care. Collaborate with the case manager to determine the appropriate setting for seamless continuing care in the community.

◆ **Evaluation: Evaluate Outcomes.** Evaluate the care of the patient with peritonitis based on the identified priority patient problems. The expected outcomes are that the patient:

- Verbalizes relief or control of pain as ***infection*** resolves
- Experiences ***fluid and electrolyte balance***

APPENDICITIS

Pathophysiology Review

Appendicitis is an acute ***inflammation*** of the vermiform appendix that occurs most often among young adults. It is the most common cause of right lower quadrant (RLQ) pain. The appendix usually extends off the proximal cecum of the colon just below the ileocecal valve. Inflammation occurs when the lumen (opening) of the appendix is obstructed (blocked), leading to ***infection*** as bacteria invade the wall of the appendix. The initial obstruction is usually a result of fecaliths (very hard pieces of feces) composed of calcium phosphate–rich mucus and inorganic salts (McCance et al., 2019).

When the lumen is blocked, the mucosa secretes fluid, increasing the internal pressure and restricting blood flow, which results in ***pain.*** If the process occurs slowly, an abscess may develop, but a rapid process may result in peritonitis. *All complications of peritonitis are serious. Gangrene and sepsis can occur within 24 to 36 hours, are life threatening, and are some of the most common indications for emergency surgery. Perforation may develop within*

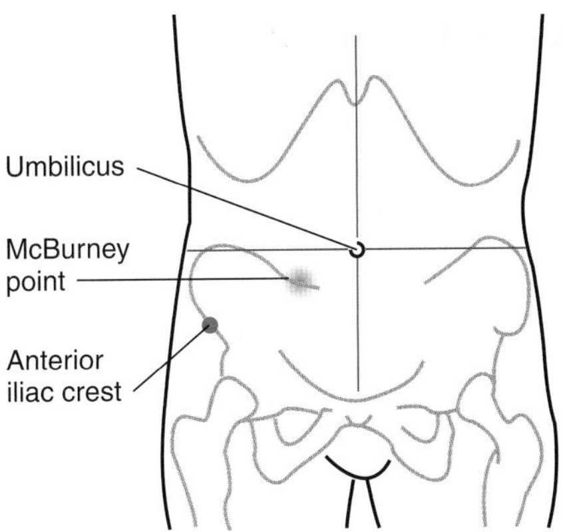

Fig. 52.1 The McBurney point is located midway between the anterior iliac crest and the umbilicus in the right lower quadrant. This is the classic area for localized tenderness during the later stages of appendicitis.

24 hours, but the risk rises rapidly after 48 hours. Perforation of the appendix results in peritonitis with a temperature of greater than 101° F (38.3° C) and a rise in pulse rate.

❖ Interprofessional Collaborative Care

◆ **Assessment: Recognize Cues.** History taking and tracking the sequence of symptoms are important because nausea or vomiting before abdominal pain can indicate gastroenteritis. Abdominal pain followed by nausea and vomiting can indicate appendicitis. Classically, patients with appendicitis have cramping ***pain*** in the epigastric or periumbilical area. Anorexia is also a frequent symptom.

Perform a complete ***pain*** assessment. Initially pain can present anywhere in the abdomen or flank area. As the ***inflammation*** and ***infection*** progress, the pain becomes more severe and shifts to the RLQ between the anterior iliac crest and the umbilicus. This area is referred to as the *McBurney point* (Fig. 52.1). *Abdominal pain that increases with cough or movement and is relieved by bending the right hip or the knees suggests perforation and peritonitis.* The primary health care provider assesses for muscle rigidity and guarding on palpation of the abdomen. The patient may report pain after release of pressure. This sensation is referred to as *rebound* tenderness.

Laboratory findings do not establish the diagnosis, but often there is a moderate elevation of the *white blood cell (WBC) count* (leukocytosis) to 10,000 to 18,000/mm^3 with a "shift to the left" (an increased number of immature WBCs). A WBC elevation to greater than 20,000/mm^3 may indicate a perforated appendix. An *ultrasound* study may show the presence of an enlarged appendix. If symptoms are recurrent or prolonged, a CT scan can be used to diagnose and may reveal the presence of a fecaloma (a small "stone" of feces) (Pagana & Pagana, 2018).

◆ **Interventions: Take Action.** All patients with suspected or confirmed appendicitis are hospitalized, and most have surgery to remove the inflamed appendix.

Nonsurgical Management. Keep the patient with suspected or known appendicitis NPO to prepare for the probability of surgery and to avoid making the ***inflammation*** worse. Be sure that the patient's ***pain*** is adequately managed before surgical intervention.

! NURSING SAFETY PRIORITY (QSEN)

Action Alert

For the patient with suspected appendicitis, administer IV fluids as prescribed to maintain ***fluid and electrolyte balance*** and replace fluid volume. If tolerated, advise the patient to maintain a semi-Fowler position so that abdominal drainage can be contained in the lower abdomen. Once the diagnosis of appendicitis is confirmed and surgery is scheduled, administer opioid analgesics and antibiotics as prescribed. *The patient with suspected or confirmed appendicitis should not receive laxatives or enemas, which can cause perforation of the appendix. Do not apply heat to the abdomen because this may increase circulation to the appendix and result in increased **inflammation** and perforation!*

Surgical Management. Surgery is required as soon as possible for most patients. An appendectomy is the removal of the inflamed appendix by one of several surgical approaches. Uncomplicated appendectomy procedures are done via laparoscopy. A laparoscopy is a minimally invasive surgery (MIS) with one or more small incisions near the umbilicus, through which a small endoscope and tools are inserted. Patients having this type of surgery for appendix removal have few postoperative complications (see Chapter 9). A procedure known as *natural orifice transluminal endoscopic surgery* (NOTES) (e.g., transvaginal endoscopic appendectomy) does not require an external skin incision. During this procedure, the surgeon places the endoscope into the vagina or other orifice and makes a small incision to enter the peritoneal space. Patients having any type of laparoscopic procedure are typically discharged the same day of surgery with less pain and few complications after discharge. Most patients can return to usual activities in 1 to 2 weeks.

If the diagnosis is not definitive but the patient is at high risk for complications from suspected appendicitis, the surgeon may perform an exploratory laparotomy. A laparotomy is an open surgical approach with a large abdominal incision.

Preoperative teaching is often limited because the patient is in ***pain*** or may be admitted quickly for emergency surgery. The patient is prepared for general anesthesia. After surgery, care of the patient who has undergone an appendectomy is the same as that required for anyone who has received general anesthesia (see Chapter 9).

If complications such as peritonitis or abscesses are found during *open* traditional surgery, wound drains are inserted and a nasogastric tube may be placed to decompress the stomach and prevent abdominal distention. Administer IV antibiotics and opioid analgesics as prescribed. Help the patient out of bed on the evening of surgery to help prevent respiratory complications, such as atelectasis. He or she may be hospitalized for as long as 3 to 5 days and return to usual activity in 4 to 6 weeks.

GASTROENTERITIS

Pathophysiology Review

Gastroenteritis is a very common health problem worldwide that causes diarrhea and/or vomiting related to ***inflammation*** of the mucous membranes of the stomach and intestinal tract. The small

TABLE 52.1 Common Types of Gastroenteritis and Their Characteristics

Type	Characteristics
Viral Gastroenteritis	
Epidemic viral	Caused by many parvovirus-type organisms Transmitted by the fecal-oral route in food and water Incubation period 10-51 hr Communicable during acute illness
Norovirus (Norwalk viruses)	Transmitted by the fecal-oral route and possibly the respiratory route (vomitus) Incubation in 48 hr Affects adults of all ages Older adults can become hypovolemic and experience electrolyte imbalances
Bacterial Gastroenteritis	
Campylobacter enteritis	Transmitted by the fecal-oral route or contact with infected animals or infants Incubation period 1-10 days Communicable for 2-7 wk
Escherichia coli diarrhea	Transmitted by fecal contamination of food, water, or fomites
Shigellosis	Transmitted by direct and indirect fecal-oral routes Incubation period 1-7 days Communicable during the acute illness to 4 wk after the illness Humans possibly carriers for months

bowel is most commonly affected and can be caused by either viral (more common) or bacterial ***infection***. Table 52.1 lists common types of gastroenteritis and their primary characteristics.

Norovirus (also known as a *Norwalk-like virus*) is the leading foodborne disease that causes gastroenteritis. It occurs most often between November and April because it is resistant to low temperatures and has a long viral shedding before and after the illness. Norovirus is transmitted (spread) through the fecal-oral route from person to person and from contaminated food and water. Infected individuals can also contaminate surfaces and objects in the environment. Vomiting may cause the virus to become airborne. The incubation time is 1 to 2 days (McCance et al., 2019).

In most cases of gastroenteritis, the illness is self-limiting and lasts about 3 days. However, in those who are immunosuppressed or in older adults, dehydration and hypovolemia can occur as complications requiring medical attention and possibly hospitalization.

Health Promotion and Maintenance. Outbreaks of norovirus have occurred in prisons, on cruise ships, and in nursing homes, college dormitories, and other places where large groups of people are in close proximity. Teach individuals that handwashing and sanitizing surfaces and other environmental items help prevent the spread of the illness. Hand sanitizers are often placed in public areas so that hands can be cleaned when washing with soap and water is inconvenient. Proper food and beverage preparation is also important to prevent contamination.

❖ Interprofessional Collaborative Care

Patients with gastroenteritis are generally cared for in the community setting and self-manage at home. Those who develop the more severe types of this condition or become extremely dehydrated during its course may be hospitalized.

◆ **Assessment: Recognize Cues.** The patient history can provide information related to the potential cause of the illness. Ask about recent travel, especially to tropical regions of Asia, Africa, Mexico, or Central or South America, because these areas historically have been a source of gastroenteritis. Inquire if the patient has eaten at any restaurant in the past 24 to 36 hours. Some people acquire gastroenteritis from eating in "fast-food" restaurants or from food items purchased at a farmer's market or grocery store. Bacterial infections have caused large outbreaks that resulted from contaminated spinach and lettuce in the United States. Raw or undercooked food such as oysters, sushi, and rare meat can also cause GI infections.

The patient who has gastroenteritis usually looks ill. Nausea and vomiting typically occur first, followed by abdominal cramping and diarrhea. For patients who are older or for those who have inadequate immune systems, weakness and cardiac dysrhythmias may occur from loss of potassium (hypokalemia) from diarrhea. Monitor for and document manifestations of hypokalemia and hypovolemia (dehydration).

! NURSING SAFETY PRIORITY (QSEN)

Action Alert

For patients with gastroenteritis, note any abdominal distention and listen for hyperactive bowel sounds. Depending on the amount of fluids and electrolytes lost through diarrhea and vomiting, patients may have varying degrees of dehydration manifested by:

- Weight loss (unintentional)
- Poor skin turgor
- Fever (not common in older adults)
- Dry mucous membranes
- Orthostatic blood pressure changes (which can cause a fall, especially for older adults)
- Hypotension
- Oliguria (decreased or absent urinary output)

In some cases, dehydration may be severe. It can occur very rapidly in older adults. Monitor mental status changes, such as acute confusion, that result from hypoxia due to dehydration in the older adult. These changes may be the only initial signs and symptoms of dehydration in older adults.

◆ **Interventions: Take Action.** For any type of gastroenteritis, encourage fluid replacement. The amount and route of fluid administration are determined by the patient's hydration status and overall health condition. Teach patients to drink extra fluids to replace fluid lost through vomiting and diarrhea. Oral rehydration therapy (ORT) may be needed for some patients to replace fluids and electrolytes. Examples of ORT solutions include sports drinks and Pedialyte. Depending on the patient's age and severity of dehydration, he or she may be treated in the hospital with IV fluids to restore hydration.

Drugs that suppress intestinal motility may not be given for bacterial or viral gastroenteritis. *Use of these drugs can prevent the infecting organisms from being eliminated from the body.* If the primary health care provider determines that antiperistaltic/antidiarrheal agents are necessary, loperamide may be recommended.

! NURSING SAFETY PRIORITY (QSEN)

Drug Alert

Diphenoxylate hydrochloride with atropine sulfate reduces GI motility but is used sparingly because of its habit-forming ability. *The drug should not be used for older adults because it also causes drowsiness and could contribute to falls.*

Treatment with antibiotics may be needed if the gastroenteritis is caused by bacterial ***infection*** with fever and severe diarrhea. Depending on the type and severity of the illness, examples of drugs that may be prescribed include ciprofloxacin or azithromycin. If the gastroenteritis is caused by shigellosis, anti-infective agents such as ciprofloxacin, ceftriaxone, or azithromycin are prescribed (Burchum & Rosenthal, 2019).

Frequent stools that are rich in electrolytes and enzymes and frequent wiping and washing of the anal region can irritate the skin. Teach the patient to avoid toilet paper and harsh soaps. Ideally, he or she can gently clean the area with warm water or an absorbent material, followed by thorough but gentle drying. Cream, oil, or gel can be applied to a damp, warm washcloth to remove stool that sticks to open skin. Special prepared skin wipes can also be used. Protective barrier cream can be applied to the skin between stools. Sitz baths for 10 minutes two or three times daily can also relieve discomfort.

If leakage of stool is a problem, the patient can use an absorbent cotton or panty liner and keep it in place with snug underwear. For patients who are incontinent, the use of incontinent pads at night instead of briefs allows air to circulate to the skin and prevents irritation. Remind assistive personnel to keep the perineal and buttock areas clean and dry and that frequent changes will be necessary.

During the acute phase of the illness, teach the patient and family about the importance of fluid replacement. Patient and family education regarding risk for transmission of gastroenteritis is also important (see the Patient and Family Education: Preparing for Self-Management: Preventing Transmission of Gastroenteritis box).

PATIENT AND FAMILY EDUCATION: PREPARING FOR SELF-MANAGEMENT

Preventing Transmission of Gastroenteritis

Advise the patient to:

- Wash hands well for at least 30 seconds with an antibacterial soap, especially after a bowel movement, and maintain good personal hygiene.
- Restrict the use of glasses, dishes, eating utensils, and tubes of toothpaste for his or her own use. In severe cases, disposable utensils may be used.
- Maintain clean bathroom facilities to avoid exposure to stool.
- Inform the primary health care provider if symptoms persist beyond 3 days.
- Do not prepare or handle food that will be consumed by others. If you (the patient) are employed as a food handler, the public health department should be consulted for recommendations about the return to work.

TABLE 52.2 Differential Features of Ulcerative Colitis and Crohn's Disease

Feature	Ulcerative Colitis	Crohn's Disease
Location	Begins in the rectum and proceeds in a continuous manner toward the cecum	Most often in the terminal ileum, with patchy involvement through all layers of the bowel
Etiology	Unknown	Unknown
Peak incidence at age	15-25 yr and 55-65 yr	15-40 yr
Number of stools	10-20 liquid, bloody stools per day	5-6 soft, loose stools per day, nonbloody
Complications	Hemorrhage Nutritional deficiencies	Fistulas (common) Nutritional deficiencies
Client need for surgery	20%-40%	75%

INFLAMMATION CONCEPT EXEMPLAR: ULCERATIVE COLITIS

Pathophysiology Review

Ulcerative colitis (UC) is a disease that creates widespread chronic ***inflammation*** of the rectum and rectosigmoid colon but can extend to the entire colon when the disease is extensive. Distribution of the disease can remain constant for years. UC is a disease that is associated with periodic remissions and exacerbations (flare-ups) and is often confused with Crohn's disease. Comparisons and differences are listed in Table 52.2.

Many factors can cause exacerbations, including intestinal ***infection***. Most patients who are affected have mild-to-moderate disease, but a small percentage of patients present with severe symptoms. Older adults with UC are at high risk for impaired ***fluid and electrolyte balance*** as a result of diarrhea, including dehydration and hypokalemia (McCance et al., 2019).

The intestinal mucosa becomes hyperemic (has increased blood flow), edematous, and reddened. In more severe inflammation, the lining can bleed and small erosions, or ulcers, occur. Abscesses can form in these ulcerative areas and result in tissue necrosis (cell death). Continued edema and mucosal thickening can lead to a narrowed colon and possibly a partial bowel obstruction. Table 52.3 lists the categories of the severity of UC.

The patient's stool typically contains blood and mucus. Patients report tenesmus (an unpleasant and urgent sensation to defecate) and lower abdominal colicky pain relieved with defecation. Malaise, anorexia, anemia, dehydration, fever, and weight loss are common. Extraintestinal manifestations such as migratory polyarthritis, ankylosing spondylitis, and erythema nodosum are present in a large number of patients. The common and extraintestinal complications of UC are listed in Table 52.4.

Etiology and Genetic Risk. The exact cause of UC is unknown, but a combination of genetic, immunologic, and environmental factors likely contributes to disease development. A genetic

TABLE 52.3 American College of Gastroenterologists Classification of Ulcerative Colitis Severity

Severity	Stool Frequency	Signs/Symptoms
Mild	<4 stools/day with/without blood	Asymptomatic Laboratory values usually normal
Moderate	>4 stools/day with/without blood	Minimal symptoms Mild abdominal pain Mild intermittent nausea Possible increased C-reactive protein[a] or ESR[b]
Severe	>6 bloody stools/day	Fever Tachycardia Anemia Abdominal pain Elevated C-reactive protein[a] and/or ESR[b]
Fulminant	>10 bloody stools/day	Increasing symptoms Anemia may require transfusion Colonic distention on x-ray

UC, Ulcerative colitis.
[a]C-reactive protein is a sensitive acute-phase serum marker that is evident in the first 6 hours of an inflammatory process.
[b]*ESR,* erythrocyte sedimentation rate; may be helpful but is less sensitive than C-reactive protein.

TABLE 52.4 Complications of Ulcerative Colitis and Crohn's Disease

Complication	Description
Hemorrhage/perforation	Lower GI bleeding results from erosion of the bowel wall.
Abscess formation	Localized pockets of ***infection*** develop in the ulcerated bowel lining.
Toxic megacolon	Massive dilation of the colon and subsequent colonic ileus that can lead to gangrene and peritonitis.
Intestinal malabsorption	Essential nutrients cannot be absorbed through the diseased intestinal wall, causing anemia and malnutrition (most common in Crohn's disease).
Nonmechanical bowel obstruction	Obstruction results from toxic megacolon or cancer.
Fistulas	In Crohn's disease in which the ***inflammation*** is transmural, fistulas can occur anywhere but usually track between the bowel and bladder, resulting in pyuria and fecaluria.
Colorectal cancer	Patients with ulcerative colitis with a history longer than 10 years have a high risk for colorectal cancer. This complication accounts for about one-third of all deaths related to ulcerative colitis.
Extraintestinal complications	Complications include arthritis, hepatic and biliary disease (especially cholelithiasis), oral and skin lesions, and ocular disorders, such as iritis. The cause is unknown.
Osteoporosis	Osteoporosis occurs, especially in patients with Crohn's disease.

basis of the disease has been supported because it is often found in families and twins. Immunologic causes, including autoimmune dysfunction, are likely the etiology of extraintestinal manifestations of the disease. Epithelial antibodies in the immunoglobulin G (IgG) class have been identified in the blood of some patients with UC (McCance et al., 2019).

With long-term disease, cellular changes can occur that increase the risk for colon cancer. Damage from proinflammatory cytokines, such as specific interleukins (ILs) (e.g., IL-1, IL-6, IL-8) and tumor necrosis factor (TNF)–alpha, have cytotoxic effects on the colonic mucosa (McCance et al., 2019).

PATIENT-CENTERED CARE: CULTURAL/SPIRITUAL CONSIDERATIONS QSEN

Ulcerative colitis is more common among Askenazki Jewish individuals than among those who are not Jewish and among whites more than non-whites (McCance et al., 2019). The reasons for these cultural differences are not known.

Incidence and Prevalence. In the United States, 1.6 million individuals are affected by chronic inflammatory bowel disease (IBD). Between the two primary types of IBD, ulcerative colitis (UC) and Crohn's disease (discussed later), the incidence is split almost equally. Although diagnosis can occur at any age, most people are diagnosed between 15 and 35 years of age (Crohn's & Colitis Foundation, 2020). Women are more often affected than men in their younger years, but men have the disease more often as middle-age and older adults (McCance et al., 2019).

❖ Interprofessional Collaborative Care

Patients with UC may be self-managed at home, cared for in the community setting, or hospitalized, depending on their immediate condition related to this chronic bowel disease.

◆ Assessment: Recognize Cues

History. Collect data on family history of IBD, previous and current therapy for the illness, and dates and types of surgery. Obtain a ***nutrition*** history, including intolerance of milk and milk products and fried, spicy, or hot foods. Ask about usual bowel ***elimination*** pattern (color, number, consistency, and character of stools); abdominal pain; tenesmus; anorexia; and fatigue. Note any relationship between diarrhea, timing of meals, emotional distress, and activity. Inquire about recent (past 2 to 3 months) exposure to antibiotics to rule out a *Clostridium difficile* infection. Has the patient traveled to or emigrated from tropical areas? Ask about recent use of NSAIDs because these can cause a flare-up of the disease. Inquire about any extraintestinal symptoms, such as arthritis, mouth sores, vision problems, and skin disorders.

Physical Assessment/Signs and Symptoms. Symptoms vary with an acuteness of onset. Vital signs are usually within normal limits in mild disease. In more severe cases, the patient may have a low-grade fever (99° to 100° F [37.2° to 37.8° C]). The physical assessment findings are usually nonspecific, and in milder cases the physical examination may be normal. Viral and bacterial infections can cause symptoms similar to those of UC.

Note any abdominal distention along the colon. Fever associated with tachycardia may indicate dehydration, peritonitis, and bowel perforation. Assess for signs and symptoms associated with extraintestinal complications, such as inflamed joints and lesions inside the mouth.

Psychosocial Assessment. Many patients are very concerned about the frequency of stools and the presence of blood. *The inability to control the disease symptoms, particularly diarrhea, can be disruptive and anxiety producing.* Severe illness may limit the patient's activities outside the home with fear of fecal incontinence resulting in feeling "tied to the toilet." Severe anxiety and depression may result. Eating may be associated with pain and cramping and an increased frequency of stools. This can make mealtimes an unpleasant experience. Frequent visits to primary health care providers and close monitoring of the colon mucosa for abnormal cell changes can be anxiety provoking.

Assess the patient's understanding of the illness and its impact on his or her lifestyle. Encourage and support the patient while exploring:

- The relationship of life events to disease exacerbations
- Stress factors that produce symptoms
- Family and social support systems
- Concerns regarding the possible genetic basis and associated cancer risks of the disease
- Internet access for reliable education information

Laboratory Assessment. Hematocrit and hemoglobin levels may be low related to chronic blood loss, which indicates anemia and a chronic disease state. *An increased WBC count, C-reactive protein, or erythrocyte sedimentation rate (ESR) is consistent with inflammatory disease.* Blood levels of sodium, potassium, and chloride may be *low* as a result of frequent diarrheal stools and malabsorption through the diseased bowel (Pagana & Pagana, 2018). Hypoalbuminemia (decreased serum albumin) is found in patients with extensive disease from losing protein in the stool.

Other Diagnostic Assessment. *Magnetic resonance enterography (MRE)* is the main examination used to study the bowel in patients who have chronic IBD. An MRE allows the primary health care provider to visualize the bowel lumen and wall, mesentery, and surrounding abdominal organs. Teach the patient that he or she will need to fast for 4 to 6 hours before the test. As part of the test the patient drinks a large amount of contrast medium; this can cause abdominal discomfort and diarrhea. Be sure that the patient has the opportunity to go to the restroom before positioning on the MRI table. The patient then lies prone while the first of two doses of glucagon are given subcutaneously. This substance helps to slow the bowel's activity and motility (Khatri et al., 2018).

An upper endoscopy and/or *colonoscopy* may be done to aid in diagnosis, but the bowel preparation ("prep") can be especially uncomfortable for patients with inflammatory bowel disease (IBD). Frequent colonoscopies are recommended when patients have longer than a 10-year history of UC involving the entire colon because they are at high risk for colorectal cancer. In some cases, a *CT scan* may be done to confirm the disease or its complications. *Barium enemas* with air contrast can show differences between UC and Crohn's disease and identify complications, mucosal patterns, and the distribution and depth of disease involvement. In early disease, the barium enema may show incomplete filling as a result of ***inflammation*** and fine ulcerations along the bowel contour, which appear deeper in more advanced disease.

◆ Analysis: Analyze Cues and Prioritize Hypotheses.

The priority collaborative problems for patients with UC include:

1. Diarrhea due to ***inflammation*** of the bowel mucosa
2. Acute or persistent ***pain*** due to ***inflammation*** and ulceration of the bowel mucosa and skin irritation
3. Potential for lower GI bleeding and resulting anemia due to UC

◆ Planning and Implementation: Generate Solutions and Take Action

Managing Diarrhea

Planning: Expected Outcomes. The major concern for a patient with ulcerative colitis is the occurrence of frequent, bloody diarrhea and fecal incontinence from tenesmus. Therefore the expected outcome of treatment is for the patient to have decreased diarrhea, formed stools, and control of bowel movements, which allow for mucosal healing.

Interventions. Many measures are used to relieve symptoms and reduce intestinal motility, decrease ***inflammation,*** and promote intestinal healing. Nonsurgical and/or surgical management may be needed.

Nonsurgical Management. Nonsurgical management includes drug and ***nutrition*** therapy. The use of physical and emotional rest is also an important consideration. Teach the patient to record color, volume, frequency, and consistency of stools, either on paper or via an electronic app, to determine severity of the problem.

Monitor the skin in the perianal area for irritation and ulceration resulting from loose, frequent stools. Stool cultures may be sent for analysis if diarrhea continues. Have the patient record their weight one or two times per week. If the patient is hospitalized, remind assistive personnel to weigh him or her on admission and daily in the morning using the same scale before breakfast and document all weights.

NCLEX EXAMINATION CHALLENGE 52.2

Physiological Integrity

The nurse is caring for an older adult client who experiences an exacerbation of ulcerative colitis with severe diarrhea and rectal bleeding that have lasted a week. For which complication(s) will the nurse assess? **Select all that apply.**

A. Increased BUN
B. Hypokalemia
C. Leukocytosis
D. Anemia
E. Hyponatremia

Drug therapy. Common drug therapy for UC includes aminosalicylates, glucocorticoids, antidiarrheal drugs, and immunomodulators. Teach patients about side effects and adverse drug events (ADEs) and when to call their primary health care provider.

The *aminosalicylates* are drugs commonly used to treat mild-to-moderate UC and/or maintain remission. Several aminosalicylic acid compounds are available. These drugs, also called *5-ASAs,* are thought to have an anti-inflammatory effect on the lining of the intestine by inhibiting prostaglandins and are usually effective in 2 to 4 weeks.

Sulfasalazine, the first aminosalicylate approved for UC, is metabolized by the intestinal bacteria into 5-ASA, which delivers the beneficial effects of the drug, and sulfapyridine, which is responsible for unwanted side effects. Teach patients to take a folic acid supplement because sulfasalazine decreases its absorption (Burchum & Rosenthal, 2019).

! NURSING SAFETY PRIORITY (QSEN)

Drug Alert

Teach patients taking sulfasalazine to report nausea, vomiting, anorexia, rash, and headache to the health care provider. With higher doses, hemolytic anemia, hepatitis, male infertility, or agranulocytosis can occur. This drug is in the same family as sulfonamide antibiotics. *Therefore, assess the patient for an allergy to sulfonamide or other drugs that contain sulfa before the patient takes the drug.* The use of a thiazide diuretic may be a contraindication for sulfasalazine (Burchum & Rosenthal, 2019).

Mesalamine is better tolerated than sulfasalazine because none of its preparations contain sulfapyridine. It may be given as a delayed-release drug in the terminal ileum and beyond within the colon, or as an extended-release drug that works throughout the colon and rectum. Mesalamine can also be given as an enema or a suppository. These preparations have minimal systemic absorption and therefore have fewer side effects (Crohn's and Colitis Foundation, 2020).

Glucocorticoids, such as prednisone and prednisolone, are corticosteroid therapies that may be prescribed during exacerbations of the disease. Prednisone is typically prescribed, and the dose may be increased as acute flare-ups occur. Once clinical improvement occurs, the corticosteroids are tapered because of the adverse effects that commonly occur with long-term steroid therapy (e.g., hyperglycemia, osteoporosis, peptic ulcer disease, increased potential for infection, adrenal insufficiency). For patients with rectal ***inflammation,*** topical steroids in the form of small retention enemas or suppositories may be prescribed. Medications such as budesonide, steroids that are thought to work mostly in the bowel, produce fewer systemic side effects (Burchum & Rosenthal, 2019).

To provide symptomatic management of diarrhea, *antidiarrheal drugs* may be prescribed. However, these drugs are given very cautiously because they can cause colon dilation and toxic megacolon (massive dilation of the colon and subsequent colonic ileus that can lead to gangrene and peritonitis). Common antidiarrheal drugs include diphenoxylate hydrochloride and atropine sulfate and loperamide.

Immunomodulators are drugs that alter an individual's immune response. Alone, they are often not effective in the treatment of UC. However, in combination with steroids, they may offer a synergistic effect to a quicker response, thereby decreasing the amount of steroids needed. Biologic response modifiers (BRMs) used for UC (and Crohn's disease, discussed later in this chapter) include infliximab and adalimumab (Humira). Although not approved as a first-line therapy for UC, infliximab may be used for refractory disease or for severe complications, such as toxic megacolon and extraintestinal manifestations. Infliximab is an immunoglobulin G (IgG) monoclonal antibody that reduces the activity of tumor necrosis factor (TNF) to decrease ***inflammation.*** Adalimumab is another monoclonal antibody approved for refractory (not responsive to other therapies) cases. BRMs are used more commonly in management of Crohn's disease. These drugs cause immunosuppression and should be used with caution. Teach the patient to report any signs of a beginning ***infection,*** including a cold, and to avoid large crowds or others who are sick.

Several newer monoclonal antibodies have recently been approved by the U.S. Food and Drug Administration (FDA) for use in patients with chronic IBD. One of these drugs, vedolizumab, is an intestinal-specific leukocyte traffic inhibitor in that it prevents white blood cells from migrating to inflamed bowel tissue (Engel et al., 2018)).

Nutrition therapy and rest. Patients with severe symptoms who are hospitalized are kept NPO to ensure bowel rest. The primary health care provider may prescribe total parenteral ***nutrition*** (TPN) for severely ill and malnourished patients during severe exacerbations. Chapter 55 describes this therapy in detail. Patients with less severe symptoms may drink elemental formulas, which have components that are absorbed in the small bowel and reduce bowel stimulation.

Diet is not a major factor in the inflammatory process, but some patients with ulcerative colitis (UC) find that caffeine and alcohol increase diarrhea and cramping. For some patients, raw vegetables and other high-fiber foods can cause GI symptoms. Lactose-containing foods may be poorly tolerated and should be reduced or eliminated. Teach patients that carbonated beverages, pepper, nuts and corn, dried fruits, and smoking are common GI stimulants that could cause discomfort. Each patient differs in his or her food and fluid tolerances.

During an exacerbation of the disease, patient activity is generally restricted because rest can reduce intestinal activity, provide comfort, and promote healing. Ensure that the patient has easy access to a bedpan, bedside commode, or bathroom in case of urgency or tenesmus.

Complementary and integrative health. In addition to dietary changes, complementary and integrative therapies may be used to supplement traditional management of UC. Examples include herbs (e.g., flaxseed), selenium, and vitamin C. Biofeedback, hypnosis, yoga, acupuncture, and ayurveda (a combination of diet, yoga, herbs, and breathing exercises) may be helpful. These therapies need further study to validate their effectiveness, but some patients find them helpful.

Surgical Management. Some patients with UC require surgery to help manage their disease when medical therapies alone are not effective. In some cases, surgery is performed for complications of UC such as toxic megacolon, hemorrhage, bowel perforation, dysplastic biopsy results, and colon cancer.

Preoperative care. General preoperative teaching related to abdominal surgery is described in Chapter 9. If a temporary or permanent ileostomy is planned, provide an in-depth explanation to the patient and family. An ileostomy is a procedure in which a loop of the ileum is placed through an opening in the abdominal wall (stoma) for drainage of fecal material into a pouching system worn on the abdomen. This *external* pouching system consists of a solid skin barrier (wafer) to protect the skin and a fecal collection device (pouch), similar to the system used for patients with colostomies (discussed in Chapter 51).

If an ileostomy is planned, the surgeon consults with a certified wound, ostomy, continence nurse (CWOCN) before surgery for recommendations on the best location of the stoma. A visit before surgery from an **ostomate** (a patient with an ostomy) may be helpful.

> **! NATIONAL PATIENT SAFETY GOALS (QSEN)**
>
> *Parenteral antibiotics are given 1 hour before surgical opening based on current best evidence.*

Operative procedures. Any one of several surgical approaches may be used for the patient with UC. Minimally invasive procedures, such as laparoscopic, laparoscopic-assisted, hand-assisted, and robotic-assisted surgery, are common for patients with UC in large tertiary care centers (Valente & Hull, 2018). Laparoscopic surgery usually involves one or several small incisions but often takes longer to perform than the open surgical approach. The natural orifice transluminal endoscopic surgery (NOTES) procedure can be performed via the anus or vagina for certain patients. The availability of this type of procedure depends greatly on the training of the surgeon. Patients may have moderate sedation or general anesthesia for minimally invasive surgical procedures. These patients are *not* typically admitted to critical care units for continuing postoperative care.

Patients who are obese, have had previous abdominal surgeries, or have dense scar tissue (adhesions) may not be candidates for laparoscopic procedures. A conventional open surgical approach involves general anesthesia and an abdominal incision. Patients with open procedures are initially admitted to critical care units for short-term stabilization.

Restorative proctocolectomy with ileo pouch–anal anastomosis (RPC-IPAA). This procedure has become the gold standard for patients with UC. In some centers, the surgery is performed via laparoscopy (laparoscopic RPC-IPAA). Typically, it is a two-stage procedure that includes the removal of the colon and most of the rectum (Fig. 52.2); the anus and anal sphincter remain intact. The surgeon then surgically creates an *internal* pouch (reservoir) using the last 1½ feet of the small intestine. The ileo-anal pouch, sometimes called a *J-pouch, S-pouch,* or *pelvic pouch,* is then connected to the anus. A *temporary* ileostomy through the abdominal skin is created to allow healing of the internal pouch and all anastomosis sites. It also allows for an increase in the capacity of the internal pouch. In the *second* surgical stage, the temporary loop ileostomy is closed. The time interval between the first and second stages varies, but many patients have the second surgical stage to close the ileostomy within 1 to 2 months of the first surgery.

Usually bowel continence is excellent after this procedure, but some patients report leakage of stool during sleep. They may take antidiarrheal drugs to help control this problem. Reassure the patient that they might have frequent stools and urgency after this procedure.

Total proctocolectomy with a permanent ileostomy. Total proctocolectomy with a *permanent* ileostomy is done for patients who are not candidates for or do not want the ileo-anal pouch. The procedure involves the removal of the colon, rectum, and anus with surgical closure of the anus (Fig. 52.3A). The surgeon brings the end of the ileum out through the abdominal wall and forms a stoma, or permanent ostomy.

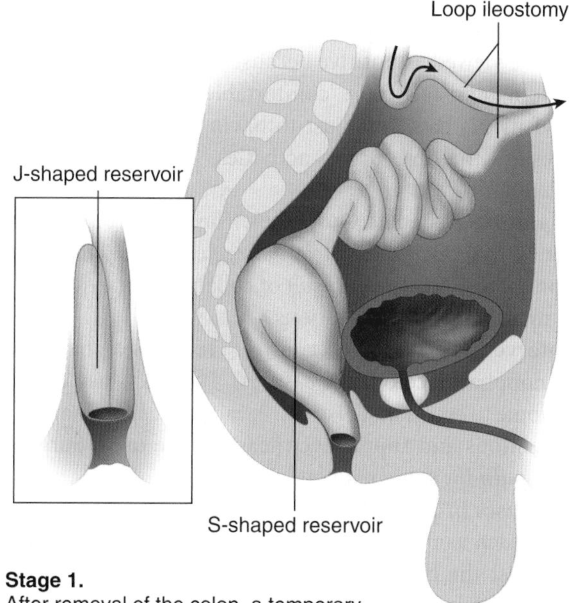

Stage 1.
After removal of the colon, a temporary loop ileostomy is created, and an ileo-anal reservoir is formed. The reservoir is created in an S-shaped reservoir (using three loops of ileum) or a J-shaped reservoir (suturing a portion of ileum to the rectal cuff, with an upward loop).

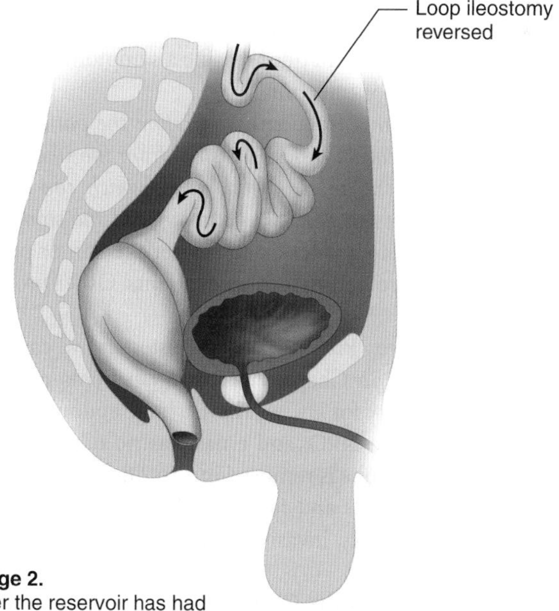

Stage 2.
After the reservoir has had time to heal—usually several months—the temporary loop ileostomy is reversed, and stool is allowed to drain into the reservoir.

Fig. 52.2 Creation of an ileo-anal reservoir.

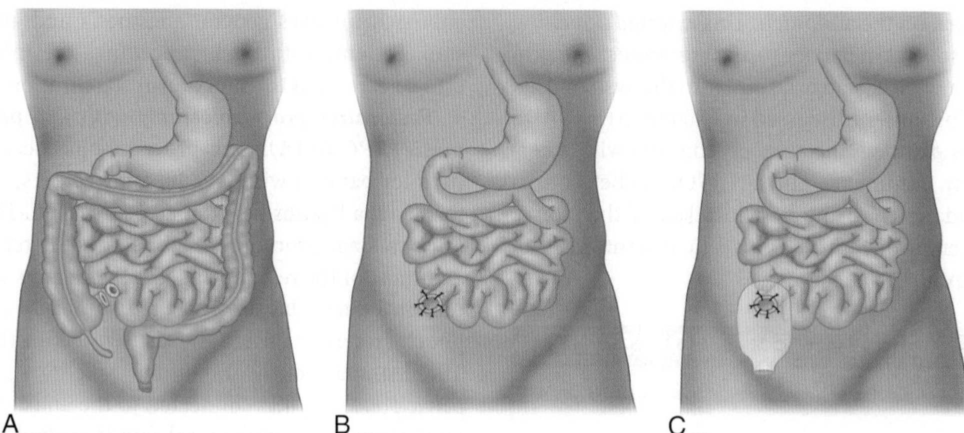

Fig 52.3 (A) Total proctocolectomy with a permanent ileostomy. This involved removal of the colon, the rectum, and the anus with closure of the anus. (B) Ileostomy surgical stoma placement. (C) Ileostomy with ostomy appliance attached.

! NURSING SAFETY PRIORITY QSEN

Critical Rescue

The ileostomy stoma (Fig. 52.3B) is usually placed in the right lower quadrant of the abdomen below the belt line. It should not be prolapsed or retract into the abdominal wall. *Assess the stoma frequently after stoma placement. Recognize that it should be pinkish to cherry red to ensure an adequate blood supply. If the stoma looks pale, bluish, or dark, respond by reporting these findings to the surgeon immediately (Stelton, 2019)!*

Initially after surgery, the output from an ileostomy is a loose, dark green liquid that may contain some blood. Over time, a process called *ileostomy adaptation* occurs. The small intestine begins to perform some of the functions that had previously been done by the colon, including the absorption of increased amounts of sodium and water. Stool volume decreases, becomes thicker (paste-like), and turns yellow-green or yellow-brown. The **effluent** (fluid material) usually has little odor or a sweet odor. Any foul or unpleasant odor may be a symptom of a problem such as blockage or infection.

The ileostomy drains frequently. *Therefore the patient must wear a pouch system at all times. The stool from the small intestine contains many enzymes and bile salts, which can quickly irritate and excoriate the skin. Skin care around the stoma is a priority!* A pouch system with a skin barrier (gelatin or pectin) provides sufficient protection for most patients. Other products are also available.

Postoperative care. Provide general postoperative care after surgery, as described in Chapter 9. The few patients requiring open-approach surgery for UC will have a large abdominal incision. Initially, they are NPO, and a nasogastric tube (NGT) is used for suction. The tube is removed in 1 to 2 days as the drainage decreases, and fluids and food are slowly introduced. The patient having minimally invasive surgery (MIS) usually does *not* have an NGT.

In collaboration with the CWOCN, help the patient adjust and learn the required care. The ileostomy usually begins to drain stool within 24 hours after surgery at more than 1 L/day. Be sure that fluids are replaced by adding 500 mL or more each day to prevent dehydration. After about a week of high-volume output, the stool drainage slows and becomes thicker. During this period, some patients need antidiarrheal drugs.

The hospital stay is usually from 1 to 4 days, depending on whether the patient has laparoscopic or conventional open surgery. Patients having MIS have less pain from surgery, fewer complications, and faster restoration of bowel function when compared with other surgical patients (Valente & Hull, 2018).

For those who have the RPC-IPAA procedure, remind them that the internal pouch can become inflamed (pouchitis). This problem is usually treated effectively with metronidazole for 7 to 10 days. Teach patients that, after the second stage of surgery, they might have burning during bowel ***elimination*** because gastric acid cannot be absorbed well by the ileum. Also, instruct them to omit foods that can cause odors or gas, such as cabbage, asparagus, brussels sprouts, and beans. Teach patients to eliminate foods that cannot be digested well, such as nuts and corn. Each patient differs in which foods he or she can tolerate.

Surgery for UC may result in altered body image. However, it may be viewed as positive because the patient will have fewer symptoms and feel more comfortable than before the procedure. Patients have to adjust to having an ostomy before they can resume their presurgery activities.

Managing Pain

Planning: Expected Outcomes. The desired outcome for the patient is that he or she will verbalize decreased ***pain*** at 2 to 3 or less on a 0 to 10 scale as a result of collaborative, evidence-based pain management interventions.

Interventions. ***Pain*** control requires pharmacologic and nonpharmacologic measures. Physical discomfort can contribute to emotional distress. A variety of symptom-reducing interventions and supportive measures are used. Surgery may reduce ***pain*** for some patients.

Increases in pain may indicate the development of complications such as **peritonitis** (see earlier discussion in this chapter). Assist the patient in reducing or eliminating factors that can cause or increase the ***pain*** experience. For example, he or she may benefit from ***nutrition*** changes to decrease abdominal discomfort such as cramping and bloating.

Antidiarrheal drugs may be needed to control diarrhea, thus reducing the discomfort. However, they must be used with caution and for a short time because toxic megacolon can develop.

Perineal skin can be irritated by contact with loose stools and frequent cleaning. Explain special measures for skin care. Use of medicated wipes is soothing if the rectal area is tender or sensitive from the use of toilet tissue. A number of ostomy manufacturers (e.g., Hollister, ConvaTec) produce a system for skin care that may help prevent and heal perineal skin irritation. These systems usually include a skin-cleaning solution, a moisturizing and healing cream, and a petroleum jelly–like barrier that prevents contact of moisture and stool with the skin.

Preventing or Monitoring for Lower GI Bleeding

Planning: Expected Outcomes. If possible, patients are expected to remain free of complications that can cause bleeding, such as perforation or anemia. For the patient experiencing lower GI bleeding, he or she is expected to have a cessation of bleeding with prompt collaborative care.

Interventions. The nursing priority is to monitor the patient closely for signs and symptoms of GI bleeding resulting from the disease or its complications. If the patient has lower GI bleeding of more than 0.5 mL/min, a *GI bleeding scan* may be useful to localize the site of the bleeding (Pagana & Pagana, 2018). However, this test cannot indicate the cause of the bleeding and may take several hours to administer. Patients in the critical care unit are not candidates for the test because they must leave the unit for it. *Keep in mind that GI bleeding is considered a medical emergency; therefore the patient should be monitored closely to prevent complications!*

! NURSING SAFETY PRIORITY QSEN

Critical Rescue

Recognize that it is important to monitor stools for blood loss for the patient with ulcerative colitis. The blood may be bright red (frank bleeding) or black and tarry (melena). Monitor hematocrit, hemoglobin, and electrolyte values and assess vital signs. Prolonged slow bleeding can lead to anemia. Observe for fever, tachycardia, and signs of fluid volume depletion. Changes in mental status may occur, especially among older adults, and may be the first indication of dehydration or anemia.

If symptoms of GI bleeding begin, respond by notifying the Rapid Response Team or primary health care provider immediately. Blood products are often prescribed for patients with severe anemia. Prepare for the blood transfusion by inserting a large-bore IV catheter if it is not already in place. Chapter 37 outlines nursing actions during blood transfusion.

Care Coordination and Transition Management

Home Care Management. The patient with ulcerative colitis provides self-management at home but may require hospitalization during severe exacerbations or after surgical intervention. In addition, those who have extraintestinal problems often need ongoing collaborative care for joint and/or skin problems.

Home care management focuses on controlling signs and symptoms and monitoring for complications. For patients returning home or transferring to nursing home or transitional care after surgery, ongoing respiratory care, incision care (if applicable), ostomy care, and pain management should be continued.

Self-Management Education. Teach the patient about the nature of ulcerative colitis, including its acute episodes, remissions, and symptom management. Stress that even though the cause is unknown, relapses can be prevented with proper health care. Teach patients taking immunosuppressive drugs, such as corticosteroids and biologic response modifiers—more commonly known as *biologics* (monoclonal antibodies), to report signs of possible ***infection*** to the primary health care provider. Remind them to avoid crowds and anyone who has an infection. Review the purpose of drug therapy, when drugs should be taken, side effects, and adverse drug events.

Instruct the patient about measures to reduce or control abdominal ***pain,*** cramping, and diarrhea. Also teach the patient and family about symptoms associated with disease exacerbation that should be reported to the primary health care provider, such as fever higher than 101°F (38.3°C), tachycardia, palpitations, and an increase in diarrhea, severe abdominal ***pain***, or nausea/vomiting. Provide written information and contact numbers for the primary health care provider.

There is no special diet for a patient with an ileostomy. However, teach the patient to avoid any foods that cause gas. Examples include high-fiber foods such as nuts, raw cabbage, corn, celery, and popcorn. The patient needs to learn which foods he or she tolerates best and adjust the diet accordingly.

If the patient has undergone a temporary or permanent surgical diversion, collaborate with the CWOCN to explain and demonstrate required care so that the patient can self-manage or the family/caregiver can assist. Teach the importance of including adequate amounts of salt and water in the diet because the diversion can increase the loss of these substances. Urge the patient to be cautious in situations that lead to heavy sweating or fluid loss, such as strenuous physical activity, high environmental heat, and episodes of diarrhea and vomiting.

Finding the best ostomy pouching system is a major issue for many patients with an ileostomy. An effective system is one that:

- Protects the skin
- Contains the effluent (drainage) and reduces odor, if any
- Remains securely attached to the skin for a dependable period of time

Most patients desire an adhesive barrier that will last for 3 to 7 days. The barrier must create a solid seal to prevent the enzymes in the drainage from irritating the skin. Solid barriers are classified as "regular wear" or "extended wear." An adult with a high output may want an extended-wear barrier. A special cream can be used to help fill any uneven skin surfaces and provide a consistent seal. Pouches can also be individualized by the patient. Large pouches can hold more but are heavy when full. Patients also have to consider the costs of the various systems and if or how much their insurance will help pay for them. The Patient and Family Education: Preparing for Self-Management: Ileostomy Care box describes the main aspects of ileostomy care, including skin care.

A patient with an ileostomy may have many concerns about management at home and about sexual and social adjustments. Considering possible sexual issues helps the patient

PATIENT AND FAMILY EDUCATION: PREPARING FOR SELF-MANAGEMENT

Ileostomy Care

Skin Protection

- Use a skin barrier to protect your skin from contact with contents from the ostomy.
- Use skin-care products, such as skin sealants and ostomy skin creams. If your skin continues to be exposed to ostomy contents, select a product to fill in problem areas and provide an even skin surface.
- Watch your skin for any irritation or redness.

Pouch Care

- Empty your pouch when it is one-third to one-half full.
- Change the pouch during inactive times, such as before meals, before retiring at night, on waking in the morning, and 2 to 4 hours after eating.
- Change the entire pouch system every 3 to 7 days.

Nutrition

- Chew food thoroughly.
- Be cautious about high-fiber and high-cellulose foods. You may need to eliminate these from the diet if they cause severe problems (diarrhea, constipation, or blockage). Examples include coconut, popcorn, tough-fiber meats, rice, cabbage, and vegetables with skins (tomatoes, corn, and peas).

Drug Therapy

- Avoid taking enteric-coated and capsule medications.
- Inform any primary health care provider who is prescribing medications for you that you have an ostomy. Before having prescriptions filled, inform your pharmacist that you have an ostomy.
- Do not take any laxative or enemas. You should usually have loose stool and should contact your primary health care provider if no stool has passed in 6 to 12 hours.

Symptoms to Watch

- Report any drastic increase or decrease in drainage to your primary health care provider.
- If stomal swelling, abdominal cramping, or distention occurs or if ileostomy contents stop draining:
  - Remove the pouch with faceplate.
  - Lie down, assuming a knee-chest position.
  - Begin abdominal massage.
  - Apply moist towels to the abdomen.
  - Drink hot tea.
- If none of these maneuvers is effective in resuming ileostomy flow or if abdominal pain is severe, call your primary health care provider right away.

identify and discuss these concerns with the sex partner. For example, a change in positioning during intercourse may alleviate apprehension. Social situations may cause anxiety related to decreased self-esteem and a disturbance in body image. Encourage the patient to discuss possible concerns in addressing and resolving these potentially stressful events. Clinical depression is common among patients with ulcerative colitis. Refer patients to appropriate mental health resources if depression is suspected.

Some hospitals provide community support groups for their patients with inflammatory bowel disease (IBD). These groups help patients and their families cope with the psychological impact of IBD and educate them about ***nutrition*** and complementary and integrative therapies.

HOME CARE CONSIDERATIONS

The Patient With Inflammatory Bowel Disease

Assess gastrointestinal function and nutritional status, including:

- Abdominal cramping or *pain*
- Bowel *elimination* pattern, specifically frequency, characteristics, and amount of stools and presence or absence of blood in stools
- Food and fluid intake (include relationship of specific foods to cramping and stools)
- Weight gain or loss
- Signs and symptoms of dehydration
- Presence or absence of fever, rectal tenesmus, or urgency
- Bowel sounds
- Condition of perianal skin, including presence or absence of perianal **fistula**, **fissure**, or **abscess**

Assess patient's and family's coping skills, including:

- Current and ongoing stress level and coping style
- Availability of support system

Assess home environment, including:

- Adequacy and availability of bathroom facilities
- Opportunity for rest and relaxation

Assess ability to self-manage therapeutic regimen, including:

- Drug therapy
- Signs and symptoms to report
- Nutrition therapy
- Availability of community resources
- Importance of follow-up care

Health Care Resources. If the patient needs assistance with self-management at home, collaborate with the case manager or social worker to arrange the services of a home care aide or nurse. A home care nurse can provide assessment and guidance in integrating ostomy care into the patient's lifestyle. The nurse may also teach about wound care, including monitoring wound healing, if needed (see the Home Care Considerations: The Patient With Inflammatory Bowel Disease box).

The patient and family need to know where to purchase ostomy supplies, along with the name, size, and manufacturer's order number.

For patients with a permanent ileostomy, locate a community ostomy support group by contacting the United Ostomy Associations of America (www.ostomy.org). The United Ostomy Association of Canada serves the needs of Canadian patients (www.ostomycanada.ca). A local support group or the Crohn's and Colitis Foundation of America (www.ccfa.org) may be helpful in obtaining supplies and providing education for ostomates. Inform the patient and family members of available ostomy ambulatory care clinics and ostomy specialists. If the patient agrees, a visit from an ostomate can be continued after discharge to home.

◆ **Evaluation: Evaluate Outcomes.** Evaluate the care of the patient with ulcerative colitis based on the identified priority patient problems. Expected outcomes may include that the patient will:

- Experience no diarrhea or a decrease in diarrheal episodes
- Verbalize decreased pain
- Have absence of lower GI bleeding
- Self-manage the ileostomy or ileo-anal pouch (temporary or permanent)

CROHN'S DISEASE

Pathophysiology Review

Crohn's disease (CD) is a chronic inflammatory disease of the small intestine (most often), the colon, or both. It can affect the GI tract from the mouth to the anus but most commonly affects the terminal ileum. CD is a slowly progressive and unpredictable disease with involvement of multiple regions of the intestine with normal sections in between (called *skip lesions* on x-rays). Like ulcerative colitis (UC), this disease is recurrent, with remissions and exacerbations.

CD presents as ***inflammation*** that causes a thickened bowel wall. Strictures and deep ulcerations (cobblestone appearance) also occur, which put the patient at risk for developing a bowel fistula (abnormal opening [tract] between two organs or structures). The result is severe diarrhea and malabsorption of vital nutrients. Anemia is common, usually from iron deficiency or malabsorption issues (McCance et al., 2019).

The complications associated with CD are similar to those of UC (see Table 52.4). Hemorrhage is more common in UC, but it can occur in CD as well. Severe malabsorption by the small intestine is more common in patients with CD versus UC that may not involve the small bowel to any significant extent. Patients with CD can become very malnourished and debilitated due to intestinal malabsorption of dietary nutrients.

Rarely, cancer of the small bowel and colon develop but can occur after the disease has been present for 15 to 20 years. Fistula formation is a common complication of CD but is rare in UC. Fistulas can occur between segments of the intestine or manifest as cutaneous fistulas (opening to the skin) or perirectal abscesses. They can also extend from the bowel to other organs and body cavities, such as the bladder or vagina (Fig. 52.4). Some patients develop intestinal obstruction, which at first is secondary to ***inflammation*** and edema. Over time, fibrosis and scar tissue develop and obstruction results from a narrowing of the bowel. Most patients with CD require surgery at some point. Chapter 51 ok discusses surgical procedures for intestinal obstruction.

Almost a million individuals in the United States have Crohn's disease, and Canada has one of the highest incidences of Crohn's disease and colitis worldwide (Crohn's and Colitis Canada, 2020). Most patients experience symptoms and are diagnosed as adolescents or young adults between 15 and 35 years of age (Crohn's and Colitis Foundation, 2020).

PATIENT-CENTERED CARE: GENETIC/GENOMIC CONSIDERATIONS (QSEN)

The exact cause of CD is unknown. A combination of genetic, immune, and environmental factors may contribute to its development. About 20% of patients have a positive family history for the disease (Cleynen et al., 2016). The discovery of a mutation in the *NOD2/CARD15* gene on chromosome 16 seems to be associated with some patients who have CD. This gene is found in monocytes that normally recognize and destroy bacteria.

Proinflammatory cytokines, such as tumor necrosis factor–alpha (TNF-alpha) and interleukins (ILs) (e.g., IL-6 and IL-8), are immunologic factors that contribute to the etiology of CD (McCance et al., 2019). Many of the drugs used for the disease inhibit or block one or more of these factors.

Other risk factors include tobacco use, Jewish ethnicity, and living in urban areas (McCance et al., 2019). CD is more common in individuals of Ashkenazi Jewish background than in any other group. Current research has found genetic markers in this population that contribute to higher rates of CD (Santos et al., 2018). It was once thought that stress and nutrition play a role in the development of CD, but these factors have not been proven. However, inadequate ***nutrition*** can exacerbate the patient's symptoms.

❖ Interprofessional Collaborative Care

Similar to patients with ulcerative colitis, patients with Crohn's disease may be self-managed at home, cared for in the community setting, or hospitalized depending on their immediate condition related to this chronic bowel disease.

◆ **Assessment: Recognize Cues.** Crohn's disease can be exacerbated by bacterial infection. A detailed history is needed to identify manifestations specific to the disease. Ask about recent unintentional weight loss, the frequency and consistency of stools, the presence of blood in the stool, fever, and abdominal pain.

Perform a thorough abdominal assessment. Assess for manifestations of the disease, and evaluate the patient's ***nutrition*** and hydration status.

When inspecting the abdomen, assess for distention, masses, or visible peristalsis. Inspection of the perianal area may reveal ulcerations, fissures, or fistulas. During auscultation, bowel sounds may be decreased or absent with severe ***inflammation*** or obstruction. An increase in high-pitched or rushing sounds

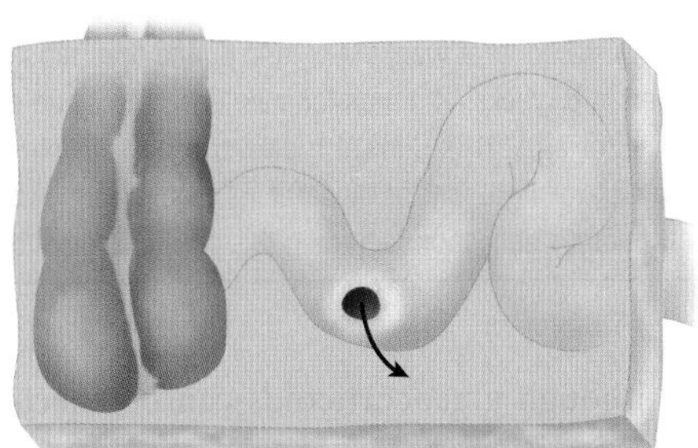

External enterocutaneous (between skin and intestine)

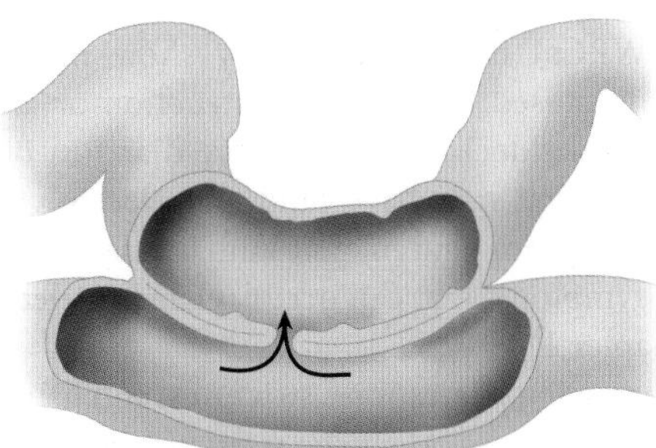

Enteroenteric (between intestine and intestine)

Fig. 52.4 Types of fistulas that are complications of Crohn's disease.

may be present over areas of narrowed bowel loops. Muscle guarding, masses, rigidity, or tenderness may be noted on palpation by the primary health care provider.

The signs and symptoms associated with Crohn's disease vary greatly from person to person. Most patients report diarrhea, abdominal ***pain,*** and low-grade fever. Fever is common with fistulas, abscesses, and severe inflammation. If the disease occurs in only the ileum, diarrhea occurs five or six times per day, often with a soft, loose stool. **Steatorrhea** (fatty diarrheal stools) is common. Stools may contain bright red blood (McCance et al., 2019).

Abdominal pain from ***inflammation*** is usually constant and often located in the right lower quadrant. The patient also may have pain around the umbilicus before and after bowel movements. If the lower colon is diseased, pain is common in both lower abdominal quadrants.

Most patients with Crohn's disease have *weight loss.* Nutritional problems are the result of increased catabolism from chronic inflammation, anorexia, malabsorption, or self-imposed dietary restrictions. These problems result in impaired ***fluid and electrolyte balance*** and vital nutrient deficiencies (see Chapter 13 for more information on fluids and electrolytes).

The patient who has Crohn's disease (CD) needs a complete psychosocial assessment. The chronic nature of the problem and the associated complications can greatly affect patients and their families. Lifestyle changes are necessary to cope with such a disruptive and painful chronic illness. Assess the patient's coping

> **! NURSING SAFETY PRIORITY QSEN**
>
> ***Action Alert***
>
> For the patient with Crohn's disease, be especially alert for signs and symptoms of **peritonitis** (discussed earlier in this chapter), small-bowel obstruction, and nutritional and fluid imbalances. Early detection of a change in the patient's status helps reduce these life-threatening complications.

skill and help identify support systems. Similar to problems associated with other chronic diseases, clinical depression and severe anxiety disorders are common among patients with CD.

Anemia is common as a result of slow bleeding and poor nutrition. Serum levels of folic acid and vitamin B_{12} are generally low because of malabsorption, further contributing to anemia. Amino acid malabsorption and protein-losing enteropathy may result in *decreased albumin* levels. C-reactive protein and ESR may be elevated to indicate inflammation. White blood cells (WBCs) in the urine may show ***infection*** (pyuria), which is caused by ureteral obstruction or an enterovesical (bowel to bladder) fistula. If severe diarrhea or fistula is present, the patient may have fluid and electrolyte losses, particularly potassium and magnesium. Assess the patient for signs and symptoms that can occur related to electrolyte losses (see Chapter 13).

X-rays show the narrowing, ulcerations, strictures, and fistulas common with Crohn's disease. *Magnetic resonance enterography (MRE)* is performed to determine bowel activity and motility as discussed under the Other Diagnostic Assessment in the Ulcerative Colitis concept exemplar.

◆ **Interventions: Take Action.** Collaborative care for patients with Crohn's disease is similar to that described in the Nonsurgical Management discussion in the Ulcerative Colitis section. Specific interventions vary with the severity of disease and the complications that are present.

Nonsurgical Management

Drug Therapy. Drugs used to manage Crohn's disease (CD) are similar to those used in the treatment of ulcerative colitis (UC). For mild-to-moderate disease, 5-ASA drugs may be effective, although research shows that their usage for CD has produced mixed results (see the Drug Therapy discussion in the Ulcerative Colitis section).

Most patients have moderate-to-severe disease and need stronger drug therapy to control their symptoms. Two agents that may be prescribed for CD are azathioprine and mercaptopurine. These drugs suppress the immune system and can lead to serious infections. Methotrexate may also be given to suppress immune activity of the disease.

A group of biologic response modifiers (BRMs), also known as *monoclonal antibody drugs,* have been approved for use in CD when other drugs have been ineffective. These drugs inhibit tumor necrosis factor (TNF)–alpha, which decreases the inflammatory response. Examples of commonly used drugs for patients with CD include infliximab, adalimumab, natalizumab, and certolizumab pegol. These agents are not given to patients with a history of cancer, heart disease, or multiple sclerosis (Winter & Burakoff, 2017).

> **! NURSING SAFETY PRIORITY QSEN**
>
> ***Drug Alert***
>
> Both infliximab and certolizumab pegol must be given in a health care setting, such as a medical office, via parenteral routes. Teach patients how to give themselves a subcutaneous injection for those drugs that come in that form. Teach them to report injection site reactions, including redness and swelling. Remind patients that headache, abdominal pain, and nausea and vomiting are common side effects. Teach them to avoid crowds and people with infection. Reinforce the need to report any ***infection,*** including a cold or sore throat, to the primary health care provider immediately (Burchum & Rosenthal, 2019).
>
> Natalizumab is given IV under medical supervision every 4 weeks for moderate-to-severe CD and when other drugs are not effective. Natalizumab can cause **progressive multifocal leukoencephalopathy** (PML), a deadly infection that affects the brain. Before giving the drug, be sure that the patient is free of all infections. Teach patients the importance of reporting any cognitive, motor, or sensory changes immediately to the primary health care provider.
>
> Vedolizumab is used for treatment of moderate-to-severe CD. This drug is administered IV at weeks 0, 2, and 6, and then the first maintenance dose is given at 8 weeks. The maintenance doses continue every 8 weeks after that (Engel et al., 2018). Clinical trials verify that vedolizumab does not increase the risk for PML, but because of its mechanism of action, the FDA strongly encourages education regarding this possible complication (Card et al., 2018).

Although glucocorticoids can be effective for patients with CD, sepsis can result from abscesses or fistulas that may be present. These drugs mask the symptoms of ***infection.*** Therefore they must be used with caution and only on a short-term basis. Monitor the patient closely for signs of infection. Teach the patient not to stop the steroids abruptly because of the potential for adrenal insufficiency. Ciprofloxacin and metronidazole have been helpful in patients with fistulas, anorectal abscesses, and ***infection*** related to CD.

Nutrition Therapy. Long-standing nutritional deficits can have severe consequences for the patient with Crohn's disease. Poor ***nutrition*** can lead to inadequate fistula and wound healing, loss of lean muscle mass, decreased immune responses, and increased morbidity and mortality. During severe exacerbations of the disease, the patient may be hospitalized to provide bowel rest and nutritional support with total parenteral nutrition (TPN). Nutritional supplements such as Ensure or Sustacal can be given to provide nutrients and more calories. Teach the patient to avoid GI stimulants, such as caffeinated beverages and alcohol.

Fistula Management. Fistulas are common with acute exacerbations of Crohn's disease. They can be between the bowel and bladder (enterovesical), between two segments of bowel (enteroenteric), between the skin and bowel (enterocutaneous), or between the bowel and vagina (enterovaginal) (see Fig. 52.4). The patient with multiple fistulas often has complications such as systemic infections, skin problems (including abscesses and fissures), and malnutrition. Treatment of the patient with an **abscess** (a localized infection in which there is a collection of pus) requires an incision and drainage (I & D) local procedure. Management of the patient with a fistula is more complicated and includes ***nutrition*** and electrolyte therapy, skin care, and prevention of infection.

! NURSING SAFETY PRIORITY (QSEN)

Action Alert

Adequate ***nutrition*** and ***fluid and electrolyte balance*** are priorities in the care of the patient with a fistula. GI secretions are high in volume and rich in electrolytes and enzymes. The patient is at high risk for malnutrition, dehydration, and hypokalemia (decreased serum potassium). Assess for these complications and collaborate with the health care team to manage them. Carefully monitor urinary output and daily weights. A decrease in either measurement indicates possible dehydration, which should be treated immediately by providing additional fluids.

The patient requires at least 3000 calories daily to promote healing of the fistula. If he or she cannot take adequate oral fluids and nutrients, total enteral nutrition (TEN) or TPN may be prescribed. For patients who do not require TEN or TPN, collaborate with the registered dietitian nutritionist to:

- Carefully monitor the patient's tolerance of the prescribed diet
- Help the patient select high-calorie, high-protein, high-vitamin, low-fiber meals
- Offer enteral supplements
- Record food intake for accurate calorie counts

Remind assistive personnel to provide enteral supplements, record accurate intake and output, and take daily weights while the patient is in the hospital. Collaborate with the certified wound, ostomy, and continence nurse (CWOCN) to select the most appropriate wound management for each patient.

! NURSING SAFETY PRIORITY (QSEN)

Action Alert

For patients with fistulas, preserving and protecting the skin are the nursing priorities. Be sure that wound drainage is not in direct contact with skin because intestinal fluid enzymes are caustic! Clean the skin promptly to prevent skin breakdown or fungal infection, which can cause major discomfort for the patient.

Enzymes and bile in the stool contribute to the problem of skin irritation and excoriation. Skin irritation needs to be prevented. This may be accomplished by using skin barriers, pouching systems, and insertion of drains (Fig. 52.5). Skin barriers or dressings are used when the fistula drainage is less than 100 mL in 24 hours. A pouch is used for heavily draining fistulas to reduce the risk for skin breakdown and measure the **effluent**. However, they are very challenging because of location and drainage amount. Treatment with an antifungal powder applied to the skin around the fistula is often very helpful to prevent or treat *Candida* infection.

For some fistulas, pouching may not be possible because of their location. Drainage may need to be managed using regulated wall suction or a negative-pressure wound therapy device. Continuous low wall suction is attached to a suction catheter in the wound bed of the fistula, not into the fistula tract. These systems are not meant for long-term management.

Negative-pressure wound therapy (e.g., vacuum-assisted closure, or wound VAC therapy) promotes wound healing by secondary intention as it prepares the wound bed for closure, reduces edema, promotes granulation and perfusion, and removes exudate and infectious material. It should not be used for patients who are at risk for bleeding or only for the purpose of drainage containment.

Patients with fistulas are also at high risk for intra-abdominal abscesses and sepsis. Antibiotic therapy is commonly prescribed. Observe for signs of sepsis (systemic infection), such as fever, abdominal pain, or a change in mental status. Monitor for increased WBC levels that could indicate a systemic infection (McCance et al., 2019).

Other helpful interventions for the patient with CD are those that relax the patient and soothe the GI tract. Such therapies may include naturopathy, herbs (e.g., ginger), acupuncture, hypnotherapy, and ayurveda (a combination of diet, herbs, yoga, and breathing exercises). The evidence supporting the use of these substances for CD is lacking, but many patients find them helpful for overall physical and emotional health. Teach patients about the availability of these therapies and recommend that they include them in their collaborative plan of care.

Surgical Management. Surgery for Crohn's disease may be performed for patients who have not improved with medical management or for those who have complications from the disease. Surgery to manage Crohn's disease is not as successful as that for ulcerative colitis because of the extent of the disease. The patient with a fistula may undergo resection of the diseased area. Other indications for surgical treatment include perforation, massive hemorrhage, intestinal obstruction or strictures, abscesses, or cancer.

CLINICAL JUDGMENT CHALLENGE 52.1

Patient-Centered Care; Evidence-Based Practice; Teamwork and Collaboration

A 28-year-old woman has had Crohn's disease for over 5 years. She is admitted today to the hospital for severe diarrhea and abdominal pain and is receiving IV fluids. The primary health care provider suspects that she has a small enteroenteric (between two segments of bowel) fistula. This client reports that she is newly married and is worried about the impacts this complication may have on her life as they are trying to get pregnant with their first child. She was taking prednisone to control her exacerbation, but now it has been discontinued. This evening, the nurse notes these assessment findings:

- Hyperactive bowel sounds × 4
- Reports abdominal pain and cramping as a 7 on a 0-10 pain intensity scale
- Severe abdominal distention
- Temperature = 101° F (38.3° C)
- Apical pulse = 88 beats/min
- Blood pressure = 124/76 mm Hg
- Respirations = 24 breaths/min
- Na = 136 mEq/L (136 mmol/L)
- K = 3.3 mEq/L (3.3 mmol/L)

1. **Recognize Cues**: What assessment information in this client situation is the most important and immediate concern for the nurse? (Hint: Identify the **relevant** information *first* to determine what is most important.)
2. **Analyze Cues:** What client conditions are consistent with the **most relevant** information? (Hint: Think about priority collaborative problems that support and contradict the information presented in this situation.)
3. **Prioritize Hypotheses:** Which possibilities or explanations are **most likely** to be present in this client situation? Which possibilities or explanations are the most serious? (Hint: Consider all possibilities and determine their urgency and risk for this client.)
4. **Generate Solutions:** What actions would most likely achieve the desired outcomes for this client? Which actions should be **avoided** or are **potentially harmful**? (Hint: Determine the desired outcomes first to decide which interventions are appropriate and those that should be avoided.)
5. **Take Action:** Which actions are the most appropriate and how should they be implemented? In what **priority order** should they be implemented? (Hint: Consider health teaching, documentation, requested health care provider orders or prescriptions, nursing skills, collaboration with or referral to health team members, etc.)
6. **Evaluate Outcomes:** What client assessment would indicate that the nurse's actions were **effective**? (Hint: Think about signs that would indicate an improvement, decline, or unchanged client condition.)

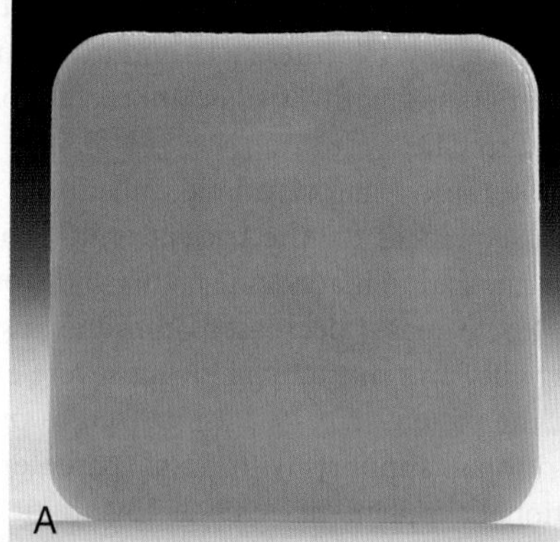

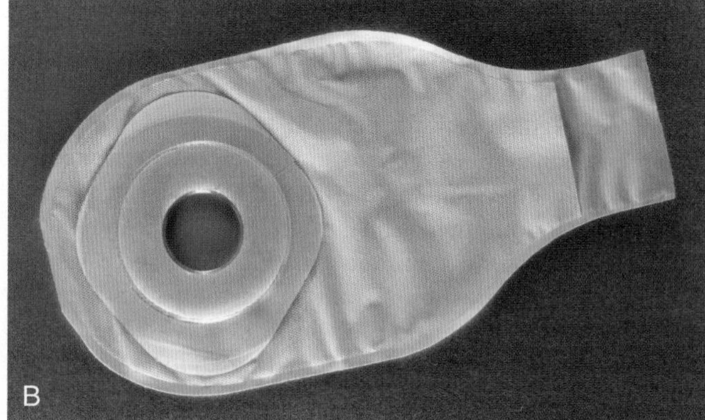

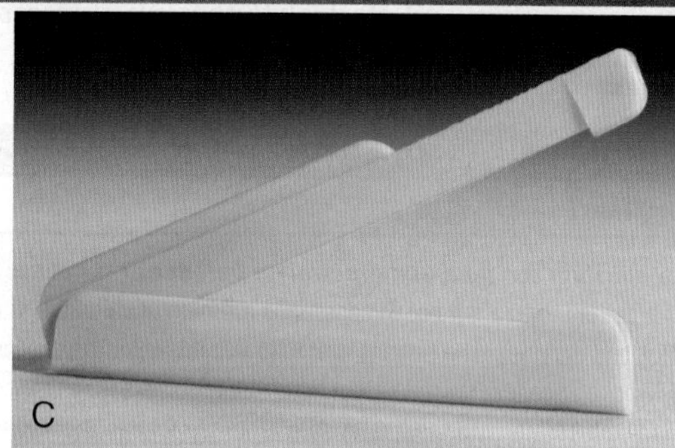

Fig. 52.5 Skin barriers, such as wafers **(A)**, are cut to fit ⅛ inch around the fistula. A drainable pouch **(B)** is applied over the wafer and clamped **(C)** until the pouch is to be emptied. Effluent should drain into the bag and not contact the skin. (Courtesy ConvaTec, a Bristol-Myers Squibb Company, Princeton, NJ.)

In some cases, a resection (removal of part of the small bowel) can be performed via minimally invasive surgery (MIS) via laparoscopy. This surgery involves one or more small incisions, less pain, and a quicker surgical recovery when compared with traditional open surgery. Both small-bowel resection (usually the ileum) and ileocecal resection can be done using this procedure. For other patients, an open surgical approach is used to allow for better visual access to the bowel.

Stricturoplasty may be performed for bowel strictures related to Crohn's disease. This procedure increases the bowel diameter. Care before and after each of these surgical procedures is similar to care for patients undergoing other types of abdominal surgery (see Chapter 9).

Care Coordination and Transition Management

Home Care Management. The discharge care plan for the patient with Crohn's disease is similar to that for the patient with ulcerative colitis (see the Care Coordination and Transition Management discussion in the Ulcerative Colitis section). Collaborate with the case manager and CWOCN or wound nurse to help the patient plan self-management.

Self-Management Education. Reinforce measures to control the disease and related symptoms and manage ***nutrition.*** Teach the patient and family to make arrangements for the patient to have easy access to the bathroom and privacy to perform fistula care, if needed.

The health teaching plan for Crohn's disease is similar to that for the patient with ulcerative colitis. Teach the patient about the usual course of the disease, symptoms of complications, and when to notify the health care provider. Provide health teaching for drug therapy, including purpose, dose, and side effects. In addition to other drugs, vitamin supplements, including monthly vitamin B_{12} injections, may be needed because of the inability of the ileum to absorb certain nutrients. In collaboration with the dietitian, instruct the patient to follow a low-residue, high-calorie diet and to avoid foods that cause discomfort, such as milk, gluten (wheat products), and other GI stimulants like caffeine.

Remind the patient to take rest periods, especially during exacerbations of the disease. If stress appears to increase symptoms of the disease, recommend stress-management techniques, counseling, and/or physical activity to improve quality of life. For long-term teaching, inform the patient about the increased risk for bowel cancer and the importance of frequent colorectal cancer screening (see Chapter 51).

If a patient has a fistula, explain and demonstrate wound care. Provide the opportunity for the patient to practice this care in the hospital. Ideally, he or she should be independent in fistula care before leaving the hospital. However, because of location of the fistula (perirectal or vaginal) or a large abdomen, assistance may be needed. If this is the case, teach a family member or other caregiver how to manage the wound. Patients may be transferred to a transitional or skilled nursing unit for collaborative care.

Health Care Resources. Patients who are discharged to home after undergoing resection and anastomosis may require visits from a home care nurse to assess the surgical wound and monitor for complications. Assess the patient's and family's ability to monitor the progress of fistula healing and to watch for indications of infection and sepsis. A home care aide or other service might be helpful for the patient who cannot meet nutritional needs or who needs help with grocery shopping and meal preparation.

In collaboration with the case manager, assist with obtaining the equipment and supplies for fistula care, such as skin barriers and wound drainage bags. A support group sponsored by the United Ostomy Associations of America (www.ostomy.org) or a local hospital in the community may also be available to help with meeting physical and psychosocial needs.

DIVERTICULAR DISEASE

Diverticula are pouchlike herniations of the mucosa through the muscular wall of any part of the gut, but most commonly the colon. Diverticulosis is the presence of many abnormal pouchlike herniations (diverticula) in the wall of the intestine. Acute diverticulitis is the inflammation or infection of diverticula.

Pathophysiology Review

Diverticula can occur in any part of the small or large intestine, but they usually occur in the sigmoid colon (Fig. 52.6). The muscle of the colon hypertrophies, thickens, and becomes rigid, and herniation of the mucosa and submucosa through the colon wall is seen. Diverticula seem to occur at points of weakness in the intestinal wall, often at areas where blood vessels interrupt the muscle layer. Muscle weakness develops as part of the aging process or because of a lack of fiber in the diet.

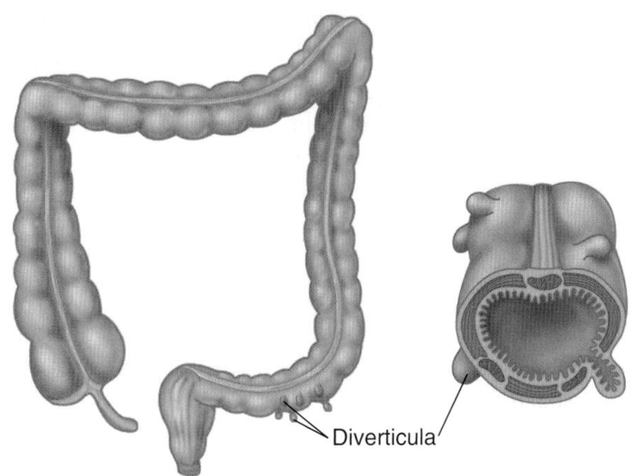

Fig. 52.6 Several abnormal outpouchings, or herniations, in the wall of the intestine, which are diverticula. These can occur anywhere in the small or large intestine but are found most often in the colon. Diverticulitis is the inflammation of a diverticulum that occurs when undigested food or bacteria become trapped in the diverticulum.

Diverticula *without* ***inflammation*** cause few problems. However, if undigested food or bacteria become trapped in a diverticulum, blood supply to that area is reduced. Bacteria invade the diverticulum, resulting in diverticulitis, which then can perforate and develop a local abscess. A perforated diverticulum can progress to an intra-abdominal perforation with peritonitis. Lower GI bleeding may also occur (see earlier discussion in this chapter under Ulcerative Colitis).

High intraluminal pressure forces the formation of a pouch in the weakened area of the mucosa. Diets low in fiber that cause less bulky stool and constipation have been implicated in the formation of diverticula. Retained undigested food in diverticula is suggested to be one cause of diverticulitis. The retained food reduces blood flow to that area and makes bacterial invasion of the sac easier (McCance et al., 2019).

The exact incidence of diverticulosis is unknown, but millions are affected by the problem. It is found in two thirds of adults older than 80 years, with more men than women affected.

❖ Interprofessional Collaborative Care

Patients with diverticular disease are self-managed at home, cared for in the community setting, or hospitalized if surgery is needed to correct a concern.

◆ **Assessment: Recognize Cues.** The patient with *diverticulosis* usually has no symptoms. Unless pain or bleeding develops, the condition may go undiagnosed. Diverticula are most often diagnosed during routine colonoscopy. Occasionally diverticulosis will cause symptoms. For the patient with uncomplicated diverticulosis, ask about intermittent ***pain*** in the left lower quadrant and a history of constipation. If diverticulitis is suspected, ask about a history of low-grade fever, nausea, and abdominal pain. Inquire about recent bowel ***elimination*** patterns because constipation may develop as a result of intestinal inflammation. Also, ask about any bleeding from the rectum.

The patient with *diverticulitis* may have abdominal ***pain,*** most often localized to the left lower quadrant. It is intermittent at first but becomes progressively steady. Occasionally, pain may be just above the pubic bone or may occur on one side. Abdominal pain is generalized if peritonitis has occurred. Nausea and vomiting are common. The patient's temperature is elevated, ranging from a low-grade fever to 101°F (38.3°C). Chills may be present. Often an increased heart rate (tachycardia) occurs with fever (Elisei & Tursi, 2016).

On examination of the abdomen, observe for distention. The patient may report tenderness over the involved area. Localized muscle spasm, guarded movement, and rebound tenderness may be present with peritoneal irritation. If generalized peritonitis is present, profound guarding occurs; rebound tenderness is more widespread; and sepsis, hypotension, or hypovolemic shock can occur. If the perforated diverticulum is close to the rectum, the health care provider may palpate a tender mass during the rectal examination. Blood pressure checks may show orthostatic changes. *If bleeding is massive, the patient may have hypovolemia and hypotension that result in shock.*

For the patient with uncomplicated diverticulosis, laboratory studies are not indicated. However, the patient with diverticulitis has an *elevated white blood cell (WBC) count. Decreased hematocrit and hemoglobin* values are common if chronic or severe bleeding occurs. Stool tests for occult blood, if requested, are sometimes positive. Abdominal x-rays may be done to evaluate for free air and fluid indicating perforation. A CT scan may be performed to diagnose an abscess or thickening of the bowel related to diverticulitis.

Abdominal ultrasonography, a noninvasive test, may also reveal bowel thickening or an abscess. The primary health care provider may recommend a colonoscopy 4 to 8 weeks *after the acute phase* of the illness to rule out a tumor in the large intestine, particularly if the patient has rectal bleeding.

◆ **Interventions: Take Action.** Patients are managed on an ambulatory care basis if the symptoms are mild. Monitor the patient for any prolonged or increased fever, abdominal ***pain,*** or blood in the stool. The patient with moderate-to-severe diverticulitis may be hospitalized, especially if he or she is older or has complications. Manifestations suggesting the need for admission are a temperature higher than 101°F (38.3°C), persistent and severe abdominal pain for more than 3 days, and/or lower GI bleeding.

Nonsurgical Management. A combination of drug and ***nutrition*** therapy with rest is used to decrease the ***inflammation*** associated with diverticular disease. Broad-spectrum antimicrobial drugs, such as metronidazole in conjunction with trimethoprim/sulfamethoxazole (TMZ) or ciprofloxacin, are often prescribed. A mild analgesic may be given for pain. The Patient-Centered Care: Older Adult Considerations: Diverticulitis box lists nursing interventions needed for care of older adults with diverticulitis.

The patient with more severe ***pain*** may be admitted to the hospital for IV fluids to correct dehydration and IV drug therapy. For patients with moderate-to-severe diverticulitis, an opioid analgesic may alleviate pain.

PATIENT-CENTERED CARE: OLDER ADULT CONSIDERATIONS QSEN

Diverticulitis

- Provide antibiotics and analgesics as prescribed. Observe older patients carefully for side effects of these drugs, especially confusion (or increased confusion), and orthostatic hypotension.
- Do not give laxatives or enemas. Teach the patient and family about the importance of avoiding these measures.
- Encourage the patient to rest and to avoid activities that may increase intra-abdominal pressure, such as straining and bending.
- While diverticulitis is active, provide a *low*-fiber diet. When the ***inflammation*** resolves, provide a *high*-fiber diet. Teach the patient and family about these diets and when they are appropriate.
- Because older patients do not always experience the typical ***pain*** or fever expected, observe carefully for other signs of active disease, such as a sudden change in mental status.
- Perform frequent abdominal assessments to determine distention and tenderness on palpation.
- Check stools for occult or frank bleeding.

Laxatives and enemas are avoided because they increase intestinal motility. Assess the patient on an ongoing basis for manifestations of impaired ***fluid and electrolyte balance.***

Teach the patient to rest during the acute phase of illness. Remind him or her to refrain from lifting, straining, coughing, or bending to avoid an increase in intra-abdominal pressure, which can result in perforation of the diverticulum. ***Nutrition*** therapy should be restricted to low fiber or clear liquids based on symptoms. The patient with more severe symptoms is NPO. A nasogastric tube (NGT) is inserted if nausea, vomiting, or abdominal distention is severe. Infuse IV fluids as prescribed for hydration. In collaboration with a dietitian, the patient increases dietary intake slowly as symptoms subside. When ***inflammation*** has resolved and bowel function returns to normal, a fiber-containing diet is introduced gradually.

Surgical Management. Diverticulitis can result in rupture of the diverticulum with peritonitis, pelvic abscess, bowel obstruction, fistula, persistent fever or ***pain,*** or uncontrolled bleeding. The surgeon performs emergency surgery if peritonitis, bowel obstruction, or pelvic abscess is present. Colon resection, with or without a colostomy, is the most common surgical procedure for patients with diverticular disease. Chapter 51 discusses the nursing care for patients with this procedure.

Care Coordination and Transition Management. Discharge plans vary according to the treatment. The patient who has surgical intervention has the added responsibilities of incision care and possibly colostomy care with temporary limitations placed on activities.

Patients with diverticular disease need education regarding a high-fiber diet. Encourage the patient with *diverticulosis* to eat a diet high in cellulose and hemicellulose types of fiber. These substances can be found in wheat bran, whole-grain breads, and cereals. Teach the patient to eat at least 25 to 35 g of fiber per day. Fresh fruits and vegetables with high fiber content are added to provide bulk to stools.

If not accustomed to eating high-fiber foods, teach the patient to add them to the diet gradually to avoid flatulence and abdominal cramping. If he or she cannot tolerate the recommended fiber requirement, a bulk-forming laxative, such as psyllium hydrophilic mucilloid, can be taken to increase fecal size and consistency. Teach the patient to drink plenty of fluids to help prevent bloating that may occur with a high-fiber diet. Alcohol should be avoided because it irritates the bowel. Foods containing seeds or indigestible material that may block a diverticulum, such as nuts, corn, popcorn, cucumbers, tomatoes, and figs, may need to be eliminated. Teach the patient that dietary fat intake should not exceed 30% of the total daily caloric intake.

The patient should be instructed to avoid all fiber when symptoms of *diverticulitis* are present, because high-fiber foods can be irritating. As ***inflammation*** resolves, fiber can gradually be added until progression to a high-fiber diet is established. The patient who has undergone surgery is usually taking solid food by the time of discharge from the hospital.

Provide oral and written instructions on incision care and the signs and symptoms to report to the health care provider for the patient who had abdominal surgery. If a colostomy was created, reinforce ostomy care as needed. Encourage the patient to express concerns about body image. Allow time and address sexual concerns regarding the changed body image.

Instruct the patient with any type of diverticular disease about the manifestations of acute diverticulitis, including fever, abdominal pain, and bloody, mahogany, or tarry stools. Instruct patients to avoid the use of laxatives (other than bulk-forming types) and enemas. Reassure them that this disorder should not cause problems if a proper diet is followed.

In collaboration with the case manager, arrange for a home care nurse, if needed, to assess wound healing and proper functioning of the ostomy and the appliance. If the patient is interested, arrange for a visit from an ostomy volunteer (**ostomate**) or an ostomy nurse. For information about other community resources, remind the patient to contact the United Ostomy Associations of America (www.ostomy.org).

NCLEX EXAMINATION CHALLENGE 52.3

Physiological Integrity

The nurse is teaching a client about nutrition and diverticulosis. Which food will the nurse teach the client to avoid?

A. Cucumber
B. Beans
C. Carrot
D. Radish

CELIAC DISEASE

Celiac disease was once thought to be a rare disease but, because of improved diagnostic testing, many cases have been diagnosed in the past 10 to 15 years. Celiac disease is a multisystem autoimmune disease with an estimated incidence as high as 1 in 250 of the world's population (McCance et al., 2019). Patients who have other autoimmune diseases, such as rheumatoid arthritis and diabetes mellitus type 1, are at the highest risk for the disease.

Celiac disease is a chronic ***inflammation*** of the small intestinal mucosa that can cause bowel wall atrophy, malabsorption, and diarrhea. Like many inflammatory disorders, it is thought to be caused by a combination of genetic, immunologic, and environmental factors. The primary complication of celiac disease is cancer, specifically non-Hodgkin lymphoma or GI cancers and ***nutrition*** deficiencies.

Patients with celiac disease have varying signs and symptoms with cycles of remission and exacerbation (flare-up), usually related to how well they monitor their diet. Classic symptoms include anorexia, diarrhea and/or constipation, steatorrhea (fatty stools), abdominal pain, abdominal bloating and distention, and weight loss. Some patients have no symptoms. Still others have atypical symptoms that affect every body system, as listed in the Key Features: Celiac Disease box. Diagnosis is usually made by obtaining a screening blood test and endoscopy.

Dietary management is the only available treatment for achieving disease remission. In most cases, a gluten-free diet (GFD) results in healing the intestinal mucosa after about 2 years. Gluten is the primary substance in wheat and wheat-based products. Teach patients to carefully check for hidden sources of gluten that are in foods, food additives, drugs, and cosmetics. Patients often take vitamin and mineral supplements to replace those lost in avoiding gluten foods. A registered dietitian nutritionist should be included in the patient's long-term planning and overall treatment.

KEY FEATURES

Celiac Disease

Classic Symptoms

- Weight loss
- Anorexia
- Diarrhea and/or constipation
- Steatorrhea
- Abdominal pain and distention
- Vomiting

Atypical Symptoms

- Osteoporosis
- Joint ***pain*** and ***inflammation***
- Lactose intolerance
- Iron deficiency anemia
- Depression
- Migraines
- Epilepsy
- Autoimmune disorders
- Stomatitis
- Early menopause
- Protein-calorie malnutrition
- Infertility

TABLE 52.5 **Comparison of Common Parasitic Infections**

	Giardiasis *(Giardia lamblia)*	Amebiasis *(Entamoeba histolytica)*	*Cryptosporidium*
Description	Occurs in cysts and trophozoites Causes superficial invasion, destruction, and ***inflammation*** of small intestine mucosa	Occurs most commonly in crowded areas with poor sanitation Invades and ulcerates large intestinal mucosa	Occurs most commonly in immunosuppressed individuals Source is often contaminated swimming pools
Common assessment findings	Diarrhea Malabsorption syndrome Weight loss Nutrient deficiencies Acute phase is self-limiting Chronic phase can last for years	Can occur without symptoms May be mild or severe symptoms if they occur, including foul-smelling stools, abdominal cramping, and weight loss Can have extraintestinal symptoms	Primarily diarrhea Self-limiting health problem in individuals with normal immune system

PARASITIC INFECTION

Pathophysiology Review

Parasites can enter and invade the gastrointestinal tract and cause ***infection.*** They commonly enter through the mouth (oral-fecal transmission) from contaminated food or water, oral-anal sexual practices, or contact with feces from a contaminated person. Common parasites that cause infection in humans are *Giardia lamblia,* which causes giardiasis; *Entamoeba histolytica,* which causes amebiasis (amoebic dysentery); and *Cryptosporidium.* The primary method for determining which parasitic infection is present is through stool analysis. The white blood cell (WBC) count can be very high when severe diarrhea (dysentery) is present. Table 52.5 differentiates these three common types of parasites.

A less common parasitic infection is increasing in the United States. Chagas disease is caused by the *Trypanosoma cruzi* parasite, which is most commonly transmitted in impoverished areas of Latin America by the triatomine (kissing) bug. Patients first develop an acute ***infection,*** followed by an intermediate asymptomatic period and a chronic infection. Patients with chronic Chagas disease often develop cardiac dysrhythmias or heart failure and colon or esophagus dilation, causing impaired digestion and bowel ***elimination.*** An estimated 300,000 individuals in the United States have the disease (most in the southern areas of the United States), which can be transmitted through blood transfusions and organ transplantations. The Centers for Disease Control and Prevention (CDC) has targeted Chagas disease as one of five neglected parasitic infections that require public health action as the number of cases is expected to increase (CDC, 2019).

❖ Interprofessional Collaborative Care

◆ **Assessment: Recognize Cues.** A thorough history can help determine potential sources of exposure to parasitic infection. A history of travel to parts of the world where such infections are prevalent increases suspicion for infection with parasites. GI symptoms related to travel might be delayed as long as 1 to 2 weeks after the return home. Immigrants (newcomers) may have the ***infection*** on entering a new country. A ***nutrition*** history is especially helpful if several people in a group become ill. Common water supplies or bodies of water may be infected with *Giardia* or *Cryptosporidium.* Trichinosis should be considered if the patient has eaten pork products.

Mild-to-moderate *E. histolytica* infestation causes the daily passage of several strongly foul-smelling stools, possibly with mucus but without blood, accompanied by abdominal cramping, flatulence (gas), fatigue, and weight loss.

The infected patient usually experiences remissions and recurrences. Severe amoebic dysentery is manifested by frequent, liquid, and foul-smelling stools with mucus *and* blood. Fever up to 104° F (40° C), **tenesmus**, generalized abdominal tenderness, and vomiting can also occur. The ulcerations of invading amebiasis that occur in the colon can cause pain, bleeding, and obstruction. Ulcerations can also occur in the rectum, resulting in formed stool with blood. Complications are rare but include appendicitis and bowel perforation.

Extraintestinal amebiasis can occur without symptoms of intestinal infection. The most common form is amoebic liver abscess, which causes symptoms of fever, pain, and an enlarged liver. The abscess can rupture, and death can result if the infection and complications are not treated.

◆ **Interventions: Take Action.** *Handwashing is the best way to prevent the spread of parasitic infections.* Treatment for all types of *amebiasis* involves the use of amebicide drugs. Metronidazole followed by a luminal agent such as paromomycin, is commonly prescribed (Houpt et al., 2016). The patient with severe amoebic dysentery requires IV fluid replacement and possibly an opiate-like drug, such as diphenoxylate hydrochloride and atropine sulfate, to control bowel motility. The patient with extraintestinal amebiasis or severe dehydration, especially the older adult, is hospitalized. The patient with asymptomatic, mild, or moderate disease is treated with drug therapy on an ambulatory care basis. Therapy effectiveness is based on the examination of at least three stools at 2- to 3-day intervals, starting 2 to 4 weeks after drug therapy has been completed. *Teach patients* *the importance of keeping their follow-up appointments and taking all drugs as prescribed.*

Treatment for *giardiasis* is drug therapy. Metronidazole is the drug of choice. Tinidazole can be used as an alternative. Stools are examined 2 weeks after treatment to assess for drug effectiveness.

Infection with *Cryptosporidium* is usually self-limiting in adults who have normal immune function. Drug therapy for patients who are immunosuppressed may include paromomycin, an aminoglycoside antibiotic. Teach patients that this drug can cause dizziness.

! NURSING SAFETY PRIORITY (QSEN)

Action Alert

Explain modes of transmission of parasitic infections and means to avoid the spread of infection and recurrent contact with parasitic organisms. *Inform the patient that the infection can be transmitted to others until amebicides effectively kill the parasites. Teach the patient to:*

- Avoid contact with stool
- Keep toilet areas clean
- Wash hands meticulously with an antimicrobial soap after bowel movements
- Maintain good personal hygiene by bathing or showering daily
- Avoid stool from dogs and beavers

Advise the patient to avoid sexual practices that allow rectal contact until drug therapy is completed. *All household and sexual partners should have stool examinations for parasites.* If the water supply is suspected as the source, a sample is obtained and sent for analysis. Multiple infections are common in households, often as a result of contaminated shared water supplies. Well water and water from areas with inadequate or no filtration equipment can be sources of contamination.

GET READY FOR THE NEXT-GENERATION NCLEX® EXAMINATION!

Key Points

Review these Key Points for each NCLEX Examination Client Needs Category.

Safe and Effective Care Environment

- Collaborate with a CWOCN, health care provider, and case manager to plan care for patients with IBD. **QSEN: Teamwork and Collaboration**
- When transitioning care, remind patients and families about community resources for IBD, including the United Ostomy Associations of America and the Crohn's and Colitis Foundation of America. **QSEN: Teamwork and Collaboration**

Health Promotion and Maintenance

- Teach patients to use ***infection*** control measures to prevent transmission of gastroenteritis. **QSEN: Safety**
- Teach patients how to self-manage an ileostomy or other surgical diversion, including skin care, pouch management, and stoma assessment. **QSEN: Patient-Centered Care**

Psychosocial Integrity

- Be aware that all IBDs (acute and chronic) are very disruptive to one's daily routine; living with IBD requires a lifetime of modifications. **QSEN: Patient-Centered Care**
- Recognize that having a chronic bowel disease or an ileostomy impacts the patient's body image and self-esteem; assess for coping strategies that the patient has previously used, and identify personal support systems, such as family members, to assist in coping. **QSEN: Patient-Centered Care**

Physiological Integrity

- Assess for the classic signs and symptoms of appendicitis, which can include abdominal pain, nausea and vomiting, and abdominal tenderness on palpation (McBurney point); some patients also have leukocytosis. **QSEN: Safety**
- Recognize that perforation (rupture) of the appendix requires prompt intervention and can result in peritonitis. **QSEN: Safety**
- Assess for signs and symptoms of dehydration and blood loss in patients who have acute and chronic inflammatory bowel disorders, such as anemia and hypotension. **QSEN: Safety**
- Administer antidiarrheal medications as prescribed to decrease stools and therefore prevent dehydration in patients with acute and chronic inflammatory bowel disorders. **QSEN: Evidence-Based Practice**
- Be alert for GI bleeding in the patient with chronic IBD. **QSEN: Safety**
- Be aware that patients with Crohn's disease are at high risk for malnutrition as a result of an inability to absorb nutrients via the small intestine. **Clinical Judgment**
- Priority problems for patients with UC include diarrhea, pain, and potential for lower GI bleeding. **Clinical Judgment**
- Teach patients with IBD to avoid GI stimulants, such as alcohol and caffeine. **QSEN: Evidence-Based Practice**
- Administer infliximab or other monoclonal antibody agent as prescribed for patients with Crohn's disease; these drugs may also be useful for those with UC in selected cases but can cause secondary ***infection.***
- Observe for signs and symptoms of lower GI bleeding in patients with chronic inflammatory and diverticular disease. **QSEN: Safety**
- Teach patients with diverticulosis to eat a high-fiber diet; diverticulitis requires a low-fiber diet. **QSEN: Evidence-Based Practice**
- Instruct patients with diverticulosis about nutrition modifications, such as avoiding nuts, foods with seeds, and GI stimulants. **QSEN: Evidence-Based Practice**
- Be aware that patients with celiac disease have various signs and symptoms; some have no symptoms, some have

classic symptoms, and some have atypical symptoms. **QSEN: Patient-Centered Care**

- Teach patients with celiac disease about the need to consume a strict gluten-free diet, which avoids wheat and wheat-based products. **QSEN: Evidence-Based Practice**
- Be aware that GI problems, including diarrhea, may be caused by parasites and contaminated or undercooked food. **QSEN: Safety**

MASTERY QUESTIONS

1. The nurse is caring for a client with peritonitis from a perforated appendix. Which abdominal assessment finding will the nurse most likely expect?
   A. Soft abdomen
   B. Board-like abdomen
   C. Slightly distended abdomen
   D. Absent bowel sounds
2. A client had a colectomy with creation of an ileo-anal pouch and temporary ileostomy yesterday morning. The nurse assesses the ostomy and its functioning. Which assessment finding will the nurse report to the primary health care provider?
   A. Client's report of abdominal pain of 3 on a 0 to 10 pain intensity scale
   B. Slight abdominal distention
   C. No drainage from the ileostomy
   D. Serosanguinous effluent from the drain

REFERENCES

Burchum, J. L. R., & Rosenthal, L. D. (2019). *Lehne's pharmacology for nursing care* (10th ed.). St. Louis: Elsevier.

Card, T., Xu, J., Liang, H., & Bhayat, F. (2018). What is the risk of progressive multifocal leukoencephalopathy in patients with ulcerative colitis or Crohn's disease treated with vedolizumab? *Inflammatory Bowel Diseases, 24*(5), 953–959.

Centers for Disease Control and Prevention (CDC). (2019). Parasites-American trypanosomiasis. http://www.cdc.gov/parasites/chagas.

Cleynen, I., Boucher, G., Jostins, L., Schumm, L. P., Zeissig, S., Ahmad, T., et al. (2016). Inherited determinants of Crohn's disease and ulcerative colitis phenotypes: A genetic association study. *Lancet, 387*, 156–167.

Crohn's and Colitis Foundation. (2020). *Crohn's disease & colitis*. http://www.crohnscolitisfoundation.org.

Crohn's and Colitis Canada. (2020). *Canada leads the fight against IBD*. http://www.crohnsandcolitis.ca.

Elisei, W., & Tursi, A. (2016). Recent advances in the treatment of colonic diverticular disease and prevention of acute diverticulitis. *Annals of Gastroenterology: Quarterly Publication of the Hellenic Society of Gastroenterology, 29*(1), 24–32.

Engel, T., Ungar, B., Yung, D. E., Ben-Horin, S., Eliakim, R., & Kopylov, U. (2018). Vedolizumab in IBD: Lessons from real-world experience; A systematic review and pooled analysis. *Journal of Crohn's and Colitis, 12*(2), 245–257.

Houpt, E., Hung, C. C., & Petri, W. (2016). *Entamoeba histolytica (Amebiasis). Infectious disease and antimicrobial agents*. http://antimicrobe.org/new/b137.asp.

Khatri, G., Coleman, J., & Levendecker, J. R. (2018). Magnetic resonance enterography for inflammatory and noninflammatory conditions of the small bowel. *Radiologic Clinics of North America, 56*(5), 671–689.

McCance, K., Huether, S., Brashers, V., & Rote, N. (2019). *Pathophysiology: The biologic basis for disease in adults and children* (8th ed.). St. Louis: Elsevier.

Pagana, K. D., & Pagana, T. J. (2018). *Manual of diagnostic and laboratory tests* (6th ed.). St. Louis: Mosby.

Ross, J. T., Matthay, M. A., & Harris, H. W. (2018). Secondary peritonitis: Principles of diagnosis and intervention. *British Medical Journal, 361*, k1407.

Santos, M. P. C., Gomes, C., & Torres, J. (2018). Familial and ethnic risk in inflammatory bowel disease. *Annals of Gastroenterology, 31*(1), 14–23.

Stelton, S. (2019). Stoma and peristomal skin care: A clinical review. *AJN, 119*(6), 38–45.

Valente, M. A., & Hull, T. L. (2018). Minimally invasive techniques for inflammatory bowel disease. In A. Pigazzi (Ed.), *Techniques in minimally invasive rectal surgery*. New York, NY: Springer Publishing.

Winter, R. W., & Burakoff, R. (2017). How should we treat mild and moderate-severe Crohn's disease in 2017? A brief overview of available therapies. *Expert Review of Gastroenterology & Hepatology, 11*(2), 95–97.

Concepts of Care for Patients With Liver Problems

Lara Carver, Jennifer Powers

http://evolve.elsevier.com/Iggy/

LEARNING OUTCOMES

1. Collaborate with the interprofessional team to manage quality care for patients with liver problems caused by impaired ***cellular regulation*** and ***infection.***
2. Identify community resources for families and patients recovering from liver problems.
3. Apply knowledge of pathophysiology of liver problems to identify common assessment findings, including actual or risk for impaired ***nutrition*** and ***fluid and electrolyte balance.***
4. Prioritize nursing and collaborative care for patients with common liver problems to manage ***pain***, control ***inflammation***, and promote ***nutrition.***
5. Plan transition management and care coordination for the patient who has a liver problem, including health teaching.

KEY TERMS

alcohol withdrawal A condition that occurs after stopping heavy and prolonged alcohol intake, which often results in tremors, acute confusion, psychotic behaviors (such as delusions and hallucinations), and autonomic symptoms including tachycardia, elevated blood pressure, and diaphoresis.

ascites The collection of free fluid within the peritoneal cavity caused by increased hydrostatic pressure from portal hypertension.

asterixis A coarse tremor characterized by rapid, nonrhythmic extensions and flexions in the wrists and fingers (hand flapping).

cirrhosis A disease characterized by widespread fibrotic (scarred) bands of connective tissue that change the liver's anatomy and physiology.

ecchymoses Large purple, blue, or yellow bruises.

esophageal varices A complication of cirrhosis in which fragile, thin-walled esophageal veins become distended and tortuous from increased pressure (portal hypertension).

fetor hepaticus The distinctive breath odor of chronic liver disease and hepatic encephalopathy that is characterized by a fruity or musty odor.

hepatic encephalopathy (also called *portal-systemic encephalopathy [PSE]*) is a complex cognitive syndrome that results from liver failure and cirrhosis.

hepatitis Widespread inflammation and infection of liver cells.

hepatomegaly Liver enlargement that commonly occurs in patients with early cirrhosis.

hepatopulmonary syndrome A complication of cirrhosis caused by excessive ascitic volume and manifested by dyspnea as a result of intraabdominal pressure, which limits thoracic expansion and diaphragmatic excursion.

hepatorenal syndrome A late complication of cirrhosis affecting the kidneys and manifested by oliguria, elevated blood urea nitrogen (BUN) and creatinine levels, and increased urine osmolarity.

icterus Yellow coloration of the eye sclerae.

jaundice Yellowish coloration of the skin caused by increased serum bilirubin.

nonalcoholic fatty liver disease (NAFLD) A rapidly growing liver disease that is associated with obesity, diabetes mellitus type 2, and metabolic syndrome.

paracentesis An invasive procedure performed to remove abdominal fluid in patients who have massive ascites.

petechiae Round, pinpoint, red-purple hemorrhagic lesions.

portal hypertension A major complication of cirrhosis resulting in persistent increase in pressure within the portal vein >5 mm Hg.

splenomegaly Spleen enlargement.

spontaneous bacterial peritonitis (SBP) An infection that results from bacteria collected in ascitic fluid.

transjugular intrahepatic portal-systemic shunt (TIPS) An interventional radiologic procedure performed for patients who have not responded to other modalities to manage hemorrhage or long-term ascites.

ultrasound transient elastography A noninvasive imaging test that measures liver stiffness, which helps the primary health care provider determine the amount of liver disease present.

PRIORITY AND INTERRELATED CONCEPTS

The priority concepts for this chapter are:
- ***Cellular Regulation***
- ***Infection***

The ***Cellular Regulation*** concept exemplar for this chapter is Cirrhosis.
The ***Infection*** concept exemplar for this chapter is Hepatitis.

The interrelated concepts for this chapter are:
- ***Fluid and Electrolyte Balance***
- ***Inflammation***
- ***Pain***
- ***Nutrition***

As the largest and one of the most vital internal organs, the liver performs more than 400 functions and affects every body system. Common problems of the liver affect ***cellular regulation, nutrition,*** and ***fluid and electrolyte balance.*** Liver diseases range in severity from mild hepatic ***inflammation*** and ***infection*** to chronic end-stage cirrhosis. Many of these problems can cause ***pain*** or discomfort. Chapter 3 briefly reviews these concepts.

CELLULAR REGULATION CONCEPT EXEMPLAR: CIRRHOSIS

Cirrhosis is extensive, irreversible scarring of the liver, usually caused by a chronic reaction to hepatic ***inflammation*** and necrosis. This scarring process directly impairs ***cellular regulation***. The disease typically develops slowly and has a progressive, prolonged, destructive course resulting in end-stage liver disease.

Pathophysiology Review

Cirrhosis is characterized by widespread fibrotic (scarred) bands of connective tissue that change the liver's anatomy and physiology. ***Inflammation*** caused by either toxins or disease results in extensive degeneration and destruction of hepatocytes (liver cells). As cirrhosis develops, the tissue becomes nodular. These nodules can block bile ducts and normal blood flow throughout the liver. Impairments in blood and lymph flow result from compression caused by excessive fibrous tissue. In early disease, the liver is usually enlarged and firm. As the pathologic process continues, the liver shrinks in size and becomes harder, resulting in decreased liver function over weeks to years. Some patients with cirrhosis have no symptoms until serious complications occur. The impaired liver function results in elevated serum liver enzymes.

Cirrhosis of the liver can be divided into several common types, depending on the cause of the disease (McCance et al., 2019):
- Postnecrotic cirrhosis (caused by viral hepatitis [especially hepatitis C] and certain drugs or other toxins)
- Laennec's or alcoholic cirrhosis (caused by chronic alcoholism)
- Biliary cirrhosis (also called *cholestatic;* caused by chronic biliary obstruction or autoimmune disease)

Complications of Cirrhosis. Common problems and complications associated with hepatic cirrhosis depend on the amount of damage sustained by the liver. In *compensated* cirrhosis, the liver is scarred and ***cellular regulation*** is impaired, but the organ can still perform essential functions without causing major symptoms. In *decompensated* cirrhosis, liver function is impaired with obvious signs and symptoms of liver failure.

The loss of hepatic function contributes to the development of metabolic abnormalities. Hepatic cell damage may lead to these common complications:
- Portal hypertension
- Ascites and esophageal varices
- Biliary obstruction
- Hepatic encephalopathy

Portal Hypertension. Portal hypertension, a persistent increase in pressure within the portal vein greater than 5 mm Hg, is a major complication of cirrhosis. It results from increased resistance to or obstruction (blockage) of the flow of blood through the portal vein and its branches. The blood meets resistance to flow and seeks collateral (alternative) venous channels around the high-pressure area.
Blood flow backs into the spleen, causing splenomegaly (spleen enlargement). Veins in the esophagus, stomach, intestines, abdomen, and rectum become dilated. Portal hypertension can result in ascites (excessive abdominal [peritoneal] fluid), esophageal varices (distended veins), prominent abdominal veins (caput medusae), and hemorrhoids.

Ascites and Gastroesophageal Varices. Ascites is the collection of free fluid within the peritoneal cavity caused by increased hydrostatic pressure from portal hypertension (McCance et al., 2019). The collection of plasma protein in the peritoneal fluid reduces the amount of circulating plasma protein in the blood. When this decrease is combined with the inability of the liver to produce albumin because of impaired liver cell functioning, the serum colloid osmotic pressure is decreased in the circulatory system. The result is a fluid shift from the vascular system into the abdomen, a form of "third spacing." As a result, the patient may have hypovolemia and edema at the same time.

Massive ascites may cause renal vasoconstriction, triggering the renin-angiotensin system. This results in sodium and water retention, which increases hydrostatic pressure and the vascular volume and leads to more ascites.
As a result of portal hypertension, the blood backs up from the liver and enters the esophageal and gastric veins. Esophageal varices occur when fragile, thin-walled esophageal veins become distended and tortuous from increased pressure. The potential for varices to bleed depends on their size; size is determined by direct endoscopic observation. Varices occur most often in the distal esophagus but can be present also in the stomach and rectum.

Decreased prothrombin production places the patient with cirrhosis at risk for bleeding. Bleeding esophageal varices are a life-threatening medical emergency. Severe blood loss may occur, resulting in shock from hypovolemia. The bleeding may present as either hematemesis (vomiting blood) or melena (black, tarry stools). Loss of consciousness may occur before

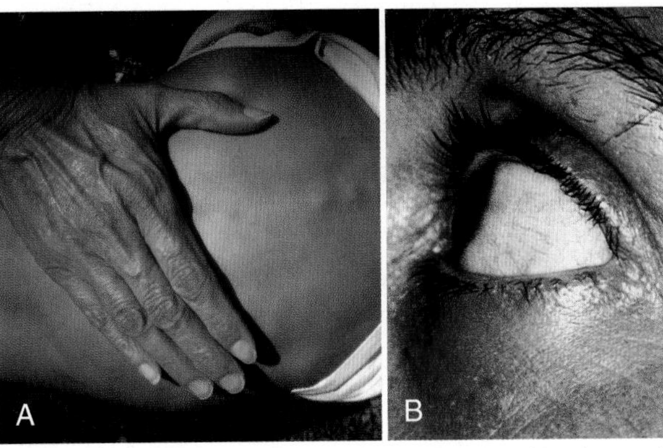

FIG. 53.1 (A and B) Jaundice as a result of liver dysfunction such as cirrhosis and hepatitis. (From Leonard PC. [2020]. *Quick & easy medical terminology* [9th ed.]. St. Louis: Elsevier.)

any observed bleeding. Variceal bleeding can occur spontaneously with no precipitating factors. However, any activity that increases abdominal pressure may increase the likelihood of a variceal bleed, including heavy lifting or vigorous physical exercise. In addition, chest trauma or dry, hard food in the esophagus can cause bleeding.

Patients with portal hypertension may also have portal hypertensive gastropathy. This complication can occur with or without esophageal varices. Slow gastric mucosal bleeding occurs, which may result in chronic slow blood loss, occult-positive stools, and anemia.

Splenomegaly results from the backup of blood into the spleen. The enlarged spleen destroys platelets, causing thrombocytopenia (low serum platelet count) and increased risk for bleeding. Thrombocytopenia is often the first clinical sign that a patient has liver dysfunction.

Biliary Obstruction. In patients with cirrhosis, the production of bile in the liver is decreased. This prevents the absorption of fat-soluble vitamins (e.g., vitamin K). Without vitamin K, clotting factors II, VII, IX, and X are not produced in sufficient quantities, and the patient is susceptible to bleeding and easy bruising. These abnormalities are confirmed by coagulation studies. Some patients have a genetic predisposition to obstruction of the bile duct that leads to biliary cirrhosis—usually from gallbladder disease or an autoimmune form of the disease called *primary biliary cirrhosis (PBC).*

Jaundice (yellowish coloration of the skin) in patients with cirrhosis is caused by one of two mechanisms: hepatocellular disease or intrahepatic obstruction (Fig. 53.1). *Hepatocellular* jaundice develops because the liver cells cannot effectively excrete bilirubin. This decreased excretion results in excessive circulating bilirubin levels. *Intrahepatic obstructive* jaundice results from edema, fibrosis, or scarring of the hepatic bile channels and bile ducts, which interferes with normal bile and bilirubin excretion. Patients with jaundice often report pruritus (itching).

Hepatic Encephalopathy. Hepatic encephalopathy (also called portal-systemic encephalopathy [PSE]) is a complex cognitive syndrome that results from liver failure and cirrhosis. Patients report sleep disturbance, mood disturbance, mental status changes, and speech problems early as this complication begins. Hepatic

TABLE 53.1 Stages of Hepatic Encephalopathy

Stage I
- Subtle manifestations that may not be recognized immediately
- Personality changes
- Behavior changes (agitation, belligerence)
- Emotional lability (euphoria, depression)
- Impaired thinking
- Inability to concentrate
- Fatigue, drowsiness
- Slurred or slowed speech
- Sleep pattern disturbances

Stage II
- Continuing mental changes
- Mental confusion
- Disorientation to time, place, or person
- Asterixis (hand flapping)

Stage III
- Progressive deterioration
- Marked mental confusion
- Stuporous, drowsy but arousable
- Abnormal electroencephalogram tracing
- Muscle twitching
- Hyperreflexia
- Asterixis (hand flapping)

Stage IV
- Unresponsiveness, leading to death in most patients progressing to this stage
- Unarousable, obtunded
- Usually no response to painful stimulus
- No asterixis
- Positive Babinski sign
- Muscle rigidity
- Fetor hepaticus (characteristic liver breath—musty, sweet odor)
- Seizures

encephalopathy may be reversible with early intervention. Later neurologic symptoms include an altered level of consciousness, impaired thinking processes, and neuromuscular problems.

Hepatic encephalopathy may develop slowly in patients with chronic liver disease and go undetected until the late stages. Symptoms develop rapidly in acute liver dysfunction. Four stages of development have been identified (Table 53.1). The patient's symptoms may gradually progress to coma or fluctuate among the four stages.

The exact mechanisms causing hepatic encephalopathy are not clearly understood but probably are the result of the shunting of portal venous blood into the central circulation, so the liver is bypassed. As a result, substances absorbed by the intestine are not broken down or detoxified and may lead to metabolic abnormalities, such as elevated serum ammonia and gamma-aminobutyric acid (GABA). Elevated serum ammonia results from the inability of the liver to detoxify protein by-products and is common in patients with hepatic encephalopathy. However, it is not a clear indicator of the presence of encephalopathy. Some patients may have major impairment without high elevations of serum ammonia, and elevations of ammonia can occur without evidence of encephalopathy.

Factors that may contribute to or worsen hepatic encephalopathy in patients with cirrhosis include:

- High-protein diet
- Infection
- Hypovolemia (decreased fluid volume)
- Hypokalemia (decreased serum potassium)
- Constipation
- GI bleeding (causes a large protein load in the intestines)
- Drugs (e.g., hypnotics, opioids, sedatives, analgesics, diuretics, illicit drugs)

The prognosis depends on the severity of the underlying cause, precipitating factors, and degree of liver dysfunction (McCance et al., 2019).

Other Complications. The development of hepatorenal syndrome indicates a poor prognosis for the patient with liver failure. It is often the cause of death in these patients. This syndrome is manifested by:

- A sudden decrease in urinary flow (<500 mL/24 hr) (oliguria)
- Elevated blood urea nitrogen (BUN) and creatinine levels with abnormally decreased urine sodium excretion
- Increased urine osmolarity

Hepatorenal syndrome often occurs after clinical deterioration from GI bleeding or the onset of hepatic encephalopathy. It may also complicate other liver diseases, including acute hepatitis and fulminant liver failure.

Patients with cirrhosis and ascites may develop acute spontaneous bacterial peritonitis (SBP). Those who are particularly susceptible are patients with very advanced liver disease. This may be the result of low concentrations of proteins; proteins normally provide some protection against bacteria.

The bacteria responsible for SBP are typically from the bowel and reach the ascitic fluid after migrating through the bowel wall and transversing the lymphatics. Symptoms vary but may include fever, chills, ***pain*** (especially in the abdomen), and tenderness. However, indications can also be minimal with only mild symptoms in the absence of fever. Worsening encephalopathy and increased jaundice may also be present without abdominal symptoms (McCance et al., 2019).

The diagnosis of SBP is made when a sample of ascitic fluid is obtained by paracentesis for cell counts and culture. An ascitic fluid leukocyte count of more than 250 polymorphonuclear (PMN) leukocytes may indicate the need for treatment (McCance et al., 2019).

Another major complication of cirrhosis is hepatopulmonary syndrome caused by excessive ascitic volume. The client experiences dyspnea as a result of intra-abdominal pressure, which limits thoracic expansion and diaphragmatic excursion.

Etiology and Genetic Risk. The most common causes for cirrhosis in the United States are chronic alcoholism, chronic viral hepatitis, and bile duct disease (Table 53.2). Hepatitis C is a leading cause of cirrhosis and liver cancer in the United States (Centers for Disease Control and Prevention, 2020b). It is an infectious bloodborne illness that usually causes chronic disease and compromises the body's immunity. ***Inflammation*** caused by ***infection*** over time leads to progressive scarring of the liver. It usually takes decades for cirrhosis to develop, although alcohol use in combination with hepatitis C may speed the process.

TABLE 53.2 Common Causes of Cirrhosis

• Alcoholic liver disease	• Drugs and chemical toxins
• Viral hepatitis	• Gallbladder disease
• Autoimmune hepatitis	• Metabolic/genetic causes
• Steatohepatitis (from fatty liver)	• Cardiovascular disease

Hepatitis B and hepatitis D are the most common causes of cirrhosis worldwide. Hepatitis B also causes ***inflammation*** and low-grade damage over decades that can ultimately lead to cirrhosis. Hepatitis D virus can infect the liver but only in people who already have hepatitis B (see discussion in **Infection** Concept Exemplar: Hepatitis).

Cirrhosis may also occur as a result of nonalcoholic fatty liver disease (NAFLD), a rapidly growing health care concern. NAFLD is associated with aging, obesity, diabetes mellitus type 2, and metabolic syndrome (Vacca, 2020). This disease can progress to liver cancer, cirrhosis, or failure, causing premature death. Up to 30% of Americans may have NAFLD (American Liver Foundation, 2020a). The Patatin-like phospholipase domain-containing 3 gene *(PNPLA3)* has been identified as a risk gene for the disease. Latinos have this gene more often than other ethnic groups and therefore are at the highest risk for NAFLD (McCance et al., 2019).

Another common cause of cirrhosis is excessive and prolonged alcohol use. Alcohol has a direct toxic effect on the hepatocytes and causes liver ***inflammation*** (alcoholic hepatitis). The liver becomes enlarged, with cellular degeneration and infiltration by fat, leukocytes, and lymphocytes. Over time, the inflammatory process decreases and the destructive phase increases. Early scar formation is caused by fibroblast infiltration and collagen formation. Damage to the liver tissue progresses as malnutrition and repeated exposure to the alcohol continue. If alcohol is withheld, the fatty infiltration and ***inflammation*** are reversible. If alcohol use continues, widespread scar tissue formation and fibrosis infiltrate the liver as a result of cellular necrosis. The long-term use of illicit drugs, such as cocaine, has similar effects on the liver.

PATIENT-CENTERED CARE: GENDER HEALTH CONSIDERATIONS QSEN

The amount of alcohol necessary to cause cirrhosis varies widely from individual to individual, and there are gender differences. In women, it may take as few as two or three drinks per day over a minimum of 10 years. In men, perhaps six drinks per day over the same time period may be needed to cause disease. However, a smaller amount of alcohol over a long period of time can increase memory loss from alcohol toxicity of the cerebral cortex. Binge drinking can increase risk for hepatitis and fatty liver (McCance et al., 2019).

Incidence and Prevalence. Approximately 3.2 million Americans have hepatitis C (American Liver Foundation, 2020b), and 1 in 7 Americans have hepatitis B, which can particularly affect Asian American and Pacific Islander-born individuals (Immunization Action Coalition, 2020).

Combined, the incidence of chronic liver disease and cirrhosis is a major common cause of death in the United States. The national prevalence of hepatitis B in Canada is 270,000 individuals (Canadian Digestive Health Association, 2020). It is more challenging to quantify the exact number of Canadians with liver disease, since these statistics are grouped with other digestive disorders; however, it is known that approximately 7000 Canadians die annually after being affected with a liver disorder (Canadian Digestive Health Association, 2020.)

❖ Interprofessional Collaborative Care

Care for the patient with cirrhosis can take place in various settings by many members of the interprofessional health care team. These patients may, at different times, self-manage at home, be hospitalized for immediate concerns, need rehabilitative care, or be cared for in the community setting, including possible hospice care.

◆ Assessment: Recognize Cues

History. Obtain data from patients with suspected cirrhosis, including age, gender, and employment history, especially history of exposure to alcohol, drugs (prescribed and illicit), use of herbal preparations, and chemical toxins. Keep in mind that all exposures are important, regardless of how long ago they occurred. Determine whether there has ever been a needle-stick injury. Sexual history and orientation may be important in determining an infectious cause for liver disease, because men having sex with men (MSM) are at high risk for hepatitis A, hepatitis B, and hepatitis C. People with hepatitis can develop cirrhosis (McCance et al., 2019).

Inquire about whether there is a family history of alcoholism and/or liver disease. Ask the patient to describe his or her alcohol intake, including the amount consumed during a given period. Is there a history of illicit drug use, including oral, IV, and intranasal forms? Is there a history of obtaining tattoos? If so, when and where were they done? Has the patient been in the military or in prison? Is the patient a health care worker, firefighter, or police officer? For patients previously or currently in an alcohol or drug recovery program, how long have they been sober? This information is sensitive and often difficult for the patient to answer. Be sure to establish why you are asking these questions and accept answers in a nonjudgmental manner. Provide privacy during the interview. For many people, the behaviors causing the liver disease occurred years before the onset of their current illness, and they are regretful and often embarrassed.

Ask the patient about previous medical conditions, such as an episode of jaundice or acute viral hepatitis, biliary tract disorders (such as cholecystitis [gallbladder ***inflammation***]), viral ***infection,*** surgery, blood transfusions, autoimmune disorders, obesity, altered lipid profile, heart failure, respiratory disorders, or liver injury.

Physical Assessment/Signs and Symptoms. Because cirrhosis has a slow onset, many of the *early* signs and symptoms are vague and nonspecific. Assess for:

- Fatigue
- Significant change in weight
- GI symptoms, such as anorexia and vomiting
- ***Pain*** in the abdominal area and liver tenderness (both of which may be ignored by the patient)

Liver function problems are often found during a routine physical examination or when laboratory tests are completed for an unrelated illness or problem. The patient with *compensated cirrhosis* may be completely unaware that there is a liver problem. The first sign may present before the onset of symptoms when routine laboratory tests, presurgical evaluations, or life and health insurance assessments show abnormalities. These tests could indicate abnormal liver function or thrombocytopenia (decreased serum platelet count), requiring a more thorough diagnostic workup.

The development of late signs of *advanced cirrhosis* (also called *end-stage liver failure*) usually causes the patient to seek medical treatment. GI bleeding, jaundice, ascites, and spontaneous bruising indicate poor liver function and complications of cirrhosis.

Thoroughly assess the patient with liver dysfunction or failure because it affects every body system. The clinical picture and course vary from patient to patient, depending on the severity of the disease. Assess for the common late disease signs and symptoms outlined in the Key Features: Late-Stage Cirrhosis box.

Abdominal Assessment. *Massive* ascites can be detected as a distended abdomen with bulging flanks (Fig. 53.2). The umbilicus may protrude, and dilated abdominal veins (caput medusae) may radiate from the umbilicus. Ascites can cause physical problems. For example, orthopnea and dyspnea from increased abdominal distention can interfere with lung expansion. The patient may have difficulty maintaining an erect body posture, and problems with balance may affect walking. Inspect and palpate for the presence of inguinal or umbilical hernias, which are likely to develop because of increased intra-abdominal pressure. *Minimal* ascites is often more difficult to detect, especially in the obese patient.

When performing an assessment of the abdomen, keep in mind that **hepatomegaly** (liver enlargement) occurs in many cases of early cirrhosis. **Splenomegaly** is common in

KEY FEATURES

Late-Stage Cirrhosis

- **Jaundice** and **icterus** (yellow coloration of the eye sclerae)
- Dry skin
- Pruritus (itchy skin)
- Rashes
- Purpuric lesions, such as **petechiae** (round, pinpoint, red-purple hemorrhagic lesions) or **ecchymoses** (large purple, blue, or yellow bruises)
- Warm and bright red palms of the hands (palmar erythema)
- Vascular lesions with a red center and radiating branches, known as spider angiomas (also called telangiectases, spider nevi, or vascular spiders), on the nose, cheeks, upper thorax, and shoulders
- **Ascites**
- Peripheral dependent edema of the extremities and sacrum
- Vitamin deficiency (especially fat-soluble vitamins A, D, E, and K)

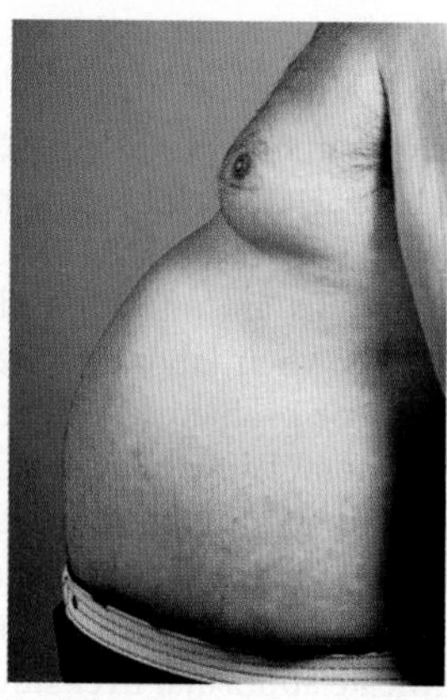

FIG. 53.2 Patient with abdominal ascites in late-stage cirrhosis. (From Leonard PC. [2020]. *Quick & easy medical terminology* [9th ed.]. St. Louis: Elsevier.)

nonalcoholic causes of cirrhosis. As the liver deteriorates, it may become hard and small.

Measure the patient's abdominal girth to evaluate the progression of ascites (see Fig. 53.2). To measure abdominal girth, the patient lies flat while the nurse or other examiner pulls a tape measure around the largest diameter (usually over the umbilicus) of the abdomen. The girth is measured at the end of exhalation. Mark the abdominal skin and flanks to ensure the same tape measure placement on subsequent readings. *However, taking daily weights is the most reliable indicator of fluid retention.*

Other Physical Assessment. Observe vomitus and stool for blood. This may be indicated by frank blood in the excrement or by a positive fecal occult blood test (FOBT). Gastritis, stomach ulceration, or oozing esophageal varices may be responsible for the blood in the stool. Note the presence of fetor hepaticus, which is the distinctive breath odor of chronic liver disease and hepatic encephalopathy and is characterized by a fruity or musty odor. Amenorrhea (no menstrual period) may occur in women, and men may exhibit testicular atrophy, gynecomastia (enlarged breasts), and impotence as a result of inactive hormones.

Continually assess the patient's neurologic function; it may also be helpful to include family members in conversations about the patient's baseline mental status if the patient is unable to effectively communicate. Subtle changes in mental status and personality often progress to coma—a late complication of hepatic encephalopathy. Monitor for asterixis—a coarse tremor characterized by rapid, nonrhythmic extensions and flexions in the wrists and fingers (hand flapping).

Psychosocial Assessment. The patient with hepatic cirrhosis may undergo subtle or obvious personality, cognitive, and behavior changes, such as agitation. He or she may experience sleep pattern disturbances or exhibit signs of emotional lability (fluctuations in emotions), euphoria (a very elevated mood), or depression. A psychosocial assessment identifies needs and helps guide care.

Repeated hospitalizations are common for patients with cirrhosis. It is a life-altering chronic disease, impacting not only the patient but also the immediate and extended family members and significant others. There are significant emotional, physical, and financial changes. Substance use may continue even as health worsens. It is important, whenever possible, to use resources available to these patients and their families. Collaborate with social workers, substance use counselors, and mental health/behavioral health care professionals as needed for patient assessment and management.

Part of the psychosocial assessment is determining if the patient is alcohol dependent. If this is the case, observe and prepare for alcohol withdrawal. Alcohol withdrawal occurs after stopping alcohol intake after heavy and prolonged use. Monitor for tremors, sometimes called the "jitters," which can begin as early as 6 to 8 hours after alcohol cessation. Cognitive and neurologic changes associated with delirium tremens (DTs) may include acute confusion, anxiety, and psychotic behaviors, such as delusions and hallucinations. Autonomic changes may include tachycardia, elevated blood pressure, and diaphoresis (Halter, 2018). Care of the patient experiencing withdrawal can be a medical emergency. Consult mental health textbooks for more information about caring for the alcohol-dependent patient.

Laboratory Assessment. Laboratory study abnormalities are common in patients with liver disease (Table 53.3). Serum levels of *aspartate aminotransferase* (AST), *alanine aminotransferase* (ALT), and *lactate dehydrogenase* (LDH) typically are elevated because these enzymes are released into the blood during hepatic ***inflammation.*** However, as the liver deteriorates, the hepatocytes may be unable to create an inflammatory response, and the AST and ALT may be normal. ALT levels are more specific to the liver, whereas AST can be found in muscle, kidney, brain, and heart. An AST/ALT ratio greater than 1.0 is usually found in alcoholic liver disease (Pagana & Pagana, 2018).

Increased *alkaline phosphatase* and gamma-glutamyl transpeptidase (GGT) levels are caused by biliary obstruction and therefore may increase in patients with cirrhosis. Alkaline phosphatase is a nonspecific bone, intestinal, and liver enzyme. However, alkaline phosphatase also increases when bone disease, such as osteoporosis, is present. Total serum *bilirubin* levels also rise. Indirect bilirubin levels increase in patients with cirrhosis because of the inability of the failing liver to excrete bilirubin. Therefore bilirubin is present in the urine (urobilinogen) in increased amounts. Fecal urobilinogen concentration is decreased in patients with biliary tract obstruction. These patients have light- or clay-colored stools.

Total serum *albumin* levels are decreased in patients with severe or chronic liver disease as a result of decreased synthesis by the liver (Pagana & Pagana, 2018). Loss of osmotic "pull" proteins such as albumin promotes the movement of intravascular fluid into the interstitial tissues (e.g., ascites). Prothrombin time/*international normalized ratio* (PT/INR) is prolonged because the liver decreases the production of prothrombin. The platelet count is low, resulting in a characteristic thrombocytopenia of cirrhosis. Anemia may be reflected by decreased red blood cell (RBC), hemoglobin, and hematocrit values. The white blood cell (WBC) count may also be decreased. *Ammonia* levels are usually elevated in patients with advanced liver disease. Serum creatinine may be elevated in patients with deteriorating kidney function. Dilutional hyponatremia (low serum sodium) may occur in patients with ascites.

TABLE 53.3 Assessment of Abnormal Laboratory Findings in Liver Disease

Abnormal Finding	Significance
Serum Enzymes	
Elevated serum aspartate aminotransferase (AST)	Hepatic cell destruction, hepatitis
Elevated serum alanine aminotransferase (ALT)	Hepatic cell destruction, hepatitis (most specific indicator)
Elevated lactate dehydrogenase (LDH)	Hepatic cell destruction
Elevated serum alkaline phosphatase	Obstructive jaundice, hepatic metastasis
Elevated gamma-glutamyl transpeptidase (GGT)	Biliary obstruction, cirrhosis
Bilirubin	
Elevated serum total bilirubin	Hepatic cell disease
Elevated serum direct conjugated bilirubin	Hepatitis, liver metastasis
Elevated serum indirect unconjugated bilirubin	Cirrhosis
Elevated urine bilirubin	Hepatocellular obstruction, viral or toxic liver disease
Elevated urine urobilinogen	Hepatic dysfunction
Decreased fecal urobilinogen	Obstructive liver disease
Serum Proteins	
Increased serum total protein	Acute liver disease
Decreased serum total protein	Chronic liver disease
Decreased serum albumin	Severe liver disease
Elevated serum globulin	Immune response to liver disease
Other Tests	
Elevated serum ammonia	Advanced liver disease or portal-systemic encephalopathy (PSE)
Prolonged prothrombin time (PT) or international normalized ratio (INR)	Hepatic cell damage and decreased synthesis of prothrombin

NCLEX EXAMINATION CHALLENGE 53.1

Physiological Integrity

The nurse is caring for a client who is diagnosed with cirrhosis. Which serum laboratory value(s) will the nurse expect to be abnormal? **Select all that apply.**

A. Prothrombin time
B. Serum bilirubin
C. Albumin
D. Aspartate aminotransferase (AST)
E. Lactate dehydrogenase (LDH)
F. Acid phosphatase

Imaging Assessment. Plain x-rays of the abdomen may show hepatomegaly, splenomegaly, or massive ascites. A CT scan may be requested.

MRI is another test used to diagnose the patient with liver disease. It can reveal mass lesions, giving additional specific information. This information is helpful in determining whether the condition is malignant or benign.

Other Diagnostic Assessment. Ultrasound (US) of the liver is often the first assessment for an adult with suspected liver disease to detect ascites, hepatomegaly, and splenomegaly. It can also determine the presence of biliary stones or biliary duct obstruction. Liver US with Doppler is useful in detecting portal vein thrombosis and evaluating whether the direction of portal blood flow is normal. **Ultrasound transient elastography** is a noninvasive test that measures liver stiffness, which helps the primary health care provider determine the amount of liver disease present. The normal amount of stiffness is 5.0 kilopascals (kPa). Higher degrees of stiffness indicate liver fibrosis. More than 11 kPa indicates that the client has cirrhosis. The imaging study may not be as reliable for patients who have excessive ascites or obesity (Chaney, 2019).

Some patients being assessed for liver disease require biopsies to determine the exact pathology and the extent of disease progression. This procedure can be problematic because a large number of patients are at risk for bleeding. Even a percutaneous (through the skin) biopsy can pose a significant risk to the patient. To minimize this risk, an interventional radiologist can perform a liver biopsy using a long sheath through a jugular vein that then is threaded into the hepatic vein and liver. A tissue sample is obtained for microscopic evaluation. If a biopsy procedure is not possible, a radioisotope liver scan may be used to identify cirrhosis or other diffuse disease.

The primary health care provider may request *arteriography* if US is not conclusive in finding portal vein thrombosis. To evaluate the portal vein and its branches, a portal venogram may be performed instead, by passing a catheter into the liver and portal vein. This procedure is described in the Transjugular Intrahepatic Portal-Systemic Shunt (TIPS) section.

The primary health care provider may perform an *esophagogastroduodenoscopy (EGD)* to directly visualize the upper GI tract to detect complications of liver failure. These complications may include bleeding or oozing esophageal varices, stomach irritation and ulceration, or duodenal ulceration and bleeding. EGD is performed by introducing a flexible fiberoptic endoscope into the mouth, esophagus, and stomach while the patient is under moderate sedation. A camera attached to the scope permits direct visualization of the mucosal lining of the upper GI tract. An *endoscopic retrograde cholangiopancreatography (ERCP)* uses the endoscope to inject contrast material via the sphincter of Oddi to view the biliary tract and allow for stone removals, sphincterotomies, biopsies, and stent placements if required. These procedures are described in more detail in Chapter 48.

◆ **Analysis: Analyze Cues and Prioritize Hypotheses.** The priority collaborative problems for patients with cirrhosis include:

1. Fluid overload due to third spacing of abdominal and peripheral fluid (ascites)
2. Potential for hemorrhage due to portal hypertension and subsequent GI varices
3. Acute confusion and other cognitive changes due to increased serum ammonia levels and/or alcohol withdrawal
4. Pruritus due to increased serum bilirubin and jaundice

◆ Planning and Implementation: Generate Solutions and Take Action

Managing Fluid Volume

Planning: Expected Outcomes. The patient with cirrhosis is expected to have less excess fluid volume as evidenced by decreased ascites and peripheral edema, as well as adequate circulatory volume.

Interventions. Fluid accumulations are minimal during the early stages of cirrhosis. Therefore nursing and interprofessional interventions are aimed at preventing the accumulation of additional fluid and decreasing any existing fluid collection. Nonsurgical treatment measures are used to treat ascites in most cases.

Supportive measures to control abdominal ascites include ***nutrition*** therapy, drug therapy, paracentesis, and respiratory support. The patient's ***fluid and electrolyte balance*** is carefully monitored during the treatment period.

Nutrition Therapy. The primary health care provider usually places the patient with early abdominal ascites on a low-sodium diet as an initial means of controlling fluid accumulation. The amount of daily sodium (Na^+) intake restriction varies, but a 1- to 2-g (2000 mg) Na^+ restriction may be tried first. In collaboration with the registered dietitian nutritionist, explain the purpose of the restriction and advise the patient and family to read the sodium content labels on all food and beverages. Table salt should be completely excluded. Low-sodium diets may be distasteful, so suggest alternative flavoring additives such as lemon, vinegar, parsley, oregano, and pepper. Remind the patient that seasoned and salty food is an acquired taste; in time, he or she will become used to the decrease in dietary sodium.

In general, patients with *late-stage* cirrhosis are malnourished and have multiple dietary deficiencies. IV vitamin supplements such as thiamine, folate, and multivitamin preparations are typically given because the liver cannot store vitamins. For patients with biliary cirrhosis, bile may not be available for fat-soluble vitamin transport and absorption. Oral vitamins are prescribed when IV fluid administration is discontinued.

Drug Therapy. The primary health care provider usually prescribes a *diuretic* to reduce fluid accumulation and prevent cardiac and respiratory problems. Monitor the effect of diuretic therapy by weighing the patient daily, measuring daily intake and output, measuring abdominal girth, documenting peripheral edema, and assessing electrolyte levels. Serious fluid and electrolyte imbalances, such as dehydration, hypokalemia (decreased potassium), and hyponatremia (decreased sodium), may occur with loop diuretic therapy. Depending on the diuretic selected, the provider may prescribe an oral or IV potassium supplement. Some clinicians prescribe furosemide and spironolactone as a combination diuretic therapy for the treatment of ascites. Because these drugs work differently, they are used for maintenance of sodium and potassium balance. For example, furosemide causes potassium loss, whereas spironolactone conserves it in the body.

All patients with ascites have the potential to develop spontaneous bacterial peritonitis (SBP) from bacteria in the collected ascitic fluid. In some patients, mild symptoms such as low-grade fever and loss of appetite occur. In others, there may be abdominal pain, fever, and change in mental status. When performing an abdominal assessment, listen for bowel sounds and assess for abdominal wall rigidity. Treatment involves IV cefotaxime or other third-generation cephalosporins or fluroquinolones.

Paracentesis. For some patients, abdominal paracentesis may be needed if ascites affects respiratory effort. A paracentesis is an invasive procedure performed to remove abdominal fluid. The procedure is performed at the bedside, in an interventional radiology department, or in an ambulatory care setting. The primary health care provider inserts a trocar catheter or drain into the abdomen to remove the ascitic fluid from the peritoneal cavity. This procedure is done using ultrasound for added safety. In some situations, a short-term ascites drain catheter may be placed while the patient is awaiting surgical intervention, or tunneled ascites drains can allow a patient or family caregiver to drain ascitic fluid at home. Nursing implications associated with this procedure are described in the Best Practice for Patient Safety & Quality Care box: The Patient Having a Paracentesis.

BEST PRACTICE FOR PATIENT SAFETY & QUALITY CARE (QSEN)

The Patient Having a Paracentesis

- Explain the procedure and answer patient questions.
- Obtain vital signs, including weight, before the procedure.
- Ask the patient to void before the procedure to prevent injury to the bladder!
- Position the patient in bed with the head of the bed elevated.
- Monitor vital signs per protocol or primary health care provider request during the procedure.
- Measure the drainage and record accurately.
- Document the characteristics of the collected fluid.
- Label and send the fluid for laboratory analysis; document in the patient health record that specimens were sent.
- After the catheter is removed, apply a dressing to the site; assess for leakage.
- Maintain bedrest per protocol.
- Take vital signs and weigh the patient after the paracentesis; document in the patient record weight both before and after paracentesis. (The patient should experience a weight loss due to fluid removal.)

If SBP is suspected, a sample of fluid is withdrawn and sent for cell count and culture. If the patient has symptoms of ***infection,*** the primary health care provider may prescribe antibiotics while awaiting the culture results.

Respiratory Support. Excessive ascitic fluid volume may cause the patient to have respiratory problems. He or she may develop *hepatopulmonary syndrome.* Dyspnea develops as a result of increased intra-abdominal pressure, which limits thoracic expansion and diaphragmatic excursion. Auscultate lungs every 4 to 8 hours for crackles that could indicate pulmonary complications, depending on the patient's overall condition.

! NURSING SAFETY PRIORITY QSEN

Action Alert

For the patient with hepatopulmonary syndrome, monitor his or her oxygen saturation with pulse oximetry. If needed, apply oxygen therapy to ease breathing. Elevate the head of the bed to at least 30 degrees or as high as the patient wants to improve breathing. This position, with his or her feet elevated to decrease dependent ankle edema, often relieves dyspnea. Remind assistive personnel to weigh the patient daily every morning before breakfast using the same scale.

Fluid and electrolyte balance problems are common as a result of the disease or treatment. Laboratory tests, such as blood urea nitrogen (BUN), serum protein, hematocrit, and electrolytes, help determine fluid and electrolyte status. An elevated BUN, decreased serum proteins, and increased hematocrit may indicate hypovolemia.

If medical management fails to control ascites, the primary health care provider may choose to divert ascites into the venous system by creating a shunt. Patients with ascites are poor surgical risks. The transjugular intrahepatic portal-systemic shunt (TIPS) is a nonsurgical procedure that is used to control long-term ascites and reduce variceal bleeding. This procedure is described in the discussion of Interventions in the Preventing or Managing Hemorrhage section that follows.

Preventing or Managing Hemorrhage

Planning: Expected Outcomes. The patient is expected to be free of bleeding episodes. However, if he or she has a hemorrhage, it is expected to be controlled by prompt, evidence-based professional interventions. Esophageal variceal bleeds are the most common cause of upper GI bleeding (also see Chapter 50 on management of upper GI bleeding).

Interventions. All patients with cirrhosis should be screened for esophageal varices by endoscopy to detect them early *before they bleed.* If patients have varices, they are placed on preventive therapy. If acute bleeding occurs, early interventions are used to manage it. *Because massive esophageal bleeding can cause rapid blood loss, emergency interventions are needed.*

The role of early drug therapy is to *prevent* bleeding and infection in patients who have varices. A nonselective *beta-blocking agent* such as propranolol is usually prescribed to prevent bleeding. By decreasing heart rate and the hepatic venous pressure gradient, the chance of bleeding may be reduced.

Up to 20% of cirrhotic patients who are admitted to the hospital as a result of upper GI bleeding have bacterial ***infection,*** and even more patients develop health care–associated infection, usually cellulitis, urinary tract infections, or pneumonia (McCance et al., 2019). Infection is one of the most common indicators that patients will have an acute variceal bleed (AVB). Therefore cirrhotic patients with GI bleeding should receive *antibiotics* when admitted to the hospital.

If bleeding occurs, the health care team intervenes quickly to control it by combining vasoactive drugs with endoscopic therapies. *Vasoactive* drugs, such as octreotide acetate and vasopressin, reduce blood flow through vasoconstriction to decrease portal pressure. Octreotide also suppresses secretion of gastrin, serotonin, and intestinal peptides, which decreases GI blood flow to help with pressure reduction within the varices (Burchum & Rosenthal, 2019). Vasopressin is used less commonly because it is a very potent drug (Pezzotti, 2020).

Endoscopic therapies include ligation of the bleeding veins or sclerotherapy. Both procedures are very effective in controlling bleeding and improving patient survival rates. Esophageal varices may be managed with *endoscopic variceal ligation (EVL) (banding).* This procedure involves the application of small "O" bands around the base of the varices to decrease their blood supply. The patient is unaware of the bands, and they cause no discomfort.

Endoscopic sclerotherapy (EST), also called *injection sclerotherapy,* may be done to stop bleeding. The varices are injected with a sclerosing agent via a catheter. This procedure is associated with complications such as mucosal ulceration, which could result in further bleeding.

If rebleeding occurs, rescue therapies are used. These procedures include a second endoscopic procedure, balloon tamponade and esophageal stents, and shunting procedures. Short-term esophagogastric balloon tamponade with esophageal stents is a very effective way to control bleeding. However, the procedure can cause potentially life-threatening complications, such as aspiration, asphyxia, and esophageal perforation. Similar to a nasogastric tube, the tube is placed through the nose and into the stomach. An attached balloon is inflated to apply pressure to the bleeding variceal area. Before this tamponade, the patient is usually intubated and placed on a mechanical ventilator to protect the airway. This therapy is used if the patient is not able to have a second endoscopy or TIPS procedure.

The **transjugular intrahepatic portal-systemic shunt (TIPS)** is a nonsurgical procedure performed in interventional radiology departments. This procedure is used for patients who have not responded to other modalities for hemorrhage or long-term ascites. If time permits, patients have a Doppler ultrasound to assess jugular vein anatomy and patency. The patient receives heavy IV sedation or general anesthesia for this procedure. The radiologist places a large sheath through the jugular vein. A needle is guided through the sheath and pushed through the liver into the portal vein. A balloon enlarges this tract, and a stent keeps it open. Most patients also have a Doppler ultrasound study of the liver after the TIPS procedure to record the blood flow through the shunt. Treating patients with TIPS who have esophageal/gastric varix hemorrhage problems may also require esophageal/gastric vein embolization as a part of the procedure. Patients with a highly cirrhotic liver usually have little flow through the liver parenchyma. These patients develop large portal-esophageal (or portal-gastric) veins diverting blood away from the diseased liver. Even after a successful TIPS, the diverting veins may persist and must be embolized (intentionally blocked) so they will not rebleed.

Serious complications of TIPS are not common. Patients are usually discharged in 1 or 2 days and are followed up with ultrasounds for the first year after the shunt is placed to ensure continued patency. Patients must also be monitored for hepatic encephalopathy, which can be caused by a TIPS. After creation of the TIPS, blood now bypasses most of the liver's filtration processes, allowing toxins to circulate throughout the body. For some patients, this can cause disturbances in consciousness and behavior. Lactulose or other medications may be given to counteract this effect, and dietary modification may also be helpful. In some cases, a TIPS may have to have the flow reduced or closed completely to reverse the encephalopathy. This is done by deploying a smaller stent or occluding device inside the original TIPS. This is a delicate decision for the health care provider to make, because reduction of flow through the shunt will likely cause the initial esophageal hemorrhaging to recur.

Patients receiving TIPS can also have significant elevation of their pulmonary artery pressure. This is a result of the sudden increase of blood flow to the right heart. Diuretics may help to treat this problem. For this reason, patients must be carefully evaluated for right heart failure before TIPS placement.

Depending on the procedure done to control esophageal bleeding, patients usually have a nasogastric tube (NGT) inserted to detect any new bleeding episodes. They often receive packed red blood cells, fresh frozen plasma, dextran, albumin, and platelets through large-bore IV catheters. Monitor vital signs every hour and check coagulation studies, including prothrombin time (PT), partial thromboplastin time (PTT), platelet count, and international normalized ratio (INR).

Preventing or Managing Confusion

Planning: Expected Outcomes. The patient is expected to be free of acute or chronic confusion. However, if it occurs, it is expected that the interprofessional health care team will intervene early to maintain patient safety and prevent further health problems or death from encephalopathy.

Interventions. Collaborative interventions are planned around the management of slowing or stopping the accumulation of ammonia in the body to improve mental status and orientation. Assess the patient's neurologic status and monitor during treatment.

Because ammonia is formed in the GI tract by the action of bacteria on protein, nonsurgical treatment measures to decrease ammonia production include dietary limitations and drug therapy to reduce bacterial breakdown. Patients with cirrhosis have increased nutritional requirements—high-carbohydrate, moderate-fat, and high-protein foods. However, the diet may be changed for those who have elevated serum ammonia levels with signs of encephalopathy. Patients should have a moderate amount of protein and fat foods and simple carbohydrates. Strict protein restrictions are not required because patients need protein for healing. In collaboration with the registered dietitian nutritionist, be sure to include family members or significant others in ***nutrition*** counseling. The patient is often weak and unable to remember complicated guidelines. Brief, simple directions regarding dietary dos and don'ts are recommended. Keep in mind any financial, cultural, or personal implications and the patient's food allergies when discussing food choices to provide optimal patient-centered care.

Drugs are used sparingly because they are difficult for the failing liver to metabolize. In particular, opioid analgesics, sedatives, and barbiturates should be restricted, especially for the patient with a history of encephalopathy.

However, several types of drugs may eliminate or reduce ammonia levels in the body. These include lactulose or lactitol and nonabsorbable antibiotics. The primary health care provider may prescribe *lactulose* (or lactitol) to promote the excretion of ammonia in the stool. This drug is a viscous, sticky, sweet-tasting liquid that is given either orally or by NG tube. The purpose is to obtain a laxative effect. Cleansing the bowels may rid the intestinal tract of the toxins that contribute to encephalopathy. It works by increasing osmotic pressure to draw fluid into the colon and prevents absorption of ammonia in the colon. The drug may be prescribed to the patient who has manifested signs of encephalopathy, regardless of the stage (Burchum & Rosenthal, 2019). The desired effect of the drug is production of two or three soft stools per day and a decrease in patient confusion caused by this complication.

Observe for response to lactulose. The patient may report intestinal bloating and cramping. Serum ammonia levels may be monitored but do not always correlate with symptoms. Hypokalemia and dehydration may result from excessive stools. Remind assistive personnel to help the patient with skin care if needed to prevent breakdown caused by excessive stools.

Several *nonabsorbable antibiotics* may be given if lactulose does not help the patient meet the desired outcome or if he or she cannot tolerate the drug. These drugs should not be given together. Older adults can become weak and dehydrated from having multiple stools. Neomycin sulfate or rifaximin, both broad-spectrum antibiotics, may be given to act as intestinal antiseptics. These drugs destroy the normal flora in the bowel, diminishing protein breakdown and decreasing the rate of ammonia production. Maintenance doses of neomycin are given orally but may also be administered as a retention enema. Long-term use has the potential for kidney toxicity and therefore is not commonly used for an extended period of time. It cannot be used for patients with existing kidney disease (Burchum & Rosenthal, 2019).

Frequently assess for changes in level of consciousness and orientation. Check for **asterixis** and **fetor hepaticus**. These signs suggest worsening encephalopathy. Thiamine supplements and benzodiazepines may be needed if the patient is at risk for alcohol withdrawal.

NCLEX EXAMINATION CHALLENGE 53.2

Physiological Integrity

The nurse is caring for a client in end-stage liver failure. Which interventions should be implemented when observing for hepatic encephalopathy? **Select all that apply.**

A. Assess the client's neurologic status as prescribed.
B. Monitor the client's hemoglobin and hematocrit levels.
C. Monitor the client's serum ammonia level.
D. Monitor the client's electrolyte values daily.
E. Prepare to insert an esophageal balloon tamponade tube.
F. Make sure the client's fingernails are short.

Managing Pruritus

Planning: Expected Outcomes. The patient is expected to experience less discomfort from pruritus as a result of comfort measures and possibly drug therapy.

Interventions. Patients frequently report pruritus and dry skin as a result of jaundice from increased levels of serum bilirubin as cirrhosis progresses. Pruritus tends to increase in warmer conditions and in the early evening and at night. Therefore comfort measures include avoiding being too warm, moisturizing the skin, and avoiding irritants to the skin. Some patients find that cool compresses and/or corticosteroids creams provide temporary relief. If these measures are not effective, drug therapy, including selective serotonin reuptake inhibitors like sertraline, may be helpful.

Care Coordination and Transition Management. If the patient with late-stage cirrhosis survives life-threatening complications, he or she is usually discharged to home or to a long-term care facility after treatment measures have managed the acute medical problems. A home care referral may be needed if the patient is discharged to home. These chronically ill patients are often readmitted multiple times, and community-based care is aimed at optimizing comfort, promoting independence, supporting caregivers, and preventing rehospitalization.

INTERPROFESSIONAL COLLABORATION

Care of Patients with Cirrhosis

For patients with moderate-to-late-stage liver disease, collaborate with the case manager (CM) or other discharge planner to coordinate interprofessional continuing care. According to the Interprofessional Education Collaborative (IPEC) Expert Panel's Competency of Roles and Responsibilities, using the unique and complementary abilities of other team members optimizes health and patient care (IPEC Expert Panel, 2016; Slusser et al., 2019). Collaborate with health care team members to help the client be as ADL independent as possible, including physical and occupational therapists. Patients with end-stage disease may benefit from hospice care.

Home Care Management. In collaboration with the patient, family, and case manager, assess physical adaptations needed to prepare the patient's home for recovery. His or her rest area needs to be close to a bathroom because diuretic and/or lactulose therapy increases the frequency of urination and stools. If the patient has difficulty reaching the toilet, additional equipment (e.g., bedside commode) is necessary. Special adult-size incontinence pads or briefs may be helpful if the patient has an altered mental status and incontinence. If the patient has shortness of breath from massive ascites, elevating the head of the bed and maintaining him or her in a semi-Fowler to high-Fowler position may help alleviate respiratory distress. Alternatively, a reclining chair with an elevated foot rest may be used.

Self-Management Education. The patient is discharged to the home setting with an individualized teaching plan that includes ***nutrition*** therapy, drug therapy, and alcohol abstinence. The patient who has a tunneled ascites drain will need to be taught how to access the drain and remove excess fluid. *Review the home care instructions that are provided with the drainage system with both the patient and family/caregiver. Remind them not to remove more than 2000 mL from the abdomen at one time to prevent hypovolemic shock.*

The patient with encephalopathy often finds that small, frequent meals are best tolerated. If his or her nutritional intake or albumin/prealbumin is decreased after discharge, multivitamin and oral nutritional supplements are usually needed. Teach patients to avoid excessive vitamins and minerals that can be toxic to the liver, such as fat-soluble vitamins, excessive iron supplements, and niacin. Remind patients to check with their primary health care provider before taking any vitamin supplement.

The patient is often discharged while receiving diuretics. Provide instructions regarding the primary health care provider's prescription for the diuretic. Teach about side effects of therapy, such as hypokalemia. The patient may need to take a potassium supplement if he or she is taking a diuretic that is not potassium sparing.

If the patient has had problems with bleeding from gastric ulcers, the primary health care provider may prescribe an H_2-receptor antagonist agent or proton pump inhibitor to reduce acid reflux (see Chapter 50). Patients who have had episodes of spontaneous bacterial peritonitis (SBP) may be on a daily low-dose maintenance antibiotic.

Teach family members how to recognize signs of encephalopathy and to contact the primary health care provider if these signs develop. Reinforce that constipation, bleeding, and ***infection*** can increase the risk for encephalopathy.

Advise the patient to avoid all over-the-counter drugs, especially NSAIDs and hepatic toxic herbs, vitamins, and minerals. Reinforce the need to keep appointments for follow-up medical care. Remind the patient and family to notify the primary health care provider immediately if any GI bleeding (overt bleeding or melena) is noted so that re-evaluation can begin quickly.

! NURSING SAFETY PRIORITY QSEN

Action Alert

One of the most important aspects of ongoing care for the patient with cirrhosis is health teaching about the need for the client to avoid acetaminophen, alcohol, smoking, and illicit drugs. By avoiding these substances, the patient may:

- Prevent further fibrosis of the liver from scarring
- Allow the liver to heal and regenerate
- Prevent gastric and esophageal irritation
- Reduce the incidence of bleeding
- Prevent other life-threatening complications

Health Care Resources. The patient with chronic cirrhosis may require a home care nurse for several visits after hospital discharge. The home care nurse can monitor the effectiveness of treatment in controlling ascites. The encephalopathic patient may need to be monitored for adherence to drug therapy and alcohol abstinence, if appropriate. Individual and group therapy sessions may be arranged to help patients deal with alcohol abstinence if they are too ill to attend a formal treatment program. Because some patients may have alienated relatives over the years because of substance use, it may be necessary to help them identify a friend, neighbor, or adult in their recovery group for support. If needed, refer the patient and family to self-help groups, such as Alcoholics Anonymous and Al-Anon. In Canada, SMART Recovery offers similar support, as well as additional services to control addictions.

The patient with cirrhosis may also desire spiritual or other psychosocial support. Finances are frequently a problem for the chronically ill patient and family; social support and community services need to be identified. The American Liver Foundation (www.liverfoundation.org) and American Gastroenterological Association (www.gastro.org) are excellent sources for more information about liver disease.

For patients who are not candidates for liver transplantation, address end-of-life issues. Discuss options such as hospice care with patients and their families (see Chapter 8). Be aware that they will go through a grieving process and will perhaps be in denial or very angry.

◆ **Evaluation: Evaluate Outcomes.** Evaluate the care of the patient with cirrhosis based on the identified priority patient problems. The expected outcomes include that the patient will:

- Have a decrease in or have no ascites
- Achieve ***fluid and electrolyte balance***
- Not have hemorrhage or will be managed immediately if bleeding occurs
- Not develop encephalopathy or will be managed immediately if it occurs
- Successfully abstain from alcohol or drugs (if disease is caused by one or more of these substances) and have adequate ***nutrition***

INFECTION CONCEPT EXEMPLAR: HEPATITIS

Pathophysiology Review

Hepatitis is the widespread ***inflammation*** and ***infection*** of liver cells. *Viral* hepatitis, which can be acute or chronic, is the most common type. Less common types of hepatitis are caused by chemicals, drugs, and some herbs. This section discusses hepatitis caused by a virus. **Viral hepatitis** results from an infection caused by one of five categories of viruses:

- Hepatitis A virus (HAV)
- Hepatitis B virus (HBV)
- Hepatitis C virus (HCV)
- Hepatitis D virus (HDV)
- Hepatitis E virus (HEV)

Some cases of viral hepatitis are not caused by any of these viruses. These patients have non–A-E hepatitis. This section focuses on the most common viral types.

Liver injury with ***inflammation*** can develop after exposure to a number of drugs and chemicals by inhalation, ingestion, or parenteral (IV) administration. *Toxic and drug-induced hepatitis* can result from exposure to hepatotoxins (e.g., industrial toxins, alcohol, and drugs). Hepatitis may also occur as a secondary ***infection*** during the course of infections with other viruses, such as Epstein-Barr, herpes simplex, varicella-zoster, and cytomegalovirus.

After the liver has been exposed to any causative agent (e.g., a virus), it becomes enlarged and congested with inflammatory cells, lymphocytes, and fluid, resulting in right upper quadrant pain and discomfort. As the disease progresses, the liver's normal lobular pattern becomes distorted as ***cellular regulation*** is compromised as a result of widespread ***inflammation,*** necrosis, and hepatocellular regeneration. This distortion increases pressure within the portal circulation, interfering with the blood flow into the hepatic lobules. Edema of the liver's bile channels results in obstructive **jaundice.**

Etiology. The five major types of acute viral hepatitis vary by etiology, mode of transmission, manner of onset, and incubation periods. Hepatitis cases must be reported to the local public health department, which then notifies the Centers for Disease Control and Prevention (CDC).

Hepatitis A. The causative agent of hepatitis A, hepatitis A virus (HAV), is a ribonucleic acid (RNA) virus of the enterovirus family. *It is a hardy virus and survives on human hands.* The virus is resistant to detergents and acids but is destroyed by chlorine (bleach) and extremely high temperatures.

Hepatitis A usually has a mild course similar to that of a typical flulike infection and often goes unrecognized. It is spread most often by the fecal-oral route by fecal contamination either from person-to-person contact (e.g., oral-anal sexual activity) or by consuming contaminated food or water. Common sources of ***infection*** include shellfish caught in contaminated water and food contaminated by food handlers infected with HAV. The incubation period of hepatitis A is usually 15 to 50 days, with a peak of 25 to 30 days. The disease is usually not life threatening, but its course may be more severe in adults older than 40 years and those with pre-existing liver disease such as hepatitis C (McCance et al., 2019).

In a small percentage of hepatitis A cases, severe illness with extrahepatic signs and symptoms can occur. Advanced age and conditions such as chronic liver disease may cause widespread damage that requires a liver transplant. In some cases when the patient's immunity is decreased, death may occur. The incidence of hepatitis A is particularly high in nonaffluent countries in which sanitation is poor; however, cases are diagnosed internationally across the globe (World Health Organization, 2017). Some adults have hepatitis A and do not know it. The course is similar to that of a GI illness, and the disease and recovery are usually uneventful.

NCLEX EXAMINATION CHALLENGE 53.3

Physiological Integrity

The nurse is caring for a client diagnosed with hepatitis A. Which transmission-based precautions are required when providing care for this client? **Select all that apply.**

A. Place client in a private room.
B. Wear a mask when handling patient bedpan.
C. Wear gloves when touching the client.
D. Wear a gown when providing personal care to this patient.
E. Wear eye goggles when providing care.

Hepatitis B. The hepatitis B virus (HBV) is not transmitted like HAV. It is a double-shelled particle containing DNA composed of a core antigen (HBcAg), a surface antigen (HBsAg), and another antigen found within the core (HBeAg) that circulates in the blood. HBV may be spread through these common modes of transmission (CDC, 2020a):

- Unprotected sexual intercourse with an infected partner
- Sharing needles, syringes, or other drug-injection equipment
- Sharing razors or toothbrushes with an infected individual
- Accidental needlesticks or injuries from sharp instruments primarily in health care workers (low incidence)
- Blood transfusions (that have not been screened for the virus, before 1992)
- Hemodialysis
- Direct contact with the blood or open sores of an infected individual
- Birth (spread from an infected mother to baby during birth)

In addition, patients whose immunity is compromised by either disease or drug therapy are more likely to develop hepatitis B. The clinical course of hepatitis B may be varied. Symptoms usually occur within 25 to 180 days of exposure.

Blood tests confirm the disease, although many individuals with hepatitis B have no symptoms. Most adults who get hepatitis B recover and clear the virus from their body and develop immunity. However, a small percentage of people do not develop immunity and become carriers. Hepatitis carriers can infect others even though they are not sick and have no obvious signs of hepatitis B. Chronic carriers are at high risk for cirrhosis and liver cancer. Because of the high number of newcomers from endemic areas, the incidence of hepatitis B has increased in the United States.

Hepatitis C. Hepatitis C (HCV) is the leading cause of end-stage liver disease in the world (Chaney, 2019). The causative virus of hepatitis C is an enveloped, single-stranded RNA virus, which is genetically unstable and has at least six known major genotypes. Transmission is blood to blood. The rate of sexual transmission is very low in a single-couple relationship but increases with multiple sex partners or in men who have unprotected sex with men. HCV is spread most commonly by (Chaney, 2019):

- Illicit IV drug needle sharing (highest incidence)
- Blood, blood products, or organ transplants received before 1992
- Baby boomers (those adults born between 1945 and 1965)
- Needlestick injury with HCV-contaminated blood (health care workers at high risk)
- Hemodialysis
- Health care workers
- People who are incarcerated (prisoners)
- Sharing of drug paraphernalia

The disease is *not* transmitted by casual contact or intimate household contact. However, those infected are advised not to share razors, toothbrushes, or pierced earrings because microscopic blood may be on these items.

The incubation period ranges from 2 weeks to 6 months. Acute infection and illness are not common. Most people are completely unaware that they have been infected. They may be asymptomatic and not diagnosed until many months or years after the initial exposure when an abnormality is detected during a routine laboratory evaluation or when liver problems occur. Unlike with hepatitis B, most people infected with hepatitis C do not clear the virus, and a chronic infection develops.

HCV usually does its damage to the body's immunity over decades by causing a chronic ***inflammation*** in the liver that eventually causes the liver cells to scar. Scarring from chronic ***infection*** with either HBV and HCV frequently leads to cirrhosis, which is a risk factor for developing primary liver cancer (McCance et al., 2019). Patients who develop liver cancer may have interventional radiologic procedures (such as transarterial chemoembolization [TACE]), cryotherapy, ablation, traditional chemotherapy, or selective radiation therapy (SIRT) (see Chapter 20 for more information on cancer management modalities and associated nursing care). Liver cancer can also occur as a metastatic disease process and is not associated with hepatitis or cirrhosis.

Hepatitis D. Hepatitis D (delta hepatitis) is caused by a defective RNA virus that needs the helper function of HBV. It occurs only with HBV to cause viral replication. This usually develops into chronic disease. The incubation period is about 14 to 56 days. As with hepatitis B, the disease is transmitted primarily by parenteral routes, especially in patients who are IV drug users. Having sexual contact with someone with HDV is also a high-risk factor (McCance et al., 2019).

Hepatitis E. The hepatitis E virus (HEV) causes a waterborne infection associated with epidemics in the Indian subcontinent, Asia, Africa, the Middle East, Mexico, and Central and South America. Many large outbreaks have occurred after heavy rains and flooding. Like hepatitis A, hepatitis E is caused by fecal contamination of food and water.

In the United States, hepatitis E has been found only in international travelers. It is transmitted via the fecal-oral route, and the clinical course resembles that of hepatitis A. Hepatitis E has an incubation period of 15 to 64 days. There is no evidence at this time of a chronic form of the disease. The disease tends to be self-limiting and resolves on its own (McCance et al., 2019).

Complications of Hepatitis. Failure of the liver cells to regenerate, with progression of the necrotic process, results in a severe acute and often fatal form of hepatitis known as *fulminant hepatitis*. Hepatitis is considered to be chronic when liver ***inflammation*** lasts longer than 6 months. *Chronic hepatitis* usually occurs as a result of hepatitis B or hepatitis C. Superimposed infection with hepatitis D virus (HDV) in patients with chronic hepatitis B may also result in chronic hepatitis. Chronic hepatitis can lead to cirrhosis and liver cancer. Many patients have multiple infections, especially a combination of HBV with HCV, HDV, or HIV infections (McCance et al., 2019).

Incidence and Prevalence. The incidence of hepatitis A and hepatitis B is declining as a result of CDC recommendations for vaccination. However, hepatitis B and hepatitis C are a concern because of their association with cirrhosis and liver cancer. Although exact numbers are not known, it is estimated that over 170 million people worldwide have the hepatitis C virus (HCV) with 3 to 4 million new cases occurring every year. It is the most common chronic bloodborne infection in the United States (Chaney, 2019; Horsley-Silva & Vargas, 2017). Most hepatitis A (HAV) infections in the United States today occur in patients who have drug abuse or those who are homeless (Heavey, 2020).

Currently there is no vaccine for HCV; however, patients may be treated with antiviral drug therapies. The desired outcome of treatment of HCV-infected patients is to reduce mortality and liver-related health adverse consequences, including end-stage liver disease and liver cancer. It is expected that the cases of HCV may rise over the next several decades as a result of increasing illicit drug use.

Health Promotion and Maintenance. Hepatitis vaccines for infants, children, and adolescents have helped to decrease the incidence of hepatitis A and hepatitis B. Teach adults the importance of obtaining immunizations for their children. These vaccines are safe and not associated with major complications. Some adults are also advised to receive these immunizations.

Measures for preventing hepatitis A in adults include:

- Proper handwashing, especially after handling shellfish
- Avoiding contaminated food or water (including tap water in countries with high incidence)
- Receiving immunoglobulin within 14 days if exposed to the virus
- Receiving the HAV vaccine before traveling to areas where the disease is common (e.g., Mexico, Caribbean)
- Receiving the vaccine if living or working in enclosed areas with others, such as college dormitories, correctional institutions, day-care centers, and long-term care facilities

Several HAV vaccines are made of inactivated hepatitis A virus and are given in the deltoid muscle. Several vaccines can also provide protection against hepatitis B virus (HBV) infection. A combination HAV and HBV vaccine is also available for adults. Examples of groups for whom immunization against HBV should be used include:

- People who have sexual intercourse with more than one partner
- People with sexually transmitted infection (STI) or a history of STI
- Men having unprotected sex with men (MSM)

BEST PRACTICE FOR PATIENT SAFETY & QUALITY CARE (QSEN)

Prevention of Viral Hepatitis in Health Care Workers

- Use Standard Precautions to prevent the transmission of disease between patients or between patients and health care staff (see Chapter 21).
- Eliminate needles and other sharp instruments by substituting needleless systems. (Needlesticks are the major source of hepatitis B transmission in health care workers.)
- Take the hepatitis B vaccine, which is given in a series of three injections. This vaccine also prevents hepatitis D by preventing hepatitis B.
- For postexposure prevention of hepatitis A, seek medical attention immediately for immunoglobulin (Ig) administration.
- Report all cases of hepatitis to the local health department.

- People with any chronic liver disease (such as hepatitis C or cirrhosis)
- Patients with human immune deficiency virus (HIV) infection
- People who are exposed to blood or body fluids in the workplace, including health care workers, firefighters, and police
- People in correctional facilities (prisoners)
- Patients needing immunosuppressant drugs
- Family members, household members, and sexual contacts of people with HBV infection

Multiple HCV genotypes have made it difficult to develop an effective vaccine against hepatitis C. Teach baby boomer adults to have a one-time screening test for HCV due to the high risk of this infection in this population (Chaney, 2019).

Additional measures to prevent viral hepatitis for health care workers and others in contact with infected patients are listed in the Best Practice for Patient Safety & Quality Care: Prevention of Viral Hepatitis in Health Care Workers box.

❖ Interprofessional Collaborative Care

Care for the patient with hepatitis can take place in various settings. These patients may, at different times, self-manage at home, be hospitalized for immediate concerns, or be cared for in the community setting.

◆ Assessment: Recognize Cues

History. Begin by asking the patient whether or not he or she has had known exposure to a person with hepatitis. For the patient who presents with few or no symptoms of liver disease but has abnormal laboratory tests (e.g., elevated alanine aminotransferase [ALT] or aspartate aminotransferase [AST] level), the history may need to include additional questions regarding risk factors.

Physical Assessment/Signs and Symptoms. Assess whether the patient has any of the signs and symptoms associated with most types of vital hepatitis as listed in the Key Features: Viral Hepatitis box. Although HCV may be asymptomatic for most adults, some patients with a new HCV ***infection*** can experience some of these signs and symptoms.

KEY FEATURES

Viral Hepatitis

- Abdominal pain
- Yellowish sclera (**icterus**)
- Arthralgia (joint pain) or myalgia (muscle pain)
- Diarrhea/constipation
- Light clay-colored stools
- Dark yellow to brownish urine
- **Jaundice**
- Fever
- Fatigue
- Malaise
- Anorexia
- Nausea and vomiting
- Dry skin
- Pruritus (itching)

Lightly palpate the right upper abdominal quadrant to assess for liver tenderness. The patient may report right upper quadrant pain with jarring movements. Inspect the skin, sclerae, and mucous membranes for **jaundice**. He or she may present for medical treatment only after jaundice appears, believing that other vague symptoms are related to a flulike syndrome.

Jaundice in hepatitis results from intrahepatic obstruction and is caused by edema of the liver's bile channels. Dark urine and clay-colored stools are often reported by the patient. If possible, obtain a urine and stool specimen for visual inspection and laboratory analysis. The patient may also have skin abrasions from scratching because of pruritus (itching).

Patients with chronic HCV infection often have extrahepatic complications. Examples include:

- Depression
- Polyarthritis
- Myalgia
- Renal insufficiency
- Cognitive impairment
- Cardiovascular problems such as vasculitis and heart disease

Psychosocial Assessment. Viral hepatitis has various presentations, but for most infected people the initial course is mild with few or no symptoms. The long-term complications of fibrosis and cirrhosis cause the more serious problem. This is especially true for patients who have chronic HBV and HCV infection.

Emotional problems for affected patients may center on their feeling sick and fatigued. General malaise, inactivity, and vague symptoms contribute to depression. Some patients often feel guilty and are remorseful about decisions made that caused the disease. These feelings are most likely to occur when the source of infection is from drug use.

Infectious diseases such as hepatitis continue to have a social stigma. (See the Evidence-Based Practice box.) The patient may feel embarrassed by the precautions that are imposed in the hospital and continue to be necessary at home. This embarrassment may cause the patient to limit social interactions. Patients may be afraid that they will spread the virus to family and friends.

EVIDENCE-BASED PRACTICE (QSEN)

Caring for Military Veterans With Hepatitis C

Phillips, F., & Barnes, D. (2016). Social support and adherence for military veterans with hepatitis C. *Clinical Nurse Specialist, 30*(1), 38–44.

This qualitative study's aim was to describe military veterans' experience of support after diagnosis of hepatitis C and how support impacted their adherence to treatment.

A convenience sample of 21 veterans was used for this phenomenological study. Inclusion criteria were composed of veterans who were older than 18 years of age; were receiving standard care for hepatitis C; and could read, write, and communicate in English. In keeping with a phenomenological design, researchers collected data during a one-time, in-depth interview with each participant. Follow-up phone calls were used to verify that the themes identified were congruent with the lived experience of subjects.

Results indicated that veterans selectively tell only certain individuals about their diagnosis due to fear of stigma. In turn, this limits the amount of people in their circle of support. Veterans found some level of support, yet some level of burden, when disclosing their status to family members, friends, and health care providers.

Level of Evidence: 3

This qualitative research was designed as a phenomenological study.

Commentary: Implications for Practice and Research

Nurses must use empathy and concern while assessing availability of support systems for patients. In absence of a personal support network, or in addition to an existing support system, nurses should recommend support groups or counseling to help the patient adhere to treatment and management of hepatitis C.

Family members are sometimes afraid of getting the disease and may distance themselves from the patient. Allow them to verbalize these feelings and explore the reasons for these fears. Educate the patient and family members about modes of transmission, and clarify information as needed.

Patients may be unable to return to work for several weeks during the acute phases of illness. The loss of wages and the cost of hospitalization for a patient without insurance coverage may produce great anxiety and financial burden. This situation may last for months or years if hepatitis becomes chronic.

Laboratory Assessment. Hepatitis A, hepatitis B, and hepatitis C are usually confirmed by acute elevations in levels of liver enzymes, indicating liver cellular damage, and by specific serologic markers.

Levels of ALT and AST may possibly rise into the thousands in acute or fulminant cases of hepatitis. Alkaline phosphatase levels may be normal or elevated. Serum total bilirubin levels are elevated and are consistent with the clinical appearance of jaundice.

The presence of *hepatitis A* is established when hepatitis A virus (HAV) antibodies (anti-HAV) are found in the blood. Ongoing ***inflammation*** of the liver by HAV is indicated by the presence of immunoglobulin M (IgM) antibodies, which persist in the blood for 4 to 6 weeks. Previous infection is identified by the presence of immunoglobulin G (IgG) antibodies. These antibodies persist in the serum and provide permanent immunity to HAV (Pagana & Pagana, 2018).

The presence of the *hepatitis B* virus (HBV) is established when serologic testing confirms the presence of hepatitis B antigen-antibody systems in the blood and a detectable viral count (HBV polymerase chain reaction [PCR] DNA). Antigens located on the surface (shell) of the virus (HBsAg) and IgM antibodies to hepatitis B core antigen (anti-HBcAg IgM) are the most significant serologic markers. The presence of these markers establishes the diagnosis of hepatitis B. *The patient is infectious as long as hepatitis B surface antigen (HBsAg) is present in the blood.* Persistence of this serologic marker after 6 months or longer indicates a carrier state or chronic hepatitis. HBsAg levels normally decline and disappear after the acute hepatitis B episode. The presence of antibodies to HBsAg in the blood indicates recovery and immunity to hepatitis B. *People who have been vaccinated against HBV have a positive HBsAg because they also have immunity to the disease (*Pagana & Pagana, 2018*).*

To detect HCV infection, blood is tested for anti-HCV antibodies to HCV recombinant core antigen, *NS3* gene, NS4 antigen, and NS5 antibody. The antibodies can be detected within 4 weeks of the infection (Pagana & Pagana, 2018). To identify the actual circulating virus, the HCV RNA test is used. This confirms active virus and can measure the viral load. A diagnostic tool called the *OraQuick HCV Rapid Antibody Test* has the advantage of providing a quick diagnosis of the disease as a point-of-care test.

The presence of *hepatitis D* virus (HDV) can be confirmed by the identification of intrahepatic delta antigen or, more often, by a rise in the hepatitis D virus antibodies (anti-HDV) titer. This increase can be seen within a few days of ***infection*** (Pagana & Pagana, 2018).

Hepatitis E virus (HEV) testing is usually reserved for travelers in whom hepatitis is present but the virus cannot be detected. Hepatitis E antibodies (anti-HEV) are found in people infected with the virus.

Other Diagnostic Assessment. *Liver biopsy* may be used to confirm the diagnosis of hepatitis and establish the stage and grade of liver damage or cancer. Characteristic changes help the pathologist distinguish among a virus, drug, toxin, fatty liver, iron, and other disease. It is usually performed in an ambulatory care setting as a percutaneous procedure (through the skin) after a local anesthetic is given. However, if coagulation is abnormal, it may be done using either a CT-guided or transjugular route to reduce the risk for pneumothorax or hemothorax. *Ultrasound* also may be used.

◆ **Analysis: Analyze Cues and Prioritize Hypotheses.** The priority collaborative problems for patients with hepatitis include:

1. Weight loss due to complications associated with ***inflammation*** of the liver
2. Fatigue due to ***infection*** and decreased metabolic energy production

◆ **Planning and Implementation: Generate Solutions and Take Action.** The patient with viral hepatitis can be mildly or acutely ill, depending on the severity of the ***inflammation*** and ***infection***. Most patients are not hospitalized, although older adults and those with dehydration may be admitted for a short-term stay. The plan of care for all patients with viral hepatitis is based on measures to rest the liver, promote hepatic regeneration, strengthen immunity, and prevent complications, if possible.

Promoting Nutrition

Planning: Expected Outcomes. The patient will maintain appropriate weight and ***nutrition*** status.

Interventions. The patient with hepatitis, especially hepatitis A, may decline food because of general malaise, anorexia, abdominal discomfort, or nausea. The patient's diet should be high in carbohydrates and calories with moderate amounts of fat and protein added after nausea and anorexia subside. Small, frequent meals are often preferable to three standard meals daily. Ask the patient about appealing food preferences because favorite foods are tolerated better than randomly selected foods. High-calorie snacks may be needed. Supplemental vitamins are often prescribed.

Managing Fatigue

Planning: Expected Outcomes. The patient will progressively exhibit increasing energy as evidenced by participation in ADLs and self-reported decrease in level of fatigue.

Interventions. During the acute stage of viral hepatitis, interventions are aimed at resting the inflamed liver to promote hepatic cell regeneration. *Rest* is an essential intervention to reduce the liver's metabolic demands and increase its blood supply. Collaborative care is generally supportive. The patient is usually tired and expresses feelings of general malaise. Complete bedrest is usually not required, but rest periods alternating with periods of activity are indicated and are often enough to promote hepatic healing. Individualize the patient's plan of care and change it as needed to reflect the severity of symptoms, fatigue, and results of liver function tests and enzyme determinations. Activities such as self-care and ambulating are gradually added to the activity schedule as tolerated.

Drugs of any kind are used sparingly for patients with hepatitis to allow the liver to rest. An antiemetic to relieve nausea may be prescribed. However, because of the life-threatening nature of chronic hepatitis B and hepatitis C, a number of drugs are given, including antiviral and immunomodulating drugs.

Two groups of drugs are approved for management of Hepatitis B—*interferon alfa preparations* and *nucleoside analogs*. Examples of interferon alfa drugs include interferon alfa-2b and Peginterferon alfa-2a. These drugs are not used as often today because newer, more effective medications are available. Examples of nucleoside analogs include lamivudine and adefovir (see the Common Examples of Drug Therapy: Chronic Hepatitis B and Hepatitis C box).

For a number of years, the standard of care for hepatitis C was pegylated (PEG) interferon alfa plus ribavirin (Burchum & Rosenthal, 2019). In the past decade, new direct-acting antiviral (DAA) drugs that target specific steps in HCV replication have been used with much more success and fewer side or adverse effects. In 2011, the U.S. Food and Drug Administration approved the first two first-generation *protease inhibitors (PIs)*. These drugs have been taken off the market in favor of better second-generation PIs (Chaney, 2019). The current standard of

COMMON EXAMPLES OF DRUG THERAPY

Chronic Hepatitis B and Hepatitis C

Drug	Nursing Implications
Chronic Hepatitis B	
Tenofovir	Monitor kidney function. *Drug is excreted through kidneys; monitoring for renal impairment is important.* Teach risk for falls to prevent fractures. *Can cause bone demineralization.*
Adefovir	Monitor kidney function. *Drug is excreted through kidneys; monitoring for renal impairment is important.*
Lamivudine	Monitor kidney function. *Drug is excreted through kidneys; monitoring for renal impairment is important.* Remind patient to not discontinue drug without consulting with primary health care provider. *Discontinuation of drug can cause flareup of HBV.*
Entecavir	Monitor kidney function. Teach the patient to avoid alcohol to prevent serious interaction. *Drug is excreted through kidneys; monitoring for renal impairment is important.*
Chronic Hepatitis C	
Second-generation protease inhibitors: • Grazoprevir • Simprevir • Paritaprevir	Monitor CBC and chemistry panel. Instruct the patient on common reactions, such as rash, itching, nausea, and headache. *Kidney and liver function may become impaired, and electrolyte imbalances may occur when taking this drug.*
NS5A inhibitors:	
• Elbasvir (also available in combination with grazoprevir)	Ask the patient if he or she has a history of or current hepatitis B. *The combination drug can reactivate hepatitis B and cause liver failure.* Teach patients that their liver enzymes must be monitored, especially ALT elevation. *The combination drug can cause liver toxicity, including an increase in liver enzymes.*
• Ledipasvir/Sofosbuvir (for hepatitis C genotype 1 only)	Ask if the patient has had any other type of hepatitis or cirrhosis. *This combination drug can reactivate hepatitis B and cause liver failure.* Do not give this drug to patients receiving amiodarone. *If this drug combination is taken with amiodarone, the patient may experience severe symptomatic bradycardia and other cardiac problems, including chest pain.*
NS5A-NS5B polymerase inhibitor:	
• Sofosbuvir/velpatasvir (for almost all main types of hepatitis C)	Ask the patient if he or she has a history of or current hepatitis B. *The combination drug can reactivate hepatitis B and cause liver failure.* Teach patients that their liver enzymes must be monitored, especially ALT elevation.

HBV, Hepatitis B virus; *HIV*, human immune deficiency virus.

practice for hepatitis C treatment is that a patient's drug regimen is determined by HCV viral genotype (AASLD, 2018). Examples of newer single and combination PIs are presented in the Common Examples of Drug Therapy: Chronic Hepatitis B and Hepatitis C box. All of these drugs can affect the immune system and make patients susceptible to ***infection***. *Teach patients to avoid crowds and people who are infected!*

Similar to patients with other chronic diseases, patients with hepatitis often use complementary and integrative therapies to promote general well-being and improve quality of life. Examples include herbs and vitamin supplements including silymarin (milk thistle plant), green tea, and vitamin E. The effectiveness of these substances has not been well researched.

Care Coordination and Transition Management. Home care management varies according to the type of hepatitis and whether the disease is acute or chronic. A primary focus in any case is preventing the spread of the infection. For hepatitis transmitted by the fecal-oral route, careful handwashing and sanitary disposal of feces are important. Therefore education is very important.

! NURSING SAFETY PRIORITY (QSEN)

Action Alert

Teach the patient with viral hepatitis and the family to use measures to prevent infection transmission. In addition, instruct the patient to avoid alcohol and check with the primary health care provider before taking any medication or vitamin, supplement, or herbal preparation.

Encourage the patient to increase activity gradually to prevent fatigue. Suggest that the patient eat small, frequent meals of high-carbohydrate foods and plan frequent rest periods.

Collaborate with the certified infection control practitioner and infectious disease specialist if needed in caring for these patients. These experts can suggest appropriate resources for the patient and family.

◆ **Evaluation: Evaluate Outcomes.** Evaluate the care of the patient with hepatitis based on the identified priority patient problems. The expected outcomes include that the patient will:

- Maintain adequate ***nutrition*** for body requirements
- Report increasing energy levels as the liver rests
- Achieve appropriate management of ***infection*** and ***inflammation***

CLINICAL JUDGMENT CHALLENGE 53.1

Patient-Centered Care; Safety

A 19-year-old woman presents at the college health clinic 3 weeks after a spring break trip to Las Vegas. She tells the nurse that the highlight of the trip was an "all-you-can-eat" seafood buffet. Since that time, she reports that she has been experiencing periodic fevers, abdominal pain, loss of appetite, nausea, vomiting, and fatigue. At first, she states that she thought she had the flu, but she now thinks that something else "must be terribly wrong" because her eyes and skin are turning yellow. She confirms that she is a nonsmoker and only drinks one to two alcoholic drinks per month.

1. **Recognize Cues:** What assessment information in this client situation is the most important and immediate concern for the nurse? (Hint: Identify the **relevant** information *first* to determine what is most important.)
2. **Analyze Cues:** What client conditions are consistent with the **most relevant** information? (Hint: Think about priority collaborative problems that support and contradict the information presented in this situation.)
3. **Prioritize Hypotheses:** Which possibilities or explanations are **most likely** to be present in this client situation? Which possibilities or explanations are the most serious? (Hint: Consider all possibilities and determine their urgency and risk for this client.)
4. **Generate Solutions:** What actions would most likely achieve the desired outcomes for this client? Which actions should be **avoided** or are **potentially harmful**? (Hint: Determine the desired outcomes first to decide which interventions are appropriate and those that should be avoided.)
5. **Take Action:** Which actions are the most appropriate and how should they be implemented? In what **priority order** should they be implemented? (Hint: Consider health teaching, documentation, requested health care providsser orders or prescriptions, nursing skills, collaboration with or referral to health team members, etc.)
6. **Evaluate Outcomes:** What client assessment would indicate that the nurse's actions were **effective**? (Hint: Think about signs that would indicate an improvement, decline, or unchanged client condition.)

LIVER TRANSPLANTATION

Pathophysiology Review

Liver transplantation has become a common procedure worldwide. The patient with end-stage liver disease or acute liver failure who has not responded to conventional medical or surgical intervention is a potential candidate for liver transplantation. Many diseases can cause liver failure. Cirrhosis (scarring of the liver) is the most common reason for liver transplants. Other common reasons are chronic hepatitis B and hepatitis C, bile duct diseases, autoimmune liver disease, alcoholic liver disease, and fatty liver disease.

Transplantation Considerations. The patient for potential transplantation has extensive physiologic and psychological assessment and evaluation by primary health care providers and transplant coordinators. Alternative treatment should be extensively explored before committing a patient for a liver transplant. Patients who are *not* considered candidates for transplantation are those with:

- Severe cardiovascular instability with advanced cardiac disease
- Severe respiratory disease
- Metastatic tumors
- Inability to follow instructions regarding drug therapy and self-management

Liver transplantation has become the most effective treatment for an increasing number of patients with acute and chronic liver diseases. Inclusion and exclusion criteria vary among transplantation centers and are continually revised as treatment options change and surgical techniques improve.

Donor livers are obtained primarily from trauma victims who have not had liver damage. They are distributed through a nationwide program, the United Network of Organ Sharing (UNOS). This system distributes donor livers based on regional considerations and patient acuity. Candidates with the highest level of acuity receive highest priority.

The donor liver is transported to the surgery center in a solution that preserves the organ for up to 8 hours. The diseased liver is removed through an incision made in the upper abdomen. The new liver is carefully put in its place and attached to the patient's blood vessels and bile ducts. The procedure can take many hours to complete and requires a highly specialized team and large volumes of fluid and blood replacement.

Living donors have also been used and are usually close family members or a spouse. This is done on a voluntary basis after careful psychological and physiologic preparation and testing. The donor's liver is resected (usually removal of one lobe) and implanted into the recipient after removal of the diseased liver. In both the donor and the recipient, the liver regenerates and grows in size to meet the demands of the body.

Transplantation Complications. Although liver transplantations are commonly performed, complications can occur. Some problems can be managed medically, whereas others require hospitalizations or removal of the transplant. The most common complications are acute graft rejection, infection, and bleeding (Lynn, 2016; McCance et al., 2019).

The success rate for transplantations has greatly improved since the introduction many years ago of cyclosporine (cyclosporin A), an immunosuppressant drug. Today, many other antirejection drugs are used. (See Chapter 18 for a discussion of rejection and preventive drug therapy for organ transplantation.)

NURSING SAFETY PRIORITY (QSEN)

Action Alert

For the patient who has undergone liver transplantation, monitor for clinical signs and symptoms of rejection, which may include tachycardia, fever, ***pain*** in the right upper quadrant or flank, decreased bile pigment and volume, and increasing jaundice. Laboratory findings include elevated serum bilirubin, rising ALT and AST levels, elevated alkaline phosphatase levels, and increased prothrombin time/international normalized ratio (PT/INR) (Pagana & Pagana, 2018).

Transplant rejection is treated aggressively with immunosuppressive drugs. As with all rejection treatments, the patient is at a greater risk for infection. If therapy is not effective, liver function rapidly deteriorates. Multisystem organ failure, including respiratory and renal involvement, develops along with diffuse coagulopathies and portal-systemic encephalopathy (PSE). The only alternative for treatment is emergency retransplantation.

Infection is another potential threat to the transplanted graft and the patient's survival. Vaccinations and prophylactic antibiotics are helpful in prevention. Immunosuppressant therapy, which must be used to prevent and treat organ rejection, significantly increases the patient's risk for infection. Other risk factors include the presence of multiple tubes and intravascular lines, immobility, and prolonged anesthesia.

In the early posttransplantation period, common infections include pneumonia, wound infections, and urinary tract infections. Opportunistic ***infections*** usually develop after the first postoperative month and include cytomegalovirus, mycobacterial infections, and parasitic infections. Latent infections such as tuberculosis and herpes simplex may be reactivated. Women, Hispanics, and patients with less than a high school education are most likely to be readmitted with transplant complications, although the cause is not known (Dols et al., 2020).

The primary health care provider prescribes broad-spectrum antibiotics for prophylaxis during and after surgery. Obtain culture specimens from all lines and tubes and collect specimens for culture at predetermined time intervals as dictated by the agency's policy. If an ***infection*** is detected, the primary health care provider prescribes organism-specific anti-infective agents. The patient should be taught to contact the primary health care provider at any time that signs of ***infection*** are present.

The biliary anastomosis is susceptible to breakdown, obstruction, and infection. If leakage occurs or if the site becomes necrotic or obstructed, an abscess can form; or peritonitis, bacteremia, and cirrhosis may develop. Observe for potential complications, which are listed in Table 53.4.

! NURSING SAFETY PRIORITY (QSEN)

Action Alert

For the patient who has had a liver transplantation, monitor the temperature frequently per hospital protocol and report elevations, increased abdominal pain, distention, and rigidity, which are indicators of peritonitis. Nursing assessment also includes monitoring for a change in neurologic status that could indicate encephalopathy from a nonfunctioning liver. Report signs of clotting problems (e.g., bloody oozing from a catheter, petechiae, ecchymosis) to the surgeon immediately because they may indicate impaired function of the transplanted liver.

❖ Interprofessional Collaborative Care

Care of the patient undergoing liver transplantation requires an interprofessional team approach. Receiving a transplant has a major psychosocial impact. Transplant complications cause patients to be very anxious. In collaboration with the members of the interprofessional health care team, assure them and their families that these problems are common and usually treated successfully.

After the patient is identified as a candidate and a donor organ is procured, the actual liver transplantation surgical procedure usually takes many hours. The length of the procedure can vary greatly.

In the immediate postoperative period, the patient is managed in the critical care unit and requires aggressive monitoring and

TABLE 53.4 Assessment and Prevention of Common Postoperative Complications Associated With Liver Transplantation

Assessment	Prevention
Acute Graft Rejection	
Occurs from the 4th to 10th postoperative day	Prophylaxis with immunosuppressant agents, such as cyclosporine
Manifested by tachycardia, fever, right upper quadrant (RUQ) or flank pain, diminished bile drainage or change in bile color, or increased jaundice	Early diagnosis to treat with more potent antirejection drugs
Laboratory changes: (1) increased levels of serum bilirubin, transaminases, and alkaline phosphatase; (2) prolonged prothrombin time	
Infection	
Can occur at any time during recovery	Antibiotic prophylaxis; vaccinations
Manifested by fever or excessive, foul-smelling drainage (urine, wound, or bile); other indicators depend on location and type of infection	Frequent cultures of tubes, lines, and drainage Early removal of invasive lines Good handwashing Early diagnosis and treatment with organism-specific anti-infective agents
Hepatic Complications (Bile Leakage, Abscess Formation, Hepatic Thrombosis)	
Manifested by decreased bile drainage, increased RUQ abdominal pain with distention and guarding, nausea or vomiting, increased jaundice, and clay-colored stools	If present, keep T-tube in dependent position and secure to patient; empty frequently, recording quality and quantity of drainage Report signs and symptoms to surgeon immediately
Laboratory changes: increased levels of serum bilirubin and transaminases	May need surgical intervention
Acute Kidney Injury	
Caused by hypotension, antibiotics, cyclosporine, acute liver failure, or hypothermia	Monitor all drug levels with nephrotoxic side effects Prevent hypotension
Indicators of hypothermia: shivering, hyperventilation, increased cardiac output, vasoconstriction, and alkalemia	Observe for early signs of acute kidney injury and report them immediately to the surgeon
Early indicators of acute kidney injury: changes in urine output, increased blood urea nitrogen (BUN) and creatinine levels, and electrolyte imbalance	

care. Monitor for signs and symptoms of complications of surgery and immediately report them to the surgeon (see Table 53.4).

Post–liver transplant patients are living longer today than ever. Teach patients to be aware of side effects of immunosuppressive drugs, such as hypertension, nephrotoxicity, drug-induced ***infection,*** and gastrointestinal disturbances. Remind them that long-term management of care includes surveillance for malignancy, metabolic syndrome, and diabetes. Teaching the patient self-examination for skin, breast, and testicular malignancies and reminders for annual Papanicolaou (Pap) smears and other cancer screening tests are important. Posttransplant patients need to maintain lifestyle changes to increase their longevity after surgery.

GET READY FOR THE NEXT-GENERATION NCLEX® EXAMINATION!

Key Points

Review these Key Points for each NCLEX Examination Client Needs Category.

Safe and Effective Care Environment

- Refer patients with liver disorders to the American Liver Foundation; refer dying patients to hospice and other community resources as needed. **QSEN: Patient-Centered Care**

Health Promotion and Maintenance

- Teach patients to take precautions to prevent viral hepatitis in the community. **QSEN: Evidence-Based Practice**
- Teach patients to avoid alcohol and illicit drugs to prevent or slow the progression of alcohol-induced cirrhosis; remind them not to take any medication (including over-the-counter drugs) without checking with their primary health care provider. **QSEN: Safety**

Psychosocial Integrity

- Recognize that patients with cirrhosis have mental and emotional changes (including confusion) due to hepatic encephalopathy. **QSEN: Patient-Centered Care**
- Be aware that patients with cirrhosis and/or chronic hepatitis may feel guilty about their disease because of past habits such as drug and alcohol use. Allow patients to express feelings openly. **Ethics**
- Be aware that patients having liver transplantation have major concerns about the possibility of complications, such as organ rejection. **QSEN: Patient-Centered Care**

Physiological Integrity

- Be aware that cirrhosis has many causes other than alcohol use.
- Observe for clinical signs and symptoms of hepatic encephalopathy (PSE) as listed in Table 53.2. **QSEN: Safety**
- Monitor laboratory values of patients suspected of or diagnosed with cirrhosis of the liver as listed in Table 53.3. **Clinical Judgment**
- Monitor the patient with cirrhosis for bleeding and neurologic changes. **QSEN: Safety**
- Administer drug therapy to decrease ammonia levels (that cause PSE) in patients with cirrhosis, such as lactulose and nonabsorbable antibiotics. **QSEN: Safety**
- Differentiate the five major types of hepatitis: A, B, C, D, and E. Hepatitis D occurs only with hepatitis B and is transmitted most commonly by blood and body fluid exposure. Hepatitis A is transmitted via the fecal-oral route. Hepatitis C is the most common type and is also transmitted via blood and body fluids. **QSEN: Evidence-Based Practice**
- Be aware that patients with chronic viral hepatitis often develop cirrhosis and cancer of the liver. **QSEN: Evidence-Based Practice**
- Recognize that potent immunomodulators and antivirals are given to treat hepatitis B and hepatitis C; teach patients on immunomodulators to avoid large crowds and people who have infections. **QSEN: Safety**
- Monitor the patient having a liver transplantation for complications, such as those described in Table 53.4. **QSEN: Safety**
- Report and document elevated temperature, increased abdominal pain and rigidity, bleeding, and/or neurologic status changes as possible indicators of liver transplantation complications. **QSEN: Safety**

MASTERY QUESTIONS

1. A client is receiving adefovir for management of hepatitis B. What health teaching will the nurse provide for the client about this drug? **Select all that apply.**

A. "Avoid places with crowds and individuals who have infection."
B. "Report increased bruising to your doctor because the drug can cause bleeding."
C. "Get your lab work done regularly because the drug can affect your kidneys."
D. "Be careful and avoid falls because the drug can cause fractures."
E. "Follow up with the dietitian to ensure that you adhere to your special diet."

2. The nurse is caring for a patient with cirrhosis who has hepatic encephalopathy. Which assessment finding should the nurse report to the primary health care provider?

A. Fatigue
B. Difficulty sleeping
C. Seizure
D. Disorientation

REFERENCES

American Association for the Study of Liver Diseases (AASLD). (2018). *Recommendations for testing, managing and treating hepatitis C.* http://hcvguidelines.org/sites/default/files/HCV-Guidance_February_2016_a1.pdf.

American Liver Foundation. (2020a). *Non-alcoholic fatty liver disease.* http://www.liverfoundation.org/abouttheliver/info/nafld/.

American Liver Foundation. (2020b). *Hepatitis C.* http://hepc.liverfoundation.org/.

Burchum, J. L. R., & Rosenthal, L. D. (2019). *Lehne's pharmacology for nursing care* (10th ed.). St. Louis: Elsevier.

Centers for Disease Control and Prevention (CDC). (2020a). *Hepatitis B FAQs for the public.* http://www.cdc.gov/hepatitis/hbv/bfaq.htm#bFAQ10.

Centers for Disease Control and Prevention (CDC). (2020b). *Liver cancer.* https://www.cdc.gov/cancer/liver/index.htm.

Chaney, A. (2019). Caring for patients with chronic hepatitis C infection. *Nursing 2019, 49*(3), 36–42.

Digestive Health Association, C. (2020). *Statistics.* http://www.cdhf.ca/en/statistics#19.

Dols, J. D., Mendoza, A., Pomerleau, T., Purcell, C. V., Gonzalez, M., et al. (2020). Causation and risk factors for 30-day readmission of patients post-liver transplant: A descriptive study. *MEDSURG Nursing, 29*(1), 27–33.

Halter, M. J. (2018). *Varcarolis' foundations of psychiatric-mental health nursing* (8th ed.). St. Louis: Elsevier.

Heavey, E. (2020). Hepatitis A takes hold in the community. *Nursing 2020, 50*(7), 24–28.

Horsley-Silva, J. L., & Vargas, H. E. (2017). New therapies for hepatitis C virus infection. *Gastroenterology and Hepatology, 13*(3), 22–31.

Immunization Action Coalition. (2020). *Hepatitis B information for Asian Americans and Pacific Islanders.* http://www.immunize.org/catg.d/p4190.pdf.

Interprofessional Education Collaborative Expert Panel. (2016). *Core competencies for interprofessional collaborative practice: Report of an expert panel* (2nd ed.). Washington, D.C: Interprofessional Education Collaborative.

Lynn, S. (2016). How to help patients with liver failure. *American Nurse Today, 11*(9), 26–29.

McCance, K., Huether, S., Brashers, V., & Rote, N. (2019). *Pathophysiology: The biologic basis for disease in adults and children* (8th ed.). St. Louis: Mosby.

Pagana, K. D., & Pagana, T. J. (2018). *Manual of diagnostic and laboratory tests* (6th ed.). St. Louis: Mosby.

Pezzotti, W. (2020). Understanding acute upper gastrointestinal bleeding in adults. *Nursing2020, 50*(5), 25–29.

Saab, S., Manne, V., Neito, J., Schwimmer, J. B., & Chalasani, N. P. (2016). Perspectives in clinical gastroenterology and hepatology: Nonalcoholic fatty liver disease in Latinos. *Clinical Gastroenterology and Hepatology, 14*, 5–12.

Slusser, M. M., Garcia, L. I., Reed, C.-R., & McGinnis, P. Q. (2019). *Foundations of interprofessional collaborative practice in health care.* St. Louis: Elsevier.

Vacca, V.M. (2020). Nonalcoholic fatty liver disease: What nurses need to know. *Nursing 2020, 50*(3), 32–39.

World Health Organization. (2017). *Global hepatitis report 2017.* http://apps.who.int/iris/bitstream/10665/255016/1/9789241565455-eng.pdf?ua=1.

54

Concepts of Care for Patients With Problems of the Biliary System and Pancreas

Lara Carver, Jennifer Powers

http://evolve.elsevier.com/Iggy/

LEARNING OUTCOMES

1. Collaborate with the interprofessional team to manage quality care for patients with biliary and pancreatic problems caused by ***inflammation.***
2. Identify community resources for families and patients recovering from biliary and pancreatic problems.
3. Apply knowledge of pathophysiology of liver problems to identify common assessment findings, including actual or risk for impaired ***nutrition*** and ***pain***.
4. Prioritize nursing and collaborative care for patients with common gallbladder or pancreatic disorders.
5. Plan transition management and care coordination for the patient who has a biliary or pancreatic problem, including health teaching.

KEY TERMS

acute pancreatitis A serious, and at times life-threatening, *inflammation* of the pancreas.

biliary colic Severe right upper abdominal pain caused by obstruction of the cystic duct or movement of one or more gallstones.

cholecystectomy The surgical removal of the gallbladder.

cholecystitis An *inflammation* of the gallbladder that may be acute or chronic.

cholelithiasis Gallstones (also known as *calculi*).

chronic pancreatitis A progressive, destructive disease of the pancreas that has remissions and exacerbations ("flare-ups").

dyspepsia An epigastric burning sensation, often referred to as "heartburn."

eructation Belching.

flatulence Gas (flatus) in the lower GI tract.

icterus Yellow coloration of the eye sclera.

jaundice Yellow coloration of the skin and mucous membranes.

pancreatic abscess Suppuration (pus formation) of pancreatic tissue caused by secondary bacterial invasion; often occurs in patients with acute or chronic pancreatitis.

pancreatic pseudocyst A condition in which infected pancreatic fluid becomes walled off by fibrous tissue.

partial pancreatectomy Surgical removal of part of the pancreas.

postcholecystectomy syndrome (PCS) A complication of cholecystectomy that causes increased abdominal or epigastric *pain* and vomiting and/or diarrhea weeks to months after surgery.

splenectomy Surgical removal of the spleen.

steatorrhea Fatty stools.

Whipple procedure (radical pancreaticoduodenectomy) Extensive surgical procedure used most often to treat cancer of the head of the pancreas; entails removal of the proximal head of the pancreas, the duodenum, a portion of the jejunum, the stomach (partial or total gastrectomy), and the gallbladder, with anastomosis of the pancreatic duct (pancreaticojejunostomy), the common bile duct (choledochojejunostomy), and the stomach (gastrojejunostomy) to the jejunum.

PRIORITY AND INTERRELATED CONCEPTS

The priority concept for this chapter is:
- ***Inflammation***

The ***Inflammation*** concept exemplars for this chapter are Cholecystitis and Acute Pancreatitis.

The interrelated concepts for this chapter are:
- ***Pain***
- ***Nutrition***

The liver, gallbladder, and pancreas make up the biliary system. This chapter focuses on common problems of the gallbladder and pancreas. Liver disorders are described in Chapter 53. The biliary system secretes enzymes and other substances that promote food digestion in the stomach and small intestine. When these organs do not work properly, adults may experience impaired *digestion,* which can result in inadequate ***nutrition.***

Disorders of the gallbladder and pancreas may extend to other organs because of the close anatomic location of these organs, if the primary health problem is not treated early. ***Inflammation*** and obstruction (blockage) can occur in the biliary system from gallstones, edema, stricture, or tumors. These problems frequently cause the patient to have moderate-to-severe acute or persistent abdominal ***pain.*** These concepts are briefly reviewed in Chapter 3.

INFLAMMATION CONCEPT EXEMPLAR: CHOLECYSTITIS

Pathophysiology Review

Cholecystitis is an ***inflammation*** of the gallbladder that affects many adults, very commonly in affluent countries. It may be either acute or chronic, although most patients have the acute type. The inflammatory process often affects the client's ***nutrition*** status.

Acute Cholecystitis. Two types of acute cholecystitis can occur: calculous and acalculous cholecystitis. The most common type is calculous cholecystitis, in which chemical irritation and inflammation result from gallstones, or calculi (cholelithiasis), that obstruct the cystic duct (most often), gallbladder neck, or common bile duct (choledocholithiasis) (Fig. 54.1). When the gallbladder is inflamed, trapped bile is reabsorbed and acts as a chemical irritant to the gallbladder wall. Reabsorbed bile, in combination with impaired circulation, edema, and distention of the gallbladder, causes ischemia and infection. The result is tissue sloughing with necrosis and gangrene within the gallbladder itself. The gallbladder wall may eventually perforate (rupture). If the perforation is small and localized, an abscess may form. Peritonitis (infection of the peritoneum) may result if the perforation is large.

The exact mechanism of gallstone formation is not clearly understood, but abnormal metabolism of cholesterol and bile salts plays an important role. The gallbladder provides an excellent environment for the production of stones because it only occasionally mixes its normally abundant mucus with its highly viscous, concentrated bile. Impaired gallbladder motility can lead to stone formation by delaying bile emptying and causing biliary stasis.

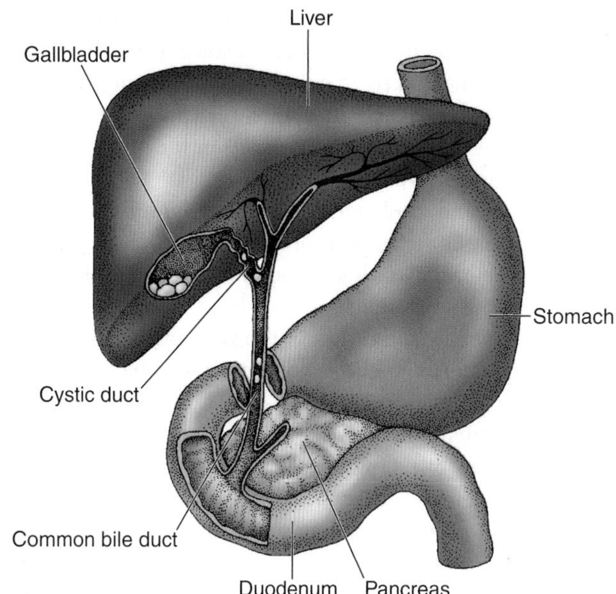

FIG. 54.1 Gallstones within the gallbladder and obstructing the common bile and cystic ducts.

Gallstones are composed of substances normally found in bile, such as cholesterol, bilirubin, bile salts, calcium, and various proteins. They are classified as either cholesterol stones or pigment stones. Cholesterol calculi form as a result of metabolic imbalances of cholesterol and bile salts. They are the most common type found in adults in the United States (McCance et al., 2019).

Bacteria can collect around the stones in the biliary system. Severe bacterial invasion can lead to life-threatening *suppurative* cholangitis when symptoms are not recognized quickly and pus accumulates in the ductal system.

Acalculous cholecystitis (***inflammation*** occurring without gallstones) is typically associated with biliary stasis caused by any condition that affects the regular filling or emptying of the gallbladder. For example, a decrease in blood flow to the gallbladder or anatomic problems such as twisting or kinking of the gallbladder neck or cystic duct can result in pancreatic enzyme reflux into the gallbladder, causing ***inflammation.*** Sphincter of Oddi dysfunction (SOD) can also occur to cause reflux and inflammation. Most cases of this type of cholecystitis occur in patients with:

- Sepsis
- Severe trauma or burns
- Long-term total parenteral ***nutrition*** (TPN)
- Multiple organ dysfunction syndrome (MODS)
- Major abdominal surgery
- Hypovolemia

Chronic Cholecystitis. Chronic cholecystitis most often results when repeated episodes of cystic duct obstruction cause chronic inflammation. Calculi are almost always present. The gallbladder becomes fibrotic and atrophied, which results in decreased motility and deficient absorption. Young thin women, especially those who are athletic (e.g., gymnasts), may experience chronic cholecystitis without calculi. In this case, the gallbladder atrophies and causes pain that is often misdiagnosed as gastritis. This problem is most likely to occur when consuming a diet low in fat, such as a vegetarian diet. In some cases, the atrophied gallbladder may adhere to nearby organs or the mesenteric wall if not surgically removed.

Pancreatitis and cholangitis (bile duct ***inflammation***) can occur as chronic complications of cholecystitis. These problems result from the backup of bile throughout the biliary tract. Bile obstruction leads to jaundice.

Jaundice (yellow coloration of the skin and mucous membranes) and icterus (yellow coloration of the eye sclera) can occur in patients with acute cholecystitis but are most commonly seen in those with the *chronic* form of the disease. Obstructed bile flow caused by edema of the ducts or gallstones contributes to *extrahepatic* obstructive jaundice. Jaundice in cholecystitis may also be caused by direct liver involvement. ***Inflammation*** of the liver's bile channels or bile ducts may cause *intrahepatic* obstructive jaundice, resulting in an increase in circulating levels of bilirubin, the major pigment of bile.

In an adult with obstructive jaundice, the normal flow of bile into the duodenum is blocked, and excessive bile salts accumulate in the skin. This accumulation of bile salts leads to pruritus (itching) or a burning sensation. The bile flow blockage also prevents bilirubin from reaching the large intestine, where it is converted to urobilinogen. Because urobilinogen accounts for the normal brown color of feces, clay-colored stools result. Water-soluble bilirubin is normally excreted by the kidneys in the urine. When an excess of circulating bilirubin occurs, the urine becomes dark because of the kidneys' effort to clear the bilirubin.

Etiology and Genetic Risk. A familial or genetic tendency appears to contribute to the development of cholelithiasis, but this may be partially related to familial ***nutrition*** habits (excessive dietary cholesterol intake) and sedentary lifestyles. Gene-environment interactions may contribute to gallstone production. For example, some gene variations program some people to make and secrete more cholesterol into bile, leading to the increase in cholesterol-containing gallstones. The highest frequency of gallstone production occurs among the American Indian and Mexican-American populations (McCance et al., 2019). Other risk factors for cholecystitis are listed in Table 54.1.

PATIENT-CENTERED CARE: GENDER HEALTH CONSIDERATIONS QSEN

Obesity is a major risk factor for gallstone formation, especially in women. Pregnancy and drugs such as hormone replacements and birth control pills alter hormone levels and delay muscular contraction of the gallbladder, decreasing the rate of bile emptying. The incidence is higher in women who have had multiple pregnancies. Therefore some clinicians continue to refer to the patient *most* at risk for acute cholecystitis and gallstones by the four *Fs*: *F*emale, *F*orty, *F*at, and *F*ertile. However, cholecystitis often occurs in younger and older women and in those who are thin.

TABLE 54.1 Risk Factors for Cholecystitis

- Women of all ages (risk of calculi increases with aging)
- American Indian, Mexican American, or Caucasian
- Obesity
- Rapid weight loss or prolonged fasting; low-fat diet
- Increased serum cholesterol and lipids
- Women on hormone replacement therapy (HRT)
- Cholesterol-lowering drugs
- Family history of gallstones
- Prolonged total parenteral nutrition
- Crohn's disease
- Gastric bypass surgery
- Sickle cell disease
- Glucose intolerance/diabetes mellitus type 2
- Pregnancy
- Genetic factors

Incidence and Prevalence. Cholecystitis and cholelithiasis most often occur in affluent countries throughout the world. The incidence is 60% to 70% in American Indians and 15% in Caucasian adults (McCance et al., 2019).

Interprofessional Collaborative Care

Care of the patient with cholecystitis primarily takes place by self-management at home, in the community, or within the same-day surgical center or hospital if surgery is required.

Assessment: Recognize Cues

History. Obtain the patient's height, weight, and vital signs; or ask that these activities be performed by assistive personnel (AP) with appropriate supervision. Ask about food preferences and determine whether excessive fat and cholesterol are part of the diet. Typically, diets high in fat, high in calories, low in fiber, and high in refined white carbohydrates place patients at high risk for developing gallstones. Consuming low-fat diets can contribute to chronic cholecystitis in young thin women.

Inquire if intake of certain foods causes pain. Question whether any GI symptoms occur when fatty food is eaten, such as flatulence (gas [flatus]in the lower GI tract), dyspepsia (an epigastric burning sensation, often referred to as "heartburn"), indigestion, eructation (belching), anorexia, nausea, vomiting, and abdominal ***pain***.

Ask patients to describe their daily activity or exercise routines to determine whether they are sedentary, a risk factor for developing gallstones. Question whether there is a family history of gallbladder disease. Ask the patient about taking current or previous hormone replacement therapy (HRT). If the patient is female, ask if she is taking or has recently been on oral contraceptives (birth control pills).

Physical Assessment/Signs and Symptoms. Patients with cholecystitis have abdominal ***pain***, although symptoms vary in intensity and frequency. Ask the patient to describe the pain, including its intensity and duration, precipitating factors, and any measures that relieve it. Pain may be described as indigestion of varying intensity, ranging from a mild, persistent ache to a steady, constant pain in the right upper abdominal quadrant. It may radiate to the right shoulder or scapula. In some cases the abdominal ***pain*** of chronic cholecystitis may be vague and nonspecific. The usual pattern is episodic. Patients often refer to acute pain episodes as "gallbladder attacks."

PATIENT-CENTERED CARE: OLDER ADULT CONSIDERATIONS QSEN

Older adults and patients with diabetes mellitus may have atypical symptoms of cholecystitis, including the absence of ***pain*** and fever. Localized tenderness may be the only presenting sign. The older patient may become acutely confused (delirium) as the first symptom of gallbladder disease.

NURSING SAFETY PRIORITY QSEN

Critical Rescue

The severe pain of **biliary colic** is produced by obstruction of the cystic duct of the gallbladder or movement of one or more gallstones. When a stone is moving through or is lodged within the duct, tissue spasm occurs in an effort to get the stone through the small duct. Biliary colic may be so severe that it occurs with tachycardia, pallor, diaphoresis, and prostration (extreme exhaustion). Assess the patient for possible shock caused by biliary colic. *Notify the health care provider or Rapid Response Team if these symptoms occur.* Stay with the patient and keep the head of the bed flat if shock occurs.

Advanced physical assessment for rebound tenderness (Blumberg sign) and deep palpation is performed only by a primary health care provider (Jarvis, 2020). To elicit rebound tenderness, the primary health care provider pushes his or her fingers deeply and steadily into the patient's abdomen and then quickly releases the pressure. Pain that results from the rebound of the palpated tissue may indicate peritoneal ***inflammation.*** Deep palpation below the liver border in the right upper quadrant may reveal a sausage-shaped mass, representing the distended, inflamed gallbladder. Percussion over the posterior rib cage worsens localized abdominal ***pain.***

In *chronic* cholecystitis, patients may have slowly developing symptoms and may not seek medical treatment until late symptoms such as **jaundice**, clay-colored stools, and dark urine occur from biliary obstruction. **Icterus** may also be present. **Steatorrhea** (fatty stools) occurs because fat absorption is decreased as a result of the lack of bile. Bile is needed for the absorption of fats and fat-soluble vitamins in the intestine. As with any inflammatory process, the patient may have an elevated temperature of 99°F to 102°F (37.2°C to 38.9°C), tachycardia, and dehydration from fever and vomiting. He or she often will decline food intake because of the resulting ***pain*** or other

KEY FEATURES

Cholecystitis

- Episodic or vague upper abdominal ***pain*** or discomfort that can radiate to the right shoulder
- Pain triggered by a high-fat or high-volume meal
- Anorexia
- Nausea and/or vomiting
- **Dyspepsia**
- **Eructation**
- **Flatulence**
- Feeling of abdominal fullness
- Rebound tenderness (Blumberg sign)
- Fever
- Jaundice, clay-colored stools, dark urine
- **Steatorrhea** (most common with chronic cholecystitis)

PATIENT-CENTERED CARE: OLDER ADULT CONSIDERATIONS QSEN

Older adults become dehydrated much more quickly than other age-groups, and they may not present with a fever. Monitor for a new onset of disorientation or acute confusion due to decreased blood volume available to oxygenate the cells of the brain (hypoxia).

symptoms that may occur. The Key Features: Cholecystitis box lists the most common signs and symptoms of cholecystitis.

Laboratory Assessment. A differential diagnosis rules out other diseases that may cause similar symptoms, such as peptic ulcer disease, hepatitis, and pancreatitis. An increased *white blood cell (WBC)* count indicates ***inflammation***. Serum levels of *alkaline phosphatase, aspartate aminotransferase (AST),* and *lactate dehydrogenase (LDH)* may be elevated, indicating abnormalities in liver function in patients with severe biliary obstruction. The direct (conjugated) and indirect (unconjugated) *serum bilirubin levels* are also elevated. If the pancreas is involved, serum amylase and lipase levels are elevated.

Other Diagnostic Assessment. Calcified gallstones are easily viewed on abdominal x-ray. Stones that are not calcified cannot be seen. *Ultrasonography (US) of the right upper quadrant is the best initial diagnostic test for cholecystitis.* It is safe, accurate, and painless. Acute cholecystitis is seen as edema of the gallbladder wall and pericholecystic fluid.

A hepatobiliary scan (sometimes called a *hepatobiliary iminodiacetic acid [HIDA] scan*) can be performed to visualize the gallbladder and determine patency of the biliary system. In this nuclear medicine test, a radioactive tracer or chemical is injected IV. About 20 minutes after the injection, a gamma camera tracks the flow of the tracer from the gallbladder to determine the ejection rate of bile into the biliary duct. A decreased bile flow indicates gallbladder disease with obstruction. Teach patients having this test to have nothing by mouth before the procedure. Remind the patient that the camera is large and close to the body for most of the procedure.

When the cause of cholecystitis or cholelithiasis is not known or the patient has symptoms of biliary obstruction (e.g., jaundice), an *endoscopic retrograde cholangiopancreatography (ERCP)* may be performed. Some patients have the less invasive and safer *magnetic resonance cholangiopancreatography (MRCP),* which can be performed by an interventional radiologist. For this procedure, the patient is given oral or IV contrast material (gadolinium) before having an MRI scan. Before the test, ask the patient about any history of urticaria (hives) or other allergy. MRI is also contraindicated in patients with a pacemaker or other incompatible devices. Gadolinium does not contain iodine, which decreases the risk for an allergic response. Chapter 48 discusses these tests in more detail.

◆ **Analysis: Analyze Cues and Prioritize Hypotheses.** The priority collaborative problems for patients with cholecystitis include:

1. Acute or persistent ***pain*** due to gallbladder ***inflammation*** and/or gallstones
2. Weight loss due to decreased intake because of pain, nausea, and anorexia

◆ **Planning and Implementation: Generate Solutions and Take Action.** If cholecystitis and its associated pain cannot be managed medically, a laparoscopic cholecystectomy is the treatment of choice for patients with acute or long-term chronic cholecystitis. ***Nutrition*** status and ***pain*** control must be addressed before and after surgery.

Managing Acute Pain

Planning: Expected Outcomes. The patient with cholecystitis is expected to report a decrease in abdominal ***pain*** as evidenced by self-report of a level of 2 or 3 level on a 0 to10 pain intensity scale.

Interventions. The priorities for patient care include providing supportive care by relieving symptoms and decreasing ***inflammation***. ***Pain*** assessment to measure the effectiveness of these interventions is an essential part of nursing care.

NCLEX Examination Challenge 54.1

Physiologic Integrity

A young adult client admitted with a diagnosis of cholecystitis from cholelithiasis has severe abdominal pain, nausea, and vomiting. Based on these assessment findings, which client problem is the **highest priority** for nursing intervention at this time?

A. Anxiety
B. Risk for dehydration
C. Acute pain
D. Malnutrition

Nonsurgical Management. Many patients with acute cholecystitis, with or without gallstones, have no symptoms. Acute ***pain*** usually occurs when gallstones partially or totally obstruct the cystic or common bile duct. Most patients find that they need to avoid fatty foods to prevent further episodes of biliary colic. Withhold food and fluids if nausea and vomiting occur. IV therapy is used to prevent dehydration. Persistent pain may occur in patients with chronic cholecystitis without gallstones, and may be misdiagnosed as gastritis.

Acute biliary pain requires opioid analgesia, such as morphine or hydromorphone (Dilaudid). All opioids may cause some degree of sphincter of Oddi spasm.

Ketorolac, a potent NSAID, may be used for mild-to-moderate ***pain***. Be sure to monitor the patient for increased pain, tachycardia, and hypotension because the drug can cause GI bleeding. The primary health care provider prescribes antiemetics to control nausea and vomiting. IV antibiotic therapy may also be given, depending on the cause of cholecystitis or as a one-time dose for surgery.

An option for a small number of patients with cholelithiasis (gallstones) is the use of oral bile acid dissolution or gallstone-stabilizing agents. Drugs such as ursodiol and chenodiol may be given as long-term therapy to dissolve or stabilize gallstones (Burchum & Rosenthal, 2019). A gallbladder ultrasound is required every 6 months for the first year of therapy to determine the effectiveness of the drug. Teach patients on this type of drug therapy to report diarrhea, vomiting, or severe abdominal pain, especially if it radiates to the shoulders, to their primary health care provider immediately. Remind them to take the medication with food and milk.

For some patients with small stones or for those who are not good surgical candidates, a treatment that is commonly used for kidney stones can be used to break up gallstones—*extracorporeal shock wave lithotripsy (ESWL).* This procedure can be used only for patients who have a normal weight, cholesterol-based stones, and good gallbladder function. The patient lies on a water-filled pad, and shock waves break up the large stones into smaller ones that can be passed through the digestive system. During the procedure, the patient might have ***pain*** resulting from the movement of the stones or duct or gallbladder spasms. A therapeutic bile acid, such as ursodeoxycholic acid (UDCA), may be used after the procedure to help dissolve the remaining stone fragments.

Another treatment option for patients who cannot have surgery is the insertion of a *percutaneous transhepatic biliary catheter* (drain) using CT or ultrasound guidance to open the blocked duct(s) so bile can flow (cholecystostomy). Catheters can be placed several ways, depending on the condition of the biliary ducts, in an internal, external, or internal/external drain. Biliary catheters usually divert bile from the liver into the duodenum to bypass a stricture. When all of the bile enters the duodenum, it is called an *internal* drain. However, in some cases a patient has an *internal/external* drain in which part of the bile empties into a drainage bag. Patients who need this drain for an extended period may have the external drain capped. If jaundice or leakage around the catheter site occurs, teach the patient to reconnect the catheter to a drainage bag and have a follow-up cholangiogram injection done by an interventional radiologist. An *external*-only catheter is connected either temporarily or permanently to a drainage bag that should be *positioned lower than the catheter insertion site* to drain by gravity. A reduction in bile drainage indicates that the drain is no longer working.

Surgical Management. **Cholecystectomy** is the surgical removal of the gallbladder. One of two procedures is performed: the laparoscopic cholecystectomy or, in rare cases, the traditional open-approach cholecystectomy.

Laparoscopic cholecystectomy. Laparoscopic cholecystectomy, a minimally invasive surgery (MIS), is the "gold standard" and is performed far more often than the traditional open approach. The advantages of MIS when compared with the open approach include:

- Complications are not common.
- The death rate is very low.
- Bile duct injuries are rare.
- Patient recovery is quicker.
- Postoperative pain is less severe.

The laparoscopic procedure (often called a "lap chole") is commonly performed on an ambulatory care basis in a same-day surgery suite or agency. The surgeon explains the procedure, and the nurse answers questions and reinforces the instructions. Reinforce what to expect after surgery and review ***pain*** management, deep-breathing exercises, incisional care, and leg exercises to prevent deep vein thrombosis. There is no special preoperative preparation other than the routine preparation for surgery under general anesthesia described in Chapter 9.

During the surgery the surgeon makes a very small midline puncture at the umbilicus. Additional small incisions may be needed, although *single-incision laparoscopic cholecystectomy (SILC)* using a flexible endoscope is often done. The abdominal cavity is insufflated with 3 to 4 L of carbon dioxide. Gasless laparoscopic cholecystectomy using abdominal wall–lifting devices are used in some centers. This technique results in improved pulmonary and cardiac function. A trocar catheter is inserted, through which a laparoscope is introduced. The laparoscope is attached to a video camera, and the abdominal organs are viewed on a monitor. The gallbladder is dissected from the liver bed, and the cystic artery and duct are closed. The surgeon aspirates the bile and crushes any large stones, if present, and then extracts the gallbladder through the umbilical puncture site.

Removing the gallbladder with the laparoscopic technique reduces the risk for wound complications. Some patients have mild-to-severe discomfort from carbon dioxide retention in the abdomen, which may be felt throughout the thorax and shoulders.

NURSING SAFETY PRIORITY (QSEN)

Action Alert

After a laparoscopic cholecystectomy, assess the patient's oxygen saturation level using pulse oximetry frequently until the effects of the anesthesia have passed. Remind the patient to perform deep-breathing exercises every hour.

Other postoperative care for the patient after a laparoscopic procedure is similar to that for any patient having minimally invasive endoscopic surgery (see Chapter 9). Offer the patient food and water when he or she is fully awake, and monitor for the nausea and/or vomiting that often results from anesthesia. If needed, administer an antiemetic drug such as ondansetron hydrochloride either IV push or as a disintegrating tablet. Several drug doses may be needed. Maintain an IV line to administer fluids until nausea and vomiting subside. Be sure to have the head of the bed elevated in the same-day surgery unit to prevent aspiration from vomiting. After nausea subsides, assist the patient to the bathroom to void. Early ambulation also promotes absorption of the carbon dioxide, which can decrease postoperative discomfort.

Administer an oral or IV push opioid and anti-inflammatory drug as needed immediately after surgery. Continuous IV pain control is usually not required because there is only one or a few small incisions, which are covered with wound closure strips (e.g., Steri-Strips) and small adhesive bandages or are surgically glued. The glue or closure strips lose their adhesiveness in about a week to 10 days and can be removed or fall off as the incision heals.

The patient is usually discharged from the hospital or surgery center the same day, although older and obese patients may stay overnight. Provide postoperative teaching regarding ***pain*** management, incision care, and follow-up appointments. Teach the patient to use ice and oral opioids for incisional pain, if needed, for a few days. For abdominal or thoracic discomfort from carbon dioxide retention, many patients report that heat application is helpful. The patient is typically allowed to bathe or shower the day after surgery.

After laparoscopic surgery the patient can return to usual activities much sooner than those having an open cholecystectomy. Instruct the patient to rest for the first 24 hours and then begin to resume usual activities Most patients are able to resume usual activities within a week.

Some patients are able to return to their usual diet after surgery, whereas others must carefully avoid high-fat foods. A large intake of fatty foods may result in abdominal ***pain*** and diarrhea, which could result in a *mild* postcholecystectomy syndrome (PCS) (see later discussion of PCS in the Traditional Cholecystectomy section). Teach patients to introduce foods high in fat one at a time to determine which foods are best tolerated.

A newer minimally invasive surgical procedure is *natural orifice transluminal endoscopic surgery (NOTES)* for removal or repair of organs. Surgery can be performed on many body organs through the mouth, vagina, and rectum. For removal of the gallbladder, the vagina is used most often in women because it can be easily decontaminated with an antiseptic and allows easy access into the peritoneal cavity. The surgeon makes a small internal incision through the cul-de-sac of Douglas between the rectum and uterine wall to access the gallbladder. The main advantages of this procedure are the lack of visible incisions and minimal, if any, postoperative complications (Roberts & Kate, 2016).

CLINICAL JUDGMENT CHALLENGE 54.1

Patient-Centered Care; Evidence-Based Practice

Today a 28-year-old woman had a scheduled laparoscopic cholecystectomy in the same-day surgical center as a result of ongoing pain intolerance to fatty foods, spices, and caffeine. Over the past few months, she has had multiple tests to rule out gastritis, peptic ulcer disease, and other GI disorders. She is currently completing graduate studies and has been on a vegetarian diet for 10 years. Her height is 5 feet 7 inches (1.7 m) and her current weight is 115 lb (52.16 kg). She has been on oral contraceptives since she turned 18 and has never been pregnant. Her immediate postoperative assessment reveals the following:

- Temperature = 98°F (36.7°C)
- Pulse = 88 beats/min
- Respirations = 22 breaths/min
- Blood pressure = 138/78 mm Hg
- Pain level = 7/10 on a 0-to-10 pain intensity scale
- Crying and states she is very nauseated
- Drowsy but easily aroused
- Wound closures intact

1. **Recognize Cues:** What assessment information in this client situation is the most important and immediate concern for the nurse? (Hint: Identify the **relevant** information *first* to determine what is most important.)
2. **Analyze Cues:** What client conditions are consistent with the **most relevant** information? (Hint: Think about priority collaborative problems that support and contradict the information presented in this situation.)
3. **Prioritize Hypotheses:** Which possibilities or explanations are **most likely** to be present in this client situation? Which possibilities or explanations are the most serious? (Hint: Consider all possibilities and determine their urgency and risk for this client.)
4. **Generate Solutions:** What actions would most likely achieve the desired outcomes for this client? Which actions should be **avoided** or are **potentially harmful**? (Hint: Determine the desired outcomes first to decide which interventions are appropriate and those that should be avoided.)
5. **Take Action:** Which actions are the most appropriate and how should they be implemented? In what **priority order** should they be implemented? (Hint: Consider health teaching, documentation, requested health care provider orders or prescriptions, nursing skills, collaboration with or referral to health team members, etc.)
6. **Evaluate Outcomes:** What client assessment would indicate that the nurse's actions were **effective**? (Hint: Think about signs that would indicate an improvement, decline, or unchanged client condition.)

Traditional cholecystectomy. Use of the open surgical approach (abdominal laparotomy) has greatly declined during the past several decades. The few patients who have this type of surgical approach usually have severe biliary obstruction, and the ducts need to be explored to ensure patency.

The nurse provides the usual preoperative care and teaching in the operating suite on the day of surgery (see Chapter 9). The surgeon removes the gallbladder through a right upper quadrant incision and explores the biliary ducts for the presence of stones or other cause of obstruction. The surgeon usually inserts a drainage tube such as a Jackson-Pratt (JP) drain. This tube is placed in the gallbladder bed to prevent fluid accumulation. The drainage is usually serosanguineous (serous fluid mixed with blood) and is stained with bile in the first 24 hours after surgery. A one-dose IV antibiotic may be given to prevent infection before or during surgery.

Nursing care for a patient who has had a traditional open cholecystectomy is similar to the care for any patient who has had abdominal surgery under general anesthesia as described in Chapter 9. Postoperative incisional ***pain*** after a traditional cholecystectomy is controlled with opioids, IV acetaminophen, and/or IV anti-inflammatory drug. Encourage the patient to use coughing and deep-breathing exercises when pain is controlled and the incision is splinted.

Antiemetics may be necessary for episodes of postoperative nausea and vomiting. Administer the antiemetic early, as prescribed, to prevent retching associated with vomiting and increased incisional ***pain.***

Provide care for the incision and the surgical drain. The surgeon typically removes the surgical dressing and drain within 24 hours after surgery.

The patient is NPO until fully awake after surgery. Document his or her level of consciousness, vital signs, and pain level. Assess the surgical incision for signs of infection, such as excessive redness or purulent drainage. Report changes to the surgeon immediately. Begin ambulation as soon as possible to prevent deep vein thrombosis and promote peristalsis.

Advance the diet from clear liquids to solid foods as peristalsis returns. The patient usually resumes solid foods and is discharged to home 1 to 2 days after surgery, depending on any complications and the patient's general condition. In the early postoperative period, if bile flow is reduced, a low-fat diet may reduce discomfort and prevent nausea.

Promoting Nutrition

Planning: Expected Outcomes. The patient will not lose weight or will regain usual weight if indicated to meet metabolic needs.

Interventions. The patient with cholecystitis may decline food because of abdominal discomfort, nausea, and anorexia. The patient's diet should be high in fiber and low in fat. Teach patients to avoid gas-producing foods. Small, frequent meals are often preferable to three standard meals daily. Ask the patient about appealing food preferences because favorite foods are tolerated more readily than randomly selected foods. Teach the patient to weigh regularly to assess for stabilization of weight or report concerns associated with weight loss. If needed, monitor laboratory results such as blood urea nitrogen (BUN), prealbumin, albumin, and total protein and transferrin levels to assess ongoing ***nutrition*** status.

TABLE 54.2 Common Causes of Postcholecystectomy Syndrome

Biliary	Nonbiliary
• Pseudocyst • Common bile duct (CBD) leak • CBD or pancreatic duct stricture or obstruction • Sphincter of Oddi dysfunction • Retained or new CBD gallstone • Pancreatic or liver mass • Primary sclerosing cholangitis • Diverticular compression	• Coronary artery disease • Intercostal neuritis • Unexplained pain syndrome • Psychiatric or neurologic disorder

Care Coordination and Transition Management. Some patients with cholecystitis may have mild-to-moderate discomfort that can be managed by nutrition intervention; others may require surgery and subsequent hospitalization. Home care preparation is individual, based on each patient's circumstances.

Education needs to be started as soon as a patient has an initial experience with cholecystitis and has appropriate pain relief. Assess the patient's and family's knowledge of the disease and provide teaching as needed. The desired outcomes for discharge planning and education are to avoid further episodes of cholecystitis.

For most patients, a special diet is not required. Advise them to eat nutritious meals and avoid excessive intake of fatty foods, especially fried food, butter, and "fast food." If the patient is obese, recommend a weight-reduction program.

Remind the patient to report repeated abdominal or epigastric pain with vomiting and/or diarrhea that may occur several weeks to months after surgery. These symptoms indicate possible postcholecystectomy syndrome (PCS). There are multiple causes of PCS, some of which are related to the biliary system, and others are not. Common causes of PCS are listed in Table 54.2.

Management depends on the exact cause but usually involves the use of endoscopic retrograde cholangiopancreatography (ERCP) to find the cause of the problem and repair it. This procedure and related nursing care are described in Chapter 48. Collaborative care includes ***pain*** management, antibiotics, ***nutrition*** and hydration therapy (possibly short-term parenteral nutrition), and control of nausea and vomiting.

◆ **Evaluation: Evaluate Outcomes.** Evaluate the care of the patient with cholecystitis based on the identified priority patient problems. The expected outcomes include that the patient will:

- Report control of abdominal pain, as indicated by self-report and pain scale measurement
- Have adequate ***nutrition*** available to meet metabolic needs

INFLAMMATION CONCEPT EXEMPLAR: ACUTE PANCREATITIS

Pathophysiology Review

Acute pancreatitis is a serious and at times life-threatening ***inflammation*** of the pancreas. This inflammatory process is caused by a premature activation of excessive pancreatic enzymes that destroy ductal tissue and pancreatic cells, resulting in autodigestion and fibrosis of the pancreas. The pathologic changes occur in different degrees. The severity of pancreatitis depends on the extent of ***inflammation*** and tissue damage. Pancreatitis can range from mild involvement evidenced by edema and inflammation to *necrotizing hemorrhagic pancreatitis (NHP)*. NHP is diffuse bleeding pancreatic tissue with fibrosis and tissue death.

The pancreas is unusual in that it functions as both an exocrine gland and an endocrine gland. The primary *endocrine* disorder is diabetes mellitus and is discussed in Chapter 59. The *exocrine* function of the pancreas is responsible for secreting enzymes that assist in the breakdown of starches, proteins, and fats. These enzymes are normally secreted in the inactive form and become activated once they enter the small intestine. Early activation (i.e., activation within the pancreas rather than the intestinal lumen) results in the inflammatory process of pancreatitis. Direct toxic injury to the pancreatic cells and the production and release of pancreatic enzymes (e.g., trypsin, lipase, elastase) result from the obstructive damage. After pancreatic duct obstruction, increased pressure may contribute to ductal rupture, allowing spillage of trypsin and other enzymes into the pancreatic parenchymal tissue. *Autodigestion* of the pancreas occurs as a result (Fig. 54.2). In *acute* pancreatitis, four major pathophysiologic processes occur: lipolysis, proteolysis, necrosis of blood vessels, and ***inflammation***.

The hallmark of pancreatic necrosis is enzymatic fat necrosis of the endocrine and exocrine cells of the pancreas caused by the enzyme *lipase*. Fatty acids are released during this *lipolytic process* and combine with ionized calcium to form a soaplike product. The initial rapid lowering of serum calcium levels is not readily compensated for by the parathyroid gland. Because the body needs ionized calcium and cannot use bound calcium, hypocalcemia occurs (McCance et al., 2019).

Proteolysis involves the splitting of proteins by hydrolysis of the peptide bonds, resulting in the formation of smaller polypeptides. Proteolytic activity may lead to thrombosis and gangrene of the pancreas. Pancreatic destruction may be localized and confined to one area or may involve the entire organ.

Elastase is activated by trypsin and causes elastic fibers of the blood vessels and ducts to dissolve. The *necrosis of blood vessels* results in bleeding, ranging from minor bleeding to massive hemorrhage of pancreatic tissue. Another pancreatic enzyme, kallikrein, causes the release of vasoactive peptides, bradykinin, and a plasma kinin known as kallidin. These substances contribute to vasodilation and increased vascular permeability, further compounding the hemorrhagic process. This massive destruction of blood vessels by necrosis may lead to generalized hemorrhage, with blood escaping into the retroperitoneal tissues. *Many deaths in patients with acute pancreatitis result from irreversible hypovolemic shock due to hemorrhage.*

The *inflammatory stage* occurs when leukocytes cluster around the hemorrhagic and necrotic areas of the pancreas. A secondary bacterial invasion may lead to suppuration (pus formation) of the pancreatic tissue called a **pancreatic abscess**. Pancreatic abscesses must be drained promptly to prevent sepsis. Mild infected lesions may be absorbed. When infected lesions are severe, calcification and fibrosis occur. If the infected

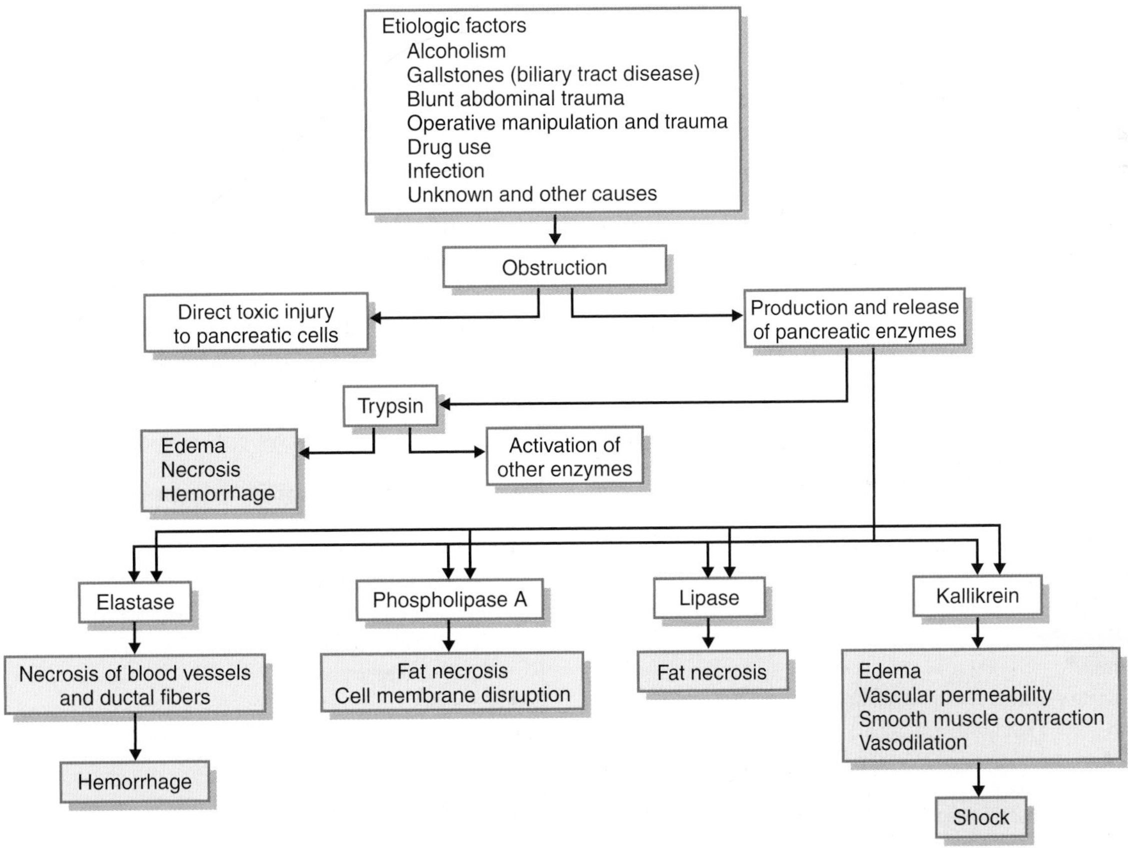

FIG. 54.2 The process of autodigestion in acute pancreatitis.

fluid becomes walled off by fibrous tissue, a pancreatic pseudocyst forms. Pseudocysts often rupture spontaneously but may require surgical removal.

Complications of Acute Pancreatitis. Acute pancreatitis may result in severe, life-threatening complications (Table 54.3). Jaundice occurs from swelling of the head of the pancreas, which slows bile flow through the common bile duct. The bile duct may also be compressed by calculi (stones) or a pancreatic pseudocyst. The resulting total bile flow obstruction causes severe jaundice. Intermittent hyperglycemia occurs from the release of glucagon, as well as the decreased release of insulin due to damage to the pancreatic islet cells. Total destruction of the pancreas may occur, leading to type 1 diabetes mellitus (McCance et al., 2019).

Left lung pleural effusions frequently develop in the patient with acute pancreatitis. *Atelectasis and pneumonia may occur also, especially in older patients.*

Multisystem organ failure is caused by necrotizing hemorrhagic pancreatitis (NHP). The patient is at risk for acute respiratory distress syndrome (ARDS). This severe form of pulmonary edema is caused by disruption of the alveolar-capillary membrane and is a serious complication of acute pancreatitis. (See Chapter 29 for a discussion of ARDS.) In acute pancreatitis, pulmonary failure accounts for more than half of all deaths that occur in the first week of the disease.

Coagulation defects are another major potential complication and may result in death. Complex physiologic changes in the pancreas cause the release of necrotic tissue and enzymes into the bloodstream, resulting in altered coagulation. Disseminated intravascular coagulation (DIC) involves hypercoagulation of the blood, with consumption of clotting factors and the development of microthrombi.

Shock in acute pancreatitis results from peripheral vasodilation from the released vasoactive substances and the retroperitoneal loss of protein-rich fluid from proteolytic digestion. Hypovolemia may result in decreased renal perfusion and acute renal failure. Paralytic (adynamic) ileus results from peritoneal irritation and seepage of pancreatic enzymes into the abdominal cavity.

Etiology and Genetic Risk. In many cases the cause of pancreatitis is not known, but many factors can injure the pancreas. The most common cause is biliary tract disease, with gallstones accounting for almost half of the cases of obstructive pancreatitis (McCance et al., 2019). Acute pancreatitis may occur as a result of trauma from surgical manipulation after biliary tract, pancreatic, gastric, and duodenal procedures, such as cholecystectomy, the Whipple procedure, and partial gastrectomy. The trauma may also occur as a complication of the diagnostic procedure *endoscopic retrograde cholangiopancreatography (ERCP),* although this rarely occurs. Additional factors that can cause acute pancreatitis are listed in Table 54.4.

TABLE 54.3 Potential Complications of Acute Pancreatitis

- Pancreatic infection (causes septic shock)
- Hemorrhage (necrotizing hemorrhagic pancreatitis [NHP])
- Acute kidney failure
- Paralytic ileus
- Hypovolemic shock
- Pleural effusion
- Acute respiratory distress syndrome (ARDS)
- Atelectasis
- Pneumonia
- Multiorgan system failure
- Disseminated intravascular coagulation (DIC)
- Type 2 diabetes mellitus

Incidence and Prevalence. Pancreatic "attacks" are especially common during holidays and vacations when alcohol consumption may be high, especially in men. Women are affected most often after having cholelithiasis and biliary tract problems. They are also most at risk for pancreatitis within several months after childbirth (McCance et al., 2019).

Death occurs in a small percentage of patients with acute pancreatitis, but with early diagnosis and treatment, mortality can be reduced. It occurs at a higher rate in *older adults* and in patients with postoperative pancreatitis. The prognosis for recovery is usually good for pancreatitis associated with biliary tract disease and poor if pancreatitis accompanies alcoholism.

❖ Interprofessional Collaborative Care

Care for the patient with acute pancreatitis usually takes place in the hospital setting for ***pain*** control and possible surgical intervention.

◆ Assessment: Recognize Cues

History. Most often the patient reports severe and constant abdominal ***pain***. Conduct the interview *after pain is controlled.* Ask whether the abdominal pain occurs when drinking alcohol or eating a high-fat meal. Obtain information about alcohol use, including the amount of alcohol consumed during what period of time (i.e., years of consumption, how much usually consumed over a particular period). Question the patient about a family or personal history of alcoholism, pancreatitis, trauma, or biliary

TABLE 54.4 Factors That Can Cause Acute Pancreatitis

- Trauma: external (blunt trauma, stab wounds, gunshot wounds [GSWs])
- Pancreatic obstruction: tumors, cysts, or abscesses; abnormal organ structure
- Metabolic problems: hyperlipidemia, hyperparathyroidism, or hypercalcemia
- Renal involvement: failure or transplantation
- Familial, inherited pancreatitis
- Penetrating gastric or duodenal ulcers, resulting in peritonitis
- Viral infections such as coxsackievirus B and human immune deficiency virus (HIV) infection
- Alcoholism
- Toxicities of drugs, including opiates, sulfonamides, thiazides, steroids, and oral contraceptives (less common)
- Cigarette smoking and tobacco use
- Cystic fibrosis
- Gallstones

tract disease. Ask whether any abdominal surgical interventions such as cholecystectomy, or diagnostic procedures such as ERCP, have been performed recently.

Ask about other medical problems known to cause pancreatitis. Inquire about recent viral infections. Ask the patient or family member to list all prescription and over-the-counter (OTC) drugs taken recently, including nutritional and herbal supplements.

Physical Assessment/Signs and Symptoms. The diagnosis of acute pancreatitis is made based on the clinical presentation combined with the results of diagnostic studies, both laboratory and imaging assessments. Symptoms of acute pancreatitis vary widely and depend on the severity of the ***inflammation.*** Typically, a patient is diagnosed after presenting with severe abdominal ***pain*** in the mid-epigastric area or left upper quadrant. Assess the intensity and quality of pain. The patient often states that the pain had a sudden onset and radiates to the back, left flank, or left shoulder. The pain is described as intense, *boring* (feeling that it is going through the body), and continuous, and is worsened by lying in the supine position. Often the patient finds relief by assuming the fetal position (with the knees drawn up to the chest and the spine flexed) or by sitting upright and bending forward. He or she may report weight loss resulting from nausea and vomiting. Obtain the patient's weight.

When performing an abdominal assessment, inspect for:

- Generalized jaundice
- Gray-blue discoloration of the abdomen and periumbilical area
- Gray-blue discoloration of the flanks, caused by pancreatic enzyme leakage to cutaneous tissue from the peritoneal cavity

Listen for bowel sounds; absent or decreased bowel sounds usually indicate paralytic (adynamic) ileus. On light palpation, note abdominal tenderness, rigidity, and guarding as a result of peritonitis. Pancreatic ascites creates a dull sound on percussion.

Monitor and record vital signs frequently to assess for elevated temperature, tachycardia, and decreased blood pressure, or assign and closely supervise this activity. Auscultate the lung fields for adventitious sounds or diminished breath sounds and observe for dyspnea or orthopnea.

! NURSING SAFETY PRIORITY QSEN

Critical Rescue

For the patient with acute pancreatitis, monitor for significant changes in vital signs that may indicate the life-threatening complication of shock. Hypotension and tachycardia may result from pancreatic hemorrhage, excessive fluid volume shifting, or the toxic effects of abdominal sepsis from enzyme damage. Observe for changes in behavior and level of consciousness (LOC) that may be related to alcohol withdrawal, hypoxia, or impending sepsis with shock.

Psychosocial Assessment. If excessive alcohol is a causative factor, tactfully explore the patient's alcohol intake history after the patient has adequate pain control. Provide patient privacy and establish a trusting relationship. Discuss the intake of alcohol and the reasons for overindulging. Using the CAGE questionnaire to assist with determining alcohol use may be beneficial. Ask the patient when increased drinking episodes occur and, in particular, whether binges occur during holidays, vacations, or weekends or revolve around particular activities, such as television viewing. Question him or her about any recent traumatic or stressful event that may have contributed to increased alcohol consumption, such as the death of a family member or a job loss.

TABLE 54.5 Causes of Serum Laboratory Abnormalities in Acute Pancreatitis

Abnormal Finding	Cause
Increased amylase	Pancreatic cell injury
Elevated lipase	Pancreatic cell injury
Elevated trypsin	Pancreatic cell injury
Elevated elastase	Pancreatic cell injury
Other Diagnostic Tests	
Elevated glucose	Pancreatic cell injury resulting in impaired carbohydrate metabolism; decreased insulin release
Decreased calcium and magnesium	Fatty acids combined with calcium; seen in fat necrosis
Elevated bilirubin	Hepatobiliary obstructive process
Elevated alanine aminotransferase (ALT)	Hepatobiliary involvement/obstruction
Elevated aspartate aminotransferase (AST)	Hepatobiliary involvement
Elevated leukocyte count and presence of C-reactive protein	Inflammatory response

Laboratory Assessment. Diagnostic laboratory abnormalities are typical in patients with acute pancreatitis (Table 54.5). A variety of pancreatic and nonpancreatic disorders can cause increased serum amylase levels. In patients with pancreatitis, *amylase* levels usually increase within 12 to 24 hours and remain elevated for 2 to 3 days. Persistent elevations may be an indicator of duct obstruction or pancreatic duct leak (Pagana & Pagana, 2018).

Lipase also helps determine the presence of acute pancreatitis. Serum levels may rise later than amylase and remain elevated for up to 2 weeks. Because these levels stay elevated for such a long time, the primary health care provider may find this test useful in diagnosing patients who are not examined until several days after the initial onset of symptoms. An increase in lipase and amylase in the urine is also expected (Pagana & Pagana, 2018).

If pancreatitis is accompanied by biliary dysfunction (biliary pancreatitis), serum *bilirubin* and *alkaline phosphatase* levels are usually elevated. A sensitive indicator of biliary obstruction in acute pancreatitis is serum *alanine aminotransferase (ALT)*. A threefold or greater rise in concentration indicates that the diagnosis of acute biliary pancreatitis is valid. Elevated *white blood cell (WBC) count and differential, erythrocyte sedimentation rate (ESR),* and serum *glucose* levels are also common in acute pancreatitis. The levels often correlate with disease severity.

Decreased serum *calcium* and *magnesium* levels are seen with fat necrosis. Calcium levels may fall and remain decreased for 7 to 10 days. Those that consistently remain below 8 mg/dL are associated with a poor prognosis. Other tests include the basic metabolic panel (BMP), complete blood count (CBC), triglycerides, serum total protein, and albumin. The blood urea nitrogen (BUN), serum glucose, and triglycerides are usually elevated. Hemoconcentration is common as a result of third-space fluid loss. Leukocytosis (elevated WBCs) and thrombocytopenia (decreased platelets) are common. Albumin levels are decreased because cytokines (e.g., tumor necrosis factor [TNF]) released as part of the inflammatory response allow it to move from the bloodstream into the extravascular space. The presence of C-reactive protein suggests possible pancreatic ***inflammation*** and necrosis (Pagana & Pagana, 2018).

Imaging Assessment. Abdominal ultrasound is the most sensitive test to diagnose causes of pancreatitis, such as gallstones, and can be performed at the bedside. However, it is not helpful in viewing the pancreas because of overlying bowel gas. Therefore *contrast-enhanced CT* provides a more reliable image and diagnosis of acute pancreatitis. This noninvasive technique may also be used to rule out pancreatic pseudocyst or ductal calculi.

An abdominal x-ray may also reveal gallstones. A chest x-ray may show elevation of the left side of the diaphragm or pleural effusion. Pancreatic stones are best diagnosed through ERCP.

◆ **Analysis: Analyze Cues and Prioritize Hypotheses.** The priority collaborative problems for patients with acute pancreatitis include:

1. Severe acute ***pain*** due to pancreatic ***inflammation*** and enzyme leakage
2. Weight loss due to inability to ingest food and absorb nutrients

NCLEX Examination Challenge 54.2

Physiologic Integrity

A client was admitted to the hospital yesterday with a diagnosis of acute pancreatitis. What assessment findings will the nurse expect for this client? **Select all that apply.**

A. Severe boring abdominal pain
B. Jaundice
C. Nausea and/or vomiting
D. Decreased serum amylase level
E. Leukocytosis
F. Dyspnea

◆ Planning and Implementation: Generate Solutions and Take Action

Managing Acute Pain

Planning: Expected Outcomes. The patient with acute pancreatitis is expected to state that he or she has a decrease in or absence of abdominal ***pain,*** as evidenced by self-report of a level of 2 or 3 on a 0 to10 pain intensity scale.

Interventions. The priorities for care for the patient with acute pancreatitis are to provide supportive care by relieving symptoms, to decrease ***inflammation,*** and to anticipate or treat complications. *As for any patient, continually assess for and support the ABCs (airway, breathing, and circulation).* In collaboration with the respiratory therapist, if available, provide oxygen and other respiratory support as needed. The collaborative plan of care depends on the severity of the illness.

Severe continuous "boring" abdominal pain is the most common symptom of pancreatitis! The main focus of nursing care is aimed at controlling ***pain*** by interventions that decrease GI tract activity, thus decreasing pancreatic stimulation. Pain assessment to measure the effectiveness of these interventions is an essential part of nursing care.

Nonsurgical Management. *Mild* pancreatitis requires hydration with IV fluids, ***pain*** control, and drug therapy. The interprofessional health care team initially attempts to relieve pain with nonsurgical interventions, which include fasting and rest, drug therapy, and comfort measures. If the patient has a life-threatening complication or requires frequent assessment, he or she is admitted to a critical care unit for invasive hemodynamic monitoring.

To rest the pancreas and reduce pancreatic enzyme secretion, withhold food and fluids (NPO) during the acute period. The primary health care provider prescribes IV isotonic fluid administration to maintain hydration. IV replacement of calcium and magnesium may also be needed. Measure and document intake and output. Some patients have an indwelling urinary catheter to obtain accurate measurements.

Nasogastric drainage and suction are reserved for more *severely ill* patients who have continuous vomiting or biliary obstruction. Gastric decompression using a nasogastric tube (NGT) prevents gastric juices from flowing into the duodenum.

! NURSING SAFETY PRIORITY QSEN

Action Alert

Because paralytic (adynamic) ileus is a common complication of acute pancreatitis, prolonged nasogastric intubation may be necessary. Assess frequently for the return of peristalsis by asking the patient if he or she has passed flatus or had a stool. The return of bowel sounds is not reliable as an indicator of peristalsis return; passage of flatus or a bowel movement is the most reliable indicator. See the discussion of intestinal obstruction in Chapter 51.

Pain management for acute pancreatitis typically begins with the administration of opioids by patient-controlled analgesia (PCA). Drugs such as morphine or hydromorphone are typically given. Other options that have been used successfully to manage acute pain include IV or transdermal fentanyl and epidural analgesia (Burchum & Rosenthal, 2019).

In *mild* pancreatitis, the pain usually subsides in 2 to 3 days. However, with *severe* acute pancreatitis, the abdominal pain and tenderness may persist for up to 2 weeks. Drug dosages and intervals are individualized according to the severity of the disease and the symptoms.

Histamine receptor antagonists (e.g., famotidine) and proton pump inhibitors (e.g., pantoprazole) help decrease gastric acid secretion. Antibiotics may be prescribed, but they are indicated primarily for patients with acute necrotizing pancreatitis or pancreatic abscess.

Helping the patient assume a side-lying position (with the legs drawn up to the chest) may help decrease the abdominal

pain of pancreatitis ("fetal position"). Sitting with the knees flexed toward the chest is also helpful.

If the patient is NPO or has an NGT, remind assistive personnel to implement frequent oral and nares hygiene measures to keep mucous membranes moist and free of inflammation or crusting. Because of the drying effect of drugs and the absence of oral fluids, the mouth and oral cavity may be extremely dry, resulting in considerable discomfort and possibly parotitis (inflammation of the parotid [salivary] glands).

! NURSING SAFETY PRIORITY QSEN

Action Alert

For the patient with acute pancreatitis, monitor his or her respiratory status every 4 to 8 hours or more often as needed and provide oxygen to promote comfort in breathing. Respiratory complications such as pleural effusions increase patient discomfort. Fluid overload can be detected by assessing for weight gain, listening for crackles, and observing for dyspnea. Carefully monitor for signs of respiratory failure.

Observe for signs and symptoms of hypocalcemia, such as muscle twitching, numbness, and irritability. Chapter 13 discusses assessment and care of patients with hypocalcemia in more detail.

Lowering the patient's anxiety level may also reduce pain. Explain all procedures and other aspects of patient care thoroughly. Provide reassurance, offer diversional activities such as music and reading material, and encourage visitors to direct attention away from the pain.

If pancreatitis was caused by gallstones, an ERCP with a sphincterotomy (opening of the sphincter of Oddi) may be performed on an urgent or emergent basis. If this procedure is not successful, surgery is required. ERCP is described in detail in Chapter 48.

Surgical Management. Surgical intervention for acute pancreatitis is usually not indicated. However, if an ERCP is not successful in removing gallstones, a laparoscopic cholecystectomy may be performed as described in the Surgical Management discussion in the section Inflammation Concept Exemplar: Cholecystitis.

Complications of pancreatitis, such as pancreatic pseudocyst and abscess, may also require surgical intervention. Laparoscopy (minimally invasive surgery [MIS]) may be done to drain an abscess or pseudocyst. For patients who are at high surgical risk, pseudocysts or abscesses can be treated by percutaneous drainage under CT guidance.

Promoting Nutrition

Planning: Expected Outcomes. The patient with acute pancreatitis is expected to have adequate ***nutrition*** to meet his or her metabolic needs.

Interventions. The patient is maintained on NPO status in the early stages of pancreatitis. Antiemetics for nausea and vomiting are prescribed as needed. Patients who have severe pancreatitis and are unable to eat for 24 to 48 hours after illness onset may begin jejunal tube feeding unless paralytic ileus is present. *Early **nutrition*** intervention enhances immune system functioning and may prevent complications and worsening ***inflammation.*** Enteral feeding is preferred over total parenteral nutrition (TPN) because it causes fewer episodes of glucose elevation and other complications associated with TPN. Be sure that the patient is weighed every day. Collaborate with the primary health care provider, registered dietitian nutritionist, and pharmacist to plan and implement the most appropriate nutrition intervention. Chapter 55 describes collaborative care of patients receiving enteral feeding and TPN.

When food is tolerated during the healing phase, the primary health care provider prescribes small, frequent, moderate- to high-carbohydrate, high-protein, low-fat meals. Food should be bland with little spice. GI stimulants such as caffeine-containing food (tea, coffee, cola, and chocolate), as well as alcohol, should be avoided. Monitor the patient beginning to resume oral food intake for nausea, vomiting, and diarrhea. *If any of these symptoms occur, notify the primary health care provider immediately.*

To boost caloric intake, commercial liquid nutritional preparations supplement the diet. The health care provider may also prescribe fat-soluble and other vitamin and mineral replacement supplements. Glutamine, omega-3 fatty acids, fiber, antioxidants, and/or nucleotides may be added to the patient's nutrition plan.

Care Coordination and Transition Management

Home Care Management. Home care preparation is individualized for each patient's circumstances. Some patients may be severely weakened from their acute illness and need to confine activity to one floor, limiting stair climbing and other strenuous activities until they regain their strength. Collaborate with the case manager (CM) to plan the best place for the patient to recover and resources that may be needed.

Self-Management Education. Education needs to be started early in the hospitalization period—as soon as the acute episodes of pain have subsided. Assess the patient's and family's knowledge of the disease.

The desired outcomes for discharge planning and education are to avoid further episodes of pancreatitis and prevent progression to a chronic disease. If the patient uses alcohol, instruct him or her to abstain from drinking to prevent further pain attacks and extension of ***inflammation*** and pancreatic insufficiency. Tell the patient that if alcohol is consumed, acute ***pain*** will return, and further autodigestion of the pancreas may lead to chronic pancreatitis.

Teach the patient to notify the primary health care provider after discharge to home if acute abdominal pain or biliary tract disease (as evidenced by jaundice, clay-colored stools, or darkened urine) occurs. These signs and symptoms are possible indicators of complications or disease progression.

Health Care Resources. Patients with acute pancreatitis may require several visits by a home care nurse if the hospital course was complicated. In these cases, home care may be needed for wound care and assistance with ADLs. The patient requires medical follow-up with the primary care provider to monitor the disease process. For those with alcoholism, provide information about groups such as Alcoholics Anonymous (AA). Family members may attend support groups such as Al-Anon and Alateen.

◆ **Evaluation: Evaluate Outcomes.** Evaluate the care of the patient with acute pancreatitis based on the identified priority patient problems. The expected outcomes include that the patient will:

- Have control of abdominal ***pain,*** as indicated by self-report and pain scale measurement
- Have adequate ***nutrition*** available to meet metabolic needs

CHRONIC PANCREATITIS

Pathophysiology Review

Chronic pancreatitis is a progressive, destructive disease of the pancreas that has remissions and exacerbations ("flare-ups"). ***Inflammation*** and fibrosis of the tissue contribute to pancreatic insufficiency and diminished function of the organ.

Chronic pancreatitis can be classified into several categories. Alcoholism is the primary risk factor for *chronic calcifying pancreatitis (CCP),* the most common type. In the early stages of the disease, pancreatic secretions precipitate as insoluble proteins that plug the pancreatic ducts and flow of pancreatic juices. As the protein plugs become more widespread, the cellular lining of the ducts changes and ulcerates. This inflammatory process causes fibrosis of the pancreatic tissue. Intraductal calcification and marked pancreatic tissue destruction (necrosis) develop in the late stages. The organ becomes hard and firm as a result of cell atrophy and pancreatic insufficiency (McCance et al., 2019).

CCP is found predominantly in men, but the incidence in women is increasing. In women, chronic pancreatitis occurs more commonly among those with biliary tract disease (cholecystitis and cholelithiasis).

Chronic obstructive pancreatitis develops from ***inflammation,*** spasm, and obstruction of the sphincter of Oddi, often from cholelithiasis (gallstones). Inflammatory and sclerotic lesions occur in the head of the pancreas and around the ducts, causing an obstruction and backflow of pancreatic secretions. (See the Complications of Acute Pancreatitis section.)

Autoimmune pancreatitis is a chronic inflammatory process in which immunoglobulins invade the pancreas. Other organs may also be infiltrated, including the lungs and liver. There is evidence to show that autoimmune pancreatitis puts the patient at risk for pancreatic cancer (Lew et al., 2017).

Idiopathic and *hereditary chronic pancreatitis* may be associated with *SPINK1* and *CFTR* gene mutations and with mutations in the *BRCA2* gene. People with hereditary pancreatitis have been shown to have a 53-fold increased risk of pancreatic cancer (Lew et al., 2017). The protein encoded by the *SPINK1* gene is a trypsin inhibitor. The *CFTR* gene is associated with cystic fibrosis. Research on these gene mutations can help in developing targeted drug therapy for treatment of these diseases.

Pancreatic insufficiency in any type of chronic pancreatitis causes loss of *exocrine* function. Most patients with chronic pancreatitis have decreased pancreatic secretions and bicarbonate. Pancreatic enzyme secretion must be greatly reduced to produce steatorrhea resulting from severe malabsorption of fats. These characteristic stools are pale, bulky, and frothy and have an offensive odor. The action of colonic bacteria on unabsorbed lipids and proteins is responsible for the extremely foul odor. On inspection of the stools, the fat content is visible.

Fat malabsorption also contributes to weight loss and muscle wasting (a decrease in muscle mass) and leads to general debilitation. Protein malabsorption results in a "starvation" edema of the feet, legs, and hands caused by decreased levels of circulating albumin.

The loss of pancreatic *endocrine* function is responsible for the development of diabetes mellitus in patients with chronic pancreatic insufficiency. (See Chapter 59 for a complete discussion of diabetes mellitus.)

The patient with chronic pancreatitis may have pulmonary complications, such as pleuritic pain, pleural effusions, and pulmonary infiltrates. Pancreatic ascites may decrease diaphragmatic excursion and lung expansion, resulting in impaired ventilation. In the ill patient with chronic pancreatitis, acute respiratory distress syndrome (ARDS) may develop.

❖ Interprofessional Collaborative Care

Care for the patient with chronic pancreatitis takes place in the home or community setting but moves to the hospital setting for ***pain*** control and possible surgical intervention.

◆ **Assessment: Recognize Cues.** Many symptoms of chronic pancreatitis differ from those of an acute ***inflammation.*** Abdominal pain is the major symptom for most types of pancreatitis. For those with chronic pancreatitis, pain is typically described as a continuous burning or gnawing dullness with periods of acute exacerbation (flare-ups). The pain is very intense and relentless. The frequency of acute exacerbations may increase as the pancreatic fibrosis develops. Key features of chronic pancreatitis are listed in the Key Features: Chronic Pancreatitis box.

Perform an abdominal assessment. Abdominal tenderness is less intense in patients with chronic pancreatitis than in those with acute pancreatitis. Massive pancreatic ascites may be present, producing dullness on abdominal percussion. Because respiratory complications can occur, auscultate the lung fields for adventitious sounds or decreased aeration and observe for dyspnea or orthopnea.

Ask the patient to collect a random stool specimen if able or ask him or her to describe the stools. The specimen may show **steatorrhea**. Assess for unintentional weight loss; muscle wasting; **jaundice**; dark urine; and the symptoms of diabetes mellitus, such as polyuria (increased urinary output), polydipsia (excessive thirst), and polyphagia (increased appetite).

Diagnosis is based on the patient's symptoms and laboratory and imaging assessment. *Endoscopic retrograde cholangiopancreatography* (ERCP) is done to visualize the pancreatic and common bile ducts. *Imaging studies* such as CT scanning, contrast-enhanced MRI, abdominal ultrasound (US), and endoscopic ultrasound (EUS) are also useful in making the diagnosis. In chronic pancreatitis, laboratory findings include normal or moderately elevated serum *amylase* and *lipase* levels. Obstruction of the intrahepatic bile duct can cause elevated

KEY FEATURES

Chronic Pancreatitis

- Intense abdominal ***pain,*** a major symptom, that is continuous and burning or gnawing
- Abdominal tenderness
- Ascites
- Possible left upper quadrant mass (if pancreatic pseudocyst or abscess is present)
- Respiratory compromise manifesting with adventitious or diminished breath sounds, dyspnea, or orthopnea
- **Steatorrhea**; clay-colored stools
- Weight loss
- **Jaundice**
- Dark urine
- Polyuria, polydipsia, polyphagia (diabetes mellitus)

serum *bilirubin* and *alkaline phosphatase* levels. Intermittent elevations in serum *glucose* levels are common and can be detected by blood glucose monitoring, both fasting and nonfasting.

◆ **Interventions: Take Action.** The focus of caring for the patient with chronic pancreatitis is to manage acute or persistent ***pain***, maintain adequate ***nutrition***, and prevent disease recurrence.

Nonsurgical Management. The primary nonsurgical interventions include drug and ***nutrition*** therapy. The major intervention for the pain of chronic pancreatitis is drug therapy. Medicate the patient as prescribed according to the assessment of the intensity of pain. Evaluate the effectiveness of the drug intervention. Initially opioid analgesia is used most frequently, but dependency may occur. Nonopioid analgesics may be tried to relieve pain. (See Chapter 5 for other interventions for acute and persistent pain.)

Pancreatic enzyme replacement therapy (PERT) is the standard of care to prevent malnutrition, malabsorption, and excessive weight loss. Pancreatic enzymes are usually prescribed in the form of capsules or tablets that contain varying amounts of amylase, lipase, and protease. Teach patients not to chew or crush pancreatic enzyme replacements that are available as delayed-release capsules or enteric tablets. Teach them to take the enzymes with all meals and snacks (Burchum & Rosenthal, 2019).

The dosage of pancreatic enzymes depends on the severity of the malabsorption. Record the number and consistency of stools per day to monitor the effectiveness of enzyme therapy. If pancreatic enzyme treatment is effective, the stools should become less frequent and less fatty.

The primary health care provider may also prescribe drug therapy to decrease gastric acid. Gastric acid destroys the lipase needed to break down fats. Controlling the acidity of the stomach with H2 blockers or proton pump inhibitors or neutralizing stomach acid with oral sodium bicarbonate may enhance the effectiveness of PERT.

> **! NURSING SAFETY PRIORITY QSEN**
>
> ***Action Alert***
>
> If the patient has diabetes, insulin or oral antidiabetic agents for glucose control are prescribed. Patients maintained on total parenteral nutrition (TPN) are particularly susceptible to elevated glucose levels and require regular insulin additives to the solution. Monitor blood glucose to control hyperglycemia. Check finger stick blood glucose (FSBG) or sugar (FSBS) levels every 2 to 4 hours. Chapter 55 describes in detail the care associated with TPN.

Protein and fat malabsorption results in significant weight loss and decreased muscle mass in the patient with chronic pancreatitis. Therefore the nutritional interventions for acute pancreatitis are also used for chronic pancreatitis. The patient often limits food intake to avoid increased pain. For this reason, nutrition maintenance is often difficult to achieve. Patients receive either total parenteral nutrition (TPN) or total enteral nutrition (TEN), including vitamin and mineral replacement.

Collaborate with the registered dietitian nutritionist to teach the patient about long-term dietary management. He or she needs an increased number of calories, up to 4000 to 6000 calories per day, to maintain weight. Food high in carbohydrates and protein also assists in the healing process. Food high in fat is avoided because it causes or increases diarrhea. Teach all patients to avoid alcohol. Alcohol-cessation programs may be recommended.

Surgical Management. Surgery is not a primary intervention for the treatment of chronic pancreatitis. However, it may be indicated for ongoing abdominal ***pain,*** incapacitating relapses of pain, or complications such as a pancreatic abscess or pancreatic pseudocyst.

The underlying pathologic changes determine the procedure indicated. Using laparoscopy, the surgeon incises and drains an abscess or pseudocyst. Laparoscopic cholecystectomy or choledochotomy (incision of the common bile duct) may be indicated if biliary tract disease is an underlying cause of pancreatitis. If the pancreatic duct sphincter is fibrotic, the surgeon performs a sphincterotomy (incision of the sphincter) to enlarge it. Endoscopic sphincterotomy may be used for patients who are poor surgical candidates.

In some cases laparoscopic distal pancreatectomy may be appropriate for resection of the distal pancreas or pancreas head. Endoscopic pancreatic necrosectomy and natural orifice transluminal endoscopic surgery (NOTES) are becoming more common for removing necrosed pancreatic tissue. Both procedures are performed through the GI wall without a visible skin incision. The NOTES procedure is discussed in Surgical Management in the Inflammation Concept Exemplar: Cholecystitis section.

In a few cases, pancreas transplantation may be done. However, this procedure is performed most often for patients with severe, uncontrolled diabetes. Chapter 59 discusses pancreas transplantation.

Care Coordination and Transition Management

Home Care Management. Collaborate with the hospital-based case manager (CM) or discharge planner about home care or follow-up in another setting. A community-based CM may continue to follow the patient after hospital discharge. If the patient is discharged to home, the living area should be limited to one floor until he or she regains strength and can increase activity. Teach patients and families that toilet facilities must be easily accessible because of chronic steatorrhea and frequent defecation. If they are not easily accessible, a bedside commode is obtained for the home.

Self-Management Education. Because there is no known cure for chronic pancreatitis, patient and family education is aimed at preventing acute episodes of the disease, providing long-term care, and promoting health maintenance. The Patient and Family Education: Preparing for Self-Management: Prevention of Exacerbations of Chronic Pancreatitis box outlines self-management to help prevent exacerbations of the disease.

> **PATIENT AND FAMILY EDUCATION: PREPARING FOR SELF-MANAGEMENT**
>
> ***Prevention of Exacerbations of Chronic Pancreatitis***
>
> - Avoid things that make your symptoms worse, such as drinking caffeinated beverages.
> - Avoid alcohol ingestion; refer to self-help group for assistance.
> - Avoid nicotine.
> - Eat bland, low-fat, high-protein, and moderate-carbohydrate meals; avoid gastric stimulants such as spices.
> - Eat small meals and snacks high in calories.
> - Take the pancreatic enzymes that have been prescribed for you with meals.
> - Rest frequently; restrict your activity to one floor until you regain your strength.

PATIENT AND FAMILY EDUCATION: PREPARING FOR SELF-MANAGEMENT

Enzyme Replacement for the Patient With Chronic Pancreatitis

- Take pancreatic enzymes with meals and snacks and follow with a glass of water.
- Administer enzymes after antacid or H_2 blockers. (Decreased pH inactivates drug.)
- Swallow the tablets or capsules without chewing, to minimize oral irritation and allow the drug to be released slowly.
- If you cannot swallow the capsule, pierce the gelatin casing and place contents in applesauce.
- Do not mix enzyme preparations in protein-containing foods.
- Wipe your lips after taking enzymes to avoid skin irritation.
- Do not crush enteric-coated preparations.
- Follow up on all scheduled laboratory testing. (Pancreatic enzyme replacements can cause an increase in uric acid levels.)

Remind the patient and family members or significant others of the importance of adhering to pancreatic enzyme replacement. The patient must take the prescribed enzymes with meals and snacks to aid in the digestion of food and promote the absorption of fats and proteins (see the Patient and Family Education: Preparing for Self-Management: Enzyme Replacement for the Patient With Chronic Pancreatitis box).

The frequency of defecation (whether continent or incontinent) poses challenging skin care problems. Instruct the patient to keep the skin dry and free of the abrasive fatty stools, which damage the skin. The skin should be cleaned thoroughly after each stool, and a moisture barrier applied to prevent breakdown and maintain skin integrity. Many products on the market actively repel stool from the skin. Remind the patient to report any skin breakdown so therapeutic interventions to promote skin integrity can be started. Abdominal fistulas are common and present a difficult challenge because pancreatic secretions irritate the skin.

If the patient develops diabetes mellitus as a result of chronic pancreatitis, management of elevated glucose levels after discharge from the hospital may require oral antidiabetic agents or insulin injections. If this is the case, collaborate with the certified diabetes educator (CDE) to provide in-depth teaching concerning diabetes, its signs and symptoms, medical management, drug therapy, nutrition therapy, blood glucose monitoring, and general care.

Chronic illnesses are devastating for families. The high costs of medical insurance, medical treatment, and drug therapy cause serious financial problems. Often the patient with chronic pancreatitis is unable to work. Collaborate with the CM about ways to assist the patient with resources for financial help.

Health Care Resources. The patient may require several home visits by nurses, depending on the severity of the chronic health problems and home maintenance and support needs. The nurse assesses the patient for pain, enzyme therapy, and psychosocial adaptation to a chronic illness. Refer him or her and the family to a counselor or a self-help group, such as Alcoholics Anonymous (www.aa.org) and Al-Anon (www.al-anon.org), if appropriate.

PANCREATIC CANCER

Pathophysiology Review

Cancer of the pancreas is a leading cause of cancer deaths each year in the United States. It is difficult to diagnose early because the pancreas is hidden and surrounded by other organs. Most often, the tumor is discovered in the late stages of development and may be a well-defined mass or diffusely spread throughout the pancreas. Treatment has limited results, and 5-year survival rates are low (American Cancer Society, 2020).

The tumor may be a primary cancer, or it may result from metastasis from cancers of the lung, breast, thyroid, kidney, or skin. Primary tumors are generally adenocarcinomas and grow in well-differentiated glandular patterns. They grow rapidly and spread to surrounding organs (stomach, duodenum, gallbladder, and intestine) by direct extension and invasion of lymphatic and vascular systems. This highly metastatic lesion may eventually invade the lung, peritoneum, liver, spleen, and lymph nodes.

Signs and symptoms depend on the site of origin or metastasis. The head of the pancreas is the most common site. The tumors are usually small lesions with poorly defined margins. Jaundice results from tumor compression and obstruction of the common bile duct and from gallbladder dilation, causing the organ to enlarge.

Cancers of the body and tail of the pancreas are usually large and invade the entire tail and body. These tumors may be palpable abdominal masses, especially in the thin patient. Through metastatic spread via the splenic vein, metastasis to the liver may cause hepatomegaly (enlargement of the liver). Regardless of where it originates, it spreads rapidly through the lymphatic and venous systems to other organs.

Venous thromboembolism is a common complication of pancreatic cancer. Necrotic products of the pancreatic tumor are believed to have thromboplastic properties resulting in the blood's hypercoagulable state. In addition, the patient is at high risk because of decreased mobility and extensive surgical manipulation.

The exact cause of pancreatic cancer is unknown. Table 54.6 highlights the major risk factors associated with the disease.

❖ Interprofessional Collaborative Care

Care for the patient with pancreatic cancer usually takes place in the hospital setting, and eventually with hospice.

TABLE 54.6 Risk Factors Associated With Pancreatic Cancer

- Diabetes mellitus
- Chronic pancreatitis
- Cirrhosis
- High intake of red meat, especially processed meat
- Long-term exposure to chemicals such as gasoline and pesticides
- Obesity
- Older age
- Male gender
- Cigarette smoking
- Family history
- Genetic mutations (e.g., *p16, BRCA2*)

KEY FEATURES

Pancreatic Cancer

- **Jaundice**
- **Icterus**
- Clay-colored (light) stools
- Dark urine
- Abdominal ***pain***, usually vague, dull, or nonspecific, that radiates into the back
- Weight loss
- Anorexia
- Nausea or vomiting
- Glucose intolerance
- Splenomegaly (enlarged spleen)
- Flatulence
- Gastrointestinal bleeding
- New-onset diabetes mellitus
- Ascites (abdominal fluid)
- Leg or calf pain (from thrombophlebitis)
- Weakness and fatigue

◆ **Assessment: Recognize Cues.** Pancreatic cancer often presents in a slow and vague manner. The presenting symptoms depend somewhat on the location of the tumor. The first sign may be jaundice, which suggests late, advanced disease (see the Key Features: Pancreatic Cancer box).

No specific blood tests are diagnostic of pancreatic cancer. Serum *amylase* and *lipase* levels and *alkaline phosphatase* and *bilirubin* levels are increased. The degree of elevation depends on the acuteness or chronicity of the pancreatic and biliary damage. Elevated *carcinoembryonic antigen* (CEA) levels occur in most patients with pancreatic cancer. This test may provide early information about the presence of tumor cells. The tumor marker CA 19-9 has been found to be a useful serologic test for monitoring a proven diagnosis and continuing surveillance for potential spread or recurrence (Pagana & Pagana, 2018).

Abdominal *ultrasound* and *contrast-enhanced CT* are the most commonly used imaging techniques for confirming a tumor and can differentiate the tumor from a cyst. Endoscopic ultrasonography can also be performed to sample tissue for diagnosis and provide information on tumor type and size (Bujanda & Herreros-Villanueva, 2017). *Endoscopic retrograde cholangiopancreatography* (ERCP) also provides visual diagnostic data. An alternative to ERCP is a percutaneous transhepatic biliary cholangiogram with placement of a percutaneous transhepatic biliary drain (PTBD). This drain decompresses the blocked biliary system by draining bile internally, externally, or both. Aspiration of pancreatic ascitic fluid by abdominal paracentesis may reveal cancer cells and elevated amylase levels.

◆ **Interventions: Take Action.** Management of the patient with pancreatic cancer is geared toward preventing tumor spread and decreasing pain. These measures are not curative, only palliative. The cancers are often metastatic and recur despite treatment.

Nonsurgical Management. As in other types of cancer, chemotherapy or radiation is used to relieve pain by shrinking the tumor. It may be used before, after, or instead of surgery. *Chemotherapy* has had limited success in increasing survival time. In most cases, combining agents has been more successful than single-agent chemotherapy. 5-Fluorouracil (5-FU), a commonly used drug, may be given alone or with gemcitabine for locally advanced, or unresectable, pancreatic cancers. Observe for adverse drug effects, such as fatigue, rash, anorexia, and diarrhea. Chapter 20 discusses nursing implications of chemotherapy in more detail.

Other targeted therapies being investigated include growth factor inhibitors, antiangiogenesis factors, and kinase inhibitors. Kinase inhibitors are a newer group of drugs that focus on cancer cells with little or no effect on healthy cells. Chapter 20 describes general nursing interventions associated with chemotherapy.

To control pain, the patient takes high doses of opioid analgesics (usually morphine) as prescribed before the pain escalates and peaks. Because of the poor prognosis, drug dependency is not a consideration. Chapter 5 describes in detail the care of the patient with chronic cancer pain.

Intensive external beam *radiation* therapy to the pancreas may offer pain relief by shrinking tumor cells, alleviating obstruction, and improving food absorption. It does not improve survival rates. The patient may experience discomfort during and after the radiation treatments. Chapter 20 describes radiation therapy in more detail.

For patients experiencing biliary obstruction who are at high surgical risk, biliary stents placed percutaneously (through the skin) can ensure patency to relieve pain. These stents are devices made of plastic materials that keep the ducts of the biliary system open. Using another approach, self-expandable stents may be inserted endoscopically to relieve obstruction.

Surgical Management. Complete surgical resection of the pancreatic tumor offers the patient with pancreatic cancer the only effective treatment, but it is done only in patients with small tumors. **Partial pancreatectomy** is the preferred surgery for tumors smaller than 3 cm in diameter, depending on location and length of time since diagnosis. Recent technologic advances have expanded the role of *minimally invasive surgery (MIS)* via laparoscopy in the staging, palliation, and removal of pancreatic cancers. The procedure selected depends on the purpose of the surgery and stage of the disease. For example, if the patient has a biliary obstruction, a laparoscopic procedure to relieve it is performed. This procedure diverts bile drainage into the jejunum.

For larger tumors, the surgeon may perform either a *radical pancreatectomy* or the *Whipple procedure (pancreaticoduodenectomy)*. These procedures have traditionally been done using an open surgical approach. Because of new advances in laparoscopic technology using a hand-assist or robotic-assist device, this method is beginning to replace the conventional method. Some surgeons are not yet trained in how to perform this technique. Therefore the traditional open surgical approach remains a common method of performing these surgeries.

Preoperative Care. The patient with pancreatic cancer may be at poor surgical risk because of malnutrition and debilitation. Specific care depends on the type of surgical approach being used.

Often, in the late stages of pancreatic cancer or before the Whipple procedure, the primary health care provider inserts a small catheter into the jejunum (jejunostomy) so enteral feedings may be given. This feeding method is preferred to prevent reflux and facilitate absorption. Feedings are started in low concentrations and volumes and gradually increased as tolerated. Provide feedings using a pump to maintain a constant volume and assess for diarrhea frequency to determine tolerance. Chapter 55 provides additional information about enteral feeding.

For optimal ***nutrition,*** TPN may be necessary in addition to tube feedings or as a single measure. When central venous access is required, a peripherally inserted central catheter (PICC) or other type of IV catheter may be necessary. Meticulous IV line care is an important nursing measure to prevent catheter sepsis. Sterile dressing changes and site observation are extremely important. Additional nursing care measures for the patient receiving TPN are given in Chapter 55. Monitor nutrition indicators such as serum prealbumin and albumin.

For the laparoscopic procedure, no bowel preparation is needed. However, either approach requires that the patient have nothing by mouth (NPO) for at least 6 to 8 hours before surgery. Surgeon preference and agency policy determine the preferred protocol for preoperative preparation.

Operative Procedures. The **Whipple procedure (radical pancreaticoduodenectomy)** is an extensive surgical procedure used most often to treat cancer of the head of the pancreas. The procedure entails removal of the proximal head of the pancreas, the duodenum, a portion of the jejunum, the stomach (partial or total *gastrectomy*), and the gallbladder, with anastomosis of the pancreatic duct (*pancreaticojejunostomy*), the common bile duct (*choledochojejunostomy*), and the stomach (*gastrojejunostomy*) to the jejunum (Fig. 54.3). In addition, the surgeon may remove the spleen (**splenectomy**).

Postoperative Care. In addition to routine postoperative care measures, the patient who has undergone an *open* radical pancreaticoduodenectomy requires intensive nursing care and is typically admitted to a surgical critical care unit. Observe for multiple potential complications of the open Whipple procedure as listed in Table 54.7.

The primary benefits of *MIS* for the patient are a shorter postoperative recovery and less pain than with traditional open procedure. The patient having the laparoscopic Whipple surgery or radical pancreatectomy is also less at risk for severe complications. For patients having one of these procedures, observe for and implement preventive measures for these common surgical complications:

- Diabetes (Check blood glucose often.)
- Hemorrhage (Monitor pulse, blood pressure, skin color, and mental status [e.g., LOC].)
- Wound infection (Monitor temperature and assess wounds for redness and induration [hardness].)
- Bowel obstruction (Check bowel sounds and stools.)
- Intra-abdominal abscess (Monitor temperature and patient's report of severe pain.)

Immediately after surgery the patient is NPO and usually has a nasogastric tube (NGT) to decompress the stomach. Monitor GI drainage and tube patency. In open surgical approaches, biliary drainage tubes are placed during surgery to remove drainage and secretions from the area and prevent stress on the anastomosis sites. Assess the tubes and drainage devices for tension or kinking and maintain them in a dependent position.

Monitor the drainage for color, consistency, and amount. The drainage should be serosanguineous. The appearance of clear,

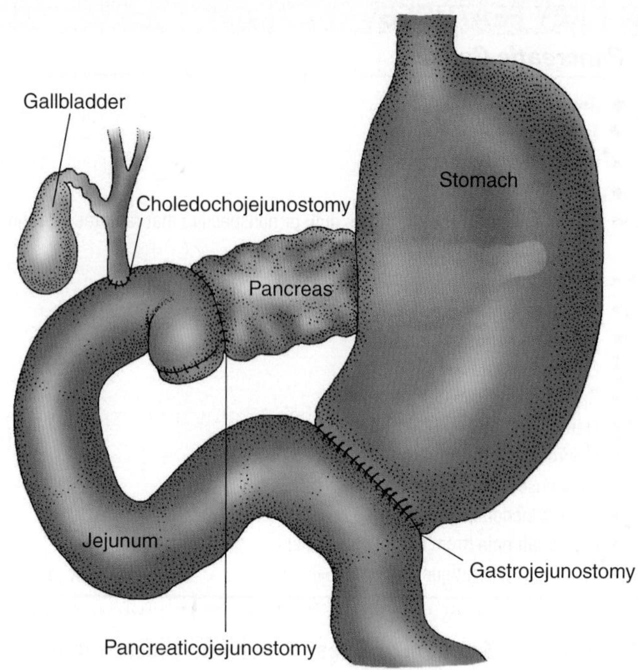

FIG. 54.3 The three anastomoses that constitute the Whipple procedure: choledochojejunostomy, pancreaticojejunostomy, and gastrojejunostomy.

TABLE 54.7 Potential Complications of the Whipple Procedure

Cardiovascular Complications	GI Complications
• Hemorrhage at anastomosis sites with hypovolemia • Myocardial infarction • Heart failure • Thrombophlebitis	• Adynamic (paralytic) ileus • Gastric retention • Gastric ulceration • Bowel obstruction from peritonitis • Acute pancreatitis • Hepatic failure • Thrombosis to mesentery
Pulmonary Complications	**Wound Complications**
• Atelectasis • Pneumonia • Pulmonary embolism • Acute respiratory distress syndrome • Pulmonary edema	• Infection • Dehiscence • Fistulas: pancreatic, gastric, and biliary
Metabolic Complications	
• Unstable diabetes mellitus • Renal failure	

colorless, bile-tinged drainage or frank blood with an increase in output may indicate disruption or leakage of an anastomosis site. Most of the disruptions of the site occur within 7 to 10 days after surgery. Hemorrhage can occur as an early or late complication.

Place the patient in the semi-Fowler position to reduce tension on the suture line and anastomosis site and to optimize lung expansion. Stress can be decreased by maintaining NGT drainage at a low or high intermittent suction level to keep the remaining stomach (if a partial gastrectomy is done) or the jejunum (if a total gastrectomy is done) free of excessive fluid buildup and pressure. The NGT also reduces stimulation of the remaining pancreatic tissue.

The development of a fistula (an abnormal passageway) is the most common and most serious postoperative complication.

Biliary, pancreatic, or gastric fistulas result from partial or total breakdown of an anastomosis site. The secretions that drain from the fistula contain bile, pancreatic enzymes, or gastric secretions, depending on which site is ruptured. *These secretions, particularly pancreatic fluid, are corrosive and irritating to the skin; and internal leakage causes chemical peritonitis.* Peritonitis (inflammation and infection of the peritoneum causing board-like abdominal rigidity) requires treatment with multiple antibiotics. *If you suspect any postoperative complications resulting from MIS or open surgical approaches, call the surgeon or Rapid Response Team immediately and provide assessment findings that support your concerns.*

Because the *open* Whipple procedure is extensive and can take many hours to complete, maintaining fluid and electrolyte balance can be difficult. Patients often have significant intraoperative blood loss and postoperative bleeding. The intestine is exposed to air for long periods, and fluid evaporates. Significant losses of fluid and electrolytes occur from the NGT and other drainage tubes. In addition, these patients may be malnourished and have low serum levels of protein and albumin, which maintain colloid osmotic pressure within the circulating system. Reduction in the serum osmotic pressure makes the patient likely to develop third spacing of body fluids, with fluid moving from the vascular to the interstitial space, resulting in shock. These problems are less likely to occur when MIS is used. Therefore, when possible, the trained surgeon prefers to perform laparoscopic Whipple procedures to shorten operating time and prevent the many complications that can occur.

! NURSING SAFETY PRIORITY (QSEN)

Action Alert

To detect early signs of hypovolemia and prevent shock, closely monitor vital signs for decreased blood pressure and increased heart rate, decreased vascular pressures with a pulmonary artery catheter (Swan-Ganz catheter) (in ICU setting), and decreased urine output. Be alert for pitting edema of the extremities, dependent edema in the sacrum and back, and an intake that far exceeds output. Maintain sequential compression devices to prevent deep vein thrombosis.

Maintenance of IV isotonic fluid replacement with colloid replacements is important. Monitor hemoglobin and hematocrit values to assess for blood loss and the need for blood transfusions. Review electrolyte values for decreased serum levels of sodium, potassium, chloride, and calcium. IV fluid concentrations must be altered to correct these electrolyte imbalances. The physician prescribes replacement of electrolytes as needed.

Immediately after the Whipple procedure, the patient may have hyperglycemia or hypoglycemia as a result of stress and surgical manipulation of the pancreas. Most of the endocrine cells (responsible for insulin and glucagon secretion) are located in the body and tail of the pancreas. In some patients, up to half of the gland remains, and diabetes does not develop. However, a large number of patients have diabetes before surgery. For patients having a radical pancreatectomy, administer insulin as prescribed because the entire pancreas is removed. Monitor glucose levels frequently during the early postoperative period and administer insulin injections as prescribed.

Care Coordination and Transition Management. The patient with pancreatic cancer is usually followed by a case manager (CM), both in the hospital and in the home or other community-based setting. Collaborate with the CM to ensure that the patient receives cost-effective treatment and that his or her needs are met.

Home Care Management. The stage of progression of pancreatic cancer and available home care resources determine whether the patient can be discharged to home or whether additional care is needed in a skilled nursing facility or with a hospice provider. Home care preparations depend on the patient's physical and activity limitations and should be tailored to his or her needs. Coordinate care with the patient, family, or whoever will be providing care after discharge from the hospital (i.e., home care provider, hospice care provider, or extended-care provider).

The patient and family need compassionate emotional support to deal with issues related to this illness. The diagnosis of pancreatic cancer can frighten and overwhelm the patient and family. Help family members look realistically and objectively at the amount of physical care required. Tell family members that their own physical and emotional health is at risk during this stressful period and that supportive counseling may be needed. If the family does not have a religious affiliation or a spiritual leader (e.g., a minister or a rabbi) to provide support, suggest alternative counseling options. Refer patients and families to the certified hospital chaplain if desired. It is appropriate for the nurse to make the initial contact or appointment according to the patient's or family's wishes.

Self-Management Education. When the patient is discharged to home, many interventions are palliative and aimed at managing symptoms such as pain. In many cases the diagnosis of pancreatic cancer is made a few months before death occurs. The patient needs time to adjust to the diagnosis, which is usually made too late for cure or prolonged survival. Help the patient identify what needs to be done to prepare for death, including end-of-life care. For example, he or she may want to write a will or see family members and friends whom he or she has not seen recently. The patient needs to make known to family members or others his or her specific requests for the funeral or memorial service. These actions help prepare for death in a dignified manner. Chapter 8 discusses in detail anticipatory grieving and preparation for death, as well as symptom management during the end of life.

Health Care Resources. Regular home care nursing and assistive personnel visits may be scheduled to assist the patient and family by providing physical, psychological, and supportive care. Supply information about local palliative and hospice care (see Chapter 8) and cancer support groups.

GET READY FOR THE NEXT-GENERATION NCLEX® EXAMINATION!

Key Points

Review these Key Points for each NCLEX Examination Client Needs Category.

Safe and Effective Care Environment

- Refer patients with end-stage pancreatic cancer for palliative and hospice care. **Ethics**
- Refer patients with pancreatitis who use alcohol to community resources such as Alcoholics Anonymous. **QSEN: Patient-Centered Care**

Health Promotion and Maintenance

- Recognize that obese, middle-age women are most likely to have gallbladder disease. **QSEN: Patient-Centered Care**
- Teach patients to avoid losing weight too quickly and to keep weight under control to help prevent gallbladder disease. **QSEN: Evidence-Based Practice**
- Teach patients to avoid alcohol consumption to help prevent alcohol-induced acute pancreatitis. **QSEN: Evidence-Based Practice**
- Instruct patients about ways to prevent exacerbations of chronic pancreatitis.

Psychosocial Integrity

- Refer patients with pancreatic cancer to support services such as spiritual leaders and counselors for coping strategies and facilitation of the grieving process. **Ethics**
- Help prepare the pancreatic cancer patient and family for the death and dying process. **Ethics**

Physiological Integrity

- Be aware that autodigestion of the pancreas causes severe ***pain*** in patients with acute pancreatitis (see Fig. 54.2). **QSEN: Patient-Centered Care**
- Monitor serum laboratory values, especially amylase and lipase (both elevated), in patients with pancreatitis (see Table 54.4). **QSEN: Evidence-Based Practice**
- Assess for common symptoms of cholecystitis including abdominal pain and intolerance to fatty foods. **Clinical Judgment**
- Provide pain management, including opioid analgesia, for patients with acute pancreatitis. **QSEN: Patient-Centered Care**
- Recognize that acute pain relief is the first priority of care for patients with acute pancreatitis. **QSEN: Evidence-Based Practice**
- Be aware that patients with biliary and pancreatic disorders are at high risk for biliary obstruction, a serious and painful complication. **QSEN: Safety**
- Document health teaching about enzyme replacement therapy. **QSEN: Informatics**
- Assess patients with symptoms of pancreatic cancer, including jaundice and abdominal ***pain.*** **QSEN: Patient-Centered Care**
- Observe for and implement interventions to prevent life-threatening complications of the Whipple procedure as outlined in Table 54.5. **QSEN: Safety**

MASTERY QUESTIONS

1. Which statement by the client who is prescribed to take pancreatic enzyme replacements indicates a need for further teaching by the nurse?
   A. "I need to take the enzymes at every meal and with snacks."
   B. "After taking the enzymes, I should drink a glass of water."
   C. "I should wipe my mouth in case any of the enzyme got on my lips."
   D. "I should chew each capsule carefully so that it works in my stomach."

2. The nurse is planning care for a client who had a laparoscopic Whipple surgery. For which complications will the nurse assess? **Select all that apply.**
   A. Bleeding
   B. Wound infection
   C. Intestinal obstruction
   D. Diabetes mellitus
   E. Abdominal abscess

REFERENCES

American Cancer Society (ACS). (2020). *Cancer facts and figures—2019*. Atlanta: Author.

Bujanda, L., & Herreros-Villanueva, M. (2017). Pancreatic cancer in Lynch syndrome patients. *Journal of Cancer*, *8*(18), 3667–3674.

Burchum, J. L. R., & Rosenthal, L. D. (2019). *Lehne's pharmacology for nursing care* (10th ed.). St. Louis: Elsevier.

Jarvis, C. (2020). *Physical examination & health assessment* (8th ed.). St. Louis: Elsevier Saunders.

Lew, D., Afghani, E., & Pandol, S. (2017). Chronic pancreatitis: Current status and challenges for prevention and treatment. *Digestive Diseases and Sciences*, *62*, 1702–1712.

McCance, K., Huether, S., Brashers, V., & Rote, N. (2019). *Pathophysiology: The biologic basis for disease in adults and children* (8th ed.). St. Louis: Mosby.

Pagana, K. D., & Pagana, T. J. (2018). *Manual of diagnostic and laboratory tests* (6th ed.). St. Louis: Mosby.

Roberts, K. E., & Kate, V. (2016). *Transvaginal cholecystectomy*. http://emedicine.medscape.com/article/1900692-overview#a5.

55

Concepts of Care for Patients With Malnutrition: Undernutrition and Obesity

Cherie R. Rebar

http://evolve.elsevier.com/Iggy/

LEARNING OUTCOMES

1. Collaborate with the interprofessional team to coordinate high-quality care for patients with malnutrition.
2. Describe factors that place a patient at high risk for malnutrition and refer to the health care provider.
3. Implement patient-centered nursing interventions to decrease the psychosocial impact of living with malnutrition.
4. Apply knowledge of anatomy, physiology, and pathophysiology to assess patients with malnutrition.
5. Use clinical judgment to analyze assessment findings and diagnostic data in the care of patients with malnutrition.
6. Prioritize evidence-based care for patients with a malnutrition problem affecting ***nutrition*** and ***fluid and electrolyte balance.***
7. Plan care coordination and transition management for patients with malnutrition.

KEY TERMS

anorexia The loss of appetite for food.

anorexia nervosa An eating disorder of self-induced starvation resulting from a fear of fatness, even though the patient is underweight.

bariatrics A branch of medicine that manages patients with obesity and its related diseases.

binge eating disorder An eating disorder that involves eating in binges with a feeling of loss of control over the eating behavior.

body mass index (BMI) A measure of nutrition status that does not depend on frame size; indirectly estimates total fat stores within the body by the relationship of weight to height.

body surface area (BSA) A calculated estimate of a person's total body surface area reflecting physiologic and metabolic processes including heat exchange, blood volume, and size of vital organs. Used as an indicator for appropriate dosage calculation, especially for anticancer agents.

bolus feeding A method of tube feeding that involves intermittent feeding of a specified amount of enteral product at specified times during a 24-hour period, typically every 4 hours.

bulimia nervosa An eating disorder characterized by episodes of binge eating in which the patient ingests a large amount of food in a short time, followed by purging behavior, such as self-induced vomiting or excessive use of laxatives and diuretics.

cachexia Extreme body wasting and malnutrition that develop from an imbalance between food intake and energy use.

continuous feeding A method of tube feeding in which small amounts of enteral product are continuously infused (by gravity drip or by a pump or controller device) over a specified time.

cyclic feeding A method of tube feeding similar to continuous feeding (see definition of continuous feeding) except the infusion is stopped for a specified time in each 24-hour period ("down time"); the down time typically occurs in the morning to allow bathing, treatments, and other activities.

dietary reference intakes (DRIs) Nutrition guide developed by the Institute of Medicine of the National Academies that provides a scientific basis for food guidelines in the United States and Canada.

dumping syndrome Vasomotor symptoms that typically occur within 30 minutes after eating, including vertigo, tachycardia, syncope, sweating, pallor, and palpitations.

enterostomal feeding tube A tube used for patients who need long-term enteral feeding.

food allergy A reaction to a food (or multiple foods), rooted in the immune system, that can cause a life-threatening complication like anaphylaxis.

food intolerance Inability to tolerate a food (or multiple foods), rooted in the gastrointestinal system when a food cannot be properly broken down.

gastric bypass A type of gastric restriction surgery in which gastric resection is combined with malabsorption surgery. The patient's stomach, duodenum, and part of the jejunum are bypassed so that fewer calories can be absorbed. Also known as a Roux-en-Y gastric bypass, or RNYGB.

gastrostomy A stoma created from the abdominal wall into the stomach.
jejunostomy Surgical creation of an opening between the jejunum and surface of the abdominal wall.
knee height caliper A device that uses the distance between the patient's patella and heel to estimate height.
kwashiorkor A lack of protein quantity and quality in the presence of adequate calories. Body weight is more normal, and serum proteins are low.
lactose intolerance A type of food intolerance when a patient has an inadequate amount of lactase enzyme, which converts lactose into absorbable glucose.
malnutrition Deficiencies, excesses, or imbalances in a person's intake of energy and/or nutrients.
marasmus A calorie malnutrition in which body fat and protein are wasted, and serum proteins are often preserved.
medical nutrition supplements Enteral products taken by patients who cannot or do not consume enough nutrients in their usual diet (e.g., Ensure, Boost).
nasoduodenal tube (NDT) A tube that is inserted through a nostril and into the small intestine.
nasoenteric tube (NET) Any feeding tube that is inserted nasally and then advanced into the gastrointestinal tract.
nasogastric (NG) tube A tube that is inserted through a nostril and into the stomach for liquid feeding or for withdrawing gastric contents.
nutrition screening An assessment of nutrition status that includes inspection, measured height and weight, weight history, usual eating habits, ability to chew and swallow, and any recent changes in appetite or food intake.
obesity An increase in body weight at least 20% above the upper limit of the normal range for ideal body weight, with an excess amount of body fat; in an adult, a body mass index greater than 30. Subdivided into Class I, II, or III.
overweight An increase in body weight for height compared with a reference standard (e.g., the Metropolitan Life height and weight tables) or 10% greater than ideal body weight. However, this weight may not reflect excess body fat, which in an adult is a body mass index of 25 to 30.
panniculectomy Surgical removal of the abdominal apron (panniculus).
percutaneous endoscopic gastrostomy (PEG) A stoma created from the abdominal wall into the stomach for insertion of a short feeding tube.
protein-energy undernutrition (PEU) A disorder of nutrition that may present in three forms: marasmus, kwashiorkor, and marasmic-kwashiorkor. Also called *protein-calorie malnutrition.*
refeeding syndrome Life-threatening metabolic complication that can occur when nutrition is restarted for a patient who is in a starvation state.
skinfold measurements Estimation of body fat, usually calculated through measurement of the triceps and subscapular skinfolds with a special caliper.
starvation A complete lack of nutrients.
total parenteral nutrition (TPN) Provision of intensive nutritional support for an extended time; delivered to the patient through access to central veins, usually the subclavian or internal jugular veins.
undernutrition A nutrition state of wasting, stunting, and being underweight

PRIORITY AND INTERRELATED CONCEPTS

The priority concept for this chapter is:
- ***Nutrition***

The ***Nutrition*** concept exemplars for this chapter are Undernutrition and Obesity.

The interrelated concept for this chapter is:
- ***Fluid and Electrolyte Balance***

Eating a balanced diet yields a strong ***nutrition*** status, which helps the body function well through growth, the maintenance of temperature, respiration, cardiac output, muscle strength, protein synthesis, and storage and metabolism of healthy food sources. In healthy adults, most energy supplied by carbohydrates, protein, and fat undergoes digestion and is absorbed from the GI tract. The relationship between energy used and energy stored is referred to as *energy balance.* Weight is gained when food intake is more than energy used, and weight loss occurs when energy used is more than intake. The body attempts to meet its calorie requirements even if it is at the expense of protein needs; when calorie intake is insufficient, body proteins are used for energy.

Influenced by personal preference, demographic location, cultural norms, spiritual observations, financial feasibility, and availability of nutrition sources, ***nutrition*** status varies for each patient. Further influencing factors include age, height, weight, gender, speed of metabolism, influence of exercise or activity, medications taken, substances used (e.g., alcohol or illicit drugs), and types of fluids consumed. The estimated energy requirement (EER) is 2000 to 3000 calories per day for healthy adult men and 1600 to 2400 calories per day for healthy adult women (Office of Disease and Health Promotion, 2020). The caloric requirement may decrease if a patient needs to lose weight or increase if the patient needs to gain weight or promote healing.

NUTRITION STANDARDS FOR HEALTH PROMOTION AND MAINTENANCE

Current focuses on ***nutrition*** are targeted toward health promotion and the prevention of disease by healthy eating and exercise. **Dietary reference intakes (DRIs)** based on age, gender, and life stage serve as a ***nutrition*** guide for more than 40 nutrients that provides a scientific basis for food guidelines in the United States and Canada (National Academies of Sciences, Engineering, & Medicine, 2020). In the United States, the *Dietary*

Guidelines for Americans are revised by the U.S. Department of Agriculture (USDA) and the U.S. Department of Health and Human Services (DHHS) every 5 years. Examples of the *2015-2020 Guidelines* (8th edition) are listed in Table 55.1. At time of publication, the *2020-2025 Dietary Guidelines for Americans* are being developed based on collected evidence in the Scientific Report of the 2020 Dietary Guidelines Advisory Committee (Dietary Guidelines for Americans, 2020).

"Start Simple with MyPlate" is an initiative that reminds users about health eating styles that are built into a lifestyle (U.S. Department of Agriculture, n.d.) (Fig. 55.1). This pictorial demonstrates how to build a healthy plate of food consisting of the right proportions of fruits, vegetables, grains, proteins, and dairy products. Canada publishes Canada's Food Guide (Government of Canada, 2020), a similar visual reference.

Common Diets

Given the variance in people's preferences, place of residence, availability of foods, financial means, cultural or spiritual observations, and financial circumstances, there is not a specific "typical (or common) diet." Some people consume a highly nutrient-rich diet and remain adequately hydrated with water. Others eat excess foods heavy in fats or carbohydrates and choose to drink soda or juice on a regular basis, which can lead to **obesity**. Others do not have adequate access to nutrient-dense food and hydration and may experience **undernutrition**. Individuals with obesity or undernutrition both experience **malnutrition** in different ways, as the state of malnutrition occurs on a continuum.

In ideal circumstances, patients should consume a diet containing complex carbohydrates, lean proteins, and monounsaturated or polyunsaturated fats that also contains necessary vitamins and minerals. The specific foods you recommend to patients to meet their nutrition needs depends on the variances mentioned earlier.

Some adults follow vegetarian diet patterns for health, environmental, religious, cultural, or spiritual reasons (Box 55.1).

People who eat a vegan diet can develop anemia as a result of vitamin B_{12} deficiency. Teach them to include a daily source of vitamin B_{12} in their diets, such as a fortified breakfast cereal, fortified soy beverage, or meat substitute. Refer those interested in vegetarianism to www.eatright.org, which contains many credible resources regarding vegetarian health (Academy of Nutrition and Dietetics (2018).

TABLE 55.1 Examples of *2015–2020 Dietary Guidelines for Americans*

- Follow a healthy eating pattern across the lifespan.
- Focus on variety, nutrient density, and amount.
- Limit calories from added sugars and saturated fats and reduce sodium intake.
- Shift to healthier food and beverage choices.
- Support healthy eating patterns for all.

From *Dietary Guidelines for Americans 2015-2020* (8th ed.). (2015). http://health.gov/dietaryguidelines/2015/resources/2015-2020_Dietary_Guidelines.pdf.

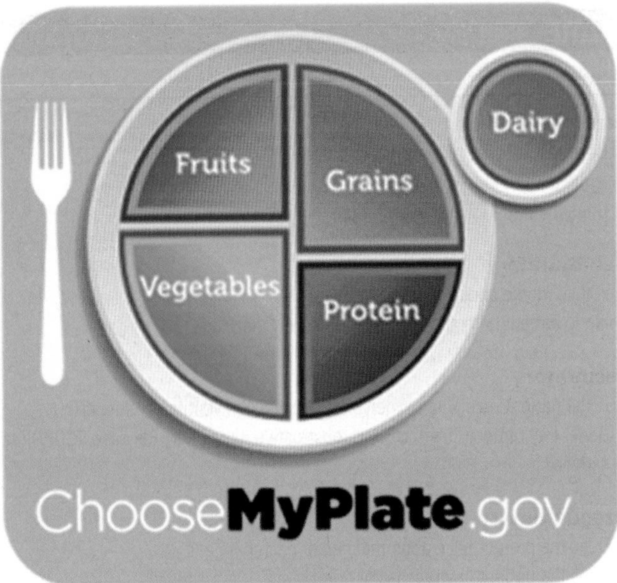

Fig. 55.1 The U.S. Department of Agriculture MyPlate. (From U.S. Department of Agriculture, 2020, www.ChooseMyPlate.gov.)

PATIENT-CENTERED CARE: CULTURAL/SPIRITUAL CONSIDERATIONS QSEN

Many adults have specific food preferences based on their ethnicity or race. Health teaching about ***nutrition*** should incorporate any cultural preferences voiced by the patient. However, *never assume that a patient eats only foods associated with his or her primary ethnicity.*

FOOD SENSITIVITIES

Some adults have food allergies or intolerances. A true **food allergy** differs from an intolerance in the sense that an allergy to a food can cause life-threatening complications like anaphylaxis. A food allergy is rooted in the immune system. The most common food allergies are milk, chocolate, eggs, soy, wheat, tree nuts, peanuts, and shellfish (McCance et al., 2019). A **food intolerance** involves the gastrointestinal system and occurs when the system cannot properly break down food (American Academy of Allergy, Asthma, and Immunology, 2020).

An example of a food allergy is shellfish, which can cause coughing; edema (face, lips, tongue, throat); shortness of breath;

BOX 55.1 Vegetarian Types

Lacto-vegetarian—allows dairy[a]; avoids meat, poultry, seafood, eggs, and foods that contain those items
Ovo-vegetarian—allows eggs; avoids meat, poultry, seafood, and dairy[a]
Lacto-ovo vegetarian—allows eggs and dairy[a]; avoids meat, poultry, seafood
Pescatarian—allows seafood; avoids meat, poultry, dairy,[a] eggs
Vegan—consumes a plant-based diet only; avoids meat, poultry, seafood, dairy,[a] and eggs, and foods that contain those items (note = some vegans also avoid honey)

[a] Dairy = milk, cheese, yogurt, butter, etc.

or anaphylaxis in certain patients. An example of a food intolerance is lactose intolerance, in which a patient has an inadequate amount of the lactase enzyme, which converts lactose into absorbable glucose. Ingesting a milk product causes bloating, diarrhea, abdominal discomfort, and flatulence. When taking a history, ask patients specifically what kind of reaction they have to certain foods; document and plan care accordingly.

PATIENT-CENTERED CARE: OLDER ADULT CONSIDERATIONS QSEN

The USDA (2015) recommends that older adults drink eight glasses of water a day and eat plenty of fiber to prevent or manage constipation. It also suggests daily calcium and vitamins D and B_{12} supplements and a reduction in sodium and cholesterol-containing foods.

NUTRITION ASSESSMENT

Nutrition status reflects the balance between nutrient requirements and intake. Evaluation of nutrition status is an important part of total patient assessment and includes:

- Review of the nutrition history
- Food and fluid intake record
- Notation of access to appropriate sources of nutrition
- Laboratory data
- Food-drug interactions
- Health history and physical assessment
- Anthropometric measurements
- Psychosocial assessment

Monitor the ***nutrition*** status of a patient during hospitalization as an important part of your initial assessment. Collaborate with the interprofessional health care team to identify patients at risk for nutrition problems.

Initial Nutrition Screening

The Joint Commission Patient Care Standards require that a nutrition screening occur within 24 hours of the patient's hospital admission, with a full nutrition assessment for patients identified as being at risk. The initial screening includes inspection, measured height and weight, weight history, usual eating habits, ability to chew and swallow, and any recent changes in appetite or food intake. The Full MNA® Form (Mini Nutrition Assessment) (Fig. 55.2) is a helpful and brief screening tool that can assist in identifying older adults who are malnourished or at risk for undernutrition. An even shorter version—the MNA®, which refers to the Mini Nutrition Assessment–Short Form (formerly the MNA®-SF) (Nestle Nutrition Institute, n.d.)—is also available for use in the clinical setting. See the Best Practice for Patient Safety & Quality Care: Nutrition Screening Assessment box for examples of questions to consider as part of the initial assessment.

Anthropometric Measurements

Anthropometric measurements are noninvasive methods of evaluating ***nutrition*** status. These measurements include obtaining height and weight and assessment of BMI. You may delegate the task of obtaining height and weight to assistive personnel (AP) under your supervision, as this is within their scope. Be sure to instruct the AP to follow up with measurements as soon as this activity is completed, as this information affects the plan of care.

Obtaining accurate measurements is important because patients tend to overestimate height and underestimate weight. Measurements taken days or weeks later may indicate an early change in nutrition status. Follow agency policy or the primary health care provider's orders for frequency of measurement.

BEST PRACTICE FOR PATIENT SAFETY & QUALITY CARE QSEN

Nutrition Screening Assessment

General

- Does the patient have conditions that cause nutrient loss (e.g., malabsorption syndromes, wounds, prolonged diarrhea)
- Does the patient have conditions that increase the need for nutrients (e.g., fever, burns, injury)
- Has the patient been NPO for 3 days or more?
- Is the patient receiving a modified diet or a diet restricted in one or more nutrients?
- Is the patient being enterally or parenterally fed?
- Does the patient describe food allergies, lactose intolerance, or limited food preferences?
- Has the patient experienced a recent unexplained weight loss?
- Is the patient on drug therapy, including prescription, over-the-counter, or herbal/natural products?

Gastrointestinal

- Does the patient have glossitis, stomatitis, or esophagitis?
- Does the patient have difficulty chewing or swallowing or have poor dentition?
- Does the patient have a partial or total GI obstruction?
- Does the patient report nausea, indigestion, vomiting, diarrhea, or constipation?
- Does the patient have an ostomy?

Cardiovascular

- Does the patient have ascites or edema?
- Is the patient able to perform ADLs?
- Does the patient have heart failure?

Genitourinary

- Is fluid intake about equal to fluid output?
- Is the patient hemodialyzed or peritoneally dialyzed?

Respiratory

- Is the patient receiving oxygen or on mechanical ventilatory support?
- Does the patient have chronic obstructive pulmonary disease (COPD) or asthma?

Integumentary

- Does the patient have abnormal nail or hair changes?
- Does the patient have rashes or dermatitis?
- Does the patient have dry or pale mucous membranes or decreased skin turgor?
- Does the patient have pressure injuries?

Musculoskeletal

- Does the patient have cachexia?

Modified Courtesy Ross Products Division, Abbott Laboratories, Columbus, OH.

Mini Nutritional Assessment MNA®

Nestlé NutritionInstitute

Last name: First name:

Sex: Age: Weight, kg: Height, cm: Date:

Complete the screen by filling in the boxes with the appropriate numbers.
Add the numbers for the screen. If score is 11 or less, continue with the assessment to gain a Malnutrition Indicator Score.

Screening

A Has food intake declined over the past 3 months due to loss of appetite, digestive problems, chewing or swallowing difficulties?
0 = severe decrease in food intake
1 = moderate decrease in food intake
2 = no decrease in food intake ☐

B Weight loss during the last 3 months
0 = weight loss greater than 3kg (6.6lbs)
1 = does not know
2 = weight loss between 1 and 3kg (2.2 and 6.6 lbs)
3 = no weight loss ☐

C Mobility
0 = bed or chair bound
1 = able to get out of bed / chair but does not go out
2 = goes out ☐

D Has suffered psychological stress or acute disease in the past 3 months?
0 = yes 2 = no ☐

E Neuropsychological problems
0 = severe dementia or depression
1 = mild dementia
2 = no psychological problems ☐

F Body Mass Index (BMI) = weight in kg / (height in m)^2
0 = BMI less than 19
1 = BMI 19 to less than 21
2 = BMI 21 to less than 23
3 = BMI 23 or greater ☐

Screening score (subtotal max. 14 points) ☐☐

12-14 points:	Normal nutritional status
8-11 points:	At risk of malnutrition
0-7 points:	Malnourished

For a more in-depth assessment, continue with questions G-R

Assessment

G Lives independently (not in nursing home or hospital)
1 = yes 0 = no ☐

H Takes more than 3 prescription drugs per day
0 = yes 1 = no ☐

I Pressure sores or skin ulcers
0 = yes 1 = no ☐

J How many full meals does the patient eat daily?
0 = 1 meal
1 = 2 meals
2 = 3 meals ☐

K Selected consumption markers for protein intake
- At least one serving of dairy products (milk, cheese, yoghurt) per day yes ☐ no ☐
- Two or more servings of legumes or eggs per week yes ☐ no ☐
- Meat, fish or poultry every day yes ☐ no ☐

0.0 = if 0 or 1 yes
0.5 = if 2 yes
1.0 = if 3 yes ☐.☐

L Consumes two or more servings of fruit or vegetables per day?
0 = no 1 = yes ☐

M How much fluid (water, juice, coffee, tea, milk...) is consumed per day?
0.0 = less than 3 cups
0.5 = 3 to 5 cups
1.0 = more than 5 cups ☐.☐

N Mode of feeding
0 = unable to eat without assistance
1 = self-fed with some difficulty
2 = self-fed without any problem ☐

O Self view of nutritional status
0 = views self as being malnourished
1 = is uncertain of nutritional state
2 = views self as having no nutritional problem ☐

P In comparison with other people of the same age, how does the patient consider his / her health status?
0.0 = not as good
0.5 = does not know
1.0 = as good
2.0 = better ☐.☐

Q Mid-arm circumference (MAC) in cm
0.0 = MAC less than 21
0.5 = MAC 21 to 22
1.0 = MAC greater than 22 ☐.☐

R Calf circumference (CC) in cm
0 = CC less than 31
1 = CC 31 or greater ☐

Assessment (max. 16 points) ☐☐.☐

Screening score ☐☐.☐

Total Assessment (max. 30 points) ☐☐.☐

Malnutrition Indicator Score

24 to 30 points	☐	Normal nutritional status
17 to 23.5 points	☐	At risk of malnutrition
Less than 17 points	☐	Malnourished

References
1. Vellas B, Villars H, Abellan G, *et al.* Overview of the MNA® - Its History and Challenges. *J Nutr Health Aging.* 2006; **10:456**-465.
2. Rubenstein LZ, Harker JO, Salva A, Guigoz Y, Vellas B. Screening for Undernutrition in Geriatric Practice: Developing the Short-Form Mini Nutritional Assessment (MNA-SF). *J. Geront.* 2001; **56A**: M366-377
3. Guigoz Y. The Mini-Nutritional Assessment (MNA®) Review of the Literature - What does it tell us? *J Nutr Health Aging.* 2006; **10**:466-487.

For more information: www.mna-elderly.com

Fig. 55.2 Full MNA® Form (Mini Nutrition Assessment). (Société des Produits Nestlé S.A., Vevey, Switzerland, Trademark Owners.)

Measure and weigh patients with the same scale and with the same amount of clothing (without shoes) each time. A sliding-blade **knee height caliper,** which uses the distance between the patient's patella and heel to estimate height, can be used for those who cannot stand. It is especially useful for patients who have knee or hip contractures.

The type of scale used depends on the patient's ability to stand or sit; wheelchairs scales or bed scales can be used for nonambulatory individuals. When using a bed scale, document the number of sheets, pillows, and blankets on the bed at the time of measurement. Lines, devices, and equipment should be lifted off the bed when the measurement is taking place. Normal weights for adult men and women are available from several reference standards, such as the Metropolitan Life tables. Online calculators are also available to calculate ideal body weight. *An unintentional weight loss of 5% in a month or 10% over a 6-month period significantly affects* ***nutrition*** *status and should be evaluated.*

NURSING SAFETY PRIORITY QSEN

Action Alert

Obtain weight at the same time each day, if possible, preferably before breakfast. Conditions such as heart failure and renal disease cause weight gain; dehydration and conditions such as cancer cause weight loss. *Weight is the most reliable indicator of fluid gain or loss!*

Assessment of body fat is usually calculated by the registered dietitian nutritionist (RDN) if in a hospital setting or by a fitness trainer or physical therapist in the community setting. The **body mass index (BMI)** indirectly estimates total fat stores within the body by the relationship of weight to height (Table 55.2). *Therefore an accurate height is as important as an accurate weight.* Online calculators can perform this computation, which divides a patient's weight in kilograms by the square of height in meters. The least risk for malnutrition is associated with scores between 18.5 and 24.9. BMIs above and below these values are associated with increased health risks (CDC, 2020a).

Limitations of BMI calculations include (Schnur, 2017, in Smith, 2019):

- Overestimation of amount of body fat in physically fit, athletic, or muscular patients
- Underestimation of body fat levels in older adults, active adults, and neurologically impaired individuals with decreased muscle mass
- Underestimated morbidity and obesity risk in Asian populations

PATIENT-CENTERED CARE: OLDER ADULT CONSIDERATIONS QSEN

Body weight and BMI usually increase throughout adulthood until about 60 years of age. As some adults get older, they often become less hungry and eat less, even if they are healthy. Others continue usual eating patterns and are at higher risk for obesity—especially older adult females (CDC, 2020a). Do not assume that an older adult automatically eats less; personalize the nutrition assessment to accurately assess eating patterns for every patient.

TABLE 55.2 Body Mass Index (BMI) Ranges

BMI	Weight Status
Below 18.5	Underweight
18.5-24.9	Normal or healthy weight
25.0-29.9	Overweight
30.0 and above	Obese

From Centers for Disease Control and Prevention (CDC). (2020b). Defining adult overweight and obesity. https://www.cdc.gov/obesity/adult/defining.html.

TABLE 55.3 Calculated BSA Averages for Adults According to Age

Age (yr)	Average BSA (m^2) for Males in United States, Rounded to Nearest Hundredth	Average BSA (m^2) for Females in United States, Rounded to Nearest Hundredth
20 and older (average)	2.09	1.86
20-39	2.09	1.85
40-59	2.11	1.90
60 and older	2.06	1.83

From Fryar, C.D., Kruszon-Moran, D., Gu, Q., & Ogden, C. L. (2018). Mean body weight, height, waist circumference, and body mass index among adults: United States, 1999–2000 through 2015–2016. National Health Statistics Reports; no 122. Hyattsville, MD: National Center for Health Statistics.

NCLEX EXAMINATION CHALLENGE 55.1

Health Promotion and Maintenance

An older adult is admitted to the hospital. The client's height is 5 feet, 6 inches (1.68 m), and weight is 250 lb (113.3 kg). The nurse calculates the client's current body mass index (BMI) as _______. **Fill in the blank. Round your answer to the nearest whole number.**

Body surface area (BSA) (Table 55.3) is an estimate of a patient's total body surface area calculated as a biometric two-dimensional measure of a person's body size (Schnur, 2017, in Smith, 2019). It reflects physiologic and metabolic processes, included heat exchange, blood volume, and size of vital organs (Weinstein & Hagle, 2014). BSA can be used as an indicator for appropriate dosage calculation for medication and IV administration, especially for anticancer agents (Eaton and Lyman, 2019).

BSA is calculated in meters squared, combining a patient's weight and height and reflecting an estimate of their total surface (outside body layer) area (Faisal et al., 2016). If a patient has a BSA of 3 m^2, it means that their skin surface could be placed into a 3-meter × 3-meter box.

Calculate BSA by the Mosteller formula, which takes the square root of the height in centimeters, multiplied by the weight in kilograms, divided by 3600. The average BSA is 2.09 m^2 for males and 1.86 m^2 for females (Fryar et al., 2018). Be aware that accurate calculation of weight is imperative, as height is unlikely to change significantly, but weight is variable.

TABLE 55.4 Common Complications of Undernutrition

Cardiovascular • Reduced cardiac output **Endocrine** • Cold intolerance **Gastrointestinal** • Anorexia • Diarrhea • Impaired protein synthesis • Malabsorption • Vomiting • Weight loss **Immunologic** • Susceptibility to infectious disease	**Integumentary** • Dry, flaky skin • Various types of dermatitis • Poor wound healing **Musculoskeletal** • Cachexia • Decreased activity tolerance • Decreased muscle mass • Impaired functional ability **Neurologic** • Weakness **Psychiatric** • Substance misuse **Respiratory** • Reduced vital capacity

Skinfold measurements estimate body fat. The *triceps and subscapular* skinfolds are most commonly measured with a special caliper. Both are compared with standard measurements and recorded as percentiles. The *midarm circumference (MAC) and calf circumference (CC)* are needed if the MNA-SF tool is used. Place a flexible tape around the upper arm (or calf) at the midpoint; wrap gently to avoid compressing the tissue, and record the findings in centimeters in the electronic health record.

NUTRITION CONCEPT EXEMPLAR: UNDERNUTRITION

Pathophysiology Review

Undernutrition is a multinutrient problem. If a patient does not, or cannot, consume calories and protein, he or she also misses intake of other healthy nutrients. Inadequate nutrient intake can also result when an adult is admitted to the hospital or long-term care facility. For example, decreased staffing may not allow time for patients who need to be fed, especially older adults, who may eat slowly. Many diagnostic tests, surgery, trauma, and unexpected medical complications require a period of NPO in which nutrients are not being consumed or cause anorexia (loss of appetite). See Table 55.4 for common complications of undernutrition and Table 55.5 for common signs and symptoms of nutrient deficiencies.

PATIENT-CENTERED CARE: CULTURAL/SPIRITUAL CONSIDERATIONS QSEN

In some cases, undernutrition results when meals provided in the health care setting differ from what the patient usually eats. Be sure to identify specific food preferences that the patient can eat and enjoy that are in keeping with his or her cultural practices.

Protein-energy undernutrition (PEU), formerly protein-calorie malnutrition (PCM), has three common forms (Morley, 2020):

- Marasmus: A calorie malnutrition in which body fat and protein are wasted. Serum proteins are often preserved.
- Kwashiorkor: A lack of protein quantity and quality in the presence of adequate calories. Body weight is more normal, and serum proteins are low.
- Starvation: A complete lack of nutrients. This problem can occur even when food is available but is most commonly seen in areas in which food is unavailable (e.g., during a time of famine or exposure to the elements).

Unrecognized or untreated PEU can lead to dysfunction or disability and increased morbidity and mortality.

Acute PEU may develop in patients who were adequately nourished before hospitalization but experience starvation while in a catabolic state from infection, stress, or injury. *Chronic* PEU can occur in those who have a chronic health condition such as cancer, end-stage kidney or liver disease, or chronic neurologic disease.

Eating disorders such as anorexia nervosa, bulimia nervosa, and binge eating disorder, which are seen most often in teens and young adults, can also lead to a state of undernutrition. Anorexia nervosa is a self-induced state of starvation resulting from a fear of fatness, even though the patient is underweight. This condition is often accompanied by a psychiatric diagnosis of *body dysmorphic disorder* (BDD). BDD is an obsessive-compulsive condition

PATIENT-CENTERED CARE: OLDER ADULT CONSIDERATIONS QSEN

Older adults are most at risk for poor ***nutrition,*** especially PEU. Risk factors include physiologic changes of aging, environmental factors, and health problems. See the Focused Assessment: Assessing for Undernutrition in the Older Adult box, which lists some of these major factors for which you will assess. If psychosocial concerns are present, collaborate with mental health and/or social work professionals who can assist. Chapter 4 discusses nutrition for older adults in more detail.

FOCUSED ASSESSMENT

Assessing for Undernutrition in the Older Adult

Physical Concerns

- Chronic conditions/illnesses
- Constipation
- Decreased appetite
- Dentition—poor dental health; poor-fitting dentures; lack of teeth or dentures
- Drugs—prescription and OTC drugs that may impair taste or appetite
- Dry mouth
- "Failure to thrive" (a combination of three of five symptoms, including weakness, slow walking speed, low physical activity, unintentional weight loss, exhaustion)
- Impaired eyesight
- Pain that is acute or persistent
- Weight loss

Psychosocial Concerns

- Ability (or inability) to prepare meals due to functional decline, fatigue, memory
- Decrease in enjoyment of meals
- Depression
- Income (ability to afford food)
- Loneliness
- Transportation access

INTERPROFESSIONAL COLLABORATION

Care of Older Adults at Risk for Undernutrition

For older adults with undernutrition, or at risk for undernutrition, assess for psychosocial concerns that can impact their desire or ability to consumer nutrient-rich foods. If any of these concerns is rooted in mental health, such as depression or loneliness, collaborate with a mental health professional, such as a counselor or psychiatric-mental health nurse practitioner who can work with the patient to enhance his or her emotional well-being. If the concerns are economic or access-related, collaborate with the case manager or social worker who can help identify ways to facilitate better access to sources of nutrition. According to the Interprofessional Education Collaborative (IPEC) Expert Panel's Competency of Roles and Responsibilities, using the unique and complimentary abilities of other team members optimizes health and patient care (IPEC, 2016; Slusser et al., 2019).

in which a patient spends an abnormal amount of time attempting to reach what he or she considers to be body perfection. In the case of a patient with anorexia nervosa, perfection is found in being thin. The condition affects the patient's ability to carry out normal ADLs and significantly impacts quality of life (Perkins, 2019). If this condition is suspected, collaborate with the primary health care provider to determine if a psychiatric consultation is needed. **Bulimia nervosa** is characterized by episodes of binge eating in which the patient ingests a large amount of food in a short time. The binge eating is followed by some form of purging behavior, such as self-induced vomiting or excessive use of laxatives and diuretics. If not treated, death can result from starvation, infection, or suicide. **Binge eating disorder** is a separate psychiatric diagnosis from bulimia nervosa. It resembles bulimia nervosa in terms of binge-eating episodes, and it involves a feeling of loss of control over the eating behavior (Kelly-Weeder et al., 2019); however, it is not accompanied by purging. Again, collaborate with the primary health care provider if this condition is suspected. Further information about eating disorders can be found in mental health nursing textbooks.

Health Promotion and Maintenance. It is estimated that 5% of hospitalized patients are diagnosed with undernutrition (Tolbert et al., 2018). This may be related to prehospitalization status, or due to lack of ***nutrition*** during a current illness or an injury. Malnourishment can increase length of stay and also be cause for readmission. Nurses can have a significant impact on patient length of stay when adequately advocating for the patient's nutrition status. (See the Systems Thinking and Quality Improvement box.)

INTERPROFESSIONAL COLLABORATION

Care of Patients With Undernutrition

For patients with undernutrition, consult with a registered dietician nutritionist (RDN) who can assist with meeting nutritional needs while the patient is hospitalized, as well as help with planning for continued nutrition health after discharge. According to the Interprofessional Education Collaborative (IPEC) Expert Panel's Competency of Roles and Responsibilities, using the unique and complementary abilities of other team members optimizes health and patient care (IPEC, 2016; Slusser et al., 2019).

TABLE 55.5 Signs and Symptoms of Nutrient Deficiencies

Sign/Symptom	Potential Nutrient Deficiency
Hair	
Alopecia	Zinc
Easy to remove	Protein
Lackluster hair	Protein
"Corkscrew" hair	Vitamin C
Decreased pigmentation	Protein
Eyes	
Dryness of conjunctiva	Vitamin A
Corneal vascularization	Riboflavin
Keratomalacia	Vitamin A
Bitot spots	Vitamin A
GI Tract	
Nausea, vomiting	Pyridoxine
Diarrhea	Zinc, niacin
Stomatitis	Pyridoxine, riboflavin, iron
Cheilosis	Pyridoxine, iron
Glossitis	Pyridoxine, zinc, niacin, folic acid, vitamin B_{12}
Magenta tongue	Vitamin A, riboflavin
Swollen, bleeding gums	Vitamin C
Fissured tongue	Niacin
Hepatomegaly	Protein
Skin	
Dry and scaling	Vitamin A
Petechiae/ecchymoses	Vitamin C
Follicular hyperkeratosis	Vitamin A
Nasolabial seborrhea	Niacin
Bilateral dermatitis	Niacin
Musculoskeletal	
Subcutaneous fat loss	Calories
Muscle wastage	Calories, protein
Edema	Protein
Osteomalacia, bone pain, rickets	Vitamin D
Hematologic	
Anemia	Vitamin B_{12}, iron, folic acid, copper, vitamin E
Leukopenia, neutropenia	Copper
Low prothrombin time, prolonged clotting time	Vitamin K, manganese
Neurologic	
Disorientation	Niacin, thiamine
Confabulation	Thiamine
Neuropathy	Thiamine, pyridoxine, chromium
Paresthesia	Thiamine, pyridoxine, vitamin B_{12}
Cardiovascular	
Heart failure, cardiomegaly, tachycardia	Thiamine
Cardiomyopathy	Selenium
Cardiac dysrhythmias	Magnesium

Courtesy Ross Products Division, Abbott Laboratories, Columbus, OH.

SYSTEMS THINKING AND QUALITY IMPROVEMENT QSEN

An Interprofessional Focus on Preventing Readmissions for Patients at High Risk for Malnutrition

Beckett, C., & Walsh, S. (2019). The malnutrition readmission prevention protocol. *American Journal of Nursing, 119*(12):60–64.

Reflecting on the fact that malnutrition affects one in three hospitalized patients, the authors of this study desired to put an evidence-based protocol in place to improve patient outcomes and avoid reduced reimbursement associated with 30-day malnutrition-related readmissions. Nurses, the clinical manager of nutrition services, physicians, care coordination staff, physical therapists, quality staff, and informatics experts were tasked together as an interprofessional team to address high hospital readmission rates due to patient malnourishment.

After a comprehensive review of evidence was accomplished, the team developed the evidence-based Malnutrition Readmission Prevention Protocol, which identifies three stages of risk for malnutrition. The Protocol was used first in one facility and then implemented across a hospital system. Informatics specialists worked to create automatic alerts within the electronic health record to flag health care professionals to use the Protocol. Using this tool, patients were identified for inpatient management of nutritional supplementation, and then referral to a registered dietician nutritionist (RDN) was made. The RDN coordinated availability of 30-day supplementation to be used in the home environment following discharge. An important part of Protocol use was involving the patient (and caregiver, as appropriate) in conversations regarding inpatient and outpatient nutrition management. Follow-up calls were made by care management nurses; home visits were conducted by paramedics; and primary care providers were notified to coordinate care after discharge.

Over a 5-year period, readmissions due to malnutrition decreased from 42% to 13.3%.

Commentary: Implications for Practice and Research

Coordinating an effort where all professions involved in patient care had input into the Protocol well before implementation facilitated a collaborative effort created with best practice and favorable patient outcomes in mind. Using the Protocol together, meeting the patient's nutrition needs in the inpatient and outpatient settings greatly decreased the readmission rate related to malnutrition. Working together facilitates better outcomes when all stakeholders, including the patient and caregiver, are involved in care processes and planning.

Incidence and Prevalence. Estimates show that 6% of outpatients, 22% of hospitalized patients, and 23.1% of patients living in an extended care facility and 29.4% of patients temporarily staying in a rehabilitation setting are undernourished (Cereda et al., 2016, in Ritchie & Yukawa, 2019).

❖ Interprofessional Collaborative Care

Care for the patient with undernutrition takes place in a variety of settings, such as the home, the community, and the hospital setting if more comprehensive management is needed.

◆ Assessment: Recognize Cues

History. See the earlier Best Practice for Patient Safety & Quality Care: Nutrition Screening Assessment box to complete the initial history. For older adults, also see the Focused Assessment: Assessing for Undernutrition in the Older Adult box. In collaboration with the registered dietitian nutritionist (RDN), also obtain information about the patient's:

- Usual daily food intake and timing of eating
- Food preferences (including cultural considerations)
- Eating behaviors/patterns
- Change in appetite
- Recent weight changes
- Economic status that may influence access to, or purchase of, food

A full ***nutrition*** history usually includes a 24-hour recall of food intake and the frequency with which foods are consumed. The adequacy of the diet can be evaluated by comparing the amount and types of foods consumed daily with the established standards. The registered dietitian nutritionist (RDN) then provides a more detailed analysis of nutrition intake. Be aware that patients who live in food deserts (i.e., urban areas where fresh, healthy food is in low supply or unaffordable) may have difficulty obtaining food that is densely nutritious. Also remember that an unintentional weight loss of 5% in 30 days, or 10% over a 6-month period, significantly affects ***nutrition*** status and should be further evaluated.

! NURSING SAFETY PRIORITY QSEN

Action Alert

Assess for difficulty or pain chewing or swallowing. Unrecognized dysphagia is a common problem among older adults and can cause undernutrition, dehydration, and aspiration pneumonia. See Chapter 49 for more information.

Physical Assessment/Signs and Symptoms. Assess for signs and symptoms of various nutrient deficiencies (see Table 55.5). Inspect hair, eyes, oral cavity, nails, and musculoskeletal and neurologic systems. Examine the condition of the skin, including any reddened or open areas. Anthropometric measurements may also be obtained. Monitors all food and fluid intake. A 3-day caloric intake may be collected and then calculated by the registered dietitian nutritionist (RDN). Delegate this activity to assistive personnel (AP) under your ongoing supervision, and direct AP to report the intake and output values back after obtaining them. Ask AP to report any signs of choking while the patient eats. Document the presence of mouth pain, difficulty chewing, nausea, vomiting, heartburn, or any other symptoms of discomfort with eating.

Psychosocial Assessment. The psychosocial history provides information about the patient's economic status, occupation, educational level, ethnicity/race, living and cooking arrangements, and emotional status. Determine whether financial resources are adequate for providing the necessary food. If resources are inadequate, the social worker or case manager may refer the patient and caregiver to available community services.

Laboratory Assessment. Interpret laboratory data carefully with regard to the total patient; focusing on an isolated value may yield an inaccurate conclusion. In general, laboratory values that may be decreased in the presence of undernourishment include (Pagana & Pagana, 2018):

- Cholesterol
- Hemoglobin

- Hematocrit
- Serum albumin
- Thyroxine-binding prealbumin (PAB)
- Transferrin

◆ **Analysis: Analyze Cues and Prioritize Hypothesis.** The priority collaborative problem for the patient with undernutrition is:

1. Weight loss due to inability to access, ingest or digest food, or absorb nutrients

◆ **Planning and Implementation: Generate Solutions and Take Action**

Improving Nutrition

Planning: Expected Outcomes. The patient with undernutrition is expected to have nutrients available to meet his or her metabolic needs.

Interventions. The preferred route for food intake is orally through the GI tract because it enhances the immune system, is safer, easier, less expensive, and more enjoyable.

Meal Management. Following the primary health care provider's and RDN's recommendation, provide high-calorie, nutrient-rich foods (e.g., milkshakes, cheese, supplement drinks such as Boost or Ensure). A feeding schedule of six small meals may be tolerated better than three large ones. A pureed or dental soft diet may be easier for those who have problems chewing or do not have teeth. Follow recommendations in the Best Practice for Patient Safety & Quality Care: Promoting Nutrition Intake box to provide a more enjoyable and productive eating experience for patients with undernutrition.

BEST PRACTICE FOR PATIENT SAFETY & QUALITY CARE (QSEN)

Promoting Nutrition Intake

Environment

- Remove bedpans, urinals, and emesis basins from the environment.
- Eliminate or decrease offensive odors as much as possible.
- Decrease environmental distractions as much as possible.
- Administer pain medication and/or antiemetics for nausea at least 1 hour before mealtime.

Comfort

- Allow the patient to toilet before mealtime.
- Provide mouth care before mealtime.
- Ensure that eyeglasses and hearing aids in place, if appropriate, during meals.
- Remind assistive personnel (AP) to have patient sit in a chair, if possible, at mealtime.

Function

- Ensure that meals are visually appealing, appetizing, and at appropriate temperatures.
- If needed, open cartons and packages and cut up food.
- Observe during meals for food intake, and document the percentage consumed.
- Encourage self-feeding (if able) or feed the patient slowly (delegate to AP, if desired).
- Eliminate or minimize interruptions during mealtime for nonurgent procedures or rounds.

Nutrition Supplements. If the patient cannot take in enough nutrients in food, fortified **medical nutrition supplements (MNSs)** (e.g., Ensure, Sustacal, Carnation Instant Breakfast [also available as a lactose-free supplement]) may be given, especially to older adults. For patients with liver and renal disease or diabetes, special products that meet these needs are available (e.g., Glucerna for patients with diabetes).

Nutrition supplements are supplied as liquid formulas, powders, soups, coffee, and puddings in a variety of flavors. Examples include Duocal for carbohydrates and fats, and Resource Beneprotein for protein. Follow the primary health care provider's prescription for nutrition supplementation.

Drug Therapy. Multivitamins, zinc, and an iron preparation are often prescribed to treat or prevent anemia in patients who are malnourished. Monitor the patient's hemoglobin and hematocrit levels for efficacy of treatment, and assess for side effects. For example, iron can cause constipation, and zinc can cause nausea and vomiting.

Total Enteral Nutrition. If a patient cannot achieve adequate ***nutrition*** via oral intake, total enteral nutrition (TEN) may be needed. Enteral tube feedings may be necessary to supplement oral intake or to provide total nutrition.

Patients likely to receive TEN can be divided into three groups:

- Those who can eat but cannot maintain adequate ***nutrition*** by oral intake of food alone
- Those with permanent neuromuscular impairment who cannot swallow
- Those who do not have permanent neuromuscular impairment but cannot eat because of their condition

Patients in the first group are often older adults or patients receiving cancer treatment. In some cases, artificial nutrition and hydration may not be desired. Check for advance directives stating whether the patient desires artificial nutrition and hydration if certain conditions exist. Legal and ethical questions often arise when patients do not have existing advance directives, are not able to make their wishes known, and do not have a designated durable power of attorney. *The decision to feed or not to feed is complex, and there is no clear right or wrong answer.* See the Ethical/Legal Considerations box for more information.

ETHICAL/LEGAL CONSIDERATIONS

Decisions about legal/ethical situations regarding feeding benefit from advice of interprofessional ethics committees in health care facilities. When clinicians are making decisions about the desirability of tube feedings in these cases, the focus should be on achieving consensus by:

- Reviewing what is known about tube feedings, especially their risks and benefits
- Reviewing the medical facts about the patient
- Investigating any available evidence that would help understand the patient's wishes
- Obtaining the input of all stakeholders in the situation
- Delaying any action until consensus is achieved

Those in the second group of patients likely to receive TEN usually have permanent swallowing problems due to a condition such as brain attack, severe head trauma, or advanced multiple sclerosis. These patients require some type of feeding tube for delivery of the enteral product on a long-term basis.

Patients in the third group receive enteral ***nutrition*** for as long as their illness lasts. The feeding is discontinued when the patient's condition improves and he or she can eat again.

A therapeutic combination of carbohydrates, fat, vitamins, minerals, and trace elements is available in liquid form. A prescription from the health care provider is required for enteral nutrition, but the RDN usually makes the recommendation and computes the amount and type of product needed for each patient.

NCLEX EXAMINATION CHALLENGE 55.2

Safe and Effective Care Environment

Total enteral nutrition (TEN) has been prescribed for a client with terminal cancer. When the nurse notes that no advanced directives are in place, yet a durable power of attorney exists, what is the appropriate action?

A. Withhold TEN indefinitely
B. Contact the durable power of attorney
C. Begin administration of TEN immediately
D. Turn over care to the interprofessional ethics committee

Methods of administering total enteral nutrition. TEN is administered as a "tube feeding" through a nasoenteric or enterostomal tube. It can be used in the patient's home or any health care setting.

A nasoenteric tube (NET) is a feeding tube inserted nasally and then advanced into the GI tract, such as a Dobbhoff tube. Commonly used NETs include the nasogastric (NG) tube, the smaller (small-bore) nasoduodenal tube (NDT) (Fig. 55.3), and the nasojejunal tube (NJT), which is used less often. All of these types of tubes are used for less than 4 weeks to provide short-term feeding.

Enterostomal feeding tubes are used for patients who need *long-term* enteral feeding. The surgeon directly accesses the GI tract using various surgical, endoscopic, and laparoscopic techniques. Under sedation, a gastrostomy—a stoma created from the abdominal wall into the stomach—is created. Then a percutaneous endoscopic gastrostomy (PEG) or dual-access gastrostomy-jejunostomy (PEG/J) tube (Fig. 55.4) is placed. A jejunostomy is used for long-term feedings when it is desirable to bypass the stomach, such as with gastric disease, upper GI obstruction, and abnormal gastric or duodenal emptying. This can be accomplished via a direct percutaneous endoscopic jejunostomy (DPEJ) (see Fig. 55.4) (Simoes et al., 2018).

Tube feedings are administered by bolus feeding, continuous feeding, and cyclic feeding. Bolus feeding is an intermittent feeding of a specified amount of enteral product at set intervals during a 24-hour period, typically every 4 hours. This method can be accomplished manually or by infusion through a mechanical pump or controller device. Continuous feeding is similar to IV therapy in that small amounts are continuously infused (by gravity drip or a pump or controller device) over a specified time. Cyclic feeding is the same as continuous feeding except that the infusion is stopped for a specified time in each 24-hour period, usually 6

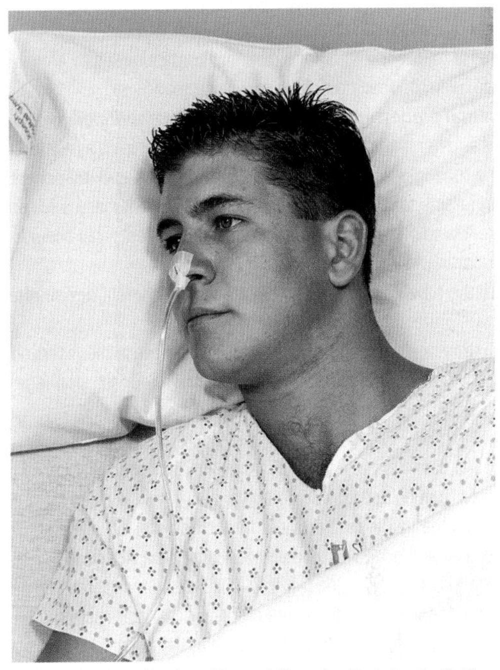

Fig. 55.3 Nasoduodenal tube. (From Lilley, L., Rainforth Collins, S., Harrington, S., & Snyder, J. [2011]. *Pharmacology and the nursing process* [6th ed.]. St. Louis: Mosby.)

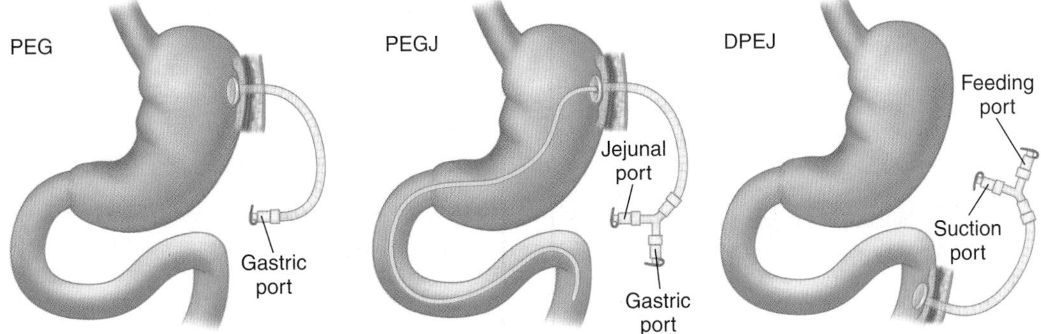

Fig. 55.4 Percutaneous endoscopic gastrostomy (PEG), dual-access gastrostomy-jejunostomy (PEG/J) tube, and direct percutaneous endoscopic jejunostomy (DPEJ). (Redrawn from Zhu, Y., Shi, L., Tang, H., & Tao, G. [2012]. Current considerations of direct percutaneous endoscopic jejunostomy. *Canadian Journal of Gastroenterology 26*[2], 92–96.)

hours or longer ("down time"). Down time typically occurs in the morning to allow bathing, treatments, and other activities. Follow the health care provider's prescription for type, rate, and method of tube feeding, as well as the amount of additional water ("free water") needed. If the patient can swallow small amounts of food, he or she may also eat orally while the tube is in place.

The nurse is responsible for the care and maintenance of the feeding tube and the enteral feeding. See the Best Practice for Patient Safety & Quality Care: Tube-Feeding Care and Maintenance box.

Complications of total enteral nutrition. The nursing priority for care of a patient receiving TEN is safety, which includes preventing, assessing, and managing complications associated with tube feeding. Some complications of therapy result from the type of tube used to administer the feeding, and others result from the enteral product itself. The most common problem is the development of an obstructed ("clogged") tube. Use the tips in the Best Practice for Patient Safety & Quality Care: Maintaining a Patent Feeding Tube box to maintain tube patency (Drummond Hayes & Drummond Hayes, 2018).

BEST PRACTICE FOR PATIENT SAFETY & QUALITY CARE QSEN

Tube-Feeding Care and Maintenance

- If nasogastric or nasoduodenal feeding is prescribed, use a soft, flexible, small-bore feeding tube (smaller than 12 Fr).
- Recognize that tubes with ports minimize contamination by eliminating the need to open the feeding system to administer drugs.
- ***The initial placement of the tube should be confirmed by x-ray study*** even if another method of confirmation is available, such as electromagnetic feeding tube–placement device (ETPD). Evidence shows that chest x-ray is still preferable to an ETPD (Bourgault et al., 2017; Metheny & Meert, 2017).
- If correct tube placement is ever in question, a chest x-ray should again be performed.
- Secure the tube with tape or a commercial attachment device after applying a skin protectant; change the tape regularly.
- If a gastrostomy or jejunostomy tube is used, assess the insertion site for signs of infection or excoriation (e.g., excessive redness, drainage). Rotate the tube 360 degrees each day and check for in-and-out play of about ¼ inch (0.6 cm).
- Check and document residual volume every 6 hours or per agency policy by aspirating stomach contents into a syringe. If residual feeding is obtained, check with the health care provider for the appropriate intervention (usually to slow or stop the feeding for a time) or consult the American Society of Parenteral and Enteral Nutrition (ASPEN) (2020) best practice recommendations.
- Check the feeding pump to ensure proper mechanical operation.
- Ensure that the enteral product is infused at the prescribed rate (mL/hr).
- Change the feeding bag and tubing every 24 to 48 hours; label the bag with the date and time of the change with your initials. Use an irrigation set for no more than 24 hours.
- For continuous or cyclic feeding, add only 4 hours of product to the bag at a time to prevent bacterial growth. *A closed system is preferred, and each set should be used no longer than 24 hours.*
- Wear clean gloves when changing or opening the feeding system or adding product; wipe the lid of the formula can with clean gauze; wear sterile gloves when caring for patients who are critically ill or immunocompromised.
- Label open cans with date and time opened; cover and keep refrigerated. Discard any unused open cans after 24 hours.
- Do not use blue (or any color) food dye in formula because it can cause serious complications.
- To prevent aspiration, keep the head of the bed elevated at least 30 degrees during the feeding and for at least 1 hour after the feeding for bolus feeding; continuously maintain the semi-Fowler position for patients receiving cyclic or continuous feeding.
- Monitor laboratory values, especially blood urea nitrogen (BUN), serum electrolytes, hematocrit, prealbumin, and glucose.
- Monitor for complications of tube feeding, especially diarrhea.
- Monitor and document the patient's weight and intake and output per the health care provider's order or agency policy.

! NURSING SAFETY PRIORITY QSEN

Action Alert

If a gastrostomy or jejunostomy tube cannot be moved while you are performing your regular assessment, notify the health care provider immediately because the retention disk may be embedded in the tissue. Cover the site with a dry, sterile dressing and change the dressing at least once a day.

BEST PRACTICE FOR PATIENT SAFETY & QUALITY CARE QSEN

Maintaining a Patent Feeding Tube

- Recognize that a tube occlusion is more easily prevented than corrected.
- Consult with the pharmacist to be sure the prescribed medications are compatible with the enteral ***nutrition*** formula.
- Consult with the pharmacist to confirm that medications and formula can be cleared from the tube with appropriate flushing.
- Collaborate with the health care provider to use liquid medications instead of crushed tablets when possible, unless the liquid form of medication causes diarrhea.
- Do not mix drugs with the feeding product before giving. Crush tablets as finely as possible and dissolve in warm water. *(Check to see which tablets are safe to crush. For example, do not crush slow-acting [SA] or slow-release [SR] drugs.)*
- Flush the tube with 30 mL of water, using at least a 30-mL syringe to prevent tube rupture:
  - At least every 4 hours
  - Before and after medication administration
  - After any interruption of enteral nutrition
- If the tube becomes clogged, use 30 mL of water for flushing, applying gentle pressure with a 50-mL piston syringe.
- *Do not use* a carbonated beverage or cranberry juice; these have an acidic pH that can worsen the occlusion by causing EN formula proteins to precipitate in the tube.
- Use warm water as the best choice for unclogging.
- Attach a 30- or 60-mL piston syringe to the feeding tube; retract the plunger to facilitate dislodging the clog. Then fill the flush with warm water, reattach it to the tube, and attempt flushing. If continued resistance is experienced, move the plunger gently back and forth. Then clamp the tube to allow the warm water to penetrate the clog for approximately 20 minutes.
- If water does not unclog the tube, an experienced nurse can use an activated pancreatic enzyme solution prescribed by the health care provider, following agency policy.
- As a final attempt, commercially available enzyme declogging kits or devices can be used by an experienced nurse, again following agency policy.
- If unclogging is unsuccessful, replacement of the tube is recommended.

Data from Boullata, J., Carrera, A., Harvey, L., et al. (2017). ASPEN safe practices for enteral nutrition therapy. *Journal of Parenteral and Enteral Nutrition, 41*(1), 15–103; Drummond Hayes, K., & Drummond Hayes, D. (2018). Best practices for unclogging feeding tubes in adults. *Nursing2018, 48*(6), 66; and University of Pittsburgh Medical Center. (2017). University of Pittsburgh Medical Center Presbyterian Shadyside Procedure: Unclogging enteral feeding tubes. Pittsburgh, PA.

Patients receiving TEN are at risk for several other complications, including refeeding syndrome; tube misplacement and dislodgment; abdominal distention and nausea/vomiting; and problems with ***fluid and electrolyte balance,*** often associated with diarrhea. These problems can be prevented if the patient is monitored carefully and complications are detected early.

Tube misplacement and dislodgment. *Misplacement or dislodgment of the tube can cause aspiration and possible death. Immediately remove any tube that you suspect is dislodged!* An x-ray is the most accurate confirmation method and should always be done on initial tube insertion. After the initial placement is confirmed, check gastric residual before each intermittent feeding or drug administration, or at least every 6 hours during feeding. Do not rely on traditional methods for checking tube placement such as auscultation; pH testing of GI contents; testing of biochemical markers, such as bilirubin, trypsin, or pepsin; or assessment for carbon dioxide using capnometry (Fan et al., 2017; Hodin & Bordeianou, 2020). Once x-ray confirmation has been made, mark the tube exit point as a baseline for visual re-evaluation of placement at each assessment.

! NURSING SAFETY PRIORITY (QSEN)

Action Alert

If enteral tubes are misplaced or become dislodged, the patient is likely to aspirate. *Aspiration pneumonia is a life-threatening complication associated with TEN, especially for older adults.* Observe for fever and signs of dehydration, such as dry mucous membranes and decreased urinary output. Auscultate lungs every 4 to 8 hours to check for diminishing breath sounds, especially in lower lobes. Patients may become short of breath and report chest discomfort. If a chest x-ray confirms this diagnosis, treatment with antibiotics is started.

Abdominal distention and nausea/vomiting. Abdominal distention, nausea, and vomiting during tube feeding are often caused by overfeeding. To *prevent* overfeeding, check gastric residual volumes every 6 hours, depending on agency policy and patient assessment. If residual feeding is obtained, check with the health care provider for the appropriate intervention (usually to slow or stop the feeding for a time) or consult the American Society of Parenteral and Enteral Nutrition (ASPEN) (2020) best practice recommendations. Follow agency policy regarding holding feeding if necessary. After a period of rest, the feeding can be restarted, usually at a lower flow rate.

Fluid and electrolyte imbalances. *Patients receiving enteral nutrition therapy, especially older adults and those with cardiac or renal problems, are at an increased risk for fluid imbalances.* Some electrolyte imbalances can be avoided. For example, a renal patient with existing high potassium levels may be prescribed a special formula lower in potassium.

Fluid imbalances associated with enteral nutrition are usually related to the body's response to increased serum osmolarity, but fluid overload from too much tube feeding can also occur. If patients do *not* have normal renal and cardiac function, expansion of the plasma volume can lead to circulatory overload and pulmonary edema, especially in older adults. Assess for signs and symptoms, such as peripheral edema, sudden weight gain, crackles, dyspnea, increased blood pressure, and bounding pulse; report these to the health care provider.

Excessive diarrhea and/or dehydration may develop when hyperosmolar enteral preparations are delivered quickly and excessive water loss is experienced. A more iso-osmolar formula may be needed. If diarrhea continues, and especially if it has a very foul odor, evaluate for *Clostridium difficile* or other infectious organisms. Contamination can occur because of repeated and often faulty handling of the feeding solution and system.

In some cases, diarrhea may be the result of administration of multiple liquid medications, such as elixirs and suspensions that have a very high osmolarity. Examples include acetaminophen, furosemide, and phenytoin. Discuss this with the health care provider to determine whether their drug regimen can be changed to prevent diarrhea or if dilution is possible.

The two most common electrolyte imbalances associated with enteral nutrition therapy are hyperkalemia and hyponatremia. Both of these conditions may be related to hyperglycemia-induced hyperosmolarity of the plasma and the resultant osmotic diuresis. Risks for disturbances in ***fluid and electrolyte balance*** are discussed in detail in Chapter 13.

Refeeding syndrome. Refeeding syndrome is a potentially life-threatening complication related to fluid and electrolyte shifts during aggressive nutrition rehabilitation of the patient in a state of starvation. Prevent this complication by carefully assessing and managing nutrition needs early before a patient is severely malnourished.

! NURSING SAFETY PRIORITY (QSEN)

Critical Rescue

Recognize signs of refeeding syndrome, which include heart failure, peripheral edema, rhabdomyolysis, seizures, and hemolysis (Mehler, 2019). Laboratory values indicate hypophosphatemia and hypokalemia. Respond by contacting the health care provider immediately. More information on ***fluid and electrolyte balance*** can be found in Chapter 13.

Parenteral Nutrition. When a patient cannot effectively use the GI tract for ***nutrition,*** either partial or total parenteral nutrition therapy may be needed. This form of nutrition is introduced into the veins and differs from standard IV therapy in that any or all nutrients (carbohydrates, proteins, fats, vitamins, minerals, electrolytes, and trace elements) can be given. Parenteral nutrition can be mixed by the pharmacist using compounded bags or delivered from a multichamber bag in which commercially premixed solutions are used (King, 2019). In a multichamber bag, dextrose, amino acids, electrolytes, and lipids are preloaded in separate chambers that are mixed together right before administration. The benefit of compounding is that mixtures can be highly personalized to each patient. However, a downfall is the rate of human error that can take place in the compounding, labeling, and administration processes (King, 2019). A benefit of the multichamber bag is that shelf life is 12 months or more (compared with a 7- to 9-day shelf life for individually compounded formulations). The downfall is lack of customization to the individual patient, as multichamber bags usually contain less protein and fewer electrolytes than personalized formulations (King, 2019). At time of publication, the American Society for Parenteral and

Enteral Nutrition (ASPEN) recommends using premixed formulations or multichamber bag solutions.

Peripheral parenteral nutrition (PPN). Peripheral parenteral nutrition (PPN) is administered through a cannula or catheter in a large distal vein of the arm on a short-term basis. It is usually used for patients who can eat but are not able to take in enough nutrients to meet their needs. PPN is fat based and does not contain all of the carbohydrates a patient needs, so it is not used on a long-term basis (Baiu & Spain, 2019). The patient must have adequate peripheral vein access and be able to tolerate large volumes of fluid to have this type of nutrition therapy. PPN has an osmolarity lower than conventional parenteral nutrition and must be administered in a high volume and/or with a high fat formulation to deliver adequate nutrients (Seres, 2020). Monitor for irritation at the site of the cannula or catheter insertion, as infusion of large volumes of PPN can be irritating to tissue.

! NURSING SAFETY PRIORITY (QSEN)

Critical Rescue

Recognize that you must monitor patients receiving fat emulsions for fever, increased triglycerides, clotting problems, and multisystem organ failure, which may indicate fat overload syndrome, especially in patients who are critically ill. Respond to any of these signs and symptoms by discontinuing the IVFE infusion and reporting the changes to the health care provider immediately.

Total parenteral nutrition. When the patient requires intensive ***nutrition*** support for an extended time, the health care provider prescribes centrally administered **total parenteral nutrition (TPN)**. TPN (Fig. 55.5) is delivered through a temporary central line inserted in the neck or chest, a long-term tunneled catheter or implanted part inserted in the chest, or via a PICC line (Baiu & Spain, 2019). (See Chapter 15 for care.) This type of nutrition is hypertonic and contains a high glucose content.

TPN solutions are administered with an infusion pump. The osmolarity of the fluid and the concentrations of the specific components make controlled delivery essential. See the Best Practice for Patient Safety & Quality Care: Care and Maintenance of Total Parenteral Nutrition box for appropriate nursing interventions.

Patients receiving parenteral nutrition fluids are at risk for a wide variety of serious and potentially life-threatening complications. Complications may result from the solutions or from the peripheral or central venous catheter (see Chapter 15).

The patient with cardiac or renal dysfunction can develop problems with ***fluid and electrolyte balance,*** including fluid overload, heart failure, and pulmonary edema. The health care provider usually requests frequent serum electrolyte levels to detect imbalances. Potassium and sodium imbalances are common, especially when insulin is also administered as part of the therapy. Calcium imbalances, particularly hypercalcemia, are associated with TPN. The risk for metabolic and electrolyte complications is reduced when the administration rate is carefully controlled and patients are closely observed. Monitor for any of these imbalances, and report any major changes or abnormalities to the health care provider immediately.

BEST PRACTICE FOR PATIENT SAFETY & QUALITY CARE (QSEN)

Care and Maintenance of Total Parenteral Nutrition

- Check each bag of total parenteral nutrition (TPN) solution for accuracy by comparing it with the original prescription.
- Administer insulin as prescribed.
- Monitor the IV pump for accuracy in delivering the prescribed hourly rate.
- If the TPN solution is temporarily unavailable, collaborate with the health care provider so that 10% dextrose/water ($D_{10}W$) or 20% dextrose/water ($D_{20}W$) can be administered until the TPN solution can be obtained.
- If the TPN administration is not on time ("behind"), do not attempt to "catch up" by increasing the rate.
- Monitor and document the patient's weight daily or according to facility protocol.
- Monitor serum electrolytes and glucose daily or per facility protocol.
- Monitor for, report, and document complications, including problems with ***fluid and electrolyte balance.***
- Monitor and carefully record the patient's intake and output.
- Assess the patient's IV site for signs of infection or infiltration (see Chapter 15).
- Change the IV tubing every 24 hours or per facility protocol.
- Change the dressing around the IV site every 48 to 72 hours or per facility protocol.
- Before administering TPN, have a second nurse check the prescription and solution to increase patient safety.

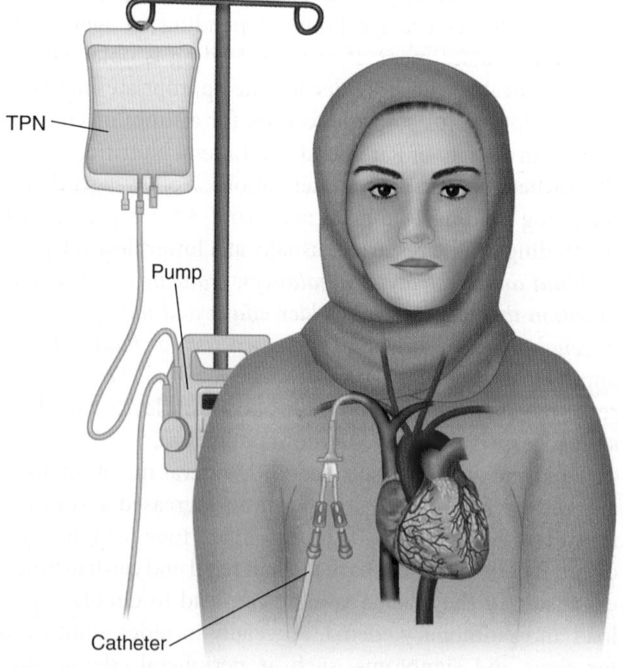

Fig. 55.5 Total parenteral nutrition.

Care Coordination and Transition Management. The patient with undernutrition, once stabilized, can be cared for in an acute care hospital, transitional care unit, nursing home, or their own home.

Home Care Management. The patient with undernutrition needs a variety of resources at home to continue consistent ***nutrition*** support. If he or she can consume food by the oral route, the case manager or other discharge planner can determine whether financial resources are available for nutrition supplements. If the hospital provides ambulatory nutrition counseling services, the patient may be scheduled for follow-up after discharge for assessment of weight gain.

Self-Management Education. The registered dietitian nutritionist (RDN) teaches the patient with undernutrition (and family, as indicated) about a high-calorie, high-protein diet and ***nutrition*** supplements. It is important for you, as the nurse, to:

- Reinforce the importance of adhering to the prescribed diet.
- Review any drugs the patient may be taking.
- Teach the importance of taking iron immediately before or during meals.
- Caution the patient that iron tends to cause constipation.
- Emphasize ways to prevent constipation, including adequate fiber intake, adequate fluids, and exercise.

Health Care Resources. The patient with undernutrition discharged to home on enteral or parenteral nutrition support needs the specialized services of a home nutrition therapy team. This team generally consists of the health care provider, nurse, registered dietitian nutritionist (RDN), pharmacist, and case manager or social worker. Several commercial companies supply these services to patients at home in addition to the feeding supplies and formulas and health teaching.

◆ **Evaluation: Evaluate Outcomes.** Evaluate the care of the patient with undernutrition based on the identified priority patient problem. The primary expected outcome is that the patient consumes available nutrients to meet the metabolic demands for maintaining weight and total protein and has adequate hydration.

NUTRITION CONCEPT EXEMPLAR: OBESITY

Pathophysiology Review

The pathophysiology of obesity is complex. A number of chemicals in the body, including hormones known as *adipokines,* work together to affect appetite and fat metabolism. Dysregulation of these chemicals can result in conditions such as appetite increase, overstimulation of the autonomic nervous system, blood vessel inflammation, and ventricular hypertrophy. Complications of obesity can affect many organ systems (Table 55.6).

TABLE 55.6 Common Complications of Obesity

Cardiovascular • Coronary artery disease (CAD) • Hyperlipidemia • Hypertension • Peripheral artery disease (PAD)	**Integumentary** • Delayed wound healing • Susceptibility to infections
Endocrine • Insulin resistance • Metabolic syndrome • Type II diabetes	**Musculoskeletal** • Chronic back and/or joint pain • Early onset of osteoarthritis
Gastrointestinal • Cholelithiasis	**Neurologic** • Stroke
Genitourinary/Reproductive • Erectile dysfunction in men • Menstrual irregularities in women • Urinary incontinence	**Psychiatric** • Depression
	Respiratory • Obesity hypoventilation syndrome • Obstructive sleep apnea

The terms *obesity* and *overweight* are often used interchangeably, but they refer to different health problems. For both problems, the patient often has not consumed enough healthy nutrients to achieve adequate ***nutrition*** and has an abnormal or excessive amount of fat accumulation (World Health Organization, 2020). Overweight is reflected by a body mass index (BMI) of 25 to 29. Obesity is reflected by a BMI of 30 or above (CDC, 2020b).

Obesity is subdivided into three categories (CDC, 2020b):

- Class I—BMI of 30 to <35
- Class II—BMI of 35 to < 40
- Class III—BMI of 40 or higher (sometimes called "extreme" or "severe" obesity)

The distribution of excess body fat rather than the degree of obesity has been used to predict increased health risks. The waist circumference (WC) is a stronger predictor of coronary artery disease (CAD) than is the BMI. A WC greater than 35 inches (89 cm) in women and greater than 40 inches (102 cm) in men indicates central obesity (National Heart, Lung, and Blood Institute; National Institutes of Health; U.S. Department of Health and Human Services, n.d.). Central obesity is a major risk factor for CAD, brain attack, type 2 diabetes, some cancers (e.g., colon, breast), sleep apnea, and early death.

The waist-to-hip ratio (WHR) is also a predictor of CAD. This measure differentiates peripheral lower body obesity from central obesity. A WHR of 0.95 or greater in men (0.8 or greater in women) indicates android obesity with excess fat at the waist and abdomen.

Etiology and Genetic Risk. The causes of obesity involve complex interrelationships of many environmental, genetic, and behavioral factors. One of the most common causes of being overweight or obese is eating *high-fat and high-cholesterol diets.* Obesity is associated with diet when it contains a significant amount of *saturated* fat, which increases low-density lipoproteins (LDL, or LDL-C for low-density lipoproteins cholesterol). *Trans* fatty acids (TFAs), saturated fats, and cholesterol are linked to a higher risk for heart disease (American Heart Association, 2017). By contrast, monounsaturated and polyunsaturated fats are healthy fats.

Physical inactivity has been identified as another cause of overweight and obesity. The major barriers to increasing physical activity include lack of time, comfort level in a sedentary lifestyle, and decreased mobility due to health conditions.

Drug therapy also contributes to obesity when prescribed medications cause weight gain when they are taken on a long-term basis. Examples include:

- Corticosteroids
- Estrogens and certain progestins
- NSAIDs

- Antihypertensives
- Antidepressants and other psychoactive drugs
- Antiepileptic drugs
- Certain oral antidiabetic agents

PATIENT-CENTERED CARE: GENETIC/GENOMIC CONSIDERATIONS QSEN

Evidence shows that genetic classifications of obesity can be (Huvenne et al., 2016):

1. Monogenic (caused by a single gene);
2. Syndromic (severe obesity associated with other phenotypes, including neurodevelopmental abnormalities like Prader-Willi syndrome);
3. Oligogenic (due to the absence of a certain phenotype); or
4. Polygenic (caused by a cumulative effect of numerous genes whose effect is increased in the environment where weight gain is prominent)

Polygenic obesity is seen most commonly. In any predisposition to obesity, environment (lifestyle) is also a strong influence. Encourage patients to focus on lifestyle modifications that are within their control, even if they believe genetics is the root cause of obesity.

Incidence and Prevalence. Worldwide, the prevalence of overweight and obesity has doubled since 1980 (Chooi et al., 2019). Approximately one third of the world's population is now classified as overweight or obese (Chooi). *This problem is a leading cause of preventable death.*

Health Promotion and Maintenance. Obesity is a major public health problem and is associated with many complications, including death. As a result of this increasing problem, the *Healthy People 2020* agenda (Office of Disease Prevention and Health Promotion, 2020) addresses the need to reduce the proportion of children, adolescents, and adults with obesity. *Healthy People 2020 Objectives for Nutrition and Weight Status* include specific population targets related to obesity and healthy ***nutrition*** habits (Table 55.7). *Healthy People 2030* includes initiatives that address:

- Reducing the proportion of adults with obesity
- Increasing the proportion of adults with obesity who receive counseling or education regarding weight reduction, nutrition, or physical therapy
- Increasing the consumption of whole grains
- Decreasing the consumption of calories from added sugars

In collaboration with the registered dietitian nutritionist (RDN), teach the importance of weight management and physical activity to improve health. Even a 5% weight loss can drastically decrease the risk for coronary artery disease (CAD) and diabetes mellitus. Teach patients that physical activity can be as simple as walking 20 min/day.

❖ Interprofessional Collaborative Care

Care for the patient with obesity takes place in a variety of settings, from the home, to the community, and in the hospital setting if more comprehensive management or surgery is needed. Members of the interprofessional team who collaborate most closely to care for this patient include the primary health care provider, surgeon if surgery is required, nurse, social worker, and registered dietitian nutritionist (RDN). For patients who experience psychological impact related to obesity, a psychologist or therapist will also have an important role in care.

NCLEX EXAMINATION CHALLENGE 55.3

Psychosocial Integrity

A client with obesity tells the nurse, "My genes are the only thing that have made me obese." What is the appropriate nursing response? **Select all that apply.**

A. "Genes can contribute to obesity."
B. "Tell me about your family history."
C. "Let's talk about your nutrition intake."
D. "Have you considered bariatric surgery?"
E. "How do you feel about physical activity?"
F. "What lifestyle modifications have you tried?"

TABLE 55.7 Meeting *Healthy People 2020* Select Objectives and Targets: Nutrition and Weight Status

- Increase the number of states that have state-level policies that incentivize food retail outlets to provide foods that are encouraged by the Dietary Guidelines for Americans (target 34 states)
- Increase the proportion of primary care physicians who regularly measure the body mass index of their adult patients (by 10%)
- Increase the proportion of physician office visits made by patients with a diagnosis of cardiovascular disease, diabetes, or hyperlipidemia that include counseling or education related to nutrition or weight (by 10%)
- Increase the proportion of physician office visits made by patients with a diagnosis of cardiovascular disease, diabetes, or hyperlipidemia that include counseling or education related to nutrition or weight (by 10%)
- Increase the proportion of adults who are at a healthy weight (by 10%)
- Reduce the proportion of adults who are obese (by 10%)

Data from Office of Disease Prevention and Health Promotion. (2020). *Nutrition and weight status.* https://www.healthypeople.gov/2020/topics-objectives/topic/nutrition-and-weight-status/objectives.

◆ Assessment: Recognize Cues

History. Patients with obesity may be embarrassed or reluctant to talk about their weight or fear judgment because of the stigma that can be attached to this condition. Approach patients with obesity by using the acronym RESPECT, created by The Ohio State University (Aycock et al, 2017). Create a rapport with them in an environment that is safe. Ensure their safety and privacy, encourage them to set realistic goals (in the planning phase), provide compassion, and use tact in conversation.

See the earlier Best Practice for Patient Safety & Quality Care: Nutrition Screening Assessment box to complete the initial history. In collaboration with the registered dietitian nutritionist (RDN), also obtain the information as noted in "History" under the concept exemplar of undernutrition.

Additionally, ask about:

- Appetite
- Attitude toward food

- Presence of any chronic diseases
- Drugs taken (prescribed and over-the-counter [OTC], including herbal preparations)
- Physical activity/functional ability
- Family history of obesity
- What forms of weight loss have been tried in the past and their results

Physical Assessment/Signs and Symptoms. Obtain an accurate height and weight. Anthropometric measurements may also be obtained.

Examine the skin for reddened or open areas. Lift skinfold areas, such as pendulous breasts and abdominal aprons *(panniculus),* to observe for *Candida* (yeast) (a condition called *intertrigo)* or other infections or lesions. Infection of the panniculus is referred to as *panniculitis.*

Psychosocial Assessment. Obtain a psychosocial history to determine the patient's circumstances and emotional factors that might prevent successful weight loss or that might be worsened by intervention. Ask about the perception of current weight and weight reduction. Some patients do not view weight as a problem, which affects planning, treatment, and outcome. Ask the patient questions about his or her health beliefs related to being overweight, such as:

- What does food mean to you?
- Do you want to lose weight?
- What prevents you from losing weight?
- What do you think will motivate you to lose weight?
- How do you think you might benefit from losing weight?
- Do you have a support system in place that will encourage you during weight loss?

Some patients become very depressed regarding their weight and/or failure of weight loss efforts. If the patient reports depressed symptoms that have occurred consistently for more than 2 weeks that impact performing ADLs, referral to a mental health professional can be helpful.

◆ **Analysis: Analyze Cues and Prioritize Hypothesis.** The priority collaborative problem for the patient with obesity is:

1. Weight gain, which stresses all vital organs due to excessive intake of calories

◆ **Planning and Implementation: Generate Solutions and Take Action.** If the patient with obesity is to be hospitalized, an appropriate bariatric care room is important in the provision of high-quality, patient-centered care whether nonsurgical or surgical management is planned. Ensure that the patient has the right room so that care can be maximized to the very best benefit. Criteria for these types of rooms are located in Table 55.8.

Improving Nutrition

Planning: Expected Outcomes. The patient with obesity is expected to return to a normal BMI, while consuming dense nutrients that meet metabolic needs without overeating.

Nonsurgical Management. Weight loss may be accomplished by nutrition modification with or without the aid of drugs and in combination with a regular exercise program. Patients who may be candidates for surgical treatment include those who have:

- Repeated failure of nonsurgical interventions
- A BMI equal to or greater than 40
- Weight more than 100% above ideal body weight

TABLE 55.8 Criteria for a Bariatric Room

Criterion	Specifications
Location	Designation specifically for bariatric care
Capacity	Single-patient
Area	Minimum clear floor area of 18 m^2
Clearance	Minimum distance of 1.5 m between sides and foot of bed and wall
Hand washing station	Mounted on wall, able to withstand downward static force of a predetermined maximum patient weight
Toilet room	Mounted to floor with at least 61 cm from wall to center of toilet line, and 112 cm of clear space on the opposite side of the toilet for wheelchair and caregiver access
Bathing facilities	Shower stalls—1.2 m x 1.8 m, with grab bars that support 450 kg Handheld spray nozzles mounted on a side wall Enclosure for privacy Must be separate from hand washing station and toilet room
Patient lift system	Built-in mechanical lift system
Airborne isolation room	At least one airborne isolation room per bariatric unit should be available

From Smigelski-Theiss, R., Gampong, M., & Kurasaki, J. (2017). Weight bias and psychosocial implications for acute care of patients with obesity. *AACN Advanced Critical Care, 28*(3), 254-262.

Diet programs. Diets for helping adults lose weight include fasting, very-low-calorie diets, nutritionally balanced diets, and unbalanced low-energy diets.

Short-term fasting programs and *very-low-calorie diets* (usually 200 to 800 calories/day) require an initial cardiac evaluation and supervision by the interprofessional health care team. Neither diet is ideal due to risks involved and the likelihood of regaining weight after completion of the diet. Ketosis is a risk of short-term fasting.

Nutritionally balanced diets generally provide about 1200 to 1800 calories/day with a conventional distribution of carbohydrate, protein, and fat. Vitamin and mineral supplements may be used. These diets adhere to conventional foods that are economical and easy to obtain.

Unbalanced low-energy diets, such as the low-carbohydrate diet, restrict one or more nutrients. Protein and vegetables are encouraged, but certain carbohydrates and high-fat foods are not. Although results are mixed per health research, these diets are extremely popular.

Nutrition therapy. ***Nutrition*** recommendations for each patient are developed through close interaction among the patient, caregiver, primary health care provider, nurse, and registered dietitian nutritionist (RDN). The diet must meet the patient's needs, habits, and lifestyle and should be realistic. At a minimum, the diet should:

- Be evidence based
- Be nutritionally balanced (see Diet Programs section)

- Have a low risk-benefit ratio
- Be practical and conducive to long-term success

Calorie estimates are easily calculated. Resting metabolic rate is determined using a gender-specific formula that incorporates the appropriate activity factor. This figure reflects the total calories needed daily for maintaining current weight. To encourage a weight loss of 1 lb (0.45 kg) a week, the registered dietitian nutritionist (RDN) subtracts 500 calories each day. To encourage a weight loss of 2 lb (0.9 kg) a week, 1000 calories each day are subtracted. The amount of weight lost varies with the patient's food intake, level of physical activity, and water losses. A reasonable expected outcome of 5% to 10% loss of body weight has been shown to improve glycemic control and reduce cholesterol and blood pressure. These benefits continue if the weight loss is sustained.

Exercise program. For most adults, adding physical activity to a healthy diet produces more weight loss than dieting alone. More of the weight lost is fat, which preserves lean body mass. An increase in exercise can reduce the waist circumference and the waist-to-hip ratio. Evidence also shows that reduction of fat in the thighs, hips, and buttocks helps to protect against cardiovascular disease and diabetes (Clifton, 2018).

A minimum-level workout should be developed so that consistency can be achieved and maintained. Encourage walking 20 minutes a day and increasing the time as endurance increases. The activity may be performed all at once or divided over the course of the day.

Drug therapy. Four medications are FDA-approved for overweight and obesity treatment. The primary health care provider will work with the patient to determine which, if any, of these drugs are appropriate. See the Common Examples of Drug Therapy: Overweight and Obesity Treatment box for information about this type of drug therapy.

Cryolipolysis. Cryolipolysis is a nonsurgical procedure also known as "fat freezing." This procedure is used to reduce fat deposits in certain body areas but is not suggested for use in patients who are overweight or have obesity (Meyer et al, 2018). Redirect patient requesting cryolipolysis to the primary health care provider for further discussion.

Behavioral management. Behavioral management of obesity helps the patient change daily eating habits to lose weight. Self-monitoring techniques include keeping a journal of foods eaten (food diary), exercise or activity patterns, and emotional and situational factors. Stimulus control involves controlling the external cues that promote overeating. Reinforcement techniques are used to self-reward the behavior change. Cognitive restructuring involves modifying negative beliefs by learning positive coping self-statements. Counseling by health care professionals must continue before, during, and after treatment. The 12-step program offered by Overeaters Anonymous (www.oa.org) has helped many adults lose weight, especially those who eat compulsively.

Complementary and integrative health. Many complementary and integrative therapies have been tested and used for obesity. These modalities aim to suppress appetite and therefore limit food intake to lose weight:

- Acupuncture
- Acupressure
- Ayurveda (a combination of holistic approaches)
- Hypnosis

Evidence about effectiveness of each of these therapies varies. Encourage the patient to speak to the primary health care provider to determine if any of these methods are recommended.

Surgical Management. Some patients seek to improve their appearance by reducing the amount of adipose tissue in selected areas of the body. A typical example of this type of surgery is

COMMON EXAMPLES OF DRUG THERAPY

Overweight and Obesity Treatment

Drug	Selected Nursing Implications
Liraglutide (activates appetite regulation in the brain)	• Monitor ALT and AST; *there is an increased risk for pancreatitis when taking this drug.* • Patients taking insulin should not take this drug; *hypoglycemia can develop.* • Teach to report taking this drug to all health care providers; *alpha$_1$-adrenergic antagonists can increase or decrease the side effects of other drugs like beta blockers, calcium channel blockers, or medications used to treat erectile dysfunction.*
Naltrexone-bupropion (combines the opioid antagonist naltrexone with the antidepressant bupropion)	• Patients with uncontrolled hypertension, seizures, anorexia nervosa, or bulimia nervosa, or who are withdrawing from drugs or alcohol, should not take this drug. • Patients taking bupropion should not take this drug; *cumulative doses can increase risks for side effects.* • Monitor for suicidal ideation; *this can develop due to the antidepressant effect.*
Orlistat Inhibits lipase; thus, fats are only partially digested and absorbed	• Monitor liver enzymes; *rare cases of liver injury have been reported.* • Teach to take a multivitamin daily; *the body may not normally absorb enough vitamins found in foods due to the effect of the drug.* • Teach that loose stools, abdominal cramps, and nausea can occur unless fat intake is reduced to less than 30% of the daily intake; *the drug mechanism facilitates GI symptoms since fats are only partially digested and absorbed.*
Phentermine-topiramate (combines short-term weight loss drug phentermine with seizure medication topiramate)	• Patients with glaucoma or hyperthyroidism should not take this medication. • Determine if patient is pregnant or planning pregnancy; *this medication can cause birth defects* (**Note:** Patient should also not use this medication if breastfeeding).

From the National Institute of Diabetes and Digestive and Kidney Disorders. (n.d.) Prescription medications to treat overweight and obesity. https://www.niddk.nih.gov/health-information/weight-management/prescription-medications-treat-overweight-obesity.

liposuction, which can be done in a health care provider's office or ambulatory surgery center. Although the patient's appearance may improve, if weight gain continues, the fatty tissue will return. This procedure is not a solution for adults with obesity.

Bariatrics is a branch of medicine that manages patients with obesity and its related diseases. Certain adults may be considered for this type of weight loss surgery. These include patients who:

- Do not respond to traditional interventions
- Have a body mass index (BMI) of 40 or greater
- Have a BMI of 35 or greater, with other health risk factors

Surgical procedures include gastric bypass, sleeve gastrectomy, adjustable gastric band and, less commonly, the biliopancreatic diversion with duodenal switch (BPD/DS) (American Society for Metabolic and Bariatric Surgery [ASMBS], 2020). Another procedure, gastrointestinal electrical stimulation (GES), involves the implantation of a vagal-blocking device (vBloc) into the abdomen (Apovian et al., 2017) that causes early satiety, and thus, reduced intake (Shikora et al., 2019).

Depending on the procedure, the surgeon may choose to use a conventional open approach or perform minimally invasive surgery (MIS). Many patients have MIS via either the laparoscopic adjustable gastric band (LAGB) procedure or laparoscopic sleeve gastrectomy (LSG). Both procedures are classified as restrictive surgeries. The decision of whether the patient is a candidate for the MIS is based on weight, body build, history of abdominal surgery, and coexisting medical complications. With any surgical approach, patients must agree to modify their lifestyle and follow stringent protocols to lose weight and keep the weight off. After successful bariatric surgery, many patients no longer have complications of obesity, such as diabetes mellitus, hypertension, depression, or sleep apnea.

Preoperative care. Preoperative care is similar to that for any patient undergoing abdominal surgery or laparoscopy (see Chapter 9). However, patients with obesity are at increased surgical risks of pulmonary and thromboembolitic complications, as well as death. Some surgeons require a specific amount of weight loss before bariatric surgery to minimize complications. Patients also have a thorough psychological assessment and testing to detect depression, substance abuse, or other mental health/behavioral health problems that could interfere with success after surgery. Cognitive ability, coping skills, development, motivation, expectations, and support systems are also assessed. Patients who are not alert and oriented or do not have sufficient strength and mobility are not considered for bariatric surgery. *The primary role of the nurse is to reinforce health teaching in preparation for surgery.* Most bariatric surgical centers provide educational sessions for groups of patients who plan to have the procedure.

Operative procedures. *Gastric restriction* surgeries, the easiest to perform, allow for normal digestion without the risk of nutritional deficiencies. In a banding procedure, the surgeon places an adjustable band to create a small proximal stomach pouch through a laparoscope (Fig. 55.6A, Fig. 55.6B). The band may or may not be inflatable. In the vertical sleeve gastroplasty (Fig. 55.6C), about ¾ of the stomach is removed, with the sleevelike remaining stomach having a much-reduced capacity. In the biliopancreatic diversion with duodenal switch (Fig. 55.6D), a lesser common bariatric surgery, almost 80% of the stomach is removed. The remaining pouch is connected to the bottom of the small intestine (bypassing the upper portion). Therefore, calories and nutrients are routed into the colon, where they are not absorbed (Phillips & Zieve, 2019).

The most common bariatric surgery performed in the United States is the *Roux-en-*Y *gastric bypass (RNYGB),* which is often done as a robotic-assistive surgical procedure. Most commonly called a **gastric bypass**, this procedure results in quick weight loss, but it is more invasive with a higher risk for postoperative complications. In this procedure, gastric resection is combined with malabsorption surgery. The patient's stomach, duodenum, and part of the jejunum are bypassed so that fewer calories can be absorbed (Fig. 55.6E).

Postoperative care. Postoperative care depends on the type of surgery performed. Patients having one of the MIS procedures have less pain, scarring, and blood loss. They typically have a faster recovery time and a faster return to daily activities. However, even patients having MIS are considered to have had major abdominal surgery along with all its risks, and their care is planned accordingly. These patients may require less than 24 hours in the hospital; some may need 1 to 2 days. Patients with open procedures may need several days to recover.

A major focus of postoperative care must be placed on patient and staff safety. Patients should be placed in a bariatric room (see Table 55.8). Always use additional personnel when moving the patient. Ensure that side rails are not touching the body because they can cause pressure injuries. Pressure between skinfolds and tubes and catheters can also cause skin breakdown. Monitor the skin in these areas and keep it clean and dry.

Care of the patient who has undergone any type of bariatric surgery is similar to that of any patient having abdominal or laparoscopic surgery (see Chapter 9). *The priority for postoperative care is airway management.* Patients with short and thick necks often have compromised airways and need aggressive respiratory support—possibly mechanical ventilation in the critical care unit.

In addition to the postoperative complications typically associated with abdominal and laparoscopic surgeries, patients who have undergone bariatric surgery are at risk for anastomotic leaks (a leak of digestive juices and partially digested food through an anastomosis). Implement measures to prevent complications as noted in the Best Practice for Patient Safety & Quality Care: Care of the Patient After Bariatric Surgery box.

All patients experience some degree of pain, but it is usually less severe when MIS is performed. Patients may use patient-controlled analgesia (PCA) with morphine for up to the first 24 hours. All patients receive oral opioid analgesic agents (liquid form when possible) as prescribed after the PCA is discontinued. Acute pain management is discussed in detail in Chapter 5.

Clear liquids are introduced slowly if the patient can tolerate water, and 1-ounce cups are used for each serving. A full liquid diet follows tolerance of the clear liquid diet; usually patients are discharged on full liquids. Pureed foods follow in about a week, with each meal consisting of about 5 tablespoons of food.

BEST PRACTICE FOR PATIENT SAFETY & QUALITY CARE (QSEN)

Care of the Patient After Bariatric Surgery

Cardiovascular/Respiratory Care

- Place the patient in semi-Fowler position to improve breathing and decrease risk for sleep apnea, pneumonia, or atelectasis.
- Monitor oxygen saturation; provide oxygen, bilevel, or continuous positive airway pressure (BiPAP or CPAP) ventilation as prescribed.
- Apply sequential compression stockings and administer prophylactic anti-coagulant therapy as prescribed to prevent venous thromboembolisms, including pulmonary embolism (PE).

Gastrointestinal Care

- Apply an abdominal binder to prevent wound dehiscence for open surgical procedures.
- Observe for signs and symptoms of **dumping syndrome** (caused by food entering the small intestine instead of the stomach) after *gastric bypass*, such as tachycardia, nausea, diarrhea, and abdominal cramping.
- Provide six small feedings (clear and then full liquids as prescribed) and plenty of fluids to prevent dehydration in collaboration with the registered dietitian nutritionist (RDN).
- Measure and record abdominal girth daily or as prescribed.

Genitourinary Care

- Remove urinary catheter within 24 hours after surgery to prevent urinary tract infection.

Integumentary Care

- Observe skin areas and folds for redness, excoriation, or breakdown, and treat these problems early.
- Use absorbent padding between folds to prevent pressure areas and skin breakdown.
- Ensure that tubes and catheters are not causing pressure on the skin.

Musculoskeletal Care

- Collaborate with the physical therapist for transfers or ambulation assistive devices, such as walkers.
- Encourage and assist with turning every 2 hours using an appropriate weight-bearing overhead trapeze.

! NURSING SAFETY PRIORITY (QSEN)

Action Alert

Some patients who have bariatric surgery have a nasogastric (NG) tube put in place, especially after open surgical procedures. In gastroplasty procedures, the NG tube drains both the proximal pouch and the distal stomach. Closely monitor the tube for patency. *Never reposition the tube because its movement can disrupt the suture line!* The NG tube is removed on the second day if the patient is passing flatus.

After several weeks of pureed foods, soft foods are introduced. Around the eighth postoperative week, solid, nutrient-dense foods are incorporated. Remind the patient to eat and drink slowly, to consume only small meals, to stop eating before feeling full, to choose foods high in protein, and to avoid foods that are fatty or have high sugar content.

Care Coordination and Transition Management. Obesity can be a chronic, lifelong problem if weight loss is not accomplished. Diets, drug therapy, exercise, and behavior modification can produce short-term weight losses with reasonable safety. However, many patients who do lose weight often regain it. Treatment of obesity should focus on the long-term reduction of health risks and problems associated with obesity, improving quality of life, and promoting a health-oriented lifestyle.

! NURSING SAFETY PRIORITY (QSEN)

Critical Rescue

Anastomotic leaks are the most common serious complication and cause of death after gastric bypass surgery. Recognize that you must monitor for symptoms of this life-threatening problem, which includes increasing back, shoulder, or abdominal pain; restlessness; and unexplained tachycardia and oliguria (scant urine). If any of these findings is present, respond by contacting the surgeon immediately!

CLINICAL JUDGMENT CHALLENGE 55.1

Safety

A 49-year-old woman had bariatric surgery 8 weeks ago. Today, she calls the telehealth nurse and reports having nausea, abdominal cramping, and ongoing diarrhea for 2 days. In addition, she says that she feels like her heart is "racing" and she wonders if she has "the stomach flu" (gastroenteritis).

1. **Recognize Cues:** What assessment information in this client situation is the most important and immediate concern for the nurse? (Hint: Identify the **relevant** information *first* to determine what is most important.)
2. **Analyze Cues:** What client conditions are consistent with the **most relevant** information? (Hint: Think about priority collaborative problems that support and contradict the information presented in this situation.)
3. **Prioritize Hypotheses:** Which possibilities or explanations are **most likely** to be present in this client situation? Which possibilities or explanations are the most serious? (Hint: Consider all possibilities and determine their urgency and risk for this client.)
4. **Generate Solutions:** What actions would most likely achieve the desired outcomes for this client? Which actions should be **avoided** or are **potentially harmful**? (Hint: Determine the desired outcomes first to decide which interventions are appropriate and those that should be avoided.)
5. **Take Action:** Which actions are the most appropriate and how should they be implemented? In what **priority order** should they be implemented? (Hint: Consider health teaching, documentation, requested health care provider orders or prescriptions, nursing skills, collaboration with or referral to health team members, etc.)
6. **Evaluate Outcomes:** What client assessment would indicate that the nurse's actions were **effective**? (Hint: Think about signs that would indicate an improvement, decline, or unchanged client condition.)

Home Care Management. In collaboration with the registered dietitian nutritionist (RDN), counsel the patient on a healthful eating pattern. The physical therapist or exercise physiologist recommends an appropriate exercise program. A psychologist may recommend cognitive restructuring approaches that help alter dysfunctional eating patterns.

For patients who have surgery, additional discharge teaching is needed. The Patient and Family Education: Preparing for Self-Management: Discharge Teaching Topics for the Patient After Bariatric Surgery box lists the important areas that should be reviewed. Patients are usually followed closely by the surgeon and registered dietitian nutritionist (RDN) for several years. Encourage patients to keep all appointments and to adhere to

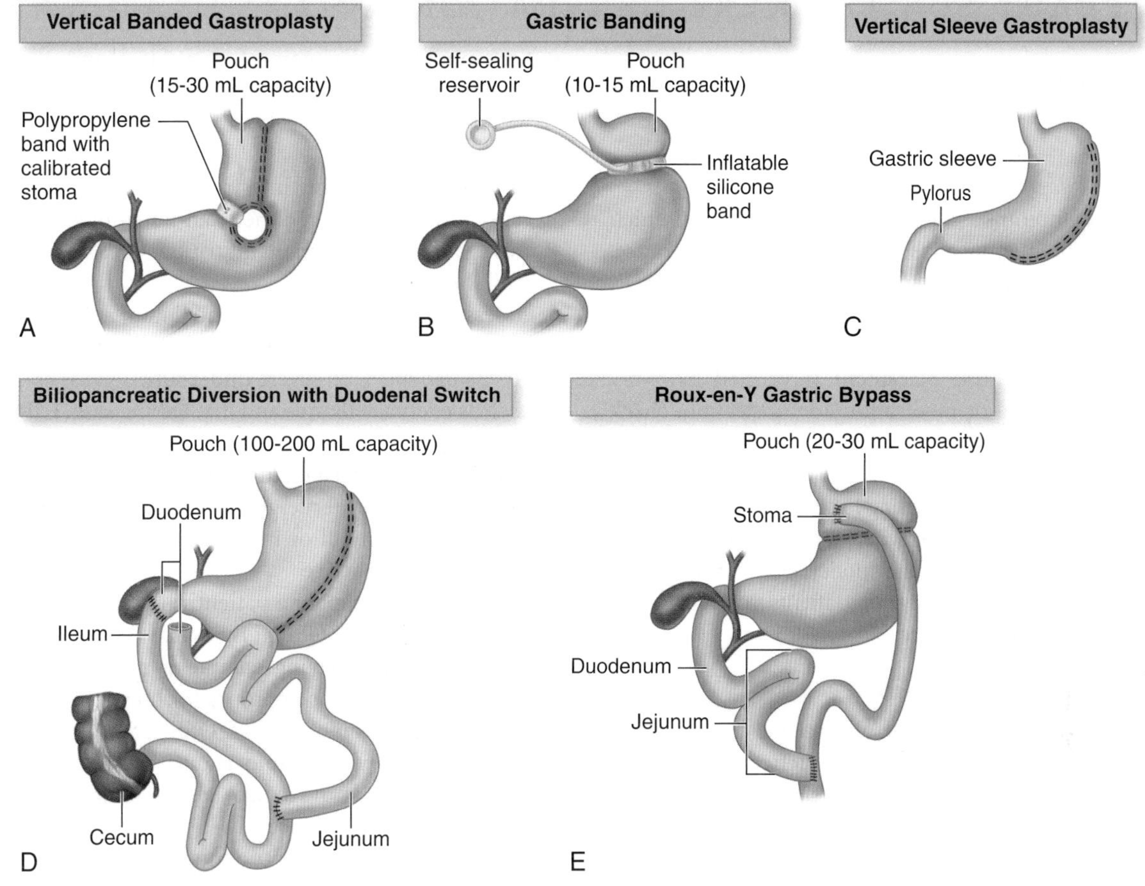

Fig. 55.6 Bariatric surgical procedures. **A**, Vertical banded gastroplasty. **B**, Gastric banding. **C**, Vertical sleeve gastroplasty. **D**, Biliopancreatic diversion with duodenal switch. **E**, Roux-en-Y gastric bypass (RNYGB). (From Silvestri, L., & Silvestri, A. [2020]. *Saunders comprehensive review for the NCLEX-RN examination* [8th ed]. St. Louis: Saunders.)

the treatment plan to ensure success. Plastic surgery, such as panniculectomy (removal of the abdominal apron, or panniculus), may be performed if needed after weight is stabilized, usually in about 18 to 24 months.

PATIENT AND FAMILY EDUCATION: PREPARING FOR SELF-MANAGEMENT

Discharge Teaching Topics for the Patient After Bariatric Surgery

Nutrition: Diet progression, nutrient (including vitamin and mineral) supplements, hydration guidelines

Drug therapy: Analgesics and antiemetic drugs, if needed; drugs for other health problems

Wound care: Clean procedure for open or laparoscopic wounds; cover during shower or bath

Activity level: Restrictions, such as avoiding lifting; activity progression; return to driving and work

Signs and symptoms to report: Fever; excessive nausea or vomiting; epigastric, back, or shoulder pain; red, hot, and/or draining wound(s); pain, redness, or swelling in legs; chest pain; difficulty breathing

Follow-up care: Health care provider office or clinic visits, support groups and other community resources, counseling for patient (and caregiver, if needed)

Continuing education: Nutrition and exercise classes; follow-up visits with registered dietitian nutritionist (RDN)

Self-Care Management. Remind patients to coordinate with their surgeon or primary health care provider to create a manageable and appropriate physical activity plan. For patients having nonsurgical management, emphasize the need to decrease overall fat intake and to avoid reliance on appetite-reducing drugs. Keeping a food journal that documents mood and events that take place with eating can be helpful to identify eating patterns.

Teach patients who have had bariatric surgery that postsurgical bowel changes are common. Vitamin and mineral supplements are prescribed after surgery, especially vitamin D, B-complex vitamins, iron, and calcium, and adherence to this regimen is important for surgical success.

Health Care Resources. Provide the patient with a list of available community resources, such as Overeaters Anonymous (www.oa.org) and the American Obesity Association (www.obesity.org). For surgical patients, the American Society for Metabolic and Bariatric Surgery (www.asmbs.org) may be helpful.

◆ **Evaluation: Evaluate Outcomes.** Evaluate the care of the patient with obesity based on the identified priority patient problem. The primary expected outcome is that the patient consumes appropriate, nutrient-dense foods to meet metabolic demands without overeating. For surgical patients, an additional expected outcome is that the patient remains free of infection after bariatric surgery.

GET READY FOR THE NEXT-GENERATION NCLEX® EXAMINATION!

Key Points

Review these Key Points for each NCLEX Examination Client Needs Category.

Safe and Effective Care Environment

- Differentiate symptoms associated with a food allergy, which can cause life-threatening anaphylaxis, and food intolerance, which involves the gastrointestinal system. **QSEN: Safety**
- Ensure that bariatric furniture and equipment are available in the agency setting. **QSEN: Safety**
- Ensure that feeding tube placement is verified by x-ray before use for feeding or medication administration; check placement thereafter per agency policy by aspirating gastric contents. **QSEN: Safety**
- Place patients receiving tube feeding in a semi-Fowler position at all times to prevent aspiration; check residual contents every 6 hours or as designated per agency policy. QSEN: **Safety**
- Maintain feeding tube patency for patients receiving total enteral nutrition. **QSEN: Safety**

Health Promotion and Maintenance

- Perform ***nutrition*** screening for all patients to determine those at risk. **QSEN: Evidence-Based Practice**
- Calculate BMI as a measure of ***nutrition*** status and/or BSA for dosage calculation purposes. **QSEN: Evidence-Based Practice**
- Implement interventions to promote healthy nutrition intake in patients with malnourishment. **QSEN: Patient-Centered Care**

Psychosocial Integrity

- Recognize that some patients with malnutrition may not view nutrition status as a problem. **QSEN: Patient-Centered Care**
- Recognize that malnutrition can contribute to psychological distress. **QSEN: Patient-Centered Care**
- Seek input from the interprofessional legal and ethics committee if questions arise regarding tube-feeding a patient. **Ethics**

Physiological Integrity

- Collaborate with the interprofessional health care team, especially the registered dietician nutritionist (RDN), when caring for patients with malnutrition. **QSEN: Teamwork and Collaboration**
- Assess serum prealbumin, hemoglobin, and hematocrit levels to identify patients at ***nutrition*** risk. **Clinical Judgment**
- Assess patients with severe undernutrition for complications such as edema, lethargy, and dry, flaking skin. **Clinical Judgment**
- Use gloves when changing feeding system tubing or adding product; use sterile gloves when working with patients who are critically ill or immunocompromised. **QSEN: Evidence-Based Practice**
- Use a feeding pump for a patient who receives continuous or cyclic tube feeding. **QSEN: Evidence-Based Practice**
- Teach patients receiving enteral or parenteral nutrition at home (and family, as appropriate) how to obtain ***nutrition*** while avoiding complications. **QSEN: Safety**
- Teach patients who are undernourished to eat high-protein, high-calorie foods and to take nutrition supplements. **QSEN: Evidence-Based Practice**
- Teach patients with obesity about the importance of a health care provider–approved diet and exercise plan for weight reduction. **QSEN: Evidence-Based Practice**
- Assess for signs and symptoms of anastomotic leak after bariatric surgery. **Clinical Judgment**
- Teach patients who have a gastric bypass how to avoid dumping syndrome. **QSEN: Patient-Centered Care**

MASTERY QUESTIONS

1. The nurse is caring for four clients who have been recommended to consider bariatric surgery. Which assessment data require immediate nursing intervention?
   A. BMI of 23 with gastrointestinal reflux
   B. BMI of 36 with hypertension
   C. BMI of 40 with type II diabetes
   D. BMI of 43 with sleep apnea

2. What discharge teaching will the nurse provide to a client who had gastric bypass surgery? **Select all that apply.**
   A. Be certain to stay hydrated by drinking water.
   B. Solid food can be introduced back into the diet in a week.
   C. Report any back, shoulder, or abdominal pain to the surgeon.
   D. You are likely to have little urine output for the first few weeks.
   E. Each of your meals should initially contain about 5 tablespoons of food.

REFERENCES

Academy of Nutrition and Dietetics. (2018). *Vegetarianism: The basic facts.* http://www.eatright.org/resource/food/nutrition/vegetarian-and-special-diets/vegetarianism-the-basic-facts.

American Academy of Allergy, Asthma, and Immunology. (2020). *Food intolerance versus food allergy*. Retrieved from https://www.aaaai.org/conditions-and-treatments/library/allergy-library/food-intolerance.

American Heart Association. (2017). *The skinny on fats.* www.heart.org/HEARTORG/Conditions/Cholesterol/PreventionTreatmentofHighCholesterol/Know-Your-Fats_UCM_305628_Article.jsp.

American Society of. (2020). *Parenteral and enteral nutrition (ASPEN).* Malnutrition Center. https://www.nutritioncare.org/Malnutrition/.

American Society for Metabolic and Bariatric Surgery (ASMBS). (2020). *Bariatric surgery procedures.* https://asmbs.org/patients/bariatric-surgery-procedures.

Apovian, C., et al. (2017). Two-Year outcomes of vagal nerve blocking (vBloc) for the treatment of obesity in the ReCharge Trial. *Obesity Surgery, 27*(1), 169–176.

Aycock, D., et al. (2017). Language sensitivity, the RESPECT model, and continuing education. *The Journal of Continuing Education in Nursing, 48*(11), 517–524.

Baiu, I., & Spain, D. (2019). Parenteral nutrition. *Journal of the American Medical Association, 321*(21), 2141.

Bourgault, A., Aguirre, L., & Ibrahim, J. (2017). CORTRAK-assisted feeding tube insertion: A comprehensive review of adverse events in the Maude database. *American Journal of Critical Care, 26*(2), 149–155.

Centers for Disease Control and Prevention (CDC). (2020a). *About adult BMI.* www.cdc.gov/healthyweight/assessing/bmi/adult_bmi/.

Centers for Disease Control and Prevention (CDC). (2020b). *Defining adult overweight and obesity.* Retrieved from https://www.cdc.gov/obesity/adult/defining.html.

Cereda, E., et al. (2016). Nutritional status in older persons according to healthcare setting: A systematic review and meta-analysis of prevalence data using MNA®. *Clinical Nutrition, 35*(6), 1282.

Chooi, Y., Ding, C., & Magkos, F. (2019). The epidemiology of obesity. *Metabolism Clinical and Experimental, 92*, 6–10.

Clifton, P. (2018). Relationship between changes in fat and lean depots following weight loss and changes in cardiovascular disease risk markers. *Journal of the American Heart Association, 7*(8), e008675.

Dietary Guidelines for Americans. (2020). *Work under way: Scientific Report of the 2020 Dietary Guidelines Advisory Committee.* https://www.dietaryguidelines.gov/2020-advisory-committee-report.

Drummond Hayes, K., & Drummond Hayes, D. (2018). Best practices for unclogging feeding tubes in adults. *Nursing2018, 48*(6), 66.

Eaton, K., & Lyman, G. (2019). Dosing of anticancer agents in adults. In P. Hesketh (Ed.), *UpToDate*. Waltham, MA.

Faisal, W., et al. (2016). Not all body surface area formulas are the same, but does it matter? *Journal of Global Oncology, 2*(6), 436–437.

Fan, E., Tan, S., & Ang, S. (2017). Nasogastric tube placement confirmation: Where we are and where we should be heading. *Proceedings of Singapore Healthcare, 26*(3), 189–195.

Fryar, C. D., Kruszon-Moran, D., Gu, Q., & Ogden, C. L. (2018). *Mean body weight, height, waist circumference, and body mass index among adults: United States, 1999–2000 through 2015–2016. National health Statistics reports; no 122.* Hyattsville, MD: National Center for Health Statistics.

Government of Canada. (2020). *Canada's food guide.* Retrieved from https://food-guide.canada.ca/en/.

Hodin, R., & Bordeianou, L. (2020). *Inpatient placement of nasogastric and nasoenteric tubes in adults.* In A. Cochran (Ed.). *UpToDate*, Waltham, MA.

Huvenne, H., et al. (2016). Rare genetic forms of obesity: Clinical approach and current treatments in 2016. *Obesity Facts, 9*(3), 158–173.

Interprofessional Education Collaborative. (2016). Core competencies for interprofessional collaborative practice: 2016 update. Retrieved from https://nebula.wsimg.com/2f68a39520b03336b-41038c370497473?AccessKeyId=DC06780E69ED19E2B3A5&disposition=0&alloworigin=1.

Kelly-Weeder, S., et al. (2019). Binge eating and loss of control in college-age women. *Journal of the American Psychiatric Nurses Association, 25*(3), 172–180.

King, K. (2019). Trends in parenteral nutrition. *Today's Dietician, 21*(1), 36–39.

McCance, K., Huether, S., Brashers, V., & Rote, N. (2019). *Pathophysiology: The biologic basis for disease in adults and children* (9th ed.). St. Louis: Mosby.

Mehler, P. (2019). Anorexia nervosa in adults and adolescents: The refeeding syndrome. In J. Yager (Ed.), *UpToDate*. Waltham, MA.

Metheny, N., & Meert, K. (2017). Update on effectiveness of an electromagnetic feeding tube-placement device in detecting respiratory placement. *American Journal of Critical Care, 26*(2), 157–161.

Meyer, P., et al. (2018). Cryolipolysis: Patient selection and special considerations. *Clinical, Cosmetic and Investigational Dermatology, 11*, 499–503.

Morley, J. (2020). *Protein-energy undernutrition: Merck manual professional version.* https://www.merckmanuals.com/professional/nutritional-disorders/undernutrition/protein-energy-undernutrition-peu.

National Academies of Sciences, Engineering, & Medicine. (2020). *Dietary reference intakes tables and applications.* Retrieved from http://www.nationalacademies.org/hmd/Activities/Nutrition/SummaryDRIs/DRI-Tables.aspx.

National Heart, Lung, and Blood Institute; National Institutes of Health; U.S. Department of Health and Human Services (n.d.). Assessing your weight and health risk. Retrieved from https://www.nhlbi.nih.gov/health/educational/lose_wt/risk.htm

Nestle Nutrition Institute (n.d.). Mini nutritional assessment - short form (MNA-SF). Retrieved from https://www.mna-elderly.com/forms/mini/mna_mini_english.pdf

Office of Disease and Health Promotion. (2020). *Dietary guidelines 2015-2020: Appendix 2, estimated calories needs per day, by age, sex, and physical activity level.* Retrieved from https://health.gov/dietaryguidelines/2015/guidelines/appendix-2/.

Pagana, K. D., & Pagana, T. J. (2018). *Mosby's manual of diagnostic and laboratory tests* (6th ed.). St. Louis: Mosby.

Perkins, A. (2019). Body dysmorphic disorder: *The drive for perfection. Nursing2019, 49*(3), 28–33.

Phillips, M., & Zieve, D. (2019). *Biliopancreatic diversion (BPD).* Retrieved from https://medlineplus.gov/ency/imagepages/19499.htm.

Ritchie, C., & Yukawa, M. (2019). Geriatric nutrition: Nutritional issues in older adults. In K. Schmader, & D. Seres (Eds.), *UpToDate*. Waltham, MA.

Schnur, M. (2017). *Body mass index and body surface area: What's the difference? Lippincott nursing center.* Retrieved from https://www.nursingcenter.com/ncblog/august-2017/body-mass-index-and-body-surface-area-what-s-the-d.

Seres, D. (2020). *Nutrition support in critically ill patients: Parenteral nutrition.* In UpToDate, & P. Parsons (Eds.). Waltham, MA.

Shikora, S., et al. (2019). *Neurologic metabolic surgery: A review. Bulletin of the American College of surgeons.* https://bulletin.facs.org/2019/03/neurologic-metabolic-surgery-a-review/.

Simoes, P., et al. (2018). Direct percutaneous endoscopic jejunostomy: Procedural and nutrition outcomes in a large patient cohort. *Journal of Parenteral and Enteral Nutrition, 42*(5), 898–906.

Slusser, M., et al. (2019). *Foundations of interprofessional collaborative practice* (1st ed.). St. Louis: Elsevier.

Smith, L. (2019). Take a deeper look into body surface area. *Nursing2019, 49*(9), 50–54.

Tolbert, C., Mott, S., & Nepple, K. (2018). Malnutrition diagnosis during adult inpatient hospitalizations: Analysis of a multi-institutional collaborative database of academic medical centers. *Journal of the Academy of Nutrition and Dietetics, 118*(1), 125–131.

U.S. Department of Agriculture (USDA). (n.d.). Start simple with MyPlate. Retrieved from https://www.choosemyplate.gov/eathealthy/start-simple-myplate

U.S. Department of Agriculture (USDA). (2015). *2015-2020 Dietary guidelines for Americans.* http://www.cnpp.usda.gov/2015-2020-dietary-guidelines-americans.

Weinstein, S., & Hagle, M. (2014). *Plumer's principles and practice of infusion therapy* (9th ed.). Philadelphia: Wolters Kluwer.

World Health Organization. (2020). *Obesity.* Retrieved from https://www.who.int/topics/obesity/en/.

56

Assessment of the Endocrine System

M. Linda Workman

http://evolve.elsevier.com/Iggy/

LEARNING OUTCOMES

1. Collaborate with the interprofessional team to perform a complete endocrine assessment, including issues with ***nutrition, elimination,*** and ***fluid and electrolyte balance***.
2. Teach adults about factors that increase the risk for endocrine problems.
3. Implement patient-centered nursing actions to help patients and families cope with the psychosocial impact caused by changes in endocrine function.
4. Apply the principles of anatomy, physiology, pathophysiology, genetics, and the aging process to perform an evidence-based assessment for the patient with a problem of the endocrine system.
5. Explain assessment findings for the patient with an endocrine problem.
6. Coordinate appropriate pretest and posttest care for patients and proper handling of specimens before, during, and after testing of the endocrine system.

KEY TERMS

gonads The male and female reproductive endocrine glands.

hormones Natural chemicals that exert their effects on specific tissues known as target tissues.

negative feedback mechanism Signals to an endocrine gland to secrete a hormone in response to a body change to cause a reaction that will result in actions to *oppose* the action of the initial condition change and restore homeostasis.

target tissues Tissues that have receptors corresponding to different hormones that when bound to the hormones respond by changing their activity.

PRIORITY AND INTERRELATED CONCEPTS

The priority concepts for this chapter are:

- ***Nutrition***
- ***Elimination***

The interrelated concept for this chapter is:

- ***Fluid and Electrolyte Balance***

The endocrine system works with the parts of the central nervous system and peripheral nervous system to provide control over all other body systems for optimal homeostasis. The organs and tissues of the endocrine system contain glandular cells that secrete **hormones**, which are natural biochemicals that exert their effects on specific target tissues. **Target tissues** have receptors corresponding to different hormones that when bound to the hormones respond by changing their activity. Endocrine glands are located in many body areas (Fig. 56.1) and affect all other body systems. These glands are ductless and have no direct connection between the glands and their target tissues, which may be located some distance from the endocrine gland. Instead, the hormones secreted from endocrine glands are secreted into the blood for transportation to the target tissues (McCance et al., 2019). The major endocrine glands are:

- Hypothalamus (a neuroendocrine gland)
- Pituitary gland
- Adrenal glands
- Thyroid gland
- Islet cells of the pancreas
- Parathyroid glands
- Gonads

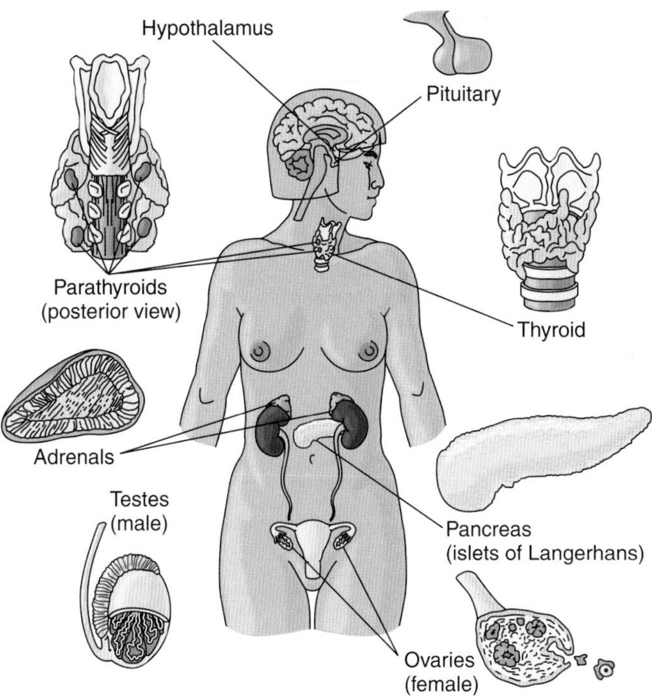

FIG. 56.1 Locations of various glands within the endocrine system.

Body functions controlled by the endocrine system for homeostasis and regulation include metabolism, ***nutrition, elimination,*** temperature, ***fluid and electrolyte balance,*** growth, and reproduction. Many interactions must occur between the endocrine system and all other body systems to ensure that each system maintains a constant normal balance *(homeostasis)* in response to environmental changes. For example, this regulation keeps the internal body temperature at or near 98.6°F (37°C), even when environmental temperatures vary. Other actions keep the serum sodium level between 136 and 145 mEq/L (mmol/L), regardless of whether a healthy adult eats 2 g or 12 g of sodium per day.

Table 56.1 lists hormones secreted by various endocrine glands. Although circulating hormones travel through the blood to all body areas, they exert their actions only on target tissues. Hormones recognize their target tissues and exert their actions by binding to receptors on or within the target tissue cells. In general, each receptor site type is specific for only one hormone. Hormone-receptor actions work in a "lock and key" manner in that only the correct hormone (key) can bind to and activate the receptor site (lock) (Fig. 56.2). Binding a hormone to its receptor causes the target tissue to change its activity, producing specific responses (Lazar & Birnbaum, 2016).

Endocrine system problems and disorders usually are related to:

- An excess of a specific hormone
- A deficiency of a specific hormone
- Poor hormone-receptor interactions resulting in decreased responsiveness of the target tissue

TABLE 56.1 Principal Hormones of the Endocrine Glands

Gland	Hormones
Hypothalamus	Corticotropin-releasing hormone (CRH) Thyrotropin-releasing hormone (TRH) Gonadotropin-releasing hormone (GnRH) Growth hormone–releasing hormone (GHRH) Growth hormone–inhibiting hormone (somatostatin GHIH) Prolactin-inhibiting hormone (PIH) Melanocyte-inhibiting hormone (MIH)
Anterior pituitary	Thyroid-stimulating hormone (TSH), also known as *thyrotropin* Adrenocorticotropic hormone (ACTH, corticotropin) Luteinizing hormone (LH), also known as *Leydig cell–stimulating hormone (LCSH)* Follicle-stimulating hormone (FSH) Prolactin (PRL) Growth hormone (GH) Melanocyte-stimulating hormone (MSH)
Posterior pituitary	Vasopressin (antidiuretic hormone [ADH]) Oxytocin
Thyroid	Triiodothyronine (T_3) Thyroxine (T_4) Calcitonin
Parathyroid	Parathyroid hormone (PTH)
Adrenal cortex	Glucocorticoids (cortisol) Mineralocorticoids (aldosterone)
Ovary	Estrogen Progesterone
Testes	Testosterone
Pancreas	Insulin Glucagon Somatostatin

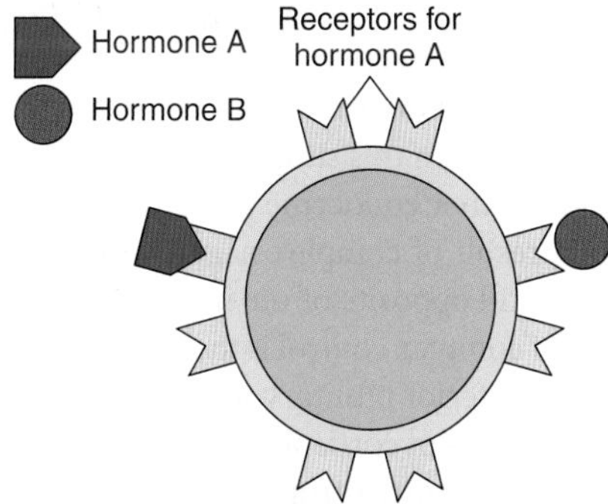

FIG. 56.2 "Lock and key" hormone-receptor binding. Hormone A fits and binds to its receptors, causing a change in cell action. Hormone B does not fit or bind to receptors; no change in cell action results.

ANATOMY AND PHYSIOLOGY REVIEW

Hormones maintain homeostasis of cellular function through a series of one or more *negative feedback control mechanisms.* Secretion of any hormone depends on the body's need for the final action of that hormone. When a body condition starts to move away from the normal range and a specific response is needed to correct this change, secretion of the hormone capable of starting the correcting action or response is stimulated until the need (demand) is met and the body condition returns to the normal range. As the correction occurs, hormone secretion decreases (and may halt). A **negative feedback mechanism** signals an endocrine

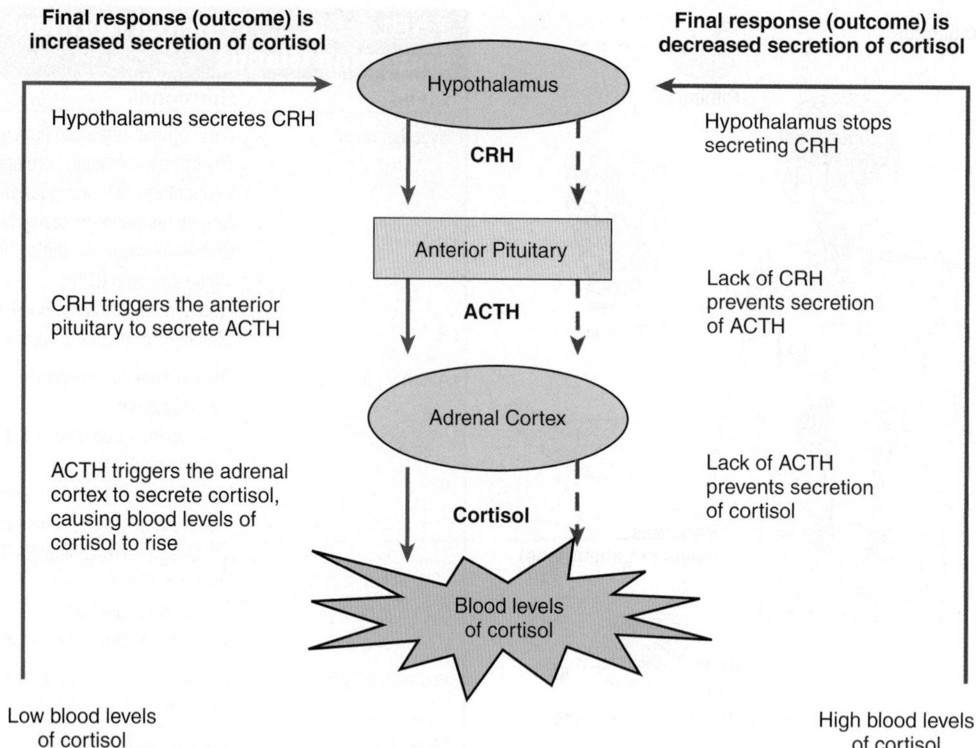

FIG. 56.3 Examples of positive and negative feedback control of hormone secretion. *ACTH,* Adrenocorticotropic hormone; *CRH,* corticotropin-releasing hormone.

gland to secrete a hormone in response to a body change to cause a reaction that will result in actions to *oppose* the action of the initial condition change and restore homeostasis.

An example of a simple negative feedback hormone response is the control of insulin secretion. When blood glucose levels start to rise above normal, the hormone *insulin* is secreted. Insulin increases glucose uptake by the cells, causing a *decrease* in blood glucose levels. Thus the action of insulin (decreasing blood glucose levels) is the opposite of or negative to the condition that stimulated insulin secretion (elevated blood glucose levels).

Some hormones have more complex interactions for negative feedback. These interactions involve a series of reactions in which more than one endocrine gland, as well as the final target tissues, are stimulated. In this situation, the first hormone in the series may have another endocrine gland or glands as the target tissue. The final result of complex negative feedback for endocrine function is still opposite of the initiating condition.

An example of complex control is the interaction of the hypothalamus and the anterior pituitary with the adrenal cortex (Fig. 56.3). Low blood levels of cortisol from the adrenal cortex stimulate the secretion of corticotropin-releasing hormone (CRH) in the hypothalamus. CRH stimulates the anterior pituitary gland to secrete adrenocorticotropic hormone (ACTH). ACTH then triggers the release of cortisol from the adrenal cortex, the final endocrine gland in this series. The rising blood levels of cortisol inhibit CRH release from the hypothalamus. Without CRH, the anterior pituitary gland stops secretion of ACTH. In response, normal blood cortisol levels are maintained.

The normal blood level range of each hormone is well defined. Excesses or deficiencies of hormone secretion can lead to pathologic conditions affecting many body systems.

Hypothalamus and Pituitary Glands

Parts of the hypothalamus are composed of glandular tissues that have many control functions for the rest of the endocrine system. It is located beneath the thalamus in the brain, and nerve fibers connect the hypothalamus to the rest of the central nervous system. The hypothalamus shares a small, closed circulatory system with the anterior pituitary gland, known as the *hypothalamic-hypophysial portal system.* This system allows hormones produced in the hypothalamus to travel directly to the anterior pituitary gland, so only very small amounts are present in systemic circulation where they are not needed.

The function of the hypothalamus is to produce regulatory hormones (see Table 56.1). Some of these hormones are released into the blood and travel to the anterior pituitary, where they either stimulate or inhibit the release of anterior pituitary hormones.

The pituitary gland is located at the base of the brain in a protective pocket of the sphenoid bone (see Fig. 56.1). It is divided into the anterior lobe *(adenohypophysis)* and the posterior lobe *(neurohypophysis).* Nerve fibers in the hypophysial stalk directly connect the hypothalamus to the posterior pituitary (Fig. 56.4).

In response to the releasing hormones of the hypothalamus, the anterior pituitary secretes some tropic (trophic) hormones that have as their target tissues other endocrine glands. Other pituitary hormones, such as prolactin, produce their effect directly on final target tissues (Table 56.2).

The hormones of the posterior pituitary—vasopressin (antidiuretic hormone [ADH]) and oxytocin—are produced in the hypothalamus and delivered to the posterior pituitary where they are stored. These hormones are released from the posterior pituitary into the blood when needed.

TABLE 56.2 Pituitary Hormones: Target Tissues and Subsequent Actions

Hormone	Target Tissue	Actions
Anterior Pituitary		
Thyroid-stimulating hormone or thyrotropin (TSH)	Thyroid	Stimulates synthesis and release of thyroid hormone
Adrenocorticotropic hormone, corticotropin (ACTH)	Adrenal cortex	Stimulates synthesis and release of corticosteroids and adrenocortical growth
Luteinizing hormone (LH) (known as *Leydig cell–stimulating hormone* in males)	Ovary Testis	Stimulates ovulation and progesterone secretion Stimulates testosterone secretion
Follicle-stimulating hormone (FSH) (known as *interstitial cell–* or *Sertoli cell–stimulating hormone* in males)	Ovary Testis	Stimulates estrogen secretion and follicle maturation Stimulates spermatogenesis
Prolactin (PRL)	Mammary glands	Stimulates breast milk production
Growth hormone (GH)	Bone and soft tissue	Promotes growth through lipolysis, protein anabolism, and insulin antagonism
Melanocyte-stimulating hormone (MSH)	Melanocytes	Promotes pigmentation
Posterior Pituitary[a]		
Vasopressin (antidiuretic hormone [ADH])	Kidney	Promotes water reabsorption
Oxytocin	Uterus and mammary glands	Stimulates uterine contractions and ejection of breast milk

[a]These hormones are synthesized in the hypothalamus and are stored in the posterior pituitary gland. They are transported from the hypothalamus down the hypothalamic stalk to the posterior pituitary while bound to proteins known as *neurophysins*.

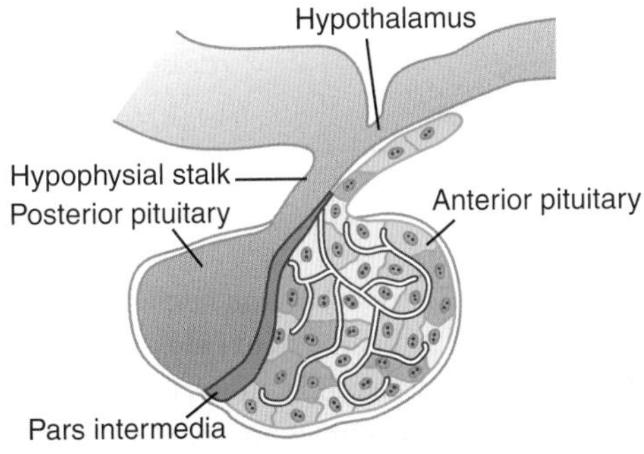

FIG. 56.4 Hypothalamus, hypophysial stalk, anterior pituitary gland, and posterior pituitary gland. (From Guyton, A., & Hall, J. [2006]. *Textbook of medical physiology* [11th ed.]. Philadelphia: Saunders.)

Other factors affect hormone release from the pituitary gland. Drugs, diet, lifestyle, and pathologic conditions can change pituitary hormone secretion (McCance et al., 2019).

Gonads

The **gonads** are the male and female reproductive endocrine glands. Male gonads are the testes, and female gonads are the ovaries. Function of the gonads is dormant until puberty when, under the influence of gonadotropic hormones secreted by the anterior pituitary, the glands and external genitalia mature. The testes are stimulated to produce testosterone, and the ovaries are stimulated to produce estrogen. These changes are responsible for the development of secondary sexual characteristics. The structure and function of the gonads are described in Chapter 64.

Adrenal Glands

The adrenal glands are vascular, tent-shaped organs on the top of each kidney. They have an outer cortex and an inner medulla (see Fig. 56.1). Adrenal hormones affect the entire body.

Adrenal Cortex. The adrenal cortex makes up about 90% of the adrenal gland and has cells divided into three layers. The main hormone types secreted by the cortex are the mineralocorticoids and the glucocorticoids. In addition, the cortex also secretes small amounts of sex hormones.

Mineralocorticoids are produced and secreted by the adrenal cortex to help control ***fluid and electrolyte balance***. *Aldosterone* is the mineralocorticoid that maintains extracellular fluid volume and electrolyte composition. It promotes sodium and water reabsorption and potassium excretion in the kidney. Aldosterone secretion is regulated by the renin-angiotensin-aldosterone system (RAAS), serum potassium ion level, and adrenocorticotropic hormone (ACTH).

Renin is produced by specialized cells of the kidney arterioles. Its release is triggered by a decrease in extracellular fluid volume from blood loss, sodium loss, or posture changes. Hypoxemia also triggers renin release. Renin converts renin substrate (angiotensinogen), a plasma protein, to angiotensin I. Angiotensin I is then converted by an enzyme to form angiotensin II, the active form of angiotensin. In turn, angiotensin II stimulates the secretion of aldosterone. Chapter 13 (see Fig. 13.7 further explains the RAAS functions. Aldosterone causes the kidney to reabsorb sodium and water to bring the plasma volume and osmolarity back to normal.

Serum potassium level also controls aldosterone secretion. It is secreted whenever the serum potassium level increases above normal by as little as 0.1 mEq/L (mmol/L). Aldosterone then enhances kidney excretion of potassium to reduce the blood potassium level back to normal.

Glucocorticoids are produced by the adrenal cortex and are essential for life. The main glucocorticoid produced by the adrenal cortex is *cortisol*. Cortisol affects:

- The body's response to stress
- Carbohydrate, protein, and fat metabolism
- Emotional stability

TABLE 56.3 Functions of Glucocorticoid Hormones

- Prevent hypoglycemia by increasing liver glucose production (gluconeogenesis) and inhibiting peripheral glucose use
- Maintain excitability and responsiveness of cardiac muscle
- Increase lipolysis, releasing glycerol and free fatty acids
- Increase protein catabolism
- Degrade collagen and connective tissue
- Increase the number of mature neutrophils released from bone marrow
- Exert anti-inflammatory effects that decrease the migration of inflammatory cells to sites of injury
- Maintain behavior and cognitive functions

- Immune function
- Sodium and water balance

Cortisol also influences other important body processes. For example, it must be present for *catecholamine* (epinephrine, norepinephrine [NE]) action and maintaining the normal excitability of the heart muscle cells (McCance et al., 2019). Glucocorticoid functions are listed in Table 56.3.

Glucocorticoid release is regulated directly by the anterior pituitary hormone *ACTH* and indirectly by the hypothalamic corticotropin-releasing hormone *(CRH)*. The release of CRH and ACTH is affected by the serum level of free cortisol, the normal sleep-wake cycle, and stress.

As described earlier and shown in Fig. 56.3, when blood cortisol levels are low, the hypothalamus secretes CRH, which triggers the pituitary to release ACTH. Then ACTH triggers the adrenal cortex to secrete cortisol. Adequate or elevated blood levels of cortisol *inhibit* the release of CRH and ACTH. This inhibitory effect is an example of a negative feedback system.

Glucocorticoid release peaks in the morning and reaches its lowest level 12 hours after the peak. Emotional, chemical, or physical stress increases the release of glucocorticoids.

Sex hormones (androgens and estrogens) are secreted in low levels by the adrenal cortex in both genders. Adrenal secretion of these hormones is usually not significant because the gonads (ovaries and testes) secrete much larger amounts of estrogens and androgens. However, in women the adrenal gland is the major source of androgens.

Adrenal Medulla. The adrenal medulla is a sympathetic nerve ganglion that has secretory cells. Stimulation of the sympathetic nervous system causes the release of adrenal medullary hormones, the catecholamines (epinephrine and norepinephrine [NE]). These hormones travel to all areas of the body through the blood and exert their effects on target cells. The adrenal medullary hormones are not essential for life because they also are secreted by other body tissues, but they do play a role in the stress response.

The adrenal medulla secretes about 15% NE and 85% epinephrine. Hormone effects vary with the specific receptor in the cell membranes of the target tissue.

These receptors are of two types: alpha adrenergic and beta adrenergic, which are further classified as $alpha_1$ and $alpha_2$ receptors and $beta_1$, $beta_2$, and $beta_3$ receptors. NE acts mainly on alpha-adrenergic receptors, and epinephrine acts mainly on beta-adrenergic receptors.

TABLE 56.4 Catecholamine Receptors and Effects of Adrenal Medullary Hormone Stimulation on Selected Organs and Tissues

Organ or Tissue	Receptors	Effects
Heart	$Beta_1$	Increased heart rate Increased contractility
Blood vessels	Alpha	Vasoconstriction
	$Beta_2$	Vasodilation
GI tract	Alpha	Increased sphincter tone
	Beta	Decreased motility
Kidneys	$Beta_2$	Increased renin release
Bronchioles	$Beta_2$	Relaxation; dilation
Bladder	Alpha	Sphincter contractions
	$Beta_2$	Relaxation of detrusor muscle
Skin	Alpha	Increased sweating
Fat cells	Beta	Increased lipolysis
Liver	Alpha	Increased gluconeogenesis and glycogenolysis
Pancreas	Alpha	Decreased glucagon and insulin release
	Beta	Increased glucagon and insulin release
Eyes	Alpha	Dilation of pupils

Catecholamines exert their actions on many target organs (Table 56.4). Activation of the sympathetic nervous system, which then releases adrenal medullary catecholamines, is an important part of the stress response. Catecholamines are secreted in small amounts at all times to maintain homeostasis. Stress triggers increased secretion of these hormones, resulting in the "fight-or-flight" response, a state of heightened physical and emotional awareness.

Thyroid Gland

The thyroid gland is in the anterior neck, directly below the cricoid cartilage (Fig. 56.5). It has two lobes joined by a thin strip of tissue *(isthmus)* in front of the trachea.

The thyroid gland is composed of follicular and parafollicular cells. Follicular cells produce the thyroid hormones *thyroxine* (T_4) and *triiodothyronine* (T_3). Parafollicular cells produce *thyrocalcitonin (TCT or calcitonin)*, which helps regulate serum calcium levels.

Control of metabolism occurs through T_3 and T_4. Both hormones increase metabolism, which causes an increase in oxygen use and heat production in all tissues. Most circulating T_4 and T_3 are bound to plasma proteins. The free hormone moves into the cell, where it binds to its receptor in the cell nucleus. Once in the cell, T_4 is converted to T_3, the most active thyroid hormone. Conversion of T_4 to T_3 is impaired by stress, starvation, dyes, and some drugs. Cold temperatures increase the conversion. Table 56.5 lists thyroid hormone functions.

Secretion of T_3 and T_4 is controlled by the hypothalamic-pituitary-thyroid gland axis negative feedback mechanism. The

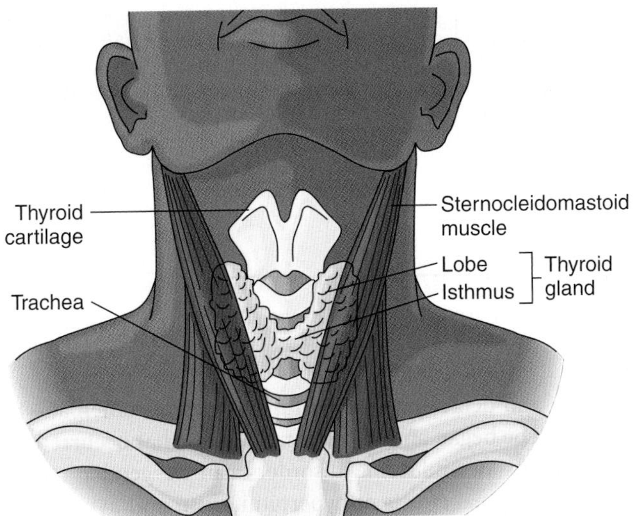

FIG. 56.5 Anatomic location of the thyroid gland.

TABLE 56.5 Functions of Thyroid Hormones in Adults

- Control metabolic rate of all cells
- Promote sufficient pituitary secretion of growth hormone and gonadotropins
- Regulate protein, carbohydrate, and fat metabolism
- Exert effects on heart rate and contractility
- Increase red blood cell production
- Affect respiratory rate and drive
- Increase bone formation and decrease bone resorption of calcium
- Act as insulin antagonists

hypothalamus secretes thyrotropin-releasing hormone (TRH). TRH triggers the anterior pituitary gland to secrete thyroid-stimulating hormone (TSH), which then stimulates the thyroid gland to make and release thyroid hormones. If thyroid hormone levels are high, release of TRH and TSH is inhibited. If thyroid hormone levels are low, TRH and TSH release is increased. Cold and stress are two factors that cause the hypothalamus to secrete TRH, which then stimulates the anterior pituitary to secrete TSH.

Dietary intake of protein and iodine is needed to produce thyroid hormones. Iodine is absorbed from the intestinal tract as iodide. The thyroid gland draws iodide from the blood and concentrates it. After iodide is in the thyroid, it combines with the amino acid *tyrosine* to form T_4 and T_3. These hormones bind to thyroglobulin and are stored in thyroid follicular cells. When stimulated, T_4 and T_3 are released into the blood. They enter all cells, where they bind to DNA receptors and turn on genes important in metabolism to regulate basal metabolic rate (BMR).

Calcium and phosphorus balance occurs partly through the actions of calcitonin (thyrocalcitonin [TCT]), which also is produced in the thyroid gland. Calcitonin lowers serum calcium and serum phosphorus levels by reducing bone resorption (release) of these minerals. Its actions are opposite of parathyroid hormone (PTH).

The serum calcium level determines calcitonin secretion. Low serum calcium levels suppress the release of calcitonin. Elevated serum calcium levels increase its secretion.

Parathyroid Glands

The parathyroid glands consist of four small glands located close to or within the back surface of the thyroid gland (see Fig. 56.1). These cells secrete parathyroid hormone (PTH).

PTH regulates calcium and phosphorus metabolism by acting on bones, the kidneys, and the GI tract (Fig. 56.6). Bone is the main storage site of calcium. PTH increases *bone resorption* (bone release of calcium into the blood from bone storage sites), thus increasing serum calcium. In the kidneys, PTH activates vitamin D, which then increases the absorption of calcium and phosphorus from the intestines. In the kidney tubules, PTH allows calcium to be reabsorbed and put back into the blood.

Serum calcium levels determine PTH secretion. Secretion decreases when serum calcium levels are high, and it increases when serum calcium levels are low. PTH and calcitonin work together to maintain normal calcium levels in the blood and extracellular fluid.

Pancreas

The pancreas has exocrine and endocrine functions. The exocrine function of the pancreas involves the secretion of digestive enzymes through ducts that empty into the duodenum. The cells in the islets of Langerhans perform the pancreatic endocrine functions (Fig. 56.7). About 1 million islet cells are found throughout the pancreas.

The islets have three distinct cell types: alpha cells, which secrete glucagon; beta cells, which secrete insulin; and delta cells, which secrete somatostatin. Glucagon and insulin affect carbohydrate, protein, and fat metabolism.

Glucagon is a hormone that increases blood glucose levels. It is triggered by decreased blood glucose levels and increased blood amino acid levels. This hormone helps prevent hypoglycemia. Chapter 59 discusses glucagon function in more detail.

Insulin promotes the movement and storage of carbohydrate, protein, and fat. It lowers blood glucose levels by enhancing glucose movement across cell membranes and into the cells of many tissues. Insulin secretion rises in response to an increase in blood glucose levels. More information on insulin is presented in Chapter 59.

Somatostatin, which is secreted not only in the pancreas but also in the intestinal tract and the brain, inhibits the release of glucagon and insulin from the pancreas. It also inhibits the release of gastrin, secretin, and other GI peptides.

NCLEX EXAMINATION CHALLENGE 56.1

Physiological Integrity

Which action **best** exemplifies the expected outcome of appropriate negative feedback control over endocrine gland hormone secretion?

A. Decreased secretion of glucagon when blood glucose approaches normal levels
B. Increased secretion of parathyroid hormone in response to a calcium-containing intravenous infusion
C. Increased secretion of thyroid-stimulating hormone in response to long-term exogenous thyroid hormone replacement therapy
D. Decreased secretion of cortisol in response to a pituitary tumor stimulating the increased secretion of adrenocorticotropic hormone

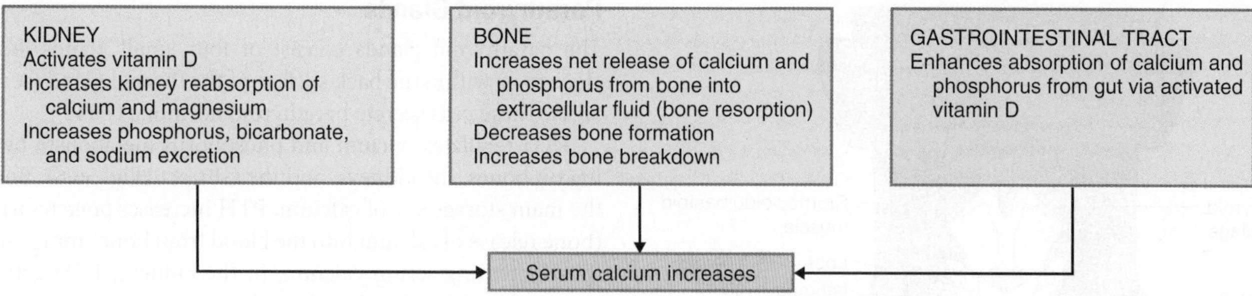

KIDNEY
Activates vitamin D
Increases kidney reabsorption of calcium and magnesium
Increases phosphorus, bicarbonate, and sodium excretion
BONE
Increases net release of calcium and phosphorus from bone into extracellular fluid (bone resorption)
Decreases bone formation
Increases bone breakdown
GASTROINTESTINAL TRACT
Enhances absorption of calcium and phosphorus from gut via activated vitamin D
Serum calcium increases

FIG. 56.6 Effects of parathyroid hormone on target tissues to maintain calcium balance.

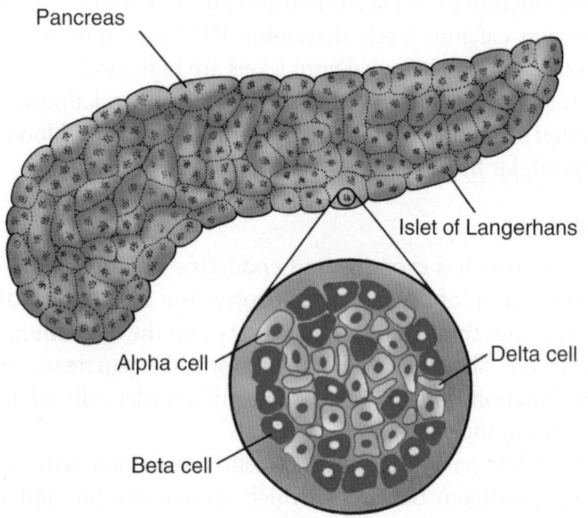

FIG. 56.7 Cells of the islets of Langerhans of the pancreas.

Endocrine Changes Associated With Aging

The effects of aging on the endocrine system vary but usually result in reduced glandular function and decreased hormone secretion. The three endocrine tissues that usually have reduced function with aging are the gonads, the thyroid gland, and the endocrine pancreas (Lamberts & van den Beld, 2016; Touhy & Jett, 2020). This reduction is normally very gradual for the thyroid glands, pancreas, and male gonads. For women, reduced function of the ovaries is somewhat faster with more noticeable changes. It is difficult to distinguish normal from abnormal endocrine activity in older adults because of chronic illness, changes in diet and activity, sleep disturbances, decreased metabolism, and the use of drugs that may affect hormone function. Consider these factors when assessing the older adult with endocrine dysfunction.

Encourage the older adult to participate in regular screening examinations, including fasting and random blood glucose checks, calcium level determinations, and thyroid function testing. The Patient-Centered Care: Older Adult Considerations: Age-Related Endocrine System Changes box lists the common endocrine changes that occur in the older adult.

ASSESSMENT: RECOGNIZE CUES

Patient History

Baseline endocrine assessment data must include age and gender because certain disorders are more common in older than in younger patients, such as diabetes mellitus, loss of ovarian function, and decreased thyroid function. Ask women at what age menarche began and whether menopause has occurred.

Symptoms of endocrine disorders can be gender related, such as the sexual effects of hyperpituitarism and hypopituitarism (see Chapter 57). Thyroid problems are more common in women (McCance et al., 2019). Assess for a history of endocrine problems, symptoms that could indicate a disorder, and hospitalizations. Ask about past and current drugs, such as cortisone, levothyroxine, oral contraceptives, and antihypertensive agents. The use of exogenous hormone drugs, when not needed for hormone replacement, can cause serious dysfunction in many endocrine glands. Use the opportunity to warn patients about the dangers of misusing hormone-based drugs such as androgens and thyroid hormones (Burchum & Rosenthal, 2019).

Nutrition History. ***Nutrition*** changes or GI tract disturbances may reflect many different endocrine problems. Ask about a history of nausea, vomiting, and abdominal pain. An increase or decrease in food or fluid intake may also indicate specific disorders. For example, diabetes insipidus triggers excessive thirst, and adrenal hypofunction triggers salt craving. Hunger and thirst also are associated with diabetes mellitus. Rapid changes in weight without diet changes are often associated with many endocrine disorders, including diabetes mellitus and thyroid problems.

Nutrition deficiencies from an inadequate diet, especially of protein and iodide-containing foods (saltwater fish and seafood, cheese and dairy products, iodized table salt), may be a cause of an endocrine disorder. Teach the patient about a well-balanced diet that includes at least 60 g of protein daily, less animal fat, and fewer concentrated simple sugars. Teach patients who do not eat saltwater fish on a regular basis to use iodized salt in food preparation.

Family History and Genetic Risk. Ask the patient about any family history of obesity, growth or development difficulties, diabetes mellitus, infertility, or thyroid disorders. These problems may have an autosomal dominant, recessive, or cluster pattern of inheritance.

Current Health Problems. Focus on the patient's reason for seeking health care, asking questions such as:

- When did symptoms begin?
- Did symptoms occur gradually, or start suddenly?
- Have you been treated for this problem in the past?
- How have the current problems affected your activities of daily living?

PATIENT-CENTERED CARE: OLDER ADULT CONSIDERATIONS QSEN

Age-Related Endocrine System Changes

Change	Nursing Considerations
Decreased Antidiuretic Hormone (ADH) Production	
Urine is more dilute and may not concentrate when fluid intake is low.	The patient is at greater risk for dehydration. Assess the older patient more frequently for dehydration. If fluids are not restricted because of another health problem, teach assistive personnel (AP) to offer fluids at least every 2 hours while the patient is awake.
Decreased Ovarian Production of Estrogen	
Bone density decreases. Skin is thinner, drier, and at greater risk for injury. Perineal and vaginal tissues become drier, and the risk for cystitis increases.	Teach the patient to engage in regular exercise and weight-bearing activity to maintain bone density. Handle the patient carefully to avoid injury from fragile fractures. Avoid pulling or dragging the patient. Use minimal tape on the skin. Help patients confined to bed or chairs change positions at least every 2 hours. Teach patients to use skin moisturizers. Perform or assist the patient to perform perineal care at least twice daily. Unless another health problem requires fluid restriction, encourage all women to drink at least 2 liters of fluids daily. Teach sexually active older women to urinate immediately after sexual intercourse. Teach sexually active women that using vaginal lubricants with sexual activity can reduce discomfort and the risk for tissue damage.
Decreased Glucose Tolerance	
Weight becomes greater than ideal, along with: • Elevated fasting blood glucose level • Elevated random blood glucose level • Slow wound healing • Frequent yeast infections • Polydipsia • Polyuria	Assess family history for obesity and type 2 diabetes. Encourage the patient to engage in regular exercise and to keep body weight within 10 lb (4.5 kg) of ideal. Teach patients the signs and symptoms of diabetes and instruct them to report any of these to the primary health care provider. Suggest diabetes testing for any patient with: • Persistent vaginal candidiasis • Failure of a foot or leg skin wound to heal in 2 weeks or less • Increased hunger and thirst • Noticeable and persistent decrease in energy level
Decreased General Metabolism	
Patient has less tolerance for cold. Appetite is decreased. Heart rate and blood pressure (BP) are decreased.	Teach patients to dress warmly in cool or cold weather. Can be difficult to distinguish from hypothyroidism. Check for additional signs and symptoms of: • Lethargy • Constipation (as a change from usual bowel habits) • Decreased cognition • Slowed speech • Body temperature consistently below 97°F (36°C) • Heart rate below 60 beats/min

These questions can provide clues to specific endocrine disorders. Also explore changes in energy levels, ***elimination*** patterns, sexual and reproductive functions, and physical features.

Energy level changes occur with many endocrine problems, especially thyroid problems (see Chapter 58) and adrenal problems (see Chapter 57). Ask the patient about any change in ability to perform ADLs, and assess his or her current energy level. For instance, has he or she been sleeping longer, or are fatigue and generalized weakness present?

Elimination is affected by the endocrine system. Identify the patient's usual and past patterns of elimination to determine deviations from the normal routine. Ask about the amount and frequency of urination. Does he or she urinate frequently in large amounts? Does the patient wake during the night to urinate *(nocturia)*? Information about the frequency of bowel movements and their consistency and color may provide clues to problems in ***fluid and electrolyte balance*** or metabolic rate (i.e., thyroid function).

Sexual and reproductive functions are greatly affected by endocrine disturbances. Ask about any changes in the menstrual cycle, such as increased flow, duration, and frequency of menses; or a change in the regularity of menses. Ask men whether they have experienced impotence. Ask men and women about a change in *libido* (sexual desire) or fertility issues.

Physical appearance changes can reflect an endocrine problem. Discuss any changes that the patient perceives in physical features. Ask about changes in:

- Hair texture and distribution
- Facial contours and eye protrusion
- Voice quality
- Body proportions
- Secondary sexual characteristics

For example, ask a man whether he is shaving less often or a woman if she has noticed an increase in facial hair. These changes may be associated with pituitary, thyroid, parathyroid, or adrenal dysfunction.

Physical Assessment

Inspection. An endocrine problem can change physical features because of its effect on growth and development, sex hormone levels, ***fluid and electrolyte balance***, and metabolism. Different clinical findings can occur with many endocrine disorders or with nonendocrine problems.

Observe the patient's general appearance, and assess height, weight, fat distribution, and muscle mass in relation to age. Heredity and age rather than health problems may be responsible for some physical features (e.g., short stature). Assess scalp and body hair growth patterns.

When examining the head, focus on abnormalities of facial structure, features, and expression, such as:

- Prominent forehead or jaw
- Round or puffy face
- Dull or flat expression
- Exophthalmos (protruding eyeballs and retracted upper lids)

Check the lower neck for a visible enlargement of the thyroid gland. Normally the thyroid tissue cannot be observed. The isthmus may be noticeable when the patient swallows. Jugular vein distention may be seen on inspection of the neck and can indicate fluid overload.

Observe skin color and look for areas of pigment loss *(hypopigmentation)* or excess *(hyperpigmentation)*. Fungal skin infections, slow wound healing, bruising, and petechiae are often seen in patients with adrenal hyperfunction. Skin infections, foot ulcers, and slow wound healing often occur with diabetes mellitus. With some types of adrenal gland dysfunction, the skin over the joints, as well as any scar tissue, may show increased pigmentation due to increased levels of adrenocorticotropic hormone (ACTH) and melanocyte-stimulating hormone.

Vitiligo (patchy areas of pigment loss) is seen with primary hypofunction of the adrenal glands and is caused by autoimmune destruction of melanocytes in the skin. It is seen most often on the face, neck, arms, hands, legs, and fold areas (Jarvis, 2020). Mucous membranes may have large areas of uneven pigmentation. Document the location, color, distribution, and size of skin color changes.

Inspect the fingernails for malformation, thickness, or brittleness, all of which may suggest thyroid gland problems. Examine the extremities and the base of the spine for edema, which suggests impaired ***fluid and electrolyte balance***.

Check the trunk for any abnormalities in chest size and symmetry. Truncal obesity and the presence of a "buffalo hump" between the shoulders on the back may indicate adrenocortical excess. Hormonal imbalance may also change secondary sexual characteristics. Inspect the breasts of men as well as women for size, symmetry, pigmentation, and discharge. Low testosterone levels in men induce breast enlargement *(gynecomastia)*. *Striae* (reddish-purple "stretch marks") on the breasts or abdomen are often seen with adrenocortical excess.

Assess the patient's hair distribution for signs of endocrine gland dysfunction. Changes can include *hirsutism* (excessive body hair growth, especially on the face, the chest, and the center abdominal line of women), excessive scalp hair loss, or changes in hair texture (Jarvis, 2020).

Examination of the genitalia may reveal a dysfunction in hormone secretion. Observe the size of the scrotum and penis or of the labia and clitoris in relation to standards for the patient's age. The distribution and quantity of pubic hair are often affected in hypogonadism.

Palpation. The thyroid gland and the testes can be examined by palpation, most often by a primary health care provider rather than a bedside nurse. Chapters 64 and 67 discuss examination of the testes. The thyroid gland is palpated for size, symmetry, general shape, and the presence of nodules or other irregularities.

The thyroid gland is palpated by standing either behind or in front of the patient (Jarvis, 2020). Having the patient swallow sips of water during the examination helps palpate the thyroid gland, which is not easily felt when normal.

The patient sits and lowers the chin. The examiner, using the posterior approach, places both thumbs on the back of the patient's neck, with the fingers curved around to the front of the neck on either side of the trachea. When the patient swallows, the thyroid is felt as it rises. The right lobe is examined with the patient's head turned to the right, and the trachea is gently displaced by the examiner's left fingers. The right lobe is palpated with the examiner's right hand. This procedure is reversed to examine the left lobe (Jarvis, 2020).

! NURSING SAFETY PRIORITY (QSEN)

Action Alert

Avoid applying pressure on or palpating the thyroid in a patient who has or is suspected to have hyperthyroidism because these actions can stimulate a sudden release of thyroid hormones and cause a thyroid storm.

Auscultation. Auscultate the chest to assess cardiac rate and rhythm to use later as a means of assessing treatment effectiveness. Some endocrine problems induce dysrhythmias. Many endocrine problems can cause dehydration and volume depletion. Document any difference in the patient's blood pressure and pulse in the lying, standing, or sitting positions (orthostatic vital signs).

When an enlarged thyroid gland is palpated, the area of enlargement is auscultated for bruits. Hypertrophy of the thyroid gland causes an increase in vascular flow, which may result in bruits.

Psychosocial Assessment

Many endocrine problems can change a patient's behaviors, personality, and psychological responses. Assess the patient's coping skills, support systems, and health-related beliefs. Ask whether the patient has noticed a change in how stress is handled, frequency of crying, or degree of patience and anger expression. Patients may not recognize these changes in themselves. Ask the family about changes in the patient's behaviors or personality.

A number of endocrine disorders affect the patient's perception of self. For example, body features can change greatly in disorders of the pituitary, adrenal, and thyroid glands. Infertility, impotence, and other changes in sexual function may result from endocrine problems. Encourage the patient to express his or her feelings and concerns about a change in appearance or in sexual function. Ask about any difficulty in coping with these changes.

Patients with endocrine problems may require lifelong drugs and follow-up care. Assess their readiness to learn and ability to carry out specific self-management skills. Patients may also face financial difficulties resulting from a prolonged medical regimen or loss of employment. A referral to social service agencies may be needed.

NCLEX EXAMINATION CHALLENGE 56.2

Safe and Effective Health Care Environment

Which assessment finding in a 40-year-old client is **most relevant** for the nurse to assess further for a possible endocrine problem?

A. He has lost 10 lb in the past month following a low-carbohydrate eating plan.
B. The client reports now needing to shave only once weekly instead of daily.
C. His new prescription for eyeglasses is for a higher strength.
D. The client's father died of a stroke at age 70 years.

CLINICAL JUDGMENT CHALLENGE 56.1

Patient-Centered Care; Safety

A 27-year-old graduate student comes to student health services with reports of feeling tired all the time and having difficulty concentrating. She has gained 30 lb (13.6 kg) in the past 10 weeks without a change in eating habits and states that she is having a hard time focusing on both her class work and laboratory work. She further states that in the past 2 weeks she has fallen asleep in class several times despite sleeping 8 to 10 hours at night.

Vital signs are:

- T = 97.0°F (36.1°C)
- P = 58 beats/min
- BP = 88/40
- R = 14/min

When the nurse asks whether any other changes have been noticed, she replies that she has not had a period in 3 months and before that they had been regular. The nurse notes that the client is wearing a heavy sweater even though the day is warm.

1. **Recognize Cues:** What assessment information in this client situation is the most important and immediate concern for the nurse? (Hint: Identify the **relevant** information *first* to determine what is most important.)
2. **Analyze Cues:** What client conditions are consistent with the **most relevant** information? (Hint: Think about priority collaborative problems that support and contradict the information presented in this situation.)

Diagnostic Assessment

Laboratory Tests. Laboratory tests are an essential part of the diagnostic process for possible endocrine problems. Fluids commonly used for these tests include blood, urine, and saliva. Salivary levels of the steroid hormones (cortisol, testosterone, progesterone, and estradiol) accurately reflect blood levels of these hormones (Sluss & Hayes, 2016). Protein hormones, such as those from the pituitary gland and thyroid gland, are not assessed using saliva. Always check with the agency's laboratory for proper collection and handling of the specimen. Specialized testing for specific disorders is described in Chapters 57 to 59. The Best Practice for Patient Safety & Quality Care: Endocrine Testing box lists correct techniques for collection of specimens for general endocrine testing.

BEST PRACTICE FOR PATIENT SAFETY & QUALITY CARE (QSEN)

Endocrine Testing

For Blood Tests

- Check your laboratory's method of handling hormone test samples for tube type, timing, drugs to be administered as part of the test, etc. For example, blood samples drawn for catecholamines must be placed on ice and taken to the laboratory immediately.
- Explain the procedure and any restrictions to the patient.
- If you are drawing blood samples from an IV line, clear the line thoroughly. Do not use a double- or triple-lumen line to obtain samples; contamination or dilution from another port is possible.
- Emphasize the importance of taking a drug prescribed for the test on time. Tell the patient to set an alarm if the drug is to be taken during the night.

For Urine Tests

- Instruct the patient to begin the urine collection (whether for 2, 4, 8, 12, or 24 hours) by first emptying his or her bladder and NOT using this specimen as part of the collection. The timing for the urine collection begins *after* this specimen is discarded.
- Tell the patient to note the time of the discarded specimen and to plan to collect all urine from this time until the end of the urine collection period.
- To end the collection, instruct the patient to empty his or her bladder at the end of the timed period, even if the urge to urinate is not felt, and add that urine to the collection.
- Check with the laboratory to determine any special handling of the urine specimen (e.g., Is a preservative needed? Does the container need to be kept cold?).
- If needed, make sure that the preservative has been added to the collection container at the beginning of the collection.
- Tell the patient about any preservative and the need to avoid splashing urine from the container because some preservatives make the urine caustic.
- If the specimen must be kept cool or cold, instruct the patient to place the container in an inexpensive cooler with ice. The specimen container should not be kept with food or drinks.

Assays. An assay measures the level of a specific hormone in blood or other body fluid. The most common assays for endocrine testing are antibody-based immunologic assays and chromatographic assays, which include mass spectrometry that measures the presence of a hormone(s) based on its molecular mass and chemical composition. These assays are very sensitive and can detect even minute quantities of a given hormone. Many different hormone concentrations can be analyzed at the same time by the mass spectrometry method.

Provocative/Suppression Tests. Measurement of specific hormone blood levels does not always distinguish between the normal and the abnormal. The wide normal range for some hormones makes it necessary to trigger responses by provocative ("stimulation") or suppression tests.

For the patient who might have an underactive endocrine gland, a stimulus may be used to determine whether the gland is capable of normal hormone production. This method is called *provocative testing.* Measured amounts of selected hormones are given to stimulate the target gland to maximum production. Hormone levels are then measured and compared with expected normal values. Failure of the hormone level to rise with provocation indicates hypofunction.

Suppression tests are used when hormone levels are high or in the upper range of normal. Drugs or other substances known to normally suppress hormone production are administered. Failure of suppression of hormone production during testing indicates hyperfunction.

Urine Tests. The levels of hormones and their metabolites in the urine can be measured to determine endocrine function. Because many of the endocrine hormones are secreted in a pulsatile fashion, measurement of a specific hormone in a 24-hour urine collection, rather than as a single blood or urine sample, better reflects the function of a specific gland, such as the adrenal gland. Teach the patient how to collect a 24-hour urine sample (see also the Best Practice for Patient Safety & Quality Care: Endocrine Testing box).

Certain hormones require additives in the container at the beginning of the collection. Instruct the patient not to discard the preservative from the container and to use caution when handling it because some are caustic. Remind him or her that this collection is timed for *exactly* 24 hours. Instruct the patient to avoid taking any unnecessary drugs during endocrine testing because some drugs can interfere with the assay.

Genetic Testing. When some hormone levels are too low to be measured, genetic testing may be performed. DNA analysis or RNA assessment can determine whether a genetic mutation is responsible for the lack of hormone production or the absence of hormone receptors (Sluss & Hayes, 2016).

Tests for Glucose. Tests for functions of the islet cells of the pancreas measure the *result* of pancreatic islet cell function. Blood glucose values and the oral glucose tolerance test help diagnose diabetes mellitus. The glycosylated hemoglobin (A1C) value indicates the *average* blood glucose level over a period of 2 to 3 months. (See Chapter 59 for diabetes mellitus testing.)

Imaging Assessment. Anterior, posterior, and lateral skull x-rays may be used to view the sella turcica, the bony pocket in the skull where the pituitary gland rests. Erosion of the sella turcica indicates invasion of the wall from an abnormal growth.

MRI with contrast is the most sensitive method of imaging the pituitary gland, although CT scans can also be used to evaluate it. The thyroid, parathyroid glands, ovaries, and testes are evaluated by ultrasound. CT scans are used to evaluate the adrenal glands, ovaries, and pancreas.

Other Diagnostic Assessment. Needle biopsy is a safe and quick ambulatory surgery procedure used to indicate the composition of thyroid nodules. It is used to determine whether surgical intervention is needed.

GET READY FOR THE NEXT-GENERATION NCLEX® EXAMINATION!

Key Points

Review these Key Points for each NCLEX Examination Client Needs Category.

Safe and Effective Care Environment

- Be aware that assessment of endocrine problems requires a systematic approach because of the variety and combination of signs and symptoms. **QSEN: Evidence-Based Practice**
- Physical, psychosocial, and laboratory findings are needed for a complete and accurate endocrine assessment to avoid overlooking any problems. **QSEN: Safety**

Health Promotion and Maintenance

- Teach all patients that abusing or misusing hormones or steroids can have an adverse effect on endocrine function. **QSEN: Patient-Centered Care**
- Explain all diagnostic procedures, restrictions, and follow-up care to the patient scheduled for endocrine tests. **QSEN: Patient-Centered Care**

Psychosocial Integrity

- Encourage the patient to express concerns about a change in appearance, sexual function, or fertility as a result of a possible endocrine problem. **QSEN: Patient-Centered Care**
- Ask family members about changes in the patient's personality or behavior. **QSEN: Patient-Centered Care**

Physiological Integrity

- Be aware that the onset of endocrine problems can be slow and insidious or abrupt and life threatening.
- The presence of excess hormone production in an older adult is more likely to be caused by an actual endocrine problem than by age-related changes.
- Ask the patient about other family members with endocrine disorders, because some problems have a genetic component. **QSEN: Evidence-Based Practice**
- Ask the patient what prescribed and over-the-counter drugs are taken on a regular basis, because some drugs can alter endocrine function. **QSEN: Patient-Centered Care**
- Follow the laboratory's procedures for collecting and handling specimens for endocrine function studies. **QSEN: Evidence-Based Practice**
- Differentiate normal from abnormal laboratory test findings and signs and symptoms for patients with possible endocrine problems. **QSEN: Patient-Centered Care**

MASTERY QUESTIONS

1. Which statement regarding trophic (tropic) hormones is true?
   A. All are categorized as catecholamines.
   B. Responses are independent of target tissue receptors.
   C. Their target tissues are always another endocrine gland.
   D. They represent the final hormone secreted in a complex negative feedback pathway.

2. Which instruction/precaution does the nurse teach a client to **prevent harm** during a 24-hour urine specimen collection?
   A. Be sure to keep the specimen cool for the entire collection period.
   B. Avoid splashing urine in the container when a preservative is present.
   C. Add the preservative to the collection container before adding any urine.
   D. Discard the first specimen that marks the beginning of the 24-hour test period.

REFERENCES

Burchum, J., & Rosenthal, L. (2019). *Lehne's pharmacology for nursing care* (10th ed.). St. Louis: Elsevier.

Jarvis, C. (2020). *Physical examination & health assessment* (8th ed.). St. Louis: Elsevier.

Lamberts, S., & van den Beld, A. (2016). Endocrinology and aging. In S. Melmed, K. Polonsky, P. R. Larsen, & H. Kronenberg (Eds.), *Williams' textbook of endocrinology* (13th ed.). Philadelphia: Elsevier.

Lazar, M., & Birnbaum, M. (2016). Principles of hormone actions. In S. Melmed, K. Polonsky, P. R. Larsen, & H. Kronenberg (Eds.), *Williams' textbook of endocrinology* (13th ed.). Philadelphia: Elsevier.

McCance, K., Huether, S., Brashers, V., & Rote, N. (2019). *Pathophysiology: The biologic basis for disease in adults and children* (8th ed.). St. Louis: Elsevier.

Sluss, P., & Hayes, F. (2016). Laboratory techniques for recognition of endocrine disorders. In S. Melmed, K. Polonsky, P. R. Larsen, & H. Kronenberg (Eds.), *Williams' textbook of endocrinology* (13th ed.). Philadelphia: Elsevier.

Touhy, T., & Jett, K. (2020). *Ebersole and Hess' toward healthy aging: Human needs and nursing response* (10th ed.) St. Louis: Mosby.

57

Concepts of Care for Patients With Pituitary and Adrenal Gland Problems

M. Linda Workman

http://evolve.elsevier.com/Iggy/

LEARNING OUTCOMES

1. Collaborate with the interprofessional team to coordinate high-quality care and promote ***fluid and electrolyte balance, cellular regulation,*** and ***immunity*** in patients who have pituitary or adrenal disorders.
2. Apply knowledge of anatomy, physiology, and pathophysiology to assess patients with impaired pituitary or adrenal gland function affecting ***fluid and electrolyte balance, cellular regulation,*** or ***immunity.***
3. Implement nursing actions to help the patient and family cope with the psychosocial impact caused by acute or chronic problems of the pituitary or adrenal gland.
4. Interpret clinical changes and laboratory data to determine the effectiveness of therapy for diabetes insipidus (DI) and for syndrome of inappropriate antidiuretic hormone (SIADH).
5. Use clinical judgment to prioritize evidence-based nursing care for the patient with acute adrenal insufficiency, hypercortisolism, and any other pituitary or adrenal problems.
6. Teach the patient and caregiver(s) about common drugs and other management strategies used for pituitary or adrenal gland problems.

KEY TERMS

acute adrenal insufficiency A life-threatening event in which the need for cortisol and aldosterone is greater than the body's supply. Also known as *adrenal crisis* or *addisonian crisis.*

diabetes insipidus (DI) Disorder of the posterior pituitary gland in which water loss is caused by either an antidiuretic hormone (ADH) deficiency or an inability of the kidneys to respond to ADH.

gynecomastia Male breast tissue development.

hyperaldosteronism Increased secretion of aldosterone with mineralocorticoid excess.

hypercortisolism (Cushing disease) The excess secretion of cortisol from the adrenal cortex, causing many problems.

hyperpituitarism Hormone oversecretion that occurs with anterior pituitary tumors or tissue hyperplasia (tissue overgrowth).

hypophysectomy Surgical removal of the pituitary gland.

hypopituitarism A deficiency of one and sometimes more than one pituitary hormone.

syndrome of inappropriate antidiuretic hormone (SIADH) A problem in which vasopressin (antidiuretic hormone [ADH]) is secreted even when plasma osmolarity is low or normal, resulting in water retention and fluid overload. (Also known as *Schwartz-Bartter syndrome.*)

virilization Presence of male secondary sex characteristics.

PRIORITY AND INTERRELATED CONCEPTS

The priority concept for this chapter is:

- ***Fluid and Electrolyte Balance***

The ***Fluid and Electrolyte Balance*** concept exemplar for this chapter is Hypercortisolism (Cushing Disease).

The interrelated concepts for this chapter are:

- ***Cellular Regulation***
- ***Immunity***

The pituitary and adrenal glands function to secrete hormones that affect the ***cellular regulation*** of the entire body, including ***fluid and electrolyte balance.*** When these hormones are secreted in either excessive or insufficient amounts, physical and psychological changes result. The anterior pituitary hormones regulate growth, metabolism, and sexual development. The posterior pituitary hormone, *vasopressin* (antidiuretic hormone [ADH]), helps maintain ***fluid and electrolyte balance.*** Adrenal gland hormones are life sustaining.

A complete assessment is performed to detect specific clinical findings. The patient also often undergoes many diagnostic tests and relies on the nurse for explanations. Surgical intervention may be indicated. Priority nursing care for the patient with pituitary or adrenal gland disorders includes assessment, patient education, evaluating patient response to therapy, and providing support.

DISORDERS OF THE PITUITARY GLAND

HYPOPITUITARISM

Pathophysiology Review

The anterior pituitary gland *(adenohypophysis)* secretes the following hormones to maintain homeostasis:

- Growth hormone (GH; somatotropin)
- Thyrotropin (thyroid-stimulating hormone [TSH])
- Corticotropin (adrenocorticotropic hormone [ACTH])
- Follicle-stimulating hormone (FSH)
- Luteinizing hormone (LH)
- Melanocyte-stimulating hormone (MSH)
- Prolactin (PRL)

Hypopituitarism is a deficiency of one and sometimes more than one pituitary hormone. Most often only one pituitary hormone is deficient, a condition known as *selective hypopituitarism.* Decreased production of *all* of the anterior pituitary hormones *(panhypopituitarism)* is rare and much more serious (Mitchell-Brown & Stephens-DiLeo, 2017).

Deficiencies of *adrenocorticotropic hormone (ACTH)* or *thyroid-stimulating hormone (TSH)* are the *most* life threatening because they cause a decrease in the secretion of vital hormones from the adrenal and thyroid glands. Adrenal gland hypofunction is discussed later in this chapter; hypothyroidism is discussed in Chapter 58.

Deficiency of the gonadotropins (luteinizing hormone [LH] and follicle-stimulating hormone [FSH]—hormones that stimulate the gonads to produce sex hormones) changes sexual function in both men and women. In men, gonadotropin deficiency results in testicular failure with decreased testosterone production that may cause sterility. In women, gonadotropin deficiency results in ovarian failure, *amenorrhea* (absence of menstrual periods), and infertility.

Growth hormone (GH) deficiency changes tissue growth patterns by reducing liver production of *somatomedins.* These substances, especially somatomedin C, trigger growth and maintain bone, cartilage, and other tissues throughout life.

GH deficiency results from decreased GH production, failure of the liver to produce somatomedins, or failure of tissues to respond to the somatomedins. In adults, GH deficiency alters ***cellular regulation*** by increasing the rate of bone destructive activity, leading to thinner bones *(osteoporosis)* and an increased risk for fractures.

The cause of hypopituitarism varies. Benign or malignant pituitary tumors can compress and destroy pituitary tissue. Pituitary function can be impaired by malnutrition or rapid loss of body fat. Shock or severe hypotension reduces blood flow to the pituitary gland, leading to hypoxia, infarction, and reduced hormone secretion. Other causes of hypopituitarism include head trauma, brain tumors or infection, radiation or surgery of the head and brain, and the last stage of human immune deficiency virus (HIV) disease, HIV-III (AIDS). *Idiopathic hypopituitarism* has an unknown cause.

Postpartum hemorrhage is the most common cause of pituitary infarction, which results in decreased hormone secretion. This clinical problem is known as *Sheehan syndrome.* The pituitary gland normally enlarges during pregnancy; if hemorrhage and hypotension occur during delivery, hemorrhage with ischemia and necrosis of the gland can occur.

❖ Interprofessional Collaborative Care

Patients with hypopituitarism require lifelong hormone replacement therapy (HRT). Such patients can be found in the community and in any care setting. It is important that HRT continues when they are admitted to an acute care setting for any reason.

◆ **Assessment: Recognize Cues.** Deficiencies of specific pituitary hormones cause changes in target organ function and even physical appearance. See the specific changes outlined in the Key Features: Pituitary Hypofunction box.

Gonadotropin (LH and FSH) deficiency changes secondary sex characteristics in men and women. Men may have facial and body hair loss. Ask about impotence and decreased *libido* (sex drive). Women may report amenorrhea, *dyspareunia* (painful intercourse), infertility, and decreased libido. Women may also have dry skin, breast atrophy, and a decrease or absence of axillary and pubic hair.

Neurologic symptoms of hypopituitarism as a result of tumor growth often first occur as changes in vision. Assess for changes in the patient's vision, especially peripheral vision. Headaches, *diplopia* (double vision), and limited eye movement are common.

Laboratory findings vary widely. Some pituitary hormone levels may be measured directly. Laboratory assessment of some pituitary hormones involves measuring the *effects* of the hormones rather than the actual hormone levels. For example, blood levels of triiodothyronine (T_3) and thyroxine (T_4) from the thyroid, testosterone and estradiol from the gonads, and prolactin levels are measured easily. If levels of any of these hormones are low, further pituitary evaluation is necessary.

Pituitary problems may cause changes in the *sella turcica* (the bony nest where the pituitary gland rests) (McCance et al., 2019). Changes include enlargement, erosion, and calcifications as a result of pituitary tumors, as well as soft-tissue lesions, seen most distinctly with CT and MRI (Pressman, 2017). An angiogram can help rule out an aneurysm or any other vascular problems in the area before surgery.

◆ **Interventions: Take Action.** Management of hypopituitarism focuses on replacement of all deficient hormones to ensure appropriate ***cellular regulation*** (Mitchell-Brown & Stephens-DiLeo, 2017). Men who have gonadotropin deficiency receive replacement therapy with androgens (testosterone), usually by the parenteral or transdermal route. Therapy begins with high-dose testosterone and is continued until **virilization** (presence of male secondary sex characteristics) is achieved. Positive responses include increases in penis size, libido, muscle mass, bone size, and bone strength, as well as increases in facial and body hair. After virilization is

KEY FEATURES

Pituitary Hypofunction

Deficient Hormone	Signs and Symptoms
Anterior Pituitary Hormones	
Growth hormone (GH)	Decreased bone density Pathologic fractures Decreased muscle strength Increased serum cholesterol levels
Gonadotropins Luteinizing hormone (LH) Follicle-stimulating hormone (FSH)	*Women:* Amenorrhea Anovulation Low estrogen levels Breast atrophy Loss of bone density Decreased axillary and pubic hair Decreased libido *Men:* Decreased facial hair Decreased ejaculate volume Reduced muscle mass Loss of bone density Decreased body hair Decreased libido Impotence
Thyroid-stimulating hormone (TSH, thyrotropin)	Decreased thyroid hormone levels Weight gain Intolerance to cold Scalp alopecia Hirsutism Menstrual abnormalities Decreased libido Slowed cognition Lethargy
Adrenocorticotropic hormone (ACTH)	Decreased serum cortisol levels Pale, sallow complexion Malaise and lethargy Anorexia Postural hypotension Headache Hypoglycemia Hyponatremia Decreased axillary and pubic hair (women)
Posterior Pituitary Hormones	
Antidiuretic hormone (ADH, vasopressin)	*Diabetes insipidus:* Greatly increased urine output Low urine specific gravity (<1.005) Hypotension Dehydration Increased plasma osmolarity Increased thirst Increased plasma electrolyte levels, especially sodium Urine output does not decrease when fluid intake decreases

achieved, the dose may be decreased, but continues throughout life. Therapy to increase fertility requires gonadotropin-releasing hormone (GnRH) injections, not testosterone therapy (Kaiser & Ho, 2016).

Androgen therapy is avoided in men with prostate cancer to prevent enhancing tumor cell growth. Side effects of therapy include **gynecomastia** (male breast tissue development), acne, baldness, and prostate enlargement.

Women who have gonadotropin deficiency receive HRT with a combination of estrogen and progesterone. The risk for hypertension or *thrombosis* (formation of blood clots in deep veins) is increased with estrogen therapy, especially among smokers and those who use nicotine in any form. Emphasize measures to reduce risk and the need for regular health visits. For inducing pregnancy, specific hormones may be given to trigger ovulation.

Adults with GH deficiency may be treated with subcutaneous injections of human growth hormone (hGH). Injections are given at night to mimic normal GH release (Kaiser & Ho, 2016).

HYPERPITUITARISM

Pathophysiology Review

Hyperpituitarism is hormone oversecretion that occurs with anterior pituitary tumors or tissue *hyperplasia* (tissue overgrowth). Tumors occur most often in the anterior pituitary cells that produce growth hormone (GH), prolactin (PRL), and adrenocorticotropic hormone (ACTH). Overproduction of PRL also may occur in response to tumors that overproduce GH and ACTH. Excess ACTH may occur with increased secretion of melanocyte-stimulating hormone (MSH).

PATIENT-CENTERED CARE: GENETIC/GENOMIC CONSIDERATIONS QSEN

One cause of hyperpituitarism is multiple endocrine neoplasia, type 1 (MEN1), in which there is inactivation of the suppressor gene *MEN1* (Online Mendelian Inheritance in Man [OMIM], 2017). MEN1 has an autosomal dominant inheritance pattern and may result in a benign tumor of the pituitary, parathyroid glands, or pancreas. In the pituitary, excessive production of growth hormone occurs and leads to acromegaly. Ask a patient with acromegaly whether either parent also has this problem or has had a tumor of the pancreas or parathyroid glands.

Most often hyperpituitarism is caused by a benign tumor *(adenoma)* within one pituitary cell type (Melmed et al., 2016). Adenomas are classified by the hormone secreted. As an adenoma gets larger and compresses brain tissue, neurologic changes, as well as endocrine problems, may occur. Symptoms may include vision changes, headache, and increased intracranial pressure (ICP). It can also be caused by a hypothalamic problem of excessive production of releasing hormones, which then overstimulate a normal pituitary gland.

Prolactin (PRL)-secreting tumors are the most common type of pituitary adenoma. Excessive PRL inhibits the secretion of gonadotropins and sex hormones in men and women, resulting in *galactorrhea* (breast milk production), amenorrhea, and infertility.

Overproduction of GH in adults results in *acromegaly* (Fig. 57.1). The onset is gradual with slow progression, and changes may remain unnoticed for years before diagnosis. Early detection and treatment are essential to prevent irreversible enlargement

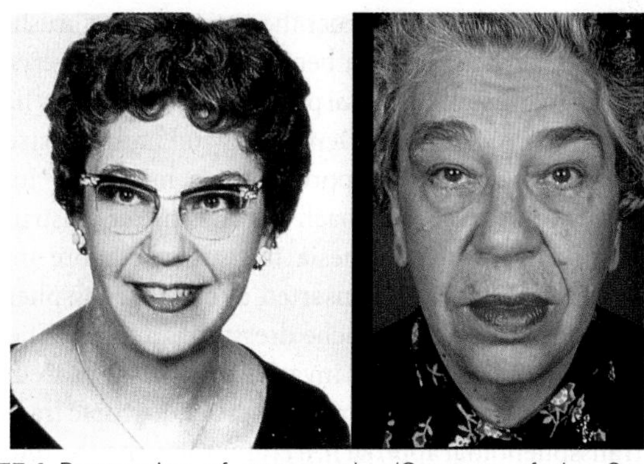

FIG. 57.1 Progression of acromegaly. (Courtesy of the Group for Research in Pathology Education [GRIPE], Oklahoma City, OK.)

of the face, hands, and feet. Other changes include increased skeletal thickness, hypertrophy of the skin, and enlargement of many organs such as the liver and heart. Some changes may be reversible after treatment, but skeletal changes are permanent.

Bone thinning and bone cell overgrowth occur slowly. Breakdown of joint cartilage and hypertrophy of ligaments, vocal cords, and eustachian tubes are common. Nerve entrapment and *hyperglycemia* (elevated blood glucose levels) are common.

Excess ACTH overstimulates the adrenal cortex. The result is excessive production of glucocorticoids, mineralocorticoids, and androgens, which leads to the development of Cushing disease or syndrome (see Fluid and Electrolyte Balance Concept Exemplar: Hypercortisolism [Cushing Disease]).

❖ Interprofessional Collaborative Care

Most care of a patient with hyperpituitarism occurs on an outpatient basis. When surgical intervention is required, hospitalization is necessary.

◆ **Assessment: Recognize Cues.** Symptoms of hyperpituitarism vary with the hormone produced in excess. Obtain the patient's age, gender, and family history. Ask about any change in hat, glove, ring, or shoe size and the presence of fatigue. The patient with high GH levels may have backache and joint pain from bone changes. Ask specifically about headaches and changes in vision.

The patient with hypersecretion of PRL often reports sexual function difficulty. Ask women about menstrual changes, decreased libido, painful intercourse, and any difficulty in becoming pregnant. Men may report decreased libido and impotence.

Usually only one hormone is produced in excess because the cell types within the pituitary gland are so individually organized and distinct. The most common hormones produced in excess with hyperpituitarism are PRL, ACTH, and GH. Changes in appearance and target organ function occur with excesses of specific anterior pituitary hormones as described in the Key Features: Anterior Pituitary Hyperfunction box.

Suppression testing can help diagnose hyperpituitarism. High blood glucose levels usually suppress the release of GH. Giving 100 g of oral glucose or 0.5 g/kg of body weight is followed by serial GH level measurements. GH levels that do not fall below 5 ng/mL (mcg/L) indicate a positive (abnormal) result associated with hyperpituitarism.

KEY FEATURES
Anterior Pituitary Hyperfunction

Prolactin (PRL)
- Hypogonadism (loss of secondary sexual characteristics)
- Decreased gonadotropin levels
- Galactorrhea
- Increased body fat
- Increased serum prolactin levels

Growth Hormone (GH), Acromegaly
- Thickened lips
- Coarse facial features
- Increasing head size
- Lower jaw protrusion
- Enlarged hands and feet
- Joint pain
- Barrel-shaped chest
- Hyperglycemia
- Sleep apnea
- Enlarged heart, lungs, and liver

Adrenocorticotropic Hormone (ACTH): Pituitary Cushing Syndrome
- Elevated plasma cortisol levels
- Weight gain
- Truncal obesity
- Moon face
- Extremity muscle wasting
- Loss of bone density
- Hypertension
- Hyperglycemia
- Striae and acne

Thyrotropin (Thyroid-Stimulating Hormone [TSH])
- Elevated plasma TSH and thyroid hormone levels
- Weight loss
- Tachycardia and dysrhythmias
- Heat intolerance
- Increased GI motility
- Fine tremors

Gonadotropins (Luteinizing Hormone [LH], Follicle-Stimulating Hormone [FSH])

Men
- Elevated LH and FSH levels
- Hypogonadism or hypergonadism

Women
- Normal LH and FSH levels

◆ **Interventions: Take Action.** The expected outcomes of management for hyperpituitarism are to return hormone levels to normal or near normal, reduce or eliminate headache and visual disturbances, prevent complications, and reverse as many of the body changes as possible.

Nonsurgical Management. Encourage the patient to express concerns about his or her altered physical appearance, such as galactorrhea, gynecomastia, and reduced sexual functioning. Reassure the patient that treatment may reverse some of these problems.

NCLEX EXAMINATION CHALLENGE 57.1

Physiological Integrity

A 30-year-old male client having an annual health physical reports that all of the following changes have developed during the past year. Which ones alert the nurse to possible pituitary hyperfunction? **Select all that apply.**

A. 15-lb weight gain
B. Decreased libido
C. Four sinus infections
D. Frequent constipation
E. Increased foot callus formation
F. Occasional dripping of clear fluid from both breasts
G. Severely sprained ankle from a volleyball injury

Drug therapy may be used alone or with surgery and/or radiation. Common drugs used are the dopamine agonists bromocriptine and cabergoline. These drugs stimulate dopamine receptors in the brain and inhibit the release of GH and PRL. Usually, small tumors decrease until the pituitary gland is of normal size and larger tumors decrease to some extent.

Side effects of bromocriptine include orthostatic (postural) hypotension, headaches, nausea, abdominal cramps, and constipation. Give bromocriptine with a meal or a snack to reduce GI side effects. Treatment starts with a low dose and is gradually increased until the desired level is reached. *If pregnancy occurs, the drug is stopped immediately.*

! NURSING SAFETY PRIORITY (QSEN)

Drug Alert

Teach patients taking bromocriptine to seek medical care immediately if chest pain, dizziness, or watery nasal discharge occurs because of the possibility of serious side effects, including cardiac dysrhythmias, coronary artery spasms, and cerebrospinal fluid leakage.

Other agents used for acromegaly are the somatostatin analogs, especially octreotide and lanreotide, and a growth hormone (GH) receptor blocker, pegvisomant (Burchum & Rosenthal, 2019). Octreotide inhibits GH release through negative feedback. Pegvisomant blocks GH receptor activity and blocks production of insulin-like growth factor (IGF). Combination therapy with monthly injections of a somatostatin analog and weekly injections of pegvisomant has provided good control of the disease.

Radiation therapy does not have immediate effects in reducing pituitary hormone excesses, and months to years may pass before a therapeutic effect can be seen. It is not recommended to manage acromegaly (Melmed & Kleinberg, 2016). The use of the Gamma Knife or stereotactic confocal radiotherapy method of delivering radiation to pituitary tumors has reduced the long-term side effects of this therapy.

Surgical Management. Surgical removal of the pituitary gland (**hypophysectomy**) along with any tumor is the most common treatment for hyperpituitarism. Successful surgery decreases hormone levels, relieves headaches, and may reverse changes in sexual functioning.

Preoperative Care. Explain that because nasal packing is present for 2 to 3 days after surgery, it will be necessary to breathe through the mouth, and a "mustache" dressing ("drip" pad) will be placed under the nose. Instruct the patient not to brush teeth, cough, sneeze, blow the nose, or bend forward after surgery. These activities can increase intracranial pressure (ICP) and delay healing.

Operative Procedures. Depending on tumor size and location, a transsphenoidal approach or a minimally invasive endoscopic transnasal approach with smaller instruments is used under general anesthesia instead of a more invasive procedure. Nasal packing is inserted after the transsphenoidal incision is closed, and a mustache dressing is applied. These are not needed for the minimally invasive transnasal procedure. If the tumor cannot be reached by either the endoscopic transnasal or the transsphenoidal approach, a craniotomy may be indicated (Melmed & Kleinberg, 2016) (see Chapter 41).

Postoperative Care. Monitor the patient's neurologic response and document any changes in vision or mental status, altered level of consciousness, or decreased extremity strength. Observe for complications such as transient diabetes insipidus (DI; discussed later in this chapter), cerebrospinal fluid (CSF) leakage, infection, and increased ICP.

Teach the patient to report any postnasal drip or increased swallowing, which may indicate leakage of cerebrospinal fluid (CSF). Keep the head of the bed elevated. Assess nasal drainage for quantity, quality, and the presence of glucose (present in CSF). A light yellow color at the edge of the clear drainage on the dressing is called the *halo sign* and indicates CSF. If the patient has persistent, severe headaches, CSF fluid may have leaked into the sinus area. Most CSF leaks resolve with bedrest, and surgical intervention is rarely needed.

Teach the patient to avoid coughing early after surgery because it increases pressure in the incision area and may lead to a CSF leak. Remind him or her to perform deep-breathing hourly while awake to prevent pulmonary problems. Instruct the patient to rinse the mouth frequently and to apply a lubricating jelly to dry lips to manage the dryness from mouth breathing.

Assess for indications of infection, especially meningitis, such as headache, fever, and nuchal (neck) rigidity. The surgeon may prescribe antibiotics, analgesics, and antipyretics.

If the entire pituitary gland has been removed, replacement of thyroid hormones and glucocorticoids is lifelong. See the Best Practice for Patient Safety & Quality Care: The Patient After Hypophysectomy box for specific nursing actions after hypophysectomy.

BEST PRACTICE FOR PATIENT SAFETY & QUALITY CARE (QSEN)

The Patient After Hypophysectomy

- Monitor the patient's neurologic status hourly for the first 24 hours and then every 4 hours.
- Monitor fluid balance, especially for output greater than intake.
- Encourage the patient to perform deep-breathing exercises.
- Instruct the patient not to cough, blow the nose, or sneeze.
- Instruct the patient to use dental floss and oral mouth rinses rather than toothbrushing until the surgeon gives permission.
- Instruct the patient to avoid bending at the waist to prevent increasing intracranial pressure.
- Monitor the nasal drip pad for the type and amount of drainage.
- Teach the patient methods to avoid constipation and subsequent "straining."
- Teach the patient self-administration of the prescribed hormones.

After surgery the patient needs daily self-management regimens and frequent checkups. Advise the patient to avoid activities that might interfere with healing or increase intracranial pressure (ICP). Teach him or her to avoid bending over from the waist to pick up objects or tie shoes because this position increases ICP. Teach the patient to bend the knees and then lower the body to pick up fallen objects. ICP also increases when the patient strains to have a bowel movement. Suggest techniques to prevent constipation, such as eating high-fiber foods, drinking plenty of fluids, and using stool softeners or laxatives.

Teach the patient to avoid toothbrushing for about 2 weeks after transsphenoidal surgery. Frequent mouth care with mouthwash and daily flossing provide adequate oral hygiene. A decreased sense of smell is expected after surgery and usually lasts 3 to 4 months.

Hormone replacement with vasopressin may be needed to maintain fluid balance (See discussion of Interventions in the Diabetes Insipidus section). If the anterior portion of the pituitary gland is removed, instruct the patient in cortisol, thyroid, and gonadal hormone replacement. Teach the patient to report the return of any symptoms of hyperpituitarism immediately to the primary health care provider.

DIABETES INSIPIDUS

Pathophysiology Review

Diabetes insipidus (DI) is a disorder of the posterior pituitary gland in which water loss is caused by either an antidiuretic hormone (ADH) deficiency or an inability of the kidneys to respond to ADH. The result of DI is the excretion of large volumes of dilute urine because the distal kidney tubules and collecting ducts do not reabsorb water; this leads to *polyuria* (excessive water loss through urination), dehydration, and disturbed ***fluid and electrolyte balance***.

Massive water loss increases plasma osmolarity and serum sodium levels, which stimulate the sensation of thirst. Thirst promotes increased fluid intake and aids in maintaining hydration. *If the thirst mechanism is poor or if the adult cannot obtain water independently, dehydration becomes more severe and can lead to death* (Robinson & Verbalis, 2016).

NURSING SAFETY PRIORITY QSEN

Action Alert

Ensure that no patient suspected of having DI is deprived of fluids for more than 4 hours because he or she cannot reduce urine output and severe dehydration can result.

ADH deficiency is classified as neurogenic (primary or secondary), nephrogenic, or drug related, depending on whether the problem is caused by insufficient production of ADH or an inability of the kidney to respond to the presence of ADH.

Primary neurogenic diabetes insipidus is caused by a defect in the hypothalamus or pituitary gland, resulting in a lack of ADH production or release. *Secondary neurogenic diabetes insipidus* is not caused by an abnormal posterior pituitary gland but is a result of tumors in or near the hypothalamus or pituitary gland, head trauma, infectious processes, or brain surgery.

Nephrogenic diabetes insipidus is a problem with the kidney's response to ADH rather than a problem with ADH production. A severe kidney injury can reduce the ability of the kidney tubules to respond to ADH. Then as long as the kidney is able to continue to produce urine, DI results. In some cases, a mutation in the gene responsible for producing the ADH receptor interferes with kidney response to ADH.

Drug-related diabetes insipidus is most often caused by lithium carbonate and demeclocycline (Robinson & Verbalis, 2016). These drugs can interfere with the response of the kidneys to ADH.

PATIENT-CENTERED CARE: GENETIC/GENOMIC CONSIDERATIONS QSEN

Nephrogenic diabetes insipidus (DI) can be a genetic disorder in which the ADH receptor (vasopressin receptor) has a defect that prevents kidney tubules from interacting with ADH. The result is poor water reabsorption by the kidney, although the actual amount of hormone produced is not deficient. This problem is most commonly inherited as an X-linked recessive disorder affecting only males (OMIM, 2019). A rarer genetic problem caused by autosomal recessive inheritance of a different mutated gene results in both males and females being affected. When assessing a patient with DI, always ask whether anyone else in the family has ever had this disorder.

❖ Interprofessional Collaborative Care

◆ **Assessment: Recognize Cues.** Most symptoms of DI are related to dehydration, as shown in the Key Features: Diabetes Insipidus box. Symptoms include an increase in urination and excessive thirst. Ask about a history of recent surgery, head trauma, or drug use (e.g., lithium). Although increased fluid intake prevents serious volume depletion, the patient who is deprived of fluids or who cannot increase oral fluid intake may develop shock from fluid loss. Symptoms of dehydration (e.g., poor skin turgor, dry or cracked mucous membranes) may be present. (See Chapter 13 for discussion of dehydration.)

Water loss changes blood and urine tests. The 24-hour fluid intake and output is measured without restricting food or fluid intake. DI is considered if urine output is more than 4 L during this period and is greater than the volume ingested. The amount of urine excreted in 24 hours by patients with DI may vary from 4 to 30 L/day. Urine is dilute with a low specific gravity (less than 1.005) and low osmolarity (50 to 200 mOsm/kg) or osmolality (50 to 200 mOsm/L).

◆ **Interventions: Take Action.** Management focuses on controlling symptoms using drug therapy with desmopressin (Burchum & Rosenthal, 2019). This drug, a synthetic form of vasopressin, replaces antidiuretic hormone (ADH) and decreases urination. It is available orally, as a sublingual "melt," or intranasally in a metered spray. The frequency of dosing varies with patient responses. Teach those patients who have mild DI that they may need only one or two doses in

KEY FEATURES
Diabetes Insipidus

Cardiovascular Symptoms
- Hypotension
- Tachycardia
- Weak peripheral pulses
- Hemoconcentration

Kidney/Urinary Symptoms
- Increased urine output
- Dilute, low specific gravity

Skin Symptoms
- Poor turgor
- Dry mucous membranes

Neurologic Symptoms
- Decreased cognition[a]
- Ataxia[a]
- Increased thirst
- Irritability[a]

[a]Occurs when access to water is limited and rapid dehydration results.

24 hours. For more severe DI, one or two metered doses two or three times daily may be needed. During severe dehydration, ADH may be given IV or IM. Ulceration of the mucous membranes, allergy, a sensation of chest tightness, and lung inhalation of the spray may occur with use of the intranasal preparations. If side effects occur or if the patient has an upper respiratory infection, oral or subcutaneous vasopressin is used.

NURSING SAFETY PRIORITY QSEN
Drug Alert

The parenteral form of desmopressin is 10 times stronger than the oral form, and the dosage must be reduced.

For the hospitalized patient with DI, nursing management focuses on early detection of dehydration and maintaining adequate hydration. Actions include accurately measuring fluid intake and output, checking urine specific gravity, and recording the patient's weight daily.

Urge the patient to drink fluids in an amount equal to urine output. If fluids are given IV, ensure the patency of the access catheter and accurately monitor the amount infused hourly.

The patient with permanent DI requires lifelong drug therapy. Check his or her ability to assess symptoms, and adjust dosages as prescribed for changes in conditions. Teach that polyuria and polydipsia indicate the need for another dose.

Drug therapy for DI induces water retention and can cause fluid overload (see Chapter 13). *Teach patients to weigh themselves daily to identify weight gain.* Stress the importance of using the same scale and weighing at the same time of day while wearing a similar amount and type of clothing. If weight gain of more than 2.2 lb (1 kg) along with other signs of water toxicity occurs (e.g., persistent headache, acute confusion, nausea, vomiting), instruct him or her to go immediately to the emergency department or call 911. Instruct the patient to wear a medical alert bracelet identifying the disorder and drug.

NCLEX EXAMINATION CHALLENGE 57.2
Safe and Effective Care Environment

Which urine characteristics indicate to the nurse that the client being managed for diabetes insipidus is responding appropriately to interventions?

A. Urine output volume increased; urine specific gravity increased
B. Urine output volume increased; urine specific gravity decreased
C. Urine output volume decreased; urine specific gravity increased
D. Urine output volume decreased; urine specific gravity decreased

SYNDROME OF INAPPROPRIATE ANTIDIURETIC HORMONE

Pathophysiology Review

The **syndrome of inappropriate antidiuretic hormone (SIADH)** or *Schwartz-Bartter syndrome* is a problem in which antidiuretic hormone (ADH, vasopressin) is secreted even when plasma osmolarity is low or normal, resulting in water retention and fluid overload. A decrease in plasma osmolarity normally inhibits ADH production and secretion. SIADH occurs with many conditions (e.g., cancer therapy, pulmonary infection or impairment) and with specific drugs, including selective serotonin reuptake inhibitors (Robinson & Verbalis, 2016). Table 57.1 lists common causes of SIADH.

In SIADH, ADH continues to be released when not needed, leading to water retention and disturbances of ***fluid and electrolyte balance***. Water retention results in dilutional *hyponatremia* (a decreased serum sodium level) and fluid overload. The increase in blood volume increases the kidney filtration and inhibits the release of renin and aldosterone, which increase urine sodium loss and results in greater hyponatremia.

Interprofessional Collaborative Care

Assessment: Recognize Cues. Ask the patient about his or her medical history, which may reveal conditions that can cause SIADH. Specifically obtain information about the conditions listed in Table 57.1.

Early symptoms of SIADH are related to the water-retention causing dilution of serum sodium levels *(hyponatremia)*. GI disturbances, such as loss of appetite, nausea, and vomiting, may occur first, as discussed in Chapter 13. Weigh the patient and document any recent weight gain. Use this information to monitor responses to therapy. In SIADH, free water (not salt) is retained and dependent edema is not usually present, even though water is retained.

Water retention, hyponatremia, and fluid shifts affect central nervous system function, especially when the serum sodium level is below 115 mEq/L (mmol/L). The patient may have lethargy, headaches, hostility, disorientation, and a change in level of consciousness. Lethargy and headaches can progress to decreased responsiveness, seizures, and coma. Assess deep tendon reflexes, which are usually decreased.

Vital sign changes include full and bounding pulse (caused by the increased fluid volume) and hypothermia (caused by

TABLE 57.1 Conditions Causing the Syndrome of Inappropriate Antidiuretic Hormone

Malignancies	CNS Disorders
• Small cell lung cancer	• Trauma
• Pancreatic, duodenal, and GU carcinomas	• Infection
• Thymoma	• Tumors (primary or metastatic)
• Hodgkin lymphoma	• Strokes
• Non-Hodgkin lymphoma	• Porphyria
	• Systemic lupus erythematosus
Pulmonary Disorders	**Drugs**
• Viral and bacterial pneumonia	• Exogenous ADH
• Lung abscesses	• Chlorpropamide
• Active tuberculosis	• Vincristine
• Pneumothorax	• Cyclophosphamide
• Chronic lung diseases	• Carbamazepine
• Mycoses	• Opioids
• Positive-pressure ventilation	• Tricyclic antidepressants
	• General anesthetics
	• Fluoroquinolone antibiotics

ADH, Antidiuretic hormone; *CNS*, central nervous system; *GU*, genitourinary.

central nervous system disturbance). Chapter 13 presents other findings that occur with hyponatremia.

Water retention causes urine volume to decrease and urine osmolarity to increase. At the same time, plasma volume increases, and plasma osmolarity decreases. Elevated urine sodium levels and specific gravity reflect increased urine concentration. Serum sodium levels decrease, sometimes to as low as 110 mEq/L (mmol/L), because of fluid retention and sodium loss.

◆ **Interventions: Take Action.** Interventions for SIADH focus on restricting fluid intake, promoting the excretion of water, replacing lost sodium, and interfering with the action of ADH. Nursing interventions include monitoring response to therapy, preventing complications, teaching the patient and family about fluid restrictions and drug therapy, and preventing injury.

Fluid restriction is essential because fluid intake further dilutes plasma sodium levels. In some cases, fluid intake may be kept as low as 500 to 1000 mL/24 hr. Use saline instead of water to dilute tube feedings, irrigate GI tubes, and give drugs by GI tube.

Measure intake, output, and daily weights to assess the degree of fluid restriction needed. A weight gain of 2.2 lb (1 kg) or more per day or a gradual increase over several days is cause for concern. A 2.2-lb (1-kg) increase is equal to a 1000-mL fluid retention (1 kg = 1 L). Prevent mouth dryness with frequent oral rinsing (warn patients not to swallow the rinses).

Drug therapy with vasopressin receptor antagonists (vaptans), such as tolvaptan or conivaptan, is used to treat SIADH when hyponatremia is present in hospitalized patients (Burchum & Rosenthal, 2019). These drugs promote water excretion without causing sodium loss. Tolvaptan is an oral drug, and conivaptan is given IV. Tolvaptan has a black box warning that rapid increases in serum sodium levels (those greater than a 12-mEq/L [mmol/L] increase in 24 hours) have been associated with central nervous system demyelination that can lead to serious complications and death. When this drug is used at higher dosages or for longer than 30 days, there is a significant risk for liver failure and death (Robinson & Verbalis, 2016).

! NURSING SAFETY PRIORITY (QSEN)

Drug Alert

Administer tolvaptan or conivaptan only in the hospital setting so serum sodium levels can be monitored closely for the development of hypernatremia and other complications.

Diuretics may be used on a limited basis to manage SIADH when sodium levels are near normal and heart failure is present. With diuretics, sodium loss can be potentiated, further contributing to the problems caused by SIADH. For milder SIADH, demeclocycline, an oral antibiotic, may help reach ***fluid and electrolyte balance***, although the drug is not approved for this problem.

Hypertonic saline (i.e., 3% sodium chloride [3% NaCl]) is used for SIADH when the serum sodium level is very low (Robinson & Verbalis, 2016). Give IV saline cautiously because it may add to existing fluid overload and promote heart failure. If the patient needs routine IV fluids, a saline solution is prescribed to prevent further sodium dilution.

Monitor the patient's response to therapy to prevent the fluid overload from becoming worse, leading to pulmonary edema and heart failure. Any patient with SIADH, regardless of age, is at risk for these complications. The older adult or one who also has cardiac, kidney, pulmonary, or liver problems is at greater risk.

Monitor for increased fluid overload (bounding pulse, increasing neck vein distention, lung crackles, dyspnea, increasing peripheral edema, reduced urine output) at least every 2 hours. *Pulmonary edema can occur very quickly and can lead to death.* Notify the primary health care provider of any change that indicates the fluid overload is not responding to therapy or is worse.

Providing a safe environment is needed when the serum sodium level falls below 120 mEq/L (mmol/L). The risk for neurologic changes and seizures increases as a result of osmotic fluid shifts into brain tissue. Observe for and document changes in the patient's neurologic status. Assess for subtle changes, such as muscle twitching, increasing irritability, or restlessness, before these progress to seizures or coma. Check orientation to time, place, and person every 2 hours because disorientation or confusion may be present as an early indication. Reduce environmental noise and lighting to prevent overstimulation.

The frequency of neurologic checks depends on the patient's status. For the patient being treated for SIADH who is hyponatremic but alert, awake, and oriented, checks every 2 to 4 hours may be sufficient. For the patient who has had a change in level of consciousness, perform neurologic checks at least every hour or as prescribed. Inspect the environment every shift, making sure that basic safety measures, such as side rails being securely in place, are observed.

DISORDERS OF THE ADRENAL GLAND

ADRENAL GLAND HYPOFUNCTION

Pathophysiology Review

Adrenal cortex production of steroid hormone may decrease as a result of inadequate secretion of adrenocorticotropic hormone (ACTH), dysfunction of the hypothalamic-pituitary control mechanism, or direct problems of adrenal gland tissue (Cole, 2018). Symptoms may develop gradually or occur quickly with stress. In acute adrenocortical insufficiency *(adrenal crisis)*, life-threatening symptoms may appear without warning.

Insufficiency of adrenocortical steroids causes problems through the loss of aldosterone and cortisol action. Decreased cortisol levels result in hypoglycemia. Gastric acid production and glomerular filtration decrease. Decreased glomerular filtration leads to excessive blood urea nitrogen (BUN) levels, which cause anorexia and weight loss.

Reduced aldosterone secretion causes disturbances of ***fluid and electrolyte balance***. Potassium excretion is decreased, causing hyperkalemia. Sodium and water excretion are increased, causing hyponatremia and hypovolemia. Potassium retention also promotes reabsorption of hydrogen ions, which can lead to acidosis.

Low adrenal androgen levels decrease body, axillary, and pubic hair, especially in women, because the adrenals produce most of the androgens in females. The severity of symptoms is related to the degree of hormone deficiency.

Acute adrenal insufficiency *(addisonian crisis)* is a life-threatening event in which the need for cortisol and aldosterone is greater than the body's supply (Cole, 2018; McCance et al., 2019). It often occurs in response to a stressful event (e.g., surgery, trauma, severe infection), especially when the adrenal hormone output is already reduced. Problems are the same as those of chronic insufficiency but are more severe. *However, unless intervention is initiated promptly, sodium levels fall, and potassium levels rise rapidly (Pereira, 2016). Severe hypotension results from the blood volume depletion that occurs with the loss of aldosterone.* Emergency care actions for patients with acute adrenal insufficiency are listed in the Best Practice for Patient Safety & Quality Care box.

Adrenal insufficiency is classified as primary or secondary. Causes of primary and secondary adrenal insufficiency are listed in Table 57.2. A common cause of secondary adrenal insufficiency is the sudden cessation of long-term glucocorticoid therapy. This therapy suppresses production of glucocorticoids through negative feedback and causes atrophy of the adrenal cortex. Glucocorticoid drugs must be withdrawn gradually to allow for pituitary production of ACTH and activation of adrenal cells to produce cortisol.

BEST PRACTICE FOR PATIENT SAFETY & QUALITY CARE (QSEN)

Emergency Management of the Patient With Acute Adrenal Insufficiency

Hormone Replacement

- Start rapid infusion of normal saline or dextrose 5% in normal saline.
- Initial higher doses of hydrocortisone sodium or dexamethasone is administered as an IV bolus.
- Administer additional hydrocortisone sodium by continuous IV infusion over the next 8 hours.
- Give an additional dose of hydrocortisone IM concomitantly with hydration every 12 hours.
- Initiate an H_2 histamine blocker (e.g., cimetidine) IV for ulcer prevention.

Hyperkalemia Management

- Administer insulin in units equal to the same number of mg of extra dextrose in normal saline intravenously to shift potassium into cells.
- Give potassium binding and excreting resin.
- Give loop or thiazide diuretics.
- Avoid potassium-sparing diuretics, as prescribed.
- Initiate potassium restriction.
- Monitor intake and output.
- Monitor heart rate, rhythm, and ECG for signs and symptoms of hyperkalemia (slow heart rate; heart block; tall, peaked T waves; fibrillation; asystole).

Hypoglycemia Management

- Administer IV glucose as prescribed.
- Prepare to administer glucagon as needed and prescribed.
- Maintain IV access.
- Monitor blood glucose level hourly.

TABLE 57.2 Causes of Primary and Secondary Adrenal Insufficiency

Primary Causes	Secondary Causes
Autoimmune disease[a]	Pituitary tumors
Tuberculosis	Postpartum pituitary necrosis
Metastatic cancer	Hypophysectomy
HIV-III (AIDS)	High-dose pituitary or whole-brain radiation
Hemorrhage	Cessation of long-term corticosteroid drug therapy[a]
Gram-negative sepsis	
Adrenalectomy	
Abdominal radiation therapy	
Drugs (mitotane) and toxins	

[a]Most common cause.

❖ Interprofessional Collaborative Care

Acute adrenal insufficiency is an emergency and managed in an acute care setting. Without appropriate management, death ensues (Amrein et al., 2018).

◆ Assessment: Recognize Cues

History. Ask about symptoms and factors that cause adrenal hypofunction. Ask about any change in activity level because lethargy, fatigue, and muscle weakness are often present.

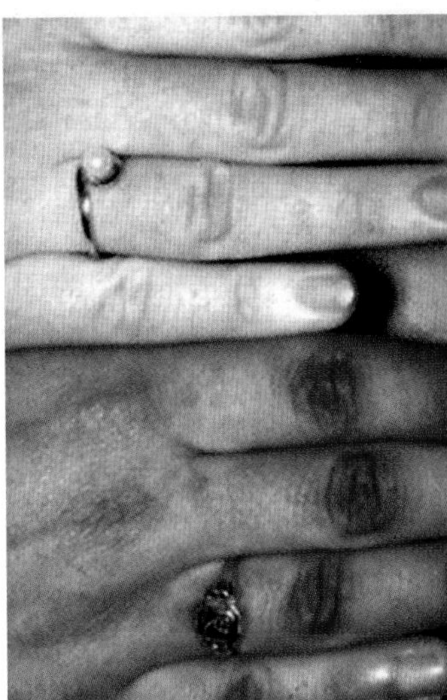

FIG. 57.2 Increased pigmentation seen in primary adrenocortical insufficiency. (From Wilson, J.D., Foster, D., Kronenberg, H., & Larsen, P.R. [1998]. *Williams' textbook of endocrinology* [9th ed.]. Philadelphia: Saunders. Courtesy Dr. H. Patrick Higgins.)

Include questions about salt intake, because salt craving often occurs with hypofunction.

GI problems, such as anorexia, nausea, vomiting, diarrhea, and abdominal pain, often occur. Ask about weight loss during the past months. Women may have menstrual changes related to weight loss, and men may report impotence.

Ask whether the patient has had radiation to the abdomen or head. Abdominal radiation could directly damage the adrenal glands, whereas cranial radiation could interfere with hypothalamic or pituitary influences on adrenal function. Document medical problems (e.g., tuberculosis or previous intracranial surgery) and all past and current drugs, especially steroids, anticoagulants, opioids, and cancer drugs.

Physical Assessment/Signs and Symptoms. Symptoms of adrenal insufficiency vary, and the severity is related to the degree of hormone deficiency as listed in the Key Features: Adrenal Insufficiency box. In patients with primary insufficiency (problem with adrenal gland function), plasma ACTH and melanocyte-stimulating hormone (MSH) levels are elevated in response to the adrenal-hypothalamic-pituitary feedback system. (Both ACTH and MSH are made from the same prehormone molecule. Anything that stimulates increased production of ACTH often also leads to increased production of MSH.) Elevated MSH levels result in areas of *increased* pigmentation (Fig. 57.2). In primary autoimmune disease, patchy areas of *decreased* pigmentation *(vitiligo)* may occur because of destruction of skin melanocytes. Body hair may also be decreased. In secondary adrenal insufficiency (problem in the hypothalamus or pituitary gland leading to decreased ACTH and MSH levels), skin pigmentation is not changed.

Assess for hypoglycemia (e.g., sweating, headaches, tachycardia, and tremors) and fluid depletion (postural hypotension and dehydration). *Hyperkalemia* (elevated blood potassium levels) can cause dysrhythmias with an irregular heart rate and result in cardiac arrest. *Hyponatremia* (low blood sodium levels) leading to hypotension and decreased

KEY FEATURES

Adrenal Insufficiency

Neuromuscular Symptoms
- Muscle weakness
- Fatigue
- Joint and/or muscle pain

Gastrointestinal Symptoms
- Anorexia
- Nausea, vomiting
- Abdominal pain
- Constipation or diarrhea
- Weight loss
- Salt craving

Skin Symptoms
- Vitiligo

or

- Hyperpigmentation

Cardiovascular Symptoms
- Anemia
- Hypotension
- Hyponatremia
- Hyperkalemia
- Hypercalcemia

cognition is often one of the first indicators of adrenal insufficiency (Pereira, 2016).

Psychosocial Assessment. Depending on the degree of imbalance, patients may appear lethargic, depressed, confused, and even psychotic. Assess the patient's orientation to person, place, and time. Families may report that the patient has wide mood swings and is forgetful.

Diagnostic Assessment. Laboratory findings are listed in the Laboratory Profile: Adrenal Gland Assessment box and include low serum sodium and low salivary cortisol levels, low fasting blood glucose, elevated potassium, and increased blood urea nitrogen (BUN) levels. In primary disease, the eosinophil count and ACTH level are elevated. Plasma cortisol levels do not rise during provocation tests (see Chapter 56).

Urinary 17-hydroxycorticosteroids are the glucocorticoid metabolites, and 17-ketosteroid levels reflect the adrenal androgen metabolites. Both levels are in the low or low-normal range in adrenal hypofunction.

An ACTH stimulation (provocative) test is the most definitive test for adrenal insufficiency. ACTH is given IV, and plasma cortisol levels are obtained at 30-minute and 1-hour intervals. In primary insufficiency, the cortisol response is absent or very decreased. In secondary insufficiency, it is increased. When acute adrenal insufficiency is suspected, treatment is started without stimulation testing (Stewart & Newell-Price, 2016).

Imaging Assessment. CT and MRI are most helpful in determining the cause of pituitary problems leading to adrenal insufficiency. CT and MRI can show adrenal gland atrophy, but not its cause.

◆ **Interventions: Take Action.** Nursing interventions focus on promoting fluid balance, monitoring for fluid deficit, and preventing hypoglycemia. Because hyperkalemia can cause dysrhythmias with an irregular heart rate and result in cardiac arrest, assessing cardiac function is a nursing priority. Assess vital signs every 1 to 4 hours, depending on the patient's condition and the presence of dysrhythmias or postural hypotension. Weigh the patient daily and record intake and output. Monitor laboratory values to identify hemoconcentration

LABORATORY PROFILE

Adrenal Gland Assessment

Test	Normal Range	Hypofunction	Hyperfunction
Sodium	136-145 mEq/L (mmol/L)	Low	High
Potassium	3.5-5.0 mEq/L (mmol/L)	High	Low
Glucose (fasting)	70-110 mg/dL (4-6 mmol/L)	Normal to low	Normal to high
Calcium	Total: 9-10.5 mg/dL (2.25-2.75 mmol/L) Ionized: 4.5-5.6 mg/dL (1.05-1.30 mmol/L)	High	Low
Bicarbonate	23-30 mEq/L (mmol/L)	High	Low
BUN	10-20 mg/dL (3.6-7.1 mmol/L)	High	Normal
Cortisol (serum)	6 a.m. to 8 a.m.: 5-23 mcg/dL (138-635 nmol/L) 4 p.m. to 6 p.m.: 3-13 mcg/dL (83-359 nmol/L)	Low	High
Cortisol (salivary)	7 a.m. to 9 a.m.: 100-750 ng/dL 3 p.m. to 5 p.m.: <401 ng/dL	Low	High

BUN, Blood urea nitrogen.
Data from Pagana, K., & Pagana, T. (2018). *Mosby's manual of diagnostic and laboratory tests* (6th ed.). St. Louis: Elsevier.

(e.g., increased hematocrit or BUN). Chapter 13 discusses dehydration in detail.

Cortisol and aldosterone deficiencies are corrected by hormone replacement therapy described in the Common Examples of Drug Therapy: Adrenal Hypofunction box. Hydrocortisone corrects glucocorticoid deficiency. Oral cortisol replacement regimens and dosages vary. The most common drug used for this purpose is prednisone. In general, divided doses are given, with two-thirds given on arising in the morning and one-third at 6:00 p.m. to mimic the normal release of this hormone.

NURSING SAFETY PRIORITY QSEN

Drug Alert

Prednisone and prednisolone are soundalike drugs, and care is needed not to confuse them. Although they are both corticosteroids, they are not interchangeable because prednisolone is more potent than prednisone.

An additional mineralocorticoid hormone, such as fludrocortisone, may be needed to maintain or restore ***fluid and electrolyte balance*** (especially sodium and potassium). Dosage adjustment may be needed, especially in hot weather when more sodium is lost because of excessive perspiration. *Salt restriction or diuretic therapy should not be started without considering whether it might lead to an adrenal crisis.*

NCLEX EXAMINATION CHALLENGE 57.3

Safe and Effective Care Environment

Which electrolyte laboratory values indicate to the nurse monitoring a client with adrenal insufficiency undergoing IV therapy with hydrocortisone that the client is responding positively to this drug therapy?

A. Serum sodium 147 mEq/L (mmol/L); serum potassium 7.1 mEq/L (mmol/L)
B. Serum sodium 137 mEq/L (mmol/L); serum potassium 4.9 mEq/L (mmol/L)
C. Serum sodium 127 mEq/L (mmol/L); serum potassium 2.8 mEq/L (mmol/L)
D. Serum sodium 119 mEq/L (mmol/L); serum potassium 6.2 mEq/L (mmol/L)

COMMON EXAMPLES OF DRUG THERAPY

Adrenal Hypofunction

Drug	Nursing Implications
Cortisone	Instruct the patient to take the drug with meals or a snack *to avoid gastric irritation.*
Hydrocortisone	Instruct the patient to report signs or symptoms of excessive drug therapy (e.g., rapid weight gain, round face, fluid retention), *which indicate Cushing syndrome and a possible need for a dosage adjustment.*
Prednisone	Instruct the patient to report illness *because the usual daily dosage may not be adequate during periods of illness or severe stress.*
Fludrocortisone	Monitor the patient's blood pressure *to assess for the potential side effect of hypertension.* Instruct the patient to report weight gain or edema *because sodium intake may need to be restricted.*

FLUID AND ELECTROLYTE BALANCE CONCEPT EXEMPLAR: HYPERCORTISOLISM (CUSHING DISEASE)

Pathophysiology Review

Hypercortisolism (Cushing disease) is the excess secretion of cortisol from the adrenal cortex, causing many problems. The disorder can be caused by a problem in the adrenal cortex itself, a problem in the anterior pituitary gland, or a problem in the hypothalamus. In addition, one of the most common causes of hypercortisolism is glucocorticoid therapy.

The presence of excess glucocorticoids, regardless of the cause, affects metabolism and all body systems. An increase in total body fat results from slow turnover of plasma fatty acids.

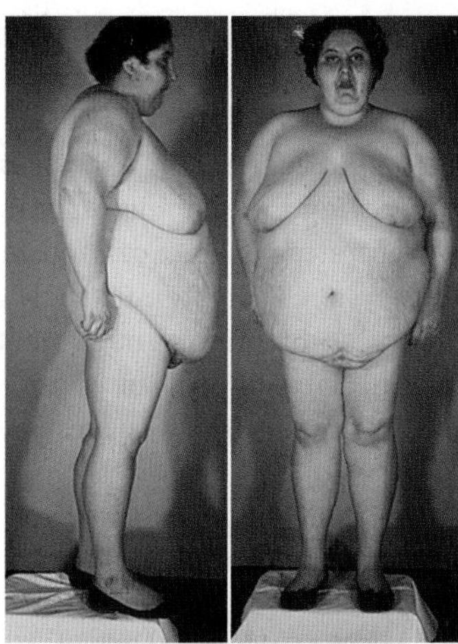

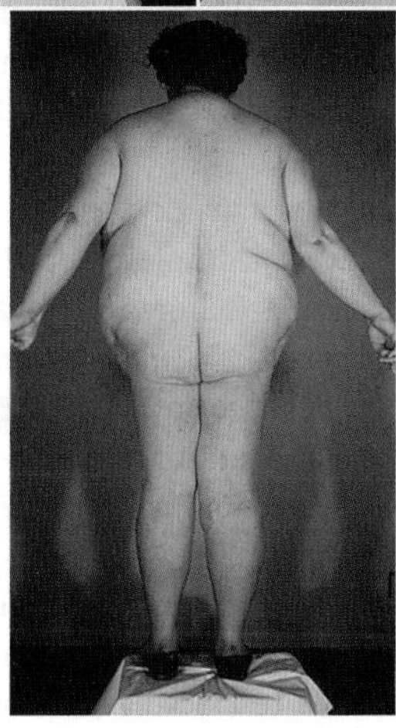

FIG. 57.3 Typical appearance of a patient with Cushing disease or syndrome. Note truncal obesity, moon face, buffalo hump, thinner arms and legs, and abdominal striae. (From Wenig, B.M., Heffess, C.S., & Adair, C.F. [1997]. *Atlas of endocrine pathology.* Philadelphia: Saunders.)

This fat is redistributed, producing truncal obesity, "buffalo hump," and "moon face" (Fig. 57.3) (Jarvis, 2020). Increases in the breakdown of tissue protein result in decreased muscle mass and muscle strength, thin skin, and fragile capillaries. Effects on minerals lead to bone density loss.

High levels of corticosteroids reduce lymphocyte production and shrink organs containing lymphocytes, such as the spleen and the lymph nodes. White blood cell (WBC) cytokine production is decreased. These changes reduce immunity and increase the risk for infection.

In most cases, increased androgen production also occurs and causes acne, *hirsutism* (increased body hair growth), and occasionally clitoral hypertrophy. Increased androgens disrupt the normal ovarian hormone feedback mechanism, decreasing the ovary's production of estrogens and progesterone. *Oligomenorrhea* (scant or infrequent menses) occurs as a result.

Etiology. Cushing disease or syndrome is a group of clinical problems caused by an excess of cortisol. Table 57.3 lists causes of cortisol excess. When the anterior pituitary gland oversecretes adrenocorticotropic hormone (ACTH), this hormone causes hyperplasia of the adrenal cortex in both adrenal glands and an excess of glucocorticoid production (shown in Fig. 56.3 in Chapter 56). This problem is *pituitary Cushing disease* because the tissue causing the problem is the pituitary, not the adrenal gland. When excess glucocorticoids are caused by a problem in the actual adrenal cortex, usually a benign tumor (adrenal adenoma), the problem is called *adrenal Cushing disease (or primary Cushing disease)* and usually occurs in only one adrenal gland. When glucocorticoid excess results from drug therapy for another health problem, it is known as *Cushing syndrome* (also called secondary Cushing syndrome).

TABLE 57.3 Conditions Causing Increased Cortisol Secretion

Endogenous Secretion (Cushing Disease)

- Bilateral adrenal hyperplasia[a]
- Pituitary adenoma increasing the production of ACTH (pituitary Cushing disease)
- Malignancies: carcinomas of the lung, GI tract, pancreas
- Adrenal adenomas or carcinomas

Exogenous Administration (Cushing Syndrome)

- Therapeutic use of ACTH or glucocorticoids—most commonly for treatment of:
  - Asthma
  - Autoimmune disorders
  - Organ transplantation
  - Cancer chemotherapy
  - Allergic responses
  - Chronic fibrosis

[a]Most common cause.
ACTH, Adrenocorticotropic hormone.

Incidence and Prevalence. The most common non–drug therapy–related cause of Cushing disease is a pituitary adenoma. Women are more likely than men to develop Cushing disease. Cushing syndrome from chronic use of exogenous corticosteroids is more common because these drugs are often used to control serious chronic inflammatory conditions (Nieman, 2018).

❖ Interprofessional Collaborative Care

◆ Assessment: Recognize Cues

History. Ask about the patient's other health problems and drug therapies because glucocorticoid drug therapy is common. Regardless of cause, the patient has many changes because of the widespread effect of excessive cortisol. He or she may report weight gain and an increased appetite. Ask about changes in activity or sleep patterns, fatigue, and muscle weakness. Ask about bone pain or a history of fractures, because osteoporosis results from hypercortisolism. Ask about a history of frequent infections and easy bruising. Women often stop menstruating. GI problems include ulcer formation from increased hydrochloric acid secretion and decreased production of protective gastric mucus.

Physical Assessment/Signs and Symptoms. The patient with hypercortisolism has specific, predictable physical changes, although

KEY FEATURES

Hypercortisolism (Cushing Disease/Syndrome)

General Appearance
- Moon face
- Buffalo hump
- Truncal obesity
- Weight gain

Cardiovascular Symptoms
- Hypertension
- Frequent dependent edema
- Bruising
- Petechiae

Immune System Symptoms
- Increased risk for infection
- Reduced immunity
- Decreased inflammatory responses
- Signs and symptoms of infection and inflammation possibly masked

Musculoskeletal Symptoms
- Muscle atrophy (most apparent in extremities)
- Osteoporosis with:
  - Fragile fractures
  - Decreased height and vertebral collapse
  - Aseptic necrosis of the femur head
  - Slow or poor healing of bone fractures

Skin Symptoms
- Thinning skin
- Increased facial and body hair
- Striae and increased pigmentation

all body systems are affected as described in the Key Features: Hypercortisolism (Cushing Disease/Syndrome) box (see Fig. 57.3). Changes in fat distribution may result in fat pads on the neck, back, and shoulders (buffalo hump); an enlarged trunk with thin arms and legs; and a round face (moon face). Other changes include muscle wasting and weakness. Assess for and document changes and use these findings to prioritize patient problems.

Skin changes result from blood vessel fragility and include bruises, thin or translucent skin, and wounds that have not healed. Reddish-purple *striae* (stretch marks) occur on the abdomen, thighs, and upper arms because of the destructive effect of cortisol on collagen.

Acne and a fine coating of hair may occur over the face and body. In women, look for the presence of hirsutism, clitoral hypertrophy, and male pattern balding related to androgen excess.

Cardiac changes occur as a result of disturbed ***fluid and electrolyte balance***. Both sodium and water are reabsorbed and retained, leading to hypervolemia and edema formation. Blood pressure is elevated, and pulses are full and bounding.

Musculoskeletal changes occur as a result of nitrogen depletion and mineral loss. Muscle mass decreases, especially in arms and legs (see Fig. 57.3). Muscle weakness increases the risk for falls. Bone is thinner, and osteoporosis is common, increasing the risk for fractures.

Glucose metabolism is affected by hypercortisolism. Fasting blood glucose levels are high because the liver releases glucose and the insulin receptors are less sensitive; therefore blood glucose does not move as easily into the tissues.

Immune changes caused by excess cortisol result in reduced ***immunity***. Excess cortisol reduces the number of circulating lymphocytes, inhibits macrophage activity, reduces antibody synthesis, and inhibits production of cytokines and inflammatory chemicals (e.g., histamine). Infection risk is increased; and the patient may not have fever, purulent exudate, or redness in the affected area when an infection is present.

Psychosocial Assessment. Hypercortisolism can result in emotional instability, and patients often say that they do not feel like themselves. Ask about mood swings, irritability, new-onset confusion, or depression. Ask the patient whether he or she has been crying or laughing inappropriately or has had difficulty concentrating. The excess hormones stimulate the central nervous system, heightening the awareness of and responses to sensory stimulation. The patient often reports sleep difficulties and fatigue. All of these changes along with the physical changes strongly suggest hypercortisolism (Nieman, 2018).

Laboratory Assessment. Laboratory tests include blood, salivary, and urine cortisol levels. These are high in patients with any type of hypercortisolism. Plasma ACTH levels vary, depending on the cause of the problem. In pituitary Cushing disease, ACTH levels are elevated. In adrenal Cushing disease or when Cushing syndrome results from chronic steroid use, ACTH levels are low.

Salivary cortisol levels may be used to detect hypercortisolism because these levels accurately reflect blood levels, especially late-night specimens. A normal salivary cortisol level is lower than 2.0 ng/mL. Higher levels indicate hypercortisolism.

Urine is tested to measure levels of free cortisol and the metabolites of cortisol and androgens (17-hydroxycorticosteroids and 17-ketosteroids). In Cushing disease, levels of urine cortisol and androgens are all elevated in a 24-hour specimen. Cortisol-to-creatinine ratios in the first specimen of the day can replace the 24-hour test for screening. A ratio greater than 25 nmol/mmol is a positive test result (Stewart & Newell-Price, 2016)

Dexamethasone suppression testing can screen for hypercortisolism and may take place overnight or over a 3-day period. Set doses of dexamethasone are given. A 24-hour urine collection follows drug administration. When urinary 17-hydroxycorticosteroid excretion and cortisol levels are suppressed by dexamethasone, Cushing disease is *not* present.

Additional laboratory findings that accompany hypercortisolism include:

- Increased blood glucose level
- Decreased lymphocyte count
- Increased sodium level
- Decreased serum calcium level

Imaging Assessment. Imaging for hypercortisolism includes CT scans, MRI, and arteriography. These images can identify lesions of the adrenal or pituitary glands, lung, GI tract, or pancreas (Mendiratta-Lala et al., 2017).

◆ **Analysis: Analyze Cues and Prioritize Hypotheses.** The priority problems for patients with Cushing disease or Cushing syndrome are:

1. Fluid overload due to hormone-induced water and sodium retention
2. Potential for injury due to skin thinning, poor wound healing, and bone density loss
3. Potential for infection due to hormone-induced reduced ***immunity***

◆ **Planning and Implementation: Generate Solutions and Take Action.** Expected outcomes of hypercortisolism management are the reduction of plasma cortisol levels, removal of tumors, and restoration of normal or acceptable body appearance. When the disorder is caused by pituitary or adrenal problems, cure is possible. When caused by drug therapy for another health problem, the focus is to prevent complications from hypercortisolism.

Restoring Fluid Volume Balance

Planning: Expected Outcomes. The patient with hypercortisolism is expected to achieve and maintain a normal or near-normal ***fluid and electrolyte balance***.

Interventions. Interventions for patients with fluid volume excess focus on ensuring patient safety, restoring ***fluid and electrolyte balance***, and providing supportive care. Depending on the cause, surgical management may be used to reduce cortisol production.

Nonsurgical interventions focus on patient safety, drug therapy, nutrition therapy, and monitoring; these interventions are the basis of nonsurgical action for hypercortisolism and fluid overload.

Patient safety includes preventing fluid overload from becoming worse, leading to pulmonary edema and heart failure. Any patient with fluid overload, regardless of age, is at risk for these complications. The older adult or one who has coexisting cardiac problems, kidney problems, pulmonary problems, or liver problems is at greater risk.

Monitor for indicators of fluid overload (bounding pulse, increasing neck vein distention, lung crackles, increasing peripheral edema, reduced urine output) at least every 2 hours. *Pulmonary edema can occur quickly and lead to death.* Notify the primary health care provider of any change that indicates fluid overload either is not responding to therapy or is worse.

The patient with fluid volume excess and dependent edema is at risk for skin breakdown. Use a pressure-reducing or pressure-relieving overlay on the mattress. Assess skin pressure areas, especially the coccyx, elbows, hips, and heels, daily for redness or open areas. For patients receiving oxygen by mask or nasal cannula, check the skin around the mask, nares, and ears and under the elastic band. Help the patient change positions every 2 hours or ensure that others assigned to perform the intervention are diligent in this action.

Drug therapy involves the use of drugs that interfere with adrenocorticotropic hormone (ACTH) production or adrenal hormone synthesis for temporary relief and are categorized as *steroidogenesis inhibitors*. Metyrapone, aminoglutethimide, ketoconazole, mitotane, and etomidate use different pathways to decrease cortisol production (Stewart & Newell-Price, 2016; Tritos & Biller, 2018). For patients with hypercortisolism resulting from increased ACTH production, cyproheptadine may be used because it interferes with ACTH production. For adults with increased ACTH production who have type 2 diabetes and who do not respond to other drug therapies, another drug is mifepristone, which is a synthetic steroid that blocks glucocorticoid receptors. Two additional drugs currently under investigation for use as steroid inhibitors are levoketoconazole and osilodrostat (Tritos & Biller, 2018).

! NURSING SAFETY PRIORITY (QSEN)

Drug Alert

Mifepristone cannot be used during pregnancy because it also blocks progesterone receptors and would cause termination of the pregnancy (Burchum & Rosenthal, 2019).

A drug to manage hypercortisolism resulting from a pituitary adenoma is pasireotide. This subcutaneous drug binds to somatostatin receptors on the adenoma and inhibits tumor production of corticotropin. Lower levels of corticotropin lead to lower levels of cortisol production in the adrenal glands. The drug is ineffective for patients whose tumors do not have somatostatin receptors.

Monitor the patient for response to drug therapy, especially weight loss and increased urine output. Observe for symptoms of problems with ***fluid and electrolyte balance***, especially changes in ECG patterns. Assess laboratory findings, especially sodium and potassium values, whenever they are drawn.

Nutrition therapy for the patient with hypercortisolism may involve restrictions of both fluid and sodium intake to control fluid volume. Often sodium restriction involves only "no added salt" to ordinary table foods when fluid overload is mild. For more pronounced fluid overload, the patient may be restricted to anywhere from 2 g/day to 4 g/day of sodium. When sodium restriction is ongoing, teach the patient and family how to check food labels for sodium content and how to keep a daily record of sodium ingested. Explain to the patient and family the reason for any fluid restriction and the importance of adhering to the prescribed restriction.

Monitor intake and output and weight to assess therapy effectiveness. Ensure that assistive personnel (AP) understand that these measurements need to be accurate, not just estimated, because treatment decisions are based on the findings. Schedule fluid offerings throughout the 24 hours. Teach AP to check urine for color and character and to report these findings. Check the urine specific gravity (a specific gravity below 1.005 may indicate fluid overload). If IV therapy is used, infuse only the amount prescribed.

Fluid retention may not be visible. Rapid weight gain is the best indicator of fluid retention and overload. Each 1 lb (about 500 g) of weight gained (after the first ½ lb) equates to 500 mL of retained water. Weigh the patient at the same time daily (before breakfast), using the same scale. Have the patient wear the same type of clothing for each weigh-in.

Surgical management of adrenocortical hypersecretion depends on the cause of the problem. When adrenal hyperfunction is due to increased pituitary secretion of ACTH, removal of a pituitary adenoma using minimally invasive techniques may be attempted. Sometimes a total *hypophysectomy* (surgical removal of the pituitary gland) is needed. (See earlier discussion of Hypophysectomy in the Hyperpituitarism section.) If hypercortisolism is caused by an adrenal tumor, an *adrenalectomy* (removal of the adrenal gland) may be needed.

Preoperative care starts with correcting disturbances of ***fluid and electrolyte balance*** before surgery. Continue to monitor blood potassium, sodium, and chloride levels. Dysrhythmias from potassium imbalance may occur, and cardiac monitoring is needed. Hyperglycemia is controlled before surgery.

The patient with hypercortisolism is at risk for complications of infections and fractures. Prevent infection with handwashing and aseptic technique. Decrease the risk for falls by raising top side rails and encouraging the patient to ask for assistance when getting out of bed. A high-calorie, high-protein diet is prescribed before surgery.

Glucocorticoid preparations are given before surgery. The patient continues to receive glucocorticoids during surgery to prevent adrenal crisis because the removal of the tumor results in a sudden drop in cortisol levels. Before surgery, discuss the need for long-term hormone replacement therapy (HRT).

Operative procedures include a unilateral adrenalectomy when one gland is involved or a bilateral adrenalectomy when ACTH-producing tumors cannot be treated by other means or when both adrenal glands are diseased. Surgery is most often performed by laparoscopic adrenalectomy, a minimally invasive surgical approach (DiDalmazi & Reincke, 2018). If necessary, an open surgery through the abdomen or the lateral flank can be performed.

Postoperative care after adrenalectomy includes monitoring in an ICU. Immediately after surgery, assess the patient every 15 minutes for shock (e.g., hypotension; a rapid, weak pulse; and a decreasing urine output) resulting from insufficient glucocorticoid replacement. Monitor vital signs, central venous pressure, pulmonary wedge pressure, intake and output, daily weights, and serum electrolyte levels.

After a bilateral adrenalectomy, patients require lifelong glucocorticoid and mineralocorticoid HRT, starting immediately after surgery. In unilateral adrenalectomy, HRT continues until the remaining adrenal gland increases hormone production. This therapy may be needed for up to 2 years after surgery.

Preventing Injury. The patient is at risk for injury from skin breakdown, bone fractures, and GI bleeding. Prevention of these injuries is a major nursing care focus.

Planning: Expected Outcomes. The patient with hypercortisolism is expected to avoid injury.

Interventions. Priority nursing interventions for prevention of injury focus on skin assessment and protection, coordinating care to ensure gentle handling, and patient teaching regarding drug therapy for prevention of GI ulcers.

Skin injury is a continuing risk even after surgery has corrected the cortisol excess because the changes induced in the skin and blood vessels remain for weeks to months. Assess the skin for reddened areas, excoriation, breakdown, and edema. If mobility is decreased, turn the patient every 2 hours and pad bony prominences.

Instruct the patient to avoid activities that can result in skin trauma. Teach him or her to use a soft toothbrush and an electric shaver. Instruct patients to keep the skin clean and dry it thoroughly after washing. Excessive dryness can be prevented by using a moisturizing lotion.

Adhesive tape often causes skin breakdown. Use tape sparingly and remove it carefully. After venipuncture, the patient may have increased bleeding because of blood vessel fragility. Apply pressure over the site until bleeding has stopped.

Fragile fractures from bone density loss and osteoporosis are possible for months to years after cortisol levels return to normal. When helping the patient move in bed, use a lift sheet instead of grasping him or her. Remind the patient to call for help when walking. Review the use of walkers or canes, if needed. Teach AP to use a gait belt when walking with a patient who has bone density loss.

Collaborate with a registered dietitian nutritionist (RDN) to teach the patient about nutrition therapy. A high-calorie diet that includes increased amounts of calcium and vitamin D is needed. Milk, cheese, yogurt, and green leafy and root vegetables add calcium to promote bone density. Advise the patient to avoid caffeine and alcohol, which increase the risk for GI ulcers and reduce bone density.

GI bleeding is common with hypercortisolism. Cortisol (1) inhibits production of the thick, gel-like mucus that protects the stomach lining, (2) decreases blood flow to the area, and (3) triggers the release of excess hydrochloric acid. Although surgery reduces cortisol levels, the normal mucus and increased blood flow may take weeks to return. Interventions focus on drug therapy to reduce irritation, protect the GI mucosa, and decrease secretion of hydrochloric acid.

Antacids buffer stomach acids and protect the GI mucosa. Teach the patient that these drugs should be taken on a regular schedule rather than on an as-needed basis.

Some agents block the H_2 receptors in the gastric mucosa. When histamine binds to these receptors, a series of actions release hydrochloric acid. Drugs that block the H_2-receptor site include cimetidine, famotidine, and nizatidine. Omeprazole and esomeprazole inhibit the gastric proton pump and prevent the formation of hydrochloric acid.

Instruct the patient to reduce alcohol or caffeine consumption, smoking, and fasting because these actions cause gastric irritation. NSAIDs and drugs that contain aspirin or other salicylates can cause gastritis and intensify GI bleeding. These should be avoided or limited.

Preventing Infection. Glucocorticoids reduce both the inflammation and the immune responses of ***immunity***, increasing the risk for infection. For the patient who is taking glucocorticoid replacement therapy, the risk is ongoing. For the patient who is recovering from surgery to prevent hypercortisolism, the infection risk continues for weeks after surgery.

Planning: Expected Outcomes. The patient with hypercortisolism is expected to remain free from infection and avoid situations that increase the risk for infection.

Interventions. Protect the patient with reduced ***immunity*** from infection. All personnel must use extreme care during all nursing procedures. Thorough handwashing is important. Anyone with an upper respiratory tract infection who enters the patient's room must wear a mask. Observe strict aseptic technique when performing dressing changes or any invasive procedure.

Continually assess the patient for possible infection. Symptoms may not be obvious because excess cortisol suppresses infection indicators caused by inflammation. Fever and pus formation depend on the presence of white blood cells (WBCs). The patient who has reduced ***immunity*** may have a severe infection without pus and with only a low-grade fever.

Monitor the patient's daily complete blood count (CBC) with differential WBC count, especially neutrophils. Inspect the mouth during every shift for lesions and mucosa breakdown. Assess the lungs every 8 hours for crackles, wheezes, or reduced breath sounds. Assess all urine for odor and cloudiness. Ask about any urgency, burning, or pain on urination.

Take vital signs at least every 4 hours to assess for fever. A temperature elevation of even 1°F (or 0.5°C) above baseline is significant for a patient who has reduced ***immunity***, and indicates infection until otherwise proven.

Perform pulmonary hygiene every 2 to 4 hours. Listen to the lungs for crackles, wheezes, or reduced breath sounds. Urge the patient to deep breathe or use an incentive spirometer every hour while awake.

NCLEX EXAMINATION CHALLENGE 57.4

Safe and Effective Care Environment

A nurse caring for a client with Cushing syndrome who must remain on continued glucocorticoid therapy for another health problem will use which of the following actions to **prevent harm**?

A. Urging the client to salt his or her food
B. Testing voided urine for the present of glucose
C. Using nonadhesive methods to secure an IV access
D. Ensuring the prescribed glucocorticoid drug is given on an empty stomach

Care Coordination and Transition Management

Home Care Management. The patient with hypercortisolism usually has muscle weakness and fatigue for some weeks after surgery and remains at risk for falls and other injury. These problems may necessitate one-floor living for a short time; and a home health aide may be needed to assist with hygiene, meal preparation, and maintenance.

Self-Management Education. The patient taking exogenous glucocorticoids who is discharged to home remains at continuing risk for impaired ***fluid and electrolyte balance***, especially fluid volume excess. Teach him or her and the family to monitor and record the patient's weight daily to show the primary health care provider at any checkups. Also instruct the patient to call the primary health care provider for weight gain of more than 3 lb in a week or more than 1 to 2 lb in a 24-hour period.

After bilateral adrenalectomy, lifelong HRT is needed to prevent adrenal insufficiency. Without the adrenal glands the patient completely depends on the exogenous drug. If the drug is stopped, even for a day or two, no other glands produce the glucocorticoids and the patient develops acute adrenal insufficiency, a life-threatening condition. Management of this problem is described in the Adrenal Gland Hypofunction section. Teach the patient and family about adherence to the drug regimen and its side effects as described in the Patient and Family Education: Preparing for Self-Management: Cortisol Replacement Therapy box.

PATIENT AND FAMILY EDUCATION: PREPARING FOR SELF-MANAGEMENT

Cortisol Replacement Therapy

- Take your medication in divided doses, as prescribed (e.g., the first dose in the morning and the second dose between 4 p.m. and 6 p.m.) for best effects.
- Take your medication with meals or snacks to prevent stomach irritation.
- Weigh yourself daily and keep a record to show your primary health care provider.
- Increase your dosage as directed by your primary health care provider for increased physical stress or severe emotional stress.
- Never skip a dose of medication. If you have persistent vomiting or severe diarrhea and cannot take your medication by mouth for 24 to 36 hours, call your primary health care provider. If you cannot reach your primary health care provider, go to the nearest emergency department. You may need an injection to take the place of your usual oral medication.
- Always wear your medical alert bracelet or necklace.
- Make regular visits for health care follow-up.
- Learn (and have a family member learn) how to give yourself an intramuscular injection of hydrocortisone in case you cannot take your oral drug.

Protecting the patient with reduced ***immunity*** from infection at home is important. Urge him or her to use proper hygiene and social distancing and to avoid crowds or others with infections. Encourage the patient and all people living in the same home with him or her to have yearly influenza vaccinations. Stress that the patient should immediately notify the primary health care provider if he or she has a fever or any other sign of infection.

Health Care Resources. Immediately after returning home, the patient may need a support person to stay and provide more attention than could be given by a visiting nurse or home care aide. Contact with the interprofessional health care team is needed for follow-up and identification of potential problems. The patient taking corticosteroid therapy may have symptoms of adrenal insufficiency if the dosage is inadequate. Suggest that the patient obtain and wear a medical alert bracelet listing the condition and the drug replacement therapy.

◆ **Evaluation: Evaluate Outcomes.** Evaluate the care of the patient with hypercortisolism based on the identified priority patient problems. The expected outcomes of interventions are that the patient will:

- Maintain fluid and electrolyte balance as indicated by blood pressure at or near the normal range, stable body weight, and normal serum sodium and potassium levels
- Remain free from injury as indicated by having intact skin, minimal bruising, absence of bone fractures, and no occult blood in vomitus, stools, or GI secretions
- Remain free from infection as indicated by absence of fever, purulent drainage, cough, pain or burning on urination
- Participate in infection prevention strategies of social distancing and obtaining appropriate immunizations
- Not experience acute adrenal insufficiency

HYPERALDOSTERONISM

Pathophysiology Review

Hyperaldosteronism is an increased secretion of aldosterone with mineralocorticoid excess. Primary hyperaldosteronism (Conn syndrome) in adults results from excessive secretion of aldosterone from one or both adrenal glands, usually caused by an adrenal adenoma. In secondary hyperaldosteronism, excessive secretion of aldosterone is caused by the high levels of angiotensin II that are stimulated by high plasma renin levels. Some causes include kidney hypoxia, diabetic nephropathy, and excessive use of some diuretics.

Increased aldosterone levels cause disturbances of ***fluid and electrolyte balance***, which then trigger the kidney tubules to retain sodium and excrete potassium and hydrogen ions. Hypernatremia, hypokalemia, and metabolic alkalosis result. Sodium retention increases blood volume, which raises blood pressure, increasing the risk for strokes, heart attacks, and kidney damage. (See Chapter 13 for discussion of specific electrolyte imbalances.)

Hypokalemia and elevated blood pressure are the most common problems that patients with hyperaldosteronism develop. He or she may have headache, fatigue, muscle weakness, dehydration, and loss of stamina. *Polydipsia* (excessive fluid intake) and *polyuria* (excessive urine output) occur less frequently. *Paresthesias* (sensations of numbness and tingling) may occur if potassium depletion is severe.

Hyperaldosteronism is diagnosed on the basis of laboratory studies and imaging with CT or MRI. Serum potassium levels are decreased, and sodium levels are elevated. Plasma renin levels are low, and aldosterone levels are high. Hydrogen ion loss leads to metabolic alkalemia (elevated blood pH). Urine has a low specific gravity and high aldosterone levels.

❖ Interprofessional Collaborative Care

Surgery is a common treatment for hyperaldosteronism, and one or both adrenal glands may be removed. The patient's potassium level must be corrected before surgery. Drugs used to increase potassium levels include spironolactone, a potassium-sparing diuretic and aldosterone antagonist. Potassium supplements may be used to increase potassium levels before surgery.

The patient who has undergone a unilateral adrenalectomy may need temporary glucocorticoid replacement; replacement is lifelong when both adrenal glands are removed. Glucocorticoids are given before surgery to prevent adrenal crisis.

When surgery cannot be performed, spironolactone therapy is continued to control hypokalemia and hypertension. Because spironolactone is a potassium-sparing diuretic, hyperkalemia can occur in patients who have impaired kidney function or excessive potassium intake. Advise the patient to avoid potassium supplements and foods rich in potassium, such as meat, fish, and many (but not all) vegetables and fruits. Hyponatremia can occur with spironolactone therapy, and the patient may need increased dietary sodium. Instruct patients to report symptoms of hyponatremia, such as muscle weakness, dizziness, lethargy, or drowsiness. Instruct them to report any additional side effects of spironolactone therapy, including gynecomastia, diarrhea, headache, rash, urticaria (hives), confusion, erectile dysfunction, hirsutism, and amenorrhea. Additional drug therapy to control hypertension is often needed.

CLINICAL JUDGMENT CHALLENGE 57.1

Patient-Centered Care, Safety, Physiological Integrity

The client is a 64-year-old man who was brought to the emergency department by his wife, who claims he is "just not acting right." When asked to elaborate, the wife explains that over the past 4 days the client has become quieter, mumbles that his head and stomach hurt, and now does not recognize the neighbor who has been coming over daily for a short visit. The wife further explains that her husband is a nuclear physicist.

On assessment, the nurse finds the client somewhat responsive to his name, although he does not talk; he is unable to lift his arm for a blood pressure measurement. His pulse is difficult to palpate and is both irregular and slow. Blood pressure is 92/50 mm Hg. He has no obvious facial drooping but appears too confused to stick out his tongue when asked or to try to shrug his shoulders. Pulse oximetry is 94% with a respiratory rate of 14 breaths/min. When the nurse asks about his medication use, the wife reports that he is very healthy and takes only aspirin 81 mg every day. Then she remembers that until 10 days ago, he was taking dexamethasone 10 mg twice daily for about 4 weeks for his back pain. He stopped taking the drug and went back to work on Monday (today is Sunday) because he was pain free.

1. **Recognize Cues:** What assessment information in this client situation is the most important and immediate concern for the nurse? (Hint: Identify the **relevant** information *first* to determine what is most important.)
2. **Analyze Cues:** What client conditions are consistent with the **most relevant** information? (Hint: Think about priority collaborative problems that support and contradict the information presented in this situation.)
3. **Prioritize Hypotheses:** Which possibilities or explanations are **most likely** to be present in this client situation? Which possibilities or explanations are the most serious? (Hint: Consider all possibilities and determine their urgency and risk for this client.)
4. **Generate Solutions:** What actions would most likely achieve the desired outcomes for this client? Which actions should be **avoided** or are **potentially harmful**? (Hint: Determine the desired outcomes first to decide which interventions are appropriate and those that should be avoided.)
5. **Take Action:** Which actions are the most appropriate and how should they be implemented? In what **priority order** should they be implemented? (Hint: Consider health teaching, documentation, requested health care provider orders or prescriptions, nursing skills, collaboration with or referral to health team members, etc.)
6. **Evaluate Outcomes:** What client assessment would indicate that the nurse's actions were **effective**? (Hint: Think about signs that would indicate an improvement, decline, or unchanged client condition.)

GET READY FOR THE NEXT-GENERATION NCLEX® EXAMINATION!

Key Points

Review these Key Points for each NCLEX Examination Client Needs Category.

Safe and Effective Care Environment

- Handle all patients with bone density loss carefully, using lift sheets whenever possible. **QSEN: Safety**
- Ensure that hormone replacement drugs are given as close to the prescribed times as possible. **QSEN: Safety**
- Teach the patient with diabetes insipidus the indicators of dehydration.

Health Promotion and Maintenance

- Instruct the patient with adrenal insufficiency to wear a medical alert bracelet and to carry simple carbohydrates with him or her at all times. **QSEN: Patient-Centered Care**
- Teach the patient and family about the symptoms of infection and when to seek medical advice. **QSEN: Patient-Centered Care**
- Teach patients who have permanent endocrine hypofunction the proper techniques and timing of hormone replacement therapy. **QSEN: Patient-Centered Care**
- Instruct patients taking bromocriptine to seek medical care immediately if chest pain, dizziness, or watery nasal discharge occurs. **QSEN: Safety**

Psychosocial Integrity

- Explain all treatment procedures, restrictions, and follow-up care to the patient. **QSEN: Patient-Centered Care**
- Allow patients who experience a change in physical appearance to mourn this change. **QSEN: Patient-Centered Care**

Physiological Integrity

- During the immediate period after a hypophysectomy, teach the patient to avoid activities that increase intracranial pressure (e.g., bending at the waist, straining to have a bowel movement, coughing). **QSEN: Patient-Centered Care**
- Measure intake and output accurately on patients who have either diabetes insipidus or syndrome of inappropriate antidiuretic hormone (SIADH). **QSEN: Evidence-Based Practice**
- Instruct patients who are taking a corticosteroid for more than a week not to stop the drug suddenly. **QSEN: Safety**
- Ensure that no patient suspected of having DI is deprived of fluids for more than 4 hours. **QSEN: Evidence-Based Practice**
- Teach patients with diabetes insipidus the proper way to self-administer desmopressin orally or by nasal spray. **QSEN: Patient-Centered Care**

MASTERY QUESTIONS

1. Which precaution is **most important** for the nurse to teach a female client to **prevent harm** while undergoing drug therapy with estrogen and progesterone for hypopituitarism?
   A. "Use a barrier method of contraception to prevent an unplanned pregnancy."
   B. "Wear a hat with a brim and use sunscreen when outdoors."
   C. "Do not smoke or use nicotine in any form."
   D. "Avoid drinking caffeinated beverages."
2. Which assessment has the **highest priority** for the nurse to perform for a client with syndrome of inappropriate antidiuretic hormone (SIADH) receiving tolvaptan therapy for 24 hours?
   A. Evaluating serum sodium levels
   B. Evaluating serum potassium levels
   C. Examining the skin and sclera for jaundice
   D. Examining the IV site for indications of phlebitis
3. Which of the following are the **priority** precautions the nurse will teach the client who remains at continuing risk for adrenal hypofunction and is taking hormone replacement therapy to **prevent harm** related to the disorder? **Select all that apply.**
   A. "Avoid crowds and people who are ill."
   B. "Check your heart rate for irregular or skipped beats twice daily."
   C. "Do not choose low-sodium versions of prepared foods."
   D. "Get up slowly from sitting or lying positions."
   E. "Keep a source of glucose, such as candy, with you at all times."
   F. "Never skip your hormone replacement drugs."
4. A client preparing for surgery to remove a cortisol-secreting tumor from the adrenal gland asks the nurse whether the physical changes from the excessive cortisol will go away as a result of the surgery so she can look like herself again. What is the nurse's **best** response?
   A. "The surgery is to remove the tumor, not reconstructive surgery."
   B. "You will notice a great difference in your appearance starting within a week after surgery."
   C. "All the changes will resolve but may take a year or longer to completely disappear."
   D. "The fatty changes and acne will resolve with time but the stretch marks only fade."

REFERENCES

Amrein, K., Martucci, G., & Hahner, S. (2018). Understanding adrenal crisis. *Intensive Care Medicine, 44*(5), 652–655.

Burchum, J., & Rosenthal, L. (2019). *Lehne's pharmacology for nursing care* (10th ed.). St. Louis: Elsevier.

Cole, S. (2018). Evaluation and treatment of adrenal dysfunction in the primary care environment. *Nursing Clinics of North America, 53*, 385–394.

Di Dalmazi, G., & Reincke, M. (2018). Adrenal surgery for Cushing's syndrome: An update. *Endocrinology and Metabolism Clinics, 47*(2), 385–394.

Jarvis, C. (2020). *Physical examination & health assessment* (8th ed.). St. Louis: Elsevier.

Kaiser, U., & Ho, K. (2016). Pituitary physiology and diagnostic evaluation. In S. Melmed, K. Polonsky, P. R. Larsen, & H. Kronenberg (Eds.), *Williams' textbook of endocrinology* (13th ed.). Philadelphia: Saunders.

McCance, K., Huether, S., Brashers, V., & Rote, N. (2019). *Pathophysiology: The biologic basis for disease in adults and children* (8th ed.). St. Louis: Mosby.

Melmed, S., & Kleinberg, D. (2016). Pituitary masses and tumor. In S. Melmed, K. Polonsky, P. R. Larsen, & H. Kronenberg (Eds.), *Williams' textbook of endocrinology* (13th ed.). Philadelphia: Saunders.

Melmed, S., Polonsky, K., Larsen, P. R., & Kronenberg, H. (Eds.). (2016). *Williams' textbook of endocrinology* (13th ed.). Philadelphia: Saunders.

Mendiratta-Lala, M., Avram, A., Turcu, A., & Dunnick, R. (2017). Adrenal imaging. *Endocrinology and Metabolism Clinics, 46*(3), 741–759.

Mitchell-Brown, F., & Stephens-DiLeo, R. (2017). Managing panhypopituitarism in adults. *Nursing, 47*(12), 26–31.

Nieman, L. (2018). Diagnosis of Cushing's syndrome in the modern era. *Endocrinology and Metabolism Clinics, 47*(2), 259–273.

Online Mendelian Inheritance in Man (OMIM). (2017). *Multiple endocrine neoplasia type 1*. www.omim.org/entry/131100.

Online Mendelian Inheritance in Man (OMIM). (2019). *Diabetes insipidus, nephrogenic, X-linked*. www.omim.org/entry/304800.

Pagana, K., & Pagana, T. (2018). *Mosby's manual of diagnostic and laboratory tests* (6th ed.). St. Louis: Elsevier.

Pereira, K. (2016). Hyponatremia signals acute adrenal insufficiency. *American Nurse Today, 11*(7), 30.

Pressman, B. (2017). Pituitary imaging. *Endocrinology and Metabolism Clinics, 46*(3), 713–740.

Robinson, A., & Verbalis, J. (2016). Posterior pituitary. In S. Melmed, K. Polonsky, P. R. Larsen, & H. Kronenberg (Eds.), *Williams' textbook of endocrinology* (13th ed.). Philadelphia: Saunders.

Stewart, P., & Newell-Price, J. (2016). The adrenal cortex. In S. Melmed, K. Polonsky, P. R. Larsen, & H. Kronenberg (Eds.), *Williams' textbook of endocrinology* (13th ed.). Philadelphia: Saunders.

Tritos, N., & Biller, B. (2018). Medical therapy for Cushing's syndrome in the twenty-first century. *Endocrinology and Metabolism Clinics, 47*(2), 427–440.

58

Concepts of Care for Patients With Problems of the Thyroid and Parathyroid Glands

M. Linda Workman

http://evolve.elsevier.com/Iggy/

LEARNING OUTCOMES

1. Collaborate with the interprofessional team to coordinate high-quality care and promote ***cellular regulation*** and optimal ***nutrition*** in patients who have thyroid or parathyroid disorders.
2. Apply knowledge of anatomy, physiology, and pathophysiology to assess patients with impaired thyroid or parathyroid function affecting ***nutrition*** or ***cellular regulation***.
3. Implement nursing interventions to help the patient and family cope with the psychosocial impact caused by acute or chronic problems of the thyroid gland or parathyroid glands.
4. Interpret clinical changes and laboratory data to determine the effectiveness of therapy for thyroid gland and parathyroid gland disorders.
5. Teach the patient and caregiver(s) about common drugs and other management strategies used for thyroid gland or parathyroid gland problems.
6. Use clinical judgment to prioritize evidence-based nursing care for the patient with severe hypothyroidism and the patient with thyroid storm.

KEY TERMS

euthyroid A condition of having normal or near-normal thyroid function.

exophthalmos Abnormal protrusion of the eyes.

goiter Visibly enlarged thyroid gland.

Graves disease Autoimmune disorder, often occurring after an episode of thyroid inflammation, in which the production of autoantibodies (thyroid-stimulating immunoglobulins [TSIs]) that attach to the thyroid-stimulating hormone (TSH) receptors on the thyroid gland greatly increases thyroid hormone production.

Hashimoto thyroiditis (HT) Autoimmune disorder in which infection and inflammation of the thyroid gland causes the production of autoantibodies to thyroglobulin and tissues within the thyroid gland, which results in extensive tissue destruction and reduced secretion of thyroid hormones.

hyperparathyroidism Disorder in which parathyroid secretion of parathyroid hormone is increased, resulting in hypercalcemia and hypophosphatemia.

hyperthyroidism (thyrotoxicosis) Excessive thyroid hormone secretion from the thyroid gland

hypoparathyroidism A rare disorder in which parathyroid function is decreased and serum calcium levels cannot be maintained.

hypothyroidism Reduced or absent hormone secretion from the thyroid gland that results in whole-body decreased metabolism from inadequate ***cellular regulation***.

myxedema coma (hypothyroid crisis) A serious complication of untreated or poorly treated hypothyroidism with dangerously reduced cardiopulmonary and neurologic functioning, although few affected adults become comatose.

pretibial myxedema Dry, waxy swelling of the front surfaces of the lower legs that resembles benign tumors or keloids; associated with hyperthyroidism.

tetany Hyperexcitability of nerves and muscles.

thyroid storm (thyroid crisis) A life-threatening event that occurs in patients with uncontrolled hyperthyroidism, most often with Graves disease.

thyroiditis An inflammation of the thyroid gland.

PRIORITY AND INTERRELATED CONCEPTS

The priority concept for this chapter is:
- ***Cellular Regulation***

The ***Cellular Regulation*** concept exemplar for this chapter is Hypothyroidism.

The interrelated concepts for this chapter are:
- ***Nutrition***
- ***Gas Exchange***

The thyroid gland and parathyroid glands secrete hormones that affect whole-body metabolism, ***cellular regulation***, ***nutrition***, ***gas exchange***, electrolyte balance, and excitable membrane activity. Problems of either gland can lead to symptoms in many body systems and can range from mild to life threatening.

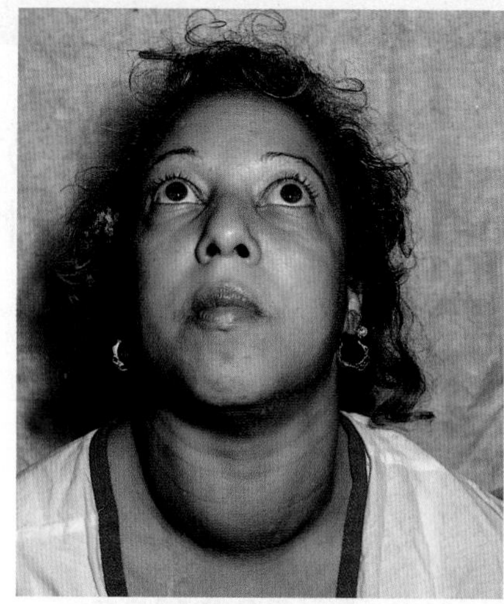

FIG. 58.1 Goiter.

CELLULAR REGULATION CONCEPT EXEMPLAR: HYPOTHYROIDISM

Hypothyroidism is reduced or absent hormone secretion from the thyroid gland that results in whole-body decreased metabolism from inadequate ***cellular regulation***. In its early stages the disorder can be missed because the onset is gradual and undramatic (Moore, 2018). Aging also affects thyroid function, as shown in the Patient-Centered Care: Older Adult Considerations box.

Pathophysiology Review

Symptoms of hypothyroidism are widespread and reflect overall decreased metabolism from low levels of thyroid hormones (THs). Thyroid cells may fail to produce sufficient levels of THs for several reasons. Sometimes the cells themselves are damaged and no longer function normally. At other times the thyroid cells are functional, but the adult does not ingest enough of the substances needed to make thyroid hormones, especially iodide and tyrosine. When the production of thyroid hormones is too low or absent, the blood levels of THs are very low, and the patient has a decreased metabolic rate. This lowered metabolism causes the hypothalamus and anterior pituitary gland to make stimulatory hormones, especially thyroid-stimulating hormone (TSH), in an attempt to trigger hormone release from the poorly responsive thyroid gland. The TSH binds to thyroid cells and causes the thyroid gland to enlarge, forming a **goiter** (visibly enlarge thyroid gland [Fig. 58.1]), although thyroid hormone production does not increase. The presence of a goiter is common to many thyroid problems and does not definitively indicate either hypothyroidism or hyperthyroidism.

Most tissues and organs are affected by the low metabolic rate and reduced ***cellular regulation*** caused by hypothyroidism. Cellular energy is decreased, and metabolites that are compounds of proteins and sugars called *glycosaminoglycans (GAGs)* build up inside cells. This GAG buildup increases the mucus and water, forms cellular edema, and changes organ texture. The edema is mucinous and called *myxedema*, rather than edema caused by water alone. This edema changes the patient's appearance (Fig. 58.2). Nonpitting edema forms everywhere, especially around the eyes, in the hands and feet, and between the shoulder blades. The tongue thickens, and edema forms in the larynx, making the voice husky. General physiologic function is decreased.

Myxedema coma, sometimes called *hypothyroid crisis*, is a serious complication of untreated or poorly treated hypothyroidism with dangerously reduced cardiopulmonary and neurologic functioning, although few affected adults become comatose (McCance et al., 2019). The decreased metabolism

PATIENT-CENTERED CARE: OLDER ADULT CONSIDERATIONS QSEN

Age-Related Change	Nursing Adaptation
Thyroid hormone secretion decreases with age, resulting in reduced circulating hormone levels.	Do not rely solely on laboratory values to assess whether and to what degree hypothyroidism may be present (or the effects of therapy). Although secretion is reduced, clearance also is reduced, allowing circulating hormones to be present longer. Use symptom changes to evaluate hormone replacement therapy effectiveness.
Muscle mass decreases and body fat increases from age-related decreased metabolism.	Avoid using change in muscle strength as an indicator of reduced thyroid function.
Age-related changes in cardiovascular and neurologic function make the older adult more sensitive to hormone replacement therapy (HRT).	When hypothyroidism is present and thyroid HRT is started, doses should be lower and increases made more slowly to avoid inducing cardiovascular and neurologic toxicities. Always assess older adults on thyroid HRT for angina, chest pain, dysrhythmias, hypertension, or indicators of increased central nervous system activity.

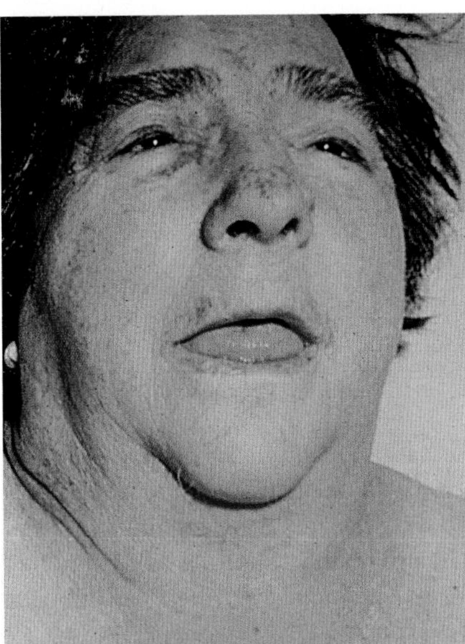

FIG. 58.2 Myxedema.

causes the heart muscle to become flabby and the chamber size to increase. The result is decreased cardiac output with decreased perfusion and ***gas exchange*** in the brain and other vital organs, which makes the already slowed cellular metabolism worse, resulting in tissue and organ failure. *The mortality rate for myxedema coma is extremely high, and this condition is a life-threatening emergency.* Myxedema coma can be caused by a variety of events, drugs, or conditions.

Etiology. Most cases of hypothyroidism in the United States occur as a result of an autoimmune problem resulting from Hashimoto thyroiditis (HT), in which infection and inflammation of the thyroid gland causes the production of autoantibodies to thyroglobulin and tissues within the thyroid gland, which results in extensive tissue destruction and reduced secretion of thyroid hormones (McCance et al., 2019). In North America, other common causes include thyroid surgery and radioactive iodine (RAI) treatment of hyperthyroidism. Worldwide, hypothyroidism is common in areas where the soil and water have little natural iodide, causing endemic goiter. Hypothyroidism is also caused by a variety of other conditions (Table 58.1).

Incidence and Prevalence. Hypothyroidism occurs most often in women between 30 and 60 years of age. Women are affected 7 to 10 times more often than men (McCance et al., 2019).

❖ Interprofessional Collaborative Care

Depending on the severity of the symptoms at the time of diagnosis, initial therapy for hypothyroidism may start in an acute care environment or in the community. When symptoms are severe or if myxedema coma is present, an intensive care environment may be required. Drug therapy is lifelong, and patients must learn to manage their disorders in the community.

TABLE 58.1 Causes of Hypothyroidism

Primary Causes

Decreased Thyroid Tissue

- Surgical or radiation-induced thyroid destruction
- Autoimmune thyroid destruction
- Congenital poor thyroid development
- Cancer (thyroidal or metastatic)

Decreased Synthesis of Thyroid Hormone

- Endemic iodine deficiency
- Drugs:
  - Lithium
  - Propylthiouracil
  - Sodium or potassium perchlorate
  - Aminoglutethimide

Secondary Causes

Inadequate Production of Thyroid-Stimulating Hormone

- Pituitary tumors, trauma, infections, or infarcts
- Congenital pituitary defects
- Hypothalamic tumors, trauma, infections, or infarcts

◆ Assessment: Recognize Cues

History. A decrease in thyroid hormones produces many symptoms related to decreased metabolism from inadequate ***cellular regulation***. However, changes may have occurred slowly, and the patient may not have noticed them. Ask him or her to compare activity now with that of a year ago. The patient often reports an increase in time spent sleeping, sometimes up to 14 to 16 hours daily. Generalized weakness, anorexia, muscle aches, and paresthesias may also be present. Constipation and cold intolerance are common. Ask whether more blankets at night or extra clothing, even in warm weather, has been needed. Some changes may be subtle and are often missed, especially in older adults.

Both men and women may report a decreased libido. Women may have had difficulty becoming pregnant or have changes in menses (heavy, prolonged bleeding or amenorrhea). Men may have problems with impotence and infertility.

Ask about current or previous use of drugs, such as lithium, thiocyanates, aminoglutethimide, sodium or potassium perchlorate, or cobalt. All of these drugs can impair thyroid hormone production. In particular, the cardiac drug amiodarone often has damaging effects on the thyroid gland (Brent & Weetman, 2016; Burchum & Rosenthal, 2019). Also ask whether the patient has ever been treated for hyperthyroidism and what specific treatment was used.

Physical Assessment/Signs and Symptoms. Observe the patient's overall appearance. Fig. 58.2 shows the typical appearance of an adult with hypothyroidism. Common changes include coarse features, edema around the eyes and face, a blank expression, and a thick tongue. The patient's overall muscle movement is slow. He or she may not speak clearly because of tongue thickening and may take a longer time to respond to questions because of reduced cognitive functioning. The Key Features: Hypothyroidism box lists common signs and symptoms of the disorder.

KEY FEATURES

Hypothyroidism

Pulmonary Symptoms
- Hypoventilation
- Pleural effusion
- Dyspnea

Cardiovascular Symptoms
- Bradycardia
- Dysrhythmias
- Enlarged heart
- Decreased activity tolerance
- Hypotension

Metabolic Symptoms
- Decreased basal metabolic rate
- Decreased body temperature
- Cold intolerance

Reproductive Symptoms

Women
- Changes in menses (amenorrhea or prolonged menstrual periods)
- Anovulation
- Decreased libido

Men
- Decreased libido
- Impotence

Gastrointestinal Symptoms
- Anorexia
- Weight gain
- Constipation
- Abdominal distention

Psychosocial Symptoms
- Apathy
- Depression
- Paranoia

Skin Symptoms
- Cool, pale or yellowish, dry, coarse, scaly skin
- Thick, brittle nails
- Dry, coarse, brittle hair
- Decreased hair growth, with loss of eyebrow hair
- Poor wound healing

Neuromuscular Symptoms
- Slowing of intellectual functions:
- Slowness or slurring of speech
- Impaired memory
- Inattentiveness
- Lethargy or somnolence
- Confusion
- Hearing loss
- Paresthesia (numbness and tingling) of the extremities
- Decreased tendon reflexes
- Muscle aches and pain

Other Symptoms
- Periorbital edema
- Facial puffiness
- Nonpitting edema of the hands and feet
- Hoarseness
- Goiter (enlarged thyroid gland)
- Thick tongue
- Increased sensitivity to opioids and tranquilizers
- Weakness, fatigue
- Decreased urine output
- Easy bruising
- Iron deficiency anemia

Cardiac and respiratory functions are decreased, leading to reduced ***gas exchange***. Heart rate may be below 60 beats/min, and respiratory rate may be slow. Body temperature is often lower than 97°F (36.1°C).

Weight gain is very common, even when the adult is not overeating. Weigh the patient and ask whether the result is the same or different from his or her weight a year ago.

Depending on the cause of hypothyroidism, the patient may have a goiter. Remember, some types of hypothyroidism do not induce a goiter, and some types of hyperthyroidism do. The presence of a goiter *suggests* a thyroid problem but does not indicate whether the problem is excessive hormone secretion or too little hormone secretion. Goiters are classified by size (Table 58.2).

Psychosocial Assessment. Hypothyroidism causes many problems in psychosocial functioning. Depression is the most common reason for seeking medical attention. Family members often bring the patient for the initial evaluation. The patient may be too lethargic, apathetic, or drowsy to recognize changes in his or her condition. Families may report that the patient is withdrawn and has reduced cognition. Assess his or her attention span and memory, both of which can be impaired by hypothyroidism. The mental slowness can contribute to social isolation.

TABLE 58.2 Goiter Classification

Goiter Grade	Description
0	There is no palpable or visible goiter.
1	Mass is not visible with neck in the normal position. Goiter can be palpated and moves up when the patient swallows.
2	Mass is visible as swelling when the neck is in the normal position. Goiter is easily palpated and is usually asymmetric.

Laboratory Assessment. Laboratory findings for hypothyroidism show a dramatic reduction of serum triiodothyronine (T_3) and thyroxine (T_4) levels. TSH levels are high in primary hypothyroidism but can be decreased or near normal in patients with secondary hypothyroidism (see the Laboratory Profile: Thyroid Function box). Patients older than 80 years may have lower-than-normal levels of thyroid hormones without symptoms of hypothyroidism, and hormone replacement is not used until other symptoms are present (Touhy & Jett, 2020).

◆ **Analysis: Analyze Cues and Prioritize Hypotheses.** The priority problems for patients who have hypothyroidism are:

1. Decreased ***gas exchange*** and oxygenation due to decreased energy, obesity, muscle weakness, and fatigue
2. Hypotension and reduced perfusion due to decreased heart rate from decreased myocardial metabolism
3. Potential for the complication of myxedema coma

◆ **Planning and Implementation: Generate Solutions and Take Action.** Respiratory and cardiac problems are serious, and their management is a priority. *The most common cause of death among patients with myxedema coma is respiratory failure.*

Improving Gas Exchange

Planning: Expected Outcomes. With appropriate management, the patient with hypothyroidism is expected to have improved ***gas exchange***.

Interventions. Observe and record the rate and depth of respirations and adequacy of ***gas exchange***. Measure oxygen saturation by pulse oximetry, and apply oxygen if the patient has hypoxemia. Auscultate the lungs for a decrease in breath sounds or presence of crackles. If hypothyroidism is severe, the patient may require ventilatory support. Severe respiratory distress occurs with myxedema coma.

Sedating a patient with hypothyroidism can make gas exchange worse and is avoided if possible. When sedation is needed, the dosage is reduced because hypothyroidism increases sensitivity to these drugs. For the patient receiving sedation, assess for adequate gas exchange.

LABORATORY PROFILE

Thyroid Function

Test	Normal Range	Hypothyroidism	Hyperthyroidism
Serum T_3	70-205 ng/dL (1.2-3.4 nmol/L)	Decreased	Increased
Serum T_4 (total)	4-12 mcg/dL (59-142 nmol/L)	Decreased	Increased
Free T_4 index	0.8-2.8 ng/dL (10-36 pmol/L)	Decreased	Increased
TSH stimulation test (thyroid stimulation test)	>10% in RAIU or >1.5 mcg/dL	No response in primary hypothyroidism Normal response in secondary hypothyroidism	Does not apply because this test is used only to differentiate primary from secondary hypothyroidism
Thyroid-stimulating immunoglobulins (TSI)	<130% of basal activity	No change	Elevated in Graves disease Normal in other types of hyperthyroidism
Thyrotropin receptor antibodies (TRAbs)	Titer: 0%	No response	80%-95% indicates Graves disease
TSH	0.3-5 mcU/mL (0.35 mU/L)	High in primary disease Low in secondary or tertiary disease	Low in Graves disease High in secondary or tertiary hyperthyroidism

RAIU, Radioactive iodine uptake; T_3, Triiodothyronine; T_4, thyroxine; *TSH,* thyroid-stimulating hormone.
Data from Pagana, K., & Pagana, T. (2018). *Mosby's manual of diagnostic and laboratory tests* (6th ed.). St. Louis: Elsevier.

Preventing Hypotension

Planning: Expected Outcomes. The patient is expected to have adequate cardiovascular function and tissue perfusion with ***gas exchange***.

Interventions. The patient may have decreased blood pressure, bradycardia, and dysrhythmias. Nursing priorities are monitoring for condition changes and preventing complications. Monitor blood pressure and heart rate and rhythm and observe for indications of shock (e.g., hypotension, decreased urine output, changes in mental status).

If hypothyroidism is chronic, the patient may have cardiovascular disease. *Instruct the patient to report episodes of chest pain or chest discomfort immediately.*

The patient requires lifelong thyroid hormone replacement. Synthetic hormone preparations are usually prescribed. The most common is levothyroxine. Therapy is started with low doses and gradually increased over a period of weeks. *The patient with more severe symptoms of hypothyroidism is started on the lowest dose of thyroid hormone replacement.* This precaution is especially important when the patient has known cardiac problems. Starting at too high a dose or increasing the dose too rapidly can cause severe hypertension, heart failure, and myocardial infarction. With myxedema coma, the drug may need to be given IV because of the severely reduced motility and absorption of the GI tract.

> **! NURSING SAFETY ALERT (QSEN)**
>
> ***Drug Alert***
>
> Teach patients and families who are beginning thyroid replacement therapy to take the drug *exactly* as prescribed and not to change the dose or schedule without consulting the primary health care provider.

Assess for chest pain and dyspnea during initiation of therapy. The final dosage is determined by blood levels of TSH and the patient's physical responses. The dosage and time required for symptom relief vary with each patient. Monitor for and teach the patient and family about the symptoms of hyperthyroidism, which can occur with replacement therapy.

Preventing Myxedema Coma. Any patient with hypo-thyroidism who has other health problem or who is newly diagnosed is at risk for myxedema coma. Factors leading to myxedema coma include acute illness, surgery, chemotherapy, discontinuation of thyroid replacement therapy, and use of sedatives or opioids. Problems that often occur with this condition include:

- Greatly reduced level of consciousness and cognition
- Respiratory failure
- Hypotension
- Hyponatremia
- Hypothermia
- Hypoglycemia

> **! NURSING SAFETY ALERT (QSEN)**
>
> ***Action Alert***
>
> Myxedema coma can lead to shock, organ damage, and death. Assess the patient with hypothyroidism at least every 8 hours for changes that indicate increasing severity, especially changes in mental status, and report these promptly to the primary health care provider.

Treatment is instituted quickly according to the patient's symptoms and without waiting for laboratory confirmation. Management interventions are listed in the Best Practice for Patient Safety & Quality Care: Emergency Care of the Patient With Myxedema Coma box.

Care Coordination and Transition Management. Hypothyroidism is usually chronic with patients living in the community and managed on an outpatient basis. Patients in acute care settings, subacute care settings, and rehabilitation centers may have long-standing hypothyroidism in addition to other

BEST PRACTICE FOR PATIENT SAFETY & QUALITY CARE QSEN

Emergency Care of the Patient With Myxedema Coma

- Maintain a patent airway.
- Replace fluids with IV normal or hypertonic saline as prescribed.
- Give levothyroxine sodium IV as prescribed.
- Give glucose IV as prescribed.
- Give corticosteroids as prescribed.
- Check the patient's temperature hourly.
- Monitor blood pressure hourly.
- Cover the patient with warm blankets.
- Monitor for changes in mental status.
- Turn every 2 hours.
- Institute Aspiration Precautions.

health problems. Ensure that whoever is responsible for overseeing the patient's daily care is aware of the condition and understands its management.

Home Care Management. The patient with hypothyroidism does not usually require changes in the home unless cognition has decreased to the point that he or she poses a danger to himself or herself. Activity intolerance and fatigue may necessitate one-floor living for a short time. If symptoms have not improved before discharge, discuss the need for extra heat or clothing because of cold intolerance. The patient may need help with the drug regimen. Discuss this issue with the family and patient and develop a plan for drug therapy. One person should be clearly designated as responsible for drug preparation and delivery so doses are neither missed nor duplicated.

Self-Management Education. *The most important educational need for the patient with hypothyroidism is about hormone replacement therapy and its side effects.* Emphasize the need for lifelong drugs, and review the symptoms of both hyperthyroidism and hypothyroidism. Teach the patient to wear a medical alert bracelet. Teach the patient and family when to seek medical interventions for dosage adjustment and the need for periodic blood tests of hormone levels. Instruct the patient not to take any over-the-counter drugs without consulting his or her primary health care provider because thyroid hormone preparations interact with many other drugs.

Advise the patient to maintain ***nutrition*** by eating a well-balanced diet with adequate fiber and fluid intake to prevent constipation. Caution him or her that use of fiber supplements may interfere with the absorption of thyroid hormone. Thyroid hormones should be taken on an empty stomach, at least 4 hours before or after a meal. Remind the patient about the importance of adequate rest.

Help the family understand that the time required for resolution of hypothyroidism varies. During this time the patient may continue to have mental slowness. Teach the family to orient the patient often and to explain everything clearly, simply, and as often as needed.

Teach the patient to monitor himself or herself for therapy effectiveness. The two easiest parameters to check are need for sleep and bowel elimination. When the patient requires more sleep and is constipated, the dose of replacement hormone may need to be increased by the primary health care provider. When the patient has difficulty getting to sleep and has more bowel movements than normal for him or her, the dose may need to be decreased.

Health Care Resources. With severe hypothyroidism, the patient at home may need a support person to stay and provide day and night attention. Contact with the interprofessional health care team is needed for follow-up and identification of potential problems. The patient taking thyroid drugs may have symptoms of hypothyroidism if the dosage is inadequate or symptoms of hyperthyroidism if the dose is too high. A home care nurse uses the guidelines listed in the Focused Assessment: The Patient With Hypothyroidism box at every home visit for the patient with hypothyroidism.

FOCUSED ASSESSMENT

The Patient With Hypothyroidism

Assess cardiovascular status:
- Vital signs, including apical pulse, pulse pressure, presence or absence of orthostatic hypotension, and the quality and rhythm of peripheral pulses
- Presence or absence of peripheral edema
- Weight gain or loss

Assess cognition and mental status:
- Level of consciousness, with orientation to time, place, and person
- Ability to accurately read a seven-word sentence containing no words greater than three syllables
- Ability to count backward from 100 by 3s

Assess condition of skin and mucous membranes:
- Moistness of skin, most reliable on chest and back
- Skin temperature and color

Assess neuromuscular status:
- Reactivity of patellar and biceps reflexes
- Oral temperature
- Handgrip strength
- Steadiness of gait
- Presence or absence of fine tremors in the hand

Ask about:
- Sleep in the past 24 hours
- Patient warm enough or too warm indoors
- 24-hour diet recall and 24-hour activity recall
- Over-the-counter and prescribed drugs taken
- Last bowel movement

Assess patient's understanding of illness and adherence with therapy:
- Symptoms to report to primary health care provider
- Drug therapy plan (correct timing and dose)

◆ **Evaluation: Evaluate Outcomes.** Evaluate the care of the patient with hypothyroidism based on the identified priority

NCLEX EXAMINATION CHALLENGE 58.1

Safe and Effective Care Environment

An assistive personnel reports that a nursing home client who has hypothyroidism has a pulse of 48 beats/min this morning. Which assessments have the highest **priority** for the nurse to perform **immediately**? **Select all that apply.**

A. Checking body temperature
B. Testing deep tendon reflex responses
C. Measuring oxygen saturation by pulse oximetry
D. Checking blood pressure, heart rate, and rhythm
E. Determining level of consciousness and cognition
F. Identifying presence or absence of the swallowing reflex
G. Examining feet and ankles for indications of peripheral edema

patient problems. The expected outcomes are that with proper management the patient should:

- Maintain normal cardiovascular function with a pulse above 60 beats/min and a blood pressure within normal limits for age and general health
- Maintain adequate respiratory function and ***gas exchange*** with SpO_2 above 90%
- Demonstrate improvement in cognition

HYPERTHYROIDISM

Pathophysiology Review

Hyperthyroidism (thyrotoxicosis) is excessive thyroid hormone secretion from the thyroid gland. The same symptoms and terms are used even if the cause is ingestion of synthetic thyroid hormones when thyroid function is normal. Excessive thyroid hormones reduce ***cellular regulation*** by increasing metabolism in all body organs, which then produces many different symptoms. Hyperthyroidism can be temporary or permanent, depending on the cause.

The excessive thyroid hormones stimulate most body systems, causing hypermetabolism and increased sympathetic nervous system activity. Symptoms are listed in the Key Features: Hyperthyroidism box.

Thyroid hormones stimulate the heart, increasing rate and stroke volume. These responses increase cardiac output, blood pressure, and blood flow (McCance et al., 2019).

KEY FEATURES
Hyperthyroidism

Cardiopulmonary Symptoms
- Palpitations
- Chest pain
- Increased systolic blood pressure
- Tachycardia
- Dysrhythmias
- Rapid, shallow respirations

Metabolic Symptoms
- Increased basal metabolic rate
- Heat intolerance
- Low-grade fever
- Fatigue

Neurologic Symptoms
- Blurred or double vision
- Eye fatigue
- Increased tears
- Injected (red) conjunctiva
- Photophobia
- Eyelid retraction, eyelid lag
- Globe lag
- Hyperactive deep tendon reflexes
- Tremors
- Insomnia

Skin Symptoms
- Diaphoresis (excessive sweating)
- Fine, soft, silky body hair
- Smooth, warm, moist skin
- Thinning of scalp hair

Gastrointestinal Symptoms
- Weight loss
- Increased appetite
- Increased stools

Reproductive Symptoms
- Amenorrhea
- Increased libido

Psychosocial Symptoms
- Decreased attention span
- Restlessness and irritability
- Emotional instability
- Manic behavior

Other Symptoms
- Goiter
- Wide-eyed or startled appearance (exophthalmos)[a]
- Enlarged spleen
- Muscle weakness and wasting

[a] Present in Graves disease only.

Elevated thyroid hormone levels affect protein, fat, and glucose metabolism. Protein buildup and breakdown are increased; but breakdown exceeds buildup, causing a net loss of body protein known as a *negative nitrogen balance.* Glucose tolerance is decreased, and the patient has *hyperglycemia* (elevated blood glucose levels). Fat metabolism is increased, and body fat decreases. Although the patient has an increased appetite, the increased metabolism causes weight loss and ***nutrition*** deficits.

Thyroid hormones are produced in response to the stimulation hormones secreted by the hypothalamus and anterior pituitary glands. Thus oversecretion of thyroid hormones changes the secretion of hormones from the hypothalamus and the anterior pituitary gland through negative feedback (see Chapter 56). Thyroid hormones also have some influence over sex hormone production. Women have menstrual problems and decreased fertility. Both men and women with hyperthyroidism have an increased *libido* (sexual interest).

Etiology and Genetic Risk. Hyperthyroidism has many causes. The most common form of the disease is Graves disease, also called *toxic diffuse goiter.* **Graves disease** is an autoimmune disorder, often occurring after an episode of thyroid inflammation, in which the production of autoantibodies (thyroid-stimulating immunoglobulins [TSIs]) that attach to the thyroid-stimulating hormone (TSH) receptors on the thyroid gland greatly increases thyroid hormone production (Davies et al., 2016; Hooley & Reagan, 2016; McCance et al., 2019). This increases the number of glandular cells, which enlarges the gland, forming a goiter, and overproduces thyroid hormones (thyrotoxicosis).

In Graves disease, all the general symptoms of hyperthyroidism are present. In addition, other changes specific to Graves disease may occur, including **exophthalmos** (abnormal protrusion of the eyes) and **pretibial myxedema** (dry, waxy swelling of the front surfaces of the lower legs that resembles benign tumors or keloids).

Hyperthyroidism caused by multiple thyroid nodules is termed *toxic multinodular goiter (TMNG).* The nodules may be enlarged thyroid tissues or benign tumors (adenomas). These patients usually have had a goiter for years. The symptoms are milder than those seen in Graves disease, and the patient does not have exophthalmos or pretibial myxedema.

Hyperthyroidism also can be caused by excessive use of thyroid replacement hormones. This type of problem is called *exogenous hyperthyroidism.*

PATIENT-CENTERED CARE: GENETIC/GENOMIC CONSIDERATIONS QSEN

Graves disease is associated with other autoimmune disorders, such as diabetes mellitus, vitiligo, and rheumatoid arthritis and often occurs in both members of identical twins (Online Mendelian Inheritance in Man [OMIM], 2016). Susceptibility to Graves disease is associated with several gene mutations *(GRD1, GRD2, GRDX1, GRDX2).* The pattern of inheritance is autosomal recessive with sex limitation to females. Ask the patient with Graves disease whether any other family members also have the problem.

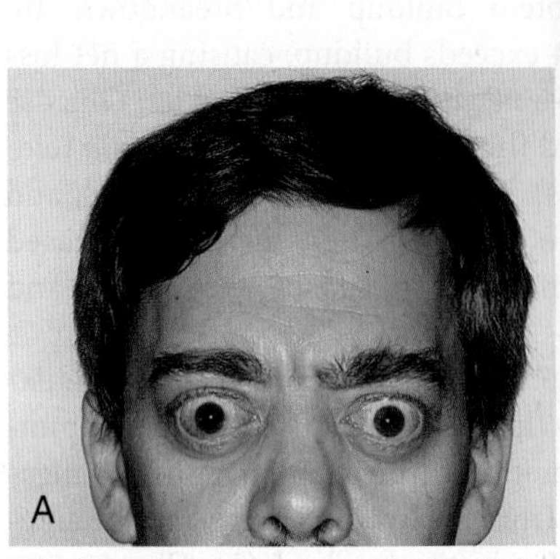

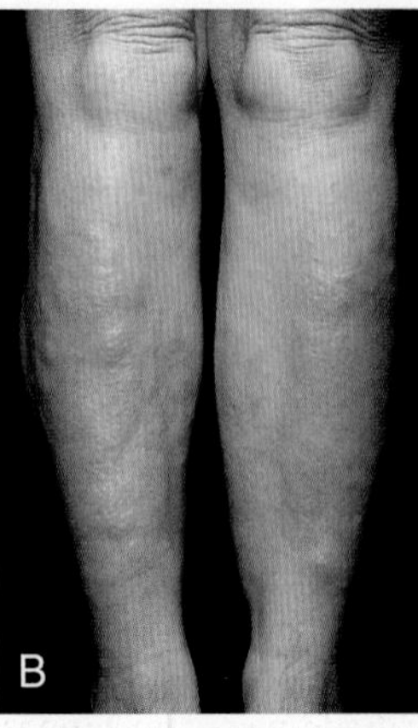

FIG. 58.3 A, Exophthalmos. B, Pretibial myxedema. (From Belchetz, P., & Hammond, P. [2003]. *Mosby's color atlas and text of diabetes and endocrinology.* Edinburgh: Mosby.)

Incidence and Prevalence. Hyperthyroidism is a common endocrine disorder. Graves disease can occur at any age but is diagnosed most often in women between 20 and 40 years of age (Davies et al., 2016). Toxic multinodular goiter usually occurs after the age of 50 years and affects women four times more often than men (McCance et al., 2019).

❖ Interprofessional Collaborative Care

◆ Assessment: Recognize Cues

History. Many changes and problems occur because the reduced ***cellular regulation*** of hyperthyroidism affects all body systems, although changes may occur over such a long period that patients may be unaware of them. Record age, gender, and usual weight. The increased metabolic rate affects ***nutrition***. The patient may report a recent unplanned weight loss, an increased appetite, and an increase in the number of bowel movements per day.

Heat intolerance is often the first symptom the patient notices. He or she may have increased sweating even when environmental temperatures are comfortable for others, and often wears lighter clothing in cold weather. The patient may also report palpitations or chest pain as a result of the cardiovascular effects. Ask about changes in breathing patterns because dyspnea (with or without exertion) is common.

Visual changes may be the earliest problem the patient or family notices, especially exophthalmos with Graves disease (Fig. 58.3). Ask about changes in vision, such as blurring or double vision and tiring of the eyes.

Ask about changes in energy level or in the ability to perform ADLs. Fatigue and insomnia are common. Families may report that the patient has become irritable or depressed.

Ask women about changes in menses, because amenorrhea or a decreased menstrual flow is common. Initially both men and women may have an increase in libido, but this changes as the patient becomes more fatigued.

Ask about previous thyroid surgery or radiation therapy to the neck, because some adults remain hyperthyroid after surgery or are resistant to radiation therapy. Ask about past and current drugs, especially the use of thyroid hormone replacement or antithyroid drugs.

Physical Assessment/Signs and Symptoms. Exophthalmos is common in patients with Graves disease. The wide-eyed or "startled" look is due to edema in the extraocular muscles and increased fatty tissue behind the eye, which pushes the eyeball forward and may cause problems with focusing. Pressure on the optic nerve may impair vision. If the eyelids fail to close completely and the eyes are unprotected, they may become dry, and corneal ulcers may develop. Observe the eyes for excessive tearing and a bloodshot appearance. Ask about sensitivity to light *(photophobia).*

Two other eye problems are common in all types of hyperthyroidism: eyelid retraction (eyelid lag) and globe (eyeball) lag. In eyelid lag, the upper eyelid fails to descend when the patient gazes slowly downward. In globe lag, the upper eyelid pulls back faster than the eyeball when the patient gazes upward. During assessment, ask the patient to look down and then up, and document the response.

Observe the size and symmetry of the thyroid gland. The generalist medical-surgical nurse does not palpate the thyroid gland although it is superficially located. In goiter, a generalized thyroid enlargement, the thyroid gland may increase to four times its normal size (see Fig. 58.1). *Not all patients with a goiter have hyperthyroidism.* Bruits (turbulence from increased blood flow) may be heard in the neck with a stethoscope.

! NURSING SAFETY PRIORITY (QSEN)

Action Alert

Do not palpate a goiter or thyroid tissue in a patient with hyperthyroid symptoms. This action can stimulate the sudden release of excessive thyroid hormones and trigger a life-threatening episode of thyroid storm (crisis).

The cardiovascular problems of hyperthyroidism include increased systolic blood pressure, tachycardia, and dysrhythmias. Usually the diastolic pressure is decreased, causing a widened pulse pressure.

Inspect the hair and skin. Fine, soft, silky hair and smooth, warm, moist skin are common. Many patients notice thinning of scalp hair. Muscle weakness and hyperactive deep tendon reflexes are common. Observe motor movements of the hands for tremors. The patient may appear restless, irritable, and fatigued.

Psychosocial Assessment. Wide mood swings, irritability, decreased attention span, and manic behavior are common. Hyperactivity often leads to fatigue because of the inability to sleep well. Some patients describe their activity as having two modes (i.e., either "full speed ahead" or "completely stopped"). Ask whether he or she cries or laughs without cause or has difficulty concentrating. Family members often report a change in the patient's mental or emotional status.

Laboratory Assessment. Testing for hyperthyroidism involves measurement of blood levels for triiodothyronine (T_3), thyroxine (T_4), and thyroid-stimulating hormone (TSH). Antibodies to the TSH receptor (thyrotropin receptor [TRAbs]) are measured to diagnose Graves disease. The most common changes in laboratory tests for hyperthyroidism are listed in the Laboratory Profile: Thyroid Function box.

Other Diagnostic Assessment. *Thyroid scan* evaluates the position, size, and functioning of the thyroid gland. Radioactive iodine (RAI [^{123}I]) is given by mouth, and the uptake of iodine by the thyroid gland (radioactive iodine uptake [RAIU]) is measured. The half-life of ^{123}I is short, and radiation precautions are not needed. Pregnancy should be ruled out before the scan is performed. The normal thyroid gland has an uptake of 5% to 35% of the given dose at 24 hours. RAIU is increased in hyperthyroidism and can be used to identify active thyroid nodules. It is no longer the most common test for thyroid function (Davies et al., 2016).

Ultrasonography of the thyroid can determine its size and general composition of any masses or nodules. This outpatient procedure takes about 30 minutes to perform and is painless.

ECG usually shows supraventricular tachycardia. Other ECG changes include atrial fibrillation, dysrhythmias, and premature ventricular contractions.

◆ **Interventions: Take Action.** Because Graves disease is the most common form of hyperthyroidism, the interventions discussed in the following sections include those specific for the problems that occur with Graves disease. In North America, the most common interventions are drug therapy and radioablation. Surgery is reserved for severe disease that is not responsive to other forms of management. Medical management is used to decrease the effect of thyroid hormone on cardiac function and to reduce thyroid hormone secretion. The priorities for nursing care focus on monitoring for complications, reducing stimulation, promoting comfort, and teaching the patient and family about therapeutic drugs and procedures.

Nonsurgical Management. *Monitoring* includes measuring the patient's apical pulse, blood pressure, and temperature at least every 4 hours. Instruct the patient to report immediately any palpitations, dyspnea, vertigo, or chest pain. Increases in temperature may indicate a rapid worsening of the patient's condition and the onset of **thyroid storm (thyroid crisis)**, a life-threatening event that occurs in patients with uncontrolled hyperthyroidism, most often with Graves disease. It presents with uncontrolled hyperthyroidism and is characterized by high fever and severe hypertension (Hooley & Reagan, 2016; Schreiber, 2017). *Immediately report a temperature increase of even 1°F.* If this task is delegated to assistive personnel (AP), instruct them to report the patient's temperature to you as soon as it has been obtained. If temperature is elevated, immediately assess the patient's cardiac status. If the patient has a cardiac monitor, check for dysrhythmias.

Reducing stimulation helps prevent increasing the symptoms of hyperthyroidism and the risk for cardiac complications. Encourage the patient to rest. Keep the environment quiet by closing the door to the room, limiting visitors, and postponing nonessential care or treatments.

Promoting comfort includes reducing the room temperature to decrease discomfort caused by heat intolerance. Instruct AP to ensure that the patient always has a fresh pitcher of ice water and to change the bed linen whenever it becomes damp from diaphoresis. Suggest that the patient take a cool shower or sponge bath several times each day. For patients with exophthalmos, prevent eye dryness by encouraging the use of artificial tears.

Drug therapy with antithyroid drugs is the initial treatment for hyperthyroidism and causes some patients to go into remission for as long as 10 years (Davies et al., 2016). The Common Examples of Drug Therapy: Hyperthyroidism box lists teaching priorities for the patient receiving drug therapy for hyperthyroidism. The preferred drugs are the thionamides, especially methimazole. Propylthiouracil is used less often because of its liver toxic effects (Davies et al., 2016; Felicilda-Reynaldo & Kenneally, 2016). These drugs block thyroid hormone production by preventing iodide binding in the thyroid gland. The response to these drugs is delayed because the patient may have large amounts of stored thyroid hormones that continue to be released.

Iodine preparations may be used for short-term therapy before surgery. They decrease blood flow through the thyroid gland, reducing the production and release of thyroid hormone. Improvement usually occurs within 2 weeks, but it may be weeks before metabolism returns to normal. This treatment can result in hypothyroidism, and the patient is monitored closely for the need to adjust the drug regimen.

Beta-adrenergic blocking drugs such as propranolol may be used as supportive therapy. These drugs relieve diaphoresis, anxiety, tachycardia, and palpitations but do not inhibit thyroid hormone production. See Chapters 32 and 33 for a discussion of the actions and nursing implications of these agents.

COMMON EXAMPLES OF DRUG THERAPY

Hyperthyroidism

Drugs	Nursing Implications
Propylthiouracil Methimazole	Teach patient to avoid crowds and people who are ill *because the drug reduces the immune response, increasing the risk for infection.* Teach patients to check for weight gain, slow heart rate, and cold intolerance, *which are indications of hypothyroidism and the need for a lower drug dose.* Teach patients taking propylthiouracil to report darkening of the urine or a yellow appearance to the skin or whites of the eyes, *which indicate possible liver toxicity or failure, a serious side effect of propylthiouracil.* Remind women taking methimazole to notify their primary health care providers if they become pregnant *because the drug causes birth defects and should not be used during pregnancy.*
Lugol solution Saturated solution of potassium iodide (SSKI)	Administer these drugs orally 1 hour *after* a thionamide has been given *because initially the iodine agents can cause an increase in the production of thyroid hormones. Giving a thionamide first prevents this initial increase in thyroid hormone production.* Check patient for a fever or rash and ask about a metallic taste, mouth sores, sore throat, or GI distress *as these are indications of iodism, a toxic effect of the drugs, and may require that the drug be discontinued.*

! NURSING SAFETY PRIORITY (QSEN)

Drug Alert

Although similar in action, methimazole and propylthiouracil are *not* interchangeable. The dosages for propylthiouracil are much higher than those for methimazole.

! NURSING SAFETY PRIORITY (QSEN)

Drug Alert

Methimazole can cause birth defects and should not be used during the first trimester of pregnancy. Instruct women to notify their primary health care provider if pregnancy occurs.

Radioactive iodine (RAI) therapy is not used in pregnant women because ^{131}I crosses the placenta and can damage the fetal thyroid gland. The patient with hyperthyroidism may receive RAI in the form of oral ^{131}I. The dosage depends on the thyroid gland's size and sensitivity to radiation. The thyroid gland picks up the RAI, and some of the cells that produce thyroid hormone are destroyed by the local radiation. Because the thyroid gland stores thyroid hormones to some degree, the patient may not have complete symptom relief until 6 to 8 weeks after RAI therapy. Additional drug therapy for hyperthyroidism is still needed during the first few weeks after RAI treatment.

RAI therapy is performed on an outpatient basis. One dose may be sufficient, although some patients need a second or third dose. The radiation dose is low and is usually completely eliminated within a month; however, the source is unsealed, and some radioactivity is present in the patient's body fluids and stool for a few weeks after therapy. Radiation precautions are needed to prevent exposure to family members and other people. Teach patients the precautions listed in the Patient and Family Education: Preparing for Self-Management: Safety Precautions for the Patient Receiving an Unsealed Radioactive Isotope box to use during the first few weeks after receiving ^{131}I.

The degree of thyroid destruction varies. Some patients become hypothyroid as a result of treatment. The patient then needs lifelong thyroid hormone replacement. All patients who have undergone RAI therapy should be monitored regularly for changes in thyroid function.

Surgical Management. Surgery to remove all or part of the thyroid gland is used to manage Graves and other types of hyperthyroidism that do not respond to nonsurgical management strategies. It is also used when a large goiter causes tracheal or esophageal compression. Removal of all *(total thyroidectomy)* or part *(subtotal thyroidectomy)* of the thyroid tissue decreases the production of thyroid hormones. After a total thyroidectomy, patients must take lifelong thyroid hormone replacement.

Preoperative Care. The patient is treated with thionamide drug therapy first to have near-normal thyroid function (**euthyroid**) before thyroid surgery. Iodine preparations also are used to decrease thyroid size and vascularity, thereby reducing the risk for hemorrhage and the potential for thyroid storm during surgery. (Thyroid storm is discussed earlier in the Nonsurgical Management section, and later in the Thyroid Storm section of Hyperthyroidism.)

PATIENT AND FAMILY EDUCATION: PREPARING FOR SELF-MANAGEMENT

Safety Precautions for the Patient Receiving an Unsealed Radioactive Isotope

- Use a toilet that is not used by others for at least 2 weeks after receiving the radioactive iodine.
- Sit to urinate (males and females) to avoid splashing urine on the seat, walls, and floor.
- Flush the toilet (with the lid closed) three times after each use.
- If urine is spilled on the toilet seat or floor, use paper tissues or towels to clean it up, bag them in sealable plastic bags, and take them to the hospital's radiation therapy department.
- Men with urinary incontinence should use condom catheters and a drainage bag rather than absorbent gel-filled briefs or pads.
- Women with urinary incontinence should use facial tissue layers in their clothing to catch the urine rather than absorbent gel-filled briefs or pads. These tissues should then be flushed down the toilet exclusively used by the patient.
- Using a laxative on the second and third days after receiving the radioactive drug helps you excrete the contaminated stool faster (this also decreases the exposure of your abdominal organs to radiation).
- Wear only machine-washable clothing and wash these items separately from others in your household.
- After washing your clothing, run the washing machine for a full cycle on empty before it is used to wash the clothing of others.
- Avoid close contact with pregnant women, infants, and young children for the first week after therapy. Remain at least 3 feet (about 1 m) away from these people and limit your exposure to them to no more than 1 hour daily.
- Some radioactivity will be in your saliva during the first week after therapy. Precautions to avoid exposing others to this contamination (both household members and trash collectors) include:
    - Not sharing toothbrushes or toothpaste tubes
    - Using disposable tissues rather than cloth handkerchiefs and either flushing used ones down the toilet or keeping them in a plastic bag and turning them in to the radiation department of the hospital for disposal

Hypertension, dysrhythmias, and tachycardia must be controlled before surgery. The patient with hyperthyroidism may need to follow a high-protein, high-carbohydrate diet for days or weeks before surgery.

Teach the patient to perform deep-breathing exercises. Stress the importance of supporting the neck when coughing or moving by placing both hands behind the neck to reduce strain on the incision.

Explain the surgery and the care after surgery to the patient. Remind him or her that a drain and a dressing may be in place after surgery.

Operative Procedures. Many thyroidectomies are now performed as minimally invasive surgeries or mini-incision surgeries. With these surgeries, as with the traditional open approach, the parathyroid glands and recurrent laryngeal nerves are avoided to reduce the risk for complications and injury.

With a subtotal thyroidectomy, the remaining thyroid tissues are sutured to the trachea. With a total thyroidectomy, the entire thyroid gland is removed, but the parathyroid glands are left with an intact blood supply to prevent causing hypoparathyroidism.

Postoperative Care. *Monitoring the patient for complications is the most important nursing action after thyroid surgery.* Monitor vital signs every 15 minutes until the patient is stable and then every 30 minutes. Increase or decrease the monitoring of vital signs based on changes in the patient's condition.

Assess the patient's level of discomfort and give prescribed drugs for pain control as needed. Use pillows to support the head and neck. Place the patient, while he or she is awake, in a semi-Fowler position. Avoid positions that cause neck extension.

Help the patient deep-breathe every 30 minutes to 1 hour. Suction oral and tracheal secretions when necessary.

Thyroid surgery can cause hemorrhage, respiratory distress with reduced ***gas exchange,*** parathyroid gland injury (resulting in *hypocalcemia* [low serum calcium levels] and tetany [hyperexcitability of nerves and muscles]), damage to the laryngeal nerves, and thyroid storm. Remain alert to the potential for complications and identify symptoms early.

Hemorrhage is most likely to occur during the first 24 hours after surgery. Inspect the neck dressing and behind the patient's neck for blood. A drain may be present, and a moderate amount of serosanguineous drainage is normal. Hemorrhage may be seen as bleeding at the incision site or as respiratory distress caused by tracheal compression.

Respiratory distress and reduced ***gas exchange*** can result from swelling, tetany, or damage to the laryngeal nerve, resulting in spasms. Laryngeal *stridor* (harsh, high-pitched respiratory sounds) is heard in acute respiratory obstruction. Keep emergency tracheostomy equipment in the patient's room. Check that oxygen and suctioning equipment are nearby and in working order.

Hypocalcemia and tetany may occur if the parathyroid glands

> **! NURSING SAFETY PRIORITY (QSEN)**
>
> ***Critical Rescue***
>
> Monitor the patient to identify symptoms of obstruction and poor ***gas exchange*** (stridor, dyspnea, falling oxygen saturation, inability to swallow, drooling) after thyroid surgery. If any indications are present, respond by immediately initiating the Rapid Response Team.

are removed, damaged, or their blood supply is impaired during thyroid surgery, resulting in decreased parathyroid hormone (PTH) levels. Ask the patient hourly about tingling around the mouth or of the toes and fingers. Assess for muscle twitching as a sign of calcium deficiency. Calcium gluconate or calcium chloride for IV use should be available in an emergency situation. (For information on the later signs of hypocalcemia, see the discussion of postoperative care in the Hyperparathyroidism section and the Assessment discussion in the Hypoparathyroidism section. Hypocalcemia is also discussed in Chapter 13.)

Laryngeal nerve damage may occur during surgery. This problem results in hoarseness and a weak voice. Assess the patient's voice at 2-hour intervals and document any changes. Reassure the patient that hoarseness is usually temporary.

Thyroid storm or **thyroid crisis** is a life-threatening event that occurs in patients with uncontrolled hyperthyroidism, most often with Graves disease. Symptoms develop quickly, and the problem is fatal if left untreated (Schreiber, 2017). It is often triggered by stressors such as trauma, infection, diabetic ketoacidosis, and pregnancy. Other conditions that can lead to thyroid storm include vigorous palpation of the goiter, exposure to iodine, and radioactive iodine (RAI) therapy. Although thyroid storm after surgery is less common because of drug therapy before thyroid surgery, it can still occur.

Symptoms of thyroid storm are caused by excessive thyroid hormone release, which dramatically increases metabolic rate. *Key symptoms include fever, tachycardia, and systolic hypertension.* The patient may have abdominal pain, nausea, vomiting, and diarrhea. Often he or she is very anxious and has tremors. As the crisis progresses, the patient may become restless, confused, or psychotic and may have seizures, leading to coma. *Even with treatment, thyroid storm may lead to death.*

> **! NURSING SAFETY PRIORITY (QSEN)**
>
> ***Critical Rescue***
>
> When caring for a patient with hyperthyroidism, even after a thyroidectomy, assess temperature often because an increase of even 1°F (1.8°C) may indicate an impending thyroid crisis. If a temperature increase occurs, respond by reporting it immediately to the primary health care provider.

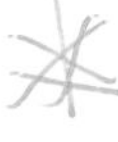

Emergency measures to prevent death vary with the intensity and type of changes. Interventions focus on maintaining airway patency, promoting adequate ventilation and ***gas exchange,*** reducing fever, and stabilizing the hemodynamic status. The Best Practice for Patient Safety & Quality Care box outlines interventions for emergency management of thyroid storm.

Eye and vision problems of Graves disease are not corrected by treatment for hyperthyroidism, and management is symptomatic. Teach the patient with mild problems to elevate the head of the bed at night and use artificial tears. If *photophobia* (sensitivity to light) is present, dark glasses may be helpful. For those who cannot close the eyelids completely, recommend gently taping the lids closed at bedtime to prevent irritation and injury.

If pressure behind the eye continues and forces the eye forward, blood supply to the eye can be compromised, leading to ischemia and blindness. In severe cases, short-term glucocorticoid therapy is prescribed to reduce swelling and halt the

> **BEST PRACTICE FOR PATIENT SAFETY & QUALITY CARE (QSEN)**
>
> ***Emergency Care of the Patient During Thyroid Storm***
>
> - Maintain a patent airway and adequate ventilation.
> - Give oral antithyroid drugs as prescribed: methimazole or propylthiouracil.
> - Administer sodium iodide solution IV daily as prescribed.
> - Give propranolol IV as prescribed, slowly over 3 minutes. The patient should be connected to a cardiac monitor, and a central venous pressure catheter should be in place.
> - Give glucocorticoids as prescribed: hydrocortisone, prednisone, or dexamethasone.
> - Monitor continually for cardiac dysrhythmias.
> - Monitor vital signs every 30 minutes.
> - Provide comfort measures, including a cooling blanket.
> - Give nonsalicylate antipyretics as prescribed.
> - Correct dehydration with normal saline infusions.
> - Apply cooling blanket or ice packs to reduce fever.

infiltrative process. Prednisone is given in high doses at first and then is tapered down according to the patient's response. Other management strategies include external radiation combined with lower-dose glucocorticoid therapy. Surgical intervention (orbital decompression) may be needed if loss of sight or damage to the eyeball is possible. Rituximab injections have been successful on a limited basis for this problem (Davies et al., 2016).

Health teaching includes reviewing with the patient and family the symptoms of hyperthyroidism and instructing the patient to report any increase or recurrence of these. Also teach about the symptoms of hypothyroidism (discussed in the next section) and the need for thyroid hormone replacement. Reinforce the need for regular follow-up because hypothyroidism can occur several years after radioactive iodine therapy.

NCLEX EXAMINATION CHALLENGE 58.2

Safe and Effective Care Environment

Which assessment finding of a client 8 hours after a subtotal thyroidectomy does the nurse consider most **relevant** as an indication of a possible complication?

A. The client's hand spasms during blood pressure measurement.
B. The respiratory rate has dropped from 18 to 14 breaths/min.
C. The dressing has a moderate amount of serosanguineous drainage.
D. The client responds to questions correctly but does not open the eyes while talking.

THYROIDITIS

Thyroiditis is an inflammation of the thyroid gland. There are three types: acute, subacute, and chronic. Chronic thyroiditis (Hashimoto disease) is the most common type.

Acute thyroiditis is caused by bacterial invasion of the thyroid gland. Symptoms include pain, neck tenderness, malaise, fever, and *dysphagia* (difficulty swallowing). It usually resolves with antibiotic therapy.

Subacute or granulomatous thyroiditis results from a viral infection of the thyroid gland after a cold or other upper respiratory infection. Symptoms include fever, chills, dysphagia, and muscle and joint pain. Pain can radiate to the ears and the jaw. The thyroid gland feels hard and enlarged on palpation. Thyroid function can remain normal, although hyperthyroidism or hypothyroidism may develop.

Chronic thyroiditis (Hashimoto thyroiditis [HT]) is a common type of hypothyroidism that affects women more often than men. HT is an autoimmune disorder that is usually triggered by a bacterial or viral infection. The thyroid is invaded by antithyroid antibodies and lymphocytes, causing selective thyroid tissue destruction. When large amounts of the gland are destroyed, hypothyroidism results.

Symptoms of Hashimoto thyroiditis include dysphagia and painless enlargement of the gland. Diagnosis is based on circulating antithyroid antibodies and needle biopsy of the thyroid gland. Serum thyroid hormone levels and TSH levels vary with disease stage and type.

CLINICAL JUDGMENT CHALLENGE 58.1

Safety; Patient-Centered Care; Evidence-Based Practice

The assistive personnel assigned to a 45-year-old client who is 1 day postoperative after a total abdominal hysterectomy reports that the client's temperature is now 102.6°F (39.2°C) and that her pulse is too fast and irregular to count accurately. The nurse assesses the client and finds the vital signs report accurate and that the client both is sweating profusely and has hand tremors. Inspection of the surgical sites reveals an intact incision with no areas of redness or drainage. When the nurse asks the client how she feels, the client reports that she is thirsty, feels jittery, can't relax, and is having a hard time focusing on the book she is trying to read. She rates her surgical site pain as a 3 on a 0 to 10 scale. She then says that she has not felt like this since she underwent radiation therapy for hyperthyroidism 8 months ago.

1. **Recognize Cues:** What assessment information in this client situation is the most important and immediate concern for the nurse? (Hint: Identify the **relevant** information *first* to determine what is most important.)
2. **Analyze Cues:** What client conditions are consistent with the **most relevant** information? (Hint: Think about priority collaborative problems that support and contradict the information presented in this situation.)
3. **Prioritize Hypotheses:** Which possibilities or explanations are **most likely** to be present in this client situation? Which possibilities or explanations are the most serious? (Hint: Consider all possibilities and determine their urgency and risk for this client.)
4. **Generate Solutions:** What actions would most likely achieve the desired outcomes for this client? Which actions should be **avoided** or are **potentially harmful**? (Hint: Determine the desired outcomes first to decide which interventions are appropriate and those that should be avoided.)
5. **Take Action:** Which actions are the most appropriate and how should they be implemented? In what **priority order** should they be implemented? (Hint: Consider health teaching, documentation, requested health care provider orders or prescriptions, nursing skills, collaboration with or referral to health team members, etc.)
6. **Evaluate Outcomes:** What client assessment would indicate that the nurse's actions were **effective**? (Hint: Think about signs that would indicate an improvement, decline, or unchanged client condition.)

THYROID CANCER

Pathophysiology Review

The four distinct types of thyroid cancer are papillary, follicular, medullary, and anaplastic (American Cancer Society, 2020; Canadian Cancer Society, 2019). The initial sign of thyroid cancer is a single, painless lump or nodule in the thyroid gland. Additional signs and symptoms depend on the presence and location of *metastasis* (spread of cancer cells).

Papillary carcinoma, the most common type of thyroid cancer, occurs most often in younger women. It is a slow-growing tumor that can be present for years before spreading to nearby lymph nodes. When the tumor is confined to the thyroid gland, the chance for cure is good with a partial or total thyroidectomy.

Follicular carcinoma occurs most often in older adults. It invades blood vessels and spreads to bone and lung tissue.

When it adheres to the trachea, neck muscles, great vessels, and skin, *dyspnea* (difficulty breathing) and *dysphagia* (difficulty swallowing) result. When the tumor involves the recurrent laryngeal nerves, the patient may have a hoarse voice.

Medullary carcinoma is most common in patients older than 50 years. It often occurs with multiple endocrine neoplasia (MEN) type 2, a familial endocrine disorder (OMIM, 2014). The tumor usually secretes a variety of hormones.

Anaplastic carcinoma is a rapidly growing, aggressive tumor that invades nearby tissues. Symptoms include stridor (harsh, high-pitched respiratory sounds), hoarseness, and dysphagia.

A hallmark of thyroid cancer is an elevated serum thyroglobulin (Tg) level. The normal Tg level is 0.5 to 53.0 ng/mL (mcg/L) for men and 0.5 to 43.0 ng/mL (mcg/L) for women.

❖ Interprofessional Collaborative Care

Radiation therapy is used most often for anaplastic carcinoma because this cancer has usually metastasized at diagnosis. The patient is treated with *ablative* (enough to destroy the tissue) amounts of RAI. (See the earlier Patient and Family Education: Preparing for Self-Management box for precautions to teach the patient receiving unsealed RAI therapy.) If spread has occurred to the neck or mediastinum, external radiation is also used. If thyroid cancer does not respond to RAI, chemotherapy is initiated.

Surgery is the treatment of choice for other types of thyroid cancer. A total thyroidectomy is usually performed with dissection of lymph nodes in the neck if regional lymph nodes are involved. (See the postoperative care discussion in the Surgical Management section for Hyperthyroidism.) Suppressive doses of thyroid hormone are usually taken for 3 months after surgery. Thyroglobulin levels are monitored after surgery. A rising level indicates probable presence of cancer cells.

The patient is hypothyroid after treatment for thyroid cancer. Nursing interventions then focus on teaching him or her about the management of hypothyroidism. (See the discussion of patient-centered collaborative care in the Cellular Regulation Concept Exemplar: Hypothyroidism section.)

HYPOPARATHYROIDISM

Pathophysiology Review

The parathyroid glands maintain calcium and phosphate balance (see Fig. 56.6 in Chapter 56). Serum calcium level is normally maintained within a narrow range. Parathyroid secretion of parathyroid hormone (PTH) act directly on the kidney, causing increased kidney reabsorption of calcium and increased phosphorus excretion.

Hypoparathyroidism is a rare disorder in which parathyroid function is decreased and serum calcium levels cannot be maintained, and *hypocalcemia* (low serum calcium levels) results. Problems are directly related to a lack of parathyroid hormone (PTH) secretion or to decreased effectiveness of PTH on target tissue.

Iatrogenic hypoparathyroidism, the most common form, is caused by the removal of all parathyroid tissue during total thyroidectomy or surgical removal of the parathyroid glands.

Idiopathic hypoparathyroidism can occur spontaneously. The exact cause is unknown, but an autoimmune basis is suspected, and it may occur with other autoimmune disorders.

Hypomagnesemia (decreased serum magnesium levels) may cause hypoparathyroidism. Low magnesium levels are seen in patients with malabsorption syndromes, chronic kidney disease (CKD), and malnutrition. Low magnesium levels suppress PTH secretion and may interfere with the effects of PTH on the bones, kidneys, and calcium regulation.

❖ Interprofessional Collaborative Care

◆ Assessment: Recognize Cues. Ask about any head or neck surgery or radiation therapy because these treatments may injure the parathyroid glands and cause hypoparathyroidism. Also ask whether the neck has ever sustained a serious injury in a car crash or by strangulation. Assess whether the patient has any symptoms of hypoparathyroidism, which may range from mild tingling and numbness to muscle tetany. Tingling and numbness around the mouth or in the hands and feet reflect mild-to-moderate hypocalcemia. Severe muscle cramps, spasms of the hands and feet, and seizures (with no loss of consciousness or incontinence) reflect a more severe hypocalcemia. The patient or family may notice mental changes ranging from irritability to psychosis.

The physical assessment may show excessive or inappropriate muscle contractions that cause finger, hand, and elbow flexion. This can signal an impending attack of tetany. Check for Chvostek and Trousseau signs; positive responses indicate potential tetany (see Figs. 13.13 and 13.14 in Chapter 13). Bands or pits may encircle the teeth, which indicates a loss of tooth calcium and enamel.

Diagnostic tests for hypoparathyroidism include electroencephalography (EEG), blood tests, and CT scans. EEG changes revert to normal with correction of hypocalcemia. Serum calcium, phosphorus, magnesium, vitamin D, and urine cyclic adenosine monophosphate (cAMP) levels may be used in the diagnostic workup for hypoparathyroidism (see the Laboratory Profile: Parathyroid Function box). The CT scan can show brain calcifications, which indicate chronic hypocalcemia.

◆ Interventions: Take Action. Nonsurgical management of hypoparathyroidism focuses on correcting hypocalcemia, vitamin D deficiency, and hypomagnesemia. For patients with acute and severe hypocalcemia, IV calcium is given as a 10% solution of calcium chloride or calcium gluconate over 10 to 15 minutes. Acute vitamin D deficiency is treated with daily oral calcitriol. Acute hypomagnesemia is corrected with IV magnesium sulfate. Long-term oral therapy for hypocalcemia involves the intake of calcium, 0.5 to 2 g daily, in divided doses.

Long-term therapy for vitamin D deficiency is replacement with oral ergocalciferol daily. The dosage is adjusted to keep the patient's calcium level in the low-normal range (slightly hypocalcemic), enough to prevent symptoms of hypocalcemia. It must also be low enough to prevent increased urine calcium levels, which can lead to stone formation.

Nursing management includes teaching about the drug regimen and interventions to reduce anxiety. Teach the patient to eat foods high in calcium but low in phosphorus. Milk, yogurt, and processed cheeses are avoided because of their high phosphorus

LABORATORY PROFILE

Parathyroid Function

Test	Normal Range	Hypoparathyroidism	Hyperparathyroidism
Serum calcium	Total: 9.0-10.5 mg/dL (2.25-2.62 mmol/L) Ionized (active): 4.5-5.6 mg/dL (1.05-1.30 mmol/L)	Decreased	Increased in primary hyperparathyroidism
Serum phosphorus	3.0-4.5 mg/dL (0.97-1.45 mmol/L)	Increased	Decreased
Serum magnesium	1.3-2.1 mEq/L (0.65-1.07 mmol/L)	Decreased	Increased
Serum parathyroid hormone	C-terminal: 50-330 pg/mL (ng/L) N-terminal: 8-24 pg/mL (ng/L) Whole: 10-65 pg/mL (ng/L)	Decreased	Increased
Vitamin D (calciferol)	25-80 ng/mL (75-200 nmol/L)	Decreased	Variable

Pagana, K., & Pagana, T. (2018). *Mosby's manual of diagnostic and laboratory tests* (8th ed.). St. Louis: Elsevier.

content. *Stress that therapy for hypocalcemia is lifelong.* Advise the patient to wear a medical alert bracelet. With adherence to the prescribed drug and diet regimen, the calcium level usually remains high enough to prevent a hypocalcemic crisis.

HYPERPARATHYROIDISM

Pathophysiology Review

Hyperparathyroidism is a disorder in which parathyroid secretion of parathyroid hormone is increased, resulting in *hypercalcemia* (excessive serum calcium levels) and *hypophosphatemia* (inadequate serum phosphorus levels). In bone, excessive PTH levels increase bone *resorption* (bone loss of calcium) by decreasing *osteoblastic* (bone production) activity and increasing *osteoclastic* (bone destruction) activity. This process releases calcium and phosphorus into the blood and reduces bone density. With chronic calcium excess and hypercalcemia, calcium is deposited in soft tissues.

Although the exact trigger is unknown, primary hyperparathyroidism results when one or more parathyroid glands do not respond to the normal feedback of serum calcium levels. Common causes of secondary hyperparathyroidism include a benign tumor in one parathyroid gland and chronic kidney disease (CKD) (Gasu & Lim, 2017). Table 58.3 lists other causes.

TABLE 58.3 Causes of Parathyroid Dysfunction

Causes of Hyperparathyroidism	Causes of Hypoparathyroidism
• Parathyroid tumor or cancer • Congenital hyperplasia • Neck trauma or radiation • Vitamin D deficiency • Chronic kidney disease with hypocalcemia • Parathyroid hormone–secreting carcinomas of the lung, kidney, or GI tract	• Surgical or radiation-induced thyroid ablation • Parathyroidectomy • Congenital dysgenesis • Idiopathic (autoimmune) hypoparathyroidism • Hypomagnesemia

❖ Interprofessional Collaborative Care

◆ **Assessment: Recognize Cues.** Symptoms of hyperparathyroidism may be related either to the effects of excessive PTH or to the effects of the accompanying hypercalcemia.

Ask about any bone fractures, recent weight loss, arthritis, or psychological stress. Ask whether the patient has received radiation treatment to the head or neck. The patient with chronic disease may have a waxy pallor of the skin, and bone deformities in the extremities and back.

High levels of PTH cause kidney stones and deposits of calcium in the soft tissue of the kidney. Bone lesions are caused by an increased rate of bone destruction and may result in fractures, bone cysts, and osteoporosis.

GI problems (e.g., anorexia, nausea, vomiting, epigastric pain, constipation, weight loss) are common when serum calcium levels are high. Elevated serum gastrin levels are caused by hypercalcemia and lead to peptic ulcer disease. Fatigue and lethargy may be present and worsen as the serum calcium levels increase. When serum calcium levels are greater than 12 mg/dL (3.0 mmol/L), the patient may have psychosis with confusion, followed by coma and death if left untreated. (See Chapter 13 for more information about hypercalcemia.)

As listed in the Laboratory Profile: Parathyroid Function box, serum PTH, calcium, and phosphorus levels and urine cyclic adenosine monophosphate (cAMP) levels are the laboratory tests used to detect hyperparathyroidism. X-rays may show kidney stones, calcium deposits, and bone lesions. Loss of bone density occurs in the patient with chronic hyperparathyroidism. Other diagnostic tests include arteriography, CT scans, venous sampling of the thyroid for blood PTH levels, and ultrasonography. Explain the procedures and care for the patient undergoing diagnostic tests.

◆ **Interventions: Take Action.** Surgical management is the treatment of choice for patients with hyperparathyroidism. For those who are not candidates for surgery, drug therapy can help control the problems. Priority nursing interventions focus on monitoring and preventing injury.

Nonsurgical Management. *Diuretic and hydration therapies* help reduce serum calcium levels in patients who have milder disease. Usually furosemide, a diuretic that increases kidney excretion of calcium, is used along with IV saline in large volumes to promote calcium excretion.

Drug therapy for patients who have more severe symptoms of hyperparathyroidism or who have hypercalcemia related to parathyroid cancer involves the use of cinacalcet, a calcimimetic. When taken orally, the drug binds to calcium-sensitive receptors on parathyroid tissue, reducing PTH production and release. The result is decreased serum calcium levels, stabilization of other minerals, and decreased progression of PTH-induced bone complications. Another drug approved for CKD-associated hyperparathyroidism in patients undergoing dialysis is etelcalcetide. It is a synthetic calcium-sensing receptor agonist given IV three times weekly at the end of a dialysis session (Hussar, 2018). Both cinacalcet and etelcalcetide require serum calcium monitoring for hypocalcemia on a regular basis for the duration of therapy.

For patients who do not respond to cinacalcet, oral phosphates are used to inhibit bone resorption and interfere with calcium absorption. IV phosphates are used only when serum calcium levels must be lowered rapidly. Calcitonin decreases the release of skeletal calcium and increases kidney excretion of calcium. It is not effective when used alone because of its short duration of action. Therapeutic effects are enhanced if calcitonin is given with glucocorticoids.

Monitor cardiac function and intake and output every 2 hours during hydration therapy. Continuous cardiac monitoring may be necessary. Compare recent ECG tracings with the patient's baseline tracings. Especially look for changes in the T waves and the QT interval, as well as changes in the rate and rhythm. Monitor serum calcium levels, and immediately report any sudden drop to the primary health care provider. Sudden drops in calcium levels may cause tingling and numbness in the muscles.

Preventing injury is important because the patient with chronic hyperparathyroidism often has significant bone density loss and is at risk for fragile fractures. Teach assistive personnel (AP) to handle the patient carefully and to use a lift sheet to reposition the patient rather than pulling him or her.

Surgical Management. Surgical management of hyperparathyroidism is a parathyroidectomy. Before surgery the patient is stabilized, and calcium levels are decreased to near normal.

The operative procedure can be performed as minimally invasive surgery or mini-incision surgery or with a traditional transverse incision in the lower neck. All four parathyroid glands are examined for enlargement. If a tumor is present on one side but the other side is normal, the surgeon removes the glands containing tumor and leaves the remaining glands on the opposite side intact. If all four glands are diseased, they are all removed.

Nursing care before and after surgical removal of the parathyroid glands is the same as that for thyroidectomy. See the Preoperative Care and Postoperative Care sections under Hyperthyroidism for specific nursing interventions.

NCLEX EXAMINATION CHALLENGE 58.3

Health Promotion and Maintenance

A client at continuing risk for hyperparathyroidism is prescribed to take furosemide 40 mg and to drink at least 3 to 4 L of fluid daily. He tells the nurse he believes taking a "water pill" and then drinking so much seems wrong. How will the nurse respond?

A. "This combination of a water pill and drinking more protects you from buildup of excess sodium in the kidney."
B. "The furosemide makes you lose water and you need to increase your intake to keep from becoming dehydrated."
C. "The drug helps you to get rid of calcium and drinking more helps dilute your blood calcium so the level doesn't get too high."
D. "You are correct. I will check with your primary health care provider to determine whether you should restrict your fluid intake."

The remaining glands, which may have atrophied as a result of PTH overproduction, require several days to several weeks to return to normal function. A hypocalcemic crisis can occur during this critical period, and the serum calcium level is assessed frequently after surgery. Check serum calcium levels whenever they are drawn until calcium levels stabilize. Monitor for indications of hypocalcemia, such as tingling and twitching in the extremities and face. Check for Trousseau and Chvostek signs, either of which indicates potential tetany (see Figs. 13.13 and 13.14 in Chapter 13).

The recurrent laryngeal nerve can be damaged during surgery. Assess the patient for changes in voice patterns and hoarseness.

When hyperparathyroidism is caused by *hyperplasia* (tissue overgrowth), three glands plus half of the fourth gland are usually removed. If all four glands are removed, a small portion of a gland may be implanted in the forearm, where it produces PTH and maintains calcium homeostasis. If all these maneuvers fail, the patient will need lifelong treatment with calcium and vitamin D because the resulting hypoparathyroidism is permanent.

GET READY FOR THE NEXT-GENERATION NCLEX® EXAMINATION!

Key Points

Review these Key Points for each NCLEX Examination Client Needs Category.

Safe and Effective Care Environment

- Keep the environment of a patient at risk for thyroid storm cool, dark, and quiet. **QSEN: Safety**
- Keep emergency suctioning and tracheotomy equipment in the room of a patient who has had thyroid or parathyroid surgery. **QSEN: Safety**
- Use a lift sheet to move or reposition a patient with hypocalcemia. **QSEN: Safety**

Health Promotion and Maintenance

- Teach all patients to take antithyroid drugs or thyroid hormone replacement therapy as prescribed. **QSEN: Patient-Centered Care**
- Teach patients to use signs and symptoms (e.g., the number of bowel movements per day, the ability to sleep) as indicators of therapy effectiveness and when the dose of thyroid hormone replacement may need to be adjusted. **QSEN: Patient-Centered Care**

Psychosocial Integrity

- Remind patients and family members that changes in cognition and behavior related to thyroid problems are usually temporary. **QSEN: Patient-Centered Care**
- Encourage the patient who has a permanent change in appearance (e.g., exophthalmia) to mourn the change. **QSEN: Patient-Centered Care**

Physiological Integrity

- Be aware that:
  - The presence of a goiter indicates a problem with the thyroid gland but can accompany either hyperthyroidism or hypothyroidism.
  - Although similar in action, methimazole and propylthiouracil are not interchangeable.
  - Methimazole can cause birth defects and should not be used during pregnancy, especially during the first trimester. Instruct women to notify their primary health care provider if pregnancy occurs.
- When stridor, dyspnea, or other symptoms of obstruction appear after thyroid surgery, notify the Rapid Response Team. **QSEN: Safety**
- When caring for a patient with hyperthyroidism, even after a thyroidectomy, immediately report a temperature increase of even 1°F because it may indicate an impending thyroid crisis. **QSEN: Evidence-Based Practice**
- Assess the cardiopulmonary status of any patient with hypothyroidism for decreased perfusion or decreased ***gas exchange*** at least every 8 hours. **QSEN: Patient-Centered Care**
- Use sedating drugs or opioids sparingly with patients who have hypothyroidism. **QSEN: Patient-Centered Care**
- Monitor the hydration status of patients who have hypercalcemia. **QSEN: Patient-Centered Care**
- Assess the patient with hypoparathyroidism for manifestations of hypocalcemia, especially numbness or tingling around the mouth and a positive Chvostek sign or Trousseau sign (see Figs. 13.13 and 13.14 in Chapter 13). **QSEN: Patient-Centered Care**

MASTERY QUESTIONS

1. Performance of which assessment is a **priority** for the nurse before giving a client the first oral dose of hormone replacement for hypothyroidism?
   A. Measuring heart rate and rhythm
   B. Checking core body temperature
   C. Asking about previous allergic drug reactions
   D. Listening to bowel sounds in all four abdominal quadrants
2. Which assessment findings in a client with hyperthyroidism indicate to the nurse that the client is in danger of thyroid storm? **Select all that apply.**
   A. Increased salivation
   B. Client report of increased palmar sweating
   C. Decreased pulse pressure from 40 mm Hg to 36 mm Hg
   D. Diminished bowel sounds in all four abdominal quadrants
   E. An increase in temperature from 99.5°F (37.5°C) to 101.3°F (38.5°C)
   F. Serum sodium level increase from 136 mEq/L (mmol/L) to 139 mEq/L (mmol/L)
   G. Increase in premature ventricular heart contractions from 4 per minute to 28 per minute
3. The nurse reviewing the laboratory values of a client with hypoparathyroidism finds a serum calcium level of 7.9 mg/dL (1.76 mmol/L). Which parameter is most important for the nurse to assess to **prevent harm**?
   A. Temperature
   B. Heart rate and rhythm
   C. Deep tendon reflexes
   D. Level of consciousness

REFERENCES

Asterisk (*) indicates a classic or definitive work on this subject.

American Cancer Society (ACS). (2020). *Cancer facts and figures-2020.* Report No. 00-300M-No. 500820. Atlanta: Author.

Brent, G., & Weetman, A. (2016). Hypothyroidism and thyroiditis. In S. Melmed, K. Polonsky, P. R. Larsen, & H. Kronenberg (Eds.), *Williams' textbook of endocrinology* (13th ed.). Philadelphia: Saunders.

Burchum, J., & Rosenthal, L. (2019). *Lehne's pharmacology for nursing care* (10th ed.). St. Louis: Elsevier.

Canadian Cancer Society, Statistics Canada. (2019). *Canadian cancer Statistics, 2019.* Toronto, ON: Canadian Cancer Society. https://www.cancer.ca/~/media/cancer.ca/CW/cancer%20information/cancer%20101/Canadian%20cancer%20statistics/Canadian-Cancer-Statistics-2019-EN.pdf?la=en.

Davies, T., Laurberg, P., & Bahn, R. (2016). Thyrotoxicosis. In S. Melmed, K. Polonsky, P. R. Larsen, & H. Kronenberg (Eds.), *Williams' textbook of endocrinology* (13th ed.). Philadelphia: Saunders.

Felicilda-Reynaldo, R., & Kenneally, M. (2016). Antithyroid drugs for hyperthyroidism. *MEDSURG Nursing, 25*(1), 50–54.

Gasu, V., & Lim, F. (2017). Secondary hyperparathyroidism in chronic kidney disease. *American Nurse Today, 12*(7), 20–23.

Hooley, J., & Reagan, S. (2016). Hyperthyroidism: A storm brewing. *American Nurse Today, 11*(10). https://www.americannursetoday.com/hyperthyroidism-a-storm-brewing/.

Hussar, D. (2018). New drugs, part 3: Drugs for hyperparathyroidism. *Nursing, 48*(10), 32–42.

McCance, K., Huether, S., Brashers, V., & Rote, N. (2019). *Pathophysiology: The biologic basis for disease in adults and children* (8th ed.). St. Louis: Elsevier.

Moore, D. (2018). Hypothyroidism and nursing care. *American Nurse Today, 13*(2), 44–46.

*Online Mendelian Inheritance in Man (OMIM). (2014). *Multiple endocrine neoplasia, Type II A; MEN2A* www.omim.org/entry/171400.

Online Mendelian Inheritance in Man (OMIM). (2016). *Graves disease, susceptibility to, 1.* www.omim.org/entry/275000.

Pagana, K., & Pagana, T. (2018). *Mosby's manual of diagnostic and laboratory tests* (6th ed.). St. Louis: Elsevier.

Schreiber, M. (2017). Thyroid storm. *MEDSURG Nursing, 26*(2), 143–145.

Touhy, T., & Jett, K. (2020). *Ebersole and Hess' toward nursing healthy aging* (10th ed.). St. Louis: Mosby.

59

Concepts of Care for Patients With Diabetes Mellitus

Sharon A. Watts

http://evolve.elsevier.com/Iggy/

LEARNING OUTCOMES

1. Collaborate with the interprofessional team to coordinate high-quality care and promote ***glucose regulation*** in patients who have diabetes mellitus (DM).
2. Teach the patient and caregiver(s) about how impaired ***glucose regulation*** from DM and its complications affect home safety.
3. Prioritize evidence-based care for patients with common complications of DM affecting ***glucose regulation***.
4. Teach the patient and caregiver(s) about common drugs and other therapies used to manage DM and its complications.
5. Teach patients with DM about self-care management when in the community.
6. Teach adults at risk for impaired ***glucose regulation*** how to prevent or delay development of type 2 DM.
7. Implement patient and family-centered nursing interventions to help adults cope with the psychosocial impact caused by DM and its complications.
8. Use clinical judgment to analyze relevant assessment data when planning care for patients who have impaired ***glucose regulation*** and DM.
9. Implement evidence-based nursing actions to improve ***glucose regulation*** and prevent complications of DM.

KEY TERMS

diabetes mellitus A common, complex, chronic disorder of impaired nutrient metabolism, especially glucose, that can affect the function of every body system.

diabetic ketoacidosis (DKA) A severe acute complication of diabetes; characterized by uncontrolled hyperglycemia, metabolic acidosis, and increased production of ketones.

diabetic peripheral neuropathy Progressive deterioration of nerve function with the loss of *sensory perception*.

gastroparesis A delay in gastric emptying.

glucagon A hormone important in glucose regulation that has balancing actions opposite those of insulin and prevents hypoglycemia.

gluconeogenesis Conversion of protein substances into glucose.

glucose regulation Process of maintaining optimal blood glucose levels; also known as *glycemic control.*

glycogenesis Production and storage of glycogen.

glycogenolysis Breakdown of stored glycogen into glucose.

glycosylated hemoglobin (A1C) A standardized test that measures how much glucose permanently attaches to the hemoglobin molecule; is often used to indicate the effectiveness of blood glucose control measures.

hyperglycemia Higher-than-normal blood glucose level.

hyperglycemic-hyperosmolar state (HHS) A severe acute hyperosmolar (increased blood osmolarity) state caused by hyperglycemia.

hypoglycemia Lower-than-normal blood glucose level.

hyperinsulinemia Chronically high blood insulin levels.

ketogenesis Conversion of fats to acid products.

ketone bodies ("ketones") Abnormal acidic breakdown products that collect in the blood when insulin is not available, leading to the *acid-base balance* problem of metabolic acidosis.

Kussmaul respiration A deep and rapid respiratory pattern triggered by acidosis to reduce blood hydrogen ion concentration by "blowing off" carbon dioxide.

lipolysis Breakdown of body fats.

metabolic syndrome Simultaneous presence of metabolic factors that increase risk for developing type 2 DM and cardiovascular disease.

proliferative diabetic retinopathy Growth of new fragile retinal blood vessels (neovascularization) that bleed easily and obscure vision.

proteolysis Breakdown of body proteins.

PRIORITY AND INTERRELATED CONCEPTS

The priority concept for this chapter is:
- ***Glucose Regulation***

The ***Glucose Regulation*** concept exemplar for this chapter is Diabetes Mellitus.

The interrelated concepts for this chapter are:
- ***Nutrition***
- ***Tissue Integrity***
- ***Sensory Perception***
- ***Perfusion***
- ***Immunity***
- ***Fluid and Electrolyte Balance***
- ***Acid-Base Balance***

GLUCOSE REGULATION CONCEPT EXEMPLAR: DIABETES MELLITUS

Diabetes mellitus (DM) is a common, chronic, complex disorder of impaired nutrient metabolism, especially glucose, that can affect the function of every body system. Although all nutrients are affected, glucose regulation is impaired first, which then changes protein and fat metabolism. *Glucose regulation* is the process of maintaining optimal blood glucose levels, also known as *glycemic control* (Fig. 59.1). With impaired glucose regulation, many acute and chronic health problems occur as life-shortening complications. In the United States and Canada the percentage of hospitalized patients who have DM is over 40%, which is much greater than the percentage of people with DM in the general population, allowing the disorder to have a large impact on health care costs and resources (Schneider et al., 2016; Watts et al., 2018). Thus a major focus of management is to identify the presence of DM to help the adult manage the disorder and maintain glycemic control for prevention of complications.

Nurses play a critical role in helping patients and families understand the disorder and actively participate in its management. As part of the team you will help plan, organize, and coordinate care with other team members to promote the patient's health and well-being. These management activities may take place in almost any setting. The desired outcome is to help patients maintain blood glucose levels in the normal range *(euglycemia)* without causing either hyperglycemia (higher than normal blood glucose level) or hypoglycemia (lower than normal blood glucose level).

Pathophysiology Review

Classification of Diabetes. Diabetes mellitus (DM) has many subtypes, and all have the main feature of chronic hyperglycemia resulting from impaired processes in ***glucose regulation*** that include reduced insulin secretion or reduced insulin action or both. The disease is classified by the underlying problem causing a lack of insulin or its action and the severity of the insulin deficiency. Table 59.1 outlines the types of DM. This chapter focuses on the two most common types of DM. Regardless of the specific type of DM, the organ-damaging consequences and complications of impaired glucose regulation are the same.

The Endocrine Pancreas. The pancreas regulates digestion through its exocrine functions and ensures ***glucose regulation*** through its endocrine functions. The endocrine pancreas has about 1 million small glands, the islets of Langerhans, scattered through the organ. Inside the islets are two types of cells important to glucose regulation. These are the *alpha* cells, which secrete glucagon, and the *beta* cells, which produce insulin and amylin (Fig. 59.2).

Glucagon is a hormone that has balancing actions opposite those of insulin. It prevents *hypoglycemia* by triggering the release of glucose from storage sites in the liver and skeletal muscle. It is sometimes called the "hormone of starvation" because it is secreted when food intake is low to release glucose from the liver to keep blood glucose levels in the normal range.

Insulin prevents *hyperglycemia* by allowing body cells to take up, use, and store carbohydrate, fat, and protein. It is sometimes called the "hormone of plenty" because it is secreted when food intake is high and works to move glucose from the blood into cells to keep blood glucose levels in the normal range. Active insulin is a protein made up of 51 amino acids. It is first produced as inactive *proinsulin,* a prohormone that is converted in the liver to active insulin. Movement of glucose into most cells requires the presence of specific membrane receptors along with insulin. Insulin is like a "key" that opens "locked" membranes to glucose, allowing blood glucose to move into cells to generate energy. Insulin starts this action by binding to membrane insulin receptors, which changes membrane permeability to glucose (Fig. 59.3).

Insulin is secreted daily in a two-step manner, with low-level secretion during fasting (basal insulin secretion) and in a two-phase release after eating *(prandial).* An early burst of insulin secretion occurs within 10 minutes of eating, followed by an increasing release that lasts until the blood glucose level returns to normal.

Glucose Regulation and Homeostasis. Although glucose is a critical nutrient, chronically high blood glucose levels cause many serious problems, and low blood glucose levels can rapidly lead to injury or death. Thus ***glucose regulation*** that maintains blood glucose levels within a relatively normal range is important (see Fig. 59.1). Several organs and hormones play a role in maintaining glucose regulation. During fasting, when the stomach is empty, blood glucose is maintained between 60 and 150 mg/dL (3.3 and 8.3 mmol/L) by a balance between glucose uptake by cells and glucose production by the liver. Insulin plays a pivotal role in this process.

Glucose is the main fuel for central nervous system (CNS) cells. Because the brain cannot produce or store much glucose, it needs a continuous supply from the blood to prevent neuron dysfunction and cell death. (Other organs can use both glucose and fatty acids to generate energy.) Glucose is stored as glycogen in the liver and skeletal muscles, and free fatty acids (FFAs) are stored as triglyceride in fat cells. During a prolonged fast or after illness, proteins are broken down, and some of the amino acids are converted into glucose.

Insulin exerts many effects on metabolism and cellular processes in all tissues and organs. The main metabolic effects of

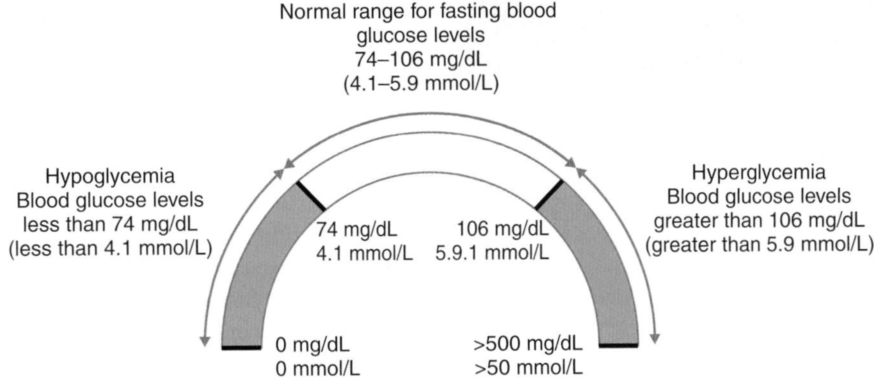

FIG. 59.1 Fasting blood glucose levels. When ***glucose regulation*** is adequate, fasting levels remain in the normal range. With insufficient insulin usage, hyperglycemia results. Excess insulin or insufficient glucose results in hypoglycemia.

TABLE 59.1 Classification of Diabetes Mellitus

Type 1 Diabetes (T1DM)
- Beta cell destruction leading to absolute insulin deficiency
- Autoimmune
- Idiopathic

Type 2 Diabetes (T2DM)

Ranges from insulin resistance with relative insulin deficiency to secretory deficit with insulin resistance

Maturity-Onset Diabetes of the Young (MODY)
- Inherited mutation in one of at least six known genes that results in loss of insulin function and hyperglycemia
- Usually diagnosed in younger adults but can be found at any time in adulthood
- Resembles type 1 DM with insulin requirements and potential for diabetic ketoacidosis (DKA)
- Is **not** an autoimmune problem

Gestational Diabetes Mellitus (GDM)
- Glucose intolerance with onset in or first recognition during pregnancy (All pregnant women should be screened.)

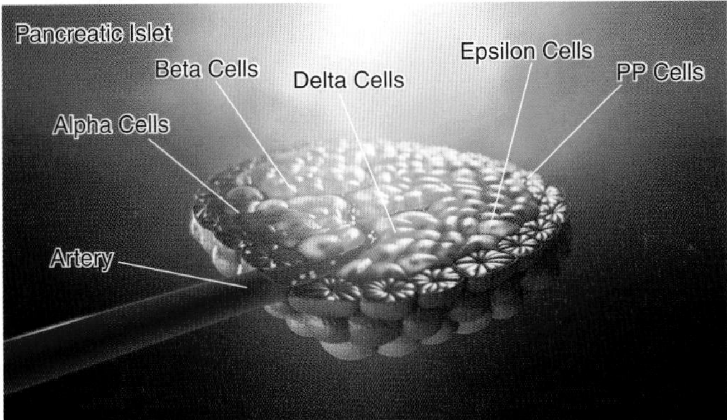

FIG. 59.2 Hormone secreting cells of the islets of Langerhans in the pancreas. Alpha cells secrete glucagon; beta cells secrete insulin. (© Elsevier Animation Collection.)

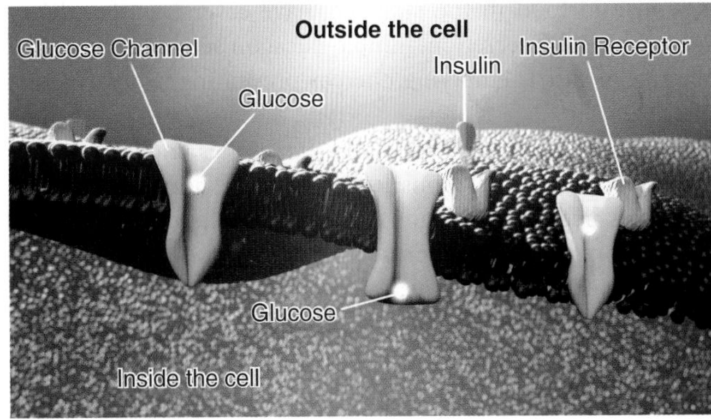

FIG. 59.3 Insulin attaches to receptors on target cells, where it promotes glucose transport into the cells through the cell membranes. (© Elsevier Animation Collection.)

insulin are to stimulate glucose uptake in skeletal muscle and heart muscle and to suppress liver production of glucose and very-low-density lipoprotein (VLDL). In the liver, insulin promotes the production and storage of glycogen (**glycogenesis**) at the same time that it inhibits glycogen breakdown into glucose (**glycogenolysis**). It increases protein and lipid (fat) synthesis and inhibits **ketogenesis** (conversion of fats to acids) and **gluconeogenesis** (conversion of proteins to glucose). In muscle, insulin promotes protein and glycogen synthesis. In fat cells, it promotes triglyceride storage. Overall, insulin keeps blood glucose levels from becoming too high and helps keep blood lipid levels in the normal range.

In the *fasting state* (not eating for 8 hours), insulin secretion is suppressed, which leads to increased gluconeogenesis in the liver and kidneys, along with increased glucose generation by the breakdown of liver glycogen. In the fed state, insulin released from pancreatic beta cells reverses this process. Instead, glycogen breakdown and gluconeogenesis are inhibited. At the same time, insulin also enhances glucose uptake and use by cells and reduces both body fat breakdown (**lipolysis**) and body protein breakdown (**proteolysis**). When more glucose is present in liver cells than can be used for energy or stored as glycogen, insulin causes the excess glucose to be converted to free fatty acids (FFAs). These extra FFAs are deposited in fat cells.

TABLE 59.2 Physiologic Responses to Insufficient Insulin

- Decreased glycogenesis (conversion of glucose to glycogen)
- Increased glycogenolysis (conversion of glycogen to glucose)
- Increased gluconeogenesis (formation of glucose from noncarbohydrate sources such as amino acids and lactate)
- Increased lipolysis (breakdown of triglycerides to glycerol and free fatty acids)
- Increased ketogenesis (formation of ketones from free fatty acids)
- Proteolysis (breakdown of protein with amino acid release in muscles)

Glucose in the blood after a meal is controlled by the emptying rate of the stomach and delivery of nutrients to the small intestine, where they are absorbed into circulation. *Incretin hormones* (e.g., *glucagon-like peptide 1 [GLP-1]*), secreted in response to food in the stomach, have several actions. They increase insulin secretion, inhibit glucagon secretion, and slow the rate of gastric emptying, thereby preventing hyperglycemia after meals.

Balancing *(counterregulatory)* hormones increase blood glucose by actions opposite those of insulin when more energy is needed. Glucagon is the main balancing hormone. Other hormones that increase blood glucose levels are epinephrine, norepinephrine, growth hormone, and cortisol. The combined actions of insulin and balancing hormones (discussed in the next section) participate in ***glucose regulation*** and keep blood glucose levels in the range of 60 to 100 mg/dL (3.3 to 5.6 mmol/L) to support brain function. When blood glucose levels fall, insulin secretion stops and glucagon is released. Glucagon causes glucose release from the liver. Liver glucose is made through breakdown of glycogen to glucose and conversion of amino acids into glucose. When liver glucose is unavailable, the breakdown of body fat and the breakdown of body proteins, especially muscle, provide acids as fuel for energy.

Absence of Insulin. ***Glucose regulation*** requires insulin to move glucose into many body tissues. The lack of insulin action in diabetes, from either a lack of production or a problem with insulin use at its cell receptors, prevents some cells from using glucose for energy. The body then breaks down fat and protein in an attempt to provide energy and increases levels of balancing hormones to make glucose from other sources. Table 59.2 outlines responses to insufficient insulin.

Without insulin, glucose builds up in the blood, causing hyperglycemia, which disturbs ***fluid and electrolyte balance***, leading to the classic symptoms of diabetes: polyuria, polydipsia, and polyphagia.

Polyuria is frequent and excessive urination and results from an osmotic diuresis caused by excess glucose in the urine. With diuresis, electrolytes are excreted in the urine, and water loss is severe. Dehydration results, and *polydipsia* (excessive thirst) occurs. Because the cells receive no glucose, cell starvation triggers *polyphagia* (excessive eating). Despite eating, the adult with diabetes remains in metabolic starvation until insulin is available to move glucose into the cells.

With insulin deficiency, the body turns to stored fat for energy, releasing free fatty acids (FFAs). When this stored fat is used for energy, small ketone bodies provide a backup energy source. **Ketone bodies** ("ketones") are abnormal acidic breakdown products that collect in the blood when insulin is not available, leading to the ***acid-base balance*** problem of metabolic acidosis.

Dehydration with DM leads to *hemoconcentration* (increased blood concentration); *hypovolemia* (decreased blood volume); poor tissue ***perfusion***; and *hypoxia* (poor tissue oxygenation), especially to the brain. Hypoxic cells do not metabolize glucose efficiently, the Krebs cycle is blocked, and lactic acid production increases, causing more acidosis.

The excess acids caused by absence of insulin increase hydrogen ion (H^+) and carbon dioxide (CO_2) levels in the blood, causing anion-gap metabolic acidosis. These products trigger the brain to increase the rate and depth of respiration in an attempt to "blow off" carbon dioxide and acid. This type of breathing is known as **Kussmaul respiration**. Acetone is exhaled, giving the breath a "rotting citrus fruit" odor. When the lungs can no longer offset acidosis, the blood pH drops. Arterial blood gas studies show a *metabolic acidosis* (decreased pH with decreased arterial bicarbonate [$HCO_3{}_-$] levels) and *compensatory respiratory alkalosis* (decreased partial pressure of arterial carbon dioxide [$Paco_2$]).

Insulin lack first causes potassium depletion. With the increased fluid loss from hyperglycemia, excessive potassium is excreted in the urine, leading to low serum potassium levels. High serum potassium levels may occur in acidosis because of the shift of potassium from inside the cells to the blood in exchange for hydrogen ions. Serum potassium levels in DM, then, may be low *(hypokalemia)*, high *(hyperkalemia)*, or normal, depending on hydration, the severity of acidosis, and the patient's response to treatment. Chapter 14 discusses ***acid-base balance*** and acidosis in more detail.

NCLEX EXAMINATION CHALLENGE 59.1

Physiological Integrity

Which hormones help **prevent** hypoglycemia? **Select all that apply.**

A. Aldosterone
B. Cortisol
C. Epinephrine
D. Growth hormone
E. Glucagon
F. Insulin
G. Norepinephrine
H. Proinsulin

Acute Complications of Diabetes. Three glucose-related emergencies can occur in patients with DM:

- Diabetic ketoacidosis (DKA) caused by absence of insulin and generation of ketoacids
- Hyperglycemic-hyperosmolar state (HHS) caused by insulin deficiency and profound dehydration
- Hypoglycemia from too much insulin or too little glucose

All three problems require emergency treatment and can be fatal if treatment is delayed or incorrect. These problems and their management are described later in this chapter.

Chronic Complications of Diabetes. Changes in large blood vessels *(macrovascular)* and small blood vessels *(microvascular)* in tissues and organs result from DM and can lead to organ complications and early death. These blood vessel changes lead to complications from poor tissue ***perfusion*** and tissue ischemia. Macrovascular complications include coronary heart disease, cerebrovascular disease, and peripheral vascular disease, all of which lead to early morbidity and mortality. Microvascular complications of blood vessel structure and function lead to *nephropathy* (kidney dysfunction), *neuropathy* (nerve dysfunction), and *retinopathy* (vision problems). Such problems are responsible for increased morbidity and reduced quality of life. Causes of these diabetic vascular complications include:

- Chronic hyperglycemia thickens basement membranes, which causes organ damage.
- Glucose toxicity directly or indirectly affects functional cell integrity.
- Chronic ischemia in small blood vessels causes tissue hypoxia and microischemia.

Chronic high blood glucose levels are the main cause of microvascular complications and allow premature development of macrovascular complications. Additional risk factors contributing to poor health outcomes for adults with DM include smoking, physical inactivity, obesity, hypertension, and high blood fat and cholesterol levels.

Hyperglycemia from poor ***glucose regulation*** leads to long-term complications of DM. Intensive therapy to maintain glycemic control with blood glucose levels as close to normal as possible delays the onset and progression of retinopathy, nephropathy, neuropathy, and macrovascular disease for patients with DM. For every percentage point decrease in A1C (glycosylated hemoglobin), a significant reduction of kidney and eye complications occurs.

Macrovascular Complications

Cardiovascular Disease. Patients with diabetes, prediabetes, or metabolic syndrome are at increased risk for cardiovascular disease (CVD) (McCance et al., 2019; Rariden, 2019; Wisnewski, 2017). Because DM is so strongly associated with CVD, it is a target for aggressive CVD risk factor reduction.

Patients with DM, especially type 2 DM, often have the traditional CVD risk factors of obesity, high blood lipid levels, hypertension, and sedentary lifestyle. Cigarette smoking and a positive family history also increase risk for CVD. Kidney disease, indicated by *albuminuria* (presence of albumin in the urine), and retinopathy are associated with increased risk for coronary heart disease and mortality from coronary artery disease.

Cardiovascular complication rates can be reduced through aggressive management of hypertension, hyperglycemia, and hyperlipidemia. The American Diabetes Association (ADA) recommends that blood pressure be maintained below 140/90 mm Hg, with a target of 130/80 mm Hg in younger adults if that level can be achieved without excessive burden. Lipid profile screening is recommended starting at first diagnosis and every 1 to 2 years thereafter. Patients with DM who do not have overt CVD are recommended to maintain low-density lipoprotein (LDL) cholesterol below 100 mg/dL (2.60 mmol/L), and patients with indications of CVD are recommended to maintain LDL at less than 70 mg/dL (1.8 mmol/L) (ADA, 2019a). Lifestyle modifications that focus on reducing saturated fat, *trans* fat, and cholesterol intake; increasing intake of omega-3 fatty acids, fiber, and plant sterols; weight loss (if indicated); and increasing physical activity are recommended (ADA, 2019e).

Priority nursing activities focus on interventions to reduce modifiable risk factors associated with CVD. Modifiable risk factors include smoking cessation, diet, exercise, blood pressure control, and maintaining prescribed lipid-lowering drug therapy and aspirin use.

Cerebrovascular Disease. The risk for stroke is two to four times higher in adults with DM compared with those who do not have the disease (McCance et al., 2019). Diabetes also increases the likelihood of severe carotid atherosclerosis. Hypertension, hyperlipidemia, nephropathy, peripheral vascular disease, and alcohol and tobacco use further increase the risk for stroke in adults with DM.

Reduced Immunity. The combination of vascular changes and hyperglycemia reduces ***immunity*** by reducing white blood cell activity, inhibiting gas exchange in tissues, and promoting the growth of microorganisms. As a result, any adult who has DM is at an increased risk for developing an infection on exposure to bacteria and other organisms. In addition, infections become serious more quickly and can lead to major complications and sepsis (McCance et al., 2019).

Microvascular Complications

Eye and Vision Complications. Blindness is 25 times more common in patients with DM. Diabetic retinopathy (DR) is strongly related to the duration of diabetes. After 20 years of DM, nearly all patients with the disease have some degree of retinopathy (ADA, 2019g). Unfortunately, DR has few symptoms until vision loss occurs.

DR is related to problems that block retinal blood vessels and cause them to leak, leading to retinal hypoxia. Nonproliferative diabetic retinopathy causes structural problems in retinal vessels with areas of poor retinal circulation, edema, hard fatty deposits in the eye, and retinal hemorrhages. Fluid and blood leak from the vessels and cause retinal edema and hard exudates. Nonproliferative DR develops slowly and rarely reduces vision to the point of blindness.

Proliferative diabetic retinopathy is the growth of new retinal blood vessels, also known as *neovascularization*. When retinal blood flow is poor and hypoxia develops, retinal cells secrete growth factors that stimulate formation of new blood vessels in the eye. These new vessels are thin, fragile, and bleed easily, leading to vision loss.

Visual ***sensory perception*** loss from DR has several mechanisms. Central vision may be impaired by macular edema with increased blood vessel permeability and deposits of hard exudates at the center of the retina. This problem is the main cause of vision loss in the adult with DM. Vision loss also occurs from macular degeneration, corneal scarring, and changes in lens shape or clarity.

Hyperglycemia may cause blurred vision, even with eyeglasses. Because hypoglycemia can cause temporary vision changes, it is important to wait until blood glucose levels are normal before assessing for refractory changes. Cataracts occur at a younger age and progress faster among patients with DM. Open-angle glaucoma also is more common in patients with DM. The management of cataracts and glaucoma is discussed in Chapter 42.

Control of blood glucose, blood pressure, and blood lipid level is important in preventing DR. Thus patients with DM should have routine ophthalmic evaluations to detect vision problems early before vision loss occurs.

PATIENT-CENTERED CARE: OLDER ADULT CONSIDERATIONS QSEN

Older patients with diabetic retinopathy also have general age-related vision changes, which reduce the ability to perform self-care. They may have blurred vision, distorted central vision, fluctuating vision, and loss of color perception. Assess the ability of patients with vision changes to measure and inject insulin and to monitor blood glucose levels to determine if adaptive devices are needed to assist in self-management (Touhy & Jett, 2020).

Diabetic Peripheral Neuropathy. Diabetic peripheral neuropathy (DPN) is a progressive deterioration of nerve function that results in loss of ***sensory perception***. It is a common complication of DM and often involves all body areas. Damage to sensory nerve fibers results first in pain, which is eventually followed by loss of sensation. Damage to motor nerve fibers results in muscle weakness. The onset is slow, affects both sides of the body, progresses, and is permanent. Late complications include foot ulcers and deformities. Damage to nerve fibers in the autonomic nervous system can cause dysfunction in every organ. The combination of factors leading to the nerve damage in diabetic neuropathy consists of:

- Hyperglycemia, long duration of DM, hyperlipidemia
- Damaged blood vessels leading to reduced neuronal oxygen and other nutrients
- Increased genetic susceptibility to nerve damage
- Smoking, nicotine, and alcohol use

Hyperglycemia leads to DPN through blood vessel changes and reduced tissue ***perfusion*** that cause nerve hypoxia, which leads to poor nerve impulse transmission. Excessive glucose is converted to sorbitol, which collects in nerves and impairs motor nerve conduction (McCance et al., 2019). Common diabetic neuropathies are listed in Table 59.3.

Diabetic Autonomic Neuropathy. Cardiovascular autonomic neuropathy (CAN) affects sympathetic and parasympathetic nerves of the heart and blood vessels. This problem is underdiagnosed in diabetes and contributes to left ventricular dysfunction, painless myocardial infarction (MI), and exercise intolerance (Wooten & Melchior, 2020). Most often, CAN leads to *orthostatic* (postural) hypotension and *syncope* (brief loss of consciousness on standing). These problems are from failure of the heart and arteries to respond to position changes by increasing heart rate and vascular tone. As a result, blood flow to the brain is interrupted briefly. Orthostatic hypotension and syncope increase the risk for falls, especially among older adults (Touhy & Jett, 2020).

TABLE 59.3 Features of Diabetic Neuropathy

	Complication	Symptom
Distal symmetric polyneuropathy	Sensory alterations	Paresthesias: burning/tingling sensations, starting in toes and moving up legs Dysesthesias: burning, stinging, or stabbing pain Anesthesia: loss of sensation
	Motor alterations in intrinsic muscles of foot	Foot deformities: high arch, claw toes, hammertoes; shift of weight bearing to metatarsal heads and tips of toes
Autonomic neuropathy	Anhidrosis	Drying, cracking of skin
	Gastrointestinal	Delayed gastric emptying, gastric retention, early satiety, bloating, nausea, vomiting, anorexia, constipation, diarrhea, diffuse sweating while eating Nocturnal diarrhea
	Neurogenic bladder	Atonic bladder, urinary retention
	Impotence	Erectile dysfunction
	Cardiovascular autonomic neuropathy (CAN)	Early fatigue, weakness with exercise, orthostatic hypotension
	Defective balancing hormones	Loss of warning signs of hypoglycemia

Autonomic neuropathy can affect the entire GI system. Common GI problems from diabetic neuropathy include gastroesophageal reflex, delayed gastric emptying and gastric retention, early satiety, heartburn, nausea, vomiting, and anorexia. Sluggish movement of the small intestine can lead to bacterial overgrowth, which causes bloating, gas, and both diarrhea and constipation. Constipation, the most common GI problem with DM, is intermittent and may alternate with bouts of diarrhea. Gastroparesis (delay in gastric emptying) is a cause of hypoglycemia related to the mismatch of nutrient absorption and insulin action.

Urinary problems from neuropathy cause incomplete bladder emptying and urine retention, which leads to urinary infection and kidney problems. Early symptoms include frequency and urgency. Later symptoms are inability to sense bladder fullness and incontinence.

Diabetic Nephropathy. *Nephropathy* is a pathologic change in the kidney that reduces kidney function and leads to kidney failure. Diabetes is the leading cause of end-stage kidney disease (ESKD) and kidney failure in the United States. Risk factors include a 10- to 15-year history of DM, poor blood glucose control, uncontrolled hypertension, and genetic predisposition. Kidney disease causes progressive albumin excretion and declining glomerular filtration rate (GFR). The onset of diabetic kidney disease may be delayed or prevented by maintaining optimum blood ***glucose regulation*** (ADA, 2019c).

Chronic high blood glucose levels cause hypertension in kidney blood vessels and excess kidney tissue ***perfusion***. The blood vessels become leakier, especially in the glomerulus, allowing filtration of albumin and other proteins that deposit in the kidney tissues and blood vessels. Narrowed blood vessels decrease kidney oxygenation,

TABLE 59.4 Differentiation of Type 1 and Type 2 Diabetes

Features	Type 1	Type 2
Former names	Juvenile-onset diabetes Ketosis-prone diabetes Insulin-dependent diabetes mellitus (IDDM)	Adult-onset diabetes Ketosis-resistant diabetes Non–insulin-dependent diabetes mellitus (NIDDM)
Age at onset	Usually younger than 30 yr	May occur at any age in adults
Symptoms	Abrupt onset, thirst, hunger, increased urine output, weight loss	Frequently none; thirst, fatigue, blurred vision, vascular or neural complications
Etiology	Viral infection, autoimmunity	Not known, genetic predisposition
Pathology	Pancreatic beta cell destruction	Insulin resistance Dysfunctional pancreatic beta cell
Antigen patterns	*HLA-DR, HLA-DQ*	None
Antibodies	Often present at diagnosis	None
Endogenous insulin and C-peptide	None to very low	Low, normal, or high
Inheritance	Complex	Autosomal dominant, multifactorial
Nutritional status	Usually nonobese	60% to 80% obese
Insulin	All dependent on insulin	Required for 20% to 30%
Medical therapy	Mandatory	Mandatory

leading to kidney cell hypoxia and cell death, which can progress to chronic kidney disease (see Chapter 63 for a detailed presentation of chronic kidney disease and end-stage kidney disease). Hypertension speeds the progression of diabetic nephropathy.

Sexual Dysfunction. Sexual dysfunction can develop in both men and women with DM as a result of damage to both nerve tissue and vascular tissue. This is made worse by poorly controlled blood glucose levels. Other factors include obesity, hypertension, tobacco use, and some prescribed drugs.

In men sexual dysfunction manifests with both erectile dysfunction (ED) and retrograde ejaculation. Women may experience deceased vaginal lubrication, uncomfortable or painful sexual intercourse, and decreases in libido and sexual response.

Cognitive Dysfunction. Older adults with DM are at higher risk for developing all types of dementia compared with adults who do not have the disease (ADA, 2019i). Chronic hyperglycemia with microvascular disease contributes to neuron damage, brain atrophy, and cognitive impairment. These problems are more frequent and more severe in patients with longer-duration DM and increase the complications of neuropathy and retinopathy.

Etiology and Genetic Risk

Type 1 Diabetes. Type 1 diabetes mellitus (DM) is an autoimmune disorder in which beta cells are destroyed in a genetically susceptible person (Table 59.4). The immune system fails to recognize normal body cells as "self," and immune system cells and antibodies take destructive actions against the insulin-secreting cells in the islets. People with certain tissue types are more likely to develop autoimmune diseases, including type 1 DM. Viral infections, such as mumps and coxsackievirus infection, may trigger autoimmune destructive actions (McCance et al., 2019).

PATIENT-CENTERED CARE: GENETIC/GENOMIC CONSIDERATIONS QSEN

Inheritance of genes encoding for the HLA-DR and HLA-DQA and DQB tissue types increases the risk for type 1 DM (McCance et al., 2019). However, inheritance of these genes only *increases the risk,* and most people with these tissue types do ***not*** develop type 1 DM. Development of DM is an interactive effect of genetic predisposition and exposure to certain environmental factors. During assessment, always ask whether any family members have been diagnosed with either type 1 or type 2 diabetes or any other autoimmune disorder.

Type 2 Diabetes and Metabolic Syndrome. Type 2 DM is a progressive disorder in which the person initially has insulin resistance that progresses to decreased beta cell secretion of insulin. *Insulin resistance* (a reduced cell receptor response to insulin) develops from obesity and physical inactivity in a genetically susceptible adult (ADA, 2019h). It occurs before the onset of type 2 DM and often is accompanied by the cardiovascular risk factors of hyperlipidemia, hypertension, and increased clot formation. Many but not all patients with type 2 DM are obese. The specific causes of type 2 DM are not known, although insulin resistance and beta cell failure have many genetic and nongenetic causes. Heredity plays a major role in the development of type 2 DM, although not all gene variations that increase the risk for type 2 DM are known.

Metabolic syndrome is the simultaneous presence of metabolic factors that increase risk for developing type 2 DM and cardiovascular disease. Features of the syndrome include:

- Abdominal obesity: waist circumference of 40 inches (100 cm) or more for men and 35 inches (88 cm) or more for women
- Hyperglycemia: fasting blood glucose level of 100 mg/dL or more or on drug treatment for elevated blood glucose levels
- Hypertension: systolic blood pressure of 130 mm Hg or more or diastolic blood pressure of 85 mg Hg or more or on drug treatment for hypertension
- Hyperlipidemia: triglyceride level of 150 mg/dL or more or on drug treatment for elevated triglycerides; high-density lipoprotein (HDL) cholesterol less than 40 mg/dL for men or less than 50 mg/dL for women

Any of these health problems also increases the rate of atherosclerosis and the risk for stroke, CVD, and early death.

Incidence and Prevalence. In the United States, more than 34 million people are living with DM, and 27.8% (7.3 million) are undiagnosed. Another 86 million have prediabetes (Centers for Disease Control and Prevention [CDC], 2020). (*Prediabetes* is defined as impaired fasting glucose [IGF], an A1C between 5.7 and 6.4, or impaired glucose tolerance [IGT]. Over a 3- to 5-year period, adults with prediabetes have a 5-fold to 15-fold higher risk for developing type 2 DM than do those with normal blood glucose levels.) In Canada, about 2.2 million adults have diabetes (Statistics Canada, 2019).

PATIENT-CENTERED CARE: VETERANS HEALTH CONSIDERATIONS QSEN

A possible additional risk factor for type 2 DM is exposure to the main component of agent orange, dioxin, which was used during the military conflicts in Korea and Viet Nam. The risk for type 2 diabetes appears higher among U.S. military members who were assigned to those geographic areas. The risk increases with higher exposures (U.S. Department of Veterans Affairs, 2016). Development of DM among veterans who served in areas where agent orange was used occurs at earlier ages and with less obesity.

Assess veterans who were exposed to agent orange at every health care visit for indications of diabetes so the disease can be identified early and interventions implemented to prevent or delay complications. Encourage veterans to use DM prevention strategies of maintaining a healthy weight and engaging in regular physical activity.

About 90% to 95% of adults with diabetes have type 2 DM (CDC, 2020). It can be diagnosed even in preadolescents but is most common among middle-age and older adults, affecting about 12.3% of adults over the age of 20 years and 25.9% of adults age 65 years or older (Touhy & Jett, 2020). With the prevalence of obesity rising in North America, diabetes is likely to become even more common (ADA, 2019h).

PATIENT-CENTERED CARE: CULTURAL/ SPIRITUAL CONSIDERATIONS QSEN

Racial and ethnic minorities have a higher prevalence and greater burden of DM compared with non-Hispanic whites. The DM rate is 13% among blacks and 12% in the Hispanic population compared with non-Hispanic white Americans. At nearly 15.1%, American Indians and Alaska Indians have the highest age-adjusted prevalence of DM among U.S. racial and ethnic groups (CDC, 2020). Be alert to the risk for DM whenever you are interviewing or assessing adults who belong to these higher-risk groups. *The increase in obesity and sedentary lifestyles in the North American population intensifies this growing problem. The ADA has identified patients who should be tested for diabetes (Table 59.5).*

Health Promotion and Maintenance. Diabetes mellitus (DM) causes many devastating complications. Control of DM and its preventable complications is a major focus for health promotion activities. No interventions prevent type 1 DM, but health promotion activities that focus on controlling hyperglycemia can reduce its long-term complications.

Adopting a healthy lifestyle that includes a low-calorie diet and increasing physical activity with weight loss improves metabolic and cardiac risk factors (ADA, 2019e; Watts & Howard, 2016) and can prevent or delay the onset of type 2 DM (ADA, 2019k). These improvements include reducing hypertension, increasing heart rate variability between resting rate and exercise rate, lowering triglyceride levels, increasing high-density lipoprotein cholesterol ("healthy" or "good" cholesterol) levels, and reducing low-density lipoprotein cholesterol ("lousy" or "bad" cholesterol) levels. Smoking cessation and avoidance of excess alcohol consumption also are important in preventing complications of DM.

Teach patients with DM that keeping their blood glucose levels within prescribed target ranges can prevent or delay complications. Urge them to regularly follow up with their primary health care provider or diabetes health care provider, to have their eyes and vision tested yearly by an ophthalmologist, and

TABLE 59.5 Indications for Testing People for Type 2 Diabetes

- Testing for diabetes is considered at any age in adults with a BMI greater than 25 kg/m^2 (or greater than 23 kg/m^2 in Asian Americans) with one or more of these additional risk factors:
  - Have a first-degree relative with diabetes
  - Are physically inactive
  - Are members of a high-risk ethnic population (e.g., African American, Hispanic American, American Indian, or Pacific Islander)
  - Give birth to a baby weighing more than 9 lb (4.1 kg) or have been diagnosed with GDM
  - Are hypertensive (>140/90 mm Hg)
  - Have a high-density lipoprotein (HDL) cholesterol level less than 35 mg/dL (0.90 mmol/L) and/or a triglyceride level greater than 250 mg/dL (2.82 mmol/L)
  - Have polycystic ovary syndrome
  - Have A1C greater than 5.7%, or IFG or IGT on previous testing
  - Have a history of vascular disease
- If the tested adult has normal glucose values at this time but other conditions and risk factors remain the same, testing should be repeated at 3-year intervals.

BMI, Body mass index; *GDM,* gestational diabetes mellitus; *IFG,* impaired fasting glucose, *IGT,* impaired glucose tolerance.
Data from American Diabetes Association (ADA). (2019b). Classification and diagnosis of diabetes: Standards of medical care in diabetes—2019. *Diabetes Care, 42*(Suppl. 1), S13-S28; and American Diabetes Association (ADA). (2019k). Prevention or delay of type 2 diabetes: Standards of medical care in diabetes—2019. *Diabetes Care, 42*(Suppl. 1), S29-S33.

to have urine albumin levels assessed yearly. Early detection of changes in the eye or kidney allows adjustments in treatment plans that can slow or halt progression of retinopathy and nephropathy. Urge adults to maintain an appropriate weight range for height and body build and to engage in physical activity at least 150 minutes per week (ADA, 2019e). Encourage daily foot inspection and the prompt reporting of ulcers or open areas to the primary health care provider to reduce the risk for deep wounds or the need for amputation.

❖ Interprofessional Collaborative Care

Although adults who have DM are often hospitalized for complications of the disease, diagnosis and management generally occur in a clinic or health care provider's office. Much of the essential education about management is performed in the community, as is the overall management of the disorder. Because DM is a chronic disorder and predisposes to other health problems, you can expect to interact with and care for these patients in any health care setting.

INTERPROFESSIONAL COLLABORATIVE CARE

The Patient With Diabetes Mellitus

The complicated and chronic nature of DM requires the coordination of an interprofessional team approach for optimum outcomes. The interprofessional team members to help patients achieve desired outcomes include primary health care providers, endocrinologists, diabetes health care providers, certified diabetes educators, ophthalmologists, other medical practitioners, registered nurses, pharmacists, registered dietitian nutritionists (RDNs), podiatrists, physical therapists, and wound care specialists.

TABLE 59.6 Criteria for the Diagnosis of Diabetes

A1C >6.5%. The test should be performed in a laboratory using a method that is NGSP certified and standardized to the DCCT assay.

AND

Fasting blood glucose greater than or equal to 126 mg/dL (7.0 mmol/L). *Fasting* is defined as no caloric intake for at least 8 hours.

OR

Two-hour blood glucose equal to or greater than 200 mg/dL (11.1 mmol/L) during oral glucose tolerance testing. The test should be performed using a glucose load containing the equivalent of 75 g anhydrous glucose dissolved in water.

OR

In a patient with classic manifestations of hyperglycemia or hyperglycemic crisis, a casual or random blood glucose concentration greater than 200 mg/dL (11.1 mmol/L). *Casual* is defined as any time of the day without regard to time since last meal. The classic symptoms of diabetes include polyuria, polydipsia, and unexplained weight loss.

NOTE: In the absence of unequivocal hyperglycemia, the first three criteria should be confirmed by repeat testing.

Data from American Diabetes Association (ADA). (2019b). Classification and diagnosis of diabetes: Standards of medical care in diabetes—2019. *Diabetes Care, 42*(Suppl. 1), S132-S28.
DCCT, Diabetes Control and Complications Trial; *NGSP,* National Glycohemoglobin Standardization Program.

◆ Assessment: Recognize Cues

History. Ask about risk factors and symptoms related to DM. Ask women how large their children were at birth, because many women who develop type 2 DM had gestational diabetes mellitus (GDM) or glucose intolerance during pregnancy (ADA, 2019b). Teach women with a history of GDM and those who have prediabetes about lifestyle changes to prevent DM (ADA, 2019b).

Assessing weight and weight change is important because excess weight and obesity are risk factors for type 2 DM. The patient with type 1 DM often has weight loss with increased appetite during the weeks before diagnosis. For both types of DM, patients usually have fatigue, polyuria, and polydipsia. Ask about recent major or minor infections and assess overall ***immunity***. Ask women about frequent vaginal yeast infections. Assess whether patients have noticed that small skin injuries become infected more easily or take longer to heal. Also ask whether they have noticed any changes in vision or in the sense of touch.

Laboratory Assessment

Diagnosis of Diabetes. Diabetes can be diagnosed by assessing the blood glucose levels listed in the Laboratory Profile: Blood Glucose Values box. A test result indicating DM should be repeated to rule out laboratory error unless symptoms of hyperglycemia or hyperglycemic crisis are also present. Table 59.6 lists criteria for the diagnosis of DM.

The diagnosis of DM includes elevated glycosylated hemoglobin levels. **Glycosylated hemoglobin (A1C)** is a standardized test that measures how much glucose permanently attaches to the hemoglobin molecule and indicates the effectiveness of blood glucose control measures. Because glucose binds to proteins, including hemoglobin, through a process called *glycosylation,* the higher the blood glucose level is over time, the more glycosylated the hemoglobin becomes.

LABORATORY PROFILE

Blood Glucose Values

Test	Normal Range	Significance of Abnormal Results
Fasting blood glucose test	100 mg/dL (5.6 mmol/L) Older adults: Levels rise 1 mg/dL per decade of age	Levels >100 mg/dL (5.6 mmol/L) but <126 mg/dL (7.0 mmol/L) indicate impaired fasting glucose (IFG). Levels >126 mg/dL (7.0 mmol/L) obtained on at least two occasions are diagnostic of diabetes, even in older adults.
Glucose tolerance test (2-hr postload result)	<140 mg/dL (7.8 mmol/L)	Levels >140 mg/dL (7.8 mmol/L) and <200 mg/dL (11.1 mmol/L) indicate impaired glucose tolerance (IGT). Levels >200 mg/dL (11.1 mmol/L) indicate provisional diagnosis of diabetes.
Glycosylated hemoglobin (A1C) test	4%-6%	Levels of 5.7% to 6.4% indicate prediabetes and an increased risk for development of diabetes. Levels >6.5% indicate diabetes. Levels >8% indicate poor diabetes control and need for adherence to regimen or changes in therapy.

Data from Pagana, K., & Pagana, T. (2018). *Mosby's manual of diagnostic and laboratory tests* (6th ed.). St. Louis: Elsevier.

Fasting plasma glucose (FPG) (fasting blood glucose [FBG]), along with A1C, is used to diagnose DM in nonpregnant adults. A diagnosis of DM is made with two separate test results greater than 126 mg/dL (7 mmol/L) (ADA, 2019b). *Random* or *casual plasma* glucose greater than 200 mg/dL (7.0 mmol/L) is used to diagnose DM in patients with classic hyperglycemia symptoms or hyperglycemic crisis.

The *oral glucose tolerance test (OGTT)* is a sensitive test for the diagnosis of DM. It is often used to diagnose gestational diabetes mellitus (GDM) during pregnancy and is not routinely used for general diagnosis (ADA, 2019f).

Other blood tests for diabetes can help determine whether a patient has type 1 or type 2 DM. Type 1 DM results from autoimmune destruction of the beta cells of the pancreas. Markers of this destruction include islet cell autoantibodies (ICAs), autoantibodies to insulin, zinc transporter antibodies (ZnT8), and autoantibodies to glutamic acid decarboxylase (GAD65). ICAs are present in 85% to 90% of patients with new-onset type 1 DM (McCance et al., 2019).

Screening for Diabetes. Testing to detect prediabetes and type 2 DM is recommended for patients older than 45 years and those defined as overweight (body mass index [BMI] greater than 25 kg/m^2) (Touhy & Jett, 2020). Testing is considered for

TABLE 59.7 Correlation Between A1C Level and Mean Blood Glucose Levels

	MEAN BLOOD GLUCOSE	
A1C (%)	mg/dL	mmol/L
6	126	7.0
7	154	8.6
8	183	10.2
9	212	11.8
10	240	13.4
11	269	14.9
12	298	16.5

younger patients who are overweight if they have additional risk factors for DM or other health problems associated with it. Screening for DM usually is done with laboratory testing of both A1C levels and fasting plasma glucose levels (ADA, 2019b).

Ongoing Assessment. *Glycosylated hemoglobin assays* are useful as a good indicator of the average blood glucose levels. Measurement of A1C shows the average blood glucose level during the previous 120 days—the life span of red blood cells. A1C testing can help assess long-term glycemic control and predict the risk for complications. *Unlike the fasting blood glucose test, A1C test results are not altered by the eating habits on the day before the test.* This testing is performed at diagnosis and at specific intervals to evaluate the treatment plan. A1C testing is recommended at least twice yearly in patients who are meeting expected treatment outcomes and have stable blood glucose control. Quarterly assessment is recommended for patients whose therapy has changed or who are not meeting prescribed glycemic levels (ADA, 2019d). Table 59.7 shows the correlation between A1C and mean blood glucose levels.

Fructosamine assays are useful for short-term follow-up of treatment changes or in patients with hemoglobin abnormalities in which A1C does not accurately reflect glucose levels. When glucose binds to amino groups on serum proteins, especially albumin, the glycosylated protein product is called fructosamine. This product increases with elevated blood glucose levels as hemoglobin does but can indicate blood glucose control over a shorter period.

NCLEX EXAMINATION CHALLENGE 59.2

Physiological Integrity

The nurse reviewing the preadmission testing laboratory values for a 62-year-old client scheduled for a total knee replacement finds an A1C value of 6.2%. How will the nurse interpret this finding?

A. The client's A1C is completely normal.
B. The client has type 1 diabetes mellitus.
C. The client has type 2 diabetes mellitus.
D. The client has prediabetes mellitus.

◆ Analysis: Analyze Cues and Prioritize Hypotheses.

The priority collaborative problems for patients with diabetes DM include:

1. Potential for injury due to hyperglycemia
2. Potential for poor wound healing due to endocrine and vascular effects of diabetes
3. Potential for injury due to diabetic neuropathy
4. Potential for kidney disease due to reduced kidney ***perfusion***
5. Potential for the complications of hypoglycemia, diabetic ketoacidosis, and hyperglycemic-hyperosmolar state (HHS) and coma

◆ Planning and Implementation: Generate Solutions and Take Action

Preventing Injury From Hyperglycemia

Planning: Expected Outcomes. The patient is expected to manage DM and prevent disease progression by maintaining blood glucose levels in his or her target range.

Interventions

Nonsurgical Management. Management of DM involves ***nutrition*** interventions, blood glucose monitoring, a planned exercise program, and often, drugs to lower blood glucose levels. Nurses, the interprofessional team members, and the patient plan, coordinate, and deliver care.

The American Diabetes Association (ADA) has proposed these treatment outcomes for glycosylated hemoglobin (A1C) and blood glucose levels (ADA, 2019d):

- A1C levels are maintained at 7.0% or below (or as prescribed).
- The majority of premeal blood glucose levels are 70 to 130 mg/dL (3.9 to 7.2 mmol/L).
- Peak after-meal blood glucose levels are less than 180 mg/dL (<10.0 mmol/L).

Drug therapy. Drug therapy is indicated when a patient with type 2 DM does not achieve blood glucose control with diet changes, regular exercise, and stress management. Several categories of drugs may be used to lower blood glucose levels. Patients with type 1 DM require insulin therapy for blood glucose control and may use other antidiabetic drugs, as well.

Drugs are started at the lowest effective dose and increased over time until the patient reaches desired blood glucose control or the maximum dosage. Glycemic control may require the use of more than one category of drug. Insulin therapy is indicated for the patient with type 2 DM when blood glucose goals cannot be met with the use of two or three different antidiabetic agents, including GLP-1 agonists (ADA, 2019j).

Antidiabetic drugs are not a substitute for dietary modification and exercise. Teach the patient about continuing dietary changes and regular exercise while taking antidiabetic drugs.

! NURSING SAFETY PRIORITY (QSEN)

Drug Alert

To avoid drug interactions, teach the patient who is taking an antidiabetic drug to consult with his or her diabetes health care provider or pharmacist before using *any* over-the-counter drugs.

Drug selection is based on cost, the patient's ability to manage multiple drug dosages, associated risks for side effects, and response to the drugs. Shorter-acting agents (e.g., glitinides) are preferred for older patients, those with irregular eating schedules, or those with liver, kidney, or cardiac problems. Longer-acting drugs (e.g., glimepiride) with once-a-day dosing are better for adherence. Beta cell function in type 2 DM declines over time, and some drugs become less effective. Management of type 2 DM may eventually require insulin therapy either alone or with other antidiabetic drugs.

Some antidiabetic drugs are oral agents, and other types require subcutaneous injection. See the Common Examples of Drug Therapy: Diabetes Mellitus box for common antidiabetic drugs in each category.

Insulin stimulators (also known as insulin secretagogues) stimulate insulin release from pancreatic beta cells and are used for patients who are still able to produce insulin. This class include sulfonylureas and meglitinide analogs.

Sulfonylurea agents lower fasting blood glucose levels by triggering the release of insulin from beta cells. Many drugs interact with sulfonylureas. Be sure to consult a drug reference source or pharmacologist when instructing patients who are prescribed a drug from this class. Meglitinide analogs are insulin stimulators and have actions and adverse effects similar to those of sulfonylureas. They tend to increase meal-related insulin secretion.

Metformin, a biguanide, decreases liver glucose production and decreases intestinal absorption of glucose. It also improves insulin sensitivity, which increases peripheral glucose uptake and utilization.

! NURSING SAFETY PRIORITY (QSEN)

Drug Alert

Metformin can cause lactic acidosis in patients with kidney impairment and should not be used by anyone with kidney disease (Burchum & Rosenthal, 2019). To prevent lactic acidosis and acute kidney injury, the drug is withheld before and after using contrast medium or any surgical procedure requiring anesthesia until adequate kidney function is established.

Insulin sensitizers, also known as thiazolidinediones (TZDs or "glitazones"), increase cellular use of glucose, which lowers blood glucose levels. These drugs are associated with an increased risk for heart-related deaths, bone fracture, and macular edema. The Food and Drug Administration (FDA) has issued a black box warning indicating that these drugs are not to be used by patients who have symptomatic heart failure or other specific types of cardiovascular disease. (A *black box warning* is a government designation indicating that a drug has a serious side effect and must be used with caution.)

Alpha-glucosidase inhibitors prevent after-meal hyperglycemia by delaying absorption of carbohydrate from the intestine. They inhibit enzymes in the intestinal tract, reducing the rate of starch digestion and glucose absorption. These actions prevent a sudden blood glucose surge after meals. These drugs do not cause hypoglycemia unless given with sulfonylureas or insulin. However, side effects of GI upset and flatulence can deter adherence to the use of these drugs.

Incretin mimetics work like the natural "gut" hormones, glucagon-like peptide-1 (GLP-1) and glucose-dependent insulinotropic polypeptide (GIP), that are released by the intestine in response to food intake and act with insulin for ***glucose regulation***. Drugs in this class include the GLP-1 agonists dulaglutide, exenatide, exenatide extended-release, liraglutide, lixisenatide, and semaglutide (Burchum & Rosenthal, 2019; Keresztes & Peacock-Johnson, 2019). These drugs are used in addition to diet and exercise to improve glycemic control in adults with type 2 DM.

! NURSING SAFETY PRIORITY (QSEN)

Drug Alert

Extended-release exenatide and dulaglutide are injected subcutaneously *once weekly*. Be sure to emphasize this dosing schedule to avoid overdoses.

Dipeptidyl peptidase-4 (DPP-4) inhibitors work by preventing the inactivation of the incretins GLP and GIP. These peptides are rapidly metabolized and inactivated by the enzyme DPP-4. Drugs that inhibit the DPP-4 enzyme allow naturally produced incretin hormones to remain available for blood ***glucose regulation***. The DPP-4 inhibitors used to control type 2 DM are sitagliptin, saxagliptin, linagliptin, and alogliptin.

! NURSING SAFETY PRIORITY (QSEN)

Drug Alert

DPP-4 inhibitors and the incretin mimetics have an increased risk for pancreatitis. Warn patients taking these drugs to immediately report to the diabetes health care provider any signs of jaundice; sudden onset of intense abdominal pain that radiates to the back, left flank, or left shoulder; or gray-blue discoloration of the abdomen or periumbilical area.

Saxagliptin and alogliptin have an increased risk for heart failure. Warn patients to report a sudden weight gain or new-onset shortness of breath.

Amylin analogs are drugs similar to amylin, a naturally occurring hormone produced by pancreatic beta cells that works with and is secreted with insulin in response to blood glucose elevation. Amylin levels are deficient in patients with type 1 DM. Pramlintide, an analog of amylin, is approved for patients with DM who are treated with insulin. It works by three mechanisms: delaying gastric emptying, reducing after-meal blood glucose levels, and triggering satiety (in the brain). (Satiety leads to decreased caloric intake and eventual weight loss.)

! NURSING SAFETY PRIORITY (QSEN)

Drug Alert

Do not mix pramlintide and insulin in the same syringe because the pH of the two drugs is not compatible.

COMMON EXAMPLES OF DRUG THERAPY

Diabetes Mellitus

Drug Category	Nursing Implications
Insulin Stimulators (Secretagogues)	
Lower blood glucose levels by triggering the release of preformed insulin from beta cells.	
Second-generation sulfonylurea agents • Glipizide • Glyburide • Glimepiride Meglitinide analogs • Repaglinide • Nateglinide	Teach patient the signs and symptoms of hypoglycemia (hunger, headache, tremors, sweating, confusion) *because these drugs lower blood glucose levels even when hyperglycemia is not present.* Instruct patients to take these drugs with or just before meals *to prevent hypoglycemia.* Instruct patients taking a sulfonylurea to check with their health care provider or a pharmacist before taking any over-the-counter drug or supplement *because these drugs interact with many other drugs.*
Biguanides	
Lower blood glucose by inhibiting liver glucose production, decreasing intestinal absorption of glucose, and increasing insulin sensitivity.	
• Metformin	Instruct patients not to drink alcohol while taking this drug *to reduce the risk for lactic acidosis.* Remind patients that this drug must be stopped before certain imaging tests using contrast agents and not started again for 48 hours after testing *because of the increased risk for kidney damage and lactic acidosis.* Warn patients that GI problems are common side effects of this drug class.
Insulin Sensitizers	
Lower blood glucose by decreasing liver glucose production and improving the sensitivity of insulin receptors.	
Thiazolidinediones (TZDs) • Pioglitazone • Rosiglitazone	Teach patients with any cardiovascular disease to weigh themselves daily and report a weight gain of more than 2 lb (1 kg) in one day or 4 lb (2 kg) in a week to the prescriber *because these drugs increase the risk for heart failure.* Instruct patients to report vision changes immediately *because these drugs increase the risk for macular edema.* Warn patients that weight gain and peripheral edema are common side effects of these drugs.
Alpha-Glucosidase Inhibitors	
Prevent after-meal hyperglycemia by inhibiting enzymes in the intestinal tract from breaking down starches into glucose. This action delays the digestion of starches and the absorption of glucose from the small intestine.	
• Acarbose • Miglitol	Teach patients to take these drugs only with a meal *because the action is in the intestinal tract.* Warn patients that abdominal discomfort and bloating, flatulence, nausea, diarrhea, and indigestion are common side effects of this drug class.
Incretin Mimetics (GLP-1 Agonists)	
Act like natural "gut" hormones that work with insulin to lower blood glucose levels by reducing pancreatic glucagon secretion, reducing liver glucose production, and delaying gastric emptying.	
• Dulaglutide • Exenatide • Exenatide extended release • Liraglutide • Lixisenatide • Semaglutide	Teach patients the signs of hypoglycemia (hunger, headache, tremors, sweating) *because these drugs lower blood glucose levels even when they are normal if used in conjunction with insulin, sulfonylureas, or meglitinides.* Instruct patient how to inject themselves *because these drugs are only available as subcutaneous formulations.* Instruct patients to read exenatide and dulaglutide pens carefully *because the extended-release form is only injected **weekly** rather than daily.* Teach patients to report persistent abdominal pain and nausea to the health care provider *because these drugs increase the risk for pancreatitis.*
DPP-4 Inhibitors	
DPP-4 is an enzyme that breaks down the natural gut hormones (GLP-1 and GIP). DPP-4 inhibitors are oral agents that prevent the enzyme DPP-4 from breaking down the natural gut hormones (GLP-1 and GIP), which then allows these natural substances to work with insulin to lower glucagon secretion from the pancreas, leading to reduced liver glucose production. These oral drugs also reduce blood glucose levels by delaying gastric emptying and slowing the rate of nutrient absorption into the blood.	
• Alogliptin • Linagliptin • Saxagliptin • Sitagliptin	Teach patient the signs and symptoms of hypoglycemia (hunger, headache, tremors, sweating, confusion) *because these drugs lower blood glucose levels even when hyperglycemia is not present if used in conjunction with insulin, sulfonylureas, or meglitinides.* Instruct patients to be alert for rash or other sign of allergic reaction *because this class of drugs is associated with a moderate incidence of drug allergy.* Teach patients to report persistent abdominal pain and nausea to the health care provider *because these drugs increase the risk for pancreatitis.* Instruct patients to notify the primary health care provider if shortness of breath, dyspnea on exertion, or cough, especially when lying down, is experienced *because this class of drugs is associated with heart failure.*

COMMON EXAMPLES OF DRUG THERAPY—Cont'd

Diabetes Mellitus

Drug Category	Nursing Implications
Amylin Analogs	
These drugs are similar to amylin, a naturally occurring hormone produced by beta cells in the pancreas that is co-secreted with insulin and lowers blood glucose levels by decreasing endogenous glucagon, delaying gastric emptying, and triggering satiety.	
• Pramlintide	Teach patient the signs and symptoms of hypoglycemia (hunger, headache, tremors, sweating, confusion) *because these drugs lower blood glucose levels even when hyperglycemia is not present when used in conjunction with insulin.*
	Instruct patient how to inject themselves *because these drugs are only available as subcutaneous formulations.*
	Warn patients that nausea and vomiting are common side effects of this drug class.
	Do not mix in the same syringe with insulin *because their pH is not compatible.*
Sodium-Glucose Cotransport Inhibitors	
Lower blood glucose levels by preventing kidney reabsorption of glucose and sodium that was filtered from the blood into the urine. This filtered glucose is excreted in the urine rather than moved back into the blood.	
• Canagliflozin • Dapagliflozin • Empagliflozin • Ertugliflozin	Teach patients the signs and symptoms of hypoglycemia (hunger, headache, tremors, sweating, confusion) *because these drugs lower blood glucose levels even when hyperglycemia is not present if used in conjunction with insulin, sulfonylureas, or meglitinides.*
	Teach the patient the signs and symptoms of dehydration (increased thirst, lightheadedness, dry mouth and mucous membranes, orthostatic hypotension) *because these drugs increase urine output and increase dehydration risk.*
	Teach patients the signs and symptoms of hyponatremia (muscle weakness, abdominal cramping, rapid heart rate, orthostatic hypotension) *because these drugs increase sodium loss.*
	Teach patients the signs and symptoms of urinary tract infection (frequency, pain and burning on urination, foul urine odor) *because the increased glucose in the urinary tract predisposes to infection.*
	Instruct women to be alert for genital itching and vaginal discharge *because these drugs increase the risk for genital yeast infection.*
	Teach patients to report any swelling, tenderness or redness of the genitals or perineal skin *because these drugs increase the risk for Fournier gangrene with perineal fasciitis.*

Sodium-glucose co-transport inhibitors lower blood glucose levels by preventing kidney reabsorption of glucose that was filtered from the blood into the urine. The filtered glucose is excreted in the urine rather than moved back into the blood. These oral drugs include canagliflozin, dapagliflozin, empagliflozin, and ertugliflozin (Hussar, 2019).

NURSING SAFETY PRIORITY QSEN

Drug Alert

The FDA has issued a warning that use of empagliflozin increases the risk for acute kidney injury and impaired renal function (Aschenbrenner, 2017). In addition, canagliflozin is associated with an increased risk for lower limb amputations. Other warnings about the sodium-glucose co-transport inhibitors include the potential for genital and perineal necrotizing fasciitis.

Combination agents combine drugs with different mechanisms of action. For example, Glucovance combines glyburide with metformin. Combining drugs with different mechanisms of action may be highly effective in maintaining desired blood glucose control. Some patients may need a combination of antidiabetic agents and insulin to control blood glucose levels.

Insulin therapy. Insulin therapy is required for type 1 DM and often is used for type 2 DM. The safety of insulin therapy in older patients may be affected by reduced vision, mobility and coordination problems, and decreased memory, increasing the risk for dosage errors.

NCLEX EXAMINATION CHALLENGE 59.3

Health Promotion and Maintenance

Which precaution is a **priority** for the nurse to teach a client prescribed semaglutide to **prevent harm**?

A. Only take this drug once weekly.
B. Report any vision changes immediately.
C. Do not mix in the same syringe with insulin.
D. This drug can only be given by a health care professional.

Many types of insulin and regimens are available to achieve normal blood glucose levels. Because insulin is a small protein that is quickly inactivated in the GI tract, it is usually injected.

Types of insulin vary with the source and manufacturing techniques. Insulin analogs are synthetic human insulins in which the structure of the insulin molecule is altered to change the rate of absorption and duration of action within the body (e.g., Lispro insulin).

Rapid-, short-, intermediate-, and long-acting forms of insulin can be injected separately, and some can be mixed in the same syringe. Insulin is available in concentrations of 100 units/mL (U-100), 200 units/mL (U-200), 300 units/mL (U-300), and 500 units/mL (U-500). Insulin concentrations above 100 units/mL are reserved for when very large doses of insulin are required.

Teach the patient that the insulin types, the injection technique, and the site of injection all affect the absorption, onset, degree, and duration of insulin activity. Reinforce that changing insulins may affect blood glucose control and should be done only under supervision of the diabetes health care provider. Table 59.8 outlines the timed activity of human insulin.

Insulin regimens try to replicate the normal insulin release pattern from the pancreas. The pancreas produces a constant *(basal)* amount of insulin that balances liver glucose production with glucose use and maintains normal blood glucose levels between meals. The pancreas also produces additional meal-time *(prandial)* insulin to prevent blood glucose elevation after meals. The insulin dose required for blood glucose control varies among patients. Starting doses may be much lower for older adults or for very thin patients. For multiple-dose regimens or continuous subcutaneous insulin infusion (CSII), basal insulin makes up about 40% of the total daily dosage, with the remainder divided into premeal doses of rapid-acting insulin analogs or regular insulin. Basal insulin coverage is provided by intermediate-acting insulin (NPH) or long-acting insulin analogs such as insulin glargine, insulin detemir, or insulin degludec. Dosages are adjusted based on the results of blood glucose monitoring.

Single daily injection protocols require insulin injection only once daily. This protocol may include one injection of intermediate- or long-acting insulin or an injection of combination short- and intermediate-acting insulin. Some patients with type 2 DM combine once-daily insulin injection for basal coverage with oral agent therapy to stimulate bolus insulin secretion.

Multiple-component insulin therapy combines short- and intermediate-acting insulin injected twice daily. Two-thirds of the daily dose is given before breakfast, and one-third before the evening meal. Ratios of intermediate-acting and regular insulin are based on results of blood glucose monitoring.

Intensified regimens include a basal dose of intermediate- or long-acting insulin and a mealtime bolus dose of short- or rapid-acting insulin designed to bring the *next* blood glucose value into the target range. Blood glucose elevations above the target range are treated with "correction" doses of short- or rapid-acting insulin. The patient's blood glucose patterns determine insulin dosage. Frequency of blood glucose monitoring is based on the timed action of insulin and may occur as often as eight times daily. Blood glucose testing 2 hours after meals and within 10 minutes before the next meal helps determine the adequacy of the previous bolus dose. The patient determines the effects of basal insulin by monitoring blood glucose levels before breakfast (fasting) and before the evening meal.

Patients on intensified insulin regimens need extensive education to achieve target blood glucose values. They need to know how to adjust insulin doses and understand ***nutrition*** therapy for dietary flexibility and meeting target blood glucose values. Patients must also be able to correctly monitor blood glucose levels so that therapy decisions are based on accurate data.

Regardless of the specific insulin regimen, adherence to insulin injection schedules is critical in achieving the glycemic control needed to reduce long-term complications. At times, skipping an occasional insulin dose may be related to an unusual meal pattern for a day or a change in exercise.

Insulin absorption is affected by many factors including injection site; timing, type, or dose of insulin used; and physical activity.

Injection site area affects the speed of insulin absorption. Fig. 59.4 shows common insulin injection areas. Absorption is fastest in the abdomen, which is, except for a 2-inch radius around the navel, the preferred injection site. Rotating injection sites allows each injection site to heal completely before the site is used again. Rotation *within* one anatomic site is preferred to rotation from one area to another to prevent day-to-day variability in absorption.

Absorption rate is determined by insulin properties. Longer duration of action makes absorption less reliable. Larger doses prolong the absorption. Factors that increase blood flow from the injection site, such as applying heat locally, massaging the area, and exercising the injected area, increase insulin absorption. Scarred areas are less sensitive to pain, but these sites usually slow insulin absorption.

Injection depth changes insulin absorption. Usually injections are made into the subcutaneous tissue. IM injection has a faster absorption and is not used for routine insulin use. Most patients lightly grasp a fold of skin and inject at a 90-degree angle; however, a 45-degree angle is used for frail older adults and those who are very thin. Aspiration for blood is not needed. Patients who are overweight can use 4-mm or 5-mm needles to inject insulin at a 90-degree angle without pinching a skinfold before injection.

Timing of injection affects blood glucose levels. The interval between premeal injections and eating, known as "lag time," affects blood glucose levels after meals. Insulins that have rapid onsets of action are given within 10 minutes before mealtime when blood glucose is in the target range. If hyperglycemia or hypoglycemia is not present, these insulins can be given at any time from 10 minutes before mealtime to just before eating or even immediately after eating. Regular insulin is given at least 20 to 30 minutes before eating when glucose levels are within the target range. When blood glucose levels are *above* the target range, lag time is increased to permit insulin to have a greater glucose-lowering effect before food enters the stomach. When blood glucose levels are *below* the target range, teach patients to inject insulin *immediately* before eating, and to delay rapid-acting insulin injection until sometime *after* eating the meal.

Mixing insulins can change the time of peak action. Mixtures of short- and intermediate-acting insulins produce a more normal blood glucose response in some patients than does a single dose. The patient's response to mixed insulin may differ from the response to the same insulins given separately.

! NURSING SAFETY PRIORITY (QSEN)

Drug Alert

Do not mix any other insulin type with insulin glargine, insulin detemir, or any of the premixed insulin formulations such as Humalog Mix 75/25.

NCLEX EXAMINATION CHALLENGE 59.4

Safe and Effective Care Environment

How will the nurse modify insulin injection technique for a client who is 5 feet 10 inches tall and weighs 106 lb (48.1 kg)?

A. Use a 6-mm needle and inject at a 90-degree angle.
B. Use a 6-mm needle and inject at a 45-degree angle.
C. Use a 12-mm needle and inject at a 90-degree angle.
D. Use a 12-mm needle and inject at a 45-degree angle.

TABLE 59.8 Timed Activity of Pharmaceutical Insulin

Preparation	Onset (hr)	Peak (hr)	Duration (hr)
Rapid-Acting Insulin Analogs			
Insulin aspart injection	0.25	1-3	3-5
Insulin glulisine injection	0.3	0.5-1.5	3-4
Human lispro injection	0.25	0.5-1.5	5
Human lispro injection U-200	0.25	0.5-1.5	5
Insulin human inhalation powder	0.25	1-1.25	2.5
Short-Acting Insulin			
Regular human insulin injection	0.5	2-4	5-12
Humulin R (Concentrated U-500)	1.5	4-12	24
Intermediate Acting Insulin			
Isophane insulin NPH injection	1-4	4-12	10-24+
70% human insulin isophane suspension/30% human insulin injection	0.5	2-12	24
70% insulin aspart protamine suspension/30% insulin aspart injection	0.25	1-4	24
75% insulin lispro protamine suspension/25% insulin lispro injection	0.25	1-2	24
Long-Acting Insulin Analogs			
Insulin glargine injection	2-4	None	24
Insulin glargine injection U-300	2-4	12	24
Insulin detemir injection	1	6-8	5.7-24
Insulin degludec injection U-100, U-200	1	9	42

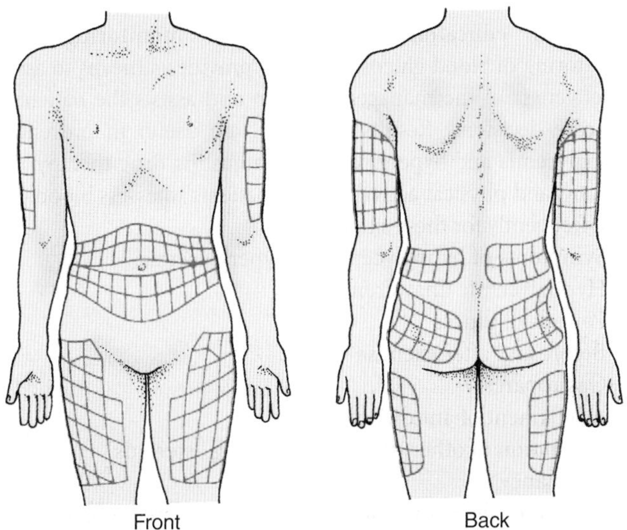

FIG. 59.4 Common insulin injection areas and sites.

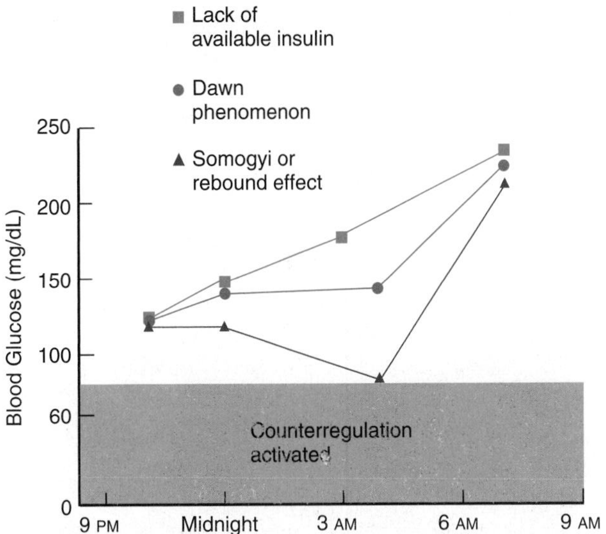

FIG. 59.5 Three blood glucose phenomena in patients with diabetes.

Hypoglycemia from insulin excess has many causes. Its effects and treatment are discussed in the Interventions for Preventing Hypoglycemia section.

Two conditions of fasting hyperglycemia (in addition to a lack of insulin) can occur (Fig. 59.5). *Dawn phenomenon* results from a nighttime release of adrenal hormones that causes blood glucose elevations at about 5 to 6 a.m. It is managed by providing more insulin for the overnight period (e.g., giving the evening dose of intermediate-acting insulin at 10 p.m. instead of with the evening meal). *Somogyi phenomenon* is morning hyperglycemia from the counterregulatory response to nighttime hypoglycemia. It is managed by ensuring adequate dietary intake at bedtime and evaluating the insulin dose and exercise programs to prevent conditions that lead to hypoglycemia. Both problems are diagnosed by blood glucose monitoring during the night. Help identify these problems and teach the patient and family about management.

Alternative methods of insulin administration are available in addition to traditional subcutaneous injections. These include continuous insulin infusion, needleless injection systems, and dry powder inhalers.

Continuous subcutaneous infusion of a basal dose of insulin (CSII) with additional insulin at mealtimes is more effective in controlling blood glucose levels than other schedules. It allows flexibility in meal timing, because if a meal is skipped, the additional mealtime dose of insulin is not given. CSII is given by an externally worn pump containing a reservoir of rapid-acting insulin and is connected to the patient by an infusion set. Teach him or her to adjust the amount of insulin based on data from blood glucose monitoring. Rapid-acting insulin analogs are used with insulin infusion pumps (Fig. 59.6).

Problems with CSII include skin infections that can occur when the infusion site is not cleaned or the infusion set is not changed every 2 to 3 days. Ketoacidosis may occur more often because of infection, obstruction of the infusion, or mechanical pump problems. Stress the need for ketone testing when blood glucose levels are greater than 300 mg/dL (16.7 mmol/L).

Patients using CSII need intensive and extensive education to operate the pump, adjust the settings, and respond appropriately to alarms. Removing the pump for any time can result

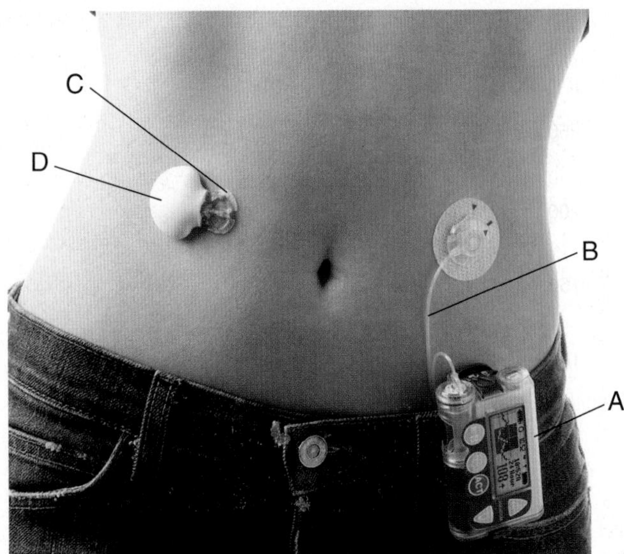

FIG. 59.6 MiniMed Paradigm REAL-Time Insulin Pump and Continuous Glucose Monitoring System. (A) Pump. (B) Injection cannula. (C) Glucose sensor. (D) Data transmitter. (Courtesy Medtronic Diabetes, Northridge, CA.)

in hyperglycemia. Provide supplemental insulin schedules for times when the pump is not operational.

Injection devices include a needleless system and an insulin pen in addition to traditional insulin syringes. With a needleless device, the needle is replaced by an ultrathin liquid stream of insulin forced through the skin under high pressure. Insulin given by jet injection is absorbed at a faster rate and has a shorter duration of action. Most types of insulin are available in pen devices, which are more convenient for multiple daily injection regimens.

A dry powder inhaler insulin delivery system with single-use cartridges is available for rapid-acting insulin. Its use is limited to adults with type 1 or type 2 DM who do not have respiratory problems and who are nonsmokers. Pulmonary testing is required before initiating this therapy. Its onset of action is about 12 minutes. Complications of this therapy include new-onset respiratory problems such as bronchospasms.

Patient education: drugs. Provide specific instructions about insulin therapy, new drug therapies, and self-monitoring of blood glucose (SMBG).

Insulin storage varies by use. Teach patients to refrigerate insulin that is not in use to maintain potency, prevent exposure to sunlight, and inhibit bacterial growth. Insulin in use may be kept at room temperature for up to 28 days to reduce injection site irritation from cold insulin.

To prevent loss of drug potency, teach the patient to avoid exposing insulin to temperatures below 36°F (2.2°C) or above 86°F° (30°C), to avoid excessive shaking, and to protect insulin from direct heat and light. Insulin should not be allowed to freeze. Teach patients to discard any unused insulin after 28 days.

Teach patients to always have a spare supply of each type of insulin used. Prefilled syringes are stable for up to 30 days when refrigerated. Store prefilled syringes in the upright position, with the needle pointing upward or flat, so insulin particles do not clog it. Teach patients to roll prefilled syringes between the hands before using to gently mix and warm the dose.

Proper dose preparation is critical for insulin effectiveness and safety. Teach patients that the person giving the insulin needs to inspect the vial before each use for changes (e.g., clumping, frosting, precipitation, or change in clarity or color) that may indicate loss in potency. Preparations containing NPH insulin are uniformly cloudy after gently rolling the vial between the hands. Other insulins should be clear. If potency is questionable, another vial or pen of the same insulin type should be used.

Syringes are usually used to inject insulin. Standard insulin syringes are marked in insulin units. They are available in 1-mL (100-U), ½-mL (50-U), and 3/10-mL (30-U) sizes. The unit scale on the barrel of the syringe differs with the syringe size and manufacturer. Insulin syringe needles are measured in 28, 29, 30, and 31 gauges and in lengths of 6 mm, 8 mm, and 12.7 mm. To ensure accurate insulin measurement, instruct the patient to always buy the same type of syringe. The Patient and Family Education: Preparing for Self-Management: Subcutaneous Insulin Administration box reviews instructions for drawing up a single insulin injection.

Disposable needles are used only once. Teach the patient to discard the syringe and needle after one use. Information on needle disposal can be obtained at www.safeneedledisposal.org.

Pen-type injectors hold small, lightweight, prefilled insulin cartridges. These devices allow greater accuracy than traditional insulin syringes, especially when measuring small doses. Discuss proper storage for prefilled insulin pens or cartridges. Ensure that the product is appropriate for the patient's unique needs. *Pen-type injectors are not designed for independent use by visually impaired patients or by those with cognitive impairment.* Ensure that the patient understands the correct use for the selected syringe or cartridge.

! NATIONAL PATIENT SAFETY GOALS

The Institute for Safe Medication Practices (ISMP) and The Joint Commission's National Patient Safety Goals identify insulin as a *High-Alert* drug. (High-Alert drugs are those that have an increased risk for causing patient harm if given in error.) The ISMP cautions that digital displays on some insulin pens can be misread. If the pen is held upside down, as a left-handed person might do, a dose of 52 units actually appears to be a dose of 25 units, and a dose of 12 units looks like a dose of 21 units.

Patient education: blood glucose monitoring. Self-monitoring of blood glucose (SMBG) provides a means to assess effectiveness of the management plan and assists the patient in self-care decisions. Results of SMBG are useful in preventing hypoglycemia and hyperglycemia by adjusting drug therapy, diet therapy, and physical activity. Teach patients to assess blood glucose frequently for these situations:

- Symptoms of hypoglycemia or hyperglycemia
- Hypoglycemic unawareness
- Periods of illness
- Before and after exercise
- Gastroparesis
- Adjustment of antidiabetes drugs
- Evaluation of other drug therapies (e.g., steroids)
- Pregnancy

Techniques for SMBG follow principles that are the same as for most self-monitoring systems. Meter systems now require a very

PATIENT AND FAMILY EDUCATION: PREPARING FOR SELF-MANAGEMENT

Subcutaneous Insulin Administration

With Vial and Syringe

- Wash your hands.
- Inspect the bottle for the type of insulin and the expiration date.
- Gently roll the bottle of intermediate-acting insulin in the palms of your hands to mix the insulin.
- Clean the rubber stopper with an alcohol swab.
- Remove the needle cover and pull back the plunger to draw air into the syringe. The amount of air should be equal to the insulin dose. Push the needle through the rubber stopper and inject the air into the insulin bottle.
- Turn the bottle upside down and draw the insulin dose into the syringe.
- Remove air bubbles in the syringe by tapping on the syringe or injecting air back into the bottle. Redraw the correct amount.
- Make certain the tip of the plunger is on the line for your dose of insulin. Magnifiers are available to assist in measuring accurate doses of insulin.
- Remove the needle from the bottle. Recap the needle if the insulin is not to be given immediately.
- Select a site within your injection area that has not been used in the past month.
- Clean your skin with an alcohol swab. Lightly grasp an area of skin and insert the needle at a 90-degree angle.
- Push the plunger all the way down. This will push the insulin into your body. Release the pinched skin.
- Pull the needle straight out quickly. Do not rub the place where you gave the shot.
- Dispose of the syringe and needle without recapping in a puncture-proof container.

With a Pen Device

- Wash your hands.
- Check the drug label to be sure it is what was prescribed.
- Remove the cap.
- Look at the insulin to be sure it is evenly mixed if it contains NPH and that there is no clumping of particles.
- Wipe the tip of the pen where the needle will attach with an alcohol swab.
- Remove the protective pull tab from the needle and screw it onto the pen until snug.
- Remove both the plastic outer cap and inner needle cap.
- Look at the dose window and turn the dosage knob to the appropriate dose.
- Holding the pen with the needle pointing upward, press the button until at least a drop of insulin appears. This is the "cold shot," "air shot," or "safety shot." Repeat this step if needed until a drop appears.
- Dial the number of units needed.
- Hold the pen perpendicular to and against the intended injection site with your thumb on the dosing knob.
- Press the dosing knob slowly all the way to dispense the dose.
- Hold the pen in place for 6 to 10 seconds, then withdraw from the skin.
- Replace the outer needle cap; unscrew until the needle is removed, and dispose of the needle in a hard plastic or metal container.
- Replace the cap on the insulin pen.

small blood sample, which allows for alternate testing sites (e.g., arm, thigh, hand). The selected site is pricked, a drop is drawn into a testing strip or disk impregnated with chemicals, and the glucose value is displayed or "spoken" (in mg/dL or mmol/L) on a screen.

Data obtained from SMBG are evaluated along with other A1C levels or periodic laboratory blood glucose test results. Even when SMBG is performed correctly, the results are affected by hematocrit values (anemia falsely elevates glucose values; polycythemia falsely depresses them) and may be unreliable in the hypoglycemic or severely hyperglycemic ranges.

Accuracy of the blood glucose monitor is ensured when the manufacturer's directions are followed. Common user errors involve failure to obtain a sufficient blood drop, poor storage of test strips, using expired strips, and not changing the code number on the meter to match the strip bottle code. Meter selection is based on cost of the meter and strips, ease of use, and availability of repair and servicing. Provide training, explain and demonstrate procedures, assess visual acuity, and check the patient's ability to perform the procedure using "teach-back" strategies. Newer meters have fewer steps, include error signals for inadequate sample size, and can store hundreds of SMBG results.

Accuracy and precision vary widely among capillary blood glucose monitoring devices. If the meter requires calibration, teach patients to properly calibrate the machine. Instruct them to recheck the calibration and retest if they obtain a test result that is unusual for them and whenever they are in doubt about test accuracy. Continued retraining of patients performing SMBG helps ensure accurate results because performance accuracy deteriorates over time. Laboratory glucose determinations are more accurate than SMBG.

Frequency of testing varies with the drug schedules, the patient's prescribed therapy, and his or her expected target outcomes. Patients taking multiple insulin injections or using insulin pump therapy may need to monitor glucose levels three or more times daily. For patients taking less-frequent injections of insulin, noninsulin therapy, or diet therapy alone, daily SMBG is useful for evaluation of therapy.

Blood glucose therapy target goals for self-management are set individually for each patient based on duration of disease, age and life expectancy, other chronic conditions, severity of cardiovascular disease, and presence of hypoglycemia unawareness (Faminu, 2018). The health care team works with him or her to reach target blood glucose levels. Recommendations for patients with type 1 DM include an A1C value less than 7%, premeal glucose levels of 70 to 130 mg/dL (3.9 to 7.2 mmol/L), and postmeal glucose levels less than 180 mg/dL (10.0 mmol/L) (ADA, 2019d). However, looser target ranges may be prescribed on the basis of age, cognitive impairment, and other health problems.

Infection control measures are needed for SMBG. The chance of becoming infected from blood glucose monitoring processes is reduced by handwashing before monitoring and by not reusing lancets. *Instruct patients to not share their blood glucose monitoring equipment* because infection can be spread by the lancet holder even when the lancet itself has been changed Regular cleaning of the meter is critical for infection control. Remind staff who perform blood glucose testing and family members who help with testing to wear gloves.

Many meters allow data to be downloaded to a computer or smart phone. Some meters allow entry of additional data such as insulin dose, amounts of carbohydrate eaten, or exercise. A radio link to an insulin pump allows automatic transfer of glucose readings to a calculator that helps the patient decide on an appropriate insulin dose. Some patients use smart phone applications to record and trend or graph serial blood glucose levels, insulin dosages, food intake, and other data.

Once the patient learns the technical aspects of meter use, help him or her use the results of SMBG to achieve glycemic control. Postmeal glucose monitoring provides information about the effects of the size and content of their meals. SMBG allows the patient to assess effects of exercise on glucose control and provides critical information to help patients who take insulin to exercise safely. Teach patients how to make agreed-on adjustments in the treatment plan when SMBG results are consistently out of range for a 3-day period when no change in meal plan, drugs, or activity has occurred.

Alternate site testing uses blood obtained from sites other than the fingertip and is available on many meters and meter-smart phone interfaces. Older meters have wider variation between fingertip and alternate sites, and variation is most evident during times when glucose levels change rapidly. Teach patients about the lag time for blood glucose levels between the fingertip and other sites when blood glucose levels are changing rapidly and that the fingertip reading is the only safe choice at those times.

! NURSING SAFETY PRIORITY (QSEN)

Action Alert

Teach patients with a history of hypoglycemic unawareness *not* to test at alternative sites.

Continuous blood glucose monitoring (CGM) systems monitor glucose levels in interstitial fluid to provide real-time glucose information to the user. Many systems consist of three parts: a disposable sensor that measures glucose levels, a transmitter that is attached to the sensor, and a receiver that displays and stores glucose information. After an initiation or warm-up period, the sensor gives glucose values every 1 to 5 minutes. Sensors may be used for 3 to 7 days, depending on the manufacturer. CGM provides information about the current blood glucose level, short-term feedback about results of treatment, and warnings when glucose readings become dangerously high or low. Most available sensors require at least two capillary glucose readings per day for calibration of the sensor. Sensor accuracy depends on these calibrations. There may be a lag time between the capillary glucose measurement and the glucose sensor value. If the blood glucose value is changing rapidly, the time between capillary and interstitial glucose values may be as long as 30 minutes. For this reason, capillary glucose readings need to be checked on all extreme values or if symptoms of hypoglycemia are present before any corrective treatment is given. *With older or less sophisticated systems, give insulin only after confirming the results of any continuous glucose monitoring system.*

Nutrition therapy. Effective self-management of DM requires that ***nutrition***, including the meal plan, education, and counseling programs, be individualized for each patient. A registered dietitian nutritionist (RDN) is a member of the interprofessional team. The nurse, RDN, patient, and family work together on a realistic and flexible meal plan. Plans that consider the patient's cultural background, financial status, and lifestyle are more likely to be successful. The desired outcomes of nutrition and diet therapy are listed in Table 59.9.

TABLE 59.9 Desired Outcomes of Nutrition Therapy for the Patient With Diabetes

- Achieving and maintaining blood glucose levels in the normal range or as close to normal as is safely possible
- Achieving and maintaining a blood lipid profile that reduces the risk for cardiovascular disease
- Achieving blood pressure levels in the normal range or as close to normal as is safely possible
- Preventing or slowing the rate of development of the chronic complications of diabetes by modifying nutrient intake and lifestyle
- Addressing patient ***nutrition*** needs, taking into account personal and cultural preferences and willingness to change
- Maintaining the pleasure of eating by limiting food choices only when indicated by scientific evidence
- Meeting the ***nutrition*** needs of unique times of the life cycle, particularly for pregnant and lactating women and for older adults with diabetes
- Providing self-management training for patients treated with insulin or insulin stimulators for exercising safely, including the prevention and treatment of hypoglycemia and managing diabetes during acute illness

Principle of medical nutrition or Medical Nutrition Management (MNT) is recommended for use with all adults with DM. For overweight or obese adults with type 2 DM, even modest weight loss through reduced caloric intake is beneficial. Blood pressure, blood glucose levels, and lipid profiles are improved by weight loss (ADA, 2019d).

The RDN develops a meal plan based on the patient's usual food intake, weight management goals, and lipid and blood glucose patterns. Consistency in the daily timing and amount of food eaten helps control blood glucose. Patients using insulin therapy need to eat at times that are coordinated with the timed action of insulin. Teach patients using intense insulin therapy to adjust premeal insulin to allow for timing and quantity changes in their meal plan.

No specific percentage of calories from carbohydrates, protein, or fat is ideal for all adults with DM. Recommendations for the distribution of these nutrients is individualized based on food preferences, eating patterns, and metabolic goals (ADA, 2019e; Watts & Howard, 2016).

Carbohydrate intake avoids nutrient deficient sources ("empty calories") and focuses on sources from vegetables, fruits, whole grains, legumes, and dairy products. Adults with diabetes should eat at least 25 g of fiber daily. Teach patients with DM or prediabetes to avoid sugar-sweetened beverages (including high fructose corn syrup) and sucrose to prevent weight gain and adverse effects on metabolism.

Dietary fat and cholesterol intake for adults with DM focuses on the quality of fat rather than on the quantity of fat. A Mediterranean-style diet rich in monounsaturated fatty acids (MUFAs) can lower cardiac risk factors. Such diets include avocados, nuts and seeds, olives, and dark chocolate. Omega-3 fatty acids, including EPA (eicosapentaenoic acid) and DHA (docosahexaenoic acid) from fish or fish oil supplements are recommended as part of a healthy diet to prevent heart disease, as is ALA (alpha-linolenic acid) derived from plant sources. Current recommendations from the ADA to limit *trans* fats, saturated fats, and cholesterol are the same as for the general population (ADA, 2019a; ADA 2019e).

Alcohol consumption affects blood glucose levels, especially with high alcohol use or when DM is poorly controlled. Teach patients that two alcoholic beverages for men and one for women can be ingested with, and in addition to, the usual meal plan. (One alcoholic beverage equals 12 ounces of beer, 5 ounces of wine, or 1½ ounces of distilled spirits.) The risk for delayed hypoglycemia is increased when drug therapy includes insulin or an insulin stimulator.

NURSING SAFETY PRIORITY QSEN

Action Alert

Because of the potential for alcohol-induced delayed hypoglycemia, instruct the patient with DM to ingest alcohol only with or shortly after meals. Even with this precaution patients must remain alert for delayed hypoglycemia following alcohol ingestion.

Patient education for nutrition is based each patient's ***nutrition*** recommendations that consider blood glucose monitoring results, total blood lipid levels, and A1C levels. These tests help determine whether current meal and exercise patterns need adjustment or whether present habits need reinforcement. A specific nutrition prescription is developed for each patient.

Reinforce nutrition information provided by the RDN. The patient with DM must understand how to adjust food intake during illness, planned exercise, social occasions, and when the usual time of eating is delayed. Share dietary information with the person who prepares the meals. The RDN sees each patient yearly to identify changes in lifestyle and make appropriate diet therapy changes. Some patients, such as those with weight-control problems or low incomes, may need more frequent dietary evaluation and counseling.

Carbohydrate (CHO) counting is a simple approach to ***nutrition*** and meal planning that uses label information of the nutritional content of packaged food items. Estimation of CHO content when dining out can be taught by the RDN. Because fat and protein have little effect on after-meal blood glucose levels, CHO counting focuses on the nutrient that has the greatest impact on these levels. It uses total grams of CHO, regardless of the food source. This method is effective in achieving blood glucose control when daily CHO intake is consistent.

Patients using intensive insulin or pump therapies can use CHO counting to determine insulin coverage. After the amount of insulin needed to cover the usual meal is determined, insulin may be added or subtracted for changes in CHO intake. An initial formula of 1 unit of rapid-acting insulin for each 15 g of CHO provides flexibility to meal plans. The patient determines the grams of CHO in a specific meal or snack by reading labels or weighing and measuring each item. The total grams of CHO are used to calculate the bolus dose of insulin based on the prescribed insulin-to-carbohydrate ratio.

Special considerations for type 1 diabetes include developing insulin regimens that conform to the patient's preferred meal routines, food preferences, and exercise patterns. Patients using rapid-acting insulin by injection or an insulin pump must learn to adjust insulin doses based on the CHO content of the meals and snacks. Insulin-to-carbohydrate ratios are developed and are used to provide mealtime insulin doses. Blood glucose monitoring before and 2 hours after meals determines whether the insulin-to-carbohydrate ratio is correct. For patients who are on fixed insulin regimens and do not adjust premeal insulin dosages, consistency in the timing of meals and the amount of CHO eaten at each meal is critical to prevent hypoglycemia.

Exercise can cause hypoglycemia if insulin is not decreased before activity. For planned exercise, hypoglycemia is prevented by a reduction in insulin dosage. For unplanned exercise, intake of additional CHO is usually needed. A 70-kg adult would need about 10 to 15 g additional CHO per hour of moderate-intensity activity. More CHO is needed for intense activity.

It is important for patients using insulin to avoid weight gain. **Hyperinsulinemia** (chronic high blood insulin levels) can occur with intensive management schedules and may result in weight gain. These patients may need to manage hyperglycemia by restricting calories rather than increasing insulin. Weight gain can be minimized by following the prescribed meal plan, getting regular exercise, and avoiding overtreatment of hypoglycemia.

Special considerations for type 2 DM focus on lifestyle changes. Many patients with type 2 DM are overweight and insulin resistant. ***Nutrition*** therapy stresses lifestyle changes that reduce calories eaten and increase calories expended through physical activity. Many patients also have abnormal blood fat levels and hypertension (metabolic syndrome), making reductions of saturated fat, cholesterol, and sodium desirable. A moderate caloric restriction (250 to 500 calories less daily) and an increase in physical activity improve ***glucose regulation*** and weight control. Decreases of more than 10% of body weight can significantly improve A1C.

When patients with type 2 DM need insulin, consistency in timing and CHO content of meals is important. Division of the total daily calories into three meals or into smaller meals and snacks is based on patient preference.

PATIENT-CENTERED CARE: OLDER ADULT CONSIDERATIONS QSEN

Factors that increase the risk for poor ***nutrition*** in older adults with DM include dental issues, finances, changes in appetite, and changes in the ability to obtain and prepare food. Older adults may have reduced awareness of hypoglycemia and hyperglycemia and dehydration, increasing the risk for hyperglycemic-hyperosmolar state (HHS) (Touhy & Jett, 2020). They may eat out or live in situations in which they have little control over meal preparation. Visits by home health nurses can help older patients follow a diabetic meal plan.

Changing the eating habits of 60 to 70 years is difficult and requires a realistic approach. The nurse, RDN, and patient assess the patient's usual eating patterns. Teach the older patient taking antidiabetic drugs the importance of eating meals and snacks at the same time every day and eating the same amount of food from day to day.

Exercise therapy. Regular exercise is an essential part of DM management and improves carbohydrate metabolism and insulin sensitivity. Increased physical activity and weight loss reduce the risk for type 2 DM in patients with prediabetes.

Plasma glucose levels remain stable during exercise in adults without DM because of the balance between glucose use by exercising muscles and glucose production by the liver. The patient with type 1 DM cannot make the hormonal changes needed to maintain stable blood glucose levels during exercise. Without an adequate insulin supply, cells cannot use glucose. Low insulin levels trigger release of glucagon and epinephrine (balancing hormones) to increase liver glucose production, further raising blood glucose levels. Without insulin, FFAs become the source of energy. Exercise in the patient with uncontrolled DM results in hyperglycemia and ketone body formation. Prolonged elevated blood glucose levels occur after vigorous exercise.

Exercise also can cause hypoglycemia because of increased muscle glucose uptake and inhibited glucose release from the liver during exercise and for up to 24 hours after exercise. Replacement of muscle and liver glycogen stores, along with increased insulin sensitivity after exercise, causes insulin requirements to drop.

Benefits of exercise include better blood ***glucose regulation*** and reduced insulin requirements for patients with type 1 DM. Exercise also increases insulin sensitivity, which enhances cell uptake of glucose and promotes weight loss.

Regular exercise decreases risk for cardiovascular disease. It decreases most blood lipid levels and increases high-density lipoproteins (HDLs, the "good" cholesterol). Exercise decreases blood pressure and improves cardiac function. Regular physical activity prevents or delays type 2 DM by reducing body weight, insulin resistance, and glucose intolerance.

PATIENT-CENTERED CARE: OLDER ADULT CONSIDERATIONS QSEN

The ability of the heart and lungs to deliver oxygen to organs declines with age. Muscle strength declines gradually. Range of motion and flexibility decrease, altering gait and increasing the risk for falls. Remaining active can limit loss of muscle mass and function.

Changes in activity levels should be gradual. Formal evaluation by a physical therapist may be needed. Emphasize that the focus for any activity program is on changing sedentary behavior to active behavior at any level. Encourage sedentary older adults to begin with low-intensity physical activity. Start low-intensity activities in short sessions (less than 10 minutes); include warm-up and cool-down components with active stretching.

Exercise adjustments are needed when some long-term DM complications are present. Vigorous aerobic or resistance exercise should be avoided in the presence of diabetic retinopathy. Teach the patient with retinopathy about activities that increase blood pressure. Heavy lifting, rapid head motion, or jarring activities can cause vitreous hemorrhage or retinal detachment. Decreased sensation in the extremities increases the risk for skin breakdown and joint damage. Teach patients with peripheral neuropathy to wear proper footwear and examine their feet daily for lesions or injury. Teach anyone with a foot injury or open sore to engage in non–weight-bearing activities such as swimming, bicycling, or arm exercises. Those with autonomic neuropathy are at increased risk for exercise-induced injury from poor temperature control, postural hypotension, and impaired thirst with risk for dehydration. Encourage high-risk patients to start with short periods of low-intensity exercise and to increase the intensity and duration slowly. Patient conditions that often require activity adjustment include:

- Uncontrolled hypertension
- Severe autonomic neuropathy
- Severe peripheral neuropathy or foot lesions
- Unstable proliferative retinopathy

In the absence of contraindications, advise adults with DM to perform at least 150 minutes per week of moderate-intensity aerobic physical activity divided into 3 days (ADA, 2019e). Teach patients to avoid going more than 2 consecutive days without aerobic physical activity. Urge patients with type 2 DM to perform resistance exercise at least twice weekly, targeting all major muscle groups.

A 5- to 10-minute warm-up period with stretching and low-intensity exercise before exercise prepares the muscles, heart, and lungs for a progressive increase in exercise intensity. After exercising, a cool-down of at least 5 to 10 minutes is performed to gradually bring the heart rate down to pre-exercise level.

Guidelines for exercise are based on blood glucose levels and urine ketone levels. Teach patients to test blood glucose before exercise, at intervals during exercise, and after exercise to determine if it is safe to exercise, and to evaluate the effects of exercise. The absence of urine ketones indicates that enough insulin is available for glucose transport. *When urine ketones are present, the patient should **NOT** exercise.* Ketones indicate that current insulin levels are not adequate and that exercise would elevate blood glucose levels. Carbohydrate foods should be ingested to raise blood glucose levels above 100 mg/dL (5.6 mmol/L) before engaging in exercise. The Patient and Family Education: Preparing for Self-Management: Exercise box lists tips to teach about exercise.

NURSING SAFETY PRIORITY QSEN

Action Alert

Teach patients with type 1 DM to perform vigorous exercise *only* when blood glucose levels are 100 to 250 mg/dL (5.6 to 13.8 mmol/L) and no ketones are present in the urine.

Blood glucose control in hospitalized patients. Hyperglycemia in hospitalized patients occurs from loss of ***glucose regulation*** caused by illness, decreased physical activity, withholding of antidiabetic drugs, use of drugs such as corticosteroids, and changes in nutrition therapy. Hyperglycemia is associated with poor outcomes.

Problems with hyperglycemia in hospitalized patients lead to higher infection rates, longer hospital stays, increased need for intensive care, and greater mortality. Admission glucose levels greater than 198 mg/dL (10.9 mmol/L) are linked with greater

PATIENT AND FAMILY EDUCATION: PREPARING FOR SELF-MANAGEMENT

Exercise

- Remember that exercise helps control blood glucose levels and blood lipid levels and helps reduce complications of diabetes.
- Perform level of exercise recommended to you by your diabetes health care provider.
- Wear appropriate footwear designed for exercise.
- Examine your feet daily and after exercising.
- Stay hydrated and do not exercise in extreme heat or cold.
- Do not exercise within 1 hour of insulin injection or near time of peak insulin action.
- Prevent hypoglycemia during exercise by:
  - Do not exercise unless blood glucose level is at least 80 and less than 250 mg/dL.
  - Have a carbohydrate snack before exercising if 1 hour has passed since the last meal or if the planned exercise is of high intensity.
  - Carry a simple sugar to eat during exercise if symptoms of hypoglycemia occur.
- Carry identification information about diabetes during exercise.
- Check your blood glucose levels more often on days you exercise and remember that extra carbohydrate and less insulin may be needed during the 24-hour period following exercise.

risk for mortality and complications. Hypoglycemia, defined as blood glucose values lower than 40 mg/dL (2.2 mmol/L), also is a risk factor for mortality.

Current guidelines recommend treatment protocols that maintain blood glucose levels between 140 and 180 mg/dL (7.8 and 10.0 mmol/L) for critically ill patients. For most non–critically ill patients, premeal glucose targets are lower than 140 mg/dL (7.8 mmol/L), with random blood glucose values less than 180 mg/dL (10.0 mmol/L). To prevent hypoglycemia, insulin regimens are reviewed if blood glucose levels fall below 100 mg/dL (5.6 mmol/L) and are modified when blood glucose levels are less than 70 mg/dL (3.9 mmol/L) (ADA, 2019d).

Continuous IV insulin solutions are the most effective method for achieving glycemic targets in the intensive care setting. Scheduled subcutaneous injection with basal, meal, and correction elements is used to maintain glucose control in non–critically ill patients. Use of correction dose or "supplemental insulin" to correct premeal hyperglycemia in addition to scheduled prandial and basal insulin is determined by the patient's insulin sensitivity and current blood glucose level.

Prevention of hypoglycemia is also part of managing blood glucose levels. Causes of inpatient hypoglycemia include an inappropriate insulin type, mismatch between insulin type and/or timing of food intake, and altered eating plan without insulin dosage adjustment. Many facilities have protocols for hypoglycemia treatment that direct staff to provide carbohydrate replacement if the patient is alert and able to swallow or to administer concentrated dextrose IV or glucagon by subcutaneous injection if the patient cannot swallow, using the 15-15 Rule (see the Nutrition Therapy section under the Interventions for Preventing Hypoglycemia heading later in this chapter for specific 15-15 rule interventions). There is confusion about whether to give or to hold insulin from a patient who is NPO. Giving rapid-acting or short-acting insulin, as well as amylin and incretin mimetics, will cause hypoglycemia if a patient is not eating. Basal insulin (often at a reduced dose) should be given when the patient is NPO because it controls baseline glucose levels. Insulin mixtures are not given because they contain some short-acting or rapid-acting insulin and will cause hypoglycemia.

Surgical Management. The most common surgical intervention for DM is pancreas transplantation. When successful, this procedure eliminates the need for insulin injections, blood glucose monitoring, and many dietary restrictions. It can eliminate the acute complications related to blood ***glucose regulation*** but is only partially successful in reversing long-term complications. Pancreatic transplant is successful when the patient no longer needs insulin therapy and all blood measures of glucose are normal.

Transplantation requires lifelong drug therapy to prevent graft rejection. These drug regimens have side effects that restrict their use to patients who have serious progressive complications from DM. Some antirejection drugs increase blood glucose levels. A pancreas-alone transplant is most often considered for patients with severe metabolic complications and for those with consistent failure of insulin-based therapy to prevent acute complications.

Pancreas transplantation is considered in patients with DM and end-stage kidney disease (ESKD) who have had or plan to have a kidney transplant. Pancreas graft survival is better when performed at the time of the kidney transplant. Pancreatic transplantation may be performed as a pancreas transplant alone (PTA), pancreas after kidney transplant (PAK), and simultaneous pancreas and kidney transplant (SPK).

The 1-year survival rate for patients receiving a whole pancreas in North America is above 95%, with most patients remaining free of insulin injection and diet restrictions. The degree of HLA tissue-type matching affects the results.

Operative procedures. Most pancreatic transplants involve cadaver donors using a whole pancreas still attached to the exit of the pancreatic duct. The recipient's pancreas is left in place, and the donated pancreas is placed in the pelvis. The insulin released by the pancreas graft is secreted into the bloodstream. The new pancreas also produces about 800 to 1000 mL of fluid daily, which is diverted to either the bladder or the bowel.

Excretion of pancreatic fluids can impair ***fluid and electrolyte balance***, and drainage of these fluids into the urinary bladder causes irritation. When the pancreas is attached to the bladder, the loss of fluid rich in bicarbonate may cause acidosis.

Rejection management. Pancreatic transplantation requires a combination of drugs to reverse and prevent rejection. Patients undergoing antirejection therapy first receive drugs to prevent viral, bacterial, and fungal infection because of the risk for opportunistic infections from overall reduced ***immunity***. When the regimen includes steroid therapy the patient will require dosage adjustments in insulin to achieve desired levels of glucose control. Long-term antirejection therapy reduces ***immunity*** and increases the risk for infection, cancer, and atherosclerosis.

Enhancing Surgical Recovery

Planning: Expected Outcomes. The patient with DM undergoing a surgical procedure is expected to recover completely without complications.

Interventions. The patient with DM is at higher risk for complications. Anesthesia and surgery cause a stress response with release of counterregulatory hormones that elevate blood glucose by suppressing insulin action and increasing the risk for ketoacidosis. Hyperglycemic-hyperosmolar state (HHS) is a complication of surgery and is associated with increased mortality. Diuresis from hyperglycemia can cause dehydration and increases the risk for acute kidney injury.

Complications of DM increase the risk for surgical problems. Patients with DM are at higher risk for hypertension, ischemic heart disease, cerebrovascular disease, myocardial infarction (MI), and cardiomyopathy. The patient with DM is at risk for acute kidney injury and urinary retention after surgery, especially if he or she has albumin in the urine (indicator of kidney damage). Nerve function to the intestinal wall and sphincters can be reduced, leading to delayed gastric emptying and reflux of gastric acid, which increases the risk for aspiration with anesthesia. Autonomic neuropathy may cause paralytic ileus after surgery.

Preoperative Care. Before surgery, blood glucose levels are optimized to reduce the risk for complications. Sulfonylureas are discontinued 1 day before surgery. Metformin is stopped at least 24 hours before surgery and restarted only after kidney function is documented as normal. All other oral drugs are stopped the day of surgery. Patients taking long-acting insulin may need to be switched to intermediate-acting insulin forms 1 to 2 days before surgery.

Preoperative blood glucose levels should be less than 200 mg/dL (11.1 mmol/L). Higher levels are associated with increased infection rates and impaired wound healing.

Intraoperative Care. IV infusion of insulin, glucose, and potassium is standard therapy for perioperative management of DM, and infusion rates are based on hourly capillary glucose testing. The object is to keep the glucose level between 140 and 180 mg/dL (7.8 and 10.0 mmol/L) during surgery to prevent hypoglycemia and reduce risks from hyperglycemia. Higher insulin doses may be needed because stress releases glucagon and epinephrine. Patients usually receive about 5 g of glucose per hour during surgery to prevent hypoglycemia, ketosis, and protein breakdown.

Postoperative Care. Hyperglycemia leads to increased mortality after surgical procedures. American Association of Clinical Endocrinologists (AACE) and ADA guidelines recommend insulin dosing to maintain blood glucose between 140 and 180 mg/dL (7.8 and 10.0 mmol/L) for critically ill patients (ADA, 2019d).

Continue glucose and insulin infusions as prescribed until the patient is stable and can tolerate oral feedings. Short-term insulin therapy may be needed after surgery for the patient who usually uses oral agents. For those receiving insulin therapy, dosage adjustments may be required until the stress of surgery subsides.

Opioid analgesics slow GI motility and alter blood glucose levels. The older patient who receives opioids is at risk for confusion, paralytic ileus, hypoventilation, hypotension, and urinary retention. Patient-controlled analgesia (PCA) systems reduce respiratory complications and confusion. (See Chapter 5 for pain interventions and Chapter 9 for general preoperative care.)

Monitoring. Patients with autonomic neuropathy or vascular disease need close monitoring to avoid hypotension or respiratory arrest. Those who take beta blockers for hypertension need close monitoring for hypoglycemia because these drugs mask symptoms of hypoglycemia. Patients with increased blood protein or nitrogen in the blood may have problems with fluid management. Check central venous pressure or pulmonary artery pressure as needed.

Balancing hormones are often activated and cause increased blood glucose levels before patients become febrile. *Hyperglycemia often occurs before a fever.*

! NURSING SAFETY PRIORITY QSEN

Action Alert

When a patient who has had reasonably controlled blood glucose levels in the hospital develops an unexpected rise in blood glucose values, check for wound infection.

Fluid and electrolyte balance is often disrupted by surgery. *Hyperkalemia* (high blood potassium level) is common in patients with mild to moderate kidney failure and can lead to cardiac dysrhythmia. In other patients, *hypokalemia* (low blood potassium level) may occur and be made worse by insulin and glucose given during surgery. Monitor the cardiac rhythm and serum potassium values.

Cardiovascular monitoring by continuous ECG is often used for older patients with DM, those with long-standing type 1 DM, and those with heart disease. Patients with DM are at higher risk for MI after surgery. Changes in ECG or potassium level may indicate a silent MI.

Kidney monitoring, especially observing fluid balance, helps detect acute kidney injury. Management of infections may require the use of nephrotoxic antibiotics. Ensure adequate hydration when these drugs are used. Check for impending kidney failure by assessing ***fluid and electrolyte balance***.

Nutrition. Patients requiring clear or full liquid diets should receive about 200 g of carbohydrate daily in equally divided amounts at meals and snack times. Initial liquids should ***not*** be sugar free. Most patients require 25 to 35 calories per kg of body weight every 24 hours. After surgery, food intake is initiated as quickly as possible, with progression from clear liquids to solid foods occurring as rapidly as tolerated to promote healing and metabolic balance. When oral foods are tolerated, make sure the patient eats at least 150 to 200 g of carbohydrate daily to prevent hypoglycemia.

If total parenteral nutrition (TPN) is used after surgery, severe hyperglycemia may occur. Monitor blood glucose often to determine the need for supplemental insulin.

Preventing Injury From Peripheral Neuropathy

Planning: Expected Outcomes. The patient with DM is expected to identify factors that increase the risk for injury, practice proper foot care, and maintain intact skin on the feet.

Interventions. Patients with DM need intensive education about foot care because foot injury is a common complication. Once a failure of ***tissue integrity*** has occurred and an ulcer has developed, there is an increased risk for wound progression that may eventually lead to amputation. Most lower extremity

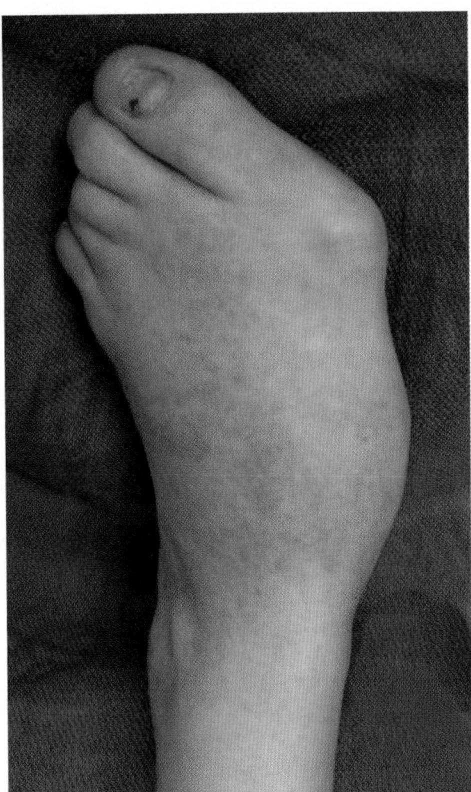

FIG. 59.7 "Charcot foot" type of diabetic foot deformity. (From Frykberg, R.G., Zgonis, T., Armstrong, D.G., Driver, V.R., Giurini, J.M., Kravitz, S.R., et al. [2006]. Diabetic foot disorders: A clinical practice guideline—2006 revision. *The Journal of Foot and Ankle Surgery, 45*[5], S1-S66.)

amputations in adults with DM are preceded by foot ulcers, and the 5-year mortality rate after leg or foot amputation is high (CDC, 2020). Neuropathy is the main factor for development of a diabetic ulcer, and inadequate ***perfusion*** is the main cause of poor healing.

Motor neuropathy damages the nerves of foot muscles, resulting in foot deformities. These deformities create pressure points that gradually reduce ***tissue integrity*** with skin breakdown and ulceration. Thinning or shifting of the fat pad under the metatarsal heads decreases cushioning and increases areas of pressure. In claw toe deformity, toes are hyperextended and increase pressure on the metatarsal heads ("ball" of the foot). These changes predispose the patient to callus formation, ulceration, and infection. The *Charcot foot* is a type of diabetic foot deformity with many abnormalities, often including a *hallux valgus* (turning inward of the great toe) (Fig. 59.7). The foot is warm, swollen, and painful. Walking collapses the arch, shortens the foot, and gives the foot a "rocker bottom" shape.

Autonomic neuropathy causes loss of normal sweating and skin temperature regulation, resulting in dry, thinning skin. Skin cracks and fissures increase the infection risk. Sensory neuropathy may cause tingling or burning, but more often it produces numbness and reduced ***sensory perception***. Without sensation, the patient does not notice injury and loss of ***tissue integrity*** in the foot. Peripheral arterial disease reduces blood flow to the foot, increasing the risk for ulcer formation and slowing ulcer healing (McCance et al., 2019).

TABLE 59.10 Foot Risk Categories

Risk Categories	Management Categories
Risk Category 0 • Has protective sensation • No evidence of peripheral vascular disease • No evidence of foot deformity or loss of ***tissue integrity***	**Management Category 0** • Comprehensive foot examination once a year • Patient education to include advice on appropriate footwear
Risk Category 1 • Does not have protective sensation • May have evidence of foot deformity	**Management Category 1** • Evaluation every 3-6 months • Consider referral to a specialist to assess need for specialized treatment and follow-up • Patient education
Risk Category 2 • Does not have protective sensation • Evidence of peripheral vascular disease **Risk Category 3** • History of ulcer or amputation	**Management Categories 2 and 3** • Evaluation every 1-3 months • Referral to a specialist • Prescription footwear • Consider vascular consultation for combined follow-up • Patient education

Foot injuries are caused by walking barefoot, wearing ill-fitting shoes, sustaining thermal injuries from heat (e.g., hot water bottles, heating pads, baths), or chemical burns from over-the-counter corn treatments. These injuries lead to loss of ***tissue integrity*** and to amputation.

Ulcers result from continued pressure. Ulcers on the sole and ball of the foot are from standing or walking. Those on the top or sides of the foot usually are from shoes. The increased pressure causes calluses. Ulcers usually form over or around the great toe, under the metatarsal heads, and on the tops of claw toes.

Loss of ***tissue integrity*** with broken skin increases the risk for infection. Skin tends to break in areas of pressure. Infection is common in diabetic foot ulcers and, once present, is difficult to treat. Infection also impairs ***glucose regulation***, leading to higher blood glucose levels and reduced ***immunity***, which further increases the risk for infection.

Prevention of High-Risk Conditions. Neuropathy of the feet and legs can be delayed by keeping blood glucose levels near normal. Poor glucose control increases the risk for neuropathy and amputation. Urge smoking cessation to reduce the risk for vascular complications.

The risk for ulcers or amputation increases with duration of diabetes. Other risk factors are male gender; poor glucose control; and cardiovascular, retinal, or kidney complications. Foot-related risks include poor gait and stepping mechanics, peripheral neuropathy, increased pressure (callus, erythema, hemorrhage under a callus, limited joint mobility, foot deformities, or severe nail pathology), peripheral vascular disease, and a history of ulcers or amputation (ADA, 2019g).

Peripheral Neuropathy Management. Foot assessment techniques are listed in the Focused Assessment: The Diabetic Foot box. A thorough assessment of the feet should be performed by a health care professional at least annually. Table 59.10 lists foot risk categories.

FOCUSED ASSESSMENT

The Diabetic Foot

Assess the patient's risk for diabetic foot problems:
- History of previous ulcer
- History of previous amputation

Assess the foot for abnormal skin and nail conditions:
- Dry, cracked, fissured skin
- Ulcers
- Toenails: thickened, long nails; ingrown nails
- Tinea pedis; onychomycosis (mycotic nails)

Assess the foot for status of circulation:
- Symptoms of claudication
- Presence or absence of dorsalis pedis or posterior tibial pulse
- Prolonged capillary filling time (greater than 25 seconds)
- Presence or absence of hair growth on the top of the foot

Assess the foot for evidence of deformity:
- Calluses, corns
- Prominent metatarsal heads (metatarsal head is easily felt under the skin)
- Toe contractures: clawed toes, hammertoes
- Hallux valgus or bunions
- Charcot foot ("rocker bottom")

Assess the foot for loss of strength:
- Limited ankle joint range of motion
- Limited motion of great toe

Assess the foot for loss of protective sensation:
- Numbness, burning, tingling
- Semmes-Weinstein monofilament testing at 10 points on each foot

Data from American Diabetes Association (ADA). (2019g). Microvascular complications and foot care: Standards of medical care in diabetes—2019. *Diabetes Care, 42*(Suppl. 1), S124-S138.

PATIENT AND FAMILY EDUCATION: PREPARING FOR SELF-MANAGEMENT

Foot Care Instructions

- Inspect your feet daily, especially the area between the toes.
- Wash your feet daily with lukewarm water and soap. Dry thoroughly.
- Apply a moisturizer to your feet (but not between your toes) after bathing.
- Change into clean cotton socks every day.
- Do not wear the same pair of shoes 2 days in a row and wear only shoes made of breathable materials, such as leather or cloth.
- Check your shoes for foreign objects (nails, pebbles) before putting them on. Check inside the shoes for cracks or tears in the lining.
- Buy shoes that have plenty of room for your toes. Buy shoes later in the day, when feet are normally larger. Break in new shoes gradually.
- Wear socks to keep your feet warm.
- Trim your nails straight across with a nail clipper and smooth them with an emery board.
- See your diabetes health care provider immediately if you have blisters, sores, or infections. Protect the area with a dry, sterile dressing. Do not use tape to secure dressing to the skin.
- Do not treat blisters, sores, or infections with home remedies.
- Do not smoke or use nicotine products.
- Do not step into the bathtub without checking the temperature of the water with your wrist or thermometer.
- Do not use very hot or cold water. Never use hot-water bottles, heating pads, or portable heaters to warm your feet.
- Do not treat corns, blisters, bunions, calluses, or ingrown toenails yourself.
- Do not go barefooted.
- Do not wear sandals with open toes or straps between the toes.
- Do not cross your legs or wear garters or tight stockings that constrict blood flow.
- Do not soak your feet.

Data from American Diabetes Association (ADA). (2019g). Microvascular complications and foot care: Standards of medical care in diabetes—2019. *Diabetes Care, 42*(Suppl. 1), S124–S138.

Sensory examination of the foot with Semmes-Weinstein monofilaments is a practical measure of loss of sensation, which increases the risk for foot ulcers. The nylon monofilament is mounted on a holder standardized to exert a 10-g force. An adult who cannot feel the 10-g pressure at any point is at increased risk for ulcers. A diabetes health care provider most often performs this examination.

Footwear. Patients with any degree of peripheral neuropathy are at risk for loss of ***tissue integrity*** and need to wear protective shoes fitted by an experienced shoe fitter, such as a certified podiatrist. The shoe should be ½ to ⅝ inch longer than the longest toe. Heels should be less than 2 inches high. Tight shoes damage tissue. Instruct the patient to change shoes by midday and again in the evening. Socks must fit properly and be appropriate for the planned activity. Socks should feel soft and have no thick seams, creases, or holes. They should pad the foot and absorb excess moisture. White socks are recommended because the presence of blood or drainage is more easily recognized than on colored socks.

Teach patients to avoid tight stockings or those that have constricting bands. Patients with toe deformities need custom shoes with high, wide toe boxes and extra depth. Those with severely deformed feet need specially molded shoes. New shoes need a long break-in period with frequent foot inspection for irritation or blistering.

Foot care. Teach patients about preventive foot care and the need for examination of the feet and legs at each visit to a diabetes health care provider or primary health care provider. A mirror placed on the floor can help the patient visually examine the plantar surface of the foot. Identify patients with high-risk foot conditions. Explain problems caused by loss of protective sensation, the importance of monitoring the feet daily, proper care of the feet (including nail and skin care), and how to select appropriate footwear.

Assess the patient's ability to inspect all areas of the foot and to perform foot care. Teach family members how to inspect and care for the patient's feet using the guidelines in the Patient and Family Education: Preparing for Self-Management: Foot Care Instructions box if the patient is unable to do this independently.

Wound care. The standards of care for diabetic ulcers are a moist wound environment, débridement of necrotic tissue, and elimination of pressure (offloading). Eliminating pressure on an infected area is essential for wound healing. Teach patients with foot ulcers to not wear a shoe on the affected foot while the ulcer is healing. Those with poor ***sensory perception*** may keep walking on an ulcer because it does not hurt, causing pressure necrosis that delays healing and increases ulcer size. Pressure is reduced by specialized orthotic devices, custom-molded shoe inserts, or shoe adjustments that redistribute weight.

Offloading redistributes force away from ulcer sites and pressure points to wider areas of the foot. Available products include total-contact casting, half shoes, removable cast walkers, wheelchairs, and crutches. Total-contact casts redistribute pressure over the bottom of the foot. Casting material is molded to the foot and leg to spread pressure along the entire surface of contact, reducing vertical force. The almost complete elimination of motion of the total-contact cast reduces plantar shear forces. *Teach the patient that foot ulcers will recur unless weight is permanently redistributed.*

Reducing the Risk for Kidney Disease

Planning: Expected Outcomes. The patient with diabetes is expected to maintain a normal urine elimination pattern.

Interventions

Prevention. Diabetic kidney disease is more likely to develop in patients with poor blood glucose control. Progression to end-stage kidney disease can be delayed or prevented by normalizing blood pressure using drugs from either the angiotensin-converting enzyme inhibitor (ACEI) class or the angiotensin receptor blocker (ARB) class. Once used to "protect" the kidney, neither class of drug is recommended for patients with DM who have normal blood pressure and normal albumin excretion (ADA, 2019c). Hypertension greatly accelerates the progression of diabetic kidney disease.

Stress the need for evaluation of kidney function according to the ADA Standards of Care. An annual test to quantify urine albumin is performed for patients who have had type 1 DM for over 5 years and in all those with type 2 DM starting at diagnosis (ADA, 2019c). Persistent albuminuria in the range of 30 to 299 mg/24 hours is the earliest stage of nephropathy in type 1 DM and a marker for the development of nephropathy in type 2 DM.

Aggressive control of blood glucose, cholesterol levels, and hypertension in patients without albuminuria can avoid nephropathy. Once albuminuria develops, management focuses on controlling blood pressure and blood glucose and avoiding nephrotoxic agents.

Control of blood pressure, cholesterol, and blood glucose levels requires the patient's participation. Prescribed drugs must be taken according to schedules, and dietary restriction must be maintained. Educate patients about the roles of blood pressure and blood glucose levels in kidney disease. Teach them about maintaining normal blood glucose and cholesterol levels and keeping blood pressure levels below 140/80 mm Hg. Stress the need for yearly screening for albuminuria.

Smoking cessation is important in halting the progression of diabetic kidney disease. Teach the patient about the risks of smoking and refer him or her to appropriate resources for assistance in smoking cessation, as described in Chapter 24.

Drugs can affect kidney function either through toxic effects on the kidney or by an acute but reversible reduction in function. The most common prescribed nephrotoxic drugs are antifungal agents and aminoglycoside antibiotics. Other common nephrotoxic drugs are NSAIDs such as ibuprofen or naproxen. Teach the patient to check with his or her diabetes health care provider or a pharmacist before taking over-the-counter drugs or herbal remedies.

Radiocontrast media can also affect kidney function, especially in patients with preexisting kidney problems. Monitor IV hydration before and after a contrast agent is used, to prevent contrast-induced nephropathy in patients with DM.

Drug Therapy. Use of angiotensin-converting enzyme inhibitors (ACEIs) or angiotensin receptor blockers (ARBs) is recommended for all patients with persistent albuminuria or advanced stages of nephropathy (ADA, 2019c). ACE inhibitors reduce the level of albuminuria and the rate of progression of kidney disease, although they do not appear to prevent albuminuria. Monitor serum potassium levels for development of hyperkalemia (ADA, 2019c).

Dialysis for patients with DM and kidney failure is the same as for patients without diabetes (see Chapter 63). The dosage of insulin needs to be adjusted when dialysis starts.

NCLEX EXAMINATION CHALLENGE 59.5

Health Promotion and Maintenance

A client with diabetes who now has chronic albuminuria asks the nurse how this change will affect his health. How will the nurse answer this question?

A. "You will need to limit your intake of dietary albumin and other proteins to reduce the albuminuria."
B. "This change indicates beginning kidney problems and requires good blood glucose control to prevent more damage."
C. "Your risk for developing urinary tract infections is greatly increased, requiring the need to take daily antibiotics for prevention."
D. "From now on you will need to limit your fluid intake to just 1 L daily and completely avoid caffeine to protect your kidneys."

Preventing Complications from Hypoglycemia, Diabetic Ketoacidosis, and Hyperglycemic-Hyperosmolar Stage (HHS)

Planning: Expected Outcomes. The patient is expected to have blood glucose levels within the normal range, avoiding levels below 70 mg/dL (3.9 mmol/L) and never higher than 200 mg/dL (11.1 mmol/L).

Interventions for Preventing Hypoglycemia. Hypoglycemia is a low blood glucose level that induces specific symptoms and resolves when blood glucose concentration is raised. Once plasma glucose levels fall below 70 mg/dl (3.9 mmol/L), a sequence of events begins with release of counterregulatory hormones, stimulation of the autonomic nervous system, and production of *neurogenic* and *neuroglycopenic* symptoms. Peripheral autonomic symptoms, including sweating, irritability, tremors, anxiety, tachycardia, and hunger, serve as an early warning system and occur before the symptoms of confusion, paralysis, seizure, and coma occur from brain glucose deprivation. *Neuroglycopenic symptoms* occur when brain glucose *gradually declines* to a low level. *Neurologic symptoms* result from autonomic nervous activity triggered by a *rapid decline* in blood glucose (Table 59.11).

Central nervous system (CNS) function depends on a continuous supply of glucose in the blood. The brain cannot make glucose and stores only a few minutes' supply as glycogen. This needed supply is not maintained when the blood glucose level falls below critical levels.

TABLE 59.11 Symptoms of Hypoglycemia

Neuroglycopenic Symptoms	Neurogenic Symptoms

• Weakness
• Fatigue
• Difficulty thinking
• Confusion
• Behavior changes
• Emotional instability
• Seizures
• Loss of consciousness
• Brain damage
• Death
	• Adrenergic:
	  • Shaky or tremulous
	  • Heart pounding
	  • Nervous or anxious
	• Cholinergic:
	  • Sweaty
	  • Hungry
	  • Tingling

The first defense against falling blood glucose levels in the adult without DM is decreased insulin secretion, decreased glucose use, and increased glucose production. Normally, insulin secretion decreases when blood glucose levels drop to about 83 mg/dL (4.5 mmol/L). Balancing (counterregulatory) hormones are activated at about 67 mg/dL (3.7 mmol/L), a level above the threshold for symptoms of hypoglycemia. The main balancing hormone is glucagon. Both glucagon and epinephrine raise blood glucose levels by stimulating liver glycogen breakdown and conversion of protein to glucose. Epinephrine also limits insulin secretion.

Type 1 DM disrupts the body's response to hypoglycemia, usually within 1 to 5 years of diagnosis, because insulin comes from an injection rather than from the pancreas. As blood glucose levels fall after the injection, insulin levels do not decrease. Over time, the pancreas loses its ability to secrete glucagon in response to hypoglycemia. Eventually the response of epinephrine to falling blood glucose levels does not occur until the blood glucose level is very low, which greatly increases the risk for severe hypoglycemia.

A second problem with long-standing type 1 DM is *hypoglycemic unawareness,* in which patients no longer have the warning symptoms of early hypoglycemia that could prompt them to take preventive action. This problem occurs most often in patients who have had type 1 DM for 30 years or longer. Hypoglycemic unawareness also can occur in patients who have had type 2 DM for many years with a long-standing history of hypoglycemia.

The blood glucose level at which symptoms of hypoglycemia occur varies among patients. Thus clinical criteria used to categorize hypoglycemia are based on symptom severity rather than blood glucose levels. In mild hypoglycemia, the patient remains alert and able to self-manage symptoms. In severe hypoglycemia, neurologic function is so impaired that he or she needs another person's help to increase blood glucose levels.

Blood Glucose Management. Monitor blood glucose levels before giving antidiabetic drugs, before meals, before bedtime, and when the patient is symptomatic. All patients who take insulin, those taking long-acting insulin stimulators (glyburide), and those taking metformin in combination with glyburide are at risk for hypoglycemia. This risk is increased if they are older, have liver or kidney impairment, or are taking drugs that enhance the effects of antidiabetic drugs. In the hospital setting, mealtime insulin *must* be coordinated with timely monitoring and food delivery to avoid episodes of hypoglycemia (Watts & Nemes, 2018). Blood glucose should be checked no more than 1 hour before a meal, and rapid-acting insulin given just before the meal to avoid hypoglycemia.

The most common causes of hypoglycemia are:

- Too much insulin compared with food intake and physical activity
- Insulin injected at the wrong time relative to food intake and physical activity
- The wrong type of insulin injected at the wrong time
- Decreased food intake resulting from missed or delayed meals
- Delayed gastric emptying from gastroparesis
- Decreased liver glucose production after alcohol ingestion
- Decreased insulin clearance due to progressive kidney failure

Nutrition Therapy. In hospitalized patients, most protocols for management of hypoglycemia follow the 15-15 rule for hypoglycemia management (Watts et al., 2020). With this rule, 15 g of CHO are given if the blood glucose level is less than 70 mg/dL (3.9 mmol/L) (or 30 g if less than 50 mg/dL [2.8 mmol/L]) or if the patient is experiencing symptoms of hypoglycemia. If the patient can swallow, give a liquid form of CHO, although any fast-acting CHO source can be used (avoid high-potassium options such as orange juice). If the blood glucose recheck within 15 minutes is still low, the same treatment is given again. If at any time the patient is unable to swallow, an IV dose of concentrated dextrose or subcutaneous glucagon is indicated. Specific recommendations are listed in the Patient and Family Education: Preparing for Self-Management box for management of hypoglycemia at home.

The blood glucose level determines the form and amount of glucose used. The response should be apparent in 10 to 20 minutes; however, test plasma glucose again in about 60 minutes because additional management may be needed. Fluid is absorbed much more quickly from the GI tract than are solids. Concentrated sweet fluids, such as chocolate, may slow absorption because of the fat content.

Management of hypoglycemia is most effective with ingestion of glucose or glucose-containing foods rather than foods containing complex carbohydrates. *Adding protein to CHO does not improve blood glucose response and does not prevent subsequent hypoglycemia.* Commercially available products provide predictable glucose absorption.

Drug Therapy. Subcutaneous or IM glucagon and concentrated IV dextrose are given to patients who cannot swallow. Glucagon is the main balancing hormone to insulin and is used as first-line therapy for severe hypoglycemia. Take care to prevent aspiration in patients receiving glucagon, because it often causes vomiting. Give concentrated dextrose carefully to avoid extravasation because it is hyperosmolar and can damage tissue. The effects of glucagon and dextrose are temporary. Evaluate response by monitoring blood glucose levels for several hours because symptoms may persist. A target blood glucose level is 70 to 110 mg/dL (3.9 to 6.2 mmol/L).

PATIENT AND FAMILY EDUCATION: PREPARING FOR SELF-MANAGEMENT

Management of Hypoglycemia at Home

For mild hypoglycemia (hungry, irritable, shaky, weak, headache, fully conscious; blood glucose usually less than 70 mg/dL [3.9 mmol/L]):

- Treat the symptoms of hypoglycemia with 15 g of carbohydrate. You may use one of these:
  - Glucose tablets or glucose gel (dosage is printed on the package)
  - A half cup (120 mL) of fruit juice or of regular (nondiet) soft drink
  - 8 ounces (240 mL) of skim milk
  - 6 to 10 hard candies
  - 4 cubes of sugar or 4 teaspoons of sugar
  - 6 saltines
  - 3 graham crackers
  - 1 tablespoon (15 mL) of honey or syrup
- Retest blood glucose in 15 minutes.
- Repeat this treatment if glucose remains less than 70 mg/dL (3.9 mmol/L). Symptoms may persist after blood glucose has normalized.
- Eat a small snack of carbohydrate and protein if your next meal is more than an hour away.

For moderate hypoglycemia (cold, clammy skin; pale; rapid pulse; rapid, shallow respirations; marked change in mood; drowsiness; blood glucose usually less than 40 mg/dL [2.2 mmol/L]):

- Treat the symptoms of hypoglycemia with 30 g of rapidly absorbed carbohydrate.
- Retest glucose in 15 minutes.
- Repeat treatment if glucose is less than 60 mg/dL (3.4 mmol/L).
- Eat additional food, such as low-fat milk, after 10 to 15 minutes.

For severe hypoglycemia (unable to swallow; unconsciousness or convulsions; blood glucose usually less than 20 mg/dL [1.0 mmol/L]):

- Treatment administered by family members:
  - Give prescribed dose of glucagon as intramuscular or subcutaneous injection.
  - Give a second dose in 10 minutes if the person remains unconscious.
  - Notify the diabetes health care provider immediately and follow instructions.
  - If still unconscious, transport the person to the emergency department.
  - Give a small meal when the person wakes up and is no longer nauseated.

! NURSING SAFETY PRIORITY (QSEN)

Critical Rescue

Assess patients to recognize the presence and severity of hypoglycemia. For the patient with *severe* hypoglycemia (unable to swallow, unconscious or convulsing, blood glucose usually less than 20 mg/dL [1.0 mmol/L]), respond by:

1. Giving prescribed dose of glucagon subcutaneously or IM.
2. Repeating the dose in 10 minutes if the patient remains unconscious
3. Notifying the diabetes health care provider immediately, and following instructions

Prevention Strategies. Teach the patient how to prevent hypoglycemia by avoiding its four common causes: (1) excess insulin, (2) deficient intake or absorption of food, (3) exercise when insulin action is peaking, and (4) alcohol intake.

Insulin excess from variable absorption of insulin can cause hypoglycemia even when insulin is injected correctly. Differences in insulin formulation can result in hypoglycemia.

Deficient food intake from inadequate or incorrectly timed meals can result in hypoglycemia. Educate about the importance of regular timing and quantity of food eaten, especially carbohydrates.

Exercise often causes blood glucose levels to fall. Prolonged exercise increases muscle glucose uptake for several hours after exercise. Teach the patient about blood glucose monitoring and carbohydrate consumption before and during exercise (if necessary). Also teach him or her to exercise at times when insulin activity is not peaking.

Alcohol inhibits liver glucose production and leads to hypoglycemia. It interferes with the hormone response to hypoglycemia and impairs glycogen breakdown. Instruct the patient to ingest alcohol only with or shortly *after* eating a meal with enough carbohydrate to prevent hypoglycemia.

Patient and Family Education. Help each patient develop a personal treatment plan for hypoglycemia. The exact glucose rise from a set amount of carbohydrate (CHO) varies; however, using the estimate that each 5 g of CHO raises blood glucose about 20 mg/dL is a good starting plan. For example, the patient may be directed to take:

- 20 to 30 g of CHO if the blood glucose level is 50 mg/dL (2.8 mmol/L) or less
- 10 to 15 g of CHO if the blood glucose level is 51 to 70 mg/dL (2.9 to 3.9 mmol/L)

Encourage the patient to wear a medical alert bracelet or have a wallet card describing how to manage diabetes emergencies. This information is helpful if the patient becomes hypoglycemic and is unable to perform self-care.

Teach the patient and family about the symptoms of hypoglycemia (see Table 59.11). Stress that delaying a meal for more than 30 minutes raises the risk for hypoglycemia when using some insulin regimens. Instruct him or her to keep a CHO source nearby at all times. Teach the patient and family how to inject glucagon. The changes in cognition associated with hypoglycemia may cause confusion among family members with those seen in severe hyperglycemia; review the differences in the common signs and symptoms of these two emergencies (Table 59.12).

PATIENT-CENTERED CARE: OLDER ADULT CONSIDERATIONS (QSEN)

Older patients are at increased risk for hypoglycemia. Age-related declines in kidney function reduce the elimination of sulfonylureas and insulin, thus potentiating their hypoglycemic effects. Older adults have reduced epinephrine and glucagon release in response to low blood glucose levels and often have hypoglycemic unawareness. The presence of impaired motor skills when glucose is low reduces the ability to take steps to return glucose levels to normal.

Instruct the older patient's family to check blood glucose values when symptoms such as unsteadiness, light-headedness, poor concentration, trembling, or sweating occur (Touhy & Jett, 2020). Remind them to make sure that sufficient foods are eaten at appropriate times. Encourage a patient with a poor appetite to eat a small snack at bedtime to prevent hypoglycemia during the night.

TABLE 59.12 Differentiation of Hypoglycemia and Hyperglycemia

Feature	Hypoglycemia	Hyperglycemia
Skin	Cool, clammy, "sweaty"	Warm, dry, vasodilated
Dehydration	Absent	Present
Respirations	No particular or consistent change	Rapid, deep[a]; Kussmaul type; acetone odor (rotten "fruity" odor) to breath
Mental status	Anxious, nervous,[a] irritable, mental confusion,[a] seizures, coma	Varies from alert to stuporous, obtunded, or frank coma
Symptoms	Weakness,[a] double vision, blurred vision, hunger, tachycardia, palpitations	None specific for DKA Acidosis; hypercapnia; abdominal cramps, nausea and vomiting Dehydration: decreased neck vein filling, orthostatic hypotension, tachycardia, poor skin turgor
Glucose	<70 mg/dL (3.9 mmol/L)	>250 mg/dL (13.8 mmol/L)
Urine or blood ketones	Negative	Positive

DKA, Diabetic ketoacidosis.
[a]Classic symptoms.

Interventions for Preventing Diabetic Ketoacidosis. Diabetic ketoacidosis (DKA) is a complication of diabetes characterized by uncontrolled hyperglycemia, metabolic acidosis, and increased production of ketones. This condition results from the combination of insulin deficiency and an increase in hormone release that leads to increased liver and kidney glucose production (Fig. 59.8). Laboratory diagnosis of DKA is shown in Table 59.13. All of these changes increase ketoacid production with resultant ketonemia and metabolic acidosis. The most common precipitating factor for DKA is infection. *Death occurs in up to 10% of these cases even with appropriate treatment.*

Hyperglycemia leads to osmotic diuresis with dehydration and electrolyte loss. Classic symptoms of DKA include polyuria, polydipsia, polyphagia, a rotting citrus fruit odor to the breath, vomiting, abdominal pain, dehydration, weakness, confusion, shock, and coma. Mental status can vary from total alertness to profound coma. As ketones rise, blood pH decreases, and acidosis occurs. Kussmaul respirations cause respiratory alkalosis in an attempt to correct metabolic acidosis by exhaling carbon dioxide. Initial serum sodium levels may be low or normal.

Blood Glucose Management. Monitor for symptoms of DKA (see Table 59.13 and Fig. 59.8). Document and use these findings to determine therapy effectiveness. *First assess the airway, level of consciousness, hydration status, electrolytes, and blood glucose level.* Check the patient's blood pressure, pulse, and respirations every 15 minutes until stable. Record urine output, temperature, and mental status every hour. When a central venous catheter is present, assess central venous pressure every 30 minutes or as prescribed. After treatment starts and these values are stable, monitor and record vital signs every 4 hours. Use blood glucose values to assess therapy and determine when to switch from saline to dextrose-containing solutions.

Fluid and Electrolyte Management. *Closely assess the patient's **fluid and electrolyte balance**.* Assess for acute weight loss, thirst, decreased skin turgor, dry mucous membranes, and oliguria with a high specific gravity. Assess for weak and rapid pulse, flat neck veins, increased temperature, decreased central venous pressure, muscle weakness, postural hypotension, and cool, clammy, and pale skin to determine if the patient is at risk for dehydration.

The first outcome of fluid therapy is to restore blood volume and maintain ***perfusion*** to vital organs. Typically initial infusion rates are 15 to 20 mL/kg/hr during the first hour.

The second outcome of replacing total body fluid losses is achieved more slowly. Usually hypotonic fluids are infused at 4 to 14 mL/kg/hr after the initial fluid bolus. When blood glucose levels reach 250 mg/dL (13.8 mmol/L), give 5% dextrose in 0.45% saline. This solution helps prevent hypoglycemia and cerebral edema, which can occur when serum osmolarity declines too rapidly.

During the first 24 hours of treatment, the patient needs enough fluids to replace the actual volume lost, as well as any ongoing losses, and the total may be as much as 6 to 10 L. Assess cardiac, kidney, and mental status to avoid fluid overload. Watch for symptoms of heart failure and pulmonary edema. Assess the status of fluid replacement by monitoring blood pressure, intake and output, and changes in daily weight.

Drug Therapy. Insulin therapy is used to lower serum glucose by about 50 to 75 mg/dL/hr (2.8 to 4.2 mmol/L/hr). Unless the episode of DKA is mild, regular insulin by continuous IV infusion is the usual management. An initial IV bolus dose is given, followed by an IV continuous infusion. Continuous insulin infusion is used because insulin half-life is short and subcutaneous insulin has a delayed onset of action (Fayfman et al., 2017). Subcutaneous insulin is started when the patient can take oral fluids and ketosis has stopped. DKA is considered resolved when blood glucose is less than 200 mg/mL (11.2 mmol/L) along with a serum bicarbonate level higher than 18 mEq/L (mmol/L), venous pH is higher than 7.30, and a calculated anion gap is less than 12 mEq/L (mmol/L). Assess therapy effectiveness by monitoring blood glucose levels and serial electrolyte levels.

Mild-to-moderate hyperkalemia is common in patients with hyperglycemia. Insulin therapy, correction of acidosis, and volume expansion decrease serum potassium concentration. To prevent hypokalemia, potassium replacement is initiated after serum levels fall below normal (5.0 mEq/L [mmol/L]). *Assess for signs of hypokalemia, including fatigue, malaise, confusion, muscle weakness, shallow respirations, abdominal distention or paralytic ileus, hypotension, and weak pulse.* An ECG shows conduction changes related to alterations in potassium. Hypokalemia is a common cause of death in the treatment of DKA.

! NURSING SAFETY PRIORITY (QSEN)

Action Alert

Before giving IV potassium-containing solutions, ensure that urine output is at least 30 mL/hr.

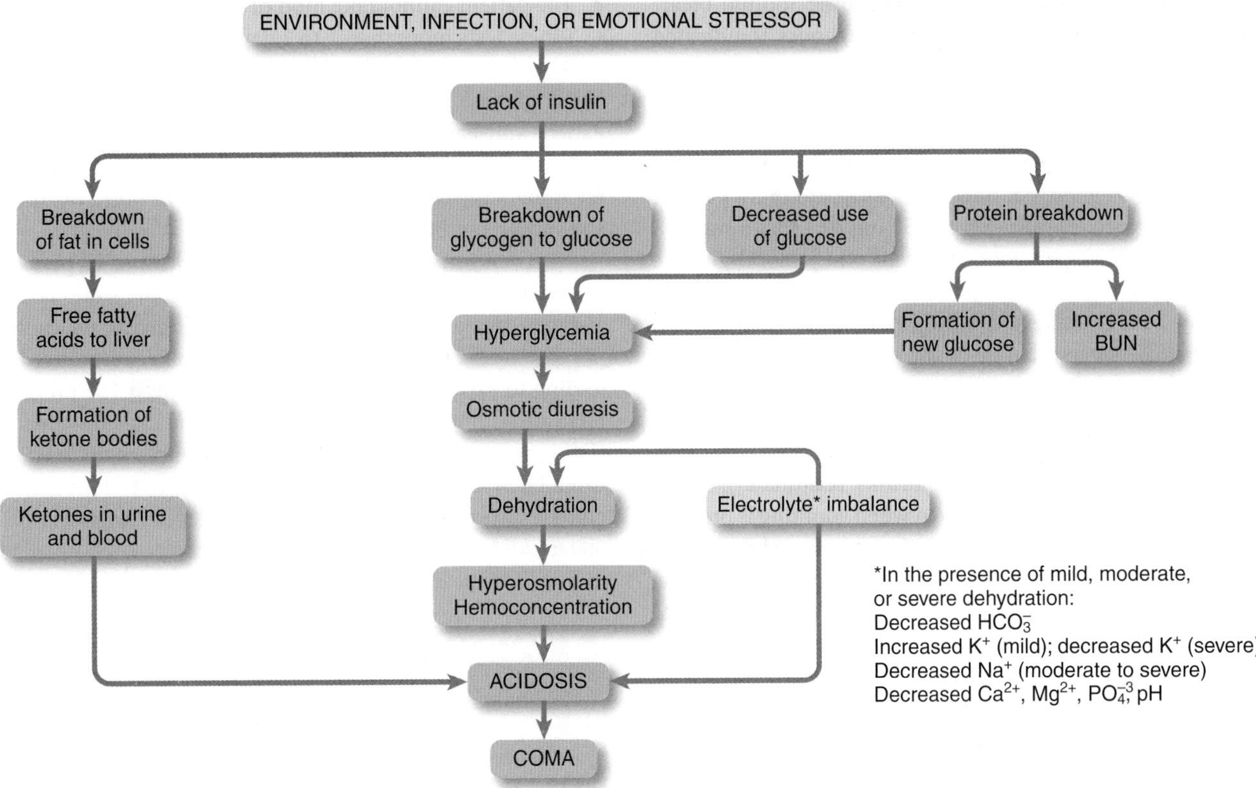

FIG. 59.8 Pathophysiologic mechanism of diabetic ketoacidosis (DKA). *BUN,* Blood urea nitrogen; *Ca^{2+}*, calcium; HCO_3^-, bicarbonate; *K^+*, potassium; *Mg^{2+}*, magnesium; *Na^+*, sodium; PO_4^{-3}, phosphate.

TABLE 59.13 Differences Between Diabetic Ketoacidosis and Hyperglycemic-Hyperosmolar State

	Diabetic Ketoacidosis (DKA)	Hyperglycemic-Hyperosmolar State (HHS)
Onset	Sudden	Gradual
Precipitating factors	Infection Other stressors Inadequate insulin dose	Infection Other stressors Poor fluid intake
Symptoms	Ketosis: Kussmaul respiration, "rotting fruit" breath, nausea, abdominal pain Dehydration or electrolyte loss: polyuria, polydipsia, weight loss, dry skin, sunken eyes, soft eyeballs, lethargy, coma	Altered central nervous system function with neurologic symptoms Dehydration or electrolyte loss: same as for DKA
Laboratory Findings		
Serum glucose	>300 mg/dL (16.7 mmol/L)	>600 mg/dL (33.3 mmol/L)
Osmolarity/osmolality	Variable	>320 mOsm/L (mOsm/kg)
Serum ketones	Positive at 1:2 dilutions	Negative
Serum pH	<7.35	>7.4
Serum HCO_3^-	<15 mEq/L (mmol/L)	>20 mEq/L (mmol/L)
Serum Na^+	Low, normal, or high	Normal or low
BUN	>30 mg/dL (10 mmol/L); elevated because of dehydration	Elevated
Creatinine	>1.5 mg/dL (60 mcmol/L); elevated because of dehydration	Elevated
Urine ketones	Positive	Negative

BUN, Blood urea nitrogen; HCO_3^-, bicarbonate; *Na^+*, sodium.

Bicarbonate is used only for severe acidosis. Sodium bicarbonate, given by slow IV infusion over several hours, is indicated when the arterial pH is 7.0 or less or the serum bicarbonate level is less than 5 mEq/L (5 mmol/L).

Patient and Family Education. Teach the patient and family to check blood glucose levels every 4 to 6 hours as long as symptoms such as anorexia, nausea, and vomiting are present and as long as glucose levels exceed 250 mg/dL (13.8 mmol/L). Teach them to check urine ketone levels when blood glucose levels exceed 300 mg/dL (16.7 mmol/L).

Teach the patient to prevent dehydration by maintaining food and fluid intake. Suggest that he or she drink at least 2 L of fluid daily and increase this amount when infection is present. When nausea is present, instruct the patient to take liquids containing both glucose and electrolytes (e.g., regular sugar-sweetened soda pop, diluted fruit juice, and sports drinks [Gatorade]). Small amounts of fluid may be tolerated even when vomiting is present. When the blood glucose level is normal or elevated, the patient should take 8 to 12 ounces (240 to 360 mL) of calorie-free and caffeine-free liquids every hour while awake to prevent dehydration.

Liquids containing carbohydrate (CHO) can be taken if the patient cannot eat solid food. Ingesting at least 150 g of CHO daily reduces the risk for starvation ketosis. After consulting the diabetes health care provider, urge the patient to take additional rapid-acting (lispro) or short-acting (regular) insulin based on blood glucose levels.

Instruct the patient and family to consult the diabetes health care provider or primary health care provider when these problems occur:

- Blood glucose exceeds 250 mg/dL (13.8 mmol/L) and does not respond to therapy.
- Ketonuria lasts for more than 24 hours.
- The patient cannot take food or fluids.
- Illness lasts more than 1 to 2 days.

Also instruct them to detect hyperglycemia by monitoring blood glucose whenever the patient is ill, as described in the Patient and Family Education: Preparing for Self-Management box for sick-day rules. Illness can result in dehydration with DKA, hyperglycemic-hyperosmolar state, or both. Insulin therapy should not be omitted during illness.

PATIENT AND FAMILY EDUCATION: PREPARING FOR SELF-MANAGEMENT

Sick-Day Rules

- Notify your primary health care provider or diabetes health care provider that you are ill.
- Monitor your blood glucose at least every 4 hours.
- Test your urine for ketones when your blood glucose level is greater than 240 mg/dL (13.8 mmol/L).
- Continue to take insulin or other antidiabetic agents, unless instructed otherwise by your primary health care provider.
- To prevent dehydration, drink 8 to 12 ounces (240 to 360 mL) of sugar-free liquids every hour that you are awake. If your blood glucose level is below your target range, drink fluids that contain sugar.
- Continue to eat meals at regular times.
- If unable to tolerate solid food because of nausea, consume more easily tolerated foods or liquids equal to the carbohydrate content of your usual meal.
- Call your diabetes health care provider for any of these problems:
  - Persistent nausea and vomiting
  - Moderate or high ketones
  - Blood glucose elevation after two supplemental doses of insulin
  - High (101.5°F [38.6°C]) temperature or increasing fever; fever for more than 24 hours
- Treat diarrhea, nausea, vomiting, fever as directed by your diabetes health care provider.
- Get plenty of rest.

Interventions for Preventing Hyperglycemic-Hyperosmolar State (HHS). Hyperglycemic-hyperosmolar state (HHS) is a hyperosmolar (increased blood osmolarity) state caused by hyperglycemia. HHS results from a sustained osmotic diuresis leading to extremely high blood glucose levels. The processes of HHS are outlined in Fig. 59.9. Both HHS and diabetic ketoacidosis (DKA) are caused by hyperglycemia and dehydration. HHS differs from DKA in that ketone levels are absent or low and blood glucose levels are much higher. Blood glucose levels may exceed 600 mg/dL (33.3 mmol/L), and blood osmolarity may exceed 320 mOsm/L. Table 59.13 lists the differences between DKA and HHS.

PATIENT-CENTERED CARE: OLDER ADULT CONSIDERATIONS QSEN

HHS occurs most often in older patients with type 2 DM, many of whom are unaware they have the disease (Touhy & Jett, 2020). Mortality rates in older patients with HHS have been reported to be as high as 16% (Fayfman et al., 2017). The onset of HHS is slow and may not be recognized. The older patient often seeks medical attention later and is sicker than the younger patient. HHS does not occur in well-hydrated patients. Older patients are at greater risk for dehydration and HHS because of age-related changes in thirst perception, poor urine-concentrating abilities, and use of diuretics. Assess all older adults for dehydration, regardless of whether they are known to have DM.

Myocardial infarction, sepsis, pancreatitis, stroke, and some drugs (glucocorticoids, diuretics, phenytoin, beta blockers, and calcium channel blockers) also may cause or contribute to HHS. Central nervous system (CNS) changes range from confusion to complete coma. Unlike DKA, patients with HHS may have seizures and reversible paralysis. The degree of neurologic impairment is related to serum osmolarity, with coma occurring once serum osmolarity is greater than 350 mOsm/L (350 mmol/L). Normal serum osmolarity is between 270 mOsm (270 mmol/L) and 300 mOsm/L (300 mmol/L).

The development of HHS rather than DKA is related to residual insulin secretion. In HHS, the patient secretes just enough insulin to prevent ketosis but not enough to prevent hyperglycemia. The hyperglycemia of HHS is more severe than that of DKA, greatly increasing blood osmolarity, leading to extreme diuresis with severe dehydration and electrolyte loss.

Fluid Therapy. The expected outcomes of therapy are to rehydrate the patient and restore normal blood glucose levels within 36 to 72 hours. The choice of fluid replacement and the rate of infusion are critical in managing HHS. The severity of the CNS problems is related to the level of blood hyperosmolarity and cellular dehydration. Re-establishing fluid balance in brain cells is a difficult and slow process, and many patients do not recover baseline CNS function until hours after blood glucose levels have returned to normal.

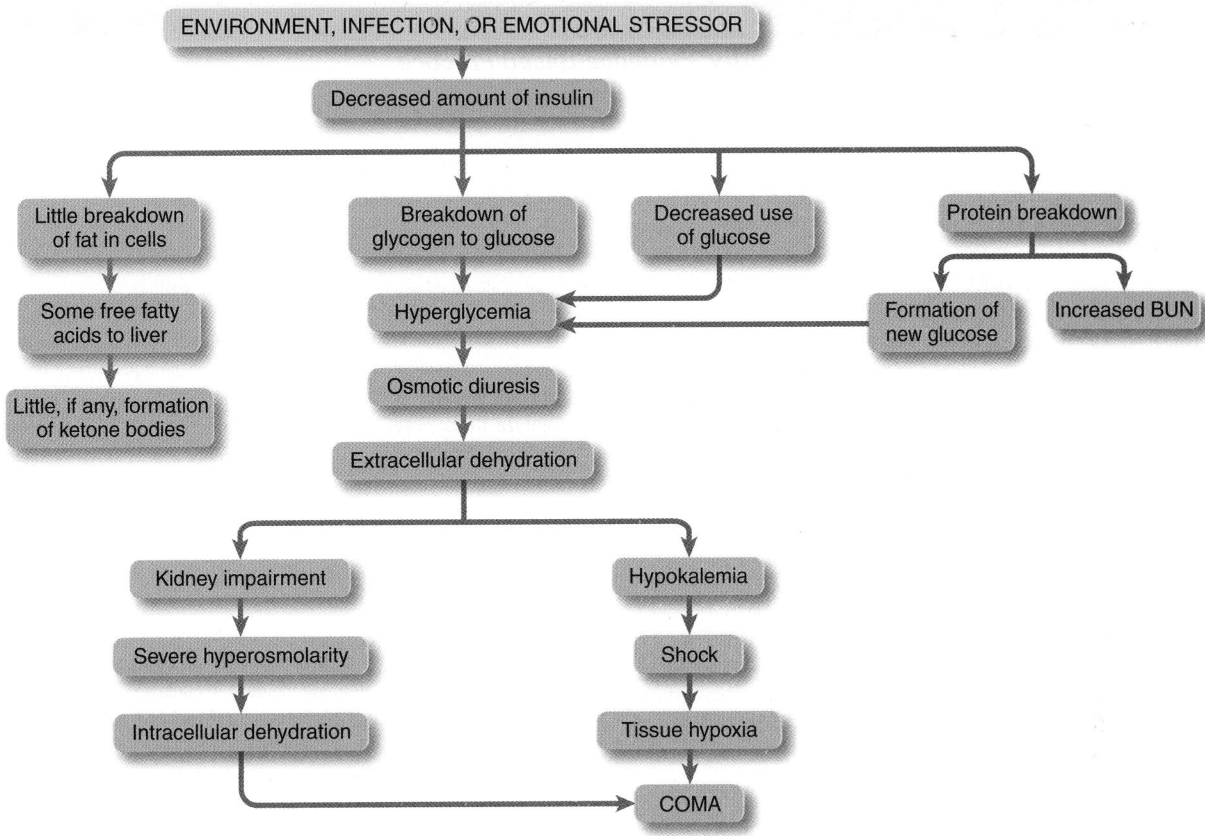

FIG. 59.9 Pathophysiologic mechanism of hyperglycemic-hyperosmolar state (HHS). *BUN,* Blood urea nitrogen.

The *first* priority for fluid replacement in HHS is to increase blood volume. In shock or severe hypotension, normal saline is used. Otherwise half-normal saline is used. Infuse fluids at 1 L/hr until central venous pressure or pulmonary capillary wedge pressure begins to rise or until blood pressure and urine output are adequate. The rate is then reduced to 100 to 200 mL/hr. Half of the estimated fluid deficit is replaced in the first 12 hours, and the rest is given over the next 36 hours. Body weight, urine output, kidney function, and the presence or absence of pulmonary congestion and jugular venous distention determine the rate of fluid infusion. *Assess the patient hourly for signs of cerebral edema (i.e., abrupt changes in mental status, abnormal neurologic signs, and coma).* Lack of improvement in level of consciousness may indicate inadequate rates of fluid replacement or reduction in plasma osmolarity. Regression after initial improvement may indicate a too-rapid reduction in plasma osmolarity. A slow but steady improvement in CNS function is the best evidence that fluid management is satisfactory.

! NURSING SAFETY PRIORITY (QSEN)

Critical Rescue

Continually monitor the patient being managed for hyperglycemic-hyperosmolar state to recognize status changes. When you notice changes in the level of consciousness; changes in pupil size, shape, or reaction; or seizures, respond by immediately notifying the diabetes health care provider.

Continuing Therapy. IV insulin is administered after adequate fluids have been replaced. Usually an initial bolus dose is given followed by continuous IV infusion until blood glucose levels fall to 250 mg/dL (13.9 mmol/L). A reduction of blood glucose of 50 to 70 mg/dL (2.8 to 4.0 mmol/L) per hour is the expected outcome. Monitor the patient closely for hypokalemia because potassium levels drop quickly with insulin therapy. Check serum electrolytes every 1 to 2 hours until stable, and monitor cardiac rhythm continuously for signs of hypokalemia or hyperkalemia. Patient education and interventions to minimize dehydration are similar to those for ketoacidosis.

Care Coordination and Transition Management

Self-Management Education. DM is a chronic disease requiring those affected to be actively involved in managing self-care. Education about blood glucose control for those with or at risk for DM occurs in a variety of health care settings. The interprofessional team of certified diabetes educators, primary health care providers, nurses, registered dietitian nutritionists (RDNs), pharmacists, social workers, and psychologists all participate in the education at every health care encounter. The patient must be an active participant at all levels for self-management to be successful (Faminu, 2019; Harris, 2019).

Assessing Learning Needs and Readiness to Learn. First assess the patient's learning needs and readiness to learn to establish what the patient already knows and what he or she needs to know. Assess the needs of both patient and family before teaching as described in Table 59.14.

CLINICAL JUDGMENT CHALLENGE 59.1

Patient-Centered Care, Physiological Integrity, Evidence-Based Practice

The client is a 69-year-old man who was brought to the emergency department by his wife because he seems confused and is not eating or drinking. He knows who she is but does not know what day it is or what else is going on in their home. When asked if he has any health problems, the wife says no—that although he has gained a lot of weight since his retirement 4 years ago from construction work, he has always been healthy. In fact, he has not seen a doctor since an at-work injury healed 28 years ago. He takes no medicine and his current hobbies include bowling and playing poker with his friends. When asked whether he smokes or drinks alcohol, the wife proudly states that he quit smoking 10 years ago but now he drinks 4 to 5 beers nightly, and sometimes more when he is with his friends. The wife reports that he has been hobbling around a little the past few days because of an infected big toe on his right foot. Yesterday he was nauseated and did not feel well enough to eat anything except a little chicken broth and only drank one cup of coffee as his liquids for the entire day. Their daughter, who lives about 3 hours away, suggested that they come to the hospital.

On assessment the nurse finds the client responsive to his name, and he keeps stating that he feels "awful." His pulse is difficult to palpate and is both irregular and very fast. Blood pressure is 90/50 mm Hg. Pulse oximetry is 96% with a respiratory rate of 24 breaths/min. Temperature is 102.2°F (39°C). His affected toe is edematous and red with a red streak extending about 3 inches up his foot. Other findings include dry skin with poor turgor (tenting of skin on the forehead is present 2 minutes after pinching it up), sunken appearance to the eyeballs, and sticky coating over tongue and teeth.

His wife says he is 5 feet 9 inches (1.75 m) tall. His weight in the emergency department is 232 lb (105.2 kg), which his wife says is about 15 lb (6.8 kg) less than his weight at home earlier this week. When asked, the wife reports that he hasn't "peed" today.

A stat blood glucose level is 720 mg/dL (40 mmol/L). When his laboratory work returns, the results are:

- Blood osmolarity = 322 mOsm/L (322 mOsm/kg)
- Electrolytes = low normal
- pH = 7.39
- Ketone bodies = negative
- Total white blood cell count = 21,000/mm^3 (21 × 10^9/L)

1. **Recognize Cues:** What assessment information in this client situation is the most important and immediate concern for the nurse? (Hint: Identify the **relevant** information *first* to determine what is most important.)
2. **Analyze Cues:** What client conditions are consistent with the **most relevant** information? (Hint: Think about priority collaborative problems that support and contradict the information presented in this situation.)
3. **Prioritize Hypotheses:** Which possibilities or explanations are **most likely** to be present in this client situation? Which possibilities or explanations are the most serious? (Hint: Consider all possibilities and determine their urgency and risk for this client.)
4. **Generate Solutions:** What actions would most likely achieve the desired outcomes for this client? Which actions should be **avoided** or are **potentially harmful**? (Hint: Determine the desired outcomes first to decide which interventions are appropriate and those that should be avoided.)
5. **Take Action:** Which actions are the most appropriate and how should they be implemented? In what **priority order** should they be implemented? (Hint: Consider health teaching, documentation, requested health care provider orders or prescriptions, nursing skills, collaboration with or referral to health team members, etc.)
6. **Evaluate Outcomes:** What client assessment would indicate that the nurse's actions were **effective**? (Hint: Think about signs that would indicate an improvement, decline, or unchanged client condition.)

TABLE 59.14 Assessment of Learning Needs for the Patient With Diabetes

- Health and medical history
- Nutrition history and practices
- Physical activity and exercise behaviors
- Prescription and over-the-counter drugs and complementary and integrative therapies and practices
- Factors that influence learning such as education and literacy levels, perceived learning needs, motivation to learn, and health beliefs
- Diabetes self-management behaviors, including experience with self-adjusting the treatment plan
- Previous diabetes self-management training, actual knowledge, and skills
- Physical factors, including age, mobility, visual acuity, hearing, manual dexterity, alertness, attention span, and ability to concentrate or special needs or limitations requiring adaptive support and use of alternative skills
- Psychosocial concerns, factors, or issues, including family and social support
- Current mental health status
- History of substance use, including alcohol, tobacco (especially smoking), and recreational drugs
- Occupation, vocation, education level, financial status, and social, cultural, and religious practices
- Access to and use of health care resources

Provide information that applies directly to the patient. Ask about his or her concerns and what specifically he or she wants to learn. Start with what the patient already knows, and build on that base. Make sure that the patient's knowledge is current and applies to his or her type of DM.

When the patient is not ready to learn needed self-management behaviors, ask his or her permission to teach a family member about DM management. Provide written materials on DM management, as well as telephone numbers for the patient to call when he or she is ready to learn.

Assessing Physical, Cognitive, and Emotional Limitations. Assessing the patient's literacy is essential in developing a plan of care and providing self-management education (Watts et al., 2017). It is important to measure the patient's ability to read and understand written materials and perform math calculations. Match the literacy level of materials to the literacy level of the patient.

Assess the patient's ability to read printed information, insulin labels, and markings on syringes and equipment. Many older adult patients have age-related vision problems that are made worse by blurred vision caused by changing blood glucose levels.

Assess manual dexterity for any physical limitations that may alter the teaching plan. A hand injury, tremors, or severe arthritis often leads to dosing errors with a standard syringe and may require a change in insulin preparation.

Learning styles vary. Successful self-management education provides written handouts, discusses steps involved in a procedure such as insulin administration or self-monitoring of blood glucose (SMBG), and encourages the learner to touch and manipulate equipment. Confirm that the patient understands your instructions by using "teach-back" techniques.

Tailor educational sessions to the time available and to the condition of the patient. Hospitalized adults require only basic education when they are acutely ill. In these situations, it is appropriate to teach basic survival skills or focused problem-solving skills while reserving more detailed education for follow-up sessions.

Survival Skills Information. The initial phase of education involves teaching just the information necessary for the survival of any adult diagnosed with DM. Survival information includes:

- Simple information on pathophysiology of DM
- Learning how to prepare and inject insulin or how to take other antidiabetic drugs
- Recognition, treatment, and prevention of hypoglycemia and hyperglycemia
- Basic diet information
- Monitoring of blood glucose and urine ketones
- Sick-day management rules
- Where to buy DM supplies and how to store them
- When and how to notify the diabetes health care provider or primary health care provider

In-Depth Education. In-depth education and counseling involve teaching more detailed information about survival skills and actions for avoiding long-term complications. Educational sessions with the patient and family are needed to individualize the DM regimen for their needs and abilities.

The adult with DM must be able to discuss the action of insulin and the effects of insulin deficiency, as well as be able to explain the effects of diet, drugs, and activity on blood glucose. The patient is expected to relate maintaining normal blood glucose levels to preventing complications. This includes relating changes in glucose level to the possible need for a change in insulin dosage.

Provide education about the symptoms of hypoglycemia along with the prescribed treatment options if the patient takes any drugs that will lower blood glucose levels. Educate patients and families about common causes of hypoglycemia described earlier. Review indications of hypoglycemia at each visit. Advise patients to check their blood glucose levels before driving and to make sure they have easy-to-reach snacks and/or fast-acting sugars with them at all times. Remind them to contact their diabetes health care provider if they experience low blood glucose levels more than twice a week.

Ask patients taking an antidiabetic drug to identify the drug(s) and describe the prescribed schedule. Determine if the patient is able to inject insulin or other injectable antidiabetic drugs accurately by having him or her demonstrate injection techniques. Ask the patient to discuss the onset, peak, and duration of the insulin used. The patient must be able to state when insulin is to be injected, where it is injected, and how it is stored. Review formulas for self-adjustment in insulin (when supported by the diabetes health care provider), and explain blood glucose monitoring requirements needed to evaluate the effects of additional insulin. Stress the dangers of skipping doses. Review drug interactions, especially with older patients taking oral antidiabetic drugs.

Teach patients receiving diet therapy alone, glucose-lowering drugs, or fixed insulin doses to eat the consistent amounts of carbohydrate (CHO) at meals and snacks. Patients who adjust mealtime doses of insulin or those on insulin pump therapy can be taught to match their insulin dose to the CHO content of their diet. The patient needs to understand what to eat, how much to eat, and when to eat. Stress the importance of eating on time, the dangers of skipping meals, and how to maintain food intake during illness. Ask the patient to describe the meal plan and explain the adjustments needed to meet diabetic diet requirements. Include the family member usually responsible for buying groceries and preparing meals in this teaching.

Teach the patient the skills needed to perform self-monitoring of blood glucose (SMBG), how to interpret results, and when to adjust behaviors and therapy based on the information. In addition, show patients who use insulin how to use SMBG to adjust dosages in order to achieve glucose control while avoiding episodes of hypoglycemia.

Teach patients sick-day procedures when initially diagnosed with DM. Hyperglycemia often develops before infection symptoms and can serve as a warning sign that infection is developing. Provide guidelines for the frequency of glucose testing, ketone testing, and insulin adjustment for those patients able to self-adjust insulin doses.

Psychosocial Preparation. The diagnosis of DM may represent a loss of control and flexibility. Life becomes ordered, and routines must be followed. Some events surrounding DM are predictable. Injecting insulin and not eating for several hours causes hypoglycemia. Poorly controlled DM leads to complications and premature death. Tight control of blood glucose prevents complications.

Patients are more likely to adhere to disease management activities when the strategies make sense and seem effective. The patient's belief that the activity is important, having confidence in himself or herself, and having support promote adherence to management strategies. Mastery of blood glucose monitoring helps the patient feel control over the disease. Knowing the effects of extra activities, extra food, or extra insulin is helpful in learning to adjust the regimen. Feeling a sense of control over the condition promotes a positive attitude about DM. Success in injecting insulin provides concrete evidence that he or she can master the disease. Teach by breaking a task into small, achievable units to ensure mastery. For example, a patient may begin learning how to inject insulin by first obtaining an accurate dose.

Devote as much teaching time as possible to insulin injection and blood glucose monitoring. Patients with newly diagnosed DM may fear giving themselves injections. After this technique is mastered, he or she may be less anxious and more able to attend to other tasks.

Home Care Management. Patients with DM self-manage their disease. Each day they decide what to eat, whether to exercise, and whether to take prescribed drugs. Maintaining blood glucose control depends on the accuracy of self-management skills. The role of the nurse is to provide support and education and to empower the patient to make informed

FOCUSED ASSESSMENT

The Insulin-Dependent Patient With Diabetes During a Home or Clinic Visit

- Assess overall mental status, wakefulness, ability to participate in a conversation.
- Take vital signs and weight:
  - Fever could indicate infection.
  - Are blood pressure and weight within target range? If not, why?
- Ask the patient about any change in vision; check current visual acuity.
- Inspect oral mucous membranes, gums, and teeth.
- Ask about injection areas used; inspect areas being used; assess whether the patient is using areas and rotating sites appropriately.
- Inspect skin for intactness, wounds that have not healed, new sores, ulcers, bruises, or burns; assess any previously known wounds for infection, progression of healing.
- Ask the patient how often and how he or she performs foot care.
- Assess lower extremities and feet for peripheral pulses, lack of or decreased sensation, abnormal sensations, breaks in skin integrity, condition of toes and nails.
- Ask about the color and consistency of stools and frequency of bowel movements; assess abdomen for bowel sounds.
- Review patient's home health diary:
  - Is blood glucose within targeted range? If not, why?
  - Is glucose monitoring being recorded often enough?
  - Is the patient's food intake adequate and appropriate? If not, why?
  - Is exercise occurring regularly? If not, why?
- Assess the patient's ability to perform self-monitoring of blood glucose.
- Assess the patient's procedures for obtaining and storing insulin and syringes, cleaning equipment, disposing of syringes and needles.
- Assess the patient's insulin preparation and injection technique.
- Assess the patient's knowledge of drug therapy and which side effects to look for.

decisions. Self-management education allows patients to identify their problems and provides techniques to help them make decisions, take appropriate actions, and adjust these actions as needed.

Provide information about resources. The patient must know whom to contact in case of emergency. Older adults who live alone need to have daily telephone contact with a friend or neighbor. The patient may also need help shopping and preparing meals. He or she may have limited access to transportation and may not have sufficient supplies of food, particularly in bad weather. Because of the likelihood of vision problems in older patients, they may need help in preparing insulin syringes for injection or in monitoring blood glucose. Make referrals to home care or public health agencies as needed. Assess the areas listed in the Focused Assessment: The Insulin-Dependent Patient With Diabetes During a Home or Clinic Visit box during any home or clinic visit.

TABLE 59.15 Outcome Criteria for Diabetes Teaching

Before self-management begins at home, the patient with diabetes or the significant other should be able to:

- Tell why insulin or a noninsulin antidiabetic drug is being prescribed
- Name which insulin or noninsulin antidiabetic drug is being prescribed, and name the dosage and frequency of administration
- Discuss the relationship between mealtime and the action of insulin or the other antidiabetic agent
- Discuss plans to follow diabetic diet instructions
- Prepare and inject insulin accurately
- Test blood for glucose or state plans for having blood glucose levels monitored
- Test urine for ketones and state when this test should be done
- Describe how to store insulin
- List symptoms that indicate a hypoglycemic reaction
- Tell which carbohydrate sources are used to treat hypoglycemic reactions
- Tell which symptoms indicate hyperglycemia
- Tell which dietary changes are needed during illness
- State when to call the diabetes health care provider or the nurse (frequent episodes of hypoglycemia, symptoms of hyperglycemia)
- Describe the procedures for proper foot care

◆ **Evaluation: Evaluate Outcomes.** Evaluate the care of the patient with DM based on the identified priority patient problems. Outcome success for diabetes education is the ability of the patient to maintain blood glucose levels within their established target range. General outcome criteria are listed below and in Table 59.15. The expected outcomes include that with successful education the patient will be able to:

- Achieve blood glucose control by following the recommended diet, following the prescribed drug regimen, and reaching and maintaining optimum body weight
- Avoid acute and chronic complications of diabetes
- Avoid injury
- Recover from surgery without infection and with good wound healing
- Experience relief of pain
- Remain free of foot lesions, infections, and deformities
- Maintain optimal vision
- Maintain a urine output in the expected range
- Have an optimal level of mental status functioning
- Have decreased episodes of hypoglycemia
- Have decreased episodes of hyperglycemia

GET READY FOR THE NEXT-GENERATION NCLEX® EXAMINATION!

Key Points

Review these Key Points for each NCLEX Examination Client Needs Category.

Safe and Effective Care Environment

- Ensure that meals are available with or immediately after the patient receives an antidiabetic drug or insulin. **QSEN: Safety**
- Collaborate with the diabetes health care provider, diabetes nurse educator, registered dietitian nutritionist, pharmacist, social worker, and case manager to individualize patient care for the adult with diabetes in any care setting. **QSEN: Patient-Centered Care**
- Never dilute or mix insulin glargine with any other insulin or solution. **QSEN: Safety**

- Instruct the patient and family about complications and when to seek assistance. **QSEN: Safety**
- Assess patients' visual acuity and peripheral tactile sensation to determine needed adjustments in teaching self-medication and self-monitoring of blood glucose levels. **QSEN: Safety**
- Teach patients with peripheral neuropathy to use a bath thermometer to test water for bathing, to avoid walking barefoot, and to inspect their feet daily. **QSEN: Safety**
- Teach the patient and family about the symptoms of infection and when to seek medical advice. **QSEN: Safety**
- Instruct patients to wear a medical alert bracelet or carry a wallet ID. **QSEN: Safety**
- Instruct patients to always carry a glucose source. **QSEN: Safety**

Health Promotion and Maintenance

- Encourage all patients to maintain weight within an appropriate range. **QSEN: Patient-Centered Care**
- Encourage patients with diabetes to participate regularly in exercise or physical activity appropriate to their health status. **QSEN: Evidence-Based Practice**
- Instruct all patients with diabetes to avoid becoming dehydrated and to drink at least 2 L of water each day unless another medical condition requires fluid restriction. **QSEN: Patient-Centered Care**
- Teach patients to self-manage hypoglycemia with 15 to 30 g of carbohydrate (especially glucose), depending on the severity of the low blood glucose level, and to avoid overtreatment. Tell them to recheck blood glucose level in 15 minutes and re-treat as needed. **QSEN: Patient-Centered Care**
- Use return demonstration with "teach-back" strategies when teaching the patient about drug regimen, insulin injection, blood glucose monitoring, and foot assessment. **QSEN: Patient-Centered Care**
- Refer patients newly diagnosed with diabetes to local resources and support groups. **QSEN: Patient-Centered Care**

Psychosocial Integrity

- Allow the patient the opportunity to express concerns about the diagnosis of diabetes or the treatment regimen. **QSEN: Patient-Centered Care**
- Pace your education sessions to match the learning needs and style of the patient. **QSEN: Patient-Centered Care**
- Urge patients newly diagnosed with DM to attend diabetes education classes to become a fully engaged partner in management of the disease. **QSEN: Patient-Centered Care**

Physiological Integrity

- Assess the patient's A1C for indications of adherence to prescribed regimens and their effectiveness. **QSEN: Evidence-Based Practice**
- Explain all procedures, restrictions, drugs, and follow-up care to the patient and family. **QSEN: Patient-Centered Care**
- Teach patients to inject an accurate dose of insulin using a prefilled or disposable insulin pen. **QSEN: Patient-Centered Care**
- Instruct patients who are taking sulfonylurea drugs or insulin stimulators about an increased risk for hypoglycemic reactions. **QSEN: Patient-Centered Care**
- Start carbohydrate replacement per the diabetes health care provider's prescription or standing protocols immediately on identifying a patient with hypoglycemia. **QSEN: Evidence-Based Practice**
- Give glucagon subcutaneously or IM or concentrated dextrose IV to patients identified with hypoglycemia who cannot swallow. **QSEN: Evidence-Based Practice**
- Use blood glucose values to assess therapy effectiveness and determine when to switch from saline to dextrose-containing solutions in a patient with diabetic ketoacidosis. **QSEN: Evidence-Based Practice**
- Immediately report indications of cerebral edema (abrupt changes in mental status; changes in level of consciousness; changes in pupil size, shape, or reaction; seizures) in a patient with HHS to the diabetes health care provider. **QSEN: Patient-Centered Care**

MASTERY QUESTIONS

1. Which physiological processes directly prevent severe hypoglycemia in a healthy adult without diabetes who is NPO for 12 hours? **Select all that apply.**
   A. Gluconeogenesis
   B. Glycogenesis
   C. Glycogenolysis
   D. Ketogenesis
   E. Lipogenesis
   F. Lipolysis
2. Which precaution is a **priority** for the nurse to teach a client prescribed pramlintide to **prevent harm**?
   A. Only take this drug once weekly.
   B. Do not drink alcohol when taking this drug.
   C. Do not mix in the same syringe with insulin.
   D. Report any genital itching to your primary health care provider.
3. Which health promotion activity(ies) will the nurse recommend to **prevent harm** in a client with type 2 diabetes? **Select all that apply.**
   A. "Avoid all dietary carbohydrate and fat."
   B. "Have your eyes and vision assessed by an ophthalmologist every year."
   C. "Reduce your intake of animal fat and increase your intake of plant sterols."
   D. "Be sure to take your antidiabetes drug right before you engage in any type of exercise."
   E. "Keep your feet warm in cold weather by using either a hot water bottle or a heating pad."
   F. "Avoid foot damage from shoe-rubbing by going barefoot or wearing flip-flops when you are at home."

4. When preparing to administer a prescribed subcutaneous dose of NPH insulin from an open vial taken from a medication drawer to a client with diabetes, the nurse notes the solution is cloudy. What action will the nurse perform to ensure client **safety**?
   A. Warm the vial in a bowl of warm water until it reaches normal body temperature.
   B. Return the vial to the pharmacy and open a fresh vial of NPH insulin.
   C. Roll the vial between the hands until the insulin is clear.
   D. Check the expiration date and draw up the insulin dose.

5. While making rounds the nurse finds a client with type 1 diabetes mellitus pale, sweaty, and slightly confused; the client can swallow. The client's blood glucose level check is 48 mg/dL (2.7 mmol/L). What is the nurse's best **first** action to **prevent harm**?
   A. Call the pharmacy and order a STAT does of glucagon.
   B. Immediately give the client 30 g of glucose orally.
   C. Start an IV and administer a small amount of a concentrated dextrose solution.
   D. Recheck the blood glucose level and call the Rapid Response Team.

REFERENCES

American Diabetes Association (ADA). (2019a). Cardiac disease and risk management: Standards of medical care in diabetes-2019. *Diabetes Care, 42*(Suppl. 1), S103–S123.

American Diabetes Association (ADA). (2019b). Classification and diagnosis of diabetes: Standards of medical care in diabetes-2019. *Diabetes Care, 42*(Suppl. 1) S132-S28.

American Diabetes Association (ADA). (2019c). Comprehensive medical evaluation and assessment of comorbidities: Standards of medical care in diabetes-2019. *Diabetes Care, 42*(Suppl. 1), S34–S45.

American Diabetes Association (ADA). (2019d). Glycemic targets: Standards of medical care in diabetes-2019. *Diabetes Care, 42*(Suppl. 1), S61–S70.

American Diabetes Association (ADA). (2019e). Lifestyle management: Standards of medical care in diabetes-2019. *Diabetes Care, 42*(Suppl. 1), S46–S60.

American Diabetes Association (ADA). (2019f). Management of diabetes in pregnancy: Standards of medical care in diabetes-2019. *Diabetes Care, 42*(Suppl. 1), S165–S172.

American Diabetes Association (ADA). (2019g). Microvascular complications and foot care: Standards of medical care in diabetes-2019. *Diabetes Care, 42*(Suppl. 1), S124–S138.

American Diabetes Association (ADA). (2019h). Obesity management for the treatment of type 2 diabetes: Standards of medical care in diabetes-2019. *Diabetes Care, 42*(Suppl. 1), S81–S89.

American Diabetes Association (ADA). (2019i). Older adults: Standards of medical care in diabetes-2019. *Diabetes Care, 42*(Suppl. 1), S139–S147.

American Diabetes Association (ADA). (2019j). Pharmacologic approaches to glycemic treatment: Standards of medical care in diabetes-2019. *Diabetes Care, 42*(Suppl. 1), S90–S102.

American Diabetes Association (ADA). (2019k). Prevention or delay of type 2 diabetes: Standards of medical care in diabetes-2019. *Diabetes Care, 42*(Suppl. 1), S29–S33.

Aschenbrenner, D. (2017). Diabetes drug receives new indication. *American Journal of Nursing, 117*(4), 24–25.

Burchum, J., & Rosenthal, L. (2019). *Lehne's pharmacology for nursing care* (10th ed.). St. Louis: Elsevier.

Centers for Disease Control and Prevention (CDC). (2020). *National diabetes statistics report-2020*. https://www.cdc.gov/diabetes/pdf/data/statistics/national-diabetes-statistics-report.pdf.

Faminu, F. (2019). Diabetes: Setting and achieving glycemic goals. *Nursing2019, 49*(3), 49–54.

Fayfman, M., Pasquel, F., & Umpierrez, G. (2017). Management of hyperglycemic crisis. *Medical Clinics of North America, 101*, 587–606.

Harris, A. (2019). Diabetes self-management education provision by an interprofessional collaborative practice team: A quality improvement project. *Nursing Clinics of North America, 54*(1), 149–158.

Hussar, D. (2019). New drugs, 2019: Part 1. *Nursing2019, 49*(2), 28–36.

Keresztes, P., & Peacock-Johnson, A. (2019). Type 2 diabetes: A pharmacologic update. *American Journal of Nursing, 119*(3), 32–40.

McCance, K., Huether, S., Brashers, V., & Rote, N. (2019). *Pathophysiology: The biologic basis for disease in adults and children* (8th ed.). St. Louis: Mosby.

Pagana, K., & Pagana, T. (2018). *Mosby's manual of diagnostic and laboratory tests* (6th ed.). St. Louis: Elsevier.

Rariden, C. (2019). Prediabetes: A wake-up call. *Nursing2019, 49*(4), 38–44.

Schneider, A., Kalyani, R., Golden, S., Stearns, S., Wruck, L., Yeh, H., et al. (2016). Diabetes and prediabetes risk of hospitalization: The atherosclerosis risk in communities (ARIC) study. *Diabetes Care, 39*(5), 772–779.

Statistics Canada. (2019). *Health: All subtopics for health-Diabetes by age-group and sex*. http://www.statcan.gc.ca/tables-tableaux/sum-som/l01/cst01/health53a-eng.htm.

Touhy, T., & Jett, K. (2020). *Ebersole & Hess' toward healthy aging* (10th ed.). St. Louis: Mosby.

U.S. Department of Veterans Affairs. (2016). *Diabetes type 2 and agent orange*. http://www.publichealth.va.gov/exposures/agentorange/conditions/diabetes.asp.

Watts, S., & Howard, J. (2016). Prediabetes: What nurses need to know. *American Journal of Nursing, 116*(7), 54–58.

Watts, S., & Nemes, D. (2018). Best practice nursing management of nosocomial hypoglycemia: Lessons learned. *Medsurg Nursing, 27*(2), 98–102.

Watts, S., Nemes, D., Davian, T., & Pensiero, A. (2020). 10 years of inpatient diabetes certification-Lessons learned. *American Nurse Journal, 15*(1), 20–23.

Watts, S., Stevenson, C., & Adams, M. (2017). Improving health literacy in patients with diabetes. *Nursing2017, 47*(1), 25–31.

Watts, S., Stevenson, C., & Russell, L. (2018). Diabetes basics for the inpatient nurse. *Medsurg Nursing, 27*(3), 161–165 185.

Wisnewski, C. (2017). Diabetes and cardiovascular disease: A deadly duo. *American Journal of Nursing, 117*(9), 12–17.

Wooton, A., & Melchior, L. (2020). Diabetes-associated cardiac autonomic neuropathy. *The Nurse Practitioner, 45*(2), 24–31.

60

Assessment of the Renal/ Urinary System

Carolyn Gersch

http://evolve.elsevier.com/Iggy/

LEARNING OUTCOMES

1. Collaborate with the interprofessional team to perform a complete urinary and renal system assessment, including ***elimination, fluid and electrolyte balance,*** and ***acid-base balance.***
2. Provide a safe environment for patients and staff when performing a physical assessment of the renal and urinary systems.
3. Explain how physiologic changes of the urinary/renal system affect ***elimination*** and the associated care of older adults.
4. Implement patient-centered nursing interventions to help patients and families cope with the psychosocial impact caused by a urinary ***elimination*** health problem.
5. Apply knowledge of anatomy and physiology to perform an evidence-based assessment for the patient with a urinary ***elimination*** health problem.
6. Use clinical judgement to analyze assessment findings for the patient with a urinary or renal system health problem.
7. Teach the patient and caregivers about diagnostic procedures associated with assessment of kidney and urinary health problems.

KEY TERMS

bruit An audible swishing sound produced when the volume of blood or the diameter of the blood vessel changes.

calculi Stone formation.

continence The ability to voluntarily control emptying of the bladder or colon.

cystitis A bladder inflammation, most often with infection.

elimination The excretion of waste from the body by the GI tract (as feces) and kidneys (as urine).

external urethral sphincter Skeletal muscle that surrounds the urethra and helps to control the exit of urine.

incontinence The involuntary loss of urine or stool.

internal urethral sphincter is smooth detrusor muscle of the bladder neck and elastic tissue that helps to control the exit of urine.

microalbuminuria The presence of very small amounts of albumin in the urine that are not measurable by usual urinalysis procedures.

nocturnal polyuria Increased urination at night.

renal threshold The point at which the kidney is overwhelmed with glucose and can no longer reabsorb; also called *transport maximum*.

proteinuria The presence of protein in the urine.

uremia The buildup of nitrogenous waste products in the blood (azotemia).

urethral meatus The opening at the endpoint of the urethra.

urgency A sense of a nearly uncontrollable need to urinate.

PRIORITY AND INTERRELATED CONCEPTS

The priority concept for this chapter is:
- ***Elimination***

The interrelated concepts for this chapter are:
- ***Fluid and Electrolyte Balance***
- ***Acid-Base Balance***

The concept of ***elimination*** is the excretion of waste from the body by the GI tract as feces and by the kidneys as urine. See Chapter 3 for an overview of the concept of elimination and how it relates to the concepts of ***fluid and electrolyte balance*** and ***acid-base balance.*** In this chapter, the focus is on elimination of waste via the renal system. The kidneys and urinary tract make up the renal system, which is responsible for urine elimination.

The kidneys are responsible for filtering water and wastes from the bloodstream. The filtered-out particles and excess fluid are excreted out of the body into the urinary tract via the ureters, bladder, and ureters ridding the body of these wastes. Structural or functional problems within the renal system may alter ***fluid and electrolyte balance*** and ***acid-base balance.***

The kidneys help maintain health in many ways. *Most important, they maintain body fluid volume and composition and create urine for waste* ***elimination.*** In addition, the kidneys help regulate blood pressure, ***acid-base balance;*** produce erythropoietin for red blood cell (RBC) synthesis; and convert vitamin D to an active form.

ANATOMY AND PHYSIOLOGY REVIEW

Kidneys

Structure. The two kidneys are located behind the peritoneum, outside of the abdominal cavity, one on either side of the spine (Fig. 60.1). The adult kidney is 4 to 5 inches (10 to 13 cm) long, 2 to 3 inches (5 to 7 cm) wide, and about 1 inch (2.5 to 3 cm) thick. The left kidney is slightly longer and narrower than the right kidney. Larger-than-usual kidneys may indicate obstruction or polycystic disease. Smaller-than-usual kidneys may indicate chronic kidney disease (CKD).

Variation in kidney shape and number is relatively common and does not always indicate a problem in kidney function. Some adults have more than two kidneys or may have only one large, horseshoe-shaped kidney. As long as tests of kidney function are normal, these variations are of no significance (Brenner, 2016).

Several layers of tissue surround the kidney, providing protection and support. The outer surface of the kidney is a layer of fibrous tissue called the *capsule* (Fig. 60.2). It covers most of the kidney except the *hilum,* which is the indented area where the kidney blood vessels and nerves enter and exit. It is also where the ureter exits. The capsule is surrounded by layers of fat and connective tissue.

Underneath the capsule fibrous layer are two layers of functional kidney tissue: the cortex and the medulla. The *renal cortex* is the outer tissue layer. The *medulla* is the medullary tissue lying below the cortex in the shape of many fans. Each "fan" is called a pyramid. Pyramids are separated by the *renal columns,* cortical tissue that dips down into the interior of the kidney.

The tip of each pyramid is called a *papilla.* The papillae drain urine into the collecting system. A cuplike structure called a *calyx* collects the urine at the end of each papilla. The calices join together to form the *renal pelvis,* which narrows to become the ureter.

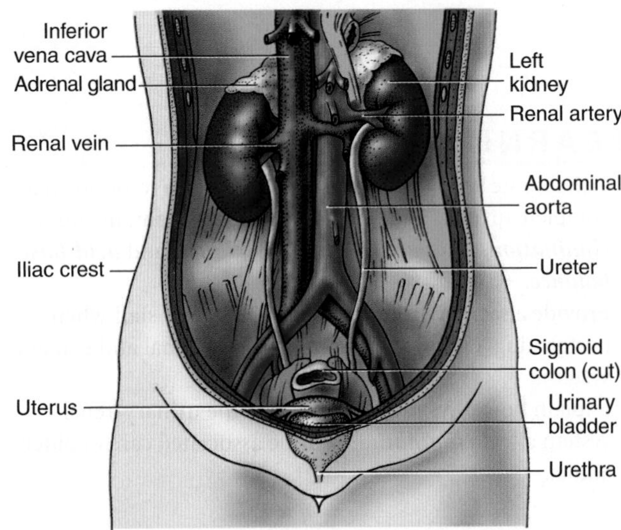

FIG. 60.1 Anatomic location of the kidneys and structures of the urinary system.

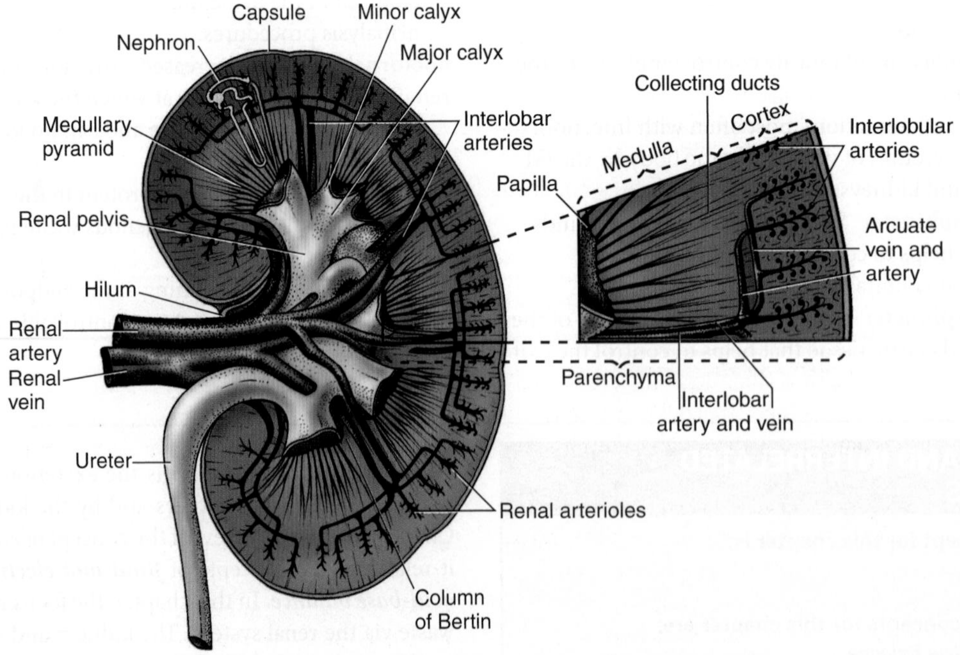

FIG. 60.2 Bisection of the kidney showing its major structures.

The kidneys have a rich blood supply and receive a blood flow from 600 to 1300 mL/min. The blood supply to each kidney comes from the renal artery, which branches off from the abdominal aorta. The renal artery divides into progressively smaller arteries, supplying blood to areas of the kidney tissue and the nephrons. The smallest arteries *(afferent arterioles)* feed the nephrons directly to form urine.

Venous blood from the kidneys starts with the capillaries surrounding each nephron. These capillaries drain into progressively larger veins, with blood eventually returned to the inferior vena cava through the renal vein.

Microscopic Anatomy. The nephron is the functional unit of the kidney and forms urine by filtering waste products and water from the blood. There are about 1 million nephrons per kidney, and each nephron separately performs filtration and makes urine from blood.

There are two types of nephrons: *cortical nephrons* and *juxtamedullary nephrons.* The cortical nephrons are short and lie totally within the renal cortex. The juxtamedullary nephrons (about 20% of all nephrons) are longer, and their tubes and blood vessels dip deeply into the medulla. The purpose of these nephrons is to concentrate urine during times of low fluid intake to allow continued excretion of body waste with less fluid loss (McCance & Huether, 2019).

Blood supply to the nephron is delivered through the *afferent arteriole* (i.e., the smallest, most distal portion of the renal arterial system). From the afferent arteriole, blood flows into the *glomerulus,* which is a series of specialized capillary loops. It is through these capillaries that water and small particles are filtered from the blood to make urine. The remaining blood leaves the glomerulus through the *efferent arteriole,* which is the first vessel in the kidney's venous system. From the efferent arteriole, blood exits into either the *peritubular capillaries* around the tube of the cortical nephrons or the *vasa recta* around the tube of juxtamedullary nephrons.

Each nephron is a tubelike structure with distinct parts (Fig. 60.3). The tube begins with the Bowman capsule, a saclike structure that surrounds the glomerulus. The tubular tissue of the Bowman capsule narrows into the *proximal convoluted tubule (PCT).* The PCT twists and turns, finally straightening into the descending limb of the *loop of Henle.* The descending loop of Henle dips in the direction of the medulla but forms a hairpin loop and comes back up into the cortex as the ascending loop of Henle.

The two segments of the ascending limb of the loop of Henle are the thin segment and the thick segment. The *distal convoluted tubule (DCT)* forms from the thick segment of the ascending limb of the loop of Henle. The DCT ends in one of many collecting ducts located in the kidney tissue. The urine in the collecting ducts passes through the papillae and empties into the renal pelvis.

Special cells in the afferent arteriole, efferent arteriole, and DCT are known as the *juxtaglomerular complex* (Fig. 60.4). These cells produce *renin,* which is a hormone that helps regulate blood flow, glomerular filtration rate (GFR), and blood pressure. Renin is secreted when sensing cells in the DCT (called the *macula densa*) sense changes in blood volume and pressure. The macula densa touches the renin-producing cells. Renin is produced when the macula densa cells sense that blood volume, blood pressure, or blood sodium level is low. Renin then converts renin substrate (angiotensinogen) into angiotensin I. This leads to a series of reactions that cause secretion of the hormone aldosterone (Fig. 60.5). Aldosterone increases kidney reabsorption of sodium and water, restoring blood pressure, blood volume, and blood sodium levels (McCance & Huether, 2019). It also promotes excretion of potassium (see Chapter 13).

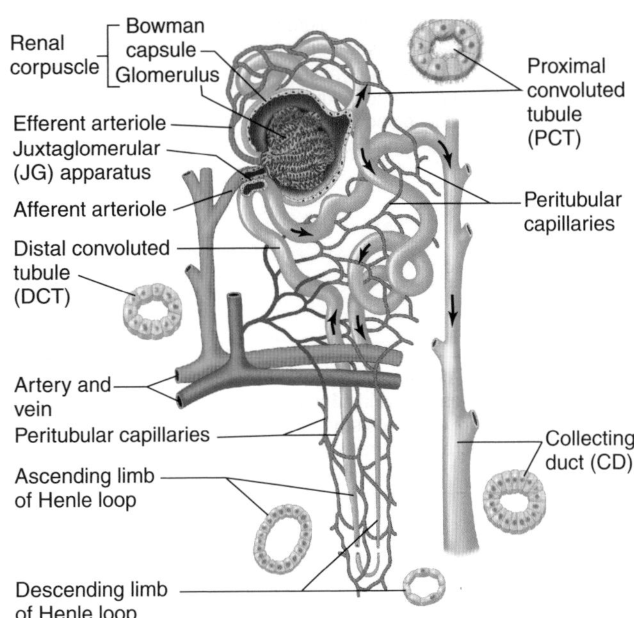

FIG. 60.3 Anatomy of the nephron—the functional unit of the kidney. The differences in appearance in tubular cells seen in a cross section reflect the differing functions of each nephron segment. Note that the particular nephron labeled here is a juxtamedullary nephron. (From Patton, K. T., & Thibodeau, G. A. [2018]. *The human body in health & disease* [7th ed.]. St. Louis: Mosby.)

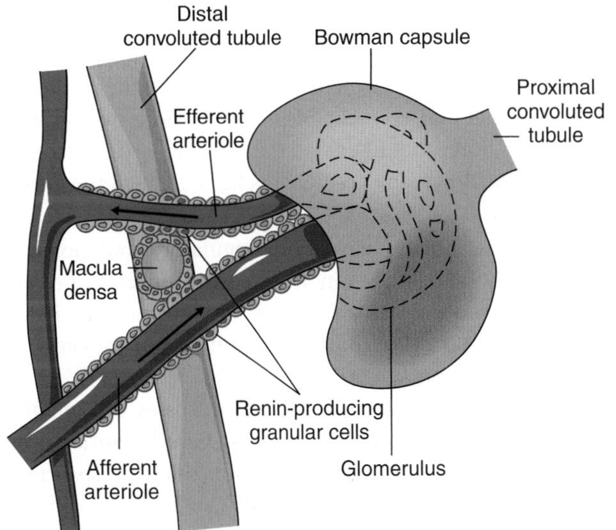

FIG. 60.4 Juxtaglomerular complex showing juxtaglomerular cells and the macula densa.

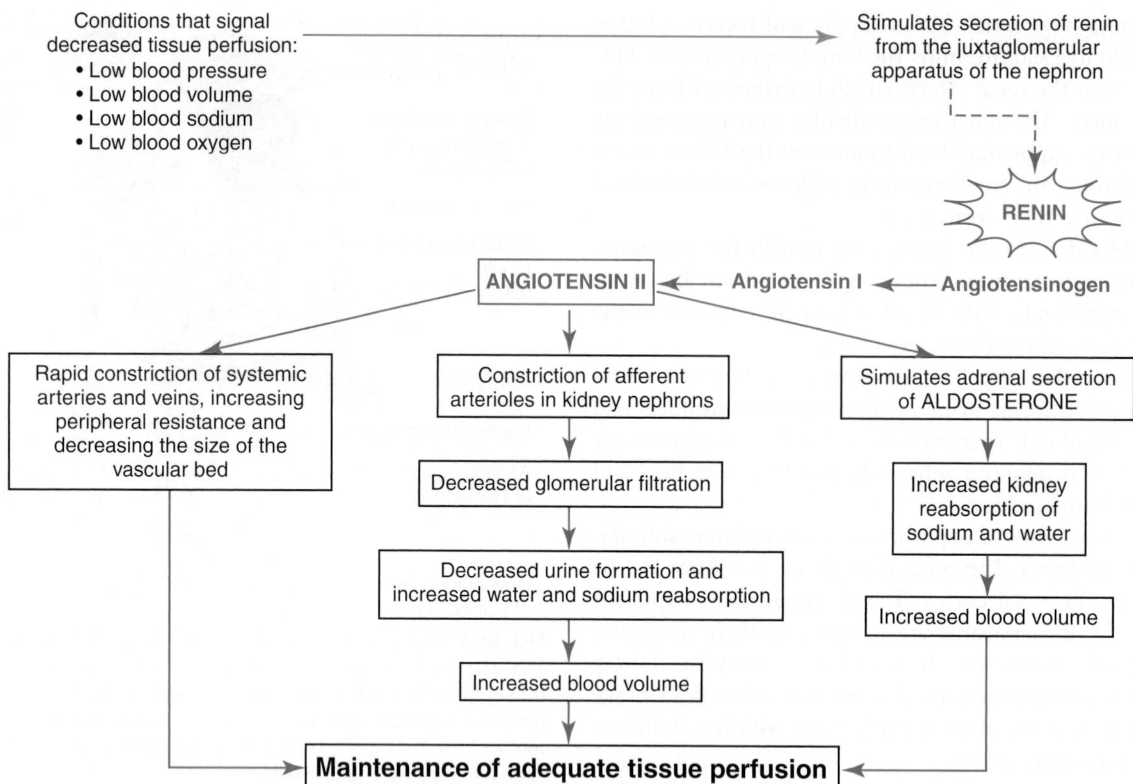

FIG. 60.5 Role of aldosterone, renin substrate (angiotensinogen), angiotensin I, and angiotensin II in the renal regulation of water and sodium.

The glomerular capillary wall has three layers (Fig. 60.6): the endothelium, the basement membrane, and the epithelium. The endothelial and epithelial cells lining these capillaries are separated by pores that filter water and small particles from the blood into the Bowman capsule. This fluid is called the *filtrate.*

Function. The kidneys have both regulatory and hormonal functions. The regulatory functions control ***fluid and electrolyte balance*** and ***acid-base balance.*** The hormonal functions control red blood cell (RBC) formation, blood pressure, and vitamin D activation.

Regulatory Functions. The kidney processes that maintain ***fluid and electrolyte balance*** and ***acid-base balance*** through urine ***elimination*** are glomerular filtration, tubular reabsorption, and tubular secretion. These processes use filtration, diffusion, active transport, and osmosis. (See Chapter 13 for a review of these actions.) Table 60.1 lists the functions of nephron tubules and blood vessels.

Glomerular filtration is the first process in urine formation. As blood passes from the afferent arteriole into the glomerulus, water, electrolytes, and other small particles (e.g., creatinine, urea nitrogen, glucose) are filtered across the glomerular membrane into the Bowman capsule to form *glomerular* filtrate. As the filtrate enters the proximal convoluted tubule (PCT), it is called *tubular filtrate* or *early urine.*

Large particles, such as blood cells, albumin, and other proteins, are too large to filter through the glomerular capillary walls. *Therefore these substances are not normally present in the excreted final urine.*

BOWMAN CAPSULE

Layer of endothelial cells

Basement membrane

Glomerular capillary lumen

Layer of epithelial cells

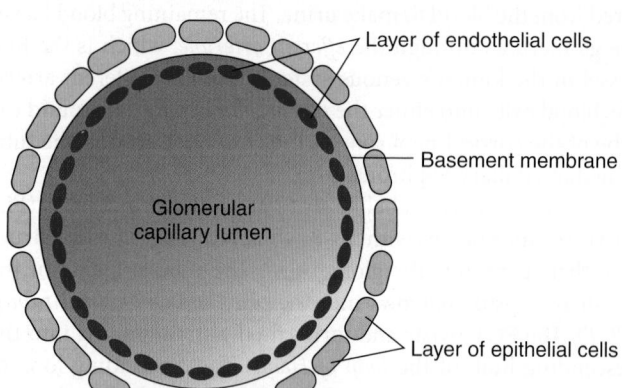

FIG. 60.6 Glomerular capillary wall.

Filtration rate is expressed in milliliters per minute. Normal glomerular filtration rate (GFR) averages 125 mL/min, totaling about 180 L daily. If the entire amount of filtrate were excreted as urine, death would occur from dehydration. Actually, only about 1 to 3 L are excreted each day as urine. The rest is reabsorbed back into the blood (McCance & Huether, 2019).

GFR is controlled by blood pressure and blood flow. The kidneys self-regulate their own blood pressure and blood flow, which keeps GFR constant. GFR is controlled by selectively constricting and dilating the afferent and efferent arterioles. When the afferent arteriole is constricted or the efferent arteriole is dilated, pressure in the glomerular capillaries falls and

TABLE 60.1 **Vascular and Tubular Components of the Nephron**

Structure	Anatomic Features	Physiologic Aspects
Vascular Components		
Afferent arteriole	Delivers arterial blood from the branches of the renal artery into the glomerulus	Autoregulation of renal blood flow via vasoconstriction or vasodilation Renin-producing granular cells
Glomerulus	Capillary loops with thin, semipermeable membrane	Site of glomerular filtration Glomerular filtration occurs when hydrostatic pressure (blood pressure) is greater than opposing forces (tubular filtrate and oncotic pressure)
Efferent arteriole	Delivers arterial blood from the glomerulus into the peritubular capillaries or the vasa recta	Autoregulation of renal blood flow via vasoconstriction or vasodilation Renin-producing granular cells
Peritubular capillaries (PTCs) and vasa recta (VR)	PTCs: surround tubular components of cortical nephrons VR: surround tubular components of juxtamedullary nephrons	Tubular reabsorption and tubular secretion allow movement of water and solutes to or from the tubules, interstitium, and blood
Tubular Components		
Bowman capsule (BC)	Thin membranous sac surrounding ⅞ of the glomerulus	Collects glomerular filtrate (GF) and funnels it into the tubule
Proximal convoluted tubule (PCT)	Evolves from and is continuous with Bowman capsule Specialized cellular lining facilitates tubular reabsorption	Site for reabsorption of sodium, chloride, water, glucose, amino acids, potassium, calcium, bicarbonate, phosphate, and urea
Loop of Henle	Continues from PTC Juxtamedullary nephrons dip deep into the medulla Permeable to water, urea, and sodium chloride	Regulation of water balance
Descending limb (DL)	Continues from the loop of Henle Permeable to water, urea, and sodium chloride	Regulation of water balance
Ascending limb (AL)	Emerges from DL as it turns and is redirected up toward the renal cortex	Potassium and magnesium reabsorption in the thick segment Thin segment is impermeable to water
Distal convoluted tubule (DCT)	Evolves from AL and twists, so the macula densa cells lie adjacent to the juxtaglomerular cells of afferent arteriole	Site of additional water and electrolyte reabsorption, including bicarbonate Potassium and hydrogen secretion
Collecting ducts	Collect formed urine from several tubules and deliver it into the renal pelvis	Receptor sites for antidiuretic hormone regulation of water balance

filtration decreases. When the afferent arteriole is dilated or the efferent arteriole is constricted, pressure in the glomerular capillaries rises and filtration increases. This way the kidney maintains a constant GFR, even when systemic blood pressure changes. When systolic pressure drops below 65 to 70 mm Hg, these self-regulation processes do not maintain GFR.

Tubular reabsorption is the second process in urine formation. Tubular reabsorption of most of the filtrate (early urine) keeps normal urine output at 1 to 3 L/day and prevents dehydration. As the filtrate passes through the tubular parts of the nephron, water and electrolytes are reabsorbed from the tubular lumen of the nephron and into the peritubular capillaries. This process returns much of the water, electrolytes, and other particles to the blood.

The tubules return about 99% of filtered water back into the body (Fig. 60.7). Most water reabsorption occurs in the proximal convoluted tubule (PCT). Water reabsorption continues as the filtrate flows down the descending loop of Henle. The thin and thick segments of the ascending loop of Henle are *not* permeable to water, and no water reabsorption occurs here.

The distal convoluted tubule (DCT) can be permeable to water, and some water reabsorption occurs as the filtrate continues to flow through the tubule. The membrane of the DCT may be made more permeable to water when *vasopressin* (antidiuretic hormone [ADH]) and aldosterone are present. Vasopressin increases tubular permeability to water, allowing water to leave the tube and be reabsorbed into the capillaries. Vasopressin also increases arteriole constriction. Arteriole constriction alters blood pressure, which then affects the amounts of fluid and particles that exit glomerular capillaries. Aldosterone promotes the reabsorption of sodium in the DCT. Water reabsorption occurs as a result of the movement of sodium (where sodium goes, water follows).

The ability of the kidneys to vary the volume or concentration of urine helps regulate water balance regardless of fluid intake. In this way, the healthy kidney can prevent dehydration when fluid intake is low and can prevent circulatory overload when fluid intake is high.

In addition to water, electrolytes are reabsorbed as needed to maintain ***fluid and electrolyte balance*** in the blood. Most sodium, chloride, and water reabsorption occurs in the proximal convoluted tubule (PCT). The collecting ducts are the other site of sodium, chloride, and water reabsorption. Here reabsorption is caused by aldosterone. Potassium is mostly reabsorbed in the PCT and thick segment of the loop of Henle.

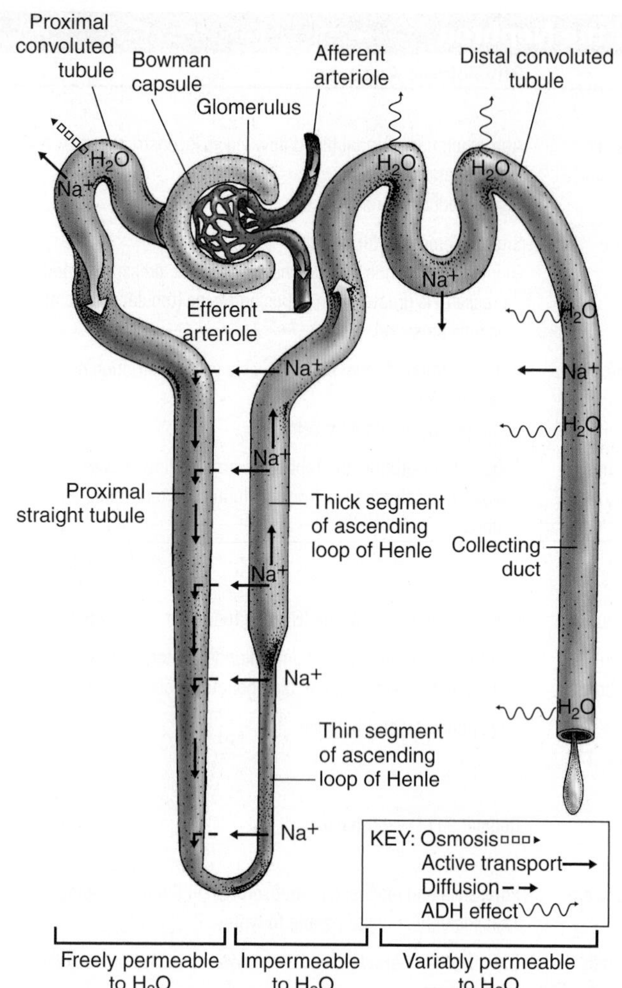

FIG. 60.7 Sodium and water reabsorption by the tubules of a cortical nephron. *ADH,* Antidiuretic hormone; *Na⁺,* sodium.

Bicarbonate, calcium, and phosphate are mostly reabsorbed in the PCT. Bicarbonate reabsorption helps ***acid-base balance*** and maintains a normal blood pH. Blood levels of calcitonin and parathyroid hormone (PTH) (see Chapters 13 and 58) control calcium balance.

Some types of particles in the tubular filtrate are also returned to the blood by *tubular reabsorption.* About 50% of all urea in the filtrate is reabsorbed; creatinine is not reabsorbed.

The kidney reabsorbs some of the glucose filtered from the blood. However, there is a limit to how much glucose the kidney can reabsorb. The point where the kidney is overwhelmed with glucose and can no longer reabsorb is called the **renal threshold** or *transport maximum* for glucose reabsorption. The renal threshold for glucose is >180 mg/dL (10 mmol/L). This means that at a blood glucose level of 180 mg/dL (10 mmol/L) or less, all glucose is reabsorbed and returned to the blood, with no glucose present in final urine. When blood glucose levels are greater than 180 mg/dL (10 mmol/L), some glucose stays in the filtrate and is present in the urine (McCulloch, 2018). Normally, almost all glucose and most proteins are reabsorbed and thus are not present in the urine.

> **! NURSING SAFETY PRIORITY (QSEN)**
>
> ***Action Alert***
>
> Report the presence of glucose or proteins in the urine of a patient undergoing a screening examination to the primary health care provider because this is an abnormal finding and requires further assessment.

Tubular secretion is the third process of urine formation. It allows substances to move from the blood into the urine. During tubular secretion, substances move from the peritubular capillaries in reverse, across capillary membranes, and into the cells that line the tubules. From the cells, these substances are moved into the urine and excreted from the body. Potassium (K^+) and hydrogen (H^+) ions are some of the substances moved in this way to maintain ***fluid and electrolyte balance*** and ***acid-base balance*** (pH).

Hormonal Functions. The kidneys produce renin, prostaglandins, erythropoietin, and activated vitamin D (Table 60.2). Other kidney products, such as the kinins, change kidney blood flow, regulate blood pressure, and influence capillary permeability. The kidneys also help break down and excrete insulin and many other drugs.

Renin, as discussed in the Microscopic Anatomy section, assists in blood pressure control. It is formed and released when there is a decrease in blood flow, blood volume, or blood pressure through the renal arterioles or when too little sodium is present in kidney blood. These conditions are detected through the receptors of the juxtaglomerular complex.

Renin release causes the production of *angiotensin II* through a series of steps (see Fig. 60.5). Angiotensin II increases systemic blood pressure with powerful blood vessel constricting effects and triggers the release of aldosterone from the adrenal glands. Aldosterone increases the reabsorption of sodium in the distal tubule of the nephron. Therefore more water is reabsorbed, which increases blood volume and blood pressure. When blood flow to the kidney is reduced, this system also prevents fluid loss and maintains circulating blood volume (see Chapter 13).

Prostaglandins are produced in the kidney and many other tissues. Those produced specifically in the kidney help regulate glomerular filtration, kidney vascular resistance, and renin production. They also increase sodium and water excretion.

Erythropoietin is produced and released in response to decreased oxygen in the kidney's blood supply. It triggers red blood cell (RBC) production in the bone marrow. When kidney function is poor, erythropoietin production decreases and anemia results.

Vitamin D activation occurs through a series of steps. Some of these steps take place in the skin when it is exposed to sunlight, and then more processing occurs in the liver. From there, vitamin D is converted to its active form in the kidney. Activated vitamin D is needed to absorb calcium in the intestinal tract and regulate calcium balance (McCance & Huether, 2019).

Ureters

Each kidney usually has a single ureter, which is a hollow tube that connects the renal pelvis with the urinary bladder. The ureter is about ½ inch (1.25 cm) in diameter and about 12 to 18 inches (30 to 45 cm) in length. The diameter of the ureter narrows in three areas:

- In the upper third of the ureter, at the point at which the renal pelvis becomes the ureter, is a narrowing known as the ureteropelvic junction (UPJ).
- The ureter also narrows as it bends toward the abdominal wall (aortoiliac bend).

TABLE 60.2 Kidney Hormones and Hormones Influencing Kidney Function

	Site	Action
Kidney Hormones		
Renin	Renin-producing granular cells	Raises blood pressure as result of angiotensin (local vasoconstriction) and aldosterone (volume expansion) secretion
Prostaglandins	Kidney tissues	Regulate intrarenal blood flow by vasodilation or vasoconstriction
Bradykinins	Juxtaglomerular cells of the arterioles	Increase blood flow (vasodilation) and vascular permeability
Erythropoietin	Kidney parenchyma	Stimulates bone marrow to make red blood cells
Activated vitamin D (1,25-dihydrocholecalciferol)	Kidney parenchyma	Promotes absorption of calcium in the GI tract
Hormones Influencing Kidney Function		
Vasopressin (antidiuretic hormone [ADH])	Released from posterior pituitary	Makes DCT and CD permeable to water to maximize reabsorption and produce a concentrated urine
Aldosterone	Released from adrenal cortex	Promotes sodium reabsorption and potassium secretion in DCT and CD; water and chloride follow sodium movement
Natriuretic hormones	Cardiac atria, cardiac ventricles, brain	Cause tubular secretion of sodium

CD, Collecting duct; *DCT*, distal convoluted tubule.

- Each ureter narrows at the point at which it enters the bladder; this point is called the ureterovesical junction (UVJ).

The ureter tunnels through bladder tissue for a short distance and then opens into the bladder at the trigone (Fig. 60.8).

The ureter has three layers: an inner lining of mucous membrane (*urothelium*), a middle layer of smooth muscle fibers, and an outer layer of fibrous tissue. The middle layer of muscle fibers is controlled by several nerve pathways from the lower spinal cord.

Contractions of the smooth muscle in the ureter move urine from the kidney pelvis to the bladder. Stretch receptors in the kidney pelvis regulate this movement. For example, a large volume of urine in the kidney pelvis triggers the stretch receptors, which respond by increasing ureteral contractions and ureter peristalsis.

Urinary Bladder

Structure. The urinary bladder is a muscular sac (see Fig. 60.8) that lies directly behind the pubic bone. In men, the bladder is in front of the rectum. In women, it is in front of the vagina.

The bladder is composed of the *body* (the rounded sac portion) and the *bladder neck* (posterior urethra), which connects to the bladder body. The bladder has three linings: an inner lining of epithelial cells *(urothelium)*, middle layers of smooth muscle *(detrusor muscle)*, and an outer lining. The *trigone* is an area on the posterior wall between the points of ureteral entry (ureterovesical junctions [UVJs]) and the urethra.

The **internal urethral sphincter** is the smooth detrusor muscle of the bladder neck and elastic tissue. The **external urethral sphincter** is skeletal muscle that surrounds the urethra. In men, the external sphincter surrounds the urethra at the base of the prostate gland. In women, the external sphincter is at the base of the bladder. The pudendal nerve from the spinal cord controls the external sphincter.

Function. The bladder stores urine, provides continence, and enables voiding. The secretions of the urothelium lining the bladder resist bacteria.

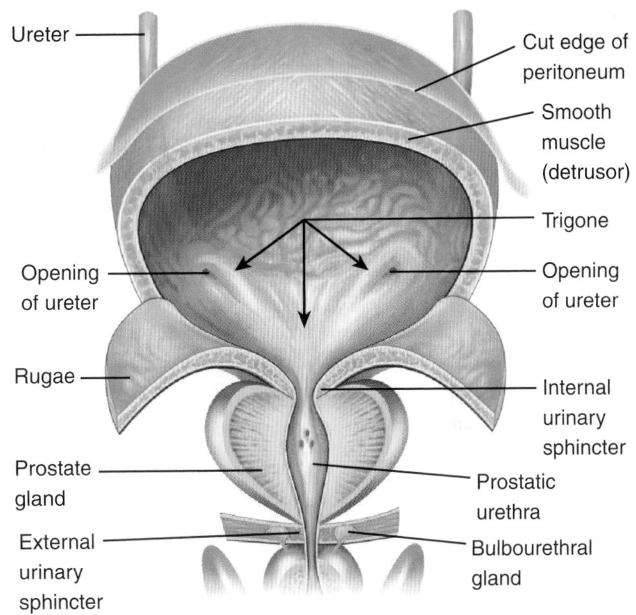

FIG. 60.8 Gross anatomy of the urinary bladder. (Modified from Patton, K.T., & Thibodeau, G.A. [2013]. *Anatomy & physiology* [8th ed.]. St. Louis: Mosby.)

Continence is the ability to voluntarily control bladder emptying. It occurs during bladder filling through the combination of detrusor muscle relaxation, internal sphincter muscle tone, and external sphincter contraction. As the bladder fills with urine, stretch sensations are transmitted to spinal sacral nerves.

Maintaining continence occurs by the interaction of the nerves that control the muscles of the bladder, bladder neck, urethra, and pelvic floor, as well as by factors that close the urethra. In the continent person, the smooth muscle of the detrusor remains relaxed during a period of urine filling and storage. Sympathetic nervous system fibers prevent detrusor muscle contraction. The control centers for voiding are located in the cerebral cortex, the brainstem, and the lower spinal cord. For urethral closure to be adequate for continence, the mucosal surfaces must be in contact and must be adhesive. Contact depends on the presence and proper function of the involved nerves and muscles. Adhesion depends on the secretion of mucus-like substances.

Micturition (voiding, urination) is a reflex of autonomic control that triggers contraction of the detrusor muscle (closing the ureter at the UVJ to prevent backflow) at the same time as relaxation of the external sphincter and the muscles of the pelvic floor. Voluntary urine ***elimination*** (voiding) occurs as a learned response and is controlled by the cerebral cortex and the brainstem. Contraction of the external sphincter inhibits the micturition reflex and prevents voiding.

Urethra

The urethra is a narrow tube lined with mucous membranes. Its purpose is to allow urine ***elimination*** from the bladder. The **urethral meatus**, or opening, is the endpoint of the urethra. In men, the urethra is about 6 to 8 inches (15 to 20 cm) long, with the meatus located at the tip of the penis. The male urethra has three sections:

- The prostatic urethra, which extends from the bladder through the prostate gland
- The membranous urethra, which extends from the prostate to the wall of the pelvic floor
- The cavernous urethra, which is external and extends through the length of the penis

In women, the urethra is 1 to 1.5 inches (2.5 to 3.75 cm) long and exits through the pelvic floor. The meatus lies slightly below the clitoris and directly in front of the vagina and rectum.

Kidney and Urinary Changes Associated With Aging

Kidney Changes. Changes occur in the kidney as a result of the aging process that can affect urine ***elimination*** and health (see the Patient-Centered Care: Older Adult Considerations: Changes in the Renal System Related to Aging box). The kidney loses cortical tissue and nephrons and gets smaller with age as a result of reduced blood flow to the kidney (Denic et al., 2016; Touhy & Jett, 2016). The medulla is not affected by aging, and the juxtamedullary nephron functions are preserved. The glomerular and tubular linings thicken. Both the number of glomeruli and their surface areas decrease with aging. Tubule length decreases. The changes reduce the older adult's ability to filter blood and excrete waste products.

PATIENT-CENTERED CARE: OLDER ADULT CONSIDERATIONS (QSEN)

Changes in the Renal System Related to Aging

Physiologic Change	Nursing Interventions	Rationales
Decreased glomerular filtration rate (GFR)	Monitor hydration status.	The ability of the kidneys to regulate water balance decreases with age.
	Ensure adequate fluid intake.	The kidneys are less able to conserve water when necessary.
	Use caution when administering potentially nephrotoxic agents or drugs	Dehydration reduces kidney blood flow and increases the nephrotoxic potential of many agents. Acute or chronic kidney failure may result.
Nocturia	Ensure adequate nighttime lighting and a hazard-free environment.	Falls and injuries are common among older patients seeking bathroom facilities.
	Ensure the availability of a bedside toilet, bedpan, or urinal.	Using these items instead of getting up to go the bathroom can help prevent falls.
	Discourage excessive fluid intake for 2-4 hr before the patient goes to bed.	Excessive fluid intake at night may increase nocturia.
	Evaluate drugs and timing.	Some drugs increase urine output and increase the risk for falling when toileting.
Decreased bladder capacity	Encourage the patient to use the toilet, bedpan, or urinal at least every 2 hr.	Emptying the bladder on a regular basis may avoid overflow urinary incontinence.
	Respond as soon as possible to the patient's indication of the need to void.	A quick response may alleviate episodes of urinary stress incontinence.
Weakened urinary sphincters and shortened urethra in women	Provide thorough perineal care after each voiding.	The shortened urethra increases the potential for bladder infections. Good perineal hygiene may prevent skin irritations and urinary tract infection (UTI).
Tendency to retain urine	Observe the patient for urinary retention (e.g., bladder distention) or urinary tract infection (e.g., dysuria, foul odor, confusion).	Urinary stasis may result in a UTI, which may lead to bloodstream infections, urosepsis, or septic shock.
	Provide privacy, assistance, and voiding stimulants such as warm water over the perineum as needed.	Nursing interventions can help initiate voiding.
	Evaluate drugs for possible contribution to retention.	Anticholinergic drugs promote urinary retention.

Blood flow to the kidney declines by about 10% per decade as blood vessels thicken. This means that blood flow to the kidney is not as adaptive in older adults, leaving nephrons more vulnerable to damage during episodes of either hypotension or hypertension.

Glomerular filtration rate (GFR) decreases with age. By age 65 years, the GFR is about 65 mL/min (half the rate of a young adult) and increases the risk for fluid overload. This decline is more rapid in patients with diabetes, hypertension, or heart failure. The combination of reduced kidney mass, reduced blood flow, and decreased GFR contributes to reduced drug clearance and a greater risk for drug reactions and kidney damage from drugs and contrast media in older adults.

Tubular changes with aging decrease the ability to concentrate urine, resulting in **urgency** (a sense of a nearly uncontrollable need to urinate) and **nocturnal polyuria** (increased urination at night). The regulation of sodium, acids, and bicarbonate is less efficient. Along with an age-related impairment in the thirst mechanism, these changes increase the risk for disturbances of ***fluid and electrolyte balance,*** such as dehydration and hypernatremia (increased blood sodium levels) in the older adult. Hormonal changes include a decrease in renin secretion, aldosterone levels, and activation of vitamin D.

Urinary Changes. Changes in detrusor muscle elasticity lead to decreased bladder capacity and reduced ability to retain urine (Touhy & Jett, 2016). The urge to void may cause immediate bladder emptying because the urinary sphincters lose tone and often become weaker with age. In women, weakened muscles in the pelvic floor shorten the urethra and promote incontinence. In men, an enlarged prostate gland makes starting the urine stream difficult and may cause urinary retention.

PATIENT-CENTERED CARE: CULTURAL/SPIRITUAL CONSIDERATIONS QSEN

African Americans have more rapid age-related decreases in GFR than do white adults. Kidney excretion of sodium is less effective in hypertensive African Americans who have high sodium intake, and the kidneys have about 20% less blood flow as a result of anatomic changes in small blood vessels and intrarenal responses to renin. Thus African-American patients are at greater risk for kidney failure than are white patients (Jarvis, 2020). Yearly health examinations should include urinalysis, checking for the presence of microalbuminuria, and evaluating serum creatinine.

ASSESSMENT: RECOGNIZE CUES

Patient History

Demographic information, such as age, gender, race, and ethnicity, is important to consider as nonmodifiable risk factors in the patient with any kidney or urinary ***elimination*** problem. A sudden onset of hypertension in patients older than 50 years suggests possible kidney disease. Clinical changes in polycystic kidney disease typically occur in patients in their 40s or 50s. In men older than 50 years, altered urine patterns accompany prostate disease.

Anatomic gender differences make some disorders worse or more common. For example, men rarely have ascending urinary tract infections. Women have a shorter urethra and more commonly develop **cystitis** (bladder inflammation, most often with infection) because bacteria pass more readily into the bladder.

Modifiable risk factors, as well as socioeconomic status, level of education, language, and health beliefs, should be considered when assessing renal function. *Socioeconomic status* may influence health care practices. Prevention, early detection, and treatment of kidney or urinary problems may be limited by inability to access to health care, lack of transportation, insufficient or no insurance, and/or reduced income. These barriers may also result in difficulty following medical advice, having prescriptions filled, adhering to dietary instructions, and keeping follow-up appointments.

Educational level may affect health-seeking practices and the patient's understanding of a disease or its symptoms. Recurring urinary tract infections can result from not completing a course of antibiotic therapy or from not following up to ensure that the infection is cleared.

The language used by patients may be different from that used by the health care professional. When obtaining a history, listen to and explore the terms used by the patient. By using the patient's own terms, you may help him or her provide a more complete description of the problem and may decrease the patient's discomfort when discussing bodily functions.

The patient's health beliefs affect the approach to health and illness. Cultural background or religious affiliation may influence the belief system, as well as comfort when discussing issues about ***elimination*** (Jackson et al., 2013).

Ask the patient about previous kidney or urologic problems, including tumors, infections, stones, or urologic surgery. A history of any chronic health problems, especially diabetes mellitus or hypertension, increases the risk for development of kidney disease because these disorders damage kidney blood vessels.

Ask the patient about environmental, food, or medication allergies. Exposure to certain contrast media during imaging can harm the kidneys. Iodinated contrast medium used for CT scans is associated with both acute and chronic kidney injury (Lambert et al., 2017). High-osmolarity contrast agents can also contribute to kidney function impairment. Exposure to gadolinium-enhanced MRI can result in nephrogenic systemic fibrosis.

Ask the patient about chemical exposures at the workplace or with hobbies. Exposure to hydrocarbons (e.g., gasoline, oil), heavy metals (especially mercury and lead), and some gases (e.g., chlorine, toluene) can impair kidney function. Use this opportunity to teach patients who come into contact with chemicals at work or during leisure-time activities to avoid direct skin or mucous membrane contact with these chemicals. Use of heroin, cocaine, methamphetamine, ecstasy, and volatile solvents (inhalants) has also been associated with kidney damage.

Specifically ask the patient whether he or she has ever been told about the presence of protein or albumin in the urine. The question, "Have you ever been told that your blood pressure is high?" may prompt a response different from the one to the question, "Do you have high blood pressure?" Ask women about health problems during pregnancy (e.g., proteinuria, high blood pressure, gestational diabetes, urinary tract infections). Obtain information about:

- Chemical or environmental toxin exposure in occupational, diagnostic, or other settings
- Recent travel to geographic regions that pose infectious disease risks
- Recent trauma or injury, particularly to the abdomen or pelvic or genital areas
- A history of altered patterns of urinary ***elimination***

Nutrition History. Ask the patient with known or suspected kidney or urologic disorders about diet and any recent dietary changes. Note any excessive intake or omission of certain food categories. Ask about food and fluid intake. Assess how much and which types of fluids the patient drinks daily, especially fluids with a high-calorie or caffeine content. Use this opportunity to teach the patient the importance of drinking sufficient fluid to cause urine to be dilute (clear or very light yellow). If another medical problem does not require fluid restriction, ingestion of about 2 L of fluid daily is recommended. If the patient has followed a diet for weight reduction, the details of the diet plan are important and collaboration with a dietitian may be needed. A high-protein intake can result in temporary kidney problems. For example, a patient at risk for calculi (stone) formation who ingests large amounts of protein or has a poor fluid intake may form new stones.

Ask about any change in appetite or taste. These symptoms can occur with the buildup of nitrogenous waste products from kidney failure. Changes in thirst or fluid intake may also cause changes in the volume of urine ***elimination.*** Endocrine disorders may also cause changes in thirst, fluid intake, and urine output. (See Chapter 56 for a discussion of endocrine influences on fluid balance.)

Medication History. Identify all of the patient's prescription drugs because many can impair kidney function (Burchum & Rosenthal, 2019). Ask about the duration of drug use and whether there have been any recent changes in prescribed drugs. Drugs for diabetes mellitus, hypertension, cardiac disorders, hormonal disorders, cancer, arthritis, and psychiatric disorders are potential causes of kidney problems. Antibiotics, such as gentamicin, may also cause acute kidney injury. Drug-drug interactions and drug–contrast media interactions also may lead to kidney dysfunction (Lambert et al., 2017).

Explore the past and current use of over-the-counter (OTC) drugs or agents, including dietary supplements, vitamins and minerals, herbal agents, laxatives, analgesics, acetaminophen, and NSAIDs. Many of these agents affect kidney function and urine ***elimination.*** For example, dietary supplementation with synthetic creatine, used to increase muscle mass, has been associated with compromised kidney function. High-dose or long-term use of NSAIDs or acetaminophen can seriously reduce kidney function. Some agents are associated with hypertension, hematuria, or proteinuria, which may occur before kidney dysfunction.

Family History and Genetic Risk. The family history of the patient with a suspected kidney or urologic problem is important because some disorders have a familial pattern. Ask whether siblings, parents, or grandparents have had kidney problems. Past terms used for kidney disease include *Bright disease, nephritis,* and *nephrosis.* Although nephritis is a current term for an inflammatory process in the kidney and nephrosis is a current term for a degenerative process in the kidney, these terms have been used by lay adults for years to describe any type of kidney problem. Polycystic kidney disease, which is a genetic disorder, can occur in either gender.

Current Health Problem. The effects of kidney failure are seen in all body systems. Document all of the patient's current health problems. Ask the patient to describe all health concerns, because some kidney disorders cause problems in other body systems. Recent upper respiratory problems, achy muscles or joints, heart disease, or GI conditions may be related to problems of kidney function.

Assess the kidney and urologic system by asking about any changes in the appearance (color, odor, clarity) of the urine, pattern of urine ***elimination,*** ability to initiate or control voiding, and other unusual symptoms. For example, urine that is reddish, rust-colored, brown or black, greenish, or different from the usual yellowish color may prompt the patient to seek health care assistance. Urine typically has a mild but distinct odor of ammonia. An increase in the intensity of color, a change in odor quality, or a decrease in urine clarity may suggest infection.

Ask about changes in urination patterns, such as incontinence (involuntary bladder emptying), nocturia (urination at night), urgency (nearly uncontrollable urge to urinate), frequency, or an increase or decrease in the amount of urine. The normal urine output for adults is about 1500 to 2000 mL/day or within 500 mL of the volume of fluid ingested daily. Ask about how closely the urine output is to the volume of fluid ingested. A bladder diary may be useful. Ask whether:

- Initiating urine flow is difficult
- A burning sensation or other discomfort occurs with urination
- The force of the urine stream is decreased
- Persistent dribbling or leaking of urine is present

The onset of pain in the flank, in the lower abdomen or pelvic region, or in the perineal area triggers concern and usually prompts the patient to seek assistance. Ask about the onset, intensity, and duration of the pain; its location; precipitating and relieving factors; and its association with any activity or event.

Pain associated with kidney or ureteral irritation is often severe and spasmodic. Pain that radiates into the perineal area, groin, scrotum, or labia is described as *renal colic.* This pain occurs with distention or spasm of the ureter, such as in an obstruction or the passing of a stone. Renal colic pain may be intermittent or continuous and may occur with pallor, diaphoresis, and hypotension. These general symptoms occur because of the location of the nerve tracts near or in the kidneys and ureters (Brenner, 2016).

Because the kidneys are close to the GI organs and the nerve pathways are similar, GI symptoms may occur with kidney problems. These renointestinal reflexes often complicate the description of the kidney problem.

Uremia is the buildup of nitrogenous waste products in the blood from inadequate ***elimination*** as a result of kidney failure. Symptoms include anorexia, nausea and vomiting, muscle cramps, *pruritus* (itching), fatigue, and lethargy.

Physical Assessment

The physical assessment of the patient with a known or suspected kidney or urologic disorder includes general appearance, a review of body systems, and specific structure and functions of the kidney and urinary system.

Assess the patient's general appearance and check the skin for the presence of any rashes, bruising, or yellowish discoloration. The skin and tissues may show edema associated with kidney disease, especially in the *pedal* (foot), *pretibial* (shin), and sacral tissues and around the eyes. Use a stethoscope to listen to the lungs to determine whether fluid is present. Weigh the patient and measure blood pressure as a baseline for later comparisons.

Assess the levels of consciousness and alertness. Record any deficits in memory, concentration, or thought processes. Family members may report subtle changes. Cognitive changes may be the result of the buildup of waste products when kidney disease is present.

Assessment of the Kidneys, Ureters, and Bladder. Assess the kidneys, ureters, and bladder during an abdominal assessment (Jarvis, 2020). Auscultate before percussion and palpation because these activities can alter bowel sounds and obscure abdominal vascular sounds.

Inspect the abdomen and the flank regions with the patient in both the supine and sitting positions. Observe the patient for asymmetry (e.g., swelling) or discoloration (e.g., bruising or redness) in the flank region, especially in the area of the costovertebral angle (CVA). The CVA is located between the lower portion of the twelfth rib and the vertebral column.

Listen for a bruit by placing a stethoscope over each renal artery on the midclavicular line. A **bruit** is an audible swishing sound produced when the volume of blood or the diameter of the blood vessel changes. It often occurs with blood flow through a narrowed vessel, as in renal artery stenosis.

Kidney palpation is usually performed by a health care provider. It can help locate masses and areas of tenderness in or around the kidney. The health care provider will lightly palpate the abdomen in all quadrants, ask about areas of tenderness or pain, and examine nontender areas first (Fig. 60.9). The outline of the bladder may be noted as high as the umbilicus in patients with severe bladder distention.

! NURSING SAFETY PRIORITY QSEN

Action Alert

Performing palpation on a patient with a suspected abdominal tumor or aneurysm may harm the patient.

Because the kidneys are located deep and posterior, palpation is easier in thin patients who have little abdominal musculature. For palpation of the right kidney, the patient is placed in a supine position while the examiner places one hand under the right flank and the other hand over the abdomen below the lower right part of the rib cage. The lower hand is used to raise the flank, and the upper hand depresses the abdomen as the patient takes a deep breath (Fig. 60.9). The left kidney is deeper and often cannot be palpated. A transplanted kidney is readily palpated in either the lower right or left abdominal quadrant. The normal kidney is smooth, firm, and nontender.

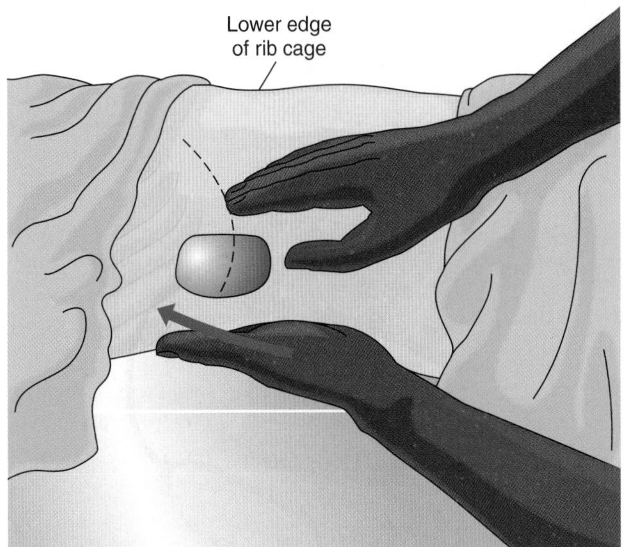

FIG. 60.9 Advanced technique for palpation of the kidney.

A distended bladder sounds dull when percussed. After gently palpating to determine the outline of the distended bladder, begin percussion on the lower abdomen and continue in the direction of the umbilicus until dull sounds are no longer produced. If you suspect bladder distention, use a portable bladder scanner (Fig. 60.10) to determine the amount of retained urine.

If the patient reports flank pain or tenderness, the nontender flank should be percussed first. For percussion, the patient is placed in a sitting, side-lying, or supine position. Percussion, generally performed by the health care provider, is done by forming one hand into a clenched fist and the other hand lies flat over the CVA of the patient. Using the hand in a fist, a quick, firm thump is administered to the hand over the CVA area (Jarvis, 2020). Costovertebral tenderness often occurs with kidney infection or inflammation. Patients with inflammation or infection in the kidney or nearby structures may describe their pain as severe or as a constant, dull ache.

Assessment of the Urethra. Using a good light source and wearing gloves, inspect the urethra by examining the meatus and the tissues around it. Record any unusual discharge such as blood, mucus, or pus. Inspect the skin and mucous membranes of surrounding tissues. Record the presence of lesions, rashes, or other abnormalities of the penis or scrotum or of the labia or vaginal opening. Urethral irritation is suspected when the patient reports discomfort with urination. Use this opportunity to remind women to clean the perineum by wiping from front to back, never from back to front. Teach them that the front-to-back technique keeps organisms in stool from coming close to the urethra and decreases the risk for infection.

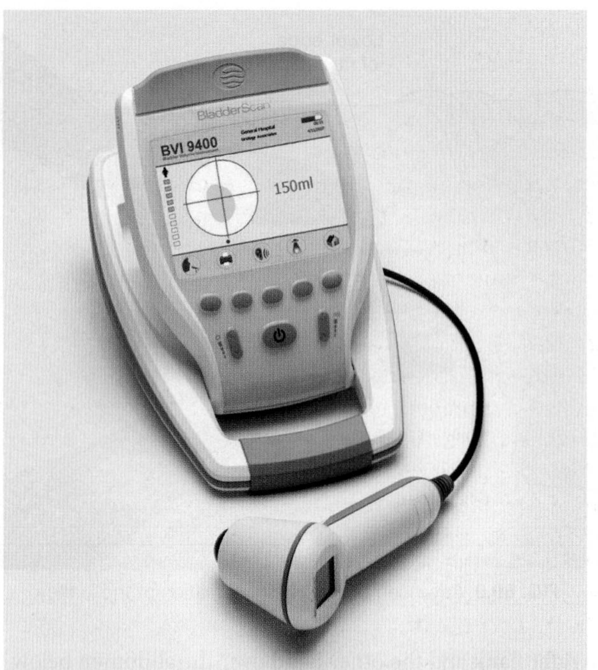

FIG. 60.10 "BladderScan" BVI 9400, a handheld portable bladder scanner. (Courtesy Verathon Corporation, Bothell, WA.)

PATIENT-CENTERED CARE: CULTURAL/ SPIRITUAL CONSIDERATIONS QSEN

Women from some cultures or religions may have undergone female circumcision. This procedure alters the appearance of the vulvar-perineal area and increases the risk for urinary tract infections. It also makes urethral inspection or catheterization difficult. Document any noted anatomic changes and ask the patient to describe hygiene practices for this area.

Psychosocial Assessment

Concerns about the urologic system may evoke fear, anger, embarrassment, anxiety, guilt, or sadness in the patient. Childhood learning often includes the idea that toileting should take place in private and not be discussed with other people. Urologic disorders may bring up forgotten memories of difficult toilet training and bedwetting or of childhood experiences of exploring one's body. The patient may ignore symptoms or delay seeking health care because of emotional responses or cultural taboos about the urogenital area.

NCLEX EXAMINATION CHALLENGE 60.1

Physiological Integrity

When obtaining a health history and physical assessment from a 68-year-old male client who has a history of an enlarged prostate, which finding does the nurse consider significant? **Select all that apply.**

A. Distended bladder
B. Absence of a bruit
C. Frequency of urination
D. Dribbling urine after voiding
E. Chemical exposure in the workplace

Diagnostic Assessment

Laboratory Assessment

Blood Tests. *Serum creatinine* is produced when muscle and other proteins are broken down. Because protein breakdown is usually constant, the serum creatinine level is a good indicator of kidney function. Serum creatinine levels are slightly higher in men than in women because men tend to have a larger muscle mass than do women. Similarly, adults with greater muscle mass or muscle mass turnover (e.g., athletes) may have a slightly higher-than-average serum creatinine level. Muscle mass and the amount of creatinine produced decrease with age. However, because of decreased rates of creatinine clearance, the serum creatinine level remains relatively constant in older adults unless kidney disease is present.

No common pathologic condition other than kidney disease increases the serum creatinine level. When the serum creatinine level is doubled, it indicates a 50% reduction in glomerular filtration rate (Pagana & Pagana, 2018); therefore *any* elevation of serum creatinine values is important and should be assessed further. Creatinine is excreted solely by the kidneys.

! NURSING SAFETY PRIORITY QSEN

Action Alert

A serum creatinine of 1.5 mg/dL (110 mcmol/L) or greater places a patient at risk for acute kidney injury (AKI) from iodinated contrast media and some drugs (Lambert et al., 2017). Monitor both baseline and trend values to recognize risk for and actual kidney damage, especially among patients exposed to agents that can cause kidney dysfunction. If indicated, respond by promptly informing the primary health care provider of increases in serum creatinine greater than 1.5 times the baseline and urine output values of less than 0.5 mL/kg/hr for 6 or more hours. Using the baseline and trending creatinine levels is important, especially in older adults and young children as they have lower creatinine levels due to reduced muscle mass than the normal adult.

Blood urea nitrogen (BUN) measures the effectiveness of kidney excretion of urea nitrogen, a by-product of protein breakdown in the liver. Urea nitrogen is produced mostly from liver metabolism of food sources of protein. The kidneys filter urea nitrogen from the blood and excrete the waste as part of urine ***elimination.***

Other factors influence the BUN level, and an elevation does not always mean that kidney disease is present (see the Laboratory Profile: Kidney Function Blood Studies box). For example, rapid cell destruction from infection, cancer treatment, or steroid therapy may elevate BUN level. In addition, blood is a protein. Blood in the tissues rather than in the blood vessels is reabsorbed as if it were a general protein. Thus reabsorbed blood protein is processed by the liver and increases BUN levels. This means that injured tissues can result in increased BUN levels even when kidney function is normal. In addition, BUN is increased by protein turnover in exercising muscle and is elevated as a result of concentration during dehydration.

The liver must function properly to produce urea nitrogen. When liver and kidney dysfunction are present, urea nitrogen levels are actually *decreased* because the liver failure limits urea production. The BUN level is not always elevated with kidney disease and is not the best indicator of kidney function. However, an elevated BUN level suggests kidney dysfunction.

Blood urea nitrogen to serum creatinine ratio can help determine whether non–kidney-related factors, such as low cardiac output or red blood cell destruction, are causing the elevated BUN level. When blood volume is deficient (e.g., dehydration) or cardiac output is low, the BUN level rises more rapidly than the serum creatinine level. As a result, the ratio of BUN to creatinine is *increased.*

When both the BUN and serum creatinine levels increase at the same rate, the BUN/creatinine ratio remains normal. However, elevations of *both* serum creatinine and BUN levels suggest kidney dysfunction that is not related to dehydration or poor perfusion.

Cystatin-C measures glomerular filtration rate. Cystatin-C is a protein produced by nucleated cells in the body. Since cystatin-C is produced at a constant rate, it can be used as an indicator of glomerular filtration rate. When the glomerular filtration rate is reduced, cystatin-C increases. Increased levels can be considered a predictor of chronic renal disease. Cystatin-C is not influenced by factors that influence BUN and creatinine levels, making it potentially a better indicator of glomerular filtration rate. Research is still in progress as to the efficacy of cystatin-C in the role of identifying renal disease and other health alterations such as cardiovascular disease and metabolic syndrome (Pagana & Pagana, 2018).

Blood osmolarity is a measure of the overall concentration of particles in the blood and is a good indicator of hydration status. The kidneys excrete or reabsorb water to keep blood osmolarity in the range of 280 to 300 mOsm/kg (mmol/kg). Osmolarity is slightly higher in older adults. When blood osmolarity is decreased, vasopressin (antidiuretic hormone [ADH]) release is inhibited. Without vasopressin, the distal tubule and collecting ducts are *not* permeable to water. As a result, water is *excreted,* not reabsorbed, and blood osmolarity increases. When blood osmolarity increases, vasopressin is released. Vasopressin increases the permeability of the distal tubule to water. Then water is reabsorbed, and blood osmolarity decreases.

Urine Tests

Urinalysis. Urinalysis is a part of any complete physical examination and is especially useful for patients with suspected kidney or urologic disorders (see the Laboratory Profile: Urinalysis box). Ideally, the urine specimen is collected at the morning's first voiding. Specimens obtained at other times may be too dilute. The specimen may be collected by several techniques (Box 60.1).

Urine color comes from urochrome pigment. Color variations may result from increased levels of urochrome or other pigments, changes in the concentration or dilution of the urine, and the presence of drug metabolites in the urine. Urine smells faintly like ammonia and is normally clear without *turbidity* (cloudiness) or haziness.

Specific gravity is the concentration of particles (i.e., electrolytes, wastes) in urine. A high specific gravity indicates concentrated urine from dehydration, decreased kidney blood flow, or excess vasopressin associated with stress, surgery, anesthetic agents, and certain drugs (e.g., morphine, some oral antidiabetic drugs) or syndrome of inappropriate antidiuretic hormone (SIADH) (see Chapter 57). Low specific gravity indicates dilute urine that may occur from high fluid intake, diuretic drugs, or diabetes insipidus (DI) (see Chapter 57).

Specific gravity of urine is compared with distilled water, which has a specific gravity of 1.000. The normal specific gravity of urine ranges from 1.005 to about 1.030. Kidney disease diminishes the concentrating ability of the kidney, and chronic kidney disease may be associated with a low (dilute) specific gravity.

pH is a measure of urine acidity or alkalinity. A pH value less than 7 is acidic, and a value greater than 7 is alkaline. Urine pH is affected by diet, drugs, systemic disturbances of ***acid-base balance,*** and kidney tubular function. For example, a high-protein diet produces acidic urine, whereas a high intake of citrus fruit produces alkaline urine. The normal pH of urine ranges from 4.6 to 8.0 with an average of 6.0 (Pagana & Pagana, 2018).

Urine specimens become more alkaline when left standing unrefrigerated for more than 1 hour, when bacteria are present,

LABORATORY PROFILE

Kidney Function Blood Studies

Test	Normal Range for Adults	Canadian Normal Range	Significance of Abnormal Findings
Serum creatinine	*Males:* 0.6-1.2 mg/dL *Females:* 0.5-1.1 mg/dL *Older adults:* may be decreased	*Males:* 53-106 mcmol/L *Females:* 44-97 mcmol/L	An *increased level* indicates kidney impairment. A *decreased level* may be caused by decreased muscle mass.
Blood urea nitrogen (BUN)	10-20 mg/dL *Older adults:* slightly higher	3.6-7.1 mmol/L	An *increased level* may indicate liver or kidney disease, dehydration or decreased kidney perfusion, a high-protein diet, infection, stress, steroid use, GI bleeding, or other situations in which blood is in body tissues. A *decreased level* may indicate malnutrition, fluid volume excess, or severe hepatic damage.
BUN/creatinine ratio (BUN divided by creatinine)	6-25 15.5 optimum level for adults	6-25	An *increased ratio* may indicate fluid volume deficit, obstructive uropathy, catabolic state, or a high-protein diet. A *decreased ratio* may indicate fluid volume excess.

Data from Pagana, K., & Pagana, T. (2018). *Mosby's manual of diagnostic & laboratory test* (6th ed.). St. Louis: Mosby; and Pagana, K., Pagana, T., & Pike-McDonald, S. (2018). *Mosby's Canadian manual of diagnostic and laboratory tests.* St. Louis: Elsevier.

LABORATORY PROFILE

Urinalysis

Test	Normal Range for Adults	Significance of Abnormal Findings
Color	Yellow	*Dark amber* indicates concentrated urine. *Very pale yellow* indicates dilute urine. *Dark red* or *brown* indicates blood in the urine. Brown may indicate increased bilirubin level. Red also may indicate the presence of myoglobin. *Other color* changes may result from diet or drugs.
Odor	Specific aroma, similar to ammonia	*Foul smell* indicates possible infection, dehydration, or ingestion of certain foods or drugs.
Turbidity	Clear	*Cloudy urine* indicates infection, sediment, or high levels of urine protein.
Specific gravity	1.005-1.030; usually 1.010-1.025 *Older adult:* decrease with age	*Increased* in decreased kidney perfusion, inappropriate ADH secretion, or heart failure. *Decreased* in chronic kidney disease, diabetes insipidus, malignant hypertension, diuretic administration, and lithium toxicity.
pH	Average: 6; range: 4.6-8	*Changes* are caused by diet, drugs, infection, age of specimen, acid-base imbalance, and kidney disease.
Glucose	Fresh specimen, negative 50-300 mg/day in a 24-hr specimen	*Presence* reflects hyperglycemia or a decrease in the kidney threshold for glucose.
Ketones	None	*Presence* occurs with diabetic ketoacidosis, prolonged fasting, and anorexia nervosa.
Protein	0-8 mg/dL (50-80 mg in 24-hr specimen at rest <250 mg in 24-hr specimen with exercise	*Increased* amounts may indicate stress, infection, recent strenuous exercise, or glomerular disorders.
Bilirubin (urobilinogen)	None	*Presence* suggests liver or biliary disease or obstruction.
Red blood cells (RBCs)	0-2 per high-power field	*Increased* is normal with catheterization or menses but may reflect tumor, stones, trauma, glomerular disorders, cystitis, or bleeding disorders.
White blood cells (WBCs)	0-4 per low-power field	*Increased* may indicate an infection or inflammation in the kidney and urinary tract, kidney transplant rejection, or exercise.
Casts	None	*Increased* indicates bacteria, protein, or urinary calculi.
Crystals	None	*Presence* may indicate that the specimen has been allowed to stand.
Bacteria	<1000 colonies/mL	*Increased* indicates the need for urine culture to determine the presence of urinary tract infection.
Parasites	None	*Presence* of *Trichomonas vaginalis* indicates infection, usually of the urethra, prostate, or vagina.
Leukocyte esterase	None	*Presence* suggests urinary tract infection.
Nitrites	None	*Presence* suggests urinary *Escherichia coli.*

Data from Pagana, K., & Pagana, T. (2018). *Mosby's manual of diagnostic & laboratory test* (6th ed.). St. Louis: Mosby; and Pagana, K., Pagana, T., & Pike-McDonald, S. (2018). *Mosby's Canadian manual of diagnostic and laboratory tests.* St. Louis: Elsevier.

or when a specimen is left uncovered. Alkaline urine increases cell breakdown; thus the presence of red blood cells may be missed on analysis. Ensure that urine specimens are covered and delivered to the laboratory promptly. Urine specimens delayed 2 or more hours require refrigerated or other specific storage and transport precautions to ensure the integrity of the urine specimen (Pagana & Pagana, 2018). During systemic acidosis or alkalosis, the kidneys, along with blood buffers and the lungs, normally respond to keep serum pH normal. Chapter 14 discusses ***acid-base balance*** and imbalance.

Protein is not normally present in the urine. Microalbumin levels greater than 80 mcg/24 hr (0.08 g/24 hr) are abnormal. Protein molecules are too large to pass through intact glomerular membranes. When glomerular membranes are not intact, protein molecules pass through and are excreted with urine ***elimination.*** Increased membrane permeability is caused by infection, inflammation, or immunologic problems. Some systemic problems cause production of abnormal proteins, such as globulin. Detection of abnormal protein types requires electrophoresis.

A random finding of **proteinuria** (usually albumin in the urine) followed by a series of negative (normal) findings does not imply kidney disease. If infection is the cause of the proteinuria, urinalyses after resolution of the infection should be negative for protein. Persistent proteinuria needs further investigation.

Microalbuminuria is the presence of albumin in the urine that is not measurable by a urine dipstick or usual urinalysis procedures. Specialized assays are used to quickly analyze a freshly voided urine specimen for microscopic levels of albumin. The normal microalbumin levels in a freshly voided specimen should be less than 2.0 mg/dL. Higher levels indicate microalbuminuria

BOX 60.1 Collection of Urine Specimens

Nursing Interventions	Rationales
Voided Urine	
Collect the first specimen voided in the morning.	Urine is more concentrated in the early morning.
Send the specimen to the laboratory as soon as possible.	After urine is collected, cellular breakdown results in more alkaline urine.
Refrigerate the specimen if a delay is unavoidable.	Refrigeration delays the alkalinization of urine. Bacteria are more likely to multiply in an alkaline environment.
Clean-Catch Specimen	
Explain the purpose of the procedure to the patient.	Correct technique is needed to obtain a valid specimen.
Instruct the patient to self-clean before voiding: Instruct the female patient to separate the labia and use the sponges and solution provided to wipe with three strokes over the urethra. The first two wiping strokes are over each side of the urethra; the third wiping stroke is centered over the urethra (from front to back). Instruct the male patient to retract the foreskin of the penis and to similarly clean the urethra, using three wiping strokes with the sponge and solution provided (from the head of the penis downward).	Surface cleaning is necessary to remove secretions or bacteria from the urethral meatus.
Instruct the patient to initiate voiding after cleaning. The patient then stops and resumes voiding into the container. At no time should any part of the patient's anatomy touch the lip or inner aspect of the container. Only 1 oz (30 mL) is needed; the remainder of the urine may be discarded into the commode.	A midstream collection further removes secretions and bacteria because urine flushes the distal portion of the internal urethra.
Ensure that the patient understands the procedure.	An improperly collected specimen may result in inappropriate or incomplete treatment.
Help the patient as needed.	The patient's understanding and the nurse's assistance ensure proper collection.
Catheterized Specimen	
For nonindwelling (straight) catheters:	The one-time passage of a urinary catheter may be necessary to obtain an uncontaminated specimen for analysis or to measure the volume of residual urine.
Use sterile technique and follow facility procedures for urinary catheterization.	These procedures minimize bacterial entry.
For indwelling catheters:	Urine is collected from an indwelling catheter or tubing when patients have catheters for continence or long-term urinary drainage.
• Apply a clamp to the drainage tubing, distal to the injection port for 15-30 minutes	Clamping allows urine to collect in the tubing at the location where the specimen is obtained.
• Clean the injection port cap of the catheter drainage tubing with an appropriate antiseptic and allow to dry. Povidone-iodine solution or alcohol is acceptable.	Surface contamination is prevented by following the cleaning procedures.
• Attach a sterile 5-mL syringe into the port and aspirate the quantity of urine required.	A minimum of 5 mL is needed for culture and sensitivity (C&S) testing.
• Inject the urine sample into a sterile specimen container.	A sterile container is used for C&S specimens.
• Remove the clamp to resume drainage.	
• Properly dispose of the syringe.	
24-Hour Urine Collection	
Instruct the patient thoroughly.	A 24-hr collection of urine is necessary to quantify or calculate the rate of clearance of a particular substance.
Provide written materials to assist in instruction. Place signs appropriately. Inform all personnel or family caregivers of test in progress.	Instructional materials for patients, signs, etc. remind patients and staff to ensure that the total collection is completed.
Check laboratory or procedure manual on proper technique for maintaining the collection (e.g., on ice, in a refrigerator, or with a preservative).	Proper technique prevents breakdown of elements to be measured.
On initiation of the collection, ask the patient to void, discard the urine, and note the time. If a Foley catheter is in use, empty the tubing and drainage bag at the start time and discard the urine. Collect all urine of the next 24 hr. Twenty-four hours after initiation, ask the patient to empty the bladder and add that urine to the container.	Proper techniques ensure that *all* urine formed within the 24-hr period is collected.
Do not remove urine from the collection container for other specimens.	Urine in the container is not considered a "fresh" specimen and may be mixed with preservative.

and could mean mild or early kidney disease, especially in patients with diabetes mellitus. In 24-hour urine specimens, levels greater than 80 mcg/24 hr (0.08 g/24 hr) indicate microalbuminuria.

Glucose in the urine may indicate a high level of glucose in the blood, typically greater than 220 mg/dL (12 mmol/L). Changes in the renal threshold for glucose may occur temporarily in patients who have infection or severe stress.

Ketone bodies are formed from the incomplete metabolism of fatty acids. Three types of ketone bodies are acetone, acetoacetic acid, and beta-hydroxybutyric acid. *Normally there are no ketones in urine.* Ketone bodies are produced when fat is used instead of glucose for cellular energy. Ketones present in the blood are partially excreted in the urine.

Leukoesterase is an enzyme found in some white blood cells, especially neutrophils. When the number of these cells increases in the urine or they are damaged (lysed), the urine then contains leukoesterase. A normal reading is no leukoesterase in the urine. A positive test (+ sign) is an indication of a urinary tract infection.

Nitrites are not usually present in urine. Many types of bacteria, when present in the urine, convert nitrates (normally found in urine) into nitrites. A positive nitrites test enhances the sensitivity of the leukoesterase test to detect urinary tract infection (Pagana & Pagana, 2018).

Sediment is precipitated particles in the urine. These particles include cells, casts, crystals, and bacteria. Normally, urine contains few, if any, cells. Types of cells abnormally present in the urine include tubular cells (from the tubule of the nephron), epithelial cells (from the lining of the urinary tract), red blood cells (RBCs), and white blood cells (WBCs). WBCs may indicate a urinary tract or kidney infection. RBCs may indicate *glomerulonephritis, acute tubular necrosis, pyelonephritis,* kidney trauma, or kidney cancer.

Casts are clumps of materials or cells. When cells, bacteria, or proteins are present in the urine, minerals and sticky materials clump around them and form a cast of the distal renal tubule and collecting duct. Casts are described by the type of particle they have surrounded (e.g., hyaline [protein-based] or cellular [from RBCs, WBCs, or epithelial cells]) or the stage of cast breakdown (whole cell or granular from cell breakdown). Although an isolated urinalysis with sediment from casts may be the result of strenuous exercise, repeated findings with sediment are more likely to be associated with disease.

Urine crystals come from mineral salts as a result of diet, drugs, or disease. Common salt crystals are formed from calcium, oxalate, urea, phosphate, magnesium, or other substances. Some drugs, such as the sulfates, can also form crystals. Crystals can form into calculi.

Bacteria multiply quickly, so the urine specimen must be analyzed promptly to avoid falsely elevated counts of bacterial colonization. Normally urine is sterile, but it can be easily contaminated by perineal bacteria during collection.

Recent advances in technology and molecular biology have led to new diagnostic tests using urine, including identification of biomarkers of disease and profiling for specific proteins. Markers such as cystatin-C are being investigated to identify early-onset kidney dysfunction, target therapy, and predict responsiveness to intervention. Other markers for angiogenesis and kidney cell adhesion, regulation, and apoptosis (i.e., connective tissue growth factor [CTGF], neutrophil gelatinase-associated lipocalin [NGAL]) will likely contribute to clinical diagnostics in the future.

Urine for Culture and Sensitivity. Urine is analyzed for the number and types of organisms present. Symptoms of infection and unexplained bacteria in a urine specimen are indications for urine culture and sensitivity testing. Bacteria from urine are placed in a medium with different antibiotics. In this way, we can know which antibiotics are effective in killing or stopping the growth of the organisms (organisms are "sensitive") and which are not effective (organisms are "resistant"). A clean-catch or catheter-derived specimen is best for culture and sensitivity testing as these procedures reduce the chance of perineal surface organisms contaminating the specimen.

Composite Urine Collections. Some urine collections are made for a specified number of hours (e.g., 24 hours) for precise analysis of urine levels of substances, such as creatinine or urea nitrogen, sodium, chloride, calcium, catecholamines, or other components (see the Laboratory Profile: 24-Hour Urine Collection box). For a composite urine specimen, *all* urine within the designated time frame must be collected. If other urine must be obtained while the collection is in progress, measure and record the amount collected but not added to the timed collection.

The urine collection may need to be refrigerated or stored on ice to prevent changes in the urine during the collection time. Follow the procedure from the laboratory for urine storage, including whether a preservative is to be added. The urine collection must be free from fecal contamination. Menstrual blood and toilet tissue also contaminate the specimen and can invalidate the results.

The collection of all urine for a 24-hour period is often challenging. With hospitalized patients, the cooperation of staff personnel, the patient, family members, and visitors is essential. Placing signs in the bathroom, instructing the patient and family, and emphasizing the need to save the urine are helpful.

Creatinine Clearance. Creatinine clearance is a measure of glomerular filtration rate (GFR) and kidney function. The patient's age, gender, height, weight, diet, and activity level influence the expected amount of excreted creatinine. Thus these factors are considered when interpreting creatinine clearance test results. Decreases in the creatinine clearance rate may require reducing drug doses and often signifies the need to further explore the cause of kidney deterioration.

Commonly, creatinine clearance is calculated from serum creatinine, age, weight, urine creatinine, gender, and race. Creatinine clearance can be based on the excretion of injected inulin or other substances that are not reabsorbed into the blood. Creatinine clearance to estimate GFR can also be based on a 24-hour urine collection, although urine can be collected for shorter periods (e.g., 8 or 12 hours). The analysis compares the urine creatinine level with the blood creatinine level; therefore a blood specimen for creatinine must also be collected. The range for normal creatinine clearance is 107 to 139 mL/min for men (1.78 to 2.32 mL/sec) and 87 to 107 mL/min (1.45 to 1.78 mL/sec) for women tested with a 24-hour urine collection (Pagana & Pagana, 2018). Values decrease

LABORATORY PROFILE

24-Hour Urine Collection

Component	Normal Range for Adults	Canadian Range for Adults	Significance of Abnormal Findings
Creatinine	*Males:* 1-2 g/24 hr *Females:* 0.6-1.8 g/24 hr *Older adults:* slightly lower	*Males:* 124-230 mcmol/kg/24 hr *Females:* 97-177 mcmol/kg/24 hr	*Decreased amounts* indicate deterioration in function caused by kidney disease. *Increased amounts* occur with infections, exercise, diabetes mellitus, and meat meals.
Urea nitrogen	12-20 g/24 hr	0.43-0.71 mmol/24 hr	*Decreased amounts* occur when kidney damage or liver disease is present. *Increased amounts* commonly result from a high-protein diet, dehydration, trauma, or sepsis.
Sodium	40-220 mEq/24 hr	40-220 mmol/day	*Decreased* in hemorrhage, shock, hyperaldosteronism, and prerenal acute kidney injury. *Increased* with diuretic therapy, excessive salt intake, hypokalemia, and acute tubular necrosis.
Chloride	110-250 mEq/24 hr	110-250 mmol/24 hr	*Decreased* in certain kidney diseases, malnutrition, pyloric obstruction, prolonged nasogastric tube drainage, diarrhea, diaphoresis, heart failure, and emphysema. *Increased* with hypokalemia, adrenal insufficiency, and massive diuresis.
Calcium	100-300 mg/24 hr	2.50-7.50 mmol/kg/24 hr	*Decreased* with hypocalcemia, hypoparathyroidism, nephrosis, and nephritis*Increased* with calcium kidney stones, hyperparathyroidism, sarcoidosis, certain cancers, immobilization, and hypercalcemia.
*Total catecholamines	<100 mcg/24 hr	<591 mmol/24 hr	*Increased* with pheochromocytoma, neuroblastomas, stress, or heavy exercise.
Protein	<80 mg/24 hr	10-150 mg/24 hr	*Increased* in glomerular disease, nephrotic syndrome, diabetic nephropathy, urinary tract malignancies, and irritations.

Data from Pagana, K., & Pagana, T. (2018). *Mosby's manual of diagnostic & laboratory test* (6th ed.). St. Louis: Mosby; Pagana, K., Pagana, T., & Pike-McDonald, S. (2018). *Mosby's Canadian manual of diagnostic and laboratory tests.* St. Louis: Elsevier; and United States Library of Medicine.

progressively per decade of life for adults older than 40 years because of age-related decline in GFR. However, these expensive and time-consuming methods are usually reserved for when a decision for starting renal replacement therapy (dialysis) is needed.

Current guidelines suggest that clinical laboratories report an estimate of GFR (eGFR) based on the Modification of Diet in Renal Disease (MDRD) study equation. The MDRD equation does not require urine to estimate GFR; the calculation requires the serum creatinine level, age, and numbers specific to gender and ethnicity. The calculation is an accurate way to measure urine creatinine clearance. The estimated GFR (eGFR) for the MDRD equation is >60 mL/min/1.73 m^2 (Pagana & Pagana, 2018).

Urine Electrolytes. Urine samples can be analyzed for electrolyte levels (e.g., sodium, chloride). Normally the amount of sodium excreted in the urine is nearly equal to that consumed. Urine sodium levels can vary depending on the amount of water and salt consumed. Normal values for a 24-hour urine sample ranges from 40 to 220 mEq/day (or 40 to 220 mmol/day). A value of greater than 20 mEq/L for a routine urine specimen is considered normal (Pagana & Pagana, 2018).

Urine Osmolarity. Osmolarity measures the concentration of particles in solution. The particles in urine contributing to osmolarity include electrolytes, glucose, urea, and creatinine.

NCLEX EXAMINATION CHALLENGE 60.2

Physiological Integrity

A client is on a 24-hour urine collection. At midpoint during the collection, the client tells the nurse that some of the urine was discarded. What action will the nurse take? **Select all that apply.**

A. No action is required.
B. Reinforce client education.
C. Notify the laboratory staff.
D. Restart the urine collection.
E. Document the discarded urine.
F. Notify the health care provider.

Urine osmolarity can vary from 50 to 1200 mOsm/kg or L (mmol/kg or L), depending on the patient's hydration status and kidney function. With average fluid intake, the range for urine osmolarity is 300 to 900 mOsm/kg or L (mmol/kg or L). Electrolytes, acids, and other normal metabolic wastes are continually produced. These particles are the solute load that must be excreted in the urine on a regular basis. This is referred to as *obligatory solute excretion.* If the patient loses excessive fluids, the kidney response is to save water while excreting wastes by excreting small amounts of highly concentrated urine. Diet, drugs, and activity can change urine osmolarity. Urine with an increased osmolarity is concentrated urine with less water and more solutes. Urine with a decreased osmolarity is dilute urine with more water and fewer solutes.

Bedside Sonography/Bladder Scanners. The use of portable ultrasound scanners in the hospital and rehabilitation setting by nurses is a noninvasive method of estimating bladder volume (see Fig. 60.10). Bladder scanners are used to screen for postvoid residual volumes and determine the need for intermittent catheterization based on the amount of urine in the bladder rather than the time between catheterizations. There is no discomfort with the scan, and no patient preparation beyond an explanation of what to expect is required.

Explain the reason the procedure is being done and what sensations the patient might experience during the procedure. For example, "This test will measure the amount of urine in your bladder. I will place a gel pad just above your pubic area and then place the probe, which is a little bigger and heavier than a stethoscope, on the gel."

Before scanning, select the male or female icon on the bladder scanner. Using the female icon allows the scanner software to subtract the volume of the uterus from any measurement. Use the male icon on all men and on women who have undergone a hysterectomy.

Place an ultrasound gel pad right above the pubic bone or moisten the round dome of the scan head area with 5 mL of conducting gel to improve ultrasound conduction. Use gel on the scanner head for obese patients and those with heavy body hair in the area to be scanned. Place the probe midline over the abdomen about 1.5 inches (4 cm) above the pubic bone. Aim the scan head so the ultrasound is projected toward the expected location of the bladder, typically toward the patient's coccyx. Press and release the scan button. The scan is complete with the sound of a beep, and a volume is displayed. Two readings are recommended for best accuracy. An aiming icon on the portable bladder scanner indicates whether the bladder image is centered on the crosshairs of the scan head. If the crosshairs on the aiming icon are not centered on the bladder, the measured volume may not be accurate.

Imaging Assessment. Many imaging procedures are used to diagnose abnormalities within the renal-urinary system (Box 60.2). Explain the procedures, prepare, and provide follow-up care to the patient. Patient education materials for many urologic tests have been developed by organizations, such as the Society for Urologic Nurses and Associates, and are freely available. Encourage the patient to use reliable and credible sources for online information.

Kidney, Ureter, and Bladder X-rays. An x-ray of the kidneys, ureters, and bladder (KUB) is a plain film of the abdomen obtained without any specific patient preparation. The KUB study shows gross anatomic features and obvious stones, strictures, calcifications, or obstructions in the urinary tract. This test identifies the shape, size, and position of the organs in relation to other parts of the urinary tract. Other tests are needed to diagnose functional or structural problems.

There is no discomfort or risk from this procedure. Tell the patient that the x-ray will be taken while in a supine position. No specific follow-up care is needed.

BOX 60.2 Radiologic and Special Diagnostic Tests for Patients With Disorders of the Kidney and Urinary System

Test	Purpose
Radiography of kidneys, ureters, and bladder (KUB) (plain film of abdomen)	To screen for the presence of two kidneys To measure kidney size To detect gross obstruction in kidneys or urinary tract
Computed tomography (CT) with contrast, CT arteriography or angiography	To measure kidney size To evaluate contour to assess for injury, masses, or obstruction in kidneys or the urinary tract To assess renal blood flow
Magnetic resonance imaging (MRI)	Similar to CT Useful for staging of cancers
Ultrasonography (US) Can be used with contrast media	To identify the urine volume in the bladder, size of the kidneys or obstruction (e.g., tumors, stones) in the kidneys or lower urinary tract Assess blood flow to and from the kidney
(Nuclear) renal scan	To evaluate renal perfusion To estimate glomerular filtration rate To provide functional information without exposing the patient to iodinated contrast medium
Cystoscopy	To identify abnormalities of the bladder wall and urethral and ureteral occlusions To treat small obstructions or lesions via fulguration, lithotripsy, or removal with a stone basket
Cystography and cystourethrography With or without retrograde studies With or without contrast medium	To outline bladder's contour when full and examine structure during voiding To examine the structure of the urethra To detect backward urine flow
Metabolic imaging with positron emission tomography (PET)	To evaluate cysts, tumors, and other lesions, eliminating the need for biopsy in some patients

Computed Tomography. Inform the patient that a CT scan provides three-dimensional information about the kidneys, ureters, bladder, and surrounding tissues. The CT scan is performed in a special room, usually in the radiology department. It can provide information about tumors, cysts, abscesses, other masses, and obstruction. CT can also be used to image the kidney's vascular system (i.e., CT angiography). Some hospitals require patients having CT scans to be NPO for some period before the scan, although there is no specific evidence guiding this practice.

Determine whether the scan requires contrast medium (often called *dye*). The most common contrast agents used for imaging of the kidney are radiopaque, contain iodine, are nonionic, and have varying osmolarity. These include iohexol, iopromide, and iodixanol. Oral or injected contrast medium is usually given before starting the imaging procedure. Dye use may be omitted in patients at risk for contrast-induced acute kidney injury, but the images produced are less distinct.

When contrast is used, ensure that there is sufficient oral or IV intake to dilute and excrete the contrast media. Typically, the radiologist will specify a total fluid intake of 1 L or a variable rate to maintain urine output at 1 to 2 mL/kg/hr for up to 6 hours. When no contrast is used, there is no special postprocedural care.

Contrast medium is potentially kidney damaging (nephrotoxic). *Contrast-induced nephropathy* is the onset of *acute kidney failure* within 48 hours after the administration of iodinated contrast medium (Lambert et al., 2017). The risk for *contrast-induced nephropathy* is greatest in patients who are older or dehydrated, have pre-existing chronic kidney disease (CKD), or have comorbidities of diabetes, heart failure, or current hypotension (Pagana & Pagana, 2018). Patients who take nephrotoxic drugs are also at risk. The best practice for patient safety and quality care lists assessment questions to ask before a patient undergoes testing with contrast material.

In addition, patients taking metformin are at risk for lactic acidosis when they receive iodinated contrast media. Metformin should be discontinued at least 24 hours before the time of a procedure and for at least 48 hours after the procedure. Kidney function should be re-evaluated before the patient resumes metformin therapy.

! NURSING SAFETY PRIORITY (QSEN)

Drug Alert

Ensure that the patient who is prescribed metformin does not receive the drug after a procedure requiring IV contrast material until adequate kidney function has been determined.

BEST PRACTICE FOR PATIENT SAFETY & QUALITY CARE (QSEN)

Assessing the Patient About to Undergo a Kidney Test or Procedure Using Contrast Medium

Before the procedure:

- Ask the patient:
  - Have you had contrast medium before? If so, did you have a reaction? If so, describe the reaction (e.g., hives, facial edema, difficulty breathing, bronchospasm). If the patient has had a reaction before, he or she is at higher risk for having another reaction.
  - Do you have a history of asthma? Patients with asthma have been shown to be at greater risk for contrast reactions than the general public. When reactions do occur, they are more likely to be severe.
  - Do you have hay fever or food or drug allergies? Contrast reactions have been reported to be as high as 15% in patients with hay fever or food or drug allergies, especially to seafood, eggs, milk, or chocolate.
  - Are you taking metformin. Metformin must be discontinued at least 24 hours before any study using contrast media because the life-threatening complication of lactic acidosis, although rare, could occur.
  - When have you last eaten or drank anything?
- Assess for a history of renal impairment and for conditions that have been implicated in increasing the chance of developing kidney injury or impairment after contrast media (e.g., diabetic nephropathy, class IV heart failure, dehydration, concomitant use of potentially nephrotoxic drugs such as the aminoglycosides or NSAIDs, and cirrhosis).
- Assess hydration status by checking blood pressure, heart and respiratory rates, mucous membranes, skin turgor, and urine concentration.

All patients at risk for contrast-induced nephrotoxicity need regular assessment and collaboration with the primary health care provider to maintain hydration and decrease the risk for kidney injury following a CT scan with IV contrast administration. IV fluids of normal saline are the most effective before the procedure to prevent contrast-induced nephrotoxic effects during radiologic procedures (Sethi et al., 2018). Diuretics may be given immediately after the contrast is injected to enhance excretion in patients who are well hydrated.

! NURSING SAFETY PRIORITY (QSEN)

Drug Alert

When a CT scan with contrast is prescribed, report the patient's history of immediate hypersensitivity reactions associated with the administration of contrast media to the radiologist and health care provider.

Magnetic Resonance Imaging. MRI provides improved imaging between normal and abnormal tissue in the renal system compared with a CT scan. As with all MRIs, the patient with metal implants (pins, pacemaker, joint replacement, aneurysmal clips, or other cosmetic or medical devices) is not eligible for this test because the magnet can move the metal implant, resulting in harm to the patient. A variation of MRI is magnetic resonance angiography (MRA). This noninvasive procedure is used to detect blockages in large arteries and can determine renal artery stenosis.

Gadolinium-based contrast agents are used with MRI similar to CT scans. The contrast agent is injected intravenously and excreted via the kidneys. These agents have been linked with nephrogenic systemic fibrosis (Pagana & Pagana, 2018) and should not be used in patients with renal impairment, usually defined as a serum creatinine above 1.5 mg/dL (110 mcmol/L) or an estimated GFR less than 45 mL/min. Adults older than 60 years should be carefully evaluated for renal impairment.

Kidney Ultrasonography. Inform the patient that ultrasonography does not cause discomfort and is without risk. This test usually requires a full bladder. Ask the patient to drink 500 to 1000 mL of water, if needed, about 2 to 3 hours before the test to help fill the bladder. The patient should not void after drinking the water until the test is complete. This test applies sound waves to structures of different densities to produce images of the kidneys, ureters, and bladder and surrounding tissues. Ultrasonography allows assessment of kidney size, cortical thickness, and status of the calices. The test can identify obstruction in the urinary tract, tumors, cysts, and other masses without the use of contrast. In addition, it can determine blood flow into and out of the kidney using Doppler color flow imaging.

The patient undergoing kidney ultrasound is usually placed in the prone position. Sonographic gel is applied to the skin over the back and flank areas to enhance sound wave conduction. A transducer in contact with and moving across the skin delivers sound waves and measures the echoes. Images of the internal structures are produced. Assisting the patient to a position of comfort and skin care to remove the gel is all that is needed after ultrasonography.

Renal Scan. This imaging test is used to examine the perfusion, function, and structure of the kidneys by the IV administration of a radioisotope. It does not use an iodinated contrast agent and thus may be used in preference to a CT scan when the patient is allergic to iodine or has impaired kidney function that places him or her at risk for kidney injury from IV contrast.

No fasting or sedation is used. A peripheral IV catheter is inserted to give the radioisotope contrast agent. While the patient lies in a prone or sitting position, a camera is passed over the kidney area and records the isotope uptake on film, minutes after the radioisotope is given. After initial images, the patient may be given furosemide or captopril to better visualize kidney function and blood flow. The isotope is eliminated 6 to 24 hours after the procedure. Encourage the patient to drink fluids to aid in excretion of the isotope. Because only tracer doses of radioisotopes are used, no precautions are needed related to radioactive exposure.

! NURSING SAFETY PRIORITY (QSEN)

Drug Alert

A renal scan is contraindicated in women who are pregnant unless the benefits outweigh the risks.

Renal Arteriography (Angiography). Renal arteriography allows visualization of the renal arteries using a radiopaque contrast medium that enters the renal blood vessels and generates images to determine blood vessel size and abnormalities. The contrast medium is injected through the femoral or brachial artery as x-ray pictures are taken. This test has largely been replaced by other imaging techniques (e.g., nuclear renal scans, ultrasonography, computed tomography) and is seldom used as a stand-alone diagnostic procedure. The most common use of renal arteriography is at the time of a renal angioplasty or other intervention.

Cystoscopy and Cystourethroscopy

Patient Preparation. Cystoscopy and cystourethroscopy are endoscopic procedures used to evaluate the bladder, urethra, and lower portions of the ureters. An endoscopy scope is inserted through the urethra into the bladder providing direct visualization. These procedures require completion of a preoperative checklist and a signed informed consent statement. The urologist provides a complete description of and reasons for the procedure, and the nurse reinforces this information. Cystoscopy may be performed for diagnosis or treatment. This test is used to examine for bladder trauma (cystoscopy) or urethral trauma (cystourethroscopy) and to identify causes of urinary tract obstruction. Cystoscopy also may be used to remove bladder tumors or plant radium seeds into a tumor, dilate the urethra and ureters with or without stent placement, stop areas of bleeding, or resect an enlarged prostate gland.

Cystoscopy may be performed under general anesthesia or under local anesthesia with sedation. The patient's age and general health and the expected duration of the procedure are considered in the decision about anesthesia. A light evening meal may be eaten. Usually the patient is NPO after midnight on the night before the cystoscopy. A bowel preparation with laxatives or enemas is performed the evening before the procedure so that bowel contents do not interfere with the procedure.

Procedure. The cystoscopy is performed in a designated cystoscopic examination room. If the procedure is performed in a surgical suite under general anesthesia, the usual surgical support personnel are present (see Chapter 9). This procedure is often performed in clinics, ambulatory surgery or short-procedure units, or a urologist's office.

Assist the patient onto a table and, after sedation, place the patient in the lithotomy position. After the anesthesia is given and the area cleansed and draped, the urologist inserts a cystoscope through the urethra into the urinary bladder. This examination commonly includes the use of both the cystoscope and urethroscope.

Follow-up Care. After this procedure with general anesthesia, the patient is returned to a postanesthesia care unit (PACU) or area. If local anesthesia and sedation were used, the patient may be returned directly to the hospital room. Patients undergoing cystoscopic examinations as outpatients are transferred to an area for monitoring before discharge to home. Monitor for airway patency and breathing, changes in vital signs (including temperature), and changes in urine output. Also observe for the complications of bladder puncture, excessive bleeding, and infection. Bladder puncture is accompanied by severe pain, including abdominal pain, nausea, and vomiting.

A catheter may or may not be present after cystoscopy. The patient without a catheter has urinary frequency as a result of irritation from the procedure. The urine may be pink tinged, but gross bleeding is not expected. Bleeding or the presence of clots may obstruct the catheter and decrease urine output. Monitor urine output and notify the urologist of obvious blood clots or a decreased or absent urine output. Irrigate the Foley catheter with sterile saline, if prescribed. Notify the urologist if the patient has a fever (with or without chills) or an elevated white blood cell (WBC) count, which suggests infection. Urge the patient to take oral fluids to increase urine output (which helps prevent clotting) and reduce the burning sensation on urination.

Cystography and Cystourethrography. These tests are a series of x-rays or a continuous radiographic visualization by fluoroscopy. During the imaging, radiopaque contrast medium fills the bladder and the bladder is emptied. Images show structure and function of the bladder and urethra. Tumors, rupture or perforation of the bladder and urethra, abnormal backflow of urine, and distortion from trauma or other pelvic masses can be seen.

Patient Preparation and Procedure. Explain the procedure to the patient. A urinary catheter is temporarily needed to instill contrast medium directly into the bladder for both procedures. The contrast medium enhances x-ray visibility of the lower urinary tract and is not absorbed into the bloodstream, reducing the risk for contrast-induced kidney injury.

After bladder filling, x-rays are taken from the front, back, and side positions. For the voiding cystourethrogram (VCUG), the patient is requested to void and x-rays are taken during the voiding. A VCUG can determine whether urine refluxes (flow backward) into the ureter. The cystogram is used in cases of trauma when urethral or bladder injury is suspected or for patients with recurrent *pyelonephritis* (kidney infection).

Follow-up Care. Monitor for infection as a result of catheter placement. In this test, the contrast medium is not nephrotoxic because it does not enter the bloodstream and does not reach the kidney. Encourage fluid intake to dilute the urine and reduce the burning sensation from catheter irritation after removal. Monitor for changes in urine output because pelvic or urethral trauma may be present.

Retrograde Procedures. *Retrograde* means going against the normal flow of urine. A retrograde examination of the ureters and pelvis *(pyelogram),* the bladder *(cystogram),* and the urethra *(urethrogram)* involves instilling radiopaque contrast medium into the lower urinary tract. Because the contrast agent is instilled directly to obtain an outline of the structures desired, the agent does not enter the bloodstream. Therefore the patient is not at risk for contrast-induced kidney injury.

The patient is prepared for retrograde procedures (retrograde pyelography, retrograde cystography, and retrograde urethrography) in the same way as for cystoscopy. Retrograde x-rays are obtained during the cystoscopy. After placement of the cystoscope by the urologist, catheters are placed into each ureter and contrast is instilled into each ureter and renal pelvis. The catheters are removed by the urologist, and x-rays are taken to outline these structures as the agent is excreted. The procedure identifies obstruction or structural abnormalities.

For patients undergoing retrograde cystoscopy or urethrography, radiopaque contrast medium is instilled similarly into the bladder or urethra. Cystography and urethrography identify structural problems, such as fistulas, diverticula, and tumors.

After retrograde procedures, monitor the patient for infection caused by placing instruments in the urinary tract. Because these procedures are performed during cystoscopic examination, follow-up care is the same as that for cystoscopy, including monitoring for bladder puncture or perforation.

Other Diagnostic Assessments

Urodynamic Studies. Urodynamic studies examine the processes of voiding and include:

- Tests of bladder capacity, pressure, and tone
- Studies of urethral pressure and urine flow
- Tests of perineal voluntary muscle function

These tests are often used along with voiding urographic or cystoscopic procedures to evaluate problems with urine flow and disorders of the lower urinary tract.

Cystometrography (CMG) can determine how well the bladder wall (detrusor) muscle functions and how sensitive it is to stretching as the bladder fills. This test provides information about bladder capacity, bladder pressure, and voiding reflexes.

Explain the procedure and inform the patient that a urinary catheter will be needed temporarily during the procedure. Ask the patient to void normally. Record the amount and time of voiding. Insert a urinary catheter to measure the residual urine volume. The cystometer is attached to the catheter, and fluid is instilled via the catheter into the bladder. The point at which the patient first notes a feeling of the urge to void and the point at which he or she notes a strong urge to void are recorded. Bladder capacity and bladder pressure readings are recorded graphically. The patient is asked to void when the bladder instillation is complete (about 500 mL). The residual urine after voiding is recorded, and the catheter is removed. Electromyography of the perineal muscles may be performed during this examination.

For any procedure that involves inserting instruments into the urinary tract, monitor for infection. Record the patient's temperature, the character of the urine, and urine output volume.

Urethral pressure profile (also called a *urethral pressure profilometry* [UPP]) can provide information about the nature of urinary incontinence or urinary retention.

Explain the procedure and inform the patient that a urinary catheter will be needed temporarily during the procedure. A special catheter with pressure-sensing capabilities is inserted into the bladder. Variations in the pressure of the smooth muscle of the urethra are recorded as the catheter is slowly withdrawn.

As with any study involving inserting instruments into the urinary tract, monitor the patient for symptoms of infection.

Urine stream testing is used to evaluate pelvic muscle strength and the effectiveness of pelvic muscles in stopping the flow of urine. It is useful in assessing urinary incontinence.

Explain the procedure and reassure the patient that efforts will be made to ensure privacy. The patient is asked to begin urinating. Three to five seconds after urination begins, the examiner gives the patient a signal to stop urine flow. The length of time required to stop the flow of urine is recorded.

Cleaning the perineal area, as after any voiding, is all that is necessary after the urine stream test.

Electromyography (EMG) of the perineal muscles tests the strength of the muscles used in voiding. This information may help identify methods of improving continence. Inform the patient that some mild, temporary discomfort may accompany placement of the electrodes.

In EMG of the perineal muscles, electrodes are placed in either the rectum or the urethra to measure muscle contraction and relaxation. After the completion of EMG, administer analgesics as prescribed to promote the patient's comfort.

NCLEX EXAMINATION CHALLENGE 60.3

Safe and Effective Care Environment

The nurse is admitting a client undergoing a CT scan with contrast. Which finding does the nurse report as a possible **immediate** hypersensitivity reaction? **Select all that apply.**

A. Nausea
B. Pruritis
C. Urticaria
D. Laryngeal stridor
E. Flushing of the skin

Kidney Biopsy

Patient Preparation. Explain that a kidney biopsy can help determine a cause of unexplained kidney problems and help direct or change therapy. Most kidney biopsies are performed **percutaneously** (through skin and other tissues) using ultrasound or CT guidance. The patient signs an informed consent. Patients are NPO for 4 to 6 hours before the procedure.

Because of the risk for bleeding after the biopsy, coagulation studies such as platelet count, activated partial thromboplastin time (aPTT), prothrombin time (PT), and bleeding time are performed before surgery. Hypertension is aggressively managed before and after the procedure because high blood pressure can make stopping the bleeding after the biopsy more difficult. Uremia also increases the risk for bleeding, and dialysis may be prescribed before a biopsy. A blood transfusion may be needed to correct anemia before biopsy.

Procedure. In a percutaneous biopsy, the nephrologist or radiologist obtains tissue samples without an incision. Patients receive sedation and are monitored throughout the procedure. The patient is placed in the prone position on the procedure table. The entry site is selected after taking preliminary images. The area is prepped and sterilely draped. A local anesthetic is injected, and the physician then inserts the biopsy device into the tissues toward the kidney. Needle depth and placement are confirmed by ultrasound or CT. While the patient holds his or her breath, the needle is advanced into the renal cortex. Samples are then taken with a spring-loaded coring biopsy needle and sent for pathologic study (Pagana & Pagana, 2018).

Follow-up Care. After a percutaneous biopsy, the major risk is bleeding into the kidney or the tissues external from the kidney at the biopsy site. For 24 hours after the biopsy, monitor the dressing site, vital signs (especially fluctuations in blood pressure), urine output, hemoglobin level, and hematocrit. Even if the dressing is dry and there is no hematoma, the patient could be bleeding from the site. An internal bleed is not readily visible but is suspected with flank pain, decreasing blood pressure, decreasing urine output, or other signs of hypovolemia or shock. With severe bleeding, some patients develop bruising along the flank and back accompanied by pain.

The patient follows a plan of strict bedrest, lying in a supine position with a back roll for additional support for 2 to 6 hours after the biopsy. The head of the bed may be elevated, and the patient may resume oral intake of food and fluids. After bedrest, the patient may have limited bathroom privileges if there is no evidence of bleeding.

Monitor for hematuria, the most common complication of kidney biopsy. Hematuria occurs microscopically in most patients, but 5% to 9% have gross hematuria. This problem usually resolves without treatment 48 to 72 hours after the biopsy but can persist for 2 to 3 weeks. In rare cases, transfusions and surgery are required. There should be no obvious blood clots in the urine.

The patient may have some local pain after the biopsy. If aching originates at the biopsy site and begins to radiate to the flank, back, and around the front of the abdomen, bleeding may have started, or a hematoma is forming around the kidney. This pattern of pain with bleeding occurs because blood in the tissues around the kidney increases pressure on local nerve tracts.

If bleeding occurs, IV fluid, packed red blood cells, or both may be needed to prevent shock. In general, a small amount of bleeding creates enough pressure to compress bleeding sites. This is called a *tamponade effect.* If tamponade does not occur and bleeding is extensive, surgery for hemostasis or even nephrectomy may be needed. A hematoma in, on, or around the kidney may become infected, requiring treatment with antibiotics and surgical drainage.

If no bleeding occurs, the patient can resume general activities after 24 hours. Instruct the patient to avoid lifting heavy objects, exercising, or performing other strenuous activities for 1 to 2 weeks after the biopsy procedure. Driving may also be restricted. Refer to Chapter 9 for general postoperative care for the patient who has undergone an open kidney biopsy.

NCLEX EXAMINATION CHALLENGE 60.4

Safe and Effective Care Environment

Which assessment finding would require the nurse to take **immediate** action in a client who is 1 hour post kidney biopsy? **Select all that apply.**

A. Pink-tinged urine
B. Nausea and vomiting
C. Increased bowel sounds
D. Reports of flank pain
E. The patient is ambulating to the bathroom

CLINICAL JUDGMENT CHALLENGE 60.1

Safety; Patient-Centered Care

The nurse is assessing a 42-year-old female client who is scheduled for surgical repair of a hip fracture from a car crash 4 hours ago. The client was traveling approximately 40 miles per hour when she struck a guard rail after a deer ran into the roadway. The client was wearing a seat belt at the time of the accident. The client reports pain in the left hip area with noted swelling. There is a 2-cm abrasion over the right eye and a contusion on the left upper forearm. When the client voids, the nurse assesses that the urine is rust colored and the client states "It burns when I urinate." The client has a history of anxiety.

1. **Recognize Cues:** What assessment information in this client situation is the most important and immediate concern for the nurse? (Hint: Identify the **relevant** information *first* to determine what is most important.)
2. **Analyze Cues:** What client conditions are consistent with the **most relevant** information? (Hint: Think about priority collaborative problems that support and contradict the information presented in this situation.)

GET READY FOR THE NEXT-GENERATION NCLEX® EXAMINATION!

Key Points

Review these Key Points for each NCLEX Examination Client Needs Category.

Safe and Effective Care Environment

- Wear gloves when handling urine or drainage from the genitourinary tract. **QSEN: Safety**
- Evaluate the patient for potential adverse or allergic reactions to radiopaque contrast agents, iodine, or gadolinium. **QSEN: Safety**
- Assess the patient for use of drugs that increase risk for kidney dysfunction. **QSEN: Safety**
- Assess the patient for bleeding, increased pain, and symptoms of perforation or infection after any invasive test of kidney/urinary function. **QSEN: Safety**
- Inform primary health care providers about any symptoms of complications following invasive or noninvasive tests of urinary and kidney structure or function. **QSEN: Safety**

Health Promotion and Maintenance

- Teach patients to clean the perineal area after voiding, after having a bowel movement, and after sexual intercourse. **QSEN: Evidence-Based Practice**
- Urge all patients to maintain an adequate fluid intake (sufficient to dilute urine to a light yellow color) unless another health problem requires fluid restriction. **QSEN: Evidence-Based Practice**

Psychosocial Integrity

- Allow the patient to express fear or anxiety about renal system diagnostic tests and renal system alterations. **QSEN: Patient-Centered Care**
- Provide privacy for patients undergoing examination or testing of the renal system. **QSEN: Patient-Centered Care**
- Use language and terminology that the patient can understand during discussions of kidney/urinary assessment. **QSEN: Patient-Centered Care**

Physiological Integrity

- Ask the patient about kidney problems in any other family members because some problems have a genetic component. **QSEN: Patient-Centered Care**
- Explain all diagnostic procedures, restrictions, and follow-up care to the patient scheduled for tests. **QSEN: Patient-Centered Care**
- Interpret laboratory data to distinguish between dehydration and kidney impairment. **QSEN: Evidence-Based Practice**
- Describe how to obtain different types of urine specimens. **QSEN: Evidence-Based Practice**
- Document renal and urinary system assessment in the patient's electronic health record. **QSEN: Patient-Centered Care**
- Assess urine and serum tests of kidney function closely after renal system diagnostic tests. **QSEN: Evidence-Based Practice**

MASTERY QUESTIONS

1. Which client being managed for dehydration does the nurse consider at greatest risk for possible reduced kidney function?
   A. An 80-year-old man who has benign prostatic hyperplasia
   B. A 62-year-old woman with a known allergy to contrast media
   C. A 48-year-old woman with established urinary incontinence
   D. A 45-year-old man receiving oral and intravenous fluid therapy
2. Which client assessment data is essential for the nurse to report to the health care provider before a renal scan is performed?
   A. Pink-tinged urine
   B. Reports pregnancy
   C. Reports claustrophobia
   D. History of an aneurysm clip
3. Which lab finding is indicative of renal function alterations and not dehydration? Select all that apply.
   A. BUN 20 mL/dL
   B. Creatinine 2.3 mL/dL
   C. Hemoglobin 14 g/dL
   D. Cystatin-c 105 mg/mL
   E. BUN/creatinine ratio 10
   F. Creatinine clearance 175 mL/min
4. Which symptom(s) in a client during the first 12 hours after a kidney biopsy indicates to the nurse a possible complication from the procedure?
   A. The client experiences nausea and vomiting after drinking juice.
   B. The biopsy site is tender to light palpation.
   C. The abdomen is distended, and the client reports abdominal discomfort.
   D. The heart rate is 118, blood pressure is 108/50, and peripheral pulses are thready.

REFERENCES

Brenner, B. M. (Ed.). (2016). *Brenner & Rector's the kidney* (10th ed.) Philadelphia: Saunders.

Burchum, J., & Rosenthal, L. (2019). *Lehne's pharmacology for nursing care* (10th ed.). St. Louis: Elsevier.

Denic, A., Glassock, R., & Rule, A. (2016). *Structural and functional changes with the aging kidney, 23*(1). https://doi.org/10.1053/j.ackd.2015.08.004.

Jackson, C., Botelho, E., Josepf, J., & Tennstedt, S. (2013). Accessing and evaluating urologic health information: Differences by race/ethnicity and gender. *Urologic Nursing, 33*(6), 282–287.

Jarvis, C. (2020). *Physical examination & health assessment* (8th ed.). St. Louis: Elsevier.

Lambert, P., Chasson, K., Horton, S., Petrin, C., Marshall, E., Bowdon, S., et al. (2017). Reducing acute kidney injury due to contrast material: How nurses can improve patient safety. *Critical Care Nurse, 37*(1), 13–26.

McCance, K., & Huether, S. (2019). *Pathophysiology: The biologic basis for disease in adults and children* (8th ed.). St. Louis: Mosby.

McCulloch, D. (2018). Estimation of blood glucose control in diabetes mellitus. In D. Nathan, & J. Wolfsdorf (Eds.), *UpToDate*. Waltham, MA.

National Institute of Diabetes and Digestive and Kidney Diseases (NIDDK). (2018). *Kidney disease*. Retrieved from https://www.niddk.nih.gov/health-information/kidney-disease.

National Kidney Foundation. (2017). *How your kidneys work*. Retrieved from https://www.kidney.org/kidneydisease/howkidneys-wrk.

Pagana, K., & Pagana, T. (2018). *Mosby's manual of diagnostic and laboratory test reference* (6th ed.). St. Louis: Mosby.

Pagana, K., Pagana, T., & Pike-McDonald, S. (2018). *Mosby's Canadian manual of diagnostic and laboratory tests*. St. Louis: Elsevier.

Sethi, A., Kohli, J., Patel, A., & Rudnick, M. (2018). Chapter 13 Contract-induced nephropathy. In E. Lerma, M. Sparks, & J. Topf (Eds.), *Nephrology secrets: First south asia edition (e-book)*.

Touhy, T., & Jett, K. (2016). *Ebersole & Hess' toward healthy aging: Human needs & nursing response*. St. Louis: Elsevier.

U.S. Renal data systems. (2018). *2018 USRDS Annual data report. Epidemiology of kidney disease in the United States*. Bethesda, MD: National Institutes of Health, National Institute of Diabetes and Digestive and Kidney Diseases. http://www.usrds.org/adr.aspx.

61

Concepts of Care for Patients With Urinary Problems

Carolyn Gersch

http://evolve.elsevier.com/Iggy/

LEARNING OUTCOMES

1. Collaborate with the interprofessional team to coordinate high-quality care and promote urinary ***elimination*** in patients who have problems in the urinary tract.
2. Teach the patient and caregiver(s) how home safety is affected by impaired ***elimination*** resulting from problems in the urinary tract.
3. Identify community resources for patients requiring assistance with incontinence or any chronic urinary tract problem.
4. Teach adults how to decrease the risk for urinary tract infections.
5. Implement nursing interventions to help patients and families cope with the psychosocial impact caused by urinary incontinence or any other chronic problem of the urinary tract.
6. Apply knowledge of anatomy and physiology to assess patients with urinary problems affecting ***elimination.***
7. Use clinical judgement to analyze information from laboratory data and assessment findings in the care of patients with urinary problems.
8. Plan evidence-based nursing care to promote ***elimination*** and prevent complications in patients with urinary problems.

KEY TERMS

anuria Absence of urine output.

bacteremia Also called *urosepsis;* spread of the infection from the urinary tract to the bloodstream.

bacteriuria Presence of bacteria in the urine.

continence Control over the time and place of urine ***elimination.***

cystitis Inflammation of the bladder.

cystocele Herniation of the bladder into the vagina.

dysuria Pain or burning with urination.

frequency Urge to urinate frequently in small amounts.

hematuria Presence of red blood cells (RBCs) in the urine; blood in the urine.

hydronephrosis Enlargement of the kidney caused by blockage of urine lower in the tract and filling of the kidney with urine.

hydroureter Enlargement of the ureter.

incontinence Involuntary loss of urine.

intracorporeal Inside the body.

intravesical Inside the bladder.

interstitial cystitis A painful inflammatory bladder condition.

lithotripsy Extracorporeal *shock wave lithotripsy* (SWL) is the use of sound, laser, or dry shock waves to break the stone into small fragments.

nephrolithiasis Formation of stones in the kidney.

oliguria Scant urine output.

pyuria Presence of white blood cells (WBCs) in the urine.

radical cystectomy Removal of the bladder and surrounding tissue.

renal colic Term used to describe the severe flank pain resulting from stones.

stent Small tube that is placed in the ureter by ureteroscopy to dilate the ureter and enlarge the passageway for the stone or stone fragments.

trabeculation Abnormal thickening of the bladder wall caused by urinary retention and obstruction.

ureterolithiasis Formation of stones in the ureter.

urethritis Inflammation of the urethra that can result from infectious and noninfectious conditions.

urgency Feeling that urination will occur immediately.

urolithiasis Presence of *calculi* (stones) in the urinary tract.

urosepsis Also called *bacteremia;* spread of the infection from the urinary tract to the bloodstream.

PRIORITY AND INTERRELATED CONCEPTS

The priority concept for this chapter is:
- ***Elimination***

The ***Elimination*** concept exemplar for this chapter is Urinary Incontinence.

The interrelated concepts for this chapter are:
- ***Pain***
- ***Immunity***
- ***Tissue Integrity***

The urinary tract includes the ureters, bladder, and urethra. Although these structures play no role in the making of urine, their functions are essential for the urine made by the kidneys to be eliminated from the body. Both infectious and noninfectious problems in the urinary tract can disrupt urinary ***elimination*** and affect control of fluids, electrolytes, nitrogenous wastes, and blood pressure.

Any urinary problem can affect the storage or ***elimination*** of urine. Both acute and chronic urinary problems are common and costly. For urinary tract infections (UTIs) there were more than 7 million office visits, 1 million emergency department visits, and more than 100,000 hospitalizations costing over $1.6 billion in the United States between 2008 and 2011 (Simmering et al., 2017). In addition, many other people sought treatment for kidney and ureter stones, urinary incontinence, urologic trauma, and cancer involving the urinary system. Although life-threatening complications are rare with urinary problems, patients may have functional, physical, and psychosocial changes that reduce quality of life. Nursing interventions are directed toward prevention, early detection, and early management of urologic disorders.

ELIMINATION CONCEPT EXEMPLAR: URINARY INCONTINENCE

Pathophysiology Review

Continence is the control over the time and place of ***elimination***. Urinary continence is specific to control over urinary elimination and is a learned behavior. Efficient bladder emptying (i.e., coordination between bladder contraction and urethral relaxation) is needed for continence. Continence occurs when pressure in the urethra is greater than pressure in the bladder. For normal voiding to occur, the urethra must relax and the bladder must contract with enough pressure and duration to empty completely. Voiding normally occurs in a smooth and coordinated manner under conscious control.

Urinary incontinence (UI) is an involuntary loss of urine severe enough to cause social or hygienic problems. It is *not* a normal consequence of aging or childbirth and often is a stigmatizing and an underreported health problem. Many adults suffer in silence, are socially isolated, and may be unaware that treatment is available. In addition, the cost of incontinence can be enormous (Zhang, 2018).

Urinary incontinence has several possible causes (Table 61.1). Except for infection, temporary causes of incontinence usually do not involve a disorder of the urinary tract. The most common types of adult urinary incontinence are stress incontinence, urge incontinence, overflow incontinence, functional incontinence, and a mixed form of incontinence.

Stress incontinence is the most common type urinary incontinence in younger women (Lukacz et al., 2017). Its main feature is the inability to retain urine when laughing, coughing, sneezing, jogging, or lifting. In the continent adult, the urethra can be relaxed and tightened under conscious control because skeletal muscles of the pelvic floor surround it. When an adult feels the urge to urinate, the conscious contraction of the urethra can override a bladder contraction if the urethral contraction is strong enough. Patients with *stress incontinence* cannot tighten the urethra enough to overcome the increased bladder pressure caused by contraction of the detrusor muscle.

Urge incontinence is the loss of urine for no apparent reason after suddenly feeling the need or urge to urinate. Normally when the bladder is full, contraction of the smooth muscle fibers of the bladder detrusor muscle signals the brain that it is time to urinate. Continent adults override that signal and relax the detrusor muscle for the time it takes to locate a toilet. Those who suffer from urge incontinence cannot suppress the signal and have a sudden strong urge to void and can leak large amounts of urine at this time. Urge incontinence is also known as an *overactive bladder (OAB)* and is more common in older women.

Overflow incontinence occurs when the detrusor muscle fails to contract and the bladder becomes overdistended. This type of incontinence (*reflex incontinence* or *underactive bladder*) occurs when the bladder has reached its maximum capacity and some urine must leak out to prevent bladder rupture. It is important to note that more than one type of incontinence can exist at the same time. This is called *mixed incontinence* and is a combination of stress and urge incontinence.

Functional incontinence occurs as a result of factors other than the abnormal function of the bladder and urethra. A common factor is the loss of cognitive function in patients affected by dementia.

Etiology. Urinary incontinence may have temporary or permanent causes (see Table 61.1) Evaluation of the patient with urinary incontinence means considering all possible causes, beginning with those that are temporary and correctable. Surgical and traumatic causes of urinary incontinence are related to procedures or surgery in the lower pelvic structures, which are areas that contain complex nerve pathways. Radical urologic, prostatic, and gynecologic procedures for treatment of pelvic cancers may result in urinary incontinence. Injury to segments S2 to S4 of the spinal cord may cause incontinence from impairment of normal nerve pathways.

Inappropriate bladder contraction may result from disorders of the brain and nervous system or from bladder irritation due to chronic infection, stones, chemotherapy, or radiation therapy. Other causes of bladder contraction failure include neuropathies associated with diabetes mellitus, syphilis, and previous treatment with neurotoxic anticancer drugs. Constipation can lead to temporary urinary incontinence. Some drugs or drug-drug interactions from polypharmacy, such as anticholinergics, calcium channel blockers, diuretics, and sedatives, can cause or worsen urinary incontinence.

TABLE 61.1 **Types of Urinary Incontinence**

Type and Description	Causes	Symptoms	Management
Stress Incontinence			
Involuntary loss of urine during activities that increase abdominal and detrusor pressure Inability to tighten the urethra sufficiently to overcome the increased detrusor pressure Leakage of urine	Weakening of bladder neck supports; associated with childbirth Intrinsic sphincter deficiency, such as epispadias (abnormal location of the urethra on the dorsum of the penis) or myelomeningocele Acquired anatomic damage to the urethral sphincter from repeated incontinence surgeries, prostatectomy, radiation therapy, and trauma Vaginal prolapse from vaginal birth or aging	Urine loss with physical exertion, cough, sneeze, or exercise Usually only small amounts of urine are lost with each exertion Normal voiding habits (≤8 times per day, ≤2 times per night) Postvoid residual usually ≤50 mL Pelvic examination shows hypermobility of the urethra or bladder neck with Valsalva maneuvers	Weight reduction for patients who are obese Smoking cessation Pelvic muscle therapy Vaginal cone therapy Bladder training Estrogen therapy for postmenopausal women Electrical stimulation Magnetic resonance therapy Pessary devices Surgery includes slings, bladder suspension, injection of bulking agents, prostatectomy Electrical stimulation device
Urge Incontinence			
Overactive bladder (OAB) Involuntary loss of urine associated with a strong desire to urinate Inability to suppress the signal from the bladder muscle to the brain that it is time to urinate	Idiopathic Neurologic disorders, such as stroke Benign prostatic hypertrophy Bladder inflammation or infection Bladder irritants, such as artificial sweeteners, caffeine, alcohol, citric intake, drugs, nicotine Bladder cancer Medications that cause increased bladder contractility	An abrupt and strong urge to void (urinary urgency) Urinary frequency Nocturia May have loss of large amounts of urine with each occurrence	Bladder training Pelvis muscle therapy Weight reduction for patients who are obese Avoid bladder irritants, such as caffeine and alcohol Smoking cessation Drug therapy if bladder training is not successful: anticholinergics, tricyclic antidepressants with anticholinergic and alpha-adrenergic agonist activity, beta-adrenergic agonist, and onabotulinumtoxinA Electrical stimulation device Surgery includes transurethral resection of the prostate or prostatectomy
Mixed Incontinence			
Combination of stress and urge incontinence	Causes associated with stress and urge incontinence	Symptoms associated with stress and urge incontinence	See management for stress and urge incontinence
Overflow Incontinence (reflex incontinence)			
Involuntary loss of urine associated with overdistention of the bladder when the bladder capacity has reached its maximum Detrusor underactivity Bladder outlet obstruction	Urethral obstruction such as benign prostatic hypertrophy or uterine prolapse Diabetic neuropathy Some neurologic disorders, such as multiple sclerosis or spinal cord damage Medication side effects	Bladder distention, Constant dribbling of urine Sense of incomplete emptying of the bladder Pelvic discomfort Palpable bladder	Bladder training Bladder compression (Credé method) Intermittent self-catheterization Drug therapy if bladder training unsuccessful: bethanechol chloride Nonsurgical treatment unless surgery is required to remove the obstruction: i.e., prostatectomy or repair of uterine prolapse
Functional Incontinence			
Leakage of urine caused by factors other than disease of the lower urinary tract	Decreased cognition such as with dementia Impaired mobility, such as paralysis or inability to walk to the toilet; some neurologic disorders	Quantity and timing of urine leakage vary Patterns difficult to discern	Habit training Prompted voiding is used to establish a predictable pattern of bladder emptying to prevent incontinence Applied devices: Intravaginal pessaries Penile clamps Condom catheter Intermittent or long-term catheterization

PATIENT-CENTERED CARE: OLDER ADULT CONSIDERATIONS QSEN

Many factors contribute to urinary incontinence in older adults (see the Patient-Centered Care: Older Adult Considerations: Factors Contributing to Urinary Incontinence box). An older adult may have decreased mobility from many causes. In inpatient settings, mobility is limited when the older patient is placed on bedrest. Vision and hearing impairments may also prevent the patient from locating a call light to notify the nurse or assistive personnel of the need to void. Assess for these factors and minimize them to prevent urinary incontinence. Getting out of bed to urinate is a common cause of falls among older adults in the home and other settings (Touhy & Jett, 2016).

PATIENT-CENTERED CARE: OLDER ADULT CONSIDERATIONS QSEN

Factors Contributing to Urinary Incontinence[a]

Drugs

- Central nervous system depressants, such as opioid analgesics, decrease the patient's level of consciousness and the urge to void and contribute to constipation.
- Diuretics cause frequent voiding, often of large amounts of urine.
- Multiple drugs can contribute to changes in mental status or mobility, and they can irritate the bladder.
- Anticholinergic drugs or drugs with anticholinergic side effects are especially challenging because they affect both cognition and the ability to void. Monitor patient responses to these drugs early in treatment.

Disease

- Stroke, Parkinson disease, dementia, and other neurologic disorders decrease mobility, sensation, or cognition.
- Arthritis decreases mobility and causes *pain.*

Depression

- Depression decreases the energy necessary to maintain continence.
- Decreased self-esteem and feelings of self-worth decrease the importance to the patient of maintaining continence.

Inadequate Resources

- Patients who need assistive devices (e.g., eyeglasses, cane, walker) may be afraid to ambulate without them or without personal assistance.
- Products that help patients manage incontinence of urine ***elimination*** are often costly.
- No one may be available to assist the patient to the bathroom or help with incontinence products.

[a]These factors are in addition to the physiologic changes of aging given in Chapter 4.

Incidence and Prevalence. Urinary incontinence is a major health problem. The incidence of UI increases with age (Milson & Gyhagen, 2018). Up to 45% of women older than 65 years report some degree of urinary incontinence (Engberg & Li, 2017).

Risk for urinary incontinence increases with chronic conditions such as diabetes mellitus, stroke, cognitive impairment, and impaired mobility. Urinary incontinence occurs not only with older age but with a history of vaginal delivery, particularly if the first child was delivered after age 30. Conditions of pelvic prolapse in women, prostate problems in men, diabetes, heart failure, spinal cord or nerve injury, and obesity also increase the risk for urinary incontinence (Lukacz et al., 2017).). Both central nervous system diseases (i.e., dementia, multiple sclerosis, Parkinson disease) and musculoskeletal disorders (i.e., osteoporosis, osteoarthritis, paresthesia, pain or paralysis) contribute to cognitive and mobility impairment, resulting in the onset and severity of urinary incontinence (Engberg & Li, 2017; McCance & Huether, 2019). Because urinary incontinence is common among older adults, routine screening for incontinence is recommended for all adults 65 years and older (Touhy & Jett, 2016). Older adults who are institutionalized with UI have a higher risk for mortality (Damien et al., 2017). Patients with mild cognitive impairment are 30% more likely to have urinary incontinence (Aoki et al., 2017).

Interprofessional Collaborative Care

Urinary incontinence can occur in any setting and is very common in the community. Usually the adult with incontinence is treated using self-management strategies. Even when surgical intervention is used, hospitalization for incontinence is rare. Because urinary incontinence carries a burden of impaired comfort, activity disruption, shame or embarrassment, and loss of ***tissue integrity,*** it has a great impact on quality of life for most adults.

Assessment: Recognize Cues

History. Incontinence may be underreported because health care professionals do not ask patients about urine loss. Ask patients about incontinence as many patients are hesitant to initiate the subject. (Lukacz et al., 2017). Effective screening includes asking patients to respond "always," "sometimes," or "never" to these questions:

- Do you ever leak urine or water when you don't want to?
- Do you ever leak urine or water when you cough, sneeze, laugh, or exercise?
- Do you ever leak urine or water on the way to the toilet?
- Do you ever use pads, tissue, or cloth in your underwear to catch urine?

If any answer is "always" or "sometimes," perform a focused assessment (see the Focused Assessment: The Patient with Urinary Incontinence box).

Physical Assessment/Signs and Symptoms. Assess the abdomen to estimate bladder fullness, rule out palpable hard stool, and evaluate bowel sounds. Urinary incontinence is confirmed by evaluating the force and character of the urine stream during voiding. Ask the patient to cough while wearing a perineal pad to assess for stress incontinence; a wet pad on forceful coughing indicates stress incontinence.

For women, inspect the external genitalia to determine whether there is apparent urethral or uterine prolapse, cystocele (herniation of the bladder into the vagina), or rectocele. These conditions occur with pelvic floor muscle weakness. A primary health care provider puts on an examination glove and inserts two fingers into the vagina to assess the strength of these muscles. Strength is described as *weak, adequate,* or *strong* based on the amount of pressure felt by the primary health care provider

FOCUSED ASSESSMENT

The Patient With Urinary Incontinence

Note the presence of risk factors for urinary incontinence:

- Age
- If female, menopausal status
- Central or peripheral neurologic disease with associated impairment in cognition or mobility
- Diabetes mellitus
- History of vaginal delivery; vaginal prolapse
- Urologic procedures
- Prescribed and over-the-counter drugs that affect cognition or mobility
- Bowel patterns; fecal impaction
- Stress/anxiety level

Detail the symptoms of urinary incontinence:

- Leakage
- Frequency
- Urgency
- Nocturia
- Sensation of full bladder before leakage

Obtain a 24-hour intake-and-output record or a voiding diary:

- Time and amount of oral intake and continent voiding
- Time and estimated amount of incontinent leakages
- Activity around the time of leakage

Assess the patient's:

- Mobility
- Self-care ability
- Cognitive ability
- Communication patterns

Assess the environment for barriers to toileting:

- Privacy
- Restrictive clothing
- Access to toilet

as the patient tightens vaginal muscles. Describe and document the color, consistency, and odor of any secretions from the genitourinary orifices. The urine stream interruption test (i.e., asking a patient to voluntarily start and stop urine flow during a void at least twice) is another method of determining pelvic muscle strength. For men, inspect the urethral meatus for any discharge.

A digital rectal examination (DRE) is performed by the primary health care provider on both male and female patients. It provides information about the nerve integrity to the bladder. The examiner determines whether there is tactile sensation in the anal area by observing whether the rectal sphincter is relaxed or contracted on digital insertion. Because nerve supply to the bladder is similar to nerve supply to the rectum, the presence of tactile sensation and a rectal sphincter that contracts suggest that the nerve supply to the bladder is intact. Impaction of stool is a cause of transient urinary incontinence and can be detected during a rectal examination. The primary health care provider assesses for prostate enlargement in men as a possible cause of incontinence.

Laboratory Assessment. A urinalysis is useful to rule out urinary tract infection. This test is the first step in the assessment of incontinent patients of any age. The presence of red blood cells (RBCs), white blood cells (WBCs), leukocyte esterase, or nitrites is an indication for culturing the urine. Any infection is treated before further assessment of incontinence.

Imaging Assessment. Determine the amount of postvoid residual urine (urine remaining in the bladder right after voiding) by portable ultrasound (bladder scanner). If prescribed, catheterizing the patient immediately after voiding can also be used to assess residual volume. Additional imaging is needed when surgery is being considered. CT is most useful for locating abnormalities in kidneys and ureters. A voiding cystourethrogram (VCUG) or urodynamic testing may be performed to assess the size, shape, support, and function of the urinary tract system. Urodynamic testing (see Chapter 60) may take several hours and more than one visit. Electromyography (EMG) of the pelvic muscles may be a part of the urodynamic studies.

◆ Analysis: Analyze Cues and Prioritize Hypotheses. The priority collaborative problems for patients with urinary incontinence include:

1. Altered urinary ***elimination*** due to incontinence
2. Potential for altered ***tissue integrity***

◆ Planning and Implementation: Generate Solutions and Take Action

Planning: Expected Outcomes. The expected outcomes for altered urinary incontinence are to maintain optimal urinary ***elimination***, ***tissue integrity***, and comfort. Nursing interventions for the management of the different types of urinary incontinence focus on restoring continence, psychosocial comfort, tissue integrity, and patient education.

Promoting Urinary Elimination. With appropriate therapy, the patient with altered urinary elimination due to incontinence is expected to develop continence of urine ***elimination.*** Indicators include that the patient consistently or often demonstrates these actions:

- Stress urinary incontinence: No urine leakage between voidings and no urine leakage with increased abdominal pressure (e.g., sneezing, laughing, lifting)
- Urge urinary incontinence: Responds to urge in a timely manner, gets to toilet between urge and passage of urine, and avoids substances that stimulate the bladder (e.g., caffeine, alcohol)
- Overflow urinary incontinence: Recognizes the urge to void, maintains a predictable pattern of voiding, empties bladder completely, and keeps urine volume in the bladder under 300 mL
- Functional urinary incontinence: Uses urine containment or collection measures to ensure dryness and manages clothing independently

Nonsurgical Management. Maintaining a diary can be beneficial for patients with stress incontinence to determine patterns of the incontinent events. Patients may use collection devices, absorbent pads, and undergarments during the often lengthy process of assessment and treatment of urinary incontinence and by patients who elect not to pursue further interventions.

Nutrition Therapy. Nutrition therapy plays a role in specific types of urinary incontinence. Nutrition therapy with weight reduction is helpful for patients who are obese because stress incontinence is made worse by increased abdominal pressure from obesity (Lukacz et al., 2017). Teach the patient to avoid bladder irritants in the diet, such as caffeine and alcohol, that can contribute to urgency and frequency. Stress the importance of maintaining an adequate fluid intake, especially water. Refer the patient to a registered dietitian as needed.

Drug Therapy. Drug therapy with topical estrogen to the perineal and vaginal orifice is used to treat postmenopausal women with stress incontinence. Estrogen may increase the blood flow and tone of the muscles around the vagina and urethra, thus improving the patient's ability to contract those muscles during times of increased intra-abdominal stress.

Because the hypertonic bladder contracts involuntarily in patients with urge incontinence, drugs that relax the smooth muscle and increase the bladder's capacity are prescribed (see the Common Examples of Drug Therapy: Urinary Incontinence box). The most commonly prescribed drugs are anticholinergics (also known as *antimuscarinics* because they target specific receptors in the cholinergic family of receptors), which include darifenacin, fesoterodine, oxybutynin, propiverine (only available in Canada), solifenacin, tolterodine, and trospium. Some of these drugs are available over the counter. This class of drugs has serious side effects, particularly for older adults, and is used along with behavioral interventions. These drugs inhibit the nerve fibers that stimulate bladder contraction. In addition, tricyclic antidepressants with anticholinergic and alpha-adrenergic agonist activity, such as imipramine, have been used successfully in younger patients for enuresis.

A beta-adrenergic agonist, mirabegron, has demonstrated effectiveness in reducing urge incontinence. The evidence comparing different drug categories for effectiveness in managing incontinence is limited, and no single drug or class is recommended over another.

Another drug therapy for urge incontinence is onabotulinumtoxinA (Botox). This drug is injected during cystoscopy into multiple areas of the detrusor muscle of the bladder. Usually 10 to 30 different sites are injected during one treatment session. This treatment relaxes the detrusor muscle and relieves the urge to urinate (Hubb et al., 2018). Some patients have relief of incontinence for as long as 6 to 9 months after injection. Side effects may include urinary retention, painful urination, and an increased incidence of urinary tract infections. For most patients who experience urinary retention, the condition is temporary but does require intermittent self-catheterization.

Drugs are prescribed for short-term management of urinary retention seen in overflow incontinence, often after surgery. They are not used in long-term management of overflow incontinence caused by a hypotonic bladder. The most commonly used drug is bethanechol chloride, an agent that increases bladder pressure.

! NURSING SAFETY PRIORITY (QSEN)

Drug Alert

Teach patients taking the extended-release forms of anticholinergic drugs to swallow the tablet or capsule whole without chewing or crushing. Chewing or crushing the tablet/capsule destroys the extended-release feature, allowing the entire dose to be absorbed quickly, which increases adverse drug side effects.

Devices. Devices can be used to assist with continence. A **pessary** (plastic device, often ring shaped, that helps hold internal organs in place) inserted into the vagina may help with a prolapsed uterus or bladder when this condition is contributing to urinary incontinence. A prolapse occurs when the supportive tissue in the vagina weakens and stretches, allowing pelvic organs to protrude into the vaginal lumen. The pessary presses against the wall of the vagina to reposition pelvic organs. Generally, a pessary is removed and cleaned with soap and water on a monthly basis by the patient, but the nurse can do it for adults with cognitive or musculoskeletal impairment.

Urethral occlusion devices (urethral plugs) can be helpful for activity-induced incontinence. One device, the Reliance insert, is like a small tampon that the patient inserts into the urethra. After insertion, the patient inflates a tiny balloon, which rests at the bladder neck and prevents the flow of urine. To void, the patient pulls a string to deflate the balloon and removes the device. The applicator is reusable, although the tampon part is disposed of after each void.

Applied devices for functional urinary incontinence include intravaginal pessaries for women and penile clamps for men. The intravaginal pessary supports the uterus and vagina and helps maintain the correct position of the bladder. (See Chapter 66 for further discussion of pessaries.) The penile clamp is applied around the outside of the penis to compress the urethra and prevent urine leakage. Adverse outcomes from pessaries and penile clamps include reduced ***tissue integrity*** with tissue damage from pressure and infection from colonization of damaged tissues. Both devices require that the patient have either manual dexterity or a caregiver to apply and remove the device. Instruct the patient or caregivers in the use of these devices.

Male patients may use an external collecting device, such as a condom catheter. In acute care settings, the Pickwick, a female external collecting device, has demonstrated promise in effectively collecting urine and preventing tissue damage due to urinary leakage (Beeson & Davis, 2018). The Pickwick female external catheter is a tube that lies between the labia next to the urethral opening and extends between the buttocks. The tube is secured to the suprapubic area and is attached to low, continuous suction to wick away urine as it leaks from the urethral opening. This external urinary collection device is effective for patients who are lying down or in the sitting position.

Electrical Stimulation. Electrical stimulation with either an intravaginal or intrarectal electrical stimulation device is available to treat urge, stress, and mixed incontinence. Treatment consists of stimulating sensory nerves to decrease the sensation of urgency. It is done as an office-based procedure one to three times weekly for 6 to 8 weeks.

Magnetic Resonance Therapy. Magnetic resonance therapy involves targeted urinary tract nerves and muscles for depolarization. The patient sits on a chair containing a magnetic device that induces depolarization and helps reduce stress-induced incontinence similar to drug-induced relaxation of muscle and nerves.

Pelvic Muscle Therapy. Pelvic muscle (Kegel) exercise therapy for women with stress incontinence strengthens the muscles of the pelvic floor (circumvaginal muscles). These muscles become strengthened, as any other skeletal muscle

COMMON EXAMPLES OF DRUG THERAPY

Urinary Incontinence

Drug Category	Nursing Implications
Hormones	
Thought to enhance nerve conduction to the urinary tract, improve blood flow, and reduce tissue deterioration of the urinary tract	
Estrogen vaginal cream daily or an estrogen-containing ring inserted monthly	Teach patients to use only a thin application of the cream *to minimize excessive absorption and distribution and avoid systemic side effects.* Teach patients that it takes 4-6 weeks to achieve continence benefits and that benefits disappear about 4 weeks after discontinuing regular use *because knowing the drug responses increases the likelihood of its correct use.*
Anticholinergics	
Suppress involuntary bladder contraction and increase bladder capacity	
Darifenacin Fesoterodine Oxybutynin Solifenacin Tolterodine Trospium	Ask whether the patient has glaucoma before starting any drugs from this class *because anticholinergics can increase intraocular pressure and make glaucoma worse.* Suggest that patients increase fluid intake and use hard candy to moisten the mouth *to reduce the dry mouth side effect.* Teach patients to increase fluid intake and the amount of dietary fiber *to prevent constipation associated with this drug category.* Teach patients to monitor urine output and to report an output significantly lower than intake to the primary health care provider *because all of these drugs can cause urinary retention, especially for men with an enlarged prostate.* Instruct patients taking the extended-release forms of these drugs not to chew or crush the tablet/capsule *to avoid both ruining the time-release feature and increasing the risk for a bolus dose with more side effects.*
Alpha-Adrenergic Agonists	
Increase contractile force of the urethral sphincter, increasing resistance to urine outflow	
Midodrine[a]	Teach the patient to monitor his or her blood pressure periodically when starting the *drug because this drug can cause severe supine hypertension and should not be used in patients with severe cardiac disease.*
Beta$_3$ Agonists	
Relax the detrusor smooth muscle to increase bladder capacity and urine storage	
Mirabegron	Teach the patient to periodically obtain a blood pressure and to inform the health care provider if the systolic or diastolic values increase more than 10 mm Hg or above 180/110 *because this drug has the potential to increase blood pressure.* If the patient is taking warfarin, avoid this drug or schedule additional blood testing for potential increased risk for bleeding *because this drug uses the same metabolic pathway as warfarin and can potentiate warfarin's effects, leading to a prolonged international normalized ratio (INR) and increase the risk for bleeding.*
Antidepressants: Tricyclics and Serotonin-Norepinephrine Reuptake Inhibitors (SNRIs)	
Increase norepinephrine and serotonin levels, which are thought to strengthen the urinary sphincters; also have anticholinergic actions	
Tricyclics: Imipramine Amitriptyline *SNRI:* Duloxetine[a]	Warn patients not to combine these drugs with other antidepressant drugs *to avoid a drug-drug interaction that can lead to a hypertensive crisis.* Instruct patients to inform their primary health care provider if they take drugs to manage hypertension. Teach patients to change positions slowly, especially in the morning *to avoid dizziness from orthostatic hypotension, which increases the risk for falls.* Teach patients the same interventions as for anticholinergic agents *because these drugs have anticholinergic activity and can produce the same side effects.*

[a]These drugs are used off label and do not have U.S. Food and Drug Administration (FDA) approval for use to treat incontinence. However, they are commonly used to manage incontinence syndromes.

does, by frequent, systematic, and repeated contractions. Pelvic floor muscle training improves not only continence but also quality of life in women with stress urinary incontinence (Aoki et al., 2017). The most important step in teaching pelvic muscle exercises is to help the patient learn which muscles to exercise. During the pelvic examination in women and the rectal examination in men or women, instruct the patient to tighten the pelvic muscles around your fingers. Then provide feedback about the strength of the contraction. Starting and stopping the urine stream or stopping the passage of flatus indicates that the patient has correctly identified the pelvic muscles. Biofeedback devices, such as electromyography or perineometers, measure the strength of contraction. A perineometer is a tampon-shaped instrument inserted into the vagina to measure the strength of pelvic muscle contractions. The graph shows the amplitude of muscle contraction to the patient for biofeedback. Alternatively, retention of a vaginal weight also shows that the patient has identified the proper muscle (see discussion on vaginal cone therapy).

Instructions for pelvic muscle exercises are provided in the Patient and Family Education: Preparing for Self-Management: Pelvic Muscle Exercises box. Although improvement may take several months, most patients notice a positive change after 6 weeks. Teach patients to continue the exercises 10 times daily to improve and maintain pelvic muscle strength.

Pelvic muscle exercises are also effective for urge incontinence and are taught in the same way as for stress incontinence. Improved urethral resistance helps the patient overcome abnormal detrusor contractions long enough to get to the toilet.

PATIENT AND FAMILY EDUCATION: PREPARING FOR SELF-MANAGEMENT

Pelvic Muscle Exercises

- The pelvic muscles are composed of a sling of muscles that support your bladder, urethra, and vagina. Like any other muscles in your body, you can make your pelvic muscles stronger by alternately contracting (tightening) and relaxing them in regular exercise periods. By strengthening these muscles, you will be able to stop your urine flow more effectively.
- To identify your pelvic muscles, sit on the toilet with your feet flat on the floor about 12 inches apart. Begin to urinate, and then try to stop the urine flow. Do not strain down, lift your bottom off the seat, or squeeze your legs together. When you start and stop your urine stream, you are using your pelvic muscles.
- To perform pelvic muscle exercises, tighten your pelvic muscles for a slow count of 10 and then relax for a slow count of 10. Do this exercise 15 times while you are lying down, sitting up, and standing (a total of 45 exercises). Repeat—and this time rapidly contract and relax the pelvic muscles 10 times. This should take no more than 10 to 12 minutes for all three positions, or 3 to 4 minutes for each set of 15 exercises.
- Begin with 45 exercises a day in three sets of 15 exercises each. You will notice faster improvement if you can do this twice a day, or a total of 20 minutes each day. Remember to exercise in all three positions so your muscles learn to squeeze effectively despite your position. At first, it is helpful to have a designated time and place to do these exercises because you will have to concentrate to do them correctly. After you have been doing them for several weeks, you will notice improvement in your control of urine. However, many people report that improvement may take as long as 3 months.

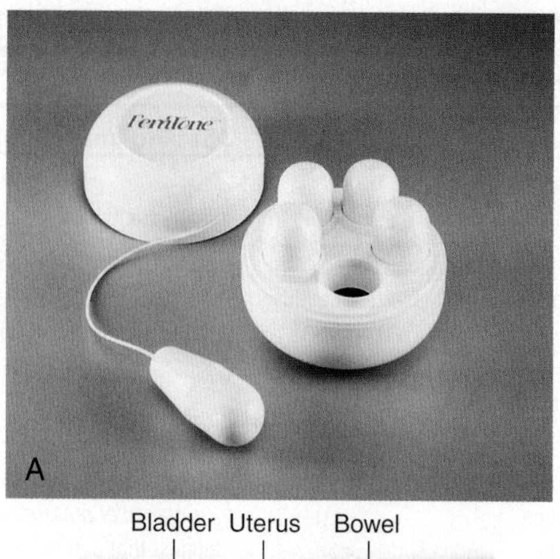

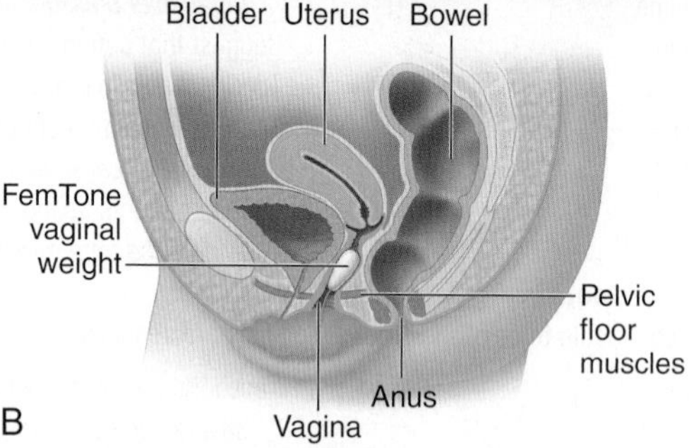

FIG. 61.1 A, FemTone vaginal weights, or cones. The number on the top of each cone represents increasing weight up to the heaviest cone, a *5*. B, Diagram showing the correct positioning of a vaginal weight, or cone, in place. (A Courtesy ConvaTec, A Bristol-Meyers Squibb Company, a Division of E.R. Squibb & Sons, Inc., Princeton, NJ.)

Vaginal Cone Therapy. *Vaginal cone weight therapy* involves using a set of five small, cone-shaped weights (Touhy & Jett, 2016). They are of equal size but of varying weights and are used together with pelvic muscle exercise. The woman inserts the lightest cone, labeled 1, into her vagina (Fig. 61.1A), with the string to the outside, for a 1-minute test period. If she can hold the first cone in place without its slipping out while she walks around, she proceeds to the second cone, labeled 2, and repeats the procedure. The patient begins her treatment with the heaviest cone she can comfortably hold in her vagina for the 1-minute test period. Treatment periods are 15 minutes twice a day. When the patient can comfortably hold the cone in her vagina for 15 minutes, she progresses to the next heaviest weight. Treatment is completed with the cone labeled 5.

Weighted vaginal cones can help strengthen the pelvic muscles and decrease stress incontinence but may not help pelvic prolapse. Vaginal cones do not require a prescription.

Behavioral Interventions. Other interventions for urinary incontinence may include behavior modification or training (i.e., bladder training [see the Best Practice for Patient Safety & Quality Care: Bladder Training and Habit Training to Reduce Urinary Incontinence box]). Bladder training involves a great deal of patient participation and often begins with a thorough explanation of the problem of urge incontinence. Instead of the bladder being in control of the patient, the patient learns to control the bladder. For the program to succeed, the patient must be alert, aware, and able to resist the urge to urinate (Aoki et al., 2017).

Start a schedule for voiding, beginning with the longest interval that is comfortable for the patient, even if the interval is only 30 minutes. Instruct the patient to void every 30 minutes and to ignore any urge to urinate between the set intervals. Once the patient is comfortable with the starting schedule, increase the interval by 15 to 30 minutes. Instruct the patient to follow the new schedule until achieving success again. As the interval increases, the bladder gradually tolerates more volume. Teach relaxation and distraction techniques to maximize success in the retraining. Provide positive reinforcement for maintaining the prescribed schedule.

Habit training (scheduled toileting) is a type of bladder training that is successful in reducing incontinence in cognitively impaired patients. To use habit training, caregivers help the patient void at specific times (e.g., every 2 hours on the even hours). The goal is to get the patient to the toilet before incontinence occurs. The focus is on reducing incontinence and resulting loss of tissue integrity. When a reduction in incontinence has been achieved, the focus may change to increasing bladder capacity by gradually lengthening the voiding intervals, but this is only secondary.

Prompted voiding, a supplement to habit training, attempts to increase the patient's awareness of the need to void and to prompt him or her to ask for toileting assistance. Habit training otherwise relies completely on a time schedule.

BEST PRACTICE FOR PATIENT SAFETY & QUALITY CARE QSEN

Bladder Training and Habit Training to Reduce Urinary Incontinence

Bladder Training

- Assess the patient's awareness of bladder fullness and ability to cooperate with training regimen.
- Assess the patient's 24-hour urine *elimination* pattern for 2 to 3 consecutive days (bladder diary).
- Base the initial interval of toileting on the voiding pattern (e.g., 45 minutes).
- Teach the patient to void every 45 minutes on the first day and to ignore or suppress the urge to urinate between the 45-minute intervals.
- Take the patient to the toilet or remind him or her to urinate at the 45-minute intervals.
- Provide privacy for toileting and run water in the sink to promote the urge to urinate at this time.
- If the patient is not consistently able to resist the urge to urinate between the intervals, reduce the intervals by 15 minutes.
- Continue this regimen for at least 24 hours or for as many days as it takes for the patient to be comfortable with this schedule and not urinate between the intervals.
- When the patient remains continent between the intervals, increase the intervals by 15 minutes daily until a 3- to 4-hour interval is comfortable for the patient.
- Praise successes. If incontinence occurs, work with the patient to re-establish an acceptable toileting interval.

Habit Training

- Assess the patient's 24-hour voiding pattern for 2 to 3 days.
- Base the initial interval of toileting on the voiding pattern (e.g., 2 hours).
- Help the patient to the toilet or provide a bedpan/urinal every 2 hours (or whatever has been determined to be an appropriate toileting interval for the individual patient).
- During the toileting, remind the patient to void and provide cues such as running water.
- If the patient is incontinent between scheduled toileting, reduce the time interval by 30 minutes until the patient is continent between voidings.
- Help the patient to toilet and prompt to void at prescribed intervals.
- Do not leave the patient on the toilet or bedpan for longer than 5 minutes.
- Ensure that all nursing staff members comply with the established toileting schedule and do not apply briefs or encourage the patient to "just wet the bed."
- Reduce toileting interval by 30 minutes if there are more than two incontinence episodes in 24 hours.
- If the patient remains continent at the toileting interval, attempt to increase the interval by 30 minutes until a 3- to 4-hour continence interval is reached.
- Praise the patient for successes and spend extra time socializing with the patient.
- Discuss daily record of continence with staff to provide reinforcement and encourage compliance with toileting schedule.
- Include assistive personnel in all aspects of the habit training.

! NURSING SAFETY PRIORITY QSEN

Action Alert

Habit training is undermined when absorbent briefs are used in place of timed toileting. Do not tell patients to "just wet the bed." A common cause of falls in health care facilities is related to patient efforts to get out of bed unassisted to use the toilet. Collaborate with all staff members, including assistive personnel (AP), to consistently implement the toileting schedule for habit training.

For overflow incontinence, the most effective common behavioral interventions are bladder compression and intermittent self-catheterization. Bladder compression uses techniques that promote bladder emptying and include the Credé method, the Valsalva maneuver, double-voiding, and splinting.

For the Credé method, teach the patient how to press over the bladder area, increasing the pressure, or to trigger nerve stimulation by tugging at pubic hair or massaging the genital area. These techniques manually help the bladder empty. In the Valsalva maneuver, breathing techniques increase chest and abdominal pressure. This increased pressure is then directed toward the bladder during exhalation. (The Valsalva maneuver is contraindicated in patients who have some cardiac problems because it can trigger a vagal response and cause bradycardia.) With the technique of double-voiding, the patient empties the bladder and then, within a few minutes, attempts a second bladder emptying.

For women who have a large cystocele (prolapse of the bladder into the vagina), a technique called splinting both compresses the bladder and moves it into a better position. The woman inserts her fingers into her vagina, gently lifts the cystocele, and begins to urinate. A pessary, described earlier, can also provide relief from cystocele-related incontinence.

Intermittent self-catheterization is often used to help patients with long-term problems of incomplete bladder emptying. It is effective, can be learned fairly easily, and remains the preferred method of bladder emptying in patients who have incontinence as a result of a neurogenic bladder (Beauchemin et al., 2018). These points are important in teaching the technique:

- Proper handwashing and cleaning of the catheter reduce the risk for infection.
- A small lumen and good lubrication of the catheter prevent urethral trauma.
- A regular schedule for bladder emptying prevents distention and mucosal trauma.

Patients must be able to understand instructions and have the manual dexterity to manipulate the catheter. Caregivers or family members in the home can also be taught to perform intermittent catheterization using clean (rather than sterile) technique with good outcomes (Beauchemin et al., 2018).

Surgical Interventions. Stress incontinence may be treated by a surgical sling or bladder suspension procedure (Table 61.2). A sling procedure creates a sling around the bladder neck and urethra using strips of body tissue or synthetic mesh. Midurethral sling procedures are particularly effective for stress urinary incontinence (Clemens, 2018). Bladder suspension procedures are more extensive than sling procedures, and the surgeon sutures tissue near the bladder neck to a pubic bone ligament to provide support and prevent sagging. A third surgical procedure is the injection of bulking agents into the urethral wall to provide resistance to urine outflow. Bulking agents include collagen, carbon-coated zirconium beads, and silicone implants. Interventions for the patient with overflow (reflex) incontinence caused by obstruction of the bladder outlet may include surgery to relieve the obstruction. The most

TABLE 61.2 Surgical Procedures for Stress Incontinence

Procedure	Purpose	Nursing Considerations
Anterior vaginal repair (colporrhaphy)	Elevates the urethral position and repairs any cystocele	Because the operation is performed by vaginal incision, it is often done in conjunction with a vaginal hysterectomy. Recovery is usually rapid, and a urethral catheter is in place for 24-48 hr.
Retropubic suspension (Marshall-Marchetti-Krantz or Burch colposuspension)	Elevates the urethral position and provides longer-lasting results	The operation requires a low abdominal incision and a urethral or suprapubic catheter for several days after. Recovery takes longer, and urinary retention and detrusor instability are the most frequent complications.
Needle bladder neck suspension (Pereyra or Stamey procedure)	Elevates the urethral position and provides longer-lasting results without a long operative time	The combined vaginal approach with a needle and a small suprapubic skin incision does not allow direct vision of the operative site; however, the high complication rates may be due to the selection of patients who, because of their medical condition, are not good candidates for longer retropubic procedures.
Pubovaginal sling procedures	A sling made of synthetic or fascial material is placed under the ureterovesical junction to elevate the bladder neck.	The operation uses an abdominal, vaginal, or combined approach to treat intrinsic sphincter deficiencies. Temporary or permanent urinary retention is common after surgery.
Midurethral sling procedures	A tensionless vaginal sling is made from polypropylene mesh (or other materials) and placed near the ureterovesical junction to increase the angle, which inhibits movement of urine into the urethra with lower intravesical pressures.	This ambulatory surgery procedure uses a vaginal approach to improve symptoms of stress incontinence. Temporary or permanent urinary retention is common after surgery.
Artificial sphincters	A mechanical device to open and close the urethra is placed around the anatomic urethra.	The operation is done more frequently in men. The most common complications include mechanical failure of the device, erosion of tissue, and infection.
Periurethral injection of collagen or Siloxane	Implantation of small amounts of an inert substance through several small injections provides support around the bladder neck.	The procedure can be done in an ambulatory care setting and can be repeated as often as needed. Certain compounds may migrate after injection; an allergy test to bovine collagen must be performed before implantation.

common procedures are prostate removal (see Chapter 67) and repair of uterine prolapse (see Chapter 66).

Preoperative Care. Teach the patient about the procedure, and clarify the surgeon's explanation of events surrounding the surgery. In contrast to stress urinary incontinence, urge urinary incontinence requires extensive preoperative testing for diagnosis and selection of surgery. The patient may need emotional support during this extensive diagnostic work-up. Surgical procedures and preoperative and postoperative management are described in Table 61.2.

Postoperative Care. After surgery, assess for and intervene to prevent or detect complications. For prevention of movement or traction on the bladder neck, secure the urethral catheter with tape or a tube holder. If a suprapubic catheter is used instead of a urethral catheter, monitor the dressing for urine leakage and other drainage. Catheters are usually in place until the patient can urinate easily and has residual urine volume of less than 50 mL after voiding. (See Chapter 9 for general care before and after surgery.)

Maintaining Tissue Integrity. A major concern with the use of wearable protective pads is the risk for skin breakdown (loss of ***tissue integrity***). Some patients develop incontinence-associated dermatitis (IAD) even when the skin is kept free of contact with urine (Gray et al., 2016). The wearable pads generate heat and sweat in the area that can cause dermatitis. Materials and costs of protective pads vary. Some are reusable; others are disposable. Avoid use of the word "diaper" when discussing these adult pants because of the association of diapers with a baby. More acceptable terms are "briefs" and "pads." Identifying patients at risk for IAD is important to prevent IAD episodes and maintain tissue integrity. Risk factors may include patients with functional, physical, cognitive, and mobility alterations (Bliss et al., 2017). See Chapter 23 for more information about IAD.

When external devices (condom catheter or female urinary collection device) or containment materials are needed, discuss the possible options and help the patient make a selection that is best for his or her lifestyle and resources. Containment is achieved with absorbent pads and briefs designed to collect urine and keep the patient's skin and clothing dry. Many types and sizes of pads are available:

- Shields or liners inserted inside a panty
- Undergarments that are full-size pads with waist straps
- Plastic-lined protective underpants
- Combination pad and pant systems
- Absorbent bed pads

Correct use of external devices and containment materials is essential to ensure ***tissue integrity*** is maintained (Beeson & Davis, 2018).

Catheterization for control of functional incontinence may be intermittent or involve a long-term catheter. Intermittent catheterization is preferred to a long-term catheter because of the reduced risk for infection (Beauchemin et al., 2018). A long-term urinary catheter is appropriate for patients with altered ***tissue integrity*** who need a dry environment for healing, for those who are terminally ill and need comfort, and for those who are critically ill and require precise measurement of urine output.

CLINICAL JUDGMENT CHALLENGE 61.1

Patient-Centered Care; Evidence-Based Practice

The client is a 45-year-old woman who reports leakage of urine when she sneezes, coughs, and laughs. She states that the problem started several years ago and it occurred only a once or twice a month but now it occurs almost daily. She is able to drive and does not have any motor or sensory dysfunctions; however, she is embarrassed and now is afraid to go anywhere in case she "wets her pants." She states that the problem is because she is getting older and asks how other woman her age handle the leakage. She currently works at home and seldom goes to church or out with her spouse because of the urine leakage. Currently, the client reports using toilet paper in her undergarments so that no one will find out she has a problem with urine leakage. Client history includes seasonal allergies, vaginal deliveries of three full-term infants, and type II diabetes mellitus.

1. **Recognize Cues:** What assessment information in this client situation is the most important and immediate concern for the nurse? (Hint: Identify the **relevant** information *first* to determine what is most important.)
2. **Analyze Cues:** What client conditions are consistent with the **most relevant** information? (Hint: Think about priority collaborative problems that support and contradict the information presented in this situation.)
3. **Prioritize Hypotheses:** Which possibilities or explanations are **most likely** to be present in this client situation? Which possibilities or explanations are the most serious? (Hint: Consider all possibilities and determine their urgency and risk for this client.)
4. **Generate Solutions:** What actions would most likely achieve the desired outcomes for this client? Which actions should be **avoided** or are **potentially harmful**? (Hint: Determine the desired outcomes first to decide which interventions are appropriate and those that should be avoided.)
5. **Take Action:** Which actions are the most appropriate and how should they be implemented? In what **priority order** should they be implemented? (Hint: Consider health teaching, documentation, requested health care provider orders or prescriptions, nursing skills, collaboration with or referral to health team members, etc.)
6. **Evaluate Outcomes:** What client assessment would indicate that the nurse's actions were **effective**? (Hint: Think about signs that would indicate an improvement, decline, or unchanged client condition.)

Care Coordination and Transition Management. Community-based care for the patient with urinary incontinence considers personal, physical, emotional, and social resources. Important personal resources for self-care include mobility and manual dexterity. When planning care, consider who will be the primary caregiver and which factors may influence the effectiveness of the plan. Nonpharmacologic and nonsurgical treatments provide significant clinical benefits with low risk for adverse effects but that these interventions are also associated with poor adherence (Clemens, 2018). Ongoing relationships with primary health care providers may improve adherence.

Home Care Management. Assess the home environment for barriers that limit access to the bathroom. Eliminate hazards that might slow walking or lead to a fall. Such hazards include throw rugs, furniture with legs that extend into the walking area, slippery waxed or polished floors, and poor lighting.

If the patient must climb stairs to reach a bathroom, handrails should be installed and stairs kept free of obstacles. Toilet seat extenders may help provide the right level and height of seating so that maximal abdominal pressure may be applied for voiding.

PATIENT AND FAMILY EDUCATION: PREPARING FOR SELF-MANAGEMENT

Urinary Incontinence

- Maintain a normal body weight to reduce the pressure on your bladder.
- Do not try to control your incontinence by limiting your fluid intake. Adequate fluid intake is necessary for kidney function and health maintenance.
- If you have a catheter in your bladder, follow the instructions given to you about maintaining the sterile drainage system.
- If you are discharged with a suprapubic catheter in your bladder, inspect the entry site for the tube daily, clean the skin around the opening gently with warm soap and water, and place a sterile gauze dressing on the skin around the tube. Report any redness, swelling, drainage, or fever to your primary health care provider.
- Do not put anything into your vagina, such as tampons, drugs, hygiene products, or exercise with weights, until you check with your primary health care provider at your 6-week checkup after surgery.
- Do not have sexual intercourse until after your 6-week postoperative checkup.
- Do not lift or carry anything heavier than 5 lb or participate in any strenuous exercise until your primary health care provider gives you postoperative clearance. In some cases, this could be as long as 3 months.
- Avoid exercises, such as running, jogging, step or dance aerobic classes, rowing, cross-country ski or stair-climber machines, and mountain biking. Brisk walking without any additional hand, leg, or body weights is allowed. Swimming is allowed after all drains and catheters have been removed and your incision is completely healed.
- If Kegel exercises are recommended, ask your nurse for specific instructions.

Portable commodes may be obtained when ambulatory access to toilets is impractical. Physical and occupational therapists are valuable resources for assisting with home care management.

Self-Management Education. Teach the patient and family about the cause of the specific type of incontinence and discuss available treatment options for its management. The teaching plan should address the prescribed drugs (purpose, dosage, method and route of administration, and expected and potential side effects). Instruct the patient and family about the importance of weight reduction and dietary modification to help control incontinence of urine ***elimination.*** Remind the patient who smokes that nicotine can contribute to bladder irritation and that coughing can cause urine leakage.

For urge urinary incontinence, teach the patient to avoid foods that irritate the bladder such as caffeine and alcohol. Spacing fluids at regular intervals throughout the day (e.g., 120 mL every hour or 240 mL every 2 hours) and limiting fluids after the dinner hour (e.g., only 120 mL at bedtime) help avoid fluid overload on the bladder and allow urine to collect at a steady pace. Remind patients that maintaining an ideal body weight helps avoid the pressure that abdominal fat places on pelvic organs, thus reducing incontinence.

For patients who require external devices or containment materials, discuss the options available and work with the patient to determine the best selection. For patients who will use intermittent catheterization or those with artificial urinary sphincters, demonstrate the correct technique to the patient or caregiver. Having the patient return demonstrate correct technique is essential to prevent complications (Beauchemin et al., 2018).

Psychosocial Preparation. The embarrassment of incontinence can be devastating to self-esteem, body image, and relationships. Sexual intimacy is often adversely affected, and the unpredictable nature of incontinence creates anxiety. Patients may be embarrassed to seek help and, even when resources are identified, they may need help to feel comfortable in using them. Buying supplies at a local store may threaten privacy.

Acknowledge the personal concerns of the patient and caregiver. Never make their concerns seem trivial. As he or she learns the specifics of the plan that will allow control of urinary incontinence, the confidence to resume social interactions should return. Many continence supplies can be purchased online and delivered to the home to maintain privacy.

Health Care Resources. Referral to home care agencies for help with personal care and to continence clinics that specialize in evaluation and treatment may be helpful. In many continence clinics, nurses collaborate with physicians and other health care professionals to evaluate and manage patients. The treatment plan is specific for each patient; supplies and products are custom selected.

Patients may benefit from education and from the support of others who experience similar concerns. The National Association for Continence (NAFC) (www.nafc.org), and the Wound, Ostomy, and Continence Nurses (www.wocn.org) publish newsletters and educational materials written with easy-to-understand explanations. The American Urological Association (www.auanet.org) provides information on many areas of urologic dysfunction. Local hospitals often have local NAFC-approved support groups.

NCLEX EXAMINATION CHALLENGE 61.1

Physiological Integrity

For which client would the nurse expect to teach intermittent catheterization?

A. 35-year-old woman who has multiple sclerosis and incontinence
B. 48-year-old man who is admitted for pneumonia and is on complete bedrest
C. 61-year-old woman who is admitted following a fall at home and has new-onset dysrhythmia
D. 74-year-old man who has lung cancer with brain metastasis and has advanced dementia

◆ **Evaluation: Evaluate Outcomes.** Evaluate the care of the patient with urinary incontinence based on the identified priority patient problems. The expected outcomes are that the patient will:

- Maintain optimal urinary elimination through a reduction in the number of urinary incontinence episodes
- Maintain tissue integrity of the skin and mucous membranes in the perineal area
- Demonstrate knowledge of proper use of drugs and correct procedures for self-catheterization, use of the artificial sphincter, or care of an indwelling urinary catheter
- Demonstrate effective use of the selected exercise or bladder-training program
- Select and use incontinence interventions, devices, and products

CYSTITIS

Pathophysiology Review

Cystitis is an inflammatory condition of the bladder. Commonly, it refers to inflammation from an infection of the bladder. However, cystitis can be caused by inflammation without infection. For example, drugs, chemicals, or local radiation therapy cause bladder inflammation without an infecting organism. Irritants, such as feminine hygiene spray, spermicidal jellies, or long-term use of a catheter can cause cystitis without infection. Cystitis may sometimes occur as a complication of other disorders, such as gynecologic cancers, pelvic inflammatory disorders, endometriosis, Crohn's disease, diverticulitis, lupus, or tuberculosis.

An infection can occur in any area of the urinary tract and the kidney. Such infections are known as *urinary tract infections* or *UTIs*. An acute UTI is the invasion of the urinary tract by an infectious organism. A recurrent UTI is defined as having two or more infections in 6 months or three or more infections in 1 year. These distinctions in UTIs are important because they have different approaches to management (Feng et al., 2018). Contributing factors associated with cystitis and other UTIs are listed in Table 61.3.

PATIENT-CENTERED CARE: GENDER HEALTH CONSIDERATIONS QSEN

Bladder infections are more common in women than men. Up to 60% of women have experienced a UTI in their lifetime with most infections being a bladder infection. Women are 30 times more likely to have a UTI than men (Tan & Chlebicki, 2016).

A UTI is further categorized as *uncomplicated* or *complicated* (Table 61.4). With an uncomplicated UTI, there is no anatomic or functional abnormality of the urinary tract or condition that increases the risk for infection or possibility of treatment failing to resolve the infection (such as the presence of a multi–drug-resistant organism or urologic dysfunction). Some factors and conditions that contribute to a diagnosis of complicated UTI are pregnancy, male gender, obstruction, diabetes, neurogenic bladder, chronic kidney disease, and reduced ***immunity*** (Nicolle, 2016). In men, a UTI is generally considered complicated even with normal structure and function because most UTIs occur in older men or in association with anal intercourse or intercourse with a female who has infectious vaginitis, resulting in exposure to potentially virulent pathogens. Complicated cystitis or other UTI requires greater vigilance to avoid or detect adverse events from the infection and a longer course of antimicrobial treatment. A diagnosis of complicated UTI may require additional testing to identify and manage other related health problems (comorbidities).

The presence of bacteria in the urine is **bacteriuria** and may occur with cystitis or any UTI. When the patient has bacteriuria but no symptoms of infection, it is called *colonization* or *asymptomatic bacteriuria (ABU)* and is more common in older adults. This problem may progress to acute infection or renal insufficiency when the patient has other conditions, and only then does it require treatment (Avelluto & Bryman, 2018).

TABLE 61.3 Factors Contributing to Urinary Tract Infections

Factor	Mechanism
Obstruction	Incomplete bladder emptying creates a continuous pool of urine in which bacteria can grow, prevents flushing out of bacteria, and allows bacteria to ascend more easily to higher structures. Bacteria have a greater chance of multiplying the longer they remain in residual urine. Overdistention of the bladder damages the mucosa and allows bacteria to invade the bladder wall.
Stones (calculi)	Large stones can obstruct urine flow. The rough surface of a stone irritates mucosal surfaces and creates a spot where bacteria can establish and grow. Bacteria can live within stones and cause reinfection.
Vesicoureteral reflux	The urethra is colonized with bacteria. These bacteria are noninfectious until they move to upstream anatomy (bladder, ureters, kidneys) and colonize or form an infection with reflux (backward-flowing urine). Reflux of sterile urine can cause kidney scarring, which may promote kidney dysfunction.
Diabetes mellitus	Excess glucose in urine provides a rich medium for bacterial growth. Peripheral neuropathy affects bladder innervation and leads to a flaccid bladder and incomplete bladder emptying.
Characteristics of urine	Urine pH can promote different species of bacterial growth. Concentrated urine allows bacterial growth and adhesion to urinary tract anatomy.
Gender	**Women** Susceptibility to urethral colonization with coliform or pathogenic bacteria is increased, especially as estrogen levels fall during menopause. Use of douches, perfumed pads or toilet tissue, diaphragms, or spermicide (including spermicide-coated condoms) in women can inflame periurethral tissue and contribute to colonization. Bladder displacement during pregnancy predisposes women to cystitis and the development of pyelonephritis. A diaphragm or pessary that is too large can obstruct urine flow or traumatize the urethra. **Men** With increased age, the prostate enlarges and may obstruct the normal flow of urine, producing stasis. With increased age, prostatic secretions lose their antibacterial characteristics and predispose to bacterial proliferation in the urine. Sexually transmitted infections may cause urethral strictures that obstruct the flow of urine and predispose to urinary stasis.
Age	Urinary stasis may be caused by incomplete bladder emptying as a result of an enlarged prostate in men and cystocele and vaginal prolapse in women. Neuromuscular conditions that cause incomplete bladder emptying, such as Parkinson disease and stroke, affect older adults more frequently. The use of drugs with intentional or unintentional anticholinergic properties in older adults contributes to delayed bladder emptying. Fecal incontinence contributes to urethral contamination. Low estrogen in menopausal women adversely affects the cells of the vagina and urethra, making them more susceptible to infections. Overall ***immunity*** declines with age, increasing the risk for uncomplicated infections to become complicated.
Sexual activity	Sexual intercourse is the strongest risk factor for uncomplicated cystitis, particularly in young women. Irritation of the perineum and urethra during intercourse can promote migration of bacteria from the perineal area to the urinary tract in some women. Inadequate vaginal lubrication may exacerbate potential urethral irritation. Bacteria may be introduced into the male urethra during anal intercourse or during vaginal intercourse with a woman who has infectious vaginitis.
Recent use of antibiotics	Antibiotics change ***immunity*** and normal protective flora, providing opportunity for pathogenic bacterial overgrowth and colonization.
Virulence factors	The more virulent the organism, the more severe the infection.

The urinary and genitourinary tracts are normally sterile, apart from the distal urethra. Several host defenses help protect against infection in the urinary tract. Mucin produced by cells lining the bladder helps maintain mucosal integrity and prevents cellular damage. Mucin also prevents bacteria from adhering to urothelial cells. Urine pH also contributes to sustaining sterile urine. White blood cells in the urinary tract are the ***immunity*** cells that engulf and destroy pathogens. Urine proteins, such as secreted antibodies, also are protective. In men, the prostate gland secretes additional protective proteins. Frequent voiding is another defense against bacterial growth and adherence by preventing urine stasis and flushing out organisms.

Etiology and Genetic Risk. UTIs, like other infections, result from interactions between a pathogen and the host. Usually a high bacterial *virulence* (ability to invade and infect) is needed to overcome normal host defenses and ***immunity.*** However, an adult with reduced immunity is more likely to become infected even with bacteria that have low virulence. With UTI, bacteria (and, infrequently, fungi) move up the urinary tract from the external

TABLE 61.4 Urinary Tract Infection Types

Type	Description
Acute uncomplicated cystitis	Acute UTI — bladder involvement only No signs/symptoms of upper UTI No anatomic or functional abnormality of the urinary tract or condition that increases the risk for infection or possibility of treatment failing to resolve the infection
Acute complicated cystitis	Involves more than the bladder Symptoms of upper UTI: fever, flank pain, chills/rigors, malaise, costovertebral angle tenderness, and pelvic and/or perineal pain in men

urethra to the bladder to cause infectious cystitis. Less commonly, spread of infection through the blood and lymph fluid can occur, although this cause of UTI is not common. Invading bacteria with special adhesions are more likely to cause ascending UTIs that start in the urethra or bladder and move up into the ureter and kidney.

Infectious cystitis is typically caused by pathogens from the bowel or, in some cases, the vagina. Greater than 80% of UTIs are caused by *Escherichia coli.* Less common organisms include *Staphylococcus saprophyticus, Klebsiella pneumoniae,* and organisms from the *Proteus* and *Enterobacter* species (McLellan & Hunstad, 2016; Nicolle, 2016). Other infecting microbes causing infectious cystitis are viruses, mycobacteria, parasites, and yeast (fungus), especially *Candida* species. Reflux from the colonized distal urethra can also contribute to UTI in vulnerable patients. Irritation, trauma, or instrumentation of the urinary tract decreases host defenses and contributes to UTIs through the ascending migration of uropathogens.

Catheters are the most common factor associated with new-onset UTIs in the hospital and long-term care settings (Conway et al., 2017; Panchisin, 2016). Within 48 hours of catheter insertion, bacterial colonization along the urethra and the catheter itself begins. Risks for infection associated with a catheter increases 3% to 10% per day the catheter is in place (Ferguson, 2018).

The way that a catheter-associated urinary tract infection (CAUTI) occurs varies between genders. Bacteria from a woman's perineal area are more likely to ascend to the bladder by moving along the urethra. The shorter urethra in women aids in the ascending organisms' migration. In men, bacteria tend to gain access to the bladder from the catheter itself (Conway et al., 2017). Any break in the closed urinary drainage system allows bacteria to move through the lumen of the catheter. The external catheter surface also provides route for migration. Best practices to reduce the risk for catheter contamination and catheter-associated UTIs are listed in the Best Practice for Patient Safety & Quality Care: Minimizing Catheter-Associated Urinary Tract Infection (CAUTI) box and in Box 61.1.

BEST PRACTICE FOR PATIENT SAFETY & QUALITY CARE QSEN

Minimizing Catheter-Associated Urinary Tract Infection (CAUTI)

- Maintain good hand hygiene during insertion and manipulation of the catheter system to avoid contamination.
- Insert urinary catheters for appropriate use only, including:
  - Acute urinary retention or bladder obstruction.
  - Accurate measurement of urine volume in critically ill patients if needed.
  - Perioperative situations only as needed, such as urogenital, gynecological, laparoscopic, and orthopedic surgeries. Avoid routine use of indwelling catheters for surgical patients.
  - To assist in healing of open sacral or perineal wounds in incontinent patients. Avoid use of indwelling catheters to manage patients who are incontinent.
  - Consider intermittent catheterization or other alternatives to indwelling catheters for patients with spinal cord injuries or conditions.
  - To provide comfort at end of life.
- Ensure that only properly trained personnel insert and maintain catheters.
- Use routine hygiene to clean periurethral area; antiseptic cleaning solutions are NOT recommended.
- Leave catheters in place only as long as needed. The strongest predictor of a CAUTI is the length of time the catheter dwells in a patient.
- Assess the need for urinary catheter daily and document patient needs or indications.
- For example, remove catheters in postanesthesia care or as soon as possible after surgery when intraoperative indications have resolved.
- Use aseptic technique and sterile equipment in the acute care setting when inserting a urinary (intermittent or indwelling) catheter.
- Maintain a closed system by ensuring that catheter tubing connections are sealed securely; disconnections can introduce pathogens into the urinary tract.
- Obtain urine samples aseptically.
- If breaks in the system occur, replace the catheter and entire collecting system.
- Maintain unobstructed urine flow:
  - Keep the catheter and collecting tube free from kinking.
  - Keep the urine collection bag below the level of the bladder and do not rest the bag on the floor.
  - Empty the bag regularly, using a separate, clean container for each patient.
  - Ensure that the drainage spigot does not come into contact with nonsterile surfaces.
- Secure the catheter to the patient's thigh (women) or lower abdomen (men); catheter movement can cause urethral friction and irritation.
- Consider the use of antiseptic or antimicrobial catheters for patients requiring urinary catheters for more than 3 to 5 days. These catheters reduce bacterial colonization (i.e., biofilm) along the catheter.
- Consider appropriate alternatives to an indwelling catheter:
  - External (condom) devices in cooperative men without obstruction or urinary retention
  - Intermittent catheterization in patients requiring drainage for neurogenic bladder or postoperative urinary retention
- Use portable ultrasound devices to assess urine volume to reduce unnecessary catheterization.
- Implement best practices in quality improvement to ensure that core recommendations for use, insertion, and maintenance are implemented. Examples of projects that improve patient care and reduce CAUTI include:
  - Nurse-initiated protocols for urinary catheter removal
  - Compliance with hand hygiene
  - Impact of educational programs on CAUTI occurrence
  - Compliance with documentation for catheter placement or maintenance
  - Number of CAUTI per 1000 catheter days or patient days on unit
  - Track number of catheters inserted

Adapted from https://www.cdc.gov/nhsn/acute-care-hospital/cauti/.

BOX 61.1 Catheter-Associated Urinary Tract Infection (CAUTI) Prevention

A catheter-associated urinary tract infection (CAUTI) is the fourth leading cause of health care–associated infections occurring in acute care settings in the United States. Up to 25% of patients admitted to an acute care setting have a catheter, which places the individual at risk for infection. The estimated cost of a CAUTI is $758 for each individual with an overall annual cost of $340 million for the United States alone. Costs associated with a CAUTI are not reimbursed. CAUTI causes harm to the patients and reduces positive outcomes. Implementing a CAUTI prevention program increases the nurses' knowledge about prevention methods, reduces the incidence of CAUTI, and improves patient outcomes (Ferguson, 2018). Implementing a CAUTI prevention program is also one way to meet the National Patient Safety Goal specific to prevention CAUTI (The Joint Commission, 2019).

PATIENT-CENTERED CARE: OLDER ADULT CONSIDERATIONS (QSEN)

In women, there is a 20% incidence of UTIs for those between ages 18 and 24 annually and 50% of women will have a UTI by 35 years of age (Simmering et al., 2017). In men, the incidence of UTI is significantly lower than in women; however, the incidence greatly increases as men become older (Lee & Le, 2018). Skin and mucous membrane changes from a lack of estrogen appear to account for much of the increased risk in older women, together with overall decreased ***immunity***. Prostate disease increases risk for UTIs in men. Often the older adult does not have the typical symptoms of UTI (i.e., flank pain, dysuria, fever). More common symptoms are grossly bloody, foul-smelling urine with increasing frequency of urination (Touhy & Jett, 2016). When UTI leads to urosepsis, mental status changes occur. Ask about these additional symptoms of UTI whenever you are assessing an older adult.

Organisms other than bacteria cause cystitis. Fungal infections, such as those caused by *Candida,* can occur during long-term antibiotic therapy because antibiotics change normal protective flora that reduce the adherence and volume of pathogenic bacteria. Patients with reduced ***immunity*** (those who are severely immunosuppressed, are receiving corticosteroids or other immunosuppressive agents, or have diabetes mellitus or acquired immune deficiency syndrome) are at higher risk for fungal UTIs.

Viral and parasitic infections are rare and usually transfer to the urinary tract from an infection at another body site. For example, *Trichomonas,* a parasite found in the vagina, can also be found in the urine. Treatment of the vaginal infection also resolves the UTI.

Noninfectious cystitis may result from chemical exposure, such as to drugs (e.g., cyclophosphamide); from radiation therapy; and from ***immunity*** problems, as with systemic lupus erythematosus (SLE).

Interstitial cystitis is a rare, chronic inflammation of the entire lower urinary tract (bladder, urethra, and adjacent pelvic muscles) that is related to genetic and ***immunity*** dysfunction rather than infection. The condition affects women more often than men, and the diagnosis is difficult to make. Symptoms are pain associated with bladder filling or voiding, usually accompanied by frequency, urgency, and nocturia (Kim, 2016). Pain occurs in suprapubic or pelvic areas, sometimes radiating to the groin, vulva, or rectum.

Although cystitis is not life threatening, infection of the urinary tract can lead to life-threatening complications, including pyelonephritis and sepsis. Severe kidney damage from an ascending UTI is a rare complication. Patients with predisposing factors, such as anatomic abnormalities, pregnancy, obstruction, reflux, calculi, or diabetes, are at greater risk for complications.

The urinary tract is often the infection source in severe sepsis or septic shock. The spread of the infection from the urinary tract to the bloodstream is termed *bacteremia* or **urosepsis**. Catheter associated urinary tract infections are the leading cause of urosepsis, which has a mortality rate of 10% (Ferguson, 2018). Sepsis, regardless of the source, is a systemic reaction to infection that prolongs hospitalization and can lead to shock, multiple organ failure, and other profound complications (see Chapter 34).

Incidence and Prevalence. The incidence of UTI is second only to upper respiratory infections in primary care and affects 150 million people worldwide annually (McLellan & Hunstad, 2016). Total costs for UTIs are estimated at $2.8 billion annually. In addition to a high prevalence in primary care, UTIs are one of the most common health care–associated infections (Feng et al., 2018).

The hallmark symptoms of UTI are **frequency** (an urge to urinate frequently in small amounts), **dysuria** (pain or burning with urination), and **urgency** (feeling that urination will occur immediately).

Health Promotion and Maintenance. Although infectious cystitis is common, in many cases it is preventable. When catheters must be used in institutional settings, strict attention to sterile technique during insertion is essential to reduce the risk for UTIs (see the Best Practice for Patient Safety & Quality Care: Minimizing Catheter-Associated Urinary Tract Infection box). Long-term placement of urinary catheters requires aseptic technique for insertion. When *intermittent catheterization* was used in home care settings, the use of clean technique resulted in a similar rate of UTI compared with sterile technique. Clean technique, using single-use catheters, for catheter insertion is recommended in home settings where multiple resistant organisms are less likely to be present. Multiuse catheters for home use are no longer recommended. Sterile technique must be used in health care facilities to reduce the risk for infection (Beauchemin et al., 2018).

NURSING SAFETY PRIORITY (QSEN)

Action Alert

Ensuring that urinary catheters are used appropriately and discontinued as early as possible is required (The Joint Commission, 2019). Do not allow catheters to remain in place for staff convenience.

Certain changes in fluid intake patterns, urinary ***elimination*** patterns, and hygiene patterns can help prevent or reduce cystitis in the general population. For example, a liberal water intake of 2.2 L for women and 3 L for men can promote general health. Another strategy to promote health is to have sufficient fluid intake to cause 1.5 L of clear or light yellow urine daily. Strategies to prevent cystitis and other UTIs are listed in the Patient and Family Education: Preparing for Self-Management: Preventing a Urinary Tract Infection box. Although some of these strategies do not have consistent evidence to support a reduced risk for UTI when followed, they are low risk and reasonable.

! NATIONAL PATIENT SAFETY GOALS

Prevention of CAUTI

The Joint Commission (2019) has implemented a national patient safety goal (NPSG) designed to decrease the incidence of indwelling catheter–associated urinary tract infections. Elements of performance include ongoing education for staff to decrease the risk and incidence of CAUTI. Each hospital should have written criteria regarding the use and care of indwelling urinary catheters. These criteria include the evidence-based guidance to minimize use when possible and limit indwelling duration. Be sure to review the facility specific protocol to minimize CAUTI.

❖ Interprofessional Collaborative Care

Cystitis and UTIs can occur in any setting and are very common in the community. Usually the adult with cystitis is treated at home using self-management strategies.

◆ Assessment: Recognize Cues

Physical Assessment/Signs and Symptoms. Frequency, urgency, and dysuria are the common symptoms of a urinary tract infection (UTI), but other symptoms may be present (see the Key Features: Urinary Tract Infection box). Urine may be cloudy, foul smelling, or blood tinged. Ask the patient about risk factors for UTI during the assessment (see Table 61.3). For noninfectious cystitis, the Pelvic Pain and Urgency/Frequency Patient Symptom Scale (PUF, 2011) can identify patients with interstitial cystitis.

PATIENT AND FAMILY EDUCATION: PREPARING FOR SELF-MANAGEMENT

Preventing a Urinary Tract Infection

- Drink fluid liberally, as much as 2 to 3 L daily if not contraindicated by health conditions.
- Be sure to get enough sleep, rest, and nutrition daily to maintain immunologic health.
- If spermicides are used, consider changing to another method of contraception.
- *[For women]* Clean your perineum (the area between your legs) from front to back.
- *[For women]* Avoid using or wearing irritating substances such as douches, scented lubricants for intercourse, bubble bath, tight-fitting underwear, and scented toilet tissue. Wear loose-fitting cotton underwear.
- *[For women]* Empty your bladder before and after intercourse.
- *[For both women and men]* Gently wash the perineal area before intercourse.
- Do not routinely delay urination because the flow of urine can help remove bacteria that may be colonizing the urethra or bladder.
- If you experience burning when you urinate, if you have to urinate frequently, or if you find it difficult to begin urinating, notify your primary health care provider right away, especially if you have a chronic medical condition (e.g., diabetes) or are pregnant.

KEY FEATURES

Urinary Tract Infection

Common Symptoms

- Frequency
- Urgency
- Dysuria
- Suprapubic pain or tenderness, low back pain
- Nocturia
- Incontinence
- Hematuria
- Pyuria
- Bacteriuria
- Retention
- Suprapubic tenderness or fullness
- Feeling of incomplete bladder emptying

Complicated Cystitis Symptoms

- Fever
- Chills and rigors
- Nausea or vomiting
- Malaise
- Flank pain and costovertebral angle tenderness

Symptoms That May Occur in the Older Adult

- Sudden or worsening: dysuria, urinary incontinence, nocturia, urgency, and frequency. A general sense of lack of well-being.
- Note: Changes in mental status and falls are not reliable predictors of UTIs. These changes need to be fully assessed to determine the underlying cause.

For patients with a urinary catheter, in addition to common signs of UTI (e.g., fever with or without chills; leukocytosis; suprapubic or flank pain; urine with sediment, blood, or foul odor), new onset of hypotension or changes in mental status can indicate a UTI. Diagnostic testing for UTIs in older adults should not be based on mental status changes alone but should be performed when UTI symptoms are present (Hooten & Gupta, 2018). If a catheter has been in place for more than 2 weeks, it may be necessary to first replace the catheter before obtaining a urine specimen for culture (McGoldrick, 2016).

Before performing the physical assessment, ask the patient to void so that the urine can be examined and the bladder emptied before palpation. Assess vital signs to help identify the presence of infection (e.g., fever, tachycardia, tachypnea). Inspect the lower abdomen and palpate the bladder. Distention after voiding indicates incomplete bladder emptying.

Using Standard Precautions, record any lesions around the urethral meatus and vaginal opening. To help differentiate between a vaginal and a urinary tract infection, note whether there is any vaginal discharge or irritation. Vaginal discharge and irritation are more indicative of vaginal infection. Women often report burning with urination when urine touches labial tissues that are inflamed or have lost ***tissue integrity*** with ulcerations by vaginal infections or sexually transmitted infections (STIs). Maintain privacy with drapes during the examination.

The prostate is palpated by digital rectal examination (DRE) by the primary health care provider for size, change in shape or consistency, and tenderness. A large prostate gland can obstruct urine outflow and contribute to urostasis and bacterial colonization of the urinary tract, contributing to the risk for a complicated UTI.

Laboratory Assessment. Laboratory assessment for a UTI begins with a clean-catch urine specimen that is divided into two containers. If the patient cannot produce a clean-catch specimen, you may need to obtain the specimen with a small-diameter (6 Fr) catheter. For a routine urinalysis, 10 mL of urine is needed; smaller quantities are sufficient for culture.

One container is used for a urinalysis. The combination of a positive leukocyte esterase and nitrate from a urinalysis is 68% to 88% sensitive in the diagnosis of a UTI. The presence of white blood cells (WBCs) (**pyuria**), red blood cells (RBCs) (**hematuria**), or casts (clumps of material or cells) also may indicate UTI (Pagana & Pagana, 2018). The presence of more than 20 epithelial cells/high-power field (HPF) suggests contamination, and a new specimen may be collected for culture and sensitivity.

If the urinalysis suggests a UTI and there are no risk factors or conditions for complicated UTI in a woman, treatment can be started. If the UTI is complicated, the second specimen is analyzed as a urine culture. A culture may also be performed when a patient with a UTI does not respond to usual therapy, when the diagnosis is uncertain, to assess for sensitivity, or to determine resolution of UTI (Hooten & Gupta, 2018). Urinalysis is less specific in diagnosing a UTI in an older adult, especially one who has a urinary catheter.

A urine culture confirms the type of organism and the number of colonies. Urine culture is expensive, and initial results take at least 24 hours. A UTI is confirmed when more than 10^5 colony-forming units/mL are in the urine from any patient. In noncatheterized patients who have symptoms of UTI (e.g., fever, dysuria, new-onset frequency or urgency, suprapubic or flank pain, or hematuria), as few as 10^3 colony-forming units/mL in a voided specimen can confirm the infection. For patients with a catheter who are symptomatic, 10^2 colony-forming units/mL are diagnostic of a complicated UTI. The presence of many different types of organisms in low colony counts usually indicates that the specimen is contaminated. Sensitivity testing follows culture results when complicating factors are present (e.g., stones or recurrent infection), when the patient is older, or to ensure that appropriate antibiotics are prescribed.

Occasionally the serum WBC count may be elevated, with the differential WBC count showing a "left shift" (see Chapter 16). This shift indicates that the number of immature WBCs is increasing and the number of mature WBCs is decreasing in response to continued infection. Thus the number of "bands," or immature WBCs, is elevated, which indicates reduced ***immunity.*** Left shift most often occurs with urosepsis and rarely occurs with uncomplicated cystitis, because cystitis is a local rather than a systemic infection.

Other Diagnostic Assessment. The diagnosis of UTI and cystitis is based on history, physical examination, and laboratory data. If urinary retention and obstruction of urine outflow are suspected, pelvic ultrasound or CT may be needed to locate the site of obstruction or the presence of calculi. Voiding cystourethrography (see Chapter 60) is needed when urine reflux is suspected.

Cystoscopy (see Chapter 60) may be performed when the patient has recurrent UTIs (more than three annually). A urine culture is performed first to ensure that no infection is present. If infection is present, the urine is sterilized with antibiotic therapy before the procedure to reduce the risk for sepsis. Cystoscopy identifies abnormalities that increase the risk for cystitis. Such abnormalities include bladder calculi, bladder diverticula, urethral strictures, foreign bodies (e.g., sutures from previous surgery), and **trabeculation** (an abnormal thickening of the bladder wall caused by urinary retention and obstruction). Retrograde pyelography, along with the cystoscopic examination, shows outlines and images of the drainage tract.

Cystoscopy is needed to accurately diagnose interstitial (noninfectious) cystitis. A urinalysis usually shows WBCs and RBCs but no bacteria. Common findings in interstitial cystitis are a small-capacity bladder, the presence of Hunner ulcers (a type of bladder lesion), and small hemorrhages after bladder distention.

◆ Interventions: Take Action

Nonsurgical Management. The expected outcome is to maintain an optimal urine ***elimination*** pattern. Nursing interventions for the management of cystitis focus on ***pain*** relief and teaching about drug therapy, fluid intake, and prevention measures. In a hospital setting, timely administration of antibiotics can prevent or reduce complications from urosepsis.

Drug Therapy. Drugs used to treat bacteriuria and relieve ***pain*** include urinary antiseptics or antibiotics, analgesics, and antispasmodics. Cure of a UTI depends on the antimicrobial levels achieved in the urine. Fluconazole is the drug of choice for treatment of *Candida* (fungal) infections. Antispasmodic drugs decrease bladder spasms and promote complete bladder emptying.

Antibiotic therapy is used for bacterial UTIs (see the Common Examples of Drug Therapy: Urinary Tract Infections box). Guidelines for uncomplicated cystitis recommend nitrofurantoin, trimethoprim/sulfamethoxazole, or fosfomycin as first-line therapy for those patients at low risk of resistance to antimicrobials (Hooten & Gupta, 2018). Longer antibiotic treatment (7 to 21 days) and sometimes different agents are required for hospitalized patients and those with complicated UTIs (e.g., men, pregnant women, and patients with anatomic, functional or metabolic derangements that affect the urinary tract).

! NURSING SAFETY PRIORITY (QSEN)

Drug Alert

Sulfamethoxazole/trimethoprim should be stopped at the first appearance of a skin rash. A rash may indicate the onset of Stevens-Johnson syndrome (aching joints and muscles; bilateral blistering skin) or toxic epidermal necrolysis (redness, blistering, and peeling skin and mucous membranes).

Antibiotics are one of the drug categories most frequently involved in the error of administration to patients who have documented allergies to these drugs.

COMMON EXAMPLES OF DRUG THERAPY

Urinary Tract Infections

Drug	Nursing Implications
Trimethoprim[a]/sulfamethoxazole	Ask patients about drug allergies, especially to sulfa drugs, before beginning drug therapy *because allergies to sulfa drugs are common and require changing drug therapy.* Teach patients to drink a full glass of water with each dose and to have an overall fluid intake of 3 L daily *because these drugs can form crystals that precipitate in the kidney tubules. Fluids can prevent this complication.* Teach patients to keep out of the sun or to wear protective clothing outdoors and use a sunscreen *because these drugs increase sun sensitivity and can lead to severe sunburn.* Caution patients to complete the drug regimen even if the symptoms improve or disappear sooner *to prevent bacterial resistance and infection recurrence.*
Ciprofloxacin, levofloxacin ofloxacin	Teach patients taking the extended-release drugs to swallow them whole and not to crush or chew the tablets *because this action ruins the extended effect.* Warn patients not to take the drug within 2 hours of taking an antacid *to prevent interference with drug absorption.* Teach patients how to take their pulse, to monitor it twice daily while on this drug, and to notify the primary health care provider if new-onset irregular heartbeats occur *to identify serious drug-induced dysrhythmias.* Teach patients to keep out of the sun or to wear protective clothing outdoors and use a sunscreen *to avoid serious sunburns from increased sun sensitivity.* Caution patients to complete the drug regimen even if the symptoms improve or disappear sooner *to reduce bacterial resistance and infection recurrence.*
Amoxicillin Amoxicillin/clavulanate	Ask patients about drug allergies to penicillin before beginning drug therapy *because allergies to this drug category are common.* Teach patients to take the drug with food *to reduce the risk for GI upset.* Instruct patients to call the primary health care provider if severe or watery diarrhea develops *to recognize the complication of pseudomembranous colitis, which may require discontinuing the drug.* Suggest that women who take oral contraceptives use an additional method of birth control while taking this drug *because these drugs may reduce the effectiveness of estrogen-containing contraceptives.* Caution patients to complete the drug regimen even if the symptoms improve or disappear sooner *to prevent bacterial resistance and infection recurrence.*
Cefdinir, cefaclor, or cefpodoxime	Ask about drug allergies to penicillin or cephalosporins before beginning drug therapy *because these drugs are structurally similar to penicillin and anyone with allergies to penicillin is likely to be allergic to the cephalosporins.* Instruct patients to call the prescriber if severe or watery diarrhea develops *to recognize the complication of pseudomembranous colitis, which may require discontinuing the drug.* Caution patients to complete the drug regimen even if the symptoms improve or disappear sooner *to prevent bacterial resistance and infection recurrence.* Instruct patients to follow the directions on the label if the medication needs to be reconstituted. Add water as directed and shake well *to ensure that all particles are mixed thoroughly and the correct dose is taken.* Avoid taking this drug when also taking metoclopramide or any other drug that increases GI motility *to prevent interference with drug absorption.* Teach patients to shake the bottle well before measuring the drug *to thoroughly mix the suspension.* Suggest that patients obtain a calibrated spoon for liquid drugs and not to use household spoons *to ensure accurate dosing.* Teach patients to drink a full glass of water with each dose and to have an overall fluid intake of at least 3 L daily *to avoid having the drug precipitate in the kidneys and cause kidney damage.* Caution patients to complete the drug regimen even if the symptoms improve or disappear sooner *to prevent bacterial resistance and infection recurrence.*
Phenazopyridine	Remind patients that this drug will not treat an infection, only the symptoms *because these drugs have no antibacterial activity.* Teach patients to take the drug with or immediately after a meal *to reduce the risk for GI upset.* Warn patients that urine will turn red or orange *to reduce anxiety about this change.*
Hyoscyamine	Teach patients to notify the primary health care provider if blurred vision or other eye problems, confusion, dizziness or fainting spells, fast heartbeat, fever, or difficulty passing urine occurs *because these symptoms indicate drug toxicity.* Teach patients to wear dark glasses in sunlight or other bright-light areas *because these drugs dilate the pupil and increase eye sensitivity to light.*

[a]Trimethoprim can be given alone to patients with a sulfa allergy.

Low-dose antibiotic therapy over 6 to 12 months is sometimes used for chronic, recurring infection caused by structural abnormalities or stones or for long-term management of the older patient with frequent UTIs. For women who have recurrent UTIs after intercourse, antibiotics may be prescribed to be taken after intercourse. The three most common drug treatment regimens are (1) one low-dose tablet of trimethoprim, (2) sulfamethoxazole/trimethoprim, or (3) nitrofurantoin.

Recent evidence demonstrates that severe UTIs leave inflammatory-related damage to the bladder wall and change the genetic material of the cells. This makes the bladder more susceptible to infection. These inflammatory changes may be controlled by COX_2 inhibitors. More research is needed to determine short and long-term efficacy (O'Brien et al., 2016).

PATIENT-CENTERED CARE: GENDER HEALTH CONSIDERATIONS (QSEN)

Pregnant women with a bacterial UTI require prompt and aggressive treatment because a UTI can lead to acute pyelonephritis during pregnancy. Pyelonephritis in pregnancy can cause preterm labor and adversely affect the fetus. Remind patients who are pregnant to contact their health care provider whenever symptoms of UTI are present.

Fluid Intake. Urge patients to drink enough fluid to maintain dilute urine throughout the day and night unless fluid restriction is needed for another health problem. Some urologists recommend sufficient fluid intake to result in at least 1.5 L of urine output or 7 to 12 voidings daily. Food can provide 20% or more of fluid intake, particularly the intake of fruits and vegetables.

Cranberry-containing products appear to decrease the ability of bacteria to adhere to the epithelial cells lining the urinary tract. In some patients, this may result in preventing UTI or decreasing the incidence of recurrent symptomatic UTIs; however, evidence is conflicting (Feng et al., 2018). Cranberry juice can be an irritant to the bladder with interstitial cystitis and should be avoided by patients with this condition. Avoiding spices, soy products, and tomato products may decrease bladder irritation and ***pain*** during cystitis (Feng et al., 2018).

Comfort Measures. A warm sitz bath two or three times a day for 20 minutes may provide ***pain*** relief and some relief of local symptoms. If burning with urination is severe or urinary retention occurs, teach the patient to sit in the sitz bath and urinate into the warm water. Urinary tract analgesics or antispasmodics may also provide comfort (see the Common Examples of Drug Therapy: Urinary Tract Infections box).

Surgical Management. Surgery for cystitis treats the conditions that increase the risk for recurrent UTIs (e.g., removal of obstructions and repair of vesicoureteral reflux). Procedures may include cystoscopy (see Chapter 60) to identify and remove calculi or obstructions.

Care Coordination and Transition Management. Assess the patient's level of understanding of the problem. The patient's knowledge about factors that promote the development of cystitis determines the teaching interventions planned.

Teach the patient how to take prescribed drugs. Stress the need for correct spacing of doses throughout the day and the need to complete all of the prescribed antibiotics. If the drug will change the color of the urine, as it does with phenazopyridine, inform the patient to expect this change.

Patients may associate discomfort with sexual activities and have feelings of guilt and embarrassment. Open and sensitive discussions with a woman who has recurrences of UTI after sexual intercourse can help her find techniques to handle the problem (see the earlier Patient and Family Education: Preparing for Self-Management: Preventing a Urinary Tract Infection box). Explore with her the factors that contribute to her infections, such as sexual penetration when the bladder is full, diaphragm use, and her general ***immunity*** responses against infection. Some positions during intercourse may reduce urethral irritation and subsequent cystitis. Remind the patient that vigorous cleaning of the perineum with harsh soaps and vaginal douching may irritate the perineal tissues and *increase* the risk for UTI. At the patient's request, discuss the problem with her and her partner to help them find ways of maintaining their intimate relationship.

NCLEX EXAMINATION CHALLENGE 61.2

Health Promotion and Maintenance

The nurse is caring for an 80-year-old female client with recurrent cystitis. Which teaching will the nurse include in the plan of care? **Select all that apply.**

A. Drink citrus juices daily.
B. Douche regularly; a minimum of two times weekly.
C. Encourage fluid intake of 2-3 L of fluid throughout the day.
D. Instruct her to always wipe the perineum from front to back after each toilet use.
E. Reinforce that she should complete the entire course of antibiotics as prescribed.
F. Instruct her to empty her bladder immediately before and after having intercourse.

URETHRITIS

Pathophysiology Review

Urethritis is an inflammation of the urethra and can result from infectious and noninfectious conditions. The incidence is highest among adults ages 20 to 24 years. The most common cause of infectious urethritis is sexually transmitted infections (STIs). These include gonorrhea or nonspecific urethritis caused by *Ureaplasma* (a gram-negative bacterium), *Chlamydia* (a sexually transmitted gram-negative bacterium), or *Trichomonas vaginalis* (a protozoan found in both the male and female genital tract). Urethritis is also known as *pyuria-dysuria syndrome, frequency-dysuria syndrome, trigonitis syndrome,* and *urethral syndrome.*

Many women with urethritis have symptoms similar to cystitis, vaginitis, or cervicitis. Men with urethritis may report symptoms of cystitis, as well as heaviness in the genitals *(orchalgia).*

Noninfectious urethritis in postmenopausal women may be related to uretero-genital tissue changes resulting from low estrogen levels.

Symptoms of urethritis include discharge of mucopurulent or purulent material, dysuria, and itching or discomfort of the area (urethral pruritus). The discharge can be any color, depending on the infecting organism or source of irritation. Additional symptoms may include fever (with or without chills) and urgent or frequent urination.

❖ Interprofessional Collaborative Care

Ask the patient about a history of STI, painful or difficult urination, discharge from the penis or vagina, and discomfort in the lower abdomen. Urinalysis may show pyuria (white blood cells [WBCs] in the urine) without a large number of bacteria. Similarly, a urethral smear may show WBCs. All patients with urethritis should be tested for *N. gonorrhoeae* and *C. trachoma* with an endourethral (in men) or endocervical (women) smear. Testing for *Chlamydia* may be done with the same sample. STI testing for VDRL serology and HIV is suggested by the Centers for Disease Control and Prevention (Barrow et al., 2020; CDC, 2016). A pregnancy test is performed for women who have had unprotected intercourse. In women, a pelvic examination may reveal tissue changes from low estrogen levels in the vagina. Urethroscopy may show low estrogen changes with inflammation of urethral tissues.

Noninfectious urethritis symptoms usually resolve spontaneously over time, regardless of treatment. Postmenopausal women often have improvement in urethral symptoms with the use of estrogen vaginal cream. Estrogen cream applied locally to the vagina increases the amount of estrogen in the urethra as well, reducing irritating symptoms. Urethritis from STIs is treated with antibiotic therapy. More information on STIs can be found in Chapter 69.

UROLITHIASIS

Pathophysiology Review

Urolithiasis is the presence of *calculi* (stones) in the urinary tract. Stones often do not cause symptoms until they pass into the lower urinary tract, where they can cause excruciating pain. **Nephrolithiasis** is the formation of stones in the kidney; formation of stones in the ureter is **ureterolithiasis**. Stones are particles in the urine that occur in amounts too high to stay dissolved (become supersaturated) in urine. As a result of supersaturation, the particles precipitate and collect to form calculi.

The most common condition associated with stone formation is dehydration. Everyone excretes crystals in the urine at some time, but less than 10% of adults form stones. Most stones contain calcium as one part of the stone complex. Struvite (15%), uric acid (8%), and cystine (3%) are more rare compositions of stones. Formation of stones involves two conditions:

1. Supersaturation of the urine with the particular element (e.g., calcium, uric acid) that first becomes crystallized and later becomes the stone
2. Formation of a *nidus* (deposit of crystals that can be the point of infection) along the lining of the kidney and urinary tract

In addition, some patients may have decreased amounts of inhibitor substances in the urine that would otherwise prevent supersaturation with crystal aggregation. This type of metabolic risk factor can be inherited.

In addition to low urine volume, high urine acidity (as with uric acid and cystine stones) or alkalinity (as with calcium phosphate and struvite stones), as well as drugs (e.g., topiramate, corticosteroids, indinavir, acetazolamide), contribute to stone formation.

One example of a metabolic problem causing stone formation begins when excessive amounts of calcium are absorbed through the intestinal tract, leading to hypercalciuria. As blood circulates through the kidneys, the excess calcium is filtered into the urine, causing supersaturation of calcium in the urine. If fluid intake is poor, such as when a patient is dehydrated, supersaturation is more likely to occur.

Any stone may result in obstruction within the urinary tract, which can threaten both glomerular filtration rate (GFR) and kidney perfusion. When the stone occludes the ureter and blocks the flow of urine, the ureter dilates. Enlargement of the ureter is called **hydroureter**.

The pain associated with ureteral spasm is excruciating and may cause the patient to go into shock from stimulation of nearby nerves. Hematuria (bloody urine) may result from damage to the urothelial lining. If the obstruction is not removed, urinary stasis can lead to infection and impair kidney function on the side of the blockage. As the blockage persists, **hydronephrosis** (enlargement of the kidney caused by blockage of urine lower in the tract and filling of the kidney with urine) and permanent kidney damage may develop.

Etiology and Genetic Risk. The vast majority of adults who form stones have a metabolic risk factor. The cause of stone formation in a susceptible adult (e.g., one who has a metabolic risk factor) is dehydration. Table 61.5 lists some metabolic problems that cause stone formation. Patients who have a family history of stones, are obese, or have diabetes or gout (hyperuricemia) have increased risk for initial stone formation (Sofia, 2016). Because a metabolic problem is so strongly associated with stone formation and is a nonmodifiable risk factor, an adult of any age who develops a stone is always at high risk for future stone development.

Diet may be considered a risk for stone formation. Increased sodium intake has been associated with stone formation (Sofia, 2016) (Table 61.6).

PATIENT-CENTERED CARE: GENETIC/GENOMIC CONSIDERATIONS QSEN

Family history has a strong association with stone formation and recurrence because of inherited metabolic variations. More than 30 genetic variations are associated with the formation of kidney stones, although single gene disorders are rare. More commonly, nephrolithiasis is a complex disease, with genetic variation in intestinal calcium absorption, kidney calcium transport, or kidney phosphate transport all associated with stone formation (Online Mendelian Inheritance in Man [OMIM], 2016). Always ask a patient with a renal stone whether other family members also have this problem.

TABLE 61.5 Metabolic Defects That Commonly Cause Kidney Stones

Metabolic Deficit	Etiology
Hypercalcemia	
Primary	Absorptive: Increased intestinal calcium absorption Renal: Decreased kidney tubular excretion of calcium
Secondary	Resorptive: Hyperparathyroidism, vitamin D intoxication, kidney tubular acidosis, prolonged immobilization
Hyperoxaluria	
Primary	Genetic: Autosomal-recessive trait resulting in high oxalate production
Secondary	Dietary: Excess oxalate from foods such as spinach, rhubarb, Swiss chard, cocoa, beets, wheat germ, pecans, peanuts, okra, chocolate, and lime peel
Hyperuricemia	
Primary	Gout is an inherited disorder of purine metabolism (20% of patients with gout have uric acid calculi)
Secondary	Increased production or decreased clearance of purine from myeloproliferative disorders, thiazide diuretics, carcinoma
Struvite	Made of magnesium ammonium phosphate and carbonate apatite; formed by urea splitting by bacteria, most commonly, *Proteus mirabilis;* needs an alkaline urine to form
Cystinuria	Autosomal-recessive defect of amino acid metabolism that precipitates insoluble cystine crystals in the urine

Incidence and Prevalence. The incidence of stone disease is high and varies with geographic location, race, and family history. About 12% of adults will have at least one episode of renal stone disease (Sofia, 2016). The incidence of most stone types is higher in men, although struvite stones are twice as common in women. This difference in struvite stone formation incidence is thought to be related to the fact that women have more UTIs and struvite stones are associated with UTI. Recurrence rates vary depending on the type of treatment, although any adult who has had a stone is much more likely to have recurrence. Recurrence of stones occurs in patients with a family history of stone disease and in those who had their first occurrence by age 25 years.

PATIENT-CENTERED CARE: CULTURAL/SPIRITUAL CONSIDERATIONS QSEN

The incidence of stone disease is most common in the southeastern United States, Japan, and western Europe. Calcium stone disease is more common in men than in women and tends to occur in young adults or during early middle adulthood. Initial onset of stone disease occurs more often in younger adults than older adults (Sofia, 2016). For patients in these higher-risk groups, nursing care includes teaching family members, as well as patients, to avoid dehydration. Collaborate with the interprofessional health care team about referring patients with recurrent stone formation to evaluate metabolic risk factors.

❖ Interprofessional Collaborative Care

◆ **Assessment: Recognize Cues.** Ask the patient about a personal or family history of urologic stones. Obtain a diet history, focusing on fluid intake patterns and supplemental vitamin or mineral intake. If he or she has a history of stone formation, ask about past treatment, whether chemical analysis of the stone was performed, and which preventive measures are followed.

TABLE 61.6 Dietary Treatment for Kidney and Urinary Stones

Stone Type	Dietary Interventions	Rationales
Calcium oxalate	Avoid oxalate sources, such as spinach, black tea, and rhubarb.	Reduction of urinary oxalate content may help prevent these stones from forming. Urinary pH is not a factor.
	Decrease sodium intake.	High sodium intake reduces kidney tubular calcium reabsorption.
Calcium phosphate	Limit intake of foods high in animal protein to 5-7 servings per week and never more than 2 per day.	Reduction of protein intake reduces acidic urine and prevents calcium precipitation.
	Some patients may benefit from a reduced calcium intake (milk, other dairy products).	Reduction of urine calcium concentration may prevent calcium precipitation and crystallization.
	Decrease sodium intake.	High sodium intake reduces kidney tubular calcium reabsorption.
Struvite (magnesium ammonium phosphate)	Limit high-phosphate foods, such as dairy products, organ meats, and whole grains.	Reduction of urinary phosphate content may help prevent these stones from forming.
Uric acid (urate)	Decrease intake of purine sources, such as organ meats, poultry, fish, gravies, red wines, and sardines.	Reduction of urinary purine content may help prevent these stones from forming.
Cystine	Limit sodium and animal protein intake (as above).	It reduces urinary cystine levels.
	Encourage oral fluid intake (500 mL every 4 hours while awake and 750 mL at night).	Increased fluid helps dilute the urine and prevents the cystine crystals from forming.

The major symptom of stones is severe pain, commonly called **renal colic.** Flank pain suggests that the stone is in the kidney or upper ureter. Flank pain that extends toward the abdomen or to the scrotum and testes or the vulva suggests that stones are in the ureters or bladder. Pain is most intense when the stone is moving or the ureter is obstructed.

Renal colic begins suddenly and is often described as "unbearable." Nausea, vomiting, pallor, and diaphoresis often accompany the pain. However, a large stationary stone in the kidney (staghorn calculus) rarely causes much pain because it is not moving. Frequency and dysuria occur when a stone reaches the bladder. **Oliguria** (scant urine output) or **anuria** (absence of urine output) suggests obstruction, possibly at the bladder neck or urethra.

NURSING SAFETY PRIORITY QSEN

Action Alert

Urinary tract obstruction is an emergency and must be treated immediately to preserve kidney function.

Assess the patient for bladder distention. He or she may appear pale, ashen, and diaphoretic and may have excruciating pain. Vital signs may be elevated with pain; body temperature and pulse are elevated with infection. Blood pressure may decrease if the severe pain causes shock.

Urinalysis is performed in patients with suspected stones. Measurement of urine specific gravity and osmolarity can provide a clue about the adequacy of fluid intake. Urine pH can help in the determination of stone type. High urine acidity (low urine pH) is associated with uric acid and cystine stones; high urine alkalinity (high urine pH) is associated with calcium phosphate and struvite stones. A 24-hour urine analysis can determine whether supersaturation of common stone particles is present. Hematuria during renal colic is common, and blood may make the urine appear smoky or rusty. RBCs are usually caused by stone-induced trauma to the lining of the ureter, bladder, or urethra. WBCs and bacteria may be present as a result of urinary stasis. Increased *turbidity* (cloudiness) and odor indicate that infection may also be present. Microscopic examination of the urine may identify possible stone-forming crystals.

The serum WBC count is elevated with infection. Increases in the serum levels of calcium, phosphate, or uric acid levels indicate that excess minerals that may contribute to stone formation are present.

The current standard for confirming urinary stones is an unenhanced helical CT scan of the abdomen and pelvis. Most stones are radiopaque; and the size, location, and surrounding anatomic structures are easily seen. In settings where a CT is not available, a routine abdominal x-ray (KUB) is useful (Fig. 61.2). Ultrasound may be used in pregnant women suspected to have stones, but it is not sensitive for ureteral stones and is not used for general screening.

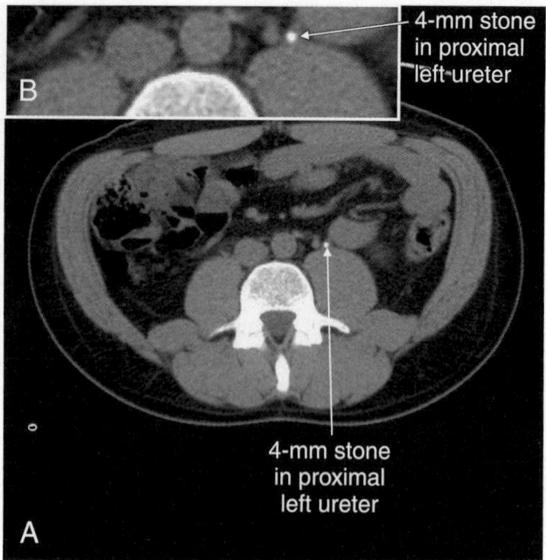

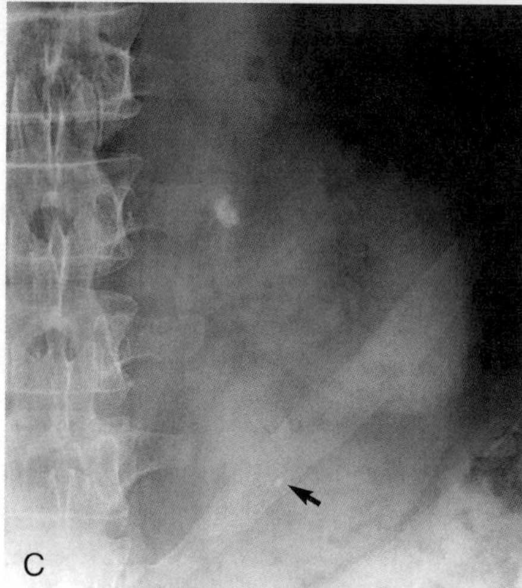

FIG. 61.2 A and B, Urinary stones on CT scan. C, Urinary stones on x-ray of the kidneys, ureters, and bladder (KUB). (A and B from Broder, J. K. [2011]. *Diagnostic imaging for the emergency physician.* Philadelphia: Saunders. C from Pollack, H. M. [2000]. *Clinical urography* [2nd ed.]. Philadelphia: Saunders.)

◆ **Interventions: Take Action.** Nursing interventions focus on ***pain*** relief and preventing infection and urinary obstruction. Most patients expel the stone without invasive procedures. Size (i.e., less than 5 mm) is the most important factor for whether a stone will pass on its own; its composition and location are also factors. The larger the stone and the higher up in the urinary tract it is, the less likely it is to pass. When the stone is passed, it should be captured and sent to the laboratory for analysis. Other interventions are needed when the stone does not pass spontaneously (Fig. 61.3).

Managing Pain. Nonsurgical and surgical approaches are used to help the patient with a kidney stone achieve an acceptable degree of ***pain*** relief.

Nonsurgical Management. Nonsurgical measures to relieve pain include strategies to enhance stone passing, as well as direct pain management.

Drug therapy is needed in the first 24 to 36 hours when pain is most severe. Opioid analgesics are used to control the severe pain caused by stones in the urinary tract and may be given IV for rapid pain relief. NSAIDs such as ketorolac or ketoprofen in the acute phase may be effective. When NSAIDs are used, there is an increased risk for kidney impairment from reduced perfusion. NSAIDs interfere with renal autoregulation, and the risk

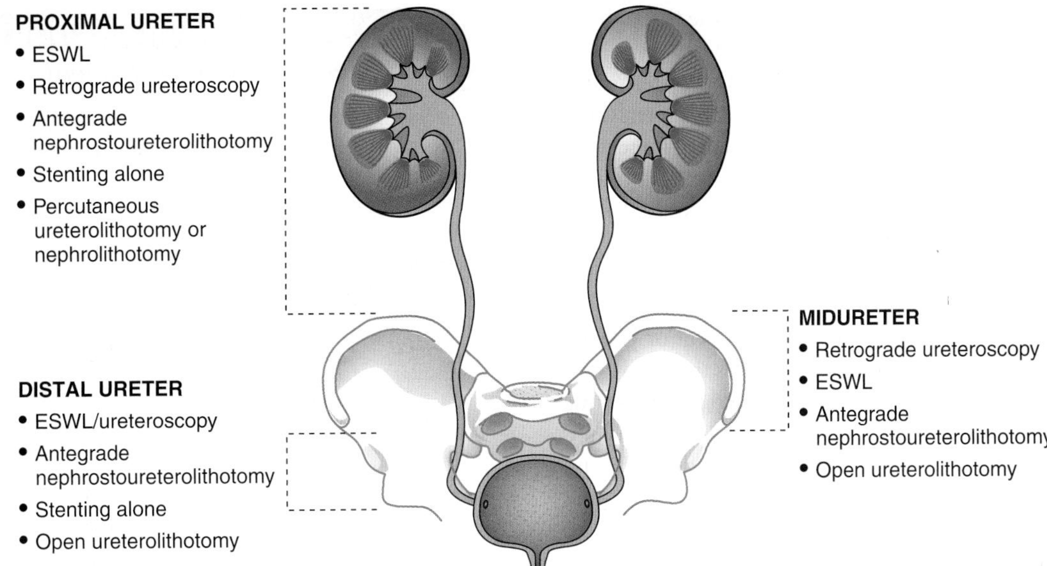

FIG. 61.3 Treatment options for ureteral stones. *ESWL,* Extracorporeal shock wave lithotripsy. (Modified from Singal, R. K., & Denstedt, J. D. [1997]. Contemporary management of ureteral stones. *The Urologic Clinics of North America, 24*[1], 59–70.)

for impairment is greater among patients with pre-existing kidney dysfunction. Risk for bleeding is also increased from platelet inhibition when NSAIDs are used. Bleeding risk is particularly concerning when surgical intervention for stones is needed.

Control of ***pain*** is more effective when drugs are given at regularly scheduled intervals or by a constant delivery system (e.g., skin patch) instead of PRN. Spasmolytic drugs, such as oxybutynin chloride and propantheline bromide, are important for control of pain. Administer the drugs as prescribed and assess the response by asking the patient to rate the discomfort on a pain-rating scale.

Other management techniques include avoiding overhydration and underhydration in the acute phase to help make the passage of a stone less painful. Strain the urine and teach the patient to strain it to monitor for stone passage. Send any stone passed to the laboratory for analysis because preventive therapy is based on stone composition.

Antibiotics may be used to manage struvite stones because these are associated with urinary infections from urease-producing organisms such as *Proteus mirabilis, Klebsiella, Enterobacter,* or *Pseudomonas.* (*E. coli* does not produce urease.) When urease-producing bacteria remain in the urine and within the stone, urine becomes alkaline, causing phosphate to precipitate and allowing staghorn-shaped struvite stones to form rapidly.

Two drugs may be used to aid in stone expulsion: a thiazide diuretic and allopurinol. These drugs, combined with a high fluid intake, increase urine volume or decrease urine pH and help increase the excretion of stones or stone fragments. Alpha-adrenergic blockers and calcium channel blockers can shorten the time to stone passage by relaxing the smooth muscle within the ureters. Citrate may be used to alkalinize urine pH and dissolve uric acid stones. Implementing oral citrate treatment cannot be done until stone composition is known. It is typically reserved for prevention and treatment of recurrent stone formation.

A stone that has not passed within 1 to 2 months is unlikely to pass spontaneously. Other options for stone intervention are considered when infection occurs, when pain cannot be well managed, or when there is an actual or increased risk for reduced kidney function. An observation period of 1 to 2 weeks may be reasonable if the patient is comfortable or has few symptoms and stones are smaller than 5 mm.

Lithotripsy or extracorporeal *shock wave lithotripsy (SWL)* is the use of sound, laser, or dry shock waves to break the stone into small fragments. The patient receives moderate sedation and lies on a flat table with the lithotriptor aimed at the stone, which is located by fluoroscopy. A local anesthetic cream is applied to the skin site over the stone 45 minutes before the procedure. During the procedure, cardiac rhythm is monitored by ECG and the shock waves are delivered in synchrony with the R wave. Shock waves at the rate of 60 to 120/min are applied over 30 to 45 minutes (Li et al., 2013). Continuous ECG monitoring for dysrhythmia and fluoroscopic observation for stone destruction are maintained.

After lithotripsy, strain the urine to monitor the passage of stone fragments. Bruising may occur on the flank of the affected side. Occasionally a stent is placed in the ureter before SWL to ease passage of the stone fragments.

Surgical Management. Minimally invasive surgical and open surgical procedures are used if urinary obstruction occurs or if the stone is too large to be passed.

Minimally Invasive Surgical Procedures. Minimally invasive surgical (MIS) procedures include stenting, ureteroscopy, percutaneous ureterolithotomy, and percutaneous nephrolithotomy.

Stenting is performed with a **stent**, a small tube that is placed in the ureter by ureteroscopy. The stent dilates the ureter and enlarges the passageway for the stone or stone fragments. This totally internal procedure prevents the passing stone from coming in contact with the ureteral mucosa, thereby reducing pain, bleeding, and infection risk, all of which could block the ureter.

A Foley catheter may facilitate passage of the stone through the urethra.

Ureteroscopy is an endoscopic procedure. The ureteroscope is passed through the urethra and bladder into the ureter. Once the stone is seen, it is removed with grasping baskets, forceps, or loops. Lithotripsy can also be performed through the ureteroscope. A Foley catheter may be placed to facilitate passage of the stone fragments through the urethra.

Percutaneous ureterolithotomy or nephrolithotomy is the removal of a stone in the ureter or kidney through the skin. The patient lies prone or on the side and receives local or general anesthesia. The urologist or radiologist identifies the ideal entry point with fluoroscopy and passes a needle into the collecting system of the kidney. Once a tract has been made in the kidney, other equipment, such as an **intracorporeal** (inside the body) ultrasonic or laser lithotriptor, can be used to break up and remove the stone. An endoscope with a special attachment to grasp and extract the stone can be used. Often a nephrostomy tube is left in place at first to prevent the stone fragments from passing through the urinary tract.

Monitor the patient for complications after the procedure. Complications include bleeding at the site or through the tube, pneumothorax, and infection. Monitor nephrostomy tube drainage for volume and the presence of blood in the urine, which is normal for the first 24 to 48 hours after tube placement. Provide routine nephrostomy tube care, with sterile dressing changes and tube flushing (if prescribed).

Open Surgical Procedures. When other stone removal attempts have failed or when risk for a lasting injury to the ureter or kidney is possible, an *open ureterolithotomy* (into the ureter), *pyelolithotomy* (into the kidney pelvis), or *nephrolithotomy* (into the kidney) procedure may be performed. These procedures are used for a large or impacted stone.

Preoperative care. Explain to the patient how, when, and where the procedure will be performed. Describe what he or she can expect to see, hear, and feel before and after the procedure. The patient is given nothing by mouth and also receives a bowel preparation before the procedure. (See Chapter 9 for routine care before surgery.)

Operative procedures. The retroperitoneal area is entered through a large flank incision, as for nephrectomy (see Chapter 62), pyelolithotomy, or nephrolithotomy and through a lower abdominal incision for ureterolithotomy. The urinary tract is entered surgically, and the stone is removed. Before closure, tubes and drains may be placed (e.g., nephrostomy tube, ureteral stent, Penrose or other wound drainage device, Foley catheter).

Postoperative care. Follow routine procedures for assessment of the patient who has received anesthesia. See Chapter 9 for routine care after surgery. Monitor the amount of bleeding from incisions and in the urine. Maintain adequate fluid intake. Strain the urine to monitor passage of stone fragments. Teach the patient how to prevent future stones with dietary changes, including consistent daily fluid intake to avoid dehydration and supersaturation.

Preventing Infection. Infection control before invasive procedures is critical for preventing urosepsis. Interventions include giving antibiotics, either to eliminate an existing infection or to prevent new infections, and maintaining nutrition and fluid intake. Because infection always occurs with struvite stone formation, the health care team plans for long-term infection prevention.

NCLEX EXAMINATION CHALLENGE 61.3

Safe and Effective Care Environment

A client with diabetes has the following assessment changes after a percutaneous nephrolithotomy procedure. Which change requires **immediate** nursing intervention?

A. Difficulty breathing and an oxygen saturation of 88% on 2 L of oxygen by nasal cannula
B. A point-of-care blood glucose of 150 mg/dL and client report of thirst
C. A decreased hematocrit by 1% (compared with preoperative values and hematuria)
D. An oral temperature of 38° C (101° F) and cloudiness of urine draining from the nephrostomy tube after IV administration of a broad-spectrum antibiotic

Drug therapy involves the use of quinolones, ampicillin, or other broad-spectrum antibiotics. When urine culture and sensitivity (C&S) results are known, more specific antibiotics may be prescribed. C&S studies are often repeated 48 hours after completion of antibiotic therapy to evaluate whether urine sterility has returned.

Urine levels of antibiotics may be measured to ensure that adequate levels have been reached. If the antibiotic is not sufficiently concentrated in urine, organisms may not be completely eliminated. Evidence of a new infection (e.g., chills, fever, altered mental status) warrants the collection of urine sample for new C&S tests.

For the patient with struvite stones, periodic and long-term monitoring of the urine for infection is needed. Urine cultures are checked monthly for as long as 1 year. Long-term use of antibiotics, while recommended, makes the development of resistant organisms more likely and antibiotic therapy less effective. Drugs that prevent bacteria from splitting urea, such as acetohydroxamic acid and hydroxyurea, are often prescribed long term for patients with struvite stones. Serum creatinine levels are monitored in patients receiving acetohydroxamic acid, and the drug is stopped if creatinine levels are above 2 mg/dL. Review interventions aimed at preventing urinary tract infection (UTI). See the earlier Patient and Family Education: Preparing for Self-Management: Preventing a Urinary Tract Infection box.

Nutrition therapy ideally includes adequate calorie intake with a balance of all food groups. Encourage a fluid intake sufficient to dilute urine to a light color throughout the 24-hour day (typically 2 to 3 L/day) unless another health problem requires fluid restriction.

Preventing Obstruction. Measures to prevent urinary obstruction by stones include a high intake of fluids (3 L/day or more) and accurate measures of intake and output. Fluid intake sufficient to provide diluted urine helps prevent dehydration, promotes urine flow, and decreases the chance of crystals forming a stone. Interventions also depend on the type of stone the patient has formed. Drugs, diet modification, and fluid intake are the major strategies used to prevent future stones.

Drug therapy to prevent obstruction depends on what is causing stone formation and the type of stone formed. Teach the patient the reason for the drug and assess for side effects or adverse drug reactions. Some drugs may need to be avoided because they may contribute to stone formation.

Drugs to treat *hypercalciuria* (high levels of calcium in the urine) include thiazide diuretics (e.g., chlorothiazide or hydrochlorothiazide). These drugs promote calcium reabsorption from the renal tubules back into the body, thereby reducing urine calcium loads. For patients with *hyperoxaluria* (high levels of oxalic acid in the urine), vitamin B_6 and thiazide diuretics may be prescribed.

Patients with hyperuricemia or chronic gout have high uric acid levels causing acidic urine and resulting in a higher risk for uric acid stone formation. Acidic urine is more likely to cause uric acid to precipitate, resulting in uric acid stones. Normal urine pH can range from 4.6 to 8.0 with the average at 6.0. Urine pH under 5.0 is considered acidic and over 8.0 alkaline. The desired urine pH range for patients with high uric acid levels and a history of uric acid stone formation is 6.5 to 7.0.

Three measures are commonly used to treat and/or prevent uric stone formation: increasing urine pH, increasing fluid intake, and decreasing uric acid production. To alkalinize the urine, drugs such as potassium citrate, 50% sodium citrate, and sodium bicarbonate are used. Drinking 2 to 3 L of water is effective in flushing out excess uric acid and reduces uric acid stone formation. Modifying the diet to restrict purines can be effective in decreasing uric acid production. Foods that contain high levels of purines include organ meats, sardines, and red meats. The use of xanthine oxidase inhibitors such as allopurinol and febuxostat can also be used to decrease the body's production of uric acid.

Cystinuria (high levels of cystine in the urine) can lead to stone formation. Cystinuria is genetic and affects children more than adults. Conservative measures are used to prevent stone formation. Drinking 2 to 3 L of water throughout the day and night is encouraged to reduce high cystine levels in the urine. Moderating sodium and protein consumption has been effective in reducing urine cystine levels. To alkalinize urine, drugs such as potassium citrate are used. However, since moderating sodium has been shown to be effective in reducing urine cystine levels, sodium bicarbonate and sodium citrate are avoided because of the sodium content in these medications. If conservative measures fail, medications such as tiopronin, D-penicillamine, and captopril are used to lower urine cystine levels (Goldfarb, 2019). *Nutrition therapy* depends on the type of stone formed (see Table 61.5). Collaborate with the registered dietitian nutritionist (RDN) to plan for and teach the appropriate diet to the patient.

Other measures can help the stone pass more quickly. Urge the patient to walk as often as possible. Walking promotes passage of stones and reduces bone calcium resorption. Check the urine pH daily and strain all urine with filter paper or a special urine sieve/strainer to collect passed stones and fragments.

Self-management education includes follow-up care to evaluate effects of intervention includes a 24-hour urine collection and serum chemical analysis. The patient often has great anxiety and fear that a stone and its pain may recur. In addition to anxiety about the pain, the risk for repeated surgical interventions or permanent and serious kidney damage may be present. Psychosocial preparation is enhanced when patients know what to expect and which actions to take if problems develop. Reassure the patient that preventive and health promotion activities help prevent recurrence. See the Patient and Family Education: Preparing for Self-Management; Urinary Calculi box.

PATIENT AND FAMILY EDUCATION: PREPARING FOR SELF-MANAGEMENT

Urinary Calculi

- Finish your entire prescription of antibiotics to ensure that you will not get a urinary tract infection.
- You may resume your usual daily activities.
- Remember to balance regular exercise with sleep and rest.
- You may return to work 2 days to 6 weeks after surgery, depending on the type of intervention, your personal tolerance, and your primary health care provider's directives.
- Depending on the type of stone you had, you may be advised to take medications or adjust your diet may to reduce the risk for further stone formation.
- Remember to drink at least 3 L of fluid a day to dilute potential stone-forming crystals, prevent dehydration, and promote urine flow.
- Monitor urine pH as directed (possibly up to three times per day).
- Expect bruising after lithotripsy. The bruising may be quite extensive and may take several weeks to resolve.
- Your urine may be bloody for several days after surgery.
- Pain in the region of the kidneys or bladder may signal the beginning of an infection or the formation of another stone. Report any pain, fever, chills, or difficulty with urination immediately to your primary health care provider or nurse.
- Keep follow-up appointments to check on infection and have repeat cultures done.

UROTHELIAL CANCER

Pathophysiology Review

Urothelial cancers are malignant tumors of the *urothelium,* which is the lining of transitional cells in the kidney, renal pelvis, ureters, urinary bladder, and urethra. Most urothelial cancers occur in the bladder, and the term *bladder cancer* describes this condition. Urothelial cancer is also known as *transitional cell carcinoma* (TCC).

In North America, most urinary tract cancers are transitional cell carcinomas of the bladder (American Cancer Society [ACS], 2019; Canadian Cancer Society, 2016). The second most common site of urinary tract cancer is the kidney and renal pelvis. Urothelial cancers are usually low grade, have multiple points of origin *(multifocal),* and are recurrent. Once the cancer spreads beyond the transitional cell layer, it is highly invasive and can spread beyond the bladder. Because of the nature of this cancer, patients may have recurrence up to 10 years after being cancer free (ACS, 2019). Less common bladder cancers include squamous cell carcinoma, adenocarcinoma, small cell carcinoma, and sarcoma (ACS, 2019).

Tumors confined to the bladder mucosa are treated by simple excision, whereas those that are deeper but not into the muscle layer are treated with excision plus **intravesical** (inside the bladder) chemotherapy. Cancer that has spread deeper into the bladder muscle layer is treated with more extensive surgery, often a **radical cystectomy** (removal of the bladder and surrounding tissue) with urinary diversion. Chemotherapy and radiation therapy are used in addition to surgery. If untreated, the tumor invades surrounding tissues; spreads to distant sites (liver, lung, and bone); and ultimately leads to death.

Exposure to toxins such as gasoline and diesel fuel, as well as to chemicals used in hair dyes and in the rubber, paint, electric cable, and textile industries, increases the risk for bladder cancer. The greatest risk factor for bladder cancer is tobacco use. Other risks include *Schistosoma haematobium* (a parasite) infection, excessive use of drugs containing phenacetin, and long-term use of cyclophosphamide.

In the United States and Canada, about 87,730 new cases of bladder cancer are diagnosed each year, and about 19,190 deaths occur each year from the disease (ACS, 2017; Canadian Cancer Society, 2016). This cancer is rare in adults younger than 40 years and is most common after 55 years of age (ACS, 2019).

As with many urologic conditions, sexual health is commonly affected by this diagnosis and treatment (ACS, 2019). To manage sexual health concerns, encourage patients to discuss sexual health and ensure that the proper interprofessional care team member provides education to patients and their partners about:

- Potential implications of treatment on sexuality
- Treatment options
- Referrals to providers who specialize in sexual dysfunction

Health Promotion and Maintenance. Many adults believe that tobacco use is associated with cancers only of organs that come into direct contact with it, such as the lungs. However, many compounds in tobacco enter the bloodstream and affect other organs, such as the bladder. Therefore encourage people who smoke to quit (see the Health Promotion and Maintenance section of Chapter 24). Just as important, encourage anyone who comes in contact with dry, liquid, or gaseous chemicals to take precautions. Some adults work with chemicals, and others may come into contact with them while engaging in hobbies. Many chemicals and fumes can enter the body through contact with skin and with mucous membranes in the respiratory tract. Use of personal protective equipment, such as gloves and masks, can reduce this contact. Also encourage anyone who works with chemicals to shower or bathe and change clothing as soon as contact is completed.

NCLEX EXAMINATION CHALLENGE 61.4

Physiological Integrity

A 68-year-old male client is seeing the primary care provider for an annual examination. Which assessment finding alerts the nurse to an increased risk for bladder cancer?

A. A 5 pack-year history of smoking 45 years ago
B. Difficulty starting and stopping the urine stream
C. A 30-year occupation as a long-distance truck driver
D. A recent colon cancer diagnosis in his 72-year-old brother

❖ Interprofessional Collaborative Care

◆ Assessment: Recognize Cues

Physical Assessment/Signs and Symptoms. Ask about the patient's perception of his or her general health. Document the gender and age of the patient. Ask about active and passive exposure to cigarette smoke. To detect exposure to harmful environmental agents, ask the patient to describe his or her occupation and hobbies in detail. Also ask the patient to describe any change in the color, frequency, or volume of urine ***elimination*** and any abdominal discomfort.

Observe the patient's overall appearance, especially skin color and nutrition status. Inspect, percuss, and palpate the abdomen for asymmetry, tenderness, and bladder distention.

Examine the urine for color and clarity. Blood in the urine is often the first indication of bladder cancer. It may be gross or microscopic and is usually painless and intermittent. Dysuria, frequency, and urgency occur when infection or obstruction is also present.

Psychosocial Assessment. Assess the patient's emotions, including the response to a tentative diagnosis of bladder cancer, and note anxiety, fear, sadness, anger, or guilt. Early symptoms are painless, and many patients ignore the blood in the urine because it is intermittent. They also may be reluctant to seek treatment if they suspect a sexually transmitted infection (STI). As a result, they may have guilt or anger about their own delays in seeking medical attention.

Assess the patient's coping methods and available support from family members. Social support may provide motivation and improve coping during recovery from treatment.

Diagnostic Assessment. The only significant finding on a routine urinalysis is gross or microscopic hematuria. Cytologic testing on voided urine specimens is usually not helpful. Bladder-wash specimens and bladder biopsies are the most specific tests for cancer.

Cystoscopy is usually performed to evaluate painless hematuria. A biopsy of a visible bladder tumor can be performed during cystoscopy. This is essential for staging and is usually performed in an ambulatory care surgery center. Cystoureterography may be used to identify obstructions, especially where the ureter joins the bladder. CT scans show tumor invasion of surrounding tissues. Ultrasonography shows masses but is less valuable for tumor staging. MRI may help assess deep, invasive tumors. See Chapter 60 for general care of the patient undergoing diagnostic testing.

◆ Interventions: Take Action. Therapy for the patient with bladder cancer usually begins with surgical removal of the tumor for diagnosis and staging of disease. For tumors extending beyond the mucosa, surgery is followed by intravesical chemotherapy or immunotherapy. High-grade or recurrent tumors are treated with more radical surgery plus intravesical chemotherapy, radiotherapy, or both. Systemic chemotherapy is reserved for patients with distant metastases. (See Chapter 20 for general care of the patient receiving chemotherapy or radiation therapy.)

Nonsurgical Management. Prophylactic immunotherapy with intravesical instillation of bacille Calmette-Guérin (BCG), a live virus compound, is used to prevent tumor recurrence of superficial cancers. This procedure is more effective than single-agent chemotherapy. Usually the agent is instilled in an outpatient cancer clinic and allowed to dwell in the bladder for a specified length of time, usually 2 hours. When the patient urinates, live virus is excreted with the urine.

Teach patients receiving this treatment to prevent contact of the live virus with other members of the household by not sharing a toilet with others for at least 24 hours after instillation. Instruct men to urinate while sitting down to avoid splashing the urine. After 24 hours, the toilet should be completely cleaned using a solution of 10% liquid bleach. If only one toilet is available in the household, teach the patient to flush the toilet after use and follow this by adding one cup of undiluted bleach to the bowl water. The bowl is then flushed after 15 minutes, and the seat and flat surfaces of the toilet are wiped with a cloth containing a solution of 10% liquid bleach. Instruct the patient to wear gloves during the cleaning and to dispose of the cloth after sealing it in a plastic bag.

Underwear or other clothing that has come in contact with the urine during the immediate 24 hours after instillation should be washed separately from other clothing in a solution of 10% liquid bleach. Sexual intercourse is avoided for 24 hours after the instillation.

Multiagent chemotherapy is successful in prolonging life after distant metastasis has occurred but rarely results in a cure. Radiation therapy is also useful in prolonging life.

Surgical Management. The type of surgery for bladder cancer depends on the type and stage of the cancer and the patient's general health. Complete bladder removal *(cystectomy)* with additional removal of surrounding muscle and tissue offers the best chance of a cure for large, invasive bladder cancers. Four alternatives for urine ***elimination*** are used after cystectomy: ileal conduit; continent pouch; bladder reconstruction, also known as *neobladder;* and ureterosigmoidostomy.

Preoperative Care. Specific patient education depends on the type and extent of the planned surgical procedure. Coordinate education before surgery with the patient, surgeon, and enterostomal therapist (ET) or wound, ostomy, and continence nurse. Discuss the type of planned urinary diversion and the selection of a site for the stoma. Including the patient in this planning improves the chances for the patient to have a positive attitude about body image and a positive self-image. Use educational counseling to ensure understanding about self-care practices, methods of pouching, control of urine drainage, and management of odor.

The site selected for the stoma should be visible to the patient and avoid folds of skin, bones, and scar tissue. When possible, the waistline or belt area is avoided to reduce the risk for reducing ***tissue integrity.*** Prepare the patient for the number and type of drains that will be present after surgery. General care before surgery is discussed in Chapter 9.

Operative Procedures. Transurethral resection of the bladder tumor (TURBT) or partial cystectomy is performed for small, early, superficial tumors. In a partial (segmental) cystectomy, a portion of the bladder is removed when there is only a single isolated bladder tumor.

When the entire bladder must be removed (complete cystectomy), the ureters are diverted into a collecting reservoir. Techniques for urinary diversion are shown in Fig. 61.4. With an ileal conduit, the ureters are surgically placed in the ileum and urine is collected in a pouch on the skin around the stoma. More often, a continent reservoir known as a "neobladder" is created from an intestinal graft to store urine and replace the surgically removed bladder. With cutaneous ureterostomy or ureteroureterostomy, the ureter opening is brought out onto the skin. The cutaneous ureterostomies may be located on either side of the abdomen or side by side.

Postoperative Care. After cutaneous ureterostomy, an external pouch covers the ostomy to collect urine and maintain ***tissue integrity.*** Collaborate with the ET to focus care on the wound, the skin, and urinary drainage. (See Chapter 51 for ostomy care.)

The patient with a Kock's pouch, a continent reservoir, may have a Penrose drain and a plastic Medena catheter in the stoma. The drain removes lymphatic fluid or other secretions; the catheter ensures urine drainage so incisions can heal. The patient with a neobladder usually requires 2 to 4 days in the ICU and will have a drain at first in the event the neobladder requires irrigation. Later, irrigation can be performed with intermittent catheterization. Irrigation is performed to ensure patency. There is no sensation of bladder fullness with a neobladder because sensory nerves are not attached. As a result, the patient will need to learn new cues to void, such as prescribed times or noticing a feeling of neobladder pressure. General care after surgery is discussed in Chapter 9.

Different types of drains and nephrostomy catheters are used, sometimes on a temporary basis, to drain urine from the kidney. Some are totally internal, with no drainage to the outside. Others may drain exclusively to the outside, and urine is collected in a pouch or bag. For this type of drainage system, urine output remains constant. Decreased or no drainage is cause for concern and must be reported to the surgeon or nephrologist, as is leakage around the catheter. Some nephrostomy tubes are connected both to the new bladder (internal drainage) and to an external drainage system. With this type of system, urine output from the external portion of the catheter varies. With any drainage system, intervention is needed if the external catheter is partially or completely pulled out accidentally. Immediately notify the surgeon or nephrologist. If the catheter remains partially in place, secure it from further movement. This action may result in a reinsertion process rather than a total replacement.

Care Coordination and Transition Management

Self-Management Education. Teach the patient and family about drugs, diet and fluid therapy, the use of external pouching systems, and the technique for catheterizing a continent reservoir.

With some procedures, the patient may need electrolyte replacement to prevent long-term deficits. Teach the patient to avoid foods that are known to produce gas if the urinary diversion uses the intestinal tract. When intestinal production of gas is excessive, flatus can induce incontinence.

Patients who have a neobladder created often have extreme weight loss during the first few weeks after surgery. Collaborate with a dietitian to develop a diet plan specific to the patient to meet his or her caloric needs.

Ureterostomies divert urine directly to the skin surface through a ureteral skin opening (stoma). After ureterostomy, the patient must wear a pouch.

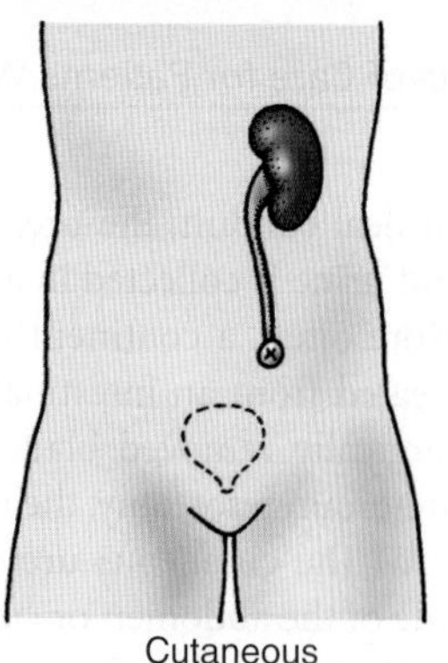

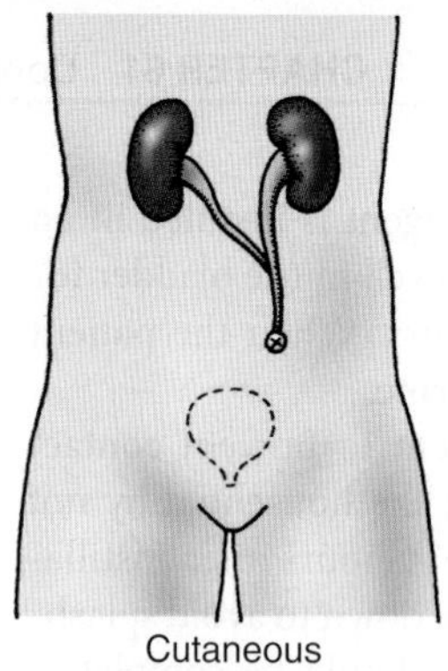

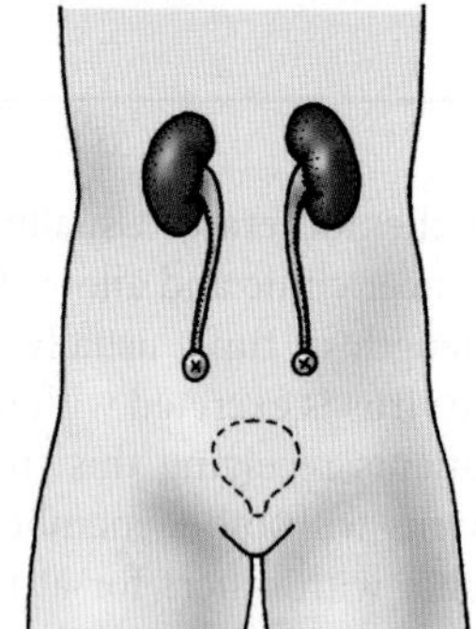

Conduits collect urine in a portion of the intestine, which is then opened onto the skin surface as a stoma. After the creation of a conduit, the patient must wear a pouch.

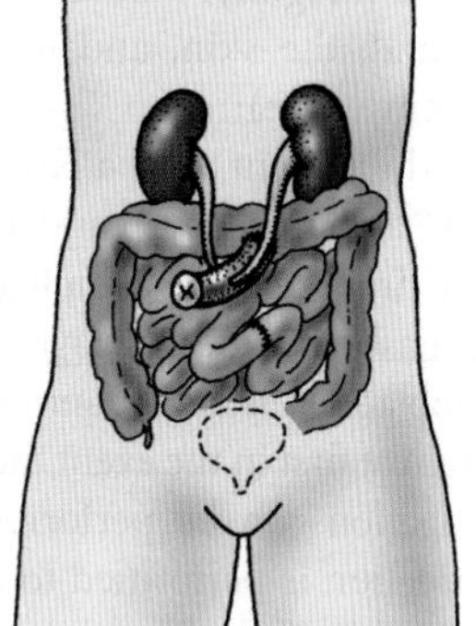

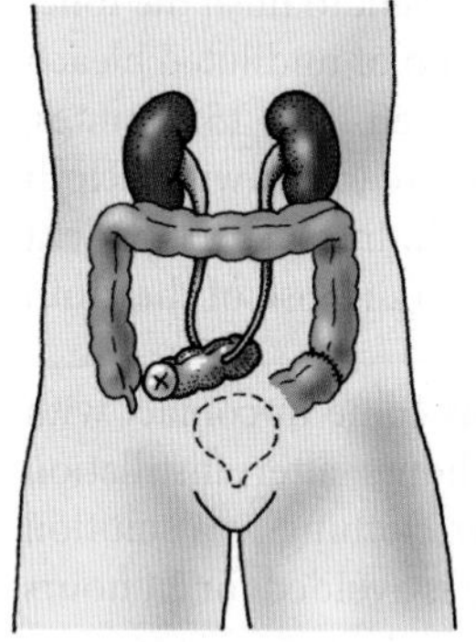

Ileal reservoirs divert urine into a surgically created pouch, or pocket, that functions as a bladder. The stoma is continent, and the patient removes urine by regular self-catheterization.

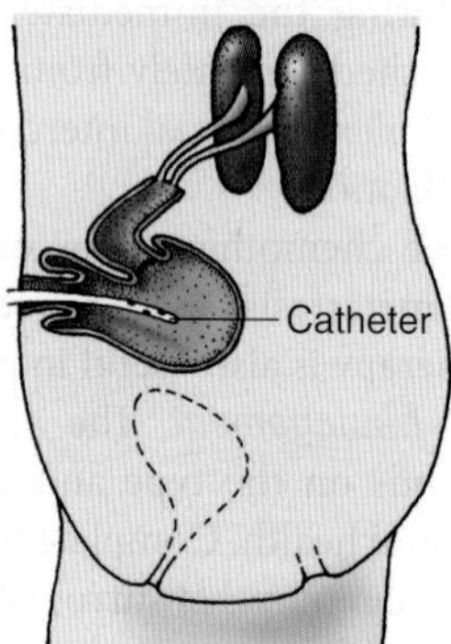

Sigmoidostomies divert urine to the large intestine, so no stoma is required. The patient excretes urine with bowel movements, and bowel incontinence may result.

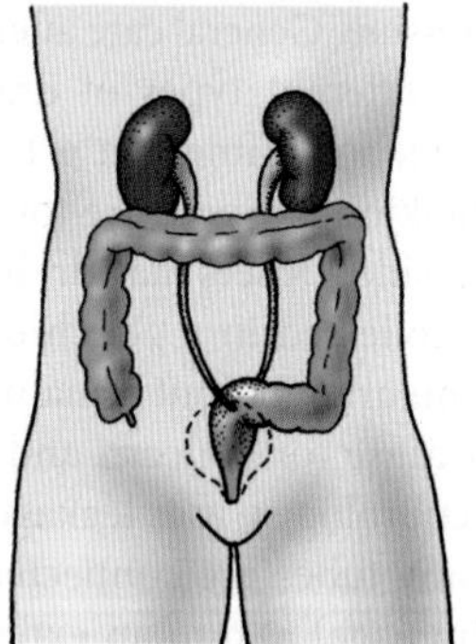

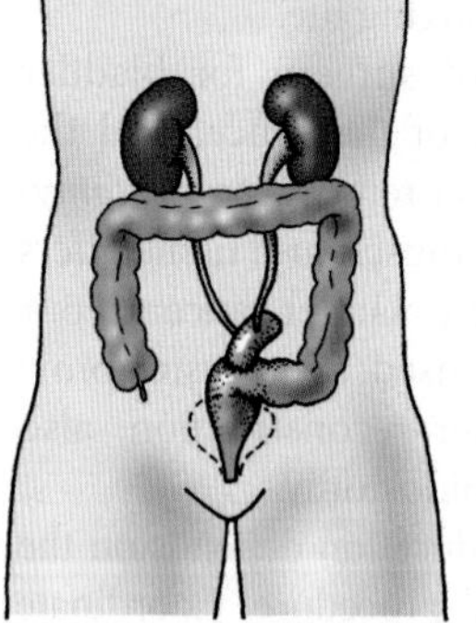

FIG. 61.4 Urinary diversion procedures used in the treatment of bladder cancer.

NURSING SAFETY PRIORITY QSEN

Action Alert

Infection is common in patients who have a neobladder. Teach patients and family members the symptoms of infection and the importance of reporting them immediately to the surgeon.

Instruct the patient and family about any changes in self-care activities related to the urinary diversion. In collaboration with the enterostomal therapist, demonstrate external pouch application, local skin care, pouch care, methods of adhesion, and drainage mechanisms. If a Kock pouch has been created, teach the patient how to use a catheter to drain the pouch. For all instruction, observe at least one return demonstration or "teach-back" session by the patient or the caregiver. Ideally the patient assumes responsibility for self-care before discharge.

Help the patient prepare for the impact of urinary diversion on self-image, body image, sexual functioning, and self-esteem. Counseling provides information and support to reduce feelings of powerlessness.

Through discussions with the patient about common social situations, help the patient gain control over new toileting practices. Men with a urinary diversion into the sigmoid colon need to learn the habit of sitting to urinate. For patients of either gender, promote confidence in social situations by encouraging frequent emptying of urinary collection devices before traveling or attending social functions. Resumption of sexual activity is a major concern for many, regardless of age. Address this topic openly and with sensitivity. Cystectomy causes impotence in men, but treatment is available (see Chapter 67).

Health Care Resources. The United Ostomy Association (https://www.ostomy.org) and the ACS have educational materials that may be useful to patients. Refer patients and family members to local chapters or units of these organizations. In some areas, local support groups have meetings to help others and to send visitors to provide peer counseling and support. Home care personnel may help with follow-up, easing the transition from hospital to home. The Wound, Ostomy, and Continence Nurses Society has educational programs and a journal for the care of patients with ostomies.

GET READY FOR THE NEXT-GENERATION NCLEX® EXAMINATION!

Key Points

Review these Key Points for each NCLEX Examination Client Needs Category.

Safe and Effective Care Environment

- Use sterile technique when inserting a catheter in the acute care environment. **QSEN: Safety**
- Use Contact Precautions with any drainage from the genitourinary tract. **QSEN: Safety**
- Teach patients with urge or stress incontinence to keep pathways to the bathroom well lighted and clear of obstacles to help prevent falls. **QSEN: Safety**

Health Promotion and Maintenance

- Teach patients to clean the perineal area daily and after voiding, having a bowel movement, and after sexual intercourse. **QSEN: Patient-Centered Care**
- Encourage all patients to maintain an adequate fluid intake. **QSEN: Evidence-Based Practice**
- Teach women who have stress incontinence the proper way to perform pelvic floor–strengthening exercises. **QSEN: Patient-Centered Care**

Psychosocial Integrity

- Allow the patient the opportunity to express feelings or concerns regarding a urinary tract disorder or a cancer diagnosis. **QSEN: Patient-Centered Care**
- Use a nonjudgmental approach in caring for patients with urinary incontinence. **QSEN: Patient-Centered Care**
- Avoid referring to protective pads, briefs, or pants as "diapers." **QSEN: Patient-Centered Care**
- Recognize the need for the patient undergoing cystectomy and urinary diversion to grieve about the body image change. **QSEN: Patient-Centered Care**

Physiological Integrity

- Identify hospitalized patients at risk for bacteriuria and urosepsis. **QSEN: Evidence-Based Practice**
- Teach patients with UTI to complete all prescribed antibiotic therapy even when symptoms of infection are absent. **QSEN: Patient-Centered Care**
- Evaluate daily the need for maintaining urinary catheters and discontinue as soon as possible. **QSEN: Evidence-Based Practice**
- Teach patients the expected side effects and any adverse reactions to prescribed drugs. **QSEN: Patient-Centered Care**

MASTERY QUESTIONS

1. Which adverse drug effects will the nurse assess for in a hospitalized client who is prescribed an anticholinergic drug to manage incontinence? (*Select all that apply.*)
   A. Insomnia
   B. Blurred vision
   C. Constipation
   D. Dry mouth
   E. Loss of sphincter control
   F. Increased sweating
   G. Worsening mental function
2. A 28-year-old female client states, "I don't know why I get cystitis every year. I don't drink much at work so that I can avoid using the public toilet." Which teaching by the nurse is most likely to reduce her risk for cystitis? *Select all that apply.*
   A. Reinforce her choice to avoid using a public toilet.
   B. Teach her to shower immediately after having sexual intercourse.
   C. Suggest that she drink at least 2 to 3 L of fluid throughout the day.
   D. Urge her to change her method of birth control from oral contraceptives to a barrier method.
   E. Instruct her to always wipe her perineum from front to back after each toilet use.
   F. Reinforce that she should complete the entire course of antibiotics as prescribed.
   G. Instruct her to empty her bladder immediately before intercourse.
3. A client is diagnosed with renal colic. What would the nurse do first?
   A. Prepare the client for lithotripsy.
   B. Encourage oral intake of fluids.
   C. Strain the urine and send for urinalysis.
   D. Administer opioids as prescribed.
4. For which hospitalized client does the nurse recommend the ongoing use of a urinary catheter?
   A. A 35-year-old woman who was admitted with a splenic laceration and femur fracture (closed repair completed) following a car crash
   B. A 48-year-old man who has established paraplegia and is admitted for pneumonia
   C. A 61-year-old woman who is admitted following a fall at home and has new-onset dysrhythmia
   D. A 74-year-old man who has lung cancer with brain metastasis and is being transitioned to hospice

REFERENCES

American Cancer Society (ACS). (2019). *About bladder cancer.* Retrieved from https://www.cancer.org/cancer/bladder/about/what-is-bladder-cancer.

American Cancer Society (ACS). (2017). *Cancer facts and figures 2017. Report No. 01-300M—No. 500817.* Atlanta: Author.

Aoki, Y., Brown, H., Brubaker, L., Comu, J., Daly, J., & Cartwright, R. (2017). Urinary incontinence in women. *National Reviews Disease Primers, 3.* https://doi.org/10.1038/nrdp.2017.42.

Avelluto, G., & Bryman, P. (2018). Asymptomatic bacteriuria vs. symptomatic urinary tract infection: Identification and treatment challenges in geriatric care. *Urologic Nursing, 38*(3). https://doi.org/10.7257/1053816X.2018.38.3.129.

Barrow, R. Y., Ahmed, F., Bolan, G. A., & Workowski, K. A. (2020). Recommendations for providing quality sexually transmitted diseases clinical services. *Morbidity and Mortality Weekly Report Recommendations and Reports, 68*(No. RR-5), 1–20. https://doi.org/10.15585/mmwr.rr6805a1.

Beauchemin, L., Newman, D., Danseur, M., Jackson, A., & Ritmiller, M. (2018). Best practices for clean intermittent catheterization. *Nursing 2018, 48*(9). https://doi.org/10.1097/01.NURSE.0000544216.23783.bc.

Beeson, T., & Davis, C. (2018). Urinary management with an external female collection device. *The Journal of Wound, Ostomy and Continence Nursing, 45*(2). https://doi.org/10.1097/WON.0000000000000417.

Bliss, D., Mathiason, M., et al. (2017). Incidence and predictors of incontinence associated skin damage in nursing home residents with new onset incontinence. *The Journal of Wound, Ostomy and Continence Nursing, 44*(2). https://doi.org/10.1097/WON.0000000000000313.

Canadian Cancer Society. (2016). *Statistics Canada. Canadian cancer Statistics, 2016.* Toronto: Canadian Cancer Society.

Centers for Disease Control and Prevention (CDC). (2016). *2015 Sexually transmitted disease treatment guidelines.* www.cdc.gov/std/tg2015.

Clemens, J. (2018). Urinary incontinence in men. In S. Calderwood (Ed.), *UpToDate,* Waltham, MA.

Conway, L., Liu, J., Harris, A., & Larson, E. (2017). Risk factors for bacteremia in patients with urinary catheter-associated bacteriuria. *American Journal of Critical Care, 26*(1), 43–52.

Damien, J., Pastor-Barriuso, R., Lopez, G., & de Pedro-Cuesta, J. (2017). Urinary incontinence and mortality among older adults residing in care homes. *Journal of Advanced Nursing, 73*(2). https://doi.org/10.1111/jan.13170.

Engberg, S., & Li, H. (2017). Urinary incontinence in frail older adults. *Urologic Nursing, 37*(3).

Feng, F., Hawks, J., Kernen, J., & Kyle, E. (2018). Recurrent urinary tract infection care: Integrating complementary and alternative medicine. *Urologic Nursing, 38*(5). https://doi.org/10.7257/1053-816X.2018.38.5.231.

Ferguson, A. (2018). Implementing a CAUTI prevention program in an acute care setting. *Urologic Nursing, 38*(6). https://doi.org/10.7257/1053816X.2018.38.6.273.

Goldfarb, D (2019). Cystine stones. In S. Goldfarb (Ed.), *UpToDate,* Waltham, MA.

Gray, M., McNichol, L., & Nix, D. (2016). Incontinence-associated dermatitis: Progress, promises, and ongoing challenges. *The Journal of Wound, Ostomy and Continence Nursing, 43*(2), 188–192.

Hooten, T., & Gupta, K. (2018). Acute simple cystitis in women. In S. Calderwood (Ed.), *UpToDate,* Waltham, MA.

Hubb, A., Stachowicz, A., & Wood, S. (2018). Onabutulinumtoxin A injections for urge incontinence. *American Family Physician, 97*(3). Online.

Kim, H. (2016). Update on the pathology and diagnosis. *International Neurology Journal, 20*(1). https://doi.org/0.5213/inj.1632522.261.

Lee, H., & Le, J. (2018). *Urinary tract infections. Infectious diseases.* Retrieved from https://www.accp.com/docs/bookstore/psap/p2018b1_sample.pdf.

Li, K., Lin, T., Zhang, C., Fan, X., Xu, K., Bi, L., et al. (2013). Optimal frequency of shock wave lithotripsy in urolithiasis treatment: A systematic review and meta-analysis of randomized controlled trials. *The Journal of Urology, 190*(4), 1260–1267.

Lukacz, E., Santiago, Y., & Albo, M. (2017). Urinary incontinence in women: A review. *Journal of American Medical Association, 318*(16). https://doi.org/10.1001/jama.2017.12137.

McCance, K., & Huether, S. (2019). *Pathophysiology: The biologic basis for disease in adults and children* (8th ed.). St. Louis: Mosby.

McGoldrick, M. (2016). Frequency for changing long-term indwelling urinary catheters. *Home Healthcare, Now, 34*(2), 105–106.

McLellan, L., & Hunstad, D. (2016). Urinary tract infection: Pathogenesis and outlook. *Trends in Molecular Medicine, 22*(11). https://doi.org/10.1016/j.molmed.2016.09.003.

Milson, I., & Gyhagen, M. (2018). The prevalence of urinary incontinence. *Climacteric.* https://doi.org/10.1080/13697137.2018.1543263.

Nicolle, L. (2016). Urinary tract infections in adults. In K. Skorecki, G. Chertow, P. Marsden, M. Taal, & A. Yu (Eds.), *Brenner and rector" the kidney* (10th ed.). Philadelphia: Elsevier.

O'Brien, V., Hannan, T., Yu, L., Robertson, E., Schwartz, D., Souza, S., et al. (2016). A mucosal imprint left by prior Escherichia coli bladder infection sensitizes to recurrent disease. *National Microbiology.* https://doi.org/10.1036/nmicrobiol.2016.196.

Panchisin, T. (2016). Improving outcomes with the ANA CAUTI prevention tool. *Nursing, 46*(3), 55–59.

Simmering, J., Tang, F., Cavannaugh, J., Polgreen, L., & Polgreen, P. (2017). The increase in hospitalizations for urinary tract infections and the associated costs in the United States, 1998-2011. *Open Forum Infectious Diseases, 4*(1). https://doi.org/10.1093/ofid/ofw281.

Tan, C., & Chlebicki, M. (2016). Urinary tract infections in adults. *Singapore Medical Journal, 57*(9). In T. Touhy & K. Jett (Vol. Ed.), *Ebersole & Hess' toward healthy aging: Human needs & nursing response.* St. Louis: Elsevier. https://doi.org/10.11622/smedj.2016153.

Zhang, N. (2018). An evolutionary concept analysis of urinary incontinence. *Urologic Nursing, 38*(6). https://doi.org/10.7257/1053-816X.2018.38.6.289.

62

Concepts of Care for Patients With Kidney Disorders

Robyn Mitchell

http://evolve.elsevier.com/Iggy/

LEARNING OUTCOMES

1. Collaborate with the interprofessional team to coordinate high-quality care and promote urinary ***elimination*** in patients who have kidney disorders.
2. Teach the patient and caregiver(s) about home safety issues affected by impaired ***elimination*** and impairment of ***fluid and electrolyte balance*** or ***acid-base balance*** resulting from kidney problems.
3. Prioritize evidence-based care for patients with kidney disorders that impair urinary ***elimination.***
4. Identify community resources for patients requiring assistance with any acute or chronic kidney problem.
5. Teach adults how to decrease the risk for kidney damage or kidney disease.
6. Implement nursing interventions to help the patient and family cope with the psychosocial impact caused by acute or chronic kidney disorders.
7. Apply knowledge of pathophysiology to assess patients with kidney disorders affecting ***elimination, fluid and electrolyte balance,*** or ***acid-base balance.***
8. Use clinical judgment to analyze information from laboratory data and assessment findings in the care of patients with kidney disorders.
9. Teach the patient and caregiver(s) about common drugs and other management strategies used for kidney disorders, including ***pain*** control.
10. Implement evidence-based nursing interventions to prevent complications of kidney disorders and their therapies.

KEY TERMS

abscess A localized collection of pus caused by an inflammatory response to bacteria in tissues and organs.

acute glomerulonephritis Inflammation of the glomerulus that develops suddenly from an excess immunity response within the kidney tissues.

dysuria Painful urination.

hydronephrosis Abnormal enlargement of the kidney.

hydroureter Abnormal distention of the ureter.

nephrectomy Surgical removal of the kidney.

nephrosclerosis Degenerative kidney disorder resulting from changes in kidney blood vessels

nephrostomy The surgical creation of an opening directly into the kidney; performed to divert urine externally and prevent further damage to the kidney when a stricture is causing hydronephrosis and cannot be corrected with urologic procedures.

nephrotic syndrome (NS) Immunologic kidney disorder in which glomerular permeability increases so larger molecules pass through the membrane into the urine and are then excreted; causes massive loss of protein into the urine and decreased plasma albumin levels.

polycystic kidney disease (PKD) Genetic disorder in which fluid-filled cysts develop in the kidneys.

pyelolithotomy Surgical removal of a stone from the kidney.

pyelonephritis A bacterial infection in the kidney and renal pelvis.

stricture Narrowing of the urinary tract.

ureteroplasty Surgical repair of the ureter.

PRIORITY AND INTERRELATED CONCEPTS

The priority concept for this chapter is:
- ***Elimination***

The ***Elimination*** concept exemplar for this chapter is Pyelonephritis.

The interrelated concepts for this chapter are:
- ***Fluid and Electrolyte Balance***
- ***Acid-Base Balance***
- ***Immunity***
- ***Pain***

Healthy kidneys are the major controllers of urinary ***elimination.*** They perform this function by filtering wastes from the blood and selectively determining which substances remain in the body and which are eliminated. Thus the kidneys maintain homeostasis by contributing to ***fluid and electrolyte balance*** and ***acid-base balance.*** Any problem that disrupts kidney function has the potential to impair general homeostasis and all aspects of urinary elimination (Fig. 62.1). Interaction with other organs and systems is necessary for the kidneys to function effectively. In addition, when the kidneys are impaired, the buildup of toxic

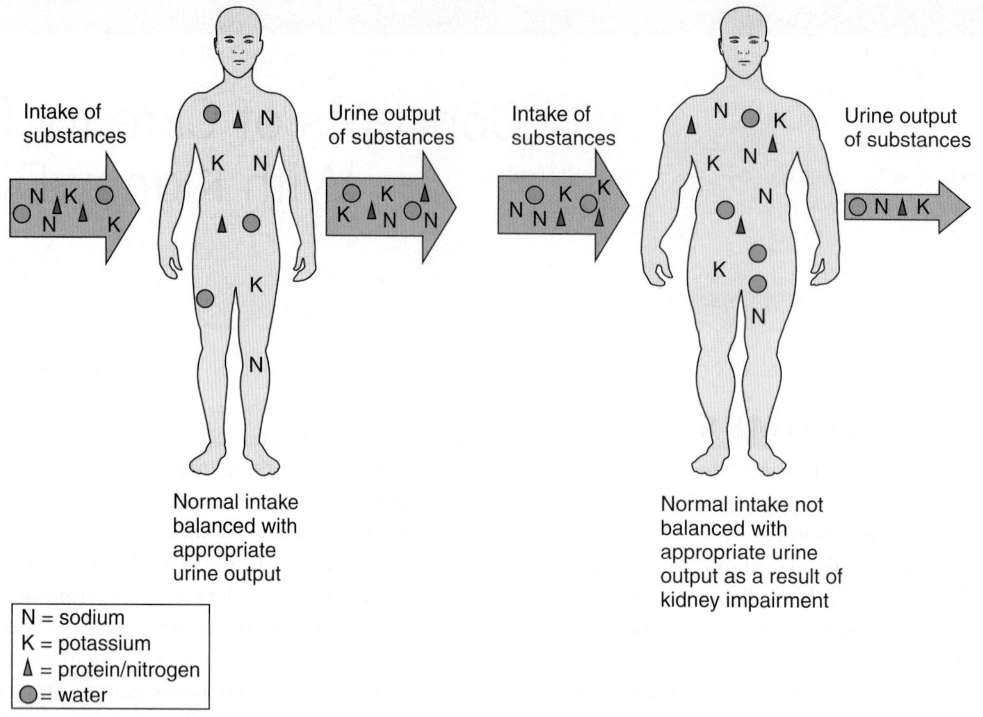

Fig. 62.1 Unbalanced body water, electrolytes, and waste products as a result of kidney problems that prevent adjustments in urinary elimination.

wastes affects all other body systems and can lead to life-threatening outcomes. This chapter describes a variety of infectious and noninfectious kidney disorders, kidney tumors, and kidney trauma. Acute kidney injury (AKI) and chronic kidney disease (CKD) are discussed in Chapter 63.

ELIMINATION CONCEPT EXEMPLAR: PYELONEPHRITIS

In the healthy adult, urine is normally sterile. Urinary tract infection (UTI) is an infection in any part of this normally sterile system. Pyelonephritis is a bacterial infection that starts in the bladder and moves upward to infect the kidneys (National Institute of Diabetes and Digestive and Kidney Diseases, 2018). It can be acute or chronic. Pyelonephritis interferes with urinary ***elimination,*** which is the excretion of waste from the body by the urinary system (as urine). Chapter 3 provides a summary of the concept of elimination in more detail.

Pathophysiology Review

Acute pyelonephritis is an active bacterial infection, whereas *chronic pyelonephritis* results from repeated or continued upper urinary tract infections that occur almost exclusively in patients who have anatomic abnormalities of the urinary tract. Bacterial infection causes local (e.g., kidney) and systemic (e.g., fever, aches, and malaise) inflammatory symptoms.

In pyelonephritis, organisms move up from the urinary tract into the kidney tissue. This is more likely to occur when urine refluxes from the bladder into the ureters and then to the kidney. Reflux is the reverse or upward flow of urine toward the renal pelvis and kidney. Infection also can be transmitted by

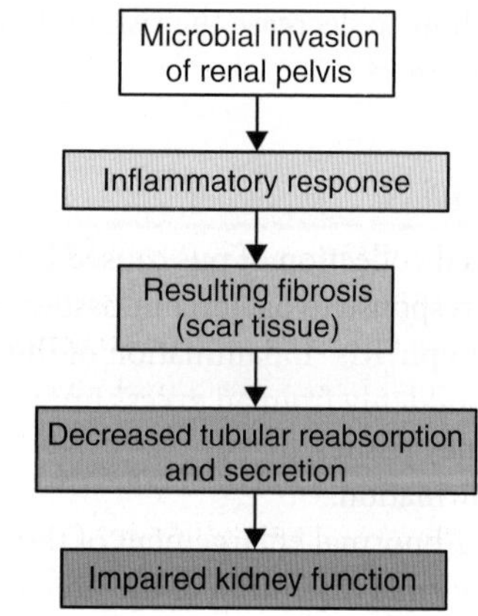

Fig. 62.2 Pathophysiology of pyelonephritis.

organisms in the blood, but this cause of pyelonephritis is rare unless the patient has impaired ***immunity.***

Acute pyelonephritis involves acute tissue inflammation, local edema, tubular cell necrosis, and possible abscess formation. Abscesses, which are pockets of infection, can occur anywhere in the kidney. The infection is scattered within the kidney; healthy tissues can lie next to infected areas. Fibrosis and scar tissue develop from chronic inflammation in the kidney glomerular and tubular structures. As a result, filtration, reabsorption, and secretion are impaired, and kidney function is reduced (Fig. 62.2).

Etiology and Genetic Risk. Single episodes of *acute pyelonephritis* result from bacterial infection, with or without obstruction or reflux. *Chronic pyelonephritis* usually occurs with structural deformities, urinary stasis, obstruction, or reflux. Conditions that lead to urinary stasis include prolonged bedrest and paralysis. Obstruction can be caused by stones, kidney cancer, scarring from pelvic radiation or surgery, recurrent infection, or injury. Reflux may occur from scarring or result from anatomic anomalies. Reflux also results from bladder tumors, prostate enlargement, or urinary stones. Reduced bladder tone from diabetic neuropathy, spinal cord injury, and neurodegenerative diseases (e.g., spina bifida, multiple sclerosis) contributes to stasis and reflux.

Pyelonephritis from an ascending infection may follow manipulation of the urinary tract (e.g., placement of a urinary catheter), particularly in patients who have reduced ***immunity*** or diabetes. In patients with chronic kidney stone disease, stones may retain organisms, resulting in ongoing infection and kidney scarring. Drugs, such as high-dose or prolonged use of NSAIDs, can lead to papillary necrosis and reflux.

The most common pyelonephritis-causing infecting organism among community-dwelling adults is *Escherichia coli. Enterococcus faecalis* is common in hospitalized patients. Both organisms are in the intestinal tract. Other organisms that cause pyelonephritis in hospitalized patients include *Proteus mirabilis, Klebsiella* species, and *Pseudomonas aeruginosa.* When the infection is bloodborne, common organisms include *Staphylococcus aureus* and *Candida* and *Salmonella* species.

Other causes of kidney scarring contributing to increased risk for pyelonephritis are inflammatory responses resulting from ***immunity*** excesses with antibody reactions, cell-mediated immunity against the bacterial antigens, or autoimmune reactions.

Incidence and Prevalence. Acute pyelonephritis is most common in women who are young and sexually active (Nicolle, 2018). Hormonal changes as well as obstruction caused by the fetus during pregnancy make acute pyelonephritis more common during the second trimester and beginning of the third trimester. Care must be taken because any febrile illness in later pregnancy can precipitate premature labor and delivery (Nicolle, 2018).

Chronic pyelonephritis is rarely characterized by infection alone, so the incidence and prevalence are linked to the underlying condition or conditions that lead to relapsing inflammatory damage of the kidney. These conditions include congenital structural abnormality, neurogenic bladder dysfunction, and primary vesicoureteral reflux (Nicolle, 2018).

❖ Interprofessional Collaborative Care

Depending on the severity of the disease, pyelonephritis may be managed in any care setting and in the community. Hospitalization becomes necessary in cases of bacteremia or hemodynamic instability and when oral medication cannot be tolerated. Bacteremia occurs in approximately 10% of cases. Bacteremia is more common in older-adult women and women with diabetes (Nicolle, 2018). The focus of care for patients with chronic pyelonephritis requires continuing attention to managing the structural or functional abnormality that contributes to recurrent infection and inflammatory fibrosis.

◆ Assessment: Recognize Cues

History. Ask about recurrent urinary tract infections (UTIs), diabetes mellitus (DM), stone disease, and known defects of the genitourinary tract. Ask about disease or treatment that results in reduced ***immunity,*** which also increases risk for pyelonephritis. Ask about kidney function; knowledgeable patients may be able to describe their stage of chronic kidney disease (CKD) if chronic pyelonephritis has led to permanent kidney damage. Ensure that a woman is not pregnant before radiographic imaging.

Physical Assessment/Signs and Symptoms. Ask about specific symptoms of acute pyelonephritis (see the Key Features: Acute Pyelonephritis box). Chronic pyelonephritis has a less dramatic presentation but similar symptoms. Ask the patient to describe any urinary symptoms or abdominal discomfort. Inquire about any history of repeated low-grade fevers. Changes in urine color or odor may accompany bacteriuria. See the Key Features: Chronic Pyelonephritis box for kidney-related effects of chronic pyelonephritis.

The objective assessment includes inspecting the flanks and gently palpating the costovertebral angle (CVA). Inspect both CVAs for enlargement, asymmetry, edema, or redness, all of which can indicate inflammation (Jarvis, 2019). If there is no tenderness to light palpation in either CVA, the primary health care provider may firmly percuss each area. Tenderness or discomfort may indicate infection or inflammation.

Psychosocial Assessment. Any infection in an older adult can lead to acute confusion. Assess the older adult who has new-onset confusion for signs and symptoms of urinary or renal infection.

The patient with any problem in the genitourinary area may have feelings of anxiety, embarrassment, or guilt. Listen for signs of anxiety or specific fears and prevent embarrassment

KEY FEATURES

Acute Pyelonephritis

- Fever
- Chills
- Tachycardia and tachypnea
- Flank, back, or loin pain
- Tenderness at the costovertebral angle (CVA)
- Abdominal, often colicky, discomfort
- Nausea and vomiting
- General malaise or fatigue
- Burning, urgency, or frequency of urination
- Nocturia
- Recent cystitis or treatment for urinary tract infection (UTI)

KEY FEATURES

Chronic Pyelonephritis

- Hypertension
- Inability to conserve sodium
- Decreased urine-concentrating ability, resulting in nocturia
- Tendency to develop hyperkalemia and acidosis

during assessment. Feelings of guilt, often associated with sexual habits or practices, may be masked through delay in seeking treatment or through vague, nonspecific responses to specific or direct questions. Encourage patients to tell their own story in familiar, comfortable language.

Laboratory Assessment. Urinalysis shows a positive leukocyte esterase and nitrite dipstick test and the presence of white blood cells (WBCs) and bacteria. Occasional red blood cells (RBCs) and protein may be present. The urine is cultured to determine the specific organisms causing the infection and the susceptibility or resistance of the specific organisms to various antibiotics. The urine sample for culture and sensitivity testing is usually obtained by the clean-catch method. In patients with recurrent pyelonephritis, more specific testing of bacterial antigens and antibodies may help determine whether the same organism is responsible for the recurrent infections.

Blood cultures may be obtained to determine the source and spread of infectious organisms. Other blood tests include the WBC count and differential of the complete blood count, as well as C-reactive protein and erythrocyte sedimentation rate (ESR) to determine ***immunity*** responses and presence of inflammation. Serum tests of kidney function, such as blood urea nitrogen (BUN) and creatinine, are used as baseline and to trend recovery or deterioration. Estimate of glomerular filtration rate (GFR) also is used to trend kidney function.

Imaging Assessment. An x-ray of the kidneys, ureters, and bladder (KUB) or CT is performed to visualize anatomy, inflammation, fluid accumulation, abscess formation, and defects in kidneys and the urinary tract. These tests also identify stones, kidney tumors or cysts, or prostate enlargement. Urine reflux caused by incompetent bladder-ureter valve closure can be seen with a cystourethrogram. (See Chapter 60 for more information on imaging assessment.)

Other Diagnostic Assessment. Other diagnostic tests include examining antibody-coated bacteria in urine, testing for certain enzymes (e.g., lactate dehydrogenase isoenzyme 5), and performing radionuclide renal scans. Examining urine for antibody-coated bacteria helps identify patients who may need long-term antibiotic therapy. High-molecular-weight enzymes in urine, such as lactate dehydrogenase isoenzyme 5, are present with any kidney tissue deterioration problem and give trend data. The renal scan can identify active pyelonephritis or abscesses in or around the kidney. A kidney biopsy may be performed to rule out less obvious causes of inflammation.

NCLEX EXAMINATION CHALLENGE 62.1

Physiological Integrity

Which assessment data would the nurse anticipate in a client with acute pyelonephritis? **Select all that apply.**

A. Urinary frequency
B. Dysuria
C. Oliguria
D. Heart rate 120 beats/min
E. Uremia
F. Costovertebral angle tenderness

◆ **Analysis: Analyze Cues and Prioritize Hypotheses.** The priority collaborative problems for the patient with pyelonephritis are:

1. ***Pain*** (flank and abdominal) due to inflammation and infection
2. Potential for chronic kidney disease (CKD) disease due to kidney tissue destruction

◆ Planning and Implementation: Generate Solutions and Take Action

Managing Pain

Planning: Expected Outcomes. With proper intervention, the patient with pyelonephritis is expected to achieve an acceptable state of comfort.

Interventions. Interventions may be nonsurgical or surgical. Interventional radiologic techniques may be used to relieve obstruction or repair a stricture of the urinary tract.

Nonsurgical Management. Interventions include the use of drug therapy, nutrition and fluid therapy, and teaching to ensure the patient's understanding of the treatment.

Drug therapy can reduce pain. Acetaminophen is preferred over NSAIDs because it does not interfere with kidney autoregulation of blood flow. Reduction of fever will also reduce ***pain.*** Some patients may require the use of opioids in the short term for pain control.

Drug therapy with antibiotics is prescribed to treat the infection. At first the antibiotics are broad spectrum. After urine and blood culture and sensitivity results are known, more specific antibiotics may be prescribed. Antibiotics are given (usually IV in hospitalized patients; orally in community-dwelling patients) to achieve adequate blood levels or sterile blood culture results. A prophylactic antibiotic is not recommended for patients with impaired voiding or chronic catheter use because it does not limit recurrence or severity of UTI (Nicolle, 2018)

Catheter replacement is supportive for a patient requiring a urinary catheter for 2 or more weeks (e.g., for neurogenic bladder or wound healing). This involves removal and replacement of the catheter and closed drainage system before starting antibiotic therapy. This intervention reduces bioburden by removing a device with a biofilm of concentrated organisms.

Nutrition therapy involves ensuring that the patient's nutrition intake has adequate calories from all food groups for healing to occur. A registered dietitian nutritionist should be part of the interprofessional team. Fluid intake is recommended at 2 L/day, sufficient to result in dilute (pale yellow) urine, unless another health problem requires fluid restriction.

Surgical Management. Surgical interventions can correct structural problems causing urine reflux or obstruction of urine outflow or can remove the source of infection. Teach the patient the nature and purpose of the proposed surgery, the expected outcome, and how he or she can participate.

The surgical procedures may be one of these: **pyelolithotomy** (stone removal from the kidney), **nephrectomy** (removal of the kidney), ureteral diversion, or reimplantation of ureter(s) to restore proper bladder drainage.

A pyelolithotomy is needed for removal of a large stone in the kidney pelvis that blocks urine flow and causes infection. Nephrectomy is a last resort when all other measures to clear the infection have failed. For patients with poor ureter valve closure or dilated ureters, ureteroplasty (ureter repair or revision) or ureteral reimplantation (through another site in the bladder wall) preserves kidney function and eliminates infections.

Preventing Chronic Kidney Disease

Planning: Expected Outcomes. The patient is expected to conserve existing kidney function. Underlying genitourinary abnormalities must be identified, and appropriate interventions taken to manage a current infection and the risk for subsequent infections. The approach by the urologist or nephrologist depends on signs and symptoms as well as on patient history.

Interventions. Specific antibiotics are prescribed to treat the infection. Stress the importance of completing the drug therapy as directed. Discuss with the patient and family the importance of regular follow-up examinations and completing the recommended diagnostic tests.

Blood pressure control slows the progression of kidney dysfunction. Ensure that the patient is able to detect adverse changes in blood pressure using community resources such as free blood pressure readings at community settings or retail pharmacies. When pyelonephritis causes or worsens CKD, ensure a referral to a nephrologist for additional assessment and management (see CKD in Chapter 63). Encourage the patient to drink sufficient fluid during waking hours to prevent dehydration because dehydration could further reduce kidney function. When dietary protein is restricted, a registered dietitian nutritionist (RDN) can help the family select appropriate food and proportions. Collaborate with the RDN and reinforce the prescribed interventions.

Care Coordination and Transition Management. Pyelonephritis may cause fear and anxiety in the patient and family. The severity of the acute process and its potential to develop into a chronic process are frightening. The patient and the family need reassurance that treatment and preventive measures can be successful.

Home Care Management. If no surgery is performed, the patient may need help with self-care, nutrition, and drug management at home. If surgery is performed, he or she may need help with incision care, self-care, and transportation for follow-up appointments.

Self-Management Education. After assessing the patient's and family's understanding of pyelonephritis and its therapy, explain:

- Drug regimen (purpose, timing, frequency, duration, and possible side effects)
- The role of nutrition and adequate fluid intake
- Best practices for chronic urinary catheter care, if needed
- The need for a balance between rest and activity, including any limitations after surgery
- The signs and symptoms of disease recurrence
- The use of previously successful coping mechanisms and community resources

Advise the patient to complete all prescribed antibiotic regimens and to report any side effects or unusual symptoms to the primary health care provider rather than stopping the drugs. Ensure that interprofessional care includes nutrition counseling, because many patients have special nutrition requirements, such as those for diabetes or pregnancy.

Health Care Resources. The patient may also briefly need a home health care nurse to help with drug or nutrition therapy at home. Housekeeping services may be helpful while he or she is regaining strength.

TABLE 62.1 Infectious Agents Associated With Glomerulonephritis

- Group A beta-hemolytic *Streptococcus*
- Staphylococcal or gram-negative bacteremia or sepsis
- Pneumococcal, *Mycoplasma*, or *Klebsiella* pneumonia
- Syphilis
- Dengue
- Hantavirus
- Varicella
- Parvovirus
- Hepatitis B and C
- Cytomegalovirus
- Parvovirus
- Epstein-Barr virus
- Human immunodeficiency virus

Adapted from Patel, N.P. (2018, November 28). Infection-induced kidney diseases. Retrieved from U.S. National Library of Medicine, National Institutes of Health. https://www.ncbi.nlm.nih.gov/pmc/articles/PMC6282040/.

◆ **Evaluation: Evaluate Outcomes.** Evaluate the care of the patient with pyelonephritis based on the identified priority patient problems. Expected outcomes may include that the patient will:

- Report that ***pain*** is controlled
- Be knowledgeable about the disease, its treatment, and interventions to prevent or reduce CKD progression

ACUTE GLOMERULONEPHRITIS

Pathophysiology Review

Glomerulonephritis (GN) is categorized into conditions that primarily involve the kidney (primary glomerular nephritis) and those in which kidney involvement is only part of a systemic disorder (secondary GN). It is a group of diseases that injure and inflame the glomerulus, the part of the kidney that filters blood. Inflamed glomeruli allow passage of protein and blood in the urine. GN is associated with high blood pressure, progressive kidney damage (leading to CKD), and edema. Anemia from reduced production of erythropoietin and high cholesterol often co-occur. GN can cause altered urinary ***elimination***.

Acute glomerulonephritis (GN) develops suddenly from an excess ***immunity*** response within the kidney tissues. Usually an infection is noticed before kidney symptoms of acute GN are present. The onset of symptoms is about 10 days from the time of infection. Usually patients recover quickly and completely from acute GN.

Many causes of primary GN are infectious (Table 62.1). Secondary GN can be caused by multisystem diseases (Table 62.2)

TABLE 62.2 Secondary Glomerular Diseases and Syndromes

- Systemic lupus erythematosus (SLE)
- Sustained liver disease (hepatitis B or C, autoimmune hepatitis, and cirrhosis)
- Amyloidosis
- Mesangiocapillary glomerulonephritis (MCGN)
- Alport syndrome
- Vasculitis
- Goodpasture syndrome
- IgA nephropathy
- Wegener granulomatosis
- HIV-associated nephropathy
- Diabetic glomerulopathy

HIV, Human immune deficiency virus.
Data from Muthu, V.R. (2018, Jan-Feb). *Clinicopathological spectrum of glomerular diseases in adolescents: a single-center experience over 4 years*. Retrieved from U.S. National Library of Medicine, National Institutes of Health. https://www.ncbi.nlm.nih.gov/pmc/articles/PMC5830804/; and Radhakrishnan, J. (2020). Glomerular disease: evaluation and differential diagnosis in adults. *UpToDate*. Retrieved from: https://www.uptodate.com/contents/glomerular-disease-evaluation-and-differential-diagnosis-in-adults.

and can manifest as acute or chronic disease. However, the division of primary and secondary GN is complex because diagnostic findings, histologic changes, and other changes are the same in both kidney and systemic disease, with both demonstrating altered ***immunity***. Drugs and inherited disorders are also implicated in GN with an acute or chronic presentation.

Interprofessional Collaborative Care

Assessment: Recognize Cues

History. Ask about recent infections, particularly of the skin or upper respiratory tract, and about recent travel or other possible exposures to viruses, bacteria, fungi, or parasites. Recent illnesses, surgery, or other invasive procedures may suggest infection. Ask about any systemic diseases that alter ***immunity***, such as systemic lupus erythematosus (SLE), which could cause acute GN.

Physical Assessment/Signs and Symptoms. Inspect the patient's skin for lesions or recent incisions, including body piercings, because these may be the source of organisms causing GN. Assess the face, eyelids, hands, and other areas for edema because edema is present in most patients with acute GN. Assess for fluid overload and pulmonary edema that may result from fluid and sodium retention occurring with acute GN. Ask about any difficulty breathing or shortness of breath. Assess for crackles in the lung fields, an S_3 heart sound (gallop rhythm), and neck vein distention.

Ask about changes in urine ***elimination*** patterns and any change in urine color, volume, clarity, or odor. The patient may describe blood in the urine as smoky, reddish brown, rusty, or cola colored. Ask about dysuria or oliguria. Weigh him or her to assess for fluid retention.

Take the patient's blood pressure and compare it with the baseline blood pressure. Mild-to-moderate hypertension occurs with acute GN as a result of impaired ***fluid and electrolyte balance*** with fluid and sodium retention. The patient may have fatigue, a lack of energy, anorexia, nausea, and/or vomiting if uremia from severe kidney impairment is present.

PATIENT-CENTERED CARE: OLDER ADULT CONSIDERATIONS QSEN

Glomerulonephritis can lead to chronic kidney disease, making it essential to prevent and treat in the older adult who is at greater risk for CKD. In the older adult, symptoms of glomerulonephritis can easily be confused with an exacerbation of heart failure. Older adults with glomerulonephritis have a higher risk of mortality than younger patients with the same diagnosis, adding to the importance of early recognition and prompt intervention (Raman, 2018).

Laboratory Assessment. Urinalysis shows red blood cells *(hematuria)* and protein *(proteinuria)*. An early morning specimen of urine is preferred for urinalysis because the urine is concentrated, most acidic, and filled with more intact formed elements at that time. Microscopic examination often shows red blood cell casts, as well as casts from other substances.

A 24-hour urine collection for total protein assay is obtained. The protein excretion rate for patients with acute GN may be increased from 500 mg/24 hr to 3 g/24 hr. Serum albumin levels are decreased because this protein is lost in the urine and fluid retention causes dilution.

Serum creatinine and BUN provide information about kidney function and may be elevated, indicating impairment of ***elimination***. The glomerular filtration rate (GFR), either estimated from a single serum and urine creatinine value or measured by the 24-hour urine test for creatinine clearance, may be decreased to 50 mL/min. Recall that the older adult has a decline in GFR, which may make GFR results challenging to interpret.

Other Diagnostic Assessment. A kidney biopsy provides a precise diagnosis of the condition, assists in determining the prognosis, and helps in outlining treatment (see Chapter 60). The specific tissue features are determined by light microscopy, immunofluorescent stains, and electron microscopy to identify cell type, the presence of immunoglobulins, or the type of tissue deposits.

Interventions: Take Action. Interventions focus on managing infection, preventing complications, and providing appropriate patient education.

Managing infection as a cause of acute GN begins with appropriate antibiotic therapy. Penicillin, erythromycin, or azithromycin is prescribed for GN caused by streptococcal infection. Check the patient's known allergies before giving any drug. Stress personal hygiene and basic infection control principles (e.g., handwashing) to prevent spread of the organism. Teach patients the importance of completing the entire course of the prescribed antibiotic.

Modifying ***immunity*** with drugs can also benefit patients with acute glomerulonephritis (GN) that is not due to acute infection but is related to excessive inflammation. Corticosteroids and cytotoxic drugs (e.g., cyclosporine, cyclophosphamide) to suppress ***immunity*** responses may be used. Patients receiving immunosuppressants need to take precautions to avoid exposure to new infections.

Preventing complications is an important nursing intervention, especially when ***fluid and electrolyte balance*** is disrupted. For patients with fluid overload, hypertension, and edema, diuretics and sodium and water restrictions are prescribed. The usual fluid allowance is equal to the 24-hour urine output plus 500 to 600 mL. Patients with oliguria usually have increased serum levels of potassium and blood urea nitrogen (BUN). Potassium and protein intake may be restricted to prevent hyperkalemia and uremia as a result of the elevated BUN. Antihypertensive drugs may be needed to control hypertension (see Chapter 33).

Nausea, vomiting, or anorexia indicates that uremia is present. Dialysis is necessary if uremic symptoms or fluid volume excess cannot be controlled with nutrition therapy and fluid management (see Chapter 63). *Plasmapheresis* (removal and filtering of the plasma to eliminate antibodies) also may be used (see Chapter 37).

Coordinate care to conserve patient energy and balance activity with rest to maintain function. Relaxation techniques and diversional activities can reduce emotional stress.

Preparing for self-management includes teaching the patient and family members about the purpose of prescribed drugs, the dosage and schedule, and potential adverse effects. Ensure that they understand diet and fluid restrictions. Advise the patient to measure weight and blood pressure daily at the same time each day. Instruct him or her to notify the primary health care provider of any sudden increase in weight or blood pressure.

If short-term dialysis is required to control ***fluid and electrolyte balance*** or uremic symptoms, explain vascular access care and dialysis schedules and routines (see Chapter 63).

Rapidly progressive glomerulonephritis (RPGN) is a primary GN also called *crescentic glomerulonephritis* because of the presence of crescent-shaped cells in the Bowman capsule. RPGN develops acutely over several weeks or months. Patients become quite ill quickly and have symptoms of kidney impairment (fluid volume excess, hypertension, oliguria, electrolyte imbalances, and uremic symptoms). Regardless of treatment, RPGN often progresses to end-stage kidney disease (ESKD).

CHRONIC GLOMERULONEPHRITIS

Pathophysiology Review

Chronic GN, or *chronic nephritic syndrome,* develops over years to decades. Mild proteinuria and hematuria, hypertension, fatigue, and occasional edema are often the only symptoms.

Although the exact cause is not known, changes in kidney tissue result from infection, hypertension, inflammation from ***immunity*** excess, or poor kidney blood flow. Kidney tissue atrophies, and functional nephrons are greatly reduced. Biopsy in the late stages of atrophy may show glomerular changes, cell loss, protein and collagen deposits, and fibrosis of the kidney tissue. Microscopic examination shows deposits of immune complexes and inflammation.

The loss of nephrons reduces glomerular filtration. Hypertension and renal arteriole sclerosis are often present. The glomerular damage allows proteins to enter the urine. Chronic GN always leads to end-stage kidney disease (ESKD) (see Chapter 63).

❖ Interprofessional Collaborative Care

◆ Assessment: Recognize Cues

History. Ask about other health problems, including systemic diseases, kidney or urologic disorders, infectious diseases (i.e., streptococcal infections), and recent exposures to infections. Ask about overall health status and whether increasing fatigue and lethargy have occurred.

Identify the patient's urine ***elimination*** pattern. Ask whether the frequency of voiding has increased or the quantity of urine has decreased. Ask about changes in urine color, odor, or clarity and whether dysuria or incontinence has occurred. Nocturia is a common symptom.

Assess the patient's general comfort and ask whether new-onset dyspnea has occurred, because fluid overload can occur with decreased urine output. Ask about and observe for changes in cognition (i.e., irritability, an inability to read, or incapacity during job-related functions) or disturbed concentration. Changes in memory and the ability to concentrate occur as waste products collect in the blood.

Physical Assessment/Signs and Symptoms. Assess for systemic circulatory overload. Auscultate lung fields for crackles, observe the respiratory rate and depth, and measure blood pressure and weight. Assess the heart rate, rhythm, and presence of an S_3 heart sound. Inspect the neck veins for venous engorgement and check for edema of the feet and ankles, on the shins, and over the sacrum.

Assess for uremic symptoms, such as slurred speech, ataxia, tremors, or asterixis (flapping tremor of the fingers or the inability to maintain a fixed posture with the arms extended and wrists hyperextended). Inspect skin for a yellowish color, texture changes, bruises, rashes, or eruptions. Ask about itching and document areas of dryness or any excoriation from scratching.

Psychosocial Assessment. A diagnosis of chronic GN is associated with psychosocial responses of uncertainty, loss, and fear of the need for lifestyle changes as the disease progresses. While obtaining the history, listen carefully for spoken and unspoken feelings of anger, resentment, futility, sadness, or anxiety, all of which may need further exploration.

Diagnostic Assessment. Urine output decreases and urinalysis shows protein, usually less than 2 g in a 24-hour collection. The specific gravity is fixed at a constant level of dilution (around 1.010) despite variable fluid intake. Red blood cells and casts may be in the urine.

The glomerular filtration rate (GFR) is low. The serum creatinine level is elevated; usually it is greater than 6 mg/dL (500 mcmol/L) but may be as high as 30 mg/dL (2500 mcmol/L) or more because of poor waste ***elimination.*** The BUN is increased, often as high as 100 to 200 mg/dL (35 to 70 mmol/L).

Decreased kidney function disturbs ***fluid and electrolyte balance.*** Sodium retention is common, but dilution of the plasma from excess fluid can result in a falsely normal serum sodium level (135 to 145 mEq/L [mmol/L]) or a low sodium level (less than 135 mEq/L [mmol/L]). When oliguria develops, potassium is not excreted, and hyperkalemia occurs when levels exceed 5.4 mEq/L (mmol/L).

Hyperphosphatemia develops with serum levels greater than 4.7 mg/dL (1.73 mmol/L). Serum calcium levels are usually low normal or are slightly below normal.

Disturbances of ***acid-base balance*** with acidosis develop from hydrogen ion retention and loss of bicarbonate. However, there may be a decrease in serum carbon dioxide (CO_2) levels as patients breathe more rapidly to compensate for the acidosis. If respiratory compensation is present, the pH of arterial blood is between 7.35 and 7.45. A pH of less than 7.35 means that the patient's respiratory system is not completely compensating for the acidosis (see Chapter 14).

The kidneys are abnormally small on x-ray or CT in chronic GN.

◆ **Interventions: Take Action.** Interventions focus on slowing the progression of the disease and preventing complications. Management is systemic and consists of diet changes, fluid intake sufficient to prevent reduced blood flow to the kidneys, and drug therapy to control the problems from uremia. Eventually ***elimination*** is so impaired that the patient requires dialysis or transplantation to prevent death. (Care for the patient requiring dialysis or transplantation is discussed in Chapter 63.)

NEPHROTIC SYNDROME

Pathophysiology Review

Nephrotic syndrome (NS) is an immunologic kidney disorder in which glomerular permeability increases so larger molecules pass through the membrane into the urine and are then excreted. This process causes massive loss of protein into the urine, edema formation, and decreased plasma albumin levels. Minimal change disease is the most common cause of NS and accounts for 90% of NS in children and 20% in adults. The name *minimal change* comes from the need to see changes in the glomerulus using an electron microscope since changes with a light microscope cannot be seen (Trachtman, 2018).

The most common cause of glomerular membrane changes is altered ***immunity*** with inflammation. Defects in glomerular filtration can also occur as a result of genetic defects of the glomerular filtering system, such as Fabry disease. Altered liver function may occur with NS, resulting in increased lipid production and hyperlipidemia.

❖ Interprofessional Collaborative Care

The main feature of NS is increased protein ***elimination*** with severe proteinuria (with more than 3.5 g of protein in a 24-hour urine sample). Patients also have low serum albumin levels of less than 3 g/dL (30 g/L), high serum lipid levels, fats in the urine, edema, and hypertension (see the Key Features: Nephrotic Syndrome box). Renal vein thrombosis often occurs at the same time as NS, either as a cause of the problem or as an effect. NS may progress to end-stage kidney disease (ESKD), but treatment can prevent progression.

Management varies, depending on which process is causing the disorder (identified by kidney biopsy). Excess ***immunity*** may improve with suppressive therapy using steroids and cytotoxic or immunosuppressive agents. Angiotensin-converting enzyme inhibitors (ACEIs) can decrease protein loss in the urine, and cholesterol-lowering drugs can improve blood lipid levels. Heparin may reduce vascular defects and improve kidney function. Diet changes are often prescribed. If the glomerular filtration rate (GFR) is normal, dietary intake of proteins is needed. If the GFR is decreased, protein intake must be decreased. Mild diuretics and sodium restriction may be needed to control edema and hypertension. Assess the patient's hydration status because vascular dehydration is common. If plasma volume is depleted, kidney problems worsen. Acute kidney injury (AKI) may be avoided if adequate blood flow to the kidney is maintained.

KEY FEATURES

Nephrotic Syndrome

Key features include sudden onset of these symptoms:

- Massive proteinuria
- Hypoalbuminemia
- Edema (especially facial and periorbital)
- Lipiduria
- Hyperlipidemia
- Delayed clotting or increased bleeding with higher-than-normal values for serum activated partial thromboplastin time (aPTT), coagulation, or international normalized ratio for prothrombin time (INR, PT)
- Reduced kidney function with elevated blood urea nitrogen (BUN) and serum creatinine and decreased glomerular filtration rate (GFR)

NEPHROSCLEROSIS

Pathophysiology Review

Nephrosclerosis is a degenerative disorder resulting from changes in kidney blood vessels. Nephron blood vessels thicken, resulting in narrowed lumens and decreased kidney blood flow. The tissue is chronically hypoxic, with ischemia and fibrosis developing over time.

Nephrosclerosis occurs with all types of hypertension, atherosclerosis, and diabetes mellitus (DM). The more severe the hypertension, the greater the risk for severe kidney damage. Nephrosclerosis is rarely seen when blood pressure is consistently below 160/110 mm Hg. The changes caused by hypertension may be reversible or may progress to end-stage kidney disease (ESKD) within months or years. Hypertension is the second leading cause of ESKD, with many patients requiring kidney replacement therapy (e.g., dialysis or transplantation).

More recent advances in genetic testing have revealed a complex pathogenesis in nephrosclerosis. Patients were often diagnosed with nephrosclerosis thought to be caused by hypertension. However, advanced genetic evidence indicated many as having genetic focal segmental glomerulosclerosis. The apolipoprotein L1 (APOL1) allele is a risk factor for glomerulosclerosis that presents with symptoms such as nephrosclerosis. People with the APOL1 allele are usually of African ancestry. Not all patients with the ALOL1 allele will develop kidney disease, suggesting that there may be environmental factors as well. The treatment of patients with genetically caused focal segmental glomerulosclerosis is evolving (Crawford, 2018).

PATIENT-CENTERED CARE: CULTURAL/ SPIRITUAL CONSIDERATIONS QSEN

Patient-Centered Care

Approximately 14% of the general population is affected by chronic kidney disease. African Americans, Native Americans, and Mexican Americans are more likely to have chronic kidney disease than Caucasians. The prevalence of end-stage renal disease (ESRD) is 3.7 times higher in African Americans and 1.4 times higher in Native Americans than in Caucasians. Hispanics are 1.5 times more likely to develop ESRD than non-Hispanics (National Institute of Diabetes and Digestive and Kidney Diseases, 2016).

❖ Interprofessional Collaborative Care

Management focuses on controlling high blood pressure and reducing albuminuria to preserve kidney function. Although many antihypertensive drugs may lower blood pressure, the patient's response is important in ensuring long-term adherence to the prescribed therapy. Factors that promote adherence include once-a-day dosing, low cost, and minimal side effects.

Lack of knowledge or misinformation about hypertension poses many challenges to health care professionals working with patients who have hypertension. When kidney disease occurs, adherence to therapy is even more important for preserving health.

Many drugs can control high blood pressure (see Chapter 33), and more than one agent may be needed for best control. Angiotensin-converting enzyme inhibitors (ACEIs) are very useful in reducing hypertension and preserving kidney function. Diuretics can maintain ***fluid and electrolyte balance*** in the presence of kidney function insufficiency. Hyperkalemia needs to be prevented when potassium-sparing diuretics, alone or in combination with other diuretics, are used to treat hypertensive patients with known kidney disease.

POLYCYSTIC KIDNEY DISEASE

Pathophysiology Review

Polycystic kidney disease (PKD) is a genetic disorder in which fluid-filled cysts develop in the nephrons (Fig. 62.3). Relentless development and growth of cysts from loss of cellular regulation and abnormal cell division result in progressive kidney enlargement. Patients with PKD often experience hypertension, abdominal fullness and pain, episodes of cyst bleeding, hematuria, kidney stone formation, infections, and systemic disease (Rizk, 2018).

The cysts look like clusters of grapes (see Fig. 62.3). Over time, growing cysts damage the glomerular and tubular membranes. Each cystic kidney enlarges, becoming the size of a football, and may weigh 10 lb or more each. As cysts fill with fluid and become larger, kidney function becomes less effective, and urine formation and waste ***elimination*** are impaired.

Most patients with PKD have high blood pressure. The cause of hypertension is related to kidney ischemia from the enlarging cysts. As the vessels are compressed and blood flow to the kidneys decreases, the renin-angiotensin system is activated, raising blood pressure. Control of hypertension is a top priority because proper treatment can disrupt the process that leads to further kidney damage, as well as avoid complications such as stroke from hypertension.

Cysts may also occur in the liver and blood vessels. The incidence of cerebral *aneurysms* (outpouching and thinning of an artery wall) is higher in patients with PKD. Aneurysms

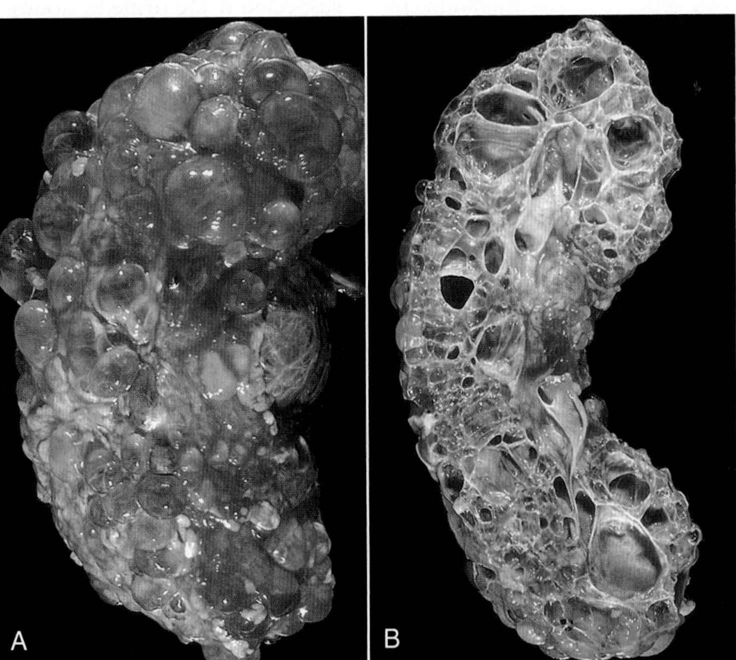

Fig. 62.3 External surface (A) and internal surface (B) of a polycystic kidney. (From Kumar, V., Abbas, A., Fausto, N., & Aster, J. [2010]. *Robbins and Cotran pathologic basis of disease* [8th ed.]. Philadelphia: Saunders.)

may rupture, causing bleeding and sudden death. For unknown reasons, kidney stones occur in many patients with PKD. Heart valve problems (e.g., mitral valve prolapse), left ventricular hypertrophy, and colonic diverticula also are common in patients with PKD.

Etiology and Genetic Risk. Kidney cysts are genetically and clinically related to many symptoms and problems. PKD can be inherited as either an autosomal dominant trait or, less often, an autosomal recessive trait. Autosomal dominant PKD is the most common inherited kidney disease, occurring in 1 in 400 to 1000 live births. People who inherit the recessive form of PKD usually die in early childhood. Rarely, a new gene mutation can cause PKD in a patient with no family history of the trait. However, the cases of gene mutation tend to be a milder form of PKD. Recent advances have made the genetic forms of cystic disorders of the kidney easier to understand. Many of the genes that cause cystic diseases of the kidney have been identified (Rizk, 2018). However, the number of genes influencing PKD is challenging and requires geneticists and genetic counselors to be a part of the interprofessional team caring for patients with or at risk for the disease.

PATIENT-CENTERED CARE: GENETIC/GENOMIC CONSIDERATIONS QSEN

Autosomal dominant PKD (ADPKD) is the most common form of the disease in adults, who have a 50% risk of passing the mutated gene to their children. Fig. 62.4 shows a pedigree for a family with ADPKD. Recent advances in molecularly targeted therapies offer new hope for improved outcomes and eventually a cure for PKD (Rizk, 2018).

Three genes have been implicated in the cause of ADPKD. Among the genes causing ADPKD, 85% of ADPKD cases are caused by mutations in the *PKD1* gene, 15% have mutations in the *PKD2* gene, and 1% have mutations in the *GANAB* gene. The *PKD1* gene mutations cause a more severe form of PKD with more kidney cysts, earlier onset of hypertension, and more instances of ESKD (Rizk, 2018).

There is no way to prevent PKD, although early detection and management of hypertension may slow the progression of kidney damage and impaired ***elimination.*** Genetic counseling may be useful for adults who have one parent with PKD. Family history analysis is used to help identify people at risk (see Fig. 62.4).

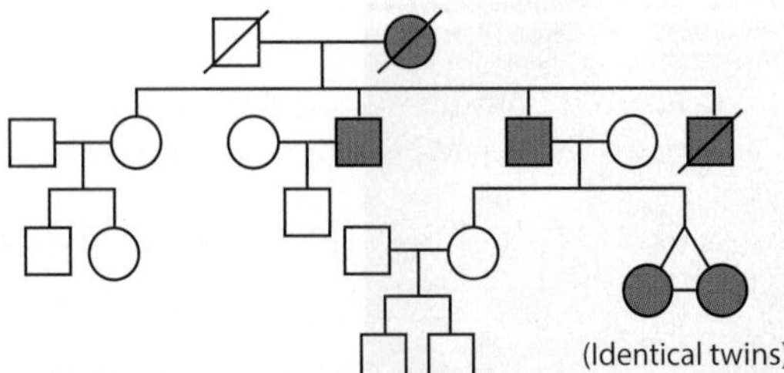

Fig. 62.4 Four-generation pedigree for autosomal dominant polycystic kidney disease (ADPKD). *Colored-in symbols* indicate family members with ADPKD. *Slashes* indicate that the person has died.

Incidence and Prevalence. PKD affects about 600,000 people of all ethnic groups in the United States and causes about 5% of kidney failure (National Kidney Foundation, 2019). Men and women have an equal chance of inheriting the disease because the gene responsible for PKD is on an autosome (see Chapter 6).

Interprofessional Collaborative Care

Assessment: Recognize Cues. Because PKD is a chronic disease with periods of acute problems, most management occurs in the community rather than in an acute care hospital. With acute problems or when surgery is needed, initial care is in a hospital setting, and continuing care can occur in any setting.

History. Explore the family history of a patient with suspected or actual PKD and ask whether either parent was known to have PKD or whether there is any family history of kidney disease. Important information to obtain is the age at which the problem was diagnosed in the parent and any related complications. Ask about ***pain,*** abdominal discomfort, constipation, changes in urine color or frequency, hypertension, headaches, and a family history of stroke or sudden death.

Physical Assessment/Signs and Symptoms. Pain is often the first symptom. Inspect the abdomen. A distended abdomen is common as the cystic kidneys swell and push the abdominal contents forward. Polycystic kidneys are easily palpated because of their increased size. Use *gentle* abdominal palpation because the cystic kidneys and nearby tissues may be tender and palpation is uncomfortable. The patient also may have flank pain as a dull ache or as a sharp and intermittent discomfort. Dull, aching pain is caused by increased kidney size with distention, abnormal stimulation of sensory neurons in the kidney, or infection within the cyst. Sharp, intermittent pain occurs when a cyst ruptures or a stone is present. When a cyst ruptures, the patient may have bright red or cola-colored urine. Infection is suspected if the urine is cloudy or foul smelling or if there is **dysuria** (pain on urination). See the Key Features: Polycystic Kidney Disease box.

Nocturia (the need to urinate excessively at night) is an early symptom and occurs because of decreased urine concentrating ability. Patients with early PKD often have hyperfiltration leading to wasting of sodium and water, which disrupts ***fluid and electrolyte balance.*** Later, as kidney function declines (i.e., reduced glomerular filtration rate [GFR]), the patient retains

KEY FEATURES

Polycystic Kidney Disease

- Abdominal or flank pain
- Hypertension
- Nocturia
- Frequent urinary tract infections
- Increased abdominal girth
- Constipation
- Hematuria (bloody urine)
- Sodium wasting and inability to concentrate urine in early stage
- Progression to kidney failure with anuria (Holt, 2018)

water and sodium, which causes hypertension, edema, and uremic symptoms such as anorexia, nausea, vomiting, pruritus, and fatigue (see Chapter 63). Because intracranial berry aneurysms often occur in patients with PKD, a severe headache with or without neurologic or vision changes requires attention.

Psychosocial Assessment. A PKD diagnosis is associated with psychosocial responses of uncertainty, loss, and fear due to the life-threatening complications that can occur (Rizk, 2018). The patient may have had a parent who died or relatives who required dialysis or transplantation. Listen for spoken and unspoken feelings of anger, resentment, futility, sadness, or anxiety. Such feelings may need further exploration. Feelings of guilt and concern for the patient's children may also complicate the issue.

Diagnostic Assessment. Ultrasound is the primary method for diagnosing PKD. The size of the kidney is measured by ultrasound as well as cysts within the kidney. MRI or CT may be used in order to confirm ultrasound findings or when a family member is being evaluated for potential kidney donation (Rizk, 2018).

Urinalysis may show proteinuria (protein in the urine), which indicates a decline in kidney function and impaired ***elimination.*** Hematuria may be gross or microscopic. Bacteria in the urine indicate infection, usually in the cysts. Obtain a urine sample for culture and sensitivity testing when there is evidence of infection. As kidney function declines, serum creatinine and blood urea nitrogen (BUN) levels rise. With further decline, creatinine clearance decreases, and the GFR is low. Changes in kidney handling of sodium may cause either sodium losses or sodium retention.

Genetic testing is not routinely performed for diagnostic assessment of PKD. It may be considered for patients who have atypical imaging findings or for those with symptoms who have no family history of PKD.

◆ **Interventions: Take Action.** Currently no treatments are effective in extending kidney function in PKD. Drug therapies to interrupt the pathways that promote malignant cyst formation such as molecular signaling for cell division or endothelial growth are being evaluated. Supportive interventions for PKD include management of hypertension and pain, reducing complications from infection and constipation, and slowing disease progression. Be attentive to the psychosocial issues of uncertainty and fear related to an inherited disorder, as well as reproductive issues. Genetic counseling is part of comprehensive care of the patient and family experiencing PKD.

When the disease progresses and the kidneys no longer function for waste ***elimination,*** care becomes similar to that needed for the patient with end-stage kidney disease (see Chapter 63).

Managing Blood Pressure. Blood pressure control and lifestyle and dietary modifications are necessary to reduce cardiovascular complications and slow the progression of kidney dysfunction. Nursing interventions include education for self-management. Dietary salt of less than 2 g/day is now advised. Calorie restriction with weight reduction has been shown to decrease blood pressure (Rizk, 2018).

Drug therapy with angiotensin-converting enzyme inhibitors (ACEIs) to reach a blood pressure below 130/80 mm Hg in all patients with PKD or 110/75 mm Hg in young adults with preserved kidney function is recommended (Rizk, 2018). These drugs also help control the cell growth aspects of PKD and reduce microalbuminuria. Additional antihypertensive drugs, such as calcium channel blockers, beta blockers, and vasodilators, may be used (see Chapter 33).

Teach the patient and family how to measure and record blood pressure. Help the patient establish a schedule for self-administering drugs, monitoring daily weights, and keeping blood pressure records (see the Patient and Family Education: Preparing for Self-Management: Polycystic Kidney Disease box). Explain the potential side effects of the drugs. Make available written materials, such as drug teaching cards and booklets. Work with the patient and a registered dietitian nutritionist to develop strategies to manage sodium and other dietary issues that contribute to hypertension.

Managing Pain. Because PKD-related pain is chronic, a multidisciplinary ***pain*** management approach is helpful. Drugs may include opioids along with acetaminophen. NSAIDs are used cautiously because they can reduce kidney blood flow. Aspirin-containing drugs are avoided to reduce bleeding risk.

Complementary therapy includes positioning and the application of dry heat to the abdomen or flank. Teach the patient methods of relaxation and comfort using deep breathing, guided imagery, or other strategies (see Chapter 5 for pain management). When pain is severe, cysts can be reduced by needle aspiration and drainage; however, they usually refill. When the quality or severity of pain abruptly increases, assess for infection.

Reducing Complications From Infection. Fever, abdominal ***pain,*** and either leukocytosis or serum markers of inflammation (e.g., elevated erythrocyte sedimentation rate [ESR] or C-reactive protein [CRP]) may be associated with cystic or systemic infection. Blood and urine cultures may or may not be positive with cyst infection. Early infection management

PATIENT AND FAMILY EDUCATION: PREPARING FOR SELF-MANAGEMENT

Polycystic Kidney Disease

- Measure and record your blood pressure daily and notify your primary health care provider about consistent changes in blood pressure.
- Take your temperature if you suspect you have a fever. If a fever is present, notify your physician or nurse.
- Weigh yourself every day at the same time of day and with the same amount of clothing; notify your primary health care provider or nurse if you have a sudden weight gain.
- Limit your intake of salt to help control your blood pressure once hyperfiltration is no longer a symptom of your disease (once chronic kidney disease [CKD] is present).
- Notify your primary health care provider or nurse if your urine smells foul or has a new occurrence of blood in it.
- Notify your primary health care provider or nurse if you have a headache that does not go away or if you have visual disturbances because these are symptoms of a stroke or bleeding in the brain.
- Monitor bowel movements to prevent constipation.

can prevent or reduce complications and acute kidney injury. Monitor serum creatinine levels because some antibiotics are nephrotoxic.

Percutaneous or surgical drainage of the cyst may be indicated. Prepare patients similarly as for kidney biopsy, described in Chapter 60.

Preventing Constipation. Teach the patient who has adequate urine output to prevent constipation by maintaining adequate fluid intake (generally 2 to 3 L daily in food and beverages), maintaining dietary fiber intake, and exercising regularly. Explain that pressure on the large intestine may occur as the polycystic kidneys increase in size. These recommendations for bowel management might change, particularly when ESKD develops. Advise the patient about the use of stool softeners and bulk agents, including careful use of laxatives, to prevent chronic constipation.

Slowing Progression of Chronic Kidney Disease. Early in the disease when patients have hyperfiltration with decreased urine concentration, nocturia, and low specific gravity, urge them to maintain adequate fluid intake to prevent dehydration, which can further reduce kidney function. Hyperfiltration may persist for several years. Maintaining adequate fluid intake can reduce the vasopressin release that reduces kidney blood flow. In patients with preserved kidney function, 3 L of fluid daily is recommended in order to slow cyst growth. Care must be taken to monitor for hyponatremia with excess water intake (Rizk, 2018).

As the disease progresses, protein intake may be limited to slow the development of ESKD. Help the patient and family understand the diet plan and why it was prescribed. Work closely with the dietitian to foster the patient's understanding.

Strategies for kidney protection include the use of a vasopressin-suppressing agent such as tolvaptan to improve blood flow, slow kidney volume growth, and sustain kidney function. Although pravastatin has shown beneficial effects on urinary albumin excretion, statins are not currently approved for treatment of PKD (Rizk, 2018).

Care Coordination and Transition Management

Health Care Resources. The PKD Foundation (www.pkdcure.org) and the National Kidney and Urologic Diseases Information Clearinghouse (NKUDIC) of the National Institute of Diabetes and Digestive and Kidney Diseases (www.niddk.nih.gov) conduct research and provide education about PKD. Many pamphlets are available; there is a fee for some materials. Chapters of the National Kidney Foundation (NKF) and the American Association of Kidney Patients (AAKP) also have resources for information and support.

HYDRONEPHROSIS AND HYDROURETER

Pathophysiology Review

Hydronephrosis and hydroureter are problems of urinary ***elimination*** with outflow obstruction. Urethral strictures obstruct urine outflow and may contribute to bladder distention, hydroureter, and hydronephrosis. Prompt recognition and treatment are crucial to preventing permanent kidney damage.

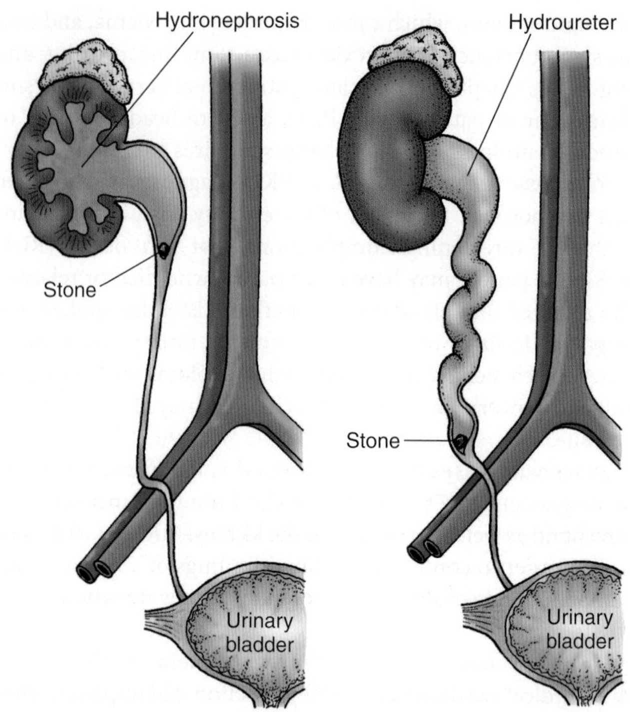

Fig. 62.5 Hydronephrosis is caused by obstruction in the upper part of the ureter. Hydroureter is caused by obstruction in the lower part of the ureter.

In **hydronephrosis**, the kidney enlarges as urine collects in the renal pelvis and kidney tissue. Because the capacity of the renal pelvis is normally 5 to 8 mL, obstruction in the renal pelvis or at the point where the ureter joins the renal pelvis quickly distends the renal pelvis. Kidney pressure increases as the volume of urine increases. Over time, sometimes in only a matter of hours, the blood vessels and kidney tubules can be damaged extensively (Fig. 62.5).

In patients with **hydroureter** (enlargement of the ureter), the effects are similar, but the obstruction is in the ureter rather than in the kidney. The ureter is most easily obstructed where the iliac vessels cross or where the ureters enter the bladder. Ureter dilation occurs above the obstruction and enlarges as urine collects (see Fig. 62.5).

Urinary obstruction causes damage when pressure builds up directly on kidney tissue. Tubular filtrate pressure also increases in the nephron as drainage through the collecting system is impaired and glomerular filtration decreases or ceases. Kidney necrosis can occur. Nitrogen waste products (urea, creatinine, and uric acid) and electrolytes (sodium, potassium, chloride, and phosphorus) are retained, and ***acid-base balance*** is impaired.

The cause of hydronephrosis or hydroureter is an obstruction, which can occur at any location between the collecting duct and the urethral meatus. Common causes of urinary obstruction include kidney stones, tumors, fibrosis, structural abnormalities, trauma, abscess, and cysts (Sutherland, 2018). With cancer, obstructed ureters may result from tumors pressing on the ureters, pelvic radiation, or surgical treatment. Early treatment of the causes can prevent ureteral problems and permanent kidney damage. The time needed to prevent permanent damage depends on the patient's kidney health. Permanent damage can occur in less than 48 hours in some patients and after several weeks in other patients.

Interprofessional Collaborative Care

Assessment: Recognize Cues. Obtain a history from the patient, focusing on known kidney or urologic disorders. A history of childhood urinary tract problems may indicate previously undiagnosed structural defects. Ask about his or her usual pattern of urinary ***elimination,*** especially amount, frequency, color, clarity, and odor. Ask about recent flank or abdominal pain. Chills, fever, and malaise may be present with a urinary tract infection (UTI).

Inspect each flank to identify asymmetry, which may occur with a kidney mass, and *gently* palpate the abdomen to locate areas of tenderness. Palpate the bladder to detect distention, or use a bedside bladder scanner (see Chapter 60). Gentle pressure on the abdomen may cause urine leakage, which reflects a full bladder and possible obstruction.

Urinalysis may show bacteria or white blood cells if infection is present. When urinary tract obstruction is prolonged, microscopic examination may show tubular epithelial cells. Blood chemistries are normal unless glomerular filtration has decreased and waste ***elimination*** is impaired. Blood creatinine and BUN levels increase with a reduced GFR. Serum electrolyte levels may be altered with elevated blood levels of potassium, phosphorus, and calcium along with a metabolic acidosis (bicarbonate deficit). Urinary outflow obstruction can be seen with ultrasound (US) or CT.

Interventions: Take Action. Urinary retention and potential for infection are the primary problems. Failure to treat the cause of obstruction leads to infection and acute kidney injury (AKI).

Urologic Interventions. If obstruction is caused by a kidney stone (calculus), it can be located and removed using cystoscopic or retrograde urogram procedures. See Chapter 61 for more information about kidney stone management. After stone removal, a plastic stent is usually left in the ureter for a few weeks to improve urine flow in the area irritated by the stone. The stent is later removed by another cystoscopic procedure.

Radiologic Interventions. When an abnormal narrowing of the urinary tract (**stricture**) causes hydronephrosis and cannot be corrected with urologic procedures, a **nephrostomy** is performed. Most nephrostomy drains provide only external drainage (diversion). Other styles of nephrostomy drains enter the kidney and extend to the bladder, draining urine out to a bag or past a ureteral obstruction and into the bladder. With these, there are both internal and external parts to the nephrostomy tubing. Externally, a fully external or an internal/external diversion drain appears the same. The urine output will fluctuate more if all urine goes to the bladder before external drainage.

Patient Preparation. If possible, the patient is kept NPO for 4 to 6 hours before the procedure. Clotting studies (e.g., international normalized ratio [INR], prothrombin time [PT], and partial thromboplastic time [PTT]) should be normal or corrected. Drugs are used to reduce hypertension. The patient receives moderate sedation for the procedure.

Procedure. The patient is placed in the prone position. The kidney is located under ultrasound or fluoroscopic guidance, and a local anesthetic is given. A needle is placed into the kidney, a soft-tipped guidewire is placed through the needle, and then a catheter is placed over the wire. The catheter tip remains in the renal pelvis, and the external end is connected to a drainage bag. The procedure immediately relieves the pressure and prevents further damage. The nephrostomy tube remains in place until the obstruction is resolved.

Follow-up Care. Assess the amount of drainage in the collection bag. The amount of drainage depends on whether a ureteral catheter is also being used (with a separate drainage bag). Patients with ureteral tubes may have all urine pass through to the bladder or may have it drain into the collection bags. The type of urine drainage system placed must be clearly communicated in the chart. If urine is expected to drain into the collection bag, assess the amount of drainage hourly for the first 24 hours. If the amount of drainage decreases and the patient has back pain, the tube may be clogged or dislodged.

Monitor the nephrostomy site for leaking urine or blood. Urine drainage may be bloody for the first 12 to 24 hours after the procedure and should gradually clear. If prescribed, the nephrostomy tube can be irrigated with 5 mL sterile saline to check patency and dislodge clots. It is common for diuresis to occur when a nephrostomy is placed for obstruction. Monitor intake and output hourly for the first several hours, and inform the surgeon if the patient begins to have symptoms of dehydration (i.e., hypotension, poor skin turgor, dry mucous membranes, increased thirst). Assess for indications of infection (i.e., fever, change in urine character).

! NURSING SAFETY PRIORITY (QSEN)

Critical Rescue

After nephrostomy, monitor the patient for indications of complications (i.e., decreased or absent drainage, cloudy or foul-smelling drainage, leakage of blood or urine from the nephrostomy site, back pain) (Martin & Baker, 2019). If any indications are present, respond by notifying the surgeon immediately.

NCLEX EXAMINATION CHALLENGE 62.2

Physiological Integrity

The nurse is reviewing the client's laboratory data prior to a nephrostomy tube insertion. Which data requires the nurse to take action?

A. White blood cells in the urine
B. INR of 2.1
C. Hematocrit 44%
D. Creatinine 0.8 mg/dL

RENOVASCULAR DISEASE

Pathophysiology Review

Processes affecting the renal arteries may severely narrow the lumen and greatly reduce blood flow to the kidney tissues. Uncorrected renovascular disease, such as renal vein thrombosis

CLINICAL JUDGMENT CHALLENGE 62.1

Patient-Centered Care; Safety

A 48-year-old client presents to the emergency department with fever, severe flank pain, and painful and restricted urinary output. The health care provider orders labs that reveal the following: creatinine 4.2 mg/dL; BUN 120 mg/dL; potassium 4.8 mEq/L; sodium 148 mEq/L. The client has a history of recurrent kidney infections and kidney stones. The client also has diabetes, anxiety, joint pain, and venous thrombosis. Current medications include metformin, escitalopram, daily vitamin supplement, and use of NSAIDs for muscular pain and associated joint pain and inflammation.

1. **Recognize Cues:** What assessment information in this client situation is the most important and immediate concern for the nurse? (Hint: Identify the **relevant** information *first* to determine what is most important.)
2. **Analyze Cues:** What client conditions are consistent with the **most relevant** information? (Hint: Think about priority collaborative problems that support and contradict the information presented in this situation.)
3. **Prioritize Hypotheses:** Which possibilities or explanations are **most likely** to be present in this client situation? Which possibilities or explanations are the most serious? (Hint: Consider all possibilities and determine their urgency and risk for this client.)
4. **Generate Solutions:** What actions would most likely achieve the desired outcomes for this client? Which actions should be **avoided** or are **potentially harmful**? (Hint: Determine the desired outcomes first to decide which interventions are appropriate and those that should be avoided.)
5. **Take Action:** Which actions are the most appropriate and how should they be implemented? In what **priority order** should they be implemented? (Hint: Consider health teaching, documentation, requested health care provider orders or prescriptions, nursing skills, collaboration with or referral to health team members, etc.)
6. **Evaluate Outcomes:** What client assessment would indicate that the nurse's actions were **effective?** (Hint: Think about signs that would indicate an improvement, decline, or unchanged client condition.)

or renal artery stenosis (RAS), atherosclerosis, or thrombosis, causes ischemia and atrophy of kidney tissue, leading to severe impairment of urinary ***elimination, fluid and electrolyte balance,*** and ***acid-base balance.***

Patients with renovascular disease, particularly those older than 50 years, often have a sudden onset of hypertension. Patients with high blood pressure but no family history of hypertension also may potentially have RAS. RAS from atherosclerosis or blood vessel hyperplasia is the main cause of renovascular disease. Other causes include thrombosis and renal vessel aneurysms.

Atherosclerotic changes in the renal artery often occur along with sclerosis in the aorta and other major vessels. Renal artery changes are often located where the renal artery and aorta meet. Fibrotic changes of the blood vessel wall occur throughout the length of the renal artery.

◆ Interprofessional Collaborative Care

◆ Assessment: Recognize Cues. Hypertension usually first occurs after age 40 to 50, and often the patient does not have a family history of hypertension (see the Key Features: Renovascular Disease box). Diagnosis is made by magnetic resonance angiography (MRA), renal ultrasound, radionuclide imaging, or renal arteriography. MRA provides an excellent image of the renal vasculature and kidney anatomy. Radionuclide imaging is

KEY FEATURES

Renovascular Disease

- Significant, difficult-to-control high blood pressure
- Poorly controlled diabetes or sustained hyperglycemia
- Elevated serum creatinine
- Decreased glomerular filtration rate (GFR)

a noninvasive way of evaluating kidney blood flow and excretory function. Combining radionuclide imaging with ingestion of an angiotensin-converting enzyme inhibitor (ACEi) such as lisinopril improves the accuracy of the test. A renal arteriogram makes the features of the renal blood vessels visible.

◆ Interventions: Take Action. Identifying the type of defect, extent of narrowing, and condition of the surrounding blood vessels is critical for treatment choice, as is the patient's overall health. Many patients with renovascular disease also have cardiovascular disease, and both conditions require treatment.

RAS may be managed by drugs to control high blood pressure and by procedures to restore the blood supply to the kidney. Drugs may control high blood pressure but may not lead to long-term preservation of kidney function. In younger adults, a lifetime of treatment with many drugs for high blood pressure makes treatment difficult and outcomes uncertain.

Endovascular techniques are nonsurgical approaches to repair RAS. Stent placement with or without balloon angioplasty is an example of an endovascular intervention (see Chapter 33). These techniques are less risky and require less time for recovery than does renal artery bypass surgery. After the procedure, the patient usually remains under close observation for 24 hours to monitor for sudden blood pressure fluctuations as the kidneys adjust to increased blood flow.

Renal artery bypass surgery is a major procedure and requires 2 or more months for recovery. A bypass may be performed for either one or both renal arteries. A synthetic blood vessel graft is inserted to redirect blood flow from the abdominal aorta into the renal artery, beyond the area of narrowing. A splenorenal bypass can also restore blood flow to the kidney. The process is similar to other arterial bypass procedures (see Chapter 35).

DIABETIC NEPHROPATHY

Diabetic nephropathy is a vascular complication of diabetes mellitus (DM) and the leading cause of chronic kidney disease in the world. Approximately 40% of patients who are diabetic will develop diabetic kidney disease (Alicic, 2017). It occurs with either type 1 or type 2 DM. Severity of diabetic kidney disease is related to the degree of hyperglycemia the patient generally experiences. With poor control of hyperglycemia, the complicating problems of atherosclerosis, hypertension, and neuropathy (which promotes loss of bladder tone, urinary stasis, and urinary tract infection) are more severe and more likely to cause kidney damage. Chapter 59 discusses diabetic nephropathy. Management of diabetic nephropathy is the same as for chronic kidney disease (see Chapter 63).

TABLE 62.3 Staging Kidney Tumors

Stage I
Tumors ≤7 cm in largest dimension in the kidney. The renal vein, perinephric fat, and adjacent lymph nodes have no tumor.
Stage II
Tumors are >7 cm in largest dimension in the kidney. However, the tumor remains in the kidney with no lymph node involvement.
Stage III
Tumor has penetrated the major veins or perinephric tissues, yet not beyond Gerota fascia. Tumors extend into the lymph nodes but do have distant metastasis.
Stage IV
Tumors include invasion of adjacent organs beyond Gerota fascia or metastasis to distant tissues.

Adapted from Gallardo, E.A. (2017, November 13). *SEOM clinical guideline for treatment of kidney cancer.* Retrieved from U.S. National Library of Medicine, National Institutes of Health. https://www.ncbi.nlm.nih.gov/pmc/articles/PMC5785618/.

RENAL CELL CARCINOMA

Pathophysiology Review

Renal cell carcinoma (RCC) or adenocarcinoma of the kidney is the most common type of kidney cancer and occurs as a result of impaired cellular regulation. Healthy kidney tissue is damaged and replaced by cancer cells, which impairs urine ***elimination*** for that kidney.

Systemic effects occurring with this cancer type are called *paraneoplastic syndromes* and include anemia, erythrocytosis, hypercalcemia, liver dysfunction with elevated liver enzymes, hormonal effects, increased sedimentation rate, and hypertension.

Anemia and erythrocytosis may seem confusing; however, most patients with this cancer have *either* anemia *or* erythrocytosis, not both at the same time. There is some blood loss from hematuria, but the small amount lost does not cause anemia. The cause of the anemia and the erythrocytosis is related to kidney cell production of erythropoietin. At times, the tumor cells produce large amounts of erythropoietin, causing erythrocytosis. At other times, the tumor cells destroy the erythropoietin-producing kidney cells and anemia results.

Parathyroid hormone produced by tumor cells can cause hypercalcemia. Other hormone changes include increased renin levels (causing hypertension) and increased human chorionic gonadotropin (hCG) levels, which decrease libido and change secondary sex features.

RCC has five distinct carcinoma cell types: clear cell, papillary cell, chromophobe cell, collecting duct carcinoma, and unclassified type (McCance et al., 2019).

Kidney tumors are classified into four stages (Table 62.3). Complications include metastasis and urinary tract obstruction. The cancer usually spreads to the adrenal gland, liver, lungs, long bones, or the other kidney. When the cancer surrounds a ureter, hydroureter and obstruction may result.

The causes of nonhereditary RCC are unknown, but the risk is slightly higher for adults who use tobacco or are exposed to cadmium and other heavy metals, asbestos, benzene, and trichloroethylene. Men are slightly more likely to acquire RCC, as are persons with obesity, those with hypertension, and African Americans.

There are 73,750 new cases of kidney cancer in the United States each year (American Cancer Society [ACS], 2020a). Approximately 14,830 people die annually from kidney cancer in the United States. Kidney cancer is among the top 10 most common cancers in men and women, with the average age at diagnosis of 64 years. Kidney cancer is not common in people younger than 45 (ACS, 2020a).

❖ Interprofessional Collaborative Care

The most common treatment for RCC is a nephrectomy. When the cancer is local (i.e., only in the kidney), a nephrectomy can provide a cure. For patients with metastasis, nephrectomy is followed by targeted chemotherapy combined with cytokine treatment. Patients with RCC are at risk for CKD and cardiovascular complications. Patients need ongoing, interprofessional care with surveillance for best outcomes. Follow-up therapy is managed on an outpatient basis.

◆ Assessment: Recognize Cues

History. Ask the patient about his or her age, known risk factors (e.g., smoking or chemical exposures), weight loss, changes in urine color, abdominal or flank discomfort, and fever. Also ask whether any other family member has ever been diagnosed with cancer of the kidney, bladder, ureter, prostate gland, uterus, or ovary.

Physical Assessment/Signs and Symptoms. Some patients with RCC have flank pain, obvious blood in the urine, and a kidney mass that can be palpated. Ask about the nature of the flank or abdominal discomfort. Patients often describe the pain as dull and aching. Pain may be more intense if bleeding into the tumor or kidney occurs. Inspect the flank area, checking for asymmetry or an obvious bulge. An abdominal mass may be felt with *gentle* palpation. A renal bruit may be heard on auscultation.

Bloody urine is a *late* common sign. Blood may be visible as bright red flecks or clots, or the urine may appear smoky or cola colored. Without gross hematuria, microscopic examination may or may not reveal red blood cells (RBCs).

Inspect the skin for pallor, darkening of the nipples, and, in men, breast enlargement *(gynecomastia)* caused by changing hormone levels. Other findings may include muscle wasting, weakness, and weight loss. All tend to occur late in the disease.

Diagnostic Assessment. Urinalysis may show RBCs. Hematologic studies show decreased hemoglobin and hematocrit values, hypercalcemia, increased erythrocyte sedimentation rate, and increased levels of adrenocorticotropic hormone, human chorionic gonadotropin (hCG), cortisol, renin, and parathyroid hormone. Elevated serum creatinine and blood urea nitrogen (BUN) levels indicate impaired kidney function.

Kidney masses may be detected by CT scan or MRI. Ultrasound is also used to detect masses or for initial screening. Kidney biopsy may be considered to help target therapy.

◆ Interventions: Take Action. Treatment for kidney cancer focuses on preventing the spread of the cancer and managing complications. Chemotherapy is not as effective when treating advanced kidney cancers. Targeted therapies that block the growth of new blood vessels that nourish cancer and immunotherapies can be effective (ACS, 2020b).

Nonsurgical Management. Microwave ablation (MWA) or cryoablation can slow tumor growth. It is a minimally invasive procedure carried out after MRI has precisely located the tumor. MWA is used most commonly for patients who have only one kidney or who are not surgical candidates.

Traditional chemotherapy has limited effectiveness against this cancer type. Use of biologic response modifiers (BRMs) such as interleukin-2 (IL-2), interferon (IFN), and tumor necrosis factor (TNF) has increased survival time (see Chapter 20) (ACS, 2020b).

Surgical Management. Renal cell carcinoma (RCC) is usually treated surgically by *nephrectomy* (kidney removal). Renal cell tumors are highly vascular, and blood loss during surgery is a major concern. Before surgery, the arteries supplying the kidney may be occluded (embolized) by the interventional radiologist to reduce bleeding during nephrectomy.

Preoperative Care. Instruct the patient about surgical routines (see Chapter 9). Explain the probable site of incision and the presence of dressings, drains, or other equipment after surgery. Reassure the patient about pain relief. Care before surgery may include giving blood and fluids IV to prevent shock.

Operative Procedures. The patient is placed on his or her side with the kidney to be removed uppermost. The trunk area is flexed to increase exposure of the kidney area. The eleventh or twelfth rib may need to be removed to provide better access to the kidney. The surgeon removes either part or all of the kidney and all visible tumor. The renal artery, renal vein, and fascia also may be removed. A drain may be placed in the wound before closure. The adrenal gland may be removed when the tumor is near this organ.

When a *radical* nephrectomy is performed, local and regional lymph nodes are also removed. The surgical approach may be transthoracic (as discussed in the previous paragraph), lumbar, or through the abdomen, depending on the size and location of the tumor. Radiation therapy may follow a radical nephrectomy.

Postoperative Care. Refer to Chapter 9 for care of the patient after surgery. Nursing priorities are focused on assessing kidney function to determine effectiveness of the remaining kidney, pain management, and preventing complications.

Monitoring includes assessing for hemorrhage and adrenal insufficiency. Inspect the patient's abdomen for distention from bleeding. Check the bed linens under the patient because blood may pool there. Hemorrhage or adrenal insufficiency causes hypotension, decreased urine output, and an altered level of consciousness.

A decrease in blood pressure is an early sign of both hemorrhage and adrenal insufficiency. With hypotension, urine output also decreases immediately. Large water and sodium losses in the urine occur in patients with adrenal insufficiency, leading to impaired ***fluid and electrolyte balance.*** As a result, a large urine output is followed by hypotension and oliguria (less than 400 mL/24 hr or less than 25 mL/hr). IV replacement of fluids and packed RBCs may be needed.

The second kidney is expected to provide adequate function, but this may take days or weeks. Assess urine output hourly for the first 24 hours after surgery (urine output of 0.5 mL/kg/hr or about 30 to 50 mL/hr is acceptable). A low urine output of less than 25 to 30 mL/hr suggests decreased blood flow to the remaining kidney and potential for acute kidney injury (AKI). The hemoglobin level, hematocrit values, and white blood cell count may be measured every 6 to 12 hours for the first day or two after surgery.

Monitor the patient's temperature, pulse rate, and respiratory rate at least every 4 hours. Accurately measure and record fluid intake and output. Weigh the patient daily.

The patient may be in a special care unit for 24 to 48 hours after surgery for monitoring of bleeding and adrenal insufficiency. A drain placed near the site of incision removes residual fluid. Because of the discomfort of deep breathing, the patient is at risk for atelectasis. Fever, chills, thick sputum, or decreased breath sounds suggest pneumonia.

Managing pain after surgery usually requires opioid analgesics given IV. The incision was made through major muscle groups used with breathing and movement. Liberal use of analgesics is needed for 3 to 5 days after surgery to manage pain. Oral agents may be tried when the patient can eat and drink.

Preventing complications focuses on infection and management of adrenal insufficiency. Antibiotics may be prescribed during and after surgery to prevent infection. The need for additional antibiotics is based on evidence of infection. Assess the patient at least every 8 hours for indications of systemic infection or local wound infection.

Adrenal insufficiency is possible as a complication of kidney and adrenal gland removal. Although only one adrenal gland may be affected, the remaining gland may not be able to secrete sufficient glucocorticoids immediately after surgery. Steroid replacements may be needed in some patients. Chapter 57 discusses the signs and symptoms of acute adrenal insufficiency in detail along with specific nursing interventions.

NCLEX EXAMINATION CHALLENGE 62.3

Physiological Integrity

The nurse is caring for a male client 8 hours after a nephrectomy. Which assessment data point requires **immediate** nursing intervention?

A. Abdominal distention
B. Urine output 38 mL in the last hour
C. Blood pressure 108/64 mm Hg
D. Hemoglobin 14 g/dL

KIDNEY TRAUMA

Pathophysiology Review

Trauma to one or both kidneys may occur with penetrating wounds or blunt injuries to the back, flank, or abdomen. Another cause of kidney trauma is urologic procedures. Blunt trauma accounts for most kidney injuries. Traumatic kidney injury is classified into five grades based on the severity of the injury. Grade 1 consists of low-grade injury in the form of kidney bruising, and grade 5 represents the most severe variety associated with shattering of the kidney and tearing of its blood

PATIENT AND FAMILY EDUCATION: PREPARING FOR SELF-MANAGEMENT

Preventing Kidney and Genitourinary Trauma

- Wear a seat belt.
- Practice safe walking habits.
- Use caution when riding bicycles and motorcycles.
- Wear appropriate protective clothing when participating in contact sports.
- Avoid all contact sports and high-risk activities if you have only one kidney.

supply. Adults of any age can sustain kidney trauma. Strategies to prevent trauma are reviewed in the Patient and Family Education: Preparing for Self-Management: Preventing Kidney and Genitourinary Trauma box.

◆ Interprofessional Collaborative Care

❖ Assessment: Recognize Cues. Obtain a history of the patient's usual health and the events involved in the trauma from the patient, a witness, or emergency personnel. Document the mechanism of injury to help determine the severity of the injury. For example, blunt trauma of the kidney from car crashes usually results in an injury of low severity. Critical information to acquire is a history of kidney or urologic disease, surgical intervention, or health problems such as diabetes or hypertension.

Ureteral or renal pelvic injury often causes diffuse abdominal pain. Urine outside of the urinary tract may be visible. Ask the patient about pain in the flank or abdomen.

Assess patients with kidney injuries carefully and thoroughly. Take the patient's blood pressure, apical and peripheral pulses, respiratory rate, and temperature. Inspect both flanks for bruising, asymmetry, or penetrating injuries. Also inspect the abdomen, chest, and lower back for bruising or wounds. Percuss the abdomen for distention. Inspect the urethra for blood.

Urinalysis shows hemoglobin or RBCs from tissue damage or kidney blood vessel rupture. Microscopic examination may also show red blood cell casts, which suggest tubular damage. Hemoglobin and hematocrit values decrease with blood loss.

Diagnostic procedures include ultrasound and CT. CT scan shows greater detail about blood vessel and tissue integrity. Hematomas within or through the kidney capsule can be seen, along with the integrity and patency of the urinary tract. If the patient is being taken to the operating room emergently, a high dose of ionic or nonionic IV contrast material can be given, followed by an abdominal x-ray (KUB) to visualize the traumatic injury and any organ damage.

❖ Interventions: Take Action

Nonsurgical Management. A combination of both drug and fluid therapy may be used to replace blood components and coagulation factors. Drug therapy is used for bleeding prevention or control. Fluid therapy is used to restore circulating blood volume and ensure adequate kidney blood flow. During fluid restoration, give fluids at the prescribed rate and monitor the patient for signs of shock. Take vital signs as often as every 5 to 15 minutes. Measure and record urine output hourly. Output should be greater than 0.5 mL/kg/hr.

The interventional radiologist may use percutaneous or other instrumentation to drain collections of fluid or to embolize (clot) an artery or artery segment or place a stent to repair the urethra or ureters.

! NURSING SAFETY PRIORITY (QSEN)

Action Alert

If the urethral opening is bleeding, consult with the urologist or primary health care provider before attempting urinary catheterization, to avoid making the injury worse.

Surgical Management. Most kidney injuries are managed without surgery. Many serious injuries can be treated with minimally invasive techniques such as angiographic embolization, which accesses the arteries of the kidneys through large blood vessels in the groin, similar to a cardiac catheterization. Surgery to explore the injured kidney occurs when the patient is in shock and may be losing a lot of blood from the kidney. Patients who have other significant abdominal injuries, such as injuries to the bowel, spleen, or liver, and require a laparotomy may also undergo inspection and repair of the injured kidney at the same time. The aim of surgical management is to repair the injured kidney and restore its ***elimination*** function. If the kidney is severely injured (grade 5 injury), a nephrectomy is performed.

Care Coordination and Transition Management. Teach the patient and family how to assess for infection and other complications following kidney trauma. The most common complications are urine leakage and delayed bleeding. Instruct the patient to check the pattern and frequency of urination and note whether the color, clarity, and amount appear normal. The development of an abscess surrounding the kidney also can occur. Instruct the patient to seek medical attention for worsening hematuria, any worrisome change, or pain with voiding. Chills, fever, lethargy, and cloudy, foul-smelling urine indicate a urinary tract infection or abscess formation. Traumatic kidney injury can also cause hypertension from changes in perfusion and activation of the renin-angiotensin-aldosterone system (see Chapter 60). Advise the patient to seek medical care promptly for all new and concerning signs or symptoms.

GET READY FOR THE NEXT-GENERATION NCLEX® EXAMINATION!

Key Points

Review these Key Points for each NCLEX Examination Client Needs Category.

Safe and Effective Care Environment

- Report any condition that obstructs urine flow. **QSEN: Safety**
- Check the blood pressure and urine output frequently in patients who have any type of kidney problem. **QSEN: Safety**
- Report immediately to the primary health care provider sudden decreases of urine output in a patient with kidney disease or trauma. Expected adult urine output is 0.5 to 1 mL/kg/hr. **QSEN: Safety**
- Teach patients with any kidney disorder about strategies to prevent kidney damage from dehydration or trauma. **QSEN: Safety**
- Instruct patients with any type of kidney problem to weigh daily and to notify the primary health care provider if there is a sudden weight gain. **QSEN: Patient-Centered Care**

Health Promotion and Maintenance

- Refer patients with polycystic kidney disease to a geneticist or a genetic counselor. **QSEN: Patient-Centered Care**
- Refer patients to community resources, support groups, and information organizations such as the National Kidney Foundation, the PKD Foundation, and the American Association of Kidney Patients. **QSEN: Patient-Centered Care**
- Encourage patients with diabetes to achieve tight glycemic control. **QSEN: Patient-Centered Care**
- Encourage patients with hypertension to follow their treatment regimens to maintain proper blood pressure **QSEN: Evidence-Based Practice**
- Teach patients to match daily urine output with fluid intake, usually at least 2 liters for kidney health unless another health problem requires fluid restriction. **QSEN: Evidence-Based Practice**

Psychosocial Integrity

- Allow the patient to express fear or anxiety regarding the potential for chronic kidney disease and end-stage kidney disease. **QSEN: Patient-Centered Care**
- Assess the patient's level of comfort in discussing issues related to ***elimination*** and the genitourinary area. **QSEN: Patient-Centered Care**
- Use language with which the patient is comfortable during assessment of the kidney and urinary system. **QSEN: Patient-Centered Care**
- Explain treatment procedures to patients and families. **QSEN: Patient-Centered Care**

Physiological Integrity

- Teach patients the expected side effects and any adverse reactions to prescribed drugs, especially as they relate to kidney function. **QSEN: Patient-Centered Care**
- Teach patients the indications of disease recurrence and when to seek medical help. **QSEN: Patient-Centered Care**
- Teach patients on antibiotic therapy for a UTI (pyelonephritis) to complete the drug regimen. **QSEN: Evidence-Based Practice**
- Explain the genetics of autosomal dominant polycystic kidney disease.
- Use laboratory data and signs and symptoms to determine the effectiveness of therapy for pyelonephritis, polycystic kidney disease, glomerulonephritis (GN), and renal cell carcinoma (RCC).
- Be aware of the signs and symptoms of hydronephrosis.
- Be aware of the relation between kidney disease and hypertension and the associated risk for cardiovascular events.

MASTERY QUESTIONS

1. Which question will the nurse ask the client who has a urinary tract infection to assess the risk for pyelonephritis?
   A. "What drugs do you take for asthma?"
   B. "How long have you had diabetes?"
   C. "How much fluid do you drink daily?"
   D. "Do you take your antihypertensive drugs at night or in the morning?"
2. When assessing a client with acute glomerulonephritis, which question will the nurse ask to determine if the client is following best practices to slow progression of kidney damage?
   A. "Do you avoid contact sports while you are taking cyclosporine?"
   B. "How are you evaluating the amount of daily fluid you drink?"
   C. "Have you contacted anyone from our dialysis support services?"
   D. "Have you increased your protein intake to promote healing of the damaged nephrons?"
3. When providing care to a client who has undergone a nephrostomy for hydronephrosis, which observation alerts the nurse to a possible complication? **Select all that apply.**
   A. Urine output of 15 mL for the first hour and then diminishing
   B. Tenderness at the surgical site
   C. Pink-tinged urine draining from the nephrostomy
   D. A hematocrit value 3% lower than the preoperative value
   E. Sudden onset of abdominal pain that worsens after abdominal palpation
   F. Blood pressure of 180/90 mm Hg that persists despite administration of pain medication

REFERENCES

Alicic, R. Z. (2017). Diabetic kidney disease. *Clinical Journal of the American Society of Nephrology*, 2032–2045.

American Cancer Society. (2020a). *Key Statistics about kidney cancer.* Retrieved from American Cancer Society: https://www.cancer.org/cancer/kidney-cancer/about/key-statistics.html.

American Cancer Society. (2020b). *Targeted therapies for kidney cancer.* Retrieved from American Cancer Society: https://www.cancer.org/cancer/kidney-cancer/treating/targeted-therapy.html.

Crawford, B. S. (2018). Genetics and kidney disease (APOL1). In S. W. Gilbert (Ed.), *Primer on kidney diseases* (pp. 356–360). Philadelphia: Elsevier.

Gallardo, E. A. (2017). *SEOM clinical guideline for treatment of kidney cancer.* Retrieved from US National Library of Medicine National Institute of Health. https://www.ncbi.nlm.nih.gov/pmc/articles/PMC5785618/.

Holt, N. (2018). Renal disease. In R. Hines (Eds.), *stoelting's anesthesia and co-existing disease* (7th ed.) (pp. 425–448). Philadelphia: Elsevier.

Jarvis, C. (2019). *Physical examination and health assessment.* Philadelphia: Elsevier.

Martin, R., & Baker, H. (2019). Nursing care and management of patients with a nephrostomy. *Nursing Times [Online], 115*(11), 40–43. Retrieved from: https://www.nursingtimes.net/clinical-archive/patient-safety/nursing-care-and-management-of-patients-with-a-nephrostomy-14-10-2019/.

McCance, K., Huether, S., Brashers, V., & Rote, N. (2019). *Pathophysiology: The biologic basis for disease in adults and children* (8th ed.). St. Louis: Mosby.

Muthu, V. R. (2018). *Clinicopathological spectrum of glomerular diseases in adolescents: A single-center experience over 4 Years.* Retrieved from US National Library of Medicine National Institute of Health. https://www.ncbi.nlm.nih.gov/pmc/articles/PMC5830804/.

National Institute of Diabetes and Digestive and Kidney Diseases. (2016). *Kidney disease Statistics for the United States.* Retrieved from https://www.niddk.nih.gov/health-information/health-statistics/kidney-disease.

National Institute of Diabetes and Digestive and Kidney Diseases. (2018). *U.S. Department of health and human services.* Retrieved from Kidney Infection (Pyelonephritis): https://www.niddk.nih.gov/health-information/urologic-diseases/kidney-infection-pyelonephritis.

National Kidney Foundation. (2019). *Polycystic kidney disease.* Retrieved from National Kidney Foundation: https://www.kidney.org/atoz/content/polycystic.

Nicolle, L. E. (2018). Urinary tract infection and pyelonephritis. In S. J. Gilbert (Ed.), *National kidney Foundation's primer on kidney diseases* (pp. 427–434). Philadelphia: Elsevier.

Patel, N. P. (2018). *Infection-induced kidney diseases.* Retrieved from US National Library of Medicine National Institute of Health. https://www.ncbi.nlm.nih.gov/pmc/articles/PMC6282040/.

Raman, M. G. (2018). Comparing the impact of older age on outcome in chronic kidney disease of different etiologies: A prospective cohort study. *Journal of Nephrology*, 931–939.

Rizk, D. R. (2018). Polycystic and other cystic kidney diseases. In S. W. Gilbert (Ed.), *National kidney Foundation's primer on kidney diseases* (pp. 375–384). Philadelphia: Elsevier.

Sutherland, R. W. (2018). Obstructive uropathy. In S. W. Gilbert (Ed.), *National kidney Foundation's primer on kidney diseases* (pp. 412–419). Philadelphia: Elsevier.

Trachtman, H. H. (2018). Minimal change nephrotic syndrome. In S. W. Gilbert (Ed.), *National kidney Foundation's primer on kidney diseases* (pp. 175–180). Philadelphia: Elsevier.

University of Pennsylvania. (2019). *Glomerular diseases.* Retrieved from Penn Medicine: https://www.pennmedicine.org/for-patients-and-visitors/find-a-program-or-service/kidney/glomerular-diseases-clinic.

63

Concepts of Care for Patients With Acute Kidney Injury and Chronic Kidney Disease

Robyn Mitchell

http://evolve.elsevier.com/Iggy/

LEARNING OUTCOMES

1. Collaborate with the interprofessional team to coordinate high-quality care and promote urinary ***elimination*** in patients who have acute kidney injury or chronic kidney disease.
2. Teach the patient and caregiver(s) about home safety issues affected by impaired ***elimination*** and impairment of ***fluid and electrolyte balance*** or ***acid-base balance*** resulting from acute kidney injury or chronic kidney disease.
3. Prioritize evidence-based care for patients with impaired urinary ***elimination*** from either acute kidney injury or chronic renal failure.
4. Identify community resources for patients requiring assistance with management of altered ***elimination*** as a result of acute kidney injury or chronic kidney disease.
5. Teach adults how to decrease the risk for acute kidney injury or chronic kidney disease.
6. Implement evidence-based nursing interventions to help patients and families cope with the psychosocial impact caused by acute kidney injury or chronic kidney disease.
7. Apply knowledge of anatomy and pathophysiology to assess patients with impaired kidney function from acute kidney injury or chronic kidney disease.
8. Teach the patient and caregiver(s) about common drugs and other strategies used for acute kidney injury and chronic kidney disease.
9. Implement evidence-based nursing interventions to prevent complications in patients undergoing kidney replacement therapy.
10. Use clinical judgment to analyze information from laboratory data and assessment findings in the care of patients with acute kidney injury and chronic kidney disease.

KEY TERMS

acute kidney injury (AKI) A rapid reduction in kidney function resulting in a failure to maintain waste *elimination, fluid and electrolyte balance,* and *acid-base balance.*

azotemia An excess of nitrogenous wastes (urea) in the blood.

cardiorenal syndrome Disorders of the kidney or heart that cause dysfunction in the other organ.

dialysate Solution used in dialysis that contains a balanced mix of electrolytes and water and that closely resembles human plasma.

diffusion Movement of molecules from an area of higher concentration to an area of lower concentration.

hyperpnea Abnormal increase in the depth of respiratory movements.

Kussmaul respiration Breathing pattern with respirations that are fast and deep; often associated with metabolic acidosis.

melena Blood in the stool with the appearance of black, tarry stool.

oliguria Urine output less than 400 mL/day.

pruritus Itching.

renal osteodystrophy Bone metabolism and structural damage caused by chronic kidney disease–induced low calcium levels and high phosphorus levels.

uremia The accumulation of nitrogenous wastes in the blood (azotemia); a result of renal failure, with clinical symptoms that include nausea and vomiting.

uremic frost Layer of urea crystals from evaporated sweat; may appear on the face, eyebrows, axillae, and groin in patients with advanced uremic syndrome.

uremic syndrome The systemic clinical and laboratory manifestations of end-stage kidney disease.

PRIORITY AND INTERRELATED CONCEPTS

The priority concept for this chapter is:
- ***Elimination***

The ***Elimination*** concept exemplar for this chapter is Chronic Kidney Disease.

The interrelated concepts for this chapter are:
- ***Acid-Base Balance***
- ***Fluid and Electrolyte Balance***
- ***Immunity***
- ***Perfusion***

The kidney function of urinary ***elimination*** includes excretion of waste, ***fluid and electrolyte balance,*** regulation of ***acid-base balance,*** and hormone secretion. These processes are greatly impaired with kidney function loss, and every organ system is affected. Acute kidney injury (AKI) is most common in the acute care setting, whereas chronic kidney disease (CKD) is more likely to be seen in community settings or as a coexisting condition in acute care settings. The features of AKI and CKD are described in Table 63.1.

Both types of kidney problems can require kidney replacement therapy (KRT; e.g., dialysis). When kidney function is permanently or persistently impaired, as with end-stage kidney disease (ESKD), dialysis or kidney transplant is a lifesaving approach for urinary ***elimination*** to maintain homeostasis, ***fluid and electrolyte balance,*** and ***acid-base balance.*** ESKD reduces independence, shortens life, and decreases quality of life. Many diseases and conditions are associated with the onset and severity of kidney function loss.

When kidney function declines gradually, it is diagnosed as CKD, formerly termed *chronic renal failure (CRF).* The patient may have many years of abnormal blood urea nitrogen (BUN) and creatinine values, sometimes called *renal insufficiency,* before ESKD develops. When kidney function decline is sudden, acute kidney injury (AKI) is diagnosed. AKI can be a temporary condition that resolves, or it can progress to CKD.

Even when AKI does not progress to CKD, AKI is associated with higher morbidity and mortality, even in young patients without other chronic diseases that increase risks (Fuhrman, 2018). AKI also can occur in a patient with established CKD. When these two conditions co-occur, the loss of kidney function and waste ***elimination*** is usually more severe and accelerated.

Acute kidney injury affects *many* body systems. Chronic kidney disease affects *every* body system. The problems that occur with kidney function loss are related to disturbances of ***fluid and electrolyte balance,*** disturbances of ***acid-base balance,*** buildup of nitrogen-based wastes (uremia), and loss of kidney hormone function.

ACUTE KIDNEY INJURY

Pathophysiology Review

Acute kidney injury (AKI) is a rapid reduction in kidney function resulting in a failure to maintain waste ***elimination, fluid and electrolyte balance,*** and ***acid-base balance.*** AKI occurs over a few hours or days. The most current definition of AKI is an increase in serum creatinine by 0.3 mg/dL (26.2 mcmol/L) or more within 48 hours; or an increase in serum creatinine to 1.5 times or more from baseline, which is known or presumed to have occurred in the previous 7 days; or a urine volume of less than 0.5 mL/kg/hr for 6 hours (Gilbert & Weiner, 2018). Criteria for staging the severity of AKI are in Table 63.2. The Kidney Disease: Improving Global Outcomes (KDIGO) classification is a universal definition and staging system for AKI.

The creatinine level is most commonly used in the recognition of AKI. However, this value is not ideal because the creatinine level takes time to increase, which can create delays in treatment. A baseline creatinine value is also necessary to evaluate for AKI, as this provides a means for comparison.

Biomarkers that are specific to kidney injury have been approved by the Food and Drug Administration (FDA) (Gilbert & Weiner, 2018). These biomarkers indicate damage earlier than the creatinine level and do not require a baseline value for comparison. These biomarkers specific to kidney injury can be used similarly to biomarkers such as troponin in cardiac injury. These biomarkers can identify patients at high risk for developing AKI during the next 12 to 24 hours and include tissue injury metalloproteinase 2 (TIMP-2) and insulin-like growth factor binding protein 7 (IGFBP-7) (Moore, 2018). Earlier identification of risk allows for earlier intervention. Although these biomarkers show significant promise, they are not yet widely used.

Glomerular filtration rate (GFR) is accepted as the best overall indicator of kidney function, but it is not accurate during acute and critical illness (Gilbert & Weiner, 2018). Estimations of GFR from serum creatinine are affected by metabolic problems and treatments during critical illnesses. Urine output is altered when diuretics or IV fluids are used. AKI also causes systemic effects and complications described in Table 63.3. These complications increase discomfort and risk for death. Duration of oliguria or anuria closely correlates with lack of recovery of kidney function; the longer the duration of oliguria or anuria, the less likely it is that the patient will return to full or baseline kidney function.

Etiology. The causes of AKI are reduced ***perfusion*** to the kidneys, damage to kidney tissue, and obstruction of urine outflow. Urine outflow obstruction along with tissue damage of the kidneys and reduction of perfusion are causes of AKI. Table 63.4 lists causes of AKI along with the diseases and associated conditions. However, the diseases listed in Table 63.3 are described in greater detail in another section of this text. Risk factors for AKI include shock, cardiac surgery, hypotension, prolonged mechanical ventilation, and sepsis. Older adults or adults with diabetes, hypertension, peripheral vascular disease, liver disease, or CKD are at higher risk of AKI if hospitalized.

AKI is categorized as prerenal, intrinsic renal (also called intrarenal), and postrenal in order to better understand and treat the disorder. Prerenal AKI is caused by a source outside of the kidney creating conditions that impair renal ***perfusion.*** Common causes include shock, dehydration, burns, and sepsis. Intrinsic renal injury occurs inside the kidney by disorders that directly affect the renal cortex or medulla. Examples of disorders causing intrinsic renal AKI include allergic disorders, embolism or thrombosis of

TABLE 63.1 Features of Acute Kidney Injury and Chronic Kidney Disease

Characteristic	Acute Kidney Injury	Chronic Kidney Disease
Onset	Sudden (hours to days)	Gradual (months to years)
Percentage of nephron involvement	50%-95%	Varies by stage; generally symptomatic with 75% loss and dialysis with 90%-95% loss
Duration	May not progress; full recovery (return to baseline) possible ESKD occurs in 10%-20% with lifetime reliance on dialysis or kidney transplant	Progressive and permanent Treatment and lifestyle can slow progression and delay onset of ESKD
Prognosis	Good when kidney function is maintained or returns High mortality associated with renal replacement therapy requirements or prolonged illness	Progression of CKD depends on stage of GFR, stage of albuminuria, and specific conditions associated with the onset of the disorder ESKD fatal without a renal replacement therapy (dialysis or transplantation) Reduced life span and potential for complex medical regimen even with optimal treatment

CKD, Chronic kidney disease; *ESKD,* end-stage kidney disease; *GFR,* glomerular filtration rate.

TABLE 63.2 The KDIGO Classification System for Severity of Acute Kidney Injury

Stage	Serum Creatinine	Urine Output
Stage 1	1.5-1.9 times baseline OR ≥0.3 mg/dL (≥26.5 mmol/L) increase over 48 hr	<0.5 mL/kg/hr for 6-12 hr
Stage 2	2.0-2.9 times baseline	<0.5 mL/kg/hr for ≥12 hr
Stage 3	1.0 times baseline OR Increase in serum creatinine to ≥4.0 mg/dL (≥353.6 mmol/L) OR Initiation of renal replacement therapy OR In patients <18 years, decrease in eGFR to <35 mL/min/1.73 m^2	Anuria lasting for ≥12 hr OR <0.3 mL/kg/hr for >24 hr

eGFR, Estimated glomerular filtration rate; *KDIGO,* Kidney Disease: Improving Global Outcomes (2012).

TABLE 63.3 Systemic Complications From Acute Kidney Injury

Metabolic
- Metabolic acidosis
- Hyperlipidemia
- Hyperkalemia
- Hyponatremia
- Hypocalcemia
- Hypophosphatemia

Cardiopulmonary
- Peripheral and pulmonary edema
- Heart failure
- Pulmonary embolism
- Pericarditis
- Pericardial effusion
- Hypertension
- Myocardial infarction

Neurologic
- Neuromuscular irritability or weakness
- Asterixis
- Seizures
- Mental status changes

Immune/Infectious
- Pneumonia
- Sepsis

Gastrointestinal
- Nausea
- Vomiting
- Decreased peristalsis
- Enteral nutrition intolerance
- Malnutrition
- Ulcer formation
- Bleeding

Hematologic
- Bleeding
- Thrombosis
- Anemia

Renal
- Chronic kidney disease (CKD)
- End-stage kidney disease (ESKD)

Other
- Hiccups
- Elevated parathyroid hormone
- Low thyroid hormone level

the renal vessels, and nephrotoxic agents. Postrenal AKI is caused by a urine flow obstruction. The obstruction can be caused by tumors, kidney stones, or strictures (McCance et al., 2019).

With prerenal or postrenal pathology, the kidney compensates with the three responses of constricting kidney blood vessels, activating the renin-angiotensin-aldosterone pathway, and releasing antidiuretic hormone (ADH). These responses increase blood volume and improve kidney ***perfusion.*** However, these same responses reduce urine ***elimination,*** resulting in **oliguria** (urine output less than 400 mL/day) and **azotemia** (the retention and buildup of nitrogenous wastes in the blood). Toxins can also cause blood vessel constriction in the kidney, leading to reduced kidney blood flow, oliguria, and azotemia.

Activated ***immunity*** and damage from kidney toxins (nephrotoxins) (Table 63.5) cause intracellular changes of the tubular system in kidney tissue. Inflammatory proteins and immune-mediated complexes can damage cells and tissues in the kidney. With extensive damage, tubular cells slough and nephrons lose the ability to repair themselves. The presence of tubular debris and sediment in urine from kidney tissue damage (intrarenal failure or *acute tubular necrosis*) is related to systemic ischemia, reduced kidney ***perfusion,*** or nephrotoxin exposure.

Even with severe AKI (i.e., stage 2 or 3 in Table 63.2), some adults return to baseline kidney function during recovery from illness. It is the responsibility of all health care professionals to be alert to the possibility of AKI and implement prevention strategies when risk factors are present. *Timely interventions to remove*

TABLE 63.4 Diseases and Conditions That Contribute to Acute Kidney Injury

Perfusion Reduction (Prerenal Causes)

- Blood or fluid loss
- Blood pressure medications
- Heart attack
- Heart disease
- Infection (e.g., sepsis, septic shock)
- Liver failure
- Use of aspirin, ibuprofen, naproxen, or other related drugs
- Severe allergic reaction (anaphylaxis)
- Severe burns
- Severe dehydration
- Renal artery stenosis
- Bleeding or clotting in the kidney blood vessels (coagulopathy)
- Atherosclerosis or cholesterol deposits that block blood flow in the kidneys

Kidney Damage (Intrinsic or Intrarenal Causes)

- Blood clots in nearby veins and arteries
- Cholesterol deposits that block blood flow in the kidneys
- Glomerulonephritis
- Hemolytic uremic syndrome
- Local infection (pyelonephritis)
- Lupus, an immune system disorder causing glomerulonephritis
- Pharmaceuticals, such as certain chemotherapy agents, antibiotics, iodinated or hyperosmolar contrast media used during imaging tests
- Scleroderma, a group of rare diseases affecting the skin and connective tissues
- Thrombotic thrombocytopenic purpura (TTP), a rare platelet disorder that increases clotting

Urine Flow Obstruction (Postrenal Causes)

- Bladder cancer
- Cervical cancer
- Colon cancer
- Prostate cancer
- Enlarged prostate
- Kidney stones
- Nerve damage involving the nerves that control the bladder
- Blood clots in the urinary tract

the cause of AKI may prevent progression to ESKD and the need for lifelong renal replacement therapy (RRT) or a renal transplant.

Incidence and Prevalence. Twenty percent of all hospitalized patients and 60% of intensive care unit patients develop AKI. AKI is increasingly recognized as an in-hospital complication that is associated with shock, heart conditions, and surgery (Pavkov et al., 2018). Patients who are older or who have chronic kidney disease or diabetes are at greater risk for AKI.

Health Promotion and Maintenance. *Keep in mind that dehydration (severe blood volume depletion) reduces* ***perfusion*** *and can lead to AKI even in adults who have no known kidney problems.* Urge all healthy adults to avoid dehydration by drinking 2 to 3 L of water daily. This is especially important for athletes or anyone who performs strenuous exercise or work and sweats heavily.

TABLE 63.5 Examples of Potentially Nephrotoxic Substances

Drugs

Antibiotics/Antimicrobials

- Amphotericin B
- Colistimethate
- Polymyxin B
- Rifampin
- Sulfonamides
- Tetracycline hydrochloride
- Vancomycin

Aminoglycoside Antibiotics

- Gentamicin
- Neomycin
- Tobramycin

Chemotherapy Agents

- Cisplatin
- Cyclophosphamide
- Methotrexate

NSAIDs

- Celecoxib
- Flurbiprofen
- Ibuprofen
- Indomethacin
- Ketorolac
- Meloxicam
- Nabumetone
- Naproxen
- Oxaprozin
- Tolmetin

Other Drugs

- Acetaminophen
- Captopril
- Cyclosporine
- Fluorinate anesthetics
- Metformin
- Quinine

Other Substances

Organic Solvents

- Carbon tetrachloride
- Ethylene glycol

Nondrug Chemical Agents

- Radiographic contrast media (e.g., iodinated media, hyperosmolar media, and gadolinium)
- Pesticides
- Fungicides
- Myoglobin (from breakdown of skeletal muscle)

Heavy Metals and Ions

- Arsenic
- Bismuth
- Copper sulfate
- Gold salts
- Lead
- Mercuric chloride

Nurses have an essential role in the prevention of AKI in hospitalized patients. Always be on the lookout for signs of impending kidney dysfunction through assessment and close monitoring of laboratory values. Early recognition and correction of problems causing reduced urinary ***elimination*** may avoid kidney tissue damage. Evaluate the patient's fluid status. Accurately measure intake and output and check body weight to identify changes in fluid balance. Note the characteristics of the urine and report new sediment, hematuria (smoky or red color), foul odor, or other worrisome changes. Report a urine output of less than 30 mL/hr for 2 hours or dark amber urine to the primary health care provider (Jarvis & Eckhardt, 2020). Waiting for 6 hours of oliguria to meet AKI criteria may allow progression of kidney damage—act early!

! NURSING SAFETY PRIORITY (QSEN)

Critical Rescue

In any acute care setting, preventing volume depletion and providing intervention early when volume depletion occurs are nursing priorities. Reduced ***perfusion*** from volume depletion is a common cause of AKI. Assess continually to recognize the signs and symptoms of volume depletion (low urine output, decreased systolic blood pressure, decreased pulse pressure, orthostatic hypotension, thirst, rising blood osmolarity). Respond by intervening early with oral fluids or, in the patient who is unable to take or tolerate oral fluid, requesting an increase in IV fluid rate from the primary health care provider to prevent permanent kidney damage.

Monitor laboratory values for any changes that reflect poor kidney function. A significant increase in creatinine, especially when the increase occurs over hours or a few days, is a concern and must be reported urgently to the primary health care provider. Other laboratory values that help monitor kidney function include serum blood urea nitrogen (BUN); serum potassium, sodium, and osmolarity; and urine specific gravity, albumin-creatinine ratio, and electrolytes. Know the baseline (steady-state) GFR because a reduced GFR makes the patient more vulnerable to AKI.

Be aware of nephrotoxic substances that the patient may ingest or be exposed to (see Table 63.5). Question any prescription for potentially nephrotoxic drugs, and validate the dose before the patient receives the drug. Many antibiotics have nephrotoxic effects. NSAIDs can cause or increase the risk for AKI. Combining two or more nephrotoxic drugs dramatically increases the risk for AKI. If a patient must receive a known nephrotoxic drug, closely monitor laboratory values, including BUN, creatinine, and drug peak and trough levels, for indications of reduced kidney function. When a nephrotoxic agent such as contrast medium will be used, additional nephrotoxic medications such as metformin should be withheld at least 24 hours before and after the procedure, if possible. Intravenous fluids should be administered before and after exposure to the contrast medium (Moore, 2018).

❖ Interprofessional Collaborative Care

AKI is managed initially in the hospital setting, most commonly in an ICU. During the acute phase of the problem, members of the interprofessional team include the nephrologist, nephrology nurse, registered dietitian nutritionist (RDN), pharmacist, and dialysis technician. The responsibilities of each of these professionals are described within the interventions sections of this chapter. When the patient is discharged before urinary ***elimination*** returns to normal, continuing management is needed as part of the transition to community care.

◆ Assessment: Recognize Cues

History. The accurate diagnosis of AKI, including its cause, depends on a detailed history. Know the risk factors for and criteria of AKI and chronic kidney disease (CKD). Ask about any change in urine appearance, frequency, or volume.

Ask about recent surgery or trauma, transfusions, allergic (hypersensitivity) reactions, or other factors that might lead to reduced kidney ***perfusion.*** Obtain a drug history, especially use of antibiotics and NSAIDs. Ask about recent imaging procedures requiring injection of a contrast medium. Coexisting conditions of advanced age, chronic kidney disease, diabetes, long-term hypertension, major or systemic infection (sepsis), peripheral vascular disease, chronic liver disease, acquired immune deficiency syndrome (AIDS [HIV-III]) and prior kidney surgery increase the risk for AKI (Gilbert & Weiner, 2018).

To identify ***immunity***-mediated AKI (i.e., acute glomerulonephritis), ask about acute illnesses such as influenza, colds, gastroenteritis, and sore throats. Allergic reactions from a drug or food allergy may result in AKI as late as 10 days after exposure. Ask about rashes, hives, or fever and evaluate the white blood cell (WBC) differential for an increased eosinophil count.

Anticipate AKI following any episode of hypotension or shock. Any problem in which the blood volume is depleted can contribute to AKI by reducing ***perfusion***. Such problems include cardiac bypass surgery, extensive bowel preparations, being NPO before surgery, or dehydration from exercise. Recent use of IV vasopressors (e.g., epinephrine or norepinephrine) may contribute to AKI when blood volume is reduced (hypovolemia).

Consider whether there is a history of urinary obstructive problems. Ask the patient about any difficulty in starting the urine stream, changes in the amount or appearance of the urine, narrowing of the urine stream, nocturia, urgency, or symptoms of kidney stones. Also ask about any cancer history that may cause urinary obstruction.

PATIENT-CENTERED CARE: OLDER ADULT CONSIDERATIONS QSEN

AKI is more common as people age. People aged 80 to 89 years of age are 55% more likely to develop AKI than people under age 50. As the kidneys age, structural and functional changes occur including fewer nephrons and sclerosis of glomeruli and the renal arteries. These changes lead to an increased risk for AKI. Older adults also have more comorbid conditions such as diabetes, hypertension, and chronic kidney disease (Johnson et al., 2019).

Further increasing the risk of AKI in the older adult is an increased exposure to nephrotoxic drugs. The use of multiple drugs is associated with drug-induced AKI, particularly in acute and critical care settings. Assess risk and take actions to reduce exposure to nephrotoxic agents, avoid hypotension and hypovolemia, evaluate drug-drug interactions for potential adverse kidney effects, and stop unnecessary drugs to maintain kidney function in older adults.

Physical Assessment/Signs and Symptoms. If a patient has a urinary catheter, assess urine output every hour after surgery until stable, during fluid resuscitation for shock or hypotension, and when the patient has a high risk for AKI following hospital admission. Even a brief period of oliguria, defined as less than 0.5 mL/kg/hr of urine output for 2 or more hours, can signal AKI.

Other symptoms of AKI are related to the buildup of nitrogenous wastes (azotemia) and decreased urine output (oliguria). As AKI progresses in severity, the patient may have symptoms of fluid overload because fluid is not eliminated. Indications of fluid overload include pulmonary crackles, dependent and generalized edema *(anasarca)*, decreased oxygenation (low peripheral oxygenation or Spo_2), confusion, increased respiratory rate, and dyspnea. See Chapter 13 for assessment of fluid overload.

Evaluate vital signs to recognize early hypoperfusion and hypoxemia. Symptoms of reduced blood volume such as mean arterial pressure (MAP) below 65 mm Hg, tachycardia, thready peripheral pulses, or decreasing cognition may indicate risk for AKI from poor ***perfusion***; an Spo_2 below 88% may indicate potential hypoxemic or ischemic damage to kidney tissue.

Laboratory Assessment. The many changes in laboratory values in the patient with AKI are similar to those occurring in chronic kidney disease (CKD). (See the Laboratory Profile:

Kidney Disease box.) Expect to see rising creatinine and BUN levels and abnormal blood electrolyte values. However, patients with AKI usually do *not* have the anemia associated with CKD unless there is blood loss from another condition (e.g., surgery, trauma) or when BUN levels are high enough to break (lyse) red blood cells (RBCs).

In early AKI, urine tests provide important information. Urine sodium levels may reflect an inability to concentrate urine. Urine may be dilute with a specific gravity near 1.000 or concentrated with a specific gravity greater than 1.030. The presence of urine sediment (e.g., RBCs, casts, and tubular cells), myoglobin, or hemoglobin may lead to nephron damage.

Imaging Assessment. Ultrasonography is useful in the diagnosis of kidney and urinary tract obstruction. Dilation of the renal calyces and collecting ducts, as well as stones, can be detected. Ultrasonography can show kidney size and patency of the ureters. Small kidney size may indicate an underlying CKD with loss of kidney tissue.

CT scans without contrast medium can determine adequacy of kidney ***perfusion*** and identify obstruction or tumors. Contrast medium is usually avoided to prevent further kidney damage (Lambert et al., 2017). An MRI may be used in place of a CT scan.

X-rays of the pelvis or kidneys, ureters, and bladder (KUB) may provide an initial view of kidneys and the urinary tract to determine the cause of AKI. Enlarged kidneys with obstruction may show hydronephrosis. X-rays can show stones obstructing the renal pelvis, ureters, or bladder. More commonly, ultrasound is used to screen for hydronephrosis.

A nuclear medicine study called *MAG3* may be used to determine the nature of the kidney failure and measure GFR. A renal scan can determine whether ***perfusion*** of the kidneys is sufficient. Cystoscopy or retrograde pyelography may be needed to identify obstructions of the lower urinary tract (see Chapter 60).

LABORATORY PROFILE

Kidney Disease

Test	Normal Range for Adults	Values in Kidney Disease
Serum creatinine	*Male:* 0.6-1.2 mg/dL (53-106 mmol/L) *Female:* 0.5-1.1 mg/dL (44-97 mmol/L) *Older adults:* May be slightly increased	**In chronic kidney disease:** May increase by 0.5-1.0 mg/dL (50-100 mcmol/L) every 1-2 yr **In acute kidney injury:** Increase of 1-2 mg/dL (100-200 mmol/L) every 24-48 hr May increase 1-6 mg/dL (100-600 mmol/L) in 1 wk or less
Serum sodium	136-145 mEq/L (136-145 mmol/L)	Normal, increased, or decreased
Serum potassium	3.5-5.0 mEq/L (3.5-5.0 mmol/L)	Increased
Serum phosphorus (phosphate)	3.0-4.5 mg/dL (0.97-1.45 mmol/L) *Older adults:* May be slightly decreased	Increased
Serum calcium	Total calcium: 9.0-10.5 mg/dL (2.25-2.62 mmol/L) Ionized calcium: 4.5-5.6 mg/dL (1.05-1.3 mmol/L) *Older adults:* Slightly decreased	Decreased
Serum magnesium	1.3-2.1 mEq/L (0.65-1.05 mmol/L)	Increased or decreased
Serum carbon dioxide combining power (bicarbonate) (venous)	23-30 mEq/L (23-30 mmol/L)	Decreased
Arterial blood pH	7.35-7.45	Decreased (in metabolic acidosis) or normal
Arterial blood bicarbonate (HCO_3^-)	21-28 mEq/L (21-28 mmol/L)	Decreased
Arterial blood Pa_{CO_2}	35-45 mm Hg	Decreased
Hemoglobin	*Female:* 12-16 g/dL (7.4-9.9 mmol/L) *Male:* 14-18 g/dL (8.7-11.2 mmol/L) *Older adults:* Slightly decreased	Decreased
Hematocrit	*Female:* 37%-47% (0.37-0.47 volume fraction) *Male:* 42%-52% (0.42-0.52 volume fraction) *Older adults:* May be slightly decreased	Decreased
Blood osmolality	285-295 mOsm/kg (285-295 mmol/kg)	Elevated in volume-depleted states, increasing the risk for acute kidney injury

Data from Pagana, K., Pagana, T. & Pagana, T. (2017). *Mosby's diagnostic and laboratory test reference* (13th ed.). St. Louis: Elsevier.

Other Diagnostic Assessments. Kidney biopsy is performed if the cause of AKI is uncertain and symptoms persist or an immunologic disease is suspected. Prepare the patient before the test, particularly managing both hypotension and hypertension. Hypertension increases the risk for intrarenal hemorrhage following needle biopsy. Provide follow-up care. Be aware of all test results and understand how they might affect the treatment regimen. (See Chapter 60 for a detailed discussion of diagnostic tests related to the kidney.)

NCLEX EXAMINATION CHALLENGE 63.1

Safe and Effective Care Environment

A 62-year-old client was admitted 2 days ago with traumatic injuries and hypovolemic shock. Which lab result is **most important** for the nurse to report to the health care provider immediately?

A. Serum sodium 132 mEq/L (mmol/L)
B. Serum potassium 6.9 mEq/L (mmol/L)
C. Blood urea nitrogen 24 mg/dL (mmol/L)
D. Hematocrit 32% (0.32 volume fraction); hemoglobin 9.2 g/dL (92 g/L)

◆ **Interventions: Take Action.** Avoid hypotension and maintain normal fluid balance *(euvolemia)* to prevent and manage AKI. A reduction in kidney ***perfusion*** may initially not be recognized when there is no associated drop in systemic blood pressure. Autoregulation and the renin-angiotensin-aldosterone system (RAAS) effectively maintain normal kidney perfusion and glomerular filtration rate. Maintaining a mean arterial pressure (MAP) of 80 to 85 mm Hg has been shown to lower rates of AKI in patients with pre-existing hypertension. However, there is an increased risk of atrial fibrillation in patients with a mean arterial pressure (MAP) of 80 to 85 mm Hg as opposed to 65 to 70 mm Hg. Accordingly, blood pressure goals are determined based on pre-existing conditions and risk versus benefit to the patient (Moore, 2018).

Reduce exposure to nephrotoxic agents and drugs that alter kidney perfusion. When such substances cannot be avoided, monitor drug levels and communicate with the pharmacist to adjust doses to minimize harm. Contrast media can have serious toxic effects on tubular cells (Lambert et al., 2017). Ensure that kidney function is assessed before an imaging test that includes contrast media. A large volume of contrast, agents with high osmolarity (>2000 mOsm/L [mmol/L]), and frequent administration (given twice in 3 months or more often) of agents are more likely to cause contrast-induced nephropathy. Ensure that kidney function is assessed before an imaging test and that both the radiologist and the requesting primary health care provider are aware of reduced kidney function before contrast medium is given.

Communicate with the radiologist so that the lowest dose of the contrast agent is used in high-risk adults. Adequate hydration is essential to prevent contrast-induced nephropathy (Honicker & Holt, 2016; Lambert et al., 2017). The patient may receive IV fluids at a rate of 1 mL/kg/hr for 12 hours before the imaging test or at 3 mL/kg/hr for 1 hour just before the procedure to ensure hydration and dilution of the contrast medium and to speed urinary ***elimination*** of the agent. A common desired outcome for patients undergoing a procedure with contrast medium is a urine output of 150 mL/hr for the first 6 hours after administration of the contrast agent.

Observations about new-onset or increased peripheral edema, increased daily weight, and reduced urine output can identify patients with a positive fluid balance from AKI who may require treatment with fluid restriction or diuretic therapy. Impairment of ***acid-base balance*** and electrolyte imbalance can occur and may require treatment, especially in older adults.

Blood sampling of patients at risk for AKI allows early recognition of elevated serum creatinine levels and trend data. Communicate observations about worsening kidney function early and often to the primary health care provider so interventions can promote kidney health and interrupt the progression of AKI when it occurs.

Not all patients with AKI experience oliguria. ***Immunity*** and inflammatory causes of AKI may allow proteins to enter the glomerulus, and these proteins can hold fluid in the filtrate, causing a *polyuria* (excess urine output) that disrupts ***fluid and electrolyte balance.*** During AKI with high-volume urine output, hypovolemia and electrolyte *loss* are the main problems. The patient in the diuretic phase of AKI needs a plan of care that focuses on fluid and electrolyte *replacement* and monitoring. Onset of polyuria can signal the start of recovery from AKI.

Surviving kidney tubule cells possess a remarkable ability to regenerate and proliferate, and early identification can stop progression of AKI, as well as aid in recovery of kidney function. Base the desired outcomes of care on collaboration and communication with interprofessional team members. Update the plan of care for either restriction (when fluid overload from new AKI is present) or liberal administration of fluid (to prevent AKI or promote elimination of contrast medium) based on timely and accurate team communication.

Frequent laboratory value monitoring, close surveillance of intake and output, drug therapy, nutrition, careful administration of fluids and minerals, and renal replacement therapy are commonly used to manage AKI.

NCLEX EXAMINATION CHALLENGE 63.2

Safe and Effective Care Environment

The nurse is caring for a 74-year-old client scheduled for a cardiac catheterization with contrast dye. What nursing action is appropriate? **Select all that apply.**

A. Assess creatinine clearance using a 24-hour urine collection test.
B. Assess for coexisting conditions of diabetes, heart failure, and kidney disease.
C. Collaborate with the provider about whether IV fluids should be infused before the test.
D. Notify the provider regarding changes in serum creatinine from 0.2 to 0.4 mg/dL in 24 hours.
E. Alert the provider to a glomerular filtration rate (GFR) below 60 mL/min/1.73 m^2.

Drug Therapy. The interprofessional team consults the inpatient pharmacist for drug adjustment based on kidney function. As kidney function changes, drug dosages are changed. It is important to be knowledgeable about the site of drug metabolism and especially careful when giving drugs. Continuously monitor the patient with AKI for adverse drug events and interactions of the drugs that he or she is receiving. Diuretics may be used to increase urine output in AKI. Diuretic-induced urine output does not preserve kidney function or stop AKI, but diuretics do rid the body of retained fluid and electrolytes in the patient with AKI that has not progressed to end-stage kidney disease (ESKD).

Fluid challenges are often used to promote kidney ***perfusion.*** In patients without fluid overload, 500 to 1000 mL of normal saline may be infused over 1 hour. It is important to assess the patient's response to fluid to prevent fluid overload. Fluid overload in critical illness has been shown to increase mortality (Moore, 2018). The term *fluid responsive* is used when identifying patients who have a positive response to fluid. There are many methods to evaluate fluid responsiveness, such as systolic pressure variation, pulse pressure variation, and stroke volume variation, which are obtained from the arterial or pulse oximetry waveforms. In patients with a method of monitoring stroke volume and cardiac output, a passive leg raise can determine if the patient is fluid responsive without the risk of giving fluids. The patient's leg is raised to 45 degrees for 30 to 90 seconds in order to temporarily move fluid by increasing venous return, and if the stroke volume or cardiac output improves, the patient will respond positively to more fluid volume (Brown & Semler, 2019).

Nutrition Therapy. Patients who have AKI often have a high rate of *catabolism* (protein breakdown). Increases in metabolism and protein breakdown may be related to the stress of illness and the increase in blood levels of catecholamines, cortisol, and glucagon. The rate of protein breakdown correlates with the severity of uremia and azotemia. Catabolism causes the breakdown of muscle protein and increases azotemia.

The interprofessional team's registered dietitian nutritionist (RDN) in the ICU setting calculates the patient's protein and caloric needs. A consultation may need to be requested for inpatients outside of the ICU or for those in community settings. Work with the RDN to establish a diet with specified amounts of protein, sodium, and fluids. For the patient who does not require dialysis, 0.6 g/kg of body weight or 40 g/day of protein is usually prescribed. For patients who require dialysis, the protein level needed ranges from 1 to 1.5 g/kg. The dietary sodium ranges from 60 to 90 mEq/kg (mmol/kg). If high blood potassium levels are present, dietary potassium is restricted to 60 to 70 mEq/kg (mmol/kg). The daily amount of fluid permitted is calculated to be equal to the urine volume plus 500 mL. Assess food intake every shift to ensure that caloric intake is adequate.

Many patients with AKI are too ill or their appetite is too poor to meet caloric goals. For these patients, nutrition support with oral supplements, enteral nutrition, or parenteral nutrition (PN or hyperalimentation) is needed. Nutrition support in AKI aims to provide sufficient nutrients to maintain or improve nutrition status, preserve lean body mass, restore or maintain fluid balance, and preserve kidney function.

There are several kidney-specific formulations of oral supplements and enteral solutions (e.g., Nepro, Suplena, and Novasource Renal). Most specialty formulas for patients with kidney problems are lower in sodium, potassium, and phosphorus and higher in calories than are standard feedings. Enteral nutrition, delivered with a nasogastric or nasojejunal tube (these tubes can also be placed orally), can be used for nutrition support. If PN is used, the IV solutions are mixed to meet the patient's specific needs. Because kidney function is unstable in AKI, continuously monitor intake and output and serum electrolyte levels to determine how the supplementation affects ***fluid and electrolyte balance.*** IV fat emulsion (Intralipid) infusions can provide a nonprotein source of calories. In uremic patients, fat emulsions are used in place of glucose to avoid the problems of excessive sugars.

Kidney Replacement Therapy. Kidney replacement therapy (KRT), also called renal replacement therapy (RRT), is used for patients with loss of kidney function and inadequate waste ***elimination.*** Indications for KRT include symptomatic uremia (e.g., pericarditis, neuropathy, decline in cognition), persistent or rapidly rising high potassium levels (i.e., greater than 6.5 mEq/L [mmol/L]), severe metabolic acidosis (pH less than 7.1), or fluid overload that inhibits tissue ***perfusion.*** When AKI occurs with drug or alcohol intoxication, KRT also can remove toxins.

Advancements in KRT over the past 10 years have led to multiple options for patients requiring treatment. Options for KRT include various types of intermittent and continuous hemodialysis (HD) as well as peritoneal dialysis (PD). Despite recent advances, the life expectancy for patients starting KRT ranges from 3 to 5 years. Mortality is highest in the first several months following dialysis (Gilbert & Weiner, 2018).

Immediate vascular access for KRT in patients with AKI is made by placement of a catheter specific for dialysis (Fig. 63.1). The temporary catheter is placed in a central vein, most often the internal jugular (Schell-Chaple, 2017), using best practices to avoid catheter-associated bloodstream infections (see Chapter 15). Placement of the catheter requires informed consent and a "time-out" similar to other surgical procedures (see Chapter 9, Care of Perioperative Patients). This catheter is not used to acquire blood samples, give drugs or fluid, or monitor central venous pressure. Provide site care in accordance with agency policy and best practices to avoid catheter-related bloodstream infection (CRBSI).

A long-term dialysis catheter may be placed in the radiology department using a tunneling technique under moderate sedation. Under ultrasound or fluoroscopic guidance, the physician makes a small incision where the internal jugular vein passes behind the clavicle. A 6- to 8-cm tunnel is created away from the site of the incision. A long-term hemodialysis (HD) catheter is inserted through the tunnel and into the jugular vein. Keeping a segment of the catheter within the subcutaneous tissues before entering the jugular vein reduces the risk for infection. This central catheter is used only for dialysis and requires aseptic dressing changes.

Dialysis catheters have two lumens—one for outflow and one for inflow. This allows the patient's blood to flow out and, once dialyzed, to be returned through the inflow lumen. Some catheters have a third lumen to sample venous blood or give drugs and fluid during dialysis.

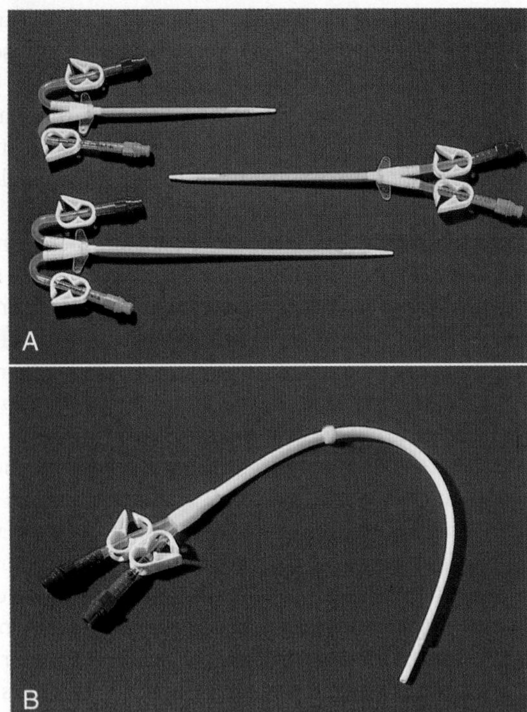

FIG. 63.1 Subclavian dialysis catheters. These catheters are radiopaque tubes that can be used for hemodialysis access. The Y-shaped tubing allows arterial outflow and venous return through a single catheter. (A) Mahurkar catheters, made of polyurethane and used for short-term access. (B) PermCath catheter, made of silicone and used for long-term access. (Courtesy Kendall Company, Bothell, WA.)

Intermittent Versus Continuous Kidney Replacement Therapy. Kidney replacement therapy (KRT) is a supportive strategy to purify blood, substituting for the normal function of the kidney. Particles are separated from blood based on the different ability of particles to pass through (diffuse) a membrane or across the peritoneal lining. KRT can be delivered intermittently, continuously, or as a hybrid of these approaches. Mortality is significant, regardless of modality, among patients who require KRT.

Intermittent KRT, sometimes called *hemodialysis,* is delivered over 3 to 6 hours. Generally a technician or dialysis nurse brings the dialysis machine to the bedside of a critically ill patient. Patients who do not need intensive care may be transported to an inpatient dialysis unit for the duration of the KRT treatment.

Intermittent KRT uses a dialysis machine to mix and monitor the *dialysate* (the fluid that helps remove the unwanted particles and waste products from blood). Dialysate is prescribed by the nephrology health care provider as an admixture to restore electrolytes and minerals to normal levels in the blood. The machine also monitors the flow of blood while it is outside of the body. Alarms are set and monitored by the dialysis technician or nurse to ensure safe and effective flow. This type of KRT is delivered three or four times weekly and requires anticoagulation in the dialysis circuit. Dialysis creates shifts of fluid and electrolytes that may not be tolerated in critically ill patients. Another form of intermittent KRT is peritoneal dialysis (PD), which is more commonly used for end-stage kidney disease. This therapy is discussed in detail in the Peritoneal Dialysis section of this chapter.

Continuous kidney replacement therapies (CKRTs), also known as continuous renal replacement therapy (CRRT), are alternative methods for removing wastes and restoring both ***acid-base balance*** and ***fluid and electrolyte balance.*** They are used in hospitalized adults who are too unstable to tolerate the changes in blood pressure that occur with intermittent conventional hemodialysis. As with hemodialysis, blood is passed through a filter to remove waste and undesired particles. Although intermittent hemodialysis occurs for 4 hours 3 days a week, CKRTs are typically prescribed for over 24 hours (Ronco et al., 2019). Some CKRT therapies use a different approach to remove particles from the blood. Hemofiltration uses ultrafiltration, whereas diffusion is used in intermittent dialysis to remove toxins and other particles. *Ultrafiltration* is the separation of particles from a suspension by passage through a filter with very fine pores. In ultrafiltration, the separation is performed by convective transport. During intermittent hemodialysis, separation depends on differential diffusion. Some approaches to CKRT combine ultrafiltration with diffusion (combined hemofiltration and hemodialysis).

CKRT occurs only in the ICU, because of the need for frequent monitoring and the specialized skill set of the nurse to maintain safety during extracorporeal circulation (blood flow outside the body). Life-threatening complications can occur if there is an error in the preparation of electrolyte solution or if the conductivity monitors fail (Ronco et al., 2019). The American Nephrology Nurses Association provides resources for intermittent and continuous KRT policies and procedures.

Several strategies can be used to provide CKRT to critically ill patients. The most commonly used CKRTs are continuous venovenous hemofiltration (CVVH) and continuous venovenous hemodialysis (CVVHD). The different CKRT modalities use the same machines, which are set up differently based on the needs of the patient. CVVH uses ultrafiltration, whereas CVVHD uses diffusion to filter the blood. CKRT is powered by a pump that drives blood from the patient catheter into the dialyzer (filter). The ultrafiltrate fluid is then collected into a bag for disposal. There may be a second pump that acts on the ultrafiltrate tubing to create negative pressure and increase fluid removal. Replacement fluid is infused via the inflow circuit in some systems. The pump increases the risk for an air embolus, and KRT systems have alarms that detect air (Ronco et al., 2019).

Another KRT modality is a hybrid of continuous and intermittent approaches. Slow continuous ultrafiltration (SCUF) provides slow removal of fluid over 12 to 24 hours and may be useful when azotemia or uremia is not a concern. Sustained low-efficiency dialysis (SLED) uses the dialysis machine to deliver prolonged dialysis for 12 to 24 hours. Lower blood flow and dialysate flow rates remove both particles and water and may be better tolerated by the unstable or critically ill patient, with fewer episodes of hypotension. A newer type of CKRT is continuous venovenous hemodiafiltration (CVVHDF), which combines the principles of hemodialysis with hemofiltration. Another new type of CKRT is continuous venovenous high-flux hemodialysis (CVVHFD), which uses high-flux membranes in the filter (Ronco et al., 2019).

Continuous KRT is expensive and resource intensive. It requires consultation and collaboration with the nephrologist and close collaboration with a dialysis nurse. Conservative management of ***fluid and electrolyte balance, acid-base balance,*** and drug therapy is an acceptable and reasonable approach to manage AKI.

Posthospital Care. Patients with AKI may have many outcomes. Some patients recover and return to baseline kidney function and general health. Others have partial recovery with mild or moderate chronic kidney disease (CKD). Still others may require permanent KRT. Some die from the acute illness.

The care for a patient with AKI after discharge from the hospital varies, depending on the status of the kidney function when the patient is discharged. Resolution of kidney injury may occur over several months, and follow-up care may be provided by a nephrologist or by the primary health care provider in consultation with the nephrologist. Frequent medical visits are necessary, as are scheduled laboratory blood and urine tests to monitor kidney function. A registered dietitian nutritionist can plan modifications to the patient's diet according to the degree of kidney function and ongoing nutrition needs. Fluid restrictions and daily weights may be advised to avoid fluid overload while kidneys are recovering.

Recovery of renal function is adversely affected by KRT, putting patients at risk for developing end-stage kidney disease (ESKD). Insult to the kidney by KRT is thought to be related to the loss of autoregulation and inflammation that occurs (Ronco et al., 2019). For patients who require dialysis at discharge following AKI, follow-up care is similar to that needed for patients with ESKD from CKD (see Care Coordination and Transition Management in the Chronic Kidney Disease section). Depending on their level of independence and family support, patients may need home care nursing or social work assistance.

NCLEX EXAMINATION CHALLENGE 63.3

Health Promotion and Maintenance

The nurse is preparing a client with stage 3 CKD for discharge. Which client statement indicates the need for further teaching?

A. "I will be sure to attend my follow-up appointment with my nephrologist."
B. "I will increase my protein intake so my body can heal."
C. "I will weigh myself daily and call the doctor if my weight increases by 2 lb or more."
D. "I will take my blood pressure each day and keep a daily log."

ELIMINATION CONCEPT EXEMPLAR: CHRONIC KIDNEY DISEASE

Pathophysiology Review

Unlike acute kidney injury (AKI), chronic kidney disease (CKD) is a progressive, irreversible disorder lasting longer than 3 months (Ferri, 2020). When kidney function and waste ***elimination*** are too poor to sustain life, CKD becomes end-stage kidney disease (ESKD). Terms used with CKD include **azotemia** (buildup of nitrogen-based wastes in the blood), **uremia** (azotemia with symptoms [see the Key Features: Uremia box]), and **uremic syndrome**. See Table 63.1 for a comparison of AKI and CKD.

KEY FEATURES

Uremia

- Metallic taste in the mouth
- Anorexia
- Nausea
- Vomiting
- Muscle cramps
- Uremic frost on skin
- Fatigue and lethargy
- Hiccups
- Edema
- Dyspnea
- Paresthesias

Stages of Chronic Kidney Disease. CKD is classified into five stages based on glomerular filtration rate (GFR) category. Direct measurement of urine creatinine (described in Chapter 60, with a 3-hour or 24-hour urine collection) is needed for the most accurate GFR estimation. The five stages of CKD are described in Table 63.6. CKD starts with a normal GFR but increased risk for kidney damage. In the first stage, the patient may have a normal GFR (>90 mL/min/1.73 m^2) but abnormal urine findings, structural abnormalities, or genetic traits that point to kidney disease. The patient is at increased risk for kidney damage from infection, ***immunity*** responses with inflammation, pregnancy, dehydration, and hypotension. Careful management of conditions such as diabetes, hypertension, and heart failure (HF) can slow the onset and progression of CKD.

In stage 2 CKD, GFR is reduced, ranging between 60 and 89 mL/min/1.73 m^2, and albuminuria may be present. Kidney nephron damage has occurred, and there may be slight elevations of metabolic wastes in the blood because of nephron loss. Levels of blood urea nitrogen (BUN), serum creatinine, uric acid, and phosphorus are not sensitive enough to define this stage. Increased output of dilute urine may occur at this stage of CKD and lead to severe dehydration.

NURSING SAFETY PRIORITY QSEN

Action Alert

Teach patients with mild chronic kidney disease (CKD) that carefully managing fluid volume, blood pressure, electrolytes, and other kidney-damaging diseases by following prescribed drug and nutrition therapies can slow progression to end-stage kidney disease (ESKD).

In stage 3 CKD, GFR reduction continues and ranges between 30 and 59 mL/min/1.73 m^2, and albuminuria is usually present. Nephron damage is greater, and azotemia reflecting poor waste ***elimination*** is present. Ongoing management of the underlying conditions that cause nephron damage is essential, especially diabetes mellitus and blood pressure control. Restriction of fluids, proteins, and electrolytes is needed. Stage 3 is further divided into 3a and 3b to more accurately assess the risk for complications from CKD as GFR decreases below 45 mL/min/1.73 m^2.

TABLE 63.6 Stages of Chronic Kidney Disease

Stage	Estimated Glomerular Filtration Rate	Intervention
Stage 1		
At risk; normal kidney function, but urine findings indicate kidney disease	>90 mL/min/1.73 m^2	Screen for risk factors and manage care to reduce risk: • Uncontrolled hypertension • Diabetes with poor glycemic control • Congenital or acquired anatomic or urinary tract abnormalities • Family history of genetic kidney diseases • Exposure to nephrotoxic substances
Stage 2		
Slightly reduced kidney function	60-89 mL/min/1.73 m^2	Focus on reduction of risk factors
Stage 3		
Moderately reduced kidney function	30-59 mL/min/1.73 m^2	Implement strategies to slow disease progression
Stage 4		
Severely reduced kidney function; a noticeable jaundice can occur, particularly around the eyes	15-29 mL/min/1.73 m^2	Manage complications. Discuss patient preferences and values. Educate about options and prepare for renal replacement therapy
Stage 5		
End-stage kidney disease (ESKD)	<15 mL/min/1.73 m^2	Implement renal replacement therapy or kidney transplantation

Over time, patients progress to stage 4 CKD and *end-stage kidney disease* (ESKD) (stage 5). Waste ***elimination*** is poor, with excessive amounts of urea and creatinine building up in the blood, and the kidneys cannot maintain homeostasis. Severe impairments of ***fluid and electrolyte balance*** and ***acid-base balance*** occur. Without kidney replacement therapy, death results from ESKD.

Three albuminuria stages also are considered in evaluating CKD. These stages are defined by the albumin-to-creatinine ratio in urine. The first stage (A1) is none to mildly increased albumin up to 29 mg/g creatinine (<3 mg/mmol) and is sometimes called *microalbuminuria.* The second (A2) stage has values of 30 to 300 mg/g creatinine (3 to 30 mg/mmol). The stage of greatest kidney damage (A3) has values >300 mg/g creatinine (>30 mg/mmol). The risk for progression of CKD, ESKD, and mortality is increased when urine albumin increases. Albumin in the urine is a marker of kidney damage, whereas GFR reflects kidney function. The combined values help identify adults at risk for progression of CKD and complications and guide interventions.

Kidney Changes. CKD with greatly reduced GFR causes many problems, including abnormal urine production, severe disruption of ***fluid and electrolyte balance,*** and metabolic abnormalities. Because healthy nephrons become larger and work harder, urine production and water ***elimination*** are sufficient to maintain essential homeostasis until about three-fourths of kidney function is lost. As the disease progresses, the ability to produce diluted urine is reduced, resulting in urine with a fixed osmolarity *(isosthenuria).* As kidney function continues to decline, the BUN increases, and urine output decreases. Extracellular volume overload can occur in CKD because the body loses the capability to excrete sodium (Johnson et al., 2019). At this point, the patient is at risk for fluid overload with edema, pulmonary crackles, shortness of breath, and pleural or pericardial effusion (with symptoms of a friction rub on auscultation and/or decreased breath sounds or heart sounds).

Metabolic Changes. *Urea and creatinine* excretion are disrupted by CKD. Creatinine comes from proteins in skeletal muscle. The rate of creatinine excretion depends on muscle mass, physical activity, and diet. Without major changes in diet or physical activity, the serum creatinine level is constant. Creatinine is partially excreted by the kidney tubules, and a decrease in kidney function leads to a buildup of serum creatinine. Urea is made from protein metabolism and is excreted by the kidneys. The BUN level normally varies directly with protein intake.

Sodium excretion changes are common. Early in CKD, the patient is at risk for *hyponatremia* (sodium depletion) because there are fewer healthy nephrons to reabsorb sodium. Thus sodium is lost in the urine. Polyuria of mild-to-moderate CKD also causes sodium loss.

In the later stages of CKD, kidney excretion of sodium is reduced as urine production decreases. Then sodium retention and high serum sodium levels *(hypernatremia)* occur with only modest increases in dietary sodium intake. This problem leads to severe disruption of ***fluid and electrolyte balance*** (see Chapter 13). Sodium retention causes hypertension and edema.

Even with sodium retention, the serum sodium level may appear normal because plasma water is retained at the same time. If fluid retention occurs at a greater rate than sodium retention, the serum sodium level is falsely low because of dilution (see the Laboratory Profile: Kidney Disease box).

Potassium excretion occurs mainly through the kidney. Any increase in potassium load during the later stages of CKD can lead to hyperkalemia (high serum potassium levels). Normal serum potassium levels of 3.5 to 5 mEq/L (mmol/L) are maintained until the 24-hour urine output falls below 500 mL. High potassium levels then develop quickly, reaching 7 to 8 mEq/L (mmol/L) or greater. Life-threatening changes in cardiac rate and rhythm result from this elevation because of abnormal depolarization and repolarization. Other factors contribute to high potassium levels in CKD, including the ingestion of potassium in drugs, failure to restrict dietary potassium, tissue breakdown, blood transfusions, and bleeding or hemorrhage. (See Chapter 13 for discussion of potassium imbalance.)

Acid-base balance is affected by CKD. In the early stages, blood pH changes little because the remaining healthy nephrons increase their rate of acid excretion. As more nephrons are lost, acid excretion is reduced and metabolic acidosis results (see Chapter 14).

Many factors lead to acidosis in CKD. First, the kidneys cannot excrete excessive hydrogen ions (acids). Normally, tubular cells move hydrogen ions into the urine for excretion, but ammonium and bicarbonate are needed for this movement to occur (Johnson et al., 2019). In patients with CKD, ammonium production is decreased and reabsorption of bicarbonate does not occur. This process leads to a buildup of hydrogen ions and reduced levels of bicarbonate *(base deficit)*. High potassium levels further reduce kidney ammonium production and excretion.

As CKD worsens and acid retention increases, increased respiratory action is needed to keep blood pH normal. The respiratory system adjusts or compensates for the increased blood hydrogen ion levels (acidosis or decreased pH) by increasing the rate and depth of breathing to excrete carbon dioxide through the lungs. This breathing pattern, called **Kussmaul respiration**, increases with worsening kidney disease. Serum bicarbonate measures the extent of metabolic acidosis (bicarbonate deficit). Patients usually need alkali replacement to counteract acidosis.

Calcium and phosphorus balance is disrupted by CKD. A complex, balanced normal reciprocal relationship exists between calcium and phosphorus (used interchangeably with phosphate) and is influenced by vitamin D (see Chapter 13). The kidney produces a hormone needed to activate vitamin D, which then enhances intestinal absorption of calcium.

Normally, excess phosphorus is excreted in the urine. In CKD, renal phosphate excretion decreases, which causes elevated phosphate levels. Bone and skeletal changes can occur when the GFR decreases to 25% or less (McCance et al., 2019).

Parathyroid hormone (PTH) controls the amount of phosphorus in the blood by causing tubular excretion of phosphorus when there is an excess. An early effect of CKD is reduced phosphorus excretion (Fig. 63.2). As plasma phosphorus levels increase *(hyperphosphatemia)*, calcium levels decrease *(hypocalcemia)*. Chronic low blood calcium levels stimulate the parathyroid glands to release more PTH. With additional PTH, calcium is released from storage areas in bones *(bone resorption)*, which results in bone density loss. The extra calcium from the bone is needed to balance the excess plasma phosphorus level. The problem of low blood calcium levels is made worse with severe CKD because kidney cell damage also reduces production of active vitamin D. Deficiencies in vitamin D lead to even further decreased calcium levels because vitamin D aids in calcium absorption (McCance et al., 2019).

The problems in bone metabolism and structure caused by CKD-induced low calcium levels and high phosphorus levels are called **renal osteodystrophy**. Bone mineral loss causes bone pain, spinal sclerosis, fractures, bone density loss, osteomalacia, and tooth calcium loss.

Crystals formed from excessive calcium or phosphorus are called *metastatic calcifications* and may precipitate in many body areas. When the plasma level of the calcium-phosphorus product (serum calcium level multiplied by the serum phosphorus level) exceeds 70 mg/dL (6 mmol/L), the crystals may lodge in the kidneys, heart, lungs, blood vessels, joints, eyes (causing conjunctivitis), and brain. Itching increases with calcium-phosphorus imbalances.

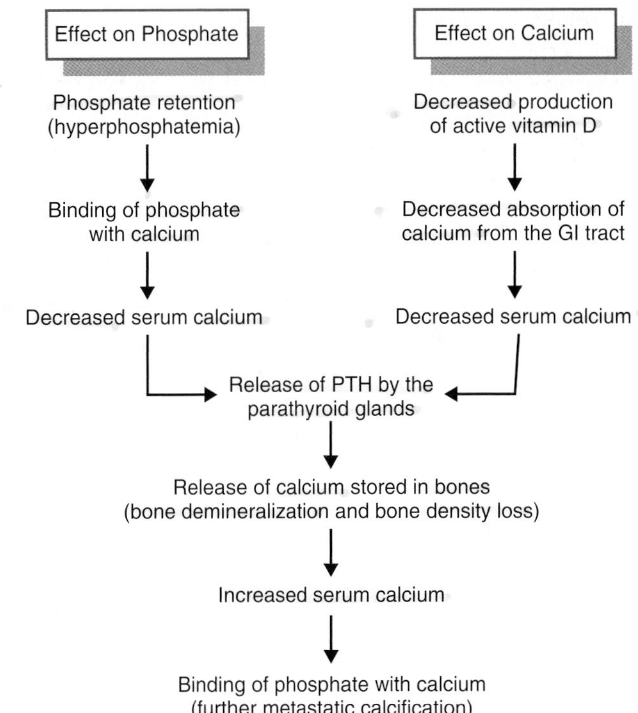

FIG. 63.2 Effects of kidney dysfunction on phosphorus and calcium balance. *PTH,* Parathyroid hormone.

Calcium is also deposited in atherosclerotic plaques in the lining of blood vessels. Vascular calcium deposits are a marker of significant risk for cardiovascular disease.

Cardiac Changes. **Cardiorenal syndrome** refers to disorders of the kidney or heart that cause dysfunction in the other organ. The kidney and the heart have a reciprocal relationship that can make an alteration in one cause an alteration in the other (Ferri, 2020).

Hypertension is common in most patients with CKD. It may be either the cause or the result of CKD. In patients who have other causes of hypertension such as atherosclerosis, the increased blood pressure damages the glomerular capillaries, and eventually ESKD results.

CKD itself elevates blood pressure by causing fluid and sodium overload and dysfunction of the renin-angiotensin-aldosterone system (RAAS). Hypertension alone can damage kidney arterioles, reducing ***perfusion.*** A decrease in kidney blood flow results in the production and release of a number of signaling chemicals, including renin, to improve blood flow to the kidney. The release of renin triggers the production of angiotensin and aldosterone. Angiotensin causes blood vessel constriction and increases blood pressure. Aldosterone stimulates kidney tubules to reabsorb sodium and water. These actions increase plasma volume and raise blood pressure. However, in the presence of CKD, an increase in blood pressure may not result in increased blood flow, and the production of renin continues, which creates a cycle of vasoconstriction in kidney arterioles and peripheral arterioles. The result is severe hypertension that is difficult to manage and worsens kidney function. Many patients with CKD have heart damage and enlargement from the long-term hypertension that results in coronary artery damage and poor coronary artery perfusion.

Hyperlipidemia occurs in CKD from changes in fat metabolism that increase triglyceride, total cholesterol, and low-density lipoprotein (LDL) levels. These changes increase the patient's risk for coronary artery disease and acute cardiac events. Problems with lipids and atherosclerosis are greatly increased for the patient with both CKD and diabetes mellitus.

Heart failure (HF) may occur in CKD because the workload on the heart is increased as a result of anemia, hypertension, and fluid overload. Left ventricular enlargement and HF are common in ESKD. Uremia may cause *uremic cardiomyopathy,* the uremic toxin effect on the myocardium. HF also may occur in these patients because of hypertension and coronary artery disease. Cardiac disease is a leading cause of death in patients with ESKD.

Pericarditis also occurs in patients with CKD. The pericardial sac becomes inflamed by uremic toxins or infection. If it is not treated, this problem leads to pericardial effusion, cardiac tamponade, and death. Symptoms include shortness of breath from low cardiac output, severe chest pain, tachycardia, narrow *pulse pressure* (close values for systolic and diastolic blood pressure), low-grade fever, and a pericardial friction rub that can be heard with a stethoscope placed over the left sternal border. Dysrhythmias may occur with uremia and uremic pericarditis. Treatment of tamponade, which is a medical emergency, requires immediate removal of pericardial fluid by placement of a needle, catheter, or drainage tube into the pericardium.

Hematologic and Immunity Changes. Anemia is common in patients in the later stages of CKD and worsens CKD symptoms. The causes of anemia include a decreased erythropoietin level with reduced red blood cell (RBC) production, decreased RBC survival time from uremia, and iron and folic acid deficiencies (Norton et al., 2017b). The patient may have increased bleeding or bruising as a result of impaired platelet function.

CKD causes reduced ***immunity,*** which increases the risk for infection. Uremia disrupts white blood cell (WBC) production and function, decreasing host defenses. Protein, fluid, and electrolyte abnormalities contribute to inflammation and further immunity impairment.

Gastrointestinal Changes. Uremia affects the entire GI system. The flora of the mouth change with uremia. The mouth contains the enzyme *urease,* which breaks down urea into ammonia. The ammonia generated remains and then causes halitosis (uremic fetor) and *stomatitis* (mouth inflammation). Anorexia, nausea, vomiting, and hiccups are common in patients with uremia. The specific cause of these problems is unknown but may be related to high BUN and creatinine levels and acidosis.

Peptic ulcer disease is common in patients with uremia, but the exact cause is unclear. Uremic colitis with watery diarrhea or constipation may also be present with uremia. Ulcers may occur in the stomach or intestine, causing erosion of blood vessels. The blood loss caused by these erosions may lead to hemorrhagic shock from severe GI bleeding.

TABLE 63.7 Selected Causes of Chronic Kidney Disease

Glomerular Disease
- Glomerulonephritis
- Basement membrane disease
- Goodpasture syndrome
- Intercapillary glomerulosclerosis

Tubular Disease
- Chronic hypercalcemia
- Chronic potassium depletion
- Fanconi syndrome
- Heavy metal (lead) poisoning

Vascular Disease of the Kidney
- Ischemic disease of the kidney
- Bilateral renal artery stenosis
- Nephrosclerosis
- Hyperparathyroidism

Inherited or Genetic Conditions
- Hypoplastic kidneys
- Medullary cystic disease
- Polycystic kidney disease

Infection
- Pyelonephritis
- Tuberculosis

Systemic Vascular Disease
- Intrarenal renovascular hypertension
- Extrarenal renovascular hypertension

Metabolic Kidney Disease
- Diabetes
- Amyloidosis
- Gout (hyperuricemic nephropathy)
- Milk-alkali syndrome
- Sarcoidosis

Connective Tissue Disease
- Progressive systemic sclerosis
- Systemic lupus erythematosus
- Polyarteritis

Urinary Tract Disease
- Obstructive uropathy

NOTE: List is not all-inclusive.

Cognitive and Functional Changes. Although CKD may be asymptomatic in the early stages, as it progresses complications include cognitive and physical impairment. There is also increased risk for systemic drug toxicity and adverse effects from interventions used to prevent or treat CKD.

Etiology and Genetic Risk. The causes of CKD are complex (Table 63.7). More than 100 different disease processes can result in progressive loss of kidney function (see also Chapter 62). Two main causes of CKD leading to dialysis or kidney transplantation are hypertension and diabetes mellitus. African-American patients are much more likely to develop ESKD and have hypertensive ESKD.

Incidence and Prevalence. The number of patients being treated for CKD is increasing, particularly among older adults. About 15% of adults in the United States (37 million people) are estimated to have CKD (Centers for Disease Control and Prevention [CDC], 2019). Most adults who have CKD (9 out of 10) do not know that they have the disease (CDC, 2019). Almost 48,000 Canadians are currently being treated for kidney failure, with 1 in 10 Canadians having CKD, and millions more at risk (Kidney Foundation of Canada, 2018). Refer to the Patient and Family Education: Preparing for Self-Management box for prevention of kidney and urinary problems.

Health Promotion and Maintenance. Health promotion activities to prevent or delay the onset of CKD focus on controlling the diseases that lead to its development, such as diabetes and hypertension. Educating and encouraging the patient to accept

PATIENT AND FAMILY EDUCATION: PREPARING FOR SELF-MANAGEMENT

Prevention of Kidney and Urinary Problems

- Be alert to the general appearance of your urine. Note any changes in its color, clarity, or odor.
- Changes in the frequency or volume of urine passage occur with changes in fluid intake. More frequent or infrequent voiding not associated with changes in fluid intake may signal health problems.
- Any discomfort or distress with the passage of urine is not normal. Pain, burning, urgency, aching, or difficulty with initiating urine flow or complete bladder emptying is of some concern. Report such symptoms to your primary health care provider.
- The kidneys need 1 to 2 L of fluid a day to flush out your body wastes. Water is the ideal flushing agent.
- Avoid sugary, high-calorie drinks; they provide low-quality calories that contribute to weight gain and sugar-induced urination.
- Changes in kidney function are often silent for many years. Periodically ask your primary health care provider to measure your kidney function with a blood test (serum creatinine) and a urinalysis.
- If you have a history of kidney disease, diabetes mellitus, or hypertension (high blood pressure) or a family history of kidney disease, you should know your serum creatinine level and your glomerular filtration rate (either estimated from serum creatinine or measured with a 24-hour creatinine urine collection). At least one checkup per year that includes laboratory blood and urine testing of kidney function is recommended.
- If you are identified as having decreased kidney function, ask about whether any prescribed drug, diagnostic test, or therapeutic procedure will present a risk to your current kidney function. Evaluate the contribution of diet to risk for kidney disease with your primary health care provider or a registered dietitian nutritionist. Check out all nonprescription drugs with your primary health care provider or pharmacist before using them.

lifestyle modifications and how to implement them are incorporated into the ongoing plan of care. Diet adjustments (e.g., sodium, protein, and cholesterol restriction), weight maintenance (i.e., achieve body mass index of 22 to 25 kg/m^2), smoking cessation, participation in 30 to 60 minutes of moderate-intensity exercise daily, and limitation of alcohol to one or two drinks daily are examples of lifestyle recommendations for the patient with CKD. Identifying patients who have diabetes or hypertension at an early stage is critical to CKD prevention (Norton et al., 2017a). Teach patients to adhere to drug and diet regimens and to engage in regular physical activity to prevent the blood vessel changes and kidney cell damage that lead to CKD. Instruct patients with diabetes to keep their blood glucose levels within the prescribed range. Teach patients with hypertension that drug therapy reduces vessel damage. Urge patients with diabetes or hypertension to have yearly testing for urine albumin-to-creatinine ratio (UACR) along with serum creatinine and BUN.

Teach adults treated for an infection anywhere in the kidney/urinary system to take all antibiotics as prescribed. Urge adults to drink at least 2 L of water daily unless a health problem requires fluid restriction. Caution adults who use NSAIDs to use the lowest dose for the briefest time period because these drugs interfere with blood flow to the kidney. High-dose and long-term NSAID use reduces kidney function.

NCLEX EXAMINATION CHALLENGE 63.4

Health Promotion and Maintenance

The nurse is caring for a 38-year-old male with hypertension and stage 1 CKD. The client reports lifestyle changes and feeling "better" and has stopped taking a prescribed diuretic. What is the appropriate nursing response?

A. "The diuretic will reduce your blood pressure, which may slow or prevent progression of your chronic kidney disease."
B. "Your primary health care provider prescribed the diuretic because it will reverse the damage caused by kidney disease."
C. "Taking medications is a personal decision, and you have the right to decline this prescription."
D. "Since you have implemented lifestyle changes, the diuretic is likely not needed."

❖ Interprofessional Collaborative Care

Although the patient with CKD may require hospitalization during exacerbation of imbalances or when other health problems require it, the vast majority of care occurs in the community. For best outcomes, the patient with CKD must be engaged in self-management. Because patients with CKD are at risk for so many adverse outcomes (not just ESKD), the interprofessional care team includes many specialists and health care professionals (e.g., nephrologists, nephrology nurses, pharmacists, registered dietitian nutritionists, mental health therapists, physical therapists, case managers, social workers, clergy or pastoral care workers). The responsibilities of these interprofessional team members are described within the interventions sections for CKD. With so many professionals involved, care coordination is essential to positive outcomes in this population (Hain, 2015). The nurse coordinates the interprofessional team to support and counsel the patient and family, often over many years of treatment. The nurse has the most contact with the patient when he or she is hospitalized or undergoing in-center dialysis treatments.

SYSTEMS THINKING AND QUALITY IMPROVEMENT (QSEN)

CKD Clinics Improving Patient Outcomes

CKD is a complex disease that affects physical, mental, and social aspects of health. This requires an understanding of available resources in order to improve patient outcomes. CKD clinics use an interprofessional approach, treating all aspects of the patient's health. Hospitals that develop and maintain clinics for patients with chronic diseases such as heart failure and CKD have fewer hospital readmissions and better patient outcomes. CKD clinics are successful because they foster care coordination and promote convenience for the patient.

The following services are recommended at a CKD clinic (Himmelfarb & Ikizler, 2018):

- Scheduling of tests (such as ultrasound and CT scans)
- Scheduling of specialist appointments as necessary
- Providing reminders for appointments and tests
- Following up with test results
- Providing a patient liaison for pharmacy and laboratory tests
- Consulting with interprofessional team members such as registered dietitian nutritionists (RDNs)
- Educating regarding disease processes, transplants, and therapies
- Referring as necessary for dialysis catheter insertion

◆ Assessment: Recognize Cues

History. When taking a history from a patient with risk for or actual CKD, document the patient's age and gender. Accurately measure weight and height and ask about usual weight and recent weight gain or loss. Weight gain may indicate fluid retention from poor kidney function with disrupted ***fluid and electrolyte balance.*** Weight loss may be the result of anorexia from uremia.

Ask about a history of kidney and urologic disorders, chronic health problems, and drug use. Chronic hypertension, diabetes, inflammatory diseases of systemic lupus erythematosus or arthritis, cancer, and tuberculosis can cause decreased kidney function. Ask the patient about family members' kidney disease, which might indicate a genetic problem.

Document the use of current and past prescribed and over-the-counter drugs because many drugs are nephrotoxic and drug interactions can cause kidney damage (Burchum & Rosenthal, 2019) (see Table 63.5). Ask whether the patient has had x-rays or CT scans with contrast medium.

Examine the patient's dietary habits and discuss any GI problems. A change in the taste of foods often occurs with CKD. Patients may report that sweet foods are not as appealing or that meats have a metallic taste. Ask about the presence of nausea, vomiting, anorexia, hiccups, diarrhea, or constipation. These symptoms may be the result of excess wastes that the body cannot eliminate because of kidney disease.

Ask about the patient's energy level and any recent injuries or bleeding. Explore changes in his or her daily routine as a possible *result* of fatigue. Fatigue is a common and often profound problem among patients with CKD, particularly among patients receiving dialysis. Weakness, drowsiness, and shortness of breath suggest impending pulmonary edema or neurologic degeneration. Ask about bruising or bleeding caused by hematologic changes from uremia.

Discuss urine ***elimination*** in detail, including frequency of urination, appearance of the urine, and any difficulty starting or controlling urination. These data can help identify urologic problems that may influence kidney function.

Physical Assessment/Signs and Symptoms. CKD causes changes in all body systems (see the Key Features: Severe, Chronic, and End-Stage Kidney Disease box). Most symptoms are related to changes in ***fluid and electrolyte balance, acid-base balance,*** and buildup of nitrogenous wastes.

Neurologic symptoms of CKD and uremic syndrome vary (see both Key Features boxes in this chapter). Observe for problems ranging from lethargy to seizures or coma, which may indicate uremic encephalopathy. Fluid overload can cause changes in cognition. Assess for sensory changes that appear in a glove-and-stocking pattern over the hands and feet *(peripheral neuropathy).* Check for weakness in upper and lower extremities *(uremic neuropathy).* Fatigue can result in decreased activity.

If untreated, encephalopathy can lead to seizures and coma. Dialysis is used emergently when neurologic problems result from CKD. The symptoms of encephalopathy may resolve with dialysis. However, improvement in neuropathy can be limited by severe or recurrent episodes of brain dysfunction. Depression may compound cognitive and neurologic problems.

KEY FEATURES

Severe, Chronic, and End-Stage Kidney Disease

Neurologic Symptoms
- Lethargy and daytime drowsiness
- Inability to concentrate or decreased attention span
- Seizures
- Coma
- Slurred speech
- Asterixis (jerky movements or "flapping" of the hands)
- Tremors, twitching, or jerky movements
- Myoclonus
- Ataxia (alteration in gait)
- Paresthesias from peripheral neuropathy

Cardiovascular Symptoms
- Cardiomyopathy
- Hypertension
- Peripheral edema
- Heart failure
- Uremic pericarditis
- Pericardial effusion
- Pericardial friction rub
- Cardiac tamponade
- Cardiorenal syndrome

Respiratory Symptoms
- Uremic halitosis
- Tachypnea
- Deep sighing, yawning
- Kussmaul respirations
- Uremic pneumonitis
- Shortness of breath
- Pulmonary edema
- Pleural effusion
- Depressed cough reflex
- Crackles

Hematologic Symptoms
- Anemia
- Abnormal bleeding and bruising
- Reduced white blood cell count
- Increased risk for infection

Gastrointestinal Symptoms
- Anorexia
- Nausea
- Vomiting
- Metallic taste in the mouth
- Changes in taste acuity and sensation
- Uremic colitis (diarrhea)
- Constipation
- Uremic gastritis (possible GI bleeding)
- Uremic fetor (breath odor)
- Stomatitis

Urinary Symptoms
- Polyuria, nocturia (early)
- Oliguria, anuria (later)
- Proteinuria
- Hematuria
- Diluted, straw-colored urine appearance (early)
- Concentrated and cloudy urine appearance (later)

Integumentary Symptoms
- Decreased skin turgor
- Yellow-gray pallor
- Dry skin
- Pruritus
- Ecchymosis
- Purpura
- Soft-tissue calcifications
- Uremic frost (late, premorbid)

Musculoskeletal Symptoms
- Muscle weakness and cramping
- Bone pain
- Fractures
- Renal osteodystrophy

Reproductive Symptoms
- Decreased fertility
- Infrequent or absent menses
- Decreased libido
- Impotence
- Sexual dysfunction

Metabolic Symptoms
- Hyperparathyroidism
- Hyperlipidemia
- Alterations in vitamin D, calcium, and phosphorus adsorption and metabolism
- Metabolic acidosis
- Hyperkalemia

Psychosocial Symptoms
- Depression
- Fatigue
- Sleep disturbances
- Sexual dysfunction
- Cognitive impairment
- Unemployment

Cardiovascular symptoms of CKD result from fluid overload, hypertension, heart failure (HF), pericarditis, potassium-induced dysrhythmias, and cholesterol/calcium (plaque, atherosclerosis) deposits in blood vessels. Assess for indications of reduced sodium and water excretion. Blood volume overload, if untreated, leads to hypertension, pulmonary edema, peripheral edema, and HF.

Assess heart rate and rhythm, listening for extra sounds (particularly an S_3), irregular patterns, or a pericardial friction rub. Unless a dialysis vascular access has been created, measure blood pressure in each arm. Assess the jugular veins for distention, and assess for edema of the feet, shins, and sacrum and around the eyes. Crackles during lung auscultation and shortness of breath with exertion and at night suggest fluid overload.

Respiratory symptoms of CKD also vary (e.g., breath that smells like urine [*uremic fetor* or uremic halitosis], deep sighing, yawning, shortness of breath). Observe the rhythm, rate, and depth of breathing. Tachypnea and **hyperpnea** (increased depth of breathing) occur with metabolic acidosis.

With severe metabolic acidosis, extreme increases in rate and depth of ventilation (Kussmaul respirations) occur. A few patients have pneumonitis, or *uremic lung*. In these patients, assess for thick sputum, reduced coughing, tachypnea, and fever. A pleural friction rub may be heard with a stethoscope. Patients often have pleuritic pain with breathing. Auscultate the lungs for crackles, which indicate fluid overload.

Hematologic symptoms of CKD include anemia and abnormal bleeding. Check for indicators of anemia (e.g., fatigue, pallor, lethargy, weakness, shortness of breath, dizziness). Check for abnormal bleeding by observing for bruising, petechiae, purpura, mucous membrane bleeding in the nose or gums, or intestinal bleeding (black, tarry stools [**melena**]).

GI symptoms of CKD include foul breath (halitosis) and mouth inflammation or ulceration. Document any abdominal pain, cramping, or vomiting. Test all stools for occult blood.

Skeletal symptoms of CKD are related to osteodystrophy from poor absorption of calcium and continuous bone calcium loss. Adults with osteodystrophy have thin, fragile bones that are at risk for fractures with even slight trauma. Vertebrae become more compact and may bend forward, leading to an overall loss of height. Ask about changes in height and bone pain. Observe for spinal curvatures and any unusual bumps or protrusions in bone areas that may indicate fractures. Handle the patient carefully during examination and care.

Urine symptoms in CKD reflect the kidneys' decreasing function. Urine amount, frequency, and appearance change. Protein, sediment, or blood may be in the urine.

The amount and composition of the urine change as kidney function decreases and waste ***elimination*** is disrupted. With the onset of mild-to-moderate CKD, the urine may be more dilute and clearer because tubular reabsorption of water is reduced. The actual urine output in a patient with CKD varies with the amount of remaining kidney function. The patient with severe CKD or ESKD usually has oliguria, but some patients continue to produce 1 L or more daily. Daily urine volume usually changes again after dialysis is started. A long duration of oliguria is an indication that recovery of kidney function is not to be expected.

Skin symptoms of CKD occur as a result of uremia. Pigment is deposited in the skin, causing a yellowish coloration, or darkening when skin is brown or bronze. The anemia of CKD causes sallowness, appearing as a faded suntan on lighter-skinned patients.

Skin oils and turgor are decreased in patients with uremia. A distressing problem of uremia is severe **pruritus** (itching). **Uremic frost**, a layer of urea crystals from evaporated sweat, may appear on the face, eyebrows, axillae, and groin in patients with advanced uremic syndrome. Assess for bruises *(ecchymosis)*, purple patches *(purpura)*, and rashes.

Psychosocial Assessment. CKD and its treatment disrupt many aspects of a patient's life. Psychosocial assessment and support are part of the nurse's role from the time that CKD is first diagnosed. With ongoing issues, a mental health professional is an important member of the care team. Ask about the patient's understanding of the diagnosis and what the treatment regimen means to him or her (e.g., diet, drugs, dialysis). Assess for anxiety and fear and for coping styles used by the patient and family. CKD affects family relations, social activity, work patterns, body image, and sexual activity. The chronic nature of severe CKD and ESKD, the many treatment options, and the uncertainties about the disease and its treatment require ongoing psychosocial assessment, psychosocial interventions, and ongoing support. Support the recommendations of the mental health professional.

Laboratory Assessment. CKD causes extreme changes in many laboratory values (see the Laboratory Profile: Kidney Disease box). Monitor these blood values: creatinine, blood urea nitrogen (BUN), sodium, potassium, calcium, phosphorus, bicarbonate, hemoglobin, and hematocrit. Also monitor GFR for trends.

A urinalysis is performed. In the early stages of CKD, urinalysis may show protein, glucose, red blood cells (RBCs) and white blood cells (WBCs), and decreased or fixed specific gravity. Urine osmolarity is usually decreased. As CKD progresses, urine output decreases dramatically, and osmolarity increases. A urine albumin-to-creatinine ratio (UACR) provides important information about kidney function and damage.

Glomerular filtration rate (GFR) can be estimated from serum creatinine levels, age, gender, race, and body size. But this type of estimation is generally used for screening rather than for staging of CKD. Estimation of GFR based on a formula that includes serum creatinine is also useful to calculate drug dose or drug frequency when reduced kidney function is a concern. However, to determine stage of CKD, a urine collection of 3 hours to 24 hours is usually done to assess creatinine clearance. A spot urine albumin-to-creatinine ratio (UACR) also is completed.

In severe CKD, serum creatinine and BUN levels may be used to determine the presence and degree of uremia. Serum creatinine levels may increase gradually over a period of years, reaching levels of 15 to 30 mg/dL (500 to 1000 mcmol/L) or more, depending on the patient's muscle mass. BUN levels are directly related to dietary protein intake. Without protein restriction, BUN levels may rise to 10 to 20 times the value of the serum creatinine level. With dietary protein restriction, BUN levels are elevated but less than those of non–protein-restricted patients. Fluid balance also affects BUN.

Imaging Assessment. Few x-ray findings are abnormal with CKD. Bone x-rays of the hand can show renal osteodystrophy. With long-term ESKD, the kidneys shrink (except for ESKD caused by polycystic kidney disease) and may be 8 to 9 cm or smaller. This small size results from atrophy and fibrosis. If CKD progresses suddenly, a kidney ultrasound or CT scan without contrast medium may be used to rule out an obstruction. (See Chapter 60 for a complete description of diagnostic tests for kidney function.)

◆ **Analysis: Analyze Cues and Prioritize Hypotheses.** The patient with CKD usually has progressive reduction of kidney function. Management generally occurs in the community setting. In the acute or long-term care setting, the focus of care is to manage problems and prevent complications of CKD. The priority collaborative problems for patients with CKD include:

1. Fluid overload due to the inability of diseased kidneys to maintain body fluid balance
2. Decreased cardiac function due to reduced stroke volume, dysrhythmias, fluid overload, and increased peripheral vascular resistance
3. Weight loss due to inability to ingest, digest, or absorb food and nutrients as a result of physiologic factors
4. Potential for injury due to effects of kidney disease on bone density, blood clotting, and drug elimination
5. Potential for psychosocial compromise due to chronic kidney disease

◆ **Planning and Implementation: Generate Solutions and Take Action**

Managing Fluid Volume

Planning: Expected Outcomes. The patient with CKD is expected to achieve and maintain an acceptable ***fluid and electrolyte balance*** and remain free of pulmonary edema.

Interventions. Management of the patient with CKD includes drug therapy, nutrition therapy, fluid restriction, and dialysis (when the patient reaches stage 5). Hemodialysis is performed intermittently for 3 to 4 hours, typically 3 days per week. Alternatively, some patients with ESKD receive peritoneal dialysis (PD). PD uses the peritoneum as the dialyzing membrane. The dialysate is infused through a catheter tunneled into the peritoneum. Dialysis for ESKD is described later in the Kidney Replacement Therapies section.

The purpose of fluid management is to attain fluid balance and prevent complications of fluid overload (see the Best Practice for Patient Safety & Quality Care: Managing Fluid Volume box). Monitor the patient's intake and output and hydration status. Assess for indications of fluid overload (e.g., lung crackles, edema, distended neck veins).

Drug therapy with diuretics is prescribed for patients with mild-to-severe CKD to increase urinary ***elimination*** of fluid. The increased urine output with this therapy helps reduce fluid overload and hypertension in patients who still have some urine output. Diuretics are seldom used in ESKD after dialysis is started, because as kidney function is reduced these drugs can accumulate and harm the remaining kidney cells and the patient's hearing. See the Common Examples of Drug Therapy: Chronic Kidney Disease box.

BEST PRACTICE FOR PATIENT SAFETY & QUALITY CARE (QSEN)

Managing Fluid Volume

- Weigh the patient daily at the same time each day, using the same scale, with the patient wearing the same amount and type of clothing, and graph the results.
- Observe the weight graph for trends (1 L of water weighs 1 kg).
- Accurately measure all fluid intake and output.
- Teach the patient and family about the need to keep fluid intake within prescribed restricted amounts and to ensure that the prescribed daily amount is evenly distributed throughout the 24 hours.
- Monitor for these symptoms of fluid overload at least every 4 hours during critical illness:
  - Decreased urine output
  - Rapid, bounding pulse
  - Rapid, shallow respirations
  - Presence of dependent edema
  - Auscultation of crackles or wheezes
  - Presence of distended neck veins in a sitting position
  - Decreased oxygen saturation
  - Elevated blood pressure
  - Narrowed pulse pressure
- Assess level of consciousness and degree of cognition.
- Ask about the presence of headache or blurred vision.

Assess fluid status by obtaining daily weights and reviewing intake and output. Daily weight gain in these patients indicates fluid retention rather than true body weight gain. Estimate the amount of fluid retained: 1 kg of weight equals about 1 L of fluid retained. Weigh the patient daily at the same time each day, on the same scale, wearing the same amount of clothing, and after voiding (if the patient is not anuric). Monitor weight for changes before and after dialysis.

Fluid restriction is often needed. Consider all forms of fluid intake, including oral, IV, and enteral sources, when calculating fluid intake. Help the patient spread oral fluid intake over a 24-hour period. Monitor his or her response to fluid restriction, and notify the primary health care provider if symptoms of fluid overload persist or worsen.

Pulmonary edema can result from left-sided heart failure (HF) related to fluid overload or from blood vessel injury. In left-sided HF, the heart is unable to eject blood adequately from the left ventricle, leading to an increased pressure in the left atrium and in the pulmonary blood vessels. The increased pressure causes fluid to cross the capillaries into the pulmonary tissue, forming edema (McCance et al., 2019). Pulmonary edema can also occur from injury to the lung blood vessels as a result of uremia. This condition causes inflammation and capillary leak. Fluid then leaks from pulmonary circulation into the lung tissue and alveoli. It may also leak into the pleural space, causing a *pleural effusion.*

Assess the patient for early indicators of pulmonary edema, such as restlessness, anxiety, rapid heart rate, shortness of breath, and crackles that begin at the base of the lungs. As pulmonary edema worsens, the level of fluid in the lungs rises. Auscultation reveals increased crackles and decreased breath sounds. The patient may have frothy, blood-tinged sputum. As cardiac and

COMMON EXAMPLES OF DRUG THERAPY

Chronic Kidney Disease

Drug	Nursing Implications
Loop Diuretics	
Increase urine output to manage volume overload when urinary elimination is still present.	
• Furosemide • Bumetanide • Dose varies with severity of kidney damage; not effective in ESKD	Monitor intake and output *to assess therapy effectiveness.* Generally the expected outcome is for output to be greater than intake by 500-1000/mL/24 hr. Monitor electrolytes *because these drugs result in loss of potassium;* this can be a desired effect in patients with hyperkalemia.
Vitamins and Minerals	
Used to replace those lost through dialysis or poorly absorbed as a result of dietary restrictions and to lower vitamin or mineral excesses that could lead to more problems.	
Phosphate binders form an insoluble calcium-phosphate complex to inhibit GI absorption to prevent hyperphosphatemia and renal osteodystrophy from hypocalcemia: • Calcium acetate • Calcium carbonate Noncalcium phosphate binders reduce blood phosphate levels without disturbing calcium levels: • Lanthanum carbonate • Sevelamer	Teach patients to take drugs with meals *to increase the effectiveness in slowing or preventing the absorption of dietary phosphorus.* Teach patients not to take these drugs within 2 hours of other scheduled drugs *to prevent the inhibited absorption of other drugs, especially cardiac drugs and antibiotics.* Monitor both serum phosphorus and calcium levels because *these drugs lower phosphorus and can cause hypercalcemia.* Monitor for constipation *because these can cause significant constipation, leading to fecal impaction or ileus.* Teach patients to report muscle weakness, slow or irregular pulse, or confusion to the prescriber *because these are symptoms of hypophosphatemia and indicate that dosage adjustment is required.*
Multivitamins and vitamin B supplements • Folic acid/folate • Cyanocobalamin (B_{12})	Teach patients to take the drugs after dialysis *to prevent the supplement from being removed from the blood during dialysis.* Teach patients to take iron supplements (ferrous sulfate) with meals *to reduce nausea and abdominal discomfort.*
Oral iron salts • Ferrous sulfate • Ferrous fumarate • Ferrous gluconate	Teach patients to take stool softeners daily while taking iron supplements, *which can cause constipation.* Remind patients that iron supplements change the color of the stool *because knowing the expected side effects decreases anxiety when they appear.*
Parenteral iron salts: • Iron dextran (IV) • Iron sucrose (IV)	A test dose of iron dextran is recommended *before IV administration because the incidence of allergic reactions is high.* Do not mix with drug with other parenteral drugs *because there are many incompatibilities.*
Vitamin D: • Calcitriol • Paricalcitol • Doxercalciferol	Monitor serum levels of calcium *because this active form of vitamin D suppresses parathyroid production and can lead to hypocalcemia.* Monitor serum levels of vitamin D *because this is a lipid-soluble vitamin that can be overingested and lead to toxicity. Serum calcium levels should stay below 10 mg/dL (Burchum & Rosenthal, 2019).*
Erythropoietin-Stimulating Agents (ESAs)	
Used to prevent or correct anemia caused by kidney disease through the stimulation of the bone marrow to increase red blood cell production and maturation.	
• Epoetin alfa • Darbepoetin alfa	Monitor hemoglobin values *because these drugs can overproduce blood cells, which increases blood viscosity and causes hypertension. This problem increases the risk for a myocardial infarction. Dosage is individualized to produce hemoglobin levels no higher than 10-11 g/dL (Burchum & Rosenthal, 2019).* Teach patients to report any of these side effects to the prescriber as soon as possible: chest pain, difficulty breathing, high blood pressure, rapid weight gain, seizures, skin rash or hives, or swelling of feet or ankles *because these symptoms indicate possible serious cardiac complications.*
Parathyroid Hormone Modulator	
Used to reduce parathyroid gland production of parathyroid hormone by decreasing the gland's sensitivity to calcium. This action helps maintain blood calcium and phosphorus levels closer to normal and can reduce renal osteodystrophy in patients with chronic kidney disease.	
• Cinacalcet	Monitor blood levels of calcium and phosphorus *to assess drug therapy effectiveness and recognize imbalances of these important electrolytes.* Teach the patient to monitor for and report diarrhea and muscle pain (myalgia), *which are indications of calcium and/or phosphorus imbalance.*

ESKD, End-stage kidney disease.

TABLE 63.8 Dietary Restrictions Needed for Severe Kidney Disease

Dietary Component	With Chronic Uremia	With Hemodialysis	With Peritoneal Dialysis
Protein	0.55-0.60 g/kg/day	1.0-1.5 g/kg/day	1.2-1.5 g/kg/day
Fluid	Depends on urine output but may be as high as 1500-3000 mL/day	500-700 mL/day plus amount of urine output	Restriction based on fluid weight gain and blood pressure
Potassium	60-70 mEq or mmol daily	70 mEq or mmol daily	Usually no restriction
Sodium	1-3 g/day	2-4 g/day	Restriction based on fluid weight gain and blood pressure
Phosphorus	700 mg/day	700 mg/day	800 mg/day

pulmonary function decrease further, the patient becomes diaphoretic and cyanotic.

The patient with pulmonary edema usually is admitted to the hospital for aggressive treatment and continuous cardiac monitoring. Place the patient in a high-Fowler position and give oxygen to improve gas exchange. Drug therapy with kidney failure and pulmonary edema is difficult because of potential adverse drug effects on the kidneys (Burchum & Rosenthal, 2019). Loop diuretics such as IV furosemide are used to manage pulmonary edema. Kidney impairment increases the risk for *ototoxicity* (ear damage with hearing loss) with furosemide; thus IV doses are given cautiously and slowly. Diuresis usually begins within 5 minutes of giving IV furosemide. Measure urine output hourly until the patient is stabilized. Monitor vital signs and assess breath sounds at least every 2 hours to evaluate the patient's response to this treatment.

IV morphine can be prescribed to reduce myocardial oxygen demand by triggering blood vessel dilation and to provide sedation. Dosage adjustments are needed to achieve the desired response and avoid respiratory depression. Monitor the patient's respiratory rate, oxygen saturation, and blood pressure hourly during this therapy. Other drugs that dilate blood vessels, such as nitroglycerin, may be given as a continuous infusion to reduce pulmonary pressure from left-sided HF. Monitor vital signs at least hourly because this drug combination may cause severe hypotension.

Monitor serum electrolyte levels daily and report abnormalities to the primary health care provider so imbalances can be corrected quickly. If using ECG monitoring, identify dysrhythmias as they occur and report changes in rhythm that affect consciousness or blood pressure immediately to the provider. Monitor oxygen saturation levels by pulse oximetry and consult with the respiratory therapist for the optimal method to deliver oxygen (e.g., facemask, nasal cannula, or noninvasive mechanical support [see Chapter 25]). Monitor the patient for worsening of the condition with indications of increasing hypoxemia (decreasing Spo_2 values, restlessness, decreased cognition, or new-onset confusion). Temporary intubation and mechanical ventilation may be needed if respiratory failure occurs.

Patients with CKD who have existing cardiac problems, high blood pressure, or chronic fluid retention are at increased risk for developing pulmonary edema. They are less likely to respond quickly to treatment and are more likely to develop problems related to drug therapy. Kidney replacement therapy with ultrafiltration or dialysis may be used to reduce fluid volume.

Improving Cardiac Function

Planning: Expected Outcomes. The patient with CKD is expected to attain and maintain adequate cardiac function.

Interventions. Many patients with long-standing hypertension are at risk for CKD and accelerated progression of kidney failure once CKD occurs. *Therefore blood pressure control is essential in preserving kidney function* (Norton et al., 2017a). To control blood pressure, diuretics (especially thiazides), calcium channel blockers, angiotensin-converting enzyme inhibitors (ACEIs), alpha-adrenergic and beta-adrenergic blockers, and vasodilators may be prescribed. ACEIs are the most effective drugs to decrease cardiovascular events when patients have CKD and hypertension. Calcium channel blockers can improve the GFR and blood flow within the kidney.

More information on the specific drugs for blood pressure control can be found in Chapter 33. Indications vary, depending on the patient, and these drugs are used carefully to avoid complications. Different dosages and combinations may be tried until blood pressure control is adequate and side effects are minimized. Although there are many blood pressure guidelines available regarding goals of treatment, in CKD (diabetic and nondiabetic) with albumin excretion greater than 30 mg/24 hr, a target blood pressure of 130/80 mm Hg or lower is recommended (Ferri, 2020).

Teach the patient and family to measure blood pressure daily. Evaluate their ability to measure and record blood pressure accurately using their own equipment. Recheck measurement accuracy on a regular basis. Teach the patient and family about the relationship of blood pressure control to diet and drug therapy. Instruct the patient to weigh daily and to bring records of blood pressure measurements and drug administration times and weights for discussion with the physician, nurse, or registered dietitian nutritionist.

Assess the patient on an ongoing basis for signs and symptoms of reduced cardiac output, heart failure (HF), and dysrhythmias. These topics are discussed in Chapters 30, 31, and 32.

Enhancing Nutrition

Planning: Expected Outcomes. The patient with CKD is expected to maintain adequate nutrition, demonstrating a protein-caloric intake appropriate for his or her weight-to-height ratio, muscle tone, and laboratory values (serum albumin, hematocrit, hemoglobin).

Interventions. The nutrition needs and diet restrictions for the patient with CKD vary according to the degree of kidney function and the type of kidney replacement therapy used (Table 63.8). The purpose of nutrition therapy is to provide the food and fluids needed to prevent malnutrition and avoid complications from CKD.

Referral to a registered dietitian nutritionist (RDN) is recommended in patients with a GFR below 50 mL/min/1.73 m^2 and is a Medicare-covered service (Ferri, 2020). Collaborate with the RDN to teach the patient about diet changes that are needed as a result of CKD. Common changes include control of protein intake; fluid intake limitation; restriction of potassium, sodium, and phosphorus intake; taking vitamin and mineral supplements; and eating enough calories to meet metabolic need.

Protein restriction early in the course of the disease prevents some of the problems of CKD and may preserve kidney function. Protein is restricted on the basis of the degree of kidney and waste ***elimination*** impairment (reduced glomerular filtration rate [GFR]) and the severity of the symptoms. Buildup of waste products from protein breakdown is the main cause of uremia.

The GFR and treatment of CKD are used to guide safe levels of protein intake. In patients with a GFR below 30 mL/min/1.73 m^2, KDIGO has recommended that protein intake should be lowered to 0.8 g/kg/day. Protein intake greater than 1.3 g/kg/day should be avoided in adults with CKD at risk of progression (Ferri, 2020). If protein is lost in the urine, it is added to the diet in amounts equal to that lost. Protein requirements are calculated by the registered dietitian nutritionist based on actual body weight (corrected for edema), not ideal body weight.

The patient with ESKD receiving dialysis needs *more* protein because some protein is lost through dialysis. Protein requirements are tailored according to the patient's postdialysis, or "dry," weight. In general, patients receiving hemodialysis are allowed about 1 to 1.3 g of protein per kilogram per day (Ferri, 2020). Suggested protein-containing foods are meat and eggs. If protein intake is not adequate, muscle wasting can occur. BUN and serum prealbumin levels are used to monitor the adequacy of protein intake. Decreased serum prealbumin levels indicate poor protein intake.

Sodium restriction is needed in patients with little or no urine output to maintain ***fluid and electrolyte balance.*** Both fluid and sodium retention cause edema, hypertension, and heart failure (HF). Most patients with CKD retain sodium; a few cannot conserve sodium.

Estimate fluid and sodium retention status by monitoring the patient's body weight and blood pressure. In uremic patients not receiving dialysis, sodium is limited to 1 to 3 g daily, and fluid intake depends on urine output. In patients receiving dialysis, the sodium restriction is 2 to 4 g daily, and fluid intake is limited to 500 to 700 mL plus the amount of any urine output. Instruct the patient not to add salt at the table or during cooking. Many foods are significant sources of sodium (e.g., processed food, fast food, potato chips, pretzels, pickles, ham, bacon, sausage) and difficult to moderate or remove from one's diet. Inattention to sodium intake can increase the duration or number of dialysis treatments and contribute to *disequilibrium syndrome* (feeling unsteady or off balance) following dialysis.

Potassium restriction may be needed because high blood potassium levels can cause dangerous cardiac dysrhythmias. Monitor the ECG for tall, peaked T waves caused by hyperkalemia. Instruct the patient with ESKD to limit potassium intake to 60 to 70 mEq (mmol) daily. Teach him or her to read labels of seasoning agents carefully for sodium and potassium content. Foods that are low in potassium and are permitted and foods that are high in potassium should be avoided (see Chapter 13). Instruct patients to avoid salt substitutes composed of potassium chloride. Those receiving peritoneal dialysis (PD) or who are producing urine may not need potassium restriction.

Phosphorus restriction for control of phosphorus levels is started early in CKD to avoid renal osteodystrophy. Monitor serum phosphorus levels. Dietary phosphorus restrictions and drugs to assist with phosphorus control may be prescribed. Phosphate binders must be taken at mealtime. Most patients with CKD already restrict their protein intake; and, because high-protein foods are also high in phosphorus, this reduces phosphorus intake. Chapter 13 lists foods high in potassium, sodium, and phosphorus. Cinacalcet, a drug to control parathyroid hormone excess, is also used to manage hyperphosphatemia and hypocalcemia.

Vitamin and mineral supplementation is needed daily for most patients with CKD. Low-protein diets are also low in vitamins, and water-soluble vitamins are removed from the blood during dialysis. Anemia also is a problem in patients with CKD because of the limited iron content of low-protein diets and decreased kidney production of erythropoietin. Thus supplemental iron is needed. Calcium and vitamin D supplements may be needed, depending on the patient's serum calcium levels and bone status.

Nutrition needs for patients undergoing peritoneal dialysis (PD) are slightly different from those for patients undergoing dialysis. Because protein is lost with the dialysate in PD, protein replacement is needed. Often 1.2 to 1.5 g of protein per kilogram of body weight per day is recommended. Patients may have anorexia and have difficulty eating enough protein. High-calorie oral supplements may also be needed (e.g., Magnacal Renal, Ensure Plus). Sodium restriction varies with fluid weight gain and blood pressure. Usually dietary potassium does not need to be restricted because the dialysate is potassium free, causing excess potassium to be removed from the blood. Any potassium restriction is determined by serum potassium levels.

Collaborate with the RDN to assess each patient's nutrition needs. Teach the patient the dietary regimen and evaluate his or her understanding of and adherence to it. Give the patient and family written examples of the diet to promote adherence. Help patients adapt diet restrictions to their budget, ethnic background, and food preferences.

Preventing Injury

Planning: Expected Outcomes. The patient with CKD is expected to remain free of injury including pathologic fractures, toxic side effects from drug therapy, infection, and bleeding.

Interventions. *Injury prevention strategies* are needed because the patient with long-standing CKD may have brittle, fragile bones that fracture easily and cause little pain. When lifting or moving a patient with fragile bones, use a lift sheet rather than pulling the patient. Teach assistive personnel (AP) the correct use of lift sheets. Observe for normal range of joint motion and for any unusual surface bumps or depressions over bony areas.

Managing drug therapy in patients with CKD is a complex clinical problem. Many over-the-counter drugs contain agents that alter kidney function. Therefore it is important to obtain a detailed drug history. Know the use of each drug, its side effects, and its site of metabolism.

Certain drugs must be avoided, and the dosages of others must be adjusted according to the degree of remaining kidney function. As the patient's kidney function decreases, consult with the nephrologist and pharmacist to determine if further dosage adjustments are necessary. Assess for side effects and indications of drug toxicity and notify the prescriber as appropriate.

! NURSING SAFETY PRIORITY QSEN

Drug Alert

Monitor the patient with severe CKD or ESKD closely for drug-related complications and ensure that dosages are adjusted as needed. Patients with CKD have complex needs due to multiple medications and comorbidities. Consult with the pharmacist to determine safe effective doses.

Drugs to control an excessively high phosphorus level include phosphate-binding agents. These drugs help prevent renal osteodystrophy and related injuries. Stress the importance of taking these agents and all prescribed drugs.

Hypophosphatemia (low serum phosphorus levels) is a complication of phosphate binding, especially in patients who do not eat adequately but continue to take phosphate-binding drugs. *Hypercalcemia* (high serum calcium levels) can occur in patients taking calcium-containing compounds to control phosphorus excess. In patients taking aluminum-based phosphate binders for prolonged periods, aluminum deposits may cause bone disease or neurologic problems. Monitor the patient for muscle weakness, anorexia, malaise, tremors, and bone pain.

Teach patients with kidney disease to avoid antacids containing magnesium. These patients cannot excrete magnesium and thus should avoid additional intake.

Some drugs, in addition to those used to treat kidney failure, require special attention because they either are normally excreted by the kidney or can further damage the kidney. These drugs include antibiotics, opioids, antihypertensives, diuretics, insulin, and heparin.

Monitor carefully for indicators of infection. These indicators include fever, lymph node enlargements, and elevated WBC counts, as well as positive cultures. For patients undergoing dialysis, inspect the vascular access site or PD catheter insertion site every shift for redness, swelling, pain, or drainage. If antibiotics are required, use caution in the patient with CKD. Many antibiotics are safe for patients with CKD, but those excreted by the kidney and those that are nephrotoxic require dose adjustment (Himmelfarb & Ikizler, 2018). To prevent complications of bloodstream infection from mouth bacteria, prophylactic antibiotics are given to patients with CKD before dental procedures.

Give opioid analgesics cautiously in patients with stage 3 or 4 CKD or ESKD because the effects often last longer. Patients with uremia are sensitive to the respiratory depressant effects of these drugs. Because opioids are broken down by the liver and not the kidneys, the dosages are often the same, regardless of the level of kidney function. Monitor the patient's reactions closely after opioids are given to determine whether adjustments are needed.

As CKD progresses, the patient with diabetes often requires reduced doses of insulin or antidiabetic drugs because the failing kidneys do not excrete or metabolize these drugs well. Thus the drugs are effective longer, increasing the risk for hypoglycemia. Monitor blood glucose levels at least four times daily to assess whether a dosage change is needed.

Poor platelet function and capillary fragility in CKD make anticoagulant therapy risky. Monitor patients receiving heparin, warfarin, or any anticoagulant every shift for bleeding. See Chapter 37 for more information on caring for patients at increased risk for bleeding.

Minimizing Psychosocial Compromise. Due to the chronic nature and impact of CKD, the patient with CKD may experience fatigue and psychosocial impact. These impacts can include anxiety, social isolation, and depression. The patient with CKD often experiences depression (Lotfaliany, 2018). Loss, such as loss of work or family roles, may contribute to depression. Depressive symptoms have been associated with nonadherence to CKD treatments. Sleep disturbances, also interrelated with depression, are common among adults receiving dialysis for ESKD.

Planning: Expected Outcomes. The goal for patients with CKD is to conserve energy by balancing activity and rest, have reduced anxiety and depression, and minimize the overall psychosocial impact of the disease.

Interventions. Perform an ongoing assessment of the patient's level of fatigue as well as reports of anxiety. Ask about sleep patterns and quality. Assess the coping mechanisms and successful methods of dealing with problems. Observe behavior for cues indicating increasing anxiety (e.g., anxious facial expressions, clenching of hands, tapping of feet, withdrawn posture, absence of eye contact) and provide interventions to decrease the anxiety level. Evaluate the support systems and the involvement of family and friends with the patient's care. Provide ongoing supportive interventions throughout therapy. Assess for indicators of depression including despair and loneliness.

Some causes of *fatigue* in the patient with CKD include vitamin deficiency, anemia, and buildup of urea. All patients are given vitamin and mineral supplements because of diet restrictions and vitamin losses from dialysis. Avoid giving these supplements right before hemodialysis (HD) treatment because they will be dialyzed out of the body and the patient will receive no benefit.

The anemic patient with CKD is treated with agents to stimulate red blood cell (RBC) production. The desired outcome of this therapy is to maintain a hemoglobin level around 10 g/dL (100 g/L). This therapy triggers bone marrow production of RBCs if the patient has adequate iron stores. Iron supplements may be needed in patients who are iron deficient. Many who receive these drugs report improved appetite and sexual function along with decreased fatigue. The increased production of all blood cells from this therapy may increase blood pressure. The improved appetite challenges patients in their attempts to maintain protein, potassium, and fluid restrictions and requires additional education.

Unfamiliar settings and lack of knowledge about treatments and tests can increase the patient's anxiety level. Explain all procedures, tests, and treatments. Identify the patient's knowledge needs about kidney disease. Provide instruction at a level that he or she can understand, using a variety of written and visual materials. Provide continuity of care, whenever possible, by using a consistent and trusting nurse-patient relationship to decrease anxiety and encourage the patient to discuss his or her thoughts and feelings about any current problems or concerns.

Encourage the patient to ask questions and discuss fears about the diagnosis, treatment strategies, and common outcomes. An open atmosphere that allows for discussion can decrease anxiety. Facilitate discussions with family members about the prognosis and the impact on lifestyle.

Identify community resources to maintain independence, including delivered meals, transportation, and financial or health care options.

In the general population, drugs are commonly used to manage depression. However, pharmacologic effects of drugs in adults with CKD or those receiving dialysis are altered, and additional monitoring may be needed with alternative approaches for effective care. Care coordination for patients with CKD is essential because multiple health care professions may be involved in delivering care. Care coordination helps to avoid adverse drug effects (and drug-drug interactions), avoid hospitalizations, and decrease problems related to depression.

Kidney Replacement Therapies. Kidney replacement therapy (KRT) is needed when the pathologic changes of stage 4 and stage 5 CKD are life threatening or pose continuing discomfort. When the patient can no longer be managed with conservative therapies, such as diet, drugs, and fluid restriction, dialysis is indicated. Transplantation may be discussed at any time.

Hemodialysis. Intermittent hemodialysis (HD) is the most common KRT used with ESKD (Table 63.9). Dialysis removes excess fluids and waste products and restores ***fluid and electrolyte balance*** and ***acid-base balance***. HD involves passing the patient's blood through an artificial semipermeable membrane to perform the kidney's filtering and excretion functions. Safe HD therapy requires technicians to provide meticulous care to the machines delivering HD and nurses to implement and supervise direct care. Technical or human error can lead to avoidable complications (e.g., hemolysis, air embolism, dialysate error, contamination, exsanguination).

Patient Selection. Any patient may be considered for intermittent HD therapy. Starting HD depends on symptoms from disruptions of ***fluid and electrolyte balance*** and waste and toxin accumulation, not the GFR alone. Normally the decision to start dialysis is made by a nephrologist who has been monitoring a patients decreasing GFR and increasing symptoms.

TABLE 63.9 Comparison of Hemodialysis and Peritoneal Dialysis

Hemodialysis	Peritoneal Dialysis
Advantages	
More efficient clearance of wastes Short time needed for treatment	Flexible schedule for exchanges Few hemodynamic changes during and following exchanges Fewer dietary and fluid restrictions
Complications	
Disequilibrium syndrome Muscle cramps and back pain Headache Itching Hemodynamic and cardiac adverse events (hypotension, cell lysis contributing to anemia, cardiac dysrhythmias) Infection Increased risk for subdural and intracranial hemorrhage from anticoagulation and changes in blood pressure during dialysis Anemia Access site complications	Protein loss Peritonitis Respiratory distress Inflammatory bowel disease Bowel perforation Infection Weight gain; discomfort from "carrying" 1-2 L in abdomen during dwell time; potential for back pain or development of hernia
Contraindications	
Hemodynamic instability or severe cardiac disease Severe vascular disease that prevents vascular access Serious bleeding disorders	Extensive peritoneal adhesions, fibrosis, or active inflammatory GI disease (e.g., diverticulitis, inflammatory bowel conditions) Ascites or massive central obesity Recent abdominal surgery
Access	
Arteriovenous (AV) fistula AV graft Central venous catheter	Intra-abdominal catheter
Procedure	
Complex; requires a second person trained in the technique whether completed at home or at a dialysis unit/center Special training for center personnel and in-home use	Simple, easier to complete at home compared with at-home hemodialysis Less complex training; typically managed by patient; can be managed by one person

Some indications for emergent dialysis include:

- Pulmonary edema
- Severe uncontrollable hypertension
- Symptomatic hyperkalemia with ECG changes
- Other severe electrolyte or acid-base disturbances
- Some overdoses
- Pericarditis

Most commonly, hemodialysis for CKD is started when uremic symptoms (e.g., intractable nausea and vomiting, confusion, seizures, or severe bleeding from platelet dysfunction) occur.

Many patients survive for years with HD therapy, and others may live only a few months. Length of survival with HD therapy depends on patient age, the cause of CKD, and the presence of other diseases, such as cardiovascular conditions or diabetes. Selection criteria include:

- Irreversible kidney failure when other therapies are unacceptable or ineffective
- No disorders that would seriously complicate HD
- Patient values and preferences
- Expected ability to continue or resume roles at home, work, or school

Dialysis Settings. Patients with CKD may receive HD treatments in many settings, depending on specific needs. Regardless of the setting for therapy, they need ongoing nursing support to maintain this complex and lifesaving treatment.

Patients may be dialyzed in a hospital-based center if they have recently started treatment or have complicated conditions that require close supervision. Stable patients not requiring intense supervision may be dialyzed in a community or freestanding dialysis center. Selected patients may participate in self-care in an ambulatory care center or with in-home HD.

In-home HD is the least disruptive treatment and allows the patient to adapt the regimen to his or her lifestyle. Newer technologies and HD equipment are making home dialysis an easier process to learn. It is growing in popularity and use. A water treatment system must be installed in the home to provide a safe, clean water supply for the dialysis process.

Procedure. Dialysis works by using the passive transfer of toxins by diffusion. **Diffusion** is the movement of molecules from an area of higher concentration to an area of lower concentration. The rate of diffusion during dialysis is most dependent on the difference in the solute concentrations between the patient's blood and the dialysate. Large molecules, such as RBCs and most plasma proteins, cannot pass through the membrane.

When HD is started, blood and **dialysate** (dialyzing solution) flow in opposite directions across an enclosed semipermeable membrane. The dialysate contains a balanced mix of electrolytes and water that closely resembles human plasma. On the other side of the membrane is the patient's blood, which contains nitrogen waste products, excess water, and excess electrolytes. During HD, the waste products move from the blood into the dialysate because of the difference in their concentrations (diffusion). Some water is also removed from the blood into the dialysate by *osmosis.* Electrolytes can move in either direction, as needed, and take some fluid with them. Potassium and sodium typically move out of the plasma into the dialysate. Bicarbonate and calcium generally move from the dialysate into the plasma. This circulating process continues for a preset length of time, removing nitrogenous wastes, reestablishing ***fluid and electrolyte balance,*** and restoring ***acid-base balance.*** Water volume may be removed from the plasma by applying positive or negative pressure to the system.

The HD system includes a dialyzer, dialysate, vascular access routes, and an HD machine. The artificial kidney, or dialyzer (Fig. 63.3), has four parts: a blood compartment, a dialysate compartment, a semipermeable membrane, and an enclosed support structure.

Dialysate is made from water and chemicals and is free of any waste products or drugs. It is usually dispensed from the

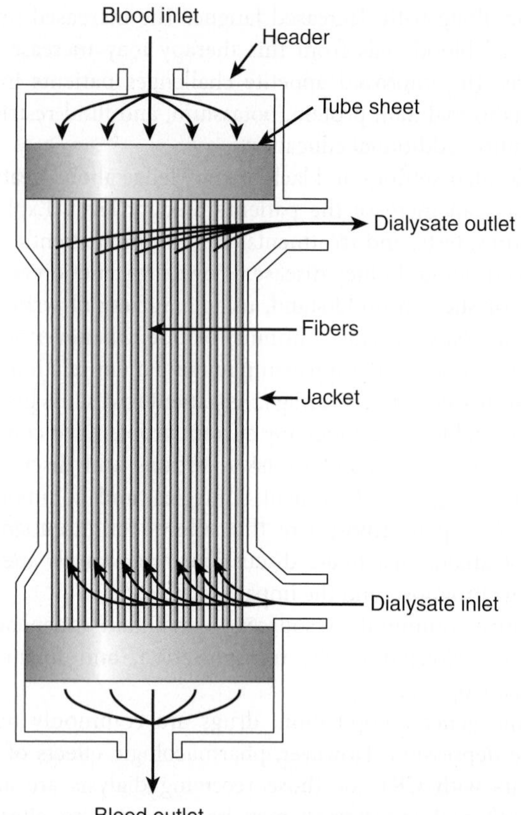

FIG. 63.3 Hollow fiber dialyzer (artificial kidney) used in hemodialysis. (From Feehally, J., Floege, J., & Johnson, R. [2007]. *Comprehensive clinical nephrology* [3rd ed.]. Philadelphia: Mosby.)

pharmacy in an acute care setting. The solution may be mixed in large or small batches by technicians in dialysis centers. Because bacteria and other organisms are too large to pass through the membrane, dialysate is not sterile. Water used in dialysate must meet specific standards and requires special treatment before mixing the dialysate. Dialysate composition may be altered for the patient's needs for management of electrolyte imbalances. During HD, the dialysate is warmed to 100°F (37.8°C) to increase the diffusion rate and prevent hypothermia.

The HD machine has built-in safety features such as the ability to record patient vital signs, blood and dialysate flows, arterial and venous pressures, delivered dialysis dose, plasma volume changes, and temperature changes. If any of these problems are detected, an alarm sounds to protect the patient from life-threatening complications.

All dialyzers function in a similar manner. Fig. 63.4 shows a comparison of fluid and particle movement across the dialyzer membranes, comparing intermittent HD with continuous kidney replacement circuits. For intermittent HD, the number and length of treatments depend on the amount of wastes and fluid to be removed, the clearance capacity of the dialyzer, and the blood flow rate to and from the machine. Fig. 63.5 shows a typical intermittent dialysis machine. Most patients receive three 4-hour treatments over the course of a week. For those with some ongoing urine production, two 5- to 6-hour treatments a week may be adequate. If the patient gains large amounts of

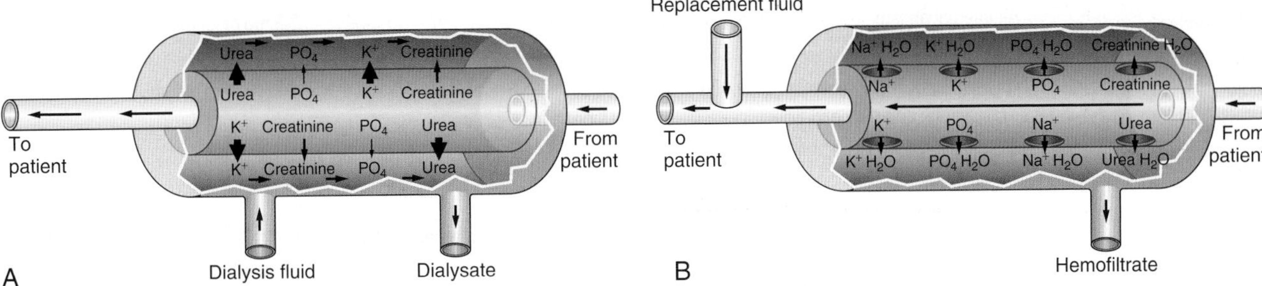

FIG. 63.4 Comparison of hemodialysis and hemofiltration fluid and solute movements across the membrane. Demonstrates this movement in hemodialysis (A) and hemofiltration (B). The *arrows* that cross the membrane indicate the predominant direction of movement of each solute through the membrane; the relative size of the *arrows* indicates the net amounts of the solute transferred. Other *arrows* indicate the direction of flow. (From Feehally, J., Floege, J., & Johnson, R. [2007]. *Comprehensive clinical nephrology* [3rd ed.]. Philadelphia: Mosby.)

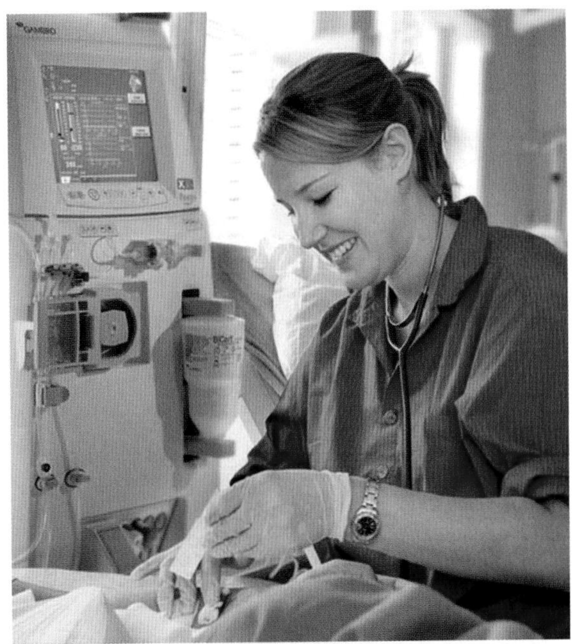

FIG. 63.5 Renal replacement therapy with an intermittent hemodialysis machine. (Courtesy Gambro Lundia AB, Lund, Sweden.)

fluid, a longer HD treatment time may be needed to remove the fluid without hypotension or other severe side effects.

Anticoagulation. Blood clotting can occur during dialysis. Anticoagulation, usually with heparin, is delivered into the blood circuit via a pump. In patients with high risk for bleeding, a reduced dose, regional anticoagulation (using citrate rather than heparin for anticoagulation or reversing heparin actions by administering protamine before returning blood to the patient), or no anticoagulation may be used. Patient response to heparin varies, and the dose is adjusted on the basis of each patient's need.

Heparin remains active in the body for 4 to 6 hours after dialysis, increasing the patient's risk for hemorrhage during and immediately after HD treatments. Invasive procedures must be avoided during that time. Monitor him or her closely for any signs of bleeding or hemorrhage. Protamine sulfate is an antidote to heparin and always should be available in the dialysis setting.

Vascular Access. Vascular access is required for hemodialysis (Table 63.10 and Fig. 63.6). The procedure requires the availability of a high blood flow: at least 250 to 300 mL/min, usually for a period of 3 to 4 hours (Norton et al., 2017b). Normal venous cannulation does not provide this high rate of blood flow.

Long-term vascular access is internal for most patients having long-term HD (see Table 63.10). The two common choices are an internal arteriovenous (AV) fistula or an AV graft (see Fig. 63.6). *AV fistulas* are formed by surgically connecting an artery to a vein. The vessels used most often are the radial or brachial artery and the cephalic vein of the nondominant arm. Fistulas increase venous blood flow to the 250 to 400 mL/min needed for effective dialysis.

Time is needed after the surgeon creates the AV fistula for it to develop into a usable access site for HD. As the AV fistula "matures," the increased pressure of the arterial blood flow into the vein causes the vessel walls to thicken. This thickening increases their strength and durability for repeated cannulation. The amount of time needed for the fistula to mature varies. Some fistulas may not be ready for use for as long as 4 months after the surgery, and a temporary vascular access (AV shunt or HD catheter) is used during this time. Fig. 63.7 shows a mature fistula.

To access a fistula, cannulate it by inserting two needles: one toward the venous blood flow and one toward the arterial blood flow. This procedure allows the HD machine to draw the blood out through the arterial needle and return it through the venous needle.

Arteriovenous grafts are used when the AV fistula does not develop or when complications limit its use. The polytetrafluoroethylene (PTFE) graft is a synthetic material (GORE-TEX). This type of graft is commonly used for older patients using HD. Figs. 63.6A and 63.7 show a patient's fistula.

Precautions. Precautions are needed to ensure the functioning of an internal AV fistula or AV graft. First assess for adequate circulation in the fistula or graft and in the lower portion of the arm. Check distal pulses and capillary refill in the arm with the fistula or graft. Then check for a bruit or a thrill by auscultation or palpation over the access site. See the Best Practice for Patient Safety & Quality Care: Caring for the Patient With an Arteriovenous Fistula or Arteriovenous Graft box.

TABLE 63.10 **Types of Vascular Access for Hemodialysis**

Access Type	Description	Location	Time to Initial Use
Permanent			
AV fistula	An internal anastomosis of an artery to a vein	Forearm Upper arm	2-3 mo or longer
AV graft	Looped plastic tubing tunneled beneath the skin, connecting an artery and a vein	Forearm Upper arm Inner thigh	1-3 wk after surgery
Temporary			
Dialysis catheter	A specially designed catheter with separate lumens for blood outflow and inflow	Subclavian vein, internal jugular, or femoral vein	Immediately after insertion and x-ray confirmation of placement
Subcutaneous catheter	An internal device with two access ports and a cuff or dual-lumen catheter inserted into a large central vein	Subclavian vein, internal jugular, or femoral vein	Dedicated use; do not access for blood sampling or drug administration

AV, Arteriovenous.

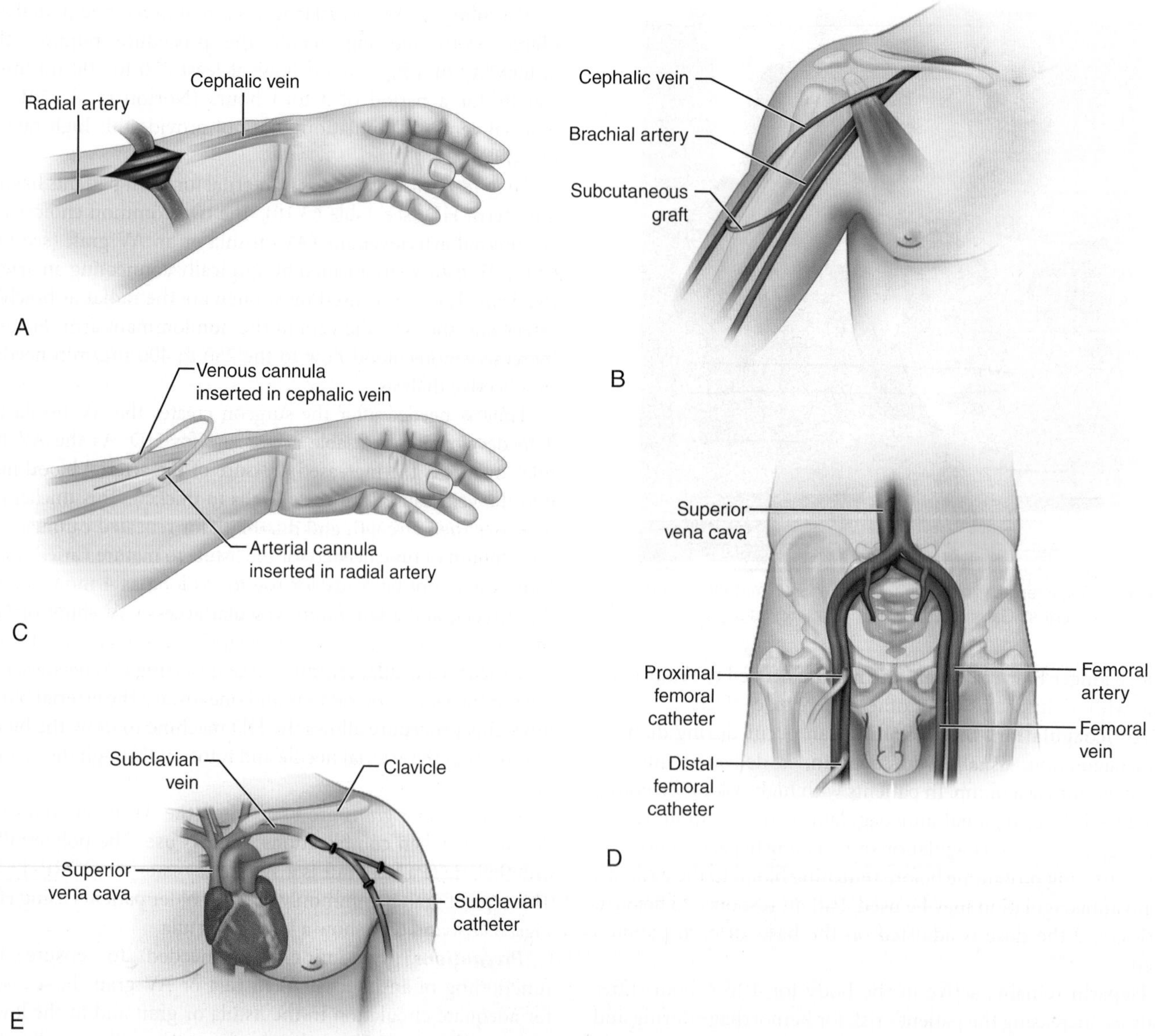

FIG. 63.6 Frequently used means for gaining vascular access for hemodialysis include arteriovenous fistula (A), arteriovenous graft (B), external arteriovenous shunt (C), femoral vein catheterization (D), and subclavian vein catheterization (E). (A) and (B) are options for long-term vascular access for hemodialysis. (C), (D), and (E) are used for short-term access for intermittent hemodialysis or for continuous renal replacement therapy in acute care.

BEST PRACTICE FOR PATIENT SAFETY & QUALITY CARE (QSEN)

Caring for the Patient With an Arteriovenous Fistula or Arteriovenous Graft

- Do not take blood pressure readings using the extremity in which the vascular access is placed.
- Do not perform venipunctures or start an IV line in the extremity in which the vascular access is placed.
- Palpate for thrills and auscultate for bruits over the vascular access site every 4 hours while the patient is awake.
- Assess the patient's distal pulses and circulation in the arm with the access.
- Elevate the affected extremity after surgery.
- Encourage routine range-of-motion exercises.
- Check for bleeding at needle insertion sites.
- Assess for indications of infection at needle sites.
- Instruct the patient not to carry heavy objects or anything that compresses the extremity in which the vascular access is placed.
- Instruct the patient not to sleep with his or her body weight on top of the extremity in which the vascular access is placed.

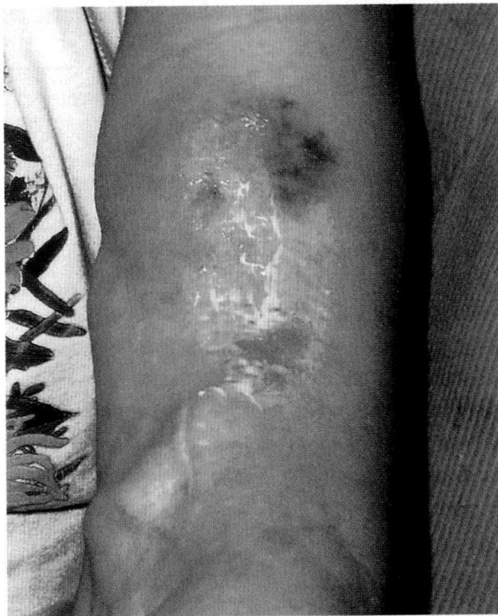

FIG. 63.7 A mature fistula for hemodialysis access. The increased pressure from the anastomosed artery forced blood into the vein. This process caused the vein to dilate enough for fistula needles to be placed for hemodialysis. When the vein is sufficiently dilated, a process that takes 8 to 12 weeks, the fistula is said to be *developed* or *mature*.

! NURSING SAFETY PRIORITY (QSEN)

Action Alert

Because repeated compression can result in the loss of the vascular access, avoid taking the blood pressure or performing venipunctures in the arm with the vascular access. Do not use an AV fistula or graft for general delivery of IV fluids or drugs.

Access Complications. Complications can occur with any type of access. Common problems include thrombosis or stenosis, infection, aneurysm formation, ischemia, and HF (Norton et al., 2017b). Table 63.11 lists strategies to prevent access complications.

Thrombosis, or clotting of the AV access, is the most frequent complication. Most grafts fail because of high-pressure arterial flow entering the venous system. The muscle layers of the veins react to this increased pressure by thickening. The venous thickening reduces or occludes blood flow. An interventional radiologist can reopen failing grafts with the injection of a thrombolytic drug to dissolve the clot. The clot usually dissolves within minutes, and often a stricture is revealed at the point where the graft and the vein connect. The stricture can be corrected by balloon angioplasty.

Most infections of the vascular access are caused by *Staphylococcus aureus* introduced during cannulation. Prepare the skin with an antibacterial agent according to agency policy before cannulation to prevent infection. When using dialysis catheters, be sure to use only the cleansing agent recommended by the catheter manufacturer. Some disinfectants can damage the catheter (Woo, 2019).

Aneurysms can form in the fistula and are caused by repeated needle punctures at the same site. Large aneurysms may cause loss of the fistula's function and require surgical repair.

Ischemia occurs in a few patients with vascular access when the fistula decreases arterial blood flow to areas below the fistula *(steal syndrome)*. Symptoms vary from cold or numb fingers to gangrene. If the collateral circulation is poor, the fistula may need to be surgically tied off, and a new one created in another area to preserve extremity circulation.

Shunting of blood directly from the arterial system to the venous system through the fistula can cause HF in patients with limited cardiac function. This complication is rare; but, if it does occur, the fistula may need to be revised to reduce arterial blood flow.

TABLE 63.11 Interventions for Preventing Complications in Hemodialysis Vascular Access

Access Type	Bleeding	Infection	Clotting
AV fistula or AV graft	Apply pressure to the needle puncture sites.	Prepare skin using best practices before cannulation. Typically 2% chlorhexidine is used, similar to central line skin preparation. Between hemodialysis sessions, the patient should wash the area with antibacterial soap and rinse with water.	Avoid constrictive devices such as blood pressure cuffs and tourniquets. Rotate needle insertion sites with each hemodialysis treatment. Assess for thrill and bruit.
Hemodialysis catheters (temporary and permanent)	Assess the access site every time you monitor vital signs.	Use aseptic technique to dress site and access catheter. Do not use catheters for blood sampling, IV fluids, or drug administration.	Place a heparin or heparin/saline dwell solution after hemodialysis treatment.

AV, Arteriovenous.

Temporary Vascular Access. Temporary access with special catheters can be used for patients requiring immediate HD. A catheter designed for HD may be inserted into the subclavian, internal jugular, or femoral vein. The lumens of these devices are much smaller than the permanent accesses, and more time (4 to 8 hours) is required to complete a dialysis session.

Subcutaneous devices may also be surgically inserted to provide temporary access for HD. Implanted beneath the skin, these devices are composed of two small metallic ports with attached catheters that are inserted into large central veins. The ports of subcutaneous devices have internal mechanisms that open when needles are inserted and close when needles are removed. Blood from one port flows from the body to the HD machine and returns to the body via the other port.

Hemodialysis Nursing Care. Many drugs are dialyzable (i.e., can be partially or completely removed from the blood during dialysis). Coordinate with the nephrology health care provider to assess the patient's drug regimen and determine which drugs should be held until after HD treatment. Table 63.12 lists common dialyzable drugs that should be given *after* rather than before HD. Consult the dialysis nurse or nephrologist to determine if antihypertensive drugs should be given before a scheduled dialysis treatment; some short-acting antihypertensives can contribute to hypotension during dialysis.

The time required to complete an HD treatment usually is at least 4 hours. During this time patients may use various distraction techniques to prevent boredom, such as reading, watching television or videos, visiting with friends or relatives, playing video games, or working puzzles. This time can be used also for brief health teaching opportunities.

Postdialysis Care. Closely monitor the patient immediately and for several hours after dialysis for any side effects from the treatment. Common problems include hypotension, headache, nausea, vomiting, dizziness, and muscle cramps.

Obtain vital signs and weight for comparison with predialysis measurements. Blood pressure and weight are expected to be reduced as a result of fluid removal. Hypotension may necessitate rehydration with IV fluids, such as normal saline. The patient's temperature may also be elevated because the dialysis machine warms the blood slightly. If he or she has a fever, sepsis may be present, and a blood sample is needed for culture and sensitivity.

The heparin or citrate required during HD increases the risk for excessive bleeding. All invasive procedures must be avoided for 4 to 6 hours after dialysis. Continually monitor the patient for hemorrhage during and for at least 1 hour after dialysis. See the Best Practice for Patient Safety & Quality Care: Caring for the Patient Undergoing Hemodialysis box.

Complications of Hemodialysis. Few adverse events occur during a 3- to 4-hour HD treatment under current practice protocols. Improved water treatment, more physiologic solutions, and improvements in HD equipment and procedures have significantly improved safe care for patients receiving this treatment. Complications during HD include hypotension, dialysis disequilibrium syndrome, cardiac events, and reactions to dialyzers (Norton et al., 2017b).

TABLE 63.12 Examples of Dialyzable Drugs

Consult the pharmacist, nephrologist, or dialysis nurse to plan the best time to administer a drug based on the dialysis schedule.

Aminoglycosides
- Amikacin
- Gentamicin
- Tobramycin

Antituberculosis Agents
- Ethambutol
- Isoniazid

Antiviral and Antifungal Agents
- Acyclovir
- Ganciclovir
- Fluconazole

Cephalosporins
- Cefaclor
- Cefazolin
- Cefoxitin
- Ceftriaxone
- Cefuroxime
- Cefepime

Anticonvulsants
- Ethosuximide
- Gabapentin
- Phenobarbital

Penicillins
- Amoxicillin
- Ampicillin
- Dicloxacillin
- Penicillin G

Miscellaneous
- Aztreonam
- Cimetidine
- Vitamins
- Clavulanic acid
- Allopurinol
- Enalapril
- Aspirin

! NURSING SAFETY PRIORITY (QSEN)

Critical Rescue

Monitor the patient closely during dialysis to recognize hypotension, which is common. Heat transfer from warm solutions can result in vasodilation and a drop in blood pressure. When this occurs, reduce the temperature of the dialysate to 35°C (95°F). Fluid shifts from the plasma volume related to differences in electrolyte concentrations between HD solutions and blood also reduce blood pressure. Respond to modest declines in blood pressure by adjusting the rate of dialyzer blood flow and placing the patient in a legs-up (Trendelenburg) position. Respond to sustained or symptomatic hypotension by giving a fluid bolus of 100 to 250 mL of normal saline, albumin, or mannitol (if prescribed). A second bolus may be needed. If hypotension persists, new-onset myocardial injury or pericardial disease may be a contributing factor; respond by applying oxygen, reducing the blood flow, and notifying the primary health care provider urgently. Discontinue HD when hypotension continues despite two bolus infusions.

BEST PRACTICE FOR PATIENT SAFETY & QUALITY CARE (QSEN)

Caring for the Patient Undergoing Hemodialysis

- Weigh the patient before and after dialysis.
- Know the patient's dry weight.
- Discuss with the nephrology health care provider or pharmacist whether any of the patient's drugs should be withheld until after dialysis.
- Be aware of events that occurred during previous dialysis treatments.
- Measure blood pressure, pulse, respirations, and temperature.
- Assess for indications of orthostatic hypotension.
- Assess the vascular access site when taking vital signs and follow agency policy for central line care and dressing changes.
- Observe for bleeding at the vascular access site and other sites where skin integrity is disrupted because anticoagulants given during dialysis and the presence of uremia increase bleeding risk.
- Assess the patient's level of consciousness.
- Assess for headache, nausea, and vomiting.
- Assess serum laboratory tests to evaluate effectiveness of treatment in removing wastes and achieving desired outcomes (e.g., ***fluid and electrolyte balance,*** reduction of uremia).

Dialysis disequilibrium syndrome may develop during HD or after HD has been completed. It is characterized by mental status changes and can include seizures or coma, although this severity of disequilibrium syndrome is rare with today's HD practice. A mild form of disequilibrium syndrome includes symptoms of nausea, vomiting, headaches, fatigue, and restlessness. It is thought to be the result of a rapid reduction in electrolytes and other particles. Reducing blood flow at the onset of symptoms can prevent this syndrome.

Cardiac events during HD are associated with underlying cardiovascular disease, especially left ventricular hypertrophy, coronary vascular disease, and a history of cardiac dysrhythmias. These conditions are described in Chapters 31, 32, and 35. Although cardiac arrest is a rare event, the setting should be equipped with an automatic defibrillator and staff or family trained in cardiopulmonary resuscitation. Often cardiac arrest is related to new-onset cardiac ischemia. This problem is managed in an acute care setting in which the presence of myocardial disease can be evaluated and cardiac treatment optimized.

Pericardial disease is a complication of patients with ESKD. Assess the patient's heart sounds for the presence of a pericardial rub before starting dialysis. Intensification of dialysis may be used to treat this complication. Other treatment might include NSAID use or surgery.

Reactions to dialyzers still occur, although more biocompatible membranes and careful attention to rinsing the dialyzer before use (to eliminate sterilizing agents) have reduced this adverse event during HD. Reactions occur during a "first-time" use of the filter and resemble an anaphylactic episode early during HD, with profound hypotension. (Chapter 18 describes anaphylactic reactions.) With suspected dialyzer reactions, do not return the blood to the patient, and discontinue HD. Corticosteroids may be used to treat the ***immunity*** reaction.

Other potential complications of HD require the nurse to monitor the level of consciousness and vital signs frequently during treatment and to slow or stop HD when symptoms occur. Hypoglycemia is a rare adverse HD event and more likely to occur when the patient has diabetes. It is managed by providing glucose and increasing dialysis glucose concentration in subsequent treatments. Hemorrhage can occur when needle dislodgment or circuit connections become loose and is amplified by anticoagulation used to maintain circuit patency. Some hemolysis occurs because of mechanical trauma to RBCs, contributing to anemia in the patient with CKD and, perhaps, to sensations of dyspnea or chest tightness.

Infectious diseases transmitted by blood transfusion are a serious complication of long-term HD. Two of the most serious blood-transmitted infections are hepatitis and human immune deficiency virus (HIV) infection. *Hepatitis B infection* and *hepatitis C infection* in patients with CKD have decreased because the use of erythropoietin-stimulating agents (ESAs) has reduced the need for blood transfusions to maintain RBC counts. Hepatitis is a problem because of the blood access and the risk for contamination during HD. The viruses can be transmitted through the use of contaminated needles or instruments, by entry of contaminated blood through open wounds in the skin or mucous membranes, or through transfusions with contaminated blood. Monitor all patients receiving HD for indications of hepatitis (see Chapter 53).

The risk for HIV transmission is reduced by the consistent practice of Standard Precautions, routine screening of donated blood for HIV, and decreased need for blood transfusions with CKD and ESKD. Patients who have been undergoing HD or who received frequent transfusions during the early to middle 1980s may have been infected at that time and are at risk for AIDS (HIV-III) (see Chapter 17).

PATIENT CENTERED CARE: OLDER ADULT CONSIDERATIONS QSEN

Adults over age 75 comprise one of the most rapidly increasing age-groups of dialysis patients. Patients should be educated about all aspects of dialysis care so that they can make an informed decision regarding dialysis initiation. In adults over age 80 with coronary artery disease in addition to other comorbid conditions, dialysis has not been shown to prolong life when compared with patients receiving more conservative treatments. Dialysis patients spend an average of 173 days per year in the hospital or at dialysis; nondialysis, medically treated patients spend an average of 16 days per year in the hospital (Himmelfarb & Ikizler, 2018).

Peritoneal Dialysis. Peritoneal dialysis (PD) allows exchanges of wastes, fluid, and electrolytes to occur in the peritoneal cavity. However, PD is slower than hemodialysis (HD), and more time is needed to achieve the same effect. Other disadvantages of PD are the protein loss in outflow fluid, risk for peritoneal injury, and potential discomfort from indwelling fluid. Advantages and complications are listed in Table 63.9. The use of PD is declining and accounts for less than 10% of the total dialysis population (Johnson et al., 2019).

Patient Selection. Most patients with CKD can select either HD or PD. For those who are unstable and those who cannot tolerate anticoagulation, PD is less hazardous than HD. For some patients, vascular access problems may eliminate HD as an option. At times a patient may use PD until a new arteriovenous (AV) fistula matures. PD is often the treatment of choice for older adults because it offers more flexibility if his or her status changes frequently.

PD *cannot* be performed if peritoneal adhesions are present or if extensive intra-abdominal surgery has been performed (Norton et al., 2017b). In these cases, the surface area of the peritoneal membrane is not sufficient for adequate dialysis exchange. Peritoneal membrane fibrosis may occur after repeated infection, which decreases membrane permeability.

Procedure. A siliconized rubber (Silastic) catheter is surgically placed into the abdominal cavity for infusion of dialysate (Fig. 63.8). Usually 1 to 2 L of dialysate is infused by gravity *(fill)* into the peritoneal space over a 10- to 20-minute period, according to the patient's tolerance. The fluid stays *(dwells)* in the cavity for a specified time prescribed for each patient individually by the nephrologist. It then flows out of the body *(drains)* by gravity into a drainage bag. The peritoneal outflow contains the dialysate and the excess water, electrolytes, and nitrogen-based waste products. The dialyzing fluid is called peritoneal *effluent* on outflow. The three phases of the process (infusion, or "fill"; dwell; and outflow, or drain) make up one PD exchange. The number and frequency of PD exchanges are prescribed by the physician, depending on symptoms and laboratory data.

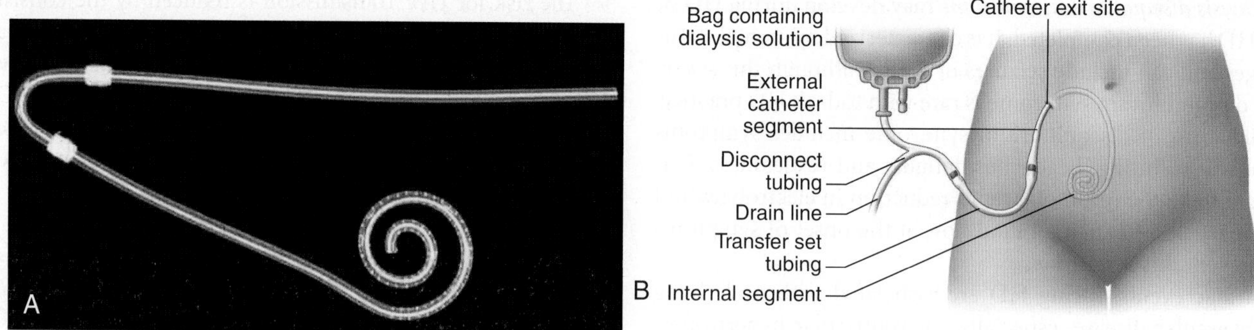

FIG. 63.8 Peritoneal dialysis catheter. (A) The actual Silastic peritoneal dialysis catheter. (B) Positioning of the Silastic catheter within the abdominal cavity. (A from Geary, D.F., & Schaefer, F. [2008]. *Comprehensive pediatric nephrology*. Philadelphia: Mosby.)

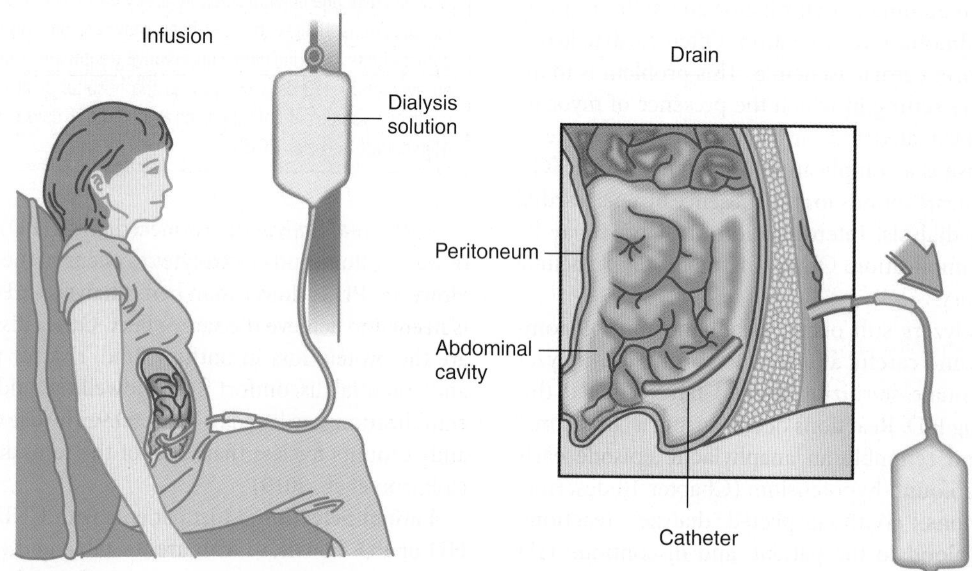

FIG. 63.9 Peritoneal dialysis exchange for control of fluids, electrolytes, nitrogenous wastes, blood pressure, and acid-base balance. The peritoneal membrane acts as the dialyzing membrane.

Process. PD occurs through diffusion and osmosis across the semipermeable peritoneal membrane and capillaries. The peritoneal membrane is large and porous. It allows particles and water to move from an area of higher concentration in the blood to an area of lower concentration in the dialyzing fluid (diffusion).

The peritoneal cavity is rich in capillaries and is a ready access to the blood supply. The fluid and waste products dialyzed from the patient move through the blood vessel walls, the interstitial tissues, and the peritoneal membrane and are removed when the dialyzing fluid is drained from the body.

PD efficiency is affected by many factors. Infection can cause scarring and reduce capillary blood flow. Vascular disease and decreased ***perfusion*** of the peritoneum reduce PD diffusion. For PD, water removal depends on the concentration of the dialysate. PD efficiency can be altered by the *tonicity* (i.e., number of particles per liter of fluid) of the dialysate. The dialysate concentration is prescribed on the basis of the patient's fluid status (Johnson et al., 2019).

Dialysate Additives. Heparin may be added to the dialysate to prevent clotting of the catheter or tubing. Usually intraperitoneal (IP) heparin is needed only after new catheter placement or if peritonitis occurs. IP heparin is not absorbed systemically and does not affect blood clotting.

Other agents that may be given in the dialysate include potassium and antibiotics. Commercially prepared dialysate does not contain potassium. Some patients need potassium added to the dialysate to prevent hypokalemia. Antibiotics may be given by the IP route when peritonitis is present or suspected. Potassium and antibiotics are not mixed in the same dialysate bag because interactions may reduce the antibiotic effect.

Types of Peritoneal Dialysis. Many types of PD are available, including continuous ambulatory PD, multiple-bag continuous ambulatory PD, automated PD, intermittent PD, and continuous-cycle PD. The type selected depends on the patient's ability and lifestyle. The two most commonly used types of PD are continuous ambulatory peritoneal dialysis and continuous cycling peritoneal dialysis.

Continuous ambulatory peritoneal dialysis (CAPD) is performed by the patient with the infusion of four 2-L exchanges of dialysate into the peritoneal cavity. Each time, the dialysate remains for 4 to 8 hours, and these exchanges occur 7 days a week (Figs. 63.9 to 63.11). During the dwell period, the patient can use a continuous connect system or disconnect and then reconnect at a later time. Most patients using PD long term prefer to complete exchanges overnight with an automated cycler (automatic peritoneal dialysis [APD]).

Automated peritoneal dialysis (APD) may be used in the acute care setting, the ambulatory care dialysis center, or the patient's home. APD uses a cycling machine for dialysate inflow, dwell, and outflow according to preset times and volumes. A warming chamber for dialysate is part of the machine (Fig. 63.12). The functions are programmed for the patient's specific needs. A typical prescription calls for 30-minute exchanges (10/10/10 for inflow, dwell, and outflow) for a period of 8 to 10 hours. The machines have many safety monitors and alarms and are relatively simple to learn to use.

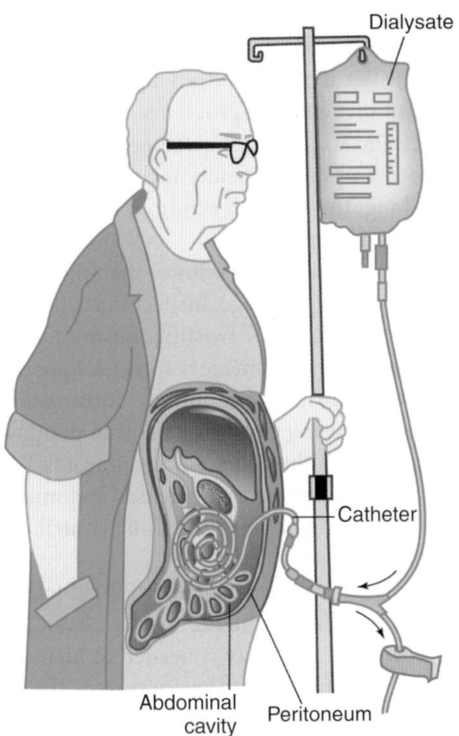

FIG. 63.10 Patient performing continuous ambulatory peritoneal dialysis (CAPD). Note that the patient can walk with this setup.

APD has advantages. It permits in-home dialysis during sleep, allowing the patient to be dialysis free during waking hours. The incidence of peritonitis is reduced with APD because fewer connections and disconnections are needed. Also, APD can be used to deliver larger volumes of dialysis solution for patients who need higher clearances.

Intermittent peritoneal dialysis (IPD) combines osmotic pressure gradients with true dialysis. The patient usually requires exchanges of 2 L of dialysate at 30- to 60-minute intervals, allowing 15 to 20 minutes of drain time. For most patients, 30 to 40 exchanges of 2 L three times weekly are needed. IPD treatments can be automated or manual.

Complications. Complications are possible with PD, but many can be prevented with meticulous care and appropriate patient education for self-management. Problems and complications are more common when evidence-based guidelines for catheter care are not followed.

Peritonitis is the major complication of PD, most commonly caused by connection site contamination. To prevent peritonitis, use meticulous sterile technique when caring for the PD catheter and when connecting and disconnecting dialysate bags. See the Best Practice for Patient Safety & Quality Care: Caring for the Patient With a Peritoneal Dialysis Catheter box.

Pain during the inflow of dialysate is common when patients are first started on PD therapy. Usually this pain no longer occurs after a week or two of PD. Cold dialysate increases discomfort. Warm the dialysate bags before instillation by using a heating pad to wrap the bag or by using the warming chamber of the automated cycling machine. *Microwave ovens are **not** recommended for warming dialysate.*

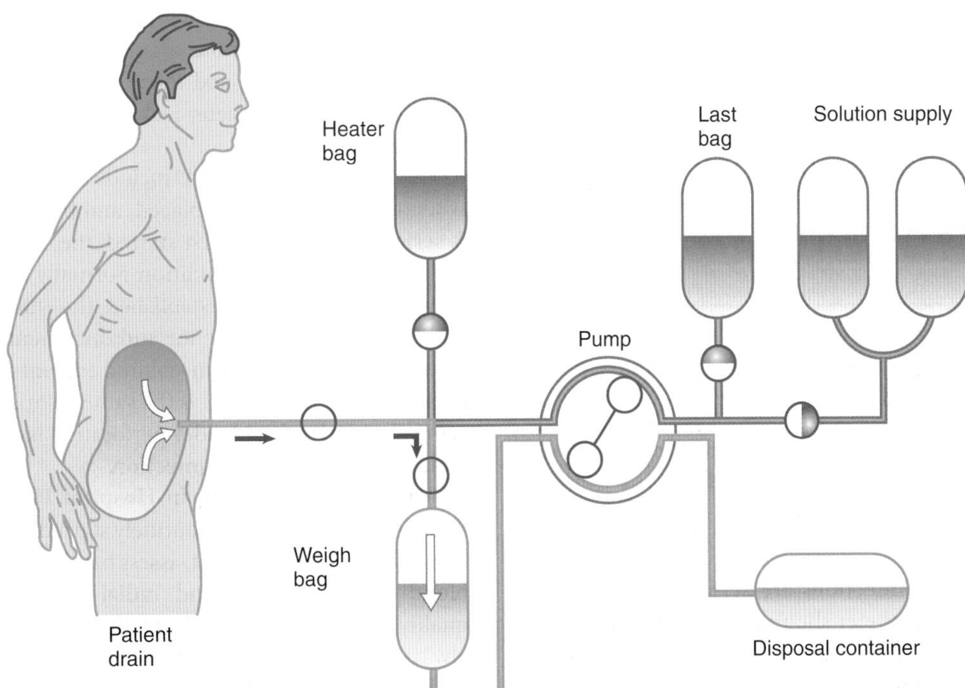

FIG. 63.11 Peritoneal dialysis machine circuit in automated peritoneal dialysis (APD).

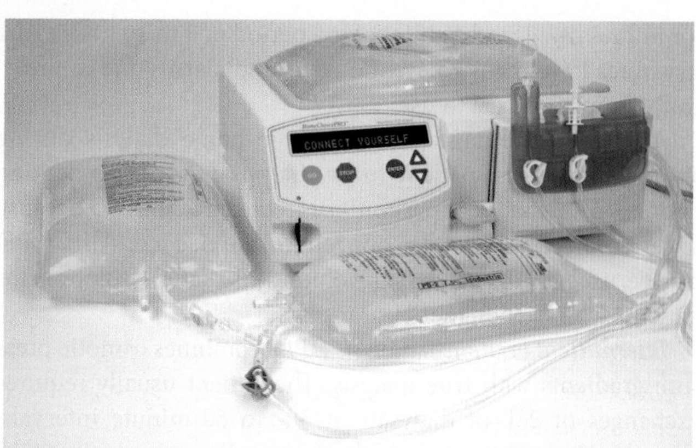

FIG. 63.12 Cycler machine for automated peritoneal dialysis at home. (Courtesy Baxter International, Inc., Deerfield, IL.)

BEST PRACTICE FOR PATIENT SAFETY & QUALITY CARE QSEN

Caring for the Patient With a Peritoneal Dialysis Catheter

- Mask yourself and your patient. Wash your hands.
- Put on sterile gloves. Remove the old dressing. Remove the contaminated gloves.
- Assess the area for signs of infection, such as swelling, redness, or discharge around the catheter site.
- Use aseptic technique:
  - Open the sterile field on a flat surface and place two precut 4 × 4–inch gauze pads on the field.
  - Place three cotton swabs soaked in povidone-iodine or other solution prescribed by the nephrology health care provider on the field. Put on sterile gloves.
  - Use cotton swabs to clean around the catheter site. Use a circular motion starting from the insertion site and moving away toward the abdomen. Repeat with all three swabs.
  - As an alternative (if recommended by the nephrology health care provider or clinic), cleanse the area with sterile gauze pads using soap and water. Use a circular motion starting from the insertion site and moving away toward the abdomen. Rinse thoroughly.
  - Apply precut gauze pads over the catheter site. Tape only the edges of the gauze pads.

! NURSING SAFETY PRIORITY QSEN

Action Alert

Monitor the patient to recognize indications of peritonitis (e.g., cloudy dialysate outflow (effluent), fever, abdominal tenderness, abdominal pain, general malaise, nausea, and vomiting). *Cloudy or opaque effluent is the earliest indication of peritonitis.* Examine all effluent for color and clarity to detect peritonitis early. When peritonitis is suspected, respond by sending a specimen of the dialysate outflow for culture and sensitivity study, Gram stain, and cell count to identify the infecting organism.

Exit site and tunnel infections are serious complications. The exit site from a PD catheter should be clean, dry, and without pain or inflammation. Exit-site infections (ESIs) can occur with any type of PD catheter. These infections are difficult to treat and can become chronic, leading to peritonitis, catheter failure, and hospitalization. Dialysate leakage and pulling or twisting of the catheter increase the risk for ESIs. A Gram stain and culture should be performed when exit sites have purulent drainage.

Tunnel infections occur in the path of the catheter from the skin to the cuff. Symptoms include redness, tenderness, and pain. ESIs are treated with antimicrobials. Deep cuff infections may require catheter removal.

Poor dialysate flow is often related to constipation. To prevent constipation, a bowel preparation is prescribed before placement of the PD. If prescribed, giving an enema before starting PD may also prevent flow problems. Teach patients to eat a high-fiber diet and to use stool softeners to prevent constipation. Other causes of flow difficulty include kinked or clamped connection tubing, the patient's position, fibrin clot formation, and catheter displacement.

Ensure that the drainage bag is lower than the patient's abdomen to enhance gravity drainage. Inspect the connection tubing and PD system for kinking or twisting. Ensure that clamps are open. If inflow or outflow drainage is still inadequate, reposition the patient to stimulate inflow or outflow. Turning the patient to the other side or ensuring that he or she is in good body alignment may help. Having the patient in a supine low-Fowler position reduces abdominal pressure. Increased abdominal pressure from sitting or standing or from coughing contributes to leakage at the PD catheter site.

Fibrin clot formation may occur after PD catheter placement or with peritonitis. Milking the tubing may dislodge the fibrin clot and improve flow. An x-ray is needed to identify PD catheter placement. If displacement has occurred, the nephrology health care provider repositions the PD catheter.

Dialysate leakage is seen as clear fluid coming from the catheter exit site. When dialysis is first started, small volumes of dialysate are used. It may take patients 1 to 2 weeks to tolerate a full 2-L exchange without leakage around the catheter site. Leakage occurs more often in obese patients, those with diabetes, older adults, and those on long-term steroid therapy. During periods of catheter leak, patients may require hemodialysis (HD) support.

Other complications of PD include bleeding, which is expected when the catheter is first placed, and bowel perforation, which is serious. When PD is first started, the outflow may be bloody or blood tinged. This condition normally clears within a week or two. After PD is well established, the effluent should be clear and light yellow. Observe for and document any change in the color of the outflow. Brown-colored effluent occurs with a bowel perforation. If the outflow is the same color as urine and has the same glucose level, a bladder perforation is probable. Cloudy or opaque effluent indicates infection.

Nursing Care During in-Hospital Peritoneal Dialysis. In the hospital setting, PD is routinely started and monitored by the nurse. Before the treatment, assess baseline vital signs, including blood pressure, apical and radial pulse rates, temperature, quality of respirations, and breath sounds. Weigh the patient, always on the same scale, before the procedure and at least every 24 hours while receiving treatment. Weight should be checked after a drain and before the next fill to monitor the patient's "dry weight." Baseline laboratory tests, such as electrolyte and glucose levels, are obtained before starting PD and repeated at least daily during the PD treatment.

In the hospital setting, especially with a new access, continually monitor the patient receiving PD fluid exchanges. Take and record vital signs every 15 to 30 minutes. Assess for respiratory distress, pain, or discomfort. Check the dressing around the catheter exit site every 30 minutes for wetness during the procedure. Monitor the prescribed dwell time and initiate outflow. Assess blood glucose levels in patients who absorb glucose.

Observe the outflow pattern (outflow should be a continuous stream after the clamp is completely open). Measure and record the total amount of outflow after each exchange. Maintain accurate inflow and outflow records when hourly PD exchanges are performed. When outflow is less than inflow, the difference is retained by the patient during dialysis and is counted as fluid intake. Weigh the patient daily to monitor fluid status.

NCLEX EXAMINATION CHALLENGE 63.5

Physiological Integrity

A client who performs continuous ambulatory peritoneal dialysis at home reports that the drainage (effluent) has become cloudy in the past 24 hours. What is the priority nursing action?

A. Remove the peritoneal catheter.
B. Notify the nephrology health care provider.
C. Obtain a sample of effluent for culture and sensitivity.
D. Teach the client that effluent should be clear or slightly yellow.

Kidney Transplantation. Dialysis and kidney transplant are life-sustaining *treatments* for end-stage kidney disease (ESKD). Kidney transplant is not considered a "cure." Each patient, in consultation with a nephrologist, determines which type of therapy is best suited to his or her physical condition and lifestyle. Approximately 17,107 kidney transplants take place annually in the United States. Just over 100,000 people are waiting for kidney transplants in the United States (National Kidney Foundation [NKF], 2019). The median wait time for a kidney transplant is 4 years (U.S. Renal Data System, 2019).

Candidate Selection Criteria. Candidates for transplantation have advanced kidney disease, have a reasonable life expectancy, and are medically and surgically fit to undergo the procedure. In the United States, patients can be added to the waiting list once the GFR is less than 20 mL/min/1.73 m^2. Absolute contraindications to transplant include active cancer, current infection, active psychiatric illness, active substance abuse, and nonadherence with dialysis or medical regimen (Himmelfarb & Ikizler, 2018).

Donors. Kidney donors may be living donors (related or unrelated to the patient), non–heart-beating donors (NHBDs), and cadaveric donors. The available kidneys are matched on the basis of tissue type similarity between the donor and the recipient. NHBDs are patients declared dead by cardiopulmonary criteria. Kidneys from NHBDs are removed (harvested) immediately after death in cases in which patients have previously given consent for organ donation. If immediate removal must be delayed, the organ is preserved by infusing a cool preservation solution into the abdominal aorta after death is declared and until surgery can be performed.

Organs from living donors have the highest rate of graft survival due to healthier donors, shorter cold ischemia times, and less ischemia-reperfusion injury. Patients who are able to find compatible kidney donors have shorter wait times for transplant. Donors must be healthy enough to undergo the procedure and be over the age of 18. Due to the benefits that have been shown, many transplant centers have relaxed their criteria and now accept donors with hypertension, obesity, and glucose intolerance, as well as a glomerular filtration rate (GFR) around the lower limits of the normal range (Himmelfarb & Ikizler, 2018). See Box 63.1.

Preoperative Care. Many issues related to patient health and the actual transplant procedure must be addressed before surgery.

Immunologic studies are needed because the major barrier to transplant success after a suitable donor kidney is available is the body's ability to reject "foreign" tissue. This immunologic process can attack the transplanted kidney and destroy it. For normal protective ***immunity*** to be overcome, tissue typing with human leukocyte antigen (HLA) studies and blood-typing are performed on all candidates. A donated kidney *must* come from a donor who is the same blood- type as the recipient. The HLAs are the main immunologic feature used to match transplant recipients with compatible donors. The more similar the antigens of the donor are to those of the recipient, the more likely the transplant will be successful, and rejection will be avoided (see Chapter 16).

Nursing actions before surgery include teaching about the procedure and care after surgery, in-depth patient assessment, coordination of diagnostic tests, and development of treatment plans. See Chapter 9 for more discussion of standard preoperative nursing care.

BOX 63.1 Never Ending Altruistic Donor Chain (NEAD)

Kidney transplants improve survival rates and lower costs compared with dialysis. The highest survival rates occur in living donor transplants (Himmelfarb & Ikizler, 2018). There are times when a patient needing a transplant has a willing donor who is not compatible and is not able to donate. Previously the patient would have had to wait until another donor was found, and the person who was willing to donate would have been denied. Fig. 63.13 shows an example of a paired exchange kidney donation, which is one option when a recipient has a donor that is not compatible.

Some transplant centers are now using Never Ending Altruistic Donor Chains (NEAD chains) that match donors with recipients. A NEAD chain begins with one nondirected donor. The nondirected donor gives to a person who has a willing but incompatible donor. That willing donor gives to the next person waiting with whom he or she is compatible, so that each living donor is giving to a stranger. The chain is kept going for as long as possible. For example, if a patient's spouse wanted to donate a kidney but was not compatible, the spouse would be matched with a compatible recipient and the patient would be matched with an acceptable donor. The NEAD chain allows for people to donate to help a specific person without having to be compatible. This simple initiative is improving countless lives (NKF, 2019).

The patient usually requires dialysis within 24 hours of the surgery and often receives a blood transfusion before surgery. Usually blood from the kidney donor is transfused into the recipient. This procedure increases graft survival of organs from living related donors (LRDs).

Operative Procedures. The donor nephrectomy procedure varies depending on whether the donor is a non–heart-beating donor (NHBD), cadaveric donor, or living donor. The NHBD or cadaveric donor nephrectomy is a sterile autopsy procedure performed in the operating room. All arterial and venous vessels and a long piece of ureter are preserved. After removal, the kidneys are preserved until time for implantation into the recipient. The technique for kidney removal from living donors is a laparoscopic procedure. Donors need postoperative nursing care and support for the psychological adjustment to loss of a body part.

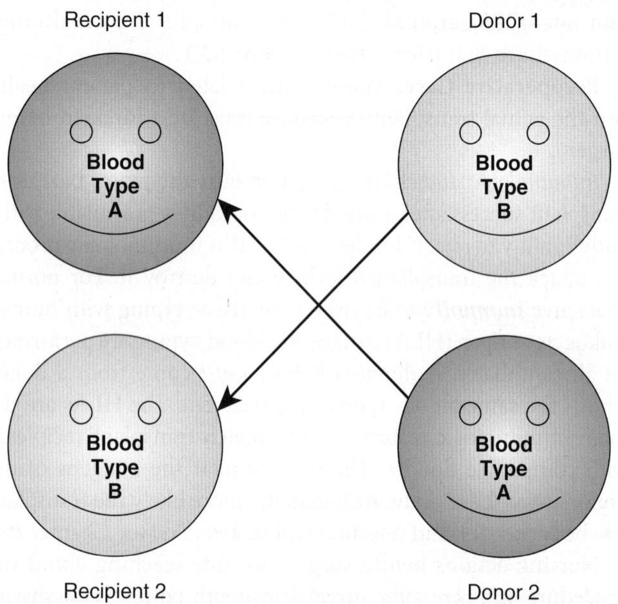

FIG. 63.13 Example of a paired exchange kidney donation. *Donor 1* is related to or acquainted with *recipient 1* and has agreed to donate a kidney but is not a blood-type or tissue-type match with *recipient 1. Donor 1* is compatible with *recipient 2* and agrees to donate a kidney to *recipient 2* if *donor 2* agrees to donate a kidney to *recipient 1 with confirmed compatibility to recipient 1.*

Transplantation surgery usually takes several hours. The new kidney is placed in the right or left anterior iliac fossa (Fig. 63.14) instead of the usual kidney position. This placement allows easier connection of the ureter and the renal artery and vein. It also allows for easier kidney palpation. The recipient's own failed kidneys are not removed unless chronic kidney infection is present or, as in the case of polycystic kidney disease, the nonfunctioning, enlarged kidneys cause pain. After surgery, the patient is taken to the postanesthesia care unit and then, when stable, to a designated unit in the transplant center or to a critical care unit.

Postoperative Care. Care of the recipient after surgery requires nurses to be knowledgeable about the expected responses and potential complications. Nursing care includes ongoing physical assessment, especially evaluation of kidney function. The most common complications occurring in patients after kidney transplant are rejection and infection (Tran & Miniard, 2017). Drug therapy used to prevent tissue rejection reduces ***immunity,*** impairs healing, and increases the risk for infection.

Urologic management is essential to graft success. A urinary catheter is placed for accurate measurements of urine output and decompression of the bladder. Decompression prevents stretch on sutures and ureter attachment sites on the bladder.

Assess urine output at least hourly during the first 48 hours. An abrupt decrease in urine output (see Table 63.2) may indicate complications such as rejection, acute kidney injury (AKI), thrombosis, or obstruction. Examine the urine color. The urine is pink and bloody right after surgery and gradually returns to normal over several days to several weeks, depending on kidney function. Obtain daily urine specimens for urinalysis, glucose measurement, the presence of acetone, specific gravity measurement, and culture (if needed).

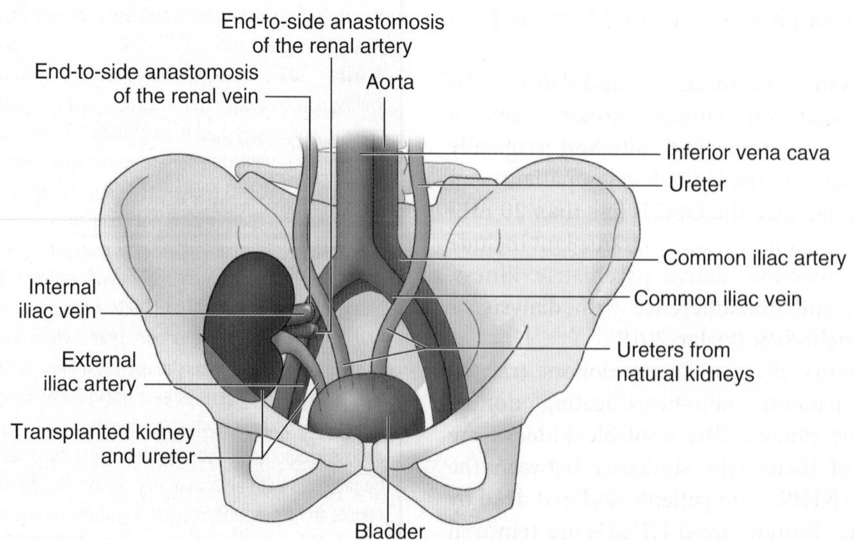

FIG. 63.14 Placement of a transplanted kidney in the right iliac fossa.

Occasionally, continuous bladder irrigation is prescribed to decrease blood clot formation, which could increase pressure in the bladder and endanger the graft. Perform routine catheter care, according to agency policy, to reduce catheter-associated urinary tract infection (CAUTI). The catheter is removed as soon as possible to avoid infection, usually 3 to 5 days after surgery. After surgery, the function of the transplanted kidney (graft) can result in either oliguria or diuresis. Oliguria may occur as a result of ischemia and acute kidney injury (AKI), rejection, or other complications. To increase urine output, the nephrology health care provider may prescribe diuretics and osmotic agents. Closely monitor the patient's fluid status because fluid overload can cause hypertension, heart failure (HF), and pulmonary edema. Evaluate his or her fluid status by weighing daily, measuring blood pressure every 2 to 4 hours, and measuring intake and output.

Instead of oliguria, the patient may have diuresis, especially with a kidney from a living related donor (LRD). Monitor intake and output and observe for disruptions of ***fluid and electrolyte balance,*** such as low potassium and sodium levels. Excessive diuresis may cause hypotension.

! NURSING SAFETY PRIORITY QSEN

Critical Rescue

Monitor the patient to recognize hypotension. If hypotension or excessive diuresis (e.g., unanticipated urine output 500 to 1000 mL greater than intake over 12 to 24 hours or other goal for intake and output) is present, respond by notifying the nephrology health care provider because hypotension reduces ***perfusion*** and oxygen to the new kidney, threatening graft survival.

Complications. Many complications are possible after kidney transplantation. Early detection and intervention improve the chances for graft survival.

Rejection is the most serious complication of transplantation and is the leading cause of graft loss. A reaction occurs between the tissues of the transplanted kidney and the antibodies and cytotoxic T-cells in the recipient's blood. These substances treat the new kidney as a foreign invader and cause tissue destruction, thrombosis, and eventual kidney necrosis.

The three types of rejection are hyperacute, acute, and chronic. Acute rejection is the most common type with kidney transplants. It is treated with increased immunosuppressive therapy and often can be reversed. Rejection is diagnosed by symptoms, a CT or renal scan, and kidney biopsy. Table 63.13 lists the features of the three types of rejection. Chapter 16 discusses their causes and treatment.

Ischemia from delayed transplantation following harvesting can contribute to acute kidney injury (AKI). Newly transplanted patients with AKI may need dialysis until adequate urine output returns and the blood urea nitrogen (BUN) and creatinine levels normalize. Biopsy can be used to determine if oliguria is the result of AKI or rejection.

Thrombosis of the major renal blood vessels may occur during the first 2 to 3 days after the transplant. A sudden decrease in urine output may signal impaired ***perfusion*** resulting from thrombosis. Ultrasound of the kidney may show decreased or absent blood supply. Emergency surgery is required to prevent ischemic damage or graft loss.

TABLE 63.13 Comparison of Hyperacute, Acute, and Chronic Posttransplant Rejection

Hyperacute Rejection	Acute Rejection	Chronic Rejection
Onset		
Within 48 hr after surgery	1 wk to any time after surgery; occurs over days to weeks	Occurs gradually during a period of months to years
Signs and Symptoms		
Increased temperature Increased blood pressure Pain at transplant site	Oliguria or anuria Temperature over 100°F (37.8°C) Increased blood pressure Enlarged, tender kidney Lethargy Elevated serum creatinine, BUN, potassium levels Fluid retention	Gradual increase in BUN and serum creatinine levels Fluid retention Changes in serum electrolyte levels Fatigue
Treatment		
Immediate removal of the transplanted kidney	Increased doses of immunosuppressive drugs	Conservative management until dialysis required

BUN, Blood urea nitrogen.

Renal artery stenosis may result in hypertension. Other signs include a bruit over the artery anastomosis site and decreased kidney function. A CT or renal scan can quantify the ***perfusion*** to the kidney. The involved artery may be repaired surgically or by balloon angioplasty in the radiology department. The decision to perform a balloon repair is determined by the amount of healing time after the surgery.

Other vascular problems include vascular leakage or thrombosis, both of which require an emergency transplant nephrectomy.

Other complications may involve the surgical wound or urinary tract. Wound problems, such as hematomas, abscesses, and lymphoceles (cysts containing lymph fluid), increase the risk for infection and exert pressure on the new kidney. Infection from reduced ***immunity*** is a major cause of death in the transplant recipient (Tran & Miniard, 2017). Prevention of infection is essential. Strict aseptic technique and handwashing must be rigorously enforced. Transplant recipients may not have the usual symptoms of infection because of the immunosuppressive therapy. Low-grade fevers, mental status changes, and vague reports of discomfort may be the only symptoms before sepsis. Always consider the possibility of infection with any patient after a kidney transplant. Urinary tract complications include ureteral leakage, fistula, or obstruction; stone formation; bladder neck contracture; and graft rupture. Surgical intervention may be required.

Immunosuppressive Drug Therapy. The success of kidney transplantation depends on changing the patient's ***immunity*** response so the new kidney is not rejected as a foreign organ. Immunosuppressive drugs protect the transplanted organ. These drugs include corticosteroids, inhibitors of T-cell proliferation and activity (azathioprine, mycophenolic acid, cyclosporine, and tacrolimus), mTOR inhibitors (to disrupt stimulatory T-cell signals), and monoclonal antibodies. Chapter 16 discusses the mechanisms of action for these agents and the associated patient responses. Patients taking these drugs are at an increased risk for death from infection. Usually, the patient receives a period of high-dose (induction) therapy followed by lower-dose maintenance immunosuppressive therapy.

Some patients do not follow the maintenance regimen correctly and are at high risk for losing the transplanted kidney. Work with the patient to ensure adherence to the drug regimen.

Despite the complexity of drug regimens following kidney transplantation, 99% of recipients of living kidneys are alive at 1 year and 95% of deceased kidney recipients are alive at 1 year. At 4 years, kidney transplant recipients have an average 70% reduction in mortality compared with patients on dialysis (Himmelfarb & Ikizler, 2018)

Although rejection is uncommon with immunosuppressive therapy, kidney transplant recipients are at risk for cardiovascular disease (the most common cause of death among kidney transplant recipients), diabetes, cancer, and infections. Prevention and management of these complications are important to maintaining the health of the transplanted kidney and prolonging patient survival. Be aware that some patient groups, including African Americans, Hispanic Americans, and Native Americans, have a greater incidence of graft failure and systemic complications (especially cardiovascular disease) after transplantation.

! NURSING SAFETY PRIORITY (QSEN)

Action Alert

Teach patients and families about the importance of adhering to the antirejection drug regimen to prevent transplant rejection.

Care Coordination and Transition Management

Home Care Management. Because of the complex nature of CKD, its progressive course, and many treatment options, a case manager is helpful in planning, coordinating, and evaluating care. As kidney disease progresses, the patient is seen by a nephrologist or nephrology nurse practitioner regularly. Together with the registered dietitian nutritionist and social worker, evaluate the home environment and determine equipment needs before discharge. Once the patient is discharged, nephrology home care nurses direct care and monitor progress.

Provide health teaching about the diet in kidney disease and the progression of disease. As CKD approaches end-stage kidney disease (ESKD), treatment with hemodialysis (HD), peritoneal dialysis (PD), or transplantation is selected. For each form of treatment, the patient and partner must learn about the procedures and consider personal lifestyle, support systems, and methods of coping. Decision making about treatment type or even whether to pursue treatment is difficult for patients and families. Provide information and emotional support to help patients with these decisions.

Teach patients who select hemodialysis (HD) about the machine and vascular access care. If in-home HD is selected, preparations are needed for the appropriate equipment, including a water-treatment system. A nephrology nurse is essential for a successful transition to at-home HD to teach the patient and monitor treatment and care. This nurse performs a home care visit before discharge to coordinate equipment setup. Family members must be available to respond to alarms during treatment. Nocturnal HD is a growing modality, and additional safety considerations must be addressed, including a plan for treatment discontinuation or generator backup during power outages. Regardless of whether the treatment occurs at home or in a center, promote independence through teaching and best practices in self-management.

The patient receiving PD needs extensive training in the procedure and help in obtaining equipment and the many supplies needed. A nephrology nurse assesses patients, monitors vital signs, assesses adherence with drug and diet regimens, and monitors for indications of peritonitis.

The nurse plays a vital role in the long-term care of the patient with a kidney transplant by facilitating acceptance and understanding of the antirejection drug regimen as a part of daily life. Carefully monitor patients for indications of graft rejection and for complications, such as infection. See the Focused Assessment: The Patient After Kidney Transplant box for care of the patient following kidney transplant.

Self-Management Education. Instruct patients and family members in all aspects of nutrition therapy, drug therapy, and complications. Teach them to report complications, such as fluid overload and infection. When a patient has a specific form of therapy, such as dialysis or transplantation, focus teaching on the chosen type of intervention. Assess the need for immunizations and request a prescription to administer needed ones before transplantation (Tran & Miniard, 2017).

Hemodialysis (HD) is the most complex form of therapy for the patient and family to understand. Even if patients receive HD in a dialysis center instead of at home, they are expected to have some knowledge of the process. Teach the patient or a family member to care for the vascular access and to report signs of infection and clotting. Teaching also includes instructing the patient to assess daily for a bruit and thrill in the vascular access. Those who plan to have in-home HD will need a partner. Both the patient and the partner must be taught the entire process of HD and must be able to perform it independently before the patient is discharged.

Peritoneal dialysis (PD) involves extensive health teaching for the patient and family. Emphasize sterile technique because peritonitis is the most common complication of PD. Instruct patients to report any symptoms of peritonitis, especially cloudy effluent and abdominal pain. If peritonitis develops, teach patients how to give themselves antibiotics by the intraperitoneal (IP) route. Stress the importance of completing the antibiotic regimen. Remind patients that repeated episodes of

FOCUSED ASSESSMENT

The Patient After Kidney Transplant

Assess cardiovascular and respiratory status, including:
- Vital signs, with special attention to blood pressure
- Presence of S_3 or pericardial friction rub
- Presence of chest pain
- Presence of edema (periorbital, pretibial, sacral)
- Jugular vein distention
- Presence of dyspnea
- Presence of crackles, beginning at the lung bases and extending upward

Assess nutritional status, including:
- Weight gain or loss
- Presence of anorexia, nausea, or vomiting

Assess kidney status, including:
- Amount, frequency, and appearance of urine (in nonanuric patients)
- Presence of bone pain
- Presence of hyperglycemia secondary to diabetes

Assess hematologic status, including:
- Presence of petechiae, purpura, ecchymosis
- Presence of fatigue or shortness of breath

Assess GI status, including:
- Presence of stomatitis
- Presence of melena

Assess integumentary status, including:
- Skin integrity
- Presence of pruritus
- Presence of skin discoloration

Assess neurologic status, including:
- Changes in mental status
- Presence of seizure activity
- Presence of sensory changes
- Presence of lower extremity weakness

Assess laboratory data, including:
- BUN
- Serum creatinine
- Creatinine clearance
- CBC
- Electrolytes

Assess psychosocial status, including:
- Presence of anxiety
- Presence of maladaptive behavior

BUN, Blood urea nitrogen; *CBC,* complete blood count.

peritonitis can reduce the effectiveness of PD, which may result in the transfer to HD.

The patient receiving a kidney transplant also needs extensive health teaching. Provide instruction about drug regimens, home monitoring, immunosuppression, symptoms of rejection, infection, and prescribed changes in the diet and activity level.

Psychosocial Preparation. In collaboration with the patient's mental health professional or counselor, provide psychosocial support for the patient and family. Help the patient adjust to the diagnosis of kidney failure and eventually accept the treatment regimens.

Many patients view dialysis as a cure instead of lifelong management. For many patients, reduction of uremic symptoms and improved ***elimination*** in the first weeks after starting dialysis treatment create a sense of well-being (the "honeymoon" period). They feel better physically, and their mood may be happy and hopeful. At this time they tend to overlook the discomfort and inconvenience of dialysis. Use this time to begin health teaching. Stress that although symptoms are reduced, they should not expect a complete return to the previous state of well-being before ESKD.

Many patients become discouraged during the first year of treatment. This mood state may last a few months to a year or longer. The difficulties of incorporating dialysis into daily life are staggering, and patients may become depressed as problems occur. They may struggle with the idea of having to be permanently dependent on a disruptive therapy. Patients may feel helpless and dependent. Some patients may deny the need for dialysis or may not adhere to drug therapy and diet restrictions. Monitor any behaviors that may contribute to nonadherence and suggest psychiatric referrals. Help the patient and family focus on the positive aspects of the treatments. Continue health education with patients as active participants and decision makers.

Most patients with CKD eventually enter a phase of acceptance or resignation. Each patient reacts differently. To make this long-term adaptation, he or she must adjust to continuous change. Concerns depend on the patient's health and specific treatment method.

After patients have accepted or become resigned to the chronic aspect of their disease, they usually attempt to return to their previous activities. However, resuming the previous level of activity may not be possible. Help patients develop realistic expectations that allow them to lead active, productive lives.

Health Care Resources. Professionals from many disciplines are resources for the patient with ESKD. Home care nurses monitor the patient's status and evaluate maintenance of the prescribed treatment regimen (HD or PD). Social services are often involved because of the complex process of applying for financial aid to pay for the required medical care. A physical therapist may be beneficial in helping to improve the patient's functional health. A registered dietitian nutritionist can help the patient and family members understand special dietary needs. A psychiatric evaluation may be needed if depressive symptoms are present. Pharmacists provide invaluable insight and teaching about drug therapy and adjustments to meet outcomes. Clergy and pastoral care specialists offer spiritual support.

Patients with CKD are routinely followed by a nephrologist. Organizations such as the National Kidney Foundation (NKF), the American Kidney Fund, and the American Association of Kidney Patients (AAKP) may be helpful to patients and families.

◆ **Evaluation: Evaluate Outcomes.** Evaluate the care of the patient with CKD based on the identified priority problems. The expected outcomes are that with appropriate management the patient should:
- Achieve and maintain appropriate fluid and electrolyte balance
- Maintain an adequate nutrition status
- Avoid infection at the vascular access site
- Use effective coping strategies
- Prevent or slow systemic complications of CKD, including osteodystrophy
- Report an absence of physical signs of anxiety or depression

CLINICAL JUDGMENT CHALLENGE 63.1

Patient-Centered Care

The nurse is performing an assessment in the outpatient clinic on a 47-year-old male client who was diagnosed with stage 4 chronic kidney disease (CKD) 4 months ago. The client had an arteriovenous fistula implanted 2 months ago. He has been undergoing hemodialysis for the last 6 weeks. However, he reports missing the last two dialysis appointments because he was "just too tired to go." The client reports that he cannot afford his medications and that following his new diet is too hard and costly. Current assessment: temperature, 102.2°F; blood pressure, 188/90 mm Hg; respirations, 28 breaths/min; and heart rate, 89 beats/min. His oxygen saturation is 88% on room air, and crackles are noted in bibasilar lung fields. He reports feeling very anxious and states, "It's all my fault that this is happening." Current labs include potassium, 5.4 mEq/L; sodium, 142 mEq/L; magnesium, 2.1 mEq/L; and WBCs, 22,000 mm^3.

1. **Recognize Cues:** What assessment information in this client situation is the most important and immediate concern for the nurse? (Hint: Identify the **relevant** information *first* to determine what is most important.)
2. **Analyze Cues:** What client conditions are consistent with the **most relevant** information? (Hint: Think about priority collaborative problems that support and contradict the information presented in this situation.)
3. **Prioritize Hypotheses:** Which possibilities or explanations are **most likely** to be present in this client situation? Which possibilities or explanations are the most serious? (Hint: Consider all possibilities and determine their urgency and risk for this client.)
4. **Generate Solutions:** What actions would most likely achieve the desired outcomes for this client? Which actions should be **avoided** or are **potentially harmful**? (Hint: Determine the desired outcomes first to decide which interventions are appropriate and those that should be avoided.)
5. **Take Action:** Which actions are the most appropriate and how should they be implemented? In what **priority order** should they be implemented? (Hint: Consider health teaching, documentation, requested health care provider orders or prescriptions, nursing skills, collaboration with or referral to health team members, etc.)
6. **Evaluate Outcomes:** What client assessment would indicate that the nurse's actions were **effective**? (Hint: Think about signs that would indicate an improvement, decline, or unchanged client condition.)

GET READY FOR THE NEXT-GENERATION NCLEX® EXAMINATION!

Key Points

Review these Key Points for each NCLEX Examination Client Needs Category.

Safe and Effective Care Environment

- Use sterile technique when initiating and providing kidney replacement therapy. **QSEN: Safety**
- Implement fall precautions and consider physical therapy referral for patients with CKD osteodystrophy to prevent fractures. **QSEN: Safety**
- Use skin protective measures to reduce injury and pressure injury in patients with CKD. **QSEN: Safety**
- Alert health care providers to patient assessments that indicate hypotension, dehydration, or hypovolemia to avoid inadequate kidney ***perfusion.*** **QSEN: Teamwork and Collaboration**
- Avoid taking blood pressure measurements or drawing blood from an arm with a vascular access. **QSEN: Safety**
- Do not use a kidney replacement vascular access device to give IV fluids. **QSEN: Safety**

Health Promotion and Maintenance

- Encourage patients with AKI, CKD, or end-stage kidney disease (ESKD) to follow fluid and dietary restrictions **QSEN: Evidence-Based Practice**
- Teach patients the expected side effects, any adverse reactions to prescribed drugs, and when to contact the prescriber. **QSEN: Safety**
- Teach patients using peritoneal dialysis the early signs and symptoms of peritonitis. **QSEN: Patient-Centered Care**
- Teach patients receiving immunosuppressive therapy for kidney transplantation to assess themselves daily for fever, general malaise, and nausea or vomiting, as well as changes in urine output and weight gain that indicate new fluid retention. **QSEN: Patient-Centered Care**

Psychosocial Integrity

- Allow patients to express concerns about the disruption of lifestyle and considerations for end-of-life care as a result of kidney failure. **QSEN: Patient-Centered Care**
- Use language and terminology that is understandable for the patient. **QSEN: Patient-Centered Care**
- Assess the patient for anxiety, depression, and nonacceptance of the diagnosis or treatment plan. **QSEN: Patient-Centered Care**
- Refer patients to community resources and support groups. **QSEN: Informatics**

Physiological Integrity

- Report immediately any condition that obstructs urine flow. **QSEN: Safety**
- Collaborate with the RDN to teach patients about dietary needs. **QSEN: Teamwork and Collaboration**
- Inform the primary health care provider immediately about hemodynamic instability, change in cognition, signs of infection, newly abnormal serum electrolytes, and urine output less than 0.5 mL/kg/hr for more than 2 to 4 hours (unless the patient is oliguric or anuric from ESKD). **QSEN: Teamwork and Collaboration**
- Teach patients in the early stages of CKD the symptoms of dehydration. **QSEN: Patient-Centered Care**
- Evaluate the patient's laboratory values, especially the metabolic panel, trends in serum creatinine, GFR, and albumin-to-creatinine ratio to assess the status of kidney problems, and communicate concerning changes to the interprofessional team. **QSEN: Teamwork and Collaboration**
- Teach patients in the later stages of CKD the indications of fluid overload and hyperkalemia. **QSEN: Patient-Centered Care**
- Avoid all invasive procedures in the 4 to 6 hours following hemodialysis. **QSEN: Evidence-Based Practice**

MASTERY QUESTIONS

1. Which client will the nurse identify as at risk for acute kidney injury? Select all that apply.
   A. 68-year-old male with diabetes mellitus
   B. 16-year-old male football player in preseason practice
   C. 27-year-old female recovering from shock following a car accident
   D. 52-year-old male with newly diagnosed hypertension
   E. 30-year-old female in intensive care receiving multiple intravenous antibiotics
2. The nurse is providing discharge teaching to a client recovering from kidney transplantation. Which client statement indicates understanding?
   A. "I can stop my medications when my kidney function returns to normal."
   B. "If my urine output decreases, I will increase my fluids."
   C. "The antirejection medications will be taken for life."
   D. "I will drink 8 ounces (236 mL) of water with my medications."
3. A client with a recently created vascular access for hemodialysis is being discharged. Which discharge teaching will the nurse include?
   A. Do not allow blood pressure measurements in the affected arm.
   B. Elevate the affected arm, allowing for total rest of the extremity.
   C. Assess for a bruit in the affected arm on a daily basis.
   D. Sleep on the affected side to protect the access device.

REFERENCES

Asterisk (*) indicates a classic or definitive work on this subject.

Brown, R. M., & Semler, M. W. (2019). Fluid management in sepsis. *Journal of Intensive Care Medicine, 34*(5), 364–373. https://doi.org/10.1177/0885066618784861.

Burchum, J., & Rosenthal, L. (2019). *Lehne's pharmacology for nursing care* (10th ed.). St. Louis: Elsevier.

Centers for Disease Control and Prevention. (2019). *Chronic kidney disease in the United States, 2019.* Atlanta, GA: US Department of Health and Human Services, Centers for Disease Control and Prevention.

Ferri, F. (2020). *Ferri's clinical advisor 2020, five books in one.* St Louis, MO: Elsevier.

Fuhrman, D. Y. -G. (2018). Acute kidney injury epidemiology, risk factors, and outcomes in critically ill patients 16–25 years of age treated in an adult intensive care unit. *Annals of Intensive Care,* 26–34.

Gilbert, S., & Weiner, D. (2018). *National kidney Foundation primer on kidney diseases* (7th ed.). St. Louis, MO: Elsevier.

Hain, D. (2015). Where's the evidence? Care coordination for adults with chronic kidney disease. *Nephrology Nursing Journal, 42*(1), 77–82.

Himmelfarb, J., & Ikizler, T. A. (2018). *Chronic kidney disease, dialysis and transplantation* (4th ed.). St. Louis: Elsevier.

Honicker, T., & Holt, K. (2016). Contrast-induced acute kidney injury: Comparison of preventive therapies. (2016). *Nephrology Nursing Journal, 43*(2), 109–116.

Jarvis, C., & Eckhardt, A. (2020). *Jarvis physical examinations and health assessment* (8th ed.). St. Louis, MO: Elsevier.

Johnson, R., Feehally, J., Floege, J., & Tonelli, M. (2019). *Comprehensive clinical nephrology* (6th ed.).

*Kidney Disease. (2012). *Improving Global outcomes (KDIGO) acute kidney injury work group. KDIGO clinical practice guideline for acute kidney injury. Kidney inter* (Vol. 2.) (pp. 1–138). https://kdigo.org/wp-content/uploads/2016/10/KDIGO-2012-AKI-Guideline-English.pdf.

Kidney Foundation of Canada. (2018). *Facing the Facts, 2018.* Retrieved from: https://www.kidney.ca/file/Facing-the-Facts-2018.pdf.

Lambert, P., Chasson, K., Horton, S., Petrin, C., Marshall, E., Bowdon, S., et al. (2017). Reducing acute kidney injury due to contrast material: How nurses can improve patient safety. *Critical Care Nurse, 37*(1), 13–26.

Lotfaliany, M. B. (2018). Depression and chronic diseases: Co-occurrence and communality of risk factors. *Journal of Affective Disorders,* 461–468.

McCance, K., Huether, S., Brashers, V., & Rote, N. (2019). *Pathophysiology: The biologic basis for disease in adults and children* (8th ed.). St. Louis: Elsevier.

Moore, P. H. (2018). Management of acute kidney injury: Core Curriculum 2018. *American Journal of Kidney Diseases,* 136–148.

National Kidney Foundation. (2019). Organ Donation And Transplantation Statistics. Retrieved from National Kidney Foundation: https://www.kidney.org/news/newsroom/factsheets/Organ-Donation-and-Transplantation-Stats

Norton, J., Newman, M., Romancito, G., Mahooty, S., Kuracina, T., & Narva, A. (2017a). Improving outcomes for patients with chronic kidney disease: Part 1. *American Journal of Nursing, 117*(2), 22–32.

Norton, J., Newman, M., Romancito, G., Mahooty, S., Kuracina, T., & Narva, A. (2017b). Improving outcomes for patients with chronic kidney disease: Part 2. *American Journal of Nursing, 117*(3), 26–35.

Pagana, K., & Pagana, T. (2018). *Mosby's manual of diagnostic and laboratory tests* (6th ed.). St. Louis: Elsevier.

Pavkov, M. E., Harding, J. L., & Burrows, N. R. (2018). Trends in hospitalizations for acute kidney injury — United States, 2000–2014. *MMWR Morb Mortal Wkly Rep, 67,* 289–293. https://doi.org/10.15585/mmwr.mm6710a2external icon.

Ronco, C., Bellomo, R., Kellum, J., & Ricci, Z. (2019). *Critical care nephrology* (3rd ed.). St. Louis: Elsevier.

Schell-Chaple, H. (2017). Continuous renal replacement therapy update: An emphasis on safe and high-quality care. *AACN Advanced Critical Care, 28*(1), 31–40.

Tran, A., & Miniard, J. (2017). Preventing infection after renal transplantation. *Nursing, 74*(1), 57–60.

United States Renal Data System. (2019). *USRDS annual data report: Epidemiology of kidney disease in the United States*. Bethesda, MD: National Institutes of Health, National Institute of Diabetes and Digestive and Kidney Diseases. 2019.

Woo, K. (2019). Hemodialysis access: Dialysis catheters. In A. P. Sidawy (Ed.), *Rutherford's vascular surgery and Endovascular therapy* (pp. 2315–2323). Philadelphia: Elsevier.

64

Assessment of the Reproductive System

Cherie R. Rebar

http://evolve.elsevier.com/Iggy/

LEARNING OUTCOMES

1. Collaborate with the interprofessional team to perform a complete reproductive assessment.
2. Prioritize evidence-based care for patients having diagnostic testing affecting the reproductive system and ***sexuality.***
3. Teach evidence-based ways for adults to protect their reproductive system.
4. Explain physiologic aging changes of the reproductive system.
5. Implement nursing interventions to decrease the psychosocial impact caused by a reproductive problem.
6. Apply knowledge of anatomy and physiology, genetic risk, and principles of aging to perform a focused reproductive system assessment.
7. Use clinical judgment to document the reproductive assessment in the electronic health record.
8. Interpret assessment findings for patients with a suspected or actual reproductive problem.

KEY TERMS

amenorrhea Absence of menses.

circumcision Surgical removal of the prepuce or foreskin of the penis.

colposcopy Examination of the cervix and vagina using a colposcope, which allows three-dimensional magnification and intense illumination of epithelium with suspected disease. This procedure can locate the exact site of precancerous and malignant lesions for biopsy.

conization Removal of a cone-shaped sample of tissue.

digital 3D mammography (digital breast tomosynthesis) Breast imaging that allows the radiologist to visualize through layers or "slices" of breast tissue, similar to a CT scan.

dilation and curettage (D&C) Procedure in which tissue is removed from inside of the uterus due to abnormal bleeding or to remove pregnancy tissue after an abortion, miscarriage or childbirth.

human papillomavirus (HPV) test Test that can identify many high-risk types of HPV infection associated with the development of cervical cancer.

hysterosalpingogram an outpatient fluoroscopy procedure that uses an injection of a contrast medium to visualize the cervix, uterus, and fallopian tubes

hysteroscopy Procedure that uses a fiberoptic camera to visualize the uterus to diagnose and treat causes of abnormal bleeding.

laparoscopy Direct examination of the pelvic cavity through an endoscope.

libido Sex drive or desire.

mammography X-ray of the soft tissue of the breast.

orchitis An acute testicular inflammation resulting from trauma or infection.

Papanicolaou test (Pap test or Pap smear) A cytologic study that is effective in detecting. precancerous and cancerous cells within the female patient's cervix.

salpingitis Fallopian tube infection.

PRIORITY AND INTERRELATED CONCEPTS

The priority concepts for this chapter are:
- ***Infection***
- ***Pain***

The interrelated concept for this chapter is:
- ***Sexuality***

The nurse is often the first health care professional to assess the patient with a reproductive system health problem. These problems typically affect physical and psychosocial aspects of ***sexuality*** and are difficult for many people to discuss. Reproductive assessment should be part of every complete physical assessment. *Respect gender identity and differences in sexual orientation and practices.* A more detailed discussion of human ***sexuality*** is found in Chapter 1.

ANATOMY AND PHYSIOLOGY REVIEW

Structure and Function of the Female Reproductive System

The female reproductive system is located outside (external) and inside (internal) the body.

External Genitalia. The external female genitalia, or vulva, extends from the mons pubis to the anal opening. The mons pubis is a pad of fat that covers the symphysis pubis and protects it during coitus (sexual intercourse).

The labia majora are two vertical folds of adipose tissue that extend posteriorly from the mons pubis to the perineum. The size of the labia majora varies, depending on the amount of fatty tissue present. The skin over the labia majora is usually darker than the surrounding skin and is highly vascular. It protects inner vulval structures and enhances sexual arousal.

The labia majora surround two thinner, vertical folds of reddish epithelium called the *labia minora.* The labia minora are highly vascular and have a rich nerve supply. Emotional or physical stimulation induces marked swelling and sensitivity. Sebaceous glands in the labia minora lubricate the entrance to the vagina. The clitoris is a small, cylindric organ that is composed of erectile tissue with a high concentration of sensory nerve endings. During sexual arousal, the clitoris becomes larger and increases sensation.

The vestibule is a longitudinal area between the labia minora, the clitoris, and the vagina that contains Bartholin glands, the urethral meatus, the opening of the Skene (paraurethral) glands, the hymen, and the vaginal opening (Jarvis, 2020). The two Bartholin glands, located deeply toward the back on both sides of the vaginal opening, secrete lubrication fluid during sexual excitement. Their ductal openings are usually not visible.

The perineum is located between the vaginal opening and the anus. The skin of the perineum covers the muscles, fascia, and ligaments that support the pelvic structures.

Internal Genitalia. The internal female genitalia are shown in Fig. 64.1. The vagina is a hollow tube that extends from the vestibule to the uterus. Ovarian hormones (primarily estrogen) influence the amounts of glycogen and lubricating fluid secreted by the vaginal cells. The normal vaginal bacteria (flora) interact with the secretions to produce lactic acid and maintain an acidic pH (3.5 to 5.0) in the vagina. This acidity helps prevent infection in the vagina.

At the upper end of the vagina, the uterine cervix projects into a cup-shaped vault of thin vaginal tissue. The recessed pockets around the cervix permit palpation of the internal pelvic organs. The posterior area provides access into the peritoneal cavity for diagnostic or surgical purposes.

The *uterus* (or "womb") is a thick-walled, pear-shaped muscular organ attached to the upper end of the vagina. This inverted pear-shaped organ is located within the true pelvis, between the bladder and the rectum. The uterus is made up of the body and the cervix. The *cervix* is a short (1 inch [2.5 cm]), narrowed portion of the uterus and extends into the vagina. The surfaces of the cervix and the canal are the sites for Papanicolaou (Pap) testing. (See discussion later in this chapter.)

The *fallopian tubes* insert into the fundus of the uterus and extend laterally close to the ovaries. They provide a duct between the ovaries and the uterus for the passage of ova and sperm. In most cases, the ovum is fertilized in these tubes up to 72 hours after release.

The *ovaries* are a pair of almond-shaped organs located near the lateral walls of the upper pelvic cavity. These small organs develop and release ova, and produce estrogen and progesterone. Adequate amounts of these hormones are needed for normal female growth and development, and to maintain a pregnancy. Women are born with *oocytes,* which are germ cells involved in reproduction; these are finite in number and do not replenish throughout the lifespan. After menopause, the ovaries become smaller.

Breasts. The female breasts are a pair of mammary glands that develop in response to secretions from the hypothalamus, pituitary gland, and ovaries, and nourish an infant after birth.

Breast tissue is composed of a network of glandular and ductal tissue, fibrous tissue, and fat. The proportion of each component of breast tissue depends on genetic factors, nutrition, age, and obstetric history. The breasts are supported by ligaments that are attached to underlying muscles. They have abundant blood supply and lymph flow that drain from an extensive network toward the axillae (Fig. 64.2).

Structure and Function of the Male Reproductive System

The primary male hormone for sexual development and function is *testosterone.* Testosterone production is fairly constant in the adult male. Only a slight and gradual reduction of testosterone production occurs in the older adult male until he is in his 80s. Low testosterone levels decrease muscle mass, reduce skin elasticity, and lead to changes in sexual performance.

External Genitalia. The male reproductive system also consists of external and internal genitalia. The penis is an organ

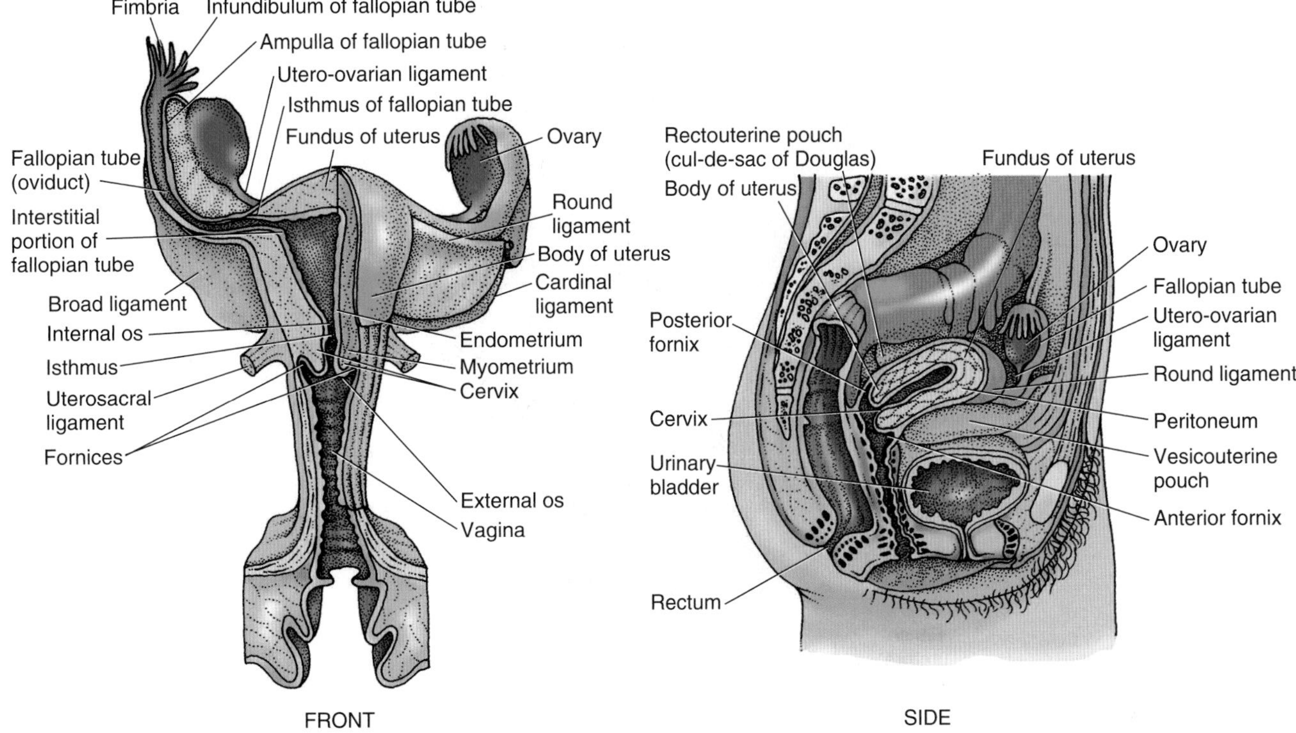

FIG. 64.1 Internal female genitalia.

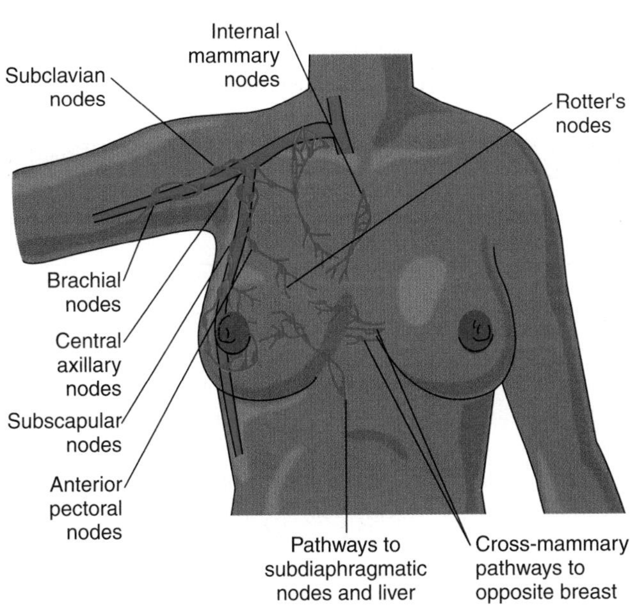

FIG. 64.2 Lymphatic drainage of the female breast.

for urination and intercourse consisting of the body or shaft and the glans penis (the distal end of the penis). The glans is the smooth end of the penis and contains the opening of the urethral meatus. Urine and semen both exit via the *urethra*. A continuation of skin covers the glans and folds to form the prepuce (foreskin). Circumcision, the surgical removal of the foreskin, is a common procedure performed in various parts of the world for cultural or religious reasons.

The scrotum is a thin-walled, fibromuscular pouch that is behind the penis and suspended below the pubic bone. This pouch protects the testes, epididymis, and vas deferens in a space that is slightly cooler than inside the abdominal cavity. The scrotal skin is darkly pigmented and contains sweat glands, sebaceous glands, and few hair follicles. It contracts with cold, exercise, tactile stimulation, and sexual excitement.

Internal Genitalia. The internal male genitalia are shown in Fig. 64.3. The major organs are the testes and prostate gland. The testes are a pair of oval organs located inside the scrotum that produce sperm and testosterone. Each testis is suspended in the scrotum by the spermatic cord, which provides blood, lymphatic, and nerve supply to the testis. Sympathetic nerve fibers are located on the arteries in the cord, and sympathetic and parasympathetic fibers are on the vas deferens. When the testes are damaged, these autonomic nerve fibers transmit signals of excruciating pain and a sensation of nausea.

The *epididymis* is the first portion of a ductal system that transports sperm from the testes to the urethra and is a site of sperm maturation. The *vas deferens,* or *ductus deferens,* is a firm, muscular tube that continues from the tail of each epididymis. The end of each vas deferens is a reservoir for sperm and tubular fluids. They merge with ducts from the seminal vesicle to form the ejaculatory ducts at the base of the prostate gland. Sperm from the vas deferens and secretions from the seminal vesicles move through the ejaculatory duct to mix with prostatic fluids in the prostatic urethra.

The *prostate gland* is a large accessory gland of the male reproductive system that can be palpated via the rectum. The gland

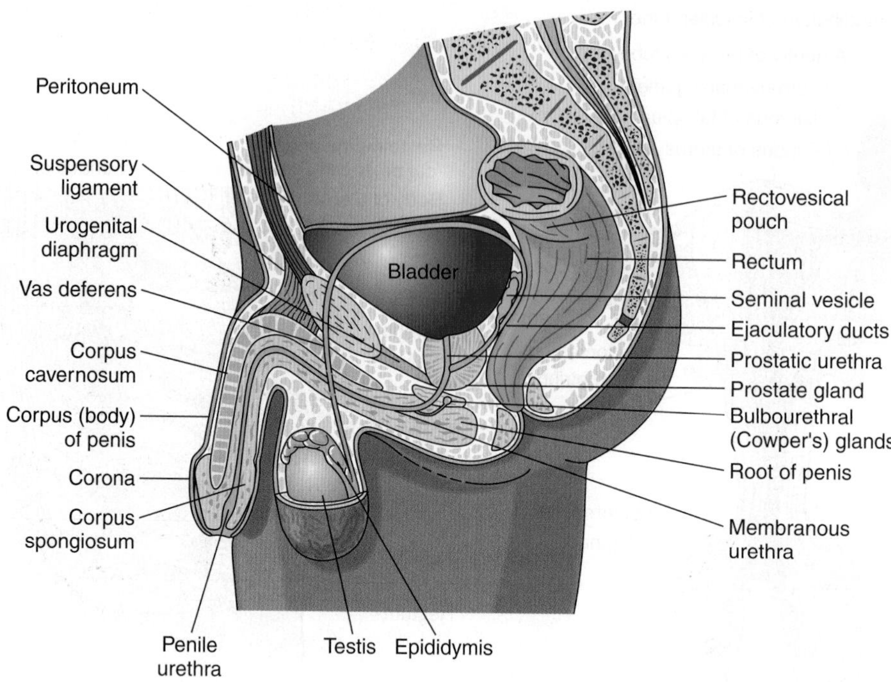

FIG. 64.3 Internal male genitalia.

secretes a milky alkaline fluid that adds bulk to the semen, enhances sperm movement, and neutralizes acidic vaginal secretions. Men older than 50 years commonly develop an enlarged prostate (benign prostatic hyperplasia [BPH]), which can cause problems such as overflow incontinence and nocturia (nighttime urination). Prostate function depends on adequate levels of testosterone.

Reproductive Changes Associated With Aging

Age brings changes to the function of the male and the female reproductive systems (see the Patient-Centered Care: Older Adult Health Considerations: Changes in the Reproductive System Related to Aging box). Teach patients the normal signs of aging, and remind them to report abnormalities to their health care provider.

PATIENT-CENTERED CARE: OLDER ADULT CONSIDERATIONS QSEN

Changes in the Reproductive System Related to Aging

Physiologic Change	Nursing Interventions	Rationales
Women		
Graying and thinning of the pubic hair Decreased size of the labia majora and clitoris	Discuss normal and expected changes (applies to all structures for both women and men).	Education helps prevent problems with body image (applies to all structures for both women and men).
Drying, smoothing, and thinning of the vaginal walls	Provide information about vaginal estrogen therapy (if desired and recommended by the health care provider) and water-soluble lubricants.	Education enables the patient to make informed decisions about the treatment of vaginal dryness, which can contribute to painful intercourse.
Decreased size of the uterus Atrophy of the endometrium Decreased size and marked convolution of the ovaries Loss of tone and elasticity of the pelvic ligaments and connective tissue	Teach Kegel exercises to strengthen pelvic muscles.	Strengthening exercises may prevent or reduce pelvic relaxation and incidences of urinary incontinence.
Increased flabbiness and fibrosis of the breasts, which hang lower on the chest wall; decreased erection of the nipples	Teach or reinforce the importance of breast self-awareness, and evidence-based recommendations for clinical breast examination and mammography based on the patient's age.	These methods can detect masses or other changes that may indicate the presence of cancer.
Men		
Graying and thinning of the pubic hair	Discuss normal and expected changes (applies to all structures for both women and men).	Education helps prevent problems with body image (applies to all structures for both women and men).
Increased drooping of the scrotum and loss of rugae	Teach or reinforce the importance of testicular self-examination (TSE).	TSE may detect changes that may indicate cancer.
Prostate enlargement, with an increased likelihood of urethral obstruction	Teach the signs of urethral obstruction and the importance of prostate cancer screening.	Education helps the patient detect enlargement or obstruction, which may indicate the presence of benign prostatic hyperplasia (BPH) or cancer.

Health Promotion and Maintenance

Many health problems of the reproductive system can be prevented through health promotion strategies and avoidance of risky lifestyle behaviors. For example, following evidence-based practices for routine preventive screenings, such as mammography and Pap tests, can detect cancer early so it can be treated with better chance for a cure. Sexually transmitted infections (STIs) and other reproductive infections can be avoided by using safer sex practices such as condoms or practicing abstinence. Teach patients about these health promotion strategies and the rationale for practicing them. Additional health promotion interventions are described under specific reproductive health problems within this unit.

ASSESSMENT: RECOGNIZE CUES

Establish a trusting relationship with the patient. Many patients find it difficult to share their reproductive history or concerns about ***sexuality.*** Provide information about why you are asking these questions, and how their answers can help inform the best approach to treatment. Respect their choice to refuse to answer questions if they state they do not wish to comment.

Patient History

Assess for chronic illnesses or surgeries that could affect reproductive function. Disorders that affect a woman's metabolism or nutrition can depress ovarian function and cause amenorrhea (absence of menses). Patients with diabetes mellitus may experience physiologic changes such as vaginal dryness or impotence. Chronic disorders of the nervous system, respiratory system, or cardiovascular system can alter the sexual response, as can psychiatric–mental health disorders.

Ask whether the patient has had infections. Pelvic inflammatory disease or a ruptured appendix followed by peritonitis in females can cause pelvic scarring and strictures or adhesions in the fallopian tubes. Salpingitis (uterine tube ***infection***) is often caused by chlamydia, a sexually transmitted infection (STI), and can result in female infertility. A history of infections or prolonged fever in males may have damaged sperm production or caused obstruction of the seminal tract, which can cause infertility.

Ask whether the patient has been treated with radiation therapy, or had prolonged use of corticosteroids, internal or external estrogen, testosterone, or chemotherapy drugs. These can all lead to reproductive system dysfunction.

Ask about childhood conditions that could have an effect on the reproductive system. A history of mumps in men may cause orchitis (painful inflammation and swelling of the testes), which can lead to testicular atrophy and (uncommonly) sterility. A history of undescended testicles can contribute to male infertility. In women, a history of untreated sexually transmitted infections can lead to infertility.

Assess general health habits, such as sleep, exercise, and diet, as the amount of body fat may be related to ovarian dysfunction in females. Determine when patients have had their last screening for reproductive concerns. Ask females about the date and result of their most recent Pap test, breast self-examination, and vulvar self-examination. Determine when male patients older than 50 years had their last prostate examination and prostate-specific antigen (PSA) test.

Document any prescribed and over-the-counter drugs, including hormones or hormone replacement therapy, the patient is taking. Certain medications can affect the reproductive system, particularly in terms of libido (sex drive) or the male patient's ability to obtain and sustain an erection. Evidence demonstrates a higher risk for adverse effects associated with taking menopausal hormone therapy (MHT) in women over the age of 60 (Martin & Barbieri, 2020). Risks are lower in younger women yet still must be recognized, particularly in women who take combination therapy including estrogen and progesterone, as MHT has been associated with cardiovascular disease and cancer (Martin & Barbieri, 2020). Inquire whether the patient takes any vitamin, mineral, or herbal supplements, as any of these can affect reproductive function.

PATIENT-CENTERED CARE: GENDER HEALTH CONSIDERATIONS QSEN

Data about sexual activity are vital parts of the patient's history. Sexual orientation and gender identity should not be assumed. Patients who are lesbian, gay, bisexual, transgender, and queer/questioning (LGBTQ) are often not fully assessed by health care professionals due to lack of education on the part of the providers of care. These patients will feel more comfortable sharing information about their reproductive health and sexual activity when approached in a caring, nonjudgmental way. Chapter 1 describes interviewing techniques that are appropriate for LGBTQ patients. Chapter 68 in this unit discusses assessment and care of transgender patients in detail.

PATIENT-CENTERED CARE: CULTURAL/ SPIRITUAL CONSIDERATIONS QSEN

Cultural, religious, and spiritual beliefs and practices influence lifestyle and ***sexuality.*** These beliefs can influence specific sexual practices, the acceptable number of sexual partners, and philosophy of contraceptive use. Be sensitive to these differences by being nonjudgmental and supportive of the patient.

Nutrition History. A nutrition history is important when assessing the reproductive system. Fatigue and low libido may occur as a result of poor diet and anemia. The American Cancer Society (ACS) estimates that 70% of uterine corpus cancers are related to overweight or obesity and lack of physical activity, rendering them preventable if people made better nutrition choices (ACS, 2019b). Ask the patient to recall his or her dietary intake for a recent 24-hour period to assess quality of nutrition.

Assess the patient's height, weight, and body mass index (BMI). The patient may be hesitant to discuss eating habits such as bingeing, purging, restricting, or excessively exercising. Teach that a certain healthy level of body fat and weight is necessary for the onset of menses and the maintenance of regular menstrual cycles. Decreased body fat results in insufficient estrogen levels.

PATIENT-CENTERED CARE: GENDER HEALTH CONSIDERATIONS QSEN

Women have special nutrition needs. Those with heavy menstrual bleeding, particularly women who have intrauterine devices, may require iron supplements. Teach women about their body's need for calcium. Although adequate calcium intake throughout life is needed, it is especially important during and after menopause to help prevent osteoporosis caused by decreased estrogen production (see Chapter 45).

Social History. Assess for alcohol, tobacco, and illicit drug use. In males, libido, sperm production, and the ability to have or sustain an erection can be affected by these substances. Females may experience alteration or cessation of the menstrual cycle. Males and females who have chronically abused drugs and/or alcohol are at higher risk for development of cancer and infectious diseases (American Addiction Centers, 2020).

Family History and Genetic Risk. The family history helps determine the patient's risk for conditions that affect reproductive function. A delayed or early development of secondary sex characteristics may be a familial pattern.

The current age and health status of family members are important. Evidence of diseases or reproductive problems in family members (e.g., diabetes, endometriosis, reproductive cancer) can be helpful in understanding a patient's current health status, or risk for development of certain conditions. For example, daughters of women who were given diethylstilbestrol (DES) to control bleeding during pregnancy are at increased risk for fertility concerns, adverse pregnancy outcomes, reproductive cancers, and breast cancer (Hatch & Karam, 2020).

Specific *BRCA1* and *BRCA2* gene mutations increase the overall risk for breast or ovarian cancer (ACS, 2019d). Men with first-degree relatives (e.g., father, brother) with prostate cancer are at two to three times the risk for development of the disease than are men in the general population (American Society of Clinical Oncology, 2019).

Current Health Problems. Patients often seek medical attention due to pain, bleeding, discharge, or masses (see the Best Practice for Patient Safety & Quality Care: Assessing the Patient With Reproductive Health Problems box). ***Pain*** related to reproductive system disorders may be confused with symptoms of GI issues (e.g., abdominal discomfort) or urinary health problems (e.g., urinary frequency). Ask the patient to describe the nature of the pain, including its type, intensity, timing and location, duration, and relationship to menstrual, sexual, urinary, or GI function. Assess the factors that exacerbate (worsen) or relieve the pain. Ask about sleeping patterns and if pain or other symptoms affect the ability to get adequate rest.

Heavy menstrual *bleeding* or a lack thereof may concern the patient. The possibility of pregnancy in any sexually active woman with amenorrhea must be considered. Postmenopausal bleeding needs to be evaluated. Ask the patient to describe the amount and characteristics of any abnormal vaginal bleeding. Assess whether the bleeding occurs in relation to the menstrual cycle or menopause, intercourse, trauma, or strenuous exercise. For male patients, ask about the presence of penile bleeding. Ask any patient who has abnormal bleeding about associated symptoms, such as ***pain,*** cramping or abdominal fullness, a change in bowel habits, urinary difficulties, and weight changes.

BEST PRACTICE FOR PATIENT SAFETY & QUALITY CARE QSEN

Assessing the Patient With Reproductive Health Problems

Patient Concern	Nursing Assessment
Pain	Type, intensity, and timing of pain Location and duration of pain Factors that relieve or worsen pain Relationship to menstrual, sexual, urinary, or GI function Relationship to sleeping and rest patterns Medications taken to address the pain
Bleeding	Presence or absence of bleeding Character and amount of bleeding Relationship of bleeding to events or other factors (e.g., menstrual cycle) Onset and duration of bleeding Presence of associated symptoms, such as pain
Discharge	Amount and character of discharge Frequency with which discharge is present (e.g., 1-2 days a month, all month) Presence of genital lesions, bleeding, itching, or pain Presence of symptoms or discharge in sexual partner
Masses	Location and characteristics of mass Presence of associated symptoms, such as pain Relationship to menstrual cycle

Discharge from the male or female reproductive tract can cause irritation of the surrounding tissues, itching, ***pain,*** embarrassment, and anxiety. Ask about the amount, color, consistency, odor, and chronicity of discharge that may be present from orifices used during sexual activity. Certain drugs (e.g., antibiotics) and clothing (e.g., tight clothing, synthetic underwear fabric) may cause or worsen genital discharge. Many types of discharge are caused by STIs or other ***infection*** (see Chapter 69).

Masses in the breasts, testes, or inguinal area must be evaluated. Ask if the patient can relate the changes in character or size of masses to menstrual cycles, heavy lifting, straining, or trauma. Ask about associated symptoms such as tenderness, heaviness, ***pain,*** dimpling, and tender lymph nodes.

Physical Assessment

Assessment of the Female Reproductive System. A Papanicolaou test (Pap test or Pap smear) should be scheduled between the patient's menstrual periods so the menstrual flow does not interfere with laboratory analysis. Teach women not to douche, use vaginal medications, powders, or deodorants, or have sexual intercourse for at least 24 hours before the test, because these may interfere with test interpretation.

The American Cancer Society (ACS, 2018) advises the following schedule for Pap testing:

- Women should begin having an annual Pap test at 21 years of age.
- Women between 21 and 29 years should have a Pap test every 3 years. Human papillomavirus (HPV) testing is not to be used for screening for this age group, although it can be used as part of a follow-up for an abnormal Pap result.
- Women between ages 30 and 65 years should have just the Pap test every 3 years.
- Women older than 65 years who have had regular cervical cancer testing with normal results in the past decade, and no serious cancers in the past 20 years, do not need further Pap testing.
- Women who have had a hysterectomy can discontinue Pap tests unless the hysterectomy was done to treat precervical or cervical cancer.
- Women with a history of cancer or precancer of the cervix should speak to their health care provider for individualized recommendations for Pap and HPV testing.

Canadian guidelines are similar. General Canadian recommendations include (Choosing Wisely Canada, 2019):

- Women should begin having an annual Pap test at 21 years of age.
- Women between 21 and 29 years who are sexually active should have a Pap test every 3 years.
- Women between ages 30 and 69 years should have a Pap test every 3 years.
- Women older than 70 years who have had three previous normal Pap tests do not need further Pap testing.
- Women with risk factors such as a history of cancer, precancerous cells in the cervix, or a weakened immune system should speak to their health care provider regarding Pap recommendations.

NCLEX EXAMINATION CHALLENGE 64.1

Health Promotion and Maintenance

A 68-year-old client who has had normal Pap results for 10 years and no history of cancer asks about scheduling a Pap smear. Which nursing response is appropriate?

A. "You will need a Pap test this year."
B. "You aren't due for a Pap test until next year."
C. "You do not need to have further Pap tests at this time."
D. "You do not need a Pap test unless you are sexually active."

The nurse generalist does not perform the comprehensive female or male reproductive examination. However, you should perform a focused physical assessment related to specific concerns of the patient. The health care provider conducts a more detailed gynecologic assessment as described in the following paragraphs; the nurse generalist often assists with the examination. The examination should be performed in a room that has adequate lighting for body inspection, has comfortable temperature, and ensures privacy. Immediately before the pelvic and breast examinations, ask the patient to empty her bladder and undress completely. Drape the patient adequately to provide as much privacy as possible throughout the examination. Remove drapes only over the region being examined and replace them after that area has been assessed. Mirrors can be used to facilitate teaching if the patient desires.

The health care provider may begin with assessing the breasts (see Chapter 65) before progressing to the abdomen and pelvic examination. The patient's arms should be at her sides or relaxed over her chest to allow better relaxation of the abdominal muscles. Assessment is conducted for symmetry, shape, skin color and temperature, and presence or absence of lesions or dimpling. Help the patient lie on her back while the health care provider performs palpation of the breast tissue (and then the abdomen). If the patient wishes to perform breast self-examinations at home, provide teaching (Chapter 65).

Inspection of the external female genitalia and the pelvic examination are usually performed at the end of a head-to-toe physical assessment. The patient may be more apprehensive about these portions of the examination than about any other part. ***Pain*** or lack of privacy during previous pelvic examinations may prevent the patient from relaxing. Stay with the patient and offer reassurance and compassion during this portion of the examination.

Assist the patient into the lithotomy position, continuously being mindful of draping for privacy. Assessment of external genitalia includes visualization of the mons pubis and vulva. Be aware that removal of pubic hair and/or piercings in this area may compromise tissue integrity and facilitate ***infection.*** In preparation for the internal genitalia examination, obtain a Graves speculum for most adult patients, or a Pederson speculum (which is narrower) for patients who are younger or postmenopausal; run warm water over it and apply a dime-sized amount of water-soluble gel lubricant (Jarvis, 2020). Teach that the plastic speculum makes a loud clicking sound when it locks and unlocks, so that this does not startle the patient (Jarvis, 2020).

Other than determining pregnancy or infertility, this portion of the examination is indicated to assess:

- Menstrual irregularities
- Unexplained abdominal or vaginal ***pain***
- Vaginal discharge, itching, sores, or ***infection***
- Rape trauma or other pelvic injury
- Physical changes in the vagina, cervix, and uterus

During the speculum examination, the health care provider palpates for symptomatic and asymptomatic abdominopelvic masses, which can be of reproductive, intestinal, or urinary tract origin. Gynecologic masses, such as ovarian masses, may be further differentiated from lesions on the body of the uterus during the bimanual portion of the pelvic examination. Several samples of cells from the cervix are obtained with a small brush or spatula during the Pap test, placed on a glass slide, and sent to the laboratory for examination. Nucleic acid amplification tests are collected to test for sexually transmitted infections, and samples for HPV testing are also obtained at this time. A bimanual examination will be performed by the health care provider to palpate the internal genitalia for location, size, mobility, and the presence of masses or tenderness (Jarvis, 2020). The health care provider may also perform a rectal examination, which can demonstrate external or internal hemorrhoids, fissures, or masses.

When the examination is complete, provide the patient with a towel to remove any residual water-soluble gel. Assist her to a sitting position, and provide privacy so that she can redress.

PATIENT-CENTERED CARE: CULTURAL/ SPIRITUAL CONSIDERATIONS QSEN

A patient's personal experiences, culture, and/or spiritual beliefs may influence thoughts about ***sexuality,*** which can affect his or her ability to enjoy a satisfactory sex life. These factors may include:

- Sexual trauma or abuse inflicted during childhood or adulthood
- Punishment for masturbation
- Psychological trauma
- Cultural influences
- Concerns about sexual partners or sexual lifestyle
- Use of alcohol or street drugs

Assessment of the Male Reproductive System. Unless a male patient seeks health care for a specific problem, the health care provider may not perform a reproductive assessment, depending on the setting and the age of the patient. Like women, men may be embarrassed and anxious when the reproductive system is assessed. The patient may be concerned about ***pain,*** the developmental stage of his genitalia, or the possibility of experiencing an erection during the examination. If he does have an erection, the examiner should assure him that this is a normal response to a tactile stimulus (touch) and should continue the examination unless the patient requests to stop the assessment.

Explain each step of the assessment procedure before it is performed. The patient needs to be reassured that the health care provider will stop and change the assessment plan or technique if requested. Provide nonjudgmental support and teach relaxation techniques that can be helpful to relieve pain, especially during the rectal examination to palpate the prostate gland.

Fears may affect the patient's satisfaction with ***sexuality*** or body image. He or she may also be concerned about the potential or actual reaction of family members to reproductive health problems (see the Best Practice for Patient Safety & Quality Care: Assessing the Patient with Reproductive Health Problems box). Use nonjudgmental listening to continue development of trust between yourself and the patient, allowing the patient to openly express feelings or concerns.

Provide privacy within a well-lit environment, and have the patient undress. As with the female patient, drape the male patient adequately to provide as much privacy as possible throughout the examination. Remove drapes only as needed for examination, and replace them after that area has been assessed.

The health care provider will conduct the physical examination, which may include a breast examination. Although men are less likely to have breast cancer than women, it is important to assess for this possibility, especially if the patient has been exposed to radiation, has a high level of estrogen, or has a family history of breast cancer (National Breast Cancer Foundation, 2019). The examination is performed by the health care provider in the same manner as for a female patient.

CLINICAL JUDGMENT CHALLENGE 64.1

Evidence-Based Practice; Patient-Centered Care

The nurse is taking a history on a 54-year-old male client who has come to the health care provider's office for an annual physical. The client reports being in good health other than "a couple of bumps in my left armpit." When asked about any pain in the left arm or breast area, the client states, "sometimes that side of my chest aches. I figure it's because I've worked out too hard."

1. **Recognize Cues:** What assessment information in this client situation is the most important and immediate concern for the nurse? (Hint: Identify the **relevant** information *first* to determine what is most important.)
2. **Analyze Cues:** What client conditions are consistent with the **most relevant** information? (Hint: Think about priority collaborative problems that support and contradict the information presented in this situation.)

An examination of the external genitalia includes visualization of the pubis, penis, and scrotum. Lesions or areas where tissue integrity is compromised can be identified during this portion of the examination. The health care provider will perform palpation to determine the presence of masses or ***pain,*** and a prostate examination. If a sexually transmitted infection is suspected, swabs may be obtained at this time by the provider. When the examination is complete, provide the patient with a towel to clean himself (if needed), and privacy while he redresses.

Psychosocial Assessment

Ask about sources of support, strengths, and coping reactions to illness or dysfunction. It is not uncommon for people with reproductive concerns to feel anxiety or fear. For patients who have few support systems in place, consider referral to community groups or social services that can be of assistance.

Diagnostic Assessment

Laboratory Assessment. The Laboratory Profile: Reproductive Assessment box summarizes important laboratory tests associated with reproductive function. The Pap test, a cytologic study, is effective in detecting precancerous and cancerous cells within the female patient's cervix.

The **human papillomavirus (HPV) test** performed on cells collected from the cervix can identify many high-risk types of HPV ***infection*** associated with development of cervical cancer. This test can be done at the same time as the Pap test for women at higher risk for HPV, or as a follow-up for those who have had an abnormal Pap test result. It does not replace the Pap test because it tests for viruses that can cause cell changes in the cervix that, if not treated, could lead to cancer. Women who have normal Pap test results and no HPV infection are at very low risk for developing cervical cancer. Conversely, women with an abnormal Pap test and a positive HPV test result are at higher risk if not treated.

Other types of laboratory testing include cytologic vaginal *cultures,* which can detect bacterial, viral, fungal, and parasitic disorders. Examination of cells from the vaginal walls can evaluate estrogen balance in female patients.

Serum levels of follicle-stimulating hormone (FSH), luteinizing hormone (LH), and prolactin are helpful in the diagnosis of male and female reproductive tract disorders. Serum testing

LABORATORY PROFILE

Reproductive Assessment

Test	Normal Range for Adults	Significance of Abnormal Findings
Serum Studies		
Follicle-stimulating hormone (FSH)	*Men:* 1.42-15.4 IU/L *Women:* • Follicular phase, 1.37-9.9 IU/L • Ovulatory peak, 6.17-17.2 IU/L • Luteal phase, 1.09-9.2 IU/L • Postmenopause, 19.3-100.6 IU/L Canadian: *Men:* 1.0-10.0 IU/L *Women:* • Follicular phase, 1.37-9.9 IU/L • Ovulatory peak, 6.17-17.2 IU/L • Luteal phase, 1.09-9.2 IU/L • Postmenopause, 40-250 IU/L	Decreased levels may indicate possible infertility, anorexia nervosa, hypothalamic failure, pituitary failure. Elevations may indicate possible ovarian or testicular dysgenesis.
Luteinizing hormone (LH)	*Men:* 1.24-7.8 IU/L *Women:* • Follicular phase, 1.68-15 IU/L • Ovulatory peak, 21.9-56.6 IU/L • Luteal phase, 0.61-16.3 IUL • Postmenopause, 14.2-52.3 IU/L Canadian: *Men:* 1.0-9.0 IU/L *Women:* • Follicular phase, 2.0-10.0 IU/L • Ovulatory peak, 15.0-65.0 IU/L • Luteal phase, 1.0-12.0 IU/L • Postmenopause, 12-65 IU/L	Decreased levels may indicate possible pituitary or hypothalamic failure, anorexia nervosa (and anovulation), or malnutrition. Elevations may indicate possible ovarian or testicular dysgenesis.
Prolactin	*Men:* 3-13 ng/mL *Women:* 3-27 ng/mL Pregnant women: 20-400 ng/mL	Decreased levels may indicate possible pituitary apoplexy or pituitary destruction from tumor. Elevations may indicate possible galactorrhea, hypothyroidism, anorexia nervosa, prolactin-secreting pituitary tumor, or amenorrhea or polycystic ovarian syndrome (in women).
Estradiol	*Men:* 10-50 pg/mL *Women:* • Follicular phase, 20-350 pg/mL • Midcycle, 150-750 pg/mL • Luteal phase, 30-450 pg/mL • Postmenopause, ≤20 pg/mL	Decreased levels may indicate possible pregnancy concerns or menopause (in women), hypopituitarism, or anorexia nervosa. Elevations may indicate possible adrenal, ovarian, or testicular tumor, or normal pregnancy development (in women).
Estriol (serum)	*Men:* N/A *Nonpregnant women:* N/A Canadian: Same	Same significance as levels of estradiol in women.
Progesterone	*Men:* 10-50 ng/dL *Women:* • Follicular phase, <50 ng/dL • Luteal phase, 300-2500 ng/dL • Postmenopausal, <40 ng/dL Canadian: *Men:* 0-1.3 nmol/L *Women:* • Follicular phase, 0.3-4.8 nmol/L • Luteal phase, 8.0-89.0 nmol/L • Postmenopausal, <1.27 nmol/L	Decreased levels in women may indicate possible preeclampsia, toxemia of pregnancy, threatened abortion, placental failure, fetal death, ovarian neoplasm, ovarian hypofunction, or amenorrhea. Elevations may indicate possible hyperadrenocorticalism or adrenocortical hyperplasia. In women, elevations indicate possible ovulation, pregnancy, or luteal cysts of the ovary.

Continued

LABORATORY PROFILE—CONT'D

Test	Normal Range for Adults	Significance of Abnormal Findings
Testosterone	*Men:* 280-1080 ng/dL *Women:* <70 ng/dL Canadian: *Men:* 275-875 ng/dL *Women:* 23-875 ng/dL	Decreased levels in men may indicate possible cryptorchidism, hypogonadism, trisomy 21, or orchidectomy. Increased levels in men may indicate possible testicular, extragonadal, or adrenocortical tumor, testosterone resistance syndrome, or hyperthyroidism. Elevations in women may indicate possible adrenal or ovarian tumor, polycystic ovaries, or idiopathic hirsutism.
Prostate-specific antigen	*Men:* • 0-2.5 ng/mL = low • 2.6-10 ng/mL = slightly to moderately elevated • 10-19.9 ng/mL = moderately elevated • 20 ng/mL = significantly elevated Canadian: *Men:* 0-4 ng/mL	Elevated levels in men may indicate prostatitis, benign prostatic hyperplasia, or prostate cancer.

1 mcg, 1 microgram or 1 millionth of a gram; *1 ng,* 1 nanogram or 1 billionth of a gram; *1 pg,* 1 picogram or 1 trillionth of a gram.
N/A, Not applicable.
Data from Pagana, K.D., & Pagana, T.J. (2018). *Mosby's manual of diagnostic and laboratory tests* (6th ed.). St. Louis: Elsevier; and Pagana, K., Pagana, T., & Pike-MacDonald, S. (2019). *Mosby's Canadian manual of diagnostic and laboratory tests* (2nd ed.). Ontario, Canada, Elsevier.

can also detect estrogen, progesterone, and testosterone levels in men and women. Teach the patient that no nutrition restrictions are necessary before having these tests performed. See the Laboratory Profile: Reproductive Assessment box for normal values and the significance of abnormal findings.

Serologic studies detect antigen-antibody reactions that occur in response to foreign organisms. This form of diagnostic testing is helpful only after an ***infection*** has become well established. Serologic testing can be used in the evaluation of exposure to organisms causing syphilis, rubella, and herpes simplex virus type 2 (HSV2). Results may be read as *nonreactive, weakly reactive,* or *reactive.* A single titer is not as revealing as serial titers, which can detect the rise in antibody reactions as the body continues to fight the ***infection.***

The *prostate-specific antigen (PSA)* test is used to screen for prostate cancer in men, and to monitor the disease after treatment. Although elevated PSA levels may be associated with prostate cancer, there is variance among health care providers in interpretation of results. Levels less than 2.5 to 4.0 ng/mL may be considered normal, depending on the resource used (Hoffman, 2020; Pagana & Pagana, 2018). Certain factors such as prostatitis, acute urinary retention, recent prostate biopsy, or transurethral resection of the prostate (TURP) can cause transient rises in PSA (Hoffman, 2020).

PATIENT-CENTERED CARE: CULTURAL/ SPIRITUAL CONSIDERATIONS QSEN

African-American men are 1.6 times as likely to develop prostate cancer and twice as likely to die from it than are white men (Research on Prostate Cancer in Men of African Ancestry, 2019). For this reason, teach African-American male patients to begin prostate cancer screening at age 40.

Imaging Assessment

Mammography. Mammography is an x-ray of the soft tissue of the breast. Mammograms assess differences in the density of breast tissue. They are especially helpful in evaluating poorly defined masses, multiple masses or nodules, nipple changes or discharge, skin changes, and ***pain.*** Mammography can detect many cancers that are not palpable by physical examination. However, false-positive and false-negative readings can occur (ACS, 2019c).

In young women's breasts, there is little difference in the density between normal glandular tissue and malignant tumors, which makes the mammogram less useful for evaluation of breast masses in these patients. For this reason, annual screening mammograms are not recommended for women younger than 40 years. In older women, it is not uncommon for the amount of fatty tissue to be higher, and the fatty tissue appears lighter than cancers. Cancer and cysts may have the same density. Cysts usually have smooth borders, and cancers often have starburst-shaped margins. Organizations such as the U.S. Preventive Services Task Force, the American Cancer Society (ACS), the American College of Obstetricians and Gynecologists (ACOG), and the American College of Physicians (ACP) have different guidelines on screening for breast cancer (Centers for Disease Control and Prevention, n.d.). Teach the patient to collaborate with her health care provider to determine the timing that is right for her to have a mammogram based on her age and risk factors.

No dietary restrictions are necessary before the mammogram. Remind the patient not to use creams, lotions, powders, or deodorant on the breasts or underarms before the study because these products may be visible on the mammogram and contribute to misdiagnosis. For women who come to their appointment and have used one of these products, provide washcloths and premoistened wipes to remove the residue. If there is any possibility that the patient is pregnant, the test should be rescheduled. Explain the purpose of the study and its anticipated discomforts. The technician or assistant provides a gown and privacy for the woman to undress above the waist. Allow the patient to express concerns about the mammogram and the presence of any lumps or breast changes that she has noticed.

When performing an analog (film) mammogram, a technician positions the patient next to the x-ray machine with one

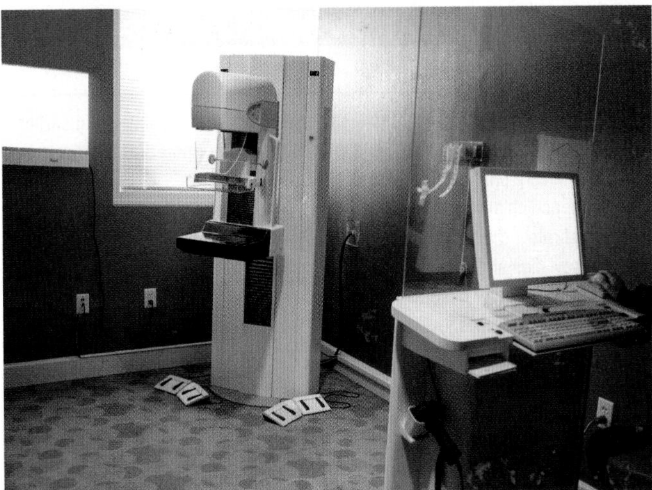

FIG. 64.4 System for digital 3D mammography, also known as digital breast tomosynthesis. (©iStock/JodiJacobson.)

breast exposed. A film plate and the platform of the machine are placed on opposite sides of the breast to be examined. The technician includes as much breast tissue as possible between the plates. The woman may experience some temporary discomfort when the breast is compressed (for about 30 seconds for each of two positions for each breast). The entire test takes less than 15 minutes. The patient usually is asked to wait until the films are reviewed in case a view needs to be repeated.

Digital imaging systems for mammography include direct radiography (DR), which is used most commonly in the United States, and computed radiography (CR). Digital mammography has been shown to have distinct advantages over analog mammography, including better resolution, the ability to detect subtle abnormalities by changing contrast and brightness of the image, and lower radiation dose (Venkataraman & Slanetz, 2020). Disadvantages include the cost of the overall system and associated higher-resolution monitors, compared to the cost of analog mammography (Venkataraman & Slanetz, 2020).

Digital 3D mammography (digital breast tomosynthesis) (Figs. 64.4 and 64.5) allows the radiologist to visualize through layers or "slices" of breast tissue, similar to a CT scan. Compared with conventional digital mammography, digital 3D mammography has been shown to increase cancer detection rates, although it does increase the radiation dose to the patient (Venkataraman & Slanetz, 2020).

Inform the patient when to expect the report of the results. Because this is a time when she may be anxious, teach or reinforce the importance of continued breast self-awareness and provide instructions as needed.

CT Scans. CT scans for reproductive system disorders involve the abdomen and the pelvis. Primary health care providers can detect and evaluate masses and identify lymphatic enlargement from metastasis. This scan can differentiate solid tissue masses from cystic or hemorrhagic structures.

MRI. MRI uses a magnetic field and radiofrequency energy to distinguish between normal and malignant tissues. MRI is used in addition to mammograms to assess for breast cancer in women who are at high risk, or for further diagnostic purposes for those who have already been diagnosed with breast cancer (ACS, 2019a). The use of MRI in evaluating patients with dense breast tissue may reduce the need for biopsy. MRI can also be used to detect pelvic tumors.

Ultrasonography. Ultrasonography (US) is a technique that is used to assess females for fibroids, cysts, ectopic pregnancy, and masses. It can be used to monitor the progress of tumor regression after medical treatment. US is also helpful in differentiating solid tumors from cysts in breast examinations. Prostate, scrotal, and rectal US can be used to detect abnormalities in these areas, such as prostate or testicular masses, varicoceles, or problems of the ejaculatory ducts, seminal vesicles and vas deferens (Pagana & Pagana, 2018).

For an external US of the abdomen, breast, or scrotum, the technician exposes the area and applies gel to the area to be scanned, which provides better transmission of sound waves from the transducer through the patient's skin. The transducer is moved in a linear pattern across the area being tested to outline and define soft-tissue masses and to differentiate tumor type, ascites, and encapsulated fluid.

For an internal *transvaginal* or *transrectal* scan, the transducer is covered with a condom-like sac onto which transmission gel has been placed. Teach the patient to report any allergies to latex, as the condom-like sac is often made of latex (Pagana & Pagana, 2018). The transducer is then inserted into the vagina or rectum as indicated. Women should have an empty bladder if they are having a transvaginal ultrasound. Patients having an internal ultrasound should be informed that they might feel some mild ***pain*** associated with pressure of the probe.

NCLEX EXAMINATION CHALLENGE 64.2

Physiological Integrity

A client has been scheduled for a transvaginal ultrasound. Which allergy does the nurse identify that should be **immediately** reported to the health care provider?

A. Eggs
B. Corn
C. Latex
D. Iodine

Hysterosalpingography. A hysterosalpingogram is an outpatient fluoroscopy procedure that uses an injection of a contrast medium to visualize the cervix, uterus, and fallopian tubes. This test is used to evaluate tubal anatomy and patency and is commonly done as part of an infertility evaluation, after placement of an internal contraception device, or after tubal ligation or tubal reversal (Lee & Kilcoyne, 2019). It can also

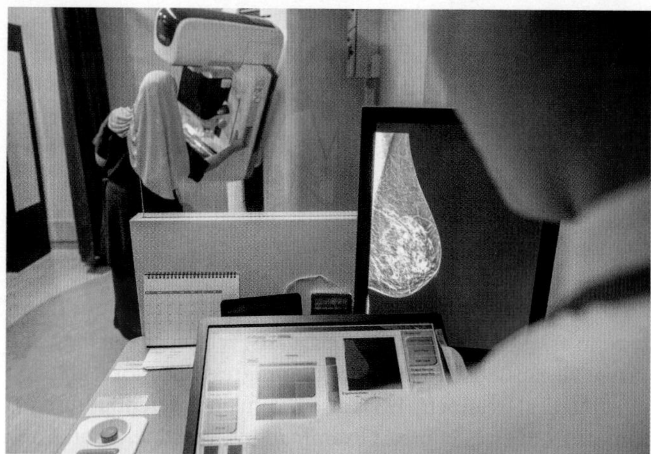

FIG. 64.5 Patient undergoing digital 3D mammography, also known as digital breast tomosynthesis. (©iStock/JohnnyGreig.)

be useful in evaluation of uterine problems such as fibroids, tumors, and fistulas. Assess the patient for pregnancy, vaginal bleeding, pelvic ***infection*** (even if taking antibiotics), and history of reaction to iodine, as these are all contraindications to this procedure.

The examination is best performed on days 6 to 11 from the patient's last menstrual cycle, which reduces the chance that the patient may be pregnant and helps to avoid menstruation (Lee & Kilcoyne, 2019). Teach that the procedure may cause some mild and self-limited pain, as well as a small amount of postprocedure bleeding; if cramping continues after the procedure, an NSAID can be used (Lee & Kilcoyne, 2019).

On the day of the examination, confirm the date of the patient's last menstrual period. Again, ask about allergies to iodine dye. The health care provider communicates benefits and risks of the procedure with the patient. As the nurse, you may witness the signed informed consent. Be aware that the patient may experience some nausea and vomiting, abdominal cramping, or faintness during the procedure. Provide support and assistance with relaxation techniques as needed.

After the patient is placed in lithotomy position, the health care provider will insert a speculum to view the cervix. Dye is injected through the cervix to fill and highlight the interior of the cervix, uterus, and fallopian tubes. If the fallopian tubes are patent, the contrast material spills into the peritoneal cavity. Usually only two or three views are obtained to show the path and distribution of the contrast medium.

As noted earlier, the patient may experience a small amount of vaginal bleeding and pelvic ***pain*** after the study, and should receive analgesic medications if prescribed. Inform her that she may also have referred pain to the shoulder because of irritation of the phrenic nerve. Provide a perineal pad after the test to prevent soiling of clothes as the dye drains from the cervix. Instruct the patient to contact the health care provider if bloody discharge continues for 4 days or longer and to immediately report any signs of ***infection,*** such as lower quadrant pain, fever, chills, malodorous discharge, or tachycardia.

NCLEX EXAMINATION CHALLENGE 64.3

Physiological Integrity

The nurse is caring for a client who underwent a hysterosalpingogram earlier in the day. Which assessment finding will the nurse **immediately** report to the health care provider? **Select all that apply.**

A. Fever and chills
B. Heart rate 120 beats/min
C. Bloody vaginal discharge
D. Pain in the lower quadrant
E. Discomfort in the shoulder

Endoscopic Studies

Colposcopy. A colposcope allows three-dimensional magnification and intense illumination of tissue of the cervix, vagina, vulva, or anus (Feltmate & Feldman, 2020). Because it provides accurate site selection, this procedure can locate the exact site of precancerous and cancerous lesions for biopsy in preparation for early treatment. Colposcopy can also be used for further diagnosis after a woman has an abnormal Pap test result or has HPV (Feltmate & Feldman, 2020).

Teach the patient that she should not douche or use vaginal preparations for 24 to 48 hours before the test. This nearly painless procedure is better tolerated if it is explained in advance and if a picture of a colposcope is shown to the patient. Explain that the health care provider may take a biopsy specimen while performing colposcopy. The provider will obtain informed consent, and you, as the nurse, may witness this.

Provide the patient with a gown and privacy, and instruct her to undress from the waist down. Help the patient to assume the lithotomy position. The health care provider locates the cervix or vaginal site through a speculum, and a visual examination is performed. After 30 to 60 seconds, acetic acid is applied to the cervix to draw moisture from the tissue, which allows large or dense nuclei (e.g., metaplastic or dysplastic cells, or cells infected with HPV) to be visualized more easily. If no abnormalities are noted, other solutions composed of iodine, potassium iodine, and distilled water are applied to the cervix (Feltmate & Feldman, 2020), and cells with glycogen turn dark brown. The health care provider may use a green or blue filter to visualize differences between the abnormal vascularities and epithelium. During the procedure, a biopsy specimen can be taken if abnormal cells are seen. (See Cervical Biopsy section later in this chapter.)

After the procedure, allow the patient to rest for a few minutes, especially if she had a biopsy performed. Provide privacy and supplies to clean the perineum and a perineal pad to absorb dye or discharge. Inform the patient that she may wish to wear a menstrual pad because mild cramping, spotting, or dark or black-colored discharge (from medication applied to the cervix to reduce bleeding) may occur for several days. Remind the patient to take pain relievers as recommended by the health care provider but to avoid aspirin to decrease the chance of bleeding. The patient should be instructed to refrain from douching, using tampons, and having sexual intercourse for 1 week (or as instructed by the health care provider).

Dilation and Curettage. A dilation and curettage (D&C) is a procedure in which tissue is removed from inside of the uterus because of abnormal bleeding or to remove pregnancy tissue after an abortion, miscarriage, or childbirth. Done through a hysteroscope (see Hysteroscopy section later in this chapter), a type of endoscope, this procedure takes approximately 15 to 30 minutes. It is done with anesthesia before and during the procedure (ACOG, 2020).

Prior to the procedure, teach patients about the anesthesia that will be used, and assess for any prior adverse reactions to anesthesia. If prescribed, teach the patient about techniques or medication that is used before the procedure to begin dilating, or softening, the cervix. Ensure that patients have someone to drive them home after the procedure is over, and teach that mild spotting, light bleeding, and/or mild pain may occur. On the day of the procedure, the health care provider will obtain informed consent, and you may witness the patient signing this. Remind the patient to report heavy bleeding, fever, abdominal pain, or foul-smelling discharge to the health care provider right away. Also, teach the patient that her next menstrual cycle may occur earlier or later than the anticipated date (ACOG, 2020).

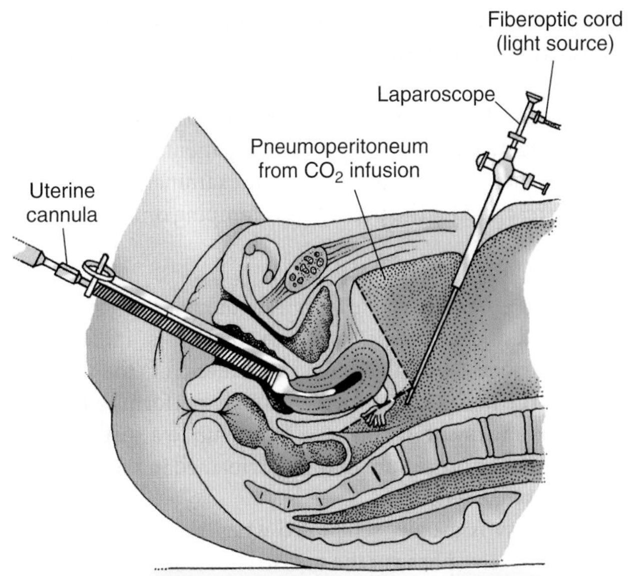

FIG. 64.6 Laparoscopy. *CO_2*, Carbon dioxide.

Laparoscopy. Laparoscopy is a direct examination of the pelvic cavity through an endoscope. This procedure can be used to rule out an ectopic pregnancy, evaluate ovarian disorders and pelvic masses, and aid in the diagnosis of infertility and unexplained pelvic ***pain.*** Laparoscopy is also used during surgical procedures such as:

- Tubal sterilization
- Ovarian biopsy
- Cyst aspiration
- Removal of endometriosis tissue or fibroids
- Lysis of adhesions around the fallopian tubes
- Retrieval of intrauterine devices that the patient cannot self-retrieve

A laparoscopy is often preferred over laparotomy for minor surgical procedures because it is less costly, sometimes requires a shorter operative time, produces smaller scars, and lends itself to a faster recovery time without formation of adhesions (Sharp, 2019).

The surgeon describes benefits and risks of the procedure to the patient. Risks include complications associated with the use of anesthesia, postoperative shoulder pain from irritation of the phrenic nerve, effects of carbon dioxide gas and/or peritoneal stretching, irritation at the incision site, and the rare occurrence of infection or electrical burns. As the nurse, you may witness the patient signing the informed consent form. A laparoscopy can be performed with use of a regional or general anesthetic depending on the patient's risk factors related to anesthesia, the type of position the patient will be placed in during the procedure, and the anticipated length of procedural time (Joshi, 2019).

After the patient is anesthetized and placed in supine or dorsal lithotomy position, a urinary catheter is inserted to drain the bladder. The operating table is placed in slight Trendelenburg position to allow the intestines to fall away from the pelvis so that the pelvic viscera can be better visualized (Sharp, 2019). The cervix is held with a cannula to allow movement of the uterus during laparoscopy (Fig. 64.6). The surgeon inserts a needle below the umbilicus to infuse carbon dioxide (CO_2) into the pelvic cavity, which distends the abdomen and permits better visualization of the organs. After the trocar and cannula are in place in the abdominal cavity, the surgeon removes the trocar and inserts the laparoscope. The surgeon can then visualize the pelvic cavity and reproductive organs. Further instrumentation is possible through one or more small incisions. The laparoscope is removed at the end of the procedure, and the abdomen is deflated. The small incision is closed with absorbable sutures and dressed with an adhesive bandage.

The patient is usually discharged on the day of the procedure. Incisional ***pain*** is managed by oral analgesics. The greatest discomfort is usually caused by referred shoulder pain. Most of these sensations disappear within 48 hours, depending on the extent of the procedure. Instruct the patient to change the small adhesive bandage as needed and to observe the incision for signs of ***infection*** or hematoma. Teach her to avoid strenuous activity for the first week after the procedure.

Hysteroscopy. Hysteroscopy is a procedure that uses a fiberoptic telescope to visualize the uterus to diagnose and treat causes of abnormal bleeding. The hysteroscope includes a fiberoptic camera that is inserted into the vagina to examine the cervix and uterus. Diagnostic hysteroscopy is used to diagnose new problems with the uterus or to confirm results from other tests. Hysteroscopy can also be used before or during other procedures (e.g., laparoscopy) for infertility and unexplained bleeding. The procedure is best performed in the proliferative stage to best visualize the uterine cavity (Bradley, 2020).

The health care provider informs the patient of benefits and risks associated with the procedure and obtains consent. You, as the nurse, may witness the patient signing the informed consent form. The preparation is the same as for a pelvic examination. After the patient is placed in lithotomy position, she may be anesthetized with a paracervical block before the cervix is dilated if the procedure will involve uterine biopsy (Bradley, 2020). The health care provider inserts the hysteroscope through the cervix. Because this distends the uterus, cells can be pushed through the fallopian tubes and into the pelvic cavity. Therefore, hysteroscopy is contraindicated in patients with suspected cervical or endometrial cancer, in those with ***infection*** of the reproductive tract, and in pregnant patients.

Care is the same as that after a pelvic examination. Analgesics may be prescribed if the patient has cramping or shoulder pain.

Biopsy Studies

Cervical Biopsy. In a cervical biopsy, cervical tissue is removed for cytologic study. A biopsy is indicated for an identifiable cervical lesion, regardless of the cytologic findings. The health care provider usually performs a biopsy in conjunction with colposcopy as a follow-up to a suspicious Pap test finding. The procedure may be performed in the health care provider's office setting.

The biopsy is usually scheduled when the woman is in the early proliferative phase of the menstrual cycle, when the cervix is least vascular. Because a biopsy evaluates potentially cancerous cells, your patient may be anxious and need time to discuss her feelings and fears. The use of relaxation techniques may address ***pain***. Assist her into the lithotomy position, recognizing that further preparation depends on the type of procedure to be performed.

The health care provider may anesthetize the patient according to the needs of the chosen procedure. The type of anesthetic used for the procedure determines the type of immediate care that is needed after the procedure.

Several techniques can be used for a cervical biopsy. If a lesion is clearly visible, an endocervical curettage can be performed as an ambulatory care procedure and with little or no anesthetic. This tissue sample is immediately placed into a formalin solution. **Conization** (removal of a cone-shaped sample of tissue) and loop electrosurgical excision procedures (LEEPs) are procedures that can be done later if there is discrepancy between the Pap test and biopsy findings (Cooper & Menifee, 2020). Conization can be done as a cold-knife procedure, a laser excision, or an electrosurgical incision.

Discharge instructions can be found in the Patient and Family Education: Preparing for Self-Management: The Patient Recovering From Cervical Biopsy box.

PATIENT AND FAMILY EDUCATION: PREPARING FOR SELF-MANAGEMENT

The Patient Recovering From Cervical Biopsy

- Do not lift any heavy objects until the site is healed (about 2 weeks).
- Rest for 24 hours after the procedure.
- Report any excessive bleeding (more than that of a normal menstrual period) to your health care provider.
- Report signs of ***infection*** (fever, increased pain, foul-smelling drainage) to your health care provider.
- Do not douche, use tampons, or have vaginal intercourse until the site is healed (about 2 weeks).
- Keep the perineum clean and dry by using antiseptic solution rinses (as directed by your health care provider) and changing pads frequently.

Endometrial Biopsy. Both endometrial biopsy and aspiration are used to obtain cells directly from the lining of the uterus to assess for cancer of the endometrium. Biopsy helps assess menstrual disturbances (especially heavy bleeding) and infertility (corpus luteum dysfunction).

When menstrual disturbances are being evaluated, the biopsy is generally done in the immediate premenstrual period to provide an index of progesterone influence and ovulation. A biopsy performed in the second half of the menstrual cycle (about days 21 and 22) evaluates corpus luteum function and the presence or absence of a persistent secretory endometrium. Postmenopausal women may undergo biopsies at any time.

An endometrial biopsy is usually done as an office procedure with or without anesthesia. Menstrual data should be obtained from the patient and are included on the specimen request for the pathologist. Confirm that the patient is not pregnant, as this is an absolute contraindication for this procedure. Prepare the patient in the same way as you would for a pelvic examination. Tell her that she may experience some cramping when the cervix is dilated. Analgesia before the procedure and relaxation and breathing techniques during the procedure may be helpful to make her more comfortable. Some providers will prescribe an NSAID 30 to 60 minutes prior to the procedure to decrease cramping; others may administer a paracervical block or administer local anesthetic via intrauterine instillation (Del Priore, 2019).

After the uterus is measured and the cervix dilated, the health care provider inserts the curette or intrauterine cannula into the uterus. A portion of the endometrium is withdrawn using either the cuplike end of the curette or suction equipment and is placed into a formalin solution to be sent for histologic examination. It is at this time that the patient is most likely to have moderate cramping. Allow her to rest on the examining table until the cramping has subsided. Provide a perineal pad and a wipe to clean the perineum. Teach her that spotting may be present for 1 to 2 days but any signs of ***infection*** or excessive bleeding should be reported to the health care provider. Instruct the patient to avoid intercourse or douching until all discharge has ceased.

Breast Biopsy. All breast masses should be evaluated for the possibility of cancer. It is important to recognize that breast cancer can occur in both men and women; less than 1% of breast cancers occur in men (National Cancer Institute, 2019). Approximately 2620 men are diagnosed with breast cancer annually in the United States, and approximately 520 die from this condition yearly (ACS, 2020).

Fibrocystic lesions, fibroadenomas, and intraductal papillomas can be differentiated by biopsy. Any discharge from the breasts is examined histologically. Prior to the procedure, provide instructions to the patient based on the type of biopsy performed and the type of anesthesia that is to be used. The patient usually will receive a local anesthetic, and the tissue will either be aspirated through a large-bore needle (core-needle biopsy) or removed using a small incision to extract multiple samples of tissue.

Aspirated fluid from benign cysts may appear clear to dark green or brown. Bloody fluid suggests cancer. These specimens undergo histologic evaluation. If cancer is found, the tissue is evaluated for estrogen receptor analysis. Chapter 65 discusses types of breast cancer and their relationship to estrogen receptors.

Teach that discomfort after the procedure is usually mild and can be controlled with analgesics or the use of ice or heat, depending on the type and extent of the biopsy. Educate the patient about how to assess the area or incision for bleeding and edema. Teach the patient to wear a supportive bra continuously for 1 week after surgery or as recommended by their surgeon. Remind the patient that numbness around the biopsy site may last several weeks. If cancer is identified, provide emotional support and reinforce information about the importance of follow-up treatment options.

Prostate Biopsy. When prostate cancer is suspected, a biopsy must be performed. This can be done by transurethral biopsy, by inserting a needle through the area of skin between the anus and scrotum, or, most commonly, by transrectal biopsy. Preparation for the procedure depends on the technique used to puncture the gland. A urinalysis should be performed prior to the procedure; if the patient has a urinary tract infection (UTI), the procedure will need to be rescheduled after the UTI has been successfully treated (Benway & Andriole, 2020).

Because the purpose of this procedure is to evaluate prostate cells for cancer, allow the patient time to discuss fears. Some health care providers will prescribe an anxiolytic to address the patient's anxiety about the procedure (Benway & Andriole, 2020). Prophylactic antibiotics are usually prescribed to lower the incidence of postbiopsy bacteriuria (Benway & Andriole, 2020). Patients taking aspirin, warfarin, or other anticoagulants should talk with the health care provider about whether to continue taking these or withholding them prior to the procedure. The health care provider will discuss benefits and risks to the procedure; you may witness the patient signing the informed consent form.

Explain to the patient that he may experience some discomfort. Teach him about breathing and relaxation techniques that may be helpful to use during the procedure. Assist the patient who is undergoing transrectal biopsy into the side-lying position with his knees pulled up toward his chest. The health care provider will cleanse the area, apply gel, and then insert a thin ultrasound probe into the patient's rectum to anesthetize (if needed) and guide the biopsy needle into place. The biopsy specimen is collected over a 5- to 10-minute period. The patient may experience a brief, uncomfortable feeling each time the needle collects a sample.

After prostate biopsy, remind the patient that he may experience slight soreness, light rectal bleeding that is bright red for a few days, and moderate hematuria that should resolve in a few days (Benway & Andriole, 2020). Tell the patient that semen may be discolored red or rust for several weeks. Pain can be treated with over-the-counter acetaminophen. NSAIDs should be avoided due to the risk for bleeding. Teach the patient to contact the health care provider if he has fever, prolonged or heavy bleeding, worsening ***pain,*** swelling in the area of biopsy, and/or difficulty urinating. Rarely, sepsis can develop after a prostate biopsy, usually in patients who did not adhere to taking prophylactic antibiotics. Teach the patient to contact the health care provider immediately if he experiences fever, pain when urinating, or penile discharge.

GET READY FOR THE NEXT-GENERATION NCLEX® EXAMINATION!

Key Points

Review these Key Points for each NCLEX Examination Client Needs Category.

Safe and Effective Care Environment

- Teach women to report symptoms of ***infection*** or bleeding to their health care provider after endoscopic procedures and biopsies of the breast, cervix, and endometrium. **QSEN: Safety**
- Instruct men to report symptoms of ***infection*** to their health care provider after a transrectal biopsy of the prostate. **QSEN: Safety**

Health Promotion and Maintenance

- Encourage women to follow recommended guidelines for early detection of cervical cancer. **QSEN: Evidence-Based Practice**
- Assess and respect cultural preferences when discussing reproductive problems and health promotion practices. **QSEN: Patient-Centered Care**

Psychosocial Integrity

- Assess the patient's comfort level in discussing issues related to reproductive health and ***sexuality.*** **QSEN: Patient-Centered Care**
- Encourage patients to express feelings of anxiety related to genital examinations, reproductive testing, or changes in function. **QSEN: Patient-Centered Care**
- Provide privacy for patients undergoing examination or testing of the reproductive system. **Ethics**

Physiological Integrity

- Teach patients with ***pain,*** bleeding, discharge, masses, or changes in reproductive function to see their health care provider. **QSEN: Safety**
- Recognize age-related reproductive changes. **QSEN: Patient-Centered Care**
- Explain diagnostic procedures, restrictions, and follow-up care associated with testing and treatment. **QSEN: Evidence-Based Practice**

MASTERY QUESTIONS

1. A client has undergone a prostate biopsy. Which postprocedure symptom will the nurse teach the client to report **immediately** to the primary health care provider?
   A. Semen discoloration 5 days after biopsy
   B. Light rectal bleeding 2 days after procedure
   C. Tenderness at the site 1 day after biopsy
   D. Pain on urination 3 days after procedure

2. A client who is scheduled for a Pap smear reports having had sexual intercourse 1 day prior and douching afterward. What is the appropriate nursing action?
   A. Reschedule the Pap smear for another week
   B. Delay the procedure until later in the afternoon
   C. Help the client prepare for the procedure at this time
   D. Hold the procedure until the client's next menstrual cycle

REFERENCES

American Addiction Centers. (2020). What Role does drug abuse Play in the health of the reproductive system? Retrieved from https://americanaddictioncenters.org/health-complications-addiction/reproductive-system.

American Cancer Society (ACS). (2020). *Key statistics for breast cancer in men*. Retrieved from https://www.cancer.org/cancer/breast-cancer-in-men/about/key-statistics.html.

American Cancer Society (ACS). (2019a). *Breast MRI scans*. Retrieved from https://www.cancer.org/cancer/breast-cancer/screening-tests-and-early-detection/breast-mri-scans.html.

American Cancer Society (ACS). (2019b). *Cancer facts and figures 2019*. https://www.cancer.org/content/dam/cancer-org/research/cancer-facts-and-statistics/annual-cancer-facts-and-figures/2019/cancer-facts-and-figures-2019.pdf.

American Cancer Society (ACS). (2019c). *Limitations of mammograms*. Retrieved from https://www.cancer.org/cancer/breast-cancer/screening-tests-and-early-detection/mammograms/limitations-of-mammograms.html.

American Cancer Society (ACS). (2019d). *Testing for BRCA gene mutation*. Retrieved from https://www.cancer.org/cancer/breast-cancer/risk-and-prevention/genetic-testing.html.

American Cancer Society (ACS). (2018). *The American Cancer Society guidelines for the prevention and early detection of cervical cancer*. Retrieved from https://www.cancer.org/cancer/cervical-cancer/prevention-and-early-detection/cervical-cancer-screening-guidelines.html.

American College of Obstetricians and Gynecologists. (2020). *Dilation and curettage*. Retrieved from https://www.acog.org/patient-resources/faqs/special-procedures/dilation-and-curettage.

American Society of Clinical Oncology. (2019). *Prostate cancer: Risk factors and prevention*. Retrieved from https://www.cancer.net/cancer-types/prostate-cancer/risk-factors-and-prevention.

Benway, B., & Andriole, G. (2020). Prostate biopsy. In J. Richie (Ed.), *UpToDate*. Waltham, MA.

Bradley, L. (2020). Overview of hysteroscopy. In T. Falcone (Ed.), *UpToDate*. Waltham, MA.

Centers for Disease Control and Prevention. (n.d.). *Breast cancer screening guidelines for women*. Retrieved from https://www.cdc.gov/cancer/breast/pdf/breastcancerscreeningguidelines.pdf

Choosing Wisely Canada. (2019). *Pap tests: When you need them and when you don't*. Retrieved from https://choosingwiselycanada.org/pap-tests/.

Cooper, D., & Menifee, G. (2020). *Conization of cervix. StatPearls*. Treasure Island, FL: StatPearls Publishing.

Del Priore, G. (2019). Endometrial sampling procedures. In B. Goff (Ed.), *UpToDate*. Waltham, MA.

Feltmate, C., & Feldman, S. (2020). Colposcopy. In B. Goff (Ed.), *UpToDate*. Waltham, MA.

Hatch, E., & Karam, A. (2020). Outcome and follow-up of diethylstilbestrol (DES) exposed individuals. In V. Berghella, & B. Goff (Eds.), *UpToDate*. Waltham, MA.

Hoffman, R. (2020). Screening for prostate cancer. In J. Elmore, & M. O'Leary (Eds.), *UpToDate*. Waltham, MA.

Jarvis, C. (2020). *Physical examination & health assessment* (8th ed.). St. Louis: Saunders.

Joshi, G. (2019). Anesthesia for laparoscopic and abdominal robotic surgery in adults. In S. Jones (Ed.), *UpToDate*. Waltham, MA.

Lee, S., & Kilcoyne, A. (2019). Hysterosalpingography. In R. Barbieri (Ed.), *UpToDate*. Waltham, MA.

Martin, K., & Barbieri, R. (2020). Menopausal hormone therapy: Benefits and risks. In P. Snyder, & W. Crowley (Eds.), *UpToDate*. Waltham, MA.

National Breast Cancer Foundation. (2019). *Male breast cancer*. Retrieved from https://www.nationalbreastcancer.org/male-breast-cancer.

National Cancer Institute at the National Institutes of Health. (2019). *General information about male breast cancer*. www.cancer.gov/cancertopics/pdq/treatment/malebreast/Patient/page1#Keypoint3.

Pagana, K. D., & Pagana, T. J. (2018). *Mosby's manual of diagnostic and laboratory tests* (6th ed.). St. Louis: Elsevier.

Research on Prostate Cancer in Men of African Ancestry: Defining the Roles of Genetics, Tumor Markers and Social Stress. (2019). *Respond: African American prostate cancer study*. Retrieved from http://respondstudy.org/Default.aspx.

Sharp, H. (2019). Overview of gynecologic laparoscopic surgery and non-umbilical entry sites. In T. Falcone (Ed.), *UpToDate*. Waltham, MA.

Venkataraman, S., & Slanetz, P. (2020). Breast imaging for cancer screening: Mammography and ultrasonography. In J. Elmore (Ed.), *UpToDate*. Waltham, MA.

65

Concepts of Care for Patients With Breast Disorders

Hannah M. Lopez, Cherie R. Rebar

http://evolve.elsevier.com/Iggy/

LEARNING OUTCOMES

1. Collaborate with the interprofessional team to coordinate high-quality care for patients with breast disorders.
2. Describe the three-pronged approach to early detection of breast masses: mammography, clinical breast examination (CBE), and breast self-awareness.
3. Describe factors that place a patient at high risk for breast cancer, and refer to the health care provider.
4. Implement nursing interventions to help patients cope with the psychosocial impact caused by a breast disorder.
5. Apply knowledge of anatomy, physiology, and pathophysiology to assess patients with breast disorders.
6. Use clinical judgment to analyze assessment findings and diagnostic data in the care of patients with breast disorders.
7. Prioritize evidence-based care for patients with a breast disorder associated with ***cellular regulation***, ***infection***, or ***pain***.
8. Plan care coordination and transition management for patients with breast disorders.

KEY TERMS

adjuvant therapy Additional treatment following an initial surgical procedure; performed to help keep cancer from recurring.

atypical hyperplasia A proliferative breast disorder that is a change in the cellular structure of a cell but is not considered cancerous.

breast augmentation Surgery to increase or improve the size, shape, or symmetry of the breasts.

breast-conserving surgery Also known as *lumpectomy* or *partial mastectomy*; procedure in which the surgeon removes part of the breast that contains cancer and some normal tissue around it.

cysts Spaces filled with fluid lined by breast glandular cells.

ductal carcinoma in situ (DCIS) An early *noninvasive* form of breast cancer; in DCIS, cancer cells are located within the duct and have not invaded the surrounding fatty breast tissue.

fibroadenoma A well-defined solid mass of connective tissue that is unattached to the surrounding breast tissue and is usually discovered by the woman herself or during mammography.

fibrocystic changes (FCCs) A range of changes involving the lobules, ducts, and stromal tissues of the breast.

fibrosis Replacement of normal cells with connective tissue and collagen.

gynecomastia A benign ridge of glandular tissue within the male breast.

inflammatory breast cancer (IBC) Aggressive type of breast cancer characterized by diffuse erythema and edema (peau d'orange).

invasive ductal carcinoma The most common type of invasive breast cancer, in which the disease originates in the mammary ducts and breaks through the walls of the ducts into the surrounding breast tissue.

lobular carcinoma in situ (LCIS) A noninvasive disease in which the cells look like cancer cells and are contained within the lobules (milk-producing glands) of the breast; LCIS is less common than DCIS and is not thought to be a precursor of invasive cancer.

prophylactic mastectomy Preventive surgical removal of one or both breasts.

prophylactic oophorectomy Removal of the ovaries.

reduction mammoplasty Breast reduction surgery in which the surgeon removes excess breast tissue and then repositions the nipple and remaining skin flaps to produce the best cosmetic effect.

triple-negative breast cancer (TNBC) A type of breast cancer that lacks expression of the estrogen receptor (ER), progesterone receptor (PR), and human epidermal growth factor receptor 2 (HER2).

PRIORITY AND INTERRELATED CONCEPTS

The priority concepts for this chapter are:
- ***Cellular Regulation***
- ***Infection***
- ***Pain***

The ***Cellular Regulation*** concept exemplar for this chapter is Breast Cancer.

The interrelated concept for this chapter is:
- ***Sexuality***

Changes in the breast tissue due to cellular regulation (in Chapter 1) can cause a great deal of anxiety for women, although many disorders of the breast are benign rather than malignant. A key nursing role is to assist patients by providing accurate information about benign breast disorders (BBDs) and breast cancer.

BENIGN BREAST DISORDERS

Benign breast disorders (BBDs) are very common, affecting more than one million women annually in the United States (Santen, 2018). Most women will experience some form of breast-related changes in their lifetime. Noncancerous changes to breast tissue can present as breast lumps, pain, and nipple changes (Mau, 2018). Table 65.1 highlights some common BBDs and the age at which these are likely to occur. BBDs are classified into three types of epithelial lesions: proliferative with atypia, proliferative without atypia, and nonproliferative. The risk of developing cancer from these breast changes varies.

PROLIFERATIVE BREAST LESION WITH ATYPIA: ATYPICAL HYPERPLASIA

Atypical hyperplasia (AH) is a proliferative breast disorder involving growth of breast cells that are abnormal. It is usually found as a result of a biopsy that was taken. AH, although not cancerous, does lead to an increased risk for development of breast cancer. The younger the woman is when diagnosed with AH, the higher the lifetime risk of developing cancer. The patient should be managed by a surgical oncologist or breast surgeon and should undergo yearly mammography and twice-yearly breast examinations (Sabel, 2018). Women with AH should be taught to stop taking oral contraceptives (under the supervision of their health care provider) and to avoid hormone replacement therapy (HRT) (Sabel, 2018). Surgical excision can also be considered as a treatment for AH.

PROLIFERATIVE BREAST LESION WITHOUT ATYPIA: FIBROADENOMA

Fibroadenomas are common benign tumors in women in their 20s and 30s, but they also may occur at any age (American Cancer Society [ACS], 2019d). A **fibroadenoma** is a well-defined solid mass of connective tissue that is unattached to the surrounding breast tissue and is usually discovered by the woman herself or during mammography. Although the immediate fear is that of breast cancer, these changes are generally not associated with an increased risk for such. On clinical examination, these tumors are oval, freely mobile, and rubbery, and vary in size.

Fibroadenomas may occur anywhere in the breast. The health care provider may request a breast ultrasound examination or may perform a needle aspiration to establish whether the lump is cystic (filled with fluid) or solid.

NONPROLIFERATIVE BREAST LESIONS: FIBROCYSTIC CHANGES (FCCS) AND CYSTS

Pathophysiology Review

Fibrocystic changes of the breast include a range of changes involving the lobules, ducts, and stromal tissues of the breast. Because these alterations affect at least half of women over the life span, they are referred to as **fibrocystic changes (FCCs)** (Fig. 65.1, normal breast tissue versus Fig. 65.2, FCCs) rather than *fibrocystic disease.* This condition most often occurs in premenopausal women between 20 and 50 years of age and is thought to be caused by an imbalance in the normal estrogen-to-progesterone ratio. Areas of fibrosis are made up of fibrous connective tissue (McCance et al., 2019). Typical symptoms include breast ***pain*** and firm, hard, tender lumps or swelling in the breasts, particularly before a woman's menstrual period. Having FCCs does not increase a woman's chance of developing breast cancer.

Cysts are spaces filled with fluid lined by breast glandular cells. They often enlarge in response to monthly hormonal changes, stretch the surrounding breast tissue, and become painful. Symptoms usually resolve after menstruation and then recur before the next menstrual period in a cyclic fashion. In postmenopausal women, symptoms often resolve because estrogen decreases. However, postmenopausal women on hormone

TABLE 65.1 Typical Presentation of Benign Breast Disorders

Breast Disorder	Description	Incidence
Fibroadenoma	Most common benign lesion; solid mass of connective tissue that is unattached to the surrounding tissue	During teenage years into the 30s (most commonly)
Fibrocystic changes (FCCs)	Breast ***pain*** and tender lumps; the lumps are rubbery, ill defined, and commonly found in the upper outer quadrant of the breast	Onset late teens and 20s; usually subsides after menopause
Ductal ectasia	Hard, irregular mass or masses with nipple discharge, enlarged axillary nodes, redness, and edema; difficult to distinguish from cancer	Women approaching menopause
Intraductal papilloma	Mass in duct that results in bloody nipple discharge; mass is usually not palpable	Women 40-55 years of age

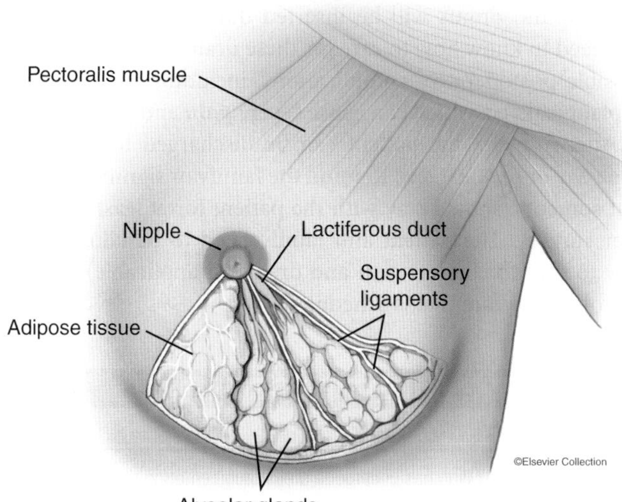

Fig. 65.1 Normal breast. (© Elsevier Collection.)

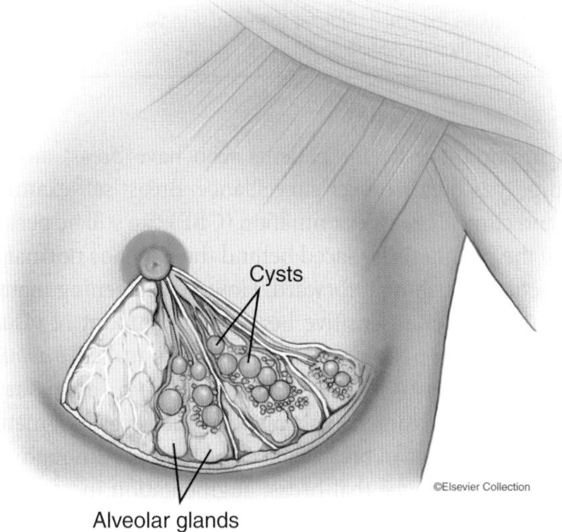

Fig. 65.2 Breast with fibrocystic changes. (© Elsevier Collection.)

replacement therapy (HRT) may not have a significant reduction in symptoms.

Breast ultrasound is used to confirm the presence of a cyst. If a lump is very firm or has other features raising a concern for cancer, mammography is indicated. A needle biopsy or surgical biopsy may also be ordered. Biopsy may be indicated in these situations:

- No fluid is aspirated.
- The mammogram shows suspicious findings.
- A mass remains palpable after aspiration.
- The aspirated fluid reveals cancer cells.

❖ Interprofessional Collaborative Care

Management of FCCs focuses on the symptoms of the condition. Teach supportive measures for women with mild discomfort. The use of analgesics can address discomfort. Limiting salt intake before menses can help decrease swelling. Many women find relief with the reduction of dietary caffeine and other stimulants. Teach patients that wearing a supportive bra, even to bed, can reduce pain by decreasing tension on the ligaments. Local application of ice or heat may provide temporary relief of pain. For a small number of women, draining the cysts by needle aspiration can help relieve painful symptoms.

In women with severe symptoms of FCCs, hormonal drugs such as oral contraceptives or selective estrogen receptor modulators (SERMs) may be prescribed to suppress oversecretion of estrogen. Diuretics may be prescribed to decrease premenstrual breast engorgement.

Encourage the patient to continue prescribed drug therapy and monitor the effectiveness of these interventions. Teach the patient to become familiar with the normal feel and texture of her breasts so she is aware of any ongoing changes.

! NURSING SAFETY PRIORITY (QSEN)

Drug Alert

Explain to women the benefits and risks associated with hormonal drug therapy for FCCs. Risks include increased chance of thrombotic events (e.g., brain attack or blood clots), and risk of development of uterine cancer. Teach them to seek medical attention immediately if any signs or symptoms of these complications occur.

LARGE BREASTS

In Men

In men, a benign ridge of glandular tissue within the breast, caused by an increase in ratio of estrogen to androgen activity, is referred to as gynecomastia (Braunstein & Anawalt, 2019). It may be bilateral or unilateral, with a palpable mass of tissue at least 0.5 cm in diameter. Most men are asymptomatic, although some may report tenderness or sensitivity when clothing touches the nipple or the affected area.

Drugs such as spironolactone can cause gynecomastia; the first line of treatment is to discontinue any drugs that may contribute to this condition. If a medical condition such as hyperthyroidism or hypogonadism contributes to the condition, treatment of the underlying issue often helps to resolve gynecomastia. Selective estrogen receptor modulators (SERMs) such as tamoxifen, aromatase inhibitors, and androgens may also be used for treatment. Surgery can be considered for men who have unresolved gynecomastia where medical intervention does not resolve the condition.

In Women

Although Western society emphasizes large breasts as a positive attribute, women with excessive breast tissue may have health problems and experience ***pain.*** A woman with large breasts may have difficulty finding clothes that fit well and in which she feels attractive, or she may feel that her breast size is out of proportion to the rest of the body. Larger bras are expensive and may need to be specially ordered. The woman may have large dents in the shoulders from bra straps, and may develop a recurrent fungal ***infection*** under the breasts, especially in hot weather, because it is difficult to keep this area dry and exposed to air.

Backaches from the added weight of larger breasts are also common. If well-fitting bras do not help and obesity is not part of the problem, the alternative for this condition may be breast reduction surgery, called **reduction mammoplasty**. This procedure can be accomplished in several ways, depending on the breast position and shape prior to surgery. Sometimes the nipples can be left intact during surgery, and in other cases they may need to be moved for cosmetic reasons (Figs. 65.3, 65.4, and 65.5). Insurance usually covers the cost of reduction mammoplasty as long as health detriments are well documented by the health care provider.

The decision to have the procedure is usually made after years of living with the discomfort of excessive breast size. Allow the woman to verbalize her feelings. Provide appropriate preoperative teaching (as in Chapter 9). Nursing care after surgery is similar to that for the woman having reconstructive surgery. (See discussion of Breast Reconstruction in the Surgical Management section under Breast Cancer.)

SMALL BREASTS

Some women choose to have **breast augmentation** surgery to increase or improve the size, shape, or symmetry of their breasts. Most health insurers do not pay for this procedure, as it is usually considered cosmetic. Most surgeries involve the implantation of saline-filled or silicone prostheses. Some are constructed from the women's own tissue in much the same way as for reconstruction after mastectomy. *Saline* implants are filled with sterile saline and can be filled with the amount needed to get the shape and firmness the woman wants. If the implant shell leaks, the saline will be safely absorbed by the body. *Silicone* implants are filled with a silicone gel, which can leak into the breast and will not be absorbed. The plastic surgeon reviews the advantages and disadvantages of each implant or surgical option with the patient.

Before breast surgery, teach the patient to stop smoking (to promote healing); avoid aspirin and other NSAIDs; and avoid herbs that can cause bleeding during the procedure. One or more wound drains will be inserted during surgery, and she will need to know how to care for these drains at home. Review possible postoperative complications, including ***infection*** and implant leakage, which can cause severe ***pain*** and fever.

After surgery, the patient can be discharged to home the same day or the next day. Remind the family or significant other that someone should stay with the patient for at least 24 hours after surgery. The patient and family need to be educated on how to care for the incision and drains (if applicable), and on the follow-up care that is scheduled.

! NURSING SAFETY PRIORITY QSEN

Action Alert

Remind the patient who has undergone breast augmentation that she should expect soreness in her chest and arms for the first few postoperative days and breast swelling for 3 to 4 weeks. Her breasts will feel tight and sensitive, and the skin over her breasts may feel warm or may itch. Teach the patient that she will have difficulty raising her arms over her head and should not lift, push, or pull anything until the surgeon permits. Teach her to avoid strenuous activity or twisting above the waist. Remind the patient to walk every few hours to prevent venous thromboembolism (VTE).

An important issue for patients who have breast augmentation surgery is breast cancer surveillance. Breast self-examination (BSE) and clinical breast examination (CBE) can still be performed because the prosthesis is placed behind the woman's normal breast tissue, actually pushing it forward. However, screening mammography may not be as sensitive because the amount of visualized breast tissue is decreased. Additional x-rays, called *implant displacement views*, may be used to examine the breast tissue more completely. Teach women desiring cosmetic breast augmentation about the differences in breast cancer screening. Although there is no conclusive evidence that breast augmentation increases breast

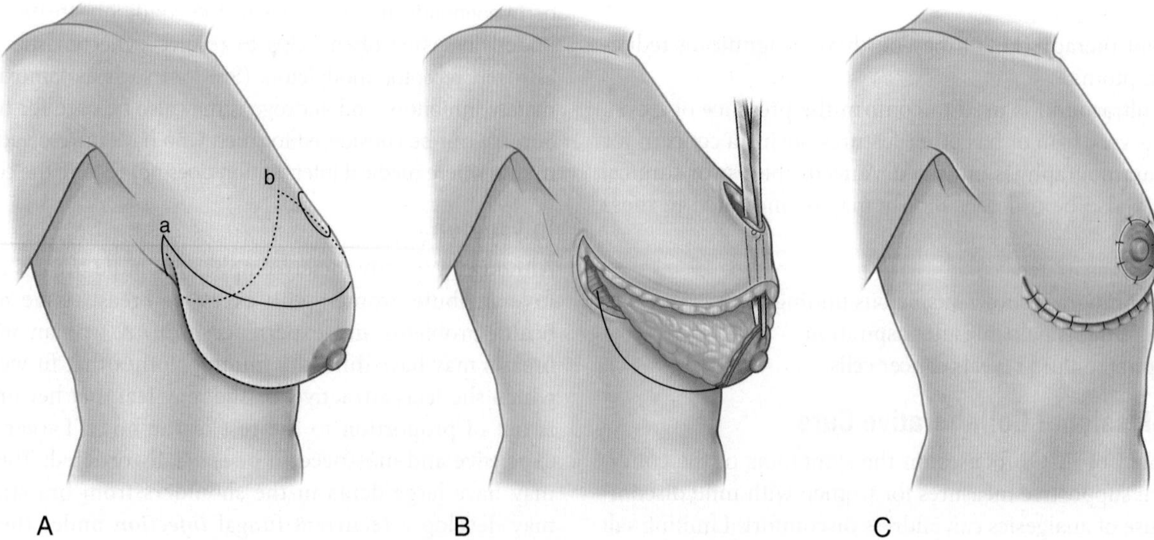

Fig. 65.3 Reduction mammoplasty: Passot technique of nipple transposition. (From Neligan P.C., & Buck D.W. [2020]. *Core procedures in plastic surgery* [2nd ed.]. Philadelphia: Elsevier.)

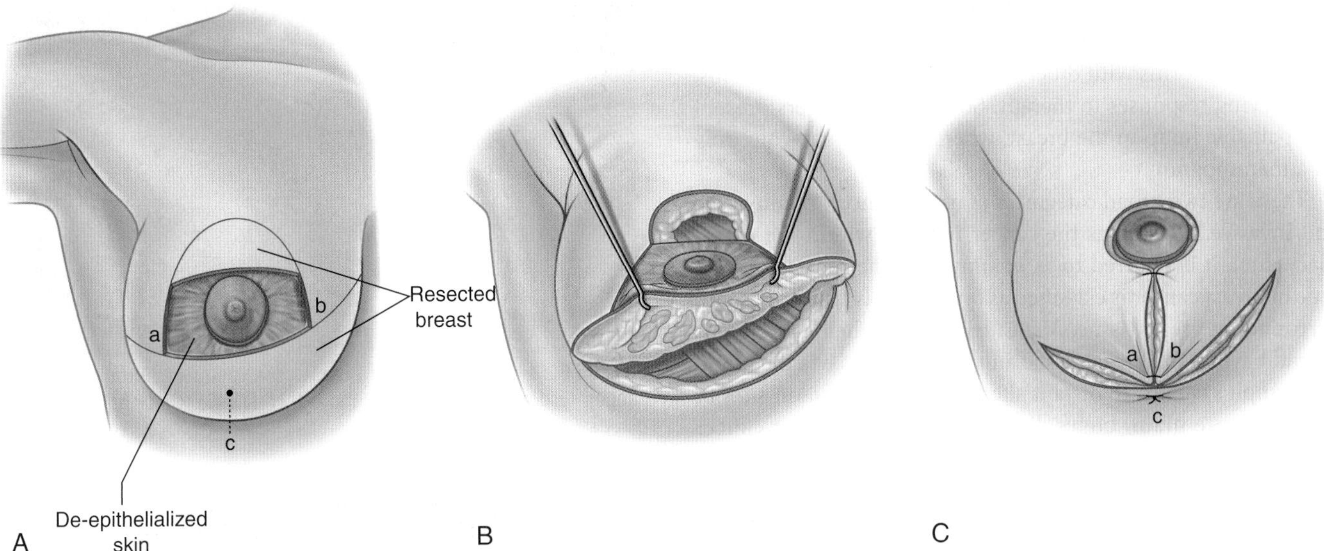

Fig. 65.4 Reduction mammoplasty: Strombeck horizontal bipedicle technique. (From Neligan P.C., & Buck D.W. [2020]. *Core procedures in plastic surgery* [2nd ed.]. Philadelphia: Elsevier.)

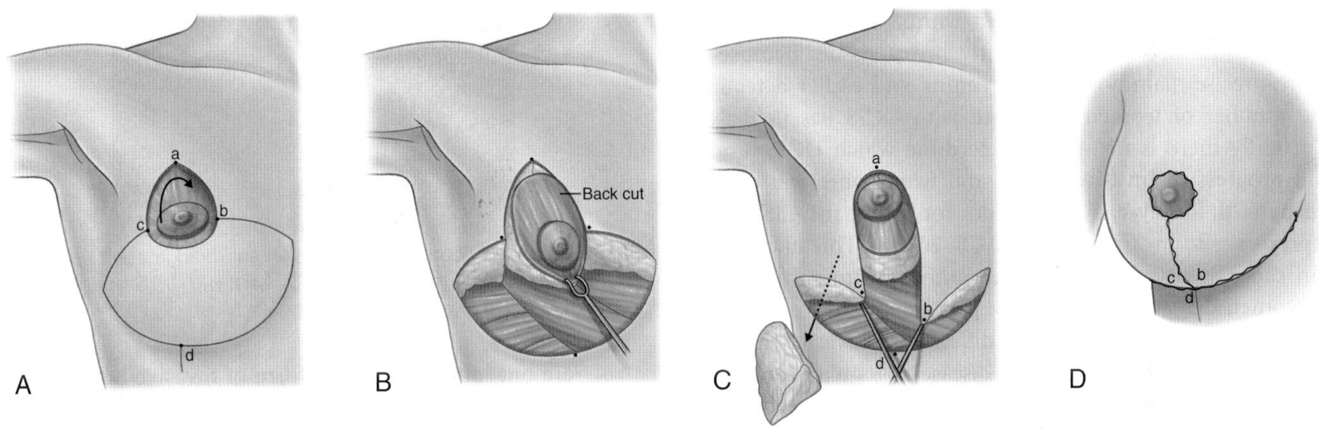

Fig. 65.5 Reduction mammoplasty: Superomedial pedicle with Wise-pattern skin closure. (From Neligan P.C., & Buck D.W. [2020]. *Core procedures in plastic surgery* [2nd ed.]. Philadelphia: Elsevier.)

cancer risk, women must be informed that there is an increased risk for development of a rare form of non-Hodgkin lymphoma called breast implant–associated anaplastic large cell lymphoma (BIA-ALCL) (U.S. Food and Drug Administration, 2019).

BREAST INFLAMMATION AND INFECTION

Breast Abscess

Nonlactational breast abscesses can occur peripherally from the nipple, or in the vicinity of the areola. These types of infections are often found in patients 18 to 50 years old who have diabetes, clogged sweat glands, acne, or trauma to the area (American Society of Breast Surgeons Foundation, 2019). Risk factors that increase the chance for nonlactational breast abscesses include smoking, obesity, and nipple piercings. Common signs and symptoms include pain and swelling in the affected region. Treatment includes broad-spectrum antibiotics, ultrasound-guided aspiration, and/or incision and drainage (American Society of Breast Surgeons Foundation, 2019).

Mastitis

Mastitis—inflammation of the breast that may be accompanied by ***infection*** and ***pain*** (Dixon & Pariser, 2020)—is often associated with lactating and breast-feeding women; however, it can occur in women who are not lactating or breast-feeding. This condition is more common in women who smoke, and in women who have nipple piercings where bacteria can enter through a milk duct. Treatment options, depending on the specific type of mastitis, include antibiotic therapy, steroid therapy, or watchful waiting (Dixon & Pariser, 2020). Women with nonlactational mastitis have a higher risk of breast cancer than women without nonlactational mastitis (Chang et al., 2019).

CELLULAR REGULATION CONCEPT EXEMPLAR: BREAST CANCER

Pathophysiology Review

Cancer is a common problem of impaired ***cellular regulation.*** Cancer of the breast begins as a single transformed cell that grows and multiplies in the epithelial cells lining one or more of the mammary ducts or lobules. It is a heterogeneous disease, having many forms with different clinical signs and symptoms, and varying responses to therapy. Some breast cancers present as a palpable lump in the breast, whereas others show up only on a mammogram.

There are two broad categories of breast cancer: noninvasive and invasive. As long as the cancer remains within the mammary duct, it is referred to as *noninvasive.* The more common type of breast cancer is classified as *invasive*; this type grows into surrounding breast tissue. *Metastasis* occurs when cancer cells spread beyond the breast tissue and lymph nodes, via the blood and lymph systems, to distant sites. The most common sites of metastasis are brain, bones, liver, and lung, but breast cancer can spread to any organ. The course and treatment of metastatic breast cancer is related to the site affected and the level of functional impairment. The processes involved in cancer development are described in Chapter 19.

Noninvasive (In Situ) Breast Cancers. Ductal carcinoma in situ (DCIS) is an early *noninvasive* form of breast cancer. In DCIS, cancer cells are located within the duct and have not invaded the surrounding fatty breast tissue. Because of more precise mammography screening and earlier detection, the number of women diagnosed with DCIS has increased. Currently there is no way to determine which DCIS lesions will progress to invasive cancer and which ones will remain unchanged; however, evidence does confirm that DCIS can be a precursor to invasive cancer (ACS, 2019c). This uncertainty can cause anxiety and conflict regarding treatment decisions in women diagnosed with DCIS. It is important to convey to patients the ways in which DCIS differs from invasive cancer.

Another type of noninvasive disease is lobular carcinoma in situ (LCIS). The cells look like cancer cells and are contained within the lobules (milk-producing glands) of the breast. LCIS is not considered cancer but does increase the patient's risk for developing invasive breast cancer (ACS, 2019e). It is usually diagnosed before menopause in women 40 to 50 years of age. Traditionally LCIS is treated with close observation only, but surgical excision is an option.

Invasive Breast Cancers. The most common type of invasive breast cancer is invasive ductal carcinoma. As the name implies, the disease originates in the mammary ducts and breaks through the walls of the ducts into the surrounding breast tissue. Once invasive, the cancer grows into the tissue around it in an irregular pattern. If a lump is present, it is felt as an irregular, poorly defined mass. As the tumor continues to grow, fibrosis (replacement of normal cells with connective tissue and collagen) develops around the cancer. This fibrosis may cause shortening of the Cooper ligaments and the resulting typical skin dimpling that is seen with more advanced disease (Fig. 65.6). Another sign, sometimes indicating late-stage breast cancer, is an edematous thickening and pitting of breast skin called *peau d'orange* (orange peel skin) (Fig. 65.7).

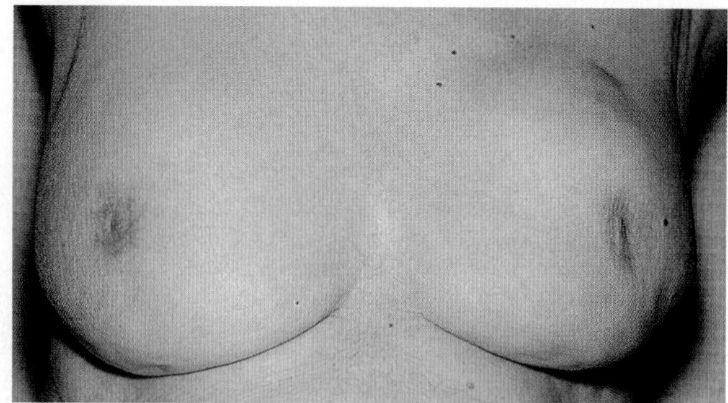

FIG. 65.6 Skin dimpling on a breast as a result of fibrosis or breast cancer. (From Mansel, R., & Bundred, N. [1995]. *Color atlas of breast disease.* St. Louis: Mosby.)

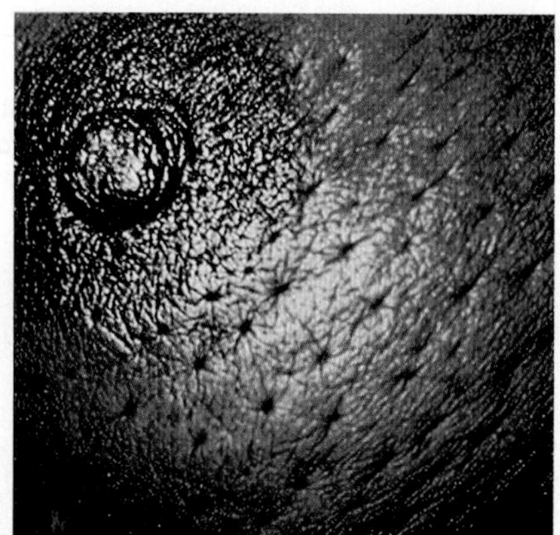

FIG. 65.7 Breast edema giving the skin an "orange peel" *(peau d'orange)* appearance. (From Gallager, H.S., Leis, H.P. Jr., Snyderman, R.K., & Urban, J.A. [1978]. *The breast.* St. Louis: Mosby.)

A rare but highly aggressive form of invasive breast cancer is inflammatory breast cancer (IBC). It is characterized by diffuse erythema and edema (peau d'orange). Patients typically report breast ***pain*** or a rapidly growing breast lump. Other common symptoms include a tender, firm, enlarged breast and breast itching. Because of its aggressive nature, IBC is usually diagnosed at a later stage than other types of breast cancer and is often harder to treat successfully (ACS, 2019f).

Other Types of Breast Cancer

Paget Disease. Paget disease of the nipple is a rare breast cancer that occurs in or around the nipple (Breastcancer.org, 2019). Although more common in women, it can also occur in men. It usually affects the nipple ducts, followed by the nipple surface, and then the areola, leaving the area scaly, red, and irritated (Breastcancer.org, 2019). It is critical to teach patients to see their health care provider if they have these symptoms, as people with Paget disease often have other types of breast cancer.

Triple-Negative Breast Cancer. Triple-negative breast cancer (TNBC) lacks expression of the estrogen receptor (ER), progesterone receptor (PR), and human epidermal growth factor receptor 2 (HER2) (Anders & Carey, 2020). This type of breast cancer grows rapidly and is often found in women with *BRCA* mutation who are premenopausal (Anders & Carey, 2020). African-American women are at higher risk for TNBC than women of other races (Anders & Carey, 2020).

PATIENT-CENTERED CARE: GENDER HEALTH CONSIDERATIONS QSEN

Male breast cancer is rare and accounts for less than 1% of all breast cancer cases (Attebery et al., 2020). Risk factors for male breast cancer include previous radiation, a family history of breast cancer (male or female), *BRCA1* and/or *BRCA2* mutation, diabetes, alcohol use and liver disease, testicular disorders, and obesity (ACS, 2020c).

Men usually present with a hard, painless, subareolar mass; gynecomastia may be present. Other symptoms include nipple discharge (often blood-stained), rash around the nipple, inverted nipple, ulceration or swelling of the chest, and possibly swollen lymph nodes. Because men usually do not suspect breast cancer, they often ignore the symptoms and postpone seeing their primary health care provider. As a result, many men are diagnosed at later stages than women. Treatment of breast cancer in men is the same as in women at a similar stage of disease.

PATIENT-CENTERED CARE: GENDER HEALTH CONSIDERATIONS QSEN

Genetic predisposition is a stronger risk factor for younger women than older women. Younger women frequently present with more aggressive forms of the disease; they are usually diagnosed at a later stage, have triple-negative breast cancer, and must receive more aggressive treatment. Screening tools can be less effective for this group because the breasts tend to be denser and mammographic recognition of breast cancer may be impaired in areas of dense tissue. Nurses should encourage women who have symptoms to seek evaluation and not watch and wait.

NCLEX EXAMINATION CHALLENGE 65.1

Health Promotion and Maintenance

When caring for four clients, which individual does the nurse identify as being at the **highest** risk for development of breast cancer?

A. 33-year-old male with gynecomastia and obesity
B. 45-year-old female whose mother has breast cancer
C. 60-year-old male whose father died from colon cancer
D. 72-year-old female who was treated for breast cancer 3 years ago

PATIENT-CENTERED CARE: CULTURAL/ SPIRITUAL CONSIDERATIONS QSEN

The rate of breast cancer in African-American women *younger than 60 years* is higher than for others in that age-group (Centers for Disease Control and Prevention [CDC], 2018). African-American women are also 40% more likely to die from breast cancer than white women (CDC, 2018). In their classic study, Ooi et al. (2011) found that American Indian, African-American, and Hispanic women were also likely to present with more aggressive breast cancer that is harder to treat, such as triple-negative breast cancer. African-American women have the highest risk for triple-negative breast cancer (Anders & Carey, 2019). These cultural disparities should be addressed with targeted interventions that are appropriate for specific cultural and ethnic groups. Nurses need to be culturally aware and competent to assist women to overcome barriers to care.

Incidence and Prevalence. One of every eight women in the United States will develop breast cancer in her lifetime (Howlader et al., 2020). It is the most common cancer diagnosis in women. Breast cancer is the second leading cause of cancer death in women aside from skin cancers (ACS, 2020a). Similar statistics can be found in Canada (Canadian Cancer Society [CCS], 2020). Early detection is the key to effective treatment and survival. The 5-year relative survival rate for localized breast cancer is 99%, whereas the rate drops to 86% when the cancer has spread to the regional lymph nodes, and to 27% for those with metastatic disease (ACS, 2020d). Metastatic cancer is not considered curable, but rather is treated as a chronic disease.

Etiology and Genetic Risk. Increased age is the primary risk factor for developing breast cancer in both women and men. Several other factors are known to increase the risk of developing breast cancer, such as family and genetic history, early menarche, and late menopause. These factors are not modifiable. Modifiable risk factors include, but are not limited to, postmenopausal obesity, physical inactivity, use of combined estrogen and progestin postmenopausal hormone replacement therapy (HRT), alcohol consumption, and lack of breast-feeding (ACS, 2019a).

According to the American Cancer Society (ACS, 2020b), breast cancer is often diagnosed late in the disease process for lesbian and bisexual women because of their fear of discrimination, negative experiences with health care professionals, and lack of health insurance. In addition, many women in these groups have no children or have a child after they are 30 years of age or older. Having several risk factors increases one's risk more than having a single risk factor. Table 65.2 lists major risk factors for breast cancer regardless of sexual orientation.

PATIENT-CENTERED CARE: GENETIC/ GENOMIC CONSIDERATIONS QSEN

Mutations in several genes, such as *BRCA1* and *BRCA2*, are related to hereditary breast cancer. People who have specific mutations in either one of these genes are at an increased risk for developing breast cancer and ovarian cancer. Encourage women to talk with a genetics counselor to carefully consider the benefits and potential consequences of genetic testing before these tests are done.

Health Promotion and Maintenance

The American Cancer Society (ACS) and the Canadian Cancer Society (CCS) establish evidence-based guidelines for breast cancer screening in women. Guidelines have not been recommended for screening men in the general population because breast cancer in men is so rare. Encourage men with a strong family history or known genetic mutations to discuss screening with their primary health care provider or request referral to a genetics counselor.

In addition to other screening and assessment methods the National Cancer Institute (n.d.) offers a Breast Cancer Risk Assessment Tool that can be used by a health care professional to estimate risk. Teach women that no single method for early detection of breast cancer is effective when used alone. The best approach for average-risk women is a screening mammogram, clinical breast examination (CBE), and breast self-awareness.

TABLE 65.2 Risk Factors for Breast Cancer

Factors	Comments
Female gender	Of all breast cancers, 99% occur in women.
Age >65 years	Risk increases across all ages until age 80 years.
Genetic factors	Inherited mutations of *BRCA1* and/or *BRCA2* increase risk.
History of a previous breast cancer	The risk for developing a cancer in the opposite breast is five times greater than for the average population at risk.
Breast density	Dense breasts contain more glandular and connective tissue, which increases the risk for developing breast cancer.
Atypical hyperplasia	Biopsy-confirmed atypical hyperplasia is a high relative risk.
Family history	Having a first-degree relative with breast or ovarian cancer increases risk.
Ionizing radiation	Women who received frequent low-level radiation exposure to the thorax have an increased risk, especially if the exposure occurred during periods of rapid breast formation or if there was high-dose radiation to the chest.
High postmenopausal bone density	High estrogen levels over time both strengthen bone and increase breast cancer risk.
Reproductive history Nulliparity *or* First child born after age 30 years	Childless women have an increased risk, as do women who bear their first child at or after age 30.
Menstrual history Early menstruation (younger than 11 years) *or* Late menopause (at or older than 55 years) *or* Both	The risk for breast cancer rises as the interval between menarche and menopause increases. Women who undergo bilateral oophorectomy before age 35 years have less risk for breast cancer than women who undergo natural menopause.
Recent oral contraceptive use	There is a slight increase in breast cancer risk in women taking oral contraceptives. The risk returns to normal 10 years after stopping the pill.
Recent hormone replacement therapy (HRT)	Use of HRT containing both estrogen and progestin increases risk; risk diminishes 5 years after discontinuation.
Obesity	Postmenopausal obesity (especially increased abdominal fat), increased body mass, insulin resistance, and hyperglycemia have been reported to be associated with an increased risk for breast cancer.
Other Risk Factors	
Alcohol consumption	Risk is dose dependent; consumption of 2-3 drinks per day is associated with a 20% increased risk; risk increases with increased consumption. This includes all forms of alcoholic beverages.
High socioeconomic status	Breast cancer incidence is greater in women of higher education and socioeconomic background. This relationship is possibly related to lifestyle differences, such as later age at first birth.
Jewish heritage	Women of Ashkenazi Jewish heritage have higher incidences of *BRCA1* and *BRCA2* genetic mutations.

Data from American Cancer Society. (2019). *Breast cancer facts & figures 2019-2020.* Atlanta: Author.

Mammography. In 2015 the American Cancer Society (ACS) updated its breast cancer screening guidelines, which now recommend that women at average risk of breast cancer begin annual screening mammography at age 45 up to age 54. Women ages 40 to 44 should have the choice to start annual mammograms after the risks and potential benefits have been explained. Women age 55 and older may switch to mammograms every 2 years, or continue annual screening mammograms if they choose to do so. Mammography should continue as long as a woman is in good health and has a life expectancy of at least 10 years (ACS, 2020a).

Canadian guidelines for mammography differ from those of the United States: no routine mammography screening is recommended until women reach 50 years of age. After 50, the recommended guidelines vary slightly across organizations but generally recommend that women after age 50 get a mammogram every 2 to 3 years until age 70 to 74 (CCS, 2020).

Breast Self-Awareness/Self-Examination. Data demonstrate that breast self-examination is not a meaningful screening tool for breast cancer (Komen, 2020). However, it is recommended that women increase breast self-awareness by becoming familiar with how their breasts look and feel so that they can report differences or abnormalities.

Teach a woman that lumps are not necessarily abnormal. For premenopausal women, lumps can come and go with the menstrual cycle. Most lumps that are detected and tested are not malignant.

Some women may want to practice regular breast self-examination (BSE) as a method for breast self-awareness. BSE should be presented as an option to women beginning in their early 20s. In addition to breast self-awareness, place emphasis on clinical breast examination (CBE) and mammogram for early detection of breast cancer. The combined approach is better than any single test. A woman who chooses to perform BSE should be taught the correct technique and have it reviewed by a health care provider during her CBE.

Use teaching models of normal and abnormal breasts when teaching BSE. Discuss the proper timing for BSE. Instruct premenopausal women to examine their breasts 1 week after the menstrual period. At this time, hormonal influence on breast tissue is decreased, so fluid retention and tenderness are reduced. Teach women whose breast tissue is no longer influenced by

BEST PRACTICE FOR PATIENT SAFETY & QUALITY CARE (QSEN)

Performing Breast Self-Examination

1. Lie on your back and place your right arm behind your head. Lying down spreads the breast tissue evenly over the chest wall, making it easier to feel all the breast tissue

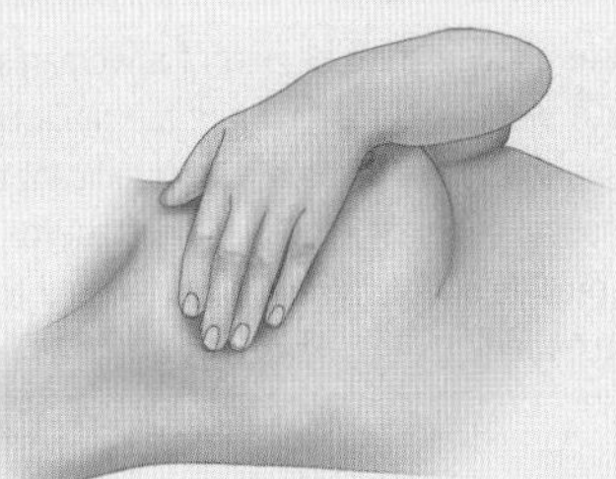

2. Use the finger pads of the three middle fingers on your left hand to feel for lumps in the right breast. Use overlapping dime-sized circular motions of the finger pads to feel the breast tissue

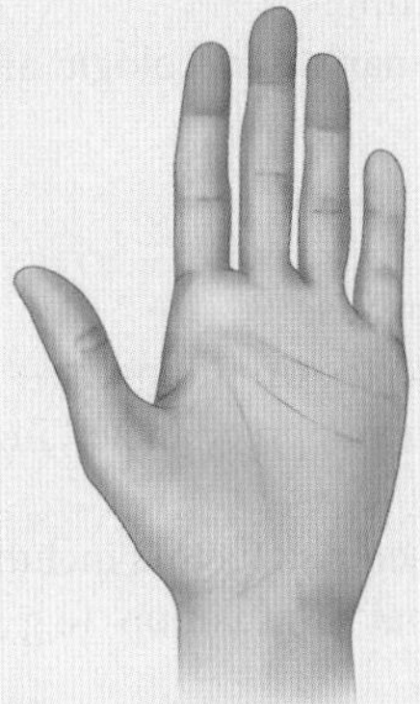

3. Use three different levels of pressure to feel all the breast tissue. Light pressure is needed to feel the tissue closest to the skin; medium pressure to feel a little deeper; and firm pressure to feel the tissue closest to the chest and ribs. It is normal to feel a firm ridge in the lower curve of each breast.
4. Move around the breast in an up-and-down pattern, starting at an imaginary line drawn straight down your side from the underarm and moving across the breast to the middle of the chest bone (sternum or breastbone). Be sure to check the entire breast area, going down until you feel only ribs and up to the neck

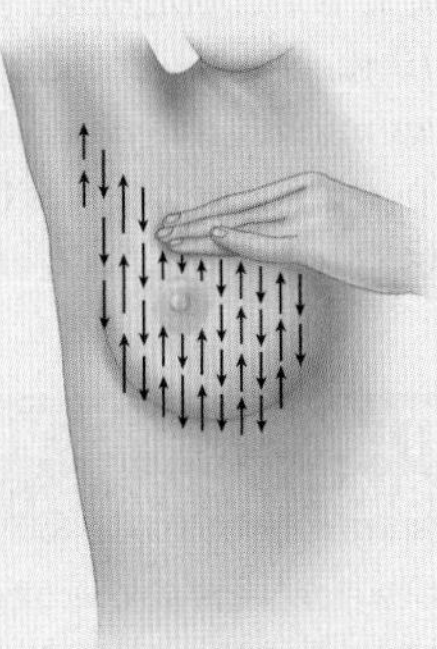

5. Repeat the examination on your left breast, putting your left arm behind your head and using the finger pads of your right hand to do the examination.
6. While standing in front of a mirror with your hands pressing firmly down on your hips, look at your breasts for any changes in size, shape, contour, or dimpling, and look at your nipples and breast skin for redness or scaling. (Pressing down on the hips contracts the chest wall muscles and enhances any breast changes.)
7. Examine each underarm while sitting up or standing and with your arm only slightly raised so you can easily feel in this area. Raising your arm straight up tightens the tissue in this area and makes it harder to examine.

hormonal fluctuations, such as after a total hysterectomy or menopause, to pick a day each month to do BSE, such as the first day of the month. The BSE technique is similar for women and men. The Best Practice for Patient Safety & Quality Care: Performing Breast Self-Examination box describes the procedure for breast self-examination and may be used as a patient resource.

Clinical Breast Examination. Clinical breast examination (CBE) is typically performed by advanced practice nurses and other health care providers. It is recommended that the CBE be part of a periodic health assessment, at least every 3 years for women in their 20s and 30s and every year for asymptomatic women at least 40 years of age (National Comprehensive Cancer Network [NCCN], 2019). Teach patients what to expect during this examination. First, they will be asked to undress from the waist up. The health care provider inspects the breasts for abnormalities in size and shape and for skin and nipple changes. Then, using the pads of the fingers, the provider palpates the breasts for any lumps and, if present, whether such lumps are attached to the skin or deeper tissues. The area under both arms is also examined.

Remind the patient to report any breast changes she may have noted during a breast self-examination to the health care provider performing the clinical breast examination.

NCLEX EXAMINATION CHALLENGE 65.2

Health Promotion and Maintenance

When caring for a 28-year-old healthy client, how frequently does the nurse recommend a clinical breast examination (CBE)?

A. Every 3 years
B. At each annual physical
C. Not until age 30, as the risks are low
D. To begin at age 40 when risks increase

PATIENT-CENTERED CARE: OLDER ADULT CONSIDERATIONS (QSEN)

As women age, the breast tissue becomes flattened and elongated and is suspended loosely from the chest wall. On palpation, the breast tissue of the older woman has a finer, more granular feel than the lobular feel in a younger woman. The inframammary ridge may be more prominent as a result of atrophy of the breast tissue. Breast examination in older adults may be easier because of tissue atrophy and relaxation of the suspensory ligaments.

Options for High-Risk Women. Those with a personal history of breast cancer are at risk for developing a recurrence or a new breast cancer. Women with known *BRCA1* and/or *BRCA2* genetic mutation have a lifetime risk of developing breast cancer by age

70 of about 55% to 60% and 45%, respectively (National Breast Cancer Foundation, 2019). Women in this category usually practice *close surveillance* as a prevention option. It is a method of *secondary prevention* and is used to detect cancer early in the initial stages. In addition to annual mammography and clinical breast examination, high-risk women are recommended to have an annual breast MRI screening (ACS, 2019a). Close surveillance may begin as early as age 30 years, but evidence is limited regarding the best age at which to start screening. *For women with a high risk for breast cancer development due to family history such as cancer in a mother or sister, it is recommended that cancer screening begin at the age that is 10 years younger than the age at which the affected cancer patient was initially diagnosed.* Encourage high-risk women to discuss their personal preferences for close surveillance with their primary health care providers.

PATIENT-CENTERED CARE: VETERANS HEALTH CONSIDERATIONS QSEN

Research shows that female veterans have a higher incidence of breast cancer than the general population, possibly due to increased exposure to risk factors or to earlier detection (McDaniel et al., 2018). Encourage women veterans to have screening done per recommended guidelines due to this increased risk.

Other options currently available for reducing a woman's breast cancer risk are **prophylactic mastectomy** (preventive surgical removal of one or both breasts), **prophylactic oophorectomy** (removal of the ovaries), and chemopreventive drugs. Although each option significantly reduces the risk for breast cancer, no option completely eliminates it. Each option has its own risks and potentially serious complications.

Even though a woman may decide to have a prophylactic mastectomy, there is a small risk that breast cancer will develop in residual breast glandular tissue because no mastectomy reliably removes all mammary tissue. Women must also understand that breast reconstruction after a prophylactic mastectomy is very different from breast augmentation. It is a more complex surgical procedure with a greater potential for complications. The decision to have this type of surgery can be a very difficult one to make. Women may find it helpful to reach out to a breast cancer support organization and talk to someone who has been through a prophylactic mastectomy.

Women undergoing prophylactic oophorectomy will likely experience menopausal symptoms, although some estrogen remains in body fat tissue. Chemoprevention drugs, such as tamoxifen, reduce breast cancer recurrence but carry other risks such as blood clots and endometrial cancer (Boucher, 2018). Encourage women to carefully consider the benefits and risks of breast cancer risk–reducing options and discuss them with their health care provider.

❖ Interprofessional Collaborative Care

◆ Assessment: Recognize Cues

History. Early breast cancer often has no symptoms (ACS, 2019a). At other times, the history is taken after a mass has been discovered but before a diagnosis has been made. For some patients, the history may be obtained at the time they are seen for treatment of an identified cancer. The interview should focus on three major areas: risk factors, the breast mass, and health maintenance practices.

PATIENT-CENTERED CARE: CULTURAL/ SPIRITUAL CONSIDERATIONS QSEN

Some cultures do not allow men to be part of a woman's care, or allow only women to care for a woman. Other cultures are male predominant, and all decisions about female care are made by the significant man in her life, who may be a father, spouse, or oldest son. It is important for the health care provider and nurse to provide culturally sensitive care and to respect the beliefs and practices of the patient.

Ask specific information about personal and family histories of breast cancer. In addition to increasing the woman's own risk, these factors also affect any sisters' or daughters' risk and should be part of later counseling.

Ask about the woman's gynecologic and obstetric (if any) history, including:

- Age at menarche
- Age at menopause
- Symptoms of menopause
- Age at first child's birth (or nulliparity—having no children)
- Number of children and pregnancies, including miscarriages or terminations

Recognize that increased risk factors include:

- Prolonged hormonal stimulation (e.g., early menses, late menopause)
- Use of contraceptives
- Birth of the first child after 30 years of age

A history of the breast mass or lump can reveal the course of the disease and information related to health care–seeking practices and health-promoting behaviors. Ask the patient about how, when, and by whom the mass was discovered and the time between discovery and seeking care. The answer to this question reveals the need for discussion and teaching about health promotion practices, regardless of whether the mass proves to be cancerous. If there was a delay between discovery and seeing the health care provider, inquire what caused the delay. These questions are linked to the psychosocial assessment but also reveal the length of time that the mass has been untreated. Review with the patient which procedures have been performed to diagnose the problem and if they have noticed any other changes in their body within the past year. This information can help determine if there will be the likelihood of metastasis. Ask especially about the presence of joint and bone pain or cognitive changes.

Assess the use of alcohol intake because this is a factor that may increase breast cancer risk. Perform an in-depth medication review, including prescribed and over-the-counter (OTC) drugs that are used. Specifically ask about hormonal supplements, such as estrogen and natural or herbal substances that stimulate hormones, and birth control use. Estrogen can be taken orally, intravaginally, or via a transdermal patch. Document the type and form of hormones (birth control pills or patches, supplements) and length of use.

BEST PRACTICE FOR PATIENT SAFETY & QUALITY CARE (QSEN)

Assessing a Breast Mass

- Identify the location of the mass by using the "face of the clock" method.
- Describe the shape, size, and consistency of the mass.
- Assess whether the mass is fixed or movable.
- Note any skin changes around the mass, such as dimpling of the skin, increased vascularity, nipple retraction, nipple inversion, or skin ulceration.
- Assess the adjacent lymph nodes, both axillary and supraclavicular nodes.
- Ask patients if they experience ***pain*** or soreness in the area around the mass.

Physical Assessment/Clinical Signs and Symptoms. Document any abnormal findings from the clinical breast examination. Describe specific information about a breast mass (as described in the Best Practice for Patient Safety & Quality Care: Assessing a Breast Mass box), such as location, using the "face of the clock" method; shape; size; consistency; and whether the mass is mobile or fixed to the surrounding tissue. Note any skin change, such as *peau d'orange,* redness and warmth, nipple retraction, or ulceration, which can indicate advanced disease. Document the location of any enlargements of axillary and supraclavicular lymph nodes. Evaluate for the presence of ***pain*** or tenderness in the affected breast.

Psychosocial Assessment. A breast cancer diagnosis is usually an unanticipated event in the life of a woman who feels physically well. It initiates a sudden and distressing transition into a potentially life-threatening illness. Feelings of fear, shock, and disbelief are predominant as a woman learns about the disease and faces numerous treatment decisions. Psychological distress is common at cancer diagnosis and at the various transitions of treatment. A previous history of mental illness, age, and life circumstances can contribute to increased psychological distress. Encourage expression of feelings, focusing on the human component of care (Mahon, 2017) and determine if a referral to a counselor would be helpful. There are also multiple community resources available for the person diagnosed with breast cancer. Talking with someone who has been through the experience is particularly helpful in dealing with the emotional aspects of the disease.

Assess the patient for concerns related to ***sexuality.*** Sexual dysfunction affects most breast cancer survivors in some way. Sometimes it is related to the loss of a breast and the threat to one's femininity, her image of herself, or how she perceives her partner's response. Lack of libido (sexual desire) related to hormonal changes, psychological distress, and anxiety are commonly experienced by women with breast cancer. If the patient does not discuss sexual concerns voluntarily, open the conversation in a nonthreatening, nonjudgmental way. Use resources that provide education about alternative expressions of intimacy and a focus on pleasure rather than performance. Refer the patient and her partner to counseling if appropriate.

Laboratory Assessment. The diagnosis of breast cancer relies on pathologic examination of tissue from the breast mass. After the diagnosis of cancer is established, laboratory tests, including pathologic study of the lymph nodes, help detect possible metastases. Elevated liver enzyme levels indicate possible liver metastases, and increased serum calcium and alkaline phosphatase levels could suggest bone metastases.

PATIENT-CENTERED CARE: GENDER HEALTH CONSIDERATIONS (QSEN)

Research about breast cancer and women who identify as lesbian or bisexual continues. Factors that are more likely to increase the risk of breast cancer in lesbian and bisexual women include nulliparity or increased age at birth of first child, use of oral contraceptives (ACS, 2020b), cigarette smoking, alcohol use, and obesity (Margolies, 2020). Lesbian and bisexual women may not seek regular care due to fear and distrust of culturally incompetent health care providers and/or health care access. Nurses' awareness and sensitivity to these issues help establish trust (Boehmer, 2018). Emphasize the importance of screening and early detection (Ceres et al., 2018). Assess the need for referrals to support organizations such as the National LGBT Cancer Network (2020).

Imaging Assessment. *Mammography* is a sensitive screening tool for breast cancer. The uniqueness of this test results from its ability to reveal preclinical lesions (masses too small to be palpated manually). Most breast centers now use *digital mammography,* a system that is able to read, file, and transmit mammograms electronically. Patient preparation and the procedure for mammography are discussed in Chapter 64. Some women may voice concern about radiation exposure with mammograms. Reassure them that the dose is very small and the risk for harm from radiation is minimal.

Digital breast tomosynthesis is technology that is similar to mammography but uses three-dimensional images (see Chapter 64; Fig. 65.8). It is useful in evaluating dense breasts and is more accurate in women younger than 50. In the United States, currently it is covered by Medicare and most other major health insurances. This advanced technology is also available in Canada.

Ultrasonography of the breast is an additional diagnostic tool used to clarify findings on mammography. If the mammogram reveals a lesion, ultrasonography is helpful in differentiating a fluid-filled cyst from a solid mass. Mammography screening combined with ultrasound may be effective for detecting cancers in women with dense breasts, but currently it is not recommended for routine breast cancer screening as a stand-alone imaging tool (ACS, 2019a).

MRI is used for screening high-risk women and better examination of suspicious areas found on a mammogram (ACS, 2019a). It is more expensive than mammography. Most insurance companies will cover a portion of the cost if the woman is shown to be at high risk. Although higher-quality images are produced, there is concern about high costs and access to quality breast MRI services for high-risk women. Most major insurances will cover a portion of MRI costs for women shown to be at higher risk (ACS, 2019a).

If the patient has an invasive breast cancer, other imaging tests may be done to rule out metastases. Positron emission tomography (PET) scan, brain MRI, and CT scans of the chest, abdomen, and pelvis can reveal distant metastases.

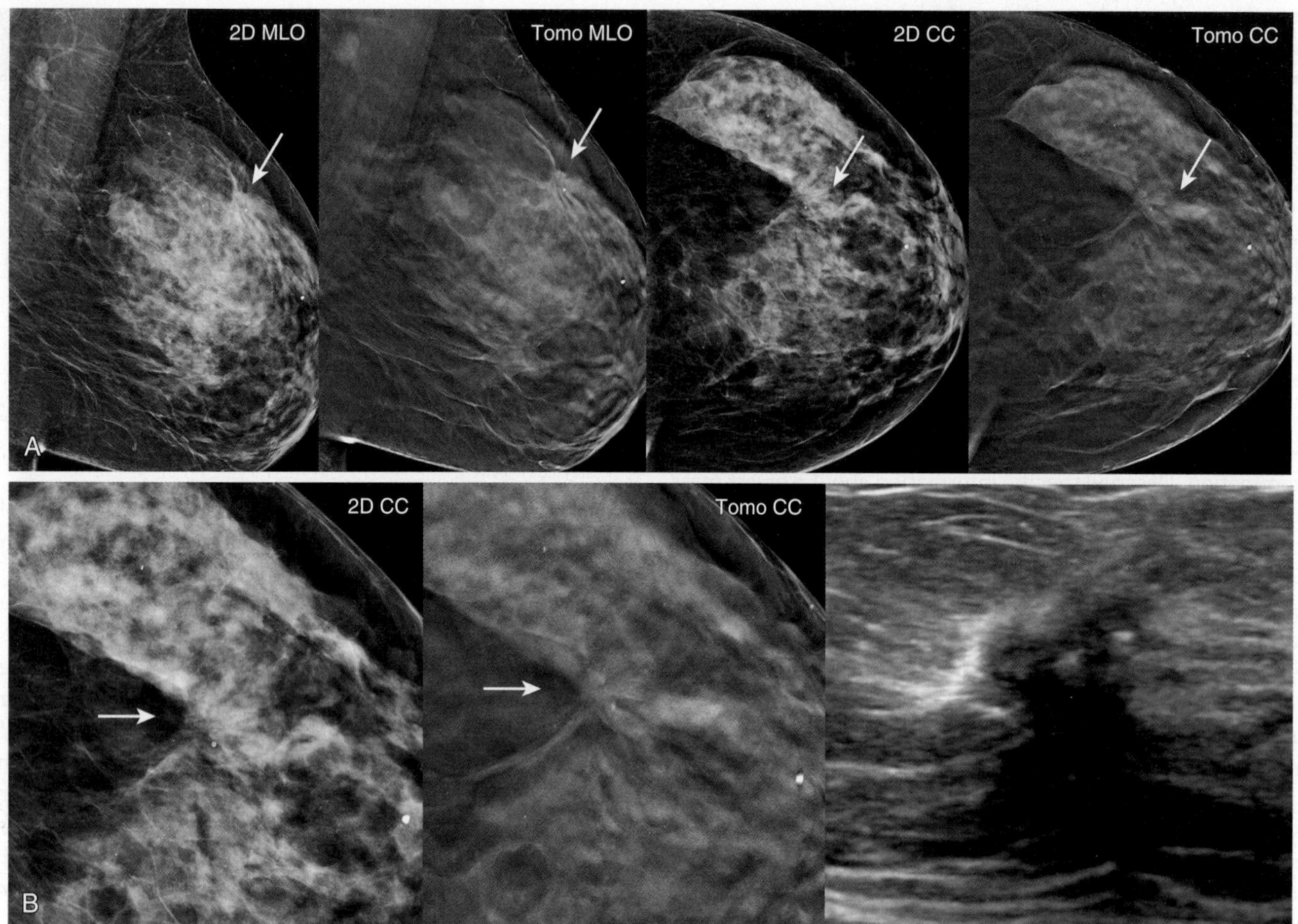

FIG. 65.8 Breast tomosynthesis. Architectural distortion (AD) seen on 2D and tomosynthesis screening mammography. A, Screening mammogram in a 50-year-old woman demonstrates an AD in the left upper outer breast *(arrows)*, which is better seen on tomosynthesis. B, Close-up craniocaudal views show the AD with associated microCa++ *(arrows)* to be very obvious on tomosynthesis. (From Philpotts, L.E., & Hooley, R.J. [2017]. *Breast tomosynthesis.* Philadelphia: Elsevier.)

Other Diagnostic Assessment. Although imaging techniques serve as tools for screening and more precise visualization of potential breast cancers, *breast biopsy (pathologic examination of the breast tissue) is the only definitive way to diagnose breast cancer* (see Chapter 64). Tissue samples are analyzed by a pathologist to determine the presence of breast cancer. If breast cancer is identified, it is classified according to the size and type of breast cancer, the histologic grade, and the type of receptors on the cells. These characteristics are used to guide treatment. For example, a small, noninvasive breast cancer may only be treated with lumpectomy and radiation, whereas a larger, aggressive tumor (one with a high histologic grade) may be treated with a mastectomy and chemotherapy, followed by radiation.

Cancer cells that contain estrogen receptors *(ER positive)* or progesterone receptors *(PR positive)* have a better prognosis and usually respond to hormonal therapy. If the type of breast cancer is *HER2 positive,* or one in which the *neu* gene is overexpressed, it may be treated successfully with trastuzumab, which is a HER2-positive breast cancer–specific *targeted therapy.*

Most women, even those with very small tumors, receive some sort of treatment in addition to surgery for breast cancer. Research has focused on ways to predict clinical outcomes so that low-risk women may avoid unnecessary treatments. Genomic tests, such as Oncotype DX and MammaPrint, have been developed to help predict clinical outcomes by analyzing genes in breast cancer tissue. Some health care providers use this information in addition to the pathologic analysis for guiding treatment decisions. These multigene tests have been shown to be accurate predictors of patient prognosis and response to therapy in breast cancer (National Comprehensive Cancer Network [NCCN] Guidelines, 2020).

◆ Analysis: Analyze Cues and Prioritize Hypotheses.

The priority collaborative problems for patients with breast cancer include:

1. Potential for cancer metastasis due to lack of, or inadequate, treatment
2. Potential for impaired coping due to breast cancer diagnosis and treatment

◆ Planning and Implementation: Generate Solutions and Take Action

Decreasing the Risk for Metastasis

Planning: Generate Solutions. The patient who is treated for breast cancer is expected to remain free of metastases or recurrence of disease, if possible. If cancer recurs, the patient will experience optimal health outcomes, including potential palliation and end-of-life care.

Interventions: Take Action. There are many surgical and nonsurgical options for breast cancer treatment. Because of the various options, the patient with breast cancer often faces difficult decisions. Although patients are living longer with metastatic disease, the 5-year survival rate remains low. Once cancer is diagnosed, the extent and location of breast cancer and metastases (if applicable) determine the overall treatment strategy. The emphasis of breast cancer treatment is on preventing or stopping the spread of tumor cells that lead to distant metastasis. Treatment is tailored specifically to each patient, taking into account other health problems and the patient's ability to tolerate a particular therapy.

Nonsurgical Management

Complementary and integrative health. Women with breast cancer often cope with distressing symptoms related to the disease itself or the side effects of treatment. Common symptoms associated with these treatments include ***pain,*** nausea/vomiting, hot flashes, anxiety, depression, and fatigue. Physical and emotional symptoms associated with breast cancer may be eased with the use of complementary and integrative therapy. Prayer is also widely used. Other types of therapies include guided imagery and massage. The most frequently used strategies are biologically based therapies such as vitamins, special cancer diets, and herbal therapy. Teach the patient that all ingested complementary agents potentially risk interaction with conventional drugs.

Encourage women to seek a practitioner with a certification or license for the specific type of integrative therapy intervention. In some states, a certification or license is required for acupuncture, chiropractic therapy, massage, and shiatsu. Some types of complementary and integrative therapy can be self-taught or done alone after a few sessions of instruction. Table 65.3 lists complementary and integrative therapies for specific symptoms associated with breast cancer and its treatments.

Although the use of complementary and integrative therapy can improve quality of life, its use does not alter the outcome of breast cancer, and it should not be used in place of standard treatment. Encourage patients who are interested in trying these therapies to check with their health care provider before using them. The website https://www.breastcancer.org/treatment/comp_med provides accurate information about complementary therapies and the extent to which they have been researched in breast cancer patients. Cost may be a factor in decision making because not all insurances provide coverage for complementary and integrative therapies. Remind the patient that it is important to disclose to the health care provider all treatments undertaken.

For patients with breast cancer at a stage for which surgery is the main treatment, follow-up with adjuvant (in addition to surgery) radiation, chemotherapy, hormone therapy, or targeted therapy is commonly prescribed. For those who cannot have surgery or whose cancer is too advanced, these therapies may be used to promote comfort (palliation). End-of-life care is discussed in Chapter 8.

Surgical Management. The management of early-stage breast cancer is surgery. A large tumor is sometimes treated with chemotherapy, called **neoadjuvant therapy**, to shrink the tumor before it is surgically removed. An advantage of this therapy is that cancer can be removed by lumpectomy rather than mastectomy. This may provide less invasive surgery and a better cosmetic outcome for the patient.

TABLE 65.3 Common Complementary and Integrative Therapies Used by Patients With Breast Cancer

Symptom	Complementary and Integrative Therapy
Physical	
Pain	Acupuncture, chiropractic therapy, hypnosis, massage, music, reiki, shiatsu
Nausea/vomiting	Acupuncture, aromatherapy, ginger, hypnosis, progressive muscle relaxation, shiatsu
Fatigue	Acupuncture, massage, meditation, reiki, tai chi, yoga
Hot flashes	Acupuncture, flaxseed, black cohosh. Use caution with all herbal and ingested supplements; there is no substantial data to support one treatment over others
Muscle tension	Aromatherapy, massage, shiatsu
Emotional	
Anxiety, stress, fear	Aromatherapy, guided imagery, hypnosis, journaling, massage, meditation, music therapy, progressive muscle relaxation, prayer, support groups, tai chi, yoga
Depression	Aromatherapy, yoga, journaling, progressive muscle relaxation

Axillary lymph nodes are analyzed for the presence of cancer and staging purposes. Axillary lymph node dissection (ALND) is usually done when there are clinically positive nodes. Sentinel lymph node biopsy (SLNB) is a much less invasive approach and is recommended by guidelines for analyzing lymph nodes in early-stage breast cancers with low-to-moderate risk for lymph node involvement. In this method, the sentinel lymph node is identified during breast surgery by injecting the breast with radioisotope and/or dye that travels via lymphatic pathways to the sentinel lymph node. The nodes that take up the dye are removed and examined for the presence of cancer cells. It is believed that if cancer cells have traveled through the lymph channels, the cells will lodge in the sentinel nodes. Travel beyond these nodes to higher-level nodes may occur as a secondary event. Therefore the absence of cancer cells in the sentinel nodes is an indicator that no other nodes in the regional area are involved.

Preoperative care. Care of the patient facing surgery for breast cancer focuses on psychological preparation and preoperative teaching. Priority nursing interventions are directed toward relieving anxiety and providing information to increase patient knowledge. Include the spouse, partner, or other family member or significant other, who may be experiencing similar stress and confusion, in the health teaching unless the patient does not desire this or the patient's culture does not permit this approach.

Review the type of procedure planned. Use open-ended questions (e.g., "What type of surgery are you having? Can you explain what will happen?") to assess the patient's current level of knowledge. Provide postoperative information, including:

- The need for a drainage tube
- The location of the incision
- Mobility restrictions
- The length of the hospital stay (if any)
- General preoperative and postoperative information needed by any surgical patient (see Chapter 9)

Supplement teaching with written or digital materials for the patient and family. This information should include whom to call in case there are any complications or questions. Address body image issues and expectations before surgery to avoid misconceptions about appearance after surgery. If available, suggest that patients and their caregivers attend classes before surgery in an ambulatory care setting, such as a breast cancer center, to promote successful early discharge from the hospital. Programs that provide emotional support, information, and opportunities for discussion related to ***sexuality,*** body image, and preoperative and postoperative care enhance the recovery of the short-stay mastectomy patient.

Operative procedures. Types of breast surgeries are shown in Fig. 65.9. During breast-conserving surgery, also known as *lumpectomy* or *partial mastectomy,* the surgeon removes part of the breast that contains cancer and some normal tissue around it. The term *margins* refers to the distance between the tumor and the edge of the surrounding tissue. The desired outcome of breast-conserving surgery is to obtain *negative margins* in which no cancer cells extend to the edge of the tissue. Patients undergoing breast conserving surgery may have drainage tubes placed if the lump is large or if axillary node dissection is performed. Typically, radiation therapy follows to kill any residual tumor cells.

Breast-conserving procedures are usually performed in same-day surgical settings. The cosmetic results of these surgeries are good to excellent, and the psychological benefits of avoiding breast removal are significant for patients who choose this option.

Typically, indications for a mastectomy include multicentric disease (tumor is present in different quadrants of the breast), inability to have radiation therapy, presence of a large tumor in a small breast, genetic testing results, and patient preference. Mastectomy does not conserve the breast; the affected breast is completely removed. A total (simple) mastectomy is surgery to remove the whole breast that has cancer. A *modified radical mastectomy* removes the breast tissue, lymph nodes, and sometimes part of the underlying chest wall muscle. During this procedure, the surgeon places one or two drainage tubes, usually Jackson-Pratt (JP) drains, under the skin flaps and attaches the tubes to a small collection chamber. These collect any fluid that accumulates under the surgical area. Reconstruction can be performed at the same time as the mastectomy. Skin flaps or expanders may be used to create a breast mound at the time of the original procedure.

Postoperative care. The hospital stay after breast surgery is short, often same day or just overnight, and recovery is usually not complicated. After surgery, avoid using the affected arm for measuring blood pressure, giving injections, or drawing blood. If lymph nodes are removed, it is critical to prevent trauma to the affected arm. The patient returns from the postanesthesia

Breast-conserving Surgery

Lumpectomy

Partial Mastectomy

Breast-conserving surgery. Dotted lines show the area containing the tumor that is removed and some of the lymph nodes that may be removed.

Total (Simple) Mastectomy

Total (simple) mastectomy. The dotted line shows where the entire breast is removed. Some lymph nodes under the arm may also be removed.

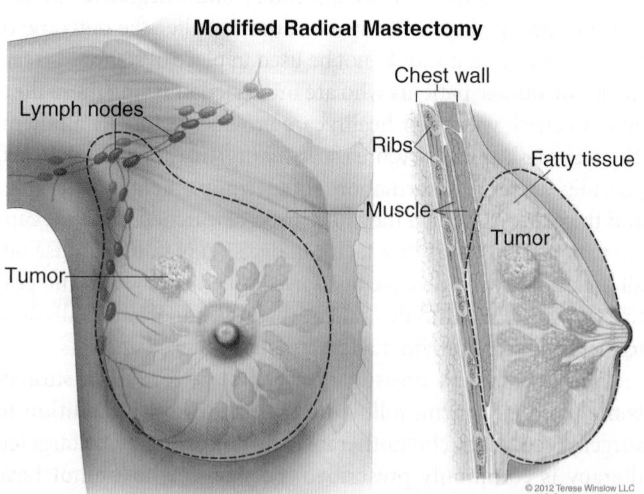

Modified radical mastectomy. The dotted line shows where the entire breast and some lymph nodes are removed. Part of the chest wall muscle may also be removed.

FIG. 65.9 Surgical treatment for breast cancer. (©2010 Terese Winslow. U.S. Govt. has certain rights.)

care unit (PACU) as soon as vital signs return to baseline levels and if no complications have occurred. Assess vital signs on a schedule of decreasing frequency, such as every 30 minutes for two times, every hour for two times, and then every 4 hours. During these checks, assess the dressing for bleeding.

When taking vital signs, monitor for the amount and color of drainage if drains are present. Document this within the intake and output section of the electronic health record.

NURSING SAFETY PRIORITY (QSEN)

Action Alert

To decrease the chance of surgical site ***infection,*** carefully observe the surgical wound after breast surgery for signs of swelling and infection throughout recovery. Assess the incision and flap of the postmastectomy patient for signs of bleeding, infection, and poor tissue perfusion. Drainage tubes are usually removed about 1 to 3 weeks after hospital discharge when the patient returns for an office visit. The drainage amount should be less than 30 mL in a 24-hour period. Inform the patient that tube removal may cause temporary ***pain.*** Provide or suggest analgesia before they are removed. Document all findings and report any abnormalities to the surgeon immediately.

Assess the patient's position to ensure that the drainage tubes or collection device is not pulled or kinked. The patient should have the head of the bed elevated at least 30 degrees, with the affected arm elevated on a pillow while awake. Keeping the affected arm elevated promotes lymphatic fluid return after removal of lymph nodes and channels. Provide other basic comfort measures, such as repositioning and analgesics as prescribed, on a regular basis until ***pain*** ceases. Patient-controlled analgesia may be used for some patients for a short time, depending on the type of surgery that was performed.

Ambulation and a regular diet are resumed by the day after surgery. While the patient is walking, the arm on the affected side may need to be supported at first. Gradually the arm should be allowed to hang straight by the side. Encourage the patient to use good posture to prevent mobility issues. Beginning exercises that do not stress the incision can usually be started on the first day after surgery. These exercises include squeezing the affected hand around a soft, round object (a ball or rolled washcloth) and flexion/extension of the elbow. The progression to more strenuous exercises depends on the subsequent procedures planned (e.g., reconstruction) and the surgeon's directions. The patient can be discharged to home after safely ambulating and when surgical ***pain*** is under control. Common instructions for exercises after mastectomy are listed in the Patient and Family Education: Preparing for Self-Management: Postmastectomy Exercises box.

Breast reconstruction. Breast reconstruction after or during mastectomy for women is common with few complications. Patients consult with the plastic surgeon to discuss the type of reconstruction, timing of the procedure, and technique desired. Many women prefer reconstruction immediately after mastectomy using their own tissue (autogenous reconstruction). Breast reconstruction at the time of mastectomy, both autogenous and prosthetic, may lessen the psychological strain associated with undergoing a mastectomy. The surgeon should offer the option of breast reconstruction before surgery is performed.

Assess her attitude by asking about future plans for restoring appearance. Although reconstruction is not appropriate for some women and others may not be interested in it, the surgeon should discuss the indications and contraindications, advantages and disadvantages, and typical recovery. If immediate reconstruction is chosen, the breast surgeon should be aware of this before surgery so plans can be coordinated with those of the plastic surgeon.

Several procedures are available for restoring the appearance of the breast (Table 65.4). Reconstruction may begin during the

PATIENT AND FAMILY EDUCATION: PREPARING FOR SELF-MANAGEMENT

Postmastectomy Exercises

The surgeon or physical therapist can provide additional stretches and exercises. Hold each stretch until you feel a gentle pulling. Exercises can be done standing, sitting or lying down.

Hand Wall Climbing

- Face the wall and put the palms of your hands flat against the wall at shoulder level.
- Flex your fingers so your hands slowly "walk" up the wall.
- Stop when your arms are fully extended.
- Slowly "walk" your hands back down the wall until they return to shoulder level.

Rope Turning

- Tie a rope to the knob of a closed door.
- Hold the other end of the rope and step back from the door until your arm is almost straight out in front of you.
- Swing the rope in a circle. Start with small circles and gradually increase to larger circles as you become more flexible.

Side Bends

- Sit in a chair.
- Clasp your hands together.
- Slowly raise your arms over your head and then gently bend to each side.

Shoulder Blade Squeeze

- Sit in chair. Do not rest your back against the chair.
- Place arms at side, elbows bent.
- Squeeze your shoulder blades together behind you. Do not lift your shoulders up toward your ears.

NCLEX EXAMINATION CHALLENGE 65.3

Physiological Integrity

The nurse has delegated care for a client with a radical left mastectomy for breast cancer to assistive personnel (AP). Which AP action requires nursing intervention? **Select all that apply.**

A. Obtains blood pressure via left arm
B. Reports client's pain level to the nurse
C. Applies gait belt prior to walking with the client
D. Records vital signs in the electronic health record
E. Assists client to administer patient-controlled analgesia

TABLE 65.4 Examples of Breast Reconstruction Procedures

Procedure	Description	Procedure	Description
Implantation	An implant matching the size of the other breast is placed under the muscle on the operative side to create a breast mound. 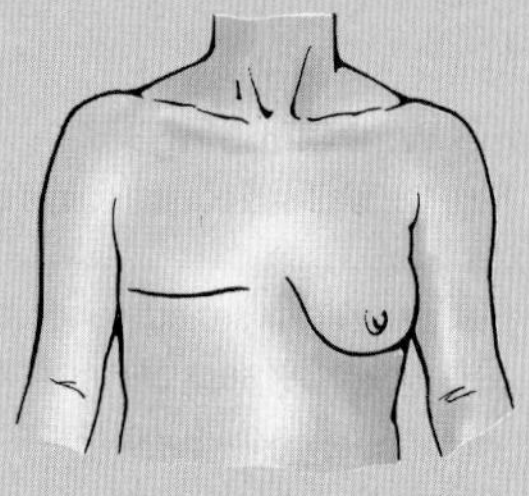 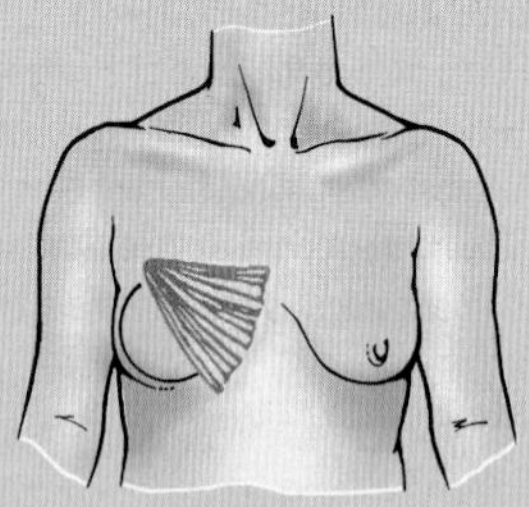	Flaps	A flap of skin, fat, and muscle is transferred from the donor site to the operative area. The flap contains an appropriate amount of fat to match the other breast and is similar in appearance to breast tissue. A blood supply is established by reanastomosis of vessels from the operative area to those with the flap when possible. A new nipple may be created with tissue from areas such as the labia or upper, inner thigh. Nipples can also be created by tattooing. Latissimus dorsi musculocutaneous flap; 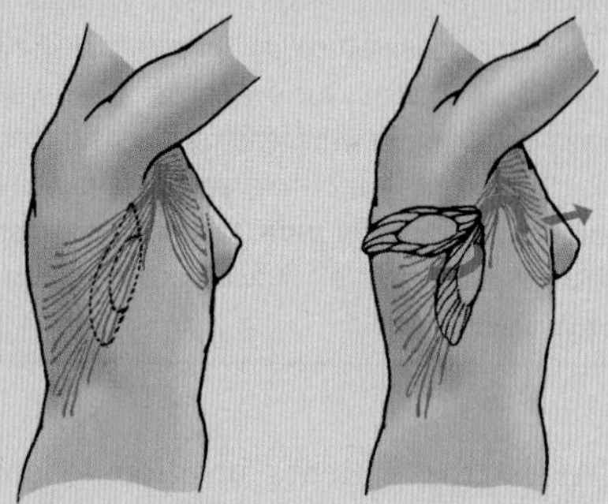 Abdominal myocutaneous flap
Tissue expansion DIEP reconstruction (deep inferior epigastric perforator flap)	A tissue expander is placed under the muscle and gradually expanded with saline to stretch the overlying skin and create a pocket. After several weeks, the tissue expander is exchanged for an implant. 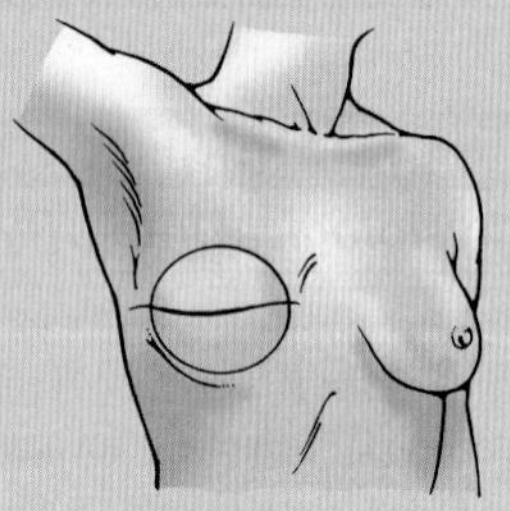		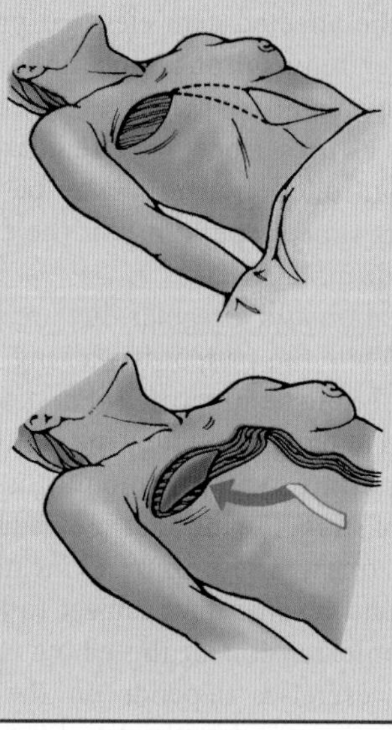

original operative procedure or later in one to several stages. Common types of breast reconstruction are:

- Breast expanders (saline or silicone)
- Autologous reconstruction using the patient's own skin, fat, and muscle

Breast expanders are the most common method of breast reconstruction used in the United States. A tissue expander is a balloon-like device with a resealable metal port that is placed under the pectoralis muscle. A small amount of normal saline is injected intraoperatively into the expander to partially inflate it. The patient then receives additional weekly saline injections for about 6 to 8 weeks until the expander is fully inflated. When full expansion is achieved, the tissue expander is then exchanged for a permanent implant during surgery in an ambulatory care center. The permanent implant is filled with either saline or silicone.

Autologous reconstruction using the patient's own skin, fat, and muscle is advantageous because the donor site tissue is similar in consistency to that of the natural breast. Therefore the results more closely resemble a real breast compared with implant reconstruction. Flap donor sites include the latissimus dorsi flap (back muscle); transverse rectus abdominis myocutaneous flap, known as the *TRAM flap* (abdominal muscle); and the gluteal flap (buttock muscle). Reconstruction of the nipple-areola complex is the last stage in the reconstruction of the breast.

BEST PRACTICE FOR PATIENT SAFETY & QUALITY CARE QSEN

Postoperative Care of the Patient After Breast Reconstruction

- Assess the incision and flap for signs of ***infection*** (excessive redness, drainage, odor) during dressing changes.
- Assess the incision and flap for signs of poor tissue perfusion (duskiness, decreased capillary refill) during dressing changes.
- Avoid pressure on the flap and suture lines by positioning the patient on her nonoperative side and avoiding tight clothing.
- Monitor and measure drainage in collection devices, such as for Jackson-Pratt (JP) drains.
- Teach the patient to return to her usual activity level gradually and to avoid heavy lifting.
- Remind the patient to avoid sleeping in the prone position.
- Teach the patient to avoid participation in contact sports or other activities that could cause trauma to the chest.
- Teach the patient to minimize pressure on the breast during sexual activity.
- Remind the patient to refrain from driving until advised by the surgeon.
- Remind the patient to ask at the 6-week postoperative visit when full activity can be resumed.
- Reassure the patient that optimal appearance may not occur for 3 to 6 months after surgery.
- If implants have been inserted, teach the proper method of breast massage to enhance expansion and prevent capsule formation (consult with the health care provider).
- Emphasize breast self-awareness; if the patient performs breast self-examination (BSE), review her technique.
- Remind the patient of the importance of clinical breast examination and follow-up surveillance by her health care provider.

Women who have had a mastectomy and breast reconstruction in one breast should have close-surveillance breast cancer screening in the contralateral (opposite) breast, including imaging with mammography or mammography and MRI. Mammography and MRI are not recommended to be done routinely in reconstructed breasts because most local recurrences of breast cancer in the residual tissue are palpable during clinical breast examination. Nursing care of the woman who has undergone breast reconstruction is outlined in the Best Practice for Patient Safety & Quality Care: Postoperative Care of the Patient After Breast Reconstruction box.

Refer the patient to the American Cancer Society's *Reach to Recovery* program. This program has trained breast cancer survivors who can help navigate the decisions needed when facing breast cancer. In this program, a volunteer who has had breast cancer visits the woman, offering information on breast forms, clothing, coping with breast cancer, and possible reconstructive options. For this intervention to be as helpful as possible, the volunteer should be about the same age as the patient and have experienced the same surgical procedure.

Adjuvant therapy. The decision to follow the original surgical procedure with additional treatment to help keep the cancer from recurring is known as ***adjuvant therapy***. This decision is based on several factors:

- Stage of the disease
- Patient's age and menopausal and functional status
- Patient preferences
- Pathologic examination
- Hormone receptor (ER/PR) status
- HER2/neu status
- Presence of a known genetic predisposition

Adjuvant therapy for breast cancer consists of systemic chemotherapy, radiation therapy, or a combination of both. The purpose of radiation therapy is to reduce the risk for local recurrence of breast cancer. The goal of systemic therapy (with chemotherapy, hormone therapy, and targeted therapy) is to reduce the risk of recurrence (locally or at distant sites) and prevent cancer-related death. These drugs destroy breast cancer cells that may be present anywhere in the body. They are typically delivered after surgery for breast cancer, although neoadjuvant chemotherapy may be given to reduce the size of a tumor before surgery. Endocrine therapy may also be used as a chemoprevention option for high-risk women with a personal history of breast cancer.

Radiation therapy. Radiation therapy is administered after breast-conserving surgery to kill breast cancer cells that may remain near the site of the original tumor. This therapy can be delivered to the whole breast or to only part of the breast. Whole-breast irradiation is delivered by external beam radiation over a period of 5 to 6 weeks. Partial breast irradiation (PBI) is an option for women with early-stage breast cancer (Siefert et al., 2018). PBI is a convenient alternative to whole-breast radiation. Less time is needed for completion, and outcomes are comparable to those of whole-breast radiation. The advantage of this type of radiation is that it is delivered over a much shorter time interval, eliminating the need for weeks of treatment. The types of methods available for delivering PBI include the following:

- Brachytherapy is a form of treatment in which an external catheter is inserted at the lumpectomy cavity and surrounding margin, and radioactive seeds are inserted into a multicatheter or balloon catheter device. Radiation is given over a period of 5 days. Ten treatments are given in total, with at least 6 hours between treatments.
- Intraoperative radiation therapy is the most accelerated form of PBI. It uses a high single dose of radiation delivered during the lumpectomy surgery.

Nursing care for the patient undergoing radiation therapy includes patient education and side effect management. Skin changes are a major side effect during this therapy (see Chapter 20). If brachytherapy is planned, instruct patients about the procedure. Assure them that they will be radioactive only while the radiation source is dwelling inside the breast tissue.

NURSING SAFETY PRIORITY QSEN

Action Alert

Teach women undergoing brachytherapy for breast cancer that radiation is contained in the temporary catheter and then removed prior to going home. The risk for others to be exposed to radiation is very small. Body fluids and items contacted by patients with brachytherapy are not radioactive. However, during the time that radiation is delivered, the patient will be alone in the room.

Drug therapy. The National Comprehensive Cancer Network (NCCN) provides a database of evidence-based practice and treatments for various cancers. *Chemotherapy* for breast cancer is a systemic treatment used to kill undetected breast cancer cells that may have left the original tumor and moved to more distant sites. Generalist nurses do not administer chemotherapy; consult your agency policies regarding the specific training and education that is needed to demonstrate and maintain competence in chemotherapy administration (Oncology Nursing Society, 2020).

Chemotherapy is recommended for treatment of invasive breast cancer after surgery (adjuvant chemotherapy). It may also be given before surgery to reduce the size of the tumor (neoadjuvant chemotherapy) and is most effective when combinations of more than one drug are used. Sometimes a patient needs to have a surgically implanted IV catheter before chemotherapy administration. Chemotherapy drugs are usually delivered in four to six cycles, with each period of treatment followed by a rest period to give the body time to recover from the adverse effects of the drugs. Each cycle is 2 to 3 weeks long. The total treatment time is 3 to 6 months, although treatment may be longer for advanced or HER2-positive breast cancer.

A common chemotherapy regimen for breast cancer treatment is doxorubicin, cyclophosphamide, and paclitaxel, which in the United States is also known as AC-T. If the patient is HER2 positive, a trastuzumab-based regimen will be used. In early-stage breast cancer, chemotherapy regimens lower the risk for breast cancer recurrence and death. In metastatic breast cancer, chemotherapy regimens reduce cancer size and slow the progression of disease.

Nurses who are qualified to give chemotherapy must be very proficient in the preparation and administration of these drugs and knowledgeable about various venous access devices. They must also be able to manage the distressing symptoms associated with side effects of these drugs. Chapter 20 discusses chemotherapy in more detail and general nursing management of alopecia, nausea and vomiting, mucositis, and bone marrow suppression.

Chemotherapy is unpleasant and expensive and can have life-threatening short-term and long-term side effects. Because more women are living longer with breast cancer, more long-term effects are emerging. For example, ovarian suppression from chemotherapy drugs can result in infertility, which can be devastating for some women of childbearing age.

NURSING SAFETY PRIORITY QSEN

Action Alert

Teach patients undergoing chemotherapy with doxorubicin and trastuzumab to be aware of cardiotoxic effects. Patients will have routine testing of their cardiac function and ejection fraction (EF) because this side effect is often asymptomatic (Morgan, 2020). Instruct them to report excessive fatigue, shortness of breath, chronic cough, and edema to the health care provider. This side effect can manifest years after treatment.

Targeted cancer therapies are drugs that target specific characteristics of cancer cells, such as a protein, an enzyme, or the formation of new blood vessels. The advantage of targeted therapy over traditional chemotherapy is that targeted therapy is less likely to harm normal, healthy cells and therefore it has fewer side effects. One of the first targeted therapies developed for breast cancer is the monoclonal antibody *trastuzumab.* This drug targets the *HER2/neu* gene product in breast cancer cells. Other targeted therapies are available.

Drugs that alter hormone levels may also be used in breast cancer prevention and treatment. The purpose of endocrine therapy is to reduce the estrogen available to breast tumors to stop or prevent their growth. *Premenopausal* women whose main estrogen source is the ovaries may benefit from drugs that inhibit estrogen synthesis. These drugs include leuprolide and goserelin, which suppress the hypothalamus from making luteinizing hormone–releasing hormone (LH-RH). When LH-RH is inhibited, the ovaries do not produce estrogen. Although the suppression of ovarian function decreases breast cancer risk, the drastic drop in estrogen causes significant menopausal symptoms. Therefore the decision to use these drugs is not made lightly.

Selective estrogen receptor modulators (SERMs), on the other hand, do not affect ovarian function. Rather, they block the effect of estrogen in women who have estrogen receptor (ER)–positive breast cancer (Burchum & Rosenthal, 2019). SERMs are also used as chemoprevention in women at high risk for breast cancer and in women with advanced breast cancer. For women with hormone receptor–positive breast cancer, tamoxifen reduces the chances of the cancer coming back by about half (ACS, 2019a). Common side effects of SERMs include hot flashes and weight gain. Rare but serious side effects of these drugs include endometrial cancer and thromboembolic events.

Aromatase inhibitors (AIs), such as letrozole and anastrozole, are used in *postmenopausal* women whose main source of estrogen is not the ovaries but, rather, body fat (Burchum & Rosenthal, 2019). AIs reduce estrogen levels by inhibiting the conversion of androgen to estrogen through the action of the enzyme *aromatase.* They are beneficial when given to postmenopausal women for up to 5 years. Newer research is recommending up to 10 years of tamoxifen or AI therapy to prevent recurrence (NCCN, 2020). A side effect of AIs, not seen with tamoxifen, is loss of bone density. Women taking AIs are candidates for bone-strengthening drugs and must be closely monitored for osteoporosis. Weight-bearing exercises and supplementation should be implemented into the daily routine.

Enhancing Coping Strategies

Planning: Generate Solutions. The patient who is treated for breast cancer will verbalize enhanced coping ability related to the diagnosis and treatment of the condition.

Interventions: Take Action. The patient with breast cancer may appear to have difficulty coping and experience anxiety related to the disease or treatment. The fear and uncertainty for the patient with breast cancer begin the moment a lump is discovered or when a mammogram reveals an abnormality. These feelings may be related to past experiences and personal associations with the disease. Assess the patient's situational perceptions. Allow the expression of feelings even if a diagnosis has not been established.

Assess the patient's need for knowledge. Some may want to read and discuss any available information. Provide accurate information and clarify any misinformation the patient may have received through the media, on the Internet, or from family and friends. If the mass has been diagnosed as cancer, many people feel a partial sense of relief to be dealing with a known entity. A feeling of shock or disbelief usually occurs. It is difficult to accept a diagnosis of cancer when one feels basically well. Patients and their families or significant others deal in individual ways with the mix of feelings. Adjust your approach to care as the patient's emotional state changes. The goal is to have the patient participate as an active partner in management of the disease.

An integral part of the plan to meet these emotional needs is the use of outside resources. For example, the patient who is worried in particular about the side effects of radiation therapy may benefit more from talking to someone who has undergone radiation than from talking to the nurse or primary health care provider. The American Cancer Society's "Reach to Recovery" program is just one community resource that connects breast cancer patients to a peer who has lived through the treatment the patient is facing. Be sure to assess her preference and place appropriate referrals.

Another helpful resource for patients who desire to receive care at one location is a full-service cancer center. Some agencies have all cancer services offered comprehensively in one location, including surgeon and provider services, counseling, nursing care, social services, nutrition services, rehabilitation, various therapies (including chemotherapy), and spiritual ministry. Obtaining all services in one familiar location can decrease the stress that the patient feels.

Care Coordination and Transition Management

Home Care Management. In collaboration with the case manager and members of the interprofessional health care team, make the appropriate referrals for care after discharge. Preoperative teaching and arrangements for home care management and referrals can be started before surgery or other treatment.

The patient who has undergone breast surgery can be discharged to the home setting unless other physical disabilities exist. Some are discharged the day after surgery with drains in place; some are discharged to home on the day of surgery. Older adults should not be sent home without a family member or friend who can stay with them for 1 to 2 days. These patients may need some assistance at home with drain care, dressings, and ADLs because of ***pain*** and impaired range of motion of the affected arm. See the Home Care Considerations: Patients Recovering From Breast Cancer Surgery box.

Teach patients that activities involving stretching or reaching for heavy objects should be avoided temporarily. This restriction can be discussed with a family member or significant other who can perform these tasks or place the objects within easy reach.

HOME CARE CONSIDERATIONS
Patients Recovering From Breast Cancer Surgery

Assess cardiovascular, respiratory, and urinary status:
- Vital signs
- Lung sounds
- Urine output patterns

Assess for ***pain*** and effectiveness of analgesics.

Assess dressing and incision site:
- Excess drainage
- Symptoms of ***infection***
- Wound healing
- Intact staples, sutures

Assess drain and site:
- Drainage around site and within drain reservoir
- Color and amount of drainage
- Symptoms of ***infection***

Review patient's recordings of drainage.

Evaluate patient's ability to care for and empty drain reservoir.

Assess status of affected extremity:
- Range of motion
- Ability to perform exercise regimen
- Lymphedema

Assess nutritional status:
- Food and fluid intake
- Presence of nausea and vomiting
- Bowel sounds

Assess functional ability:
- ADLs
- Mobility and ambulation

Assess home environment:
- Safety
- Structural barriers

Assess patient's compliance and knowledge of illness and treatment plan:
- Follow-up appointment with surgeon
- Symptoms to report to health care provider
- Hand and arm care guidelines

Self-Management Education. The teaching plan for the patient after surgery includes:
- Care of the incision and drainage device
- Exercises to regain full range of motion
- Measures to avoid lymphedema
- Measures to improve body image, coping, and self-esteem
- Information about interpersonal relationships and roles

See the Patient and Family Education: Preparing for Self-Management: Recovery From Breast Cancer Surgery box for additional important patient teaching.

Postoperative Mastectomy Teaching. Teach incisional care to the patient, family, and/or other caregiver. The patient may wear a light dressing to prevent irritation. Although swelling and redness of the scar itself are normal for the first few weeks, swelling, redness, increased heat, and tenderness of the surrounding area indicate ***infection*** and should be reported to the surgeon immediately. If a lymph node dissection was performed, instruct the patient to elevate the affected arm on a pillow and to use interventions to decrease risk of lymphedema. Encourage the patient to dress in comfortable street clothes at home, not pajamas, to further enhance a positive self-image.

PATIENT AND FAMILY EDUCATION: PREPARING FOR SELF-MANAGEMENT

Recovery From Breast Cancer Surgery

- There may be a dry gauze dressing over the incision when you leave the hospital. You may change this dressing if it becomes soiled.
- A small, dry dressing will be around the site where a drain is placed. Often there is some leakage of fluid around the drain. Check the gauze dressing for drainage and change it if it becomes soiled. Some leakage is normal, but if the dressing becomes soaked more than once a day, call your health care provider.
- You have been taught how to empty the reservoir from your drain and how to measure the volume of drainage. You should empty the reservoir twice a day and record the measurements.
- Drains are generally removed when drainage is less than 30 mL/day for 3 consecutive days.
- You may take sponge baths or tub baths, making certain that the area of the drain and incision stays dry. You may shower after the stitches, staples, and drains are removed.
- You can begin using your arm for normal activities, such as eating or combing your hair. Exercises involving the wrist, hand, and elbow, such as flexing your fingers, circular wrist motions, and touching your hand to your shoulder, are very good. You can usually resume more strenuous exercises after the drains have been removed.
- You can expect mild pain after surgery; but within 4 to 5 days, most patients have no need for pain medication or require medication only at bedtime.
- Numbness in the area of the surgery and along the inner side of the arm from the armpit to the elbow occurs in almost all patients owing to injury to the nerves. Patients have described sensations of heaviness, pain, tingling, burning, and "pins and needles." This is neuropathic pain, and short-acting analgesics may be given. These sensations may change over the next several months, becoming less and less noticeable, and may resolve entirely by the end of the first year following surgery.
- Pamphlets on exercises, hand and arm care, and general facts about breast cancer are available from your hospital or from a volunteer visitor of the local or national office on cancer or breast cancer. The American Cancer Society has volunteers who have had surgery similar to yours and are available to visit you.

Teach the patient to continue performing the exercises that began in the hospital. Active range-of-motion exercises should begin 1 week after surgery and should be continued after sutures and drains are removed. Emphasize that reaching and stretching exercises should continue only to the point of ***pain*** or pulling, never beyond that. Some YWCA locations have a free postmastectomy program that supports patients following breast cancer surgery.

Patients should be screened for mobility and provided education on exercises to perform after surgery. Referral to physical therapy prior to surgery allows for education and assessment to be done in a nonhurried environment. Additionally, if the patient is unable to raise her arm over her head, positioning for radiation therapy will be difficult.

Lymphedema (Fig. 65.10), an abnormal accumulation of protein fluid in the subcutaneous tissue of the affected limb after a mastectomy, is a commonly overlooked topic in health teaching. Risk factors include injury or ***infection*** of the extremity, obesity, presence of extensive axillary disease, and radiation treatment. Once lymphedema develops, it can be very difficult to manage, and *lifelong measures must be taken to prevent it.* Nurses play a vital role in educating patients about this complication. Teach patients, especially those who have had axillary lymph nodes removed, that measures to prevent lymphedema are lifelong and include avoiding trauma to the arm on the side of the mastectomy. Teach your patient to immediately report symptoms of lymphedema such as sensations of heaviness, aching, fatigue, numbness, tingling, and/or swelling in the affected arm, as well as swelling in the upper chest (Mehrara, 2020).

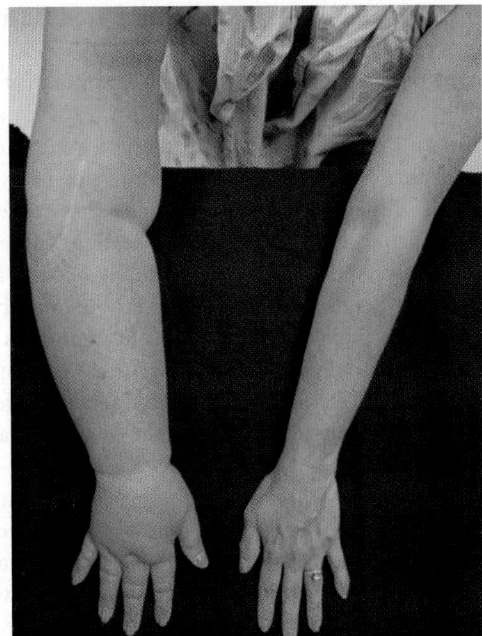

FIG. 65.10 Lymphedema of the arm. (From Song, D.H., & Neligan, P.C. [2018]. *Plastic surgery. Volume 4. Lower extremity, trunk, and burns* [4th ed.]. Philadelphia: Elsevier.)

Nurses should not assume that women with lymphedema are disabled; they are able to live full lives within this limitation. A referral to a lymphedema specialist may be necessary for the patient to be fitted for a compression sleeve and/or glove, to be taught exercises and manual lymph drainage, and to discuss ways to modify daily activities to avoid worsening the problem. Management is directed toward measures that promote drainage of the affected arm.

! NURSING SAFETY PRIORITY QSEN

Action Alert

Teach the patient how to avoid ***infection*** and subsequent lymphedema of the affected arm after the mastectomy. Teach the importance of **avoiding** having blood pressure measurements taken on, having injections in, or having blood drawn from the arm on the side of the mastectomy, especially if lymph node dissection has occurred. Instruct the patient to wear a mitt when using the oven, wear gloves when gardening, and treat cuts and scrapes appropriately. If lymphedema occurs, early intervention provides the best chance for control.

Psychosocial Preparation. Concerns about appearance after surgery are common and are often a threat to the patient's self-concept as a woman. Before breast surgery, the woman and her partner can benefit from an explanation of the expected postoperative appearance. After a modified radical mastectomy, the chest wall is fairly smooth and has a horizontal incision from the axilla to the mid-chest area. After breast-conserving surgery, scars vary according to the amount of breast tissue removed. Emphasize that scars will fade and edema will lessen with time. Scars may be red and raised at first, but these features lessen in the first few months. After surgery, encourage the woman to look at her incision when she is ready. Do not push her to accept this body image change immediately.

Much of one's body image is a reflection of how others respond. Therefore the response of the patient's partner or family members to the surgery impacts the effect on self-esteem. These people may also need the support of the nurse. They may have concerns about their ability to accept the changes and need to discuss these feelings with an objective listener. They may also need help with communicating their feelings, both negative and positive, to their loved one. Involving them in teaching, if the patient desires, may also help reinforce learning and increase retention.

Discuss sexual concerns before discharge. Most surgeons recommend avoiding sexual intercourse for 4 to 6 weeks. Patients may prefer to lay a pillow over the surgical site or to wear a bra, camisole, or T-shirt to prevent contact with the surgical site during intercourse. He or she may be embarrassed to discuss the topic of ***sexuality.*** Be sensitive to possible concerns and approach the subject first.

For young women, issues related to childbearing may be a concern. Chemotherapy and radiation are considered serious teratogenic (birth defect–causing) agents. Advise sexually active patients receiving chemotherapy or radiotherapy to use birth control during therapy. The method and length of birth control should be discussed with the health care provider. Patients with hormone ER/PR–positive breast cancer need to avoid estrogen, including contraceptives.

Health Care Resources. Resources available to the patient after discharge include personal support and community programs. After discharge, the spouse or partner may need help in planning support for home responsibilities. This caregiver may be assuming additional duties at home and work, and may feel stressed. Discussing the need for ongoing emotional support is also beneficial to both the patient and caregiver. Leaving the hospital and appearing normal do not end the anxiety and fear. Identifying a support person with whom the patient or couple can explore these feelings and discussing the need to ventilate feelings enhance personal and family recovery.

Numerous support and educational resources are available to those diagnosed with breast cancer. Nurses must provide accurate and current information to patients who may have obtained inaccurate information from various outlets. There are over 3.8 million breast cancer survivors in the United States (ACS, 2019a), and many men and women are active in breast cancer support and advocacy organizations. National breast cancer organizations are accessible online, and many of them have local affiliates. Examples of such organizations are Susan G. Komen for the Cure, the National Breast Cancer Coalition, Sisters Network, and Young Survival Coalition. Local support organizations can be found and accessed through the health care provider, the local hospital, wellness centers, or home care agencies; by word of mouth; or by Internet search.

The American Cancer Society (ACS) is a comprehensive resource for information and support in the United States. Breastcancer.org provides evidence-based information in language a lay person can understand.

The Canadian Cancer Society offers information, resources, and support services for breast cancer patients and their families. The Breast Cancer Society of Canada conducts research on breast cancer in Canada.

Helping patients diagnosed with breast cancer to be active participants in their care, to find resources to help them cope, and to gain support with physical and emotional changes are priorities for the nurse and members of the interprofessional team.

◆ **Evaluation: Evaluate Outcomes.** Evaluate the care of the patient with breast cancer based on the identified priority patient problems. The expected outcomes include that the patient:

- Has no recurrence or metastasis of breast cancer after completion of treatment; if metastasis occurs, have optimal palliative and end-of-life care
- Reports adequately coping with the uncertainty of having breast cancer and its treatment

CLINICAL JUDGMENT CHALLENGE 65.1

Safety

The telehealth nurse receives a call from a client who is home recovering from a right mastectomy 2 days prior. The client reports swelling in the right upper chest, and swelling in the right arm. When asked if she is in pain, the client says her right arm aches, but she is not in any other pain. She says she feels more fatigued each day following surgery, and just wants to know if this is normal.

1. **Recognize Cues:** What assessment information in this client situation is the most important and immediate concern for the nurse? (Hint: Identify the **relevant** information *first* to determine what is most important.)
2. **Analyze Cues:** What client conditions are consistent with the **most relevant** information? (Hint: Think about priority collaborative problems that support and contradict the information presented in this situation.)
3. **Prioritize Hypotheses:** Which possibilities or explanations are **most likely** to be present in this client situation? Which possibilities or explanations are the most serious? (Hint: Consider all possibilities and determine their urgency and risk for this client.)
4. **Generate Solutions:** What actions would most likely achieve the desired outcomes for this client? Which actions should be **avoided** or are **potentially harmful**? (Hint: Determine the desired outcomes first to decide which interventions are appropriate and those that should be avoided.)
5. **Take Action:** Which actions are the most appropriate and how should they be implemented? In what **priority order** should they be implemented? (Hint: Consider health teaching, documentation, requested health care provider orders or prescriptions, nursing skills, collaboration with or referral to health team members, etc.)
6. **Evaluate Outcomes:** What client assessment would indicate that the nurse's actions were **effective**? (Hint: Think about signs that would indicate an improvement, decline, or unchanged client condition.)

GET READY FOR THE NEXT-GENERATION NCLEX® EXAMINATION!

Key Points

Review these Key Points for each NCLEX Examination Client Needs Category.

Safe and Effective Care Environment

- Collaborate with the interprofessional health care team to reduce risk for lymphedema **QSEN: Safety; Teamwork and Collaboration**
- Notify the health care team that the arm of the surgical mastectomy side should not be used for blood pressures, blood drawing, IV therapy, or injections. **QSEN: Safety**

Health Promotion and Maintenance

- Identify and educate patients at high risk for breast cancer. **QSEN: Patient-Centered Care**
- Teach women the importance of breast self-awareness, and teach breast self-examination (BSE) to women who wish to learn. **QSEN: Patient-Centered Care**
- Encourage women to have a screening mammography and clinical breast examinations (CBE) according to recommended guidelines. **QSEN: Evidence-Based Practice**
- Observe for and report complications of breast surgery, especially ***infection*** and inadequate vascular perfusion. **QSEN: Safety**

Psychosocial Integrity

- Allow patients to express feelings about a cancer diagnosis and treatment on body image and ***sexuality***. **QSEN: Patient-Centered Care**
- Teach women ways to minimize surgical area changes and enhance body image **QSEN: Patient-Centered Care**
- Provide support, education, and community referrals to the patient with breast cancer and their significant others. **QSEN: Patient-Centered Care**

Physiological Integrity

- Assess benign lumps as mobile and round or oval; assess possible malignant lumps as fixed and irregularly shaped. **Clinical Judgment**
- After breast surgery, assess vital signs, dressings, drainage tubes, amount of drainage, and return of arm and shoulder mobility. **Clinical Judgment**
- Teach self-management after breast surgery. **QSEN: Patient-Centered Care**

MASTERY QUESTIONS

1. Which nursing intervention is appropriate when caring for a female client who has undergone a mastectomy and will receive chemotherapy? **Select all that apply.**
   A. Encourage client to accept her new body image.
   B. Provide self-care resources to the primary caretaker.
   C. Teach client about birth control options that are available.
   D. Refer to support groups for people who have had mastectomy.
   E. Involve partner in discussions about sexuality if client desires.
2. Which assessment finding in a client who recently had a right mastectomy 2 days ago will the home health nurse report to the health care provider?
   A. Temperature of 99°F
   B. Tingling sensation in the right arm
   C. Impaired range of motion in the right arm
   D. Drainage of 20 mL collected over 24 hours

REFERENCES

Asterisk (*) indicates a classic or definitive work on this subject.

American Cancer Society (ACS). (2020a). *American Cancer Society recommendations for the early detection of breast cancer*. https://www.cancer.org/cancer/breast-cancer/screening-tests-and-early-detection/american-cancer-society-recommendations-for-the-early-detection-of-breast-cancer.html.

American Cancer Society (ACS). (2020b). *Cancer facts for lesbians and bisexual women*. https://www.cancer.org/healthy/find-cancer-early/womens-health/cancer-facts-for-lesbians-and-bisexual-women.html.

American Cancer Society (ACS). (2020c). *How common is breast cancer*. https://www.cancer.org/cancer/breast-cancer/about/how-common-is-breast-cancer.html.

American Cancer Society (ACS). (2020d). *Survival rates for breast cancer*. https://www.cancer.org/cancer/breast-cancer/understanding-a-breast-cancer-diagnosis/breast-cancer-survival-rates.html.

American Cancer Society (ACS). (2019a). *Breast cancer facts and figures 2019-2020*. https://www.cancer.org/content/dam/cancer-org/research/cancer-facts-and-statistics/breast-cancer-facts-and-figures/breast-cancer-facts-and-figures-2019-2020.pdf.

American Cancer Society (ACS). (2019b). *Cancer facts and figures*. 2019 https://www.cancer.org/content/dam/cancer-org/research/cancer-facts-and-statistics/annual-cancer-facts-and-figures/2019/cancer-facts-and-figures-2019.pdf.

American Cancer Society (ACS). (2019c). *Ductal carcinoma in situ (DCIS)*. https://www.cancer.org/cancer/breast-cancer/understanding-a-breast-cancer-diagnosis/types-of-breast-cancer/dcis.html.

American Cancer Society (ACS). (2019d). *Fibroadenomas of the breast*. https://www.cancer.org/cancer/breast-cancer/non-cancerous-breast-conditions/fibroadenomas-of-the-breast.html.

American Cancer Society (ACS). (2019e). *Lobular carcinoma in situ*. https://www.cancer.org/cancer/breast-cancer/non-cancerous-breast-conditions/lobular-carcinoma-in-situ.html.

American Cancer Society (ACS). (2019f). *Treatment of inflammatory breast cancer*. https://www.cancer.org/cancer/breast-cancer/treatment/treatment-of-inflammatory-breast-cancer.html.

American Cancer Society (ACS). (2017). *Breast cancer screening guideline*. https://www.cancer.org/research/infographics-gallery/breast-cancer-screening-guideline.html.

American Society of Breast Surgeons Foundation. (2019). *Breast abscess*. Retrieved from: https://breast360.org/topic/2017/01/01/breast-abscess/.

Anders, C., & Carey, L. (2020). ER/PR negative, HER2-negative (triple-negative) breast cancer. In D. Hayes, & H. Burstein (Eds.), *UpToDate*. Waltham, MA.

Attebery, L., Adams, J., & Weiss, M. (2020). *Male breast cancer*. Retrieved from: https://www.breastcancer.org/symptoms/types/male_bc.

Boehmer, U. (2018). LGBT populations' barrier to cancer care. *Seminars in Oncology Nursing*, *34*(1), 21–29. https://doi.org/10.1016/j.soncn.2017.11.002.

Boucher, J. E. (2018). Chemoprevention: An Overview of Pharmacologic agents and nursing Considerations. *CJON*, *22*(3), 350–353. https://doi.org/10.1188/18.CJON.350-353.

Braunstein, G., & Anawalt, B. (2019). *Clinical features, diagnosis, and evaluation of gynecomastia in adults*. In A. Matsumoso (Ed.). *UpToDate*. Waltham, MA.

Breastcancerorg. (2019). *Paget's disease of the nipple*. Retrieved from: https://www.breastcancer.org/symptoms/types/pagets.

Burchum, J. L. R., & Rosenthal, L. D. (2019). *Lehne's pharmacology for nursing care* (9th ed.). St. Louis: Elsevier.

Canadian Cancer Society. (2020). *Breast cancer statistics*. Retrieved from: https://www.cancer.ca/en/cancer-information/cancer-type/breast/statistics/?region=on.

Centers for Disease Control and Prevention (CDC). (2018). *Breast cancer rates among black women and white women*. Retrieved from: https://www.cdc.gov/cancer/dcpc/research/articles/breast_cancer_rates_women.htm.

Ceres, M., Quinn, G. P., Loscalzo, M., & Rice, D. (2018). Cancer screening considerations and cancer screening uptake for lesbian, gay, bisexual and transgender persons. *Seminars in Oncology Nursing*, *34*(1), 37–51. https://doi.org/10.1016/j.soncn.2017.12.001.

Chang, C., Lin, M., & Yin, W. (2019). Risk of breast cancer in women with non-lactational mastitis. *Scientific Reports*, *9*, 15587. https://doi.org/10.1038/s41598-019-52046-3.

Dixon, J., & Pariser, K. (2020). Nonlactational mastitis in adults. In Sexton, D. (Ed.), *UpToDate*. Waltham, MA.

Howlader, N., Noone, A., Krapcho, M., et al. (Eds.). (2020). *SEER cancer statistics review, 1975-2016*. Bethesda, MD: National Cancer Institute. https://seer.cancer.gov/csr/1975_2016/.

Komen, S. G. (2020). *Breast self-exam*. Retrieved from: https://ww5.komen.org/BreastCancer/BreastSelfExam.html.

Mahon, S. M. (2017). Genetics and Genomics: An Oncology nurse's Journey in practice. *CJON 2017*, *21*(6), 715–721. https://doi.org/10.1188/17.CJON.715-721.

Margolies, S. (2020). *Lesbians and breast cancer risk*. National LGBT Cancer Network. Retrieved from: https://cancer-network.org/cancer-information/lesbians-and-cancer/lesbians-and-breast-cancer-risk/.

Mau, K. (2018). Benign breast diseases: An introduction for the advanced practice nurse. *CJON 2018*, *22*(5), 493–495. https://doi.org/10.1188/18.CJON.493-495.

McCance, K., Huether, S., Brashers, V., & Rote, N. (2019). *Pathophysiology: The biologic basis for disease in adults and children* (8th ed.). St. Louis: Mosby.

McDaniel, J., et al. (2018). Breast cancer screening and outcomes: An ecological study of county-level female veteran population density and social vulnerability. *Journal of Military, Veteran, and Family Health*, *4*(1). https://doi.org/10.3138/jmvfh.2017-0023.

Mehrara, B. (2020). Patient education: Lymphedema after cancer surgery (beyond the basics). In P. Ganz, & E. Bruera (Eds.), *UpToDate*. Waltham, MA.

Morgan, J. (2020). *Cardiotoxicity of trastuzumab and other HER-2 targeted agents*. In Hayes, D. (Ed.), *UpToDate*. Waltham, MA.

National Breast Cancer Foundation. (2019). *BRCA: The breast cancer gene*. Retrieved from: https://www.nationalbreastcancer.org/what-is-brca.

National Cancer Institute. (n.d). Breast Cancer Risk Assessment Tool. Bethesda, MD. Retrieved from: https://bcrisktool.cancer.gov/calculator.html.

National Comprehensive Cancer Network. (2020). *NCCN clinical practice guidelines in Oncology (NCCN Guidelines®)*. [v.3.2017]. Retrieved from: https://www.nccn.org/professionals/physician_gls/default.aspx.

National Comprehensive Cancer Network. (2019). *Breast cancer screening and diagnosis*. https://www.nccn.org/professionals/physician_gls/pdf/breast-screening.pdf.

National LGBT Cancer Network. (2020). https://cancer-network.org/.

Oncology Nursing Society. (2020). Which RN is competent in chemotherapy administration? https://voice.ons.org/news-and-views/which-rn-is-competent-in-chemotherapy-administration.

*Ooi, S., Martinez, M., & Li, C. (2011). Disparities in breast cancer characteristics and outcomes by race/ethnicity. *Breast Cancer Research and Treatment*, *127*(3), 729–738.

Sabel, M. (2018). Overview of benign breast disease. In Chagpar, A. (Ed.), *UpToDate*. Waltham, MA.

Santen, R. J. (2018). Benign breast disease in women. In Feingold, K., Anawalt, B., Boyce, A. et al., (Eds.), *Endotext [Internet]*. South Dartmouth (MA): MDText.com, Inc.; 2000-. Available from: https://www.ncbi.nlm.nih.gov/books/NBK278994/.

Siefert, M. L., Fennie, K., & Knobf, M. T. (2018). Partial breast irradiation: A longitudinal study of symptoms and quality of life. *Clinical Journal of Oncology Nursing*, *22*(6), 635–642. https://doi.org/10.1188/18.CJON.635-642.

U.S. Food and Drug Administration. (2019). *Questions and answers about breast implant-associated anaplastic large cell lymphoma (BIA-ALCL)*. https://www.fda.gov/medical-devices/breast-implants/questions-and-answers-about-breast-implant-associated-anaplastic-large-cell-lymphoma-bia-alcl.

Concepts of Care for Patients With Gynecologic Problems

Cherie R. Rebar

http://evolve.elsevier.com/Iggy/

LEARNING OUTCOMES

1. Collaborate with the interprofessional team to coordinate high-quality care for patients with a gynecologic problem.
2. Describe factors that place a patient at high risk for a gynecologic cancer, and refer to the health care provider.
3. Implement patient-centered nursing interventions to decrease the psychosocial impact of living with a gynecologic problem.
4. Apply knowledge of anatomy, physiology, and pathophysiology to assess patients with a gynecologic problem.
5. Use clinical judgment to analyze assessment findings and diagnostic data in the care of patients with a gynecologic problem.
6. Prioritize evidence-based care for patients with gynecologic problems affecting ***elimination, infection, sexuality,*** or ***reproduction,*** or that induce ***pain.***
7. Plan care coordination and transition management for patients with a gynecologic problem.

KEY TERMS

anterior colporrhaphy Surgery for severe symptoms of cystocele in which the pelvic muscles are tightened for better bladder support.

bilateral salpingo-oophorectomy (BSO) Surgical removal of both fallopian tubes and both ovaries.

colposcopy Examination of the cervix and vagina using a colposcope, which allows three-dimensional magnification and intense illumination of epithelium with suspected disease. This procedure can locate the exact site of precancerous and malignant lesions for biopsy.

concurrent chemoradiation The use of chemotherapy and radiation together at the same time.

cystocele Protrusion of the bladder through the vaginal wall (urinary bladder prolapse).

dyspareunia Painful intercourse.

endometrial cancer Cancer of the inner uterine lining.

fibroid See *leiomyoma.*

leiomyoma Benign, slow-growing solid tumor of the uterine myometrium.

loop electrosurgical excision procedure (LEEP) Diagnostic procedure or treatment in which a thin loop-wire electrode that transmits a painless electrical current is used to cut away affected cervical cancer tissue.

myoma See *leiomyoma.*

myomectomy Removal of leiomyomas from the uterus.

pelvic organ prolapse (POP) Condition in which the sling of muscles and tendons that support the pelvic organs becomes weak and is no longer able to hold them in place.

posterior colporrhaphy Surgery to repair a rectocele by strengthening pelvic supports and reducing the bulging.

rectocele Protrusion of the rectum through a weakened vaginal wall (rectal prolapse).

stress urinary incontinence (SUI) Loss of urine during activities that increase intra-abdominal pressure, such as laughing, coughing, sneezing, or lifting heavy objects.

total hysterectomy Removal of the uterus and cervix; the procedure may be vaginal or abdominal.

uterine artery embolization Use of a percutaneous catheter by a radiologist, inserted through the femoral artery to inject polyvinyl alcohol pellets into the uterine artery. The resulting blockage starves the tumor of circulation, allowing it (or them) to shrink.

uterine fibroid embolization See *uterine artery embolization.*

uterine prolapse The most common kind of pelvic organ prolapse (POP); the downward displacement of the uterus into the vagina.

vulvovaginitis inflammation of the lower genital tract resulting from a disturbance of the balance of hormones and flora in the vagina and vulva.

PRIORITY AND INTERRELATED CONCEPTS

The priority concepts for this chapter are:

- ***Sexuality***
- ***Infection***
- ***Pain***

The ***Sexuality*** concept exemplar for this chapter is Uterine Leiomyoma.

The interrelated concepts for this chapter are:

- ***Elimination***
- ***Reproduction***

Pain, vaginal discharge, abnormal bleeding, and urinary ***elimination*** problems are common gynecologic symptoms that are reported by adult women. These problems can impair her feelings about ***sexuality*** and intimacy with others, as well as ***reproduction.*** Because of the private nature of these concerns, women may be hesitant to seek medical attention. Create an open, nonjudgment, and therapeutic environment in which the patient can feel comfortable expressing her concerns. See Chapter 1 to review these concepts.

Nurses provide whole-person, patient-centered care to women across the lifespan. Sexual health is an important part of each woman's life, and the ability to discuss something this private allows the nurse and patient to work together to agree on a plan of care regardless of stage of life. Evidence shows that nurses must continue to learn more about entry-level competencies to provide this type of care, particularly for women who have cancer. (See the Evidence-Based Practice box.)

EVIDENCE-BASED PRACTICE QSEN

Sexual Health Care Provision in Cancer Nursing Care: A Systematic Review on the State of Evidence and Deriving International Competencies Chart for Cancer Nurses

Papadopoulou, C., Sime, C., Rooney, K., & Kotronoulas, G. (2019). Sexual health care provision in cancer nursing care: A systematic review on the state of evidence and deriving international competencies chart for cancer nurses. *International Journal of Nursing Studies, 100,* 103405.

The authors conducted a systematic review of research aligned with Preferred Reporting Items for Systematic Reviews and Meta-Analyses (PRISMA) guidelines for the evidence-based minimum set of items for report. An extensive literature review of nine databases, spanning from 2008 to 2018, yielded 31 unique studies to include in the review. Diverse research methods were represented in these studies, including randomized controlled trials, and single-arm before-and-after trials.

Evidence demonstrates that intrapersonal, interpersonal, societal, and organizational factors affect the nurse's professional confidence in providing sexual health care to women with cancer. The review demonstrated that this disconnect in care provision is often linked to the nurse's assumptions and prejudices about sexuality.

Level of Evidence: 1

The study was a systematic review, which is a strong source of evidence.

Implications for Research and Practice

As a result of this systematic review, a two-level chart was created to promote development of nurse competence. Containing competencies at the entry level and champion level, this educational approach can help nurses to be better prepared to provide sexual health care to women with cancer. In this chapter, a number of gynecologic cancers are covered; any patient with one of these disorders could benefit from nurse intervention to address ***sexuality*** concerns.

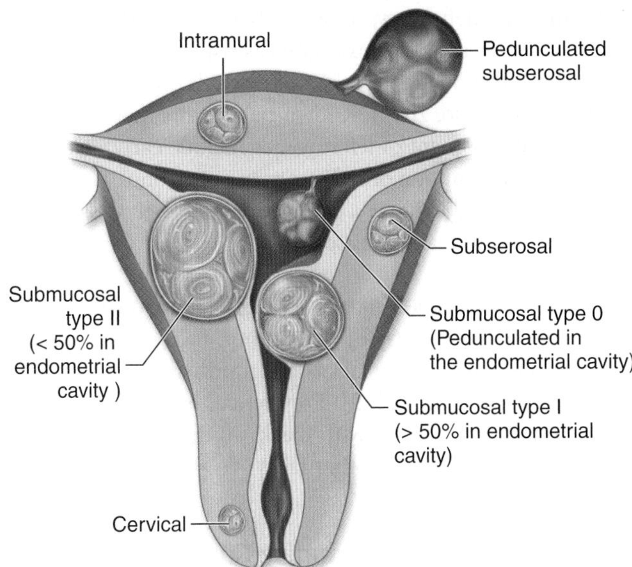

FIG. 66.1 Classification of uterine leiomyomas. (From Fielding, J.R., Brow, D.L., & Thrumond, A.S. [2011]. *Gynecologic Imaging.* Philadelphia: Elsevier.)

SEXUALITY CONCEPT EXEMPLAR: UTERINE LEIOMYOMA

Pathophysiology Review

Leiomyomas, also called **fibroids** or **myomas**, are very commonly found in women. These are benign, slow-growing solid tumors of the uterine myometrium (muscle layer) that develop from excessive local growth of smooth muscle cells. The growth of leiomyomas may be related to stimulation by estrogen, progesterone, and growth hormone. They are classified according to their position in the layers of the uterus (Fig. 66.1) (Stewart & Laughlin-Tommaso, 2019) :

- *Intramural* leiomyomas are contained in the uterine wall within the myometrium.
- *Submucosal* leiomyomas protrude into the cavity of the uterus and can cause bleeding and disrupt pregnancy.
- *Subserosal* leiomyomas protrude through the outer surface of the uterine wall and may extend to the broad ligament, pressing other organs. These may have a broad or pedunculated base.

Although most fibroids develop within the uterine wall, a few may appear in the cervix, called *cervical* leiomyomas. Pedunculated leiomyomas are attached by a pedicle (stalk) to the outside of the uterus and occasionally break off and attach to other tissues (parasitic fibroids).

Etiology and Genetic Risk. The etiology of leiomyomas is not fully understood. Researchers continue to search for answers, recognizing that most are diagnosed at a peak time within a women's early 40s (McWilliams & Chennathukuzhi, 2017). The incidence of leiomyomas is two to three times greater in black women than white women, although again, the reason for this disparity is not known (Stewart & Laughlin-Tommaso, 2019).

Vitamin D deficiency, reproductive tract infection, and African ancestry are being examined as risk factors through the Study of Environment, Lifestyle, and Fibroids (SELF) (Stewart & Laughlin-Tommaso, 2019). Known risk factors that are associated with development of leiomyomas include early menarche, significant consumption of red meats, use of alcohol, and hypertension. Gene studies show a connection between development of leiomyomas and family history of such.

Incidence and Prevalence. Although leiomyomas are the most commonly diagnosed pelvic tumor, incidence is difficult to determine based on the lack of longitudinal studies (Stewart & Laughlin-Tommaso, 2019). Prevalence, based on a 10-year population study, is 9.6%, with black women having a higher prevalence than women of other races (Yu et al., 2018).

❖ Interprofessional Collaborative Care

◆ Assessment: Recognize Cues

History. Some women with fibroids do not experience ***pain,*** but others do. She may experience ***dyspareunia*** (painful intercourse) depending on the location of the leiomyoma. Acute discomfort may occur with twisting of the fibroid on its stalk. Many women with leiomyomas report painful menstruation, often with heavy flow and the presence of clots (Stewart & Laughlin-Tommaso, 2019).

The patient often seeks medical attention because of heavy vaginal bleeding. Ask about how many tampons or menstrual pads she uses in a day. Establish whether she has a predictable menstrual pattern, if she experienced intermenstrual bleeding (between periods), and if she has prolonged bleeding (periods that exceed the normal 5 to 6 days). Determine if she has a feeling of pelvic pressure and altered ***elimination*** patterns, including constipation and urinary frequency or retention. These symptoms result when the enlarged fibroid presses on other organs.

Physical Assessment/Signs and Symptoms. The patient may notice that her abdomen has increased in size. Assess the woman's abdomen for distention or enlargement. Abdominal, vaginal, and rectal examinations performed by the health care provider usually reveal the presence of a uterine enlargement. Further diagnostic procedures are needed to differentiate benign tumors from cancerous ones.

Psychosocial Assessment. Symptoms such as dyspareunia may significantly impact the patient's quality of life. A woman may fear that she has cancer or may have anxiety about abnormal bleeding or her failure to conceive. She may also be concerned if surgery is recommended if she desires to become pregnant in the future. Assess the woman's feelings and concerns. If hysterectomy is recommended, explore the significance of the loss of the uterus for the woman and her partner, including its effects on ***sexuality*** and ***reproduction*** plans.

Diagnostic Assessment. Laboratory testing is usually limited to a hematocrit (in the case of heavy bleeding), a thyroid-stimulating hormone (TSH) test (to rule out hypothyroidism), and a pregnancy test to determine whether pregnancy is the cause of the uterine enlargement. An endometrial biopsy may be performed to evaluate for endometrial cancer.

Transvaginal ultrasound (US), a procedure in which the ultrasound probe is placed into the vagina for visualization, is the diagnostic study of choice (Stewart & Laughlin-Tommaso, 2019). Saline infusion sonography, hysteroscopy, and MRI (which can differentiate between benign and malignant tumors) may also be ordered if the transvaginal ultrasounds results are inconclusive.

◆ Analysis: Analyze Cues and Prioritize Hypothesis. The priority collaborative problem for patients with uterine leiomyoma is:

- Potential for prolonged or heavy bleeding due to abnormal uterine growth

◆ Planning and Implementation: Generate Solutions and Take Action

Managing Bleeding

Planning: Expected Outcomes. The expected outcome for the patient with the diagnosis of uterine leiomyoma is that she will not experience or continue to experience heavy (severe) or prolonged bleeding following treatment.

Interventions. Asymptomatic leiomyomas may not require treatment. Leiomyomas in menopausal women usually shrink, so surgery may not be necessary. Management depends on the size and location of the tumor, as well as the woman's desire for future pregnancy. Women who want to become pregnant may be prescribed drug therapy or have a myomectomy procedure to remove the tumor. Uterine artery embolization, endometrial ablation, and hysterectomy are choices for women who no longer desire pregnancy.

Nonsurgical Management. If the woman has few symptoms or desires childbearing, the health care provider may recommend intermittent observation and examination. Mild leiomyoma symptoms can be managed with hormonal therapies. The choice of oral contraceptive is based on the woman's risk factors, co-occurring disorders, and personal symptoms associated with the leiomyoma (Stewart, 2020).

Myolysis is a laparoscopic thermal, radiofrequency, or cryoablation of leiomyoma tissue. Most women report an increased quality in life after this procedure, although it does bear risk of adhesion formation.

An alternative to surgery for the woman who does not desire pregnancy is **uterine artery embolization** (also called *uterine fibroid embolization [UFE]*) performed under local anesthesia, or with sedation if the patient requests it (van der Kooij & Hehenkamp, 2020). The interventional radiologist uses a percutaneous catheter inserted through the femoral artery to inject polyvinyl alcohol and gelatin-like pellets into the uterine artery. The uterine artery then carries these materials into the blood vessels that feed the leiomyoma. The resulting blockage starves the tumor of circulation, allowing it (or them) to shrink.

Common concerns reported following uterine artery embolization include pelvic pain, which is most severe in the first 24 hours, and vaginal discharge, which is self-limiting and can last for months (van der Kooij & Hehenkamp, 2020). Teach her to resume usual activities slowly and avoid strenuous activity until the surgeon recommends it. Most patients can return to work or daily routine within a week.

NURSING SAFETY PRIORITY QSEN

Action Alert

After uterine artery embolization, the woman may have severe cramping within the first 24 hours owing to tissue necrosis. Cramping can last from a few days to 2 weeks. Patient-controlled analgesia (PCA) is often used before transition to oral pain medication. Remind the patient how to use PCA most effectively while hospitalized. If she experiences fever, nausea, and malaise with the pain (known as *postembolization syndrome*) or if severe pain or indication of ***infection*** is present (such as purulent vaginal drainage and fever), a continued hospital stay or readmission may be needed.

Surgical Management. When possible, minimally invasive surgery (MIS) techniques are performed, such as a myomectomy, to prevent removing the uterus. If not, a hysterectomy is the procedure of choice.

Uterus-sparing surgeries. If the woman desires children, the surgeon may perform a laparoscopic or hysteroscopic myomectomy (the removal of leiomyomas from the uterus). Laparoscopic myomectomy, performed on an outpatient basis or with a 1-day hospital stay, is used to remove leiomyomas that are intramural or subserosal; hysteroscopic myomectomy is done to remove intracavity leiomyomas (Bradley, 2020). During this procedure, a laser may be used to remove the tumors. This MIS procedure is usually performed in the early phase of the menstrual cycle to minimize blood loss and avoid the possibility of interrupting an unsuspected pregnancy. A small percentage of leiomyomas recur after surgery. The health care provider, when obtaining informed consent, will share that scarring makes the uterus more likely to rupture during labor. Depending on the type of leiomyoma extracted, a planned cesarean delivery may be advised; other women can be offered a trial of labor.

Normal activities can resume as quickly as the woman is comfortable after the laparoscopic procedure. She can return to work, daily activities, and sexual activity whenever she is ready. Other nursing care is similar to that for a woman undergoing a hysterectomy, as discussed in the following paragraphs.

NURSING SAFETY PRIORITY QSEN

Critical Rescue

Monitor for rare but potential complications of hysteroscopic surgery, which include:

- Fluid overload (fluid used to distend the uterine cavity can be absorbed)
- Embolism
- Hemorrhage
- Perforation of the uterus, bowel, or bladder and ureter injury
- Persistent increased menstrual bleeding
- Incomplete suppression of menstruation

*Monitor for any indications of these problems and report signs and symptoms, such as severe **pain** and heavy bleeding, to the surgeon or Rapid Response Team immediately.*

Hysterectomy. Leiomyomas are very common reason that a hysterectomy is performed. Hysterectomies may be performed abdominally, vaginally, or with laparoscopic or robotic assistance (Fig. 66.2) based on the patient's clinical reason for hysterectomy and the surgeon's area of technical expertise. Table 66.1 defines common terminology associated with common gynecologic surgeries.

Preoperative care. Preoperative teaching typically begins in the surgeon's office or surgical clinic. Explain procedures that routinely take place before surgery, including laboratory tests and expected drugs such as a prophylactic antibiotic. Depending on the type of surgical technique planned, teach about the need for turning, coughing, and deep-breathing exercises; incentive spirometry; early ambulation; and ***pain*** relief. (See Chapter 9 for a discussion of general patient care before surgery.) Correct any misperceptions about the effects of hysterectomy, such as association with masculinization and weight gain.

Psychological assessment is essential. Assess the significance of the surgery for the woman and her partner related to ***sexuality*** and ***reproduction.*** Many women relate their uterus to self-image, femininity, and/or sexuality. Although surgically induced menopause can contribute to a loss of libido and vaginal changes if the ovaries are also removed, teach the patient that vaginal estrogen cream, lubricants, and gentle dilation can help with these issues.

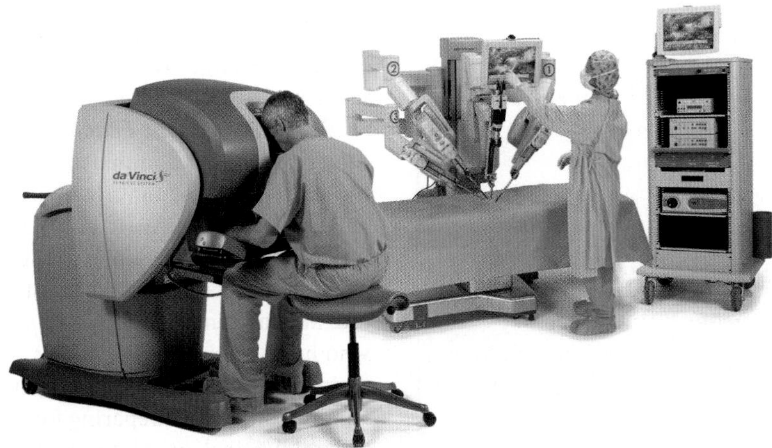

FIG. 66.2 Operating room layout for robotic surgery with da Vinci Robotic Surgery System. (©2016 Intuitive Surgical, Inc.)

Assess the patient's support system and recognize that she may fear rejection by her sexual partner. To be patient-centered, include the partner in all teaching sessions *unless this practice is not culturally acceptable or the patient prefers not to do so for other reasons.*

TABLE 66.1 Common Gynecologic Surgeries

Total Hysterectomy
- The entire uterus, including the cervix, is removed. The procedure may be performed via the vagina or abdominally, with laparoscopic or robotic assistance.

Supracervical Hysterectomy (Also Called "Subtotal" or "Partial" Hysterectomy)
- The upper part of the uterus is removed; however, the cervix is left in place. This procedure is performed laparoscopically or abdominally.

Salpingo-Oophorectomy (BSO)
- Fallopian tubes and ovaries are removed. This can be done on one side of the body, or both (termed *bilateral salpingo-oophorectomy*).
- If only the fallopian tubes are removed, it is a *salpingectomy.*
- If only the ovaries are removed, it is an *oophorectomy.*
- For patients at risk of ovarian or breast cancer who choose to have both ovaries removed (even if healthy) in order to decrease their risk of developing cancer, it is a *risk-reducing bilateral salpingo-oophorectomy.*

Radical Hysterectomy
- The uterus, cervix, adjacent lymph nodes, upper third of the vagina, and surrounding tissues (parametrium) are removed.

Data from American College of Obstetricians and Gynecologists. (2018). *Hysterectomy.* https://www.acog.org/Patients/FAQs/Hysterectomy.

FOCUSED ASSESSMENT

Postoperative Nursing Care of the Patient After Open Total Abdominal Hysterectomy

Focus assessment on:
- Vital signs, including pain level
- Activity tolerance level
- Temperature and color of the skin
- Heart, lung, and bowel sounds
- Incision characteristics
  - Presence or absence of bleeding at the site (a small amount is normal)
  - Intactness of incision
  - Pain at site of incision
- Dressing and drains for color and amount of drainage
- Fluid intake (IVs until peristalsis returns and patient is tolerating oral intake)
- Urine output
  - Provide catheter care for patients with open surgery (catheter will be removed in approximately 24 hours)
- Red blood cell, hemoglobin, and hematocrit levels
- *For patients with vaginal hysterectomy:*
  - Perineal care
  - Perineal pads for vaginal bleeding and clots (should be less than one saturated perineal pad in 4 hours)

Operative procedures. Hysterectomy can be performed in several ways: vaginally, abdominally, laparoscopically, or via robotic-assisted laparoscopy. The choice of route is based on (Walters, 2020):
- Best approach to treatment of the underlying condition
- Risks and benefits of route
- The need (or lack thereof) to treat additional conditions
- Patient preference
- Surgeon's skill set, preference, and facility availability.

Postoperative care. Nursing care of the woman who has undergone a total abdominal hysterectomy is similar to that of any patient who has had laparoscopic or traditional open abdominal surgery. See the Focused Assessment: Postoperative Nursing Care of the Patient After Open Total Abdominal Hysterectomy box for specific information.

NCLEX EXAMINATION CHALLENGE 66.1

Physiological Integrity

The nurse is caring for a client who just had a laparoscopic total abdominal hysterectomy. Which assessment finding requires **immediate** nursing intervention?

A. Temperature of 99.2°F (37.3°C)
B. One saturated perineal pad per hour
C. Decreased bowel sounds in all quadrants
D. Report of pain level of 5 on a scale of 0 to 10

Care Coordination and Transition Management. Discharge teaching, including activity restrictions, depends on the type of surgical procedure performed.

Home Care Management. Patients who have *uterus-sparing surgeries* usually go home the same day of surgery or after a 1-day hospital stay. They usually experience less postprocedural ***pain*** and fewer complications than patients who have their uterus and cervix removed. See Chapter 9 for postoperative teaching points.

If the patient had a *laparoscopic hysterectomy,* few limitations in activity are needed. Teach patients who had a *vaginal hysterectomy* or *traditional open hysterectomy* to limit stair climbing for several weeks. If women live alone and are not permitted to drive for several weeks, they may need to arrange for transportation for follow-up surgical visits.

Self-Management Education. Teach the woman who has undergone an abdominal hysterectomy about the expected physical changes, any activity restrictions, diet, sexual activity, wound care (if any), complications, and the need for follow-up care. Some women experience abdominal or shoulder discomfort because of the introduction of carbon dioxide gas during a *laparoscopic* procedure. Teach patients who had a *vaginal* hysterectomy to promptly report excessive or increasing bleeding to their surgeon. See the Patient and Family Education: Preparing for Self-Management: Care After a Total Vaginal or Abdominal Hysterectomy box for more specific health teaching.

PATIENT AND FAMILY EDUCATION: PREPARING FOR SELF-MANAGEMENT

Care After a Total Vaginal or Abdominal Hysterectomy

Expected Physical Changes
- You will no longer have a period, although you may have some vaginal discharge for a few days after you go home.
- It will not be possible for you to become pregnant, and birth control methods are no longer needed. (Condoms should still be used to decrease the chance of getting a sexually transmitted infection [STI].)
- If your ovaries were removed, you may experience menopause symptoms such as hot flushes, night sweats, and vaginal dryness.
- It is normal to tire more easily and require more sleep and rest during the first few weeks after surgery.

Activity (Typically for Vaginal and Traditional Open Surgeries)
- Limit stair climbing to fewer than five times per day.
- Do not lift anything heavier than 5 to 10 lb.
- Gradually increase walking as exercise, but stop before you become fatigued.
- Avoid sitting position for extended periods. When you sit, do not cross your legs at the knees.
- Avoid strenuous activity and exercise for 2 to 6 weeks, depending on which type of surgical procedure was performed.
- Do not drive until your surgeon has told you that it's alright.

Sexual Activity
- Do not engage in sexual intercourse for 6 weeks or as prescribed by your surgeon.
- If you had a vaginal "repair" as part of your surgery, you may experience some tenderness or ***pain*** the first time you have intercourse because the vaginal walls are tighter. Careful intercourse and the use of water-based lubricants can help reduce this discomfort. It usually goes away with time and stretching of the vagina.

Complications
- Take your temperature twice each day for the first 3 days after surgery. Report fevers of over 100°F (38°C).
- Check any incisions daily for signs of infection (increasing redness, open areas, drainage that is thick or foul smelling, incision ***pain***).

Symptoms to Report to Your Surgeon
- Increased vaginal drainage or change in drainage (bloodier, thicker, foul-smelling)
- Signs of infection at an incision site
- Temperature over 100°F (38°C)
- ***Pain***, tenderness, redness, or swelling in your calves
- ***Pain*** or burning on urination

Health Care Resources. Loss of female reproductive organs causes many women to go through the grieving process. Psychological reactions can occur months to years after surgery, particularly if sexual functioning and libido are diminished. Intermittent sadness is normal, but continued feelings of low self-esteem or loss of interest or pleasure in usual activities and pastimes is not expected and should be evaluated.

If desired and culturally appropriate, refer the woman to a religious or spiritual leader, or a community support group, to discuss feelings of sadness. Women identified as being at high risk for psychological problems may need long-term follow-up care or referral to a mental health counselor or clinical psychologist, particularly if they exhibit symptoms of depression.

◆ **Evaluation: Evaluate Outcomes.** Evaluate the care of the patient with leiomyomas on the basis of the identified priority problem. The expected outcomes are that she:
- Has relief of bleeding after effective management

PELVIC ORGAN PROLAPSE

Pathophysiology Review

The pelvic organs are supported by a sling of muscles and tendons, which sometimes become weak and no longer able to hold an organ in place. **Uterine prolapse**, the most common type of **pelvic organ prolapse (POP)**, can be caused by neuromuscular damage of childbirth; increased intra-abdominal pressure related to pregnancy, obesity, or physical exertion; or weakening of pelvic support caused by decreased estrogen. The stages of uterine prolapse are described by the degree of descent of the uterus through the pelvic floor.

Whenever the uterus is displaced, other structures such as the bladder, rectum, and small intestine can protrude through the vaginal walls (Fig. 66.3). A **cystocele** is a protrusion of the bladder through the vaginal wall (urinary bladder prolapse), which can lead to stress urinary incontinence (SUI) and urinary tract infections (UTIs). A **rectocele** is a protrusion of the rectum through a weakened vaginal wall (rectal prolapse).

❖ Interprofessional Collaborative Care

◆ **Assessment: Recognize Cues.** Patients with suspected uterine prolapse may report a feeling of "something falling out," dyspareunia, backache, and/or heaviness or pressure in the pelvis. A pelvic examination performed by the health care provider may reveal a protrusion of the cervix or anterior vaginal wall when the woman is asked to bear down. Listen to her concerns and note signs of anxiety or depression from having long-term symptoms.

Ask the patient whether she has urinary ***elimination*** problems, such as difficulty emptying her bladder, urinary frequency and urgency, a urinary tract ***infection*** (UTI), or **stress urinary incontinence (SUI)** (loss of urine during activities that increase intra-abdominal pressure, such as laughing, coughing, sneezing, or lifting heavy objects). These symptoms may be associated with a **cystocele** (bladder prolapse).

Diagnostic assessment methods performed by the health care provider may include (Fashokun & Rogers, 2020):
- Speculum and bimanual examination
- Rectovaginal examination
- Pelvic floor muscle testing—accomplished by palpating through the vagina or rectum to determine pelvic floor strength
- Pelvic Organ Prolapse Quantification (POP-Q) system assessment—a staging system that helps to guide surgical planning (if needed)

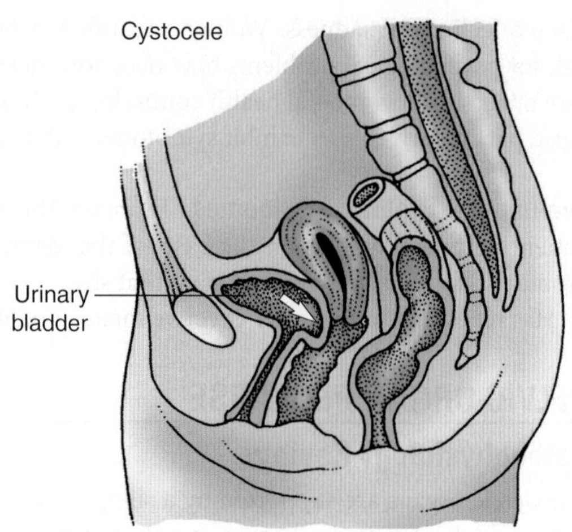

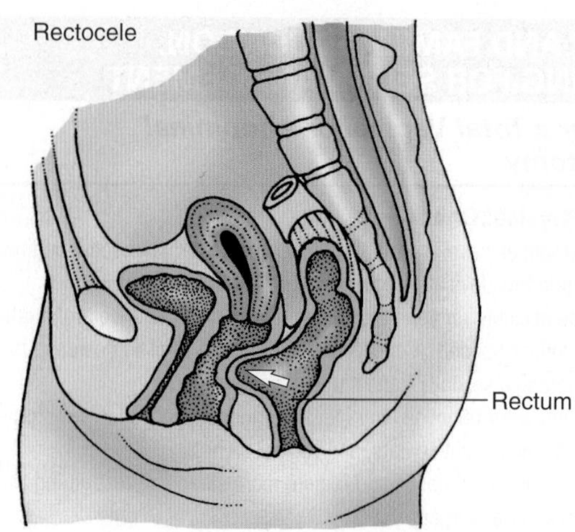

FIG. 66.3 In cystocele, the urinary bladder is displaced downward, causing bulging of the anterior vaginal wall. In rectocele, the rectum is displaced, causing bulging of the posterior vaginal wall.

The health care provider may also order a perineal ultrasound and/or a postvoid residual urine volume (PRUV) test.

◆ **Interventions: Take Action.** Interventions are based on the degree of the POP. Conservative treatment is preferred over surgical treatment when possible.

Nonsurgical Management. Teach women to improve pelvic support and tone by doing pelvic floor muscle exercises (PFMEs, or Kegel exercises). Space-filling devices such a vaginal pessary can be worn to elevate the uterine prolapse. Women with bladder symptoms may benefit from bladder training and attention to complete emptying. Management of a rectocele focuses on promoting bowel ***elimination.*** The primary health care provider usually prescribes a high-fiber diet, stool softeners, and laxatives.

Surgical Management. Various surgical approaches may be considered for severe symptoms of POP, with preference given to the least invasive approach. Most women with symptomatic POP are treated with a reconstructive procedure, which may or may not include hysterectomy (Jelovsek, 2020). Synthetic mesh is often used in transabdominal POP repair; mesh intended for *transvaginal* surgical repair was discontinued in the United States in 2019 because of complications associated with this procedure (Trabuco & Gebhart, 2020; U.S. Food and Drug Administration [FDA], 2019). Follow preoperative assessment processes as in Chapter 9.

! NURSING SAFETY PRIORITY (QSEN)

Action Alert

To be certain that the patient is fully educated about a surgical procedure using mesh, provide information for her to review before the surgeon discusses and obtains informed consent. The surgeon will ultimately obtain informed consent after reviewing details about benefits and risks of the procedure, specifically about complications that may arise when using synthetic mesh. Reinforce information about possible adverse events, the signs and symptoms of ***infection,*** and when she should contact her surgeon. Provide the patient with the manufacturer's labeling and written information.

Teach patients who have just had the mesh procedure to avoid strenuous exercise, heavy lifting, and sexual intercourse for 6 weeks. After 6 weeks, the patient may gradually begin to return to regular activities but must be educated about prevention of increasing intra-abdominal pressure (e.g., constipation, weight lifting, cigarette smoking) for a minimum of 3 months to allow proper healing and prevent POP recurrence.

If caring for a patient who previously underwent a transvaginal mesh procedure prior to discontinuation of this product, advise her to see her health care provider if she has any concerns or complications. There is no additional action that is needed, unless complications have arisen since the time of implantation (FDA, 2019).

Alternatives to minimally invasive surgery (MIS) are open surgical techniques. An **anterior colporrhaphy** (anterior repair) tightens the pelvic muscles for better *bladder* support, and is usually performed only after the patient has unsuccessfully tried conservative management and continues to have bothersome symptoms. This procedure is usually deferred until the woman no longer wishes to have children. Teach the patient to adhere to preoperative teaching (as in Chapter 9) and to consult her surgeon about the possible use of transvaginal estrogen prior to the procedure, which helps to maximize vaginal mucosal thickening (Mahajan, 2020).

A vaginal surgical approach is used and may be done as a laparoscopic-assisted procedure. Nursing care for a woman undergoing an anterior repair is similar to that for a woman undergoing a vaginal hysterectomy.

After surgery, the woman will have a urinary catheter in place for approximately 24 hours. Provide appropriate catheter care, and follow other postoperative care recommendations as in Chapter 9. Instruct the patient in how to splint her abdomen to protect sutures, and teach her to limit activities. She should *avoid lifting anything heavier than 5 lb (2.27 kg), strenuous exercises, straining with bowel movements, and sexual intercourse for up to 6 weeks* (Mahajan, 2020). If she is prescribed postoperative vaginal estrogen, teach her how to administer this. Tell the woman to notify her surgeon if she has signs of ***infection,*** such as fever, persistent ***pain,*** or purulent, foul-smelling discharge, and to be sure to keep her follow-up appointment after surgery.

Although there are a number of approaches to managing posterior vaginal defects, traditional **posterior colporrhaphy**, which reduces *rectal* bulging, is used most commonly. If both a cystocele and a rectocele are present, an *anterior and posterior colporrhaphy* (A&P repair) is performed. In this case, the woman may return from surgery with a urinary catheter in place to keep the surgical area clean and dry.

The nursing care after a posterior repair is similar to that after any rectal surgery. After surgery, a low-residue (low-fiber) diet is usually prescribed to decrease bowel movements and allow time for the incision to heal. Instruct the patient to avoid straining when she does have a bowel movement so she does not put pressure on the suture line. Bowel movements are often painful, and she may need pain medication before having a stool. Provide sitz baths or delegate this activity to assistive personnel (AP) to relieve the woman's ***pain***; this is a task that the AP can easily perform, and he or she can then report outcomes back to you. Health teaching for the patient undergoing a posterior repair is similar to that for the patient undergoing an anterior repair.

NCLEX EXAMINATION CHALLENGE 66.2

Safe and Effective Care Environment

A client is scheduled for a transvaginal surgical repair this morning. Which assessment finding requires **immediate** nursing intervention?

A. Notation of surgery type with mesh
B. Expression of fear prior to procedure
C. Blood pressure 140/92 mm Hg, P 88, R 20, T 98.8°F
D. Client request for caregiver to come to PACU

ENDOMETRIAL CANCER

Pathophysiology Review

Cancer can affect any organ in the reproductive tract. This chapter covers very common gynecologic cancers. **Endometrial cancer** (cancer of the uterine lining) is the most common gynecologic malignancy; its incidence continues to rise in the United States, with an estimated 65,620 new cases diagnosed annually (American Cancer Society [ACS], 2020b).

Endometrial cancer grows slowly in most cases, and early symptoms of vaginal bleeding generally lead to prompt evaluation and treatment. As a result, this type of cancer has a generally favorable prognosis. *Adenocarcinoma* of the endometrium is the most common type of uterine cancer. Abnormal uterine bleeding (AUB) is the most common symptom, resulting from estrogen exposure that leads to endometrial hyperplasia (McCance et al., 2019).

The initial growth of the cancer is within the uterine cavity, followed by extension into the myometrium and the cervix. Staging reflects the location of the cancer and whether it has spread. Categorized by histology, type I uterine tumors (the most common) result from endometrial hyperplasia (described above). Type II, which reflect 10% of endometrial cancers, are likely to invade the uterine muscle and metastasize (McCance et al., 2019).

Endometrial cancer is strongly associated with conditions causing prolonged exposure to estrogen without the protective effects of progesterone. Although most cases of endometrial cancer do not involve a genetic predisposition, it is more common in families that have gene mutations for hereditary nonpolyposis colon cancer (HNPCC) (McCance et al., 2019). Other risk factors are listed in Table 66.2.

TABLE 66.2 Risk Factors for Endometrial Cancer

- Early menarche or late menopause
- Use of estrogen after menopause
- Use of birth control pills or tamoxifen
- Use of an intrauterine device (IUD)
- Nulliparity
- History of type 2 diabetes, polycystic ovarian syndrome (PCOS), breast or ovarian cancer, or endometrial hyperplasia
- Treatment of the pelvis with radiation therapy
- Obesity; especially if body mass index at age 18 was high

Data from American Cancer Society. (2019). *Endometrial cancer risk factors.* https://www.cancer.org/cancer/endometrial-cancer/causes-risks-prevention/risk-factors.html; Katz, A. (2019). Obesity-related cancer in women: A clinical review. *American Journal of Nursing, 119*(8), 34-40; and McCance, K., Huether, S., Brashers, V., & Rote, N. (2019). *Pathophysiology: The biologic basis for disease in adults and children* (8th ed.). St. Louis: Mosby.

❖ Interprofessional Collaborative Care

◆ **Assessment: Recognize Cues.** *The main symptom of endometrial cancer is abnormal uterine bleeding [AUB], especially postmenopausal bleeding. Ask the patient how many tampons or menstrual pads she uses each day.* Some women also have a watery, bloody vaginal discharge or low back, low pelvis, or abdominal ***pain*** (caused by pressure of the enlarged uterus). Ask the patient to describe the exact location and intensity of her discomfort. A pelvic examination performed by the health care provider may reveal the presence of a palpable uterine mass or uterine polyp. The uterus is enlarged if the cancer is advanced.

Several laboratory tests are used to determine the overall condition of the woman with possible or confirmed endometrial cancer. A complete blood count may shows anemia due to heavy bleeding. Serum tumor markers to assess for metastasis include CA 125 (cancer antigen 125) and alpha fetoprotein (AFP), both of which may be elevated when ovarian cancer is present (Pagana & Pagana, 2018). A human chorionic gonadotropin (hCG) level may be obtained to rule out pregnancy before treatment for cancer begins.

Transvaginal ultrasound and *endometrial biopsy* are the gold standard diagnostic tests to determine the presence of endometrial thickening and cancer. Saline may be infused during the ultrasound to improve the image of the uterine cavity. This allows for careful evaluation of the uterine cavity and any small lesions that may be missed on other diagnostic tests (Feldman, 2020).

Other diagnostic tests to determine the patient's overall health status and the presence of metastasis (cancer spread) include (Campos & Cohn, 2020; Feldman, 2020):

- Dilation and curettage (when the patient cannot tolerate an endometrial biopsy)
- Hysteroscopy (for better visualization of the endometrial cavity)
- Chest x-ray
- Whole-body imaging of chest, abdomen, and pelvis (CT, MRI, positron emission tomography [PET], or combined PET/CT can be used)
- Liver and bone scans to assess for distant metastasis

During the diagnostic phase, the woman may express fears and concerns about having the disease and the effect on her ***sexuality*** and/or ***reproduction.*** After the diagnosis is confirmed, she may express disbelief, anger, depression, anxiety, or withdrawal behaviors. Assess these emotional reactions, and encourage the patient to discuss her feelings. Ask her about how she copes with other stressful events, and assess her support systems.

◆ **Interventions: Take Action.** Surgical removal and cancer staging of the tumor with adjacent lymph nodes are the most important interventions for endometrial cancer. Cancer staging is often done using minimally invasive techniques, such as laparoscopic or robotic-assisted procedures.

Nonsurgical Management. Nonsurgical interventions (radiation therapy and chemotherapy) are typically used after surgery and depend on the surgical staging.

Radiation Therapy. The oncologist may prescribe radiation therapy to be delivered by external beam and/or brachytherapy depending on stage and grade.

The purpose of *brachytherapy* is to prevent disease recurrence. This procedure is used for women who have had their uterus and cervix removed (ACS, 2019). The upper part of the vagina is treated when a cylinder is placed inside it by the radiologist. In high-dose-rate (HDR) brachytherapy, each treatment takes about 10 to 20 minutes. While the radioactive implant is in place, radiation is emitted that can affect other people, so others will not be in the room. Inform the patient that she is restricted to bedrest during the treatment session to prevent dislodgment of the radioactive source. At the completion of treatment, the woman may go home the same day. There are no restrictions for the woman to stay away from her family or the public between treatments. Depending on the oncologist's determination, treatments may be given weekly or daily for at least three doses (ACS, 2019).

The Best Practice for Patient Safety & Quality Care: Health Teaching for the Patient Having Brachytherapy for Gynecologic Cancer box lists additional health teaching for the patient having brachytherapy for gynecologic cancer.

BEST PRACTICE FOR PATIENT SAFETY & QUALITY CARE (QSEN)

Health Teaching for the Patient Having Brachytherapy for Gynecologic Cancer

Teach the patient to report any of these signs and symptoms to the health care provider immediately:

- Heavy vaginal bleeding
- Urethral burning for more than 24 hours
- Blood in the urine
- Extreme fatigue
- Severe diarrhea
- Fever over 100°F (38°C)
- Abdominal ***pain***

External beam radiation therapy (*EBRT*) may be used to treat any stage of endometrial cancer in combination with surgery, brachytherapy, and/or chemotherapy. The treatment is given on an ambulatory care basis usually 5 days a week for 4 to 6 weeks, with each session taking less than 30 minutes (ACS, 2019). Tissue around the tumor and pelvic wall nodes also is treated. *Teach the patient to monitor for signs of skin breakdown, especially in the perineal area; to avoid sunbathing; and to avoid washing the markings outlining the treatment site.*

Reactions to radiation therapy vary. Some women feel "radioactive" or "unclean" after treatments and may exhibit withdrawal behaviors. Reassure them by correcting any misconceptions. Chapter 20 discusses nursing care of patients receiving radiation therapy in more detail.

Drug Therapy. Multiagent *chemotherapy* is used as palliative treatment in advanced and recurrent disease when it has spread to distant parts of the body, but it is not always effective (Campos & Cohn, 2020). For that reason, it is important to also consider other methods of palliative care (see Chapter 8).

A common side effect of chemotherapy used to treat endometrial cancer is **alopecia** (hair loss). Remind the patient of this possibility before treatment starts. Chapter 20 describes chemotherapy and general nursing care during treatment.

Complementary and Integrative Health. Every woman experiences cancer differently. Many complementary and integrative therapies have evidence of benefit in decreasing the side effects of drug therapy and boosting the immune system. Provide your patient with information that will help her make informed, evidence-based decisions. Encourage her to check with her oncologist and/or pharmacist because some integrative therapies can be harmful or interfere with cancer treatment. Current evidence-based information is available at the American Cancer Society (www.cancer.org) and Canadian Cancer Society (www.cancer.ca) websites about mind-body therapies, healing touch, herbs, vitamins, nutrition, and biologic therapies.

Surgical Management. The most common surgical procedure to address endometrial cancer involves the removal of the uterus, fallopian tubes, and ovaries (**total hysterectomy** and **bilateral salpingo-oophorectomy** [**BSO**]). Laparoscopy or robotic-assisted surgery is preferred when the disease is confined to the uterus (Cohn, 2020), as these surgeries are usually less expensive and have fewer complications and shorter hospital stays. If minimally invasive surgery is not possible, laparotomy can be considered. Vaginal or abdominal hysterectomy are also options.

Care Coordination and Transition Management. Home care after surgery for endometrial cancer is the same as that after a hysterectomy. Patients who are receiving chemotherapy or radiation therapy are treated on an ambulatory care basis. Most women are surprised by the fatigue caused by radiation and chemotherapy. Help the patient and her family plan daily activities around treatment requirements so that she can effectively pace herself.

High doses of radiation cause sterility, and vaginal shrinkage can occur. Vaginal dilators can be used with water-soluble lubricants for 10 minutes three to four times weekly until sexual activity resumes, generally within 4 weeks (ACS, 2020c).

Often patients experience emotional crises because of the physical effects of cancer treatments. Radical hysterectomy may be seen as mutilating. Both radiation and chemotherapy have side effects that change physical appearance and body image. Women may have a grief reaction to these changes. The feelings of loss depend on the visibility of the loss and the perception or reality of loss of function. Help the patient adapt to the body changes. Using a calm and accepting approach, encourage self-management as soon as her physical condition is stable.

Encourage patients and their families to discuss their feelings. Refer to support services such as a certified hospital chaplain or other spiritual leader, social worker, or counselor. In the United States, local American Cancer Society chapters provide written materials about endometrial cancer and information about local support groups. Each province in Canada also has a division of the Canadian Cancer Society (www.cancer.ca).

Death can occur with or without treatment. The goal is for the patient to meet and exceed the 5-year survival mark without a recurrence of disease. If the tumor recurs and cure is not likely, the woman and her family need to consider hospice care and whether she can be cared for in the home. If nursing care is needed at home, the hospital nurse or case manager makes referrals to a home health care agency. A referral to a social services agency may be needed if the patient needs financial assistance for treatment and long-term follow-up.

OVARIAN CANCER

Pathophysiology Review

Ovarian cancer is the leading cause of gynecologic cancer death, and the second most common type of gynecologic cancer (Chen & Berek, 2019). Most ovarian cancers are epithelial tumors that grow on the surface of the ovaries. These tumors grow rapidly, spread quickly, and are often bilateral. Tumor cells spread by direct extension into nearby organs and through blood and lymph circulation to distant sites (McCance et al., 2019). Free-floating cancer cells also spread through the abdomen to seed new sites, usually accompanied by ascites (abdominal fluid).

Ovarian cancer seems to be disordered growth in response to excessive exposure to estrogen. This would explain the protective effects of pregnancies and oral contraceptive use, both of which interrupt the monthly estrogen exposure.

Risk factors include older age, obesity, nulliparity, use of estrogen alone (without progesterone), and certain infertility diagnoses (ACS, 2020a; Centers for Disease Control and Prevention [CDC], 2019b). Women with genetic mutations of *BRCA1* or *BRCA2* are at higher risk (National Ovarian Cancer Coalition, 2020a). Of these, some choose to have a *risk-reducing bilateral salpingo-oophorectomy* (BSO) (see Table 66.1) to prevent ovarian cancer. For many years, the use of talcum powder was associated with development of ovarian cancer; the most current research shows that this correlation is not statistically significant (O'Brien et al., 2020). Table 66.3 lists known and suspected risk factors for ovarian cancer.

TABLE 66.3 Risk Factors for Ovarian Cancer

- Middle to older age
- *BRCA1* or *BRCA2* gene mutations
- Infertility
- Difficulty getting pregnant
- Nulliparity
- History of endometriosis
- History of breast, uterine, or colorectal (colon) cancer (especially Lynch syndrome, hereditary nonpolyposis colorectal cancer [HNPCC])
- Of Eastern European or Ashkenazi Jewish background

Data from Centers for Disease Control and Prevention (CDC). (2019). What are the risk factors for ovarian cancer? https://www.cdc.gov/cancer/ovarian/basic_info/risk_factors.htm; and Lu, K., & Schmeler, K. (2020). Lynch syndrome (Hereditary nonpolyposis colorectal cancer): Screening and prevention of endometrial and ovarian cancer. In *UpToDate*. Goff, B. (Ed.). Waltham, MA.

Formerly, it was thought that ovarian cancer was a "silent" disease where symptoms did not present until the late stages of the disease. Evidence now shows that common symptoms of bloating, urinary urgency or frequency, difficulty eating, feeling full, and pelvic pain are often experienced very early (Chen & Berek, 2019). Caught early, ovarian cancer is treatable in the early stages (ACS, 2020a). However, many women do not seek care because they associate those and other vague symptoms (weight gain, constipation, bloating) with menopause (Bohnenkamp et al., 2019). Survival rates are low, therefore, because it is often not detected until its late stages (ACS, 2020a).

❖ Interprofessional Collaborative Care

◆ **Assessment: Recognize Cues.** As a matter of prevention, it is important for nurses to teach women to *"think ovarian"* even at the onset of vague abdominal and GI symptoms. Most women with ovarian cancer have had mild symptoms for several months but may have thought they were caused by normal perimenopausal changes or stress. They may report abdominal ***pain*** or swelling or have vague GI disturbances such as indigestion and gas. Ask the patient if she has had urinary frequency or incontinence, unexpected weight loss, and/or vaginal bleeding.

Complications of advanced metastatic cancer include (Chen & Berek, 2019):

- Pleural effusion
- Venous thromboembolism (VTE)
- Bowel obstruction

On pelvic examination, an abdominal mass may not be palpable until it reaches a size of 4 to 6 inches (10 to 15 cm). Any enlarged ovary found after menopause should be evaluated as though it were malignant.

A cancer antigen test, *CA 125,* measures the presence of damaged endometrial and uterine tissue in the blood. It may be elevated if ovarian cancer is present, but it can also be elevated in patients with endometriosis, fibroids, pelvic inflammatory disease, pregnancy, and even menses (Pagana & Pagana, 2018). It is also useful for monitoring a patient's progress during and after treatment. Abdominal and pelvic CT scans or MRI is most commonly used to evaluate for metastasis. A chest x-ray is obtained to evaluate for the presence of pleural effusion, metastases, and mediastinal lymphadenopathy (Chen & Berek, 2019). A liver profile may be ordered if there is ascites.

The woman with ovarian cancer has concerns similar to those described for the patient with other gynecologic cancers. Because the cancer is often diagnosed in an advanced stage, thoughts of death and dying, menopause, and loss of fertility may come as a shock.

NCLEX EXAMINATION CHALLENGE 66.3

Psychosocial Integrity

The nurse is preparing a client for surgery related to ovarian cancer. When the client states, "I'm just going to die anyway; why do I even need this surgery?" what is the appropriate nursing response?

A. "We don't know that you will die from this."
B. "Are you thinking of canceling the surgery?"
C. "Ovarian cancer has an unfavorable prognosis."
D. "If the condition is fatal, hospice can provide care."

◆ **Interventions: Take Action.** Nursing care of the patient with ovarian cancer is similar to that for the patient with endometrial or cervical cancer. The options for treatment depend on the extent of the cancer and usually include surgery first, followed by chemotherapy. Radiation may be used for treatment of metastasis, but is not used often for ovarian cancer alone as a treatment method (National Ovarian Cancer Coalition, 2020b).

Diagnosis depends on findings during surgical exploration and diagnostic testing. A total abdominal hysterectomy, bilateral salpingo-oophorectomy (BSO; removal of the ovaries and fallopian tubes), and pelvic and para-aortic lymph node dissection are usually performed. Tumors are staged during surgery. Very large tumors that cannot be removed are debulked (reduced). These procedures can be performed via laparoscopic technique or robotic-assisted laparoscopy to decrease recovery time, minimize ***pain,*** and reduce postoperative complications.

Nursing care of the patient is similar to that for any patient having abdominal surgery (see Chapter 9). As for any patient after abdominal surgery, assess vital signs and ***pain*** and maintain catheters and drains. Teach her the importance of antiembolism stockings, incentive spirometry, and early ambulation. Evaluate for respiratory or urinary ***infection.*** Assess vital signs and monitor the quantity and quality of urine output.

After removing and staging ovarian cancer, *chemotherapy* is used often. See Chapter 20 for care of the patient with cancer for more information. Chemotherapeutic agents may be given IV and/or intraperitoneally. Intraperitoneal (IP) therapy is described in Chapter 15.

Care Coordination and Transition Management. Teach patients discharged to home to avoid tampons, douches, and sexual intercourse for at least 6 weeks or as instructed by the surgeon. Remind them to keep their follow-up surgical appointment and to follow the surgeon's other recommendations about resuming usual activities.

Refer patients and their families to Gilda's Club within their local demographic (e.g., www.gildasclubnyc.org) and the National Ovarian Cancer Coalition (NOCC) (www.ovarian.org) for more information and support groups. In Canada, Ovarian Cancer Canada (www.ovariancanada.org) is available for the same purpose.

Ovarian cancer has a high recurrence rate. After recurrence, the cancer is treatable but no longer curable. A once-daily oral pill, Zejula (niraparib), is now approved for *maintenance therapy,* which is a type of treatment given after a favorable response to chemotherapy to keep ovarian cancer from recurring (GSK, 2020). If the patient refuses maintenance therapy, or if maintenance therapy is unsuccessful, the patient may deny symptoms at first or express feelings of anger and grief. The patient and family are often fearful of the outcome. Provide encouragement and support during this difficult time and refer to grief counseling, spiritual leaders (if desired), and community support groups. For patients with advanced metastatic disease, collaborate with members of the interprofessional team for possible referral to hospice. Chapter 8 discusses end-of-life care.

CERVICAL CANCER

Pathophysiology Review

The uterine cervix is covered with squamous cells on the outer cervix and columnar (glandular) cells that line the endocervical canal. Papanicolaou (Pap) tests sample cells from both areas as a screening test for cervical cancer. The squamocolumnar junction is the *transformation zone* where most cell abnormalities occur. The adolescent has more columnar cells exposed on the outer cervix, which may be one reason that she is more vulnerable to sexually transmitted infections (STIs) and human immune deficiency virus (HIV). In contrast, in the menopausal woman the squamocolumnar junction may be higher up in the endocervical canal, making it difficult to sample for a Pap test.

Premalignant changes are classified on a continuum from cervical intraepithelial neoplasia (dysplasia) to cervical carcinoma in situ (where the full epithelial thickness of the cervix is involved) to invasive carcinoma (McCance & Huether, 2019).

Most cervical cancers arise from the squamous cells on the outside of the cervix. The other cancers arise from the mucus-secreting glandular cells (adenocarcinoma) in the endocervical canal. The disease spreads by direct extension to the vaginal mucosa, lower uterine segment, parametrium, pelvic wall, bladder, and bowel. Metastasis is usually confined to the pelvis, but distant spread can occur through lymphatic spread and the circulation to the liver, lungs, or bones.

TABLE 66.4 Risk Factors for Cervical Cancer

- Infection with human papillomavirus (HPV)
- Infection with chlamydia
- Smoking
- Being immunocompromised (e.g., having HIV, or taking immunosuppressant drugs for an autoimmune condition)
- Multiparity (multiple births)
- Obesity
- Women whose mothers took diethylstilbestrol (DES; a hormone to prevent miscarriage) between 1940 and 1971
- Long-term use of oral contraceptives
- Use of an intrauterine device (IUD)
- Having multiple full-term pregnancies
- Having a first full-term pregnancy earlier than age 17
- Having a family history of cervical cancer

Data from Centers for Disease Control and Prevention (CDC). (2020). *Risk factors for cervical cancer.* https://www.cancer.org/cancer/cervical-cancer/causes-risks-prevention/risk-factors.html; and Katz, A. (2019). Obesity-related cancer in women: A clinical review. *American Journal of Nursing, 119*(8), 34-40.

Human papillomavirus ***infection*** (HPV) is the most common type of sexually transmitted infection (STI) in the United States (CDC, 2019a). Almost all women will have HPV sometime in their life, but not all types lead to cancer. Most cases of cervical cancer are caused by certain types of HPV. The high-risk HPV types 16 and 18 are responsible for 70% of cervical cancers (World Health Organization [WHO], 2019). They impair the tumor-suppressor gene and cause most of the cervical cancers. The unrestricted tissue growth can spread, becoming invasive and metastatic (McCance et al., 2019). Risk factors for cervical cancer are listed in Table 66.4. Teach patients how to reduce their risk of sexual exposure to HPV by being immunized with an HPV vaccine, and using condoms during sexual intimacy.

Health Promotion and Maintenance

Girls and young women should be immunized with one of the HPV vaccines:

- *Gardasil* (available in Canada)—available for ages 9 through 26
- *Gardasil 9* (available in the United States and Canada)—available for ages 9 to 26; can be administered until age 45
- *Cervarix* (available in Canada)—available for ages 9 through 25

In addition to being immunized, women should be taught to follow the U.S. Preventive Services Task Force recommendations on Papanicolaou (Pap) tests and HPV testing (U.S. Preventive Services Task Force, 2018). See Chapter 69 for a thorough discussion of the importance of HPV vaccination; Pap and HPV testing recommendations; and associated patient teaching.

Canadian guidelines for cervical cancer screening were last established in 2013, as of this writing. These recommend no screening for women age 19 years and younger, or older than 70 years (if she has had three negative Pap tests over the past 10 years) (Canadian Task Force on Preventive Health Care, 2013). For women ages 20 to 24, no routine screening is recommended. For women ages 25 to 69, screening is recommended every 3 years.

❖ Interprofessional Collaborative Care

◆ Assessment: Recognize Cues

Physical Assessment/Signs and Symptoms. The patient who has preinvasive cancer is often asymptomatic. The classic symptoms of invasive cancer include painless vaginal bleeding, which may be irregular or heavy, and bleeding after sexual intercourse. As the cancer grows, bleeding increases in frequency, duration, and amount and may become continuous. Other symptoms may include pelvic or back pain, hematuria, hematochezia, or vaginal passage of stool or urine, which accompanies advanced disease (Frumovitz, 2020).

A physical examination may not reveal any abnormalities regarding early preinvasive cervical cancer. The internal pelvic examination may identify late-stage disease.

CLINICAL JUDGMENT CHALLENGE 66.1

Safety; Patient-Centered Care

A 39-year-old female client reports that she has heavy menstrual periods that have been irregular in nature for the last couple of years. For the last 3 months, the frequency of the periods has increased, and she has noticed that she has begun bleeding after sexual intercourse. She says she wants to have a hysterectomy so that she will not bleed anymore, because she had a friend who had that procedure and is very happy not having periods.

1. **Recognize Cues:** What assessment information in this client situation is the most important and immediate concern for the nurse? (Hint: Identify the **relevant** information *first* to determine what is most important.)
2. **Analyze Cues:** What client conditions are consistent with the **most relevant** information? (Hint: Think about priority collaborative problems that support and contradict the information presented in this situation.)
3. **Prioritize Hypotheses:** Which possibilities or explanations are **most likely** to be present in this client situation? Which possibilities or explanations are the most serious? (Hint: Consider all possibilities and determine their urgency and risk for this client.)
4. **Generate Solutions:** What actions would most likely achieve the desired outcomes for this client? Which actions should be **avoided** or are **potentially harmful**? (Hint: Determine the desired outcomes first to decide which interventions are appropriate and those that should be avoided.)
5. **Take Action:** Which actions are the most appropriate and how should they be implemented? In what **priority order** should they be implemented? (Hint: Consider health teaching, documentation, requested health care provider orders or prescriptions, nursing skills, collaboration with or referral to health team members, etc.)
6. **Evaluate Outcomes:** What client assessment would indicate that the nurse's actions were **effective**? (Hint: Think about signs that would indicate an improvement, decline, or unchanged client condition.)

Diagnostic Assessment. Taken during the Pap test, an *HPV-typing DNA test* of the cervical sample can determine the presence of one or more high-risk types (CDC, 2020e; Emory Winship Cancer Institute, 2020). The health care provider may perform a colposcopic examination to view the transformation zone. **Colposcopy** is a procedure in which application of an acetic acid solution is applied to the cervix. The cervix is then examined under magnification with a bright filter light that enhances the visualization of the characteristics of dysplasia or cancer. If abnormal tissue is recognized, multiple biopsies of the cervical tissue are performed.

If atypical glandular cells are suspected, the health care provider may perform a cervical biopsy in the form of a punch biopsy, a cone biopsy, or *endocervical curettage* (scraping of the endocervix wall) as well. Inform her that a small amount of bleeding is expected for several days after this procedure, and that she should not douche, use tampons, or have sexual intercourse for at least a week.

◆ **Interventions: Take Action.** Interventions for the woman with cervical cancer are similar to those for endometrial cancer: surgery, which is possibly followed by radiation and chemotherapy for late-stage disease.

Nonsurgical Management. *Radiation therapy* can be used to treat certain stages of cervical cancer, or cervical cancer that has spread to other organs. Brachytherapy and external beam radiation therapy (EBRT) are the two types used.

A combination of chemotherapy and radiation, referred to as ***concurrent chemoradiation,*** may also be used. This treatment modality has been shown to be effective because the chemotherapy enhances the effect of the radiation. See Chapter 20 for more information about the general nursing care for the patient on chemotherapy and radiation.

Surgical Management. Choice of surgical management approach is dependent on the patient's overall health, desire for future childbearing, tumor size and stage, cancer cell type, degree of lymph node involvement, and patient preference.

The **loop electrosurgical excision procedure (LEEP)** is short (10 to 30 minutes) and is performed in a health care provider's office or an ambulatory care setting with a local anesthetic injected into the cervix. A thin loop-wire electrode that transmits a painless electrical current is used to cut away affected tissue. LEEP (Fig. 66.4) is both a diagnostic procedure and a treatment because it provides a specimen that can be examined by a pathologist to ensure that the lesion was completely removed. Spotting (very scant bleeding) and slight ***pain*** after the procedure is common. Teach patients to adhere for 3 weeks, or the time frame recommended by the health care provider, to the restrictions listed in the Patient and Family Education: Preparing for Self-Management: Care After Local Cervical Ablation Therapies box.

Laser surgery is also an office procedure done under local anesthesia to address early cancers. A laser beam is directed through the vagina to vaporize abnormal cells. A small amount of bleeding occurs with the procedure, and the woman may have a slight vaginal discharge. Healing occurs in 6 to 12 weeks. A disadvantage of this procedure is that no specimen is available for study.

PATIENT AND FAMILY EDUCATION: PREPARING FOR SELF-MANAGEMENT

Care After Local Cervical Ablation Therapies

- Refrain from sexual intercourse.
- Do not use tampons.
- Do not douche.
- Take showers rather than tub baths.
- Avoid lifting heavy objects.
- Report any heavy vaginal bleeding, foul-smelling drainage, or fever.

Cryosurgery involves freezing of the cancer, causing subsequent necrosis. The procedure is usually painless, although some women have slight cramping after it. Teach the patient that she will have heavy, watery brown discharge for several weeks after the procedure. Instruct her to follow the restrictions in the Patient and Family Education: Preparing for Self-Management: Care After Local Cervical Ablation Therapies box.

In cases of microinvasive cancer, a *conization* can remove the affected tissue while still preserving fertility. This procedure is done when the lesion cannot be visualized by colposcopic examination. A cone-shaped area of cervix is removed surgically and sent to the laboratory to determine the extent of the cancer. Potential complications from this procedure include hemorrhage and uterine perforation. Long-term follow-up care is needed because new cancers can develop.

For women who may wish to become pregnant in the future, a *radical trachelectomy* can be done. Going through the vagina or abdomen (sometimes laparoscopically), the cervix and upper part of the vagina are removed, leaving the body of the uterus intact (ACS, 2020d). A "purse-string" stitch is made, which then functions as an artificial opening of the cervix, and close lymph nodes are removed. This procedure can help some women to carry a pregnancy to term and deliver by cesarean section, although the risk of miscarriage still exists (ACS, 2016b).

A *total hysterectomy* may be performed as treatment of microinvasive cancer if the woman does not wish to become pregnant in the future. A laparoscopic approach is commonly used, although evidence shows that women who have the open approach have a lesser chance of recurrence of cancer, and live longer lives (ACS, 2020d). Lymph node dissection can be performed at the same time, if needed. Care for patients undergoing hysterectomy is discussed in the Sexuality Concept Exemplar: Uterine Leiomyoma section earlier in this chapter.

Care Coordination and Transition Management. As with all patients who have undergone treatment, provide discharge teaching that is congruent with the procedure used. Refer to psychosocial support as needed, and encourage the patient to keep all follow-up appointments.

VULVOVAGINITIS

Pathophysiology Review

Vaginal discharge and itching are two common problems experienced by most women at some time in their lives. Vaginal infections may be transmitted sexually and nonsexually. Gonorrhea, syphilis, chlamydia, and herpes simplex virus infections are sexually transmitted infections (STIs) discussed in Chapter 69.

Vulvovaginitis is inflammation of the lower genital tract resulting from a disturbance of the balance of hormones and flora in the vagina and vulva. It may be characterized by itching, change in vaginal discharge, odor, or lesions. Pediculosis pubis, known as crab lice or "crabs," and scabies are parasitic infections of the vulvar skin that are *sexually* transmitted. The most common causes of *nonsexually* transmitted infections include (U.S. National Library of Medicine, 2020):

- Infections
  - Yeast infections

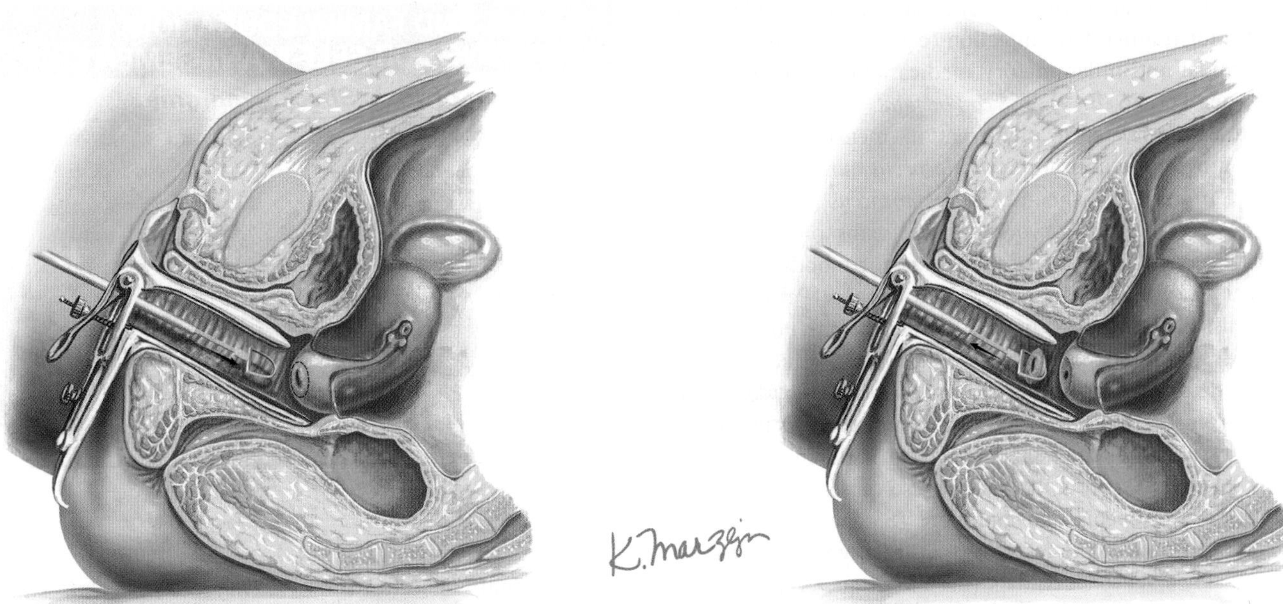

FIG. 66.4 Loop electrosurgical excision procedure (LEEP). (From Smith, R.P. [2018]. *Netter's Obstetrics and Gynecology* [3rd ed.]. Philadelphia: Elsevier.)

- Chemicals
  - Spermicide
  - Vaginal sponges
  - Feminine hygiene sprays
  - Bubble baths and soaps
  - Use of new or different laundry detergent
- Other causes
  - Wearing tight-fitting clothing
  - Wiping from back to front, introducing bacteria from stool into the vagina

Some women may have an *itch-scratch-itch cycle,* in which the itching leads to scratching, which causes excoriation that then must heal. As healing takes place, itching occurs again. If the cycle is not interrupted, the chronic scratching may lead to the white, thickened skin of lichen planus. This dry, leathery skin cracks easily, increasing the risk for ***infection.***

❖ Interprofessional Collaborative Care

Assess for vulvovaginitis by asking questions about the symptoms, assisting with a pelvic examination, and obtaining vaginal smears for laboratory testing. Ask if the patient is experiencing an itching or burning sensation, erythema (redness), edema, and/or superficial skin ulcers. Use a nonjudgmental approach and provide reassurance during the assessment because the patient may be embarrassed or afraid to discuss her symptoms. Encourage her to talk about her problem and its effect on ***sexuality.***

Interventions for vulvovaginitis depend on the specific vaginal ***infection.*** Proper health habits can benefit treatment. Instruct the patient to get enough rest and sleep, observe good dietary habits, exercise regularly, and use good personal hygiene. Teach her about how to manage the condition and prevent further infections per the instructions in the Patient and Family Education: Preparing for Self-Management: Prevention of Vulvovaginitis box.

Cold compresses can be recommended, as can a lukewarm sitz bath for 5 to 10 minutes several times a day. Topical drugs such as estrogens and lidocaine may be prescribed to relieve itching. Encourage the patient to wear breathable fabrics such as cotton and to avoid irritants or allergens in products such as laundry detergents or bath products.

PATIENT AND FAMILY EDUCATION: PREPARING FOR SELF-MANAGEMENT

Prevention of Vulvovaginitis

- Wear cotton underwear.
- Avoid wearing tight clothing, such as pantyhose or tight jeans, because it can cause chafing. You can also get hot and sweaty, which can increase the risk for ***infection.***
- Always wipe front to back after having a bowel movement or urinating.
- Use fragrance-free laundry detergent.
- During a bath or shower, cleanse inner labial mucosa with water, not soap.
- Do not douche or use feminine hygiene sprays.
- Choose other methods of contraception instead of spermicide or vaginal sponges, which can irritate the condition
- If your sexual partner has an ***infection*** of the sex organs, do not have intercourse with him or her until he or she has been treated.
- You are more likely to get an ***infection*** if you are pregnant, have diabetes, take oral contraceptive drugs, or are menopausal.
- Practice vulvar self-examination monthly.
- If irritation is due to a yeast infection, fully take the prescribed drug treatment as ordered by the primary health care provider.

Treatment of pediculosis and scabies is used if needed and includes:

- Applying a topical pediculicide to the affected area as prescribed
- Cleaning affected clothes, bedding, and towels
- Disinfecting the home environment (Lice cannot live for more than 24 hours away from the body.)

TOXIC SHOCK SYNDROME

Pathophysiology Review

Toxic shock syndrome (TSS) can result from leaving a tampon, contraceptive sponge, or diaphragm in the vagina. Other conditions associated with TSS include surgical wound ***infection,*** minor trauma, viral infection (e.g., varicella), and use of nonsteroidal anti-inflammatory medications (NSAIDs) (Bush & Vazquez-Pertejo, 2019). *TSS can be fatal.*

In infection related to menstruation, menstrual blood provides a growth medium for *Staphylococcus aureus* (or, less frequently, group A beta-hemolytic *Streptococcus* [GABHS], also known as *Streptococcus pyogenes*). Exotoxins produced from the bacteria cross the vaginal mucosa to the bloodstream via a mucosal break or via the uterus (Bush & Vazquez-Pertejo, 2019).

TSS usually develops within 5 days after the onset of menstruation. Most common symptoms include fever (which remains elevated despite treatment), diffuse macular rash, myalgias, and hypotension. The rash associated with TSS often looks like a sunburn, and patients often develop broken capillaries in the eyes and skin. TSS due to *Staphylococcus aureus* also causes vomiting, diarrhea, thrombocytopenia, and confusion; TSS due to streptococcal infection can cause acute respiratory distress syndrome (ARDS), coagulopathy, and hepatic damage (Bush & Vazquez-Pertejo, 2019).

❖ Interprofessional Collaborative Care

Educate all women on prevention of TSS as covered in the Patient and Family Education: Preparing for Self-Management: Prevention of Toxic Shock Syndrome box.

PATIENT AND FAMILY EDUCATION: PREPARING FOR SELF-MANAGEMENT

Prevention of Toxic Shock Syndrome

- Wash your hands before inserting a tampon.
- Do not use a tampon if it is dirty.
- Insert the tampon carefully to avoid injuring the delicate tissue in your vagina.
- Change your tampon every 3 to 6 hours.
- Do not use superabsorbent tampons.
- Use perineal pads ("sanitary napkins") (instead of tampons) at night.
- Avoid use of insertable contraceptive devices
- Call your primary health care provider if you experience a sudden onset of high temperature, vomiting, or diarrhea.
- Do not use tampons at all if you have had toxic shock syndrome.

Treatment includes removal of the ***infection*** source, such as a tampon; restoring fluid and electrolyte balance; administering drugs to manage hypotension; and IV antibiotics. Other measures may include transfusions to reverse low platelet counts and corticosteroids to treat skin changes.

GET READY FOR THE NEXT-GENERATION NCLEX® EXAMINATION!

Key Points

Review these Key Points for each NCLEX Examination Client Needs Category.

Safe and Effective Care Environment

- Collaborate with the interprofessional team when planning care for patients with gynecologic problems. **QSEN: Teamwork and Collaboration**
- Perform a focused physical assessment for patients reporting gynecologic problems. **QSEN: Patient-Centered Care**
- Remind patients wanting to use complementary and integrative therapies to check with their health care provider first. **QSEN: Safety**
- Teach patients receiving external beam radiation therapy how to preserve skin integrity. **QSEN: Safety**

Health Promotion and Maintenance

- Teach women to follow the American Cancer Society's screening guidelines for prevention and early detection of gynecologic cancers. **QSEN: Evidence-Based Practice**
- Teach women methods of practicing safer sex to prevent ***infection*** of the reproductive tract. **QSEN: Evidence-Based Practice**
- Teach women at risk for gynecologic cancer to be screened and to follow early detection guidelines. **QSEN: Evidence-Based Practice**
- Teach women methods to prevent toxic shock syndrome (TSS). **QSEN: Safety**

Psychosocial Integrity

- Explain all tests, procedures, and treatments, especially if they cause ***pain.*** **Ethics**
- Assess patient's understanding regarding the fact that some procedures related to reproductive problems cause infertility. **Ethics**
- Assess the patient's anxiety before surgery and allow expression of feelings of fear or grief. **QSEN: Patient-Centered Care**
- Assess the patient's reaction to the possible loss of ***reproduction*** ability, and concerns about ***sexuality*** and changes in body image. **QSEN: Patient-Centered Care**
- Refer patients with gynecologic cancer to resources that can provide support. **QSEN: Patient-Centered Care**

Physiological Integrity

- Coordinate postoperative care for women having gynecologic surgery. **QSEN: Teamwork and Collaboration**
- Provide self-care health teaching for the woman who had gynecologic surgery. **QSEN: Patient-Centered Care**
- When caring for a patient who has a radioactive implant, use best safety practices. **QSEN: Evidence-Based Practices**
- Observe for and report complications after surgery, including ***infection, pain,*** and ***elimination*** problems. **Clinical Judgment**
- Assess for and report symptoms associated with toxic shock syndrome. **Clinical Judgment**

MASTERY QUESTIONS

1. What teaching will the nurse provide to a 30-year-old female client who has never been sexually active about decreasing her risk of developing cervical cancer? **Select all that apply.**
   A. "You cannot lower the risk for cervical cancer."
   B. "You cannot receive the Gardasil-9 immunization."
   C. "Use condoms when you plan to be sexually intimate."
   D. "Over-the-counter contraceptive methods can be used to prevent HPV."
   E. "Having an annual Pap test will decrease your chances of cervical cancer."

2. The nurse has provided teaching to a client with vulvovaginitis. Which client statement indicates that nursing intervention is required? **Select all that apply.**
   A. "I will wipe from the front to the back."
   B. "I will wash with fragranced soap to prevent odor."
   C. "I am going to the store now to buy cotton underwear."
   D. "I will use fragrance-free laundry detergents in the future."
   E. "I am going to take all of the medicine the provider prescribed."

REFERENCES

Asterisk (*) indicates a classic or definitive work on this subject.

American Cancer Society (ACS). (2019). *Radiation therapy for endometrial cancer*. Retrieved from https://www.cancer.org/cancer/endometrial-cancer/treating/radiation.html.

American Cancer Society (ACS). (2020a). *About ovarian cancer*. Retrieved from https://www.cancer.org/cancer/ovarian-cancer/about/what-is-ovarian-cancer.html.

American Cancer Society (ACS). (2020b). *Key statistics for endometrial cancer*. Retrieved from https://www.cancer.org/cancer/endometrial-cancer/about/key-statistics.html.

American Cancer Society (ACS). (2020c). *Radiation therapy can affect the sex life of females with cancer*. Retrieved from http://www.cancer.org/treatment/treatments-and-side-effects/physical-side-effects/fertility-and-sexual-side-effects/sexuality-for-women-with-cancer/pelvic-radiation.html.

American Cancer Society (ACS). (2020d). *Surgery for cervical cancer*. Retrieved from https://www.cancer.org/cancer/cervical-cancer/treating/surgery.html.

American Cancer Society (ACS). (2020e). *The HPV DNA test*. Retrieved from https://www.cancer.org/cancer/cervical-cancer/prevention-and-early-detection/hpv-test.html.

Bohnenkamp, S., McClurg, E., & Bohnenkamp, Z. (2019). What medical-surgical nurses need to know about caring for patients with epithelial ovarian cancer: Part I. *Medsurg Nursing*, *28*(5), 334–338.

Bradley, L. (2020). Uterine fibroids (leiomyomas): Hysteroscopic myomectomy. In T. Falcone (Ed.), *UpToDate*. Waltham, MA.

Bush, L., & Vazquez-Pertejo, M. (2019). *Toxic shock syndrome*. https://www.merckmanuals.com/professional/infectious-diseases/gram-positive-cocci/toxic-shock-syndrome-tss.

Campos, S., & Cohn, D. (2020). Treatment of metastatic endometrial cancer. In B. Goff, & D. Dizon (Eds.), *UpToDate*. Waltham, MA.

*Canadian Task Force on Preventive Health Care. (2013). Cervical Cancer: Summary of recommendations for clinical and policy-makers. Retrieved from https://canadiantaskforce.ca/guidelines/published-guidelines/cervical-cancer/.

Centers for Disease Control and Prevention (CDC). (2019a). *Genital HPV infection: Fact sheet*. www.cdc.gov/std/hpv/stdfact-hpv.htm.

Centers for Disease Control and Prevention (CDC). (2019b). What are the risk factors for ovarian cancer? Retrieved from https://www.cdc.gov/cancer/ovarian/basic_info/risk_factors.htm.

Chen, L., & Berek, J. (2019). Epithelial carcinoma of the ovary, fallopian tube, and peritoneum: Clinical features and diagnosis. In B. Goff, & D. Dizon (Eds.), *UpToDate*. Waltham, MA.

Cohn, D. (2020). Endometrial carcinoma: Staging and surgical treatment. In B. Goff (Ed.), *UpToDate*. Waltham, MA.

Emory Winship Cancer Institute. (2020). *HPV DNA test*. https://www.cancerquest.org/patients/detection-and-diagnosis/hpv-dna-test.

Fashokun, T., & Rogers, R. (2020). Pelvic organ prolapse in women: Diagnostic evaluation. In L. Brubaker (Ed.), *UpToDate*. Waltham, MA.

Feldman, S. (2020). Overview of evaluation of the endometrium for malignant or premalignant disease. In D. Levine, & B. Goff (Eds.), *UpToDate*. Waltham, MA.

Frumovitz, M. (2020). Invasive cervical cancer: Epidemiology, risk factors, clinical manifestations, and diagnosis. In B. Goff, & D. Dizon (Eds.), *UpToDate*. Waltham, MA.

GSK. (2020). *Benefits of Zejula*. https://www.zejula.com/en/benefits-of-ZEJULA.

Jelovsek, J. (2020). Pelvic organ prolapse in women: Choosing a primary surgical procedure. In L. Brubaker (Ed.), *UpToDate*. Waltham, MA.

Johnson, C., George, M., & Fader, A. (2017). Distress screening: Evaluating a protocol for gynecologic cancer survivors. *Clinical Journal of Oncology Nursing*, *21*(3), 353–361.

Mahajan, S. (2020). Pelvic organ prolapse in women: Surgical repair of anterior vaginal wall prolapse. In L. Brubaker (Ed.), *UpToDate*. Waltham, MA.

McCance, K., Huether, S., Brashers, V., & Rote, N. (2019). *Pathophysiology: The biologic basis for disease in adults and children* (8th ed.). St. Louis: Mosby.

McWilliams, M., & Chennathukuzhi, V. (2017). Recent advances in uterine fibroid etiology. *Seminars in Reproductive Medicine*, *35*(2), 181–189.

National Ovarian Cancer Coalition (NOCC). (2020a). Do I have a genetic predisposition to ovarian cancer? Retrieved from http://ovarian.org/about-ovarian-cancer/am-i-at-risk/do-i-have-a-genetic-predisposition

National Ovarian Cancer Coalition. (2020b). *Radiation*. Retrieved from http://ovarian.org/about-ovarian-cancer/treatment/14-iii.

O'Brien, K., et al. (2020). Association of powder use in the genital area with risk of ovarian cancer. *Journal of the American Medical Association*, *323*(1), 49–59.

Pagana, K. D., & Pagana, T. J. (2018). *Mosby's manual of diagnostic and laboratory tests* (6th ed.). St. Louis: Mosby.

Stewart, E. (2020). Uterine fibroids (leiomyomas): Treatment overview. In R. Barbieri (Ed.), *UpToDate*. Waltham, MA.

Stewart, E., & Laughlin-Tommaso, S. (2019). Uterine Fibroids: Epidemiology, clinical features, diagnosis, and natural history. In R. Barbieri, & D. Levine (Eds.), *UpToDate*. Waltham, MA.

Trabuco, J., & Gebhart, E. (2020). Transvaginal synthetic mesh: Complications and risk factors. In K. Brubaker (Ed.), *UoToDate*. Waltham, MA.

U.S. Food and Drug Administration (FDA). (2019). *Urogynecologic surgical mesh implants*. Retrieved from https://www.fda.gov/medical-devices/implants-and-prosthetics/urogynecologic-surgical-mesh-implants.

U.S. National Library of Medicine. (2020). Vulvovaginitis. Retrieved from https://medlineplus.gov/ency/article/000897.htm.

U.S. Preventive Services Task Force. (2018). *Cervical cancer: Screening*. Retrieved from. https://www.uspreventiveservicestaskforce.org/uspstf/recommendation/cervical-cancer-screening.

van der Kooij, S., & Hehenkamp, W. (2020). Uterine leiomyomas (fibroids): Treatment with uterine artery embolization. In D. Levine, & R. Barbieri (Eds.), *UpToDate*. Waltham, MA.

Walters, M. (2020). Choosing a route of hysterectomy for benign uterus disease. In H. Sharp (Ed.), *UpToDate*. Waltham, MA.

World Health Organization (WHO). (2019). *Human papillomavirus (HPV) and cervical cancer*. Retrieved from https://www.who.int/news-room/fact-sheets/detail/human-papillomavirus-(hpv)-and-cervical-cancer.

Yu, O., et al. (2018). A US population-based study of uterine fibroid diagnosis incidence, trends, and prevalence: 2005 to 2014. *American Journal of Obstetrics and Gynecology*, *219*(6), 591.e1–591.e8.

67

Concepts of Care for Patients With Male Reproductive Problems

Cherie R. Rebar

http://evolve.elsevier.com/Iggy/

LEARNING OUTCOMES

1. Collaborate with the interprofessional team to coordinate high-quality care for patients with a male reproductive problem.
2. Describe factors that place a patient at high risk for a male reproductive cancer, and refer to the health care provider.
3. Implement patient-centered nursing interventions to decrease the psychosocial impact of living with a male reproductive problem.
4. Apply knowledge of anatomy, physiology, and pathophysiology to assess patients with a male reproductive problem.
5. Use clinical judgment to analyze assessment findings and diagnostic data in the care of patients with a male reproductive problem.
6. Prioritize evidence-based care for patients with a male reproductive problem affecting ***elimination, infection, cellular regulation, sexuality,*** or ***reproduction.***
7. Plan care coordination and transition management for patients with a male reproductive problem.

KEY TERMS

active surveillance (AS) Observation for cancer without immediate active treatment.

azoospermia The absence of living sperm in the semen.

bilateral orchiectomy The surgical removal of both testes, typically performed as palliative surgery in patients with prostate cancer. It is not intended to cure the prostate cancer but to arrest its spread by removing testosterone.

cryptorchidism Failure of the testes to descend into the scrotum.

erectile dysfunction (ED) The inability to achieve or maintain a penile erection sufficient for sexual intercourse.

gynecomastia Abnormal enlargement of the breasts in men.

hematuria Blood in the urine.

hydronephrosis Abnormal enlargement of the kidney caused by a blockage of urine lower in the tract and filling of the kidney with urine.

hydroureter Abnormal distention of the ureter.

hyperplasia Growth that causes tissue to increase in size by increasing the number of cells; abnormal overgrowth of tissue.

libido Sexual desire.

lower urinary tract symptoms (LUTS) Symptoms that occur as a result of prostatic hyperplasia, such as urinary retention and overflow incontinence, or urinary leaking.

nocturia The need to urinate excessively at night. Also called *nocturnal polyuria.*

oligospermia Low sperm count.

orchiectomy The surgical removal of one or both testes.

overflow urinary incontinence The involuntary loss of urine when the bladder is overdistended. In males, urine "leaks" around an enlarged prostate, causing dribbling.

prostate artery embolization A procedure in which the interventional radiologist threads a small vascular catheter into the prostate's arteries and injects particles blocking some of the blood flow to shrink the prostate gland.

prostate-specific antigen (PSA) A glycoprotein produced solely by the prostate.

prostatitis Inflammation and possible infection of the prostate.

radiation proctitis Rectal mucosa inflammation that results from external beam radiation therapy.

retrograde ejaculation A condition where semen flows backward into the bladder so only a small amount will be ejaculated from the penis; usually is a result of nerve damage during surgery.

transurethral resection of the prostate (TURP) The traditional "closed" surgical procedure for removal of the prostate. In this procedure, the surgeon inserts a resectoscope (an instrument similar to a cystoscope, but with a cutting and cauterizing loop) through the urethra. The enlarged portion of the prostate gland is then resected in small pieces.

tumescence Swelling; vascular congestion in erectile tissue.

PRIORITY AND INTERRELATED CONCEPTS

The priority concepts for this chapter are:
- ***Elimination***
- ***Cellular Regulation***
- ***Infection***

The ***Elimination*** concept exemplar for this chapter is Benign Prostatic Hyperplasia.

The ***Cellular Regulation*** concept exemplar for this chapter is Prostate Cancer.

The interrelated concepts for this chapter are:
- ***Sexuality***
- ***Reproduction***

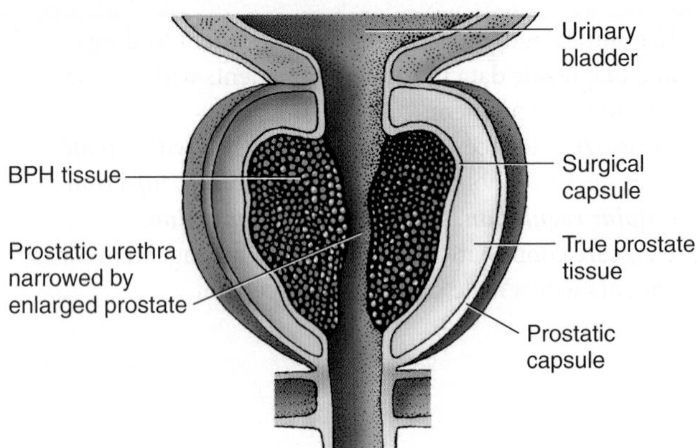

FIG. 67.1 Benign prostatic hyperplasia (BPH) grows inward, causing narrowing of the urethra.

The nurse's role in caring for men with reproductive problems is to be open, supportive, and nonjudgmental. Male reproductive problems are very personal and can range from short-term infections to long-term health care problems that require end-of-life care. These conditions can affect the human need for ***sexuality, elimination,*** and ***reproduction,*** all of which can impact the man's physiological and psychosocial sense of well-bring. See Chapter 1 for a review of the nursing concepts applied in this chapter.

ELIMINATION CONCEPT EXEMPLAR: BENIGN PROSTATIC HYPERPLASIA

Pathophysiology Review

With aging and increased dihydrotestosterone (DHT) levels, the glandular units in the prostate undergo nodular tissue hyperplasia (an increase in the number of cells; an abnormal overgrowth of tissue). This altered tissue promotes local inflammation by attracting cytokines and other substances (McCance et al., 2019).

As the prostate gland enlarges, it extends upward into the bladder and inward, causing bladder outlet obstruction (BOO) (Fig. 67.1). In response, urinary ***elimination*** is affected in several ways, causing lower urinary tract symptoms (LUTS)—an umbrella term that includes problems such as urinary retention, urinary leaking, or incontinence. First, the detrusor (bladder) muscle thickens to help urine push past the enlarged prostate gland (McCance et al., 2019). In spite of the bladder muscle change, the patient has increased residual urine (stasis) and chronic urinary retention. The increased volume of residual urine often causes overflow urinary incontinence, in which the urine "leaks" around the enlarged prostate, causing dribbling. Urinary stasis can also result in urinary tract infections and bladder calculi (stones).

In a few patients the prostate becomes very large and the man cannot void (acute urinary retention [AUR]). The patient with this problem requires *emergent* care. In other patients, chronic urinary retention may result in a backup of urine and cause a gradual, abnormal distention of the ureters (hydroureter) and enlargement of the kidneys (hydronephrosis) if benign prostatic hyperplasia (BPH) is not treated. These urinary ***elimination*** problems can lead to chronic kidney disease as described in Chapter 63.

Etiology and Genetic Risk. BPH is a very common male health problem, but the exact cause is unclear. Its relationship to aging is the only known factor (McCance et al., 2019). Other unmodifiable risk factors include (McVary, 2019):

- Race—Black men younger than 65 need treatment earlier than white men; also, LUTS is more common in black men than white men.
- Genetic susceptibility—Variants in the *GATA3* gene have been associated with development of BPH/LUTS.
- Family history of cancer—Men with a family history of bladder cancer (not prostate cancer) are at higher risk to develop BPH.

Modifiable risk factors include (McVary, 2019):

- Obesity and metabolic syndrome—Obesity, glucose intolerance, dyslipidemia, and hypertension are associated with higher risk for development of BPH.
- Beverage consumption—Coffee and caffeine intake have been associated with an increase in risk for progression of existing BPH.

Incidence and Prevalence. Benign prostatic hyperplasia affects 40% to 50% of men between the ages of 51 and 60, and over 80% of men older than 80 years (McVary, 2019).

Health Promotion and Maintenance. Teach men that BPH is a common occurrence and that sexual frequency does not cause this condition. Current evidence does not show that there are absolute specific actions that prevent the development of BPH; however, teach men that addressing modifiable risk factors can improve their overall health.

Interprofessional Collaborative Care

Assessment: Recognize Cues

History. When taking a history, several standardized assessment tools are used to help the health care provider determine the severity of lower urinary tract symptoms (LUTS) associated with prostatic enlargement. One of the most commonly used assessments is the International Prostate Symptom Score (I-PSS) (Fig. 67.2). This tool incorporates the American Urological Association Symptom Index (AUA-SI) as questions 1 through 7 and asks an eighth question about the implication of the patient's urinary symptoms on quality of life.

International Prostate Symptom Score (I-PSS)

Patient Name: ______________ **Date of Birth:** ______________ **Date Completed** ______________

In the past month:	Not at All	Less Than 1 in 5 Times	Less Than Half the Time	About Half the Time	More Than Half the Time	Almost Always	Your Score
1. Incomplete Emptying How often have you had the sensation of not emptying your bladder?	0	1	2	3	4	5	
2. Frequency How often have you had to urinate less than every 2 hours?	0	1	2	3	4	5	
3. Intermittency How often have you found you stopped and started again several times when you urinated?	0	1	2	3	4	5	
4. Urgency How often have you found it difficult to postpone urination?	0	1	2	3	4	5	
5. Weak Stream How often have you had a weak urinary stream?	0	1	2	3	4	5	
6. Straining How often have you had to strain to start urination?	0	1	2	3	4	5	
	None	**1 Time**	**2 Times**	**3 Times**	**4 Times**	**5 Times**	
7. Nocturia How many times do you typically get up at night to urinate?	0	1	2	3	4	5	
Total I-PSS Score							

Score: 1-7: Mild 8-19: Moderate 20-35: Severe

Quality of Life Due to Urinary Symptoms	Delighted	Pleased	Mostly Satisfied	Mixed	Mostly Dissatisfied	Unhappy	Terrible
If you were to spend the rest of your life with your urinary condition just the way it is now, how would you feel about that?	**0**	**1**	**2**	**3**	**4**	**5**	**6**

FIG. 67.2 The International Prostate Symptom Score (I-PSS). (Adapted from the American Urological Association Practice Guidelines Committee. [2003]. Guideline on the management of benign prostatic hyperplasia [BPH]. *Journal of Urology, 170*[2 Pt 1], 530–547.)

Continued

About the I-PSS

The International Prostate Symptom Score (I-PSS) is based on the answers to seven questions concerning urinary symptoms and one question concerning quality of life. Each question concerning urinary symptoms allows the patient to choose one out of six answers indicating increasing severity of the particular symptom. The answers are assigned points from 0 to 5. The total score can therefore range from 0 to 35 (asymptomatic to very symptomatic).

The questions refer to the following urinary symptoms:

Questions	Symptom
1	Incomplete emptying
2	Frequency
3	Intermittency
4	Urgency
5	Weak Stream
6	Straining
7	Nocturia

Question 8 refers to the patient's perceived quality of life.

The first seven questions of the I-PSS are identical to the questions appearing on the American Urological Association (AUA) Symptom Index, which currently categorizes symptoms as follows:

Mild (symptom score less than or equal to 7)
Moderate (symptom score range 8 to 19)
Severe (symptom score range 20 to 35)

The International Scientific Committee (SCI), under the patronage of the World Health Organization (WHO) and the International Union Against Cancer (UICC), recommends the use of only a single question to assess the quality of life. The answers to this question range from "delighted" to "terrible," or 0 to 6. Although this single question may or may not capture the global impact of benign prostatic hyperplasia (BPH) symptoms or quality of life, it may serve as a valuable starting point for a doctor-patient conversation.

The SCI has agreed to use the symptom index for BPH, which has been developed by the AUA Measurement Committee, as the official worldwide symptoms assessment tool for patients suffering from prostatism.

The SCI recommends that physicians consider the following components for a basic diagnostic workup: history; physical examination; appropriate labs such as U/A, creatinine, etc.; and DRE or other evaluation to rule out prostate cancer.

FIG. 67.2 Cont'd

Most patients complete the questions as a self-administered tool because it is available in many languages. If the patient cannot read, or does not wish to read, the nurse or health care provider can ask the questions to complete the assessment.

Physical Assessment/Signs and Symptoms. Ask about the patient's current urinary ***elimination*** pattern, and ask if it has changed recently. Assess for urinary frequency and urgency. Determine the number of times the patient awakens during the night to void (**nocturia**). Also assess for:

- Difficulty in starting (hesitancy) and continuing urination
- Reduced force and size of the urinary stream ("weak" stream)
- Sensation of incomplete bladder emptying
- Straining to begin urination
- Postvoid (after voiding) dribbling or leaking

The patient is also at risk to develop an ***infection*** or other bladder problem. Ask whether the patient has had **hematuria** (blood in the urine) when starting the urine stream or at the end of voiding. BPH is a common cause of hematuria in older men due to ***infection.***

Remind the patient to void before the physical examination. Inspect and palpate the abdomen. If the patient has a sense of urgency when gentle pressure is applied, the bladder may be distended. Patients with obesity are best assessed by percussion (done by the health care provider) or bedside ultrasound bladder scanner rather than by inspection or palpation.

Prepare the patient for the prostate gland examination, which will be conducted by the health care provider. Tell him that he may feel the urge to urinate as the prostate is palpated. Because the prostate is close to the rectal wall, it is easily examined by *digital rectal examination* (DRE). If needed, help the patient bend over the examination table or assume a side-lying fetal position, whichever is the easiest position for him. The health care provider assesses for size and consistency of the prostate. BPH presents as a uniform, elastic, nontender enlargement; whereas cancer of the prostate gland feels like a stony-hard nodule. Advise the patient that after the prostate gland is palpated, it may be massaged to obtain a fluid sample for examination to rule out prostatitis (inflammation and possible ***infection*** of the prostate), a common problem that can occur with BPH. If the patient has bacterial prostatitis, he is treated with broad-spectrum antibiotic therapy to prevent the spread of infection (McCance et al., 2019).

Psychosocial Assessment. Patients who have nocturia and other LUTS may be frustrated or depressed as a result of interrupted sleep and ongoing visits to the bathroom. Assess the effect of sleep interruptions on the patient's mood and mental status. Ask him about the impact of symptoms on ***sexuality*** and libido (sexual desire).

Postvoid dribbling and overflow incontinence may cause embarrassment and prevent the patient from socializing or leaving the home. For some patients, this social isolation can affect quality of life and lead to clinical depression and/or severe anxiety. Provide time for the patient to express his feelings about these concerns.

Laboratory Assessment. A *urinalysis* and urine *culture* are typically obtained to diagnose urinary tract infection and microscopic hematuria. If ***infection*** is present, the urinalysis measures the number of white blood cells (WBCs).

Other laboratory studies that may be performed include:

- A *complete blood count* (CBC) to evaluate any evidence of systemic infection (elevated WBCs) or anemia (decreased red blood cells [RBCs]) from hematuria.
- *Blood urea nitrogen* (BUN) and *serum creatinine* levels to evaluate renal function (both are usually elevated with kidney disease).
- A *prostate-specific antigen* (PSA) test for screening purposes (the most commonly used and valuable test for early detection of prostate cancer [Kantoff et al., 2020]).
- A *serum acid phosphatase* level if metastatic prostate cancer is suspected (this is typically elevated in patients who have prostate cancer that has metastasized).
- A biopsy, which may be performed if life expectancy is greater than 5 to 10 years, and if needed to confirm a histologic diagnosis; usually transrectal ultrasound (TRUS) or MRI is performed first (Kantoff et al., 2020); see Other Diagnostic Assessment (next section).
- *Culture and sensitivity* of prostatic fluid (if expressed during the examination).

Other Diagnostic Assessment. Imaging studies that are typically performed are *transrectal ultrasound (TRUS)* (more common in the United States) and *MRI* (more common in other countries) (Kantoff et al., 2020). The patient having a TRUS lies on his side while the transducer is inserted into the rectum for viewing the prostate and surrounding structures. A tissue biopsy may also be done during this procedure.

In some cases, cystoscopy may be ordered to view the interior of the bladder, the bladder neck, and the urethra. This procedure is used to study the presence and effect of bladder neck obstruction and is usually done in an ambulatory care setting. Residual urine can also be measured when the cystoscope is inserted. See Chapter 60 for a detailed description of *cystoscopy* and the nursing care needed for patients having this procedure.

Residual urine may be determined by *bladder ultrasound* immediately after the patient voids. *Urodynamic pressure-flow studies* can be helpful in determining if there is urine blockage or weakness of the detrusor muscle.

◆ **Analysis: Analyze Cues and Prioritize Hypotheses.** The priority collaborative problems for the patient with benign prostatic hyperplasia (BPH) are:

1. Urinary retention due to bladder outlet obstruction (BOO)
2. Decreased self-esteem due to overflow urinary incontinence and possible sexual dysfunction

CLINICAL JUDGMENT CHALLENGE 67.1

Evidence-Based Practice; Patient-Centered Care

A 61-year-old male client presents to the emergency department reporting that he has not fully urinated other than dribbling in the past 13 hours. He reports difficulty emptying his bladder and having an intermittent urinary stream for the past several months. He also admits to rising two to three times nightly to urinate. He states that he usually has no pain on urination, but does report increasing abdominal discomfort today after being unable to urinate.

1. **Recognize Cues:** What assessment information in this client situation is the most important and immediate concern for the nurse? (Hint: Identify the **relevant** information *first* to determine what is most important.)
2. **Analyze Cues:** What client conditions are consistent with the **most relevant** information? (Hint: Think about priority collaborative problems that support and contradict the information presented in this situation.)
3. **Prioritize Hypotheses:** Which possibilities or explanations are **most likely** to be present in this client situation? Which possibilities or explanations are the most serious? (Hint: Consider all possibilities and determine their urgency and risk for this client.)
4. **Generate Solutions:** What actions would most likely achieve the desired outcomes for this client? Which actions should be **avoided** or are **potentially harmful**? (Hint: Determine the desired outcomes first to decide which interventions are appropriate and those that should be avoided.)
5. **Take Action:** Which actions are the most appropriate and how should they be implemented? In what **priority order** should they be implemented? (Hint: Consider health teaching, documentation, requested health care provider orders or prescriptions, nursing skills, collaboration with or referral to health team members, etc.)
6. **Evaluate Outcomes:** What client assessment would indicate that the nurse's actions were **effective**? (Hint: Think about signs that would indicate an improvement, decline, or unchanged client condition.)

◆ Planning and Implementation: Generate Solutions and Take Action

Improving Urinary Elimination

Planning: Generate Solutions. The patient with BPH is expected to have a normal urinary ***elimination*** pattern without lower urinary tract symptoms (LUTS) or ***infection.***

Interventions: Take Action. Treatment for BPH ranges from careful monitoring to surgery, depending on the degree of impairment the patient is experiencing. If the patient is not experiencing complications or discomfort, behavioral modification may be recommended. Patients with symptomatic BPH are usually first treated with nonsurgical interventions, such as drug therapy.

Nonsurgical Management

Behavioral modification. Teach patients with BPH to avoid drinking large amounts of fluid in a short time, especially before going out or at bedtime (Cunningham & Kadmon, 2019). Caffeine and alcohol consumption should be limited, as these have a diuretic effect. Caution patients to avoid drugs that can cause urinary retention, especially anticholinergics, antihistamines, antipsychotics, and muscle relaxants (Cunningham & Kadmon, 2019). *Emphasize the importance of telling any health care provider about the diagnosis of BPH so these drugs are not prescribed.*

Drug therapy. *Alpha$_1$-adrenergic antagonists,* which act to relax smooth muscle in the bladder neck, and *5-alpha-reductase inhibitors* (5-ARIs), which act to reduce prostate size, are often prescribed in combination, as evidence shows that they work better in combination (Burchum & Rosenthal, 2019). See the Common Examples of Drug Therapy: Drug Therapy Used to Treat Benign Prostatic Hyperplasia (BPH) box for an overview of drug therapy used to treat BPH.

The most effective drug therapy approach used for many patients is a combination of a 5-ARI drug and an alpha$_1$-adrenergic antagonist. Two commonly prescribed drug regimens include finasteride and doxazosin, and dutasteride and tamsulosin.

COMMON EXAMPLES OF DRUG THERAPY

Drug Therapy Used to Treat Benign Prostatic Hyperplasia (BPH)

Drug Category	Selected Nursing Implications
Alpha$_1$-Adrenergic Antagonists	
Common examples of alpha$_1$-adrenergic antagonists: • Alfuzosin • Doxazosin • Prazosin • Tamsulosin • Silodosin	Monitor blood pressure, and teach to move slowly from sitting to standing; *orthostatic hypotension can occur.* Monitor for side effects such as ongoing dizziness, headache and weakness; *these side effects may require dose reduction or discontinuation of the drug.* Teach patient to report taking this drug to all health care providers; *Alpha$_1$-adrenergic antagonists can increase or decrease the side effects of other drugs such as beta blockers, calcium channel blockers, or medications used to treat erectile dysfunction (ED).*
5-Alpha-Reductase Inhibitors	
Common examples of 5-alpha-reductase inhibitors: • Dutasteride • Finasteride	Monitor blood pressure, and teach to move slowly from sitting to standing; *orthostatic hypotension can occur.* Teach about possible side effect of gynecomastia; *men taking a 5-alpha-reductase inhibitor are three times more likely to develop this condition.* Teach about the increased risk for development of prostate cancer; *men taking a 5-alpha-reductase inhibitor are at higher risk for development of prostate cancer.* Teach to keep medications stored away from pregnant women or women who may become pregnant; *these drugs are teratogenic and can be absorbed through the skin; therefore, pregnant women should not touch dutasteride nor finasteride.* Teach patients taking dutasteride to take the capsule with a full glass of water, and to refrain from opening the capsule to sprinkle on food; *dutasteride irritates oropharyngeal mucosa.*
Erectogenic	
• Tadalafil	Teach that this drug is usually given to treat erectile dysfunction, but can also be used to improve lower urinary tract symptoms (LUTS); *the patient needs to know the mechanism of action as it relates to treatment of BPH and LUTS.* Teach that the duration of action is up to 36 hours, and to avoid taking more than once daily; *this duration of action is much longer than that of most phosphodiesterase-5 (PDE5) inhibitor medications that the patient may have used in the past, which have only a 4-hour duration of action.* Teach to refrain from taking this drug with grapefruit juice or grapefruits. *Drinking grapefruit juice or eating grapefruit while taking tadalafil can increase the amount of drug in the body.*

Other information taken from Burchum, J.L.R., & Rosenthal, L.D. (2016). *Lehne's pharmacology for nursing care* (9th ed.). St. Louis: Elsevier.
Data from Hagberg, K., et al. (2017). Risk of gynecomastia and breast cancer associated with the use of 5-alpha reductase inhibitors for benign prostatic hyperplasia. *Clinical Epidemiology, 9,* 83-91.

! NURSING SAFETY PRIORITY (QSEN)

Drug Alert

Remind patients taking a 5-ARI for BPH that they may need to take it for as long as 6 months before improvement is noticed. Remind them to keep all follow-up appointments for laboratory testing, because liver damage can occur. Teach about possible side effects including erectile dysfunction (ED), decreased libido, and dizziness due to orthostatic hypotension. *Remind them to change positions carefully and slowly!*

! NURSING SAFETY PRIORITY (QSEN)

Drug Alert

Teach patients taking a 5-ARI to keep these drugs stored away from pregnant women or women who may become pregnant. These drugs are absorbed through the skin, and are teratogenic.

! NURSING SAFETY PRIORITY (QSEN)

Drug Alert

If giving alpha blockers in an inpatient setting, assess for orthostatic (postural) hypotension, tachycardia, and syncope ("blackout"), especially after the first dose is given to older men. If the patient is taking the drug at home, *teach him to be careful when changing position and to report any weakness, light-headedness, or dizziness to the health care provider immediately.* Bedtime dosing may decrease the risk for problems related to hypotension.

Other drugs may be helpful in managing specific urinary symptoms. For example, low-dose oral desmopressin, a synthetic antidiuretic analog, has been used successfully for nocturia (Burchum & Rosenthal, 2019).

Complementary and integrative health. Saw palmetto (*Serenoa repens*) has been shown in some studies to be useful in treating BPH. However, other studies have demonstrated no benefit, or benefit that is similar to placebo effect. Remind patients who are interested in taking saw palmetto to talk with their health care provider before taking this herb because of potential interactions with prescribed drugs such as anticoagulants and NSAIDs. Side effects of saw palmetto are rare, and are usually limited to mild nausea and headache (Burchum & Rosenthal, 2019).

Other nonsurgical interventions. Frequent sexual intercourse can reduce obstructive symptoms because it causes the release of prostatic fluid. This approach is helpful for the man whose obstructive symptoms result from an enlarged prostate with a large amount of retained prostatic fluid.

If drug therapy or other measures are not helpful in relieving urinary symptoms, several noninvasive techniques are available to shrink or destroy excess prostate tissue. The minimally invasive **prostate artery embolization** is performed by an interventional radiologist (IR) who threads a small vascular catheter into an artery in the wrist or groin. An arteriogram (dye injected in the blood vessels) allows the IR to see the vessels that feed the prostate, into which particles are injected to reduce some of the blood flow. In turn, this shrinks the prostate gland. This procedure has a low side effect profile for development of incontinence or erectile dysfunction (ED), so it is preferred by many patients. Local anesthesia is used rather than general anesthesia (Abt et al., 2018), which allows a typical discharge from the hospital in as little as 3 hours after the procedure. Select other procedures that treat BPH are included in Table 67.1.

All of these minimally invasive treatments use local or regional anesthesia. Some, but not all, require an indwelling urinary catheter for a short period after the procedure. They are also associated with less risk for complications such as intraoperative bleeding and erectile dysfunction when compared with traditional surgical approaches. Patients can return to their usual activities in a short time as prescribed by their provider.

Surgical Management. For patients who are not candidates for nonsurgical management or are not interested in medication or other less invasive options, surgery may be performed. Some or all of these criteria indicate the need for surgery:

- Acute urinary retention (AUR) due to obstruction
- Chronic urinary tract infections secondary to residual urine in the bladder
- Hematuria
- Hydronephrosis
- Persistent pain with decrease in urine flow

If a lesser invasive procedure is not indicated or desired, the historical gold standard surgery has been a **transurethral resection of the prostate (TURP)**, in which the enlarged part of the prostate is removed through an endoscopic instrument. A similar procedure is the transurethral incision of the prostate (TUIP) in which small cuts are made into the prostate to relieve pressure on the urethra. This alternate technique is used for smaller prostates.

The holmium laser enucleation of the prostate (HoLEP) procedure, laparoscopic prostatic adenomectomy, and robotic-assisted simple prostatectomy (RASP) are safer minimally invasive surgeries (MISs) that may be performed for BPH. Open, laparoscopic, or robotic-assisted simple prostatectomy (entire prostate removal) may also be considered (see discussion of Surgical Management in the section Cellular Regulation Concept Exemplar: Prostate Cancer). Very little blood is lost during these procedures, and patient recovery is faster than that for the more traditional TURP.

Preoperative care. When planning surgical interventions, the patient's general physical condition, the size of the prostate gland, and the man's preferences are considered. The patient may have fears and misconceptions about prostate surgery, such as believing that automatic loss of sexual functioning or permanent incontinence will occur. Assess the patient's anxiety, correct any misconceptions about the surgery, and provide accurate information to him and his family. Regardless of the type of surgery to be performed, reinforce information about anesthesia (see Chapter 9). Remind patients taking anticoagulants that the drugs will be discontinued several days prior to the TURP or

TABLE 67.1 Other Procedures Used to Treat Benign Prostatic Hyperplasia (BPH)

Procedure	Description	Nursing Implications
Photoselective vaporization (PVP)—GreenLight Laser Therapy	Laser energy is used to vaporize the prostate tissue	Teach: • A catheter will be in place following the procedure, and removed in a day. • Retrograde ejaculation may occur.
Transurethral needle ablation (TUNA)	Low radiofrequency energy is used to shrink the prostate	Teach: • The patient will need someone to drive him home from the procedure. • A catheter will be in place following the procedure, and removed in several days. • Take the full course of antibiotics prescribed to prevent a urinary tract infection (UTI) from the catheter.
Transurethral microwave therapy (TUMT)	An antenna is inserted through the penis toward the prostate to deliver a dose of microwave energy that heats and destroys prostate tissue	Teach: • A urinary catheter will be needed after the procedure for approximately 1 week. • It may take up to several months to experience the best procedural benefit, as this is dependent on how long the body needs to absorb the overgrown prostate that has been destroyed • Have continued digital rectal examinations (DREs) and screenings for prostate cancer annually, even after the procedure.
Transurethral electro-vaporization of the prostate (TUEVAP)	Involves the use of a *roller ball* to heat the prostate tissue, reducing it to vapor	Teach: • Avoid heavy lifting; avoid straining when having a bowel movement. • Drink 8 cups of water daily. • It may take several months before fully normal urination occurs, although the stream will likely be stronger right after the procedure.
Transurethral water vapor therapy (Rezum)	A radiofrequency current is applied to an *inductive coil heater,* which produces water vapor that is delivered to the transition zone of the prostate; this produces necrosis in targeted cell tissue (Westwood et al., 2018)	Teach: • Dysuria, hematuria, hematospermia, and urgency may last several weeks, and usually resolve. • A favorable change will begin in about 2 weeks following the procedure, with full benefit noticed around 3 months postprocedure.
Urolift	A delivery device is placed through the obstructed urethra; small implants are placed to lift and hold the enlarged prostate tissue, which increases the urethral opening (NeoTract, 2020).	Teach: • Relief will be felt in as little as 2 weeks. • Dysuria, hematuria, and urgency may be experienced postprocedure; these usually resolve in 2-4 weeks.

open prostate surgery to prevent postoperative bleeding. Other general preoperative care is described in Chapter 9.

The patient may have other medical problems that increase the risk for complications of general anesthesia and may be advised to have spinal anesthesia. Because the patient is conscious during spinal anesthesia, it is easier to assess for hyponatremia (low serum sodium), fluid overload, and water intoxication, which can result from large-volume bladder irrigations.

After a TURP, all patients have an indwelling urethral catheter. *Be sure that they know that they will feel the urge to void while the catheter is in place.* Tell the patient that he will likely have traction on the catheter that may cause discomfort, and reassure him that analgesics will be prescribed to relieve pain. Explain that it is normal for the urine to be blood-tinged after surgery. Small blood clots and tissue debris may pass while the catheter is in place and immediately after it is removed. Some patients also have continuous bladder irrigation (CBI), depending on the procedure performed.

Operative procedures. The traditional TURP is a "closed" surgery. To perform the procedure, the surgeon inserts a resectoscope (an instrument similar to a cystoscope, but with a cutting and cauterizing loop) through the urethra. The enlarged portion of the prostate gland is then removed in small pieces (prostate chips). The estimated blood loss during TURP is less than 500 mL (Schreiber, 2017). A fibrinolytic inhibitor such as tranexamic acid may be used during surgery to prevent bleeding and excess clotting. This does not prevent the need for blood transfusions, nor is it effective in increasing hemoglobin levels, after surgery. However, it does assist in preventing perioperative blood loss (Mina & Garcia-Perdomo, 2018; Qian-Qian et al., 2019).

The disadvantage of a TURP is that only small pieces of the gland are removed. Remaining prostate tissue may continue to grow and cause urinary obstruction, requiring additional TURPs. Urethral trauma from the resectoscope with resulting urethral strictures is also possible.

Postoperative care. During any surgical procedure for BPH, a urinary catheter is placed into the bladder. Traction is often applied on the catheter by pulling it taut and taping it to the patient's abdomen or thigh. If the catheter is taped to the patient's thigh, instruct him to keep his leg straight. The patient who had a TURP may have a catheter and continuous bladder irrigation (CBI) in place for several days. For the CBI, a three-way urinary catheter is used to allow drainage of urine and inflow of a

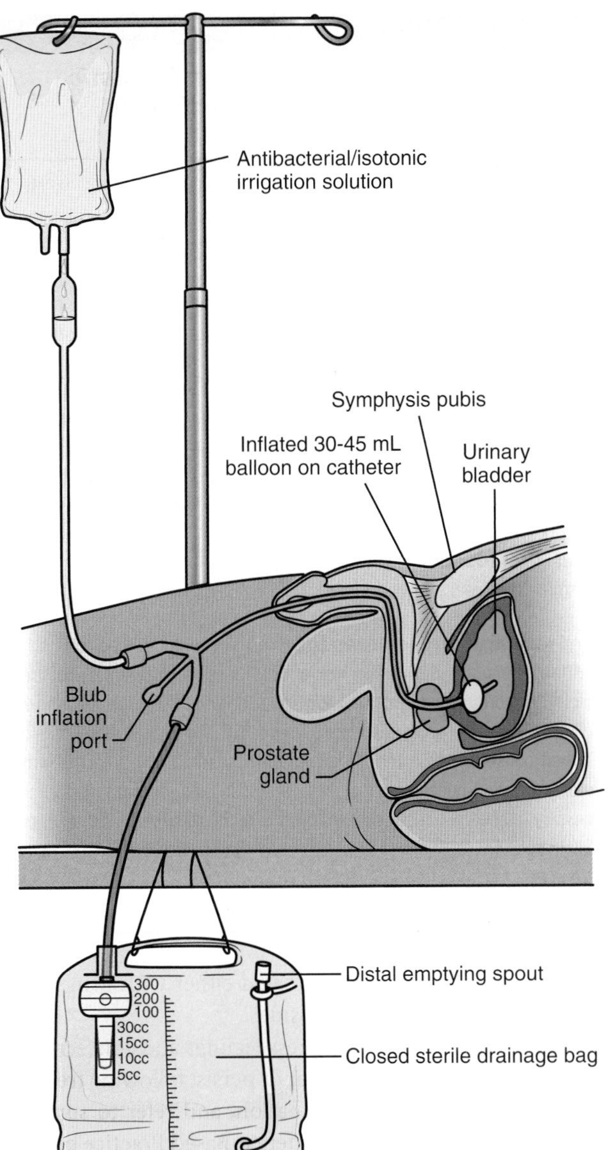

FIG. 67.3 Continuous bladder irrigation system after a TURP. *TURP,* Transurethral resection of the prostate.

bladder irrigating solution (Fig. 67.3). Be sure to maintain the flow of the irrigant to keep the urine clear. When measuring the fluid in the urinary drainage bag, subtract the amount of irrigating solution that was used, to determine actual urinary output.

NCLEX EXAMINATION CHALLENGE 67.1

Physiological Integrity

A client has continuous bladder irrigation after surgery yesterday. The amount of bladder irrigating solution that has infused over the past 12 hours is 1100 mL. The amount of fluid in the urinary drainage bag is 1950 mL. The nurse records that the client had ________ mL urinary output in the past 12 hours. **Fill in the blank.**

Remind the patient that because of the urinary catheter's large diameter and the pressure of the retention balloon on the internal sphincter of the bladder, he will feel the urge to void continuously. This is a normal sensation, not a surgical complication. Advise him not to try to void around the catheter, which causes the bladder muscles to contract and may result in painful spasms.

The Best Practice for Patient Safety & Quality Care: Care of the Patient After Transurethral Resection of the Prostate box summarizes the nursing care for patients having a TURP.

BEST PRACTICE FOR PATIENT SAFETY & QUALITY CARE QSEN

Care of the Patient After Transurethral Resection of the Prostate

- Monitor the patient closely for signs of ***infection.*** Older men undergoing prostate surgery often also have underlying chronic diseases (e.g., cardiovascular disease, chronic lung disease, diabetes).
- Help the patient out of the bed to the chair as soon as permitted to prevent complications of immobility. Provide assistance, especially for patients with underlying changes in the musculoskeletal system (e.g., decreased range of motion, stiffness in joints). These patients are at *high risk* for falls.
- Assess the patient's pain every 2 to 4 hours and intervene as needed to control pain.
- Provide a safe environment for the patient. Anticipate a temporary change in mental status for the older patient in the immediate postoperative period as a result of anesthetics and unfamiliar surroundings. Reorient the patient frequently. Keep catheter tubes secure.
- Maintain the rate of the continuous bladder irrigation to ensure clear urine without clots and bleeding.
- Use normal saline solution (which is isotonic) for the intermittent bladder irrigant unless otherwise prescribed.
- Monitor and document the color, consistency, and amount of urine output.
- Check the drainage tubing frequently for external obstructions (e.g., kinks) and internal obstructions (e.g., blood clots, decreased output).
- Assess the patient for reports of severe bladder spasms with decreased urinary output, which may indicate obstruction.
- If the urinary catheter is obstructed, irrigate it per agency or surgeon protocol.
- Notify the surgeon immediately if the obstruction does not resolve by hand irrigation or if the urinary return looks like ketchup.

PATIENT-CENTERED CARE: OLDER ADULT CONSIDERATIONS QSEN

When caring for older men who may become confused after surgery, reorient them frequently and remind them not to pull on the catheter. If the patient is restless or "picks" at tubes, provide a familiar object such as a family picture for him to hold for distraction and a feeling of security. Do not restrain the patient unless all other alternatives have failed.

! NURSING SAFETY PRIORITY QSEN

Critical Rescue

Monitor the patient for the rare, yet critical, complication of TURP syndrome. If irrigation fluid is over-absorbed into the body in addition to blood transfusions and bleeding, stress can be placed on the heart. Signs and symptoms include headache, dizziness, and/or shortness of breath; the patient is likely to also have hypertension, bradycardia, and an altered level of consciousness. ECG findings include wide QRS, elevated ST, and inverted T wave (Schreiber, 2017). Notify the surgeon immediately, as the patient will likely need intensive care while diuresing.

NURSING SAFETY PRIORITY QSEN

Critical Rescue

After a TURP, monitor the patient's urine output every 2 to 4 hours and vital signs (including pain assessment) every 4 hours for the first postoperative day or according to agency or surgeon protocol. Assess for postoperative bleeding. *Patients who undergo a TURP are at risk for severe bleeding or hemorrhage after surgery. Although rare, bleeding is most likely within the first 24 hours.* Bladder spasms or movement may trigger fresh bleeding from previously controlled vessels. This bleeding may be arterial or venous, but venous bleeding is more common.

NURSING SAFETY PRIORITY QSEN

Critical Rescue

If *arterial* bleeding occurs, the urinary drainage is bright red or ketchup-like with numerous clots. *Notify the surgeon immediately and irrigate the catheter with normal saline solution per surgeon or hospital protocol.* Surgical intervention may be needed to clear the bladder of clots and stop bleeding.

If the bleeding is *venous,* the urine output is burgundy, with or without any change in vital signs. *Inform the surgeon of any bleeding.* Closely monitor the patient's hemoglobin (Hgb) and hematocrit (Hct) levels for anemia as a result of blood loss.

Observe for other possible but uncommon complications of TURP, such as ***infection*** and incontinence. Teach the patient that sexual function should not be affected after surgery but that retrograde ejaculation is possible, wherein semen flows backward into the bladder so only a small amount will be ejaculated from the penis.

NCLEX EXAMINATION CHALLENGE 67.2

Physiological Integrity

The nurse notes bright red urinary drainage from a client who had a transurethral resection of the prostate (TURP) with continuous bladder irrigation yesterday. What is the appropriate **initial** nursing action?

A. Calculate intake and output.
B. Monitor hemoglobin and hematocrit.
C. Increase the rate of the bladder irrigation.
D. Document findings in the electronic health record.

Improving Self-Esteem

Planning: Generate Solutions. The expected outcome is that the patient will experience improved self-esteem through incontinence management and avoidance of sexual dysfunction.

Interventions: Take Action. The patient with BPH typically has frequent urges to void and may have overflow incontinence at times because of urinary retention. Teach him to keep the surrounding area clean and dry to prevent skin breakdown. Remind him to toilet when he feels the urge and, if needed, to wear a small absorbent pad to prevent undergarment soiling. Involve the patient's sexual partner, if the patient agrees, in teaching about the cause of the incontinence and any prescribed treatment. Once the patient is treated either with drug therapy or surgery, the incontinence subsides.

Encourage the patient to express feelings and concerns about sexual dysfunction that may occur or persist following treatment. Provide objective, factual information, and refer to supportive resources as needed. (see the Evidence-Based Practice box).

EVIDENCE-BASED PRACTICE QSEN

Can Surgical Treatment for Benign Prostatic Hyperplasia Improve Sexual Function? A Systematic Review

Soans, J., Vazirian-Zadeh, M., Kum, F., Dhariwal, R., Breish, M.O., Singh, S., et al. (2019). Can surgical treatment for benign prostatic hyperplasia improve sexual function? A systematic review. *The Aging Male,* 1-10.

This systematic review focused on the effect of surgery for benign prostatic hyperplasia (BPH) on sexual function following the procedure. A total of 16 studies were reviewed, with a total of 2087 cases. Various surgical methods of treatment were represented in the studies, with emphasis on TURP. Most studies reported their outcomes based on the International Index of Erectile Function (IIEF). The findings revealed that in the majority of studies, patients experienced no changes in erectile function (from baseline) after surgery. Some patients even reported improvement in erectile function following surgery.

Level of Evidence: 1

A systematic review was performed.

Commentary: Implications for Practice and Research

Erectile dysfunction is a known risk of any operative procedure that treats BPH. It is important that patients know the risks and benefits associated with any procedure. The surgeon will cover these with the patient when obtaining informed consent, which the nurse can witness. If at any time the patient expresses further concern or fear, the nurse can listen to the patient and, if necessary, place the patient back in touch with the surgeon for clarification. It is also important for the nurse to be aware of the evidence available demonstrating that most men experience no changes in erectile function (from baseline) after surgery.

Care Coordination and Transition Management. The patient with benign prostatic hyperplasia (BPH) is typically managed at home. Patients who have surgery are also discharged to their home or other setting from where they were admitted.

Home Care Management. Depending on the procedure performed, some patients may be discharged with a urinary catheter in place for a short period of time. Teach patients not to take a bath or swim, to prevent a urinary tract ***infection*** while the catheter is in place. When the urinary catheter is removed, the patient may experience burning on urination and some urinary frequency, dribbling, and leakage. Reassure him that these symptoms are normal and will decrease. Instruct him to increase fluid intake to at least 2000 to 2500 mL daily, which helps decrease dysuria and keep the urine clear. *Be aware that an older patient who has renal disease or who is at risk for heart failure may not be able to tolerate this much fluid.*

Self-Management Education. Some patients, especially those who have had a TURP, may have temporary loss of control of urination or a dribbling of the urine. Reassure the patient that these symptoms are almost always temporary and will resolve. Also remind him that ***reproduction*** ability should not be affected by surgery.

Help the patient and his family find ways to keep his clothing dry until sphincter control returns. Instruct him to contract and relax his sphincter frequently to re-establish urinary ***elimination*** control (Kegel exercises). External urinary (condom) catheters are not used except in extreme cases because they may give the patient a false sense of security and delay urinary control.

Health Care Resources. Patients being managed for BPH usually do not require extensive follow-up care or health care resources. Older men may need one or two visits from a home health care agency to ensure that they are not experiencing postsurgical complications and can provide safe self-care.

Teach patients to have follow-up care as recommended by the surgeon. After prostatic surgery, some men experience a return of LUTS and/or erectile dysfunction, which can decrease their quality of life.

◆ **Evaluation: Evaluate Outcomes.** Evaluate the care of the patient with BPH based on the identified priority patient problem. The primary expected outcome is that the patient will:

- Have improved urinary ***elimination*** as a result of appropriate and effective interprofessional management
- Experience improved self-esteem as a result of effective BPH management

CELLULAR REGULATION CONCEPT EXEMPLAR: PROSTATE CANCER

Pathophysiology Review

Testosterone and dihydrotestosterone (DHT) are the major androgens (male hormones) in the adult male. Testosterone is produced by the testis and circulates in the blood. DHT is a testosterone derivative in the prostate gland. In some patients, the prostate grows very rapidly, leading to noncancerous high-grade prostatic intraepithelial neoplasia (PIN). This impairment of ***cellular regulation*** causes men to be at a higher risk for developing prostate cancer than men who do not have that growth pattern.

Many prostate tumors are androgen sensitive (McCance et al., 2019). Most are adenocarcinomas and arise from epithelial cells located in the posterior lobe or outer portion of the gland (Fig. 67.4).

Of all malignancies, prostate cancer is one of the slowest growing, and it metastasizes in a predictable pattern. Common sites of metastasis are the nearby lymph nodes, and bones (McCance et al., 2019), although it can also metastasize to the lungs or liver. The bones of the pelvis, sacrum, and lumbar spine are most often affected. Chapter 19 describes staging categories of localized and advanced cancers.

Etiology and Genetic Risk. Advanced age is the leading risk factor for development of prostate cancer (Centers for Disease Control and Prevention [CDC], 2019). The risk increases for men who have a first-degree relative (father, brother, son) with the disease, and for African-American men (CDC, 2019).

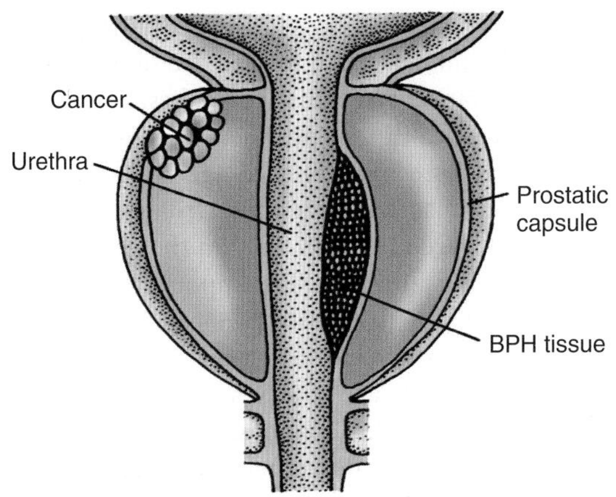

FIG. 67.4 Prostate gland with cancer and benign prostatic hyperplasia (BPH). Note that cancer normally arises in the periphery of the gland, whereas BPH occurs in the center of the gland.

PATIENT-CENTERED CARE: CULTURAL/SPIRITUAL CONSIDERATIONS QSEN

Prostate cancer affects African Americans more often than other ethnic/racial groups (McCance et al., 2019). Males of African descent who live in the Caribbean have the highest mortality rates in the world (McCance et al., 2019). Mortality is increasing in Asia as well as in Central and Eastern European countries, whereas it has decreased in Australia, Canada, Italy, Norway, the United Kingdom, and the United States (McCance et al., 2019). Be aware of epidemiologic factors to best teach your patient.

Studies are ongoing regarding what role, if any, that diet has in the risk for development of prostate cancer, or the progression once it has been diagnosed. The hypothesis for the current Men's Eating and Living (MEAL) Study is that consuming more fruits and vegetables (versus animal fat) will slow the progression of aggressive prostate cancer.

PATIENT-CENTERED CARE: GENETIC/GENOMIC CONSIDERATIONS QSEN

Many gene mutations play a role in various types of prostate cancer. Some men with the most aggressive prostate cancers have *BRCA2* mutations similar to those women who have *BRCA2*-associated breast and ovarian cancers. The most common genetic factor that increases the risk for prostate cancer is a mutation in the glutathione *S*-transferase *(GSTP1)* gene. This gene is normally part of the pathway that helps to protect against carcinogen damage (McCance et al., 2019).

Incidence and Prevalence. Prostate cancer is the most commonly diagnosed nonskin cancer in men in the United States (McCance et al., 2019). If found and treated early, has a nearly 100% cure rate. Men older than 65 years have the greatest risk for the disease (McCance et al., 2019), with the average age at diagnosis being 66 (American Cancer Society, 2019a). In the United States, one in every nine men will be diagnosed with prostate cancer in his lifetime (American Cancer Society, 2020).

Health Promotion and Maintenance. Teach men about the most current evidence-based guidelines for prostate cancer screening and early detection. The current recommendations from the U.S. Preventive Services Task Force (2018) are that men aged 55 to 69 should make an informed decision about whether to have prostate cancer screening. This is best accomplished by talking with their health care provider. This same agency recommends against screening for men age 70 and older. Other organizations such as the American Urological Association, the American College of Physicians, and the American Cancer Society have varying guidelines. It is important to note that:

- Men at a high risk for prostate cancer, including African Americans or men who have a first-degree relative with prostate cancer before the age of 65 years, should talk with their provider at the age of 45 about possible screening.
- Men with multiple first-degree relatives with prostate cancer at an early age should discuss screening at age 40 (American Cancer Society, 2010).

Although a family history of prostate cancer cannot be changed, certain nutritional habits can be modified to possibly decrease the risk for the disease. First, teach men to eat a healthy, balanced diet, including decreasing animal fat (e.g., red meat) and the intake of dairy product (Sartor, 2020). Also reinforce the need to increase fruits and vegetables—especially tomatoes, which are high in lycopene (Sartor, 2020). Soy contains phytoestrogens that are thought to be helpful in reducing the risk for prostate cancer (Sartor, 2020).

❖ Interprofessional Collaborative Care

◆ Assessment: Recognize Cues

History. Assess the patient's age, race/ethnicity, and family history of prostate cancer. Ask about his nutritional habits, especially focusing on the intake of red meat and dairy products as a source of concern. Recognize that in early prostate cancer, there are often no signs or symptoms experienced by the patient.

Assess whether the patient has existing or new problems with urinary ***elimination.*** Take a drug history to determine if he is taking any medication that could affect voiding. The first symptoms that the man may notice and report are related to bladder outlet obstruction (BOO), such as difficulty in starting urination, frequent bladder infections, and urinary retention. Ask about urinary frequency, **hematuria** (blood in the urine), and nocturia. Ask if he has had any pain during intercourse, especially when ejaculating. Inquire if he has had or currently has any other pain (particularly bone pain in the hips and legs), a symptom associated with advanced prostate cancer. Ask him if he has had any recent unexpected weight loss.

Take a sexual history for recent changes in ***sexuality,*** including libido or function. Ask about current or previous sexually transmitted infections, penile discharge, or scrotal pain or swelling.

Physical Assessment/Signs and Symptoms. Most *early* cancers are diagnosed while the patient is having a routine physical examination or is being treated for benign prostatic hyperplasia (BPH). Gross blood in the urine (hematuria) is a common sign of *late* prostate cancer. Pain in the pelvis, hips, spine, or ribs, and swollen nodes indicate advanced disease that has spread. Take and record the patient's weight because unexpected weight loss is also common when the disease is advanced.

Prepare the patient for a digital rectal examination (DRE) by the health care provider. A prostate that is stony hard and with palpable irregularities or indurations is suspected to be malignant.

Psychosocial Assessment. A diagnosis of any type of cancer causes fear and anxiety for most people. Some men, particularly African Americans, develop the disease in their 40s and 50s (Richie, 2020) when they are putting their children through college, looking toward retirement in the coming years, and/or enjoying their middle years. Assess the reaction of the patient and family to the diagnosis. Men may describe their feelings as shock, fear, or anger, or a combination of these. Expect that patients usually go through the grieving process and may be in denial or depressed. Determine what support systems they have, such as family, friends, spiritual leaders, or community group support, to help them through diagnosis, treatment, and recovery.

One of the biggest concerns the patient may have is his ability for sexual function after cancer treatment. Tell him that function will depend on the type of treatment he has. Common surgical techniques used today do not involve cutting the perineal nerves that are needed for an erection. A dry climax may occur if the prostate is removed because it produces most of the fluid in the ejaculate. Refer the patient to his surgeon (urologist), sex therapist, or intimacy counselor if available.

Laboratory Assessment. **Prostate-specific antigen (PSA)** is a glycoprotein produced by the prostate. If the patient and health care provider have agreed to screening, *PSA analysis can be used as a screening test for prostate cancer. Because other prostate problems also increase the PSA level, it is not specifically diagnostic for cancer.* However, it is commonly used in an effort to detect cancer early (Kantoff et al., 2020). If the test is performed, the specimen should be drawn before the DRE because the examination can cause an increase in PSA as a result of prostate irritation.

Most authoritative sources agree that the normal blood level of PSA in men younger than 50 years is less than 2.5 ng/mL. PSA levels increase to as high as 6.5 ng/mL when men reach their 70s (Pagana & Pagana, 2018). *African-American men between the ages of 50 and 59 have a slighter higher normal value than men who are Caucasian or Asian, but the reason for this difference is not known.* However, levels greater than 4 ng/mL have been noted in more than 80% of men with prostate cancer (Pagana & Pagana, 2018).

An elevated PSA level should decrease a few days after a prostatectomy for cancer. An increase in the PSA level several weeks after surgery may indicate that the disease has recurred (Pagana & Pagana, 2018).

Because PSA is not absolutely specific to prostate cancer, another blood test, *early prostate cancer antigen (EPCA-2),* may be a serum marker for prostate cancer. It can reveal changes in the prostate gland early and is a very sensitive test.

Other Diagnostic Assessment. After assessments by DRE and PSA, most patients have a *transrectal ultrasound (TRUS)* of the prostate in an ambulatory care or imaging setting. Before the procedure, the health care provider uses lidocaine jelly on the ultrasound probe and/or injects lidocaine into the prostate gland to promote patient comfort. The provider inserts a small probe into the rectum and obtains a view of the prostate using sound waves. If prostate cancer is suspected, a *biopsy* is usually performed at that time to obtain an accurate diagnosis.

TABLE 67.2 Prostate Cancer Staging

Stage	Description	Metastasis
0	No evidence of a primary tumor	N/A
I	Tumor not detectable by digital rectal examination (DRE); cannot be seen on imaging studies	No
II	Tumor detected by DRE; present only in prostate	No
III	Tumor extends outside of prostate and possibly to seminal vesicles	No
IV	Tumor has spread to tissues near prostate and beyond seminal vesicles, such as bladder or pelvis wall	Yes

Adapted from Prostate Conditions Education Council. (2020). https://www.prostateconditions.org/images/about/Tumor_Chart.jpg; and American Cancer Association. (2019). https://www.cancer.org/cancer/prostate-cancer/detection-diagnosis-staging/staging.html.

! NURSING SAFETY PRIORITY (QSEN)

Action Alert

After a transrectal ultrasound with biopsy, instruct the patient about possible complications, although rare, including hematuria with clots, signs of ***infection,*** and perineal pain. Teach him to report fever, chills, bloody urine, and any difficulty voiding. Advise him to avoid strenuous physical activity and to drink plenty of fluids, especially in the first 24 hours after the procedure. Teach him that a small amount of bleeding turning the urine pink is expected during this time. However, bright red bleeding should be reported to the health care provider immediately.

After prostate cancer is diagnosed, the patient has additional imaging and blood studies to determine the extent of the disease. Common tests include lymph node biopsy, CT of the pelvis and abdomen, and MRI to assess the status of the pelvic and para-aortic lymph nodes. A radionuclide bone scan may be performed to detect metastatic bone disease. An enlarged liver or abnormal liver function study results indicate possible liver metastasis.

Patients with advanced prostate cancer often have *elevated* levels of *serum acid phosphatase.* Most men with bone metastasis have *elevated serum alkaline phosphatase* levels and severe pain.

As with any cancer, accurate staging and grading of prostate tumors guide monitoring and treatment planning during the course of the disease. Based on diagnostic assessment results, the cancer is staged, which can help to guide treatment choices. Table 67.2 shows how prostate cancer is staged.

◆ **Analysis: Analyze Cues and Prioritize Hypotheses.** The priority collaborative problem for the patient with prostate cancer is:

1. Potential for cancer metastasis due to lack of, or inadequate, treatment

◆ Planning and Implementation: Generate Solutions and Take Action

Preventing Metastasis

Planning: Generate Solutions. The patient with prostate cancer is expected to remain free of metastases or recurrence of disease, if possible. If cancer recurs, the patient will experience optimal health outcomes, including potential palliation and end-of-life care.

Interventions: Take Action. Patients are faced with several treatment options. A urologist and an oncologist usually collaborate to help patients make the best decision.

Active Surveillance. Because prostate cancer is slow growing with late metastasis, older men who are asymptomatic and have other illnesses may choose observation without immediate active treatment, especially if the cancer is at an early stage. This option is known as **active surveillance (AS)**. This form of treatment involves initial surveillance with active treatment only if the symptoms become bothersome. The average time from diagnosis to start of treatment is up to 10 years. During the AS period, men are monitored at regular intervals through DRE and PSA testing. Factors that are considered in choosing AS include potential side effects of treatment (e.g., urinary incontinence, erectile dysfunction), estimated life expectancy, the presence of comorbid medical conditions, and the risk for increased morbidity and mortality from not seeking active treatment.

Patients who have very early–stage cancer of the prostate who choose AS require close follow-up by their primary health care provider. If obstruction occurs, a transurethral resection of the prostate (TURP) may be done. The care of patients having this procedure is described in the discussion of Surgical Management in the section Elimination Concept Exemplar: Benign Prostatic Hyperplasia.

Specific management is based on the extent of the disease and the patient's physical condition. The patient may undergo surgery for a biopsy (if not previously done), staging and removal of the tumor, or palliation to control the spread of disease or relieve distressing symptoms. As with AS, the health care provider and patient must weigh the benefits of treatment against potential adverse effects such as incontinence and erectile dysfunction (ED).

Nonsurgical Management. Nonsurgical management may be an adjunct to surgery or alternative intervention if the cancer is widespread or the patient's condition or age prevents surgery. Available modalities include radiation therapy, hormone therapy, and chemotherapy (less often).

Radiation therapy. External or internal radiation therapy may be used in the treatment of prostate cancer or as salvage treatments when cancer recurs. It may also be done for palliation of the patient's symptoms.

External beam radiation therapy (EBRT) comes from a source outside the body. Patients are usually treated 5 days a week for a minimum of several weeks. EBRT can also be used to relieve pain from bone metastasis. Three-dimensional conformal radiation therapy (*3D-CRT*) can more accurately target prostate tissue and reduce damage to nearby organs and tissue. An advanced type of 3D-CRT radiation is *intensity-modulated radiation therapy,* which provides very high doses to the prostate. It is the most commonly used type of external beam radiation therapy for prostate cancer (American Cancer Society, 2019b).

Teach patients that external beam radiation causes ED in many men well after the treatment is completed. Remind the

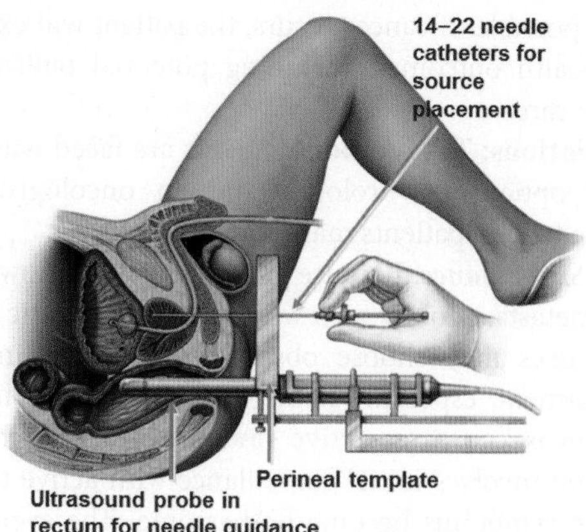

FIG. 67.5 Patient position and vital component of prostate brachytherapy with transrectal ultrasound guidance. (From Stish, B.J., Davis, B.J., Mynderse, L.A., Deufel, C.L., & Choo, R. [2017]. Brachytherapy in the management of prostate cancer. *Surgical Oncology Clinics of North America, 26*[3], 491–513. https://doi.org/10.1016/j.soc.2017.01.008.)

patient that other complications from EBRT include urinary frequency, diarrhea, and *acute radiation cystitis,* which causes persistent pain and hematuria. Symptoms are usually mild to moderate and subside 6 weeks after treatment, although there is a rare chance that this will not go away. Teach the patient to avoid caffeine and continue drinking plenty of water and other fluids.

Radiation proctitis may also develop but is less likely with 3D-CRT. Radiation that has irritated the rectum can cause urgency and cramping, which leads to rectal leakage (American Cancer Society, 2019b). Teach him to report these symptoms to the health care provider. Like cystitis, this problem usually resolves 4 to 6 weeks after the treatment stops, although in rare cases it is permanent. If proctitis occurs, teach patients to limit spicy or fatty foods, caffeine, and dairy products.

Low-dose brachytherapy is a type of internal radiation (Fig. 67.5) that is delivered by implanting low-dose radiation "seeds" (the size of a grain of rice) directly into the prostate gland. This treatment involves transrectal ultrasound, CT scans, or MRI, which are used to guide implantation of the seeds. These procedures are usually done on an ambulatory care basis under spinal or general anesthesia, and are the most cost-effective treatment for early-stage prostate cancer. Reassure the patient that the dose of radiation is low and that the radiation will not pose a hazard to him or others. Teach him that ED, urinary incontinence, and rectal problems do occur in a small percentage of cases. Fatigue is also common and may last for several months after the treatment stops. Chapter 20 describes general nursing care for patients having radiation therapy.

Drug therapy. Drug therapy may consist of either hormone therapy (androgen deprivation therapy [ADT]) or chemotherapy. Because most prostate tumors are hormone dependent, patients with extensive tumors or those with metastatic disease may be managed by androgen deprivation. *Luteinizing hormone–releasing hormone (LHRH) agonists* or antiandrogens can be used.

LHRH agonists available in the United States include leuprolide, goserelin, histrelin, and triptorelin. These drugs first stimulate the pituitary gland to release luteinizing hormone (LH). After about 3 weeks, the pituitary gland is depleted of LH, which reduces testosterone production by the testes (Burchum & Rosenthal, 2019). Leuprolide is used most commonly for advanced prostate cancer with the goal of palliation (Burchum & Rosenthal, 2019).

! NURSING SAFETY PRIORITY QSEN

Drug Alert

Teach patients taking LHRH agonists that side effects include "hot flashes," which usually decrease as treatment progresses. The subsequent reduction in testosterone may contribute to erectile dysfunction and decreased **libido** (desire to have sex). Some men also develop **gynecomastia** (abnormal enlargement of the breasts in men.). These drugs can also increase the patient's risk for osteoporosis and fractures. Teach the patient to take calcium and vitamin D and to engage in regular weight-bearing exercise. Bisphosphonates can be prescribed to prevent bone fractures.

Antiandrogen drugs, also known as *androgen deprivation therapy (ADT),* work differently in that they block the body's ability to use the available androgens (Burchum & Rosenthal, 2019). These drugs are the major treatment for metastatic disease. Examples include flutamide, bicalutamide, and nilutamide. They inhibit tumor progression by blocking the uptake of testicular and adrenal androgens at the prostate tumor site. Patients should be taught to follow closely with their health care provider and to undergo all laboratory testing as prescribed. These medications increase the risk for liver toxicity. Regular liver functions tests will be ordered at baseline, monthly during the first 4 months, and periodically thereafter (Burchum & Rosenthal, 2019).

Antiandrogens may be used alone or in combination with LHRH agonists for total or maximal androgen blockade (hormone ablation).

Systemic *chemotherapy* may be an option for patients whose cancer has spread and for whom other therapies have not worked. For example, small cell prostate cancer is rare and is more responsive to chemotherapy than to hormone therapy. The goal of therapy is not curative; it is to slow the cancer's growth so that the patient experiences a better quality of life. Chapter 20 describes general nursing care for patients receiving chemotherapy.

Surgical Management. *Surgery is the most common intervention for a cure.* Minimally invasive surgery (MIS) or, less commonly, an open surgical technique for radical prostatectomy (prostate removal) can be performed. A **bilateral orchiectomy** (removal of both testicles) is another palliative surgery that slows the spread of cancer by removing the main source of testosterone.

Preoperative care. Preoperative care depends on the type of surgery that will be done. Minimally invasive surgery (MIS) is most appropriate for localized prostate cancer and is used as a curative intervention. The most common procedure is the *laparoscopic radical prostatectomy (LRP),* often done with robotic assistance. Other procedures include transrectal high-intensity focused ultrasound (HIFU) and cryotherapy.

Patients who qualify for LRP must have a PSA less than 10 ng/mL and have had no previous hormone therapy or abdominal surgeries. Remind the patient that the advantages of this procedure over open surgery include:

- Decreased hospital stay (1 to 2 days)
- Minimal bleeding
- Smaller or no incisions and less scarring
- Less postoperative discomfort
- Decreased time for urinary catheter placement (usually removed on third postoperative day)
- Fewer complications
- Faster recovery and return to usual activities
- Nerve-sparing advantages

For the patient undergoing an *open* radical prostatectomy, provide preoperative care as for any patient having surgery (see Chapter 9).

Operative procedures. For the *LRP procedure,* the patient is placed in lithotomy positioning with steep Trendelenburg. The urologist makes one or more small punctures or incisions into the abdomen. A laparoscope with a camera on the end is inserted through one of the incisions while other instruments are inserted into the other incisions. The robotic system may be used to control the movement of the instruments by a remote device. The prostate is removed along with nearby lymph nodes, but perineal nerves are not affected.

The *open* radical prostatectomy can be performed via several surgical approaches, depending on the patient's desired outcomes and the staging of the disease. The perineal and retropubic (nerve-sparing) approaches are most commonly used. The surgeon removes the entire prostate gland along with the prostatic capsule, the cuff at the bladder neck, the seminal vesicles, and the regional lymph nodes. The remaining urethra is connected to the bladder neck. The removal of tissue at the bladder neck allows the seminal fluid to travel upward into the bladder rather than down the urethral tract, resulting in retrograde ejaculation.

Postoperative care. Provide postoperative care of the patient after *open* radical prostatectomy as summarized in the Best Practice for Patient Safety & Quality Care: Care of the Patient After an Open Radical Prostatectomy box. Nursing interventions include all the typical care for a patient undergoing major surgery. Maintaining hydration, caring for wound drains (open procedure), managing pain, and preventing pulmonary complications are important aspects of nursing care. (See general postoperative care in Chapter 9.)

Assess the patient's pain level and monitor the effectiveness of pain management with opioids given as patient-controlled analgesia (PCA), a common method of delivery during the first 24 hours after surgery. Administer a stool softener if needed to prevent possible constipation from the drugs.

The patient has an indwelling urinary catheter to straight drainage to promote urinary ***elimination.*** Monitor intake and output every shift and record or delegate this activity to assistive personnel (AP), as this is a task that is within an AP's scope that can effectively and quickly be reported back to the nurse. An antispasmodic may be prescribed to decrease bladder spasm induced by the indwelling urinary catheter. The time for catheter removal depends on the type of procedure that is performed and overall patient condition. Those who undergo the laparoscopic prostatectomy usually have the catheter in place until the third postoperative day. Those who had open surgical procedures use the catheter for 7 to 10 days or longer.

Ambulation should begin no later than the day after surgery. Provide assistance in walking the patient when he first gets out of bed. Assess for scrotal or penile swelling from the disrupted pelvic lymph flow. If this occurs, elevate the scrotum and penis and apply ice to the area intermittently for the first 24 to 48 hours.

Many patients who have the minimally invasive techniques are discharged 1 to 2 days after surgery and can resume usual activities in about a week or two. Those who have open procedures are discharged in 2 to 3 days or longer, depending on their progress.

Remind patients that common potential long-term complications of open radical prostatectomy are erectile dysfunction (ED) and urinary incontinence. For ED, drugs such as sildenafil may be effective. *Urge incontinence* may occur because the internal and external sphincters of the bladder lie close to the prostate gland and are often damaged during the surgery. Kegel perineal exercises may reduce the severity of urinary incontinence after radical prostatectomy. Teach the patient to contract and relax the perineal and gluteal muscles in several ways. For one of the exercises, teach him to:

1. Tighten the perineal muscles for 3 to 5 seconds as if to prevent voiding, and then relax
2. Bear down (but not to strain) as if having a bowel movement
3. Relax and repeat the exercise

Show him how to inhale through pursed lips while tightening the perineal muscles and how to exhale when he relaxes. He may also sit on the toilet with the knees apart while voiding and start and stop the stream several times.

BEST PRACTICE FOR PATIENT SAFETY & QUALITY CARE (QSEN)

Care of the Patient After an Open Radical Prostatectomy

- Encourage the patient to use patient-controlled analgesia (PCA) as needed.
- Help the patient get out of bed into a chair on the night of surgery and ambulate by the next day.
- Maintain the sequential compression device until the patient begins to ambulate.
- Monitor the patient for venous thromboembolism and pulmonary embolus.
- Keep an accurate record of intake and output, including drainage from a Jackson-Pratt or other drainage device.
- Keep the urinary meatus clean using soap and water.
- Avoid rectal procedures or treatments.
- Teach the patient how to care for the urinary catheter because he may be discharged with the catheter in place.
- Teach the patient how to use a leg bag.
- Emphasize the importance of not straining during a bowel movement yet to avoid suppositories or enemas.
- Remind the patient about the importance of follow-up appointments with the surgeon and oncologist to monitor progress.

Care Coordination and Transition Management. Interprofessional collaborative care of the man with prostate cancer should include his partner, if he agrees. The diagnosis and treatment of cancer greatly affect couples who survive the disease. Recognize that the patient and partner have specific physical and psychosocial needs that should be addressed before hospital discharge, and management should continue in the community setting.

Patients with prostate cancer may require care in a wide variety of settings at any stage of the disease process: at the hospital, the radiation therapy department, the oncologist's office, or home. Specific interventions depend on which treatment the patient had or if he had a combination of treatments. Regardless of treatment, coordination to effectively manage transitions in care is essential. This section focuses on the needs of those who had a *radical prostatectomy.*

Home Care Management. Discharge planning and health teaching start early, even before surgery. A patient can better plan home care management when he knows what to expect. Collaborate with the case manager to coordinate the efforts of various health care providers, surgical unit nursing staff, and possibly a home nurse. *As specified by The Joint Commission and other accrediting agencies, continuity of care is essential when caring for this patient because he may need weeks or months of therapies.*

Self-Management Education. An important area of teaching for the patient going home is urinary catheter care. An indwelling urinary catheter may be in place for 3 days for the patient who had an LRP, or up to several weeks for the patient who underwent an open radical prostatectomy. Teach him and his partner how to care for the catheter, use a leg bag, and identify signs and symptoms of ***infection*** and other complications. See the Patient and Family Education: Preparing for Self-Management: Urinary Catheter Care at Home box.

Encourage the patient to walk short distances. Lifting may be restricted to no more than a milk jug for up to 6 weeks if an open procedure was done. Remind him to maintain an upright position and not to walk bent or flexed. Vigorous exercise such as running or jumping should be avoided for at least 6 weeks and then gradually introduced. By contrast, patients having the minimally invasive laparoscopic surgery can usually return to work or usual activities in about a week.

Teach the patient not to strain to defecate. A stool softener may be prescribed to reduce the need for straining. If an opioid is prescribed for pain management, encourage the patient to drink adequate water to prevent constipation.

If the patient had an *open* radical prostatectomy, teach him to adhere to the surgeon's recommendation for when he can first shower and to continue showering for the first 2 to 3 weeks rather than soak in a bathtub. Patients who had a *laparoscopic* procedure can usually shower in 1 to 2 days. Teach them to remove the small bandage but leave the wound closure tape in place and allow it to fall off naturally in about a week. Show patients how to inspect the incision or puncture site(s) daily for signs of ***infection.*** Remind them to keep all follow-up appointments. PSA blood tests are performed 6 weeks after surgery and then every 4 to 6 months to monitor progress.

Health Care Resources. Refer the patient and partner to agencies or support groups such as the American Cancer Society's *Man-to-Man* program to help cope with prostate cancer. This program provides one-on-one education, personal visits, educational presentations, and the opportunity to engage in open and candid discussions. Another prostate cancer support group is *Us TOO International* (https://www.ustoo.org/Support-Group-Near-You) sponsored by the Prostate Cancer Education and Support Network. This group provides education and support with national and international chapters. Information can also be obtained from the Prostate Cancer Foundation (www.prostatecancerfoundation.org) or the National Alliance of State Prostate Cancer Coalitions (www.naspcc.org). In Canada, the Canadian Cancer Society (www.prostatecancer.ca) is dedicated to research and support for this disease. Other personal and community support services such as spiritual leaders or churches, synagogues, or mosques are also important to many patients.

For same-sex couples surviving prostate cancer, *Malecare* (http://malecare.org) is an excellent resource. This nonprofit organization provides support groups for gay and bisexual men and their partners.

Some men have erectile dysfunction (ED) for the first 3 to 18 months after a prostatectomy. Refer them to a specialist who can help with this problem. (ED is discussed later in this chapter.) Refer patients with urinary incontinence to a urologist who specializes in this area. Chapter 61 discusses incontinence management in detail.

PATIENT AND FAMILY EDUCATION: PREPARING FOR SELF-MANAGEMENT

Urinary Catheter Care at Home

- Once a day, gently wash the first few inches of the catheter, starting at the penis and washing outward with mild soap and water.
- Rinse and dry the catheter well.
- If you have not been circumcised, push the foreskin back to clean the catheter site; when finished, push the foreskin forward.
- Change the drainage bag at least once a week as needed:
  - Hold the catheter with one hand and the tubing with the other hand and twist in opposite directions to disconnect.
  - Place the end of the catheter in a clean container to catch leakage of urine.
  - Remove the rubber cap from the tubing of the leg bag or clean drainage bag.
  - Clean the end of the new tubing with alcohol swabs.
  - Insert the end of the new tubing into the catheter and twist to connect securely.
  - Clean the drainage bag just removed by pouring a solution of one part vinegar to two parts water through the tubing and bag. Rinse well with water and allow the bag to dry.

◆ **Evaluation: Evaluate Outcomes.** Evaluate the care of the patient with prostate cancer based on the identified priority patient problem. The primary expected outcome is that the patient with prostate cancer is expected to remain free of metastases or recurrence of disease, if possible. If cancer recurs, the patient will experience optimal health outcomes, including potential palliation and end-of-life care.

TESTICULAR CANCER

Pathophysiology Review

Testicular cancer, which can occur in one or both testicles, is a rare cancer that most often affects men between 20 and 35 years of age but can affect men of any age. It usually strikes men at a productive time of life and thus has significant economic, social, and psychological impact on the patient and his family and/or partner. With early detection by testicular self-examination (TSE) (see the Patient and Family Education: Preparing for Self-Management: Testicular Self-Examination box and Fig. 67.6) and treatment, testicular cancer has a greater than 95% cure rate (McCance et al., 2019).

Primary testicular cancers fall into two major groups:

- Germ cell tumors (GCTs) arising from the sperm-producing cells (account for most testicular cancers)
- Non–germ cell tumors arising from the stromal, interstitial, or Leydig cells that produce testosterone (account for a very small percentage of testicular cancers)

Testicular germ cell tumors are classified into two broad categories: germ cell tumors (GCTs) and others (Table 67.3). The most common type of testicular tumor is *seminoma.* Patients with seminomas have the most favorable prognoses because the tumors are usually localized, metastasize late, and respond to treatment. They often are diagnosed when they are still confined to the testicles and retroperitoneal lymph nodes.

The risk for testicular tumors is higher in males who have an undescended testis (cryptorchidism); human immune deficiency virus (HIV) infection or acquired immune deficiency syndrome (AIDS [HIV-III]); frequent use of marijuana; or history of testicular cancer (McCance et al., 2019; Michaelson & Oh, 2020).

PATIENT-CENTERED CARE: GENETIC/GENOMIC CONSIDERATIONS QSEN

Men are at a higher risk for testicular cancer if they have a family history of the disease (Michaelson & Oh, 2020). The incidence is higher among identical twins, brothers, and other close male relatives. Caucasian men are at a higher risk for testicular cancer than men of other races or ethnicities (Michaelson & Oh, 2020). The reason for these differences is not known.

PATIENT AND FAMILY EDUCATION: PREPARING FOR SELF-MANAGEMENT

Testicular Self-Examination

- Examine your testicles monthly immediately after a bath or a shower, when your scrotal skin is relaxed.
- Examine each testicle by gently rolling it between your thumbs and fingers. Testicular tumors tend to appear deep in the center of the testicle.
- Look and feel for any lumps; smooth rounded masses; or any change in the size, shape, or consistency of the testes.
- Report any lump or swelling to your primary health care provider as soon as possible.

Synchronous bilateral testicular cancer is extremely rare; many men have metastatic disease versus those who experience primary testicular cancer (in one testicle) (Campobasso et al., 2017).

❖ Interprofessional Collaborative Care

◆ Assessment: Recognize Cues

History. When taking a history from a patient with a suspected testicular tumor, assess for risk factors including a history or presence of an undescended testis and a family history of testicular cancer.

The most common report is a painless, hard swelling or enlargement of the testicle, although a small portion of patients do report pain. Patients with testicular pain, lymph node swelling, bone pain, abdominal masses or aching, sudden hydrocele (fluid in the scrotum), or gynecomastia may have metastatic disease. Determine and document how long any signs and symptoms have been present.

Questions about sexuality and ***reproduction*** are important. If the man has one healthy testis, he can function sexually. If he has a retroperitoneal lymph node dissection (RPLND) or chemotherapy, he may become sterile because of treatment effects on the sperm-producing cells or surgical trauma to the sympathetic nervous system resulting in retrograde ejaculation. Therefore, collect information regarding whether the patient is sexually active, whether he wishes to have children in the future, and if so, if he would be interested in learning about sperm storage in a sperm bank.

Physical Assessment/Signs and Symptoms. The testes, lymph nodes, and abdomen should be examined thoroughly. Patients may feel embarrassed about having this examination. Provide privacy and explain the procedure to the patient. Inspect the testicles for swelling or a lump that the patient reports is painless. A health care provider will palpate the testes for lumps and swelling that are not visible.

Psychosocial Assessment. Because testicular cancer and its treatment can lead to sexual dysfunction, pay close attention to the psychosocial aspects of the disease. ***Sexuality*** is likely to be a prime concern for any patient, yet it may be even concerning for younger men who may have a fear of not being able to perform sexually, or father children. Assess the man's support systems, and refer to community support resources as necessary.

TABLE 67.3 Classification of Testicular Tumors

Germ Cell Tumors (GCTS)	Non–Germ Cell Tumors	Mixed Tumors

• Seminomas
  • Classic
  • Spermatocytic
• Nonseminomas
  • Embryonal carcinoma
  • Yolk sac carcinoma
  • Choriocarcinoma
  • Teratoma
	• Leydig cell
	• Sertoli cell
	• Granulosa cell
	• Thecal cell
		• Teratocarcinoma
		• Other

Adapted from McCance, K., Huether, S., Brashers, V., & Rote, N. (2019). *Pathophysiology: The biologic basis for disease in adults and children* (8th ed.). St. Louis: Mosby.

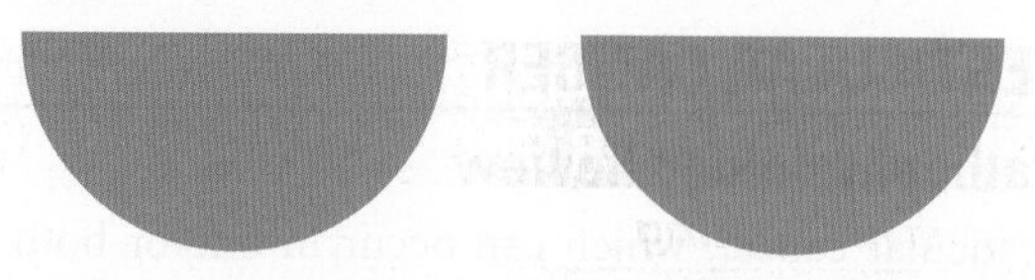

Monthly Self-Exam

HOW TO PERFORM A MONTHLY SELF EXAM.

Always perform monthly self-exams and ask your doctor for a testicular exam at your annual appointment, or sports physical.

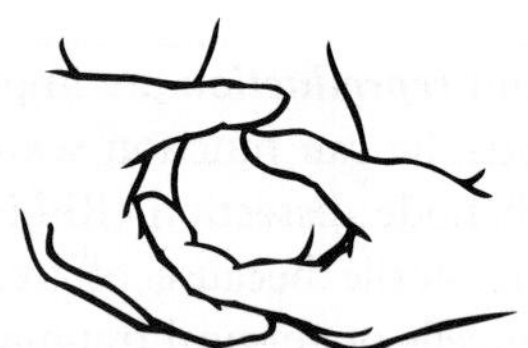

One.

Cup one testicle at a time using both hands.
This is best performed during or after a warm shower.

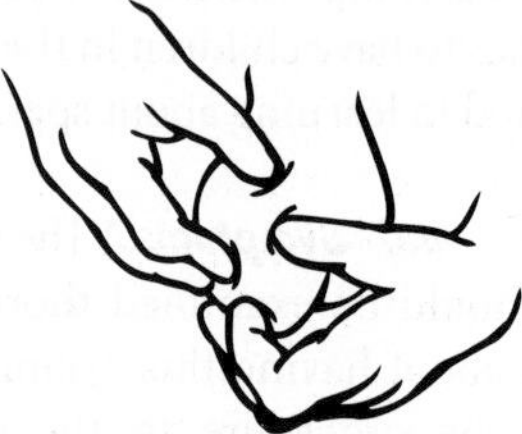

Two.

Examine by rolling the testicle between thumb and fingers.
Use slight pressure.

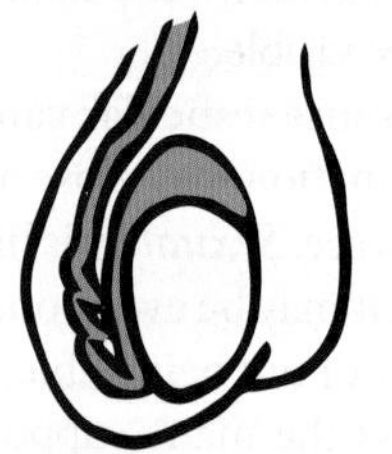

Three.

Familiarize yourself with the spermatic cord and epididymis.
The tube like structures connected on the back side of each testicle.

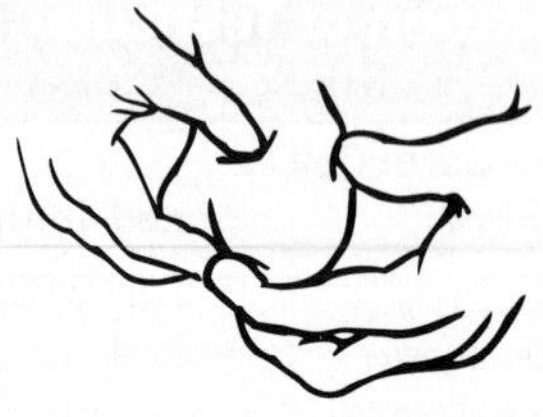

Four.

Feel for lumps, changes in size, or irregularities.
It is normal for one testis to be slightly larger than the other.

KNOW THE FACTS ABOUT TESTICULAR CANCER

- *Leading cancer in men 15-44*
- *Early detection is key*
- *Every hour a male is diagnosed*
- *Every day a life is lost*

RISK FACTORS

- *Undescended testicles (cryptorchidism)*
- *Family history*
- *Personal history of TC*
- *Intratubular germ cell neoplasia*

SIGNS & SYMPTOMS

- *A painless lump, change in size or any irregularity*
- *Pain or discomfort in the scrotum or testicle*
- *A dull ache or sense of pressure in the lower abdomen, back or groin*

ADVANCED SIGNS

- *Significant weight loss*
- *Back and/or abdominal pain*
- *Chest pain, coughing or difficulty breathing*
- *Headaches*
- *Enlarged lymph nodes in abdomen and/or neck*

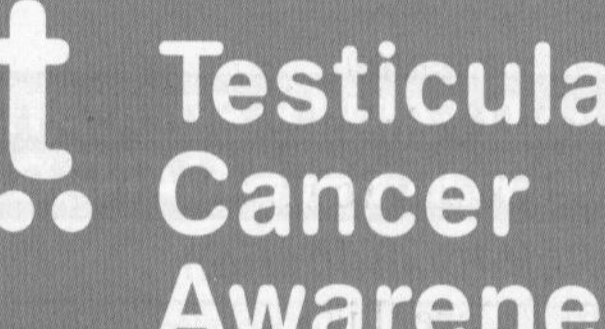

Awareness •• Support •• Survivorship

FIG. 67.6 Monthly self-examination of testicles. (Courtesy of Testicular Cancer Awareness Foundation.)

PATIENT AND FAMILY EDUCATION: PREPARING FOR SELF-MANAGEMENT

Sperm Banking

- You may want to investigate sperm storage (called "cryopreservation") in a sperm bank as a way to preserve your sperm for future use.
- No one knows how long sperm can be stored successfully, but pregnancies have resulted from sperm stored for longer than 40 years (Szell et al., 2013).
- Check with the sperm bank to see how much it charges to process and store your sperm and whether you must pay when the service is provided.
- Investigate whether your health insurance company will reimburse you for sperm collection and storage.

Diagnostic Assessment. Common serum tumor markers and other diagnostic methods that are used when formulating a diagnosis of testicular cancer are:

- Alpha fetoprotein (AFP)
- Beta human chorionic gonadotropin (hCG)
- Lactate dehydrogenase (LDH)
- Scrotal ultrasound
- Chest x-ray
- CT of the chest (if metastasis is suspected)
- CT scan of the abdomen and pelvis
- MRI of the brain (if metastasis is suspected)

◆ **Interventions: Take Action.** The incidence of oligospermia (low sperm count) and azoospermia (absence of living sperm) is common in patients diagnosed with testicular cancer. In the pretreatment phase, review the normal reproductive function, as well as possible effects of cancer and its treatment on reproductive function. Explore with the patient various reproductive options if desired (see the Patient and Family Education: Preparing for Self-Management: Sperm Banking box). A sperm bank facility provides comprehensive information on semen collection, storage of semen, the storage contract, costs, and the insemination process.

Nonsurgical Management. Chemotherapy or radiation therapy may be used depending on the tumor staging, whether surgery is performed, and based on the degree of adherence to treatment that is anticipated (Oh, 2020). The specific treatment, including frequency, cycling, and duration, will vary from patient to patient, depending on the extent of the disease and the protocol being followed. Chapter 20 discusses the general nursing care for the patient receiving chemotherapy.

Surgical Management. Surgery is the main treatment for testicular cancer. For localized disease, the surgeon performs a unilateral orchiectomy to remove the affected testicle, which is usually curative (Oh, 2020).

Preoperative Care. Like most patients with cancer, the man with testicular cancer may be very apprehensive. Offer support and reinforce the teaching provided by the surgeon. Teach the patient and his family or partner about what to expect after surgery.

Operative Procedures. Most patients with seminoma have only one surgery to remove the diseased testicle through the groin (inguinal) for a cure. A frozen section of the tumor is examined to confirm the type and stage of the cancer. A saline-filled silicone prosthesis may be surgically implanted into the scrotum at the time of the orchiectomy or later if the patient desires. This type of reconstructive surgery gives the appearance of having two testes. With one functioning testicle, the man is still able to achieve an erection for sexual intercourse.

Some men have more advanced disease or tumor types that are more aggressive. The preferred method to address this is laparoscopic retroperitoneal lymph node dissection (RPLND), which is a minimally invasive surgery (MIS). This technique is much shorter than the traditional open surgical approach, which is much more complicated and requires more postoperative hospital recovery time. In laparoscopic RPLND, very small skin incisions in the abdomen are made by a laparoscope, through which the nodes are dissected for examination. Bleeding, postoperative pain, and postoperative complications are minimized. The patient who has had laparoscopic RPLND can still achieve an erection, yet if there has been nerve damage during surgery, he may experience retrograde ejaculation. Newer nerve-sparing surgeries have shown to be very successful when performed by experienced surgeons (American Cancer Society, 2018). Research continues on robotic-assisted laparoscopic RPLND (R-RPLND) regarding whether it is superior to laparoscopic RPLND (Schwen et al., 2018).

Postoperative Care. Nursing care for the patient after surgery depends on the type of surgical procedure that was performed and the extent of the disease process. The patient is usually hospitalized for multiple days after an *open* radical retroperitoneal lymph node dissection. The patient having the laparoscopic procedure may have a urinary catheter in place following the procedure, which is removed before discharge 1 to 2 days later. Refer to Chapter 9 for general postoperative care.

NCLEX EXAMINATION CHALLENGE 67.3

Physiological Integrity

Which assessment finding will the nurse report to the health care provider for a client who had an orchiectomy and laparoscopic radical retroperitoneal lymph node dissection this morning?

A. BP 130/80 mm Hg, T 98.9°F, R 16, P 70
B. Urinary catheter draining clear yellow urine
C. Expresses fearfulness of inability to perform sexually
D. Reports pain of 9 on a 0-10 scale after receiving pain medication

Care Coordination and Transition Management. After an open *orchiectomy*, the patient is discharged without a dressing on the inguinal incision (as long as there is no wound complication). A scrotal support may be needed for several days. He may want to wear a dry dressing to prevent clothing from rubbing on the sutures and causing irritation. Tell him that the sutures will be removed in the health care provider's office 7 to 10 days after surgery.

Patients who also had an *open* RPLND recover even more slowly. They should not lift anything over 15 lb (6.8 kg), should avoid stair climbing, and should not drive a car for several weeks. Be sure that bathroom facilities are on the first floor of the house where he can easily access them.

Teach the patient who had a laparoscopic procedure that he will be able to resume most of his usual activities within 1 week after discharge. He can take a shower 1 or 2 days after surgery, but be sure that he does not remove the wound closure tape. These strips of tape will loosen and fall off about a week after surgery.

! NURSING SAFETY PRIORITY (QSEN)

Action Alert

For the patient who has undergone testicular surgery, emphasize the importance of scheduling a follow-up visit with the surgeon to examine the incision for proper healing. Instruct him to notify the surgeon immediately if chills, fever, vomiting, increasing incisional pain, drainage, or dehiscence of the incision occurs. These signs and symptoms may indicate ***infection*** for which antibiotics are needed.

Explain the importance of performing monthly testicular self-examination (TSE) on the remaining testis and scheduling follow-up examinations with the health care provider. The patient who has had testicular cancer should be seen regularly by his health care provider for follow-up care and testing.

For the patient who has reproductive concerns, refer to the American Society for Reproductive Medicine (www.reproductivefacts.org) or RESOLVE: The National Infertility Association (www.resolve.org).

ERECTILE DYSFUNCTION

Pathophysiology Review

Erectile dysfunction (ED), also known as *impotence,* is the inability to achieve or maintain an erection for sexual intercourse. It affects millions of men throughout the world. There are two major types of ED: organic and psychogenic.

Organic ED is a gradual deterioration of function. The man may first notice diminishing firmness and a decrease in frequency of erections. Causes include (McCance et al., 2019; Schreiber, 2019):

- Vascular, endocrine, or neurologic disease
- Chronic disease (e.g., diabetes mellitus, renal failure)
- Penile disease or trauma
- Surgery or pharmaceutical therapies
- Obesity
- Psychological conditions

If the patient has episodes of ED, it usually has a *psychogenic* cause. Men with this type of ED usually still have normal nocturnal (nighttime) and morning erections. Onset is usually sudden and follows a period of high stress.

❖ Interprofessional Collaborative Care

The health care provider will attempt to determine the cause of the ED through a variety of diagnostic tests. These may include evaluating glycated hemoglobin, a lipid panel for cardiac risk factors, thyroid-stimulating hormone (TSH) to rule out thyroid disease, and serum total testosterone (Khera, 2020a). Doppler ultrasonography can be used to determine blood flow to the penis. Treatment depends on the underlying cause, and may include (Khera, 2020b):

- Lifestyle modifications (e.g., smoking cessation, weight loss, management of hypertension)
- Management of medications that may cause ED (e.g., antidepressants)
- Penile self-injection with prostaglandin E1
- Phosphodiesterase-5 (PDE5) drug therapy
- Psychotherapy
- Testosterone and PDE5 drug therapy (for men with hypogonadism)
- Surgery (prosthesis)
- Vacuum-assisted erection devices

See Table 67.4 for select treatment options for ED.

! NURSING SAFETY PRIORITY (QSEN)

Drug Alert

Instruct patients taking PDE-5 inhibitors to abstain from alcohol before sexual intercourse because it could impair the ability to have an erection. Common side effects of these drugs include dyspepsia (heartburn), headaches, facial flushing, and stuffy nose. If more than one pill a day is being taken, leg and back cramps, nausea, and vomiting also may occur. *Teach men who take nitrates to avoid PDE-5 inhibitors because the vasodilation effects can cause a profound hypotension and reduce blood flow to vital organs* (Burchum & Rosenthal, 2019).

VASECTOMY

Vasectomy is the most effective mode of male contraception. It involves interruption or occlusion of each vas deferens (Viera, 2019). The preferred procedure is the "no-scalpel" vasectomy, performed with local anesthetic (without epinephrine) in an outpatient setting.

Teach the patient to leave the bandaging in place for at least 48 hours post-procedure, and to apply an ice pack intermittently to the scrotum for 24 to 48 hours to minimize pain and swelling. Remind the patient that mild pain, swelling, and bruising are normal, however, for the first few days. Teach him to report increasing pain, incisional bleeding, increased swelling, or fever to the health care provider (Viera, 2019).

The patient is usually instructed by the health care provider to rest for 1 to 2 days, and then he can return to light work. Heavy lifting, sports, and sexual intercourse should be avoided for at least 1 week. Teach the patient and partner to use an alternate form of contraception until a 3-month follow-up. At that time, a semen analysis will be performed to determine if the procedure was effective.

Although this procedure is performed with the intention of permanent sterilization, vasectomy can be reversed microsurgically in approximately 50% to 70% of cases (Viera, 2019).

OTHER CONDITIONS AFFECTING THE MALE REPRODUCTIVE SYSTEM

Other conditions that can affect the male reproductive system include inflammation, infection, swelling, trauma, and torsion. Table 67.5 lists select examples of these common conditions with nursing implications.

TABLE 67.4 Select Treatment Options for Erectile Dysfunction

Procedure	Description	Nursing Implications
Phosphodiesterase-5 (PDE5) inhibitors (drug therapy)	Work by relaxing the smooth muscles in the corpora cavernosa so blood flow to the penis is increased. The veins exiting the corpora are compressed, limiting outward blood flow and resulting in penile **tumescence** (swelling).	Teach: • Any PDE5 drug can lower blood pressure; teach to be aware of safety precautions before taking the drug. • When taking avanafil, sexual stimulation is needed within 15 minutes to promote an erection. Take pill about 15 minutes before intercourse. • When taking sildenafil or vardenafil, sexual stimulation is needed within ½ to 1 hour to promote the erection. Take pill about 1 hour before intercourse. • When taking tadalafil, an erection can be stimulated over several hours; take pill at least 2 hours before intercourse. Effects can last up to 36 hours. • When taking any PDE5 drug, refrain from eating grapefruit or drinking grapefruit juice.
Penile injections	Self-injection into the shaft of the penis. Patient uses an insulin syringe with prostaglandin E1.	Teach: • Use a condom due to increased risk for infection created at injection site. • Ibuprofen can be used to treat penile pain.
Penile prostheses	Semirigid or inflatable options. • Semirigid option results in permanent erection. • Inflatable option involves placement of two hollow cylinders in the corpora cavernosa, and a saline reservoir. Use of a pump moves the saline from behind the cylinders to the front of the eates an erection.	Teach: • Report any signs of infection immediately to the health care provider.
Vacuum-assisted erection device	A cylinder is placed over the penis, sitting firmly against the body. Using a pump, a vacuum is created to draw blood into the penis to maintain an erection. A rubber ring (tension band) is placed around the base of the penis to maintain the erection, and the cylinder is removed.	Teach: • Do not apply vacuum for more than 30 minutes • The vacuum device can be used in tandem with PDE5 inhibitors

TABLE 67.5 Select Conditions Affecting the Male Reproductive System

Condition Type	Examples of Condition	Description	Signs and Symptoms	Nursing Implications
"Cele"	Hydrocele	Swelling in the scrotum where fluid has collected around one or both testicles	Painless testicle swelling; often the sensation is described as "heaviness" of the scrotum	Teach: • Treatment is usually not needed unless the condition becomes painful or too large for comfort; at that time, surgery may be recommended. • If pain does occur, acetaminophen or ibuprofen can be taken. • Report any changes involving pain, fever, redness, or swelling.
	Spermatocele	A cyst that develops in the epididymis; usually is painless	Is usually asymptomatic; sometimes there is pain and/or heaviness in the affected testicle	Teach: • Treatment is usually not needed unless the condition becomes painful or too large for comfort; at that time, surgery may be recommended. • If pain does occur, acetaminophen or ibuprofen can be taken.
	Varicocele	Vein enlargement inside the scrotum (usually on the left side), which can cause low sperm production	Is often asymptomatic; pain, if experienced, may be dull or sharp, and worsens with activity and throughout the day	Teach: • Treatment is usually not needed unless the condition becomes painful or too large for comfort; at that time, surgery may be recommended, particularly if the condition has left the patient infertile.

Continued

TABLE 67.5 Select Conditions Affecting the Male Reproductive System—cont'd

Condition Type	Examples of Condition	Description	Signs and Symptoms	Nursing Implications
Emergent	Paraphimosis	The foreskin (of an uncircumcised male) cannot be pulled over the penis tip, resulting in the foreskin becoming stuck, impeding blood flow to the penile tip and lymphatic drainage	Enlargement and congestion of glans and foreskin, with a band of constrictive tissue that prevents moving the foreskin forward over the penile tip (glans)	Teach: • This is a *urologic emergency;* seek emergency care immediately. • Treatment can be manual or surgical in nature. • Topical antibiotic ointment may be prescribed following reduction of the paraphimosis; this should be applied as directed. • The foreskin should not be retracted for a week following reduction.
	Priapism		Persistent, painful erection (usually >4 hr) not associated with sexual stimulation; is common in patients with sickle cell disease, and can be caused by certain drugs	Recognize: • Treatment varies depending on underlying cause; medical therapy involves injection of a sympathomimetic drug into the penis, with or without aspiration of blood to decompress the corpora. Surgical intervention includes placement of a shunt. • Patients with sickle cell disease may require additional treatment including a simple red blood cell transfusion. Monitor: • Patients with sickle cell disease should receive venous thromboembolism prophylaxis. • See Chapter 9 for postoperative procedures.
	Testicular torsion	Twisting of the spermatic cord that results in ischemia from decreased arterial inflow and venous outflow obstruction; can occur spontaneously or as a result of trauma	Nausea Vomiting Lower abdominal pain A tender mass or knot above the testis	Teach: • This is a *urologic emergency;* seek emergency care immediately. Damage may be irreversible after 8 hours. • Surgery is usually performed urgently; manual detorsion is attempted if surgery is not available immediately Monitor: • See Chapter 9 for postoperative procedures.
Infection	Epididymitis	Inflammation or infection of the epididymis; often caused by *Neisseria gonorrhoeae* or *Chlamydia trachomatis* in men under 35; in older men, it often occurs in association with obstructive uropathy from benign prostatic hyperplasia (BPH)	Localized testicular pain Tenderness and swelling on palpation of the epididymis May have scrotal erythema	Teach: • Take the full course of antibiotics, even if you begin to feel better. • Ibuprofen can be used for pain. • Elevate the scrotum and apply ice intermittently. • Refrain from sexual intercourse until treatment is completed. • Always use a condom when engaging in sexual intercourse. • Report development of fever, chills, and/or lower urinary tract symptoms (LUTS) to the health care provider right away.
	Phimosis	Tightness that results in the inability to retract the foreskin	Swelling and pain at the head of the penis, causing difficulty in retraction of the foreskin Is often associated with hygienic concerns (neglecting to replace the foreskin after cleaning, intercourse, or urination), or body piercing of the glans or foreskin	Teach: • Proper hygiene is important. • Topical corticosteroids may be prescribed. • Circumcision may be recommended by the health care provider.

Information adapted from Bragg, B., & Leslie, S. (2019). *Paraphimosis.* StatPearls Publishing, LLC. Treasure Island, FL; Deveci, S. (2019). Priapism. Evaluation of acute scrotal pain in adults. In *UpToDate,* O'Leary, M. (Ed.). Waltham, MA; Eyre, R. (2020). Evaluation of acute scrotal pain in adults. In *UpToDate,* O'Leary, M. (Ed.). Waltham, MA; Eyre, R. (2020). Evaluation of nonacute scrotal conditions in adults. In *UpToDate,* O'Leary, M. (Ed.). Waltham, MA; Field, J. et al. (2019). Priapism and erectile dysfunction in sickle cell disease. In *UpToDate,* Mahoney, D., & Vichinsky, E. (Eds.). Waltham, MA.

GET READY FOR THE NEXT-GENERATION NCLEX® EXAMINATION!

Key Points

Review these Key Points for each NCLEX Examination Client Needs Category.

Safe and Effective Care Environment

- Perform a focused physical assessment for patients reporting lumps or swelling in their genital area; inspect and palpate bladder and scrotum. **QSEN: Safety**
- Teach patients to not lift more than 15 lb (6.8 kg) after open prostate surgery. **QSEN: Safety**
- Teach patients to report signs of ***infection*** when caring for a urinary catheter in the home. **QSEN: Safety**

Health Promotion and Maintenance

- Teach patients to eat a well-balanced diet including fish, fruits, and vegetables to help prevent prostate cancer. **QSEN: Evidence-Based Practice**
- Teach men at risk for prostate cancer to be screened and follow early detection guidelines. **QSEN: Evidence-Based Practice**
- Teach men how to perform testicular self-examination **QSEN: Evidence-Based Practice**
- Teach men who are uncircumcised about the importance of keeping the penis clean to prevent penile cancer. **QSEN: Evidence-Based Practice**

Psychosocial Integrity

- Assess the patient's understanding regarding the fact that some procedures and drugs related to reproductive problems cause temporary or permanent erectile dysfunction and/or incontinence. **Ethics**
- Assess the patient's anxiety before surgery and allow expression of feelings of fear or grief. **QSEN: Patient-Centered Care**
- Assess the patient's reaction to the possible loss of ***reproduction*** ability, and concerns about ***sexuality*** and changes in body image. **QSEN: Patient-Centered Care**
- Teach patients with male reproductive cancer about resources available to provide support. **QSEN: Patient-Centered Care**

Physiological Integrity

- Remind patients wanting to use complementary and integrative therapies to check with their health care provider first. **QSEN: Safety**
- Maintain traction on the urinary catheter and continuous bladder irrigation after a TURP. **QSEN: Safety**
- Observe for and report complications after surgery, including ***infection,*** severe pain, urinary infection, ***elimination*** problems, bloody urine with clots, and/or erectile dysfunction. **Clinical Judgment**
- Teach patients with BPH to avoid drugs that can cause urinary retention. **QSEN: Evidence-Based Practice**
- Teach patients about hormone therapies used to treat prostate cancer. **QSEN: Evidence-Based Practice**
- Teach patients with a urinary catheter how to properly care for it at home. **QSEN: Safety**

MASTERY QUESTIONS

1. The nurse is teaching a client with erectile dysfunction about taking sildenafil to achieve an erection. Which client statement demonstrates an understanding of this drug?
   A. "I can have sex up to 8 hours after taking the drug."
   B. "I might get a headache or stuffy nose when this drug is used."
   C. "Taking this with a drink or two of alcohol will enhance my performance."
   D. "If one pill doesn't work, it is acceptable for me to quickly take another pill."
2. A client with a history of BPH calls the telehealth nurse reporting the sudden onset of testicular pain after moving heavy furniture. What is the appropriate nursing response?
   A. "Taking ibuprofen may help alleviate the pain."
   B. "Please go to your closest emergency department right away."
   C. "This is a common reaction when performing labor; the pain will go away."
   D. "Your BPH is probably giving you difficulty because you were moving furniture."

REFERENCES

Asterisk (*) indicates a classic or definitive work on this subject.

Abt, D., et al. (2018). Comparison of prostatic artery embolisation (PAE) versus transurethral resection of the prostate (TURP) for benign prostatic hyperplasia: Randomised, open label, non-inferiority trial. *British Medical Journal [BMJ], 361*, k2338.

*American Cancer Society (ACS). (2010). *American Cancer Society guideline for the early detection of prostate cancer: Update 2010.* Retrieved from https://onlinelibrary.wiley.com/doi/full/10.3322/caac.20066.

American Cancer Society (ACS). (2018). *Surgery for testicular cancer.* Retrieved from https://www.cancer.org/cancer/testicular-cancer/treating/surgery.html.

American Cancer Society (ACS). (2019a). *About prostate cancer.* Retrieved from https://www.cancer.org/content/dam/CRC/PDF/Public/8793.00.pdf.

American Cancer Society (ACS). (2019b). *Radiation therapy for prostate cancer.* Retrieved from https://www.cancer.org/cancer/prostate-cancer/treating/radiation-therapy.html.

American Cancer Society (ACS). (2020). *Key statistics for prostate cancer.* Retrieved from https://www.cancer.org/cancer/prostate-cancer/about/key-statistics.html.

Burchum, J. L. R., & Rosenthal, L. D. (2016). *Lehne's pharmacology for nursing care* (9th ed.). St. Louis: Elsevier.

Campobasso, D., Ferretti, S., & Frattini, A. (2017). Synchronous bilateral testis cancer: Clinical and oncological management. *Contemporary Oncology, 21*(1), 70–76.

Centers for Disease Control and Prevention. (2019). *Who is at risk for prostate cancer?* Retrieved from https://www.cdc.gov/cancer/prostate/basic_info/risk_factors.htm.

Cunningham, G., & Kadmon, D. (2019). Medical treatment of benign prostatic hyperplasia. In M. O'Leary (Ed.), *UpToDate*. Waltham, MA.

Hagberg, K., et al. (2017). Risk of gynecomastia and breast cancer associated with the use of 5-alpha reductase inhibitors for benign prostatic hyperplasia. *Clinical Epidemiology, 9*, 83–91.

Kantoff, P., Taplin, M., & Smith, J. (2020). Clinical presentation and diagnosis of prostate cancer. In N. Vogelzang, W. Lee, & J. Richie (Eds.), *UpToDate*. Waltham, MA.

Khera, M. (2020a). Evaluation of male sexual dysfunction. In P. Snyder, A. Matsumoto, & M. O'Leary (Eds.), *UpToDate*. Waltham, MA.

Khera, M. (2020b). Treatment of male sexual dysfunction. In P. Snyder, & M. O'Leary (Eds.), *UpToDate*. Waltham, MA.

McCance, K., Huether, S., Brashers, V., & Rote, N. (2019). *Pathophysiology: The biologic basis for disease in adults and children* (8th ed.). St. Louis: Elsevier.

McVary, K. (2019). Epidemiology and pathophysiology of benign prostatic hyperplasia. In M. O'Leary (Ed.), *UpToDate*. Waltham, MA.

Michaelson, M., & Oh, W. (2020). Epidemiology of and risk factors for testicular germ cell tumors. In P. Kantoff (Ed.), *UpToDate*. Waltham, MA.

Mina, S., & Garcia-Perdomo, H. (2018). Effectiveness of tranexamic acid for decreasing bleeding in prostate surgery: A systematic review and meta-analysis. *Central European Journal of Urology, 71*(1), 72–77.

Neotract. (2020). *What is urolift?* https://www.urolift.com/what-is-urolift?.

Oh, W. (2020). Overview of the treatment of testicular germ cell tumors. In P. Kantoff (Ed.), *UpToDate*. Waltham, MA.

Pagana, K. D., & Pagana, T. J. (2018). *Mosby's manual of diagnostic and laboratory tests* (6th ed.). St. Louis: Mosby.

Qian-Qian, M., et al. (2019). Tranexamic acid is beneficial for reducing perioperative blood loss in transurethral resection of the prostate. *Experimental and Therapeutic Medicine, 17*(1), 943–947.

Richie, J. (2020). Active surveillance for men with clinically localized prostate cancer. In N. Vogelzang & J. Richard (Eds.). *UpToDate*, Waltham, MA.

Sartor, A. (2020). Risk factors for prostate cancer. In N. Vogelzang, et al. (Ed.), *UpToDate*. Waltham, MA.

Schreiber, M. (2017). Postoperative nursing considerations: Transurethral resection of the prostate. *Medsurg Nursing, 26*(6), 419–422.

Schreiber, M. (2019). Erectile dysfunction. *MedSurg Nursing*, 28(5), 327–330.

Schwen, Z., Gupta, M., & Pierorazio, P. (2018). A review of outcomes and technique for the robotic-assisted laparoscopic retroperitoneal lymph node dissection for testicular cancer. *Advances in Urology, 214680*, 1–7. https://doi.org/10.1155/2018/2146080.

Szell, A., et al. (2013). Live births from frozen human semen stored for 40 years. *Journal of Assisted Reproduction and Genetics, 30*(6), 743–744.

U.S. Preventive Services Task Force. (2018). Final recommendation statement: *Prostate cancer: Screening*. Retrieved from https://www.uspreventiveservicestaskforce.org/Page/Document/RecommendationStatementFinal/prostate-cancer-screening.

Viera, A. (2019). Vasectomy. In M. O'Leary (Ed.), *UpToDate*. Waltham, MA.

Westwood, J., et al. (2018). Rezum: A new transurethral water vapour therapy for benign prostatic hyperplasia. *Therapeutic Advances in Urology, 10*(11), 327–333.

68

Concepts of Care for Transgender Patients

Donna D. Ignatavicius, Stephanie M. Fox

http://evolve.elsevier.com/Iggy/

LEARNING OUTCOMES

1. Collaborate with the interprofessional team to provide evidence-based care to transgender patients.
2. Explain the role of the nurse in providing high-quality care and minimizing ***health care disparities*** for transgender patients.
3. Discuss how to use culturally sensitive terminology when providing care for transgender patients.
4. Identify appropriate health care resources for transgender patients.
5. Identify major sources of stress that contribute to transgender health issues.
6. Prioritize evidence-based care for patients having male-to-female or female-to-male genital surgery, or feminizing or masculinizing genital surgery.
7. Develop a health teaching plan for transgender patients who take hormone therapy and/or have gender-affirming surgery.

KEY TERMS

female-to-male (FtM) An adjective to describe people who were born with anatomically female parts but identify as and/or live as male; FtM persons are also referred to as *transmen.*

gender dysphoria Emotional or psychological distress caused by an incongruence between one's natal (birth) sex and gender identity.

gender identity A person's inner sense of being a male, a female, or an alternative gender (e.g., genderqueer); not related to *reproduction* anatomy.

gender-affirming surgery (GAS) A group of surgical procedures that change primary and/or secondary sex characteristics to affirm a person's gender identity; also called *gender reassignment surgery (GRS)* or *gender-confirming surgery.*

LGBTQ An acronym referring to lesbian, gay, bisexual, transgender, and queer/questioning individuals (people who do not feel they belong in any other subgroup).

LGBTQIA+ An acronym referring to lesbian, gay, bisexual, transgender, queer, intersex, and asexual people, as well as those who identify with other sexualities, sexes, and genders not included in the acronym.

male-to-female (MtF) An adjective to describe people who were born with anatomically male parts but identify as and/or live as female; MtF persons are also known as *transwomen.*

sex A person's genital anatomy present at birth; also called *biological* or *natal sex.*

transgender An adjective that describes persons who self-identify as the opposite gender or a gender that does not match their natal sex.

PRIORITY AND INTERRELATED CONCEPTS

The priority concepts for this chapter are:

- ***Patient-Centered Care***
- ***Health Care Disparities***

The interrelated concepts for this chapter are:

- ***Sexuality***
- ***Reproduction***

The American Nurses Association (ANA) Code of Ethics states that the nurse practices with compassion and respect for the dignity and worth of every patient (ANA, 2015). The Institute of Medicine (IOM; now the National Academies of Sciences, Engineering, and Medicine) and the Quality and Safety Education for Nurses (QSEN) Institute further have identified the need for nurses to be competent in ***patient-centered care*** (see Chapter 1). This competency ensures that nurses provide care with sensitivity and respect for diverse patients, even if those patients have values and preferences different from their own (ANA, 2015). Diversity is often discussed as ethnicity and race, but other cultural aspects such as sexual orientation and gender identity are part of the diverse human experience.

People of minority sexual and gender identities are often grouped under one umbrella population category described by the acronym LGBTQ—lesbian, gay, bisexual, transgender, and queer/questioning individuals (people who do not feel they belong in any other subgroup). Another similar acronym used is LGBTQIA+, encompassing lesbian, gay, bisexual, transgender, queer, intersex, and asexual people, as well as those who identify as other sexualities, sexes, and genders not included in the acronym. Some literature includes only the letters "LGBT." These evolving labels are misleading regarding people who identify as transgender. The grouping of ***sexuality*** (sexual attraction and behavior) and gender identity (the sense of self as male, female, a blend of both, or neither) (Human Rights Campaign, 2020) suggests that these two concepts are related or dependent on one another, but they are very different. *LGB* refers to specific sexual orientation. However, transgender people may identify as heterosexual, homosexual, bisexual, or neither.

Nurses and other health care professionals should not assume that transgender patients have the same experiences or health care needs as those who identify as lesbian, gay, or bisexual; this misconception leads to inequality in care. Since 2016, people in the sexual and gender minorities have been designated (for research purposes) as populations who experience differences in access to or availability of appropriate health care services, called ***health care disparities*** (IOM, 2011; Margolies & Brown, 2019). It is important for the nurse to remember that members of these populations are extremely diverse and represent many ethnicities, religions, and socioeconomic statuses (Landry, 2017) and that care must be personalized according to each individual.

PATIENT-CENTERED TERMINOLOGY

Commonly, gender is categorized with one of two terms: *male* and *female.* For the majority of people, these descriptors are accurate. However, some people do not clearly fit into either category and may define themselves as *transgender.* Identifying oneself as transgender is not a choice or lifestyle, but rather an inner sense of being born in the wrong body. When transgender people pursue ways of making their physical body and appearance affirm their gender identity, their interaction with the health care system requires knowledge, respect, compassion, and specialized ***patient-centered care.***

Use of appropriate terminology is essential to demonstrating respect. Of utmost importance is the distinction between gender and sex. Gender, also known as gender identity, describes a person's inner sense of being a male, a female, an alternative gender (e.g., genderqueer), or neither (Human Rights Campaign, 2020) and is not related to ***reproduction*** anatomy. Sex, also known as *biological* or *natal sex*, refers to a person's genital anatomy present, designated, or assigned at birth.

When babies are born, the gender of the child is determined by the genitalia present, but there is no way of knowing the child's true sense of gender. Transgender people report feeling a mismatch between their gender identity and natal sex, often extending back into early childhood. The sense of gender and feelings toward maleness or femaleness can develop in children as early as age 2 years and is usually present in most people during the early elementary years. When this incongruence occurs, the person can experience gender dysphoria, or the emotional or psychological distress caused by an incongruence between one's natal (birth) sex and gender identity. Some people who have gender dysphoria may seek interventions to transition to the identified gender.

The term *transgender* is often used as an umbrella description for all people whose gender identity and presentation do not conform to social expectations. In this text, transgender describes people who self-identify as the opposite gender or a gender that does not match their natal sex (Rosendale et al., 2018). For proper usage, the term *transgender* should be used only in adjective form. For example, a patient "is transgender," "identifies as transgender," or "is a transgender patient." Note that "transgender" never ends in "-ed." The term *transgender* should not be used as a noun, and a patient should never be described as "*a* transgender."

The most recent data on the transgender population indicate that there are approximately 1 to 1.4 million adults in the United States who identify as transgender (Flores et al., 2016; Meerwijk & Sevelius, 2017). Most scholars suggest that the prevalence is much higher, and more research is needed to collect accurate demographic data for this population.

An aging term that is less commonly used is *transsexual,* which originated from the medical and psychological communities (GLAAD, 2020). This term has historically been used to describe a person who has modified his or her natal body to match the appropriate gender identity, through cosmetic, hormonal, or surgical means. In some populations, this term is considered offensive (The Trevor Project, 2020). *As with other terms, use terminology* ***only*** *if the patient identifies as such.* If used, the word "transsexual" is an adjective. People who were born with anatomically male parts but identify as and/or live as female are known as male-to-female (MtF). Male-to-female people are also known as "transwomen," with the gender descriptor indicating the current-lived gender identity. Conversely, "transmen" are natal females who identify as and/or live as men. They are described as female-to-male (FtM).

Transgender people are sometimes inaccurately described as "transvestites" or "cross-dressers," often in a judgmental or negative manner. These terms should **not** be used unless the patient identifies as such. It is also important to note that people who practice *transvestism* or *cross-dressing* (dressing as a member of the opposite sex at chosen times, while living in public as the natal gender) should not be confused with people who are transgender.

Other terms, such as *tranny, he-she,* or *shemale,* are inappropriate, offensive, and hurtful. These terms and other negative comments should *never* be used.

A patient may self-identify with certain terms or choose not to be defined at all. Become familiar with appropriate terms and concepts, but do not force definitions on your patients. *Instead, if you are unsure how to address patients, during your nursing assessment ask them how they define their gender identity* (Margolies & Brown, 2019) *and what terms they prefer to be used.*

TRANSGENDER HEALTH ISSUES

Transgender people (also referred to as *transpeople*) encounter frequent discrimination and are faced with numerous stressful situations related to their identity. Sources of stress such as job discrimination and bias-related harassment can have an impact on patients' physical and psychological health. In the most recent large-scale national survey on discrimination, the majority of transgender people had experienced mistreatment in the workplace (James et al., 2016). Also, approximately one-third of transgender respondents reported loss of job or denial of promotion because of their transgender identity (James et al., 2016). Loss of income may result in homelessness, with one in five transgender people reporting homelessness at one point in their lives (National Center for Transgender Equality, 2020). In some cases, they may turn to sex work (prostitution) as a mechanism for survival (James et al., 2016). Only a small subset of primarily MtF transgender people engage in sex work, which can expose them to human immune deficiency virus (HIV) and sexually transmitted infection (STI).

Transgender people are also vulnerable to bias-related violence and verbal harassment, including threats and intimidation. In the most recent national survey, 45% of transgender people had been physically attacked at least once in the past year, with 16% reporting four or more physical attacks (James et al., 2016). Nearly half of transgender people experience sexual assault in their lifetime, with 10% experiencing a sexual assault in the previous year (James et al., 2016). MtF people are more likely to experience physical violence and discrimination than nontranswomen; the likelihood of harassment is even greater for transwomen of color (James et al., 2016). Factors that increase this risk for violence include poverty, homelessness, and sex work.

Having an identity that puts a person at risk for violence and mistreatment can lead to emotional distress, particularly if the person has been victimized directly. Transgender people who have experienced traumatic situations may demonstrate symptoms of posttraumatic stress disorder (PTSD) and/or depression. Risks for psychological distress are even higher for transgender people living in poverty and those with disabilities. They may turn to a variety of coping strategies to deal with distress, some of which can negatively affect physical health. In a large-scale national survey, 29% of transgender people reported illicit drug use in the previous month and 27% reported binge-drinking in the previous month (James et al., 2016). Most important, major life stressors, emotional distress, and lack of resources can lead to suicidal ideation or suicide attempts when all other methods of coping have failed. In a sample of over 27,000 transgender adults in all 50 states in the United States, 40% reported at least one suicide attempt in their lifetime (James et al., 2016). Data support similar trends in Canada, reflecting the fact that individual, systemic, and structural factors affect the complexity of suicide among people who are transgender (Bauer & Scheim, 2015; McNeil et al., 2017).

Stress and Transgender Health

Several risk factors for poor health outcomes have been identified in the transgender population, with greater risks for those who have housing and economic instability, lower educational status, and lack of family support (James et al., 2016). Transgender people have additional sources of stress when attempting to access health care, such as lack of health insurance due to unemployment and lack of knowledge of health care professionals. This barrier to health care—one of many ***health care disparities***—causes them to postpone acute as well as preventive medical care. For people who are insured, coverage for health care related to gender transition, such as hormone use and surgery, is often denied.

When transgender people gain access to health care, they are often fearful and anxious about the providers and setting. In particular, they may be hesitant to disclose their transgender status because of fear of discrimination or ridicule. They may also fear that this information will be documented in health records and shared with family members. This reluctance is increased if they have had previous negative experiences with primary health care providers. One national survey found that 33% of transgender adults who saw a primary health care provider in the previous year had a negative experience, including being refused treatment or receiving verbal abuse (James et al., 2016). Male-to-female transgender people were more likely to encounter discrimination and avoid health care because of these experiences (James et al., 2016). Another study demonstrated that transgender people of racial/ethnic minorities experienced negative health care experiences related to race/ethnicity as well as gender identity (Howard et al., 2019). A primary concern of this population is that health care providers do not understand the transgender experience (Halloran, 2015). Even with providers who seem tolerant and caring with transgender patients, there is still a risk for patients overhearing jokes in the hallway and defamatory comments. Consequently, up to 25% of transgender people may not seek necessary medical care owing to a fear of mistreatment (James et al., 2016), which again leads to ***health care disparities.***

When health care professionals do not have knowledge about the needs of the population (James et al., 2016), transgender patients are put in a position of acting as their own health care experts, which can limit the quality of their care. Although most transgender patients generally expect their providers to have some level of knowledge or know where to seek answers, a majority of them find that they have to teach their providers. When they encounter primary health care providers who are unfamiliar with the specific health care needs of their population, patient confidence can diminish drastically and affect desire for future health care.

Although transgender patients may encounter health care professionals who do not understand or who overlook their gender identity, some may encounter those who over-focus on it. Although it is important to be generally knowledgeable about a patient's gender status and understand how it may affect health care needs, this factor is not always relevant for every health problem. For example, transgender patients with fractures or influenza do not need to be questioned extensively about their gender identity. Although there are instances in which the presenting problems require transgender-specific care, many other instances require the same health care that all patients receive. At these times, most transgender patients prefer to be treated as any other patient. Use sound clinical judgment to decide if gender identity impacts patient assessment and care at each encounter.

Transgender Aging

Many nurses are not knowledgeable about culturally competent care of older adults or the LGBTQ population. Estimates have indicated that there are between 217,000 and 700,000 transgender adults who are 65 or older in the United States (Dragon et al., 2017). Many of them lived through the acquired immune deficiency syndrome (AIDS [HIV-III]) crisis of the 1980s and experienced the loss of friends at an early age when life expectancy was much lower; this generation is now included in today's population of older adults (Pfeifer, 2019). Up to 60% of respondents to a 2018 survey of LGBT adults age 45 years and older expressed concerns with neglect, abuse, and harassment in long-term care agencies (Houghton, 2018, in Pfeifer, 2019). This is compelling evidence that nurses need to understand how to meet the special needs of aging transgender people. They may have avoided seeking health care due to fear of ridicule and social stigma. Many of these people may not have had an opportunity to seek gender-affirming hormones or surgeries and feel isolated or alone.

Older transgender adults may be at greater risk for health problems because they may have used ineffective coping strategies such as heavy drinking and smoking for a longer period of time compared with their younger counterparts (Kraus & Duhamel, 2018). This population has been shown to face greater risks for disability, anxiety, depression, victimization, and stigma in comparison with older adults who are not transgender (Johnson et al., 2018).

As a result of these factors, older transgender patients often do not trust health care professionals or the health care system. They may fear staff mistreatment, abuse and neglect, and discrimination, especially when admitted to an acute or long-term care facility. Advocate for older transgender patients and support their gender identity and right to dignity and respect. Seek and refer to long-term care agencies that hire LGBT staff, advertise LGBT friendliness, and display welcoming signs online and inside the facility (Pfeifer, 2019) (see Fig. 68.1). Reassure all patients that they are safe, which is a primary component of culturally competent care (Kraus & Duhamel, 2018).

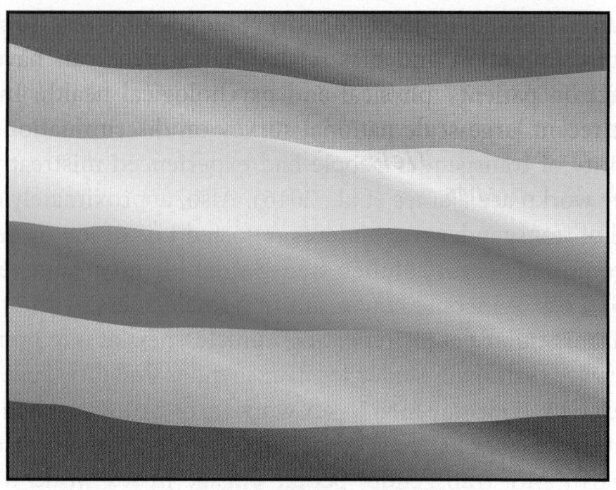

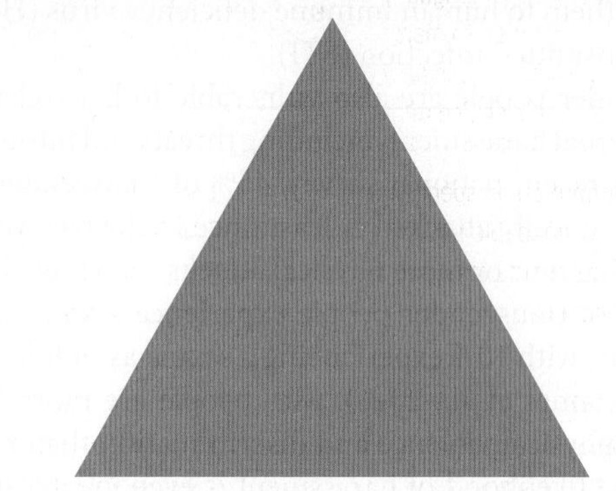

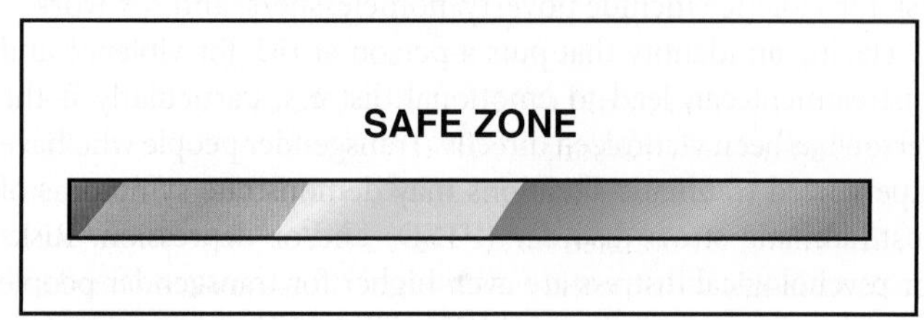

FIG. 68.1 The Safe Zone—rainbow or pink triangle signs welcome LGBTQ patients in a health care agency.

The Need to Improve Transgender Health Care

During the past few years, several national documents have been published by the U.S. Department of Health and Human Services and private health care organizations that call for improvement in LGBTQ health care to reduce ***health care disparities.*** These important publications include:

- *Healthy People 2020* and *Healthy People 2030*
- The Institute of Medicine of the National Academies (now the National Academies of Sciences, Engineering, and Medicine) report on LGBT health
- The Joint Commission (TJC) Field Guide for care of LGBT patients
- World Professional Association for Transgender Health (WPATH) Standards of Care (SOC)

The U.S. Department of Health and Human Services' *Healthy People 2010* publication did *not* include the need to improve health care for LGBT people. As a result of this omission, a companion document was developed by the Gay and Lesbian Medical Association (GLMA) to address special health care needs of this population across the life span. Ten common health problems affecting the LGBT group were identified, including cancer, nutrition and weight, and sexually transmitted infection (STI).

The *Healthy People 2020* agenda added objectives for improving the health of LGBT people, including the need to recognize and address the special health needs of transgender patients of all ages. *Healthy People 2030* continues to focus on these objectives. Select proposed objectives include increasing national surveys that collect data on or for transgender populations, and increasing health questions about sexual orientation and gender identity that could improve patient outcomes (Office of Disease Prevention and Health Promotion, 2020).

The IOM LGBT health report calls for the need for more research to identify the special health care concerns of LGBT people of all ages. To help meet this outcome, the document outlined the need to collect more demographic data to better

BEST PRACTICE FOR PATIENT SAFETY & QUALITY CARE QSEN

The Joint Commission Recommendations for Creating a Safe, Welcoming Environment for LGBTQ Patients

- Post the *Patients' Bill of Rights* and nondiscrimination policies in a visible place.
- Make waiting rooms inclusive for LGBTQ patients and families, such as posting *Safe Zone*, rainbow, or pink triangle signs.
- Designate unisex or single-stall restrooms.
- Ensure that visitation policies are equitable for families of LGBTQ patients.
- Avoid assumptions about any patient's sexual orientation and gender identity.
- Include gender-neutral language on all medical forms and documents (e.g., "partnered" in addition to married, single, or divorced categories).
- Do not limit gender options on medical forms to "male" and "female."
- Reflect the patient's choice of terminology in communication and documentation.
- Provide information on special health concerns for LGBTQ patients.
- Become knowledgeable about LGBTQ health needs and care.
- Refer LGBTQ patients to qualified health care professionals as needed.
- Provide community resources for LGBTQ information and support as needed.

Adapted from The Joint Commission (TJC). (2011). *Advancing effective communication, cultural competence, and patient- and family-centered care for the lesbian, gay, bisexual, and transgender community.* www.jointcommission.org/lgbt.

identify this population. LGBTQ people need to feel safe when disclosing this very personal information.

In 2011, the World Professional Association for Transgender Health (WPATH) updated its Standards of Care (Coleman et al., 2012). As of this writing, the 2011 edition of the Standards of Care (SOC) remains the most current. The SOC document outlines core principles that nurses and other health care professionals should follow when caring for transgender patients (Table 68.1).

Also in 2011, The Joint Commission (TJC) published a similar document recommending ways for health care agencies to create a welcoming and safe environment for LGBT patients. In response to growing attention to the need for cultural competence for all health care professionals and to provide high-quality health care for sexual and gender minority patients, TJC published a classic field guide for health care agencies to improve LGBT patient care (TJC, 2011). The Best Practice for Patient Safety & Quality Care: The Joint Commission Recommendations for Creating a Safe, Welcoming Environment for LGBTQ Patients box lists the recommendations for health care agencies in designing a safe environment for this population.

Fig. 68.1 shows an example of a "safe zone" image that should be used to reassure these patients that they are in a safe place where they can receive respectful and knowledgeable high-quality care.

Further resources for creating an inclusive environment for LGBT patients can be found through the National LGBT Health Education Center, a program of the Fenway Institute. Part of the Fenway Health, this organization's mission is "to enhance well-being of the LGBTQIA+ community and all people in [their] neighborhoods and beyond through access to the highest quality health care, education, research, and advocacy" (Fenway Health, 2020).

TABLE 68.1 Core Principles for Health Care Professionals Who Care for Transgender Patients

- Become knowledgeable about the health care needs of transgender and other gender-nonconforming people.
- Become knowledgeable about the treatment options for transgender patients and required follow-up care.
- Do not assume that all transgender patients are the same; treat each one as an individual and develop an individualized plan of care.
- Demonstrate respect for patients with nonconforming gender identities.
- Provide culturally sensitive care and use appropriate terminology that affirms the patient's gender identity.
- Facilitate patient access to appropriate and knowledgeable health care providers.
- Seek informed consent before providing treatment.
- Offer continuity of care or refer patients for ongoing quality health care.
- Advocate for patients within their families and communities.

Data from Coleman, E., et al. (2012). Standards of care for the health of transsexual, transgender, and gender-nonconforming people, Version 7, *International Journal of Transgenderism, 13*(4), 165–232. DOI: 10.1080/15532739.2011.700873; and Makadon, H., Goldhammer, H., & Davis, J. (2015). *Fenway guide to lesbian, gay, bisexual, and transgender health* (2nd ed.). Philadelphia, PA: American College of Physicians.

Interprofessional Collaborative Care

Assessment: Recognize Cues. As with any patient, ask during the nursing history and physical assessment how he or she prefers to be addressed. For example, for nontransgender patients, some people may use a nickname or their middle name and prefer to be addressed as such. For transgender patients, it is not uncommon for driver's licenses, insurance cards, and other forms of identification to retain their birth names (and by extension, birth sex) because it can be difficult to change this information, particularly if a person is in the process of transitioning. Therefore nurses may receive patient documentation with misleading patient data, such as health care record listing a male name and birth sex while caring for a patient who presents as female in appearance. It can be offensive and embarrassing for the patient who clearly identifies as female to be called "Mister" or "sir" or by the male birth name. Not only does it communicate disrespect, it also signals to the patient that she may receive inadequate care or that the environment is unsafe.

In addition to preferred names, correct pronoun usage is also important. Each patient has his or her own pronoun preference. A MtF patient may visit a clinic during lunch hour at work. Because the patient has not disclosed the transgender identity at work, this patient maintains male dress and demeanor at the office. Although the patient may identify as female and live as female at home, the patient may request the nurse to use male pronouns (he, him, his) to match the patient's current presentation and may not disclose the transgender identity to the nurse. Conversely, even though the patient presents at the time as male, the patient may ask the nurse to use female pronouns (she, her, hers) because the patient identifies with a female gender identity.

In general, use pronouns that match the patient's physical presentation and dress unless the patient requests otherwise. Even though the biologic sex may not match, patients presenting as female should be addressed as female, and patients presenting as male should be addressed as male. With changing clothing styles and trends, do not rely on clothing cues alone. However, it is most appropriate to address a patient as male whose birth sex is listed as female yet presents in traditionally male attire, facial hair, and a men's hairstyle. Understandably, the clinical setting can be fast paced, and nurses may encounter multiple patients at a time; however, taking time to use clinical judgment is important. Appropriately interacting with a transgender patient can sometimes mean the difference between the patient continuing to seek health care or not.

In some cases you might notice that patients may not identify as male or female and prefer not to use male or female pronouns. These patients often feel that the binary gender system in which a person must fit clearly into one category or the other is too limiting. Although this is a small subset of the transgender population, it is important to be aware of this subculture in case you encounter a patient who does not identify with a specific gender. Some patients may request the use of gender-neutral pronouns, or they may use these pronouns in the nurse's presence. Some examples of gender-neutral pronouns are "they/them/their/theirs/themself," "sie/hir/hirs/hirself," and "zie/zir/zirs/zirself" (University of Southern California, 2020).

Getting used to addressing the patient by the correct name or pronoun can take some time. Occasionally, nurses recognize the cues and know their patient's preferred name or pronoun, but accidentally say the wrong one. Transgender patients encounter this situation often and typically anticipate an occasional error. When this error occurs, simply self-correct and continue with care rather than make a prolonged apology. Focusing too much on the error may make the patient more uncomfortable because more attention has been drawn to the situation. Most transgender patients, particularly those who live full time in their gender-affirming role, wish to be treated like any other patient.

History. Transgender people who experience gender dysphoria (discomfort with one's natal sex) may have had one or more of these interventions (Coleman et al., 2012):

- Changes in gender expression that may involve living part-time or full-time in another gender role
- Psychotherapy to explore gender identity and expression, improve body image, or strengthen coping mechanisms
- Hormone therapy to feminize or masculinize the body
- Surgery to change primary and/or secondary sex characteristics (e.g., the breasts/chest, facial features, internal and/or external genitalia)

During the health history, inquire about which interventions the patient has had, if any, or if there are plans to have them in the future. Ask about current use of *drug therapy,* including hormones, and other feminizing or masculinizing agents, including silicone injections. These medications are usually prescribed by endocrinologists or other specialists in transgender health care, but some patients may obtain them from nonmedical sources, including the Internet.

Exogenous hormone therapy can cause adverse health problems and requires careful patient monitoring, including laboratory testing. Estrogen therapy can increase health risks such as increased blood clotting causing venous thromboembolism (VTE), elevated blood glucose, hypertension, estrogen-dependent cancers, and fluid retention. Smoking and obesity increase these risks. The risks also increase with higher doses of the medication. Ask the patient about a history of these problems.

Inquire about the patient's *surgical history.* For the MtF patient, ask about breast surgery and any surgical changes to the genitalia, such as a penectomy (removal of the penis), orchiectomy (removal of one or both testes), and vaginoplasty (creation of a vagina). The MtF patient still has a prostate gland. For older patients, ask about any problems with prostate health problems, such as urinary dribbling and retention. For the FtM patient, ask whether a hysterectomy, bilateral salpingo-oophorectomy (BSO), mastectomy, phalloplasty (creation of a penis), and/or scrotoplasty (creation of a scrotum) was performed.

Keep in mind that health insurance usually does not cover the cost of the transition process and patients may seek alternative care. Hormones may be obtained illegally or from countries that do not have quality controls for medication. "Gray market pharmacies," secondary wholesalers that are unauthorized by drug manufacturers, offer many of these products at significantly higher costs. Other products can also be purchased through venues that are not regulated. The risk for hepatitis C and silicone complications increases significantly when products are obtained through these channels. Ask patients about the use of these alternatives as a part of their transition process.

Physical Assessment. Be sure to review the patient's health record carefully before performing a physical assessment. To help increase the patient's comfort with examinations and the purpose of the assessment, explain why the information or examination is important to their health care. Be culturally sensitive, nonjudgmental, and respectful during the assessment. Recognize that transgender patients may be young, middle-age, or older adults.

When assessing transgender patients, be aware that they may be in varying stages of transition. Some patients present with no obvious physical signs that they are in the process of transitioning. Others have had gender-confirming surgery such that their new appearance matches their gender identity. Realize that a transgender patient's genitalia may not match his or her physical appearance.

Psychosocial Assessment. If gender and/or ***sexuality*** are relevant to the patient's presenting health problem, ask specific questions to determine how these factors may impact care. Again, it is helpful to share with patients why this information is relevant to their treatment. Reassure patients that their responses are confidential and will not be shared with any family, friends, or significant others without the patient's permission. However, evidence of abuse must be reported as mandated by law. Appropriate screening questions about psychosocial functioning related to gender and ***sexuality*** include:

- Are you experiencing any challenges, concerns, or anxiety related to your sexuality?

- Related to your gender, how do you identify?
- Are you experiencing sadness, depression, or thoughts of hurting yourself?
- Have you experienced violence or discrimination in your personal or work life?
- Are you currently being seen by a counselor or psychologist related to your sexuality and gender identity? If so, would you wish to share the reason?

If the responses to these questions indicate that the patient has potential or actual mental health concerns, consult with the primary health care provider for further evaluation by a qualified mental health care professional, such as a licensed counselor or clinical psychologist.

◆ **Interventions: Take Action.** Nurses may care for transgender patients of any age who are transitioning or have completed gender confirmation. They may care for them for health problems related to their transition process or for problems that are unrelated to the patient's ***sexuality*** or gender identity. In general, care for transgender patients with most health problems is the same as for any other patient. However, some interventions such as hormone therapy may affect nursing assessment and care. As a leader in health care, advocate for transgender patients and provide health teaching to promote their health. Encourage them to include their partner, if desired, in discussions about the transition process.

Nonsurgical Management. The primary nonsurgical interventions for transgender patients include drug (hormone) therapy, counseling about ***reproduction*** and reproductive health, and vocal therapy. The type of intervention depends on whether the patient is transitioning from male to female (MtF) or from female to male (FtM).

Drug Therapy. Drug therapy may be started after completing a psychosocial assessment by a qualified mental health care professional and informed consent has been obtained. According to WPATH's most recent Standards of Care (Coleman et al., 2012), the criteria for gender-affirming hormonal therapy include:

- Continuing and well-documented gender dysphoria
- Patient ability to make a fully informed decision and give consent to treatment
- Patient older than 18 years
- Well-controlled existing medical or mental health problems, if any

Feminizing Drug Therapy. Patients transitioning from male to female (MtF) typically take a combination of estrogen therapy and androgen-reducing medications to achieve feminizing effects. Expected physical changes from *estrogen therapy* are listed in Table 68.2. Additional measures to eliminate facial hair may be needed, such as laser treatment or electrolysis (Ettner et al., 2016). Aesthetic fillers and neurotoxins are also used to achieve facial changes (Ginsberg, 2017).

Because oral estrogen can increase the risk for venous thromboembolism (VTE), transdermal estrogen or injectable estradiol is preferred for use in transgender patients. Progesterone may also be prescribed to be used during a portion of each month (Burchum & Rosenthal, 2019).

TABLE 68.2 Feminizing Drug Therapy for MtF Patients: Expected Changes

- Breast tissue development
- Reduced or absent sperm count and ejaculatory fluid
- Reduced muscle mass
- Change in emotions
- Change in sweat and odor patterns
- Decreased testicular size
- Reduced erectile function
- Decreased libido (sex drive)
- Decreased body hair growth
- Softening of skin

! NURSING SAFETY PRIORITY (QSEN)

Drug Alert

Before the first dose of transdermal estrogen, teach the patient to apply the patch to an area that is hairless to ensure good contact with the skin. When changing to a new patch, wash any excess drug and adhesive from the skin where the previous patch was applied.

Teach patients taking any form of estrogen about side effects such as headache, breast tenderness, nausea/vomiting, and weight gain (often due to fluid retention) or loss. Tell them to report increased feelings of anxiety or depression to their primary health care provider. Estrogens can also cause estrogen-dependent cancers, hypertension (due to fluid retention), venous thromboembolism (VTE) such as deep vein thrombosis (DVT), and gallbladder disease. Teach patients to follow up with their primary health care provider to monitor for these potential adverse drug effects.

NCLEX EXAMINATION CHALLENGE 68.1

Physiological Integrity

The nurse provides health teaching for a transgender woman receiving estrogen therapy. Which statement by the client indicates a **need for further teaching**?

A. "I'll call my doctor if I have any redness or swelling in my legs."
B. "I'll have less hair on my body after taking this drug."
C. "I know that the drug will make my breasts bigger."
D. "I think I will have more sex drive when taking this drug."

In addition to estrogen therapy, androgen-reducing agents (also called androgen blockers or antiandrogens) are often given to block the effects of testosterone, including (Burchum & Rosenthal, 2019; Deutsch, 2016):

- Spironolactone (the most commonly used androgen blocker), a low-cost diuretic that also inhibits testosterone secretion and androgen binding to androgen receptors
- 5-alpha-reductase inhibitors (e.g., finasteride and dutasteride), drugs typically used to treat benign prostatic hyperplasia (BPH) (These drugs block the conversion of testosterone to a more active ingredient to decrease the hair loss associated with estrogen therapy and shrink prostate tissue.)

! NURSING SAFETY PRIORITY (QSEN)

Drug Alert

Teach patients taking *spironolactone* to monitor their blood pressure for hypotension. Remind them to expect polyuria and possible polydipsia. Periodic laboratory tests to assess for hyperkalemia may be needed for patients with renal insufficiency (Burchum & Rosenthal, 2019; Deutsch, 2016). Remind those patients that increased serum potassium can cause cardiac dysrhythmias and skeletal muscle spasticity.

Common side effects of finasteride and other *5-alpha reductase inhibitors* include dizziness, cold sweats, and chills. These symptoms typically decrease over time. If patients continue to have them, instruct them to contact their health care provider.

Masculinizing Drug Therapy. Testosterone is the primary drug used for achieving masculinizing effects in transgender people transitioning from female to male; however, much of the available drug converts to estrogen in the body. This drug can be taken orally, transdermally (topical gel or patch), or parenterally (IM). Buccal and implantable forms of testosterone are also available. Oral testosterone is the least effective form of the drug. Depo-Testosterone, the most common IM preparation, is usually started at a low dose and increased every 1 to 2 weeks (Burchum & Rosenthal, 2019). Teach patients the importance of not sharing needles to prevent bloodborne diseases such as hepatitis C.

Testosterone gel and the testosterone patch are topical forms that are more expensive than other testosterone preparations but may provide more consistent (although slower) results. A newer topical form of the drug, testosterone axillary gel, can be applied to the armpits to increase serum testosterone levels. For all topical testosterone preparations, be sure that the patient washes his hands between applications and covers the area with clothing.

Expected effects of testosterone therapy are listed in Table 68.3. Teach the patient taking testosterone that some of these changes take up to a year to occur. If menses does not stop in the first few months of drug therapy, the patient may be placed on progesterone until the testosterone becomes effective.

Common undesirable effects of testosterone therapy include edema, acne, seborrhea (oily skin), headaches, weight gain,

TABLE 68.3 Masculinizing Drug Therapy for FtM Patients: Expected Changes

- Voice deepening
- Body hair growth (hirsutism), but possibly hairline recession and male pattern baldness
- Increased muscle mass
- Increased libido
- Increased aggression
- Vaginal dryness
- Clitoral growth
- Redistribution of fat
- Cessation of menses

and possible psychosis. Before taking this medication, the patient must be screened for a history of liver and heart disease. Testosterone therapy can cause increased liver enzymes, increased low-density lipoproteins (LDLs, or "bad" cholesterol), and decreased high-density lipoproteins (HDLs, or "good" cholesterol). Increased blood glucose and decreased clotting factors can also occur when taking the drug. Teach patients that these changes can lead to diabetes, heart disease, and stroke. Remind patients that they need to follow up with their health care providers for careful monitoring for these complications, including having extensive diagnostic and laboratory testing.

Reproductive Health Options. Using feminizing or masculinizing hormone therapy affects reproductive health, especially fertility. Ensure that patients know their options for ***reproduction,*** if desired, *before* transition begins. MtF patients may want to consider sperm banking before drug therapy or gender-confirming surgery if they desire to have a biologic child. FtM patients may want to consider oocyte (egg) or embryo freezing. These frozen gametes or embryos could be implanted in a surrogate woman to become pregnant and carry to birth. Inform patients that these options are expensive, but are still available to them. Be sure to include the patient's partner, if the patient desires, in discussions related to reproductive options.

Voice and Communication Therapy. Communication is an essential aspect of human behavior and gender expression. Voice deepening for transgender people who are transitioning from female to male is accomplished by taking masculinizing hormones, such as testosterone. However, feminizing hormones have no effect on the adult MtF voice.

MtF patients may undergo surgery to change the voice (Schwarz et al., 2017). Others may seek assistance from a voice and communication specialist to help them modify certain vocal characteristics, such as pitch and intonation. Vocal therapy can assist in management of gender dysphoria and be a positive step in the transition process. Remind patients to seek a speech-language pathologist (SLP) who is knowledgeable in transgender health, and has specialized training in assessment and development of vocal health and therapy for transgender patients.

The purpose of vocal therapy is to help patients adapt their voice and communication such that it is authentic and reflects their gender identity. The SLP should take the patient's communication preferences and style into consideration as part of the assessment process to develop an individualized treatment plan. Vocal therapy can also be completed after surgery.

Surgical Management. Many transgender people are satisfied with their gender identity, role, and self-expression without surgery. Surgery, particularly procedures that affect the external or internal genitalia, is usually the last and most carefully considered option for transitioning from one's natal sex to one's inner gender identity. These procedures are often referred to as **gender-affirming surgery (GAS)** but are also known as gender-confirming surgery or gender reassignment surgery. The patient may have a number of surgeries that change primary and/or secondary sex characteristics to confirm a person's gender identity. These procedures achieve either feminizing or masculinizing effects. Regardless of the procedure(s) performed, the nurse collaborates with the patient, family, and health care team to promote positive outcomes for the transition process.

Gender-affirming surgeries are procedures that alter anatomically healthy structures. Not all surgeons feel comfortable in performing procedures that could "harm" transgender patients. However, these procedures help treat gender dysphoria. Some patients elect to undergo the full range of surgeries, whereas others choose to have only some or none of them, typically because of the profound medical expense.

Surgeries that remove or create breasts are often referred to as "top surgery." Genital surgeries "below the waist," often called "bottom surgery," are the most invasive procedures. The criteria for genital surgery depend on the type of surgery being requested. For example, most surgeons (usually urologists or plastic surgeons) require 12 months of hormone therapy plus one or two referrals from qualified psychotherapists for MtF patients who desire an orchiectomy. The same requirements may be needed for FtM patients who desire a hysterectomy (uterus removal) and bilateral salpingo-oophorectomy (BSO), or removal of both fallopian tubes and ovaries.

The psychotherapist assesses the patient's readiness for genital surgery and hormone therapy, including a discussion of risks and out-of-pocket costs. The patient's support system is assessed to ensure that the patient makes the best possible decision and achieves the desired outcomes.

For MtF patients requesting a vaginoplasty (creation of a vagina) or FtM patients desiring a phalloplasty (creation of a penis), the required criteria include 12 continuous months of living in a gender role that is congruent with the patient's gender identity. Prior to any surgical procedure, the surgeon ensures that coexisting medical health problems are well managed and monitored. The patient is advised to discontinue all hormonal therapy at least 2 weeks prior to surgery (Ettner et al., 2016). Current evidence shows that GAS is associated with multiple, significant psychological benefits for those who had gender dysphoria (Wernick et al., 2019) despite other evidence showing prosthesis complications in up to one-third of patients (Rooker et al., 2019).

Feminizing Surgeries for MtF Patients. Feminizing surgeries are performed for MtF patients to create a functional and/or aesthetic (cosmetic) female anatomy, including:

- *Breast/chest surgeries,* such as breast augmentation (mammoplasty to increase breast tissue)
- Other surgeries, such as *facial feminizing surgery* (to achieve feminine facial contour); liposuction (fatty tissue removal), often from the waist or abdominal area; *vocal feminizing surgery*; and other body-contouring procedures
- *Genital surgeries,* such as partial penectomy (removal of the penis), orchiectomy (removal of the testes), vaginoplasty and labiaplasty/vulvoplasty (creation of a vagina and labia/vulva), and clitoroplasty (creation of a clitoris)

Breast augmentation creates breast tissue for the MtF patient through the use of silicone gel-filled implants or saline implants. Although not a prerequisite, it is recommended that MtF patients take feminizing hormones for 12 months before surgery for the best results. Feminizing breast augmentation procedures require small incisions and are therefore usually performed as same-day surgeries. Teach patients that they may have swelling, soreness, and mild bruising for several weeks after surgery, but complications are rare (Ettner et al., 2016).

Voice feminizing surgery, such as reduction thyroid chondroplasty, is performed to decrease the size of the "Adam's apple" (Schwarz et al., 2017). This procedure is performed through a bronchoscope for cosmetic purposes. Nursing care of the patient having a bronchoscopy is discussed in Chapter 24.

The most common *genital surgeries* for MtF patients are bilateral *orchiectomy* to remove the testes and vaginoplasty with partial penectomy. Orchiectomy procedures and associated nursing care are the same for the transgender patient as they are for other natal males (see Chapter 67 for a detailed discussion).

A *vaginoplasty* is the construction of a neovagina (new vagina), usually with inverted penile tissue (obtained during a partial penectomy) and scrotal, skin, or colon graft. This complex surgical procedure also usually includes creating a clitoris and labia (clitoro-labioplasty) using scrotal or penile tissue and skin grafts.

Preoperative Care. In addition to the required criteria to qualify for a vaginoplasty (also called *transvaginal surgery*), the transgender patient is medically evaluated like any other presurgical patient. Patients who have poorly controlled diabetes with vascular complications, coronary artery disease, or other systemic disease that limits functional ability are not candidates for major gender-affirming surgery. Chapter 9 describes general preoperative care for any patient.

The surgeon explains the options for selected procedures, postoperative care expectations, and potential for complications after surgery. Postoperative recovery for transvaginal surgery takes a long time and has a high complication rate. As seen after any surgery, patients with obesity have a higher incidence of surgical infection and often have problems with adequate ventilation (breathing) and ambulation (see Chapter 9).

Written and verbal preoperative instructions are provided by the surgeon, including optional methods of body hair removal. A bowel preparation may be started 24 hours before surgery and may include a clear liquid diet, laxatives, and sodium phosphate/saline enemas. Increased fluids are recommended until the patient goes to bed the night before surgery because the bowel preparation can be very dehydrating. Antimicrobials are typically given on the day of surgery to minimize the risk for infection.

Some surgeons require that the patient take supplements to prevent bruising and promote tissue healing, such as vitamin C. Patients who are very thin are encouraged to eat a high-protein diet. A powdered protein supplement with arginine (an amino acid) may also be prescribed to promote wound healing.

Patients undergo a number of laboratory tests to ensure that they are healthy before surgery. Adequate hemoglobin and hematocrit (H&H) levels are especially important because some blood is lost during surgery. For patients who have low H&H levels, an erythropoietin such as epoetin alfa or IM testosterone with iron is given. Most patients choose testosterone because it is a lower-cost drug.

Operative Procedures. Because surgery requires multiple procedures to create a female anatomy, the patient is on the operating table for many hours. The surgery may be performed in a hospital or specialized center for transgender surgeries. After general or epidural anesthesia is administered, the patient is placed in a lithotomy position (feet in stirrups) for the procedure. Epidural anesthesia is preferred for patients with asthma or obesity. The patient is transferred to the postanesthesia care unit (PACU) with a perineal dressing and packing, Jackson-Pratt drain, and indwelling urinary catheter.

Postoperative Care. Provide general postoperative care as described in Chapter 9. In addition, starting immediately after surgery, to decrease pain and bruising apply an ice pack to the perineum for 20 minutes every hour and continue for the first postoperative week (Deutsch, 2016). Monitor the patient's pain level carefully and offer analgesia as needed. *Genital surgery is very painful because there is a high concentration of nerve endings in the perineum.*

Although not a common postoperative complication, monitor the patient for bleeding. Observe the surgical dressing and surrounding area for oozing or bright red blood. Always look under the patient in case blood has pooled there. Report and document any indication of active bleeding immediately to the surgeon and keep the patient in bed.

! NURSING SAFETY PRIORITY (QSEN)

Action Alert

Patients are in a lithotomy position for an extended period during surgery. After surgery, monitor lower extremity neurovascular status and encourage the patient to move the legs often during the first 24 hours after surgery to help prevent compartment syndrome. Report and document any unexpected findings, such as continued numbness, inability to move the lower legs or feet, or leg pain and swelling. Patients who had epidural anesthesia are not able to move their legs for several hours after surgery until the effect of the drug diminishes.

All patients stay in the hospital for at least 1 night after genital surgery, but some patients may stay much longer, depending on the number and complexity of the surgical procedures. Patients who have the inverted skin flap technique for a *vaginoplasty* usually remain on bedrest for at least 4 to 5 days with a dilator or gauze packing in the neovagina. Subcutaneous fractionized heparin is given during this time to prevent venous thromboembolism (VTE) (Ettner et al., 2016).

After the bedrest period, the dilator or gauze packing is removed to allow the patient to ambulate. The patient is taught how to cleanse the new vagina with an antiseptic solution and given careful instructions on how to follow the strict dilator protocol. Other postoperative instructions are listed in the Best Practice for Patient Safety & Quality Care: Postoperative Teaching for Patients Who Have a Vaginoplasty box (Deutsch, 2016).

The Jackson Pratt drain is removed when drainage is less than 15 to 20 mL in a 24-hour period. About 7 to 10 days after surgery, the surgical pressure dressing and external sutures are removed. The urinary catheter is removed between postoperative days 7 and 12. Early removal can cause urinary retention, but prolonged placement can lead to catheter-associated urinary tract infection (CAUTI).

Patients should continue follow-up visits with their primary health care provider for signs and symptoms of complications. One of the worst complications is a vaginal-rectal fistula, which is caused by rectal perforation during surgery. Teach patients to report any leakage of stool into the vagina immediately to their surgeon. The treatment for this complication is a temporary colostomy and fistula wound management for many months. Other surgical complications of vaginoplasty are listed in Table 68.4.

Some MtF patients are not satisfied with the quality of the results of feminizing surgeries. For example, the neovagina may not be functional for sexual intercourse. Some patients request another surgery to achieve more satisfying results.

BEST PRACTICE FOR PATIENT SAFETY & QUALITY CARE (QSEN)

Postoperative Teaching for Patients Who Have a Vaginoplasty

- Resume taking showers after the first postoperative follow-up visit.
- Do not take baths (submerged in water) for 8 weeks after surgery.
- Avoid strenuous activities for at least 6 weeks.
- Avoid swimming or bike riding for 3 months.
- Expect minimal vaginal bleeding/spotting and/or a brownish-yellow drainage for 6 to 8 weeks; use a soap and water douche to minimize these problems.
- Avoid tobacco or smoking for at least a month after surgery to promote healing.
- Take stool softeners as prescribed to help prevent constipation.
- Take acetaminophen as prescribed for pain control at home.
- Carefully follow the prescribed individualized dilator protocol.
- Do not have sexual intercourse until at least 3 months after surgery.

NCLEX EXAMINATION CHALLENGE 68.2

Physiological Integrity

The nurse is caring for a client who had a vaginoplasty yesterday. Which assessment finding will the nurse report to the health care provider?

A. Perineal pain
B. Lower extremity swelling
C. Constipation
D. Urinary retention

Masculinizing Surgeries for FtM Patients. Masculinizing surgeries are performed for FtM patients to create a functional and/or aesthetic male anatomy, including:

- Breast/chest surgeries, usually a bilateral mastectomy (removal of both breasts) and chest reconstruction and contouring
- Genital surgeries, such as a hysterectomy and bilateral BSO, vaginectomy (removal of the vagina), phalloplasty (creation of an average-size male penis) with ureteroplasty (creation of a urethra) or metoidioplasty (creation of a small penis using hormone-enhanced clitoral tissue), and scrotoplasty (creation of a scrotum) with insertion of testicular prostheses
- Other surgeries, such as liposuction, pectoral muscle implants, and other facial or body-contouring procedures

Care of transgender patients having a mastectomy, hysterectomy, and bilateral salpingo-oophorectomy (BSO) is similar

TABLE 68.4 Postoperative Complications of Vaginoplasty Surgery

Most Serious Complications

- Vaginal-rectal fistula
- Rectal perforation
- Lower extremity compartment syndrome
- Bleeding (early but rare)

Other Complications

- Surgical wound infection
- Urinary leakage/incontinence
- Chronic urinary tract infections
- Urinary meatus stenosis (late but rare)
- Vaginal stenosis
- Vaginal collapse
- Labial hematoma
- Inadequate vaginal length or width
- Lack of sensation
- Lack of sexual pleasure

to care for any patient having these procedures as described elsewhere in this text. Some FtM patients are not satisfied with the results of mastectomy and chest reconstruction due to complications, which can include scarring, nipple-areola misplacement or size, and contour abnormalities (Deutsch, 2016). As an alternative to breast surgery, use of a binder to constrict and hide the breasts may be preferred (Ettner et al., 2016). Remind the patient that long-term use of a binder can result in lax or drooping breast tissue. If the patient has not had previous abdominal surgery, a laparoscopic procedure is preferred for the hysterectomy and BSO surgery.

Procedures to create a male anatomy for FtM patients are not performed as often as for MtF patients who desire a female anatomy. Phalloplasties are the most difficult reconstructive genital surgeries to perform and usually require several stages. Skin flaps from the radial forearm, anterior lateral thigh, or back are used to create the penis. Fat grafts may be needed to increase penile girth, and buccal mucosal tissue may be used to create the urethra. A penile prosthesis or implant is not inserted until months after surgery when the initial surgical healing has occurred.

Complications from phalloplasty include:

- Urethral complications
- Bleeding
- Wound infections
- Donor graft site scarring or loss
- Rectal injury

In addition to these physical problems, the patient may not be satisfied with the results of the surgery, such as an inadequate length of the penis. For these reasons, many FtM patients do not have this procedure and prefer to have only a laparoscopic hysterectomy and BSO.

Care Coordination and Transition Management. Transgender patients often take hormone therapy for many years. Teach them that ongoing follow-up with a qualified health care professional is needed to maintain health and detect any complications, such as diabetes or cardiovascular problems, as early as possible.

Long-term follow-up with the surgeon after gender-affirming surgery is essential to detect and treat the frequent complications that occur. Assess the patient's support systems and coping strategies, including financial status and health insurance benefits. Collaborate with the case manager to ensure a smooth transition into the community, including the possible need for any ongoing mental health counseling or therapy.

Urogenital care is also needed for patients who have gender-affirming surgery. FtM patients usually do not have a vaginectomy and therefore may experience vaginal atrophy causing itching and burning. Recommend that they seek gynecologic care to treat this problem, although the examination can be physically and emotionally painful.

MtF patients may need counseling about ***sexuality,*** genital hygiene, and prevention of sexually transmitted diseases. They are also at a high risk for frequent urinary tract infections as a result of a shortened urethra and urinary incontinence if they have had genital surgery. Teach patients the importance of having follow-up care for these problems.

Preventive health care screenings for transgender patients are also important. The MtF patient requires prostate health care screenings that natal males need. Mammograms are also recommended to monitor for early signs of cancer in the augmented breast. FtM patients who have not undergone a hysterectomy and BSO need gynecologic care to minimize risk for cervical and ovarian cancer, as well as mammograms if the breasts have not been removed.

A number of community resources and organizations are available for transgender support and information, such as:

- National Coalition for LGBT Health (https://healthlgbt.org/)
- Advocacy and Services for LGBT Elders (www.sageusa.org)
- Transgender Health Information Program (http://www.phsa.ca/our-services/programs-services/trans-care-bc)
- University of California San Francisco Center of Excellence for Transgender Health (www.transhealth.ucsf.edu)
- Vancouver Coastal Health Transgender Health Program (http://www.vch.ca/locations-services/result?res_id=1342)
- Canadian Professional Association for Transgender Health (www.cpath.ca)
- World Professional Association for Transgender Health (www.wpath.org)

CLINICAL JUDGMENT CHALLENGE 68.1

Evidence-Based Practice; Patient-Centered Care

A client who is well-known to the nurse has come to see the primary care provider. The client, a natal sex female, asks the nurse to be addressed by the name "Marc" but to keep the name "Michelle" on the electronic health record. While bringing the history up-to-date and asking the reason for today's visit, the nurse notices that the client makes only intermittent eye contact. The client responds, "I want to talk with the provider about hormones."

1. **Recognize Cues:** What assessment information in this client situation is the most important and immediate concern for the nurse? (Hint: Identify the **relevant** information *first* to determine what is most important.)
2. **Analyze Cues:** What client conditions are consistent with the **most relevant** information? (Hint: Think about priority collaborative problems that support and contradict the information presented in this situation.)
3. **Prioritize Hypotheses:** Which possibilities or explanations are **most likely** to be present in this client situation? Which possibilities or explanations are the most serious? (Hint: Consider all possibilities and determine their urgency and risk for this client.)
4. **Generate Solutions:** What actions would most likely achieve the desired outcomes for this client? Which actions should be **avoided** or are **potentially harmful**? (Hint: Determine the desired outcomes first to decide which interventions are appropriate and those that should be avoided.)
5. **Take Action:** Which actions are the most appropriate and how should they be implemented? In what **priority order** should they be implemented? (Hint: Consider health teaching, documentation, requested health care provider orders or prescriptions, nursing skills, collaboration with or referral to health team members, etc.)
6. **Evaluate Outcomes:** What client assessment would indicate that the nurse's actions were **effective**? (Hint: Think about signs that would indicate an improvement, decline, or unchanged client condition.)

GET READY FOR THE NEXT-GENERATION NCLEX® EXAMINATION!

Key Points

Review these Key Points for each NCLEX Examination Client Needs Category.

Safe and Effective Care Environment

- Depending on identified health care needs, collaborate with multiple members of the interprofessional team when caring for the transgender patient. **QSEN: Teamwork and Interprofessional Collaboration**
- Monitor for expected, side, and adverse effects of hormone therapy, including effects on ***sexuality*** and ***reproduction***, as described in Tables 68.2 and 68.3. **QSEN: Safety**

Health Promotion and Maintenance

- Advocate for the transgender patient who may be distrustful of health care professionals and fearful when seeking care. **QSEN: Patient-Centered Care**
- Refer the transgender patient and partner, as appropriate, to local and national resources for information and support. **QSEN: Patient-Centered Care**

Psychosocial Integrity

- Use culturally sensitive and accurate language and pronouns when communicating with transgender patients. **QSEN: Patient-Centered Care**
- Provide ***patient-centered care*** for the transgender patient with dignity and respect. **Ethics**
- Be aware that transgender people may experience gender dysphoria. **QSEN: Patient-Centered Care**
- Assess transgender patients for sources of stress that can lead to health issues. **Clinical Judgment**
- Be aware that transgender patients may experience ***health care disparities*** due to lack of insurance or other circumstances. **QSEN: Patient-Centered Care**

Physiological Integrity

- Recognize that patients receiving hormone therapy need periodic laboratory testing to monitor for adverse drug events and complications. **QSEN: Evidence-Based Practice**
- Provide thorough preoperative and postoperative care for patients having gender affirming surgery. **QSEN: Evidence-Based Practice**
- Monitor for potentially life-threatening complications of vaginoplasty, such as fistula development, bleeding, and wound infection after surgery (see Table 68.4). **Clinical Judgment**

MASTERY QUESTIONS

1. The nurse is caring for a client who reports beginning to transition from male to female. Which nursing action is appropriate regarding pronoun use?
   A. Ask the patient which pronouns are preferred and use those.
   B. Implement use of "he/him" pronouns as the client's natal sex is male.
   C. Use "Miss" or" Mrs.," since the client has begun the transition to female.
   D. Document that male or female pronouns are appropriate to use at this time.

2. Which nursing action decreases the risk for health care disparities for transgender clients? **Select all that apply.**
   A. Refer to the client's identification card for name.
   B. Determine gender identity based on clothing worn.
   C. Seek to understand the experience of the transgender client.
   D. Apologize several times if the wrong name is used for the client.
   E. On meeting the client, ask what name and which pronouns are desired.
   F. Explain how the health history and assessment are affected by gender identity.

REFERENCES

Asterisk (*) indicates a classic or definitive work on this subject.

*American Nurses Association (ANA). (2015). *Code of ethics for nurses.* Washington, DC: Author.

*Bauer, G. R., & Scheim, A. I. (2015). *Transgender people in Ontario, Canada: Statistics from the Trans PULSE Project to inform human rights policy.* London, ON: Canadian Institute of Health Research.

Burchum, J. L. R., & Rosenthal, L. D. (2019). *Lehne's pharmacology for nursing care* (10th ed.). St. Louis: Elsevier.

*Coleman, E., Bockting, W., Botzer, M., Cohen-Kettenis, P., DeCuypere, G., Fladman, J., et al. (2012). Standards of care for the health of transsexual, transgender, and gender-nonconforming people (Version 7). *International Journal of Transgenderism, 13,* 165–232.

Deutsch, M. B. (2016). *Guidelines for the primary and gender-affirming care of transgender and gender nonbinary people.* Center of Excellence for Transgender Health. University of California San Francisco. http://transhealth.ucsf.edu/trans?page=guidelines-home.

Dragon, C. N., Guerino, P., Ewald, E., & Laffan, A. M. (2017). Transgender Medicare beneficiaries and chronic conditions: Exploring fee-for-service claims data. *LGBT Health, 4*(6), 404–411.

Ettner, R., Monstrey, S., & Coleman, E. (2016). *Principles of transgender medicine and surgeries* (2nd ed.). New York: NY: Routledge.

Fenway Health. (2020). *Your care, your community.* https://fenwayhealth.org/about/history/.

Flores, A. R., Herman, J. L., Gates, G. J., & Brown, T. N. T. (2016). *How many adults identify as transgender in the United States?* Los Angeles, CA: The Williams Institute. https://williamsinstitute.law.ucla.edu/publications/trans-adults-united-states/.

Ginsberg, B. (2017). Dermatologic care of the transgender patient. *International Journal of Women's Dermatology, 3*(1), 65–67.

GLAAD. (2020). *GLAAD media reference guide: Transgender.* https://www.glaad.org/reference/transgender.

Halloran, L. (2015). Caring for transgender patients. *The Journal for Nurse Practitioners, 11*(9), 915–916.

Houghton, A. (2018). *Maintaining dignity: Understanding and responding to the challenges facing older LGBT Americans.* Washington, DC: AARP Research. https://doi.org/10.26419/res.00217.001. March 2018.

Howard, S., et al. (2019). Healthcare experiences of transgender people of color. *Journal of General Internal Medicine, 34*(10), 2068–2074.

Human Rights Campaign. (2020). *Sexual orientation and gender identity definitions.* https://www.hrc.org/resources/sexual-orientation-and-gender-identity-terminology-and-definitions.

*Institute of Medicine (IOM). (2015). *The health of LGBT people: Building a foundation for better understanding.* Washington, DC: National Academies Press.

James, S. E., Herman, J. L., Rankin, S., Keisling, M., Mottet, L., & Anafi, M. (2016). *The report of the 2015 U.S. transgender survey.* Washington, DC: National Center for Transgender Equality.

Johnson, K., et al. (2018). Gay and gray session: An interdisciplinary approach to transgender aging. *American Journal of Geriatric Psychiatry, 6*(7), 719–738.

Kraus, S., & Duhamel, K. V. (2018). Culturally competent care for older LGBTQ patients. *Nursing, 48*(8), 48–53.

Landry, J. (2017). Delivering culturally sensitive care to LGBTQI patients. *The Journal for Nurse Practitioners, 13*(5), 342–347.

Margolies, L., & Brown, C. G. (2019). Increasing cultural competence with LGBTQ patients. *Nursing, 49*(6), 34–40.

McNeill, J., Ellis, S., & Eccles, S. (2017). Suicide in trans populations: A systematic review of prevalence and correlates. *Psychology of Sexual Orientation.* https://doi.org/10.1037/sgd0000235.

Meerwijk, K. E., & Sevelius, J. M. (2017). Transgender population size in the United States: A meta-regression of population-based probability samples. *American Journal of Public Health, 107*(2), 1–8.

National Center for Transgender Equality. (2020). *Issues: Housing and homelessness.* Retrieved from https://transequality.org/issues/housing-homelessness.

Office of Disease Prevention and Health Promotion. (2020). *Healthy people 2030 Framework.*

Pfeifer, G. (2019). Panel convened to discuss end-of-life care concerns in the LGBT community. *American Journal of Nursing, 119*(9), 14.

Rooker, S., et al. (2019). The rise of the neophallus: A systematic review of penile prosthetic outcomes and complications in gender-affirming surgery. *The Journal of Sexual Medicine, 16*(5), 661–672.

Rosendale, N., Goldman, S., Ortiz, G. M., & Haber, L. A. (2018). Acute clinical care for transgender patients: A review. *JAMA Internal Medicine, 178*(11), 1535–1542.

Schwarz, K., et al. (2017). Laryngeal surgical treatment in transgender women: A systematic review and meta-analysis. *The Laryngoscope, 127,* 2596–2603.

*The Joint Commission (TJC). (2011). *Advancing effective communication, cultural competence, and patient- and family-centered care for the lesbian, gay, bisexual, and transgender community.* www.jointcommission.org/lgbt.

The Trevor Project. (2020). *Trans + gender identity.* https://www.thetrevorproject.org/trvr_support_center/trans-gender-identity/.

University of Southern California. (2020). Gender neutral pronouns. https://lgbtrc.usc.edu/trans/transgender/pronouns/

Wernick, J., et al. (2019). A systematic review of the psychological benefits of gender-affirming surgery. *Urologic Clinics, 46*(4), 475–486.

Concepts of Care for Patients With Sexually Transmitted Infections

Cherie R. Rebar

http://evolve.elsevier.com/Iggy/

LEARNING OUTCOMES

1. Collaborate with the interprofessional team to coordinate high-quality care for patients with sexually transmitted infections (STIs).
2. Provide a safe, private environment for patients when assessing and discussing STIs.
3. Teach evidence-based ways for adults to protect themselves from acquiring a sexually transmitted ***infection.***
4. Teach patients with STIs and their partners self-care measures, including the role of expedited partner therapy.
5. Implement nursing interventions to help patients cope with the psychosocial impact caused by an STI and/or ***reproduction*** concern associated with an STI.
6. Apply knowledge of anatomy, physiology, and pathophysiology to assess patients with STIs.
7. Use clinical judgment to analyze assessment findings and diagnostic data in the care of patients with STIs.
8. Plan care coordination and transition management for patients with STIs.
9. Describe ***health care disparities*** associated with the incidence and management of STIs.
10. Maintain patient confidentiality and privacy related to STIs.
11. Respect patients' personal values and beliefs regarding ***sexuality.***

KEY TERMS

chancre The ulcer that is the first sign of syphilis. It develops at the site of entry (inoculation) of the organism, usually 3 weeks after exposure. The lesion may be found on any area of the skin or mucous membranes but occurs most often on the genitalia, lips, nipples, and hands and in the oral cavity, anus, and rectum.

dyspareunia Painful sexual intercourse.

dysuria Painful urination.

endometritis Endometrial infection.

expedited partner therapy (EPT) The practice of treating sexual partners of patients diagnosed with chlamydia infection or gonorrhea by providing prescriptions or medication to the patient, which they can take to their partner(s), without the primary health care provider examining the partner(s). Also called *patient-delivered partner therapy.*

genital herpes (GH) An acute, recurring incurable viral disease of the genitalia caused by the herpes simplex virus and transmitted through contact with an infected person.

pelvic inflammatory disease (PID) An acute syndrome resulting in tenderness in the Fallopian tubes and ovaries (adnexa) and, typically, dull pelvic pain.

safer sex practices Interventions that reduce the risk of nonintact skin or mucous membranes coming in contact with infected body fluids and blood, such as using a condom.

salpingitis Fallopian tube infection.

sexually transmitted disease (STD) Term used by the Centers for Disease Control and Prevention for sexually transmitted infection.

sexually transmitted infection (STI) Infectious organisms that have been passed from one person to another through intimate contact.

syphilis A complex sexually transmitted disease that can become systemic and cause serious complications and even death.

PRIORITY AND INTERRELATED CONCEPTS

The priority concepts for this chapter are:

- ***Sexuality***
- ***Infection***
- ***Pain***

The ***Sexuality, Infection,*** and ***Pain*** concept exemplar for this chapter is Pelvic Inflammatory Disease.

The interrelated concepts for this chapter are:

- ***Reproduction***
- ***Health Care Disparities***

INTRODUCTION TO SEXUALLY TRANSMITTED INFECTIONS

Infectious organisms that have been passed from one person to another through intimate contact—usually oral, vaginal, or anal intercourse—are considered sexually transmitted infections (STIs). Some organisms that cause these diseases are transmitted only through sexual contact. Others are transmitted also by parenteral exposure to infected blood, fecal-oral transmission, intrauterine transmission to the fetus, and perinatal transmission from mother to neonate. The term sexually transmitted disease (STD) is used by the Centers for Disease Control and Prevention (CDC, 2020b). The CDC provides best practice guidelines for treatment of STIs (CDC, 2015). This includes information, treatment standards, and counseling recommendations to help decrease the spread of these diseases and their complications.

The reported numbers of cases of STIs are influenced by improved diagnostic techniques, increased knowledge about organisms that can be sexually transmitted, and changes in ***sexuality*** (see Chapter 1) and sexual practices. Other factors such as an increasing population, cultural practices, political and economic policies, incidences of sexual abuse and human trafficking, and international travel and migration also affect the prevalence of STIs.

The prevalence of STIs is a major public health concern worldwide. People at greatest risk for acquiring an STI include those who (American College of Obstetricians and Gynecologists, 2017; U.S. Department of Health and Human Services, 2020a):

- Have more than one sexual partner (especially anonymous partners)
- Have had more than one sexual partner in the past
- Engage in sexual activity with someone who has an STI
- Have a history of having an STI
- Use intravenous drugs
- Have or had a partner who uses (used) intravenous drugs
- Engage in anal, vaginal, or oral sex without a condom
- Have sex while using drugs or alcohol

There are populations that are more affected than others, and a key nursing role is to ensure that all people are equally assessed for, and educated about, STIs. It is important to not assume that certain groups are less vulnerable than others, as sexual practices and knowledge about self-protection vary greatly.

PATIENT-CENTERED CARE: OLDER ADULT CONSIDERATIONS QSEN

Older adults may not realize their risk for STIs or feel comfortable discussing ***sexuality*** with health care providers. Provide a safe and private environment to teach older adults who are sexually active about their risk for developing STIs, and how to protect themselves.

One of the greatest factors associated with STI prevalence is the interest in ***sexuality,*** sexual behaviors, and intimacy in the American culture. The stigma of STIs in the United States has been associated with higher rates of these infections compared with rates in other developed countries. The prevalence of STIs is also affected by changing human physiology patterns such as earlier onset of menarche, comorbidities associated with human immune deficiency virus (HIV) and diabetes, and ***health care disparities*** (see Chapter 1). Misuse of substances has also been identified as a significant risk factor because of the effects that drugs have on decision making and risk-taking behavior.

STIs cause complications that can contribute to severe physical and emotional pain, including infertility, ectopic pregnancy, cancer, and death. Some of the most common complications caused by sexually transmitted organisms are listed in Table 69.1.

Certain types of STIs must be reported to local health authorities. Check requirements in your state, and communicate incidences of reportable STIs accordingly (see the Ethical/Legal Considerations: Reporting Sexually Transmitted Infections [STIs] box).

ETHICAL/LEGAL CONSIDERATIONS

Reporting Sexually Transmitted Infections (STIs)

Chlamydia ***infection,*** gonorrhea, syphilis, chancroid, and HIV infection (through HIV Stage III—acquired immune deficiency syndrome [AIDS]) are notifiable to local health authorities in every state (CDC, 2020a). Other STIs such as genital herpes (GH) may or may not be reported, depending on local legal requirements. Positive results can be reported by clinicians and laboratories. Reports are kept strictly confidential.

Nurses in all environments of care have a responsibility to recognize patients who are at risk for or who have STIs, possibly while being treated for another unrelated health problem. Sexual issues, particularly those involving suspected or actual STIs, are sensitive, personal, and sometimes controversial. As a patient advocate, demonstrate a nonjudgmental attitude when caring for people who have concerns related to ***sexuality.*** Providing confidentiality and privacy is essential for patients to receive correct information, make informed decisions, and obtain evidence-based care.

Recognize that 88% of victims of human trafficking have had to seek medical care at some point (The Joint Commission, 2019). In any clinical setting, you are in a key position to identify and assist victims. Signs of trafficking can be found in Chapter 10. Best practices for identifying and caring for people who may need assistance include (The Joint Commission, 2019):

- Interviewing the patient without the presence of a partner or other person who accompanies them
- Providing professional interpreters, if needed; never rely on the partner or others to speak for the patient
- Collaborating with social workers, sexual assault nurse examiners (SANEs), and other members of the interprofessional team, as indicated
- Ensuring that documentation is consistent if there are concerns regarding trafficking

PATIENT-CENTERED CARE: GENDER HEALTH CONSIDERATIONS QSEN

Because of the very vascular and large surface area of the mucous membranes of the vagina, women are more easily infected with STIs and are at greater risk for STI-related health problems than are men. Women are also more vulnerable to infections because of the exposure of cervical basal epithelium cells. Lesbian women who exclusively have had sex with women have a *lower* risk for STIs than women who have had sex with men (Molin et al., 2016). Transgender women have a *higher* rate of HIV infection (Neumann et al., 2017; Raiford et al., 2016) than others.

Changing social relationships later in life affect risk for exposure to STIs. Women who are no longer concerned with pregnancy may be at risk for STIs if they do not use barrier methods. Physiologic changes experienced by postmenopausal women such as mucosal tears from vaginal atrophy increase risk.

Women have more asymptomatic infections, which may delay diagnosis and treatment. Many infectious organisms reside in the cervical os and cause little change in vaginal discharge or vulvar tissue, so women are not aware that they are infected. This delay increases the risk for complications, including ascending infections that may cause reproductive organ damage and illness. Embarrassment, denial, or fear about STIs may further delay treatment, increasing the potential for serious complications.

Health Promotion and Maintenance

A *Healthy People 2020* objective is to reduce sustained domestic transmission of primary and secondary syphilis (U.S. Department of Health and Human Services, 2020b) (Table 69.2). *Healthy People 2030,* in development at the time of publication, also contains proposed objectives to reduce syphilis specifically in women, as well as to reduce congenital syphilis (U.S. Department of Health and Human Services, 2019). One of the primary tools for prevention of sexually transmitted infections (STIs), including syphilis, is education. All people, regardless of age, natal gender, gender identity, ethnicity, socioeconomic status, education level, or sexual orientation, are susceptible to these diseases. Health literacy, motivation, and perceived risk can affect the health status of any patient. Do not assume that a person is not sexually active because of age, education, marital status, profession, culture, or religion.

STIs are largely preventable through safer sex practices. Discuss prevention methods, including safer sex, with all patients who are or may become sexually active. **Safer sex practices** are those that reduce the risk for nonintact skin or mucous membranes coming in contact with infected body fluids and blood. These practices include:

- Using a latex or polyurethane condom for genital and anal intercourse
- Using a condom or latex barrier (dental dam) over the genitals or anus during oral-genital or oral-anal sexual contact

TABLE 69.1 Complications Caused by Sexually Transmitted Organisms

Complication	Causative Organisms
Salpingitis, infertility, and ectopic pregnancy	*Neisseria gonorrhoeae* *Chlamydia trachomatis* *Mycoplasma hominis* *Ureaplasma urealyticum*
Puerperal infection	*N. gonorrhoeae* *C. trachomatis*
Perinatal infection	Hepatitis B virus HIV Human papillomavirus *N. gonorrhoeae* *C. trachomatis* Herpes simplex virus *Treponema pallidum* Cytomegalovirus Group B streptococci
Cancer of genital area	Human papillomavirus
Male urethritis	*M. hominis* Herpes simplex virus *N. gonorrhoeae* *C. trachomatis* *U. urealyticum*
Vulvovaginitis	Herpes simplex virus *Trichomonas vaginalis* Bacterial vaginosis *Candida albicans*
Cervicitis	*N. gonorrhoeae* *C. trachomatis* Herpes simplex virus
Proctitis	*N. gonorrhoeae* *C. trachomatis* Herpes simplex virus *Campylobacter jejuni* *Shigella* species *Entamoeba histolytica*
Hepatitis	*T. pallidum* Hepatitis A, hepatitis B, and hepatitis C viruses
Dermatitis	*Sarcoptes scabiei* *Phthirus pubis*
Genital ulceration or warts	*C. trachomatis* Herpes simplex virus Human papillomavirus *T. pallidum* *Haemophilus ducreyi* *Calymmatobacterium granulomatis*

TABLE 69.2 Meeting *Healthy People 2020* Objectives and Targets for Improvement: Sexually Transmitted Infections/Diseases

- Reduce the proportion of adolescents and young adults with *Chlamydia trachomatis* infections
- Increase the proportion of sexually active females aged 24 years and under enrolled in Medicaid plans who are screened for genital *Chlamydia* infections during the measurement year
- Increase the proportion of sexually active females aged 24 years and younger enrolled in commercial health insurance plans who are screened for genital *Chlamydia* infections during the measurement year
- Reduce gonorrhea rates
- Reduce sustained domestic transmission of primary and secondary syphilis
- Reduce the proportion of females with human papillomavirus (HPV) infection
- Reduce the proportion of young adults with genital herpes due to herpes simplex type 2

Data from https://www.healthypeople.gov/2020/topics-objectives/topic/sexually-transmitted-diseases/objectives.

- Wearing gloves for finger or hand contact with the vagina or rectum
- Practicing abstinence
- Practicing mutual monogamy
- Decreasing the number of sexual partners

GENITAL HERPES

Pathophysiology Review

Genital herpes (GH) is an acute, recurring, common viral disease. Although preventative and therapeutic vaccines are still under investigation, at this time, GH is still considered incurable (American Sexual Health Association, 2020). Two serotypes of herpes simplex virus (HSV) affect the genitalia: type 1 (HSV-1) and type 2 (HSV-2) (McCance et al., 2019). Most *nongenital* lesions such as cold sores are caused by HSV-1, transmitted via oral-oral contact. Historically, HSV-2 caused most of the genital lesions. However, either type can produce oral or genital lesions through oral-genital or genital-genital contact with an infected person. HSV-2 recurs and sheds asymptomatically more often than HSV-1. Many people with GH have not been diagnosed because they have mild symptoms and shed the virus intermittently.

The incubation period of genital herpes is 2 to 20 days (average is 1 week). Many people do not have symptoms during the primary outbreak. The virus remains dormant and recurs periodically, even if the patient is asymptomatic. Recurrences are not caused by reinfection; they are related to *viral shedding, and the patient is infectious.* Long-term complications of GH include the risk for neonatal transmission and an increased risk for acquiring HIV ***infection*** (McCance et al., 2019).

HSV-1 is highest in prevalence among Mexican Americans, and HSV-2 is highest in prevalence among non-Hispanic blacks (National Center for Health Statistics [NCHS], 2018). The overall prevalence of HSV-1 and HSV-2 in the United States has continued to decrease over time since 2000 (NCHS, 2018).

FOCUSED ASSESSMENT

The Patient With a Sexually Transmitted Infection

Assess history of present illness:
- Chief concern
- Time of onset
- Symptoms by quality and quantity, precipitating and palliative factors
- Any treatments taken (self-prescribed or over-the-counter products), and whether they have been helpful

Assess past medical history:
- Major health problems, including any history of STIs, PID, or immunosuppression
- Surgeries: obstetric and gynecologic; circumcision

Assess current health status:
- Menstrual history for irregularities
- Sexual history:
  - Type and frequency of sexual activity
  - Number of lifetime and past 6 months sexual contacts/partners; or monogamous
  - Sexual orientation
  - Contraception history
- Medications
- Allergies
- Lifestyle risks: drugs, alcohol, tobacco

Assess preventive health care practices:
- Papanicolaou (Pap) tests
- Regular STI screening
- Use of barrier contraceptives to prevent STIs and/or pregnancy

Assess physical examination findings:
- Vital signs
- Oropharyngeal findings
- Abdominal findings
- Genital or pelvic findings
- Anorectal findings

Assess laboratory data:
- Urinalysis
- Hematology
- ESR or CRP if PID is being considered
- Cervical, urethral, oral, rectal specimens
- Lesion samples for microbiology and virology
- Pregnancy testing

CRP, C-reactive protein; *ESR,* erythrocyte sedimentation rate; *PID,* pelvic inflammatory disease; *STI,* sexually transmitted infection.

Interprofessional Collaborative Care

Assessment: Recognize Cues. The diagnosis of GH is based on the patient's history and physical examination (see the Focused Assessment: The Patient With a Sexually Transmitted Infection box).

Ask the patient if he or she felt itching or a tingling sensation in the skin 1 to 2 days before the outbreak, known as the *prodrome.* These sensations are usually followed by the appearance of **vesicles** (blisters) in a typical cluster on the vulva (Fig. 69.1), vagina, cervix, scrotum, penis (Fig. 69.2), or perianal region at the site of inoculation. The blisters rupture spontaneously in a

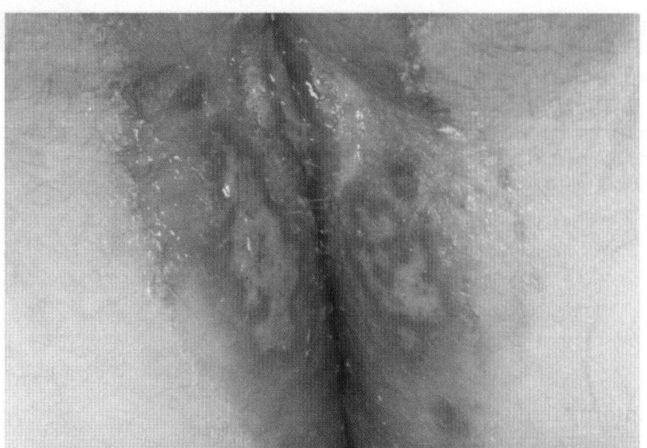

FIG. 69.1 Herpes simplex virus type 2 (HSV-2) infection; blisters on the vulva. (From Jarvis, C. [2020]. *Physical examination and health assessment* [8th ed.]. St. Louis: Elsevier.)

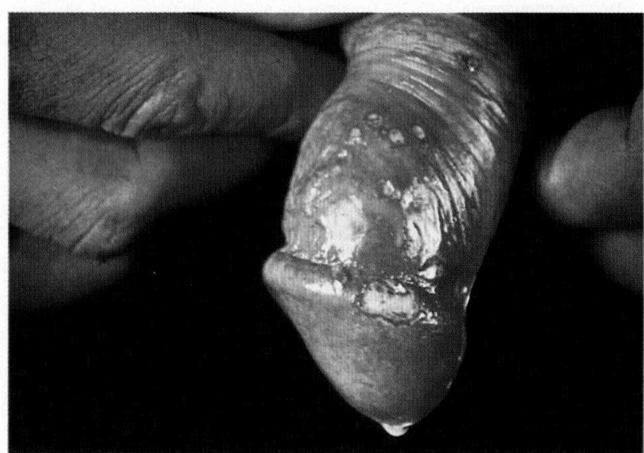

FIG. 69.2 Herpes simplex virus type 2 (HSV-2) infection; blisters on the penis. (From Jarvis, C. [2020]. *Physical examination and health assessment* [8th ed.]. St. Louis: Elsevier.)

day or two and leave ulcerations that can become extensive and cause ***pain.***

Assess for other symptoms such as headaches, fever, general malaise, and swelling of inguinal lymph nodes. Ask if urination is painful. External dysuria is a painful symptom when urine passes over the eroded areas. Patients with urinary retention may need to be catheterized. Lesions resolve within 2 to 6 weeks. After the lesions heal, the virus remains in a dormant state in the sacral nerve ganglia.

Periodically the virus activates, and symptoms recur. These recurrences can be triggered by stress, fever, sunburn, poor nutrition, menses, and sexual activity. Provide anticipatory guidance regarding stressor management to prevent outbreaks.

GH is usually confirmed through a viral culture or polymerase chain reaction (PCR) assays of the lesions (Albrecht, 2018). Fluid from inside the blister obtained within 48 hours of the first outbreak will yield the most reliable results because accuracy decreases as the blisters begin to heal. Direct fluorescent antibody can also be used. Serology testing, which is glycoprotein G antibody based, can identify the HSV type, either 1 or 2. Antibodies may take up to 12 weeks to develop, so false-negative results can occur if testing is performed too soon after the initial infection (Albrecht, 2018).

BEST PRACTICE FOR PATIENT SAFETY & QUALITY CARE

Care of or Self-Management for the Patient With Genital Herpes (GH)

- Administer oral analgesics as prescribed.
- Apply local anesthetic sprays or ointments as prescribed.
- Apply ice packs or warm compresses to lesions.
- Administer sitz baths three or four times a day.
- Encourage increase in fluid intake to replace fluid lost through open lesions.
- Encourage frequent urination.
- Pour water over genitalia while voiding or encourage voiding while standing in a shower.
- Catheterize as necessary and prescribed.
- Encourage genital hygiene, and teach to keep the skin clean and dry.
- Wear gloves when applying ointments or making any direct contact with lesions.
- Wash hands thoroughly after contact with lesions
- Launder towels that have had direct contact with lesions.
- Teach avoidance of sexual activity when lesions are present.
- Teach use of latex or polyurethane condoms during all sexual exposures.
- Teach about the use, side effects, and risks versus benefits of antiviral agents.
- Encourage discussion of the diagnosis of GH with current and new partners.

◆ **Interventions: Take Action.** The desired outcomes of treatment for patients infected with GH are to decrease ***pain*** from ulcerations, promote healing without secondary infection, decrease viral shedding, and prevent ***infection*** transmission (see the Best Practice for Patient Safety & Quality Care: Care of or Self-Management for the Patient With Genital Herpes [GH] box).

Drug Therapy. Antiviral drugs are used to treat GH. The drugs decrease the severity, promote healing, and decrease the frequency of recurrent outbreaks, but do not cure the ***infection.***

Drug therapy should be offered to anyone with an initial outbreak of GH regardless of the severity of the symptoms. The CDC (2015) recommends treatment with acyclovir, famciclovir, or valacyclovir. Intravenous acyclovir and hospitalization may be indicated for patients with severe HSV and possibly fatal infections, such as disseminated (systemic) disease or encephalitis (brain infection) (Albrecht, 2019).

Dosage and length of treatment differ and can be discussed between the patient and health care provider. Intermittent therapy for recurrent outbreaks is most beneficial if it is started within 1 day of the appearance of lesions or during the period of itching or tingling before lesions appear. Daily antiviral therapy (called *chronic suppressive therapy*) can also be offered to patients (Albrecht, 2019; Burchum & Rosenthal, 2019). Suppression reduces recurrences in most patients, but it does not prevent viral shedding, even when symptoms are absent. Encourage patients on chronic suppressive therapy to follow up at least annually with their provider.

Self-Management Education. Nursing interventions focus on ***pain*** control by treatment of the underlying problem, and patient education. Teach about the ***infection,*** modes of sexual transmission, potential for recurrent episodes, and correct use and possible side effects of antiviral therapy. Clear discussion about sexual activity, including whether the patient has new or multiple partners, is an essential component of the nurse's intervention.

Assess the patient's and partner's emotional responses to the diagnosis of GH. Many people are initially shocked and need reassurance that they can manage the disease. Patients who are infected may have feelings of disbelief, uncleanness, isolation, and loneliness. They may be angry at their partner(s) for transmitting the ***infection*** or fear rejection because they have it. Help patients cope with the diagnosis by being nonjudgmental, sensitive, and supportive during assessments and interventions. Encourage social support and refer patients to support groups (e.g., local support groups of the Herpes Resource Center [http://www.ashasexualhealth.org/stdsstis/herpes/]) and therapists. Symptomatic care may include oral analgesics, topical anesthetics, sitz baths, and increased oral fluid intake. People who have tested serology positive for HSV-1 or HSV-2 but have never had GH symptoms should be counseled with the same information as those who have symptoms.

! NURSING SAFETY PRIORITY QSEN

Action Alert

Remind patients to abstain from sexual activity while GH lesions are present. Sexual activity can cause ***pain,*** and likelihood of viral transmission is higher. Urge condom use during all sexual encounters because of the increased risk for HSV transmission from viral shedding, which can occur even when lesions are not present. Teach the patient how to properly use condoms (see the Patient and Family Education: Preparing for Self-Management: Use of Condoms box).

PATIENT AND FAMILY EDUCATION: PREPARING FOR SELF-MANAGEMENT

Use of Condoms

- Use latex or polyurethane condoms; avoid natural membrane condoms as they provide much less protection.
- Use a new condom with every sexual encounter (including oral, vaginal, and anal).
- Internal condoms ("female condoms")—polyurethane or nitrile sheaths in the vagina—are thought to be somewhat protective against STIs, but have not been studied as closely as traditional male condoms (Hoke et al., 2020).
- Condoms can break during sexual intercourse. If a condom breaks, replace it immediately.
- Keep condoms (especially latex) in a cool, dry place, out of direct sunlight.
- Do not use condoms that are in damaged packages or are brittle or discolored.
- Always handle a condom with care to avoid damaging it with fingernails, teeth, or other sharp objects.
- Put condoms on before any genital contact. Hold the condom by the tip and unroll it on the penis. Leave a space at the tip to collect semen.
- Ensure that lubricant, if used, is water based and washes away with water. Oil-based products damage latex condoms.
- Use of spermicide (nonoxynol-9) with condoms, either lubricated condoms or vaginal application, has *not* been proven to be more or less effective against STIs than use without spermicide. Nonoxynol-9 may increase risk for transmission of HIV in women during vaginal and anal intercourse, so its use is discouraged (Bartz, 2019; World Health Organization, 2020).
- After ejaculation, withdraw the erect penis carefully, holding the condom at the base of the penis to prevent the condom from slipping off.
- Never use a condom more than once.

STI, Sexually transmitted infection.
Modified from Centers for Disease Control and Prevention (CDC). (2015). Sexually transmitted diseases treatment guidelines, 2015. *Morbidity and Mortality Weekly Report Recommendations and Reports, 64*(RR-3), 1-137.

SYPHILIS

Pathophysiology Review

Syphilis is a complex sexually transmitted **infection** (STI) that can become systemic and cause serious complications, including death. The causative organism is a spirochete called *Treponema pallidum.* The infection is usually transmitted by sexual contact and blood exposure, but transmission can occur through close body contact such as touching or kissing where there are open lesions (e.g., on the breast, genitals, or lips, or in the oral cavity) (Hicks & Clement, 2020a).

Untreated syphilis is divided into two categories—early and late—and progresses through four stages: primary (localized chancre), secondary (systemic illness), early latent (seropositive yet without symptoms), and tertiary (symptomatic infection). Neurosyphilis can occur at any time in any stage; patients with this form of the disease may experience meningitis, vision or hearing loss, and brain and spinal cord dysfunction.

The appearance of an ulcer called a chancre is the first sign of *primary* syphilis (Fig. 69.3). It develops at the site of entry (inoculation) of the organism from 12 days to 12 weeks days after exposure (3 weeks is average) (McCance et al., 2019). Chancres may be found on any area of the skin or mucous membranes but occur most often on the genitalia (Hicks & Clement, 2020a).

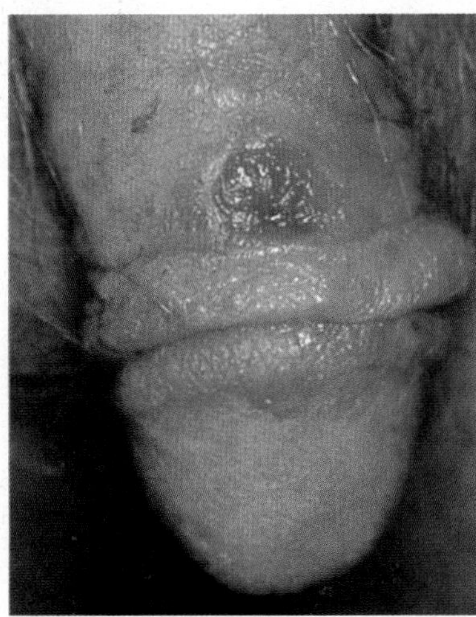

FIG. 69.3 Syphilitic chancre on the penis. (From Jarvis, C. [2020]. *Physical examination and health assessment* [8th ed.]. St. Louis: Elsevier.)

During this highly infectious stage, the chancre begins as a small papule, approximately 1 to 2 cm in diameter with a raised margin (Hicks & Clement, 2020a). Within 3 to 7 days, it breaks down into its typical appearance: a painless, indurated, smooth, weeping lesion. Regional lymph nodes enlarge, feel firm, and are not painful. Without treatment, the chancre usually disappears within 3 to 6 weeks (Hicks & Clement, 2020a). However, the organism spreads throughout the body, and the patient is still infectious.

Secondary syphilis develops in approximately 25% of untreated infected persons within a few months (Hicks & Clement, 2020a). During this stage, syphilis is a systemic disease because the spirochetes circulate throughout the bloodstream. Commonly mistaken for influenza, signs and symptoms include malaise, low-grade fever, headache, muscular aches, sore throat, hoarseness, generalized adenopathy, joint pain, and a generalized rash (McCance et al., 2020a). There is no typical appearance of this rash, but it usually appears on the palm, soles, trunk, and mucous membranes. It can appear as diffuse macules (reddish brown), papules (usually less than 5 mm) or pustules, scaly psoriasis-like lesions (Fig. 69.4), or gray-white wartlike lesions (condylomata lata). *All of these lesions are highly contagious and should not be touched without gloves.* Patchy alopecia on the scalp or facial hair (missing part of the eyebrow, "moth-eaten" appearance) is another symptom. The rash subsides without treatment in 4 to 12 weeks (McCance et al., 2019), and the patient enters the early latent stage, during which he or she is seropositive but asymptomatic. The stage may last as little as a year, or as long as a lifetime (McCance et al., 2019).

Tertiary, or late, syphilis is uncommon because of the widespread availability of antibiotics (McCance et al., 2019). If experienced, this occurs after a highly variable period, from 4 to 20 years. This stage develops in untreated cases and can mimic other conditions because any organ system can be affected. Signs and symptoms of late syphilis include (McCance et al., 2019):

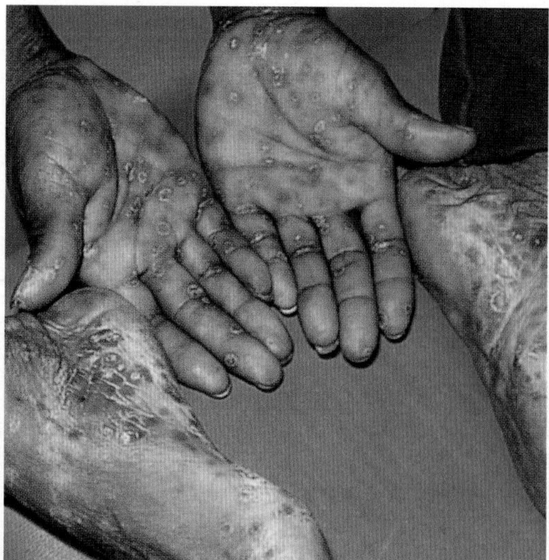

FIG. 69.4 Palmar and plantar secondary syphilis. (From Morse, S., Ballard, R., Holmes, K., & Moreland, A. [2003]. *Atlas of sexually transmitted diseases and AIDS* [3rd ed.]. Edinburgh: Mosby.)

- Cardiovascular infection with *T. pallidum,* which may cause aneurysms, heart valve insufficiencies, and heart failure
- Neurosyphilis, including progressive dementia and locomotor ataxia
- Gummatous syphilis (uncommon) lesions on the skin, bones, or internal organs

PATIENT-CENTERED CARE: CULTURAL/SPIRITUAL CONSIDERATIONS QSEN

Health care disparities exist between racial and ethnic groups in the incidence of primary and secondary syphilis. In recent reports from the CDC (2020b, 2018c), the prevalence of syphilis was highest among blacks and Native Hawaiians/Other Pacific Islanders (NHOPI). The reason for these differences is unclear, but access to high-quality health care is thought to be a factor (CDC, 2018b).

PATIENT-CENTERED CARE: GENDER HEALTH CONSIDERATIONS QSEN

Identify unique needs regarding sexual health and prevention and treatment of STIs for lesbian, gay, bisexual, transgender, and questioning (LGBTQ) patients. Discrimination, ***health care disparities,*** and health care provider lack of understanding can greatly affect the health status of this population (Fenway Health, 2020). People who identify as LGBTQ may have difficulty finding health care providers who ask about and address their particular needs, risks, and concerns. Taking a health history that provides opportunity for the patient to identify sexual orientation, gender identity, and sexual activity is crucial.

Especially among transgender people, opportunities for health assessment may be avoided by the patient or missed by the provider because of fears of being misunderstood or inadequately prepared to give or receive appropriate care. Chapter 1 describes recommendations for communicating with this population. Chapter 68 discusses the special health care needs of transgender patients.

PATIENT-CENTERED CARE: GENDER HEALTH CONSIDERATIONS QSEN

Gay, bisexual, and other men who have sex with men (MSM) are at greatest risk for contracting primary and secondary syphilis and made up 79.6% of cases of these diseases in 2017 (CDC, 2018b). Assuming that gay men or lesbian women have sex only with same-gender partners or similarly assuming that heterosexual patients never have sexual encounters with partners of the same sex limits the accuracy of the nurse's risk assessment.

❖ Interprofessional Collaborative Care

◆ **Assessment: Recognize Cues.** Assessment of the patient with signs and symptoms of syphilis begins with gathering a history about ulcers or rash. Take a sexual history and conduct a risk assessment to include whether previous testing or treatment for syphilis or other STDs has ever been done (see the Focused Assessment: The Patient With a Sexually Transmitted Infection box). Ask about allergic reactions to drugs, especially penicillin. A woman may report inguinal lymph node enlargement resulting from a chancre in the vagina or cervix that is not easily visible to her. She may report a history of contact with a male partner who had an ulcer that she noticed during a sexual encounter. Men usually discover the chancre on the penis or scrotum.

Conduct a physical examination, including inspection and palpation. *Wear gloves while palpating any lesions because of the highly contagious treponemes that are present.* Observe for and document rashes of any type because of the variable presentation of secondary syphilis.

The health care provider will obtain a specimen of the chancre for examination under a darkfield microscope. Diagnosis of primary or secondary syphilis is confirmed if *T. pallidum* is present.

Nontreponemal blood tests include the *Venereal Disease Research Laboratory (VDRL)* serum test, the more sensitive *rapid plasma reagin (RPR)* test, and the *toluidine red unheated serum test (TRUST)*. These tests are based on an antibody-antigen reaction that determines the presence and amount of antibodies produced by the body in response to an ***infection*** by *T. pallidum*. False-positive and false-negative results are a downfall of these types of tests.

Treponemal tests detect antibodies directed against treponemal antigens; they are more reliable than nontreponemal tests (Hicks & Clement, 2020a). These include:

- Fluorescent treponemal antibody absorption (FTA-ABS) test
- Microhemagglutination test for antibodies to *T. pallidum* (MHA-TP)
- *T. pallidum* particle agglutination assay (TPPA)
- *T. pallidum* enzyme immunoassay (TP-EIA)
- Chemiluminescence immunoassay (CIA)

Patients who are shown to be reactive to one of these nontreponemal tests will have this positive result for their entire life, even after treatment. This may be surprising news for a patient who denies a history of or does not know that he or she had syphilis. Use therapeutic communication skills and a nonjudgmental attitude to objectively discuss this finding.

◆ Interventions: Take Action

Drug Therapy. Interprofessional collaborative care includes drug therapy and health teaching to resolve the ***infection*** and prevent transmission to others. Benzathine penicillin G given IM as a single dose at the time of the initial visit with the health care provider is the evidence-based treatment for primary, secondary, and early latent syphilis (CDC, 2015). Patients in the latent stage receive weekly treatment for a longer time (CDC, 2015). A different regimen, found in the CDC's *2015 STD Treatment Guidelines,* is recommended for patients who are pregnant or have HIV.

! NURSING SAFETY PRIORITY (QSEN)

Drug Alert

Allergic reactions to benzathine penicillin G can occur. Monitor for allergic signs and symptoms (e.g., rash, edema, shortness of breath, chest tightness, anxiety). Penicillin desensitization is recommended for penicillin-allergic patients. *Keep all patients at the health care agency for at least 30 minutes after they have received the antibiotic so signs and symptoms of an allergic reaction can be detected and treated. The most severe reaction is anaphylaxis. Treatment should be available and implemented immediately if symptoms occur.* Chapter 18 describes the management of drug allergies in detail.

The *Jarisch-Herxheimer reaction* may also follow antibiotic therapy for syphilis. This reaction is caused by the rapid release of products from the disruption of the cells of the organism. Symptoms include fever, generalized aches, rigors, vasodilation, diaphoresis, hypotension, and worsening of any rash that was present. These symptoms are usually benign and begin within 24 hours after therapy, and are treated symptomatically with analgesics and antipyretics (Hicks & Clement, 2020b).

Self-Management Education. To provide teaching, choose a setting that offers privacy and encourages open discussion. Discuss the importance of partner notification and treatment, including the risk for reinfection if the partner goes untreated. All sexual partners must be prophylactically treated as soon as possible, preferably within 90 days of the syphilis diagnosis.

Inform the patient that the disease will be reported to the local health authority and that all information will be held in strict confidence. Urge the patient to keep follow-up appointments. For primary and secondary syphilis, drug therapy is provided at the first visit, which may suggest to the patient that no further visits are indicated or important. Remind the patient that follow-up for self and partner(s) is critical, and that sexual abstinence is recommended until full treatment is complete. After the initial antibiotic, the CDC recommends follow-up evaluation, including blood tests at 6, 12, and 24 months. Repeat treatment may be needed if the patient does not respond to the initial antibiotic.

The emotional responses to syphilis vary and may include feelings of fear, depression, guilt, and anxiety. Patients may experience guilt if they have infected others or anger if a partner has infected them. If further psychosocial interventions are needed, encourage the patient to discuss these feelings or refer him or her to other resources such as psychotherapy, self-help support groups, or STI/STD clinics.

NCLEX EXAMINATION CHALLENGE 69.1

Physiological Integrity

The nurse is caring for a client who has just been diagnosed with primary syphilis. Which client statement reflects that teaching has been effective? **Select all that apply.**

A. "I can resume having intercourse right after this injection."
B. "At least this infection is not as serious as gonorrhea or chlamydia."
C. "I'm afraid, but I'm going to tell my partners about my diagnosis."
D. "After my treatment, I still need several follow-up appointments."
E. "I can take acetaminophen if I get a fever and chills after this shot."
F. "I am going to wait here in the clinic 30 minutes after treatment."

CONDYLOMATA ACUMINATA (GENITAL WARTS)

Pathophysiology Review

Condylomata acuminata (genital warts) are caused by certain types of *human papillomavirus (HPV)*. Genital warts are a very common viral disease that is sexually transmitted and often coexist with other infections. Most of these infections

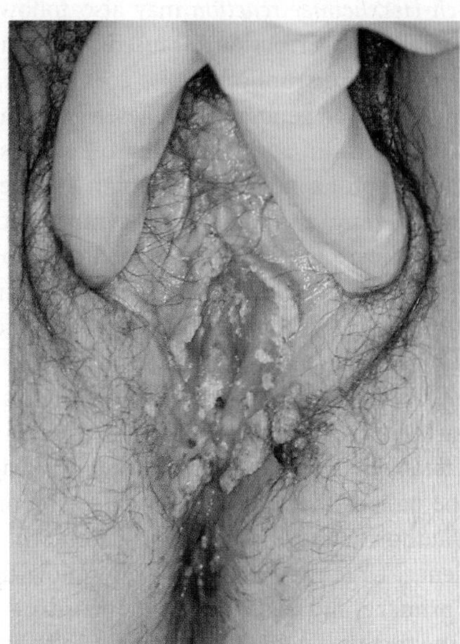

FIG. 69.5 Genital warts on the vulva. (From Jarvis, C. [2020]. *Physical examination and health assessment* [8th ed.]. St. Louis: Elsevier.)

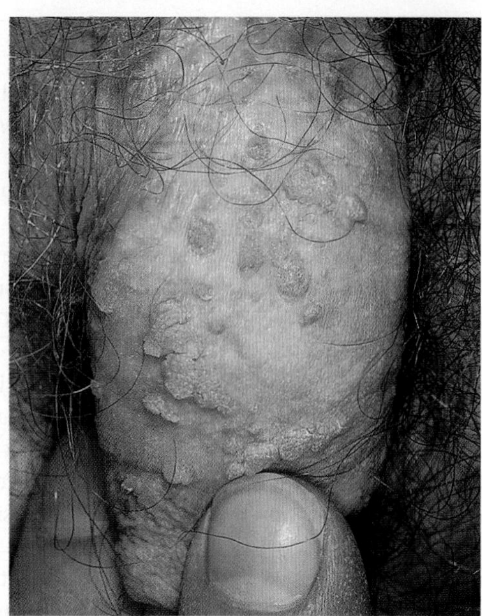

FIG. 69.6 Genital warts on the penis. (From Jarvis, C. [2020]. *Physical examination and health assessment* [8th ed.]. St. Louis: Elsevier.)

originate from HPV types 6 and 11, which cause 90% of genital warts (Palefsky, 2019). HPV types 16, 18, 31, 33, 45, 52, and 58 are associated with precancerous or dysplastic lesions, as well as cervical, vulvar, vaginal, and anal cancers (Merck Sharp & Dohme Corp., 2019). HPV infection has been established as the primary risk factor for development of cervical cancer. Evidence shows that HPV can also cause cancer of the penis and the oropharynx (throat, tongue, and tonsils) (CDC, 2019). High-risk HPV (strains that cause cancer) ***infection*** may coexist with low-risk HPV (strains that cause warts). The presence of one strain increases the risk for acquiring other strains.

❖ Interprofessional Collaborative Care

◆ **Assessment: Recognize Cues.** The diagnosis of condylomata acuminata is made by examination of the lesions. They are initially small, papillary growths that are white or resemble the color of the patient's skin (Figs. 69.5 and 69.6) and may grow into large cauliflower-like masses (Fig. 69.7). Multiple warts usually occur in the same area. Bleeding may occur if the wart is disturbed. Warts may disappear or resolve on their own without treatment. They may occur once or recur at the original site. Warts can occur on the external or internal surfaces of the genitalia, including the mucosal surfaces of the vagina and urethra. Screening for HPV and dysplasia of the cervix is done by obtaining cervical specimens for Papanicolaou (Pap) and HPV DNA testing.

Identifying high-risk strains of HPV and correlating with abnormal Pap smear findings are the standard of care (CDC, 2015). The diagnosis should include consideration of condyloma lata (which occurs in secondary syphilis) because STIs frequently coexist. Blood tests, an HIV test, and cultures for chlamydia and gonorrhea infections are done. If a wartlike lesion bleeds easily, appears infected, is atypical, or persists, a biopsy of the lesion is performed to rule out other pathologic problems such as cancer. A biopsy of warts that are seen on the cervix should be performed before any treatment to eradicate them.

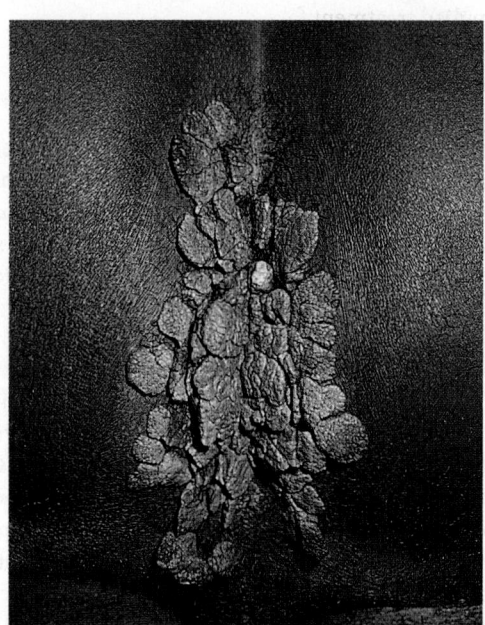

FIG. 69.7 Perianal condylomata acuminata. (From Morse, S., Ballard, R., Holmes, K., & Moreland, A. [2003]. *Atlas of sexually transmitted diseases and AIDS* [3rd ed.]. Edinburgh: Mosby.)

◆ **Interventions: Take Action.** The outcome of treatment is to remove the warts. No current therapy eliminates the HPV ***infection,*** and recurrences after treatment are likely. It is not known whether removal of visible warts decreases the risk for disease transmission.

Nonsurgical Management. Patients may be prescribed cryodestructive therapies such as podophyllotoxin, podophyllum resin, or trichloroacetic acid (TCA) as personally applied topical applications for treatment of warts (Carusi, 2019). Immune-mediated therapies include imiquimod (topical), sinecatechins (topical), and interferons (available as a topical treatment, as well as through IM and subcutaneous injections). Patients taking imiquimod should be taught to minimize exposure to the sun and tanning beds, wear protective clothing, and use sunscreen, as this medication increases sensitivity to ultraviolet radiation (Burchum & Rosenthal, 2019). These treatments are less expensive than those performed in the health care provider's office, but they take longer for healing. *Teach patients that over-the-counter (OTC) wart treatments should not be used on genital tissue.*

Surgical Management. Surgical excision, cryoablation, laser ablation, electrocautery, and ultrasonic aspiration are treatment options that the health care provider can perform (Carusi, 2019). Extensive warts have been treated with carbon dioxide laser procedures, intralesion interferon injections, and surgical removal (CDC, 2015). The choice of treatment is based on the patient's individualized presentation, including number, size, and location of warts; preference of the patient; cost; adverse effects; the skills of the clinician; and treatment availability.

Self-Management Education. The priority nursing intervention is patient and sexual partner education about the mode of transmission, incubation period, treatment, and complications, especially the association with various types of cancer. Teach about local care for postsurgical lesions or patient-applied treatment for self-management.

! NURSING SAFETY PRIORITY QSEN

Drug Alert

Teach patients that, after treatment with podophyllotoxin, podophyllum resin, or trichloroacetic acid (TCA), they may experience ***pain,*** bleeding, or discharge from the site or sloughing of parts of warts. Teach to keep the area clean and dry, and to be alert for any signs or symptoms of further ***infection*** or side effects of the treatment.

Inform patients that recurrence is likely, especially in the first 3 months, and that repeated treatments may be needed. Urge all patients to have complete STI testing, since exposure to one STI increases the risk for contracting another. Sexual partners should also be evaluated and offered treatment if warts are present. Teach patients to avoid intimate sexual contact until external lesions are healed, and to use condoms to help reduce transmission even after warts have been treated (see the Patient and Family Education: Preparing for Self-Management: Use of Condoms box). Teach women to follow the U.S. Preventive Services Task Force (2018) recommendations on Pap and HPV testing:

- If 21 to 29 years old, get a Pap test every 3 years.
- If 30 to 65 years old, get:
  - A Pap test every 3 years, or
  - An HPV test every 5 years, or
  - A Pap test and HPV test together (called co-testing) every 5 years
- If older than 65, ask the health care provider whether Pap tests and HPV tests can be stopped.

Vaccination to protect patients against HPV is one of the most important interventions available, especially for MSM and immunocompromised young adults (CDC, 2015). Teach patients about the various vaccinations available (Table 69.3), and encourage them to be immunized.

TABLE 69.3 Human Papillomavirus (HPV) Vaccines

Vaccination	HPV Type	Gender and Age Recommended
Gardasil (available in Canada)	6, 11 16, 18	Males 9-26 yr Females 9-26 yr
Gardasil 9 (available in Canada and the United States)	6, 11, 16, 18, 31, 33, 45, 52, 58	Males and females 9-26 yr (can be administered up to age 45 yr)
Cervarix (available in Canada)	16, 18	Males 9-25 yr Females 9-25 yr

[a]From Merck. (2019). https://www.gardasil9.com/about-gardasil9/schedule/.
[b]From FDA.gov. https://www.fda.gov/media/78013/download.

CHLAMYDIA INFECTION

Pathophysiology Review

Chlamydia trachomatis is an intracellular bacterium and the causative agent of cervicitis (in women), urethritis, and proctitis. It invades the epithelial tissues in the reproductive tract. The incubation period ranges from 1 to 3 weeks, but the pathogen may be present in the genital tract for months without producing symptoms.

C. trachomatis is reportable to local health departments in all states. In the United States, it is the most frequently reported bacterial sexually transmitted ***infection*** (CDC, 2018a; CDC, 2016). Diagnosed cases continue to increase yearly, which reflects more sensitive screening tests and increased public health efforts to screen high-risk people. Because it is frequently asymptomatic, the estimated incidence is approximately double what is reported.

PATIENT-CENTERED CARE: CULTURAL/ SPIRITUAL CONSIDERATIONS QSEN

Significant ***health care disparities*** exist between racial/ethnic groups. Prevalence among non-Hispanic blacks is 5.6 times greater than the prevalence among non-Hispanic whites (CDC, 2018a). There is also a high prevalence of rectal and pharyngeal chlamydial ***infection*** among men who have sex with men (MSM) (CDC, 2018a).

❖ Interprofessional Collaborative Care

◆ Assessment: Recognize Cues. As with all interviews concerning ***sexuality,*** use a nonjudgmental approach and provide privacy and confidentiality. Obtain a complete history, including a genitourinary system review, psychosocial history, and sexual history (see the Focused Assessment: The Patient With a Sexually Transmitted Infection box). In particular, ask about:

- Presence of symptoms, including vaginal or urethral discharge, dysuria (painful urination), pelvic ***pain,*** and any irregular bleeding (for women)

- A history of sexually transmitted diseases (STIs)
- Whether current or past sexual partners have had symptoms or a history of STIs
- Whether the patient has had a new partner, or multiple sexual partners
- Whether the patient or a current or recent partner has had unprotected intercourse

Evidence shows that incidence is higher among black, Native Alaskan, and American Indian populations (U.S. Department of Health and Human Services, Indian Health Services, U.S. Centers for Disease Control and Prevention, 2015).

PATIENT-CENTERED CARE: GENDER HEALTH CONSIDERATIONS QSEN

Ask men about about dysuria, frequent urination, or discharge, which may indicate urethritis. He may report a mucoid discharge that is more watery and less copious than what is expected with a gonorrheal discharge. Some men have the discharge only in the morning on arising. Complications of untreated chlamydia in men include epididymitis, prostatitis, infertility, and Reiter syndrome, a type of connective tissue disease.

Men may report penile discharge, urinary frequency, and dysuria. In contrast, many women have no symptoms. Those with symptoms may report mucopurulent vaginal discharge (typically yellow and opaque), urinary frequency, and abdominal discomfort or ***pain.*** Cervical bleeding, from infected, fragile tissue, may present as spotting or bleeding between menses and frequently after intercourse. Complications of ***infection*** with chlamydia include salpingitis (inflammation of the fallopian tubes), pelvic inflammatory disease (PID), and ***reproduction*** problems including infertility, ectopic pregnancy, and complications with a newborn that is delivered. These health problems are discussed in detail in maternal-child textbooks.

Diagnosis is made by sampling cells from the endocervix, urethra, or both, easily obtained with a swab. Because chlamydiae can reproduce only inside cells, cervical (or host) cells that harbor the organism (or parts of it) are required in the sample. Tissue culture obtained from the cervical os during the female pelvic examination or from male urethral examination obtained by swabbing has been replaced by genetic tests. Nucleic acid amplification tests (NAATs) are the most common method of detecting chlamydia in endocervical samples, urethral swabs, and urine. Samples can be obtained by swab by the examining clinician or by a patient-collected swab or urine specimen. Retesting after 3 months is advised in order to detect repeat ***infection*** (CDC, 2015; Johnson-Mallard et al., 2018).

All sexually active women 25 years old or younger and all women older than 25 years with a new partner, multiple partners, or a partner with an STI should be screened annually for chlamydia (CDC, 2018a). Routine screening is not recommended for men; however, screening should be done for sexually active younger men, especially those who have sex with men (MSM) (CDC, 2018a).

◆ Interventions: Take Action

Drug Therapy. The treatment of choice for chlamydia infections is azithromycin (usually given in a single dose at the time of the initial visit with the health care provider) or doxycycline. The one-dose course, although more expensive, is preferred because of the ease in completing the treatment. Directly observing the patient taking the medication in the health care setting will assure you of adherence. Alternative treatments that are prescribed for patients with allergies to these drugs include erythromycin, ofloxacin, and levofloxacin (CDC, 2015).

Sexual partners should be treated and tested for other STIs. Expedited partner therapy (EPT), or patient-delivered partner therapy, shows signs of reducing chlamydia ***infection*** rates (CDC, 2015). Expedited partner therapy (EPT) involves treating sexual partners of patients diagnosed with chlamydia infection or gonorrhea by providing prescriptions or medication to the patient, which they can take to their partner(s), without the partner(s) having to be examined by a provider of care. Evidence shows that when the patient gives the drug to their partner(s), rates of infection decrease, and more partners report receiving treatment (CDC, 2015).

Self-Management Education. As with all STI diagnoses, patient and partner education is a crucial nursing intervention geared toward effectively treating the condition and reducing the risk of reinfection. Teach about:

- The sexual mode of transmission
- The incubation period
- The high possibility of asymptomatic infections and the usual symptoms, if present
- The need for antibiotic treatment of ***infection*** and the need to complete all medications, even if feeling better
- The need for abstinence from sexual intercourse until the patient and partner(s) have all completed treatment (7 days from the start of treatment, including if treated with the single-dose regimen)
- The need for women to be rescreened for reinfection 3 to 12 months after treatment because of the high risk for PID; also, the fact that there is less evidence of the need for rescreening of treated men, but it should be considered
- The need to return for evaluation if symptoms recur or new symptoms develop (most recurrences are reinfections from a new or untreated partner)
- Complications of untreated or inadequately treated ***infection,*** which may include PID, infertility, ectopic pregnancy, or newborn complications

GONORRHEA

Pathophysiology Review

Gonorrhea is a sexually transmitted bacterial ***infection*** caused by *Neisseria gonorrhoeae,* a gram-negative intracellular diplococcus. It is transmitted by direct sexual contact with mucosal surfaces (vaginal intercourse, orogenital contact, or anogenital contact) (McCance et al., 2019).

The first symptoms of gonorrhea may appear within a week after sexual contact with an infected person. The disease can be present without symptoms and can be transmitted or progress without warning. In women, ascending spread of the organism can cause pelvic infection (pelvic inflammatory disease [PID]), **endometritis** (endometrial infection), **salpingitis** (fallopian tube infection), and pelvic peritonitis. In men, gonorrhea can cause epididymitis, which can lead to infertility if left untreated.

❖ Interprofessional Collaborative Care

◆ **Assessment: Recognize Cues.** Establish a trusting relationship and use a nonjudgmental approach to gather complete information. A complete history includes a review of the genitourinary system, and colleting a sexual history. Sites of sexual exposure or intercourse should be elicited, because gonorrhea can affect the genitals, rectum, and throat. Assess for allergies to antibiotics.

The ***infection*** can be asymptomatic in both men and women, but women have asymptomatic, or "silent," infections more often than do men. If symptoms are present, men usually notice dysuria and a penile discharge that can be either profuse yellowish-green fluid or scant clear fluid. The urethra, epididymis, seminal vesicles, and prostate can become infected. Men seek curative treatment sooner, usually because they have symptoms, and thereby avoid some of the serious complications.

Women may report a change in vaginal discharge (yellow, green, profuse, odorous), urinary frequency, or dysuria. The cervix and urethra are the most common sites of ***infection.***

Anal signs and symptoms may include itching and irritation, rectal bleeding or diarrhea, and painful bowel movements. Assess the mouth for a reddened throat, ulcerated lips, tender gingivae, and lesions in the throat. Fig. 69.8 shows common sites of gonococcal infections.

Fever may be a sign of an ascending (PID or epididymitis) or systemic (disseminated gonococcal) ***infection.*** Symptoms often include joint pain of the shoulder, wrist, and lower extremities, and a rash of several days' duration (Schweon, 2019).

Clinical symptoms of gonorrhea can resemble those of chlamydia ***infection*** and need to be differentiated. Nucleic acid amplification tests (NAATs) are the most common type of testing for the initial microbiologic diagnosis of gonorrhea; culture is also used when antibiotic resistance is suspected (Ghanem, 2020). During examination, the health care provider can swab the male urethra or female cervix to obtain specimens. Patient-collected urine or vaginal swabs can also be used to diagnose both gonorrhea and chlamydia infections, allowing for testing without a full examination.

All patients with gonorrhea should be tested for syphilis, chlamydia, hepatitis B and hepatitis C, and HIV infection and, if possible, examined for HSV and HPV because they may have been exposed to these STIs as well. Sexual partners who have been exposed in the past 30 days should be examined, and specimens should be obtained.

◆ **Interventions: Take Action.** Uncomplicated gonorrhea is treated with antibiotics. Chlamydia ***infection,*** which is four times more common, is frequently found in patients with gonorrhea. Because of this, patients treated for gonorrhea should also be managed with drugs that treat chlamydia infection.

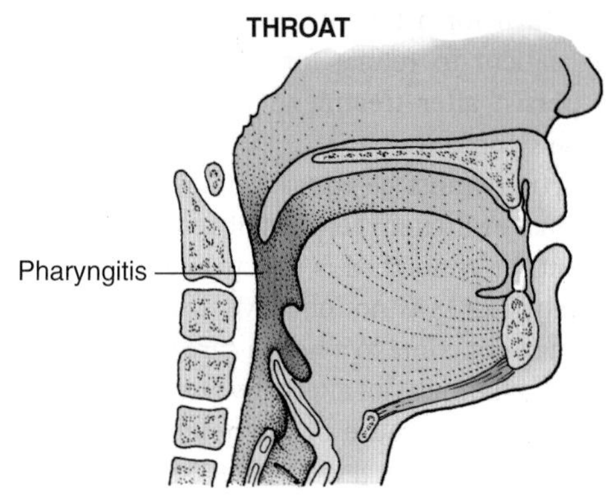

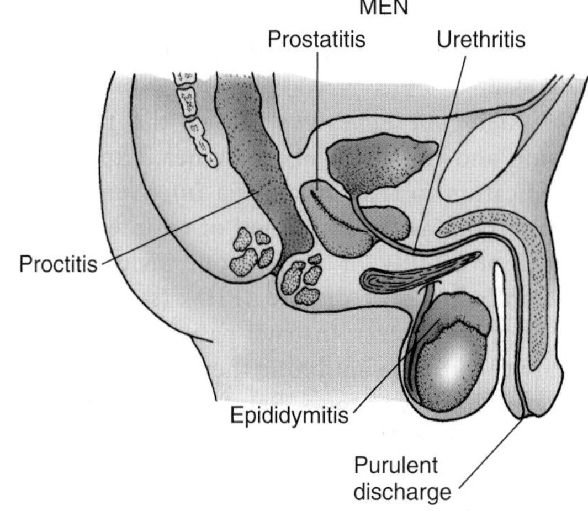

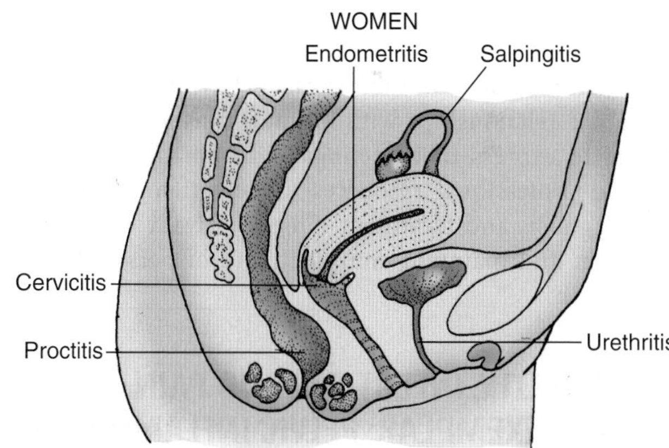

FIG. 69.8 Areas of involvement of gonorrhea in men and women.

Drug Therapy. Drug therapy recommended by the CDC is IM ceftriaxone *plus* oral azithromycin in a single dose at the time of the initial visit with the health care provider *or* oral doxycycline for a longer period of time to treat a presumed co-infection with chlamydia (unless a negative chlamydia result has been obtained). These combinations seem to be effective for all mucosal gonorrheal infections; treatment failure is rare (CDC, 2015). A test-of-cure is not required for treatment of uncomplicated urogenital or rectal gonorrhea treated with ceftriaxone and azithromycin; patients with oropharyngeal gonorrhea treated with any alternative treatment should be advised to return for a test-of-cure in 14 days (CDC, 2015). Advise any patient to return for a follow-up examination if symptoms persist after treatment. Reinfection is usually the cause of these symptoms.

Sexual partners must be education about the ***infection*** and treated (not just evaluated) to prevent reinfection. Because the best treatment for gonorrhea is injected ceftriaxone, expedited partner therapy (EPT) is not effective. If there is concern that the partner may not come to a health care facility for treatment, providing oral cefixime as an alternative has been recommended by the CDC (2015). Because of the potential for resistance of gonorrhea to cefixime, a test-of-cure is recommended after treatment is completed.

Gonorrhea ***infection*** can become disseminated, requiring hospitalization and IV or IM ceftriaxone. If symptoms resolve within 24 to 48 hours, the patient may be discharged to home to continue cefixime as oral antibiotic therapy while recovering (CDC, 2015).

Self-Management Education. Teach the patient about transmission and treatment of gonorrhea. Explain that the use of medication to treat chlamydia ***infection*** at the same time is important, as the likelihood of co-infection is high. Discuss the possibility of reinfection, including the risk for pelvic inflammatory disease (PID) (see discussion of PID later in this chapter). Instruct patients to abstain from sexual activity until the antibiotic therapy is completed and they no longer have symptoms. Reinforce the need for use of condoms at all times. Explain that gonorrhea is a reportable disease.

Patients with gonorrhea (or any other STI) may have feelings of fear or guilt. They may be concerned that they have contracted other STIs or consider the disease a religious or spiritual punishment for their sexual behaviors. Such feelings can impair relationships with intimate partners. Encourage patients to express their feelings and offer other information and professional resources to help them understand their diagnosis and treatment. Ensure privacy during your discussion and maintain confidentiality of personal health information.

SEXUALITY, INFECTION, AND PAIN CONCEPT EXEMPLAR: PELVIC INFLAMMATORY DISEASE

Pathophysiology Review

Pelvic inflammatory disease (PID) is an acute syndrome resulting in tenderness in the tubes and ovaries (adnexa) and, typically, dull pelvic ***pain.*** Some women experience only mild discomfort or menstrual irregularity, whereas others have acute ***pain,*** which can affect their gait (Table 69.4). Others experience no symptoms at all (i.e., so-called "silent" or "subclinical" PID).

This infectious process involves movement of organisms from the endocervix upward through the uterine cavity into the fallopian tubes. Usually multiple pathogens are involved in the development of PID. Sexually transmitted organisms are most often responsible, especially *C. trachomatis, N. gonorrhoeae,* and *Mycoplasma genitalium* (Ross & Chacko, 2020). Bacterial vaginosis has also been shown to be a causative agent (Ross & Chacko, 2020).

TABLE 69.4 Diagnostic Criteria for Pelvic Inflammatory Disease (PID)

Minimum Criteria for Initiating Empiric Treatment for Pelvic Inflammatory Disease

- Sexually active woman and at risk for sexually transmitted infections (STIs)
- Pelvic or lower abdominal pain
- Cervical motion, uterine, or adnexal tenderness on examination
- No other cause for illness can be found (e.g., appendicitis)

Additional Criteria to Increase the Specificity of the Diagnosis of PID

- Oral temperature >101°F (>38.3°C)
- Abnormal cervical or vaginal mucopurulent discharge, or cervical friability
- Abundance of white blood cells (WBCs) on saline microscopy of vaginal secretions
- Laboratory documentation of cervical infection with *Neisseria gonorrhoeae* or *Chlamydia trachomatis*

Definitive Criteria for Diagnosing PID, Warranted in Selected Cases

- Histopathologic evidence of endometritis on endometrial biopsy
- Transvaginal sonography or MRI techniques showing thickened, fluid-filled tubes with or without free pelvic fluid or tubo-ovarian complex, or Doppler studies suggesting pelvic infection
- Laparoscopic abnormalities consistent with PID

Modified from Centers for Disease Control and Prevention (CDC). (2015). Sexually transmitted diseases treatment guidelines, 2015. *Morbidity and Mortality Weekly Report Recommendations and Reports, 64*(RR-3), 1-137; and Ross, J., & Chacko, M. (2020). Pelvic inflammatory disease: Clinical manifestations and diagnosis. In *UpToDate,* Marrozzo, J. (Ed.). Waltham, MA.

The spread of ***infection*** to other organs and tissues of the upper genital tract occurs from direct contact with mucosal surfaces or through the fimbriated ends of the tubes to the ovaries, parametrium, and peritoneal cavity (Fig. 69.9). This may involve one or more pelvic structures, including the uterus, fallopian tubes, and adjacent pelvic structures. The most common site is the fallopian tube (salpingitis). Complications of PID include chronic pelvic pain, infertility, risk for ectopic pregnancy, and tubo-ovarian abscess (TOA), a serious short-term condition requiring hospitalization in which an inflammatory mass arises on the fallopian tube, ovary, and/or other pelvic organs (CDC, 2017). These complications are discussed in maternal-newborn textbooks. Perihepatitis—inflammation of the liver capsule and peritoneal surfaces of the anterior right upper quadrant—occurs in 10% of women with acute PID (Ross & Chacko, 2020). This condition is characterized by right upper quadrant pain with a pleuritic component (often the right shoulder) (Ross & Chacko, 2020).

Infections can be spread during sexual intercourse, during childbirth (including the postpartum period), and after abortion. *Sepsis and death can occur, especially if treatment is delayed or inadequate.*

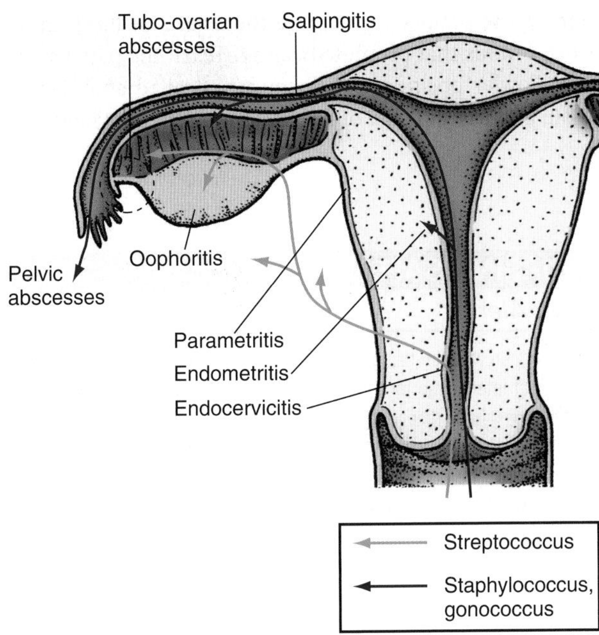

FIG. 69.9 The spread of pelvic inflammatory disease.

❖ Interprofessional Collaborative Care

◆ Assessment: Recognize Cues

History. Obtain a complete history of the symptoms with menstrual, obstetric, sexual, and family history. Inquire about any history of previous episodes of pelvic inflammatory disease (PID) or other sexually transmitted infections (see Focused Assessment: The Patient With A Sexually Transmitted Infection). Assess for contraceptive use, a history of reproductive surgery, and other risk factors previously discussed. Ask the patient if sexual abuse has occurred. If so, encourage her to discuss what happened and whether she was seen by a health care provider.

Many of the same factors that place women at risk for STIs also place them at risk for PID. Risk factors for sexually active women include (CDC, 2017):

- Being younger than 26 years old
- Having a new sexual partner, or having multiple sexual partners
- Having a sexual partner who has other concurrent sexual partners
- Practicing inconsistent use of condoms
- Having a history of PID
- Having a concurrent chlamydial or gonococcal ***infection,*** or having bacterial vaginosis
- Practicing vaginal douching
- Having a history of sexually transmitted diseases (STIs)
- Having had an intrauterine device (IUD) placed within the previous 3 weeks (this is noted as a small risk)

Physical Assessment/Signs and Symptoms. One of the most frequent symptoms of PID is lower abdominal or pelvic ***pain.*** Conduct a complete pain assessment. Other symptoms include irregular vaginal bleeding (spotting or bleeding between periods), dysuria (painful urination), an increase or change in vaginal discharge, dyspareunia (painful sexual intercourse), malaise, fever, and chills.

Observe whether the patient has pain with movement. She may bend forward to guard her abdomen. She may find it difficult to independently get on the examination table or stretcher. Assess for lower abdominal tenderness, possibly with rigidity or rebound tenderness. A pelvic examination by the health care provider may reveal yellow or green cervical discharge and a reddened or friable cervix (a cervix that bleeds easily). Criteria for accurate diagnosis of PID are listed in Table 69.4. The diagnosis of PID is based on health history, physical assessment, and laboratory tests. Imaging studies and laparoscopy are not generally used to make the diagnosis.

CLINICAL JUDGMENT CHALLENGE 69.1

Patient-Centered Care; Evidence-Based Practice

The nurse is caring for a 19-year-old female client who reports lower abdominal ***pain,*** a low-grade fever, and burning on urination. She states that she "must have gotten the flu" from a co-worker, and "probably has a urinary tract infection." On assessment, the client states that she became sexually active for the first time 6 months ago, and has noticed recently that intercourse is uncomfortable. When a pelvic examination is recommended by the health care provider, the client states she does not understand why she needs that type of assessment when she is certain she has a urinary tract infection (UTI) and influenza. She asks for a prescription to treat these conditions, and says she does not want to have the pelvic examination.

1. **Recognize Cues:** What assessment information in this client situation is the most important and immediate concern for the nurse? (Hint: Identify the **relevant** information *first* to determine what is most important.)
2. **Analyze Cues:** What client conditions are consistent with the **most relevant** information? (Hint: Think about priority collaborative problems that support and contradict the information presented in this situation.)
3. **Prioritize Hypotheses:** Which possibilities or explanations are **most likely** to be present in this client situation? Which possibilities or explanations are the most serious? (Hint: Consider all possibilities and determine their urgency and risk for this client.)
4. **Generate Solutions:** What actions would most likely achieve the desired outcomes for this client? Which actions should be **avoided** or are **potentially harmful**? (Hint: Determine the desired outcomes first to decide which interventions are appropriate and those that should be avoided.)
5. **Take Action:** Which actions are the most appropriate and how should they be implemented? In what **priority order** should they be implemented? (Hint: Consider health teaching, documentation, requested health care provider orders or prescriptions, nursing skills, collaboration with or referral to health team members, etc.)
6. **Evaluate Outcomes:** What client assessment would indicate that the nurse's actions were **effective**? (Hint: Think about signs that would indicate an improvement, decline, or unchanged client condition.)

Psychosocial Assessment. The woman who has symptoms of PID may be anxious and fearful of the examination and unknown diagnosis. She may need reassurance and support during the examination because of pelvic ***pain.*** Explain what is taking place in real time to help promote understanding.

Because PID is often associated with an STI, the woman may feel embarrassed or uncomfortable discussing symptoms or history. Use a nonjudgmental approach and encourage expression of feelings and concerns. Assessing the patient's ability to follow through with the interprofessional collaborative plan of care is essential in deciding whether hospitalization should be considered.

Laboratory Assessment. The health care provider obtains specimens from the cervix, urethra, and rectum to determine the presence of *N. gonorrhoeae* or *C. trachomatis.* The white blood cell (WBC) count may be elevated but is not specific for PID. A sensitive test that detects human chorionic gonadotropin (hCG) in urine or blood should be performed to determine whether the patient is pregnant (Pagana & Pagana, 2018). Microscopic examination of vaginal discharge is done to evaluate for the presence of WBCs.

Other Diagnostic Assessment. Abdominal *ultrasonography* may be used to determine the presence of appendicitis and tubo-ovarian abscesses (TOAs) that need to be ruled out when the diagnosis of PID is made. Ultrasound can be used to visualize the upper genital tract. CT or MRI can be helpful in determining if there is gastrointestinal pathology (Ross & Chacko, 2020).

◆ **Analysis: Analyze Cues and Prioritize Hypotheses.** The priority collaborative problem for a patient with pelvic inflammatory disease (PID) is:

1. ***Infection*** due to invasion of pelvic organs by sexually transmitted pathogens

◆ Planning and Implementation: Generate Solutions and Take Action

Managing Infection and Pain

Planning: Expected Outcomes. The patient with PID is expected to have the ***infection*** resolved, be free of abdominal ***pain,*** and prevent reinfection.

Interventions. Interprofessional collaborative care includes antibiotic therapy and self-management measures. Uncomplicated PID is usually treated on an ambulatory care basis. The CDC recommends oral and/or parenteral antibiotics for PID (CDC, 2015). The CDC (2015) recommends hospitalization for the patient with PID if:

- A surgical emergency (e.g., appendicitis) has not been excluded as a diagnosis
- The patient is pregnant
- She cannot follow or tolerate treatment as an outpatient
- There is severe illness, nausea and vomiting, or high fever
- A tubo-ovarian abscess (TOA) has been diagnosed
- There has been no clinical response to earlier oral antimicrobial treatment

Inpatient therapy involves a combination of several IV antibiotics until the woman shows signs of improvement (e.g., decreased pelvic tenderness for at least 24 hours). Then oral antibiotics are continued at home until the course of treatment has lasted 14 days.

Antibiotic therapy relieves ***pain*** by destroying the pathogens and decreasing the inflammation caused by ***infection.*** Other measures to treat pain include taking mild analgesics and applying heat to the lower abdomen or back. As with any infection, encourage the patient to increase the intake of fluids and eat nutritious foods that promote healing. Teach the patient to rest in semi-Fowler position and encourage limited ambulation to promote gravity drainage of the infection that may help relieve ***pain.***

> **! NURSING SAFETY PRIORITY (QSEN)**
>
> ***Action Alert***
>
> Instruct women who are being treated for PID on an ambulatory care basis to avoid sexual intercourse for the full course of antibiotic treatment and until their symptoms have resolved. Teach them to check their temperature twice daily, and to report an increase in temperature to their health care provider. Remind them to be seen by the health care provider within 72 hours from starting antibiotic treatment and then 1 and 2 weeks from the time of the initial diagnosis.

Laparoscopy can confirm the presence of PID, but it is uncommonly performed for this purpose (Ross & Chacko, 2020). It is more frequently performed if the patient has not responded to outpatient treatment and the health care provider is considering alternative causes for symptoms, or if the patient's symptoms are not improving or are worsening after 72 hours of inpatient treatment (Ross & Chacko, 2020). Before surgery, provide information about the procedure. After surgery, the care of the woman with PID is similar to that of any patient after laparoscopic abdominal surgery. One difference is that she may have a wound drain for drainage of abscess fluid if an abscess was removed during the procedure. Observe, measure, and record wound drainage every 4 to 8 hours as requested.

Care Coordination and Transition Management. Establish an atmosphere of trust that encourages the woman to return frequently, if needed, for education or reassurance. Teach the patient with PID to see her health care provider for follow-up to assess for complications and to confirm that the ***infection*** has resolved. If the woman is hospitalized, collaborate with the case manager or discharge planner before she is discharged to home.

Home Care Management. Parenteral antibiotic therapy may be given at home, but usually the health care provider changes the treatment regimen to oral antibiotics before hospital discharge. Home care for the patient who had laparoscopic surgery is discussed in Chapter 9.

Self-Management Education. Patient teaching focuses on providing information about PID, identifying symptoms of persistent or recurrent ***infection*** (persistent pelvic ***pain,*** dysmenorrhea, low backache, fever), and teaching about the importance of completion of treatment, rest, and healthy nutrition. Teach specifically about oral antibiotic therapy (see the Patient and Family Education: Preparing for Self-Management: Oral Antibiotic Therapy for Sexually Transmitted Infections box).

PATIENT AND FAMILY EDUCATION: PREPARING FOR SELF-MANAGEMENT

Oral Antibiotic Therapy for Sexually Transmitted Infections

- Take medicine for the number of times a day that it is prescribed and until it is completed, even if you begin to feel better.
- Take your antibiotics on an empty stomach unless your health care provider instructs you to take them with food.
- Do not take antacids containing calcium, magnesium, or aluminum, such as Tums, Maalox, or Mylanta, with your antibiotics. They may decrease the effectiveness of the antibiotic.
- Your sexual partner must be treated if you have a sexually transmitted infection (STI). Expedited partner therapy is one way to ensure that partners are treated.
- Do not have sex until after you and your partner complete your antibiotic therapy. Wait 7 days to resume intimacy if treatment was delivered in one dose.
- Drink at least 8 to 10 glasses of fluid a day while taking your antibiotics.
- Be sure to return for your follow-up appointment after completing your antibiotic treatment.
- Call if you have any questions or concerns.

NCLEX EXAMINATION CHALLENGE 69.2

Physiological Integrity

Which teaching will the nurse provide to a client who has been prescribed antibiotics for pelvic inflammatory disease (PID)? **Select all that apply.**

A. "Finish all of the prescribed drug even if you begin to feel better."
B. "If you feel nauseated from the antibiotics, take a dose of Tums or Maalox."
C. "Take antibiotics with food to decrease the chance of stomach irritation."
D. "You may resume intercourse once you have been on the antibiotic for 48 hours."
E. "You will need to return to see the health care provider after finishing drug therapy."

Teach the patient to contact her sexual partner(s) for examination and treatment. All sexual partners should be treated for gonorrhea and chlamydia ***infection*** regardless of whether they have symptoms. Remind the patient about follow-up care, and counsel her about the complications that can occur after an occurrence of PID, including recurrence, chronic pelvic ***pain***, ectopic pregnancy, and infertility.

Discuss contraception and the patient's feelings about this. Teach about the use of condoms that can provide contraception and decrease the risk for future episodes of PID. Help the patient understand that having sexual intercourse with multiple partners increases the risk for recurrent episodes. Douching has also been suggested as a risky behavior for development of PID and/or infection with chlamydia or *N. gonorrhoeae.*

Psychosocial concerns may require counseling. A patient who has PID may exhibit a variety of feelings (guilt, disgust, anger) about having a condition that may have been transmitted to her sexually. These feelings may affect her relationship with significant others and future sexual partners. She may also have concerns about future fertility if PID has damaged or scarred the fallopian tubes and other reproductive organs. Provide nonjudgmental emotional support and allow time for her to discuss her feelings. Collaborate with a mental health care provider as a longer-term method of support for the patient.

Health Care Resources. The cost of antibiotics for patients with PID and other STIs may be a concern for those who are uninsured, underinsured, or impoverished. Ask the patient directly if she has the ability to pay for the drug and her follow-up visits, regardless of her apparent financial status. Collaborate with the case manager or social worker, as these professionals can help to locate free or reduced-cost drugs and community resources for women who cannot afford them.

If infertility is a result of PID, the patient may need referral to a clinic specializing in infertility treatment and counseling. She can also contact infertility support groups, which exist in many local communities.

◆ **Evaluation: Evaluate Outcomes.** Evaluate the care of the patient with PID based on the identified priority patient problem(s). The expected outcomes include that the patient should:

- Show evidence that the ***infection*** has resolved
- Report or demonstrate that ***pain*** is relieved or reduced and that she feels more comfortable
- Articulate a plan for ensuring treatment of her partner, obtaining antibiotics, and returning for follow-up care

GET READY FOR THE NEXT-GENERATION NCLEX® EXAMINATION!

Key Points

Review these Key Points for each NCLEX Examination Client Needs Category.

Safe and Effective Care Environment

- Use gloves when examining genitalia and oral or skin lesions. **QSEN: Safety**

Health Promotion and Maintenance

- Teach to refrain from sexual intercourse during treatment for sexually transmitted ***infection*** (STI). **QSEN: Safety**
- Assume that all adult patients may be sexually active, regardless of age or stage of life. **QSEN: Patient-Centered Care**
- Educate people who are most vulnerable about risk for STIs. **QSEN: Safety**
- Teach about the availability of expedited partner therapy. **QSEN: Evidence-Based Practice**
- Encourage adults who are sexually active to use condoms. **QSEN: Evidence-Based Practice**
- Teach sexually active adults to have STI screenings at least annually. **QSEN: Safety**
- Respect the sexual choices and practices of all patients. **QSEN: Patient-Centered Care**

Psychosocial Integrity

- Maintain patient and partner confidentiality and privacy at all times. **QSEN: Patient-Centered Care**
- Treat all patients, regardless of diagnosis, gender identity, or sexual orientation, with respect. **QSEN: Patient-Centered Care**
- Provide privacy for patients undergoing examination or testing for STIs. **QSEN: Patient-Centered Care**
- Encourage expression of feelings regarding a diagnosis of STI. **QSEN: Patient-Centered Care**
- Refer patients newly diagnosed with an STI to local resources and support groups. **QSEN: Teamwork and Collaboration**

Physiological Integrity

- Assess patients with an STI using best practice guidelines. **QSEN: Evidence-Based Practice**
- Recognize that some STIs progress in stages and over various periods of time. **QSEN: Evidence-Based Practice**
- Understand that patients without symptoms may still be infected with an STI. **QSEN: Evidence-Based Practice**
- Teach about the importance of completing the entire antiinfective drug regimen, even when feeling better. **QSEN: Evidence-Based Practice**
- Teach the expected side effects of and possible adverse reactions to prescribed drugs. **QSEN: Safety**
- Teach about the short-term and long-term complications of STIs. **QSEN: Safety**
- Encourage all patients who have an STI to inform their sexual partner(s). **QSEN: Safety**

MASTERY QUESTIONS

1. The nurse hears a patient tell her partner that condoms with spermicide are important to protect themselves from sexually transmitted infections (STIs). What is the appropriate nursing response?
   A. Teach that spermicide has not been shown to be effective in STI prevention.
   B. Do nothing because the nurse should not be listening to the client's conversation.
   C. Educate that spermicide must be used with water-based lubricant to be effective.
   D. Affirm that spermicide helps to block transfer of sexually transmitted organisms.

2. The nurse is caring for a 33-year-old female client who has been intimate with women and men. What teaching will the nurse provide regarding the Gardisil 9 vaccine?
   A. "Patients older than 26 cannot receive an HPV vaccine."
   B. "You will need three doses of the vaccine instead of two."
   C. "I will give you a single dose and you will be protected from future HPV."
   D. "HPV vaccines must be administered to people who have never had intercourse."

REFERENCES

Albrecht, M. (2018). Epidemiology, clinical manifestations, and diagnosis of genital herpes simplex virus infection. In M. Hirsch (Ed.), *UpToDate*. Waltham, MA.

Albrecht, M. (2019). Treatment of genital herpes simplex infection. In M. Hirsch (Ed.), *UpToDate*. Waltham, MA.

American College of Obstetricians and Gynecologists. (2017). *How to prevent sexually transmitted infections (STIs)*. https://www.acog.org/Patients/FAQs/How-to-Prevent-Sexually-Transmitted-Infections-STIs?IsMobileSet=false#risk.

American Sexual Health Association. (2020). *Diagnosing and managing genital herpes*. http://www.ashasexualhealth.org/?s=herpes.

Barrow, R., Ahmed, F., Bolan, G., & Workowski, K. (2020). Recommendations for providing quality sexually transmitted diseases clinical services, 2020. *Morbidity and Mortality Weekly Report Recommendations and Reports*, *68*(No. RR-5), 1–20.

Bartz, D. (2019). Pericoital contraception: Diaphragm, cervical cap, spermicide, and sponge. In C. Schreiber (Ed.), *UpToDate*. Waltham, MA.

Burchum, J. L. R., & Rosenthal, L. D. (2019). *Lehne's pharmacology for nursing care* (10th ed.). St. Louis: Elsevier.

Carusi, D. (2019). Condylomata acuminate (anogenital warts): Treatment of vulvar and vaginal warts. In R. Barbieri (Ed.), *UpToDate*. Waltham, MA.

Centers for Disease Control and Prevention (CDC). (2015). Sexually transmitted diseases treatment guidelines, 2015. *Morbidity and Mortality Weekly Report Recommendations and Reports*, *64*(RR–3), 1–137.

Centers for Disease Control and Prevention. (2016). *Chlamydia – CDC fact sheet*. https://www.cdc.gov/std/chlamydia/stdfact-chlamydia-detailed.htm.

Centers for Disease Control and Prevention. (2017). *Pelvic inflammatory disease (PID) – CDC fact sheet*. https://www.cdc.gov/std/pid/stdfact-pid-detailed.htm.

Centers for Disease Control and Prevention. (2018a). *Sexually transmitted disease surveillance, 2017*. Atlanta, GA: Department of Health and Human Services.

Centers for Disease Control and Prevention. (2018b). *STDs in racial and ethnic minorities*. https://www.cdc.gov/std/stats17/minorities.htm.

Centers for Disease Control and Prevention. (2018c). Syphilis. https://www.cdc.gov/std/stats17/syphilis.htm.

Centers for Disease Control and Prevention. (2019). *Genital HPV infection – fact sheet*. https://www.cdc.gov/std/hpv/stdfact-hpv.htm.

Centers for Disease Control and Prevention. (2020a). *2020 national notifiable conditions*. https://wwwn.cdc.gov/nndss/conditions/notifiable/2019/.

Centers for Disease Control and Prevention. (2020b). *Sexually transmitted diseases*. https://www.cdc.gov/std/default.htm.

Fenway Health. (2020). *The national LGBT health education Center*. https://fenwayhealth.org/the-fenway-institute/education/the-national-lgbt-health-education-center/.

Ghanem, K. (2020). Clinical manifestations and diagnosis of Neisseria gonorrhoeae infection in adults and adolescents. In J. Marrazzo (Ed.), *UpToDate*. Waltham, MA.

Hicks, C., & Clement, M. (2020a). Syphilis: Epidemiology, pathophysiology, and clinical manifestations in patients without HIV. In J. Marrazzo (Ed.), *UpToDate*. Waltham, MA.

Hicks, C., & Clement, M. (2020b). Syphilis: Treatment and monitoring. In J. Marrazzo (Ed.), *UpToDate*. Waltham, MA.

Hoke, T., et al. (2020). Female condoms. In C. Schreiber (Ed.), *UpToDate*. Waltham, MA.

Johnson-Mallard, V., et al. (2018). Managing sexually transmitted infections: Beyond the 2015 guidelines. *The Nurse Practitioner Journal*, *43*(8), 28–34.

McCance, K., Huether, S., Brashers, V., & Rote, N. (2019). *Pathophysiology: The biologic basis for disease in adults and children* (8th ed.). St. Louis: Elsevier.

Merck Sharp & Dohme Corp. (2019). Why 9 HPV types? https://www.merckvaccines.com/Products/Gardasil9/hpv-types.

Molin, S. B., De Blasio, B. F., & Olsen, A. O. (2016). Is the risk for sexually transmissible infections (STI) lower among women with exclusively female sexual partners compared with women with male partners? A retrospective study based on attendees at a Norwegian STI clinic from 2004 to 2014. *Sexual Health*, *13*(3), 257–264.

National Center for Health Statistics (NCHS). (2018). *Data brief number 304*. https://www.cdc.gov/nchs/products/databriefs/db304.htm#hsv1_prevalence_by_race_comparision.

Neumann, M., Finlayson, T., Pitt, N., & Keatley, J. (2017). Comprehensive HIV prevention for transgender persons. *American Journal of Public Health*, *107*(2), 207–212.

Pagana, K. D., & Pagana, T. J. (2018). *Mosby's manual of diagnostic and laboratory tests* (6th ed.). St. Louis: Elsevier.

Palefsky, J. (2019). Human papillomavirus infections: Epidemiology and disease associations. In M. Hirsch (Ed.), *UpToDate*. Waltham, MA.

Raiford, J., Hall, G., Taylor, R., Bimbi, D., & Parsons, J. (2016). The role of structural barriers in risky sexual behavior, victimization, and readiness to change HIV/STI-related risk behavior among transgender women. *AIDS Behaviors*, *20*(10), 2212–2221.

Ross, J., & Chacko, M. (2020). Pelvic inflammatory disease: Clinical manifestations and diagnosis. In J. Marrazzo (Ed.), *UpToDate*. Waltham, MA.

Schweon, S. (2019). Disseminated gonococcal infection. *Nursing2019*, *49*(3), 15–16.

The Joint Commission. (2019). *Why clinicians struggle with identifying human trafficking victims*. https://www.jointcommission.org/resources/news-and-multimedia/blogs/dateline-tjc/2019/06/why-clinicians-struggle-with-identifying-human-trafficking-victims/.

U.S. Department of Health and Human Services, Indian Health Service, US Centers for Disease Control and Prevention (2015). *2015 Indian health surveillance report: Sexually transmitted diseases*. https://www.cdc.gov/std/stats/ihs/18IHS-DEDP102_REPORT_STD_M_508.pdf.

U.S. Department of Health and Human Services. (2019). *Proposed objectives for inclusion in Healthy People 2030*. https://www.healthypeople.gov/sites/default/files/ObjectivesPublicComment508_1.17.19.pdf

U.S. Department of Health and Human Services. (2020a). *HIV and sexually transmitted diseases (STDs)*. https://aidsinfo.nih.gov/understanding-hiv-aids/fact-sheets/26/98/hiv-and-sexually-transmitted-diseases--stds-.

U.S. Department of Health and Human Services (USDHHS), Office of Disease Prevention and Health Promotion. (2020b). *Healthy people 2020*. https://www.healthypeople.gov/.

U.S. Preventive Services Task Force. (2018). *Cervical cancer: Screening*. https://www.uspreventiveservicestaskforce.org/uspstf/recommendation/cervical-cancer-screening.

World Health Organization. (2020). *Nonoxynol-9 ineffective in preventing HIV infection*. https://www.who.int/mediacentre/news/notes/release55/en/.

NCLEX® EXAMINATION CHALLENGES ANSWER KEY

Chapter 1
1. B, E
2. A, D, E

Chapter 2
1. A, B, C, E
2. A, B, C, D, E

Chapter 3
1. A, C, F
2. A
3. B

Chapter 4
1. A, B, C, D, E
2. C
3. B

Chapter 5
1. A
2. A

Chapter 6
1. A
2. C
3. D
4. B, F

Chapter 7
1. C
2. A, C, E
3. C

Chapter 8
1. D
2. A, B, D, F

Chapter 9
1. B
2. C, D
3. A, C, D, E
4. A
5. A
6. A
7. C, D, E

Chapter 10
1. D
2. B, E
3. C

Chapter 11
1. A, D, E
2. D
3. A, B, C, D, E, F, G

Chapter 12
1. B
2. A, C, D
3. A, B, C, D, F, G

Chapter 13
1. A
2. A, D, F
3. C
4. D
5. C
6. C

Chapter 14
1. C
2. D
3. C, D

Chapter 15
1. C
2. B

Chapter 16
1. D
2. C
3. C, D

Chapter 17
1. C
2. C
3. A
4. C
5. B, F, G
6. B

Chapter 18
1. A, E
2. C

Chapter 19
1. C
2. A, D, E, F
3. C, D, G

Chapter 20
1. A
2. B, C, F
3. B
4. B
5. C, D, E

Chapter 21
1. A, B, D
2. A, B, C, D, E

Chapter 22
1. B, C, D
2. D

Chapter 23
1. C
2. A, C, D, E
3. D
4. C

Chapter 24
1. C, F, G
2. B
3. D

Chapter 25
1. D, F, H
2. C
3. D
4. B, C

Chapter 26
1. A
2. B, C, G, H
3. D
4. B

Chapter 27
1. C
2. B
3. A
4. D, F, G
5. B

Chapter 28
1. C
2. B
3. A, G

Chapter 29
1. B
2. A, C, D
3. C
4. A

Chapter 30
1. A, D, E, G
2. C
3. B

Chapter 31
1. C
2. D
3. C, D, B, A, E

Chapter 32
1. B, C, E, F
2. B
3. C
4. B

Chapter 33
1. C, D, E
2. A
3. D
4. C
5. A, D, E

Chapter 34
1. A, B, D, E, H
2. C
3. D
4. B, C

Chapter 35
1. A, C, D, E
2. B, D, F
3. A

Chapter 36
1. D
2. A, C, E
3. A

Chapter 37
1. C
2. A, C, E
3. C
4. C

Chapter 38
1. A, B, D, E
2. A
3. D

Chapter 39
1. A, F
2. C
3. A, C, D, E
4. B, C, D, E, F

Chapter 40
1. B, C, D, E, F
2. C
3. A

Chapter 41
1. A
2. B
3. C
4. B

Chapter 42
1. D
2. A
3. B, C, D, E
4. C
5. C

Chapter 43
1. D
2. A, C, D
3. C, E

Chapter 44
1. A, B, C, D, E, F
2. C

Chapter 45
1. A, B, C, F
2. C
3. C

Chapter 46
1. B, C, D
2. A, B, D, E
3. C
4. A, D, F

Chapter 47
1. A, B, C, D
2. B, C, E
3. D
4. C

Chapter 48
1. A, B, E, G
2. C
3. A, D, E

Chapter 49
1. B
2. A
3. A, E
4. B, F
5. B
6. D, F

Chapter 50
1. B, C, E
2. A

Chapter 51
1. A, B, C, D, E, F
2. A
3. C

Chapter 52
1. B, C
2. A, B, C, D, E
3. A

Chapter 53
1. A, B, C, D, E
2. A, C
3. C, D

Chapter 54
1. C
2. A, B, C, E, F

Chapter 55
1. 40.0
2. B
3. A, B, C, E, F

Chapter 56
1. A
2. B

Chapter 57
1. A, B, F
2. C
3. B
4. C

Chapter 58
1. C, D
2. A
3. C

Chapter 59
1. B, C, D, E, G
2. D
3. A
4. B
5. B

Chapter 60
1. A, C, D
2. B, C, E, F
3. B, C, D, E
4. A

Chapter 61
1. A
2. C, D, E, F
3. A
4. C

Chapter 62
1. A, B, D, F
2. B
3. A

Chapter 63
1. B
2. B, C, E
3. B
4. A
5. C

Chapter 64
1. C
2. C
3. A, B, D

Chapter 65
1. B
2. A
3. A, E

Chapter 66
1. B
2. A
3. B

Chapter 67
1. 850 mL.
2. C
3. D

Chapter 68
1. D
2. B

Chapter 69
1. C, D, E, F
2. A, E

MASTERY QUESTIONS ANSWER KEY

Chapter 1
1. A
2. A, D, E

Chapter 2
1. C
2. D
3. D

Chapter 3
1. A, B, D, F
2. A

Chapter 4
1. D
2. A, B, C, D, E

Chapter 5
1. A
2. B

Chapter 6
1. C
2. A, B, F, G
3. A
4. B, D

Chapter 7
1. A, D, F
2. C

Chapter 8
1. B
2. B

Chapter 9
1. A, C, D
2. B

Chapter 10
1. A
2. A

Chapter 11
1. B
2. D

Chapter 12
1. D
2. C

Chapter 13
1. A, D
2. D
3. B
4. B

Chapter 14
1. A
2. C

Chapter 15
1. D
2. C

Chapter 16
1. A, B, C, F
2. C
3. A

Chapter 17
1. B
2. D
3. A
4. D

Chapter 18
1. B, C, G
2. C
3. B

Chapter 19
1. B
2. D
3. C, D

Chapter 20
1. B
2. A, D, E
3. B

Chapter 21
1. A, B, C, D, E
2. B

Chapter 22
1. B, C
2. A, C, E

Chapter 23
1. C
2. D
3. C

Chapter 24
1. C
2. A

Chapter 25
1. D
2. A
3. C

Chapter 26
1. D
2. C
3. D
4. B, D, F

Chapter 27
1. B
2. C
3. A
4. A, B, E, F
5. B

Chapter 28
1. B
2. C
3. B, C, D, E

Chapter 29
1. D
2. C, D, G
3. A, C, E, F

Chapter 30
1. A, C, E, F
2. A
3. B

Chapter 31
1. B
2. D
3. C

Chapter 32
1. A, B, C, D, E
2. C
3. A

Chapter 33
1. D
2. B
3. B

Chapter 34
1. D
2. A
3. A, C, D

Chapter 35
1. A, D, E, F
2. C
3. A
4. B

Chapter 36
1. B
2. D
3. C

Chapter 37
1. A, C, E
2. D
3. A, F

Chapter 38
1. C
2. B

Chapter 39
1. D
2. A, B, C, D
3. A, B, C, D, E

Chapter 40
1. D
2. B
3. D

Chapter 41
1. A, D, E
2. D

Chapter 42
1. A, B, C
2. A, C, D, E

Chapter 43
1. A
2. C, E
3. D

Chapter 44
1. A, B, C, D, E
2. D

Chapter 45
1. A
2. A, B

Chapter 46
1. A
2. D
3. B, D, E

Chapter 47
1. B
2. C
3. B, C, D, E

Chapter 48
1. C, D
2. A, B, D, E

Chapter 49
1. A, B, D
2. A, B, D
3. B

Chapter 50
1. B
2. A, B, D, E

Chapter 51
1. A, D, E
2. C

Chapter 52
1. B
2. C

Chapter 53
1. A, C
2. C

Chapter 54
1. D
2. A, B, C, D, E

Chapter 55
1. A
2. A, C, E

Chapter 56
1. C
2. B

Chapter 57
1. C
2. A
3. A, B, C, D, E, F
4. D

Chapter 58
1. A
2. B, E, G
3. C

Chapter 59
1. A, C
2. C
3. B, C
4. D
5. B

Chapter 60
1. A
2. B
3. B, D, F
4. D

Chapter 61
1. B, C, D, G
2. C, E, F, G
3. D
4. D

Chapter 62
1. B
2. B
3. A, D, E, F

Chapter 63
1. B, C, E
2. C
3. A

Chapter 64
1. D
2. A
3. D

Chapter 65
1. B, C, D, E
2. B

Chapter 66
1. B, C
2. B

Chapter 67
1. B
2. B

Chapter 68
1. A
2. C, E, F

Chapter 69
1. A
2. B

INDEX

Page numbers followed by f indicate figures; t, tables; b, boxes

F

H

O

P

Q

R

T

V